CLINICAL ANESTHESIA

CLINICAL ANESTHESIA

FIFTH EDITION

Edited By

Paul G. Barash, MD

Professor, Department of Anesthesiology
Yale University School of Medicine
Attending Anesthesiologist
Yale–New Haven Hospital
New Haven, Connecticut

Bruce F. Cullen, MD

Professor, Department of Anesthesiology
University of Washington School of Medicine
Attending Anesthesiologist
Harborview Medical Center
Seattle, Washington

Robert K. Stoelting, MD

Emeritus Professor and Chair, Department of Anesthesia
Indiana University School of Medicine
Indianapolis, Indiana

LIPPINCOTT WILLIAMS & WILKINS
A Wolters Kluwer Company
Philadelphia • Baltimore • New York • London
Buenos Aires • Hong Kong • Sydney • Tokyo

Acquisitions Editor: Brian Brown
Developmental Editor: Grace Caputo, Dovetail Content Solutions
Production Editor: Dave Murphy
Manufacturing Manager: Ben Rivera
Creative Director: Doug Smock
Cover Designer: Joseph DePinho
Compositor: TechBooks
Printer: Courier-Westford

Printed in the USA

Library of Congress Cataloging-in-Publication Data

Clinical anesthesia / edited by Paul G. Barash, Bruce F. Cullen, Robert K. Stoelting. — 5th ed.
p. ; cm.
Includes bibliographical references and index.
ISBN 0-7817-5745-2 (alk. paper)
1. Anesthesiology. 2. Anesthesia. I. Barash, Paul G. II. Cullen, Bruce F. III. Stoelting, Robert K.
[DNLM: 1. Anesthesia. 2. Anesthesiology. 3. Anesthetics.
WO 200 C6398 2006]
RD81.C58 2006
617.9′6—dc22

2005017173

To purchase additional copies of this book, call our customer service department at (800) 638-3030 or fax orders to (301) 824-7390. International customers shoud call (301) 714-2324.

Visit Lippincott Williams & Wilkins on the Internet: at LWW.com. Lippincott Williams & Wilkins customer service representatives are available from 8:30 am to 6 pm, EST.

10 9 8 7 6 5 4 3 2

The Image of the Tracheal Bronchial Tree on the Cover is Courtesy of Cook, Bloomington, Indiana.

THIS EDITION OF CLINICAL ANESTHESIA IS DEDICATED TO THE MEMORY AND SPIRIT OF DANIEL BERNARD BARASH

CONTRIBUTING AUTHORS

Stephen E. Abram, MD
Professor
Department of Anesthesiology
Medical College of Wisconsin
Staff Anesthesiologist
Froedtert Memorial Hospital
Milwaukee, Wisconsin

J. Jeffrey Andrews, MD
Professor and Vice-Chair for Education
Department of Anesthesiology
University of Alabama School of Medicine
Birmingham, Alabama

Douglas R. Bacon, MD, MA
Professor of Anesthesiology and Medical History
Mayo Clinic College of Medicine
Consultant Anesthesiologist
Mayo Clinic
Rochester, Minnesota

Robert L. Barkin, MBA, PharmD, FCP
Rush University Medical College
Clinical Pharmacologist
Rush Pain Center
Chicago, Illinois
Clinical Pharmacologist
The Rush North Shore Pain Center
Skokie, Illinois

Audrée A. Bendo, MD
Professor and Vice Chair for Education
Department of Anesthesiology
State University of New York
Downstate Medical Center
Brooklyn, New York

Christopher M. Bernards, MD
Virginia Mason Medical Center
Clinical Professor
Department of Anesthesiology
University of Washington
Staff Anesthesiologist
Seattle, Washington

Arnold J. Berry, MD, MPH
Professor
Department of Anesthesiology
Emory University
Staff Anesthesiologist
Emory University Hospital
Atlanta, Georgia

Frederic A. Berry, MD
Professor Emeritus of Pediatrics and Anesthesiology
Department of Anesthesiology
The University of Virginia
Charlottesville, Virginia

David R. Bevan, MB
Professor and Chair
Department of Anesthesia
University of Toronto
Anesthesiologist-in-Chief
University Health Network
Toronto, Ontario, Canada

Barbara W. Brandom, MD
Professor
Department of Anesthesiology
University of Pittsburgh
Attending Physician
Department of Anesthesiology
Children's Hospital of Pittsburgh
Pittsburgh, Pennsylvania

Ferne R. Braverman, MD
Professor
Department of Anesthesiology
Director, Section of Obstetric Anesthesiology
Yale University School of Medicine
New Haven, Connecticut

Russell C. Brockwell, MD
Associate Professor
University of Alabama School of Medicine
Chief of Anesthesiology Birmingham Veterans Affairs Medical Center
Birmingham, Alabama

Levon M. Capan, MD
Professor of Anesthesiology
Department of Anesthesiology
New York University School of Medicine
Associate Director
Department of Anesthesiology
Bellevue Hospital Center
New York, New York

Barbara A. Castro, MD
Associate Professor of Anesthesiology and Pediatrics
University of Virginia School of Medicine
University of Virginia Health System
Charlottesville, Virginia

Frederick W. Cheney, Jr., MD
Professor and Chair
Department of Anesthesiology
University of Washington School of Medicine
Attending Anesthesiologist
University of Washington Medical Center
Seattle, Washington

Barbara A. Coda, MD
Clinical Associate Professor
Department of Anesthesiology
University of Washington School of Medicine
Seattle, Washington
Staff Anesthesiologist
McKenzie Anesthesia Group
McKenzie-Willamette Hospital
Springfield, Oregon

Edmond Cohen, MD
Professor of Anesthesiology
The Mount Sinai School of Medicine
Director of Thoracic Anesthesia
The Mount Sinai Medical Center
New York, New York

James E. Cottrell, MD
Professor and Chairman
Department of Anesthesiology
State University of New York
Downstate Medical Center
Brooklyn, New York

Joseph P. Cravero, MD
Associate Professor of Anesthesiology
Dartmouth Hitchcock Medical Center
Lebanon, New Hampshire

C. Michael Crowder, MD, PhD
Associate Professor of Anesthesiology and Molecular Biology/Pharmacology
Washington University School of Medicine
Attending Anesthesiologist
Division of Neuroanesthesia
Barnes-Jewish Hospital
St. Louis, Missouri

Marie Csete, MD, PhD
Associate Professor and John E. Steinhaus Professor of Anesthesiology
Emory University
Director, Liver Transplant Anesthesiology
Department of Anesthesiology
Emory University Hospital
Atlanta, Georgia

Anthony J. Cunningham, MD
Professor/Clinical Vice Dean
Department of Anaesthesia
Royal College of Surgeons in Ireland
Consultant and Professor
Department of Anaesthesia
Beaumont Hospital
Dublin, Ireland

Jacek B. Cywinski, MD
Department of General Anesthesiology
The Cleveland Clinic Foundation
Cleveland, Ohio

Steven Deem, MD
Associate Professor of Anesthesiology and Medicine (Adjunct, Pulmonary and Critical Care)
University of Washington
Harborview Medical Center
Seattle, Washington

Stephen F. Dierdorf, MD
Professor
Department of Anesthesia
Medical University of South Carolina
Charleston, South Carolina

François Donati, PhD, MD, FRCPC
Professor
Department of Anesthesiology
University of Montreal
Staff Anesthesiologist
Hospital Maisonneuve-Rosemont
Montreal, Quebec, Canada

John C. Drummond, MD, FRCPC
Professor of Anesthesiology
University of California, San Diego
Staff Anesthesiologist
VA Medical Center, San Diego
La Jolla, California

Thomas J. Ebert, MD, PhD
Professor
Department of Anesthesiology
Medical College of Wisconsin
Staff Anesthesiologist
VA Medical Center
Milwaukee, Wisconsin

Jan Ehrenwerth, MD
Professor
Department of Anesthesiology
Yale University School of Medicine
Attending Anesthesiologist
Yale–New Haven Hospital
New Haven, Connecticut

John H. Eichhorn, MD
Professor
Department of Anesthesiology
University of Kentucky College of Medicine
Department of Anesthesiology
UK Chandler Medical Center
Lexington, Kentucky

James B. Eisenkraft, MD
Professor of Anesthesiology
Mount Sinai School of Medicine
Attending Anesthesiologist
The Mount Sinai Hospital
New York, New York

John E. Ellis, MD
Professor
Department of Anesthesia and Critical Care
Pritzker School of Medicine
The University of Chicago
Section Chief
Anesthesia for Vascular, Thoracic, and General Surgery
University of Chicago Hospitals
Chicago, Illinois

Alex S. Evers, MD
Henry E. Mallinckrodt Professor and Chairman
Department of Anesthesiology
Washington University School of Medicine
Anesthesiologist-in-Chief
Barnes-Jewish Hospital
St. Louis, Missouri

Lynne R. Ferrari, MD
Associate Professor of Anesthesiology
Harvard Medical School
Medical Director, Perioperative Services
Department of Anesthesia, Perioperative and Pain Medicine
Children's Hospital
Boston, Massachusetts

Mieczyslaw Finster, MD
Professor of Anesthesiology and Obstetrics and Gynecology
Columbia University College of Physicians and Surgeons
New York Presbyterian Hospital
New York, New York

Jeffrey E. Fletcher, PhD
Clinical Publications Lead
Medical Communications
AstraZeneca
Wilmington, Deleware

J. Sean Funston, MD
Assistant Professor
Department of Anesthesiology
University of Texas Medical Branch
Galveston, Texas

Steven I. Gayer, MD, MBA
Associate Professor
Departments of Anesthesiology and Ophthalmology
University of Miami Miller School of Medicine
Director of Anesthesia Services
Bascom Palmer Eye Institute
Miami, Florida

Kathryn Glas, MD
Assistant Professor
Department of Anesthesiology
Associate Director
Cardiothoracic Anesthesiology
Director, Intra-Operative Echo Service
Emory University School of Medicine
Atlanta, Georgia

Alexander W. Gotta, MD
Emeritus Professor of Anesthesiology
State University of New York
Downstate Medical Center
Brooklyn, New York

John Hartung, PhD
Associate Editor
Journal of Neurosurgical Anesthesiology
State University of New York
Brooklyn, New York

Tara M. Hata, MD
Associate Professor
Department of Anesthesia
University of Iowa
Roy J. and Lucille A. Carver College of Medicine
University of Iowa Hospitals and Clinics
Iowa City, Iowa

Laurence M. Hausman, MD
Assistant Professor
Department of Anesthesiology
Mount Sinai School of Medicine
Vice Chair, Academic Affiliations
Department of Anesthesiology
Mount Sinai Hospital
New York, New York

Thomas K. Henthorn, MD
Professor and Chair
Department of Anesthesiology
University of Colorado Health Sciences Center
Denver, Colorado

Simon C. Hillier, MB, ChB
Associate Professor
Department of Anesthesia
Indiana University School of Medicine
Staff Anesthesiologist
Riley Hospital for Children
Indianapolis, Indiana

Terese T. Horlocker, MD
Professor
Departments of Anesthesiology and Orthopedics
Mayo Clinic College of Medicine
Rochester, Minnesota

Robert J. Hudson, MD, FRCPC
Clinical Professor
Department of Anesthesiology and Pain Medicine
University of Alberta
Attending Anesthesiologist
University of Alberta Hospitals
Edmonton, Alberta, Canada

Anthony D. Ivankovitch, MD
Professor and Chair
Department of Anesthesiology
Rush University Medical Center
Chicago, Illinois

Joel O. Johnson, MD, PhD
Professor and Chair
Department of Anesthesiology
University of Missouri-Columbia Hospitals and Clinics
Columbia, Missouri

Raymond S. Joseph Jr., MD
Staff Anesthesiologist
Virginia Mason Medical Center
Seattle, Washington

Zeev N. Kain, MD, MBA
Professor and Executive Vice-Chairman
Department of Anesthesiology
Yale University School of Medicine
Anesthesiologist-in-Chief
Yale–New Haven Children's Hospital
New Haven, Connecticut

Ira S. Kass, MD
Professor
Departments of Anesthesiology, Physiology, and Pharmacology
Downstate Medical Center
Brooklyn, New York

Jonathan D. Katz, MD
Clinical Professor of Anesthesiology
Yale University School of Medicine
New Haven, Connecticut

Brian S. Kaufman, MD
Associate Professor
Departments of Anesthesiology, Medicine, and Neurosurgery
New York University School of Medicine
Co-Director, Critical Care
Tisch Hospital
New York, New York

Charbel A. Kenaan, MD
Chief Resident in Anesthesiology
Department of Anesthesiology, Perioperative Medicine, and Pain Management
Jackson Memorial Hospital
University of Miami Miller School of Medicine
Miami, Florida

Donald A. Kroll, MD, PhD
Staff Anesthesiologist
Veterans Affairs Medical Center
Biloxi, Mississippi

Carol L. Lake, MD, MBA, MPH
CEO
Verefi Technologies, Inc.
Elizabethtown, Pennsylvania

Noel W. Lawson, MD
Professor
Department of Anesthesiology
University of Missouri-Columbia
Staff Anesthesiologist
University of Missouri-Columbia Hospitals and Clinics
Columbia, Missouri

Wilton C. Levine, MD
Instructor in Anesthesia
Harvard Medical School
Department of Anesthesia and Critical Care
Massachusetts General Hospital
Boston, Massachusetts

Jerrold H. Levy, MD
Professor and Deputy Chair of Research
Department of Anesthesiology
Emory University School of Medicine
Director of Cardiothoracic Anesthesiology
Emory Healthcare
Atlanta, Georgia

Adam D. Lichtman, MD
Assistant Professor of Anesthesiology
Department of Anesthesiology
Weill Cornell Medical Center
New York Presbyterian Hospital
New York, New York

J. Lance Lichtor, MD
Professor
Department of Anesthesia
University of Iowa
Iowa City, Iowa

Spencer S. Liu, MD
Clinical Professor of Anesthesiology
Department of Anesthesiology
University of Washington
Staff Anesthesiologist
Department of Anesthesiology
Virginia Mason Medical Center
Seattle, Washington

Richard L. Lock, MD
Associate Professor
Department of Anesthesiology
University of Kentucky College of Medicine
University of Kentucky Chandler Medical Center
Lexington, Kentucky

David A. Lubarsky, MD, MBA
Emanuel M. Papper Professor and Chair
Department of Anesthesiology, Perioperative Medicine, and Pain Management
University of Miami Miller School of Medicine
Chief of Service
Department of Anesthesiology
Jackson Memorial Hospital
Miami, Florida

Timothy R. Lubenow, MD
Professor of Anesthesiology
Rush Medical College
Director, Section of Pain Medicine
Department of Anesthesiology
Rush University Medical Center
Chicago, Illinois

Srinivas Mantha, MD
Professor of Anesthesiology
Department of Anesthesiology and Intensive Care
Sub-Dean, Nizam's Institute of Medical Sciences
Hyberabad, India

Joseph P. Mathew, MD
Associate Professor
Department of Anesthesiology
Chief, Division of Cardiothoracic Anesthesia
Duke University Medical Center
Durham, North Carolina

Michael S. Mazurek, MD
Assistant Professor of Clinical Anesthesia
Department of Anesthesia
Indiana University School of Medicine
Staff Anesthesiologist
Riley Hospital for Children
Indianapolis, Indiana

Kathryn E. McGoldrick, MD
Professor and Chair
Department of Anesthesiology
New York Medical College
Director
Department of Anesthesiology
Westchester Medical Center
Valhalla, New York

Roger S. Mecca, MD
Chairman
Department of Anesthesiology
Danbury Hospital
Danbury, Connecticut
Clinical Associate Professor of Anesthesiology
New York Medical College
New York, New York

Sanford M. Miller, MD
Clinical Associate Professor
New York University School of Medicine
Assistant Director of Anesthesiology
Bellevue Hospital Center
New York, New York

Terri G. Monk, MD, MS
Professor
Department of Anesthesiology
Duke University Medical Center
Faculty, Department of Anesthesia
VA Hospital
Durham, North Carolina

John R. Moyers, MD
Professor
Department of Anesthesia
University of Iowa
Roy J. and Lucille A. Carver College of Medicine
University of Iowa Hospitals and Clinics
Iowa City, Iowa

Michael F. Mulroy, MD
Clinical Professor
Department of Anesthesiology
University of Washington School of Medicine
Staff Anesthesiologist
Department of Anesthesiology
Virginia Mason Medical Center
Seattle, Washington

Stanley Muravchick, MD, PhD
Professor
Department of Anesthesia
University of Pennsylvania School of Medicine
Vice Chair for Clinical Operations
Department of Anesthesia
Hospital of the University of Pennsylvania
Philadelphia, Pennsylvania

Glenn S. Murphy, MD
Assistant Professor
Department of Anesthesiology
Feinberg School of Medicine
Northwestern University
Director, Cardiac Anesthesia
Department of Anesthesiology
Evanston Northwestern Healthcare
Evanston, Illinois

Michael J. Murray, MD, PhD
Professor and Chair
Department of Anesthesiology
Mayo Clinic College of Medicine
Jacksonville, Florida

Steven M. Neustein, MD
Associate Professor
Department of Anesthesiology
Mount Sinai School of Medicine
Attending Anesthesiologist
Mount Sinai Hospital
New York, New York

Cathal Nolan, MB
Lecturer in Anaesthesia
Department of Anaesthesia
Beaumont Hospital
Royal College of Surgeons in Ireland
Dublin, Ireland

Babatunde O. Ogunnaike, MD
Associate Professor
Director of Anesthesia Surgical Services
Parkland Memorial Hospital
Department of Anesthesiology and Pain Management
University of Texas Southwestern Medical Center
Dallas, Texas

Jerome F. O'Hara, Jr., MD
Associate Professor
Head, Section of Urological Anesthesiology
Department of General Anesthesiology
Cleveland Clinic Foundation
Cleveland, Ohio

Charles W. Otto, MD, FCCM
Professor of Anesthesiology
Associate Professor of Medicine
University of Arizona College of Medicine
Director of Critical Care Medicine
Department of Anesthesiology
Arizona Health Sciences Center
Tucson, Arizona

Nathan Leon Pace, MD, MStat
Professor
Department of Anesthesiology
University of Utah
Staff Anesthesiologist
University of Utah Health Sciences Center
Salt Lake City, Utah

Charise T. Petrovitch, MD
Professor of Anesthesiology
George Washington University
Washington, DC

Mihai V. Podgoreanu, MD
Assistant Professor
Department of Anesthesiology
Duke University Medical Center
Durham VA Hospital
Durham, North Carolina

Karen L. Posner, PhD
Research Associate Professor
Department of Anesthesiology
University of Washington
Seattle, Washington

Donald S. Prough, MD
Professor and Chair
Department of Anesthesiology
University of Texas Medical Branch
Galveston, Texas

J. David Roccaforte, MD
Assistant Professor
Department of Anesthesiology
New York University
Co-Director, SICU
Bellevue Hospital Center
New York, New York

Michael F. Roizen, MD
Professor and Chairman
Division of Anesthesiology, Critical Care Medicine, and Comprehensive Pain Management
Cleveland Clinical Foundation
Cleveland, Ohio

Gladys Romero, MD
Visiting Assistant Professor
Department of Anesthesiology and Pain Management
University of Texas Southwestern Medical Center
Dallas, Texas

Stanley H. Rosenbaum, MD
Professor of Anesthesiology, Internal Medicine, and Surgery
Vice Chairman for Academic Affairs
Department of Anesthesiology
Yale University School of Medicine
Director of Perioperative and Adult Anesthesia
Yale–New Haven Hospital
New Haven, Connecticut

Henry Rosenberg, MD
Professor of Anesthesiology
Mount Sinai School of Medicine
New York, New York
Director
Department of Medical Education and Clinical Research
Saint Barnabas Medical College
Livingston, New Jersey

Meg A. Rosenblatt, MD
Associate Professor
Department of Anesthesiology
Director of Orthopedic and Regional Anesthesia
Mount Sinai School of Medicine
New York, New York

William H. Rosenblatt, MD
Professor of Anesthesia and Surgery
Yale University School of Medicine
Attending Physician
Department of Anesthesiology
Yale–New Haven Hospital
New Haven, Connecticut

Carl E. Rosow, MD, PhD
Professor
Department of Anaesthesia
Harvard Medical School
Anesthetist
Department of Anesthesia and Critical Care
Massachusetts General Hospital
Boston, Massachusetts

Nyamkhishig Sambuughin, PhD
Senior Biologist
Clinical Neurogenetics Unit
National Institute of Neurological Disorders and Stroke
National Institute of Health
Bethesda, Maryland

Alan C. Santos, MD, MPH
Chairman of Anesthesiology
Ochsner Clinic Foundation
New Orleans, Louisiana

Jeffrey J. Schwartz, MD
Associate Professor
Department of Anesthesiology
Yale University School of Medicine
Attending Physician
Yale–New Haven Hospital
New Haven, Connecticut

Margaret L. Schwarze, MD
Clinical Associates
Vascular Surgery
University of Chicago
Chicago, Illinois

Harry A. Seifert, MD, MSCE
Adjunct Assistant Professor of Clinical Anesthesiology
Department of Anesthesiology and Critical Care
Children's Hospital of Philadelphia
Adjunct Assistant Professor of Epidemiology
Department of Biostatistics and Epidemiology
University of Pennsylvania School of Medicine
Philadelphia, Pennsylvania

Aarti Sharma, MD
Assistant Professor
Department of Anesthesiology
Assistant Director of Pediatric Anesthesia
Weill Cornell Medical Center
New York Presbyterian Hospital
New York, New York

Nikolaos Skubas, MD
Assistant Professor
Department of Anesthesiology
Weill Cornell Medical Center
New York Presbyterian Hospital
New York, New York

Hugh M. Smith, MD, PhD
Resident
Department of Anesthesiology
Mayo Clinic College of Medicine
Mayo Clinic
Rochester, Minnesota

Karen J. Souter, MBBS, MSc, FRCA
Assistant Professor
Department of Anesthesia
University of Washington Medical Center
Seattle, Washington

M. Christine Stock, MD, FCCM, FACP
James E. Eckenhoff Professor and Chair
Department of Anesthesiology
Feinberg School of Medicine
Northwestern University
Chicago, Illinois

Christer H. Svensén, MD, PhD, DEAA, MBA
Associate Professor
Department of Anesthesiology
University of Texas Medical Branch
Galveston, Texas

Stephen J. Thomas, MD
Topkin-Van Poznak Professor and Vice-Chair
Department of Anesthesiology
Weill Medical College of Cornell University
New York Presbyterian Hospital
New York, New York

Miriam M. Treggiari, MD, MPH
Associate Professor
Department of Anesthesiology
University of Washington School of Medicine
Harborview Medical Center
Seattle, Washington

Jeffery S. Vender, MD, FCCM, FCCP
Professor
Department of Anesthesiology
Feinberg School of Medicine
Northwestern University
Chairman
Department of Anesthesiology
Evanston Northwestern Healthcare
Evanston, Illinois

J. Scott Walton, MD
Associate Professor
Department of Anesthesia
Medical University of South Carolina
Charleston, South Carolina

Mark A. Warner, MD
Professor and Chair
Department of Anesthesiology
Mayo Clinic College of Medicine
Rochester, Minnesota

Denise J. Wedel, MD
Professor of Anesthesiology
Mayo Clinic College of Medicine
Rochester, Minnesota

Paul F. White, PhD, MD, FANZCA
Professor and Holder of the Margaret Milam McDermott Distinguished Chair
Department of Anesthesiology and Pain Management
University of Texas Southwestern Medical Center
Dallas, Texas

Charles W. Whitten, MD
Professor and Vice President of Resident Affairs
M.T. "Pepper" Jenkins Professor in Anesthesiology
Department of Anesthesiology and Pain Management
University of Texas Southwestern Medical Center
Dallas, Texas

Scott W. Wolf, MD
Assistant Professor
Department of Anesthesiology
University of Texas Medical Branch
Galveston, Texas

James R. Zaidan, MD, MBA
Professor and Chair
Department of Anesthesiology
Associate Dean for GME
Emory University School of Medicine
Atlanta, Georgia

PREFACE

Transformation in the delivery of patient care, combined with changes in education, is the new paradigm for anesthesiology in the 21st century. Minimizing costs while improving efficiency and enhancing patient safety are the goals of contemporary anesthesia practice. To ensure that practitioners have incorporated the most-up-to-date information in their practice, certifying and licensing authorities have mandated continual education and testing both at the trainee and at the practicing anesthesiologist level. These changes are coupled with the need for ongoing innovation as the anesthesiologist continues to be challenged to adapt clinical management to new surgical procedures and technologies. These developments are an extension of the observation we made in the first edition of *Clinical Anesthesia*: "The major achievements of modern surgery would not have taken place without the accompanying vision of the pioneers in anesthesiology."

Anesthesiology is recognized as the specialty that has done the most to ensure patient safety. Despite these advances, the specialty's own leadership, in addition to outside agencies, has mandated further improvement. No longer does the anesthesiologist have the luxury of admitting the patient to the hospital a day or more before the surgical procedure and of performing a leisurely workup and preoperative assessment. In the ambulatory surgery unit, for example, the patient may be available only minutes before the operation, and decisions must be made immediately as to adequacy of the preanesthetic evaluation and treatment plan. In the inpatient setting, care is perceived as being even more fragmented. For example, the health care professional performing the preoperative evaluation may not be the caregiver in the operating room. In the operating room, where costs can reach $40 to $50 per minute, "production pressure" has been noted to get "the case going." This occurs in a setting of diminished resources, equipment, drugs, and personnel, with the simultaneous requirement to improve patient safety in the OR. Thus, the anesthesiologist must have information immediately available for the appropriate integration of care in the preincision period. In fact, the American Board of Anesthesiology, in its *Booklet of Information,* emphasizes the importance of this facet of clinical management by stating, "The ability to independently acquire and process information in a timely manner is central to assure individual responsibility for all aspects of anesthesiology care."

Simultaneous with these clinical requirements are significant changes in the educational process for trainees and established practioners. Responsibility and accountability for one's education have increased. Certifying boards use a framework, such as Maintenance of Certification in Anesthesiology (MOCA), to ensure that the practitioner is current in aspects of patient care. This concept is based on lifelong learning, assessment of professional standing, assessment of clinical practice performance, and a written examination testing cognitive expertise. These changes require a significant shift in the manner in which textbooks present knowledge. With the advent of electronic publishing, clinicians cannot rely solely on a single textbook to supply the "answers" to a clinical conundrum or a board recertification question. As a result, *Clinical Anesthesia* remains faithful to its original goal: *To develop a textbook that supports efficient and rapid acquisition of knowledge.* However, to meet this objective, the editors have also developed a multifaceted, systematic approach to this target. *Clinical Anesthesia* serves as the foundation and reference source for the other educational tools in the Clinical Anesthesia series: *The Handbook of Clinical Anesthesia, Clinical Anesthesia for the PDA, Review of Clinical Anesthesia,* and *The Lippincott Interactive Anesthesia Library on CD-ROM* (LIAL). Each of these provides a bridge to clinical care and education.

To recognize these requirements, in this the first edition of *Clinical Anesthesia* of the 21st century, we have totally redesigned the textbook, from its cover to chapter format and inclusion of new and relevant material. To enhance access to information, as well as align chapters with contemporary educational goals, each chapter starts with a detailed outline and Key Points. To meet the realities of the world we live in, we have added new chapters on disaster preparedness and weapons of mass destruction, genomics, obesity (bariatric surgery), and office-based anesthesia. We have encouraged contributors to develop clinically relevant themes and prioritize various clinical options considered by many the definitive strength of previous editions. In addition, each contributor emphasizes applicable areas of importance to patient safety. On occasion, redundancy between chapters may exist. We have made every effort to reduce repetition or even disagreement between chapters. Different approaches to a clinical problem also represent the realities of consultant-level anesthesia practice, however, so this diversity in approach remains in certain instances.

Finally, we wish to express our gratitude to the individual authors whose hard work, dedication, and timely submissions have expedited the production of the fifth edition. In addition, we acknowledge the contributions of colleagues and readers for their constructive comments. We also thank our secretaries, Gail Norup, Ruby Wilson and Deanna Walker, each of whom gave unselfishly of their time to facilitate the editorial process. We would also like to take this opportunity to recognize the continuing support of Lippincott Williams & Wilkins. It was more than 25 years ago that Lewis Reines, the former CEO of J.B. Lippincott, recognized the need for a major American anesthesiology textbook focused on education and clinical care. Throughout the intervening years, he has been a trusted colleague, an advisor, and, most importantly, a friend. In addition, we have been blessed with executive editors who have made singular contributions to the success of *Clinical Anesthesia*: Susan Gay, Mary Kay Smith, and Craig Percy. The enduring commitment to excellence in medical publishing continues from Lippincott Williams & Wilkins with Brian Brown, Senior Acquisitions Editor, and David Murphy, Production Manager, with the assistance of Grace Caputo, Project Director, Dovetail Content Solutions, and Chris Miller, Project Manager, TechBooks.

Paul G. Barash, MD
Bruce F. Cullen, MD
Robert K. Stoelting, MD

CONTENTS

SECTION VI ■ POSTANESTHESIA AND CONSULTANT PRACTICE

SECTION I ■ INTRODUCTION TO ANESTHESIA PRACTICE

CHAPTER 1 ■ THE HISTORY OF ANESTHESIA

HUGH M. SMITH AND DOUGLAS R. BACON

KEY POINTS

1. Anesthesiology is a young specialty historically, especially when compared to surgery or internal medicine.
2. Discoveries in anesthesiology have taken decades to build upon the observations and experiments of many people, and in some instances we are still searching. For example, the ideal volatile anesthetic has yet to be discovered.
3. Regional anesthesia is the direct outgrowth of a chance observation by an intern who would go on to become a successful ophthalmologist.
4. Pain medicine began as an outgrowth of regional anesthesia.
5. Much of our current anesthesia equipment is the direct result of anesthesiologists being unhappy with and needing better tools to properly anesthetize patients.
6. Many safety standards have been established through the work of anesthesiologists who were frustrated by the status quo.
7. Organizations of anesthesia professionals have been critical in establishing high standards in education and proficiency, which in turn has defined the specialty.
8. Respiratory critical care medicine started as the need by anesthesiologists to use positive pressure ventilation to help polio victims.
9. Surgical anesthesia, and physician specialization in its administration, has allowed for increasingly complex operations to be performed on increasingly ill patients.

Surgery without adequate pain control may seem cruel to the modern reader, yet this was the common practice throughout most of history. While anesthesia is considered a relatively new field, surgery predates recorded human history. Human skull trephinations occurred as early as 10,000 BC, with archaeologic evidence of post-procedure bone infection and healing, proving these primitive surgeries were performed on living humans. Juice from coca leaves may have been dribbled onto the scalp wound but the recipient of these procedures was almost certainly awake while a hole was bored into his or her skull with a sharp flake of volcanic glass. This was a unique situation in anesthesia; there are no other instances in which both the operator and his patient share the effects of the same drug.

In contemporary practice, we are prone to forget the realities of pre-anesthesia surgery. Fanny Burney, a well-known literary artist from the early nineteenth century, described a mastectomy she endured after receiving a "wine cordial" as her sole anesthetic. As seven male assistants held her down, the surgery commenced: "When the dreadful steel was plunged into the breast-cutting through veins-arteries-flesh-nerves-I needed no injunction not to restrain my cries. I began a scream that lasted unintermittently during the whole time of the incision—& I almost marvel that it rings not in my Ears still! So excruciating was the agony. Oh Heaven!—I then felt the knife racking against the breast bone-scraping it! This performed while I yet remained in utterly speechless torture."[1] Burney's description reminds us that it is difficult to overstate the impact of anesthesia on the human condition. An epitaph on a monument to William T. G. Morton, one of the founders of anesthesia, summarizes the contribution of anesthesia: "BEFORE WHOM in all time Surgery was Agony."[2] Although most human civilizations evolved some method for diminishing patient discomfort, *anesthesia*, in its modern and effective meaning, is a comparatively recent discovery with traceable origins in the mid-nineteenth century. How we have changed perspectives from one in which surgical pain was terrible and expected to one where patients may fairly presume they will be safe, pain free, and unaware during extensive operations is a fascinating story.

Anesthesiologists are like no other physicians: we are experts at controlling the airway and at emergency resuscitation; we are real-time cardiopulmonologists achieving hemodynamic and respiratory stability for the anesthetized patient; we are pharmacologists and physiologists, calculating appropriate doses and desired responses; we are gurus of postoperative care and patient safety; we are internists performing perianesthetic medical evaluations; we are the pain experts across all medical disciplines and apply specialized techniques in pain clinics and labor wards; we manage the severely sick or injured in critical care units; we are neurologists, selectively blocking sympathetic, sensory, or motor functions with our regional techniques; we are trained researchers exploring scientific mystery and clinical phenomenon.

Anesthesiology is an amalgam of specialized techniques, equipment, drugs, and knowledge that, like the growth rings of a tree, have built up over time. Current anesthesia practice is the summation of individual effort and fortuitous discovery of centuries. Every component of modern anesthesia was at some point a new discovery and reflects the experience, knowledge, and inventiveness of our predecessors. Historical examination enables understanding of how these individual components of anesthesia evolved. A knowledge of the history of anesthesia enhances our appreciation of current practice and intimates where our specialty might be headed.

ANESTHESIA BEFORE ETHER

Today, major surgery without adequate anesthesia would be unthinkable, and probably constitute grounds for malpractice
1 litigation. And yet this paradigm, this way of seeing anesthesia as a necessary part of surgery, is a fairly recent development dating back only 160 years. Scholars have sought to explain the comparatively late arrival of anesthesia. In addition to limitations in technical knowledge, cultural attitudes toward pain are often cited as reasons humans endured centuries of surgery without effective anesthesia. For example, it is known that the Roman writer Celsius encouraged "pitilessness" as an essential characteristic of the surgeon, an attitude that prevailed for centuries. While there is some proof for this perspective, closer inspection reveals that most cultures were, in fact, sensitive to the suffering caused by surgical operations and developed methods for lessening pain. Various techniques and plant-based agents in many parts of the world were employed to alter consciousness or as analgesics. Examination of the methods of managing pain before ether anesthesia is useful for what it illuminates about the historical roots and principal advances of our specialty.

Physical and Psychological Anesthesia

The Edwin Smith Surgical Papyrus, the oldest known written surgical document, describes 48 cases performed by an Egyptian surgeon from 3000 to 2500 BC. While this remarkable surgical treatise contains no direct mention of measures to lessen patient pain or suffering, Egyptian pictographs from the same era show a surgeon compressing a nerve in a patient's antecubital fossa while operating on the patient's hand. Another image displays a patient compressing his own brachial plexus while a procedure is performed on his palm.[3] In the sixteenth century, military surgeon Ambroise Paré became adept at nerve compression as a means of creating anesthesia.

Building upon the technique of Paré, James Moore described in 1874 the combined use of nerve compression and opium. In his book *A Method of Preventing or Diminishing Pain in Several Operations of Surgery*, Moore described a machine devised to apply continuous pressure on nerves and how, with the administration of a grain of opium, surgical pain might be lessened. Surgeon John Hunter used Moore's technique at St. Georges Hospital during the amputation of a leg below the knee following compression of the sciatic and anterior crural nerves.[4] The pain control during the surgery was judged better than without the technique.

Medical science has benefited from the natural refrigerating properties of ice and snow as well. For centuries anatomical dissections were performed only in winter because colder temperatures delayed deterioration of the cadaver, and in the Middle Ages the anesthetic effects of cold water and ice were recognized. It is unclear how frequently cold might have been used during this era but in the seventeenth century, Marco Aurelio Severino documented "refrigeration anesthesia" in some detail. By placing snow in parallel lines across the incisional plane, he was able to render a surgical site insensate within minutes. The technique never became popular, probably because of the challenge of maintaining stores of snow year-round.[5] Severino is also known to have saved numerous lives during an epidemic of diphtheria by performing tracheostomies and inserting trochars to maintain patency of the airway.[6]

Formal manipulation of the psyche to relieve surgical pain was undertaken by French physicians Charles Dupotet and Jules Cloquet in the late 1820s with hypnosis, then called *mesmerism*. Although the work of Anton Mesmer was discredited by the French Academy of Science after formal inquiry several decades earlier, proponents like Dupotet and Cloquet continued to make mesmeric experiments and pleaded to the Academie de Medicine to reconsider its utility.[7] In a well-attended demonstration in 1828, Cloquet removed the breast of a 64-year-old patient while she reportedly remained in a calm, mesmeric sleep. This demonstration made a lasting impression upon British physician John Elliotson who became a leading figure of the mesmeric movement in England in the 1830s and 1840s. Innovative and quick to adopt new advances, Elliotson performed mesmeric demonstrations and in 1843 published *Numerous Cases of Surgical Operations without Pain in the Mesmeric State*. In this work, Elliotson used the term "anaesthesia," and again 5 years later when he gave the Harveian Oration before the Royal College of Physicians in London. This was 2 years before Oliver Wendell Holmes, who is often credited for introducing the term, but many centuries after Dioscorides first used the word "anesthesia." Elliotson was roughly criticized by his colleagues for his unorthodox practices. Support for mesmerism faded when in 1846 renowned surgeon Robert Liston performed the first operation under ether anesthesia in England and remarked, "This Yankee dodge beats mesmerism all hollow."[8]

Despite its inevitable demise, the mesmeric movement was an attempt to cope with surgical pain by manipulation of mental and emotional states. In modern obstetrics, the psychoprophylaxis of Lamaze classes and support provided to parturients by midwives and doulas represent forms of "psychological anesthesia" shown to reduce pharmacologic analgesia requirements and the need for regional anesthesia.

Early Analgesics and Soporifics

Dioscorides, a Greek physician from the first century AD, commented on the analgesia of mandragora, a drug prepared from the bark and leaves of the mandrake plant. He stated that the plant substance could be boiled in wine, strained, and used "in the case of persons . . . about to be cut or cauterized, when they wish to produce anesthesia."[9] Mandragora was still being used to benefit patients as late as the seventeenth century. From the ninth to the thirteenth centuries, the *soporific sponge* was a dominant mode of providing pain relief during surgery. Mandrake leaves, along with black nightshade, poppies, and other herbs, were boiled together and cooked onto a sponge. The sponge was then reconstituted in hot water and placed under the patient's nose before surgery. Prior to the hypodermic syringe and routine venous access, ingestion and inhalation were the only known routes of administering medicines to gain systemic effects. Prepared as indicated by published reports of the time, the sponge generally contained morphine and scopolamine in varying amounts—drugs used in modern anesthesia.[10]

Alcohol was another element of the pre-ether armamentarium because it was thought to induce stupor and blunt the impact of pain. Although alcohol is a central nervous system depressant, in the amounts administered it produced little analgesia in the setting of true surgical pain. Fanny Burney's account, mentioned previously, demonstrates the ineffectiveness of alcohol as an anesthetic. Not only did the alcohol provide minimal pain control, it did nothing to dull her recollection of events. Laudanum was an alcohol-based solution of opium first compounded by Paracelsus in the sixteenth century. It was wildly popular in the Victorian and Romantic periods, and prescribed for a wide variety of ailments from the common cold to tuberculosis. Although appropriately used as an analgesic in some instances, it was frequently misused and abused. Laudanum was given by nursemaids to quiet wailing infants and abused by many upper-class women, poets, and artists who were unaware of its addictive potential.

Inhaled Anesthetics

The discovery of surgical anesthetics, in the modern era, remains linked to inhaled anesthetics. The compound now known as *diethyl ether* had been known for centuries; it may have been compounded first by an eighth-century Arabian philosopher Jabir ibn Hayyam, or possibly by Raymond Lully, a thirteenth-century European alchemist. But diethyl ether was certainly known in the sixteenth century, both to Valerius Cordus and Paracelsus, who prepared it by distilling sulfuric acid (oil of vitriol) with fortified wine to produce an *oleum vitrioli dulce* (sweet oil of vitriol). One of the first "missed" observations of the effects of inhaled agents, Paracelsus observed that ether caused chickens to fall asleep and awaken unharmed. He must have been aware of its analgesic qualities, because he reported that it could be recommended for use in painful illnesses.

For three centuries thereafter, this simple compound remained a therapeutic agent with only occasional use. Some of its properties were examined but without sustained interest by distinguished British scientists Robert Boyle, Isaac Newton, and Michael Faraday, none of whom made the conceptual leap to surgical anesthesia. Its only routine application came as an inexpensive recreational drug among the poor of Britain and Ireland, who sometimes drank an ounce or two of ether when taxes made gin prohibitively expensive.[11] An American variation of this practice was conducted by groups of students who held ether-soaked towels to their faces at nocturnal "ether frolics."

Like ether, nitrous oxide was known for its ability to induce lightheadedness and was often inhaled by those seeking a thrill. It was not used as frequently as ether because it was more complex to prepare and awkward to store. It was made by heating ammonium nitrate in the presence of iron filings. The evolved gas was passed through water to eliminate toxic oxides of nitrogen before being stored. Nitrous oxide was first prepared in 1773 by Joseph Priestley, an English clergyman and scientist, who ranks among the great pioneers of chemistry. Without formal scientific training, Priestley prepared and examined several gases, including nitrous oxide, ammonia, sulfur dioxide, oxygen, carbon monoxide, and carbon dioxide.

At the end of the eighteenth century in England, there was a strong interest in the supposed wholesome effects of mineral waters and gases. Particular waters and gases were believed to prevent and treat disease, and there was great interest in the potential use of gases as remedies for scurvy, tuberculosis, and other diseases. Thomas Beddoes opened his Pneumatic Institute close to the small spa of Hotwells, in the city of Bristol, to study the effect of inhaled gases. He hired Humphry Davy in 1798 to conduct research projects for the Institute. Davy performed brilliant investigations of several gases but focused much of his attention on nitrous oxide. He measured the rate of uptake of nitrous oxide, its effect on respiration, and other central nervous system actions. His human experimental results, combined with research on the physical properties of the gas, were published in *Nitrous Oxide,* a 580-page book published in 1800.

This impressive treatise is now best remembered for a few incidental observations. Davy commented that nitrous oxide transiently relieved a severe headache, obliterated a minor headache, and briefly quenched an aggravating toothache. The most frequently quoted passage was a casual entry: "As nitrous oxide in its extensive operation appears capable of destroying physical pain, it may probably be used with advantage during surgical operations in which no great effusion of blood takes place."[12] This is perhaps the most famous of the "missed opportunities" to discover surgical anesthesia. Davy's lasting nitrous oxide legacy was coining the phrase "laughing gas" to describe its unique property.

Almost Discovery: Hickman, Clarke, Long, and Wells

2 As the nineteenth century wore on, societal attitudes toward pain changed, perhaps best exemplified by the romantic poets.[13] Thus, the discovery of a means to relieve pain may have become more accepted, and several more near-breakthroughs occurred that are worthy of mention. An English surgeon named Henry Hill Hickman searched intentionally for an inhaled anesthetic to relieve pain in his patients.[14] Hickman used high concentrations of carbon dioxide in his studies on mice and dogs. Carbon dioxide has some anesthetic properties, as shown by the absence of response to an incision in the animals of Hickman's study, but it was never determined if the animals were insensate because of hypoxia rather than anesthesia. Hickman's concept was magnificent; his choice of agent, regrettable.

William E. Clarke, a medical student from Rochester, New York, may have given the first ether anesthetic in January 1842. From techniques learned as a chemistry student in 1839, Clarke entertained his companions with nitrous oxide and ether. Emboldened by these experiences, in January 1842, he administered ether, from a towel, to a young woman named Hobbie. One of her teeth was then extracted without pain by a dentist named Elijah Pope.[15] A second indirect reference to Clarke's anesthetic suggested that it was believed that her unconsciousness was due to hysteria. Clarke was advised to conduct no further anesthetic experiments.[16]

There is no doubt that 2 months later, on March 30, 1842, Crawford Williamson Long administered ether with a towel for surgical anesthesia in Jefferson, Georgia. His patient, James M. Venable, was a young man who was already familiar with ether's exhilarating effects, for he reported in a certificate that he had previously inhaled it and was fond of its use. Venable had two small tumors on his neck but refused to have them excised because he feared the pain that accompanied surgery. Knowing that Venable was familiar with ether's action, Dr. Long proposed that ether might alleviate pain and gained his patient's consent to proceed. After inhaling ether from the towel and having the procedure successfully completed, Venable reported that he was unaware of the removal of the tumors.[17] In determining the first fee for anesthesia and surgery, Long settled on a charge of $2.00.[18]

Crawford Long, although limited by a rural surgical practice, conducted the first comparative trial of an anesthetic. He wished to prove that insensibility to pain was caused by ether and was not simply a reflection of the individual's pain threshold or the result of self-hypnosis. When ether was withheld during amputation of the second of two fingers, his experimental patient, a slave boy, and a second patient, a woman from whom he removed two tumors without ether and one with, caused Long to observe that surgery was painless with ether.[19] For Long to gain recognition as the initial discoverer of anesthesia he needed to publish his findings. Long remained silent until 1849, when ether anesthesia was already well known. He explained that he practiced in an isolated environment and had few opportunities for surgical or dental procedures.

Mid-nineteenth-century dentists practiced on the horns of a dilemma. Patients refused beneficial treatment of their teeth for fear of the pain inflicted by the procedure. From a dentist's perspective, pain was not so much life threatening as it was livelihood threatening. A few dentists searched for new ways to relieve pain and one of the first to "discover" a solution was Horace Wells of Hartford, Connecticut, whose great moment of discovery came on December 10, 1844. He observed a lecture-exhibition on nitrous oxide by an itinerant "scientist," Gardner Quincy Colton, who encouraged members of the audience to inhale the gas. Wells observed a young man injure his leg without pain while under the influence of nitrous oxide. Sensing that nitrous oxide might provide pain relief during dental procedures, Wells contacted Colton and boldly proposed an experiment in which Wells was to be the subject. The following day, Colton gave Wells nitrous oxide before a fellow dentist, William Riggs, extracted a tooth.[20] When Wells awoke, he declared that he had not felt any pain and deemed the experiment a success. Colton taught Wells to prepare nitrous oxide, which the dentist administered with success in his practice. His apparatus probably resembled that used by Colton, a wooden tube placed in the mouth through which nitrous oxide was breathed from a small bag filled with the gas.

A few weeks later, in January 1845, Wells attempted a public demonstration in Boston at the Harvard Medical School. He had planned to anesthetize a patient for an amputation, but, when the patient refused surgery, a dental anesthetic for a medical student was substituted. Wells, perhaps influenced by a large and openly critical audience, began the extraction without an adequate level of anesthesia, and the trial was judged a failure. The exact circumstances of Wells' lack of success are not known. His patient may not have cooperated fully or the dose of anesthetic may have been inadequate. Moreover, Wells may not yet have learned that nitrous oxide lacks sufficient potency to serve predictably as an anesthetic without supplementation. In any event, the patient cried out, and Wells was jeered by his audience. No one offered Wells even conditional encouragement. No one recognized that, even though the presentation had been flawed, nitrous oxide might possess significant therapeutic potential. The disappointment disturbed Wells deeply, and while profoundly distressed, he committed suicide in 1848.

Public Demonstration of Ether Anesthesia

Another New Englander, William Thomas Green Morton, briefly shared a dental practice with Horace Wells in Hartford. Wells' daybook shows that he gave Morton a course of instruction in anesthesia, but Morton apparently moved to Boston without paying for the lessons.[21] In Boston, Morton continued his interest in anesthesia and sought instruction from chemist and physician Charles T. Jackson. After learning that ether dropped on the skin provided analgesia, he began experiments with inhaled ether, an agent that proved to be much more versatile than nitrous oxide. Bottles of liquid ether were easily transported, and the volatility of the drug permitted effective inhalation. The concentrations required for surgical anesthesia were so low that patients did not become hypoxic when breathing ether vaporized in air. It also possessed what would later be recognized as a unique property among all inhaled anesthetics: the quality of providing surgical anesthesia without causing respiratory depression. These properties, combined with a slow rate of induction, gave the patient a significant margin of safety, even in the hands of relatively unskilled anesthetists.[22]

After anesthetizing a pet dog, Morton became confident of his skills and anesthetized patients in his dental office. Encouraged by his success, Morton gained an invitation to give a public demonstration in the Bullfinch amphitheater of the Massachusetts General Hospital, the same site as Wells' failed demonstration. Many details of the October 16, 1846, demonstration are well known. Morton secured permission to provide an anesthetic to Edward Gilbert Abbott, a patient of surgeon John Collins Warren. Warren planned to excise a vascular lesion from the left side of Abbott's neck and was about to proceed when Morton arrived late. He had been delayed because he was obliged to wait for an instrument maker to complete a new inhaler (Fig. 1-1). It consisted of a large glass bulb containing a sponge soaked with colored ether and a spout that was placed in the patient's mouth. An opening on the opposite side of the bulb allowed air to enter and be drawn over the ether-soaked sponge with each breath.[23]

The conversations of that morning were not accurately recorded; however, popular accounts state that the surgeon responded testily to Morton's apology for his tardy arrival by remarking, "Sir, your patient is ready." Morton directed his

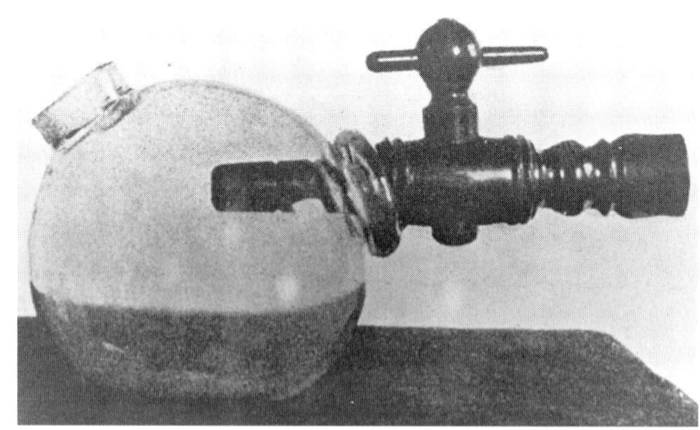

FIGURE 1-1. Morton's ether inhaler (1846).

attention to his patient and first conducted a very abbreviated preoperative evaluation. He inquired, "Are you afraid?" Abbott responded that he was not and took the inhaler in his mouth. After a few minutes, Morton is said to have turned to the surgeon to respond, "Sir, your patient is ready." Gilbert Abbott later reported that he was aware of the surgery but had experienced no pain. When the procedure ended, Warren immediately turned to his audience and uttered that famous line, "Gentlemen, this is no humbug."[24]

What would be recognized as America's greatest contribution to nineteenth-century medicine had been realized, but Morton, wishing to capitalize on his "discovery," refused to divulge what agent was in his inhaler. Some weeks passed before Morton admitted that the active component of the colored fluid, which he had called "Letheon," was diethyl ether. Morton, Wells, Jackson, and their supporters soon became drawn into in a contentious, protracted, and fruitless debate over priority for the discovery. This debate has subsequently been termed "the ether controversy." In short, Morton had applied for a patent for Letheon, and when it was granted, tried to receive royalties for the use of ether as an anesthetic. Eventually, the matter came before the U.S. Congress where the House of Representatives voted to grant Morton a large sum of money for the discovery; however, the Senate quashed the deal.

When the details of Morton's anesthetic technique became public knowledge, the information was transmitted by train, stagecoach, and coastal vessels to other North American cities, and by ship to the world. As ether was easy to prepare and administer, anesthetics were performed in Britain, France, Russia, South Africa, Australia, and other countries almost as soon as surgeons heard the welcome news of the extraordinary discovery. Even though surgery could now be performed with "pain put to sleep," the frequency of operations did not rise rapidly, and several years would pass before anesthesia was universally recommended.

Chloroform and Obstetrics

James Young Simpson was a successful obstetrician of Edinburgh, Scotland, and among the first to use ether for the relief of labor pain. Yet he became dissatisfied with ether and sought a more pleasant, rapid-acting anesthetic. He and his junior associates conducted a bold search by inhaling samples of several volatile chemicals collected for Simpson by British apothecaries. David Waldie suggested chloroform, which had first been prepared in 1831. Simpson and his friends inhaled it after dinner at a party in Simpson's home on the evening of November 4, 1847. They promptly fell unconscious and, when they awoke, were delighted with their success. Simpson quickly set about encouraging the use of chloroform. Within 2 weeks, he submitted his first account of its use to *The Lancet*. Although Simpson introduced chloroform with boldness, and enthusiasm, and defended its use for women in labor, he gave few anesthetics himself. His goal was simply to improve patient comfort during his operative or obstetric activities.

In the nineteenth century, the relief of obstetrical pain had significant social ramifications and made anesthesia during childbirth a controversial subject. Simpson argued against the prevailing view, which held that relieving labor pain was contrary to God's will. The pain of the parturient was perceived as both a component of punishment, and a means of atonement for the Original Sin. Less than a year after administering the first anesthesia during childbirth, Simpson addressed these concerns in a pamphlet entitled *Answers to the Religious Objections Advanced against the Employment of Anaesthetic Agents in Midwifery and Surgery and Obstetrics*. In this work, Simpson recognized the Book of Genesis as being the root of this sentiment, and noted that God promised to relieve the descendants of Adam and Eve of the curse. Additionally, Simpson asserted that labor pain was a result of scientific and anatomic causes, and not the result of religious condemnation. He stated that the upright position of humans necessitated strong pelvic muscles to support the abdominal contents. As a result, he argued, the uterus necessarily developed strong musculature to overcome the resistance of the pelvic floor and that great contractile power caused great pain. All in all, Simpson's pamphlet probably did not have much impact in terms of changing the prevailing viewpoints about controlling labor pain, but he did articulate many concepts that his contemporaries were debating at the time.[25]

Chloroform gained considerable notoriety after John Snow used it during the deliveries of Queen Victoria. The Queen's consort, Prince Albert, interviewed John Snow before he was called to Buckingham Palace to administer chloroform at the request of the Queen's obstetrician. During the monarch's labor, Snow gave analgesic doses of chloroform on a folded handkerchief. This technique was soon termed *chloroform à la reine*. Victoria abhorred the pain of childbirth and enjoyed the relief that chloroform provided. She wrote in her journal, "Dr. Snow gave that blessed chloroform and the effect was soothing, quieting, and delightful beyond measure."[26] When the Queen, as head of the Church of England, endorsed obstetric anesthesia, religious debate over the appropriateness of anesthesia for labor pain terminated abruptly. Four years later, Snow was to give a second anesthetic to the Queen, who was again determined to have chloroform. Snow's daybook states that by the time he arrived, Prince Albert had begun the anesthetic and had given his wife "a little chloroform."

John Snow, already a respected physician, took an interest in anesthetic practice and was soon invited to work with many leading surgeons of the day. In 1848, John Snow introduced a chloroform inhaler. He had recognized the versatility of the new agent and came to prefer it in his practice. At the same time, he initiated what was to become an extraordinary series of experiments that were remarkable in their scope and for anticipating sophisticated research performed a century later. Snow realized that successful anesthetics must not only abolish pain but also prevent movement. He anesthetized several species of animals with varying concentrations of ether and chloroform to determine the concentration required to prevent movement in response to sharp stimuli. Despite the limitations of mid-nineteenth-century technology, this work approximated the modern concept of minimum alveolar concentration (MAC).[27] Snow assessed the anesthetic action of a large number of potential anesthetics but did not find any to rival chloroform or ether. His studies led him to recognize the relationship between solubility, vapor pressure, and anesthetic potency, which was not fully appreciated until after World War II. He also fabricated an experimental closed-circuit device in which the subject (Snow himself) breathed oxygen while the exhaled carbon dioxide was absorbed by potassium hydroxide. Snow published two remarkable books, *On the Inhalation of the Vapour of Ether* (1847) and *On Chloroform and Other Anaesthetics* (1858). The latter was almost completed when he died of a stroke at the age of 45.

THE SECOND GENERATION OF INHALED ANESTHETICS

Throughout the second half of the nineteenth century, other compounds were examined for their anesthetic potential. The pattern of fortuitous discovery that brought nitrous oxide, diethyl ether, and chloroform forward between 1844 and 1847 continued. The next inhaled anesthetics to be used routinely, ethyl chloride and ethylene, were also discovered as a result of unexpected observations. Ethyl chloride and ethylene were first formulated in the eighteenth century. Ethyl chloride was used as a topical anesthetic and counterirritant; it was so volatile that the skin transiently "froze" after ethyl chloride was sprayed on it. Its rediscovery as an anesthetic came in 1894, when a Swedish dentist named Carlson sprayed ethyl chloride into a patient's mouth to "freeze" a dental abscess. Carlson was surprised to discover that his patient suddenly lost consciousness.

As the mechanisms to deliver drugs were refined, entirely new classes of medications were also developed, with the intention of providing safer, more pleasant pain control. Ethylene gas was the first alternative to ether and chloroform, but it had some major disadvantages. The rediscovery of ethylene in 1923 also came from a serendipitous observation. After it was learned that ethylene gas had been used to inhibit the opening of carnation buds in Chicago greenhouses, it was speculated that a gas that put flowers to sleep might also have an anesthetic action on humans. Arno Luckhardt was the first to publish a clinical study in February 1923. Within a month, Isabella Herb in Chicago and W. Easson Brown in Toronto presented two other independent studies. Ethylene was not a successful anesthetic because high concentrations were required and it was explosive. An additional significant shortcoming was a particularly unpleasant smell, which could only be partially disguised by the use of oil of orange or a cheap perfume. When cyclopropane was introduced, ethylene was abandoned.

Cyclopropane's anesthetic action was inadvertently discovered in 1929.[28] Brown and Henderson had previously shown that propylene had desirable properties as an anesthetic when freshly prepared; but after storage in a steel cylinder, it deteriorated to create a toxic material that produced nausea and cardiac irregularities in humans. Velyien Henderson, a professor of pharmacology at the University of Toronto, suggested that the toxic product be identified. After a chemist, George Lucas, identified cyclopropane among the chemicals in the tank, he prepared a sample in low concentration with oxygen and administered it to two kittens. The animals fell asleep quietly but quickly recovered unharmed. Rather than being a toxic contaminant, Lucas saw that cyclopropane was a potent anesthetic. After its effects in other animals were studied and cyclopropane proved to be stable after storage, human experimentation began.

Henderson was the first volunteer; Lucas followed. They then arranged a public demonstration in which Frederick Banting, a Nobel laureate for the discovery of insulin, was anesthetized before a group of physicians. Despite this promising beginning, further research was abruptly halted. Several anesthetic deaths in Toronto had been attributed to ethyl chloride, and concern about Canadian clinical trials of cyclopropane prevented human studies from proceeding. Rather than abandon the study, Henderson encouraged an American friend, Ralph Waters, to use cyclopropane at the University of Wisconsin. The Wisconsin group investigated the drug thoroughly and reported their clinical success in 1934.[29]

In 1930, Chauncey Leake and MeiYu Chen performed successful laboratory trials of vinethene (divinyl ether) but were thwarted in its further development by a professor of surgery in San Francisco. Ironically, Canadians, who had lost cyclopropane to Wisconsin, learned of vinethene from Leake and Chen in California and conducted the first human study in 1932 at the University of Alberta, Edmonton. International research collaboration enabled early anesthetic use of both cyclopropane and divinyl ether, advances that may not have occurred independently in either the United States or Canada.

All potent anesthetics of this period were explosive save for chloroform, whose hepatic and cardiac toxicity limited use in America. Anesthetic explosions remained a rare but devastating risk to both anesthesiologist and patient. To reduce the danger of explosion during the incendiary days of World War II, British anaesthetists turned to trichloroethylene. This nonflammable anesthetic found limited application in America, as it decomposed to release phosgene when warmed in the presence of soda lime. By the end of World War II, however, another class of noninflammable anesthetics was prepared for laboratory trials. Ten years later, fluorinated hydrocarbons revolutionized inhalation anesthesia.

FLUORINATED ANESTHETICS

Fluorine, the lightest and most reactive halogen, forms exceptionally stable bonds. These bonds, although sometimes created with explosive force, resist separation by chemical or thermal means. For that reason, many early attempts to fluorinate hydrocarbons in a controlled manner were frustrated by the marked chemical activity of fluorine. In 1930, the first commercial application of fluorine chemistry came in the form of the refrigerant, Freon. This was followed by the first attempt to prepare a fluorinated anesthetic by Harold Booth and E. May Bixby in 1932. Although their drug, monochlorodifluoromethane, was devoid of anesthetic action, as were other drugs studied that decade, their report predicted future developments. "A survey of the properties of 166 known gases suggested that the best possibility of finding a new noncombustible anesthetic gas lay in the field of organic fluoride compounds. Fluorine substitution for other halogens lowers the boiling point, increases stability, and generally decreases toxicity."[30]

The secret demands of the Manhattan Project for refined uranium-235 served as an impetus to better understanding of fluorine chemistry. Researchers learned that uranium might be refined through the creation of an intermediate compound, uranium hexafluoride. Earl McBee of Purdue University, who had a long-standing interest in the fluoridation of hydrocarbons, undertook part of this project. McBee also held a grant from the Mallinckrodt Chemical Works, a manufacturer of ether and cyclopropane, to prepare new fluorinated compounds, for anesthesia testing. By 1945, the Purdue team had created small amounts of 46 fluorinated ethanes, propanes, butanes, and an ether.

The anesthetic value of these chemicals would not have been appreciated, however, if Mallinckrodt had not also provided financial support for research in pharmacology at Vanderbilt University. The chair, Benjamin Robbins, was a pharmacologist, and was better able to assess the new drugs than could most other anesthesiologists of that period. Robbins tested McBee's compounds in mice, and selected the most promising for evaluation in dogs. Unfortunately, none of these compounds found a place as an anesthetic but Robbins' conclusions on the effects of fluorination, bromination, and chlorination in his landmark report of 1946 encouraged later successful studies.[31]

A team at the University of Maryland under Professor of Pharmacology John C. Krantz Jr. investigated the anesthetic properties of dozens of hydrocarbons over a period of several years, but only one, ethyl vinyl ether, entered clinical use in 1947. Because it was flammable, Krantz requested that it be fluorinated. In response, Julius Shukys prepared several fluorinated analogs. One of these, trifluoroethyl vinyl ether, or fluroxene, became the first fluorinated anesthetic. Fluroxene was marketed from 1954 until 1974. However, it was withdrawn when a delayed discovery showed a metabolite to be toxic to lower animals. Fluroxene is important for its historical interest as the first fluorinated anesthetic gas but our experience with it also underscores the need for continual surveillance of anesthetic drug actions and adverse effects.[32]

In 1951, Charles Suckling, a British chemist of Imperial Chemical Industries, was asked to create a new anesthetic. Suckling, who already had an expert understanding of fluorination, began by asking clinicians to describe the properties of an ideal anesthetic. He learned from this inquiry that his search must consider several limiting factors, including the volatility, inflammability, stability, and potency of the compounds. After 2 years of research and testing, Charles Suckling created halothane. He first determined that halothane possessed anesthetic action by anesthetizing mealworms and houseflies before he forwarded it to pharmacologist James Raventos. Suckling also made accurate predictions as to the concentrations required for anesthesia in higher animals. After Raventos completed a favorable review, halothane was offered to Michael Johnstone, a respected anesthetist of Manchester, England, who recognized its great advantages over other anesthetics available in 1956. After Johnstone's endorsement, halothane use spread quickly and widely within the practice of anesthesia.[33]

Halothane was followed in 1960 by methoxyflurane, an anesthetic that remained popular for a decade. By 1970, however, it was learned that dose-related nephrotoxicity following protracted methoxyflurane anesthesia was caused by inorganic fluoride. Similarly, because of persisting concern that rare cases of hepatitis following anesthesia might be a result of a metabolite of halothane, the search for newer inhaled anesthetics focused on the resistance to metabolic degradation.

Two fluorinated liquid anesthetics, enflurane and its isomer isoflurane, were results of the search for increased stability. They were synthesized by Ross Terrell in 1963 and 1965, respectively. Because enflurane was easier to create, it preceded isoflurane. Its application was restricted after it was shown to be a marked cardiovascular depressant and to have some convulsant properties. Isoflurane was nearly abandoned because of difficulties in its purification, but after Louise Speers overcame this problem, several successful trials were published in 1971. The release of isoflurane for clinical use was delayed again for more than half a decade by calls for repeated testing in lower animals, owing to an unfounded concern that the drug might be carcinogenic. As a consequence, isoflurane received more thorough testing than any other drug heretofore used in anesthesia. The era when an anesthetic could be introduced following a single fortuitous observation had given way to a cautious program of assessment and reassessment. Remarkably, no anesthetics were introduced into clinical use for another 20 years. Finally, desflurane was released in 1992, and sevoflurane was released in 1994. Xenon, a gas having many properties of the ideal anesthetic, was administered to a few patients in the early 1950s but it never gained popularity because of the extreme costs associated with its removal from air. However, interest in xenon has been renewed now that gas concentrations can be accurately measured when administered at low flows, and devices are available to scavenge and reuse the gas.

REGIONAL ANESTHESIA

3 Cocaine, an extract of the coca leaf, was the first effective local anesthetic. After Albert Niemann refined the active alkaloid and named it *cocaine,* it was used in experiments by a few investigators. It was noted that cocaine provided topical anesthesia and even produced local insensibility when injected, but Carl Koller, a Viennese surgical intern, first recognized the utility of cocaine in clinical practice.

In 1884, Carl Koller was completing his medical training at a time when many operations on the eye were performed without general anesthesia. Almost four decades after the discovery of ether, general anesthesia by mask still had limitations for ophthalmic surgery: lack of patient cooperation, interference of the anesthesia apparatus with surgical access, and the high incidence of postoperative nausea and vomiting. At that time, since fine sutures were not available and surgical incisions of the eye were not closed, postoperative vomiting threatened the extrusion of the globe's contents, putting the patient at risk for irrevocable blindness.[34]

While a medical student, Koller had worked in a Viennese laboratory in a search of a topical ophthalmic anesthetic to overcome the limitations of general anesthesia. Unfortunately, the suspensions of morphine, chloral hydrate, and other drugs that he had used had been ineffectual. In 1884, Koller's friend, Sigmund Freud, became interested in the cerebral-stimulating effects of cocaine and gave him a small sample in an envelope, which he placed in his pocket. When the envelope leaked, a few grains of cocaine stuck to Koller's finger and he absentmindedly licked his tongue. When his tongue became numb, Koller instantly realized that he had found the object of his search. In his lab, he made a suspension of cocaine crystals that he and a lab associate tested in the eyes of a frog, a rabbit, and a dog. Satisfied with the anesthetic effects seen in the animal models, Koller dropped the solution onto his own cornea. To his amazement, his eyes were insensitive to the touch of a pin.[35] As an intern, Carl Koller could not afford to attend a Congress of German Ophthalmologists in Heidelberg on September 15, 1884. However, a friend presented his article at the meeting and a revolution in ophthalmic surgery and other surgical disciplines began. Within the next year, more than 100 articles supporting the use of cocaine appeared in European and American medical journals. In 1888, Koller immigrated to New York, where he practiced ophthalmology for the remainder of his career.

American surgeons quickly developed new applications for cocaine. Its efficacy in anesthetizing the nose, mouth, larynx, trachea, rectum, and urethra was described in October 1884. The next month, the first reports of its subcutaneous injection were published. In December 1884, two young surgeons, William Halsted and Richard Hall, described blocks of the sensory nerves of the face and arm. Halsted even performed a brachial plexus block but did so under direct vision while the patient received an inhaled anesthetic.[36] Unfortunately, self-experimentation with cocaine was hazardous, as both surgeons became addicted.[37] Addiction was an ill-understood but frequent problem in the late nineteenth century, especially when cocaine and morphine were present in many patent medicines and folk remedies.

Other regional anesthetic techniques were attempted before the end of the nineteenth century. The term "spinal anesthesia" was coined in 1885 by Leonard Corning, a neurologist who had observed Hall and Halsted. Corning wanted to assess the action of cocaine as a specific therapy for neurologic problems. After first assessing its action in a dog, producing a blockade of rapid onset that was confined to the animal's rear legs, he performed a neuraxial block using cocaine on a man "addicted to masturbation." Corning administered one dose without effect, then after a second dose, the patient's legs "felt sleepy." The man had impaired sensibility in his lower extremity after about 20 minutes and left Corning's office "none the worse for the experience."[38] Although Corning did not describe escape of cerebrospinal fluid (CSF) in either case, it is likely that the dog had a spinal anesthetic and that the man had an epidural anesthetic. No therapeutic benefit was described, but Corning closed his account and his attention to the subject by suggesting that cocainization might in time be "a substitute for etherization in genito-urinary or other branches of surgery."[39]

Two other authors, August Bier and Theodor Tuffier, described authentic spinal anesthesia, with mention of cerebrospinal fluid, injection of cocaine, and an appropriately short onset of action. In a comparative review of the original articles by Bier, Tuffier, and Corning, it was concluded that Corning's injection was extradural, and Bier merited the credit for introducing spinal anesthesia.[40]

SPINAL ANESTHESIA

Fourteen years passed before spinal anesthesia was performed for surgery. In the interval, Heinrich Quincke of Kiel, Germany, had described his technique of lumbar puncture. He offered the valuable observation that it was most safely performed at the level of the third or fourth lumbar interspace, because entry at that level was below the termination of the spinal cord. Quincke's technique was used in Kiel for the first deliberate cocainization of the spinal cord in 1899 by his surgical colleague, August Bier. Six patients received small doses of cocaine intrathecally, but, because some cried out during surgery while others vomited and experienced headaches, Bier considered it necessary to conduct further experiments before continuing this technique for surgery.

Professor Bier permitted his assistant, Dr. Hildebrandt, to perform a lumbar puncture, but, after the needle penetrated the dura, Hildebrandt could not fit the syringe to the needle and a large volume of the professor's spinal fluid escaped. They were at the point of abandoning the study when Hildebrandt volunteered to be the subject of a second attempt. Their persistence was rewarded with an astonishing success. Twenty-three minutes after the spinal injection, Bier noted: "A strong blow with an iron hammer against the tibia was not felt as pain. After 25 minutes: Strong pressure and pulling on a testicle were not painful."[40] They celebrated their success with wine and cigars. That night, both developed violent headaches, which they attributed at first to their celebration. Bier's headache was relieved after 9 days of bedrest. Hildebrandt, as a house officer, did not have the luxury of continued rest. Bier postulated that their headaches were a result of the loss of large volumes of CSF and urged that this be avoided if possible. The high incidence of complications following lumbar puncture with wide-bore needles and the toxic reactions attributed to cocaine explain his later loss of interest in spinal anesthesia.[41]

Surgeons in several other countries soon practiced spinal anesthesia and progress occurred by many small contributions to the technique. Theodor Tuffier published the first series of 125 spinal anesthetics from France and he later counseled that the solution should not be injected before CSF was seen. The first American report was by Rudolph Matas of New Orleans, whose first patient developed postanesthetic meningismus, a frequent complication that was overcome in part by the use of hermetically sealed sterile solutions recommended by E. W. Lee of Philadelphia and sterile gloves as advocated by Halsted. During 1899, Dudley Tait and Guidlo Caglieri of San Francisco performed experimental studies in animals and therapeutic spinals for orthopedic patients. They encouraged the use of fine needles to lessen the escape of CSF and urged that the skin and deeper tissues be infiltrated beforehand with local anesthesia.[42] This had been suggested earlier by William Halsted and the foremost advocate of infiltration anesthesia, Carl Ludwig Schleich of Berlin. An early American specialist in anesthesia, Ormond Goldan, published an anesthesia record appropriate for recording the course of "intraspinal cocainization" in 1900. In the same year, Heinrich Braun learned of a newly described extract of the adrenal gland, epinephrine, which he used to prolong the action of local anesthetics with great success. Braun developed several new nerve blocks, coined the term "conduction anesthesia," and is remembered by European writers as the "father of conduction anesthesia." Braun was the first person to use procaine, which, along with stovaine, was one of the first synthetic local anesthetics produced to reduce the toxicity of cocaine. Further advances in spinal anesthesia followed the introduction of these and other synthetic local anesthetics.

Before 1907, anesthesiologists were sometimes disappointed to observe that their spinal anesthetics were incomplete. Most believed that the drug spread solely by local diffusion before the property of baricity was investigated by Arthur Barker, a London surgeon.[43] Barker constructed a glass tube shaped to follow the curves of the human spine and used it to demonstrate the limited spread of colored solutions that he had injected through a T-piece in the lumbar region. Barker applied this observation to use solutions of stovaine made hyperbaric by the addition of 5% glucose, which worked in a more predictable fashion. After the injection was complete, Barker placed his patient's head on pillows to contain the anesthetic below the nipple line. Lincoln Sise acknowledged Barker's work in 1935 when he introduced the use of hyperbaric solutions of pontocaine. John Adriani advanced the concept further in 1946 when he used a hyperbaric solution to produce "saddle block," or perineal anesthesia. Adriani's patients remained seated after injection as the drug descended to the sacral nerves.

Tait, Jonnesco, and other early masters of spinal anesthesia used a cervical approach for thyroidectomy and thoracic procedures, but this radical approach was supplanted in 1928 by the lumbar injection of hypobaric solutions of "light" nupercaine by G. P. Pitkin. Although the use of hypobaric solutions is now limited primarily to patients positioned in the jackknife position, their former use for thoracic procedures demanded skill and precise timing. The enthusiasts of hypobaric anesthesia devised formulas to attempt to predict the time in seconds needed for a warmed solution of hypobaric nupercaine to spread in patients of varying size from its site of injection in the lumbar area to the level of the fourth thoracic dermatome.

The recurring problem of inadequate duration of single-injection spinal anesthesia led a Philadelphia surgeon, William Lemmon, to devise an apparatus for continuous spinal anesthesia in 1940.[44] Lemmon began with the patient in the lateral position. The spinal tap was performed with a malleable silver needle, which was left in position. As the patient was turned supine, the needle was positioned through a hole in the mattress and table. Additional injections of local anesthetic could be performed as required. Malleable silver needles also found a less cumbersome and more common application in 1942 when Waldo Edwards and Robert Hingson encouraged the use of Lemmon's needles for continuous caudal anesthesia in obstetrics. In 1944 Edward Tuohy of the Mayo Clinic introduced two important modifications of the continuous spinal techniques. He developed the now familiar Tuohy needle[45] as a means of improving the ease of passage of lacquered silk ureteral catheters through which he injected incremental doses of local anesthetic.[46]

In 1949, Martinez Curbelo of Havana, Cuba, used Tuohy's needle and a ureteral catheter to perform the first continuous epidural anesthetic. Silk and gum elastic catheters were difficult to sterilize and sometimes caused dural infections before being superseded by disposable plastics. Yet deliberate single-injection peridural anesthesia had been practiced occasionally for decades before continuous techniques brought it greater popularity. At the beginning of the twentieth century, two French clinicians experimented independently with caudal anesthesia. The neurologist Jean Athanase Sicard applied the technique for a nonsurgical purpose, the relief of back pain. Fernand Cathelin used caudal anesthesia as a less dangerous alternative to spinal anesthesia for hernia repairs. He also demonstrated that the epidural space terminated in the neck by injecting a solution of India ink into the caudal canal of a dog. The lumbar approach was first used solely for multiple paravertebral nerve blocks before the Pagés-Dogliotti single-injection technique became accepted. As they worked separately, the technique carries the names of both men. Captain Fidel Pagés prepared an elegant demonstration of segmental single-injection peridural anesthesia in 1921, but died soon after his paper appeared in a Spanish military journal.[47] Ten years later, Achille M. Dogliotti of Turin, Italy, wrote a classic study that made the epidural technique well known.[48] Whereas Pagés used a tactile approach to identify the epidural space, Dogliotti identified it by the loss-of-resistance technique.

Surgery on the extremities lent itself to other regional anesthesia techniques. In 1902, Harvey Cushing coined the phrase "regional anesthesia" for his technique of blocking either the brachial or sciatic plexus under direct vision during general anesthesia to reduce anesthesia requirements and provide postoperative pain relief.[49] Fifteen years before his publication, George Crile advanced a similar approach to reduce the stress and shock of surgery. Crile, a dedicated advocate of regional and infiltration techniques during general anesthesia, coined the term "anoci-association."[50]

An intravenous regional technique with procaine was reported in 1908 by August Bier, the surgeon who had pioneered spinal anesthesia. Bier injected procaine into a vein of the upper limb between two tourniquets. Even though the technique is termed the "Bier block," it was not used for many decades until it was reintroduced 55 years later by Mackinnon Holmes, who modified the technique by exsanguination before applying a single proximal cuff. Holmes used lidocaine, the very successful amide local anesthetic synthesized in 1943 by Lofgren and Lundquist of Sweden.

Several investigators achieved upper extremity anesthesia by percutaneous injections of the brachial plexus. In 1911, based on his intimate knowledge of the anatomy of the axillary area, Hirschel promoted a "blind" axillary injection. In the same year, Kulenkampff described a supraclavicular approach in which the operator sought out paresthesias of the plexus while keeping the needle at a point superficial to the first rib and the pleura. The risk of pneumothorax with Kulenkampff's approach led Mulley to attempt blocks more proximally by a lateral paravertebral approach, the precursor of what is now popularly known as the "Winnie block."

Heinrich Braun wrote the earliest textbook of local anesthesia, which appeared in its first English translation in 1914. After 1922, Gaston Labat's *Regional Anesthesia* dominated the American market. Labat migrated from France to the Mayo Clinic in Minnesota, where he served briefly before taking a permanent position at the Bellevue Hospital in New York. He formed the first American Society for Regional Anesthesia.[51] After Labat's death, Emery A. Rovenstine was recruited to Bellevue to continue Labat's work, among other responsibilities. Rovenstein created the first American clinic for the treatment of chronic pain, where he and his associates refined techniques of lytic and therapeutic injections and used the American Society of Regional Anesthesia to further the knowledge of pain management across the United States.[52]

4 The development of the multidisciplinary pain clinic was one of many contributions to anesthesiology made by John J. Bonica, a renowned teacher of regional techniques. During his periods of military, civilian, and university service at the University of Washington, Bonica formulated a series of improvements in the management of patients with chronic pain. His classic text *The Management of Pain,* now in its third edition, is regarded as a classic of the literature of anesthesia.

ANESTHESIA MACHINES AND MECHANICAL VENTILATION

Early Anesthesia Delivery Systems

5 The transition from ether inhalers and chloroform-soaked handkerchiefs to more sophisticated anesthesia delivery equipment occurred gradually, with incremental advances supplanting older methods. One of the earliest anesthesia apparatus designs was that of John Snow, who had realized the inadequacies of ether inhalers through which patients rebreathed via a mouthpiece. After practicing anesthesia for only 2 weeks, Snow created the first of his series of ingenious ether inhalers.[53] His best-known apparatus featured unidirectional valves within a malleable, well-fitting mask of his own design, which closely resembles the form of a modern face mask. The face piece was connected to the vaporizer by a breathing tube, which Snow deliberately designed to be wider than the human trachea so that even rapid respirations would not be impeded. A metal coil within the vaporizer ensured that the patient's inspired breath was drawn over a large surface area to promote the uptake of ether. The device also incorporated a warm water bath to maintain the volatility of the agent (Fig. 1-2). Snow did not attempt to capitalize on his creativity, in contrast to William Morton; he closed his account of its preparation with the generous observation, "There is no restriction respecting the making of it."[54]

Joseph Clover, another British physician, was the first anesthetist to administer chloroform in known concentrations through the "Clover bag." He obtained a 4.5% concentration of chloroform in air by pumping a measured volume of air with a bellows through a warmed evaporating vessel containing a known volume of liquid chloroform.[55] Although it was realized that nitrous oxide diluted in air often gave a hypoxic mixture, and that the oxygen-nitrous oxide mixture was safer, Chicago surgeon Edmund Andrews complained about the physical limitations of delivering anesthesia to patients in their homes. The

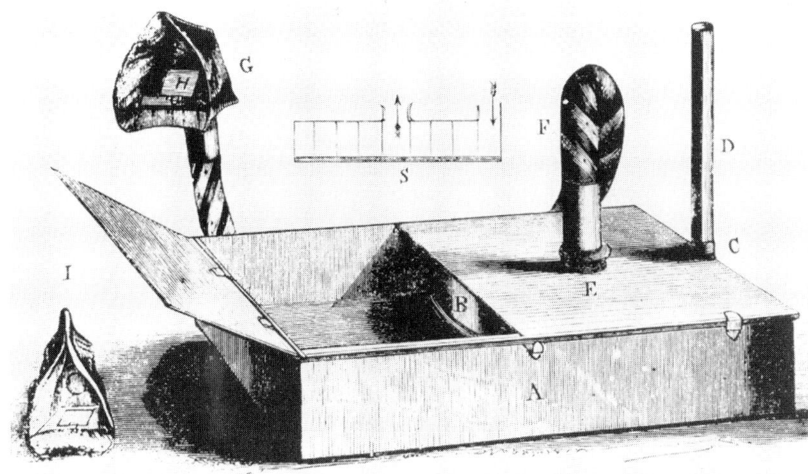

FIGURE 1-2. John Snow's ether inhaler (1847). The ether chamber *(B)* contained a spiral coil so that the air entering through the brass tube *(D)* was saturated by ether before ascending the flexible tube *(F)* to the face mask *(G)*. The ether chamber rested in a bath of warm water *(A)*.

large bag was conspicuous and awkward to carry along busy streets. He observed that, "In city practice, among the higher classes, however, this is no obstacle as the bag can always be taken in a carriage, without attracting attention."[56] In 1872, Andrews was delighted to report the availability of liquefied nitrous oxide compressed under 750 pounds of pressure, which allowed a supply sufficient for three patients to be carried in a single cylinder.

Critical to increasing patient safety was the development of a machine capable of delivering a calibrated amount of gas and volatile anesthetic. In the late nineteenth century, demands in dentistry instigated development of the first freestanding anesthesia machines. Three American dentist-entrepreneurs, Samuel S. White, Charles Teter, and Jay Heidbrink, developed the original series of U.S. instruments that used compressed cylinders of nitrous oxide and oxygen. Before 1900, the S. S. White Company modified Frederick Hewitt's apparatus and marketed its continuous-flow machine, which was refined by Teter in 1903. Heidbrink added reducing valves in 1912. In the same year, physicians initiated other important developments. Water-bubble flow meters, introduced by Frederick Cotton and Walter Boothby of Harvard University, allowed the proportion of gases and their flow rate to be approximated. The Cotton and Boothby apparatus was transformed into a practical portable machine by James Tayloe Gwathmey of New York. The Gwathmey machine caught the attention of a London anesthetist Henry E. G. "Cockie" Boyle, who acknowledged his debt to the American when he incorporated Gwathmey's concepts in the first of the series of "Boyle" machines that were marketed by Coxeter and British Oxygen Corporation. During the same period in Lubeck, Germany, Heinrich Draeger and his son, Bernhaard, adapted compressed-gas technology, which they had originally developed for mine rescue equipment, to manufacture ether and chloroform-oxygen machines.

In the years after World War I, several U.S. manufacturers continued to bring forward widely admired anesthesia machines. Some companies were founded by dentists, including Heidbrink and Teter. Karl Connell and Elmer Gatch were surgeons. Richard von Foregger was an engineer who was exceptionally receptive to clinicians' suggestions for additional features for his machines. Elmer McKesson became one of the country's first specialists in anesthesiology in 1910 and developed a series of gas machines. In an era of flammable anesthetics, McKesson carried nonflammable nitrous oxide anesthesia to its therapeutic limit by performing inductions with 100% nitrous oxide and thereafter adding small volumes of oxygen. If the resultant cyanosis became too profound, McKesson depressed a valve on his machine that flushed a small volume of oxygen into the circuit. Even though his techniques of primary and secondary saturation with nitrous oxide are no longer used, the oxygen flush valve is part of McKesson's legacy.

Carbon Dioxide Absorption

Carbon dioxide (CO_2) absorbance is a basic element of modern anesthetic machines. It was initially developed to allow rebreathing of gas and minimize loss of flammable gases into the room, thereby reducing the risk of explosion. In current practice, it permits decreased utilization of anesthetic and reduced cost. The first CO_2 absorber in anesthesia came in 1906 from the work of Franz Kuhn, a German surgeon. His use of canisters developed for mine rescues by Draeger was innovative, but his circuit had unfortunate limitations. The exceptionally narrow breathing tubes and a large dead space explain its very limited use, and Kuhn's device was ignored.

A few years later, the first American machine with a CO_2 absorber was independently fabricated by a pharmacologist named Dennis Jackson. In 1915, Jackson developed an early technique of CO_2 absorption that permitted the use of a closed anesthesia circuit. He used solutions of sodium and calcium hydroxide to absorb CO_2. As his laboratory was located in an area of St. Louis, Missouri, heavily laden with coal smoke, Jackson reported that the apparatus allowed him the first breaths of absolutely fresh air he had ever enjoyed in that city. The complexity of Jackson's apparatus limited its use in hospital practice, but his pioneering work in this field encouraged Ralph Waters to introduce a simpler device using soda lime granules 9 years later. Waters positioned a soda lime canister (Fig. 1-3) between a face mask and an adjacent breathing bag to which was attached the fresh gas flow. As long as the mask was held against the face, only small volumes of fresh gas flow were required and no valves were needed.[57]

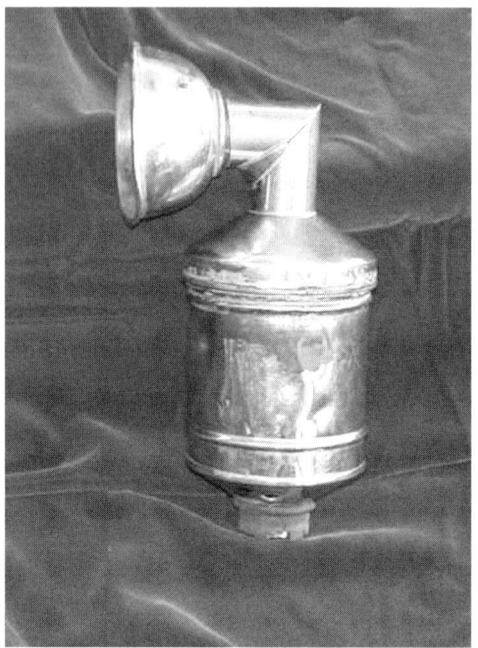

FIGURE 1-3. Waters' carbon dioxide absorbance canister.

When Waters made his first "to-and-fro" device, he was attempting to develop a specialist practice in anesthesia in Sioux City, Iowa, and had achieved limited financial success. Waters believed that his device had advantages for both clinician and patient. Economy of operation was crucial when private patients and insurance companies were reluctant to pay for specialist's services, drugs, and supplies. Waters estimated that his new canister would reduce costs for gases and soda lime to less than $.50 per hour. This portable apparatus could be easily carried to private residences and hospital settings, preventing contamination of the operating environments with the malodorous and explosive vapors of ethylene. Waters even recognized that the canister supplied the added benefits of conserving body heat and humidifying inspired gases.

Waters' device featured awkward positioning of the canister close to the patient's face. Brian Sword overcame this limitation in 1930 with a freestanding machine with unidirectional valves to create a circle system and an in-line CO_2 absorber.[58] James Elam and his co-workers at the Roswell Park Cancer Institute in Buffalo, New York, further refined the CO_2 absorber, increasing the efficiency of CO_2 removal with a minimum of resistance for breathing.[59] Consequently, the circle system introduced by Sword in the 1930s, with a few refinements, became the standard anesthesia circuit in North America.

Alternative Circuits

A valveless device, the Ayre's T-piece, has found wide application in the management of intubated patients. Phillip Ayre practiced anesthesia in England when the limitations of equipment for pediatric patients produced what he described as "a protracted and sanguine battle between surgeon and anaesthetist, with the poor unfortunate baby as the battlefield."[60] In 1937, Ayre introduced his valveless T-piece to reduce the effort of breathing in neurosurgical patients. The T-piece soon became particularly popular for cleft palate repairs, as the surgeon had free access to the mouth. Positive pressure ventilation could be achieved when the anesthetist obstructed the expiratory limb. In time, this ingenious, lightweight, nonrebreathing device evolved through more than 100 modifications for a variety of special situations. A significant alteration was Gordon Jackson Rees' circuit, which permitted improved control of ventilation by substituting a breathing bag on the outflow limb.[61] An alternative method to reduce the amount of equipment near the patient is provided by the coaxial circuit of the Bain-Spoerel apparatus.[62] This lightweight tube-within-a-tube has served very well in many circumstances since its Canadian innovators described it in 1972.

Flow Meters

As closed and semiclosed circuits became practical, gas flow could be measured with greater accuracy. Bubble flow meters were replaced with dry bobbins or ball-bearing flow meters, which, although they did not leak fluids, could cause inaccurate measurements if they adhered to the glass column. In 1910, M. Neu had been the first to apply rotameters in anesthesia for the administration of nitrous oxide and oxygen, but his machine was not a commercial success, perhaps because of the great cost of nitrous oxide in Germany at that time. Rotameters designed for use in German industry were first employed in Britain in 1937 by Richard Salt; but as World War II approached, the English were denied access to these sophisticated flow meters. After World War II rotameters became regularly employed in British anesthesia machines, although most American equipment still featured nonrotating floats. The now universal practice of displaying gas flow in liters per minute was not a customary part of all American machines until more than a decade after World War II. Some anesthesiologists still in practice learned to calculate gas flows in the cumbersome proportions of gallons per hour.

Vaporizers

The art of a smooth induction with a potent anesthetic was a great challenge, particularly if the inspired concentration could not be determined with accuracy. This limitation was particularly true of chloroform, as an excessive rate of administration produced a lethal cardiac depression. Even the clinical introduction of halothane after 1956 might have been similarly thwarted except for a fortunate coincidence: the prior development of calibrated vaporizers. Two types of calibrated vaporizers designed for other anesthetics had become available in the half decade before halothane was marketed. The prompt acceptance of halothane was in part because of an ability to provide it in carefully titrated concentrations.

The Copper Kettle was the first temperature-compensated, accurate vaporizer. It had been developed by Lucien Morris at the University of Wisconsin in response to Ralph Waters' plan to test chloroform by giving it in controlled concentrations.[63] Morris achieved this goal by passing a metered flow of oxygen through a vaporizer chamber that contained a porex disk to separate the oxygen into minute bubbles. The gas became fully saturated with anesthetic vapor as it percolated through the liquid. The concentration of the anesthetic inspired by the patient could be calculated by knowing the vapor pressure of the liquid anesthetic, the volume of oxygen flowing through the liquid, and the total volume of gases from all sources entering the anesthesia circuit. Although experimental models of Morris' vaporizer used a water bath to maintain stability, the excellent thermal conductivity of copper was substituted in later models. When first marketed, the Copper Kettle did not feature a mechanism to indicate changes in the temperature (and vapor pressure) of the liquid. Shuh-Hsun Ngai proposed the incorporation of a thermometer, a suggestion that was later added to all vaporizers of that class.[64]

The Copper Kettle (Foregger Company) and the Vernitrol (Ohio Medical Products) were universal vaporizers—a property that remained a distinct advantage as new anesthetics were marketed. Universal vaporizers could be charged with any anesthetic liquid, and, provided that its vapor pressure and temperature were known, the inspired concentration could be calculated quickly. This feature gave an unanticipated advantage to American investigators. They were not dependent on the construction of new agent-specific vaporizers.

When halothane was first marketed in Britain, an effective temperature-compensated, agent-specific vaporizer had recently been placed in clinical use. The TECOTA (TEmperature COmpensated Trichloroethylene Air) vaporizer had been created by engineers who had been frustrated by a giant corporation's unresponsiveness. Their vaporizer featured a bimetallic strip composed of brass and a nickel–steel alloy, two metals with different coefficients of expansion. As the anesthetic vapor cooled, the strip bent to move away from the orifice, thereby permitting more fresh gas to enter the vaporizing chamber. This maintained a constant inspired concentration despite changes in temperature and vapor pressure. After their TECOTA vaporizer was accepted into anesthetic practice, the technology was used to create the "Fluotec," the first of a series of agent-specific "tec" vaporizers for use in the operating room.

Ventilators

Mechanical ventilators are now an integral part of the anesthesia machine. Patients are ventilated during general anesthesia by electrical or gas-powered devices that are simple to control yet sophisticated in their function. The history of mechanical positive pressure ventilation began with attempts to resuscitate victims of drowning by a bellows attached to a mask or tracheal tube. These experiments found little role in anesthetic care for many years. At the beginning of the twentieth century, however, several modalities were explored before intermittent positive pressure machines evolved.

A series of artificial environments were created in response to the frustration experienced by thoracic surgeons who found that the lung collapsed when they incised the pleura. Between 1900 and 1910, continuous positive or negative pressure devices were created to maintain inflation of the lungs of a spontaneously breathing patient once the chest was opened. Brauer (1904) and Murphy (1905) placed the patient's head and neck in a box in which positive pressure was continually maintained. Sauerbruch (1904) created a negative-pressure operating chamber encompassing both the surgical team and the patient's body and from which only the patient's head projected.[66]

In 1907, the first intermittent positive-pressure device, the Draeger "Pulmotor," was developed to rhythmically inflate the lungs. This instrument and later American models such as the E & J Resuscitator were used almost exclusively by firefighters and mine rescue workers. A few European medical workers had an early interest in rhythmic inflation of the lungs. In 1934 a Swedish team developed the "Spiropulsator," which C. Crafoord later modified for use during cyclopropane anesthesia.[65] Its action was controlled by a magnetic control valve called the flasher, a type first used to provide intermittent gas flow for the lights of navigational buoys. When Trier Morch, a Danish anesthesiologist, could not obtain a Spiropulsator during World War II, he fabricated the Morch "Respirator," which used a piston pump to rhythmically deliver a fixed volume of gas to the patient.[66]

A major stimulus to the development of ventilators came as a consequence of a devastating epidemic of poliomyelitis that struck Copenhagen, Denmark, in 1952. As scores of patients were admitted, the only effective ventilatory support that could be provided to patients with bulbar paralysis was continuous manual ventilation via a tracheostomy employing devices such as Waters' "to-and-fro" circuit. This succeeded only through the dedicated efforts of hundreds of volunteers. Medical students served in relays to ventilate paralyzed patients. The Copenhagen crisis stimulated a broad European interest in the development of portable ventilators in anticipation of another epidemic of poliomyelitis. At this time, the common practice in North American hospitals was to place polio patients with respiratory involvement in "iron lungs," metal cylinders that encased the body below the neck. Inspiration was caused by intermittent negative pressure created by an electric motor acting on a piston-like device occupying the foot of the chamber.

Some early American ventilators were adaptations of respiratory-assist machines originally designed for the delivery of aerosolized drugs for respiratory therapy. Two types employed the Bennett or Bird "flow-sensitive" valves. The Bennett valve was designed during World War II when a team of physiologists at the University of Southern California encountered difficulties in separating inspiration from expiration in an experimental apparatus designed to provide positive pressure breathing for aviators at high altitude. An engineer, Ray Bennett, visited their laboratory, observed their problem, and resolved it with a mechanical flow-sensitive automatic valve. A second valving mechanism was later designed by an aeronautical engineer, Forrest Bird.

The use of the Bird and Bennett valves gained an anesthetic application when the gas flow from the valve was directed into a rigid plastic jar containing a breathing bag or bellows as part of an anesthesia circuit. These "bag-in-bottle" devices mimicked the action of the clinician's hand as the gas flow compressed the bag, thereby providing positive pressure inspiration. Passive exhalation was promoted by the descent of a weight on the bag or bellows.

SAFETY STANDARDS

6 The introduction of safety features was coordinated by the American National Standards Institute (ANSI) Committee Z79, which was sponsored from 1956 until 1983 by the American Society of Anesthesiologists. Since 1983, representatives from industry, government, and healthcare professions have met on Committee Z79 of the American Society for Testing and Materials. They establish voluntary goals that may become accepted national standards for the safety of anesthesia equipment.

Ralph Tovell voiced the first call for standards during World War II while he was the U.S. Army Consultant in Anesthesiology for Europe. Tovell found that, as there were four different dimensions for connectors, tubes, masks, and breathing bags, supplies dispatched to field hospitals might not match their anesthesia machines. As Tovell observed, "When a sudden need for accessory equipment arose, nurses and corpsmen were likely to respond to it by bringing parts that would not fit."[67] Although Tovell's reports did not gain an immediate response, after the war Vincent Collins and Hamilton Davis took up his concern and formed the ANSI Committee Z79. One of the committee's most active members, Leslie Rendell-Baker, wrote an account of the committee's domestic and international achievements.[68] He reported that Tovell encouraged all manufacturers to select the now uniform orifice of 22 mm for all adult and pediatric face masks and to make every tracheal tube connector 15 mm in diameter. For the first time, a Z79-designed mask-tube elbow adapter would fit every mask and tracheal tube connector.

The Z79 Committee introduced other advances. Tracheal tubes of nontoxic plastic bear a Z79 or IT (Implantation Tested) mark. The committee also mandated touch identification of oxygen flow control at Roderick Calverley's suggestion, which reduced the risk that the wrong gas would be selected before internal mechanical controls prevented the selection of an hypoxic mixture.[69] Pin indexing reduced the hazard of attaching a wrong cylinder in the place of oxygen. Diameter indexing of connectors prevented similar errors in high-pressure tubing. For many years, however, errors committed in reassembling hospital oxygen supply lines led to a series of tragedies before polarographic oxygen analyzers were added to the inspiratory limb of the anesthesia circuit.

Control of the Airway

Prior to development of techniques and equipment for safely and effectively intubating the trachea, airway management left much to be desired. Inhalers, drop techniques, and mask anesthesia functioned equally when inducing unconsciousness, but unfortunately, were equally incapable of preventing obstruction of airways. Definitive control of the airway, a skill anesthesiologists now consider paramount, developed only after many harrowing and apneic episodes spurred the development of safer airway management techniques. Preceding tracheal intubation, however, several important techniques were proposed toward the end of the nineteenth century that remain integral to anesthesiology education and practice.

Joseph Clover was the first Englishman to urge the now universal practice of thrusting the patient's jaw forward to overcome obstruction of the upper airway by the tongue. Clover also published a landmark case report in 1877 in which he performed a surgical airway. Once his patient was asleep, Clover discovered that his patient had a tumor of the mouth that obstructed the airway completely, despite his trusted jaw thrust maneuver. He averted disaster by inserting a small curved cannula of his design through the cricothyroid membrane. He continued anesthesia via the cannula until the tumor was excised. Clover, the model of the prepared anesthesiologist, remarked, "I have never used the cannula before although it has been my companion at some thousands of anaesthetic cases."[70]

Tracheal Intubation in Anesthesia

The development of techniques and instruments for intubation ranks among the major advances in the history of anesthesiology. The first tracheal tubes were developed for the resuscitation of drowning victims, but were not used in anesthesia until 1878. The first use of elective oral intubation for an anesthetic was undertaken by Scottish surgeon William Macewan. He had practiced passing flexible metal tubes through the larynx of a cadaver before attempting the maneuver on an awake patient with an oral tumor at the Glasgow Royal Infirmary, on July 5, 1878.[71] Because topical anesthesia was not yet known, the experience must have demanded fortitude on the part of Macewan's patient. Once the tube was correctly positioned, an assistant began a chloroform–air anesthetic via the tube. Once anesthetized, the patient soon stopped coughing. Unfortunately, Macewan abandoned the practice following a fatality in which a patient had been successfully intubated while awake but the tube became dislodged once the patient was asleep. After the tube was removed, an attempt to provide chloroform by mask anesthesia was unsuccessful and the patient died.

Although there was a sporadic interest in tracheal anesthesia in Edinburgh and other European centers after Macewan, an American surgeon named Joseph O'Dwyer is remembered for his extraordinary dedication to the advancement of tracheal intubation. In 1885, O'Dwyer designed a series of metal laryngeal tubes, which he inserted blindly between the vocal cords of children suffering a diphtheritic crisis. Three years later, O'Dwyer designed a second rigid tube with a conical tip that occluded the larynx so effectively that it could be used for artificial ventilation when applied with the bellows and T-piece tube designed by George Fell. The Fell-O'Dwyer apparatus, as it came to be known, was used during thoracic surgery by Rudolph Matas of New Orleans. Matas was so pleased with it that he predicted, "The procedure that promises the most benefit in preventing pulmonary collapse in operations on the chest is . . . the rhythmical maintenance of artificial respiration by a tube in the glottis directly connected with a bellows."

After O'Dwyer's death, the outstanding pioneer of tracheal intubation was Franz Kuhn, a surgeon of Kassel, Germany. From 1900 until 1912, Kuhn published several papers and a classic monograph, "*Die perorale Intubation,*" which were not well known in his lifetime but have since become widely appreciated.[72] His work might have had a more profound impact if it had been translated into English. Kuhn described techniques of oral and nasal intubation that he performed with flexible metal tubes composed of coiled tubing similar to those now used for the spout of metal gasoline cans. After applying cocaine to the airway, Kuhn introduced his tube over a curved metal stylet that he directed toward the larynx with his left index finger. While he was aware of the subglottic cuffs that had been used briefly by Victor Eisenmenger, Kuhn preferred to seal the larynx by positioning a supralaryngeal flange near the tube's tip before packing the pharynx with gauze. Kuhn even monitored the patient's breath sounds continuously through a monaural earpiece connected to an extension of the tracheal tube by a narrow tube.[68]

Intubation of the trachea by palpation was an uncertain and sometimes traumatic act. For some years, surgeons even believed that it would be anatomically impossible to visualize the vocal cords directly. This misapprehension was overcome in 1895 by Alfred Kirstein in Berlin who devised the first direct-vision laryngoscope.[73] Kirstein was motivated by a friend's report that a patient's trachea had been accidentally intubated during esophagoscopy. Kirstein promptly fabricated a hand-held instrument that at first resembled a shortened cylindrical esophagoscope. He soon substituted a semicircular blade that opened inferiorly. Kirstein could now examine the larynx while standing behind his seated patient, whose head had been placed in an attitude approximating the "sniffing position." Although Alfred Kirstein's "autoscope" was not used by anesthesiologists, it was the forerunner of all modern laryngoscopes. Endoscopy was refined by Chevalier Jackson in Philadelphia, who designed a U-shaped laryngoscope by adding a handgrip that was parallel to the blade. The Jackson blade has remained a standard instrument for endoscopists but was not favored by anesthesiologists. Two laryngoscopes that closely resembled modern L-shaped instruments were designed in 1910 and 1913 by two American surgeons, Henry Janeway and George Dorrance, but neither instrument achieved lasting use despite their excellent designs.[74]

Anesthesiologist-Inspired Laryngoscopes

Before the introduction of muscle relaxants in the 1940s, intubation of the trachea could be challenging. This challenge was made somewhat easier, however, with the advent of laryngoscope blades specifically designed to increase visualization of the vocal cords. Robert Miller of San Antonio, Texas, and Robert Macintosh of Oxford University created their respectively named blades within an interval of 2 years. In 1941, Miller brought forward the slender, straight blade with a slight curve near the tip to ease the passage of the tube through the larynx. Although Miller's blade was a refinement, the technique of its use was identical to that of earlier models as the epiglottis was lifted to expose the larynx.[75]

The Macintosh blade, which is placed in the vallecula, rather than under the epiglottis, was invented as an incidental result of a tonsillectomy. Sir Robert Macintosh later described the circumstances of its discovery in an appreciation of the career of his technician, Mr. Richard Salt, who constructed the blade. As Sir Robert recalled, "A Boyle-Davis gag, a size larger than intended, was inserted for tonsillectomy, and when the mouth was fully opened the cords came into view. This was a surprise since conventional laryngoscopy, at that depth of anaesthesia, would have been impossible in those pre-relaxant days. Within a matter of hours, Salt had modified the blade of the Davis gag and attached a laryngoscope handle to it; and streamlined (after testing several models), the end result came into widespread use."[76] Macintosh underestimated the popularity of the blade as more than 800,000 have been produced, and many special-purpose versions have been marketed.

The most distinguished innovator in tracheal intubation was the self-trained British anesthetist Ivan (later, Sir Ivan) Magill.[77] In 1919, while serving in the Royal Army as a general medical officer, Magill was assigned to a military hospital near London. Although he had only rudimentary training in anesthesia, Magill was obliged to accept an assignment to the anesthesia service, where he worked with another neophyte, Stanley Rowbotham.[78] Together, Magill and Rowbotham attended casualties disfigured by severe facial injuries who underwent repeated restorative operations. These procedures required that the surgeon, Harold Gillies, have unrestricted access to the face and airway. These patients presented formidable challenges, but both Magill and Rowbotham became adept at tracheal intubation and quickly understood its current limitations. Because they learned from fortuitous observations, they soon extended the scope of tracheal anesthesia.

They gained expertise with blind nasal intubation after they learned to soften semirigid insufflation tubes for passage through the nostril. Even though their original intent was to position the tips of the nasal tubes in the posterior pharynx, the slender tubes frequently ended up in the trachea. Stimulated by this chance experience, they developed techniques of deliberate nasotracheal intubation. In 1920, Magill devised an aid to manipulating the catheter tip, the "Magill angulated forceps," which continue to be manufactured according to his original design of 75 years ago.

With the war over, Magill entered civilian practice and set out to develop a wide-bore tube that would resist kinking but be conformable to the contours of the upper airway. While in a hardware store, he found mineralized red rubber tubing that he cut, beveled, and smoothed to produce tubes that clinicians around the world would come to call "Magill tubes." His tubes remained the universal standard for more than 40 years until rubber products were supplanted by inert plastics. Magill also rediscovered the advantage of applying cocaine to the nasal mucosa, a technique that greatly facilitated awake blind nasal intubation.

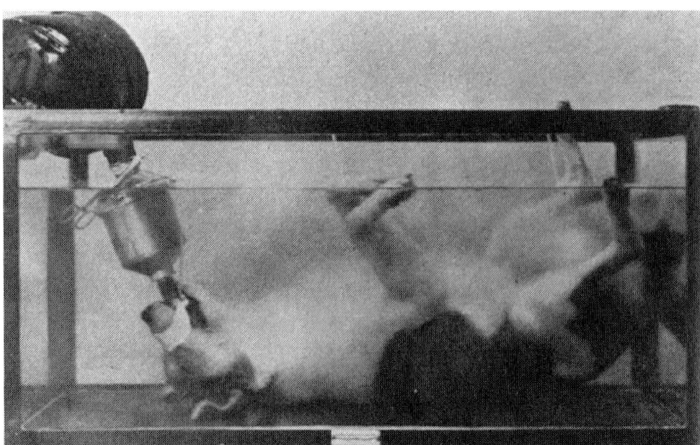

FIGURE 1-4. "The dunked dog." Arthur Guedel demonstrated the safety of endotracheal intubation with a cuffed tube by submerging his anesthetized pet, Airway, in an aquarium while the animal breathed an ethylene-oxygen anesthetic through an underwater Waters' "to-and-fro" anesthesia circuit.

In 1926, Arthur Guedel began a series of experiments that led to the introduction of the cuffed tube. His goal was to combine the safety of tracheal intubation with the safety and economy of the closed-circuit anesthesia, recently refined by his close friend Ralph Waters.[79] Guedel transformed the basement of his Indianapolis home into a laboratory, where he subjected each step of the preparation and application of his cuffs to a vigorous review.[80] He fashioned cuffs from the rubber of dental dams, condoms, and surgical gloves that were glued onto the outer wall of tubes. Using animal tracheas donated by the family butcher as his model, he considered whether the cuff should be positioned above, below, or at the level of the vocal cords. He recommended that the cuff be positioned just below the vocal cords to seal the airway. Waters later recommended that cuffs be constructed of two layers of soft rubber cemented together. These detachable cuffs were first manufactured by Waters' children, who sold them to the Foregger Company.

Guedel sought ways to show the safety and utility of the cuffed tube. He first filled the mouth of an anesthetized and intubated patient with water and showed that the cuff sealed the airway. Even though this exhibition was successful, he searched for a more dramatic technique to capture the attention of those unfamiliar with the advantages of intubation. He reasoned that if the cuff prevented water from entering the trachea of an intubated patient, it should also prevent an animal from drowning, even if it were submerged under water. To encourage physicians attending a medical convention to use his tracheal techniques, Guedel prepared the first of several "dunked dog" demonstrations (Fig. 1-4). An anesthetized and intubated dog, Guedel's own pet, "Airway," was immersed in an aquarium. After the demonstration was completed, the anesthetic was discontinued before the animal was removed from the water. Airway awoke promptly, shook water over the onlookers, saluted a post, then trotted from the hall to the applause of the audience.

Endobronchial Tubes—The Next Step

After a patient experienced an accidental endobronchial intubation, Ralph Waters reasoned that a very long cuffed tube could be used to ventilate the dependent lung while the upper lung was being resected.[81] On learning of his friend's success with intentional one-lung anesthesia, Arthur Guedel proposed an important modification for chest surgery, the double-cuffed single-lumen tube, which was introduced by Emery Rovenstine. These tubes were easily positioned, an advantage over bronchial blockers that had to be inserted by a skilled bronchoscopist.

Following World War II, several double-cuffed single-lumen tubes were used for thoracic surgery, but after 1953, these were supplanted by double-lumen endobronchial tubes. The double-lumen tube currently most popular was designed by Frank Robertshaw of Manchester, England, and is prepared in both right- and left-sided versions. Robertshaw tubes were first manufactured from mineralized red rubber but are now made of extruded plastic, a technique refined by David Sheridan. Sheridan was also the first person to embed centimeter markings along the side of tracheal tubes, a safety feature that reduced the risk of the tube's being incorrectly positioned.

Airway Management Devices

Conventional laryngoscopes proved inadequate for patients with "difficult airways." A few clinicians credit harrowing intubating experiences as the incentive for invention. In 1928, a rigid bronchoscope was specifically designed for examination of the large airways. Rigid bronchoscopes were refined and used by pulmonologists. Although it was known in 1870 that a thread of glass could transmit light along its length, technological limitations were not overcome until 1964 when Shigeto Ikeda developed the first flexible fiberoptic bronchoscope. Fiberoptic-assisted tracheal intubation has become a common approach in the management of patients with difficult airways having surgery.

Roger Bullard desired a device to simultaneously examine the larynx and intubate the vocal cords. He had been frustrated by failed attempts to visualize the larynx of a patient with Pierre-Robin syndrome. In response, he developed the Bullard laryngoscope, whose fiberoptic bundles lie beside a curved blade. Similarly, the Wu-scope was designed by Tzu-Lang Wu in 1994 to combine and facilitate visualization and intubation of the trachea in patients with difficult airways.[82]

The passage of flexible fiberoptic bronchoscopes has been aided by "intubating airways" such as those designed by Berman, Ovassapian, Augustine, Williams, Luomanen, and Patil. Patients requiring continuous-oxygen administration during fiberoptic bronchoscopy may breathe through the Patil face mask, which features a separate orifice through which the scope is advanced. The Patil face mask is only one of an extensive series of aides to intubation created by the innovative "Vijay" Patil.

Dr. A. I. J. "Archie" Brain first recognized the principle of the laryngeal mask airway (LMA) in 1981 when, like many British clinicians, he provided dental anesthesia via a Goldman nasal mask. However, unlike any before him, he realized that just as the dental mask could be fitted closely about the nose, a comparable mask attached to a wide-bore tube might be positioned around the larynx. He not only conceived of this radical departure in airway management, which he first described in 1983,[83] but also spent years in single-handedly fabricating and testing scores of incremental modifications. Scores of Brain's prototypes are displayed in the Royal Berkshire Hospital, Reading, England, where they provide a detailed record of the evolution of the LMA. He fabricated his first models from Magill tubes and Goldman masks, then refined their shape by performing postmortem studies of the hypopharynx to determine the form of cuff that would be most functional. Before silicone rubber was selected, Brain had even mastered the technique of forming masks from liquid latex. Every detail of the LMA, the number and position of the aperture bars, the shape and the size of the masks, required repeated modification.

PATIENT MONITORING

In many ways, the history of late-nineteenth- and early-twentieth-century anesthesiology is the quest for the safest anesthetic. The discovery and widespread use of electrocardiography, pulse oximetry, blood gas analysis, capnography, and neuromuscular blockade monitoring have reduced patient morbidity and mortality and revolutionized anesthesia practice. While safer machines assured clinicians that appropriate gas mixtures were delivered to the patient, monitors provided an early warning of acute physiologic deterioration before patients suffered irrevocable damage.

Joseph Clover was one of the first clinicians to routinely perform basic hemodynamic monitoring. Clover developed the habit of monitoring his patients' pulse but surprisingly, this was a contentious issue at the time. Prominent Scottish surgeons scorned Clover's emphasis on the action of chloroform on the heart. Baron Lister and others preferred that senior medical students give anesthetics and urged them to "strictly carry out certain simple instructions, among which is that of never touching the pulse, in order that their attention may not be distracted from the respiration."[84] Lister also counseled, "it appears that preliminary examination of the chest, often considered indispensable, is quite unnecessary, and more likely to induce the dreaded syncope, by alarming the patients, than to avert it."[84] Little progress in anesthesia could come from such reactionary statements. In contrast, Clover had observed the effect of chloroform on animals and urged other anesthetists to monitor the pulse at all times and to discontinue the anesthetic temporarily if any irregularity or weakness was observed in the strength of the pulse.

Two American surgeons, George W. Crile and Harvey Cushing, developed a strong interest in measuring blood pressure during anesthesia. Both men wrote thorough and detailed examinations of blood pressure monitoring; however, Cushing's contribution is better remembered because he was the first American to apply the Riva Rocci cuff, which he saw while visiting Italy. Cushing introduced the concept in 1902 and had blood pressure measurements recorded on anesthesia records.[85] In 1894, Cushing and a fellow student at Harvard Medical School, Charles Codman, initiated a system of recording patients' pulses to assess the course of the anesthetics they administered. In 1902, Cushing continued the practice of monitoring and recording patient blood pressures and pulses. The transition from manual to automated blood pressure devices, which first appeared in 1936 and operate on an oscillometric principle, has been gradual. The development of inexpensive microprocessors has enabled routine use of automatic cuffs in clinical settings.

The first precordial stethoscope was believed to have been used by S. Griffith Davis at Johns Hopkins University.[65] He adapted a technique developed by Harvey Cushing in a laboratory in which dogs with surgically induced valvular lesions had stethoscopes attached to their chest wall so that medical students might listen to bruits characteristic of a specific malformation. Davis' technique was forgotten but was rehabilitated by Dr. Robert Smith, an energetic pioneer of pediatric anesthesiology in Boston. A Canadian contemporary, Albert Codesmith, of the Hospital for Sick Children, Toronto, became frustrated by the repeated dislodging of the chest piece under the surgical drapes and fabricated his first esophageal stethoscope from urethral catheters and Penrose drains. His brief report heralded its clinical role as a monitor of both normal and adventitious respiratory and cardiac sounds.[86] An additional benefit was that the stethoscope could protect against the risk of disconnection of a paralyzed patient from the anesthesia circuit. In the era before audible circuit disconnect alarms, the patient's survival depended upon the anesthesiologist's recognition of the sudden disappearance of breath sounds.

Electrocardiography, Pulse Oximetry, and Capnography

Clinical electrocardiography began with Willem Einthoven's application of the string galvanometer in 1903. Within two decades, Thomas Lewis had described its role in the diagnosis of disturbances of cardiac rhythm, while James Herrick and Harold Pardee first drew attention to the changes produced by myocardial ischemia. After 1928, cathode ray oscilloscopes were available, but the risk of explosion owing to the presence of flammable anesthetics forestalled the introduction of the electrocardiogram into routine anesthetic practice until after World War II. At that time, the small screen of the heavily shielded "bullet" oscilloscope displayed only 3 seconds of data, but that information was highly prized.

Pulse oximetry, the optical measurement of oxygen saturation in tissues, is one of the more recent additions to the anesthesiologist's array of routine monitors. Severinghaus states, "Pulse oximetry is arguably the most important technological advance ever made in monitoring the well-being and safety of patients during anesthesia, recovery, and critical care."[87] Although research in this area began in 1932, its first practical application came during World War II. An American physiologist, Glen Millikan, responded to a request from British colleagues in aviation research. Millikan set about preparing a series of devices to improve the supply of oxygen that was provided to pilots flying at high altitude in unpressurized aircraft. To monitor oxygen delivery and to prevent the pilot from succumbing to an unrecognized failure of his oxygen supply, Millikan created an oxygen-sensing monitor worn on the pilot's earlobe, and coined the name *oximeter* to describe its action. Before his tragic death in a climbing accident in 1947, Millikan had begun to assess anesthetic applications of oximetry.

For the next three decades, oximetry was rarely used by anesthesiologists, and then primarily in research studies such as those of Albert Faulconer and John Pender. Refinements of oximetry by a Japanese engineer, Takuo Aoyagi, led to the development of pulse oximetry. As John Severinghaus recounted the episode, Aoyagi had attempted to eliminate the changes in a signal caused by pulsatile variations when he realized that this fluctuation could be used to measure both the pulse and oxygen saturation.[87]

Although pulse oximetry gives second-by-second data about oxygen saturation, anesthesiologists have recognized a need for breath-by-breath measurement of respiratory and anesthetic gases. After 1954, infrared absorption techniques gave immediate displays of the exhaled concentration of CO_2. Clinicians quickly learned to relate abnormal concentrations of CO_2 to threatening situations such as the inappropriate placement of a tracheal tube in the esophagus, abrupt alterations in pulmonary blood flow, and other factors. More recently, infrared analysis has been perfected to enable breath-by-breath measurement of anesthetic gases as well. This technology has largely replaced mass spectrometry, which initially had only industrial applications before Albert Faulconer of the Mayo Clinic first used it to monitor the concentration of an exhaled anesthetic in 1954.

The ability to confirm endotracheal intubation and monitor ventilation, as reflected by concentrations of CO_2 in respired gas, began in 1943. At that time, K. Luft described the principle of infrared absorption by CO_2 and he developed an apparatus for measurement.[88] Routine application of capnography in anesthesia practice was pioneered by Dr. Bob Smalhout and Dr. Zden Kalenda in the Netherlands. Breath-to-breath continuous monitoring and a waveform display of CO_2 levels help anesthesiologists recognize abnormalities in metabolism, ventilation, and circulation.

INTRAVENOUS MEDICATIONS IN ANESTHESIA

Prior to William Harvey's description of a complete and continuous intravascular circuit in *De Motu Cordis* (1628), it was widely held that blood emanated from the heart and was propelled to the periphery where it was consumed. The idea that substances could be injected intravascularly and travel systemically probably originated with Christopher Wren. In 1657, Wren injected aqueous opium into a dog through a goose quill attached to a pig's bladder, rendering the animal "stupefied."[89] Wren similarly injected intravenous *crocus mettalorum*, an impure preparation of antimony, and observed the animals to vomit and then die. Knowledge of a circulatory system and intravascular access spurred investigations in other areas, and Wren's contemporary, Richard Lower, performed the first blood transfusions of lamb's blood into dogs and other animals.

In the mid-nineteenth century, equipment necessary for effective intravascular injections was conceived. Vaccination lancets were used in the 1830s to puncture the skin and force morphine paste subcutaneously for analgesia.[90] The hollow needle and hypodermic syringe were developed in the following decades but were not initially designed for intravenous use. In 1845, Dublin surgeon Francis Rynd created the hollow needle for injection of morphine into nerves in the treatment of "neuralgias." Similarly, Charles Gabriel Pravaz designed the first functional syringe in 1853 for perineural injections. Alexander Wood, however, is generally credited with perfecting the hypodermic glass syringe. In 1855, Wood published a paper on the injection of opiates into painful spots by use of hollow needle and his glass syringe.[91]

In 1872, Pierre Oré of Lyons performed what is perhaps the first successful intravenous surgical anesthetic by injecting chloral hydrate immediately prior to incision. His 1875 publication describes its use in 36 patients but several postoperative deaths lent little to recommend this method to other practitioners.[92] In 1909, Ludwig Burkhardt produced surgical anesthesia by intravenous injections of chloroform and ether in Germany. Seven years later, Elisabeth Bredenfeld of Switzerland reported the use of intravenous morphine and scopolamine. The trials failed to show an improvement over inhaled techniques. Intravenous anesthesia found little application or popularity, primarily because of a lack of suitable drugs. In the following decades, this would change.

INDUCTION AGENTS

The first barbiturate, barbital, was synthesized in 1903 by Fischer and von Mering. Phenobarbital and all other successors of barbital had very protracted action and found little use in anesthesia. After 1929, oral pentobarbital was used as a sedative before surgery, but when it was given in anesthetic concentrations, long periods of unconsciousness followed. The first short-acting oxybarbiturate was hexobarbital (Evipal), available clinically in 1932. Hexobarbital was enthusiastically received by the anesthesia communities in Europe and North America because its abbreviated induction time was unrivaled by any other technique. A London anesthetist, Ronald Jarman, found that it had a dramatic advantage over inhalation inductions for minor procedures. Jarman instructed his patients to raise one arm while he injected hexobarbital into a vein of the opposite forearm. When the upraised arm fell, indicating the onset of hypnosis, the surgeon could begin. Patients were also amazed in that many awoke unable to believe they had been anesthetized.[93] (Soon after Evipal was introduced, Robert Macintosh administered it to Sir William Morris, the manufacturer of the Morris Garages [MG] automobiles. When Morris awoke, he learned that his surgery was completed, and was amazed by this "magic experience," which he contrasted with his vivid recollections of the terror of undergoing a mask induction as a child in a dentist's office. Morris [later, Viscount Nuffield] insisted, over the objections of Oxford's medical establishment, on endowing a department of anesthesia for the university as a precondition of his support for a postgraduate medical center. In 1937, Sir Robert Macintosh became Oxford's first professor of anesthesiology. He led the growth of the first university department in Europe from the first fully endowed Chair of Anaesthesia and helped establish one of the most distinguished anesthesia centers in the world.)

Even though the prompt action of hexobarbital had a dramatic effect on the conduct of anesthesia, it was soon replaced by two thiobarbiturates. In 1932, Donalee Tabern and Ernest H. Volwiler of the Abbott Company synthesized thiopental (Pentothal) and thiamylal (Surital). The sulfated barbiturates proved to be more satisfactory, potent, and rapid acting than were their oxybarbiturate analogs. Thiopental was first administered to a patient at the University of Wisconsin in March 1934, but the successful introduction of thiopental into clinical practice followed a thorough investigation conducted by John Lundy and his colleagues at the Mayo Clinic in June 1934.

When first introduced, thiopental was often given in repeated increments as the primary anesthetic for protracted procedures. Its hazards were soon appreciated. At first, depression of respiration was monitored by the simple expedient of observing the motion of a wisp of cotton placed over the nose. Only a few skilled practitioners were prepared to pass a tracheal tube if the patient stopped breathing. Such practitioners realized that thiopental without supplementation did not suppress airway reflexes, and they therefore encouraged the prophylactic provision of topical anesthesia of the airway beforehand. The vasodilatory effects of thiobarbiturates were widely appreciated only when thiopental caused cardiovascular collapse in hypovolemic burned civilian and military patients in World War II. In response, fluid replacement was used more aggressively and thiopental administered with greater caution.

In 1962, ketamine was synthesized by Dr. Calvin Stevens at the Parke Davis laboratories in Ann Arbor, Michigan. One of the cyclohexylamine compounds that includes phencyclidine (PCP), ketamine was the only drug of this group that gained clinical utility. The other compounds produced undesirable postanesthetic delirium and psychomimetic reactions. In 1966, the neologism "dissociative anesthesia" was created by Guenter Corrsen and Edward Domino to describe the trance-like state of profound analgesia produced by ketamine.[94] It was released for use in 1970 and although it remains primarily an agent for anesthetic induction, its analgesic properties are increasingly studied and utilized by pain specialists.

Etomidate was first described by Paul Janssen and his colleagues in 1964, and originally given the name Hypnomidate. Its key advantages, minimal hemodynamic depression and lack of histamine release, account for its ongoing utility in clinical practice. It was released for use in 1974 and despite its drawbacks (pain on injection, myoclonus, postoperative nausea and vomiting, and inhibition of adrenal steroidogenesis), etomidate is often the drug of choice for anesthetizing hemodynamically unstable patients.

Propofol, or 2,-6 di-isopropyl phenol, was first synthesized by Imperial Chemical Industries and tested clinically in 1977. Investigators found that it produced hypnosis quickly with minimal excitation and that patients awoke promptly once the drug was discontinued. In addition to its excellent induction characteristics, propofol's antiemetic action made it an agent of choice in patient populations prone to nausea and emesis. Regrettably, Cremophor EL, the solvent with which it was formulated, produced several severe anaphylactic reactions and it was withdrawn from use. Once propofol was reformulated with egg lecithin, glycerol, and soybean oil, the drug reentered clinical practice and gained great success. Its popularity in Britain coincided with the introduction of the LMA, and it was soon noted that propofol suppressed pharyngeal reflexes to a degree that permitted the insertion of an LMA without a need for either muscle relaxants or potent inhaled anesthetics.

Opioids

Opioids (historically referred to as narcotics, although semantically incorrect—see Chapter 14) remain the analgesic workhorse in anesthesia practice. They are used routinely in the perioperative period, in the management of acute pain, and in a variety of terminal and chronic pain states. The availability of short-, medium-, and long-acting opioids, as well as the many routes of administration, gives physicians considerable flexibility in the use of these agents. The analgesic and sedating properties of opium have been known for over two millennia. Certainly the Greeks and Chinese civilizations harnessed these properties in medical and cultural practices. Opium is derived from the seeds of the poppy (Papaver somniferum), and is an amalgam of over 25 pharmacologic alkaloids. The first alkaloid isolated, morphine, was extracted by Prussian chemist Freidrich A.W. Sertürner in 1803. He named this alkaloid after the Greek god of dreams, Morpheus. Morphine became commonly used as a supplement to inhaled anesthesia and for postoperative pain control during the latter half of the nineteenth century. Codeine, another alkaloid of opium, was isolated in 1832 by Robiquet but its relatively weaker analgesic potency and nausea at higher doses limits its role in managing moderate to severe perioperative surgical pain.

Meperidine was the first synthetic opioid and was developed in 1939 by two German researchers at IG Farben, Otto Eisleb and O. Schaumann. Although many pharmacologists are remembered for the introduction of a single drug, one prolific researcher, Paul Janssen, has since 1953 brought forward more than 70 agents from among 70,000 chemicals created in his laboratory. His products have had profound effects on disciplines as disparate as parasitology and psychiatry. The pace of productive innovation in Janssen's research laboratory is astonishing. Chemical R4263 (fentanyl), synthesized in 1960, was followed only a year later by R4749 (droperidol), and then etomidate in 1964. Innovar, the fixed combination of fentanyl and droperidol, is less popular now but Janssen's phenylpeperidine derivatives, fentanyl, sufentanil and alfentanil, are staples in the anesthesia pharmacopoeia. Remifentanil, an ultra short-acting opioid introduced by Glaxo-Wellcome in 1996, is a departure from other opioids in that it has very rapid onset and equally rapid offset due to metabolism by nonspecific tissue esterases. Ketorolac, a nonsteroidal antiinflammatory drug (NSAID) approved for use in 1990, was the first parenteral NSAID indicated for postoperative pain. With a 6- to 8-mg morphine equivalent analgesic potency, Ketorolac provides significant postoperative pain control, and has particular use as a sole intravenous agent in minor procedures, or for pain attenuation when an opioid-sparing approach is essential. Ketorolac use is limited by side effects and may be inappropriate in patients with underlying renal dysfunction, bleeding problems, or compromised bone healing.

Antiemetics

Effective treatment for postoperative nausea and vomiting (PONV) evolved relatively recently and has been driven by incentives to limit hospitalization expenses and improve patient satisfaction. But PONV is an old problem for which late-nineteenth-century practitioners recognized many causes including anxiety, severe pain, sudden changes in blood pressure, ileus, ingestion of blood, and the residual effects of opioids and inhalational anesthetics. Risk of pulmonary aspiration of gastric contents and subsequent death from asphyxia or aspiration pneumonia was a feared consequence of anesthetics, especially those preceding use of cuffed endotracheal tubes. Vomiting and aspiration during anesthesia led to the practice of maintaining an empty stomach preoperatively, a policy that continues today despite evidence that clear fluids up to 3 hours before surgery do not increase gastric volumes, change gastric pH, or increase the risk of aspiration.

A variety of treatments for nausea and vomiting were proposed by early anesthetists. James Gwathemy's 1914 publication, *Anesthesia*, commented that British surgeons customarily gave tincture of iodine in a teaspoonful of water every half hour for three or four doses. Inhalation of vinegar fumes, and rectal injection of 30 to 40 drops of tincture of opium with 60 grains of sodium bromide were also felt to quiet the vomiting center.[95] Other practitioners attempted olfactory control by placing a piece of gauze moistened with essence of orange or an aromatic oil on the upper lip of the patient.[96] A 1937 anesthesia textbook encouraged treatment of PONV with lateral positioning, "iced soda water, strong black coffee, and chloretone."[97] Counterirritation, such as mustard leaf on the epigastrium, was also believed useful in limiting emesis.[98] As late as 1951, anesthesia texts recommended oxygen administration, whiffs of ammonia spirits, and control of blood pressure and positioning.[99] The complex central mechanisms of nausea and vomiting were largely unaffected by most of these treatments. Newer drugs capable of intervening at specific pathways were needed to have an impact on PONV. As more short-acting anesthetics were developed, the problem received sharper focus in awake postoperative patients in the recovery room. The nausea attending use of newer chemotherapy agents provided additional impetus to the development of antiemetic medications.

In 1955, a nonrandomized study using the antihistamine cyclizine showed a reduction in PONV from 27% to 21% in a group of 3,000 patients. The following year, a more rigorous study by Knapp and Beecher reported a significant benefit from prophylaxis with the neuroleptic chlorpromazine. In 1957, promethazine (Phenergan) and chlorpromazine were both found to reduce PONV when used prophylactically. Thirteen years later, a double-blind study evaluating metoclopramide was published and it became a first-line drug in the management of PONV. Droperidol, released in the early 1960s, became widely used until 2001 when concerns regarding prolongation of QT intervals prompted a warning from the Food and Drug Administration about its continued use.

The antiemetic effects of corticosteroids were first recognized by oncologists treating intracranial edema from tumors.[100] Subsequent studies have borne out the antiemetic properties of this class of drugs in treating PONV. Recognition of the serotonin 5-HT3 pathway in PONV has led to a unique class of drugs devoted only to addressing this particular problem. Ondansetron, the first representative of this drug class, was FDA approved in 1991. Additional serotonin 5-HT3 antagonists have been approved and are available today.

Muscle Relaxants

Muscle relaxants entered anesthesia practice nearly a century after inhalational anesthetics. (See Table 1-1.) Curare, the first known neuromuscular blocking agent, was originally used in hunting and tribal warfare by native peoples of South America. The curares are alkaloids prepared from plants native to equatorial rain forests. The refinement of the harmless sap of several species of vines into toxins that were lethal only when injected was an extraordinary triumph introduced by paleopharmacologists in loincloths. Their discovery was the more remarkable because it was independently repeated on three separate continents—South America, Africa, and Asia. These jungle tribes also developed nearly identical methods of delivering the toxin by darts, which, after being dipped in curare, maintained their potency indefinitely until they were propelled through blowpipes to strike the flesh of monkeys and other animals of the treetops. Moreover, the American Indians knew of the juice of an herb that would counteract the effects of the poison if administered in time.[101]

Accounts from sixteenth-century explorers of South America include reports of the poison-arrow darts used by the natives. In 1564, Sir Walter Raleigh described the effects of curare upon their targets, as well as the use of an antidote. Later, explorers brought home samples of the poison-tipped darts to Europe and Great Britain where scientific studies were undertaken. Early experiments on birds, cats, rabbits, and dogs in the 1780s verified that the poison worked by abolishing muscle function, including respiratory muscles, and that direct insertion into nerves had no effect. In 1811, Benjamin C. Brodie demonstrated that large animals such as horses and donkeys treated with curare could be kept alive if ventilated for several hours through a bellows sewn directly to the trachea.[101]

The earliest clinical use of curare in humans was to ameliorate the tortuous muscle spasms of infectious tetanus. In 1858, New York physician Louis Albert Sayres reported two cases in which he attempted to treat severe tetanus with curare at the Bellevue Hospital. Both of his patients died. Similar efforts were undertaken to use muscle relaxants to treat epilepsy, rabies, and choreaform disorders. Treatment of Parkinson-like rigidity and the prevention of trauma from seizure therapy also preceded the use of curare in anesthesia.[102]

Interestingly, curare antagonists were developed well before muscle relaxants were ever used in surgery. In 1900, Jacob Pal, a Viennese physician, recognized that curare could be antagonized by physostigmine. This substance had been isolated from the calabar bean some 36 years earlier by Scottish pharmacologist Sir T.R. Fraser. Neostigmine methylsulphate was synthesized in 1931 and was significantly more potent in antagonizing the effects of curare.[103]

TABLE 1-1

EVENTS IN THE DEVELOPMENT OF MUSCLE RELAXANTS

YEAR	EVENT
1516	Peter Martyr d'Anghera, *De orbe novo*, published account of South American Indian arrow poisons
1596	Sir Walter Raleigh provides detailed account of arrow poison effects and antidote
1745	Charles-Marie de la Condamine returns from Ecuador and conducts curare experiments with chickens and attempted to use sugar as an antidote
1780	Abbe Felix Fontana inserts curare directly into exposed sciatic nerve of rabbit without effect, concludes that mechanism is the destruction of the irritability of voluntary muscles. Publishes *On the American Poison Ticunas* (name of South American tribe)
1811	Benjamin Collins Brodie demonstrates that animals mechanically ventilated may survive significant doses of curare
1812	William Sewell suggests use of curare in "hydrophobia" (rabies) and tetanus
1844	Claude Bernard determines that death occurs by respiratory failure, motor nerves are unable to transmit stimuli from higher centers, differential effect on muscles with peripheral and thoracic muscles being affected before respiratory muscles. Bernard concludes that the site of action is the junction between muscles and nerves, neuromuscular junction
1858	Louis Albert Sayres, New York physician, uses curare to treat tetanus in two patients
1864	Physostigmine isolated from Calabar beans by Sir T.R. Fraser, a Scottish pharmacologist
1886–1897	R. Boehm, a German chemist, demonstrated three separate classes of alkaloids in each of three types of indigenous containers: tube-curares, pot-curares, and calabash-curares
1900	Jacob Pal recognizes that physostigmine can antagonize the effects of curare
1906	Succinylcholine prepared by Reid Hunt and R. Taveau, experimented on rabbits pretreated with curare to learn of cardiac effects and so paralysis went unrecognized
1912	Arthur Lawen uses curare in surgery but report published in German and goes largely unrecognized
1938	Richard and Ruth Gill bring large quantity of curare to New York for further study by pharmaceutical company
1939	Abram E. Bennett uses curare in children with spastic disorders and to prevent trauma from metrazol therapy (precursor to ECT)
1942	Harold Griffith and Enid Johnson use curare for abdominal relaxation in surgery
1942	H. A. Halody develops Rabbit drop head Assay for standardization and large-scale production of curare and d-tubocurarine
1948	Decamethonium, a depolarizing relaxant, is synthesized
1949	Succinylcholine prepared by Daniel Bovet, the following year by J.C. Castillo and Edwin de Beer
1956	Distinction between depolarizing and nondepolarizing neuromuscular blockade is made by William D. M. Paton
1964	Pancuronium released for use in humans, synthesized by Savage and Hewett
1979	Vecuronium introduced, specifically designed to be more hepatically metabolized than pancuronium
1993	Mivacurium released for clinical use
1994	Rocuronium introduced to clinical practice

In 1938, Richard and Ruth Gill returned to New York from South America, bringing with them 11.9 kg of crude curare collected near their Ecuadorian ranch. Their motivation was a mixture of personal and altruistic goals. Some months before, while on an earlier visit to the United States, Richard Gill learned that he had multiple sclerosis. His physician, Dr. Walter Freeman, mentioned the possibility that curare might have a therapeutic role in the management of spastic disorders. When the Gills returned to the United States with their supply of crude curare, they encouraged scientists at E. R. Squibb & Co. Squibb to take an interest in its unique properties. Squibb soon offered semirefined curare to two groups of American anesthesiologists, who assessed its action but quickly abandoned their studies when it caused total respiratory paralysis in two patients and the death of laboratory animals.

The earliest effective clinical application of curare in medicine occurred in physiatry. After A. R. McIntyre refined a portion of the raw curare in 1939, Abram. E. Bennett of Omaha, Nebraska, injected it into children with spastic disorders. While no persistent benefit could be observed in these patients, he next administered it to patients about to receive metrazol, a precursor to electroconvulsive therapy. Because it eliminated seizure-induced fractures, they termed it a "shock absorber." By 1941, other psychiatrists followed this practice and, when they found that the action of curare was protracted, occasionally used neostigmine as an antidote.

Curare was used initially in surgery by Arthur Lawen in 1912, but the published report was written in German and was ignored for decades. Lawen, a physiologist and physician from Leipzig, used curare in his laboratory before boldly producing abdominal relaxation at a light level of anesthesia in a surgical patient. Lawen's efforts were not appreciated for decades, and while his pioneering work anticipated later clinical application, safe use would have to await the introduction of regular intubation of the trachea and controlled ventilation of the lungs.[104]

Thirty years after Lawen, Harold Griffith, the chief anesthetist of the Montreal Homeopathic Hospital, learned of A. E. Bennett's successful use of curare and resolved to apply it in anesthesia. As Griffith was already a master of tracheal intubation, he was much better prepared than were most of his contemporaries to attend to potential complications. On January 23, 1942, Griffith and his resident, Enid Johnson, anesthetized and intubated the trachea of a young man before injecting curare early in the course of his appendectomy. Satisfactory abdominal relaxation was obtained and the surgery proceeded without incident. Griffith and Johnson's report of the successful use of curare in the 25 patients of their series launched a revolution in anesthetic care.[105]

Anesthesiologists who practiced before muscle relaxants recall the anxiety they felt when a premature attempt to intubate the trachea under cyclopropane caused persisting laryngospasm. Before 1942, abdominal relaxation was possible only if the patient tolerated high concentrations of an inhaled anesthetic, which might bring profound respiratory depression and protracted recovery. Curare and the drugs that followed transformed anesthesia profoundly. Because intubation of the trachea could now be taught in a deliberate manner, a neophyte could fail on a first attempt without compromising the safety of the patient. For the first time, abdominal relaxation could be attained when curare was supplemented by light planes of inhaled anesthetics or by a combination of intravenous agents providing "balanced anesthesia." New frontiers opened. Sedated and paralyzed patients could now successfully undergo the major physiologic trespasses of cardiopulmonary bypass, deliberate hypothermia, or long-term respiratory support after surgery.

Credit for successful and safe introduction of curare and d-tubocurarine into anesthesia must in part be given to a Squibb researcher named H. A. Holaday. Crude, unstandardized preparations of curare produced uncertain clinical effects and undesirable side effects related to various impurities. Isolation of d-tubocurarine in 1935 renewed clinical interest but a method for standardizing "Intocostrin" and its purer derivative, d-tubocurarine, had yet to be devised. In the early 1940s, in part as a result of Griffith and Johnson's successful trials, Squibb embarked upon wide-scale production. Holaday developed a reliable, easily reproducible method for standardizing curare doses that became known as the Rabbit head drop assay (Fig. 1-5). The assay consisted of aqueous curare solution injected intravenously in 0.1-mL doses every 15 seconds until the endpoint, when the rabbit became unable to raise its head, was reached.[106]

Successful clinical use of curare led to the introduction of other muscle relaxants. By 1948, gallamine and decamethonium had been synthesized. Metubine, a curare "rediscovered" in the 1970s, was used clinically in the same year. Succinylcholine was prepared by the Nobel laureate Daniel Bovet in 1949 and was in wide international use before historians noted that the drug had been synthesized and tested long beforehand.

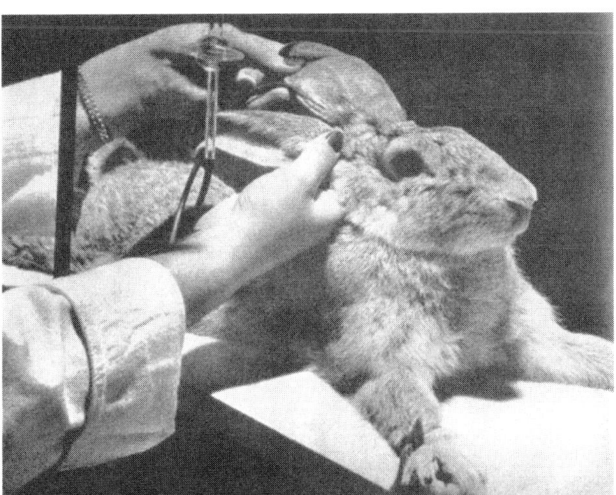

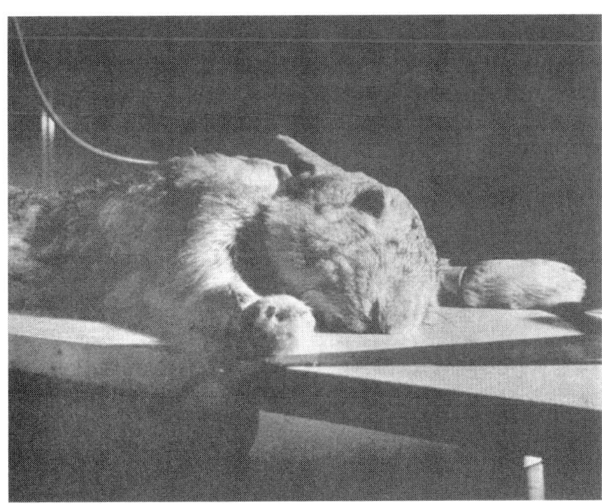

FIGURE 1-5. The rabbit head drop assay. H. A. Halloday of Squibb pharmaceutical company developed a method for standardizing doses of curare and d-tubocurarine by injecting 0.1 mL of aqueous curare solution every 15 seconds until the rabbit could no longer raise its head.

In 1906, Reid Hunt and R. Taveaux prepared succinylcholine among a series of choline esters, which they had injected into rabbits to observe their cardiac effects. If their rabbits had not been previously paralyzed with curare, the depolarizing action of succinylcholine might have been recognized decades earlier.

The ability to monitor intraoperative neuromuscular blockade with nerve stimulators began in 1958. Working at St. Thomas' Hospital in London, T. H. Christie and H. Churchill-Davidson developed a method for monitoring peripheral neuromuscular blockade during anesthesia. It was not until 1970, however, that H. H. Ali and colleagues devised the technique of delivering four supramaximal impulses delivered at 2 Hz (0.5 seconds apart), or a "Train of Four," as a method of quantifying the degree of residual neuromuscular blockade.[107]

Research in relaxants was rekindled in 1960, when researchers became aware of the action of maloetine, a relaxant from the Congo basin. It was remarkable in that it had a steroidal nucleus. Investigations of maloetine led to pancuronium in 1968. In the 1970s and 1980s, research shifted toward identification of specific receptor biochemistry and development of receptor-specific drugs. From these isoquinolones, four related products emerged: vecuronium, pipecuronium, rocuronium, and rapacuronium. Rapacuronium, released in the early 1990s, was withdrawn from clinical use after several cases of intractable bronchospasm led to brain damage or death. Four clinical products based upon the steroid parent drug d-tubocurarine (atracurium, mivacurium, doxacurium, and cis-atracurium) also made it to clinical use. Recognition that atracurium and cis-atracurium undergo spontaneous degradation by Hoffmann elimination has defined a role for these muscle relaxants in patients with liver and renal insufficiency.

BLOOD, FLUIDS, AND HEMODYNAMIC CONTROL

Paleolithic cave drawings found in France depict a bear losing blood from multiple spear wounds, indicating that primitive man understood the simple relationship between blood and life.[108] Over 10,000 years later, modern anesthesiologists attempt to preserve this intimate relationship by replacing fluids and blood products when faced with intravascular volume depletion or diminished oxygen-carrying capacity from blood loss. Interestingly, knowledge of blood and volume deficits related to symptomatic hypovolemia and anemia was probably first understood and connected with the ancient art of phlebotomy, or bloodletting. Since before Hippocrates in the fifth century BC, bloodletting was practiced to restore balance to the body's four humors: blood, phlegm, black and yellow bile. From the middle ages, Barbers performing venesection advertised their services with the red (blood) and white (tourniquet) striped pole that patients squeezed and used to steady their arms during the procedure. One to four pints of blood was typically drained at a time and the procedure was stopped if the patient became faint. This amount is intriguing in that it is consistent with current understanding of acute blood loss and the volume necessary to produce symptoms secondary to anemic hypovolemic states. Recognition that phlebotomizing more than 3 to 4 pints of blood led to undesirable symptoms undoubtedly occurred by process of trial and error.[109] The obvious problem with bloodletting, erroneous therapeutic assumptions aside, was that overzealous phlebotomy could lead to hypovolemia and shock with no method available for restoring fluids to the intravascular compartment. Unrestrained venesection killed U.S. president George Washington when in 1799 he was drained of nine pints of blood in 24 hours following a throat infection.

The technique that might have saved Washington from this fate, blood transfusion, was first attempted in 1667 by physician to Louis XIV, Jean Baptiste Denis. Denis had learned of Richard Lower's transfusion of lamb's blood into a dog the previous year. Lamb's blood was most frequently used because the donating animal's essential qualities were thought to be transferred to the recipient. Despite this dangerous trans-species transfusion, Denis' first patient got better. His next two patients were not as fortunate, however, and Denis avoided further attempts. Given the poor outcomes of these early blood transfusions, and heated religious controversy regarding the implications of transferring animal-specific qualities across species, blood transfusion in humans was banned for over a hundred years in both France and England beginning in 1670.[90]

In 1900, Karl Landsteiner and Samuel Shattock independently helped lay the scientific basis of all subsequent transfusions by recognizing that blood compatibility was based upon different blood groups. Landsteiner, an Austrian physician, originally organized human blood into three groups based upon substances present on the red blood cells. The fourth type, AB group, was identified in 1902 by two students, A. Decastrello and A. Sturli. Based upon these findings, Reuben Ottenberg performed the first type-specific blood transfusion in 1907.

Transfusion of physiologic solutions occurred in 1831, independently performed by O'Shaughnessy and Lewins in Great Britain. In his letter to *The Lancet*, Lewins described transfusing large volumes of saline solutions into patients with cholera. He reported that he would inject into adults from 5 to 10 pounds of saline solution and repeat as needed.[110] Despite its publication in a prominent journal, Lewins' technique was apparently overlooked for decades and balanced physiologic solution availability would have to await the coming of analytical chemistry.

ANESTHESIA ORGANIZATION AND EDUCATION

7 Anesthesiology evolved slowly as a medical specialty in the United States. While ether remained the dominant anesthetic in America, the provision of anesthesia was often a service relegated to medical students, junior house officers, nurses, and nonprofessionals. The subordinate status of anesthesia was reflected in American art. Thomas Eakins' great studies, "The Gross Clinic" of 1876 and "The Agnew Clinic" of 1889, both present the surgeon as the focus of attention, whereas the person administering the anesthetic is seen among the supporting figures. During the late nineteenth century, small communities were often served by a single physician, who assigned a nurse to "drop" ether under his direction. In larger towns, doctors practiced independently and did not welcome being placed in what they perceived to be the subordinate role of anesthetist while their competitors enhanced their surgical reputations and collected the larger fees. Many American surgeons recalled the simple techniques they had practiced as junior house officers and regarded anesthesia as a technical craft that could be left to anyone. Some hospitals preferred to pay a salary to an anesthesia nurse while gaining a profit from the fees charged for that person's services. The most compelling argument to be advanced in favor of nurse anesthesia was that of skill: a trained nurse who administered anesthetics every working day was to be preferred to a physician who gave anesthesia infrequently.

Before the beginning of the twentieth century, Mary Botsford and Isabella Herb[111] were among the first Americans to become specialists in anesthesia. Both women were highly regarded as clinicians and also were influential in the formation of specialty societies. Dr. Botsford is believed to have been the first woman to establish a practice as a specialist in anesthesia. In 1897, she became the anesthesiologist at a children's hospital in San Francisco. Following her example, several other Californian female physicians entered the specialty. Botsford later received the first academic appointment in anesthesia in the western United States when she became clinical professor of anesthesia at the University of California, San Francisco. Dr. Botsford also served as the president of the Associated Anesthetists of the United States and Canada.[112]

One of the first physicians to actually declare himself a "specialist in anesthesia" was Sydney Ormond Goldan of New York, who published seven articles in 1900, including an early description of the use of cocaine for spinal anesthesia. After studying Goldan's early career, Raymond Fink recognized in him some of the qualities of many modern anesthesiologists: "He was brimful of enthusiasm for anesthesia, an excellent communicator and a prolific writer, a gadgeteer and the owner of several patents of anesthesia equipment."[113] At a time when many surgeons considered that spinal anesthesia did away with their need for an anesthesiologist, Goldan was particularly bold in his written opinions. He called for equality between surgeon and anesthesiologist and was among the first to state that the anesthesiologist had a right to establish and collect his own fee. Goldan regarded the anesthesiologist as being more important than the surgeon to the welfare of the patient.

Since the training of physician anesthetists around the turn of the century lacked uniformity, many prominent surgeons preferred nurse anesthetists and directed the training of the most able candidates they could recruit. At the Mayo Clinic, there were no medical students or residents to give anesthetics in the early 1890s. The Mayo brothers turned to Edith Graham to administer anesthesia. After she married Charles Mayo, Alice Magaw became their personal anesthetist. In turn, Magaw trained Florence Henderson and many others in the art of anesthesia.[114] George W. Crile relied on the skills of Agatha Hodgins. During World War I, Agatha Hodgins, Geraldine Gerrard, Ann Penland, and Sophie Gran were among the more than 100 nurse anesthetists who attended thousands of American and Allied casualties in France. On their return to the United States, many developed schools of nurse anesthesia.[115]

ORGANIZED ANESTHESIOLOGY

Physician anesthetists sought to obtain respect among their surgical colleagues by organizing professional societies and improving the quality of training. The first American organization was founded by nine members on October 6, 1905, and called the Long Island Society of Anesthetists with annual dues of $1.00. In 1911, the annual assessment rose to $3.00 when the Long Island Society became the New York Society of Anesthetists. Although the new organization still carried a local title, it drew members from several states and had a membership of 70 physicians in 1915.[116]

One of the most noteworthy figures in the struggle to professionalize anesthesiology was Francis Hoffer McMechan. McMechan had been a practicing anesthesiologist in Cincinnati until 1911, when he suffered a severe first attack of rheumatoid arthritis, which eventually left him confined to a wheelchair and forced his retirement from the operating room in 1915. McMechan had been in practice only fifteen years, but he had written eighteen clinical articles in this short time. A prolific researcher and writer, McMechan did not permit his crippling disease to sideline his career. Instead of pursuing goals in clinical medicine, he applied his talents to establishing anesthesiology societies.[117]

McMechan supported himself and his devoted wife through editing the *Quarterly Anesthesia Supplement* from 1914 until August 1926. He became editor of the first journal devoted to anesthesia, *Current Researches in Anesthesia and Analgesia*, the precursor of *Anesthesia and Analgesia*, the oldest journal of the specialty. As well as fostering the organization of the International Anesthesia Research Society (IARS) in 1925, McMechan and his wife, Laurette, became overseas ambassadors of American anesthesia. Since Laurette was French, it was understandable that McMechan combined his own ideas about anesthesiology with concepts from abroad.[118]

In 1926, McMechan held the Congress of Anesthetists in a joint conference with the Section on Anaesthetics of the British Medical Association. Subsequently, he traveled throughout Europe, giving lectures and networking physicians in the field. Upon his final return to America, he was gravely ill and was confined to bed for 2 years. His hard work and constant travel paid dividends, however: in 1929, the IARS, which McMechan founded in 1922, had members not only from North America, but also from several European countries, Japan, India, Argentina, and Brazil.[119]

In the 1930s, McMechan expanded his mission from organizing anesthesiologists to promoting the academic aspects of the specialty. In 1931, work began on what would become the International College of Anesthetists. This body began to award fellowships in 1935. For the first time, physicians were recognized as specialists in anesthesiology. The certification qualifications were universal, and fellows were recognized as specialists in several countries. Although the criteria for certification were not strict, the College was a success in raising the standards of anesthesia practice in many nations.[120] In 1939, McMechan finally succumbed to illness, and the anesthesia world lost its tireless leader.

Other Americans promoted the growth of organized anesthesiology. Ralph Waters and John Lundy, among others, participated in evolving organized anesthesia. Waters' greatest contribution to the specialty was raising its academic standards. After completing his internship in 1913, he entered medical practice in Sioux City, Iowa, where he gradually limited his practice to anesthesia. His personal experience and extensive reading were supplemented by the only postgraduate training available, a 1-month course conducted in Ohio by E. I. McKesson. At that time, the custom of becoming a self-proclaimed specialist in medicine and surgery was not uncommon. Waters, who was frustrated by low standards and who would eventually have a great influence on establishing both anesthesia residency training and the formal examination process, recalled that before 1920, "The requirements for specialization in many Midwestern hospitals consisted of the possession of sufficient audacity to attempt a procedure and persuasive power adequate to gain the consent of the patient or his family."[121]

In an effort to improve anesthetic care, Waters regularly corresponded with Dennis Jackson and other scientists. In 1925, he relocated to Kansas City with a goal of gaining an academic post at the University of Kansas, but the professor of surgery failed to support his proposal. The larger city did allow him to initiate his freestanding outpatient surgical facility, "The Downtown Surgical Clinic," which featured one of the first postanesthetic recovery rooms.[122] In 1927, Erwin Schmidt, professor of surgery at the University of Wisconsin's medical school, encouraged Dean Charles Bardeen to recruit Waters.

In accepting the first American academic position in anesthesia, Waters described four objectives that have been since adopted by many other academic departments. His goals were as follows: "(1) to provide the best possible service to patients of the institution; (2) to teach what is known of the principles of Anesthesiology to all candidates for their medical degree; (3) to help long-term graduate students not only to gain a fundamental knowledge of the subject and to master the art of administration, but also to learn as much as possible of the effective methods of teaching; (4) to accompany these efforts with the encouragement of as much cooperative investigation as is consistent with achieving the first objectives."[123]

Waters' personal and professional qualities impressed talented young men and women who sought residency posts in his department. He encouraged residents to initiate research interests in which they collaborated with two pharmacologists whom Waters had known before arriving in Wisconsin, Arthur Loevenhart and Chauncey Leake, as well as others with whom he became associated in Madison. Clinical concerns were also investigated. As an example, anesthesia records were coded onto punch cards to form a database that was used to analyze departmental activities. Morbidity and mortality meetings, now a requirement of all training programs, also originated in Madison. Members of the department and distinguished visitors from other centers attended them. As a consequence of their critical reviews of the conduct of anesthesia, responsibility for an operative tragedy gradually passed from the patient to the physician. In more casual times, a practitioner could complain, "The patient died because he did not take a good anesthetic." Alternatively, the death might be attributed to a mysterious force such as "status lymphaticus," of which Arthur Guedel, a master of sardonic humor, observed, "Certainly status lymphaticus is at times a great help to the anesthetist. When he has a fatality under anesthesia with no other cleansing explanation he is glad to recognize the condition as an entity."[123]

In 1929, John Lundy at the Mayo Clinic organized the Anaesthetists' Travel Club, whose members were leading American or Canadian teachers of anesthesia. Each year one member was the host for a group of 20 to 40 anesthesiologists who gathered for a program of informal discussions. There were demonstrations of promising innovations for the operating room and laboratory, which were all subjected to what is remembered as a "high-spirited, energetic, critical review."[124] The Travel Club would be critical in the upcoming battle to form the American Board of Anesthesiology.

Even during the lean years of the Depression, international guests also visited Waters' department. For Geoffrey Kaye of Australia, Torsten Gordh of Sweden, Robert Macintosh and Michael Nosworthy of England, and scores of others, Waters' department was their "mecca of anesthesia." Ralph Waters trained 60 residents during the 22 years he was the "Chief." From 1937 onward, the alumni, who declared themselves the "Aqualumni" in his honor, returned annually for a professional and social reunion. Thirty-four "Aqualumni" took academic positions, and, of these, 14 became chairpersons of departments of anesthesia. They maintained Waters' professional principles and encouraged teaching careers for many of their own graduates.[125] His enduring legacy was once recognized by the dean who had recruited him in 1927, Charles Bardeen, who observed, "Ralph Waters was the first person the University hired to put people to sleep, but, instead, he awakened a world-wide interest in anesthesia."[127]

Waters and Lundy along with Paul Wood, of New York City, had an important role in establishing organized anesthesia, and the definition of the specialty. In the heart of the Great Depression, these three physicians realized that anesthesiology needed to have a process to determine who was an anesthetic specialist with American Medical Association (AMA) backing. Using the New York Society of Anesthetists, of which Paul Wood was secretary-treasurer, a new class of members, "Fellows," was created. The "Fellows" criteria followed established AMA guidelines for specialty certification. However, the AMA wanted a national organization to sponsor a specialty board. The New York Society of Anesthetists changed its name to the American Society of Anesthetists (ASA) in 1936. Combined with the American Society of Regional Anesthesia, whose president was Emery Rovenstein, the American Board of Anesthesiology (ABA) was organized as a subordinate board to the American Board of Surgery in 1938. With McMechan's death in 1939, the AMA favored independence for the ABA, and in 1940, independence was granted.[122,127]

A few years later, the officers of the American Society of Anesthetists were challenged by Dr. M. J. Seifert, who wrote, "An Anesthetist is a technician and an Anesthesiologist is the specific authority on anesthesia and anesthetics. I cannot understand why you do not term yourselves the American Society of Anesthesiologists."[126] Ralph Waters was declared the first president of the newly named ASA in 1945. In that year, when World War II ended, 739 (37%) of 1,977 ASA members were in the armed forces. In the same year, the ASA's first Distinguished Service Award (DSA) was presented to Paul M. Wood for his tireless service to the specialty, one element of which can be examined today in the extensive archives preserved in the Society's Wood Library Museum at ASA headquarters, Park Ridge, Illinois.[127]

After World War II, specialties within the realm of anesthesiology began to thrive. Kathleen Belton was a superb pediatric specialist. In 1948, while working in Montreal, Belton and her colleague, Digby Leigh, wrote the classic text *Pediatric Anesthesia*. At the same time, a second pediatric anesthesiologist, Margot Deming, was the Director of Anesthesia at the Children's Hospital of Philadelphia. Pediatric anesthesia also figured in the career of Doreen Vermeulen-Cranch, who had earlier initiated thoracic anesthesia in The Netherlands and pioneered hypothermic anesthesia. Obstetric anesthesia also figured prominently in the career of Virginia Apgar. After encountering severe financial and professional frustrations during her training and while serving as Director of the Division of Anesthesia at Columbia University, Apgar turned to obstetric anesthesia in 1949. She dedicated the next decade of her multifaceted career to the care of mothers and their infants.[128]

ANESTHESIA PRACTICE TODAY AND TOMORROW

This overview of the development of anesthesiology could be extended almost indefinitely by an exploration of each subspecialty area, but an assessment of our current roles can be seen by a personal survey of the areas in which anesthesiologists serve in hospitals, clinics, and laboratories. The operating room and obstetric delivery suite remain the central interest of most specialists. Aside from being the location where the techniques described in this chapter find regular application, service in these areas brings us into regular contact with new advances in pharmacology and bioengineering.

After surgery, patients are transported to the postanesthesia care unit or recovery room, an area that is now considered the anesthesiologist's "ward." Fifty years ago, patients were carried directly from the operating room to a surgical ward to be at-
8 tended only by a junior nurse. That person lacked both the skills and equipment to intervene when complications occurred. After the experiences of World War II taught the value of centralized care, physicians and nurses created recovery rooms, which were soon mandated for all major hospitals. By 1960 the evolution of critical care progressed through the use of mechanical ventilators. Patients who required many days of intensive medical and nursing management were cared for in a curtained corner of the recovery room. In time, curtains drawn about one or two beds gave way to fixed partitions and the relocation of those areas to form intensive care units. The principles of resuscitative and supportive care established by anesthesiologists transformed critical care medicine.

9 The future of anesthesiology is a bright one. The safer drugs that once revolutionized the care of patients undergoing surgery are constantly being improved upon. The role of

the anesthesiologist continues to broaden, as physicians with backgrounds in the specialty have developed clinics for chronic pain control and outpatient surgery. Anesthesia practice will continue to increase in scope, both inside and outside of the operating suite, such that anesthesiologists will become even more of an integral part of the entire perioperative experience.

References

1. Joyce H: The Journals and Letters of Fanny Burney. Oxford, Clarendon 1975, As quoted in: Papper EM: Romance, Poetry, and Surgical Sleep. Westport, CT, p 12. Greenwood Press, 1995
2. Epitaph to W.T.G. Morton on a memorial from the Mt. Auburn Cemetery, Cambridge, Massachusetts.
3. These Egyptian Pictographs are dated approximately 2500 B.C. See Ellis ES: Ancient Anodynes: Primitive Anaesthesia and Allied Conditions, p 80. London, WM Heinemann Medical Books, 1946
4. Ellis ES: Ancient Anodynes: Primitive Anaesthesia and Allied Conditions, p 9. London, WM Heinemann Medical Books, 1946
5. Bacon DR: Regional anesthesia and chronic pain therapy: A history. In: Brown DL (ed): Regional Anesthesia and Analgesia, p 11. Philadelphia, WB Saunders, 1996
6. Rutkow I: Surgery, An Illustrated History, p 215. St. Louis, Mosby, 1993
7. Winter A: Mesmerized: Powers of Mind in Victorian Britain. Chicago, p 42. University of Chicago Press, 1998
8. Marmer MJ: Hypnosis in Anesthesiology, p 10. Springfield, IL, Charles C. Thomas, 1959
9. Dioscorides: On mandragora. In: Dioscorides Opera Libra. Quoted in: Bergman N: The Genesis of Surgical Anesthesia, p 11. Park Ridge, IL, Wood Library-Museum of Anesthesiology, 1998
10. Infusino M, Viole O'Neill Y, Calmes S: Hog beans, poppies, and mandrake leaves—A test of the efficacy of the soporific sponge. In: The History of Anaesthesia, p 31. London, Parthenon Publishing Group, 1989
11. Strickland RA: Ether drinking in Ireland. Mayo Clinic Proceedings, 71(10):1015, 1996
12. Davy H: Researches Chemical and Philosophical Chiefly Concerning Nitrous Oxide or Dephlogisticated Nitrous Air, and Its Respiration, p 533. London, J Johnson, 1800
13. Papper EM: Romance, Poetry, and Surgical Sleep. Westport, CT, Greenwood Press, 1995
14. Hickman HH: A letter on suspended animation, containing experiments showing that it may be safely employed during operations on animals, with the view of ascertaining its probable utility in surgical operations on the human subject, addressed to T.A. Knight, Esq. Imprint Ironbridge, W. Smith, 1824
15. Lyman HM: Artificial Anaesthesia and Anaesthetics, p 6. New York, William Hood, 1881
16. Stetson JB, William E: Clarke and the discovery of anesthesia. In: Fink BR, Morris L, Stephen ER (eds.): The History of Anesthesia: Third International Symposium Proceedings, p 400. Park Ridge, IL, Wood Library-Museum of Anesthesiology, 1992
17. Long CW: An account of the first use of sulphuric ether by inhalation as an anaesthetic in surgical operations. South Med Surg J 5:705, 1849
18. Robinson V: Victory Over Pain, p 91. New York, Henry Schuman, 1946
19. Raper HR: Man Against Pain, p 286. New York, Prentice-Hall, Inc., 1945
20. Smith GB, Hirsch NP: Gardner Quincy Colton: Pioneer of nitrous oxide anesthesia. Anesth Analg 72:382, 1991
21. Menczer LF: Horace Wells's "day book A": a transcription and analysis. Wolfe RJ, Menczer LF (eds.): I Awaken to Glory, p 112. Boston, Boston Medical Library, 1994
22. Greene NM: A consideration of factors in the discovery of anesthesia and their effects on its development. Anesthesiology 35:515, 1971
23. Fenster J: Ether Day. New York, Harper Collins, 2001
24. Duncum BM: The Development of Inhalation Anaesthesia, p 86. London, Oxford University Press, 1947
25. Caton D: What a Blessing She had Chloroform, p 103. New Haven, Yale University Press, 1999
26. Journal of Queen Victoria. In: Strauss MB (ed): Familiar Medical Quotations, p 17. Boston, Little Brown, 1968
27. Snow J: On Chloroform and Other Anesthetics (reprinted by the Wood Library-Museum of Anesthesiology.), p 58. London, J Churchill, 1858
28. Lucas GH: The discovery of cyclopropane. Curr Res Anesth Analg 40:15, 1961
29. Seevers MH, Meek WJ, Rovenstine EA, Stiles JA: Cyclopropane study with espical reference to gas concentration, respiratory and electrocardiographic changes. Journal of Pharmacology and Experimental Therapeutics 51:1, 1934
30. Calverley RK: Fluorinated anesthetics: I. The early years. Surv Anesth 29:170, 1986
31. Robbins BH: Preliminary studies of the anesthetic activity of the fluorinated hydrocarbons. J Pharmacol Exp Ther 86:197, 1946
32. Calverley RK: Fluorinated anesthetics: II. Fluroxene. Surv Anesth 30:126, 1987
33. Suckling CW: Some chemical and physical factors in the development of Fluothane. Br J Anaesth 29:466, 1957
34. Koller C: Personal reminiscences of the first use of cocaine as local anesthetic in eye surgery. Current Researches in Anesthesia and Analgesia 7:9, 1928
35. Becker HK: Carl Koller and cocaine. Psychoanal Q 32:309, 1963
36. Halstead WS: Practical comments on the use and abuse of cocaine; suggested by its in variably successful employment in more than a thousand minor surgical operations. NY Med J 42:294, 1885
37. Olch PD, William S: Halstead and local anesthesia: Contributions and complications. Anesthesiology 42:479, 1975
38. Marx G: The first spinal anesthesia: Who deserves the laurels? Reg Anesth 19:429, 1994
39. Corning JL: Spinal anaesthesia and local medication of the cord. NY Med J 42:483, 1885
40. Bier AKG: Experiments in cocainization of the spinal cord, 1899. In: Faulconer A, Keys TE (trans): Foundations of Anesthesiology, p 854. Springfield, IL, Charles C Thomas, 1965
41. Goerig M, Agarwal K, Schulte am Esch J: The versatile August Bier (1861–1949), father of spinal anesthesia. J Clin Anesth 12:561, 2000
42. Larson MD: Tait and Caglieri. The first spinal anesthetic in America. Anesthesiology. 85(4):913, 1996
43. Lee JA: Arthur Edward James Barker, 1850–1916: British pioneer of regional anaesthesia. Anaesthesia 34:885, 1979
44. Lemmon WT: A method for continuous spinal anesthesia: A preliminary report. Ann Surg 111:141, 1940
45. Martini JA, Bacon DR, Vasdev GM: Edward Tuohy: The man, his needle, and its place in obstetric anesthesia. Reg Anesth Pain Med 27:520, 2002
46. Tuohy EB: Continuous spinal anesthesia: Its usefulness and technique involved. Anesthesiology 5:142, 1944
47. Pagés F: Metameric anesthesia, 1921. In: Faulconer A, Keys TE (trans): Foundations of Anesthesiology, p 927. Springfield, IL, Charles C Thomas, 1965
48. Fink BR: History of local anesthesia. In: Cousins MJ, Bridenbaugh PO (eds.): Neural Blockade, p 12. Philadelphia, JB Lippincott, 1980
49. Cushing H: On the avoidance of shock in major amputations by cocainization of large nerve trunks preliminary to their division: With observations on blood-pressure changes in surgical cases. Ann Surg 36:321, 1902
50. Crile GW, Lower WE: Anoci-Association. Philadelphia, W.B. Saunders Company, 1915
51. Brown DL, Winnie AP: Biography of Louis Gaston Labat, M.D. Regional Anesthesia 17(5):248, 1992
52. Bacon DR, Darwish H: Emery Rovenstine and regional anesthesia. Reg Anesth 22:273, 1997
53. Calverley RK: An early ether vaporizer designed by John Snow, a Treasure of the Wood Library-Museum of Anesthesiology. In: Fink BR, Morris LE, Stephen CR (eds): The History of Anesthesia, p 91. Park Ridge, IL, Wood Library-Museum of Anesthesiology, 1992
54. Snow J: On the Inhalation of the Vapour of Ether (reprinted by the Wood Library-Museum of Anesthesiology), p 23. London, J Churchill, 1847
55. Calverley RK, J. T. Clover: A giant of Victorian anaesthesia. In: Rupreht J, van Lieburg MJ, Lee JA, Erdmann W (eds.): Anaesthesia: Essays on Its History, p 21. Berlin, Springer-Verlag, 1985
56. Andrews E: The oxygen mixture, a new anaesthetic combination. Chicago Medical Examiner 9:656, 1868
57. Waters RM: Clinical scope and utility of carbon dioxide filtration in inhalation anesthesia. Curr Res Anesth Analg 3:20, 1923
58. Sword BC: The closed circle method of administration of gas anesthesia. Curr Res Anesth Analg 9:198, 1930
59. Sands RP, Bacon DR: An inventive mind: The career of James O. Elam, M.D. (1918–1995). Anesthesiology 88:1107, 1998
60. Obituary of T. Philip Ayre. Br Med J 280:125, 1980
61. Rees GJ: Anaesthesia in the newborn. Br Med J 2:1419, 1950
62. Bain JA, Spoerel WE: A stream-lined anaesthetic system. Can Anaesth Soc J 19:426, 1972
63. Morris LE: A new vaporizer for liquid anesthetic agents. Anesthesiology 13:587, 1952
64. Sands R, Bacon DR: The copper kettle: A historical perspective. J Clin Anesth 8:528, 1996
65. Shephard DAE: Harvey Cushing and anaesthesia. Can Anaesth Soc J 12:431, 1965
66. Mushin WW, Rendell-Baker L: Thoracic Anaesthesia Past and Present (reprinted by the Wood Library Museum of Anesthesiology 1991), p 44. Springfield, IL, Charles C Thomas, 1953
67. Tovell RM: Problems in supply of anesthetic gases in the European theater of operations. Anesthesiology 8:303, 1947
68. Rendell-Baker L: History of standards for anesthesia equipment. In: Rupreht J, van Lieburg MJ, Lee JA, Erdmann W (eds.): Anaesthesia: Essays on Its History, p 161. Berlin, Springer-Verlag, 1985
69. Calverley RK: A safety feature for anaesthesia machines: Touch identification of oxygen flow control. Can Anaesth Soc J 18:225, 1971
70. Clover JT: Laryngotomy in chloroform anesthesia. Br Med J 1:132, 1877
71. Macewan W: Clinical observations on the introduction of tracheal tubes by the mouth instead of performing tracheotomy or laryngotomy. Br Med J 2:122, 163, 1880

72. Kuhn F: Nasotracheal intubation (trans). In: Faulconer A, Keys TE (eds.): Foundations of Anesthesiology, p 677. Springfield, IL, Charles C Thomas, 1965
73. Hirsch NP, Smith GB, Hirsch PO: Alfred Kirstein, pioneer of direct laryngoscopy. Anaesthesia 41:42, 1986
74. Burkle CM, Zepeda FA, Bacon DR, Rose SH: A historical perspective on use of the laryngoscope as a tool in anesthesiology. Anesthesiology. 100(4):1003, 2004
75. Miller RA: A new laryngoscope. Anesthesiology 2:317, 1941
76. Macintosh RR: Richard Salt of Oxford, anaesthetic technician extraordinary. Anaesthesia 31:855, 1976
77. Thomas KB: Sir Ivan Whiteside Magill, KCVO, DSc, MB, BCh, BAO, FRCS, FFARCS (Hon), FFARCSI (Hon), DA: A review of his publications and other references to his life and work. Anaesthesia 33:628, 1978
78. Condon HA, Gilchrist E: Stanley Rowbotham: twentieth century pioneer anaesthetist. Anaesthesia 41:46, 1986
79. Calverley RK: Arthur E Guedel (1883–1956). In: Ruprecht J, van Lieburg MJ, Lee JA, Erdmann W (eds.): Anaesthesia: Essays on Its History, p 49. Berlin, Springer-Verlag, 1985
80. Calverley RK: Classical file. Surv Anesth 28:70, 1984
81. Gale JW, Waters RM: Closed endobronchial anesthesia in thoracic surgery: Preliminary report. Curr Res Anesth Analg 11:283, 1932
82. Wu TL, Chou HC: A new laryngoscope: the combination intubating device (letter). Anesthesiology 81:1085, 1994
83. Brain AIJ: The laryngeal mask: A new concept in airway management. Br J Anaesth 55:801, 1983
84. Duncum BM: The Development of Inhalation Anaesthesia, p 538. London, Oxford University Press, 1947
85. Cushing H: On the avoidance of shock in major amputations by cocainization of large nerve trunks preliminary to their division: With observations on blood-pressure changes in surgical cases. Ann Surg 36:321, 1902
86. Codesmith A: An endo-esophageal stethoscope. Anesthesiology 15:566, 1954
87. Severinghaus JC, Honda Y: Pulse oximetry. Int Anesthesiol Clin 25:205, 1987
88. Luft K. Methode der registrieren gas analyse mit hilfe der absorption ultraroten Strahlen ohne spectrale Zerlegung. Z Tech Phys 1943;24:97.
89. Wren PC: Philosophical Transactions,Vol I. London, Anno, 1665 and 1666
90. Keys TE: The History of Surgical Anesthesia, p 38. New York, Dover Publications, 1945
91. Dundee J, Wyant G: Intravenous Anesthesia, p 1. Hong Kong, Churchill Livingstone, 1974
92. Oré PC: Etudes, cliniques sur l'anesthésie chirurgicale par la methode des injection de choral dans les veines. Paris,: JB Balliere et Fils 1875, As quoted in: Hemelrijck JV, Kissin I: History of Intravenous Anesthesia. In: PF White (ed): Textbook of Intravenous Anesthesia, p 3. Baltimore, Williams & Wilkins, 1997
93. Macintosh RR: Modern anaesthesia, with special reference to the chair of anaesthetics in Oxford. In, Ruprecht J, van Lieburg MJ, Lee JA, Erdmann W (eds.): Anaesthesia: Essays on Its History, p 352. Berlin, Springer-Verlag, 1985
94. Hemelrijck JV, Kissin I: History of Intravenous Anesthesia. In: White PF (ed): Textbook of Intravenous Anesthesia, p 3. Baltimore, Williams & Wilkins, 1997
95. Gwathmey JT: Anesthesia, p 379. New York, D. Appleton and Company, 1914
96. Flagg PJ: The Art of Anaesthesia, p 80. Philadelphia, JB Lippincott Company, 1918
97. Chloretone (chlorobutanol) is prepared by mixing chloroform and acetone, and has a camphor-like odor that some find pleasant. Chloretone is now commonly used for euthanizing reptiles and amphibians
98. Hewer CL: Recent Advances in Anaesthesia and Analgesia, p 237. Philadelphia: P Blakiston's Son & Co. Inc., 1937
99. Collins VJ: Principles and Practice of Anesthesiology, p 327. Philadelphia, Lea & Febiger, 1952
100. Raeder J: History of Postoperative Nausea and Vomiting. Int Anesthesiol Clin 41(4):1, 2003
101. McIntyre AR: Curare, Its History, Nature, and Clinical Use, p 6, 131. Chicago, University of Chicago Press, 1947
102. Thomas BK: Curare: Its History and Usage, p 90. Philadelphia, JB Lippincott Company, 1963
103. Rushman GB, Davies NJH, Atkinson RS: A Short History of Anaesthesia, p 78. Oxford, Butterworth-Heinemann, 1996
104. Knoefel PK: Felice Fontana: Life and Works, p 284. Trento, Societa de Studi Trentini, 1985
105. Griffith HR, Johnson GE: The use of curare in general anesthesia. Anesthesiology 3:418, 1942
106. McIntyre AR: Historical background, early use and development of muscle relaxants. Anesthesiology 20: 412, 1959
107. Ali HH, Utting JE, Gray C: Quantitative assessment of residual antidepolarizing block (part II). Br J Anaesth 43:478, 1971
108. Gottlieb AM: A Pictorial History of Blood Practices and Transfusion, p 2. Scottsdale, AZ, Arcane Publications, 1992
109. For further details regarding bloodletting, see CK Wilbur: Antique Medical Instruments, 1987, or G. Pendergraph: Handbook of Phlebotomy. Philadelphia Lea and Febiger, 1984
110. Jenkins MT: Epochs in intravenous fluid therapy: from the goose quill and pig bladder to balanced salt solutions, p 4. The Lewis H. Wright Memorial Lecture, Wood Library-Museum Collection, Park Ridge, IL, 1993
111. Strickland RA: Isabella Coler Herb, MD: an early leader in anesthesiology. Anesth Analg. 80(3):600, 1995
112. Calmes SH: Anesthesiology in California: the early years. Bulletin of the History of Anesthesiology 17(1):8, 1999
113. Fink BR: Leaves and needles: the introduction of surgical local anesthesia. Anesthesiology 63:77, 1985
114. Harris NA, Hunziker-Dean J: Florence Henderson. Nursing History Review 9:159, 2001
115. Bankert M: Watchful Care: A History of America's Nurse Anesthetists. New York, Continuum, 1989
116. Betcher AM, Ciliberti BJ, Wood PM, Wright LH: The jubilee year of organized anesthesia. Anesthesiology 17:226, 1956
117. Bacon DR: The promise of one great anesthesia society. Anesthesiology 80:929, 1994
118. Seldon TH: Francis Hoeffer McMechan. In: Volpitto PP, Vandam LD (eds): Genesis of American Anesthesiology, p 5. Springfield, IL, Charles C Thomas, 1982
119. Bacon DR: The world federation of societies of anesthesiologists: McMechan's final legacy? Anesth Analg 84:1131, 1997
120. Bacon DR, Lema MJ: To define a specialty: A brief history of the American Board of Anesthesiology's first written examination. J Clin Anesth 1992;4:489
121. Waters RM: Pioneering in anesthesiology. Postgrad Med 4:265, 1948
122. Waters RM: The down-town anesthesia clinic. Am J Surg 33:71, 1919
123. Guedel AE: Inhalation Anesthesia: A Fundamental Guide, p 129. New York: MacMillan, 1937
124. MacKenzie RA, Bacon DR, Martin DP: Anaesthetists' Travel Club: a transformation of the society of clinical surgery? Bull Anesth Hist Jul;22(3):7, 2004
125. Bacon DR, Ament R: Ralph Waters and the beginnings of academic anesthesiology in the United States: the Wisconsin template. J Clin Anesth 7:534, 1995
126. Little DM Jr, Betcher AM: The Diamond Jubilee 1905–1980, p 8. Park Ridge, IL, American Society of Anesthesiologists, 1980
127. Bamforth BJ, Siebecker KL: Ralph M. Waters. In: Volpitto PP, Vandam LD (eds): Genesis of American Anesthesiology,. Springfield, IL: Charles C Thomas, 1982
128. Calmes SH: Development of the Apgar Score. In: Ruprecht J, van Leigurgh MJ, Lee JA, Erdman W (eds.): Anaesthesia: Essays on Its History, p 45. Berlin, Springer-Verlag, 1985

CHAPTER 2 ■ PRACTICE AND OPERATING ROOM MANAGEMENT

RICHARD L. LOCK AND JOHN H. EICHHORN

KEY POINTS

1. Anesthesiology residents, and many postgraduates also, tend to lack sufficient knowledge (with sometimes unfortunate results) about practice structures, financial matters of all types, and contracting in particular. They must educate themselves and also seek expert advice and counsel to survive (and hopefully flourish) in today's exceedingly complex medical practice milieu.
2. There are several very helpful detailed information resources on practice and OR management available from the American Society of Anesthesiologists (ASA) and other sources.
3. Securing hospital privileges is far more than a bureaucratic annoyance and must be taken seriously by anesthesiologists.
4. Anesthesiologists need to be involved, concerned, active participants and leaders in their institution and community to enhance their practice function and image.
5. Anesthesiology is the leading medical specialty in establishing and promulgating standards of practice, which have significantly positively influenced practice.
6. The immediate response to a major adverse anesthesia event is critical to the eventual result and an extremely valuable protocol is available at www.apsf.org, "Resources: Clinical Safety."
7. Managed care's influence waxes, wanes, and changes but it must always be considered by modern anesthesiologists. While cost, value, outcome, and quality issues are certainly central to all anesthesiology practices, difficulties in constructing and applying definitive measurements and rigorous statistical analysis of these parameters have prevented, so far at least, some of the potential negative influences of the core features of fully managed health care on anesthesiology practice in most circumstances.
8. Anesthesiologists must participate in operating room (OR) management in their facilities and should play a central leadership role. Operating room scheduling, staffing, utilization, and patient flow issues are complex and anesthesiologists should work hard to both thoroughly understand and positively influence them.
9. Anesthesiology personnel issues involve an elaborate balancing act and groups/departments should give these issues, as well as their constituent personnel, more attention and energy than has been traditional in the past or the anesthesia provider shortage will likely continue to worsen.
10. Attention to the many often-underemphasized details of infrastructure, organization, and administration can transform a merely endurable anesthesia practice into one that is efficient, effective, productive, collegial, and even fun.

Ongoing evolution of medical practice in the United States has accelerated to such a pace that considerations of organization, administration, and management require constant updating. Functions and details across the whole spectrum of the health care "system" or "enterprise," from the briefest and simplest primary care encounter of a single patient, through the administration and management of an anesthesiology practice group and its environment, all the way up to national policies for financing the care of the entire population, demand more attention and effort than ever before.

In the past, anesthesiologists traditionally were little involved in the management of many components of their practice beyond the strictly medical elements of applied physiology and pharmacology, pathophysiology, and therapeutics. This was, perhaps, somewhat understandable because anesthesiologists traditionally spent the vast majority of their usually very long work hours in a hospital OR. Business matters were often left to the one or two group members interested or willing to deal with an outside contractor billing agency. Often there were few if any support personnel (sometimes no office base at all other than a corner desk in the 'doctors' lounge). In many circumstances, there was little or no time to even consider or attempt management functions. Reluctant compliance with critical mandatory processes such as credentialing was secured only by the insistence of a hospital staff administrator. In that era, very little formal teaching of or training in practice management of any kind occurred in anesthesiology residency programs. Word-of-mouth handing down of what was mostly folklore was often all an anesthesiology resident had to go on after completing training and beginning practice. Interestingly in this regard, the Anesthesiology Residency Review Committee of the Accreditation Council on Graduate Medical Education now requires that the didactic curricula of anesthesiology residencies include material on practice management. Today, most residency programs offer at least a cursory introduction to issues of practice management, but these can be insufficient to prepare satisfactorily the resident being graduated for the real infrastructure, administrative, business, and management challenges of the modern practice of anesthesiology.

This chapter, which draws significantly from its predecessor[1] and also incorporates concepts from a related chapter[2]
1 in the previous edition, presents a wide variety of topics that, until very recently, were not in anesthesiology textbooks. Several basic components of the administrative, organizational (including daily functioning of the OR), and financial aspects of anesthesiology practice are outlined. Included is mention of some of the issues associated with practice arrangements in the modern environment heavily influenced by various types of managed care and its permutations and combinations. Although certain of these issues are undergoing almost constant change, it is important to understand the basic vocabulary and principles in this dynamic universe. Lack of understanding of these issues may put anesthesiologists at a disadvantage when attempting to maximize the efficiency and impact of their daily activities, to create and execute practice arrangements, and to secure fair compensation in an increasingly complex health care system with greater and greater competition for scarcer and scarcer resources.

ADMINISTRATIVE COMPONENTS OF ANESTHESIOLOGY PRACTICE

Operational and Information Resources

While it may be relatively rare, there are still situations in which a brand-new anesthesiology practice is created and there is no previously existing infrastructure, protocol, organization, habits, or tradition to draw on for guidance. Likewise, mergers and spin-offs of anesthesiology practices occur, just as in the business world. How can anesthesiologists and the administrative/support personnel they hire learn from the collective experience of the profession and thus avoid having to "reinvent the wheel" in facilitating their practice? Similarly, practicing anesthesiologists frequently recognize the need to examine and, it is hoped, improve the function of their practices through comparable efforts.

Overview summaries such as this chapter are intended as an introduction. Further, fortunately, the American Society of Anesthesiologists (ASA), the professional association for physician anesthesiologists in the United States, for many years has made available to its members extensive resource material regarding practice in general and specific arrangements for its execution. Citation and availability of this material can be found on the ASA website, www.asahq.org. Elements are updated periodically by the ASA through its physician officers,
2 committees, task forces, administrative and support staff, and various offices. Although many of the documents generated and even the advice given in response to members' questions contain broad-brush generalities that must be interpreted in each individual practice situation, these nonetheless stand as a solid foundation on which anesthesiology practice can be formulated. In the past, many ASA members were unaware of the existence of these resources and discovered them only when referred to them during an appeal to the ASA for help resolving some significant practice or financial problem. Prospective familiarity with the principles outlined in the ASA material likely could help avoid some of the problems leading to calls for help. Selected key documents are compiled and bound into a volume that can be purchased.[3] Each spring, the ASA offers a Practice Management Conference, following which the lecture materials are published in an annual volume (see www.asahq.org, "Publications and Services," "Publications on Practice Management").

Background

The current atmosphere in American medicine, which creates the impression that "all of a sudden, all the rules and understandings are changing," makes it virtually mandatory that anesthesiologists be familiar with the fundamental background of their profession. The ASA "Guidelines for the Ethical Practice of Anesthesiology"[3] includes sections on the principles of medical ethics; the definition of medical direction of nonphysician personnel (including the specific statement that an anesthesiologist engaged in medical direction should not personally be administering another anesthetic); the anesthesiologist's relationship to patients and other physicians; the anesthesiologist's duties, responsibilities, and relationship to the hospital; and the anesthesiologist's relationship to nurse anesthetists and other nonphysician personnel. Further, the ASA publishes "The Organization of an Anesthesia Department"[3] and states through it that the ASA "has adopted a Statement of Policy, which contains principles that the Society urges its members to consider in structuring their own individual medical practices." This document has sections on physician responsibilities for medical care and on medical-administrative organization and responsibilities. The ASA has been particularly proactive in helping its members keep up with rapidly changing areas of both managed care and government programs with all the myriad financial implications of the evolving rules and requirements. In the past, some (probably many) anesthesiology residents finishing training felt unprepared, in a business and organizational sense, to enter the job and practice markets. They had to learn complex difficult lessons through a self-taught crash course during negotiations for a position, sometimes to their detriment. Beyond summaries such as this chapter, reference to the considerable body of material created and presented by the ASA (which includes a thick volume specifically on the details of business arrangements[4]) is an excellent starting point to help young anesthesiologists during residency prepare for the increasing rigors of starting and managing a career in practice. Likewise, there is a great deal of information on the ASA website concerning the most recent governmental regulations, rulings, and billing codes. The ASA *Newsletter* distributed to all members now contains the monthly columns "Washington Report" and

"Practice Management," which disseminate related current developments.

Of course, the Internet is a very important source of information. In addition to the ASA, most other anesthesiology subspecialty societies and interest groups have Web locations, as do most journals. Certain anesthesiology and other journals that exist only on the Internet are now in existence, and more will likely be developed. Particularly, the website of the Anesthesia Patient Safety Foundation, www.apsf.org, has been cited as especially useful in promoting safe clinical practice. Electronic bulletin boards allow anesthesiology practitioners from around the world to immediately exchange ideas on diverse topics, both medical and administrative. Traditionally, the ASA has not maintained one. However, one of the original sites that remains very popular is www.gasnet.org and a web search ("anesthesiology + bulletin board") using a search engine such as www.google.com reveals a great number of sites that contain a variety of discussions about all manner of anesthesiology-related topics, including practice organization, administration, and management. Additionally, references to the entirety of the medical literature are readily accessible to any practitioner (such as by starting with www.nlm.nih.gov to access Medline). A modern anesthesiology practice cannot reasonably exist without readily available high-speed Internet connections.

The Credentialing Process and Clinical Privileges

The system of credentialing a health care professional and
3 granting clinical privileges in a health care facility is motivated by a fundamental assumption that appropriate education, training, and experience, along with the absence of excessive numbers of bad patient outcomes, increase the chances that the individual will deliver acceptable-quality care. As a result, the systems have received considerably increased emphasis in recent years.[5] The process of credentialing health care professionals has been the focus of considerable public attention (particularly in the mass media), in part the result of very rare incidents of untrained persons (impostors) infiltrating the health care system and sometimes harming patients. The more common situation, however, involves health professionals who exaggerate past experience and credentials or fail to disclose adverse past experiences. There has been some justified publicity concerning physicians who lost their licenses sequentially in several states and simply moved on each time to start practice elsewhere (which should be much, much more difficult now).

The patient–physician relationship also has changed radically, with a concomitant increase in suspicion directed toward the medical profession. There is now a pervasive public perception that physicians are inadequately policed, particularly by their own professional organizations and hospitals. Intense public and political pressure has been brought to bear on various law-making bodies, regulatory and licensing agencies, and health care institution administrations to discover and purge both (1) fraudulent, criminal, and deviant health care providers, and (2) incompetent or simply poor-quality practitioners whose histories show sufficient poor patient outcomes to attract attention, usually through malpractice suits. Identifying and avoiding or correcting an incompetent practitioner is the goal. Verification of appropriate education, training, and experience on the part of a candidate for a position rendering anesthesia care assumes special importance in light of the legal doctrine of *vicarious liability,* which can be described as follows: if an individual, group, or institution hires an anesthesia provider or even simply approves of that person (e.g., by granting clinical privileges through a hospital medical staff), those involved in the decision may later be held liable in the courts, along with the individual, for the individual's actions. This would be especially true if it were later discovered that the offending practitioner's past adverse outcomes had not been adequately investigated during the credentialing process.

Out of these various long-standing concerns has arisen the sometimes cumbersome process of obtaining state licenses to practice and of obtaining hospital privileges. It is somewhat analogous to passing through screening and metal detection devices at airports, which is tolerated by the individual in the interest of the safety of all, with the presumption that danger will be detected and eliminated. The stringent credentialing process is intended both to protect patients and to safeguard the integrity of the medical profession. Recently, central credentialing systems have been developed, including those affiliated with the American Medical Association, American Osteopathic Association, and, particularly, the Federation Credentials Verification Service of the Federation of State Medical Boards. These systems verify a physician's basic credentials (identity, citizenship or immigration status, medical education, postgraduate training, licensure examination history, prior licenses, board actions, etc.) once and then, thereafter, can certify the validity of these credentials to a state licensing board or medical facility. Some states do not yet accept this verification and most states seek specific supplemental information.

There are checklists of the requirements for the granting of medical staff privileges by hospitals (see the American Hospital Association Resource Center, www.aharc.library.net). In addition, the National Practitioner Data Bank and reporting system administered by the U.S. government now has many years' worth of information in it. This data bank is a central repository of licensing and credentials information about physicians. Many adverse situations involving a physician—particularly instances of substance abuse, malpractice litigation, or the revocation, suspension, or limitation of that physician's license to practice medicine or to hold hospital privileges—must be reported (via the state board of medical registration/licensure) to the National Practitioner Data Bank. It is a statutory requirement that all applications for hospital staff privileges be cross-checked against this national data bank. The potential medicolegal liability on the part of a facility's medical staff, and the anesthesiology group in particular, for failing to do so is significant. The Data Bank, however, is not a complete substitute for direct documentation and background checking. Often, practitioners reach negotiated solutions following quality-driven medical staff problems, thereby avoiding the mandatory reporting. In such cases, a suspect physician may be given the option to resign medical staff privileges and avoid Data Bank reporting rather than undergo full involuntary privilege revocation.

Documentation

The documentation for the credentialing process for each anesthesia practitioner must be complete. Privileges to administer anesthesia must be officially granted and delineated in writing.[3] This can be straightforward or it can be more complex to accommodate institutional needs to identify practitioners specially qualified to practice in designated anesthesia subspecialty areas such as cardiac, infant/pediatric, obstetric, intensive care, or pain management. Specific documentation of the process of granting or renewing clinical privileges is required and, unlike some other records, the documentation likely is protected as confidential peer review information. Any questions about complex sensitive issues such as this should be referred to an experienced attorney familiar with applicable federal and state law. Verification of an applicant's credentials and experience is mandatory. Because of another type of legal case, some examples of which have been highly publicized, medical practitioners may be hesitant to give an honest evaluation (or any evaluation at all) of individuals known to them who are seeking a professional position elsewhere. Obviously, someone writing a reference for a current or former coworker should be honest. Sticking to clearly documentable facts is advisable. Stating a fact that is in the public record (such as a malpractice case lost at trial) should not justify an objection from the subject of the reference. Whether omitting such a fact is dishonest on the part of the reference writer is more of a gray area. Including positive opinions and enthusiastic recommendations, of course, is no problem. Some fear that including facts that may be perceived as negative (e.g., the lost malpractice case or personal problems such as a history of treatment for substance abuse) and negative opinions will provoke retaliatory lawsuits (such as for libel, defamation of character, or loss of livelihood) from the subject. As a result, many reference writers in these questionable situations confine their written material to brief, simple facts such as dates employed and position held. As always, questions about complex sensitive issues such as this should be referred to an experienced attorney familiar with applicable federal and state law.

Because there should be no hesitation for a reference writer to include positive opinions, receipt of a reference that includes nothing more than dates worked and position held should be a suggestion that there may be more to the story. Receipt of such a reference about a person applying for a position should always lead to a telephone call to the writer. A telephone call is likely advisable in all cases, independent of whatever the written reference contains. Frequently, pertinent questions over the telephone can elicit more candid information. In rare instances, there may be dishonesty through omission by the reference giver even at this level. This may involve an applicant who an individual, a department or group, or an institution would like to see leave. The subject applicant may have poor-quality practice, but there may also be reluctance by the reference giver(s) to approach licensing or disciplinary authorities (because of the unpleasantness and also out of concern about retaliatory legal action). This type of "sandbagging" is fortunately infrequent. The best way to avoid it is to telephone an independent observer or source (such as a former employer or associate who no longer has a personal stake in the applicant's success or even the head nurse of an OR in which the applicant worked) when any question exists. Because the ultimate goal is optimum patient care, the subjects applying for positions generally should not object to such calls being made. Discovery of a history of unsafe practices and/or habits or of causing preventable anesthesia morbidity or mortality should elicit careful evaluation as to whether the applicant can be appropriately assigned, trained, and/or supervised to be maximally safe in the proposed new environment.

In all cases, new personnel in an anesthesia practice environment must be given a thorough orientation and checkout. Policy, procedures, and equipment may be unfamiliar to even the most thoroughly trained, experienced, and safe practitioner. This may occasionally seem tedious, but it is both sound and critically important safety policy. Being in the midst of a crisis situation caused by unfamiliarity with a new setting is not the optimal orientation session.

After the initial granting of clinical privileges to practice anesthesia, anesthesiologists must periodically renew their privileges within the institution or facility (e.g., annually or every other year). There are moral, ethical, and societal obligations on the part of the privilege-granting entity to take this process seriously. State licensing bodies often become aware of problems with health professionals very late in the evolution of the difficulties. An anesthesia provider's peers in the hospital or facility are much more likely to notice untoward developments as they first appear. However, privilege renewals are often essentially automatic and receive little of the necessary attention. Judicious checking of renewal applications and awareness of relevant peer review information is absolutely necessary. The physicians or administrators responsible for evaluating staff members and reviewing their practices and privileges may be justifiably concerned about retaliatory legal action by a staff member who is censured or denied privilege renewal. Accordingly, such evaluating groups must be thoroughly objective (totally eliminating any hint of political or financial motives) and must have documentation that the staff person in question is in fact practicing below the standard of care. Court decisions have found liability by a hospital, its medical staff group, or both when the incompetence of a staff member was known or should have been known and was not acted upon.[6] Again, questions about complex sensitive issues such as this should be referred to an experienced attorney familiar with applicable federal and state law.

A major issue in the granting of clinical privileges, especially in procedure-oriented specialties such as anesthesiology, is whether it is reasonable to continue the common practice of "blanket" privileges. This process in effect authorizes the practitioner to attempt any treatment or procedure normally considered within the purview of the applicant's medical specialty. These considerations may have profound political and economic implications within medicine, such as which type of surgeon should be doing carotid endarterectomies or lumbar discectomies. More important, however, is whether the practitioner being evaluated is qualified to do everything traditionally associated with the specialty. Specifically, should the granting of privileges to practice anesthesia automatically approve the practitioner to handle pediatric cardiac cases, critically ill newborns (such as a day-old premature infant with a large diaphragmatic hernia), ablative pain therapy (such as an alcohol celiac plexus block under fluoroscopy), high-risk obstetric cases, and so forth? This question raises the issue of procedure-specific or limited privileges. The quality assurance (QA) and risk management considerations in this question are weighty if inexperienced or insufficiently qualified practitioners are allowed or even expected, because of peer or scheduling pressures, to undertake major challenges for which they are not prepared. The likelihood of complications and adverse outcome will be higher, and the difficulty of defending the practitioner against a malpractice claim in the event of catastrophe will be significantly increased.

There is no clear answer to the question of procedure-specific credentialing and granting of privileges. Ignoring issues regarding qualifications to undertake complex and challenging procedures has clear negative potential. On the other hand, stringent procedure-specific credentialing is impractical in smaller groups, and in larger groups encourages many small "fiefdoms," with a consequent further atrophy of the clinical skills outside of the practitioner's specific area(s). Each anesthesia department or group needs to address these issues. At the very least, the common practice of every applicant for privileges (new or renewal) checking off every line on the printed list of anesthesia procedures should be reviewed. Additionally, board certification is now essentially a standard of quality assurance of the minimum skills required for the consultant practice of anesthesiology. Subspecialty boards, such as those in pain management, critical care, and transesophageal echocardiography, further objectify the credentialing process. This is now significant because initial board certification after the year 2000 by the American Board of Anesthesiology is time limited and subject to periodic testing and recertification. Clearly, this will encourage an ongoing process of continuing medical education (CME). Many states, some institutions, even some regulatory bodies have requirements for a minimum number of hours of CME. Documentation of meeting such a standard again acts as one type of quality assurance mechanism for the individual practitioner, while providing another objective credentialing measurement for those granting licenses or privileges.

Medical Staff Participation and Relationships

All medical care facilities and practice settings depend on their medical staffs, of course, for daily activities of the delivery of health care; but, very importantly, they also depend on those staffs to provide administrative structure and support. Medical staff activities are increasingly important in achieving favorable accreditation status (e.g., from the Joint Commission for
4 the Accreditation of Healthcare Organizations [JCAHO]) and in meeting a wide variety of governmental regulations and reviews. Principal medical staff activities involve sometimes time-consuming efforts, such as duties as a staff officer or committee member. Anesthesiologists should be participants in—in fact, should play a significant role in—credentialing, peer review, tissue review, transfusion review, OR management, and medical direction of same-day surgery units, postanesthesia care units (PACUs), intensive care units (ICUs), and pain management units. Also, it is very important that anesthesiology personnel be involved in fund-raising activities, benefits, community outreach projects sponsored by the facility, and social events of the facility staff.

The role these and related activities play in anesthesia practice management may not be obvious at first glance, but this is a reflection of the unfortunate fact that, all too often, anesthesiologists have in the past chosen to have very little or no involvement in such efforts. Of course, there are exceptions in specific settings. However, it is an unmistakable reality that anesthesiologists as a group have a reputation for lack of involvement in medical staff and facility issues because of a lack of time (because of long hours in the OR) or simply a lack of interest. In fact, anesthesiology personnel are all too often perceived in a facility as the ones who slip in and out of the building essentially anonymously (often dressed very casually or even in the pajama-like comfort of scrub suits) and virtually unnoticed. This is an unfortunate state of affairs, and it has frequently come back in various painful ways to haunt those who have not been involved, or even noticed. Anesthesiology personnel sometimes respond that the demands for anesthesiology service are so great that they simply never have the time or the opportunity to become involved in their facility and with their peers. If this is really true, it is clear that more providers of anesthesia care must be added at that facility, even if doing so slightly reduces the income of those already there.

In any case, anesthesiologists simply must make the time to be involved in medical staff affairs, both in health care facility administration and also as part of the organization, administration, and governance of the comparatively large multispecialty physician groups that provide entities with which managed care organizations (MCOs) and health care facilities can negotiate for physician services. The types and styles of these organizations vary widely and are discussed later. The point here is simple. If anesthesiologists are not involved and not perceived as interested, dedicated "team players," they will be shut out of critical negotiations and decisions. Although one obvious instance in which others will make decisions for anesthesiologists is the distribution of capitated or bundled practice fee income collected by a central "umbrella" organization, there are many such situations, and the anesthesiologists will have to comply with the resulting mandates. In the most basic terms, absence from the bargaining table and/or being seen as uninvolved in the welfare of the large group virtually ensure that anesthesiologists will not participate in key decisions or receive their "fair share of the pie."

Similarly, involvement with a facility, a medical staff, or a multispecialty group goes beyond formal organized governance and committee activity. Collegial relationships with physicians of other specialties and with administrators are central to maintenance of a recognized position and avoidance of the situation of exclusion described above. Being readily available for formal and informal consults, particularly regarding preoperative patient workup and the maximally efficient way to get surgeons' patients to the OR in a timely, expedient manner, is extremely important. No one individual can be everywhere all the time, but an anesthesiology group or department should strive to be always responsive to any request for help from physicians or administrators. It often appears that anesthesiologists fail to appreciate just how great a positive impact a relatively simple involvement (starting an intravenous line for a pediatrician, helping an internist manage an ICU ventilator, or helping a facility administrator unclog a jammed recovery room) may have. Unfortunately, anesthesiologists in a great many locations have a negative stereotype built up over years to overcome and must work hard to maintain the perception that they deserve an equal voice regarding the impact of the current changes in the health care system.

Establishing Standards of Practice and Understanding the Standard of Care

Given all the current and future changes in the anesthesiology practice environment, it is more important than ever that anesthesiologists genuinely understand what is expected of them in their clinical practice. The increasing frequency and intensity of "production pressure,"[7] with the tacit (or even explicit) directive to anesthesia personnel to "go fast" no matter what and to "do more with less," creates situations in which anesthesiologists may conclude that they must cut corners and compromise maximally safe care just to stay in business. This type of pressure has become even greater with the implementation of more and more protocols or parameters for practice, some from professional societies such as the ASA and some mandated by or developed in conjunction with purchasers of health care (government, insurance companies, or MCOs). Many of these protocols are devised to fast-track patients through the medical care system, especially when an elective procedure is involved, in as absolutely little time as possible, thus minimizing costs. Do these fast-track protocols constitute standards of care that health care providers are mandated to implement? What are the implications of doing so? Of not doing so?

To better understand answers to such questions, it is important to have a basic background in the concept of the *standard of care*. Anesthesiology personnel are fortunate in this regard because for nearly 20 years American anesthesiology has been recognized as one of the significant leaders in establishing practice standards intended to maximize the quality of patient care and help guide personnel at times of difficult decisions, including the risk–benefit and cost–benefit decisions of specific practices. Another important component of this issue is the unique legal system in the United States, in which the potential liability implications of most decisions must be considered. Businesses, groups, and individuals have had their entire public existences destroyed by staggering legal settlements and judgments allowed by the U.S. legal system. Major attempts at reform of this system have occurred and will continue to occur. However, although a very positive restructuring of the tort liability system could alleviate some of the catecholamine-generating "sword over the head" mentality exhibited by some physicians, it will not relieve anesthesiology personnel of the responsibility to provide maximally safe care for their patients. Integration of systems and protocols to help maximize the quality of patient care, whether from formal standards or not, is an important component of managing an anesthesiology practice.

The standard of care is the conduct and skill of a prudent practitioner that can be expected by a reasonable patient. This is a very important medicolegal concept because a bad medical result due to a failure to meet the standard of care is malpractice. Extensive discussions have attempted to establish exactly the applicable standard of care. Courts have traditionally relied on medical experts knowledgeable about the point in question to give opinions as to what is the standard of care and if it has been met in an individual case. This type of standard is somewhat different from the standards promulgated by various standard-setting bodies regarding, for example, the color of gas hoses connected to an anesthesia machine or the inability to open two vaporizers on that machine simultaneously. However, ignoring the equipment standards and tolerating an unsafe situation is a violation of the standard of care. Promulgated standards, such as the various safety codes and anesthesia machine specifications, rapidly become the standard of care because patients (through their attorneys, in the case of an untoward event) expect the published standards to be observed by the prudent practitioner.

Understanding the concept of the standard of care is the key to integrating the numerous standards, guidelines, statements, practice parameters, and suggested protocols applicable to American anesthesiology practice in the unfortunately necessary constant undercurrent of concern about potential legal liability. Ultimately, the standard of care is what a jury says it is. However, it is possible to anticipate, at least in part, what knowledge and actions will be expected. There are two main sources of information as to exactly what is the expected standard of care. Traditionally, the beliefs offered by expert witnesses in medical liability lawsuits regarding what was being done in real life (de facto standards of care) were the main input juries had in deciding what was reasonable to expect from the defendant. The resulting problem is well known: except in the most egregious cases, it is usually possible for the lawyers to find experts who will support each of the two opposing sides, making the process more subjective than objective. (Because of this, there is the ASA *Guidelines for Expert Witness Qualifications and Testimony*.) Of course, there can be legitimate differences of opinion among thoughtful, insightful experts, but even in these cases the jury still must decide who is more believable, looks better, or sounds better. The second, much more objective, source for defining certain component parts of the standard of care has developed since the mid 1980s in American anesthesiology. It is the published standards of care, guidelines, practice parameters, and protocols now becoming more common. These serve as hard evidence of what can be reasonably expected of practitioners and can make it easier for a jury evaluating whether a malpractice defendant failed to meet the applicable standard of care. Several types of documents exist and have differing implications.

Leading the Way

Anesthesiology may be the medical specialty most involved with published standards of care. It has been suggested that the nature of anesthesia practice (having certain central critical
5 functions relatively clearly defined and common to all situations and having an emphasis on technology) makes it the most amenable of all the fields of medicine to the use of published standards. The original intraoperative monitoring standards[8] are a classic example. The ASA first adopted its own set of basic intraoperative monitoring standards in 1986 and has modified them several times (Table 2-1).

This document includes clear specifications for the presence of personnel during an anesthetic episode and for continual evaluation of oxygenation, ventilation, circulation, and temperature. The rationale for these monitoring standards is simple; it was felt that functionally mandating certain behaviors oriented toward providing the earliest, maximum possible warning of threatening developments during an anesthetic should help minimize intraoperative catastrophic patient injury. These ASA monitoring standards very quickly became part of the accepted standard of care in anesthesia practice. This means they are important to practice management because they have profound medicolegal implications: a catastrophic accident occurring while the standards are being actively ignored is very difficult to defend in the consequent malpractice suit, whereas an accident that occurs during well-documented full compliance with the standards will automatically have a strong defense because the standard of care was being met. Several states in the United States have made compliance with these ASA standards mandatory under state regulations or even statutes. Various malpractice insurance companies offer discounts on malpractice insurance policy premiums for compliance with these standards, something quite natural to insurers because they are familiar with the idea of managing known risks to help minimize financial loss to the company. The ASA monitoring standards have been widely emulated in other medical specialties and even in fields outside of medicine. Although there are definite parallels in these other efforts (such as in obstetrics and gynecology), no other group has pursued the same degree of definition.

Many of the same management questions that led to the intraoperative monitoring standards have close parallels in the immediate preoperative and postoperative periods in the PACU. With many of the same elements of thinking, the ASA adopted Basic Standards for Preanesthesia Care (Table 2-2). This was supplemented significantly by another type of document, the ASA Practice Advisory for Preanesthesia Evaluation (www.asahq.org, "Publications and Services, Practice Parameters"), a 40-page meta-analysis of clinical aspects of preoperative evaluation. Also, the ASA adopted Standards for Postanesthesia Care (Table 2-3) in which there was consideration of and collaboration with the very detailed standards of practice for PACU care published by the American Society of Post Anesthesia Nurses (another good example of the sources of standards of care). This also was later supplemented by an extensive Practice Guideline.[9]

A slightly different situation exists with regard to the standards for conduct of anesthesia in obstetrics. These standards were originally passed by the ASA in 1988, in the same manner as the other ASA standards, but the ASA membership eventually questioned whether they reflected a realistic and desirable standard of care. Accordingly, the obstetric anesthesia standards were downgraded in 1990 to guidelines (Table 2-4), specifically to remove the mandatory nature of the document. Because there was no agreement as to what should be prescribed as the standard of care, the medicolegal imperative of published standards has been temporarily set aside. From a management perspective, this makes the guidelines no less valuable, because the intent of optimizing care through the avoidance of complications is no less operative. However, in the event of the need to defend against a malpractice claim in this area, it is clear from this sequence of events that the exact standard of care is debatable and not yet finally established. A different ASA document, *Practice Guidelines for Obstetrical Anesthesia*, with more detail and specificity as well as an emphasis on the meta-analytic approach has been generated.[10]

Practice Guidelines

The newest type of related ASA document is the Practice Guideline (formerly "Practice Parameter"). This has some of the same elements as a standard of practice but is more intended to guide judgment, largely through algorithms with some element of guidelines, in addition to directing the details of specific procedures as would a formal standard. A good example of a set

TABLE 2-1

AMERICAN SOCIETY OF ANESTHESIOLOGISTS STANDARDS FOR BASIC ANESTHETIC MONITORING

These Standards apply to all anesthesia care, although, in emergency circumstances, appropriate life-support measures take precedence. These standards may be exceeded at any time based on the judgment of the responsible anesthesiologist. They are intended to encourage quality patient care, but observing them cannot guarantee any specific patient outcome. They are subject to revision from time to time, as warranted by the evolution of technology and practice. They apply to all general anesthetics, regional anesthetics, and monitored anesthesia care. This set of standards addresses only the issue of basic anesthetic monitoring, which is one component of anesthesia care. In certain rare or unusual circumstances, (1) some of these methods of monitoring may be clinically impractical, and (2) appropriate use of the described monitoring methods may fail to detect untoward clinical developments. Brief interruptions of continual[a] monitoring may be unavoidable. Under extenuating circumstances, the responsible anesthesiologist may waive the requirements marked with an asterisk (*); it is recommended that when this is done, it should be so stated (including the reasons) in a note in the patient's medical record. These standards are not intended for application to the care of the obstetrical patient in labor or in the conduct of pain management.

■ STANDARD I

Qualified anesthesia personnel shall be present in the room throughout the conduct of all general anesthetics, regional anesthetics, and monitored anesthesia care.

Objective

Because of the rapid changes in patient status during anesthesia, qualified anesthesia personnel shall be continuously present to monitor the patient and provide anesthesia care. In the event there is a direct known hazard, for example, radiation, to the anesthesia personnel that might require intermittent remote observation of the patient, some provision for monitoring the patient must be made. In the event that an emergency requires the temporary absence of the person primarily responsible for the anesthetic, the best judgment of the anesthesiologist will be exercised in comparing the emergency with the anesthetized patient's condition and in the selection of the person left responsible for the anesthetic during the temporary absence.

■ STANDARD II

During all anesthetics, the patient's oxygenation, ventilation, circulation, and temperature shall be continually evaluated.

■ OXYGENATION

Objective

To ensure adequate oxygen concentration in the inspired gas and the blood during all anesthetics.

Methods

1. Inspired gas: During every administration of general anesthesia using an anesthesia machine, the concentration of oxygen in the patient breathing system shall be measured by an oxygen analyzer with a low oxygen concentration limit alarm in use.*
2. Blood oxygenation: During all anesthetics, a quantitative method of assessing oxygenation such as pulse oximetry shall be employed.* Adequate illumination and exposure of the patient are necessary to assess color.*

■ VENTILATION

Objective

To ensure adequate ventilation of the patient during all anesthetics.

Methods

1. Every patient receiving general anesthesia shall have the adequacy of ventilation continually evaluated. Qualitative clinical signs such as chest excursion, observation of the reservoir breathing bag, and auscultation of breath sounds are useful. Continual monitoring for the presence of expired carbon dioxide shall be performed unless invalidated by the nature of the patient, procedure, or equipment. Quantitative monitoring of the volume of expired gas is strongly encouraged.*
2. When an endotracheal tube or laryngeal mask is inserted, its correct positioning must be verified by clinical assessment and by identification of carbon dioxide in the expired gas. Continual end-tidal carbon dioxide analysis, in use from the time of endotracheal tube/laryngeal mask placement, until extubation/removal or initiating transfer to a postoperative care location, shall be performed using a quantitative method such as capnography, capnometry, or mass spectroscopy.*
3. When ventilation is controlled by a mechanical ventilator, there shall be in continuous use a device that is capable of detecting disconnection of components of the breathing system. The device must give an audible signal when its alarm threshold is exceeded.
4. During regional anesthesia and monitored anesthesia care, the adequacy of ventilation shall be evaluated, at least, by continual observation of qualitative clinical signs.

■ CIRCULATION

Objective

To ensure the adequacy of the patient's circulatory function during all anesthetics.

Methods

1. Every patient receiving anesthesia shall have the electrocardiogram continuously displayed from the beginning of anesthesia until preparing to leave the anesthetizing location.*
2. Every patient receiving anesthesia shall have arterial blood pressure and heart rate determined and evaluated at least every 5 minutes.*
3. Every patient receiving general anesthesia shall have, in addition to the above, circulatory function continually evaluated by at least one of the following: palpation of a pulse, auscultation of heart sounds, monitoring of a tracing of intra-arterial pressure, ultrasound peripheral pulse monitoring, or pulse plethysmography or oximetry.

■ BODY TEMPERATURE

Objective

To aid in the maintenance of appropriate body temperature during all anesthetics.

Methods

Every patient receiving anesthesia shall have temperature monitored when clinically significant changes in body temperature are intended, anticipated, or suspected.

[a]Note that *continual* is defined as "repeated regularly and frequently in steady rapid succession," whereas *continuous* means "prolonged without any interruption at any time."

Approved by House of Delegates on October 21, 1986, and last affirmed on October 15, 2003.

of practice parameters came some years ago from the cardiologists and addressed the indications for cardiac catheterization. Beyond the details of the minimum standards for carrying out the procedure, these practice parameters set forth algorithms and guidelines for helping to determine under what circumstances and with what timing to perform it. Understandably, purchasers of health care (government, insurance companies, and MCOs) with a strong desire to limit the costs of medical care have great interest in practice parameters as potential vehicles for helping to eliminate "unnecessary" procedures and limit even the necessary ones.

The ASA has been very active in creating and publishing practice guidelines. The first published parameter (since revised) concerned the use of pulmonary artery (PA) catheters.[11] It considered the clinical effectiveness of PA catheters, public policy issues (costs and concerns of patients and providers), and recommendations (indications and practice settings). The next month, the ASA Difficult Airway Algorithm was published (also since revised).[12] This thoughtful document synthesized a strategy summarized in a decision tree diagram for dealing acutely with airway problems. It has great clinical value, and it is reasonable to anticipate that it will be used to help many patients. However, all these documents are readily noticed by plaintiffs' lawyers, the difficult airway parameter from the ASA being an excellent example. An important and so-far undecided question is whether guidelines and practice parameters from recognized entities such as the ASA *define* the standard of care. There is no simple answer. This will be decided over time by practitioners' actions, debates in the literature, mandates from malpractice insurers, and, of course, court decisions. Some guidelines, such as the FDA preanesthetic apparatus checkout, are accepted as the standard of care. There will be debate among experts, but the practitioner must make the decision as to how to apply practice parameters such as those from the ASA. Practitioners have incorrectly assumed that they *must* do everything specified. This is clearly not true, yet there is a valid concern that these will someday be held up as defining the standard of care. Accordingly, prudent attention within the bounds of reason to the principles outlined in guidelines and parameters will put the practitioner in at least a reasonably defensible position, whereas radical deviation from them should be based on obvious exigencies of the situation at that moment or clear, defensible alternative beliefs (with documentation).

The ASA has many other task forces charged with the development of practice parameters. Several aspects of pain management, transesophageal echocardiography, policies for sedation by nonanesthesia personnel, preoperative fasting, avoidance of peripheral neuropathies, and others have been published and will likely have at least the same impact as those noted above.

On the other hand, practice protocols, such as those for the fast-track management of coronary artery bypass graft patients, that are handed down by MCOs or health insurance companies are a different matter. Even though the desired implication is that practitioners must observe (or at least strongly consider) them, they do not have the same implications in defining the standard of care as the other documents. Practitioners must avoid getting trapped. It may well not be a valid legal defense to justify action or the lack of action because of a company protocol. Difficult as it may be to reconcile with the payer, the practitioner still is subject to the classic definitions of standard of care.

The other type of standards associated with medical care are those of the JCAHO, the best-known medical care quality regulatory agency. As noted earlier, these standards were for many years concerned largely with structure (e.g., gas tanks chained down) and process (e.g., documentation complete), but in recent years they have been expanded to include reviews of the outcome of care. JCAHO standards also focus on credentialing and privileges, verification that anesthesia services are of uniform quality throughout an institution, the qualifications of the director of the service, continuing education, and basic guidelines for anesthesia care (need for preoperative and postoperative evaluations, documentation, and so forth). Full JCAHO accreditation of a health care facility is usually for 3 years. Even the best hospitals and facilities receive some citations of problems or deficiencies that are expected to be corrected, and an interim report of efforts to do so is required. If there are enough problems, accreditation can be conditional for 1 year, with a complete reinspection at that time. Preparing for JCAHO inspections starts with verification that essential group/department structure is in place; excellent examples exist.[3] The process ultimately involves a great deal of work, but because the standards usually do promote high-quality care, the majority of this work is highly constructive and of benefit to the institution and its medical staff.

TABLE 2-2

AMERICAN SOCIETY OF ANESTHESIOLOGISTS BASIC STANDARDS FOR PREANESTHESIA CARE

These Standards apply to all patients who receive anesthesia or monitored anesthesia care. Under unusual circumstances, for example, extreme emergencies, these standards may be modified. When this is the case, the circumstances shall be documented in the patient's record.

Standard I: An anesthesiologist shall be responsible for determining the medical status of the patient, developing a plan of anesthesia care, and acquainting the patient or the responsible adult with the proposed plan.

The development of an appropriate plan of anesthesia care is based upon:

1. Reviewing the medical record.
2. Interviewing and examining the patient to:
   a. Discuss the medical history, previous anesthetic experiences, and drug therapy.
   b. Assess those aspects of the physical condition that might affect decisions regarding perioperative risk and management.
3. Obtaining and/or reviewing tests and consultations necessary to the conduct of anesthesia.
4. Determining the appropriate prescription of preoperative medications as necessary to the conduct of anesthesia.

The responsible anesthesiologist shall verify that the above has been properly performed and documented in the patient's record.

Approved by House of Delegates on October 14, 1987, and affirmed on October 18, 1998.
Reprinted with permission of the American Society of Anesthesiologists, Park Ridge, Illinois 60068-5586.

Review Implications

Another type of regulatory agency is the peer review organization. Professional standards review organizations (PSROs) were established in 1972 as utilization review/QA overseers of the care of federally subsidized patients (Medicare and Medicaid). Despite their efforts to deal with quality of care, these groups were seen by all involved as primarily interested in cost containment. Various negative factors led to the PSROs' being replaced in 1984 with the peer review organization (PRO).[13] There is a PRO in each state, many being associated with a state medical association. The objectives of a PRO include 14 goals related to hospital admissions (e.g., to shift care to an outpatient basis as much as possible) and 5 related to quality

TABLE 2-3

AMERICAN SOCIETY OF ANESTHESIOLOGISTS STANDARDS FOR POSTANESTHESIA CARE

These Standards apply to postanesthesia care in all locations. These Standards may be exceeded based on the judgment of the responsible anesthesiologist. They are intended to encourage quality patient care, but cannot guarantee any specific patient outcome. They are subject to revision from time to time as warranted by the evolution of technology and practice. Under extenuating circumstances, the responsible anesthesiologist may waive the requirements marked with an asterisk (*); it is recommended that when this is done, it should be so stated (including the reasons) in a note in the patient's medical record.

STANDARD I

All patients who have received general anesthesia, regional anesthesia, or monitored anesthesia care shall receive appropriate postanesthesia management.[a]

1. A Postanesthesia Care Unit (PACU) or an area that provides equivalent postanesthesia care shall be available to receive patients after anesthesia care. All patients who receive anesthesia care shall be admitted to the PACU or its equivalent except by specific order of the anesthesiologist responsible for the patient's care.
2. The medical aspects of care in the PACU shall be governed by policies and procedures that have been reviewed and approved by the Department of Anesthesiology.
3. The design, equipment, and staffing of the PACU shall meet requirements of the facility's accrediting and licensing bodies.

STANDARD II

A patient transported to the PACU shall be accompanied by a member of the anesthesia care team who is knowledgeable about the patient's condition. The patient shall be continually evaluated and treated during transport with monitoring and support appropriate to the patient's condition.

STANDARD III

Upon arrival in the PACU, the patient shall be reevaluated and a verbal report provided to the responsible PACU nurse by the member of the anesthesia care team who accompanies the patient.

1. The patient's status on arrival in the PACU shall be documented.
2. Information concerning the preoperative condition and the surgical/anesthetic course shall be transmitted to the PACU nurse.
3. The member of the Anesthesia Care Team shall remain in the PACU until the PACU nurse accepts responsibility for the nursing care of the patient.

STANDARD IV

The patient's condition shall be evaluated continually in the PACU.

1. The patient shall be observed and monitored by methods appropriate to the patient's medical condition. Particular attention should be given to monitoring oxygenation, ventilation, circulation, and temperature. During recovery from all anesthetics, a quantitative method of assessing oxygenation such as pulse oximetry shall be employed in the initial phase of recovery.* This is not intended for application during the recovery of the obstetrical patient in whom regional anesthesia was used for labor and vaginal delivery.
2. An accurate written report of the PACU period shall be maintained. Use of an appropriate PACU scoring system is encouraged for each patient on admission, at appropriate intervals prior to discharge, and at the time of discharge.
3. General medical supervision and coordination of patient care in the PACU should be the responsibility of an anesthesiologist.
4. There shall be a policy to assure the availability in the facility of a physician capable of managing complications and providing cardiopulmonary resuscitation for patients in the PACU.

STANDARD V

A physician is responsible for the discharge of the patient from the PACU.

1. When discharge criteria are used, they must be approved by the Department of Anesthesiology and the medical staff. They may vary depending upon whether the patient is discharged to a hospital room, to the Intensive Care Unit, to a short stay unit, or home.
2. In the absence of the physician responsible for the discharge, the PACU nurse shall determine that the patient meets the discharge criteria. The name of the physician accepting responsibility for discharge shall be noted on the record.

[a]Refer to *Standards of Post Anesthesia Nursing Practice 1992*, published by American Society of Post Anesthesia Nurses (ASPAN), for issues of nursing care.
Approved by House of Delegates on October 12, 1988, and last amended on October 19, 1994.
Reprinted with permission of the American Society of Anesthesiologists, Park Ridge, Illinois 60068-5586.

of care (e.g., to reduce avoidable deaths and avoidable complications). The PROs comprise full-time support staff and physician reviewers paid as consultants or directors. Ideally, PRO monitoring will discover suboptimal care, and this will lead to specific recommendations for improvement in quality. There is a perception that quality of care efforts are hampered by the lack of realistic objectives and also that these PRO groups, like others before them, will largely or entirely function to limit the cost of health care services.

The practice management implications have become clear. Aside from the as-yet unrealized potential for quality improvement efforts and the occasional denial of payment for a procedure, the most likely interaction between the local PRO and anesthesiology personnel will involve a request for perioperative admission of a patient whose care is mandated to be outpatient surgery (this could also occur dealing with a managed care organization). If the anesthesiologist feels, for example, that either (1) preoperative admission for treatment to optimize cardiac, pulmonary, diabetic, or other medical status or (2) postoperative admission for monitoring of labile situations such as uncontrolled hypertension will reduce clear anesthetic risks for the patient, an application to the PRO for approval

TABLE 2-4

AMERICAN SOCIETY OF ANESTHESIOLOGISTS GUIDELINES FOR REGIONAL ANESTHESIA IN OBSTETRICS

These guidelines apply to the use of regional anesthesia or analgesia in which local anesthetics are administered to the parturient during labor and delivery. They are intended to encourage quality patient care but cannot guarantee any specific patient outcome. Because the availability of anesthesia resources may vary, members are responsible for interpreting and establishing the guidelines for their own institutions and practices. These guidelines are subject to revision from time to time as warranted by the evolution of technology and practice.

■ GUIDELINE I

Regional anesthesia should be initiated and maintained only in locations in which appropriate resuscitation equipment and drugs are immediately available to manage procedurally related problems.

Resuscitation equipment should include, but is not limited to: sources of oxygen and suction, equipment to maintain an airway and perform endotracheal intubation, a means to provide positive-pressure ventilation, and drugs and equipment for cardiopulmonary resuscitation.

■ GUIDELINE II

Regional anesthesia should be initiated by a physician with appropriate privileges and maintained by or under the medical direction[a] of such an individual.

Physicians should be approved through the institutional credentialing process to initiate and direct the maintenance of obstetric anesthesia and to manage procedurally related complications.

■ GUIDELINE III

Regional anesthesia should not be administered until: (1) the patient has been examined by a qualified individual[b] and (2) a physician with obstetrical privileges to perform operative vaginal or cesarean delivery, who has knowledge of the maternal and fetal status and the progress of labor and who approves the initiation of labor anesthesia, is readily available to supervise the labor and manage any obstetric complications that may arise.

Under circumstances defined by department protocol, qualified personnel may perform the initial pelvic examination. The physician responsible for the patient's obstetrical care should be informed of her status so that a decision can be made regarding present risk and further management.[b]

■ GUIDELINE IV

An intravenous infusion should be established before the initiation of regional anesthesia and maintained throughout the duration of the regional anesthetic.

■ GUIDELINE V

Regional anesthesia for labor and/or vaginal delivery requires that the parturient's vital signs and the fetal heart rate be monitored and documented by a qualified individual. Additional monitoring appropriate to the clinical condition of the parturient and the fetus should be employed when indicated. When extensive regional blockade is administered for complicated vaginal delivery, the standards for basic anesthetic monitoring[c] should be applied.

■ GUIDELINE VI

Regional anesthesia for cesarean delivery requires that the standards for basic anesthetic monitoring[c] be applied and that a physician with privileges in obstetrics be immediately available.

■ GUIDELINE VII

Qualified personnel, other than the anesthesiologist attending the mother, should be immediately available to assume responsibility for resuscitation of the newborn.[b]

The primary responsibility of the anesthesiologist is to provide care to the mother. If the anesthesiologist is also requested to provide brief assistance in the care of the newborn, the benefit to the child must be compared to the risk to the mother.

■ GUIDELINE VIII

A physician with appropriate privileges should remain readily available during the regional anesthetic to manage anesthetic complications until the patient's postanesthesia condition is satisfactory and stable.

■ GUIDELINE IX

All patients recovering from regional anesthesia should receive appropriate postanesthesia care. Following cesarean delivery and/or extensive regional blockade, the standards for postanesthesia care[d] should be applied.

1. A postanesthesia care unit (PACU) should be available to receive patients. The design, equipment, and staffing should meet requirements of the facility's accrediting and licensing bodies.
2. When a site other than the PACU is used, equivalent postanesthesia care should be provided.

■ GUIDELINE X

There should be a policy to assure the availability in the facility of a physician to manage complications and to provide cardiopulmonary resuscitation for patients receiving postanesthesia care.

[a] The Anesthesia Care Team (approved by ASA House of Delegates October 6, 1982, and last amended October 17, 2001).
[b] Guidelines for Perinatal Care (American Academy of Pediatrics and American College of Obstetricians and Gynecologists, 1988).
[c] Standards for Basic Anesthetic Monitoring (approved by ASA House of Delegates October 21, 1986, and last amended October 21, 1998).
[d] Standards for Postanesthesia Care (approved by ASA House of Delegates October 12, 1988, and last amended October 19, 1994).
Approved by House of Delegates on October 12, 1988, and last amended on October 18, 2000.

of admission must be made and vigorously supported. All too often, however, such issues surface a day or so before the scheduled procedure in a preanesthesia screening clinic or even in a preoperative holding area outside the OR on the day of surgery. This will continue to occur until anesthesia providers educate their constituent surgeon community as to what types of associated medical conditions may disqualify a proposed patient from the outpatient (ambulatory) surgical schedule. If adequate notice is given by the surgeon, such as at the time an elective case is booked for the OR, the patient can be seen far enough in advance by an anesthesiologist to allow appropriate planning.

In the circumstance in which the first knowledge of a questionable patient comes 1 or 2 days before surgery, the anesthesiologist can try to have the procedure postponed, if possible, or can undertake the time-consuming task of multiple telephone calls to get the surgeon's agreement, get PRO approval, and make the necessary arrangements. Because neither alternative is particularly attractive, especially from administrative and reimbursement perspectives, there may be a strong temptation to "let it slide" and try to deal with the patient as an outpatient even though this may be questionable. In almost all cases, it is likely that there would be no adverse result (the "get away with it" phenomenon). However, the patient might well be exposed to an avoidable risk. Both because of the workings of probability and because of the inevitable tendency to let sicker and sicker patients slip by as lax practitioners repeatedly "get away with it" and are lulled into a false sense of security, sooner or later there will be an unfortunate outcome or some preventable major morbidity or even mortality.

The situation is worsened when the first contact with a questionable ambulatory patient is preoperatively (possibly even already in the OR) on the day of surgery. There may be intense pressure from the patient, the surgeon, or the OR administrator and staff to proceed with a case for which the anesthesia practitioner believes the patient is poorly prepared. The arguments made regarding patient inconvenience and anxiety are valid. However, they should not outweigh the best medical interests of the patient. Although this is a point in favor of screening all outpatients before the day of surgery, the anesthesiologist facing this situation on the day of operation should state clearly to all concerned the reasons for postponing the surgery, stressing the issue of avoidable risk and standards of care, and then help with alternative arrangements (including, if necessary, dealing with the PRO or MCO).

Potential liability exposure is the other side of the standard of care issue. Particularly regarding questions of postoperative admission of ambulatory patients who have been unstable in some worrisome manner, it is an extremely poor defense against a malpractice claim to state that the patient was discharged home, only later to suffer a complication because the PRO/MCO deemed that operative procedure outpatient and not inpatient surgery. As bureaucratically annoying as it may be, it is a prudent management strategy to admit the patient if there is any legitimate question, thus minimizing the chance for complications, and later haggle with the PRO or directly with the involved third-party payer (MCO).

Policy and Procedure

Management of an anesthesiology practice involves business, organizational, and clinical issues. One important organizational point that is often overlooked is the need for a complete policy and procedure manual. Such a compilation of documents is necessary for all practices, from the largest departments covering multiple hospitals to a single-room outpatient facility with one anesthesia provider. Contemplation of this compilation of documents may evoke a collective groan from anesthesiology personnel, and maintaining this manual may be misperceived as a bureaucratic chore. Quite the contrary, such a manual can be extraordinarily valuable, as, for example, when it provides crucial information during an emergency. Some suggestions for the content of this compendium exist,[14] but, at minimum, organizational and procedural elements must be included.

The organizational elements that should be present include a chart of organization and responsibilities that is not just a call schedule but a clear explanation of who is responsible for what functions of the department and when, with attendant details such as expectations for the practitioner's presence within the institution at designated hours, telephone availability, pager availability, the maximum permissible distance from the institution, and so forth. Experience suggests it is especially important for there to be an absolutely clear specification of the availability of qualified anesthesiology personnel for emergency cesarean section, particularly in practice arrangements in which there are several people on call covering multiple locations. Sadly, these issues often are only considered after a disaster has occurred that involved miscommunication and the mistaken belief by one or more people that someone else would take care of an acute problem.

The organizational component of the policy and procedure manual should also include a clear explanation of the orientation and checkout procedure for new personnel, continuing medical education requirements and opportunities, the mechanisms for evaluating personnel and for communicating this evaluation to them, disaster plans (or reference to a separate disaster manual or protocol), QA activities of the department, and the format for statistical record keeping (number of procedures, types of anesthetics given, types of patients anesthetized, number and types of invasive monitoring procedures, number and type of responses to emergency calls, complications, or whatever the group/department decides).

The procedural component of the policy and procedure manual should give both handy practice tips and specific outlines of proposed courses of action for particular circumstances; it also should store little-used but valuable information. Reference should be made to the statements, guidelines, practice parameters, and standards appearing on the ASA website. Also included should be references to or specific protocols for the areas mentioned in the JCAHO standards: preanesthetic evaluation, immediate preinduction reevaluation, safety of the patient during the anesthetic period, release of the patient from any PACU, recording of all pertinent events during anesthesia, recording of postanesthesia visits, guidelines defining the role of anesthesia services in hospital infection control, and guidelines for safe use of general anesthetic agents. Other appropriate topics include the following:

1. Recommendations for preanesthesia apparatus checkout, such as from the U.S. Food and Drug Administration (FDA)[15] (see Chapter 21)
2. Guidelines for minimal monitoring and duration of stay of an infant, child, or adult in the PACU
3. Procedures for transporting patients to/from the OR, PACU, or ICU
4. Policy on ambulatory surgical patients—for example, screening, use of regional anesthesia, discharge home criteria
5. Policy on evaluation and processing of same-day admissions
6. Policy on recovery room admission and discharge
7. Policy on ICU admission and discharge
8. Policy on physicians responsible for writing orders in recovery room and ICU
9. Policy on informed consent and its documentation
10. Policy on the use of patients in clinical research

11. Guidelines for the support of cadaver organ donors and its termination
12. Guidelines on environmental safety, including pollution with trace gases and electrical equipment inspection, maintenance, and hazard prevention
13. Procedure for change of personnel during an anesthetic
14. Procedure for the introduction of new equipment, drugs, or clinical practices
15. Procedure for epidural and spinal narcotic administration and subsequent patient monitoring (e.g., type, minimum time, nursing units)
16. Procedure for initial treatment of cardiac or respiratory arrest
17. Policy for handling patient's refusal of blood or blood products, including the mechanism to obtain a court order to transfuse
18. Procedure for the management of malignant hyperthermia
19. Procedure for the induction and maintenance of barbiturate coma
20. Procedure for the evaluation of suspected pseudocholinesterase deficiency
21. Protocol for responding to an adverse anesthetic event
22. Policy on resuscitation of DNR patients in the OR.

Individual departments will add to the suggestions listed here as dictated by their specific needs. A thorough, carefully conceived policy and procedure manual is a valuable tool. The manual should be reviewed and updated as needed but at least annually, with a particularly thorough review preceding each JCAHO inspection. Each member of a group or department should review the manual at least annually and sign off in a log indicating familiarity with current policies and procedures.

Meetings and Case Discussion

There must be regularly scheduled departmental or group meetings. Although didactic lectures and continuing education meetings are valuable and necessary, there also must be regular opportunities for open clinical discussion about interesting cases and problem cases. Also, the JCAHO requires that there be at least monthly meetings at which risk management and QA activities are documented and reported. Whether these meetings are called case conferences, morbidity and mortality conferences, or deaths and complications, the entire department or group should gather for an interchange of ideas. More recently these gatherings have been called QA meetings. An open review of departmental statistics should be done, including all complications, even those that may appear trivial. Unusual patterns of small events may point toward a larger or systematic problem, especially if they are more frequently associated with one individual practitioner.

A problem case presented at the departmental meeting might be an overt accident, a near accident (critical incident), or an untoward outcome of unknown origin. Honest but constructive discussion, even of an anesthesiologist's technical deficiencies or lack of knowledge, should take place in the spirit of constructive peer review. The classic question "What would you do differently next time?" is a good way to start the discussion. There may be situations in which inviting the surgeon or the internist involved in a specific case would be advantageous. The opportunity for each type of provider to hear the perspective of another discipline not only is inherently educational, but also can promote communication and cooperation in future potential problem cases.

Records of these meetings must be kept for accreditation purposes, but the enshrining of overly detailed minutes (potentially subject to discovery by a plaintiff's attorney at a later date) may inhibit true educational and corrective interchanges about untoward events. In the circumstance of discussion of a case that seems likely to provoke litigation, it is appropriate to be certain that the meeting is classified as official "peer review" and possibly even invite the hospital attorney or legal counsel from the relevant malpractice insurance carrier (to guarantee the privacy of the discussion and minutes).

Support Staff

There is a fundamental need for support staff in every anesthesia practice. Even independent practitioners rely in some measure on facilities, equipment, and services provided by the organization maintaining the anesthetizing location. In large, well-organized departments, reliance on support staff is often very great. The need for adequate staff and the inadvisability of scrimping on critical support personnel to cut costs is obvious. What is often overlooked, however, is a process analogous to that of credentialing and privileges for anesthesiologists, although at a slightly different level. The people expected to provide clinical anesthesia practice support must be qualified and must at all times understand what they are expected to do and how to do it. It is singularly unfortunate to realize only after an anesthesia catastrophe has occurred that basic details of simple work assignments, such as the changing of carbon dioxide absorbent, were routinely ignored. This indicates the need for supervision and monitoring of the support staff by the involved practitioners. Further, such support personnel are favorite targets of cost-cutting administrators who do not understand the function of anesthesia technicians or their equivalent. In the modern era, many administrators seem driven almost exclusively by the "bottom line" and cannot appreciate the connection between valuable workers such as these and the "revenue stream." Even though it is obvious to all who work in an OR that the anesthesia support personnel make it possible for there to be patients flowing through the OR, it is their responsibility to convince the facility's fiscal administrator that elimination of such positions is genuinely false economy because of the attendant loss in efficiency, particularly in turning over the room between surgeries. Further, it is also false economy to reduce the number of personnel below that are genuinely needed to retrieve, clean, sort, disassemble, sterilize, reassemble, store, and distribute the tools of daily anesthesia practice. Inadequate attention to all these steps truly creates the environment of "an accident waiting to happen." When there is threatened loss of budget funding from a health care facility for the salaries of needed anesthesia support personnel, the practitioners involved must not simply stand by and see the necessary functions thrown into a "hit-or-miss" status by a few remaining heavily overburdened workers. Vigorous defense (or initiation of and agitation for new positions if the staff is inadequate) by the anesthesia practitioners should be undertaken, always with the realization that it may be necessary in some circumstances for them to supplement the budget from the facility with some of their practice income to guarantee an adequate complement of competent workers.

Business and organizational issues in the management of an anesthesia practice are also critically dependent on the existence of a sufficient number of appropriately trained support staff. One frequently overlooked issue that contributes to the negative impression generated by some anesthesiology practices centers on being certain there is someone available to answer the telephone at all times during the hours surgeons, other physicians, and OR scheduling desks are likely to telephone. This seemingly trivial component of practice management is very important to the success of an anesthesiology practice as a business whose principal customers are the surgeons.

Certainly there is a commercial server–client relationship both with the patient and the purchaser of health care; however, the uniquely symbiotic nature of the relationship between surgeons and anesthesiologists is such that availability even for simple "just wanted to let you know" telephone calls is genuinely important. The person who answers the telephone is the representative of the practice to the world and must take that responsibility seriously. From a management standpoint, significant impact on the success of the practice as a business often hinges on such details. Further, anesthesiologists should always have permanent personal electronic pagers and reliable mobile telephones (or the radio equivalent) to facilitate communications from other members of the department or group and from support personnel. This may sound intrusive, but the unusual position of anesthesiologists in the spectrum of physicians mandates this feature of managing an anesthesiology practice. Anesthesiology personnel should have no hesitation about spending their own practice income to do so. The symbolism alone is obvious.

Anesthesia Equipment and Equipment Maintenance

Problems with anesthesia equipment have been discussed for some time.[16,17] However, compared to human error, overt equipment failure very rarely causes intraoperative critical incidents[18] or deaths resulting from anesthesia care.[19] Aside from the obvious human errors involving misuse of or unfamiliarity with the equipment, when the rare equipment failure does occur, it appears often that correct maintenance and servicing of the apparatus has not been done. These issues become the focus of anesthesia practice management efforts, which could have significant liability implications, because there can often be confusion or even disputes about precisely who is responsible for arranging maintenance of the anesthesia equipment—the facility or the practitioners who use it and collect practice income from that activity. In many cases, the facility assumes the responsibility. In situations in which that is not true, however, it is necessary for the practitioners to recognize that responsibility and seek help securing a service arrangement, because this is likely an unfamiliar obligation for clinicians.

Programs for anesthesia equipment maintenance and service have been outlined.[3,20] A distinction is made between failure as a result of progressive deterioration of equipment, which should be preventable because it is observable and should provoke appropriate remedial action, and catastrophic failure, which, realistically, often cannot be predicted. Preventive maintenance for mechanical parts is critical and involves periodic performance checks every 4 to 6 months. Also, an annual safety inspection of each anesthetizing location and the equipment itself is necessary. For equipment service, an excellent mechanism is a relatively elaborate cross-reference system (possibly kept handwritten in a notebook but ideal for maintenance on an electronic spreadsheet program) to identify both the device needing service and also the mechanism to secure the needed maintenance or repair.

Equipment handling principles are straightforward. Before purchase, it must be verified that a proposed piece of equipment meets all applicable standards, which will usually be true when dealing with recognized major manufacturers. (The recent renewed efforts of some facility administrators to save money by attempting to find "refurbished" anesthesia machines and monitoring systems should provoke thorough review by the involved practitioners of any proposed purchases of used equipment. Unlike refurbished computers, used anesthesia equipment has many moving mechanical parts that are subject to wear and eventual mechanical failure.) On arrival, electrical equipment must be checked for absence of hazard (especially leakage current) and compliance with applicable electrical standards. Complex equipment such as anesthesia machines and ventilators should be assembled and checked out by a representative from the manufacturer or manufacturer's agent. There are potential adverse medicolegal implications when relatively untrained personnel certify a particular piece of new equipment as functioning within specification, even if they do it perfectly. It is also very important to involve the manufacturer's representative in pre- and in-service training for those who will use the new equipment. On arrival, a sheet or section in the departmental master equipment log must be created with the make, model, serial number, and in-house identification for each piece of capital equipment. This not only allows immediate identification of any equipment involved in a future recall or product alert, but also serves as the permanent repository of the record of every problem, problem resolution, maintenance, and servicing occurring until that particular equipment is scrapped. This log must be kept up to date at all times. There have been rare but frightening examples of potentially lethal problems with anesthesia machines leading to product alert notices requiring immediate identification of certain equipment and its service status.

Service

Beyond the administrative liability implications, precisely what type of support personnel should maintain and service major anesthesia equipment has been widely debated. There are significant management implications. Equipment setup and checkout have been mentioned. After that, some groups or departments rely on factory service representatives from the equipment manufacturers for all attention to equipment, others engage independent service contractors, and still other (often larger) departments have access to personnel (either engineers and/or technicians) permanently within their facility. Needs and resources differ. The single underlying principle is clear: the person(s) doing preventive maintenance and service on anesthesia equipment must be qualified. Anesthesia practitioners may wonder how they can assess these qualifications. The best way is to unhesitatingly ask pertinent questions about the education, training, and experience of those involved, including asking for references and speaking to supervisors and managers responsible for those doing the work. Whether an engineering technician who spent a week at a course at a factory can perform the most complex repairs depends on a variety of factors, which can be investigated by the practitioners ultimately using the equipment in the care of patients. Failure to be involved in this oversight function exposes the practice to increased liability in the event of an untoward outcome associated with improperly maintained or serviced equipment.

Determining when anesthesia equipment becomes obsolete and should be replaced is another question that is difficult to answer. Replacement of obsolete anesthesia machines and monitoring equipment is a key element of a risk modification program. Ten years is often cited as an estimated useful life for an anesthesia machine, but although an ASA statement repeats that idea, it also notes that the ASA promulgated a Policy for Assessing Obsolescence in 1989 that does not subscribe to any specific time interval. Anesthesia machines considerably more than 15 years old likely do not meet certain of the safety standards now in force for new machines (such as vaporizer lockout, fresh gas ratio protection, and automatic enabling of the oxygen analyzer) and, unless extensively retrofitted, do not incorporate the new technology that advanced very rapidly during the 1980s, much of it directly related to the effort to prevent untoward incidents. Further, it appears that this technology will continue to advance, particularly because of the adoption of anesthesia workstation standards by the European

Economic Union that are affecting anesthesia machine design worldwide. Note that some anesthesia equipment manufacturers, anxious to minimize their own potential liability, have refused to support (with parts and service) some of the oldest of their pieces (particularly gas machines) still in use. This disowning of equipment by its own manufacturer is a very strong message to practitioners that such equipment must be replaced as soon as possible.

Should a piece of equipment fail, it must be removed from service and a replacement substituted. Groups, departments, and facilities are obligated to have sufficient backup equipment to cover any reasonable incidence of failure. The equipment removed from service must be clearly marked with a prominent label (so it is not returned into service by a well-meaning technician or practitioner) containing the date, time, person discovering, and the details of the problem. The responsible personnel must be notified so they can remove the equipment, make an entry in the log, and initiate the repair. As indicated in the protocol for response to an adverse event, a piece of equipment involved or suspected in an anesthesia accident must be immediately sequestered and not touched by anybody—particularly not by any equipment service personnel. If a severe accident occurred, it may be necessary for the equipment in question to be inspected at a later time by a group consisting of qualified representatives of the manufacturer, the service personnel, the plaintiff's attorney, the insurance companies involved, and the practitioner's defense attorney. The equipment should thus be impounded following an adverse event and treated similarly to any object in a forensic "chain of evidence," with careful documentation of parties in contact with and responsible for securing the equipment in question following such an event. Also, major equipment problems may, in some circumstances, reflect a pattern of failure as a result of a design or manufacturing fault. These problems should be reported to the FDA's Medical Device Problem Reporting system[21] via MedWatch on Form 3500 (at www.fda.gov/medwatch/index.html, or telephone 800-FDA-1088). This system accepts voluntary reports from users and requires reports from manufacturers when there is knowledge of a medical device being involved in a serious incident. Whether or not filing such a report will have a positive impact in subsequent litigation is impossible to know, but it is a worthwhile practice management point that needs to be considered in the unlikely but important instance of a relevant event involving equipment failure.

Malpractice Insurance

All practitioners need liability insurance coverage specific for the specialty and role in which they are practicing. Premium rates depend on specialty, subspecialty, and whether the insured performs procedures that the insurance company's experience suggests may be more likely to result in a malpractice lawsuit. It is absolutely critical that applicants for medical liability insurance be completely honest in informing the insurer what duties and procedures they perform. Failure to do so, either from carelessness or from a foolishly misguided desire to reduce the resulting premium, may well result in retrospective denial of insurance coverage in the event of an untoward outcome from an activity the insurer did not know the insured engaged in.

Proof of adequate insurance coverage is usually required to secure or renew privileges to practice at a health care facility. The facility may specify certain minimum policy limits in an attempt to limit its own liability exposure. It is difficult to suggest specific dollar amounts for policy limits because the details of practice vary so much among situations and locations. The malpractice crisis of the 1980s eased significantly in the early 1990s for anesthesiologists, largely because of the decrease in number and severity of malpractice claims resulting from anesthesia catastrophes as anesthesia care in the United States became safer.[22–24] The exact analysis of this phenomenon can be debated,[25,26] but it is a simple fact that malpractice insurance risk ratings have been decreased and premiums for anesthesiologists have not been increased at the same rate as for other specialties over the past decade and, in many cases, have actually decreased. This does not mitigate the need for adequate coverage, however. In the early 2000s, coverage limits of $1 million to $3 million would seem the bare minimum advisable. This policy specification usually means that the insurer will cover up to $1 million liability per claim and up to $3 million total per year, but this terminology is not necessarily universal. Therefore, anesthesiology personnel must be absolutely certain what they are buying when they apply for malpractice insurance. In parts of the United States known for a pattern of exorbitant settlements and jury verdicts, liability coverage limits of $2 million to $5 million may be prudent and well worth the moderate additional cost. An additional feature in this regard is the potential to employ "umbrella" liability coverage above the limits of the base policy, as noted later.

Background

The fundamental mechanism of medical malpractice insurance changed significantly in the last two decades because of the need for insurance companies to have better ways to predict what their losses (amounts paid in settlements and judgments) might be. Traditionally, medical liability insurance was sold on an "occurrence" basis, meaning that if the insurance policy was in force at the time of the occurrence of an incident resulting in a claim, whenever that claim might be filed, the practitioner would be covered. Occurrence insurance was somewhat more expensive than the alternative "claims made" policies, but was seen as worth it by some (many) practitioners. These policies created some open-ended exposure for the insurer that sometimes led to unexpected large losses, even some large enough to threaten the existence of the insurance company. As a result, medical malpractice insurers have converted almost exclusively to claims-made insurance, which covers claims that are filed while the insurance is in force. Premium rates for the first year a physician is in practice are relatively low because there is less likelihood of a claim coming in (a majority of malpractice suits are filed 1 to 3 years after the event in question). The premiums usually increase yearly for the first 5 years and then the policy is considered "mature." The issue comes when the physician later, for whatever reason, must change insurance companies (e.g., because of relocation to another state). If the physician simply discontinues the policy and a claim is filed the next year, there will be no insurance coverage. Therefore, the physician must secure "tail coverage," sometimes for a minimum number of years (e.g., 5) or sometimes indefinitely to guarantee liability insurance protection for claims filed after the physician is no longer primarily covered by the insurance policy. It may be possible in some circumstances to purchase tail coverage from a different insurer than was involved with the primary policy, but by far the most common thing done is to simply extend the existing insurance coverage for the period of the tail. This very often yields a bill for the entire tail coverage premium, which can be quite sizable, potentially staggering a physician who simply wants to move to another state where his existing insurance company is not licensed to or refuses to do business. The issue of how to pay this premium is appropriately the subject of management attention and effort within the anesthesia practice. Individual situations will vary widely, but it is reasonable for anesthesiologists organized into a fiscal entity to consider this issue at the time of the inception of the group and record their policy decisions in writing, rather than facing the potentially difficult question of how to treat one individual later. Other strategies have occasionally been employed when insuring the tail period, including converting the previous policy to part-time status for a period of years, and purchasing "nose" coverage from the new insurer—that is, paying an initial higher yearly premium with the new insurer, who then will cover claims that may occur during the tail period. Whatever strategy is adopted, it is critical that the individual practitioner be absolutely certain through personal verification that he or she is thoroughly covered at the time of any transition. The potential stakes are much too great to leave such important issues solely to an office clerk. Further, a practitioner arriving in a new location is often filling a need or void and is urged to begin clinical work as soon as humanly possible by others who have been shouldering an increased load. It is essential that the new arrival verify with confirmation in writing (often called a "binder") that malpractice liability insurance coverage is in force before any patient contact.

Another component to the liability insurance situation is consideration of the advisability of purchasing yet another type of insurance called "umbrella coverage," which is activated at the time of the need to pay a claim that exceeds the limits of coverage on the standard malpractice liability insurance policy. Because such an enormous claim is extremely unlikely, many practitioners are tempted to forgo the comparatively modest cost of such insurance coverage in the name of economy. As before, it is easy to see that this is potentially a very false economy—if there is a huge claim. Practitioners should consult with their financial managers, but it is likely that it would be considered wise management to purchase "umbrella" liability insurance coverage.

Medical malpractice insurers are becoming increasingly active in trying to prevent incidents that will lead to insurance claims. They often sponsor risk-management seminars to teach practices and techniques to lessen the chances of liability claims and, in some cases, suggest (or even mandate) specific practices, such as strict documented compliance with the ASA Standards for Basic Anesthetic Monitoring. In return for attendance at such events and/or the signing of contracts stating that the practitioner will follow certain guidelines or standards, the insurer often gives a discount on the liability insurance premium. Clearly, it is sound practice management strategy for practitioners to participate maximally in such programs. Likewise, some insurers make coverage conditional on the consistent implementation of certain strategies such as minimal monitoring, even stipulating that the practitioner will not be covered if it is found that the guidelines were being consciously ignored at the time of an untoward event. Again, it is obviously wise from a practice management standpoint to cooperate fully with such stipulations.

Response to an Adverse Event

In spite of the decreased incidence of anesthesia catastrophes, even with the very best of practice, it is statistically likely that
6 each anesthesiologist at least once in his or her professional life will be involved in a major anesthesia accident. (See Chapter 5.) Precisely because such an event is rare, very few are prepared for it. It is probable that the involved personnel will have no relevant past experience regarding what to do. Although an obvious resource is another anesthetist who has had some exposure or experience, one of these may not be available either. Various authors have discussed what to do in that event.[27–29] Cooper et al. have thoughtfully presented the appropriate immediate response to an accident in a straightforward, logical, compact format[30] that should periodically be reviewed by all anesthesiology practitioners and should be included in all anesthesia policy and procedure manuals. This "adverse events protocol" is also always immediately available at www.apsf.org, "Resources: Clinical Safety." Unfortunately, however, the principal personnel involved in a significant untoward event may react with such surprise or shock as to temporarily lose sight of logic. At the moment of recognition that a major anesthetic complication has occurred or is occurring, help must be called. A sufficient number of people to deal with the situation must be assembled on site as quickly as possible. For example, in the unlikely but still possible event that an esophageal intubation goes unrecognized long enough to cause a cardiac arrest, the immediate need is for enough skilled personnel to conduct the resuscitative efforts, including making the correct diagnosis and replacing the tube into the trachea. Whether the anesthesiologist apparently responsible for the complication should direct the immediate remedial efforts will depend on the person and the situation. In such a circumstance, it would seem wise for a senior or supervising anesthesiologist quickly to evaluate the scenario and make a decision. This person becomes the "incident supervisor" and has responsibility for helping prevent continuation or recurrence of the incident, for investigating the incident, and for ensuring documentation while the original and helping anesthesiologists focus on caring for the patient. As noted, involved equipment must be sequestered and not touched until such time as it is certain that it was not involved in the incident.

If the accident is not fatal, continuing care of the patient is critical. Measures may be instituted to help limit damage from brain hypoxia. Consultants may be helpful and should be called without hesitation. If not already involved, the chief of anesthesiology must be notified as well as the facility administrator, risk manager, and the anesthesiologist's insurance company. These latter are critical to allow consideration of immediate efforts to limit later financial loss. (Likewise, there are often provisions in medical malpractice insurance policies that might limit or even deny insurance coverage if the company is not notified of any reportable event immediately.) If there is an involved surgeon of record, he or she probably will first notify the family, but the anesthesiologist and others (risk manager, insurance loss control officer, or even legal counsel) might appropriately be included at the outset. Full disclosure of facts as they are best known—with no confessions, opinions, speculation, or placing of blame—is currently still believed to be the best presentation. Any attempt to conceal or shade the truth will later only confound an already difficult situation. Obviously, comfort and support should be offered, including, if appropriate, the services of facility personnel such as clergy, social workers, and counselors. There is a new movement in medical risk management and insurance advocating immediate full disclosure to the victim or survivors, including "confessions" of medical judgment and performance errors with attendant sincere apologies. If indicated, early offers of reasonable compensation may be included. There have been instances when this overall strategy has prevented the filing of a malpractice lawsuit and has been applauded by all involved as an example of a shift from the "culture of blame" with punishment to a "just culture" with restitution. Laudable as this approach may sound, it would be mandatory for an individual practitioner to check with the involved liability insurance carrier, the practice group, and the facility administration before attempting it.

The primary anesthesia provider and any others involved must document relevant information. Never, ever change any existing entries in the medical record. Write an amendment note if needed with careful explanation of why amendment is necessary, particularly stressing explanations of professional judgments involved. State only facts as they are known. Make no judgments about causes or responsibility and do not "point fingers." The same guidelines hold true for the filing of the incident report in the facility, which should be done as soon as is practical. Further, all discussions with the patient or family should be carefully documented in the medical record. Recognizing that detailed memories of the events may fade in the 1 to

3 years before the practitioner may face deposition questions about exactly what happened, it is possible that it will be recommended, immediately after the incident, that the involved clinical personnel sit down as soon as practical and write out their own personal notes, which will include opinions and impressions as well as maximally detailed accounts of the events as they unfolded. These personal notes are not part of the medical record or the facility files. These notes should be written in the physical presence of an involved attorney representing the practitioner, even if this is not yet the specific defense attorney secured by the malpractice insurance company, and then that attorney should take possession of and keep those notes as case material. This strategy is intended to make the personal notes "attorney–client work product," and thus not subject to forced "discovery" (revelation) by other parties to the case.

Follow-up after the immediate handling of the incident will involve the primary anesthesiologist but should again be directed by a senior supervisor, who may or may not be the same person as the incident supervisor. The "follow-up supervisor" verifies the adequacy and coordination of ongoing care of the patient and facilitates communication among all involved, especially with the risk manager. Lastly, it is necessary to verify that adequate postevent documentation is taking place.

Of course, it is expected that such an adverse event will be discussed in the applicable morbidity and mortality meeting. This is good and appropriate. It is necessary, however, to coordinate this activity with the involved risk manager and attorney so as to be completely certain that the contents and conclusions of the discussion are clearly considered peer review activity, and thus are shielded from discovery by the plaintiffs' attorney.

Unpleasant as this is to contemplate, it is better to have a clear plan and execute it in the event of an accident causing injury to a patient. Vigorous immediate intervention may improve the outcome for all concerned.

PRACTICE ESSENTIALS

The "Job Market" for Anesthesiologists

While it is true that in the mid 1990s, for the first time, uncertainty faced residents finishing anesthesiology training because of a perception that there were not enough jobs available, that concept faded relatively quickly. Somewhat of a manageable balance between supply and demand developed, but with a significant ongoing component of the idea that there is an overall shortage of anesthesia providers. It is likely that this fundamental paradigm will persist in the next decade.

Factors governing the issues of supply of and demand for anesthesiologists are complex and evolving. Before about 1993, with the exception of a very few of the most popular cities, finishing residents could first decide where they wanted to live and then seek an anesthesiology practice there to join or simply start one themselves. Although a maldistribution of anesthesiologists in the United States existed (and still exists, with underserved rural and inner-city areas that may have few or no physician anesthesia services), there were enough finishing residents coming into the system to populate practices across the country in a manner that created a more "normal" marketplace system in which candidates for anesthesiology jobs faced most of the same considerations as all other professionals. Another factor of historical significance (but also with potential application in the future) was the proposal in 1993 by the U.S. federal administration to restructure radically American health care delivery. Although this proposal was abandoned as too radical, it introduced an element of uncertainty that persisted long after the idea had been dismissed. This element of uncertainty led many anesthesiologists and facilities to adopt a "wait and see" attitude about hiring new anesthesiologists at that time.

Later, there was an element of "pent up demand" that opened many anesthesiologist positions later in the decade of the 1990s. Another factor is the marketplace forces that have been and continue to induce significant changes in the U.S. health care system independent of any government proposal for change. Put as simply as possible, the business community, employers who provide health care insurance for their employees, and government entities that fund programs such as Medicare and Medicaid have suggested that it may be impossible for them to continue to fund the rapidly increasing expenditures necessary to provide health care coverage. As a result, an entire new industry, managed health care, appeared. The managed care concept is built on the idea that traditional fee-for-service health care has no incentive for health care providers, principally physicians, to limit expenditures. In fact, physicians, health care workers, and health care facilities were financially rewarded the more health care was "consumed" or rendered to patients. Accordingly, MCOs came into being, declaring to business and government that a new administrative layer was needed to control (reduce) what physicians and health care facilities spend. This management of care by outside, independent reviewers and decision makers who determine what care can and should be rendered to the patient was intended to replace the traditional fee-for-service indemnity system (bills submitted by physicians based on what they decide is necessary that are then paid after the fact by a health plan or insurance company) and thereby significantly reduce the cost for health care to employers and governments. One of the main themes of managed care plans was that there would be much less surgery. This idea led logically to questions about how many anesthesiologists really were needed in this country. Discussions occurred both outside and within organized anesthesiology about such questions,[31–34] but, predictably, no definitive answers were or are possible.

By 2001, the situation had largely reversed with the marketplace declaring a shortage of anesthesia providers and multiple attractive job offers for most residents being graduated. Senior medical students very quickly realized this and the number of highly qualified American graduates applying to anesthesiology residencies increased dramatically in the first years of the twenty-first century.[35] The situation is evolving and fluid,[36] and it is important to remember that there will always be surgery, no matter what health system changes take place. Even in the face of new potential health system reforms and also continued clinical innovation with "nonoperative procedures" replacing some traditional surgical operations, it seems likely that, again, any predictions of less need for OR anesthesia simply will not come true and there may well be, in fact, ongoing increases in demand. Moreover, anesthesiologists do more than just OR anesthesia (and likely increasingly so in the future). Accordingly, at the time of this writing, prospects for finishing anesthesiology residents are extremely bright and they must be armed with knowledge about the practice world.

Types of Practice

With the "alphabet soup" of new practice arrangements for physicians (IPA, PPO, PHO, MCO, MSO, HMO) and the rapidly evolving forces of the health care marketplace, as well as the intermittent appearance of major governmental initiatives to institute radical reform of the health care system, it is difficult to outline the details of all the possible types of opportunities for anesthesiologists. Rather, it is reasonable to provide basic background information and also suggestions of sources of further information.

At least through the first decade of the twenty-first century, residents finishing anesthesiology training will still need to choose among three fundamental possibilities: academic practice in a teaching hospital environment; a practice exclusively of patient care in the private practice marketplace; and a practice exclusively of patient care as an employee of a health care system, organization, or facility.

Teaching hospitals with anesthesiology residency programs constitute only a very small fraction of the total number of facilities requiring anesthesia services. These academic departments tend to be among the largest, but the aggregate fraction of the entire anesthesiologist population is small. It is interesting, however, that by the nature of the system, most residents finishing their training have almost exclusively been exposed only to academic anesthesiology. Accordingly, finishing residents in the past often were comparatively unprepared to evaluate and enter the anesthesiology job market. As noted, the Anesthesiology Residency Review Committee now requires teaching of job acquisition skills and practice management as part of the residency didactic curriculum.

Specialty certification by the American Board of Anesthesiology (ABA) should be the goal of all anesthesia residency graduates. Some graduating residents who know they are eventually headed for private practice have started their attending careers as junior faculty. This allows them to obtain some clinical practice and supervisory experience and offers them the opportunity to prepare for the ABA examinations in the nurturing, protected academic environment with which they are familiar. Most residents, however, do not become junior faculty; they accept practice positions immediately. But such newly trained residents should take into account the need to become ABA-certified and build into their new practice arrangements the stipulation that there will be time and consideration given toward this goal. The hectic and unsettling time of embarking on a new career, possibly moving one's home and family, and getting acclimated to a new professional and financial environment may inhibit optimum performance on the examinations. The possibilities to avoid this disruption may be comparatively limited, but awareness of the problem can help. At the very least, it may lead to the forging of initial practice arrangements that will maximize the probability of success.

Academic Practice

For those who choose to stay in academic practice, the first question is whether to consider staying at one's training institution. On the one hand, "the devil you know is better than the devil you don't know." On the other hand, however, fear of the unknown should not inhibit investigation of all possibilities. Aside from obvious personal preferences such as area of the country, size of city, and climate, a number of specific characteristics of academic anesthesia departments can be used as screening questions.

How big is the department? Junior faculty sometimes can get lost in very big departments and be treated as little better than glorified senior residents. On the other hand, the availability of subspecialty service opportunities and significant research and educational resources can make large departments extremely attractive. In smaller academic departments, there may be fewer resources, but the likelihood of being quickly accepted as a valued, contributing member of the teaching faculty (and research team, if appropriate) may be higher. In very small departments, the number of expectations, projects, and involvements could potentially be overwhelming. Additionally, a small department may lack a dedicated research infrastructure, so it may be necessary for the faculty in this situation to collaborate with other, larger departments to accomplish meaningful academic work.

What exactly is expected of junior faculty? If teaching one resident class every other week is standard, the candidate must enthusiastically accept that assignment and the attendant preparation work and time up front. Likewise, if it is expected that junior faculty will, by definition, be actively involved in publishable research, specific plans for projects to which the candidate is amenable must be made. In such situations, clear stipulations about startup research funding and nonclinical time to carry out the projects should be obtained as much as possible. Particularly important is determining what the expectation is concerning outside funding—it can be a rude shock to realize that projects will suddenly halt after, for example, 2 years if extramural funding has not been secured.

What are the prospects for advancement? Many new junior faculty directly out of residency start with medical school appointments as instructors unless there is something else in their background that immediately qualifies them as assistant professors. It is wise to understand from the beginning what it takes in that department and medical school to facilitate academic advancement. There may be more than one academic "track;" the tenure track, for example, is usually dependent on published research whereas the clinical or teacher track relies more heavily on one's value in patient care and as a clinical educator. The criteria for promotion may be clearly spelled out by the institution—number of papers needed, involvement and recognition at various levels, grants submitted and funded, and so on—or the system may be less rigid and depend more heavily on the department chairman's and other faculty evaluations and recommendations. In either case, careful inquiry before accepting the position can avert later surprise and disappointment.

How much does it pay? Traditionally, academic anesthesiologists have not earned quite as much as those in private practice—in return for the advantage of more predictable (and maybe less strenuous) schedules, continued intellectual stimulation, and the intangible rewards of academic success. There is now great activity and attention concerning reimbursement of anesthesiologists, and it is difficult to predict future income for any anesthesiology practice situation. However, all of the forces influencing payment for anesthesia care may significantly diminish the traditional income differential between academic and private practice. This is not a small issue. Anesthesiologists justifiably can expect to live reasonably well. Income is also a valid consideration both because anesthesiologists are frequently at least 30 years old when they finish training and are thus starting well behind their age-mates in lifetime earnings and because most physicians have substantial educational loans to repay when finishing residency. The compensation arrangements in academic practice vary widely in structure. In some cases, a faculty member is exclusively an employee of the institution, which bills and collects or negotiates group contracts for the patient care rendered by the faculty member, and then pays a negotiated amount (either an absolute dollar figure or a floating amount based on volume and/or collections—or a combination of the two) that constitutes the faculty person's entire income. Under other less common arrangements, faculty members themselves may be able to bill and collect or negotiate contracts for their clinical work. Some institutions have a (comparatively small) academic salary from the medical school for being on the faculty, but many do not; some channel variable amounts of money (from so-called Part A clinical revenue) into the academic practice in recognition of teaching and administration or simply as a subsidy for needed service. A salary from the medical school, if extant, is then supplemented significantly by the practice income. Usually, the faculty will be members of some type of group or practice plan (either for the anesthesia department alone or the entire faculty as a whole) that bills and collects or negotiates contracts and then distributes the practice income to the faculty under an arrangement that must be examined by the candidate. In most academic institutions, practice expenses such as all overhead and malpractice insurance as well as reasonable benefits, including discretionary funds for meetings, subscriptions, books, dues, and so on, are automatically part of the compensation package, which often may not be true in private practice and must be counted in making any comparison. An important corollary issue is that of the source of the salaries of the department's primary anesthesia providers—residents and, in some cases, nurse anesthetists. Although the hospital usually pays for at least some of these, arrangements vary, and it is important to ascertain whether the faculty practice income is also expected to cover the cost of the primary providers. Overall, it is reasonable to sound out faculty, both anesthesiology and others, regarding the past and likely future commitment of the institution to the establishment and maintenance of reasonable compensation for the expected involvement.

Private Practice in the Marketplace

As noted, some residents finish their anesthesia training never having seen a private practice anesthesia setting or even talked to an anesthesiologist who has been in private practice. These candidates are ill-equipped to seek a position in the private practice marketplace. Obviously, rotations to a private practice hospital in the final year of anesthesia residency could help greatly in this regard, but not all residency programs offer such opportunities. In that case, the finishing resident who is certain about going into private practice must seek information on career development and mentors from the private sector.

Armed with as much information as possible, one fundamental initial choice is between independent individual practice and a position with a group (either a sole proprietorship, partnership, or corporation) that functions as a single financial entity. Independent practice may become increasingly less viable in many locations because of the need to be able to bid for contracts with managed care entities. However, where independent practice is possible, it usually first involves attempting to secure clinical privileges at a number of hospitals or facilities in the area in which one chooses to live. This may not always be easy, and this issue has been the subject of many (frequently unsuccessful) antitrust suits over recent years (see Antitrust Considerations). Then the anesthesiologist makes it known to the respective surgeon communities that he or she is available to render anesthesia services and waits until there is a request for his or her services. The anesthesiologist obtains the requisite financial information from the patient and then either individually bills and collects for services rendered or employs a service to do billing and collection for a percentage fee (which will vary depending on the circumstances, especially the volume of business; for billing [without scheduling services] it would be unlikely to be more than 7% or, at the most, 8% of actual collections). How much of the needed equipment and supplies will be provided by the hospital or facility and how much by the independent anesthesiologist varies widely. If an anesthesiologist spends considerable time in one operating suite, he or she may purchase an anesthesia machine exclusively for his or her own use and move it from room to room as needed. It is likely to be impractical to move a fully equipped anesthesia machine from hospital to hospital on a day-to-day basis. Among the features of this style of practice are the collegiality and relationships of a genuine private practice based on referrals and also the ability to decide independently how much time one wants to be available to work. The downside is the potential unpredictability of the demand for service and the time needed to establish referral patterns and obtain bookings sufficient to generate a livable income.

Acknowledging that the issues presented earlier may at some times render components of these suggestions moot, it is reasonable for the graduating resident to know that when seeking a position with a private group, the applicant should search for potential practice opportunities through word of mouth, recruiting letters sent to the training program supervisor, journal advertisements, and placement services (either commercial or professional, such as that provided at the ASA annual meeting). Some of the screening questions are the same as for an academic position, but there must be even more emphasis on the exact details of clinical expectations and financial arrangements. Some residents finish residency (or fellowship training to an even greater extent) very highly skilled in complex, difficult anesthesia procedures. They can be surprised to find that in some private practice group situations, the junior-most anesthesiologist must wait some time, perhaps even years, before being eligible to do, for example, cardiac anesthesia and in the meantime will mostly be assigned more routine or less challenging anesthetics. Of course, this is not always the circumstance, but the applicant needs to investigate thoroughly to be certain that the opportunity satisfies the desire for professional challenge.

Financial arrangements in private group practices vary widely. Some groups are loose organizational alliances of independent practitioners who bill and collect separately and rotate clinical assignments and call for mutual convenience. Many groups act also as a fiscal entity, and there are many possible variations on this theme. In many circumstances in the past, new junior members started out as functional employees of the group for a probationary interval before being considered for full membership or partnership. This is not a classic employment situation because it is intended to be temporary as a prelude to full financial participation in the group. However, there have been enough instances of established groups abusing this arrangement that the ASA includes in its fundamental Statement of Policy the proviso: "Exploitation of anesthesiologists by other anesthesiologists is improper."[3] This goes on to say that after a reasonable trial period, income should reflect services rendered. Unfortunately, these statements may have little meaning or impact on groups in the marketplace. Some groups have a history of demanding excessively long trial periods during which the junior anesthesiologist's income is artificially low and then denying partnership and terminating the relationship to go on to employ a new probationer and start the cycle over again. Accordingly, new junior staff attempting to join groups should try to have such an arrangement spelled out carefully in the agreement drafted by an expert representing the anesthesiologist. Another variation of this, in an attempt to disguise the fundamentally unethical nature of the practice, is to employ anesthesiologists on a fixed salary with the false incentive of no night or weekend call. This is disingenuous, as the vast majority of income is usually generated during routine scheduled day work, for which the anesthesiologist-employee is poorly compensated. Yet another usurious scheme is for a group to employ an anesthesiologist for a period of years at a low salary and then require a further cash outlay to purchase partnership in the corporation. As the cash outlay can be quite substantial, it is frequently borrowed from the corporation, leading to a sophisticated form of indentured servitude. Sadly, when the job market conditions are poor as they were some years ago, the tendency is for there to be less likelihood of securing a prospective commitment of partnership at a specified future time. This is especially true in the more desirable areas of the United States where stories of abuse of junior "partners" have been more common. Whether this should substantially affect an applicant's interest in or willingness to accept a position is a highly individual matter that must be evaluated by each applicant. As the market turned and the demand often exceeded the supply of new anesthesiologists, such abuses appeared less likely. In all cases, the applicant must utilize resources[4] that allow them to enter the negotiating process armed with maximum information and reasonable expectations.

Private Practice as an Employee

There has been some trend toward anesthesiologists becoming permanent employees of any one of various fiscal entities. The key difference is that there is no intention or hope of achieving an equity position (share of ownership, usually of a partnership, thus becoming a full partner). Hospitals, outpatient surgery centers, multidisciplinary clinics, other facilities tied to a specific location where surgery is performed, physician groups that have umbrella fiscal entities specifically created to serve as the employer of physicians, and even surgeons may seek to hire anesthesiologists as permanent employees. The common thread in this system is that these fiscal entities see the anesthesiologists as additional ways of generating profits. Again, in many cases it would appear that employees are not paid a salary that is commensurate with their production of receivables. That is, the fiscal entity will pay a salary substantially below collections generated plus appropriate overhead. These arrangements are particularly favored by some large managed care organizations in certain cities that view anesthesiologists simply as expensive necessities that prevent hospitals from realizing maximum profit (although sometimes there is a promise of a lighter or more manageable schedule in these positions compared to marketplace private practice). At the height of the managed care mania of the mid to late 1990s, there were predictions that this trend would continue to grow, and that eventually most physicians in the support specialties of anesthesiology, radiology, pathology, and emergency medicine would be outright permanent employees of an organized entity of some type. While clearly this did not happen and the managed care bubble has deflated somewhat, it is impossible to speculate on the future in this regard. Many anesthesiologists believe that the future is extraordinarily bright and that anesthesiology will expand its role, predicting that anesthesiologists will increasingly assume positions of central authority in managed care and other practice entities, making decisions about the hiring and firing of physicians of other specialties.

Negotiating for a position as a permanent employee is somewhat simpler and more straightforward than it is in marketplace private practice. It parallels the usual understandings that apply to most regular employer–employee situations: job description, role expectations, working conditions, hours, pay, and benefits. The idea of anesthesiologists functionally becoming shift workers disturbs many in the profession because it contradicts the traditional professional model. On the other hand, major upheaval in the health care delivery system has sometimes led to reorganization that, until very recently, was unheard of. Again, the complex nature and multiple levels of such considerations make it a personal issue that must be carefully evaluated by each individual with full awareness and consideration of the issues outlined here.

Billing and Collecting

In practices in which anesthesiologists are directly involved with the financial management, they need to understand as much as possible about the complex world of health care reimbursement. This significant task has been made easier by the ASA, which some time ago added a significant component to its Washington, D.C., office by adding a practice management coordinator to the staff. One of the associated assignments is helping ASA members understand and work with the sometimes confusing and convoluted issues of effective billing for anesthesiologists' services. There are often updates with the latest information and codes in the monthly ASA *Newsletter*.

There continue to be proposals for significant changes in billing for anesthesiology care. However, the basics have changed only slightly in recent years. It is important to understand that many of the most contentious issues, such as the requirement for physician supervision of nurse anesthetists and the implications of that for reimbursement, apply in many circumstances mostly to Medicare and, in some states, Medicaid. Thus, the fraction of the patient population covered by these government payers is important in any consideration. Different practice situations have different arrangements regarding the financial relationships between anesthesiologists and nurse anesthetists, and this can affect the complex situation of who bills for what. The nurses may be employees of a hospital, of the anesthesiologists who medically direct them, or of no one in that they are independent contractors billing separately (even in cases in which physician supervision—not medical direction—is required but where those physicians do not bill for that component). In 1998, Medicare mandated that an anesthesia care team of a nurse anesthetist medically directed by an anesthesiologist could bill as a team no more than 100% of the fee that would apply if the anesthesiologist did the case alone. The implications of this change are complex and variable among anesthesiology practices, particularly because there is another trend—for health care facilities that traditionally had employed nurse anesthetists to seek to shift total financial responsibility for them to the anesthesiologist practice group. Also, complex related issues played out in the early 2000 years. The federal government issued a new regulation allowing individual states to "opt out" of the requirement that nurse anesthetists be supervised by physicians and several states did so. This was opposed by the ASA. Because perioperative patient care, one component of which is administering anesthesia, is traditionally considered the practice of medicine, the implications of this change as far as the role of surgeons supervising nurse anesthetists and the malpractice liability status of nurse anesthetists practicing independently were unclear. Further, the implications of all this for billing insurers other than Medicare and Medicaid are exceedingly complex. Obviously, careful consideration of these issues and seeking out advice from knowledgeable resources (such as the ASA Washington office) is critical to fiscal stability in modern anesthesiology practice.

There has been significant consideration of the mechanism of billing for anesthesiology. There have been some suggestions that so-called schedule fees (a single predetermined fee for an anesthetic, independent of its length or complexity) will become more common. Further, there is pressure from some quarters to bundle together all the physicians' fees for one procedure into a single global professional fee that would pay the surgeon, anesthesiologist, radiologist, pathologist, and so on for one case, such as a laparoscopic cholecystectomy. However, all of this concern about billing for specific procedures could become irrelevant in systems with prospective capitated payments for large populations of patients, in which each group of involved physicians in a system would receive a fixed amount per enrolled member per month (PMPM) and agree, except in the most unusual circumstances, to provide whatever care is needed by that population for that prospective payment. These are intended to be large-scale operations involving at least tens of thousands of people ("covered lives") in each organization. There was a trend in this direction in the late 1990s, but, as with so many aspects of managed care, the actual implantation of the ideas in real life did not work out smoothly or as planned and there was a resulting retrenchment into more blended models of facility reimbursement based on DRG (diagnosis related group) codes and professional reimbursement based on a negotiated multiple (or fraction) of the corresponding Medicare payment for that service.

Classic Methodology

Because there is still widespread application of the traditional method of billing for anesthesiology services, understanding it is very important for anesthesiologists starting practice. In this system, each anesthetic generates a value of so many "units," which represent effort and time. A conversion factor (dollars per unit) that can vary widely multiplied by the number of units generates an amount to be billed. Each anesthetic has a base value number of units (e.g., 8 for a cholecystectomy) and then the time taken for the anesthetic is divided into units, usually 15 minutes per unit. Thus, a cholecystectomy with anesthesia time of 1 hour and 50 minutes would have 8 base units and 7.33 time units for a total of 15.33 units. In some practice settings, it may be allowed to add modifiers, such as extra units for complex patients with multiple problems as reflected by an ASA physical status classification of 3 to 5 and/or E ("emergency") or for insertion of an arterial or pulmonary artery catheter. The sum is the total billing unit value. Determining the base value for an anesthetic in units depends on full and correct understanding of what operation was done. Although this sounds easy, it is the most difficult component of traditional anesthesia billing. The process of determining the procedure done is known as coding because the procedure name listed on the anesthesia record is assigned an identifying code number from the universally used CPT-4 coding book. This code is then translated through the ASA Relative Value Guide, which assigns a base unit value to the type of procedure identified by the CPT-4 code. In the past, some anesthesiologists failed to understand the importance of correct coding to the success of the billing process. Placing this task in the hands of someone unfamiliar with the system and with surgical terminology can easily lead to incorrect coding. This can fail to capture charges and the resulting income to which the anesthesiologist is entitled or, worse, can systematically overcharge the payers, which will bring sanctions, penalties and, in certain cases, criminal prosecution. In recent years a prevailing official attitude has been that there are no simple, innocent coding errors. All upcoding (charging for more expensive services than were actually delivered) is considered to be prima facie evidence of fraud and subject to severe disciplinary and legal action. All practices should have detailed compliance programs in place to ensure correct coding for services rendered.[37] Outside expert help (such as from a health care law firm that specializes in compliance programs) is highly desirable for the process of formulating and implementing a compliance plan.

Assembly and transfer of the information necessary to generate bills must be efficient and complete. Traditionally, this involved depositing in a secure central location a paper extra copy of the anesthesia record and often a "billing sheet" with it, on which was inscribed the names of all the involved personnel and any additional information about other potentially billable services, such as invasive monitors. Any practice involved with a comprehensive electronic perioperative information management system in the facility should be using that to assemble this "front end" billing information. Short of that, some practices collect electronic information specifically generated by the anesthesia providers for that purpose. They have equipped each staff member with a hand-held organizer into which data are entered and then the device is synched with a departmental computer at the end of the day. If the OR suite has "wi-fi" (wireless electronic connection), the same function could be accomplished in real time with the providers entering the requisite information into a miniprogram on a laptop computer affixed to each anesthesia machine (or one carried by each staff member). Of course, the universal use of hand-helds or laptops could have significant other benefits to the members of the group/department. Overall, while achieving full compliance with such a protocol of billing data entry by the group's staff may take significant in-service education and training, it will only take one reduced or, better, missed paycheck to achieve full compliance by any given member. Once the information has been secured, a mechanism must be employed to generate the actual bill and communicate it to the payer (on paper, on disk, or, usually, directly computer-to-computer: "electronic claims submission"). The possible precise arrangements for doing this vary widely. Ultimately, the entity actually submitting the bill will verify that it has been paid (posting of receipts) and may or may not actually handle the incoming money. Very often, anesthesia practices or individuals who use a billing service will arrange that the payments go directly to a bank lockbox, which is a post office box (better individual than shared, even if more expensive) to which the payments come and then go directly into a bank account. This system avoids the situation of having the people who generate the bill actually handle the incoming receipts, a practice that has led to theft and fraud in a few cases. Eventual decisions about how hard to try to collect from payers who deny coverage and then from patients directly will depend on the circumstances, including local customs.

Detailed summary statistics of the work done by an anesthesiology practice group are critical for logistic management of personnel, scheduling, and financial analysis. Spreadsheet and database computer programs customized for an individual practice's characteristics will be invaluable. A summary of the types of data an anesthesia practice should track is shown in Table 2-5. Once all the data are assembled and reviewed, at least monthly analysis by a business manager or equivalent as well as officers/leaders of the practice group can spot trends very early in their development and allow appropriate correction or planning. Often the responsible members of an anesthesiology group question how effective their financial services operation is, particularly regarding net collections. This is a complex issue[38] that, again, often requires outside help. Routine internal audits can be useful but could be self-serving. No billing office or company that is honest and completely above board should ever object to a client, in this case the anesthesiology practice group, engaging an independent outside auditor to come in and thoroughly examine both the efficiency of the operation and also "the books" concerning correctness and completeness of collections.

Anesthesia billing and collecting are among the most complex challenges in the medical reimbursement field. Traditional anesthesia reimbursement is unique in all of medicine. The experience of many people over the years has suggested that it often is well advised to deal with an entity that is not only very experienced in anesthesia billing, but also does anesthesia billing exclusively or as a large fraction of its efforts. It is very difficult for an anesthesiologist or a family member to do billing and collecting as a side activity to a normal life. This has led to inefficient and inadequate efforts in many cases, illustrating the value of paying a reasonable fee to a professional who will devote great time and energy to this challenging endeavor.

Antitrust Considerations

Although it is true that there are many potential antitrust implications of business arrangements involving anesthesiologists—particularly with all the realignments, consolidations, mergers, and contracts associated with the advent of managed care—it is also true that the applicable statutes and regulations are poorly understood. Contrary to popular belief, the antitrust laws do not involve the rights of individuals to engage in business. Rather, the laws are concerned solely with the preservation of competition within a defined marketplace and the

TABLE 2-5

TYPES OF DATA AN ANESTHESIOLOGY GROUP SHOULD TRACK AND MAINTAIN CONCERNING ITS OWN PRACTICE

Types of Data the Anesthesiology Group's Computer System Should Track

1. Transaction-based system (track each case and charge as separate record)
   - Track individual charges by CPT-4 code
   - Track individual payments by payer
2. Track all data elements on an interrelated basis
   - By place of service
   - By charge, broken down
     —by number of units (time and base)
     —by ASA modifiers
     —by number of lines
   - By CPT-4 code
   - By payer
   - By payment code (full payment, discount, write-off, or refund)
   - By diagnosis (ICD-9 code)
   - By surgeon
   - By anesthesiologist
   - By anesthesia care team provider
   - By start and stop times
   - By age
   - By gender
   - By employer
   - By ZIP code

Type of Information to Generate from These Data

1. Aggregate number of cases per year for the group
2. Total number of cases per year for each provider within the group
   - Number of cases performed by anesthesiologists
   - Number of cases performed by the anesthesia care team
3. Average number of units per case (as one measure of intensity per case)
4. Average number of units per CPT-4 code
5. Average time units per case and per CPT-4 code
   - Group should be able to calculate time units per individual surgeon
6. Average line charge per case
7. Charges per case by CPT-4 code
8. Payments per case by payer
9. Patient mix
   - Percent traditional indemnity
   - Percent managed care (broken down by each MCO for which services are provided)
   - Percent self-pay
   - Percent Medicare
   - Percent Medicaid
10. Collection rate for each population served
11. Overall collection rate
12. Costs per unit (total costs, excluding compensation ÷ total units) (costs include liability insurance, rent, collection costs, and legal and accounting fees)
13. Compensation costs per unit (total compensation ÷ total units) for MCO populations, utilization patterns by age, gender, and diagnosis

Reprinted with permission from American Society of Anesthesiologists. *Managed Care Reimbursement Mechanisms: A Guide for Anesthesiologists*. Park Ridge, IL: ASA; 1994.

rights of the consumer, independent of whether any one vendor or provider of service is involved. This misunderstanding has been the source of confusion. When an anesthesiologist has been excluded from a particular hospital's staff or anesthesia group and then sues based on an alleged antitrust violation, the anesthesiologist loses virtually automatically. This is because there is still significant competition in the relevant marketplace and competition in that market is not threatened by the exclusion of one physician from one staff.

In essence, if there are *several* hospitals offering relatively similar services to an immediate community (the market), denial of privileges to one physician by one hospital is not anticompetitive. If, on the other hand, there is only *one* hospital in a smaller market, then the same act, the same set of circumstances, could be seen very differently. In that case, there would be a limitation of competition because the hospital dominates and, in fact, may control the market for hospital services. Exclusion of one physician, then, would limit access by the consumers to alternative competing services and hence would likely be judged an antitrust violation.

The Sherman Antitrust Act is a federal law more than 100 years old. Section 1 deals with contracts, combinations, conspiracy, and restraint of trade. By definition, two or more separate economic entities must be involved in an agreement that is challenged as illegal for this section to apply. Section 2 prohibits monopolies or conspiracy to create a monopoly, and it is possible that this could apply to a single economic entity that has illegally gained domination of a market. Consideration of possible monopolistic domination of a market involves a situation in which a single entity controls at least 50% of the business in that market. The stakes are high in that the antitrust legislation provides for triple damages if a lawsuit is successful. The U.S. Department of Justice and the Federal Trade Commission are keenly interested in the current rapid evolution in the health care industry, and thus are actively involved in evaluating situations of possible antitrust violations. There are two ways to judge violations. Under the per se rule, which is applied relatively rarely, conduct that is obviously limiting competition in a market is automatically illegal. The other type of violation is based on the rule of reason, which involves a careful analysis of the market and the state of competition. The majority of complaints against physicians are judged by this rule. The more competitors there are in a market, the less likely that any one act is anticompetitive. In a community with two hospitals, one smaller than the other, with an anesthesiology group practice exclusively at each, if the larger anesthesiology practice group buys out and absorbs the smaller, leaving only one group for the only two hospitals in the community, that may be anticompetitive, particularly if a new anesthesiologist seeks to practice solo at those hospitals.

Legal Implications

In the current era of rapidly evolving managed care arrangements, the antitrust laws are important. If physicians (individuals or groups) who normally would be competitors because they are separate economic entities meet and agree on the prices they will charge or the terms they will seek in a managed care contract, that can be anticompetitive, monopolistic, and hence possibly illegal. Note that sharing a common office and common billing service alone is not enough to constitute a true group. If, on the other hand, the same physicians join in a true economic partnership to form a new group (total integration) that is a single economic entity (and meets certain other criteria) that will set prices and negotiate contracts, that is perfectly legal. The other criteria are critical. There must be capital investment and also risk sharing (if there is a profit or loss, it is distributed among the group members)—that is, total integration into a genuine partnership. This issue is very important in considering the drive for new organizations to put together networks of physicians that then seek contracts with major employers to provide medical care. Sometimes, hospitals or clinics attempt to form a network comprising all the members of the medical staff so that the resulting entity can bid globally for total care contracts. Any network is a joint venture of independent practitioners. If the participating physicians of one specialty in a network are separate economic entities and the network advertises one price for their services, this would seem to suggest an antitrust violation (horizontal price fixing). In the past, if a network involved fewer than 20% of one type of medical specialist in a market, that was called a "safe harbor," meaning that it was permissible for nonpartners to get together and negotiate prices. The federal government has tried to encourage formation of such networks to help reduce health care costs and, as a result, made some relevant exceptions to the application of these rules. As long as the network is nonexclusive (other nonnetwork physicians of a given specialty are free to practice in the same facilities and compete for the same patients), the network can comprise up to 30% of the physicians of one specialty in a market. Note specifically that this does not allow a local specialty society in a big city to serve as a bargaining agent on fees for its members, because it is very likely that more than 30% of the specialists in an area will be members of the society. The only real exception to this provision is in thinly populated rural areas where there may be just one physician network. In such cases (which are, so far, rare because the major managed care and network activity has occurred mainly in heavily populated urban areas), there is no limit on how many of one specialty can become network members and have the network negotiate fees, as long as the network is nonexclusive.

Clearly, these issues are very complex. Relevant legislation, regulations, and court actions all happen rapidly and often. Mergers among anesthesiology groups in a market area for the purposes of both efficiency and strength in negotiating fees have been very popular as a response to the rapidly changing marketplace. A list of questions must be answered to determine if such a merger would have anticompetitive implications. Although compendia of relevant information are available to anesthesiologists,[39–41] they cannot substitute for expert advice and help.

Obviously, anesthesiologists contemplating a merger or facing any one of a great number of other situations in the modern health care arena must secure assistance from professional advisors, usually attorneys, whose job it is to be aware of the most recent developments, how they apply, and how best to forge agreements in formal contracts. Anesthesiologists hoping to find reputable advisors can start their search with word-of-mouth referrals from colleagues who have used such services. Local or state medical societies frequently know of attorneys who specialize in this area. Finally, the ASA Washington, D.C., office has compiled a state-by-state list of advisors who have worked successfully with anesthesiologists in the past.

Exclusive Service Contracts

Often, one of the larger issues faced by anesthesiologists seeking to define practice arrangements concerns the desirability of considering an exclusive contract with a health care facility to provide anesthesia services. An exclusive contract states that anesthesiologists seeking to practice at a given facility must be members of the group holding the exclusive contract and, usually, that members of the group will practice nowhere else. A hospital may want to give an exclusive contract in return for a guarantee of coverage as part of the contract. Also, the hospital may believe that such a contract can help ensure the quality of the practitioner because the contract can contain credentialing and performance criteria. It is important to understand that the hospital likely will exercise a degree of control over the anesthesiologists with such a contract in force, such as requiring them to participate as providers in any contracts the hospital makes with third-party payers and also tying hospital privileges to the existence of the contract (the so-called "clean sweep provision" that bypasses any due process of the medical staff should the hospital terminate the contract). Certain of these types of provisions constitute *economic credentialing,* which is defined as the use of economic criteria unrelated to the quality of care or professional competency of physicians in granting or renewing hospital privileges (such as the acceptance of below-market fees associated with a hospital-negotiated care contract or even requiring financial contributions in some form to the hospital). The ASA in 1993 issued a statement condemning economic credentialing.[3] The anesthesiologists involved may accept such an exclusive services contract to guarantee that they alone will get the business from the surgeons on staff at that hospital, and hence the resulting income. There may be other considerations on both sides, and these have been outlined in extensive relevant ASA publications that also include a sample contract for information purposes only.[37,40] Although many exclusive contracts with anesthesiology groups are in force, the sentiment, particularly from the ASA, is against them. As has been stated, it is critical that anesthesiologists faced with important practice management decisions such as whether to enter into an exclusive contract must seek outside advice and counsel. There are a great many nuances to these issues,[40–43] and anesthesiologists are at risk attempting to negotiate such complex matters alone, just as patients would be at risk if a contract attorney attempted to induce general anesthesia.

Denial of hospital privileges as a result of the existence of an exclusive contract with the anesthesiologists in place at the facility has been the source of many lawsuits, including the well-known Louisiana case of *Hyde v. Jefferson Parish.* In that case, the court found for the defendant anesthesiologists and the hospital, saying that there was no antitrust violation because there was no real adverse effect on competition as far as patients were concerned because there were several other hospitals within the market to which they could go, and therefore they could exercise their rights to take advantage of competition in the relevant market. Thus, existence of an exclusive contract only in the rare setting where anticompetitive effects on patients can be proved might lead to a legitimate antitrust claim by a physician denied privileges. This was proven true in the more recent *Kessel v. Monongalia County General Hospital* case in West Virginia in which an exclusive anesthesiology contract was held illegal. Therefore, again, these arrangements are by definition complex and fraught with hazard. Accordingly, outside advice and counsel are always necessary.

Hospital Subsidies

Modern economic realities have forced a significant number of anesthesiology practice groups (in both private and academic settings) to recognize that their patient care revenue, after overhead is paid, does not provide sufficient compensation to attract and retain the number and quality of staff necessary to provide the expected clinical service (and fulfill any other group/department missions). Attempting to do the same (or more) work with fewer staff may temporarily provide increased financial compensation. Cutting benefits (discretionary personal professional expenses, retirement contributions, or even insurance coverage) may also be a component of a response to inadequate practice revenue. However, the resulting decrements in personal security, in convenience, and in quality of life as far as acute and chronic fatigue, decreased family and recreation time, and tension among colleagues fearful someone else is getting a "better deal" will quickly overcome any brief advantage of a somewhat higher income. Therefore, many practice groups in such situations are requesting their hospital (or other health care facility where they practice) to pay them a direct cash subsidy that is used to augment practice revenue to maintain benefits and amenities while increasing the pay of staff members, hopefully to a market-competitive level that will promote recruitment and retention of group members.

Obviously, requests by a practice group for a direct subsidy must be thoroughly justified to the facility administration receiving the petition. The group's business operation should already have been examined carefully for any possible defects or means to enhance revenue generation. Explanation of the general trend of declining reimbursements for anesthesia services should be carefully documented. Facts and figures on that and also the shortage of anesthesia providers can be obtained from journal articles and ASA publications, particularly the *Newsletter*. Demand for anesthesia coverage for the surgical schedule is a key component of this proposal. Scheduling and utilization, particularly if early-morning staffing is required for many operating rooms that are routinely unused later during the traditional work day, is a major issue to be understood and presented. Any other OR inefficiencies created by hospital support staff and previous efforts to deal with them should also be highlighted. Unfavorable payer mix impact of contracts and programs initiated by the hospital also often is a major factor in situations of inadequate practice revenue. Always, the group's good will with the surgeons and the community in general should be emphasized, as well as of the indirect or "behind the scenes" services and benefits the anesthesiology group provides to the hospital.

Clearly, any request for a subsidy must be reasonable. An overly aggressive effort beyond the bounds of logic could provoke the facility to consider alternative arrangements, even up to the point of putting out a request for proposal from other anesthesiology practice groups. Therefore, thoughtful calculations are required and a careful balance must be sought, seeking enough financial support to supplement practice revenues so that members' compensation is competitive but not so much as to be excessive. Supporting statements about offers and potential earnings elsewhere must be completely honest and not exaggerated or credibility and good faith will be lost. Further, part of any agreement will be the full sharing of the group's detailed financial information with the facility administration, both at the time of the request and on an ongoing basis if the payment is more than a one-time "bail out." Plans for review and renewal should be made once a subsidy is paid.

Any subsidy will likely require a formal contract. There may be concern about malpractice liability implications for the hospital even though the practice group stays an independent entity as before. There may be "inurement" or "private benefit" concerns that could be perceived as a threat to the tax-exempt status of a nonprofit hospital. Lack of understanding of the applicable laws may lead to fears that a subsidy could be an illegal "kickback" or a violation of the Stark II self-referral prohibition. As is almost always the case, expert outside professional consultant advice, usually from an attorney who specializes exclusively in health care finance contracting, is mandatory in such circumstances. The ASA Washington, D.C., office maintains lists of consultants who have helped other anesthesiologists or groups in the past on various subjects and, also, the ASA has some basic information on subsidies to anesthesiology practice groups.[44,45]

Managed Care and New Practice Arrangements

As noted, managed care systems for health care delivery fundamentally exist as a mechanism to control and then reduce health care costs by having independent reviewers and decision makers who are not the physicians rendering the care limit the health care services delivered to large groups of patients. These ideas represent a huge change for American physicians. For a time, these changes appeared inescapable, not necessarily
7 because of government initiatives, but because of marketplace forces that result from the business community and government entities simply refusing to continue to pay ever-increasing sums for health care. However, there was a dramatic public backlash against the limitations on medical care services, so much so that several states passed laws outlining for certain circumstances what MCOs must pay for. This led to decreased expansion of managed care and to some easing of the restrictions on services in many plans. The overall impact was to slow (but not stop) the adoption of rigidly managed health care and to rekindle anew many of the concerns about how to structure and fund the health care system in this country. Some MCOs were forced to retool their operations and some went out of business entirely. However, many continued operations, albeit more quietly. The degree of penetration of managed care into market areas around the country has been highly variable. Areas such as Minneapolis, San Diego, San Francisco, eastern Massachusetts, and several other northern cities were the first to become mature managed care markets with a significant majority of the population enrolled in one or another managed care health plan. Other parts of the country with very sparsely populated areas such as sections of the Deep South and the West were not much affected because the population density was insufficient to support MCO requirements. An MCO attempts to secure health care provision contracts with employers who provide health plan coverage for their workers and with government agencies (e.g., Medicaid) responsible for the health care of large populations. Each worker or covered head of a household may have dependents covered by the plan. Each person covered in the plan is referred to as a *covered life*. An MCO probably needs contracts for at least 10,000 covered lives and preferably many more to make a legitimate entry into the marketplace. The MCO then enrolls physicians or physician groups and hospitals as providers and contracts to send its enrolled patients (the covered lives) to the health care providers under contract. The central issue is finances. The MCO seeks to enroll covered lives by offering the lowest prices possible. In turn, it seeks to contract with providers (individuals and facilities) for the lowest possible fees for medical care in return for sending large volumes of patient business to those providers.

In the initial stages of the evolution of a managed care marketplace, the MCOs usually seek contracts with providers based on discounted fee-for-service arrangements. This preserves the basic traditional idea of production-based physician reimbursement (do more, bill more) but the price of each act of services is lower (the providers are induced to give deep discounts with the promise of significant volumes of patients) and, also, the MCO gatekeeper primary care physicians and the MCO reviewers are strongly encouraged to limit complex and costly services as much as possible. There are other features intermittently along the way, such as global fees and negotiated fee schedules (agreed-upon single prices for individual procedures, independent of length or complexity). Further, another element is introduced to encourage the providers, both gatekeepers and specialists, to reduce costs. In an application of the concept of risk-sharing (spend too much for patient care and lose income), this usually is initially manifest in the form of "withholds," the practice of the MCO holding back a fraction of the agreed-upon payment to the providers (e.g., 10 or 15%) and keeping this money until the end of the fiscal year. At that time, if there is any money left in the risk pool or withhold account after all the (partial) provider fees and MCO expenses are paid, it is distributed to the providers in proportion to their degree of participation during the year. This is a clever and powerful incentive to providers to reduce health care expenses. It is not as powerful as the stage of full risk sharing, however. As the managed care marketplace matures and MCOs grow and succeed, the existing organizations and, especially, any new ones, shift to prospective capitated payments for providers.

Prospective Payments

This eventual reimbursement arrangement constitutes an entirely new world to the providers, involving prospective capitated payments for large populations of patients, in which each group of providers in the MCO receives a fixed amount per enrolled covered life per month (PMPM) and agrees, except in the most unusual circumstances, to provide whatever care is needed by that population for that prospective payment. The most unusual circumstances involve "carve-out" arrangements in which specific very costly and unusual conditions or procedures (such as the birth of a child with disastrous multiple congenital anomalies) are covered separately on a discounted fee-for-service basis. With full capitation, the entire financial underpinning of American medical care does a complete about-face from the traditional rewards for giving more care and doing more procedures to new rewards for giving and doing less. Some managed care contracts contain other features intended to protect the providers against unexpected overutilization by patients that would stretch the providers beyond the bounds of the original contract with the MCO. The provisions setting the boundaries are called "risk corridors," and the "stop-loss clauses" add some discounted fee-for-service payment for the excess care beyond the risk corridor (capitated contract limit). Providers who were used to getting paid more for doing more suddenly find themselves getting paid a fixed amount no matter how much or how little they do with regard to a specified population—hence the perceived incentive to do, and consequently spend, less. If the providers render too much care within the defined boundary of the contract, they essentially will be working for free, the ultimate in risk-sharing. There are clearly potential internal conflicts in such a system,[46] and how patients reacted initially to this radical change in attitude on the part of physicians demonstrated that this overall mechanism is unlikely to be readily embraced by the general public. This has forced some "return to the drawing board" thinking and it is not clear how fully managed care as it was originally constituted will evolve. What is clear is that nothing is settled and there will be ongoing debate about and experimentation in the American health care system.

Health care providers (physicians, health care workers, and facilities), in turn, allied themselves in a wide variety of organizations to create strength and desirable resources to present to the MCOs in contract negotiations. Some of these alliances were formed very quickly, almost in a panic, because of fears by providers that they might get left out of the managed care marketplace and thus deprived of major sources of income or, someday, any income at all. Management service organizations (MSOs) are joint venture network arrangements that do not involve true economic integration among the practitioners, but merely offer common services to physicians who may, as a loosely organized informal group, elect to seek MCO contracts. Preferred provider organizations (PPOs) are network arrangements of otherwise economically independent physicians who form a new corporate entity to seek managed care contracts in which there are significant financial incentives to patients to use the network providers and financial penalties for going to out-of-network providers. This has proved a relatively popular model and appears to be gaining wide acceptance. Physician–hospital organizations (PHOs) are similar entities but involve understandings between groups of physicians and a hospital so that a large package or bundle of services can be constructed as essentially one-stop points of care. Independent practice associations (IPAs) are like PPOs but are specifically oriented toward capitated contracts for covered lives with significant risk-sharing by the providers. Groups (or clinics) without walls are collections of practitioners who fully integrate economically into a single fiscal entity (true partnership) and then compete for MCO contracts on the basis of risk-sharing incentives among the partners. Fully integrated groups or health maintenance organizations (HMOs) house the group of partner provider physicians and associated support staff at a single location for the convenience of patients, a big selling point when they seek MCO contracts.

Changing Paradigm

The questions anesthesiologists face when addressing this alphabet soup of organizations are many and complex, even more complex than those faced by office-based primary care or specialty physicians, because of the interdependent relationships with health care facilities as practice locations and with surgeons. The era of solo independent practitioners may be ending in some locations where MCOs dominate. Small groups of anesthesiologists may find themselves at a competitive disadvantage unless they become part of a vertically integrated (multispecialty) or horizontally integrated (with other anesthesiologists) organization. An extensive compendium of relevant information has been prepared by the ASA.[39] Because it appears likely that many anesthesiologists in the United States will be affected by managed care, the information in this and related publications[47] is very important. Negotiations with MCOs require expert advice, probably even more so than even the traditional exclusive contracts with hospitals noted earlier. Before any negotiation can even be considered, the MCO must provide significant amounts of information about the covered patient population. The projected health care utilization pattern of a large group of white-collar workers (and their families) from major upscale employers in an urban area will be quite different from that of a rural Medicaid population. Specific demographics and past utilization histories are absolutely mandatory for each proposed population to be covered, and this information should go directly to the advising experts for evaluation, whether the proposed negotiation is for discounted fee-for-service, a fee schedule, global bundled fees, or full capitation.

A component of the shifting thinking in the 1990s was consideration of "value-based anesthesia practice,"[2] an attempt to balance reasonably the relationship of the cost of care and ultimate patient outcomes (with a very strong emphasis on controlling costs). Elaborate modeling was employed to attempt to calculate applicable cost-benefit ratios and thus define the point on a hypothetical curve of care at which the least resource investment would yield the highest quality. A systems approach was carefully applied to attempt to define and track the component elements of both cost and outcome, which would lead to models of the larger concepts of value and quality. Understanding effectiveness and efficiency of the involved processes was essential. Quantifiable outcomes and costs were compared to national benchmarks found in the literature or from surveys. The ultimate goal was application of outcome data to the management (reduction) of costs. Medication choice and utilization by anesthesiologists was a frequently cited example of the potential beneficial application of the tenets of value-based anesthesia practice. Attempts to apply this type of analysis to overall anesthesia morbidity and mortality were complicated by the (fortunate) extreme rarity of significant adverse outcomes and the difficulty of calculating the associated actual incrementally increased costs, as well as of definitively identifying remediable causes that could be prevented through system change. Attempts to assess the relative value of different anesthetic techniques (e.g., regional vs. general) for specific surgical procedures were complicated by problems discovering the true cost of different scenarios. Analysis of the cost of monitoring revealed the difficulty of determining the total costs saved or incurred by, for example, the insertion of a TEE in a specific patient, and, further, the belief that pulse oximetry has never been "statistically proven" to influence anesthesia outcome provoked questions about its cost and "value" in direct conflict with the fact that it is a universal standard of care. Overall, because "hard number" data readily amenable to rigorous statistical analysis for both the actual costs and the outcomes of anesthesia care have been very difficult, if not impossible, to generate, the widespread applicability of this approach in everyday anesthesia practice remains to be developed.

Significant questions were raised about the reimbursement implications for anesthesiologists of the putative managed care revolution. Again, the ASA assembled a great deal of relevant information, the understanding of which is essential to successful negotiations.[39] Table 2-5 has a list of information an anesthesia practice should have about its activities. Initial consideration of a capitated contract should involve an attempt to take all the data about the existing practice and the proposed MCO-covered population from a "capitation checklist"[39] and translate back from the proposed capitated rate to income figures that would correlate with the existing practice structure, to allow a comparison and an understanding of the relationship of the projected work in the contract to the projected income from it. It is, of course, impossible to suggest dollar values for capitated rates for anesthesiology care because details and conditions vary so widely. One ASA publication[39] used examples, purely for illustrative purposes, involving $2.50 or $4.00 PMPM, but there were unconfirmed reports at the peak of the managed care activities of capitated rates as low as $0.75 PMPM for anesthesiology. Discounted fee-for-service arrangements are easier for anesthesiologists to understand because these are directly referable to existing fee structures. Reports of groups instituting 10 to 50% discounts off the starting point of 80% of usual and customary reimbursement in various practice circumstances were circulated at national meetings of anesthesiologists. Were rigidly controlled fully mature managed care to dominate the practice community, it would be likely that the average income for anesthesiologists would decrease from past levels. However, it likely also would be true that anesthesiologists would continue to have incomes still above average among all physicians in that market.

Health Insurance Portability and Accountability Act (HIPAA)

All health care professionals in active practice were aware of the April 2003 implementation of the Privacy Rule of the Health Insurance Portability and Accountability Act of 1996 (HIPAA), because of the required significant changes in how medical records and patient information are handled in the day-to-day delivery of health care. The impact on and requirements for anesthesiologists are summarized in a comprehensive publication from the ASA[48] that followed two educational summaries.[49,50]

Attention is focused on "protected health information" (identifiable as from a specific patient by name). Patients must be notified of their privacy rights. Usually this will be covered by the health care facility in which anesthesiologists work, but if separate private records are maintained, separate notification may be necessary. Privacy policies must be created, adopted, and promulgated to all practitioners, all of whom then must be trained in application of those policies. Often, anesthesiology groups can combine with the facilities in which they practice as an "organized health care arrangement" so that the anesthesia practitioners can be covered in part by the HIPAA compliance activities of the facility. A "privacy officer" must be appointed for the practice group. Finally, and most importantly, medical records containing protected health information must be secured so they are not readily available to those who do not need them to render care.

One of the most obvious applications for many anesthesiologists is concern about the assembled preoperative information and charts for tomorrow's cases that frequently were placed prominently in the OR holding area at the end of one work day in readiness for the next day's cases. HIPAA provisions require that all that patient information be locked away overnight. Another classic example is what many ORs refer to as "the board." Often, a large white marker board occupies a prominent wall near the front desk of an operating room suite and the rooms, cases, and personnel assignments are inscribed thereon at the beginning of the day and modified or crossed off as the day progresses. Under HIPAA, patients' names may not be used on such a board if there is any chance that anyone not directly involved in their care could see them. The same is true for similar boards in holding areas and PACUs. Many anesthesiology practices also must apply HIPAA provisions to their billing operations; the details will vary depending on the mechanisms used and a great deal will depend on which type of electronic claims submission software is being used by the billing entity actually submitting the claims.[51] Telephone calls and faxes into offices must be handled specially if containing identifiable patient information. Presentation of patient information for quality assurance or teaching purposes must be free of all identifiers unless specific individual permission has been obtained on prescribed printed forms. Requests for patient information from a wide variety of outside entities, including insurance companies and collection agencies, must be processed in HIPAA-compliant ways. HIPAA policy and actions, as well as enforcement activities, are being developed over time and as situations develop. Particularly because this system depends on patient complaints for both enforcement and policy evolution, it is likely that it will be at least several years until a well-accepted smoothly functioning system is established.

Expansion into Perioperative Medicine, Hospital Care, and Hyperbaric Medicine

As the role of the anesthesiologist changes, new opportunities should be explored. One set of ideas that has been circulating for some time led to serious suggestions that the name of the profession of anesthesiology be changed to "perioperative medicine and pain management." This suggestion illustrates that one prospective significant anesthesiology practice management strategy can be more formal organization of responsibilities for patients in the pre- and postoperative periods.

Some anesthesiologists now function at least some of the time in preoperative screening clinics because of the great fraction care of OR patients who do not spend the night before surgery in the hospital or who do not come to a hospital at all. In such settings, these anesthesiologists frequently assume a role analogous to that of a primary care physician, planning and executing a workup of one or more significant medical or surgical problems before the patient can reasonably be expected to undergo surgery. More formalized arrangements of this type would involve the creation of designated perioperative clinics operated and staffed by anesthesiologists. Ophthalmologists and orthopedists, for example, would no longer need to try to manage their surgical patients' medical problems themselves or send their patients proposed for surgery to an internist or other primary care provider for "preop clearance" that often has little value in a complex patient facing specific anesthesia challenges that only an experienced anesthesiologist would, by definition, understand. The anesthesiologist would assume that role at the same time the patient is undergoing preoperative evaluation for anesthesia care.

Likewise, this concept would be excellent for the postoperative period. An anesthesiologist, completely free of OR or other duties, could not only make at least twice-daily rounds on patients after surgery and provide exceedingly comprehensive pain management service, but also could follow the surgical progress and make virtually continuous reports (likely via an electronic medical record or e-mail) to the surgeon's office or alphanumeric pocket communicator. Surgeons would have a much better handle on their patients' progress while having more time to tend to other new patients in the office or the OR. The utilization review and "fast-track protocol" administrators would have a contact person who is not tied up in an OR or office continuously available. Patients would receive much more physician attention and perceive this as actually a significant improvement in their care. Equivalent outpatient or recuperative center services could easily be established. In this regard, some anesthesiologists function as hospitalists for the care of both surgical and medical patients. A fundamental aspect of the practice of anesthesiology is the management of acute problems in the hospital setting. It is logical that anesthesiologists would be among the physicians best suited to provide primary care for patients in the hospital setting. Although the comfort level of anesthesiologists varies in the fields of internal medicine and pediatrics, it is likely that this trend will continue among those anesthesiologists interested and competent in hospital care.

Finally, anesthesiologists have become increasingly involved in the practice of hyperbaric medicine and wound care. This is likely related to the familiarity of anesthesiologists with concepts of gas laws and physics, along with their constant presence in the hospital. The treatment of various medical conditions by the application of oxygen under increased pressure, usually 2 to 3 atmospheres absolute, at one time was one of the most rapidly growing hospital services. Anesthesiologists are among the leaders of this field, with unlimited opportunities for clinical care, teaching, and research. Even a brief discussion of this field is outside the scope of this chapter and interested readers are referred to the Undersea and Hyperbaric Medical Society, www.uhms.org.

Creative exploration of new opportunities involving these and other ideas will open new avenues for anesthesiology (or whatever the specialty is eventually called) practice.

OPERATING ROOM MANAGEMENT

The role of anesthesiologists in OR management has changed dramatically in the past few years. While not that long ago, most anesthesiologists avoided any responsibilities of administrative duties (contributing significantly to a potentially nega-
8 tive professional image, as noted earlier), more recently many anesthesia practices have pleaded for an expanded role in OR management, both to promote efficiency and also to protect their interests. With the current climate of a considerable shortage of anesthesia providers, hospitals subsidizing many anesthesiology group practices, and an increasing workload, participation in OR management is essentially mandatory. The profession needs to move beyond exclusive attention to what is and always will be the mainstay of our practice, the administration of anesthetics for surgery. The current emphasis on cost containment and efficiency will force anesthesiologists to take an active role in eliminating many dysfunctional aspects of OR practice that were previously ignored. First-case morning start times have changed from a suggestion to a mandate. Delays of any sort are now carefully scrutinized to eliminate waste and inefficiency. While a helpful cooperative approach from the anesthesiologists may have sufficed in the past, today's anesthesiologists should take an extremely active role in OR management. Real life has demonstrated and management courses teach that strong leadership is necessary for any group to achieve their stated goals. Anesthesiologists should adopt a leading role among the other constituent personnel in the OR team. Together, anesthesiologists, surgeons, OR nurses and technicians, and, increasingly, professional administrators/managers need to determine who is best qualified to be a leader in the day-to-day management of the operating room. Clearly, different groups have different perspectives. However, anesthesiologists are in the best position to see the "big picture," both overall and on any given day. Surgeons are commonly elsewhere before and after their individual cases; nurses and administrators may lack the medical knowledge to make appropriate, timely decisions, often "on the fly." It is the anesthesiologist with the insight, overview, and unique perspective who is best qualified to provide leadership in an OR community. Anesthesiologists must step forward and aggressively seek involvement at the highest level possible in the OR at which they practice. The subsequent recognition and appreciation from the other groups (especially hospital administration) will clearly establish the anesthesiologists as concerned physicians genuinely interested in the welfare of the OR and the institution. Failure to be involved in any leadership role not only negates the desired image of anesthesiologists as concerned physicians, but also may result in a loss of autonomy in practice or a loss of support from the other groups in the OR and the institution overall.

By nature, an OR is a society unto itself with its various constituent groups, interdepartmental dynamics, and uniquely high levels of stress all defining the ebb and flow of the workplace. The essential groups: anesthesia providers, surgeons, OR staff (usually comprising nursing, scrub technicians and other support personnel), hospital administrators and/or professional managers need to develop a working relationship to survive. As diverse as the priorities of these various groups seem, it is imperative that these groups move beyond simple cooperation and construct a friendly efficient work environment that provides high-quality patient care. Because the spectrum of operating rooms varies significantly from the largest regional teaching hospital to the smallest freestanding ambulatory care center, it is difficult to provide anything but the broadest of guidelines for OR management. However, despite each facility's distinct characteristics, many of these principles can be implemented at virtually all institutions.

Organization

Traditionally (although exceptions may be increasing), in virtually every OR setting, neither the anesthesia providers nor the surgeons have been employees of the institution housing the OR. Rarely did either group/service report to a central authority. Even when one or both constituents were employees, they reported through their respective chiefs/chairmen to the chief of the medical staff, not to a hospital administration. Consequently, a natural division existed between the hospital (OR) staff and the physicians practicing there. Anesthesia providers were commonly thrust into a position of being the arbitrator between the surgeons and the OR staff, balancing what both those parties considered reasonable, desirable, and possible.

The symbiotic relationship between anesthesia providers and surgeons remains unchanged. Both groups recognize this fact and also the common goal of having the operating room function in a safe, expeditious manner. The age-old question "Who is in charge of the Operating Room?" still confronts most hospitals/institutions. Because some anesthesia groups are subsidized by the hospital, the OR organization in such cases has changed accordingly. Many hospital administrators want to have input regarding "Who's in charge of the OR?" with an eye to increasing efficiency and throughput while reducing cost. Their wishes have an even added significance when more of their dollars are involved through the anesthesiology group subsidy. Sometimes there can be no real answer to "Who's in charge?" because of the complexity of the interpersonal relationships in the OR. Some institutions have a professional manager (often a former OR RN) whose sole job is to organize and run the OR. This individual may be vested with enough authority to be recognized by all as the person in charge. Other institutions ostensibly have a "medical director of the OR." However, the implications to the surgeons that an anesthesiologist is in charge, or vice versa, have caused many institutions to abandon the title or retain the position but assign no authority to it. In such instances, institutions usually resolve disputes through some authority with a physician's perspective. If there is no medical director with authority to make decisions stick, central authority usually resides with the Operating Room Committee, most often populated by physicians, senior nurses, and administrators. Every operating room has this forum for major policy and fiscal decisions. As part of committee function, the standard practices of negotiation, diplomacy, and lobbying for votes are regularly carried out. The impact of such an OR committee varies widely among institutions.

Despite the constantly changing dynamics of the OR management and the frequent major frustrations, anesthesiologists should pursue a greater role in day-to-day management in every possible applicable practice setting. An anesthesiologist who is capable of facilitating the start of cases with minimal delays and solving problems "on the fly" as they arise will be in an excellent position to serve his or her department. Succeeding in this role will have a dramatic positive impact on all the OR constituents. The surgeons will be less concerned about "Who's in charge?" because their cases are getting done. The hospital administration will welcome the effort because they want something extra in return for any money they are now giving to the anesthesiology groups as a subsidy. Furthermore, the OR Committee (or whatever system for dispute resolution is in place) is still functional and has not been circumvented (and will be thankful for the absence of disputes needing resolution).

Some institutions use the term "clinical director of the OR." The person awarded this designation should be a senior-level individual with firsthand knowledge of the OR environment and function. Anesthesiologists have a better understanding of the perioperative process. They possess the medical knowledge to make appropriate decisions. Their intimate association with surgeons and their patients allows them to best allocate resources. According to a survey conducted by the American Association of Clinical Directors (AACD) in 2002, 71% of the respondents reported that an anesthesiologist was designated as the clinical director of the OR.[52]

Those in lines of authority must possess the corresponding responsibility. Who has power over who will determine a great deal about the function of an individual OR. A classic example involves pefusionists for cardiac surgery. In some circumstances, they are employed by the hospital; in others, by the cardiac surgeons; in a few, by the anesthesia group; and some are independent contractors. The organizational logistics of each of the above scenarios need to fulfill the standard functions regarding call, work shifts, policy and procedure for cardiac bypass operations, equipment purchasing, and so forth. Each institution develops its own method for dealing with these issues. Sometimes the system utilized falters and one of the constituents out of power offers to step in (or just seizes control) to rectify the deteriorated situation. Then the process begins anew, under new management. These changes are frequently viewed as healthy for the perfusionists in that previous unresolved issues can be settled (including often a pay raise). The OR that has no such cyclical changes because a very strong central authority prevents them is commonly an unappealing place to work. Problems get brushed aside or ignored until they seem to explode with vengeance onto the scene. The nature of surgery and working in an operating room creates significant stress on the people employed there. This fact remains underappreciated by the outside world but also becomes commonplace for those who work there because the stress is constant and therefore routine. Until an individual steps aside and reflects for a moment, he or she may never realize the odd nature of their workplace and changes they've been through. Because of this burnout-prone, high-stress environment, those in charge need to be understanding, sympathetic, facilitative, and often somewhat parental to all involved. The resulting collegial and supportive work environment will pay many dividends over the long run for all involved.

Other aspects that involve lines of authority also impact the daily function of the OR. Almost always, the OR staff are employees of the hospital/facility. Frequently, the hospital is perceived as being primarily concerned with containing cost and generating more revenue regardless of the situation. From a purely business perspective, paying overtime is more cost efficient than hiring additional staff to open more operating rooms at 7 AM. This fact often works against the desires of surgeons and anesthesiologists who want more flexibility in their scheduling ability. The topic of adequate nursing and technical support personnel and function frequently dominates many OR committees. The anesthesiologist, whether clinical director or not, who has established his or her reputation as one who has the operating room's best interest in mind is in a good position to help resolve these disputes. Gone are the days when many anesthesia groups/departments have surplus funds to hire additional anesthesia technicians from their budget to help the hospital, demonstrating team spirit, promoting efficiency, and thus ensuring a healthy working relationship with administration. Sometimes, still, surgeons who feel constrained by the lack of institutional support may be able to get together and fund positions (usually dedicated scrub technicians) from their practice income. Regardless of the source of the problem, or its ultimate solution, it remains imperative that all members of the OR "family," led by the responsible anesthesiologists, practice a spirit of cooperation.

Contact and Communication

An important issue for the anesthesia providers in any OR setting is who among the group will be the contact person to interact with the OR and its related administrative functions. In situations where everyone is an independent contractor, there may be a titular chief who by design is the contact person. The anesthesiologist in this role commonly changes yearly to spread the duties among all the members. Large groups or departments that function as the sole providing entity for that hospital/facility often identify an individual as the contact person to act as the voice for the department. Furthermore, these same groups delineate someone on a daily basis to be the clinical director, or the person "running the board." Frequently, this position is best filled by one of a small dedicated fraction of the group (three people, for example) rather than rotating the responsibility among every member of the group. Experienced "board runners" have an instinctually derived better perspective on the nuances of managing the operating schedule in real time. Certain procedures may require specific training (e.g., TEE skills) that not all members of the group possess. Clearly, changes sometimes have to be made to match the ability of the anesthesia provider and the requirements of the procedure when urgent or emergent cases are posted. Another benefit of a very small number of daily clinical directors is a relative consistency in the application of OR policies, particularly in relationship to the scheduling of cases, especially add-ons. One of the most frustrating aspects to both surgeons and OR personnel is unpredictability and inconsistency in the decisions made by the anesthesia group/department members. A patient deemed unacceptable for surgery by anesthesiologist X on Monday may be perfectly acceptable, in the same medical condition, for anesthesiologist Y on Tuesday. Disagreements are inevitable in any large group. However, day-to-day OR function may be hampered by a large number of these types of circumstances. Having one member of a very small group in charge will lead to more consistency in this process, especially if the "board runner/clinical director" has the authority to switch personnel to accommodate the situation. Without stifling individual practices, philosophies, and comfort levels, a certain amount of consistency applied to similar clinical scenarios will improve OR function immeasurably. These few dedicated directors should be able to accomplish both goals better than a large rotating group.

Another important aspect of OR organization is materials management. The availability of the required supplies for the safe administration of anesthesia needs to be maintained at all times. Usually, the institutional component of the anesthesia service staffs and maintains a location containing the specific supplies unique to the practice of anesthesia ("the workroom"). Objectives necessary for efficient materials management include the standardization of equipment, drugs, and supplies. Avoidance of duplication, volume purchasing, and inventory reduction are also worthwhile. There needs to be coordination with the OR staff as to who is responsible for acquisition of routine hospital supplies such as syringes, needles, tubing, and intravenous fluids. Decisions as to which brands of which supplies to purchase ideally should be made as a group. Often, when several companies compete against each other in an open market, lower prices are negotiable. These negotiations may occur between the anesthesia providers and the hospital administration, or by the physician components of the OR Committee. In many cases, however, hospitals belong to large buying groups that determine what brands and models of equipment and supplies will be available, with no exceptions possible except at greatly increased cost. Sometimes, this is false economy if the provided items are inferior (cheap) or annoying and, for example, if it routinely takes opening three or four IV cannulae in the process of starting a preop IV as opposed to the higher quality and reliable single one that may cost more per cannula but is less expensive overall because so many fewer will be used. Dispassionate presentation of such logic by a respected "team-player" senior anesthesiologist to the OR Committee or director of materials management may help resolve such conundrums.

Scheduling Cases

Anesthesiologists need to participate in the OR scheduling process at their facility or institution. In some facilities the scheduling office and the associated clerical personnel work under the anesthesia group. Commonly, scheduling falls under the OR staff's responsibility. Direct control of the schedule usually resides with the OR supervisor or charge person, frequently a nurse. Whatever the arrangements, the anesthesia group must have a direct line of communication with the scheduling system. The necessary number of anesthesia providers that must be supplied often changes on a daily basis per the caseload and sometimes due to institutional policy decisions. After-hours calls must be arranged, policy changes factored in, and additions/subtractions to the surgical load (day to day, week to week, and long term as surgical practices come and go in that OR) dealt with as well. These issues are important even when all the anesthesia providers are independently contracted and are not affiliated with each other. In such situations, the titular chief of anesthesia should be the one to act as the link to the scheduling system. When the anesthesia group/department functions as a single entity, the chairman/chief, clinical director, or appointed spokesperson will be the individual who represents his or her group at meetings where scheduling decisions are made in conjunction with the OR supervisors, surgeons, and hospital administrators.

There are as many different ways to create scheduling policies as there are operating room suites. Most hospitals/facilities follow patterns established over the years. Despite all the efforts directed toward its creation, the OR schedule, both weekly time allotments and day-to-day scheduling of specific cases, remains one of the most contentious subjects for the Operating Room Committee or whatever body presides over the operating room. Recognizing the fact that it is impossible to satisfy completely even a moderate percentage of the surgeons involved, the anesthesia group should endeavor to facilitate the process as much as possible. Initially, anesthesiologists need to be sympathetic toward all the surgeons' desires/demands (stated or implied) and attempt to coordinate these requests with the institution's ability to provide rooms, equipment, and staff. Second, the anesthesia group should make every possible effort to provide enough anesthesia services and personnel to meet realistically the goals of the institution. In light of the current shortage of anesthesia providers in this country, these efforts need to be made with a great deal of open communication among all contingencies of the OR Committee as well as every member of the anesthesia group. Failure to do so will result in hard feelings, misunderstandings, and resignations among the anesthesia providers. "After all," they may claim, "the hospital across town will pay me more money for fewer hours!"

Regarding scheduling, surgeons essentially fall into one of three groups. One group wants to operate any time they can get their cases scheduled. This group wants the operating room open 24/7 and doesn't understand why they can't do their case whenever they want to. Another larger group wants "first case of the day" as often as possible so they can get to their offices. A smaller third group wants either the first time slot or an opening following that time slot, a several-hour hiatus, then to return to the OR after office hours to complete additional cases; usually starting after 5 PM. Clearly a compromise among these disparate constituencies must be reached. Obviously, none of these groups can be completely satisfied at the same institution. Anesthesiologists who approach the OR Committee regarding this dilemma with a nonconfrontational attitude will greatly facilitate agreement on a compromise. There will always be a certain amount of both overt and covert politicking by surgeons regarding scheduling.

Types of Schedules

The majority of operating rooms utilize either block scheduling (preassigned guaranteed OR time for a surgeon or surgical service to schedule cases prior to an agreed upon cutoff time, e.g., 24 or 48 hours before) or open scheduling (first come, first serve). Most large institutions have a combination of both. Block scheduling inherently contains several advantageous aspects for creating a schedule. Block scheduling allows for more predictability in the daily OR function as well as an easy review of utilization of allotted time. Historic utilization data should be reviewed with surgeons, OR staff, and the OR Committee to determine its validity. Many operating suites have found it useful to assemble rather comprehensive statistics about what occurs in each OR. Some computerized scheduling systems (see below) are part of a larger computerized perioperative information management system that automatically generates statistics. Graphic examples are 13-month "statistical control charts" or "run charts" that show the number of cases, number of OR minutes used for those cases (and when: in block, exceeding block, evenings, nights, weekends, etc.), number of cancellations (and multiple other related parameters if desired) by service, by individual surgeon, and total for the current month and the 12 prior months, always with "control limits" (usually two standard deviations from the 13-month moving average) clearly indicated. All these data are valuable in that they generate a clear picture of what is actually going on in the OR rather than just listening to surgeons claim they are busier than ever or supervisors claim they have staff who sit around idle half the day. It is also extremely valuable in that block time allocation should be reviewed periodically and adjusted based on changes, degree of utilization, and projected needs. Inflexible block time scheduling can create a major point of contention if the assigned blocks are not regularly reevaluated. The surgeon or surgical service with the early starting block that habitually runs beyond his or her block time will create problems for the following cases. If this surgeon were made to schedule into the later block on a rotating basis, delays in his or her start caused by others may provoke improved accuracy of his or her subsequent early case postings. Adjustments in availability of block time can also be made in the setting of the "release time," the time prior to the operative date that a given block is declared not full and becomes available for open scheduling. Surgeons prefer as late a release time as possible to maintain their access to their OR block time. However, unused reserved block time wastes resources and prevents another service from scheduling. While a single "release time" rarely fits all circumstances, negotiating service-specific "release times" may lead to improved satisfaction for all. In the ideal system, enough OR time and equipment should exist to provide for each surgical service's genuine needs, while retaining the ability to add to the schedule (via open scheduling) as needed. Such an environment does not exist. Invariably, surgical demand exceeds available block and open time, leading services to request additional block time. When this time is not granted, services perversely then schedule procedures in open time before filling their block time. Surgeons who prefer open time would then be shut out of OR time. Open scheduling may reward those surgeons who run an efficient service, but it also may be a source of problems to those surgeons who have a significant portion of their service arrive unscheduled, for example, orthopedic surgeons. Some degree of flexibility will be necessary whichever system is used. The anesthesia group should adopt a neutral position in these discussions while being realistic about what can be accomplished given the number of operating rooms and the length of the normal operating day.

The handling of the urgent/emergent case posting precipitates a great deal of discussion in most OR environments. There are as many methods to handle this dilemma as there are institutions that provide emergency services. No studies allow determination of exactly what rate of OR utilization is the most cost-effective. However, many institutions subscribe to the following parameters: adjusted utilization rates averaging below 70% are not associated with full use of available block time, wasting resources, while rates above 90% are frequently associated with the need for overtime hours.[53] Different OR constituencies have different comfort zones for degrees of utilization (see Table 2-6). Most institutions cannot afford to have one or two operating rooms staffed and waiting unless there is a reliable steady supply of late open-schedule additions, that is, urgents/emergencies, during the regular work day. A previously agreed upon, clear algorithm for the acceptance and ordering of these cases will need to be adopted. In general, critical life-threatening emergencies and elective add-ons are fairly straightforward and at the two ends of the spectrum. The critical emergency goes in the next available room whereas the elective case gets added to the end of the schedule. The so-called "urgent" patient requires the most judgment. Individual services should provide guidelines and limitations for their expected "urgent cases." These "add-on case policy" guidelines[54] should be common knowledge to everyone involved in running the operating room. Consequently, these cases, such as ectopic pregnancies, open fractures, the patient with obstructed bowels, and eye injuries, can then be triaged and inserted into the elective schedule as needed with minimal discussion from the delayed surgeon. The surgeons whose "urgent" case is presented as one that must immediately bump another service's patient, yet could wait several hours if it is their own patient that will be delayed, will have to face their own previously agreed-upon standards in a future OR Committee meeting. A simple way to express one logical policy for "urgent" cases (e.g., acute appendicitis, unruptured ectopic pregnancy, intestinal obstruction) is: (1) bump the same surgeon's elective scheduled case; (2) if none, bump a scheduled case on the same service (GYN, General A, etc.); (3) if none, bump a scheduled case from an open-schedule surgical service; and (4) if none, bump a scheduled case from a block-schedule service.[54] Some institutions require the attending surgeon of the posted urgent/emergent patient to speak personally with the surgeon of any bumped case, as opposed to letting the anesthesiologist board runner or charge nurse take the heat for delaying a scheduled case.

Another area of burgeoning growth that must be accounted for in the daily work schedule is the non–operating room "off-site" diagnostic test, or therapeutic intervention that requires anesthesia care. In many instances these procedures replace operations that, in the recent past, would have been posted on the OR schedule as urgent/emergency cases. For example, cerebral aneurysm coiling and CT guided abscess drainage, among other procedures, are done in imaging suites. However, they do require anesthesia care from anesthesia personnel, albeit in a new

TABLE 2-6

OR UTILIZATION "COMFORT ZONES" OF THE OR PERSONNEL CONSTITUENCIES

	■ FACILITY ADMINISTRATION	■ ANESTHESIOLOGY GROUP	■ OR STAFF	■ SURGEONS
Block time utilization				
>100%	++	−−	−−−	−−−−
85–100%	++++	++	−	−−−
70–84%	+++	++++	+	+/−
55–69%	+	+++	+++	++
<55%	−−	−	++	++++

"+" = favorable; "−" = unfavorable
Reprinted with permission from American Society of Anesthesiologists: Mazzei WJ. *OR management: state of the art. 2003 conference on practice management*. Park Ridge, IL: American Society of Anesthesiologists; 2003:65.

location. Additionally, depending on distances involved and logistics, it may even be necessary to assign two people, a primary provider and an attending, exclusively to that remote location when, had the case come to the OR, the attending may have been able to cover another or other cases also. Hospital administration or the OR Committee may try to view these cases as unrelated to OR function and, thus, purely a problem for the anesthesia group to solve. These cases must be treated with the same methodology regarding access and prioritization as all other OR procedures. To apportion hospital-based anesthesia resources reasonably, these "off-site" procedures should be subject to the same guidelines and processes as any other OR posting. Most institutions have added at least one extra anesthetizing location to their formal operating schedule to designate these "off-site" procedures (occasionally with an imaginative name such as "road show," "outfield," or "safari"). For many of these "off-site" cases, there is little or no reimbursement for anesthesia care. Most government plans and insurance carriers will probably not pay for the claustrophobic adult to receive a MAC or even a general anesthetic for an obviously needed diagnostic MRI, as much as the patient, the surgeon, and the hospital benefit from the test results. The anesthesia group, the OR Committee, and the hospital administration need to reach compromises regarding "off-site" procedures, regarding scheduling, allocation of anesthesia resources that would otherwise go to the OR, and even subsidization of the personnel costs to continue this obviously beneficial service.

Computerization

Computerized scheduling will likely benefit every operating room regardless of size. Computerization allows for a faster more efficient method of case posting than any handwritten system. Changes to the schedule can be made quickly without any loss of information. Rearranging the daily schedule is much simpler on a computer than erasing and rewriting on a ledger. Furthermore, most hospitals have adopted a computer-determined time for a given surgical procedure for that particular surgeon. Commonly, this time is the average of the last 10 of the specific procedure (e.g., total knee replacement) with the potential to add a modifier (e.g., it is a redo) that shows a material difference in the projected time length (almost always longer) for one particular patient. Suppose surgeon X has a block time of 8 hours on a given day and wants to schedule four procedures in that allotted time. The computerized scheduling program looks at surgeon X's past performances and determines a projected length for each of the procedures that are identified to the computer, usually by CPT-4 codes or possibly some other code developed locally for frequent procedures done by surgeon X. (Note that the recorded time length includes the turnover time, thus making the case time definition from the time the patient enters the OR until the time any following patient enters that OR [unless an "exception" is entered specifically for an unusual circumstance].) The use of agreed-upon codes instead of just text descriptions helps ensure accuracy because it eliminates any need for the scheduling clerk to guess what the surgeon intends to do. Bookings should not be taken without the accompanying codes. The computer then decides whether surgeon X will finish the four procedures in the allotted block time. If the computer concludes that the fourth case would finish significantly (the definition of which can be determined and entered into the program) beyond the available block time, it will not accept the fourth case into that room's schedule on that particular day. The surgeon will accept the computer's assigned times and adjust accordingly, planning only three cases, or appeal for an "exception" based on some factor not in the booking that is claimed will materially decrease the time needed for at least one of the four cases, which the surgeon must explain to the "exception czar" (anesthesiology clinical director or OR charge nurse) of the day. Note that, routinely, surgeons generally object to having actual past turnover times counted in the case length average. An alternative method has the computer simply add (to each case except the last) a projected turnover time that is agreed upon by all involved at an (often contentious) OR committee meeting. Computerizing the scheduling process significantly reduces any personal biases and smoothes out the entire operating day. The long-standing ritual of late-afternoon disputes between the surgeons and the anesthesia group and/or OR staff whether to start the last case or not may be eliminated or at least reduced by this more realistic prospective OR scheduling method.

There are many variables to consider in any OR scheduling system. The patient population served and the nature of the institution dictate the overall structure of the OR schedule. Inner-city Level 1 Trauma Centers must accommodate emergencies on a regular basis, 24 hours a day. These centers are unlikely to create a workable schedule more than a day in advance. An ambulatory surgery center serving plastic surgery patients may see only the rare emergency bring-back bleeding patient. Their schedule may be accurate many days in advance with a high degree of expectation that the patient will arrive on time properly prepared for surgery. The anesthesia group at this ambulatory center may rarely have to make changes to the schedule, allowing them to proceed with a fairly predictable daily workload. At the inner-city trauma hospital, a great deal of flexibility and constant communication with the surgeons will be required in an attempt to get the cases done in a reasonable time frame with the inherent constraints placed on the OR staff's resources and the time available. These two extreme examples from opposite ends of the scheduling-process spectrum can provide guidelines for the majority of the institutions that fall somewhere in between. Independent of where an individual operating theater falls in this spectrum, open communication and an honest discussion among the three principle groups involved in OR scheduling is critical in maintaining a smooth functioning operating room. Avoiding the anesthesia–surgery "us versus them" mentality helps keep the schedule on track. Surgeons are frequently viewed as having totally unrealistic expectations of what the operating room is capable of accomplishing. Anesthesiologists are sometimes accused of trying to avoid work when a case is canceled for legitimate medical reasons or turnover between cases is perceived as too slow. The OR staff often feels they are being pushed too hard. These conflicting and contentious attitudes should not and need not dominate the operating room environment. When each of the three contingencies genuinely appreciates the others' points of view and everyone starts working toward a logical common goal—safe, efficient, expedient patient care—then the already stressful OR environment will be a much better place to work.

Beyond open communication, how best to work toward this mutual understanding depends on the particulars of the people involved and the environment, but some ORs report benefits from team-building exercises, leadership retreats, and even OR-wide social events. ORs with a particularly malignant history of finger-pointing and bad feelings among the personnel groups may constitute one of the few instances an outside consultant really may be valuable in that there are workplace psychologists who specialize in analyzing dysfunctional work environments and implementing changes to improve the situation for all involved.

Anesthesia Preoperative Evaluation Clinic

An anesthesia preoperative evaluation clinic (APEC) that provides a comprehensive perioperative medical evaluation usually results in a more efficient running of the operating room schedule.[55,56] Unanticipated cancellations or delays are avoided when the anesthesia group evaluates complex patients prior to surgery. Even if the patient arrives to the OR on time the day of surgery, inadequate preoperative clearance mandating the ordering of additional tests will consume precious OR time during the delay waiting for results. Cancellations or delays adversely affect the efficiency of any operating room. Subsequent cases in that room, whether for the same or a different surgeon, may get significantly delayed or forced to be squeezed into an already busy schedule on another day. The financial impact of delays or cancellations on the institution is considerable. Revenue is lost with no offsetting absence of expenses. Worse, expenses may actually increase when overtime has to be paid, or the sterile equipment has to be repackaged after having been opened for the canceled procedure. Even worse, the inconvenienced patient and/or surgeon go to another facility.

Optimal timing for preoperative evaluation should be related to the institution's scheduling preferences, patient convenience, and the overall health of the patient. Earlier completion of the preop evaluation may not reduce the overall cancellation rate when compared to a more proximate evaluation. However, an early evaluation and clearance may well provide a larger pool of patients available to place on the OR schedule (block or open), resulting in a more efficient use of OR time. Additionally, a protocol-driven evaluation process can anticipate possible need for time-consuming investigations (such as a cardiology evaluation for the patient with probable angina). Early recognition of a failed preoperative test allows time for another patient to be moved into the now-vacant time slot. Also, early identification of certain problems requiring special care on the day of surgery (for example, preoperative epidural or PA catheter placement) should lead to fewer unanticipated delays. Unfortunately, many issues precipitating delays are discovered on the day of surgery. Some of these preventable delays are unrelated to the patients' health status. Seemingly simple issues such as verification of a ride home, or incomplete financial information also contribute to unexpected delays. A properly functioning APEC may be able to eliminate a majority of these annoying causes of unnecessary delays.

Regardless of the institutional specifics surrounding the service provided by the APEC, further cost savings can be obtained through its proper usage by the anesthesia group. With only a basic protocol to go on, commonly a full "shotgun" battery of tests is ordered by surgeons to "cover all the bases" for every patient from a specific surgeon or surgical service in the hopes of avoiding last-minute delays on the day of surgery. The APEC frequently reduces dramatically the number of pre-op tests performed by focusing on which diagnostic tests and medical consults are really required for any specific patient. In some circumstances, the APEC may also function as an additional source of revenue for the anesthesia group when a formal preop consult on a complicated patient is ordered well in advance by the surgeon, in the same manner as would have otherwise been directed to a primary care physician for "clearance for surgery." Securing a genuinely relevant medical evaluation of the patient prior to anesthesia and surgery with its subsequent reduction of wasted OR resources and cost containment are not the only benefits of an APEC. The ability to centralize pertinent information including admission precertification/clearance, financial data, diagnostic and laboratory results, consult reports, and preoperative recommendations improves OR function by decreasing the time spent searching for all these items after changes have been made to the schedule. Patient and family education performed by the APEC frequently leads to an increase in patients' overall satisfaction of the perioperative experience. In addition, patient anxiety may be reduced secondary to the more in-depth contact possible inherent in the APEC process when compared to anesthesia practitioners meeting an ambulatory outpatient for the first time in an OR holding area immediately prior to surgery. The APEC model enables the anesthesia group to be more active and proactive in the perioperative process, improving their relations with the other OR constituents. By taking a leading role in establishing and running an APEC, the anesthesia group enhances its reputation as a cooperative, concerned entity by significantly contributing to high-quality patient care as well as the overall efficiency of the operating room function.

Anesthesiology Personnel Issues

In light of the current and future shortage of anesthesia care providers, managing and maintaining a stable supply of anesthesia practitioners promises to dominate the OR landscape for years to come. The 2002 shortfall of anesthesiologists was calculated at 100 to 3,800 and the estimate for 2005 was 500 to 3,900, the range dependent on service demand growth.[34] A survey of hospital administrators revealed that nearly 60% of them are actively recruiting anesthesiologists; over half of them have done so for more than six months.[57] The lean resident recruiting years of the mid- to late 1990's continue to impact the profession. Even though applications to anesthesiology residencies rebounded significantly, it will take many years of relatively large numbers of anesthesia residency graduates to reverse this trend. Furthermore, the supply of nonphysician anesthesia providers is also dwindling. With the aging population of nurse anesthetists and the limited number of applications to schools in that profession, as well as the very limited number of training facilities for anesthesiology assistants, the overall supply of anesthesia providers remains inadequate to meet current and, at least, short-term future demands. The need for anesthesia groups to create a flexible, attractive work environment to retain providers who might leave or retire will continue to increase.

A related issue is consideration of what is a reasonable work load for an anesthesiologist and how best to measure,
9 if possible, the clinical productivity of an anesthesia group/department. These questions have been the subject of considerable discussion.[58–61] Subjects involve comparisons among members of the anesthesiology group, both against outside benchmarks and also against each other as well as the group as a whole against others, if possible. Beyond the simple number of FTEs, cases, and OR minutes, consideration of factors such as the nature of the facility, types of surgical practice, patient acuity, and speed of the surgeons must be incorporated to allow fair comparisons. Thoughtful filtering of resulting data should take place before dissemination of the aggregate information to all members of a group because of the understandable extreme sensitivity among stressed and fatigued anesthesiologists to a suggestion that they are not working as hard as their group/department peers.

Except in highly unusual circumstances, flexible scheduling of anesthesia providers and also fulfilling the demands placed on the group by the institution continues to be a constant balancing act. This demand assumes added significance because institutions now subsidize many anesthesia groups. Even when a majority of providers in a facility are independent contractors where it is required that a specific surgeon request their services, there are time conflicts ranging from no one at all being available to unwanted downtime. When the anesthesia group/department accepts the responsibility of providing anesthesia services for an institution, they must schedule enough providers for that OR suite on each given day. Ideally, a sufficient number of providers would be hired so that there would always be enough personnel to staff the minimum number of rooms scheduled on any given day, as well as after-hours call duty. This situation rarely exists because it would be financially disadvantageous to have an excess number of providers with no clinical activity. Having exactly the right number of anesthesia providers in a group for the clinical load works well until one (or more) of them is out with an unplanned absence such as an extended illness or a family emergency. Many academic departments have a natural buffer with some clinicians assigned intervals of nonclinical time for research, teaching, or administrative duties. However, repeated loss of these nonclinical days because of inadequate clinical staffing in the OR leads to undermining the academic/research mission of the department. Continued loss of this time will eventually lead to resignations, thus eliminating the original buffer. Consequently, anesthesia groups/departments need to anticipate available clinical personnel and match them to the operating room demands. Ideally, this information should be accurate for several months into the future. Meeting this specification has become more difficult in the recent past. With sudden major realignments of insurance carriers, changes in managed care, and the constant bidding war for anesthesia providers, predicting both personnel availability and the corresponding operating room case load any length of time into the future may require a crystal ball. There is no easy answer to this dilemma and no clear solution presents itself, except to acknowledge that the situation exists and is likely to continue for the foreseeable future. Hospital administrators must offer reasonable assurances to the anesthesia group providing service that a given OR utilization rate is likely, as well as accurate data regarding reimbursement (payer mix and any package contracts negotiated by the hospital). This data must be provided accurately and updated frequently if a health care institution is to acquire and retain an anesthesia group staffed with the personnel to meet the expected demands.

Timing

Each operating environment has its own personnel scheduling system and expectations for the anesthesia group. Daily coordination between the anesthesia group's clinical director and the OR supervisor permits the construction of a reasonable schedule showing the number of operating rooms that day and when the schedule expects each of them to finish. Invariably, some cases take longer than anticipated, or add-ons are posted requiring the OR to run into the late afternoon or early evening. Many anesthesia providers accept this occurrence as a matter of course. Few anesthesia providers will tolerate this sequence of events as an essentially daily routine whether they are paid overtime or not. These practitioners become exhausted and resent the burdens continuously placed on them. If the OR schedule is such that add-ons frequently occur and elective cases run well into the evening, many anesthesia providers will opt to protect their personal and family time and cut back their working hours or resign. Neither would be welcome in such a tight market. Under these circumstances, hiring additional personnel who are scheduled to arrive at a later time, for example, 11:00 AM, and then providing lunch relief and staying late (e.g., 7:30 PM or later if needed) to finish the schedule may well be a very worthwhile investment.

Another possible solution to the demands of an extended OR schedule on an anesthesia group's personnel may revolve around employing part-time anesthesia providers. Part-time opportunities could enhance a group's ability to attract additional staff. According to a *New York Times* survey, many medical practitioners (12% of male physicians and 25% of female physicians) currently work fewer than 40 hours a week.[57] In the past, a disproportionately high percentage of women chose anesthesiology as a career. In 1970, women represented 7.6% of the physician population but were 14% of anesthesiologists; much more recently, they make up 45% of the physician population and only 20% of anesthesiologists, proportionately a significant reduction.[62] Beyond the basic demographic shift among all physicians, one likely partial explanation for the decreased number of women anesthesiologists may be the lack of part-time positions, which will hamper an anesthesia groups' ability to attract and keep at least some of the female anesthesia providers.

Scheduling after-hours coverage also adds to the personnel difficulties facing the anesthesia group. The variations of call schemes are endless. The nature of the institution and the workload determine the degree of late night coverage. Major referral centers and Level 1 trauma centers require in-house primary providers. If these providers include residents and/or nurse anesthetists, then the supervising attending staff will also be in-house 24 hours a day. In other less intense settings, the primary provider will be in house with the attending taking call from home (within the boundary of a predetermined maximum arrival time, usually 30 minutes). The number of providers required to take call (in-house or back-up) is always a never-ending topic of animated discussion. Should the call team staff for a minimum, average, or potentially possible number of cases, with a call-in list as further backup? A common solution employed at many institutions is to staff the evening/night call shifts for an average workload, recognizing that on some occasions there will be idle operating rooms, and on other nights, the surgical demand will exceed the call team's numbers, resulting in a scramble. Obviously if this occurs frequently, changes are needed in the number of staff on call.

There are also medicolegal issues surrounding the call team's availability. At a small community hospital with a limited number of independent attending practitioners, the practitioners may agree to cover call on a rotating basis. The individuals not on call are usually not obligated to the OR and may well be truly unreachable. What happens then when the on-call anesthesiologist is administering an anesthetic and another true emergency case arrives in the OR suite and the remaining staff anesthesiologists are legitimately unavailable? Does that anesthesiologist leave his or her current patient under the care of an operating room nurse and go next door to tend to a more acutely (possibly critically) ill patient? Should the patient be transferred from the ER to another (hopefully nearby) hospital? These questions have no easy answers. Clearly, those practitioners on the scene have to assess in real time the relative risks and benefits and make the difficult decisions. This example is but one of the many issues facing any call scheme, whatever the size of the facility and the number of people involved, and the possible scenarios that exist in staffing an operating suite.

A related scheduling issue regarding the evening and night call assignments revolves around what to do with the call team that has worked the previous night. Should they provide anesthesia care the next day? As always, the answers to this question are as varied as there are health care facilities. If the call duty requires the practitioner(s) frequently to work much or all of the night, leaving the individual(s) stressed and fatigued, they should not be required to work the next day during normal working hours. However, if that call team normally works most of the night, but they have not had any cases to do and were able to sleep, it is not unreasonable to expect such individuals to remain in the OR in the morning and help out as long as needed. A more complicated answer involves what to do when the call assignment rarely requires a long night's work and the on-call anesthesia providers routinely have rooms assigned to them the next day, but at least one person has just finished a difficult 24-hour shift being awake working all night. Does the group wish the practitioner to continue the scheduled daytime assignment with the intent of being relieved as soon as possible? Alternatively, should the practitioner go home, with the result of closing or delaying a lineup of scheduled cases, which will bring significant negative feedback to the anesthesiology group? Common sense and reason should guide everyone in such a circumstance. Anesthesia groups need to decide how to handle the possible call shift scenarios, with permutations and combinations, and clearly communicate prospectively their decisions to the OR Committee before any difficult decision has to be made one morning. As always, the medicolegal aspects of any decision such as this need to be taken into consideration. Whether or not fatigue was a factor, the practitioner who worked throughout the night before and appeared to contribute to an anesthetic catastrophe the next morning would have a very difficult defense in court. Further, the anesthesiology group may also be held liable in that their practice/policy was in place, allegedly authorizing the supposedly dangerous conduct.

Cost and Quality Issues

One of the more pervasive aspects of American medical care in today's environment is the drive to maintain and improve high-quality health care while reducing the cost of that care. Health care accounts for approximately 14% of the Gross Domestic Product, nearly triple the fraction a generation ago. Consequently, all physicians, including anesthesiologists, are urged constantly to include cost-consciousness in decisions balancing the natural desire to provide the highest possible quality of care with the overall priorities of both the health care system and the individual patient, all while facing increasingly limited resources.[63] Anesthesiologists remain a target for limiting health care expenditures. Anesthesia providers (directly and indirectly) have represented 3 to 5% of the total health care costs in the country.[64] Anesthesiologists are under more and more pressure to limit expenses. Complicated decisions are required regarding which patients are suitable for ambulatory surgery, what preoperative studies to order, what anesthetic drugs or technique is best for the patient, what monitors or equipment are reasonably required to run an OR, and the list goes on and on. Additionally, anesthesiologists must not lose sight of maintaining the quality of care in this ever-increasing cost-conscious environment in which there is intense production pressure to cut corners that is fueled by the "get away with it" mentality in which it is noted that the vast, vast majority of the time one does something inherently unsafe, nothing bad happens to the patient—setting up some subsequent patient for a potentially catastrophic adverse event when the pressured anesthesiologist does not "get away with it." With this as background, anesthesiologists legitimately can include economic considerations in their decision processes. When presented with multiple options to provide for therapeutic intervention or patient assessment, one should not automatically choose the more expensive approach (just to "cover all the bases") unless there is compelling evidence proving its value. Decisions that clearly materially increase cost should only be pursued when the benefit outweighs the risk. In anesthesia care as well as medicine in general, such decisions can be difficult regarding interventions that provide marginal benefit but contain significant cost increases.[65] To deliver high-quality anesthesia care, anesthesiologists are obliged to consider the goals of the planned intervention, the expectations of all of their customers (patients, surgeons, colleagues, hospital administrators, payers, etc.), and the costs of the anticipated care. Because cost containment initially requires accurate cost awareness, anesthesiologists need to find out in an organized manner, more than ever before, the actual costs and benefits of their anesthesia care techniques. Details will be unique to each practice setting. Because they will be excited that the anesthesiologists actually care, usually it is possible to get the cooperation of the facility administration's financial department members in researching and calculating the actual cost of anesthesia care so that thoughtful evaluations of potential reductions can be initiated.

Anesthesia drug expenses represent a small portion of the total perioperative costs. However, the great number of doses actually administered contributes substantially to aggregate total cost to the institution in actual dollars. Prudent drug selection combined with appropriate anesthetic technique can result in substantial savings. Reducing fresh gas flow from 5 L/minute to 2 L/minute wherever possible would save approximately $100 million annually in the United States.[66] While a majority of anesthesia providers usually attempt a practical approach to cost savings, they are more frequently faced with difficult choices regarding methods of anesthesia that likely produce similar outcomes but at substantially different cost. When comparing the total costs of more expensive anesthetic drugs and techniques to lesser expensive ones, many variables need to be added to the formula. The cost of anesthetic drugs needs to include the costs of additional equipment such as special vaporizers or extra infusion pumps and the associated maintenance. There are other indirect costs that may be difficult to quantitate and are commonly overlooked. Some of these indirect costs include: increased setup time, possibly increasing room turnover time, extended PACU recovery time, and additional expensive drugs required to treat side effects. Sometimes, more expensive techniques reduce indirect costs. A propofol infusion, while more expensive than vapor, commonly results in a decreased PACU stay for a short noninvasive procedure. If fewer PACU staff are needed or patient throughput is increased, the more expensive drug can reduce overall cost. Conversely, using comparatively expensive propofol for a long procedure definitely requiring postop admission to an ICU is hardly justified. The impact of shorter-acting drugs and those with fewer side effects is context specific. During long surgical procedures, such drugs may offer limited benefits over older less expensive longer-acting alternatives.[67] Under these conditions, advocating cost containment using educational efforts may decrease drug expenditures for several categories of drugs.[68] Drugs in the same therapeutic class have widely varying costs. The acquisition expenses may vary as much as 50-fold in some pharmacological categories. It is estimated that the 10 highest expenditure drugs account for more than 80% of the anesthetic drug costs at some institutions.[69] While newer more expensive drugs may be easier to use, no data exists to support or refute the hypothesis that these drugs provide a "better" anesthetic experience when compared to carefully titrated older less expensive longer-acting drugs in the same class. Many experienced clinicians feel that patients can awaken promptly using a wide variety of general anesthetic techniques when the agents are utilized optimally.

Understanding the cost–benefit ratio for many aspects of and around anesthesia care can be difficult at best. Even when published studies provide information evaluating the outcome of a particular new therapy or intervention, determination of the specific clinical relevance remains easier said than done. Sample size, statistics, methodology, and other analytic issues often confuse the reader, making it complex and difficult to scrutinize the study results and place them in their proper perspective. What may appear a large clinically relevant difference may assume lesser importance if the sample size was too small to achieve statistical significance. Furthermore, seemingly small changes may grow to high statistical significance if the sample size is large enough. Careful attention must be devoted to any study proposing a reduction in relative risk to the patient. For example, if intervention A is associated with a 25% actual reduction in the incidence of a complication, and intervention B is associated with a 4% actual reduction in the incidence of another complication, both could still be described as producing the same relative improvement despite different clinical application. This approach has profound importance for the analysis of cost-effectiveness. A specific anesthetic or antiemetic might need to be administered to just four patients to decrease one episode of postop nausea/vomiting (intervention A). On the other hand, one would have to use more than 100 costly new spinal needles to prevent one case of postdural puncture headache (intervention B). Calculating the minimum number required to achieve the reported effect helps the clinician determine cost-effectiveness of clinical alternatives.[2,70]

Independent of costs involved, analysis of patient outcomes relevant to the practice of anesthesia permits the anesthesiologist to establish which aspects of care deserve attention. Outcome measures are typically defined as those changes, either favorable or adverse, that occur in actual or potential health status after prior or concurrent care.[71] Health status changes include both physical and physiological parameters (such as death, cardiac arrest, length of PACU stay, postop myocardial infarction, or unexpected intensive care admission), as well as psychosocial functions (patient satisfaction, family issues, or resumption of normal life). Historically, a great deal of attention and money has been dedicated to reducing adverse clinical events. While limiting severe/catastrophic adverse effects remains a noble and worthy cause, anesthesia groups would be well served devoting a significant effort towards reducing common, non–life-threatening adverse events related to everyday OR anesthesia.[72,73] Improved quality of care and better patient satisfaction is a legitimate yardstick upon which to measure the value of anesthesia services. Focused efforts to avoid major adverse events may dominate an anesthesia group's attention, but it must be acknowledged that other factors, such as attitude and friendliness of the staff, may be equally if not more important than some clinical outcomes.[74] A reduction of serious adverse anesthetic outcomes has a variable economic impact on total costs, depending on different assumptions regarding case mix, the added expense of improving perioperative care and/or preventing complications, the frequency of adverse complications, and the relative costs of the uncomplicated surgery.[75] Nonetheless, reducing minor but common perioperative anesthesia related incidents and complications theoretically can be economically beneficial, since these are significant predictors of PACU utilization in terms of length of PACU stay.[76]

Evaluation of outcomes and their subsequent application to cost analysis can be derived from two principal sources, data published in the literature and data collected from experience. As noted, computerized information management systems are useful tools to track outcomes and analyze the impact on the cost–benefit ledger. Using the collated data, in the same manner as for OR utilization and case load, practitioners can readily apply a statistical process to evaluate outcomes in their practice, possibly including correlation with cost.[2] This information may take on added importance in that published incidence studies may not exist for the specific outcome an anesthesia group is searching for. Cause and effect diagrams can track the parameters involved in the process and relate them to the various outcomes desired. Multiple pertinent examples could be constructed from the now extensive body of literature on the factors contributing to postop nausea and vomiting and the various possible preventions and treatments, many of which involve very expensive medications. Of course, this can be done locally within an institution. Information would be collected and stored in the database. Ideally, the database would identify and track as many variables as needed/possible to delineate sources for possible improvement and its ultimate cost analysis. Once these sources for improvement and the ensuing cost impact are known, the anesthesia group can determine whether or not to pursue changing their practice. Outcomes related to adverse effects can also be monitored. If analysis reveals a significant difference in an adverse outcome among practitioners, after all the other variables such as surgeon, patient mix, and so on, are eliminated, the outcome database can investigate the anesthetic technique utilized by that practitioner. If significant variations are identified, that practitioner would be able to learn of these variations in a non-threatening manner since computer-derived data are used as opposed to a specific case analysis, which might lead that practitioner to feel singled out for public criticism.

Another relevant application of such statistical outcome analysis is its use to improve the quality of a health care process (e.g., the perioperative experience[2]) in general. The principles of continuous quality improvement promoted by Deming[77] are being applied widely in the health care industry. Deming's approach focuses on statistical analysis of quality assessment, specifically evaluating variations in outcome parameters that are deemed meaningful to the target population (e.g. patients anesthetized). Addressing the etiologies of outcome variations rather than indicting the health care process as a whole can help resolve problematical outcome issues discovered in the analysis. If the data reveal an outcome change for the worse, prompt evaluation of the processes involved should immediately ensue with the intention of identifying the cause. Steps to eliminate or reduce the undesired outcomes can be investigated and implemented. If a beneficial change appears, the process variations then responsible for the subsequent improvement should be identified and implemented in other areas if possible. The application of the spirit of this type of beneficial continuous quality assessment and resulting improvement, with or without elaborate statistical analysis, should be an integral ongoing component of every anesthesia practice.

CONCLUSION

Practice and operating room management in anesthesiology today is more complex and more important than ever before. Attention to details that previously either did not exist or were perceived as unimportant can likely make the difference between success and failure in anesthesiology practice.

Outlined here are basic descriptions and understandings of many different administrative, organizational, financial, and
10 personnel components and factors in the practice of anesthesiology. Ongoing significant changes in the health care system will provide a continuing array of challenges. Application of the principles presented here will allow anesthesiologists to extrapolate creatively from these basics to their own individual circumstances and then forge ahead in anesthesiology practice that is efficient, effective, productive, collegial, and even fun.

References

1. Mychaskiw G, Eichhorn JH: Practice Management. In Barash PG, Cullen BF, Stoelting RK (eds): Clinical Anesthesia (4th edition), p 25–50. Philadelphia, Lippincott Williams & Wilkins, 2001
2. Tuman KJ, Ivankovich AD: Value-Based Anesthesia Practice, Resource Utilization, and Operating Room Management. In Barash PG, Cullen BF, Stoelting RK (eds): Clinical Anesthesia (4th edition), p 97–118. Philadelphia, Lippincott Williams and Wilkins, 2001
3. American Society of Anesthesiologists: 2003–04 Manual for Anesthesia Department Organization and Management. Park Ridge, IL, ASA, 2003
4. American Society of Anesthesiologists: Anatomy of the Bargain: Sword, Shield, or Shackle? Park Ridge, IL, ASA, 1999

5. Gilbert B: Relating quality assurance to credentials and privileges. In Chapman-Cliburn G (ed): Risk Management and Quality Assurance: Issues and Interactions, p 79–83. Chicago, Joint Commission on the Accreditation of Hospitals, 1986
6. Peters JD, Fineberg KS, Kroll DA *et al*: Anesthesiology and the Law. Ann Arbor, MI, Health Administration Press, 1983
7. Gaba DM, Howard SK, Jump B: Production pressure in the work environment. Anesthesiology 81: 488, 1994
8. Eichhorn JH, Cooper JB, Cullen DJ *et al*: Anesthesia practice standards at Harvard: A review. J Clin Anesth 1: 56, 1988
9. American Society of Anesthesiologists Task Force on Postanesthetic Care: Practice Guidelines for Postanesthetic Care. Anesthesiology 96: 742, 2002
10. Hawkins JL (Chair) *et al*: Practice guidelines for obstetrical anesthesia. Anesthesiology 90: 600, 1999
11. American Society of Anesthesiologists Task Force on Pulmonary Artery Catheterization: Practice guidelines for pulmonary artery catheterization: an updated report by the American Society of Anesthesiologists Task Force on Pulmonary Artery Catheterization. Anesthesiology 99: 988, 2003
12. American Society of Anesthesiologists Task Force on Management of the Difficult Airway: Practice guidelines for management of the difficult airway: an updated report by the American Society of Anesthesiologists Task Force on Management of the Difficult Airway. Anesthesiology 98: 1269, 2003
13. Dans PE, Weiner JP, Otter SE: Peer review organizations: Promises and potential pitfalls. N Engl J Med 313: 1131, 1985
14. American Society of Anesthesiologists: Peer Review in Anesthesiology, p 105. Park Ridge, IL, ASA, 1993
15. Eichhorn JH: Anesthesia equipment: Checkout and quality assurance. In Ehrenwerth J, and Eisenkraft JB (eds.): Anesthesia Equipment: Principles and Applications, p 473–491. St. Louis, Mosby–Yearbook, 1992
16. Spooner RB, Kirby RR: Equipment-related anesthetic incidents. In Pierce EC, Cooper JB (eds): Analysis of Anesthetic Mishaps. International Anesthesiology Clinics 22(2): 133, 1984
17. Cooper JB, Newbower RS, Kitz RJ: An analysis of major errors and equipment failures in anesthesia management: considerations for prevention and detection. Anesthesiology 60: 34, 1984
18. Cooper JB, Newbower RS, Long CD *et al*: Preventable anesthesia mishaps: A study of human factors. Anesthesiology 49: 399, 1978
19. Lunn JN, Mushin WW: Mortality Associated with Anaesthesia. London, Nuffield Provincial Hospitals Trust, 1982
20. Duberman S, Wald A: An integrated quality control program for anesthesia equipment. In Chapman-Cliburn G (ed): Risk Management and Quality Assurance: Issues and Interactions, p 105–112. Chicago, Joint Commission on the Accreditation of Hospitals, 1986
21. HHS Publication No. (FDA) 85-4196. Food and Drug Administration, Center for Devices and Radiologic Health, Rockville, MD 20857, p 10
22. Eichhorn JH: Influence of practice standards on anesthesia outcome. In Desmonts JM (ed): Outcome After Anesthesia and Surgery. Bailliere's Clinical Anaesthesiology—International Practice and Research 6: 663, 1992
23. Eichhorn JH: Prevention of intraoperative anesthesia accidents and related severe injury through safety monitoring. Anesthesiology 70: 572, 1989
24. Keats AS: Anesthesia mortality in perspective. Anesth Analg 71: 113, 1990
25. Lagasse RS: Anesthesia safety: model or myth? Anesthesiology 97: 1609, 2002
26. Cooper JB, Gaba DM: No myth: anesthesia is a model for addressing patient safety. Anesthesiology 97: 1335, 2002
27. Bacon AK: Death on the table: Some thoughts on how to handle an anaesthetic-related death. Anaesthesia 44: 245, 1989
28. Runciman WB, Webb RK, Klepper ID *et al*: Crisis management: Validation of an algorithm by analysis of 2000 incident reports. Anaesth Intensive Care 21: 579, 1993
29. Davies JM, Webb RK: Adverse events in anaesthesia: The wrong drug. Can J Anaesth 41: 83, 1994
30. Cooper JB, Cullen DJ, Eichhorn JH *et al*: Administrative guidelines for response to an adverse anesthesia event. J Clin Anesth 5: 79, 1993
31. Weiner JP: Forecasting the effects of health reform on U.S. physician workforce requirements. JAMA 272: 222, 1994
32. Cullen BF: Anesthesia workforce requirements: Are there too many anesthesiologists? ASA Newsletter 58(11): 27, 1994
33. Schubert A, Eckhout G, Cooperider T, Kuhel A: Evidence of a current and lasting national anesthesia personnel shortfall: scope and implications. Mayo Clin Proc. 76: 995, 2001
34. Schubert A, Eckhout G Jr, Tremper K: An updated view of the national anesthesia personnel shortfall. Anesth Analg 96: 207, 2003
35. Grogono AW: National Resident Matching Program Results for 2004: Slight Decline in Recruitment. ASA Newsletter 68(5): 18, 2004
36. Eckhout GV: Where Are Those Anesthesiologists? Deciphering the Numbers. ASA Newsletter 68(5): 13, 2004
37. American Society of Anesthesiologists: Practice Management: Compliance with Medicare and Other Payor Billing Requirements. Park Ridge, IL, ASA, 1997
38. Locke J: The Net Collections Fallacy and Other Performance Metric Myths. American Society of Anesthesiologists 2003 Conference on Practice Management, 141. Park Ridge, IL, ASA, 2003
39. American Society of Anesthesiologists: Managed Care Reimbursement Mechanisms: A Guide for Anesthesiologists. Park Ridge, IL, ASA, 1994
40. American Society of Anesthesiologists: Contracting Issues: A Primer for Anesthesiologists. Park Ridge, IL, ASA, 1999
41. Willett DE: Exclusive Contracts: Update on Legal Issues. American Society of Anesthesiologists 2001 Conference on Practice Management, 8–1. Park Ridge, IL, ASA, 2001
42. Scott SJ, Blough GG: Exclusive Contracts: Survey of Hospital Contracts. American Society of Anesthesiologists 2001 Conference on Practice Management, 9–1 Park Ridge, IL, ASA, 2001
43. American Society of Anesthesiologists: Practice Management: Managed Care Contracting. Park Ridge, IL, ASA, 1996
44. Everett, PC: Securing a Hospital Stipend: the Business-Like Approach. American Society of Anesthesiologists 2003 Conference on Practice Management, 189. Park Ridge, IL, ASA, 2003
45. Semo, JJ: Hospital Stipend Negotiations: Practical and Legal Issues. American Society of Anesthesiologists 2004 Conference on Practice Management, 51. Park Ridge, IL, ASA, 2004
46. Rodin MA: Conflicts in managed care. N Eng J Med 332: 604, 1995
47. Hetrick WD: Health care reform: Implications for the anesthesiologist. Adv Anesth 12: 1, 1995
48. American Society of Anesthesiologists: The HIPAA Privacy Rule in Anesthesia and Pain Medicine Practices. Park Ridge, IL, ASA, 2003
49. Semo JJ: HIPAA Privacy: What You Need to Know, What You Need to Do. American Society of Anesthesiologists 2003 Conference on Practice Management, 96. Park Ridge, IL, ASA, 2003
50. Semo JJ: HIPAA Privacy Update. American Society of Anesthesiologists 2004 Conference on Practice Management, 123. Park Ridge, IL, ASA, 2004
51. Johnson JF: Questions to Ask Your Billing Software Vendor. American Society of Anesthesiologists 2003 Conference on Practice Management, 130. Park Ridge, IL, ASA, 2003
52. Szokol JW: Administrative Support Survey Results. Association of Anesthesia Clinical Directors Newsletter, Summer 2002 1
53. Mazzei WJ: OR Management. American Society of Anesthesiologists 2001 Conference on Practice Management, 12–1. Park Ridge, IL, ASA, 2001
54. Malhotra V: Practical Issues in OR Management: The Obvious and the Not So Obvious. American Society of Anesthesiologists 2004 Conference on Practice Management, 43. Park Ridge, IL, ASA, 2004
55. Pollard JB, Zboray AL, Mazze RI: Economic benefits attributed to opening a preoperative evaluation clinic for outpatients. Anesth Analg 83: 407, 1996
56. Fischer SP: Development and effectiveness of an anesthesia preoperative evaluation clinic in a teaching hospital. Anesthesiology 85: 196, 1996
57. Blough GG, Scott SJ: Creative Scheduling for Anesthesiologists: Physician Retention in a Tight Market. American Society of Anesthesiologists 2003 Conference on Practice Management, 71. Park Ridge, IL, ASA, 2003
58. Abouleish AE, Prough DS, Zornow MH *et al*: Designing meaningful industry metrics for clinical productivity for anesthesiology departments. Anesth Analg 93: 309, 2001
59. Abouleish AE, Prough DS, Whitten CW *et al*: Comparing clinical productivity of anesthesiology departments. Anesthesiology 97: 608, 2002
60. Abouleish AE, Prough DS, Barker SJ *et al*: Organizational factors affect comparisons of clinical productivity of academic anesthesiology departments. Anesth Analg 96: 802, 2003
61. Abouleish AE: Working Hard: Hardly Working; Comparing Clinical Productivity of Anesthesiology Groups. American Society of Anesthesiologists 2004 Conference on Practice Management, 195. Park Ridge, IL, ASA, 2004
62. Calmes SH: Anesthesiology Demographics: Women's Changing Specialty Choices and Implications for Anesthesiology Workforce Shortage. American Society of Anesthesiologists Newsletter 65(8): 2001, 22
63. Tuman KJ, Ivankovich AD: High cost, high tech medicine—are we getting our money's worth? J Clin Anesth 5: 168, 1993
64. Johnstone RE, Martinec CL: Costs of anesthesia. Anesth Analg 76: 840, 1993
65. Eddy DM: Applying cost-effectiveness analysis: The inside story. JAMA 268: 2575, 1992
66. Baum JA: Low flow anaesthesia: The sensible and judicious use of inhalation anaesthetics. Acta Anaesthiol Scand 111: 264, 1997
67. Szocik JF, Learned DW: Impact of a cost containment program on the use of volatile anesthetics and neuromuscular blocking drugs. J Clin Anesth 6: 378, 1994
68. Barclay LP, Hatton RC, Doering PL, Shands JW: Physicians' perceptions and knowledge of drug costs: Results of a survey. Formulary 30: 268, 1995
69. Johnstone R, Jozefczyk KG: Costs of anesthetic drugs: Experiences with a cost education trial. Anesth Analg 78: 766, 1994
70. Davidson RA: Does it work or not? Clinical vs. statistical significance. Chest 106: 932, 1994
71. Donabedian A: Explorations in Quality Assessment and Monitoring. Vol 3. The Methods and Findings of Quality Assessment and Monitoring: An Illustrated Analysis. Ann Arbor, MI, Health Administration Press, 1985

72. Macario A, Weinger M, Truong P, Lee M: Which clinical anesthesia outcomes are both common and important to avoid? The perspective of a panel of expert anesthesiologists. Anesth Analg 88: 1085, 1999
73. Tarazi E, Philip B: Friendliness of OR staff is top determinant of patient satisfaction with outpatient surgery. Am J Anesth 25: 154, 1998
74. Dexter F, Tinker JH: The cost efficacy of hypothetically eliminating adverse anesthetic outcomes from high-risk, but neither low- nor moderate-risk, surgical operations. Anesth Analg 81: 939, 1995
75. Bothner U, Georgieff M, Schwilk B: The impact of minor perioperative anesthesia-related incidents, events, and complications on postanesthesia care unit utilization. Anesth Analg 89: 506, 1999
76. Deming WE: Out of the Crisis. Cambridge, MA, MIT, Center for Advanced Engineering Study, 1986

CHAPTER 3 ■ EXPERIMENTAL DESIGN AND STATISTICS

NATHAN LEON PACE

KEY POINTS

1. Statistics and mathematics are the language of scientific medicine.
2. Good research planning includes a clear biologic hypothesis, the specification of outcome variables, the choice of anticipated statistical methods, and sample size planning.
3. To avoid bias in the performance of clinical research, the crucial elements of good research design include concurrent control groups; random allocation of subjects to treatment groups; and blinding of random allocation, patients, caregivers, and outcome assessors.
4. Descriptive (mean, standard deviation, etc.) and inferential statistics (*t* test, confidence interval, etc.) are both essential methods for the presentation of research results.
5. The central limit theorem allows the use of parametric statistics for most statistical testing.
6. Systematic review and meta-analysis can synthesize and summarize the results of smaller, nonsignificant individual studies and permit more powerful inferences.

INTRODUCTION

1 Medical journals are replete with numbers. These include weights, lengths, pressures, volumes, flows, concentrations, counts, temperatures, rates, currents, energies, and forces. The analysis and interpretation of these numbers require the use of statistical techniques. The design of the experiment to acquire these numbers is also part of statistical competence. The need for these statistical techniques is mandated by the nature of our universe, which is both orderly and random at the same time. Probability and statistics have been formulated to solve concrete problems, such as betting on cards, understanding biologic inheritance, and improving food processing. Studies in anesthesia have even inspired new statistics. The development of statistical techniques is manifest in the increasing use of more sophisticated research designs and statistical tests in anesthesia research.

If a physician is to be a practitioner of scientific medicine, he or she must read the language of science to be able to independently assess and interpret the scientific report. Without exception, the language of the medical report is increasingly statistical. Readers of the anesthesia literature, whether in a community hospital or a university environment, cannot and should not totally depend on the editors of journals to banish all errors of statistical analysis and interpretation. In addition, there are regularly questions about simple statistics in examinations required for anesthesiologists. Finally, certain statistical methods have everyday applications in clinical medicine. This chapter briefly scans some elements of experimental design and statistical analysis.

DESIGN OF RESEARCH STUDIES

The scientific investigator should view himself or herself as an experimenter and not merely as a naturalist. The naturalist goes out into the field ready to capture and report the numbers that flit into view; this is a worthy activity, typified by the *case report*. Case reports engender interest, suspicion, doubt, wonder, and, one hopes, the desire to experiment; however, the case report is not sufficient evidence to advance scientific medicine. The experimenter attempts to constrain and control, as much as possible, the environment in which he or she collects numbers to test a hypothesis.

Sampling

Two words of great importance to statisticians are *population* and *sample*. In statistical language, each has a specialized meaning. Instead of referring only to the count of individuals in a geographic or political region, population refers to any target group of things (animate or inanimate) in which there is interest. For anesthesia researchers, a typical target population might be mothers in the first stage of labor or head-trauma victims undergoing craniotomy. A target population could also be cell cultures, isolated organ preparations, or hospital bills. A sample is a subset of the target population. Samples are taken because of the impossibility of observing the entire population; it is generally not affordable, convenient, or practical to examine more than a relatively small fraction of the population. Nevertheless, the researcher wishes to generalize from the results of the small sample group to the entire population.

Although the subjects of a population are alike in at least one way, these population members are generally quite diverse in other ways. Since the researcher can work only with a subset of the population, he or she hopes that the sample of subjects in the experiment is representative of the population's diversity. Head-injury patients can have open or closed wounds, a variety of coexisting diseases, and normal or increased intracranial pressure. These subgroups within a population are called *strata*. Often the researcher wishes to increase the sameness or homogeneity of the target population by further restricting it to just a few strata; perhaps only closed and not open head injuries will be included. Restricting the target population to eliminate too much diversity must be balanced against the desire to have the results be applicable to the broadest possible population of patients.

The best hope for a representative sample of the population would be realized if every subject in the population had the same chance of being in the experiment; this is called *random sampling*. If there are several strata of importance, random sampling from each stratum would be appropriate. Unfortunately, in most clinical anesthesia studies researchers are limited to using those patients who happen to show up at their hospitals; this is called *convenience sampling*. Convenience sampling is also subject to the nuances of the surgical schedule, the goodwill of the referring physician and attending surgeon, and the willingness of the patient to cooperate. At best, the convenience sample is representative of patients at that institution, with no assurance that these patients are similar to those elsewhere. Convenience sampling is also the rule in studying new anesthetic drugs; such studies are typically performed on healthy, young volunteers.

Performance

The researcher must define the conditions to which the sample members will be exposed. Particularly in clinical research, one must decide whether these conditions should be rigidly standardized or whether the experimental circumstances should be adjusted or individualized to the patient. In anesthetic drug research, should a fixed dose be given to all members of the sample or should the dose be adjusted to produce an effect or to achieve a specific end point? Standardizing the treatment groups by fixed doses simplifies the research work. There are risks to this standardization, however: (1) a fixed dose may produce excessive numbers of side effects in some patients; (2) a fixed dose may be therapeutically insufficient in others; and (3) a treatment standardized for an experimental protocol may be so artificial that it has no broad clinical relevance, even if demonstrated to be superior. The researcher should carefully choose and report the adjustment/individualization of experimental treatments.

Control Groups

Even if a researcher is studying just one experimental group,
2 the results of the experiment are usually not interpreted solely in terms of that one group but are also contrasted and compared with other experimental groups. Examining the effects of a new drug on blood pressure during anesthetic induction is important, but what is more important is comparing those results with the effects of one or more standard drugs commonly used in the same situation. Where can the researcher obtain these comparative data? There are several possibilities: (1) each patient could receive the standard drug under identical experimental circumstances at another time; (2) another group of patients receiving the standard drug could be studied simultaneously; (3) a group of patients could have been studied previously with the standard drug under similar circumstances; and (4) literature reports of the effects of the drug under related but not necessarily identical circumstances could be used. Under the first two possibilities, the control group is contemporaneous—either a *self-control* (crossover) or *parallel control* group. The second two possibilities are examples of the use of *historical controls*.

Because historical controls already exist, they are convenient and seemingly cheap to use. Unfortunately, the history of medicine is littered with the "debris" of therapies enthusiastically accepted on the basis of comparison with past experience. A classic example is operative ligation of the internal mammary artery for the treatment of angina pectoris—a procedure now known to be of no value. Proposed as a method to improve coronary artery blood flow, the lack of benefit was demonstrated in a trial where some patients had the procedure and some had a sham procedure; both groups showed benefit.[1] There is now firm empirical evidence that studies using historical controls usually show a favorable outcome for a new therapy, whereas studies with concurrent controls, that is, parallel control group or self-control, less often reveal a benefit.[2] Nothing seems to increase the enthusiasm for a new treatment as much as the omission of a concurrent control group. If the outcome with an old treatment is not studied simultaneously with the outcome of a new treatment, one cannot know if any differences in results are a consequence of the two treatments, or of unsuspected and unknowable differences between the patients, or of other changes over time in the general medical environment. One possible exception would be in studying a disease that is uniformly fatal (100% mortality) over a very short time.

Random Allocation of Treatment Groups

Having accepted the necessity of an experiment with a control group, the question arises as to the method by which each subject should be assigned to the predetermined experimental groups. Should it depend on the whim of the investigator, the day of the week, the preference of a referring physician, the wish of the patient, the assignment of the previous subject, the availability of a study drug, a hospital chart number, or some other arbitrary criterion? All such methods have been used and are still used, but all can ruin the purity and usefulness of the experiment. It is important to remember the purpose of sampling: by exposing a small number of subjects from the target population to the various experimental conditions, one hopes to make conclusions about the entire population. Thus, the experimental groups should be as similar as possible to each other in reflecting the target population; if the groups are different, this introduces a bias into the experiment. Although randomly allocating subjects of a sample to one or another of the experimental groups requires additional work, this principle prevents selection bias by the researcher, minimizes (but cannot always prevent) the possibility that important differences exist among the experimental groups, and disarms the critics' complaints about research methods. Random allocation is most commonly accomplished by the use of computer-generated random numbers.

Blinding

Blinding refers to the masking from the view of patient and experimenters the experimental group to which the subject has been or will be assigned. In clinical trials, the necessity for blinding starts even before a patient is enrolled in the research study; this is called the concealment of random allocation. There is good evidence that, if the process of random allocation is accessible to view, the referring physicians, the research team members, or both are tempted to manipulate the entrance of specific patients into the study to influence their assignment to a specific treatment group[3]; they do so having formed a personal opinion about the relative merits of the treatment groups and desiring to get the "best" for someone they favor. This creates bias in the experimental groups.

Each subject should remain, if possible, ignorant of the assigned treatment group after entrance into the research protocol. The patient's expectation of improvement, a placebo effect, is a real and useful part of clinical care. But when studying a new treatment, one must ensure that the fame or infamy of the treatments does not induce a bias in outcome by changing patient expectations. A researcher's knowledge of the treatment assignment can bias his or her ability to administer the research protocol and to observe and record data faithfully; this is true for clinical, animal, and in vitro research. If the treatment group is known, those who observe data cannot trust themselves to record the data impartially and dispassionately. The appellations *single-blind* and *double-blind* to describe blinding are commonly used in research reports, but often applied inconsistently; the researcher should carefully plan and report exactly who is blinded.

Types of Research Design

Ultimately, research design consists of choosing what subjects to study, what experimental conditions and constraints to enforce, and which observations to collect at what intervals. A few key features in this research design largely determine the strength of scientific inference on the collected data. These key features allow the classification of research reports (Table 3-1). This classification reveals the variety of experimental approaches and indicates strengths and weaknesses of the same design applied to many research problems.

The first distinction is between *longitudinal* and *cross-sectional* studies. The former is the study of changes over time, whereas the latter describes a phenomenon at a certain point in time. For example, reporting the frequency with which certain drugs are used during anesthesia is a cross-sectional study, whereas investigating the hemodynamic effects of different drugs during anesthesia is a longitudinal one.

TABLE 3-1

CLASSIFICATION OF BIOMEDICAL RESEARCH REPORTS

- I. Longitudinal studies
  - A. Prospective (cohort) studies
    - 1. Studies of deliberate intervention
      - a. Concurrent controls
      - b. Historical controls
    - 2. Observational studies
  - B. Retrospective (case-control) studies
- II. Cross-sectional studies

Longitudinal studies are next classified by the method with which the research subjects are selected. These methods for choosing research subjects can be either *prospective* or *retrospective;* these two approaches are also known as *cohort* (prospective) or *case-control* (retrospective). A prospective study assembles groups of subjects by some input characteristic that is thought to change an output characteristic; a typical input characteristic would be the opioid drug administered during anesthesia, for example, remifentanil or fentanyl. A retrospective study gathers subjects by an output characteristic; an output characteristic is the status of the subject after an event, for example, the occurrence of a myocardial infarction. A prospective (cohort) study would be one in which a group of patients undergoing neurological surgery was divided in two groups, given two different opioids (remifentanil or fentanyl), and followed for the development of a perioperative myocardial infarction. In a retrospective (case-control) study, patients who suffered a perioperative myocardial infarction would be identified from hospital records; a group of subjects of similar age, gender, and disease who did not suffer a perioperative myocardial infarction also would be chosen, and the two groups would then be compared for the relative use of the two opioids (remifentanil or fentanyl). Retrospective studies are a primary tool of epidemiology. A case-control study can often identify an association between an input and output characteristic, but the causal link or relationship between the two is more difficult to specify.

Prospective studies are further divided into those in which the investigator performs a deliberate intervention and those in which the investigator merely observes. In a study of *deliberate intervention,* the investigator would choose several anesthetic maintenance techniques and compare the incidence of postoperative nausea and vomiting. If it was performed as an *observational study,* the investigator would observe a group of patients receiving anesthetics chosen at the discretion of each patient's anesthesiologist and compare the incidence of postoperative nausea and vomiting among the anesthetics used. Obviously, in this example of an observational study, there has been an intervention; an anesthetic has been given. The crucial distinction is whether the investigator controlled the intervention. An observational study may reveal differences among treatment groups, but whether such differences are the consequence of the treatments or of other differences among the patients receiving the treatments will remain obscure.

Studies of deliberate intervention are further subdivided into those with concurrent controls and those with historical controls. Concurrent controls are either a simultaneous parallel control group or a self-control study; historical controls include previous studies and literature reports. A *randomized controlled trial* is thus a longitudinal, prospective study of deliberate intervention with concurrent controls.

Although most of this discussion about experimental design has focused on human experimentation, the same principles apply and should be followed in animal experimentation. The randomized, controlled clinical trial is the most potent scientific tool for evaluating medical treatment; randomization into treatment groups is relied upon to equally weight the subjects of the treatment groups for baseline attributes that might predispose or protect the subjects from the outcome of interest.

Hypothesis Formulation

3 Whether the research subjects are tissue preparations, animals, or people, the researcher is constantly faced with finding both similarities and differences among the diversities of a group of subjects. The researcher starts the work with some intuitive feel for the phenomenon to be studied. Whether stated explicitly or not, this is the *biologic hypothesis;* it is a statement of experimental expectations to be accomplished by the use of experimental tools, instruments, or methods accessible to the research team. An example would be the hope that isoflurane would produce less myocardial ischemia than fentanyl; the experimental method might be the electrocardiographic determination of ST segment changes. The biologic hypothesis of the researcher becomes a *statistical hypothesis* during research planning. The researcher measures quantities that can vary—variables such as heart rate or temperature or ST segment change. In a statistical hypothesis, statements are made about the relationship among parameters of one or more populations. A *parameter* is a number describing a variable of a population; Greek letters are used to denote parameters. The typical statistical hypothesis can be established in a somewhat rote fashion for every research project, regardless of the methods, materials, or goals. The most frequently used method of setting up the algebraic formulation of the statistical hypothesis is to create two mutually exclusive statements about some parameters of the study population (Table 3-2); estimates for the values for these parameters are acquired by sampling data. In the hypothetical example comparing isoflurane and fentanyl, ϕ_1 and ϕ_2 would represent the ST segment changes with isoflurane and with fentanyl. The *null hypothesis* is the hypothesis of no difference of ST segment changes between isoflurane and fentanyl. The *alternative hypothesis* is usually nondirectional, that is, either $\phi_1 < \phi_2$ or $\phi_1 > \phi_2$; this is known as a two-tail alternative hypothesis. This is a more conservative alternative hypothesis than assuming that the inequality can only be either less than or greater than.

Logic of Proof

One particular decision strategy is used almost universally to choose between the null and alternative hypothesis. The decision strategy is similar to a method of indirect proof used in mathematics called *reductio ad absurdum*. If a theorem cannot be proved directly, assume that it is not true; show that the falsity of this theorem will lead to contradictions and absurdities; thus, reject the original assumption of the falseness of the theorem. For statistics, the approach is to assume that the null hypothesis is true even though the goal of the experiment is to show that there is a difference. One examines the consequences of this assumption by examining the actual sample values obtained for the variable(s) of interest. This is done by calculating what is called a *sample test statistic*; sample test statistics are calculated from the sample numbers. Associated with a sample test statistic is a *probability.* One also chooses the *level of significance;* the level of significance is the probability level considered too low to warrant support of the null hypothesis being tested. If sample values are sufficiently unlikely to have occurred by chance (i.e., the probability of the sample test statistic is less than the chosen level of significance), the null hypothesis is rejected; otherwise, the null hypothesis is not rejected.

Because the statistics deal with probabilities, not certainties, there is a chance that the decision concerning the null hypothesis is erroneous. These errors are best displayed in table form (Table 3-3); Condition 1 and Condition 2 could be different drugs, two doses of the same drug, or different patient groups. Of the four possible outcomes, two are clearly undesirable. The error of wrongly rejecting the null hypothesis (false-positive) is called the *type I* or *alpha error.* The experimenter should choose a probability value for alpha before collecting data; the experimenter decides how cautious to be about falsely claiming a difference. The most common choice for the value of alpha is 0.05. What are the consequences of choosing an alpha of 0.05? Assuming that there is, in fact, no difference between the two conditions and that the experiment is to be repeated 20 times, then during one of these experimental replications (5% of 20) a mistaken conclusion that there is a difference would be made. The probability of a type I error depends on the chosen level of significance and the existence or nonexistence of a difference between the two experimental conditions. The smaller the chosen alpha, the smaller will be the risk of a type I error.

The error of failing to reject a false null hypothesis (false-negative) is called a *type II* or *beta error.* The power of a test is 1 minus beta. The probability of a type II error depends on four factors. Unfortunately, the smaller the alpha, the greater the chance of a false-negative conclusion; this fact keeps the experimenter from automatically choosing a very small alpha. Second, the more variability there is in the populations being compared, the greater the chance of a type II error. This is analogous to listening to a noisy radio broadcast; the more static there is, the harder it will be to discriminate between words. Next, increasing the number of subjects will lower the probability of a type II error. The fourth and most important factor is the magnitude of the difference between the two experimental conditions. The probability of a type II error goes from very high, when there is only a small difference, to extremely low, when the two conditions produce large differences in population parameters.

TABLE 3-2

ALGEBRAIC STATEMENT OF STATISTICAL HYPOTHESES

$H_0 : \phi_1 = \phi_2$ (null hypothesis)
$H_a : \phi_1 \neq \phi_2$ (alternative hypothesis)
ϕ_1 = Parameter estimated from sample of first population
ϕ_2 = Parameter estimated from sample of second population

Sample Size Calculations

Discussion of hypothesis testing by statisticians has always included mention of both type I and type II errors, but researchers have typically ignored the latter error in experimental design. The practical importance of worrying about type II errors reached the consciousness of the medical research community several decades ago.[4] Some controlled clinical trials that claimed to find no advantage of new therapies compared with standard therapies lacked sufficient statistical

TABLE 3-3

ERRORS IN HYPOTHESIS TESTING: THE TWO-WAY TRUTH TABLE

		■ REALITY (POPULATION PARAMETERS)	
		■ CONDITIONS 1 AND 2 EQUIVALENT	■ CONDITIONS 1 AND 2 NOT EQUIVALENT
Conclusion from Observations (Sample Statistics)	Conditions 1 and 2 equivalent[a]	Correct conclusion	False-negative type II error (beta error)
	Conditions 1 and 2 not equivalent[b]	False-positive type I error (alpha error)	Correct conclusion

[a]Do not reject null hypothesis: Condition 1 = Condition 2.
[b]Reject null hypothesis: Condition 1 ≠ Condition 2.

power to discriminate between the experimental groups and would have missed an important therapeutic improvement. There are four options for decreasing type II error (increasing statistical power): (1) raise alpha, (2) reduce population variability, (3) make the sample bigger, and (4) make the difference between the conditions greater. Under most circumstances, only the sample size can be varied. Sample size planning has become an important part of research design for controlled clinical trials. Some published research still fails the test of adequate sample size planning.

STATISTICAL TESTING

Statistics is a method for working with *sets* of numbers, a set being a group of objects. Statistics involves the description of number sets, the comparison of number sets with theoretical models, comparison between number sets, and comparison of recently acquired number sets with those from the past. A typical scientific hypothesis asks which of two methods (treatments), *X* and *Y*, is better. A statistical hypothesis is formulated concerning the sets of numbers collected under the conditions of treatments *X* and *Y*. Statistics provides methods for deciding if the set of values associated with *X* are different from the values associated with *Y*. Statistical methods are necessary because there are sources of variation in any data set, including random biologic variation and measurement error. These errors in the data cause difficulties in avoiding bias and in being precise. Bias keeps the true value from being known and fosters incorrect decisions; precision deals with the problem of the data scatter and with quantifying the uncertainty about the value in the population from which a sample is drawn. These statistical methods are relatively independent of the particular field of study. Regardless of whether the numbers in sets *X* and *Y* are systolic pressures, body weights, or serum chlorides, the approach for comparing sets *X* and *Y* is usually the same.

Data Structure

Data collected in an experiment include the defining characteristics of the experiment and the values of events or attributes that vary over time or conditions. The former are called *explanatory variables* and the latter are called *response variables*. The researcher records his or her observations on data sheets or case record forms, which may be one to many pages in length, and assembles them together for statistical analysis. Variables such as gender, age, and doses of accompanying drugs reflect the variability of the experimental subjects. Explanatory variables, it is hoped, explain the systematic variations in the response variables. In a sense, the response variables are dependent on the explanatory variables.

Response variables are also called *dependent variables*. Response variables reflect the primary properties of experimental interest in the subjects. Research in anesthesiology is particularly likely to have repeated measurement variables, that is, a particular measurement recorded more than once for each individual. Some variables can be both explanatory and response; these are called *intermediate response variables*. Suppose an experiment is conducted comparing electrocardiographic and myocardial responses between five doses of an opioid. One might analyze how ST segments depended on the dose of opioids; here, maximum ST segment depression is a response variable. Maximum ST segment depression might also be used as an explanatory variable to address the more subtle question of the extent to which the effect of an opioid dose on postoperative myocardial infarction can be accounted for by ST segment changes. The mathematical characteristics of the possible values of a variable fit into five classifications (Table 3-4). Properly assigning a variable to the correct data type is essential for choosing the correct statistical technique. For *interval variables*, there is equal distance between successive intervals; the difference between 15 and 10 is the same as the difference between 25 and 20. *Discrete interval data* can have only integer values, for example, age in years, number of live children, or papers rejected by a journal. *Continuous interval data* are measured on a continuum and can be a decimal fraction; for example, blood pressure can be described as accurately as desired (e.g., 136, 136.1, or 136.14 mm Hg). The same statistical techniques are used for discrete and continuous data.

Putting observations into two or more discrete categories derives *categorical variables*; for statistical analysis, numeric values are assigned as labels to the categories. *Dichotomous data* allow only two possible values, for example, male versus female. *Ordinal data* have three or more categories that can logically be ranked or ordered; however, the ranking or ordering of the variable indicates only relative and not absolute differences between values; there is not necessarily the same difference between American Society of Anesthesiologists Physical Status score I and II as there is between III and IV. Although ordinal data are often treated as interval data in choosing a statistical technique, such analysis may be suspect; alternative techniques for ordinal data are available. *Nominal variables* are placed into categories that have no logical ordering. The eye colors blue, hazel, and brown might be assigned the numbers 1, 2, and 3, but it is nonsense to say that blue < hazel < brown.

TABLE 3-4

DATA TYPES

DATA TYPE	DEFINITION	EXAMPLES
INTERVAL		
Discrete	Data measured with an integer only scale	Parity, number of teeth
Continuous	Data measured with a constant scale interval	Blood pressure, temperature
CATEGORICAL		
Dichotomous	Binary data	Mortality, gender
Nominal	Qualitative data that cannot be ordered or ranked	Eye color, drug category
Ordinal	Data ordered, ranked, or measured without a constant scale interval	ASA physical status score, pain score

Descriptive Statistics

4 A typical hypothetical data set could be a sample of ages (the variable) of 12 residents in an anesthesia training program (the population). Although the results of a particular experiment might be presented by repeatedly showing the entire set of numbers, there are concise ways of summarizing the information content of the data set into a few numbers. These numbers are called *sample* or *summary statistics;* summary statistics are calculated using the numbers of the sample. By convention, the symbols of summary statistics are Roman letters. The two summary statistics most frequently used for interval variables are the *central location* and the *variability,* but there are other summary statistics. Other data types have analogous summary statistics. Although the first purpose of descriptive statistics is to describe the sample of numbers obtained, there is also the desire to use the summary statistics from the sample to characterize the population from which the sample was obtained. For example, what can be said about the age of all anesthesia residents from the information in a sample? The population also has measures of central location and variability called the parameters of the population; as previously mentioned, population parameters are denoted by Greek letters. Usually, the population parameters cannot be directly calculated, because data from all population members cannot be obtained. The beauty of properly chosen summary statistics is that they are the best possible estimators of the population parameters.

These sampling statistics can be used in conjunction with a probability density function to provide additional descriptions of the sample and its population. Also commonly described as a probability distribution, a probability density function is an algebraic equation, $f(x)$, which gives a theoretical percentage distribution of x. Each value of x has a probability of occurrence given by $f(x)$. The most important probability distribution is the *normal* or *Gaussian function.* There are two parameters (population mean and population variance) in the equation of the normal function that are denoted μ and σ^2. Often called the normal equation, it can be plotted and produces the familiar bell-shaped curve. Why are the mathematical properties of this curve so important to biostatistics? First, it has been empirically noted that when a biologic variable is sampled repeatedly, the pattern of the numbers plotted as a histogram resembles the normal curve; thus, most biologic data are said to follow or to obey a normal distribution. Second, if it is reasonable to assume that a sample is from a normal population, the mathematical properties of the normal equation can be used with the sampling statistic estimators of the population parameters to describe the sample and the population. Third,
5 a mathematical theorem (the central limit theorem) allows the use of the assumption of normality for certain purposes, even if the population is not normally distributed.

Central Location

The three most common summary statistics of central location for interval variables are the arithmetic *mean,* the *median,* and the *mode.* The mean is merely the average of the numbers in the data set. Being a summary statistic of the sample, the arithmetic mean is denoted by the Roman letter x under a bar:

$$\bar{x} = \sum_{i=1}^{n} x_i \qquad (3\text{-}1)$$

If all values in the population could be obtained, then the population mean μ could be calculated similarly. Because all values of the population cannot be obtained, the sample mean is used. (Statisticians describe the sample mean as the unbiased, consistent, minimum variance, sufficient estimator of the population mean. Estimators are denoted by a hat over a roman letter, for example $\hat{x}$. Thus, the sample mean $\bar{x}$ is the estimator $\hat{x}$ of the population mean μ.)

The median is the middlemost number or the number that divides the sample into two equal parts. The median is obtained by first ranking the sample values from lowest to highest and then counting up halfway. The concept of ranking is used in nonparametric statistics. A virtue of the median is that it is hardly affected by a few extremely high or low values. The mode is the most popular number of a sample, that is, the number that occurs most frequently. A sample may have ties for the most common value and be bi- or polymodal; these modes may be widely separated or adjacent. The raw data should be inspected for this unusual appearance. The mode is always mentioned in discussions of descriptive statistics, but it is rarely used in statistical practice.

Spread or Variability

Any set of interval data has variability unless all the numbers are identical. The range of ages from lowest to highest expresses the largest difference. This spread, diversity, and variability can also be expressed in a concise manner. Variability is specified by calculating the *deviation* or *deviate* of each individual x_i from the center (mean) of all the x_i's. The *sum of the squared deviates* is always positive unless all set values are identical. This sum is then divided by the number of individual measurements. The result is the *averaged squared deviations;* the average squared deviation is ubiquitous in statistics.

The concept of describing the spread of a set of numbers by calculating the average distance from each number to the center of the numbers applies to both a sample and a population; this average squared distance is called the *variance*. The population variance is a parameter and is represented by σ^2. As with the population mean, the population variance is not usually known and cannot be calculated. Just as the sample mean is used in place of the population mean, the sample variance is used in place of the population variance. The sample variance is:

$$s^2 = \frac{\sum_{i=1}^{n} (x_i - \bar{x})^2}{(n-1)} \tag{3-2}$$

Statistical theory demonstrates that if the divisor in the formula for s^2 is $(n-1)$ rather than n, the sample variance is an unbiased estimator of the population variance. While the variance is used extensively in statistical calculations, the units of variance are squared units of the original observations. The square root of the variance has the same units as the original observations; the square roots of the sample and population variances are called the *sample* and *population standard deviations*.

It was previously mentioned that most biologic observations appear to come from populations with normal distributions. By accepting this assumption of a normal distribution, further meaning can be given to the sample summary statistics (mean and standard deviation) that have been calculated. This involves the use of the expression $\bar{x} \pm k \times s$, where $k = 1, 2, 3$, etc. If the population from which the sample is taken is unimodal and roughly symmetric, then the bounds for 1, 2, and 3 encompasses roughly 68%, 95%, and 99% of the sample and population members.

Confidence Intervals

A confidence interval describes how likely it is that the population parameter is estimated by any particular sample statistic such as the mean. (The technical definition of confidence interval is more rigorous. A 95% confidence interval implies that if the experiment were done over and over again, then 95 of each 100 confidence intervals would be expected to contain the true value of the mean.) Confidence intervals are a range of the following form: summary statistic ± (confidence factor) × (precision factor).

The *precision factor* is derived from the sample itself, whereas the *confidence factor* is taken from a probability distribution and also depends on the specified confidence level chosen. For a sample of interval data taken from a normally distributed population for which confidence intervals are to be chosen for $\bar{x}$, the precision factor is called the *standard error of the mean* and is obtained by dividing s by the square root of the sample size:

$$SE = \frac{s}{\sqrt{n}} = \sqrt{\sum_{i=1}^{n} (x_i - \bar{x})^2 \Big/ n(n-1)} \tag{3-3}$$

The confidence factors are the same as those used for the dispersion or spread of the sample and are obtained from the normal distribution. The confidence intervals for confidence factors 1, 2, and 3 have roughly a 68%, 95%, and 99% chance of containing the population mean. Strictly speaking, when the standard deviation must be estimated from sample values, the confidence factors should be taken from the *t distribution*, another probability distribution. These coefficients will be larger than those used above. This is usually ignored if the sample size is reasonable, for example, $n > 25$. Even when the sample size is only five or greater, the use of the coefficients 1, 2, and 3 is simple and sufficiently accurate for quick mental calculations of confidence intervals on parameter estimates.

Almost all research reports include the use of SE, regardless of the probability distribution of the populations sampled. This use is a consequence of the central limit theorem—one of the most remarkable theorems in all of mathematics. The central limit theorem states that the SE can always be used, if the sample size is sufficiently large, to specify confidence intervals around the sample mean containing the population mean. These confidence intervals are calculated as described above. This is true even if the population distribution is so different from normal that s cannot be used to characterize the dispersion of the population members. Only rough guidelines can be given for the necessary sample size; for interval data, 25 and above is large enough and 4 and below is too small.

Although the SE is discussed along with other descriptive statistics, it is really an inferential statistic. Standard error and standard deviation are mentioned together because of their similarities of computation and because of the confusion of their use in research reports. This use is most often of the form "mean ± number;" some confusion results from the failure of the author to specify whether the number after the ± sign is the one or the other. More important, the choice between using s and using SE has become controversial; because SE is always less than s, it has been argued that authors seek to deceive by using SE to make the data look better than they really are. The choice is actually simple. When describing the spread, scatter, or dispersion of the sample, use the standard deviation; when describing the precision with which the population center is known, use the standard error.

Proportions

Categorical binary data, also called *enumeration data,* provide counts of subject responses. Given a sample of subjects of whom some have a certain characteristic (e.g., death, female sex), a ratio of responders to the number of subjects can be easily calculated as $p = x/n$; this ratio or rate can be expressed as a decimal fraction or as a percentage. It should be clear that this is a measure of central location of a binary data in the same way that μ was a measure of central location for continuous data. In the population from which the sample is taken, the ratio of responders to total subjects is a population parameter, denoted π; π is the measure of central location for the population. This is not related to the geometry constant pi (π = 3.14159K). As with other data types, π is usually not known but must be estimated from the sample. The sample ratio p is the best estimate of π. The probability of binary data is provided by the *binomial distribution function.*

Since the population is not generally known, the experimenter usually wishes to estimate π by the sample ratio p and to specify with what confidence π is known. If the sample is sufficiently large ($n \times p \geq 5; n \times (1-p) \geq 5$), advantage is taken of the central limit theorem to derive a standard error analogous to that derived for interval data:

$$SE = \sqrt{\frac{p \times (1-p)}{n}} \tag{3-4}$$

This sample standard error is exactly analogous to the sample standard error of the mean for interval data, except that it is a standard error of the proportion. Just as a 95% confidence limit of the mean was calculated, so may a confidence limit on the proportion may be obtained. Larger samples and rates closer to 0.5 will make the confidence intervals more and more precise.

Inferential Statistics

There are two major areas of statistical inference: the estimation of parameters and the testing of hypotheses. The use of the SE to create confidence intervals is an example of *parameter estimation.* The testing of hypotheses or *significance testing* is the main focus of inferential statistics. Hypothesis testing allows the experimenter to use data from the sample to make inferences about the population. Statisticians have created formulas that use the values of the samples to calculate test statistics. Statisticians have also explored the properties of various theoretical probability distributions. Depending on the assumptions about how data are collected, the appropriate probability distribution is chosen as the source of critical values to accept or reject the null hypothesis. If the value of the test statistic calculated from the sample(s) is greater than the critical value, the null hypothesis is rejected. The critical value is chosen from the appropriate probability distribution after the magnitude of the type I error is specified.

There are parameters within the equation that generate any particular probability distribution; for the normal probability distribution, the parameters are μ and σ^2. For the normal distribution, each set of values for μ and σ^2 will generate a different shape for the bell-like normal curve. All probability distributions contain one or more parameters and can be plotted as curves; these parameters may be discrete (integer only) or continuous. Each value or combination of values for these parameters will create a different curve for the probability distribution being used. Thus, each probability distribution is actually a family of probability curves. Some additional parameters of theoretical probability distributions have been given the special name *degrees of freedom* and are represented by the letters *m, n, p,* and *s.*

Associated with the formula for computing a test statistic is a rule for assigning integer values to the one or more parameters called degrees of freedom. The number of degrees of freedom and the value for each degree of freedom depend on (1) the number of subjects, (2) the number of experimental groups, (3) the specifics of the statistical hypothesis, and (4) the type of statistical test. The correct curve of the probability distribution from which to obtain a critical value for comparison with the value of the test statistic is obtained with the values of one or more degrees of freedom.

To accept or reject the null hypothesis, the following steps are performed: (1) confirm that experimental data conform to the assumptions of the intended statistical test; (2) choose a significance level (alpha); (3) calculate the test statistic; (4) determine the degree(s) of freedom; (5) find the critical value for the chosen alpha and the degree(s) of freedom from the appropriate probability distribution; (6) if the test statistic exceeds the critical value, reject the null hypothesis; (7) if the test statistic does not exceed the critical value, do not reject the null hypothesis. There are general guidelines that relate the variable type and the experimental design to the choice of statistical test (Table 3-5).

Dichotomous Data

In the experiment negating the value of mammary artery ligation, 5 of 8 patients (62.5%) having ligation showed benefit while 5 of 9 patients (55.6%) having sham surgery also had benefit.[1] Is this difference real? This experiment sampled patients from two populations—those having the real procedure and those having the sham procedure; the display of such results is usually presented as a contingency table (Table 3-6). A variety of statistical techniques allow a comparison of the success rate. These include *Fishers exact test* and *(Pearson's) chi-square test.* The chi-square test offers the advantage of being computationally simpler; it can also analyze contingency tables with more than two rows and two columns; however, certain assumptions of sample size and response rate are not achieved by this experiment. Fishers exact test fails to reject the null hypothesis for this data.

The results of such experiments are often presented as rate ratios. The ratio of improvement for the experimental group (62.5%) is divided by the ratio of improvement for the control group (55.6%). A rate ratio of 1.00 (100%) fails to show a difference of benefit or harm between the two groups. In this example the rate ratio is 1.125. Thus the experimental group had a 112.5% chance of improvement compared to the control group. A confidence interval can be calculated for the rate ratio; in this example it is widely spread to either side of the 1—a confidence interval of no difference.

Interval Data

Parametric statistics are the usual choice in the analysis of interval data, both discrete and continuous. The purpose of such analysis is to test the hypothesis of a difference between population means. The population means are unknown and are estimated by the sample means. A typical example would be

TABLE 3-5

WHEN TO USE WHAT

■ VARIABLE TYPE	■ ONE-SAMPLE TESTS	■ TWO-SAMPLE TESTS	■ MULTIPLE-SAMPLE TESTS
Dichotomous or nominal	Binomial distribution	chi-square test, Fisher's Exact test	chi-square test
Ordinal	chi-square test	chi-square test, nonparametric tests	chi-square test, nonparametric tests
Continuous or discrete	*z* distribution or *t* distribution	Unpaired *t* test, paired *t* test, nonparametric tests	Analysis of variance, nonparametric analysis of variance

TABLE 3-6

MAMMARY ARTERY LIGATION FOR ANGINA PECTORIS

OUTCOMES	TREATMENT: ACTUAL LIGATION	TREATMENT: SHAM LIGATION
Improved	5 (62.5%)	5 (55.6%)
Not improved	3 (37.5%)	4 (44.4%)

Fishers exact test: $p >> 0.05$.
Rate Ratio = 62.5%/55.6% = 1.125, 95% Confidence Interval (0.47 to 2.7); $p >> 0.05$.

the comparison of the mean heart rates of patients receiving and not receiving atropine. Parametric test statistics have been developed by using the properties of the normal probability distribution and two related probability distributions, the t and the F distributions. In using such parametric methods, the assumption is made that the sample or samples is/are drawn from population(s) with a normal distribution. The parametric test statistics that have been created for interval data all have the form of a ratio. In general terms, the numerator of this ratio is the variability of the means of the samples; the denominator of this ratio is the variability among all the members of the samples. These variabilities are similar to the variances developed for descriptive statistics. The test statistic is thus a ratio of variabilities or variances. All parametric test statistics are used in the same fashion; if the test statistic ratio becomes large, the null hypothesis of no difference is rejected. The critical values against which to compare the test statistic are taken from tables of the three relevant probability distributions. By definition, in hypothesis testing, at least one of the population means is unknown, but the population variance(s) may or may not be known. Parametric statistics can be divided into two groups according to whether or not the population variances are known. If the population variance is known, the test statistic used is called the z score; critical values are obtained from the normal distribution. In most biomedical applications, the population variance is rarely known and the z score is little used.

t Test

An important advance in statistical inference came early in the twentieth century with the creation of *Student's t test statistic* and the *t distribution*, which allowed the testing of hypotheses when the population variance is not known. The most common use of Student's t test is to compare the mean values of two populations. There are two types of t test. If each subject has two measurements taken, for example, one before (x_i) and one after a drug (y_i), then a one sample or *paired t test* procedure is used; each control measurement taken before drug administration is paired with a measurement in the same patient after drug administration. Of course, this is a self-control experiment. This pairing of measurements in the same patient reduces variability and increases statistical power. The difference $d_i = x_i - y_i$ of each pair of values is calculated and the average $\bar{d}$ is calculated. In the formula for Student's t statistic, the numerator is $\bar{d}$, whereas the denominator is the standard error of $\bar{d}$ ($SE_{\bar{d}}$):

$$t = \frac{\bar{d}}{SE_{\bar{d}}} \tag{3-5}$$

All t statistics are created in this way; the numerator is the difference of two means, whereas the denominator is the standard error of the two means. If the difference between the two means is large compared with their variability, then the null hypothesis of no difference is rejected. The critical values for the t statistic are taken from the t probability distribution. The t distribution is symmetric and bell-shaped but more spread out than the normal distribution. The t distribution has a single integer parameter; for a paired t test, the value of this single degree of freedom is the sample size minus one. There can be some confusion about the use of the letter t. It refers both to the value of the test statistic calculated by the formula and to the critical value from the theoretical probability distribution. The critical t value is determined by looking in a t table after a significance level is chosen and the degree of freedom is computed.

More commonly, measurements are taken on two separate groups of subjects. For example, one group receives blood pressure treatment (x_i), whereas no treatment is given to a control group (y_i). The number of subjects in each group might or might not be identical; regardless of this, in no sense is an individual measurement in the first group matched or paired with a specific measurement in the second group. An *unpaired* or *two-sample t test* is used to compare the means of the two groups. The numerator of the t statistic is $\bar{x} - \bar{y}$. The denominator is a weighted average of the SEs of each sample. The degree of freedom for an unpaired t test is calculated as the sum of the subjects of the two groups minus two. As with the paired t test, if the t ratio becomes large, the null hypothesis is rejected.

Multiple Comparisons and Analysis of Variance

Experiments in anesthesia, whether they are with humans or with animals, may not be limited to one or two groups of data for each variable. It is very common to follow a variable longitudinally; heart rate, for example, might be measured five times before and during anesthetic induction. These are also called repeated measurement experiments; the experimenter will wish to compare changes between the initial heart rate measurement and those obtained during induction. The experimental design might also include several groups receiving different induction drugs, for example, comparing heart rate across groups immediately after laryngoscopy. Researchers have mistakenly handled these analysis problems with the t test. If heart rate is collected five times, these collection times could be labeled A, B, C, D, and E. Then A could be compared with B, C, D, and E; B could be compared with C, D, and E; and so forth. The total of possible pairings is ten; thus, ten paired t tests could be calculated for all the possible pairings of A, B, C, D, and E. A similar approach can be used for comparing more than two groups for unpaired data.

The use of t tests in this fashion is inappropriate. In testing a statistical hypothesis, the experimenter sets the level of type I error; this is usually chosen to be 0.05. When using many t tests, as in the example given earlier, the chosen error rate for performing all these t tests is much higher than 0.05, even though the type I error is set at 0.05 for each individual comparison. In fact, the type I error rate for all t tests simultaneously, that is, the chance of finding at least one of the multiple t test statistics significant merely by chance, is given by the formula $\alpha = 1 - 0.95^k$. If 13 *t* tests are performed ($k = 13$), the real error rate is 49%. Applying *t* tests over and over again to all the possible pairings of a variable will misleadingly identify statistical significance when there is, in fact, none.

The most versatile approach for handling comparisons of means between more than two groups or between several measurements in the same group is called *analysis of variance* and is frequently cited by the acronym ANOVA. Analysis of variance consists of rules for creating test statistics on means when there are more than two groups. These test statistics are called *F ratios,* after Ronald Fisher; the critical values for the *F* test statistic are taken from the *F* probability distribution that Fisher derived.

Suppose that data for three groups are obtained. What can be said about the mean values of the three target populations? The *F* test is actually asking several questions simultaneously: is group 1 different from group 2; is group 2 different from group 3; and is group 1 different from group 3? As with the *t* test, the *F* test statistic is a ratio; in general terms, the numerator expresses the variability of the mean values of the three groups, whereas the denominator expresses the average variability or difference of each sample value from the mean of all sample values. The formulas to create the test statistic are computationally elegant but are rather hard to appreciate intuitively. The *F* statistic has two degrees of freedom, denoted *m* and *n;* the value of *m* is a function of the number of experimental groups; the value for *n* is a function of the number of subjects in all experimental groups. The analysis of multigroup data is not necessarily finished after the ANOVAs are calculated. If the null hypothesis is rejected and it is accepted that there are differences among the groups tested, how can it be decided where the differences are? A variety of techniques are available to make what are called multiple comparisons after the ANOVA test is performed.

Robustness and Nonparametric Tests

Most statistical tests depend on certain assumptions about the nature of the distribution of values in the underlying populations from which experimental samples are taken. For the parametric statistics, that is, *t* tests and analysis of variance, it is assumed that the populations follow the normal distribution. However, for some data, experience or historical reasons suggest that these assumptions of a normal distribution do not hold; some examples include proportions, percentages, and response times. What should the experimenter do if he or she fears that the data are not normally distributed?

The experimenter might choose to ignore the problem of nonnormal data and inhomogeneity of variance, hoping that everything will work out. Such insouciance is actually a very practical and reasonable approach to the problem. Parametric statistics are called "robust" statistics; they stand up to much adversity. To a statistician, robustness implies that the magnitude of type I errors is not seriously affected by ill-conditioned data. Parametric statistics are sufficiently robust that the accuracy of decisions reached by means of *t* tests and analysis of variance remains very credible, even for moderately severe departures from the assumptions.

Another possibility would be to use statistics that do not require any assumptions about probability distributions of the populations. Such statistics are known as *nonparametric tests;* they can be used whenever there is very serious concern about the shape of the data. Nonparametric statistics are also the tests of choice for ordinal data. The basic concept behind nonparametric statistics is the ability to rank or order the observations; nonparametric tests are also called *order statistics.*

Most nonparametric statistics still require the use of theoretical probability distributions; the critical values that must be exceeded by the test statistic are taken from the binomial, normal, and chi-square distributions, depending on the nonparametric test being used. The *nonparametric sign test, Mann-Whitney rank sum test,* and *Kruskal-Wallis one-way analysis of variance* are analogous to the paired *t* test, unpaired *t* test, and one-way analysis of variance, respectively. The currently available nonparametric tests are not used more commonly because they do not adapt well to complex statistical models and because they are less able than parametric tests to distinguish between the null and alternative hypotheses if the data are, in fact, normally distributed.

Interpretation of Results

Scientific studies do not end with the statistical test. The experimenter must submit an opinion as to the generalizability of his or her work to the rest of the world. Even if there is a statistically significant difference, the experimenter must decide if this difference is medically or physiologically important. Statistical significance does not always equate with biologic relevance. The questions an experimenter should ask about the interpretation of results are highly dependent on the specifics of the experiment. First, even small, clinically unimportant differences between groups can be detected if the sample size is sufficiently large. On the other hand, if the sample size is small, one must always worry that identified or unidentified confounding variables may explain any difference; as the sample size decreases, randomization is less successful in assuring homogenous groups. Second, if the experimental groups are given three or more doses of a drug, do the results suggest a steadily increasing or decreasing dose-response relationship? Suppose the observed effect for an intermediate dose is either much higher or much lower than that for both the highest and lowest dose; a dose-response relationship may exist, but some skepticism about the experimental methods is warranted. Third, for clinical studies comparing different drugs, devices, and operations on patient outcome, are the patients, clinical care, and studied therapies sufficiently similar to those provided at other locations to be of interest to a wide group of practitioners? This is the distinction between *efficacy*—does it work under the best (research) circumstances—and *effectiveness*—does it work under the typical circumstances of routine clinical care. Finally, in comparing alternative therapies, the confidence that a claim for a superior therapy is true depends on the study design. The strength of the evidence concerning efficacy will be least for an anecdotal case report; next in importance will be a retrospective study, then a prospective series of patients compared with historical controls, and finally a randomized, controlled clinical trial. The greatest strength for a therapeutic claim is a series of randomized, controlled clinical trials confirming the same hypothesis. There is now considerable enthusiasm for the formal synthesis and combining of results from two or more trials.

READING JOURNAL ARTICLES

Thousands of words are written each year in journal articles relevant to anesthesia. No one can read them all. How should the clinician determine which articles are useful? All that is possible is to learn to rapidly skip over most articles and concentrate on the few selected for their importance to the reader. Those few should be chosen according to their relevance and credibility. Relevance is determined by the specifics of one's anesthetic practice. Credibility is a function of the merits of the research methods, the experimental design, and the statistical analysis; the more proficient one's statistical skills, the more rapidly one can accept or reject the credibility of a research article.

Guidelines

Six easily remembered appraisal criteria for clinical studies can be fashioned from the words WHY, HOW, WHO, WHAT, HOW MANY, and SO WHAT: (1) WHY: Is the biologic hypothesis clearly stated? (2) HOW: What is the research design? (3) WHO: Is the target population clearly defined? (4) WHAT: How was the therapy administered and the data collected? (5) HOW MANY: Are the test statistics convincing? (6) SO WHAT: Is it clinically relevant to my patients? Although the statistical knowledge of most physicians is limited, these skills of critical appraisal of the literature can be learned and can tremendously increase the efficiency and benefit of journal reading.

Resources in journal reading, print and electronic, are now widely available. For example, The Evidenced-Based Medicine Working Group—a group of mainly Canadian physicians and statisticians from McMaster University, Ontario, Canada—has been organized to de-emphasize a foundation of unsystematic clinical experience, clinical intuition, and pathophysiologic rationale as the basis for medical decision and to teach the systematic evaluation of published evidence. Now combined in a single volume, detailed topics range from "How to Use an Article about Therapy or Prevention" to "How to Use an Article about Disease Probability for Differential Diagnosis."[5] This material is also available interactively (http://ugi.usersguides.org/UGI/default.asp accessed 30-JUL-2004).

Statistical Resources

Accompanying the exponential growth of medical information since World War II has been the creation of a wealth of biostatistical knowledge. Textbooks with expositions of basic, intermediate, and advanced statistics abound.[6–8] There are new journals of biomedical statistics, including *Clinical Trials, Statistics in Medicine,* and *Statistical Methods in Medical Research,* whose audiences are both statisticians and biomedical researchers. Some medical journals, for example, the *British Medical Journal,* regularly publish expositions of both basic and newer advanced statistical methods. Extensive Internet resources can be linked from the home page of the long established American Statistical Association (http://www.amstat.org/ accessed 30-JUL-2004) and at the StatLib (http://lib.stat.cmu.edu/ accessed 30-JUL-2004) of Carnegie Mellon University including electronic textbooks of basic statistical methods, online statistical calculators, standard data sets, reviews of statistical software, and so on.

Example of Newer Statistics

6 Reports using a new type of research method—the systematic review—have become commonplace over the last 15 years in anesthesia journals. (As of July 2004, a literature search for "systematic review AND anesthesia" in PubMed at the National Library of Medicine returned 695 citations out of a total of 82,484 citations for systematic reviews [www.ncbi.nlm.nih.gov/entrez accessed 15-JUL-2004].) In systematic reviews, a focused question drives the research, for example, (1) *Transient neurologic symptoms (TNS) following spinal anaesthesia with lidocaine versus other local anaesthetic*[9] or (2) *Ventilation with lower tidal volumes versus traditional tidal volumes in adults for acute lung injury and acute respiratory distress syndrome.*[10] These titles reveal some of the research design of a systematic review. There is a population of interest: (1) patients having *spinal anesthesia* and (2) *adults* [with] *acute lung injury and acute respiratory distress syndrome.* There is an intervention versus a comparison group: (1) *lidocaine versus other local anaesthetics* and (2) *ventilation with lower tidal volumes versus traditional tidal volumes.* There is an outcome for choosing success or failure: (1) occurrence of *transient neurologic symptoms (TNS)* and (2) *28-day mortality* (listed in text).

To answer the experimental question, data are obtained from randomized controlled trials already in the medical literature rather than from direct experimentation; the basic unit of analysis of this observational research is the published study. The researchers, also called the reviewers, proceed through a structured protocol, which includes in part: (1) choice of study inclusion/exclusion criteria, (2) explicitly defined literature searching, (3) abstraction of data from included studies, (4) appraisal of data quality, (5) systematic pooling of data, and (6) discussion of inferences. Binary outcomes (yes/no, alive/dead, presence/absence) within a study are usually compared by the relative risk (rate ratio) statistic. If there is sufficient clinical similarity among the included studies, a summary relative risk of the overall effect of the comparison treatments is estimated by meta-analysis; meta-analysis is a set of statistical techniques for combining results from different studies. The calculations for the statistical analyses of a meta-analysis are unfamiliar to most, but are not difficult. The results of a meta-analysis are usually present in a figure called a forest plot (see Fig 3-1).[9] The left-most column identifies the included studies and the observed data. The horizontal lines and diamond shapes are graphical representations of individual study relative risk and summary relative risk, respectively; the right-most column of the figure lists the relative risks with 95% Confidence Intervals for the individual studies and the summary statistics. There are also descriptive and inferential statistics concerning the statistical heterogeneity of the meta-analysis and the significance of the summary statistics.

An examination of Figure 3-1 shows that many of the individual studies (8 of 12) had wide, nonsignificant confidence intervals that touch or cross the relative risk of identity (RR = 1). In this systematic review of TNS there were three subgroup comparisons: spinal lidocaine versus bupivacaine, prilocaine, and procaine; for each subgroup the relative risk of TNS was 6 to 7 times higher for lidocaine and the overall relative risk calculated from all studies was 7.13 with a 95% Confidence Interval [3.92, 12.95]. The power of summary statistics to combine evidence is clear. The reviewers concluded: "Lidocaine can cause transient neurologic symptoms (TNS) in every seventh patient who receives spinal anaesthesia. The relative risk of developing TNS is about seven times higher for lidocaine than for bupivacaine, prilocaine, and procaine. These painful symptoms disappear completely by the tenth postoperative day."[9]

The promotion of systematic reviews comes from several sources. Many come from the individual initiative of researchers who publish their results as stand alone reports in the journals of medicine and anesthesia. The American Society of Anesthesiologists has developed a process for the creation of practice parameters that includes among other things a variant form of systematic reviews. The most prominent proponent of systematic reviews is the Cochrane Collaboration, Oxford, UK. "The Cochrane Collaboration is an international non-profit and independent organization, dedicated to making up-to-date, accurate information about the effects of health care readily available worldwide. It produces and disseminates systematic reviews of health care interventions and promotes the search

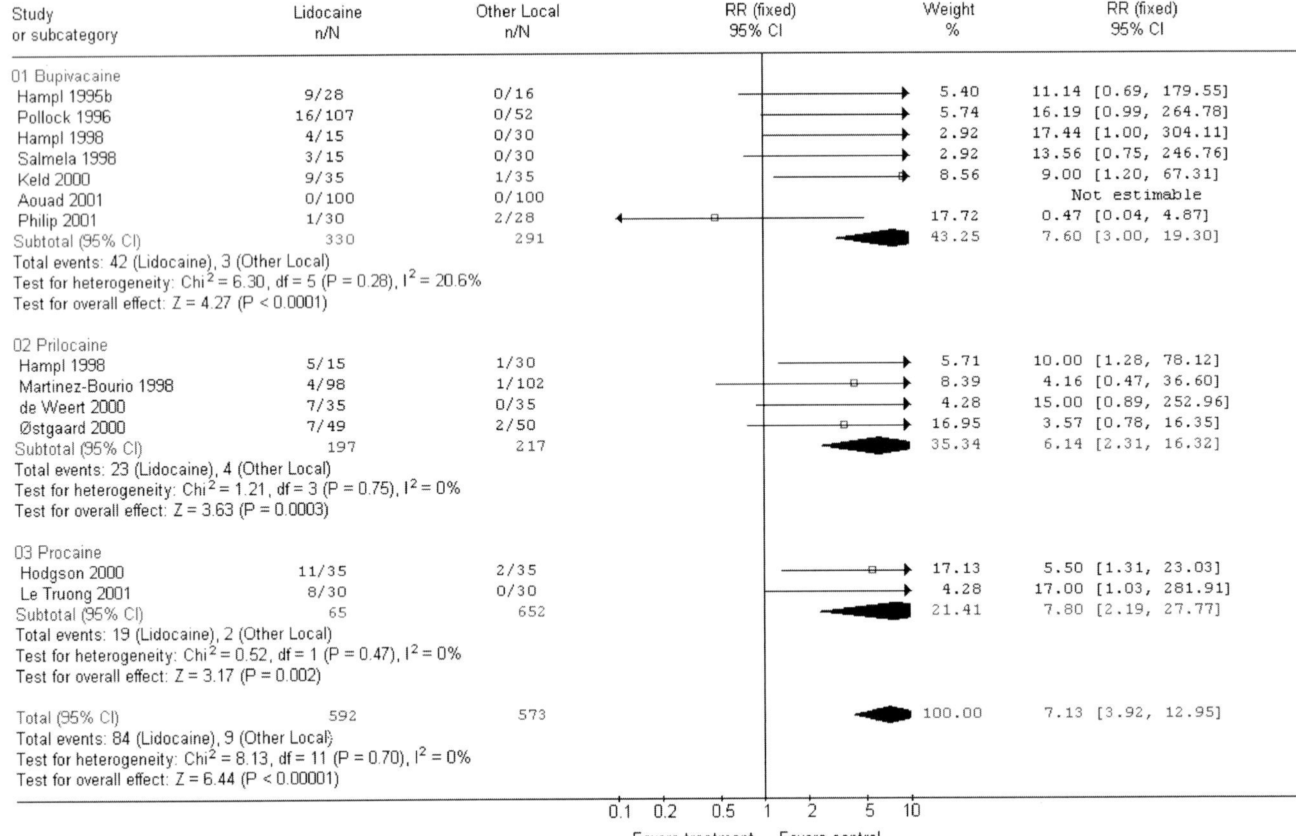

FIGURE 3-1. Forest plot modified from Graph 02/01 in Zaric D, Christiansen C, Pace NL, Punjasawadwong Y. Transient neurologic symptoms (TNS) following spinal anaesthesia with lidocaine versus other local anaesthetics (Cochrane Review). In: *The Cochrane Library*, Issue 3. Chichester, UK: John Wiley & Sons, Ltd., 2004. Copyright Cochrane Library, reproduced with permission.

for evidence in the form of clinical trials and other studies of interventions. The Cochrane Collaboration was founded in 1993 and named for the British epidemiologist, Archie Cochrane" (www.cochrane.org, accessed July 31, 2004).

There are more than 50 collaborative review groups that provide the editorial control and supervision of systematic reviews; one of these, located in Copenhagen, prepares and maintains the accessibility of systematic reviews of the effects of health care interventions in the areas of anesthesia, perioperative medicine, intensive care medicine, and so on (www.cochrane-anaesthesia.suite.dk, accessed July 31, 2004). The Cochrane Collaboration has extensive documentation available electronically explaining the techniques of systematic reviews and meta-analysis. Introductory textbooks of biostatistics now include expositions on systematic reviews also.[5]

CONCLUSION

One intent of this chapter is to present the scope of support that the discipline of statistics can provide to anesthesia research. Although an intuitive understanding of certain basic principles is emphasized, these basic principles are not necessarily simple and have been developed by statisticians with great mathematical rigor. Academic anesthesia needs more workers to immerse themselves in these statistical fundamentals. Having done so, these statistically knowledgeable academic anesthesiologists will be prepared to improve their own research projects, to assist their colleagues in research, to efficiently seek consultation from the professional statistician, to strengthen the editorial review of journal articles, and to expound to the clinical reader the whys and wherefores of statistics. The clinical reader also needs to expend his or her own effort to acquire some basic statistical skills. Journals are increasingly difficult to understand without some basic statistical understanding. Some clinical problems can be best understood with a perspective based on probability. Finally, understanding principles of experimental design can prevent premature acceptances of new therapies from faulty studies.

References

1. Cobb LA, Thomas GI, Dillard DH, Merendino KA, Bruce RA: An evaluation of internal-mammary-artery ligation by a double-blind technic. N Engl J Med 260:1115–1118,1959
2. Sacks H, Chalmers TC, Smith HJ: Randomized versus historical controls for clinical trials. Am J Med 72:233–240,1982
3. Schulz KF, Chalmers I, Hayes RJ, Altman DG: Empirical evidence of bias. Dimensions of methodological quality associated with estimates of treatment effects in controlled trials. JAMA 273:408–412, 1995
4. Freiman JA, Chalmers TC, Smith HJ, Kuebler RR: The importance of beta, the type II error and sample size in the design and interpretation of the randomized control trial. Survey of 71 "negative" trials. N Engl J Med 299:690–694, 1978

5. Rennie D, Guyatt G: Users Guides Manual for Evidence-Based clinical Practice. Chicago, AMA Press, 2002
6. Altman DG, Trevor B, Gardner MJ, Machin D: Statistics with Confidence. London, BMJ Books, 2000
7. Dawson B, Trapp R: Basic & Clinical Biostatistics. New York, McGraw-Hill/Appleton & Lange, 2004
8. Glantz S: Primer of Biostatistics. New York, McGraw-Hill/Appleton & Lange, 2001
9. Zaric D, Christiansen C, Pace NL, Punjasawadwong Y: Transient neurologic symptoms (TNS) following spinal anaesthesia with lidocaine versus other local anaesthetics (Cochrane Review), In: The Cochrane Library. Chichester, UK, John Wiley & Sons, Ltd, Issue 3, 2004
10. Petrucci N, Iacovelli W: Ventilation with lower tidal volumes versus traditional tidal volumes in adults for acute lung injury and acute respiratory distress syndrome (Cochrane Review), In: The Cochrane Library. Chichester, UK, John Wiley & Sons, Ltd, Issue 3, 2004

CHAPTER 4 ■ OCCUPATIONAL HEALTH

ARNOLD J. BERRY AND JONATHAN D. KATZ

KEY POINTS

1. With the use of scavenging equipment, routine machine maintenance, and appropriate work practices, exposure to waste anesthetic gases can be reduced to levels below those recommended by National Institute for Occupational Safety and Health (NIOSH).
2. Twenty-four percent of anesthesia personnel manifest evidence of contact dermatitis in response to latex exposure and approximately 15% are sensitized and vulnerable to allergic reactions.
3. Vigilance is one of the most critical tasks performed by anesthesiologists. The vigilance task is adversely affected by several factors including poor equipment engineering and design, excessive noise in the operating room, impediments to interpersonal communication, production pressure, and fatigue.
4. Sleep deprivation and fatigue are common among anesthesiologists. Sleep deprivation can have deleterious effects on cognition, performance, mood, and health.
5. The risk of exposure to infectious pathogens can be reduced by the routine use of standard precautions, appropriate isolation precautions for infected patients, and safety devices designed to prevent needlestick injuries.
6. Hepatitis B vaccine is recommended for all anesthesia personnel because of the increased risk for occupational transmission of this bloodborne pathogen.
7. Many consider chemical dependency to be the primary occupational hazard among anesthesiologists. An incidence of 1 to 2% of controlled substance abuse has been repeatedly reported within anesthesia training programs.
8. It remains controversial whether anesthesiologists are, on average, vulnerable to premature death. However, by correcting for the fact that living anesthesiologists are, on average, younger than most other specialists, it is apparent that anesthesiologists do not die younger.

Anesthesia personnel spend long hours, in fact, most of their waking days, in an environment filled with many potential hazards—the operating room. This setting is unique among workplaces as a result of the potential exposure to chemical vapors, ionizing radiation, and infectious agents. Additionally, anesthesia personnel are subject to heightened levels of psychological stress engendered by the high-stakes nature of the practice. Although such physical hazards as fires and explosions from flammable anesthetic agents are currently of limited concern, occupational illnesses, such as alcohol and drug abuse, are well recognized as significant within the anesthesia community. Some hazards, such as exposure to trace levels of waste anesthetic gases, have been extensively studied. Others, like suicide, have been recognized but not adequately pursued. Only within the past few decades have epidemiologic surveys been conducted to assess the health of anesthesia personnel. In general, the potential health risks to those working in the operating room may be significant, but with awareness of the problems and the use of proper precautions, they are not formidable.

PHYSICAL HAZARDS

Anesthetic Gases

Although the inhalation anesthetics diethyl ether, nitrous oxide, and chloroform were first used in the 1840s, the biologic effects of occupational exposure to anesthetic agents were not investigated until the 1960s. Reports on the effects of chronic environmental exposure to anesthetics have included epidemiologic surveys, in vitro studies, cellular research, and studies in laboratory animals and humans. Areas addressed include the potential influence of trace anesthetic concentrations on the incidence in affected populations of the following: death, infertility, spontaneous abortion, congenital malformations, cancer, hematopoietic diseases, liver disease, neurologic disease, psychomotor, and behavioral changes.

Anesthetic Levels in the Operating Room

Early investigators established that significant levels of ether were present in the operating room when the open drop technique was used, but the first report of occupational exposure to modern anesthetics was by Linde and Bruce in 1969.[1] They sampled air at various distances from the "pop-off" valve of anesthesia machines and noted an average concentration of halothane of 10 parts per million (ppm) and of nitrous oxide of 130 ppm. (Parts per million is a volume-per-volume unit of measurement; 10,000 ppm equals 1%.) End-expired air samples taken from 24 anesthesiologists after work revealed 0 to 12 ppm of halothane. It was later demonstrated that with appropriate scavenging equipment and adequate air exchange in the operating room, levels of waste anesthetic gases could be significantly reduced.

Waste anesthetic concentrations in modern operating rooms where routine scavenging is performed are considerably less than those found in the early studies.[2,3] This raises the questions of whether chronic exposure to these low levels of waste anesthetic gases actually constitutes a significant occupational hazard and whether results from studies performed in "unscavenged" operating rooms are applicable to current practice.

Epidemiologic Studies

Epidemiologic surveys were among the first studies to suggest the possibility of a hazard resulting from exposure to trace levels of anesthetics. Although epidemiologic studies may be useful in assessing problems of this type, they have the potential for errors associated with the collection of data and their interpretation. Valid epidemiologic studies require appropriate design strategies including the presence of an appropriate control group for the cohort being studied. When questionnaires are used to obtain personal medical information, the data may be misleading because individuals may knowingly or unknowingly give incorrect information based solely on remembered data. Cause-and-effect relationships or causality cannot be documented by epidemiologic studies unless all other possible etiologies (confounders) can be ruled out or other lines of evidence are used for substantiation. Few epidemiologic studies on the effects of occupational exposure to waste anesthetic gases fulfill these design criteria.

Reproductive Outcome. One of the largest epidemiologic studies to assess the effects of trace anesthetics on reproductive outcome was conducted by the American Society of Anesthesiologists (ASA).[4] Questionnaires were sent to 49,585 operating room personnel who had potential exposure to waste anesthetic gases (members of the ASA, the American Association of Nurse Anesthetists, the Association of Operating Room Nurses, and the Association of Operating Room Technicians). A nonexposed group of 23,911 from the American Academy of Pediatrics and the American Nurses' Association served as controls. Analyses of these data indicated that there was an increased risk of spontaneous abortion and congenital abnormalities in children of women who worked in the operating room and an increased risk of congenital abnormalities in offspring of unexposed wives of male operating room personnel. Several reviews have identified inconsistencies in the data used to compare exposed and unexposed groups and to make within-group comparisons. Expected levels of anesthetic exposure did not correlate with reproductive outcome.

The ASA subsequently commissioned a group of epidemiologists and biostatisticians to evaluate and assess conflicting data from published epidemiologic surveys.[5] After analysis of methods, they found only five studies on spontaneous abortion and congenital abnormalities in offspring of anesthesia personnel that were free of errors in study design or statistical analysis. From these studies, the relative risks (the ratio of the rate of disease among those exposed to that found in those not exposed) of spontaneous abortion for female physicians and female nurses working in the operating room were 1.4 and 1.3, respectively (a relative risk of 1.3 represents a 30% increase in risk when compared with the risk of the control population). The increased relative risk for congenital abnormalities was of borderline statistical significance for exposed physicians only. Although they found a statistically significant relative risk of spontaneous abortion and congenital abnormalities in women working in the operating room, the relative risk was small compared with other, better-documented environmental hazards. They also pointed out that duration and level of anesthetic exposure were not measured in any of the studies and that other confounding factors, such as stress, infections, and radiation exposure, were not considered.

Because personnel working in some dental operatories have exposure to nitrous oxide, the dental literature has also addressed these issues. One pertinent study used data collected via telephone interviews with 418 female dental assistants to assess the effect of nitrous oxide exposure on fertility.[6] Fecundability (the ability to conceive, which is measured by the time to pregnancy during periods of unprotected sexual intercourse) was significantly reduced in women with 5 or more hours of exposure to unscavenged nitrous oxide per week. In another study of 7,000 female dental assistants, questionnaires were used to determine rates of spontaneous abortion.[7] There was an increased rate of spontaneous abortion among women who worked for 3 or more hours per week in offices not using scavenging devices for nitrous oxide (relative risk [RR] = 2.6, adjusted for age, smoking, and number of amalgams prepared per week). These findings must be viewed with caution because the estimates of nitrous oxide exposure were based solely on respondents' reports, and measurements of nitrous oxide concentrations in the work space were not performed. Therefore, dose–effect relationships cannot be confirmed. It is important to note that in both studies of female dental assistants, use of nitrous oxide in offices with scavenging devices was not associated with an increased risk for adverse reproductive outcomes.[6,7]

A meta-analysis of 19 epidemiologic studies, which included hospital workers, dental assistants, and veterinarians and veterinary assistants, demonstrated an increased risk of spontaneous abortion in women with occupational exposure to anesthetic gases (RR = 1.48; 95% confidence interval, 1.40 to 1.58).[8] Additional analysis demonstrated that the relative risk of 1.48 corresponded to an increased absolute risk of abortion of 6.2%. Stratification by job category indicated that the relative risk was greatest for veterinarians (RR = 2.45), followed by dental assistants (RR = 1.89) and hospital workers (RR = 1.30). When the meta-analysis was confined to five studies that controlled for several nonoccupational confounding variables, had appropriate control groups, and had sufficient response rate, the relative risk for spontaneous abortion was 1.90 (95% confidence interval, 1.72 to 2.09). The author noted that the routine use of scavenging devices has been implemented since the time that most of the studies in this analysis were performed and that there was no risk of spontaneous abortion in studies of personnel that worked in scavenged environments.

Retrospective surveys of large numbers of women who worked during pregnancy indicate that negative reproductive outcomes may be related to job-associated conditions other than exposure to trace anesthetic gases. A survey of 3,985 Swedish midwives demonstrated that night work was significantly associated with spontaneous abortions after the twelfth week of pregnancy (OR = 3.33), while exposure to nitrous oxide appeared to have no effect.[9] Using a case-control study design, Luke et al[10] found that increased work hours, hours worked while standing, and occupational fatigue were associated with preterm birth in obstetric and neonatal nurses. These and other studies have provided data that link spontaneous abortion in women working in health care to job-related factors other than exposure to trace anesthetic gases. This casts doubt on the validity of earlier studies that did not control for occupational stresses such as fatigue, long work hours, and night shifts.

Although many of the existing epidemiologic studies have potential flaws in design, the evidence taken as a whole suggests that there is a slight increase in the relative risk of spontaneous abortion and congenital abnormalities in offspring for female physicians working in the operating room.[11] Whether these findings are attributable to anesthetic exposure or other work-related conditions cannot be definitely determined from this type of investigation. Well-designed surveys of large numbers of personnel and appropriate control groups, controlled for other factors such as work hours and night shifts, are necessary to link trace anesthetic exposures to adverse reproductive outcomes. The routine use of scavenging techniques has generally lowered environmental anesthetic levels in the operating room and may make it more difficult to prove any adverse reproductive effects using epidemiologic data. Although it is easy to measure and quantify the levels of anesthetic in the operating room air, it is harder to measure and assess the effect of other possible factors, such as stress, alterations in working schedule, and fatigue.

Neoplasms and Other Nonreproductive Diseases. One of the first surveys enumerating causes of death among anesthesiologists was reported by Bruce et al in 1968.[12] The authors compared the death rates of members of the ASA from 1947 to 1966 with those for American men and male policyholders of a large insurance company. There was a higher death rate among male anesthesiologists from malignancies of the lymphoid and reticuloendothelial tissues and from suicide, but a lower death rate from lung cancer and coronary artery disease.

In a subsequent prospective study, Bruce et al[13] compared the causes of death in ASA members during the years 1967 to 1971 with those of men insured by one company. The overall death rate for ASA members was lower than for the controls, and contrary to the previous results, there was no increase in death rates from malignancies of lymphoid and reticuloendothelial tissues. The authors concluded that their data provided no evidence to support the speculation that lymphoid malignancies were an occupational hazard for anesthesiologists.

An ASA-sponsored study, published in 1974, found no differences in cancer rates between men exposed and those not exposed to trace concentrations of anesthetic gases.[4] For women respondents, there was a 1.3-fold to 2-fold increase in the occurrence of cancer in the exposed group, resulting predominantly from an increase in leukemia and lymphoma. The analysis of Buring et al[5] of these data confirmed an increase in relative risk of cancer in exposed women (1.4) but attributed the increase solely to cervical cancer[2,8]. They also noted that the ASA study did not assess the effect of confounding variables, such as sexual history or smoking, that may have contributed to the findings. It is doubtful that the carcinogenic effect of anesthetics would be sex related, and the conflicting results for men and women, especially in light of the low statistical significance of the data, cast doubt that anesthetics were the causative agents.

Another ASA-sponsored mortality study of anesthesiologists, covering the period from 1976 to 1995, utilized data on cause of death from the National Death Index.[14] The mortality risks of a cohort of 40,242 anesthesiologists were compared to a matched cohort of internists. There was no difference between the two groups in overall mortality risk or mortality because of cancer or heart disease, but the mean age at death for decedents was significantly lower for anesthesiologists compared to internists (66.5 years versus 69.0 years). In a subsequent study, Katz[15] used data from the American Medical Association (AMA) to conclude that there was no statistical difference in age-specific mortality among anesthesiologists, internists, and other physicians when ages of the living members of the physician groups were considered in the analyses.

Epidemiologic studies are useful tools for attempting to identify adverse effects of the operating room environment, including exposure to many substances, of which waste anesthetic gases comprise but one factor. The data from epidemiologic surveys can, at best, suggest associations but can never prove cause-and-effect relationships between an exposure to a condition or substance and a disease process. There are shortcomings in many surveys that attempt to assess the effects of waste anesthetic gases, and these have resulted in conflicting conclusions. Overall, there appears to be some evidence that the operating room environment produces a slight increase in the rate of spontaneous abortion and cancer in female anesthesiologists and nurses.[5] Mortality risks from cancer and heart disease for anesthesiologists do not differ from those for other medical specialists.

Laboratory Studies

Along with epidemiologic studies, investigators have been active in the laboratory, assessing the effects of anesthetic agents on cell, tissue, and animal models. It is thought that this work might provide the scientific evidence linking anesthetic exposure to the adverse effects that have been suggested by some epidemiologic surveys.

Cellular Effects. Nitrous oxide administered in clinically useful concentrations affects hematopoietic and neural cells by irreversibly oxidizing the cobalt atom of vitamin B_{12} from an active to inactive state. This inhibits methionine synthetase and prevents the conversion of methyltetrahydrofolate to tetrahydrofolate, which is required for DNA synthesis, assembly of the myelin sheath, and methyl substitutions in neurotransmitters. Inhibition of methionine synthetase in individuals exposed to high concentrations of nitrous oxide may result in anemia and polyneuropathy, but chronic exposure to trace levels does not appear to produce these effects.[16]

Many studies have been performed in animals to assess the carcinogenicity of anesthetics. A preliminary study suggested that isoflurane produced hepatic neoplasia when administered to mice during gestation and early life, but a subsequent, well-controlled study failed to reproduce these results.[17] Research using mice and rats found no carcinogenic effect of halothane, nitrous oxide, or enflurane.

Several investigators have used the Ames bacterial assay system for studying the mutagenicity of anesthetics. This assay is rapid, inexpensive, and has a high true-positive rate when compared with in vivo tests. Halothane, enflurane, methoxyflurane, isoflurane, and urine from patients anesthetized with these agents was not mutagenic using this assay.[18] Urine from people working in scavenged or unscavenged operating rooms was also negative for mutagens.[19]

Other studies have used analyses of sister chromatid exchanges (SCE) or formation of micronucleated lymphocytes to assess for genotoxicity in association with anesthetic exposure. These tests may be of interest because there may be an association between these genetic changes and cancer. The majority of studies using SCE testing have been negative for enflurane, isoflurane, and sevoflurane exposure.[20] Anesthetists at an institution where waste gas scavenging was not used had an increased fraction of micronucleated lymphocytes compared to those practicing in a hospital where waste anesthetic gases were scavenged.[21] Low-level exposure as occurs in scavenged operating rooms is not associated with increased formation of micronucleated lymphocytes. The predictive value for the association of this test to the incidence of cancer is unclear.

The data from several lines of evidence indicate that occupational exposure to the low levels of anesthetics found with effective waste gas scavenging is not associated with significant cellular effects.

Reproductive Outcome. Because of the suggestion from epidemiologic data that occupational exposure to waste anesthetic gases may have resulted in an increased rate of spontaneous abortion and congenital abnormalities, numerous studies have been performed in laboratory animals to assess reproductive outcome. Most animal experiments fail to demonstrate alterations in female or male fertility or reproduction with exposure to subanesthetic concentrations of the currently used anesthetic agents. It is important to realize that data from laboratory investigations in animals may not be directly applicable to humans.

Effects of Trace Anesthetic Levels on Psychomotor Skills

Several studies have been conducted to attempt to clarify whether low concentrations of anesthetics alter the psychomotor skills required for providing high-quality care. In one investigation, psychomotor tests were used to assess the effect of nitrous oxide (500, 50, or 25 ppm) alone or with halothane (10, 1.0, or 0.5 ppm).[22] After exposure to the highest concentrations of nitrous oxide and halothane, subjects' performance declined on four of the seven tests. Interestingly, there was a decrease in ability in six of seven tests after exposure to the same level of nitrous oxide alone. Exposure to the lowest concentrations studied, 25 ppm nitrous oxide and 0.5 ppm halothane, produced no effects as measured by this battery of tests.

Other investigators, using similar protocols, have found no effect on psychomotor test performance after exposure to trace concentrations of halothane or nitrous oxide. The reason for differences in outcome between studies is unclear, but Bruce, one of the original investigators, has attributed the psychological effects of low levels of anesthetics to unusual sensitivity in the group of paid volunteers used in the study.[23]

Recommendations of the National Institute for Occupational Safety and Health

The National Institute for Occupational Safety and Health is the federal agency responsible for ensuring that workers have a safe and healthful working environment. It meets these goals through the conduct and funding of research, through education of employers and employees about occupational illnesses, and through establishing occupational health standards. A second federal agency, the Occupational Safety and Health Administration (OSHA), is responsible for enacting job health standards, investigating work sites to detect violation of standards, and enforcing the standards by citing violators. In 1977, NIOSH published a criteria document that recommended that waste anesthetic exposure should not exceed 2 ppm (1-hour ceiling) of halogenated anesthetic agents when used alone, or 0.5 ppm of a halogenated agent and 25 ppm of nitrous oxide (time-weighted average during use).[24] In addition, it stated that operating room employees should be advised of the potential harmful effects of anesthetics. The guidelines proposed that annual medical and occupational histories be obtained from all personnel and that any abnormal outcomes of pregnancies should be documented. The publication also included information on scavenging procedures and equipment and methods for monitoring concentrations of waste anesthetic gases in the air.

The 1977 NIOSH criteria document has not been adopted by OSHA, which currently does not have a standard for waste anesthetic gases. Some states, however, have instituted regulations calling for routine measurement of ambient nitrous oxide in operating rooms and have mandated that levels not exceed an arbitrary maximum.

In 1994, NIOSH published an alert to warn health care personnel that exposure to nitrous oxide may produce "harmful effects."[25] In this document, NIOSH recommends the following to reduce nitrous oxide exposure: (1) monitoring the air in operating rooms; (2) implementation of appropriate engineering controls, work practices, and equipment maintenance procedures; and (3) institution of a worker education program.

Since publication of the NIOSH criteria document, several volatile anesthetic agents (enflurane, isoflurane, sevoflurane, and desflurane) have been introduced into clinical practice. Although the NIOSH document addressed halogenated agents (halothane), the agents most commonly used in current practice have potencies, chemical characteristics, and rate and products of metabolism that differ significantly from older anesthetics. One must question whether the exposure thresholds cited by NIOSH in 1977 should also apply to agents that were not available at the time. It is important to note that other organizations and agencies in the United States and Europe have set occupational exposure limits for waste anesthetic gases and in most cases, these are greater than those recommended by NIOSH (Table 4-1).

In view of the conflicting scientific data and published recommendations, it is reasonable to ask what is an acceptable exposure level for waste anesthetic gases. Although it may be difficult to be certain of a threshold concentration below which

TABLE 4-1

EXAMPLES OF RECOMMENDED THRESHOLD LIMITS[a] FOR OCCUPATIONAL EXPOSURE TO ANESTHETIC AGENTS

COUNTRY	NITROUS OXIDE	HALOTHANE	ENFLURANE	ISOFLURANE
U.S. (NIOSH)	25	2	2	2
U.S. (ACGIH)	50	50	75	N
Great Britain	100	10	50	50
Norway	100	5	2	2
Sweden	100	5	10	10

[a]Time-weighted average in parts per million.
NIOSH, National Institute of Occupational Safety and Health; **ACGIH**, American Conference of Governmental Industrial Hygienists; **N**, not determined.

chronic exposure is "safe," it is prudent to institute measures that reduce waste anesthetic levels in the operating room environment without compromising patient safety. Methods for reducing and monitoring waste gases in the operating room have
1 been suggested.[3] Through the use of scavenging equipment, equipment maintenance procedures, altered anesthetic work practices, and efficient operating room ventilation systems, the environmental anesthetic concentration can be reduced to minimal levels. To ensure reduced occupational exposure, departmental programs should incorporate the ability to monitor for detection of leaks in the high- and low-pressure systems of anesthetic machines, contamination as a result of faulty anesthetic techniques such as poor mask fit or leaks around the cuffs of endotracheal tubes and laryngeal mask airways, and scavenging system malfunctions (Table 4-2). When there have been leaks of anesthetic gases, dispersion and removal of the pollutants are dependent on the adequacy of room ventilation. Standards for operating room construction from the American Institute of Architects require 15 to 21 air exchanges per hour with 3 bringing in outside air.[26] Environmental levels of anesthetics can be measured using instantaneously collected samples, continuous air monitoring, or time-weighted averages.[3] With appropriate care, environmental levels of anesthetics in the operating room can be reduced to comply with those suggested by NIOSH.

TABLE 4-2

SOURCES OF OPERATING ROOM CONTAMINATION

■ ANESTHETIC TECHNIQUES

- failure to turn off gas flow control valves at the end of an anesthetic
- turning gas flow on before placing mask on patient
- poorly fitting masks, especially with mask induction of anesthesia
- flushing of the circuit
- filling of anesthesia vaporizers
- uncuffed or leaking tracheal tubes (e.g., pediatric) or poor-fitting laryngeal mask airways
- pediatric circuits (e.g., Jackson-Rees version of the Mapleson D system)
- sidestream sampling carbon dioxide and anesthetic gas analyzers

■ ANESTHESIA MACHINE DELIVERY SYSTEM AND SCAVENGING SYSTEM

- open/closed system
- occlusion/malfunction of hospital disposal system
- maladjustment of hospital disposal system vacuum
- leaks
  - high-pressure hoses or connectors
  - nitrous oxide tank mounting
  - O rings
  - CO_2 absorbent canisters
  - low-pressure circuit

■ OTHER SOURCES

- cryo surgery units
- cardiopulmonary bypass circuits

Modified from Task Force on Trace Anesthetic Gases of the Committee on Occupational Health of Operating Room Personnel: *Waste Anesthetic Gases: Information for Management in Anesthetizing Areas and the Postanesthesia Care Unit (PACU).* Park Ridge, Ill, American Society of Anesthesiologists, 1999, with permission from the American Society of Anesthesiologists. A copy of the full text can be obtained from the ASA, 520 N. Northwest Highway, Park Ridge, Illinois 60068-2573.

Anesthetic Levels in the Postanesthesia Care Unit

As patients awaken from general anesthesia in the postanesthesia care unit (PACU), waste anesthetic gases are released into this environment. In a 1998 study, the time-weighted average concentrations for isoflurane, desflurane, and nitrous oxide were 1.1 ppm, 2.1 ppm, and 29 ppm, respectively, in the breathing zone of PACU nurses.[27] Half of the patients were intubated on arrival in the PACU, suggesting that they were still partially anesthetized and were exhaling a greater concentration of anesthetic gases than if they had already awakened. In contrast, other investigators reported time-weighted nitrous oxide levels less than 2.0 ppm from two PACUs.[28] The practice in these institutions was to routinely discontinue nitrous oxide at the end of surgery, approximately 5 minutes before the patient left the operating room. Also, there was adequate ventilation documented in the PACUs. NIOSH threshold limits for anesthetic gases can be obtained in the PACU by ensuring adequate room ventilation and fresh gas exchange and by discontinuing the anesthetic gases in sufficient time prior to leaving the operating room.

Chemicals

Methyl Methacrylate

Methyl methacrylate is commonly used to cement prostheses to bone or to repair bone defects. Known cardiovascular complications of methyl methacrylate in surgical patients include hypotension, bradycardia, and cardiac arrest. The effects of occupational exposure are less well documented. Reported risks from repeated occupational exposure to methyl methacrylate include allergic reactions and asthma, dermatitis, eye irritation including possible corneal ulceration, headache, and neurological signs. In one report, a health care worker suffered significant lower limb neuropathy after repeated occupational exposure to methyl methacrylate.[29]

OSHA has established an 8-hour, time-weighted average allowable exposure of 100 ppm. Concentrations as high as 280 ppm have been measured when methyl methacrylate is prepared for use in the operating room, but peak environmental concentration can be decreased by 75% when scavenging devices are properly used.

Allergic Reactions

In addition to concerns about toxic effects associated with exposure to volatile anesthetics or chemicals, anesthesiologists may develop sensitivities or allergic reactions to substances found in the health care environment.

Halothane. Repeated bouts of hepatitis in a small number of anesthesiologists have been attributed to hypersensitivity reactions rather than to a direct toxic effect of halothane. Analyses of sera from pediatric and general anesthesiologists demonstrated that exposure to halothane was associated with an increased prevalence of autoantibodies to cytochrome P450 2E1 and hepatic endoplasmic reticulum protein (ERp58).[30] Despite the presence of these autoantibodies, only 1 of 105 pediatric anesthesiologists had symptoms of hepatic injury. These data suggest that although autoantibodies may occur in anesthesiologists exposed to volatile anesthetics, they do not appear to be the cause of anesthetic-induced hepatitis.

Latex. Latex in surgical and examination gloves has be-
2 come a common source of allergic reactions among operating room personnel. In many cases, health care workers who are allergic to latex experience their first adverse reactions while they are patients undergoing surgery. The prevalence of latex

TABLE 4-3

TYPES OF REACTIONS TO LATEX GLOVES

REACTION	SIGNS/SYMPTOMS	CAUSE	MANAGEMENT
Irritant Contact Dermatitis	Scaling, drying, cracking of skin	Direct skin irritation by gloves, powder, soaps	Identify reaction, avoid irritant, possible use of glove liner, use of alternative product
Type IV—Delayed Hypersensitivity	Itching, blistering, crusting (delayed 6–72 hours)	Chemical additives used in manufacturing (such as accelerators)	Identify offending chemical, possible use of alternative product without chemical additive, possible use of glove liner
Type I—Immediate Hypersensitivity		Proteins found in latex	Identify reaction, avoid latex-containing products, use of nonlatex or powder-free, low-protein gloves by coworkers
A. Localized Contact Urticaria	A. Itching, hives in area of contact with latex (immediate)		Antihistamines, topical/systemic steroids
B. Generalized Reaction	B. Runny nose, swollen eyes, generalized rash or hives, bronchospasm, anaphylaxis		Anaphylaxis protocol

Reproduced from "Natural Rubber Latex Allergy: Considerations for Anesthesiologists," copyrighted 1999, Task Force on Latex Sensitivity of the Committee on Occupational Health of Operating Room Personnel. Park Ridge, Illinois, American Society of Anesthesiologists. http://www.asahq.org/publicationsAndServices/physician.htm, with permission from the American Society of Anesthesiologists. A copy of the full text can be obtained from the ASA, 520 N. Northwest Highway, Park Ridge, Illinois 60068-2573.

sensitivity among anesthesiologists is estimated to be 12.5 %[31] to 15.8%.[32]

Latex is a complex substance composed of polyisoprenes, lipids, phospholipids, and proteins. A number of additional substances, including preservatives, accelerators, antioxidants, vulcanizing compounds, and lubricating agents (such as cornstarch or talc), are added in the manufacture of the final product. The protein content of latex is responsible for the vast majority of generalized allergic reactions to latex-containing surgical gloves. These reactions are exacerbated by the presence of powder that enhances the potential of latex particles to aerosolize and to spread to the respiratory system of personnel and to environmental surfaces during the donning or removal of gloves.

Irritant or contact dermatitis accounts for approximately 80% of reactions resulting from wearing latex-containing gloves (Table 4-3). In the study reported by Brown et al,[31] 24% of anesthesia personnel were found to manifest evidence of contact dermatitis. True allergic reactions present as T-cell mediated contact dermatitis (Type IV) or as an IgE-mediated anaphylactic reaction.

Anesthesiologists who believe that they are allergic to latex should take immediate steps to assess this possibility.[33] A careful clinical history combined with laboratory evaluation helps to correlate the allergic symptoms with latex exposure. Once the diagnosis of allergy has been established, the affected anesthesiologist must avoid all direct contact with latex-containing products. It is also important that coworkers wear nonlatex or powderless, low latex-allergen gloves to limit the levels of ambient allergens. Because sensitization is an irreversible process, limited exposure and primary prevention of allergy is the best overall strategy.[33] Anaphylactic reactions to latex can be life threatening.

Radiation

Many modern surgical procedures rely heavily on fluoroscopic guidance techniques. As a result, anesthesiologists are at risk for being exposed to an excessive dose of radiation. The magnitude of radiation absorbed by anesthesia personnel is a function of three variables: (1) total radiation exposure intensity and time, (2) distance from the source of radiation, and (3) the use of radiation shielding. The latter two are amenable to modification by the individual. Unfortunately, the lead aprons and thyroid collars commonly worn in operating rooms leave exposed many vulnerable sites, such as the long bones of the extremities, the cranium, the skin of the face, and the eyes. Because radiation exposure is inversely proportional to the square of the distance from the source, increasing this distance is more universally protective. Radiation exposure becomes minimal at a distance greater than 36 inches from the source, a distance that is easily attainable in most anesthetizing locations.

The U.S. Regulatory Commission has established an occupational exposure limit of 5,000 mrem/year. Occupational exposure among anesthesia personnel have been reported to be considerably below this limit.[34] However, these studies were conducted before the introduction of many of the modern surgical procedures that rely heavily on fluoroscopic guidance techniques, such as major spine surgery, endovascular repair of aortic aneurysms, and invasive cardiology procedures. Pregnant workers present special concerns, and the dose to the fetus should be less than 500 mrem during the gestation period.

Oncogenesis, teratogenesis, and long-term genetic defects can occur with sufficiently high exposure to radiation. However, even low levels of radiation exposure are not inconsequential. The stochastic biologic effects of radiation are cumulative and permanent. (A *stochastic* effect is one for which the probability of the occurrence increases with an increasing dose but the severity of the resulting disease does not depend on the magnitude of the dose.) There are no published data that define the lower threshold for radiation-induced disease. Therefore, the general admonition regarding occupational radiation exposure and the basis of protection programs is as low as reasonably achievable (ALARA).

Radiation exposure should be monitored with film badges or pocket dosimeters in anesthesia personnel at risk. Monthly documentation allows for recognition of personnel with high levels of exposure. When warranted, work practices can be evaluated and reassignment to work areas with less radiation exposure considered. Educational programs on the effects of radiation and techniques for preventing exposure are important parts of radiation safety programs.

Noise Pollution

A potential health hazard that is virtually uncontrolled in the modern hospital and specifically in the operating room is noise pollution. Noise pollution is quantified by determining both the intensity of the sound in decibels (dB) and the duration of the exposure. NIOSH has established a maximum level for safe noise exposure of 90 dB for 8 hours.[35] Each increase in noise of 5 dB halves the permissible exposure time, so that 100 dB is acceptable for just 2 hours per day. The maximum allowable exposure in an industrial setting is 115 dB.

The noise level in many operating rooms is surprisingly close to what constitutes a health hazard.[36] Ventilators, suction equipment, music, and conversation produce background noise at a level of 75 to 90 dB. Superimposed on this are sporadic and unexpected noises as dropped equipment, surgical saws and drills, and monitor alarms. Resultant noise levels frequently exceed those of a freeway and even of a rock-and-roll band.

Excessive levels of noise can have an adverse influence on the anesthesiologist's capacity to perform his or her chores. Noise can interfere with an anesthesiologist's ability to discern conversational speech and even to hear auditory alarms. Mental efficiency and short-term memory are diminished by exposure to excess noise.[36] Complex psychomotor tasks associated with anesthesiology, such as monitoring and vigilance, are particularly sensitive to the adverse influences of noise pollution.

There are also chronic ramifications of long-term exposure to excessive noise in the workplace. At the very least, noise pollution is an important factor in decreased worker productivity. At higher noise levels, workers are likely to show signs of irritability and demonstrate evidence of stress, such as elevated blood pressure. Ultimately, hearing loss may ensue.

Conversely, music can provide beneficial effects as a different kind of "background noise." Music has proved advantageous as a supplement to sedation for awake patients during surgery. Self-selected background music can contribute to reducing autonomic responses in surgeons and improving their performance. The beneficial effects are less pronounced when the music is chosen by a third party. Unfortunately, this is often the case for the anesthesiologist.

Human Factors

The work performed by an anesthesiologist is intricate and includes a number of complex tasks. A large body of research has evolved with the goal of applying high-technology solutions to assist the anesthesiologist in managing this demanding workload. Less attention has been given to applying human factor technology to improve our workplace and ensure patient safety. Human error has been identified as a cause of patient morbidity and mortality.[37]

A number of human factor problems potentially exist in the operating room. For example, the design and positioning of equipment can be an impediment to the successful completion of all of an anesthesiologist's obligatory tasks. Anesthesia monitors are frequently placed so that attention is directed away from the patient. Indeed, nearly half of the anesthesiologist's time is spent performing tasks away from the patient–surgeon field and not directly related to patient care.[38] This was well demonstrated by observations that revealed that the insertion and monitoring of a transesophageal echocardiograph added significantly to the anesthesiologist's workload and diverted attention away from other patient-specific tasks. The ability to respond to critical incidents and to sustain complex monitoring tasks, such as maintaining vigilance (vigilance is the ability to detect changes in a stimulus during prolonged monitoring tasks when the subject has no prior knowledge of whether or when any changes might occur), are among those tasks that are most vulnerable to the distractions created by poor equipment design or placement. The critical importance of the "vigilance" task to the practice of anesthesiology is evidenced by the fact that the seal of the American Society of Anesthesiologists bears as its only motto, "Vigilance" (Fig. 4-1), and the official motto of the Australian Society of Anaesthetists is "*Vigila et Ventila.*"

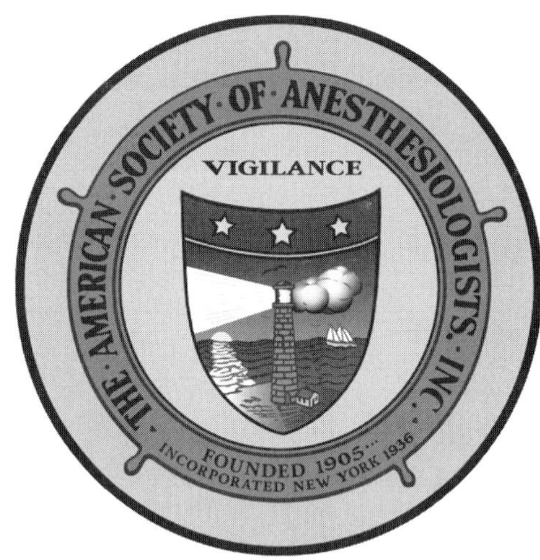

FIGURE 4-1. Official Seal of the American Society of Anesthesiologists. "VIGILANCE" has always been recognized as the most critical of the anesthesiologist's tasks.

Several aspects of the vigilance task deserve attention. By
3 definition, this function is repetitive and monotonous. The task does not fully occupy the anesthesiologist's mental activity, but neither does it leave him or her free to perform other mental functions. Finally, the task is complex, requiring visual attention as well as manual dexterity.

Vigilance tasks are generally performed at the level of 90% accuracy.[39] In a setting where the stakes are as high as that of anesthesia, this leaves an unacceptable margin of error. In fact, human error, in part resulting from lapses in attention, accounts for a large proportion of the preventable deaths and serious injuries resulting from anesthetic mishaps in the United States annually.

In addition to poor equipment design, a number of other factors conspire to hamper the ability of the anesthesiologist to perform multiple tasks that demand cognitive skills. Any factor that requires the expenditure of excessive energy to perform a given task produces a predictable decrement in performance. Even the most trivial aspect of an operator's performance plays a significant role over the course of time. For example, if the anesthesiologist must make frequent rapid changes in observation from a dim, distant screen to a bright, nearby one, the continuous muscular activity required for pupil dilation and constriction and lens accommodation promotes fatigue and hinders performance.

Excessive energy expenditure need not be entirely physical. As more functions are monitored and more data processed during the course of a surgical procedure, increasingly larger amounts of mental work are expended. The mental work varies directly with the difficulty encountered in extracting information from the monitors and displays competing for the anesthesiologist's attention. Engineering of the monitor displays, such as signal frequency and strength, as well as the mode of presentation of the input also significantly influence the operator's performance.

Even the alarms that have been developed with the specific goal of supplementing the task of vigilance have considerable drawbacks. In general, alarms are nonspecific (the same alarm signaling as many as 12 different deviations from "normal") and can be a source of frustration and confusion. They are also susceptible to artifacts and frequent false-positive alarms that can distract the observer from more clinically significant information and, therefore, it is not unusual for frequently distractive alarms to be inactivated.

Noise can have a detrimental influence on the anesthesiologist working at multiple tasks. The average noise level of 77 decibels found in operating rooms can reduce mental efficiency and short-term memory. In general, obtrusive noises, such as loud talking, excessive clanging of instruments, and "broadband" noise, are associated with decrements in performance.

Organizational issues, such as communication among team members, can have a detrimental effect on the ability of the anesthesiologist to perform well. The potential for disaster as a result of poor communication has been well illustrated in a number of airline catastrophes. The possibility for miscommunication and resultant accident is heightened in the operating room where, in contrast to the structure inherent in an airline crew, there is an absence of a well-defined hierarchical organization and there are overlaps in areas of expertise and responsibility.

"Production pressure" is an organizational concern that has the potential to create an environment in which issues of productivity supercede those of safety.[40] Production pressure has been associated with the commission of errors resulting from haste and/or deliberate deviations from known safe practices.

The application of simulation technology has proven to be very useful in the study of human performance issues in anesthesiology.[41] Much remains to be done in bringing human factor research to the anesthesiologist's work environment.

Work Hours and Night Call

Prolonged work hours that result in sleep deprivation and fatigue are a ubiquitous component of many anesthesiologists' professional lives. Ten- to 12-hour workdays are common. Additional emergency and on-call coverage frequently result in 24- to 32-hour shifts. Gravenstein reported the average anesthesiologist's work week was 56 hours.[42] Seventy-four percent of the study respondents reported that they had worked without a break for longer periods than they personally thought was safe and 64% attributed an error in anesthetic management to fatigue.

Long hours of work and night call are especially challenging for the aging anesthesiologist. Older individuals are particularly sensitive to disturbances of the sleep–wake cycle and are in general better suited to phase advances (morning work) than phase delays (nocturnal work).[43] Demands associated with night call have been identified as the most stressful aspect of practice and most frequently cited impetus toward retirement.[43]

Sleep deprivation and circadian disruption have deleterious effects on cognition, performance, mood, and health.[44] Both acute sleep loss (24 hours of on-call duty) and chronic partial sleep deprivation (less than 6 hours of sleep) result in a similar degree of neurobehavioral impairment. The nature and degree of impairment with acute sleep deprivation bears a striking similarity to that seen with alcohol intoxication.[45]

The deleterious effect of sleep loss and fatigue on work efficiency and accuracy is well documented in many industries.[41,46] Sleep deprivation has been implicated as a contributing factor in many well-publicized industrial accidents such as those that occurred at Chernobyl and Three Mile Island. Complex cognitive tasks that are specific to anesthesiology, such as monitoring and accurate clinical decision making, may be adversely affected by sleep deprivation. Surveys of anesthesia personnel have linked fatigue and anesthetic errors, but these contain self-reported data that may not be verifiable.[42,47] In a study of performance on an anesthesia simulator, residents in the sleep-deprived condition demonstrated progressive impairment of alertness, mood, and performance and had longer response latency to vigilance probes.[41] In spite of this, there were no significant differences in the clinical management of the simulated patients between the rested and sleep-deprived groups. Additional studies should be performed in this area to determine the role of sleep deprivation in adverse clinical events.

Subsequent to a period of sleep deprivation, performance does not return to normal levels until 24 hours of rest and recovery has occurred. An interesting phenomenon is the "end-spurt," in which previously deteriorated performance shows improvement when the subject realizes that the task is 90% completed. The converse undoubtedly also occurs, a "letdown" with additional deterioration in performance when the procedure is unexpectedly prolonged.

An additional area of concern is the potential effect of sleep deprivation and chronic fatigue on health and psychosocial adjustment. Work schedules that disrupt circadian rhythms are associated with impaired health, emotional problems, and a decline in performance. Howard et al[48] demonstrated that residents in their routine, non–post-call state suffered from chronic sleep deprivation and had the same degree of sleepiness as measured in residents finishing 24 hours of in-house call.

The sleep-loss pattern experienced by anesthesiologists who take night call is complex and includes elements of each of the three general classes of sleep deprivation: total, partial, and selective sleep deprivation. Selective sleep deprivation resulting from frequent interruptions is most disruptive to important components of sleep including slow wave sleep (associated with "body repair") and rapid eye movement sleep ("mind repair"). Indicators of psychosocial distress, including irritability, displaced anger, depression, and anxiety, have all been identified in house officers suffering from sleep deprivation.[49]

National attention was focused on the problems associated with sleep-deprived medical housestaff by the well-publicized Libby Zion case.[50] A large portion of this claim hinged on the allegation that fatal, avoidable mistakes were made by exhausted, unsupervised residents. A number of medical organizations and state legislatures subsequently took action to limit excessive work hours and resultant sleep deprivation among physicians, especially trainees. For example, the Accreditation Council for Graduate Medical Education (ACGME) has set universal standards that limit resident duty hours to an average of 80 hours per week and no more than 30 hours at any one time, limit the frequency of in-house call, and mandate that "off-duty" time be provided. Unfortunately, no regulations pertain to the practicing anesthesiologist or nurse anesthetist. In this area, medicine remains significantly behind other industries, most notably the transport and airline industries, in identifying and regulating work practices that permit excessively long shifts.[44]

Until changes can be made in staffing patterns, there are several strategies that can be used to prevent fatigue and the effects of sleep deprivation during long work periods.[44] Personnel should be educated on the problems associated with poor sleep habits outside the hospital. Naps prior to the start of call as well as the use of caffeine can improve alertness during long shifts.

INFECTION HAZARDS

Anesthesia personnel are at risk for acquiring infections both from patients and from other personnel.[51] Viral infections, reflecting their prevalence in the community, are the most significant threat to health care workers. Most commonly, these are spread through the respiratory route—a mechanism that is, unfortunately, the most difficult to control effectively with environmental alterations. Other infections are propagated by hand-to-hand transmission, and hand washing is considered the single most important intervention for protection against this form of contagion.[52] Immunity against some viral pathogens can be provided through vaccination.[53] Bloodborne pathogens such as hepatitis and human immunodeficiency virus cause serious infections, but transmission can be prevented with mechanical barriers blocking portals of entry or, in the case of hepatitis B, by producing immunity by vaccination.[54] Current recommendations from the Centers for Disease Control and Prevention (CDC) for preemployment screening, infection control practices, vaccination, postexposure treatment, and work restrictions for infected personnel should be consulted for specific information related to each pathogen.[54–56]

Respiratory Viruses

Respiratory viruses, which are responsible for many community-acquired infections, are usually transmitted by two routes. Small-particle aerosols produced by coughing, sneezing, or talking can propel viruses over large distances. The influenza and measles viruses are spread in this way. The second mechanism involves large droplets produced by coughing or sneezing, contaminating the donor's hands or an inanimate surface, whereupon the virus is transferred to the oral, nasal, or conjunctival mucous membranes of a susceptible person by self-inoculation. Rhinovirus and respiratory syncytial virus (RSV) are spread by this process.

Influenza Viruses

Because influenza viruses are easily transmitted, community epidemics of influenza are common, with large outbreaks occurring annually. Acutely ill patients shed virus through small-particle aerosols by coughing or sneezing for as long as 5 days after the onset of symptoms. Respiratory isolation precautions can be used for the duration of the clinical illness in an attempt to prevent spread to susceptible individuals. Because of their contact with nasopharyngeal secretions, anesthesiologists can play a role in the spread of influenza virus in hospitals.

Influenza rarely produces significant morbidity in healthy health care workers but can result in high rates of absenteeism. Hospital staff, especially those who care for patients in high-risk groups, should be immunized annually (October or November) with the inactivated (killed virus) influenza virus vaccine.[56] Antigenic variation of influenza viruses occurs over time, so that new viral strains (usually two Type A and one Type B) are selected for inclusion in each year's vaccine. During hospital outbreaks of influenza A, the antiviral agents amantadine and rimantadine are reasonably effective in preventing influenza A infection in unvaccinated hospital personnel and, if administered within 48 hours of the onset of illness, can reduce the duration and severity of illness.[57] The neuraminidase inhibitors zanamivir and oseltamivir have been shown to be effective in preventing and treating both influenza A and B.[57] Because of possible morbidity to hospitalized patients and to hospital personnel, it is recommended that during community influenza epidemics, hospitals should consider limiting elective admissions and surgery.

Respiratory Syncytial Virus

Respiratory syncytial virus is the most common cause of serious bronchiolitis and lower respiratory tract disease in infants and young children worldwide. During periods when RSV is prevalent in the community (usually late November through May in the United States), many hospitalized infants and children may carry the virus. Large numbers of virus are present in respiratory secretions of infected children, and although viable virus can be recovered for up to 6 hours on contaminated environmental surfaces, it is readily inactivated with soap and water and disinfectants. Infection of susceptible people occurs by self-inoculation when RSV in secretions is transferred to the hands, which then contact the mucous membranes of the eyes or nose.[58] Although most children have been exposed to RSV early in life, immunity is not permanent and reinfection is common.

Respiratory syncytial virus is shed for approximately 7 days after infection. Hospitalized patients with the virus should be isolated, but during seasonal outbreaks large numbers of patients may make isolation impractical.[59] Careful hand washing and the use of gowns, gloves, masks, and goggles (standard precautions) have all been shown to reduce RSV infection in hospital personnel.

Herpes Viruses

Varicella-zoster virus (VZV), herpes simplex virus Types 1 and 2, and cytomegalovirus (CMV) are members of the Herpetoviridine family. Close personal contact is required for transmission of all the herpes viruses except for VZV, which is spread by direct contact or small-particle aerosols. After primary infection with herpes viruses, the organism becomes latent and may reactivate at a later time. Most people in the United States have been infected with all of the herpes viruses by middle age. Therefore, nosocomial transmission is uncommon except in the pediatric population and in immunosuppressed patients.

Varicella-Zoster Virus. Varicella-zoster virus produces both chicken pox and herpes zoster (shingles). Although the primary infection (chicken pox) is usually uncomplicated in healthy children, VZV infection in adults may be associated with major morbidity or death. Infection during pregnancy may result in fetal death or, rarely, in congenital defects. Health care workers with active VZV infection can transmit the virus to others.

After the primary infection, VZV remains latent in dorsal root or extramedullary cranial ganglia. Herpes zoster results from reactivation of the VZV infection and produces a painful vesicular rash in the innervated dermatome. Anesthesiologists working in pain clinics may be exposed to VZV when caring for patients who have discomfort from herpes zoster.

Varicella-zoster virus is highly contagious, especially from patients with chicken pox or disseminated zoster. The CDC estimates that the period of communicability begins 1 to 2 days before the onset of the rash and ends when all the lesions are crusted, usually 4 to 6 days after the rash appears.[60] Because VZV may be spread through airborne transmission, respiratory isolation should be used for patients with chicken pox or disseminated herpes zoster.[59] Use of gloves to avoid contact with vesicular fluid is adequate to prevent VZV spread from patients with localized herpes zoster.

Most adults in the United States have protective antibodies to VZV. Because there have been many reports of nosocomial transmission of VZV, it is recommended that all health care workers (HCW) have immunity to the virus. Anesthesia personnel should be questioned about prior VZV infection, and those with a negative or unknown history of such infection should be serologically tested.[55] All employees with negative titers should be restricted from caring for patients with active VZV infection and should consider immunization with live, attenuated varicella vaccine.[60] Susceptible personnel with a significant exposure to people with VZV infection are candidates for varicella zoster immune globulin (VZIG), which is most effective when administered within 96 hours after exposure.[60] Personnel without VZV immunity should be reassigned to alternative locations so that they do not care for patients who have active VZV infections.

Herpes Simplex. Herpes simplex virus (HSV) infection is quite common in adults. After viral entry through the mucous membranes of the mouth, the primary infection with HSV Type 1 is usually clinically inapparent but may involve severe oral lesions, fever, and adenopathy. In healthy people, the primary infection subsides and the virus persists in a latent state within the sensory nerve ganglion innervating the site of infection. Any of several mechanisms can reactivate the virus to produce recurrent infection, which manifests in the vicinity of the primary lesion.

A second HSV, Type 2, is usually associated with genital infections and is spread by sexual contact. Newborns may become infected with HSV Type 2 during vaginal delivery.

Health care personnel may be inoculated by direct contact with body fluids carrying either herpes simplex virus Type 1 or 2.

Herpetic infection of the finger, herpetic paronychia or herpetic whitlow, is an occupational hazard for anesthesia personnel. The infection usually begins at the portal of viral entry, a site on the distal finger where the integrity of the skin has been broken, and results in vesicle formation. Within 3 weeks, the throbbing pain lessens, and the lesions begin to heal. Use of acyclovir, an antiviral drug that inhibits replication of HSV, may shorten the course of the primary cutaneous viral infection. Personnel with HSV infections of the fingers or hands should not contact patients until their lesions are healed.

Cytomegalovirus. Cytomegalovirus (CMV) infects between 50 and 85% of individuals in the United States before age 40, with most infections producing minimal symptoms. After the primary infection, the virus remains dormant, and recurrent disease only occurs with compromise of the individual's immune system. Transmission of CMV can take place through close contact with an individual excreting the virus or through contact with contaminated saliva or urine. It is unlikely that aerosols or small droplets play a role in CMV transmission.

Primary or recurrent CMV infection during pregnancy results in fetal infection in up to 2.5% of occurrences. Congenital CMV syndrome may be found in up to 10% of infected infants. Thus, although CMV infection usually does not result in morbidity in healthy adults, it may have significant sequelae in pregnant women. CMV infection can also be deadly in immunocompromised patients, such as those undergoing bone marrow transplantation.

The two major populations with CMV infection in the hospital include infected infants and immunocompromised patients, such as those who have undergone organ transplants or those on oncology units. Routine infection control procedures (standard precautions) are sufficient to prevent CMV infection in health care workers (Tables 4-4 and 4-5).[55] Pregnant personnel should be made aware of the risks associated with CMV infection during pregnancy and of appropriate infection control precautions to be used when caring for high-risk patients. There is no evidence to indicate that it is necessary to reassign pregnant women from patient care areas in which they may have contact with CMV-positive patients.

TABLE 4-4

PREVENTION OF OCCUPATIONALLY ACQUIRED INFECTIONS[55,59,62]

INFECTIOUS AGENT	PREVENTIVE MEASURES[a]
Cytomegalovirus	Standard precautions
Hepatitis B	Vaccine; hepatitis B immune globulin, standard precautions
Hepatitis C	Standard precautions
Herpes simplex	Standard precautions; contact precautions if disseminated disease
Human immunodeficiency virus	Standard precautions; postexposure prophylactic antiretrovirals
Influenza	Vaccine; prophylactic antiretrovirals; droplet precautions
Measles	Vaccine; airborne infection isolation precautions
Rubella	Vaccine; droplet precautions
Severe acute respiratory syndrome (SARS)	Standard precautions; airborne infection isolation precautions
Tuberculosis	Airborne infection isolation precautions; isoniazid ± ethambutol for PPD conversion
Varicella-zoster	Vaccine; varicella-zoster immune globulin; airborne infection isolation and contact precautions; standard precautions if localized disease

[a]Isolation precautions outlined in Table 4-5.

Rubella

Outbreaks of rubella, or German measles, in hospital personnel have resulted in significant loss in employee working time, employee morbidity, and cost to the hospital. Although most adults in the United States are immune to rubella, up to 20% of women of childbearing age are still susceptible. Rubella infection during the first trimester of pregnancy is associated with congenital malformations or fetal death.

Rubella is transmitted by contact with nasopharyngeal droplets spread by infected individuals coughing or sneezing. Patients are most contagious while the rash is erupting but can transmit the virus from 1 week before to 5 to 7 days after the onset of the rash. Droplet precautions should be used to prevent transmission (Table 4-5).[55]

Ensuring immunity at the time of employment (evidence of prior vaccination with live rubella vaccine or serologic confirmation) should prevent nosocomial transmission of rubella to personnel. It has been shown that history is a poor indicator of immunity. A live, attenuated rubella virus vaccine, contained in measles, mumps, rubella vaccine (MMR), is available to produce immunity in susceptible personnel.[53,61] Many state or local health departments mandate rubella immunity for all HCW, and local regulations should be consulted.

Measles (Rubeola)

Measles virus is highly transmissible both by large droplets and by the airborne route. The virus is found in the mucus of the nose and pharynx of the infected individual and is spread by coughing and sneezing. The disease can be transmitted from

TABLE 4-5

HOSPITAL ISOLATION PRECAUTIONS[59]

■ STANDARD PRECAUTIONS

5 These are to be used for the care of all patients regardless of their diagnosis or presumed infection status.
Standard precautions should be used in conjunction with other forms of isolation precautions (see below) for the care of specific patients.

1. *Hand washing*
   After touching blood, body fluids, or contaminated items even if gloves are worn.
2. *Gloves*
   Wear gloves when touching blood, body fluids, or contaminated items.
   Change gloves between tasks on the same patient when there is likely to be a high concentration of organisms.
   Remove gloves after use, before touching noncontaminated items and environmental surfaces.
3. *Mask, eye protection, face shield*
   Use during procedures likely to generate splashes of blood or body fluids that may contaminate face or mucous membranes.
4. *Gown*
   Use during procedures likely to generate splashes of blood or body fluids that may contaminate clothing or arms.
5. *Patient-care equipment*
   Handle soiled equipment in a manner that prevents skin, mucous membrane, clothing, or environmental contamination.
6. *Environmental control*
   Contaminated environmental surfaces should routinely be cleaned and/or disinfected.
7. *Linen*
   Soiled linen should be handled in a manner that prevents contamination of personnel, other patients, and environmental surfaces.
8. *Occupational health and bloodborne pathogens*
   Use care to prevent injuries when using or disposing of needles and sharp devices.
   Contaminated needles should not be recapped or manipulated by using both hands. If recapping is necessary for the procedure being performed, a one-handed scoop technique or mechanical device for holding the needle sheath should be used.
   Contaminated needles should not be removed from disposable syringes by hand.
   Do not break or bend contaminated needles before disposal.
   After use, disposable syringes and needles and other sharp devices should be placed in appropriate puncture-resistant containers located as close as practical to the area in which the items were used.
   Mouthpieces, resuscitation bags, or other ventilation devices should be available for use as an alternative to mouth-to-mouth ventilation.
9. *Patient placement*
   Private rooms should be used for patients who are likely to contaminate the environment.

■ TRANSMISSION-BASED PRECAUTIONS

These should be used along with standard precautions for patients known or suspected to be infected or colonized with highly transmissible pathogens requiring additional precautions.

■ AIRBORNE INFECTION ISOLATION PRECAUTIONS

These should be used for patients known or suspected to be infected with microorganisms transmitted by airborne droplet nuclei (particles 5 μm or smaller in size) that can be dispersed over large distances by air currents.

1. *Patient placement*
   The patient should be placed in a private room with (1) documented negative air pressure relative to surrounding areas, (2) 6 to 12 air changes per hour, (3) discharge of air outdoors or monitored high-efficiency filtration of room air before the air is circulated to other areas in the hospital.
   The door to the room should be kept closed and the patient should remain in the room.
2. *Respiratory protection*
   Respiratory protection should be worn when entering the room of a patient with known or suspected infectious pulmonary tuberculosis.
   Susceptible personnel should not enter the room of patients known or suspected to have measles or varicella if other immune caregivers are available. If susceptible persons must enter the room of a patient known or suspected to have measles or varicella, they should wear respiratory protection. Persons immune to measles or varicella need not wear respiratory protection.
3. *Patient transport*
   Patients should be transported from the isolation room only for essential purposes. When transport is necessary, a surgical mask should be placed on the patient to prevent dispersal of droplet nuclei.
4. *Patients with tuberculosis*
   Current CDC guidelines should be consulted for additional precautions.[81]

■ DROPLET PRECAUTIONS

These should be used for patients known or suspected to be infected with microorganisms transmitted by large-particle droplets (particles larger than 5 μm) that can be generated during coughing, sneezing, talking, or by performing certain procedures.

1. *Patient placement*
   The patient should be placed in a private room.
2. *Respiratory protection*
   Personnel should wear a mask when working within 3 feet of the patient.

(*continued*)

TABLE 4-5

(CONTINUED)

3. *Patient transport*
   Patients should be transported from the isolation room only for essential purposes. When transport is necessary, a surgical mask should be placed on the patient to prevent dispersal of droplets.

■ CONTACT PRECAUTIONS

These should be used for patients known or suspected to be infected or colonized with epidemiologically important microorganisms transmitted by direct contact with the patient or indirect contact with environmental surfaces or patient-care items.

1. *Patient placement*
   The patient should be placed in a private room.
2. *Gloves and hand washing*
   In addition to wearing gloves as outlined under standard precautions, gloves (nonsterile) should be worn when entering the patient's room.
   Gloves should be changed after contacting infective material that may contain high concentrations of microorganisms.
   Gloves should be removed before leaving the patient's environment and hands should be washed immediately with an antimicrobial agent or a waterless antiseptic agent.
   After removal of gloves and hand washing, care should be taken so that contaminated environmental surfaces should not be touched to avoid transfer of microorganisms to other patients.
3. *Gown*
   In addition to wearing a gown as outlined under standard precautions, a gown (nonsterile) should be worn when entering the room when it is anticipated that clothing will have contact with the patient, environmental surfaces, or contaminated items or if the patient is incontinent or has diarrhea, an ileostomy, a colostomy, or wound drainage not contained by a dressing.
   The gown should be removed before leaving the patient's environment.
   Clothing should not contact potentially contaminated surfaces after removal of the gown.
4. *Patient transport*
   The patient should be transported from the room for only essential purposes.
   If it is necessary to transport the patient, precautions should be maintained to minimize the risk of transmission of microorganisms to other patients and contamination of environmental surfaces or equipment.
5. *Patient-care equipment*
   Dedicate the use of noncritical patient-care equipment (e.g., blood pressure cuffs) to a single patient to avoid transmission of microorganisms to another patient. If use of common equipment is unavoidable, then items should be adequately cleaned or disinfected before use on another patient.

4 days prior to the onset of the rash to 4 days after its onset. Airborne precautions should be used for infected patients (Table 4-5).[55] Introduction of the measles vaccine in the United States has successfully eliminated indigenous cases of measles but importation of measles from other countries continues to occur.

Health care workers are at increased risk for acquiring measles and transmitting the virus to susceptible coworkers and patients. The CDC recommends that medical personnel have adequate immunity to measles, as documented by one of the following: evidence of two doses of live measles vaccine, a record of physician-diagnosed measles, or serologic evidence of measles immunity (Table 4-4).[55] Susceptible personnel born in or after 1957 should receive two doses of the live measles vaccine at the time of employment.[61]

Severe Acute Respiratory Syndrome

Severe acute respiratory syndrome (SARS) is an emerging respiratory tract infection produced by a coronavirus, SARS-associated coronavirus (SARS-CoV). After the first cases were reported from Asia in late 2002, the disease quickly spread globally in 2003 before being controlled. SARS typically presents with a high fever, greater than 38.0°C, and is followed with symptoms of headache, generalized aches, and cough. Severe pneumonia may lead to acute respiratory distress syndrome (ARDS) and death.

SARS is spread by close person-to-person contact through virus carried in large respiratory droplets and possibly by airborne transmission. The virus can also be spread when an individual touches a contaminated object and then inoculates their mouth, nose, or eyes. Aerosolization of respiratory secretions during coughing or endotracheal suctioning has been associated with transmission of the disease to HCW, including anesthesiologists and critical care nurses. It appears that some infected individuals are "super-shedders" of the virus and present a greater risk for transmission to contacts.

One of the most important interventions to prevent the spread of SARS in the health care setting is early detection and isolation of patients who may be infected with SARS-CoV.[62] Standard and Droplet Precautions should be used when contacting patients with symptoms of a respiratory illness (Table 4-5) until it is determined that the cause of the pneumonia is not contagious. Contact and Airborne Infection Isolation (AII) should be used for patients with laboratory evidence of SARS or those strongly suspected of having SARS-CoV infection. Gloves, gown, respiratory protection (as a minimum, use a NIOSH-certified N-95 filtering respirator), and eye protection should be donned before entering a SARS patient's room or during procedures likely to generate respiratory aerosols.[62]

Viral Hepatitis

Although many viruses may produce hepatitis, the most common are Type A or infectious hepatitis, Type B (HBV) or serum hepatitis, and Type C (HCV), which is responsible for most cases of parenterally transmitted non-A, non-B hepatitis (NANBH) in the United States. Delta hepatitis, caused by an incomplete virus, occurs only in people infected with HBV. Outbreaks of an enterically transmitted NANBH (hepatitis E) have been reported from outside the United States and are usually caused by contaminated water. The greatest risks of occupational transmission to anesthesia personnel are associated with HBV and HCV.

Hepatitis A

About 20 to 40% of viral hepatitis in adults in the United States is caused by the Type A virus. Hepatitis A is usually a self-limited illness, and no chronic carrier state exists. Spread is predominantly by the fecal–oral route, either by person-to-person contact or by ingestion of contaminated food or water. Outbreaks are usually found in institutions or other closed groups where there has been a breakdown in normal sanitary conditions. Hospital personnel do not appear to be at increased risk for hepatitis A and nosocomial transmission is rare.

Personnel exposed to patients with hepatitis A should receive immune globulin intramuscularly as soon as possible but not greater than 2 weeks after the exposure to reduce the likelihood of infection.[63] Immune globulin provides protection against hepatitis A through passive transfer of antibodies and is used for postexposure prophylaxis. Hepatitis A vaccine is not routinely recommended for HCW except for those that may be working in countries where hepatitis A is endemic.[53,63]

Hepatitis B

Hepatitis B is a significant occupational hazard for nonimmune anesthesiologists and other medical personnel who have frequent contact with blood and blood products. The prevalence (the proportion of people who have or have had the condition at the time of the survey) of hepatitis B in the general population of the United States is 3 to 5%, and the carrier rate is 0.2 to 0.9% based on serologic screening. Serosurveys including more than 2400 unvaccinated anesthesia personnel conducted in the United States and several other countries demonstrated a mean prevalence of HBV serologic markers of 17.8% (range, 3.2–48.6%).[64] The range of seropositive findings in anesthesia personnel in various locations probably reflects the prevalence of HBV carriers in the referral population for the area. Within the United States, studies conducted before the widespread usage of hepatitis B vaccine indicated that the prevalence of hepatitis B serologic markers in anesthesia personnel ranged from 19 to 49%.

Acute HBV infection may be asymptomatic and usually resolves without significant hepatic damage. Less than 1% of acutely infected patients develop fulminant hepatitis. Approximately 10% become chronic carriers of HBV (i.e., serologic evidence demonstrated for more than 6 months). Within 2 years, half of the chronic carriers resolve their infection without significant hepatic impairment. Chronic active hepatitis, which may progress to cirrhosis and is linked to hepatocellular carcinoma, is found most commonly in individuals with chronic viral infection for more than 2 years. The implementation of routine vaccination, use of standard precautions, use of safety devices, and postexposure prophylaxis have significantly reduced the risk of occupationally acquired HBV infection and its sequelae in HCW.

The diagnosis and classification of the stage of HBV infection can be made on the basis of serologic testing. Antibody to the surface antigen (anti-HBs) appears with resolution of the acute infection and confers lasting immunity against subsequent HBV infections. Chronic HBV carriers are likely to have hepatitis B surface antigen (HBsAg) and antibody to the core antigen (anti-HBc) present in serum samples. The presence of hepatitis B e antigen (HBeAg) in serum is indicative of active viral replication in hepatocytes.

Anesthesia personnel are at risk for occupationally acquired HBV infection as a result of accidental percutaneous or mucosal contact with blood or body fluids from infected patients. Patient groups with a high prevalence of HBV include immigrants from endemic areas, users of illicit parenteral drugs, homosexual men, and patients on hemodialysis.[54] Carriers are frequently not identified during hospitalization because the clinical history and routine preoperative laboratory tests may be insufficient for diagnosis. The risk for infection after an HBV-contaminated percutaneous exposure, such as an accidental needle stick, is 37 to 62% if the source patient is HBeAg-positive and 23 to 37% if HBeAg-negative. HBV can be found in saliva, but the rate of transmission is significantly less after mucosal contact with infected oral secretions than after percutaneous exposures to blood. HBV is a hardy virus that may be infectious for at least 1 week in dried blood on environmental surfaces.

Hepatitis B Vaccine. Use of hepatitis B vaccine is the pri-
6 mary strategy to prevent occupational transmission of HBV to anesthesia personnel and other HCW at increased risk.[54] Administration of three doses of vaccine into the deltoid muscle results in the production of protective antibodies (anti-HBs) in more than 90% of healthy HCW. Hospitals or anesthesia departments should have policies for educating, screening, and counseling personnel about their risk of acquiring HBV infection and should make vaccination available for susceptible personnel.[54,65]

To ensure adequate postvaccination immunity, serologic testing for anti-HBs should take place within 1 to 2 months after the third dose of vaccine.[54] Protective antibodies develop in 30 to 50% of nonresponders (i.e., anti-HBs <10 mIU/mL) with a second 3-dose vaccine series. Nonresponders to vaccination, who are HBsAg-negative, remain at risk for HBV infection and should be counseled on strategies to prevent infections and the need for postexposure prophylaxis.

Vaccine-induced antibodies decline over time, with maximum titers after vaccination correlating directly with duration of antibody persistence. The CDC states that for vaccinated adults with normal immune status, routine booster doses are not necessary and periodic monitoring of antibody concentration is not recommended.[54]

When susceptible or nonvaccinated anesthesia personnel have a documented exposure to a contaminated needle or to blood from an HBsAg-positive patient, postexposure prophylaxis with HBV hyperimmune globulin (HBIG) is recommended.[54] Hepatitis B vaccine should be offered to any unvaccinated, susceptible person who sustains a blood or body fluid exposure.

Hepatitis C

Hepatitis C virus causes most cases of parenterally transmitted NANBH and is a leading cause of chronic liver disease in the United States. Although antibody to HCV (anti-HCV) can be detected in most patients with hepatitis C, its presence does not correlate with resolution of the acute infection or progression of hepatitis, and it does not confer immunity against HCV infection.[66] Seropositivity for HCV RNA, using polymerase chain reaction, is a marker of chronic infection and continued viral presence.

Most cases of acute HCV infection are asymptomatic, but infected individuals have a high rate of progression to chronic hepatitis. Up to 60% of HCV-infected patients will have biopsy-proven chronic hepatitis, with many developing cirrhosis. HCV RNA can still be detected in more than 75% of patients after resolution of acute hepatitis C.[66] Combination therapy with interferon and ribavirin has been effective in the treatment of some cases of chronic hepatitis C. In a limited clinical trial, interferon alfa-2b was effective in preventing chronic hepatitis C in patients with acute infection.[67]

Like HBV, HCV is transmitted through blood and sexual contact, but the rate of occupational HCV infection is less than for HBV. Although HCV transmission has been documented in health care settings, the prevalence of anti-HCV in HCW in the

United States is not greater than that found in the general population. The greatest risk of occupational HCV transmission is associated with exposure to blood from an HCV-positive source, and the average rate of seroconversion after accidental percutaneous exposure is 1.8%.[54] HCV has been transmitted through blood splashes to the eye and with exposure via nonintact skin. HCV in dried blood on environmental surfaces may remain infectious for up to 16 hours, but environmental contamination does not appear to be a common route of transmission. Although HCV can be found in the saliva of infected individuals, it is not believed to represent a great risk for occupational transmission.[54]

There is no vaccine or effective postexposure prophylaxis available to prevent HCV infection, and use of immune globulin is no longer recommended after a known exposure.[54] The effectiveness of interferon has not been documented as effective prophylaxis after occupational exposure. Prevention of exposures remains as the primary strategy for protecting HCW against HCV infection. Personnel who have had a percutaneous or mucosal exposure to HCV-positive blood should have serologic testing for anti-HCV and alanine aminotransferase and counseling at the time of the exposure and at 6 months.[54]

Pathogenic Human Retroviruses

HIV Infection and AIDS

The agent that produces acquired immunodeficiency syndrome (AIDS) is the human immunodeficiency virus (HIV), one of several pathogenic human retroviruses. Current estimates suggest that 650,000 to 900,000 people in the United States are infected with HIV. According to CDC data, from 1981 through December 2002 there have been 859,000 cases of AIDS in the United States.[68]

The initial infection with HIV presents clinically as a mononucleosis-like syndrome with lymphadenopathy and rash. Although the patient then enters an asymptomatic period, monocyte-macrophage cells serve as a reservoir for the virus throughout the body, and CD4+ T cells harbor the virus in the blood. Within a few weeks after infection, an antibody may be detected by the enzyme-linked immunosorbent assay (ELISA) and is confirmed using the more specific Western blot test. After a variable length period of asymptomatic HIV infection, there is an increase in viral titer and impaired host immunity, resulting in opportunistic infections and malignancies characteristic of AIDS. As the use of highly active antiretroviral therapy became widespread in the United States in 1996, the average length of survival after HIV infection increased.

HIV is spread by sexual contact (especially homosexual males), perinatally from infected mother to neonate, and through infected blood (transfusion or shared needles) and blood products. Although the virus can be found in saliva, tears, and urine, these body fluids have a low risk for viral transmission. Many HIV-infected patients in health care settings may not be identified as such by their initial or presenting diagnosis.

Risk of Occupational Human Immunodeficiency Virus Infection. Although there are several modes of transmission for HIV infection in the community, the most important source for occupational transmission of HIV to HCW is blood contact.[54] The rate of seroconversion in health care workers sustaining a percutaneous exposure (needle stick injury) to HIV-infected blood is estimated to be 0.3%,[69] while the rate after a mucous membrane exposure is 0.09%.[70] Transmission has occurred after blood exposure to nonintact skin, but although the rate is unknown, it is likely less than for mucous membrane exposure.

A case-control study has demonstrated that specific factors are associated with an increased rate of HIV transmission after a percutaneous injury.[71] Increased risk was associated with a deep injury, visible blood on the device producing the injury, a procedure in which the needle was placed in an artery or vein, and terminal illness (death from AIDS within 2 months) in the source patient. Therefore, the risk of occupational HIV transmission is greatest after a deep injury with a blood-filled, large-gauge, hollow-bore needle used on a patient in the terminal phase of AIDS.

The occupational risk of HIV infection is a function of the annual number of blood exposures, the rate of HIV transmission with each exposure to infected blood, and the prevalence of HIV infection in the specific patient population. Greene et al prospectively collected data on 138 contaminated percutaneous injuries to anesthesia personnel.[72] The rate of contaminated percutaneous injuries per year per full-time equivalent anesthesia worker was 0.42, and the average annual risk of HIV and HCV infection was estimated to be 0.0016 and 0.015%, respectively.

Anesthesia personnel are frequently exposed to blood and body fluids during invasive procedures such as insertion of vascular catheters, arterial punctures, and endotracheal intubation.[51,72,73] Although many exposures are mucocutaneous and can be prevented by the use of gloves and protective clothing, these barriers do not prevent percutaneous exposures such as needle stick injuries, which carry a greater risk for pathogen transmission. Because of the tasks they perform, anesthesia personnel are likely to use and be injured by large-bore, hollow needles such as IV catheter stylets and needles on syringes.[72,74] Needleless or protected needle safety devices can be used to replace standard devices to reduce the risk of needle stick injuries. Although safety devices usually are more expensive than a comparable nonsafety item, they may be more cost-effective when the cost of needle stick injury investigation and medical care for infected personnel is considered.

Percutaneous injuries have now been accepted as a significant occupational risk for health care workers.[51] The Needlestick Safety and Prevention Act of 2000 mandated that OSHA update its Bloodborne Pathogen Standard to require that exposure control plans include a process for evaluating and implementing the use of commercially available safety medical devices.[65] Employers were also required to maintain a "sharps" injury log to collect data to evaluate exposure risks and the effectiveness of safety devices. Because federal regulations require the use of safety devices, as new technologies become available, clinicians must assess these within their practice to determine which are most effective for specific tasks.

Postexposure Treatment and Prophylactic Antiretroviral Therapy. When personnel have been exposed to patients' blood or body fluids, the incident should immediately be reported to the employee health service or the designated individual within the institution. Based on the nature of the injury, the exposed worker and the source individual should be tested for serologic evidence of HIV, HBV, and HCV infection.[54] Current local laws must be consulted to determine policies for testing the source patient, and confidentiality must be maintained. When the source patient is found to be HIV-positive, the employee should be retested for HIV antibodies at 6 and 12 weeks and at 6 months after exposure, although most infected people are expected to undergo seroconversion within the first 6 to 12 weeks. During this period, the exposed employee should follow CDC recommendations for preventing transmission of HIV to family members and patients.[54] If the source patient is found to be HIV-negative, no additional treatment is required.

The U.S. Public Health Service recommends that antiretroviral postexposure prophylaxis (PEP) be offered to HCW who have incurred a significant percutaneous exposure to HIV-infected blood.[54] The specific antiretroviral regimen is based on the severity of exposure and the source patient. Because protocols for chemoprophylaxis are likely to change with additional research and the introduction of new antiretroviral drugs, the most current recommendations, such as those provided on the CDC website (http://www.cdc.gov/niosh/topics/bbp), should be consulted prior to instituting postexposure prophylactic therapy. To be most effective, PEP should be initiated as soon as possible after exposure (less than 24 hours) and continued for 4 weeks. HCW should be counseled on the potential toxic effects of antiretrovirals so that they can make an informed decision on the risks associated with PEP. Failure of PEP has been attributed to large viral inoculum, use of a single antiviral agent, drug resistance in the virus from the source patient, and delayed initiation or short duration of PEP therapy.

Occupational Safety and Health Administration Standards, Universal Precautions, and Isolation Precautions

In the late 1980s the CDC formulated recommendations, or universal precautions, for preventing transmission of bloodborne infections (including HIV, HBV, and HCV) to HCW. The guidelines were based on the epidemiology of HBV as a worst-case model for transmission of bloodborne infections and current knowledge of the epidemiology of HIV and HCV. Because some carriers of bloodborne viruses could not be identified, universal precautions were recommended for use during all patient contact. Although exposure to blood carries the greatest risk of occupationally related transmission of HIV, HBV, and HCV, it was recognized that universal precautions should also be applied to semen, vaginal secretions, human tissues, and the following body fluids: cerebrospinal, synovial, pleural, peritoneal, pericardial, and amniotic. Subsequently, the CDC synthesized the major features of universal precautions into standard precautions, a single set of precautions that should be applied to all patients (Table 4-5).[59] Standard precautions were included in a more complete set of isolation precautions, which contain guidelines (airborne precautions, droplet precautions, and contact precautions) to reduce the risk of transmission of bloodborne and other pathogens in health care settings.[59]

Standard precautions include the use of gloves when an HCW contacts mucous membranes and oral fluids, such as during endotracheal intubation and pharyngeal suctioning. The selection of specific barriers or personal protective equipment should be commensurate with the task being performed. Gloves may be all that is necessary during insertion of a peripheral intravenous catheter, whereas gloves, gown, mask, and face shield may be required during endotracheal intubation in a patient with hematemesis. Gloves should be removed after they become contaminated to prevent dissemination of blood or body fluids to equipment or other items that may be contacted by ungloved personnel. Waterless antiseptics should be available to permit anesthesia personnel to wash their hands after glove removal without leaving the operating room.

OSHA has promulgated Standards to protect employees from occupational exposure to bloodborne pathogens.[65] Employers subject to OSHA must comply with these federal regulations. The Standard requires that there must be an Exposure Control Plan specifically detailing the methods that the employer is providing to reduce employees' risk of exposure. The employer must evaluate engineering controls such as needleless devices to eliminate hazards. Work practice controls are encouraged to reduce blood exposures by altering the manner in which personnel perform tasks (e.g., an instrument rather than fingers should be used to handle needles). The employer must furnish appropriate personal protective equipment (e.g., gloves, gowns) in various sizes to permit employees to comply with universal precautions. The HBV vaccine must be offered at no charge to personnel. A mechanism for postexposure treatment and follow-up must be provided. An annual educational program should inform employees of their risk for bloodborne infection and the resources available to prevent blood exposures. Implementation of standard precautions and OSHA regulations have been effective in decreasing the number of exposure incidents that result in HCW contact with patient blood and body fluids.

Creutzfeldt-Jakob Disease

Creutzfeldt-Jakob disease (CJD), caused by an infectious protein or prion, may be unsuspected in patients presenting with dementia.[75] More recently, it has been recognized that the prion strain associated with bovine spongiform encephalopathy has infected humans to produce a variant CJD. Iatrogenic transmission of CJD to patients has taken place through contaminated biologic products and surgical instruments and via blood transfusion. The risk of transmission to hospital personnel is unknown because surveillance is complicated by the long period from the time of infection until the onset of symptoms. Universal precautions should be used. Tissues with greatest risk of infectivity are brain, spinal cord, and eyes.

The prion is difficult to eradicate from equipment, and special sterilization methods are required for instruments that come into contact with high-infectivity tissues. The World Health Organization has developed infection control and sterilization guidelines for CJD (http://www.who.int/emc-documents/tse/docs/whocdscsraph2003.pdf). The prion is not transmitted through respiratory routes.

Tuberculosis

The incidence of tuberculosis in the United States has declined since 1992, reversing the increase in reported cases that had begun in 1986. Although most individuals infected with tuberculosis are treated on an outpatient basis, undiagnosed patients may be hospitalized for the workup of pulmonary pathology. Hospital personnel are especially at risk for infection from unrecognized cases.[76,77] Groups with a higher prevalence of tuberculosis include (1) personal contacts of people with active tuberculosis; (2) people from countries with a high prevalence of tuberculosis; and (3) alcoholics, homeless people, and intravenous drug users.[76]

Mycobacterium tuberculosis is transmitted through viable bacilli carried on airborne particles, 1 to 5 μm in size, by coughing, speaking, or sneezing. Airborne infection isolation should be used for hospitalized patients suspected of having tuberculosis until they are confirmed as nontransmitters by sputum examination that demonstrates no bacilli.[76] Appropriate chemotherapy is the most effective means to prevent spread of tuberculous infection.[78] Elective surgery should be postponed until infected patients have had an adequate course of chemotherapy. If surgery is required, filters should be used on the anesthetic breathing circuit for patients with tuberculosis.[76,79]

Several hospital outbreaks of multidrug-resistant *M. tuberculosis* infection have been reported.[77,80] Mortality associated with these outbreaks is high. Factors responsible for nosocomial transmission include delayed diagnosis of tuberculosis so that multiple patients and personnel were exposed and delayed recognition of drug resistance resulting in inadequate initial drug therapy.

Effective prevention of spread to HCW requires early identification of infected patients and immediate initiation of airborne infection isolation (negative-pressure rooms with air vented outside; see Table 4-5).[76,79] Patients must remain in isolation until adequate treatment is documented. If patients with tuberculosis must leave their rooms, they should wear face masks to prevent spread of organisms into the air. HCW should wear respiratory protective devices when they enter an isolation room or when performing procedures that may induce coughing, such as endotracheal intubation or tracheal suctioning.[76] The CDC recommends that respiratory protective devices worn to protect against *M. tuberculosis* should be able to filter 95% of particles 1 mm in size at flow rates of 50 liters per minute and should fit the face with a leakage rate around the seal of less than 10% documented by fit testing.[76] High-efficiency particulate air respirators (classified as N95) are NIOSH-approved devices that meet the CDC criteria for respiratory protective devices against *M. tuberculosis*.[81]

Routine periodic screening of employees for tuberculosis should be included as part of a hospital's employee health policy with the frequency of screening dependent on the prevalence of infected patients in the hospitalized population. When a new conversion is detected by skin testing, a history of exposure should be sought to determine the source patient. Treatment or preventive therapy is based on the drug-susceptibility pattern of the *M. tuberculosis* in the source patient, if known. Personnel who have been exposed to a patient with active tuberculosis should be followed by skin testing.

Viruses in Smoke Plumes

The laser is commonly used for vaporizing carcinomatous and viral tumors. Use of lasers and electrosurgical devices is associated with several hazards, both to patients and to operating room personnel. Risks include thermal burns, eye injuries, electrical hazards, and fires and explosions. There is evidence that the smoke plumes resulting from tissue vaporization contain toxic chemicals such as benzene and formaldehyde, and in 1996, NIOSH released a Health Hazard Alert on the dangers of smoke plumes.[82]

Clinical and laboratory studies have demonstrated that when the carbon dioxide laser is used to treat verrucae (papilloma and warts), intact viral DNA could be recovered from the plume. Viable viruses can be found in plumes produced by both carbon dioxide and argon laser vaporization of a virus-loaded culture plate, but viable viruses are carried on larger particles that travel less than 100 mm from the site being vaporized.[83]

A case report describes laryngeal papillomatosis in a surgeon who had used a laser to remove anogenital condylomas from several patients.[84] Although DNA analysis of the surgeon's papillomas revealed a viral type similar to that of the condylomas, proof of transmission is lacking.

To protect operating room personnel from exposure to the viral and chemical content of the laser plume, it is recommended that a smoke evacuation system be utilized with the suction nozzle being held as close as possible to the tissue being vaporized.[85] In addition, operating room personnel working in the vicinity of the laser plume should wear gloves, goggles, and high-efficiency filter masks.[73]

EMOTIONAL CONSIDERATIONS

Stress

Stress is a well-recognized element of the operating room workplace. However, there is very little objective information specifically directed toward understanding the nature of job-related stress among anesthesiologists.[86]

Stress is a nonspecific response to any change, demand, pressure, challenge, threat, or trauma.[87] There are three distinct components of the stress response: the initiating stressors, the psychological filters that process and evaluate the stressors, and the coping mechanisms that are employed in an attempt to control the stressful situation.

Stress on the job is unavoidable and to a certain degree is desirable. A moderate, manageable level of stress is the fuel necessary for individual achievement. Hans Seyle, one of the pioneering scientists in the modern study of stress, described a beneficial effect resulting from mild, brief and controllable episodes of stress.[88] In Seyle's words, "The absence of stress is death." On the other hand, extreme degrees of stress can be associated with disorders of the psychological homeostatic mechanism and consequently can lead to physical or mental disease. Exactly how an individual responds to a particular stressor is the product of a series of factors, including age, gender, experience, preexisting personality style, available defense and coping mechanisms, support systems, and concomitant events (such as sleep deprivation).

A number of circumstances that classically define a stressful workplace are characteristic of the practice of anesthesiology. There is a background of chronic, low-level stress punctuated by intermittent episodes of extreme stress. The demands are externally paced, usually out of the anesthesiologist's control. Habituation to the demands is difficult. Perturbations are intermittently but continuously inserted into the system. Finally, failure to meet the demands imposed by the workplace produces grave consequences.

Certain stressors are specific to the practice of anesthesiology. Concerns about liability, long working hours and night call, production pressures, economic uncertainty, and interpersonal relations are frequently cited as sources of chronic stress for anesthesiologists. The process of inducing anesthesia (particularly with a difficult airway) can be among the most profound sources of acute stress to anesthesiologists. Physiologic changes, including heart rate and rhythm, elevations in blood pressure, and myocardial ischemia, are not uncommon. One study reported increases in the blood pressure and heart rate of anesthesiologists during all stages of the anesthetic procedure, especially during the induction.[89] There was an inverse relationship between the years of experience of the anesthesiologist and the degree of stress as manifested by heart rate change.

Interpersonal relationships impose a set of demands that can be a major source of stress to an anesthesiologist. The operating room is unique as one of the few hospital sites where two co-equal physicians simultaneously share responsibility for the care of a patient. This creates a situation in which there are overlapping realms of clinical responsibility that can upset the customary hierarchy of command. To many anesthesiologists, as well as surgeons, this shared responsibility is the source of greatest conflict and professional stress. Other workplace settings, most notably the airline industry, have made better progress in identifying and correcting sources of interpersonal friction that facilitate stress and lead to professional errors.[90]

Several personality traits, in many cases identifiable before entrance to medical school, can be predictive of the potential toward maladaptive responses to stress. Prominent among these is the obsessive-compulsive, dependent character structure. These individuals typically manifest pessimism, passivity, self-doubt, and feelings of insecurity. Commonly they respond to stress by internalizing anger and becoming hypochondriacal and depressed. Undergraduate students who demonstrate these characteristics were more likely to have their medical careers disrupted by alcoholism or drug abuse, psychiatric illness, and marital disturbances.[91] McDonald et al[92] applied some of these considerations in an attempt to identify psychological attributes that may be of value in the selection process for anesthesiology residents. A large number of adaptive coping functions have been advocated for successful stress management.[87] Only when appropriate coping mechanisms become overwhelmed by the magnitude of the stress do the defenses tend to become inappropriate. This situation may give rise to maladaptive behavior and the personal and professional deterioration that can lead to disorders such as drug addiction, professional burnout, and suicide.

Substance Use, Abuse, and Dependence

Illicit drug use remains one of our society's major afflictions. It is estimated that 20 million Americans are drug abusers, with some 5 million addicted. *Substance abuse* is characterized by significant adverse consequences resulting from the repeated use of a substance.[93] With *chemical dependence*, the individual continues to use a substance in spite of having significant substance-related problems including symptoms of withdrawal, the need for larger amounts of the substance, unsuccessful attempts to control its use, and the need to spend increasing amounts of time seeking the substance. With time, chemical dependence leads to health, social, and economic problems.

Epidemiology

The abuse of drugs and consequent chemical dependency by physicians has attracted considerable media attention and notoriety. Recognition of the problem of substance dependence among physicians is not new. In the first edition of *The Principles and Practice of Medicine*, edited by Sir William Osler and published in 1892, it is stated: "The habit (morphia) is particularly prevalent among women and physicians who use the hypodermic syringe for the alleviation of pain, as in neuralgia or sciatica."

It is debatable whether substance abuse is more prevalent among physicians than the general population. Hughes et al[94] found that physicians abused alcohol, minor opiates, and benzodiazepine tranquilizers more frequently than the general population. In many cases, the prescription drugs were self-prescribed and were considered by the physician to be "self-treatment." On the other hand, physicians were less likely to use tobacco or illicit substances. A report from the National Institute on Drug Abuse concludes that HCW suffer from chemical dependency (including alcohol abuse) at a rate roughly equivalent to that of the general population (8 to 12%).[95]

In the event that a drug-related problem does exist, physicians are less likely than the population in general to seek professional assistance. Denial plays a major role in this reluctance to undergo counseling or therapy. Medical students learn early in their education to utilize denial to enable them to endure long, sleepless nights and the personal shortcomings that inevitably accompany the practice of medicine. These well-developed denial mechanisms enable the physician-addict to conclude that his or her problem is minor and that self-treatment is possible. Physicians typically enter programs for treatment only after they have reached the end stages of their illness.

7 It is commonly reported that chemical dependency is a specific problem for the specialty of anesthesiology and represents its primary occupational hazard.[96] One example of the increased incidence of substance abuse reported among anesthesiologists comes from the Medical Association of Georgia Disabled Doctors' Program.[97] Anesthesiologists constituted 12% of physician patients treated at the center although they represented only 3.9% of American physicians. On the other hand, other studies have failed to identify an overall excess prevalence of substance abuse among anesthesiologists with the notable exception of major opiates.[98,99]

One very troubling aspect of this problem is the increased incidence of substance abuse reported among anesthesiology residents. In the report from the Medical Association of Georgia Disabled Doctors' Program,[97] anesthesiology residents constituted 33.7% of the resident population of the treatment group, despite representing only 4.6% of the resident population.

The incidence of controlled substance abuse within anesthesiology training programs is estimated to be 1 to 2%.[100] This statistic is particularly troubling because it has persisted despite the increased emphasis placed on education and accountability of controlled substances in the recent decade. ACGME requirements mandate that anesthesiology residency programs have a written policy and an educational program regarding substance abuse, but these efforts have not successfully addressed the problem of substance abuse in training programs.

The Disease of Substance Dependence

What accounts for this unacceptably high prevalence of substance dependence among anesthesiologists? To answer this, it is important to understand substance dependence as a chronic psychosocial, biogenetic disease.[101] Addiction shares many characteristics with other common chronic illnesses: (1) it is a primary condition (not a symptom), (2) it has established etiologies, (3) it is associated with specific anatomic and physiologic changes, (4) it has a set of recognizable signs and symptoms, and (5) if left untreated, it has a predictable, progressive course.

The causative factors in this disease process involve a genetic predisposition as well as the environment. The disease results from a dynamic interplay between a susceptible host and a "favorable" environment. Vulnerability in the host is an important factor. What constitutes an instigating exposure to a drug in one person may have absolutely no effect on another. Unfortunately, there is not a predictive tool to identify the susceptible individual until he or she gets the disease.

Causative factors thought to be specific to certain anesthesiologists include job stress, an orientation toward self-medication, lack of external recognition and self-respect, the availability of addicting drugs, and a susceptible premorbid personality. Self-prescription and recreational use of drugs are commonly seen as a prelude to more extensive substance abuse and dependence. Of concern are the increasing recreational use of drugs among younger physicians and medical students and the choice of more potent drugs with enhanced potential for addiction, such as cocaine, the synthetic opioids, propofol, and some of the newer inhalation anesthetics.

Anesthesiologists work in a climate in which large quantities of powerful psychoactive drugs are freely available. Anesthesiologists are unique because they usually prescribe as well as personally administer these drugs in contrast to most other physicians who prescribe while others administer. The experience from soldiers in the United States Army in Vietnam suggests that when there is easy access to narcotics, alcohol use declines in favor of use of opiates. As each new synthetic opioid, anesthetic induction agent, and inhalation anesthetic has become available for clinical use, it has also become a drug of choice of abusing anesthesiologists. Because availability of drugs does play a role in the onset of this disease, attention has been directed toward programs to enforce increased accountability and regulation of controlled substances.[102] However, despite widespread application of protocols to enforce greater accountability, such as satellite pharmacies for operating suites, the frequency of substance abuse has changed little, if at all, in recent years.[100]

There is an apparent association between behavior before entering medical school and subsequent development of

TABLE 4-6

SIGNS OF SUBSTANCE ABUSE AND DEPENDENCE

■ WHAT TO LOOK FOR OUTSIDE THE HOSPITAL

1. Addiction is a disease of loneliness and isolation. Addicts quickly withdraw from family, friends, and leisure activities.
2. Addicts have unusual changes in behavior, including wide mood swings and periods of depression, anger, and irritability alternating with periods of euphoria.
3. Unexplained overspending, legal problems, gambling, extramarital affairs, and increased problems at work are commonly seen in addicts.
4. An obvious physical sign of alcoholism is the frequent smell of alcohol on the breath.
5. Domestic strife, fights, and arguments may increase in number and intensity.
6. Sexual drive may significantly decrease.
7. Children may develop behavioral problems.
8. Some addicts frequently change jobs over a period of several years in an attempt to find a "geographic cure" for their disease, or to hide it from coworkers.
9. Addicts need to be near their drug source. For a health care professional, this means long hours at the hospital, even when off duty. For alcoholics, it means calling in sick to work. Alcoholics may disappear without any explanation to bars or hiding places to drink secretly.
10. Addicts may suddenly develop the habit of locking themselves in the bathroom or other rooms while they are using drugs.
11. Addicts frequently hide pills, syringes, or alcohol bottles around the house.
12. Persons who inject drugs may leave bloody swabs and syringes containing blood-tinged liquid in conspicuous places.
13. Addicts may display evidence of withdrawal, especially diaphoresis (sweating) and tremors.
14. Narcotic addicts often have pinpoint pupils.
15. Weight loss and pale skin are also common signs of addiction.
16. Addicts may be seen injecting drugs.
17. Tragically, some addicts are found comatose or dead before any of these signs have been recognized by others.

■ WHAT TO LOOK FOR INSIDE THE HOSPITAL

1. Addicts sign out ever-increasing quantities of narcotics.
2. Addicts frequently have unusual changes in behavior, such as wide mood swings and periods of depression, anger, and irritability alternating with periods of euphoria.
3. Charting becomes increasingly sloppy and unreadable.
4. Addicts often sign out narcotics in inappropriately high doses for the operation being performed.
5. They refuse lunch and coffee relief.
6. Addicts like to work alone in order to use anesthetic techniques without narcotics, falsify records, and divert drugs for personal use.
7. They volunteer for extra cases, often where large amounts of narcotics are available (e.g., cardiac cases).
8. They frequently relieve others.
9. They're often at the hospital when off duty, staying close to their drug supply to prevent withdrawal.
10. They volunteer frequently for extra call.
11. They're often difficult to find between cases, taking short naps after using.
12. Addicted anesthesia personnel may insist on personally administering narcotics in the recovery room.
13. Addicts make frequent requests for bathroom relief. This is usually where they use drugs.
14. Addicts may wear long-sleeved gowns to hide needle tracks and also to combat the subjective feeling of cold they experience when using narcotics.
15. Narcotic addicts often have pinpoint pupils.
16. An addict's patients may come into the recovery room complaining of pain out of proportion to the amount of narcotic charted on the anesthesia records.
17. Weight loss and pale skin are also common signs of addiction.
18. Addicts may be seen injecting drugs.
19. Untreated addicts are found comatose.
20. Undetected addicts are found dead.

Adapted from Farley WJ, Arnold WP: Videotape: Unmasking addiction: Chemical Dependency in Anesthesiology. Produced by Davids Productions, Parsippany, NJ, funded by Janssen Pharmaceutica, Piscataway, New Jersey, 1991.
Reprinted with permission from American Society of Anesthesiologists: Task Force on Chemical Dependence of the Committee on Occupational Health of Operating Room Personnel: Chemical Dependence in Anesthesiologists: What You Need to Know When You Need to Know It. Park Ridge, Illinois, American Society of Anesthesiologists, 1998.

substance abuse.[103] Personality profiles of anesthesiologists have suggested that a disturbingly high proportion that may be associated with a predisposition toward maladaptive behavior. Talbott et al[97] have observed that many of the anesthesia residents in their treatment program specifically chose the specialty of anesthesiology because of the known availability of powerful drugs.

The consequences of untreated chemical dependence are ultimately devastating. There is a gradual and inexorable deterioration in professional, family, and social relationships. The substance abuser becomes increasingly withdrawn and isolated, first in his or her personal life, and ultimately in his or her professional existence (Table 4-6). Every attempt is made to maintain a facade of normality at work, because discovery means isolation from the source of the abused drug. When professional conduct is finally impaired such that it is apparent to the physician's colleagues, the disease is approaching its end stage.

TABLE 4-7

POLICY STATEMENT OF THE AMERICAN BOARD OF ANESTHESIOLOGY (ABA)

The Americans with Disabilities Act (ADA) protects individuals with a history of alcohol abuse or substance abuse who are not currently abusing alcohol or using drugs illegally. The ABA supports the intent of the ADA.

The ABA will admit qualified applicants and candidates with a history of alcohol abuse to its examination system and to examination if, in response to its inquiries, the ABA receives acceptable documentation that they do not currently pose a direct threat to the health and safety of others.

The ABA will admit qualified applicants and candidates with a history of illegal use of drugs to its examination system and to examination if, in response to its inquiries, the ABA receives acceptable documentation that they are not currently engaged in the illegal use of drugs.

After a candidate with a history of alcohol abuse or illegal use of drugs satisfies the examination requirements for certification, the ABA will determine whether it should defer awarding its certification to the candidate for a period of time to avoid certifying a candidate who poses a direct threat to the health and safety of others. If the ABA determines that deferral of the candidate's certification is appropriate because the candidate does currently pose a threat to the health and safety of others, the ABA will assess the specific circumstances of the candidate's history of alcohol abuse or illegal use of drugs to determine when the candidate should write the Board to request issuance of its certification.

Reprinted with permission from Booklet of Information, Board Policies 6.01: Alcohol and Substance Abuse. Raleigh, North Carolina, American Board of Anesthesiology, March 2004.

In its end stage, substance dependence is often a fatal illness. Alexander et al[14] calculated a relative risk of 2.75 for drug-related deaths among anesthesiologists compared to internists. In their study of substance abuse in anesthesiologists, Ward et al[104] reported that among the 334 confirmed drug abusers, 27 died of drug overdose and in another 3, abuse was discovered at death. Gravenstein et al[105] reported 7 deaths among 44 confirmed drug abusers. Menk et al[106] found 14 drug-related deaths among the 79 drug abusers who had been reenrolled in anesthesiology residencies after treatment.

In addition to health hazards, there are significant legal and medicolegal considerations that may affect chemically dependent physicians.[96] Laws and regulations vary by state but they detail the necessary steps for handling the drug-abusing physician. In many states disciplinary action and criminal penalties can be imposed on physicians who knowingly fail to report an impaired colleague. Disciplinary action taken against an impaired physician must also be reported to the National Practitioner Data Bank to be in compliance with federal law. State medical societies often have "wellness committees," and when chemically dependent physicians seek treatment through this venue, the legal impact may be mitigated.

Debate continues regarding the issue of compulsory random drug testing of physicians.[107] Preemployment and/or random drug screening is already well established in various industries, especially those with high public health profiles (nuclear, aviation, military). Many chairs of academic anesthesiology programs have indicated a willingness to initiate a program of random drug screening of their staff.[100] Although random drug testing is an established element of most reentry contracts for recovering anesthesiologists, serious questions remain about the legality of this approach and its effectiveness in preventing substance abuse. Because fentanyl and sufentanil are the drugs abused by many chemically dependent anesthesiologists and because routine drug screens do not detect these agents, tests that effectively identify their use are expensive and have limited availability.

When there is sufficient data to identify an anesthesiologist as having chemical dependence, an intervention should be conducted by an experienced individual. The purpose of the intervention is to demonstrate to the anesthesiologist that they have the disease and to immediately have them enter a facility for evaluation and treatment. Treatment usually begins with inpatient therapy progressing to outpatient sessions. The family is actively involved with treatment, and the individual begins association with Alcoholics Anonymous (AA) or Narcotics Anonymous (NA).

Controversy remains about the ultimate career path of the anesthesiologist in recovery from chemical dependency. Within the general population, the recidivism rate approaches 60% for patients who have been treated for drug dependency. However, physicians are highly motivated and better rehabilitation rates might be expected. Reports by Talbott et al[97] and Ward et al[104] provided early optimism that in many cases anesthesiologists could be successfully rehabilitated and safely returned to their practices. In a study that examined relapse in addicted physicians, the rate of relapse among anesthesiologists was 40% and that of control physicians was 44%.[108] Sustained recovery for longer than 2 years occurred in 81% and 86%, respectively. Although these data suggested that the outcome for recovering anesthesiologists was similar to other physicians, a study by Menk and colleagues[106] drew a different conclusion. Among 79 opioid-dependent anesthesiology residents, there was a 66% (52 of 79) failure rate for successful rehabilitation and return to practice. Even more discouraging, there were 14 suicide or overdose deaths among the 79 returning trainees. Their conclusion was that redirection into another specialty is the safer course after rehabilitation of narcotic-dependent residents.

Because of the contradictory data, no universal recommendations can be made about reentry into the practice of anesthesia after treatment. The American Board of Anesthesiology has established a policy for candidates with a history of alcoholism or illegal use of drugs (Table 4-7). To reenter practice, the recovering physician must qualify for a valid license to practice medicine and must be recredentialed at their medical facility. This must be done in compliance with their state laws and regulations that detail the circumstances under which a recovering physician can return to practice. Federal laws, such as the Americans with Disabilities Act, impose additional considerations. Additionally, a carefully worded contract is an important first step in the reentry process to define the obligations of the physician and the department.[96,109] There should also be regular meetings with the departmental supervisor to monitor the return process. It is also generally recommended that the returning anesthesiologist not take night or weekend call or handle opioids without direct supervision for at least the first 3 months. Despite all of these precautions, the potential for relapse must be anticipated.

Guidelines from physician treatment centers may be helpful to assist in the decisions surrounding reentry.[93] Individuals who, in most situations, can successfully return to the practice of anesthesiology immediately after treatment (Category I) accept and understand their disease and have no evidence of accompanying psychiatric disorders. They have strong support from their family, demonstrate a balanced lifestyle, are committed to their recovery contract, and bond with AA or NA. Their anesthesiology department and hospital must be supportive of their return, and the individual must have a sponsor that supports their return to anesthesiology.

Category II includes those individuals who could possibly return to anesthesiology within a few years. They must have no or minimal denial regarding their disease and have no other psychiatric diagnoses. Their recovery skills are continually improving and they are involved, but not necessarily bonded, with AA/NA. Although their family situation may be characterized as dysfunctional, there should be tangible evidence of improvement.

Individuals who should not return to anesthesiology and would best be redirected into another medical specialty are included in Category III. These individuals may have had a history of prolonged intravenous substance use and have experienced relapses and prior treatment failures. Their disease remains active, and they have coexisting severe psychiatric diagnoses. Often, these individuals entered anesthesiology with an expectation of being able to readily obtain drugs.

Impairment

Substance abuse probably accounts for the majority of the cases of impairment among physicians. (An impaired physician is defined as one "whose performance as a professional person and as a practitioner of the healing arts is impaired because of alcoholism, drug abuse, mental illness, senility, or disabling disease."[110]) Other factors that may lead to impairment include physical or mental illness and deterioration associated with aging. Some authorities include unwillingness or inability to keep up with current literature and techniques as a form of impairment.

Data regarding the prevalence of these disabling disorders are more difficult to obtain than are those on drug abuse. Physicians are admitted to psychiatric facilities for organic psychoses, personality disorders, schizophrenia, neuroses, and affective, disorders, particularly depression.

It is not surprising that depression should figure prominently among the personality characteristics of emotionally impaired physicians. One survey noted that approximately 30% of medical interns were clinically depressed.[111] Indeed, when exaggerated, many of the personality traits that ensure success in the physician's world, such as self-sacrifice, competitiveness, achievement orientation, denial of feelings, and intellectualization of emotions, may also serve as risk factors for depression. Several studies on alcoholic physicians have provided some insight into this link between achievement orientation and emotional disturbance. In one study, more than half of the alcoholic physicians graduated in the upper one third of their medical school class, 23% were in the upper one tenth, and only 5% were in the lower one third of their class.[112] Similarly, a report on alcohol use in medical school demonstrated better first-year grades and higher scores on Part I National Board of Medical Examiners tests among those students identified as alcohol abusers.[113] Alcohol abuse is likely a manifestation of psychological disturbance resulting from excessive degrees of stress among some students who are most determined to have flawless records.

It can be difficult to appropriately respond to the problems imposed by the impaired or unsafe anesthesiologist.[114] Fortunately, most state legislatures and medical societies have formal protocols that address the impaired physician. These programs are usually therapeutic and nonpunitive in nature and provide for a relatively nonthreatening environment for intervention for the impaired physician. The license suspension power of the State Board of Medical Examiners is exercised only in cases in which a real risk to the public welfare exists and the involved physician is unwilling to voluntarily suspend practice and accept assistance. Management protocols for dealing with the impaired physician are covered in a series of articles by Canavan.[115]

The Aging Anesthesiologist

Little research has been directed toward the challenges faced by older anesthesiologists.[43] This is in contrast to the situation in most other industries where strict attention is paid to the competence and well-being of older workers. For example, commercial pilots are required to take regular medical examinations and conform to policies regarding hours of work.

There are no age-specific conditions placed on state medical licensure or on the practice of anesthesiology. In most cases, the decision to limit practice or retire remains at the discretion of the individual anesthesiologist based on his or her self-evaluation. Since 2000, diplomates of the American Board of Anesthesiologists have time-limited certification and must successfully complete the Maintenance of Certification in Anesthesiology program every 10 years to document continuing qualifications and to maintain certification.

As a result of a number of demographic factors, including the smaller residency class sizes observed during the mid 1990s, the mean age of the anesthesiology workforce is increasing. The greatest number (30%) of anesthesiologists are between age 45 and 54 years of age, and 56% are age 45 and older (up from 49% 10 years ago).[15]

Several physiologic changes frequently associated with aging have the potential of impacting on an individual's ability to practice anesthesiology. Potential sources of impairment including decrements in hearing, vision, short-term memory, strength, and endurance may often be compensated by other advantages conferred by older age, including the experience acquired by a lifelong practice of the specialty.

One area of particular difficulty for anesthesiologists is maintaining the stamina required for long work shifts and night call. Superimposed on a propensity to sleep disturbance, the demands of night call and associated sleep deprivation are particularly difficult for older anesthesiologists. Night call is considered one of the most stressful aspects of practice and is often cited as a reason for retirement among older anesthesiologists.

Aging among anesthesiologists raises interesting legal issues. A number of federal laws potentially impact the aging anesthesiologist's and his or her colleagues' decisions whether to continue to work and under what arrangements. These include the Age Discrimination Act, Title VII of the Civil Rights Act ("Equal Pay Act"), the Medical and Family Leave Act, the Fair Labor Standards Act, and the Employee Retirement Income Security Act (ERISA). An anesthesiologist's decision to retire must fit within the complex framework of federal and state laws and regulations. Anesthesiologists tend to retire at a younger age than do many other specialists.[116]

Mortality Among Anesthesiologists

8 It is debatable whether anesthesiologists are subject to premature death compared to other physicians. Early studies of anesthesiologists in the United States[13] and studies conducted in Europe[117] have demonstrated death rates among anesthesiologists less than that seen in their control groups. However, contrary results have been reported in other studies both from the United States[14] and Europe.[118] As an example, data

from Alexander et al[14] demonstrated a significant difference in the mean age at death among anesthesiologists, 66.5 ± 14.7 years, compared to their control group (internists), 69.0 ± 14.5 years. In a subsequent study, Katz[15] concluded that there was no statistical difference in age-specific mortality among anesthesiologists, internists, and other physicians when ages of the living members of the physician groups were considered in the analyses.

Suicide

Perhaps one of the most alarming of the potential occupational hazards for anesthesiologists is a frequently cited excess rate of suicide. It has been well established that among physicians in general, the rate of suicide ranks disproportionately high as a cause of death.[119] Early reports singled out anesthesiologists as being particularly vulnerable. However, this conclusion has been questioned as the result of the methodological difficulties in collecting accurate data on suicide and the frequent failure to adequately correct for confounding variables in the study populations.

Why might there be a high rate of suicide among anesthesiologists? A partial explanation lies with the high degree of stress that is an integral part of the job. The relationship between generalized stress and suicide is not direct. But, in susceptible people, feelings of inability to cope resulting from overwhelming stress can give way to despair and suicide ideation.

Extensive personality profiles collected from suicide-susceptible individuals indicate characteristics such as high anxiety, insecurity, low self-esteem, impulsiveness, and poor self-control. It is disturbing to note that in Reeve's study of personality traits of anesthesiologists,[120] some 20% manifested psychological profiles that reflected a predisposition to behavioral disintegration and attempted suicide when placed under extremes of stress. This study raises the discomforting notion that "premorbid" personality characteristics exist before entering specialty training and are not being identified in the admissions process.

One specific type of stress, that resulting from a malpractice lawsuit, may have a direct causative association with suicide among physicians in general and anesthesiologists in particular. Newspaper reports have described the emotional deterioration and ultimate suicide of experienced physicians who have become involved in a malpractice suit. One study reported that 4 of 185 anesthesiologists being sued for medical malpractice attempted or committed suicide.[121]

Substance abuse among anesthesia personnel is another potential contributor to the increased suicide rate. Individuals with chemical dependence, who are not identified and are in the end stages of the disease, may die of drug overdose, a cause of death that may be difficult to distinguish from suicide. Physicians who are impaired from chemical dependence and whose privileges to practice medicine are revoked are also at heightened risk for attempting suicide. Crawshaw et al[122] reported eight successful and two near-miss suicide attempts among 43 physicians placed on probation for drug-related disability.

References

1. Linde HW, Bruce DL: Occupational exposure of anesthetists to halothane, nitrous oxide and radiation. Anesthesiology 30:363, 1969
2. Panni MK, Corn SB: Scavenging in the operating room. Current Opinion in Anaesthesiology 16:611, 2003
3. Task Force on Trace Anesthetic Gases of the Committee on Occupational Health of Operating Room Personnel: Waste Anesthetic Gases: Information for Management in Anesthetizing Areas and the Postanesthesia Care Unit (PACU). Park Ridge, Illinois, American Society of Anesthesiologists, 1999
4. American Society of Anesthesiologists Ad Hoc Committee on the Effect of Trace Anesthetics on the Health of Operating Room Personnel: Occupational disease among operating room personnel: A national study. Anesthesiology 41:321, 1977
5. Buring JE, Hennekens CH, Mayrent SL *et al*: Health experiences of operating room personnel. Anesthesiology 62:325, 1985
6. Rowland AS, Baird D, Weinberg CR *et al*: Reduced fertility among women employed as dental assistants exposed to high levels of nitrous oxide. N Engl J Med 327:993, 1992
7. Rowland AS, Baird DD, Shore DL *et al*: Nitrous oxide and spontaneous abortion in female dental assistants. Am J Epidemiol 141:531, 1995
8. Boivin JF: Risk of spontaneous abortion in women occupationally exposed to anaesthetic gases: A meta-analysis. Occup Environ Med 54:541, 1997
9. Axelsson G, Ahlborg G, Bodin L: Shift work, nitrous oxide exposure, and spontaneous abortion among Swedish midwives. Occup Environ Med 53:374, 1996
10. Luke B, Mamelle N, Keith L *et al*: Obstetrics. The association between occupational factors and preterm birth: A United States nurses' study. Am J Obstet Gynecol 173:849, 1995
11. Ebi KL, Rice SA: Reproductive and developmental toxicity of anesthetics in humans. In Rice SA, Fish KJ (eds): Anesthetic Toxicity. New York, Raven Press, 1994
12. Bruce DL, Eide KA, Linde HW *et al*: Causes of death among anesthesiologists: A 20-year survey. Anesthesiology 29:565, 1968
13. Bruce DL, Eide KA, Smith NJ *et al*: A prospective survey of anesthesiologist mortality, 1967–1971. Anesthesiology 41:71, 1974
14. Alexander BH, Checkoway H, Nagahama SI, Domino KB: Cause-specific mortality risks of anesthesiologists. Anesthesiology 93:922, 2000
15. Katz JD: Do anesthesiologists die at a younger age than other physicians? Age-adjusted death rates. Anesth Analg 98:1111, 2004
16. Nunn JF, Sharer N: Serum methionine and hepatic enzyme activity in anaesthetists exposed to nitrous oxide. Br J Anaesth 54:593, 1982
17. Eger EI, White AE, Brown CL *et al*: A test of the carcinogenicity of enflurane, isoflurane, halothane, methoxyflurane and nitrous oxide in mice. Anesth Analg 57:678, 1978
18. Baden JM, Kelley M, Wharton RS *et al*: Mutagenicity of halogenated ether anesthetics. Anesthesiology 46:346, 1977
19. Baden JM, Kelley M, Cheung A *et al*: Lack of mutagens in urines of operating room personnel. Anesthesiology 53:195, 1980
20. Byhahn C, Wilke HJ, Westphal K: Occupational exposure to volatile anaesthetics: Epidemiology and approaches to reducing the problem. CNS Drugs 15:197, 2001
21. Wiesner G, Hoerauf K, Schroegendorfer K, Sobczynaki P, Harth M, Ruediger HW: High-level, but not low-level, occupational exposure to inhaled anesthetics is associated with genotoxicity in the micronucleus assay. Anesth Analg 92:118, 2001
22. Bruce DL, Bach MJ: Effects of trace anaesthetic gases on behavioural performance of volunteers. Br J Anaesth 48:871, 1976
23. Bruce DL, Stanley TH: Research replication may be subject specific (letter). Anesth Analg 62:617, 1983
24. National Institute for Occupational Safety and Health (NIOSH): Criteria for a Recommended Standard . . . Occupational Exposure to Waste Anesthetic Gases and Vapors. Cincinnati, Ohio, Department of Health, Education, and Welfare (NIOSH), Publication No. 77-140
25. NIOSH Alert: Request for assistance in controlling exposures to nitrous oxide during anesthetic administration. Cincinnati, Ohio, DHHS (NIOSH) Publication No. 94-100, 1994
26. American Institute of Architects Academy of Architecture for Health, U.S. Department of Health and Human Services: 1996–1997 Guidelines for design and construction of hospital and health care facilities. Washington, DC, The American Institute of Architects Press, 1996
27. Sessler DI, Badgwell JM: Exposure of postoperative nurses to exhaled anesthetic gases. Anesth Analg 87:1083, 1998
28. McGregor DG, Senjem DH, Mazze RI: Trace nitrous oxide levels in the postanesthesia care unit. Anesth Analg 89:472, 1999
29. Sadoh DR, Sharief MK, Howard RS: Occupational exposure to methyl-methacrylate monomer induces generalized neuropathy in a dental technician. Br Dent J 186:380, 1999
30. Njoku DB, Greenberg RS, Bourdi M *et al*: Autoantibodies associated with volatile anesthetic hepatitis found in the sera of a large cohort of pediatric anesthesiologists. Anesth Analg 94:243, 2002
31. Brown RH, Schauble JF, Hamilton RG: Prevalence of latex allergy among anesthesiologists. Anesthesiology 89:292, 1998
32. Konrad C, Fieber T, Gerber H: The prevalence of latex sensitivity among anesthesiology staff. Anesth Analg 84:629, 1997
33. Task Force on Latex Sensitivity of the Committee on Occupational Health of Operating Room Personnel: Natural Rubber Latex Allergy: Considerations for Anesthesiologists. Park Ridge, Illinois, American Society of Anesthesiologists, 1999. http://www.asahq.org/publicationsAndServices/physician.htm
34. McGowan C, Heaton B, Stephenson RN: Occupational x-ray exposure of anaesthetists. Br J Anaesth 76:868, 1996
35. NIOSH recommendations for occupational safety and health standard. MMWR 37(suppl 5–7):1, 1988

36. Murthy VSSN, Malhotra SK, Bala I, Raghunathan M: Detrimental effects of noise on anaesthetists. Can J Anaesth 42:608, 1995
37. Gaba D: Human error in anesthetic mishaps. Int Anesthesiol Clin 27:137, 1989
38. Weinger MB, Herndon OW, Gaba DM: The effect of electronic record keeping and transesophageal echocardiography on task distribution, workload, and vigilance during cardiac anesthesia. Anesthesiology 87:144, 1997
39. Paget NS, Lambert TF, Sridhar K: Factors affecting an anaesthetist's work: Some findings on vigilance and performance. Anaesth Intensive Care 9:359, 1981
40. Gaba DM, Howard SK, Jump B: Production pressure in the work environment: California anesthesiologists' attitudes and experiences. Anesthesiology 81:488, 1994
41. Howard SK, Gaba DM, Smith BE *et al*: Simulation study of rested versus sleep-deprived anesthesiologists. Anesthesiology 98:1345, 2003
42. Gravenstein JS, Cooper JB, Orkin FK: Work and rest cycles in anesthesia practice. Anesthesiology 72:737, 1990
43. Katz JD: Issues of concern for the aging anesthesiologist. Anesth Analg 92:1487, 2001
44. Howard SK, Rosekind MR, Katz JD, Berry AJ: Fatigue in anesthesia: implications and strategies for patient and provider safety. Anesthesiology 97:1281, 2002
45. Dawson D, Reid K: Fatigue, alcohol and performance impairment. Nature 388:235, 1997
46. Weinger MB, Ancoli-Israel S: Sleep deprivation and clinical performance. JAMA 287:955, 2002
47. Gander PH, Merry A, Millar MM, Weller J: Hours of work and fatigue-related error: A survey of New Zealand anaesthetists. Anaesthesia and Intensive Care 28:178, 2000
48. Howard SK, Gaba DM, Rosekind MR, Zarcone VP. The risks and implications of excessive daytime sleepiness in resident physicians. Acad Med 77:1019, 2002
49. Veasey S, Rosen R, Barzansky B, Rosen I, Owens J: Sleep loss and fatigue in residency training: a reappraisal. JAMA 288:1116, 2002
50. Asch DA, Parker RM: The Libby Zion case. One step forward or two steps backward? N Engl J Med 318:771, 1988
51. Berry AJ: Needle stick and other safety issues. Anesthesiology Clinics of North America 22:493, 2004
52. Katz JD: Hand washing and disinfection: More than your mother taught you. Anesthesiology Clinics of North America 22:457, 2004
53. Centers for Disease Control and Prevention: Immunization of health-care workers: Recommendations of the Advisory Committee on Immunization Practices (ACIP) and the Hospital Infection Control Practices Advisory Committee (HICPAC). MMWR 46(no. RR-18):1, 1997
54. Centers for Disease Control and Prevention: Updated U.S. Public Health Service guidelines for the management of occupational exposures to HBV, HCV, and HIV and recommendations for postexposure prophylaxis. MMWR 50(no. RR-11):1, 2001
55. Bolyard EA, Tablan OC, Williams WW *et al*: The Hospital Infection Control Practices Advisory Committee: Guideline for infection control in health care personnel, 1998. Am J Infect Control 26:289, 1998
56. Centers for Disease Control and Prevention: Prevention and control of influenza: Recommendations of the Advisory Committee on Immunization Practices (ACIP). MMWR 53(no. RR-6):1, 2004
57. Couch RB: Prevention and treatment of influenza. N Engl J Med 343:1778, 2000
58. Centers for Disease Control and Prevention: Guidelines for preventing health-care-associated pneumonia, 2003. Recommendations of the CDC and the Healthcare Infection Control Practices Advisory Committee. MMWR 53(no. RR-3):1, 2004
59. Garner JS: Hospital Infection Control Practices Advisory Committee: Guidelines for isolation precautions in hospitals. Infect Control Hosp Epidemiol 17:56, 1996
60. Centers for Disease Control and Prevention: Prevention of varicella: Recommendations of the Immunization Practices Advisory Committee (ACIP). MMWR 45(no. RR-11):1, 1996
61. Centers for Disease Control and Prevention: Measles, mumps, and rubella—Vaccine use and strategies for elimination of measles, rubella, and congenital rubella syndrome and control of mumps: Recommendations of the Immunization Practices Advisory Committee (ACIP). MMWR 47(no. RR-8):1, 1998
62. Centers for Disease Control and Prevention: Severe acute respiratory syndrome. Public health guidance for community-level preparedness and response to severe acute respiratory syndrome (SARS) Version 2. Supplement I: Infection control in healthcare, home, and community settings. III. Infection control in healthcare facilities. CDC website: http://www.cdc.gov/ncidod/sars/guidance/index.htm
63. Centers for Disease Control and Prevention: Protection of hepatitis A through active or passive immunization: Recommendations of the Immunization Practices Advisory Committee (ACIP). MMWR 48(no. RR-12):1, 1999
64. Berry AJ, Greene ES: The risk of needlestick injuries and needlestick-transmitted diseases in the practice of anesthesiology. Anesthesiology 77:1007, 1992
65. Department of Labor, Occupational Safety and Health Administration: Occupational exposure to bloodborne pathogens: Needle-sticks and other sharp injuries: Final rule (29 CFR Part 1910.1030). Federal Register 66:5318, 2001
66. Alter MJ, Margolis HS, Krawczynski K *et al*: The natural history of community-acquired hepatitis C in the United States. N Engl J Med 327:1899, 1992
67. Jaeckel E, Comberg M, Wedemeyer H *et al*: Treatment of acute hepatitis C with interferon alfa-2b. N Engl J Med 345:1452, 2001
68. Centers for Disease Control and Prevention: HIV/AIDS surveillance report. Vol. 14, 2002. http://www.cdc.gov/hiv/stats/hasr1402.htm
69. Bell DM: Occupational risk of human immunodeficiency virus infection in healthcare workers: An overview. Am J Med 102(suppl 5B):9, 1997
70. Ippolito G, Puro V, De Carli G. Italian Study Group on Occupational Risk of HIV Infection: The risk of occupational human immunodeficiency virus infection in health care workers: Italian multicenter study. Arch Intern Med 153:1451, 1993
71. Cardo DM, Culver DH, Clesielski CA *et al*: A case-control study of HIV seroconversion in health care workers after percutaneous exposure. N Engl J Med 337:1485, 1997
72. Greene ES, Berry AJ, Jagger J *et al*: Multicenter study of contaminated percutaneous injuries in anesthesia personnel. Anesthesiology 89:1362, 1998
73. Task Force on Infection Control of the Committee on Occupational Health of Operating Room Personnel: Recommendations for Infection Control for the Practice of Anesthesiology, 2nd ed. Park Ridge, Illinois, American Society of Anesthesiologists, 1998
74. Greene ES, Berry AJ, Arnold WP, Jagger J: Percutaneous injuries in anesthesia personnel. Anesth Analg 83:273, 1996
75. Johnson RT, Gibbs CJ: Creutzfeldt-Jakob disease and related transmissible spongiform encephalopathies. N Engl J Med 339:1994, 2001
76. Centers for Disease Control and Prevention: Guidelines for preventing the transmission of *Mycobacterium tuberculosis* in health care facilities, 1994. MMWR 43(no. RR-13):1, 1994
77. Menzies D, Fanning A, Yuan L, Fitzgerald M: Tuberculosis among health care workers. N Engl J Med 332:92, 1995
78. American Thoracic Society, Centers for Disease Control and Prevention, Infectious Diseases Society of America: Treatment of tuberculosis. Am J Respir Crit Care Med 167:603, 2003
79. Tait AR: Occupational transmission of tuberculosis: Implications for anesthesiologists. Anesth Analg 85:444, 1997
80. Jereb JA, Klevens RM, Privett TD *et al*: Tuberculosis in health care workers at a hospital with an outbreak of multidrug-resistant *Mycobacterium tuberculosis*. Arch Intern Med 155:854, 1995
81. United States Department of Health and Human Services: 42 CRF Part 84: Respiratory protective devices; final rule and notice. Federal Register 60:30336, 1995
82. Control of Smoke from Laser/Electric Surgical Procedures, DHHS (NIOSH) Publication No. 96-128, National Institute for Occupational Safety and Health, Cincinnati, Ohio September 1996
83. Matchette LS, Faaland RW, Royston DD *et al*: In vitro production of viable bacteriophage in carbon dioxide and argon laser plumes. Lasers Surg Med 11:380, 1991
84. Hallmo P, Naess O: Laryngeal papillomatosis with human papilloma virus DNA contracted by a laser surgeon. Eur Arch Otorhinolaryngol 248:425, 1991
85. Recommended Practices Committee of the Association of Operating Room Nurses: Recommended practices for electrosurgery. AORN Journal 79:432, 2004
86. Nyssen AS, Hansez I, Baele P, Lamy M, De Keyser V: Occupational stress and burnout in anaesthesia. Br J Anaesth 90:333, 2003
87. Jackson SH: The role of stress in anaesthetists' health and well-being. Acta Anaesthesiol Scand 43:583, 1999
88. Seyle H: The Stress of Life. New York, McGraw-Hill, 1984
89. Kain ZN, Chan KM, Katz JD *et al*: Anesthesiologists and acute perioperative stress: A cohort study. Anesth Analg 95:177, 2002
90. Sexton JB, Thomas EJ, Helmreich RL: Error, stress, and teamwork in medicine and aviation: cross sectional surveys. BMJ 320:745, 2000
91. Vaillant GE, Brighton JR, McArthur C: Physicians' use of mood-altering drugs. N Engl J Med 282:365, 1970
92. McDonald JS, Lingam RP, Gupta B *et al*: Psychologic testing as an aid to selection of residents in anesthesiology. Anesth Analg 78:542, 1994
93. Angres DH, Talbott GD, Bettinardi-Angres K: Anesthesiologist's Return to Practice, in Healing the Healer: The Addicted Physician. Madison, CT, Psychosocial Press, 1998
94. Hughes PH, Brandenburg N, Baldwin DC *et al*: Prevalence of substance use among US physicians. JAMA 267:2333, 1992
95. Prescription Drugs: Abuse and Addiction. Bethesda, MD, National Institute on Drug Abuse, 2001
96. Silverstein JH, Silva DA, Iberti TJ: Opioid addiction in anesthesiology. Anesthesiology 79:354, 1993
97. Talbott DG, Gallegos KV, Wilson PO, Porter TL: The Medical Association of Georgia's impaired physicians program review of the first 1000 physicians: Analysis of specialty. JAMA 257:2927, 1987
98. Lutsky I, Hopwood M, Abram SE *et al*: Use of psychoactive substances in three medical specialties: Anaesthesia, medicine and surgery. Report of investigation. Can J Anaesth 41:561, 1994

99. Hughes PH, Storr CL, Brandenburg NA, Baldwin DC, Anthony JC, Sheehan DV: Physician substance use by medical specialty. J Addict Dis 18:23, 1999
100. Booth JV, Grossman D, Moore J *et al*: Substance abuse among physicians: A survey of academic anesthesiology programs. Anesth Analg 95:1024, 2002
101. Cami J, Farre M: Drug addiction. N Engl J Med 349:975, 2003
102. Klein RL, Stevens WC, Kingston HGG: Controlled substance dispensing and accountability in United States anesthesiology residency programs. Anesthesiology 77:806, 1992
103. Moore RD, Mead L, Pearson TA: Youthful precursors of alcohol abuse in physicians. Am J Med 88:332, 1990
104. Ward CG, Ward GC, Saidman LJ: Drug abuse in anesthesia training programs. JAMA 250:922, 1983
105. Gravenstein JS, Kory WP, Marks RG: Drug abuse by anesthesia personnel. Anesth Analg 62:467, 1983
106. Menk EJ, Baumgarten RK, Kingsley CP, Culling RD, Middaugh R: Success of reentry into anesthesiology training programs by residents with a history of substance abuse. JAMA 263:3060, 1990
107. Scott M, Fisher KS: The evolving legal context for drug testing programs. Anesthesiology 73:1022, 1990
108. Paris RT, Canavan DI: Physician substance abuse impairment: Anesthesiologists vs. other specialties. J Addict Dis 18:1, 1999
109. Task Force on Chemical Dependence of the Committee on Occupational Health of Operating Room Personnel: Chemical Dependence in Anesthesiologists: What You Need to Know When You Need to Know It. Park Ridge, Illinois, American Society of Anesthesiologists, 1998
110. Canavan DJ: The impaired physician program: The subject of impairment. J Med Soc NJ 80:47, 1983
111. Clark DC, Salazar-Grueso E, Grabler P, Fawcett J: Predictors of depression during the first 6 months of internship. Am J Psychiatry 141:1095, 1984
112. Bissell L, Jones R: The alcoholic physician: A survey. Am J Psychiatry 133:1142, 1976
113. Clark DC, Eckenfels EJ, Daugherty SR *et al*: Alcohol-use patterns through medical school. A longitudinal study of one class. JAMA 257:2921, 1987
114. Atkinson RS: The problem of the unsafe anaesthetist. Br J Anaesth 73:29, 1994
115. Canavan DI, Baxter LE: The twentieth anniversary of the Physicians' Health Program of the Medical Society of New Jersey. J Med Soc NJ 100:27, 2003
116. Grauer H, Campbell NM: The aging physician and retirement. Can J Psychiatry 28:552, 1983
117. Carpenter LM, Swerdlow AJ, Fear NT: Mortality of doctors in different specialties: Findings from a cohort of 20,000 NHS hospital consultants. Occup Environ Med 54:388, 1997
118. Svardsudd K, Wedel H, Gordh T: Mortality rates among Swedish physicians: a population-based nationwide study with special reference to anesthesiologists. Acta Anaesthesiol Scand 46:1187, 2002
119. Center C, Davis M, Detre T *et al*: Confronting depression and suicide in physicians: A consensus statement. JAMA 289:3161, 2003
120. Reeve PE: Personality characteristics of a sample of anaesthetists. Anaesthesia 35:559, 1980
121. Birmingham PK, Ward RJ: A high risk suicide group: The anesthesiologist involved in litigation. Am J Psychiatry 142:1225, 1985
122. Crawshaw R, Bruce JA, Eraker PL *et al*: An epidemic of suicide among physicians on probation. JAMA 243:1915, 1980

CHAPTER 5 ■ PROFESSIONAL LIABILITY, QUALITY IMPROVEMENT, AND ANESTHETIC RISK

KAREN L. POSNER, FREDERICK W. CHENEY Jr., AND DONALD A. KROLL

KEY POINTS

1. Medical malpractice refers to the legal concept of professional negligence. The patient-plaintiff must prove that the anesthesiologist owed the patient a duty, failed to fulfill this duty, that the anesthesiologist's actions caused an injury, and that the injury resulted from a breach in the standard of anesthesia care.
2. The court establishes the standard of care in a particular case by the testimony of expert witnesses. The standard of care may also be determined from published sources such as hospital policies, textbooks, and standards adopted by the American Society of Anesthesiologists.
3. Risk management programs are broadly oriented toward reducing the liability exposure of the organization. Risk management programs complement quality improvement programs in minimizing liability exposure while maximizing quality of patient care.
4. Quality improvement programs are generally guided by the requirements of the Joint Commission on Accreditation of Healthcare Organizations (JCAHO). Quality improvement programs focus on improving the structure, process, and outcome of care.
5. Continuous quality improvement (CQI) is a systems approach to identifying and improving quality of care.
6. Anesthetic mortality has decreased recently but accidental deaths and disabling complications still occur.

In anesthesia, as in other areas of life, everything does not always go as planned. Undesirable outcomes occur regardless of the quality of care provided. The legal aspects of American medical practice have become increasingly important as the public has turned to the courts for economic redress when their expectations of medical treatment are not met. Payers such as Medicare are increasingly depending on accreditation through bodies such as the Joint Commission on Accreditation of Healthcare Organizations (JCAHO) to ensure that mechanisms are in place to deliver quality care to all patients. An anesthesia risk management program can work in conjunction with a program for quality improvement to minimize the liability risk of practice while assuring the highest quality of care for patients.

This chapter provides background for the practitioner about how the legal system handles malpractice claims and the role of risk management activity in minimizing and managing liability exposure. An introduction to the concepts of quality improvement (formerly called quality assurance) extends the discussion to the broader arena of quality of care in anesthesia practice. Finally, there is a discussion of anesthetic mortality and some anesthetic complications frequently associated with malpractice litigation.

PROFESSIONAL LIABILITY

This section addresses the basic concepts of medical liability. A more detailed discussion of the steps of the lawsuit process and appropriate actions for physicians to take when sued is available from the American Society of Anesthesiologists (ASA).[1]

Tort System

Although physicians may become involved in the criminal law system in a professional capacity, they more commonly become involved in the legal system of civil laws. Civil law is broadly divided into *contract law* and *tort law.* A tort may be loosely defined as a civil wrongdoing; negligence is one type of tort. *Malpractice* actually refers to any professional misconduct but its use in legal terms typically refers to professional negligence.

1 To be successful in a malpractice suit, the patient–plaintiff must prove four things:

1. Duty: that the anesthesiologist owed the patient a duty;
2. Breach of duty: that the anesthesiologist failed to fulfill his or her duty;

3. Causation: that a reasonably close causal relation exists between the anesthesiologist's acts and the resultant injury; and
4. Damages: that actual damage resulted because of a breach of the standard of care.

Failure to prove any one of these four elements will result in a decision for the defendant–anesthesiologist.

Duty

As a physician, the anesthesiologist establishes a duty to the patient when a doctor–patient relationship exists. When the patient is seen preoperatively, and the anesthesiologist agrees to provide anesthesia care for the patient, a duty to the patient has been established. In the most general terms, the duty the anesthesiologist owes to the patient is to adhere to the *standard of care* for the treatment of the patient. Because it is virtually impossible to delineate specific standards for all aspects of medical practice and all eventualities, the courts have created the concept of the *reasonable and prudent* physician. For all specialties, there is a national standard which has displaced the local standard.

There are certain general duties that all physicians have to their patients, and breaching these duties may also serve as the basis for a lawsuit. One of these general duties is that of obtaining informed consent for a procedure. Consent may be written, verbal, or implied. Oral consent is just as valid, albeit harder to prove years after the fact, as written consent. Implied consent for anesthesia care may be present in circumstances in which the patient is unconscious or unable, for any reason, to give his or her consent, but where it is presumed that any reasonable and prudent patient would give consent.

Although there are exceptions to the requirement that consent be obtained, anesthesiologists should be sure to obtain consent whenever possible. Failure to do so could, in theory, expose the anesthesiologist to possible prosecution for battery.

The requirement that the consent be *informed* is somewhat more opaque. The guideline is determining whether the patient received a fair and reasonable account of the proposed procedures and the risks inherent in these procedures. The duty to disclose risks is not limitless, but it does extend to those risks that are reasonably likely in any patient under the circumstances and to those that are reasonably likely in particular patients because of their condition. For example, it would be prudent to inform the patient of possible sore throat or dental damage associated with tracheal intubation, but not about an unlikely complication such as vocal cord paralysis.

Breach of Duty

In a malpractice action, expert witnesses will review the medical records of the case and determine whether the anesthesiologist acted in a reasonable and prudent manner in the specific situation and fulfilled his or her duty to the patient. If they find that the anesthesiologist either did something that should not have been done or failed to do something that should have been done, then the duty to adhere to the standard of care has been breached. Therefore, the second requirement for a successful suit will have been met.

Causation

Judges and juries are interested in determining whether the breach of duty was the *proximate cause* of the injury. If the odds are better than even that the breach of duty led, however circuitously, to the injury, this requirement is met.

There are two common tests employed to establish causation. The first is the *but for* test, and the second is the *substantial factor* test. If the injury would not have occurred but for the action of the defendant-anesthesiologist, or if the act of the anesthesiologist was a substantial factor in the injury despite other causes, then proximate cause is established.

Although the burden of proof of causation ordinarily falls on the patient-plaintiff, it may, under special circumstances, be shifted to the physician-defendant under the doctrine of *res ipsa loquitur* (literally, "the thing speaks for itself"). Applying this doctrine requires proving that:

1. the injury is of a kind that typically would not occur in the absence of negligence,
2. the injury must be caused by something under the exclusive control of the anesthesiologist,
3. the injury must not be attributable to any contribution on the part of the patient,
4. the evidence for the explanation of events must be more accessible to the anesthesiologist than to the patient.

Because anesthesiologists render patients insensible to their surroundings and unable to protect themselves from injury, this doctrine may be invoked in anesthesia malpractice cases. All that needs to be proved is that the injury typically would not occur in the absence of negligence. At this point, the anesthesiologist is put in the position of having to prove that he or she was not negligent.

Damages

The law allows for three different types of damages. *General damages* are those such as pain and suffering that directly result from the injury. *Special damages* are those actual damages that are a consequence of the injury, such as medical expenses, lost income, and funeral expenses. *Punitive damages* are intended to punish the physician for negligence that was reckless, wanton, fraudulent, or willful. Punitive damages are exceedingly rare in medical malpractice cases. More likely in the case of gross negligence is a loss of the license to practice anesthesia. In extreme cases, criminal charges may be brought against the physician. Determining the dollar amount of damages is the job of the jury, and the determination is usually based on some assessment of the plaintiff's condition versus the condition he or she would have been in had there been no negligence. Plaintiffs' attorneys generally charge a percentage of the damages and will, therefore, seek to maximize the award given.

Standard of Care

2 Because medical malpractice usually involves issues beyond the comprehension of lay jurors and judges, the court establishes the standard of care in a particular case by the testimony of *expert witnesses*. These witnesses differ from factual witnesses mainly in that they may give opinions. The trial court judge has sole discretion in determining whether a witness may be qualified as an expert. Although any licensed physician may be an expert, information will be sought regarding the witness's education and training, the nature and scope of the person's practice, memberships and affiliations, and publications. The purpose in gathering this information is not only to establish the qualifications of the witness to provide expert testimony, but also to determine the weight to be given to that testimony by the jury. In many cases the success of a suit depends primarily on the stature and believability of the expert witnesses.

In certain circumstances, the standard of care may also be determined from published societal guidelines, written policies of a hospital or department, or textbooks and monographs. Some medical specialty societies have carefully avoided applying the term "standards" to their guidelines in the hope that no binding behavior or mandatory practices have been created. In 1986 the ASA, for the first time, published *Standards for Basic Intra-Operative Monitoring* (now entitled *Standards for Basic Anesthetic Monitoring*). These standards have been updated several times since their initial adoption and are more binding than guidelines. The essential difference between standards and guidelines is that guidelines *should* be adhered to and standards *must* be adhered to. Currently, the ASA also publishes standards on preanesthesia care and postanesthesia care, as well as guidelines for a variety of anesthesia-related activities.[2]

Causes of Suits

Since 1985, the principal cause of suits against anesthesiologists is patient injury. The ASA Committee on Professional Liability has conducted a nationwide analysis of malpractice claims against anesthesiologists.[3,4] The leading injuries in malpractice claims in the 1990s were death (22%), nerve damage (21%), and brain damage (10%). The causes of death and permanent brain damage were predominantly problems in airway management, such as inadequate ventilation, difficult intubation, premature extubation, and multifactorial and other cardiovascular events such as arrhythmia, stroke, and myocardial infarction. Nerve damage, especially to the ulnar nerve, often occurs despite apparently adequate positioning.[5,6] Spinal cord injury was the most common cause of nerve damage claims against anesthesiologists in the 1990s.[5] Chronic pain management is an increasing source of malpractice claims against anesthesiologists.[7]

Because death and brain damage are high-cost injuries, anesthesia practice is clearly a high-risk endeavor. The anesthesiologist is likely to be the target of a law suit if an untoward outcome occurs because the physician–patient relationship is usually tenuous at best. That is the patient rarely chooses the anesthesiologist, the preoperative visit is brief, and the anesthesiologist who sees the patient preoperatively may not actually anesthetize the patient. Communication between anesthesiologists and surgeons about complications is often lacking and the tendency is for the surgeon to "blame anesthesia."

Supervision of nurse anesthetists is another endeavor that puts the anesthesiologist in a high-risk category. The more nurse anesthetists supervised by any one anesthesiologist, the greater the exposure to the possibility of patient injury. Anesthesiologists are liable not only for the nurse anesthetists they employ but also for those they supervise who are employed by the hospital.

Because anesthesiologists are involved in the care of patients undergoing high-risk surgical procedures, they are often sued along with the surgeon in the case of an adverse outcome. This may occur even if the outcome was in no way related to the anesthetic care.

What to Do When Sued

A lawsuit begins when the patient–plaintiff's attorney files a complaint and demand for jury trial with the court. The anesthesiologist is then served with the complaint and a summons requiring an answer to the complaint. Until this happens, no lawsuit has been filed. Insurance carriers must be notified immediately after the receipt of the complaint. The anesthesiologist will need assistance in answering the complaint, and there is a time limit placed on the response.

Specific actions at this point include the following:

1. Do not discuss the case with anyone, including colleagues who may have been involved, operating room personnel, or friends.
2. Never alter any records.
3. Gather together all pertinent records, including a copy of the anesthetic record, billing statements, and correspondence concerning the case.
4. Make notes recording all events recalled about the case.
5. Cooperate fully with the attorney provided by the insurer.

The first task the anesthesiologist must perform with an attorney is to prepare an answer to the complaint. The complaint contains certain facts and allegations with which the defense may either agree or disagree. Defense attorneys rely on the frank and totally candid observations of the physician in preparing an answer to the complaint. Physicians should be willing to educate their attorneys about the medical facts of the case, although most medical malpractice attorneys will be knowledgeable and medically sophisticated.

The next phase of the malpractice suit is called *discovery*. The purpose of discovery is the gathering of facts and clarification of issues in advance of the trial. Another purpose of discovery is to assess or harass the defendant to determine how good a witness he or she will make. This occurs at several points in the discovery process, and by several mechanisms.

In all likelihood the anesthesiologist will receive a written interrogatory, which will request factual information. In consultation with the defense attorney, the interrogatory should be answered in writing, because carelessly or inadvertently misstated facts can become troublesome later.

Depositions are a second mechanism of discovery. The defendant–anesthesiologist will be deposed as a fact witness, and depositions will be obtained from other anesthesiologists who will act as expert witnesses. The defendant–anesthesiologist may be asked to suggest other anesthesiologists who would provide expert review of the medical records. A nationally recognized expert in the area in question who is not a personal friend but agrees with the defense position may be very valuable.

The plaintiff's attorney, not the defense attorney, will depose the anesthesiologist. Most often, the deposition will occur at a place and time convenient for the anesthesiologist, typically in the defense attorney's office. Despite the apparent informality of the deposition, the anesthesiologist must be constantly aware that what is said during the deposition carries as much weight as what would be said in court. It is important to be factually prepared for the deposition. A review of personal notes, the anesthetic record, and the medical record is necessary. The physician should dress conservatively and professionally because appearance and image are very important. The opposition is assessing the physician to see how he or she will appear to a jury. Answer only the question asked, and do not volunteer information. Occasionally, physicians will be asked leading questions that are impossible to answer without qualifications. In this case, the physician may qualify his or her answer but should avoid giving lengthy opinion answers.

There will be depositions from expert witnesses, both for the plaintiff and for the defense. The anesthesiologist should work with his or her attorney to suggest questions and rebuttals. The better educated the attorney is about the medical facts, the reasons the anesthesiologist did what was done, and the alternative approaches, the better able the attorney will be to conduct these expert depositions.

If there is some merit in the case but the damages are minimal, or if proof of innocence will be difficult, there will probably be a settlement offer. There is a high cost incurred by both plaintiffs and defendants in pursuing a malpractice claim up through a jury trial. Unless there is a strong probability of a large dollar award, reputable plaintiffs' attorneys are not likely to pursue the claim. Thus, even if physicians believe that they are totally innocent of any wrongdoing, they should not be offended or angered about settling of the case: this is solely a matter of money, not medicine.

If a settlement is not reached during the discovery phase, a trial will occur. Only about 1 in 20 malpractice cases ever reaches the point of a jury trial. It usually becomes clear during discovery whether the suit has a solid chance of being successfully prosecuted. Only those cases in which both sides feel they can win, and which are likely to have significant financial impact, will proceed to trial.

The discussion of deposition testimony also applies to testimony in court, but there are a few additional points to consider during the trial. The members of the jury will not be as sophisticated medically as the attorneys who deposed the anesthesiologist during discovery. A tendency to overuse specific medical terms should be corrected by learning to explain answers in lay terms for the benefit of the jury. Do not underestimate the intelligence of the jury, however, because talking down to them will create an unfavorable impression. If the answer to a question is not known, avoid guessing. If specific facts cannot be remembered, say so. Nobody expects total recall of events that may have occurred years before.

The defendant–physician should be present during the entire trial, even when not testifying, and should dress conservatively, neatly, and professionally. Displays of anger, remorse, relief, or hostility will hurt the physician in court. When giving testimony, the anesthesiologist must give clear answers to all questions asked. The physician should be able to give his or her testimony without using notes or documents. When it is necessary to refer to the medical record, it will be admitted into evidence. The anesthesiologist's goal is to convince the jury that he or she behaved in this case as any other competent and prudent anesthesiologist would have behaved.

It is important to keep in mind that *proof* in a malpractice case means only "more likely than not." The patient–plaintiff must "prove" the four elements of negligence, not to absolute certainty, but only to a probability greater than 50%. On the positive side, this means that the defendant–anesthesiologist must only show that his or her actions were, more likely than not, within an acceptable standard of care.

RISK MANAGEMENT AND QUALITY IMPROVEMENT

Risk management and quality improvement programs work
3 hand in hand in minimizing liability exposure while maximizing quality of patient care. Although the functions of these programs vary from one institution to another, they overlap in their focus on patient safety. They can generally be distinguished by their basic difference in orientation. A hospital risk management program is broadly oriented toward reducing the liability exposure of the organization. This includes not only professional liability (and therefore patient safety) but also contracts, employee safety, public safety, and any other liability exposure of the institution. Quality improvement programs have as their main goal the continuous maintenance and improvement of the quality of patient care. These programs may be broader in their patient safety focus than strictly risk management.

Risk Management

Those aspects of risk management that are most directly relevant to the liability exposure of the anesthesiologist include prevention of patient injury, adherence to standards of care, documentation, and patient relations.

The key factors in the prevention of patient injury are vigilance, up-to-date knowledge, and adequate monitoring.[8] Physiologic monitoring of cardiopulmonary function, combined with monitoring of equipment function, might be expected to reduce anesthetic injury to a minimum. This was the rationale for the adoption of the ASA *Standards for Basic Anesthetic Monitoring*.[2]

The ASA website should be reviewed yearly for any changes in ASA *Standards of Practice*. It would also be reasonable to review the ASA *Guidelines and Statements* published on the ASA website. It should be noted that, although membership in the ASA is not required for the practice of anesthesiology, expert witnesses will, with virtual certainty, hold any practitioner to the ASA standards. It is also possible that, as a risk management strategy, a professional liability insurer or hospital may hold an individual anesthesiologist to standards higher than those promulgated by the ASA.

Another risk management tool is the use of checklists prior to each case, or at least daily, in an attempt to reduce equipment-related mishaps.[9–11] A regular schedule of equipment maintenance should be established as well as procedures to follow whenever equipment malfunction is suspected of contributing to patient injury. If equipment malfunction is suspected to have contributed to a complication, the device should be impounded and examined concurrently by the representatives of the hospital, the anesthesiologist, and the manufacturer.

Although it may seem obvious, qualified anesthesia personnel should be in continuous attendance during the conduct of all anesthetics. The only exceptions should be those that lay people (i.e., judge and jury) can understand, such as radiation hazards or an unexpected life-threatening emergency elsewhere. Even then, provisions should be made for monitoring the patient adequately. Adequate supervision of nurse anesthetists and residents is also important, as is good communication with surgeons when adverse anesthetic outcomes occur.

Informed consent should be documented with a general consent, which should include a statement to the effect that, "I understand that all anesthetics involve risks of complications, serious injury, or, rarely, death from both known and unknown causes." In addition, there should be a note in the patient's record that the risks of anesthesia and alternatives were discussed, and that the patient accepted the proposed anesthetic plan. A brief documentation in the record that the common complications of the proposed technique were discussed is helpful. If it is necessary to change the agreed-on anesthesia plan significantly after the patient is premedicated or anesthetized, the reasons for the change should be documented in the record.

Good records can form a strong defense if they are adequate, however records can be disastrous if inadequate. The anesthesia record itself should be as accurate, complete, and as neat as possible. The use of automated anesthesia records may be helpful in the defense of malpractice cases.[12] In addition to documenting vital signs every 5 minutes, special attention should be paid to ensure that the patient's ASA classification, the monitors utilized, fluids administered, and doses and times of all administered drugs are accurately charted. Because the principal causes of hypoxic brain damage and death during anesthesia are related to ventilation and/or oxygenation, all respiratory variables that are monitored should be documented accurately. It is important to note when there is a change of anesthesia personnel during the conduct of a case. Sloppy, inaccurate anesthesia records, when enlarged and placed before a jury, can be damaging to the defense.

If a critical incident occurs during the conduct of an anesthetic, the anesthesiologist should document, in narrative form, what happened, which drugs were used, the time sequence, and who was present. This should be documented in the patient's progress notes, as catastrophic intra-anesthetic event cannot be summarized adequately in a small amount of space on the usual anesthesia record. The critical incident note should be written as soon as possible. The report should be as consistent as possible with concurrent records, such as the anesthesia, operating room, recovery room, and cardiac arrest records. If significant inconsistencies exist, they should be explained. Records should never be altered after the fact. If an error is made in record keeping, a line should be drawn through the error, leaving it legible, and the correction should be initialed and timed. Litigation is a lengthy process, and a court appearance to explain the incident to a jury may be years away, when memories have faded.

If anesthetic complications occur, the anesthesiologist should be honest with both the patient and family about the cause. Whenever an anesthetic complication becomes apparent postoperatively, appropriate consultation should be obtained quickly, and the departmental or institutional risk management group should be notified. If the complication is apt to lead to prolonged hospitalization or permanent injury, the liability insurance carrier should be notified. The patient should be followed closely while in the hospital, with telephone follow-up, if indicated, after discharge. Also, the anesthesiologist and surgeon should be consistent in their explanations to the patient or the patient's family as to the cause of any complication.

Jehovah's Witnesses and Other Treatment Obligations

It is important to recognize that patients have well-established rights, and that among these is the right to refuse specific treatments because of religious beliefs. In the case of Jehovah's Witnesses, the treatment refused is the administration of blood or blood products. This is a central part of their religious beliefs, which hold that the faithful will be forbidden the pleasures of the afterlife if they receive blood or blood products. Thus, for them to receive a transfusion is a mortal sin, and many Jehovah's Witnesses would actually rather die in grace than live with no possibility of salvation. Anesthesiologists recognize and respect these beliefs but are also cognizant that these convictions may conflict with the physicians' personal, religious, or ethical codes.

Minor children of Jehovah's Witness parents represent a special group for consideration. Although the U.S. Supreme Court has upheld the right of an adult to become a martyr by refusing treatments based on religious convictions, no court has extended to parents the right to martyr their children.[13] Obtaining a proper court order is of critical importance in the care of a minor child of Jehovah's Witness parents when the parents refuse to authorize a blood transfusion.

As a general rule, physicians are not obligated to treat all patients who apply for treatment in elective situations. It is well within the rights of a physician to decline to care for any patient who wishes to place burdensome constraints on the physician or to unacceptably limit the physician's ability to provide optimal care. When presented with the opportunity to provide elective care for a Jehovah's Witness, the physician may decline to provide any care or may limit, by mutual consent with the patient, his or her obligation to adhere to the patient's religious beliefs. If such an agreement is reached, it must be documented clearly in the medical record, and it is desirable to have the patient co-sign the note. Not all Jehovah's Witnesses have identical beliefs regarding blood transfusions or which methods of blood preservation or sequestration will be allowed. Some patients will not allow any blood that has left the body to be reinfused, yet others will accept autotransfusion if their blood remains in constant contact with the body (via tubing). Therefore, it is important to reach a clear understanding of which techniques for blood preservation are to be used and to document this plan in the record.

Emergency medical care imposes greater constraints on the treating physician, as there is no opportunity to decline the care of a patient with an immediately life-threatening condition. If the patient is an adult and is conscious and mentally competent, he or she has the right to refuse blood transfusion. The exceptions to patients' rights in this regard include pregnant women and adults who are the sole support of minor children. In these circumstances, the interests of the fetus in surviving may supersede the rights of the mother, as may the interests of the state in not being obligated to provide for the welfare of dependent children.[13] In either case, obtaining a court order is the best plan if time permits. If the problem concerns blood products and there is insufficient time to obtain a court order, pregnant women should be given a transfusion to save the life of the fetus, but parents of minor children should not receive transfusions against their wishes unless the dependency of the children is obvious.

When the patient is a minor, it is important to ascertain the true wishes of the parents. Some parents know that a court order can be obtained and view this as a relief from the onerous burden of having to decide whether they are willing to let their child die. However, some parents are adamant that blood not be given, and there have been cases in which children have been ostracized by their parents and religious community for having received a court-ordered transfusion. Reaching an understanding about the consequences for the child who receives a court-ordered transfusion is therefore vital for the determination of what risks will be taken before ordering a transfusion.

The procedure for obtaining a court order may vary, depending on the specific state laws. Typically, an order may be obtained over the telephone. This call initiates the issue of a written order, which will arrive several days later. Although not a totally automatic procedure, it would be very rare for a judge to deny this order for a minor.

National Practitioner Data Bank

It is usually the obligation of the hospital risk management department to make reports and inquiries to the National Practitioner Data Bank (NPDB), a nationwide information system that theoretically would allow licensing boards and hospitals a means of detecting adverse information about physicians.[14] Simply moving into another state would no longer provide safe haven for incompetent physicians.

The NPDB requires input from five sources: (1) medical malpractice payments, (2) license actions by medical boards, (3) professional review or clinical privilege actions taken by hospitals and other health care entities (including professional societies), (4) actions taken by the Drug Enforcement Agency (DEA), and (5) Medicare/Medicaid exclusions. There has been a great deal of effort to establish a minimum reporting dollar value below which no report is necessary, but to date, any payment made on behalf of a physician in response to a written complaint or claim must be reported. Settlements made by cancellation of bills or settlements made on verbal complaints are not considered a reportable payment.

Once a report has been submitted, the physician is notified and has 60 days from the date the data bank processed the report to dispute the input. At this time, the reporting entity may correct the form or void it. Failing that, the physician has the option of putting a brief statement in the file or appealing to the U.S. Secretary of Health and Human Services, who may also either correct or void the form. Once it is entered, there is no means of purging the form. A practitioner may make a query about his or her file at any time. The existence of the NPDB reporting requirements has made physicians reluctant to allow settlement of nuisance suits because it will cause their names to be added to the data bank.

QUALITY IMPROVEMENT IN ANESTHESIA PRACTICE

Quality is a concept that has continued to elude precise definition in medical practice. However, it is generally accepted that attention to quality will improve patient safety and satisfaction

with anesthesia care. The field of quality assurance or quality improvement is continually evolving, as is the terminology used to describe such efforts. The term "quality assurance" has
4 gone out of fashion, being replaced by "quality improvement" in an effort to emphasize a change in underlying philosophy. Although quality improvement programs in anesthesia are generally guided by requirements of the JCAHO, they are basically oriented toward improvement of the structure, process, and outcome of health care delivery programs. An understanding of the fundamental principles of quality improvement may clarify the relationship between the continually evolving JCAHO requirements and mandated quality improvement activities.

Structure, Process, and Outcome: The Building Blocks of Quality

Although quality of care is difficult to define, it is generally accepted that it is composed of three components: structure, process, and outcome.[15] *Structure* refers to the setting in which care was provided, for example, personnel and facilities used to provide health care services and the manner in which they are organized. This includes the qualifications and licensing of personnel, ratio of practitioners to patients, standards for the facilities and equipment used to provide care, and the organizational structure within which care is delivered. The *process* of care includes the sequence and coordination of patient care activities, that is, what was actually done. Was a preanesthetic evaluation performed and documented? Was the patient continuously attended and monitored throughout the anesthetic? *Outcome* of care refers to changes in health status of the patient following the delivery of medical care. A quality improvement program focuses on measuring and improving these basic components of care.

5 *Continuous quality improvement* (CQI) takes a systems approach to identifying and improving quality of care.[16,17] The operator is just one part of a complex system. An important underlying premise is that poor results may be a result of either random or systematic error. Random errors are inherently difficult to prevent and programs focused in this direction are misguided. System errors, however, should be controllable and strategies to minimize them should be within reach. CQI is basically the process of continually evaluating anesthesia practice to identify systematic problems (opportunities for improvement) and implementing strategies to prevent their occurrence.

A CQI program may focus on undesirable outcomes as a way to identify opportunities for improvement in the structure and process of care. The focus is not on blame but rather on identification of the causes of undesirable outcomes. Instead of asking which practitioners have the highest patient mortality rates, a CQI program may focus on the relationship between the process of care and patient mortality. What proportion of deaths was related to the patient's disease process or debilitated condition? Are these patients being appropriately evaluated for anesthesia and surgery? Were there any controllable causes, such as a lack of hands during resuscitation? The latter may lead to a modification of personnel resources (structure) or assignments (process) to be sure that adequate personnel are available at all times.

Formally, the process of CQI involves the identification of opportunities for improvement through the continual assessment of important aspects of care. Peer review and input are critical to this process. It is a process that is instituted from the bottom up, by those who are actually involved in the process to be improved, rather than from the top down by administrators. Identification of opportunities for improvement may be carried out by various means, from brainstorming sessions focusing on a systematic evaluation of care activities to the careful measurement of indicators of quality (such as morbidity and mortality). In any event, once areas are identified for improvement, their current status is measured and documented. This may involve measurement of outcomes, such as delayed recovery from anesthesia or peripheral nerve injury. The process of care leading to these problems is then analyzed. If a change is identified that should lead to improvement, it is implemented. After an appropriate time period, the status is then measured again to determine whether improvement actually resulted. Attention may then be directed to continuing to improve this process or turning to a different process to target for improvement.

An extension of the CQI method is *total quality management* (TQM). A TQM program would extend beyond patient care to apply CQI methods to all aspects of the patient care delivery system. This would include such things as billing and housekeeping, for example. With the expectation of continuing changes in the structure and financing of health care in the United States, CQI programs in anesthesia can be incorporated into TQM of the entire hospital system to maintain the quality of patient care as practice changes are implemented in response to a changing environment.

Difficulty of Outcome Measurement in Anesthesia

Improvement in quality of care is often measured by a reduction in the rate of adverse outcomes. However, adverse outcomes are relatively rare in anesthesia making measurement of improvement difficult. For example, if an institution lowers its mortality rate of surgery patients from 1 in 1,000 to 0.5 in 1,000, this difference may not be statistically significant. Many adverse outcomes in anesthesia are even more rare.

To complement outcome measurement, anesthesia CQI programs can focus on critical incidents, sentinel events, and human errors. *Critical incidents* are events that cause, or had the potential to cause, patient injury if not noticed and corrected in a timely manner. For example, a partial disconnect of the breathing circuit may be corrected before patient injury occurs, yet has the potential for causing hypoxic brain injury or death. Critical incidents are more common than adverse outcomes. Measurement of the occurrence rate of important critical incidents may serve as a proxy measure for rare outcomes in anesthesia in a CQI program designed to improve patient safety and prevent injury.

Sentinel events are single, isolated events that may indicate a systemic problem. JCAHO has a specific definition of sentinel events that will be discussed later. In general, a sentinel event may be a significant or alarming critical incident that did not result in patient injury, such as a syringe swap and administration of a potentially lethal dose of medication that was noted and treated promptly, avoiding catastrophe. Or a sentinel event may be an unexpected significant patient injury such as intraoperative death. In either case, a CQI program may investigate sentinel events in an attempt to uncover systemic problems in the delivery of care that can be corrected. For example, a syringe swap may be analyzed for confusing or unclear labeling of medications or unnecessary medications routinely stocked on the anesthesia cart, setting the scene for unintended mix-up. In the case of death, all aspects of the patient's hospital course from selection for surgery to anesthetic management may be analyzed to determine if similar deaths can be prevented by a change in the care delivery system.

Human error has garnered much attention since a government report that 98,000 Americans may die annually from medical errors in hospitals.[18] Human errors are inevitable yet potentially preventable by appropriate system safeguards.

Errors of planning involve use of a wrong plan to achieve an aim.[19] Errors of execution are the failure of a planned action to be completed as intended. [19] Modern anesthesia equipment is designed with safeguards such as alarm systems to detect errors that could lead to patient injury. Other anesthesia care processes are also amenable to human factors design principles, such as color coding of drug labels. A quality improvement program may identify human errors and institute safety systems to aid in error prevention.

JCAHO Requirements for Quality Improvement

JCAHO requirements for quality improvement activities are updated on an annual basis. In general, a hospital must adopt a method for systematically assessing and improving important functions and processes of care and their outcomes in a cyclical fashion. The general outline for this CQI cycle is the design of a process or function, measurement of performance, assessment of performance measures through statistical analysis or comparison with other data sources, and improvement of the process or function. Then the cycle repeats. JCAHO provides specific standards that must be met, with examples of appropriate measures of performance. The goal of this cycle of design, measurement, assessment, and improvement of performance of important functions and processes is to improve patient safety and quality of care.

Anesthesia care is one important function of the care of patients monitored by JCAHO. It is important that policies and procedures for administration of anesthesia be consistent in all locations within the organization.

In 2004, JCAHO adopted patient safety goals for accredited organizations. These include improved accuracy of patient identification, improved effectiveness of communication among caregivers, elimination of wrong site/wrong patient/wrong procedure surgery, improved safety of infusion pumps, and improved effectiveness of clinical alarm systems. JCAHO also requires all sentinel events (any unexpected occurrences involving death or serious physical or psychological injury or risk thereof) to undergo Root Cause Analysis.[20] A Root Cause Analysis is typically facilitated by the hospital and includes everyone involved in the care of the affected patient in reconstructing the events to identify system process flaws that facilitated medical error. Any surgery on the wrong patient or wrong body part is included in this policy. JCAHO publishes a Sentinel Event Alert so health care organizations can learn from the experiences of others and prevent future medical errors.

Measuring Quality: Approaches to Data Collection

There are various methods in use for collection of CQI data in anesthesia. These include retrospective records review as well as self-reporting by providers of care. Checklists to report adverse events or outcomes are sometimes used. Important considerations include compliance with reporting requirements, standardization of definitions, and appropriate sampling.

Retrospective records review usually involves a random sample of anesthesia records. The actual review may be done by an anesthesia provider or by a trained medical records specialist. Explicit definitions of quality indicators would be provided, such as "hypotension = blood pressure <80% of baseline for 5 minutes or more." Such *indicators* of possible quality problems and opportunities for improvement are restricted to data that are normally included in the anesthesia record for every patient. Records review is an especially appropriate technique for gathering data on adequacy of documentation. An asset of automated anesthesia records is that they can be programmed to screen all records for quality indicators.

For collection of data on events or outcomes that may not normally be charted, a self-reporting system may be used. This is an especially good mechanism for tracking critical incidents and sentinel events. For example, a syringe swap that was noted and corrected before drug administration is a critical incident that would not normally be included in an anesthetic record but could be reported by an anesthesia provider in a self-report system. Many self-report systems provide a checklist of events and outcomes that is completed by the provider for each anesthetic. Other systems provide general guidelines of critical incident reporting without specific check-off items.[21,22] The relevant clinical information is then obtained from the practitioner by quality improvement personnel.

Whatever system is used, it is important that it be in compliance with current JCAHO standards. Standardized definitions must be provided. In general, definitions that take into account the context of care (patient status, type of anesthetic) while maintaining explicit criteria for inclusion in the CQI system will most clearly reflect quality issues (rather than, for example, complications related purely to patient physical condition). For example, blood loss and replacement of 8 units would be considered excessive and indicative of a problem during a knee arthroscopy but would be considered minimal during a liver transplant. A strict definition of "excessive blood loss = >5 units" would identify both cases as quality issues where it would only be appropriate for the arthroscopy. Contextualization of definitions will help avoid the frustration of providers when presented with data that otherwise may be irrelevant to improving the process of anesthesia care.

Peer Review

Peer review, which refers to the review of cases by members of one's specialty, is an integral part of quality improvement programs. Peer review is commonly integrated into a quality improvement program in the context of the morbidity and mortality conference. This provides a forum for review of case management by all members of the department, integrating an educational component into the quality improvement process as differing knowledge bases and clinical experiences are shared. Peer review can provide a mechanism to analyze the structure and process of care and opportunities for improvement.

Peer review can also be incorporated into the analysis of critical incidents, sentinel events, and trends in measured outcomes of care. Peer review has the distinct advantage of credibility and an aura of fairness in a democratic system. Although personal bias in clinical care may be recognized, adherence to the "reasonable man" principle provides a basis for analysis that reflects generally accepted principles of care. It provides a basis for analysis of trends and incidents, suggesting hypotheses for their causes and changes in the system that might improve the structure, process, and outcome of care.

However, peer review is subject to bias that may not be recognized by the participants. This is a tendency of anesthesiologists to judge care as less than appropriate if severe patient injury occurs.[23] In a study of anesthesiologists presented with identical case scenarios with differing outcomes, they were more likely to judge the care as appropriate if the injury was temporary and to judge care as less than appropriate if the injury was permanent. In conducting peer review for a CQI system, this tendency toward assessments biased by case outcome should be recognized and resisted. Careful attention to the process of care and opportunities for improvement should be made regardless of the extent of patient injury. Critical incidents resulting in no injury should be as carefully analyzed for opportunities for improvement in the structure and process of care as incidents with adverse outcomes.

Even though anesthesiologists may be biased in their assessment of case management by outcome, they exhibit only moderate levels of general agreement in their assessments.[24,25] When reviewing identical case histories, different anesthesiologists may not always agree on whether the care was appropriate. Although this disagreement may be because of differences in individually held standards and practices, it must be recognized in any analysis of case management for a CQI program. Incorporation of multiple anesthesiologists into the process of case review will compensate for this lack of agreement. Although a consensus may not be reached, decisions will not be subject to the variability of individual judgments. Incorporation of multiple peer reviewers will compensate for differences in assessments and strengthen the process by improving reliability.[25]

The Future of Quality Improvement: A Multidisciplinary Focus

JCAHO is moving toward a focus on the patient's hospital course in a multidisciplinary emphasis rather than departmental quality improvement programs. The shift in emphasis is toward an analysis of the entirety of each patient's care as the process to be improved. Each department's role is just one part of this process, and the care provided by various departments is often not the relevant unit of analysis. This shift in focus may require movement from departmental reliance on standing committees to increased use of ad hoc study groups. Comparison of outcomes of care across institutions, with adjustments for case mix, has long been the goal but has proven to be difficult to implement.

MORTALITY AND MAJOR MORBIDITY RELATED TO ANESTHESIA

Estimates of anesthesia-related morbidity and mortality are difficult to quantify. Not only are there difficulties obtaining data on complications, but different methodologies yield different estimates of anesthesia risk. Studies differ in their definitions of complications, length of follow-up, and especially in approaches to evaluation of the contribution of anesthesia care to patient outcomes. A comprehensive review of anesthesia complications is beyond the scope of this chapter. A sampling of studies of anesthesia mortality and morbidity will be presented to provide historical perspective plus a limited overview of relatively recent findings.

Early studies estimated the anesthesia-related mortality rate
6 as 1 per 1,560 anesthetics.[26] More recent studies using data from the 1990s estimate the anesthesia-related death rate in the United States to be <1 per 10,000 anesthetics.[27,28] Some examples of modern estimates of anesthesia-related death from throughout the world are provided in Table 5-1. Differences in estimates may be influenced by different reporting methods, definitions, anesthesia practices, patient population, as well as actual differences in underlying complication rates.

TABLE 5-1

RECENT ESTIMATES OF ANESTHESIA-RELATED DEATH

REFERENCE	COUNTRY	TIME PERIOD	DATA SOURCES/METHODS	RATE OF DEATH
Newland et al.[27]	USA	1989–1999	Cardiac arrests within 24 hrs of surgery (n=72,959 anesthetics) in a teaching hospital	Death related to anesthesia-attributable perioperative cardiac arrest = 0.55/10,000 anesthetics
Lagasse[28]	USA	(a) 1992–1994 (b) 1995–1999	(a) suburban teaching hospital (n=115 deaths; n=37,924 anesthetics) (b) urban teaching hospital (n=232 deaths; n=146,548 anesthetics)	Anesthesia-related death = (a) 0.79/10,000 anesthetics; (b) 0.75/10,000 anesthetics
Arbous et al.[37]	Holland	1995–1997	All deaths within 24 hrs or patients who remained unintentionally comatose 24 hrs postanesthesia (n=811 in 869,483 anesthetics)—64 hospitals	Anesthesia-related death = 1.4/10,000 anesthetics
Eagle, Davis[38]	Western Australia	1990–1995	Deaths within 48 hrs or deaths in which anesthesia was considered a contributing factor (n=500 deaths)	Anesthesia-related death = 1/40,000 anesthetics
Davis, ed.[39]	Australia	1994–1996	Deaths reported to the committee (n=8,500,000 anesthetics)	Anesthesia-related death = 0.16/10,000 anesthetics
Irita et al.[40]	Japan	1999–2002	Deaths as a result of life-threatening events in the operating room (n=3,855,384 anesthetics) in training hospitals	Death totally attributable to anesthetic management = 0.1/10,000 anesthetics
Kawashima et al.[41]	Japan	1994–1998	Questionnaires to training hospitals (n=2,363,038 anesthetics)	Death totally attributable to anesthesia = 0.21/10,000 anesthetics
Biboulet et al.[42]	France	1989–1995	ASA 1–4 patients undergoing anesthesia (n=101,769 anesthetics)—cardiac arrest within 12 hrs postanesthesia (n=24)	Anesthesia-related death = 0.6/10,000 anesthetics
Morray et al.[43]	USA	1994–1997	Pediatric patients from 63 hospitals (n=1,089,200 anesthetics)	Anesthesia-related death = 0.36/10,000 anesthetics

TABLE 5-2

RATES OF SELECTED ANESTHESIA COMPLICATIONS

COMPLICATION	REFERENCE	COUNTRY	TIME PERIOD	SPECIFIC COMPLICATION	RESULTS
Nerve injury	Warner et al.[44]	USA	1995	Ulnar neuropathy in adults following noncardiac surgery	0.5%
	Warner et al.[45]	USA	1957–1991	Persistent ulnar neuropathy following diagnostic or noncardiac procedures with anesthesia	1/2,729 patients
	Alvine et al.[46]	USA	1980–1981	Ulnar neuropathy after general anesthesia	0.26%
	Warner et al.[29]	USA	1957–1991	Lower extremity motor neuropathy following surgery in lithotomy position	1/3,608 procedures
Awareness and recall	Sandin et al.[30]	Sweden	1997–1998	Awareness and recall associated with general anesthesia	18/11,785 procedures
	Lui et al.[31]	Great Britain	1990	Awareness with recall in adults following surgery	0.2%
	Ranta et al.[32]	Finland	1994–1995	Awareness in patients >12 yrs old having general anesthesia	0.4%
Eye injuries and visual changes	Warner et al.[34]	USA	1999	New onset blurred vision lasting ≥3 days	4.2%
	Warner et al.[35]	USA	1986–1998	New onset visual loss or visual changes lasting >30 days after noncardiac surgery	1/125,234 patients
	Roth et al.[33]	USA	1988–1992	Eye injury after nonocular surgery	0.056%
Dental injury	Warner et al.[36]	USA	1987–1997	Dental injuries within 7 days of anesthesia that required intervention	1/4,537 patients

Nevertheless, it is generally accepted that anesthesia safety has improved over the past 50+ years.

Other complications related to anesthesia that have received relatively recent attention include postoperative nerve injury, awareness and recall, eye injuries and visual deficits, and dental injury. Ulnar neuropathy is one of the most common nerve injuries leading to anesthesia malpractice claims in the United States.[5] The incidence of ulnar neuropathy has been estimated between 3.7 and 50 per 10,000 patients (Table 5-2). Lower extremity neuropathy following surgery in the lithotomy position was observed in 2.7/10,000 patients (Table 5-2).[29] Awareness with recall after general anesthesia has been estimated to occur in 15 to 40 per 10,000 patients.[30–32]

Eye injuries are a risk of anesthesia, including corneal abrasions as well as more rare complications such as blindness from ischemic optic neuropathy or central retinal artery occlusion (Table 5-2). Eye injury after nonocular surgery was observed in 5.6/10,000 patients.[33] New onset blurred vision has been observed in 4.2% of patients (Table 5-2).[34] New onset visual loss or changes lasting more than 30 days after noncardiac surgery were observed in 1/125,234 patients.[35]

Damage to teeth or dentures is perhaps the most common injury leading to anesthesia malpractice claims. Dental injury complaints are usually resolved by a hospital risk management department. Dental injuries requiring intervention were observed in 1/4537 patients.[36]

Unlike studies of anesthesia mortality, most studies of nonfatal complications do not attempt to assess the relationship between the complication and anesthesia care. Many of these complications are known risks of anesthesia. Such risks vary according to the specific surgical and anesthesia plan as well as the patient's physical characteristics. Risk management and quality improvement programs generally focus on local experience with postoperative complications in targeting emphasis areas for improvement.

References

1. Kroll DA: Professional Liability and the Anesthesiologist. Park Ridge, IL, American Society of Anesthesiologists, 1992 at www.asahq.org/publicationsAndServices/professional.pdf (last viewed 8/12/04)
2. www.asahq.org/publicationsAndServices/sgstoc.htm (last viewed 8/12/04)
3. Cheney FW, Posner K, Caplan RA *et al:* Standard of care and anesthesia liability. JAMA 261:1599, 1989
4. Cheney FW: The American Society of Anesthesiologists Closed Claims Project: What have we learned, how has it affected practice, and how will it affect practice in the future? Anesthesiology 91:552, 1999
5. Cheney FW, Domino KB, Caplan RA *et al:* Nerve injury associated with anesthesia. A closed claims analysis. Anesthesiology 90:1062, 1999
6. Warner MA, Warner ME, Martin JT: Ulnar neuropathy. Incidence, outcome and risk factors in sedated or anesthetized patients. Anesthesiology 81:1332, 1994
7. Fitzgibbon DR, Posner KL, Domino KB *et al:* Chronic Pain Management: American Society of Anesthesiologists Closed Claims Project. Anesthesiology 100:98, 2004
8. Gaba DM, Maxwell M, DeAnda A: Anesthetic mishaps: Breaking the chain of accident evolution. Anesthesiology 66:670, 1987

9. Petty C: The Anesthesia Machine, p 213. New York; Churchill-Livingstone, 1987
10. Spooner RB, Kirby RR: Equipment-related anesthetic incidents. Int Anesthesiol Clin 22:133, 1984
11. Food and Drug Administration: Anesthesia Apparatus Checkout Recommendations, 1993. Rockville, MD; Food and Drug Administration, 1994
12. Kroll DA: The medicolegal aspects of automated anaesthesia records. Bailliere's Clin Anaesthesiol 4:237, 1990
13. Benson KT: The Jehovah's Witness patient: Considerations for the anesthesiologist. Anesth Analg 69:647, 1989
14. Baldwin LM, Hart LG, Oshel RE *et al:* Hospital peer review and the National Practitioner Data Bank: Clinical privileges action reports. JAMA 282:349, 1999
15. Donabedian A: The quality of care. How can it be assessed? JAMA 260:1743, 1988
16. Deming WE: Out of the Crisis. Cambridge, MA, Massachusetts Institute of Technology, 1986
17. Juran JM: Juran on Planning for Quality. New York, Free Press, 1988
18. Kohn LT, Corrigan JM, Donaldson MS (eds). Committee on Quality of Health Care in America, Institute of Medicine. To Err is Human: Building a Safer Health System. Washington, DC; National Academy Press, 1999.
19. Reason JT. Human Error. Cambridge; Cambridge University Press, 1990.
20. JCAHO. Sentinel Event Policy and Procedures Revised: July 2002. http://www.jcaho.org/accredited+organizations/ambulatory + care/sentinel +events/se-pp.htm (accessed 3/15/2004)
21. Posner KL, Kendall-Gallagher D, Wright IH *et al:* Linking process and outcome of care in a continuous quality improvement program for anesthesia services. Am J Med Qual 9:129, 1994
22. Posner KL, Freund PR: Trends in quality of anesthesia care associated with changing staffing patterns, productivity, and concurrency of case supervision in a teaching hospital. Anesthesiology 91:839, 1999
23. Caplan RA, Posner KL, Cheney FW: Effect of outcome on physician judgments of appropriateness of care. JAMA 265:1957, 1991
24. Posner KL, Sampson PD, Caplan RA *et al:* Measuring interrater reliability among multiple raters: An example of methods for nominal data. Stat Med 9:1103, 1990
25. Posner KL, Caplan RA, Cheney FW: Variation in expert opinion in medical malpractice review. Anesthesiology 85:1049, 1996
26. Beecher HK, Todd DP: A study of the deaths associated with anesthesia and surgery: based on a study of 599,548 anesthesias in 10 institutions 1948–1952, inclusive. Ann Surg 140:2, 1954.
27. Newland MC, Ellis SJ, Lydiatt CA, Peters KR, Tinker JH, Romberger DJ, Ullrich FA, Anderson JR: Anesthetic-related cardiac arrest and its mortality. A report covering 72,959 anesthetics over 10 years from a US teaching hospital. Anesthesiology 97:108, 2002
28. Lagasse , RS: Anesthesia safety: model or myth?: a review of the published literature and analysis of current original data. Anesthesiology 97:1609, 2002
29. Warner MA, Martin JT, Schroeder DR, Offord KP, Chute CG: Lower-extremity motor neuropathy associated with surgery performed on patients in a lithotomy position. Anesthesiology 81:6, 1994
30. Sandin RH, Enlund G, Samuelsson P, Lennmarken C: Awareness during anaesthesia: a prospective case study. Lancet 355:707, 2000
31. Lui WH, Thorp TA, Graham SG, Aitkenhead AR: Incidence of awareness with recall during general anaesthesia. Anaesthesia 46:435, 1991
32. Ranta SO, Laurila R, Saario J, Ali-Melkkila T, Hynynen M: Awareness with recall during general anesthesia: incidence and risk factors. Anesth Analg 86:1084, 1998
33. Roth S, Thisted RA, Erickson JP, Black S, Schreider BD. Eye injuries after nonocular surgery. A study of 60,965 anesthetics from 1988 to 1992. Anesthesiology 85:1020, 1996
34. Warner ME, Fronapfel PJ, Hebl JR, Herman DC, Warner DO, Decker P, Warner MA: Perioperative visual changes. Anesthesiology 96:855, 2002
35. Warner ME, Warner MA, Garrity JA, MacKenie RA, Warner DO: The frequency of perioperative vision loss. Anesth Analg 93:1417, 2001
36. Warner ME, Benenfeld SM, Warner MA, Schroeder DR, Maxson PM: Perianesthetic dental injuries: frequency, outcomes, and risk factors. Anesthesiology 90:302, 1999
37. Arbous MS, Grobbee DE, van Kleef JW, deLange JJ, Spoormans HHAJM, Touw P, Werner FM, Meursing AEE. Mortality associated with anaesthesia: a qualitative analysis to identify risk factors. Anaesthesia 56:1141, 2001
38. Eagle CCP, Davis NJ. Report of the Anaesthetic Mortality Committee of Western Australia 1990–1995. Anaesth Intens Care 25:51, 1997
39. Davis NJ (editor).Anaesthesia related mortality in Australia 1994–1996. Report of the Committee convened under the auspices of the Australian and New Zealand College of Anaesthetists. Capitol Press, 1999.
40. Irita K, Kawashima Y, Iwao Y, Seo N, Tsuzaki K, Morita K, Obara H. Annual mortality and morbidity in operating rooms during 2002 and summary of morbidity and mortality between 1999 and 2002 in Japan: A brief review. Masui 53:320, 2004
41. Kawashima Y, Takahashi S, Suzuki M, Morita K, Irita K, Iwao Y, Seo N, Tsuzaki K, Dohi S, Kobayashi T, Goto Y, Suzuki G, Fujii A, Suzuki H, Yokoyama K, Kugimiya T. Anesthesia-related mortality and morbidity over a 5-year period in 2,363,038 patients in Japan. Acta Anaesthesiol Scand 47:809, 2003
42. Biboulet P, Aubas P, Dubourdieu J, Rubenovitch J, Capdevila X, d'Athis F. Fatal and non-fatal cardiac arrests related to anesthesia. Can J Anaesth 48:326, 2001
43. Morray JP, Geiduschek JM, Ramamoorthy C, Haberkern CM, Hackel A, Caplan RA, Domino KB, Posner K, Cheney FW. Anesthesia-related cardiac arrest in children: initial findings of the Pediatric Perioperative Cardiac Arrest (POCA) Registry. Anesthesiology 93:6, 2000
44. Warner MA, Warner DO, Matsumoto JY, Harper CM, Schroeder DR, Maxson PM. Ulnar neuropathy in surgical patients. Anesthesiology 90:54, 1999
45. Warner MA, Warner ME, Martin JT. Ulnar neuropathy. Incidence, outcome, and risk factors in sedated or anesthetized patients. Anesthesiology 81:1332, 1994
46. Alvine FG, Schurrer ME. Postoperative ulnar-nerve palsy. Are there predisposing factors? J Bone Joint Surg 69:255, 1987.

SECTION II ■ BASIC PRINCIPLES OF ANESTHESIA PRACTICE

CHAPTER 6 ■ CELLULAR AND MOLECULAR MECHANISMS OF ANESTHESIA

ALEX S. EVERS AND C. MICHAEL CROWDER

KEY POINTS

1. Despite the importance of general anesthetics, the molecular mechanisms responsible for anesthetic actions remain one of the unsolved mysteries of pharmacology.
2. The spinal cord is probably the site at which anesthetics act to inhibit purposeful responses to noxious stimulation (end point for measurements of equal potency, MAC).
3. Inhalational anesthetics can depress the excitability of thalamic neurons, potentially resulting in the loss of consciousness.
4. Synaptic function is considered a likely subcellular site of general anesthetic action. Nevertheless, the effects of anesthetics on synaptic function differ among various anesthetic agents, neurotransmitters, and neuronal preparations.
5. Ion channels (especially $GABA_A$ receptors) are a likely molecular targets of anesthetic action.
6. Direct anesthetic–protein-binding interactions may be responsible for anesthetic effects on ion channels in the central nervous system (CNS) (stereoselectivity is the strongest argument in favor of this mechanism).
7. Genetic techniques provide the most reliable and versatile methods for changing the structure of putative anesthetic targets.
8. The unitary theory of anesthesia is incorrect and there are several molecular mechanisms (anesthetics act via selective effects on specific molecular targets).

1 The introduction of general anesthetics into clinical practice 150 years ago stands as one of the seminal innovations of medicine. This single discovery facilitated the development of modern surgery and spawned the specialty of anesthesiology. Despite the importance of general anesthetics and despite over 100 years of active research, the molecular mechanisms responsible for anesthetic action remain one of the unsolved mysteries of pharmacology.

Why have mechanisms of anesthesia been so difficult to elucidate? Anesthetics, as a class of drugs, are challenging to study for three major reasons:

1. Anesthesia, by definition, is a change in the responses of an *intact animal* to external stimuli. Making a definitive link between anesthetic effects observed in vitro and the anesthetic state observed and defined in vivo has proven difficult.

2. No structure–activity relationships are apparent among anesthetics; a wide variety of structurally unrelated compounds, ranging from steroids to elemental xenon, are capable of producing clinical anesthesia. This suggests that there are multiple molecular mechanisms that can produce clinical anesthesia.
3. Anesthetics work at very high concentrations in comparison to drugs, neurotransmitters, and hormones that act at specific receptors. This implies that if anesthetics do act by binding to specific receptor sites, they must bind with very low affinity and probably stay bound to the receptor for very short periods of time. Low-affinity binding is much more difficult to observe and characterize than high-affinity binding.

Despite these difficulties, molecular and genetic tools are now available that should allow for major insights into anesthetic mechanisms in the next decade. The aim of this chapter is to provide a conceptual framework for the reader to catalog current knowledge and integrate future developments about mechanisms of anesthesia. Five specific questions will be addressed in this chapter:

1. What is anesthesia and how do we measure it?
2. What is the anatomic site of anesthetic action in the central nervous system?
3. What are the cellular neurophysiologic mechanisms of anesthesia (e.g., effects on synaptic function versus effects on action potential generation) and what anesthetic effects on ion channels and other neuronal proteins underlie these mechanisms?
4. What are the molecular targets of anesthetics?
5. How are the molecular and cellular effects of anesthetics linked to the behavioral effects of anesthetics observed in vivo?

WHAT IS ANESTHESIA?

General anesthesia can broadly be defined as a drug-induced reversible depression of the central nervous system resulting in the loss of response to and perception of all external stimuli. Unfortunately, such a broad definition is inadequate for two reasons. First, the definition is not actually broad enough. Anesthesia is not simply a deafferented state; amnesia and unconsciousness are important aspects of the anesthetic state. Second, the definition is too broad, as all general anesthetics do not produce equal depression of all sensory modalities. For example, barbiturates are considered to be anesthetics, but they are not particularly effective analgesics. These conflicting problems with definition can be bypassed by a more practical description of the anesthetic state as a collection of "component" changes in behavior or perception. The components of the anesthetic state include unconsciousness, amnesia, analgesia, immobility, and attenuation of autonomic responses to noxious stimulation.

Regardless of which definition of anesthesia is used, essential to anesthesia are drug-induced changes in behavior or perception. As such, anesthesia can only be defined and measured in the intact organism. Changes in behavior such as unconsciousness or amnesia can be intuitively understood in higher organisms such as mammals, but become increasingly difficult to define as one descends the phylogenetic tree. Thus, while anesthetics have effects on organisms ranging from worms[1] to man, it is difficult to map with certainty the effects of anesthetics observed in lower organisms to any of our behavioral definitions of anesthesia. This contributes to the difficulty of using simple organisms as models in which to study the molecular mechanisms of anesthesia. Similarly, any cellular or molecular effects of anesthetics observed in higher organisms can be extremely difficult to link with the constellation of behaviors that constitute the anesthetic state. The absence of a simple and concise definition of anesthesia is clearly one of the stumbling blocks to elucidating the mechanisms of anesthesia at a molecular and cellular level.

HOW IS ANESTHESIA MEASURED?

To study the pharmacology of anesthetic action, quantitative measurements of anesthetic potency are absolutely essential. To this end, Eger and colleagues have defined the concept of MAC, or minimum alveolar concentration. MAC is defined as the alveolar partial pressure of a gas at which 50% of humans do not respond to a surgical incision.[2] In animals, MAC is defined as the alveolar partial pressure of a gas at which 50% of animals do not respond to a noxious stimulus, such as tail clamp,[3] or at which they lose their righting reflex. The use of MAC as a measure of anesthetic potency has two major advantages. First, it is an extremely reproducible measurement that is remarkably constant over a wide range of species.[2] Second, the use of end-tidal gas concentration provides an index of the "free" concentration of drug required to produce anesthesia since the end-tidal gas concentration is in equilibrium with the free concentration in plasma. The MAC concept has several important limitations, particularly when trying to relate MAC values to anesthetic potency observed in vitro. First, the end point in a MAC determination is quantal: a subject is either anesthetized or unanesthetized; it cannot be partially anesthetized. Furthermore, MAC represents the average response of a whole population of subjects rather than the response of a single subject. The quantal nature of the MAC measurement makes it very difficult to compare MAC measurements to concentration-response curves obtained in vitro, where the graded response of a single preparation is measured as a function of anesthetic concentration. The second limitation of MAC measurements is that they can only be directly applied to anesthetic gases. Parenteral anesthetics (barbiturates, neurosteroids, propofol) cannot be assigned a MAC value, making it difficult to compare the potency of parenteral and volatile anesthetics. A MAC equivalent for parenteral anesthetics is the free concentration of the drug in plasma required to prevent response to a noxious stimulus in 50% of subjects; this value has been estimated for several parenteral anesthetics.[4] A third limitation of MAC is that it is highly dependent on the anesthetic end point used to define it. For example, if loss of response to a verbal command is used as an anesthetic end point, the MAC values obtained (MAC_{awake}) will be much lower than classic MAC values based on response to a noxious stimulus. Indeed, each behavioral component of the anesthetic state will likely have a different MAC value. Despite its limitations, MAC remains the most robust measurement and the standard for determining the potency of volatile anesthetics.

The foregoing discussion of MAC brings forth an important and somewhat controversial question. What drug concentration should be measured when determining anesthetic potency? When measuring potency of intravenous anesthetics, the answer to this question is relatively simple. One would like to relate the free concentration of the drug at its site of action (the biophase) to the drug's effect. It is, of course, not practical to measure the drug's concentration in the extracellular fluid of the brain, so free concentration in plasma is used as an approximation of the biophase concentration. This allows one to compare the concentration of drug required to produce anesthesia in humans to the concentrations required to produce specific effects in vitro. With the volatile anesthetics, potency is defined by MAC, which is measured in units of partial pressure. Because the partial pressure of a dissolved gas is directly proportional to the free concentration of that gas in a liquid, alveolar partial pressures are accurate reporters of the free anesthetic concentrations in plasma and in brain tissue.

WHERE IN THE CENTRAL NERVOUS SYSTEM DO ANESTHETICS WORK?

In principle, general anesthesia could result from interruption of nervous system activity at myriad levels. Plausible targets include peripheral sensory receptors, spinal cord, brainstem, and cerebral cortex. Of these potential sites, only peripheral sensory receptors can be eliminated as an important site of anesthetic action. Animal studies have shown that fluorinated volatile anesthetics have no effect on cutaneous mechanosensors in cats[5] and can even sensitize nociceptors in monkeys.[6] Furthermore, selective perfusion studies in dogs have shown that MAC for isoflurane is unaffected by the presence or absence of isoflurane at the site of noxious stimulation, provided that the central nervous system is perfused with blood containing isoflurane.[7]

Spinal Cord

2 Clearly, anesthetic actions on the spinal cord cannot produce either amnesia or unconsciousness. However, several lines of evidence indicate that the spinal cord is probably the site at which anesthetics act to inhibit purposeful responses to noxious stimulation. This is, of course, the end point used in most measurements of anesthetic potency. Rampil and colleagues have shown that MAC values for fluorinated volatile anesthetics are unaffected in the rat by either decerebration[8] or cervical spinal cord transection.[9] Antognini and colleagues have used the strategy of isolating the cerebral circulation of goats to explore the contribution of brain and spinal cord to the determination of MAC. They found that when isoflurane is administered only to the brain, MAC is 2.9%, whereas when it is administered to the entire body, MAC is 1.2%.[10] Surprisingly, when isoflurane was preferentially administered to the body and not to the brain, isoflurane MAC was reduced to 0.8%.[11] The actions of volatile anesthetics in the spinal cord are mediated, at least in part, by direct effects on the excitability of spinal motor neurons. This conclusion has been substantiated by experiments in rats,[12] goats,[13] and humans,[14] showing that volatile anesthetics depress the amplitude of the F wave in evoked potential measurements (F-wave amplitude correlates with motor neuron excitability). These provocative results suggest not only that anesthetic actions at the spinal cord underlie the determination of MAC, but also that anesthetic actions on the brain may actually sensitize the cord to noxious stimuli. The plausibility of the spinal cord as a locus for anesthetic immobilization is also supported by several electrophysiological studies showing inhibition of excitatory synaptic transmission in the spinal cord.[15–18]

Reticular Activating System

The reticular activating system, a diffuse collection of brainstem neurons involved in arousal behavior, has long been speculated to be a site of general anesthetic action on consciousness. Evidence to support this notion came from early whole animal experiments showing that electrical stimulation of the reticular activating system could induce arousal behavior in anesthetized animals.[19] A role for the brainstem in anesthetic action is also supported by studies examining somatosensory evoked potentials. Generally, these studies show that anesthetics produce increased latency and decreased amplitude of cortical potentials, indicating that anesthetics inhibit information transfer through the brainstem.[20] In contrast, studies using brainstem auditory evoked potentials have shown variable effects ranging from depression to enhancement of information transfer through the reticular formation.[21–23] While there is evidence that the reticular formation of the brainstem is a locus for anesthetic effects, it cannot be the only anatomic site of anesthetic action for two reasons. First, as discussed earlier, the brainstem is not even required for anesthetics to inhibit responsiveness to noxious stimuli. Second, the reticular formation can be largely ablated without eliminating awareness.[24]

Within the reticular formation is a set of pontine noradrenergic neurons called the locus coeruleus (LC). The LC innervates a number of targets in basal forebrain and cortex including a set of GABAergic hypothalamic neurons called the ventrolateral preoptic nucleus (VLPO). The VLPO in turn innervates the tuberomammillary nucleus (TMN). The LC-VLPO-TMN pathway has been shown to be critical for non-REM sleep. Given that EEG patterns under anesthesia and non-REM sleep are quite similar, this pathway is a particularly good candidate for a site of anesthetic action. Using stereotactic techniques, Maze and colleagues tested this hypothesis by measuring whether application of a GABAergic antagonist directly onto the TMN altered the efficacy of anesthetics.[25] Indeed, discrete application of the GABAergic antagonist gabazine onto the TMN markedly reduced the duration of sedation produced by systemically administered propofol or pentobarbital. This effect is unlikely to be a consequence of a nonspecific increase in arousal state because systemically administered gabazine did not antagonize the potency of ketamine whereas it did antagonize propofol and pentobarbital in a manner similar to application directly onto the TMN. This result strongly implicates the TMN as a site for the sedative action of GABAergic anesthetics like propofol and barbiturates.

Cerebral Cortex

The cerebral cortex is the major site for integration, storage, and retrieval of information. As such, it is a likely site at which anesthetics might interfere with complex functions like memory and awareness. Anesthetics clearly alter cortical electrical activity, as evidenced by the changes in surface EEG patterns recorded during anesthesia. Anesthetic effects on patterns of cortical electrical activity vary widely among anesthetics,[26] providing an initial suggestion that all anesthetics are not likely to act through identical mechanisms. More detailed in vitro electrophysiological studies examining anesthetic effects on different cortical regions support the notion that anesthetics can differentially alter neuronal function in various cortical preparations. For example, volatile anesthetics have been shown to inhibit excitatory transmission at some synapses in the olfactory cortex[27] but not at others.[28] Similarly, whereas volatile anesthetics inhibit excitatory transmission in the dentate gyrus of the hippocampus,[29] these same drugs can actually enhance excitatory transmission at other synapses in the hippocampus.[30] Anesthetics also produce a variety of effects on inhibitory transmission in the cortex. A variety of parenteral and inhalational anesthetics have been shown to enhance inhibitory transmission in olfactory cortex[28] and in the hippocampus.[31] Conversely, volatile anesthetics have also been
3 reported to depress inhibitory transmission in hippocampus.[32] One area of the brain that has been postulated as a potential site of anesthetic action is the thalamus. The thalamus is

important in relaying sensory modalities and motor information to the cortex *via* thalamocortical pathways. A developing body of evidence indicates that inhalational anesthetics can depress the excitability of thalamic neurons, thus blocking thalamocortical communication potentially resulting in loss of consciousness.[33]

Summary

Anesthetics are able to produce effects on a variety of anatomic structures in the CNS, including spinal cord, brainstem, and cerebral cortex. Whereas certain anesthetic effects may be attributable to specific anatomic locations (e.g., purposeful response to noxious stimulation maps to the spinal cord), existing evidence provides no basis for a single anatomic site responsible for anesthesia. This difficulty in identifying a site for anesthesia might plausibly result from the various components of the anesthetic state being produced by anesthetic effects on different regions of the CNS. Nevertheless, despite the difficulty in identifying a common anatomic site for anesthesia, investigators have continued to look for other unifying principles in anesthetic action. Specifically, attention has been focused on identifying common cellular or molecular anesthetic targets that may have a wide anatomic distribution, explaining the ability of anesthetic to affect nervous system function in an anatomically diffuse manner.

HOW DO ANESTHETICS INTERFERE WITH THE ELECTROPHYSIOLOGIC FUNCTION OF THE NERVOUS SYSTEM?

In the simplest terms anesthetics inhibit or "turn off" vital central nervous system functions. They must do this by acting at specific physiologic "switches." A great deal of investigative effort has been devoted to identifying these switches. In principle, the CNS could be switched off by several means:

1. By depressing those neurons or pattern generators that subserve a pacemaker function in the CNS,
2. By reducing overall neuronal excitability; either by changing resting membrane potential or by interfering with the processes involved in generating an action potential,
3. By reducing communication between neurons—specifically, by either inhibiting excitatory synaptic transmission or enhancing inhibitory synaptic transmission.

Pattern Generators

Information concerning the effects of anesthetics on pattern-generating neuronal circuits in the CNS is limited, but clinical concentrations of anesthetics are likely to have significant effects on these circuits. The simplest evidence for this is the observation that most anesthetics exert profound effects on respiratory rate and rhythm, strongly suggesting an effect on respiratory pattern generators in the brainstem. Invertebrate studies suggest that volatile anesthetics can selectively inhibit the spontaneous (pacemaker) firing of specific neurons. As shown in Fig. 6-1, halothane (1.0 MAC) completely inhibits spontaneous action potential generation by one neuron in the right parietal ganglion of the great pond snail while producing no observable effect on the firing frequency of adjacent neurons.[34]

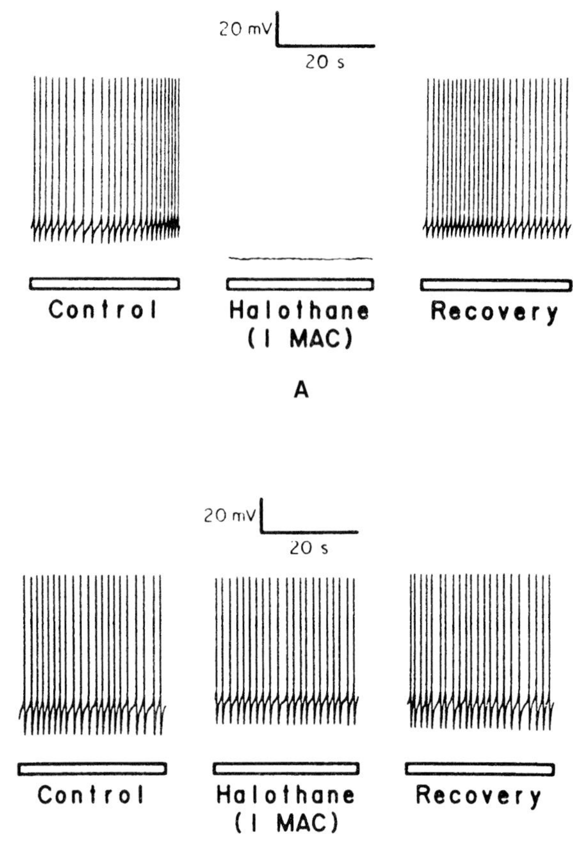

FIGURE 6-1. Selectivity of volatile anesthetic inhibition of neuronal automaticity. Halothane (1 MAC) reversibly inhibits the spontaneous firing activity of a neuron from the parietal ganglion of *Lymnaea stagnalis* (**A**). The same concentration of halothane has no effect on the firing activity of an adjacent, and apparently identical, neuron (**B**). Note that in (**A**) halothane markedly reduces resting membrane potential in addition to inhibiting firing. (From Franks NP, Lieb WR. Mechanisms of general anesthesia. *Environ Health Perspect.* 1990;87:204.)

Neuronal Excitability

The ability of a neuron to generate an action potential is determined by three parameters: resting membrane potential, the threshold potential for action potential generation, and the function of voltage-gated sodium channels. Anesthetics can hyperpolarize (create a more negative resting membrane potential) both spinal motor neurons and cortical neurons,[35,36] and this ability to hyperpolarize neurons correlates with anesthetic potency. In general, the increase in resting membrane potential produced by anesthetics is small in magnitude and is unlikely to have an effect on axonal *propagation* of an action potential. Small changes in resting potential may, however, inhibit the *initiation* of an action potential either at a postsynaptic site or in a spontaneously firing neuron. Indeed, hyperpolarization is responsible for the inhibition of spontaneous action potential generation shown in Fig. 6-1. Recent evidence also indicates that isoflurane hyperpolarizes thalamic neurons, leading to an inhibition of tonic firing of action potentials.[33] There is no evidence indicating that anesthetics alter the threshold potential of a neuron for action potential generation.

However, the data is conflicting on whether the size of the action potential, once initiated, is diminished by general anesthetics. A classic paper by Larrabee and Posternak demonstrated that concentrations of ether and chloroform that completely block synaptic transmission in mammalian sympathetic ganglia have no effect on presynaptic action potential amplitude.[37] Similar results have been obtained with fluorinated volatile anesthetics in several mammalian brain preparations.[27,29] This dogma that the action potential is relatively resistant to general anesthetics has been challenged by more recent reports that volatile anesthetics at clinical concentrations produce a small but significant reduction in the size of the action potential in mammalian neurons.[38,39] In one case, the reduction in the action potential was shown to be amplified at the presynaptic terminal resulting in a large reduction in neurotransmitter release.[39] Thus, while current data still support the prevailing view that neuronal excitability is only slightly affected by general anesthetics, this small effect may nevertheless contribute significantly to the clinical actions of volatile anesthetics.

Synaptic Function

4 Synaptic function is widely considered to be the most likely subcellular site of general anesthetic action. Neurotransmission across both excitatory and inhibitory synapses has been found to be markedly altered by general anesthetics. General anesthetics have been shown to inhibit excitatory synaptic transmission in a variety of preparations, including sympathetic ganglia,[37] olfactory cortex,[27] hippocampus,[29] and spinal cord.[17] However, not all excitatory synapses appear to be equally sensitive to anesthetics; indeed, transmission across some hippocampal excitatory synapses has been shown to be enhanced by inhalational anesthetics.[30] In a similar fashion, general anesthetics have been shown both to enhance and depress inhibitory synaptic transmission in various preparations. In a classic paper in 1975, Nicoll and colleagues showed that barbiturates enhanced inhibitory synaptic transmission by prolonging the decay of the GABAergic inhibitory postsynaptic current.[40] Enhancement of inhibitory transmission has also been observed with many other general anesthetics, including etomidate,[41] propofol,[42] inhalational anesthetics,[28] and neurosteroids.[43] Although anesthetic enhancement of inhibitory currents has received a great deal of attention as a potential mechanism of anesthesia,[4] it is important to note that there is also a large body of experimentation showing that clinical concentrations of general anesthetics can depress inhibitory postsynaptic potentials in the hippocampus[32,44,45] and in the spinal cord.[18] Anesthetics do appear to have preferential effects on synapses, but there is a great deal of heterogeneity in the manner in which anesthetic agents affect different synapses. This is not surprising given the large variation in synaptic structure, function (i.e., efficacy), and chemistry (neurotransmitters, modulators) extant in the nervous system.

Presynaptic Effects

General anesthetics affect synaptic transmission both pre- and postsynaptically. However, the magnitude and even the type of effect vary according to the type of synapse and the particular anesthetic. Presynaptically, neurotransmitter release from glutamatergic synapses has consistently been found to be inhibited by clinical concentrations of volatile anesthetics. For example, a study by Perouansky and colleagues conducted in mouse hippocampal slices showed that halothane inhibited excitatory postsynaptic potentials elicited by presynaptic electrical stimulation, but not those elicited by direct application of glutamate. This indicates that halothane must be acting to prevent the release of glutamate, the major excitatory neurotransmitter in the brain.[46] MacIver and colleagues extended these observations by providing evidence that the inhibition of glutamate release from hippocampal neurons is not due to effects at GABAergic synapses that could indirectly decrease transmitter release from glutamatergic neurons. Effects of intravenous anesthetics on glutamate release have also been demonstrated but the evidence is more limited and the effects potentially indirect.[47,48] The data for anesthetic effects on inhibitory neurotransmitter release is mixed. Inhibition,[49] stimulation,[50,51] and no effect[52] have been reported for volatile anesthetic and intravenous anesthetic action on GABA release. In a brain synaptosomal preparation where effects on both GABA and glutamate release could be studied simultaneously, Hemmings and coworkers found that glutamate and, to a lesser degree, GABA release were inhibited by clinical concentrations of isoflurane.[53] The mechanism underlying anesthetic effects on transmitter release have not been established. The effects of anesthetics on neurotransmitter release do not appear to be mediated by reduced neurotransmitter synthesis or storage, but rather by a direct effect on the process of neurosecretion. A variety of evidence argues that at some synapses the majority of the anesthetic effect is upstream of the transmitter release machinery, perhaps on presynaptic sodium channels (see discussion later). However, genetic data in *C. elegans* shows that the transmitter release machinery strongly influences volatile anesthetic sensitivity;[54,55] at present, it is unclear whether these findings represent species differences or different aspects of the same mechanism.

Postsynaptic Effects

Anesthetics also alter the postsynaptic response to released neurotransmitter. The effects of general anesthetics on excitatory neurotransmitter receptor function vary depending on neurotransmitter type, anesthetic agent, and preparation. Richards and Smaje examined the effects of several anesthetic agents on the response of olfactory cortical neurons to application of glutamate, the major excitatory neurotransmitter in the CNS.[56] They found that while pentobarbital, diethyl ether, methoxyflurane, and alphaxalone depressed the electrical response to glutamate, halothane was without effect. In contrast, when acetylcholine was applied to the same olfactory cortical preparation, halothane and methoxyflurane stimulated the electrical response whereas pentobarbital had no effect; only alphaxalone depressed the electrical response to acetylcholine.[57] The effects of anesthetics on neuronal responses to inhibitory neurotransmitters are more consistent. A wide variety of anesthetics, including barbiturates, etomidate, neurosteroids, propofol, and the fluorinated volatile anesthetics, have been shown to enhance the electrical response to exogenously applied GABA (for a review, see [58]). For example, Fig. 6-2 illustrates the ability of enflurane to increase both the amplitude and the duration of the current elicited by application of GABA to hippocampal neurons.[59]

Summary

Attempts to identify a physiologic "switch" at which anesthetics act have suffered from their own success. Anesthetics produce a variety of effects on many physiologic processes that might logically contribute to the anesthetic state, including neuronal automaticity, neuronal excitability, and synaptic function. The synapse is generally thought to be the most likely relevant site of anesthetic action. Existing evidence indicates that even at this one site, anesthetics produce various effects, including presynaptic inhibition of neurotransmitter release, inhibition of excitatory neurotransmitter effect, and

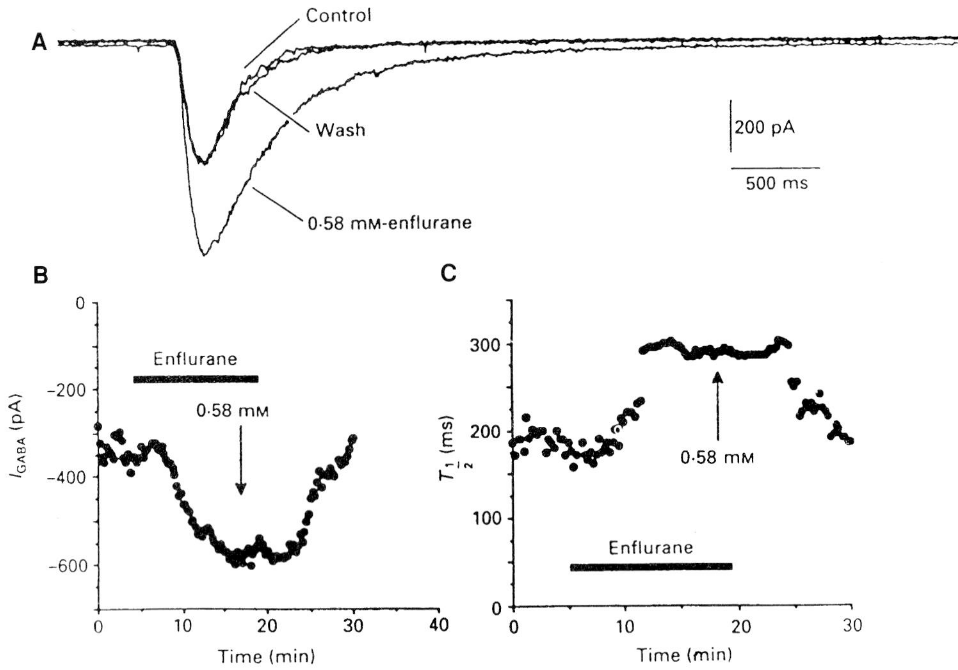

FIGURE 6-2. Enflurane potentiates the ability of GABA to activate a chloride current in cultured rat hippocampal cells. This potentiation is rapidly reversed by removal of enflurane (wash) (**Panel A**). Enflurane increases both the amplitude of the current (**Panel B**) and the time ($\tau_{1/2}$) it takes for the current to decay (**Panel C**). (Reproduced with permission from Jones MV, Brooks PA, Harrison L. Enhancement of γ-aminobutyric acid-activated Cl^- currents in cultured rat hippocampal neurones by three volatile anaesthetics. *J Physiol.* 1992;449:289.)

enhancement of inhibitory neurotransmitter effect. Furthermore, the effects of anesthetics on synaptic function differ among various anesthetic agents, neurotransmitters, and neuronal preparations.

ANESTHETIC ACTIONS ON ION CHANNELS

5 Ion channels are one likely target of anesthetic action. The advent of patch clamp techniques in the early 1980s made it possible to directly measure the currents from single ion channel proteins. It was attractive to think that anesthetic effects on a small number of ion channels might help to explain the complex physiologic effects of anesthetics that we have already described. Accordingly, during the 1980s and 1990s a major effort was directed at describing the effects of anesthetics on the various kinds of ion channels. The following section summarizes and distills this effort. For the purposes of this discussion, ion channels are cataloged according to the stimuli to which they respond by opening or closing (i.e., their mechanism of gating).

Anesthetic Effects on Voltage-Dependent Ion Channels

A variety of ion channels can sense a change in membrane potential and respond by either opening or closing their pore. These channels include voltage-dependent sodium, potassium, and calcium channels, all of which share significant structural homologies. Voltage-dependent sodium and potassium channels are largely involved in generating and shaping action potentials. The effects of anesthetics on these channels have been extensively studied by Haydon and colleagues in the squid giant axon.[60,61] These studies show that these invertebrate sodium channels and potassium channels are remarkably insensitive to volatile anesthetics. For example, 50% inhibition of the peak sodium channel current required halothane concentrations 8 times those required to produce anesthesia. The delayed rectifier potassium channel was even less sensitive, requiring halothane concentrations more than 20 times those required to produce anesthesia. Similar results have been obtained in a mammalian cell line (GH_3 pituitary cells) where both sodium and potassium currents were inhibited by halothane only at concentrations greater than 5 times those required to produce anesthesia.[62] However, a number of studies with volatile anesthetics have challenged the notion that voltage-dependent sodium channels are insensitive to anesthetics. Rehberg and colleagues expressed rat brain IIA sodium channels in a mammalian cell line and showed that clinically relevant concentrations of a variety of inhalational anesthetics suppressed voltage-elicited sodium currents.[63] Hemmings and coworkers showed that sodium flux mediated by rat brain sodium channels was significantly inhibited by clinical concentrations of halothane.[64] Harris and colleagues documented the effects of isoflurane on a variety of sodium channel subtypes and found that several but not all subtypes are sensitive to clinical concentrations.[65] Finally as described above, in a rat brainstem neuron Wu and colleagues found that a small inhibition of sodium currents by isoflurane resulted in a large inhibition of synaptic activity.[39] Thus, sodium channel activity not only appears to be inhibited by volatile anesthetics, but this inhibition results in a significant reduction in synaptic function, at least at some mammalian synapses. Intravenous anesthetics have also been shown to inhibit sodium channels, but the concentrations for this effect are supraclinical.[66–68]

Voltage-dependent calcium channels (VDCC) serve to couple electrical activity to specific cellular functions. In the nervous system, VDCCs located at presynaptic terminals respond to action potentials by opening. This allows calcium to enter the cell, activating calcium-dependent secretion of neurotransmitter into the synaptic cleft. At least six types of calcium channels (designated L, N, P, Q, R, and T) have been identified on the basis of electrophysiological properties and a larger number based on amino acid sequence similarities.[69] N-, P-, Q-, and R-type channels, as well as some of the untitled channels, are preferentially expressed in the nervous system and are thought to play a major role in synaptic transmission. L-type calcium channels, although expressed in the brain, have been best studied in their role in excitation–contraction coupling in cardiac, skeletal, and smooth muscle and are thought to be less important in synaptic transmission. The effects of anesthetics on L- and T-type currents have been well characterized,[62,70,71] and there are some reports concerning the effects of anesthetics on N- and P-type currents.[72–74] As a general rule, these studies have shown that volatile anesthetics inhibit VDCCs (50% reduction in current) at concentrations 2 to 5 times those required to produce anesthesia in humans, with less than a 20% inhibition of calcium current at clinical concentrations of anesthetics (Fig. 6-3). However, some studies have found VDCCs that are extremely sensitive to anesthetics. Takenoshita and Steinbach reported a T-type calcium current in dorsal root ganglion neurons that was inhibited by subanesthetic concentrations of halothane.[75] Additionally, ffrench-Mullen and colleagues have reported a VDCC of unspecified type in guinea pig hippocampus that is inhibited by pentobarbital at concentrations identical to those required to produce anesthesia.[76] Thus, VDCCs could well mediate some actions of general anesthetics, but their general insensitivity makes them unlikely to be major targets.

Potassium channels are the most diverse of the ion channel types and include voltage-gated, second messenger and ligand-activated, and so-called inward rectifying channels; some channels fall into more than one category. High concentrations of both volatile anesthetics and intravenous anesthetics are required to significantly affect the function of voltage-gated K^+ channels.[61,77,78] Similarly, classic inward rectifying K^+ channels are relatively insensitive to sevoflurane and barbiturates.[79–81] However, some ligand-gated K^+ channels are reasonably sensitive to volatile anesthetics as discussed below.

Summary

Existing evidence suggests that most VDCCs are modestly sensitive or insensitive to anesthetics, but some reports argue for significant heterogeneity in the anesthetic sensitivity of specific channel types and subtypes. In particular, some sodium channel subtypes are inhibited by volatile anesthetics and this effect may be responsible in part for a reduction in neurotransmitter release at some synapses. Additional experimental data will be required to establish whether anesthetic-sensitive VDCCs are localized to specific synapses at which anesthetics have been shown to inhibit neurotransmitter release.

Anesthetic Effects on Ligand-Gated Ion Channels

Fast excitatory and inhibitory neurotransmission is mediated by the actions of ligand-gated ion channels. Synaptically released glutamate or GABA diffuse across the synaptic cleft and bind to channel proteins that open as a consequence of neurotransmitter release. The channel proteins that bind GABA ($GABA_A$ receptors) are members of a superfamily of structurally related ligand-gated ion channel proteins that include nicotinic acetylcholine receptors, glycine receptors, and 5-HT_3 receptors.[82] Based on the structure of the nicotinic acetylcholine receptor, each ligand-gated channel is thought to be composed of five nonidentical subunits. The glutamate receptors also comprise a family, each receptor thought to be a tetrameric protein composed of structurally related subunits.[83] The ligand-gated ion channels provide a logical target for anesthetic action because selective effects on these channels could inhibit fast excitatory synaptic transmission and/or facilitate fast inhibitory synaptic transmission. The effects of anesthetic

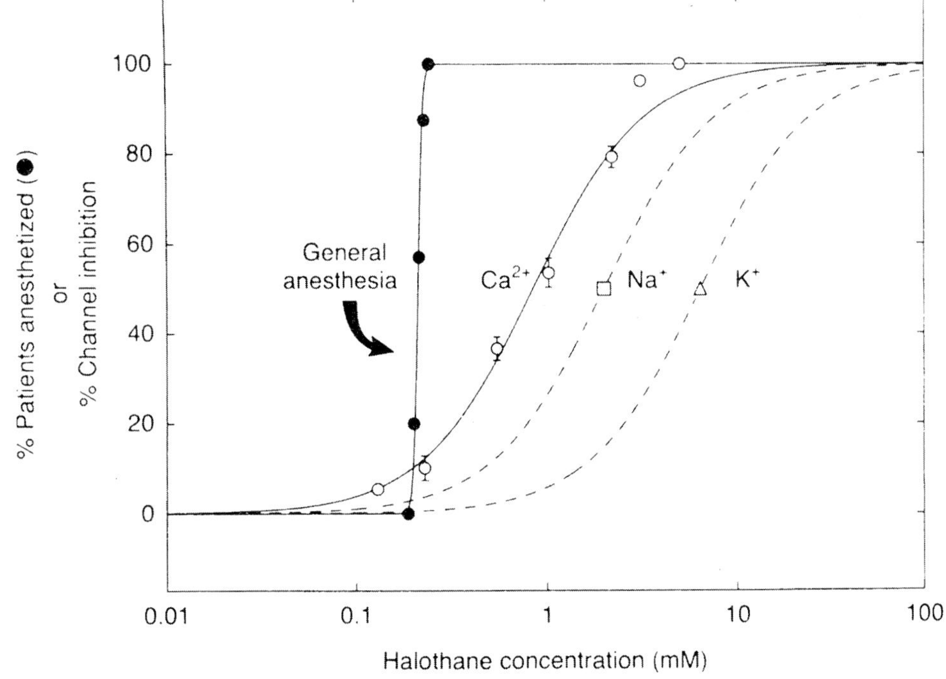

FIGURE 6-3. Halothane inhibition of voltage-dependent Ca^{2+}, Na^+, and K^+ currents. The Ca^{2+} channels are L-type channels from GH_3 cells, and the Na^+ and K^+ channels are from the squid giant axon. The closed circles show the concentrations of halothane required to anesthetize humans. Note that the Ca^{2+} currents are inhibited about 20% by clinical concentrations of halothane whereas the Na^+ and K^+ currents are not inhibited at all. (Reproduced by permission from Franks NP, Lieb WR. Molecular and cellular mechanisms of anesthesia. *Nature*. 1994;367:607, Macmillan Magazines Ltd.)

agents on ligand-gated ion channels are thoroughly cataloged in a review by Krasowski and Harrison.[58] The following section provides a brief summary of this large body of work.

Glutamate-Activated Ion Channels

Glutamate-activated ion channels have been classified, based on selective agonists, into three categories: AMPA receptors, kainate receptors, and NMDA receptors. Molecular biologic studies indicate that a large number of structurally distinct glutamate receptor subunits can be used to form each of the three categories of glutamate receptors.[84] This structural heterogeneity is reflected in functional heterogeneity within each category of glutamate receptor. AMPA and kainate receptors are relatively nonselective monovalent cation channels involved in fast excitatory synaptic transmission, whereas NMDA channels conduct not only Na^+ and K^+ but also Ca^{++} and are involved in long-term modulation of synaptic responses (long-term potentiation). Studies from the early 1980s in mouse and rat brain preparations showed that AMPA- and kainate-activated currents are insensitive to clinical concentrations of halothane,[85] enflurane,[86] and the neurosteroid allopregnanolone.[87] In contrast, kainate- and AMPA-activated currents were shown to be sensitive to barbiturates; in rat hippocampal neurons, 50 μM pentobarbital (pentobarbital produces anesthesia at approximately 50 μM) inhibited kainate and AMPA responses by 50%.[87] More recent studies using cloned and expressed glutamate receptor subunits show that submaximal agonist responses of GluR3 (AMPA-type) receptors are inhibited by fluorinated volatile anesthetics whereas agonist responses of GluR6 (kainate-type) receptors are enhanced.[88] In contrast both GluR3 and GluR6 receptors are inhibited by pentobarbital. The directionally opposite effects of the volatile anesthetics on different glutamate receptor subtypes may explain the earlier inconclusive effects observed in tissue, where multiple subunit types are expressed. These opposite effects have also been used as a strategy to identify critical sites on the molecules involved in anesthetic effect. By producing GluR3/GluR6 receptor chimeras (receptors made up of various combinations of sections of the GluR3 and GluR6 receptors) and screening for volatile anesthetic effect, specific areas of the protein required for volatile anesthetic potentiation of GluR6 have been identified. Subsequent site-directed mutagenesis studies have identified a specific glycine residue (Gly-819) as critical for volatile anesthetic action on GluR6-containing receptors.[89]

NMDA-activated currents also appear to be sensitive to a subset of anesthetics. Electrophysiological studies show virtually no effects of clinical concentrations of volatile anesthetics,[85,86] neurosteroids, or barbiturates[87] on NMDA-activated currents. It should be noted that there is some evidence from flux studies that volatile anesthetics may inhibit NMDA-activated channels. A study in rat brain microvesicles showed that anesthetic concentrations (0.2–0.3 mM) of halothane and enflurane inhibited NMDA-activated calcium flux by 50%.[90] In contrast, ketamine is a potent and selective inhibitor of NMDA-activated currents. Ketamine stereoselectively inhibits NMDA currents by binding to the phencyclidine site on the NMDA receptor protein.[91–93] The anesthetic effects of ketamine in intact animals show the same stereoselectivity as that is observed in vitro,[94] suggesting that the NMDA receptor may be the principal molecular target for the anesthetic actions of ketamine. Two other recent findings suggest that NMDA receptors may be an important target for nitrous oxide and xenon. These studies show that N_2O[95,96] and xenon[97] are potent and selective inhibitors of NMDA-activated currents. This is illustrated in Fig. 6-4, showing that N_2O inhibits NMDA-elicited, but not GABA-elicited, currents in hippocampal neurons.

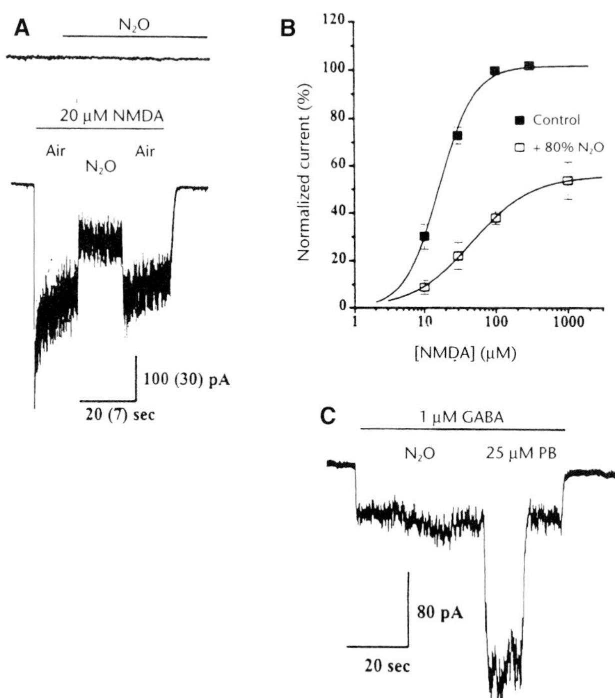

FIGURE 6-4. Nitrous oxide inhibits NMDA-elicited, but not GABA-elicited, currents in rat hippocampal neurons. (**Panel A**) 80% N_2O has no effect on holding current (upper trace), but inhibits the current elicited by NMDA. (**Panel B**) N_2O causes a rightward and downward shift of the NMDA concentration-response curve, indicating a mixed competitive/noncompetitive antagonism. (**Panel C**) 80% N_2O has little effect on GABA-elicited currents. In contrast, an equipotent anesthetic concentration of pentobarbital markedly enhances the GABA-elicited current. (Reproduced with permission from Jevtovic-Todorovic V, Todorovic SM, Mennerick S, *et al.* Nitrous oxide (laughing gas) is an NMDA antagonist, neuroprotectant, and neurotoxin. *Nature Medicine*. 1998;4:460.)

GABA-Activated Ion Channels

GABA is the most important inhibitory neurotransmitter in the mammalian central nervous system. GABA-activated ion channels ($GABA_A$ receptors) mediate the postsynaptic response to synaptically released GABA by selectively allowing chloride ions to enter and thereby hyperpolarizing neurons. $GABA_A$ receptors are multisubunit proteins consisting of various combinations of α, β, γ, δ, and ε subunits, and there are many subtypes of each of these subunits. The function of $GABA_A$ receptors is modulated by a wide variety of pharmacological agents including convulsants, anticonvulsants, sedatives, anxiolytics, and anesthetics.[98] The effects of these various drugs on $GABA_A$ receptor function varies across brain regions and cell types. The following section briefly reviews the effects of anesthetics on $GABA_A$ receptor function.

Barbiturates, anesthetic steroids, benzodiazepines, propofol, etomidate, and the volatile anesthetics all modulate $GABA_A$ receptor function.[59,98–101] These drugs produce three kinds of effects on the electrophysiological behavior of the $GABA_A$ receptor channels: potentiation, direct gating, and inhibition. *Potentiation* refers to the ability of anesthetics to increase markedly the current elicited by low concentrations of GABA, but to produce no increase in the current elicited by a maximally effective concentration of GABA.[85,102] Potentiation is illustrated in Fig. 6-5, showing the effects of halothane on currents elicited by a range of GABA concentrations in dissociated cortical neurons. Anesthetic potentiation of $GABA_A$

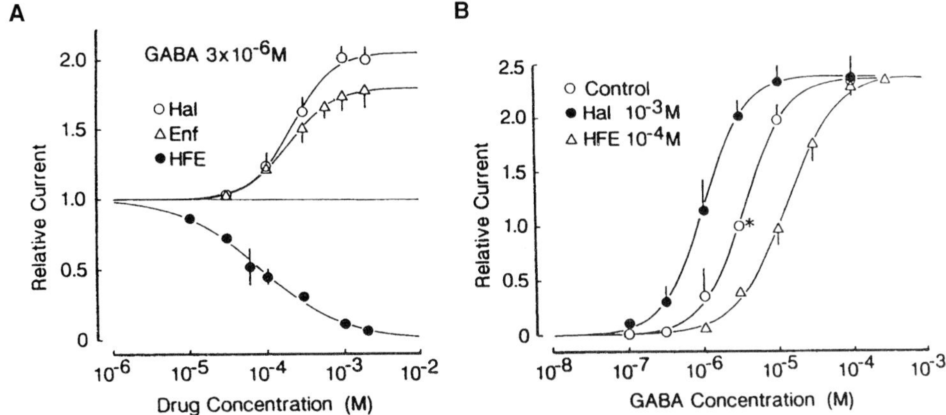

FIGURE 6-5. The effects of halothane (Hal), enflurane (Enf), and fluorothyl (HFE) on GABA-activated chloride currents in dissociated rat CNS neurons. **(Panel A)** Clinical concentrations of halothane and enflurane potentiate the ability of GABA to elicit a chloride current. The convulsant fluorothyl antagonizes the effects of GABA. **(Panel B)** GABA causes a concentration-dependent activation of a chloride current. Halothane shifts the GABA concentration-response curve to the left (increases the apparent affinity of the channel for GABA) whereas fluorothyl shifts the curve to the right (decreases the apparent affinity of the channel for GABA). (Reproduced with permission from Wakamori M, Ikemoto Y, Akaike N. Effects of two volatile anesthetics and a volatile convulsant on the excitatory and inhibitory amino acid responses in dissociated CNS neurons of the rat. *J Neurophysiol.* 1991;66:2014.)

currents generally occurs at concentrations of anesthetics within the clinical range. *Direct gating* refers to the ability of anesthetics to activate $GABA_A$ channels in the absence of GABA. Generally, direct gating of $GABA_A$ currents occurs at anesthetic concentrations higher than those used clinically, but the concentration-response curves for potentiation and for direct gating can overlap. It is not known whether direct gating of $GABA_A$ channels is either required for or contributes to the effects of anesthetics on GABA-mediated inhibitory synaptic transmission in vivo. In the case of anesthetic steroids, strong evidence indicates that potentiation, rather than direct gating of $GABA_A$ currents, is required for producing anesthesia.[103] Anesthetics can also inhibit GABA-activated currents. *Inhibition* refers to the ability of anesthetics to prevent GABA from initiating current flow through $GABA_A$ channels and has generally been observed at high concentrations of both GABA and anesthetic.[104,105] Inhibition of $GABA_A$ channels may help to explain why volatile anesthetics have, in some cases, been observed to inhibit rather than facilitate inhibitory synaptic transmission.[32]

Effects of anesthetics have also been observed on the function of single $GABA_A$ channels. These studies show that barbiturates,[99] propofol,[101] and volatile anesthetics[106] do not alter the conductance (rate at which ions traverse the open channel) of the channel, but that they increase the frequency with which the channel opens and/or the average length of time that the channel remains open. Collectively, the whole cell and single channel data are most consistent with the idea that clinical concentrations of anesthetics produce a change in the conformation of $GABA_A$ receptors that increases the affinity of the receptor for GABA. This is consistent with the ability of anesthetics to increase the duration of inhibitory postsynaptic potentials (IPSPs), because higher affinity binding of GABA would slow the dissociation of GABA from postsynaptic $GABA_A$ channels. It would not be expected that anesthetics would increase the peak amplitude of a GABAergic IPSP because synaptically released GABA probably reaches very high concentrations in the synapse. Higher concentrations of anesthetics can produce additional effects, either directly activating or inhibiting $GABA_A$ channels. Consistent with these ideas, a study by Banks and Pearce showed that isoflurane and enflurane simultaneously increased the duration and decreased the amplitude of GABAergic inhibitory postsynaptic currents in hippocampal slices.[107]

Despite the similar effects of many anesthetics on $GABA_A$ receptor function, there is significant evidence that the various anesthetics do not act by binding to a single common binding site on the channel protein. First, even anesthetics that directly activate the channel probably do not bind to the GABA binding site. This is most clearly demonstrated by molecular biologic studies in which the GABA binding site is eliminated from the channel protein but pentobarbital can still activate the channel.[108] Direct radioligand binding studies have demonstrated that benzodiazepines bind to the $GABA_A$ receptor at nanomolar concentrations and that other anesthetics can modulate binding but do not bind directly to the benzodiazepine site.[98,109] A series of more complex studies examining the interactions between barbiturates, anesthetic steroids, and benzodiazepines indicates that these three classes of drugs cannot be acting at the same sites.[98] The actions of anesthetics on $GABA_A$ receptors are further complicated by the observation that steroid anesthetics can produce different effects on $GABA_A$ receptors in different brain regions.[110] This suggests the possibility that the specific subunit composition of a $GABA_A$ receptor may encode pharmacological selectivity. This is well illustrated by benzodiazepine sensitivity, which requires the presence of the γ_2 subunit subtype.[111] Similarly, sensitivity to etomidate has been shown to require the presence of a β_2 or β_3 subunit.[112] More recently, it has been shown that the presence of a δ or ε subunit in a $GABA_A$ receptor confers insensitivity to the potentiating effects of some anesthetics.[113,114]

Interestingly, $GABA_A$ receptors composed of ρ-type subunits (referred to as $GABA_C$ receptors) have been shown to be inhibited rather than potentiated by volatile anesthetics.[115] This property has been exploited, using molecular biologic techniques, by constructing chimeric receptors composed of part of the ρ receptor coupled to part of an α, β, or glycine receptor subunit. By screening these chimeras for anesthetic sensitivity, regions of the α, β, and glycine subunits responsible for anesthetic sensitivity have been identified. Based on the results of these chimeric studies, site-directed mutagenesis studies were performed to identify the specific amino acids responsible for conferring anesthetic sensitivity. These studies revealed two critical amino acids, near the extracellular regions of transmembrane domains 2 and 3 (TM2, TM3) of the glycine and $GABA_A$ receptors that are required for volatile anesthetic potentiation of agonist effect.[116] It is not yet clear if these amino acids represent a volatile anesthetic binding site, or whether they are sites critical to transducing anesthetic-induced conformational changes in the receptor molecule. Interestingly, one of the amino acids shown to be critical to volatile anesthetic effect (TM3 site) has also been shown to be required (in the β_2/β_3 subunit) for the potentiating effects of etomidate.[117] In contrast, the TM2 and TM3 sites do not appear to be required for the actions of propofol, barbiturates, or neurosteroids.[118] Interestingly, a distinct amino acid in the TM3 region of the β_1 subunit of the $GABA_A$ receptor has been shown to selectively modulate the ability of propofol to potentiate GABA agonist effects.[118] Collectively, these molecular biologic data provide strong evidence that there are multiple unique binding sites for anesthetics on the $GABA_A$ receptor protein.

Other Ligand-Activated Ion Channels

Other members of the ligand-gated receptor superfamily include the nicotinic acetylcholine receptors (muscle and neuronal types), glycine receptors, and 5-HT_3 receptors. A large body of work has gone into examining the effects of anesthetics on nicotinic acetylcholine receptors. The muscle type of nicotinic receptor has been shown to be inhibited by anesthetic concentrations in the clinical range[119] and to be desensitized by higher concentrations of anesthetics.[120] The muscle nicotinic receptor is an informative model to study because of its abundance and the wealth of knowledge about its structure. It is, however, not expressed in the central nervous system and hence not involved in the mechanism of anesthesia. However, a neuronal type of nicotinic receptor, which is widely expressed in the nervous system, might plausibly be involved in anesthetic mechanisms. Older studies looking at neuronal nicotinic receptors in molluscan neurons[121] and in bovine chromaffin cells[122] indicate that these channels are inhibited by clinical concentrations of volatile anesthetics. More recent studies using cloned and expressed neuronal nicotinic receptor subunits have shown a high degree of subunit and anesthetic selectivity. Acetylcholine-elicited currents are inhibited, in receptors composed of various combinations of α_2, α_4, β_2, and β_4 subunits, by *subanesthetic* concentrations of halothane[123] or isoflurane.[124] In contrast, these receptors are relatively insensitive to propofol. Most interestingly, receptors composed of α_7 subunits are completely insensitive to both isoflurane and propofol.[124,125] Subsequent pharmacological experiments using selective inhibitors of neuronal nicotinic receptors led to the conclusion that these receptors are unlikely to have a major role in immobilization by volatile anesthetics.[126,127] However, they might play a role in the amnestic or hypnotic effects of volatile anesthetics.[128]

Glycine is an important inhibitory neurotransmitter, particularly in the spinal cord and brainstem. The glycine receptor is a member of the ligand-activated channel superfamily that, like the $GABA_A$ receptor, is a chloride-selective ion channel. A large number of studies have shown that clinical concentrations of volatile anesthetics potentiate glycine-activated currents in intact neurons[85] and in cloned glycine receptors expressed in oocytes.[129,130] The volatile anesthetics appear to produce their potentiating effect by increasing the affinity of the receptor for glycine.[130] Propofol,[101] alphaxalone, and pentobarbital also potentiate glycine-activated currents, whereas etomidate and ketamine do not.[129] Potentiation of glycine receptor function may contribute to the anesthetic action of volatile anesthetics and some parenteral anesthetics. 5-HT_3 receptors are also members of the genetically related superfamily of ligand-gated receptor channels. Clinical concentrations of volatile anesthetics potentiate currents activated by 5-hydroxytryptamine in intact cells[131] and in cloned receptors expressed in oocytes.[132] In contrast, thiopental inhibits 5-HT_3 receptor currents[131] and propofol is without effect on these receptor channels.[132] 5-HT_3 receptors may play some role in the anesthetic state produced by volatile anesthetics and may also contribute to some unpleasant anesthetic side effects such as nausea and vomiting.

Summary

Several ligand-gated ion channels are modulated by clinical concentrations of anesthetics. Ketamine, N_2O, and xenon inhibit NMDA-type glutamate receptors, and this effect may play a major role in their mechanism of action. A large body of evidence shows that clinical concentrations of many anesthetics potentiate GABA-activated currents in the central nervous system. This suggests that $GABA_A$ receptors are a probable molecular target of anesthetics. Other members of the ligand-activated ion channel family, including glycine receptors, neuronal nicotinic receptors, and 5-HT_3 receptors, are also affected by clinical concentrations of anesthetics and remain plausible anesthetic targets.

Anesthetic Effects on Second Messenger–Activated Ion Channels

Ion channels can be activated by ligands present in the cytoplasm as well as by ligands present in the extracellular space. The intracellular ligands that activate these channels are generally chemical second messengers, including cyclic nucleotides, Ca^{2+} or H^+ ions, inositol phosphates, and ATP. The structure of second messenger–activated ion channels is not as well understood as that of the voltage- or ligand-activated channels, and there is little information about anesthetic effects on these channels.

A potassium-selective channel (referred to as $I_{K(an)}$), found in snail neurons, that has many of the properties of a second messenger–activated channel is activated by clinical concentrations of volatile anesthetics.[121,133,134] $I_{K(AN)}$ shares many biophysical properties with a second messenger–activated potassium channel found in *Aplysia* neurons that is referred to as the S channel. Recent work by Yost and colleagues has shown that the S channel is also activated by clinical concentrations of volatile anesthetics.[135] The importance of volatile anesthetic activation of second messenger–activated potassium channels in invertebrates has now become apparent with the discovery of a large family of so-called "background potassium channels" in mammals. These mammalian potassium channels have a unique structure with two pore-forming domains in tandem plus four transmembrane segments (2P/4TM; Fig. 6-6C).[136] TOK1, a member of this family, was first shown by Yost and colleagues to be activated by volatile anesthetics.[137] The laboratory of Michel Lazdunski has studied the effects of a variety of volatile anesthetics on several members of the 2P/4TM family. They found that TREK-1 channels were activated by clinical concentrations of chloroform, diethyl ether, halothane, and isoflurane (Fig. 6-6B). In contrast, closely related TRAAK channels were insensitive to all the volatile anesthetics, and TASK channels were activated by halothane and isoflurane, inhibited by diethyl ether, and unaffected by chloroform. These authors went on to show that the C-terminal regions of TASK and TREK-1 contained amino acids essential for anesthetic actions

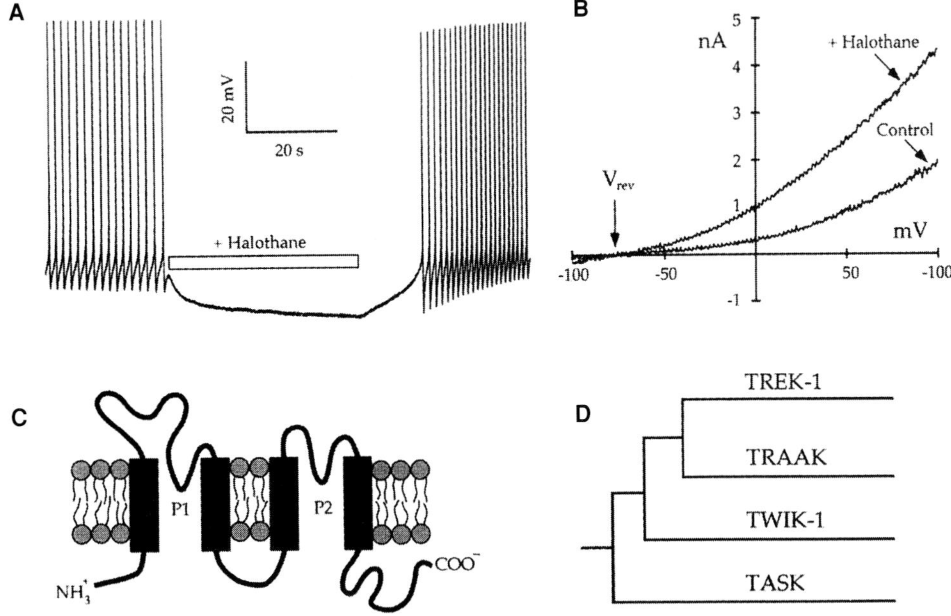

FIGURE 6-6. Volatile anesthetics activate background K^+ channels. (**Panel A**) Halothane reversibly hyperpolarizes a pacemaker neuron from *Lymnaea stagnalis* (the pond snail) by activating I_{Kan}. (**Panel B**) Halothane (300 μM) activates human recombinant TREK-1 channels expressed in COS cells. The figure shows current–voltage relationships with reversal potential (V_{rev}) of −88 mV, indicative of a K^+ channel. (**Panel C**) Predicted structure of a typical subunit of the mammalian background K^+ channels. Note the four transmembrane spanning segments *(in black)* and the two pore-forming domains (P1 and P2). Some but not all of these 2P/4TM K^+ channels are activated by volatile anesthetics. (**Panel D**) Phylogenetic tree for the 2P/4TM family. (Reproduced with permission from Franks NP, Lieb WR. Background K^+ channels: An important target for anesthetics? *Nature Neurosci.* 1999;2:395.)

on TASK and TREK-1 channels.[138] More recently, TREK-1 but not TASK was found to be activated by clinical concentrations of the gaseous anesthetics—xenon, nitrous oxide, and cyclopropane.[139] Thus, activation of background K^+ channels in mammalian vertebrates could be an important and general mechanism through which inhalational anesthetics regulate neuronal resting membrane potential and thereby excitability; this effect could plausibly be a significant contributor to some components of the anesthetic state.

One type of second messenger–activated channel, the calcium-dependent potassium channels, has been shown to be inhibited by clinical concentrations of anesthetics.[140] These large conductance potassium channels open in response to increases in cytoplasmic Ca^{2+} concentration and are important in modulating the shape and frequency of action potentials in the central nervous system. While a wide variety of anesthetics inhibit channel opening, this would tend to excite neurons and is thus unlikely to be important in the depressant effects of anesthetics. Anesthetic effects on these channels may contribute to the excitatory effects of low concentrations of anesthetics and to the convulsant properties of some anesthetic agents. Several other potassium-selective ion channels are also activated by second messengers, including ATP-activated channels and channels activated by muscarinic acetylcholine receptors, but the effects of anesthetics on these channels has not been delineated.

Summary

Second messenger–activated ion channels are a plausible target for anesthetic action. Recent evidence suggests that members of the 2P/4TM family of background potassium channels may be important in producing some components of the anesthetic state.

WHAT IS THE CHEMICAL NATURE OF ANESTHETIC TARGET SITES?

The Meyer-Overton Rule

Almost 100 years ago, Meyer and Overton independently observed that the potency of gases as anesthetics was strongly correlated with their solubility in olive oil (Fig. 6-7).[141,142] This observation has significantly influenced thinking about anesthetic mechanisms in two ways. First, because a wide variety of structurally unrelated compounds obey the Meyer-Overton rule, it has been reasoned that all anesthetics are likely to act at the same molecular site. This idea is referred to as the *Unitary Theory of Anesthesia*. Second, it has been argued that since solubility in a specific solvent strongly correlates with anesthetic potency, the solvent showing the strongest correlation between anesthetic solubility and potency is likely to most closely mimic the chemical and physical properties of the anesthetic target site in the CNS. Based on this reasoning, the anesthetic target site was assumed to be hydrophobic in nature.

The Meyer-Overton correlation suffers from two limitations: (1) it only applies to gases and volatile liquids because olive oil/gas partition coefficients cannot be determined for liquid anesthetics; (2) olive oil is a poorly characterized mixture of oils. To circumvent these limitations, attempts have been made to correlate anesthetic potency with water/solvent partition

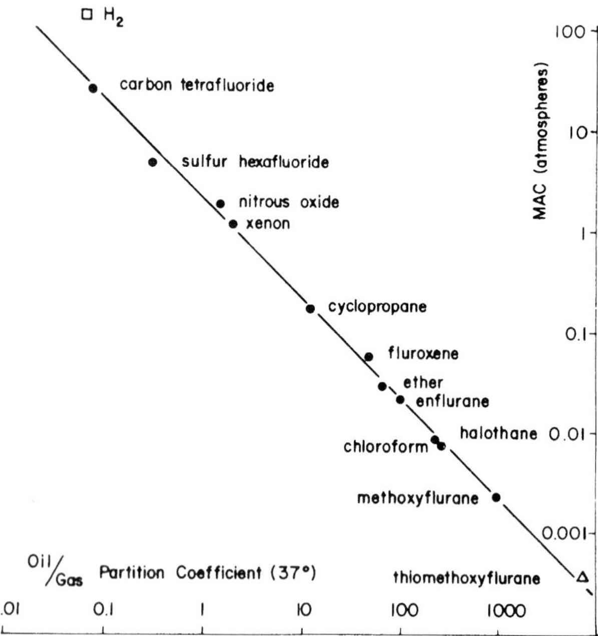

FIGURE 6-7. The Meyer-Overton rule. There is a linear relationship (on a log–log scale) between the oil/gas partition coefficient and the anesthetic potency (MAC) of a number of gases. The correlation between lipid solubility and MAC extends over a 70,000-fold difference in anesthetic potency. (Reproduced with permission from Tanfiuji Y, Eger EI, Terrell RC. Some characteristics of an exceptionally potent inhaled anesthetic: thiomethoxyflurane. *Anesth Analg.* 1977;56:387.)

coefficients. To date, the octanol/water partition coefficient best correlates with anesthetic potency. This correlation holds for a variety of classes of anesthetics and spans a 10,000-fold range of anesthetic potencies.[143] The properties of the solvent octanol suggest that the anesthetic site is likely to be amphipathic, having both polar and nonpolar characteristics.

Exceptions to the Meyer-Overton Rule

Halogenated compounds exist that are structurally similar to the inhaled anesthetics yet are convulsants rather than anesthetics.[144] There are also convulsant barbiturates[145] and neurosteroids.[146] One convulsant compound, fluorothyl (hexafluorodiethylether), has been shown to cause seizures in 50% of mice at 0.12 vol%, but to produce anesthesia at higher concentrations (EC_{50} = 1.22 vol%).[147] The concentration of fluorothyl required to produce anesthesia is approximately predicted by the Meyer-Overton rule. In contrast, several polyhalogenated alkanes have been identified that are convulsants but that do not produce anesthesia. Based on the olive oil/gas partition coefficients of these compounds, anesthesia should have been achieved within the range of concentrations studied.[148] The end point used to determine the anesthetic effect of these compounds was movement in response to a noxious stimulus (MAC). Interestingly, some of these polyhalogenated compounds do produce amnesia in animals.[149] These compounds are thus referred to as *nonimmobilizers* rather than as nonanesthetics. Several polyhalogenated alkanes have also been identified that anesthetize mice, but only at concentrations 10 times those predicted by their oil/gas partition coefficients;[148] these compounds are referred to as *transitional* compounds. The nonimmobilizers and transitional compounds have been proposed as a "litmus test" for the relevance of anesthetic effects observed in vitro to those observed in the whole animal.

In several homologous series of anesthetics, anesthetic potency increases with increasing chain length until a certain critical chain length is reached. Beyond this critical chain length, compounds are unable to produce anesthesia, even at the highest attainable concentrations. In the series of *n*-alkanols, for example, anesthetic potency increases from methanol through dodecanol; all longer alkanols are unable to produce anesthesia.[150] This phenomenon is referred to as the *cutoff effect.* Cutoff effects have been described for several homologous series of anesthetics including *n*-alkanes, *n*-alkanols, cycloalkanemethanols,[151] and perfluoroalkanes.[152] While the anesthetic potency in each of these homologous series of anesthetics shows a cutoff, a corresponding cutoff in octanol/water or oil/gas partition coefficients has not been demonstrated. Therefore, compounds above the cutoff represent a deviation from the Meyer-Overton rule.

A final deviation from the Meyer-Overton rule is the observation that enantiomers of anesthetics differ in their potency as anesthetics. Enantiomers (mirror-image compounds) are a class of stereoisomers that have identical physical properties, including identical solubility in solvents such as octanol or olive oil. Animal studies with the enantiomers of barbiturate anesthetics,[153,154] ketamine,[94] neurosteroids,[103] etomidate,[155] and isoflurane[156] all show enantioselective differences in anesthetic potency. These differences in potency range in magnitude from a >10-fold difference between the enantiomers of etomidate or the neurosteroids to a 60% difference between the enantiomers of isoflurane. It is argued that a *major* difference in anesthetic potency between a pair of enantiomers could only be explained by a protein binding site (see Protein Theories of Anesthesia); this appears to be the case for etomidate and the neurosteroids. Enantiomeric pairs of anesthetics have also been used to study anesthetic actions on ion channels. It is argued that if an anesthetic effect on an ion channel contributes to the anesthetic state, the effect on the ion channel should show the same enantioselectivity as is observed in whole animal anesthetic potency. Early studies showed that the (+)-isomer of isoflurane is 1.5 to 2 times more potent than the (−)-isomer in eliciting an anesthetic-activated potassium current, in potentiating $GABA_A$ currents, and in inhibiting the current mediated by a neuronal nicotinic acetylcholine receptor.[105,121] In contrast, the stereoisomers of isoflurane are equipotent in their effects on a voltage-activated potassium current and in their effects on lipid phase-transition temperature.[121] Studies with the neurosteroids[103] and etomidate[155] show that these anesthetics exert enantioselective effects on $GABA_A$ currents that parallel the enantioselective effects observed for anesthetic potency.

The exceptions to the Meyer-Overton rule do not obviate the importance of the rule. They do, however, indicate that the properties of a solvent such as octanol describe some, but not all, of the properties of an anesthetic binding site. Compounds that deviate from the Meyer-Overton rule suggest that anesthetic target site(s) are also defined by other properties including size and shape.

In defining the molecular target(s) of anesthetic molecules one must be able to account both for the Meyer-Overton rule and for the well-defined exceptions to this rule. It has sometimes been suggested that a correct molecular mechanism of anesthesia should also be able to account for pressure reversal. *Pressure reversal* is a phenomenon whereby the concentration of a given anesthetic needed to produce anesthesia is greatly increased if the anesthetic is administered to an animal under hyperbaric conditions. The idea that pressure reversal is a useful tool for elucidating mechanisms of anesthesia is based on the assumption that pressure reverses the specific physicochemical actions of the anesthetic that are responsible for producing anesthesia; that is to say, pressure and anesthetics act on the same molecular targets. However, recent evidence suggests that pressure reverses anesthesia by producing excitation that physiologically counteracts anesthetic depression, rather than by acting as an anesthetic antagonist at the anesthetic site of action.[157] Therefore, in the following discussion of molecular targets of anesthesia, pressure reversal will not be further discussed.

Lipid vs. Protein Targets

Anesthetics might interact with several possible molecular targets to produce their effects on the *function* of ion channels and other proteins. Anesthetics might dissolve in the *lipid* bilayer, causing physicochemical changes in membrane structure that alter the ability of embedded membrane proteins to undergo conformational changes important for their function. Alternatively, anesthetics could bind directly to *proteins* (either ion channel proteins or modulatory proteins), thus either (1) interfering with binding of a ligand (e.g., a neurotransmitter, a substrate, a second messenger molecule) or (2) altering the ability of the protein to undergo conformational changes important for its function. The following section summarizes the arguments for and against lipid theories and protein theories of anesthesia.

Lipid Theories of Anesthesia

The elucidation of the Meyer-Overton rule suggested that anesthetics interact with a hydrophobic target. To investigators in the early part of the twentieth century, the most logical hydrophobic target was a lipid. In its simplest incarnation, the lipid theory of anesthesia postulates that anesthetics dissolve in the lipid bilayers of biological membranes and produce anesthesia when they reach a critical concentration in the membrane. Consistent with this hypothesis, the membrane/gas partition coefficients of anesthetic gases in pure lipid bilayers correlate strongly with anesthetic potency.[158] This simple theory can account for anesthetics that obey the Meyer-Overton rule, but cannot account for anesthetics that deviate from this rule. For example, the cutoff effect cannot be explained by this theory because compounds above the cutoff can achieve membrane concentrations equal to those of compounds below the cutoff.[159] Similarly, enantioselectivity cannot be explained by this theory. Most importantly, this simplest version of the lipid theory does not explain how the presence of the anesthetic in the membrane is translated into an effect on the function of the embedded proteins.

Membrane Perturbation

More sophisticated versions of the lipid theory require that the anesthetic molecules dissolved in the lipid bilayer cause a change or perturbation in one or more physical properties of the membrane. According to this theory, anesthesia is a function of both the concentration of anesthetic in the membrane and the effectiveness of that anesthetic as a perturbant. This potentially could explain deviations from the Meyer-Overton rule, because nonanesthetics could achieve high concentrations in the membrane, but might not be effective perturbants. In examining this theory it is important to define explicitly the perturbation caused by an anesthetic. One can then test the relevance of a specific perturbation to the mechanism of anesthesia by measuring the perturbation caused by various compounds (anesthetics and nonanesthetics) and correlating perturbation with anesthetic potency. The specific perturbations of membrane structure that have been proposed to be causally related to the anesthetic state are briefly explored in the following section.

Membrane Expansion

Anesthetics dissolved in membranes do increase membrane volume. This occurs both because the anesthetic molecules occupy space and, in principle, because they produce changes in lipid packing and/or protein folding. The *critical volume hypothesis* is an attempt to correlate changes in membrane volume with anesthesia. This hypothesis predicts that anesthesia occurs when anesthetic dissolved in the membrane produces a critical change in membrane volume. Changes in membrane volume could compress ion channels and thus alter their function. Alternatively, increases in membrane thickness could alter neuronal excitability by changing the potential gradient across the plasma membrane.[160] Several studies have shown that anesthetics can produce changes in membrane volume.[161] However, the amount of expansion caused by clinical concentrations of anesthetics is probably very small. One study of erythrocyte membranes showed that halothane (0.27 mM = 1.0 MAC) expanded the membranes by only 0.1%.[162] Another study of erythrocyte membranes showed that both anesthetics and nonanesthetics (long-chain *n*-alkanols above the anesthetic cutoff) produced similar degrees of membrane expansion.[163] While clinical concentrations of anesthetics clearly produce membrane expansion, the small magnitude of anesthetic-induced membrane expansion, coupled with the inability of this theory to account for the cutoff effect, makes it unlikely that membrane expansion is the correct mechanism of anesthesia. A recent study by Cantor revisits this topic.[164] Based on thermodynamic modeling, he argues that anesthetics in biologic membranes preferentially distribute to the interface between lipid and aqueous phases. This distribution results in increased lateral pressure, which could alter the function of membrane-embedded ion channels. His calculations also suggest that nonimmobilizers should not show the same interfacial distribution. There is some experimental evidence showing that anesthetics, but not nonimmobilizers, do preferentially distribute to the lipid/aqueous interface in a membrane.[165] The relationship between these recent observations and anesthetic effects on protein function remains to be determined.

Membrane Disordering

Studies using nuclear magnetic resonance (NMR) spectroscopy[166] and electron spin resonance (ESR) spectroscopy[167] have shown that a variety of anesthetics can disorder the packing of phospholipids in lipid bilayers and in biological membranes. The decrease in membrane order (often referred to as an increase in membrane fluidity) can, in principle, alter the function of ion channels embedded in the lipid bilayer. The ability of anesthetics to fluidize lipid bilayers does show a modest correlation with anesthetic potency.[168] Membrane disordering can also account for the cutoff effect. Studies on synaptic membranes have shown that anesthetic alkanols (octanol, decanol, dodecanol) fluidize membranes, whereas nonanesthetic alkanols have either no effect on fluidity (tetradecanol) or a rigidifying effect (hexadecanol, octadecanol) on the membranes.[169] Unfortunately, the degree of fluidization produced by clinical concentrations of anesthetics is quite small.[168] While it is unclear how much fluidization would be required to affect ion channel function, anesthetics produce changes in membrane fluidity that can be mimicked by changes in temperature of less than 1°C. Clearly, a 1°C increase in temperature does not cause anesthesia, or even increase anesthetic potency. It is highly unlikely that changes in the fluidity of bulk membrane lipid are responsible for general anesthesia.

Lipid Phase Transitions

Another lipid perturbation that has been proposed to account for general anesthesia is a change in lipid phase-transition behavior. In its original version this theory proposed that anesthetics promote a transition of the lipids in neuronal membranes between a solid (gel) phase and a liquid-crystalline phase. Indeed, in pure lipid systems clinical concentrations of anesthetics do decrease the temperature at which such a transition occurs.[170] A second version of this theory, the *lateral phase-separation theory,* proposed that anesthetics *prevent* phase transitions between the liquid-crystalline and the gel phase.[171] According to this theory, liquid-crystalline to gel phase transition is required for normal ion channel function; inhibition of this phase transition causes anesthesia. There is little evidence to support the phase-transition theories. Anesthetic-induced phase changes have not been observed in biologic membranes, lipid phase transitions are not known to be required for normal ion channel function, and the changes in phase-transition temperature observed in pure lipid systems are less than 1°C.

Protein Theories of Anesthesia

6 The Meyer-Overton rule could also be explained by the direct interaction of anesthetics with hydrophobic sites on proteins. Three types of hydrophobic sites on proteins might interact with anesthetics:

1. Hydrophobic amino acids comprise the core of water-soluble proteins. Anesthetics could bind in hydrophobic pockets that are fortuitously present in the protein core.
2. Hydrophobic amino acids also form the lining of binding sites for hydrophobic ligands. For example, there are hydrophobic pockets in which fatty acids tightly bind on proteins such as albumin and the low–molecular-weight fatty acid–binding proteins. Anesthetics could compete with endogenous ligands for binding to such sites on either water-soluble or membrane proteins.
3. Hydrophobic amino acids are major constituents of the α-helices, which form the membrane-spanning regions of membrane proteins; hydrophobic amino acid side chains form the protein surface that faces the membrane lipid. Anesthetic molecules could interact with the hydrophobic surface of these membrane proteins, disrupting normal lipid–protein interactions and possibly directly affecting protein conformation. This last possibility would involve the interaction of many anesthetic molecules with each membrane protein molecule and would probably be a nonselective interaction between anesthetic molecules and *all* membrane proteins.

Direct interactions of anesthetic molecules with proteins would not only satisfy the Meyer-Overton rule, but would also provide the simplest explanation for compounds that deviate from this rule. Any protein-binding site is likely to be defined by properties such as size and shape in addition to its solvent properties. Limitations in size and shape could reduce the binding affinity of compounds beyond the cutoff, thus explaining their lack of anesthetic effect. Enantioselectivity is also most easily explained by a direct binding of anesthetic molecules to defined sites on proteins; a protein-binding site of defined dimensions could readily distinguish between enantiomers on the basis of their different shape. Protein-binding sites for anesthetics could also explain the convulsant effects of some polyhalogenated alkanes. Different compounds binding (in slightly different ways) to the same binding pocket can produce different effects on protein conformation and hence on protein function. For example, there are three kinds of compounds that can bind at the benzodiazepine binding site on the $GABA_A$ channel: *agonists,* which potentiate GABA effects and produce sedation and anxiolysis; *inverse-agonists,* which promote channel closure and produce convulsant effects; and *antagonists,* which produce no effect on their own but can competitively block the effects of agonists and inverse-agonists. By analogy, polyhalogenated alkanes could be inverse-agonists, binding at the same protein sites at which halogenated alkane anesthetics are agonists. The evidence for direct interactions between anesthetics and proteins is briefly reviewed in the following section.

Evidence for Anesthetic Binding to Proteins

One of the initial approaches to probing anesthetic interactions with proteins was to observe the effects of anesthetics on the function of a protein and to try to make inferences about binding from the functional behavior. It is entirely reasonable to assume that direct anesthetic–protein interactions are responsible for functional effects of anesthetics on purified water-soluble proteins because no lipid or membrane is present in the preparations studied. Firefly luciferase is a water-soluble, light-emitting protein, which is inhibited by a wide variety of anesthetic molecules. Numerous studies have extensively characterized anesthetic inhibition of firefly luciferase activity and have revealed the following:[172,173]

1. Anesthetics inhibit firefly luciferase activity at concentrations very similar to those required to produce clinical anesthesia.
2. The potency of anesthetics as inhibitors of firefly luciferase activity correlates strongly with their potency as anesthetics, in keeping with the Meyer-Overton rule.
3. Halothane inhibition of luciferase activity is competitive with respect to the substrate D-luciferin.
4. Inhibition of firefly luciferase activity shows a cutoff in anesthetic potency for both *n*-alkanes and *n*-alkanols.

Based on these studies it can be inferred that a wide variety of anesthetics can bind in the luciferin-binding pocket of firefly luciferase. The fact that anesthetic inhibition of luciferase activity is consistent with the Meyer-Overton rule, occurs at clinical anesthetic concentrations, and explains the cutoff effect suggests that the luciferin-binding pocket may have physical and chemical characteristics similar to those of a putative anesthetic binding site in the CNS.

More direct approaches to study anesthetic binding to proteins have included NMR spectroscopy and photoaffinity labeling. Based on early studies by Wishnia and Pinder, it was suspected that anesthetics could bind to several fatty acid–binding proteins, including β-lactoglobulin and bovine serum albumin (BSA).[174,175] ^{19}F-NMR spectroscopic studies confirmed[176] this, and demonstrated that isoflurane binds to approximately three saturable binding sites on BSA. Isoflurane binding is eliminated by co-incubation with oleic acid, suggesting that isoflurane binds to the fatty acid–binding sites on albumin. Other anesthetics, including halothane, methoxyflurane, sevoflurane, and octanol, compete with isoflurane for binding to BSA.[177] The studies with BSA provide direct evidence that a variety of anesthetics can compete for binding to the same site on a protein. Using this BSA model, it was subsequently shown that anesthetic binding sites could be identified and characterized using a photoaffinity labeling technique. The anesthetic halothane contains a carbon–bromine bond. This bond can be broken by ultraviolet light generating a free radical. That free radical allows the anesthetic to permanently (covalently) label the anesthetic binding site. Eckenhoff and colleagues used ^{14}C-labeled halothane to photoaffinity-label anesthetic binding sites on BSA[178] and obtained results virtually identical to those obtained using NMR spectroscopy. Eckenhoff subsequently has identified the specific amino acids that are photoaffinity-labeled by [^{14}C]halothane.[179] NMR and photoaffinity-labeling techniques have also been applied to several other proteins. For example, saturable binding of halothane to the luciferin-binding site on firefly luciferase has been directly confirmed using NMR and photoaffinity-labeling techniques.[180] Both NMR and photoaffinity-labeling techniques are also being applied to membrane proteins. At the current time these techniques can only be applied to purified proteins available in relatively large quantity. The muscle-type nicotinic acetylcholine receptor is one of the few membrane proteins that can be purified in large quantity. Eckenhoff has used photoaffinity labeling to show that halothane binds to this protein. The pattern of photoaffinity labeling is complex, suggesting multiple binding sites.[181] Most recently, Miller and colleagues have developed a general anesthetic that is an analog of octanol and functions as a photoaffinity label. This compound, 3-diazyrinyloctanol, also binds to specific sites on the nicotinic acetylcholine receptor.[182]

Although NMR and photoaffinity techniques can provide extensive information about anesthetic binding sites on proteins, they cannot reveal the details of the three-dimensional structure of these sites. X-ray diffraction crystallography can provide this kind of three-dimensional detail and has been used to study anesthetic interactions with a small number of proteins. To date, it has been difficult to crystallize membrane proteins; thus, these studies have been limited to water-soluble proteins. In 1965, Schoenborn and colleagues first used x-ray diffraction techniques to examine the interactions of several anesthetics with crystalline myoglobin.[183,184] These studies demonstrated that at a partial pressure of 2.5 atm (xenon MAC = 1 atm), a single molecule of xenon binds to a specific pocket in the hydrophobic core of the myoglobin molecule. The anesthetics cyclopropane and dichloromethane also bind in this pocket, but larger anesthetics do not. It should be noted that xenon occupies a small empty space in the hydrophobic core of myoglobin and that even dichloromethane is a tight fit in this space. These data provided a clear demonstration that anesthetic molecules can bind in the hydrophobic core of a water-soluble protein and that the size of the hydrophobic binding pocket can account for a cutoff in the size of anesthetic molecules that can bind in that pocket. However, myoglobin cannot bind most anesthetic molecules (because of their size) and is therefore not a good model for the actual anesthetic binding site(s) in the central nervous system.

X-ray diffraction has also been used to demonstrate that a single molecule of halothane binds in a hydrophobic pocket deep within the enzyme adenylate kinase.[185] Halothane binding was localized to the binding site for the adenine moiety of AMP (adenine monophosphate), a substrate for adenylate kinase. Consistent with this finding, halothane was found to inhibit adenylate kinase in a manner that is competitive with respect to AMP. Unfortunately, halothane binding to adenylate kinase only occurs at concentrations well beyond the clinically useful range. More recently, firefly luciferase has been crystallized in the presence and absence of the anesthetic bromoform. X-ray diffraction studies of these crystals showed that the anesthetic does bind in the luciferin-binding pocket, as had been inferred from functional studies. Interestingly, two molecules of bromoform bind in the luciferin pocket—one that is likely to compete directly with luciferin for binding and one that is not.[186] The binding data with firefly luciferase and adenylate kinase are of particular interest because they demonstrate that anesthetics can bind to endogenous ligand binding sites and that this binding strongly correlates with anesthetic inhibition of protein function. The same group has also crystallized human serum albumin in the presence of either propofol or halothane. The x-ray crystallographic data demonstrate binding of both anesthetics to preformed pockets that had been shown previously to bind fatty acids.[187] Given that both of these anesthetics bind to serum albumin at clinical concentrations, these data give the best insight yet into the structure of an anesthetic binding pocket.

A recent approach to study anesthetic interactions with proteins has been to employ site-directed mutagenesis of candidate anesthetic targets, coupled with molecular modeling to make predictions about the location and structure of anesthetic binding sites. For example, Harris, Trudell, and colleagues have used this approach to predict the location and structure of the alcohol binding site on $GABA_A$ and glycine receptors.[188] A related approach has been to develop model proteins to define the structural requirements for an anesthetic binding site. Using this approach, Johansson has shown that a four–α-helix bundle with a hydrophobic core can bind volatile anesthetics at concentrations (K_D) similar to those required to produce anesthesia.[189]

Summary

Unequivocal evidence from studies using water-soluble proteins demonstrates that anesthetics can bind to hydrophobic pockets on proteins. Functional and binding studies with firefly luciferase demonstrate that anesthetics can bind to a protein site at clinically relevant concentrations in a manner that can account for the Meyer-Overton rule and deviations from it. Evidence that direct anesthetic–protein-binding interactions may be responsible for anesthetic effects on ion channels in the CNS remains indirect; stereoselectivity currently offers the strongest indirect argument.

Overall, current evidence strongly indicates protein rather than lipid as the molecular target for anesthetic action. While the long-standing controversy between lipid and protein theories of anesthesia may be behind us, numerous unanswered questions remain about the details of anesthetic–protein interactions including:

1. What is the stoichiometry of anesthetic binding to a protein? (i.e., Do many anesthetic molecules interact with a single protein molecule or only a few?)
2. Do anesthetics compete with endogenous ligands for binding to hydrophobic pockets on protein targets or do they bind to fortuitous cavities in the protein?
3. Do all anesthetics bind to the same pocket on a protein or are there multiple hydrophobic pockets for different anesthetics?
4. How many proteins have hydrophobic pockets in which anesthetics can bind at clinically used concentrations?

HOW ARE THE EFFECTS OF ANESTHETICS ON MOLECULAR TARGETS LINKED TO ANESTHESIA IN THE INTACT ORGANISM?

The previous sections have described how anesthetics affect the function of a number of ion channels and signaling proteins, probably via direct anesthetic–protein interactions. It is unclear which, if any, of these effects of anesthetics on protein function are necessary and/or sufficient to produce anesthesia in an intact organism. A number of approaches have been employed to try to link anesthetic effects observed at a molecular level to anesthesia in intact animals. These approaches and their pitfalls are briefly explored in the following section.

Pharmacological Approaches

An experimental paradigm frequently used to study anesthetic mechanisms is to administer a drug thought to act specifically at a putative anesthetic target (e.g., a receptor agonist or antagonist, an ion channel activator or antagonist), then determine whether the drug has either increased or decreased the animal's sensitivity to a given anesthetic. The underlying assumption is that if a change in anesthetic sensitivity is observed, then the anesthetic is likely to act via an action on the specific target of the administered drug. This is a largely flawed strategy that has nonetheless produced a huge literature. The drugs used to modulate anesthetic sensitivity usually have their own direct effects on central nervous system excitability and thus *indirectly* affect anesthetic requirements. For example, while α_2-adrenergic agonists decrease halothane MAC,[190] they are profound CNS depressants in their own right and produce anesthesia by mechanisms distinct from those used by volatile anesthetics. Thus, the "MAC-sparing" effects of α_2-agonists provide little insight into how halothane works. A more useful pharmacological strategy would be to identify drugs that have no effect on CNS excitability but prevent the effects of given anesthetics. Currently, however, there are no such anesthetic antagonists. Development of specific antagonists for anesthetic agents would provide a major tool for linking anesthetic effects at the molecular level to anesthesia in the intact organism, and might also be of significant clinical utility.

An alternative pharmacological approach is to develop "litmus tests" for the relevance of anesthetic effects observed in vitro. One such test takes advantage of compounds that are nonanesthetic despite the predictions of the Meyer-Overton rule. It is argued that "a site affected by these nonanesthetic compounds is unlikely to be relevant to the production of anesthesia."[148] A similar argument uses stereoselectivity as the discriminator and argues that a site that does not show the same stereoselectivity as that observed for whole animal anesthesia is unlikely to be relevant to the production of anesthesia.[191] Although these tests may be useful, they are very dependent on the assumption that anesthesia is produced via drug action at a *single* site. For example, a nonanesthetic might depress CNS excitability via its actions on an important anesthetic target site while simultaneously producing counterbalancing excitatory effects at a second site. In this case the "litmus test" would incorrectly eliminate the anesthetic site as irrelevant to whole animal anesthesia. This example is quite plausible given the convulsant effects of many of the nonanesthetic polyhalogenated hydrocarbons. Another sort of litmus test is to selectively antagonize the putative anesthetic target so that this target is no longer functional. If anesthetic effects are mediated through this target, inactivation of the target by the antagonist should result in anesthetic resistance. Using this logic, the MAC-sparing effects of $GABA_A$ and glycine receptor antagonists were used to argue that both $GABA_A$ and glycine receptors mediate some but not all of the immobilizing effects of volatile anesthetics in rodents.[192,193] This same group used the lack of effect of neuronal nicotinic antagonists on isoflurane MAC to conclude that these receptors had no role in volatile anesthetic immobilization.[127] As with many pharmacological results, the issues of specificity and efficacy of the antagonists prevent these experiments from being definitive. Nevertheless, these results are consistent with the findings that volatile anesthetics affect the function of a large number of important neuronal proteins and no one target is likely to mediate all of the effects of these drugs.

Genetic Approaches

7 An alternative approach to study the relationship between anesthetic effects observed in vitro and whole animal anesthesia is to alter the structure of putative anesthetic targets and determine how this affects whole animal anesthetic sensitivity. Genetic techniques provide the most reliable and versatile methods for changing the structure of putative anesthetic targets. Toward this end, a variety of approaches have been taken that can be methodologically categorized as selective breeding, forward genetics, and reverse genetics. Selective breeding makes use of existing genetic variance among strains that are presumably because of differences in multiple genes and attempts to breed and select for enhanced differences in the trait of interest—in this case general anesthetic sensitivity. Koblin and colleagues have successfully used this strategy to breed two strains of mice (HI and LO) that differ in their sensitivity to N_2O by almost 1.0 atm.[194] A similar strategy has been used to breed mice that have differential sensitivity to the hypnotic effects of the benzodiazepine, diazepam. The two strains of mice (DR and DS) show some modest, but consistent, differences in their sensitivity to volatile anesthetics.[195] Both sets of strains have differences in sensitivities to drugs other than general anesthetics;[196] thus, it seems likely that the genetic differences in these strains may be more general differences in brain function/excitability rather than specific differences in an anesthetic target. Nevertheless, the HI/LO and DS/DR strains demonstrated that in principle genes controlling anesthetic sensitivity, perhaps encoding anesthetic targets, could be discovered. These strains have not led as yet to the identification of the responsible genetic loci. Even under the best of circumstances, mapping genes to the point of their identification in mice is exceedingly difficult, time-consuming, and expensive. In the particular cases of mapping the anesthetic sensitivity loci in these strains, the task is made even more difficult because the phenotype being mapped requires special testing and there is overlap in anesthetic sensitivity between the strains. Further, at least for the HI/LO strains, multiple genetic loci are contributing to the differences in anesthetic sensitivity.[196] Multiple loci are much more complex to identify because typically the contribution of each to the phenotype is small and therefore easily lost in the environmental noise. Forward genetics refers to the classical approach of starting from a phenotype of interest, for example, altered anesthetic sensitivity, and moving "forward" ultimately to identify the gene of interest. Strictly speaking, selective breeding is one form of forward genetics although it rarely proceeds all the way to identification of the genes responsible for the phenotype. More commonly, forward genetics involves inducing random mutations throughout the genome of a pool of animals, then identifying the rare individual that carries a mutation producing the phenotype of interest. This approach requires screening through large numbers of animals and can be effectively accomplished only in lower organisms with a large number of offspring and short generation times. This typically means invertebrate models such as the fruit fly or nematode.

The first true forward genetic screen for mutants with altered general anesthetic sensitivity was performed in the nematode *C. elegans* by Phil Morgan and Margaret Sedensky.[197,198] They screened for altered sensitivity to supraclinical concentrations of halothane. High halothane concentrations were used because they are required to immobilize *C. elegans*. The first mutant isolated had a three-fold reduction in its EC_{50} for halothane. Interestingly, this mutant was hypersensitive to chloroform, methoxyflurane, and thiomethoxyflurane but not to less lipophilic anesthetics such as isoflurane and enflurane.[198] This selective hypersensitivity argues that a generalized nervous system dysfunction is unlikely to account for the halothane hypersensitivity. The mutation was genetically mapped and found to be a loss-of-function allele of the *unc-79* gene, which encodes a neuronal protein that is most similar in amino acid sequence to a large human protein encoded by a gene on chromosome 14.[199] The cellular function of either the *C. elegans* or human protein is unknown. To attempt to understand the function of *unc-79*, a search for mutations that return the halothane hypersensitivity of the *unc-79* mutants toward normal levels was undertaken. Mutations in genes encoding stomatin-like proteins, an integral membrane protein first identified in erythrocytes, were found to suppress *unc-79*.[200] Genetic evidence suggested that the *C. elegans* stomatins might control halothane sensitivity by regulating the function of a mechanically gated sodium channel.[201] Additional mutant screens identified a gene, called *gas-1*, which encodes a highly conserved mitochondrial protein functioning in the electron transport chain.[202] *gas-1* mutants were hypersensitive to all halogenated volatile anesthetics tested. The mechanistic relationship between *gas-1* and *unc-79* and its suppressors genes is unclear.

Clinical concentrations of volatile anesthetics do not immobilize *C. elegans*, but they do produce behavioral effects including loss of coordinated movement.[203] Crowder and colleagues have screened for mutants that are resistant to anesthetic-induced uncoordination and found that mutations in a set of genes encoding proteins regulating neurotransmitter release control anesthetic sensitivity. The gene with the largest effect encoded syntaxin 1A, a neuronal protein highly conserved from *C. elegans* to humans and essential for fusion of neurotransmitter vesicles with the presynaptic membrane.[54] Importantly some syntaxin mutations produced hypersensitivity to volatile anesthetics while others conferred resistance. These allelic differences in anesthetic sensitivity could not be accounted for by effects on the process of transmitter release itself;[54,55] rather, the genetic data argued that syntaxin interacts with a protein critical for volatile anesthetic action, perhaps an anesthetic target. This putative target has not yet been identified.

In *Drosophila*, clinical concentrations of volatile anesthetics disrupt negative geotaxis behavior and response to a noxious light or heat stimulus.[204–206] Using one or more of these anesthetics effects, Nash and colleagues performed a forward genetic screen for halothane resistance. Several *har* (*ha*lothane *r*esistance) mutants were isolated. One set of mutants, *har38* and *har85*, was found to have mutations in a gene encoding a putative cation channel with predicted structural similarities to both sodium and calcium channels.[207] Interestingly, halothane was shown to reduce glutamatergic transmission at the Drosophila larval neuromuscular junction, most likely by inhibiting glutamate release, and the *har38* and *har85* mutants were resistant to this presumed presynaptic halothane action.[208] As the identification of the syntaxin mutants suggested in *C. elegans*, this result suggests that inhibition of excitatory neurotransmitter release may be a consequential action of volatile anesthetics in disrupting behavior in *Drosophila*.

At anesthetic concentrations 1.5- to 2-fold higher than MAC, volatile anesthetics ablate response of *Drosophila* to touch.[209] Using this anesthetic end point, Gamo and colleagues have extensively screened for *Drosophila* mutants with altered sensitivity to diethyl ether. Mutated genes in two of the strains have been identified. A partial-loss-of-function mutation in the α subunit of the major neuronal sodium channel mediating action potentials (*para*) was one of the mutants. This *para* Na^+ channel mutant had about a 50% reduction in its ether EC_{50}.[210,211] A mutation in the *Drosophila* calreticulin gene was also found to produce similar hypersensitivity to ether.[212] Interestingly, this calreticulin mutant was mildly resistant to isoflurane and normally sensitive to halothane. Calreticulin is a highly conserved protein localized to the endoplasmic reticulum of all cell types and is involved in Ca^{2+} buffering and protein folding in the ER.[213] Because of this broad role in cellular function, calreticulin's role in anesthetic sensitivity could be indirect.

As with all model organisms, a critical question to ask is how do the anesthetic mechanisms implicated in nematode and fruit fly relate to mechanisms of anesthesia in humans? Even if a similar gene exists in humans, the evolutionary divergence of the molecules and the very different nervous systems makes the relevance question impossible to answer without additional experiments. Thus, a more practical question is which of the implicated invertebrate genes deserves a potentially more arduous and expensive examination in a vertebrate species? A few criteria seem reasonable. First, is the gene involved in a process known to be affected by general anesthetics in vertebrates? Certainly, the genes in *C. elegans* and *Drosophila* encoding proteins regulating neurotransmitter release and the sodium channel fit this criterion. While mitochondrial electron transport has generally not been implicated in vertebrate anesthetic action, a case report of four children who are hypersensitive to sevoflurane by processed EEG criteria and found to carry defects in the same mitochondrial protein complex implicated in *C. elegans* is an intriguing observation that would likely not have been made without the work in *C. elegans*.[214] Second, is the gene conserved in vertebrates and does it function in the nervous system? In this regard, both the mitochondrial protein and syntaxin 1A are very highly conserved and both function in the nervous system with syntaxin 1A expressed exclusively in neurons; however, for each of these proteins one must explain the enigma of neuron-subtype-specific effects of anesthetics by a protein that functions in all neurons. A third criterion is anesthetic concentration. Do the genes regulate sensitivity to clinical concentrations of anesthetics? However, in this case, some latitude should be given for the possibility that the binding sites on the anesthetic targets are partially diverged and therefore the affinity of the target could be reduced. Certainly, experiments with $GABA_A$ receptors and model anesthetic binding proteins have shown that single amino acid changes can drastically alter anesthetic potency or affinity.[116,215–218] Thus, anesthetic concentration criteria should not be used to exclude mechanisms as is reasonably done in more closely related species such as rodents; rather, the "correct concentration" neither rules in or out the mechanism in question but simply makes it more plausible. Finally, one should keep in mind that even if a particular anesthetic mechanism identified in invertebrates is operant in humans, it may not be the only mechanism of anesthetic action in humans and indeed it may not even be involved in anesthesia at all but rather in anesthetic side effects in other tissues such as myocardium or vascular smooth muscle. Thus, invertebrate genetics should be viewed as a means to pose novel hypotheses, some of which may be compelling enough to test in vertebrates.

Reverse genetics refers to altering the sequence of a known gene and then observing the effects of this mutation on the process of interest. In other words, reverse genetics moves from gene to phenotype as opposed to classical forward genetics that starts with a phenotype and then proceeds to identify the responsible gene(s). Reverse genetics is used typically to test a well-established hypothesis, although occasionally surprising phenotypes produce novel hypotheses. While reverse genetics is employed in both invertebrate and vertebrate models, in terms of anesthetic sensitivity, reverse genetics has been most instructive in mice.

The $GABA_A$ receptor has been extensively studied using reverse genetic techniques.[219] The genes encoding for various subunits of the $GABA_A$ receptor have been mutated so that they are either nonfunctional (gene knockouts) or so that they have altered amino acids that might produce altered function (gene knockins). Knockouts of two α subunits of the $GABA_A$ receptor have been tested for their anesthetic sensitivity. Lack of the $\alpha 1$ subunit was not found to alter sensitivity of the animal to the hypnotic effects of pentobarbital.[220] Similarly, $\alpha 6$ subunit knockout mice were normally sensitive to halothane and enflurane.[221] Knockin mouse strains have been generated for several of the α-subunits, primarily for examining benzodiazepine action. The loss of various aspects of benzodiazepine action in these strains demonstrated that the $\alpha 1$ subunit mediates the sedative and amnestic actions, and is partially required for its anticonvulsant properties. Similarly, the $\alpha 2$ subunit was found to be essential for anxiolysis by diazepam, and $\alpha 3$ and $\alpha 5$ knockin strains were partially resistant to its myorelaxant effects. However, none of these α-subunit knockin strains have been reported to be abnormally sensitive to any complete general anesthetics. In contrast, knockout of the $\beta 3$ subunit produced mice with a markedly decreased sensitivity to the hypnotic action of both midazolam and etomidate and a mildly decreased sensitivity to halothane and enflurane in tail clamp response assays.[222] The interpretation of these data was complicated by a variety of behavioral and neurological abnormalities in these mice that suggested the possibility of an indirect effect of the mutation on anesthetic sensitivity.

In vitro electrophysiological experiments had shown that a specific $\beta 3$ subunit point mutation, $\beta 3$(N265M), blocked the action of etomidate and propofol on the $GABA_A$ receptor without greatly altering receptor function in the absence of drug;[117,223] this result suggested a means to circumvent the problems produced by knocking out $\beta 3$. Thus, a mouse $\beta 3$(N265M) knockin strain was generated and found to be insensitive to the immobilizing effects of etomidate and propofol.[224] However, the $\beta 3$(N265M) mice were not completely resistant to the loss-of-righting reflex by etomidate and propofol, indicating that other targets mediated this behavioral effect. Volatile anesthetic sensitivity was modestly reduced in the $\beta 3$(N265M) mice suggesting that the $\beta 3$ subunit may play some role in their action. A similar approach was taken to show that the $\beta 2$ subunit is critical for the sedating but not anesthetic action of etomidate.[225,226] Finally, strains carrying a knockout mutation of the δ subunit of the $GABA_A$ receptor were found to have a shorter duration of neurosteroid-induced loss-of-righting reflex, whereas their sensitivity was normal to other intravenous and volatile anesthetics.[227] Thus, the δ subunit may play a relatively specific role in neurosteroid action.

Summary

Overall, genetic studies provide a powerful tool for determining which genes and gene products are important in producing anesthesia in an intact organism. Forward genetics has the potential to identify anesthetic mechanisms/targets that may not have been implicated by vertebrate biochemical and electrophysiological studies that are biased toward abundant ion channels. However, particularly for invertebrate genetics, the genetically identified mechanisms may not be operant in humans or may be operant in a different physiological context. Reverse genetics has strengths and weaknesses complementary to those of forward genetics. Reverse genetics rarely generates novel hypotheses or fundamental breakthroughs, but it can confirm definitively the in vivo role of a gene product. Indeed, the demonstration that the action of the general anesthetics etomidate and propofol can be blocked by a single missense mutation in a subunit of the $GABA_A$ receptor is at the same time not surprising and yet one of the most important results thus far in anesthetic mechanism research.

CONCLUSION

8 In this chapter evidence has been reviewed concerning the anatomic, physiologic, and molecular loci of anesthetic action. It is clear that all anesthetic actions cannot be localized to a specific anatomic site in the central nervous system; indeed, some evidence suggests that different components of the anesthetic state may be mediated by actions at disparate anatomic sites. The actions of anesthetics also cannot be localized to a specific physiologic process. While there is consensus that anesthetics ultimately affect synaptic function as opposed to intrinsic neuronal excitability, the effects of anesthetics are dependent on the agent and synapse studied and can affect presynaptic and/or postsynaptic function. At a molecular level, anesthetics show some selectivity, but still affect the function of multiple ion channels and signaling proteins. Although it is likely that these effects are mediated via direct protein–anesthetic interactions, it appears that there are numerous proteins that can

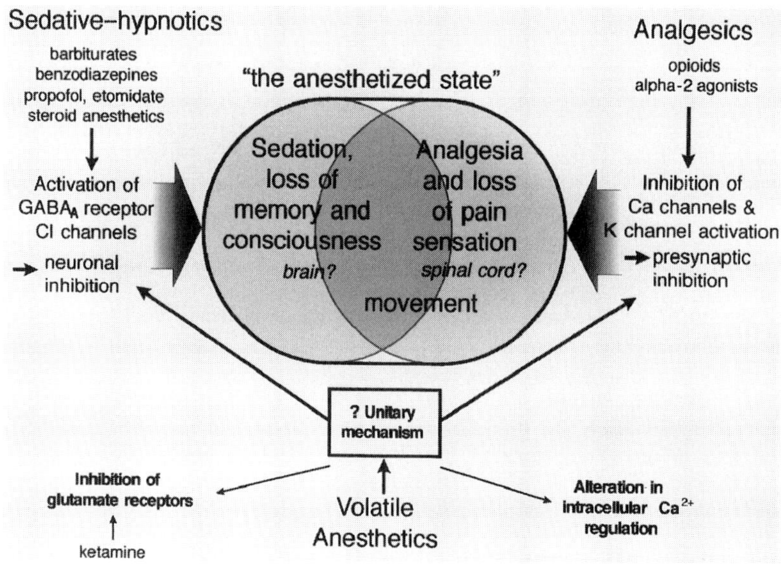

FIGURE 6-8. A multisite model for anesthesia. The model proposes that presynaptic inhibition (Ca^{2+} channel inhibition, K^+ channel activation) is responsible for analgesic effects, whereas postsynaptic $GABA_A$ receptor activation is responsible for sedation and amnesia. As indicated by the overlapping circles, the behavioral effects of Ca^{2+} channel inhibition and $GABA_A$ receptor activation are not mutually exclusive. The model suggests that some anesthetic agents predominantly affect Ca^{2+} and K^+ channels, other anesthetic agents predominantly affect $GABA_A$ receptors, and volatile anesthetics affect both. As illustrated at the bottom of the model, inhibition of glutamate receptor function is an alternative pathway by which ketamine and perhaps the volatile anesthetics produce anesthesia. (Reproduced with permission from Pancrazio JJ, Lynch C. Snails, spiders, and stereospecificity—Is there a role for calcium channels in anesthetic mechanisms? *Anesthesiology.* 1994;81:3.)

directly interact with anesthetics. All of these data suggest that the unitary theory of anesthesia is incorrect and that there are at least several molecular mechanisms of anesthesia.

In keeping with the idea that anesthesia can be produced in a variety of ways, Pancrazio and Lynch have suggested that different anesthetic targets may mediate different components of the anesthetic state.[228] As illustrated in Fig. 6-8, they suggest that the analgesic effects of opiates, α_2-agonists, and volatile anesthetics are mediated *via* inhibition of calcium currents and/or activation of potassium currents. Sedation and amnesia, they propose, are mediated by potentiation or activation of $GABA_A$ receptors. In this model, anesthetic states can also be produced by totally independent mechanisms such as the inhibition of glutamate receptors by ketamine. Although there may be many more important anesthetic targets than those suggested by Pancrazio and Lynch, their proposal illustrates the idea that different molecular targets may mediate the various components of the anesthetic state, and that volatile anesthetics are complete anesthetics because they can interact with several of these molecular targets.

Although the precise molecular interactions responsible for producing anesthesia have not been fully elucidated, it has become clear that anesthetics do act via selective effects on specific molecular targets. The technologic revolutions in molecular biology, genetics, and cell physiology make it likely that the next decade will provide the answers to the century-old pharmacological puzzle of the molecular mechanism of anesthesia.

References

1. Sedensky MM, Meneely PM: Genetic analysis of halothane sensitivity in *Caenorhabditis elegans*. Science 236:952, 1987
2. Quasha AL, Eger EI, Tinker JH: Determination and applications of MAC. Anesthesiology 53:315, 1980
3. White PF, Johnston RR, Eger EI II: Determination of anesthetic requirement in rats. Anesthesiology 40:52, 1974
4. Franks NP, Lieb WR: Molecular and cellular mechanisms of general anesthesia. Nature 367:607, 1994
5. De Jong RH, Nace RA: Nerve impulse conduction and cutaneous receptor responses during general anesthesia. Anesthesiology 28:851, 1967
6. Campbell JN, Raja SN, Meyer RA: Halothane sensitizes cutaneous nociceptors in monkeys. J Neurophysiol 52:762, 1984
7. Antognini JF, Kien ND: Potency (minimum alveolar anesthetic concentration) of isoflurane is independent of peripheral anesthetic effects. Anesth Analg 81:69, 1995
8. Rampil IJ, Mason P, Singh H: Anesthetic potency (MAC) is independent of forebrain structures in the rat. Anesthesiology 78:707, 1993
9. Rampil IJ: Anesthetic potency is not altered after hypothermic spinal cord transection in rats. Anesthesiology 80:606, 1994
10. Antognini JF, Schwartz K: Exaggerated anesthetic requirements in the preferentially anesthetized brain. Anesthesiology 79:1244, 1993
11. Borges M, Antognini JF: Does the brain influence somatic responses to noxious stimuli during isoflurane anesthesia? Anesthesiology 81:1511, 1994
12. Rampil IJ, King BS: Volatile anesthetics depress spinal motor neurons. Anesthesiology 85(1):129, 1996
13. Antognini JF, Carstens E, Buzin V: Isoflurane depresses motoneuron excitability by a direct spinal action: An F-wave study. Anesth Analg 88:681, 1999
14. Zhou HH, Mehra M, Leis AA: Spinal cord motoneuron excitability during isoflurane and nitrous oxide anesthesia. Anesthesiology 86:302, 1997
15. Zorychta E, Esplin DW, Capek R: Action of halothane on transmitter release in the spinal monosynaptic pathway. Fed Proc Am Soc Exp Biol 34:2999, 1975
16. Fujiwara N, Higashi H, Fujita S: Mechanism of halothane action on synaptic transmission in motoneurons of the newborn rat spinal cord *in vitro*. J Physiol 412:155, 1988
17. Kullmann DM, Martin RL, Redman SJ: Reduction by general anaesthetics of group Ia excitatory postsynaptic potentials and currents in the cat spinal cord. J Physiol (Lond) 412:277, 1989
18. Takenoshita M, Takahashi T: Mechanisms of halothane action on synaptic transmission in motoneurons of the newborn rat spinal cord *in vitro*. Brain Res 402:303, 1987
19. French JD, Verzeano M, Magoun HW: A neural basis of the anesthetic state. Arch Neurol Psychiatry 69:519, 1953
20. Angel A: Central neuronal pathways and the process of anaesthesia. Br J Anaesth 71:148, 1993
21. Mori K, Winters WD: Neural background of sleep and anesthesia. Int Anesthesiol Clin 13:67, 1975
22. Darbinjan TM, Golovchinsky VB, Plehotinka SI: The effects of anesthetics on reticular and cortical activity. Anesthesiology 34:219, 1971
23. Thornton C, Heneghan CP, James MF *et al*: Effects of halothane or enflurane with controlled ventilation on auditory evoked potentials. Br J Anaesth 56:315, 1984
24. Feldman SM, Waller HJ: Dissociation of electrocortical activation and behavioral arousal. Nature 196:1320, 1962
25. Nelson LE, Guo TZ, Lu J *et al*: The sedative component of anesthesia is mediated by $GABA_A$ receptors in an endogenous sleep pathway. Nat Neurosci 5:979., 2002
26. Frost EAM: Electroencephalography and evoked potential monitoring. In Saidman LJ, Smith NT (ed): Monitoring in Anesthesia, p 203. Boston, Butterworth-Heinemann, 1993
27. Richards CD, Russel WJ, Smaje JC: The action of ether and methoxyflurane on synaptic transmission in isolated preparations of the mammalian cortex. J Physiol (Lond) 248:121, 1975
28. Nicoll RA: The effects of anaesthetics on synaptic excitation and inhibition in the olfactory bulb. J Physiol (Lond) 223:803, 1972
29. Richards CD, White AN: The actions of volatile anaesthetics on synaptic transmission in the dentate gyrus. J Physiol (Lond) 252:241, 1975
30. MacIver MB, Roth SH: Inhalational anaesthetics exhibit pathway-specific and differential actions on hippocampal synaptic responses *in vitro*. Br J Anaesth 60:680, 1988
31. Gage PW, Robertson B: Prolongation of inhibitory postsynaptic currents by pentobarbitone, halothane and ketamine in CA1 pyramidal cells in rat hippocampus. Br J Pharmacol 85:675, 1985
32. Fujiwara M, Higashi H, Nishi S *et al*: Changes in spontaneous firing patterns of rat hippocampal neurones induced by volatile anaesthetics. J Physiol (Lond) 402:155, 1988
33. Ries CR, Puil E: Mechanism of anesthesia revealed by shunting actions of isoflurane on thalamocortical neurons. J Neurophysiol 81:1795, 1999
34. Franks NP, Lieb WR: Mechanisms of general anesthesia. Environ Health Perspect 87:199, 1990
35. Madison DV, Nicoll RA: General anesthetics hyperpolarize neurons in the vertebrate central nervous system. Science 217:1055, 1982
36. MacIver MB, Kendig JJ: Anesthetic effects on resting membrane potential are voltage-dependent and agent-specific. Anesthesiology 74:83, 1991
37. Larrabee MG, Posternak JM: Selective action of anesthetics on synapses and axons in mammalian sympathetic ganglia. J Neurophysiol 15:91, 1952
38. Langmoen IA, Larsen M, Berg-Johnsen J: Volatile anaesthetics: Cellular mechanisms of action. Eur J Anaesthesiol 12:51, 1995
39. Wu XS, Sun JY, Evers AS *et al*: Isoflurane inhibits transmitter release and the presynaptic action potential. Anesthesiology 100:663, 2004
40. Nicoll RA, Eccles JC, Oshima T *et al*: Prolongation of inhibitory postsynaptic potentials by barbiturates. Nature 258:625, 1975
41. Proctor WR, Mynlieff M, Dunwiddie TV: Facilitatory action of etomidate and pentobarbital on recurrent inhibition in rat hippocampal pyramidal neurons. J Neurosci 6:3161, 1986
42. Collins GG: Effects of the anaesthetic 2,6-diisopropylphenol on synaptic transmission in the rat olfactory cortex slice. Br J Pharmacol 95:939, 1988
43. Harrison NL, Vicini S, Barker JL: A steroid anesthetic prolongs inhibitory postsynaptic currents in cultured rat hippocampal neurons. J Neurosci 7:604, 1987
44. Yoshimura M, Higashi H, Fujita S *et al*: Selective depression of hippocampal inhibitory postsynaptic potentials and spontaneous firing by volatile anesthetics. Brain Res 340:363, 1985
45. Mui P, Puil E: Isoflurane-induced impairment of synaptic transmission in hippocampal neurons. Exp Brain Res 75:354, 1989
46. Perouansky M, Baranov D, Salman M *et al*: Effects of halothane on glutamate receptor-mediated excitatory post-synaptic currents: A patch-clamp study in adult mouse hippocampal slices. Anesthesiology 83:109, 1995
47. Buggy DJ, Nicol B, Rowbotham DJ *et al*: Effects of intravenous anesthetic agents on glutamate release: a role for $GABA_A$ receptor-mediated inhibition. Br J Pharmacol 95:939, 1988
48. Kendall TJ, Minchin MC: The effects of anaesthetics on the uptake and release of amino acid neurotransmitters in thalamic slices. Br J Pharmacol 75:219, 1982
49. Larsen M, Haugstad TS, Berg-Johnsen J *et al*: Effect of isoflurane on release and uptake of gamma-aminobutyric acid from rat cortical synaptosomes. Br J Anaesth 80:634, 1998
50. Collins GGS: Release of endogenous amino acid neurotransmitter candidates from rat olfactory cortex slices: possible regulatory mechanisms and the effects of pentobarbitone. Brain Res 190:517, 1980
51. Murugaiah KD, Hemmings HC Jr: Effects of intravenous general anesthetics on [^{3}H]GABA release from rat cortical synaptosomes. Anesthesiology 89:919, 1998
52. Mantz J, Lecharny JB, Laudenbach V *et al*: Anesthetics affect the uptake but not the depolarization-evoked release of GABA in rat striatal synaptosomes. Anesthesiology 82:502, 1995
53. Westphalen RI, Hemmings HC Jr: Selective depression by general anesthetics of glutamate versus GABA release from isolated cortical nerve terminals. J Pharmacol Exp Ther 304:1188, 2003
54. van Swinderen B, Saifee O, Shebester L *et al*: A neomorphic syntaxin

mutation blocks volatile-anesthetic action in *Caenorhabditis elegans*. Proc Natl Acad Sci USA 96:2479, 1999
55. Hawasli AH, Saifee O, Liu C *et al*: Resistance to volatile anesthetics by mutations enhancing excitatory neurotransmitter release in *Caenorhabditis elegans*. Genetics 168:831, 2004
56. Richards CD, Smaje JC: Anaesthetics depress the sensitivity of cortical neurones to L-glutamate. Br J Pharmacol 58:347, 1976
57. Smaje JC: General anaesthetics and the acetylcholine-sensitivity of cortical neurones. Br J Pharmacol 58:359, 1976
58. Krasowski MD, Harrison NL: General anaesthetic actions on ligand-gated ion channels. Cell Mol Life Sci 55:1278, 1999
59. Jones MV, Brooks PA, Harrison NL: Enhancements of gamma-aminobutyric acid-activated Cl^- currents in cultured rat hippocampal neurones by three volatile anesthetics. J Physiol 449:279, 1992
60. Haydon DA, Urban BW: The effects of some inhalation anesthetics on the sodium current of the squid giant axon. J Physiol 341:429, 1983
61. Haydon DA, Urban BW: The actions of some general anaesthetics on the potassium current of the squid giant axon. J Physiol 373:311, 1986
62. Herrington J, Stern RC, Evers AS *et al*: Halothane inhibits two components of calcium current in clonal (GH_3) pituitary cells. J Neurosci 11:2226, 1991
63. Rehberg B, Xiao YH, Duch DS: Central nervous system sodium channels are significantly suppressed at clinical concentrations of volatile anesthetics. Anesthesiology 84:1223, 1996
64. Ratnakumari L, Hemmings HC Jr: Inhibition of presynaptic sodium channels by halothane. Anesthesiology 88:1043, 1998
65. Shiraishi M, Harris RA: Effects of alcohols and anesthetics on recombinant voltage-gated Na^+ channels. J Pharmacol Exp Ther 309:987, 2004
66. Frenkel C, Duch DS, Urban BW: Effects of i.v. anaesthetics on human brain sodium channels. Br J Anaesth 71:15, 1993
67. Frenkel C, Weckbecker K, Wartenberg HC *et al*: Blocking effects of the anaesthetic etomidate on human brain sodium channels. Neurosci Lett 249:131, 1998
68. Rehberg B, Duch DS: Suppression of central nervous system sodium channels by propofol. Anesthesiology 91:512, 1999
69. Varadi G, Mori Y, Mikala G *et al*: Molecular determinants of calcium channel function and drug action. Trends Pharmacol Sci 16:43, 1995
70. Eskinder H, Rusch NJ, Supan FD *et al*: The effects of volatile anesthetics on L- and T-type calcium channel currents in canine cardiac Purkinje cells. Anesthesiology 74:919, 1991
71. Terrar DA: Structure and function of calcium channels and the actions of anaesthetics. Br J Anaesth 71:39, 1993
72. Hall AC, Lieb WR, Franks NP: Insensitivity of P-type calcium channels to inhalational and intravenous general anesthetics. Anesthesiology 81:117, 1994
73. Study RE: Isoflurane inhibits multiple voltage-gated calcium currents in hippocampal pyramidal neurons. Anesthesiology 81:104, 1994
74. Gundersen CB, Umbach JA, Swartz BE: Barbiturates depress currents through human brain calcium channels studied in Xenopus oocytes. J Pharmacol Exp Ther 247:824, 1988
75. Takenoshita M, Steinbach JH: Halothane blocks low-voltage-activated calcium current in rat sensory neurons. J Neurosci 11:1404, 1991
76. ffrench-Mullen JMH, Barker JL, Rogawski MA: Calcium current block by (−)-pentobarbital, phenobarbital, and CHEB but not (+)-pentobarbital in acutely isolated hippocampal CA1 neurons: Comparison with effects on GABA-activated Cl^- current. J Neurosci 13:3211, 1993
77. Correa AM: Gating kinetics of Shaker K^+ channels are differentially modified by general anesthetics. Am J Physiol 275:C1009, 1998
78. Friederich P, Urban BW: Interaction of intravenous anesthetics with human neuronal potassium currents in relation to clinical concentrations. Anesthesiology 91:1853, 1999
79. Gerstin KM, Gong DH, Abdallah M *et al*: Mutation of KCNK5 or Kir3.2 potassium channels in mice does not change minimum alveolar anesthetic concentration. Anesth Analg 96:1345, 2003
80. Gibbons SJ, Nunez-Hernandez R, Maze G *et al*: Inhibition of a fast inwardly rectifying potassium conductance by barbiturates. Anesth Analg 82:1242, 1996
81. Stadnicka A, Bosnjak ZJ, Kampine JP *et al*: Effects of sevoflurane on inward rectifier K^+ current in guinea pig ventricular cardiomyocytes. Am J Physiol 273:H324, 1997
82. Schofield PR, Darlsion NG, Fujita N *et al*: Sequence and functional expression of a $GABA_A$ receptor shows a ligand-gated receptor super-family. Nature 328:221, 1987
83. Rosenmund C, Stern-Bach Y, Stevens CR: The tetrameric structure of a glutamate receptor channel. Science 280:1596, 1998
84. Seeburg PH: The TiPS/TINS lecture: the molecular biology of mammalian glutamate receptor channels. Trends Pharmacol Sci 14:297, 1993
85. Wakamori M, Ikemoto Y, Akaike N: Effects of two volatile anesthetics and a volatile convulsant on the excitatory and inhibitory amino acid responses in dissociated CNS neurons of the rat. J Neurophysiol 66:2014, 1991
86. Lin L, Chen LL, Harris RA: Enflurane inhibits NMDA,AMPA and kainate-induced currents in *Xenopus* oocytes expressing mouse and human brain mRNA. FASEB J 7:479, 1992
87. Weight FF, Lovinger DM, White G *et al*: Alcohol and anesthetic actions on excitatory amino acid-activated ion channels. Ann N Y Acad Sci 625:97, 1991
88. Dildy-Mayfield JE, Eger EI 2nd, Harris RA: Anesthetics produce subunit-selective actions on glutamate receptors. J Pharmacol Exp Ther 276:1058, 1996
89. Minami K, Wick MJ, Stern-Bach Y *et al*: Sites of volatile anesthetic action on kainate (glutamate receptor 6) receptors. J Biol Chem 273:8248, 1998
90. Aronstam RS, Martin DC, Dennison RL: Volatile anesthetics inhibit NMDA-stimulated ^{45}Ca uptake by rat brain microvesicles. Neurochem Res 19:1515, 1994
91. Lodge D, Anis NA, Burton NR: Effects of optical isomers of ketamine on excitation of cat and rat spinal neurons by amino acids and acetylcholine. Neurosci Lett 29:281, 1982
92. Anis NA, Berry SC, Burton NR *et al*: The dissociative anaesthetics, ketamine and phencyclidine, selectively reduce excitation of central mammalian neurones by N-methyl-aspartate. Br J Pharmacol 79:565, 1983
93. Zeilhofer HU, Swandulla D, Geisslinger G *et al*: Differential effects of ketamine enantiomers on NMDA receptor currents in cultured neurons. Eur J Pharmacol 213:155, 1992
94. Ryder S, Way WL, Trevor AJ: Comparative pharmacology of the optical isomers of ketamine in mice. Eur J Pharmacol 49:15, 1978
95. Mennerick S, Jevtovic-Todorovic V, Todorovic SM *et al*: Effect of nitrous oxide on excitatory and inhibitory synaptic transmission in hippocampal cultures. J Neurosci 18(23):9716, 1998
96. Jevtovic-Todorovic V, Todorovic SM, Mennerick S *et al*: Nitrous oxide (laughing gas) is an NMDA antagonist, neuroprotectant and neurotoxin. Nat Med 4:460, 1998
97. Franks NP, Dickinson R, de Sousa SL *et al*: How does xenon produce anaesthesia? [letter]. Nature 396:324, 1998
98. Macdonald RL, Olsen RW: $GABA_A$ receptor channels. Annu Rev Neurosci 17:569, 1994
99. Macdonald RL, Rogers CJ, Twyman RE: Barbiturate regulation of kinetic properties of the $GABA_A$ receptor channels of mouse spinal neurones in culture. J Physiol 417:483, 1989
100. Barker JL, Harrison NL, Lange GD *et al*: Potentiation of gamma-aminobutyric-acid-activated chloride conductance by a steroid anesthetic in cultured rat spinal neurons. J Physiol 386:485, 1987
101. Hales TH, Lambert JJ: Modulation of the $GABA_A$ receptor by propofol. Br J Pharmacol 93:84P, 1988
102. Parker I, Gundersen CB, Miledi RJ: Actions of pentobarbital on rat brain receptors expressed in *Xenopus* oocytes. J Neurosci 6:2290, 1986
103. Wittmer LL, Hu Y, Kalkbrenner M *et al*: Enantioselectivity of steroid-induced gamma-aminobutyric acid A receptor modulation and anesthesia. Mol Pharmacol 50:1581, 1996
104. Nakahiro M, Yeh JZ, Brunner E *et al*: General anesthetics modulate GABA receptor channel complex in rat dorsal root ganglion neurons. FASEB J 3:1850, 1989
105. Hall AC, Lieb WR, Franks NP: Stereoselective and non-stereoselective actions of isoflurane on the $GABA_A$ receptor. Br J Pharmacol 112:906, 1994
106. Yeh JZ, Quandt FN, Tanguy J *et al*: General anesthetic action on gamma-aminobutyric acid-activated channels. Ann N Y Acad Sci 625:155, 1991
107. Banks MI, Pearce RA: Dual actions of volatile anesthetics on $GABA_A$ IPSCs: Dissociation of blocking and prolonging effects. Anesthesiology 90:120, 1999
108. Amin J, Weiss DS: $GABA_A$ receptors need two homologous domains of the beta-subunit for activation by GABA but not by pentobarbital. Nature 366:565, 1993
109. Tanelian DL, Kosek P, Mody I *et al*: The role of the $GABA_A$ receptor/chloride channel complex in anesthesia. Anesthesiology 78:757, 1993
110. Sapp DW, Witte U, Turner DM *et al*: Regional variation in steroid anesthetic modulation of [^{35}S]TBPS binding to gamma-aminobutyric acid receptors in rat brain. J Pharmacol Exp Ther 262:801, 1992
111. Pritchett DB, Sontheimer H, Shivers BD: Importance of a novel $GABA_A$ receptor subunit for benzodiazepine pharmacology. Nature 338:582, 1989
112. Hill-Venning C, Belelli D, Paters JA *et al*: Subunit-dependent interaction of the general anesthetic etomidate with the gamma-aminobutyric acid type A receptor. Br J Pharmacol 120:749, 1997
113. Zhu WJ, Wang JF, Krueger KE *et al*: Delta subunit inhibits neurosteroid modulation of $GABA_A$ receptors. J Neurosci 16:6648, 1996
114. Davies PA, Hanna MC, Hales TG *et al*: Insensitivity to anaesthetic agents conferred by a class of $GABA_A$ receptor subunit. Nature 385:820, 1997
115. Mihic SJ, Harris RA: Inhibition of rho1 receptor GABAergic currents by alcohols and volatile anesthetics. J Pharmacol Exp Ther 277:411, 1996
116. Mihic SJ, Ye Q, Wick MJ *et al*: Sites of alcohol and volatile anaesthetic action on $GABA_A$ and glycine receptors. Nature 389:385, 1997
117. Belelli D, Lambert JJ, Peters JA *et al*: The interaction of the general anesthetic etomidate with the gamma-aminobutyric acid type A receptor is influenced by a single amino acid. Proc Natl Acad Sci USA. 92:11031, 1997
118. Krasowski MD, Koltchine VV, Rick C *et al*: Propofol and other intravenous anesthetics have sites of action on the gamma-aminobutyric acid type A receptor distinct from that for isoflurane. Mol Pharmacol 53:530, 1998
119. Dilger JP, Vidal AM, Mody HI *et al*: Evidence for direct actions of general anesthetics on an ion channel protein. A new look at a unified mode of action. Anesthesiology 81:431, 1994
120. Firestone LL, Sauter JF, Braswell LM *et al*: Actions of general anesthetics on acetylcholine receptor-rich membranes from *Torpedo californica*. Anesthesiology 64:694, 1986
121. Franks NP, Lieb WR: Stereospecific effects of inhalational general anesthetic optical isomers on nerve ion channels. Science 254:427, 1991

122. Charlesworth P, Richards CD: Anaesthetic modulation of nicotinic ion channel kinetics in bovine chromaffin cells. Br J Pharmacol 114:909, 1995
123. Violet JM, Downie DL, Nakisa RC *et al*: Differential sensitivities of mammalian neuronal and muscle nicotinic acetylcholine receptors to general anesthetics. Anesthesiology 86:866, 1997
124. Flood P, Ramirez-Latorre J, Role L: Alpha 4 beta 2 neuronal nicotinic acetylcholine receptors in the central nervous system are inhibited by isoflurane and propofol, but alpha 7-type nicotinic acetylcholine receptors are unaffected. Anesthesiology 86:859, 1997
125. Evers AS, Steinbach JH: Supersensitive sites in the central nervous system: Anesthetics block brain nicotinic receptors. Anesthesiology 86:760, 1997
126. Wong SM, Sonner JM, Kendig JJ: Acetylcholine receptors do not mediate isoflurane's actions on spinal cord *in vitro*. Anesth Analg 94:1495, 2002
127. Eger II EI, Zhang Y, Laster M *et al*: Acetylcholine receptors do not mediate the immobilization produced by inhaled anesthetics. Anesth Analg 94:1500, 2002
128. Raines DE, Claycomb RJ, Forman, SA. Nonhalogenated anesthetic alkanes and perhalogenated nonimmobilizing alkanes inhibit alpha(4)beta(2) neuronal nicotinic acetylcholine receptors. Anesth Analg 95:573, 2002
129. Mascia MP, Machu TK, Harris RA: Enhancement of homomeric glycine receptor function by long-chain alcohols and anaesthetics. Br J Pharmacol 119(7):1331, 1996
130. Downie DL, Hall AC, Lieb WR *et al*: Effects of inhalational general anaesthetics on native glycine receptors in rat meduallary neurons and recombinant glycine receptors in *Xenopus oocytes*. Br J Pharmacol 118:493, 1996
131. Jenkins A, Franks NP, Lieb WR: Actions of general anaesthetics on 5-HT3 receptors in N1E-115 neuroblastoma cells. Br J Pharmacol 117:1507, 1996
132. Machu TK, Harris RA: Alcohols and anesthetics enhance the function of 5-HT3 receptors expressed in *Xenopus laevis* oocytes. J Pharmacol Exp Ther 271:898, 1994
133. Franks NP, Lieb WR: Volatile general anaesthetics activate a novel neuronal K^+ current. Nature 333:662, 1988
134. Lopes CM, Franks NP, Lieb WR: Actions of general anaesthetics and arachidonic pathway inhibitors on K^+ currents activated by volatile anaesthetics and FMRFamide in molluscan neurones. Br J Pharmacol 125:309, 1998
135. Winegar BD, Yost CS: Volatile anesthetics directly activate baseline S K^+ channels in aplysia neurons. Brain Res 807:255, 1998
136. Franks NP, Lieb WR: Background K^+ channels: An important target for volatile anesthetics? Nat Neurosci 2(5):395, 1999
137. Gray AT, Winegar BD, Leonoudakis DJ *et al*: TOK1 is a volatile anesthetic stimulated K^+ channel. Anesthesiology 88:1076, 1998
138. Patel AJ, Honore E, Lesage F *et al*: Inhalational anesthetics activate two-pore-domain background K^+ channels. Nat Neurosci 2:422, 1999
139. Gruss M, Bushell TJ, Bright DP *et al*: Two-pore-domain K^+ channels are a novel target for the anesthetic gases xenon, nitrous oxide, and cyclopropane. Mol Pharmacol 65:443, 2004
140. Pancrazio JJ, Park WK, Lynch C: Inhalational anesthetic actions on voltage-gated ion currents of bovine adrenal chromaffin cells. Mol Pharmacol 43:783, 1993
141. Overton CE: Studies of Narcosis, 1st ed. London, Chapman and Hall
142. Meyer H: Theorie der alkoholnarkose. Arch Exp Pathol Pharmakol 42:109, 1899
143. Franks NP, Lieb WR: Where do general anaesthetics act? Nature 274:339, 1978
144. Larsen ER: Fluorine compounds in anesthesiology. 1, 1960
145. Andrews PR, Jones JG, Pulton DB: Convulsant, anticonvulsant and anaesthetic barbiturates. In vivo activities of oxo- and thiobarbiturates related to pentobarbitone. Eur J Pharmacol 79:61, 1982
146. Paul SM, Purdy RH: Neuroactive steroids. FASEB J 6:2311, 1992
147. Koblin DD, Eger EI II, Johnson BH *et al*: Are convulsant gases also anesthetics? Anesth Analg 60:464, 1981
148. Koblin DD, Chortkoff BS, Laster MJ *et al*: Polyhalogenated and perfluorinated compounds that disobey the Meyer-Overton hypothesis. Anesth Analg 79:1043, 1994
149. Kandel L, Chortkoff BS, Sonner J *et al*: Nonanesthetics can suppress learning. Anesth Analg 82:321, 1996
150. Alifimoff JK, Firestone LL, Miller KW: Anaesthetic potencies of primary alkanols: Implications for the molecular dimensions of the anaesthetic site. Br J Pharmacol 96:9, 1989
151. Raines DE, Korten SE, Hill WAG *et al*: Anesthetic cutoff in cycloalkanemethanols. A test of current theories. Anesthesiology 78:918, 1993
152. Liu J, Laster MJ, Koblin DD *et al*: A cutoff in potency exists in the perfluoroalkanes. Anesth Analg 79:238, 1994
153. Andrews PR, Mark LC: Structural specificity of barbiturates and related drugs. Anesthesiology 57:314, 1982
154. Richter JA, Holtman JR: Barbiturates: their *in vivo* effects and potential biochemical mechanisms. Prog Neurobiol 18:275, 1982
155. Tomlin SL, Jenkins A, Lieb WR *et al*: Stereoselective effects of etomidate optical isomers on gamma-aminobutyric acid type A receptors and animals. Anesthesiology 88:708, 1998
156. Lysko GS, Robinson JL, Casto R *et al*: The stereospecific effects of isoflurane isomers *in vivo*. Eur J Pharmacol 263:25, 1994
157. Kendig JJ, Grossman Y, MacIver MB: Pressure reversal of anaesthesia: a synaptic mechanism. Br J Anaesth 60:806, 1988
158. Smith RA, Porter EG, Miller KW: The solubility of anesthetic gases in lipid bilayers. Biochim Biophys Acta 645:327, 1981
159. Franks NP, Lieb WR: Partitioning of long-chain alcohols into lipid bilayers: implications for mechanisms of general anesthesia. Proc Natl Acad Sci USA 83:5116, 1986
160. Elliot JR, Haydon DA, Hendry BM *et al*: Inactivation of the sodium current in squid giant axons by hydrocarbons. Biophys J 48:617, 1985
161. Seeman P: The membrane actions of anesthetics and tranquilizers. Pharmacol Rev 24:583, 1972
162. Franks NP: Is membrane expansion relevant to anaesthesia? Nature 292:248, 1981
163. Bull MH, Brailsford JD, Bull BS: Erythrocyte membrane expansion due to the volatile anesthetics, the 1-alkanols, and benzyl alcohol. Anesthesiology 57:399, 1982
164. Cantor RS: The lateral pressure profile in membranes: a physical mechanism of general anesthesia. Biochemistry 36:2339, 1997
165. North C, Cafiso DS: Contrasting membrane localization and behavior of halogenated cyclobutanes that follow or violate the Meyer-Overton hypothesis of general anesthetic potency. Biophys J 72:1754, 1997
166. Metcalfe JC, Seeman P, Burgen ASV: The proton relaxation of benzyl alcohol in erythrocyte membranes. Mol Pharmacol 4:87, 1967
167. Miller KW, Pang KY: General anaesthetics can selectively perturb lipid bilayer membranes. Nature 263:253, 1976
168. Pang KY, Braswell LM, Chang L *et al*: The perturbation of lipid bilayers by general anesthetics: a quantitative test of the disordered lipid hypothesis. Mol Pharmacol 18:84, 1980
169. Miller KW, Firestone LL, Alifimoff JK *et al*: Nonanesthetic alcohols dissolve in synaptic membranes without perturbing their lipids. Proc Natl Acad Sci USA 86:1084, 1986
170. Mountcastle DB, Biltonen RL, Halsey MJ: Effect of anesthetics and pressure on the thermotropic behavior of multilamellar dipalmitoylphosphatidylcholine liposomes. Proc Natl Acad Sci USA 75:4906, 1978
171. Trudell JR: A unitary theory of anesthesia based on lateral phase separations in nerve membranes. Anesthesiology 46:5, 1977
172. Franks NP, Lieb WR: Do general anaesthetics act by competitive binding to specific receptors? Nature 310:599, 1984
173. Franks NP, Lieb WR: Mapping of general anaesthetic target sites provides a molecular basis for cutoff effects. Nature 316:149, 1985
174. Wishnia A, Pinder TW: Hydrophobic interactions in proteins. The alkane binding site of B-lactoglobulins A and B. Biochemistry 5:1534, 1966
175. Wishnia A, Pinder T: Hydrophobic interactions in proteins: Conformation changes in bovine serum albumin below pH 5. Biochemistry 3:1377, 1964
176. Dubois BW, Evers AS: An ^{19}F-NMR spin-spin relaxation (T_2) method for characterizing volatile anesthetic binding to proteins. Analysis of isoflurane binding to serum albumin. Biochemistry 31:7069, 1992
177. Dubois BW, Cherian SF, Evers AS: Volatile anesthetics compete for common binding sites on bovine serum albumin: a ^{19}F-NMR study. Proc Natl Acad Sci USA 90:6478, 1993
178. Eckenhoff RG, Shuman H: Halothane binding to soluble proteins determined by photoaffinity labeling. Anesthesiology 79:96, 1993
179. Eckenhoff RG: Amino acid resolution of halothane binding sites in serum albumin. J Biol Chem 271:15521, 1996
180. Burris KE, Dubois BW, Evers AS: Direct observation of saturable halothane binding to firefly luciferase: a photoaffinity labeling and ^{19}F-NMR study. Anesthesiology 79:A700, 1993
181. Eckenhoff RG: An inhalational anesthetic binding domain in the nicotinic acetylcholine receptor. Proc Natl Acad Sci USA 93:2807, 1996
182. Husain SS, Forman SA, Kloczewiak MA *et al*: Synthesis and properties of 3-(2-hydroxyethyl)-3-n-pentyldiazirine, a photoactivable general anesthetic. J Med Chem 41:3300, 1999
183. Schoenborn BP, Watson HC, Kendrew JC: Binding of xenon to sperm whale myoglobin. Nature 207:28, 1965
184. Schoenborn BP: Binding of cyclopropane to sperm whale myoglobin. Nature 14:1120, 1967
185. Sachsenheimer W, Pai EF, Schulz GE *et al*: Halothane binds in the adenine specific niche of crystalline adenylate kinase. FEBS Lett 79:310, 1977
186. Franks NP, Jenkins A, Conti E *et al*: Structural basis for the inhibition of firefly luciferase by a general anesthetic. Biophys J 75:2205, 1998
187. Bhattacharya AA, Curry S, Franks NP: Binding of the general anesthetics propofol and halothane to human serum albumin. High resolution crystal structures. J Biol Chem 275:38731, 2000
188. Wick MJ, Mihic SJ, Ueno S *et al*: Mutations of gamma-aminobutyric acid and glycine receptors change alcohol cutoff: evidence for an alcohol receptor? Proc Natl Acad Sci USA 95:6504, 1998
189. Johansson JS, Gibney BR, Rabanal F *et al*: A designed cavity in the hydrophobic core of a four-alpha-helix bundle improves volatile anesthetic binding affinity. Biochemistry 37:1421, 1998
190. Segal IS, Vickery RG, Walton JK *et al*: Dexmedetomidine diminishes halothane anesthetic requirements in rats through a postsynaptic alpha 2 adrenergic receptor. Anesthesiology 69:818, 1988
191. Moody EJ, Harris BD, Skolnick P: The potential for safer anaesthesia using stereoselective anaesthetics. Trends Pharmacol Sci 15:387, 1994
192. Zhang Y, Laster MJ, Hara K *et al*: Glycine receptors mediate part of the immobility produced by inhaled anesthetics. Anesth Analg 96:97, 2003
193. Zhang Y, Wu S, Eger EI II *et al*: Neither GABA(A) nor strychnine-sensitive

glycine receptors are the sole mediators of MAC for isoflurane. Anesth Analg 92:123, 2001

194. Koblin DD, Dong DE, Deady JE *et al*: Selective breeding alters murine resistance to nitrous oxide without alteration in synaptic membrane lipid composition. Anesthesiology 52:401, 1980
195. McCrae AF, Gallaher EJ, Winter PM *et al*: Volatile anesthetic requirements differ in mice selectively bred for sensitivity or resistance to diazepam—implications for the site of anesthesia. Anesth Analg 76:1313, 1993
196. Koblin DD, Eger EI II: Cross-mating of mice selectively bred for resistance or susceptibility to nitrous oxide anesthesia: potencies of nitrous oxide in offspring. Anesth Analg 60:646, 1981
197. Morgan PG, Cascorbi HF: Effect of anesthetics and a convulsant on normal and mutant *Caenorhabditis elegans*. Anesthesiology 62:738, 1985
198. Morgan PG, Sedensky MM, Meneely PM, *et al*: The effect of two genes on anesthetic response in the nematode *Caenorhabditis elegans*. Anesthesiology 69:246, 1988
199. Humphrey JA, Sedensky MM, Morgan PG: A novel protein alters sensitivity to specific volatile anesthetics. Anesthesiology 99:A107, 2003
200. Rajaram S, Sedensky MM, Morgan PG: Unc-1: A stomatin homologue controls sensitivity to volatile anesthetics in *Caenorhabditis elegans*. Proc Natl Acad Sci USA 95:8761, 1998
201. Rajaram S, Spangler TL, Sedensky MM *et al*: A stomatin and a degenerin interact to control anesthetic sensitivity in *Caenorhabditis elegans*. Genetics 153:1673, 1999
202. Kayser EB, Morgan PG, Sedensky MM: GAS-1: a mitochondrial protein controls sensitivity to volatile anesthetics in the nematode *Caenorhabditis elegans*. Anesthesiology 90:545, 1999
203. Crowder CM, Shebester LD, Schedl T: Behavioral effects of volatile anesthetics in *Caenorhabditis elegans*. Anesthesiology 85:901, 1996
204. Krishnan KS, Nash HA: A genetic study of the anesthetic response: mutants of *Drosophila melanogaster* altered in sensitivity to halothane. Proc Natl Acad Sci USA 87:8632, 1990
205. Campbell DB, Nash HA: Use of *Drosophila* mutants to distinguish among volatile general anesthetics. Proc Natl Acad Sci USA 91:2135, 1994
206. Campbell JL, Nash HA: The visually-induced jump response of *Drosophila melanogaster* is sensitive to volatile anesthetics. Proc Natl Acad Sci USA 12:241, 1998
207. Nash HA, Scott RL, Lear BC *et al*: An unusual cation channel mediates photic control of locomotion in *Drosophila*. Curr Biol 12:2152, 2002
208. Nishikawa K, Kidokoro Y: Halothane presynaptically depresses synaptic transmission in wild-type *Drosophila* larvae but not in halothane-resistant (har) mutants. Anesthesiology 90:1691, 1999
209. Gamo S, Ogaki M, Nakashima-Tanaki E: Strain differences in minimum anesthetic concentrations in *Drosophila melanogaster*. Anesthesiology 54:289, 1981
210. Gamo S, Dodo K, Matakatsu H *et al*: Molecular genetical analysis of *Drosophila* ether sensitive mutants. Toxicol Lett 100-101:329, 1998
211. Gamo S, Tanaka Y, Yamamoto H *et al*: Ether anesthesia and a sodium channel in *Drosophila melanogaster*. Hiroshima J Anesthesia 28:279, 1992
212. Gamo S, Tomida J, Dodo K *et al*: Calreticulin mediates anesthetic sensitivity in *Drosophila melanogaster*. Anesthesiology 99:867, 2003
213. Gelebart P, Opas M, Michalak M: Calreticulin, a Ca^{2+}-binding chaperone of the endoplasmic reticulum. Int J Biochem Cell Biol 37:260, 2005
214. Morgan PG, Hoppel CL, Sedensky MM: Mitochondrial defects and anesthetic sensitivity. Anesthesiology 96:1268, 2002
215. Jenkins A, Greenblatt EP, Faulkner HJ *et al*: Evidence for a common binding cavity for three general anesthetics within the $GABA_A$ receptor. J Neurosci 21:RC136, 2001
216. Koltchine VV, Finn SE, Jenkins A *et al*: Agonist gating and isoflurane potentiation in the human gamma-aminobutyric acid type A receptor determined by the volume of a second transmembrane domain residue. Mol Pharmacol 56:1087, 1999
217. Manderson GA, Johansson JS: Role of aromatic side chains in the binding of volatile general anesthetics to a four-alpha-helix bundle. Biochemistry 41:4080, 2002
218. Johansson JS, Scharf D, Davies LA *et al*: A designed four-alpha-helix bundle that binds the volatile general anesthetic halothane with high affinity. Biophys J 78:982, 2000
219. Rudolph U, Mohler H: Analysis of $GABA_A$ receptor function and dissection of the pharmacology of benzodiazepines and general anesthetics through mouse genetics. Annu Rev Pharmacol Toxicol 44:475, 2004
220. Blednov YA, Jung S, Alva H *et al*: Deletion of the alpha1 or beta2 subunit of $GABA_A$ receptors reduces actions of alcohol and other drugs. J Pharmacol Exp Ther 304:30, 2003
221. Homanics GE, Ferguson C, Quinlan JJ *et al*: Gene knockout of the alpha6 subunit of the gamma-aminobutyric acid type A receptor: lack of effect on responses to ethanol, pentobarbital, and general anesthetics. Mol Pharmacol 51:588, 1997
222. Quinlan JJ, Homanics GE, Firestone LL: Anesthesia sensitivity in mice that lack the beta3 subunit of the gamma-aminobutyric acid type A receptor. Anesthesiology 88:775, 1998
223. Siegwart R, Jurd R, Rudolph U: Molecular determinants for the action of general anesthetics at recombinant alpha(2)beta(3)gamma(2)gamma-aminobutyric acid(A) receptors. J Neurochem 80:140, 2002
224. Jurd R, Arras M, Lambert S *et al*: General anesthetic actions in vivo strongly attenuated by a point mutation in the $GABA_A$ receptor beta3 subunit. FASEB J 17:250, 2003
225. O'Meara GF, Newman RJ, Fradley RL *et al*: The $GABA_A$ beta3 subunit mediates anaesthesia induced by etomidate. Neuroreport 15:1653, 2004
226. Reynolds DS, Rosahl TW, Cirone J *et al*: Sedation and anesthesia mediated by distinct $GABA_A$ receptor isoforms. J Neurosci 23:8608, 2003
227. Mihalek RM, Banerjee PK, Korpi ER *et al*: Attenuated sensitivity to neuroactive steroids in gamma-aminobutyrate type A receptor delta subunit knockout mice. Proc Natl Acad Sci USA 96(22):12905, 1999
228. Lynch C III, Pancrazio JJ: Snails, spiders, and stereospecificity: Is there a role for calcium channels in anesthetic mechanisms? Anesthesiology 81:1, 1994

CHAPTER 7 ■ GENOMIC BASIS OF PERIOPERATIVE MEDICINE

MIHAI V. PODGOREANU AND JOSEPH P. MATHEW

KEY POINTS

1. *Functional genomics* employs large-scale experimental methodologies and statistical analyses to investigate the regulation of gene expression in response to physiological, pharmacological, and pathological changes.
2. Most of genetic diversity in the population is attributable to widespread DNA sequence variations (*polymorphisms*).
3. Specific genotypes are associated with a variety of organ-specific perioperative adverse outcomes, including neurocognitive dysfunction, renal compromise, vein graft restenosis, postoperative thrombotic complications, vascular reactivity, severe sepsis, transplant rejection, and death.
4. Risk stratification based on clinical, procedural, and biological markers explains only a small part of the variability in incidence of perioperative complications. Specific genotypes may improve prediction of adverse perioperative outcomes in otherwise healthy individuals.
5. Several genes predictive of perioperative vascular response have been identified.
6. Variability in the reported incidence of both early and late neurological deficits remains poorly explained by procedural risk factors, suggesting that environmental (operative) and genetic factors may interact to determine disease onset, progression, and recovery.
7. Genetics polymorphisms are associated with acute renal injury following coronary artery bypass graft (CABG) surgery.
8. Genetic variants in the renin–angiotensin pathway and in proinflammatory cytokine genes have been associated with respiratory complications post-cardiopulmonary bypass.
9. The term "pharmacogenomics" describes how inherited variations in genes modulating drug actions are related to interindividual variability in drug response. Such variability in drug action may be *pharmacokinetic* or *pharmacodynamics*.
10. Malignant hyperthermia (MH) susceptibility results from a complex interaction between multiple genes and environment.
11. A genetic basis for increased anesthetic requirements is beginning to emerge, suggested, for instance, by the observation that desflurane requirements are increased in subjects with red hair versus dark hair.
12. In addition to the genetic control of peripheral nociceptive pathways, considerable evidence exists for genetic variability in the descending central pain modulatory pathways, potentially explaining the interindividual variability in analgesic responsiveness.
13. The large interindividual variability in the magnitude of response to injury, including activation of inflammatory and coagulation cascades, apoptosis, and fibrosis, suggests the involvement of genetic regulatory factors.
14. The standard "single gene" paradigm is insufficient to adequately describe the tissue response to severe systemic stimuli. Instead, organ injury might better be defined by patterns of altered gene and protein expression.

GENETIC BASIS OF DISEASE

Human biological diversity involves interindividual variability in morphology, behavior, physiology, development, susceptibility to disease, response to stressful stimuli and drug therapy (i.e., *phenotypes*). This phenotypic variation is determined, at least in part, by differences in the specific genetic makeup (i.e., *genotype*) of an individual. In 2003, the fiftieth anniversary of Watson and Crick's description of the DNA double helix structure also marked the completion of the Human Genome Project.[1] This major accomplishment provides the discipline of genomics with basic resources to study the functions and interactions of all genes in a systematic fashion, including their interaction with environmental factors, and translate the findings into clinical and societal benefits.
1 *Functional genomics* employ large-scale experimental methodologies and statistical analyses to investigate the regulation of gene expression in response to physiological, pharmacological, and pathological changes. It also uses genetic information from clinical studies to examine the impact of genetic variability on disease characterization and outcome.[2] To integrate this new generation of genetic results into clinical practice, perioperative physicians need to understand the patterns of human genome variation, the methods of population-based genetic investigation, and the principles of gene and protein expression analysis.

Overview of Human Genetic Variation

Although the human DNA sequence is 99.9% identical between individuals, the variations may greatly affect a person's disease risk. In elucidating the genetic basis of disease, much of what has been investigated to date has focused on rare genetic variants (*mutations*) responsible for monogenic disorders such as hypertrophic cardiomyopathy, long-QT syndrome, sickle cell anemia, or familial hypercholesterolemia, which are highly penetrant (carriers of the mutant gene will likely have the disease) and inherited in mendelian fashion (hence,
2 termed mendelian diseases). However, most of the genetic diversity in the population is attributable to more widespread DNA sequence variations (*polymorphisms*), which can be either nucleotide base substitutions (*single nucleotide polymorphisms*, SNPs), short sequence repeats (*microsatellites*), or insertion/deletion of one or more nucleotides (*indels*), and may or may not be associated with a specific phenotype (Fig. 7-1). To be classified as a polymorphism, the DNA sequence alternatives (i.e., *alleles*) must exist with a frequency of at least 1% in the population. About 10 million SNPs are estimated to exist in the human genome, approximately once every 300 base pairs, located in genes as well as in the surrounding regions of the genome. Polymorphisms may directly alter the amino acid sequence and therefore potentially alter protein function, or alter regulatory DNA sequences that modulate protein expression. Sets of nearby SNPs on a chromosome are inherited in blocks, referred to as *haplotypes*. As it will be shown later, haplotype analysis is a useful way of applying genotype information in disease gene discovery.

Many common diseases like atherosclerosis, coronary artery disease, hypertension, diabetes, cancer, asthma and our responses to injury, drugs, and nonpharmacological therapies are genetically complex, characteristically involving an interplay of many genetic variations in molecular and biochemical pathways (i.e., *polygenic*) and genetic-environmental interactions (i.e., *multifactorial*). Therefore, complex phenotypes can be viewed as the integrated effect of many susceptibility genes and many environmental exposures (Fig. 7-2). The proportion

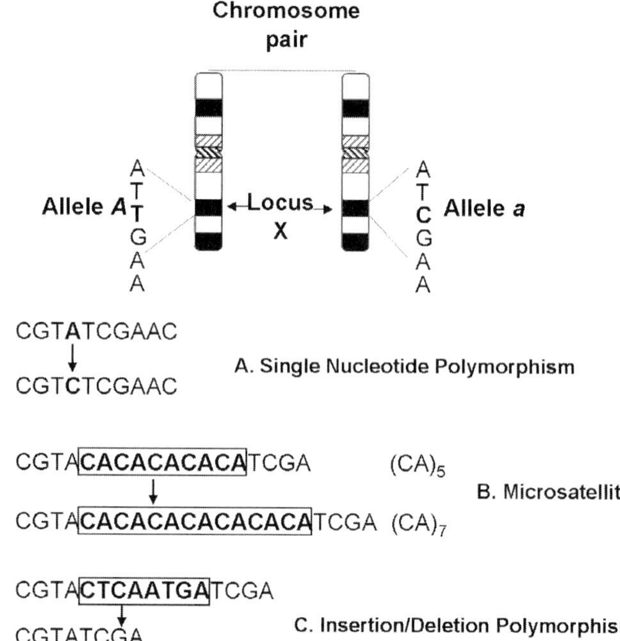

FIGURE 7-1. Categories of genetic polymorphisms. **A.** *Single nucleotide polymorphisms (SNP)* can be silent or have functional consequences ranging from changes in amino acid sequence or premature termination of protein synthesis (if they occur in the coding regions of the gene) to alterations in the expression of the gene, resulting in more or less protein (if they occur in regulatory regions of the gene such as the promoter region or the intron/exon boundaries). **B.** *Microsatellite polymorphism* with varying number of dinucleotide $(CA)_n$ repeats. **C.** *Insertion-deletion polymorphism*. NOTE: *locus*—the location of a gene/genetic marker in the genome; *alleles*—alternative forms of a gene/genetic marker; *genotype*—the observed alleles for an individual at a genetic locus; *heterozygous*—two different alleles are present at a locus; *homozygous*—two identical alleles are present at a locus. An SNP at position 1691 of a gene, with alleles G and A would be written as 1691G>A.

of phenotypic variance that is the result of genetic factors is referred to as *heritability* and can be estimated by examining the increased similarity of a phenotype in related as compared to unrelated individuals. One of the major challenges and ongoing research efforts facing the postgenomic period is to connect the nearly 30,000 protein-coding genes of mammalian organisms to the genetic basis of complex polygenic diseases and the integrated function of complex biological systems. According to the "common-variants/common-disease hypothesis,"[3] it is the common functional polymorphisms that modulate individual susceptibility to common complex diseases and the manifestation, severity, and prognosis of the disease process. In the next section, we review the common strategies used to incorporate genetic analysis into clinical studies.

Genetic Analysis of Complex Disease

Most ongoing research on complex disorders focuses on identifying genetic polymorphisms that enhance susceptibility to given conditions. Often the design of such studies is complicated by the presence of multiple risk factors, gene–environment interactions, and a lack of even rough estimates of the number of genes underlying such complex traits. Two broad strategies are being employed to identify complex trait loci. The *candidate gene* approach is motivated by what is

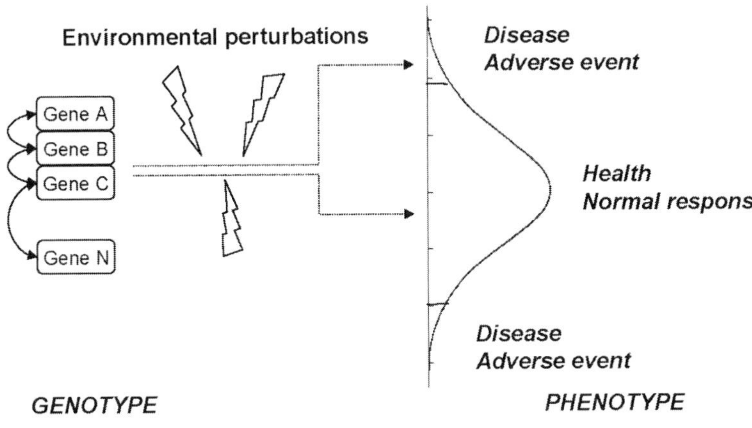

FIGURE 7-2. Common diseases (e.g., coronary artery disease, hypertension, diabetes, cancer) and individual responses to various perturbations (e.g., drug administration, hemodynamic challenge, surgical stress, trauma) are complex, involving multiple gene–gene interactions (*polygenic*) and gene–environment interactions (*multifactorial*) to produce a final clinical outcome, or *phenotype*. In these instances, rather than directly causing the disease, genetic variability may contribute to disease onset and/or progression.

known about the trait biologically and can be characterized as a hypothesis-testing approach. The second strategy is a *genome scan*, in which thousands of markers uniformly distributed throughout the genome are used to locate genomic regions that may harbor genes influencing the phenotypic variability. This is a hypothesis-generating approach, allowing the detection of previously unknown trait loci.[4] Both the candidate gene and genome scan approaches can be implemented using one of two fundamental methods of identifying polymorphisms affecting common diseases: linkage analysis or association studies in human populations.

Linkage Analysis

Linkage analysis is used to identify the chromosomal location of gene variants related to a given disease. This approach has been used successfully to map hundreds of genes for rare, monogenic disorders. However, the nature of complex diseases precludes the use of extended families wherein the same disease allele acts in most affected individuals throughout a pedigree. Rather, in complex disease a multitude of genes with rare and/or common alleles create an apparently chaotic pattern of heterogeneity within and between families. The overall effect of this heterogeneity, together with the potentially weak influence of many loci, places a heavy burden on the statistical power needed to detect individual contributing genes, and may be the reason why very few genome scans so far have yielded disease loci that meet genome-wide significance criteria.[5] However, a few positive findings have emerged using this approach. Combining linkage analysis with advanced molecular genetic techniques, the chromosomal location (5q12) of a gene influencing stroke was identified,[6] and risk of myocardial infarction was mapped to a single region on chromosome 14.[7] Additionally, many determinants of complex cardiovascular and renal function have been mapped in the rat,[8] providing the first rough approximation of genomic regions linked to homeostatic control of sodium–water excretion and arterial pressure. However, within these broad regions reside hundreds of genes that may act alone or in concert to influence homeostasis. Narrowing the regions of genetic interest and identifying specific genes that participate in homeostatic control using techniques of chromosomal substitution coupled with gene expression analysis and physiological profiling is the object of intense research effort.[9]

Genetic Association Studies

As mentioned earlier, genetic effects on complex disorders are likely to involve multiple susceptibility markers of individually modest importance, thereby limiting the application of linkage analysis. Association studies examine the frequency of specific genetic polymorphisms in a population-based sample of unrelated diseased individuals and appropriately matched unaffected controls. The increased statistical power to uncover small clinical effects of multiple genes[10] and the fact that they do not require family based sample collections are the main advantages of this approach over linkage analysis. Most significant information has been gathered so far from association studies in which prior knowledge of the gene or its protein product existed. This candidate gene approach has been widely used to analyze possible associations between genetic variants and disease progression or outcome, with genes selected because of a priori hypotheses about their potential etiological role in disease, based on current understanding of the disease pathophysiology.[11] For example, genetic variants within the renin–angiotensin system,[12] nitric oxide synthase,[13] and β_2-adrenergic receptors,[14] known to modulate vascular tone, were tested and found to be associated with hypertension. Similarly, the possible effects of polymorphisms on genetic predisposition for coronary artery disease[15–17] or restenosis after angioplasty[18,19] have been extensively investigated, and recently, two large-scale association studies have identified gene variants that might affect suscep-
3 tibility to myocardial infarction.[20,21] Accumulating evidence suggests that specific genotypes are associated with a variety of organ-specific perioperative adverse outcomes, including neurocognitive dysfunction,[22,23] renal compromise,[24,25] vein graft restenosis,[26] postoperative thrombosis,[27] vascular reactivity,[28] severe sepsis,[29] transplant rejection,[30] and death (for a review, see Ziegeler et al.[31]).

One of the main weaknesses of the association approach is that, unless the marker of interest "travels" (i.e., is in *linkage disequilibrium*) with a functional variant, or the marker allele *is* the actual functional variant, the power to detect and map complex trait loci will be reduced. Other known limitations of genetic association studies include potential false-positive findings resulting from population stratification (i.e., admixture of different ethnic or genetic backgrounds in the case and control groups)[32] and multiple comparison issues when large numbers of candidate genes are being assessed.[33] Replication of findings across different populations or related phenotypes remains the most reliable method of validating a true relationship between genetic polymorphisms and disease,[11] but poor reproducibility in subsequent studies is one of the main criticisms of the candidate gene association approach.[34] However, a recent meta-analysis suggested that lack of statistical power may be the main contributor to this inconsistent replication and proposed more stringent statistical criteria to exclude false-positive results and the design of large collaborative association studies.[35] Ongoing efforts to develop high-resolution maps of genetic variation and haplotypes (the International HapMap Project) should facilitate the fine localization of causal genetic variants for common diseases and variable drug responses and increase the power of future association studies.

Large-Scale Gene and Protein Expression Profiling

Genomic approaches are anchored in the "central dogma" of molecular biology, the concept of transcription of messenger RNA (mRNA) from a DNA template, followed by translation of RNA into protein (Fig. 7-3). Since transcription is a key regulatory step that may eventually signal many other cascades of events, the study of RNA levels in a cell or organ (i.e., quantifying gene expression) can improve the understanding of a wide variety of biological systems. Furthermore, while the human genome contains only about 30,000 genes, functional variability at the protein level is far more diverse, resulting from extensive posttranscriptional, translational, and posttranslational modifications. It is believed that there are approximately 200,000 distinct proteins in humans, which are further modified posttranslationally by phosphorylation, glycosylation, oxidation, and disulfide structures.[36] Thus, in addition to the assessment of genetic variability at the DNA level using various genotyping techniques, analysis of large-scale variability at the RNA and protein level using microarray and proteomic approaches provides a better understanding of the overall regulatory networks involved in complex phenotypes.

Microarray technologies have revolutionized the analysis of gene expression changes in biological events and in complex diseases, by simultaneously examining on a genome-wide scale the expression of many thousands of transcripts in a single experiment. Some have even called microarray analysis "the essence of genomics."[37] Special algorithms used in the computational analyses of the vast amounts of data thus generated enable the identification of global patterns of gene expression and grouping genes into expression clusters. Investigating the relationship between such clusters of candidate genes provides greater insight into their potential biological relevance than simple comparisons of up- and down-regulated genes. In perioperative medicine, DNA microarrays may be applied to evaluate and catalog organ-specific responses to surgical stress and severe systemic stimuli such as cardiopulmonary bypass and endotoxemia, which can be subsequently used to identify and validate targets for therapeutic intervention.[38] Several studies have profiled myocardial gene expression in the ischemic heart, demonstrating alterations in the expression of immediate-early genes (c-*fos*, *jun*B),[39] genes coding for calcium-handling proteins (calsequestrin, phospholamban), and extracellular matrix and cytoskeletal proteins.[40] Upregulation of transcripts mechanistically involved in cytoprotection (heat shock proteins), resistance to apoptosis, and cell growth has been found in stunned myocardium.[41] Furthermore, cardiac gene expression profiling after cardiopulmonary bypass and cardioplegic arrest has identified the upregulation of inflammatory and transcription activators, apoptotic genes, and stress genes,[42] which appear to be age-related.[43] Microarray technology has also been utilized in the quest for novel cardioprotective genes, with the ultimate goal of designing strategies to activate these genes and prevent myocardial injury. Preconditioning is one of such well-studied models of cardioprotection, which can be induced by various triggers including intermittent ischemia, osmotic or redox stress, heat shock, toxins, and interestingly, inhaled anesthetics. The main functional categories of genes identified as potentially involved in cardioprotective pathways include a host of transcription factors, heat shock proteins, antioxidant genes (heme-oxygenase, glutathione peroxidase), and growth factors,[44] but different gene programs appear to be activated in ischemic versus anesthetic preconditioning, resulting in two distinct cardioprotective phenotypes.[45]

Identification of genes displaying significant changes in expression (differentially expressed) by microarray analysis can be used as an unbiased method to select candidate genes for future association studies. However, before such use, quality assurance protocols are required to validate the microarray

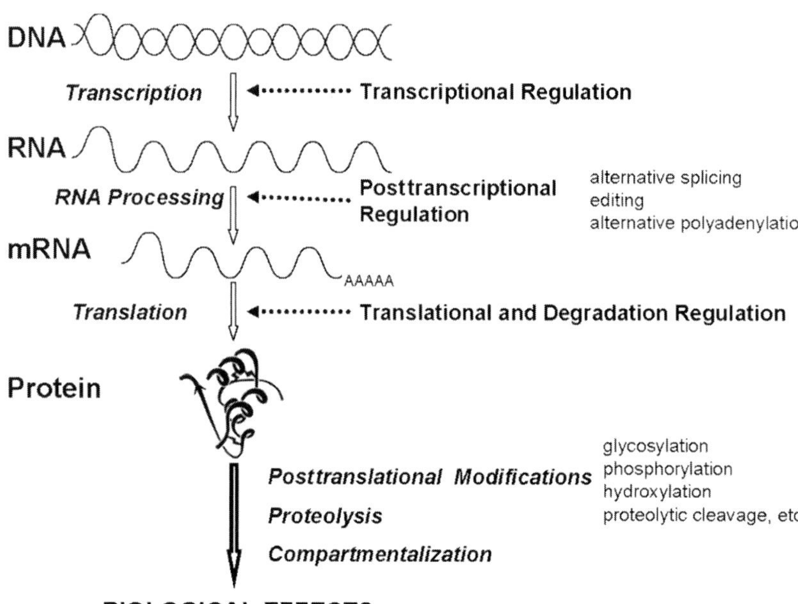

FIGURE 7-3. Central dogma of molecular biology. Protein expression involves two main processes, RNA synthesis (*transcription*) and protein synthesis (*translation*), with many intermediate regulatory steps. A single gene can give rise to multiple protein products (isoforms) via alternative splicing and RNA editing. Thus functional variability at the protein level, ultimately responsible for biological effects, is the cumulative result of genetic variability as well as extensive posttranscriptional, translational, and posttranslational modifications.

results. These include experiment replication, selection of cutoff values used to identify differentially expressed genes, and confirmation of findings by alternative methods (quantitative reverse transcriptase polymerase chain reaction, Northern blotting, or in situ hybridization).[5] It is important to realize that expression studies alone cannot prove function. To establish a causal relationship between the change in gene expression and the disease, every new hypothesis has to be further tested through either gain- or loss-of-function studies in biological systems (such as transgenic overexpression, dominant negative, antisense, or gene targeting strategies).[46] In spite of their limitations and only when coupled with richly annotated comparative databases, DNA microarrays have the potential to become useful tools in complex disease classification, prediction of response to treatment and prognosis, and identification of novel therapeutic targets.

The *transcriptome* (the complete collection of transcribed elements of the genome) is not fully representative of the *proteome* (the complete complement of proteins encoded by the genome), since many transcripts are not targeted for translation, as evidenced recently with the concept of gene silencing by RNA interference. Alternative splicing, a wide variety of posttranslational modifications, and protein–protein interactions responsible for biological function would remain therefore undetected by gene expression profiling. This has led to the emergence of a new field, *proteomics*, studying the sequence, modification, and function of all proteins in a biological system at a given time. Rather than focusing on "static" DNA, proteomic studies examine dynamic protein products, with the goal of identifying proteins that undergo changes in abundance, modification, or localization in response to a particular disease state, trauma, stress, or therapeutic intervention.[47] Thus, proteomics offers a more global and integrated view of biology, complementing other functional genomic approaches. Currently available methods for proteomic analysis include protein extraction, separation by two-dimensional gel electrophoresis or chromatography, followed by identification using mass spectrometry. Although rapidly improving, these methods are currently limited by sensitivity, specificity, and throughput.[36] The development of protein arrays has the potential to become a versatile and rigorous high-throughput method for proteomic analysis and is the object of intense investigation.

Integrated genomic and proteomic data analysis may be applied in perioperative medicine to elucidate individual responses to surgical injury and provide useful prognostic information. Recently, such a combined genomic and proteomic approach was used to determine the outcome in patients undergoing thoracoabdominal aortic aneurysm repair. Expression patterns of 138 genes from peripheral blood leukocytes and the concentrations of 7 circulating plasma proteins discriminated between the patients who developed multiple organ dysfunction syndrome (MODS) and those who did not. More importantly, these patterns of genome-wide gene expression and plasma protein concentration were observed before surgical trauma and visceral ischemia-reperfusion injury, suggesting that patients who developed MODS differed in either their genetic predisposition or their preexisting inflammatory state.[48]

GENOMICS AND PERIOPERATIVE RISK PROFILING

Recognizing the significant increase in surgical burden because of accelerated aging of the population and increased reliance on surgery for treatment of disease, the National Heart, Blood and Lung Institute has recently convened a Working Group on perioperative medicine. The group concluded that perioperative complications are significant, costly, variably reported, and often imprecisely detected, and identified a critical need for accurate comprehensive perioperative outcome databases. Furthermore, presurgical risk profiling is inconsistent and deserves further attention, especially for noncardiac, nonvascular surgery and older patients.[49]

One of the hallmarks of perioperative medicine is the striking variability in patient responses to surgical procedures, anesthetic agents, hemodynamic challenge, and the pharmacopoeia used in the perioperative period. Although many preoperative predictors have been identified and are constantly being refined, risk stratification based on clinical, procedural, and biological markers explains only a small part of the variability
4 in the incidence of perioperative complications. It is becoming increasingly recognized that specific genotypes may also predict adverse perioperative outcomes in otherwise healthy individuals. Such adverse outcomes will develop only in patients whose combined burden of genetic and environmental risk factors exceeds a certain threshold, which may vary with age. Identification of such genetic contributions not only to disease causation and susceptibility, but also to influencing the *response* to disease and drug therapy, and incorporation of genetic risk information in clinical decision making may lead to improved health outcomes and reduced costs. For instance, understanding the gene–environment interactions involved in atherosclerotic cardiovascular disease and neurological injury may facilitate preoperative patient optimization and resource utilization. Furthermore, understanding the role of genotypic variation in thrombosis and inflammation, the main pathophysiological mechanisms responsible for perioperative complications, may contribute to the development of target-specific therapies, thereby limiting the incidence of adverse events in high-risk patients.

Genetic Susceptibility to Adverse Perioperative Cardiovascular Outcomes

As part of the preoperative evaluation, anesthesiologists are involved in assessing the risks of perioperative complications. It is commonly accepted that patients who have underlying cardiovascular disease are at risk for adverse cardiac events after surgery, and several multifactorial risk indices have been developed and validated for patients undergoing both noncardiac surgical procedures (such as the Goldman[50] or the Lee Cardiac Risk Index[51]), as well as cardiac surgery (such as the Hannan[52] or Sergeant[53] scores). However, identifying patients at the highest risk of perioperative infarction remains difficult, and risk scores, while potentially valuable for population studies, are not an ideal tool for directing care in an individual patient.[54] Genomic approaches have been used in the search for a better assessment of the individual coronary risk profile. Numerous reports from animal models; linkage analysis; family, twin, and population association studies have definitely proven the role of genetic influences in the incidence and progression of coronary artery disease (CAD). Recent twin studies report a heritability of death from CAD as high as 0.58. Genetic factors associated with CAD mortality are in operation throughout the entire lifespan, although they seem to be particularly important in early phases of life, as manifested by a decrease in heritability with age. Moreover, comprehensive linkage analysis[7] and association studies[20,21] have reemphasized the role of genetic variability in myocardial infarction. While these studies do not directly address the heritability of adverse perioperative myocardial events, they do suggest a strong genetic contribution to the risk of adverse cardiovascular outcomes in general. Indeed, given similar known risk factors, many patients still manifest differences in the incidence of both early and late adverse myocardial events. Like most common diseases, perioperative cardiovascular complications involve an interplay of many genetic variations of molecular and biochemical pathways and their interactions with environmental factors (e.g., surgical procedural, pharmacological), and can therefore be classified as complex disease phenotypes. On a genetic level, functional allelic variations likely modulate, each with a small overall contribution and relative risk, individual susceptibility to develop such adverse myocardial events, and the manifestation, severity, and prognosis of the disease process. Unfortunately, although the effects of genetic predisposition for CAD or restenosis after angioplasty have been extensively investigated, only a paucity of studies exist regarding genetic risk factors directly associated with perioperative myocardial outcomes, mainly following surgical revascularization.[26,55,56] However, an increasing body of evidence has linked various genotypes to mechanistic pathways known to be involved in triggering or modulating the severity of perioperative myocardial injury, including thrombosis, inflammatory response, or vascular reactivity.

The acute phase response or stress response to surgery is characterized by an increase in fibrinogen concentration, platelet adhesiveness, and plasminogen activator inhibitor-1 (PAI-1) production. During cardiac surgery, alterations in the hemostatic system are even more complex and multifactorial, including the effects of hypothermia, hemodilution, and cardiopulmonary bypass (CPB)-induced activation of coagulation, fibrinolytic, and inflammatory pathways. Perioperative thrombotic outcomes following cardiac surgery (e.g., coronary graft thrombosis, myocardial infarction, stroke, pulmonary embolism) represent one extreme on a continuum of coagulation dysfunction, with coagulopathy at the other end of the spectrum. Pathophysiologically, the balance between bleeding, normal hemostasis, and thrombosis is markedly influenced by the rate of thrombin formation and platelet activation. Recent evidence suggests genetic variability modulates the activation of each of these mechanistic pathways,[57] suggesting significant heritability of the prothrombotic state. Several genotypes have been associated with increased risk of coronary graft thrombosis and myocardial injury following CABG. Plasminogen activator inhibitor-1 gene is an important negative regulator of fibrinolytic activity; a genetic variant in the promoter of the PAI-1 gene, consisting of an insertion (5G)/deletion (4G) polymorphism at position −675, has been consistently associated with changes in the plasma levels of PAI-1. The 4G allele was associated with increased risk of early graft thrombosis after CABG,[58] and a recent meta-analysis showed a significant effect of PAI-1 genotype on incidence of myocardial infarction.[59] Similarly, a polymorphism in the platelet glycoprotein IIIa, resulting in increased platelet aggregation (Pl^{A2} polymorphism), was found to be a risk factor for thrombotic coronary graft occlusion, myocardial infarction, and death following CABG.[60] Furthermore, the Pl^{A2} allele has been associated with higher postoperative concentrations of troponin I following CABG, suggesting that this platelet polymorphism contributes to perioperative myocardial injury.[61] One of the most common inherited prothrombotic risk factors is a point mutation in coagulation factor V (1691G>A) resulting in resistance to activated protein C, and referred to as factor V Leiden (FVL). FVL has been associated with various postoperative thrombotic complications following noncardiac surgery (for a review, see Donahue[27]), but interestingly, also associated with a significant reduction in postoperative blood loss and overall risk of transfusion in cardiac surgery patients.[62]

Genetic variants modulating the magnitude of postoperative inflammatory response have been identified. Polymorphisms in the promoter of the interleukin 6 (*IL6*) gene (−572G>C and −174G>C) significantly increase the inflammatory response after heart surgery with cardiopulmonary bypass (CPB)[63] and have been associated with length of hospitalization after CABG.[64] Furthermore, both apolipoprotein E genotype (the ε4 allele)[65] and several variants in the tumor necrosis factor genes (*TNFA*−308G>A, *LTA*+250G>A) have been associated with proinflammatory effects in patients undergoing CPB.[66] Conversely, a genetic variant modulating the release of the anti-inflammatory cytokine interleukin 10 (*IL10*) in response to CPB has been reported (*IL10*-1082G>A), with high levels of IL10 being associated with postoperative cardiovascular dysfunction.[67]

5 Several genes predictive of perioperative vascular response have been identified. Significantly increased vascular responsiveness to alpha-adrenergic stimulation (phenylephrine) was found both in patients carrying the endothelial nitric oxide synthase 894G>T polymorphism[68] and in patients homozygous for *D* allele of the angiotensin converting enzyme insertion/deletion (*I/D*) polymorphism.[28,69] Also, variability in the β_2-adrenergic receptor gene has been associated with increased mean arterial blood pressure to the stress stimuli of tracheal intubation.[70]

Genetic Variability and Perioperative Event-Free Survival

Several large randomized clinical trials examining the benefits of CABG surgery and percutaneous coronary interventions relative to medical therapy and/or to one another have refined our knowledge of early and long-term survival after CABG. While these studies have helped define the subgroups of patients who benefit from surgical revascularization, they also demonstrated a substantial variability in long-term survival after CABG, altered by important demographic and environmental risk factors. Increasing evidence suggests that the angiotensin converting enzyme (ACE) gene indel polymorphism may influence post-CABG complications. In a recent study, carriers of the *D* allele had higher mortality and restenosis rates after CABG surgery compared with the *I* allele.[56] Similarly, a functionally important amino acid alteration in the β_3-integrin chain of the glycoprotein IIb/IIIa platelet receptor (the Pl^{A2} polymorphism) was associated with an increased risk (odds ratio of 4.7) for major adverse cardiac events (a composite of myocardial infarction, coronary bypass graft occlusion, or death) following CABG surgery. Mechanistically, this may be related to a genetically modulated prothrombotic tendency, as Pl^{A2} results in increased fibrinogen-binding and epinephrine-induced platelet aggregation,[71] and has been previously identified as a risk factor for acute coronary thrombosis.[72] We have found preliminary evidence for association between two functional polymorphisms modulating β_2-adrenergic receptor activity (Arg16Gly and Gln27Glu) and incidence of death or major adverse cardiac events following cardiac surgery.[73]

Genetic Susceptibility to Adverse Perioperative Neurologic Outcomes

Despite advances in surgical and anesthetic techniques, significant neurologic morbidity continues to occur following cardiac surgery, ranging in severity from coma and focal stroke (incidence up to 6%) to more subtle cognitive deficits (incidence up to 69%), with a substantial impact on the risk of perioperative death, quality of life, and resource utilization.
6 Variability in the reported incidence of both early and late

neurological deficits remains poorly explained by procedural risk factors, suggesting that environmental (operative) and genetic factors may interact to determine disease onset, progression, and recovery.[74] Thus, cardiac surgery represents a unique clinical paradigm where, in addition to genetic predispositions, certain procedural events (such as aortic manipulation) may lead to the embolization of material to the brain. The pathophysiology of perioperative neurological injury is thought to involve complex interactions between primary pathways associated with atherosclerosis and thrombosis, and secondary response pathways like inflammation, vascular reactivity, and direct cellular injury. Many functional genetic variants have been reported in each of these mechanistic pathways involved in modulating the magnitude and the response to neurological injury, which may have implications in chronic as well as acute perioperative neurocognitive outcomes. Our group has demonstrated a significant association between the apolipoprotein E (*APOE*) E4 genotype and adverse cerebral outcomes in cardiac surgery patients.[22,74] This is consistent with other studies, suggesting a role for the *APOE* genotype in recovery from acute brain injury, such as intracranial hemorrhage,[75] closed head injury,[76] and stroke,[77] as well as experimental models of cerebral ischemia-reperfusion injury.[78] Unlike adult cardiac surgery patients, infants carrying the *APOE* $\varepsilon 2$ allele have recently been found at increased risk for developing adverse neurodevelopmental sequelae following cardiac surgery.[79] Mechanistically, the role of *APOE* genotypes in modulating the inflammatory response,[65] extent of aortic atheroma burden,[80] risk for coronary atherosclerosis,[81] and cerebral blood flow and autoregulation may explain the observed associations with impaired neurological outcomes.

Recent studies have suggested a role for platelet activation in the pathophysiology of adverse neurological sequelae. Genetic variants in surface platelet membrane glycoproteins, important mediators of platelet adhesion and platelet–platelet interactions, have been shown to increase the susceptibility to prothrombotic events. Among these, the Pl^{A2} polymorphism in glycoprotein IIb/IIIa has been related to various adverse thrombotic outcomes, including acute coronary thrombosis[72] and atherothrombotic stroke.[82] We found the Pl^{A2} allele to be associated with more severe neurocognitive decline after cardiopulmonary bypass,[23] which could represent an exacerbation of platelet-dependent thrombotic processes associated with plaque embolism.

Identifying novel predictors for risk of neurological and neurocognitive dysfunction and the molecular mechanisms underlying such risk will allow improved patient informed consent, stratification and resource allocation, development of neuroprotective agents, and therapeutic modalities tailored to the yet-to-be-discovered molecular abnormalities.

Genetic Susceptibility to Adverse Perioperative Renal Outcomes

Acute renal dysfunction is a common, serious complication of cardiac surgery; about 8 to 15% of patients develop moderate renal injury (>1.0 mg/dL peak creatinine rise), and up to 5% of them develop renal failure requiring dialysis.[83,84] Acute renal failure is independently associated with in-hospital mortality rates,[85] exceeding 60% in patients requiring dialysis.[84]
7 Recent studies have demonstrated that inheritance of genetic polymorphisms in the apolipoprotein E gene ($\varepsilon 4$ allele)[25] in the promoter region of the *IL6* gene (−174C allele[86] and −572C allele[143]) and angiotensinogen gene (842C allele)[143] are associated with acute renal injury following CABG surgery. Further identification of genotypes predictive of adverse perioperative renal outcomes may facilitate individually tailored therapy, risk stratify the patients for interventional trials targeting the gene product itself, and aid in medical decision making (e.g., selecting medical over surgical management).

Genetic Variants and Risk for Prolonged Postoperative Mechanical Ventilation

Prolonged mechanical ventilation (inability to extubate patient by 24 hours postoperatively) is a significant complication following cardiac surgery, occurring in 5.6% and 10.5% of patients undergoing first and repeat CABG surgery, respectively.[87] Several pulmonary and nonpulmonary causes have been identified, and scoring systems based on preoperative and procedural
8 risk factors have been proposed and validated. Recently, genetic variants in the renin–angiotensin pathway and in proinflammatory cytokine genes have been associated with respiratory complications post–cardiopulmonary bypass. The *D* allele of a common functional insertion/deletion (*I/D*) polymorphism in the *ACE* gene, accounting for 47% of variance in circulating ACE levels,[88] has been associated with prolonged mechanical ventilation following CABG[89] and with susceptibility to and prognosis of ARDS.[90] Furthermore, a hyposecretor haplotype in the neighboring genes tumor necrosis factor alpha (*TNFA*) and lymphotoxin alpha (*LTA*) on chromosome 6 (*TNFA-308G/LTA+250G* haplotype)[91] and a functional polymorphism modulating postoperative interleukin 6 levels (*IL6-174G>C*)[86] have been independently associated with higher risk of prolonged mechanical ventilation post-CABG. The association was more dramatic in patients undergoing conventional CABG than in those undergoing off-pump CABG (OPCAB), suggesting that in high-risk patients identified by preoperative genetic screening OPCAB may be the optimal surgical procedure.

A next crucial step in understanding the complexity of adverse perioperative outcomes is to assess the contribution of variations in many genes simultaneously and their interaction with traditional risk factors to the longitudinal prediction of outcomes in individual patients. The use of such outcome predictive models incorporating genetic information may help stratify mortality and morbidity in surgical patients. It may also improve prognostication, direct medical decision making both intraoperatively and during postoperative follow-up, and even suggest novel targets for therapeutic intervention in the perioperative period.

PHARMACOGENOMICS AND ANESTHESIA

Variability in response to drug therapy, both in terms of efficacy and safety, is a rule by which anesthesiologists live. In fact, much of the art of anesthesiology is the astute clinician being
9 prepared to deal with outliers. The term "pharmacogenomics" is used to describe how inherited variations in genes modulating drug actions are related to interindividual variability in drug response. Such variability in drug action may be *pharmacokinetic* or *pharmacodynamic* (Fig. 7-4). Pharmacokinetic variability refers to variability in a drug's absorption, distribution, metabolism, and excretion that mediates its efficacy and/or toxicity. The molecules involved in these processes include drug-metabolizing enzymes (such as members of the cytochrome P450, or CYP, superfamily) and drug transport molecules that mediate drug uptake into, and efflux from, intracellular sites. Pharmacodynamic variability refers to variable drug effects despite equivalent drug delivery to molecular sites of action. This may reflect variability in the function of the molecular target of the drug, or in the pathophysiological context in which the

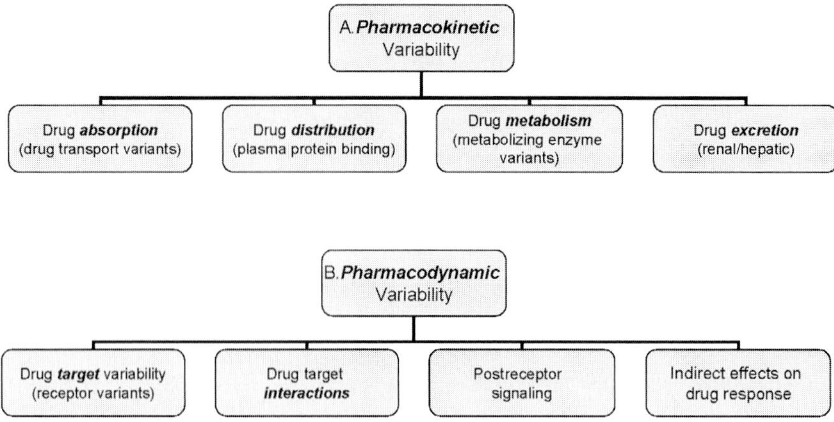

FIGURE 7-4. Pharmacogenomic determinants of individual drug response operate by pharmacokinetic and pharmacodynamic mechanisms. **A.** Genetic variants in *drug transporters* (e.g., ATP-binding cassette subfamily B member 1 or *ABCB1* gene) and *drug-metabolizing enzymes* (e.g., cytochrome P450 2D6 or *CYP2D6* gene, *CYP2C9* gene, N-acetyltransferase or *NAT2* gene, plasma cholinesterase or *BCHE* gene) are responsible for *pharmacokinetic* variability in drug response. **B.** Polymorphisms in *drug targets* (e.g., β_1 and β_2-adrenergic receptor *ADRB1*, *ADRB2* genes; angiotensin-I converting enzyme *ACE* gene), *postreceptor signaling molecules* (e.g., guanine nucleotide–binding protein *β3* or *GNB3* gene), or *molecules indirectly affecting drug response* (e.g., various ion channel genes involved in drug-induced arrhythmias) are sources of *pharmacodynamic* variability.

drug interacts with its receptor target (e.g., affinity, coupling, expression).[92] Thus, pharmacogenomics investigates complex, polygenically determined phenotypes of drug efficacy or toxicity, with the goal of identifying novel therapeutic targets and customizing drug therapy.

Pseudocholinesterase Deficiency

Historically, characterization of the genetic basis for plasma pseudocholinesterase deficiency in 1956 was of fundamental importance to anesthesia and the further development and understanding of genetically determined differences in drug response.[93] Individuals with an atypical form of pseudocholinesterase resulting in a markedly reduced rate of drug metabolism are at risk for excessive neuromuscular blockade and prolonged apnea. More than 20 variants have since been identified in the butyrylcholinesterase gene (*BCHE*), the most common of which are the A-variant (209A>G) and the K-variant (1615G>A), with various and somewhat poorly defined phenotypic consequences on prolonged neuromuscular blockade. Therefore, pharmacogenetic testing is currently not recommended in the population at large, but only as an explanation for an adverse event.[94]

Genetics of Malignant Hyperthermia

Malignant hyperthermia (MH) is a rare autosomal dominant genetic disease of skeletal muscle calcium metabolism, triggered by administration of general anesthesia with volatile anesthetic agents or succinylcholine in susceptible individuals. The clinical MH syndrome is characterized by skeletal muscle hypermetabolism and manifested as skeletal muscle rigidity, tachycardia, tachypnea, hemodynamic instability, increased oxygen consumption and CO_2 production, lactic acidosis, and fever, progressing to malignant ventricular arrhythmias, disseminated intravascular coagulation, and myoglobinuric renal failure. MH susceptibility has been initially linked to the ryonadine receptor (*RYR1*) gene locus on chromosome 19q.[95] However, subsequent studies have shown that MH may represent a common severe phenotype that originates not only from point mutations in the *RYR1* gene (Arg614Cys), but also within its functionally and/or structurally associated proteins regulating excitation–contraction coupling (such as *α1DHPR*
10 and *FKBP12*). It is becoming increasingly apparent that MH susceptibility results from a complex interaction between multiple genes and environment (such as environmental toxins), suggested by the heterogeneity observed in the clinical MH syndrome and the variable penetrance of the MH phenotype.[96] Current diagnostic methods (the caffeine-halothane contracture test) are invasive and potentially nonspecific. Unfortunately, because of the polygenic determinism and variable penetrance, direct DNA testing in the general population for susceptibility to MH is currently not recommended; in contrast, testing in individuals from families with affected individuals has the potential to greatly reduce mortality and morbidity.[94] Furthermore, genomic approaches may help elucidate the molecular mechanisms involved in altered RYRI-mediated calcium signaling and identify novel, more specific therapeutic targets.

Genetic Variability and Response to Anesthetic Agents

Anesthetic potency, defined by the minimum alveolar concentration (MAC) of an inhaled anesthetic that abolishes purposeful movement in response to a noxious stimulus, varies among individuals, with a coefficient of variation (the ratio of standard deviation to the mean) of approximately 10%.[97] This observed variability may be explained by interindividual differences in multiple genes that underlie responsiveness to anesthetics, by environmental or physiological factors (brain temperature,
11 age), or by measurement errors. Evidence of a genetic basis for increased anesthetic requirements is beginning to emerge, suggested, for instance, by the observation that desflurane requirements are increased in subjects with red hair versus

dark hair.[98] Recent studies evaluating the genetic control of anesthetic responses, coupled with molecular modeling, neurophysiology, and pharmacologic approaches, have provided important developments in our understanding of general anesthetic mechanisms. Triggered by the seminal work of Franks and Lieb,[99,100] research shifted from the membrane lipid bilayer to protein receptors (specifically ligand- and voltage-gated ion channels) as potential anesthetic targets, ending a few decades of stagnation that were primarily a result of an almost universal acceptance of the dogma of nonspecific anesthetic action (the so-called "lipid theory"). Some of the genes responsible for phenotypic differences in anesthetic effects have been mapped in various animal models, including the fruit fly *Drosophila melanogaster*,[101] the nematode *Caenorhabditis elegans*,[102] and the mouse. Later, we summarize the three broad categories of genetic approaches that have been used in mammalian models to provide mechanistic insight into the molecular basis of anesthetic action in humans, with an emphasis on genetically altered animal models. First, classical genetics studies identify mutations in single genes that result in individuals qualitatively different from the nonmutant (i.e., *wild type*) individuals. Numerous inbred mouse strains and several spontaneously arising mutants have been demonstrated to differ in response to anesthetics.[103] The second approach, quantitative genetics, studies the inheritance of continuously varying, quantitative traits (such as height, weight, IQ, blood pressure, response to drugs, nociceptive sensitivity). These traits are controlled by multiple genes (called *quantitative trait loci*, QTL), each contributing quantitatively to the net trait and also affected by the environment to varying degrees. Specific chromosomal regions that control sensitivity to propofol[104] and alcohol[105] have been identified using the QTL mapping technique. Because of the many potential anesthetic targets, quantitative genetics, with its ability to examine multiple genes simultaneously, holds great promise for identifying the genetic control mechanisms of anesthetic response. The classic and quantitative genetic approaches are examples of *forward genetics* in which the line of investigation progresses from an altered phenotype to the genetic basis for that observed difference (i.e., from phenotype to genotype). In contrast, *reverse genetics* explores the functional consequences of directly mutating or altering the expression of a known gene (i.e., from genotype to phenotype). Specifically, genomic manipulation of plausible candidate receptors is used to investigate their function in vitro and, through the use of genetically engineered (e.g., transgenic, knockout, and knockin) animals (Fig. 7-5), to evaluate in vivo their relationship to various anesthetic end points, such as immobility (i.e., MAC), hypnosis, amnesia, and analgesia (for reviews, see Homanics et al[106] and Sonner et al[107]).

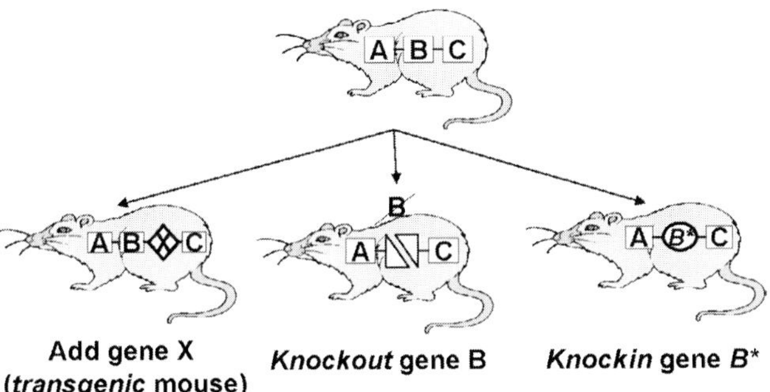

FIGURE 7-5. Genetically engineered animals used in functional genomic studies. *Transgenic* animals—gene X is introduced at random somewhere in the genome; *knockout* animals—gene B is inactivated by a direct mutation; *knockin* animals—gene B^* is introduced at a specific locus to replace gene B.

Transgenic animals overexpress or misexpress an additional gene that has been deliberately inserted into their genome. The foreign gene (i.e., *transgene*) is constructed using recombinant DNA methodology and used either to transfect embryonic stem cells growing in culture or microinjected into the pronucleus of a fertilized egg. However, the random insertion of the transgene in the genome that affects its expression pattern and the need for the transgene to have a dominant effect over the endogenous gene are major disadvantages of this technique. The process of gene targeting has enabled scientists to replace virtually any specific gene with an inactive allele (i.e., *gene knockouts*) and circumvent some of the limitations of transgenic technology. *Knockout* animals are created by inserting a vector containing the disrupted gene into mouse embryonic stem cells, with the goal of inactivating both alleles so that the gene is nonfunctional in all cells for the animal's lifetime (*global knockout*). Several thousand different strains of knockout mice have been created and are used to investigate specific functions of particular genes and mechanisms of drug action, including the sensitivity to general anesthetic in mice lacking the β_3 subunit[108] or the α_6 subunit[109] of the $GABA_A$ receptor. These studies have identified two potential downfalls of the global knockout approach: the genome has enough redundancy to compensate for the missing pair of alleles by altering the expression of other genes (developmental compensation) and second, because the knockout affects all neurons, it is impossible to attribute a phenotype (such as MAC) to a specific neural region or circuit. To eliminate some of these confounding problems, *conditional knockouts* seek to delete a gene in a particular cell type or tissue at specific stages of development.

Knockin animals express a site-directed mutation in the targeted gene that remains under the control of endogenous regulatory elements, allowing the mutated gene to be expressed in the same amount, at the same time, and in the same tissues as the normal gene. This method has provided remarkable insight into the mechanisms of action of benzodiazepines[110] and intravenous anesthetics. In a seminal study by Jurd et al, a point mutation in the gene encoding the β_3 subunit of the $GABA_A$ receptor previously known to render the receptor insensitive to etomidate and propofol in vitro[111] was validated in vivo by creating a knockin mouse strain that proved also essentially insensitive to the immobilizing actions of etomidate and propofol.[112] A point mutation in the β_2 subunit of the $GABA_A$ receptor results in a knockin mouse with reduced sensitivity to the sedative[113] and hypothermic effects[114] of etomidate. Knockin mice harboring point mutations in the α_{2A}-adrenergic receptor have enabled the elucidation of the role of this receptor in anesthetic-sparing, analgesic, and sedative responses to dexmedetomidine.[115]

The situation is far more complex for inhaled anesthetics, which appear to mediate their effects by acting on several receptor targets. Based on combined pharmacologic and genetic in vivo studies to date, several receptors are unlikely to be direct mediators of MAC, including the $GABA_A$ (despite their compelling role in intravenous anesthetic-induced immobility), 5-HT_3, AMPA, kainate, acetylcholine and α_2-adrenergic receptors, and potassium channels.[116] Glycine, NMDA receptors, and sodium channels remain likely candidates.[107] These conclusions, however, do not apply to other anesthetic end points, such as hypnosis, amnesia, and analgesia. Such genomic approaches have the potential to evolve into preoperative screening profiles useful in guiding therapeutic decisions, such as prevention of anesthetic awareness in patients with a genetic predisposition to increased anesthetic requirements.

Genetic Variability and Response to Pain

Similar to the observed variability in anesthetic potency, the response to painful stimuli and analgesic manipulations varies among individuals. The sources of variability in the report and experience of pain and analgesia are multifactorial, including factors extrinsic to the organism (such as cultural factors, or circadian rhythms) and intrinsic factors (such as age, gender, hormonal status, or genetic makeup). Increasing evidence suggests that pain behavior in response to noxious stimuli and its modulation by the central nervous system in response to drug administration or environmental stimuli may be strongly influenced by genetic factors.[117]

Results from studies in twins[118] and inbred mouse strains[119] indicate a moderate heritability for chronic pain and nociceptive sensitivity, which appears to be mediated by multiple genes. Furthermore, QTL for hot-plate sensitivity and formalin test have been mapped to mouse chromosomes 4 (near the δ-opioid receptor gene), 2, and 10, respectively.[120] Various strains of knockout mice lacking target genes like neurotrophins and their receptors (e.g., nerve growth factor), peripheral mediators of nociception and hyperalgesia (e.g., substance P), opioid and nonopioid transmitters and their receptors, and intracellular signaling molecules have significantly contributed to the understanding of pain-processing mechanisms.[121]

12 In addition to the genetic control of peripheral nociceptive pathways, considerable evidence exists for genetic variability in the descending central pain modulatory pathways, potentially explaining the interindividual variability in analgesic responsiveness. One good example relevant to analgesic efficacy is cytochrome P450D6 (*CYP2D6*), a member of the superfamily of microsomal enzymes that catalyze phase I drug metabolism and is responsible for the metabolism of a large number of therapeutic compounds. The relationship between the *CYP2D6* genotype and the enzyme metabolic rate has been extensively characterized, with at least 12 known mutations leading to a tetramodal distribution of CYP2D6 activity: ultrarapid metabolizers (5 to 7% of the population), extensive metabolizers (60%), intermediate metabolizers (25%), and poor metabolizers (10%). Currently, pharmacogenomic screening tests predict CYP2D6 phenotype with >95% reliability. The consequences of inheriting an allele that compromises CYP2D6 function include the inability to metabolize codeine (a prodrug) to morphine by O-demethylation, leading to lack of analgesia but increased side effects from the parent drug (e.g., fatigue) in poor metabolizers.[94,117]

Animal studies have mapped other polymorphic genes involved in various analgesic modalities. A QTL responsible for 28% of phenotypic variance in magnitude of systemic morphine analgesia in mice has been mapped to chromosome 10, in or near the *OPRM* (μ-opioid receptor) gene, and several putative QTL mediating nitrous oxide analgesias have been identified. The μ-opioid receptor is also subject to pharmacodynamic variability; polymorphisms in the promoter region of the *OPRM* gene modulating interleukin4-mediated gene expression have been correlated with morphine antinociception. Furthermore, an *OPRM*188A>G polymorphism associated with decreased responses to morphine-6-glucuronide was identified in humans, with implications in reduced risks of toxicity in renal failure patients.[94] A sex-specific locus on chromosome 8 has been associated with nonopioid stress-induced analgesia in females only and may be related to κ-opioid analgesia, providing a possible mechanism for sex-genetic interactions in regulating analgesic response.[117]

Genetic Variability in Response to Other Drugs Used Perioperatively

A wide variety of drugs used in the perioperative period display significant pharmacokinetic or pharmacodynamic variability that is genetically modulated, some listed in Table 7-1. Although such genetic variation in drug-metabolizing enzymes or drug targets mainly result in unusually variable drug response, genetic markers associated with rare but life-threatening side effects have also been described. Of note, the most commonly cited categories of drugs involved in adverse drug reactions include cardiovascular, antibiotic, psychiatric, and analgesic medications, and interestingly, each category has a known genetic basis for increased risk of adverse reactions.[122]

There are more than 30 families of drug-metabolizing enzymes in humans, most with genetic polymorphisms shown to influence enzymatic activity. Of special importance to the anesthesiologists is the *CYP2D6*, one of the most intensively studied and best understood examples of pharmacogenetic variation, involved in the metabolism of several drugs including analgesics (codeine, dextromethorphan), β-blockers (Fig. 7-6), antiarrhythmics (flecainide, propafenone, quinidine), and diltiazem. Another important pharmacogenetic variation has been described in cytochrome P450C9 (*CYP2C9*), involved in metabolizing anticoagulants (warfarin), anticonvulsants (phenytoin), antidiabetic agents (glipizide, tolbutamide), and nonsteroidal anti-inflammatory drugs (celecoxib, ibuprofen), among others. Three known *CYP2C9* variant alleles result in different enzyme activities (extensive, intermediate, and slow metabolizer phenotypes) and have clinical implications in the increased risk of life-threatening bleeding complications in slow metabolizers during standard warfarin therapy. This illustrates the concept of "high-risk pharmacokinetics," which applies to drugs with low therapeutic ratios eliminated by a single pathway (in this case CYP2C9-mediated oxidation); genetic variation in that pathway may lead to large changes in drug clearance, concentrations, and effects.[92] Dose adjustments based on the pharmacogenetic phenotype have been proposed for drugs metabolized via both CYP2D6 and CYP2C9 pathways.[94]

Genetic variation in drug targets (receptors) can have a profound effect on drug efficacy, and over 25 examples have already been identified. Functional polymorphisms in the β_2-adrenoreceptor (Arg16Gly, Gln27Glu) influencing the bronchodilator and vascular responses to β-agonists have been described, as well as in the β_1-adrenoreceptor (Arg389Gly), modulating the response to β-blockers.

Finally, clinically important genetic polymorphisms with indirect effects on drug response have been described. These include variants in candidate genes like sodium (*SCN5A*) and potassium ion channels (*KCNH2*, *KCNE2*, *KCNQ1*), which alter susceptibility to drug-induced long-QT syndrome and ventricular arrhythmias (torsade de pointes) associated with the use of drugs like erythromycin, terfenadine, disopyramide, sotalol, cisapride, or quinidine. Carriers of such susceptibility alleles have not manifest a QT-interval prolongation or family history of sudden death until QT-prolonging drug challenge is superimposed.[92] Predisposition to QT-interval prolongation (considered a surrogate for risk of life-threatening ventricular arrhythmias) has been responsible for more drug withdrawals from the market than any other category of adverse events in recent times, so understanding genetic predisposing factors constitutes one of the highest priorities of current pharmacogenomic efforts.

TABLE 7-1

EXAMPLES OF GENETIC POLYMORPHISMS INVOLVED IN VARIABLE RESPONSES TO DRUGS USED IN THE PERIOPERATIVE PERIOD

■ DRUG CLASS	■ GENE NAME (GENE SYMBOL)	■ EFFECT OF POLYMORPHISM
■ PHARMACOKINETIC VARIABILITY		
β-blockers	Cytochrome P450 2D6 (*CYP2D6*)	Enhanced drug effect
Codeine, dextromethorphan	*CYP2D6*	Decreased drug effect
Ca channel blockers	Cytochrome P450 3A4 (*CYP3A4*)	Uncertain
Alfentanil	*CYP3A4*	Enhanced drug response
Angiotensin-II receptor type 1 blockers	Cytochrome P450 2C9 (*CYP2C9*)	Enhanced blood pressure response
Warfarin	*CYP2C9*	Enhanced anticoagulant effect, risk of bleeding
Phenytoin	*CYP2C9*	Enhanced drug effect
ACE inhibitors	Angiotensin-I converting enzyme (*ACE*)	Blood pressure response
Procainamide	N-acetyltransferase 2 (*NAT2*)	Enhanced drug effect
Succinylcholine	Butyrylcholinesterase (*BCHE*)	Enhanced drug effect
Digoxin	P-glycoprotein (*ABCB1, MDR1*)	Increased bioavailability
■ PHARMACODYNAMIC VARIABILITY		
β-blockers	β_1 and β_2 adrenergic receptors (*ADRB1, ADRB2*)	Blood pressure and heart rate response, airway responsiveness to β_2-agonists
QT-prolonging drugs (antiarrhythmics, cisapride, erythromycin, etc.)	Sodium and potassium ion channels (*SCN5A, KCNH2, KCNE2, KCNQ1*)	Long QT-syndrome, risk of torsade de pointes
Aspirin, glycoprotein IIb/IIIa inhibitors	Glycoprotein IIIa subunit of platelet glycoprotein IIb/IIIa (*ITGB3*)	Variability in antiplatelet effects
Phenylephrine	Endothelial nitric oxide synthase (*NOS3*)	Blood pressure response

Pharmacogenomics is emerging as an additional modifying component to anesthesia along with age, gender, comorbidities, and medication use. Specific testing and treatment guidelines allowing clinicians to appropriately modify drug utilization (e.g., adjust dose or change drug) already exist for a few compounds[94] and will likely be expanded to all relevant therapeutic compounds, together with identification of novel therapeutic targets.

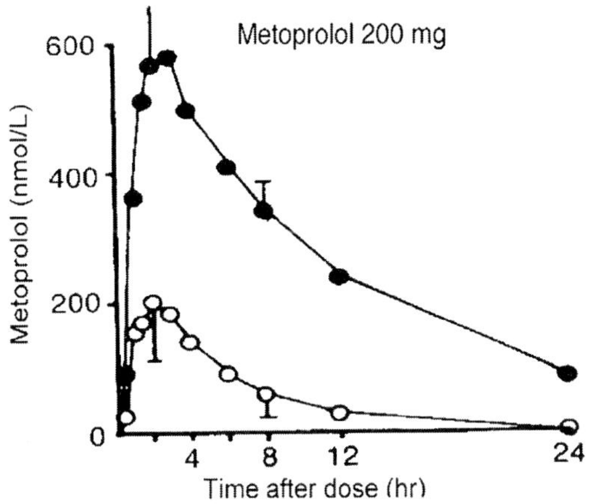

FIGURE 7-6. Genetically mediated variation in plasma metoprolol concentrations in CYP2D6 poor (•) versus extensive metabolizers (○), following a single oral dose of metoprolol tartrate (200 mg). Beta$_1$-blocking effects occur at metoprolol plasma concentrations in the 30 to 540 nmol/L range. The concentration-effect curve begins reaching a plateau between 200 and 300 nmol/L, and higher plasma levels produce little additional beta$_1$-blocking effect and diminished relative beta$_1$-selectivity with increased beta$_2$-blocking effects. (Reprinted from Bukaveckas BL, Valdes R, Linder MW: Pharmacogenetics as related to the practice of cardiothoracic and vascular anesthesia. J Cardiothorac Vasc Anesth 18:353, 2004, with permission.)

GENOMICS AND CRITICAL CARE

Genetic Variability in Response to Injury

Systemic injury (including trauma and surgical stress), shock, or infection trigger physiological responses of fever, tachycardia, tachypnea, and leukocytosis that collectively define the systemic inflammatory response syndrome. This can progress to severe sepsis, septic shock, and multiple organ dysfunction syndrome, the pathophysiology of which remains poorly understood. With the genomic revolution, a new paradigm has emerged in critical care medicine: outcomes of critical illness are determined by the interplay between the *injury* and *repair* processes triggered by the initial insults.[123] Negative outcomes are thus the combined result of direct tissue injury, the side effects of resulting repair processes, and secondary injury mechanisms leading to suboptimal repair. Regulation of these repair mechanisms is currently being extensively investigated at the genomic, proteomic, and pharmacogenomic levels, aiming to model adaptive and maladaptive responses to injury, aid in development of diagnostic indices predictive of injury, monitor progress of repair, and eventually design novel therapeutic modalities that take into account the individual genetic makeup.

13 The large interindividual variability in the magnitude of response to injury, including activation of inflammatory and coagulation cascades, apoptosis,[124] and fibrosis, suggests the involvement of genetic regulatory factors. Several functional genetic polymorphisms in molecules involved in various components of the inflammatory response have been associated with differences in susceptibility to and mortality from sepsis

of different etiologies, including postoperative sepsis (for review, see Lin et al[125]). These include polymorphisms in bacterial recognition molecules like lipopolysaccharide-binding protein (*LBP*), bactericidal/permeability increasing protein (*BPI*), *CD14*, toll-like receptors (*TLR4*), and pro-inflammatory cytokines like tumor necrosis alpha (*TNFA*),[126,127] lymphotoxin alpha (*LTA*),[29,128] interleukin-1 (*IL1*) and IL1 receptor antagonist (*IL1RN*),[129] and interleukin-6 (*IL6*).[130] Similarly, functional genetic variants in the PAI-1[131] and ACE[90,132] genes have been associated with poor outcomes in sepsis, reflecting the complex interaction between inflammation, coagulation, endothelial function, and vascular tone in the pathogenesis of sepsis-induced organ dysfunction.

This continuing effort to identify initial SNP-disease associations is followed by a process of selecting reliable predictive SNPs by validation in independent populations and determining which and how many markers will maximize the power to predict risk for sepsis or mortality following injury.

Functional Genomics of Injury

At a cellular level, injurious stimuli trigger adaptive stress responses determined by quantitative and qualitative changes in interdigitating cascades of biological pathways interacting in complex, often redundant ways. As a result, numerous clinical trials attempting to block single inflammatory mediators, such as TNFα in sepsis, have been largely unsuccessful.[133]
14 Given these complex interconnections, the standard "single gene" paradigm is insufficient to adequately describe the tissue response to severe systemic stimuli. Instead, organ injury might better be defined by patterns of altered gene and protein expression.[134] DNA microarray technology has become a powerful high-throughput method of analyzing changes induced by various injuries on a genome-wide scale, by quantifying mRNA abundance and generating an expression profile (the *transcriptome*) for the cell or tissue of interest. Several studies have reported the gene expression profiles in both critically ill patients and in animal models of sepsis,[135,136] acute lung injury,[137] and burn injury.[138] Furthermore, two large-scale national programs are using gene and protein expression profiles in circulating leukocytes to investigate the biological reasons behind the extreme variability in patient outcomes after similar traumatic insults (the NIH-funded Trauma Glue Grant; www.gluegrant.org) and to elucidate regulatory mechanisms in response to septic challenge in high-risk patients (the German National Genome Research Network).[134]

Since only less than half of the changes at mRNA level are usually translated into changes in protein expression, transcriptional profiling has to be complemented by characterizing the injury proteome for a more complete understanding of the host response to injury. Although the protein arrays are evolving rapidly, the main technology for proteomic analysis remains two-dimensional gel electrophoresis followed by mass spectrometry. Such integrated analysis of neutrophils transcriptome and proteome in response to lipopolysaccharide stimulation has identified upregulation of a variety of genes including transcriptional regulators (NF-κB), cytokines (TNFα, IL6, IL1β), and chemokines (MCP-1, MIP-3α) and confirmed the poor concordance between transcriptional and translational responses.[139]

Modeling disease entities like sepsis and multiple organ dysfunction syndrome, which are complex, nonlinear systems, requires the ability not only to measure many diverse molecular events simultaneously, but also to integrate the data using novel analytical tools based on complex systems theory and nonlinear dynamics.[140] Such analysis might help identify the key signaling nodes against which therapeutics can be directed.

FUTURE DIRECTIONS

Integration of "Omic" Information: System Biology Approaches

The Human Genome Project provides the sequence of nucleotides, localization of genes, and amino acid sequence in encoded proteins. However, less than 5% of the human genome represents DNA whose sequence ultimately encodes a protein. Although regulatory sequences and boundaries between the coding (i.e., *exons*) and noncoding (i.e., *introns*) regions of the genes are now being recognized and investigated, reaching the goals of functional genomics would require detailed knowledge of regulatory networks of gene expression as well as developmental and metabolic pathways. As mentioned earlier, microarray studies have revealed that many concurrently regulated genes share the same biochemical pathway and that cellular states can be ascribed to distinct and unique transcriptional profiles. These studies have provided a framework on which proteome analyses are based. Proteomics complements genome-based approaches by enabling the identification and characterization of differential protein expression, turnover and localization, posttranslational modifications (e.g., addition of sugar moieties or lipid attachments to a protein), and interaction with other biological molecules, thus providing new insights into the complex cellular processes involved in the response to anesthesia and surgical injury. The potential for "protein chips" to function as versatile and rigorous high-throughput methods for proteomic analyses is the object of intense investigation. Other more recent functional genomic and proteomic approaches include protein–protein, protein-DNA, or other "component–component" interaction mapping (*interactome*); systematic phenotypic analyses (*phenome*); and transcript or protein three-dimensional localization mapping (*localizome*).[141] To overcome the intrinsic limitations of all individual "omic" approaches, integration of data obtained from several distinct approaches using systems biology strategies has been proposed. This may lead to better functional annotations for the gene products and functional relationships between them and allow the formulation of relevant biological hypotheses, which can subsequently be tested using either synthetic biology or mathematical modeling of complex signaling networks.[141] Such integrative approaches to specifically study cardiovascular function (the Cardiome Project) have already been outlined. Furthermore, the scientific community needs to wrap the profiling data within the biological phenomenology, the so-called *"phenome"* in which the model under study is completely characterized in terms of the changes at the cellular, biochemical, organ and system level (Fig. 7-7).[5]

Targeted Drug Development

Genomic and proteomic approaches are rapidly becoming platforms for all aspects of drug discovery and development, from target identification and validation to individualization of drug therapy. As mentioned earlier, the human genome contains about 30,000 genes encoding for approximately 200,000 proteins, which represent potential drug targets. However, only about 120 drug targets are currently being marketed, thus making identification of novel therapeutic targets an area of intense research. Following gene identification, its therapeutic potential needs to be validated by defining the sequence function and its role in disease and demonstrating that the gene product can be manipulated with beneficial effect and no toxic effects. A developing field, *toxicogenomics*, studies the influence of toxic or potentially toxic substances on different model organisms

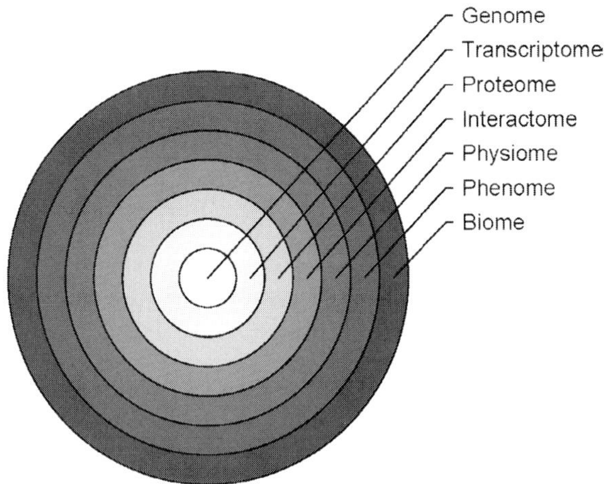

FIGURE 7-7. Integration of "omic" information. Cellular function is organized as a multilayered set of interdependent processes controlled at the level of the *genome* (DNA), *transcriptome* (messenger RNA), *proteome* (the collection of all proteins encoded within the DNA of a genome), *physiome* (regulatory networks and signaling pathways), and *phenome* (the quantitative description of the integrated functions of the living organism and its interactions both with the environment and within the phenotype itself). Relating genome variability to complex traits requires integrative systems biology approaches that will provide quantitative and mechanistic descriptions that unify signaling networks and identify critical regulatory nodes for therapeutic manipulation.

by evaluating the gene expression changes induced by novel drugs in a given tissue.

Sponsored by the National Institutes of Health, a nationwide collaborative effort called the Pharmacogenetics Research Network (http://www.nigms.nih.gov/pharmacogenetics/) is aiming to establish a strong pharmacogenomics knowledge base (http://www.pharmgkb.org/) as well as create a shared computational and experimental infrastructure required to connect human sequence variation with drug responses and translate information into novel therapeutics.

Ethical Considerations

Although one of the aims of the Human Genome Project is to improve therapy through genome-based prediction, there is a risk for discrimination against individuals who are genetically predisposed for a medical disorder. Such discrimination may include barriers to obtaining health, life, or long-term care insurance or obtaining employment. Thus, extensive efforts are made to protect patients participating in genetic research from prejudice, discrimination, or uses of genetic information that will adversely affect them. To address the concerns of both biomedical research and health communities, the U.S. Senate approved in 2003 the Genetic Information and Nondiscrimination Act, which provides the strong safeguards required to protect the public participating in human genome research.

Another ethical concern is the transferability of genetic tests across ethnic groups, particularly in the prediction of adverse drug responses. It is known that most polymorphisms associated with variability in drug response show significant differences in allele frequencies among populations and racial groups. Furthermore, the patterns of linkage disequilibrium are markedly different between ethnic groups, which may lead to spurious findings when markers, instead of causal variants, are used in diagnostic tests extrapolated across populations. In exploring racial disparities in health and disease outcomes, considerable debate has focused on whether race and ethnic identity are primarily social or biological constructs and the contribution of genetic variability in explaining observed differences in the rates of disease between racial groups. With the goal of personalized medicine being the prediction of risk and treatment of disease on the basis of an individual's genetic profile, some have argued that biologic consideration of race will become obsolete. However, in this discovery phase of the postgenome era, continuing to incorporate racial information in genetic studies should improve our understanding of the architecture of the human genome, and its implications for novel strategies aiming at identifying variants protecting against, or conferring susceptibility to, common diseases and modulating drug effects.[142]

CONCLUSION

The Human Genome Project has revolutionized all aspects of medicine, allowing us to assess the impact of genetic variability on disease taxonomy, characterization, and outcome and individual responses to various drugs and injuries. Mechanistically, information gleaned through genomic approaches is already unraveling long-standing mysteries behind general anesthetic action and adverse responses to drugs used perioperatively. However, a strong need remains for prospective, well-powered genetic studies in highly phenotyped surgical populations, which require the development of multidimensional perioperative databases. For the anesthesiologist, this may soon translate into prospective risk assessment incorporating genetic profiling of markers important in thrombotic, inflammatory, vascular, and neurologic responses to perioperative stress, with implications ranging from individualized additional preoperative testing and physiological optimization, to choice of perioperative monitoring strategies and critical care resource utilization. Furthermore, genetic profiling of drug-metabolizing enzymes, carrier proteins, and receptors, using currently available high-throughput molecular technologies, will enable personalized choice of drugs and dosage regimens tailored to suit a patient's pharmacogenetic profile. At that point, perioperative physicians will have far more robust information to use in designing the most appropriate and safest anesthetic plan for a given patient.

Future trends and challenges in perioperative genomics are still being defined but mainly concern interdisciplinary studies designed to combine an analytical system approach, mathematical modeling, and engineering principles with the multiple molecular and genetic factors and stimuli, and the macroscale interactions that determine the pathophysiological response to surgery.

References

1. Collins FS, Green ED, Guttmacher AE *et al*: A vision for the future of genomics research. Nature 422:835, 2003
2. Schwinn DA, Booth JV: Genetics infuses new life into human physiology: implications of the human genome project for anesthesiology and perioperative medicine. Anesthesiology 96:261, 2002
3. Lander ES: The new genomics: Global views of biology. Science 274:536, 1996
4. Borecki IB, Suarez BK: Linkage and association: Basic concepts. In Rao DC, Province MA (eds): Genetic Dissection of Complex Traits, p 45. San Diego, Academic Press, 2001
5. Podgoreanu MV, Schwinn DA: Genomics and the circulation. Br J Anaesth 93:140, 2004
6. Gretarsdottir S, Sveinbjornsdottir S, Jonsson HH *et al*: Localization of a susceptibility gene for common forms of stroke to 5q12. Am J Hum Genet 70:593, 2002
7. Broeckel U, Hengstenberg C, Mayer B *et al*: A comprehensive linkage analysis for myocardial infarction and its related risk factors. Nat Genet 30:210, 2002

8. Stoll M, Cowley AW Jr, Tonellato PJ *et al*: A genomic-systems biology map for cardiovascular function. Science 294:1723, 2001
9. Cowley AW Jr: Genomics and homeostasis. Am J Physiol Regul Integr Comp Physiol 284:R611, 2003
10. Risch N, Merikangas K: The future of genetic studies of complex human diseases. Science 273:1516, 1996
11. Tabor HK, Risch NJ, Myers RM: Opinion: Candidate-gene approaches for studying complex genetic traits: practical considerations. Nat Rev Genet 3:391, 2002
12. Zhu X, Chang YP, Yan D *et al*: Associations between hypertension and genes in the renin-angiotensin system. Hypertension 41:1027, 2003
13. Jachymova M, Horky K, Bultas J *et al*: Association of the Glu298Asp polymorphism in the endothelial nitric oxide synthase gene with essential hypertension resistant to conventional therapy. Biochem Biophys Res Commun 284:426, 2001
14. Tomaszewski M, Brain NJ, Charchar FJ *et al*: Essential hypertension and beta2-adrenergic receptor gene: linkage and association analysis. Hypertension 40:286, 2002
15. Tang Z, Tracy RP: Candidate genes and confirmed genetic polymorphisms associated with cardiovascular diseases: a tabular assessment. J Thromb Thrombolysis 11:49, 2001
16. Winkelmann BR, Hager J: Genetic variation in coronary heart disease and myocardial infarction: Methodological overview and clinical evidence. Pharmacogenomics 1:73, 2000
17. McCarthy JJ, Parker A, Salem R *et al*: Large scale association analysis for identification of genes underlying premature coronary heart disease: cumulative perspective from analysis of 111 candidate genes. J Med Genet 41:334, 2004
18. Agema WR, Jukema JW, Pimstone SN *et al*: Genetic aspects of restenosis after percutaneous coronary interventions: towards more tailored therapy. Eur Heart J 22:2058, 2001
19. Zee RY, Hoh J, Cheng S *et al*: Multi-locus interactions predict risk for post-PTCA restenosis: an approach to the genetic analysis of common complex disease. Pharmacogenomics J 2:197, 2002
20. Ozaki K, Ohnishi Y, Iida A *et al*: Functional SNPs in the lymphotoxin-alpha gene that are associated with susceptibility to myocardial infarction. Nat Genet 32:650, 2002
21. Yamada Y, Izawa H, Ichihara S *et al*: Prediction of the risk of myocardial infarction from polymorphisms in candidate genes. N Engl J Med 347:1916, 2002
22. Tardiff BE, Newman MF, Saunders AM *et al*: Preliminary report of a genetic basis for cognitive decline after cardiac operations. The Neurologic Outcome Research Group of the Duke Heart Center. Ann Thorac Surg 64:715, 1997
23. Mathew JP, Rinder CS, Howe JG *et al*: Platelet PlA2 polymorphism enhances risk of neurocognitive decline after cardiopulmonary bypass. Multicenter Study of Perioperative Ischemia (McSPI) Research Group. Ann Thorac Surg 71:663, 2001
24. Chew ST, Newman MF, White WD *et al*: Preliminary report on the association of apolipoprotein E polymorphisms, with postoperative peak serum creatinine concentrations in cardiac surgical patients. Anesthesiology 93:325, 2000
25. MacKensen GB, Swaminathan M, Ti LK *et al*: Preliminary report on the interaction of apolipoprotein E polymorphism with aortic atherosclerosis and acute nephropathy after CABG. Ann Thorac Surg 78:520, 2004
26. Ortlepp JR, Janssens U, Bleckmann F *et al*: A chymase gene variant is associated with atherosclerosis in venous coronary artery bypass grafts. Coron Artery Dis 12:493, 2001
27. Donahue BS: Factor V Leiden and perioperative risk. Anesth Analg 98:1623, 2004
28. Lasocki S, Iglarz M, Seince PF *et al*: Involvement of renin-angiotensin system in pressure-flow relationship: role of angiotensin-converting enzyme gene polymorphism. Anesthesiology 96:271, 2002
29. Stuber F, Petersen M, Bokelmann F *et al*: A genomic polymorphism within the tumor necrosis factor locus influences plasma tumor necrosis factor-alpha concentrations and outcome of patients with severe sepsis. Crit Care Med 24:381, 1996
30. Slavcheva E, Albanis E, Jiao Q *et al*: Cytotoxic T-lymphocyte antigen 4 gene polymorphisms and susceptibility to acute allograft rejection. Transplantation 72:935, 2001
31. Ziegeler S, Tsusaki BE, Collard CD: Influence of genotype on perioperative risk and outcome. Anesthesiology 99:212, 2003
32. Cardon LR, Palmer LJ: Population stratification and spurious allelic association. Lancet 361:598, 2003
33. Cardon LR, Bell JI: Association study designs for complex diseases. Nat Rev Genet 2:91, 2001
34. Hirschhorn JN, Lohmueller K, Byrne E *et al*: A comprehensive review of genetic association studies. Genet Med 4:45, 2002
35. Lohmueller KE, Pearce CL, Pike M *et al*: Meta-analysis of genetic association studies supports a contribution of common variants to susceptibility to common disease. Nat Genet 33:177, 2003
36. Loscalzo J: Proteomics in cardiovascular biology and medicine. Circulation 108:380, 2003
37. Tefferi A, Bolander ME, Ansell SM *et al*: Primer on medical genomics. Part III: Microarray experiments and data analysis. Mayo Clin Proc 77: 927, 2002
38. Hughes TR, Marton MJ, Jones AR *et al*: Functional discovery via a compendium of expression profiles. Cell 102:109, 2000
39. Deindl E, Schaper W: Gene expression after short periods of coronary occlusion. Mol Cell Biochem 186:43, 1998
40. Sehl PD, Tai JT, Hillan KJ *et al*: Application of cDNA microarrays in determining molecular phenotype in cardiac growth, development, and response to injury. Circulation 101:1990, 2000
41. Depre C, Tomlinson JE, Kudej RK *et al*: Gene program for cardiac cell survival induced by transient ischemia in conscious pigs. Proc Natl Acad Sci U S A 98:9336, 2001
42. Ruel M, Bianchi C, Khan TA *et al*: Gene expression profile after cardiopulmonary bypass and cardioplegic arrest. J Thorac Cardiovasc Surg 126:1521, 2003
43. Konstantinov IE, Coles JG, Boscarino C *et al*: Gene expression profiles in children undergoing cardiac surgery for right heart obstructive lesions. J Thorac Cardiovasc Surg 127:746, 2004
44. Onody A, Zvara A, Hackler L Jr *et al*: Effect of classic preconditioning on the gene expression pattern of rat hearts: A DNA microarray study. FEBS Lett 536:35, 2003
45. Sergeev P, da Silva R, Lucchinetti E *et al*: Trigger-dependent gene expression profiles in cardiac preconditioning: Evidence for distinct genetic programs in ischemic and anesthetic preconditioning. Anesthesiology 100:474, 2004
46. Schinke M, Riggi L, Butte AJ *et al:* Large scale expression profiling in cardiovascular disease using microarrays: Prospects and pitfalls. In Van Eyk JE, Dunn MJ (eds): Proteomic and Genomic Analysis of Cardiovascular Disease, p 3. Weinheim, WILEY-VCH Verlag GmbH & Co. KgaA, 2003
47. Tyers M, Mann M: From genomics to proteomics. Nature 422:193, 2003
48. Feezor RJ, Baker HV, Xiao W *et al*: Genomic and proteomic determinants of outcome in patients undergoing thoracoabdominal aortic aneurysm repair. J Immunol 172:7103, 2004
49. Mangano DT: Perioperative medicine: NHLBI working group deliberations and recommendations. J Cardiothorac Vasc Anesth 18:1, 2004
50. Goldman L, Caldera DL, Nussbaum SR *et al*: Multifactorial index of cardiac risk in noncardiac surgical procedures. N Engl J Med 297:845, 1977
51. Lee TH, Marcantonio ER, Mangione CM *et al*: Derivation and prospective validation of a simple index for prediction of cardiac risk of major noncardiac surgery. Circulation 100:1043, 1999
52. Hannan EL, Kilburn H Jr, Racz M *et al*: Improving the outcomes of coronary artery bypass surgery in New York State. JAMA 271:761, 1994
53. Sergeant P, Blackstone E, Meyns B: Validation and interdependence with patient-variables of the influence of procedural variables on early and late survival after CABG. K.U. Leuven Coronary Surgery Program. Eur J Cardiothorac Surg 12:1, 1997
54. Howell SJ, Sear JW: Perioperative myocardial injury: individual and population implications. Br J Anaesth 93:3, 2004
55. Delanghe J, Cambier B, Langlois M *et al*: Haptoglobin polymorphism, a genetic risk factor in coronary artery bypass surgery. Atherosclerosis 132:215, 1997
56. Volzke H, Engel J, Kleine V *et al*: Angiotensin I-converting enzyme insertion/deletion polymorphism and cardiac mortality and morbidity after coronary artery bypass graft surgery. Chest 122:31, 2002
57. Voetsch B, Loscalzo J: Genetic determinants of arterial thrombosis. Arterioscler Thromb Vasc Biol 24:216, 2004
58. Rifon J, Paramo JA, Panizo C *et al*: The increase of plasminogen activator inhibitor activity is associated with graft occlusion in patients undergoing aorto-coronary bypass surgery. Br J Haematol 99:262, 1997
59. Iacoviello L, Burzotta F, Di Castelnuovo A *et al*: The 4G/5G polymorphism of PAI-1 promoter gene and the risk of myocardial infarction: A meta-analysis. Thromb Haemost 80:1029, 1998
60. Zotz RB, Klein M, Dauben HP *et al*: Prospective analysis after coronary-artery bypass grafting: Platelet GP IIIa polymorphism (HPA-1b/PIA2) is a risk factor for bypass occlusion, myocardial infarction, and death. Thromb Haemost 83:404, 2000
61. Rinder CS, Mathew JP, Rinder HM *et al*: Platelet PlA2 polymorphism and platelet activation are associated with increased troponin I release after cardiopulmonary bypass. Anesthesiology 97:1118, 2002
62. Donahue BS, Gailani D, Higgins MS *et al*: Factor V Leiden protects against blood loss and transfusion after cardiac surgery. Circulation 107:1003, 2003
63. Brull DJ, Montgomery HE, Sanders J *et al*: Interleukin-6 gene −174g>c and −572g>c promoter polymorphisms are strong predictors of plasma interleukin-6 levels after coronary artery bypass surgery. Arterioscler Thromb Vasc Biol 21:1458, 2001
64. Burzotta F, Iacoviello L, Di Castelnuovo A *et al*: Relation of the −174 G/C polymorphism of interleukin-6 to interleukin-6 plasma levels and to length of hospitalization after surgical coronary revascularization. Am J Cardiol 88:1125, 2001
65. Grocott HP, Newman MF, El-Moalem H *et al*: Apolipoprotein E genotype differentially influences the proinflammatory and anti-inflammatory response to cardiopulmonary bypass. J Thorac Cardiovasc Surg 122:622, 2001
66. Roth-Isigkeit A, Hasselbach L, Ocklitz E *et al*: Inter-individual differences in cytokine release in patients undergoing cardiac surgery with cardiopulmonary bypass. Clin Exp Immunol 125:80, 2001
67. Galley HF, Lowe PR, Carmichael RL *et al*: Genotype and interleukin-10 responses after cardiopulmonary bypass. Br J Anaesth 91:424, 2003

68. Philip I, Plantefeve G, Vuillaumier-Barrot S *et al*: G894T polymorphism in the endothelial nitric oxide synthase gene is associated with an enhanced vascular responsiveness to phenylephrine. Circulation 99:3096, 1999
69. Henrion D, Benessiano J, Philip I *et al*: The deletion genotype of the angiotensin I-converting enzyme is associated with an increased vascular reactivity in vivo and in vitro. J Am Coll Cardiol 34:830, 1999
70. Kim NS, Lee IO, Lee MK *et al*: The effects of beta2 adrenoceptor gene polymorphisms on pressor response during laryngoscopy and tracheal intubation. Anaesthesia 57:227, 2002
71. Vijayan KV, Goldschmidt-Clermont PJ, Roos C *et al*: The Pl(A2) polymorphism of integrin beta(3) enhances outside-in signaling and adhesive functions. J Clin Invest 105:793, 2000
72. Weiss EJ, Bray PF, Tayback M *et al*: A polymorphism of a platelet glycoprotein receptor as an inherited risk factor for coronary thrombosis. N Engl J Med 334:1090, 1996
73. Podgoreanu MV, Booth JV, White WD *et al*: Beta adrenergic receptor polymorphisms and risk of adverse events following cardiac surgery. Circulation 108:IV, 2003
74. Newman MF, Booth JV, Laskowitz DT *et al*: Genetic predictors of perioperative neurological and cognitive injury and recovery. Best Pract Res Clin Anesthesiol 15:247, 2001
75. Alberts MJ, Graffagnino C, McClenny C *et al*: ApoE genotype and survival from intracerebral haemorrhage. Lancet 346:575, 1995
76. Teasdale GM, Nicoll JA, Murray G *et al*: Association of apolipoprotein E polymorphism with outcome after head injury. Lancet 350:1069, 1997
77. Slooter AJ, Tang MX, van Duijn CM *et al*: Apolipoprotein E epsilon4 and the risk of dementia with stroke. A population-based investigation. JAMA 277:818, 1997
78. Sheng H, Laskowitz DT, Bennett E *et al*: Apolipoprotein E isoform-specific differences in outcome from focal ischemia in transgenic mice. J Cereb Blood Flow Metab 18:361, 1998
79. Gaynor JW, Gerdes M, Zackai EH *et al*: Apolipoprotein E genotype and neurodevelopmental sequelae of infant cardiac surgery. J Thorac Cardiovasc Surg 126:1736, 2003
80. Ti LK, Mackensen GB, Grocott HP *et al*: Apolipoprotein E4 increases aortic atheroma burden in cardiac surgical patients. J Thorac Cardiovasc Surg 125:211, 2003
81. Newman MF, Laskowitz DT, White WD *et al*: Apolipoprotein E polymorphisms and age at first coronary artery bypass graft. Anesth Analg 92:824, 2001
82. Carter AM, Catto AJ, Bamford JM *et al*: Platelet GP IIIa PlA and GP Ib variable number tandem repeat polymorphisms and markers of platelet activation in acute stroke. Arterioscler Thromb Vasc Biol 18:1124, 1998
83. Conlon PJ, Stafford-Smith M, White WD *et al*: Acute renal failure following cardiac surgery. Nephrol Dial Transplant 14:1158, 1999
84. Mangano CM, Diamondstone LS, Ramsay JG *et al*: Renal dysfunction after myocardial revascularization: risk factors, adverse outcomes, and hospital resource utilization. The Multicenter Study of Perioperative Ischemia Research Group. Ann Intern Med 128:194, 1998
85. Chertow GM, Levy EM, Hammermeister KE *et al*: Independent association between acute renal failure and mortality following cardiac surgery. Am J Med 104:343, 1998
86. Gaudino M, Di Castelnuovo A, Zamparelli R *et al*: Genetic control of postoperative systemic inflammatory reaction and pulmonary and renal complications after coronary artery surgery. J Thorac Cardiovasc Surg 126:1107, 2003
87. Yende S, Wunderink R: Causes of prolonged mechanical ventilation after coronary artery bypass surgery. Chest 122:245, 2002
88. Rigat B, Hubert C, Alhenc-Gelas F *et al*: An insertion/deletion polymorphism in the angiotensin I-converting enzyme gene accounting for half the variance of serum enzyme levels. J Clin Invest 86:1343, 1990
89. Yende S, Quasney MW, Tolley EA *et al*: Clinical relevance of angiotensin-converting enzyme gene polymorphisms to predict risk of mechanical ventilation after coronary artery bypass graft surgery. Crit Care Med 32:922, 2004
90. Marshall RP, Webb S, Bellingan GJ *et al*: Angiotensin converting enzyme insertion/deletion polymorphism is associated with susceptibility and outcome in acute respiratory distress syndrome. Am J Respir Crit Care Med 166:646, 2002
91. Yende S, Quasney MW, Tolley E *et al*: Association of tumor necrosis factor gene polymorphisms and prolonged mechanical ventilation after coronary artery bypass surgery. Crit Care Med 31:133, 2003
92. Roden DM: Cardiovascular pharmacogenomics. Circulation 108:3071, 2003
93. Lehmann H, Ryan E: The familial incidence of low pseudocholinesterase level. Lancet 271:124, 1956
94. Bukaveckas BL, Valdes R Jr, Linder MW: Pharmacogenetics as related to the practice of cardiothoracic and vascular anesthesia. J Cardiothorac Vasc Anesth 18:353, 2004
95. McCarthy TV, Healy JM, Heffron JJ *et al*: Localization of the malignant hyperthermia susceptibility locus to human chromosome 19q12–13.2. Nature 343:562, 1990
96. Pessah IN, Allen PD: Malignant hyperthermia. Best Pract Res Clin Anesthesiol 15:277, 2001
97. Eger EI 2nd. Anesthetic Uptake and Action. Baltimore, Williams and Wilkins, 1974
98. Liem EB, Lin CM, Suleman MI *et al*: Anesthetic requirement is increased in redheads. Anesthesiology 101:279, 2004
99. Franks NP, Lieb WR: Do general anaesthetics act by competitive binding to specific receptors? Nature 310:599, 1984
100. Franks NP, Lieb WR: Molecular and cellular mechanisms of general anaesthesia. Nature 367:607, 1994
101. Campbell DB, Nash HA: Use of Drosophila mutants to distinguish among volatile general anesthetics. Proc Natl Acad Sci USA 91:2135, 1994
102. Sedensky MM, Meneely PM: Genetic analysis of halothane sensitivity in Caenorhabditis elegans. Science 236:952, 1987
103. Sonner JM, Gong D, Eger EI 2nd: Naturally occurring variability in anesthetic potency among inbred mouse strains. Anesth Analg 91:720, 2000
104. Simpson VJ, Rikke BA, Costello JM *et al*: Identification of a genetic region in mice that specifies sensitivity to propofol. Anesthesiology 88:379, 1998
105. Markel PD, Bennett B, Beeson M *et al*: Confirmation of quantitative trait loci for ethanol sensitivity in long-sleep and short-sleep mice. Genome Res 7:92, 1997
106. Homanics GE, Quinlan JJ, Mihalek RM *et al*: Alcohol and anesthetic mechanisms in genetically engineered mice. Front Biosci 3:D548, 1998
107. Sonner JM, Antognini JF, Dutton RC *et al*: Inhaled anesthetics and immobility: mechanisms, mysteries, and minimum alveolar anesthetic concentration. Anesth Analg 97:718, 2003
108. Wong SM, Cheng G, Homanics GE *et al*: Enflurane actions on spinal cords from mice that lack the beta3 subunit of the GABA(A) receptor. Anesthesiology 95:154, 2001
109. Homanics GE, Ferguson C, Quinlan JJ *et al*: Gene knockout of the alpha6 subunit of the gamma-aminobutyric acid type A receptor: lack of effect on responses to ethanol, pentobarbital, and general anesthetics. Mol Pharmacol 51:588, 1997
110. Rudolph U, Crestani F, Benke D *et al*: Benzodiazepine actions mediated by specific gamma-aminobutyric acid(A) receptor subtypes. Nature 401:796, 1999
111. Belelli D, Lambert JJ, Peters JA *et al*: The interaction of the general anesthetic etomidate with the gamma-aminobutyric acid type A receptor is influenced by a single amino acid. Proc Natl Acad Sci U S A 94:11031, 1997
112. Jurd R, Arras M, Lambert S *et al*: General anesthetic actions in vivo strongly attenuated by a point mutation in the GABA(A) receptor beta3 subunit. Faseb J 17:250, 2003
113. Reynolds DS, Rosahl TW, Cirone J *et al*: Sedation and anesthesia mediated by distinct GABA(A) receptor isoforms. J Neurosci 23:8608, 2003
114. Cirone J, Rosahl TW, Reynolds DS *et al*: Gamma-aminobutyric acid type A receptor beta 2 subunit mediates the hypothermic effect of etomidate in mice. Anesthesiology 100:1438, 2004
115. Lakhlani PP, MacMillan LB, Guo TZ *et al*: Substitution of a mutant alpha2a-adrenergic receptor via "hit and run" gene targeting reveals the role of this subtype in sedative, analgesic, and anesthetic-sparing responses in vivo. Proc Natl Acad Sci U S A 94:9950, 1997
116. Gerstin KM, Gong DH, Abdallah M *et al*: Mutation of KCNK5 or Kir3.2 potassium channels in mice does not change minimum alveolar anesthetic concentration. Anesth Analg 96:1345, 2003
117. Sternberg WF, Mogil JF: Genetic and hormonal basis of pain states. Best Pract Res Clin Anesthesiol 15:229, 2001
118. Bengtsson B, Thorson J: Back pain: A study of twins. Acta Genet Med Gemellol (Roma) 40:83, 1991
119. Mogil JS, Wilson SG, Bon K *et al*: Heritability of nociception I: Responses of 11 inbred mouse strains on 12 measures of nociception. Pain 80:67, 1999
120. Mogil JS, Richards SP, O'Toole LA *et al*: Genetic sensitivity to hot-plate nociception in DBA/2J and C57BL/6J inbred mouse strains: Possible sex-specific mediation by delta2-opioid receptors. Pain 70:267, 1997
121. Mogil JS, Grisel JE: Transgenic studies of pain. Pain 77:107, 1998
122. Phillips KA, Veenstra DL, Oren E *et al*: Potential role of pharmacogenomics in reducing adverse drug reactions: A systematic review. JAMA 286:2270, 2001
123. Lin LH, Hopf HW: Paradigm of the injury-repair continuum during critical illness. Crit Care Med 31:S493, 2003
124. Ayala A, Lomas JL, Grutkoski PS *et al*: Pathological aspects of apoptosis in severe sepsis and shock? Int J Biochem Cell Biol 35:7, 2003
125. Lin MT, Albertson TE: Genomic polymorphisms in sepsis. Crit Care Med 32:569, 2004
126. Mira JP, Cariou A, Grall F *et al*: Association of TNF2, a TNF-alpha promoter polymorphism, with septic shock susceptibility and mortality: a multicenter study. JAMA 282:561, 1999
127. Stuber F: Effects of genomic polymorphisms on the course of sepsis: Is there a concept for gene therapy? J Am Soc Nephrol 12(suppl 17):S60, 2001
128. Kahlke V, Schafmayer C, Schniewind B *et al*: Are postoperative complications genetically determined by TNF-beta NcoI gene polymorphism? Surgery 135:365, 2004
129. Fang XM, Schroder S, Hoeft A *et al*: Comparison of two polymorphisms of the interleukin-1 gene family: Interleukin-1 receptor antagonist polymorphism contributes to susceptibility to severe sepsis. Crit Care Med 27:1330, 1999
130. Schluter B, Raufhake C, Erren M *et al*: Effect of the interleukin-6 promoter polymorphism (−174 G/C) on the incidence and outcome of sepsis. Crit Care Med 30:32, 2002

131. Menges T, Hermans PW, Little SG *et al*: Plasminogen-activator-inhibitor-1 4G/5G promoter polymorphism and prognosis of severely injured patients. Lancet 357:1096, 2001
132. Harding D, Baines PB, Brull D *et al*: Severity of meningococcal disease in children and the angiotensin-converting enzyme insertion/deletion polymorphism. Am J Respir Crit Care Med 165:1103, 2002
133. Zeni F, Freeman B, Natanson C: Anti-inflammatory therapies to treat sepsis and septic shock: a reassessment. Crit Care Med 25:1095, 1997
134. Cobb JP, O'Keefe GE: Injury research in the genomic era. Lancet 363:2076, 2004
135. Prucha M, Ruryk A, Boriss H *et al*: Expression profiling: toward an application in sepsis diagnostics. Shock 22:29, 2004
136. Cobb JP, Laramie JM, Stormo GD *et al*: Sepsis gene expression profiling: Murine splenic compared with hepatic responses determined by using complementary DNA microarrays. Crit Care Med 30:2711, 2002
137. Leikauf GD, McDowell SA, Wesselkamper SC *et al*: Acute lung injury: functional genomics and genetic susceptibility. Chest 121:70S, 2002
138. Dasu MR, Cobb JP, Laramie JM *et al*: Gene expression profiles of livers from thermally injured rats. Gene 327:51, 2004
139. Fessler MB, Malcolm KC, Duncan MW *et al*: A genomic and proteomic analysis of activation of the human neutrophil by lipopolysaccharide and its mediation by p38 mitogen-activated protein kinase. J Biol Chem 277:31291, 2002
140. Buchman TG, Cobb JP, Lapedes AS *et al*: Complex systems analysis: A tool for shock research. Shock 16:248, 2001
141. Ge H, Walhout AJ, Vidal M: Integrating 'omic' information: A bridge between genomics and systems biology. Trends Genet 19:551, 2003
142. Phimister EG: Medicine and the racial divide. N Engl J Med 348:1081, 2003
143. Stafford-Smith M, Podgoreanu M, Swaminathan M, et al.: Association of genetic polymorphisms with risk of renal injury after coronary bypass graft surgery. Am J Kidney Dis 45(3):519, 2005

CHAPTER 8 ■ ELECTRICAL AND FIRE SAFETY

JAN EHRENWERTH AND HARRY A. SEIFERT

KEY POINTS

1. A basic principle of electricity is known as Ohm's law.
2. To have the completed circuit necessary for current flow, a closed loop must exist and a voltage source must drive the current through the impedance.
3. To receive a shock, one must contact the electrical circuit at two points, and there must be a voltage source that causes the current to flow through an individual.
4. In electrical terminology, grounding is applied to two separate concepts: the grounding of electrical power and the grounding of electrical equipment.
5. To provide an extra measure of safety from gross electrical shock (macroshock), the power supplied to most operating rooms is ungrounded.
6. The line isolation monitor (LIM) is a device that continuously monitors the integrity of an isolated power system.
7. The ground fault circuit interrupter (GFCI) is another popular device used to prevent individuals from receiving an electrical shock in a grounded power system.
8. An electrically susceptible patient (i.e., one who has a direct, external connection to the heart) they may be at risk from very small currents; this is called microshock.
9. Problems can arise if the electrosurgical return plate is improperly applied to the patient or if the cord connecting the return plate to the electrosurgical unit (ESU) is damaged or broken.
10. Fires in the operating room are just as much a danger today as they were 100 years ago when patients were anesthetized with flammable anesthetic agents.
11. The fire triad consists of a heat or ignition source, a fuel, and an oxidizer.
12. The two major ignition sources for OR fires are the ESU and the laser.
13. It is known that desiccated carbon dioxide absorbent can, in rare circumstances, react with sevoflurane to produce a fire.
14. All OR personnel should be familiar with the location and operation of the fire extinguishers.

The myriad of electrical and electronic devices in the modern operating room greatly improve patient care and safety. However, these devices also subject both the patient and operating room personnel to increased risks. To reduce the risk of electrical shock, most operating rooms have electrical systems that incorporate special safety features. It is incumbent upon the anesthesiologist to have a thorough understanding of the basic principles of electricity and an appreciation of the concepts of electrical safety applicable to the operating room environment.

PRINCIPLES OF ELECTRICITY

1 A basic principle of electricity is known as *Ohm's law,* which is represented by the equation:

$$E = I \times R$$

where E is electromotive force (in volts), I is current (in amperes), and R is resistance (in ohms). Ohm's law forms the basis for the physiologic equation BP = CO × SVR; that is, blood pressure (BP) is equal to the cardiac output (CO) times the systemic vascular resistance (SVR). In this case, the blood pressure of the vascular system is analogous to voltage, the cardiac output to current, and systemic vascular resistance to the forces opposing the flow of electrons. Electrical power is measured in watts. Wattage (W) is the product of the voltage (E) and the current (I), as defined by the formula:

$$W = E \times I$$

The amount of electrical work done is measured in watts multiplied by a unit of time. The watt-second (a joule, J) is a common designation for electrical energy expended in doing work. The energy produced by a defibrillator is measured in watt-seconds (or joules). The kilowatt-hour is used by electrical utility companies to measure larger quantities of electrical energy.

Wattage can be thought of as a measure not only of work done but also of heat produced in any electrical circuit. Substituting Ohm's law in the formula

$$W = E \times I$$
$$W = (I \times R) \times I$$
$$W = I^2 \times R$$

Thus, wattage is equal to the square of the current I^2 (amperage) times the resistance R. Using these formulas, it is possible to calculate the number of amperes and the resistance of a given device if the wattage and the voltage are known. For example, a 60-watt light bulb operating on a household 120-volt circuit would require 0.5 ampere, of current for operation. Rearranging the formula so that

$$I = W/E$$

we have

$$I = (60 \text{ watts})/(120 \text{ volts})$$
$$I = 0.5 \text{ ampere}$$

Using this in Ohm's law

$$R = E/I$$

the resistance can be calculated to be 240 ohms:

$$R = (120 \text{ volts})/(0.5 \text{ ampere})$$
$$R = 240 \text{ ohms}$$

It is obvious from the previous discussion that 1 volt of electromotive force (EMF) flowing through a 1-ohm resistance will generate 1 ampere of current. Similarly, 1 ampere of current induced by 1 volt of electromotive force will generate 1 watt of power.

Direct and Alternating Currents

Any substance that permits the flow of electrons is called a *conductor.* Current is characterized by electrons flowing through a conductor. If the electron flow is always in the same direction, it is referred to as *direct current* (DC). However, if the electron flow reverses direction at a regular interval, it is termed *alternating current* (AC). Either of these types of current can be pulsed or continuous in nature.[1]

The previous discussion of Ohm's law is accurate when applied to DC circuits. However, when dealing with AC circuits, the situation is more complex because the flow of the current is opposed by a more complicated form of resistance, known as *impedance.*

Impedance

Impedance, designated by the letter Z, is defined as the sum of the forces that oppose electron movement in an AC circuit. Impedance consists of resistance (ohms) but also takes capacitance and inductance into account. In actuality, when referring to AC circuits, Ohm's law is defined as

$$E = I \times Z$$

An *insulator* is a substance that opposes the flow of electrons. Therefore, an insulator has a high impedance to electron flow, whereas a conductor has a low impedance to electron flow.

In AC circuits the capacitance and inductance can be important factors in determining the total impedance. Both capacitance and inductance are influenced by the frequency (cycles per second or hertz, Hz) at which the AC current reverses direction. The impedance is directly proportional to the frequency (f) times the inductance (IND):

$$Z \propto (f \times \text{IND})$$

and the impedance is inversely proportional to the product of the frequency (f) and the capacitance (CAP):

$$Z \propto 1/(f \times \text{CAP})$$

As the AC current increases in frequency, the net effect of both capacitance and inductance increases. However, because impedance and capacitance are inversely related, total impedance decreases as the product of the frequency and the capacitance increases. Thus, as frequency increases, impedance falls and more current is allowed to pass.[2]

Capacitance

A *capacitor* consists of any two parallel conductors that are separated by an insulator (Fig. 8-1). A capacitor has the ability to store charge. *Capacitance* is the measure of that substance's ability to store charge. In a DC circuit the capacitor plates are charged by a voltage source (i.e., a battery) and there is only a momentary current flow. The circuit is not completed and no further current can flow unless a resistance is connected between the two plates and the capacitor is discharged.[3]

In contrast to DC circuits, a capacitor in an AC circuit permits current flow even when the circuit is not completed by a resistance. This is because of the nature of AC circuits, in which the current flow is constantly being reversed. Because current flow results from the movement of electrons, the capacitor plates are alternately charged—first positive and then negative with every reversal of the AC current direction—resulting in an effective current flow as far as the remainder of the circuit is concerned, even though the circuit is not completed.[4]

Because the effect of capacitance on impedance varies directly with the AC frequency (Hz), the greater the AC frequency, the lower the impedance. Therefore, high-frequency currents (0.5 to 2 million Hz), such as those used by electrosurgical units (ESUs), will cause a marked decrease in impedance. For example, a 20-million–ohm impedance in a 60-Hz AC circuit will be reduced to just a few hundred ohms when the frequency is increased to 1 million Hz.[5]

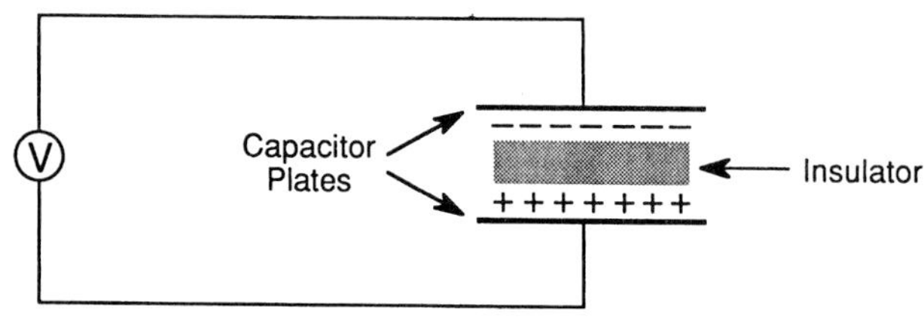

FIGURE 8-1. A capacitor consists of two parallel conductors separated by an insulator. The capacitor is capable of storing charge supplied by a voltage source.

Electrical devices use capacitors for various beneficial purposes. There is, however, a phenomenon known as *stray capacitance*—capacitance that was not designed into the system but is incidental to the construction of the equipment.[6] All AC-operated equipment produces stray capacitance. An ordinary power cord, for example, consisting of two insulated wires running next to each other will generate significant capacitance simply by being plugged into a 120-volt circuit, even though the piece of equipment is not turned on. Another example of stray capacitance is found in electric motors. The circuit wiring in electric motors generates stray capacitance to the metal housing of the motor.[7] The clinical importance of capacitance will be emphasized later in the chapter.

Inductance

Whenever electrons flow in a wire, a magnetic field is induced around the wire. If the wire is coiled repeatedly around an iron core, as in a transformer, the magnetic field can be very strong. *Inductance* is a property of AC circuits in which an opposing EMF can be electromagnetically generated in the circuit. The net effect of inductance is to increase impedance. Because the effect of inductance on impedance is also dependent on AC frequency, increases in frequency will increase the total impedance. Therefore, the total impedance of a coil will be much greater than its simple resistance.[4]

ELECTRICAL SHOCK HAZARDS

Alternating and Direct Currents

Whenever an individual contacts an external source of electricity, an electrical shock is possible. An electrical current can stimulate skeletal muscle cells to contract, and thus can be used therapeutically in devices such as pacemakers or defibrillators. However, casual contact with an electrical current, whether AC or DC, can lead to injury or death. Although it takes approximately three times as much DC as AC to cause ventricular fibrillation,[3] this by no means renders DC harmless. Devices such as an automobile battery or a DC defibrillator can be sources of direct current shocks.

In the United States, utility companies supply electrical energy in the form of alternating currents of 120 volts at a frequency of 60 Hz. The 120 volts of EMF and 1 ampere of current are the effective voltage and amperage in an AC circuit. This is also referred to as RMS (root-mean-square). It takes 1.414 amperes of peak amperage in the sinusoidal curve to give an effective amperage of 1 ampere. Similarly, it takes 170 volts (120×1.414) at the peak of the AC curve to get an effective voltage of 120 volts. The 60 Hz refers to the number of times in 1 second that the current reverses its direction of flow.[8] Both the voltage and current waveforms form a sinusoidal pattern (Fig. 8-2).

2 To have the completed circuit necessary for current flow, a closed loop must exist and a voltage source must drive the current through the impedance. If current is to flow in the electrical circuit, there has to be a *voltage differential,* or a drop in the driving pressure across the impedance. According to Ohm's law, if the resistance is held constant, then the greater the current flow, the larger the voltage drop must be.[9]

The power company attempts to maintain the line voltage constant at 120 volts. Therefore, by Ohm's law the current flow is inversely proportional to the impedance. A typical power cord consists of two conductors. One, designated as *hot* carries the current to the impedance; the other is *neutral,* and it returns the current to the source. The potential difference between the two is effectively 120 volts (Fig. 8-3). The amount of current flowing through a given device is frequently referred to as the *load.* The load of the circuit is dependent on the impedance. A very high impedance circuit allows only a small current to flow and thus has a small load. A very low impedance circuit will draw a large current and is said to be a large load. A *short circuit* occurs when there is a zero impedance load with a very high current flow.[10]

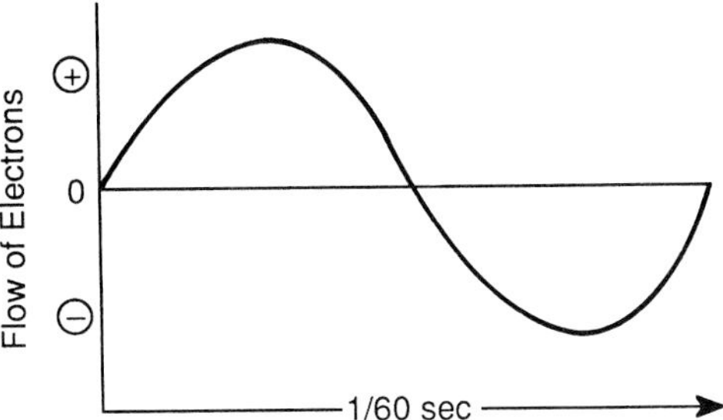

FIGURE 8-2. Sine wave flow of electrons in a 60-Hz alternating current.

Source of Shocks

To practice electrical safety it is important for the anesthesiologist to understand the basic principles of electricity and be aware of how electrical accidents can occur. Electrical accidents or shocks occur when a person becomes part of or completes
3 an electrical circuit. To receive a shock, one must contact the electrical circuit at two points, and there must be a voltage source that causes the current to flow through an individual (Fig. 8-4).

When an individual contacts a source of electricity, damage occurs in one of two ways. First, the electrical current can disrupt the normal electrical function of cells. Depending on its magnitude, the current can contract muscles, alter brain function, paralyze respiration, or disrupt normal heart function, leading to ventricular fibrillation. The second mechanism involves the dissipation of electrical energy throughout the body's tissues. An electrical current passing through any resistance raises the temperature of that substance. If enough thermal energy is released, the temperature will rise sufficiently to produce a burn. Accidents involving household currents usually do not result in severe burns. However, in accidents involving very high voltages (i.e., power transmission lines), severe burns are common.

The severity of an electrical shock is determined by the amount of current (number of amperes) and the duration of the current flow. For the purposes of this discussion, electrical

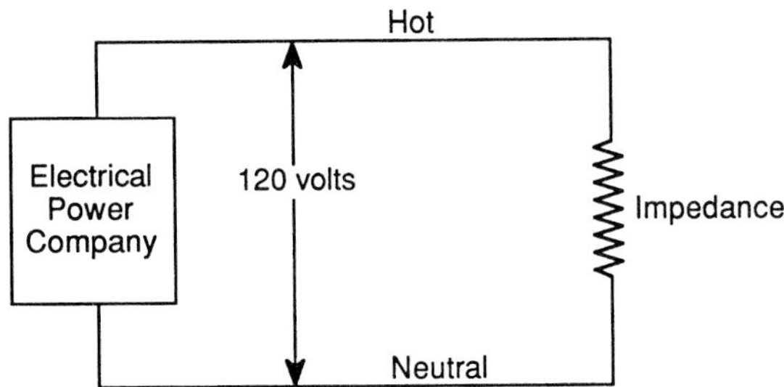

FIGURE 8-3. A typical AC circuit where there is a potential difference of 120 volts between the hot and neutral sides of the circuit. The current flows through a resistance, which in AC circuits is more accurately referred to as impedance, and then returns to the electrical power company.

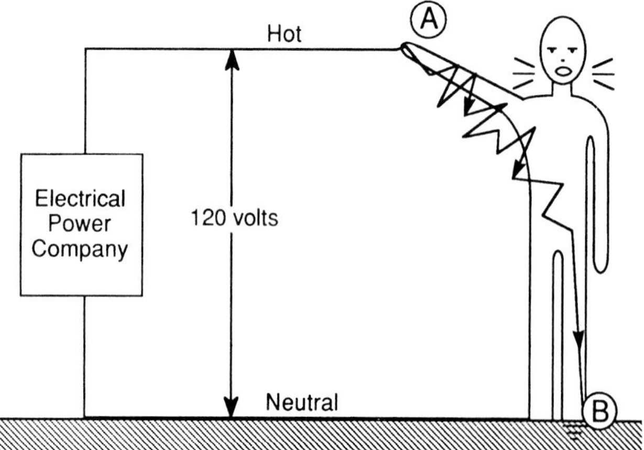

FIGURE 8-4. An individual can complete an electric circuit and receive a shock by coming in contact with the hot side of the circuit (point *A*). This is because he or she is standing on the ground (point *B*) and the contact point *A* and the ground point *B* provide the two contact points necessary for a completed circuit. The severity of the shock that the individual receives is dependent on his or her skin resistance.

shocks are divided into two categories. *Macroshock* refers to large amounts of current flowing through a person, which can cause harm or death. *Microshock* refers to very small amounts of current and applies only to the electrically susceptible patient. This is an individual who has an external conduit that is in direct contact with the heart. This can be a pacing wire or a saline-filled catheter such as a central venous or pulmonary artery catheter. In the case of the electrically susceptible patient, even minute amounts of current (microshock) may cause ventricular fibrillation.

Table 8-1 shows the effects typically produced by various currents following a 1-second contact with a 60-Hz current. When an individual contacts a 120-volt household current, the severity of the shock will depend on his or her skin resistance, the duration of the contact, and the current density. Skin resistance can vary from a few thousand to 1 million ohms. If a person with a skin resistance of 1,000 ohms contacts a 120-volt circuit, he or she would receive 120 milliamperes (mA) of current, which would probably be lethal. However, if that same person's skin resistance is 100,000 ohms, the current flow would be 1.2 mA, which would barely be perceptible.

$$I = E/R = (120\,\text{volts})/(1,000\,\text{ohms}) = 120\,\text{mA}$$
$$I = E/R = (120\,\text{volts})/(100,000\,\text{ohms}) = 1.2\,\text{mA}$$

The longer an individual is in contact with the electrical source, the more dire the consequences because more energy will be released and more tissue damaged. Also, there will be a greater chance of ventricular fibrillation from excitation of the heart during the vulnerable period of the electrocardiogram (ECG) cycle.

Current density is a way of expressing the amount of current that is applied per unit area of tissue. The diffusion of current in the body tends to be in all directions. The greater the current or the smaller the area to which it is applied, the higher the current density. In relation to the heart, a current of 100 mA (100,000 μA) is generally required to produce ventricular fibrillation when applied to the surface of the body. However, only 100 μA (0.1 mA) is required to produce ventricular fibrillation when that minute current is applied directly to the myocardium through an instrument having a very small contact area, such as a pacing wire electrode. In this case, the current density is 1,000-fold greater when applied directly to the heart; therefore, only 1/1,000 of the energy is required to cause ventricular fibrillation. In this case, the electrically susceptible patient can be electrocuted with currents well below 1 mA, which is the threshold of perception for humans. The frequency at which the current reverses is also an important factor in determining the amount of current an individual can safely contact. Utility companies in the United States produce electricity at a frequency of 60 Hz. They use 60 Hz because higher frequencies cause greater power loss through transmission lines and lower frequencies cause a detectable flicker from light sources.[11] The "let-go" current is defined as that current above which sustained muscular contraction occurs and at which an individual would be unable to let go of an energized wire. The let-go current for a 60-Hz AC power is 10 to 20 mA,[10,12,13] whereas at a frequency of 1 million Hz, up to 3 amperes (3,000 mA) is generally considered safe.[3] It should be noted that very high frequency currents do not excite contractile tissue; consequently, they do not cause cardiac arrhythmias.

It can be seen that Ohm's law governs the flow of electricity. For a completed circuit to exist, there must be a closed loop with a driving pressure to force a current through a resistance, just as in the cardiovascular system there must be a blood pressure to drive the cardiac output through the peripheral resistance. Figure 8-5 illustrates that a hot wire carrying a 120-volt pressure through the resistance of a 60-watt light bulb produces a current flow of 0.5 ampere. The voltage in the neutral wire is approximately 0 volts, while the current in the neutral wire remains at 0.5 ampere. This correlates with our cardiovascular analogy, where a mean blood pressure decrease of 80 mm Hg between the aortic root and the right atrium forces a cardiac output of 6 L/min^{-1} through a systemic vascular resistance of 13.3 resistance units. However, the flow (in this case, the cardiac output, or in the case of the electrical model, the current) is still the same everywhere in the circuit. That is, the cardiac output on the arterial side is the same as the cardiac output on the venous side.

TABLE 8-1

EFFECTS OF 60-Hz CURRENT ON AN AVERAGE HUMAN FOR A 1-SECOND CONTACT

CURRENT	EFFECT
MACROSHOCK	
1 mA (0.001 A)	Threshold of perception
5 mA (0.005 A)	Accepted as maximum harmless current intensity
10–20 mA (0.01–0.02 A)	"Let-go" current before sustained muscle contraction
50 mA (0.05 A)	Pain, possible fainting, mechanical injury; heart and respiratory functions continue
100–300 mA (0.1–0.3 A)	Ventricular fibrillation will start, but respiratory center remains intact
6,000 mA (6 A)	Sustained myocardial contraction, followed by normal heart rhythm; temporary respiratory paralysis; burns if current density is high
MICROSHOCK	
100 μA (0.1 mA)	Ventricular fibrillation
10 μA (0.01 mA)	Recommended maximum 60-Hz leakage current

A, amperes; mA, milliamperes; μA, microamperes.

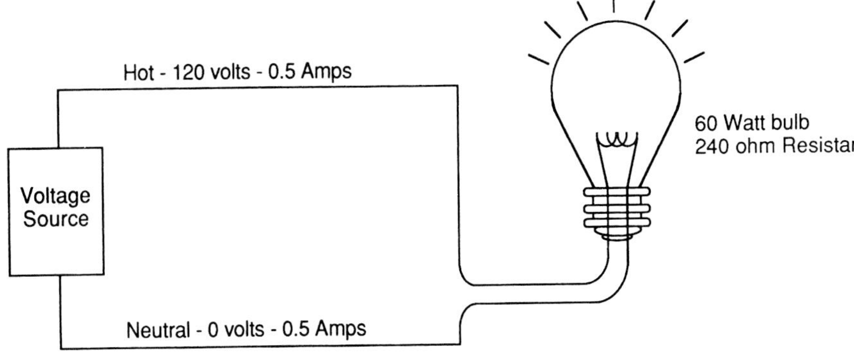

FIGURE 8-5. A 60-watt light bulb has an internal resistance of 240 ohms and draws 0.5 ampere of current. The voltage drop in the circuit is from 120 in the hot wire to 0 in the neutral wire, but the current is 0.5 ampere in both the hot and neutral wires.

Grounding

To fully understand electrical shock hazards and their prevention, one must have a thorough knowledge of the concepts of grounding. These concepts of grounding probably constitute the most confusing aspects of electrical safety because the same term is used to describe several different principles.
4 In electrical terminology, grounding is applied to two separate concepts. The first is the grounding of electrical *power,* and the second is the grounding of electrical *equipment*. Thus, the concepts that (1) power can be grounded or ungrounded and that (2) power can supply electrical devices that are themselves grounded or ungrounded are not mutually exclusive. It is vital to understand this point as the basis of electrical safety (Table 8-2). Whereas electrical *power* is grounded in the home, it is usually ungrounded in the operating room. In the home, electrical *equipment* may be grounded or ungrounded, but it should always be grounded in the operating room.

ELECTRICAL POWER: GROUNDED

Electrical utilities universally provide power that is grounded (by convention, the earth–ground potential is zero, and all voltages represent a difference between potentials). That is, one of the wires supplying the power to a home is intentionally connected to the earth. The utility companies do this as a safety measure to prevent electrical charges from building up in their wiring during electrical storms. This also prevents the very high voltages used in transmitting power by the utility from entering the home in the event of an equipment failure in their high-voltage system.[3]

The power enters the typical home via two wires. These two wires are attached to the main fuse or the circuit breaker box at the service entrance. The "hot" wire supplies power to the "hot" distribution strip. The neutral wire is connected to the neutral distribution strip and to a service entrance ground (i.e., a pipe buried in the earth) (Fig. 8-6). From the fuse box, three wires leave to supply the electrical outlets in the house. In the United States, the "hot" wire is color-coded black and carries a voltage 120 volts above ground potential. The second wire is the neutral wire color-coded white; the third wire is the ground wire, which is either color-coded green or is uninsulated (bare wire). The ground and the neutral wires are attached at the same point in the circuit breaker box and then further connected to a cold-water pipe (Figs. 8-7 and 8-8). Thus, this grounded power system is also referred to as a neutral grounded power system. The black wire is not connected to the ground, as this would create a short circuit. The black wire is attached to the "hot" (i.e., 120 volts above ground) distribution strip on which the circuit breakers or fuses are located. From here, numerous branch circuits supply electrical power to the outlets in the house. Each branch circuit is protected by a circuit breaker or fuse that limits current to a specific maximum amperage. Most electrical circuits in the house are 15- or 20-ampere circuits. These typically supply power to the electrical outlets and lights in the house. Several higher amperage circuits are also provided for devices such as an electric stove or an electric clothes dryer. These devices are powered by 240-volt circuits, which can draw from 30 to 50 amperes of current. The circuit breaker or fuse will interrupt the flow of current on the hot side of the line in the event of a short circuit or if the demand placed on that circuit is too high. For example, a 15-ampere branch circuit will be capable of supporting 1,800 watts of power.

$$W = E \times I$$
$$W = 120 \text{ volts} \times 15 \text{ amperes}$$
$$W = 1{,}800 \text{ watts}$$

Therefore, if two 1,500-watt hair dryers were simultaneously plugged into one outlet, the load would be too great for a 15-ampere circuit, and the circuit breaker would open (trip) or the fuse would melt. This is done to prevent the supply wires in the circuit from melting and starting a fire. The amperage of the circuit breaker on the branch circuit is determined by the thickness of the wire that it supplies. If a 20-ampere breaker is used with wire rated for only 15 amperes, the wire could melt and start a fire before the circuit breaker would trip. It is important to note that a 15-ampere circuit breaker does not protect an individual from lethal shocks. The 15 amperes of current that would trip the circuit breaker far exceeds the 100 to 200 mA that will produce ventricular fibrillation.

The wires that leave the circuit breaker supply the electrical outlets and lighting for the rest of the house. In older homes the electrical cable consists of two wires, a hot and a neutral, which supply power to the electrical outlets (Fig. 8-9). In newer homes, a third wire has been added to the electrical cable (Fig. 8-10). This third wire is either green or uninsulated (bare)

TABLE 8-2

DIFFERENCES BETWEEN POWER AND EQUIPMENT GROUNDING IN THE HOME AND THE OPERATING ROOM

	POWER	EQUIPMENT
Home	+	±
Operating room	–	+

+, grounded; –, ungrounded; ±, may or may not be grounded.

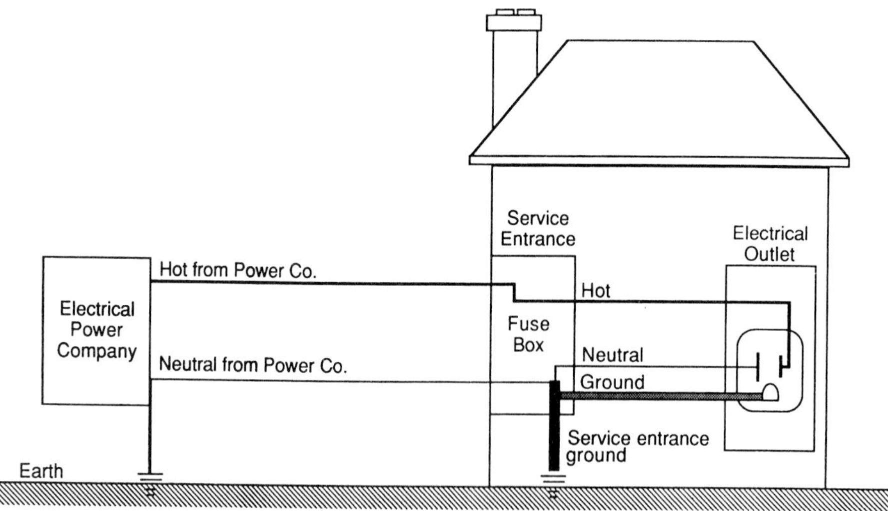

FIGURE 8-6. In a neutral grounded power system, the electric company supplies two lines to the typical home. The neutral is connected to ground by the power company and again connected to a service entrance ground when it enters the fuse box. Both the neutral and ground wires are connected together in the fuse box at the neutral bus bar, which is also attached to the service entrance ground.

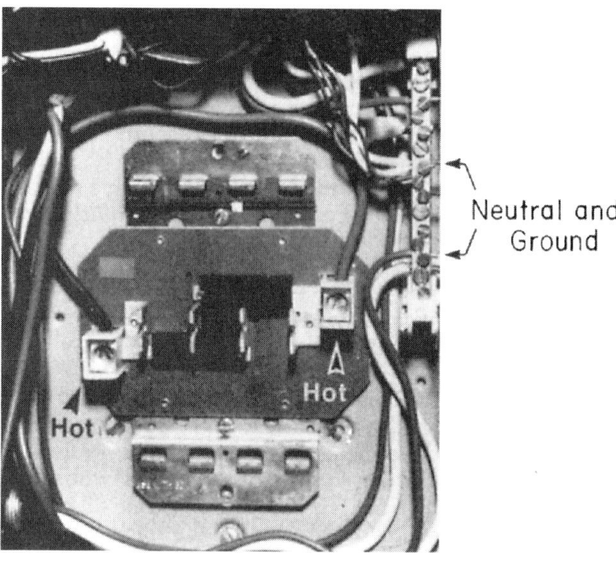

FIGURE 8-7. Inside a fuse box with the circuit breakers removed. The *arrowheads* indicate the hot wires energizing the strips where the circuit breakers are located. The *arrows* point to the neutral bus bar where the neutral and ground wires are connected.

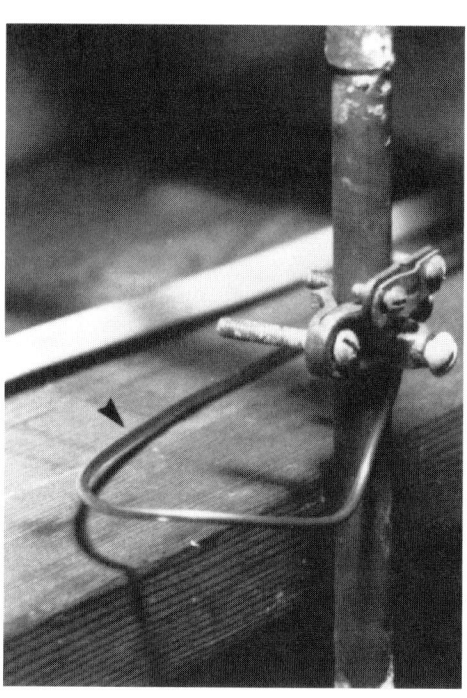

FIGURE 8-8. The *arrowhead* indicates the ground wire from the fuse box attached to a cold-water pipe.

FIGURE 8-9. An older style electrical outlet consisting of just two wires (a hot and a neutral). There is no ground wire.

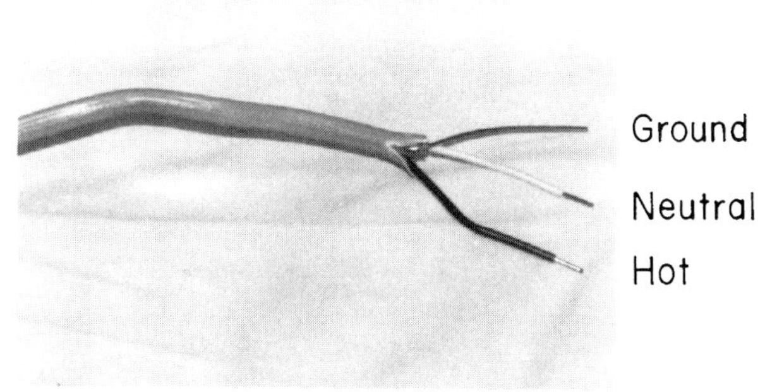

FIGURE 8-10. Modern electrical cable in which a third, or ground, wire has been added.

FIGURE 8-11. Modern electrical outlet in which the ground wire is present. The *arrowhead* points to the part of the receptacle where the ground wire connects.

and serves as a ground wire for the power receptacle (Fig. 8-11). On one end, the ground wire is attached to the electrical outlet (Fig. 8-12); on the other, it is connected to the neutral distribution strip in the circuit breaker box along with the neutral (white) wires (Fig. 8-13).

It should be realized that in both the old and new situations, the power is grounded. That is, a 120-volt potential exists between the hot (black) and the neutral (white) wire and between the hot wire and ground. In this case, the ground is the earth (Fig. 8-14). In modern home construction, there is still a 120-volt potential difference between the hot (black) and the neutral (white) wire as well as a 120-volt difference between the equipment ground wire (which is the third wire), and between the hot wire and earth (Fig. 8-15).

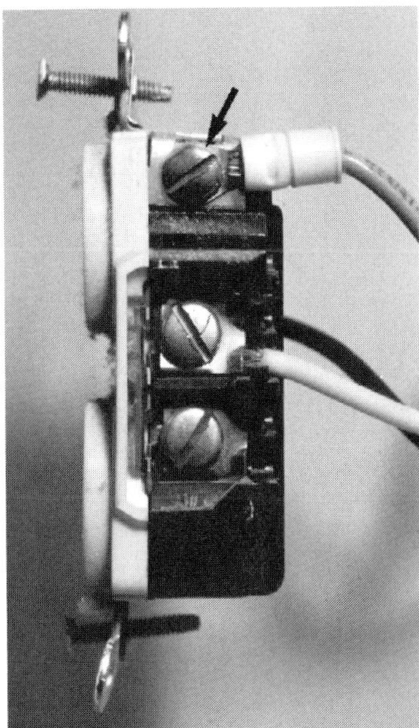

FIGURE 8-12. Detail of modern electrical power receptacle. The *arrow* points to the ground wire, which is attached to the grounding screw on the power receptacle.

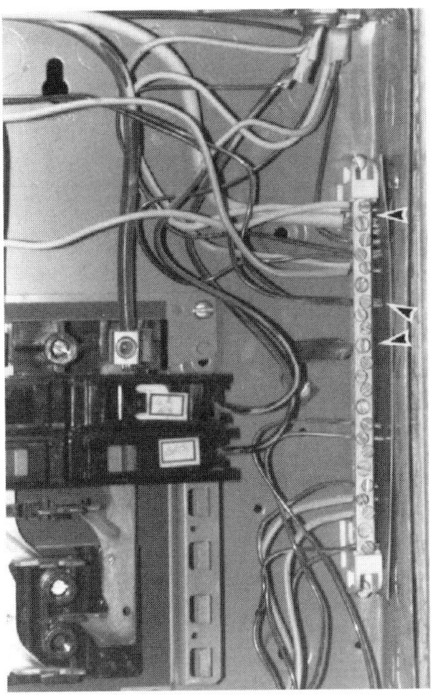

FIGURE 8-13. The ground wires from the power outlet are run to the neutral bus bar, where they are connected with the neutral wires (*arrowheads*).

A 60-watt light bulb can be used as an example to further illustrate this point. Normally, the hot and neutral wires are connected to the two wires of the light bulb socket, and throwing the switch will illuminate the bulb (Fig. 8-16). Similarly, if the hot wire is connected to one side of the bulb socket and the other wire from the light bulb is connected to the equipment ground wire, the bulb will still illuminate. If there is no equipment ground wire, the bulb will still light if the second wire is connected to any grounded metallic object such as a water pipe or a faucet. This illustrates the fact that the 120-volt potential difference exists not only between the hot and the neutral wires but also between the hot wire and any grounded object. Thus, in a grounded power system, the current will flow between the hot wire and any conductor with an earth ground.

As previously stated, current flow requires a closed loop with a source of voltage. For an individual to receive an electric shock, he or she must contact the loop at two points. Because we may be standing on ground or be in contact with an object that is referenced to ground, only one additional contact point is necessary to complete the circuit and thus receive an electrical shock. This is an unfortunate and inherently dangerous consequence of grounded power systems. Modern wiring systems have added the third wire, the equipment ground wire, as a safety measure to reduce the severity of a potential electrical shock. This is accomplished by providing an alternate, low-resistance pathway through which the current can flow to ground.

Over time the insulation covering wires may deteriorate. It is then possible for a bare, hot wire to contact the metal case or frame of an electrical device. The case would then become energized and constitute a shock hazard to someone coming in contact with it. Figure 8-17 illustrates a typical short circuit, where the individual has come in contact with the hot case of an instrument. This illustrates the type of wiring found in older homes. There is no ground wire in the electrical outlet, nor is the electrical apparatus equipped with a ground wire. Here, the individual completes the circuit and receives a severe shock. Figure 8-18 illustrates a similar example, except that now the

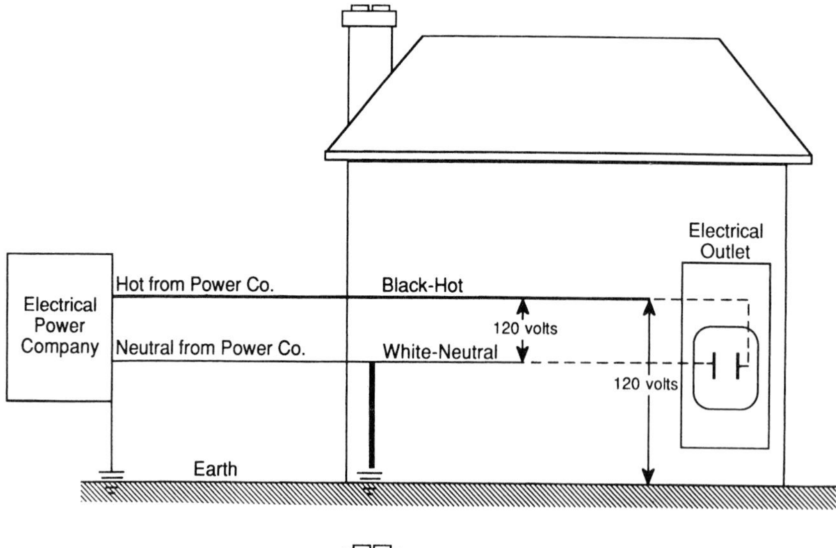

FIGURE 8-14. Diagram of a house with older style wiring that does not contain a ground wire. A 120-volt potential difference exists between the hot and the neutral wire, as well as between the hot wire and the earth.

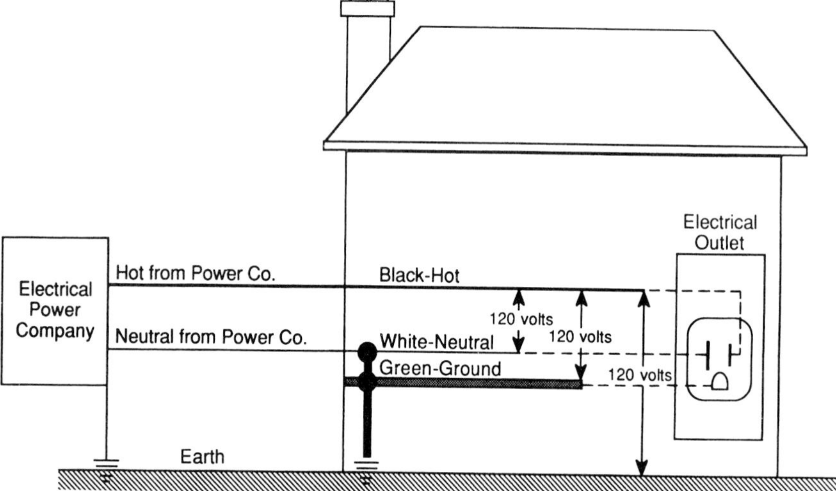

FIGURE 8-15. Diagram of a house with modern wiring in which the third, or ground, wire has been added. The 120-volt potential difference exists between the hot and neutral wires, the hot and the ground wires, and the hot wire and the earth.

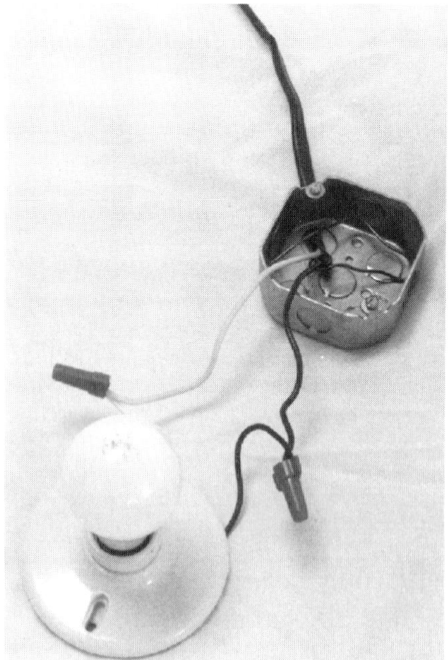

FIGURE 8-16. A simple light bulb circuit in which the hot and neutral wires are connected with the corresponding wires from the light bulb fixture.

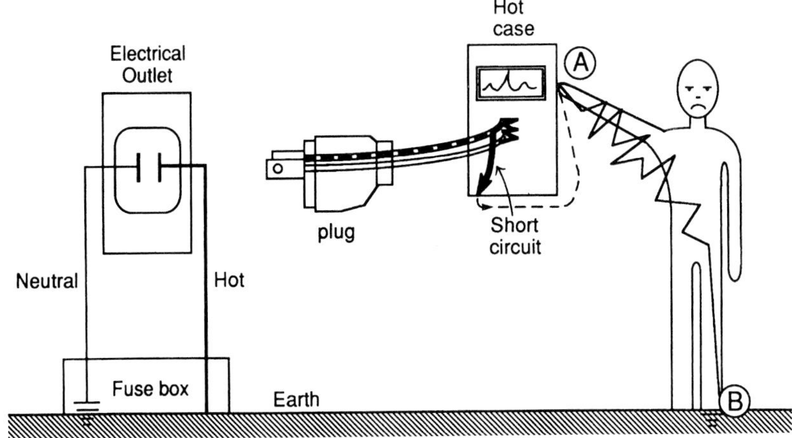

FIGURE 8-17. When a faulty piece of equipment without an equipment ground wire is plugged into an electrical outlet not containing a ground wire, the case of the instrument will become hot. An individual touching the hot case (point *A*) will receive a shock because he or she is standing on the earth (point *B*) and completes the circuit. The current (*dashed line*) will flow from the instrument through the individual touching the hot case.

equipment ground wire is part of the electrical distribution system. In this example, the equipment ground wire provides a pathway of low impedance through which the current can travel; therefore, most of the current would travel through the ground wire. In this case, the person may get a shock, but it is unlikely to be fatal.

The electrical power supplied to homes is always grounded. A 120-volt potential always exists between the hot conductor and ground or earth. The third or equipment ground wire used in modern electrical wiring systems does not normally have current flowing through it. In the event of a short circuit, an electrical device with a three-prong plug (i.e., a ground wire connected to its case) will conduct the majority of the short-circuited or "fault" current through the ground wire and away from the individual. This provides a significant safety benefit to someone accidentally contacting the defective device. If a large enough fault current exists, the ground wire also will provide a means to complete the short circuit back to the circuit breaker or fuse, and this will either melt the fuse or trip the circuit breaker. Thus, in a grounded power system, it is possible to have either grounded or ungrounded equipment, depending on when the wiring was installed and whether the electrical device is equipped with a three-prong plug containing a ground wire. Obviously, attempts to bypass the safety system of the equipment ground should be avoided. Devices such as a "cheater plug" (Fig. 8-19) should never be used because they defeat the safety feature of the equipment ground wire.

ELECTRICAL POWER: UNGROUNDED

Numerous electronic devices, together with power cords and puddles of saline solutions on the floor, make the operating room an electrically hazardous environment for both patients and personnel. Bruner et al[14] found that 40% of electrical accidents in hospitals occurred in the operating room. The complexity of electrical equipment in the modern operating room demands that electrical safety be a factor of paramount importance. 5 To provide an extra measure of safety from macroshock, the power supplied to most operating rooms is ungrounded. In this ungrounded power system, the current is isolated from ground potential. The 120-volt potential difference exists only between the two wires of the isolated power system, but no circuit exists between the ground and either of the isolated power lines.

Supplying ungrounded power to the operating room requires the use of an *isolation transformer* (Fig. 8-20). This device uses electromagnetic induction to induce a current in the ungrounded or secondary winding of the transformer from energy supplied to the primary winding. There is no direct electrical connection between the power supplied by the utility company on the primary side and the power induced by the transformer on the ungrounded or secondary side. Thus, the power supplied to the operating room is isolated from ground (Fig. 8-21). Because the 120-volt potential exists only between

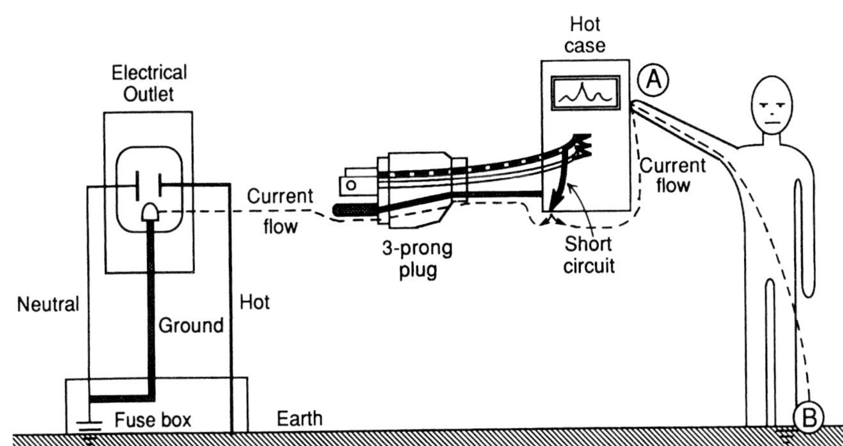

FIGURE 8-18. When a faulty piece of equipment containing an equipment ground wire is properly connected to an electrical outlet with a grounding connection, the current (*dashed line*) will preferentially flow down the low-resistance ground wire. An individual touching the case (point *A*) while standing on the ground (point *B*) will still complete the circuit; however, only a small part of the current will go through the individual.

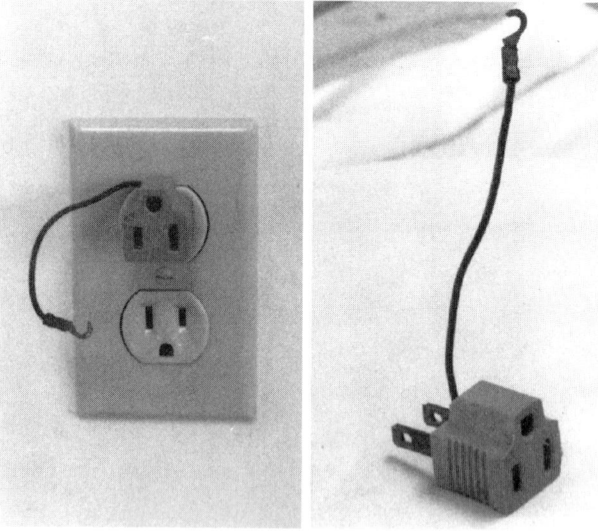

FIGURE 8-19. *Right.* A "cheater plug" that converts a three-prong power cord to a two-prong cord. *Left.* The wire attached to the cheater plug is rarely connected to the screw in the middle of the outlet. This totally defeats the purpose of the equipment ground wire.

the two wires of the isolated circuit, neither wire is hot or neutral with reference to ground. In this case, they are simply referred to as line 1 and line 2 (Fig. 8-22). Using the example of the light bulb, if one connects the two wires of the bulb socket to the two wires of the isolated power system, the light will illuminate. However, if one connects one of the wires tot one side of the isolated power and the other wire to ground, the light will not illuminate. If the wires of the isolated power system are connected, the short circuit will trip the circuit breaker. In comparing the two systems, the standard grounded power has a direct connection to ground, whereas the isolated system imposes a very high impedance to any current flow to ground.

The added safety of this system can be seen in Figure 8-23. In this case, a person has come in contact with one side of the isolated power system (point *A*). Because standing on ground (point *B*) does not constitute a part of the isolated circuit, the individual does not complete the loop and will not receive a shock. This is because the ground is part of the primary circuit (*solid lines*), and the person is contacting only one side of the isolated secondary circuit (*cross-hatched lines*). The person does not complete either circuit (i.e., have two contact points); therefore, this situation does not pose an electric shock hazard. Of course, if the person contacts both lines of the isolated power system (an unlikely event), he or she would receive a shock.

If a faulty electrical appliance with an intact equipment ground wire is plugged into a standard household outlet, and the home wiring has a properly connected ground wire, then the amount of electrical current that will flow through the individual is considerably less than what will flow through the low-resistance ground wire. Here, an individual would be fairly well protected from a serious shock. However, if that ground wire were broken, the individual might receive a lethal shock. No shock would occur if the same faulty piece of equipment were plugged into the isolated power system, even if the equipment ground wire were broken. Thus, the isolated power system provides a significant amount of protection from macroshock. Another feature of the isolated power system is that the faulty piece of equipment, even though it may be partially short-circuited, will not usually trip the circuit breaker. This is an important feature because the faulty piece of equipment may be part of a life-support system for a patient. It is important to note that even though the power is isolated from ground, the case or frame of all electrical equipment is still connected to an equipment ground. The third wire (equipment ground wire) is necessary for a total electrical safety program.

Figure 8-24 illustrates a scenario involving a faulty piece of equipment connected to the isolated power system. This does not represent a hazard; it merely converts the isolated power back to a grounded power system as exists outside the

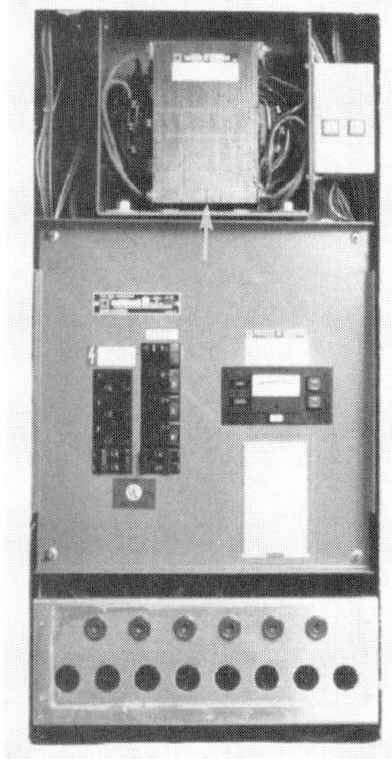

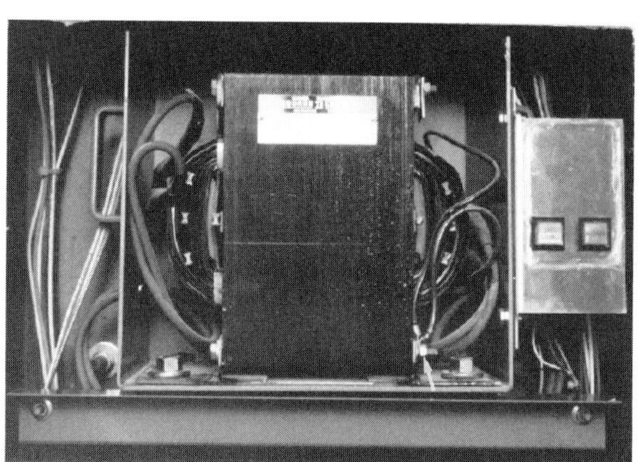

FIGURE 8-20. **A.** Isolated power panel showing circuit breakers, LIM, and isolation transformer (*arrow*). **B.** Detail of an isolation transformer with the attached warning lights. The arrow points to ground wire connection on the primary side of the transformer. Note that no similar connection exists on the secondary side of the transformer.

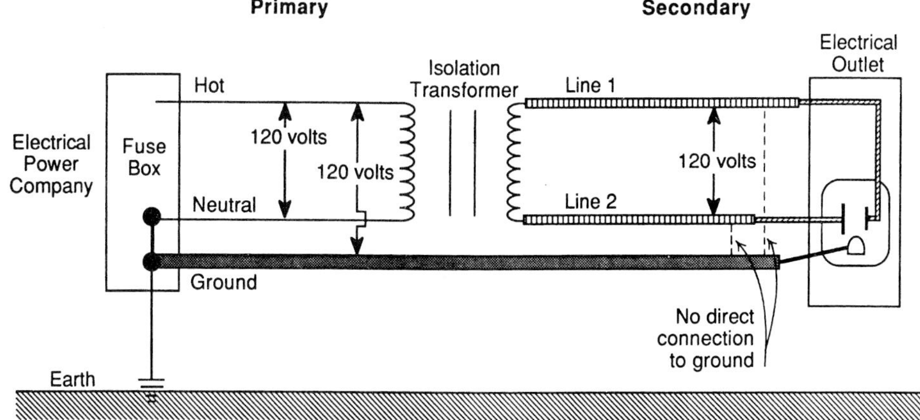

FIGURE 8-21. In the operating room, the isolation transformer converts the grounded power on the primary side to an ungrounded power system on the secondary side of the transformer. A 120-volt potential difference exists between line 1 and line 2. There is no direct connection from the power on the secondary side to ground. The equipment ground wire, however, is still present.

operating room. In fact, a *second* fault is necessary to create a hazard.

The previous discussion assumes that the isolated power system is perfectly isolated from ground. Actually, perfect isolation is impossible to achieve. All AC-operated power systems and electrical devices manifest some degree of capacitance. As previously discussed, electrical power cords, wires, and electrical motors exhibit capacitive coupling to the ground wire and metal conduits and "leak" small amounts of current to ground (Fig. 8-25). This so-called *leakage current* partially ungrounds the isolated power system. This does not usually amount to more than a few milliamperes in an operating room. So an individual coming in contact with one side of the isolated power system would receive only a very small shock (1 to 2 mA). Although this amount of current would be perceptible, it would not be dangerous.

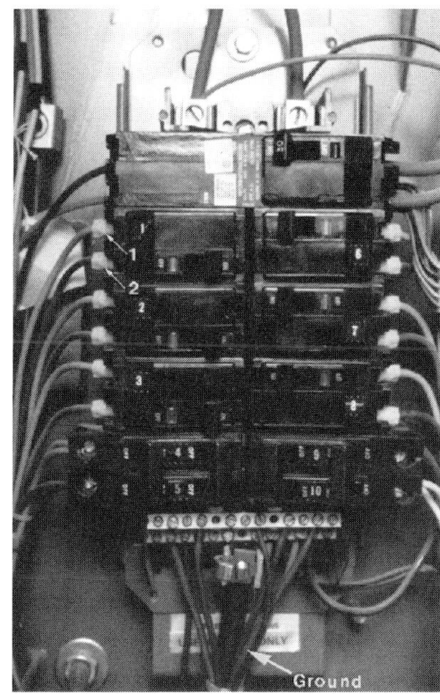

FIGURE 8-22. Detail of the inside of a circuit breaker box in an isolated power system. The *bottom arrow* points to ground wires meeting at the common ground terminal. *Arrows 1 and 2* indicate lines 1 and 2 from the isolated power circuit breaker. Neither line 1 nor line 2 is connected to the same terminals as the ground wires. This is in marked contrast to Figure 8-13, where the neutral and ground wires are attached at the same point.

THE LINE ISOLATION MONITOR

6 The *line isolation monitor* (LIM) is a device that continuously monitors the integrity of an isolated power system. If a faulty piece of equipment is connected to the isolated power system, this will, in effect, change the system back to a conventional grounded system. Also, the faulty piece of equipment will continue to function normally. Therefore, it is essential that a warning system be in place to alert the personnel that the power is no longer ungrounded. The LIM continuously monitors the isolated power to ensure that it is indeed isolated from ground, and the device has a meter that displays a continuous indication of the integrity of the system (Fig. 8-26). The LIM is actually measuring the impedance to ground of each side of the isolated power system. As previously discussed, with perfect isolation, impedance would be infinitely high and there would be no current flow in the event of a first fault situation ($Z = E / I$; if $I = 0$, then $Z = \infty$). Because all AC wiring and all AC-operated electrical devices have some capacitance, small leakage currents are present that partially degrade the isolation of the system. The meter of the LIM will indicate (in milliamperes) the total amount of leakage in the system resulting from capacitance, electrical wiring, and any devices plugged into the isolated power system.

The reading on the LIM meter does not mean that current is actually flowing; rather, it indicates how much current would flow in the event of a first fault. The LIM is set to alarm at 2 or 5 mA, depending on the age and brand of the system. Once this preset limit is exceeded, visual and audible alarms are triggered to indicate that the isolation from ground has been degraded beyond a predetermined limit (Fig. 8-27). This does not necessarily mean that there is a hazardous situation, but rather that the system is no longer totally isolated from ground. It would require a second fault to create a dangerous situation.

For example, if the LIM were set to alarm at 2 mA, using Ohm's law, the impedance for either side of the isolated power system would be 60,000 ohms:

$$Z = E/I$$
$$Z = (120\,\text{volts})/(0.002\,\text{ampers})$$
$$Z = 60,000\,\text{ohms}$$

Therefore, if either side of the isolated power system had less than 60,000 ohms impedance to ground, the LIM would trigger an alarm. This might occur in two situations. In the first, a faulty piece of equipment is plugged into the isolated power system. In this case, a true fault to ground exists from one line to ground. Now the system would be converted to the equivalent of a grounded power system. This faulty piece of equipment

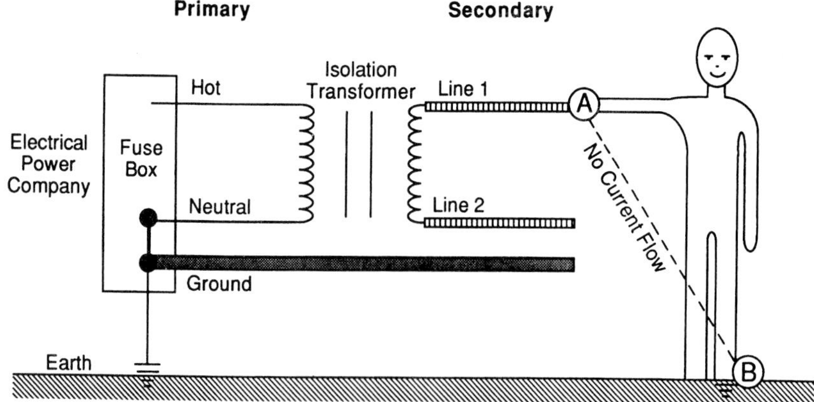

FIGURE 8-23. A safety feature of the isolated power system is illustrated. An individual contacting one side of the isolated power system (point *A*) and standing on the ground (point *B*) will not receive a shock. In this instance, the individual is not contacting the circuit at two points and thus is not completing the circuit. Point *A* (*cross-hatched lines*) is part of the isolated power system, and point *B* is part of the primary or grounded side of the circuit (*solid lines*).

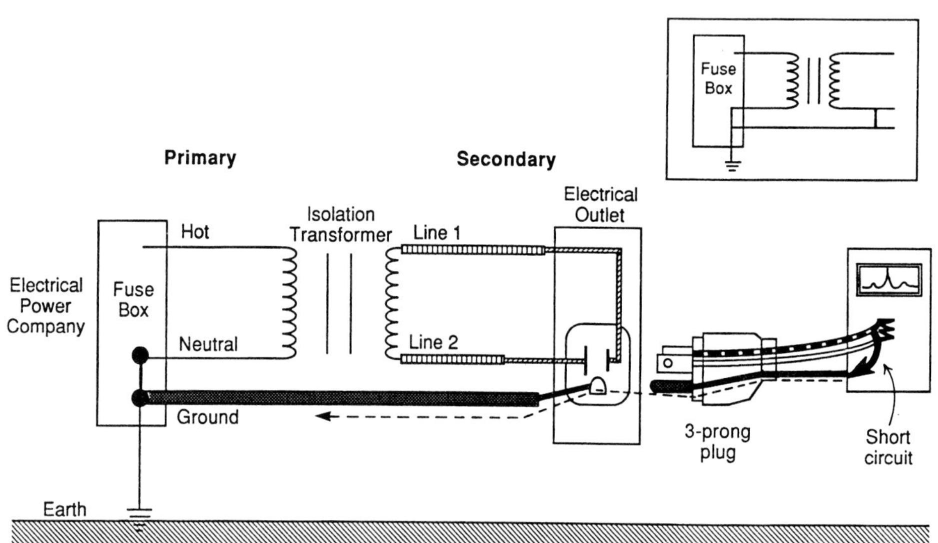

FIGURE 8-24. A faulty piece of equipment plugged into the isolated power system does not present a shock hazard. It merely converts the isolated power system into a grounded power system. The figure insert illustrates that the isolated power system is now identical to the grounded power system. The *dashed line* indicates current flow in the ground wire.

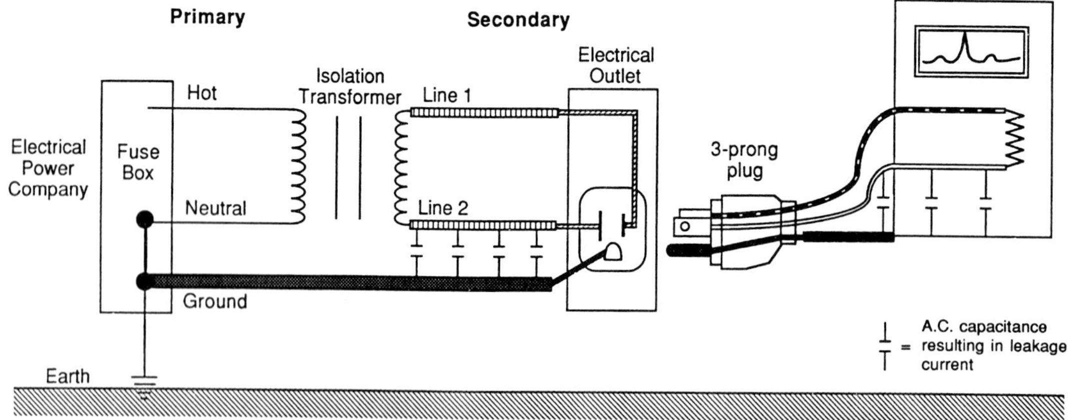

FIGURE 8-25. The capacitance that exists in AC power lines and AC-operated equipment results in small "leakage currents" that partially degrade the isolated power system.

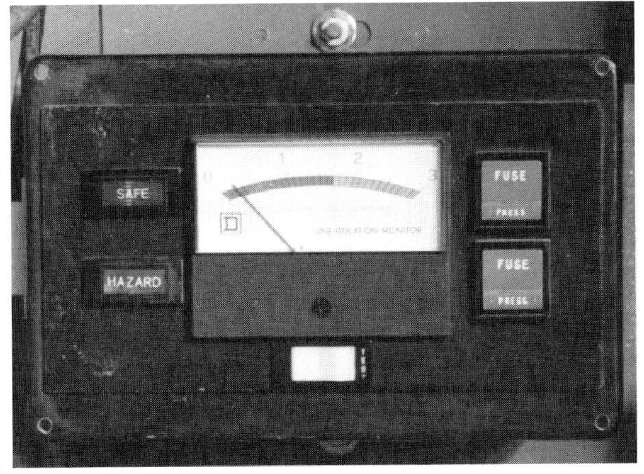

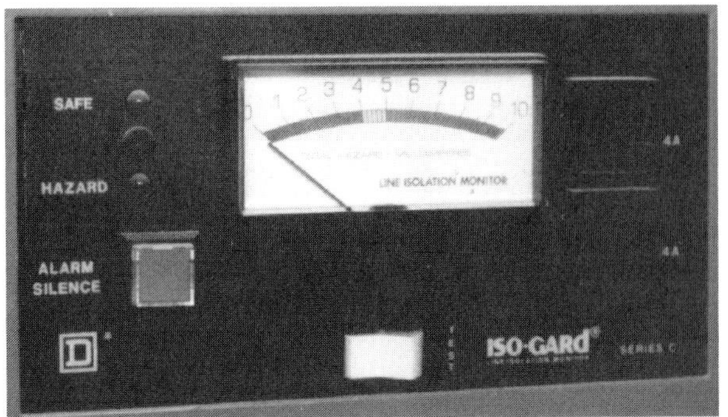

A B

FIGURE 8-26. The meter of the line isolation monitor is calibrated in milliamperes. If the isolation of the power system is degraded such that >2 mA (5 mA in newer systems) of current could flow, the hazard light will illuminate and a warning buzzer will sound. Note the button for testing the hazard warning system. **A.** Older LIM that will trigger an alarm at 2 mA. **B.** Newer line isolation monitor that will trigger an alarm at 5 mA.

should be removed and serviced as soon as possible. However, this piece of equipment could still be used safely if it were essential for the care of the patient. It should be remembered, however, that continuing to use this faulty piece of equipment would create the potential for a serious electrical shock. This would occur if a second faulty piece of equipment were simultaneously connected to the isolated power system.

The second situation involves connecting many perfectly normal pieces of equipment to the isolated power system. Although each piece of equipment has only a small amount of leakage current, if the total leakage exceeds 2 mA, the LIM will trigger an alarm. Assume that in the same operating room there are 30 electrical devices, each having 100 μA of leakage current. The total leakage current (30 × 100 μA) would be 3 mA. The impedance to ground would still be 40,000 ohms (120/0.003). The LIM alarm would sound because the 2-mA set point was violated. However, the system is still safe and represents a state significantly different from that in the first situation. For this reason, the newer LIMs are set to alarm at 5 mA instead of 2 mA.

The newest LIMs are referred to as third-generation monitors. The first-generation monitor, or static LIM, was unable to detect balanced faults (i.e., a situation in which there are equal faults to ground from both line 1 and line 2). The second-generation, or dynamic, LIM did not have this problem but could interfere with physiologic monitoring. Both of these monitors would trigger an alarm at 2 mA, which led to annoying "false" alarms. The third-generation LIM corrects the problems of its predecessors and has the alarm threshold set at 5 mA.[15] Proper functioning of the LIM is dependent on having both intact equipment ground wires as well as its own connection to ground. First- and second-generation LIMs could not detect the loss of the LIM ground connection. The third-generation LIM can detect this loss of ground to the monitor. In this case the LIM alarm would sound and the red hazard light would illuminate, but the LIM meter would read zero. This condition will alert the staff that the LIM needs to be repaired. However, the LIM still cannot detect broken equipment ground wires. An example of the third-generation LIM is the *Iso-Gard* ™ made by the Square D Company (Monroe, NC).

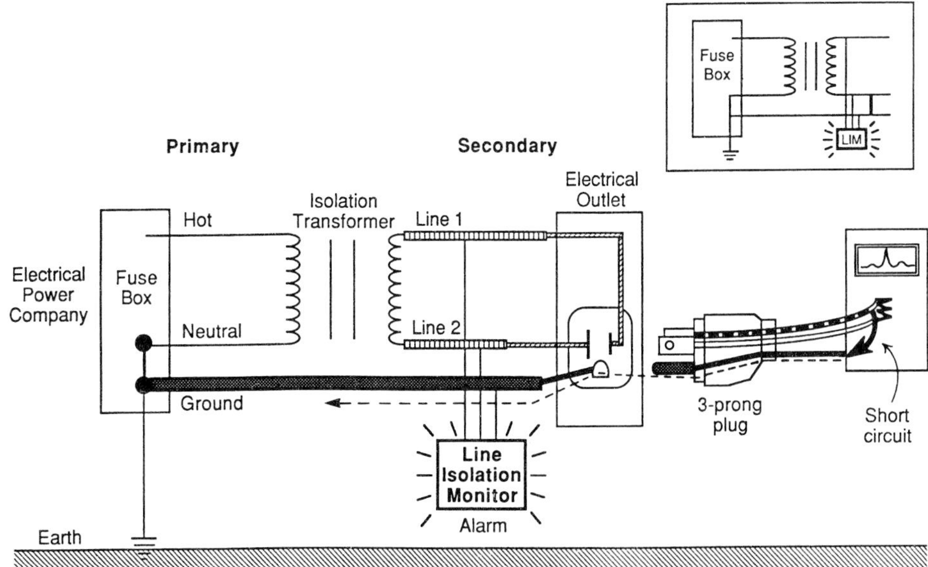

FIGURE 8-27. When a faulty piece of equipment is plugged into the isolated power system, it will markedly decrease the impedance from line 1 or line 2 to ground. This will be detected by the LIM, which will sound an alarm.

The equipment ground wire is again an important part of the safety system. If this wire is broken, a faulty piece of equipment that is plugged into an outlet would operate normally, but the LIM would not alarm. A second fault could therefore cause a shock, without any alarm from the LIM. Also, in the event of a second fault, the equipment ground wire provides a low-resistance path to ground for most of the fault current (see Fig. 8-24). The LIM will only be able to register leakage currents from pieces of equipment that are connected to the isolated power system and have intact ground wires.

If the line isolation monitor alarm is triggered, the first thing to do is to check the gauge to determine if it is a true fault. The other possibility is that too many pieces of electrical equipment have been plugged in and the 2-mA limit has been exceeded. If the gauge is between 2 and 5 mA, it is probable that too much electrical equipment has been plugged in. If the gauge reads >5 mA, most likely there is a faulty piece of equipment present in the operating room. The next step is to identify the faulty equipment, which is done by unplugging each piece of equipment until the alarm ceases. If the faulty piece of equipment is not of a life-support nature, it should be removed from the operating room. If it is a vital piece of life-support equipment, it can be safely used. However, it must be remembered that the protection of the isolated power system and the line isolation monitor is no longer operative. Therefore, if possible, no other electrical equipment should be connected during the remainder of the case, or until the faulty piece of equipment can be safely removed.

GROUND FAULT CIRCUIT INTERRUPTER

7 The ground fault circuit interrupter (GFCI, or occasionally abbreviated to GFI) is another popular device used to prevent individuals from receiving an electrical shock in a grounded power system. Electrical codes for most new construction require that a GFCI circuit be present in potentially hazardous (e.g., wet) areas such as bathrooms, kitchens, or outdoor electrical outlets. The GFCI may be installed as an individual power outlet (Fig. 8-28) or may be a special circuit breaker to which all the individual protected outlets are connected at a single point. The special GFCI circuit breaker is located in the main fuse/circuit breaker box and can be distinguished by its red test button (Fig. 8-29). As Figure 8-5 demonstrates, the current flowing in both the hot and neutral wires is usually equal. The GFCI monitors both sides of the circuit for the equality of current flow; if a difference is detected, the power is immediately interrupted. If an individual should contact a faulty piece of equipment such that current flowed through the individual, an imbalance between the two sides of the circuit would be created, which would be detected by the GFCI. Because the GFCI can detect very small current differences (in the range of 5 mA), the GFCI will open the circuit in a few milliseconds, thereby interrupting the current flow before a significant shock occurs. Thus, the GFCI provides a high level of protection at a very modest cost.

The disadvantage of using a GFCI in the operating room is that it interrupts the power without warning. A defective piece of equipment could no longer be used, which might be a problem if it were of a life-support nature, whereas if the same faulty piece of equipment were plugged into an isolated power system, the LIM would alarm, but the equipment could still be used.

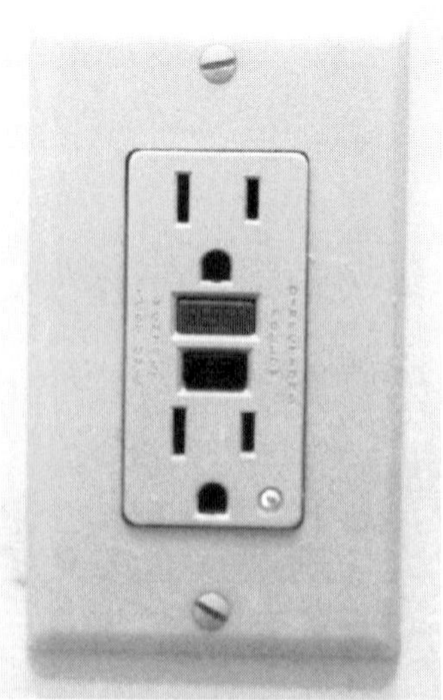

FIGURE 8-28. A GFCI electrical outlet with integrated test and reset buttons.

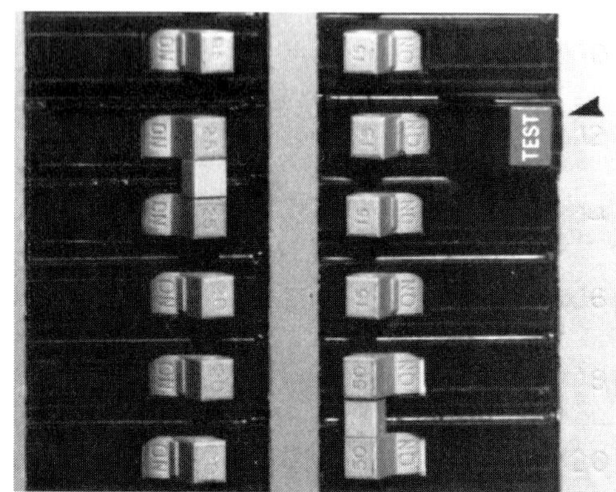

FIGURE 8-29. Special GFCI circuit breaker. The *arrowhead* points to the distinguishing red test button.

MICROSHOCK

As previously discussed, macroshock involves relatively large amounts of current applied to the surface of the body. The current is conducted through all the tissues in proportion to their conductivity and area in a plane perpendicular to the current. Consequently, the "density" of the current (amperes per meter squared) that reaches the heart is considerably less than what is
8 applied to the body surface. However, an electrically susceptible patient (i.e., one who has a direct, external connection to the heart, such as through a CVP catheter or transvenous cardiac pacing wires) may be at risk from very small currents; this is called *microshock*.[16] The catheter orifice or electrical wire with a very small surface area in contact with the heart produces a relatively large current density at the heart.[17] Stated another way, even very small amounts of current applied directly to the myocardium will cause ventricular fibrillation. Microshock is a particularly difficult problem because of the insidious nature of the hazard.

In the electrically susceptible patient, ventricular fibrillation can be produced by a current that is below the threshold of human perception. The exact amount of current necessary to cause ventricular fibrillation in this type of patient is unknown. Whalen et al[18] were able to produce fibrillation with 20 μA of current applied directly to the myocardium of dogs. Raftery

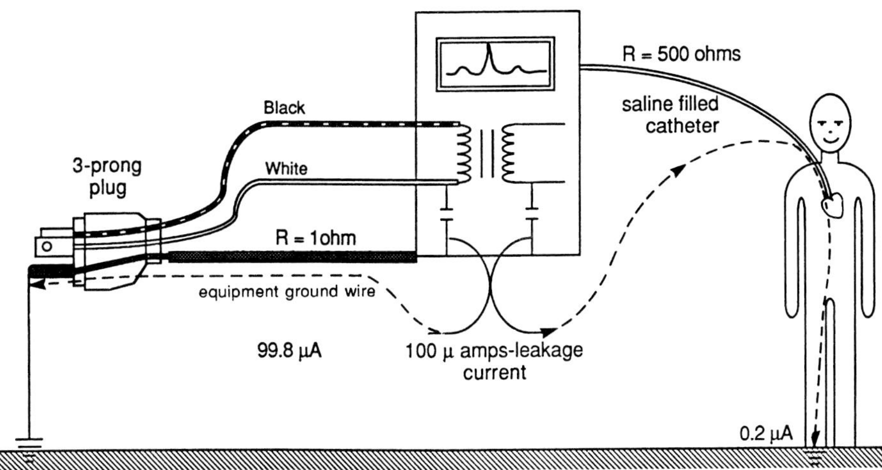

FIGURE 8-30. The electrically susceptible patient is protected from microshock by the presence of an intact equipment ground wire. The equipment ground wire provides a low-impedance path in which the majority of the leakage current (*dashed lines*) can flow.

et al[19] produced fibrillation with 80 μA of current in some patients. Hull[20] used data obtained by Watson et al[21] to show that 50% of patients would fibrillate at currents of 200 μA. Because 1,000 μA (1 mA) is generally regarded as the threshold of human perception with 60-Hz AC, the electrically susceptible patient can be electrocuted with one-tenth the normally perceptible currents. This is not only of academic interest but also of practical concern because many cases of ventricular fibrillation from microshock have been reported.[22–27]

The stray capacitance that is part of any AC-powered electrical instrument may result in significant amounts of charge buildup on the case of the instrument. If an individual simultaneously touches the case of an instrument where this has occurred and the electrically susceptible patient, he or she may unknowingly cause a discharge to the patient that results in ventricular fibrillation. Once again, the equipment ground wire constitutes the major source of protection against microshock for the electrically susceptible patient. In this case, the equipment ground wire provides a low-resistance path by which most of the leakage current is dissipated instead of stored as a charge.

Figure 8-30 illustrates a situation involving a patient with a saline-filled catheter in the heart with a resistance of ~500 ohms. The ground wire with a resistance of 1 ohm is connected to the instrument case. A leakage current of 100 μA will divide according to the relative resistances of the two paths. In this case, 99.8 μA will flow through the equipment ground wire, and only 0.2 μA will flow through the fluid-filled catheter. This extremely small current does not endanger the patient. If, however, the equipment ground wire were broken, the electrically susceptible patient would be at great risk because all 100 μA of leakage current could flow through the catheter and cause ventricular fibrillation (Fig. 8-31).

Modern patient monitors incorporate another mechanism to reduce the risk of microshock for electrically susceptible patients. This mechanism involves electrically isolating all direct patient connections from the power supply of the monitor by placing a very high impedance between the patient and any device. This limits the amount of internal leakage through the patient connection to a very small value. Currently the standard is <10 μA. For instance, the output of an ECG monitor's power supply is electrically isolated from the patient by placing a very high impedance between the monitor and the patient's ECG leads.[6,28] Isolation techniques are designed to inhibit hazardous electrical pathways between the patient and the monitor while allowing the passage of the physiologic signal.

An intact equipment ground wire is probably the most important factor in preventing microshock. There are, however, other things that the anesthesiologist can do to reduce the incidence of microshock. One should never simultaneously touch an electrical device and a saline-filled central catheter or external pacing wires. Whenever one is handling a central catheter or pacing wires, it is best to insulate oneself by wearing rubber gloves. Also, one should never let any external current source, such as a nerve stimulator, come into contact with the catheter or wires. Finally, one should be alert to potential sources of energy that can be transmitted to the patient. Even stray

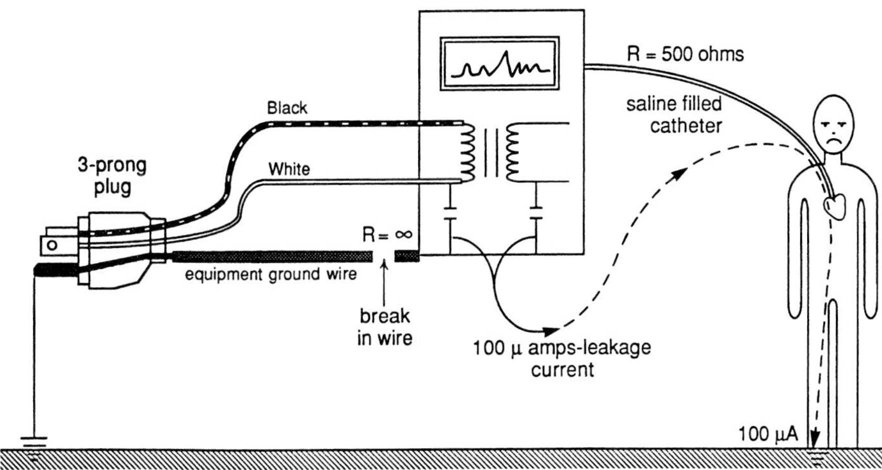

FIGURE 8-31. A broken equipment ground wire results in a significant hazard to the electrically susceptible patient. In this case, the entire leakage current can be conducted to the heart and may result in ventricular fibrillation.

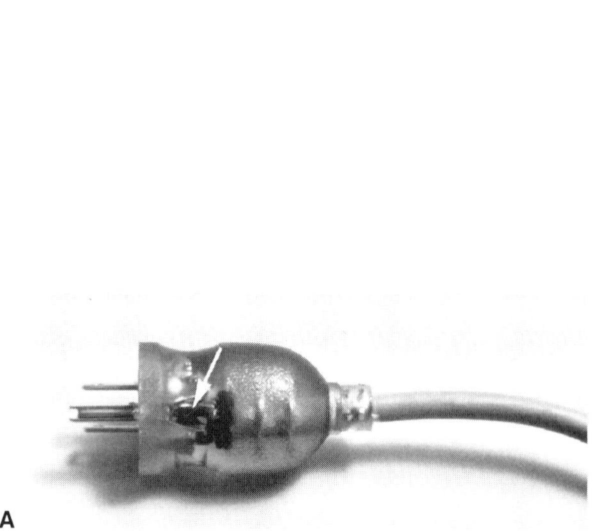
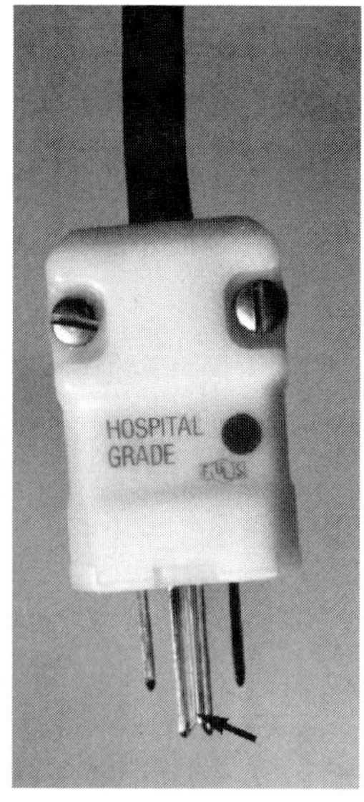

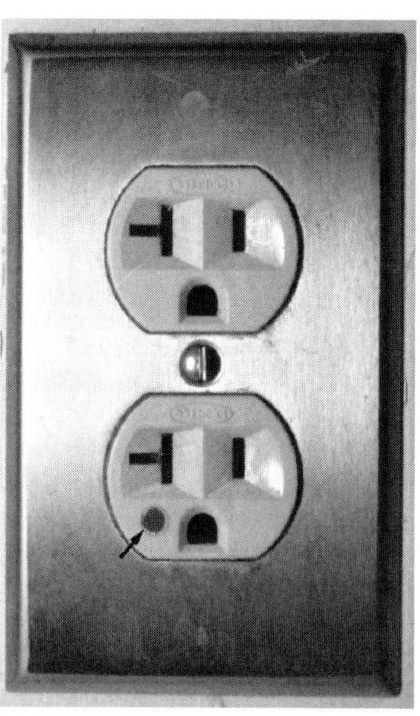

FIGURE 8-32. **A.** A hospital-grade plug that can be visually inspected. The *arrow* points to the equipment ground wire whose integrity can be readily verified. **B.** A hospital-grade plug that can be easily disassembled for inspection. Note that the prong for the ground wire (*arrow*) is longer than the hot or neutral prong, so that it is the first to enter the receptacle. **C.** The *arrow* points to the green dot denoting a hospital-grade power outlet.

radiofrequency current from the electrosurgical unit (cautery) can, with the right conditions, be a source of microshock.[29]

It must be remembered that the LIM is not designed to provide protection from microshock. The microampere currents involved in microshock are far below the LIM threshold of protection. In addition, the LIM does not register the leakage of individual monitors, but rather indicates the status of the total system. The LIM reading indicates the total amount of leakage current resulting from the entire capacitance of the system. This is the amount of current that would flow to ground in the event of a first-fault situation.

The essence of electrical safety is a thorough understanding of all the principles of grounding. According to Bruner, "Grounding is neither safe nor unsafe. Its significance is dependent on what is grounded and in what context."[9] The objective of electrical safety is to make it difficult for electrical current to pass through people. For this reason, both the patient and the anesthesiologist should be isolated from ground as much as possible. That is, their resistance to current flow should be as high as is technologically feasible. In the inherently unsafe electrical environment of an operating room, several measures can be taken to help protect against contacting hazardous current flows. First, the grounded power provided by the utility company can be converted to ungrounded power by means of an isolation transformer. The LIM will continuously monitor the status of this isolation from ground and warn that the isolation of the power (from ground) has been lost in the event that a defective piece of equipment is plugged into one of the isolated circuit outlets. In addition, the shock that an individual could receive from a faulty piece of equipment is determined by the capacitance of the system and is limited to a few milliamperes. Second, all equipment plugged into the isolated power system has an equipment ground wire that is attached to the case of the instrument. This equipment ground wire provides an alternative low-resistance pathway enabling potentially dangerous currents to flow to ground. Thus, the patient and the anesthesiologist should be as insulated from ground as possible and all electrical equipment should be grounded.

The equipment ground wire serves three functions. First, it provides a low-resistance path for fault currents to reduce the risk of macroshock. Second, it dissipates leakage currents that are potentially harmful to the electrically susceptible patient. Third, it provides information to the LIM on the status of the ungrounded power system. If the equipment ground wire is broken, a significant factor in the prevention of electrical shock is lost. Additionally, the isolated power system will appear safer than it actually is, because the LIM is unable to detect broken equipment ground wires.

Because power cord plugs and receptacles are subjected to greater abuse in the hospital than in the home, the Underwriters Laboratories (Melville, NY) has issued a strict specification for special "hospital-grade" plugs and receptacles (Fig. 8-32). The plugs and receptacles that conform to this specification are marked by a green dot.[30] The hospital-grade plug is one that can be visually inspected or easily disassembled to ensure the integrity of the ground wire connection. Molded opaque plugs are not acceptable. Edwards reported that of 3,000 nonhospital-grade receptacles installed in a new hospital building, 1,800 (60%) were defective after 3 years.[31] When 2,000 of the nonhospital-grade receptacles were replaced with ones of hospital grade, no failures had occurred after 18 months of use.

ELECTROSURGERY

On that fateful October day in 1926 when Dr. Harvey W. Cushing first used an electrosurgical machine invented by Professor William T. Bovie to resect a brain tumor, the course of modern surgery and anesthesia was forever altered.[32] The ubiquitous use of electrosurgery attests to the success of Professor Bovie's invention. However, this technology was not adopted without a cost. The widespread use of electrocautery has, at the very least, hastened the elimination of explosive anesthetic agents from the operating room. In addition, as every anesthesiologist is aware, few things in the operating room are immune to interference from the "Bovie." The high-frequency electrical energy generated by the electrosurgery unit (ESU) interferes with everything from the ECG signal to cardiac output computers, pulse oximeters, and even implanted cardiac pacemakers.[33]

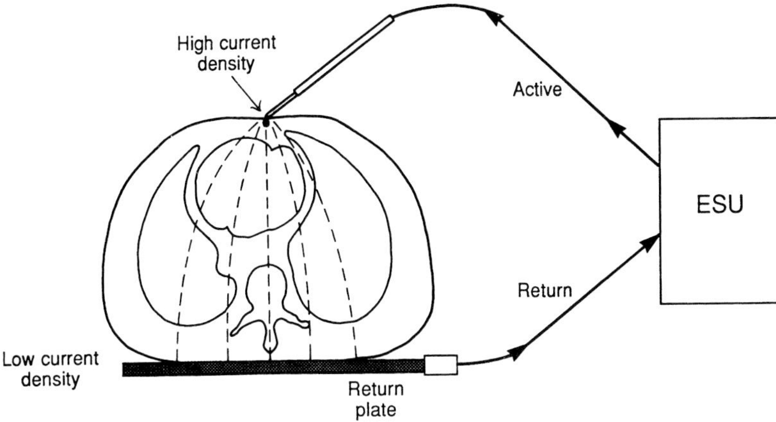

FIGURE 8-33. A properly applied ESU return plate. The current density at the return plate is low, resulting in no danger to the patient.

The ESU operates by generating very–high-frequency currents (radiofrequency range) of anywhere from 500,000 to 1 million Hz. Heat is generated whenever a current passes through a resistance. The amount of heat (H) produced is proportional to the square of the current and inversely proportional to the area through which the current passes ($H = I^2/A$).[34] By concentrating the energy at the tip of the "Bovie pencil," the surgeon can produce either a cut or a coagulation at any given spot. This very high frequency current behaves differently from the standard 60-Hz AC current and can pass directly across the precordium without causing ventricular fibrillation.[34] This is because high-frequency currents have a low tissue penetration and do not excite contractile cells.

The large amount of energy generated by the ESU can pose other problems to the operator and the patient. Dr. Cushing became aware of one such problem. He wrote, "Once the operator received a shock which passed through a metal retractor to his arm and out by a wire from his headlight, which was unpleasant to say the least."[35] The ESU cannot be safely operated unless the energy is properly routed from the ESU through the patient and back to the unit. Ideally, the current generated by the active electrode is concentrated at the ESU tip constituting a very small surface area. This energy has a high current density and is able to generate enough heat to produce a therapeutic cut or coagulation. The energy then passes through the patient to a dispersive electrode of large surface area that returns the energy safely to the ESU (Fig. 8-33).

One unfortunate quirk in terminology concerns the return (dispersive) plate of the ESU. This plate, often incorrectly referred to as a *ground plate*, is actually a dispersive electrode of large surface area that safely returns the generated energy to the ESU via a low current density pathway. When inquiring whether the dispersive electrode has been attached to the patient, operating room personnel frequently ask, "Is the patient grounded?" Because the aim of electrical safety is to isolate the patient from ground, this expression is worse than erroneous; it can lead to confusion. Because the area of the return plate is large, the current density is low; therefore, no harmful heat is generated and no tissue destruction occurs. In a properly functioning system, the only tissue effect is at the site of the active electrode that is held by the surgeon.

9 Problems can arise if the electrosurgical return plate is improperly applied to the patient or if the cord connecting the return plate to the ESU is damaged or broken. In these instances, the high-frequency current generated by the ESU will seek an alternate return pathway. Anything attached to the patient, such as ECG leads or a temperature probe, can provide this alternate return pathway. The current density at the ECG pad will be considerably higher than normal because its surface area is much less than that of the ESU return plate. This may result in a serious burn at this alternate return site. Similarly, a burn may occur at the site of the ESU return plate if it is not properly applied to the patient or if it becomes partially dislodged during the operation (Fig. 8-34). This is not merely a theoretical possibility but is evidenced by the numerous case reports involving patients who have received ESU burns.[36–41]

The original ESUs were manufactured with the power supply connected directly to ground by the equipment ground wire. These devices made it extremely easy for ESU current to return by alternate pathways. The ESU would continue to operate normally even without the return plate connected to the patient. In most modern ESUs, the power supply is isolated from

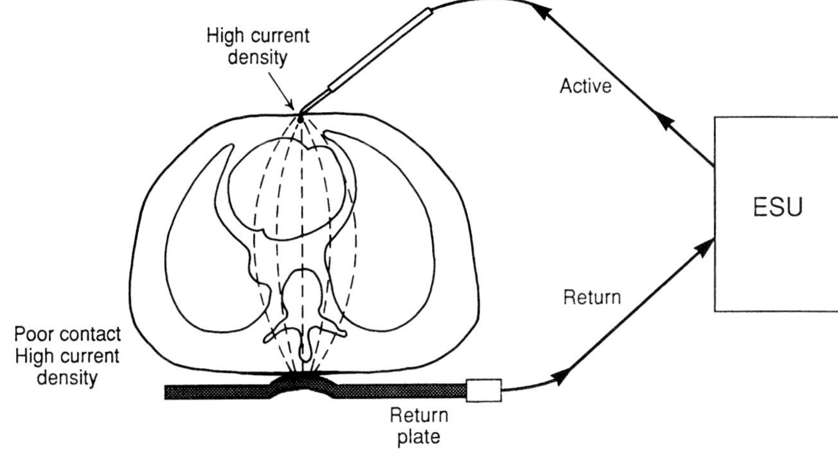

FIGURE 8-34. An improperly applied ESU return plate. Poor contact with the return plate results in a high current density and a possible burn to the patient.

ground to protect the patient from burns. It was hoped that by isolating the return pathway from ground, the only route for current flow would be via the return electrode. Theoretically, this would eliminate alternate return pathways and greatly reduce the incidence of burns.[5] However, Mitchell found two situations in which the current could return via alternate pathways, even with the isolated ESU circuit.[42] If the return plate were left either on top of an uninsulated ESU cabinet or in contact with the bottom of the operating room table, then the ESU could operate fairly normally and the current would return via alternate pathways. It will be recalled that the impedance is inversely proportional to the capacitance times the current frequency. The ESU operates at 500,000 to >1,000,000 Hz, which greatly enhances the effect of capacitive coupling and causes a marked reduction in impedance. Therefore, even with isolated ESUs, the decrease in impedance allows the current to return to the ESU by alternate pathways. In addition, the isolated ESU does not protect the patient from burns if the return electrode does not make proper contact with the patient. Although the isolated ESU does provide additional patient safety, it is by no means foolproof protection against the patient receiving a burn.

Preventing patient burns from the ESU is the responsibility of all professional staff in the operating room. Not only the circulating nurse, but also the surgeon and the anesthesiologist must be aware of proper techniques and be vigilant to potential problems. The most important factor is the proper application of the return plate. It is essential that the return plate have the appropriate amount of electrolyte gel and an intact return wire. Reusable return plates must be properly cleaned after each use, and disposable plates must be checked to ensure that the electrolyte has not dried out during storage. In addition, it is prudent to place the return plate as close as possible to the site of the operation. ECG pads should be placed as far from the site of the operation as is feasible. Operating room personnel must be alert to the possibility that pools of flammable "prep" solutions such as ether and acetone can ignite when the ESU is used. If the ESU must be used on a patient with a demand pacemaker, the return electrode should be located below the thorax, and preparations for treating potential dysrhythmias should be available, including a magnet to convert the pacemaker to a fixed rate, a defibrillator, and an external pacemaker. The ESU has also caused other problems in patients with pacemakers, including reprogramming and microshock.[43,44] If the surgeon requests higher than normal power settings on the ESU, this should alert both the circulating nurse and the anesthesiologist to a potential problem. The return plate and cable must be immediately inspected to ensure that it is functioning and properly positioned. If this does not correct the problem, the return plate should be replaced. If the problem remains, the entire ESU should be taken out of service. Finally, an ESU that is dropped or damaged must be removed immediately from the operating room and thoroughly tested by a qualified biomedical engineer. Following these simple safety steps will prevent most patient burns from the ESU.

The previous discussion concerned only *unipolar* ESUs. There is a second type of ESU, in which the current passes only between the two blades of a pair of forceps. This type of device is referred to as a *bipolar* ESU. Because the active and return electrodes are the two blades of the forceps, it is not necessary to attach another dispersive electrode to the patient, unless a unipolar ESU is also being used. The bipolar ESU generates considerably less power than the unipolar and is mainly used for ophthalmic and neurologic surgery.[2]

In 1980 Mirowski et al[45] reported the first human implantation of a device to treat intractable ventricular tachyarrhythmias. This device, known as the *automatic implantable cardioverter-defibrillator* (AICD), is capable of sensing ventricular tachycardia (VT) and ventricular fibrillation (VF) and then automatically defibrillating the patient. Since 1980 thousands of patients have received AICD implants.[46,47] Because some of these patients may now present for noncardiac surgery, it is important that the anesthesiologist be aware of potential problems.[48] The use of a unipolar ESU may cause electrical interference that could be interpreted by the AICD as a ventricular tachyarrhythmia. This would trigger a defibrillation pulse to be delivered to the patient and would likely cause an actual episode of VT or VF. The patient with an AICD is also at risk for VF during electroconvulsive therapy.[48] In both cases, the AICD should be disabled by placing a magnet over the device. Although most AICDs can be disabled with a magnet, some require a special device or specific magnet to shut them off. Therefore, it is best to consult with someone experienced with the device before starting surgery. The device can be reactivated by reversing the process. Also, an external defibrillator and a noninvasive pacemaker should be in the operating room whenever a patient with an AICD is anesthetized.

Electrical safety in the operating room is a matter of combining common sense with some basic principles of electricity. Once operating room personnel understand the importance of safe electrical practice, they are able to develop a heightened awareness to potential problems. All electrical equipment must undergo routine maintenance, service, and inspection to ensure that it conforms to designated electrical safety standards. Records of these test results must be kept for future inspection because human error can easily compound electrical hazards. Starmer et al[49] cited one case concerning a newly constructed laboratory where the ground wire was not attached to a receptacle. In another study Albisser et al[50] found a 14% (198/1,424) incidence of improperly or incorrectly wired outlets. Furthermore, potentially hazardous situations should be recognized and corrected before they become a problem. For instance, electrical power cords are frequently placed on the floor where they can be crushed by various carts or the anesthesia machine. These cords could be located overhead or placed in an area of low traffic flow. Multiple-plug extension boxes should not be left on the floor where they can come in contact with electrolyte solutions. These could easily be mounted on a cart or the anesthesia machine. Pieces of equipment that have been damaged or have obvious defects in the power cord must not be used until they have been properly repaired. If everyone is aware of what constitutes a potential hazard, dangerous situations can be prevented with minimal effort.

Sparks generated by the ESU may provide the ignition source for a fire with resulting burns to the patient and operating room personnel. This is a particular risk when the ESU is used in an oxygen-enriched environment as may be present in the patient's airway or in close proximity to the patient's face. Most plastics such as tracheal tubes and components of the anesthetic breathing system that would not burn in room air will ignite in the presence of oxygen and/or nitrous oxide. Tenting of the drapes to allow dispersion of any accumulated oxygen and/or its dilution by room air or use of a circle anesthesia breathing system with minimal to no leak of gases around the anesthesia mask will decrease the risk of ignition from a spark generated by a nearby ESU.

Conductive Flooring

Conductive flooring was mandated for operating rooms where flammable anesthetic agents were being administered. The conductive floor was specified to have a resistance of between 25,000 and 1 million ohms. This would minimize the buildup of static charges that could cause a flammable anesthetic agent to ignite. The standards have been changed to eliminate the necessity for conductive flooring in anesthetizing areas where flammable agents are no longer used.

ENVIRONMENTAL HAZARDS

There are a number of potential electrically related hazards in the operating room that are of concern to the anesthesiologist. There is the potential for electrical shock not only to the patient but also to operating room personnel. In addition, cables and power cords to electrical equipment and monitoring devices can become hazardous. Finally, all operating room personnel should have a plan of what to do in the event of a power failure.

In today's operating room, there are literally dozens of pieces of electrical equipment. It is not uncommon to have numerous power cords lying on the floor, where they are vulnerable to damage. If the insulation on the power cable becomes damaged, it is fairly easy for the hot wire to come in contact with a piece of metal equipment. If the operating room did not have isolated power, that piece of equipment would become energized and a potential electrical shock hazard.[51] Having isolated power minimizes the risk to the patient and operating room personnel. Clearly, getting electrical power cords off the floor is desirable. This can be accomplished by having electrical outlets in the ceiling or by having ceiling-mounted articulated arms that contain electrical outlets. Also, the use of multioutlet extension boxes that sit on the floor can be hazardous. These can be contaminated with fluids, which could easily trip the circuit breaker. In one case, it apparently tripped the main circuit breaker for the entire operating room, resulting in a loss of all electrical power except for the overhead lights.[52]

Modern monitoring devices have many safety features incorporated into them. Virtually all of them have isolated the patient input from the power supply of the device. This was an important feature that was lacking from the original ECG monitors. In the early days, patients could actually become part of the electrical circuit of the monitor. There have been relatively few problems with patients and monitoring devices since the advent of isolated inputs. However, between 1985 and 1994, the Food and Drug Administration (FDA) received approximately 24 reports where infants and children had received an electrical shock including five children who died by electrocution.[53,54] These electrical accidents occurred because the electrode lead wires from either an ECG monitor or an apnea monitor were plugged directly into a 120-volt electrical outlet instead of the appropriate patient cable. In 1997, the FDA issued a new performance standard for electrode lead wires and patient cables that requires that the exposed male connector pins from the electrode lead wires must be eliminated. Therefore, the lead wires must have female connections and the connector pins must be housed in a protected patient cable (Fig. 8-35). This effectively eliminates the possibility of the patient being connected directly to an alternating current source since there are no exposed connector pins on the lead wires.

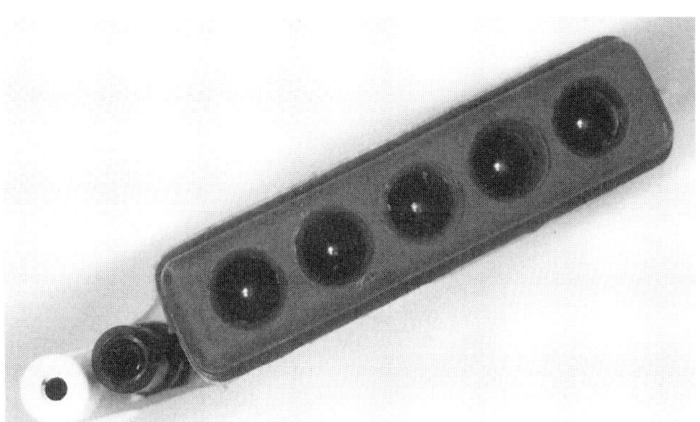

FIGURE 8-35. The current standard for patient lead wires (*left*) requires a female connector. The patient cable (*right*) has shielded connector pins that the lead wires plug into.

All health care facilities are required to have a source of emergency power. This generally consists of one or more electrical generators. These generators are configured to start up automatically and provide power to the facility within a few seconds after detecting the loss of power from the utility company. The facility is required to test these generators on a regular basis. However, not all health care facilities test them under actual load. There are numerous anecdotal reports of generators not functioning properly during an actual power failure. If the generators are not tested under actual load, it is possible that many years will pass before a real power outage puts a severe demand on the generator. If the facility has several generators and one of them fails, the increased demand on the others may be enough to cause them to fail in rapid succession.

Other situations may also cause unexpected power outages. In our facility, a construction crew was remodeling an existing operating room. They accidentally caused a short circuit in the power supply when they were working on an electrical panel. This caused the GFI in the basement to trip, thus shutting off power to a whole section of the operating room. Consequently, several operating rooms were suddenly without power at crucial junctures in surgery. The operating room personnel were waiting for the emergency generators to come on. Obviously, this was not going to happen because there was no interruption of power from the electrical utility. It took approximately 20 to 30 minutes until the source of the problem could be identified and corrected.

It is vitally important that each operating room have a contingency plan for a power failure. In most cases, the emergency generator will take over, but that is not always going to happen. There should be a supply of battery-operated light sources available in each operating room. A laryngoscope can serve as a readily available source of light that allows one to find flashlights and other pieces of equipment. The operating room's overhead lights should also be connected to some sort of battery-operated lighting system. A supply of battery-operated monitoring devices and pneumatically powered ventilators and anesthesia machines would enable life-support functions to continue. The cost of these contingencies is relatively small but the benefits can be incomparably great in an emergency.

Electromagnetic Interference (EMI)

Rapid advances in technology have led to an explosion in the number of wireless communication devices in the marketplace. These devices include cellular telephones, cordless telephones, walkie-talkies, and even wireless Internet access devices. All of these devices have something in common: they emit EMI. This most commonly manifests itself when traveling on airplanes. Most airlines require that these devices be turned off when the plane is taking off or landing or, in some cases, during the entire flight. There is concern that the EMI emitted by these devices may interfere with the plane's navigation and communication equipment.

In recent years, the number of people who own these devices has increased exponentially. Indeed, in some hospitals, they form a vital link in the regular or emergency communication system. It is not uncommon for physicians, nurses, paramedics, and other personnel to have their own cellular telephones. In addition, patients and visitors may also have cellular telephones and other types of communication devices. Hospital maintenance and security personnel frequently have walkie-talkie–type radios and some hospitals have even instituted an in-house cellular telephone network that augments or replaces the paging system. There has been concern that the

EMI emitted by these devices may interfere with implanted pacemakers or various types of monitoring devices in critical care areas.

Several studies have been done to find out if cellular telephones cause problems with cardiac pacemakers. One study by Hayes et al looked at 980 patients with five different types of cellular telephones.[55] They conducted more than 5,000 tests and found that in more than 20% of the cases they could detect some interference from the cellular telephone. Patients were symptomatic in 7.2% of the cases, and clinically significant interference occurred in 6.6% of the cases. When the telephone was held in the normal position over the ear, clinically significant interference was not detected. In fact, the interference that caused clinical symptoms occurred only if the telephone was directly over the pacemaker. Other studies have demonstrated changes such as erroneous sensing and pacer inhibition.[56,57] Again, these occurred only when the telephone was close to the pacemaker. The changes were temporary, and the pacemaker reverted to normal when the cellular telephone was moved to a safe distance. Currently, the FDA guidelines are that the cellular telephones be kept at least 6 inches from the pacemaker. Therefore, the cellular telephone should not be carried in the shirt pocket, which is adjacent to the pacemaker.

Automatic implantable cardioverter-defibrillators comprise another group of devices of concern to biomedical engineers. Fetter et al conducted a study of 41 patients who had AICDs.[58] They had a 0% incidence of oversensing and concluded that the cellular telephones did not interfere with the AICDs that they tested. They did, however, recommend keeping the cellular telephone at least 6 inches from the device.

Electromagnetic interference extends well beyond that of cellular telephones. Walkie-talkies, which are frequently used by hospital maintenance and security personnel; paging systems; police radios; and even televisions all emit EMI, which could potentially interfere with medical devices of any nature. Although there are many anecdotal reports, the amount of available scientific information on this problem is scanty. Reports of interference include ventilator and infusion pumps that have been shut down or reprogrammed, interference with ECG monitors, and even an electronic wheelchair that was accidentally started because of EMI. It is a difficult problem to study because there are many different types of devices that emit EMI and a vast array of medical equipment that has the potential to interact with these devices. Even though a device may seem "safe" in the medical environment, if two or three cellular telephones or walkie-talkies are brought together in the same area at the same time, there may be unanticipated problems or interference.

Any time a cellular telephone is turned on, it is actually communicating with the cellular network, even though a call is not in progress. Therefore, the potential to interfere with devices exists. The Emergency Care Research Institute (ECRI) reported in October 1999 that walkie-talkies were far more likely to cause problems with medical devices than cellular telephones.[59] This is because they operate on a lower frequency than cellular telephones and have a higher power output. The ECRI recommends that cellular telephones be maintained at a distance of 1 meter from medical devices, while walkie-talkies be kept at a distance of 6 to 8 meters.

Some hospitals have made restrictive policies on the use of cellular telephones, particularly in critical care areas.[60] These policies are supported by little scientific documentation and are nearly impossible to enforce. The ubiquitous presence of cellular telephones carried by hospital personnel and visitors makes enforcing a ban virtually impossible. Even when people try to comply with the ban, failure is nearly inevitable because the general public is usually unaware that a cellular telephone in the standby mode is still communicating with the tower and generating EMI.

The real solution is to "harden" devices against electromagnetic interference. This is difficult to do because of the many different frequencies on which these devices operate. Education of medical personnel is essential. When working in an operating room or critical care area, all personnel must be alert to the fact that electronic devices and pacemakers can be interfered with by EMI. Creating a restrictive policy would certainly irritate personnel and visitors, and, in some cases, may actually compromise emergency communications.[61]

CONSTRUCTION OF NEW OPERATING ROOMS

Frequently, an anesthesiologist is asked to consult with hospital administrators and architects in designing new, or remodeling older, operating rooms. In the past a strict electrical code was enforced because of the use of flammable anesthetic agents. This code included a requirement for isolated power systems and LIMs. The National Fire Protection Association (NFPA) revised its standard for health care facilities in 1984 (NFPA 99-1984). These standards do not require isolated power systems or LIMs in areas designated for use of nonflammable anesthetic agents only.[62,63] Although not mandatory, NFPA standards are usually adopted by local authorities when revising their electrical codes.

This change in the standard creates a dilemma. The NFPA 99—Standard for Health Care Facilities, 1990 Edition, mandates that "wet location patient care areas be provided with special protection against electrical shock." Section 3-4.1.2.6 further states that "this special protection shall be provided by a power distribution system that inherently limits the possible ground fault current due to a first fault to a low value, without interrupting the power supply; or by a power distribution system in which the power supply is interrupted if the ground fault current does, in fact, exceed a value of 6 milliamperes."

The decision of whether to install isolated power hinges on two factors. The first is whether or not the operating room is considered a wet location, and, if so, whether an interruptible power supply is tolerable. Where power interruption is tolerable, a GFCI is permitted as the protective means. However, the standard also states that "the use of an isolated power system (IPS) shall be permitted as a protective means capable of limiting ground fault current without power interruption."

Most people who have worked in an operating room would attest to its being a wet location. The presence of blood, body fluids, and saline solutions spilled on the floor all contribute to making this a wet environment. The cystoscopy suite serves as a good example.

Once the premise that the operating room is a wet location is accepted, it must be determined whether a GFCI can provide the means of protection. The argument against using GFCIs in the operating room is illustrated by the following example. Assume that during an open heart procedure the cardiopulmonary bypass pump and the patient monitors are plugged into outlets on the same branch circuit. Also assume that during bypass, the circulating nurse now plugs in a faulty headlight. If there is a GFCI protecting the circuit, the fault will be detected and the GFCI will interrupt all power to the pump and the monitors. This undoubtedly would cause a great deal of confusion and consternation among the operating room personnel and may place the patient at risk for injury. The pump would have to be manually operated while the problem was being resolved. In addition, the GFCI could not be reset (and power restored) until the headlight was identified as the cause of the fault and unplugged from the outlet. However, if the operating room were protected with an isolated power system and LIM, the same scenario would cause the LIM to alarm, but the pump and patient monitors would continue to operate normally. There would be no interruption of power, and the problem could be resolved without risk to the patient.

It should be realized that a GFCI is an active system. That is, a potentially hazardous current is already flowing and must be actively interrupted, whereas the isolated power system (with LIM) is designed to be safe during a first-fault situation. Thus, it is a passive system because no mechanical action is required to activate the protection.[64]

It is likely that hospital administrators may want to eliminate isolated power systems in new operating room construction as a cost-saving measure. Others,[64–66] however, have advocated the retention of isolated power systems. Not to do this would be a short-sighted, foolhardy measure. This is especially true because the cost of adding isolated power is estimated to be 1% of the cost of constructing an operating room.[64] Although not perfect,[67] the isolated power system and LIM do provide both the patient and operating room personnel with a significant amount of protection in an electrically hazardous environment. The value of the isolated power system is illustrated in a report by Day in 1994.[68] He reported four instances of electrical shock to operating room personnel in a 1-year period. The operating suite had been renovated and the isolated power system removed, and it was not until the operating room personnel received a shock that a problem was discovered.

Anesthesiologists need to be aware of this cost-saving attitude and strongly encourage that new operating rooms be constructed with isolated power systems. The relatively small cost savings that the alternative would represent do not justify the elimination of such a useful safety system, and the use of GFCIs is not practical in the operating room environment.

Electrical safety should be the concern of everyone in the operating room. Accidents can be prevented only if proper installation and maintenance of the appropriate safety equipment in the operating room have occurred and the operating room personnel understand the concepts of electrical safety and are vigilant in their efforts to detect new hazards.[69]

FIRE SAFETY

10 Fires in the operating room are just as much a danger today as they were 100 years ago when patients were anesthetized with flammable anesthetic agents.[70,71] For more than 100 years, the practice of anesthesia throughout the world involved the use of flammable and explosive inhalational anesthetics such as ether and cyclopropane. It is only in the last 30 to 40 years that these agents have been phased out of use in the developed countries. Of the early inhalational anesthetics, only nitrous oxide was nonflammable, yet it is similar to oxygen in that it can readily support combustion. Since the potential consequences of a fire or explosion with ether or cyclopropane could be so devastating, everyone who worked in the operating room actively observed fire safety practices on a daily basis.[72,73]

Today, the risk of an operating room fire is probably as great or greater than the days when ether and cyclopropane were used. This is because of the routine use of potential sources of ignition (such as electrosurgical cauteries and fiberoptic light sources) in an environment rich in flammable materials (i.e., fuels). The problem is compounded by a markedly decreased awareness of the potential for an operating room fire. With the possible exception of laser surgery in or around the airway, there is rarely any special attention paid to fire safety. However, ESUs, and not lasers, are probably responsible for starting the majority of operating room fires. In fact, ESUs were implicated in the vast majority of the 146 device-associated surgical fires reported to the FDA between January 1995 and June 1998.[74]

11 For a fire to start, three elements are necessary. This is called the *Fire Triad*. The first part of the triad is a heat or ignition source, the second part is fuel, and the third part is an oxidizer.[75] A fire occurs when there is a chemical reaction of a fuel rapidly combining with an oxidizer to release energy in the form of heat and light. In the operating room there are many heat or ignition sources and these include the ESU, lasers, electrical tools such as drills, and the ends of fiberoptic light cords. The main oxidizers in the operating room are air, oxygen, and nitrous oxide. Oxygen and nitrous oxide function equally well as oxidizers, so a combination of 50% oxygen and 50% nitrous oxide would support combustion as well as 100% oxygen. Fuel for a fire can be found everywhere in the operating room. Paper drapes have largely replaced cloth drapes and these are much easier to ignite and they can burn with greater intensity.[76,77] Other sources of fuel include gauze dressings, endotracheal (ET) tubes, gel mattress pads, and even facial or body hair[78] (Table 8-3).

Fire prevention is accomplished by not allowing all three of the elements to come together at the same time.[79] The problem in the operating room is that frequently each of the limbs of the fire triad is controlled by a different individual. For instance, the surgeon is frequently in charge of the ignition source, the anesthesiologist is usually administering the oxidizer, and the OR nurse frequently controls the fuel sources. It is not always evident to any one individual that all of these elements may be coming together at the same time. This is especially true in any case where there is the possibility of oxygen or an oxygen–nitrous oxide mixture being delivered around the surgical site. In these circumstances, the risk of an OR fire is markedly increased and the need for communication among the surgeon, the anesthesiologist, and the OR nurses is especially important.

There are several dangers that may result from an operating room fire. The most obvious is that the patient and operating room personnel can suffer severe burns. However, a less obvious but potentially more deadly risk can be posed by the products of combustion (called "toxicants"). When materials, especially plastics, are burned, a variety of injurious compounds can be produced. These include carbon monoxide, ammonia, hydrogen chloride, and even cyanide. Toxicants can produce injury by damaging airways and lung tissue, and can cause asphyxia. Operating room fires can often produce significant amounts of smoke and toxicants, but may not cause enough heat to activate overhead sprinkler systems. If enough smoke is produced, the operating room personnel may have to evacuate the operating room. Thus, it is essential to have a prearranged evacuation plan for both the OR personnel and the patient.

Operating room fires can be divided into two different types. The more common type of fire occurs *in* or *on* the patient. These would include endotracheal tube fires, fires during laparoscopy or bronchoscopy, or a fire in the oropharynx, which may occur during a tonsillectomy Fires occurring on the patient mainly involve head and neck surgery done under regional anesthesia or monitored anesthesia care when the patient is receiving high flows of supplemental oxygen via a face mask or nasal prongs. Since these fires occur in an oxygen-enriched environment, items such as surgical towels, drapes, or even the body hair can be readily ignited and produce a severe burn (Fig. 8-36). The other type of operating room fire is one that is remote from the patient. This would include an electrical fire in a piece of equipment or a CO_2 absorber fire.

12 Although major ignition sources for OR fires are the ESU and the laser, the ends of some fiberoptic light cords can also become hot enough to start a fire if they are placed on paper drapes. And although the ESU is responsible for igniting the majority of the fires,[74] it is the laser that has generated the most attention and research. Laser is the acronym that stands for light amplification by stimulated emission of radiation. A laser consists of an energy source and material that the energy

TABLE 8-3

FUEL SOURCES COMMONLY FOUND IN THE OPERATING ROOM

- "Prep" Agents
  - Alcohol
  - Degreasers (acetone, ether)
  - Adhesives (tincture of benzoin, Aeroplast™)
  - Chlorhexidine digluconate (Hibitane™)
  - Iodophor (Dura-Prep™)
- Drapes and Covers
  - Patient drapes (paper, plastic, cloth)
  - Equipment drapes (paper, plastic, cloth)
  - Blankets and sheets
  - Pillows, mattresses, and padding
  - Gowns
  - Masks
  - Shoe covers
  - Gloves (latex, nonlatex)
  - Clothing
  - Compression (anti-embolism) stockings
- Patient
  - Hair
  - Alimentary tract gases (methane, hydrogen)
  - Desiccated tissue
- Dressings
  - Gauze and sponges
  - Petrolatum-impregnated dressings
  - Xeroform™
  - Adhesive tape (cloth, plastic, paper)
  - Elastic bandages
  - Stockinettes
  - Sutures
  - Steri-Strips
  - Collodion
- Ointments
  - Petrolatum
  - Antibiotics (bacitracin, neomycin, polymyxin B)
  - Nitropaste (Nitro-Bid™)
  - EMLA™
  - Lip balms
- Anesthesia Equipment
  - Breathing circuit hoses
  - Masks
  - Endotracheal tubes
  - Oral and nasal airways
  - Laryngeal mask airways
  - Nasogastric tubes
  - Suction catheters and tubing
  - Scavenger hoses
  - Volatile anesthetics
  - CO_2 absorbers
  - Intravenous tubing
  - Pressure monitor tubing and plastic transducers
- Other Equipment
  - Charts and records
  - Cardboard, wooden, and particleboard boxes and cabinets
  - Packing materials [cardboard, expanded polystyrene (Styrofoam™)]
  - Fiberoptic cable covers
  - Wire covers and insulation
  - Fiberoptic endoscope coverings
  - Sphymomanometer cuffs and tubing
  - Pneumatic tourniquet cuffs and tubing
  - Stethoscope tubing
  - Vascular shunts (Gore-tex™, Dacron™)
  - Dialysis and extracorporeal circulation circuits
  - Wound drains and collection systems
  - Mops and brooms
  - Textbooks and instruction manuals

excites to emit light.[80–82] The material that the energy excites is called the "lasing medium" and provides the name of the particular type of laser. The important property of laser light is that it is coherent, meaning that is monochromatic (or even of a single wavelength). This coherent light can be focused into very small spots that have very high power density.

There are many different types of medical lasers, and each has a specific application. The *argon laser* is used in eye and dermatologic procedures, as it is absorbed by hemoglobin and has a modest tissue penetration of between 0.05 and 2.0 mm. The potassium-titanyl-phosphate (KTP) or frequency-doubled *yttrium aluminum garnet* (YAG) lasers are also absorbed by hemoglobin and have tissue penetrations similar to that of the argon laser. The *Dilaser* has a wavelength that is easily changed and can be used in different applications, particularly in dermatologic procedures. The *neodymium-doped yttrium aluminum garnet* (Nd-YAG) laser is the most powerful of the medical lasers. Since the tissue penetration is between 2 and 6 mm, it can be used for tumor debulking, particularly in the trachea and main-stem bronchi, or in the upper airway. The energy can be transmitted through a fiberoptic cable that is placed down the suction port of a fiberoptic bronchoscope. The laser can then be used in a contact mode to treat a tumor mass. The *carbon dioxide* (CO_2) laser has very little tissue penetration and can be used where great precision is needed. It is also absorbed by water, so that minimal heat is dispersed to surrounding tissues. The CO_2 laser is used primarily for procedures in the oropharynx and in and around the vocal cords. The *helium-neon* laser (He-Ne) produces an intense red light and thus can be used for aiming the CO_2 and the Nd-YAG lasers. It has very low power and thus will present no significant danger to OR personnel.

One of the most devastating types of OR fires occurs when an endotracheal tube is ignited *in* the patient.[83–88] If the patient is being ventilated with oxygen and/or nitrous oxide, the endotracheal tube will essentially emit a blowtorch type of flame that can result in severe injury to the trachea, lungs, and surrounding tissues. In 1987 Wolf and Simpson showed that red rubber, polyvinyl chloride, and silicone endotracheal tubes all have oxygen flammability indices (defined as "the minimum O_2 fraction in N_2 that will just support a candle-like flame for a given fuel source using a standard ignition source") of less than 26%.[89] Because these tubes will combust at such low concentrations of oxygen, they are not the best choice when using lasers or electrocautery in or around the airway.

To prevent airway fires and their potentially devastating consequences, "laser-resistant" endotracheal tubes have been developed.[90–92] Before the advent of these tubes, anesthesiologists often wrapped red rubber or polyvinyl chloride tubes with some sort of reflective tape. Today, this practice is discouraged because taped-wrapped tubes can be easily kinked, gaps in the tape can expose areas of the tube to the laser, and nonlaser-resistant tape might be unintentionally used. Instead, anesthesiologists are encouraged to use an endotracheal tube that is designed to be resistant to the specific laser that will be used during surgery. For instance, when using the carbon dioxide laser, the LaserFlex™ (Mallinckrodt, Pleasanton, CA) is an excellent choice. This is a flexible metal tube that has two cuffs that can be inflated with saline colored with methylene blue. The methylene blue enables the surgeon to easily recognize if he or she has accidentally penetrated one of the cuffs. The LaserFlex™ tube is highly resistant to being struck by the laser. If the Nd-YAG laser is being used, then the Lasertubus™ (Rüsch Inc., Duluth, GA) can be used. The Lasertubus™ has a soft rubber shaft that is covered by a corrugated silver foil, which is, in turn, covered in a Merocel™ sponge jacket. To provide maximum protection, the Merocel™ must be kept moist with saline. If everything is done properly, the tube will resist ignition even with several strikes from the laser.

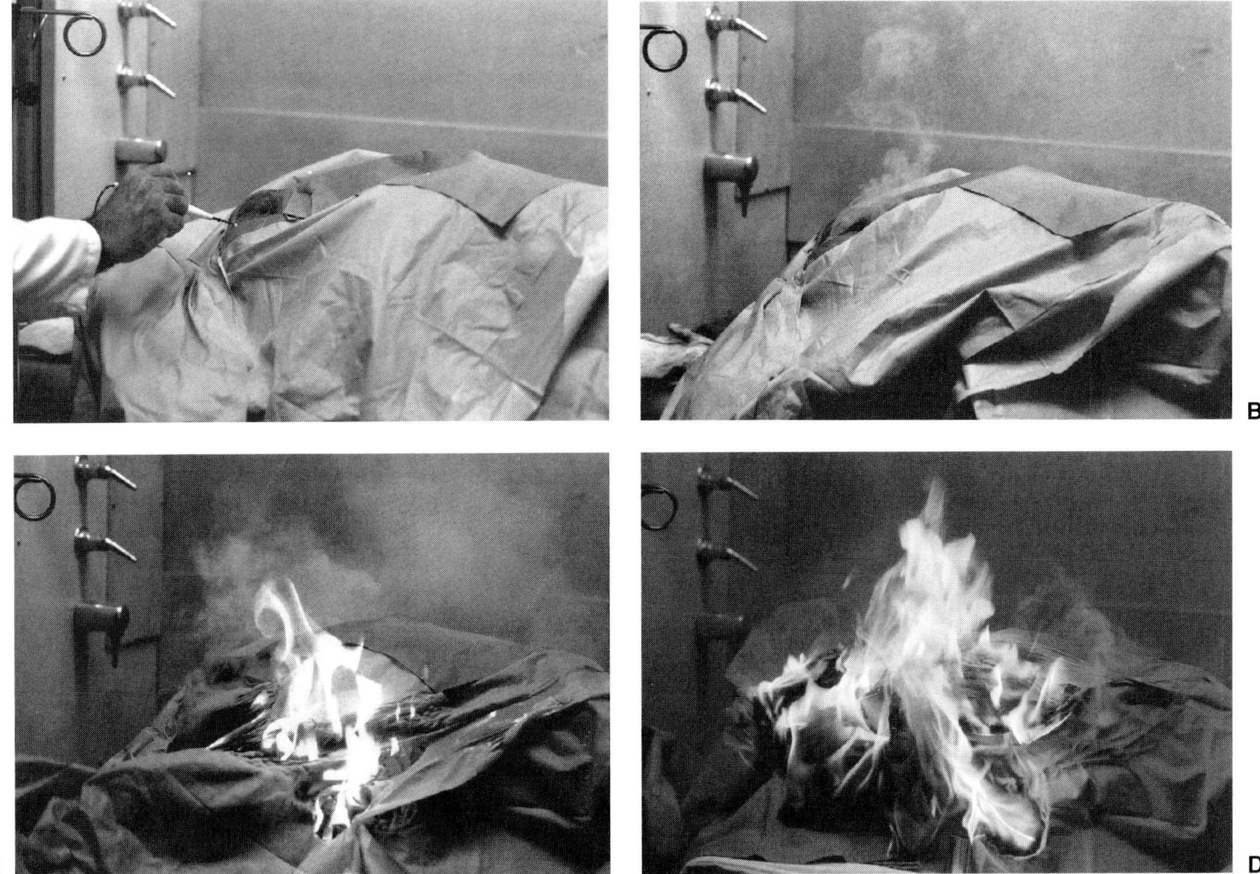

FIGURE 8-36. Simulation of fire caused by electrode during surgery. **A.** Mannequin prepared and draped for surgery. Electrosurgical unit monopolar pencil electrode applied to operative site at start of surgery. **B.** Six seconds after electrosurgical unit application. Smoke appears from under the drapes. **C.** Fourteen seconds after electrosurgical unit application. Flames burst through the drapes. **D.** Twenty-four seconds after electrosurgical unit application. Entire patient head and drapes in flames. (From Barker SJ, Polson JS. Fire in the operating room: A case report and laboratory study. Anesth Analg 93:960–965, 2001, with permission.)

As previously stated the ESU is a frequent ignition source for an OR fire.[93,94] A typical example of how an ESU could cause ignition would be during a tonsillectomy in a child where the anesthesiologist was using an uncuffed, flammable endotracheal tube. In this case, the oxygen or oxygen–nitrous oxide mixture could leak around the endotracheal tube and pool at the operative site, providing an oxygen-enriched environment. When the surgeon uses the ESU (or laser) to cauterize the tonsil bed, the combination of high concentration of oxidizer (oxygen or oxygen–nitrous oxide mixture), fuel (endotracheal tube), and ignition source (the ESU) could easily start a fire.[95,96]

The best way to prevent this type of fire is to take steps to prevent the three legs of the fire triad from coming together. For example, mixing the oxygen with air to keep the inspired oxygen concentration as low as possible, thus reducing the available oxidizer. Another possibility would be to place wet pledgets around the endotracheal tube, which would prevent the escape of oxygen or oxygen–nitrous oxide mixture from the trachea into the operative field. This reduces the available oxidizer and would keep the endotracheal tube and tissues from becoming desiccated, thus reducing their suitability as fuel sources. However, the pledgets must be kept moist, or they will dry out and become an additional source of fuel for a fire.

A related situation that requires a different solution can arise when a critically ill patient requires a tracheostomy.[97,98] These patients may require very high concentrations of inspired oxygen to maintain tissue oxygenation, so that any decrease in F_iO_2 or interruption of ventilation would not be tolerated. In this circumstance, the best option for preventing a fire would be to avoid the use of electrocautery (ignition source) when opening the trachea.

The Nd-YAG laser can be used to treat tumors of the lower trachea and main-stem bronchi. Most commonly, the surgeon will use a fiberoptic bronchoscope (FOB) and pass the laser fiber through the suction port of the bronchoscope. The FOB can be used in conjunction with a rigid metal bronchoscope or passed through an 8.5 or 9.0 mm polyvinyl chloride (PVC) endotracheal tube. A special laser resistant tube would not be used in this circumstance, because the FOB and laser fiber pass through the endotracheal tube and focus on tissue distal to the tube. Fire safety precautions available in this setting include titrating the concentration of inspired oxygen to as low as the patient can tolerate while maintaining a saturation of between 90 and 95% (ideally keeping the inspired oxygen below 30%), keeping the tip of the endotracheal tube and FOB away from the site of surgery and out of the "line of fire" of the laser, and removing charred and desiccated tissue from the surgical field. The use of a rigid metal bronchoscope instead of an endotracheal tube will eliminate the possibility of setting the tube on fire but does not eliminate the possibility of setting the fiberoptic bronchoscope on fire. This would also necessitate the use of a jet venturi system to ventilate the patient, which would, in turn, deliver oxygen at a concentration between 40 and 60%.

There are a number of basic safety precautions that should be taken whenever a laser is used in surgery. Since laser light can be reflected off any metal surface, it is important that all OR personnel wear protective goggles that are specific to the type of laser being used. The anesthesiologist needs to be aware that the laser goggles may make it difficult to read certain monitor displays. In addition, it is important that the patient's eyes be covered with wet gauze or eye packs. Operating room personnel should also wear high-filtration masks since the laser "plume" may contain vaporized virus particles or chemical toxins. Finally, all doors to the OR should have warning signs that a laser is in use, and all windows should be covered with black window shades.

Laparoscopic surgery in the abdomen is another potential risk for a fire in the patient. In 1993, Newman et al showed that nitrous oxide administered to the patient as part of their anesthetic can, over 30 minutes, diffuse into the abdominal cavity and attain a level that could support combustion.[99] In fact, when sampling the abdominal gas contents after 30 minutes, the mean nitrous oxide concentration was 36%; however, in certain patients it reached a concentration of 47%. Both methane and hydrogen are flammable gases that are frequently present in bowel gas in significant concentrations. Methane concentration in bowel gas can be up to 56% and hydrogen has been reported as high as 69%. With the maximum abdominal concentration of 47% nitrous oxide mixed with carbon dioxide, it would require the maximum of 56% of methane to be flammable. Therefore, this represents a relatively small hazard. In contrast, a concentration of 69% hydrogen is flammable if the nitrous oxide concentration is greater than 29%. Therefore, a fire is possible if the surgeon, while using the ESU, enters the bowel with a high concentration of hydrogen, and the intra-abdominal nitrous oxide content is greater than 29%.

Today, it is routine to use carbon dioxide to inflate the abdomen during laparoscopic surgery. Carbon dioxide is an excellent choice as it does not support combustion. However, a serious fire risk could occur if a mixture of carbon dioxide and oxygen was accidentally substituted for the carbon dioxide cylinder. Greilich reported such a case in 1995 in which the abdomen was inflated using a tank containing 14% carbon dioxide and 86% oxygen.[100] A flash fire occurred when the surgeon used the ESU. This was possible because all tanks with a CO_2 concentration greater than 7% have the same pin index as a tank with 100% CO_2.

In recent years, fires *on* the patient seem to have become the most frequent type of OR fire. These cases occur most often during surgery in and around the head and neck where the patient is receiving monitored anesthesia care (MAC) and supplemental oxygen is being administered by either a face mask or nasal cannula.[101–105] In these cases, the oxygen can collect under the drapes if not properly vented, and when the surgeon uses the ESU or the laser, a fire can easily start. There are many things that can act as fuel such as the surgical towels, paper drapes, disinfecting "prep" solutions, sponges, plastic tubing from the oxygen face mask, and even the body hair. These fires start very quickly and in only a few seconds can turn into an intense blaze. Even if the fire is quickly extinguished, the patient will usually sustain a significant burn.

The most important principle that the anesthesiologist has to keep in mind is to titrate the inspired oxygen concentration to a level that is low, yet safe for the patient. Oxygen should be treated just as any other drug and should be administered to provide optimum benefits and minimal side effects. If the anesthesia machine has the ability to deliver air, then the nasal cannula or face mask can be attached to the anesthesia circuit by using a small #3 or #4 15-mm ET tube adapter. This is attached to the right angle elbow of the circuit. If the anesthesia machine is equipped with an auxiliary oxygen flowmeter that has a removable nipple adaptor, then a humidifier can be installed in place of the nipple adaptor. The humidifier has a Venturi mechanism through which room air is entrained and thus the oxygen concentration that is delivered to the face mask can be varied from 28 to 100%. Finally, if this machine has a common gas outlet that is easily accessible, then a nasal cannula or face mask can be attached at this point using the same small 3- or 4-mm endotracheal tube adaptor. If it is not possible to dilute the oxygen with air, then it is important that the drapes be arranged in such a manner that there is no oxygen buildup beneath them. Tenting the drapes and having the surgeon use an adhesive sticky drape that seals the operative site from the oxygen flow are steps that will help reduce the risk of a fire.

It is potentially possible to discontinue the use of oxygen before the surgeon plans to use the ESU or laser. This would have to be done several minutes beforehand to allow any oxygen that has built up to dissipate. If the surgeon is planning to use the ESU or laser during the entire case, then this may not be practical.

In recent years, newer surgical prep solutions have been introduced into the OR. These typically come prepackaged in a "paint stick" applicator with a sponge on the end. DuraPrep™ is one of these prep solutions. It consists of Iodophor™ mixed with isopropyl alcohol. The concentration of alcohol in this solution is 74%, which is highly flammable and can easily be the fuel for an OR fire. In 2001, Barker and Polson reported just such a case.[101] In a laboratory re-creation of the case, he found that if the DuraPrep™ had been allowed to dry completely (4 to 5 minutes), then the fire did not occur. The other problem with these types of prep solutions is that small pools of the solution can accumulate if the person doing the prep is not careful. The alcohol in these small puddles will continue to evaporate for a period of time and the alcohol vapors are also extremely flammable.

It is important to bear in mind that halogenation of hydrocarbon anesthetics confers relative, but not absolute, resistance to combustion. Even the newer, "nonflammable" volatile anesthetics can, under certain circumstances, present fire hazards. For example, sevoflurane is nonflammable in air, but can serve as a fuel at concentrations as low as 11% in oxygen and 10% in nitrous oxide.[106] In addition, sevoflurane and desiccated CO_2 absorbent (either soda lime or Baralyme®) can undergo exothermic chemical reactions that have been implicated in several fires that involved the anesthesia breathing circuit.[107–110] At least some of these fires have injured patients. To prevent future fires, the manufacturer of sevoflurane has recommended that anesthesiologists employ several measures, including avoiding the use of desiccated CO_2 absorbent and monitoring the temperature of the absorber and the inspired concentration of sevoflurane. If an elevated temperature or an inspired sevoflurane concentration that differed unexpectedly from the vaporizer setting is detected, it is recommended that the patient be disconnected from the anesthesia circuit and monitored for signs of thermal or chemical injury and that the CO_2 absorbent be removed from the circuit and/or replaced.

Another way to prevent this type of fire is to use a CO_2 absorbent that does not contain a strong alkali, as do soda lime and Baralyme^R^. Amsorb^R^ is a CO_2 absorbent that contains calcium hydroxide and calcium chloride, but no strong alkali.[111] In experimental studies, Amsorb^R^ is unreactive with currently used volatile anesthetics and does not produce carbon monoxide or Compound A with desiccated absorbent. Therefore, it would not interact with sevoflurane and undergo an exothermic chemical reaction.

13 It is known that desiccated carbon dioxide absorbent can in rare circumstances react with sevoflurane to produce a fire. This seems to be a unique property of sevoflurane and would be highly unlikely with isoflurane or desflurane. Laster et al published an experimental report that compared the thermal effects of the three agents in desiccated Baralyme^R^.[112] They found that with both isoflurane and desflurane the temperature

transiently increased to about 100°C, then spontaneously decreased. However, with sevoflurane the temperature continued to increase to more than 200°C (and in one case to over 300°C). Two of the five sevoflurane experiments resulted in fires, illustrating the importance of the sevoflurane–desiccated Baralyme[R] combination as a potential source of fire in the operating room.

If a fire does occur, it is important to extinguish it as soon as possible. The first step is to interrupt the fire triad by removing one component. This is best accomplished by removing the oxidizer from the fire. Therefore, if an endotracheal tube is on fire, disconnecting the anesthetic circuit from the tube, or disconnecting the inspiratory limb of the circuit, will usually result in the fire immediately going out. It is not recommended to remove a burning endotracheal tube because this may cause even greater harm to the patient. Once the fire is extinguished, the endotracheal tube can be safely removed, the airway inspected via bronchoscopy, and the patient's trachea reintubated.

If the fire is on the patient, extinguishing it with a basin of saline may be the most rapid and effective method to put it out. Use of a sheet or towel may also extinguish the fire. If the drapes are burning, particularly if they are paper drapes, they must be removed and placed on the floor. Paper drapes are impervious to water, thus throwing water or saline on them will do little to extinguish the fire. Once the burning drapes are removed from the patient, the fire can then be extinguished with a fire extinguisher. In most operating room fires, the sprinkler system is not activated. This is because sprinklers are usually not located directly over the OR table and OR fires seldom get hot enough to activate the sprinklers.

4 All operating room personnel should be familiar with the location and operation of fire extinguishers in the area. These extinguishers are divided into three classes, termed A, B, and C. Class A extinguishers are used on paper, cloth, and plastic materials. Class B extinguishers are used for fires when liquids or grease are involved, and Class C extinguishers are used for energized electrical equipment. A single fire extinguisher may be useful for any one, two, or all three types of fires. Probably the best fire extinguisher for the operating room is the carbon dioxide extinguisher. This can be used on Class B and Class C fires and some Class A fires. Other extinguishers are water mist, or new environmentally friendly fluorocarbon extinguishers that replaced the Halon fire extinguisher. Finally, many operating rooms are equipped with a fire hose, which is pressurized water that is delivered at a rate of 50 gallons/minute. Such equipment is best left to the fire department to use, unless there is a need to rescue someone from a fire. To effectively use a fire extinguisher, the acronym PASS can be used. This stands for Pull the pin to activate the fire extinguisher, Aim at the base of the fire, Squeeze the trigger, and Sweep the extinguisher back and forth across the base of the fire. When responding to a fire the acronym RACE is useful. This stands for Rescue, Alarm, Confine, Extinguish. Clearly, having a plan that everyone is familiar with will greatly facilitate extinguishing the fire and minimize the harm to the patient and equipment. Fire drills are an important part of the plan and can help personnel become familiar with the exits, evacuation routes, and location of fire extinguishers and how to shut off gas and electrical supplies. If all of the OR personnel communicate with each other, the risk of a fire will be greatly reduced. It is important to never assume that others know what you are doing. Verbally confirm that the heat source has been placed in standby and not on the drapes. Lasers and ESUs should have their own holders and the surgeon needs to be sure which control activates the laser and which control activates the ESU. It is important that all prep solutions with alcohol be dry before surgery begins. During head and neck surgery, the anesthesiologist should inform the surgeon that there is an open source of oxygen being administered to the patient. Only through heightened awareness, continuing education, and communication can the legs of the fire triad be kept apart and the risk of an OR fire minimized.

References

1. Bruner JMR: Hazards of electrical apparatus. Anesthesiology 28:396, 1967
2. Hull CJ: Electrical hazards in monitoring. Int Anesthesiol Clin 19:177, 1981
3. Leonard PF, Gould AB: Dynamics of electrical hazards of particular concern to operating-room personnel. Surgical Clin North Am 45:817, 1965
4. Miller F: College Physics, 2nd ed, p 457. New York, Harcourt Brace and World, 1967
5. Uyttendaele K, Grobstein S, Svetz P: Monitoring instrumentation—isolated inputs, electrosurgery filtering, burns protection: What does it mean? Acta Anaesthesiol Belg 29:317, 1978
6. Leonard PF: Characteristics of electrical hazards. Anesth Analg 51:797, 1972
7. Taylor KW, Desmond J: Electrical hazards in the operating room, with special reference to electrosurgery. Can J Surg 13:362, 1970
8. Leonard PF: Apparatus and appliances: Current thinking. III. Alternating current, the isolation transformer, and the differential-transformer pressure transducer. Anesth Analg 45:814, 1966
9. Bruner JMR: Fundamental concepts of electrical safety. In Hershey SG (ed): ASA Refresher Courses in Anesthesiology, p 11. Philadelphia, JB Lippincott, 1974
10. Harpell TR: Electrical shock hazards in the hospital environment: Their causes and cures. Can Hosp 47:48, 1970
11. Buczko GB, McKay WPS: Electrical safety in the operating room. Can J Anaesth 34:315, 1987
12. Wald A: Electrical safety in medicine. In Skalak R, Chien S (eds): Handbook of Bioengineering, p 34.1. New York, McGraw-Hill, 1987
13. Dalziel CF, Massoglia FP: Let-go currents and voltages. AIEE Trans 75:49, 1956
14. Bruner JMR, Aronow S, Cavicchi RV: Electrical incidents in a large hospital: A 42 month register. JAAMI 6:222, 1972
15. Bernstein MS: Isolated power and line isolation monitors. Biomed Instrum Technol 24:221, 1990
16. Weinberg DI, Artley JL, Whalen RE, McIntosh HD: Electric shock hazards in cardiac catheterization. Circ Res 11:1004, 1962
17. Starmer CF, Whalen RE: Current density and electrically induced ventricular fibrillation. Med Instrum 7:158, 1973
18. Whalen RE, Starmer CF, McIntosh HD: Electrical hazards associated with cardiac pacemaking. Ann NY Acad Sci III:922, 1964
19. Raftery EB, Green HL, Yacoub MH: Disturbances of heart rhythm produced by 50-Hz leakage currents in human subjects. Cardiovasc Res 9:263, 1975
20. Hull CJ: Electrocution hazards in the operating theatre. Br J Anaesth 50:647, 1978
21. Watson AB, Wright JS, Loughman J: Electrical thresholds for ventricular fibrillation in man. Med J Aust 1:1179, 1973
22. Furman S, Schwedel JB, Robinson G, Hurwitt ES: Use of an intracardiac pacemaker in the control of heart block. Surgery 49:98, 1961
23. Noordijk JA, Oey FJI, Tebra W: Myocardial electrodes and the danger of ventricular fibrillation. Lancet 1:975, 1961
24. Pengelly LD, Klassen GA: Myocardial electrodes and the danger of ventricular fibrillation. Lancet 1:1234, 1961
25. Rowe GG, Zarnstorff WC: Ventricular fibrillation during selective angiocardiography. JAMA 192:947, 1965
26. Hopps JA, Roy OS: Electrical hazards in cardiac diagnosis and treatment. Med Electr Biol Eng 1:133, 1963
27. Mody SM, Richings M: Ventricular fibrillation resulting from electrocution during cardiac catheterization. Lancet 2:698, 1962
28. Leeming MN: Protection of the electrically susceptible patient: A discussion of systems and methods. Anesthesiology 38:370, 1973
29. McNulty SE, Cooper M, Staudt S: Transmitted radiofrequency current through a flow directed pulmonary artery catheter. Anesth Analg 78:587, 1994
30. Cromwell L, Weibell FJ, Pfeiffer EA: Biomedical Instrumentation and Measurements, 2nd ed, p 430. Englewood Cliffs, NJ: Prentice-Hall, 1980
31. Edwards NK: Specialized electrical grounding needs. Clin Perinatol 3:367, 1976
32. Goldwyn RM: Bovie: The man and the machine. Ann Plast Surg 2:135, 1979
33. Lichter I, Borrie J, Miller WM: Radio-frequency hazards with cardiac pacemakers. Br Med J 1:1513, 1965
34. Dornette WHL: An electrically safe surgical environment. Arch Surg 107: 567, 1973
35. Cushing H: Electro-surgery as an aid to the removal of intracranial tumors: With a preliminary note on a new surgical-current generator by W.T. Bovie. Surg Gynecol Obstet 47:751, 1928
36. Meathe EA: Electrical safety for patients and anesthetists. In Saidman LJ, Smith NT (eds): Monitoring in Anesthesia, 2nd ed, p 497. Boston, Butterworth, 1984

37. Rolly G: Two cases of burns caused by misuse of coagulation unit and monitoring. Acta Anaesthesiol Belg 29:313, 1978
38. Parker EO: Electrosurgical burn at the site of an esophageal temperature probe. Anesthesiology 61:93, 1984
39. Schneider AJL, Apple HP, Braun RT: Electrosurgical burns at skin temperature probes. Anesthesiology 47:72, 1977
40. Bloch EC, Burton LW: Electrosurgical burn while using a battery-operated doppler monitor. Anesth Analg 58:339, 1979
41. Becker CM, Malhotra IV, Hedley-Whyte J: The distribution of radiofrequency current and burns. Anesthesiology 38:106, 1973
42. Mitchell JP: The isolated circuit diathermy. Ann R Coll Surg Engl 61:287, 1979
43. Titel JH, El Etr AA: Fibrillation resulting from pacemaker electrodes and electrocautery during surgery. Anesthesiology 29:845, 1968
44. Domino KB, Smith TC: Electrocautery-induced reprogramming of a pacemaker using a precordial magnet. Anesth Analg 62:609, 1983
45. Mirowski M, Reid PR, Mower MM *et al:* Termination of malignant ventricular arrhythmias with an implanted automatic defibrillator in human beings. N Engl J Med 303:322, 1980
46. Crozier IG, Ward DE: Automatic implantable defribrillators. Br J Hosp Med 40:136, 1988
47. Elefteriades JA, Biblo LA, Batsford WP *et al:* Evolving patterns in the surgical treatment of malignant ventricular tachyarrhythmias. Ann Thorac Surg 49:94, 1990
48. Carr CME, Whiteley SM: The automatic implantable cardioverter-defibrillator. Anaesthesia 46:737, 1991
49. Starmer CF, McIntosh HD, Whalen RE: Electrical hazards and cardiovascular function. N Engl J Med 284:181, 1971
50. Albisser AM, Parson ID, Pask BA: A survey of the grounding systems in several large hospitals. Med Instrum 7:297, 1973
51. McLaughlin AJ, Campkin NT: Electrical safety: A reminder (letter). Anaesthesia 53:608, 1998
52. Nixon MC, Ghurye M: Electrical failure in theatre—A consequence of complacency? Anaesthesia 52(1):88, 1997
53. Medical Devices; Establishment of a Performance Standard for Electrode Lead Wires and Patient Cables, Federal Register 62(90):25477, May 9, 1997
54. Emergency Care Research Institute: FDA establishes performance standards for electrode lead wires. Health Devices 27:34, 1998
55. Hayes DL, Wang PJ, Reynolds DW *et al:* Interference with cardiac pacemakers by cellular telephones. N Engl J Med 336:1473, 1997
56. Schlegel RE, Grant FH, Raman S, Reynolds D: Electromagnetic compatibility study of the in-vitro interaction of wireless phones with cardiac pacemakers. Biomed Instrum Technol 32:645, 1998
57. Chen WH, Lau CP, Leung SK *et al:* Interference of cellular phones with implanted permanent pacemakers. Clin Cardiol 19:881, 1996
58. Fetter JG, Ivans V, Benditt DG, Collins J: Digital cellular telephone interaction with implantable cardioverter-defibrillators. J Am Coll Cardiol 21:623, 1998
59. Emergency Care Research Institute: Cell phones and walkie-talkies: Is it time to relax your restrictive policies? Health Devices 28:409, 1999
60. Adler D, Margulies L, Mahler Y, Israeli A: Measurements of electromagnetic fields radiated from communication equipment and of environmental electromagnetic noise: Impact on the use of communication equipment within the hospital. Biomed Instrum Technol 32(6):581, 1998
61. Schwartz JJ, Ehrenwerth J: Electrical safety: In Lake CL, Hines RH, Blitt C (eds): Clinical Monitoring: Practical Applications for Anesthesia and Critical Care, ch 5. Philadelphia, WB Saunders, 2000
62. Kermit E, Staewen WS: Isolated power systems: Historical perspective and update on regulations. Biomed Tech Today 1:86, 1986
63. National Fire Protection Association: National electric code (ANSI/NFPA 70-1984). Quincy, MA, National Fire Protection Association, 1984
64. Bruner JMR, Leonard PF: Electricity, Safety and the Patient, p 300. Chicago, Year Book Medical Publishers, 1989
65. Matjasko MJ, Ashman MN: All you need to know about electrical safety in the operating room. In Barash PG, Deutsch S, Tinker J (eds): ASA Refresher Courses in Anesthesiology, vol 18, p 251. Philadelphia, JB Lippincott, 1980
66. Lennon RL, Leonard PF: A hitherto unreported virtue of the isolated power system (letter). Anesth Analg 66:1049, 1987
67. Gilbert TB, Shaffer M, Matthews M: Electrical shock by dislodged spark gap in bipolar electrosurgical device. Anesth Analg 73:355, 1991
68. Day FJ: Electrical safety revisited: A new wrinkle. Anesthesiology 80:220, 1994
69. Litt L, Ehrenwerth J: Electrical safety in the operating room: Important old wine, disguised in new bottles. Anesth Analg 78:417, 1994
70. Seifert HA: Fire safety in the operating room. In Eisenkraft JB (ed): Progress in Anesthesiology. Philadelphia, WB Saunders, 1994
71. Neufeld GR: Fires and explosions. In Orkin K, Cooperman LH (eds): Complications in Anesthesiology, p 671. Philadelphia, Lippincott, 1983
72. Moxon MA: Fire in the operating room. Anaesthesia 41:543, 1986
73. Vickers MD: Fire and explosion hazards in operating theatres. Br J Anaesth 50:659, 1978
74. Food and Drug Administration: Surgical Fires Reported January 1995–June 1998. FDA Databases MDR/MAUDE, 1999
75. de Richemond AL: The patient is on fire! Health Devices 21:19, 1992
76. Cameron BG, Ingram GS: Flammability of drape materials in nitrous oxide and oxygen. Anesthesiology 26:218, 1971
77. Johnson RM, Smith CV, Leggett K: Flammability of disposable surgical drapes. Arch Ophthalmol 94:1327, 1976
78. Simpson JI, Wolf GL: Flammability of esophageal stethoscopes, nasogastric tubes, feeding tubes, and nasopharyngeal airways in oxygen- and nitrous oxide-enriched atmospheres. Anesth Analg 67:1093, 1988
79. Ponath RE: Preventing surgical fires. JAMA 252:1762, 1984
80. Rampil IJ: Anesthetic considerations for laser surgery. Anesth Analg 74:424, 1992
81. Pashayan AG, Ehrenwerth J: Lasers and electrical safety in the operating room. In Ehrenwerth J, Eisenkraft JB (eds): Anesthesia Equipment: Principles and Applications. St. Louis, Mosby, 1993
82. Emergency Care Research Institute: Lasers in medicine—An introduction. Health Devices 13:151, 1984
83. Casey KR, Fairfax WR, Smith SJ *et al*: Intratracheal fire ignited by the Nd:YAG laser during treatment of tracheal stenosis. Chest 84:295, 1983
84. Burgess GE, LeJeune FE: Endotracheal tube ignition during laser surgery of the larynx. Arch Otolaryngol 105:561, 1979
85. Cozine K, Rosenbaum LM, Askanazi J *et al*: Laser induced endotracheal tube fire. Anesthesiology 55:583, 1981
86. Geffin B, Shapshay SM, Bellack GS *et al*: Flammability of endotracheal tubes during Nd:YAG laser application in the airway. Anesthesiology 65:511, 1986
87. Hirshman CA, Smith J: Indirect ignition of the endotracheal tube during carbon dioxide laser surgery. Arch Otolaryngol 106:639, 1980
88. Krawtz S, Mehta AC, Weidemann HP *et al*: Nd:YAG laser-induced endobronchial burn. Chest 95:916, 1989
89. Wolf GL, Simpson JI: Flammability of endotracheal tubes in oxygen and nitrous oxide enriched atmosphere. Anesthesiology 67:236, 1987
89a. Goldblum UB: Oxygen index: Key to precise flamibility ratings. Society of Plastic engineers Journal 25:50–52, 1969.
90. de Richemond AL: Laser resistant endotracheal tubes—Protection against oxygen-enriched airway fires during surgery? In Stoltzfus JM, McIlroy K (eds): Flammability and Sensitivity of Material in Oxygen-Enriched Atmospheres, vol 5, p 157 (ASTM STP 1111). Philadelphia, American Society for Testing and Materials, 1991
91. Emergency Care Research Institute: Airway fires: Reducing the risk during laser surgery. Health Devices 19:109, 1990
92. Emergency Care Research Institute: Laser-resistant tracheal tubes (evaluation). Health Devices 21:4, 1992
93. Aly A, McIlwain M, Ward M: Electrosurgery-induced endotracheal tube ignition during tracheotomy. Ann Otol Rhinol Laryngol 100:31, 1991
94. Simpson JI, Wolf GL: Endotracheal tube fire ignited by pharyngeal electrocautery. Anesthesiology 65:76, 1986
95. Gupte SR: Gauze fire in the oral cavity: A case report. Anesth Analg 51:645, 1972
96. Snow JC Norton ML, Saluja TS *et al*: Fire hazard during CO_2 laser microsurgery on the larynx and trachea. Anesth Analg 55:146, 1975
97. Lew EO, Mittleman RE, Murray D: Tube ignition by electrocautery during tracheostomy: Case report with autopsy findings. J Forensic Sci 36:1586, 1991
98. Marsh B, Riley DH: Double-lumen tube fire during tracheostomy. Anesthesiology 76:480, 1992
99. Neuman GG, Sidebotham G, Negoianu E *et al*: Laparoscopy explosion hazards with nitrous oxide. Anesthesiology 78:875, 1993
100. Greilich NB, Froelich EG *et al*: Intraabdominal fire during laparoscopic cholecystectomy. Anesthesiology 83:871, 1995
101. Barker SJ, Polson JS: Fire in the operating room: A case report and laboratory study. Anesth Analg 93:960, 2001
102. Bruley ME, Lavanchy C: Oxygen-enriched fires during surgery of the head and neck. In Symposium on Flammability and Sensitivity of Material in Oxygen-Enriched Atmospheres, p 392 (ASTM STP 1040). Philadelphia, American Society for Testing and Materials, 1989
103. de Richemond AL, Bruley ME: Head and neck surgical fires. In Eisele DW (ed): Complications in Head and Neck Surgery. St. Louis, Mosby, 1993
104. Emergency Care Research Institute: Fires during surgery of the head and neck area (hazard). Health Devices 9:50, 1979
105. Ramanathan S, Capan L, Chalon J *et al*: Mini-environmental control under the drapes during operations on eyes of conscious patients. Anesthesiology 48:286, 1978
106. Wallin RF, Regan BM, Napoli MD, Stern IJ: Sevoflurane: A new inhalational anesthetic agent. Anesth Analg 54:758, 1975
107. Fatheree RS, Leighton BL: Acute respiratory syndrome after an exothermic baralymeR-sevoflurane reaction. Anesthesiology 101:531, 2004
108. Castro BA, Freedman LA, Craig WL, Lynch C: Explosion within an anesthesia machine: BaralymeR, high fresh gas flows and sevoflurane concentration. Anesthesiology 101:537, 2004
109. Wu J, Previte JP, Adler E *et al*: Spontaneous ignition, explosion and fire with sevoflurane and barium hydroxide lime. Anesthesiology 101:534, 2004
110. Abbott A: Dear healthcare provider (letter). November 17, 2003. [www.fda.gov/medwatch/SAFETY/2003/ultane_deardoc.pdf]
111. Murray JM, Renfrew CW, Bedi A, *et al*: Amsorb: A new carbon dioxide absorbent for use in anesthetic breathing systems. Anesthesiology 91:1342, 1999
112. Laster M, Roth P, Eger EI: Fires from the interaction of anesthetics with desiccated absorbent. Anesth Analg 99:769, 2004

CHAPTER 9 ■ ACID-BASE, FLUIDS, AND ELECTROLYTES

DONALD S. PROUGH, SCOTT W. WOLF, J. SEAN FUNSTON, AND CHRISTER H. SVENSÉN

KEY POINTS

1. The Henderson–Hasselbalch equation describes the relationship between pH, $PaCO_2$, and serum bicarbonate. The Henderson equation defines the previous relationship but substitutes hydrogen concentration for pH.
2. The pathophysiology of metabolic alkalosis is divided into generating and maintenance factors. A particularly important maintenance factor is renal hypoperfusion, often a result of hypovolemia.
3. Metabolic acidosis occurs as a consequence of the use of bicarbonate to buffer endogenous organic acids or as a consequence of external bicarbonate loss. The former causes an increase in the anion gap ($Na^+ - [Cl^- + [HCO_3^-]]$).
4. When substituting mechanical ventilation for spontaneous ventilation in a patient with severe metabolic acidosis, it is important to maintain an appropriate level of ventilatory compensation, pending effective treatment of the primary cause for the metabolic acidosis.
5. Sodium bicarbonate, never proved to alter outcome in patients with lactic acidosis, should be reserved for those patients with severe acidemia.
6. The addition of iatrogenic respiratory alkalosis to metabolic alkalosis can produce severe alkalemia.
7. Tight control of blood glucose in critically ill patients has been associated with substantial improvements in mortality.
8. In patients undergoing moderate surgical procedures, generous administration of fluids is associated with fewer minor complications, such as nausea, vomiting, and drowsiness.
9. In patients undergoing colon surgery, careful perioperative fluid restriction has been associated with lower mortality and better wound healing.
10. Homeostatic mechanisms are usually adequate for the maintenance of electrolyte balance. However, critical illnesses and their treatment strategies can cause significant perturbations in electrolyte status, possibly leading to worsened patient outcome.
11. Calcium, phosphorus, and magnesium are all essential for maintenance and function of the cardiovascular system. In addition, they also provide the milieu that ensures neuromuscular transmission. Disorders affecting any one of these electrolytes may lead to significant dysfunction and possibly result in cardiopulmonary arrest.
12. Disorders of the concentration of sodium, the principal extracellular cation, are dependent on the total body water concentration and can lead to neurologic dysfunction. Disorders of potassium, the principal intracellular cation, are influenced primarily by insults that result in increased total body losses of potassium or changes in distribution.

As a consequence of underlying diseases and of therapeutic manipulations, surgical patients may develop potentially harmful disorders of acid-base equilibrium, intravascular and extravascular volume, and serum electrolytes. Precise perioperative management of acid-base status, fluids, and electrolytes may limit perioperative morbidity and mortality.

ACID-BASE INTERPRETATION AND TREATMENT

To facilitate management of perioperative acid-base disturbances, this chapter reviews the pathogenesis, major complications, physiologic compensatory mechanisms, and treatment of the four simple acid-base disorders: metabolic alkalosis, metabolic acidosis, respiratory alkalosis, and respiratory acidosis.

Overview of Acid-Base Equilibrium

1 The conventional approach to describing acid-base equilibrium is the Henderson–Hasselbalch equation:

$$pH = 6.1 + \log\frac{[HCO_3^-]}{0.03 \times PaCO_2} \quad (9\text{-}1)$$

where 6.1 = the pK_a of carbonic acid and 0.03 is the solubility coefficient in blood of carbon dioxide (CO_2). Conventional acid-base terminology defines acid-base disturbances as metabolic (i.e., those in which the bicarbonate concentration $[HCO_3^-]$ is primarily increased or decreased) and respiratory (i.e., those in which $PaCO_2$ is primarily increased or decreased). pH, the term used to define the acidity or alkalinity of solutions or blood, is the negative logarithm of the hydrogen ion concentration ($[H^+]$). The simpler Henderson equation (the origins of which precede the Henderson–Hasselbalch equation)[1] clearly expresses the relationship between the three major variables measured or calculated in blood gas samples:

$$[H^+] = \frac{24 \times PaCO_2}{[HCO_3^-]} \quad (9\text{-}2)$$

To convert pH to $[H^+]$, assume that $[H^+]$ is 40 mmol/L at a pH of 7.4; that an increase in pH of 0.10 pH units reduces $[H^+]$ to 0.8 × the starting $[H^+]$ concentration; that a decrease in pH of 0.10 pH units increases the $[H^+]$ by a factor of 1.25; and that small changes (i.e., <0.05 pH units) produce approximately a 1.0 mmol/L increase in $[H^+]$ for each 0.01 decrease in pH or a decrease in $[H^+]$ of one mmol/L per 0.01 increase in pH. These rules-of-thumb only approximate the logarithmic relationship between pH and $[H^+]$. The more the pH deviates from 7.4, the less accurate the rules become.

The alternative Stewart approach to acid-base interpretation distinguishes between the independent variables and dependent variables that define pH.[1,2] The independent variables are $PaCO_2$, the strong (i.e., highly dissociated) ion difference (SID), and the concentration of proteins, which usually are not strong ions. The strong ions include sodium (Na^+), potassium (K^+), chloride (Cl^-), and lactate. The SID, calculated as ($Na^+ + K^+ - Cl^-$), under normal circumstances is approximately 42 mEq/L. In general, the Stewart approach provides more insight into the mechanisms underlying acid-base disturbances, in contrast to the Henderson–Hasselbalch approach, which is more descriptive. However, the clinical interpretation or treatment of common acid-base disturbances is rarely handicapped by the simpler constructs of the conventional Henderson–Hasselbalch or Henderson equations.

Metabolic Alkalosis

Metabolic alkalosis, usually characterized by an alkalemic pH
2 (>7.45) and hyperbicarbonatemia (>27.0 mEq/L), is the commonest acid-base abnormality in critically ill patients and is associated with increased cost, morbidity, and mortality.[3] Factors that generate metabolic alkalosis include nasogastric suction and diuretic administration (Table 9-1).[4] Maintenance of metabolic alkalosis is dependent on a continued stimulus, such as renal hypoperfusion, hypokalemia, hypochloremia, or hypovolemia, for distal tubular reabsorption of $[HCO_3^-]$.

Metabolic alkalosis exerts multiple physiologic effects. Metabolic alkalosis is associated with hypokalemia, ionized hypocalcemia, secondary ventricular arrhythmias, increased digoxin toxicity, and compensatory hypoventilation (hypercarbia), although $PaCO_2$ rarely exceeds 55 mmHg (Table 9-2).[4] Alkalemia also increases bronchial tone and, through a combination of increased bronchial tone and decreased ventilatory effort, may promote atelectasis. Alkalemia may reduce tissue oxygen availability by shifting the oxyhemoglobin dissociation curve to the left and by decreasing cardiac output. During anesthetic management, inadvertent addition of iatrogenic respiratory alkalosis to preexisting metabolic alkalosis may produce cardiovascular depression, dysrhythmias, and the other complications of severe alkalemia (Table 9-3).

In patients in whom arterial blood gases have not yet been obtained, serum electrolytes and a history of major risk factors, such as vomiting, nasogastric suction, or chronic diuretic use, can suggest metabolic alkalosis. Total "CO_2" (usually abbreviated on electrolyte reports as CO_2) should be about 1.0 mEq/L greater than $[HCO_3^-]$ calculated on simultaneously obtained arterial blood gases. If either calculated $[HCO_3^-]$ on the arterial blood gases or "CO_2" on the serum electrolytes exceeds normal (24 and 25 mEq/L, respectively) by

TABLE 9-1

GENERATION AND MAINTENANCE OF METABOLIC ALKALOSIS

GENERATION	EXAMPLE	MAINTENANCE
I. Loss of acid from extracellular space		
A. Loss of gastric fluid	Vomiting; nasogastric drainage	↓ effective arterial volume (EAV)
B. Loss of acid into urine; continued Na^+ delivery to the distal tubule in presence of hyperaldosteronism	1. Primary aldosteronism 2. Diuretic administration	1. K^+ depletion + aldosterone excess 2. ↓ EAV + K^+ depletion
II. Excessive HCO_3^- loads		
A. Absolute		
1. HCO_3^-	$NaHCO_3$ administration	↓EAV
	Lactate, acetate, citrate administration	↓EAV
2. Metabolic conversion of salts of organic acid anions to HCO_3^-	Alkali administration to patients with renal failure	Renal failure
B. Relative		
1. Alkaline loads in renal failure		
III. Posthypercapnic state	Abrupt correction of chronic hypercapnia	↓EAV

TABLE 9-2

RULES OF THUMB FOR RESPIRATORY COMPENSATION IN RESPONSE TO METABOLIC ALKALOSIS AND METABOLIC ACIDOSIS

Metabolic alkalosis

1. $PaCO_2$ increases approximately 0.5 to 0.6 mmHg for each 1.0 mEq/L increase in $[HCO_3^-]$
2. The last two digits of the pH should equal the $[HCO_3^-] + 15$

Metabolic acidosis

1. $PaCO_2 = [HCO_3^-] \times 1.5 + 8$
2. $PaCO_2$ decreases 1.2 mmHg for every 1.0 mEq/L in $[HCO_3^-]$ to a minimum of 10 to 15 mmHg
3. The last two digits of the pH equal $[HCO_3^-] + 15$

>4.0 mEq/L, either the patient has a primary metabolic alkalosis or has conserved bicarbonate in response to chronic hypercarbia. Recognition of hyperbicarbonatemia on the preoperative serum electrolytes justifies arterial blood gas analysis and should alert the anesthesiologist to the likelihood of factors that generate or maintain metabolic alkalosis.

Treatment of metabolic alkalosis consists of etiologic and nonetiologic therapy. Etiologic therapy consists of measures such as expansion of intravascular volume or the administration of potassium. To restore intravascular volume, administration of 0.9% saline tends to increase serum $[Cl^-]$ and decrease serum $[HCO_3^-]$.[5] Although hypoproteinemia can cause a mild metabolic alkalosis,[6] such changes usually require no specific treatment. Nonetiologic therapy includes administration of acetazolamide (a carbonic anhydrase inhibitor that causes renal bicarbonate wasting) or $[H^+]$ as ammonium chloride, arginine hydrochloride, or 0.1 N hydrochloric acid (100 mmol/L), or acid dialysis. Of the preceding, 0.1 N hydrochloric acid most rapidly corrects life-threatening metabolic alkalosis but must be infused into a central vein; peripheral infusion will cause severe tissue damage.

Metabolic Acidosis

Metabolic acidosis, usually characterized by an acidemic pH (<7.35) and hypobicarbonatemia (<21 mEq/L), can be innocu-
3 ous or reflect a life-threatening emergency.[7] Metabolic acidosis occurs as a consequence of buffering by bicarbonate of endogenous or exogenous acid loads or as a consequence of abnormal external loss of bicarbonate. Approximately 70 mmol of acid metabolites are produced, buffered, and excreted daily; these include about 25 mmol of sulfuric acid from amino acid metabolism, 40 mmol of organic acids, and phosphoric and other acids.[8] Extracellular volume (ECV) in a 70-kg adult contains 336 mmol of bicarbonate buffer (24 mEq/L × 14 l of ECV). Glomerular filtration of plasma volume necessitates reabsorption of 4,500 mmol of bicarbonate daily, of which 85% is reabsorbed in the proximal tubule and 10% in the thick ascending limb, and the remainder is titrated by proton secretion in the collecting duct.[8]

Calculation of the anion gap ($Na^+ - [Cl^-] + [HCO_3^-]$) distinguished between two types of metabolic acidosis (Table 9-4).[9] The anion gap is normal (<13 mEq/L) in situations, such as diarrhea, biliary drainage, and renal tubular acidosis, in which bicarbonate is lost externally. The anion gap also is normal or reduced in hyperchloremic acidosis associated with perioperative infusion of substantial quantities of 0.9% saline.[5,10,11] Metabolic acidosis associated with a high anion gap (>13 mEq/L) occurs because of production of excess lactic acid or ketoacids, increased retention of waste products (such as sulfate and phosphate) that are inadequately excreted in uremic states, and ingestion of toxic quantities of substances such as aspirin, ethylene glycol, and methanol. In those circumstances, bicarbonate ions are consumed in buffering hydrogen ions, while the associated anion replaces bicarbonate in serum. Because three-quarters of the normal anion gap consists of albumin, the calculated anion gap should be corrected for hypoalbuminemia by adding to the calculated anion gap the difference between measured serum albumin and a normal albumin concentration of 4.0 g/dL multiplied by 2.0 to 2.5.[12,13]

Sufficient reductions in pH may reduce myocardial contractility, increase pulmonary vascular resistance, decrease systemic vascular resistance, and impair the response of the cardiovascular system to endogenous or exogenous catecholamines. It is
4 particularly important to note that failure of a patient to appropriately hyperventilate in response to metabolic acidosis is physiologically equivalent to respiratory acidosis and suggests impending deterioration. If a patient with metabolic acidosis requires mechanical ventilation, every attempt should be made to maintain an appropriate level of ventilatory compensation until the primary process can be corrected (see Table 9-2). Table 9-5 illustrates failure to maintain compensatory hyperventilation.

The anesthetic implications of metabolic acidosis are proportional to the severity of the underlying process. Although a patient with hyperchloremic metabolic acidosis may be relatively healthy, those with lactic acidosis, ketoacidosis, uremia, or toxic ingestions will be chronically or acutely ill.

TABLE 9-3

METABOLIC ALKALOSIS PLUS HYPERVENTILATION

	NORMAL	CHRONIC DIURETIC ADMINISTRATION	INTRAOPERATIVE HYPERVENTILATION
BLOOD GASES			
pH	7.40	7.47	7.62
$PaCO_2$ (mmHg)	40	45	30
$[HCO_3^-]$ (mEq/L)	24	32	29
ELECTROLYTES			
"CO_2" (mEq/L)	25	33	30

Note: Respiratory alkalosis, produced by an inappropriately high minute ventilation, has been added to the previously compensated metabolic alkalosis induced by chronic diuretic administration. "CO_2", Total CO_2.

TABLE 9-4

DIFFERENTIAL DIAGNOSIS OF METABOLIC ACIDOSIS

■ ELEVATED ANION GAP	■ NORMAL ANION GAP
Three diseases	
1. Uremia	1. Renal tubular acidosis
2. Ketoacidosis	2. Diarrhea
3. Lactic acidosis	3. Carbonic anhydrase inhibition
Toxins	4. Ureteral diversions
1. Methanol	5. Early renal failure
2. Ethylene glycol	6. Hydronephrosis
3. Salicylates	7. HCl administration
4. Paraldehyde	8. Saline administration

Correction of the anion gap for hypoalbuminemia is essential for effective perioperative use.

Preoperative assessment should emphasize volume status and renal function. If shock is the etiology, direct arterial pressure monitoring and preload may require assessment via echocardiography or pulmonary arterial catheterization. Intraoperatively, one should be concerned about the possibility of exaggerated hypotensive responses to drugs and positive pressure ventilation. Preoperative compensatory hyperventilation should be maintained during anesthesia and monitored using capnography and arterial blood gases. In planning intravenous fluid therapy, consider that balanced salt solutions tend to increase $[HCO_3^-]$ and pH and 0.9% saline tends to decrease $[HCO_3^-]$ and pH.[5,10]

The treatment of metabolic acidosis consists of the treatment of the primary pathophysiologic process (i.e., hypoperfusion, hypoxia, and if pH is severely decreased, administration of $NaHCO_3^-$). Hyperventilation, though an important compensatory response to metabolic acidosis, is not definitive therapy for metabolic acidosis. The initial dose of $NaHCO_3$ can be calculated as:

$$NaHCO_3(\text{mEq/L}) = \frac{\text{Wt (kg)} \times 0.3 \times (24\ \text{mEq/L} - \text{Actual } HCO_3^-)}{2} \quad (9\text{-}3)$$

where 0.3 = the assumed distribution space for bicarbonate and 24 mEq/L is the normal value for $[HCO_3^-]$ on arterial blood gas determination. The calculation markedly underestimates dosage in severe metabolic acidosis. In infants and children, an appropriate initial dose is 1.0 to 2.0 mEq/kg of body weight.

5 One continuing controversy is the use of $NaHCO_3$ to treat acidemia induced by lactic acidosis. In critically ill patients with lactic acidosis, there were no important differences between the physiologic effects (other than changes in pH) of 0.9 M $NaHCO_3$ and 0.9 M sodium chloride.[14] Importantly, $NaHCO_3$ did not improve the cardiovascular response to catecholamines and actually reduced plasma ionized calcium.[14] Although many clinicians continue to administer $NaHCO_3$ to patients with persistent lactic acidosis and ongoing deterioration, neither $NaHCO_3$ nor dichloroacetate[15] has improved outcome. The buffer THAM (tris-hydroxymethyl aminomethane) is effective at reducing $[H^+]$ and does not generate CO_2 as a byproduct of buffering[16]; however, there is no generally accepted indication for THAM.

Respiratory Alkalosis

6 Respiratory alkalosis, usually characterized by an alkalemic pH (>7.45) and always characterized by hypocarbia ($PaCO_2 \leq 35$ mmHg), describes an increase in minute ventilation that is greater than that required to excrete metabolic CO_2 production. Because respiratory alkalosis may be a sign of pain, anxiety, hypoxemia, central nervous system (CNS) disease, or systemic sepsis, the development of spontaneous respiratory alkalosis in a previously normocarbic patient requires prompt evaluation. The hyperventilation syndrome, a diagnosis of exclusion, is most often encountered in the emergency department.[17]

Respiratory alkalosis, like metabolic alkalosis, may produce hypokalemia, hypocalcemia, cardiac dysrhythmias, bronchoconstriction, and hypotension, and may potentiate the toxicity of digoxin. In addition, both brain pH and cerebral blood flow are tightly regulated and respond rapidly to changes in systemic pH.[18] Doubling minute ventilation reduces $PaCO_2$ to 20 mmHg and halves cerebral blood flow; conversely, halving minute ventilation doubles $PaCO_2$ and doubles cerebral blood flow. Acute hyperventilation may be useful in neurosurgical procedures to reduce brain bulk and to control intracranial pressure (ICP) during emergent surgery for noncranial injuries associated with acute closed head trauma. In those situations, intraoperative monitoring of arterial blood gases, correlated with capnography, will document adequate reduction of $PaCO_2$. Acute profound hypocapnia (<20 mmHg) may produce EEG evidence of cerebral ischemia. If $PaCO_2$ is maintained at abnormally high or low levels for 8 to 24 hours, cerebral blood flow will return toward previous levels, associated with a return of cerebrospinal fluid $[HCO_3^-]$ toward normal.[19]

Treatment of respiratory alkalosis per se is often not required. In most patients, the most important steps are recognition and treatment of the underlying etiology.[17] For instance, correction of hypoxemia or hypoperfusion-induced lactic acidosis should result in resolution of the associated increases in respiratory drive. Preoperative recognition of chronic hyperventilation necessitates intraoperative maintenance of a similar $PaCO_2$.

TABLE 9-5

FAILURE TO MAINTAIN APPROPRIATE VENTILATORY COMPENSATION FOR METABOLIC ACIDOSIS

		■ SPONTANEOUS VENTILATION		■ MECHANICAL VENTILATION
Arteria 1 blood gases	pH	7.29		7.13
	$PaCO_2$ (mmHg)	29	→→→→→→→→	49
	$[HCO_3^-]$ (mEq/L)	14		16

In the presence of metabolic acidosis, an otherwise innocuous increase in $PaCO_2$ may create a life-threatening decrease in pH.

Respiratory Acidosis

Respiratory acidosis, usually characterized by a low pH (<7.35) and always characterized by hypercarbia ($PaCO_2 \geq 45$ mmHg), occurs because of a decrease in minute alveolar ventilation ($\dot{V}_A$), an increase in production of carbon dioxide ($\dot{V}_{CO2}$), or both, from the equation:

$$PaCO_2 = K\frac{\dot{V}_{CO2}}{\dot{V}_A} \quad (9\text{-}4)$$

where K = constant (rebreathing of exhaled, carbon dioxide-containing gas may also increase $PaCO_2$). Respiratory acidosis may be either acute, without compensation by renal $[HCO_3^-]$ retention, or chronic, with $[HCO_3^-]$ retention offsetting the decrease in pH (Table 9-6). A reduction in $\dot{V}_A$ may be because of an overall decrease in minute ventilation ($\dot{V}_E$) or to an increase in the amount of wasted ventilation ($\dot{V}_D$), according to the equation:

$$\dot{V}_A = \dot{V}_E - \dot{V}_D \quad (9\text{-}5)$$

Decreases in $\dot{V}_E$ may occur because of central ventilatory depression by drugs or central nervous system injury, because of increased work of breathing, or because of airway obstruction or neuromuscular dysfunction. Increases in $\dot{V}_D$ occur with chronic obstructive pulmonary disease, pulmonary embolism, and most acute forms of respiratory failure. $\dot{V}_{CO2}$ may be increased by sepsis, high-glucose parenteral feeding, or fever.

Patients with chronic hypercarbia because of intrinsic pulmonary disease require careful preoperative evaluation. The ventilatory restriction imposed by upper abdominal or thoracic surgery may compound ventilatory insufficiency. Administration of opioids and sedatives, even in small doses, may cause hazardous ventilatory depression. Preoperative evaluation should consider direct arterial pressure monitoring and frequent intraoperative blood gas determinations, as well as postoperative pain management. Intraoperatively, a patient with chronic hypercapnia should be ventilated to maintain a normal pH. An abrupt increase in minute ventilation may result in profound alkalemia (analogous to the addition of hyperventilation to metabolic alkalosis described in Table 9-3). Postoperatively, prophylactic ventilatory support may be required for selected patients with severe lung disease and chronic hypercarbia. Epidural opioid administration represents one potential alternative that may provide adequate postoperative analgesia without undue depression of ventilatory drive.

The treatment of respiratory acidosis depends on whether the process is acute or chronic. Acute respiratory acidosis may require mechanical ventilation unless a simple etiologic factor (i.e., narcotic overdosage or residual muscular blockade) can be treated quickly. Bicarbonate administration rarely is indicated unless severe metabolic acidosis is also present or unless mechanical ventilation is ineffective in reducing acute hypercarbia. In contrast, chronic respiratory acidosis is rarely managed with ventilation. Rather, efforts are made to improve pulmonary function to permit more effective elimination of carbon dioxide. In patients requiring mechanical ventilation for acute respiratory failure, ventilation with a lung-protective strategy may result in hypercapnia, which in turn has been managed with alkalinization.

TABLE 9-6

RULES OF THUMB FOR $[HCO_3^-]$ AND pH CHANGES IN RESPONSE TO ACUTE AND CHRONIC CHANGES IN $PaCO_2$

Decreased $PaCO_2$
1. pH increases 0.10 for every 10 mmHg decrease in $PaCO_2$.
2. $[HCO_3^-]$ decreases 2 mEq/L for every 10 mmHg decrease in $PaCO_2$.
3. pH will nearly normalize if hypocarbia is sustained.
4. $[HCO_3^-]$ will decrease 5 to 6 mEq/L for each chronic 10 mmHg ↓ in $PaCO_2$.[a]

Increased $PaCO_2$
1. pH will decrease 0.05 for every acute $PaCO_2$ increase of 10 mmHg.
2. $[HCO_3^-]$ will increase 1.0 mEq/L for every $PaCO_2$ increase of 10 mmHg.
3. pH will return toward normal if hypercarbia is sustained.
4. $[HCO_3^-]$ will increase 4 to 5 mEq/L for each chronic 10 mmHg increase in $PaCO_2$.

[a]Hospitalized patients rarely develop chronic compensation for hypocarbia because of stimuli that enhance distal tubular reabsorption of sodium.

PRACTICAL APPROACH TO ACID-BASE INTERPRETATION

Rapid interpretation of a patient's acid-base status involves the integration of three sets of data: arterial blood gases, electrolytes, and history. A systematic, sequential approach facilitates interpretation (Table 9-7). Acid-base assessment usually can be completed before initiating therapy; however, the first step in interpretation may disclose disturbances (e.g., respiratory acidosis or metabolic acidosis with pH <7.1) that require immediate attention.

The next step is to determine whether a patient is acidemic (pH <7.35) or alkalemic (pH >7.45). The pH status will usually indicate the predominant primary process, that is, acidosis produces acidemia; alkalosis produces alkalemia. (Note that the suffix "-osis" indicates a primary process that, if unopposed, will produce the corresponding pH change. The suffix "-emia" refers to the pH. A compensatory process is not considered an "-osis.") Of course, a patient may have mixed "-oses," that is, more than one primary process.

The next step is to determine whether the entire arterial blood gas picture is consistent with a simple acute respiratory alkalosis or acidosis (see Table 9-6). For example, a patient with acute hypocapnia ($PaCO_2$ 30 mmHg) would have a pH increase of 0.10 units to a pH of 7.50 and a calculated $[HCO_3^-]$ of 22.

If changes in $PaCO_2$, pH, and $[HCO_3^-]$ are not consistent with a simple acute respiratory disturbance, chronic respiratory acidosis (≥24 hours) or metabolic acidosis or alkalosis should be considered. In chronic respiratory acidosis, pH

TABLE 9-7

SEQUENTIAL APPROACH TO ACID-BASE INTERPRETATION

1. Is the pH life threatening, requiring immediate intervention?
2. Is the pH acidemic or alkalemic?
3. Could the entire arterial blood gas picture represent only an acute increase or decrease in $PaCO_2$?
4. If the answer to question #3 is "No," is there evidence of a chronic respiratory disturbance or of an acute metabolic disturbance?
5. Are appropriate compensatory changes present?
6. Is an anion gap present?
7. Do the clinical data fit the acid-base picture?

becomes nearly normal as bicarbonate is retained by the kidneys (see Table 9-6), usually at a ratio of 4 to 5 mEq/L per 10 mmHg chronic increase in $PaCO_2$.[20] For example, chronic hypoventilation at a $PaCO_2$ of 60 mmHg would be associated with an increase in $[HCO_3^-]$ of 8 to 10 mEq/L ($[HCO_3^-]$ of 32 to 34 mEq/L) and a pH of 7.35 to 7.38. If neither an acute nor chronic respiratory change could have resulted in the arterial blood gas measurements, then a metabolic disturbance must also be present.

Respiratory compensation for metabolic disturbances occurs more rapidly than renal compensation for respiratory disturbances (see Table 9-2). Several general rules describe compensation. First, overcompensation is rare. Second, inadequate or excessive compensation suggests an additional primary disturbance. Third, hypobicarbonatemia associated with an increased anion gap is never compensatory.

The next question, whether an anion gap is present, should be assessed even if the arterial blood gases appear straightforward. The simultaneous occurrence of metabolic alkalosis and metabolic acidosis (as a consequence of pathophysiology producing a high anion gap) may result in an unremarkable pH and $[HCO_3^-]$; the combined abnormality may only be appreciated by examining the anion gap.[21] As noted previously, correct assessment of the anion gap requires correction for hypoalbuminemia.[12,13] Metabolic acidoses associated with increased anion gaps require specific treatments, thus necessitating a correct diagnosis. This is particularly important in managing hyperchloremic metabolic acidosis after administration of large volumes of 0.9% saline perioperatively or even in critically ill hospitalized patients.[22] In these circumstances, no anion gap would be expected and no specific treatment of metabolic acidosis would be required.[5,23]

The final question is whether the clinical data are consistent with the arterial blood gas data. Failure to consider clinical status also may lead to serious errors in gas acid-base interpretation.

Examples

The foregoing has summarized an approach that simplifies interpretation. The following two hypothetical cases will be approached using the algorithm and rules discussed earlier.

Example #1

A 65-year-old female has undergone 12 hours of an expected 16-hour radical neck dissection and flap construction. Estimated blood loss is 1,000 mL. She has received three units of packed red blood cells and nine liters of 0.9% saline. Her blood pressure and heart rate have remained stable while anesthetized with 0.5% to 1.0% isoflurane in 70:30 nitrous oxide and oxygen. Urinary output is adequate. Arterial blood gas levels are shown in Table 9-8.

The step-by-step interpretation is as follows:

1. The pH is not life threatening.
2. The pH is <7.40 but is not frankly acidemic.
3. The arterial blood gases cannot be adequately explained by acute hypocarbia. The predicted pH would be 7.48 and the predicted $[HCO_3^-]$ would be 22 mEq/L (see Table 9-6).
4. A metabolic acidosis appears to be present.
5. The question of compensation is not pertinent during general anesthesia with controlled mechanical ventilation, given that $PaCO_2$ is not determined by the patient's ventilatory control. However, spontaneous hypocapnia of this magnitude would represent slight overcompensation (see Table 9-2) and should prompt a search for a reason for primary respiratory alkalosis.
6. During prolonged anesthesia and surgery, one might assume the presence of lactic acidosis and provide additional fluid therapy or otherwise attempt to improve perfusion. However, serum electrolytes reveal an anion gap that is slightly less than normal (see Table 9-8), indicating that the metabolic acidosis is probably the result of dilution of the extracellular volume with a high-chloride fluid.[5] Correction of the anion gap for the serum albumin of 2.0 g/dl only increases the anion gap to 10 to 11 mEq/L, again consistent with a hyperchloremic metabolic acidosis.[10] A random urine sample could help confirm this etiology (Table 9-9).[8] Hyperchloremic acidosis secondary to infusion of high-chloride fluid requires no treatment. The arterial blood gases and serum electrolytes are compatible with the clinical picture.

TABLE 9-8

HYPOBICARBONATEMIA AND HYPERCHLOREMIC ACIDOSIS DURING PROLONGED SURGERY

Arterial blood gases	pH	7.38
	$PaCO_2$	32 mmHg
	$[HCO_3^-]$	17 mEq/L
Electrolytes	Na^+	140 mEq/L
	Cl^-	116 mEq/L
	CO_2	18 mEq/L
	Anion Gap	6 mEq/L
Serum albumin		2.0 g/dL

Example #2

A 35-year-old male, 3 days after appendectomy, develops nausea with recurrent emesis persisting for 48 hours. An arterial blood gas reveals the results shown in the middle column of Table 9-10.

1. The pH of 7.50 requires no immediate intervention.
2. The pH is alkalemic, suggesting a primary alkalosis.

TABLE 9-9

EVALUATION OF HYPERCHLOREMIC ACIDOSIS

	URINARY SOLUTES			
	NH_4^+	CL^-	A^-	NA^+
GI tract HCO_3^- loss	↑ (a)	↓ (b)	↔	↓ (c)
Generated/ingested organic acids	↑ (a)	↔	↑ (d)	↑ (e)
HCI intake or equivalent[a]	↑ (a)	↑ (f)	↔	↑ (e)
Inadequate renal HCO_3^-	↓ (g)	↔	↔	↔
Renal HCO_3^- loss	↓ (g)	↔	↔	↔

[a] NH_4Cl, chloride salts of amino acids or dilutional acidosis; ↔ designates normal: (a) NH_4^+ >1 mmol/kg daily; (b) FE_{Cl} <1 mmol/kg daily. FE = fractional excretion of a solute. Urinary unmeasured anion concentration (sum of urinary K^+, NH_4^+, and Na^+ less Cl^-) estimates sum of urinary sulphate and organic anion concentrations.
From Gluck SL: Acid-base. Lancet 352:474, 1998.

TABLE 9-10

METABOLIC ALKALOSIS SECONDARY TO NAUSEA AND VOMITING WITH SUBSEQUENT LACTIC ACIDOSIS SECONDARY TO HYPOVOLEMIA

		NORMAL	METABOLIC ALKALOSIS	METABOLIC ACIDOSIS
Blood gases	pH	7.40	7.50	7.40
	$PaCO_2$ (mmHg)	40	46	40
	$[HCO_3^-]$ (mEq/L)	24	35	24
Serum electrolytes	Na^+ (mEq/L)	140	140	140
	Cl^- (mEq/L)	105	94	94
	CO_2 (mEq/L)	25	36	25
	Anion gap (mEq/L)	10	10	21

3. An acute $PaCO_2$ of 46 mmHg would yield a pH of approximately 7.37; therefore, this is not simply an acute ventilatory disturbance.
4. The patient has a primary metabolic alkalosis as suggested by the $[HCO_3^-]$ of 35 mEq/L.
5. The limits of respiratory compensation for metabolic alkalosis are wide and difficult to predict for individual patients. The rules of thumb, summarized in Table 9-2, suggest that $[HCO_3^-] + 15$ should equal the last two digits of the pH and that the $PaCO_2$ should increase 5 to 6 mmHg for every 10 mEq/L change in serum $[HCO_3^-]$, that is, pH = 7.50 and $PaCO_2$ = 46 mmHg.
6. The anion gap is 12 mEq/L.
7. The diagnosis of a primary metabolic alkalosis with compensatory hypoventilation is consistent with the history of recurrent vomiting. Consider how the arterial blood gases would change if vomiting were sufficiently severe to produce hypovolemic shock and lactic acidosis (third column, Table 9-10).

This sequence illustrates the important concept that the final pH, $PaCO_2$, and $[HCO_3^-]$ represent the result of all of the vectors operating on acid-base status. Complex, or "triple disturbances," can only be interpreted using a thorough, stepwise approach.

FLUID MANAGEMENT

Physiology

Body Fluid Compartments

Accurate replacement of fluid deficits necessitates an understanding of the distribution spaces of water, sodium, and colloid. Intracellular volume (ICV), which constitutes 40% of total body weight, and extracellular volume (ECV), which constitutes 20% of body weight, comprise total body water (TBW), which therefore constitutes 60% of total body weight. Plasma volume (PV) equals about one-fifth of ECV, the remainder of which is interstitial fluid volume (IFV). Red cell volume, approximately 2 liters, is part of ICV.

The distribution volume of sodium-free water is TBW. The distribution volume of infused sodium is ECV, which contains equal sodium concentrations ($[Na^+]$) in the PV and IF. Plasma $[Na^+]$ is approximately 140 mEq/L. The predominant intracellular cation, potassium, has an intracellular concentration ($[K^+]$) approximating 150 mEq/L. Albumin, the most important oncotically active constituent of ECV, is unequally distributed in PV (~4 g/dL) and IFV (~1 g/dL). The IFV concentration of albumin varies greatly among tissues; however, ECV is the distribution volume for colloid solutions.

Distribution of Infused Fluids

Conventionally, clinical prediction of plasma volume expansion (PVE) after fluid infusion assumes that body fluid spaces are static. Kinetic analysis of PVE replaces the static assumption with a dynamic description. As an example of the static approach, assume that a 70-kg patient has suffered an acute blood loss of 2,000 mL, approximately 40% of the predicted 5-liter blood volume. The formula describing the effects of replacement with 5% dextrose in water (D5W), lactated Ringer's solution, or 5% or 25% human serum albumin is as follows:

$$\text{Expected PV increment} = \text{volume infused} \times \text{normal PV/distribution volume} \quad (9\text{-}6)$$

Rearranging the equation yields the following:

$$\text{Volume infused} = \text{expected PV increment} \times \text{distribution volume/normal PV} \quad (9\text{-}7)$$

To restore blood volume using D5W requires 28 liters:

$$28 \text{ liters} = 2 \text{ liters} \times 42 \text{ liters}/3 \text{ liters} \quad (9\text{-}8)$$

where 2 liters is the desired PV increment, 42 liters = TBW in a 70-kg person, and 3 liters is the normal estimated PV.

To restore blood volume using lactated Ringer's solution requires 9.1 liters:

$$9.1 \text{ liters} = 2 \text{ liters} \times 14 \text{ liters}/3 \text{ liters} \quad (9\text{-}9)$$

where 14 liters = ECV in a 70-kg person.

If 5% albumin, which exerts colloid osmotic pressure similar to plasma, were infused, the infused volume initially would remain in the PV, perhaps attracting additional interstitial fluid intravascularly. Twenty-five percent human serum albumin, a concentrated colloid, expands PV by approximately 400 mL for each 100 mL infused.

However, in kinetic terms, these analyses are simplistic. Infused fluid does not simply equilibrate throughout an assumed distribution volume, but is added to a highly regulated system that attempts to maintain intravascular, interstitial, and intracellular volume. Kinetic models of intravenous fluid therapy allow clinicians to predict more accurately the time course of volume changes produced by infusions of fluids of various compositions. Kinetic analysis permits estimation of peak volume expansion and rates of clearance of infused fluid and complements analysis of "pharmacodynamic" effects, such as changes in cardiac output or cardiac filling pressures.

Figure 9-1 illustrates the conceptual kinetic model proposed by Svensén and Hahn.[24] A practical physiologic tracer for

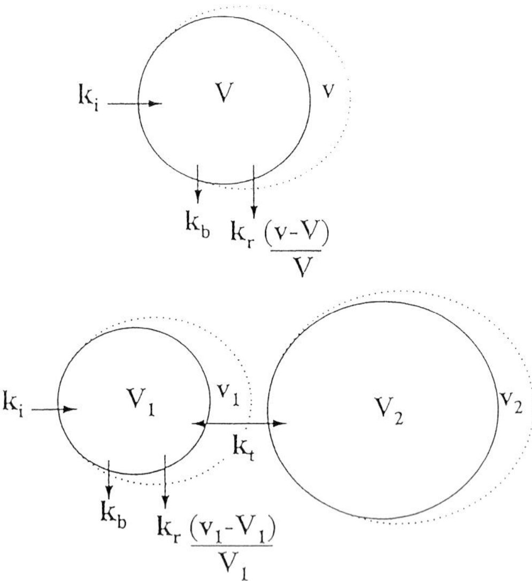

FIGURE 9-1. Schematic drawing of the kinetic model used to calculate the size of the body fluid spaces expanded by intravenous infusions of fluid in humans. Data are fitted to a one-volume or two-volume-of-fluid-space (VOFS) model. The assumptions underlying the one-compartment VOFS model (**top**) are as follows: (1) during fluid infusion, fluid enters an expandable space of volume v at a constant rate k_i; (2) the expandable fluid space has a target volume V, which the body strives to maintain; (3) volume v changes by fluid being eliminated from the fluid space at a basal rate, k_b (perspiration and basal diuresis), and at a controlled rate. The controlled rate is proportional by a constant k_r to the relative deviation of v from the target volume V. The assumptions behind the two-compartment VOFS model (**bottom**) are similar: (1) during fluid infusion, fluid enters an expandable space of volume v_1 at a constant rate k_i; (2) there is a secondary expandable fluid space of volume v_2 exchanging fluid with the primary fluid space; (3) volume v_1 changes through exchange with the secondary fluid space and as a result of fluid being eliminated from the primary fluid space at a basal rate, k_b (perspiration and basal diuresis), and at a controlled rate; (4) the primary and secondary fluid spaces have target volumes V_1 and V_2, which the system strives to maintain by acting on the controlled elimination mechanism k_r, which is proportional to the relative deviation from the target volume of the primary fluid space, and by acting on the fluid exchange mechanism; (5) the net rate of fluid exchange between the two spaces is proportional to the difference in relative deviations from the target volumes by a constant k_t. (From Svensén C, Hahn RG: Volume kinetics of Ringer solution, dextran 70, and hypertonic saline in male volunteers. Anesthesiology 87: 204, 1997.)

kinetic analysis should permit frequent measurements to define clearance curves more completely. Svensén and Hahn[24] evaluated three endogenous tracers—blood water concentration, serum albumin concentration, and hemoglobin concentration [Hb]—in volunteers who received infusions of acetated Ringer's solution, 6% dextran 70, or 7.5% saline. Although much less tedious than blood water calculations, [Hb] provided similar estimates of volumes of distribution and elimination rate constants. After infusing the test fluids, Svensén and Hahn fitted the results to one-volume and two-volume-of-fluid-space (VOFS) models. The two-compartment VOFS model is most likely to be superior to the one-compartment model when urinary excretion in response to infusion is small.[25]

Figure 9-2 shows the mean plasma volume dilution curves obtained with the infusion of Ringer's solution or dextran 70. All dextran infusions were consistent with a one-VOFS model, suggesting that the colloid infusion remained in the PV. Hypertonic crystalloid, like isotonic crystalloid, was associated in individual instances with a mixture of one- and two-VOFS models

Using this approach, the effects of common physiologic and pharmacologic influences can be examined in experimental animals or humans. For example, in chronically instrumented sheep, isoflurane anesthesia was associated with similar kinetics of PV expansion after fluid infusion, but reduced urinary output in anesthetized in comparison to conscious sheep, demonstrated that expansion of extravascular volume was actually greater during anesthesia[26]; subsequent experiments demonstrated that this effect was attributable to isoflurane and not to mechanical ventilation during anesthesia.[27] Isoflurane is associated with extravascular fluid accumulation, although these observations must be confirmed in anesthetized humans and other anesthetics must be examined.

Regulation of Extracellular Fluid Volume

Total body water content is regulated by the intake and output of water. Water intake includes ingested liquids plus an average of 750 mL ingested in solid food and 350 mL that is generated metabolically. Insensible losses are normally 1 L/day and GI losses are 100 to 150 mL/day. Thirst, the primary mechanism of controlling water intake, is triggered by an increase in body fluid tonicity or by a decrease in extracellular volume.

Reabsorption of filtered water and sodium is enhanced by changes mediated by the hormonal factors antidiuretic hormone (ADH), atrial natriuretic peptide (ANP), and aldosterone. Renal water handling has three important components: (1) delivery of tubular fluid to the diluting segments of the nephron; (2) separation of solute and water in the diluting segment; and (3) variable reabsorption of water in the collecting ducts. In the descending loop of Henle, water is reabsorbed while solute is retained to achieve a final osmolality of tubular fluid of approximately 1,200 mOsm/kg (Fig. 9-3). This concentrated fluid is then diluted by the active reabsorption of electrolytes in the ascending limb of the loop of Henle and in the distal tubule, both of which are relatively impermeable to water. As fluid exits the distal tubule and enters the collecting duct, osmolality is approximately 50 mOsm/kg. Within the collecting duct, water reabsorption is modulated by ADH (also called vasopressin). Vasopressin binds to V_2 receptors along the basolateral membrane of the collecting duct cells, then stimulates the synthesis and insertion of the aquaporin-2 water channel into the luminal membrane of collecting duct cells.[28]

Plasma hypotonicity suppresses ADH release, resulting in excretion of dilute urine. Hypertonicity stimulates ADH secretion, which increases the permeability of the collecting duct to water and enhances water reabsorption. In response to changing plasma [Na^+], changing secretion of ADH can vary urinary osmolality from 50 to 1,200 mOsm/kg and urinary volume from 0.4 to 20 L/day (Fig. 9-4). Other factors that stimulate ADH secretion, though none as powerfully as plasma tonicity, include hypotension, hypovolemia, and nonosmotic stimuli such as nausea, pain, and medications, including opiates.

Two powerful hormonal systems regulate total body sodium. The natriuretic peptides, ANP, brain natriuretic peptide, BNP, and C-type natriuretic peptide, defend against sodium overload[29] and the renin-angiotensin-aldosterone axis defends against sodium depletion and hypovolemia. ANP, released from the cardiac atria in response to increased atrial stretch, exerts vasodilatory effects and increases the renal excretion of sodium and water. ANP secretion is decreased during hypovolemia. Even in patients with chronic (nonoliguric) renal insufficiency, infusion of ANP in low, nonhypotensive doses increased sodium excretion and augmented urinary losses of retained solutes.[30]

Aldosterone is the final common pathway in a complex response to decreased effective arterial volume, whether decreased effective arterial volume is true or relative (edematous states or hypoalbuminemia). In this pathway, decreased

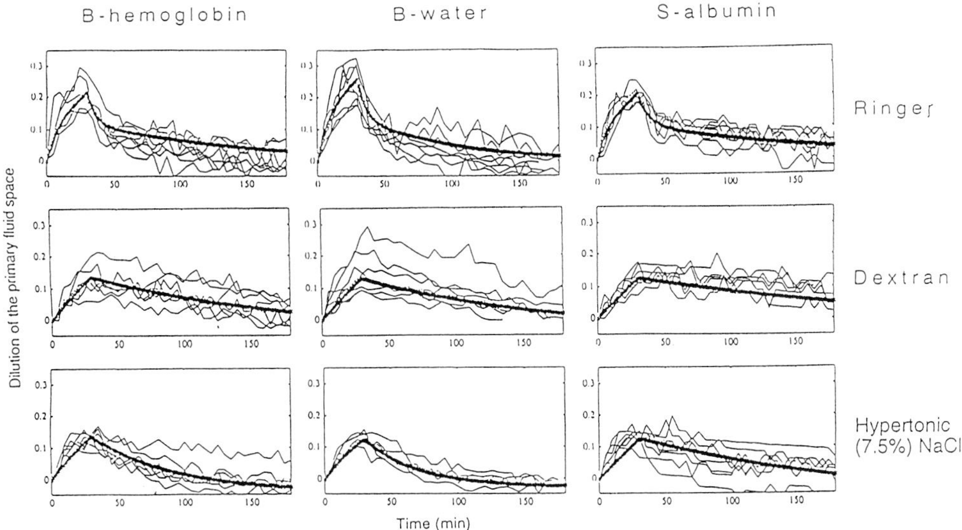

FIGURE 9-2. Kinetic curves obtained after infusion in adult male volunteers of 25 mL/kg of acetated Ringer' s solution (Ringer) or 5 mL/kg of dextran 70 over 30 minutes. Dilution of plasma volume is calculated from changes in hemoglobin concentration (B-hemoglobin), blood water (B-water) concentration, and serum albumin (S-albumin) concentration. (From Svensén C, Hahn RG: Volume kinetics of Ringer solution, dextran 70, and hypertonic saline in male volunteers. Anesthesiology 87: 204, 1997.)

stretch in the baroreceptors of the aortic arch and carotid body and stretch receptors in the great veins, pulmonary vasculature, and atria result in increased sympathetic tone. Increased sympathetic tone, in combination with decreased renal perfusion, leads to renin release and formation of angiotensin I from angiotensinogen. Angiotensin-converting enzyme (ACE) converts angiotensin I to angiotensin II, which stimulates the adrenal cortex to synthesize and release aldosterone.[31,32] Acting primarily in the distal tubules, high concentrations of aldosterone cause sodium reabsorption and may reduce urinary excretion of sodium nearly to zero. Intrarenal physical factors are also important in regulating sodium balance. Sodium loading decreases colloid osmotic pressure, thereby increasing the glomerular filtration rate (GFR), decreasing net sodium

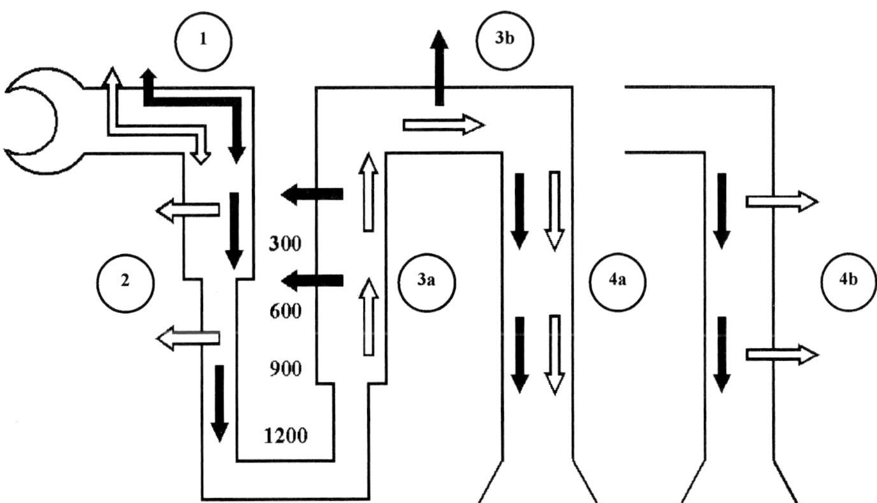

FIGURE 9-3. Renal filtration, reabsorption, and excretion of water. *Open arrows* represent water and *solid arrows* represent electrolytes. Water and electrolytes are filtered by the glomerulus. In the proximal tubule (*1*), water and electrolytes are absorbed isotonically. In the descending loop of Henle (*2*), water is absorbed to achieve osmotic equilibrium with the interstitium while electrolytes are retained. The numbers (300, 600, 900, and 1,200) between the descending and ascending limbs represent the osmolality of the interstitium in mOsm/kg. The delivery of solute and fluid to the distal nephron is a function of proximal tubular reabsorption; as proximal tubular reabsorption increases, delivery of solute to the medullary (*3a*) and cortical (*3b*) diluting sites decreases. In the diluting sites, electrolyte-free water is generated through selective reabsorption of electrolytes while water is retained in the tubular lumen, generating a dilute tubular fluid. In the absence of vasopressin, the collecting duct (*4a*) remains relatively impermeable to water and a dilute urine is excreted. When vasopressin acts on the collecting ducts (*4b*), water is reabsorbed from these vasopressin-responsive nephron segments, allowing the excretion of a concentrated urine. (From Fried LF, Palevsky PM: Hyponatremia and hypernatremia. Med Clin North Am 81(3):585, 1997.)

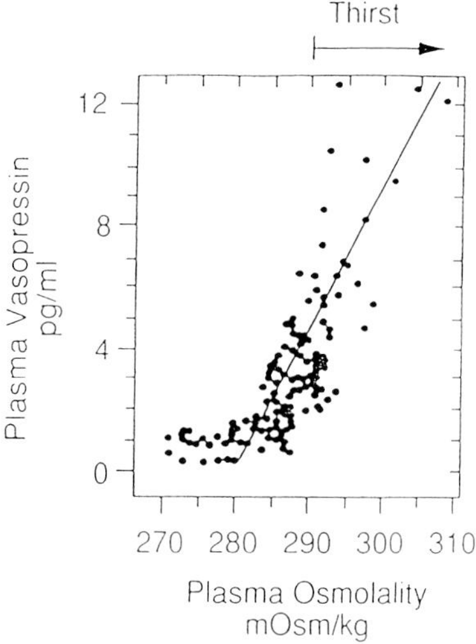

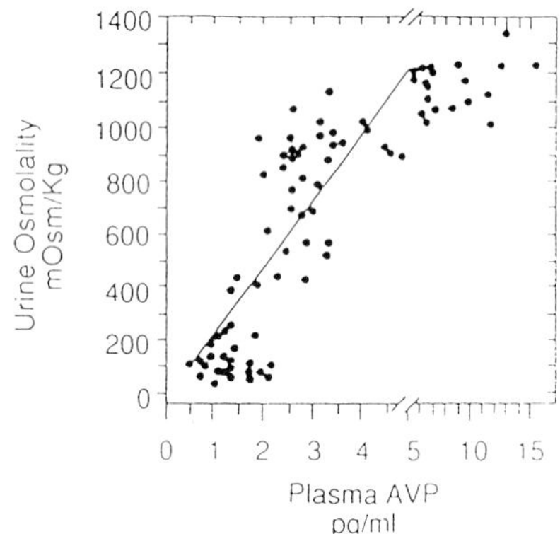

FIGURE 9-4. **Top:** Relationship between plasma osmolality and plasma vasopressin (AVP; also referred to as ADH). **Bottom:** Relationship between plasma AVP and urinary osmolality. (From Fried LF, Palevsky PM: Hyponatremia and hypernatremia. Med Clin North Am 81(3):585, 1997.)

reabsorption and increasing distal sodium delivery, which, in turn, suppresses renin secretion.

Fluid Replacement Therapy

Maintenance Requirements for Water, Sodium, and Potassium

Two simple formulas are used interchangeably to estimate maintenance water requirements (Table 9-11). In healthy adults, sufficient water is required to balance gastrointestinal losses of 100 to 200 mL/day, insensible losses of 500 to 1,000 mL/day (half of which is respiratory and half is cutaneous), and urinary losses of 1,000 mL/day. Urinary losses exceeding 1,000 mL/day may represent an appropriate physiologic response to ECV expansion or an inability to conserve salt or water.

Daily requirements for sodium and potassium are approximately 75 mEq/L and 40 mEq/L, respectively, although wider ranges of sodium intake than potassium intake are physiologically tolerated because renal sodium conservation and excretion are more efficient than potassium conservation and excretion. Therefore, healthy, 70-kg adults require 2,500 mL/day of water containing a [Na^+] of 30 mEq/L and a [K^+] of 15 to 20 mEq/L. Intraoperatively, fluids containing sodium-free water (i.e., [Na^+] $<$130 mEq/L) are rarely used in adults, because of the necessity for replacing isotonic losses and the risk of postoperative hyponatremia.

Dextrose

Traditionally, glucose-containing intravenous fluids have been given in an effort to prevent hypoglycemia and limit protein catabolism. However, because of the hyperglycemic response associated with surgical stress, only infants and patients receiving insulin or drugs that interfere with glucose synthesis are at risk for hypoglycemia. Iatrogenic hyperglycemia can limit the effectiveness of fluid resuscitation by inducing an osmotic diuresis and, in animals, may aggravate ischemic neurologic injury.[33] Although associated with worse outcome after subarachnoid hemorrhage[34] and traumatic brain injury[35] in humans, hyperglycemia may also constitute a hormonally medi-
7 ated response to more severe injury. In critically ill patients, evidence strongly suggests that tight control of plasma glucose (maintenance of plasma glucose between 80 and 110 mg/dL) is associated with reduced mortality and morbidity.[36–39] Evidence also suggests that glucose control improves outcome in surgical patients.[40]

Surgical Fluid Requirements

Water and Electrolyte Composition of Fluid Losses. Surgical patients require replacement of PV and ECV losses secondary to wound or burn edema, ascites, and gastrointestinal secretions. Wound and burn edema and ascitic fluid are protein rich and contain electrolytes in concentrations similar to plasma. Although gastrointestinal secretions vary greatly in composition, the composition of replacement fluid need not be closely matched if ECV is adequate and renal and cardiovascular functions are normal. Substantial loss of gastrointestinal fluids requires more accurate replacement of electrolytes (i.e., potassium, magnesium, phosphate). Chronic gastric losses may produce hypochloremic metabolic alkalosis that can be corrected with 0.9% saline; chronic diarrhea may produce hyperchloremic metabolic acidosis that may be prevented or corrected by infusion of fluid containing bicarbonate or bicarbonate substrate (e.g., lactate). If cardiovascular or renal function is impaired, more precise replacement may require frequent assessment of serum electrolytes.

TABLE 9-11

MAINTENANCE WATER REQUIREMENTS

■ WEIGHT (kg)	■ mL/kg/hr	■ mL/kg/d
1–10	4	100
11–20	2	50
21–n	1	20

Fluid Shifts During Surgery. Replacement of intraoperative fluid losses must include consideration of fluid that accumulates extravascularly in surgically manipulated tissue. Therefore, guidelines have been developed for replacement of fluid losses during surgical procedures. The simplest formula provides, in addition to maintenance fluids and replacement of estimated blood loss, 4 mL/kg/h for procedures involving minimal trauma, 6 mL/kg/h for those involving moderate trauma, and 8 mL/kg/h for those involving extreme trauma.

However, formulas for intraoperative fluid replacement will no doubt undergo considerable debate and reformulation over the next few years. Clinical trials suggest that perioperative fluid management may strongly influence both minor and major morbidity and that the influence may be specific to the type of surgery and to the types of fluid used. Yogendran et al[41]
3 randomized 200 ASA I–III, ambulatory surgical patients to receive either 20 mL/kg or 2 mL/kg of Plasmalyte as a bolus over 30 minutes before surgery; patients receiving the higher dose had less postoperative thirst, drowsiness, dizziness, and nausea. Holte et al[42] randomized 48 ASA I–II patients undergoing laparoscopic cholecystectomy to receive either 15 mL/kg or 40 mL/kg of lactated Ringer's solution intraoperatively; the higher dose of fluid was associated with improved postoperative pulmonary function and exercise capacity, reduced neurohumoral stress response, and improvements in nausea, general sense of well-being, thirst, dizziness, drowsiness, fatigue, and balance function. In marked contrast, Brandstrup et al[43] randomized 172 elective colon surgery patients to either restrictive perioperative fluid management or standard perioperative fluid management with the primary goal of maintaining preoperative body weight in the fluid-restricted group. By design, the fluid-restricted group received less perioperative fluid
9 and acutely gained <1 kg in contrast to >3 kg in the standard therapy group. More importantly, total postoperative complications were significantly fewer in the fluid-restricted group (Table 9-12). Cardiopulmonary and tissue-healing complications were also significantly reduced in association with fluid restriction.

Mobilization of Expanded Interstitial Fluid

An important corollary of perioperative IFV expansion is the mobilization and return of accumulated fluid to the ECV and the PV, colloquially termed "deresuscitation." In most patients, mobilization occurs on approximately the third postoperative day. If the cardiovascular system and kidneys cannot effectively transport and excrete mobilized fluid, such as in the patient with borderline cardiac function, hypervolemia and pulmonary edema may occur.

Colloids, Crystalloids, and Hypertonic Solutions

Physiology and Pharmacology

Osmotically active particles attract water across semipermeable membranes until equilibrium is attained. The *osmolarity* of a solution refers to the number of osmotically active particles per *liter* of solvent; *osmolality,* a measurement of the number of osmotically active particles per *kilogram,* can be estimated as follows:

$$\text{Osmolality} = ([\text{Na}^+] \times 2) + (\text{Glucose}/18) + (\text{BUN}/2.3) \quad (9\text{-}10)$$

where osmolality is expressed in mOsm/kg, $[\text{Na}^+]$ is expressed in mEq/L, serum glucose is expressed in mg/dL, and BUN is blood urea nitrogen expressed in mg/dL. Sugars, alcohols, and radiographic dyes increase measured osmolality, generating an increased "osmolal gap" between the measured and calculated values.

A hyperosmolar state occurs whenever the concentration of osmotically active particles is high. Both uremia (increased BUN) and hypernatremia (increased serum sodium) increase serum osmolality. However, because urea distributes throughout TBW, an increase in BUN does not cause *hypertonicity.* Sodium, largely restricted to the ECV, causes hypertonicity, that is, osmotically mediated redistribution of water from ICV to ECV. The term "tonicity" is also used colloquially to compare the osmotic pressure of a parenteral solution to that of plasma.

Although only a small proportion of the osmotically active particles in blood consist of plasma proteins, those particles are essential in determining the equilibrium of fluid between the interstitial and plasma compartments of ECV. The reflection coefficient (σ) describes the permeability of capillary membranes to individual solutes, with 0 representing free permeability and 1.0 representing complete impermeability. The reflection coefficient for albumin ranges from 0.6 to 0.9 in various capillary beds. Because capillary protein concentrations exceed interstitial concentrations, the osmotic pressure exerted by plasma proteins (termed *colloid osmotic pressure* or *oncotic*

TABLE 9-12

NUMBER OF PATIENTS WITH COMPLICATIONS (PER-PROTOCOL ANALYSIS)

	BLINDED ASSESSMENT			UNBLINDED ASSESSMENT		
	RESTRICTED GROUP	STANDARD GROUP	*P* VALUE	RESTRICTED GROUP	STANDARD GROUP	*P* VALUE
Overall complications	21	40	0.003	21	43	0.000
Major complications[a]	8	18	0.040	8	19	0.026
Minor complications[a]	15	36	0.000	15	37	0.000
Tissue-healing complications[a]	11	22	0.040	10	24	0.009
Cardiopulmonary complications[a]	5	17	0.007	4	18	0.002

n = 69 in restricted group and n = 72 in standard group.
[a] Number of patients in subgroups does not add up to number of overall complications because some patients had more than one complication.
From Brandstrup B, Tonnesen H, Beier-Holgersen R *et al*: Effects of intravenous fluid restriction on postoperative complications: Comparison of two perioperative fluid regimens—A randomized assessor-blinded multicenter trial. Ann Surg 238:641, 2003.

pressure) is higher than interstitial oncotic pressure and tends to preserve PV. The filtration rate of fluid from the capillaries into the interstitial space is the net result of a combination of forces, including the gradient from intravascular to interstitial colloid osmotic pressures and the hydrostatic gradient between intravascular and interstitial pressures. The net fluid filtration at any point within a systemic or pulmonary capillary is represented by Starling's law of capillary filtration, as expressed in the equation:

$$Q = \underline{k}\underline{A}[(P_c - P_i) + \sigma(\pi_i - \pi_c)] \qquad (9\text{-}11)$$

where Q = fluid filtration, $\underline{k}$ = capillary filtration coefficient (conductivity of water), $\underline{A}$ = the area of the capillary membrane, P_c = capillary hydrostatic pressure, P_i = interstitial hydrostatic pressure, σ = reflection coefficient for albumin, π_i = interstitial colloid osmotic pressure, and π_c = capillary colloid osmotic pressure.

The IFV is determined by the relative rates of capillary filtration and lymphatic drainage. P_c, the most powerful factor promoting fluid filtration, is determined by capillary flow, arterial resistance, venous resistance, and venous pressure. If capillary filtration increases, the rates of water and sodium filtration usually exceed protein filtration, resulting in preservation of π_c, dilution of π_i, and preservation of the oncotic pressure gradient, the most powerful factor opposing fluid filtration. When coupled with increased lymphatic drainage, preservation of the oncotic pressure gradient limits the accumulation of IF. If P_c increases at a time when lymphatic drainage is maximal, then IFV accumulates, forming edema.

Clinical Implications of Choices Between Alternative Fluids

If membrane permeability is intact, colloids such as albumin or hydroxyethyl starch preferentially expand PV rather than IFV. Concentrated colloid-containing solutions (e.g., 25% albumin) exert sufficient oncotic pressure to translocate substantial volumes of IFV into the PV. Plasma volume expansion unaccompanied by IFV expansion offers apparent advantages: lower fluid requirements, less peripheral and pulmonary edema accumulation, and reduced concern about the cardiopulmonary consequences of later fluid mobilization.

However, exhaustive research has failed to establish the superiority of either colloid-containing or crystalloid-containing fluids (Table 9-13). Systematic reviews of available comparisons of colloid versus crystalloid[44] and albumin versus crystalloid[45] suggest unchanged mortality associated with colloid use, although crystalloid may be superior in multiply traumatized patients.[46] Despite the lack of compelling evidence suggesting that perioperative use of colloid influences mortality, Moretti et al[47] reported that patients who were randomized to receive 6% hetastarch had less postoperative nausea and vomiting than those who received lactated Ringer's solution without colloid. In addition, colloid administration appears to have been an essential component of perioperative management strategies that demonstrated improved morbidity after colon surgery[43] and after major surgery in conjunction with goal-directed fluid challenges.[48,49]

Although hydroxyethyl starch, the most commonly used synthetic colloid, is less expensive than albumin, large doses (exceeding 20 mL/kg/d) produce laboratory evidence of coagulopathy.[50] Recently, a new hydroxyethyl starch formulation has been introduced that contains a different mix of molecular sizes and is dissolved in a base consisting of a balanced salt solution rather than 0.9% saline. Proposed advantages of the new formulation include less risk of inducing coagulopathy and of hyperchloremic metabolic acidosis.[51] However, lower molecular weight hetastarch formulations appear to influence coagulation less.[50] Further refinement is likely to occur in the distinctions among various clinically available colloids.[52]

Implications of Crystalloid and Colloid Infusions on Intracranial Pressure

Because the cerebral capillary membrane, the blood-brain barrier, is highly impermeable to sodium, abrupt changes in serum osmolality produced by changes in serum sodium produce reciprocal changes in brain water. In anesthetized rabbits, reducing plasma osmolality from 295 mOsm/kg to 282 mOsm/kg (which decreases plasma osmotic pressure by ~250 mmHg) increased cortical water content and ICP; in contrast, reducing colloid osmotic pressure from 20 to 7 mmHg produced no significant change in either variable.[53] Similar independence of brain water and ICP from colloid osmotic pressure has been demonstrated with prolonged hypoalbuminemia[54] and in animals after forebrain ischemia[55] and focal cryogenic injury.[56] In contrast, after fluid percussion brain injury, increasing colloid oncotic pressure with hetastarch reduced brain water in comparison to infusion of 0.9% saline (Fig. 9-5).[57]

TABLE 9-13

CLAIMED ADVANTAGES AND DISADVANTAGES OF COLLOID VS. CRYSTALLOID INTRAVENOUS FLUIDS

SOLUTION	ADVANTAGES	DISADVANTAGES
Colloid	Smaller infused volume Prolonged increase in plasma volume Greater peripheral edema Less cerebral edema	Greater cost Coagulopathy (dextran > HES) Pulmonary edema (capillary leak states) Decreased GFR Osmotic diuresis (low molecular weight dextran)
Crystalloid	Lower cost Greater urinary flow Replaces interstitial fluid	Transient hemodynamic improvement Peripheral edema (protein dilution) Pulmonary edema (protein dilution plus high PAOP)

HES, hydroxyethyl starch; GFR, glomerular filtration rate; PAOP, pulmonary arterial occlusion pressure.

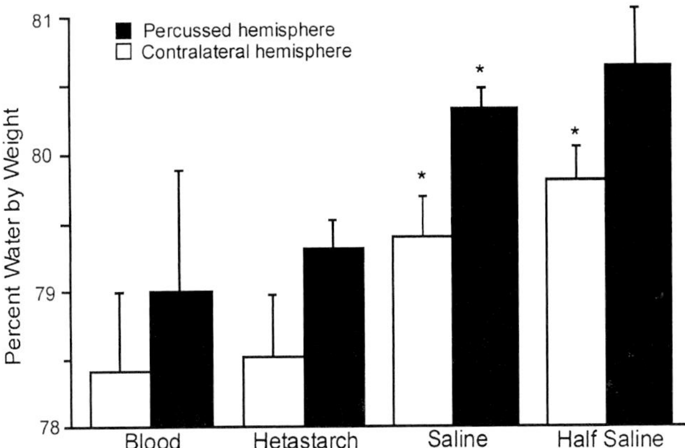

FIGURE 9-5. The percentage of water content (mean ± SD; wet-dry method) of the percussed (*right*) hemisphere and in the contralateral (*left*) hemisphere in animals that underwent isovolemic exchange with whole blood, hetastarch, normal saline, or half-normal saline. Within each group, the water content of the percussed hemisphere was greater than the water content of the contralateral hemisphere. *$P < 0.05$ versus the corresponding hemisphere in the whole blood and hetastarch groups. (From Drummond JC, Patel PM, Cole DJ *et al*: The effect of the reduction of colloid oncotic pressure, with and without reduction of osmolality, on post-traumatic cerebral edema. Anesthesiology 88:993, 1998.)

Clinical Implications of Hypertonic Fluid Administration

An ideal alternative to conventional crystalloid and colloid fluids would be inexpensive, would produce minimal peripheral or pulmonary edema, would generate sustained hemodynamic effects, and would be effective even if administered in small volumes. Hypertonic, hypernatremic solutions appear to fulfill some of these criteria (Table 9-14).

Current enthusiasm for hypertonic resuscitation was stimulated by the work of Velasco et al[58] who successfully used small volumes (6.0 mL/kg) of 7.5% hypertonic saline as the sole resuscitative measure in dogs after severe hemorrhage. Hypertonic solutions exert favorable effects on cerebral hemodynamics, in part because of the reciprocal relationship between plasma osmolality and brain water.[53] ICP increased during resuscitation from hemorrhagic shock with lactated Ringer's solution but remained unchanged if 7.5% saline was infused in a sufficient volume to comparably improve systemic hemodynamics.[59] However, improvements in ICP gradually are lost. Delayed increases in ICP were reported after hypertonic resuscitation from hypovolemic shock accompanied by an intracranial mass lesion.[60] In addition, systemic hemodynamic improvement produced by hypertonic resuscitation is short lived.[59] Strategies to prolong the therapeutic effects beyond 30 to 60 minutes include continued infusion of hypertonic saline, subsequent infusion of blood or conventional fluids, or addition of colloid to hypertonic resuscitation.

Despite concerns about central nervous system dysfunction because of hypertonicity and hypernatremia associated with hypertonic saline, acute increases in serum sodium from 155 to 160 mEq/L produced no apparent harm in humans resuscitated with hypertonic saline.[61] Central pontine myelinolysis, which follows rapid correction of severe, chronic hyponatremia, has not been observed in clinical trials of hypertonic resuscitation. Despite theoretical considerations favoring the use of hypertonic saline in resuscitation of patients with traumatic brain injury, a randomized trial failed to demonstrate an improvement in outcome.[62]

Will clinicians routinely use hypertonic or combination hypertonic/hyperoncotic fluids for resuscitation in the future? Pending further preclinical work, the theoretical advantages of such fluids appear most attractive in the acute resuscitation of hypovolemic patients who have decreased intracranial compliance.[63]

Fluid Status: Assessment and Monitoring

Assessment of Hypovolemia and Tissue Hypoperfusion

For most surgical patients, conventional clinical assessment of the adequacy of intravascular volume is appropriate. For high-risk patients, goal-directed hemodynamic management may be superior.

Conventional Clinical Assessment. Clinical quantification of blood volume and ECV begins with recognition of deficit-generating settings, such as bowel obstruction, preoperative bowel preparation, chronic diuretic use, sepsis, burns, and trauma. Physical signs that suggest hypovolemia include oliguria, supine hypotension, and a positive tilt test. Oliguria

TABLE 9-14

HYPERTONIC RESUSCITATION FLUIDS: ADVANTAGES AND DISADVANTAGES

SOLUTION	ADVANTAGES	DISADVANTAGES
Hypertonic crystalloid	Inexpensive Promotes urinary flow Small initial volume Improved myocardial contractility? Arteriolar dilation Reduced peripheral edema Lower intracranial pressure	Hypertonicity Subdural hemorrhage Transient effect
Hypertonic crystalloid plus colloid (in comparison to hypertonic crystalloid alone)	Sustained hemodynamic response Reduced subsequent volume requirements	Added expense Coagulopathy (dextran > HES) Osmotic diuresis Impaired crossmatch (dextran) Hypertonicity

HES, hydroxyethyl starch.
From Prough DS, Johnston WE: Fluid resuscitation in septic shock: No solution yet. Anesth Analg 69:699, 1989.

implies hypovolemia, although hypovolemic patients may be nonoliguric and normovolemic patients may be oliguric because of renal failure or stress-induced endocrine responses.[64] Supine hypotension implies a blood volume deficit exceeding 30%, although arterial blood pressure within the normal range could represent relative hypotension in an elderly or chronically hypertensive patient.

In the tilt test, a positive response is defined as an increase in heart rate ≥20 beats/min and a decrease in systolic blood pressure ≥20 mmHg when the subject assumes the upright position. However, young, healthy subjects can withstand acute loss of 20% of blood volume while exhibiting only postural tachycardia and variable postural hypotension. In contrast, orthostasis may occur in 20 to 30% of elderly patients despite normal blood volume.[65] In volunteers, withdrawal of 500 mL of blood[66] was associated with a greater increase in heart rate on standing than before blood withdrawal but no significant difference in the response of blood pressure or cardiac index.

Laboratory evidence that suggests hypovolemia or ECV depletion includes azotemia, low urinary sodium, metabolic alkalosis (if hypovolemia is mild), and metabolic acidosis (if hypovolemia is severe). Hematocrit is virtually unchanged by acute hemorrhage until fluids are administered or until fluid shifts from the interstitial to the intravascular space. BUN, normally 8.0 to 20 mg/dL, is increased by hypovolemia, high protein intake, gastrointestinal bleeding, or accelerated catabolism and decreased by severe hepatic dysfunction. Serum creatinine (SCr), a product of muscle catabolism, may be misleadingly low in elderly adults, females, and debilitated or malnourished patients. In contrast, in muscular or acutely catabolic patients, SCr may exceed the normal range (0.5 to 1.5 mg/dL) because of more rapid muscle breakdown. A ratio of BUN:SCr exceeding the normal range (10 to 20) suggests dehydration. In prerenal oliguria, enhanced sodium reabsorption should reduce urinary [Na^+] to ≤20 mEq/L and enhanced water reabsorption should increase urinary concentration (i.e., urinary osmolality >400; urine/plasma creatinine ratio >40:1). However, the sensitivity and specificity of measurements of urinary variables may be misleading. Although hypovolemia does not generate metabolic alkalosis, ECV depletion is a potent stimulus for the maintenance of metabolic alkalosis. Severe hypovolemia may result in systemic hypoperfusion and lactic acidosis.

Intraoperative Clinical Assessment. Visual estimation, the simplest technique for quantifying intraoperative blood loss, assesses the amount of blood absorbed by gauze squares and laparotomy pads and adds an estimate of blood accumulation on the floor and surgical drapes and in suction containers. Both surgeons and anesthesiologists tend to underestimate losses.

Assessment of the adequacy of intraoperative fluid resuscitation integrates multiple clinical variables, including heart rate, blood pressure, urinary output, arterial oxygenation, and pH. Tachycardia is an insensitive, nonspecific indicator of hypovolemia. In patients receiving potent inhalational agents, maintenance of a satisfactory blood pressure implies adequate intravascular volume. Preservation of blood pressure, accompanied by a CVP of 6 to 12 mmHg, more strongly suggests adequate replacement. During profound hypovolemia, indirect measurements of blood pressure may significantly underestimate true blood pressure. In patients undergoing extensive 10
procedures, direct arterial pressure measurements are more accurate than indirect techniques and provide convenient access for obtaining arterial blood samples. An additional advantage of direct arterial pressure monitoring may be recognition of increased systolic blood pressure variation accompanying positive pressure ventilation in the presence of hypovolemia.[67,68]

Urinary output usually declines precipitously during moderate to severe hypovolemia. Therefore, in the absence of glycosuria or diuretic administration, a urinary output of 0.5 to 1.0 mL/kg/h during anesthesia suggests adequate renal perfusion. Arterial pH may decrease only when tissue hypoperfusion becomes severe. Cardiac output can be normal despite severely reduced regional blood flow. Mixed venous hemoglobin desaturation, a specific indicator of poor systemic perfusion, reflects average perfusion in multiple organs and cannot supplant regional monitors such as urinary output.

Oxygen Delivery as a Goal of Management. No intraoperative monitor is sufficiently sensitive or specific to detect hypoperfusion in all patients. One key variable that has been associated with improved outcome in high-risk surgical patients and critically ill patients is a systemic oxygen delivery (Do_2)≥600 mL O_2/m^2/min (equivalent to a CI of 3.0 L/m^2/min, a [Hgb] of 14 g/dL, and 98% oxyhemoglobin saturation). Boyd et al randomized 107 patients to conventional treatment or fluid plus dopexamine to maintain oxygen delivery ≥600 mL O_2/m^2/min and demonstrated a decrease in mortality and in the number of complications in the patients managed at the higher level of oxygen delivery.[69] Based on these results, the authors calculated that the cost of obtaining a survivor was 31% lower in the protocol group.[70] Wilson et al randomized 138 patients undergoing major elective surgery into three groups.[71] One group received routine perioperative care; one received fluid and dopexamine preoperatively, intraoperatively, and postoperatively to maintain oxygen delivery ≥600 mL O_2/m^2/min; and the third received fluid plus epinephrine preoperatively, intraoperatively, and postoperatively to achieve the same end points. In the two groups in which oxygen delivery was supported, only 3 of 92 died, compared to 8 of 46 control patients. However, the complication rate was significantly lower in the dopexamine group than in the epinephrine group. In contrast, Hayes et al, who randomized 109 patients to conventional treatment or oxygen delivery ≥600 mL O_2/m/min using a combination of volume and dobutamine, demonstrated an increase in mortality in the treatment group maintained at the higher levels and speculated that aggressive elevations in Do_2 actually may have been harmful.[72]

At present, available data are consistent with several inferences. First, there is no apparent benefit for patients other than surgical patients[73] and patients undergoing initial resuscitation from septic shock in the emergency room.[74] In surgical patients, early initiation of goal-directed resuscitation is associated with better outcome than delayed initiation.[75] Second, outcome may be strongly influenced by the choice of inotropic agents. Third, increased fluid given as part of goal-oriented resuscitation has been associated with an increased incidence of abdominal compartment syndrome in trauma patients.[76]

Several studies have reported improved outcome based on adjustment of perioperative fluids through the use of an esophageal Doppler monitor that estimates descending aortic blood flow and quantifies the duration of systole.[77] Using the esophageal Doppler to guide administration of colloid boluses, Venn et al[48] and Gan et al[49] have reported shortened length of hospital stay after hip surgery and major surgery, respectively. Horowitz and Kumar[78] have speculated that the infusion of colloid and not the monitor-driven algorithm were responsible for the improved results.

ELECTROLYTES

Sodium

Physiologic Role

Na^+, the principal extracellular cation and solute, is essential for generation of action potentials in neurologic and cardiac tissue. Disorders (pathological increases or decreases) of *total body sodium* are associated with corresponding increases or

TABLE 9-15

REGULATION OF ELECTROLYTES

■ ELECTROLYTE	■ REGULATED BY
Sodium	Aldosterone ANP $[Na^+]$ altered by ADH
Potassium	Aldosterone Epinephrine Insulin Intrinsic renal mechanisms
Calcium	PTH Vitamin D
Phosphorus	Primarily renal mechanisms Minor: PTH
Magnesium	Primarily renal mechanisms Minor: PTH, vitamin D

ANP, atrial natriuretic peptide; $[Na^+]$, sodium concentration; ADH, antidiuretic hormone; PTH, parathyroid hormone.

11 decreases of ECV and PV. Disorders of sodium *concentration*, that is, hyponatremia and hypernatremia, usually result from relative excesses or deficits, respectively, of water. Regulation of total body sodium and $[Na^+]$ is accomplished primarily by the endocrine and renal systems (Table 9-15). Secretion of aldosterone and ANP control *total body sodium*. ADH, which is secreted in response to increased osmolality or decreased blood pressure, primarily regulates $[Na^+]$.

Hyponatremia

Hyponatremia, defined as $[Na^+]$ <130 mEq/L, is the most common electrolyte disturbance in hospitalized patients. In the majority of hyponatremic, hospitalized patients, total body sodium is normal or increased. The most common clinical associations with hyponatremia include the postoperative state, acute intracranial disease, malignant disease, medications, and acute pulmonary disease. Hyponatremia is associated with substantially increased mortality,[79] both as a direct effect of hyponatremia and because hyponatremia is associated with severe systemic disease.

The signs and symptoms of hyponatremia depend on both the rate and severity of the decrease in plasma $[Na^+]$. Symptoms that can accompany severe hyponatremia ($[Na^+]$ <120 mEq/L) include loss of appetite, nausea, vomiting, cramps, weakness, altered level of consciousness, coma, and seizures.

Acute CNS manifestations relate to brain overhydration. Because the blood-brain barrier is poorly permeable to sodium but freely permeable to water, a rapid decrease in plasma $[Na^+]$ promptly increases both extracellular and intracellular brain water. Because the brain rapidly compensates for changes in osmolality, acute hyponatremia produces more severe symptoms than chronic hyponatremia. The symptoms of chronic hyponatremia probably relate to depletion of brain electrolytes. Once brain volume has compensated for hyponatremia, rapid increases in $[Na^+]$ may lead to abrupt brain dehydration.

Hyponatremia is classified as pseudohyponatremia or true hyponatremia. Pseudohyponatremia was an artifact associated with the use of flame photometry, now an obsolete technique, to measure plasma $[Na^+]$ in severely hyperproteinemic or hyperlipidemic patients. The current analytic method, direct potentiometry, directly measures $[Na^+]$ and is uninfluenced by nonaqueous components such as proteins and lipids.

In true hyponatremia, serum osmolality may be normal, high, or low (Fig. 9-6). Hyponatremia with a normal or high serum osmolality results from the presence of a nonsodium solute, such as glucose or mannitol, which holds water within the extracellular space and results in dilutional hyponatremia. The presence of a nonsodium solute (or of factitious hyponatremia) may be inferred if measured osmolality exceeds calculated osmolality by >10 mOsm/kg. For example, plasma $[Na^+]$ decreases approximately 2.4 mEq/L for each 100-mg/dL rise in glucose concentration, with perhaps even greater decreases as glucose concentration >400 mg/dL.[80] In anesthesia practice,

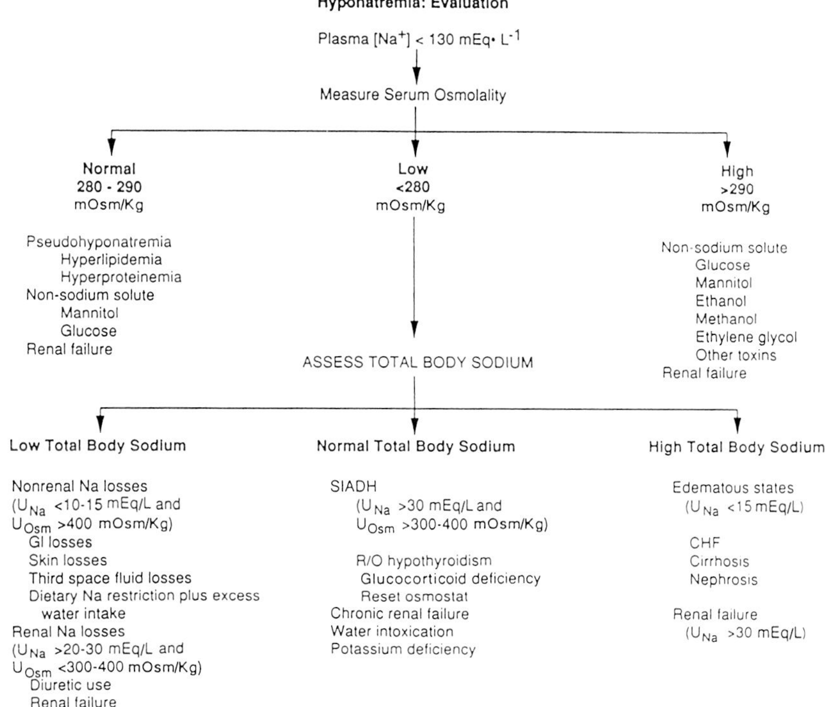

FIGURE 9-6. Algorithm by which hyponatremia can be evaluated.

a common cause of hyponatremia associated with a normal osmolality is the absorption of large volumes of sodium-free irrigating solutions (containing mannitol, glycerine, or sorbitol as the solute) during transurethral resection of the prostate.[81] Neurologic symptoms are minimal if mannitol is employed because the agent does not cross the blood-brain barrier and is excreted with water in the urine. In contrast, as glycine or sorbitol is metabolized, hypoosmolality will gradually develop and cerebral edema may appear as a late complication, that is, hypoosmolality is more important in generating symptoms than hyponatremia per se.[81] True hyponatremia with a normal or elevated serum osmolality also may accompany renal insufficiency. BUN, included in the calculation of total osmolality, distributes throughout both ECV and ICV. Calculation of *effective* osmolality ($2[Na^+] + glucose/18$) excludes the contribution of urea to tonicity and demonstrates true hypotonicity.

True hyponatremia with low serum osmolality may be associated with a high, low, or normal total body sodium and PV. Therefore, hyponatremia with hypoosmolality (see Fig. 9-6) is evaluated by assessing total body sodium content, BUN, SCr, urinary osmolality, and urinary $[Na^+]$. Hyponatremia with increased total body sodium is characteristic of edematous states, that is, congestive heart failure, cirrhosis, nephrosis, and renal failure. Aquaporin 2, the vasopressin-regulated water channel, is upregulated in experimental congestive heart failure[82] and cirrhosis[83] and decreased by chronic vasopressin stimulation.[84] In patients with renal insufficiency, reduced urinary diluting capacity can lead to hyponatremia if excess free water is given.

The underlying mechanism of hypovolemic hyponatremia is secretion of ADH in response to volume contraction in association with ongoing oral or intravenous intake of hypotonic fluid.[85] Angiotensin II also decreases renal free water clearance. Thiazide diuretics, unlike loop diuretics, promote hypovolemic hyponatremia by interfering with urinary dilution in the distal tubule.[85] Hypovolemic hyponatremia associated with a urinary $[Na^+] \geq 20$ mmol/L suggests mineralocorticoid deficiency, especially if serum $[K^+]$, BUN, and SCr are increased.[85]

The cerebral salt-wasting syndrome is an often severe, symptomatic salt-losing diathesis that appears to be mediated by brain natriuretic peptide[86] and is independent of *the syndrome of inappropriate antidiuretic hormone (SIADH) secretion*; patients at risk include those with cerebral lesions as a result of trauma, subarachnoid hemorrhage, tumors, and infection.[87–89]

Euvolemic hyponatremia most commonly is associated with nonosmotic vasopressin secretion, for example, glucocorticoid deficiency, hypothyroidism, thiazide-induced hyponatremia, SIADH, and the reset osmostat syndrome. Total body sodium and ECV are relatively normal and edema is rarely evident. SIADH may be idiopathic but also is associated with diseases of the central nervous system and with pulmonary disease (Table 9-16). Euvolemic hyponatremia is usually associated with exogenous ADH administration, pharmacologic potentiation of ADH action, drugs that mimic the action of ADH in the renal tubules or excessive ectopic ADH secretion. Tissues from some small-cell lung cancers, duodenal cancers, and pancreatic cancers increase ADH production in response to osmotic stimulation.[90]

At least 4% of postoperative patients develop plasma $[Na^+]$ <130 mEq/L.[91] Although neurologic manifestations usually do not accompany postoperative hyponatremia, signs of hypervolemia are occasionally present.[91] Much less frequently, postoperative hyponatremia is accompanied by mental status changes seizures and transtentorial herniaton,[92] attributable in part to intravenous administration of hypotonic fluids, secretion of ADH, and other factors, including drugs and altered renal function, that influence perioperative water balance.[93] Menstruating women may be particularly vulnerable to brain damage secondary to postoperative hyponatremia.[94] Smaller patients change plasma $[Na^+]$ more in response to similar

TABLE 9-16

CAUSES OF THE SYNDROME OF INAPPROPRIATE SECRETION OF ANTIDIURETIC HORMONE (SIADH)

Neoplasms
- Bronchogenic carcinoma
- Pancreatic carcinoma
- Carcinoma of the duodenum
- Prostate carcinoma
- Thymoma
- Lymphoma
- Mesothelioma

Central nervous system diseases
- Head trauma
- Subdural hematoma
- Subarachnoid hemorrhage
- Cerebrovascular accident
- Meningitis
- Encephalitis
- Brain abscess
- Hydrocephalus
- Brain tumors
- Guillain-Barré
- Acute intermittent porphyria
- Delirium tremens

Pulmonary diseases
- Tuberculosis
- Pneumonia
- Bronchiectasis
- Aspergillosis
- Cystic fibrosis
- Positive pressure ventilation

Medications
- Opiates
- Chlorpropamide
- Carbamazepine
- Phenothiazines
- Tricyclic antidepressants
- Clofibrate
- Vincristine
- Cyclophosphamide
- Oxytocin

Miscellaneous
- General surgery
- Pain
- Nausea
- Psychosis

From Fried LF, Palevsky PM: Hyponatremia and hypernatremia. Med Clin North Am 81(3):585, 1997.

volumes of hypotonic fluids. In an editorial accompanying a report[95] of apparent postoperative SIADH in a 30-kg, 10-year-old girl, Arieff [96] suggested that children receive no sodium-free water perioperatively. Postoperative hyponatremia can develop even with infusion of isotonic fluids if ADH is persistently increased. Twenty-four hours after surgery, mean plasma $[Na^+]$ in 22 women (mean age 42 years) undergoing uncomplicated gynecologic surgery had decreased from 140 ± 1 mEq/L to 136 ± 0.5 mEq/L.[97] Although the patients retained sodium perioperatively, they retained proportionately more water (an
12 average of 1.1 L of electrolyte-free water). Careful postoperative attention to fluid and electrolyte balance may minimize the occurrence of symptomatic hyponatremia.

If both $[Na^+]$ and measured osmolality are below the normal range, hyponatremia is further evaluated by first assessing volume status using physical findings and laboratory data. In hypovolemic patients or edematous patients, the ratio of BUN to SCr should be $>20:1$. Urinary $[Na^+]$ is generally <15 mEq/L in edematous states and volume depletion is >20 mEq/L in hyponatremia secondary to renal salt wasting or renal failure with water retention.

The criteria for the diagnosis of SIADH include hypotonic hyponatremia; urinary osmolality >100 to 150 mOsm/kg; absence of extracellular volume depletion; normal thyroid and adrenal function; and normal cardiac, hepatic, and renal function. Urinary $[Na^+]$ should be >30 mEq/L unless fluids have been restricted. Arieff [96] has argued that the diagnosis of SIADH may be inaccurately applied to functionally hypovolemic postoperative patients in whom, by definition, ADH secretion would be "appropriate."

Treatment of hyponatremia associated with a normal or high serum osmolality requires reduction of the elevated concentrations of the responsible solute. Uremic patients are treated by free water restriction or dialysis. Treatment of edematous (hypervolemic) patients necessitates restriction of both sodium and water (Fig. 9-7). Therapy is directed toward improving cardiac output and renal perfusion and using diuretics

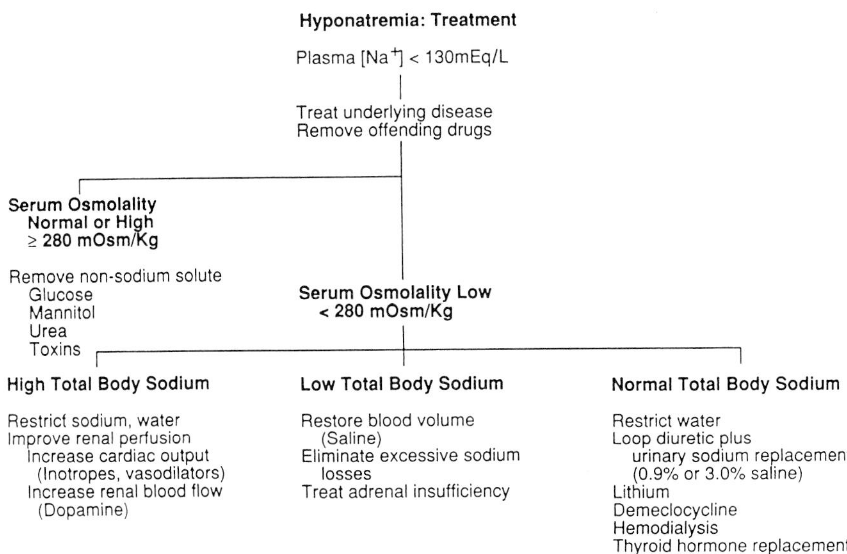

FIGURE 9-7. Hyponatremia is treated according to the etiology of the disturbance, the level of serum osmolality, and a clinical estimation of total body sodium.

to inhibit sodium reabsorption. In hypovolemic, hyponatremic patients, blood volume must be restored, usually by infusion of 0.9% saline, and excessive sodium losses must be curtailed. Correction of hypovolemia usually results in removal of the stimulus for ADH release, accompanied by a rapid water diuresis.

The cornerstone of SIADH management is free water restriction and elimination of precipitating causes. Water restriction, sufficient to decrease TBW by 0.5 to 1.0 L/d, decreases ECV even if excessive ADH secretion continues. The resultant reduction in GFR enhances proximal tubular reabsorption of salt and water, thereby decreasing free water generation, and stimulates aldosterone secretion. As long as free water losses (i.e., renal, skin, gastrointestinal) exceed free water intake, serum $[Na^+]$ will increase. During treatment of hyponatremia, increases in plasma $[Na^+]$ are determined both by the composition of the infused fluid and by the rate of renal free water excretion.[98] Free water excretion can be increased by administering furosemide.

Neurologic symptoms or profound hyponatremia ($[Na^+]$ <115 to 120 mEq/L) requires more aggressive therapy. Hypertonic (3%) saline is most clearly indicated in patients who have seizures or patients who acutely develop symptoms of water intoxication secondary to intravenous fluid administration. In such cases, 3% saline may be administered at a rate of 1 to 2 mL/kg/h, to increase plasma $[Na^+]$ by 1 to 2 mEq/L/h; however, this treatment should not continue for more than a few hours. Three percent saline may only transiently increase plasma $[Na^+]$ because ECV expansion results in increased urinary sodium excretion. Intravenous furosemide, combined with quantitative replacement of urinary sodium losses with 0.9% or 3.0% saline, can rapidly increase plasma $[Na^+]$, in part by increasing free water clearance.

The rate of treatment of hyponatremia continues to generate controversy, extending from "too fast, too soon" to "too slow, too late." Although delayed correction may result in neurologic injury, inappropriately rapid correction may result in abrupt brain dehydration (Fig. 9-8) or permanent neurologic sequelae (i.e., osmotic demyelination syndrome),[99] cerebral hemorrhage, or congestive heart failure. The symptoms of the osmotic demyelination syndrome vary from mild (transient behavioral disturbances or seizures) to severe (including pseudobulbar palsy and quadriparesis).[100]

The principal determinants of neurologic injury appear to be the magnitude and chronicity of hyponatremia and the rate of correction. The osmotic demyelination syndrome is more likely when hyponatremia has persisted >48 hours.[101] Most patients in whom the osmotic demyelination syndrome is fatal have undergone correction of plasma $[Na^+]$ of more than 20 mEq/L/day. Other risk factors for the development of the osmotic demyelination syndrome include alcoholism, poor nutritional status, liver disease, burns, and hypokalemia.

The clinician faces formidable difficulties in predicting the rate at which plasma $[Na^+]$ will increase because increases in plasma $[Na^+]$ are determined both by the composition of the infused fluid and by the rate of renal free water excretion.[98] The expected change in plasma $[Na^+]$ resulting from 1 liter of selected infusate can be estimated using the following equation:[102]

$$\Delta[Na^+]_s = \frac{[Na^+]_{inf} - [Na^+]_s}{TBW + 1} \qquad (9\text{-}12)$$

where $\Delta[Na^+]_s$ = the change in the patient's serum $[Na^+]$, $[Na^+]_{inf}$ = $[Na^+]$ of the infusate, $[Na^+]_s$ = the patient's serum $[Na^+]$, TBW = the patient's estimated total body water in liters, and 1 = a factor added to take into account the volume of infusate.

Treatment should be interrupted or slowed when symptoms improve. Frequent determinations of $[Na^+]$ are important to prevent correction at a rate >10 mEq/L/24hr.[101] Initially, plasma $[Na^+]$ may be increased by 1 to 2 mEq/L/hr; however, plasma $[Na^+]$ should not be increased more than 10 mEq/L in 24 hours or 25 mEq/L in 48 hours.[100] Another proposed sequence for treating symptomatic hyponatremia is to increase $[Na^+]$ promptly by about 10 mmol, then to proceed more slowly. The rationale is that cerebral water is increased by approximately 10% in chronic hyponatremia.[85] Hypernatremia should be avoided. Once the plasma $[Na^+]$ exceeds 120 to 125 mEq/L, water restriction alone is usually sufficient to normalize $[Na^+]$. As acute hyponatremia is corrected, CNS signs and symptoms usually improve within 24 hours, although 96 hours may be necessary for maximal recovery.

For patients who require long-term pharmacologic therapy of hyponatremia, demeclocycline is now the drug of choice.[85] Although better tolerated than lithium, demeclocycline may induce nephrotoxicity, a particular concern in patients with hepatic dysfunction. Hemodialysis is occasionally necessary in severely hyponatremic patients who cannot be adequately managed with drugs or hypertonic saline. Once hyponatremia has

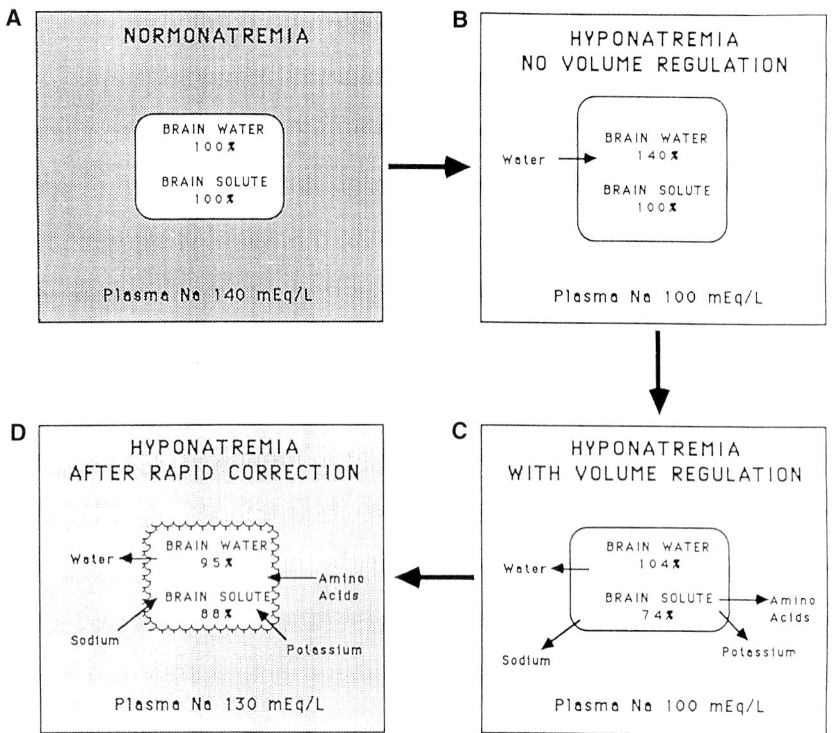

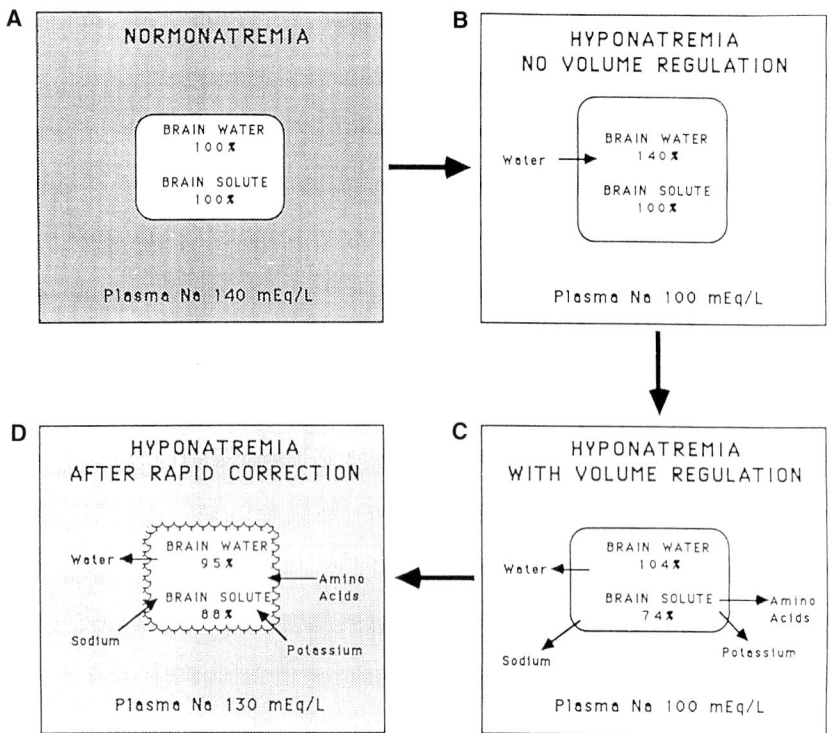

FIGURE 9-8. Brain water and solute in concentrations in hyponatremia. If normal plasma sodium (Na) (A) suddenly decreased, the increase in brain water theoretically would be proportional to the decrease in plasma Na (B). However, because of adaptive loss of cerebral intracellular solute, cerebral edema is minimized in chronic hyponatremia (C). Once adaptation has occurred, a rapid return of plasma Na concentration toward a normal level results in brain dehydration (D). (From Sterns RH: Vignettes in clinical pathophysiology. Neurological deterioration following treatment for hyponatremia. Am J Kidney Dis 13:434, 1989.)

improved, careful fluid restriction is necessary to avoid recurrence of hyponatremia. In the future, vasopressin receptor antagonists may be used to treat hyponatremia.[103]

Hypernatremia

Hypernatremia ($[Na^+]$ >150 mEq/L) indicates an absolute or relative water deficit. Normally, slight increases in tonicity or $[Na^+]$ stimulate thirst and ADH secretion. Therefore, severe, persistent hypernatremia occurs only in patients who cannot respond to thirst by voluntary ingestion of fluid, that is, obtunded patients, anesthetized patients, and infants.

Hypernatremia produces neurologic symptoms (including stupor, coma, and seizures), hypovolemia, renal insufficiency (occasionally progressing to renal failure), and decreased urinary concentrating ability.[104,105] Because hypernatremia frequently results from diabetes insipidus (DI) or osmotically induced losses of sodium and water, many patients are hypovolemic or bear the stigmata of renal disease. Postoperative neurosurgical patients who have undergone pituitary surgery are at particular risk of developing transient or prolonged DI. Polyuria may be present for only a few days within the first week of surgery, may be permanent, or may demonstrate a triphasic sequence: early DI, return of urinary concentrating ability, then recurrent DI.

The clinical consequences of hypernatremia are most serious at the extremes of age and when hypernatremia develops abruptly. Geriatric patients are at increased risk of hypernatremia because of decreased renal concentrating ability and thirst.[106] Brain shrinkage secondary to rapidly developing hypernatremia may damage delicate cerebral vessels, leading to subdural hematoma, subcortical parenchymal hemorrhage, subarachnoid hemorrhage, and venous thrombosis. Polyuria may cause bladder distention, hydronephrosis, and permanent renal damage. At the cellular level, restoration of cell volume occurs remarkably quickly after tonicity is altered (Fig 9-9).[107] Although the mortality of hypernatremia is 40 to 55%, it is unclear whether hypernatremia is the cause or a marker of severe associated disease.

Surprisingly, if plasma $[Na^+]$ is initially normal, moderate acute increases in plasma $[Na^+]$ do not appear to precipitate central pontine myelinolysis. However, larger accidental increases in plasma $[Na^+]$ have produced severe consequences in children. In experimental animals, acute severe hypernatremia (acute increase from 146 to 170 mEq/L) caused neuronal damage at 24 hours, suggestive of early central pontine myelinolysis.[108]

By definition, hypernatremia indicates an absolute or relative water deficit and is always associated with hypertonicity. Hypernatremia can be generated by hypotonic fluid loss, as in burns, GI losses, diuretic therapy, osmotic diuresis, renal disease, mineralocorticoid excess or deficiency, and iatrogenic causes, or can be generated by isolated water loss, as in central or nephrogenic DI (Fig. 9-10). The acquired form of nephrogenic DI is more common and usually less severe than the congenital form. As chronic renal failure advances, most patients have defective concentrating ability, resulting in resistance to ADH associated with hypotonic urine. Because hypovolemia accompanies most pathologic water loss, signs of hypoperfusion also may be present. In many patients, before the development of hypernatremia, an increased volume of hypotonic urine suggests an abnormality in water balance. Although uncommon as a cause of hypernatremia, isolated sodium gain occasionally occurs in patients who receive large quantities of sodium, such as treatment of metabolic acidosis with 8.4% sodium bicarbonate, in which $[Na^+]$ is approximately 1,000 mEq/L, or perioperative or prehospital treatment with hypertonic saline resuscitation solutions.

Hypernatremic patients can be separated into three groups, based on clinical assessment of ECV (see Fig. 9-10). Note that plasma $[Na^+]$ does not reflect total body sodium, which must be estimated separately based on signs of the adequacy of ECV. In polyuric, hypernatremic patients, the next differential diagnostic decision is between solute diuresis and DI. Measurement of urinary sodium and osmolality can help to differentiate the

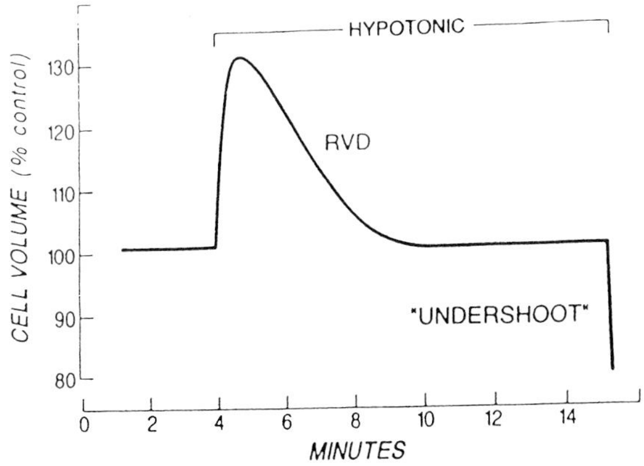

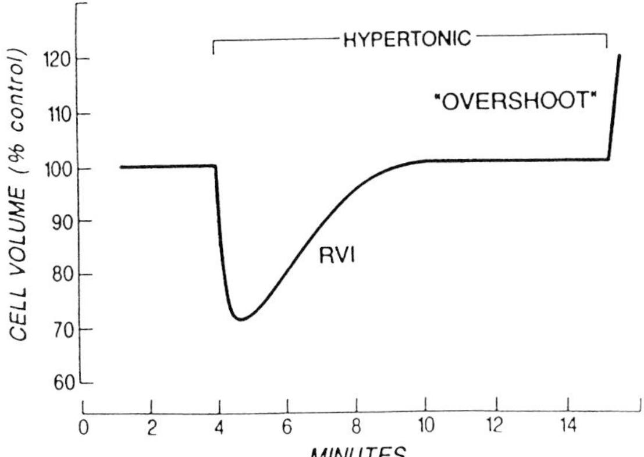

FIGURE 9-9. Activation of mechanisms regulating cell volume in response to acute osmotic stress. Regulatory volume decrease and regulatory volume increase refer to compensatory losses and gains of solutes. Although the course of these regulatory volume decreases and increases varies with the type of cell and experimental conditions, typically the responses occur over a period of minutes. Returning volume-regulated cells to normotonic conditions causes shrinkage or swelling. (From McManus ML, Churchwill KB, Strange K: Regulation of cell volume in health and disease. N Engl J Med 333:1260, 1995.)

various causes. A urinary osmolality <150 mOsm/kg in the setting of hypertonicity and polyuria is diagnostic of DI.

Treatment of hypernatremia produced by water loss consists of repletion of water as well as associated deficits in total body sodium and other electrolytes (Table 9-17). Common errors in treating hypernatremia include excessively rapid correction as well as failing to appreciate the magnitude of the water deficit and failing to account for ongoing maintenance requirements and continued fluid losses in planning therapy.

The first step in treating hypernatremia is to estimate the TBW deficit, which can be accomplished by inserting the measured plasma $[Na^+]$ into the equation:

$$\text{TBW deficit} = 0.6 \times \text{body weight (kg)} \times [([Na^+] - 140)/140] \qquad (9\text{-}13)$$

where 140 is the middle of the normal range for $[Na^+]$.

Hypernatremia must be corrected slowly because of the risk of neurologic sequelae such as seizures or cerebral edema (Fig. 9-11).[109] At the cellular level, restoration of cell volume occurs remarkably quickly after tonicity is altered; as a consequence, acute treatment of hypertonicity may result in overshooting the original, normotonic cell volume.[107,109] The water deficit should be replaced over 24 to 48 hours, and the plasma $[Na^+]$ should not be reduced by more than 1 to 2 mEq/L/h. Reversible underlying causes should be treated. Hypovolemia should be corrected promptly with 0.9% saline. Although the $[Na^+]$ of 0.9% saline is 154 mEq/L, the solution is effective in treating volume deficits and will reduce $[Na^+]$ that exceeds 154 mEq/L. Once hypovolemia is corrected, water can be replaced orally or with intravenous hypotonic fluids, depending on the ability of the patient to tolerate oral hydration. In the occasional sodium-overloaded patient, sodium excretion can be accelerated using loop diuretics or dialysis.

The management of hypernatremia secondary to DI varies according to whether the etiology is central or nephrogenic (see Table 9-17). The two most suitable agents for correcting central DI (an ADH deficiency syndrome) are desmopressin (DDAVP) and aqueous vasopressin. DDAVP, given subcutaneously in a dose of 1 to 4 μg or intranasally in a dose of 5 to 20 μg every 12 to 24 hours, is effective in the vast majority of patients. DDAVP is less likely than vasopressin to produce vasoconstriction and abdominal cramping.[110] Incomplete ADH deficits (partial DI) often are effectively managed with pharmacologic agents that stimulate ADH release or enhance the renal

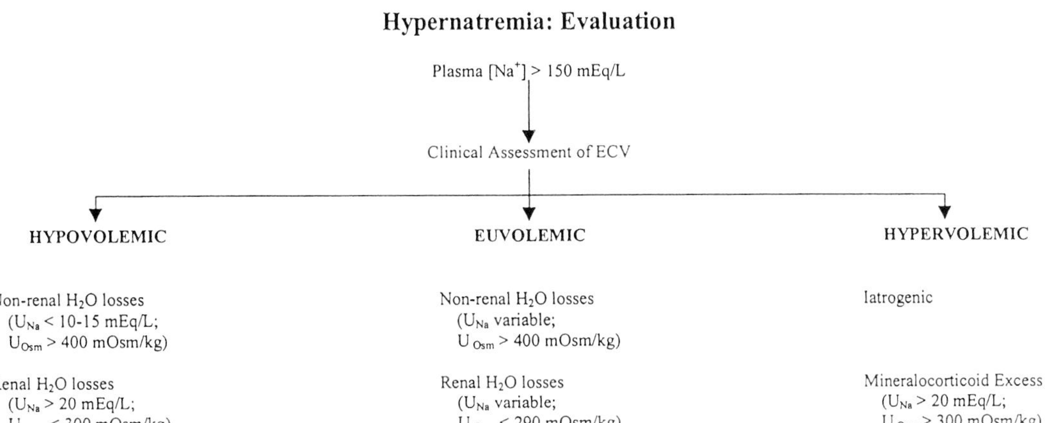

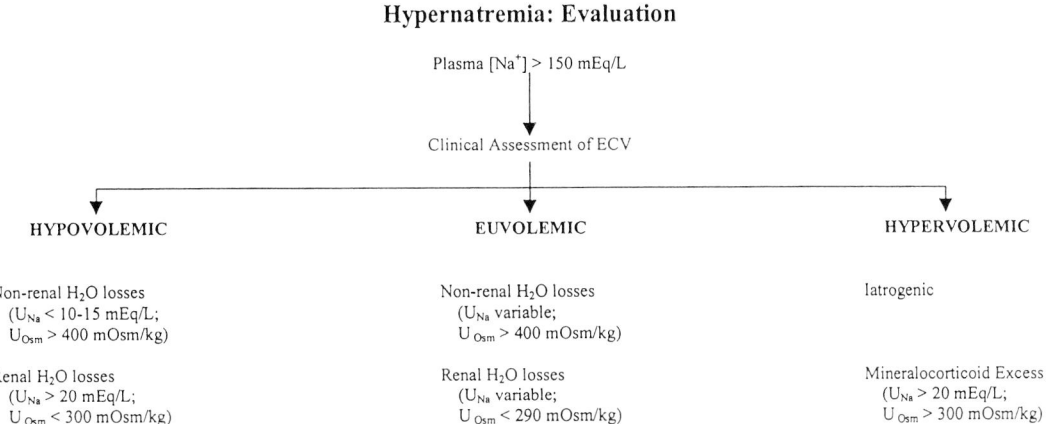

FIGURE 9-10. Severe hypernatremia is evaluated by first separating patients into hypovolemic, euvolemic, and hypervolemic groups based on assessment of extracellular volume (ECV). Next, potential etiologic factors are diagnostically assessed. $[Na^+]$, serum sodium concentration; U_{Na}, urinary sodium concentration; U_{Osm}, urinary osmolality.

TABLE 9-17

HYPERNATREMIA: ACUTE TREATMENT

Sodium depletion (hypovolemia)
Hypovolemia correction (0.9% saline)
Hypernatremia correction (hypotonic fluids)

Sodium overload (hypervolemia)
Enhance sodium removal (loop diuretics, dialysis)
Replace water deficit (hypotonic fluids)

Normal total body sodium (euvolemia)
Replace water deficit (hypotonic fluids)
Control diabetes insipidus
- Central diabetes insipidus:
  - DDAVP, 10–20 μg intranasally; 2–4 μg sc
  - Aqueous vasopressin, 5 U q 2–4 hours im or sc
- Nephrogenic diabetes insipidus:
  - Restrict sodium, water intake
  - Thiazide diuretics

response to ADH. Chlorpropamide, which potentiates the renal effects of vasopressin, and carbamazepine, which enhances vasopressin secretion, have been used to treat partial central DI, but are associated with clinically important side effects. In nephrogenic DI, salt and water restriction or thiazide diuretics induce contraction of ECV, thereby enhancing fluid reabsorption in the proximal tubules. If less filtrate passes through into the collecting ducts, less water will be excreted.

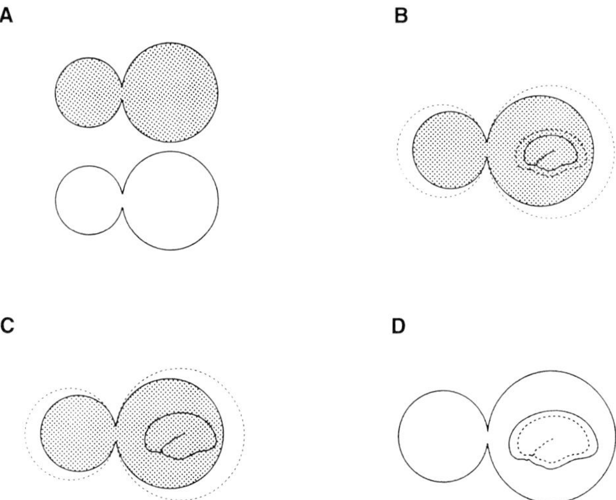

FIGURE 9-11. **A.** The concentration of sodium is reflected in the intensity of the stippling: the upper figure, representing extracellular volume (smaller circle) and intracellular volume (larger circle), is more heavily stippled, that is, serum sodium is higher. **B.** In response to an acute increase in serum sodium resulting from water loss, both intracellular and extracellular volume substantially decrease. The brain (schematically illustrated) shrinks in proportion to the reduction in intracellular volume in other tissues. **C.** However, owing to the production of idiogenic osmoles, the brain rapidly restores its intracellular volume, despite the persistent reduction in intracellular volume in other tissues and in extracellular volume. **D.** With excessively rapid correction of hypernatremia (the reduction in serum sodium is reflected in the decrease in the intensity of stippling), the brain expands to greater than its original size. The resulting increase in cerebral edema and intracranial pressure can cause severe neurologic damage. (Modified from Feig PU: Hypernatremia and hypertonic syndromes. Med Clin North Am 65:271, 1981.)

Potassium

Physiologic Role

Potassium plays an important role in cell membrane physiology, especially in maintaining resting membrane potentials and in generating action potentials in the central nervous system and heart. Potassium is actively transported into cells by a Na/K ATPase pump, which maintains an intracellular [K^+] that is at least 30-fold greater than extracellular [K^+]. Intracellular potassium concentration ([K^+]) is normally 150 mEq/L, while the extracellular concentration is only 3.5 to 5.0 mEq/L. Serum [K^+] measures about 0.5 mEq/L higher than plasma [K^+] because of cell lysis during clotting. Total body potassium in a 70-kg adult is approximately 4,256 mEq, of which 4,200 mEq is intracellular; of the 56 mEq in the ECV, only 12 mEq is located in the PV. The ratio of intracellular to extracellular potassium contributes to the resting potential difference across cell membranes and therefore to the integrity of cardiac and neuromuscular transmission. The primary mechanism that maintains potassium inside cells is the negative voltage created by the transport of three sodium ions out of the cell for every two potassium ions transported in (Fig. 9-12).[111] Both insulin and β-adrenergic agonists promote potassium entry into cells.[111,112] In contrast, α-adrenergic agonists impair cellular potassium uptake.[113] Metabolic acidosis tends to shift potassium out of cells, while metabolic alkalosis favors movement into cells.

Usual potassium intake is between 50 and 150 mEq/day. Freely filtered at the glomerulus, most potassium excretion is urinary, with some fecal elimination. Most filtered potassium is reabsorbed; usually, excretion is approximately equal to daily intake. As long as GFR is >8 mL/kg, dietary potassium intake, unless greater than normal, can be excreted. Assuming a plasma [K^+] of 4.0 mEq/L and a normal GFR of 180 L/day, 720 mEq of potassium is filtered daily, of which 85 to 90% is reabsorbed in the proximal convoluted tubule and loop of Henle. The remaining 10 to 15% reaches the distal convoluted tubule, which is the major site at which potassium excretion is regulated. Excretion of potassium ions is a function of open potassium channels and the electrical driving force in the cortical collecting duct.[111]

The two most important regulators of potassium excretion are the plasma [K^+] and aldosterone, although there is some evidence to suggest involvement of the central nervous system and of an enteric reflex mediated by potassium-rich meals.[114] Potassium secretion into the distal convoluted tubules and cortical collecting ducts is increased by hyperkalemia, aldosterone, alkalemia, increased delivery of Na^+ to the distal tubule and collecting duct, high urinary flow rates, and the presence in luminal fluid of nonreabsorbable anions such as carbenicillin,

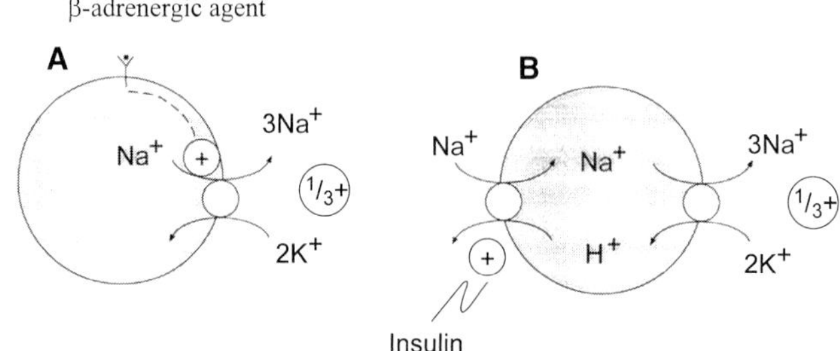

FIGURE 9-12. Hormones shifting potassium into cells. Major hormones involved are: (**A**) insulin and (**B**) β-2 adrenergic agents. (From Halperin ML, Kamel KS: Potassium. Lancet 352:135, 1998.)

phosphates, and sulfates. As sodium reabsorption increases, the electrical driving force opposing reabsorption of potassium is increased. Aldosterone increases sodium reabsorption by inducing a more open configuration of the epithelial sodium channel[115]; potassium-sparing diuretics (amiloride and triamterene) and trimethroprim block the epithelial sodium channel, thereby increasing potassium reabsorption.[116] Magnesium depletion contributes to renal potassium wasting.

Hypokalemia

Uncommon among healthy persons, hypokalemia ($[K^+]$ <3.0 mEq/L) is a frequent complication of treatment with diuretic drugs and occasionally complicates other diseases and treatment regimens (Table 9-18).[113] As a general rule, a chronic decrement of 1.0 mEq/L in the plasma $[K^+]$ corresponds to a total body deficit of approximately 200 to 300 mEq. In uncomplicated hypokalemia, the potassium deficit exceeds 300 mEq if plasma $[K^+]$ is <3.0 mEq/L and 700 mEq if plasma $[K^+]$ is <2.0 mEq/L. Plasma $[K^+]$ poorly reflects total body potassium; hypokalemia may occur with normal, low, or high total body potassium.

Hypokalemia causes muscle weakness and, when severe, may even cause paralysis. With chronic potassium loss, the ratio of intracellular to extracellular $[K^+]$ remains relatively stable; in contrast, acute redistribution of potassium from the extracellular to the intracellular space substantially changes resting membrane potentials.

Cardiac rhythm disturbances are among the most dangerous complications of potassium deficiency. Acute hypokalemia causes hyperpolarization of the cardiac cell and may lead to ventricular escape activity, re-entrant phenomena, ectopic tachycardias, and delayed conduction. In patients taking digoxin, hypokalemia increases toxicity by increasing myocardial digoxin binding and pharmacologic effectiveness. Hypokalemia contributes to systemic hypertension, especially when combined with a high-sodium diet.[117] In diabetic patients, hypokalemia impairs insulin secretion and end-organ sensitivity to insulin. Although no clear threshold has been defined for a level of hypokalemia below which safe conduct of anesthesia is compromised, $[K^+]$ <3.5 mEq/L has been associated with an increased incidence of perioperative dysrhythmias, especially atrial fibrillation/flutter, in cardiac surgical patients.[118]

Potassium depletion also induces defects in renal concentrating ability, resulting in polyuria and a reduction in GFR. Potassium replacement improves GFR, although the concentrating deficit may not improve for several months after treatment. If hypokalemia is sufficiently prolonged, chronic renal interstitial damage may occur. In experimental animals, hypokalemia was associated with intrarenal vasoconstriction and a pattern of renal injury similar to that produced by ischemia.[119]

Hypokalemia may result from chronic depletion of total body potassium or from acute redistribution of potassium from the ECV to the ICV. Redistribution of potassium into cells occurs when the activity of the sodium–potassium ATPase pump is acutely increased by extracellular hyperkalemia or increased intracellular concentrations of sodium, as well as by insulin, carbohydrate loading (which stimulates release of endogenous insulin), β_2-adrenergic agonists, and aldosterone.[111] Both metabolic and respiratory alkalosis lead to decreases in plasma $[K^+]$.[111,117]

Causes of chronic hypokalemia include those etiologies associated with renal potassium conservation (extrarenal potassium losses; low urinary $[K^+]$) and those with renal potassium wasting (Fig. 9-13).[111,117] A low urinary $[K^+]$ suggests inadequate dietary intake or extrarenal depletion (in the absence of recent diuretic use). Diuretic-induced urinary potassium losses are frequently associated with hypokalemia, secondary to increased aldosterone secretion, alkalemia, and increased renal tubular flow. Aldosterone does not cause renal potassium wasting unless sodium ions are present; that is, aldosterone primarily controls sodium reabsorption, not potassium excretion. Renal tubular damage because of nephrotoxins such as aminoglycosides or amphotericin B may also cause renal potassium wasting.

Initial evaluation of hypokalemia includes a medical history (e.g., diarrhea, vomiting, diuretic or laxative use), physical examination (e.g., hypertension, cushingoid features, edema),

TABLE 9-18

CAUSES OF RENAL POTASSIUM LOSS

Drugs	Bicarbonaturia
Diuretics	Distal renal tubular acidosis
Thiazide diuretics	Treatment of proximal renal tubular acidosis
Loop diuretics	Correction phase of metabolic alkalosis
Osmotic diuretics	Magnesium deficiency
Antibiotics	Other less common causes
Penicillin and penicillin analogues	Cisplatin
Amphotericin B	Carbonic anhydrase inhibitors
Aminoglycosides	Leukemia
Hormones	Diuretic phase of acute tubular necrosis
Aldosterone	Intrinsic renal transport defects
Glucocorticoid-excess states	Barter's syndrome
	Gitelman's syndrome

Modified from Weiner ID, Wingo CS: Hypokalemia consequences, causes, and correction. J Am Soc Nephrol 8:1179, 1997.

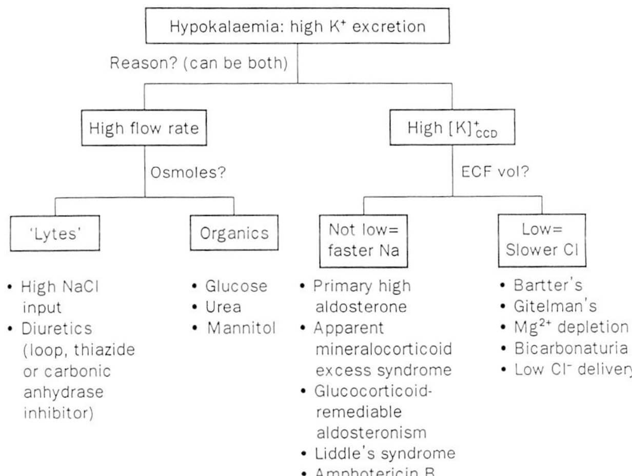

FIGURE 9-13. Approach to managing hypokalemia. Causes for excessive excretion of potassium (>15 mmol/day) despite hypokalemia are too high a flow rate in the cortical collecting duct ([CCD], left limb) and/or too high a concentration of potassium [K+] in lumen of the CCD (right limb). Both flow rate and CCD [K+] should be evaluated. Final considerations are shown by bullets. A relatively slower Cl^- reabsorption in CCD is suggested by high plasma renin activity and NaCl wasting despite low extracellular fluid volume; the converse applies for relatively faster Na^+ reabsorption. (From Halperin ML, Kamel KS: Potassium. Lancet 352:135, 1998.)

measurement of serum electrolytes (e.g., magnesium), arterial pH assessment, and evaluation of the electrocardiogram (ECG). A majority of trauma patients develop hypokalemia that returns to normal within 24 hours without specific therapy.[113] Measurement of 24-hour urinary excretion of sodium and potassium may distinguish extrarenal from renal causes. Magnesium deficiency, associated with aminoglycoside and cisplatin therapy, can generate hypokalemia that is resistant to replacement therapy. Plasma renin and aldosterone levels may be helpful in the differential diagnosis. Characteristic electrocardiographic changes associated with hypokalemia include flat or inverted T waves, prominent U waves, and ST segment depression.

The treatment of hypokalemia consists of potassium repletion, correction of alkalemia, and removal of offending drugs (Table 9-19). Hypokalemia secondary only to acute redistribution may not require treatment. There is no urgent need for potassium replacement therapy in mild to moderate hypokalemia (3 to 3.5 mEq/L), especially if it is a chronic state and the patient has no symptoms. If total body potassium is decreased, oral potassium supplementation is preferable to intravenous replacement. Potassium is usually replaced as chloride salt because coexisting chloride deficiency may limit the ability of the kidney to conserve potassium.

Potassium repletion must be performed cautiously (i.e., usually at a rate $\leq$10 to 20 mEq/h) because the magnitude of potassium deficits is unpredictable. The plasma [K^+] and the ECG must be monitored during rapid repletion (10 to 20 mEq/h) to avoid hyperkalemic complications.[113,120] The plasma [K^+] and ECG should be monitored to detect inadvertent hyperkalemia. Particular care should be taken in patients who have concurrent acidemia, type IV renal tubular acidosis, or diabetes mellitus, or in those patients receiving nonsteroidal anti-inflammatory agents, ACE inhibitors, or β-blockers, all of which delay movement of extracellular potassium into cells.

However, in patients with life-threatening dysrhythmias secondary to hypokalemia, serum [K^+] must be rapidly increased. Assuming that PV in a 70-kg adult is 3.0 L, administration of 6.0 mEq/L of potassium in 1.0 minute will increase serum [K^+] by no more than 2.0 mEq/L because redistribution into interstitial fluid will decrease the quantity remaining in the plasma volume.[111]

Hypokalemia associated with hyperaldosteronemia (e.g., primary aldosteronism, Cushing syndrome) usually responds favorably to reduced sodium intake and increased potassium intake. Hypomagnesemia, if present, aggravates the effects of hypokalemia, impairs potassium conservation, and should be treated. Potassium supplements or potassium-sparing diuretics should be given cautiously to patients who have diabetes mellitus or renal insufficiency, which limit compensation for acute hyperkalemia. In patients, such as those who have diabetic ketoacidosis, who are both hypokalemic and acidemic, potassium administration should precede correction of acidosis to avoid a precipitous decrease in plasma [K^+] as pH increases.

In patients with normal serum potassium accompanied by symptoms of potassium depletion (e.g., muscle fatigue), history of potassium loss or insufficient intake, or in patients in whom potassium depletion may be of special threat, for example, patients on diuretics, digitalis, or β-2 adrenergic agonists, muscle biopsy with measurement of muscle potassium concentration may be a useful procedure to detect and quantify potassium depletion.

TABLE 9-19

HYPOKALEMIA: TREATMENT

Correct precipitating factors
Increased pH
Decreased [Mg^{2+}]
Drugs

Mild hypokalemia ([K^+] >2.0 mEq/L)
Intravenous KCl infusion $\leq$10 mEq/h

Severe hypokalemia ([K^+] $\leq$2.0 mEq/L, paralysis, or electrocardiographic [ECG] changes)
Intravenous KCl infusion $\leq$40 mEq/h
Continuous ECG monitoring
If life threatening, 5–6 mEq bolus

Hyperkalemia

The most lethal manifestations of hyperkalemia ([K^+] >5.0 mEq/L) involve the cardiac conducting system and include dysrhythmias, conduction abnormalities, and cardiac arrest. In anesthesia practice, the classic example of hyperkalemic cardiac toxicity is associated with the administration of succinylcholine to paraplegic, quadriplegic, or severely burned [121] patients. If plasma [K^+] is <6.0 mEq/L, cardiac effects are negligible. As the concentration increases further, the electrocardiogram shows tall, peaked T waves, especially in the precordial leads. With further increases, the PR interval becomes prolonged, followed by a decrease in the amplitude of the P wave. Finally, the QRS complex widens into a pattern resembling a sine wave, as a prelude to cardiac standstill (Fig. 9-14).[122] Hyperkalemic cardiotoxicity is enhanced by hyponatremia, hypocalcemia, or acidosis. Because progression to fatal cardiotoxicity is unpredictable and often swift, the presence of hyperkalemic ECG changes mandates immediate therapy. The life-threatening cardiac effects usually require more urgent treatment than other manifestations of hyperkalemia. However, ascending muscle weakness appears when plasma [K^+] approaches 7.0 mEq/L, and may progress to flaccid paralysis, inability to phonate, and respiratory arrest.

The most important diagnostic issues are medical history, emphasizing recent drug therapy, and assessment of renal function. Although the ECG may provide the first suggestion of hyperkalemia in some patients, and despite the well-described effects of hyperkalemia on cardiac conduction and rhythm, the ECG is an insensitive and nonspecific method of detecting hyperkalemia.[123] If hyponatremia is also present, adrenal function should be evaluated.

Hyperkalemia may occur with normal, high, or low total body potassium stores. A deficiency of aldosterone, a major regulator of potassium excretion, leads to hyperkalemia in adrenal insufficiency and hyporeninemic hypoaldosteronism, a state associated with diabetes mellitus, renal insufficiency, and advanced age. Because the kidneys excrete potassium, severe renal insufficiency commonly causes hyperkalemia. Patients with chronic renal insufficiency can maintain normal plasma [K^+] despite markedly decreased GFR because urinary potassium excretion depends on tubular secretion rather than glomerular filtration if GFR exceeds 8 mL/min.

Drugs are now the most common cause of hyperkalemia, especially in elderly patients.[124] Drugs that may limit potassium excretion include nonsteroidal anti-inflammatory drugs, ACE inhibitors, cyclosporin, and potassium-sparing diuretics such as triamterene. Drug-induced hyperkalemia most commonly occurs in patients with other predisposing factors, such as diabetes mellitus, renal insufficiency, advanced age, or hyporeninemic hypoaldosteronism. ACE inhibitors are particularly likely to produce hyperkalemia in patients who have congestive heart failure.[125]

In patients who have normal total body potassium, hyperkalemia may accompany a sudden shift of potassium from the ICV to the ECV because of acidemia, increased catabolism, or

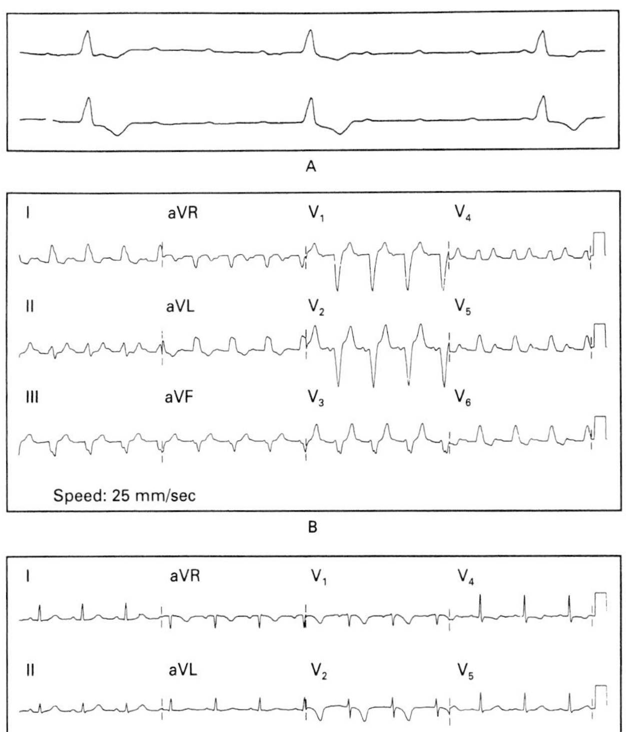

FIGURE 9-14. Electrocardiographic changes as a result of hyperkalemia occurring in a 42-year-old woman undergoing placement of an arteriovenous fistula for permanent hemodialysis access to treat end-stage renal disease. **A.** During dissection of the brachial artery under local anesthesia, her cardiac rhythm converted from normal sinus rhythm to complete heart block with ventricular escape (approximately 25 beats per minute). Two ampules of calcium gluconate (9.2 mEq) were administered intravenously. **B.** An electrocardiogram revealed sinus tachycardia with profound prolongation of the QRS interval (left bundle-branch morphology), first-degree atrioventricular block, and "peaked" T waves. The serum potassium concentration was 8.6 mmol/L. **C.** After reduction of the serum potassium concentration, the electrocardiogram showed sinus rhythm with normalization of the PR and QRS intervals. Anteroseptal ST wave and T wave changes were noted on subsequent electrocardiograms. A cardiac exercise imaging study did not show ischemia. (From Kuvin JT: Electrocardiographic changes of hyperkalemia. N Engl J Med 338:662, 1998.)

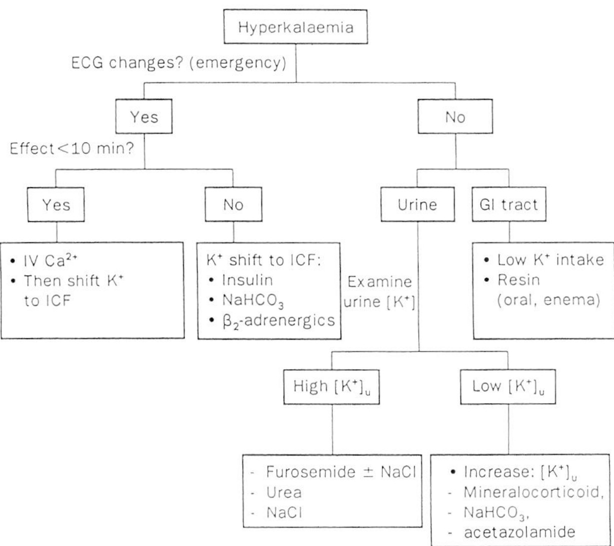

FIGURE 9-15. Treatment of patient with hyperkalemia. If an emergency is present (usually cardiac), intravenous Ca^{2+} must be given. This treatment should be given promptly. Efforts are also taken to shift potassium into cells with insulin with or without $NaHCO_3$. Longer term strategies are to limit intake of potassium, prevent its absorption in the gastrointestinal tract, and promote its excretion; the latter includes measuring urine $[K^+]$ and flow rate to decide leverage for therapy. (From Halperin ML, Kamel KS: Potassium. Lancet 352:135, 1998.)

rhabdomyolysis. Metabolic acidosis and respiratory acidosis tend to cause an increase in plasma $[K^+]$. However, organic acidoses (i.e., lactic acidosis, ketoacidosis) have little effect on $[K^+]$, whereas mineral acids cause significant cellular shifts. In response to increased hydrogen ion activity because of addition of acids, potassium will increase if the anion remains in the extracellular volume.[111] Neither lactate nor ketoacids remain in the extracellular fluid. Therefore, hyperkalemia in these circumstances reflects tissue injury or lack of insulin.[111] Pseudohyperkalemia, which occurs when potassium is released from cells in blood collection tubes, can be diagnosed by comparing serum and plasma K^+ levels from the same blood sample. Hyperkalemia usually accompanies malignant hyperthermia.

The treatment of hyperkalemia is aimed at eliminating the cause, reversing membrane hyperexcitability, and removing potassium from the body (Fig. 9-15).[111,125] Emergent management of severe hyperkalemia is listed in detail in Table 9-20.[125] Mineralocorticoid deficiency can be treated with 9-α-fludrocortisone (0.025 to 0.10 mg/day). Hyperkalemia secondary to digitalis intoxication may be resistant to therapy because attempts to shift potassium from the ECV to the ICV are often ineffective. In this situation, use of digoxin-specific antibodies has been successful.

Membrane hyperexcitability can be antagonized by translocating potassium from the ECV to the ICV, removing excess potassium, or (transiently) by infusing calcium chloride to depress the membrane threshold potential. Pending definitive treatment, rapid infusion of calcium chloride (one gram of $CaCl_2$ over 3 minutes, or two to three ampules of 10% calcium gluconate over 5 minutes) may stabilize cardiac rhythm (see Fig. 9-14). Calcium should be given cautiously if digitalis intoxication is likely. Acute alkalinization using sodium

TABLE 9-20

SEVERE HYPERKALEMIA:[a] TREATMENT

Reverse membrane effects
Calcium (10 mL of 10% calcium chloride IV over 10 min)
Transfer extracellular $[K^+]$ into cells
Glucose and insulin (D10W + 5–10 U regular insulin per 25–50 g glucose)
Sodium bicarbonate (50 to 100 mEq over 5–10 min)
β-2 agonists
Remove potassium from body
Diuretics, proximal or loop
Potassium-exchange resins (sodium polystyrene sulfonate)
Hemodialysis
Monitor ECG and serum $[K^+]$ level

[a]Potassium concentration ($[K^+]$) >7.0 mEq/L or electrocardiographic (ECG) changes.

bicarbonate (50 to 100 mEq over 5 to 10 minutes in a 70-kg adult) transiently promotes movement of potassium from the ECV to the ICV. Bicarbonate can be administered even if pH exceeds 7.40; however, it should not be administered to patients with congestive cardiac failure or hypernatremia. Insulin, in a dose-dependent fashion, causes cellular uptake of potassium by increasing the activity of the sodium/potassium ATPase pump. However, when used alone, bicarbonate is relatively ineffective and is no longer favored.[125] Insulin increases cellular uptake of potassium best when high insulin levels are achieved by intravenous injection of 5 to 10 U of regular insulin, accompanied by 50 mL of 50% glucose.[125] β-2 adrenergic drugs such as salbutamol and albuterol also increase potassium uptake by skeletal muscle and reduce plasma $[K^+]$, an action that may explain hypokalemia with severe, acute illness. β-2 agonists have been used to treat hyperkalemia.[126] Salbutamol, a selective β-2 agonist, decreases serum potassium acutely when given by inhalation or intravenously. In 15 pediatric patients with baseline serum $[K^+]$ of 6.6 mEq/L, a single infusion of salbutamol (5 μg/kg over 15 minutes) reduced serum $[K^+]$ to 5.7 mEq/L after 30 minutes and 4.9 mEq/L after 120 minutes.[127] When using β-2 adrenergic agents to reduce serum $[K^+]$, the potential for generating cardiac dysrhythmias should be recognized.[128]

Potassium may be removed from the body by the renal or gastrointestinal routes. Furosemide promotes kaliuresis in a dose-dependent fashion. Sodium polystyrene sulfonate resin (Kayexalate), which exchanges sodium for potassium, can be given orally (30 g) or as a retention enema (50 g in 200 mL of 20% sorbitol). However, sodium overload and hypervolemia are potential risks. Rarely, when temporizing measures are insufficient, emergency hemodialysis may remove 25 to 50 mEq/h. Peritoneal dialysis is less efficient.

Calcium

Physiologic Role

Calcium is a divalent cation found primarily in the extracellular fluid. The free calcium concentration $[Ca^{2+}]$ in ECV is approximately 1 mM, whereas the free $[Ca^{2+}]$ in the ICV approximates 100 mM, a gradient of 10,000 to 1. Circulating calcium consists of a protein-bound fraction (40%), a chelated fraction (10%), and an ionized fraction (50%), which is the physiologically active and homeostatically regulated component.[129] Acute acidemia increases and acute alkalemia decreases ionized calcium. Because mathematical formulae that "correct" total calcium measurements for albumin concentration are inaccurate in critically ill patients,[130] ionized calcium should be directly measured.

In general, calcium is essential for all movement that occurs in mammalian systems. Essential for normal excitation-contraction coupling, calcium is also necessary for proper function of muscle tissue, ciliary movement, mitosis, neurotransmitter release, enzyme secretion, and hormonal secretion. Cyclic AMP (cAMP) and phosphoinositides, which are major second messengers regulating cellular metabolism, function primarily through the regulation of calcium movement. Activation of numerous intracellular enzyme systems requires calcium. Calcium is important both for generation of the cardiac pacemaker activity and for generation of the cardiac action potential, and therefore is the primary ion responsible for the plateau phase of the action potential. Calcium also plays vital functions in membrane and bone structure.

Serum $[Ca^{2+}]$ is regulated by multiple factors (Fig. 9-16),[131] including a calcium receptor[132,133] and several hormones. Parathyroid hormone (PTH) and calcitriol, the most important neurohumoral mediators of serum $[Ca^{2+}]$[134] (see Table 9-15), mobilize calcium from bone, increase renal tubular reabsorption of calcium, and enhance intestinal absorption of calcium. Vitamin D, after ingestion or cutaneous manufacture under the stimulus of ultraviolet light, is 25-hydroxylated to calcidiol in the liver and then is 1-hydroxylated to calcitriol, the active metabolite, in the kidney. Even in the absence of dietary calcium intake, PTH and vitamin D can maintain a normal circulating $[Ca^{2+}]$ by mobilizing calcium from bone.

Hypocalcemia

Hypocalcemia (ionized $[Ca^{2+}]$ <4.0 mg/dL or <1.0 mmol/L) occurs as a result of failure of PTH or calcitriol action or because of calcium chelation or precipitation, not because of calcium deficiency alone. PTH deficiency can result from surgical damage or removal of the parathyroid glands or from suppression of the parathyroid glands by severe hypo- or hypermagnesemia. Burns, sepsis, and pancreatitis may suppress parathyroid function and interfere with vitamin D action.

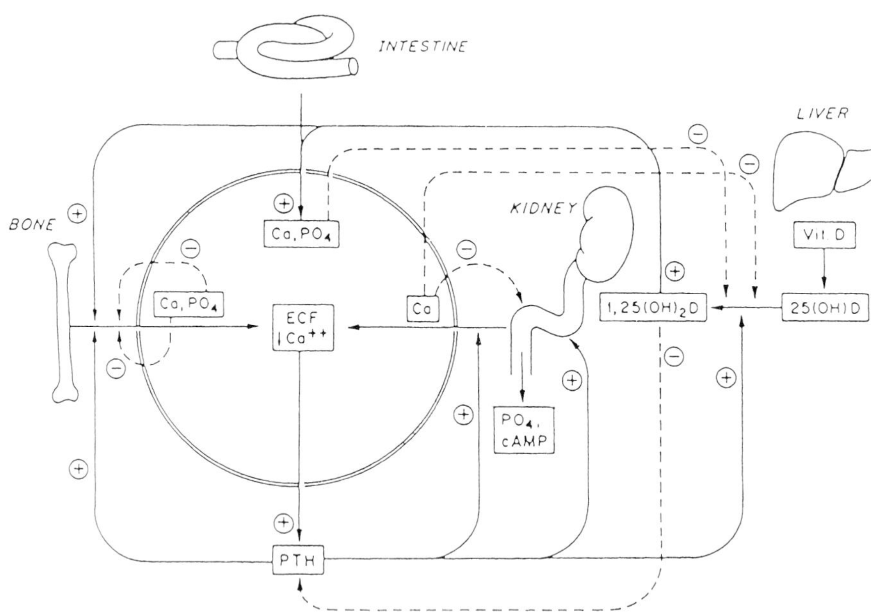

FIGURE 9-16. Schematic representation of the regulatory system maintaining Ca_o^{2+} homeostasis. The *solid arrows* and *lines* delineate effects of parathyroid hormone and 1,25 $(OH)_2D_3$ on their target tissues; *dashed arrows* and *lines* show examples of how extracellular Ca^{2+} or phosphate ions act directly on tissues regulating mineral ion metabolism. Ca, calcium; PO_4, phosphate; ECF, extracellular fluid; PTH, parathyroid hormone; 1,25 $(OH)_2D_3$, 1,25 dihydroxyvitamin D; 25(OH)D, 25-hydroxyvitamin D; negative signs indicate inhibitory actions and plus signs indicate stimulatory effects. (From Brown EM, Pollak M, Hebert SC: The extracellular calcium-sensing receptor: Its role in health and disease. Annu Rev Med 49:15, 1998.)

Vitamin D deficiency may result from lack of dietary vitamin D or vitamin D malabsorption in patients who lack sunlight exposure. Hyperphosphatemia-induced hypocalcemia may occur as a consequence of overzealous phosphate therapy, from cell lysis secondary to chemotherapy, or as a result of cellular destruction from rhabdomyolysis. Precipitation of $CaHPO_4$ complexes occurs with hyperphosphatemia. However, ionized $[Ca^{2+}]$ only decreases approximately 0.019 mM for each 1.0 mM increase in phosphate concentration. In massive transfusion, citrate may produce hypocalcemia by chelating calcium; however, decreases are usually transient and produce no cardiovascular effects. A healthy, normothermic adult who has intact hepatic and renal function can metabolize the citrate present in 20 units of blood per hour without becoming hypocalcemic.[135] However, when citrate clearance is decreased (e.g., by hepatic or renal disease or hypothermia) and when blood transfusion rates are rapid (e.g., >0.5 to 2 mL/kg/min), hypocalcemia and cardiovascular compromise may occur. Alkalemia resulting from hyperventilation or sodium bicarbonate injection can acutely decrease $[Ca^{2+}]$.

The hallmark of hypocalcemia is increased neuronal membrane irritability and tetany (Table 9-21). Early symptoms include sensations of numbness and tingling involving fingers, toes, and the circumoral region. In frank tetany, tonic contraction of respiratory muscles may lead to laryngospasm, bronchospasm, or respiratory arrest. Smooth muscle spasm can result in abdominal cramping and urinary frequency. Mental status alterations include irritability, depression, psychosis, and dementia. Hypocalcemia may impair cardiovascular function and has been associated with heart failure, hypotension, dysrhythmias, insensitivity to digitalis, and impaired β-adrenergic action.

Reduced *ionized* serum calcium occurs in as many as 88% of critically ill patients, 66% of less severely ill ICU patients, and 26% of hospitalized non-ICU patients.[136] Patients at particular risk include patients after multiple trauma and cardiopulmonary bypass. In most such patients, ionized hypocalcemia is clinically mild ($[Ca^{2+}]$ 0.8 mmol/L to 1.0 mmol/L).

Initial diagnostic evaluation should concentrate on history and physical examination, laboratory evaluation of renal function, and measurement of serum phosphate concentration. Latent hypocalcemia can be diagnosed by tapping on the facial nerve to elicit Chvostek's sign or by inflating a sphygmomanometer to 20 mmHg above systolic pressure, which produces radial and ulnar nerve ischemia and causes carpal spasm known as Trousseau's sign. The differential diagnosis of hypocalcemia can be approached by addressing four issues: age of the patient, serum phosphate concentration, general clinical status, and duration of hypocalcemia.[137] High phosphate concentrations suggest renal failure or hypoparathyroidism. In renal insufficiency, reduced phosphorus excretion results in hyperphosphatemia, which down-regulates the 1α-hydroxylase responsible for the renal conversion of calcidiol to calcitriol. This, in combination with decreased production of calcitriol secondary to reduced renal mass, causes reduced intestinal absorption of calcium and hypocalcemia.[134] Low or normal phosphate concentrations imply vitamin D or magnesium deficiency. An otherwise healthy patient with chronic hypocalcemia probably is hypoparathyroid. Chronically ill adults with hypocalcemia often have disorders such as malabsorption, osteomalacia, or osteoblastic metastases. Clinical diagnosis of hypocalcemia in the patient receiving multiple transfusions, because of citrate excess, is often difficult. The only manifestation may be hypotension as a result of poor cardiac function, which is difficult to differentiate from hypotension as a result of hypovolemia.

The definitive treatment of hypocalcemia necessitates identification and treatment of the underlying cause (Table 9-22). Symptomatic hypocalcemia usually occurs when serum ionized $[Ca^{2+}]$ is <0.7 mM. The clinician should carefully consider whether mild, asymptomatic ionized hypocalcemia requires therapy, particularly in ischemic and septic states in which experimental evidence suggests that calcium may increase cellular damage.

Unnecessary offending drugs should be discontinued. Hypocalcemia resulting from hypomagnesemia or hyperphosphatemia is treated by repletion of magnesium or removal of phosphate. Treatment of a patient who has tetany and hyperphosphatemia requires coordination of therapy to avoid the consequences of metastatic soft tissue calcification.[138] Potassium and other electrolytes should be measured and abnormalities should be corrected. Hyperkalemia and hypomagnesemia potentiate hypocalcemia-induced cardiac and neuromuscular irritability. In contrast, hypokalemia protects against hypocalcemic tetany; therefore, correction of hypokalemia without correction of hypocalcemia may provoke tetany.

Mild, ionized hypocalcemia should not be overtreated. For instance, in most patients after cardiac surgery, administration of calcium only increases blood pressure[139] and actually attenuates the β-adrenergic effects of epinephrine.[139] In normocalcemic dogs, calcium chloride primarily acts as a peripheral vasoconstrictor, with transient reduction of myocardial contractility; in hypocalcemic dogs, calcium infusion significantly improves contractile performance and blood pressure (Table 9-23).[140] Therefore, calcium infusions should be of

TABLE 9-21

HYPOCALCEMIA: CLINICAL MANIFESTATIONS

Cardiovascular	**Respiratory**
Dysrhythmias	Apnea
Digitalis insensitivity	Laryngeal spasm
ECG changes	Bronchospasm
Heart failure	**Psychiatric**
Hypotension	Anxiety
Neuromuscular	Dementia
Tetany	Depression
Muscle spasm	Psychosis
Papilledema	
Seizures	
Weakness	
Fatigue	

ECG, electrocardiographic.

TABLE 9-22

HYPOCALCEMIA: ACUTE TREATMENT

Administer calcium
- IV: 10 mL 10% calcium gluconate[a] over 10 min, followed by elemental calcium 0.3–2.0 mg/kg/h
- Oral: 500–100 mg elemental calcium q 6 hours

Administer vitamin D
- Ergocalciferol, 1,200 μg/day ($T_{1/2}$ = 30 days)
- Dihydrotachysterol, 200–400 μg/day ($T_{1/2}$ = 7 days)
- 1,25-dihydroxycholecalciferol, 0.25–1.0 μg/day ($T_{1/2}$ = 1 day)

Monitor electrocardiogram

[a]Calcium gluconate contains 93 mg elemental calcium per 10-mL vial.
$T_{1/2}$, half-life.

TABLE 9-23

SERUM IONIZED [Ca^{2+}] CONCENTRATION AND HEMODYNAMIC VARIABLES ONE MINUTE AFTER CALCIUM ADMINISTRATION (5 mg/kg INTRAVENOUS BOLUS) INNORMOCALCEMIC AND HYPOCALCEMIC (PRODUCED BY CPD ADMINISTRATION) DOGS

	NORMOCALCEMIC		HYPOCALCEMIC		
	BASELINE	1 MIN	BASELINE	CPD	1 MIN
Ca^{2+} (mmol/L)	1.24 ± 0.04	1.47 ± 0.06[a]	1.24 ± 0.03	0.76 ± 0.03[a]	1.42 ± 0.22[b]
E_{lves} (mmHg/mL)	4.06 ± 1.00	2.16 ± 0.90[a]	5.03 ± 0.47	3.76 ± 0.61[a]	4.87 ± 0.64[b]
HR (beats/min)	159 ± 8	260 ± 9	154 ± 6	144 ± 7[a]	148 ± 6[a]
PAOP (mmHg)	9 ± 2	9 ± 1	7 ± 1	10 ± 2	9 ± 2
MAP (mmHg)	120 ± 6	137 ± 8[a]	157 ± 6	131 ± 6[a]	154 ± 6[b]
SVR (dyne/s/cm)	3,858 ± 458	4,347 ± 596[a]	4,067 ± 550	3,697 ± 479	4,548 ± 904
CO (L/min)	2.7 ± 0.4	2.7 ± 0.4	3.4 ± 0.2	3.0 ± 0.3	3.1 ± 0.4

Values are mean ± SEM (n = 6); E_{lves}, slope of the left ventricular end-systolic pressure–volume relationship; CPD, citrate-phosphate-dextrose; HR, heart rate; PAOP, pulmonary arterial occlusion pressure; MAP, mean arterial pressure; SVR, systemic vascular resistance; CO, cardiac output.
[a]P <0.05 vs. baseline.
[b]p <0.05 vs CPD.
From Mathru M, Rooney MW, Goldberg SA *et al*: Separation of myocardial versus peripheral effects of calcium administration in normocalcemic and hypocalcemic states using pressure-volume (conductance) relationships. Anesth Analg 77:250, 1993.

limited value in surgical patients unless there is demonstrable evidence of hypocalcemia.[140] Calcium salts appear to confer no benefit to patients already receiving inotropic or vasoactive agents.

The cornerstone of therapy for confirmed, symptomatic, ionized hypocalcemia ([Ca^{2+}] <0.7 mM) is calcium administration. In patients who have severe hypocalcemia or hypocalcemic symptoms, calcium should be administered intravenously. In emergency situations, in an averaged-sized adult, the "rule of 10s" advises infusion of 10 mL of 10% calcium gluconate (93 mg elemental calcium) over 10 minutes, followed by a continuous infusion of elemental calcium, 0.3 to 2 mg/kg/h (i.e., 3 to 16 mL/h of 10% calcium gluconate for a 70-kg adult). Calcium salts should be diluted in 50 to 100 mL D5W (to limit venous irritation and thrombosis), should not be mixed with bicarbonate (to prevent precipitation), and must be given cautiously to digitalized patients because calcium increases the toxicity of digoxin. Continuous ECG monitoring during initial therapy will detect cardiotoxicity (e.g., heart block, ventricular fibrillation). During calcium replacement, the clinician should monitor serum calcium, magnesium, phosphate, potassium, and creatinine. Once the ionized [Ca^{2+}] is stable in the range of 4 to 5 mg/dL (1.0 to 1.25 mM), oral calcium supplements can substitute for parenteral therapy. Urinary calcium should be monitored in an attempt to avoid hypercalciuria (>5 mg/kg per 24 hours) and urinary tract stone formation.

When supplementation fails to maintain serum calcium within the normal range, or if hypercalciuria develops, vitamin D may be added. Although the principal effect of vitamin D is to increase enteric calcium absorption, osseous calcium resorption is also enhanced. When rapid changes in dosage are anticipated or an immediate effect is required (e.g., postoperative hypoparathyroidism), shorter acting calciferols such as dihydrotachysterol may be preferable. Because the effect of vitamin D is not regulated, the dosages of calcium and vitamin D should be adjusted to raise the serum calcium into the low normal range.

Adverse reactions to calcium and vitamin D include hypercalcemia and hypercalciuria. If hypercalcemia develops, calcium and vitamin D should be discontinued and appropriate therapy given. The toxic effects of vitamin D metabolites persist in proportion to their biologic half-lives (ergocalciferol, 20 to 60 days; dihydrotachysterol, 5 to 15 days; calcitriol, 2 to 10 days). Glucocorticoids antagonize the toxic effects of vitamin D metabolites.

Hypercalcemia

Although ionized [Ca^{2+}] most accurately demonstrates hypercalcemia (ionized [Ca^{2+}] >1.5 mmol/L or total serum calcium >10.5 mg/dL), hypercalcemia customarily is defined in terms of total serum calcium. In hypoalbuminemic patients, total serum calcium can be estimated by assuming an increase of 0.8 mg/dL for every 1 g/dL of albumin concentration below 4.0 g/dL. Patients in whom total serum calcium is less than 11.5 mg/dL are usually asymptomatic. Patients with moderate hypercalcemia (total serum calcium 11.5 to 13 mg/dL) may show symptoms of lethargy, anorexia, nausea, and polyuria. Severe hypercalcemia (total serum calcium >13 mg/dL) is associated with more severe neuromyopathic symptoms, including muscle weakness, depression, impaired memory, emotional lability, lethargy, stupor, and coma. The cardiovascular effects of hypercalcemia include hypertension, dysrhythmias, heart block, cardiac arrest, and digitalis sensitivity. Skeletal disease may occur secondary to direct osteolysis or humoral bone resorption.

Hypercalcemia impairs urinary concentrating ability and renal excretory capacity for calcium by irreversibly precipitating calcium salts within the renal parenchyma and by reducing renal blood flow and GFR. In response to hypovolemia, renal tubular reabsorption of sodium enhances renal calcium reabsorption. Effective treatment of severe hypercalcemia is necessary to prevent progressive dehydration and renal failure leading to further increases in total serum calcium, because volume depletion exacerbates hypercalcemia.[141] Hypercalcemia occurs when calcium enters the extracellular volume more rapidly than the kidneys can excrete the excess. Clinically, hypercalcemia most commonly results from an excess of bone resorption over bone formation, usually secondary to malignant disease, hyperparathyroidism, hypocalciuric hypercalcemia, thyrotoxicosis, immobilization, and granulomatous diseases. Granulomatous diseases produce hypercalciuria and hypercalcemia because of conversion by granulomatous tissue of calcidiol to calcitriol.[134]

Malignancy may produce hypercalcemia either through bone destruction or secretion by malignant tissue of hormones that promote hypercalcemia.[142] Although weakness, weight loss, and anemia associated with primary hyperparathyroidism may suggest malignancy, these may result simply from the primary disease process. Hypercalcemia associated with granulomatous diseases (e.g., sarcoidosis) results from the production of calcitriol by granulomatous tissue. To compensate for increased gut absorption or bone resorption of calcium, renal excretion can readily increase from 100 to more than 400 mg/day. Factors that promote hypercalcemia may be offset by coexisting disorders, such as pancreatitis, sepsis, or hyperphosphatemia, that cause hypocalcemia.

Although definitive treatment of hypercalcemia requires correction of underlying causes, temporizing therapy may be necessary to avoid complications and to relieve symptoms. Total serum calcium exceeding 14 mg/dL represents a medical emergency. General supportive treatment includes hydration, correction of associated electrolyte abnormalities, removal of offending drugs, dietary calcium restriction, and increased physical activity. Because anorexia and antagonism by calcium of ADH action invariably lead to sodium and water depletion, infusion of 0.9% saline will dilute serum calcium, promote renal excretion, and can reduce total serum calcium by 1.5 to 3 mg/dL. Urinary output should be maintained at 200 to 300 mL/h. As GFR increases, sodium ions increase calcium excretion by competing with calcium ions for reabsorption in the proximal renal tubules and loop of Henle.

Furosemide further enhances calcium excretion by increasing tubular sodium. Patients who have renal impairment may require higher doses of furosemide. During saline infusion and forced diuresis, careful monitoring of cardiopulmonary status and electrolytes, especially magnesium and potassium, is required. Intensive diuresis and saline administration can achieve net calcium excretion rates of 2,000 to 4,000 mg per 24 hours, a rate eight times greater than saline alone, but still somewhat less than the rate of removal achieved by hemodialysis (i.e., 6,000 mg every 8 hours). Patients treated with phosphates should be well hydrated.

Bone resorption, the primary cause of hypercalcemia, can be minimized by increasing physical activity and initiating drug therapy.[131,143] Bisphosphonates, currently the first-line therapy for acute hypercalcemia, inhibit osteoclast function and viability. Bisphosphonates are the principal drugs for the management of hypercalcemia mediated by osteoclastic bone resorption.[144] Pamidronate, unlike earlier biphosphonates, does not appear to worsen renal insufficiency. More recently released biphosphonates include alendronate, risendronate, and zolecronic acid. Risendronate has been associated with less gastrointestinal morbidity than alendronate.[145,146] Zoledronic acid has the most rapid onset of action among the biphosphonates and prolongs the duration before relapse of hypercalcemia; however, zoledronic acid has been associated with compromised renal function.[143]

Other osteoclast-inhibiting agents used to treat hypercalcemia include mithramycin and calcitonin.[147] Mithramycin, a cytotoxic agent, lowers serum calcium primarily by inhibiting bone resorption, probably because of toxicity to osteoclasts. The hypocalcemic effect, usually seen within 12 to 24 hours following a single intravenous dose of 25 μg/kg, peaks at 48 to 72 hours, and persists for 5 to 7 days. Major toxic effects of mithramycin, more likely to occur in patients with renal insufficiency, include thrombocytopenia, nephrotoxicity, and hepatotoxicity. Calcitonin lowers serum calcium within 24 to 48 hours and is more effective when combined with glucocorticoids.[143] Usually calcitonin reduces total serum calcium by only 1 to 2 mg/dL. Although calcitonin is relatively nontoxic, more than 25% of patients may not respond. Thus, calcitonin is unsuitable as a first-line drug during life-threatening hypercalcemia.

Hydrocortisone is effective in treating hypercalcemic patients with lymphatic malignancies, vitamin D or A intoxication, and diseases associated with production by tumor or granulomas of 1,25$(OH)_2$D or osteoclast-activating factor. Glucocorticoids rarely improve hypercalcemia secondary to malignancy or hyperparathyroidism. In the near future, calcium receptor agonists may become the treatments of choice for suppressing primary and secondary hyperparathyroidism. Currently undergoing initial clinical trials, these agents also reduce inorganic phosphate concentration (Pi) and the calcium × phosphate produce.[148]

Phosphates lower serum calcium by causing deposition of calcium in bone and soft tissue. Because the risk of extraskeletal calcification of organs such as the kidneys and myocardium is less if phosphates are given orally, the intravenous route should be reserved for patients with life-threatening hypercalcemia or patients in whom other measures have failed.

Phosphate

Physiologic Role

Phosphorus, in the form of inorganic phosphate (Pi), is distributed in similar concentrations throughout intracellular and extracellular fluid. Of total body phosphorus, 90% exists in bone, 10% is intracellular, and the remainder, <1%, is found in the extracellular fluid. Phosphate circulates as the free ion (55%), complexed ion (33%), and in a protein-bound form (12%). Blood levels vary widely: the normal total Pi ranges from 2.7 to 4.5 mg/dL in adults.

Control of Pi is achieved by altered renal excretion and redistribution within the body compartments. Absorption occurs in the duodenum and jejunum and is largely unregulated. Phosphate reabsorption in the kidney is primarily regulated by PTH, dietary intake, and insulin-like growth factor.[149] Phosphate is freely filtered at the glomerulus and its concentration in the glomerular ultrafiltrate is similar to plasma. The filtered phosphate is then reabsorbed in the proximal tubule where it is cotransported with sodium.[149] Proximal tubular reabsorption of phosphorus occurs by passive cotransport with sodium.[150] Cotransport is regulated by phosphorus intake and PTH.[151] Phosphate excretion is increased by volume expansion and decreased by respiratory alkalosis.

Phosphates provide the primary energy bond in ATP and creatine phosphate. Therefore, severe phosphate depletion results in cellular energy depletion. Phosphorus is an essential element of second-messenger systems, including cAMP and phosphoinositides, and a major component of nucleic acids, phospholipids, and cell membranes. As part of 2,3-diphosphoglycerate, phosphate promotes release of oxygen from the hemoglobin molecule. Phosphorus also functions in protein phosphorylation and acts as a urinary buffer.

Hypophosphatemia

Hypophosphatemia is characterized by low levels of phosphate-containing cellular components, including ATP, 2,3-diphosphoglycerate, and membrane phospholipids. Serious life-threatening organ dysfunction may occur when the serum Pi falls below 1 mg/dL. Neurologic manifestations of hypophosphatemia include paresthesias, myopathy, encephalopathy, delirium, seizures, and coma.[152] Hematologic abnormalities include dysfunction of erythrocytes, platelets, and leukocytes. Because hypophosphatemia limits the chemotactic, phagocytic, and bactericidal activity of granulocytes, associated immune dysfunction may contribute to the susceptibility of hypophosphatemic patients to sepsis.[153] Muscle weakness and malaise are common. Respiratory muscle failure and myocardial dysfunction are potential problems of particular concern to anesthesiologists. Rhabdomyolysis is a complication of severe hypophosphatemia.[154]

Common in postoperative and traumatized patients, hypophosphatemia (Pi <2.5 mg/dL) is caused by three primary abnormalities in Pi homeostasis: an intracellular shift of Pi, an increase in renal Pi loss, and a decrease in gastrointestinal Pi absorption. Carbohydrate-induced hypophosphatemia (*refeeding syndrome*),[155] mediated by insulin-induced cellular Pi uptake, is the type most commonly encountered in hospitalized patients. Hypophosphatemia may also occur as catabolic patients become anabolic, and during medical management of diabetic ketoacidosis. Acute alkalemia, which may reduce serum Pi to 1 to 2 mg/dL, increases intracellular consumption of Pi by increasing the rate of glycolysis. Hyperventilation significantly reduces Pi and, importantly, the effect is progressive after cessation of hyperventilation.[156] Acute correction of respiratory acidemia may also result in severe hypophosphatemia. Respiratory alkalosis probably explains the hypophosphatemia associated with gram-negative bacteremia and salicylate poisoning. Excessive renal loss of Pi explains the hypophosphatemia associated with hyperparathyroidism, hypomagnesemia, hypothermia, diuretic therapy, and renal tubular defects in Pi absorption. Excess gastrointestinal loss of Pi is most commonly secondary to the use of Pi-binding antacids or to malabsorption syndromes.

Measurement of urinary Pi aids in differentiation of hypophosphatemia as a result of renal losses from that because of excessive gastrointestinal losses or redistribution of Pi into cells. Extrarenal causes of hypophosphatemia cause avid renal tubular Pi reabsorption, reducing urinary excretion to <100 mg/day.

Patients who have severe (<1 mg/dL) or symptomatic hypophosphatemia require intravenous phosphate administration (Table 9-24).[152,156] In chronically hypophosphatemic patients, 0.2 to 0.68 mmol/kg (5 to 16 mg/kg elemental phosphorus) should be infused over 12 hours. For moderately hypophosphatemic adult patients suffering from critical illness, the use of 15 mmol boluses (465 mg) mixed with 100 mL of 0.9% sodium chloride and given over a 2-hour period safely repletes phosphate.[157] The dosage is then adjusted as indicated by the serum Pi level, because the cumulative deficit cannot be predicted accurately. Oral therapy can be substituted for parenteral Pi once the serum Pi level exceeds 2.0 mg/dL. Continued therapy with Pi supplements is required for 5 to 10 days to replenish body stores.

Phosphate should be administered cautiously to hypocalcemic patients because of the risk of precipitating more severe hypocalcemia. In hypercalcemic patients, Pi may cause soft-tissue calcification. Phosphorus must be given cautiously to patients with renal insufficiency because of impaired excretory ability. During treatment, close monitoring of serum Pi, calcium, magnesium, and potassium is essential to avoid complications.

Hyperphosphatemia

The clinical features of hyperphosphatemia (Pi >5.0 mg/dL) relate primarily to the development of hypocalcemia and ectopic calcification. Hyperphosphatemia is caused by three basic mechanisms: inadequate renal excretion, increased movement of Pi out of cells, and increased Pi or vitamin D intake. Rapid cell lysis from chemotherapy, rhabdomyolysis, and sepsis can cause hyperphosphatemia, especially when renal function is impaired. Renal failure is the most common cause of hyperphosphatemia.[151] Renal excretion of Pi remains adequate until the GFR falls below 20 to 25 mL/min.

Measurements of BUN, creatinine, GFR, and urinary Pi are helpful in the differential diagnosis of hyperphosphatemia. Normal renal function accompanied by high Pi excretion (>1,500 mg/day) indicates an oversupply of Pi. An elevated BUN, elevated creatinine, and low GFR suggest impaired renal excretion of Pi. Normal renal function and Pi excretion less than 1,500 mg/day suggest increased Pi reabsorption (i.e., hypoparathyroidism).

Hyperphosphatemia is corrected by eliminating the cause of the Pi elevation and correcting the associated hypocalcemia. Calcium supplementation of hypocalcemic patients should be delayed until serum phosphate has fallen below 2.0 mmol/L (6.0 mg/dL).[134] The serum concentration of Pi is reduced by restricting intake, increasing urinary excretion with saline and acetazolamide (500 mg every 6 hours), and increasing gastrointestinal losses by enteric administration of aluminum hydroxide (30 to 45 mL every 6 hours). Aluminum hydroxide absorbs Pi secreted into the bowel lumen and increases Pi loss even if none is ingested. Hemodialysis and peritoneal dialysis are effective in removing Pi in patients who have renal failure.

TABLE 9-24

HYPOPHOSPHATEMIA: ACUTE TREATMENT

Parenteral phosphate, 0.2 mM–0.68 mM/kg (5–16 mg/kg) over 12 hours
Potassium phosphate (93 mg/mL of phosphate)
Sodium phosphate (93 mg/mL of phosphate)

Magnesium

Physiologic Role

Magnesium is an important, multifunctional, divalent cation located primarily in the intracellular space (intracellular magnesium ~2,400 mg; extracellular magnesium ~280 mg). Approximately 50% of magnesium is located in bone, 25% is found in muscle, and less than 1% of total body magnesium circulates in the serum. Of the normal circulating total magnesium concentration (1.5 to 1.9 mEq/L or 0.75 to 0.95 mmol/L or 1.5 to 1.9 mg/dL),[151] there are three components: protein bound (30%), chelated (15%), and ionized (55%), of which only ionized magnesium is active.

Magnesium is necessary for enzymatic reactions involving DNA and protein synthesis, energy metabolism, glucose utilization, and fatty acid synthesis and breakdown.[158,159] As a primary regulator or cofactor in many enzyme systems, magnesium is important for the regulation of the sodium-potassium pump, Ca-ATPase enzymes, adenyl cyclase, proton pumps, and slow calcium channels. Magnesium has been called an endogenous calcium antagonist, because regulation of slow calcium channels contributes to maintenance of normal vascular tone, prevention of vasospasm, and perhaps to prevention of calcium overload in many tissues. Because magnesium partially regulates PTH secretion and is important for the maintenance of end-organ sensitivity to both PTH and vitamin D, abnormalities in ionized magnesium concentration ([Mg^{2+}]) may result in abnormal calcium metabolism. Magnesium functions in potassium metabolism primarily through regulating sodium–potassium ATPase, an enzyme that controls potassium entry into cells, especially in potassium-depleted states, and controls reabsorption of potassium by the renal tubules. In addition, magnesium functions as a regulator of membrane excitability and serves as a structural component in both cell membranes and the skeleton.

Because magnesium stabilizes axonal membranes, hypomagnesemia decreases the threshold of axonal stimulation and increases nerve conduction velocity. Magnesium also influences the release of neurotransmitters at the neuromuscular junction by competitively inhibiting the entry of calcium into the presynaptic nerve terminals. The concentration of calcium required to trigger calcium release and the rate at which calcium is released from the sarcoplasmic reticulum are inversely related to the ambient magnesium concentration. Thus, the net effect of hypomagnesemia is muscle that contracts more in response to stimuli and is tetany prone.

Magnesium is widely available in foods and is absorbed through the GI tract, although dietary consumption appears to have decreased over several decades.[159] The distal tubule is the major site of magnesium regulation. Plasma [Mg^{2+}] regulates magnesium reabsorption through the Ca^{2+}/Mg^{2+}–sensing receptor, located on the capillary side of cells in the thick ascending limb.[160] While both magnesium and Pi are primarily regulated by intrinsic renal mechanisms,[158] PTH exerts a greater effect on renal loss of Pi.

Magnesium has been used to help manage an impressive array of clinical problems in patients who are not hypomagnesemic.[161] Therapeutic hypermagnesemia is used to treat patients with premature labor, preeclampsia, and eclampsia. Because magnesium blocks the release of catecholamines from adrenergic nerve terminals and the adrenal glands, magnesium has been used to reduce the effects of catecholamine excess in patients with tetanus and pheochromocytoma. Magnesium administration may influence dysrhythmias by direct effects on myocardial membranes, by altering cellular potassium and sodium concentrations, by inhibiting cellular calcium entry, by improving myocardial oxygen supply and demand, by prolonging the effective refractory period, by depressing conduction, by antagonizing catecholamine action on the conducting system, and by preventing vasospasm. Administration of magnesium reduces the incidence of dysrhythmias after myocardial infarction and in patients with congestive heart failure.[162] In humans with ischemic myocardium, magnesium prevented ischemic increases in action potential duration and membrane repolarization.[163] After acute myocardial infarction, intravenous magnesium administration decreased short-term mortality.[164] In addition, magnesium may be useful as treatment for a torsades de pointes ventricular dysrhythmia, even in normomagnesemic patients.[165]

Hypomagnesemia

The clinical features of hypomagnesemia ([Mg^{2+}] <1.8 mg/dL), like those of hypocalcemia, are characterized by increased neuronal irritability and tetany (Table 9-25).[166] Symptoms are rare when the serum [Mg^{2+}] is 1.5 to 1.7 mg/dL; in most symptomatic patients serum [Mg^{2+}] is <1.2 mg/dL. Patients frequently complain of weakness, lethargy, muscle spasms, paresthesias, and depression. When severe, hypomagnesemia may induce seizures, confusion, and coma. Cardiovascular abnormalities include coronary artery spasm, cardiac failure, dysrhythmias, and hypotension. Severe hypomagnesemia may reduce the response of adenylate cyclase to stimulation of the PTH receptor.[167] Hypomagnesemia can aggravate digoxin toxicity and congestive heart failure.

Rarely resulting from inadequate dietary intake, hypomagnesemia most commonly is caused by inadequate gastrointestinal absorption, excessive magnesium losses, or failure of renal magnesium conservation. Excessive magnesium loss is associated with prolonged nasogastric suctioning, gastrointestinal or biliary fistulas, and intestinal drains. Inability of the renal tubules to conserve magnesium complicates a variety of systemic and renal diseases, although advanced renal disease with a decreased GFR may lead to magnesium retention. Polyuria, whether secondary to ECV expansion or to pharmacologic or pathologic diuresis, may result in excessive urinary magnesium excretion. Various drugs, including aminoglycosides,

TABLE 9-25

MANIFESTATIONS OF ALTERED SERUM MAGNESIUM CONCENTRATIONS

MAGNESIUM LEVEL			
mg/dL	mEq/L	mmol/L	MANIFESTATION
<1.2	<1	<0.5	Tetany Seizures Arrhythmias
1.2–1.8	1.0–1.5	0.5–0.75	Neuromuscular irritability Hypocalcemia Hypokalemia
1.8–2.5	1.5–2.1	0.75–1.05	Normal magnesium level
2.5–5.0	2.1–4.2	1.05–2.1	Typically asymptomatic
5.0–7.0	4.2–5.8	2.1–2.9	Lethargy Drowsiness Flushing Nausea and vomiting Diminished deep tendon reflex
7.0–12	5.8–10	2.9–5	Somnolence Loss of deep tendon reflexes Hypotension ECG changes
>12	>10	>5	Complete heart block Cardiac arrest Apnea Paralysis Coma

From Topf JM, Murray PT: Hypomagnesemia and hypermagnesemia. Rev Endocr Metab Disord 4:195, 2003.

cis-platinum, cardiac glycosides, and diuretics, enhance urinary magnesium excretion. Intracellular shifts of magnesium as a result of thyroid hormone or insulin administration may also decrease serum [Mg^{2+}].

Because the sodium-potassium pump is magnesium dependent, hypomagnesemia increases myocardial sensitivity to digitalis preparations and may cause hypokalemia as a result of renal potassium wasting. Attempts to correct potassium deficits with potassium replacement therapy alone may not be successful without simultaneous magnesium therapy. Magnesium is important in the regulation of potassium channels. The interrelationships of magnesium and potassium in cardiac tissue have probably the greatest clinical relevance in terms of arrhythmias, digoxin toxicity, and myocardial infarction. Both severe hypomagnesemia and hypermagnesemia suppress PTH secretion and can cause hypocalcemia. Severe hypomagnesemia may also impair end-organ response to PTH.

Hypomagnesemia is associated with hypokalemia, hyponatremia, hypophosphatemia, and hypocalcemia. The reported prevalence of hypomagnesemia in hospitalized and critically ill patients varies from 11 to 61%, with the variability attributable to differences in measurement technique.[168] Development of a specific electrode to measure ionized [Mg^{2+}] has demonstrated an association between hypomagnesemia, use of diuretics, and development of sepsis.[168] Patients who develop hypomagnesemia while in intensive care have an increased mortality.[168] Of alcoholic patients admitted to the hospital, 30% are hypomagnesemic.[169] Serum [Mg^{2+}] may not reflect intracellular magnesium content. Peripheral lymphocyte magnesium concentration correlates well with skeletal and cardiac magnesium content.

Measurement of 24-hour urinary magnesium excretion is useful in separating renal from nonrenal causes of hypomagnesemia. Normal kidneys can reduce magnesium excretion to less than 1 to 2 mEq/day in response to magnesium depletion. Hypomagnesemia accompanied by high urinary excretion of magnesium (>3 to 4 mEq/day) suggests a renal etiology. In the magnesium-loading test, urinary Mg^{2+} excretion is measured for 24 hours after an intravenous magnesium load.[170]

Magnesium deficiency is treated by the administration of magnesium supplements (Table 9-26). One gram of magnesium sulfate provides approximately 4 mmol (8 mEq, or 98 mg) of elemental magnesium. Mild deficiencies can be treated with diet alone. Replacement must be added to daily magnesium requirements (0.3 to 0.4 mEq/kg/day). Symptomatic or severe hypomagnesemia ([Mg^{2+}] <1.0 mg/dL) should be treated with parenteral magnesium: 1 to 2 g (8 to 16 mEq) of magnesium sulfate as an intravenous bolus over the first hour, followed by a continuous infusion of 2 to 4 mEq/h. Therapy should be guided subsequently by the serum magnesium level. The rate of infusion should not exceed 1 mEq/min, even in emergency situations, and the patient should receive continuous cardiac monitoring to detect cardiotoxicity. Because magnesium antagonizes calcium, blood pressure and cardiac function should be monitored, although blood pressure and cardiac output usually change little during magnesium infusion. Treatment of hypomagnesemia during cardiopulmonary bypass decreased the incidence of postoperative ventricular tachycardia from 30 to 7% and increased the frequency of continuous sinus rhythm from 5 to 34%.[171]

During repletion, patellar reflexes should be monitored frequently and magnesium withheld if they become suppressed. Patients who have renal insufficiency have a diminished ability to excrete magnesium and require careful monitoring during therapy. Repletion of systemic magnesium stores usually requires 5 to 7 days of therapy, after which daily maintenance doses of magnesium should be provided. Magnesium can be given orally, usually in a dose of 60 to 90 mEq/day of magnesium oxide. Hypocalcemic, hypomagnesemic patients should receive magnesium as the chloride salt, because the sulfate ion can chelate calcium and further reduce the serum [Ca^{2+}].

TABLE 9-26

HYPOMAGNESEMIA: ACUTE TREATMENT

Intravenous Mg^a: 8–16 mEq (1–2 g $MgSO_4$) bolus over 1 hour, followed by 2–4 mEq/h (250–500 mg/h $MgSO_4$) as continuous infusion

Intramuscular Mg^a: 10 mEq q 4–6 hours

[a] $MgSO_4$: 1 g = 8 mEq Mg; $MgCl_2$: 1 g = 10 mEq Mg.

Hypermagnesemia

Most cases of hypermagnesemia ([Mg^{2+}] >2.5 mg/dL) are iatrogenic, resulting from the administration of magnesium in antacids, enemas, or parenteral nutrition, especially to patients with impaired renal function. Other rarer causes of mild hypermagnesemia are hypothyroidism, Addison's disease, lithium intoxication, and familial hypocalciuric hypercalcemia. Hypermagnesemia is rarely detected in routine electrolyte determinations.[166,172,173] Hypermagnesemia antagonizes the release and effect of acetylcholine at the neuromuscular junction. The result is depressed skeletal muscle function and neuromuscular blockade. Magnesium potentiates the action of nondepolarizing muscle relaxants and decreases potassium release in response to succinylcholine. The clinical features of progressive hypermagnesemia are listed in Table 9-25.[166]

The neuromuscular and cardiac toxicity of hypermagnesemia can be acutely, but transiently, antagonized by giving intravenous calcium (5 to 10 mEq) to delay toxicity while more definitive therapy is instituted.[166] All magnesium-containing preparations must be stopped. Urinary excretion of magnesium can be increased by expanding ECV and inducing diuresis with a combination of saline and furosemide. In emergency situations and in patients with renal failure, magnesium may be removed by dialysis.

References

1. Corey HE: Stewart and beyond: New models of acid-base balance. Kidney Int 64:777, 2004
2. Moviat M, van Haren F, van der Hoeven H: Conventional or physicochemical approach in intensive care unit patients with metabolic acidosis. Crit Care 7:219, 2003
3. Webster NR, Kulkarni V: Metabolic alkalosis in the critically ill. Crit Rev Clin Lab Sci 36:497, 1999
4. Khanna A, Kurtzman NA: Metabolic alkalosis. Respir Care 46:354, 2001
5. Scheingraber S, Rehm M, Sehmisch C *et al*: Rapid saline infusion produces hyperchloremic acidosis in patients undergoing gynecologic surgery. Anesthesiology 90:1265, 1999
6. Figge J, Mydosh T, Fencl V: Serum proteins and acid-base equilibria: A follow-up. J Lab Clin Med 120:713, 1992
7. Swenson ER: Metabolic acidosis. Respir Care 46:342, 2001
8. Gluck SL: Acid-base. Lancet 352:474, 1998
9. Moe OW, Fuster D: Clinical acid-base pathophysiology: Disorders of plasma anion gap. Best Pract Res Clin Endocrinol Metab 17:559, 2003
10. McFarlane C, Lee A: A comparison of plasmalyte 148 and 0.9% saline for intra-operative fluid replacement. Anaesthesia 49:779, 1994
11. Waters JH, Bernstein CA: Dilutional acidosis following hetastarch or albumin in healthy volunteers. Anesthesiology 93:1184, 2000
12. Carvounis CP, Feinfeld DA: A simple estimate of the effect of the serum albumin level on the anion gap. Am J Nephrol 20:369, 2000
13. Figge J, Jabor A, Kazda A *et al*: Anion gap and hypoalbuminemia. Crit Care Med 26:1807, 1998
14. Cooper DJ, Walley KR, Wiggs BR *et al*: Bicarbonate does not improve hemodynamics in critically ill patients who have lactic acidosis. A prospective, controlled clinical study. Ann Intern Med 112:492, 1990

15. Stacpoole PW, Wright EC, Baumgartner TG *et al*: A controlled clinical trial of dichloroacetate for treatment of lactic acidosis in adults. N Engl J Med 327:1564, 1992
16. Nahas GG, Sutin KM, Fermon C *et al*: Guidelines for the treatment of acidaemia with THAM. Drugs 55:191, 1998
17. Foster GT, Vaziri ND, Sassoon CSH: Respiratory alkalosis. Respir Care 46:384, 2001
18. Chesler M: Regulation and modulation of pH in the brain. Physiol Rev 83:1183, 2003
19. Christensen MS: Acid-base changes in cerebrospinal fluid and blood, and blood volumes changes following prolonged hyperventilation in man. Br J Anaesth 46:348, 1974
20. Martinu T, Menzies D, Dial S: Re-evaluation of acid-base prediction rules in patients with chronic respiratory acidosis. Can Respir J 10:311, 2003
21. Elisaf MS, Tsatsoulis AA, Katopodis KP *et al*: Acid-base and electrolyte disturbances in patients with diabetic ketoacidosis. Diabetes Res Clin Pract 34:23, 1996
22. Jaber BL, Madias NE: Marked dilutional acidosis complicating management of right ventricular myocardial infarction. Am J Kidney Dis 30:561, 1997
23. Prough DS, Bidani A: Hyperchloremic metabolic acidosis is a predictable consequence of intraoperative infusion of 0.9% saline. Anesthesiology 90:1247, 1999
24. Svensén C, Hahn RG: Volume kinetics of Ringer solution, dextran 70, and hypertonic saline in male volunteers. Anesthesiology 87:204, 1997
25. Hahn RG, Svensén C: Plasma dilution and the rate of infusion of Ringer's solution. Br J Anaesth 79:64, 1997
26. Brauer KI, Svensén C, Hahn RG *et al*: Volume kinetic analysis of the distribution of 0.9% saline in conscious versus isoflurane-anesthetized sheep. Anesthesiology 96:442, 2002
27. Connolly CM, Kramer GC, Hahn RG *et al*: Isoflurane but not mechanical ventilation promotes extravascular fluid accumulation during crystalloid volume loading. Anesthesiology 98:670, 2003
28. Harris HW, Jr., Strange K, Zeidel ML: Current understanding of the cellular biology and molecular structure of the antidiuretic hormone-stimulated water transport pathway. J Clin Invest 88:1, 1991
29. Levin AR, Gardner DG, Samson WK: Natriuretic peptides. N Engl J Med 339:321, 1998
30. Conte G, Bellizzi V, Cianciaruso B *et al*: Physiologic role and diuretic efficacy of atrial natriuretic peptide in health and chronic renal disease. Kidney Int 51:S28, 1997
31. Laragh JH: The endocrine control of blood volume, blood pressure and sodium balance: atrial hormone and renin system interactions. J Hypertens 4(suppl 2):S143, 1986
32. Silveira PF, Gil J, Casis L *et al*: Peptide metabolism and the control of body fluid homeostasis. Curr Med Chem Cardiovasc Hematol Agents 2:219, 2004
33. Baughman VL: Brain protection during neurosurgery. Anesthesiol Clin North America 20:315, 2002
34. Lanzino G, Kassell NF, Germanson T *et al*: Plasma glucose levels and outcome after aneurysmal subarachnoid hemorrhage. J Neurosurg 79:885, 1993
35. Rovlias A, Kotsou S: The influence of hyperglycemia on neurological outcome in patients with severe head injury. Neurosurgery 46:335, 2000
36. Van Den BG: How does blood glucose control with insulin save lives in intensive care? J Clin Invest 114:1187, 2004
37. Van Den BG, Wouters PJ, Bouillon R *et al*: Outcome benefit of intensive insulin therapy in the critically ill: Insulin dose versus glycemic control. Crit Care Med 31:359, 2003
38. Van den Berghe G, Wouters P, Weekers F *et al*: Intensive insulin therapy in critically ill patients. N Engl J Med 345:1359, 2001
39. Pittas AG, Siegel RD, Lau J: Insulin therapy for critically ill hospitalized patients: A meta-analysis of randomized controlled trials. Arch Intern Med 164:2005, 2004
40. Clement S, Braithwaite SS, Magee MF *et al*: Management of diabetes and hyperglycemia in hospitals. Diabetes Care 27:553, 2004
41. Yogendran S, Asokumar B, Cheng DCH *et al*: A prospective randomized double-blinded study on the effect of intravenous fluid therapy on adverse outcomes on outpatient surgery. Anesth Analg 80:682, 1995
42. Holte K, Klarskov B, Christensen DS *et al*: Liberal versus restrictive fluid administration to improve recovery after laparoscopic cholecystectomy: A randomized, double-blind study. Ann Surg 240:892, 2004
43. Brandstrup B, Tonnesen H, Beier-Holgersen R *et al*: Effects of intravenous fluid restriction on postoperative complications: Comparison of two perioperative fluid regimens—A randomized assessor-blinded multicenter trial. Ann Surg 238:641, 2003
44. Roberts I, Alderson P, Bunn F *et al*: Colloids versus crystalloids for fluid resuscitation in critically ill patients. Cochrane Database Syst Rev 18:CD000567, 2004
45. The Albumin Reviewers, Alderson P, Bunn F *et al*: Human albumin solution for resuscitation and volume expansion in critically ill patients. Cochrane Database Syst Rev 18:CD001208, 2004
46. Choi PT, Yip G, Quinonez LG *et al*: Crystalloids vs. colloids in fluid resuscitation: A systematic review. Crit Care Med 27:200, 1999
47. Moretti EW, Robertson KM, El Moalem H *et al*: Intraoperative colloid administration reduces postoperative nausea and vomiting and improves postoperative outcomes compared with crystalloid administration. Anesth Analg 96:611, 2003
48. Venn R, Steele A, Richardson P *et al*: Randomized controlled trial to investigate influence of the fluid challenge on duration of hospital stay and perioperative morbidity in patients with hip fractures. Br J Anaesth 88:65, 2002
49. Gan TJ, Soppitt A, Maroof M *et al*: Goal-directed intraoperative fluid administration reduces length of hospital stay after major surgery. Anesthesiology 97:820, 2002
50. Boldt J, Haisch G, Suttner S *et al*: Effects of a new modified, balanced hydroxyethyl starch preparation (Hextend) on measures of coagulation. Br J Anaesth 89:722, 2002
51. Gan TJ, Bennett-Guerrero E, Phillips-Bute B *et al*: Hextend, a physiologically balanced plasma expander for large volume use in major surgery: A randomized phase III clinical trial. Anesth Analg 88:992, 1999
52. Boldt J: Fluid choice for resuscitation of the trauma patient: A review of the physiological, pharmacological, and clinical evidence. Can J Anaesth 51:500, 2004
53. Zornow MH, Todd MM, Moore SS: The acute cerebral effects of changes in plasma osmolality and oncotic pressure. Anesthesiology 67:936, 1987
54. Kaieda R, Todd MM, Warner DS: Prolonged reduction in colloid oncotic pressure does not increase brain edema following cryogenic injury in rabbits. Anesthesiology 71:554, 1989
55. Warner DS, Boehland LA: Effects of iso-osmolal intravenous fluid therapy on post-ischemic brain water content in the rat. Anesthesiology 68:86, 1988
56. Zornow MH, Scheller MS, Todd MM *et al*: Acute cerebral effects of isotonic crystalloid and colloid solutions following cryogenic brain injury in the rabbit. Anesthesiology 69:180, 1988
57. Drummond JC, Patel PM, Cole DJ *et al*: The effect of the reduction of colloid oncotic pressure, with and without reduction of osmolality, on post-traumatic cerebral edema. Anesthesiology 88:993, 1998
58. Velasco IT, Pontieri V, Rochae Silva M, Jr. *et al*: Hyperosmotic NaCl and severe hemorrhagic shock. Am J Physiol 239:H664, 1980
59. Prough DS, Whitley JM, Taylor CL *et al*: Regional cerebral blood flow following resuscitation from hemorrhagic shock with hypertonic saline: Influence of a subdural mass. Anesthesiology 75:319, 1991
60. Prough DS, Whitley JM, Taylor CL *et al*: Rebound intracranial hypertension in dogs after resuscitation with hypertonic solutions from hemorrhagic shock accompanied by an intracranial mass lesion. J Neurosurg Anesth 11:102, 1999
61. Vassar MJ, Fischer RP, O'Brien PE *et al*: A multicenter trial for resuscitation of injured patients with 7.5% sodium chloride: The effect of added dextran 70. Arch Surg 128:1003, 1993
62. Cooper DJ, Myles PS, McDermott FT *et al*: Prehospital hypertonic saline resuscitation of patients with hypotension and severe traumatic brain injury: A randomized controlled trial. JAMA 291:1350, 2004
63. Chesnut RM: Avoidance of hypotension: Condition sine qua non of successful severe head-injury management. J Trauma 42:S4, 1997
64. Zaloga GP, Hughes SS: Oliguria in patients with normal renal function. Anesthesiology 72:598, 1990
65. Lipsitz LA: Orthostatic hypotension in the elderly. N Engl J Med 321:952, 1989
66. Wong DH, O'Connor D, Tremper KK *et al*: Changes in cardiac output after acute blood loss and position change in man. Crit Care Med 17:979, 1989
67. Perel A: Assessing fluid responsiveness by the systolic pressure variation in mechanically ventilated patients. Anesthesiology 89:1309, 1998
68. Stoneham MD: Less is more . . . using systolic pressure variation to assess hypovolaemia. Br J Anaesth 83:550, 1999
69. Boyd O, Grounds RM, Bennett ED: A randomized clinical trial of the effect of deliberate perioperative increase of oxygen delivery on mortality in high-risk surgical patients. JAMA 270:2699, 1993
70. Guest JF, Boyd O, Hart WM *et al*: A cost analysis of a treatment policy of a deliberate perioperative increase in oxygen delivery in high risk surgical patients. Intensive Care Med 23:85, 1997
71. Wilson J, Woods I, Fawcett J *et al*: Reducing the risk of major elective surgery: Randomised controlled trial of preoperative optimisation of oxygen delivery. BMJ 318:1099, 1999
72. Hayes MA, Timmins AC, Yau EHS *et al*: Elevation of systemic oxygen delivery in the treatment of critically ill patients. N Engl J Med 330:1717, 1994
73. Heyland DK, Cook DJ, King D *et al*: Maximizing oxygen delivery in critically ill patients: A methodologic appraisal of the evidence. Crit Care Med 24:517, 1996
74. Rivers E, Nguyen B, Havstad S *et al*: Early goal-directed therapy in the treatment of severe sepsis and septic shock. N Engl J Med 345:1368, 2001
75. Kern JW, Shoemaker WC: Meta-analysis of hemodynamic optimization in high-risk patients. Crit Care Med 30:1686, 2002
76. Balogh Z, McKinley BA, Cocanour CS *et al*: Supranormal trauma resuscitation causes more cases of abdominal compartment syndrome. Arch Surg 138:637, 2003
77. DiCorte CJ, Latham P, Greilich PE *et al*: Esophageal Doppler monitor determinations of cardiac output and preload during cardiac operations. Ann Thorac Surg 69:1782, 2000

78. Horowitz P, Kumar A: It's the colloid, not the esophageal doppler monitor (letter). Anesthesiology 99:238, 2003
79. Tierney WM, Martin DK, Greenlee MC *et al*: The prognosis of hyponatremia at hospital admission. J Gen Intern Med 1:380, 1986
80. Kashyap AS: Hyperglycemia-induced hyponatremia: Is it time to correct the correction factor? Arch Intern Med 159:2745, 1999
81. Gravenstein D: Transurethral resection of the prostate (TURP) syndrome: A review of the pathophysiology and management. Anesth Analg 84:438, 1997
82. Xu DL, Martin PY, Ohara M *et al*: Upregulation of aquaporin-2 water channel expression in chronic heart failure rat. J Clin Invest 99:1500, 1997
83. Fujita N, Ishikawa SE, Sasaki S *et al*: Role of water channel AQP-CD in water retention in SIADH and cirrhotic rats. Am J Physiol 269:F926, 1995
84. Ecelbarger CA, Nielsen S, Olson BR *et al*: Role of renal aquaporins in escape from vasopressin-induced antidiuresis in rat. J Clin Invest 99:1852, 1997
85. Kumar S, Beri T: Sodium. Lancet 352:220, 1998
86. Berendes E, Walter M, Cullen P *et al*: Secretion of brain natriuretic peptide in patients with aneurysmal subarachnoid haemorrhage. Lancet 349:245, 1997
87. Kroll M, Juhler M, Lindholm J: Hyponatremia in acute brain disease. J Intern Med 232:291, 1992
88. Wijdicks EFM, Ropper AH, Hunnicutt EJ *et al*: Atrial natriuretic factor and salt wasting after aneurysmal subarachnoid hemorrhage. Stroke 22:1519, 1991
89. Yamaki T, Tano-oka A, Takahashi A *et al*: Cerebral salt wasting syndrome distinct from the syndrome of inappropriate secretion of antidiuretic hormone (SIADH). Acta Neurochir 115:156, 1992
90. Kim JK, Summer SN, Wood WM *et al*: Osmotic and non-osmotic regulation of arginine vasopressin (AVP) release, mRNA, and promoter activity in small cell lung carcinoma (SCLC) cells. Mol Cell Endocrinol 123:179, 1996
91. Chung H, Kluge R, Schrier RW *et al*: Postoperative hyponatremia. A prospective study. Arch Intern Med 146:333, 1986
92. Fraser CL, Arieff AI: Fatal central diabetes mellitus and insipidus resulting from untreated hyponatremia: A new syndrome. Ann Intern Med 112:113, 1990
93. Ayus JC, Arieff AI: Symptomatic hyponatremia: Making the diagnosis rapidly. J Crit Illn 5:846, 1990
94. Ayus JC, Arieff AI: Brain damage and postoperative hyponatremia: The role of gender. Neurology 46:323, 1996
95. Gomola A, Cabrol S, Murat I: Severe hyponatraemia after plastic surgery in a girl with cleft palate, medial facial hypoplasia and growth retardation. Paediatr Anaesth 8:69, 1998
96. Arieff AI: Postoperative hyponatraemic encephalopathy following elective surgery in children. Paediatric Anesthesia 8:1, 1998
97. Steele A, Gowrishankar M, Abrahamson S *et al*: Postoperative hyponatremia despite near-isotonic saline infusion: a phenomenon of desalination. Ann Intern Med 126:20, 1997
98. Karmel KS, Bear RA: Treatment of hyponatremia: A quantitative analysis. Am J Kidney Dis 21:439, 1994
99. Sterns RH, Riggs JE, Schochet SS, Jr: Osmotic demyelination syndrome following correction of hyponatremia. N Engl J Med 314:1535, 1986
100. Brown WD: Osmotic demyelination disorders: Central pontine and extrapontine myelinolysis. Curr Opin Neurol 13:691, 2000
101. Laureno R, Karp BI: Myelinolysis after correction of hyponatremia. Ann Intern Med 126:57, 1997
102. Adrogué HJ, Madias NE: Aiding fluid prescription for the dysnatremias. Intensive Care Med 23:309, 1997
103. Kitiyakara C, Wilcox CS: Vasopressin V2-receptor antagonists: Panaceas for hyponatremia? Curr Opin Nephrol Hypertens 6:461, 1997
104. Hall J, Robertson G: Diabetes insipidus. Prob Crit Care 4:342, 1990
105. Ober KP: Endocrine crises: Diabetes insipidus. Crit Care Clin 7:109, 1991
106. Rowe JW, Shock NW, DeFronzo RA: The influence of age on the renal response to water deprivation in man. Nephron 17:270, 1976
107. McManus ML, Churchwill KB, Strange K: Regulation of cell volume in health and disease. N Engl J Med 333:1260, 1995
108. Ayus JC, Armstrong DL, Arieff AI: Effects of hypernatraemia in the central nervous system and its therapy in rats and rabbits. J Physiol 492:243, 1996
109. Adrogué HJ, Madias NE: Hypernatremia. N Engl J Med 342:1493, 2000
110. Chanson P, Jedynak CP, Dabrowski G *et al*: Ultralow doses of vasopressin in the management of diabetes insipidus. Crit Care Med 15:44, 1987
111. Halperin ML, Kamel KS: Potassium. Lancet 352:135, 1998
112. Williams ME, Gervino EV, Rosa RM *et al*: Catecholamine modulation of rapid potassium shifts during exercise. N Engl J Med 312:823, 1985
113. Mandal AK: Hypokalemia and hyperkalemia. In Saklayen MG (ed): The Medical Clinics of North America. Renal Disease, p 611. Philadelphia, WB Saunders, 1997
114. Rabinowitz L: Aldosterone and potassium homeostasis. Kidney Int 49: 1738, 1996
115. Rossier BC: Cum grano salis: The epithelial sodium channel and the control of blood pressure. J Am Soc Nephrol 8:980, 1997
116. Schreiber M, Schlanger LE, Chen CB *et al*: Antikaluretic action of trimethoprim is minimized by raising urine pH. Kidney Int 49:82, 1996
117. Weiner ID, Wingo CS: Hypokalemia consequences, causes, and correction. J Am Soc Nephrol 8:1179, 1997
118. Wahr JA, Parks R, Boisvert D *et al*: Preoperative serum potassium levels and perioperative outcomes in cardiac surgery patients. JAMA 281:2203, 1999
119. Suga SI, Phillips MI, Ray PE *et al*: Hypokalemia induces renal injury and alterations in vasoactive mediators that favor salt sensitivity. Am J Physiol Renal Physiol 281:F620, 2001
120. Gennari FJ: Hypokalemia. N Engl J Med 339:451, 1998
121. Gronert GA: Succinylcholine hyperkalemia after burns. Anesthesiology 91:320, 1999
122. Kuvin JT: Electrocardiographic changes of hyperkalemia. N Engl J Med 338:662, 1998
123. Wrenn KD, Slovis CM, Slovis BS: The ability of physicians to predict hyperkalemia from the ECG. Ann Emerg Med 20:1229, 1991
124. Nates JL, Lloyd PJ, Verklan T: Iatrogenic brain ischemia after head injury in USA Level I trauma centers. Crit Care Med 28:A52(83), 2000
125. Kim HJ, Han SW: Therapeutic approach to hyperkalemia. Nephron 92 Suppl 1:33, 2002
126. Allon M, Dunlay R, Copkney C: Nebulized albuterol for acute hyperkalemia in patients on hemodialysis. Ann Intern Med 110:426, 1989
127. Kemper MJ, Harps E, Müller-Wiefel DE: Hyperkalemia: Therapeutic options in acute and chronic renal failure. Clin Nephrol 46:67, 1996
128. Salem MM, Rosa RM, Batlle DC: Extrarenal potassium tolerance in chronic renal failure: Implications for the treatment of acute hyperkalemia. Am J Kidney Dis 18:421, 1991
129. Zaloga GP: Hypocalcemia in critically ill patients. Crit Care Med 20:251, 1992
130. Slomp J, van der Voort PHJ, Gerritsen RT *et al*: Albumin-adjusted calcium is not suitable for diagnosis of hyper-and hypocalcemia in the critically ill. Crit Care Med 31:1389, 2003
131. Edelson GW, Kleerekoper M: Hypercalcemia crisis. Med Clin North Am 79:79, 1995
132. Brown EM, Pollak M, Hebert SC: The extracellular calcium-sensing receptor: Its role in health and disease. Annu Rev Med 49:15, 1998
133. Brown EM, Pollak M, Seidman CE *et al*: Calcium-ion-sensing cell-surface receptors. N Engl J Med 333:234, 1995
134. Bushinsky DA, Monk RD: Calcium. Lancet 352:306, 1998
135. Rutledge R, Sheldon GF, Collins ML: Massive transfusion. Crit Care Clin 2:791, 1986
136. Zivin JR, Gooley T, Zager RA *et al*: Hypocalcemia: A pervasive metabolic abnormality in the critically ill. Am J Kidney Dis 37:689, 2001
137. Guise TA, Mundy GR: Evaluation of hypocalcemia in children and adults. J Clin Endocrinol Metab 80:1473, 1995
138. Sutters M, Gaboury CL, Bennett WM: Severe hyperphosphatemia and hypocalcemia: A dilemma in patient management. J Am Soc Nephrol 7:2055, 1996
139. Zaloga GP, Strickland RA, Butterworth JF IV *et al*: Calcium attenuates epinephrine's β-adrenergic effects in postoperative heart surgery patients. Circulation 81:196, 1990
140. Mathru M, Rooney MW, Goldberg SA *et al*: Separation of myocardial versus peripheral effects of calcium administration in normocalcemic and hypocalcemic states using pressure-volume (conductance) relationships. Anesth Analg 77:250, 1993
141. Bilezikian JP: Clinical review 51: Management of hypercalcemia. J Clin Endocrinol Metab 77:1445, 1993
142. Mundy GR, Guise TA: Hypercalcemia of malignancy. Am J Med 103:134, 1997
143. Ariyan CE, Sosa JA: Assessment and management of patients with abnormal calcium. Crit Care Med 32:S146, 2004
144. Berenson JR, Lichtenstein A, Porter L *et al*: Efficacy of pamidronate in reducing skeletal events in patients with advanced multiple myeloma. Myeloma Aredia Study Group. N Engl J Med 334:488, 1996
145. Kane S, Borisov NN, Brixner D: Pharmacoeconomic evaluation of gastrointestinal tract events during treatment with risedronate or alendronate: A retrospective cohort study. The American Journal of Managed Care 10:S216, 2004
146. Miller RG, Bolognese M, Worley K *et al*: Incidence of gastrointestinal events among bisphosphonate patients in an observational setting. Am J Manage Care 10:S207, 2004
147. Chan FKW, Koberle LMC, Thys-Jacobs S, Bilezikian JP: Differential diagnosis, causes, and management of hypercalcemia. Curr Probl Surg 34:449, 1997
148. Urena P, Frazao JM: Calcimimetic agents: Review and perspectives. Kidney Int Suppl S91, 2003
149. Murer H, Werner A, Reshkin S *et al*: Cellular mechanisms in proximal tubular reabsorption of inorganic phospate. Am J Physiol (Cell Physiol) 260:C885, 1991
150. Murer H, Markovich D, Biber J: Renal and small intestinal sodium-dependent symporters of phosphate and sulphate. J Exp Biol 196:167, 1994
151. Weisinger JR, Bellorin-Font E: Magnesium and phosphorus. Lancet 352:391, 1998
152. Peppers MP, Geheb M, Desai T: Hypophosphatemia and hyperphosphatemia. Crit Care Clin 7:201, 1991
153. Giovannini I, Chiarla C, Nuzzo G: Pathophysiologic and clinical correlates of hypophosphatemia and the relationship with sepsis and outcome in postoperative patients after hepatectomy. Shock 18:111, 2002

154. Knochel JP: Hypophosphatemia and rhabdomyolysis. Am J Med 92:455, 1992
155. Brooks MJ, Melnik G: The refeeding syndrome: an approach to understanding its complications and preventing its occurrence. Pharmacology 15:713, 1995
156. Paleologos M, Stone E, Braude S: Persistent, progressive hypophosphataemia after voluntary hyperventilation. Clin Sci (Lond) 98:619, 2000
157. Rosen GH, Boullata JI, O'Rangers EA *et al*: Intravenous phosphate repletion regimen for critically ill patients with moderate hypophosphatemia. Crit Care Med 23:1204, 1995
158. Whang R, Hampton EM, Whang DD: Magnesium homeostasis and clinical disorders of magnesium deficiency. Ann Pharmacother 28:220, 1997
159. Gums JG: Magnesium in cardiovascular and other disorders. Am J Health Syst Pharm 61:1569, 2004
160. Quamme GA: Renal magnesium handling: New insights in understanding old problems. Kidney Int 52:1180, 1997
161. McLean RM: Magnesium and its therapeutic uses: A review. Am J Med 96:63, 1994
162. Sueta CA, Clarke SW, Dunlap SH *et al*: Effect of acute magnesium administration on the frequency of ventricular arrhythmia in patients with heart failure. Circulation 89:660, 1994
163. Redwood SR, Taggart PI, Sutton PM *et al*: Effect of magnesium on the monophasic action potential during early ischemia in the in vivo human heart. J Am Coll Cardiol 28:1765, 1996
164. Teo KK, Yusuf S, Collins R *et al*: Effects of intravenous magnesium in suspected acute myocardial infarction: Overview of randomised trials. BMJ 303:1499, 1991
165. Tzivoni D, Banai S, Schuger C *et al*: Treatment of torsade de pointes with magnesium sulfate. Circulation 77:392, 1988
166. Topf JM, Murray PT: Hypomagnesemia and hypermagnesemia. Rev Endocr Metab Disord 4:195, 2003
167. Abbott LG, Rude RK: Clinical manifestations of magnesium deficiency. Miner Electrolyte Metab 19:314, 1993
168. Soliman HM, Mercan D, Lobo SS *et al*: Development of ionized hypomagnesemia is associated with higher mortality rates. Crit Care Med 31:1082, 2003
169. Elisaf M, Merkouropoulos M, Tsianos EV *et al*: Pathogenetic mechanisms of hypomagnesemia in alcoholic patients. J Trace Elem Med Biol 9:210, 1995
170. Hebert P, Mehta N, Wang J *et al*: Functional magnesium deficiency in critically ill patients identified using a magnesium-loading test. Crit Care Med 25:749, 1997
171. Wilkes NJ, Mallett SV, Peachey T *et al*: Correction of ionized plasma magnesium during cardiopulmonary bypass reduces the risk of postoperative cardiac arrhythmia. Anesth Analg 95:828, table, 2002
172. Whang R, Ryder KW: Frequency of hypomagnesemia and hypermagnesemia. Requested vs routine. JAMA 263:3063, 1990
173. Wong ET, Rude RK, Singer FR *et al*: A high prevalence of hypomagnesemia and hypermagnesemia in hospitalized patients. Am J Clin Pathol 79:348, 1983
174. Prough DS, Johnston WE: Fluid resuscitation in septic shock: No solution yet. Anesth Analg 69:699, 1989
175. Fried LF, Palevsky PM: Hyponatremia and hypernatremia. In Saklayen MG (ed): The Medical Clinics of North America. Renal Disease, p 585 Philadelphia, WB Saunders, 1997
176. Sterns RH: Vignettes in clinical pathophysiology. Neurological deterioration following treatment for hyponatremia. Am J Kidney Dis XIII:434, 1989
177. Feig PU: Hypernatremia and hypertonic syndromes. Med Clin North Am 65:271, 1981

CHAPTER 10 ■ HEMOTHERAPY AND HEMOSTASIS

JOHN C. DRUMMOND AND CHARISE T. PETROVITCH

KEY POINTS

1. In terms of the transfusion-transmitted infectious diseases, the American blood supply has never been safer than it is today.
2. The three leading causes of transfusion-related death in the United States are ABO incompatibility, transfusion-related acute lung injury (TRALI), and sepsis caused by bacterial infections.
3. In the setting of massive transfusion, assuming maintenance of isovolemia, critical dilution of clotting factors and platelets will occur after an average replacement of 140% and 230% of blood volume, respectively.
4. Coagulation factor and platelet replacement should be determined by laboratory assessment and/or observation of clinical coagulopathy and *not* EBL-driven formulas.
5. The red blood cell (RBC) transfusion "trigger" for most patients will lie between hemoglobin values of 7 and 10 g/dL.
6. Platelet administration thresholds relevant to anesthesiologists will lie usually between 50,000 and 100,000/uL.
7. Normal coagulation can be achieved with clotting factor levels of 20 to 30% of normal. Those levels can usually be achieved by administration of 10 to 15 mL/kg of fresh frozen plasma (FFP).
8. A patient who has received 10 to 12 units of group O RBCs should not be switched back to his or her own ABO group unless testing has been performed to confirm that significant titers of Anti-A or Anti-B antibodies are not present.
9. The classical, dual-cascade (intrinsic and extrinsic pathway) model of coagulation is an inadequate representation of coagulation, as it occurs in vivo.
10. In vivo, coagulation is initiated principally by contact of factor VII with extravascular tissue factor leading first to platelet activation followed by the generation of large amounts of thrombin by activated clotting factors acting on the phospholipid surface provided by activated platelets.
11. Von Willebrand's disease is the most common hereditary bleeding disorder and some form of the disease, which may be subclinical prior to surgery, is present in approximately 1% of the population.
12. Factors II, VII, IX, and X and Proteins C and S are dependent on vitamin K for their synthesis. Vitamin K deficiency occurs frequently in hospitalized patients because of dietary insufficiency, gut sterilization, and malabsorption. A high index of suspicion should be maintained.
13. As many as 5% of patients who receive heparin therapy for 5 days will develop heparin-induced thrombocytopenia/thrombosis. The clinical manifestations are more often the result of thrombosis and thromboembolism than thrombocytopenia.

The knowledge that the human immunodeficiency virus (HIV) is transmissible by blood generated public fear of transfusion and led to dramatic changes in the approach to the patient requiring blood products. While the transfusion-related risk of acquiring HIV is now vanishingly small, there remain numerous other hazards associated with blood products. The administration of blood products should be undertaken only with a complete understanding of those hazards and of the potential benefits. Accordingly, this chapter begins with a review of the risks associated with the administration of blood products, followed by a discussion of the factors that determine the necessity for the administration of the three most commonly used components, packed red blood cells (RBCs), fresh frozen plasma (FFP), and platelets, and then a discussion of conservation techniques for minimizing the necessity for transfusion.

The remainder of the chapter presents a description of the preparation of blood products, a discussion of the physiology of hemostasis, a description of tests of the hemostatic mechanism, and finally a review of common bleeding disorders, including discussion of the effects of pharmacologic agents on hemostasis.

THE RISKS OF BLOOD PRODUCT ADMINISTRATION

The risks can be subdivided into those of infectious and noninfectious etiologies. An excellent review has been provided by Kleinman et al.[1] Transfusion-transmissible infections, in particular viral infections, have had the highest profile and will therefore be addressed first. However, in reality, the morbidity and mortality associated with nonviral hazards is far greater.

Infectious Risks Associated with Blood Product Administration

The potentially transmittable diseases/agents are numerous and include several viruses: hepatitis A, B, C, D, and E; the human T-cell lymphotropic viruses (HTLV-1, HTLV-2); the human immunodeficiency viruses 1 and 2; cytomegalovirus; West Nile virus (WNV); the Epstein-Barr virus; parvovirus B19; the GBV-C virus (also called hepatitis G); transfusion-transmitted virus (TTV); the SEN virus; prions (Creutzfeldt-Jakob and variant Creutzfeldt-Jakob); Lyme disease; contaminating bacteria; parasites (malaria, Chagas disease, ehrlichiosis, babesiosis); and syphilis.[1] Several of these will not be considered further. While GBV-C, TTV, and SENV are transmitted by transfusion, they do not appear to cause clinical disease; the rate of transmission of Parvovirus B19 is very low and clinical disease is extremely infrequent;[1] there have been no reported instances of transfusion-transmitted Lyme disease and only one instance of ehrlichiosis.[2]

Estimates of the frequency of infectious agents in the North American blood supply are presented in Table 10-1. The rate of viral infectivity has decreased dramatically in the last two decades. It is in particular the advent of universal (in the United States) nucleic acid testing (NAT) for HIV and the hepatitis C virus (HCV) that has reduced the frequency of transmission of those agents to very low levels, that is, about one in two
1 million. Hepatitis B virus (HBV) remains the greatest risk, currently about 1/350,000 donor exposures.[3] All of these estimates are derived from the observed rates of seropositivity among donors and the statistical likelihood of administration of blood from donors whose infection is in the "window period" between contracting the virus and detectability by the available

TABLE 10-1

ESTIMATES OF THE RATE (PER DONOR EXPOSURE) OF TRANSFUSION-TRANSMITTED INFECTIOUS DISEASE

• Hepatitis B[3] (HBV)	1/350,000
• Hepatitis C[3] (HCV)	1/2,000,000
• Human immunodeficiency virus[3] (HIV)	1/2,000,000
• Human T-cell lymphotrophic virus[5] (HTLV)	1/2,900,000
• Bacterial sepsis/endotoxin reaction[5]	
RBC	1/30,000
Platelets	1/2,000

assays. Using NAT testing, the window periods for HIV and HCV are 13 and 12 days, respectively.[1] For HBV, using HbsAg testing, the window period is 59 days. A NAT test for HBV is available[4] and will probably be implemented by or before 2008.

Hepatitis C Virus

The significance of HCV is that, despite its commonly mild initial presentation, in 85% of patients it progresses to a chronic state with significant associated morbidity and mortality. Twenty percent of chronic carriers develop cirrhosis and 1 to 5% develop hepatocellular carcinoma.[6,7]

Hepatitis B Virus

It is estimated that only 35% of HBV-exposed patients will develop acute disease,[8] although approximately 1% will develop fulminant acute hepatitis. In approximately 85% of patients, the disease resolves spontaneously, 9% develop chronic persistent hepatitis, 3% develop chronic active hepatitis, 1% develop cirrhosis with or without chronic active hepatitis, and 1% develop hepatocellular carcinoma.[9] The current estimate of risk in the United States is 1 HBV infection per 350,000 donor exposures.

Hepatitis A Virus

Transmission of hepatitus A virus (HAV) by transfusion has been very rare. Blood banks screen for HAV by history only and there is no carrier state for this virus. The infectious period is limited to 1 to 2 weeks. The diagnosis depends on hepatitis antibody seroconversion.

Human Immunodeficiency Virus

The most feared complication of a blood transfusion is the transmission of HIV, the causative agent of the acquired immunodeficiency syndrome (AIDS). It is a retrovirus, so called because its propagation requires translation of RNA to DNA. Current screening tests are directed at both HIV 1 and HIV 2, though the latter has been an extremely infrequent cause of human disease. The incidence of transfusion-related HIV infection has fallen dramatically and progressively with the implementation of a series of serologic screening tests of donors, including, very recently, NAT testing. The current estimate of risk in the United States is 1 HIV infection per 1.5 to 2 million donor exposures. For reference, that risk was approximately 1:100 in the early 1980s and 1:400,000 in 1997.[10]

Human T-Cell Lymphotropic Virus

HTLV-1 and HTLV-2 belong to the same retrovirus family as HIV. The incidence of clinical disease resulting from transmitted virus appears to be very low. They are associated with T-cell leukemia and lymphoma rather than the generalized immunodeficiency of AIDS. In the United States, all donor units are screened for the presence of antibody to HTLV-I and HTLV-2.

Cytomegalovirus

Transfusion-associated CMV infections are usually benign and self-limited. However, CMV may cause serious, even fatal, infections in the immunocompromised. Patients at risk include premature neonates, solid organ and bone marrow transplant recipients, and those patients with severely depressed immune function. CMV pneumonia is an important infectious cause of death in allogenic bone marrow transplant recipients.[11] Leukoreduction reduces, but does not prevent, CMV transmission.[12] Restriction of immunocompromised patients to blood from CMV seronegative donors is required in many centers.

Parasitic Diseases

Transfusion-transmitted malaria is relatively common in regions where the disease is endemic but has been rare in the United States.[1] Because the parasite resides within the red cell, the hazard is associated almost exclusively with RBC transfusion. Chagas disease is caused by a protozoan (Trypanosoma cruzi) that is endemic to South and Central America (including Mexico). Significant clinical disease has been rare in North America and has occurred almost exclusively in immunocompromised transfusion recipients.

Bacterial Contamination of Blood Components

Bacterial contamination occurs at a much higher frequency (Table 10-1) than any of the other infections discussed in this section and is associated with substantial mortality.[13] Fatalities are estimated to occur at the rate of between 1: 1-6,000,000 transfused units[5], with the rate being substantially greater with platelet than RBC administration because the former are stored at room temperature and because platelet administration commonly involves pools of 6 to 10 units. A psoralen-based photochemical process that inactivates the DNA and RNA of bacteria (as well as viruses and protozoa) has recently shown efficacy without causing material impairment of platelet function and may serve to address this problem of bacterial contamination of platelets.[14] The source of the bacteria can be donor blood, donor skin flora, or contaminants introduced during collection, processing, and storage. Numerous Gram-positive and -negative organisms can occur in platelets. Goodnough et al identified the organisms in order of frequency as Staphylococcus aureus, Klebsiella pneumoniae, Serratia marcescens, and Staphylococcus epidermidis.[8] Only a limited number of bacteria, including Yersinia enterocolitica and certain Serratia and Pseudomonas species can grow at RBC storage temperatures.[1]

The patient who receives contaminated blood transfusion will rapidly experience some combination of fever, chills, tachycardia, emesis, and shock and may develop disseminated intravascular coagulation (DIC) and acute renal failure. The reactions are variable in severity and an index of suspicion should be maintained in order to distinguish these reactions from other major and minor transfusion reactions. The transfusion should be stopped immediately and blood cultures obtained.

West Nile Virus

WNV is a mosquito-borne flavivirus (as is dengue fever) that became epidemic, principally in Midwestern states, including Nebraska, Colorado, and Kansas, in 2002. Although the majority of infected individuals are either asymptomatic or develop only a mild illness, encephalitis/meningitis can occur and the death rate among confirmed cases is 5–10%.[3,15] Transmission by blood transfusion and organ transplantation has been confirmed. Fortunately, the window period between infection and clinical symptoms is short, at around 3 days, and the period of infectivity also appears to be relatively brief. Individual donor NAT testing for WNV is being performed in areas of high incidence.[3]

Prion-Related Diseases

Prions are the causative agents of Creutzfeldt-Jakob disease (CJD) and variant Creutzfeldt-Jakob disease (vCJD). The latter is the human disease caused by the agent responsible for bovine spongiform encephalitis (BSE). All three are fatal, degenerative neurologic diseases caused by an abnormally folded variant of a protein that is constitutively present. Between the beginning of the BSE epidemic in England in 1984 and February 2004, 156 cases of vCJD had been reported, with all but 10 occurring in the United Kingdom.[16] The risk of transfusion-related vCJD is undefined. CJD has never been known to have been transmitted by transfusion and there has been only a single reported case of apparently transfusion related vCJD.[17] However, the incubation period of vCJD may be as long as 6 years so the true transmission rate may be, as yet, underrecognized. Nonetheless, it is to be hoped that changes in animal husbandry practices combined with exclusion of donors who have sojourned in high-risk areas will minimize whatever risk exists.

Noninfectious Risks Associated with Blood Product Administration

The noninfectious risks associated with blood product administration, the majority of which are immunologically mediated, and their approximate incidences are presented in Table 10-2.

Immunologically Mediated Transfusion Reactions

Reactions to transfused blood products can occur as a result of the presence of antibodies that are either constitutive (e.g., Anti-A, Anti-B) or that have been formed as a result of prior exposure to donor RBCs, white blood cells, platelets, and/or proteins, or as a consequence of the effects of transfused white cells.

Reactions to RBC Antigens

Acute Hemolytic Transfusion Reactions. The most feared of the immune reactions is the immediate acute hemolytic

TABLE 10-2

THE NONINFECTIOUS ADVERSE REACTIONS ASSOCIATED WITH BLOOD PRODUCT ADMINISTRATION AND THEIR APPROXIMATE INCIDENCES[1,5,10]

ADVERSE REACTION	INCIDENCE
Acute hemolytic transfusion reactions	1/25,000–50,000
Delayed hemolytic transfusion reactions	1/2,500
Minor allergic reactions	1/200–250
Anaphylactic/-toid reactions	1/25,000–50,000
Febrile reactions	1/200
Transfusion-related acute lung injury (TRALI)	1/5,000
Graft-versus-Host Disease	Rare
Immunomodulation	(?) 1/1

transfusion reaction (AHTR) against foreign RBCs. Hemolysis of the donor RBCs often leads to acute renal failure, disseminated intravascular coagulation, and death. There are more than 300 different antigens on human red cells, but many are weak immunogens that usually do not elicit a clinically detectable antibody response. The antibodies that fix complement and commonly produce immediate intravascular hemolysis include anti-A, anti-B, anti-Kell, anti-Kidd, anti-Lewis, and anti-Duffy.[18]

The incidence of AHTRs is estimated to be on the order of 1 per 12,000 units transfused.[1] ABO incompatibility is among the three leading causes of transfusion-related deaths in the United States with a frequency in recent years slightly less than TRALI and narrowly greater than bacterial contamination (L. Holness, MD, personal communication, November 2004). In one jurisdiction (Canada), clerical/care provider errors were responsible for the majority of the incompatible blood transfusions that resulted in patient death.[1] It is an uncomfortable irony that, at the time of this writing, one of the principal hazards to the patient resides not in the blood supply per se, but rather in the process that delivers it to the patient.

When incompatible blood is administered, antibodies and complement in recipient plasma attack the corresponding antigens on donor RBCs. Hemolysis ensues. The hemolytic reaction may take place in the intravascular space and/or it may occur extravascularly within the endoplasmic reticulum. The antigen–antibody complexes activate Hageman factor (factor XII), which in turn acts on the kinin system to produce bradykinin. The release of bradykinin increases capillary permeability and dilates arterioles, both of which contribute to hypotension. Activation of the complement system results in the release histamine and serotonin from mast cells, resulting in bronchospasm. Thirty to fifty percent of patients develop DIC.[18]

Hemolysis releases hemoglobin into the blood. Initially it is bound to haptoglobin and albumin until the binding sites are saturated, then it circulates unbound in the blood until it is excreted by the kidneys. Renal damage occurs for several reasons. Blood flow to the kidneys is reduced in the presence of systemic hypotension and renal vasoconstriction. Free hemoglobin in the form of acid hematin or red cell stroma may precipitate in the renal tubules causing mechanical obstruction.[18] Antigen–antibody complexes may be deposited in the glomeruli. If the patient develops DIC, fibrin thrombi will also be deposited in the renal vasculature, further compromising perfusion.

The signs and symptoms of a hemolytic transfusion reaction include fever, chills, nausea, vomiting, diarrhea, and rigors. The patient is hypotensive and tachycardic (bradykinin effects) and may appear flushed and dyspneic (histamine). Chest and back pains result from diffuse intravascular occlusion by agglutinated red cells. The patient is often restless and has a headache and a sense of impending doom. Hemoglobinuria will occur as well as diffuse bleeding with the development of DIC. With renal failure, oliguria develops. During general anesthesia, many of the signs are masked. Hypotension and hemoglobinuria and diffuse bleeding be may the only clues that a hemolytic transfusion reaction has occurred. However, hypotension and bleeding are nonspecific and fairly common in the operating room environment and the diagnosis may not be suspected until hemoglobinuria is observed. A reasonable index of suspicion should be maintained during administration of RBCs to anesthetized patients in order to avoid critical delay in diagnosis.

If a reaction is suspected, the transfusion should be stopped and the identity of the patient and the labeling of the blood rechecked. Management has three main objectives—maintenance of systemic blood pressure, preservation of renal function, and the prevention of DIC. Systemic blood pressure should be supported by administration of volume, pressors, and inotropes as required. Urine output should be promoted by administration of fluids and the use of diuretics, either mannitol or furosemide, or both. Sodium bicarbonate can be administered to alkalinize the urine. There currently is no specific therapy to prevent the development of DIC. However, preventing hypotension and supporting cardiac output to prevent stasis and hypoperfusion, both of which contribute to the evolution of DIC, are important.

Laboratory tests should include (1) a repeat crossmatch and (2) a direct antiglobulin (Coombs) test. The direct antiglobulin test is the definitive test for an acute hemolytic transfusion reaction. It examines recipient RBCs for the presence of surface immunoglobulins and complement. Patient serum is also examined for the presence of antibodies that react with the donor cells. Serum haptoglobin level, plasma, and urine hemoglobin and bilirubin assays are usually performed. However, these are evidence only of hemolysis, not specifically of an immune reaction.[18] Laboratory tests to establish baseline coagulation status including platelet count, PT, aPTT, TT, fibrinogen level, and fibrin degradation products should be performed.

Examination of the patient's plasma after brief centrifugation for the pinkish discoloration caused by free hemoglobin is a simple, rapid screening test when a hemolytic transfusion reaction is suspected.[18] Hemolysis can be a result of other causes, including overheating prior to transfusion or inadvertent use of a hypotonic solution as a diluent. However, hemolysis should be assumed to indicate a hemolytic transfusion reaction until proven otherwise.

Delayed Hemolytic Transfusion Reactions. Numerous instances have been reported in which transfused red cells are rapidly eliminated from the circulation at a short interval (days) after an apparently "compatible" crossmatch. Many of these events are delayed hemolytic transfusion reactions (DHTRs).[19] These reactions occur when the donor RBCs bear an antigen to which the recipient has previously been exposed by either transfusion or pregnancy. Over time, the recipient antibodies fall to levels too low to be detected by compatibility testing. When re-exposure occurs, the recipient undergoes an anamnestic response and produces more antibody that eventually lyses the foreign RBCs. Typically the antibody-coated RBC is sequestered extravascularly and lysis occurs in the spleen and reticuloendothelial system. Because the red cell destruction occurs extravascularly, symptoms are less severe and the reaction is less likely to be fatal. Unlike AHTRs, which usually involve antibodies in the ABO system, DHTRs commonly involve antibodies against Rhesus (Rh), Kell, Duffy, and Kidd antigens. The frequency of delayed hemolytic reactions is reported to be 1 per 800 to 2,500 transfusions.[18,20]

Evidence of hemolysis is usually detected by the first or second week following transfusion. The reaction may be undetected or may be identified because of the combination of a low-grade fever, increased bilirubin with or without mild jaundice, and/or an unexplained reduction in hemoglobin concentration. The diagnosis is confirmed by a positive direct antiglobulin test (Coombs test). Serum haptoglobin is also decreased. The reaction is self-limiting and the clinical manifestations resolve as the transfused cells are removed from the circulation.[18]

Reactions to Donor Proteins

Minor Allergic Reactions. Allergic reactions to proteins in donor plasma cause urticarial reactions in 0.5% of all transfusions.[1,5,10] The reaction is almost always associated with the transfusion of fresh frozen plasma, but because there is a small volume of donor plasma present in other blood products

(RBCs, platelets), allergic reactions can occur with transfusion of these components as well. The patient may have itching, swelling, and a rash as a result of the release of histamine. These mild symptoms can be treated with diphenhydramine. Patients who experience severe urticarial reactions may benefit from the use of saline washed cells.[18]

Anaphylactic Reactions. Infrequently a more severe form of allergic reaction involving anaphylaxis will occur in which the patient experiences dyspnea, bronchospasm, hypotension, laryngeal edema, chest pain, and shock. Anaphylaxis precipitated by a transfusion is a rare, but potentially fatal, event. It occurs when patients with hereditary IgA deficiency who have been sensitized by previous transfusions or pregnancy are exposed to blood with "foreign" IgA protein. Treatment consists of discontinuation of the transfusion and epinephrine and methylprednisolone. Washed red cells, frozen deglycerolized red cells, or red cells from IgA-deficient donors should subsequently be used for these patients.[18]

White Cell–Related Transfusion Reactions

Febrile Reactions. Patients who receive multiple transfusions of RBCs or platelets often develop antibodies to the HLA antigens on the passenger leukocytes in these products. During subsequent RBC transfusions, febrile reactions may occur as a result of antibody attack on donor leukocytes. The febrile response occurs in about 1% of all red blood cell transfusions. Typically, the patient experiences a temperature increase of more than 1 degree centigrade within 4 hours of a blood transfusion and defervesces within 48 hours.[18] Patients may experience fever only but they may also develop chills, respiratory distress, anxiety,[21] headache, myalgias, nausea, and a nonproductive cough. Febrile reactions can be treated with acetaminophen. A leukocyte-mediated febrile transfusion reaction should be distinguished from a hemolytic transfusion reaction (direct Coombs test). Leukoreduction (see later) reduces or prevents these reactions.

Transfusion-Related Acute Lung Injury. Transfusion-related acute lung injury (TRALI) is a noncardiogenic form of pulmonary edema associated with blood product administration. It has been associated with administration of all blood components but occurs most frequently with RBCs (whole blood or packed cells), FFP, and platelets. The incidence is frequently estimated to be 1:5,000 units transfused. However, it is likely that TRALI is both underrecognized and underreported. TRALI, with a mortality of 5 to 8%, was the most common cause of transfusion-related death reported to the FDA for the years 2001 to 2003, although but it was only narrowly ahead of ABO incompatibility and bacterial contamination (L. Holness, MD, personal communication, November 2004).

Detailed reviews of TRALI are available.[22,23] In most instances, TRALI occurs when agents present in the plasma phase of donor blood activate leukocytes in the host.[24] Those agents are probably most often antileukocyte antibodies in donor blood formed as a result of previous transfusion or pregnancy. In some instances, the opposite reaction, aggregation of donor leukocytes and recipient antibodies, may be the cause when the recipient has been alloimmunized against WBC antigens. Because antigranulocyte antibodies can be demonstrated in most but not all instances of TRALI, it is suspected that biologically active lipids can also be the initiator of the pulmonary insult. Those lipids are thought to be derived from the breakdown over time of the membranes of the cellular elements in stored blood products. It also appears that TRALI requires the presence of some preexisting and predisposing inflammatory condition in the recipient, for example, sepsis, trauma, surgery.

The clinical appearance is very similar to the adult respiratory distress syndrome (ARDS), though the mortality rate is substantially less than that associated with the latter. Beginning within 6 hours after transfusion, and often more rapidly, the patient develops dyspnea, chills, fever, and noncardiogenic pulmonary edema. Chest x-ray reveals bilateral infiltrates. Severe pulmonary insufficiency can develop. Treatment is largely supportive. The transfusion should be stopped if the reaction is recognized in time. The patient should be given supplemental oxygen and ventilatory support as necessary, ideally using the same low tidal volume lung protective strategies that are employed in ARDS.[25] The pulmonary edema is noncardiogenic. Accordingly, diuretics are not warranted. Glucocorticoids have been administered but there are no data to support that practice.

Patients who have experienced this reaction previously may benefit from the use of washed PRBCs. Multiparous female donors have been identified as frequent sources of antileukocyte antibodies and it has been proposed that these "femmes fatales"[26] be excluded from the donor pool.[27]

Graft-versus-Host Disease (GVHD). Packed RBCs and platelet concentrates both contain a significant number of viable donor lymphocytes. When transfused ("transplanted") into immunocompromised patients, the donor lymphocytes may become engrafted, proliferate, and establish an immune response against the recipient. In essence, the engrafted lymphocytes reject the host.[28]

Patients at risk for GVHD include organ transplant recipients, neonates who have undergone a blood-exchange transfusion,[18] and patients immunocompromised by many other disease processes. GVHD typically progresses rapidly to pancytopenia and the fatality rate is very high. Transfusion-associated GVHD has also been reported in apparently immunocompetent patients when a genetic relationship exists between the donor and the recipient. In these circumstances, the recipient may share HLA antigen haplotypes with the donor lymphocytes. The patients, although immunologically competent, fail to reject the transfused cells because they do not recognize them as foreign. The transfused donor lymphocytes, however, recognize the host as foreign and a GVHD reaction takes place.[29] Because of this phenomenon, the American Association of Blood Banks has recommended that directed donations from first-degree relatives be irradiated to inactivate donor lymphocytes.

GVHD has been reported only after the transfusion of cellular blood components. It has not occurred following transfusion of FFP, cryoprecipitate, or frozen red cells.[29] Ideally, cellular blood products intended for immunocompromised patients and directed donor units from relatives should always be irradiated.[21] Leukoreduction may reduce the incidence of GVHD, but it does not prevent it.[1] Irradiation remains the
2 only effective means for preventing GVHD.[30]

Immunomodulation. Alteration of immune function has been associated with allogenic transfusion. The initial observations were of decreased rates of transplant rejection[31] and decreased rates of spontaneous abortion in patients who had received homologous transfusions. Alteration in immune surveillance was inferred. Numerous adverse effects of transfusion, presumed to reflect this attenuation of immunocompetence, have been reported, including increased mortality, accelerated recurrence of malignancy, increased risk of infection, and more rapid progression of HIV/AIDS.[32] The studies addressing cancer, infection, and mortality have been very thoroughly reviewed by Vamvakas et al. Those authors questioned the validity of the conclusions on the basis of the failure, in most reports, to control for compounding variables.[33] The issue, in short, is: patients with more severe illness are more likely to require transfusion and are at increased risk of complications independent of the transfusion. Subsequent reports of an adverse effect of allogenic blood, with allowance made for confounding variables, have appeared.[34]

TABLE 10-3

BENEFITS OF LEUKOREDUCTION

■ CONFIRMED BENEFITS
Decreased alloimmunization/platelet refractoriness in multiply transfused leukemics[35]
Prevention of febrile reactions to RBC transfusions[36]
Reduction of CMV transmission[12]
■ REPORTED BUT UNCONFIRMED BENEFITS[37]
Decreased postoperative infections
Decreased postoperative mortality[38]
Shortened hospitalization
Prevention of transfusion-related HIV acceleration[39]
Prevention of transfusion-related increase in tumor recurrence
Reduced incidence/severity of GVHD

Transfused white cells are thought to be the mediators of the immunity attenuating effects, although the precise mechanisms have not been defined. These observations have led to the development and application of techniques for leukocyte depletion of donor blood products.

Leukoreduction. Many countries including Canada, France, Portugal, and the United Kingdom and certain states and regions within the United States have already adopted the practice of leukoreduction of 100% of their blood supplies, and the entire United States is moving toward that objective. There are several well-confirmed benefits of leukoreduction including reduction in the development of alloimmunization and platelet refractoriness,[35] reduction in the incidence of febrile nonhemolytic transfusion reactions,[36] and reduction in (but not prevention of[12]) the transmission of CMV. However, selective leukoreduction could readily be applied for the patients to whom these benefits are relevant. The advocacy of universal leukoreduction is based on the premise that it might serve to accomplish the various benefits listed as "Reported but unconfirmed" in Table 10-3.

While many of the putative benefits are unconfirmed, additional reports of benefits attributable to leukoreduction are being added to the literature.[38,40] Although skepticism persists, the common view is that, in spite of the associated costs, because the hazards of leukoreduction are minimal, the possible benefits justify proceeding with universal leukoreduction.[41,42]

Universal leukoreduction, when fully implemented, will employ prestorage depletion to prevent the release of mediators from WBCs during storage. This is especially relevant to platelets, which are stored at room temperature. In the interim, clinicians using bedside filtering should appreciate that the available filters are less efficient at higher temperatures and filtering should therefore ideally be performed before blood warms to room temperature. Clinicians should also be attentive to the possibility of severe, apparently bradykinin-mediated, hypotension in patients who receive bedside filtered blood. The reaction appears to occur more frequently, though not exclusively, in patients receiving angiotensin converting enzyme inhibitors (which reduce breakdown of bradykinin).[43]

Other Noninfectious Risks Associated with Transfusion

Massive Transfusion

The rapid transfusion of large volumes of stored blood can have several consequences. Some of these are functions of properties of the blood itself, of the agents used to preserve and anticoagulate it, and of the biochemical reactions that occur during storage. There are other complications that are not unique to blood transfusions, but which may occur with the rapid transfusion of any large volume of fluid.

Hypothermia. The administration of one unit of PRBCs at 4 degrees centigrade will reduce the core temperature of a 70-kg patient approximately 0.25 degrees C. Hypothermia slows coagulation (as it does all enzymatically mediated reactions) and causes sequestration of platelets. At 29°C (at which temperature the risk of cardiac dysrhythmias is critical), PT and aPTT will increase approximately 50% over normothermic values and platelet count will decrease by approximately 40%.[44] Dysrhythmias may be seen at higher core temperatures if unwarmed blood is administered rapidly, in particular through central access catheters. While there is a general conviction that "cold patients bleed," there have been no quantitative correlations of temperature and bleeding in the clinical setting. Temperatures of 33°C are commonly used in elective neurosurgery without clinically apparent coagulopathy. However, Ferrara et al[45] reviewed the clinical course of 45 patients who received massive transfusion following trauma. The duration of hypotension was similar in patients who survived and those who did not. However, the degree of acidosis and hypothermia was more extreme in the nonsurvivors and the nonsurvivors developed coagulopathies despite adequate blood, plasma, and platelet replacement. In studies of this nature, it is difficult to separate the effects of the common clinical concomitants of hypothermia, for example, acidosis, shock, massive transfusion, massive tissue injury, from those of hypothermia per se. Furthermore, the significance of hypothermia may lie in the interaction with other variables. In spite of the ambiguity, hypothermia should be carefully avoided and aggressively corrected in the patient receiving massive transfusion. Accordingly, transfusions administered rapidly or in substantial volume should be warmed, to prevent hypothermia. With decreasing body temperature, cardiac output declines, tissue perfusion is impaired (as a consequence of both vasoconstriction and a left shifting of the O2-Hb dissociation curve), and metabolic acidosis may develop. Shivering on emergence can increase oxygen consumption by 400%. Hypothermia has been associated with increased postoperative morbidity and mortality including increased rates of postoperative infection.[46,47]

Volume Overload. Circulatory volume overload occurs when blood or fluid is transfused too rapidly for compensatory
3 fluid redistribution to take place.

Dilutional Coagulopathy. Administration of large volumes of fluid deficient in platelets and clotting factors will predictably lead to the development of a coagulopathy as a consequence of dilution. There has been considerable discussion of whether, in the face of massive transfusion of blood products, patients will first manifest deficiencies of platelets or clotting factors. The initial conclusion was that thrombocytopenia would develop first. In retrospect, that clinical conclusion may have been the consequence of a wider use of whole blood than prevails today. In spite of the lability of factors V and VIII, sufficient concentrations of these factors probably remain in banked whole blood to maintain coagulation function even in the face of very large transfusions. The same is probably *not* true when patients receive only the small residual plasma volume present with packed RBCs. Investigations of patients receiving large volume isovolemic transfusions suggest that clinically significant dilution of fibrinogen; factors II, V, and VIII; and platelets will occur after volume exchanges of approximately 140%, 200 to 230%, and 230% (i.e., 1.4, 2, and 2.3 blood volumes), respectively.[48] Resuscitation from hypovolemia will result in reaching these thresholds at smaller percentage volume exchanges. However, calculations of this nature should not be used as a guide to blood product administration but merely as a means of

anticipating clinically relevant occurrences. The decision to administer fresh frozen plasma or platelets will depend on clin-
4 ical and laboratory evidence of coagulopathy.

Decreases in 2,3-Diphosphoglycerate (2,3-DPG). Storage of red blood cells is associated with a progressive decrease in intracellular ATP and 2,3-DPG with a resultant left shifting of the O2-Hb dissociation curve. Accordingly, transfusion of the 2,3-DPG–depleted blood while increasing the patient's hemoglobin value will result in less efficient oxygen delivery than would occur with native hemoglobin at the same hematocrit. After transfusion, 2,3-DPG levels return toward normal over 12 to 24 hours.[49]

Acid-Base Changes. When CPD solution is added to a unit of freshly drawn blood, pH decreases to approximately 7.0 to 7.1. Further reduction of pH will occur during storage as a consequence of ongoing metabolism of glucose to lactate. At the end of 21 days, the pH may be as low as 6.9, but much of this is the result of the production of CO2 that is rapidly eliminated following the transfusion. Whether rapid infusion of this acidic bank blood leads to metabolic acidosis is debated. In the past, some clinicians have administered sodium bicarbonate empirically to patients on a fixed schedule (e.g., sodium bicarbonate 44.6 mEq after each 5 units of bank blood infused). Others contend that the citrate from the CPD solution is metabolized by the patient to endogenous bicarbonate and that acid-base disturbance is therefore self-correcting. Clinically, in the injured patient who is hypotensive and poorly perfused and has inadequate tissue oxygenation, it will be difficult to differentiate what portion of the metabolic acidosis is because of rapid transfusion and what portion is because of the production of lactic acid.[46] The appropriate course is to base bicarbonate therapy on blood gas analysis.

Hyperkalemia. During storage, potassium moves out of the RBCs, in part to maintain electrochemical neutrality as hydrogen ions generated during storage redistribute. The potassium concentration in plasma may reach levels variously reported to be between 17 and 24 mEq/L at 21 to 35 days or 19 to 35 mEq/L in blood stored for 21 days. Hazard exists if large volumes of stored blood are administered rapidly. Rates in excess of 90 to 120 mL/min have been associated with hyperkalemia. Furthermore, while there are only 20 to 60 mL of plasma in a unit of packed RBCs, contemporary infusion devices allow blood to be transfused at rates of 500 to 1,000 mL/min. At these infusion rates, critical hyperkalemia can occur and intraoperative arrests have been documented.[50] ECG changes associated with hyperkalemia include peaked T waves, a prolonged PR interval, and a widened QRS complex. If ECG changes are observed, the transfusion should be stopped and intravenous calcium should be administered. Bicarbonate, dextrose, and insulin may also be appropriate according to the severity of the episode.

Citrate Intoxication. Commonly used additive solutions contain citrate, which anticoagulates by chelation of ionized calcium. When large volumes of stored blood (> one blood volume) are administered rapidly, the citrate can cause a temporary reduction in ionized calcium levels. Citrate is normally metabolized efficiently by the liver and decreased ionized calcium levels should not occur unless the rate of transfusion exceeds 1 mL/kg per minute or about 1 unit of blood per 5 minutes in an average-sized adult. Note that the now common Additive Solution (AS) preservative blood has a much smaller citrate content than citrate-phosphate-dextrose-adenine (CPDA) blood. However, most of the citrate administered during massive transfusion is in the FFP rather than the PRBCs. Impaired liver function or perfusion will lower the rate threshold for developing citrate intoxication. Note that critical cardiac consequences occur before hypocalcemia has significant implications for coagulation. Signs of citrate intoxication (hypocalcemia) include: hypotension, narrow pulse pressure, and elevated intraventricular end-diastolic pressure and central venous pressure, prolonged Q-T interval, widened QRS complexes, and flattened T waves.

Microaggregate Delivery. Stored blood contains microaggregates. Platelet aggregates form during the second to fifth day of storage and after approximately 10 days, larger aggregates composed of fibrin, degenerated white cells, and platelets appear. Macroaggregates of RBCs also develop. Standard fluid administration sets contain 170 micron filters, which will remove these larger "clots." Micropore filters, typically with a 40-micron pore size, have been advocated but both their efficiency at removing the microaggregates and the significance to patient well-being is uncertain. Microaggregates have been implicated in the pathogenesis of pulmonary insufficiency and the development of ARDS, which often follows large volume transfusions (defined as >10 to 12 units in 24 hrs).[21,51] However, the available data do not confirm this suspicion and suggest that pulmonary injury and the occurrence of ARDS are more often related to the type of injury and the magnitude or severity of the injury than to the volume of blood transfused. Hypotension and sepsis may play a much greater role in the development of ARDS than microaggregates and some of what has been attributed to microaggregates may in fact be TRALI. A practical consideration nonetheless frequently prompts clinicians to introduce a micropore filter between the blood unit and the administration set. Unfiltered blood may clog the 170-micron filter of the standard set and it is less time-consuming to change the 40-micron filter periodically, for example, after every fourth RBC unit, than to exchange the entire administration set.

RBCs are frequently diluted with crystalloid solutions to increase the rate at which the blood can be transfused. Normal saline is commonly recommended in preference to lactated Ringer's solution (LR). In fact, the amount of citrate present in stored blood is more than sufficient to bind the small amounts of calcium in the 100 to 300 cc of LR typically used for dilution.[52] There is no evidence that any clinically significant sequelae have resulted from the use of LR as an RBC diluent.[51]

BLOOD PRODUCTS AND TRANSFUSION THRESHOLDS

Red Blood Cells

The question level of what hemoglobin/hematocrit level justifies the risks associated with the administration of blood has been widely discussed (Table 10-4). The once all but inviolable "10 to 30" rule has been abandoned. Experience with several patient subpopulations (renal failure, military casualties, Jehovah's Witnesses) and systematic study has revealed that considerable greater degrees of anemia can be well tolerated

TABLE 10-4

HAZARDS ASSOCIATED WITH MASSIVE TRANSFUSION

Hypothermia
Volume overload
Dilutional coagulopathy
Reduced O_2 carrying capacity (decreased 2,3-DPG)
Metabolic acidosis
Hyperkalemia
Citrate intoxication
Microaggregate delivery

TABLE 10-5

CONDITIONS THAT MAY DECREASE TOLERANCE FOR ANEMIA AND INFLUENCE THE RBC TRANSFUSION THRESHOLD

Increased oxygen demand
Hyperthermia
Hyperthyroidism
Sepsis
Pregnancy
Limited ability to increase cardiac output
Coronary artery disease
Myocardial dysfunction (infarction, cardiomyopathy)
Beta adrenergic blockade
Inability to redistribute CO
Low SVR states
—Sepsis
—Postcardiopulmonary bypass
—Occlusive vascular disease (cerebral, coronary)
Left shift of the O_2–Hb curve
Alkalosis
Hypothermia
Abnormal hemoglobins
Presence of recently transfused Hb (decreased 2,3-DPG)
HbS (sickle cell disease)
Acute anemia (limited 2,3-DPG compensation)
Impaired oxygenation
Pulmonary disease
High altitude
Ongoing or imminent blood loss
Traumatic/surgical bleeding
Placenta previa or accreta, abruption, uterine atony
Clinical coagulopathy

and that, in many situations, morbidity and mortality rates did not increase until hemoglobin levels fell below 7 g/dL.[53,54] The contemporary transfusion trigger for general medical-surgical patients is now 21%/7.0 g/dL (Hgb/Hct). However, there is evidence that the threshold for patients with cardiac disease should be higher.[53] That evidence includes a well-conducted study supporting a threshold of 30%/10 g/dL (Hgb/Hct) in patients who have suffered a recent acute myocardial infarction[55] and an observational study suggesting better outcomes in patients with several cardiac diagnoses (cardiac and vascular surgery, ischemic heart disease, dysrhythmias) above a threshold of 9.5 g/dL.[56] *The Practice Guidelines for Blood Component Therapy* developed by the American Society of Anesthesiologists (ASA) state that "red blood cell transfusion is rarely indicated when the hemoglobin concentration is greater than 10 g/dL and is almost always indicated when it is less than 6 g/dL. The indications for autologous transfusion my be more liberal than for allogeneic (homologous) transfusion."[57]

The clinician's responsibility is to anticipate, on a patient-
5 by-patient basis, the minimum hemoglobin level (probably in the range of 7 to 10 g/dL) that will avoid organ damage as a result of oxygen deprivation. Determining this individual transfusion trigger requires reference to the many elements of patient condition that determine demand for the delivery of oxygen and the physiologic reserve (Table 10-5). Ultimately the decision to transfuse red blood cells should be made based on the clinical judgment that the oxygen-carrying capacity of the blood must be increased to prevent oxygen consumption from outstripping oxygen delivery.

Compensatory Mechanisms during Anemia

When anemia develops, but blood volume is maintained (isovolemic hemodilution), four compensatory mechanisms serve to maintain oxygen delivery: (1) an increase in cardiac output, (2) a redistribution of blood flow to organs with greater oxygen requirements, (3) increases in the extraction ratios of some vascular beds, and (4) alteration of oxygen–hemoglobin binding to allow the hemoglobin to deliver oxygen at lower oxygen tensions.

1. Increased cardiac output.
   With isovolemic hemodilution, cardiac output increases primarily because of an increase in stroke volume brought about by reductions in systemic vascular resistance (SVR). There are two principal determinants of SVR: vascular tone and the viscosity of blood.[58] As hematocrit decreases, reduction of blood viscosity decreases SVR. This decrease in SVR increases stroke volume and consequently cardiac output and blood flow to the tissues. Over a wide range of hematocrits, isovolemic hemodilution is self-correcting. Linear decreases in the oxygen carrying capacity of the blood are matched by improvements in oxygen transport. Because oxygen transport is optimal at hematocrits of 30%, oxygen delivery may remain constant between the hematocrits of 45 and 30%.[58] Further reductions in hematocrit are accompanied by increases in cardiac output, which reach 180% of control as the hematocrit approaches 20%. The exact hemoglobin value at which cardiac output rises varies among individuals and is influenced by age and whether the anemia is acute or develops slowly.[59]
2. Redistribution of cardiac output.
   With isovolemic hemodilution, blood flow to the tissues increases but this increased blood flow is not distributed equally to all tissue beds. Organs with higher extraction ratios (brain and heart) receive disproportionately more of the increase in blood flow than organs with low extraction ratios (muscle, skin, viscera).
   The redistribution of blood flow to the coronary circulation is the principal means by which the healthy heart compensates for anemia.[58] Coronary blood flow may increase by 400 to 600%. Because the heart under basal conditions already has a high extraction ratio (between 50 and 70% vs. 30% in most tissues) and the primary compensation for anemia involves cardiac work (increasing CO), the heart must rely on redistributing blood flow to increase oxygen supply.[60] These factors make the heart the organ at greatest risk under conditions of isovolemic hemodilution. When the heart can no longer increase either cardiac output or coronary blood flow, the limits of isovolemic hemodilution are reached. Further decreases in oxygen delivery will result in myocardial injury.
3. Increased oxygen extraction.
   Increasing oxygen extraction ratio (ER) is thought to play an important adaptive role when the normovolemic hematocrit drops below 25%. Increased oxygen extraction in multiple tissue beds leads to an increase in the whole body ER and consequently to a decrease in mixed venous oxygen saturation. One investigation demonstrated that as hematocrit decreases to 15%, whole body oxygen ER increases from 38 to 60%, and the SvO2 decreases from 70 to 50% or less.[46] Some organs (brain and heart) already have high extraction ratios under basal conditions and have a limited capacity to increase oxygen delivery by this mechanism. The heart, under basal conditions, extracts between 55 and 70% of the oxygen delivered.[61,62] In contrast, in kidney and skin, the ER is 7 to 10%. In clinical practice, we cannot measure the extraction ratios of the various organs. Because the heart has the highest ER, it is the organ at greatest risk under conditions of normovolemic anemia.[46]

4. Changes in oxygen–hemoglobin affinity.

The affinity of hemoglobin for oxygen is described by the sigmoid shaped oxygen–hemoglobin dissociation curve. This curve relates the partial pressure of oxygen in the blood to the percentage saturation of the hemoglobin molecule with oxygen. The partial pressure of oxygen at which the hemoglobin molecule is 50% saturated with oxygen and 50% unsaturated is termed the P50. P50 for normal adult hemoglobin at 37 degrees C and a pH of 7.4 is 27 mmHg. Changes in acid-base status or temperature can shift the oxyhemoglobin dissociation curve to the left or right, lowering or raising the P50 value respectively. When the curve is shifted to the left as with hypothermia or alkalosis, the P50 is lowered. With a lower P50, the hemoglobin molecule is more "stingy" and requires lower oxygen partial pressures to release oxygen to the tissues, that is, the hemoglobin molecule does not release 50% of its oxygen until an ambient PO_2 less than 27 mmHg is reached. This may impair tissue oxygenation. By contrast, right shifting of the oxygen-hemoglobin dissociation curve, as occurs with increases in temperature or acidosis, results in an increase of P50, decreased hemoglobin affinity for the oxygen molecule, and release of oxygen to tissues at higher partial pressures of oxygen.

When anemia develops slowly, the affinity of hemoglobin for oxygen may be decreased, that is, the curve is right shifted, as a result of the accumulation in red blood cells of 2,3-phosphoglycerate (2,3-DPG). Synthesis of supranormal levels of 2,3-DPG begins at a Hb of 9 g/dL. At Hb levels of 6.5 the curve is shifted more prominently. Stored red blood cells become depleted of 2,3-DPG. Temperature reduction and storage-related pH decreases also reduce the P50 of stored blood. These changes, however, are reversed in vivo but the resynthesis of 2,3-DPG by red blood cells may require from 12 to 36 hours.[60]

Isovolemic Anemia versus Acute Blood Loss

Although the same compensatory mechanisms are operative in acute and chronic anemias, they have different degrees of importance and occur at different levels of hemoglobin. With acute blood loss, hypovolemia induces stimulation of the adrenergic nervous system, leading to vasoconstriction and tachycardia. Increased cardiac output does not contribute. In chronically anemic patients, cardiac output increases as the hemoglobin decreases to approximately 7–8 g/dL.[59] In these patients, the accumulation of 2,3-DPG in the red blood cells, thereby increasing the P50 of Hb, is the important first mechanism for compensation.[63]

Platelets

While published guidelines for platelet administration are available, there is once again a substantial requirement for clinician judgment. The indications for platelet administration presented in Table 10-6 are an amalgam of recommendations presented by the ASA in 1996 and the British Committee for Standards in Haematology in 2003.[57,64]

Table 10-6 makes it apparent that the platelet administration thresholds that will most often be relevant to anesthesiologists will lie between 50,000 and 100,000/uL. The threshold within that range at which platelets are administered should be based on the likelihood of the intended procedure to cause bleeding, the hazard of bleeding should it occur. For example, intracranial neurosurgery > peripheral orthopaedics and

TABLE 10-6

INDICATIONS FOR THE ADMINISTRATION OF PLATELETS

Nonbleeding patients without other abnormalities of hemostasis[65]	<10,000/uL
Lumbar puncture, epidural anesthesia, central line placement, endoscopy with biopsy, liver biopsy, or laparotomy in patients without other abnormalities of hemostasis	<50,000/uL
Intended procedures in which closed cavity bleeding might be especially hazardous, for example, neurosurgery	<100,000/uL
To maintain platelets during ongoing bleeding and transfusion not less than	50,000/uL
To maintain platelets during DIC with ongoing bleeding not less than	50,000/uL
Microvascular bleeding attributed to platelet dysfunction, for example, uremia,[a] postcardiopulmonary bypass, or in association with massive transfusion	Clinician judgment

[a] After a trial of DDAVP if permitted by the clinical situation.[66]

the presence or possibility of additional causes of coagulation disturbance, for example, recent administration of antiplatelet agents, cardiopulmonary bypass, DIC, dilution as a result of large volume administration. Bleeding manifestations can vary substantially from patient to patient in the face of similar platelet counts. This occurs because some platelets are more effective than others. When thrombocytopenia results from peripheral destruction of platelets, the bone marrow continues to produce normal, young, large platelets that are hemostatically very effective. A patient with these platelets may have more effective primary hemostasis than a patient with the same platelet count but whose platelets were produced by a less active, less

6 healthy bone marrow.

One platelet unit will typically increase platelet count by 5 to 10,000/uL. However, the increase must be verified by platelet count, especially in patients who may have been alloimmunized by frequent platelet administration.

Fresh Frozen Plasma

7 In spite of the fact that over 2,000,000 units of FFP are administered annually in the United States there is remarkably little systematically derived evidence of efficacy.[67] Nonetheless, the use of FFP to restore coagulation factor levels is inevitably valid in many clinical circumstances. The indications for fresh frozen plasma administration presented in Table 10-7 are an amalgam of recommendations presented by the ASA in 1996 and the British Committee for Standards in Haematology in 2004.[57,68]

Cryoprecipitate

Cryoprecipitate contains factor VIII, the von Willebrand factor (vWF), fibrinogen, fibronectin, and factor XIII. Virally inactivated Factor VIII coagulation factor concentrates, some of which contain clinically effective concentrations of vWF (Antihemophilic Factor, e.g., Humate P®, Alphanate®) are now available. As a result, hemophilia A and von Willebrand's disease (vWD) are usually treated (in consultation with a hematologist) with those concentrates rather than cryoprecipitate.

TABLE 10-7

INDICATIONS FOR THE ADMINISTRATION OF FRESH FROZEN PLASMA

Correction of single coagulation factor deficiencies for which specific concentrates are not available (principally Factor V)
Correction of multiple coagulation factor deficiencies, for example, DIC, with evidence of microvascular bleeding and PT and/or aPTT >1.5 times normal
Urgent reversal of warfarin therapy[a]
Correction of microvascular bleeding during massive transfusion (>1 blood volume) when PT/aPTT cannot be obtained in a timely manner

[a]Prothrombin complex concentrate (II, VII, IX, X) is an alternative that has been reported to be more effective than FFP.[69]

The remaining indications for cryoprecipitate are presented in Table 10-8.[5]

BLOOD CONSERVATION STRATEGIES

Because of the many hazards of blood product administration, numerous techniques and alternatives have been explored (Table 10-9).

Autologous Donation

Preoperative donation and perioperative salvage of autologous blood have been used extensively as part of programs to reduce homologous blood administration. Autologous blood may be collected days to weeks prior to surgery (predonation); it may be donated immediately prior to surgery (isovolemic hemodilution); or it may be salvaged from the surgical field or wound drains and reinfused (blood salvage). Deciding whether any of these options is appropriate for individual patients presents another challenge in transfusion medicine.

Preoperative Autologous Donation

Preoperative autologous donation (PAD) of blood has been applied principally in patients undergoing major orthopaedic procedures (total hip and knee replacement, scoliosis procedures) and prostatic and cardiac surgery.[70,71] However, the systematic experience has frequently failed to confirm a reduction in allogenic blood exposure[72–74] and utilization is declining.[75] Effectiveness has probably been limited because the patients' erythropoietic response is often not vigorous, in which case the process may simply result in an anemia at the time of surgery. PAD has other disadvantages. The PAD procedure is more expensive than the collection of homologous blood. In addition, if autologous blood is unused, most institutions discard it and do not permit "crossover" to other patients. Practices with respect to infectious agent testing also vary. Some institutions will store and permit return to the donor of HIV-, hepatitis-, or CMV-infected blood while others discard it. Note also that the transfusion of autologous blood does not eliminate the chance of either human error during blood collection, processing, and reinfusion or the risk of bacterial contamination. Some institutions perform a crossmatch prior to return of blood to the donor and others do not. This underscores the caveat that no transfusion is without risk.

The medical condition of the patient must be considered prior to recommending PAD.[71] Severe aortic stenosis, significant coronary disease or myocardial dysfunction, and low initial hematocrit and blood volume (body weight less than 110 pounds) are relative contraindications to PAD.[76] If the patient's hemoglobin level, cardiac status, and general condition permit, blood can be donated at weekly intervals prior to surgery. Four units is typically the maximum donation because of the shelf life of the first unit collected.

Patients making PAD should receive supplemental iron, for example, 2 mg/kg/day for 3 weeks. In addition, PAD can be supplemented with administration of recombinant erythropoietin (Epo).

TABLE 10-8

INDICATIONS FOR THE ADMINISTRATION OF CRYOPRECIPITATE

Prophylaxis before surgery or treatment of bleeding in patients with congenital dysfibrinogenemias
Microvascular bleeding when there is a disproportionate decrease in fibrinogen, e.g., DIC and very massive transfusion,[a] with fibrinogen <80–100 mg/dL (or assay result not available)
Prophylaxis before surgery or treatment of bleeding in hemophilia A or vWD if concentrates are unavailable or ineffective
Bleeding because of uremia that is unresponsive to DDAVP

[a]FFP is the first-line component for the factor depletion associated with massive transfusion.

TABLE 10-9

BLOOD CONSERVATION TECHNIQUES

Preoperative autologous donation
Acute normovolemic hemodilution
Intraoperative blood salvage
Postoperative blood salvage
Pharmacologic agents
Erythropoietin
Blood substitutes (hemoglobin and nonhemoglobin based)
DDAVP (Section VII)
Antifibrinolytics (Section VII)

Erythropoietin

The effectiveness of Epo in hastening recovery of hematocrit in conjunction with PAD and in improving hematocrit in patients not submitted to PAD has been demonstrated.[77–80] However, the practice has not become widespread in part because of the expense of the agent (not less than 500 to 1,600 USD/patient depending on the regimen used) and in part because of the necessity for frequent (e.g., weekly times 3 weeks and 2 additional injections in the final week) parenteral (subcutaneous or iv) administration of Epo. Selective administration of Epo to anemic patients has resulted in more obvious reduction in allogenic blood administration[81,82] than has administration to "all comers."[83,84] Epo, a recombinant product, is usually accepted by Jehovah's Witnesses and its efficacy in that population has been demonstrated.[85] The recent demonstration of the reduction of transfusion requirements in critically ill patients by Epo[86] may increase awareness and encourage its systematic use in anemic elective surgical patients. An alternative erythropoietic agent, darbopoietin alpha, has recently been developed. Its longer half-life results in a more sustained erythropoietic effect than occurs with Epo.[87]

Acute Normovolemic Hemodilution

Acute normovolemic hemodilution (ANH) entails withdrawal of the patient's blood early in the intraoperative period with concurrent administration crystalloids or colloids to maintain normovolemia. The rationale is that during the ensuing surgery, the patient will lose blood of low hematocrit and the withdrawn blood will be available for reinfusion at the end of the operation. The end point for the initial withdrawal is a hematocrit of 27 to 33%, depending on the patient's cardiovascular and respiratory reserve. Selection for this technique should rely on careful evaluation of the patient for coronary or cerebral vascular disease. This procedure evolved in the anticipation that it would reduce total red cell loss and homologous blood administration. However, both mathematical modeling and empiric experience have revealed only a modest benefit with respect to reducing the necessity for homologous RBCs.[80,88–91] By way of example, Goodnough[92] calculated that, in a 100-kg patient from whom three units of blood is withdrawn and replaced by asanguinous fluid, if the subsequent blood loss is 2,800 mL, 215 mL of RBCs (about one unit) will be saved. For patients of limited body size, low starting hematocrit, or blood loss less than 70% of one blood volume,[93] avoidance of allogenic blood or patient benefit might be difficult to achieve. A recent meta-analysis, while confirming that reduction of allogenic blood on the order of one unit per patient was common among the reported investigations, on the basis of the modest savings and the scientific merit of the investigations, concluded that "the literature supports only modest benefits from preoperative ANH. Widespread adoption of ANH cannot be encouraged."[94] Nonetheless, there are reports of favorable experiences in liver resection, prostatectomy, total hip arthroplasty, and abdominal aortic surgery.[80,95–97] It is possible that in the future the efficacy of ANH will be enhanced by administration of preoperative erythropoietics and/or by the use of either hemoglobin-based oxygen-carrying compounds or perflourocarbon emulsions to permit withdrawal of larger volumes of blood.

ANH has also been employed for the purpose of making fresh autologous blood at the end of procedures in which either a dilutional or cardiopulmonary bypass-related coagulopathy may occur. The efficacy in this context has not been confirmed by systematic study. Blood collected and reinfused for this purpose should not be passed through a 40-micron filter to avoid platelet elimination.

Perioperative Blood Salvage

Perioperative blood salvage refers to the recovery of shed blood from the surgical field or wound drains and readministration to the patient. In most instances, the process involves "washing" of the salvaged material with return of only the RBC component of blood. In some instances, usually those involving wound drainage, blood is returned filtered but otherwise unprocessed.

Intraoperative Blood Salvage

Intraoperative blood salvage (IBS) is employed with many surgical procedures that have the potential to require homologous transfusion. Contemporary "cell saver" devices anticoagulate the salvaged blood as it leaves the surgical field, separate the RBCs from other liquid and cellular elements by centrifugation, and then wash the salvaged RBCs extensively with saline. The RBCs are typically returned to the patient suspended in saline in aliquots of 125 or 225 mL with a hematocrit of 45 to 65%[98]. Higher hematocrits can be achieved at the expense of the additional time required for slower filling of the centrifuge chamber.

IBS has been used commonly during cardiovascular surgical procedures, aortic reconstruction, spinal instrumentation, joint arthroplasty, liver transplantation, resection of arteriovenous malformations,[99] and occasionally in the management of trauma patients.[100] There have been numerous demonstrations that IBS can reduce the use of homologous RBCs.[101,102] The presence of infection, malignant cells, urine, bowel contents, and amniotic fluid in the operative field have been viewed as contraindications. However, though malignant cells are known to be retained with RBCs after the washing process, IBS has been applied in the management of hepatic and urologic malignancies without evidence of metastasis.[103,104] At least one IBS washing device has also been shown to remove the critical procoagulant factors present in amniotic fluid[105] and IBS has been employed successfully in Cesarean section.[106] However, the safety of IBS use in that context is unconfirmed and should not be routine.[107]

The potential complications of IBS are largely a function of the reinfusion of materials that might remain after the washing process. These include fat, microaggregates such as platelets and leukocytes, air, red cell stroma, free hemoglobin, heparin, bacteria, and debris from the surgical field. Most of these are in fact removed quite efficiently by contemporary cell salvage equipment. Bacteria are the exception and contamination of cell saver return with skin organisms is relatively common.[101] Leukocyte reduction filters have been shown to remove most bacteria[108] and may be relevant to the use of IBS in trauma. Massive air embolism has occurred as a result of user error. Direct return from the cell saver apparatus has now been largely abandoned in favor of return via an intermediary bag under the control of the anesthesiologist. Care should still be taken in the event that pressure infuser devices are applied to these bags.

A dilutional coagulopathy in association with large volume IBS is to be expected because essentially all clotting factors and most platelets are removed by the washing process. Management is the same as for a dilutional coagulopathy occurring with administration of homologous or PAD blood. A DIC-like coagulopathy, the "salvaged blood syndrome,"[109] has also been associated with IBS. However, it seems likely that this syndrome was the result of inadequate preparation of blood by older cell salvage devices. Unwashed, salvaged blood has been shown to contain numerous constituents that influence the coagulation process: thromboplastic material, interleukins, complement, fibrin degradation products, and factors released from activated leukocytes and platelets.[99] The majority of these, however, are quite efficiently removed by contemporary processing devices and their presence is used as an argument against the return of unprocessed blood (see later).[110]

An additional coagulopathy risk arises with the use of thrombin and microfibrillar collagen or cellulose products in the surgical field.[111] These agents are not reliably removed by the washing process and suction of blood to the IBS device should be discontinued during the use of these agents and resumed after the field has been irrigated.

The clinician should appreciate that the recovery of shed RBCs by the IBS process is on the order of 50%. Allogenic blood will therefore frequently be necessary in spite of the IBS and blood and fluid replacement calculations should take this into account.[112,113]

Postoperative Blood Salvage

Postoperative recovery of blood from mediastinal chest tubes and wound drains after hip and knee replacement with immediate reinfusion of "unwashed" blood has been employed quite commonly. The many substances present in the unprocessed blood (previous section) suggest that coagulation dysfunction might result and many are skeptical regarding the wisdom of this practice.[98,110] However, there have been only occasional reports of apparent adverse consequences.[114] This may reflect the fact that the recovered and reinfused volumes are usually small.

Hemoglobin-Based Oxygen Carrying Solutions

It seems possible that hemoglobin-based oxygen carrying solutions (HBOCs) will become available in the near future. Hemopure® (Biopure, Inc) has been approved for clinical use in South Africa. However, although numerous polymerized hemoglobin products have been studied only one, PolyHeme®, Northfield Laboratories, is currently in phase III trial in the United States. The many products studied use bovine, outdated human, or recombinant hemoglobin that has been entirely separated from red cell membranes (stroma) and polymerized to increase half-life. The initial difficulties with renal failure caused by stroma and excessive free hemoglobin have been overcome. However, there are several residual difficulties with which clinicians will probably have to contend including methemoglobinemia, interference with some calorimetrically based laboratory assays (including creatinine, total bilirubin and LDH), some degree of vasoconstriction caused by nitric oxide binding by free Hb, and a relatively short half-life. Polymerization increases half-life to 18 to 36 hours but that period is sufficiently short that O_2-carrying capacity will usually become inadequate before native reticulocytosis can compensate.[115,116] Perflourocarbon emulsions[116] appear to be further from potential clinical application than HBOCs and will not be discussed here.

The Jehovah's Witness

In general, Jehovah's Witnesses will accept neither administration of homologous blood products nor the readministration of autologous products that have left the circulation. However, their faith allows significant personal discretion and the wishes of each patient must be clarified. Few will permit the administration of the common whole blood components and the majority will decline PAD. However, many will accept procedures that maintain extracorporeal blood in continuity with the circulation. The acceptability of cardiopulmonary bypass, acute normovolemic hemodilution, and perioperative cell salvage must be clarified with each patient individually. Most will permit administration of Epo.

COLLECTION AND PREPARATION OF BLOOD PRODUCTS FOR TRANSFUSION

Red Blood Cells

In the preparation of red blood cells for transfusion, whole blood is first collected in bags containing citrate-phosphate-dextrose-adenine (CPDA) or CPD solution. The citrate chelates the calcium present in blood and prevents coagulation. PRBCs are prepared by centrifugation. The two common preparations ultimately delivered to the clinician have either CPDA or so-called Additive Solution as the preservative. CPDA blood has a hematocrit of about 70 to 75%, contains 50 to 70 mL of residual plasma in a total volume of 250 to 275 mL, and has a shelf life of 35 days. With the Additive Solution preparation, the original preservative and most of the plasma (10 to 15 mL residual) is removed and replaced with 100 mL of Additive Solution. This results in a lower hematocrit, 60%, in a total volume of 250 to 350 mL; less citrate per unit, 75 to 80% fewer microaggregates; and a longer shelf life, 42 days. Additive Solution RBCs are thought to regenerate 2,3-DPG more rapidly. The pH and K+ content of the two preparations are similar. The smaller plasma volume in Additive Solution blood results in smaller amounts of coagulation factors in PRBCs but also a potentially lesser risk of allergic reactions and TRALI.

Sequential centrifugation at various spin speeds and durations is used to separate whole blood into components; including packed RBCs, platelet concentrates, cryoprecipitate, leukocyte-poor RBCs, and cell-free plasma. For preparation of platelet concentrates, centrifugation is first performed at room temperature. This separates the platelet-rich plasma fraction from the red blood cells. To separate all other blood components, centrifugation is carried out between 1 degree and 6 degrees C.

There are alternative RBC preparations that eliminate the various "passengers." Saline-washed RBCs may be used for patients who experience reactions to foreign proteins. White cells can be removed by washing, irradiation, or leukofiltration. The administration of one unit of packed RBCs will increase the Hb and Hct of a 70-kg adult by approximately 1 g/dL and 3%, respectively.

RBCs can be frozen and stored indefinitely. However, preservatives to prevent freeze-thaw associated damage must be added and subsequently removed before administration, which must occur within 24 hours of thawing. The process is expensive and therefore not widely used.

Compatibility Testing

Compatibility testing involves three separate procedures involving both donor and recipient blood: ABO, Rh blood type identification, antibody screening of donor plasma, and the donor/recipient crossmatch.

ABO, Rhesus Typing

The first step is to determine the ABO blood group type and the Rh status of both donor and recipient blood. This is a critical step because most of the fatal hemolytic transfusion reactions result from the transfusion of ABO-incompatible blood. Blood types are defined according to the antigens present on the surface of the RBCs. Patients with type A blood have type A antigens on the surface of their red cells. Type B blood has B antigens. When both antigens are present the patient is said to have type AB blood and when both are lacking, the patient is said to have type O blood. The serum constitutively contains antibodies to the AB antigens that are lacking on the RBC. Patients with type A blood have antibodies against the B antigen and vice versa. Patients with no antigens on their cells, type O blood, will have both anti-A and anti-B antibodies in the plasma. The approximate frequencies of ABO blood types in the U.S. are presented in Table 10-10.

Patients with the Rhesus (D) antigen are said to be Rh-positive and those who lack the D antigen are termed Rh-negative. Approximately 85% of the population is Rh-positive. In contrast to the A and B blood groups, anti-D antibodies are not constitutively present in the serum of an Rh-negative patient. However, 60 to 70% of Rh-negative patients exposed to donor Rh-positive RBCs will develop anti-D antibodies. There is a latency before these antibodies are synthesized. As a consequence, the reaction between the Rh-positive donor cells and

TABLE 10-10

MAJOR RBC SURFACE ANTIGEN INCIDENCE (%) IN THE U.S. POPULATION[117]

GROUP	WHITES	BLACKS
O	45	49
A	40	27
B	11	20
AB	4	4
Rh (D)	85	92

the anti-D evolves slowly and may not be clinically apparent on first exposure. This process, whereby a foreign antigen stimulates the synthesis of the corresponding antibody, is termed "alloimmunization." Subsequent exposure of these Rh-negative individuals to Rh-positive cells may result in an acute hemolytic reaction.

In determining what donor blood group types may be compatible for transfusion to a particular recipient, it is useful to focus on which antibodies will be present in the recipient plasma. It is the reaction of these antibodies with donor RBC antigens that can activate complement and lead to intravascular hemolysis of the red cell. Type O+ recipients [type O, Rh(D)-positive] will have both anti-A and anti-B antibodies, but not the anti-D antibody in their plasma. These patients must not receive either type A, type B, or type AB blood. They must receive type O blood but it may be Rh-positive or Rh-negative. In contrast, patients with blood type AB− (Type AB, Rh-negative), will lack both the A and B antibodies in their plasma and may or may not have the anti-D antibody in their plasma. They can receive A−, B−, AB−, or O− blood. Individuals with the greatest number of antigens on their RBCs have the fewest constitutive antibodies in their plasma and can receive all blood types (Types A+, A−, B+, B−, AB+, AB−, O+, and O−), and are referred to as universal recipients. Individuals with the fewest antigens on their cells (type O-negative) have the greatest number of antibodies in their plasma. Type O-negative RBCs can be administered to all ABO, Rh types and these individuals are referred to as universal donors.

The Antibody Screen

The antibody screen, an indirect Coombs test, is performed to identify recipient antibodies against RBC antigens. Commercially supplied RBCs, selected for the panel of antigens they possess, are mixed with both donor and recipient serum to screen for the presence of unexpected antibodies. Only about 4 in 1,000 blood donations demonstrate unexpected antibodies. The likelihood that the antibody screen will miss a potentially dangerous antibody has been estimated to be no more than 1 in 10,000. If the recipient plasma screen is positive, the antibody must be identified and appropriate antigen negative donor units selected. The antibody screening of recipient plasma should be repeated if the patient has been transfused since the last antibody screening test.

The Crossmatch

Donor RBCs are mixed with recipient serum. This test requires about 45 minutes and is carried out in three phases: (1) the immediate phase, (2) incubation phase, and (3) antiglobulin phase.

The immediate phase serves primarily to ensure that there have been no errors in ABO-Rh typing. The test entails examination of a mixture of donor RBCs and patient serum for macroscopic agglutination. This immediate phase crossmatch requires only 1 to 5 minutes and detects ABO incompatibilities and those caused by antibodies in the MN, P, and Lewis systems.

The second phase, the incubation phase, requires 30 to 45 minutes and detects antibodies primarily in the Rh system.

The third phase, the antiglobulin phase, also called the antiglobulin crossmatch or the indirect antiglobulin test, entails the addition of antiglobulin sera at the end of the incubation phase. This phase is performed only on blood yielding a positive antibody screen and requires 60 to 90 minutes. The test identifies the presence of antibodies attached to antigens on the surface of the donor red blood cells. This phase is an attempt to identify the most incomplete antibodies (i.e., those that do not cause agglutination) from all blood group systems, including Rh, Kell, Kidd, and Duffy systems.

In patients who have been transfused previously or who may have been exposed to foreign red blood cell antigens during pregnancy, only 1 in 100 will have an antibody other than the anti-A, anti-B, and/or anti-Rh antibodies and many of these are not reactive at physiologic temperatures. Determining the ABO blood group type and Rh status alone yields the probability that the transfusion will be compatible in 99.8% of instances. The addition of the 30- to 45-minute antibody screen improves the likelihood of a compatible transfusion to 99.94%; the addition of a complete crossmatch increases this to 99.95%.[63] In patients who have not previously been transfused or pregnant, the odds that an incompatible transfusion will occur when uncrossmatched blood is administered is only 1 in 1,000. For those who have previously been exposed to foreign red blood cell antigens, the likelihood that they will have developed an antibody is about 1 in 100. Nonetheless, all blood banks perform the crossmatch. However, these data reveal that the administration, in emergency situations, of uncrossmatched blood to patients with no history of pregnancy or transfusion should entail relatively low risk.

Type and Screen Orders

When blood is ordered preoperatively for surgical cases in which it is unlikely that the blood will actually be transfused, the orders should be for "type and screen" only. The ABO, Rh status of the patient is determined and the antibody screen (see earlier) is performed to determine the presence of antibodies other than ABO in the potential recipient's plasma. If the antibody screen is negative, type specific uncrossmatched blood will result in a hemolytic reaction in less than 1/50,000 units[5]. If the screen is positive, the blood bank proceeds to identify a pool of potentially compatible units.

Emergency Transfusions

The exsanguinating patient may require RBCs before complete compatibility testing can be performed. If testing is to be abbreviated, there is a preferred order for selecting partially tested blood. The first choice is to transfuse type-specific, partially crossmatched blood. In urgent situations in which a patient needs blood before compatibility testing can be completed, the use of uncrossmatched blood is indicated. If the patient's ABO and Rh type is unknown or has not been tested on a current sample, group O RBCs should be administered until there is time to complete ABO and Rh testing. Rh-negative blood is preferable if the patient's Rh type is unknown or if the patient is a woman of child-bearing age. If Rh-negative blood is not available for a critically ill, bleeding Rh-negative patient, Rh-positive blood should not be withheld. If the blood bank has time to test a current sample, then ABO and Rh type-specific uncrossmatched RBCs can be administered. In either case, the blood bank will begin compatibility tests as soon as possible if a current pretransfusion sample is available. If a non group O patient receives a large volume of group O red cells, the combined amount of anti-A and/or anti-B present in the small amounts in the residual plasma each PRBC unit may react with the patient's own A, B, or AB red cells and cause some hemolysis. For this reason, non group O patients who have received group O red cells approximating one patient blood volume (10 to 12 units) during the period of acute blood loss should not be switched back to their own ABO group[118] unless testing has been performed to confirm that significant titers of anti-A or anti-B antibodies are not present. The decision as to whether or not to switch to type-specific blood should be made, in conjunction with the blood bank, on the basis of that result and administration of type O blood should continue in the interim.

Platelets

Platelets are separated from plasma by centrifugation. They are commonly supplied as single-donor units with the platelets suspended in a small quantity of residual plasma. One unit of platelets will increase the platelet count of a 70-kg recipient by 5 to 10,000/mm^3. A common practice is to administer one unit/10 kg of body weight. Accordingly, platelet transfusion will often entail exposure to multiple donors. Donor exposure can be minimized by the use of single-donor platelet pheresis packs that contain the platelet equivalent of approximately six single units in a volume of 200 to 400 mL. These are obtained by serial blood withdrawals from a single donor followed by centrifugation and return of the RBCs to the donor.

Platelet viability is optimal at 22°C but storage is limited to 4 to 5 days. The short shelf time means that platelets are usually administered before the results of the newly introduced nucleic acid antigen (NAT) testing for viral agents are available.

Platelets bear both ABO and human leukocyte antigens (HLA). ABO compatibility is ideal because incompatibility shortens the life span of the platelet. However, it is not required. ABO/HLA-matched platelets are indicated for patients who become refractory to random donor platelets. Platelets do not carry the Rh antigen. However, administration of platelets from an Rh-positive donor to an Rh-negative female of child-bearing age should be avoided in order to prevent sensitization as a result of passenger RBCs in the platelet preparation. If it occurs, Rh-immune globulin should be administered.

Platelets should be administered through a filter. The standard 170-micron filter is sufficient and there is no advantage or necessity to use the 40-micron filters typically used for RBC administration.[5]

Fresh Frozen Plasma

Plasma is separated from the RBC component of whole blood by centrifugation. One unit has a volume of 200 to 250 mL. It will contain the preservative added at the time of collection, usually CPD-adenine. To preserve the two labile clotting factors (V and VIII), it is frozen promptly and thawed only immediately prior to administration. FFP must be ABO compatible. Rh-positive plasma can be given to an Rh-negative recipient but ideally this should be avoided in young females because of the possibility of alloimmunization to the Rh antigen on passenger RBCs in the FFP.

Solvent Detergent Plasma

One of the principal hazards of FFP administration has been virus transmission. Three procedures, pasteurization, photochemical treatment, and solvent detergent (SD) treatment, have been used to inactivate viruses. The SD technique is highly effective in inactivating all of the lipid encapsulated viruses, for example, HIV, HCV, HBV, and HTLV. The disadvantage of the SD technique is that the process involves pooling of large numbers of single FFP units (>1,000) and is not effective against nonlipid enveloped viruses (HAV, parvovirus) or the agent of Creutzfeldt-Jakob disease. The concern with SD plasma is that the pooling process might result in wide dissemination of an infectious agent. The incidence of parvovirus viremia among donors is estimated to be between 0.03 and 0.6%.[119] Parvovirus infection has been reported as a consequence of transfusion. While the disease is usually self-limited, significant morbidity, for example, red cell aplasia, meningitis, especially in immunocompromised patents, can occur.[119] The future of SD plasma is not clear to the authors of this review.

Cryoprecipitate

Cryoprecipitate is the precipitate that remains when FFP is thawed slowly at 4°C. It is a concentrated source of factor VIII, factor XIII, vWF, and fibrinogen. One unit of cryoprecipitate (the yield from one unit of FFP) contains sufficient fibrinogen to increase fibrinogen level 5 to 7 mg/dL.[120] Accordingly, it is usually provided in bags that contain 10 or 20 units. ABO compatibility is not essential because of the limited antibody content of the associated plasma vehicle (10 to 20 mL). Viruses can be transmitted with cryoprecipitate. It is stored at −20°C and thawed immediately prior to use.

Factor VIII and IX

Recombinant and virally inactivated FVII concentrates are available.

Antithrombin III

Virus-treated antithrombin III (ATIII) concentrates are available. They have been employed in the treatment of congenital and acquired ATIII deficiencies.[121] The latter include DIC and fulminant hepatic failure.

THE HEMOSTATIC MECHANISM

Normal "hemostasis" involves a series of physiologic checks and balances that assure that blood remains in an invariably liquid state as it circulates throughout the body but, once the vascular network is violated, transforms rapidly to a solid state. That transformation to a solid state, that is, coagulation, must inevitably be complemented by processes for eliminating clot that is no longer needed for hemostasis. The latter is accomplished by fibrinolysis

The Nomenclature of Coagulation

Understanding the coagulation process has been made more difficult by the complexity of the nomenclature. An early attempt was made to standardize it by assigning Roman numerals to each of the 12 known clotting factors. Unfortunately, the factors were numbered in the order in which they were discovered and not in the sequence in which they interact. To complicate matters, the first 4 of the original 12 factors are usually referred to by their common names, fibrinogen,

TABLE 10-11

FACTOR NOMENCLATURE AND HALF-LIVES

FACTOR	SYNONYMS	IN VIVO HALF-LIFE (HOURS)
I	Fibrinogen	100–150
II	Prothrombin	50–80
III	Tissue thromboplastin, tissue factor (TF)	
IV	Calcium ion	
V	Proaccelerin, labile factor	24
VII	Serum prothrombin conversion accelerator (SPCA), stable factor	6
VIII	Antihemophilic factor (AHF)	12
vWF	von Willebrand factor	24
IX	Christmas factor	24
X	Stuart-Power factor, Stuart factor, autoprothrombin	25–60
XI	Plasma thromboplastin antecedent (PTA)	40–80
XII	Hageman factor	50–70
XIII	Fibrin stabilizing factor (FSF)	150
Prekallikrein	Fletcher factor	35
HMW kininogen	Fitzgerald, Flaujeac, or Williams factor; contact-activation cofactor	150

prothrombin, tissue thromboplastin (tissue factor), and calcium, and not by their Roman numerals. Factor VI no longer exists; it proved to be activated factor V. The more recently discovered clotting factors, for example, prekallikrein and high–molecular-weight kininogen, have not been assigned Roman numerals. They too are identified by common names, and to further complicate matters, some have more than one name (Table 10-11).

The Coagulation Mechanism

The classical, dual-cascade (intrinsic and extrinsic pathway) model of coagulation (Figs. 10-1 and 10-2) is now recognized to be an inadequate representation of in vivo coagulation. It failed to explain several clinical phenomena. First, persons lacking factor XII, prekallikrein, or high–molecular-weight kininogen do not bleed abnormally, suggesting that contact activation is not critical for normal hemostasis. Second, patients with only trace quantities of factor XI withstand major trauma without unusual bleeding and those completely lacking factor XI have only a mild hemorrhagic disorder. Factor XI therefore appears to have a more minor role in coagulation than ascribed to it by classical theory. Next, deficiencies of factor VIII (an extrinsic pathway factor) and factor IX (an intrinsic pathway factor) lead to Hemophilia A and B, respectively. The classical

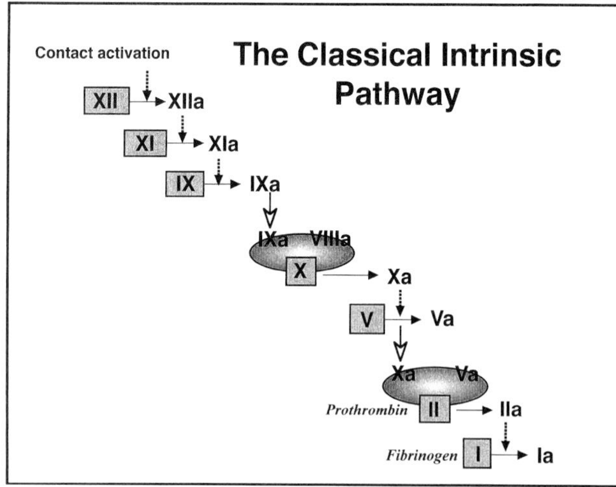

FIGURE 10-1. The classical intrinsic pathway of coagulation. A cascade initiated by contact with a foreign surface leads to the formation of the fibrin (Ia) necessary for the generation of a fibrin clot. The *dotted arrows* indicate the occurrence of an enzymatically mediated conversion of an inactive factor to its active form. The *open-headed arrows* indicate the translocation of an activated factor to participate in a subsequent reaction. The *shaded spheroids* represent the phospholipid surfaces (usually provided by activated platelets).

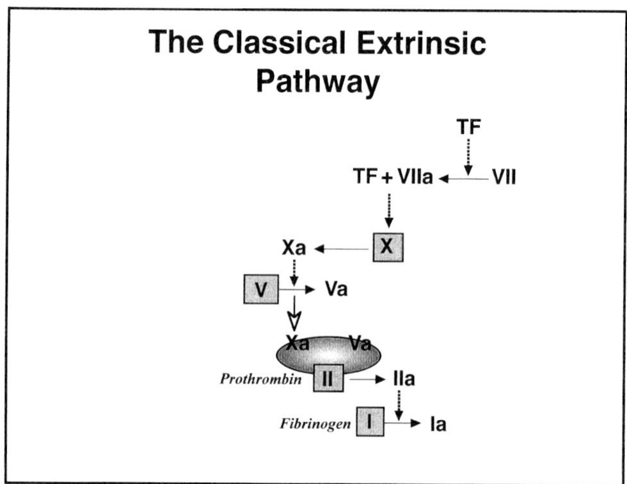

FIGURE 10-2. The classical extrinsic pathway of coagulation. This pathway is depicted as it was originally thought to occur, that is, largely extravascularly and independent of the classical intrinsic pathway (compare Fig. 10-1). The *dotted arrows* indicate the occurrence of an enzymatically mediated conversion of an inactive factor to its active form. The *open-headed arrows* indicate the translocation of an activated factor to a phospholipid surface to participate in a reaction complex. The *shaded spheroid* represents the phospholipid surface (usually provided by activated platelets).

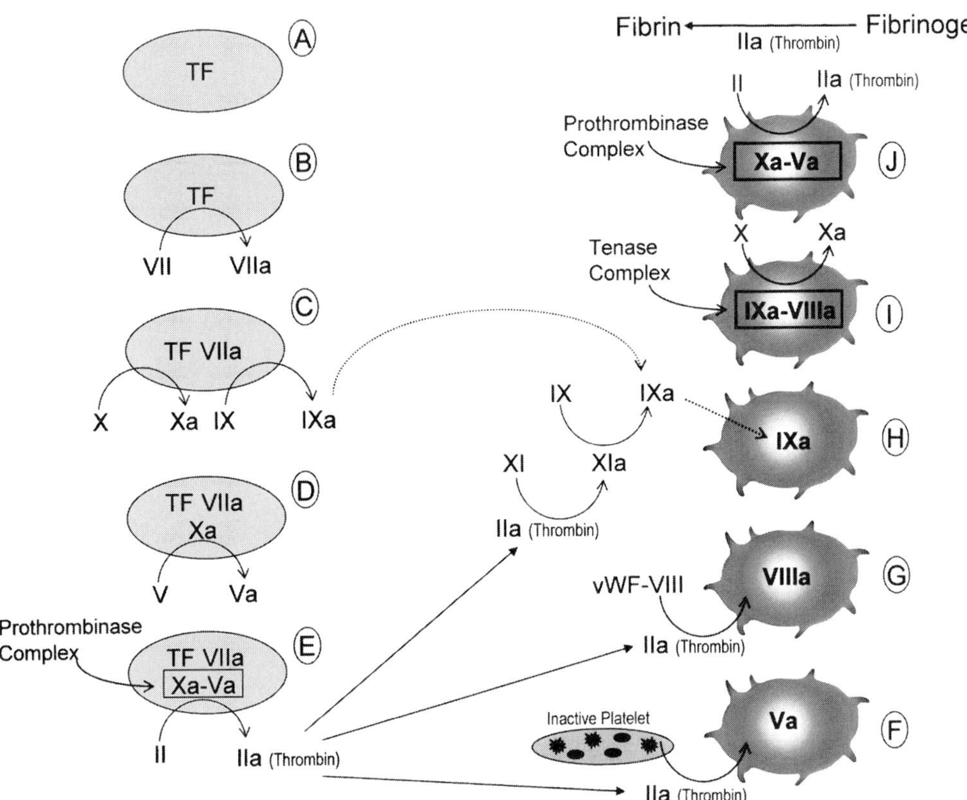

FIGURE 10-3. The coagulation mechanism. See text. TF, membrane-bound tissue factor on a extravascular cell surface; vWF-VIII:C, circulating factor VIII bound to its carrier protein, the von Willebrand factor.

description of two pathways of coagulation leaves it unclear why either type of hemophiliac could not simply clot via the unaffected pathway. Most importantly it is now appreciated that while the classical theories may provide a reasonable model of in vitro coagulation tests, that is, the aPTT and PT, they fail to incorporate the central role of cell-based phospholipid surfaces in the in vivo coagulation process. The three stages of that process, which has been thoroughly defined and described by Hoffman, are summarized in the next sections and
9 in Figure 10-3.[122]

Activation

Activation of the coagulation process begins when a breach in the vascular endothelium exposes blood to the membrane-bound protein, tissue factor (TF) (Fig. 10-3A). TF activates circulating FVII to yield a complex of TF and activated (a) FVII (FVIIa) (Fig. 10-3B). The TF-VIIa complex in turn activates factors IX and X (Fig. 10-3C). Xa then activates FV (Fig. 10-3D), resulting in the formation of the "prothrombinase complex," composed of Xa and Va, on the phospholipid surface provided by membrane bound TF. The prothrombinase complex catalyzes the conversion of prothrombin (FII) to thrombin (FIIa) (Fig. 10-3E). It is this initial formation of thrombin in small amounts that advances the coagulation process to the more efficient "amplification" phase that follows. (For those in need of a mnemonic, it is the "nickel-dime," Va-Xa prothrombinase complex that is responsible for the initial, modest thrombin generation.)

Amplification

While it was the phospholipid surface provided by membrane-bound TF that initiated the coagulation process, it is now the phospholipid surface provided by platelets that serves to perpetuate it. The breach in the vascular tree that began the activation process also exposed platelets to collagen to which they become bound by vWF via the GPIb receptor on the platelet surface (Fig 10-4). The thrombin just generated by the TF-bound prothrombinase complex supports the amplification of the coagulation process in four ways. First, it further activates the adjacent platelets (Fig. 10-3F). That activation results in platelet surface changes, most notably the appearance of the GPIIIb/IIa receptor, and in the release of the contents of platelet granules (Fig. 10-5). Among those contents are ADP, a powerful platelet activator and proaggregant that rapidly recruits other platelets to the growing platelet mass, and Factor V. Thrombin's second effect is to promote the activation FV to FVa (Fig. 10-3F). Third, thrombin releases circulating FVIII from its carrier molecule (vWF) and activates it (Fig. 10-3G); and fourth, thrombin activates FXI (Fig. 10-3H). FXIa in turn activates FIX (Fig. 10-3H), further adding to the pool of IXa that first formed during the activation phase above (Fig. 10-3C). The net result of this amplification stage is the availability of activated platelets and activated factors V, VIII, and IX.

Propagation

The platelet then provides the phospholipid surface on which two coagulation factor complexes form and act to produce the explosive generation of thrombin. First, VIIIa and IXa form the "tenase complex," which activates FX (Fig. 10-3I). The resultant Xa forms additional prothrombinase complex (Xa–Va) and large amounts of thrombin are elaborated (Fig. 10-3J). (For mnemonic purposes it is "eight-nine and nickel-dime" that together are responsible for the thrombin burst.) Thrombin (IIa) catalyzes the formation of fibrin from

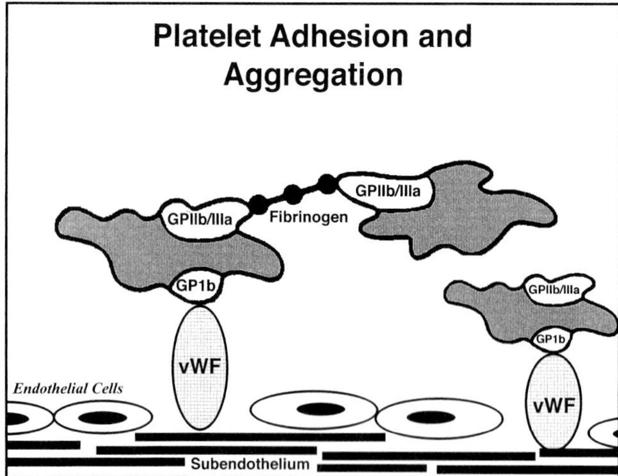

FIGURE 10-4. Platelet adhesion and aggregation. When the endothelium is denuded, von Willebrand factor (vWF) binds to collagen in the subendothelial layer. Platelets patrolling the blood vessel lining adhere via their glycoprotein (GP) 1b receptors to vWF. The binding of vWF to the GP1b receptors initiates platelet activation. Platelets change their shape from discoid to spheroid and extrude multiple pseudopods. Platelets aggregate to one another by crosslinking via fibrinogen (or vWF, not shown) between glycoprotein IIb/IIIa receptors expressed on the platelet surface during the process of platelet activation.

fibrinogen and fibrin acts to crosslink the platelets to reinforce the friable platelet plug (see Fig. 10-4). Thrombin also activates thrombin activatable fibrinolysis inhibitor (TAFI) and FXIII (neither shown), both of which serve to stabilize the fibrin clot. Fibrin monomers initially aggregate relatively loosely to form a clot composed of fibrin S (soluble), which is held together only by hydrogen bonds. FXIII (fibrin stabilizing factor) mediates the formation of covalent peptide bonds between the fibrin monomers to yield a stable (insoluble) fibrin
10 clot.

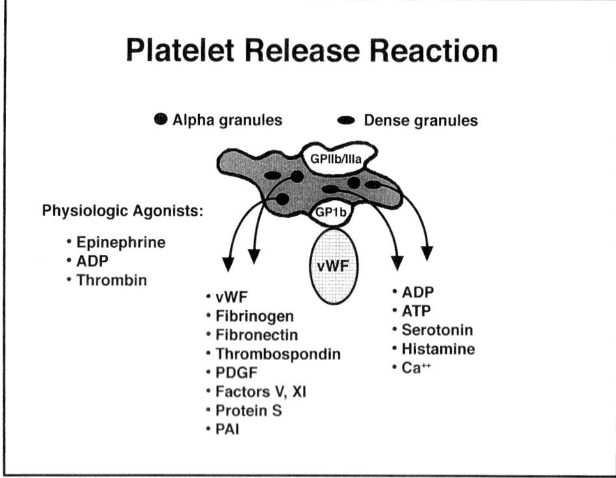

FIGURE 10-5. Platelet release reaction. Platelets undergo a release reaction coincident with shape change or in response to physiologic agonists including epinephrine, ADP, and thrombin. The numerous substances released from the alpha and dense granules of platelets contribute to platelet aggregation (fibrinogen), to the activation and adhesion of additional platelets (ADP, epinephrine, thrombin, vWF) and to clot formation (vWF, fibrinogen, thrombin, calcium, Factors V and XI, fibronectin).

Additional Principles of Coagulation

A few additional facts will aid in achieving a broader understanding of coagulation:

1. Most clotting factors circulate in an inactive form.
   Most of the clotting factors circulate as inactive proenzymes. During the process of coagulation, a portion of the molecule is cleaved off, resulting in active enzymes (designated by the addition of a lower case "a" after the Roman numeral, e.g., Xa), most of which are serine proteases.
2. Most clotting factors are synthesized by the liver.
   Accordingly, their normal structure and function are dependent on normal hepatic activity. One possible exception is factor VIII, which probably also has some extrahepatic synthesis.
3. Factor VIII is actually a large, two-molecule complex (vWF and coagulant factor VIII).
   Factor VIII circulates as a very large complex of two distinct protein components. The high–molecular-weight portion (VIIIR:Ag) encompasses both the factor VIII antigen (used to identify "factor VIII" in the laboratory assay) and the vWF. The vWF portion serves as a carrier protein for the second and smaller component of this macromolecular complex, VIIIC, which contains the factor VIII coagulant activity. The vWF has a second function in addition to its role as carrier protein. During the process of primary hemostasis when the endothelial lining has been denuded, vWF mediates adhesion of platelets to collagen. Absence of the smaller portion of the factor VIII complex (VIII:C) results in hemophilia A. Absence of vWF causes two hemostatic abnormalities: (1) a defect in primary hemostasis because of a failure of platelet adhesion to the sites of vascular injury and (2) clinical hemophilia A because of an absence of circulating factor VIII:C. Restoration of vWF levels restores normal hemostasis. Synthesis of the vWF occurs in endothelial cells and megakaryocytes. The site of synthesis of the coagulant portion of factor VIII is unknown but may be located in the hepatic sinusoidal endothelial cells.
4. Four clotting factors are vitamin K dependent.
   Four of the clotting factors, II, VII, IX, and X, require vitamin K for completion of their synthesis in the liver. Each undergoes a final enzymatic addition of a carboxyl group that requires the presence of vitamin K. The carboxyl group enables these factors to bind (with calcium as a cofactor) to phospholipid surfaces. Without vitamin K, factors II, VII, IX, and X are produced in normal amounts but are nonfunctional.
   The anticoagulant action of vitamin K antagonists is the result to their ability to inhibit this final carboxylation step. The warfarin-like drugs compete with vitamin K for binding sites on the hepatocyte. With sufficient warfarin administration, vitamin K is displaced and the vitamin K–dependent factors are not carboxylated. Of the four vitamin K–dependent factors, factor VII has the shortest half-life. It is the first clotting factor to disappear from the circulation when a patient is placed on warfarin or begins to develop vitamin K deficiency.
5. Factors V and VIII have short storage half-lives.
   Factors V and VIII are also referred to as the "labile factors" because their coagulant activity is not durable in stored blood. While packed RBCs contains residual plasma with clotting factors, massive transfusion with stored blood will nonetheless lead to a dilutional coagulopathy because of diminished activity of factors V and VII.

Fibrinolysis

The process of fibrinolysis leads to the dissolution of fibrin clots. Fibrinolysis serves to remodel fibrin clots and "recanalize" vessels that have been occluded by thrombosis.

The Formation of Plasmin

Fibrinolysis involves primarily the production of plasmin, an active fibrinolytic enzyme. Plasmin is formed by the conversion of plasminogen to plasmin (Fig. 10-6). Plasmin does not circulate freely because it is rapidly degraded by circulating antiplasmins. Instead, plasminogen, the precursor to plasmin, circulates and when it comes into contact with fibrin binds to it. In fact, when a fibrin clot is forming, plasminogen is incorporated into the growing fibrin clot together with tissue plasminogen activator (t-PA). Once bound to the fibrin surface, plasminogen is converted to plasmin by t-PA. The bound plasmin is protected from attack by circulating antiplasmins because the binding site by which the plasmin binds to the fibrin is the same site to which the antiplasmins bind.[123] When plasmin is released into the bloodstream (with its binding site exposed), it is immediately neutralized by alpha-2 antiplasmin. Thus, like the coagulation cascade, the fibrinolytic system relies on surface-mediated reactions both for the production of plasmin and for the localization of fibrinolysis to the site of vascular injury.

Tissue Plasminogen Activator

Tissue plasminogen activator, which converts plasminogen to plasmin, is produced by vascular endothelial cells. This site of synthesis is important to the maintenance of the "nonthrombogenic" endothelial surface. If a clot begins to form on the normal endothelial surface, several mechanisms, including the elaboration of t-PA from endothelial cells, will rapidly inhibit clot formation or lead to its dissolution. t-PA release from endothelial cells can be stimulated by several factors. If sufficient thrombin has been synthesized, thrombin will form a complex with thrombomodulin and activate protein C. Activated protein C (APC) then stimulates the release of t-PA from endothelial cells. t-PA is also released from the endothelium in response to venous occlusion, physical activity, stress, or vasoactive drugs (such as epinephrine, vasopressin, and DDAVP).[124] t-PA, once released from endothelial cells, selectively binds to fibrin, much like plasminogen, which also selectively binds to fibrin. Bound to fibrin, the t-PA converts plasminogen to plasmin.

t-PA does not activate circulating plasminogen. This has important implications. Because t-PA activates only plasminogen bound to fibrin, the process of fibrinolysis by plasmin is localized to the fibrin clot. Therefore, under normal circumstances, widespread, uncontrolled fibrinolysis is prevented. The vascular endothelium and platelets also synthesize an inhibitor of t-PA, plasminogen activator inhibitor (PAI-1), which reduces the amount of plasmin formed and serves to slow the fibrinolytic process (Fig. 10-6). Some patients with thrombotic disorders have been found to have increased levels of this inhibitor.[124] A similar inhibitor is found in placental tissue. It may be that the progressive "hypercoagulable state" associated with pregnancy is related to increased levels of this t-PA inhibitor.[124]

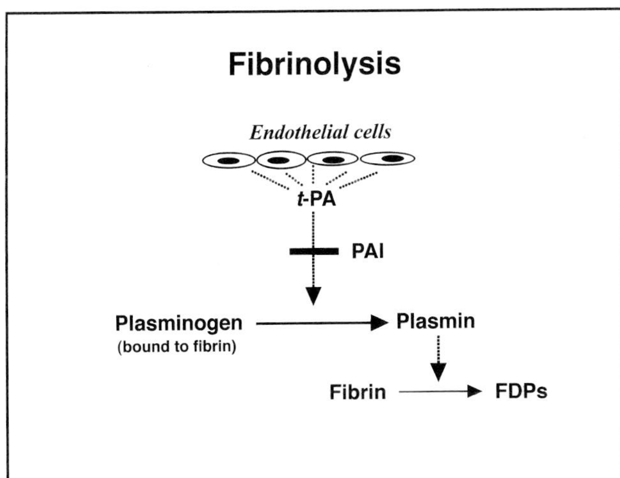

FIGURE 10-6. Control of fibrinolysis. Normal endothelial cells release tissue plasminogen activator (t-PA), which activates plasminogen, leading to the breakdown of fibrin to its various degradation products (FDPs) in areas remote from sites of vascular injury. The action of t-PA can be inhibited by plasminogen activator inhibitor (see text).

Plasminogen Activators

There are plasminogen activators in addition to t-PA. Urokinase is present in the urine but unlike t-PA, it has no affinity for fibrin and is not present in circulating blood.[123] Physiologic activators of the fibrinolytic system include vigorous exercise, anoxia, and stress, in addition to factor XIIa and thrombin. Exogenous plasminogen activators include streptokinase, urokinase, and recombinant t-PA. These fibrinolytic agents all differ with respect to their action, clot specificity, systemic fibrinolytic effect, antigenic effect, and efficacy. Proteins derived from streptococci and staphylococci have also been found to be activators of the fibrinolytic system. The therapeutic fibrinolytic agents, streptokinase and urokinase, differ from t-PA in that they will activate circulating plasminogen. These lead to more widespread fibrinolysis. Fibrinolytic therapy has been used in the treatment of unstable angina, acute peripheral arterial occlusions, deep vein thrombosis, and pulmonary embolism, and in occluded indwelling catheters and arteriovenous shunts.

Fibrin Degradation Products

The primary action of plasmin is to degrade fibrin clots. The degradation products produced are called fibrin degradation products (FDPs) or fibrin split products (FSPs). Their structure varies according to whether plasmin cleaves fibrinogen, fibrin that is crosslinked, or fibrin that is not crosslinked.[125] Under normal circumstances, FDPs are removed from the blood by the liver, kidney, and reticuloendothelial system. They normally have half-lives of about 9 hours. However, if the FDPs are produced at a rate that exceeds their normal clearance, they will accumulate. This happens when the fibrinolytic system is excessively active. In high concentrations, FDPs impair platelet function, inhibit thrombin, and prevent the crosslinking of fibrin strands.[126] The defective polymerization of the fibrin monomers results in a clot that is more readily degraded by plasmin.[124] In such high concentrations, FDPs lead to bleeding because FDPs are "inhibitors" of both platelets and coagulation.

Excess Circulating Plasmin

Under normal circumstances, once plasmin has degraded fibrin clot and escapes from the fibrin surface, it is rapidly inactivated by antiplasmins. Deficiency of alpha-2 antiplasmin leads to a bleeding tendency because, with reduced levels of antiplasmin in the circulation, plasmin can circulate. In addition, in pathologic conditions in which the fibrinolytic system produces large quantities of plasmin (primary fibrinolysis), the antiplasmin capacity may be exceeded and plasmin may circulate. This can also happen when fibrinolysis is stimulated in response to disseminated intravascular coagulation (secondary fibrinolysis). Excess plasmin can lead to a coagulopathy. This is because plasmin primarily degrades fibrin; but because it is a serine protease, it can also degrade other coagulation factors, for example, fibrinogen, factor V, factor VIII, factor XIII, and also vWF.[124] Plasmin can also digest the platelet receptor, GPIb. Accordingly, circulating plasmin inhibits platelet function and disrupts coagulation.

Summary of the Control of Fibrinolysis

Under normal conditions, plasmin is generated only at the site of clot formation, is protected from degradation while attached to fibrin, and is destroyed rapidly once released into the circulation.

Control of Coagulation—The Checks and Balances

Coagulation must be precisely regulated to prevent rampant, uncontrolled clotting, such as that which occurs with DIC. Several mechanisms regulate and control coagulation.

Endothelial Inhibition

The first line of defense is the vascular endothelium. The intact endothelial has properties that serve to limit both platelet aggregation and coagulation and to induce fibrinolysis should a clot begin to form on normal endothelium. They are summarized in Table 10-12.

The Thromboxane–Prostacyclin Balance. Primary hemostasis is, in part, controlled by the balance between the actions of two prostaglandins, thromboxane A_2 and prostacyclin. Thromboxane A_2 (TxA_2) is synthesized at the site of vascular damage by activated platelets. TxA_2 has two hemostatic effects: (1) it is a potent vasoconstrictor that causes blood vessels to constrict locally and shunt blood flow away from the site of injury, and (2) it stimulates additional ADP release from platelets and thereby causes recruitment of additional platelets.[127]

Remote from the site of vascular damage, normal endothelial cells synthesize prostacyclin (PGI2). PGI2, which is also synthesized from arachidonic acid, has actions opposite those of TxA_2. PGI2 inhibits platelet activation, secretion, and aggregation and is a potent vasodilator. It therefore serves to prevent platelet aggregation and clot formation on the endothelial surface beyond the site of injury.

TABLE 10-12

ENDOTHELIAL CONTROL OF PLATELET AGGREGATION, COAGULATION, AND FIBRINOLYSIS

Endothelial control of platelet aggregation
Synthesis of prostacyclin
Synthesis of ADPases and nitric oxide
Endothelial inhibition of coagulation
Synthesis of thrombomodulin
Synthesis of heparan sulfate
Endothelial control of fibrinolysis
Synthesis of t-PA

Nitric Oxide and ADPase. The effects of prostacyclin are potentiated by nitric oxide (formerly called endothelium-dependent relaxing factor, EDRF), which is constitutively synthesized by normal endothelium and which also has vasodilatory and platelet antiaggregant effects.[128] As an additional means of preventing clot formation on the surface of normal endothelium, ADPases are expressed on the outer membrane of endothelial cells and serve to degrade "surplus" ADP that might otherwise initiate platelet aggregation on normal surfaces.

Inhibition of Coagulation

Many factors serve to limit and localize clot formation. First, the clotting factors themselves circulate in an inactive form. Once they do become activated, normal blood flow dilutes their concentration and washes them away from sites of injury, limiting clot formation. Activated clotting factors are preferentially removed from the circulation by the liver and the reticuloendothelial system. And finally, the fact that some interactions of the coagulation pathway require the presence of a phospholipid surface localizes clot formation to these phospholipid surfaces. Several specific coagulation inhibiting systems exist. Three of them are depicted in Figure 10-7 and described later.

Thrombin, Thrombomodulin, and Protein C and Protein S. Thrombin, in a negative feedback manner, can decrease its own synthesis by inhibition of factors V and VIII. That inhibition is accomplished via protein C, a vitamin K–dependent anticoagulant protein. Protein C circulates in plasma as an inactive precursor until it is activated by thrombin. Thrombomodulin is a protein located on the vascular endothelial cell surface. The binding of thrombin to thrombomodulin alters the thrombin molecule such that it can no longer directly activate clotting factors V and VIII or catalyze the conversion of fibrinogen to fibrin (Fig. 10-3). Instead, the thrombin–thrombomodulin complex rapidly converts protein C to active protein C (APC). APC, with protein S as a cofactor, cleaves and inactivates factors Va and VIIIa. Like protein C, protein S is vitamin K dependent. The location of thrombomodulin on the endothelial surface is strategic. Where the endothelium is intact, the thrombomodulin-thrombin-protein C interaction will inhibit coagulation and

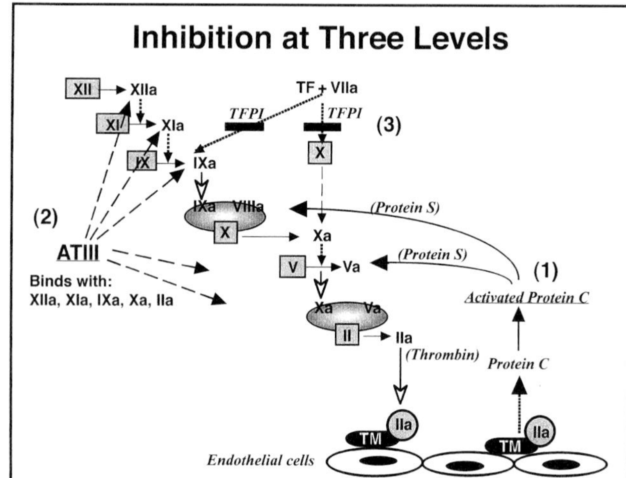

FIGURE 10-7. Inhibition of coagulation at three levels. Three important mechanisms that serve to prevent unrestrained coagulation are depicted. (1) A complex of thrombomodulin (TM) and thrombin (IIa) activates protein C, which, with protein S as a cofactor, inhibits activated factors V and VIII. (2) Antithrombin III (AT III) binds, and thereby inhibits, several activated clotting factors (XIIa, XIa, IXa, Xa, IIa). (3) Tissue factor pathway inhibitor (TFPI) inhibits both of the pathways that lead to the activation of Factor X (see text).

maintain the "nonthrombogenic" property of the endothelial lining. Where the endothelium has been stripped away or damaged, this anticoagulant mechanism will be absent and clotting can continue unopposed.

Thrombin and Antithrombin III. ATIII is a circulating serine protease inhibitor that binds to thrombin and thereby inactivates it. ATIII can bind and inactivate each of the activated clotting factors of the classical "intrinsic" coagulation cascade—factors XIIa, XIa, IXa, and Xa[129] (see Fig. 10-7). By virtue of its broad inhibitory action, ATIII plays a central role in the regulation of hemostasis in vivo. The ATIII molecule has two critical binding sites, one of which reacts with thrombin (and the other activated clotting factors), and a second to which heparin can bind. In the absence of heparin, ATIII has a relatively low affinity for thrombin. However, when heparin is bound to ATIII, the efficiency of binding of ATIII to thrombin and the other factors increases dramatically. Congenital ATIII deficiency (levels 40 to 50% of normal) can lead to dangerous thrombotic events. Acquired deficiencies of ATIII may occur in a number of conditions, including liver disease, prolonged heparin administration, nephrotic syndrome, DIC, sepsis, preeclampsia, fatty liver of pregnancy, and following surgery.[130] Plasma ATIII levels are sometimes depressed by oral contraceptive use. ATIII concentrates have been used in ATIII deficiency states, including heparin resistance.[131,132]

Tissue Factor Pathway Inhibitor (TFPI). Superficially, the description of the cell-based coagulation mechanism still leaves in place one of the inadequacies of the classical cascade theories of coagulation, that is, if activated factor Xa can be formed via the direct action of the VIIa/TF complex, why is it that hemophiliacs bleed? Why do they appear to be dependent on both factors VIII and IX to produce activated factor X (Xa)? The answer lies in the existence of a feedback inhibitor of the extrinsic pathway known as tissue factor pathway inhibitor (TFPI) (see Fig. 10-7). TFPI, which is generated in a factor Xa-dependent fashion, is a potent inhibitor of the formation of factor Xa by both VIIa/TF-initiated sequences.[133] In the presence of TFPI, further activation of factor X becomes entirely dependent on the reaction sequences of the classical intrinsic pathway. The TF pathway can initiate the first flurry of thrombin generation—enough to activate platelets and stimulate cofactors V and VIII. Thereafter, continued thrombin production appears to require the action of factors VIIIa and IXa.[122]

Heparan Sulfate. There is a fourth native anticoagulant mechanism. The endothelial surface is coated with a mucopolysaccharide referred to as the glycocalyx. One of the constituents of this glycocalyx is a naturally occurring heparin-like component, heparan sulfate. Much like heparin, heparan has the ability to accelerate the binding of ATIII to thrombin and the other activated clotting factors of the classical intrinsic pathway. This heparan sulfate is well positioned because it is at this blood-endothelial interface that activated factors of the coagulation cascade are being generated. The presence of heparan sulfate on the endothelial surface further helps to promote the "antithrombotic" property of the normal endothelial lining.

The Complexities of the Hemostatic Mechanism

The preceding sections reveal that many mechanisms interact to maintain the liquid state of the blood under normal circumstances and to transform blood into a solid clot when injury occurs. These mechanisms include numerous feedback processes. The complexity is revealed by the existence of "double agents," which act at some times as procoagulants and at other times as anticoagulants. Chief among them is thrombin. Thrombin is primarily a procoagulant. Under normal circumstances, it promotes primary hemostasis by activating platelets and promotes coagulation by direct activation of factors V, VIII, and XIII. Thrombin, in the final step of the coagulation cascade, cleaves fibrinogen to fibrin. However, it also has anticoagulant effects. As described in the coagulation section earlier, when thrombin is first synthesized, it stimulates production of TFPI, which slows coagulation via the tissue factor pathway and makes continued coagulation dependent on the reaction complex formed by factors VIII and IXa. Thrombin also inhibits coagulation through its interaction with thrombomodulin and protein C. Activated protein C stimulates the release of t-PA from endothelial cells and by this mechanism it has a fibrinolytic effect. Recall, however, that the thrombin generated as part of the thrombin burst at the end of the propagation phase of coagulation also causes the release of the fibrinolysis inhibitor TAFI. Accordingly, thrombin acts at different loci as a procoagulant, an anticoagulant, a profibrinolytic, and an antifibrinolytic.

The Hemostatic Mechanism: Summary

Under normal circumstances, the hemostatic mechanism is quiescent with many of the potential participants circulating in an inactive form. Only when the endothelial lining is breached is the hemostatic mechanism set in motion. With collagen and tissue factor exposed, the intertwined processes of platelet-mediated primary hemostasis and factor-mediated coagulation begin and rapidly the vascular injury is sealed by a platelet mass into which are incorporated fibrinogen, thrombin, plasminogen, and t-PA. The completion of the coagulation process converts fibrinogen into fibrin and the platelet plug is transformed into a fibrin clot. Simultaneously, several properties of adjacent intact endothelium (elaboration of ADPases, prostacyclin, thrombomodulin, heparans, and t-PA) serve to prevent extension of the clot beyond the site of injury. Within the clot, plasmin, generated from the trapped plasminogen and t-PA, begins the process of fibrinolysis. Over time, the entire fibrin clot dissolves, new endothelial cells line the vessel, and flow is restored.

LABORATORY EVALUATION OF THE HEMOSTATIC MECHANISM

Laboratory Evaluation of Primary Hemostasis

Platelet Count

A platelet count should be the first test ordered in the evaluation of primary hemostasis. The platelet count is quick, accurate, and reproducible. However, it reveals only platelet numbers and gives no information regarding their function. Normal platelet counts range between 50,000 and 440,000/mm^3. Counts below 150,000/mm^3 are defined as thrombocytopenia. Spontaneous bleeding is unlikely in patients with platelet counts >10 to 20,000/mm^3.[65] With counts from 40 to 70,000/mm^3, bleeding induced by surgery may be severe.

Bleeding Time

The Ivy bleeding time is the most widely accepted clinical test of platelet function. Both poor platelet function and thrombocytopenia can prolong the bleeding time. A blood pressure cuff is placed around the upper arm and inflated to 40 mmHg. A cut is made on the volar surface of the forearm and the wound blotted at 30-second intervals until bleeding stops. The

Simplate Bleeding Time (BT) device, which utilizes a spring-loaded lancet, standardizes the size and depth of the cut. The normal range for the Ivy BT is 2 to 9 minutes. Variations in venous pressure, blotting technique, and patient cooperation result in a lack of precision and reproducibility that make this test somewhat less reliable than other coagulation tests. The BT is purported to evaluate the time necessary for a platelet plug to form following vascular injury. This requires a normal number of circulating platelets, platelets with normal function (which can adhere and aggregate) and an appropriate platelet interaction with the blood vessel wall. A prolongation of the BT may be a result of (1) thrombocytopenia, (2) platelet dysfunction (adhesion, aggregation), and (3) vascular abnormalities such as scurvy or the Ehlers-Danlos syndrome. BTs are prolonged in patients with many conditions that cause platelet dysfunction, for example, use of aspirin or uremia. However, prolonged BTs have been observed with numerous disorders that are not associated with platelet dysfunction, for example, vitamin K deficiency of the newborn, amyloidosis, congenital heart disease, the presence of factor VIII inhibitors.[134] Whether or not the BT test represents a specific measure of in vivo platelet function is debated. The test is unpleasant for the patient and leaves a small scar. In spite of the correlation of BT with conditions known to influence platelet function, and in spite of BT quite reliably becoming progressively prolonged as platelet count falls below 80,000/uL, there are no convincing data to confirm that bleeding time is a reliable predictor of the bleeding that will occur in association with surgical procedures.

Platelet Function Analyser

The PFA-100 is a point-of-care device. The test is based on variation in the resistance to passage of platelets through a standard aperture in the presence of platelet activators, for example, collagen and ADP. Its predictive value has not been well confirmed and it is not yet used widely.[135]

Platelet Aggregometry

The ability of platelets to aggregate can be assessed quantitatively by observing the response to stimulation with ADP, epinephrine, collagen, or ristocetin. The platelet aggregometer measures platelet aggregation spectrophotometrically. Clot retraction is another function of platelets that can be assessed grossly. When maintained at 37°C, a clot should begin to retract within 2 to 4 hours. This test is difficult to quantify and only qualitative results (retraction vs. no retraction) are usually reported.

Laboratory Evaluation of Coagulation

Evolution of the Prothrombin Time (PT) and the Partial Thromboplastin Time (PTT)

When blood is placed in a glass test tube, clot formation occurs in response to contact with the foreign surface. No exogenous reagents are required because all of the factors necessary for contact to initiate coagulation are "intrinsic" to blood. The time to formation of a clot via this pathway can be prolonged by deficiencies of any factors in the classical intrinsic pathway. However, the observation that, even in hemophiliacs, the addition of thromboplastin (now more commonly called tissue factor) to the test tube could shorten the time to clot formation suggested the presence of an alternative pathway of fibrin formation. That pathway required the addition of something "extrinsic to blood" and did not require the presence of factors VIII or IX. In 1936, when Quick introduced the PT to clinical medicine, sufficient "thromboplastin" was used to yield a clotting time of approximately 12 seconds. Under these circumstances, even patients lacking factors VIII or IX showed normal clotting times.[136] However, when "dilute" thromboplastin (or a "partial" thromboplastin) was used in lieu of the "12-second reagent," hemophiliacs showed much longer clotting times than did healthy controls. The two different pathways could be tested individually simply by varying the amount and type of thromboplastin added to blood. With "complete thromboplastin," coagulation could proceed via reactions that were independent of factors VIIIa and IXa. With a lesser thromboplastin stimulus, coagulation would proceed via a sequence of reactions that required the presence of factors VIIIa and IXa.

Basic Elements of the PT and PTT

The PT and the PTT differ primarily by the type of thromboplastin that is used. Calcium must also be added because of the chelating agent in the blood specimen container. The time to fibrin strand formation is then measured.

Prothrombin Time

The PT evaluates the coagulation sequence initiated by TF and leading to the formation of fibrin without the participation of factors VIII or IX, that is, the classical extrinsic pathway (see Fig. 10-2). The PT measures the time to fibrin strand formation via a short sequence of reactions involving only TF, and factors VII, X, V, II (prothrombin), and I (fibrinogen). Tissue factor forms a complex with VIIa and together this complex activates factor X. From that point, coagulation proceeds via the common pathway of coagulation. The test does not evaluate the coagulation process that is initiated by the classical intrinsic pathway or that sequence of reactions initiated by tissue factor that generate Xa via the reaction complex formed by factors IXa and VIIIa.

The normal PT is 10 to 12 seconds. The PT will be prolonged if deficiencies, abnormalities, or inhibitors of factors VII, X, V, II, or I are present. The PT test has limitations. First, it is not very sensitive to deficiencies of any of these factors. In fact, the coagulant activity of these factors must drop to 30% of normal before the PT is prolonged. The PT is most sensitive to a decrease in factor VII and least sensitive to changes in prothrombin (factor II). When prothrombin levels are only 10% of normal, the increase in the PT may be only 2 seconds. Also, PT will not be prolonged until the fibrinogen level is below 100 mg/dL. A prolonged PT does not define the exact hemostatic defect. However, if the aPTT (see later) is normal, then a prolonged PT is most likely to represent a deficiency or abnormality of factor VII. Because factor VII has the shortest half-life of the clotting factors synthesized in the liver, factor VII is the clotting factor that first becomes deficient with liver disease, vitamin K deficiency, or warfarin therapy. Prolongation of the PT may also occur because of deficiencies of multiple factors. However, when multiple factor deficiencies coexist, the PTT or activated PTT (see later) will usually be prolonged as well.

International Normalized Ratio. Another difficulty with the PT test is that many different thromboplastin reagents are used. This results in wide variation in normal values, which makes comparison of PT results between laboratories difficult. The International Normalized Ratio was introduced to circumvent this difficulty.[137] Each thromboplastin is compared with an internationally accepted standard thromboplastin and assigned an International Sensitivity Index (ISI). If the test thromboplastin is equivalent to the international standard, it will have an ISI index of 1. Once the ISI number has been determined, PT test times obtained with that reagent are normalized and reported as an International Normalized Ratio.[138]

Partial Thromboplastin Time

The PTT assesses the function of the classical intrinsic and final common pathways (see Fig. 10-1). It entails the addition of a "partial thromboplastin" (usually a phospholipid extracted from rabbit brain or human placenta) and calcium to citrated plasma. The PTT reflects the time to fibrin strand formation via the classical "intrinsic pathway" of coagulation. The PTT will reveal deficiencies, abnormalities, or inhibitors to one or more coagulation factors—high–molecular-weight kininogen (HMWK), prekallikrein, XII, XI, IX, VIII, X, V, II, and I. The normal values for PTT vary widely. However, the PTT has been made more reproducible and the range of normal values narrower by the addition of contact activator in addition to the partial thromboplastin; hence the name "activated" partial thromboplastin time (aPTT).[139] Surface activation in the laboratory parallels the contact-activation phase involving factors XII and XI, prekallikrein, and high–molecular-weight kininogen that are thought to initiate the intrinsic pathway in vivo. Diatomaceous earth, kaolin, celite, and ellagic acid are used as surface activators. The aPTT is much faster than the PTT, which may be as long as 120 seconds, because it eliminates the lengthy "natural" contact-activation phase. Normal aPTT values are between 25 and 35 seconds.[140] The aPTT is prolonged when there is a deficiency, abnormality, or inhibitor of factors XII, XI, IX, VIII, X, V, II, and I (i.e., all factors except VII and XIII). The aPTT is most sensitive to deficiencies of factors VIII and IX, but, as is the case with the PT, levels of these factors must be reduced to approximately 30% of normal values before the test is prolonged. Heparin prolongs the aPTT but with high levels will also prolong PT. As with the PT, the level of fibrinogen must also be reduced to 100 mg/dL before the aPTT is prolonged. FXII deficiency, which is a relatively common cause of aPTT prolongation, does not cause a clinical coagulopathy. aPTT results (like those of the PT) vary from laboratory to laboratory because of nonstandardization of the phospholipids and activators.

Activated Clotting Time

The activated clotting time (ACT) is similar to the aPTT in that it tests the ability of blood to clot in a test tube and is dependent on factors that are all "intrinsic" to blood (the classical intrinsic pathway of coagulation). Fresh whole blood is added to a test tube that contains a particulate surface activator of factors XII and XI. The time to clot formation is measured. Partial thromboplastin or a platelet phospholipid substitute is not added. Coagulation is therefore dependent on adequate amounts of platelet phospholipid being present in the blood sample. The automated ACT is widely used to monitor heparin therapy in the operating room. Normal values are in the range of 90 to 120 seconds.[139] The ACT is far less sensitive than the aPTT to factor deficiencies in the classical intrinsic coagulation pathway. In fact, the ACT may not be prolonged until the coagulant activity of some of the factors is reduced to 1% of normal.

Thrombin Time

Thrombin time (TT), also called the "thrombin clotting time," is a measure of the ability of thrombin to convert fibrinogen to fibrin. This test, which is performed by adding exogenous thrombin to citrated plasma, bypasses all the preceding reactions. The thrombin time may be prolonged because of conditions that effect either the substrate, fibrinogen, or the action of the enzyme thrombin. The TT is prolonged when there is an inadequate amount of fibrinogen (<100 mg/dL) or when the fibrinogen molecules that are present are abnormal (dysfibrinogenemia), for example, advanced liver disease. Thrombin's enzymatic function can be inhibited by inhibitors such as heparin (complexed to ATIII), FDPs, or by inhibitors that may be seen in patients with plasma cell myeloma and other immunoproliferative conditions.[141] The normal TT is <30 seconds.

Reptilase Time

When the thrombin time is prolonged, the reptilase time can be used to differentiate between the effects of heparin and FDPs. Reptilase, which is derived from a snake venom, converts fibrinogen to fibrin. The action of reptilase is unaffected by heparin but is inhibited by FDPs. A prolonged TT and a normal reptilase time suggest the presence of heparin. Prolongation of both TT and reptilase time will occur in the presence of FDPs, or when fibrinogen level is low. The normal reptilase time is 14 to 21 seconds.

Ecarin Clotting Time

Direct thrombin inhibitors (DTI) (hirudin, argatroban, bivalirudin, lepirudin) are frequently used in patients with heparin-induced thrombocytopenia. At low DTI concentrations, TT and ACT provide reasonable correlations with DTI concentrations, but with the concentrations required for cardiopulmonary bypass the correlation becomes poor and the risk of overdose with these agents, for which there are no antagonists, becomes significant. The ecarin clotting time (ECT) provides a better correlation and can be used for monitoring in this context.[142] The test employs the venom of the Saw-Scaled (a.k.a. Sawtooth) Viper (Echis carinatus). A metalloprotease in the venom converts normal prothrombin to a form that is inhibited by the DTIs in a dose-dependent manner.

Fibrinogen Level

Normal values are between 160 and 350 mg/dL. Below 100 mg/dL, fibrinogen may be inadequate to produce a clot. Fibrinogen is rapidly depleted during DIC. A marked increase in fibrinogen may occur in response to stress including surgery and trauma. Levels in excess of 700 mg/dL may occur. Because of this increase, in spite of rapid fibrinogen consumption during a hypercoagulable state such as DIC, the fibrinogen level may still appear to be "normal."

Laboratory Evaluation of Fibrinolysis

Fibrin Degradation Products and D-Dimer

The fibrin degradation products (FDP) test identifies the breakdown products of fibrin (crosslinked or uncrosslinked) and fibrinogen itself. The D-dimer assay is specific for breakdown products of crosslinked fibrin. FDPs will be increased in any state of accelerated fibrinolysis, including advanced liver disease, fibrinolysis associated with cardiopulmonary bypass, administration of exogenous thrombolytics, for example, streptokinase, and DIC. D-dimer is specific to conditions in which extensive lysis of the crosslinked fibrin of mature thrombus is occurring, in particular DIC but also DVT and PE.

The Thromboelastogram

Thromboelastography provides a measure of the mechanical properties of evolving clot as a function of time. A principal advantage of this test is that the processes it measures require the integrated action of all the elements of the hemostatic process: platelet aggregation, coagulation, and fibrinolysis. The thromboelastogram (TEG®) is obtained by placing a specimen of blood in a rotating cuvette into which a "piston" is lowered. As clot formation begins, the piston rotates as function of the adherence of the evolving fibrin clot to the piston. The piston

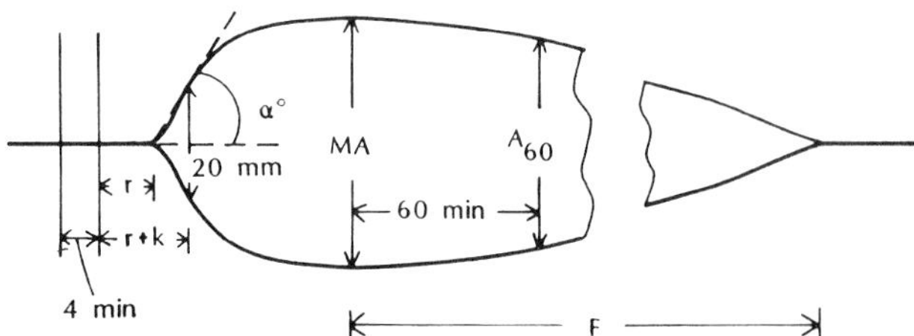

FIGURE 10-8. The normal thromboelastogram and the variables commonly derived from it. See text for explanation. (From Kang et al, Epsilon-aminocaproic acid for treatment of fibrinolysis during liver transplantation. Anesthesiology 66:766, 1987, with permission.)

is connected to a recorder and the rotation of the piston results in a to and fro excursion of the stylus, the amplitude of which is proportional to the speed of piston rotation.

Figure 10-8 depicts a normal thromboelastogram. Several parameters are derived from the TEG®. The most commonly used ones and their interpretation are as follows.[144]

R, the reaction time, is the interval until initial clot formation. It requires thrombin formation, and prolongation is usually indicative of an intrinsic pathway factor deficiency.

K, the clot formation time, is the interval required after R for the thromboelastogram to achieve a width of 20 mm. Prolongation occurs with deficiencies of thrombin formation or generation of fibrin from fibrinogen.

The alpha angle, like K, is a measure of the speed of clot formation. A decrease of the alpha angle has similar significance to a prolongation of K.

MA, the maximum amplitude, is a measure of the strength of the fully formed clot. It reflects primarily platelet number and function, although it also requires proper fibrin formation to achieve normal values. MA typically occurs between 30 and 60 minutes.

The (MA + x)/ MA, the ratio of the amplitude at a specific time interval (x) after MA divided by MA, is used as a measure of the rate of fibrinolysis. The (MA +60)/MA ratio has been used most widely.[145] A ratio of less than 0.85 is evidence of abnormal fibrinolysis.[146] In clinical practice, particularly in liver transplantation, a nonquantitative appreciation of the typical tear drop shape (Fig. 10-9) is used more often to support a diagnosis of increased fibrinolysis than are specific numerical values. F, the interval from MA to return to a zero amplitude, is a measure of the rate of fibrinolysis. F is sufficiently long in normal subjects that often the test is usually terminated before this time elapses.

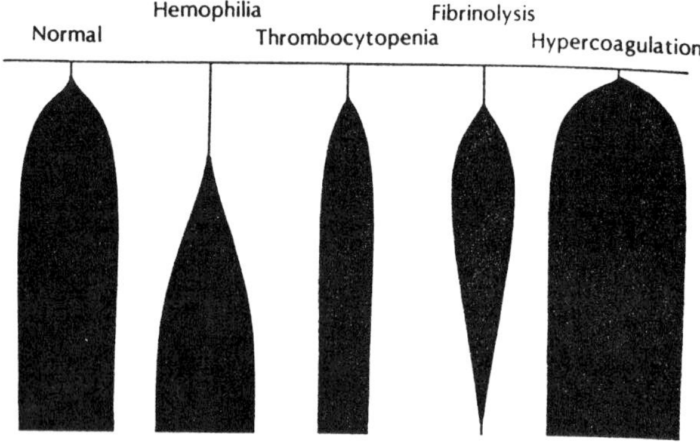

FIGURE 10-9. Thromboelastogram patterns seen in normal subjects and in subjects with four abnormalities of hemostasis. (From Kang YG: Monitoring and treatment of coagulation. Winter KM, Kang YG: Hepatic Transplantation: Anesthetic and Periperative management, p. 151. New York, Praeqer, 1986, with permission.)

The thromboelastogram has been employed in cardiac surgery, major trauma, and hepatic transplantation. It is in the latter that it is used most frequently. Commonly, in that context, an increased R prompts the administration of FFP, a decreased MA leads to platelet administration, and the tear drop configuration of fibrinolysis to the administration of antifibrinolytics. The use of the thromboelastogram in liver transplantation has been shown to decrease both the amount of RBCs and FFP transfused as compared with transfusion guided by routine coagulation tests.[148]

Interpretation of Tests of the Hemostatic Mechanism

An effective approach to the interpretation of coagulation tests is to appreciate in advance the constellation of test results (the coagulation "profile") that is likely to occur with each of the common bleeding disorders (Table 10-13). The most commonly ordered coagulation tests are the platelet count, PT, aPTT, and occasionally BT. When a greater disruption of the hemostatic mechanism is suspected, further tests including fibrinogen, TT, and assays for fibrin degradation products and the D-dimer may be ordered.

Because the coagulation defects that appear most often are revealed as abnormal values of PT and/or aPTT, Figure 10-10 provides an algorithm for the evaluation of those abnormalities.

Common Coagulation Profiles

Platelet Count Decreased (Normal aPTT and PT). Differential diagnosis: causes (see later) of decreased platelet production, excess consumption, platelet destruction, or sequestration in the spleen (see bleeding disorders, thrombocytopenia).

Prolonged BT (Normal Platelet Count, aPTT, PT). Differential diagnosis: antiplatelet drug ingestion (NSAIDs, ASA, clopidogrel, etc.), uremia, vWD (although the factor VIII:C levels may be decreased with vWD [type 1], only 25 to 30% of VIII:C coagulant activity is necessary to produce a normal aPTT).

Prolonged aPTT (Normal Platelet Count and PT). Differential diagnosis: heparin, the lupus anticoagulant or other antiphospholipid antibodies, for example, anticardiolipin and anti-B2-GPI antibodies, deficiency of factor XII, HMWK, or prekallikrein, Hemophilia A or B, vWD, acquired factor inhibitors, poor collection technique.

Disorders that produce this combination affect factors of the intrinsic pathway (prekallikrein, HMWK, factors XII, XI, IX, VIII) and/or the common pathway (X, V, II, and I). With heparin therapy, initially only the aPTT is prolonged. At higher doses both the aPTT and PT are prolonged. The lupus "anticoagulant" and other antiphospholipid antibodies are common causes of a prolonged aPTT. That prolongation is the result of the binding of the phospholipid used to initiate coagulation in vitro. The patients do not have a bleeding diathesis. In fact, they have a prothrombotic tendency. This laboratory abnormality is not corrected when the patient's plasma is mixed with normal plasma because of the presence of inhibitors. Deficiencies of factor XII, HMWK, or prekallikrein, in particular FXII, are also common causes of aPTT prolongation. However, they are not usually associated with a significant clinical hemostatic defect. Collection technique can prolong the aPTT either by heparin contamination or because factors V and VIII, the labile factors, may be consumed if the blood becomes partially clotted prior to delivery to the laboratory.[149] The aPTT is very sensitive to factor VIII deficiency.

TABLE 10-13

INTERPRETATION OF COAGULATION TESTS

PLATELET COUNT	BLEEDING TIME	aPTT	PT	TT	FIBRINOGEN	FDPs	POSSIBLE CAUSE	EXAMPLE
↓	N or ↓	N	N	N	N	N	↓ Production sequestration ↑ Consumption Immune destruction	Radiation, chemotherapy Splenomegaly Extensive tissue damage HIT
N	↑	N	N	N	N	N	Platelet dysfunction	Drugs: ASA, NSAIDs, Clopidogrel, IIb/IIIa inhibitors; uremia; mild vWD
N	↑	↑	N	N	N	N	Severe vWF deficiency	vWD
N	N	↑	N	N	N	N	Factor deficiency Factor inhibition Antiphospholipid antibody	Hemophilia A or B Low-dose heparin, LMWH[a] Poor collection technique Lupus anticoagulant
N	N	N	↑	N	N	N	Factor VII deficiency	Early liver disease Early vitamin K deficiency Early Coumadin therapy
N	N	↑	↑	↑	N	N	Multiple factor deficiencies	Late vitamin K deficiency Late Coumadin therapy Heparin therapy[b]
↓	↑	↑	↑	↑	↓	N	Dilution of factors and platelets	Massive transfusion
↓	↑	↑	↑	↑	↓	↑	Hypercoagulable state ± ↓ production of factors	DIC[c] Advanced liver disease

↑, increased; ↓, decreased; N, normal; aPTT, "activated" partial thromboplastin time; PT, prothrombin time; TT, thrombin time; FDPs, fibrin degradation products; HIT, heparin-induced thrombocytopenia; vWF, von Willebrand factor; vWD, von Willebrand's disease; LMWH, low-molecular-weight heparin; NSAIDs, nonsteroidal anti-inflammatory drugs; DIC, disseminated intravascular coagulation.

[a] aPTT prolongation is more likely to occur with LMWHs with lower Xa/IIa effect ratios, for example, tinzaparin, than with greater ratios, for example, enoxaparin.

[b] Bleeding time may also be prolonged in association with a marked aPTT increase.

[c] DIC may be distinguished by the presence of D-dimers.

When a PTT is prolonged in isolation, is it less likely to be because of a bleeding disorder that involves multiple factor deficiencies (such as liver disease, vitamin K deficiency, the administration of warfarin, or the coagulopathy associated with massive transfusion or DIC). Heparin therapy or congenital disorders of hemostasis are more probable.

Prolonged PT (Normal Platelet Count and aPTT). Differential diagnosis: vitamin K deficiency, warfarin administration, early liver dysfunction, FVII deficiency, acquired coagulation factor inhibitors.

Because of the vitamin K–dependent factors, factor VII has the shortest half-life, depletion of the vitamin K–dependent factors will first prolong the PT and later the aPTT as well. Similarly, the development of liver disease will lead to deficiencies of factor VII first and initially prolong only the PT. With further deterioration of liver function, both the PT and the aPTT

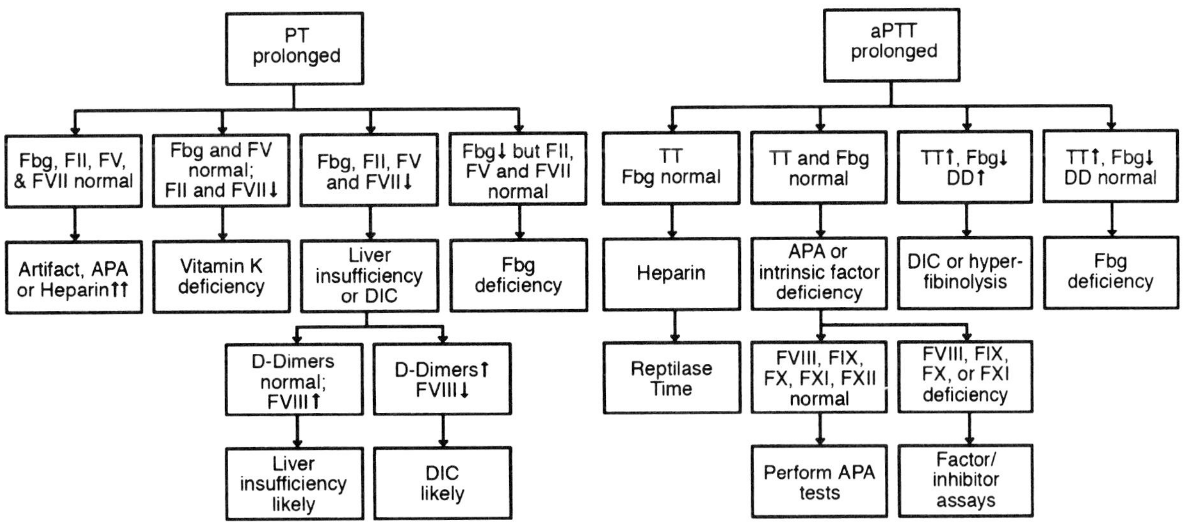

FIGURE 10-10. An approach to the evaluation of prolonged PT and/or aPTT. APA, antiphospholipid antibody (e.g., lupus anticoagulant, anticardiolipin and anti-B2-GPI antibodies); DD, D-dimers; DIC, disseminated intravascular coagulation. (Reproduced [with modification] from Bombeli T, Spahn DR: Updates in perioperative coagulation: Physiology and management of thromboembolism and haemorrhage. Br J Anaesth 93:275, 2004, with permission.)

will be prolonged. Liver disease can also lead to thrombocytopenia and platelet dysfunction. Acquired coagulation factor inhibitors are rare but can occur in patients with lymphoma or collagen vascular disease.

Prolonged PT and aPTT (Normal Platelet Count). Differential diagnosis: vitamin K deficiency, warfarin, heparin.

Although liver disease can produce multiple factor deficiencies and this pattern, the platelet count is usually decreased. FDPs will also be elevated (see later).

Prolonged PT, aPTT, and TT (Normal Platelet Count). Differential diagnosis: heparin, DTIs or FDPs, hypofibrinogenemia, dysfibrinogenemia.

Simultaneous prolongation of the TT makes the diagnosis of simple vitamin K deficiency or warfarin therapy unlikely. TT is sensitive to minute levels of heparin. Addition of protamine or reptilase time will identify heparin. FDPs may be elevated with fibrinolytic therapy, DIC, or liver disease. DIC and liver disease usually result in thrombocytopenia as well. A normal platelet count makes heparin or extensive fibrinolysis more likely.

Prolonged PT, aPTT, TT (Decreased Platelet Count). Differential diagnosis: DIC, dilution by massive transfusion, liver disease, heparin therapy.

FDPs and D-dimer are elevated in DIC and allow differentiation from dilutional effects and excess heparin. Heparin causes thrombocytopenia only when prolonged exposure results in HIT. FDPs, but not D-dimer, are elevated in severe liver disease.

The interpretation of coagulation tests may be made more difficult by the fact that patients who develop a bleeding diathesis in the perioperative period may have more than one bleeding disorder (e.g., DIC and coagulopathy as a result of massive transfusion) and may also have a surgical cause for bleeding.

DISORDERS OF HEMOSTASIS: DIAGNOSIS AND TREATMENT

The hemostatic mechanism involves an intricate balance that serves to limit blood loss in the event of vascular injury while maintaining the liquid character of blood at other times. Under normal circumstances, an equilibrium between clotting and bleeding is maintained with the help of multiple activators, inhibitors, cofactors, and feedback loops, both positive and negative. Under pathologic circumstances, that equilibrium may be lost, leading to either hemorrhagic or thrombotic complications. Accordingly, disorders of hemostasis can be broadly classified into those that lead to abnormal bleeding and those that lead to abnormal clotting. The disorders may be further categorized according to whether they involve platelets, clotting factors, and/or the presence or absence of inhibitors (such as FDPs). Finally, disorders may be hereditary or acquired. These organizational frameworks will be helpful in reaching a diagnosis on the basis of the results of coagulation tests. The treatment that follows from diagnosis may require administration of hemostatic agents (platelets and/or clotting factors) or the use of pharmacologic agents. The latter may be chosen for effects on platelets (desmopressin, antiplatelet drugs), on clotting factors (vitamin K, warfarin, heparin), or on naturally occurring inhibitors (antifibrinolytic agents, protamine, fibrinolytics).

The preoperative history is invaluable in the identification of disorders of hemostasis. Abnormalities of primary hemostasis, usually caused by reduced platelet number or function, will be revealed by evidence of "superficial" (skin and mucosal) bleeding including easy bruising, petechiae, prolonged bleeding from minor skin lacerations, recurrent epistaxis, and menorrhagia. Coagulation abnormalities are associated with "deep" bleeding events including hemarthroses or hematomas after blunt trauma.

Hereditary Disorders of Hemostasis

Von Willebrand's Disease

Von Willebrand's disease is the most common hereditary bleeding disorder. Some form of the disease is present in approximately 1% of the general population, though it is overtly symptomatic in only about 10% of those afflicted.[151] vWD is the result of abnormal synthesis of the von Willebrand factor (vWF). The vWF, a protein synthesized by endothelial cells, megakaryoctyes, and platelets, is important for both primary hemostasis, that is, the binding of platelets to sites of vascular injury, and coagulation, the latter through its role as a carrier protein/stabilizer for FVIII. The vWF has several distinct binding domains responsible for its several hemostatic functions. Those domains include sites that are specific for collagen (for adherence to the subendothelium), the platelet GPIb receptor (for platelet adhesion to collagen), the platelet GPIIb/IIIa receptor (for platelet aggregation), and factor VIII:C (for its carrier protein function). There are at least 50 genetic variations of vWD, which accounts for its phenotypic heterogeneity. There are three principal subtypes. Type 1, which comprises 70 to 80% of vWD, is a quantitative defect. vWF is present but is secreted in reduced amount. Patients with Type 1 vWD present with a pattern of bleeding that is characteristic of abnormalities of primary hemostasis. Type 2 vWD, which comprises 20 to 30% of patients with vWD, includes a host of qualitative defects of vWF. Some mutations affect the platelet interactions of vWF and others the factor VIII interaction. Type 2 is subdivided into four subtypes. 2B is characterized by a variant of the vWF that causes abnormal aggregation of platelets and thrombocytopenia. The abnormal vWF has a high affinity for the platelet GPIb receptor. The bleeding diathesis is probably the result of formation and clearance of vWF-platelet complexes and the resultant thrombocytopenia. In the subtype 2N (Normandy) vWD, the vWF has a markedly reduced affinity for factor VIII. These patients demonstrate normal platelet function, but bleed because of decreased factor VIII coagulant activity. These patients are readily misdiagnosed as having mild hemophilia A. Type 3, which is very rare, entails a complete absence of vWF, resulting in a severe abnormality of both primary hemostasis and coagulation.

The Role of vWF in Hemostasis. vWF is essential for platelet plug formation. It mediates platelet adhesion to the subendothelial surface of blood vessels. After binding to the subendothelium, the vWF undergoes a conformational change that allows platelets to adhere via their glycoprotein GPIb receptors (Fig. 10-4). This binding can only occur after the conformational change and in solution, platelets will not spontaneously bind to vWF. The antibiotic ristocetin can induce the platelet GPIb-vWF interaction and, accordingly, is the basis for one laboratory test of platelet function. vWF also participates in platelet to platelet aggregation. Platelet aggregation occurs by binding of vWF molecules to the GPIIb/IIIa receptors on the surface of several platelets. The vWF also acts as a carrier protein for the coagulant activity of factor VIII, referred to as VIII:C, with which it circulates in a complexed form that prolongs VIII:C's circulation time.

Diagnosis and Treatment of vWD. History will commonly reveal abnormal bleeding from mucosal surfaces. Sixty percent of the patients will report epistaxis, 50% report menorrhagia, and 35% will acknowledge gingival bleeding, easy bruising, and hematomas.[152] vWD should be considered in patients who give a history of unexplained postoperative bleeding, particularly following tonsillectomy or dental extraction. Although this is a hereditary disease, a clear family history is not always evident because disease severity varies substantially.

Specialized laboratory tests, ideally directed by a hematologist, may be required to confirm the diagnosis and type of vWD. One or more vWF markers including vWF factor antigen (vWF:Ag), vWF ristocetin cofactor activity (vWF:RCo), or vWF collagen binding activity (vWF:CB) will be diminished or absent. Because vWD is a carrier protein/stabilizer of FVIII, FVIII half-life is diminished and FVIII levels are characteristically also decreased.[151] What is important for the anesthesiologist to appreciate is that the results of the most commonly ordered coagulation tests, the platelet count, the aPTT, and the PT, may be normal in the patient with vWD. While the half-life of VIII:C is diminished in vWD there is usually sufficient VIII:C to yield a normal aPTT in basal conditions.

The two established treatments for vWD are DDAVP and factor concentrates.[153] DDAVP (1-deamino-8-D-arginine vasopressin), which promotes release of vWF, is effective first-line therapy for the large majority (approximately 80%) of patients with vWD, including those with type 1 and type 2A disease. However the recognition of subtype 2B (see earlier) is important because DDAVP will cause thrombocytopenia in these patients.[154] DDAVP, given intravenously in a dose of 0.3 ug/kg, increases factor VIII:C and vWF two- to fivefold in most patients. Its effect is maximal after 30 minutes and elevated levels persist for 6 to 8 hours[152] (see Pharmacologic Therapy: Desmopressin section). For the 20% of patients who do not respond adequately to DDAVP, factor concentrates, for example, Haemate-P, will be appropriate. Their efficacy is well confirmed.[155,156] Antifibrinolytic agents, epsilon-aminocaproic acid, and tranexamic acid are sometimes used in combination with DDAVP to manage these patients during the perioperative period.[154] They may be given intravenously or orally. They have also been administered topically, as mouthwashes, in patients with vWD undergoing dental extractions. Oral contraceptives (estrogens) have been used to treat patients with vWD and menorrhagia or who are undergoing elective surgery.[154] The mechanism of action of the estrogens is not well understood, although a connection with vWF synthesis is suspected. Antiplatelet drugs should be avoided in patients with vWD.

The Hemophilias

Hemophilia A results from mutations that lead to either deficient or functionally defective factor VIII:C. Hemophilia B (Christmas disease) and hemophilia C are caused by deficiency or abnormality of factors IX and XI, respectively.[157] The relative frequencies of the three hemophilias are factor VIII:C, 85%; factor IX, 14%; and factor XI, 1%. Rare inherited deficiencies of factors II, VII, V, and XI also occur.[157] Both hemophilia A and B are sex-linked recessive disorders, which therefore occur almost exclusively in males. Hemophilia C is an autosomal recessive disorder that occurs almost exclusively in Ashkenazi Jews.[157] About 50% of operations in hemophiliacs are orthopaedic procedures required for treatment of the arthritic consequences of hemarthroses.

Hemophilia A. Factor VIII is a very large macromolecule with two components, the coagulant factor VIII (VIII:C) and the von Willebrand factor. The VIII:C molecule circulates bound to and protected by vWF. In hemophilia A, patients have normal levels of vWF, but have reduced or defective factor VIII:C. Hemophilia A occurs in approximately 1 in 10,000 males.

Hemophiliacs experience deep tissue bleeding, hemarthroses, and hematuria most commonly. Clinically, hemophilia A can be classified as mild, moderate, and severe. Patients with mild disease have factor levels of 5 to 30% of normal and usually bleed abnormally only following trauma. Patients with moderate disease have factor levels of 1 to 5% and occasionally bleed spontaneously as well as following trauma. The great majority of hemophiliacs have the severe form of the disease. Factor VIII:C levels are less than 1% of normal and they frequently experience spontaneous bleeding episodes. The severity of clinical symptoms usually correlates with the level of clotting factor activity. Like the patient with vWD, hemophiliacs should avoid aspirin and other platelet inhibiting agents.

Diagnosis and treatment of hemophilia A. Patients with hemophilia A will commonly report a history that reveals the X-linked recessive pattern of disease inheritance. Diagnosis of hemophilia A is made on the basis of a prolonged aPTT and specific factor assays demonstrating a deficiency of factor VIII coagulant activity with normal levels of vWF, factor IX, and factor XI. The patient will have a normal PT and BT. Hemophilia A is treated with plasma-derived concentrates that have been treated by viral attenuation procedures or, now more commonly, with recombinant factor VIII.[157]

If a hemophiliac presents for elective surgery, the patient's hematologist should be consulted. The required factor replacement will be dependent on (1) the patient's plasma volume and (2) the desired procoagulant activity. The patient's plasma volume can be assumed to be equal to 40 mL of plasma per kilogram of body weight. A 60-kg person would have a plasma volume of 2,400 mL. One unit of procoagulant activity per milliliter of plasma is defined as a plasma procoagulant level of 100%. A procoagulant level of 25% is a common target for achieving control of a bleeding episode. This would mean that a total of 600 units (25% × 2,400 mL) of factor VIII:C would be required. For elective surgery, the level of factor VIII:C activity is usually raised to 50 to 100% of normal. Many hemophiliacs develop inhibitors to factor VIII:C. The presence of the inhibitor increases the amount of factor VIII:C that must be administered to manage a given hemostatic challenge. Recombinant activated FVIIa (see later) may be required for the patient with inhibitors.

DDAVP will also increase plasma factor VIII:C and vWF concentrations and may be effective in mild hemophilia A. DDAVP is thought to cause the release of factor VIII:C from liver endothelial cells. There is a large variation in patient response to DDAVP and it is most effective in patients with factor VIII:C levels greater than 5%.[66,158] It is given iv in a dose of 0.3 ug/kg in 50 mL of saline over 15 to 30 minutes. It causes a prompt increase in factor VIII:C. However, tachyphylaxis does develop, which limits its usefulness.

The antifibrinolytics epsilon aminocaproic acid and tranexamic acid have been used to treat hemophiliac patients prior to dental procedures. The agents are contraindicated in bleeding episodes involving joints or the urinary tract because the clots that do form may not be lysed for a long period of time.

Hemophilia B. Factor IX deficiency is also an X-linked recessive disorder, occurring in ca. 1/25,000 males,[157] that produces a bleeding diathesis that is clinically indistinguishable from hemophilia A. A recombinant FIX factor concentrate is now available. Typically, minor hemorrhage is managed by achieving FIX levels of 20 to 30% of normal. Levels of 50 to 100% are sought for more severe hemorrhage and in anticipation of surgery. Factor IX complex concentrates, also known as prothrombin complex concentrates (II, VII, IX, X), have been used in the face of resistance to FIX concentrates. However, they convey an infectious hazard and may entail a risk of thrombosis and DIC because of the presence of activated factors.

Protein C and Protein S Deficiency

Hereditary deficiencies of protein C and protein S are associated with thromboembolic events originating on the venous side of the circulation, for example, DVT, PE, and stroke as a consequence of paradoxical embolization. The complete absence of protein C is associated with death in infancy. Patients who experience thromboembolic events and have decreased levels of protein C or protein S should remain on anticoagulant therapy indefinitely.

Acquired Disorders of Hemostasis

For mnemonic purposes, it is helpful to classify bleeding disorders according to which of the three hemostatic processes are involved: primary hemostasis (platelet disorders), coagulation (clotting factor disorders), fibrinolysis (production of inhibitors such as FDPs), or some combination of the three. Similarly, it is useful to use the results of coagulation tests to determine whether the clinical problem involves primary hemostasis (decreased platelet count, increased bleeding time, etc.), coagulation (prolonged PT and aPTT, decreased factor levels, etc.), fibrinolysis (increased FDPs, increased D-dimer), or some combination of the three. Ultimately, therapeutic decisions (e.g., administration of platelets, FFP, or an antifibrinolytic agent) will similarly be oriented to treatment of one or more of these processes.

Acquired Disorders of Platelets

The clinical conditions that cause an isolated disorder of primary hemostasis typically involve abnormalities of either platelet number or function.

Thrombocytopenia. Platelets are derived from megakaryocytes in the bone marrow in response to thrombopoietin, which is synthesized by the liver. The causes of thrombocytopenia may be categorized as follows: (1) inadequate production by the bone marrow, (2) increased peripheral consumption or destruction (nonimmune mediated), (3) increased peripheral destruction (immune mediated), (4) dilution of circulating platelets, and (5) sequestration (Fig. 10-11).

1. Bone marrow production of platelets can be impaired in many ways. Physical and chemical agents (radiation and chemotherapy), various drugs (thiazide diuretics, sulfonamides, diphenylhydantoin, alcohol), infectious agents (hepatitis B, TB, overwhelming sepsis), and chronic disease states (uremia, liver disease) can all cause bone marrow suppression. Infiltration of the bone marrow by cancer cells or replacement by fibrosis will also result in inadequate platelet production.
2. Accelerated nonimmunologically mediated consumption can occur in many conditions that cause extensive activation of coagulation with or without the occurrence of DIC. After extensive tissue damage such as occurs with burns or massive crush injuries, which denude vascular endothelium, the normal process of hemostasis activates platelets, leading to their consumption and to thrombocytopenia. In a similar fashion, the interaction of platelets with nonendothelialized structures such as large vascular grafts can also lead to a transient thrombocytopenia. Platelets are consumed in patients with an extensive vasculitis such as occurs with toxemia of pregnancy. The many conditions that cause DIC (see later) will also cause platelets to be consumed or destroyed faster than they can be produced.
3. Immunologically mediated consumption can be caused by various drugs (heparin, quinidine, cephalosporins) and autoimmune disorders (systemic lupus erythematosis, rheumatoid arthritis, thrombotic thrombocytopenic purpura). Alloimmunization resulting from previous blood transfusions or pregnancy can cause refractoriness to platelet transfusions.
4. Dilution of platelets will occur in the context of massive transfusion (see later and Collection and Preparation of Blood Products for Transfusion section).
5. Under normal conditions, approximately one-third of platelets are sequestered in the spleen. When the spleen enlarges, an increasing number are sequestered and thrombocytopenia may result. This may occur with the splenomegaly associated with myelodysplastic syndromes and cirrhosis of the liver, though in the latter condition decreased production also contributes to thrombocytopenia.

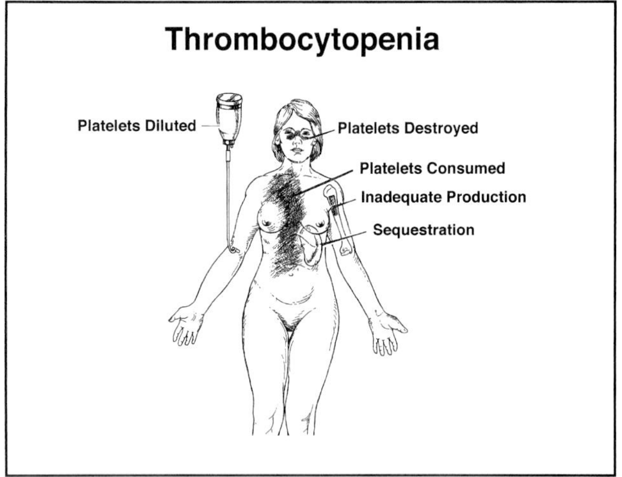

FIGURE 10-11. Thrombocytopenia. The figure depicts the five processes that can lead to thrombocytopenia. They include platelet destruction, as occurs immunologically in lupus erythematosus; platelet consumption, as occurs with burns or other massive tissue injury conditions; inadequate production, as can occur with marrow infiltration, chemotherapy, or radiation; sequestration, as can occur in the presence of splenomegaly; and dilution, occurring during massive transfusion.

Disorders of Platelet Function

Uremia. Platelet dysfunction is common in uremic patients. The accumulation of guanidino succinic acid and hydroxy phenolic acid is thought to contribute to this dysfunction through interference with the platelet's ability to expose the PF3 phospholipid surface. These compounds are dialysable and, accordingly, dialysis frequently improves the hemostatic defect associated with uremia. An additional abnormality involving the interaction of vWF with platelet receptors is also suspected. DDAVP (desmopressin), which among other effects induces immediate release of vWF from endothelial cells, rapidly improves platelet adhesiveness.[159] However, the mechanism of this effect is not understood. It is not simply a matter of restoring vWF levels because circulating vWF is typically present in normal levels in uremia. Administration of erythropoietin and conjugated estrogens have also been observed to cause gradual improvement of the hemostatic defect associated with uremia. The mechanisms of these effects are similarly not known. Cryoprecipitate will also improve the platelet dysfunction of uremia but, given the efficacy of DDAVP, the associated risks are not justified. When life-threatening bleeding occurs in the uremic patient, platelet concentrates should be administered.

Antiplatelet agents. Numerous medications are administered expressly for the purpose of platelet inhibition in order to reduce the risk of myocardial infarction, stroke, and other thromboembolic complications. They induce platelet dysfunction by several mechanisms, which include inhibition of cyclooxygenase, inhibition of phosphodiesterase, ADP receptor antagonism, and blockade of the glycoprotein IIb/IIIa receptor.

Cyclooxygenase inhibitors. Aspirin is the prototype. Aspirin produces irreversible inhibition of platelet cyclooxygenase (cox), which prevents synthesis of thromboxane A_2, a potent platelet proaggregant and vasoconstrictor. In moderate doses, there is selective sparing of the synthesis of prostacyclin (antiaggregant, vasodilator), which results in "tilting" the balance substantially in favor of platelet inhibition. Indomethacin, phenylbutazone, and all the nonsteroidal anti-inflammatory agents similarly inhibit cyclooxygenase. However, their inhibition is promptly reversible with clearance of the drug. The recently introduced cox-2 inhibitors selectively inhibit the cox-2 isoform, the isoform responsible for generating the mediators of pain and inflammation, while sparing the cox-1 isoform, inhibition of which causes both gastric damage, decreased renal blood flow, and inhibition of platelet thromboxane A_2. Accordingly, platelet function should not be impaired. However, there has been concern that cox-2 inhibitors, which should reduce prostacyclin generation by vascular endothelial cells, may thereby actually tilt the natural balance toward platelet aggregation.[160] That concern has been reinforced by the report in 2004 of an increased rate of myocardial ischemic events in patients taking cox-2 inhibitors, and the withdrawal of certain cox-2 inhibitors from the market.

Phosphodiesterase inhibitors. Cyclic AMP is an inhibitor of platelet aggregation and levels are increased by inhibition of phosphodiesterase. Dipyridamole, which is used for stroke prophylaxis alone or more commonly in combination with aspirin, and cilostazol appear to act primarily by this mechanism. Caffeine, aminophylline, and theophylline will also similarly produce mild, reversible platelet inhibition.

ADP receptor antagonists. Ticlopidine and clopidogrel, which are administered for stroke prophylaxis, block the ADP receptor, activation of which leads to expression of the IIb/IIIa receptor. They noncompetitively and irreversibly inhibit ADP-induced platelet aggregation. Ticlopidine has been withdrawn from the market because of the occurrence of neutropenia and thrombotic thrombocytopenic purpura.

Glycoprotein IIb/IIIa receptor antagonists. These agents block platelet aggregation by blocking the GPIIb/IIIa receptor. The IIb/IIIa site, by which fibrinogen crosslinks platelets, is the final common pathway for platelet aggregation. The IIb/IIIa antagonists have been used principally for the management of acute coronary syndromes. They include abciximab, a monoclonal antibody, tirofiban, and eptifibatide. These agents all require iv administration. Their effect is reversible. The half-lives are approximately 2.5 hours for tirofiban and eptifibatide and 12 hours for abciximab.[161] However, abciximab has a relatively high affinity for the IIb/IIIa receptor and platelet dysfunction may be longer (ca. 48 hours) than implied by half-life. All of these agents have also been associated with thrombocytopenia, the incidence of which has been greater for abciximab (2.5%) than tirofiban and eptifibatide (0.5%).[162] Note that these agents cause prolongation of the ACT.[161]

Herbal Medication and Vitamins. Several herbal medications, including ginkgo biloba, ginseng, garlic, and ginger, may cause inhibition of platelet function. Because the actual risks are not well defined, they should be discontinued before surgery, and in particular, before cardiac, neurologic, and cosmetic surgical procedures. Vitamin E is also a platelet inhibitor and should similarly be discontinued.[163]

Other Conditions. Myeloproliferative and myelodysplastic syndromes can produce intrinsic defects in platelets. In these disorders, the platelets may be abnormal in both morphology and function. Platelet dysfunction occurs in conjunction with conditions that also cause other hemostatic abnormalities (liver disease, fibrinolytic states including DIC, storage defects) and is discussed in the following section.

Acquired Disorders of Clotting Factors (Including Anticoagulant Therapy)

Vitamin K Deficiency

Hepatic synthesis of clotting factors II, VII, IX, and X, as well as protein C and protein S requires the presence of vitamin K. Vitamin K is necessary for the enzymatic carboxylation of the vitamin K–dependent clotting factors. The carboxyl group enables these factors to bind via a calcium bridge to phospholipid surfaces during the coagulation process. When vitamin K deficiency occurs, these factors are depleted in an order determined by their individual half-lives. Factor VII has the shortest half-life and is the first to be depleted, then factors IX and X, and finally factor II.

"Vitamin K" actually refers to a group of vitamins.[164] Vitamin K_1 (phylloquinone) is found in leafy green vegetables. The greatest quantities occur in Brussels sprouts. Vitamin K_2 (menaquinone) is synthesized by the normal intestinal flora. It is uncommon for patients to develop vitamin K deficiency solely because of dietary deficiency but it may occur in patients who are receiving parenteral nutrition without vitamin K supplementation and who are being treated concurrently with broad-spectrum antibiotics that destroy the gut flora. Because the body has no appreciable stores of vitamin K, deficiencies can develop in roughly 1 week. Newborns, who have a sterile gut at birth, have been noted to develop vitamin
12 K deficiency.

Vitamin K is a fat-soluble vitamin and therefore requires bile salts for absorption from the jejunum. Patients with biliary obstruction, pancreatic insufficiency, malabsorption syndromes, GI obstruction, or rapid GI transit can develop vitamin K deficiency as a result of inadequate absorption.

Diagnosis and Treatment of Vitamin K Deficiency. Vitamin K deficiency will cause prolongation of the PT. This occurs because factor VII is depleted first. With more prolonged deficiency, the aPTT will also be increased because of declining levels of factors IX and X. Platelet count will be normal. Vitamin K may be administered orally, intramuscularly, or intravenously. Urgent treatment of vitamin K deficiency is best accomplished by the intramuscular or intravenous administration of vitamin K (Aquamephyton), usually in doses 1 to 5 mg. Vitamin K should be administered slowly to avoid the occurrence of hypotension. Improvement of the coagulation disturbance will begin to be apparent within 6 to 8 hours.

Warfarin Therapy

Warfarin produces its anticoagulant effect by competition with vitamin K for the carboxylation binding sites. Administration of warfarin leads to the depletion of factors II, VII, IX, X, protein C, and protein S. As with vitamin K deficiency, FVII is the first factor to be depleted. Subsequently, FIX and FX are depleted, and then FII. Accordingly, initially only the PT will be prolonged. With higher doses, the aPTT will be affected as well.

Warfarin is administered for the prevention of deep venous thrombosis and pulmonary embolism and to patients with atrial fibrillation, some prosthetic heart valves, and ventricular mural thrombi in the setting of acute myocardial. Patients with protein S or protein C deficiency may also be treated with long-term anticoagulation with warfarin. Warfarin therapy is adjusted according to the international internalized ratio (INR) (see tests of the hemostatic mechanism). The primary untoward effect of warfarin therapy is bleeding. Rapid reversal (12 to

24 hours) of warfarin effect[69] can be accomplished by administration of vitamin K, 5 mg iv. Smaller doses, 0.5 to 3 mg, should be used in less-urgent situations when the objective is to lower rather than normalize INR. INR should be rechecked at 6-hour intervals. Vitamin K administration may have to be repeated at 12-hour intervals. In situations of greater urgency, FFP has been administered. However, as noted in Disorders of Hemostasis: Diagnosis and Treatment section, prothrombin complex concentrate, which contains FII, VII, IX, X, is an alternative that has been reported to be more effective than FFP[165,166] because FFP administration frequently fails to achieve adequate concentrations of FIX[165] and because some patients cannot tolerate the requisite volume, that is, ca. 15 mL/kg. If FFP or concentrates are administered for rapid reversal and sustained reversal is desired, vitamin K should be administered simultaneously because of FVII's short (6 hours) half-life. Recombinant FVIIa (see later) has also been used to achieve rapid normalization of INR.[167]

Heparin Therapy

Heparin is used widely for anticoagulation in vascular surgery and in procedures requiring cardiopulmonary bypass (CPB). It inhibits coagulation principally through its interaction with one of the body's natural anticoagulant proteins, antithrombin III (ATIII). Heparin binds to ATIII and in so doing causes a conformational change that greatly increases ATIII's inhibitory activity. In spite of its name, anti-"thrombin" III, ATIII also inhibits several activated factors including, in addition to IIa (thrombin), Xa, IXa, Xia, and XIIa. It is most active against thrombin and Xa. Heparin also increases the activity of a second native antithrombin, heparin cofactor II. Heparin cofactor II inhibits thrombin and not the other activated factors. Its contribution to the clinical effects of heparin is not clear. Resistance to heparin can occur in patients who are deficient in ATIII on either a hereditary or an acquired basis. The latter may occur in patients on sustained heparin therapy or in the presence of depletion by a consumptive coagulopathy. Heparin responsiveness can be restored by administration of ATIII (ATIII concentrates[131,132] or FFP).

Low–Molecular-Weight Heparin (LMWH). Low–molecular-weight fractions of heparin have been employed principally for deep vein thrombosis prophylaxis and treatment and are supplanting subcutaneous unfractionated heparin and coumadin for these indications.[168] There are several available agents: including certoparin, dalteparin, danaparoid, enoxaparin, reviparin, and tinzaparin. These agents do not appear to differ in their efficacy[150] and enoxaparin is used most widely in the United States. LMWHs, which also act via ATIII, have greater activity against factor Xa than thrombin (IIa). However, the ratio of that activity varies among the agents, for example, enoxaparin 3.8:1; tinzaparin 1.9:1.[169] Accordingly, the effect of these agents on standard coagulation tests will vary (minimal for enoxaparin[170]) as will the effect of protamine neutralization, which is very incomplete for enoxaparin. Monitoring is usually not required or performed. If it is deemed necessary, the anti-Xa level is the appropriate test. The LMWHs cause less platelet inhibition and are associated with a lesser incidence of heparin induced thrombocytopenia.[171] There has been considerable discussion of optimal dose regimens. European practitioners have often started prophylaxis 12 to 24 hours preoperatively. However, there is little evidence that that practice is superior to postprocedure initiation.[150] While twice-daily dosing with enoxaparin has been common in North America, once-daily regimens are usually sufficient. Because of the relatively long half-life of enoxaparin, twice-daily dosing poses a problem with respect to removal of epidural catheters because there is no anticoagulant nadir (see Chapter 40).

Heparin-Induced Thrombocytopenia/Thrombosis.[172] As many as 5% of patients who receive heparin therapy for 5 days will develop thrombocytopenia as a result of antibodies (usually IgG) directed against platelet factor 4-heparin complexes on the platelet surface. Onset requires several days in the heparin-naïve patient but can occur much more quickly (10 to 12 hours) in those who have been exposed within the preceding 100 days.[173] Occurrence appears to be dose related and is more common with bovine than porcine heparin. Heparin-induced thrombocytopenia/thrombosis (HITT) is relatively uncommon with LMWH and requires longer periods of exposure.[174] While HITT is most often identified because of thrombocytopenia, not all patients become markedly thrombocytopenic. Thrombotic and thromboembolic events, including DVT, PE, limb or acral ischemia, MI, stroke, not infrequently reveal the occurrence of HITT.[172] Diagnosis is complicated by the fact that not all patients who develop antiplatelet antibodies have clinical HITT. A hematologist should be consulted. Treatment entails withdrawal of heparin after instituting an alternate anticoagulant, for example, a DTI (hirudin, argatroban, lepirudin, bivalirudin) or a heparinoid, for example, danaparoid (but not a LMWH). Warfarin is contraindicated because the combination of protein C and S inhibition by warfarin in the face of ongoing platelet clumping may aggravate thrombosis. Platelets similarly should not be administered unless thrombocytopenia
13 is extreme.

Heparin in Cardiopulmonary Bypass. A comprehensive discussion of the use and monitoring of heparin therapy in CPB is beyond the scope of this chapter. Extensive reviews are available.[175,176] In brief, the common practice is to maintain ACT >480 to 500 seconds for the duration of bypass. There is substantial variation in the heparin–ACT dose-response relationship, probably because of variability in heparin binding to many native surfaces including platelets, WBCs, endothelium, and plasma proteins including the vWF and ATIII.[175,176] While there is controversy, it appears that there is greater hazard in allowing ACT to be on the "low side" than in maintaining more complete heparinization.[177] Evidence of platelet activation is less apparent when longer ACTs are maintained. Whether this is a function of direct inhibition of platelets, which are subject to contact activation by the CPB circuit, binding of vWF, or the result of reduced formation of thrombin and inhibition of platelets by its breakdown products (FDPs) is not apparent to the authors of this review. Protamine is administered for reversal of heparin effect. Many clinicians employ an "mL-for-mL" technique. However, a more careful titration of protamine against ACT is ideal to avoid excessive administration of protamine, which has inherent anticoagulant effects including platelet inhibition, stimulation of t-PA release from endothelium, and inhibition of fibrinogen cleavage by thrombin.[178]

Various alternatives have been considered for the patient with HIT who requires CPB. Plasmaphereis prior to surgery with subsequent use of heparin has been employed.[179] The nonheparin alternatives for anticoagulation include specific inhibitors of thrombin (see later) and the defibrinogenating agent Ancrod (from the venom of the Malaysian pit viper). The contact activation of platelets is not inhibited and it may be appropriate to administer platelet inhibitors simultaneously. Experience is limited and well-defined protocols are not established.

Direct Thrombin Inhibitors

The agents most commonly used CPB when there are contraindications to heparin are the DTIs. This group includes hirudin, argatroban, lepirudin, and bivalirudin. Hirudin is a recombinant product and the others are synthetic. There are disadvantages to their use in CPB. The first is that there is no antidote. Termination of effect is largely dependent on renal elimination. The exception is bivalirudin, which is in part cleared by proteolysis by thrombin. In the patient with renal failure or in urgent situations, elimination can be accomplished by dialysis or hemofiltration.[180]

Ximelagatran is a direct thrombin inhibitor that can be taken orally. It has no relevance to CPB but has undergone phase three trial in the prevention of recurrent venous thromboembolism with favorable results.[181] It has a relatively short half-life (ca. 4 hours) and is largely eliminated by the kidneys. Because of predictable bioavailability, coagulation monitoring is usually not employed. Like other DTIs, it will prolong TT, aPTT, PT, and ACT, but not in a well dose-related manner. As with the other DTIs, if monitoring is required, the ecarin clotting time (see earlier) is probably the preferred method.[181]

Inhibitors of Xa

These agents (fondaparinux, idraparinux) act via antithrombin to inhibit FXa. The prototype is fondaparinux. It is an increasingly popular alternative for DVT prophylaxis,[168] in part because its very predictable uptake (after once-daily subcutaneous administration) and kinetics make monitoring and dosage adjustment unnecessary.[181,182] However, these agents have long half-lives (fondaparinux, 17 hours; idraparinux, 80 hours[181]) and there is no antidote. Excretion is via the kidneys. Therapeutic doses do not cause changes in PT, aPTT, or ACT.[181]

Acquired Combined Disorders of Platelets and Clotting Factors with Increased Fibrinolysis

Liver Disease. Chronic liver disease is associated with abnormalities of all three phases of hemostasis: primary hemostasis, coagulation, and fibrinolysis.[183] Table 10-14 provides an overview of these abnormalities.

Impaired primary hemostasis. Impaired primary hemostasis occurs as a result of both thrombocytopenia and impaired platelet function. The former is largely the result of decreased production, which in turn is probably the result of decreased thrombopoietin secretion by the liver. Hypersplenism may also contribute but its role has been overemphasized. Platelet dysfunction can occur when liver disease is sufficiently advanced that clearance of FDPs is impaired or when DIC complicates the coagulation disturbance. The FDPs coat the surface of platelets and impair aggregation. Ethanol can also directly contribute to platelet dysfunction by inhibition of the synthesis of ADP, ATP, and thromboxane A_2. Accordingly, when faced with a patient with liver disease who is bleeding, a normal platelet count cannot be assurance of intact primary hemostasis. DDAVP may be helpful, but transfusion of platelet concentrates may be necessary.

Disturbances of coagulation. With liver disease, factor production decreases and consumption increases. The liver synthesizes all of the clotting factors (with the probable exception of factor VIII). As with vitamin K deficiency, hepatic disease first leads to a deficiency of factor VII since it has the shortest half-life. Thereafter, deficiencies will develop in factors II, IX, and X. Dietary deficiency of vitamin K, as may occur in alcoholics, and with diminished secretion of bile salts leading to malabsorption, will exaggerate these deficiencies. If impaired coagulation is the result of vitamin K deficiency and not hepatic damage, then parenteral vitamin K may be helpful in restoring factor levels of II, VII, IX, and X. Further deterioration of hepatic function will affect the remaining factors, I, V, XI, and XII. Impaired liver function can also cause a thrombotic tendency, which leads to increased consumption of clotting factors. This occurs for two reasons. First, synthesis of the natural anticoagulants, antithrombin III, protein C, and protein S, may be diminished thereby altering the balance of pro- and anticoagulant forces, and second, clearance of activated clotting factors from the circulation may be impaired thereby allowing persistent activation of the coagulation cascade.

Increased fibrinolysis. Increased fibrinolysis occurs as a result of decreased clearance of t-PA from the circulation by the impaired liver and decreased hepatic synthesis of alpha-2 antiplasmin.[184] For uncertain reasons, the production of the natural inhibitor of the plasmin system, PAI-1, is diminished.[185] The combination of accelerated coagulation and increased fibrinolysis in patients with advanced liver disease can lead to a persistent, low-grade DIC. The release into the circulation of the breakdown products of necrotic hepatocytes may contribute to the development of DIC.[164]

Diagnosis and treatment of coagulation abnormalities associated with liver disease. The initial laboratory evaluation should include platelet count, PT, aPTT, fibrinogen level, and D-dimer. In the event of thrombocytopenia and clinical bleeding or pending surgery, platelet transfusions are appropriate. If the PT is prolonged (>1.5 times control), vitamin K should be administered speculatively. In the absence of a response to vitamin K (which requires a minimum of 8 hours), factor deficiencies should be treated with FFP with attention to the possibility of volume overload. Cryoprecipitate is appropriate in the event of hypofibrinogenemia (fibrinogen <100 to 125 g/dL). However, cryoprecipitate does not contain the vitamin K–dependent factors. While antifibrinolytics have been applied in the context of liver transplantation, they should not otherwise be used for bleeding associated with liver disease because of the catastrophic consequences of administering these agents in the face of an unrecognized DIC.[186]

Diagnosis of DIC (see later) is often difficult because the laboratory tests used to identify DIC are already abnormal in patients with liver dysfunction. Thrombocytopenia, prolonged PT and aPTT, decreased fibrinogen level, and circulating FDPs will commonly occur in the absence of DIC. Elevated D-dimer is somewhat more specific for the occurrence of DIC.

Disseminated Intravascular Coagulation. Detailed reviews of DIC are available.[187,188] DIC is characterized by excessive deposition of fibrin throughout the vascular tree, with simultaneous depression of the normal coagulation inhibitory mechanisms and impaired fibrin degradation. It is triggered by the appearance of procoagulant material (tissue factor or equivalent) in the circulation in amounts sufficient to overwhelm the mechanisms that normally restrain and localize clot

TABLE 10-14

THE ETIOLOGY OF HEMOSTATIC ABNORMALITIES IN LIVER DISEASE

- Thrombocytopenia
  - Decreased production
  - Hypersplenism
  - Increased consumption (DIC)
- Impaired platelet function
  - Decreased FDP clearance
- Decreased factor synthesis
  - Decreased hepatocyte function
  - Vitamin K deficiency (diet, malabsorption)
- Increased factor consumption
  - Decreased clearance of activated factors
  - Decreased synthesis of inhibitors (protein C, protein S)
- Increased fibrinolysis
  - Decreased synthesis of alpha-2 antiplasmin
  - Decreased clearance of t-PA
  - Decreased synthesis of PAI-1

TABLE 10-15

CLINICAL CONDITIONS ASSOCIATED WITH DISSEMINATED INTRAVASCULAR COAGULOPATHY

Sepsis (Gram + or −)
Viremias
Obstetric conditions
  Amniotic fluid embolus
  Fetal death in utero
  Abruptio placentae
  Preeclampsia
Extensive tissue damage
  Burns
  Trauma
Liver failure
Extensive cerebral injury
  Head injury
  Stroke
Extensive vascular endothelial damage
  Vasculitis
  Preeclampsia
Hemolytic transfusion reactions
Metastatic malignancies
Leukemia
Snake venoms

formation. That appearance may be the result of either extensive endothelial injury, which exposes tissue factor of fibroblastic origin, or the release of TF into the circulation as occurs with amniotic fluid embolus, extensive soft tissue damage, severe head injury, or any cause of a systemic inflammatory response. Table 10-15 lists the numerous clinical conditions that have been associated with DIC. For reasons not entirely clear, the native pathways that inhibit coagulation, antithrombin III and the protein C pathway are simultaneously inhibited. The accelerated process of clot formation causes both tissue ischemia and, ultimately, critical depletion of platelets and factors. Simultaneously, the fibrinolytic system is activated and plasmin is generated to lyse the extensive fibrin clots. Fibrin degradation products appear in the circulation. FDPs stimulate release of plasminogen activator inhibitor, type 1 (PAI-1), from the endothelium and thrombolysis becomes impaired. The FDPs also inhibit platelet aggregation and prevent the normal crosslinking of fibrin monomers. Depleted of platelets and clotting factors and inhibited by FDPs, the coagulation system fails and the patient bleeds. Simultaneously, the microvascular occlusion by fibrin causes tissue ischemia, contributing to multiorgan failure.

Table 10-15 reveals that several clinical entities that are encountered frequently in anesthetic and critical care practice are associated with the development of DIC. Sepsis is the most common cause. Endotoxins or lipopolysaccharide break down products from Gram-negative and -positive bacteria, respectively, incite an inflammatory response that includes the generation of cytokines (tumor necrosis factor alpha, various interleukins). These cytokines in turn stimulate the release or expression of TF by endothelial cells, macrophages, and monocytes, and the DIC sequence is initiated.

Several obstetric conditions can cause DIC. Amniotic fluid embolism, placental abruption, and fetal death in utero result in the direct release of TF-equivalent material into the circulation. Preeclampsia is characterized by a systemic vasculitis. The associated endothelial damage causes an initially low-grade DIC that accelerates as vasculitis-related damage leads to release of TF from ischemic tissues, in particular placenta.

Large burns, extensive traumatic soft tissue injuries, severe brain injury, and hemolytic transfusion reactions can also liberate TF-equivalent material into the circulation and incite DIC. Certain malignancies, most notably promyelocytic leukemia and adenocarcinomas, are associated with DIC. However, with malignancy–associated DIC, thrombotic manifestations are more likely to appear first, whereas with the others mentioned earlier, the hemorrhagic diathesis is often the first clinical manifestation.

A few general conditions such as acidosis, shock, and hypoxia are associated with DIC. Shock promotes coagulation because one of the control mechanisms (rapid blood flow) is compromised. Clearance of activated clotting factors is reduced when blood flow is decreased. Acidosis and hypoxia may contribute to both tissue and endothelial damage.

The clinical manifestations of DIC are a consequence of both thrombosis and bleeding. Bleeding is a more common clinical presentation in patients with acute, fulminant DIC. Petechiae, ecchymoses, epistaxis, gingival/mucosal bleeding, hematuria, and bleeding from wounds and puncture sites may be evident. With the chronic forms of DIC, thrombotic manifestations are more likely. Organs with the greatest blood flow, for example, kidney and brain, typically sustain the greatest damage. Pulmonary function may deteriorate as a consequence microthrombus accumulation.

Diagnosis of DIC. There is no absolutely consistent constellation of laboratory findings among routine tests.[187] Increased PT, aPTT, thrombocytopenia, a decreased fibrinogen level, and the presence of FDPs and D-dimer may all be noted. The peripheral smear may reveal schistocytes (fragmented RBCs reflecting the microangiopathy that occurs as a consequence of widespread fibrin deposition). Thrombocytopenia (<100,00/uL) is not always evident early in the process, but true DIC without sequential reduction in platelet count is very unlikely. PT and aPTT may remain normal in spite of decreasing factor levels because of the presence of high levels of activated factors including thrombin and Xa. Fibrinogen level may not be decreased, that is, <100 mg/dL, initially. Fibrinogen is an "acute phase reactant," which increases in response to stress and the early consumption of fibrinogen may simply reduce its levels to "normal." FDPs are a sensitive measure of fibrinolytic activity although they not specific for DIC. D-dimer (which is a breakdown product of the crosslinked fibrin in a mature clot) is somewhat more specific for DIC, but not entirely so, and should be measured when that diagnosis is suspected.

Various other laboratory assays have been employed to support a diagnosis of DIC,[187] but should probably not be considered part of the anesthesiologist's routine. They include levels of prothrombin fragments F1+F2 (a marker of prothrombin conversion to thrombin-increased), thrombin-ATIII (TAT) complexes (increased), ATIII (decreased), alpha-2 antiplasmin (decreased by binding to excess plasmin), protein C (decreased), plasminogen (decreased), and factor VIII (decreased in DIC but normal with hepatic failure without DIC).

Treatment of DIC. Treatment should focus on management of the underlying condition. Septicemia will require antibiotic therapy. The obstetric conditions are frequently self-limited, although evacuation of the uterus or hysterectomy may be warranted. Hypovolemia, acidosis, and hypoxemia should be corrected to prevent their contribution to the DIC process. When bleeding is or may become life threatening, the consumptive coagulopathy must be treated. Platelets will be required for thrombocytopenia, for example, $<50{,}000/mm^3$. FFP will replace the clotting factor deficiencies. Fibrinogen level should be raised to >100 mg/dL. When hypofibrinogenemia is severe (<50 mg/dL) cryoprecipitate may be required. Six units of cryoprecipitate will increase fibrinogen level by approximately 50 mg/dL in a 70-kg patient.[189]

Heparin has been advocated. However, the contemporary practice is to restrict its use to only those situations where thrombosis is clinically problematic, principally DIC associated with malignancies. There is no proven benefit in situations in which bleeding is the predominant manifestation. Antifibrinolytics have been considered. However, their use in the face of widespread thrombosis is potentially disastrous and they should not be used. Antithrombin III concentrates have been administered. The hope is that its administration will serve to slow the runaway coagulation process. However, a beneficial effect on outcome from DIC has not been confirmed (see data review by Levi[188]) and its use should be viewed as experimental. An insufficiency in the protein C endogenous coagulation inhibition system is thought to contribute to the prothrombotic state in DIC. Activated protein C has been shown to decrease mortality and organ failure in patients with sepsis and that improvement is also evident among patients with sepsis with overt DIC.[190] Its use should be considered in any sustained episode of DIC.[190]

Cardiopulmonary Bypass and Coagulation. The management of anticoagulation and post-CPB bleeding are addressed in the chapter on Cardiac Anesthesia.

Pharmacologic Therapy

Recombinant Factor VIIa (rFVIIa, NovoSeven®, Novo Nordisk, Bagsvaerd, Denmark)

Recombinant FVIIa was developed for, and its only current "on-label" use is, the treatment of patients with hemophilia A or B and inhibitors to exogenous FVIII or FIX preparations. However, it is fast becoming the hemostatic agent of last (and sometimes earlier) resort in many clinical situations. Its use has been reported in trauma, hepatic failure, and in cardiac, prostatic, hepatic, spinal, neurologic, and hepatic transplantation surgery. It has been used to reverse the anticoagulant effect of warfarin and selective Xa inhibitors. It has been administered to patients with thrombocytopenia and both congenital (Bernard Soulier syndrome, Glanzmann's thrombasthenia) and acquired (uremia, aspirin, ADP and IIb/IIIa antagonists) platelet abnormalities.[167]

The mechanism of action is uncertain. It is clearly more than an augmentation of the native functions of FVII. Were that the case, it would not be effective in hemophilia. However, FVIIa, whose preferred ligand is TF, also undergoes low affinity binding to activated platelets. In the concentrations achieved with typical rVIIa dosing, the serum levels are several hundred times those achieved physiologically and are probably sufficient to activate Xa on the platelet surface and to achieve the "thrombin burst" necessary to support the propagation phase of coagulation (Fig. 10-3).[122] Because rVIIa is an active procoagulant only when it is in contact with TF or activated platelets, unwanted coagulation has been very infrequent. However, it should be viewed as relatively contraindicated in clinical states in which TF may be circulating freely, that is, in most of the conditions associated with DIC.

The appropriate dosing of this expensive agent (1,020 USD for 1.2 mg at UCSD) is not well defined. The dose used most often in hemophilia has been 90 ug/kg. However, doses as low as 20 ug/kg have been effective in some reports.[191] The current, somewhat arbitrary, algorithm in place at the University of California, San Diego, provides for the administration of 60 ug/kg for profuse bleeding unresponsive to conventional therapy specifies. That dose is rounded to the nearest 1,200 ug in recognition that the agent is supplied in vials of 1.2 mg. The half-life is ca. 2.5 hours and repeat dosing at 2-hour intervals may be required.

Desmopressin

Desmopressin (DDAVP, 1-deamino-8-D-arginine vasopressin) is a synthetic analogue off the natural hormone vasopressin. The actions of vasopressin are thought to mediated by two general classes of receptors: V1 receptors, which mediate smooth muscle contraction in the peripheral vasculature, and V2 receptors, which regulate water resorption in the collecting ducts of the nephron. Desmopressin has no activity at the V1 receptors and accordingly has virtually no vasoconstrictor effect. It does, however, act at V2 receptors. In fact, desmopressin is a more potent antidiuretic than vasopressin and has a more prolonged activity. Desmopressin was used primarily for clinical conditions such as diabetes insipidus until its hemostatic effects were recognized. The hemostatic effects of desmopressin are thought to be mediated by "low-affinity, extra-renal V2-like" receptors.[159] Desmopressin causes release of coagulation factor VIII:C, vWF, and tissue plasminogen activator. Desmopressin is thought to release VIII:C from the sinusoidal liver endothelial cells and the vWF from endothelial cells. In mild hemophilia A, desmopressin can increase the circulating factor VIII:C concentration two- to sixfold. Desmopressin also increases platelet adhesiveness and shortens the bleeding time, though the mechanism of these effects is not fully understood. It appears to entail more than a simple increase in the plasma vWF level.

Indications. Desmopressin has proven effective treatment for certain types of vWD and mild hemophilia (see earlier). Desmopressin has been shown to reduce the bleeding time in a variety of conditions associated with platelet dysfunction. It produces rapid and temporary correction of prolonged bleeding times in uremic patients following intravenous or intranasal administration. In cirrhotics, desmopressin increases the concentrations of larger vWF multimers and shortens prolonged bleeding times. Desmopressin also decreases the prolonged bleeding times caused by many drugs including aspirin, nonsteroidal anti-inflammatory drugs (NSAIDs), dextran, clopidogrel, and heparin.[159]

The prophylactic use of desmopressin in cardiac surgical patients has been controversial. Because platelet dysfunction and thrombocytopenia are common, numerous studies have been performed. Those that have revealed decreased blood loss or blood product administration have involved principally patients who were predisposed to blood loss, for example, redo procedures[192–195] and patients receiving aspirin.[196]

Dosage Recommendations. Desmopressin is commonly administered intravenously in a dose of 0.3 mg/kg. The effect of desmopressin is almost immediate. Peak levels of factor VIII:C and vWF are achieved within 30 to 60 minutes and the effect lasts for several hours.[159] Desmopressin administration may be repeated after 8 to 12 hours. When used in cardiac surgery, the drug should be administered after termination of cardiopulmonary bypass. Water balance should be monitored. However, while congestive cardiac failure and hyponatremia and seizures in children have been reported, clinically significant water retention is relatively uncommon. Desmopressin may be administered as a nasal spray and is available for home use for both mild hemophiliacs and patients with vWD (type 1). Intravenous administration causes a more rapid rise in VIII:C levels and is therefore preferable for acute hemostatic challenges.

Antifibrinolytics

Antifibrinolytic agents have been used frequently in situations in which exaggerated fibrinolysis is suspected of contributing to intraoperative bleeding. The situations in which favorable effects on blood loss and replacement have been reported include cardiopulmonary bypass procedures, hepatic transplantation, scoliosis surgery, total joint replacement, and prostate surgery.[197–201] The use of antifibrinolytic mouthwashes in the context of dental procedures in patients with hemophilia has been mentioned elsewhere in this chapter. There are three commonly available antifibrinolytics. They are the lysine analogues, epsilon-aminocaproic acid and tranexamic acid, and the serine protease inhibitor aprotinin.

Epsilon-Aminocaproic Acid (EACA) and Tranexamic Acid (TXA). EACA and TXA bind to and produce a structural change in both plasminogen and plasmin. That structural change prevents the conversion of plasminogen to plasmin and also prevents plasmin from degrading fibrinogen and fibrin. The dual action of these agents results in two effects on the hemostatic mechanism. First, decreased synthesis of plasmin from plasminogen results in reduced fibrinolysis. The second effect of these drugs, the inactivation of plasmin, decreases the formation of degradation products of fibrinogen and fibrin. These FDPs have anticoagulant effects, including the inhibition of platelet aggregation and the inhibition of the crosslinking of fibrin strands, which are thereby avoided.

Aprotinin. Aprotinin produces its antifibrinolytic effect by a different mechanism. It is an inhibitor of numerous serine protease enzymes including plasmin and kallikrein. The latter participates in the process of contact activation of Factor XII. As a consequence of its inhibition of plasmin, aprotinin, like EACA and TXA, prevents degradation of fibrinogen and fibrin. As is the case with EACA and TXA, the reduction in FDPs should improve both platelet and coagulation function. However, aprotinin is believed to have additional beneficial effects on the inflammatory response to CPB, in general, and on platelets, in particular.[202,203] The mechanism of these effects is not known with certainty. However, thrombin is a serine protease that can activate platelets via a "protease activated receptor" (PAR) on the platelet surface.[202] Better preservation of the GP1b receptor (which is necessary for initial platelet adhesion to vascular defects) has been reported during CPB in patients who received aprotinin.[204] Aprotinin also appears to reduce neutrophil activation and transmigration across capillary endothelium, perhaps via an effect on an endothelial PAR[205] and may therefore also blunt the neutrophil mediated component of the response to endothelial injury.

Use of antifibrinolytics in cardiac surgery. Meta-analyses of the many studies of these agents performed in the context of CPB confirm that, overall, blood loss and the administration of allogeneic blood is diminished by the use of all three agents.[197,206,207] Concern has been expressed that antifibrinolysis might lead to an increased rate of graft occlusion, myocardial infarction, and renal failure. However, the meta-analyses have not borne out those concerns.[197,206,207] There does not appear to be a clear consensus as to which of the three agents is most appropriate in the context of CPB. Various authors have argued that EACA and TXA are preferable to aprotinin because they are less expensive and have apparently similar efficacy.[208,209] However, the most recent of those meta-analyses reported a trend toward a reduced incidence of atrial fibrillation and a reduced incidence of stroke in patients receiving aprotinin[207] and this result may well create a stronger bias in favor of aprotinin.

The patterns of use of antifibrinolytic agents in cardiac surgery vary substantially among institutions. Few appear to use these agents routinely for all CPB procedures. Some reserve their use for situations more likely to be associated with post-CPB bleeding, for example, redo procedures, circulatory arrest procedures. Still others appear to reserve antifibrinolytics for refractory bleeding postcardiopulmonary bypass. The latter seems less logical because much of the activation of the hemostatic mechanism occurs during CPB.

There is a small but finite rate of allergic responses to aprotinin. Accordingly, a test dose has been recommended for patients who have had prior exposure to aprotinin. The potential for developing sensitivity has been used as a rationale for avoiding administration of aprotinin in circumstances where it is not clearly indicated, for example, first time coronary artery bypass graft (CABG), so that it may be used safely in the event of a redo procedure. The risk of an anaphylactic/toid response appears to decline very substantially with reexposure intervals greater than six months.[210]

Use of antifibrinolytics in liver transplantation. Accelerated fibrinolysis occurs commonly in patients undergoing hepatic transplantation. This is probably, in part, the consequence of decreased clearance of activated clotting factors by the diseased liver. More importantly, hepatic clearance ceases entirely during the anhepatic phase. In addition, with reperfusion of the donor liver, there is an "explosive" release of t-PA into the systemic circulation.[211] Aprotinin, EACA, and TXA have all been used and reported to reduce blood loss in hepatic transplantation.[143,200,211–213] Some advocate prophylactic administration for all patients,[200] while others administer these agents only in response to the demonstration, typically by thromboelastography, of hyperfibrinolysis.[143,214]

Use of antifibrinolytics in orthopaedic and other surgery. There have been numerous reports of reduction of transfusion requirement in scoliosis and joint replacement surgery[198,199,201] However, meta-analysis has not confirmed the efficacy in noncardiac surgery and the available data do not permit a determination of the relative efficacy of EACA, TXA, and aprotinin.[197]

CONCLUSIONS

The approach to the bleeding patient requires a knowledge of the basic hemostatic mechanism and common bleeding disorders, an ability to interpret coagulation tests, and an appreciation of the risks involved with blood component therapy. The hemostatic balance is delicate and complex and it is the responsibility of the anesthesiologist to anticipate, prevent, and treat disturbances of that balance. Preoperative evaluation must identify those patients whose inherited or acquired medical conditions or whose current medications may influence these processes. With respect to medications, there are a rapidly increasing number of agents that are administered specifically for the purpose of altering the hemostatic balance, for example, clopidogrel, t-PA, low–molecular-weight heparin. As the patient proceeds through surgery and the postoperative period, the anesthesiologist must determine whether bleeding is surgical in nature or the result of a preexisting or evolving hemostatic defect that will require the transfusion of hemostatic blood components—platelets, fresh frozen plasma, or cryoprecipitate—or the administration of pharmacologic agents.

References

1. Kleinman S, Chan P, Robillard P: Risks associated with transfusion of cellular blood components in Canada. Transfus Med Rev 17:120, 2003
2. Cable RG, Leiby DA: Risk and prevention of transfusion-transmitted babesiosis and other tick-borne diseases. Curr Opin Hematol 10:405, 2003
3. Alter HJ: Emerging, re-emerging and submerging infectious threats to the blood supply. Vox Sang 87(suppl 2):56, 2004
4. Marshall DA, Kleinman SH, Wong JB *et al*: Cost-effectiveness of nucleic acid test screening of volunteer blood donations for hepatitis B, hepatitis C and human immunodeficiency virus in the United States. Vox Sang 86:28, 2004
5. Lane TA: UCSD Medical Center Blood Bank Handbook. http://health.ucsd.edu/labref/ 2003
6. Conry-Cantilena C, VanRaden M, Gibble J *et al*: Routes of infection, viremia, and liver disease in blood donors found to have hepatitis C virus infection. N Engl J Med 334:1691, 1996
7. Tong MJ, el-Farra NS, Reikes AR *et al*: Clinical outcomes after transfusion-associated hepatitis C. N Engl J Med 332:1463, 1995

8. Goodnough LT, Brecher ME, Kanter MH *et al*: Transfusion medicine. First of two parts—blood transfusion. N Engl J Med 340:438, 1999
9. Carson JL, Willett LR: Is a hemoglobin of 10 g/dL required for surgery? Med Clin North Am 77:335, 1993
10. Shander A: Emerging risks and outcomes of blood transfusion in surgery. Semin Hematol 41:117, 2004
11. Bowden RA, Slichter SJ, Sayers MH *et al*: Use of leukocyte-depleted platelets and cytomegalovirus-seronegative red blood cells for prevention of primary cytomegalovirus infection after marrow transplant. Blood 78:246, 1991
12. Nichols WG, Price TH, Gooley T *et al*: Transfusion-transmitted cytomegalovirus infection after receipt of leukoreduced blood products. Blood 101:4195, 2003
13. Blajchman MA: Bacterial contamination of cellular blood components: Risks, sources and control. Vox Sang 87(suppl 1):98, 2004
14. McCullough J, Vesole DH, Benjamin RJ *et al*: Therapeutic efficacy and safety of platelets treated with a photochemical process for pathogen inactivation: The SPRINT Trial. Blood 104:1534, 2004
15. Stephenson J: Investigation probes risk of contracting West Nile virus via blood transfusions. JAMA 288:1573, 2002
16. Knight R: Prion diseases. Vox Sang 87(suppl 1):104, 2004
17. Bird SM: Recipients of blood or blood products "at vCJD risk." BMJ 328:118, 2004
18. Welborn JL, Hersch J: Blood transfusion reactions. Which are life-threatening and which are not? Postgrad Med 90:125-8, 131-2, 135 passim, 1991
19. Perrotta PL, Snyder EL: Non-infectious complications of transfusion therapy. Blood Rev 15:69, 2001
20. Jain R: Use of blood transfusion in management of anemia. Med Clin North Am 76:727, 1992
21. Klapper EB, Goldfinger D: Leukocyte-reduced blood components in transfusion medicine. Current indications and prospects for the future. Clin Lab Med 12:711, 1992
22. Silliman CC, Boshkov LK, Mehdizadehkashi Z *et al*: Transfusion-related acute lung injury: Epidemiology and a prospective analysis of etiologic factors. Blood 101:454, 2003
23. Looney MR, Gropper MA, Matthay MA: Transfusion-related acute lung injury: A review. Chest 126:249, 2004
24. Silliman CC: Transfusion-related acute lung injury. Transfus Med Rev 13:177, 1999
25. ARDSNetwork: Ventilation with lower tidal volumes as compared with traditional tidal volumes for acute lung injury and the acute respiratory distress syndrome. The Acute Respiratory Distress Syndrome Network. N Engl J Med 342:1301, 2000
26. Popovsky MA, Davenport RD: Transfusion-related acute lung injury: Femme fatale? Transfusion 41:312, 2001
27. Insunza A, Romon I, Gonzalez-Ponte ML *et al*: Implementation of a strategy to prevent TRALI in regional blood centre. Transfus Med 14:157, 2004
28. Ferrara JL, Krenger W: Graft-versus-host disease: the influence of type 1 and type 2 T cell cytokines. Transfus Med Rev 12:1, 1998
29. Harrison CR, Sawyer PR: Special issues in transfusion medicine. Clin Lab Med 12:743, 1992
30. Lane TA: Leukocyte depletion of cellular blood components. Curr Opin Hematol 1:443, 1994
31. Opelz G, Sengar DP, Mickey MR *et al*: Effect of blood transfusions on subsequent kidney transplants. Transplant Proc 5:253, 1973
32. Hillyer CD, Lankford KV, Roback JD *et al*: Transfusion of the HIV-seropositive patient: Immunomodulation, viral reactivation, and limiting exposure to EBV (HHV-4), CMV (HHV-5), and HHV-6, 7, and 8. Transfus Med Rev 13:1, 1999
33. Vamvakas EC, Blajchman MA: Deleterious clinical effects of transfusion-associated immunomodulation: fact or fiction? Blood 97:1180, 2001
34. Taylor RW, Manganaro L, O'Brien J *et al*: Impact of allogenic packed red blood cell transfusion on nosocomial infection rates in the critically ill patient. Crit Care Med 30:2249, 2002
35. TRAPSGroup: Leukocyte reduction and ultraviolet B irradiation of platelets to prevent alloimmunization and refractoriness to platelet transfusions. The Trial to Reduce Alloimmunization to Platelets Study Group. N Engl J Med 337:1861, 1997
36. Patterson BJ, Freedman J, Blanchette V *et al*: Effect of premedication guidelines and leukoreduction on the rate of febrile nonhaemolytic platelet transfusion reactions. Transfus Med 10:199, 2000
37. van de Watering L: What has universal leukodepletion given us: Evidence from clinical trials? Vox Sang 87(suppl 2):139, 2004
38. Hebert PC, Fergusson D, Blajchman MA *et al*: Clinical outcomes following institution of the Canadian universal leukoreduction program for red blood cell transfusions. JAMA 289:1941, 2003
39. Vamvakas E, Kaplan HS: Early transfusion and length of survival in acquired immune deficiency syndrome: Experience with a population receiving medical care at a public hospital. Transfusion 33:111, 1993
40. Fergusson D, Hebert PC, Lee SK *et al*: Clinical outcomes following institution of universal leukoreduction of blood transfusions for premature infants. JAMA 289:1950, 2003
41. Corwin HL, AuBuchon JP: Is leukoreduction of blood components for everyone? JAMA 289:1993, 2003
42. Carson JL, Berlin JA: Will we ever know if leukoreduction of red blood cells should be performed? Can J Anaesth 51:407, 2004
43. Nightingale S: Hypotension and bedside leukocyte reduction filters. JAMA 281:1978, 1999
44. McLoughlin TM, Greilich PE: Preexisting hemostatic defects and bleeding disorders. In Lake CL, Moore RA (eds): Blood: Hemostasis, Transfusion, and Alternatives in the Perioperative Period, p 25. New York, Raven Press, 1995
45. Ferrara A, MacArthur JD, Wright HK *et al*: Hypothermia and acidosis worsen coagulopathy in the patient requiring massive transfusion. Am J Surg 160:515, 1990
46. Crosby ET: Perioperative haemotherapy: I. Indications for blood component transfusion. Can J Anaesth 39:695, 1992
47. Sessler DI: Mild perioperative hypothermia. N Engl J Med 336:1730, 1997
48. Hiippala ST, Myllyla GJ, Vahtera EM: Hemostatic factors and replacement of major blood loss with plasma-poor red cell concentrates. Anesth Analg 81:360, 1995
49. AuBuchon JP: Minimizing donor exposure in hemotherapy. Arch Pathol Lab Med 118:380, 1994
50. Jameson LC, Popic PM, Harms BA: Hyperkalemic death during use of a high-capacity fluid warmer for massive transfusion. Anesthesiology 73:1050, 1990
51. Crosby ET: Perioperative haemotherapy: II. Risks and complications of blood transfusion. Can J Anaesth 39:822, 1992
52. Rock G, Tittley P, Fuller V: Effect of citrate anticoagulants on factor VIII levels in plasma. Transfusion 28:248, 1988
53. Hebert PC, Wells G, Blajchman MA *et al*: A multicenter, randomized, controlled clinical trial of transfusion requirements in critical care. Transfusion Requirements in Critical Care Investigators, Canadian Critical Care Trials Group. N Engl J Med 340:409, 1999
54. Hebert PC, McDonald BJ, Tinmouth A: Overview of transfusion practices in perioperative and critical care. Vox Sang 87(suppl 2):209, 2004
55. Wu WC, Rathore SS, Wang Y *et al*: Blood transfusion in elderly patients with acute myocardial infarction. N Engl J Med 345:1230, 2001
56. Hebert PC, Wells G, Tweeddale M *et al*: Does transfusion practice affect mortality in critically ill patients? Transfusion Requirements in Critical Care (TRICC) Investigators and the Canadian Critical Care Trials Group. Am J Respir Crit Care Med 155:1618, 1997
57. American Society of Anesthesiologists: Practice Guidelines for blood component therapy: A report by the American Society of Anesthesiologists Task Force on Blood Component Therapy. Anesthesiology 84:732, 1996
58. Robertie PG, Gravlee GP: Safe limits of isovolemic hemodilution and recommendations for erythrocyte transfusion. Int Anesthesiol Clin 28:197, 1990
59. Stehling L, Simon TL: The red blood cell transfusion trigger. Physiology and clinical studies. Arch Pathol Lab Med 118:429, 1994
60. Welch HG, Meehan KR, Goodnough LT: Prudent strategies for elective red blood cell transfusion. Ann Intern Med 116:393, 1992
61. Fluit CR, Kunst VA, Drenthe-Schonk AM: Incidence of red cell antibodies after multiple blood transfusion. Transfusion 30:532, 1990
62. Tuman K: Tissue oxygen delivery—the physiology of anemia. Anesthesiology Clinics of North America 8:451, 1990
63. Irving GA: Perioperative blood and blood component therapy. Can J Anaesth 39:1105, 1992
64. Guidelines for the use of platelet transfusions. Br J Haematol 122:10, 2003
65. Rebulla P, Finazzi G, Marangoni F *et al*: The threshold for prophylactic platelet transfusions in adults with acute myeloid leukemia. Gruppo Italiano Malattie Ematologiche Maligne dell'Adulto. N Engl J Med 337:1870, 1997
66. Levi MM, Vink R, de Jonge E: Management of bleeding disorders by prohemostatic therapy. Int J Hematol 76(suppl 2):139, 2002
67. Stanworth SJ, Brunskill SJ, Hyde CJ *et al*: Is fresh frozen plasma clinically effective? A systematic review of randomized controlled trials. Br J Haematol 126:139, 2004
68. O'Shaughnessy DF, Atterbury C, Bolton Maggs P *et al*: Guidelines for the use of fresh-frozen plasma, cryoprecipitate and cryosupernatant. Br J Haematol 126:11, 2004
69. Makris M, Watson HG: The management of coumarin-induced over-anticoagulation Annotation. Br J Haematol 114:271, 2001
70. Leveque CM, Yawn DH: Limiting homologous blood exposure. Clin Lab Med 12:771, 1992
71. Goodnough LT, Brecher ME: Autologous blood transfusion. Intern Med 37:238, 1998
72. Billote DB, Glisson SN, Green D *et al*: A prospective, randomized study of preoperative autologous donation for hip replacement surgery. J Bone Joint Surg Am 84-A:1299, 2002
73. Couvret C, Tricoche S, Baud A *et al*: The reduction of preoperative autologous blood donation for primary total hip or knee arthroplasty: the effect on subsequent transfusion rates. Anesth Analg 94:815, 2002
74. Waters JH, Potter PS: Cell salvage in the Jehovah's Witness patient. Anesth Analg 90:229, 2000
75. Goldman M, Savard R, Long A *et al*: Declining value of preoperative autologous donation. Transfusion 42:819, 2002
76. Spiess BD, Sassetti R, McCarthy RJ *et al*: Autologous blood donation: hemodynamics in a high-risk patient population. Transfusion 32:17, 1992
77. Goodnough LT: The use of erythropoietin in the enhancement of autologous transfusion therapy. Curr Opin Hematol 2:214, 1995

78. Laupacis A, Fergusson D: Erythropoietin to minimize perioperative blood transfusion: A systematic review of randomized trials. The International Study of Peri-operative Transfusion (ISPOT) Investigators. Transfus Med 8:309, 1998
79. Milbrink J, Birgegard G, Danersund A *et al*: Preoperative autologous donation of 6 units of blood during rh-EPO treatment. Can J Anaesth 44:1315, 1997
80. Monk TG, Goodnough LT, Brecher ME *et al*: A prospective randomized comparison of three blood conservation strategies for radical prostatectomy. Anesthesiology 91:24, 1999
81. Pierson JL, Hannon TJ, Earles DR: A blood-conservation algorithm to reduce blood transfusions after total hip and knee arthroplasty. J Bone Joint Surg Am 86-A:1512, 2004
82. Couvret C, Laffon M, Baud A *et al*: A restrictive use of both autologous donation and recombinant human erythropoietin is an efficient policy for primary total hip or knee arthroplasty. Anesth Analg 99:262, 2004
83. Marchetti M, Barosi G: Cost-effectiveness of epoetin and autologous blood donation reducing allogeneic blood transfusions in coronary artery bypass graft surgery. Transfusion 40:673, 2000
84. Avall A, Hyllner M, Bengtson JP *et al*: Recombinant human erythropoietin in preoperative autologous blood donation did not influence the haemoglobin recovery after surgery. Acta Anaesthesiol Scand 47:687, 2003
85. Rosengart TK, Helm RE, Klemperer J *et al*: Combined aprotinin and erythropoietin use for blood conservation: Results with Jehovah's Witnesses. Ann Thorac Surg 58:1397, 1994
86. Corwin HL, Gettinger A, Pearl RG *et al*: Efficacy of recombinant human erythropoietin in critically ill patients: A randomized controlled trial. JAMA 288:2827, 2002
87. Egrie JC, Dwyer E, Browne JK *et al*: Darbepoetin alfa has a longer circulating half-life and greater in vivo potency than recombinant human erythropoietin. Exp Hematol 31:290, 2003
88. Feldman JM, Roth JV, Bjoraker DG: Maximum blood savings by acute normovolemic hemodilution. Anesth Analg 80:108, 1995
89. Bryson GL, Laupacis A, Wells GA: Does acute normovolemic hemodilution reduce perioperative allogeneic transfusion? A meta-analysis. The International Study of Perioperative Transfusion. Anesth Analg 86:9, 1998
90. Boldt J, Weber A, Mailer K *et al*: Acute normovolaemic haemodilution vs controlled hypotension for reducing the use of allogeneic blood in patients undergoing radical prostatectomy. Br J Anaesth 82:170, 1999
91. Ness PM, Bourke DL, Walsh PC: A randomized trial of perioperative hemodilution versus transfusion of preoperatively deposited autologous blood in elective surgery. Transfusion 32:226, 1992
92. Goodnough LT: Acute normovolemic hemodilution. Vox Sang 83(suppl 1):211, 2002
93. Weiskopf RB: Efficacy of acute normovolemic hemodilution assessed as a function of fraction of blood volume lost. Anesthesiology 94:439, 2001
94. Segal JB, Blasco-Colmenares E, Norris EJ *et al*: Preoperative acute normovolemic hemodilution: a meta-analysis. Transfusion 44:632, 2004
95. Matot I, Scheinin O, Jurim O *et al*: Effectiveness of acute normovolemic hemodilution to minimize allogeneic blood transfusion in major liver resections. Anesthesiology 97:794, 2002
96. Goodnough LT, Despotis GJ, Merkel K *et al*: A randomized trial comparing acute normovolemic hemodilution and preoperative autologous blood donation in total hip arthroplasty. Transfusion 40:1054, 2000
97. Wolowczyk L, Lewis DR, Nevin M *et al*: The effect of acute normovolaemic haemodilution on blood transfusion requirements in abdominal aortic aneurysm repair. Eur J Vasc Endovasc Surg 22:361, 2001
98. Williamson KR, Taswell HF: Intraoperative blood salvage: A review. Transfusion 31:662, 1991
99. Ereth MH, Oliver WC Jr., Santrach PJ: Perioperative interventions to decrease transfusion of allogeneic blood products. Mayo Clin Proc 69:575, 1994
100. Hughes LG, Thomas DW, Wareham K *et al*: Intra-operative blood salvage in abdominal trauma: a review of 5 years' experience. Anaesthesia 56:217, 2001
101. Desmond MJ, Thomas MJ, Gillon J *et al*: Consensus conference on autologous transfusion. Perioperative red cell salvage. Transfusion 36:644, 1996
102. Huet C, Salmi LR, Fergusson D *et al*: A meta-analysis of the effectiveness of cell salvage to minimize perioperative allogeneic blood transfusion in cardiac and orthopedic surgery. International Study of Perioperative Transfusion (ISPOT) Investigators. Anesth Analg 89:861, 1999
103. Fujimoto J, Okamoto E, Yamanaka N *et al*: Efficacy of autotransfusion in hepatectomy for hepatocellular carcinoma. Arch Surg 128:1065, 1993
104. Hart OJ 3rd, Klimberg IW, Wajsman Z *et al*: Intraoperative autotransfusion in radical cystectomy for carcinoma of the bladder. Surg Gynecol Obstet 168:302, 1989
105. Bernstein HH, Rosenblatt MA, Gettes M *et al*: The ability of the Haemonetics 4 Cell Saver System to remove tissue factor from blood contaminated with amniotic fluid. Anesth Analg 85:831, 1997
106. Potter PS, Waters JH, Burger GA *et al*: Application of cell-salvage during cesarean section. Anesthesiology 90:619, 1999
107. Weiskopf RB: Erythrocyte salvage during cesarean section. Anesthesiology 92:1519, 2000
108. Waters JH, Tuohy MJ, Hobson DF *et al*: Bacterial reduction by cell salvage washing and leukocyte depletion filtration. Anesthesiology 99:652, 2003
109. Silvergleid AJ: Safety and effectiveness of predeposit autologous transfusions in preteen and adolescent children. JAMA 257:3403, 1987
110. Tawes RL, Jr., Sydorak GR, DuVall TB: Postoperative salvage: A technological advance in the 'washed' versus 'unwashed' blood controversy. Semin Vasc Surg 7:98, 1994
111. McKie JS, Herzenberg JE: Coagulopathy complicating intraoperative blood salvage in a patient who had idiopathic scoliosis. A case report. J Bone Joint Surg Am 79:1391, 1997
112. Waters JH, Lee JS, Karafa MT: A mathematical model of cell salvage efficiency. Anesth Analg 95:1312, 2002
113. Drummond J, Petrovitch C: Intraoperative blood salvage: Fluid replacement calculations. Anesth Analg 100:645, 2005
114. Griffith LD, Billman GF, Daily PO *et al*: Apparent coagulopathy caused by infusion of shed mediastinal blood and its prevention by washing of the infusate. Ann Thorac Surg 47:400, 1989
115. Vlahakes GJ: Haemoglobin solutions in surgery. Br J Surg 88:1553, 2001
116. Spahn DR, Kocian R: The place of artificial oxygen carriers in reducing allogeneic blood transfusions and augmenting tissue oxygenation. Can J Anaesth 50:S41, 2003
117. AABB: American Association of Blood Banks Technical Manual. 1999
118. Brecher M: Technical Manual. Bethesda, The American Association of Blood Banks, 2002
119. Azzi A, Morfini M, Mannucci PM: The transfusion-associated transmission of parvovirus B19. Transfus Med Rev 13:194, 1999
120. Reiner A: Massive transfusion. In Spiess B, Counts R, Gould S (eds): Perioperative Transfusion Medicine, p 351. Baltimore, Williams & Wilkins, 1998
121. Vinazzer H: Clinical use of antithrombin III concentrations. Vox Sang 53:193, 1997
122. Hoffman M: A cell-based model of coagulation and the role of factor VIIa. Blood Rev 17 (Suppl 1):S1, 2003
123. Diethorn ML, Weld LM: Physiologic mechanisms of hemostasis and fibrinolysis. J Cardiovasc Nurs 4:1, 1989
124. Nilsson IM: Coagulation and fibrinolysis. Scand J Gastroenterol suppl 137:11, 1987
125. Bone RC: Modulators of coagulation. A critical appraisal of their role in sepsis. Arch Intern Med 152:1381, 1992
126. Bick RL: Disseminated intravascular coagulation. Objective criteria for diagnosis and management. Med Clin North Am 78:511, 1994
127. Bennett JS: Disorders of platelet function: evaluation and treatment. Cleve Clin J Med 58:413, 1991
128. Wu KK: Endothelial cells in hemostasis, thrombosis, and inflammation. Hosp Pract (Off Ed) 27:145, 152, 163, 1992
129. Mehta JL, Kitchens CS: Pharmacology of platelet-inhibitory drugs, anticoagulants, and thrombolytic agents. Cardiovasc Clin 18:163, 1987
130. Buller HR, ten Cate JW: Acquired antithrombin III deficiency: Laboratory diagnosis, incidence, clinical implications, and treatment with antithrombin III concentrate. Am J Med 87:44S, 1989
131. Bucur SZ, Levy JH, Despotis GJ *et al*: Uses of antithrombin III concentrate in congenital and acquired deficiency states. Transfusion 38:481, 1998
132. Lemmer JH Jr, Despotis GJ: Antithrombin III concentrate to treat heparin resistance in patients undergoing cardiac surgery. J Thorac Cardiovasc Surg 123:213, 2002
133. Broze GJ Jr: The role of tissue factor pathway inhibitor in a revised coagulation cascade. Semin Hematol 29:159, 1992
134. Rodgers RP, Levin J: A critical reappraisal of the bleeding time. Semin Thromb Hemost 16:1, 1990
135. Greaves M: Assessment of haemostasis. Vox Sang 87(suppl 1):47, 2004
136. Nemerson Y: The tissue factor pathway of blood coagulation. Semin Hematol 29:170, 1992
137. Poller L: The British system for anticoagulant control. Thromb Diath Haemorrh 33:157, 1975
138. Henriksen R: Instrumentation and quality control of hemostasis. In Lotspiech-Steininger C, Koepke J (eds): Clinical Hematology, p 695. Baltimore, J.B. Lippincott, 1992
139. Ellison N, Silberstein LE: Hemostasis in the perioperative period. In Stoelting RK, Gallagher TJ (eds): Advances in Anesthesia, 1st ed, p 67, St. Louis, Year Book Medical Publishers, Inc., 1986
140. Freiberger JJ, Lumb PD: How to manage intraoperative bleeding. In Vaughn RW (ed): Problems in Anesthesia: Perioperative Problems/Catastrophes, p 161, Baltimore, Lippincott, 1987
141. Triplett DA: Overview of hemostasis. Menitove JE, McCarthy LJ (eds): Hemostatic Disorders and the Blood Bank, p 1. Arlington, American Association of Blood Banks, 1984
142. Casserly IP, Kereiakes DJ, Gray WA *et al*: Point-of-care ecarin clotting time versus activated clotting time in correlation with bivalirudin concentration. Thromb Res 113:115, 2004
143. Kang Y, Lewis JH, Navalgund A *et al*: Epsilon-aminocaproic acid for treatment of fibrinolysis during liver transplantation. Anesthesiology 66:766, 1987
144. Traverso CI, Caprini JA, Arcelus JI: The normal thromboelastogram and its interpretation. Semin Thromb Hemost 21(suppl 4):7, 1995
145. Tuman KJ, Spiess BD, McCarthy RJ *et al*: Effects of progressive blood loss on coagulation as measured by thrombelastography. Anesth Analg 66:856, 1987

146. Kang W: Blood coagulation during liver, kidney, and pancreas transplantation. In Lake CL, Moore RA (eds): Blood: Hemostasis, Transfusion, and Alternatives in the Perioperative Period, p 529. New York, Raven Press, 1995
147. Kang YG: Monitoring and treatment of coagulation. Winter KM, Kang YG: Hepatic Transplantation (eds): Anesthetic and Periperative Management, p 151. New York, Praeger, 1986
148. Zuckerman L, Cohen E, Vagher JP *et al*: Comparison of thrombelastography with common coagulation tests. Thromb Haemost 46:752, 1981
149. Colon-Otero G, Cockerill KJ, Bowie EJ: How to diagnose bleeding disorders. Postgrad Med 90:145, 1991
150. Bombeli T, Spahn DR: Updates in perioperative coagulation: Physiology and management of thromboembolism and haemorrhage. Br J Anaesth 93:275, 2004
151. Ewenstein BM: Von Willebrand's disease. Annu Rev Med 48:525, 1997
152. Vischer UM, de Moerloose P: von Willebrand factor: From cell biology to the clinical management of von Willebrand's disease. Crit Rev Oncol Hematol 30:93, 1999
153. Federici AB, Mazurier C, Berntorp E *et al*: Biologic response to desmopressin in patients with severe type 1 and type 2 von Willebrand disease: Results of a multicenter European study. Blood 103:2032, 2004
154. Mannucci PM: Treatment of von Willebrand's Disease. N Engl J Med 351:683, 2004
155. Michiels JJ, Berneman ZN, van der Planken M *et al*: Bleeding prophylaxis for major surgery in patients with type 2 von Willebrand disease with an intermediate purity factor VIII-von Willebrand factor concentrate (Haemate-P). Blood Coagul Fibrinolysis 15:323, 2004
156. Franchini M, Gandini G, Veneri D *et al*: Safety and efficacy of subcutaneous bolus injection of deferoxamine in adult patients with iron overload: An update. Blood 103:747, 2004
157. Lee J-W: von Willebrand disease, hemophilia A and B, and other factor deficiencies. Int Anesthesiol Clin 42:59, 2004
158. Warrier AI, Lusher JM: DDAVP: A useful alternative to blood components in moderate hemophilia A and von Willebrand disease. J Pediatr 102:228, 1983
159. Lethagen S: Desmopressin—a haemostatic drug: state-of-the-art review. Eur J Anaesthesiol suppl 14:1, 1997
160. DeWitt DL: Cox-2-selective inhibitors: The new super aspirins. Mol Pharmacol 55:625, 1999
161. Kam PC, Egan MK: Platelet glycoprotein IIb/IIIa antagonists: Pharmacology and clinical developments. Anesthesiology 96:1237, 2002
162. Merlini PA, Rossi M, Menozzi A *et al*: Thrombocytopenia caused by abciximab or tirofiban and its association with clinical outcome in patients undergoing coronary stenting. Circulation 109:2203, 2004
163. Szuwart T, Brzoska T, Luger TA *et al*: Vitamin E reduces platelet adhesion to human endothelial cells in vitro. Am J Hematol 65:1, 2000
164. Staudinger T, Locker GJ, Frass M: Management of acquired coagulation disorders in emergency and intensive-care medicine. Semin Thromb Hemost 22:93, 1996
165. Makris M, Greaves M, Phillips WS *et al*: Emergency oral anticoagulant reversal: The relative efficacy of infusions of fresh frozen plasma and clotting factor concentrate on correction of the coagulopathy. Thromb Haemost 77:477, 1997
166. Lubetsky A, Hoffman R, Zimlichman R *et al*: Efficacy and safety of a prothrombin complex concentrate (Octaplex) for rapid reversal of oral anticoagulation. Thromb Res 113:371, 2004
167. Ghorashian S, Hunt BJ: "Off-license" use of recombinant activated factor VII. Blood Rev 18:245, 2004
168. Geerts WH, Pineo GF, Heit JA *et al*: Prevention of venous thromboembolism: The Seventh ACCP Conference on Antithrombotic and Thrombolytic Therapy. Chest 126:338S, 2004
169. Groce JB 3rd: Treatment of deep vein thrombosis using low-molecular-weight heparins. Am J Manag Care 7:S510; discussion S515, 2001
170. Boneu B, de Moerloose P: How and when to monitor a patient treated with low molecular weight heparin. Semin Thromb Hemost 27:519, 2001
171. Schwarz RP: The preclinical and clinical pharmacology of Novastan (Argatroban). In Pifarre R (ed): New Anticoagulants for the Cardiovascular Patient, p 231. Philadelphia, Hanley & Belfus, 1997
172. Warkentin TE, Greinacher A: Heparin-induced thrombocytopenia and cardiac surgery. Ann Thorac Surg 76:2121, 2003
173. Warkentin TE, Kelton JG: Temporal aspects of heparin-induced thrombocytopenia. N Engl J Med 344:1286, 2001
174. Gruel Y, Pouplard C, Nguyen P *et al*: Biological and clinical features of low-molecular-weight heparin-induced thrombocytopenia. Br J Haematol 121:786, 2003
175. Despotis GJ, Gravlee G, Filos K *et al*: Anticoagulation monitoring during cardiac surgery: A review of current and emerging techniques. Anesthesiology 91:1122, 1999
176. Despotis GJ, Joist JH: Anticoagulation and anticoagulation reversal with cardiac surgery involving cardiopulmonary bypass: An update. J Cardiothorac Vasc Anesth 13:18; discussion 36, 1999
177. Okita Y, Takamoto S, Ando M *et al*: Coagulation and fibrinolysis system in aortic surgery under deep hypothermic circulatory arrest with aprotinin: The importance of adequate heparinization. Circulation 96:II-376, 1997
178. Body SC, Morse DS: Coagulation, transfusion and cardiac surgery. In Spiess BD, Counts RB, Gould SA (eds): Perioperative Transfusion Medicine, p 419. Baltimore, Williams & Wilkins, 1998
179. Messmore H, Upadhyay G, Farid S *et al*: Heparin-induced thrombocytopenia and thrombosis in cardiovascular surgery. In Pifarre R (ed): New Anticoagulants for the Cardiovascular Patient, p 83. Philadelphia, Hanley & Belfus, Inc., 1997
180. Koster A, Chew D, Grundel M *et al*: An assessment of different filter systems for extracorporeal elimination of bivalirudin: An in vitro study. Anesth Analg 96:1316, table of contents, 2003
181. Weitz JI: New anticoagulants for treatment of venous thromboembolism. Circulation 110:I19, 2004
182. Nutescu EA, Helgason CM: Evolving concepts in the treatment of venous thromboembolism: The role of factor Xa inhibitors. Pharmacotherapy 24:82S, 2004
183. DeLoughery TG: Management of bleeding with uremia and liver disease. Curr Opin Hematol 6:329, 1999
184. Mammen EF: Coagulation defects in liver disease. Med Clin North Am 78:545, 1994
185. Kahl B, Schwartz B, Mosher D: Profound imbalance of pro-fibrinolytic and anti-fibrinolytic factors (tissue plasminogen activator and plasminogen activator inhibitor type 1) and severe bleeding diathesis in a patient with cirrhosis: Correction by liver transplantation. Blood Coagulation and Fibrinolysis 14:741, 2003
186. Bakker CM, Knot EA, Stibbe J *et al*: Disseminated intravascular coagulation in liver cirrhosis. J Hepatol 15:330, 1992
187. Bick RL: Disseminated intravascular coagulation current concepts of etiology, pathophysiology, diagnosis, and treatment. Hematol Oncol Clin North Am 17:149, 2003
188. Levi M: Current understanding of disseminated intravascular coagulation. Br J Haematol 124:567, 2004
189. Carey MJ, Rodgers GM: Disseminated intravascular coagulation: Clinical and laboratory aspects. Am J Hematol 59:65, 1998
190. Dempfle CE: Coagulopathy of sepsis. Thromb Haemost 91:213, 2004
191. Friederich PW, Henny CP, Messelink EJ *et al*: Effect of recombinant activated factor VII on perioperative blood loss in patients undergoing retropubic prostatectomy: A double-blind placebo-controlled randomised trial. Lancet 361:201, 2003
192. Cattaneo M, Harris AS, Stromberg U *et al*: The effect of desmopressin on reducing blood loss in cardiac surgery—a meta-analysis of double-blind, placebo-controlled trials. Thromb Haemost 74:1064, 1995
193. Salzman EW, Weinstein MJ, Weintraub RM *et al*: Treatment with desmopressin acetate to reduce blood loss after cardiac surgery. A double-blind randomized trial. N Engl J Med 314:1402, 1986
194. Czer LS, Bateman TM, Gray RJ *et al*: Treatment of severe platelet dysfunction and hemorrhage after cardiopulmonary bypass: reduction in blood product usage with desmopressin. J Am Coll Cardiol 9:1139, 1987
195. Mongan PD, Hosking MP: The role of desmopressin acetate in patients undergoing coronary artery bypass surgery. A controlled clinical trial with thromboelastographic risk stratification. Anesthesiology 77:38, 1992
196. Gratz I, Koehler J, Olsen D *et al*: The effect of desmopressin acetate on postoperative hemorrhage in patients receiving aspirin therapy before coronary artery bypass operations. J Thorac Cardiovasc Surg 104;1417, 1992
197. Henry D: Anti-fibrinolytic use for minimising perioperative allogeneic blood transfusion. The Cochrane Library 2002
198. Khoshhal K, Mukhtar I, Clark P *et al*: Efficacy of aprotinin in reducing blood loss in spinal fusion for idiopathic scoliosis. J Pediatr Orthop 23:661, 2003
199. Lemay E, Guay J, Cote C *et al*: Tranexamic acid reduces the need for allogenic red blood cell transfusions in patients undergoing total hip replacement. Can J Anaesth 51:31, 2004
200. Porte RJ, Molenaar IQ, Begliomini B *et al*: Aprotinin and transfusion requirements in orthotopic liver transplantation: A multicentre randomised double-blind study. EMSALT Study Group. Lancet 355:1303, 2000
201. Zohar E, Fredman B, Ellis MH *et al*: A comparative study of the postoperative allogeneic blood-sparing effects of tranexamic acid and of desmopressin after total knee replacement. Transfusion 41:1285, 2001
202. Cirino C, Napoli C, Bucci M *et al*: Inflammation-coagulation network: Are serine protease receptors the knot? Trends Pharmacologic Sci 21:170, 2000
203. Landis CR, Haskard DO, Taylor KM: New antiinflammatory and platelet-preserving effects of aprotinin. Ann Thorac Surg 72:S1808, 2001
204. van Oeveren W, Harder MP, Roozendaal KJ *et al*: Aprotinin protects platelets against the initial effect of cardiopulmonary bypass. J Thorac Cardiovasc Surg 99:788; discussion 796, 1990
205. Landis RC, Asimakopoulos G, Poullis M *et al*: The antithrombotic and antiinflammatory mechanisms of action of aprotinin. Ann Thorac Surg 72:2169, 2001
206. Levi M, Cromheecke ME, de Jonge E *et al*: Pharmacological strategies to decrease excessive blood loss in cardiac surgery: A meta-analysis of clinically relevant endpoints. Lancet 354:1940, 1999
207. Sedrakyan A, Treasure T, Elefteriades JA: Effect of aprotinin on clinical outcomes in coronary artery bypass graft surgery: A systematic review and meta-analysis of randomized clinical trials. J Thorac Cardiovasc Surg 128:442, 2004
208. Munoz JJ, Birkmeyer NJ, Birkmeyer JD *et al*: Is epsilon-aminocaproic acid as effective as aprotinin in reducing bleeding with cardiac surgery?:A meta-analysis. Circulation 99:81, 1999

209. Casati V, Guzzon D, Oppizzi M *et al*: Hemostatic effects of aprotinin, tranexamic acid and epsilon-aminocaproic acid in primary cardiac surgery. Ann Thorac Surg 68:2252; discussion 2256, 1999
210. Dietrich W, Spath P, Zuhlsdorf M *et al*: Anaphylactic reactions to aprotinin reexposure in cardiac surgery: Relation to antiaprotinin immunoglobulin G and E antibodies. Anesthesiology 95:64; discussion 5A, 2001
211. Porte RJ, Bontempo FA, Knot EA *et al*: Systemic effects of tissue plasminogen activator-associated fibrinolysis and its relation to thrombin generation in orthotopic liver transplantation. Transplantation 47:978, 1989
212. Grosse H, Lobbes W, Frambach M *et al*: The use of high dose aprotinin in liver transplantation: The influence on fibrinolysis and blood loss. Thromb Res 63:287, 1991
213. Carlier M, Veyckemans F, Scholtes JL *et al*: Anesthesia for pediatric hepatic transplantation: Experience of 33 cases. Transplant Proc 19:3333, 1987
214. Kufner RP: Antifibrinolytics and orthotopic liver transplantation. Transplant Proc 30:692, 1998

SECTION III ■ BASIC PRINCIPLES OF PHARMACOLOGY IN ANESTHESIA PRACTICE

CHAPTER 11 ■ BASIC PRINCIPLES OF CLINICAL PHARMACOLOGY

ROBERT J. HUDSON AND THOMAS K. HENTHORN

KEY POINTS

1. Most drugs must pass through cell membranes to reach their sites of action. Consequently, drugs tend to be relatively lipophilic, rather than hydrophilic.
2. Most drugs are either organic bases or organic acids. A greater extent of ionization at physiologic pH will limit the rapidity of drug uptake and distribution.
3. The liver is the most important organ for metabolism of drugs. Hepatic drug clearance depends on three factors: the intrinsic ability of the liver to metabolize a drug, hepatic blood flow, and the extent of binding of the drug to blood components.
4. The kidneys eliminate hydrophilic drugs and relatively hydrophilic metabolites of lipophilic drugs. Renal elimination of lipophilic compounds is negligible.
5. The cytochrome P450 (CYP) superfamily is the most important group of enzymes involved in drug metabolism. It and other drug-metabolizing enzymes exhibit genetic polymorphism.
6. In pharmacokinetic models, the volume of distribution quantifies the extent of drug distribution. The greater the affinity of tissues for the drug, relative to blood, the greater the volume of distribution.
7. Generally, more lipophilic drugs are more highly bound to plasma proteins and have greater volumes of distribution.
8. In pharmacokinetic models, the elimination clearance quantifies the ability of drug-eliminating organs to irreversibly remove drugs from the body. High values for elimination clearance indicate efficient drug elimination.
9. All else being equal, an increase in the volume of distribution of a drug will increase its elimination half-life; an increase in elimination clearance will decrease elimination half-life.
10. Pharmacologic effects can be analyzed by both dose-response curves and concentration-response relationships. A disadvantage of dose-response curves is the inability to distinguish between pharmacokinetic and pharmacodynamic variability.
11. Many drugs bind to specific receptors. Receptors are dynamic entities that adapt to their environment by changing in response to exposure their agonists or antagonists.
12. During continuous infusions of drugs that partition rapidly and extensively into body tissues, the rate of rise to the eventual steady-state plasma drug concentration is determined primarily by the half-lives of the early distribution phases,

not the elimination half-life. Thus, drug concentrations rapidly approach the steady-state concentration during the first minutes, and then rise much more slowly after the first hour, of the infusion.

13 Target-controlled infusions are achieved with computer-controlled infusion pumps in Europe and Asia (not yet FDA-approved in the United States), and permit clinicians to make use of the drug concentration–effect relationship, optimally accounting for pharmacokinetics, and predicting the offset of drug effect.

Over four decades ago, Dr. E. M. Papper[1] emphasized the importance of understanding the pharmacology of anesthetics:

> Clinical anaesthetists have administered millions of anaesthetics during more than a century with little precise information of the uptake, distribution, and elimination of inhalational and non-volatile anaesthetic agents. Considering how serious is the handicap of not knowing those fundamental and important facts about the drugs they have used so often, the record of success and safety in clinical anaesthesia is an extraordinary accomplishment indeed. It can in some measure be attributed to the accumulated experience and successful teaching of a highly developed sense of intuition from generation to generation of anaesthetists. It can also be attributed in part to the ability to learn by error after observing patients come uncomfortably close to injury and even to death.
>
> In the last few years, however, sufficient fundamental information has become available to explain these clinical successes. The empirical process of giving an anaesthetic can be better understood because of the specific data provided by the studies reported in this symposium and by the work of others which has preceded them.

Knowledge of the principles of pharmacology and specific properties of individual drugs is even more important today. New anesthetics, opioids, and neuromuscular blockers have recently become available. We do not have the benefit of decades of experience with new drugs, so we must depend on carefully conducted investigations for the information needed to use them optimally. As Dr. Papper wrote:

> If the anaesthetist studies the pharmacology of these agents and understands their pharmacokinetic properties, he can with reasonable certainty predict which of these newer anaesthetic agents will hold promise for clinical utility ... the clinician can spare his patients much danger and his own work many hardships if he is aware of the physicochemical and pharmacological [properties] of new agents.

Our patients are also changing. Many have comorbidities that were once considered contraindications to anesthesia and surgery. Therefore, we must consider the impact of chronic diseases and associated pharmacotherapy on the responses to drugs administered during the perioperative period. Comprehensive knowledge of clinical pharmacology is a prerequisite to the practice of anesthesiology.

The first sections of this chapter discuss the biologic and pharmacologic factors that influence drug absorption, distribution, and elimination. Quantitative analysis of these processes is discussed in the section on pharmacokinetics. The next section presents the fundamentals of pharmacodynamics—those factors that determine the relationship between drug concentration and pharmacologic effects. Mechanisms of drug interactions are then reviewed. The final section discusses clinical application of pharmacokinetics and pharmacodynamics, and systems for delivery of intravenous drugs. Although specific properties of drugs are used to illustrate basic pharmacologic principles, detailed information regarding the pharmacology of drugs used in anesthesiology is presented in succeeding chapters.

TRANSFER OF DRUGS ACROSS MEMBRANES

Drug absorption, distribution, metabolism, and excretion of drugs all require transfer of drugs across cell membranes. Most drugs must also traverse cell membranes to reach their sites of
1 action. Biologic membranes consist of a lipid bilayer with a nonpolar core and polar elements on their surfaces. Proteins are embedded in the lipid bilayer and are oriented similarly, with ionic, polar groups on the membrane surfaces and hydrophobic groups in the membrane interior. The nonpolar core hinders the passage of water-soluble molecules, so that only lipid-soluble molecules easily traverse cell membranes.

Transport Processes

Drugs can cross cell membranes either by passive processes or by active transport. *Passive diffusion* occurs when a concentration gradient exists across a membrane. The rate of passive transfer is directly proportional to the concentration gradient and the lipid solubility of the drug. Passage of water-soluble drugs is restricted to small aqueous channels through the membrane. These channels are so small that only molecules less than 200 D pass through them readily. Capillary endothelial cells, except those in the central nervous system (CNS), permit transfer of much larger molecules, such as albumin (molecular weight ~67,000 D). Because of these unique features, diffusion of drugs across capillary membranes outside the CNS is limited by blood flow, not by lipid solubility.[2]

Some drugs are transferred through cell membranes of hepatocytes, renal tubular cells, and others by *active transport.* This is an energy-requiring process that is both specific and saturable. Active transport can move compounds against concentration gradients. *Facilitated diffusion* shares some characteristics with active transport. It is also carrier mediated, specific, and saturable, but does not require energy and cannot overcome a concentration gradient.[2]

Effects of Molecular Properties

Most drugs are too large to pass through aqueous membrane channels and must traverse the lipid component of membranes.
2 Almost all drugs are either weak acids or weak bases, and are present in both ionized and nonionized forms at physiologic pH. The nonionized form is more lipid soluble and able easily to traverse cell membranes. The nonionized fraction of weak acids, such as salicylates and barbiturates, is greater at low pH values, so acidic drugs become more lipid soluble as pH decreases. The nonionized fraction of weak bases like opioids and local anesthetics increases as the pH becomes more alkaline. The pK_a is the pH at which exactly 50% of a weak acid or base is present in each of the ionized and nonionized forms. The closer the pK_a is to the ambient pH, the greater the change in the degree of ionization for a given change in pH. If there is a pH gradient across a membrane, drug will be trapped on the side that has the higher ionized fraction, because only the

nonionized drug is diffusible. This phenomenon is known as *ion trapping*. The total drug concentration is greater on the side of the membrane with the higher ionized fraction. However, at equilibrium, the concentration of nonionized drug will be the same. In most situations, the range of pH values is too small to cause major changes in the degree of ionization. However, there are major pH changes in the upper gastrointestinal (GI) tract, which can affect drug absorption.

DRUG ABSORPTION

Except after intravenous (iv) injections, drugs must be absorbed into the circulation before they can be delivered to their sites of action. Therefore, absorption is an important determinant of both the intensity and duration of drug action. Incomplete absorption limits the amount of drug reaching the site of action, reducing the peak pharmacologic effect. Rapid absorption is a prerequisite for rapid onset of action. In contrast, slow absorption permits a sustained duration of action because of the "depot" of drug at the absorptive site. The speed of absorption depends on the solubility and concentration of drug. All drugs must dissolve in water to reach the circulation. Consequently, drugs in aqueous solutions are absorbed faster than those in solid formulations, suspensions, or organic solvents, such as propylene glycol. A high concentration of drug facilitates absorption. Increased blood flow to the site of injection increases the rate of absorption. Decreased blood flow secondary to hypotension, vasoconstrictors, or other factors slows drug absorption. Vasoconstrictors added to local anesthetics delay absorption after subcutaneous injection. This prolongs the duration of action at the site of injection and lessens the chance of systemic toxicity.

Route of Administration

In general medical practice, drugs are most commonly administered orally. The advantages of oral administration are convenience, economy, and safety. Disadvantages include the requirement for a cooperative patient, incomplete absorption, and metabolism of the drug in the GI tract and liver before it reaches the systemic circulation.[2] In anesthesia, drugs are most frequently administered via iv and inhalational routes. Both permit rapid and reasonably predictable attainment of the desired blood concentration.

Oral Administration

Absorption from the GI tract is highly variable because of the multiple factors involved. Tablets and capsules must disintegrate before the drug can dissolve in the GI lumen. The drug must then cross the GI epithelium and pass into the portal circulation. The most important site of absorption of all drugs is the small intestine, because of its large surface area and the anatomic characteristics of its mucosa. The nonionized fraction of weak acids such as barbiturates is higher at low pH values, which favors absorption from the stomach. However, the effect of pH on ionization of acidic drugs in the stomach is offset by the small surface area and thickness of the gastric mucosa and the rapidity of gastric emptying. Basic drugs are highly ionized at low pH, so they cannot cross the gastric mucosa. The more alkaline pH of the small intestine increases the nonionized fraction of basic drugs such as opioids, facilitating their absorption.

Once drugs enter the portal circulation, they must traverse the liver before reaching the systemic circulation. Some drugs are extensively metabolized during this initial pass through the liver, so that only a small fraction of the drug reaches the systemic circulation. This is called the *first-pass effect*. Depending on the magnitude of the first-pass effect, the oral dose must be proportionately larger than the iv dose to achieve the same pharmacologic response. Metabolism of some drugs by the GI mucosa also contributes to the first-pass effect.[3]

Sublingual Administration

Drug absorbed from the oral mucosa passes directly into the systemic circulation, eliminating the first-pass effect. Because of the small surface area for absorption, this route is efficacious only for nonionized, highly lipid-soluble drugs, such as nitroglycerin.

Transcutaneous Administration

Only lipid-soluble drugs can penetrate intact skin sufficiently to produce systemic effects. Drug "patches" applied to the skin are now widely used. These systems consist of an adhesive containing a reservoir of drug that is slowly released after the patch is applied, producing a stable pharmacologic effect. Drugs currently administered in this fashion include scopolamine (for motion sickness) and nitroglycerin. Opioid patches are used for treatment of chronic pain. Transcutaneous absorption of drugs from patches is passive, so the onset time is delayed. This disadvantage can be overcome by using an electric current to "drive" ionized drugs into the skin, a process is called *iontophoresis*. Transcutaneous iontophoretic administration of fentanyl has been described.[4]

Intramuscular and Subcutaneous Injection

Absorption of drugs from subcutaneous tissue is relatively slow, permitting a sustained effect. The rate of absorption can be altered by changes in the drug formulation. Examples of such manipulations are the various preparations of insulin and the addition of vasoconstrictors to local anesthetic solutions. Uptake of drugs after intramuscular injection is more rapid than after subcutaneous administration because of greater blood flow. Drugs in aqueous solution are very readily absorbed. The effect of drugs in nonaqueous solutions, such as diazepam in propylene glycol, is less predictable because of erratic absorption.[5]

Intrathecal, Epidural, and Perineural Injection

Intrathecal injection of local anesthetics or other drugs close to their sites of action in the spinal cord permits the use of very low doses, eliminating the risk of adverse systemic drug effects. This is not an advantage of epidural anesthesia or major perineural regional anesthesia because of the greater total dose required. The major disadvantage of these routes of injection is the expertise they require.

Inhalational Administration

Uptake of inhalational anesthetics from the pulmonary alveoli to the blood is exceedingly rapid because of their low molecular weight and high lipid solubility, and the large total alveolar surface area, and because alveolar blood flow is almost equal to cardiac output.

Intravenous Injection

Intravenous injection eliminates the need for absorption, so that therapeutic blood concentrations are rapidly attained. This is especially advantageous when rapid onset of action is desired. It also simplifies titration of the dose to individual patients' responses. Unfortunately, rapid onset also has its hazards; should an adverse drug reaction or overdose occur, the effects are immediate and potentially severe.

Bioavailability

Bioavailability is defined as the fraction of the total dose that reaches the systemic circulation. Bioavailability is reduced by factors such as incomplete absorption from the site of injection or GI tract, the first-pass effect, or pulmonary uptake of drugs.

Even after iv injection, the bioavailability of drugs formulated in lipid suspensions may be less than 100%. These suspensions contain small lipid droplets. Some, but not all, of the drug diffuses from the lipid droplets into the plasma. These droplets are taken up by the liver and metabolized. Presumably, some drug is also metabolized before it is released back into the circulation. The bioavailability of the lecithin suspension of diazepam is 30% less than that of diazepam in propylene glycol, even with direct iv injection.[6]

DRUG DISTRIBUTION

After absorption or injection into the systemic circulation, drugs are distributed throughout the body. Highly perfused organs, such as the brain, heart, lungs, liver, and kidneys, receive most of the drug soon after injection. Delivery to muscle, skin, fat, and other less well perfused tissues is slower, and equilibration of distribution into these tissues may take several hours or even days.

Capillary membranes are freely permeable in most tissues, so drugs pass quickly into the extracellular space. Subsequent distribution varies according to the physicochemical properties of the drug. Distribution of highly polar, water-soluble drugs such as the neuromuscular blockers is essentially limited to extracellular fluid. Lipid-soluble drugs like propofol easily cross cell membranes and are therefore distributed much more extensively.

Distribution of drugs into the CNS is unique. Brain capillaries do not have the large aqueous channels typical of capillaries in other tissues. Consequently, diffusion of water-soluble drugs into the brain is severely restricted—hence the term *blood-brain barrier*. In contrast, distribution of highly lipid-soluble drugs into the CNS is limited only by cerebral blood flow. For more polar compounds, the rate of entry into the brain is proportional to the lipid solubility of the nonionized drug.

Drugs accumulate in tissues because of binding to tissue components, pH gradients, or uptake of lipophilic drugs into fat. These tissue stores can act as reservoirs that prolong the duration of drug action, either in the same tissue, or by delivery to the site of action elsewhere after reabsorption into the circulation.

Binding of drugs to plasma proteins and erythrocytes influences distribution to other tissues. Only free, unbound drug can cross capillary membranes. The extent of tissue uptake of drugs depends on the affinity of drug binding to blood constituents, relative to the overall affinity of binding to tissue components.

Redistribution

The rapid entry and equally rapid egress of lipophilic drugs from richly perfused organs such as the brain and heart is referred to as *redistribution*. This phenomenon is illustrated by the events that follow an injection of thiopental. The brain concentration of thiopental peaks within 1 minute because of high blood flow to the brain and the high lipid solubility of thiopental. As the drug is taken up by other, less well perfused tissues, the plasma level rapidly decreases. This creates a concentration gradient from cerebral tissue to the blood, so that thiopental quickly diffuses back into the blood, where it is redistributed to other tissues that are still taking up the drug. Ultimately, adipose tissue contains much of the drug remaining in the body because of the high lipid solubility of thiopental. However, recovery from a single dose of thiopental depends predominantly on redistribution of thiopental from the brain to muscle, because of the larger mass and greater perfusion of muscle compared to adipose tissue.[7,8]

A single moderate dose of thiopental (<5 to 6 mg/kg) has a very short duration of action because of redistribution. If repeated injections are given, the concentration of thiopental builds up in the peripheral tissues, and termination of drug action becomes increasingly dependent on the much slower process of drug elimination. Termination of the pharmacologic effects of other lipophilic drugs, such as fentanyl and its derivatives, and propofol, is also governed by these factors.

Placental Transfer

Most drugs cross the placenta by simple diffusion, so propofol and other lipid-soluble drugs with low molecular weights are most readily transferred. Highly polar, water-soluble compounds such as the neuromuscular blocking drugs do not cross the placenta to a significant extent. Fetal pH is slightly lower than maternal pH. This pH gradient causes the ionized fraction of weak bases, such as opioids and local anesthetics, to be higher in the fetus. Therefore, the fetal total drug level may be higher than predicted from the maternal total drug level because of ion trapping.[9] Different total drug concentrations can also result from differences between mother and fetus in the extent of drug binding to plasma proteins. However, regardless of the effects of pH and protein binding, the concentration of free, nonionized drug is the same on both sides of the placenta once equilibrium is reached. For most drugs, this is the most important form, because it has the most pharmacologic activity.

DRUG ELIMINATION

Elimination is an inclusive term referring to all the processes that remove drugs from the body. Elimination occurs either by excretion of unchanged drug or by metabolism (biotransformation) and subsequent excretion of metabolites. The liver and kidneys are the most important organs for drug elimination. The liver eliminates drugs primarily by metabolism to less active compounds and, to a lesser extent, by hepatobiliary excretion of drugs or their metabolites. The primary role of the kidneys is the excretion of water-soluble, polar compounds. Drugs having these properties, such as some nondepolarizing neuromuscular blockers, undergo renal excretion intact.[10] The kidneys also excrete water-soluble metabolites of drugs that initially undergo biotransformation. Pulmonary excretion is the major route for elimination of anesthetic gases and vapors.

The term "drug clearance," or "elimination clearance," describes the ability to remove drug from the blood. Drug clearance is the theoretical volume of blood from which drug is completely and irreversibly removed in a given time interval. It is analogous to creatinine clearance, which quantitatively describes the ability of the kidneys to eliminate creatinine. Like creatinine clearance, drug clearance has units of flow, milliliters per minute (mL/min). Many drugs are cleared by more than one route, and multiple elimination pathways are additive. Consequently, total drug clearance is equal to the sum of the clearances of all of the elimination pathways.

Total drug clearance can be calculated with pharmacokinetic models of blood concentration versus time data. However, clearance by individual organs and the biologic factors influencing drug elimination cannot be estimated from blood concentration data alone. Additional data, such as the hepatic arteriovenous drug concentration difference or the rate of urinary excretion of the drug, are needed to determine the contribution of a specific organ to total drug clearance.

Hepatic Drug Clearance

Drug clearance by the liver is dependent on three factors: (1) hepatic blood flow, (2) the intrinsic ability of the liver to irreversibly eliminate the drug from the blood, and (3) the extent of drug binding to plasma proteins or other blood constituents. The interrelationships between these factors have been described with the *venous equilibration model* of hepatic drug clearance.[11,12] According to this model, the unbound concentration of drug in hepatic venous blood is in equilibrium with the unbound concentration in hepatocytes. This unbound drug within the liver is available for elimination by biotransformation or biliary excretion.

The venous equilibration model is based on two assumptions: that hepatic drug clearance is limited by delivery of drug to the liver, and that elimination is a first-order process.[11] By definition, *first order* means that a constant fraction of the drug is eliminated per unit time. The fraction of the drug removed from the blood passing through the liver is the hepatic extraction ratio, *E*:

$$E = \frac{C_a - C_v}{C_a} \quad (11\text{-}1)$$

where C_a is the mixed hepatic arterial–portal venous drug concentration and C_v is the mixed hepatic venous drug concentration. The total hepatic drug clearance, Cl_H, is:

$$Cl_H = Q \cdot E \quad (11\text{-}2)$$

where Q is hepatic blood flow. Therefore, hepatic clearance is a function of hepatic blood flow and the ability of the liver to extract drug from the blood. The ability to extract drug depends on the activity of drug-metabolizing enzymes and the capacity for hepatobiliary excretion.

The concept of *intrinsic clearance* was developed to account for the effects of blood flow and drug binding in the blood on elimination.[11] Intrinsic clearance represents the ability of the liver to remove drug from the blood in the absence of any limitations imposed by blood flow or drug binding. The relationship of total hepatic drug clearance to the extraction ratio and intrinsic clearance, Cl_I, is:

$$Cl_H = Q \cdot E = Q\left(\frac{Cl_I}{Q + Cl_I}\right) \quad (11\text{-}3)$$

The right-hand side of Equation 11-3 indicates that if intrinsic clearance is very high (many times larger than hepatic blood flow), total hepatic clearance approaches hepatic blood flow. On the other hand, if intrinsic clearance is very small, hepatic clearance will be similar to intrinsic clearance. These relationships are shown in Figure 11-1.

Thus, hepatic drug clearance and extraction are determined by two independent variables, intrinsic clearance and hepatic blood flow. Changes in either will change hepatic clearance. However, the extent of the change depends on the initial intrinsic clearance. If the inherent ability of the liver to eliminate a drug (intrinsic clearance) is doubled, then the extraction ratio also increases, but not necessarily to the same extent. The extraction ratio and intrinsic clearance do not have a simple, linear relationship:

$$E = \frac{Cl_I}{Q + Cl_I} \quad (11\text{-}4)$$

If the initial intrinsic clearance is small relative to hepatic blood flow, then the extraction ratio is also small, and Equation 11-4 indicates that doubling intrinsic clearance will produce an almost proportional increment in the extraction ratio, and, consequently, clearance. However, if intrinsic clearance is much greater than hepatic blood flow, a twofold change in intrinsic clearance has a negligible effect on the extraction ratio and drug clearance. In nonmathematical terms, high intrinsic clearance indicates efficient hepatic elimination. It is hard to enhance an already efficient process, whereas it is relatively easy to improve on inefficient drug clearance because of low intrinsic clearance.

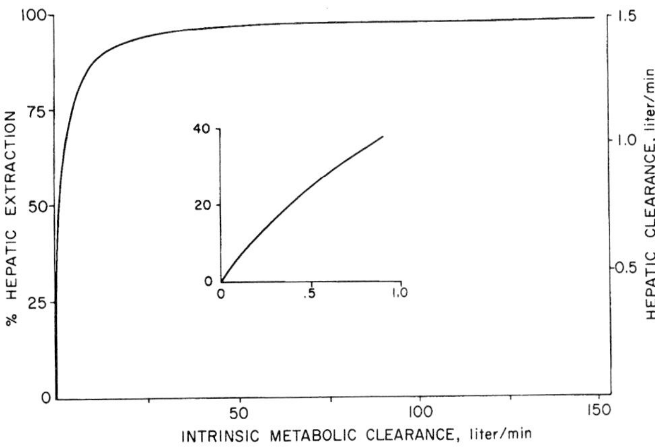

FIGURE 11-1. The relationship between hepatic extraction ratio, intrinsic clearance, and hepatic clearance at the normal hepatic blood flow of 1.5 L/min. For drugs with high intrinsic clearance (>25 L/min), increasing intrinsic clearance has little effect on hepatic extraction and total hepatic clearance. The inset demonstrates the relationship at low values of intrinsic clearance on an expanded scale. (Reprinted with permission from Wilkinson GR, Shand DG: A physiologic approach to hepatic drug clearance. Clin Pharmacol Ther 18:377, 1975.)

The effect of changes in hepatic blood flow also depends on the magnitude of intrinsic clearance. If extraction and intrinsic clearance are high, a decrease in hepatic blood flow causes a small increase in the extraction ratio (Fig. 11-2) that is insufficient to offset the effects of reduced hepatic flow (Eq. 11-4). Consequently, changes in hepatic blood flow produce virtually proportional changes in clearance of drugs with high extraction ratios (Fig. 11-3). For drugs having a low intrinsic clearance, a decrease in hepatic blood flow is associated with a larger, almost proportional increase in the extraction ratio (see Fig. 11-2). This largely offsets the effects of changes in blood flow, so that clearance of drugs with low extraction ratios is essentially independent of hepatic blood flow (see Fig. 11-3).

Hepatic clearance of drugs with extraction ratios $\leq$30% is independent of changes in liver blood flow, but very sensitive to the liver's ability to metabolize the drug, which can vary as a result of pathologic conditions, inhibition or induction of drug-metabolizing enzymes, or interindividual differences. In contrast, variations of hepatic clearance of drugs with high extraction ratios (>70%) are determined primarily by liver blood flow. Drugs with intermediate extraction ratios, between 30 and 70%, share characteristics with both the other groups. Drugs can be classified as having either high, intermediate, or low extraction ratios (Table 11-1).

Binding of drugs to plasma proteins and other blood components may also affect drug clearance. Whether or not drug binding influences drug clearance depends on the extraction ratio and the extent of binding. Three classes of hepatic clearance can be defined by integrating the effects of drug binding in the blood and the extraction ratio.[13] Clearance of drugs with high extraction ratios is *flow limited* because it depends only on

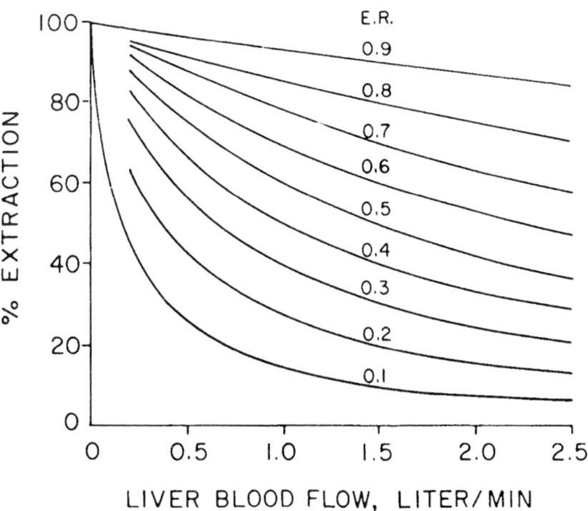

FIGURE 11-2. The effect of changes in hepatic blood flow on extraction of drugs with different extraction ratios. The extraction ratios at the normal hepatic blood flow of 1.5 L/min are above the corresponding curves. (Reprinted with permission from Wood AJJ: Drug disposition and pharmacokinetics. In Wood M, Wood AJJ [eds]: Drugs and Anesthesia—Pharmacology for Anesthesiologists, p 27. Baltimore, Williams & Walkins, 1990. After Wilkinson GR, Shand DG: A physiologic approach to hepatic drug clearance. Clin Pharmacol Ther 18:377, 1975.)

TABLE 11-1

CLASSIFICATION OF DRUGS ENCOUNTERED IN ANESTHESIOLOGY ACCORDING TO HEPATIC EXTRACTION RATIOS

LOW	INTERMEDIATE	HIGH
diazepam	alfentanil	alprenolol
lorazepam	methohexital	bupivacaine
methadone	midazolam	diltiazem
phenytoin	vecuronium	fentanyl
rocuronium		ketamine
theophylline		lidocaine
thiopental		meperidine
		metoprolol
		morphine
		naloxone
		nifedipine
		propofol
		propranolol
		sufentanil
		verapamil

Drugs eliminated primarily by other organs are not included in this table.

hepatic perfusion and is not affected by changes in drug binding or intrinsic clearance. The combination of a low extraction ratio and a high free fraction results in *capacity-limited, binding-insensitive* clearance, which is affected by changes in intrinsic clearance but is not significantly influenced by binding or hepatic perfusion. Drugs with low extraction ratios and low free fractions have *capacity-limited, binding-sensitive* clearance, which is not greatly affected by changes in hepatic blood flow but depends on both intrinsic clearance and the free drug concentration. Elimination of drugs with intermediate extraction ratios and binding is influenced by all three biologic factors—hepatic blood flow, intrinsic clearance, and the free drug concentration in the blood. The relative importance of these three factors cannot be predicted unless the extraction ratio and the unbound fraction in the blood are known.

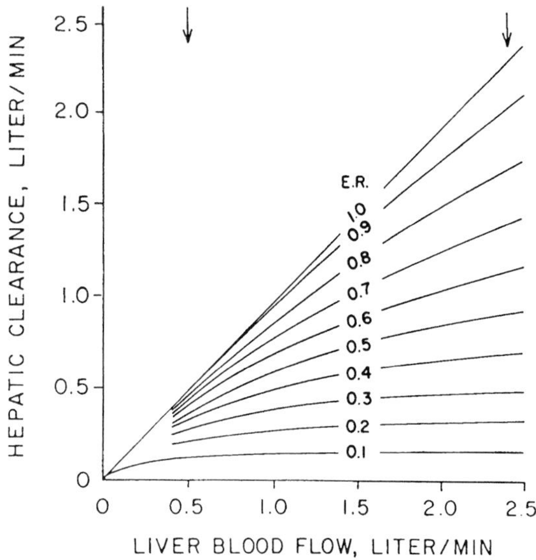

FIGURE 11-3. The effect of changes in hepatic blood flow on hepatic clearance of drugs with different extraction ratios. The extraction ratios for each curve at 1.5 L/min flow are indicated. The *arrows* indicate the normal physiologic range of hepatic blood flow. (Reprinted with permission from Wood AJJ: Drug disposition and pharmacokinetics. In Wood M, Wood AJJ [eds]: Drugs and Anesthesia—Pharmacology for Anesthesiologists, p 27. Baltimore, Williams & Wilkins, 1990. After Wilkinson GR, Shand DG: A physiologic approach to hepatic drug clearance. Clin Pharmacol Ther 18:377, 1975.)

Physiologic, Pathologic, and Pharmacologic Alterations in Hepatic Drug Clearance

At rest, approximately 30% of cardiac output perfuses the liver. The hepatic artery provides roughly 25% of total hepatic flow, with the remainder supplied via the portal vein. Many physiologic and pathologic conditions alter hepatic blood flow, but there is little information regarding the effect of these changes in blood flow on hepatic drug clearance. The splanchnic circulation responds to a variety of stimuli, and splanchnic flow is often sacrificed to meet the demands of other tissues.

Moving from the supine to the upright position decreases cardiac output, which produces a reflex increase in systemic vascular resistance. The splanchnic circulation participates in this generalized vasoconstriction, which decreases hepatic blood flow by 30 to 40%.[12] Clearance of aldosterone, which has a high hepatic extraction ratio, is decreased in the upright position.[12] Postural changes probably also influence clearance of drugs with high hepatic extraction ratios, but this has not been systematically investigated.

Exercise, heat stress, and hypovolemia all decrease splanchnic blood flow in proportion to the associated increase in heart rate, which suggests that these responses are mediated by the sympathetic nervous system.[12] As expected, these conditions decrease clearance of indocyanine green, which has a high hepatic extraction ratio. In contrast, the clearance of antipyrine, a drug with a low extraction ratio, is not affected by these conditions.[14]

Decreases in cardiac output cause reflex splanchnic vasoconstriction, which reduces hepatic blood flow in proportion to the reduction in cardiac output.[15] Lidocaine clearance is reduced in patients with congestive cardiac failure.[16] Consequently, if usual doses of lidocaine are given to patients with heart failure, the risk of lidocaine toxicity is increased. Marked reduction in hepatic blood flow causes hepatocellular dysfunction; therefore, severe congestive heart failure decreases drug clearance by reducing both intrinsic clearance and hepatic blood flow.[17] Cardiovascular collapse severely compromises both liver blood flow and hepatocellular function.[12] In experimental hemorrhagic shock, clearance of lidocaine was decreased by 40%, whereas hepatic blood flow declined by 30%.[18] The reduction in clearance is too large to be caused solely by decreased hepatic perfusion, implying a concomitant reduction in intrinsic clearance secondary to hepatic ischemia.

Liver disease can decrease drug clearance because of hepatocellular dysfunction, altered hepatic blood flow, or both.[12] Cirrhosis reduces clearance of drugs with high extraction ratios, including lidocaine,[16] meperidine,[19,20] and propranolol.[21] This is secondary to decreased hepatic perfusion, which can be the result of reduced total liver blood flow, intrahepatic shunting, or extrahepatic shunting of portal venous blood.[12] Portosystemic shunting increases the bioavailability of orally administered drugs with high extraction ratios.[12] Cirrhosis also decreases clearance of drugs with low extraction ratios, such as diazepam,[22,23] because of impaired hepatocellular function, which decreases intrinsic clearance. Acute viral hepatitis reduces the clearance of drugs with both high (meperidine,[24] lidocaine[25]) and low (diazepam[22]) hepatic extraction ratios. These observations indicate that both acute and chronic liver diseases affect liver function and blood flow in a parallel fashion. Consequently, in chronic therapy, doses of any drug cleared by the liver should be reduced in patients with hepatic disease.

Drugs that alter splanchnic hemodynamics affect clearance of highly extracted drugs. Propranolol decreases hepatic blood flow, thus decreasing its own clearance[12] and the clearance of concomitantly administered lidocaine.[26] The volatile anesthetics all decrease hepatic blood flow, although isoflurane does so to a lesser extent than halothane or enflurane.[27,28] Intra-abdominal surgery causes a further decrease in hepatic perfusion.[27] Hypotension produced by spinal anesthesia reduces splanchnic blood flow.[29] In contrast to the volatile anesthetics, nitrous oxide, opioids, and barbiturates have little effect on hepatic blood flow.[12] Although they are potentially of great clinical importance, the effects of these hemodynamic alterations have not been thoroughly investigated. It is logical to assume that the clearance of drugs with high hepatic extraction ratios will be reduced during anesthesia and surgery.

Renal Drug Clearance

Although the kidneys do metabolize drugs, their major function in drug elimination is to excrete water-soluble drugs, and metabolites produced elsewhere (primarily the liver), into the urine. Renal clearance of drugs is determined by the net effects of three processes: glomerular filtration, tubular secretion, and tubular reabsorption.[30,31]

Glomerular filtration cannot eliminate drugs efficiently. The glomerular filtration rate (GFR) is approximately 20% of renal plasma flow.[32] Consequently, even if none of the drug is bound to plasma proteins, only about 20% can be removed by glomerular filtration. Drug binding to plasma proteins and erythrocytes reduces the amount filtered, because only unbound drug can pass through the glomerular membrane into the renal tubule. If a drug is neither secreted nor reabsorbed by the renal tubules, then renal drug clearance will be equal to glomerular clearance. Drugs and metabolites excreted in this fashion have low renal extraction ratios, and their renal clearance depends on the degree of binding to blood constituents. Therefore, protein binding is a major determinant of both hepatic and renal clearance of drugs with low extraction ratios.

Proximal renal tubular cells have two discrete mechanisms for secreting acidic and basic organic compounds.[30] These processes are carrier mediated, so they are saturable. Drugs with similar physicochemical characteristics compete for available carrier molecules and interfere with each other's secretion. If a drug is very avidly secreted by tubular cells and not subsequently reabsorbed, it will have a high renal extraction ratio. Renal clearance of such drugs is largely determined by the magnitude of renal blood flow.[30] This is analogous to the importance of liver blood flow in the clearance of drugs with high hepatic extraction ratios.

Clearance of drugs filtered by the glomeruli or secreted by the proximal renal tubule may be decreased by subsequent reabsorption from the renal tubule. If this is extensive, the drug will have a very low renal extraction ratio and negligible renal clearance. Tubular reabsorption occurs by active, carrier-mediated transport that is similar to active secretion. Drugs can also be reabsorbed by passive diffusion across the tubular epithelium. The progressive reabsorption of water from the renal tubule facilitates passive reabsorption of drugs by creating a tubule-to-plasma concentration gradient for the drug. Consequently, oliguria can decrease renal drug clearance.[31] Passive reabsorption is determined by the lipid solubility and degree of ionization of a drug. Highly lipophilic drugs like propofol are almost completely reabsorbed and have virtually no renal clearance. For less lipophilic drugs, the degree of ionization is a major determinant of the extent of passive reabsorption because only the nonionized drug readily diffuses across the renal tubular epithelium. Urine pH can range from 4.5 to 8.0, which can cause large changes in the ionized fraction of weak acids and bases, particularly if the pK_a is close to or within this range. Urine pH can be manipulated to increase renal drug clearance after overdoses.

Physiologic, Pharmacologic, and Pathologic Alterations in Renal Drug Clearance

In adults, renal blood flow is approximately 1,200 mL/min, so renal plasma flow is approximately 700 mL/min. About one-fifth of the plasma is filtered by the glomerulus, resulting in an average GFR of 125 mL/min. Renal blood flow and GFR are autoregulated, so they remain fairly constant as long as mean arterial pressure is between 70 and 160 mmHg.[32] Consequently, renal drug clearance is more constant than hepatic clearance, because renal blood flow usually varies less than hepatic blood flow.

The capacity for excreting endogenous and exogenous compounds depends on the number of functionally intact nephrons. Decreased glomerular filtration is accompanied by a parallel loss of renal tubular function. Therefore, clearance of endogenous creatinine, which is essentially equivalent to the GFR, can be used to estimate overall renal function. It follows that renal drug clearance is proportional to creatinine clearance, even for drugs eliminated primarily by tubular secretion. This principle has been used to develop nomograms for reducing drug doses according to the creatinine clearance in the presence of renal dysfunction.[33] Many drugs, including lidocaine,[34] pancuronium,[35] and meperidine,[36] have pharmacologically active metabolites that are excreted by the kidneys. Therefore, both parent drugs and their metabolites can contribute to drug toxicity in patients with renal failure.

Renal function decreases progressively with age. By age 80 years, creatinine clearance is reduced by about 50%.[37] Despite the age-related decrease in glomerular filtration rate, serum creatinine is not elevated in healthy elderly patients because muscle mass, the primary source of creatinine, also decreases with age. Therefore, even if serum creatinine is normal, renal clearance of drugs is reduced in elderly patients.

The kidneys eliminate many drugs encountered in anesthetic practice (Table 11-2). In renal failure, doses of these drugs must be reduced to avoid adverse effects. In addition to renal

TABLE 11-2

DRUGS WITH SIGNIFICANT RENAL EXCRETION ENCOUNTERED IN ANESTHESIOLOGY

Aminoglycosides	Pancuronium
Atenolol	Penicillins
Cephalosporins	Pipecuronium
Digoxin	Procainamide
Doxacurium	Pyridostigmine
Edrophonium	Rocuronium
Nadolol	Quinolones
Neostigmine	

disease, other pathologic processes can impair kidney function. Low cardiac output states reduce renal blood flow, glomerular filtration, and, consequently, renal drug clearance.[30] Advanced hepatic cirrhosis also interferes with renal function,[30] and this combination, the *hepatorenal syndrome,* reduces elimination of almost all drugs.

DRUG METABOLISM

Unless tolerance develops, termination of drug action depends on removal of the drug from its sites of action. (Tolerance is defined as decreasing pharmacologic effect with sustained exposure to a drug. It results in higher doses [or concentrations] being required to maintain a given effect. The mechanisms responsible for tolerance are diverse. They include adaptive or reflex responses to drug effects that alter the observed effects and alterations in the number or sensitivity of receptors.) Most operations are completed within a relatively short period (duration of anesthesia <2 to 3 hours). In such cases, drug redistribution is the primary mechanism responsible for reducing drug concentrations in the blood. This, in turn, establishes the concentration gradient required for removal of drugs from their sites of action. Drug metabolism is more important in terminating effects of drugs that are not extensively redistributed, or when larger, or repeated, doses are administered. This could occur after prolonged anesthesia (>4 to 5 hours). Consideration of drug metabolism is also important in the therapeutics of critical care and pain therapy.

Drugs must usually cross biologic membranes to reach their sites of action, so most are relatively lipid soluble. This property makes their excretion difficult, because lipophilic compounds are readily reabsorbed from the gut and the distal renal tubule. Metabolism, or *biotransformation* of drugs to more polar, water-soluble compounds, facilitates the ultimate excretion of metabolites in the bile and urine. Biotransformation is a protective mechanism for preventing the accumulation and resultant toxicity of various lipophilic compounds acquired from the environment.

Metabolites are usually less active pharmacologically than the parent drug. However, this is not always true. Many benzodiazepines have metabolites that have similar pharmacologic effects.[5] The analgesic effects of codeine are a result of its biotransformation to morphine. Metabolites can also be toxic. The major metabolite of meperidine is normeperidine, which can cause seizures.[36] If metabolites are pharmacologically active or toxic, further biotransformation or excretion is required for termination of their effects.

Metabolism of drugs and other exogenous compounds, known collectively as *xenobiotics,* occurs primarily in the liver. Other organs, including the kidneys, lungs, gut, and skin, also metabolize drugs, but extrahepatic biotransformation is quantitatively unimportant in most instances.

Biotransformation Reactions

Biotransformation reactions have classically been divided into two groups. *Phase I* reactions alter the molecular structure of xenobiotics by modifying an existing functional group of the drug, by adding a new functional chemical group to the compound, or by splitting the original molecule into two fragments. These changes in molecular structure result from oxidation, reduction, or hydrolysis of the parent compound. *Phase II* reactions consist of the coupling, or conjugation, of a variety of endogenous compounds to polar chemical groups. The polar chemical group at which conjugation occurs is frequently the result of a previous Phase I reaction, hence the "Phase I–Phase II" nomenclature. However, not all drugs are eliminated by this sequential pathway of biotransformation. Oxidation of thiopental produces its major metabolite, thiopental carboxylic acid,[38] which undergoes renal excretion without undergoing a Phase II biotransformation. Morphine is directly conjugated to form morphine glucuronide without first undergoing a Phase I reaction.

Phase I Reactions

Phase I reactions may hydrolyze, oxidize, or reduce the parent compound. *Hydrolysis* is the insertion of a molecule of water into another molecule, which forms an unstable intermediate compound that subsequently splits apart. Thus, hydrolysis cleaves the original substance into two separate molecules. Hydrolytic reactions are the primary way amides, such as lidocaine and other amide local anesthetics, and esters, such as succinylcholine, are metabolized.

Many drugs are biotransformed by oxidative reactions. *Oxidations* are defined as reactions that remove electrons from a molecule. The common element of most, if not all, oxidations is an enzymatically mediated reaction that inserts a hydroxyl group (OH) into the drug molecule.[39] In some instances, this produces a chemically stable, more polar hydroxylated metabolite. However, hydroxylation usually creates unstable compounds that spontaneously split into separate molecules. Many different biotransformations are effected by this basic mechanism. Dealkylation (removal of a carbon-containing group), deamination (removal of nitrogen-containing groups), oxidation of nitrogen-containing groups, desulfuration, dehalogenation, and dehydrogenation all follow an initial hydroxylation.[39] Hydrolysis and hydroxylation are comparable processes. Both have an initial, enzymatically mediated step that produces an unstable compound that rapidly dissociates into separate molecules.

Some drugs are metabolized by *reductive reactions,* that is, reactions that add electrons to a molecule. In contrast to oxidations, where electrons are transferred from NADPH to an oxygen atom, the electrons are transferred to the drug molecule. Oxidation of xenobiotics requires oxygen, but reductive biotransformation is inhibited by oxygen, so it is facilitated when the intracellular oxygen tension is low.[40]

The Cytochromes P450. The cytochromes P450 (CYP) are enzymes that catalyze most biotransformations. These hemoproteins, when reduced by carbon monoxide, have an absorption spectrum with a peak at the 450-nm wavelength, hence their name. CYP are incorporated into the smooth endoplasmic reticulum of hepatocytes. The endoplasmic reticulum is an intracellular network of tubules similar in ultrastructure to cellular membranes. Other tissues, including the lungs, kidneys, and skin, also contain CYP, but in much smaller amounts.[41] Upper intestinal enterocytes contain high concentrations of CYP, which contributes to the first-pass effect by metabolizing drugs absorbed from the GI tract before they reach the systemic circulation.[3,41,42] CYP are capable of metabolizing hundreds of compounds, including endogenous substances such as steroids and amines, as well as drugs and other exogenous compounds acquired from the environment.[42] CYP isoenzymes oxidize their substrates primarily by the insertion of an atom of oxygen in the form of a hydroxyl group, while another oxygen atom is reduced to water.

5 CYP is a superfamily of related enzymes.[43] More than 2,000 CYP isoenzymes have been identified in plants, animals, and microbiologic species.[44] In humans, 57 CYP members, grouped into 42 subfamilies and 18 families according to amino acid sequences, have been identified.[45] CYP families share ≥40% sequence identity and are denoted by an Arabic numeral (i.e., CYP2, CYP3). Subfamilies share ≥55% identity and are designated sequentially using a letter (CYP3A, CYP3B, etc.). Individual members of a family are assigned a second numeral (such as CYP3A4, CYP3A5).[45]

Several constitutive CYPs are involved in the production of various endogenous compounds, such as cholesterol, steroid hormones, prostaglandins, and eicosanoids.[45] In addition to the constitutive forms, production of various CYPs can be induced by a wide variety of xenobiotics.[46] CYP drug-metabolizing activity increases after exposure to various exogenous chemicals, including many drugs.[44,47] The number and type of CYPs present at any time depends on exposure to different xenobiotics. The CYP system is able to protect the organism from the deleterious effects of accumulation of exogenous compounds because of its two fundamental characteristics—broad substrate specificity and the capability to adapt to exposure to different substances by induction of different CYP isoenzymes.

Biotransformations can be inhibited if different substrates compete for the drug-binding site on the same CYP member. The effect of two competing substrates on each other's metabolism depends on their relative affinities for the enzyme. Biotransformation of the compound with the lower affinity is inhibited to a greater degree. This is the mechanism by which the H_2 receptor antagonist cimetidine inhibits the metabolism of many drugs, including meperidine, propranolol, and diazepam.[48–50] The newer H_2 antagonist ranitidine has a different structure and causes fewer clinically significant drug interactions.[51] Other drugs, notably calcium channel blockers and antidepressants, also inhibit oxidative drug metabolism in humans.[52,53] Information regarding both induction and inhibition of different CYP isoenzymes by specific compounds has become available.[53] This information allows clinicians to predict which combinations of drugs are more likely to lead to clinically significant interactions because of altered drug metabolism by the cytochrome P450 system.

CYP isoenzymes from families 1, 2, and 3 effect 70 to 80% of all Phase I metabolism of all clinically used drugs.[54] CYP3A4 is the single most important enzyme, accounting for 40 to 45% of all CYP-mediated drug metabolism.[54] The CYP2 family accounts for a similar percentage of CYP-mediated biotransformation.[54] Tables 11-3 and 11-4 group drugs encountered in anesthetic practice according to the CYP isoenzymes responsible for their biotransformation.[41,55] Some drugs are metabolized by more than one CYP isoenzyme.

Induction and inhibition of hepatic drug-metabolizing enzyme systems change the intrinsic hepatic clearance of drugs. This is most important for drugs with low hepatic extraction ratios, because intrinsic clearance is the primary determinant of their hepatic clearance. Altered drug-metabolizing enzyme activity has little effect on drugs with high hepatic extraction ratios because their clearance depends primarily on hepatic blood flow.

Phase II Reactions

Phase II reactions are also known as *conjugation* or *synthetic reactions*. Many drugs do not have a polar chemical group suitable for conjugation, so conjugation occurs only after a Phase I reaction. Other drugs, such as morphine, already have a polar group that serves as a "handle" for conjugation, and they undergo these reactions directly. Various endogenous compounds can be attached to parent drugs or their Phase I metabolites to form different conjugation products.[56] These endogenous substrates include glucuronic acid, acetate, and amino acids. Mercapturic acid conjugates result from the binding of exogenous compounds to glutathione. Other conjugation reactions produce sulfated or methylated derivatives of drugs or their metabolites. Like the cytochrome P450 system, the enzymes that catalyze Phase II reactions are inducible.[47] Phase II reactions produce conjugates that are polar, water-soluble compounds. This facilitates the ultimate excretion of the drug via the kidneys or hepatobiliary secretion. Like CYP, there are different families and superfamilies of the enzymes that catalyze Phase II biotransformations.[56]

TABLE 11-3

SUBSTRATES OF CYP3A4 ENCOUNTERED IN ANESTHESIOLOGY

Acetaminophen	Lidocaine
Alfentanil	Methadone
Alprazolam	Midazolam
Bupivacaine	Nicardipine
Cisapride	Nifedipine
Codeine	Omeprazole
Cortisol	Pantoprazole
Diazepam	Ropivacaine
Digitoxin	Statins
Diltiazem	Sufentanil
Felodipine	Verapamil
Fentanyl	Warfarin
Granisetron	

Compiled from references 41 and 55.

Factors Affecting Biotransformation

Drug metabolism varies substantially between individuals because of variability in the genes controlling the numerous enzymes responsible for biotransformation. For most drugs, individual subjects' rates of metabolism have a unimodal

TABLE 11-4

SUBSTRATES OF THE CYP2 FAMILY ENCOUNTERED IN ANESTHESIOLOGY

CYP2D6	captopril codeine hydrocodone metoprolol ondansetron propranolol timolol
CYP2C9	diclofenac ibuprofen indomethacin
CYP2C19	diazepam omeprazole propranolol warfarin

Compiled from references 41 and 55.

distribution. However, distinct subpopulations with different rates of elimination of some drugs have been identified. The resulting multimodal distribution of individual rates of metabolism is known as *polymorphism*. For example, different genotypes result in either normal, low, or (rarely) absent plasma pseudocholinesterase activity, accounting for the well-known differences in individuals' responses to succinylcholine, which is hydrolyzed by this enzyme. Many drug-metabolizing enzymes exhibit genetic polymorphism, including CYP and various transferases that catalyze phase II reactions.[54,56–59]

Drug metabolism also varies with age. The fetus and neonate have less capacity for most biotransformations, especially those catalyzed by the CYP superfamily.[60] Neonates also have less capacity for most phase II biotransformation, with the exception of sulfate conjugation.[60] Impaired conjugation of bilirubin causes "physiologic jaundice." Biotransformation capacities rapidly in the postpartum period, reaching adult capacity by 1 year of age.[60]

Metabolism of some drugs may also be decreased in geriatric patients, although it is difficult to separate the effects of age per se from the effects of organ dysfunction, which is more prevalent in the elderly. Some, but not all, investigations suggest decreased CYP activity in the elderly.[61] Conjugation capacity has little or no age-related changes.[61]

Men have greater capacity for most Phase II reactions, and for Phase I reactions catalyzed by CYP2E1.[62,63] There do not appear to be any sex-related differences in CYP2C9 or CYP2C19 activity.[62,63] CYP3A isoenzymes metabolize the largest number of medications. Whether there are any clinically relevant differences between men and women in CYP3A activity is controversial.[62,63]

Exposure to various foreign compounds can alter drug-metabolizing enzyme activity. Barbiturates, phenytoin, macrolide antibiotics, imidazole antifungal agents, and corticosteroids can cause drug interactions secondary to induction of hepatic drug-metabolizing enzymes.[47] Chronic ethanol consumption induces enzyme activity, but acute intoxication inhibits the biotransformation of some drugs.[64] Smoking increases the metabolism of many drugs secondary to enzyme induction by polycyclic hydrocarbons in tobacco smoke.[65]

Liver disease profoundly affects drug disposition. It is difficult to distinguish the impact of altered biotransformation per se from other effects of liver disease: altered binding of drugs to plasma proteins and decreased liver blood flow. Nonetheless, hepatic disease decreases clearance of drugs with low hepatic extraction ratios,[13,66] which implies impaired biotransformation. Decreased in vitro activity in cirrhotic livers of some, but not all, CYP isoforms has been reported, although this also depends on the severity of the hepatic impairment.[67] Congestive heart failure decreases metabolism of lidocaine and theophylline.[17] Renal failure decreases CYP activity not only in the kidneys, but also in the intestines and liver.[68] This is primarily because of downregulation of CYP gene expression.[68] Hepatic Phase II biotransformation is also reduced by renal failure. Presumably, substances that decrease biotransformation enzyme activity and downregulate gene expression accumulate in patients with renal failure.[68]

Effects of Anesthesia and Surgery on Biotransformation

Drug disposition is altered in the perioperative period. Although many other factors are probably also involved, biotransformation reactions are affected by anesthesia and surgery. In dogs anesthetized with halothane, the intrinsic hepatic clearance of propranolol is decreased, which implies that hepatic drug-metabolizing ability is impaired.[69] Halothane inhibits demethylation of aminopyrine in a dose-dependent fashion. Isoflurane has less effect, and enflurane does not affect aminopyrine biotransformation.[70]

Many investigators have studied the effects of anesthesia and surgery on antipyrine clearance. Antipyrine, an antipyretic that is no longer used therapeutically, does not bind to plasma proteins, has a low hepatic extraction ratio, and is not cleared by the kidneys. Therefore, clearance of antipyrine is solely dependent on the activity of hepatic drug-metabolizing enzymes. This permits the use of antipyrine clearance as an indicator of hepatic drug-metabolizing activity.[71] Clearance of antipyrine is generally increased after surgery conducted with a wide variety of general anesthetic techniques,[72,73] although there are exceptions to this rule. General anesthesia with enflurane does not appear to increase antipyrine clearance.[74] After operations lasting more than 4 hours, antipyrine clearance is decreased.[75] Presumably, major surgical trauma interferes with drug metabolism, although the precise mechanisms are not known. Antipyrine clearance is also increased after spinal anesthesia.[73] Therefore, general anesthesia is not a prerequisite for increased rates of biotransformation in the postoperative period, and other perioperative factors also affect drug metabolism. For example, the caloric source of iv nutritional regimens influences antipyrine clearance. It is decreased when the only caloric source is 5% dextrose, and increased when amino acids are substituted for dextrose.[76]

Factors other than altered rates of biotransformation, such as decreased hepatic blood flow during surgery,[27,28] can affect drug elimination in the perioperative period. In many patients the magnitude of these changes is too small to cause any clinically evident problems. However, in some patients clinically significant changes in drug elimination could occur. Decreased drug clearance can result in higher concentrations of drugs and increase the risk of adverse effects, especially after prolonged surgery. Clinicians must be aware of the potential for excessive pharmacologic effects and must tailor doses accordingly.

BINDING OF DRUGS TO PLASMA PROTEINS

Drugs are present in the blood in two fractions. Some are simply dissolved in plasma water; the rest is bound to various components of whole blood, such as plasma proteins and red blood cells. Ideally, drug concentrations should be measured in whole blood because drugs are transported in blood, not plasma, and drugs equilibrate between erythrocytes and plasma very quickly.[77] Unfortunately, measurement of total drug levels and drug binding in whole blood is technically more difficult than in plasma or serum, so few investigators have directly measured whole blood binding. As a compromise, the blood:plasma concentration ratio can be used to estimate whole blood binding.

Drugs bind to plasma proteins in a reversible fashion that obeys the law of mass action. The rate constants of the association and dissociation reactions are k_1 and k_2, respectively. These reactions are very rapid, having half-lives of a few milliseconds. Binding of drugs to blood constituents other than proteins, such as erythrocytes, proceeds in an analogous fashion. The equilibrium dissociation constant, k_d, quantifies the affinity of drug-protein binding:

$$K_a = \frac{k_2}{k_1} = \frac{[\text{unbound drug}] \times [\text{protein}]}{[\text{drug-protein complex}]} \qquad (11\text{-}5)$$

The dissociation constant has units of moles per liter (mol/L), and is the drug concentration at which 50% of the binding sites are occupied. The degree of binding is dependent on the affinity of the protein for the drug, the protein concentration, and the concentration of drug available for binding.

The extent of plasma drug binding can be expressed as the *percentage of drug bound*, which is the percentage of the total drug present that is bound to plasma proteins. Alternatively, the *free fraction*, which is the percentage of drug not bound to plasma proteins, can be used. For example, approximately 83% of fentanyl is bound to plasma proteins—thus, the free fraction is about 17%.[78,79]

Protein binding is affected by many factors, including temperature and pH.[77] At high drug concentrations, binding sites become saturated and the free fraction increases. There are also qualitative differences between species in plasma proteins that affect drug binding, and binding to purified human albumin may not correlate with binding in plasma.[77] Consequently, to provide clinically useful information, in vitro measurement of drug binding must be conducted at physiologic temperature and pH, with human plasma, and at concentrations within the usual therapeutic range.

Drug–protein binding has important pharmacologic implications, because only unbound drug can cross cell membranes to reach its sites of action. Also, free drug is more readily available for elimination. This has led to the frequently held misconception that drug bound to plasma proteins and other blood constituents is pharmacologically inert. This is not the case. As soon as unbound drug leaves circulation, the law of mass action dictates that some drug will dissociate from binding sites, which tends to restore the free drug concentration. This occurs almost instantaneously, so that the bound fraction of drug serves as a dynamic reservoir that buffers acute changes in the free drug concentration.

As discussed earlier, clearance of some drugs depends on the degree of protein binding. The extent of distribution of drugs throughout the body also depends on the degree of binding. At equilibrium, the portion of the total drug in the body that is in extravascular sites is determined by the relative affinity of blood binding versus binding to all other tissues. A drug that is highly bound to plasma proteins or erythrocytes cannot be extensively distributed unless it has even greater affinity for extravascular binding sites.

Binding Proteins

Two plasma proteins are primarily responsible for drug binding: albumin and α_1-acid glycoprotein (AAG). Drugs also bind to other plasma proteins, such as globulins or lipoproteins, and to erythrocytes. Drugs can bind to more than one protein. For example, fentanyl and sufentanil bind to albumin, AAG, globulins, and also to red blood cells.[79]

Albumin is the most important drug-binding protein. In addition to a wide range of drugs, including barbiturates, benzodiazepines, and penicillins, albumin binds endogenous compounds such as bilirubin. Many drugs bind to more than one site on the albumin molecule, and most drugs have one or two high-affinity, primary binding sites and a variable number of secondary, low-affinity sites. Studies with radioactively labeled drugs indicate that albumin has at least three discrete, high-affinity drug-binding sites. Diazepam, digitoxin, and warfarin each bind to a different site. The sites at which other drugs bind to albumin and the affinity of the drug–albumin bond can be determined by using these three markers.[80] This permits prediction of the likelihood of drug interactions as a result of one drug displacing another. Drugs that compete for the same binding site are more likely to displace one another than drugs that bind at different sites, and the drug with the lower affinity for the binding site will be more easily displaced.

Factors Affecting Drug Binding

The physicochemical properties of drugs influence binding to plasma proteins. Albumin is the major binding protein for organic acids, such as penicillins and barbiturates. Basic drugs also bind to albumin, but to a lesser extent. The primary binding protein for many basic drugs is AAG (Table 11-5). Basic drugs also bind to lipoproteins and globulins. AAG is an acute phase reactant, and its concentration increases in many acute and chronic illnesses.

In general, the greater the lipid solubility of a drug, the greater the binding to plasma proteins (Table 11-6).[79,81–99] Water-soluble drugs, such as neuromuscular blocking agents, are bound to a substantially lesser extent than lipid-soluble drugs, like propofol. This is also true for drugs that belong to the same class. The degree of binding of opioids parallels their lipid solubility: morphine is the least bound, fentanyl and its derivatives are highly bound, and meperidine is intermediate.

TABLE 11-5

DRUGS BINDING TO α_1-ACID GLYCOPROTEIN

Alfentanil	Methadone
Alprenolol	Propranolol
Bupivacaine	Quinidine
Disopyramide	Ropivacaine
Fentanyl	Sufentanil
Lidocaine	Verapamil
Meperidine	

TABLE 11-6

PLASMA PROTEIN BINDING OF SOME DRUGS USED IN ANESTHESIOLOGY

CLASS/DRUG	PERCENT BOUND	REFERENCE
Opioids		
Alfentanil	92	79
Fentanyl	84	79
Meperidine	53–63	81
Methadone	60–90	82
Morphine	20–35	82,83,84
Sufentanil	92	79
Intravenous Anesthetics		
Methohexital	73	85
Propofol	98	86
Thiopental	85	87
Neuromuscular Blockers		
Pancuronium	11–29	88,89
Rocuronium	46	90
Vecuronium	30	88
Local Anesthetics[a]		
Bupivacaine	95	91
Lidocaine	70	91
Ropivacaine	94	92
Benzodiazepines		
Diazepam	97–99	93
Lorazepam	88–92	94
Midazolam	96	95
Cardiovascular Drugs		
Digoxin	20–30	96
Diltiazem	77–80	97
Esmolol	55	98
Nifedipine	96–98	97
Propranolol	89	99
Verapamil	84–91	97

[a] At nontoxic concentrations. At toxic plasma concentrations, binding of local anesthetic decreases, leading to a marked increase in the free drug concentration.

Similarly, bupivacaine is bound to a greater extent than lidocaine.

Many physiologic and pathologic states cause quantitative and qualitative changes in the primary drug-binding plasma proteins, albumin and AAG. Drug binding may also be affected by acid-base disturbances that alter the degree of ionization of drugs and proteins, and by accumulation of endogenous compounds that compete for drug-binding sites.

Maternal and Neonatal Drug Binding

Binding of drugs in pregnancy and in the fetus or neonate has received much attention because of its impact on placental drug transfer. Pregnant women have reduced levels of albumin, and the binding of many organic acids, such as phenytoin, is decreased at term.[100] Although thiopental is also an organic acid, unlike phenytoin, the free fraction of thiopental is not increased in patients undergoing cesarean section,[101] so that usual doses of thiopental do not result in excessive free drug levels. This is fortunate, because high free drug levels would increase the risk of side effects and enhance placental transfer of the drug. The free fraction of diazepam, which binds primarily to albumin, is increased at term.[102] AAG levels are not changed during pregnancy.[102] However, the free fractions of lidocaine and propranolol are, nonetheless, increased at term.[102]

Neonates have decreased levels of albumin and AAG,[100–103] and neonatal albumin has less affinity for some drugs.[100,103] Consequently, the free fraction of many drugs, especially those that bind to AAG, is higher in the neonate than in the mother.[103] Although binding of many drugs is decreased in neonates, this does not affect the unbound concentration of drugs transferred across the placenta. Under near steady-state conditions, maternal and fetal free drug concentrations are the same, although the total fetal level is lower. Because the free drug is the more pharmacologically active species, the decrease in maternal plasma protein drug binding is of greater consequence as far as placental transfer of drugs is concerned. Decreased drug binding must be considered in neonatal therapeutics.[60]

Age and Sex

The plasma concentrations of the primary drug-binding proteins change with increasing age: albumin decreases slightly, whereas AAG tends to increase.[104–106] The free fractions of lidocaine, meperidine, and propranolol, all of which bind to AAG, are not changed in the elderly.[81,106,107] Similarly, binding of drugs to albumin is minimally altered. The binding of midazolam does not change,[95] and diazepam binding may decrease slightly.[22,104,108] The typical magnitude of age-associated decreases in drug binding is illustrated by thiopental. The average free fraction of thiopental of 18% in young adults only increases to 22% in geriatric patients.[109] Clinically significant changes in drug binding in elderly patients are more often caused by pathologic processes than by age per se. Age-related changes in drug–protein binding are usually not clinically significant.[110]

Studies comparing drug binding in men and women have not found any clinically significant differences between the sexes. This is not surprising, because the concentrations of albumin and AAG in men and women do not differ significantly.[105]

Hepatic Disease

The plasma albumin concentration is often decreased in patients with liver disease. Drug binding may also be affected by qualitative changes in the albumin molecule that decrease affinity for drugs, and by accumulation of endogenous substances, such as bilirubin, that compete for drug-binding sites.[13] Although hepatic diseases vary widely in pathophysiology and severity, it is possible to make some generalizations regarding their impact on drug binding. The free fractions of drugs that bind primarily to albumin are increased. This is true for organic bases such as diazepam[22,111] and morphine,[83] and for the organic acids phenytoin[83] and thiopental.[112,113] The free fractions of basic drugs, such as meperidine[24] and lidocaine,[25] are not increased in patients with acute viral hepatitis, which suggests that drug binding to AAG is minimally affected by liver disease.

Renal Disease

Albumin levels tend to decrease in all types of renal disease. However, even when albumin levels are normal, binding of phenytoin[83] and thiopental[87] is decreased. The free fraction of phenytoin is correlated with both the albumin concentration and the severity of renal dysfunction.[83] This indicates that renal failure reduces the affinity of albumin for organic acids. Dialysis does not restore the affinity of albumin for thiopental or phenytoin.[83,87] The plasma–protein binding of many other organic acids is also decreased in renal failure.[114]

The effect of renal disease on the binding of basic drugs depends on whether the drug binds primarily to albumin or to AAG, and on the type of renal disease. The free fraction of diazepam, which binds primarily to albumin, is increased in the nephrotic syndrome, renal failure, and after renal transplantation.[115] Similarly, binding of morphine is decreased in uremia.[83] Binding of other basic drugs varies according to the changes in AAG in different types of renal disease. Lidocaine binding increases in renal failure and after renal transplantation, conditions associated with increased AAG levels.[115] Likewise, propranolol binding is increased in patients with renal disease and elevated concentrations of AAG.[99] Lidocaine binding is not altered in nephrotic patients who have normal levels of AAG.[115]

Other Diseases, Surgery, and Trauma

Patients with inflammatory diseases, such as rheumatoid arthritis and Crohn's disease, have increased levels of AAG and, consequently, decreased free fractions of drugs that bind to this protein.[99,116] Malignant disease is also associated with elevated levels of AAG, and increased binding of lidocaine, propranolol, and other basic drugs has been demonstrated in patients with cancer.[117] In contrast, albumin tends to decrease in patients with malignancies, which can decrease binding of acidic drugs.[116] After acute myocardial infarction, AAG levels double and remain elevated for about 3 weeks.[118] Consequently, the binding of lidocaine and propranolol is increased.[118,119]

The catabolic state that follows surgery and trauma decreases plasma albumin levels.[120] In contrast, the concentration of AAG increases after trauma[121] and surgery[122] and remains elevated for several weeks. These changes result in alterations in drug binding. The free fraction of phenytoin increases after surgery, probably secondary to decreased levels of albumin, although the contemporaneous increase in free fatty acids may result in competition for binding sites.[120] Higher AAG levels increase binding of basic drugs, such as lidocaine and propranolol, after trauma[121] and surgery.[123,124]

PHARMACOKINETIC PRINCIPLES

The concentration of a drug at its site or sites of action is a fundamental determinant of its pharmacologic effects. Because drugs are transported to and from their sites of action in the blood, the concentration at the active site is in turn a function of the concentration in the blood. The change in drug concentration over time in the blood, at the site of action, and in other tissues is a result of complex interactions of multiple biologic factors with the physicochemical characteristics of the drug. Together, these factors determine the rate, extent, and pattern of drug absorption, distribution, metabolism, and excretion. The term "pharmacokinetics," derived from the Greek words *pharmakon* (medicine) and *kinesis* (movement), refers to the quantitative analysis of the relationship between the dose of a drug and the ensuing changes in drug concentration in the blood and other tissues.

Early pharmacokinetic studies of intravenous and inhalational anesthetics used physiologic or perfusion models. In these models, body tissues are classified according to similarities in perfusion and affinity for drugs.[125] Highly perfused tissues, including the brain, heart, lungs, liver, and kidneys, make up the vessel-rich group. Muscle and skin comprise the lean tissue group, and fat is considered as a separate group. The vessel-poor group, which has minimal effect on drug distribution and elimination, is composed of bone and cartilage. Physiologic pharmacokinetic models made major contributions to understanding the factors influencing recovery from thiopental. These models established that awakening after a single dose was primarily the result of redistribution of thiopental from the brain to muscle and skin.[7,8] Distribution to other tissues and metabolism played minor roles. This fundamental concept, *redistribution,* also applies to all lipophilic drugs. Physiologic models have also contributed greatly to our understanding of the uptake and distribution of inhalational anesthetics.[126]

Physiologic pharmacokinetic models provide much insight into factors affecting drug action. They can predict the effects of physiologic changes, such as altered regional blood flows or reduced cardiac output, on drug distribution and elimination. The disadvantage of perfusion-based models is their complexity. Verification of these models requires measurement of drug concentrations in many different tissues, which is rarely practical.[125] Because of these disadvantages, simpler pharmacokinetic models have been developed. In these models the body is envisaged as composed of one or more *compartments.* Drug concentrations in the blood are used to define the relationship between dose and the time course of changes of the drug concentration.[127] It is critically important to understand that the different "compartments" of a compartmental pharmacokinetic model cannot be equated with the tissue groups that make up physiologic pharmacokinetic models. Compartments are theoretical entities that are used to derive pharmacokinetic parameters, such as clearance, volume of distribution, and half-lives. These parameters quantify drug distribution and elimination.

Although the simplicity of compartmental models, compared to physiologic pharmacokinetic models, has its advantages, it also has some disadvantages. For example, cardiac output is not a parameter of compartmental models, and compartmental models therefore cannot be used to predict directly the effect of cardiac failure on drug disposition. However, compartmental pharmacokinetic models can still quantify the effects of reduced cardiac output on the disposition of a drug if a group of patients with cardiac failure is compared to a group of otherwise healthy subjects.

The discipline of pharmacokinetics is, to the despair of many, mathematically based. In the succeeding sections, formulas are used to illustrate the concepts needed to understand and interpret pharmacokinetic studies. Readers are encouraged to concentrate on the concepts, not the formulas.

Pharmacokinetic Concepts

Rate Constants and Half-Lives

The disposition of most drugs follows *first-order* kinetics. A first-order kinetic process is one in which a constant fraction of the drug is removed during a finite period of time. This fraction is equivalent to the rate constant of the process. Rate constants are usually denoted by the letter k and have units of "inverse time," such as min^{-1} or h^{-1}. If 10% of the drug is eliminated per minute, then the rate constant is 0.1 min^{-1}. Because a constant fraction is removed per unit of time in first-order kinetics, the absolute amount of drug removed is proportional to the concentration of the drug. It follows that, in first-order kinetics, the rate of change of the concentration at any given time is proportional to the concentration present at that time. When the concentration is high, it will fall faster than when it is low. First-order kinetics apply not only to elimination, but also to absorption and distribution.[127]

Rather than using rate constants, the rapidity of pharmacokinetic processes is often described with half-lives—the time required for the concentration to change by a factor of 2. Half-lives are calculated directly from the corresponding rate constants with this simple equation:

$$t_{1/2} = \frac{(\ln 2)}{k} = \frac{0.693}{k} \qquad (11\text{-}6)$$

Thus, a rate constant of 0.1 min^{-1} translates into a half-life of 6.93 minutes. The half-life of any first-order kinetic process, including drug absorption, distribution, and elimination, can be calculated. First-order processes asymptotically approach completion, because a constant fraction of the drug, not an absolute amount, is removed per unit of time. However, after five half-lives, the process will be almost 97% complete (Table 11-7). For practical purposes, this is close enough to 100% and can be considered as such.

Volumes of Distribution

6 The volume of distribution quantifies the extent of drug distribution. The physiologic factor that governs the extent of drug distribution is the overall capacity of tissues versus the capacity of blood for that drug. Overall tissue capacity for uptake of a drug is in turn a function of the total mass of the tissues into which a drug distributes and their average affinity for the drug. In compartmental pharmacokinetic models, drugs are envisaged as distributing into one or more "boxes," or compartments. These compartments cannot be equated directly with specific tissues. Rather, they are hypothetical entities that permit analysis of drug distribution and elimination and description of the drug concentration versus time profile.

The volume of distribution is an "apparent" volume because it represents the size of these hypothetical boxes, or compartments, that is necessary to explain the concentration of drug in a reference compartment, usually called the *central* or *plasma compartment.* The volume of distribution, Vd, relates the total amount of drug present to the concentration observed in the central compartment:

$$Vd = \frac{\text{total amount of drug present}}{\text{concentration}} \qquad (11\text{-}7)$$

TABLE 11-7

HALF-LIVES AND PERCENT OF DRUG REMOVED

NUMBER OF HALF-LIVES	PERCENT OF DRUG REMAINING	PERCENT OF DRUG REMOVED
0	100	0
1	50	50
2	25	75
3	12.5	87.5
4	6.25	93.75
5	3.125	96.875

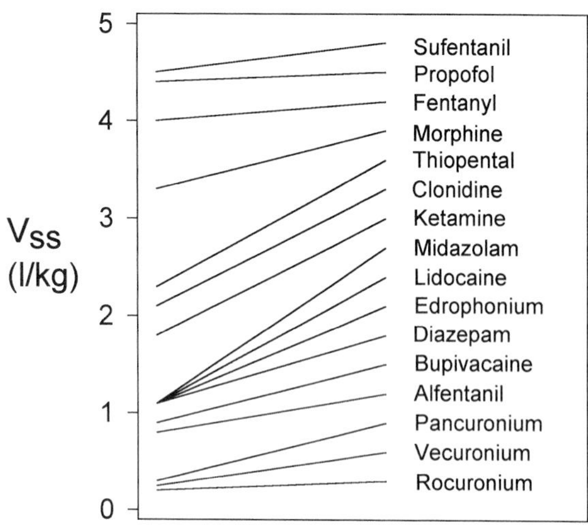

FIGURE 11-4. The volume of distribution of some drugs used in anesthesiology.

This formula is logical. If a drug is extensively distributed, then the concentration will be lower relative to the amount of drug present, which equates to a larger volume of distribution. For example, if a total of 10 mg of drug is present and the concentration is 2 mg/L, then the apparent volume of distribution is 5 L. On the other hand, if the concentration was 4 mg/L, then the volume of distribution would be 2.5 L.

Simply stated, the apparent volume of distribution is a numeric index of the extent of drug distribution that does not have any relationship to the actual volume of any tissue or group of tissues. It may be as small as plasma volume, or, if overall tissue uptake is extensive, the apparent volume of distribution may
7 greatly exceed the actual total volume of the body (Fig. 11-4). In general, lipophilic drugs have larger volumes of distribution than hydrophilic drugs (see Fig. 11-4). Because the volume of distribution is a mathematical approximation, it cannot be directly correlated with the anatomic and physiologic factors that influence drug distribution. Determination of the volume of distribution from a compartmental model does not provide any information regarding the tissues into which the drug actually distributes or the concentrations in those tissues. Despite these limitations, the volume of distribution provides useful information. For example, an increase in the volume of distribution means that a larger loading dose will be required to "fill up the box" and achieve the same concentration. Various pathologic conditions can alter the volume of distribution, necessitating therapeutic adjustments.

Total Drug Clearance

In compartmental pharmacokinetic models, the ability of the system as a whole to irreversibly eliminate a drug is quantified by the *total drug clearance* or *elimination clearance*.
8 Elimination clearance is the portion of the volume of distribution from which drug is completely and irreversibly removed during a given time interval. It is analogous to creatinine clearance, and, like creatinine clearance, drug clearance has units of flow. Drug clearance is often corrected for weight or body surface area, in which case the units are mL/min/kg or mL/min/m^2, respectively.

Elimination clearance, *Cl*, can be calculated from the declining blood levels observed after an iv injection, as follows:

$$Cl = \frac{\text{dose}}{\text{area under the concentration versus time curve}} \tag{11-8}$$

Again, this formula is intuitively logical. If a drug is rapidly removed from the plasma, its concentration will fall more quickly than the concentration of a drug that is less readily eliminated. This results in a smaller area under the concentration versus time curve, which equates to greater clearance.

A significant limitation of calculating elimination clearance from compartmental pharmacokinetic models is that the relative contribution of different organs to drug elimination cannot be determined. Nonetheless, estimation of drug clearance with these models has made important contributions to clinical pharmacology. In particular, these models have provided a great deal of clinically useful information regarding altered drug elimination in various pathologic conditions.

Compartmental Pharmacokinetic Models

One-Compartment Model

Although for most drugs the one-compartment model is an oversimplification, it does serve to illustrate the basic relationships among clearance, volume of distribution, and the elimination half-life. In this model, the body is envisaged as a single homogeneous compartment. Drug distribution after injection is assumed to be instantaneous, so there are no concentration gradients within the compartment. The concentration can decrease only by elimination of drug from the system. The plasma concentration versus time curve for a hypothetical drug with one-compartment kinetics is shown in Figure 11-5. With the concentration plotted on a logarithmic scale, the concentration versus time curve becomes a straight line. The slope of the logarithm of concentration versus time is equal to the first-order elimination rate constant.

Immediately after injection, before any drug can be eliminated, the amount of drug present is equal to the dose. Therefore, by modifying Equation 11-7, the volume of distribution can be calculated:

$$Vd = \frac{\text{dose}}{\text{initial concentration}} \tag{11-9}$$

In the one-compartment model, drug clearance, *Cl*, is equal to the product of the elimination rate constant, k_e, and the volume

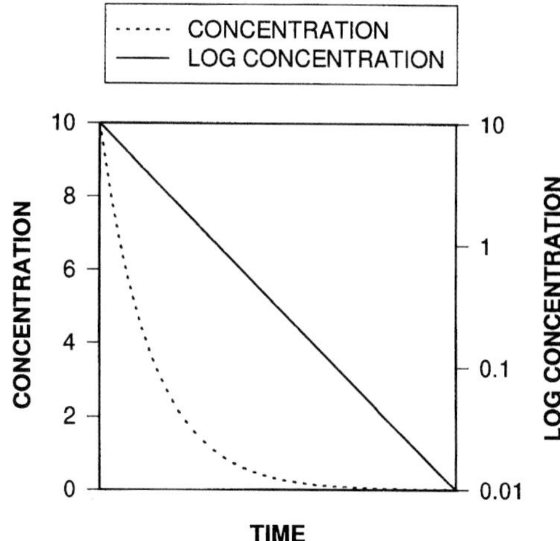

FIGURE 11-5. The plasma concentration, plotted on both linear (—, *left vertical axis*) and logarithmic (- - -, *right vertical axis*) scales, versus time for a hypothetical drug exhibiting one-compartment, first-order pharmacokinetics.

of distribution:

$$Cl = k_e \cdot Vd \quad (11\text{-}10)$$

Combining Equations 11-6 and 11-10 yields:

$$Cl = \frac{0.693 \cdot Vd}{t_{1/2}}; \text{thus}: \frac{0.693 \cdot Vd}{Cl} \quad (11\text{-}11)$$

Therefore, the greater the clearance, the shorter the elimination half-life, which is easy to understand. Less obvious is the impact of the volume of distribution on the elimination half-life. It is easiest to understand if the physiologic correlate of a large volume of distribution is considered. A large volume of distribution reflects extensive tissue uptake of a drug, so that only a small fraction of the total amount of drug is in the blood and accessible to the organs of elimination. Consequently, the greater the volume of distribution, the longer the elimination half-life. For drugs that exhibit multicompartment pharmacokinetics, the relationship among clearance, volume of distribution, and the elimination half-life is not a simple linear one such as Equation 11-11. However, the same principles apply. All else being equal, the greater the clearance, the shorter the elimination half-life; the larger the volume of distribution, the longer the elimination half-life. Thus, the elimination half-life depends on two other variables, clearance and volume of distribution, that characterize, respectively, the extent of drug distribution and efficiency of drug elimination.

Two-Compartment Model

For many drugs, a graph of the logarithm of the plasma concentration versus time after an iv injection is similar to the schematic graph shown in Figure 11-6. There are two discrete phases in the decline of the plasma concentration. The first phase after injection is characterized by a very rapid decrease in concentration. The rapid decrease in concentration during this "distribution phase" is largely caused by passage of drug from the plasma into tissues. The distribution phase is followed by a slower decline of the concentration owing to drug elimination. Elimination also begins immediately after injection, but its contribution to the drop in plasma concentration is initially much smaller than the fall in concentration because of drug distribution.

To account for this biphasic behavior, one must consider the body to be made up of two compartments, a central (or plasma) compartment and a peripheral compartment (Fig. 11-7). This two-compartment model assumes that it is the central compartment into which the drug is injected and from which the blood samples for measurement of concentration are obtained,

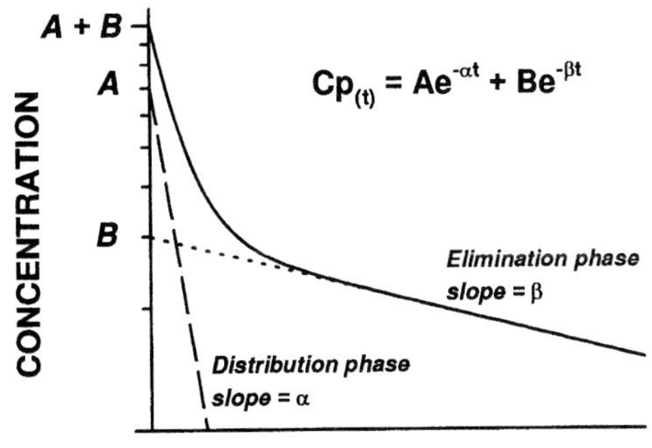

FIGURE 11-6. A schematic graph of the plasma concentration, on a logarithmic scale, versus time for a drug with a distribution phase preceding the elimination phase (two-compartment or biexponential kinetics). See text for explanation.

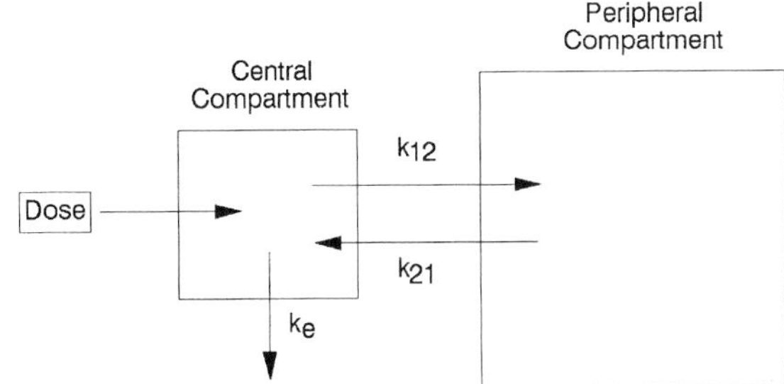

FIGURE 11-7. A two-compartment pharmacokinetic model. See text for explanation.

and that drug is eliminated only from the central compartment. Drug distribution within the central compartment is considered to be instantaneous. In reality, this last assumption cannot be true. However, drug uptake into some of the highly perfused tissues is so rapid that it cannot be detected as a discrete phase on the plasma concentration versus time curve.

The distribution and elimination phases can be characterized by graphic analysis of the plasma concentration versus time curve, as shown in Figure 11-6. The elimination phase line is extrapolated back to time zero (the time of injection). At any time, the difference between the total concentration and the concentration on the extrapolated elimination phase line is equal to a corresponding point, at that time, on the distribution phase line. In Figure 11-6, the zero time intercepts of the distribution and elimination lines are points A and B, respectively. The *hybrid rate constants*, α and β, are equal to the slopes of the two lines, and are used to calculate the distribution and elimination half-lives; α and β are called hybrid rate constants because they depend on both distribution and elimination processes.

At any time after an iv injection, the plasma concentration of drugs with two-compartment kinetics is equal to the sum of two exponential terms:

$$Cp_{(t)} = Ae^{-\alpha t} + Be^{-\beta t}, \quad (11\text{-}12)$$

where t = time, $Cp_{(t)}$ = plasma concentration at time t, A = y-axis intercept of the distribution phase line, α = hybrid rate constant of the distribution phase, B = y-axis intercept of the elimination phase line, and β = hybrid rate constant of the elimination phase. The first term characterizes the distribution phase and the second term characterizes the elimination phase. Immediately after injection, the first term represents a much larger fraction of the total plasma concentration than the second term. After several distribution half-lives, the value of the first term approaches zero, and the plasma concentration is essentially equal to the value of the second term (see Fig. 11-6).

In multicompartment models, the drug is initially distributed only within the central compartment. Therefore, the initial apparent volume of distribution is the volume of the central compartment. Immediately after injection, the amount of drug present is the dose, and the concentration is the extrapolated concentration at time $t = 0$, which is equal to the sum of the intercepts of the distribution and elimination lines. The volume of the central compartment, $V1$, is calculated by modifying Equation 11-7:

$$V1 = \frac{\text{dose}}{\text{initial plasma concentration}} = \frac{\text{dose}}{A + B} \quad (11\text{-}13)$$

The volume of the central compartment is important in clinical anesthesiology because it is the pharmacokinetic parameter that determines the peak plasma concentration after an iv bolus injection. Hypovolemia, for example, reduces the volume of the central compartment. If doses are not correspondingly reduced, the higher plasma concentrations will increase the incidence of adverse pharmacologic effects.

Immediately after iv injection, all of the drug is in the central compartment. Simultaneously, three processes begin. Drug moves from the central to the peripheral compartment, which also has a volume, $V2$. This intercompartmental transfer is a first-order process, and its magnitude is quantified by the rate constant k_{12}. As soon as drug appears in the peripheral compartment, some passes back to the central compartment, a process characterized by the rate constant k_{21}. The transfer of drug between the central and peripheral compartments is quantified by the *distributional* or *intercompartmental clearance:*

$$\text{Intercompartmental clearance} = V1 \cdot k_{12} = V2 \cdot k_{21} \quad (11\text{-}14)$$

The third process that begins immediately after administration of the drug is irreversible removal of drug from the system via the central compartment. As in the one-compartment model, the elimination rate constant is k_e, and *elimination clearance* is:

$$\text{Elimination clearance} = V1 \cdot k_e \quad (11\text{-}15)$$

The rapidity of the decrease in the central compartment concentration after iv injection depends on the magnitude of the compartmental volumes, the intercompartmental clearance, and the elimination clearance.

At equilibrium, the drug is distributed among the central and the peripheral compartment, and by definition, the concentrations in the compartments are equal. Therefore, the ultimate volume of distribution, termed the volume of distribution at steady-state (V_{ss}), is the sum of $V1$ and $V2$. Extensive tissue uptake of a drug is reflected by a large volume of the peripheral compartment, which, in turn, results in a large V_{ss}. Consequently, V_{ss} can greatly exceed the actual volume of the body.

As in the single-compartment model, in multicompartment models the elimination clearance is equal to the dose divided by the area under the concentration versus time curve. This area, as well as the compartmental volumes and intercompartmental clearances, can be calculated from the intercepts and hybrid rate constants, without having to reach steady-state conditions.[128]

Three-Compartment Model

After iv injection of some drugs, the initial, rapid distribution phase is followed by a second, slower distribution phase before the elimination phase becomes evident. Therefore, the plasma concentration is the sum of three exponential terms:

$$Cp_{(t)} = Ae^{-\alpha t} + Be^{-\beta t} + G^{-\gamma t}, \quad (11\text{-}16)$$

where t = time, $Cp_{(t)}$ = plasma concentration at time t, A = intercept of the rapid distribution phase line, α = hybrid rate constant of the rapid distribution phase, B = intercept of the slower distribution phase line, α = hybrid rate constant of the slower distribution phase, G = intercept of the elimination phase line, and β = hybrid rate constant of the elimination phase. This triphasic behavior is explained by a three-compartment pharmacokinetic model (Fig. 11-8). As in the two-compartment model, the drug is injected into and eliminated from the central compartment. Drug is reversibly transferred between the central compartment and two peripheral compartments, which accounts for two distribution phases. Drug transfer between the central compartment and the more rapidly equilibrating, or "shallow," peripheral compartment is characterized by the first-order rate constants k_{12} and k_{21}. Transfer in and out of the more slowly equilibrating, "deep" compartment is characterized by the rate constants k_{13} and k_{31}. In this model, there are three compartmental volumes: $V1$, $V2$, and $V3$, whose sum equals V_{ss}; and three clearances: the rapid intercompartmental clearance, the slow intercompartmental clearance, and elimination clearance.

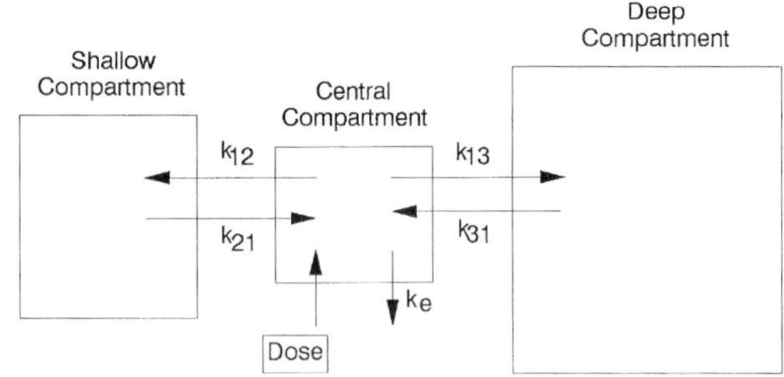

FIGURE 11-8. A three-compartment pharmacokinetic model. See text for explanation.

The pharmacokinetic parameters of interest to clinicians, such as clearance, volumes of distribution, and distribution and elimination half-lives, are determined by calculations analogous to those used in the two-compartment model. Accurate estimates of these parameters depend on accurate characterization of the measured plasma concentration versus time data. A frequently encountered problem is that the duration of sampling is not long enough to define accurately the elimination phase.[129] Similar problems arise if the assay cannot detect low concentrations of the drug. Whether a drug exhibits two- or three-compartment kinetics is of no clinical consequence. In fact, some drugs have two-compartment kinetics in some patients and three-compartment kinetics in others.[108,130] In selecting a pharmacokinetic model, the most important factor is that it accurately characterize the measured concentrations. In general, the model with the smallest number of compartments or exponents that accurately reflects the data is used.

Almost all earlier pharmacokinetic studies used *two-stage modeling*. With this technique, pharmacokinetic parameters were estimated independently for each subject and then averaged to provide estimates of the typical parameters for the population. One problem with this approach is that if outliers are present, averaging parameters could result in a model that does not accurately predict typical drug concentrations. Currently, most pharmacokinetic models are developed using *population pharmacokinetic modeling*, which has been made feasible because of advances in modeling software and increased computing power. With these techniques, the pharmacokinetic parameters are estimated using all the concentration versus time data from the entire group of subjects in a single stage, using sophisticated nonlinear regression methods. This modeling technique provides single estimates of the typical parameter values for the population.

Effects of Hepatic or Renal Disease on Pharmacokinetic Parameters

As discussed earlier, hepatic and renal disease not only affect the ability to eliminate drugs, but also change the binding of drugs to plasma proteins. Consequently, the effects of altered protein binding and the effects of impaired organ function must be considered to understand fully the impact of hepatic or renal disease on pharmacokinetic variables.

The extent of drug distribution depends on the relative affinity of blood versus tissues for the drug. Therefore, if the free fraction in plasma increases, the volume of distribution must also increase. The magnitude of the change depends on the initial free fraction and volume of distribution. An increase in the free fraction will produce the greatest increase in the volume of distribution for drugs that are highly bound to plasma proteins and have small volumes of distribution. In contrast, changes in plasma protein binding of drugs with large volumes of distribution have minimal effects on the volume of distribution, because so little of the total amount of drug is in the plasma.[131]

In theory, a parallel change in tissue binding would cancel the effect of changes in plasma binding. However, this appears to be uncommon. Increased volumes of distribution of diazepam[22] and propranolol[132] associated with increased free fractions have been observed in patients with hepatic disease. Decreased binding of thiopental in patients with renal failure also increases the volume of distribution.[87]

The effect of altered protein binding on total drug clearance also depends on the initial magnitude of the clearance. Increases in the free fraction of drugs with low hepatic extraction ratios and drugs eliminated primarily by glomerular filtration cause a proportional increase in clearance. In contrast, altered protein binding has little effect on drugs with high hepatic or renal clearance. The effect of an increased free fraction on elimination depends on the net effect on clearance and the volume of distribution.[131] The elimination half-life will increase if increased volume of distribution is the paramount change, or decrease if increased clearance predominates.

Diverse pathophysiologic changes preclude precise prediction of the pharmacokinetics of a given drug in individual patients with hepatic or renal disease. However, some generalizations can be made. Binding of drugs to albumin is decreased, so that doses of drugs given as an iv bolus, such as thiopental, should be reduced. In patients with hepatic disease, the elimination half-life of drugs metabolized or excreted by the liver is often increased because of decreased clearance, and, possibly, increased volume of distribution. Repeated doses of such drugs as benzodiazepines, opioids, and barbiturates may accumulate, leading to excessive and prolonged pharmacologic effects. Recovery from small doses of drugs such as thiopental and fentanyl is largely the result of redistribution, so recovery from conservative doses will be minimally affected. In patients with renal failure, similar concerns apply to the administration of drugs excreted by the kidneys. It is almost always better to underestimate a patient's dose requirement, observe the response, and give additional drug if necessary.

Nonlinear Pharmacokinetics

The physiologic and compartmental models thus far discussed are based on the assumption that drug distribution and elimination are first-order processes. Therefore, their parameters, such as clearance and elimination half-life, are independent of the dose or concentration of the drug. However, the rate of elimination of a few drugs is dose dependent, or *nonlinear.*

Elimination of drugs involves interactions with either enzymes catalyzing biotransformation reactions or carrier proteins for transmembrane transport. If sufficient drug is present, the capacity of the drug-eliminating systems can be exceeded. When this occurs, it is no longer possible to excrete a constant fraction of the drug present to the eliminating system, and a constant amount of drug is excreted per unit time. Phenytoin is a well-known example of a drug that exhibits nonlinear elimination at therapeutic concentrations. In theory, all drugs are cleared in a nonlinear fashion. In practice, the capacity to eliminate most drugs is so great that this is usually not evident, even with toxic concentrations.

PHARMACODYNAMIC PRINCIPLES

In its broadest sense, pharmacodynamics is the study of the effects of drugs on the body. Classically, pharmacologic effects have been quantified by dose-response studies. Advances in drug assay techniques and data analysis now allow definition of the relationship between the drug concentration and the associated pharmacologic effect in vivo. As a result, the term "pharmacodynamics" has acquired a more specific definition: the quantitative analysis of the relationship between the drug concentration in the blood, or at the site of action, and the resultant effects of the drug on physiologic processes.[133]

Dose-Response Curves

10 Dose-response studies determine the relationship between increasing doses of a drug and the ensuing changes in pharmacologic effects. Schematic dose-response curves are shown in Figure 11-9, with the dose plotted on both linear and logarithmic scales. There is a curvilinear relationship between dose and the intensity of response. Low doses produce little pharmacologic effect. Once effects become evident, a small increase in dose produces a relatively large change in effect. At near-maximal response, large increases in dose produce little change in effect. Usually the dose is plotted on a logarithmic scale (see Fig. 11-9, right panel), which demonstrates the linear relationship between the logarithm of the dose and the intensity of the response between 20 and 80% of the maximum effect.

Dose-response curves provide information regarding four aspects of the relationship of dose and pharmacologic effect. The *potency* of the drug—the dose required to produce a given effect—is determined. Potency is usually expressed as the dose required to produce a given effect in 50% of subjects, the *ED50*. The *slope* of the curve between 20 and 80% of the maximal effect indicates the rate of increase in effect as the dose is increased. The maximum effect is referred to as the *efficacy* of the drug. Finally, if curves from multiple subjects are generated, the *variability* in potency, efficacy, and the slope of the dose-response curve can be estimated.

The dose needed to produce a given pharmacologic effect varies considerably, even in "normal" patients. The patient most resistant to the drug usually requires a dose two- to threefold greater than the patient with the lowest dose requirements. This variability is caused by differences between individuals in the relationship between drug concentration and pharmacologic effect, superimposed on differences in pharmacokinetics.

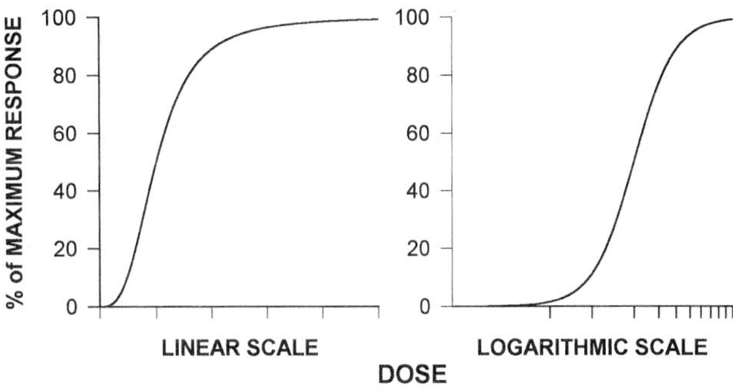

FIGURE 11-9. **Left panel:** A schematic curve of the effect of a drug plotted against dose. **Right panel:** The same curve, replotted with dose on a logarithmic scale. This yields the familiar sigmoid dose-response curve, which is linear between 20 and 80% of the maximal effect.

Dose-response studies have the disadvantage of not being able to determine whether variations in pharmacologic response are caused by differences in pharmacokinetics, pharmacodynamics, or both.

Concentration-Response Relationships

Ideally, the concentration of drug at its site of action should be used to define the concentration-response relationship. Unfortunately, these data are rarely available, so the relationship between the concentration of drug in the blood and pharmacologic effect is studied instead. This relationship is easiest to understand if the changes in pharmacologic effect that occur during and after an iv infusion of a hypothetical drug are considered. If a drug is infused at a constant rate, the plasma concentration initially increases rapidly and asymptotically approaches a steady-state level after approximately five elimination half-lives have elapsed (Fig. 11-10). The effect of the drug initially increases very slowly, then more rapidly, and eventually also reaches a steady state. When the infusion is discontinued, indicated by point C in Figure 11-10, the plasma concentration immediately decreases because of drug distribution and elimination. However, the effect stays the same for a short period, and then also begins to decrease—there is always a time lag between changes in plasma concentration and changes in pharmacologic response. Figure 11-10 also demonstrates that the same plasma concentration is associated with different responses if the concentration is changing. At points *A* and *B* in Figure 11-10, the plasma concentrations are the same, but the effects at each time differ. When the concentration is increasing, there is a concentration gradient from blood to the site of action. When the infusion is discontinued, the concentration gradient is reversed. Therefore, at the same plasma concentration, the concentration at the site of action is higher after, compared to during, the infusion. This is associated with a correspondingly greater effect.

In theory, there must be some degree of temporal disequilibrium between plasma concentration and drug effect for all drugs with extravascular sites of action. However, for some drugs, the time lag may be so short that it cannot be demonstrated. The magnitude of this temporal disequilibrium depends on several factors:

1. perfusion of the organ on which the drug acts
2. the tissue:blood partition coefficient of the drug
3. the rate of diffusion or transport of the drug from the blood to the cellular site of action
4. the rate and affinity of drug–receptor binding
5. the time required for processes initiated by the drug-receptor interaction to produce changes in cellular function

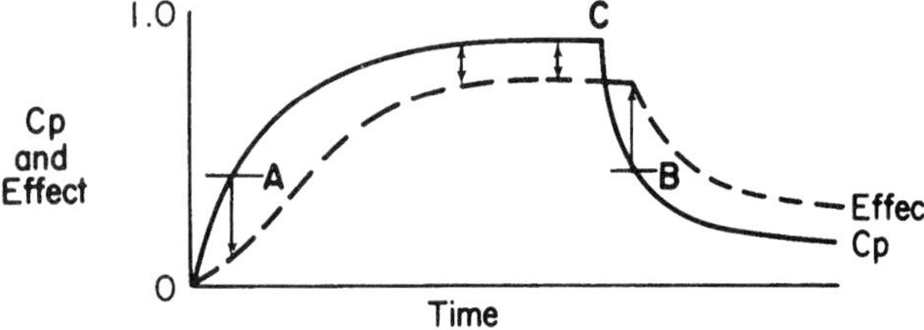

FIGURE 11-10. The changes in plasma drug concentration and pharmacologic effect during and after an intravenous infusion. See text for explanation. (Reprinted with permission from Stanski DR, Sheiner LB: Pharmacokinetics and pharmacodynamics of muscle relaxants. Anesthesiology 51:103, 1979.)

The consequence of this time lag between changes in concentration and changes in effects is that the plasma concentration will have an unvarying relationship with pharmacologic effect only under steady-state conditions. At steady state, the plasma concentration is in equilibrium with the concentrations throughout the body, and is thus directly proportional to the steady-state concentration at the site of action. Plotting the logarithm of the steady-state plasma concentration versus response generates a curve identical in appearance to the dose-response curve shown in the right panel of Figure 11-9. The $Cp_{ss}50$, the steady-state plasma concentration producing 50% of the maximal response, is determined from the concentration-response curve. Like the ED50, the $Cp_{ss}50$ is a measure of sensitivity to a drug, but the $Cp_{ss}50$ has the advantage of being unaffected by pharmacokinetic variability. Because it takes five elimination half-lives to approach steady-state conditions, it is not practical to determine the $Cp_{ss}50$ directly. For drugs with long elimination half-lives, the pseudoequilibrium during the elimination phase can be used to approximate steady-state conditions, because the concentrations in plasma and at the site of action are changing very slowly.

The onset and duration of pharmacologic effects depend not only on pharmacokinetic factors but also on the pharmacodynamic factors governing the degree of temporal disequilibrium between changes in concentration and changes in effect. The magnitude of the pharmacologic effect is a function of the amount of drug present at the site of action, so increasing the dose increases the peak effect. Larger doses have a more rapid onset of action because pharmacologically active concentrations at the site of action occur sooner. Increasing the dose also increases the duration of action because pharmacologically effective concentrations are maintained for a longer time.

Integrated pharmacokinetic–pharmacodynamic models fully characterize the relationships between time, dose, plasma concentration, and pharmacologic effect.[133] This is accomplished by adding an "effect compartment" to a standard compartmental pharmacokinetic model. The effect compartment is also called the *biophase*. Transfer of drug between central compartment and the effect compartment, or biophase, is assumed to be a first-order process, and the pharmacologic effect is assumed to be directly related to the concentration in the biophase. By quantifying the time lag between changes in plasma concentration and changes in pharmacologic effect, these models can also define the $Cp_{ss}50$, even without steady-state conditions. These models have contributed greatly to our understanding of factors influencing the response to intravenous anesthetics,[134,135] opioids,[136,137] and nondepolarizing muscle relaxants[138,139] in humans.

Dose-response and concentration-response relationships can be altered by many factors, such as drug interactions or pathologic conditions. They are also affected by the development of tolerance, which increases the ED50 and $Cp_{ss}50$. When tolerance develops rapidly, it is referred to as *tachyphylaxis*, or *acute tolerance*.

Drug–Receptor Interactions

The biochemical and physiologic effects of drugs, neurotransmitters, and hormones result from the binding of these compounds to receptors, which initiates changes in cellular function. In addition to the well-known muscarinic and nicotinic cholinergic receptors, and α- and β-adrenoceptors, there are specific receptors for histamine, serotonin, dopamine, eicosanoids, peptide hormones, steroid hormones, endorphins and exogenous opiates, benzodiazepines, and calcium channel blockers, to name a few. Subtypes of many of these receptors have been characterized. Most receptors are protein molecules situated in the cell membrane, although some are located within the cell.

Binding of drugs to receptors, like the binding of drugs to plasma proteins, is usually reversible, and follows the law of mass action:

$$[drug] + [receptor] \equiv [drug\text{–}receptor\ complex] \quad (11\text{-}17)$$

The higher the concentration of free drug or unoccupied receptor, the greater the tendency to form the drug-receptor complex. Plotting the percentage of receptors occupied by a drug against the logarithm of the concentration of the drug yields a sigmoid curve, as shown in Figure 11-11.

It is often assumed that the percentage of the maximal effect observed at any given drug concentration is equal to the percentage of receptors occupied by the drug. However, this is not always the case. At the neuromuscular junction, only 20 to 25% of the postjunctional nicotinic cholinoceptors need to bind acetylcholine to produce contraction of all the fibers in the muscle.[140] Thus, 75 to 80% of the receptors can be considered "spare receptors." The presence of spare receptors has two important consequences. Equation 11-17 indicates that the higher the concentration of unoccupied receptors, the greater the tendency to form the drug–receptor complex. Therefore, spare receptors permit near-maximal effects at very low concentrations of drugs or neurotransmitters.[141] The other corollary of the existence of spare receptors is that most of the receptors must be occupied by an antagonist before transmission is affected. This accounts for the "margin of safety" of neuromuscular transmission.[140]

The binding of drugs to receptors and the resulting changes in cellular function are the last two steps in the complex series of events between administration of the drug and production of its pharmacologic effects. There are two primary mechanisms by which the binding of an agonist to a receptor changes cellular function: receptor-linked membrane ion channels called *ionophores,* and guanine nucleotide binding proteins, referred to as *G-proteins.* The nicotinic cholinoceptor in the neuromuscular postsynaptic membrane is one example of a receptor-ionophore complex. Binding of acetylcholine opens the cation ionophore, leading to an influx of Na^+ ions, propagation of an action potential, and, ultimately, muscle contraction.[142] The β-amino butyric acid (GABA) receptor–chloride ionophore complex is another example of this type of effector mechanism. Binding of either endogenous neurotransmitters (GABA) or exogenous agonists (benzodiazepines and iv anesthetics) increases Cl^- conductance, which hyperpolarizes the neuron and decreases its excitability.[143] α-Adrenoceptors are the prototypical receptors that alter cellular function via G-proteins. G-proteins change the intracellular concentrations of various so-called *second messengers,* such as Ca^{2+} and cyclic AMP.[144]

Receptors are not static entities. Rather, they are dynamic cellular components that adapt to their environment. For example, administration of α-adrenergic agonists leads to desensitization of α-adrenoceptors.[145] This occurs by several mechanisms: reduced ability to combine with G-proteins; *sequestration,* which is the removal of receptors from the cell membrane so they are no longer accessible to agonists; and by *downregulation,* a decrease in the total number of receptors. Administration of adrenoceptor antagonists increases the number of receptors.[145]

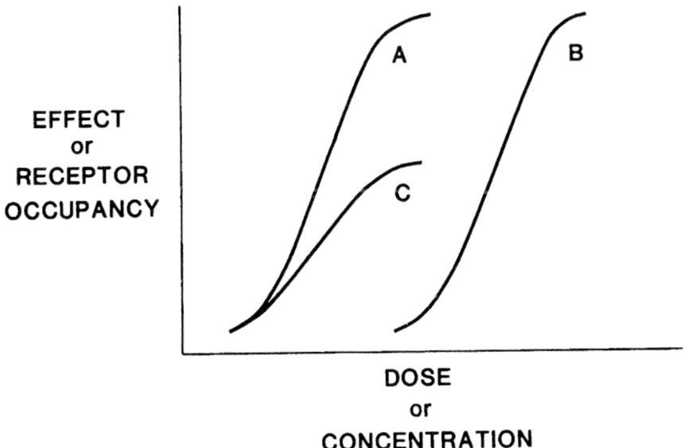

FIGURE 11-11. Schematic dose-response curves representing various conditions. Either dose or concentration is plotted on the *x*-axis, and either effect or the number of receptors occupied on the *y*-axis. Curve *A* is a typical dose-response curve. Curve *B* is a parallel rightward shift of the curve and represents a drug that is less potent than the drug depicted by curve *A*, but is a full agonist and thus capable of producing the same maximal effect. Curve *B* would also result if the drug used to generate curve *A* was studied in the presence of a competitive antagonist. Curve *C* is shifted to the right, with a reduction in slope and the maximal effect. This is the curve observed with partial agonists and also when a full agonist (curve *A*) is studied in the presence of a noncompetitive antagonist.

Agonists, Partial Agonists, and Antagonists

11 Drugs that bind to receptors and produce an effect are called *agonists.* Drugs may be capable of producing the same maximal effect, although they may differ in potency. Agonists that differ in potency but bind to the same receptors will have parallel concentration-response curves (curves *A* and *B* in Fig. 11-11). Differences in potency of agonists reflect differences in affinity for the receptor. *Partial agonists* are drugs that are not capable of producing the maximal effect, even at very high concentrations (curve C in Fig. 11-11).

Compounds that bind to receptors without producing any changes in cellular function are referred to as *antagonists.* Binding of agonists to receptors is inhibited by antagonists. Competitive antagonists bind reversibly to receptors, and their blocking effect can be overcome by high concentrations of an agonist. Therefore, *competitive antagonists* produce a parallel shift in the dose-response curve, but the maximum effect is not altered (see Fig. 11-11, curves *A* and *B*). *Noncompetitive antagonists* bind irreversibly to receptors. This has the same effect as reducing the number of receptors and shifts the dose-response curve downward and to the right, decreasing both the slope and the maximum effect (curves *A* and *C* in Fig. 11-11). The effect of noncompetitive antagonists is reversed only by synthesis of new receptor molecules.

Agonists produce a structural change in the receptor molecule that initiates changes in cellular function. Partial agonists may produce a qualitatively different change in the receptor, whereas antagonists bind without producing a change in the receptor that results in altered cellular function. The underlying mechanisms by which different compounds that bind to the same receptor act as agonists, partial agonists, or antagonists are not fully understood.

DRUG INTERACTIONS

Taking into account premedication, perioperative antibiotics, iv agents used for induction or maintenance, inhalational anesthetics, opioids, muscle relaxants, the drugs used to restore neuromuscular transmission, and postoperative analgesics, 10 or more drugs may be given for a relatively "routine" anesthetic. Consequently, thorough understanding of the mechanisms of drug interactions and knowledge of specific interactions with drugs used in anesthesia are essential to the safe practice of anesthesiology. Indeed, anesthesiologists often deliberately take advantage of drug interactions. For example, when cholinesterase inhibitors are given to reverse the effects of neuromuscular blockers on nicotinic cholinoceptors, atropine or glycopyrrolate is administered concomitantly to avoid such undesirable side effects as bradycardia and bronchospasm, which would result from increased acetylcholine binding to muscarinic cholinoceptors.

Drug interactions because of physicochemical properties can occur in vitro. Mixing acidic drugs, such as thiopental, and basic drugs, such as opioids or muscle relaxants, results in the formation of insoluble salts that precipitate.[146] Another type of in vitro reaction is absorption of drugs by plastics. Examples include the uptake of nitroglycerin by polyvinyl chloride infusion sets[147] and the absorption of fentanyl by the apparatus used for cardiopulmonary bypass.[148]

Drugs can alter each other's absorption, distribution, and elimination. Absorption from the GI tract is altered by drugs like ranitidine, which alters gastric pH,[51] and metoclopramide, which speeds gastric emptying.[149] Vasoconstrictors are added to local anesthetic solutions to prolong their duration of action at the site of injection and to decrease the risk of systemic toxicity from rapid absorption.

Drugs that compete for binding sites on plasma proteins have complex interactions.[77] Displacement of a drug from plasma proteins affects its distribution. The increase in the free drug concentration increases tissue uptake of the drug, increasing the volume of distribution. The extent of the effect on drug distribution depends on the fraction of the total drug in the body that is bound to plasma proteins. The change in distribution will be greatest when drugs with relatively large bound fractions and small volumes of distribution are displaced. Displacement of one drug by another may produce toxic-free-drug concentrations. When a steady state is reestablished, the effect of decreased binding on total and free drug concentrations depends on the rate of clearance of the drug. For drugs with low extraction ratios, clearance varies with the degree of binding, and clearance increases proportionately to the increase in free fraction. Therefore, when a steady state is reestablished, the total drug concentration will be lower, but the free drug level will be the same as the level before displacement. Clearance of drugs with high extraction ratios is not restricted to the free fraction and is not affected by changes in binding. Consequently, when a new steady state is reached, the total drug concentration is unchanged, and the higher free drug level will persist. Adverse interactions are thus most likely to occur if the displaced drug has high (nonrestrictive) clearance, a small volume of distribution, and relatively high binding to plasma proteins.

Drugs that inhibit or induce the enzymes that catalyze biotransformation reactions can affect clearance of other concomitantly administered drugs. Clearance can also be affected by drug-induced changes in hepatic blood flow. Drugs that are cleared by the kidneys and have similar physicochemical characteristics compete for the transport mechanisms involved in renal tubular secretion.

Pharmacodynamic interactions fall into two broad classifications. Drugs can interact, either directly or indirectly, at the same receptors. Opioid antagonists directly displace opioids from opiate receptors. Cholinesterase inhibitors indirectly antagonize the effects of neuromuscular blockers by increasing the amount of acetylcholine, which displaces the blocking drug from nicotinic receptors. Pharmacodynamic interactions can also occur if two drugs affect a physiologic system at different sites. Benzodiazepines and opioids, each acting on their own specific receptors, appear to interact synergistically.[150,151] Although receptors and mechanisms are not as well defined as for the benzodiazepine–opioid interaction, this is presumably how volatile anesthetics increase sensitivity to neuromuscular blocking drugs[138] and also how premedication increases sensitivity to inhalational anesthetics.[152]

CLINICAL APPLICATION OF PHARMACOKINETICS AND PHARMACODYNAMICS TO ADMINISTRATION OF INTRAVENOUS AGENTS

While no new inhaled anesthetics have been synthesized since the 1960s, intravenous drugs that act on the central nervous system continue to be developed. Anesthesiologists have become accustomed to the exquisite control of anesthetic blood (and effect site) concentrations afforded by modern volatile anesthetic agents and their vaporizers, coupled to end-tidal anesthetic gas monitoring. To achieve similar degrees of control of intravenously administered anesthetic drug concentrations in blood and in the central nervous system, new technologies aimed at improving intravenous infusion devices, as well as new software to manage the daunting pharmacokinetic principles involved, are needed. This section examines the current state of infusion devices and the pharmacokinetic and pharmacodynamic principles specifically required for precise delivery of anesthetic agents.

Infusion Pumps

Originally designed over 30 years ago to control intravenous nutrition, infusion pumps have been developed for the large intensive care unit (ICU) and hospital-based market for an ever-widening variety of drugs. Anesthesia-specific pumps remain a relative rarity because the overall market is smaller. Anesthesia is the only arena in which a highly trained individual continuously monitors both the infusion pump and the patient. Optimally, the control interface for infusion pumps would be analogous to the switches, knobs, and dials found on anesthesia machines, allowing for rapid adjustments with a minimum number of steps to actuate the new infusion rate.[153] However, most pumps currently available in hospitals are designed for safe management by personnel with varying skill levels and protection from those with no skill level, that is, patients, family members, and so on. These systems often feature time-consuming, menu-driven, double-checked programming; detection of minute air bubbles; and alarms when the pump is left on "pause" or "standby" mode, none of which are necessarily required or desired by anesthesiologists.[153]

Since the therapeutic indices and the need to accurately predict emergence are largely similar for inhaled and intravenous agents, similar precision in the drug delivery systems is required. Table 11-8 lists the theoretical attributes of an ideal anesthesia-specific infusion pump. While elimination of the aforementioned "safety" features is desirable, in many ways such pumps should be more sophisticated than generic infusion pumps. Specifically, they should display information relevant to the conduct of an anesthetic, including assurance that the correct drug is being delivered precisely as programmed. The latter is a particular problem with most currently used pumps, resulting in underdosing and patient awareness, as well as other misadventures.[154–157] Other improvements from standard hospital pumps should include a different set of alarm conditions, the ability to variably set air detection limits, and a mechanism for rapidly effecting changes in pump programming. A pump with these specifications would obviously require the continuous presence of a highly trained individual. However, drugs being delivered via an anesthesia-specific pump would likely not be acceptable in other units within the hospital unless a pump were to have dual settings, one for anesthesia and one for the rest of the hospital. Drugs delivered by an anesthesia-specific

TABLE 11-8

DESIRABLE FEATURES FOR INTRAVENOUS INFUSION DEVICES

Low acquisition and operating costs
Accuracy over a wide range of flow rates to allow use with multiple drug formulations in adult and pediatric patients
Small size and battery backup for transporting patients
Controls that allow rapid changes in drug delivery
Pause function without alarm
Programmability:
 Drug identification
 Ability to enter patient weight and drug concentration, allowing user to set dose in mass units rather than volumes (i.e., mg/h or μg/kg/min instead of mL/h)
 Preset bolus dose in mass units or volume, with reversion to continuous infusion rate after completion of bolus
 Computer interface for data acquisition and control
 Target-controlled infusion capability
Displays:
 All programmed parameters
 Current infusion rate and cumulative dose
 Visible in low ambient light
Safety features:
 Drug identification (analogous to vaporizer)
 Audio and visual alarms for empty drug reservoir, air inline, occlusion, impending battery depletion, nonspecific malfunction
 Variable air detection limits
 Sensing and control circuits to detect discrepancies between programmed and actual flow rates
 Microprocessor-based integration of drug identification, patient weight, and set dose to alert user of potential overdoses

pump that would continue to be infused outside of the OR, for example, anesthetic agents and vasoactive drugs, would then need to be switched to another infusion device upon arrival at another care setting.

Pharmacokinetic and Pharmacodynamic Principles of Drug Infusions

While pharmacokinetic and pharmacodynamic principles and data have contributed greatly to our understanding of drug action in anesthesia, their primary utility and ultimate purpose are to determine optimal dosing with as much mathematical precision and clinical accuracy as possible. In most pharmacotherapeutic scenarios outside of anesthesia care, the time scales for onset of drug effect, its maintenance, and its offset are measured in days, weeks, or even years. In such cases, global pharmacokinetic variables such as total volume of distribution (V_{SS}), elimination clearance (Cl_e), and half-life ($t_{1/2}$) are sufficient and utilitarian parameters for calculating dose regimens.[158] However, in the OR and ICU, the temporal tolerances for onset and offset of desired drug effects are measured in minutes. Consequently, these global variables are insufficient to describe the details of kinetic behavior of drugs in the minutes following intravenous administration. This is particularly true of lipid-soluble hypnotics and opioids that rapidly and extensively distribute throughout the various tissues of the body, because distribution processes dominate pharmacokinetic behavior during the time frame of most anesthetics. Additionally, the therapeutic indices of many intravenous anesthetic drugs are small and two-tailed (i.e., an underdose, resulting in awareness, is a "toxic" effect). Optimal dosing in these situations requires use of all the variables of a multicompartmental pharmacokinetic model to account for drug distribution in blood and other tissues.

It is not easy to intuit the pharmacokinetic behavior of a multicompartmental system by simple examination of the kinetic variables.[159] Computer simulation is required to meaningfully interpret dosing or to accurately devise new dosing regimens. In addition, there are several pharmacokinetic concepts that are uniquely applicable to intravenous administration of drugs with multicompartmental kinetics and must be taken into account when administering intravenous infusions.

Rise to Steady-State Concentration

The drug concentration versus time profile for the rise to steady state is the mirror image of its elimination profile. In a one-compartment model with a decline in concentration versus time that is mono-exponential following a single dose, the rise of drug concentration to the steady-state concentration (C_{SS}) is likewise mono-exponential during a continuous infusion. That is, in one elimination half-life an infusion is halfway to its eventual steady-state concentration, in another half-life it reaches half of what remains between halfway and steady state (i.e., 75% of the eventual steady state is reached in two elimination half-lives), and so on for each half-life increment. The equation describing this behavior is:

$$Cp_{(t)} = C_{SS}\left[1 - e^{-kt}\right] \qquad (11\text{-}18)$$

where $Cp_{(t)}$ = the concentration at time t, k is the rate constant related to the elimination half-life, and t is the time from the start of the infusion. This relationship can also be described by:

$$Cp_{(n)} = C_{SS}\left[1 - (1/2)^{n}\right] \qquad (11\text{-}19)$$

in which $Cp(n)$ is the concentration at n half-lives. Equation 11-19 indicates that during a constant infusion, the concentration reaches 90% of C_{SS} after 3.3 half-lives, which is usually deemed close enough for clinical purposes.

However, for a drug such as propofol, which partitions extensively to pharmacologically inert body tissues (e.g., muscle, gut), a mono-exponential equation, or single-compartment model, is insufficient to describe the time course of propofol concentrations in the first minutes and hours after beginning drug administration. Instead, a multicompartmental or multiexponential model must be used.[158] With such a model, the picture changes drastically for the plasma drug concentration rise toward steady state. The rate of rise toward steady state is determined by the distribution rate constants to the degree that their respective exponential terms contribute to the total area under the concentration versus time curve. Thus, for the three-compartment model describing the pharmacokinetics of propofol, Equation 11-18 becomes:

$$Cp_{(t)}=C_{SS}\left[\frac{A}{A+B+G}\left(1-e^{-\alpha t}\right) + \frac{B}{A+B+G}\left(1-e^{-\beta t}\right) + \frac{G}{A+B+G}\left(1-e^{-\gamma t}\right)\right] \qquad (11\text{-}20)$$

in which t = time; $Cp_{(t)}$ = plasma concentration at time; A = coefficient of the rapid distribution phase and α = hybrid rate constant of the rapid distribution phase; B = coefficient of the slower distribution phase and β = hybrid rate constant of the slower distribution; and G = coefficient of elimination phase and γ = hybrid rate constant of the elimination phase. $A + B + G$ is the sum of the coefficients of all the exponential terms. For most lipophilic anesthetics and opioids, A is typically one order of magnitude greater than *B*, and *B* is in turn an order of magnitude greater than *G*. Therefore, distribution-phase kinetics for intravenous anesthetics have a much greater influence on the time to reach C_{SS} than do elimination-phase kinetics.

For example, with propofol having an elimination half-life of approximately 6 hours,[160] the simple one-compartment rule in Equation 11-19 tells us that it would take 6 hours from the start of a constant rate infusion to reach even 50% of the eventual steady-state propofol plasma concentration and 12 hours to reach 75%. In contrast, with a full three-compartment propofol kinetic model,[160] Equation 11-20 accurately predicts that 50% of steady state is reached in less than 30 minutes and 75% will be reached in less than 4 hours. This example emphasizes the necessity of using multicompartment models to describe the clinical pharmacokinetics of intravenous anesthetics.

Concentration-Effect Relationship

The fundamental goal driving the advances in pharmacokinetics and pharmacodynamics during the past three decades has been to better understand and predict drug concentration–effect relationships. For inhaled anesthetics, end-tidal concentration measurements allow a very close approximation of this goal in the clinical setting. For drugs that are not inhaled, clinicians must operate at the level of the dose-effect relationship, that is, clinicians observe the effect resulting from an administered because it is not possible to know the drug concentration at the time of the observed effect. Dose-effect relationships are inherently more difficult to interpret and control because of the multiple pharmacokinetic factors affecting the relationship between the dose of drug administered and the concentration at the effect site. For this reason anesthesiologists have not generally been able to take full advantage of the advances in our understanding of the clinical pharmacology of intravenous anesthetics.

Isoconcentration Nomogram

The rise toward steady state described by a multicompartmental system can be both visualized and put to clinical use by a concept introduced by Shafer in 1994 called an isoconcentration nomogram (Fig. 11-12).[161] This graphical tool allows users to employ concentration-effect, rather than dose-effect, relationships when determining optimal dosing of intravenous anesthetic agents. The nomogram is constructed by calculating the plasma drug concentration versus time curve for a constant-rate infusion from a set of pharmacokinetic variables for a particular drug. From this single simulation, one can readily visualize (and estimate) the rise toward steady-state plasma drug concentration described by the drug's pharmacokinetic model. By simulating a range of potential infusion rates a series of curves of identical shape are then plotted on a single graph with drug concentrations at any time that are directly proportional to the infusion rate.

By placing a horizontal line at the desired plasma drug concentration (*y*-axis) the times (*x*-axis) at which the horizontal intersects the line for a particular infusion rate will represent the times at which the infusion rate should be set to the rate on the intercepting line.[162] In the example shown (see Fig. 11-12) with 25 μg/kg/min increments, the predicted plasma propofol concentrations remain within 10% of the target from 2 minutes onward with a bias of underestimation. If never allowing the estimated concentration to fall below the target is desired, then the time to decrease to the next lower infusion should be at the midpoint of the subsequent interval. Extending the infusions to the subsequent midpoint times will introduce a maximum overestimation bias of approximately 17% with the illustrated infusion increments (Fig. 11-13). Biases would be

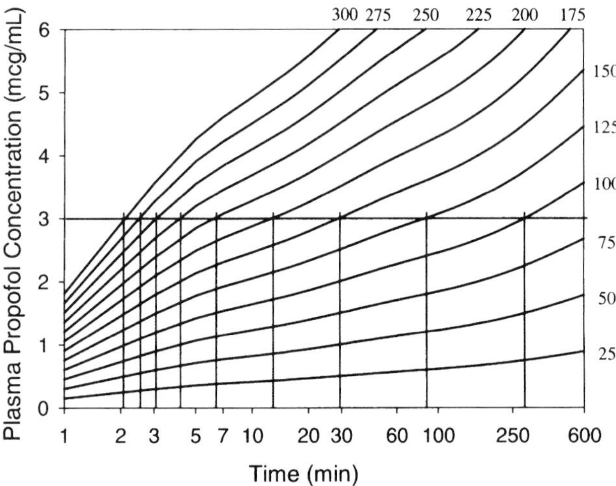

FIGURE 11-12. Isoconcentration nomogram for determining propofol infusion rates designed to maintain a desired plasma propofol concentration. This nomogram is based on the pharmacokinetics of Schnider et al[160] and plotted on a log–log scale to better delineate the early time points. Curved lines represent the plasma propofol concentration versus time plots, resulting from the various continuous infusion rates indicated along the right and upper borders (units in μg/kg/min). A horizontal line is placed at the desired target plasma propofol concentration (3 μg/mL in this case) and vertical lines are placed at each intersection of a curved concentration-time plot. The vertical lines indicate the times that the infusion rate should be set to the one represented by the next intersected curve as one moves from left to right along the horizontal line drawn at 3 μg/mL. In this example the infusion rate would be reduced from 300 μg/kg/min to 275 μg/kg/min at 2.5 minutes, to 250 μg/kg/min at 3 minutes, to 225 μg/kg/min at 4.5 minutes, and so on until it is turned to 100 μg/kg/min at 260 minutes.

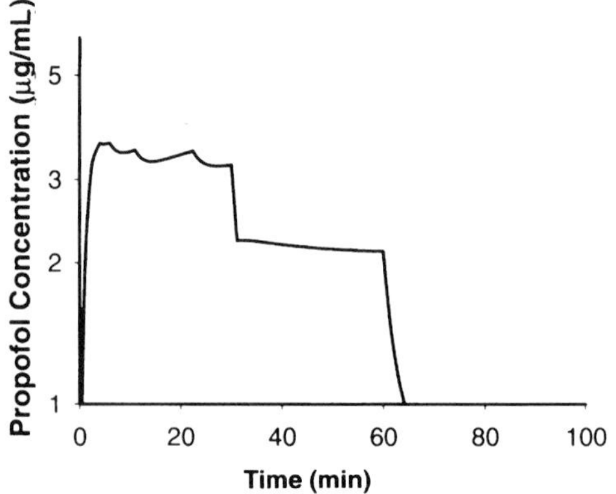

FIGURE 11-13. Simulated plasma propofol concentration history resulting from the information in the isoconcentration nomogram in Figure 11-12 and extending the times to switch the infusion to the next lower increment to the midpoint of the subsequent time segment (i.e., the switch from 250 to 225 μg/kg/min was at 5 minutes, rather than at 4.5 minutes). Note that for the first 30 minutes, this sequence predicts plasma propofol concentrations that are always slightly above 3 μg/mL (see text). At 30 minutes the target is adjusted to 2 μg/mL and so the infusion is stopped for 1 minute and 10 seconds to allow for the concentration to fall by one-third (see text) before resuming an infusion at 75 μg/kg/min. The infusion is stopped at 60 minutes in this case.

increased or decreased by constructing nomograms with larger or smaller infusion increments, respectively.

The nomogram can also be used to increase or reduce the targeted plasma propofol concentration. To target a new plasma drug concentration, a new horizontal line can be drawn at the desired concentration. The infusion rate that is closest to the current time intersect is the one that should be used initially, followed by the decremental rates dictated by the subsequent intercept times. For best results when increasing the target concentration, a bolus equal to the product of V1 (the central compartment volume) and the incremental change in concentration should be administered. Likewise, when decreasing the concentration the best strategy is to turn off the infusion for the duration predicted by the applicable context-sensitive decrement time and resume the infusion rate predicted for the current time plus the context-sensitive decrement time. For instance, if after 30 minutes one wishes to decrease the target plasma propofol concentration from 3 μg/mL to 2 μg/mL (a 33% decrement at a time context of 30 minutes), one would shut off the infusion for 1 minute and 10 seconds to let the concentration fall by 33% and then restart at 75 μg/kg/min. The estimated plasma propofol concentrations from this nomogram-guided dosing scheme is shown in Figure 11-13.

Target-Controlled Infusions

A more comprehensive means of bridging the gap between dose-effect and concentration-effect came with the introduction of the concept of target-controlled infusions (TCI), which was first described by Schwilden et al[163,164] in early 1980s. Other software systems were developed in North America by groups at Stanford University[165] and Duke University.[166] By the late 1990s a commercially available TCI system for propofol (Diprifusor®) was introduced. This greatly increased both anesthesiologists' interest in this mode of delivery and their understanding of the concentration-effect relationships for hypnotics and opioids.

2 To accomplish target-controlled infusions, the mathematical calculations of the pharmacokinetic events that convert a dose into a plasma or effect site concentration are interfaced between the anesthesia provider and the infusion pump by means of a computer. With TCI, the clinician prescribes a desired concentration (the target) and the computer-controlled pump calculates and produces the drug infusion rates required to reach and maintain the desired concentration. The success of this approach is influenced by the extent to which the drug pharmacokinetic and pharmacodynamic parameters programmed into the computer match those of the particular patient at hand. While this same limitation applies to the more rudimentary (non-TCI) dosing done routinely in every clinical setting, we must examine the special ramifications of pharmacokinetic–pharmacodynamic model misspecification with TCI in any discussion of its future importance in the clinical setting.

The mathematical principles governing TCI are actually quite simple. For a computer-control pump to produce and maintain a plasma drug concentration it must first administer a dose equal to the product of the central compartment V1 and the target concentration. Then for each moment after that, the amount of drug to be administered into the central compartment to maintain the target concentration is equal to drug eliminated from the central compartment *plus* drug distributed from the central compartment to peripheral compartments *minus* drug returning to the central compartment from peripheral compartments. The software keeps track of the estimated drug in each compartment over time and applies the rate constants for intercompartmental drug transfer from the pharmacokinetic model to these amounts to determine drug movement at any given time. It then matches the estimated concentrations to the target concentration at any time to determine the amount of drug that should be infused. The software can also predict future concentrations, usually with the assumption that the infusion will be stopped so that emergence from anesthesia or the dissipation of drug effect will occur optimally according to the context-sensitive recovery time, or half-life.[167,168]

Because there is a delay or hysteresis between the attainment of a drug concentration in the plasma and the production of a drug effect, it is advantageous to have the mathematics of this delay incorporated into TCI. By adding the kinetics of the effect site it is possible to target effect site concentrations as would be in keeping with the principle of working as closely to the relevant concentration-effect relationship as possible. A dose scheme that targets concentrations in a compartment remote from the central compartment (i.e., the effect site) has no closed form solution for calculating the infusion rate(s) needed. Instead, the solution is solved numerically and involves some additional concepts that must be considered, namely the time to peak effect, T_{MAX}, and the volume of distribution at peak effect, V_{DPE}. These are discussed later. In principle, targeting the effect site necessitates producing an overshoot in plasma drug concentrations during induction and for subsequent target increases. This is similar in concept to overpressurizing inhaled anesthetic concentrations to achieve a targeted end-tidal concentration. However, unlike the inspiratory limb of an anesthesia circuit, the plasma compartment seems to be closely linked to cardiovascular effects, and large overshoots in plasma drug concentration may produce unwanted side effects.

The performance of TCI is influenced by the variance between pharmacokinetic parameters determined from group or population studies and the individual patient. Median absolute performance errors for fentanyl,[165] alfentanil,[169] sufentanil,[170] midazolam,[171,172] and propofol[172,173] are in the range of ±30% when literature values for pharmacokinetic parameters are used to drive the TCI device and fall to approximately ±7% when the average kinetics of the test subjects themselves are used.[169] Divergence (the percentage change of the absolute performance error) is generally quite low (approximately 1%) when target concentrations remain relatively stable, but increase to nearly 20% when the frequency of concentration steps is as frequent as every 12 minutes.[173] These data suggest that while a considerable error may exist (±30%) between the targeted drug concentration and the one actually achieved in a patient, the concentration attained will not vary much over time. Thus, incremental adjustments in the target should result in incremental and stable new concentrations in the patient as long as the incremental adjustments are not too frequent.

In Europe and Asia, devices for delivering propofol by TCI are commercially available from at least three companies (Graseby, Alaris, and Fresenius) with similar performance parameters.[174] In the United States, there are still no FDA-approved devices. For investigational purposes, STANPUMP (developed by Steve Shafer at Stanford University) can be interfaced via an RS232 port to an infusion pump. STANPUMP currently provides pharmacokinetic parameters for 19 different drugs, but has the ability to accept any kinetic model for any drug provided by the user. (Information regarding STANPUMP is available at *http://anesthesia.stanford.edu/pkpd/*. Accessed August 27, 2004.) RUGLOOP© is TCI software (developed by Michel Struys of Ghent University), which is similar to STANPUMP but operates in Windows® rather than DOS® and is capable of controlling multiple drug infusions simultaneously. (Information regarding RUGLOOP is available at *http://www.anesthesia-uzgent.be/rugloop.htm*. Accessed August 27, 2004.)

While the pharmacologic principle of relating a concentration rather than a dose is scientifically sound, few studies have actually attempted to determine whether TCI improves clinical performance or outcome. Only a few limited studies have actually compared manual infusion control versus TCI. Some have shown better control and a more predictable emergence with TCI,[175,176] whereas others have simply shown no advantage.[177,178]

TCI principles continue to be developed beyond the scope of intravenous anesthesia techniques. TCI has been used to provide postoperative analgesia with alfentanil.[179,180] In this system a desired target plasma alfentanil concentration was set in the range of 40 to 100 ng/mL. A demand by the patient automatically increased the target level by 5 ng/mL. Lack of a demand caused the system to gradually reduce the targeted level. The quality of analgesia was judged to be superior to standard morphine PCA.

Similarly, TCI has been used to provide patient-controlled sedation with propofol.[181] The TCI was set to 1 μg/mL and a demand by the patient increased the level by 0.2 μg/mL. As with the TCI analgesia system, the lack of a demand caused the system to gradually reduce the targeted plasma propofol concentration. The timing and increment of the decrease were adjusted by the clinician. Over 90% of patients were satisfied with this method of sedation.

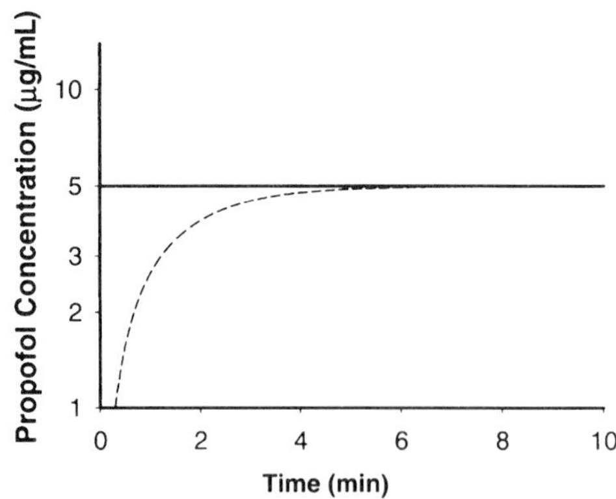

FIGURE 11-14. This is a simulation of a target-controlled infusion (TCI) in which the plasma concentration is targeted at 5 μg/mL. The *solid line* represents the predicted plasma propofol concentration of 5 μg/mL, which in theory is attained at time t = 0 and is then maintained by a variable rate infusion. The *dashed line* is the predicted effect site concentration under the conditions of a constant pseudo–steady-state plasma concentration. Note that 95% of the target concentration is reached in the effect site at approximately 4 minutes.

Time to Maximum Effect Compartment Concentration (T_{MAX})

Earlier in this chapter, the delay between attaining a plasma concentration and an effect site concentration was described. This delay, or hysteresis, is presumed to be a result of transfer of drug between the plasma compartment, V1, and an effect compartment, V_e. By simultaneously modeling the plasma drug concentration versus time data (pharmacokinetics) and the measured drug effect (pharmacodynamics), an estimate of the drug transfer rate constant, k_{e0}, between plasma and the putative effect site can be estimated.[138] However, estimates of k_{e0}, like all rate constants, are model specific.[182] That is, k_{e0} cannot be transported from one set of kinetic parameters determined in one specific pharmacokinetic–pharmacodynamic study to any another set of pharmacokinetic parameters. Likewise, it is not valid to compare estimates of k_{e0} among studies of the same drug or across different drugs and, therefore, one should not be surprised that reported values for k_{e0} for the same drug vary markedly among studies. The model-independent parameter that characterizes the delay between the plasma and effect site is the time to maximal effect, or T_{MAX}.[182] Accordingly, if the T_{MAX} and the pharmacokinetics for a drug are known from independent studies, a k_{e0} can be estimated by numeric techniques for the independent kinetic set that would produce the known effect site T_{MAX}.

The concept of a transportable, model-independent parameter that characterizes the kinetics of the effect site is important for robust effect site–targeted, computer-controlled infusions. This is because there many more pharmacokinetic studies characterizing a wider variety of patient types and groups in the literature than there are complete pharmacokinetic–pharmacodynamic studies. By making the generally valid assumption that intraindividual differences are small in a drug's rate of effect site equilibration, it is possible with a known T_{MAX} to estimate effect site kinetics for a drug across a wide variety of patient groups where only the pharmacokinetics are known. This cannot be done in a valid manner using k_{E0} or $t^1/_{2KE0}$ alone.[182]

V_{DPE}

While the plasma concentration can be brought rapidly to the targeted drug concentration by administering a bolus dose to the central compartment (C · V1) and then held there by a computer-controlled infusion (Fig. 11-14), the time for the effect site to reach the target concentration will be much longer than T_{MAX} (4 minutes for propofol effect site concentration to reach 95% of that targeted). It is possible to calculate a bolus dose that will attain the estimated effect site concentration at T_{MAX} without overshoot in the effect site. However, plasma drug concentration will overshoot (Fig. 11-15). This is done by combining the concept of describing drug distribution as an expanding volume of distribution that starts at V1 and approaches V_β (the apparent volume of distribution during the elimination phase) over time with the concept of T_{MAX}.[183,184]

Volume of distribution over time is calculated by dividing the total amount of drug remaining in the body by the plasma

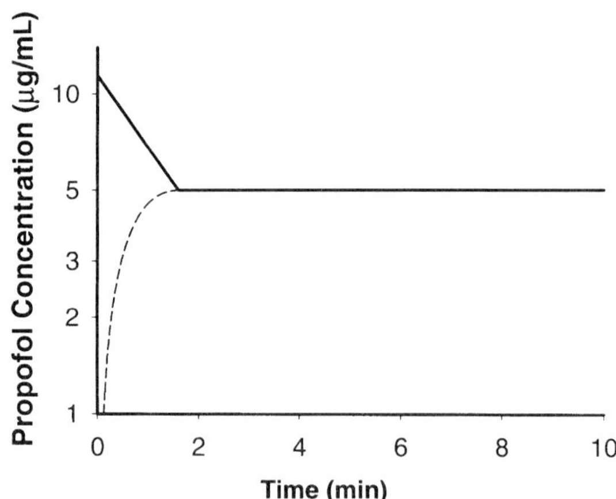

FIGURE 11-15. This is a simulation of a target controlled infusion (TCI) in which the effect site concentration is targeted at 5 μg/mL. The *solid line* represents the predicted plasma propofol concentration that results from a bolus dose, given at time t = 0, that is predicted to purposely overshoot the plasma propofol concentration target until time t = T_{MAX} (1.6 minutes). At T_{MAX} pseudo-equilibration between the effect site and the plasma occurs and both concentrations are then predicted to be the same until the target is changed. Note that the effect site attains the target in less than half the time with effect site targeting compared to the plasma concentration targeting seen in Figure 11-14.

drug concentration at each time t. The time-dependent volume at the time of peak effect (or T_{MAX}) is V_{DPE}. The product of the targeted effect site concentration and V_{DPE} plus the amount lost to elimination in the time to T_{MAX} becomes the proper bolus dose that will attain the target concentration at the effect site as rapidly as possible without overshoot. In practical terms this bolus is given at time $t = 0$, after which the infusion stops until time $t = T_{MAX}$. It then resumes infusing drug in its normal "stop loss" manner.

Some software programs for controlling target-controlled infusions include this concept in their algorithms. In the case of the propofol kinetics used to construct the isoconcentration nomogram in Figure 11-13, the pharmacokinetic–pharmacodynamic parameter set of Schnider et al[160] predicts a T_{MAX} of 1.6 minutes, a V_{DPE} of 16.62 L, and an elimination loss of 23.8% of the dose over 1.6 minutes in a 70-kg man. Thus the proper propofol bolus for a targeted effect site propofol concentration of 5 μg/mL is 109 mg. The computer-controlled infusion pump will deliver this dose as rapidly as possible and then begin a targeted infusion for 5 μg/mL at t = 1.6 minutes (see Fig. 11-15).

Frontend Pharmacokinetics

The term "frontend pharmacokinetics" refers to the intravascular mixing, pulmonary uptake, and recirculation events that occur in the first few minutes during and after intravenous drug administration.[185] These kinetic events and the drug concentration versus time profile that results are important because the peak effect of rapidly acting drugs occurs during this temporal window.[186,187] Although it has been suggested that frontend pharmacokinetics be utilized to guide drug dosing,[188] current TCI does not incorporate frontend kinetics into the models from which drug infusion rates are calculated. Not doing so may introduce further error.[189]

TCI relies on pharmacokinetic models that are based on the simplifying assumption of instantaneous and complete mixing within V1. However, the determination of V1 is routinely overestimated in most pharmacokinetic studies. Overestimation of V1, when used to calculate TCI infusion rates, results in plasma drug concentrations that overshoot the desired target concentration, especially in the first few minutes after beginning TCI. Furthermore, correct description of drug distribution to tissues is dependent on an accurate V1 estimate, so inaccuracies caused by not taking frontend pharmacokinetics into account may be persistent and result in undershoot as well as overshoot. Simulation indicates that pharmacokinetic parameters derived from studies in which the drug is administered by a short (approximately 2 minutes) infusion better estimate V1 and tissue-distribution kinetics than those from a rapid intravenous bolus infusion.[189] When the latter drug administration method is used, full characterization of the frontend recirculatory pharmacokinetics is required to obtain valid estimates of V for use in TCI.[189]

Closed-Loop Infusions

When a valid, and nearly continuous, measure of drug effect is available, drug delivery can be automatically titrated by feedback control. Such systems have been used experimentally for control of blood pressure,[190] oxygen delivery,[191] blood glucose,[192] neuromuscular blockade,[193] and depth of anesthesia.[193–199] A target value for the desired effect measure (the output of the system) is selected and the rate of drug delivery (the input into the system) is dependent on whether the effect measure is above, below, or at the target value. Thus the output feeds back and controls the input. Standard controllers (referred to as *proportional-integral-derivative* [or PID] *controllers*) adjust drug delivery based on both the integral, or magnitude, of the deviation from target and the rate of deviation, or the derivative.

Under a range of responses, standard PID controllers work quite well. However, they have been shown to develop unstable characteristics in situations where the output may vary rapidly and widely. Schwilden et al[200] have proposed a controller in which the output (measured response) controls not only the input (drug infusion rate), but also the pharmacokinetic model driving the infusion rate. This is a so-called *model-driven* or *adaptive* closed-loop system. Such a system has performed well in clinical trials,[201] and in a simulation of extreme conditions it was demonstrated to outperform a standard PID controller.[196]

Closed-loop systems for anesthesia are the most difficult to design and implement because the precise definition of "anesthesia" remains elusive, as does a robust monitor for "anesthetic depth." Because modification of consciousness must accompany anesthesia, processed EEG parameters that correlate with level of consciousness, such as the Bispectral Index (BIS),[201,202] electroencephalographic entropy,[203] and auditory evoked potentials,[198] make it possible to undertake closed-loop control of anesthesia. There is keen interest in further developing these tools to make them more reliable because, advances in pharmacokinetic modeling, including the effect compartment, the implementation of such models into drug delivery systems, and the creation of adaptive controllers based on these models, has made routine closed-loop delivery of anesthesia imaginable.[204] So far it has been difficult to bring a true closed-loop system to market in medical applications, because of the regulatory agency hurdles. From a regulatory point of view, an open-loop TCI system is much easier to attain and offers many of the benefits of actual closed-loop systems. Unless there is a regulatory or a design "breakthrough," closed-loop systems for anesthesia will likely remain in the theoretical and experimental realms.

References

1. Papper EM: The pharmacokinetics of inhalation anaesthetics: Clinical applications. Br J Anaesth 36:124, 1964
2. Wilkinson GR: Pharmacokinetics: The dynamics of drug absorption, distribution and elimination. In Hardman JG, Limbird LE, Gilman AG (eds): The Pharmacological Basis of Therapeutics, 10th ed, p 3. New York, McGraw Hill, 2001
3. Ding X, Kaminsky LS: Human extrahepatic cytochromes P450: Function in xenobiotic metabolism and tissue-selective chemical toxicity in the respiratory and gastrointestinal tracts. Ann Rev Pharmacol Toxicol 43:149, 2003
4. Ashburn MA, Streisand J, Zhang J *et al:* The iontophoresis of fentanyl citrate in humans. Anesthesiology 82:1146, 1995
5. Greenblatt DJ, Shader RI, Abernethy DR: Current status of benzodiazepines. N Engl J Med 309:354, 410, 1983
6. Fee JPH, Collier PS, Dundee JW: Bioavailability of three formulations of intravenous diazepam. Acta Anaesthesiol Scand 30:337, 1986
7. Price HL, Kovnat PJ, Safer JN *et al:* The uptake of thiopental by body tissues and its relationship to the duration of narcosis. Clin Pharmacol Ther 1:16, 1960
8. Saidman LJ, Eger EI II: The effect of thiopental metabolism on duration of anesthesia. Anesthesiology 27:118, 1966
9. Brown WU Jr, Bell GC, Alper MH: Acidosis, local anesthetics and the newborn. Obstet Gynecol 48:27, 1976
10. Shanks CA: Pharmacokinetics of the nondepolarizing neuromuscular relaxants applied to calculation of bolus and infusion dosage regimens. Anesthesiology 64:72, 1986
11. Wilkinson GR, Shand DG: A physiological approach to hepatic drug clearance. Clin Pharmacol Ther 18:377, 1975
12. Nies AS, Shand DG, Wilkinson GR: Altered hepatic blood flow and drug disposition. Clin Pharmacokinet 1:135, 1976
13. Blaschke TF: Protein binding and kinetics of drugs in liver diseases. Clin Pharmacokinet 2:32, 1977
14. Swartz RD, Sidell FR, Cucinell SA: Effects of physical stress on the disposition of drugs eliminated by the liver in man. J Pharmacol Exp Ther 188:1, 1974

15. Stenson RE, Constantino RT, Harrison DC: Interrelationships of hepatic blood flow, cardiac output, and blood levels of lidocaine in man. Circulation 43:205, 1971
16. Thomson PD, Melmon KL, Richardson JA *et al:* Lidocaine pharmacokinetics in advanced heart failure, liver disease, and renal failure in humans. Ann Intern Med 78:499, 1973
17. Benowitz NL, Meister W: Pharmacokinetics in patients with cardiac failure. Clin Pharmacokinet 1:389, 1976
18. Benowitz NL, Forsyth RP, Melmon KL *et al:* Lidocaine disposition kinetics in monkey and man: II. Effects of hemorrhage and sympathomimetic drug administration. Clin Pharmacol Ther 16:99, 1974
19. Klotz U, McHorse TS, Wilkinson GR *et al:* The effect of cirrhosis on the disposition and elimination of meperidine in man. Clin Pharmacol Ther 16:667, 1974
20. Neal EA, Meffin PJ, Gregory PB *et al:* Enhanced bioavailability and decreased clearance of analgesics in patients with cirrhosis. Gastroenterology 77:96, 1979
21. Wood AJJ, Kornhauser DM, Wilkinson GR *et al:* The influence of cirrhosis on steady-state blood concentrations of unbound propranolol after oral administration. Clin Pharmacokinet 3:478, 1978
22. Klotz U, Avant GR, Hoyumpa A *et al:* The effects of age and liver disease on the disposition and elimination of diazepam in adult man. J Clin Invest 55:347, 1975
23. Klotz U, Antonin KH, Brugel H *et al:* Disposition of diazepam and its major metabolite desmethyldiazepam in patients with liver disease. Clin Pharmacol Ther 21:430, 1977
24. McHorse TS, Wilkinson GR, Johnson RF *et al:* Effect of acute viral hepatitis in man on the disposition and elimination of meperidine. Gastroenterology 68:775, 1975
25. Williams RL, Blaschke TF, Meffin PJ *et al:* Influence of viral hepatitis on the disposition of two compounds with high hepatic clearance: Lidocaine and indocyanine green. Clin Pharmacol Ther 20:290, 1976
26. Branch RA, Shand DG, Wilkinson GR *et al:* The reduction of lidocaine clearance by *dl*-propranolol: An example of hemodynamic drug interaction. J Pharmacol Exp Ther 184:515, 1973
27. Gelman S: Disturbances in hepatic blood flow during anesthesia and surgery. Arch Surg 111:881, 1976
28. Gelman S, Fowler KC, Smith LR: Liver circulation and function during isoflurane and halothane anesthesia. Anesthesiology 61:726, 1984
29. Cooperman LH: Effects of anaesthetics on the splanchnic circulation. Br J Anaesth 44:967, 1972
30. Duchin KL, Schrier RW: Interrelationship between renal haemodynamics, drug kinetics, and drug action. Clin Pharmacokinet 3:58, 1978
31. Garrett ER: Pharmacokinetics and clearances related to renal processes. Int J Clin Pharmacol 16:155, 1978
32. Stanton A, Koeppen BM: Elements of renal function. In Berne RM, Levy MN (eds): Physiology, 4th ed, p 677. St. Louis, Mosby, 1998
33. Lam YW, Banerji S, Hatfield C, Talbert RL: Principles of drug administration in renal insufficiency. Clin Pharmacokinet 32:30, 1997
34. Collinsworth KA, Strong JM, Atkinson AJ *et al:* Pharmacokinetics and metabolism of lidocaine in patients with renal failure. Clin Pharmacol Ther 18:59, 1975
35. Miller RD, Agoston S, Booij LHDJ *et al:* The comparative potency and pharmacokinetics of pancuronium and its metabolites in anesthetized man. J Pharmacol Exp Ther 207:539, 1978
36. Szeto HH, Inturrisi CE, Houde R *et al:* Accumulation of normeperidine, an active metabolite of meperidine, in patients with renal failure or cancer. Ann Intern Med 86:738, 1977
37. Bennett WM: Geriatric pharmacokinetics and the kidney. Am J Kidney Dis 26:283, 1990
38. Stanski DR, Watkins WD: Drug Disposition in Anesthesia, p 76. New York, Grune & Stratton, 1982
39. Hollenberg PF: Mechanisms of cytochrome P450 and peroxidase-catalyzed xenobiotic metabolism. Fed Am Soc Exp Biol J 6:686, 1992
40. de Groot H, Sies H: Cytochrome P-450, reductive metabolism, and cell injury. Drug Metab Rev 20:275, 1989
41. Anzenbacher P, Anzenbackerová E: Cytochromes P450 and metabolism of xenobiotics. Cell Mol Life Sci 58:737, 2001
42. Hall SD, Thummel KE, Watkins PB *et al:* Molecular and physical mechanisms of first-pass extraction. Drug Metab Dispos 27:161, 1999
43. Nelson DR, Koymans L, Kamataki T *et al*: P450 superfamily: update on new sequences, gene mapping, accession numbers and nomenclature Pharmacogenetics 6:1, 1996
44. Lewis DFV: Human cytochromes P450 associated with the phase I metabolism of drugs and other xenobiotics: A compilation of substrates and inhibitors of the CYP1, CYP2, and CYP3 families. Curr Med Chem 10:1955, 2003
45. Nebert DW, Russell DW: Clinical importance of the cytochromes P450. Lancet 360:1155, 2002
46. Gonzalez FJ, Nebert DW: Evolution of the P-450 gene superfamily: Animal–plant warfare, molecular drive and human genetic differences in drug oxidation. Trends Genet 6:182, 1990
47. Okey AB: Enzyme induction in the cytochrome P-450 system. Pharmacol Ther 45:241, 1990
48. Guay DRP, Meatherall RC, Chalmers JL *et al:* Cimetidine alters pethidine disposition in man. Br J Clin Pharmacol 18:907, 1984
49. Feely J, Wilkinson GR, Wood AJJ: Reduction of liver blood flow and propranolol metabolism by cimetidine. N Engl J Med 304:692, 1981
50. Klotz U, Reimann I: Delayed clearance of diazepam due to cimetidine. N Engl J Med 302:1012, 1980
51. Smith SR, Kendall MJ: Ranitidine *versus* cimetidine: A comparison of their potential to cause clinically important drug interactions. Clin Pharmacokinet 15:44, 1988
52. Schlanz KD, Myre SA, Bottoroff MB: Pharmacokinetic interactions with calcium channel antagonists (Parts I and II). Clin Pharmacokinet 21:344, 448, 1991
53. Cupp MJ, Tracy TS: Cytochrome P450: New nomenclature and clinical implications. Am Fam Physician 57:107, 1998
54. Ingelman-Sundberg M: Pharmacogenetics of cytochrome P450 and its applications in drug therapy: The past, present and future. Trend Pharmacol Sci 25:193, 2004
55. Venkatakrishnan K, von Moltke LL, Greeblatt DJ: Human drug metabolism and the cytochromes P450: Application and relevance of *in vitro* models. J Clin Pharmacol 41:1149, 2001
56. Daly AK: Pharmacogenetics of the major polymorphic metabolizing enzymes. Fund Clin Pharmacol 17:27, 2003
57. Wormhoudt LW, Commandeur JNM, Vermeulen NPE: Genetic polymorphisms of human *N*-acetyltransferase, cytochrome P450, glutathione-*S*-transferase, and epoxide hydrolase enzymes: Relevance to xenobiotic metabolism and toxicity. Crit Rev Toxicol 29:59, 1999
58. Ingelman-Sundberg M: Polymorphism of cytochrome P450 and xenobiotic toxicity. Toxicology 181–182:447, 2002
59. Pirmohamed M, Park BK: Cytochrome P450 enzyme polymorphisms and adverse drug reactions. Toxicology 192:23, 2003
60. Alcorn J, McNamara PJ: Ontogeny of hepatic and renal systemic clearance pathways in infants (Parts I and II). Clin Pharmacokinet 41:959 and 1077, 2002
61. Hämmerlein A, Derendorf H, Lowanthal DT: Pharmacokinetic and pharmacodynamic changes in the elderly. Clin Pharmacokinet 35:49, 1998
62. Meibohm B, Beierle I, Derendorf H: How important are gender differences in pharmacokinetics? Clin Pharmacokinet 41:329, 2002
63. Schwartz JB: The influence of sex on pharmacokinetics. Clin Pharmacokinet 42:107, 2003
64. Lane EA, Guthrie S, Linnoila M: Effects of ethanol on drug and metabolite pharmacokinetics. Clin Pharmacokinet 10:228, 1985
65. Miller LG: Recent developments in the study of the effects of cigarette smoking on clinical pharmacokinetics and clinical pharmacodynamics. Clin Pharmacokinet 17:90, 1989
66. Williams RL, Mamelok RD: Hepatic disease and drug pharmacokinetics. Clin Pharmacokinet 5:528, 1980
67. Rodighiero V. Effects of liver disease on pharmacokinetics (An update). Clin Pharmacokinet 37:399, 1999
68. Pinchette V, Leblond FA: Drug metabolism in renal failure. Curr Drug Metab 4:91, 2003
69. Reilly CS, Wood AJJ, Koshakji RP *et al:* The effect of halothane on drug disposition: Contribution of changes in intrinsic drug metabolizing capacity and hepatic blood flow. Anesthesiology 63:70, 1985
70. Wood M, Wood AJJ: Contrasting effects of halothane, isoflurane, and enflurane on in vivo drug metabolism in the rat. Anesth Analg 63:709, 1984
71. Vesell ES: The antipyrine test in clinical pharmacology: Conceptions and misconceptions. Clin Pharmacol Ther 26:275, 1979
72. Duvaldestin P, Mazze RI, Nivoche Y *et al:* Enzyme induction following surgery with halothane and neurolept anesthesia. Anesth Analg 60:319, 1981
73. Loft S, Boel J, Kyst A *et al:* Increased hepatic microsomal enzyme activity after surgery under halothane or spinal anesthesia. Anesthesiology 62:11, 1985
74. Duvaldestin P, Mauge F, Desmonts JM: Enflurane anesthesia and antipyrine metabolism. Clin Pharmacol Ther 29:61, 1981
75. Pessayre D, Allemand H, Benoist C *et al:* Effect of surgery under general anaesthesia on antipyrine clearance. Br J Clin Pharmacol 6:505, 1978
76. Pantuck EJ, Pantuck CB, Weismann C *et al:* Effects of parenteral nutrition regimens on oxidative drug metabolism. Anesthesiology 60:534, 1984
77. Wood M: Plasma drug binding—Implications for anesthesiologists. Anesth Analg 65:786, 1986
78. McLain DA, Hug CC: Intravenous fentanyl kinetics. Clin Pharmacol Ther 28:106, 1980
79. Meuldermans WEG, Hurkmans RMA, Heykants JJP: Plasma protein binding and distribution of fentanyl, sufentanil, alfentanil and lofentanil in blood. Arch Int Pharmacodynam 257:4, 1982
80. Sjoholm I, Ekman B, Kober A *et al:* Binding of drugs to serum albumin: XI. Mol Pharmacol 16:767, 1979
81. Holmberg L, Odar-Cederlof I, Nilsson JLG *et al:* Pethidine binding to blood cells and plasma proteins in old and young subjects. Eur J Clin Pharmacol 23:457, 1982
82. Säwe J: High-dose morphine and methadone in cancer patients. Clinical pharmacokinetic considerations of oral treatment. Clin Pharmacokinet 11:87, 1986
83. Olsen GD, Bennett WM, Porter GA: Morphine and phenytoin binding to plasma proteins in renal and hepatic failure. Clin Pharmacol Ther 17:677, 1975

84. Patwardhan RV, Johnsson RJ, Hoyumpa A *et al:* Normal metabolism of morphine in cirrhosis. Gastroenterology 81:1006, 1981
85. Brand L, Mark LC, Snell MM *et al:* Physiologic disposition of methohexital in man. Anesthesiology 24:331, 1963
86. Kirkpatrick T, Cockshott ID, Douglas EJ, Nimmo WS: Pharmacokinetics of propofol (Diprivan) in elderly patients. Br J Anaesth 60:146, 1988
87. Burch PG, Stanski DR: Decreased protein binding and thiopental kinetics. Clin Pharmacol Ther 32:212, 1982
88. Duvaldestin P, Henzel D: Binding of tubocurarine, fazadinium, pancuronium, and Org NC45 to serum proteins in normal man and in patients with cirrhosis. Br J Anaesth 54:513, 1982
89. Wood M, Stone WJ, Wood AJJ: Plasma binding of pancuronium: Effects of age, sex, and disease. Anesth Analg 62:29, 1983
90. Roy JJ, Varin F: Physicochemical properties of neuromuscular blocking agents and their impact on the pharmacokinetic-pharmacodynamic relationship. Br J Anaesth 93:241, 2004
91. Tucker GT, Mather LM: Pharmacokinetics of local anaesthetic agents. Br J Anaesth 47:213, 1975
92. Lee A, Fagan D, Lamont M *et al:* Disposition kinetics of ropivacaine in humans. Anesth Analg 69:763, 1989
93. Mandelli M, Tognoni G, Garattini S: Clinical pharmacokinetics of diazepam. Clin Pharmacokinet 3:72, 1978
94. Greenblatt DJ: Clinical pharmacokinetics of oxazepam and lorazepam. Clin Pharmacokinet 6:89, 1981
95. Greenblatt DJ, Abernethy DR, Locniskar A *et al:* Effect of age, gender, and obesity on midazolam kinetics. Anesthesiology 61:27, 1984
96. Mooradian AD: Digitalis: An update of clinical pharmacokinetics, therapeutic monitoring techniques and treatment recommendations. Clin Pharmacokinet 15:165, 1988
97. Echizen H, Eichelbaum M: Clinical pharmacokinetics of verapamil, nifedipine and diltiazem. Clin Pharmacokinet 11:425, 1986
98. Lowenthal DT, Porter RS, Saris SD *et al:* Clinical pharmacology, pharmacodynamics and interactions with esmolol. Am J Cardiol 56:14F, 1985
99. Piafsky KM, Borga O, Odar-Cederlof I *et al:* Increased plasma protein binding of propranolol and chlorpromazine mediated by disease-induced elevations of plasma alpha$_1$-acid glycoprotein. N Engl J Med 299:1435, 1978
100. Notarianni LJ: Plasma protein binding of drugs in pregnancy and in neonates. Clin Pharmacokinet 18:20, 1990
101. Morgan DJ, Blackman GL, Paull JD *et al:* Pharmacokinetics and plasma binding of thiopental: II. Studies at cesarean section. Anesthesiology 54:474, 1981
102. Wood M, Wood AJJ: Changes in plasma drug binding and alpha$_1$-acid glycoprotein in mother and newborn infant. Clin Pharmacol Ther 29:522, 1981
103. Hill MD, Abramson FP: The significance of plasma protein binding on the fetal/maternal distribution of drugs at steady-state. Clin Pharmacokinet 14:156, 1988
104. Davis D, Grossman SH, Ketchell BB *et al:* The effects of age and smoking on the plasma protein binding of lignocaine and diazepam. Br J Clin Pharmacol 19:261, 1985
105. Verbeeck RK, Cardinal J-A, Wallace SM: Effect of age and sex on the plasma binding of acidic and basic drugs. Eur J Clin Pharmacol 27:91, 1984
106. Wallace S, Whiting B: Factors affecting drug binding in plasma of elderly patients. Br J Clin Pharmacol 3:327, 1976
107. Herman RJ, McAllister CB, Branch RA *et al:* Effect of age on meperidine disposition. Clin Pharmacol Ther 37:19, 1985
108. Greenblatt DJ, Allen MD, Harmatz JS *et al:* Diazepam disposition determinants. Clin Pharmacol Ther 27:301, 1980
109. Jung D, Mayersohn M, Perrier D *et al:* Thiopental disposition as a function of age in female patients undergoing surgery. Anesthesiology 56:263, 1982
110. Grandison MK, Boudinot FD: Age-related changes in protein binding of drugs: Implications for therapy. Clin Pharmacokinet 38:271, 2000
111. Thiessen JJ, Sellers EM, Denbeigh P *et al:* Plasma protein binding of diazepam and tolbutamide in chronic alcoholics. J Clin Pharmacol 16:345, 1976
112. Ghoneim MM, Pandya H: Plasma protein binding of thiopental in patients with impaired renal or hepatic function. Anesthesiology 42:545, 1975
113. Pandale G, Chaux F, Salvadori C *et al:* Thiopental pharmacokinetics in patients with cirrhosis. Anesthesiology 59:123, 1983
114. Reidenberg MM, Drayer DE: Alteration of drug–protein binding in renal disease. Clin Pharmacokinet 9(suppl 1):18, 1984
115. Grossman SH, Davis D, Kitchell BB *et al:* Diazepam and lidocaine plasma protein binding in renal disease. Clin Pharmacol Ther 31:350, 1982
116. Zini R, Riant P, Barré J, Tillement J-P: Disease-induced variations in plasma protein levels. Implications for drug dosage regimens. Clin Pharmacokinet 19:147, 218, 1990
117. Jackson PR, Tucker GT, Woods HF: Altered plasma drug binding in cancer: Role of alpha$_1$-acid glycoprotein and albumin. Clin Pharmacol Ther 32:295, 1982
118. Routledge PA, Stargel WW, Wagner GS *et al:* Increased alpha$_1$-acid glycoprotein and lidocaine disposition in myocardial infarction. Ann Intern Med 93:701, 1980
119. Routledge PA, Stargel WW, Wagner GS et al: Increased plasma protein binding in myocardial infarction. Br J Clin Pharmacol 9:438, 1980
120. Elfstrom J: Drug pharmacokinetics in the postoperative period. Clin Pharmacokinet 4:16, 1979
121. Edwards DJ, Lalka D, Cerra F *et al:* Alpha$_1$-acid glycoprotein concentration and protein binding in trauma. Clin Pharmacol Ther 31:62, 1982
122. Fremstad D, Bergerud K, Haffner JFW *et al:* Increased plasma binding of quinidine after surgery: A preliminary report. Eur J Clin Pharmacol 10:441, 1976
123. Feely J, Forrest A, Gunn A *et al:* Influence of surgery on plasma propranolol levels and protein binding. Clin Pharmacol Ther 28:579, 1980
124. Holley FO, Ponganis KV, Stanski DR: Effects of cardiac surgery with cardiopulmonary bypass on lidocaine disposition. Clin Pharmacol Ther 35:617, 1984
125. Balant LP, Gex-Fabry M: Physiological pharmacokinetic modelling. Xenobiotica 20:1241, 1990
126. Eger EI II: Anesthetic Uptake and Action, p 79. Baltimore, Williams & Wilkins, 1974
127. Gibaldi M, Perrier D: Pharmacokinetics, 2nd ed, p 45. New York, Marcel Dekker, 1982
128. Wagner JH: Linear pharmacokinetic equations allowing direct calculation of many needed pharmacokinetic parameters from the coefficients and exponents of polyexponential equations which have been fitted to the data. J Pharmacokinet Biopharm 4:443, 1976
129. Gibaldi M, Weintraub H: Some considerations as to the determination and significance of biologic half-life. J Pharm Sci 60:624, 1971
130. Hudson RJ, Stanski DR, Burch PG: Pharmacokinetics of methohexital and thiopental in surgical patients. Anesthesiology 59:215, 1983
131. Rowland M: Protein binding and drug clearance. Clin Pharmacokinet 9(suppl 1):10, 1984
132. Branch RA, James J, Read AE: A study of factors influencing drug disposition in chronic liver disease, using the model drug (+)-propranolol. Br J Clin Pharmacol 3:243, 1976
133. Holford NHG, Sheiner LB: Understanding the dose–effect relationship: Clinical application of pharmacokinetic–pharmacodynamic models. Clin Pharmacokinet 6:429, 1981
134. Stanski DR, Hudson RJ, Homer TD *et al:* Pharmacodynamic modelling of thiopental anesthesia. J Pharmacokinet Biopharm 12:223, 1984
135. Stanski DR, Maitre PO: Population pharmacokinetics and pharmacodynamics of thiopental: The effect of age revisited. Anesthesiology 72:412, 1990
136. Scott JC, Ponganis KV, Stanski DR: EEG quantitation of narcotic effect: The comparative pharmacodynamics of fentanyl and alfentanil. Anesthesiology 62:234, 1985
137. Scott JC, Cooke JE, Stanski DR: Electroencephalographic quantitation of opioid effect: Comparative pharmacodynamics of fentanyl and sufentanil. Anesthesiology 74:34, 1991
138. Stanski DR, Ham J, Miller RD *et al:* Pharmacokinetics and pharmacodynamics of *d*-tubocurarine during nitrous oxide–narcotic and halothane anesthesia in man. Anesthesiology 51:235, 1979
139. Fisher DM, O'Keeffe C, Stanski DR *et al:* Pharmacokinetics and pharmacodynamics of *d*-tubocurarine in infants, children, and adults. Anesthesiology 57:203, 1982
140. Waud BE, Waud DR: The margin of safety of neuromuscular transmission in the muscle of the diaphragm. Anesthesiology 37:417, 1972
141. Norman J: Drug–receptor reactions. Br J Anaesth 51:595, 1979
142. Feldman S: Neuromuscular blocking agents. In Feldman SA, Paton W, Scurr C (eds): Mechanisms of Drugs in Anaesthesia, 2nd ed, p 340. London, Hodder & Stoughton, 1993
143. Ooi R: Effects of drugs on ion channels and transmembrane signalling. In Feldman SA, Paton W, Scurr C (eds): Mechanisms of Drugs in Anaesthesia, 2nd ed, p 32. London, Hodder & Stoughton, 1993
144. Ooi R: Effects of drugs on ion channels and transmembrane signalling. In Feldman SA, Paton W, Scurr C (eds): Mechanisms of Drugs in Anaesthesia, 2nd ed, p 34. London, Hodder & Stoughton, 1993
145. Jenkinson DH: An introduction to receptors and their actions. In Feldman SA, Paton W, Scurr C (eds): Mechanisms of Drugs in Anaesthesia, 2nd ed, p 14. London, Hodder & Stoughton, 1993
146. Cullen BF, Miller MG: Drug interactions in anesthesia. Anesth Analg 58:413, 1979
147. Mutch WAC, Thomson IR: Delivery systems for intravenous nitroglycerin. Can Anaesth Soc J 30:98, 1983
148. Koren G, Goresky G, Crean P *et al:* Pediatric fentanyl dosing based on pharmacokinetics during cardiac surgery. Anesth Analg 63:577, 1984
149. Rawlins MD: Drug interactions and anaesthesia. Br J Anaesth 50:689, 1978
150. Vinik HR, Bradley EL Jr, Kissin I: Midazolam–alfentanil synergism for anesthetic induction in patients. Anesth Analg 69:213, 1989
151. Kissin I, Vinik HR, Castillo R, Bradley EL Jr: Alfentanil potentiates midazolam-induced unconsciousness in subanalgesic doses. Anesth Analg 71:65, 1990
152. Quasha AL, Eger EI II, Tinker JH: Determinations and applications of MAC. Anesthesiology 53:315, 1980
153. Schlotterbeck D: Infusion pumps and their safety in the OR. Anesthesia Patient Safety Foundation Newsletter 15:15, 2000
154. McLeskey C: Drug recognition. Infusion pumps and their safety in the OR. Anesthesia Patient Safety Foundation Newsletter 15:14, 2000
155. Tong D, Chung F: Recall after total intravenous anaesthesia due to an equipment misuse. Can J Anaesth 44:73, 1997
156. Hee HI, Lim SL, Tan SS: Infusion technology: A cause for alarm. Paediatr Anaesth 12:780, 2002

157. Kelly D, Brull SJ: The cost of modern technology. J Clin Anesth 7:80, 1995
158. Roland M, Tozer T: Time to reach plateau. In Roland M, Tozer T (eds): Clinical Pharmacokinetics, 2nd ed, p 311. Philadelphia, Lea & Febiger, 1989
159. Shafer SL, Stanski DR: Improving the clinical utility of anesthetic drug pharmacokinetics. Anesthesiology 76:327, 1992
160. Schnider TW, Minto CF, Gambus PL *et al*: The influence of method of administration and covariates on the pharmacokinetics of propofol in adult volunteers. Anesthesiology 88:1170, 1988
161. Shafer S: Towards optimal intravenous dosing strategies. Semin Anesth 12:222, 1994
162. Han T, Kim D, Kil H, Inagaki Y: The effects of plasma fentanyl concentrations on propofol requirement, emergence from anesthesia, and postoperative analgesia in propofol-nitrous oxide anesthesia. Anesth Analg 90:1365, 2000
163. Schwilden H: A general method for calculating the dosage scheme in linear pharmacokinetics. Eur J Clin Pharmacol 20:379, 1981
164. Schwilden H, Schuttler J, Stoekel H: Pharmacokinetics as applied to total intravenous anaesthesia. Theoretical considerations. Anaesthesia 38 (suppl):51, 1983
165. Shafer SL, Varvel JR, Aziz N *et al*: Pharmacokinetics of fentanyl administered by computer-controlled infusion pump. Anesthesiology 73:1091, 1990
166. Alvis JM, Reves JG, Govier AV *et al*: Computer-assisted continuous infusions of fentanyl during cardiac anesthesia: Comparison with a manual method. Anesthesiology 63:41, 1985
167. Shafer SL, Varvel JR: Pharmacokinetics, pharmacodynamics, and rational opioid selection. Anesthesiology 74:53, 1991
168. Hughes MA, Glass PS, Jacobs JR: Context-sensitive half-time in multicompartment pharmacokinetic models for intravenous anesthetic drugs. Anesthesiology 76:334, 1992
169. Barvais L, Cantraine F, D'Hollander A *et al*: Predictive accuracy of continuous alfentanil infusion in volunteers: Variability of different pharmacokinetic sets. Anesth Analg 77:801, 1993
170. Barvais L, Heitz D, Schmartz D *et al*: Pharmacokinetic model-driven infusion of sufentanil and midazolam during cardiac surgery: Assessment of the prospective predictive accuracy and the quality of anesthesia. J Cardiothorac Vasc Anesth 14:402, 2000
171. Barvais L, D'Hollander AA, Cantraine F *et al*: Predictive accuracy of midazolam in adult patients scheduled for coronary surgery. J Clin Anesth 6:297, 1994
172. Veselis RA, Glass P, Dnistrian A *et al*: Performance of computer-assisted continuous infusion at low concentrations of intravenous sedatives. Anesth Analg 84:1049, 1997
173. Vuyk J, Engbers FH, Burm AG *et al*: Performance of computer-controlled infusion of propofol: An evaluation of five pharmacokinetic parameter sets. Anesth Analg 81:1275, 1995
174. Schraag S, Flaschar J: Delivery performance of commercial target-controlled infusion devices with Diprifusor module. Eur J Anaesthesiol 19:357, 2002
175. Passot S, Servin F, Allary R *et al*: Target-controlled versus manually-controlled infusion of propofol for direct laryngoscopy and bronchoscopy. Anesth Analg 94:1212, 2002
176. Russell D, Wilkes MP, Hunter SC *et al*: Manual compared with target-controlled infusion of propofol. Br J Anaesth 75:562, 1995
177. Suttner S, Boldt J, Schmidt C *et al*: Cost analysis of target-controlled infusion-based anesthesia compared with standard anesthesia regimens. Anesth Analg 88:77, 1999
178. Gale T, Leslie K, Kluger M: Propofol anaesthesia via target controlled infusion or manually controlled infusion: Effects on the bispectral index as a measure of anaesthetic depth. Anaesth Intensive Care 29:579, 2001
179. Checketts MR, Gilhooly CJ, Kenny GN: Patient-maintained analgesia with target-controlled alfentanil infusion after cardiac surgery: a comparison with morphine PCA. Br J Anaesth 80:748, 1998
180. van den Nieuwenhuyzen MC, Engbers FH, Burm AG *et al*: Target-controlled infusion of alfentanil for postoperative analgesia: Contribution of plasma protein binding to intra-patient and inter-patient variability. Br J Anaesth 82:580, 1999
181. Irwin MG, Thompson N, Kenny GN: Patient-maintained propofol sedation. Assessment of a target-controlled infusion system. Anaesthesia 52:525, 1997
182. Minto CF, Schnider TW, Gregg KM *et al*: Using the time of maximum effect site concentration to combine pharmacokinetics and pharmacodynamics. Anesthesiology 99:324, 2003
183. Shafer SL, Gregg KM: Algorithms to rapidly achieve and maintain stable drug concentrations at the site of drug effect with a computer-controlled infusion pump. J Pharmacokinet Biopharm 20:147, 1992
184. Henthorn TK, Krejcie TC, Shanks CA *et al:* Time-dependent distribution volume and kinetics of the pharmacodynamic effector site [letter]. J Pharm Sci 81:1136, 1992
185. Krejcie TC, Avram MJ: What determines anesthetic induction dose? It's the front-end kinetics, doctor! Anesth Analg 89:541, 1999
186. Kuipers JA, Boer F, Olofsen E *et al:* Recirculatory and compartmental pharmacokinetic modeling of alfentanil in pigs: The influence of cardiac output. Anesthesiology 90:1146, 1999
187. Kuipers JA, Boer F, Olofsen E *et al*: Recirculatory pharmacokinetics and pharmacodynamics of rocuronium in patients: the influence of cardiac output. Anesthesiology 94:47, 2001
188. Wada DR, Ward DS: The hybrid model: A new pharmacokinetic model for computer-controlled infusion pumps. IEEE Trans Biomed Eng 41:134, 1994
189. Avram MJ, Krejcie TC: Using front-end kinetics to optimize target-controlled drug infusions. Anesthesiology 99:1078, 2003
190. Woodruff EA, Martin JF, Omens M: A model for the design and evaluation of algorithms for closed-loop cardiovascular therapy. IEEE Trans Biomed Eng 44:694, 1997
191. Tehrani F, Rogers M, Lo T *et al*: Closed-loop control if the inspired fraction of oxygen in mechanical ventilation. J Clin Monit Comput 17:367, 2002
192. Renard E: Implantable closed-loop glucose-sensing and insulin delivery: the future for insulin pump therapy. Curr Opin Pharmacol 2:708, 2002
193. O'Hara DA, Hexem JG, Derbyshire GJ *et al*: The use of a PID controller to model vecuronium pharmacokinetics and pharmacodynamics during liver transplantation. Proportional-integral-derivative. IEEE Trans Biomed Eng 44:610, 1997
194. Schwilden H, Schuttler J, Stoeckel H: Closed-loop feedback control of methohexital anesthesia by quantitative EEG analysis in humans. Anesthesiology 67:341, 1987
195. Absalom AR, Kenny GN: Closed-loop control of propofol anaesthesia using bispectral index: Performance assessment in patients receiving computer-controlled propofol and manually controlled remifentanil infusions for minor surgery. Br J Anaesth 90:737, 2003
196. Struys MM, De Smet T, Greenwald S *et al*: Performance evaluation of two published closed-loop control systems using bispectral index monitoring: A simulation study. Anesthesiology 100:640, 2004
197. Allen R, Smith D: Neuro-fuzzy closed-loop control of depth of anaesthesia. Artif Intell Med 21:185, 2001
198. Kenny GN, Mantzaridis H: Closed-loop control of propofol anaesthesia. Br J Anaesth 83:223, 1999
199. Westenskow DR: Closed-loop control of blood pressure, ventilation, and anesthesia delivery. Int J Clin Monit Comput 4:69, 1987
200. Tzabazis A, Ihmsen H, Schywalsky M *et al*: EEG-controlled closed-loop dosing of propofol in rats. Br J Anaesth 92:564, 2004
201. Mortier E, Struys M, De Smet T *et al*: Closed-loop controlled administration of propofol using bispectral analysis. Anaesthesia 53:749, 1998
202. Absalom AR, Sutcliffe N, Kenny GN: Closed-loop control of anesthesia using Bispectral index: performance assessment in patients undergoing major orthopedic surgery under combined general and regional anesthesia. Anesthesiology 96:67, 2002
203. Vanluchene AL, Vereecke H, Thas O *et al*: Spectral entropy as an electroencephalographic measure of anesthetic drug effect: A comparison with bispectral index and processed midlatency auditory evoked response. Anesthesiology 101:34, 2004
204. Struys MM, De Smet T, Depoorter B *et al*: Comparison of plasma compartment versus two methods for effect compartment-controlled target-controlled infusion for propofol. Anesthesiology 92:399, 2000

CHAPTER 12 ■ AUTONOMIC NERVOUS SYSTEM: PHYSIOLOGY AND PHARMACOLOGY

NOEL W. LAWSON AND JOEL O. JOHNSON

KEY POINTS

1. The autonomic nervous system (ANS) participates in nearly all of the physiologic processes of the human body and an understanding of its function is essential for anesthesiologists.
2. The function of the ANS is intimately tied to neurohumeral mechanisms covered elsewhere in the text.
3. Perioperative β-blockade has been proven to be beneficial in certain patients with compromised cardiovascular function.
4. Knowledge of the effects of prescribed oral medication on the ANS is essential in the perioperative management of the surgical patient.
5. Angiotensin-converting enzyme (ACE) inhibitors may precipitate hypotension in the perioperative patient.

AUTONOMIC PHARMACOLOGY

Anesthesiology is the practice of autonomic medicine. Drugs that produce anesthesia also produce potent autonomic side effects. The greater part of our training and practice is spent acquiring skills in averting or utilizing the autonomic nervous system (ANS) side effects of anesthetic drugs under a variety of pathophysiologic conditions. The success of any anesthetic depends on how well homeostasis is maintained. The numbers that we faithfully record during the course of anesthesia reflect ANS function and not necessarily the presence of surgical anesthesia.

AUTONOMIC NERVOUS SYSTEM PURPOSE

1 The ANS includes that part of the central and peripheral nervous system concerned with involuntary regulation of cardiac muscle, smooth muscle, glandular, and visceral functions. ANS activity refers to visceral reflexes that function essentially below the conscious level. The term autonomic remains the best description of this ubiquitous system, as opposed to automatic. ANS implies self-controlling, whereas automatic implies nonreflexic or intrinsic responses; however, the use of "autonomy" to describe this nervous system is illusory. The ANS is also

responsive to changes in somatic motor and sensory activities of the body. The physiologic evidence of visceral reflexes as a result of somatic events is abundantly clear. Psychosomatic disease is an expression of this connection. The ANS is therefore not as distinct an entity as the term suggests. Neither somatic nor ANS activity occurs in isolation.[1] The ANS organizes visceral support for somatic behavior and adjusts body states in anticipation of emotional behavior or responses to the stress of disease (i.e., fight or flight).

Traditionally, the ANS has been viewed as strictly a peripheral, efferent (motor) system. This concept is no longer tenable. Afferent fibers from visceral structures are the first link in the reflex arcs of the ANS, whether relaying visceral pain or changes in vessel stretch. Most ANS efferent fibers are accompanied by sensory fibers that are now commonly recognized as components of the ANS. However, the afferent components of the ANS cannot be as distinctively divided as can the efferent nerves. ANS visceral sensory nerves are anatomically indistinguishable from somatic sensory nerves. The clinical importance of visceral afferent fibers is more closely associated with chronic pain management.

FUNCTIONAL ANATOMY

The ANS falls into two divisions by anatomy, physiology, and pharmacology. Langley divided this nervous system into two parts in 1921. He retained the term "sympathetic" (SNS) introduced by Willis in 1665 for the first part and introduced the term parasympathetic (parasympathetic nervous system, PNS) for the second. The term "autonomic nervous system" was adopted as a comprehensive name for both. Ordinarily, activation of the SNS produces expenditure of body energy, whereas the PNS produces conservation or accumulation of energy resources. Table 12-1 lists the complementary effects of SNS (adrenergic) and PNS (cholinergic) activity of organ systems.

Central Autonomic Organization

Pure central ANS or somatic centers are not known. An extensive overlap of function occurs. Integration of ANS activity occurs at all levels of the cerebrospinal axis. Efferent ANS

TABLE 12-1

HOMEOSTATIC BALANCE BETWEEN ADRENERGIC AND CHOLINERGIC EFFECTS

ORGAN SYSTEM	RESPONSE	
	ADRENERGIC	CHOLINERGIC
HEART		
Sinoatrial node	Tachycardia	Bradycardia
Atrioventricular node	Increased conduction	Decreased conduction
His-purkinje	Increased automaticity and conduction velocity	Minimal
Myocardium	Increased contractility, conduction velocity, automaticity	Minimal decrease in contractility
Coronary vessels	Constriction (α_1) and dilation (β_1)	Dilation and constriction?[a]
BLOOD VESSELS		
Skin and mucosa	Constriction	Dilation
Skeletal muscle	Constriction (α_1) > dilation (β_2)	Dilation
Pulmonary	Constriction	?Dilation
BRONCHIAL SMOOTH MUSCLE	Relaxation	Contraction
GASTROINTESTINAL TRACT		
Gallbladder and ducts	Relaxation	Contraction
Gut motility	Decreased	Increased
Secretions	Decreased	Increased
Sphincters	Constriction	Relaxation
BLADDER		
Detrusor	Relaxes	Contracts
Trigone	Contracts	Relaxes
GLANDS		
Nasal Lacrimal Parotid Submandibular Gastric Pancreatic	Vasoconstriction and reduced secretion	Stimulation of secretions
SWEAT GLANDS	Diaphoresis (cholinergic)	None
APOCRINE GLANDS	Thick, odiferous secretion	None
EYE		
Pupil	Mydriasis	Miosis
Ciliary muscle	Relaxation for far vision	Contraction for near vision

[a] See the Interaction of Autonomic Nervous System Receptors section.

TABLE 12-2

HYPOTHALAMIC NUCLEI

■ ANTERIOR	■ POSTERIOR
PARAVENTRICULAR NUCLEUS Oxytocin release Water conservation **MEDIAL PREOPTIC AREA** Bladder contraction Decreased heart rate Decreased blood pressure **SUPRAOPTIC NUCLEUS** Water conservation **POSTERIOR PREOPTIC AND ANTERIOR HYPOTHALAMIC AREA** Body temperature regulation Panting Sweating Thyrotropin inhibition	**POSTERIOR HYPOTHALAMUS** Increased blood pressure Pupillary dilation Shivering Corticotropin **DORSOMEDIAL NUCLEUS** Gastrointestinal stimulation **PERIFORNICAL NUCLEUS** Hunger Increased blood pressure Rage **VENTROMEDIAL NUCLEUS** Satiety **MAMMILLARY BODY** Feeding reflexes **LATERAL HYPOTHALAMIC AREA** Thirst and hunger

activity can be initiated locally and by centers located in the spinal cord, brainstem, and hypothalamus. The cerebral cortex is the highest level of ANS integration. Fainting at the sight of blood is an example of this higher level of somatic and ANS integration. ANS function has also been successfully modulated through conscious, intentional efforts demonstrating that somatic responses are always accompanied by visceral responses and vice versa.

The principal site of ANS organization is the hypothalamus. SNS functions are controlled by nuclei in the posterolateral hypothalamus. Stimulation of these nuclei results in a massive discharge of the sympathoadrenal system (Table 12-2). PNS functions are governed by nuclei in the midline and some anterior nuclei of the hypothalamus. The anterior hypothalamus is involved with regulation of temperature. The supraoptic hypothalamic nuclei regulate water metabolism and are anatomically and functionally associated with the posterior lobe of the pituitary (see Interaction of Autonomic Nervous System Receptors section). This hypothalamic–neurohypophyseal connection represents a central ANS mechanism that affects the kidney by means of antidiuretic hormone. Long-term blood pressure control, reactions to physical and emotional stress, sleep, and sexual reflexes are regulated through the hypothalamus.

The medulla oblongata and pons are the vital centers of acute ANS organization. Together, they integrate momentary hemodynamic adjustments and maintain the sequence and automaticity of ventilation. Integration of afferent and efferent ANS impulses at this central nervous system (CNS) level is responsible for the tonic activity exhibited by the ANS. Control of peripheral vascular resistance and blood pressure is an example of this tonic activity. Tonicity holds visceral organs in a state of intermediate activity that can either be diminished or be augmented by altering the rate of nerve firing. The nucleus tractus solitarius, located within the medulla, is the primary area for relay of afferent chemoreceptor and baroreceptor information from the glossopharyngeal and vagus nerves. Increased afferent impulses from these two nerves inhibit peripheral SNS vascular tone, producing vasodilation, and increase vagal tone, producing bradycardia. High spinal cord transection eliminates the medulla and results in hypotension. Studies of patients with high spinal cord lesions show that a number of reflex changes are mediated at the spinal or segmental level. ANS hyperreflexia is an example of spinal cord mediation of ANS reflexes without integration of function from higher inhibitory centers.[1]

Peripheral Autonomic Nervous System Organization

The peripheral ANS is the efferent (motor) component of the ANS and consists of two complementary parts: the SNS and the PNS. Most organs receive fibers from both divisions (Fig. 12-1). In general, activities of the two systems produce opposite but complementary effects (see Table 12-1). Actions of the two subdivisions are supplementary in some tissues such as the salivary glands. A few tissues, such as sweat glands and spleen, are innervated by only SNS fibers. Although the anatomy of the somatic and ANS sensory pathways is identical, the motor pathways are characteristically different. The efferent somatic motor system, like somatic afferents, is composed of a single (unipolar) neuron with its cell body in the ventral gray matter of the spinal cord. Its myelinated axon extends directly to the voluntary striated muscle unit. In contrast, the efferent (motor) ANS is a two-neuron (bipolar) chain from the CNS to the effector organ (Fig. 12-2). The first neuron of both the SNS and PNS originates within the CNS but does not make direct contact with the effector organ. Instead, it relays the impulse to a second station known as an ANS ganglion, which contains the cell body of the second ANS (postganglionic) neuron. Its axon contacts the effector organ. Thus, the motor pathways of both divisions of the ANS are schematically a serial, two-neuron chain consisting of a preganglionic neuron and a postganglionic effector neuron (Fig. 12-3).

Preganglionic fibers of both subdivisions are myelinated with diameters of less than 3 mm.[1] Impulses are conducted at a speed of 3 to 15 m/s The postganglionic fibers are unmyelinated and conduct impulses at slower speeds of less than 2 m/s. They are similar to unmyelinated visceral and somatic afferent C fibers (Table 12-3). Compared with the myelinated somatic nerves, the ANS conducts impulses at speeds that preclude its participation in the immediate phase of a somatic response.

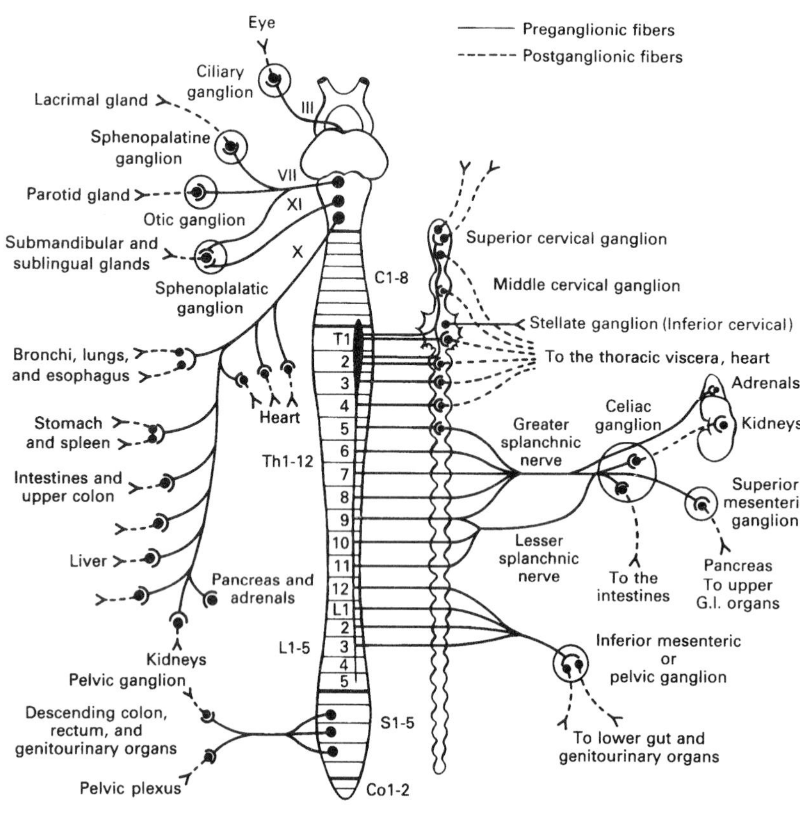

FIGURE 12-1. Schematic distribution of the craniosacral (parasympathetic) and thoracolumbar (sympathetic) nervous systems. Parasympathetic preganglionic fibers pass directly to the organ that is innervated. Their postganglionic cell bodies are situated near or within the innervated viscera. This limited distribution of parasympathetic postganglionic fibers is consistent with the discrete and limited effect of parasympathetic function. The postganglionic sympathetic neurons originate in either the paired sympathetic ganglia or one of the unpaired collateral plexuses. One preganglionic fiber influences many postganglionic neurons. Activation of the SNS produces a more diffuse physiologic response rather than discrete effects.

Sympathetic Nervous System or Thoracolumbar Division

The efferent SNS is referred to as the thoracolumbar nervous system. The origin of its preganglionic fibers provides the anatomic basis for this designation. Figure 12-1 demonstrates the distribution of the SNS and its innervation of visceral organs.

The preganglionic fibers of the SNS (thoracolumbar division) originate in the intermediolateral gray column of the 12 thoracic (T1-12) and the first three lumbar segments (L1-3) of the spinal cord. The myelinated axons of these nerve cells leave the spinal cord with the motor fibers to form the white (myelinated) communicating rami (Fig. 12-4). The rami enter one of the paired 22 sympathetic ganglia at their respective segmental levels. On entering the paravertebral ganglia of the lateral sympathetic chain, the preganglionic fiber may follow

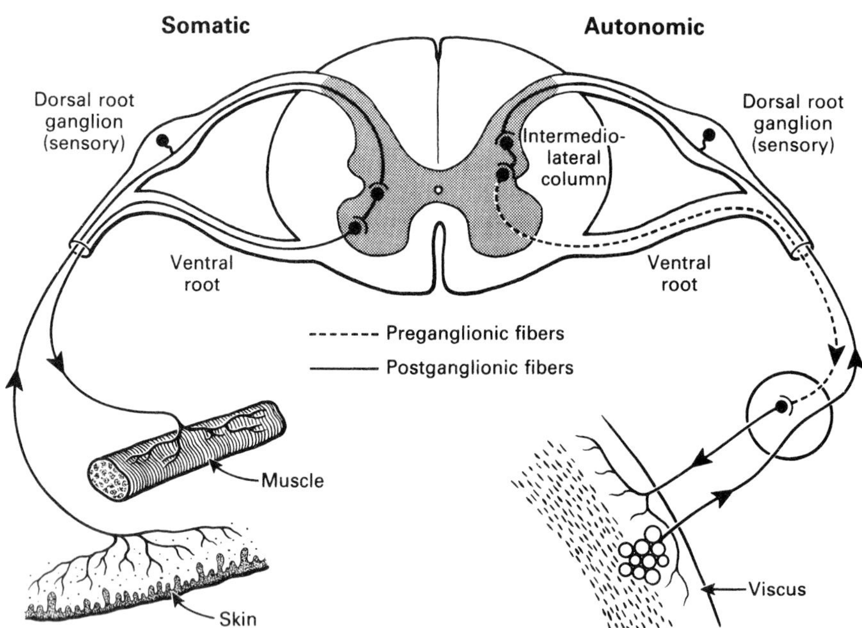

FIGURE 12-2. Comparison of somatic and autonomic reflex arcs. Somatic arcs are unipolar and autonomic arcs are bipolar.

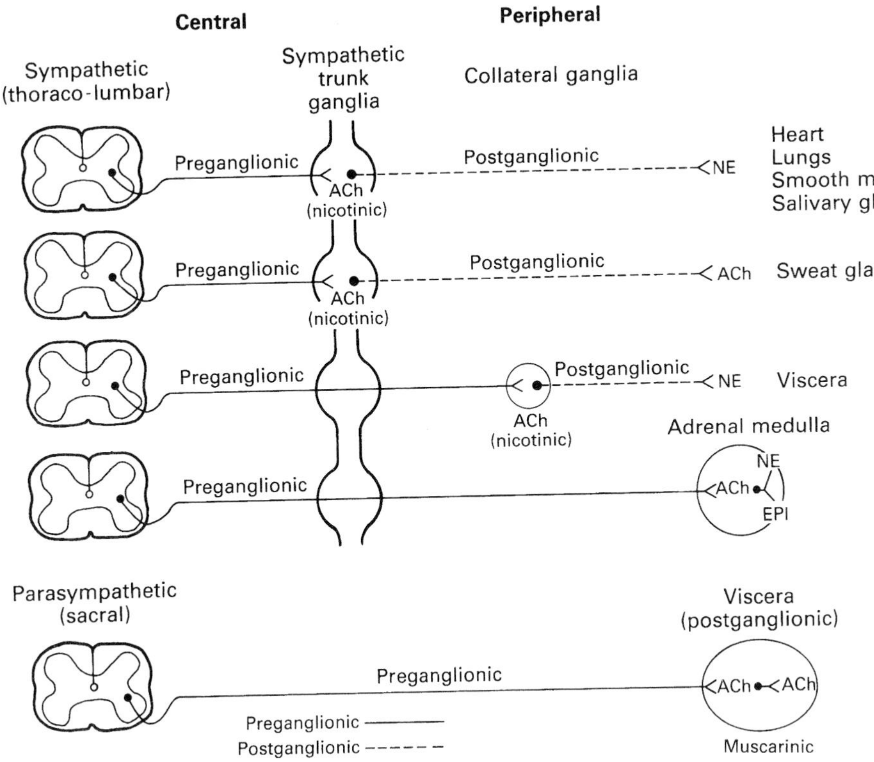

FIGURE 12-3. Schematic diagram of the efferent ANS. Afferent impulses are integrated centrally and sent reflexly to the adrenergic and cholinergic receptors. Sympathetic fibers ending in the adrenal medulla are preganglionic, and acetylcholine (ACh) is the neurotransmitter. Stimulation of the chromaffin cells, acting as postganglionic neurons, releases epinephrine (EPI) and norepinephrine (NE).

one of three courses: (1) synapse with postganglionic fibers in ganglia at the level of exit, (2) course upward or downward in the trunk of the SNS chain to synapse in ganglia at other levels, or (3) track for variable distances through the sympathetic chain and exit without synapsing to terminate in an outlying, unpaired, SNS collateral ganglion (see Fig. 12-4). The adrenal gland is an exception to the rule. Preganglionic fibers pass directly into the adrenal medulla without synapsing in a ganglion (see Fig. 12-3). The cells of the medulla are derived from neuronal tissue and are analogous to postganglionic neurons.

The sympathetic postganglionic neuronal cell bodies are located in ganglia of the paired lateral SNS chain or unpaired collateral ganglia in more peripheral plexuses. Collateral ganglia, such as the celiac and inferior mesenteric ganglia (plexus), are formed by the convergence of preganglionic fibers with many postganglionic neuronal bodies. SNS ganglia are almost always located closer to the spinal cord than to the organs they innervate. The sympathetic postganglionic neuron can therefore originate in either the paired lateral paravertebral SNS ganglia or one of the unpaired collateral plexus. The unmyelinated postganglionic fibers then proceed from the ganglia to terminate within the organs they innervate.

Many of the postganglionic fibers pass from the lateral SNS chain back into the spinal nerves, forming the gray (unmyelinated) communicating rami at all levels of the spinal cord (see Fig. 12-4). They are distributed distally to sweat glands, pilomotor muscle, and blood vessels of the skin and muscle. These nerves are unmyelinated C type fibers (see Table 12-3) and are carried within the somatic nerves. Approximately 8% of the fibers in the average somatic nerve are sympathetic.[1]

The first four or five thoracic spinal segments generate preganglionic fibers that ascend in the neck to form three special paired ganglia. These are the superior cervical, middle cervical, and cervicothoracic ganglia. The last is known as the stellate ganglion and is actually formed by the fusion of the inferior cervical and first thoracic SNS ganglia. These ganglia provide sympathetic innervation of the head, neck, upper extremities, heart, and lungs. Afferent pain fibers also travel with these nerves, accounting for chest, neck, or upper extremity pain with myocardial ischemia.

TABLE 12-3

CLASSIFICATION OF NERVE FIBERS

DESCRIPTION OF NERVE FIBERS	GROUP		DIAMETER (μm)	CONDUCTION VELOCITY (m/s)
Myelinated somatic	A	Alpha α	20	120
		Beta β		
		Gamma γ		5–40 (pain fibers)
		Delta δ	3–4	5–40 (pain fibers)
		Epsilon ϵ	2	5
Myelinated visceral (preganglionic autonomic)	B		<3	3–15
Unmyelinated somatic	C		<2	0.5–2 (pain fibers)

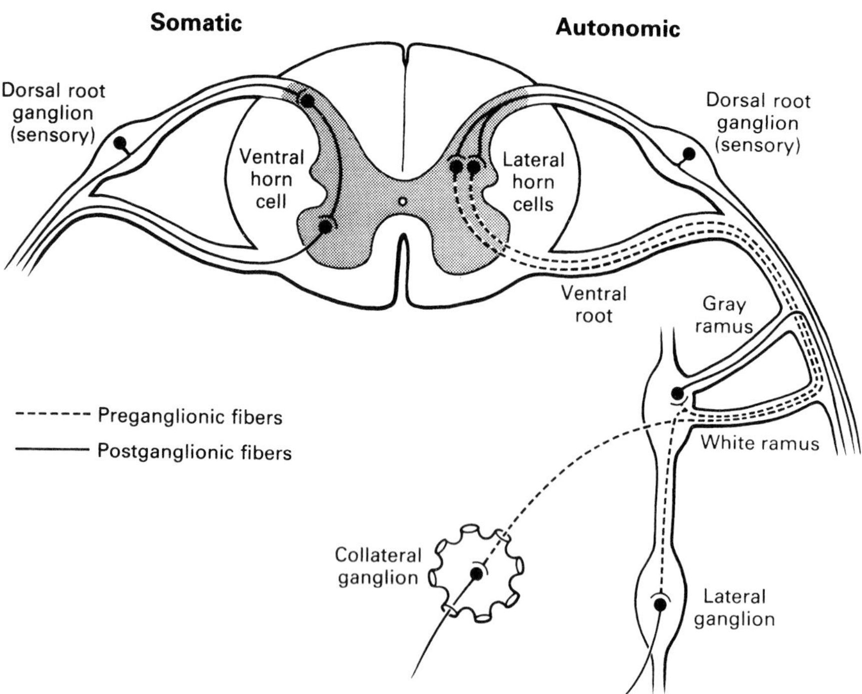

FIGURE 12-4. The spinal reflex arc of the somatic nerves is shown on the left. The different arrangements of neurons in the sympathetic system are shown on the right. Preganglionic fibers coming out through white rami may make synaptic connections following one of three courses: (1) synapse in ganglia at the level of exit, (2) course up or down the sympathetic chain to synapse at another level, or (3) exit the chain without synapsing to an outlying collateral ganglion.

Activation of the SNS produces a diffused physiologic response (mass reflex) rather than discrete effects. Function follows design. SNS postganglionic neurons outnumber the preganglionic neurons in an average ratio of 20:1 to 30:1.[2] One preganglionic fiber influences a larger number of postganglionic neurons, which are dispersed to many organs. In addition, the SNS response is augmented by the hormonal release of epinephrine (EPI) from the adrenal medulla.

Parasympathetic Nervous System or Craniosacral Division

The PNS, like the SNS, has both preganglionic and postganglionic neurons. This division is sometimes called the craniosacral outflow because the preganglionic cell bodies originate in the brainstem and sacral segments of the spinal cord. PNS preganglionic fibers are found in cranial nerves III (oculomotor), VII (facial), IX (glossopharyngeal), and X (vagus). The sacral outflow originates in the intermediolateral gray horns of the second, third, and fourth sacral nerves. Figure 12-1 shows the distribution of the PNS division and its innervation of visceral organs.

The vagus (cranial nerve X) nerve has the most extensive distribution of all the PNS, accounting for more than 75% of PNS activity. The paired vagus nerves supply PNS innervation to the heart, lungs, esophagus, stomach, small intestine, proximal half of the colon, liver, gallbladder, pancreas, and upper portions of the ureters. The sacral fibers form the pelvic visceral nerves, or nervi erigentes. These nerves supply the remainder of the viscera that are not innervated by the vagus. They supply the descending colon, rectum, uterus, bladder, and lower portions of the ureters and are primarily concerned with emptying. Various sexual reactions are also governed by the sacral PNS. The PNS is responsible for penile erection, but SNS stimulation governs ejaculation.

In contrast to the SNS division, PNS preganglionic fibers pass directly to the organ that is innervated. The postganglionic cell bodies are situated near or within the innervated viscera and generally are not visible. The proximity of PNS ganglia to or within the viscera provides a limited distribution of postganglionic fibers. The ratio of postganglionic to preganglionic fibers in many organs appears to be 1:1 to 3:1, compared with the 20:1 found in the SNS system. Auerbach's plexus in the distal colon is the exception, with a ratio of 8,000:1. The fact that PNS preganglionic fibers synapse with only a few postganglionic neurons is consistent with the discrete and limited effect of PNS function. For example, vagal bradycardia can occur without a concomitant change in intestinal motility or salivation. Mass reflex action is not a characteristic of the PNS. The effects of organ response to PNS stimulation are outlined in Table 12-1.

Autonomic Innervation

Heart

The heart is well supplied by the SNS and PNS. These nerves affect cardiac pumping in three ways: (1) by changing the rate (chronotropism), (2) by changing the strength of contraction (inotropism), and (3) by modulating coronary blood flow. The PNS cardiac vagal fibers approach the stellate ganglia and then join the efferent cardiac SNS fibers; therefore, the vagus nerve to the heart and lungs is a mixed nerve containing both PNS and SNS efferent fibers. The PNS fibers are distributed mainly to the sinoatrial and atrioventricular (AV) nodes and to a lesser extent to the atria. There is little or no distribution to the ventricles. Therefore, the main effect of vagal cardiac stimulation to the heart is chronotropic. Vagal stimulation decreases the rate of sinoatrial node discharge and decreases excitability of the AV junctional fibers, slowing impulse conduction to the ventricles. A strong vagal discharge can completely arrest sinoatrial node firing and block impulse conduction to the ventricles.[3]

The physiologic importance of the PNS on myocardial contractility is not as well understood as that of the SNS. Cholinergic blockade can double the heart rate (HR) without altering contractility of the left ventricle. Vagal stimulation of the heart can reduce left ventricular maximum rate of tension development (dP/dT) and decrease contractile force by as much as 10 to

20%. However, PNS stimulation is relatively unimportant in this regard compared with its predominant effect on HR.

The SNS has the same supraventricular distribution as the PNS, but with stronger representation to the ventricles. SNS efferents to the myocardium funnel through the paired stellate ganglia. The right stellate ganglion distributes primarily to the anterior epicardial surface and the interventricular septum. Right stellate stimulation decreases systolic duration and increases HR. The left stellate ganglion supplies the posterior and lateral surfaces of both ventricles. Left stellate stimulation increases mean arterial pressure and left ventricular contractility without causing a substantial change in HR. Normal SNS tone maintains contractility approximately 20% above that in the absence of any SNS stimulation.[4] Therefore, the dominant effect of the ANS on myocardial contractility is mediated primarily through the SNS. Intrinsic mechanisms of the myocardium, however, can maintain circulation quite well without the ANS, as evidenced by the success of cardiac transplants (see Denervated Heart).[5]

Early investigations, performed in anesthetized, open-chest animals, demonstrated that cardiac ANS nerves exert only slight effects on the coronary vascular bed; however, more recent studies on chronically instrumented, intact, conscious animals show considerable evidence for a strong SNS regulation of the small coronary resistance and larger conductance vessels.[6] (See Adrenergic Receptors section.)

Different segments of the coronary arterial tree react differently to various stimuli and drugs. Large conductance vessels, the primary location for atheromatous plaques, are found on the epicardial surface, whereas the small, precapillary resistance vessels are found within the myocardium. Normally, the large conductance vessels contribute little to overall coronary vascular resistance. Fluctuations in resistance reflect changes in lumen size of the small, precapillary vessels. Blood flow through the resistance vessels is regulated primarily by the local metabolic requirements of the myocardium. The larger conductance vessels, however, can constrict markedly with neurogenic stimulation. Neurogenic influence also assumes a greater role in the resistance vessels when they become hypoxic and lose autoregulation. There is a strong interaction between SNS and PNS nerves in organs with dual, antagonistic innervation.

Peripheral Circulation

The SNS nerves are by far the most important regulators of the peripheral circulation. The PNS nerves play only a minor role in this regard. The PNS dilates vessels, but only in limited areas such as the genitals. SNS stimulation produces both vasodilation and vasoconstriction, with vasoconstrictor effects predominating. The effect is determined by the type of receptors on which the SNS fiber terminates (see Receptors). SNS constrictor receptors are distributed to all segments of the circulation. This distribution is greater in some tissues than in others. Blood vessels in the skin, kidneys, spleen, and mesentery have an extensive SNS distribution, whereas those in the heart, brain, and muscle have less SNS innervation. SNS stimulation of the coronary arteries may produce vasoconstriction or vasodilation, depending on the predominant receptor activity at the time of stimulation (see Table 12-1). Vagal stimulation may also produce coronary vasoconstriction (see β-Adrenergic Receptors section). However, local autoregulatory factors usually have the predominant influence on coronary vascular tone.

Basal vasomotor tone is maintained by impulses from the lateral portion of the vasomotor center in the medulla oblongata that continually transmits impulses through the SNS, maintaining partial arteriolar and venular constriction. Circulating EPI from the adrenal medulla has additive effects. This basal ANS tone maintains arteriolar constriction at an intermediate diameter.[7] The arteriole, therefore, has the potential for either further constriction or dilation. If the basal tone were not present, the SNS could only effect vasoconstriction and not vasodilation.[1] The SNS tone in the venules produces little resistance to flow compared with the arterioles and the arteries. The importance of SNS stimulation of veins is to reduce or increase their capacity. By functioning as a reservoir for approximately 80% of the total blood volume, small changes in venous capacitance produce large changes in venous return and, thus, cardiac preload.

Lungs

The lungs are innervated by both the SNS and PNS. Postganglionic SNS fibers from the upper thoracic ganglia (stellate) pass to the lungs to innervate the smooth muscles of the bronchi and pulmonary blood vessels. PNS innervation of these structures is from the vagus nerve.

SNS stimulation produces bronchodilation and pulmonary vasoconstriction.[8] Little else has been proven conclusively about the vasomotor control of the pulmonary vessels other than that they adjust to accommodate the output of the right ventricle. The effect of stimulation of the pulmonary SNS nerves on pulmonary vascular resistance is not great but may be important in maintaining hemodynamic stability during stress and exercise by balancing right and left ventricular output. Stimulation of the vagus nerve produces almost no vasodilation of the pulmonary circulation. The phenomenon of hypoxic pulmonary vasoconstriction appears to be an important force in regulation of pulmonary blood flow. Hypoxic pulmonary vasoconstriction is a local phenomenon capable of providing a faster adjustment to needs.

Both the SNS and the vagus nerve provide active bronchomotor control. SNS stimulation causes bronchodilation, whereas vagal stimulation produces constriction. PNS stimulation may also increase secretions of the bronchial glands. Vagal receptor endings in the alveolar ducts also play an important role in the reflex regulation of the ventilation cycle.[9] The lung has important nonventilatory activity as well. It serves as a metabolic organ that removes local mediators such as norepinephrine (NE) from the circulation and converts others, such as angiotensin 1, to active compounds.[10] (See Interaction with Other Regulatory Systems section.)

AUTONOMIC NERVOUS SYSTEM: NEUROTRANSMISSION

Transmission of excitation across the terminal junctional sites (synaptic clefts) of the peripheral ANS occurs through the mediation of liberated chemicals (Fig. 12-5). Transmitters interact with a receptor on the end organ to evoke a biologic response. The ANS can be pharmacologically subdivided by the neurotransmitter secreted at the effector cell. Pharmacologic parlance designates the SNS and PNS as adrenergic and cholinergic, respectively. The terminals of the PNS postganglionic fibers release acetylcholine (ACh). With the exception of sweat glands, NE is considered the principal neurotransmitter released at the terminals of the sympathetic postganglionic fibers (see Fig. 12-3). Co-transmission of ATP, neuropeptide Y (NPY), and NE has been demonstrated at vascular sympathetic nerve terminals in a number of different tissues including muscle, intestine, kidney, and skin (see SNS Neurotransmission section). The preganglionic neurons of both systems secrete ACh.

The terminations of the postganglionic fibers of both ANS subdivisions are anatomically and physiologically similar. The terminations are characterized by multiple branchings called terminal effector plexuses, or reticulae. These filaments surround the elements of the effector unit "like a mesh stocking."[11] Thus, one SNS postganglionic neuron, for example, can

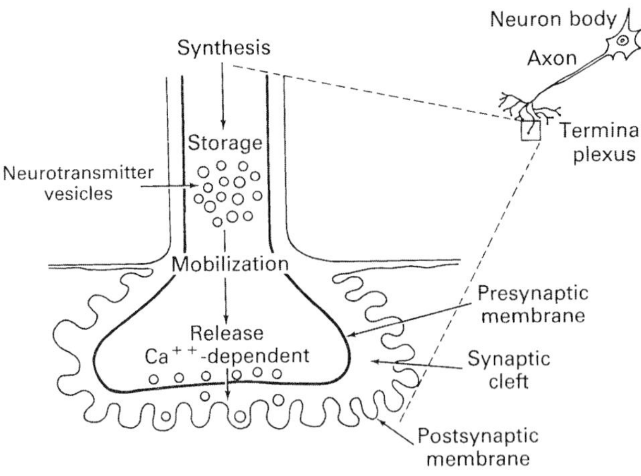

FIGURE 12-5. The anatomy and physiology of the terminal postganglionic fibers of sympathetic and parasympathetic fibers are similar.

innervate ~25,000 effector cells (e.g., vascular smooth muscle). The terminal filaments end in presynaptic enlargements called varicosities. Each varicosity contains vesicles, ~500 μ in diameter, in which the neurotransmitters are stored (see Fig. 12-5). The varicosities are also heavily populated with mitochondria, which relates to the increased energy (adenosine triphosphate, ATP) requirements of ACh and NE synthesis. The rate of synthesis depends on the level of ANS activity and is regulated by local feedback. The distance between the varicosity and the effector cell (synaptic or junctional cleft) varies from 100 μ in ganglia and arterioles to as much as 20,000 μ in large arteries. This distance determines the amount of transmitter required to stimulate and the time it takes to diffuse to the effector cell. The time for diffusion is directly proportional to the width of the synaptic gap. Depolarization releases the vesicular contents into the synaptic cleft by exocytosis.

Parasympathetic Nervous System Neurotransmission

Synthesis

ACh is considered the primary neurotransmitter of the PNS. ACh is formed in the presynaptic terminal by acetylation of choline with acetyl coenzyme A. This step is catalyzed by choline acetyl transferase (Fig. 12-6). ACh is then stored in a concentrated form in presynaptic vesicles. A continual release of small amounts of ACh, called quanta, occurs during the resting state. Each quantum results in small changes in the electrical potential of the synaptic end plate without producing depolarization. These are known as miniature end-plate potentials. Arrival of an action potential causes a synchronous release of hundreds of quanta, resulting in depolarization of the end plate. Release of ACh from the vesicles is dependent on influx of calcium (Ca2+) from the interstitial space. Drugs that alter Ca2+ binding or influx may decrease ACh release and affect end-organ function. ACh is not reused like NE; therefore, it must be synthesized constantly.

Metabolism

The ability of a receptor to modulate function of an effector organ is dependent on rapid recovery to its baseline state after stimulation. For this to occur, the neurotransmitter must be quickly removed from the vicinity of the receptor. ACh removal occurs by rapid hydrolysis by acetylcholinesterase (see Fig. 12-6). This enzyme is found in neurons, at the neuromuscular junction, and in various other tissues of the body. A similar enzyme, pseudocholinesterase or plasma cholinesterase, is also found throughout the body but only to a limited extent in nervous tissue. It does not appear to be physiologically important in termination of the action of ACh. Both acetylcholinesterase and pseudocholinesterase hydrolyze ACh, as well as other esters (such as the ester-type local anesthetics), but they may be distinguished by specific biochemical tests.[3]

Sympathetic Nervous System Neurotransmission

Traditionally, the catecholamines EPI and NE were considered the exclusive mediators of peripheral SNS activity. Evidence accumulated over the past two decades, though, suggests roles for ATP as an additional sympathetic neurotransmitter. NE is released from localized presynaptic vesicles of nearly all postganglionic sympathetic nerves. Vascular SNS nerve terminals, though, also release ATP. Thus, ATP and NE are co-neurotransmitters. They are released directly into the site where they act. Their postjunctional effects appear to be synergistic in tissues studied to date.

The SNS fibers ending in the adrenal medulla are preganglionic, and ACh is the neurotransmitter (see Fig. 12-3). It interacts with the chromaffin cells in the medulla, causing release of EPI and NE. The chromaffin cells take the place of the postganglionic neurons. Stimulation of the sympathetic nerves to the adrenal medulla, however, causes the release of large

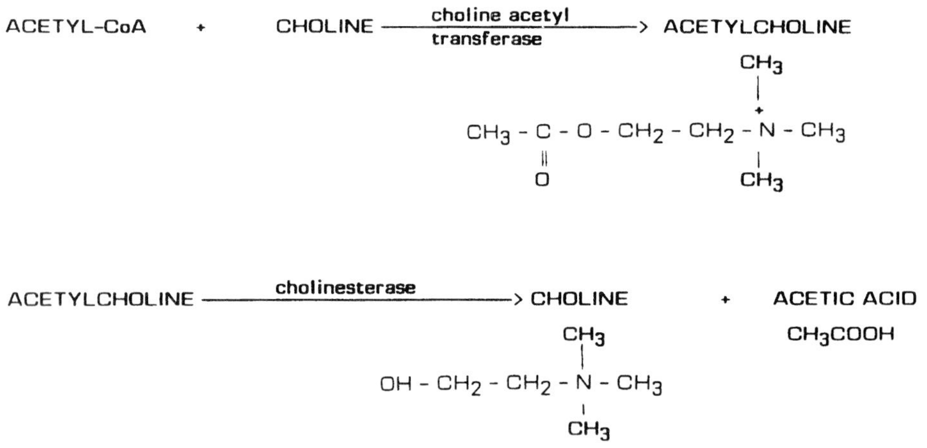

ACETYL-CoA + CHOLINE —(choline acetyl transferase)→ ACETYLCHOLINE

$$CH_3-\underset{\underset{O}{\|}}{C}-O-CH_2-CH_2-\overset{\overset{CH_3}{|}}{\underset{\underset{CH_3}{|}}{\overset{+}{N}}}-CH_3$$

ACETYLCHOLINE —(cholinesterase)→ CHOLINE + ACETIC ACID

$$OH-CH_2-CH_2-\overset{\overset{CH_3}{|}}{\underset{\underset{CH_3}{|}}{N}}-CH_3 \qquad CH_3COOH$$

FIGURE 12-6. Synthesis and metabolism of acetylcholine.

quantities of a mixture of EPI and NE into the circulation to become neurotransmitter hormones. The greater portion of this hormonal surge is normally EPI. EPI and NE, when released into the circulation, are classified as hormones in that they are synthesized, stored, and released from the adrenal medulla to act at distant sites.

Hormonal EPI and NE have almost the same effects on effector cells as those caused by local direct sympathetic stimulation; however, the hormonal effects, although brief, last about 10 times as long as those caused by direct stimulation.[12] EPI has a greater metabolic effect than NE. It can increase the metabolic rate of the body as much as 100%.[1] It also increases glycogenolysis in the liver and muscle with glucose release into the blood. These functions are all necessary to prepare the body for fight or flight. Some of the overall vascular tone results from the basal resting secretion of the adrenal medulla in addition to the tone that is maintained directly through stimulation from central vasomotor centers in the medulla.

Catecholamines: The First Messenger

The endogenous catecholamines in humans are dopamine (DA), NE, and EPI. Dopamine is a neurotransmitter in the CNS. It is primarily involved in coordinating motor activity in the brain. It is the precursor of NE. NE is synthesized and stored in nerve endings of postganglionic SNS neurons. It is also synthesized in the adrenal medulla and is the chemical precursor of EPI. Stored EPI is located chiefly in chromaffin cells of the adrenal medulla. Eighty to 85% of the catecholamine content of the adrenal medulla is EPI and 15 to 20% is NE. The brain contains both noradrenergic and dopaminergic receptors, but circulating catecholamines do not cross the blood-brain barrier. The catecholamines present in the brain are synthesized there. Endogenous catecholamines are unique in that several intermediates in the synthesis function as neurotransmitters.

A catecholamine is any compound of a catechol nucleus (a benzene ring with two adjacent hydroxyl groups) and an amine-containing side chain.[13] The chemical configuration of six of the more common catecholamines in clinical use is demonstrated in Figure 12-7. A true catecholamine must possess this basic structure. Catecholamines are often referred to as adrenergic drugs because their effector actions are mediated through receptors specific for the SNS. Synthetic catecholamines can activate these same receptors because of their structural similarity. For example, clonidine is an α-2 receptor agonist that does not possess a catechol nucleus and even has two ring systems that are aplanar to each other (Fig. 12-8). However, clonidine enjoys a remarkable spatial similarity to NE that allows it to activate the receptor.[14] Drugs that produce sympathetic-like effects but lack the basic catecholamine structure are defined as sympathomimetics. All clinically useful catecholamines are sympathomimetics, but not all sympathomimetics are catecholamines (Table 12-4).

The effects of endogenous or synthetic catecholamines on adrenergic receptors can be direct or indirect (see Table 12-4). Indirect-acting catecholamines (i.e., ephedrine) have little intrinsic effect on adrenergic receptors but produce their effects by stimulating release of the stored neurotransmitter from SNS nerve terminals. Some synthetic and endogenous catecholamines stimulate adrenergic receptor sites directly, whereas others have a mixed mode of action. The actions of direct-acting catecholamines are independent of endogenous NE stores; however, the indirect-acting catecholamines are totally dependent on adequate neuronal stores of endogenous NE.

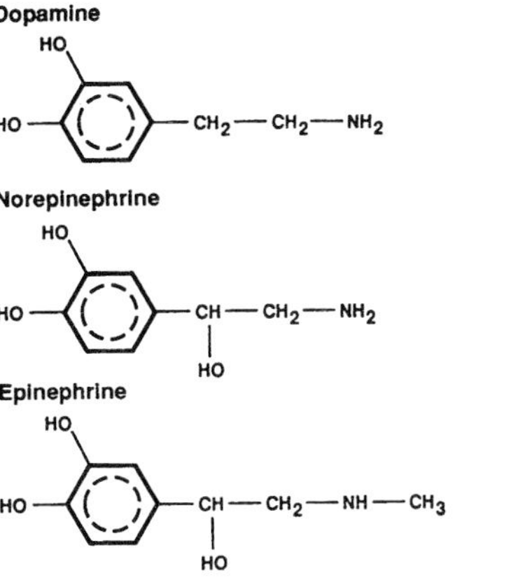

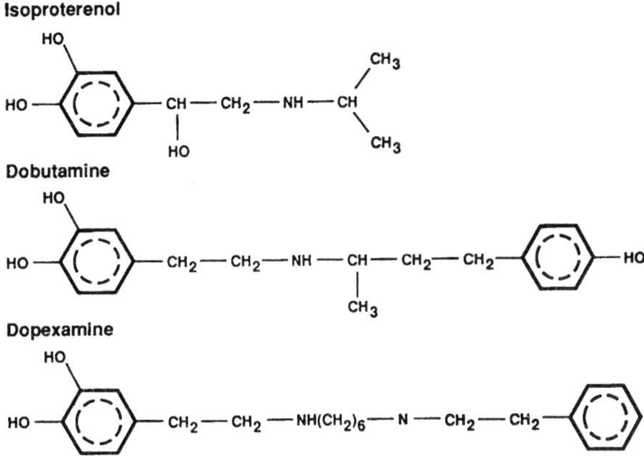

FIGURE 12-7. The chemical configurations of three endogenous catecholamines are compared with those of three synthetic catecholamines. Sympathomimetic drugs differ in their hemodynamic effects largely because of differences in substitution of the amine group on the catechol nucleus.

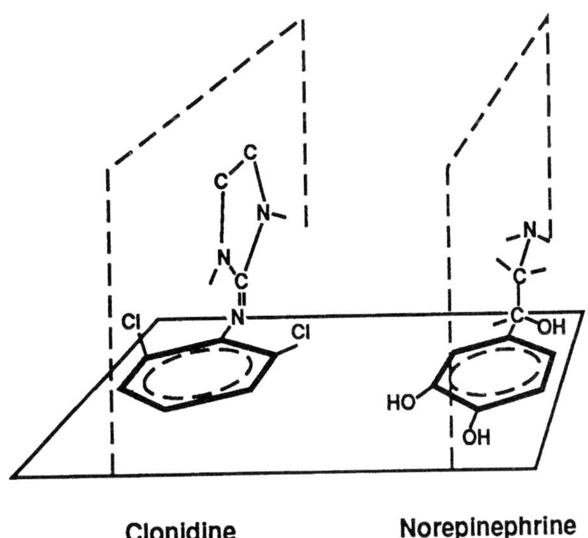

FIGURE 12-8. The spatial similarity of clonidine and NE allows it to activate presynaptic α-2 receptors inhibiting NE release.

TABLE 12-4

SYMPATHOMIMETIC DRUGS

DRUG	TRADE NAME
ADRENERGIC AMINES	
Catecholamines	
Epinephrine	Adrenalin
Norepinephrine	Levophed
Dopamine[a]	Inotropin
Dobutamine	Dobutrex
Dopexamine	
Isoproterenol	Isuprel
Noncatecholamines	
Metaraminol[a,b]	Aramine
Mephentermine[b]	Wyamine
Ephedrine[b]	Ephedrine
Methoxamine	Vasoxyl
Phenylephrine	Neo-Synephrine
Clonidine	
NONADRENERGICS	
Xanthines	Aminophylline
Glucagon	Glucagon
Digitalis	Lanoxin
Calcium salts	
Naloxone	Narcan
Amrinone	Inocor

[a] Direct-acting catecholamine with some indirect action.
[b] Primarily indirect-acting with some direct action. Adrenergic amines produce sympathomimetic effects via adrenergic receptors. Nonadrenergics produce sympathomimetic effects exclusive of the adrenergic receptor.

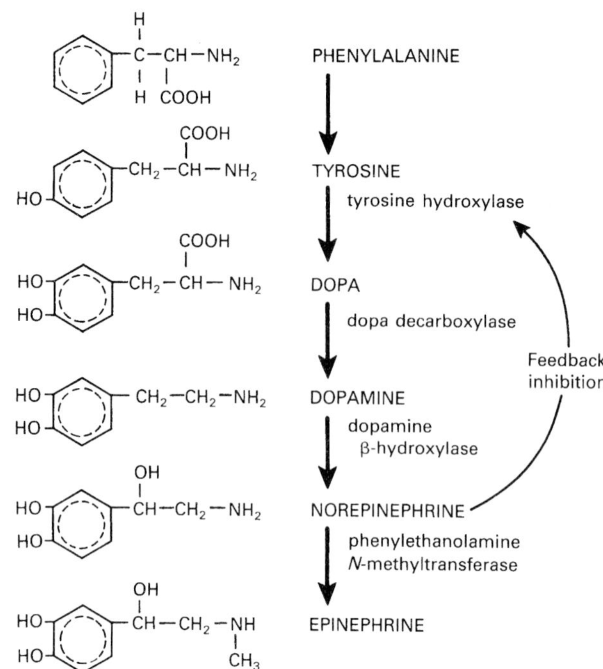

FIGURE 12-9. Schematic of the synthesis of catecholamines. The conversion of tyrosine to DOPA by tyrosine hydroxylase is inhibited by increased NE synthesis. Epinephrine is shown in these steps but is primarily synthesized in the adrenal medulla.

Synthesis

The main site of NE synthesis is in or near the postganglionic nerve endings. Some synthesis does occur in vesicles near the cell body that pass to the nerve endings.[15] Phenylalanine or tyrosine is taken up into the axoplasm of the nerve terminal and synthesized into either NE or EPI. Figure 12-9 demonstrates this synthesis cascade. Tyrosine hydroxylase catalyzes the conversion of tyrosine to dihydroxyphenylalanine. This is the rate-limiting step at which NE synthesis is controlled through feedback inhibition.[16] Dihydroxyphenylalanine and the subsequent compounds in this cascade are catecholamines.

Dopamine synthesis occurs in the cytoplasm of the neuron. Dopamine then enters the storage vesicles. Synthesis stops at this point where dopamine is the neurotransmitter. The vesicles of peripheral postganglionic neurons contain the enzyme dopamine-b-hydroxylase, which converts dopamine to NE. The adrenal medulla additionally contains phenylethanolamine-N-methyltransferase, which converts NE to EPI. This reaction takes place outside the medullary vesicles, and the newly formed EPI then enters the vesicle for storage (Fig. 12-10). All the endogenous catecholamines are stored in presynaptic vesicles and released on arrival of an action potential. Excitation-secretion coupling in sympathetic neurons is Ca2+-dependent.

Regulation

Increased SNS nervous activity, as in congestive heart failure (CHF) or chronic stress, stimulates the synthesis of catecholamines.[17] Glucocorticoids from the adrenal cortex stimulate an increase in phenylethanolamine-N-methyltransferase that methylates NE to EPI.

The release of NE is dependent on depolarization of the nerve and an increase in calcium ion permeability.[17] This release is inhibited by colchicine and prostaglandin E2, suggesting a contractile mechanism. Blockade of prostaglandin synthesis enhances NE release. NE inhibits its own release by stimulating presynaptic (prejunctional) α-2 receptors. Phenoxybenzamine

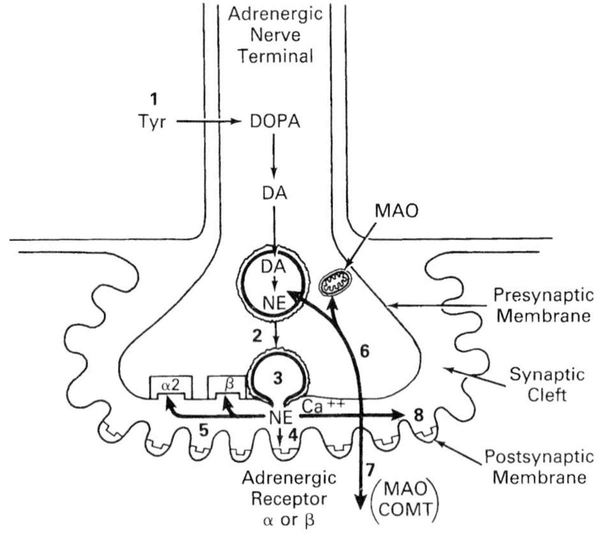

FIGURE 12-10. Schematic of the synthesis and disposition of NE in adrenergic neurotransmission. (1) Synthesis and storage in neuronal vesicles; (2) action potential permits calcium entry with (3) exocytosis of NE into synaptic gap. (4) Released NE reacts with receptor on effector cell. NE (5) may react with presynaptic α-2 receptor to inhibit further NE release or with presynaptic β receptor to enhance reuptake of NE (6) (uptake 1). Extraneuronal uptake (uptake 2) absorbs NE into effector cell (7) with overflow occurring systemically (8). MAO, monoamine oxidase; COMT, catechol-O-methyltransferase; Tyr, tyrosine; DOPA, dihydroxyphenylalanine; NE, norepinephrine.

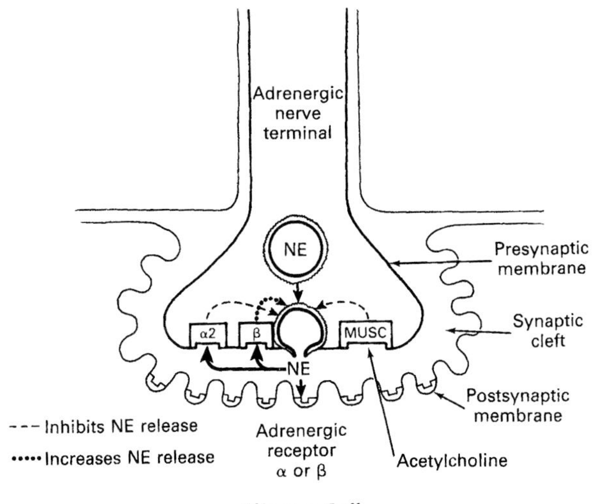

FIGURE 12-11. This schematic demonstrates just a few of the presynaptic adrenergic receptors thought to exist. Agonist and antagonist drugs are clinically available for these receptors (see Table 12-5). The α-2 receptors serve as a negative feedback mechanism whereby NE stimulation inhibits its own release. Presynaptic β stimulation increases NE uptake, augmenting its availability. Presynaptic muscarinic (MUSC) receptors respond to ACh diffusing from nearby cholinergic terminals. They inhibit NE release and can be blocked by atropine.

and phentolamine, α-receptor antagonists, increase the release of NE by blocking inhibitory presynaptic α-2 receptors (Fig. 12-11). Other receptors may also be important in NE regulation. (See Other Receptors section.)

Inactivation

The catecholamines are removed from the synaptic cleft by three mechanisms (see Fig. 12-10). These are reuptake into the presynaptic terminals, extraneuronal uptake, and diffusion. Termination of NE at the effector site is almost entirely by reuptake of NE into the terminals of the presynaptic neuron (uptake 1) for reuse. Uptake 1 is an active, energy-requiring, temperature-dependent process.

The reuptake of NE in the presynaptic terminals is also a stereospecific process. Structurally similar compounds (guanethidine, metaraminol) may enter the vesicles and displace the neurotransmitter. Tricyclic antidepressants and cocaine inhibit the reuptake of NE, resulting in high synaptic NE concentrations and accentuated receptor response. In addition, evidence suggests that NE reuptake is mediated by a presynaptic β-adrenergic mechanism because β-blockade causes marked elevations of EPI and NE[18] (see Figs. 12-10 and 12-11), whereas a blockade does not. Extraneuronal uptake (uptake 2) is a minor pathway for inactivating NE. NE is taken up by effector cells and other extraneuronal tissues. The NE that is taken up by the extraneuronal tissue is metabolized by monoamine oxidase and by catechol-O-methyltransferase to form vanillylmandelic acid (Fig. 12-12). The minute amount of catecholamine that escapes uptake 1 and uptake 2 diffuses into the circulation (uptake 3), where it is similarly metabolized in the liver and kidney. The importance of uptake 1 and uptake 2 is diminished when sympathomimetics are given exogenously. EPI is inactivated by the same enzymes. Whereas uptake 1 is the predominant pathway for inactivation of the endogenous catecholamines, uptake 3 is the predominant pathway for catecholamines given exogenously and is clinically important. This accounts for the longer duration of action by exogenous catecholamines than that noted at the local synapse. The former is slow (liver metabolism) and the latter is fast (uptake 1).

The final metabolic product of the catecholamines is vanillylmandelic acid. Vanillylmandelic acid constitutes the major metabolite (80 to 90%) of NE found in the urine. Less than 5% of released NE appears unchanged in the urine. The metabolic products excreted in the urine provide a gross estimate of SNS activity and can facilitate the clinical diagnosis of pheochromocytoma.

RECEPTORS

An agonist is a substance that interacts with a receptor to evoke a biologic response. ACh, NE, EPI, DA, and ATP are the major agonists of the ANS. An antagonist is a substance that interferes

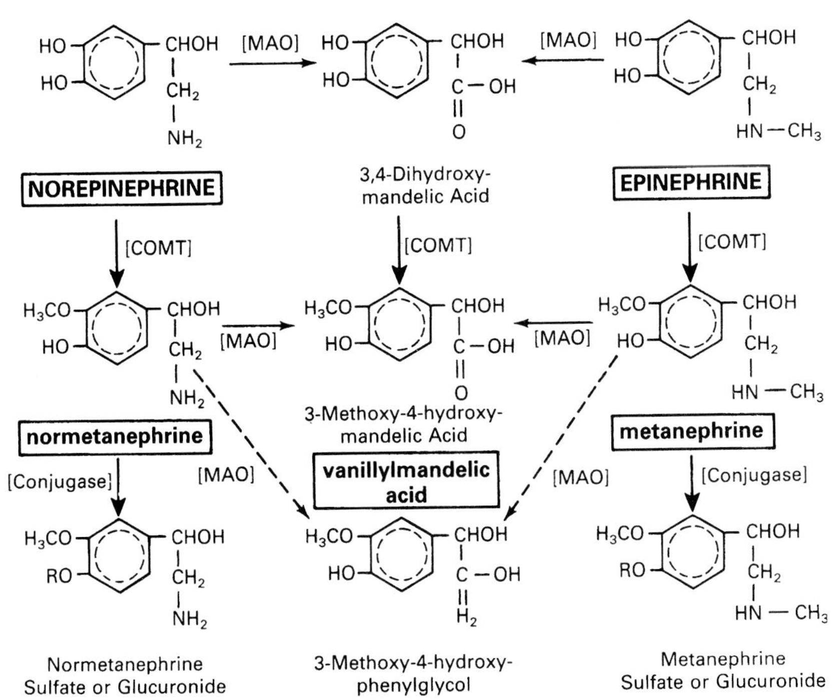

NOREPINEPHRINE — [MAO] → 3,4-Dihydroxymandelic Acid ← [MAO] — EPINEPHRINE

[COMT]

normetanephrine — [MAO] → 3-Methoxy-4-hydroxymandelic Acid (vanillylmandelic acid) ← [MAO] — metanephrine

[Conjugase] [MAO] [MAO] [Conjugase]

Normetanephrine Sulfate or Glucuronide

3-Methoxy-4-hydroxyphenylglycol

Metanephrine Sulfate or Glucuronide

FIGURE 12-12. Catabolism of NE and EPI.

with the evocation of a response at a receptor site by an agonist. Receptors are therefore regarded as target sites that when activated by an agonist will lead to a response by the effector cell. Receptors are protein macromolecules and are located in the plasma membrane. Several thousand receptors have been demonstrated in a single cell. The enormity of this network is realized when it is considered that ~25,000 single cells can be innervated by a single neuron.[19]

Cholinergic Receptors

ACh is the neurotransmitter at three distinct classes of receptors. These receptors can be differentiated by their anatomic location and their affinity to bind various agonists and antagonists.[20] ACh mediates the "first messenger" function of transmitting impulses in the PNS, the ganglia of the SNS, and the neuroeffector junction of striated, voluntary muscle (see Fig. 12-3). The receptors are referred to as cholinoceptive or cholinergic receptors. The PNS is referred to as the cholinergic system.

Cholinergic receptors are further subdivided into muscarinic and nicotinic receptors because muscarine and nicotine stimulate them selectively.[3] However, both muscarinic and nicotinic receptors respond to ACh (see Cholinergic Drugs section). Muscarine activates cholinergic receptors at the postganglionic PNS junctions of cardiac and smooth muscle throughout the body. Muscarinic stimulation is characterized by bradycardia, decreased inotropism, bronchoconstriction, miosis, salivation, gastrointestinal (GI) hypermotility, and increased gastric acid secretion (see Table 12-1). Muscarinic receptors can be blocked by atropine without effect on nicotinic receptors (see Cholinergic Drugs section).

Muscarinic receptors are known to exist in sites other than PNS postganglionic junctions. They are found on the presynaptic membrane of sympathetic nerve terminals in the myocardium, coronary vessels, and peripheral vasculature (see Fig. 12-11). These are referred to as adrenergic muscarinic receptors because of their location; however, they are stimulated by ACh. Stimulation of these receptors inhibits release of NE in a manner similar to α-2 receptor stimulation.[6] Muscarinic blockade removes inhibition of NE release, augmenting SNS activity. Atropine, the prototypical muscarinic blocker, may produce sympathomimetic activity in this manner as well as vagal blockade. Neuromuscular blocking drugs that cause tachycardia are thought to have a similar mechanism of action.

ACh acting on presynaptic adrenergic muscarinic receptors is a potent inhibitor of NE release.[18] The prejunctional muscarinic receptor may play an important physiologic role because several autonomically innervated tissues (e.g., the heart) possess ANS plexuses in which the SNS and PNS nerve terminals are closely associated.[3] In these plexuses, ACh, released from the nearby PNS nerve terminals (vagus nerve), can inhibit NE release by activation of presynaptic adrenergic muscarinic receptors (see Fig. 12-11).

Nicotinic receptors are found at the synaptic junctions of both SNS and PNS ganglia. Because both junctions are cholinergic, ACh or ACh-like substances such as nicotine will excite postganglionic fibers of both systems (see Fig. 12-3). Low doses of nicotine produce stimulation of ANS ganglia, whereas high doses produce blockade. This dualism is referred to as the nicotinic effect (see Ganglionic Drugs section). Nicotinic stimulation of the SNS ganglia produces hypertension and tachycardia by causing the release of EPI and NE from the adrenal medulla. Adrenal hormone release is mediated by ACh in the chromaffin cells, which are analogous to postganglionic neurons (see Fig. 12-3). A further increase in nicotine concentration produces hypotension and neuromuscular weakness as it becomes a ganglionic blocker. The cholinergic neuroeffector junction of skeletal muscle also contains nicotinic receptors, although they are not identical to the nicotinic receptors in ANS ganglia.

Adrenergic Receptors

Von Euler differentiated the physiologic effects of EPI and NE in 1946.[14] The adrenergic receptors were termed adrenergic or noradrenergic, depending on their responsiveness to EPI or NE. The dissimilarities of these two drugs led Ahlquist in 1948 to propose two types of opposing adrenergic receptors, termed alpha (α) and beta (β). This postulation implied that selective antagonism of these receptors was possible. The receptors can be classified according to the order of potency by which they are affected by SNS agonists and antagonists. Receptors that respond with an order of potency of NE $\geq$ EPI > isoproterenol are called α receptors. Those responding with an order of potency of isoproterenol > EPI $\geq$ NE are called β receptors (Table 12-5). The development of new agonists and antagonists with relatively selective activity allowed subdivision of the β receptors into β_1 and β_2. α receptors were subsequently divided into α_1 and α_2. The concept of relative selective activity arises from differential potencies among tissue groups to the same drug, such that two dose-response curves are obtained (Fig. 12-13). The sympathomimetic adrenergic drugs in current use differ from one another in their effects largely because of differences in substitution on the amine group, which influences the relative α or β effect (see Fig. 12-7).[13]

Another major peripheral adrenergic receptor specific for dopamine is termed the dopaminergic (DA) receptor. Further studies have revealed not only subsets of the α and β receptors but also the DA receptor. These DA receptors have been identified in the CNS and in renal, mesenteric, and coronary vessels. The physiologic importance of these receptors is a matter of controversy because there are no identifiable *peripheral* DA neurons. Dopamine measured in the circulation is assumed to result from spillover from the brain.

The function of dopamine in the CNS has long been known, but the peripheral DA receptor has been elucidated only within the past 25 years. The presence of the peripheral DA receptor was obscured because dopamine does not affect the DA receptor exclusively. It also stimulates α and β receptors in a dose-related manner.[21] However, DA receptors function independently of α or β blockade and are modified by DA antagonists such as haloperidol, droperidol, and phenothiazines. Thus, there is a necessity for the addition of the DA receptor and its subsets (DA1 and DA2).

The anatomic location and amino acid structure of receptor binding sites have been made possible through radioligand studies. The distribution of adrenoreceptors in organs and tissues is not uniform and their function differs not only by their location but also in their numbers and/or distribution.[22] Adrenoceptors are found in two loci in the sympathetic neuroeffector junction. They are found in both the presynaptic (prejunctional) and postsynaptic (postjunctional) sites as well as extrasynaptic sites (Fig. 12-14). Table 12-6 is a review of the function and synaptic location of some of the clinically important sites.

Prejunctional receptors are considered innervated in that they are in the immediate vicinity of the neurotransmitter released by a sympathetic action potential. Postjunctional receptors are considered to be innervated or noninnervated depending on their proximity to the synaptic cleft.[23] Receptors located directly on postjunctional membranes are considered to be innervated. However, most postsynaptic α-2 and β-2 receptors are extrasynaptic and considered noninnervated even though they are located in the vicinity of the postsynaptic membrane. These receptors are influenced more by hormonal catecholamines (EPI) than by neurotransmitter (NE).

TABLE 12-5

ADRENERGIC RECEPTORS: ORDER OF POTENCY OF AGONISTS AND ANTAGONISTS

RECEPTOR		AGONISTS[a]	ANTAGONISTS	LOCATION	ACTION
α_1	++++	Norepinephrine	Phenoxybenzamine[b]	Smooth muscle (vascular, iris, radial, ureter, pilomotor, uterus, trigone, gastrointestinal, and bladder sphincters)	Contraction Vasoconstriction
	+++	Epinephrine	Phentolamine[b]		
	++	Dopamine	Ergot alkaloids[b]		
	+	Isoproterenol	Prazosin		
			Tolazoline[b]	Brain	Neurotransmission
			Labetalol[b]	Smooth muscle (gastrointestinal)	Relaxation
				Heart	Glycogenolysis
				Salivary glands	Increased force,[c] glycolysis
				Adipose tissue	Secretion (K^+, H_2O)
				Sweat glands (localized)	Glycogenesis
				Kidney (proximal tubule)	Secretion
					Gluconeogenesis Na^+ reabsorption
α_2	++++	Clonidine	Yohimbine	Adrenergic nerve endings	Inhibition norepinephrine release
	+++	Norepinephrine	Piperoxan	Presynaptic—CNS	
	++	Epinephrine	Phentolamine[b]		
	++	Norepinephrine	Phenoxybenzamine[b]	Platelets	Aggregation, granule release
	+	Phenylephrine	Tolazoline[b]		
			Labetalol[b]	Adipose tissue	Inhibition lypolysis
				Endocrine pancrease	Inhibition insulin release
				Vascular smooth muscle—?	Contraction
				Kidney	Inhibition renin disease
				Brain	Neurotransmission
β_1	++++	Isoproterenol[b]	Acebutolol	Heart	Increased rate, contractility, conduction velocity
	+++	Epinephrine	Practolol		
	++	Norepinephrine	Propranolol[b]		Coronary vasodilation
	+	Dopamine	Alprenolol[b]	Adipose tissue	Lipolysis
			Metoprolol		
			Esmolol		
β_2	++++	Isoproterenol[a]	Propranolol[b]	Liver	Glycogenolysis, gluconeogenesis
	+++	Epinephrine	Butoxamine		
	+++	Norepinephrine	Alprenolol		
	+	Dopamine	Esmolol	Skeletal muscle	Glyogenolysis, lactate release
			Nadolol		
			Timolol	Smooth muscle (bronchi, uterus, vascular, gastrointestinal, detrusor, spleen capsule)	Relaxation
			Labetalol		
				Endocrine pancreas	Insulin secretion
				Salivary glands	Amylase secretion
DA_1	++++	Fenoldopam		Vascular smooth muscle	Vasodilation
	++	Dopamine	Haloperidol	Renal and mesentery	
	+	Epinephrine	Droperidol		
	+	Metaclopramide	Phenothiazines		
DA_2	++	Dopamine	Domperidone	Presynaptic—adrenergic nerve endings	Inhibits norepinephrine release
	+	Bromocriptine			

[a]Listed in decreasing order of potency.
[b]Nonselective.
[c]β_1-adrenergic responses are greater.
Pluses indicate strength of potency.

Extrasynaptic receptors also seem to be less influenced by factors causing the "up or down" regulation of receptor numbers and sensitivity. This may explain the clinical observation of why EPI may work where other agonists, which work on synaptic receptors, may be ineffective. The agonist–receptor interaction of noninnervated receptors is of slower onset and longer duration as well.

α-Adrenergic Receptors

Two classes of clinically important α receptors have been demonstrated, α-1 and α-2. This classification is based on their response to the α antagonists yohimbine and prazosin. Prazosin is a more potent antagonist of α-1 receptors, whereas α-2 receptors are more sensitive to yohimbine. The α-1- adrenergic receptors are found in the smooth muscle cells of the peripheral

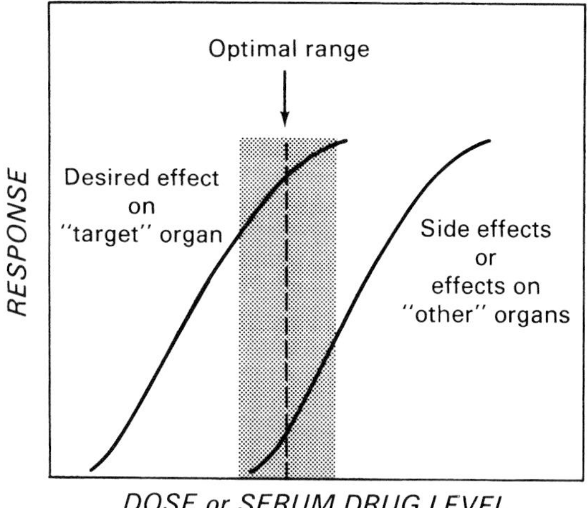

FIGURE 12-13. Relative dose-response relationship on target and other organs. Relative selectivity is illustrated by showing the relationship between two dose-response curves. The curve on the left represents the desired response of bronchodilation using a relatively selective β-2 agonist. The unwanted effects on other organs that occur at higher doses are represented by the curve on the right. For example, an increased HR (β-1 effect) may occur with higher doses of a relatively select β-2 agonist. The optimal range is that concentration of drug that will give the maximal desired response with minimal effects on other organs. The size of the optimal range is dependent on the therapeutic index, or the distance between the two curves. These are usually established in vitro where drug concentration can be precisely controlled. For many cardiovascular drugs, the optimal range is small, and wide fluctuations in serum level of the drug are common; therefore, secondary or side effects are often seen during drug therapy.

vasculature of the coronary arteries, skin, uterus, intestinal mucosa, and splanchnic beds (see Table 12-5). The α-1 receptors serve as postsynaptic activators of vascular and intestinal smooth muscle as well as of endocrine glands. Their activation results in either decreased or increased tone, depending on the effector organ. The response in resistance and capacitance vessels is constriction, whereas in the intestinal tract it is relaxation. There is now a large body of evidence documenting the presence of postjunctional α-1 adrenoreceptors in the mammalian heart. α-1 adrenoreceptors have been shown to have a positive inotropic effect on cardiac tissues from most mammals studied, including humans.[24] Experimental work strongly supports the concept that enhanced myocardial α-1 responsiveness plays a primary role in the genesis of malignant arrhythmias induced by catecholamines during myocardial ischemia and reperfusion. Drugs possessing potent α-1 antagonist activity such as prazosin and phentolamine provide significant antiarrhythmic activity. The clinical mechanism and significance of these findings are not yet clear.[25] However, there is no doubt that α-1 adrenergic antagonists prevent catecholamine-induced ventricular arrhythmias.[26] In contrast, studies of the effects of β-antagonists in experimental and clinical myocardial infarction have provided conflicting results.

The discovery of presynaptic α-adrenoreceptors and their role in the modulation of NE transmission provided the stimulus for the subclassification of α receptors into α-1 and α-2 subtypes.[27] Presynaptic α-1 receptors have not been identified and appear confined to the postsynaptic membrane. α-2 receptors are found on both presynaptic and postsynaptic membranes of the adrenergic neuroeffector junction. Table 12-6 reviews these sites. Postsynaptic membranes contain a near equal mix of α-1 and α-2 receptors.

The α-2 adrenoreceptors may be subdivided even further into as many as four possible subtypes. Many actions have been attributed to the postsynaptic α-2 receptor, including arterial and venous vasoconstriction, platelet aggregation, inhibition of insulin release, inhibition of bowel motility, stimulation of growth hormone release, and inhibition of antidiuretic hormone release.

α-2 receptors can be found in cholinergic pathways as well as in adrenergic pathways. They can significantly modulate parasympathetic activity as well. Current research implies that α-2 stimulation in parasympathetic pathways plays a role in the modulation of the baroreceptor reflex (increased sensitivity),

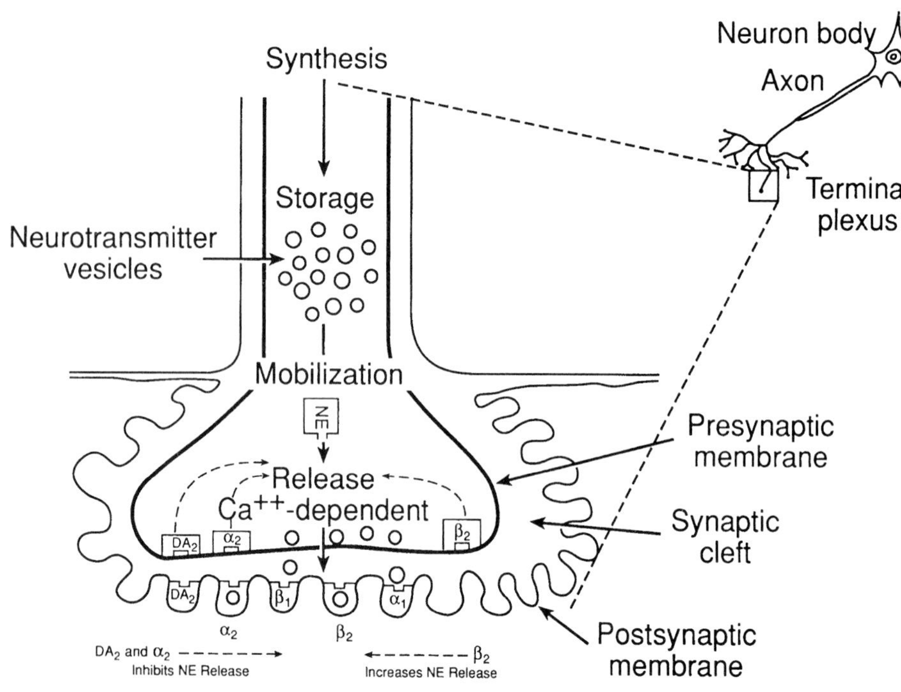

FIGURE 12-14. Loci of several known adrenergic receptors. The presynaptic α-2 and DA receptors serve as a negative feedback mechanism, whereby stimulation of NE inhibits its own release. Presynaptic β-2 stimulation increases NE uptake, augmenting its availability. Postsynaptic α-2 and β-2 receptors are extrasynaptic and are considered noninnervated hormonal receptors.

TABLE 12-6

ADRENERGIC RECEPTORS

RECEPTOR	SYNAPTIC SITE	ANATOMIC SITE	ACTION	LV FUNCTION AND STROKE VOLUME
α_1	Postsynaptic	Peripheral vascular smooth muscle	Constriction	Decreased
		Renal vascular smooth muscle	Constriction	
		Coronary arteries, epicardial	Constriction	
		Myocardium	Positive inotropism	Improved
		30–40% of resting tone		
		Renal tubules	Antidiuresis	
α_2	Presynaptic	Peripheral vascular smooth muscle release	Inhibit NE	
			Secondary vasodilation	Improved
		Coronaries	?	
		CNS	Inhibition of CNS activity Sedation Decrease MAC	
	Postsynaptic	Coronaries, endocardial	Constriction	Decreased
		CNS	Inhibition of insulin release Decreased bowel motility Inhibition of antidiuretic hormone Analgesia	
		Renal tubule	Promotes Na^{2+} and H_2O excretion	
β_1	Postsynaptic NE sensitive	Myocardium	Positive inotropism and chronotropism	Improved
		Sinoatrial (SA) node		
		Ventricular conduction		
		Kidney	Renin release	
		Coronaries	Relaxation	
β_2	Presynaptic NE sensitive	Myocardium	Accelerates NE release	Improved
		SA node ventricular conduction vessels	Opposite action to presynaptic α_2 agonism	
			Constriction	
	Postsynaptic (extrasynaptic) (EPI sensitive)	Myocardium	Positive inotropism and chronotropism	
		Vascular smooth muscle	Relaxation	Improved
		Bronchial smooth muscle	Relaxation	Improved
		Renal vessels	Relaxation	Improved
DA_1	Postsynaptic	Blood vessels (renal, mesentery, coronary)	Vasodilation	Improved
		Renal tubules	Natriuresis Diuresis	
		Juxtaglomerular cells	Renin release (modulates diuresis)	
		Sympathetic ganglia	Minor inhibition	
DA_2	Presynaptic	Postganglionic sympathetic nerves	Inhibit NE release	Improved
			Secondary vasodilation	
	Postsynaptic	Renal and mesenteric vasculature	? Vasoconstriction	

vagal mediation of heart rate (bradycardia), bronchoconstriction, and salivation (dry mouth). However, cholinergic receptors can also be found in adrenergic pathways; thus, muscarinic and nicotinic receptors have been found in presynaptic and postsynaptic locations, where they in turn modulate sympathetic activity (see Fig. 12-11). Maze speculates that although the functional role of the postsynaptic α-2 receptor in the CNS has not been well characterized, it is probable that the features that are so desirable to the anesthesiologist, such as sedation, anxiolysis, analgesia, and hypnosis, are mediated through this site.

Stimulation of presynaptic α-2 receptors mediates inhibition of NE release into the synaptic cleft, serving as a negative feedback mechanism.[28] The central effects are primarily related to a reduction in sympathetic outflow with a concomitantly enhanced parasympathetic outflow (e.g., enhanced baroreceptor activity). This results in a decreased systemic vascular resistance, decreased cardiac output (CO), decreased inotropic state in the myocardium, and decreased HR. The peripheral presynaptic α-2 effects are similar, and NE release is inhibited in postganglionic neurons. However, stimulation of postsynaptic α-2 receptors, like the α-1 postsynaptic receptor, affects vasoconstriction.

NE acts on both α-1 and α-2 receptors. Thus, NE not only activates smooth muscle vasoconstriction (postsynaptic α-1 and α-2 receptors) but also stimulates presynaptic α-2 receptors and inhibits its own release. Selective stimulation of the presynaptic α-2 receptor could produce a beneficial reduction of peripheral vascular resistance. Unfortunately, most known presynaptic α-2 agonists also stimulate the postsynaptic α-2 receptors, causing vasoconstriction. Blockade of α-2 presynaptic receptors, however, ablates normal inhibition of NE, causing vasoconstriction. Vasodilation occurs with the blockade of postsynaptic α-1 and α-2 receptors.

α Receptors in the Cardiovascular System. The presence of postsynaptic α-1 and α-2 receptors in the mammalian myocardium and coronary arteries as well as the peripheral vasculature are known.[25]

Coronary Arteries. The presence of postsynaptic α-1 and α-2 receptors in the coronary arteries of humans has not been established with certainty, but other mammalian models have demonstrated their presence. Sympathetic nerves cause coronary vasoconstriction, which is mediated more by postsynaptic α-2 than α-1 receptors. The larger epicardial arteries possess mainly α-1 receptors, whereas α-2 receptors and some α-1 receptors are present in the small coronary artery resistance vessels.[29] Epicardial vessels contribute only 5% to the total resistance of the coronary circulation; therefore, α-1 agonists such as phenylephrine have little influence on coronary resistance.[30]

Myocardial ischemia has been shown to increase α-2 receptor density in the coronary arteries. Ischemia has also been shown to cause a reflex increase in sympathetic activity mediated by α mechanisms. This cascade may further increase coronary constriction. Postsynaptic α-1 receptors do not rely on extracellular $Ca2+$ to constrict the vessel, whereas the α-2–constrictor response is highly dependent on extracellular influx and exquisitely sensitive to calcium channel inhibitors.[31]

Myocardium. The role of β receptors in mediating catecholamine-induced inotropism and arrhythmogenesis is known. Studies have shown the presence of postsynaptic myocardial α-1 receptors, which also exert a major, facilatory, positive inotropic effect on the myocardium of several species of mammals including humans. Their contribution to malignant reperfusion arrhythmogenesis has also been recognized.

Phenylephrine, an α-1 agonist, can increase myocardial contractility two- to threefold compared with a six- to sevenfold increase produced by isoproterenol, a pure β agonist.[32] Myocardial postsynaptic α-1 receptors mediate perhaps as much as 30 to 50% of the basal inotropic tone of the normal heart. The inotropic response of the normal myocardium is more sensitive to β agonists.

Postsynaptic myocardial α-1 receptors play a more prominent inotropic role in the failing heart by serving as reserve to the normally predominant β-1 receptors. Although the response to both α-1 and β-1 agonists is reduced in the failing myocardium, the interaction between the two receptors is more apparent. Chronic heart failure is known to produce a reduced density (down-regulation) of myocardial β-1 receptors as a result of high levels of circulating catecholamines. However, there is no evidence of down-regulation of either α-1 or β-2 receptors with failure.[33]

The increase in density of myocardial α-1 adrenoreceptors shows a relative increase with failure and myocardial ischemia.[33] Thus, enhanced myocardial α-1 receptor numbers, and sensitivity, may contribute to positive inotropism seen during ischemia as well as to the malignant arrhythmias that occur with reperfusion. Intracellular mobilization of cytosolic $Ca2+$ by the activated α-1 myocardial receptors during ischemia appears to contribute to these arrhythmias.[33] The α-1 receptor also increases the sensitivity of the contractile elements to $Ca2+$. Drugs possessing potent α-1 antagonism such as prazosin and phentolamine have been shown to possess significant antiarrhythmic activity, although of limited usefulness because of hypotension. Enhanced α-1 activity with myocardial ischemia may explain why the antiarrhythmic benefits of β antagonists in patients with acute myocardial infarction are far from certain. The contribution of β receptors to positive inotropism and arrhythmogenesis during ischemia and reperfusion may be overshadowed by the α receptors during acute failure and ischemia.

Peripheral Vessels. Activation of the presynaptic α-2 vascular receptors produces vasodilation, whereas the postsynaptic α-1 and α-2 vascular receptors subserve vasoconstriction. Presynaptic vascular α-2 receptors inhibit NE release. This represents a negative feedback mechanism by which NE inhibits its own release via the prejunctional receptor. Presynaptic α-2 agonists, such as clonidine, inhibit NE release at the neurosympathetic junction producing vasodilatation. The effects of selective presynaptic α-2 receptor agonists to ameliorate coronary vasoconstriction in humans are unclear. Excitation of the inhibitory presynaptic α-2 receptors by endogenous or synthetic catecholamines also inhibits NE release. However, most sympathomimetics are nonselective α agonists that will excite equally presynaptic α-2 vasodilators and vasoconstrictive postsynaptic α-1 and α-2 receptors.

Postsynaptic α-1 and α-2 receptors coexist in both the arterial and venous sides of the circulation with the relative distribution of α-2 receptors being greater on the venous side.[34] This may explain why pure α-1 agonists, such as methoxamine, produce little venoconstriction, whereas many nonselective agonists such as phenylephrine produce significant venoconstriction. NE is the most potent venoconstrictor of all the catecholamines. Clinically, venoconstriction would have the effect of preloading by shifting venous capacitance centrally, whereas stimulation of *arterial* postsynaptic α-1 and α-2 receptors would effect afterloading by increasing arterial resistance.

α Receptors in the Central Nervous System. All subtypes of the α, β, and DA receptors have been found in various regions of the brain and spinal cord. The functional role of the cerebral α and β receptors suggests a close association with blood pressure and HR control. Cerebral and spinal cord presynaptic α-2 receptors are also involved in inhibition of presynaptic NE release. Although the brain contains adrenergic and dopaminergic receptors, circulating catecholamines do not cross the blood-brain barrier. The catecholamines in the brain are synthesized there. Many actions have been attributed to the cerebral postsynaptic α-2 receptor. This includes inhibition of insulin release, inhibition of bowel motility, stimulation of growth hormone release, and inhibition of antidiuretic hormone release. Central neuraxis injection of α-2 agonists, such as clonidine, act to produce analgesia, sedation, and cardiovascular depression. The increased duration of epidural or intrathecal anesthesia by the addition of nonselective α agonists to the local anesthetic may also produce additional analgesia through this mechanism.

α Receptors in the Kidney. The kidney has an extensive and exclusive adrenergic innervation of the afferent and efferent glomerular arterioles, proximal and distal renal tubules, ascending loop of Henle, and juxtaglomerular apparatus. The greatest density of innervation is in the thick ascending loop of Henle, followed by the distal convoluted tubules and proximal tube. Both α-1 and α-2 subtypes are found in the kidney with the α-2 receptor dominating. The α-1 receptor is predominant in the renal vasculature and elicits vasoconstriction, which modulates renal blood flow. Tubular α-1 receptors enhance sodium and water resorption, leading to antinatriuresis, whereas tubular α-2 receptors promote sodium and water excretion.

β-Adrenergic Receptors

The β-adrenergic receptors, like the α receptor, have been divided into subtypes. They are designated as the β-1 and β-2 subtypes. The β-1 receptors predominate in the myocardium, the sinoatrial node, and the ventricular conduction system. The β-1 receptors also mediate the effects of the catecholamines on the myocardium. These receptors are equally sensitive to EPI and NE, which distinguishes them from the β-2 receptors. Effects of β-1 stimulation are outlined in Table 12-5. Table 12-6 outlines their effects specifically on the cardiovascular system.

The β-2 receptors are located in the smooth muscles of the blood vessels in the skin, muscle, and mesentery, and in bronchial smooth muscle. Stimulation produces vasodilation and bronchial relaxation. The β-2 receptors are more sensitive to EPI than NE. The β-1 receptors are suggested to be innervated receptors responding to neuronally released NE, whereas β-2 receptors are "normal" receptors responding primarily to circulating EPI.[35]

β receptors are found in both presynaptic and postsynaptic membranes of the adrenergic neuroeffector junction (see Table 12-6). β-1 receptors are distributed to postsynaptic sites and have not been identified on the presynaptic membrane. Presynaptic β receptors are mostly of the β-2 subtype. The effects of activation of the presynaptic β-2 receptor are diametrically opposed to those of the presynaptic α-2 receptor. The presynaptic β-2 receptor accelerates endogenous NE release, whereas blockade of this receptor will inhibit NE release. Antagonism of the presynaptic β-2 receptors produces a physiological result similar to activation of the presynaptic α-2 receptor.

The postsynaptic β-1 receptors are located on the synaptic membrane and are innervated receptors responding primarily to neuronal NE. The postsynaptic β-2 receptors, like the postsynaptic α-2 receptor, are considered noninnervated, extrasynaptic, normal receptors responding primarily to circulating EPI.

β Receptors in the Cardiovascular System

Myocardium. Myocardial β receptors were originally classified as β-1 receptors. Those in the vascular and bronchial smooth muscle were called the β-2 subtype. However, studies have confirmed the coexistence of β-1 and β-2 receptors in the myocardium.[35] Both β-1 and β-2 receptors are functionally coupled to adenyl cyclase, suggesting a similar involvement in the regulation of inotropism and chronotropism.

Postsynaptic β-1 receptors are distributed predominantly to the myocardium, the sinoatrial node, and the ventricular conduction system. The β-2 receptors have the same distribution but are presynaptic. Activation of the presynaptic β-2 receptor accelerates the release of NE into the synaptic cleft. The β-2 receptor approximates 20 to 30% of the β receptors in the ventricular myocardium and up to 40% of the β receptors in the atrium.

The increased catecholamine levels associated with heart failure lead to a proportionally greater down-regulation of the β-1 receptor density with a relative sparing of the β-2 subtype and an increase in the α-1 subtype. The β-2 receptors increasingly mediate the inotropic response to catecholamines during heart failure and are facilitated by the α-1 receptor.

The effect of NE on inotropism in the normal heart is mediated entirely through the postsynaptic β-1 receptor, whereas the inotropic effects of EPI are mediated through both the β-1 and β-2 myocardial receptors. The β-2 receptors may also mediate the chronotropic responses to EPI because selective β-1 antagonists are less effective in suppressing induced tachycardia than the nonselective β-1 antagonist propranolol.

Peripheral Vessels. The postsynaptic vascular β receptors are virtually all of the β-2 subtype. The β-2 receptors are located in the smooth muscle of the blood vessels of the skin, muscle, mesentery, and bronchi. Stimulation of the postsynaptic β-2 receptor produces vasodilation and bronchial relaxation. Modest vasoconstriction occurs when subjected to blockade because the actions of the vascular postsynaptic β-2 receptors no longer oppose the actions of the α-1 and α-2 postsynaptic receptors.

β Receptor in the Kidney. The kidney contains both β-1 and β-1 receptors, with the β-1 being predominant. Renin release from the juxtaglomerular apparatus is enhanced by β stimulation. β-blockers inhibit this response. The β-1 receptor evokes renin release in humans. Renal β-2 receptors also appear to regulate renal blood flow at the vascular level. They have been identified pharmacologically and mediate a vasodilatory response.

Dopaminergic Receptors

Dopamine, synthesized in 1910, was recognized in 1959 not only as a vasopressor and the precursor of NE and EPI, but also as an important central and peripheral neurotransmitter. Dopamine receptors (DA) have been localized in the CNS, on blood vessels, and on postganglionic sympathetic nerves (see Table 12-6). Two clinically important types of DA receptors have been recognized. These are the DA1 and DA2 receptors. The DA1 receptors are postsynaptic, whereas the DA2 receptors are both presynaptic and postsynaptic. The presynaptic DA2 receptors, like the presynaptic α-2 receptor, inhibit NE release and can produce vasodilatation.[36] The postsynaptic DA2 receptor may subserve vasoconstriction similar to that of the postsynaptic α-2 receptor.[37] This effect is opposite to that of the postsynaptic DA1 renal vascular receptor. Unpublished data suggest that dopamine may be the intrinsic regulator of renal function.[38] The zona glomerulose of the adrenal cortex also contains DA2 receptors, which inhibit release of aldosterone.

Myocardium. Defining specific dopaminergic receptors has been difficult because dopamine also exerts effects on the α and β receptors.[39] DA receptors have not been described in the myocardium. Effects of dopamine are those related to activation of β-1 receptors, which promote positive inotropism and chronotropism. β-2 activation would produce *some* systemic vasodilatation.

Peripheral Vessels. The greatest numbers of DA1-postsynaptic receptors are found on vascular smooth muscle cells of the kidney and mesentery, but are also found in the other systemic arteries including coronary, cerebral, and cutaneous arteries. The vascular receptors are, like the β-2 receptors, linked to adenyl cyclase and mediate smooth muscle relaxation. Activation of these receptors produces vasodilatation, increasing blood flow to these organs. Concurrent activation of vascular presynaptic DA2 receptors also inhibits NE release at presynaptic α-2 receptors, which may also contribute to peripheral vasodilatation. Higher doses of dopamine can mediate vasoconstriction via the postsynaptic α-1 and α-2 receptors. The constrictive effect is relatively weak in the cardiovascular system where the action of dopamine on adrenergic receptors is 1/35 and 1/50 as potent as that of EPI and NE, respectively.[40]

Central Nervous System. DA receptors have been identified in the hypothalamus where they are involved in prolactin release. They are also found in the basal ganglia where they coordinate motor function.[39] Degeneration of dopaminergic neurons of the substantia nigra is the source of Parkinson's disease. Another central action of dopamine is to stimulate the chemoreceptor trigger zone of the medulla, producing nausea and vomiting. Dopamine antagonists such as haloperidol and droperidol are clinically effective in countering this action.

Kidney and Mesentery. Apart from their effect on the vessels of the kidney and mesentery, DA receptors on the smooth muscle of the esophagus, stomach, and small intestine enhance secretion production and reduce intestinal motility.[40]

Metoclopramide, a dopamine antagonist, is useful for aspiration prophylaxis by promoting gastric emptying.

The distribution of DA receptors in the renal vasculature is well known, but DA receptors have other functions within the kidney. DA1 receptors are located on renal tubules, which inhibit sodium resorption with subsequent natriuresis and diuresis. The natriuresis may be the result of a combined renal vasodilatation, improved CO, and tubular action of the DA1 receptors. Juxtaglomerular cells also contain DA1 receptors, which increase renin release when activated. This action modulates the diuresis produced by DA1 activation of the tubules.

Dopamine has unique autonomic effects by activating specific peripheral dopaminergic receptors, which promote natriuresis and reduce afterload via dilatation of the renal and mesenteric arterial beds. Peripheral dopaminergic activity serves as a natural antihypertensive mechanism.[41] Its actions are overshadowed by the opposite effect of its main biologic partner, NE.[42] Plasma NE levels are known to increase with aging, likely the result of reduced clearance. Peripheral dopaminergic activity is known to diminish. Subtle changes in the DA–NE balance with aging may account for the diminished ability of the aged kidney to excrete a salt load. This may also contribute to the uniform finding of increasing systolic blood pressure in societies with high salt consumption.

Other Receptors

Adenosine Receptors

Adenosine produces inhibition of NE release. The effect of adenosine is blocked by caffeine and other methylxanthines. The physiologic and pharmacologic roles of adenosine-mediated inhibition of NE release are not clearly defined. The physiologic function of these receptors may be the reduction of sympathetic tone under hypoxic conditions when adenosine production is enhanced. As a consequence of reduced NE release, cardiac work would be decreased and oxygen demand reduced. Adenosine has been effectively used to produce controlled hypotension.[42]

Serotonin

Serotonin (5-hydroxytryptamine) depresses the response of isolated blood vessels to SNS stimulation and decreases release of labeled NE in these preparations. This inhibitory action of serotonin is antagonized by raising the external calcium ion concentration. Thus, serotonin may inhibit neuronal NE release by a mechanism that limits the availability of calcium ions at the nerve terminal.

Prostaglandin E2, Histamine, and Several Opioids

Prostaglandin E2, histamine, and several opioids have been reported to act on prejunctional receptor sites to inhibit NE release in certain sympathetically innervated tissue. However, these inhibitory receptors are unlikely to play a physiologic role in limiting NE release because inhibitors of cyclo-oxygenase, histamine antagonists, and naloxone produce no increase in NE release.

Histamine acts in a manner similar to the neurotransmitters of the SNS. It has membrane receptors specific for histamine, with the individual response being determined by the type of cell being stimulated. Two receptors for histamine have been determined. These have been designated H1 and H2, for which it has been possible to develop specific agonists and antagonists. Stimulation of the H1 receptors produces bronchoconstriction and intestinal contraction. The major role of the H2 receptors is related to acid production by the parietal cells of the stomach; however, histamine is present in relatively high concentrations in the myocardium and cardiac conducting tissue, where it exerts positive inotropic and chronotropic effects while depressing dromotropism. The positive inotropic and chronotropic effects of histamine are H2 receptor effects that are not blocked by β antagonism. These effects are blocked by H2 antagonists, such as cimetidine, which accounts for the occasional report of cardiovascular collapse following the use of cimetidine.[43] The negative dromotropic effect and that of coronary spasm caused by histamine are H1 receptor effects.

Adrenergic Receptor Numbers or Sensitivity

Receptors, once thought to be static entities, are now thought to be dynamically regulated by a variety of conditions and in a constant state of flux. Receptors are synthesized in the sarcoplasmic reticulum (SR) of the parent cell, where they may remain extrasynaptic or externalize to the synaptic membranes where they may cluster. Membrane receptors may be removed or internalized to intracellular sites for either dehydration or recycling.

The number and sensitivity of adrenergic receptors can be influenced by normal, genetic, and developmental factors. Changes in the number of receptors alter the response to catecholamines. Alteration in the number, or density, of receptors is referred to as either up-regulation or down-regulation. As a rule, the number of receptors is inversely proportional to the ambient concentration of the catecholamines. Extended exposure of receptors to their agonists markedly reduces, but does not ablate, the biologic response to catecholamines.[44] For example, increased adrenergic activity occurs in response to reduced perfusion as a result of acute or chronic myocardial dysfunction. Plasma catecholamines are increased. As a result, myocardial postsynaptic β-1 receptors "downregulate." This is thought to explain the diminished inotropic and chronotropic response to β-1 agonists and exercise in patients with chronic heart failure. However, calcium-induced inotropism is not impaired because β-2 receptor (extrasynaptic) numbers remain relatively intact.[45] The β-2 receptors may account for up to 40% of the inotropism of the failing heart compared with 20% in the normal heart.[46] Tachyphylaxis to infused catecholamines is also thought to be the result of acute down-regulation of receptor numbers. There appears to be a reduction in numbers or sensitivity of β receptors in hypertensive patients who also have elevated plasma catecholamines. Down-regulation is the presumptive explanation for the lack of correlation between plasma catecholamine levels and the blood pressure elevation in patients with pheochromocytoma. Chronic use of β agonists such as terbutaline, isoproterenol, or EPI for the treatment of asthma can result in tachyphylaxis because of down-regulation. Even short-term use (1 to 6 hours) of β agonists may cause down-regulation of receptor numbers.

Down-regulation is reversible on termination of the agonist. Chronic treatment of animals with nonselective β-blockade causes a 100% increase in the number of β receptors.[47] This accounts for the propranolol withdrawal syndrome in which the acute discontinuation of the β antagonist leaves the α receptors unopposed plus an increased number of β receptors. Clonidine withdrawal can be explained by the same mechanism.[48] Acute discontinuation of the α-2- inhibitory agonist would permit a resumption of stimulation of adrenoreceptors that upregulated during the time NE release was inhibited.

Up- or down-regulation of receptor numbers may not alter sensitivity of the receptor. Likewise, sensitivity may be increased or decreased in the presence of normal numbers of receptors. The pharmacologic factors affecting up- or down-regulation of the α and β receptors are similar.

AUTONOMIC NERVOUS SYSTEM REFLEXES AND INTERACTIONS

The ANS reflex has been compared to the computer circuit. This control system, as in all reflex systems, has (1) sensors, (2) afferent pathways, (3) CNS integration, and (4) efferent pathways to the receptors and efferent organs. Fine adjustments are made at the local level according to positive and negative feedback mechanisms. The baroreceptor is an example. The variable to be controlled (blood pressure) is sensed (carotid sinus), integrated (medullary vasomotor center), and adjusted through specific effector–receptor sites. Drugs or disease can interrupt this circuit at any point. β-blockers may attenuate the effector response, whereas an α agonist such as clonidine may alter both the effector and the integrator functions of blood pressure control (see Antihypertensives section).[48]

Baroreceptors

Several reflexes in the cardiovascular system help control arterial blood pressure, CO, and HR. Cardiovascular ANS reflexes are an anachronism. The business of circulation is to provide blood flow. Yet the most important controlled variable to which the sensors are attuned is blood pressure, a product of flow and resistance.

Etienne Marey noted in 1859 that the pulse rate is inversely proportional to the blood pressure, and this is known as Marey's law. Subsequently, Hering, Koch, and others demonstrated that the alterations in HR evoked by changes in blood pressure stretch are dependent on baroreceptors located in the aortic arch and the carotid sinuses. These pressure sensors react to alterations in stretch caused by blood pressure. Compliance of the stretch receptors and their sensitivity may be altered by carotid sinus atherosclerosis. Thus, carotid artery disease may be one source of hypertension rather than the result.

Impulses from the carotid sinus and aortic arch reach the medullary vasomotor center by the glossopharyngeal and vagus nerves, respectively. Increased sensory traffic from the baroreceptors, caused by increased blood pressure, inhibits SNS effector traffic. The relative increase in vagal tone produces vasodilation, slowing of the HR, and a lowering of blood pressure. Real increases in vagal tone occur when blood pressure exceeds normal limits.[49]

The arterial baroreceptor reflex can best be demonstrated by the Valsalva maneuver (Fig. 12-15). The Valsalva maneuver raises the intrathoracic pressure by forced expiration against a closed glottis. The arterial blood pressure rises momentarily as the intrathoracic blood is forced into the heart (preload). Sustained intrathoracic pressure diminishes venous return, reduces the CO, and drops the blood pressure. Reflex vasoconstriction and tachycardia ensue. Blood pressure returns to normal with release of the forced expiration, but then briefly "overshoots" because of the vasoconstriction and increased venous return. A slowing of the HR accompanies the overshoot in pressure, according to Marey's law.

The cardiovascular responses to the Valsalva maneuver require an intact ANS circuit from peripheral sensor to peripheral adrenergic receptors. The Valsalva maneuver has been used to identify patients at risk for anesthesia because of ANS instability (see Fig. 12-15). This was once a major concern in patients receiving drugs that depleted catecholamines, such as reserpine. Dysfunction of the SNS is implicated if exaggerated and prolonged hypotension develops during the forced expiration phase (50% from resting mean arterial pressure).[4] In addition, the overshoot at the end of the Valsalva maneuver is absent. Dysfunction of the PNS can be assumed if the HR does not

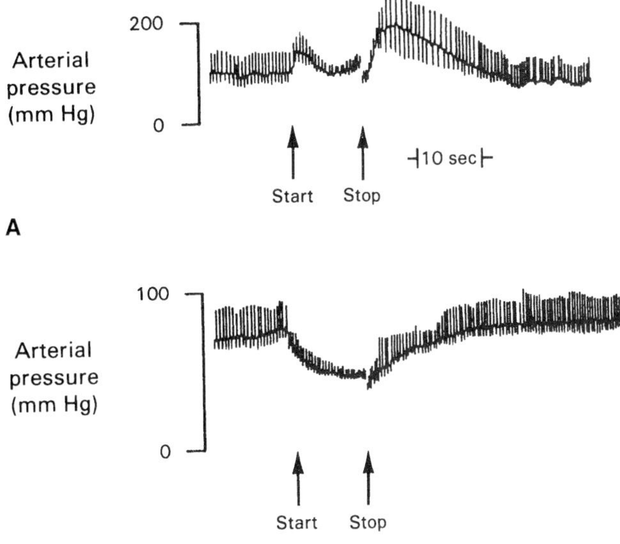

FIGURE 12-15. A. The normal blood pressure response to the Valsalva maneuver is demonstrated. Pulse rate moves in a reciprocal direction according to Marey's law of the heart. B. An abnormal Valsalva response is shown in a patient with C5 quadriplegia.

respond appropriately to the blood pressure changes. The Valsalva maneuver may still be a valid clinical preoperative test for detecting the autonomic dysautonomia that accompanies diabetes.

Venous baroreceptors may be more dominant in the moment-to-moment regulation of CO. Baroreceptors in the right atrium and great veins produce an increase in HR when stretched by increased right atrial pressure.[50] Reduced venous pressure decreases HR. Unlike the arterial baroreceptors, venous sensors are not thought to alter vascular tone; however, venoconstriction is postulated to occur when atrial pressures decline. Stretch of the venous receptors produces changes in HR opposite to those produced when the arterial pressure sensors are stimulated. The arterial and venous pressure receptors are separately monitoring two of the four major determinants of CO: afterload and preload, respectively. Venous baroreceptors sample preload by stretch of the atrium. Arterial baroreceptors survey resistance, or afterload, as reflected in the mean arterial pressure. Afterload and preload produce opposite effects on CO; thus, one should not be surprised that the venous and arterial baroreceptors produce effects opposite those of a similar stretch stimulus, pressure.

Bainbridge described the venous baroreceptor reflex and demonstrated that it can be abolished by vagal resection. Numerous investigators have confirmed the acceleration of the HR in response to volume. However, the magnitude and direction of the HR response are dependent on the prevailing HR at the time of stimulation. The denervated, transplanted mammalian heart also accelerates in response to volume loading. HR, like CO, can apparently be adjusted to the quantity of blood entering the heart.[51]

The Bainbridge reflex relates to the characteristic but paradoxical slowing of the heart seen with spinal anesthesia. Blockade of the SNS levels of T1-4 ablates the efferent limb of the cardiac accelerator nerves. This source of cardiac deceleration is obvious, as the vagus nerve is unopposed. However, bradycardia during spinal anesthesia is more related to the development of arterial hypotension than to the height of the block. The primary defect in the development of spinal hypotension is a decrease in venous return. Theoretically, the arterial

TABLE 12-7

DRUG EFFECTS ON THE DENERVATED HEART

DRUG	SINUS RATE		ATRIOVENTRICULAR CONDUCTION VELOCITY	INTRAVENTRICULAR CONDUCTION VELOCITY	BLOOD PRESSURE	CARDIAC OUTPUT	SYSTEMIC VASCULAR RESISTANCE
	RECIPIENT	DONOR					
Resting	Normal	↑[a]	Normal	Normal	Normal	Normal or low	Normal
Exercise	↑	Slow ↑			↑	↑	
Atropine	↑	—	—				
Norepinephrine	↓	↑ ↑[a]	↑	—	↑	— or ↑	↑↑
Methoxamine	↓	—			↑	↓	↑↑
Isoproterenol	↑	↑ ↑	↑		↓	↑↑	↓
Glucagon	↑	↑			—	↑	
Propranolol	↓	↓	↓	—	— or ↓	↓	↑
Amyl nitrite	↑	—			↓		↓
Digoxin							
Acute	↓	—	—[a]	—	—	— or ↑[b]	
Chronic	↓	—	↓				
Quinidine	↑	↓[a]	↓[a]	↓			
Edrophonium	↓	—[a]	—[a]				
Increased preload		↑				↑ or ↓[b]	

↑, increase; ↓, decrease; — , no change.
[a]Opposite from normals.
[b]Response depends on contractile state related to rejection.
Reprinted with permission from Lawson NW, Wallfisch HK: Cardiovascular pharmacology: A new look at the "pressors." In Stoelting RK, Barash PG, Gallagher TJ (eds): Advances in Anesthesia, p 195. Chicago, Year Book Medical Publishers, 1986.

hypotension should reflexly produce a tachycardia through the arterial baroreceptors. Instead, bradycardia is more common. Greene suggests that in the unmedicated person, the venous baroreceptors are dominant over the arterial. A reduced venous pressure, therefore, slows HR.[52] In contrast, humorally mediated tachycardia is the usual response to hypotension or acidosis from other causes.

Denervated Heart

Reflex modulation of the adrenergic agonists is best seen in the denervated transplant heart, which retains the recipient's innervated sinoatrial node and the donor's denervated sinoatrial node.[53] Table 12-7 is a summary of drug effects on the transplanted heart. NE simultaneously activates α and β receptors of the intact heart and vessels. NE infusion in the transplanted heart produces a slowing of the recipient's atrial rate through vagal feedback as the blood pressure rises. In the unmodulated donor heart, atrial rate increases. Methoxamine-induced hypertension and nitrite-induced hypotension fail to induce deceleration and acceleration of the donor atrial rate. The baroreceptors are therefore not operant in the transplanted heart. Isoproterenol, a pure β agonist, increases the discharge rate of both the recipient and donor node by direct action, with the donor rate near doubling that of the recipient node. Atropine accelerates the recipient's atrial rate, whereas no effect is seen on the donor rate, which now controls HR. Hypersensitivity to β cardiac stimulation in denervated dog hearts has been demonstrated. Patients who have undergone chemical sympathectomy with bretylium or guanethidine are known to be hyperreactive to the usual doses of catecholamines.

β-blockade produces comparable slowing of the sinoatrial node of both recipient and donor. The exercise capability of the denervated heart is conspicuously reduced by β-blockade, presumably because of its reliance on circulating catecholamines. Propranolol has also been demonstrated to reduce the β response to chronotropic effects of NE and isoproterenol in the transplanted heart. The CO of the transplanted heart varies appropriately with changes in preload and afterload.

Interaction of Autonomic Nervous System Receptors

Strong interactions have been noted between SNS and PNS nerves in organs that receive dual, antagonistic innervation. Release of NE at the presynaptic terminal is modified by the PNS. For example, vagal inhibition of left ventricular contractility is accentuated as the level of SNS activity is raised. This interaction is termed "accentuated antagonism" and is mediated by a combination of presynaptic and postsynaptic mechanisms. The coronary arteries present an example of this phenomenon and deserve special attention. The concept of accentuated antagonism has yet to be clearly defined because it is unusual for high SNS and PNS activity to coexist, except during anesthesia. The importance of accentuated antagonism in the intact, conscious human has yet to be demonstrated; however, it may explain the clinical observation that angina and myocardial infarction owing to coronary spasm in humans are not often related to cardiac work, as is angina caused by sclerotic coronary disease. Attacks of angina usually occur at rest, often waking the patient from sleep. This diurnal variation also corresponds to the greatest activity of the PNS system. The mechanism by which coronary arterial spasm occurs remains unknown, but this continues to be an exciting area of investigation.

The myocardium and coronary vessels are abundantly supplied with adrenergic and cholinergic fibers. Strong activity of both α and β receptors has been demonstrated in the coronary vascular bed. Selective stimulation of both the α-1 and postsynaptic α-2 receptors increases coronary vascular resistance, whereas selective α blockade eliminates this effect. Therefore, both β-1 and α-1adrenoreceptors are present on coronary arteries and accessible to NE from sympathetic nerves.[54]

The close anatomic proximity of the postganglionic vagal and SNS nerve endings in coronary arteries provides the morphologic basis for strong interaction. SNS and PNS nerve terminals are found in such close proximity that transmitters from one can easily reach the other and affect transmitter release. In addition, the presynaptic adrenergic terminals of the myocardium and coronary vessels, like all blood vessels examined, contain muscarinic receptors.[18] Recent observations confirm that muscarinic agents and vagal stimulation, acting on the presynaptic, SNS muscarinic receptor, inhibit the release of NE in a manner similar to that of the presynaptic α-2 and DA2 receptors (see Fig. 12-11). Conversely, blockade of the muscarinic receptors with atropine markedly augments the positive inotropic responses to catecholamines.[3] Suppression of NE release explains, in part, vagal-induced attenuation of the inotropic response to strong SNS stimulation (accentuated antagonism) and only a weak negative inotropic effect of vagal stimulation when there is low background SNS activity. This may also explain why vagal activity reduces the vulnerability of the myocardium to fibrillation during infusions of NE.

ACh may cause coronary spasm during periods of high SNS tone.[6] Inhibition of NE release by presynaptic adrenergic muscarinic receptors of the smooth muscle of coronary vessels would lessen the coronary relaxation normally produced by NE on the β-1 receptor (see Fig. 12-11). In anesthetized dogs, the rate of NE outflow into the coronary sinus blood, evoked by cardiac SNS stimulation, is markedly diminished by simultaneous vagal efferent stimulation.[55] This action is known to be prevented by atropine, which also causes coronary vasodilation. Methacholine, a muscarinic parasympathomimetic agent, has been reported to cause coronary vasoconstriction.[56] However, it simultaneously reduces ventricular irritability by reducing NE release in myocardial fibers.[3]

Interaction with Other Regulatory Systems

2 The ANS is integrally related to several endocrine systems that ultimately summate to control blood pressure and regulate homeostasis. These include the renin–angiotensin system, antidiuretic hormone, glucocorticoids, and insulin.

Antidiuretic hormone or vasopressin is formed in the hypothalamus and released from nerve endings in the posterior pituitary gland. It causes vasoconstriction and increased resorption of water in the distal collecting ducts of the kidney. It therefore affects not only central blood volume but also plasma osmolality. The primary regulator of antidiuretic hormone release is plasma osmolality; however, several other stimuli may outweigh this control in stressful situations. Release is also triggered by decreased central blood volume via low-pressure atrial receptors and hypotension via the carotid baroreceptors. Stress, pain, hypoxia, anesthesia, and surgery also stimulate release of antidiuretic hormone. Infusion of catecholamines may alter its release, but these effects appear to be mediated by the carotid baroreceptors. ANS drugs that induce hypotension or decrease cardiac filling may induce release of antidiuretic hormone and thus affect plasma osmolality.

Both α and β receptors have been found in the endocrine pancreas and modulate insulin release (see Table 12-5). β stimulation increases insulin release, whereas α stimulation decreases it. The overall importance of this interaction is not entirely clear, but decreased tolerance to glucose and potassium has been noted in subjects taking β-blocking drugs.[57]

The renin–angiotensin system is a complex endocrine system that modulates both blood pressure and water-electrolyte homeostasis (Fig. 12-16). Renin is a proteolytic enzyme contained within the cells of the juxtaglomerular apparatus of the renal cortex. When released, it acts on plasma angiotensinogen to form angiotensin I. Angiotensin I is then converted to angiotensin II by converting enzyme in the lung. Angiotensin II is a powerful direct arterial vasoconstrictor. It also acts on the adrenal cortex to release aldosterone and on the adrenal medulla to release EPI. In addition to its direct effects on vascular smooth muscle, angiotensin II augments NE release via presynaptic receptors, thus enhancing peripheral SNS tone. A group of drugs called angiotensin-converting enzyme (ACE) inhibitors act by interfering with the formation or function of angiotensin II. These drugs have been found useful in the treatment of essential and renovascular hypertension and of congestive heart failure. Captopril, enalapril, and lisinopril inhibit the action of converting enzyme, thus preventing the conversion of angiotensin I to angiotensin II.[58] They have supplanted diuretics and β-blockers as first-line agents in the treatment of hypertension.

Renin is released in response to hyponatremia, decreased renal perfusion pressure, and ANS stimulation via β receptors on juxtaglomerular cells. Changes in sympathetic tone may thus alter renin release and affect homeostasis in a variety

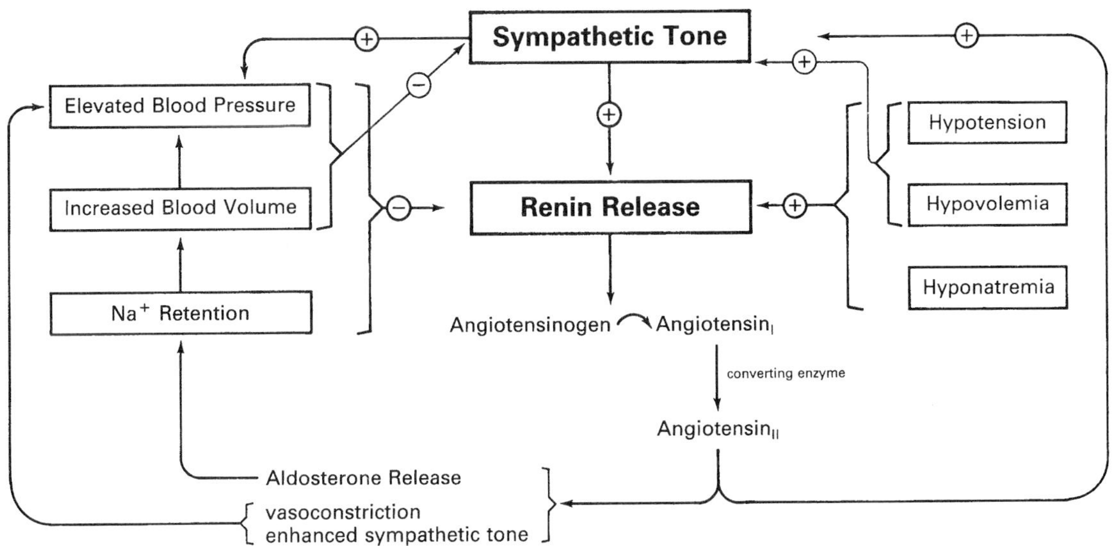

FIGURE 12-16. The interactions of the renin–angiotensin and SNS in regulating homeostasis are shown schematically along with the physiologic variables that modulate their function. Arrows with a plus sign (+) represent stimulation, and those with a minus sign (−) represent inhibition.

of ways. The ANS is also intimately related to adrenocortical function. As outlined earlier, glucocorticoid release modulates phenylethanolamine-N-methyltransferase formation and thus synthesis of EPI. Glucocorticoids are also important in regulating the response of peripheral tissues to changes in SNS tone. Thus, the ANS is intimately related to other homeostatic mechanisms.

CLINICAL AUTONOMIC NERVOUS SYSTEM PHARMACOLOGY

The clinical application of ANS pharmacology is based on knowledge of ANS anatomy, physiology, and molecular pharmacology. Drugs that modify ANS activity can be classified by their site of action, mechanism of action, or pathology for which they are most commonly used. Antihypertensive drugs are an example of the third category. This classification is a matter of degree because considerable functional overlap occurs. An example of classification by site relates to the ganglionic agonists or blocking agents. ANS drugs can be further categorized as those that act at the prejunctional membrane and those acting postjunctionally. They can then be more specifically classified by the predominant receptor or receptors on which they act.

Mode of Action

ANS drugs may be broadly classified by mode of action according to their mimetic or lytic actions. This may also be termed agonist or antagonist. A sympathomimetic, such as ephedrine, mimics SNS sympathetic activity by stimulation of adrenergic receptor sites both directly and indirectly. Sympatholytic drugs cause dissolution of SNS activity at these same receptor sites. β receptor blockers are examples of sympatholytic drugs. The terms "parasympathomimetic" and "parasympatholytic" are self-explanatory and may be further divided by their site of action on the muscarinic or nicotinic receptors.

Several modes of ANS drug action become evident when one follows the cascade of neurotransmission. The mode is related to site. Drugs that act on prejunctional membranes may therefore (1) interfere with transmitter synthesis (α-methyl paratyrosine), (2) interfere with transmitter storage (reserpine), (3) interfere with transmitter release (clonidine), (4) stimulate transmitter release (ephedrine), or (5) interfere with reuptake of transmitter (cocaine). Drugs may also modify metabolism of the neurotransmitter in the synaptic cleft (anticholinesterase). Drugs acting at postjunctional sites may directly stimulate postjunctional receptors and interfere with transmitter agonist at the postjunctional receptor.

The ultimate response of an effector organ to an agonist or antagonist depends on (1) the drug, (2) its plasma concentration, (3) the number of receptors in the effector organ, (4) binding by the receptor, (5) the concurrent activities of other drugs and hormones, (6) the cellular metabolic status, and (7) reflex adjustments by the organism. This is the source of conflicting results for drugs used in differing clinical circumstances.

Ganglionic Drugs

SNS and PNS ganglia are pharmacologically similar in that transmission through these ANS ganglia is affected by ACh (see Fig. 12-3). Most ganglionic agonists and antagonists are not selective and affect SNS and PNS ganglia equally. This nonselective property creates many undesirable and unpredictable side effects, which have limited the clinical usefulness of this category of drugs.

Agonists

There are essentially no clinically useful ganglionic agonists. Nicotine is the prototypical ganglionic agonist. In low doses, it stimulates ANS ganglia and the neuromuscular junction of striated muscle. High doses produce ganglionic and neuromuscular blockade. Low-dose stimulation and high-dose blockade are referred to as nicotinic effects in describing any drug with similar effects. Most ganglionic agonists and antagonists produce their effects through their nicotinic effects. The protean side effects of nicotinic stimulation render it useful only as an investigative tool.

Despite its lack of clinical usefulness, nicotine is widely used in the form of tobacco. The novice tobacco user can often describe the overlap of SNS and PNS side effects of nicotinic stimulation, which appear as nausea and vomiting, tachycardia, bradycardia, diarrhea, and sometimes fainting as a result of high-dose ganglionic blockade.[3]

Antagonists

Drugs that interfere with neurotransmission at ANS ganglia are known as ganglionic blocking agents. Nicotine, in high doses, is the prototypical ganglionic blocking agent also; however, early stimulatory nicotinic activity can be blocked at the ganglia and muscle end plates with other ganglionic blockers and muscle relaxants, respectively, without blocking muscarinic effects. Ganglionic blockers produce their nicotinic effects by competing, mimicking, or interfering with ACh metabolism. Hexamethonium, trimethaphan, and pentolinium produce a selective nondepolarizing blockade of neurotransmission at ANS ganglia without producing nicotinic neuromuscular blockade. They compete with ACh in the ganglia without stimulating the receptors. The introduction of drugs that produce vasodilation directly or by action on the SNS vasomotor center has made the ganglionic blockers obsolete. d-Tubocurare (dTC) produces a competitive nondepolarizing block of both motor end plates and ANS ganglia. The action of motor paralysis predominates, but the concomitant ganglionic blockade at higher doses explains part of the hypotensive effect often seen with the use of dTC for muscle relaxation. Histamine release is the major hypotensive factor that is common to dTC and other ganglionic blockers. Anticholinesterase drugs may produce nicotinic type ganglionic blockade by competition with ACh as well as by persistent depolarization via accumulated ACh.

Trimethaphan is the only ganglionic blocker available in the United States. Trimethaphan produces blockade by competition with ACh for receptors, thus stabilizing the postsynaptic membrane. However, side effects and rapid onset tachyphylaxis have markedly reduced its use in anesthesia.[59] The patient's pupils become fixed and dilated during administration, which obscures eye signs, an important consideration for neurosurgery. In this regard, it is distinctly inferior to nitroprusside. The major advantage of trimethaphan is its short duration of action, which is the result of pseudocholinesterase hydrolysis.

Cholinergic Drugs

Cholinergic drugs may be classified by the following outline, which follows physiologic response and site of action.

I. Cholinergic drugs: agonists[3]

  A. Nicotinic

1. ANS ganglionic transmission
2. Neuromuscular transmission

B. Muscarinic
1. Direct acting
2. Indirect acting

II. Cholinolytic agents: antagonists

A. Nicotinic
1. ANS ganglionic transmission
2. Neuromuscular transmission

B. Muscarinic

Muscarinic Agonists

The cholinomimetic muscarinic drugs act at sites in the body where ACh is the neurotransmitter of the nerve impulse. These drugs may be divided into three groups, the first two of which are direct muscarinic agonists.[60] The third group acts indirectly. These groups are choline esters (ACh, methacholine, carbamylcholine, bethanechol), alkaloids (pilocarpine, muscarine, arecoline), and anticholinesterases (physostigmine, neostigmine, pyridostigmine, edrophonium, echothiophate).

Direct Cholinomimetics. ACh has virtually no therapeutic applications because of its diffuse action and rapid hydrolysis by cholinesterase (see Fig. 12-6). One may encounter the use of topical ACh (1%) drops during cataract extraction when a rapid miosis is desired. Systemic effects are not usually seen because of the rapidity of ACh hydrolysis.

Other choline esters have been synthesized, mostly derivatives of ACh, which possess more selective muscarinic activity than ACh. They differ from ACh in being more resistant to inactivation by cholinesterase and thus having a more prolonged and useful action. They also differ from ACh in their relative muscarinic and nicotinic activities. The best studied of these drugs are methacholine, bethanechol, and carbamylcholine.[3] The chemical structures of ACh and these choline esters are shown in Figure 12-17. Their pharmacologic actions are compared with those of ACh in Table 12-8. These are not important drugs in anesthesiology but anesthesiologists may encounter patients who are receiving them. They may be useful in the postoperative period to alleviate cardiac tachydysrhythmias, urinary retention, and ileus.

ACh is a quaternary ammonium compound that interacts with postsynaptic receptors, causing conformational membrane changes. This results in increased permeability to small ions and, thus, depolarization. All the receptors translate the reversible binding of ACh into openings of discrete channels in excitable membranes, allowing Na+ and K+ ions to flow along their electrochemical gradients. Structure–activity relationships point to the presence of two important binding sites on the receptor, an esteractic site that binds the ester end of the molecule and an ionic site that binds the quaternary amine portion (see Fig. 12-6). Subtle changes in the structure of the compound can markedly alter the responses among different tissue groups. The degree of muscarinic activity falls if the acetyl group is replaced, but this confers a resistance to enzymatic hydrolysis. Carbamylcholine is synthesized by replacing the acetyl group with carbamyl (see Fig. 12-17). It possesses both muscarinic and nicotinic actions but is virtually resistant to esterase hydrolysis (see Table 12-8). Bethanechol is also resistant to hydrolysis but possesses mainly muscarinic activity. β-methyl substitution produces methacholine, which is less resistant to hydrolysis but is primarily a muscarinic agonist.

Methacholine slows the heart and dilates peripheral blood vessels. It is used to terminate supraventricular tachydysrhythmias, especially paroxysmal tachycardia, when other measures have failed. It also increases intestinal tone. Methacholine should not be given to patients with asthma. Hypertensive patients may also develop marked hypotension. Side effects are those of PNS stimulation such as nausea, vomiting, and flushed sweating. Overdose is treated with atropine.

Choline Esters: Choline, Acetylcholine, Carbamylcholine, Metacholine, Bethanechol

Alkaloids: Pilocarpine, Muscarine, Arecoline

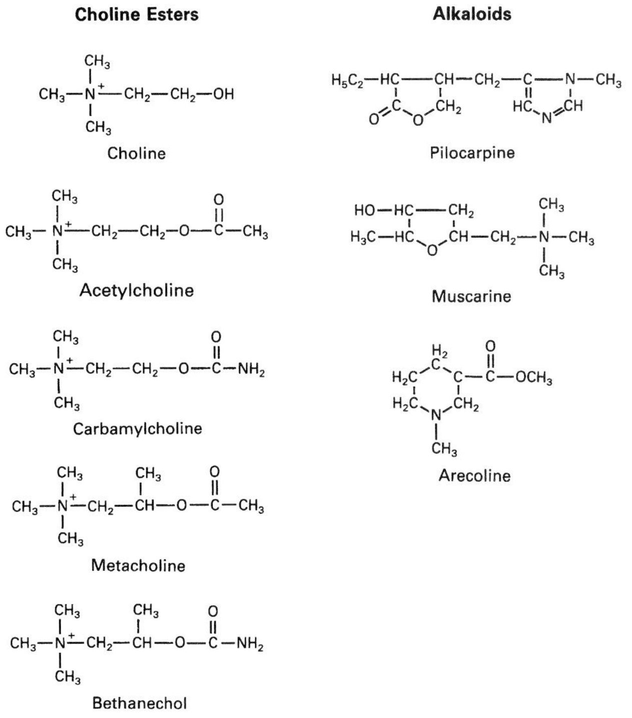

FIGURE 12-17. Chemical structures of direct-acting cholinomimetic esters and alkaloids.

Bethanechol is relatively selective for the gastrointestinal and urinary tracts. In usual doses it does not slow the heart or lower the blood pressure, as does methacholine. Bethanecol is of value in treating postoperative abdominal distention (nonobstructive paralytic ileus), gastric atony following bilateral vagotomy, congenital megacolon, nonobstructive urinary retention, and some cases of neurogenic bladder. It is not a parenteral drug. Precautions are as for methacholine.

Direct-acting cholinomimetic alkaloids include muscarine, pilocarpine, and arecoline. They act at the same sites as ACh, and their effects are similar to those of ACh as described in Table 12-8. There are no uses for these drugs in anesthesiology. Pilocarpine is the only drug of this group used therapeutically in the United States. Its sole use is for the treatment of glaucoma, for which it is the standard. It is used as a topical miotic drug in ophthalmologic practice to reduce intraocular pressure in glaucoma.

Common side effects of cholinomimetic alkaloids are those of intense PNS stimulation, which include gastrointestinal cramping, hypotension, diaphoresis, salivation, diarrhea, and bladder pain.[3] Muscarinic agonists are particularly dangerous in patients with myasthenia gravis (who are receiving anticholinesterases), bulbar palsy, cardiac disease, asthma, peptic ulcer, progressive muscular atrophy, or mechanical intestinal obstruction or urinary retention.[61]

Indirect Cholinomimetics. The indirect-acting cholinomimetic drugs are of greater importance to the anesthesiologist than are the direct-acting drugs. These drugs produce cholinomimetic effects indirectly as a result of inhibition or inactivation of the enzyme acetylcholinesterase, which normally destroys ACh by hydrolysis. They are referred to as cholinesterase inhibitors or anticholinesterases. Table 12-9 lists therapeutic cholinesterase inhibitors and their major indications. Most of these drugs inhibit both acetylcholinesterase and pseudocholinesterase. Inhibition of acetylcholinesterase

TABLE 12-8

COMPARATIVE MUSCARINIC ACTIONS OF DIRECT CHOLINOMIMETIC AGENTS

	SYSTEMIC				
	ACETYLCHOLINE	METHACHOLINE	CARBAMYLCHOLINE	BETHANECHOL	PILOCARPINE
Esterase Hydrolysis	+++	+	0	0	0
Eye (Topical)					
Iris	++	++	+++	+++	+++
Ciliary	++	++	+++	+++	++
Heart					
Rate	---	---	–	–	?
Contractility	–	–	–	–	
Conduction	--	---	–	–	
Smooth Muscle					
Vascular	--	---	–	–	--
Bronchial	++	++	+	+	++
Gastrointestinal motility	++	++	+++	+++	++
Gastrointestinal sphincters	--	–	---	---	++
Biliary	++	++	+++	+++	++
Bladder					
Detrusor	++	++	+++	+++	++
Sphincter	--	–	---	---	--
Exocrine Glands					
Respiratory	+++	++	+++	++	++++
Salivary	++	++	++	++	+++++
Pharyngeal	++	++	++	++	++++
Lacrimal	++	++	++	++	++++
Sweat	++	++	++	++	+++++
Gastrointestinal acid and secretions	++	++	++	++	++++
Nicotinic Actions	+++	+	+++	–	+++

+, stimulation; –, inhibition.

permits the accumulation of ACh transmitter in the synapse, resulting in intense PNS activity similar to that of the direct cholinomimetic agents. The action of ACh is therefore potentiated and prolonged. Their effects can be predicted from a knowledge of ANS pharmacology previously presented. Some of the acetylcholinesterase drugs (i.e., edrophonium) may also stimulate cholinergic receptors by direct action. The accumulation of ACh by the anticholinesterases potentially can produce all of the following: (1) stimulation of muscarinic receptors at ANS effect organs, (2) stimulation followed by depression of all ANS ganglia and skeletal muscle (nicotinic), and (3) stimulation with later depression of cholinergic receptor sites in the CNS. All of these effects may be seen with lethal doses of anticholinesterase drugs, but therapeutic doses only produce the first two.

Actions of therapeutic significance of the anticholinesterase drugs to the anesthesiologist concern the eye, the intestine, and the neuromuscular junction. The effects of anticholinesterases are useful in the treatment of myasthenia gravis, glaucoma, and atony of the gastrointestinal and urinary tracts. Anticholinesterase drugs are used routinely in anesthesia to reverse nondepolarizing neuromuscular block.

The most prominent pharmacologic effects of the anticholinesterase drugs are muscarinic. Their most useful actions are their nicotinic effects.[3] Muscarinic activity is evoked by lower concentrations of ACh than are necessary to produce the desired nicotinic effect. For example, the anticholinesterase neostigmine reverses neuromuscular blockade by increasing ACh concentration at the muscle end plate, a nicotinic receptor. Nicotinic reversal of neuromuscular blockade can usually be produced safely only when the patient has been protected by atropine or other muscarinic blockers. This prevents the untoward muscarinic effects of bradycardia, hypotension, bronchospasm, or intestinal spasm. Conversely, neuromuscular paralysis may be produced or increased if excessive anticholinesterase is used. Excess accumulation of ACh at the motor end plates produces a depolarizing block similar to that produced by succinylcholine or nicotine.

Reversal of neuromuscular blockade in patients who have had bowel anastomosis was at one time a major controversy. Some thought that the muscarinic effects of anticholinesterase drugs (hypermotility) increased the risk of anastomotic leakage[62] whereas others found no association between their use and subsequent breakdown.[63] National experience has favored the latter opinion.

Clinically, anticholinesterase drugs may be divided into two types: the reversible and nonreversible cholinesterase inhibitors.[60] Reversible cholinesterase inhibitors delay the hydrolysis of ACh from 1 to 8 hours. Nonreversible drugs are so named because their inhibitory effects may last from days to weeks. The differences in duration of various anticholinesterases apparently depend on whether they inhibit the anionic or esteratic site of acetylcholinesterase. Therefore, the anticholinesterase drugs have also been pharmacologically

TABLE 12-9

CHOLINESTERASE INHIBITORS

DRUG	TRADE NAME	ROUTE	DURATION	INDICATIONS
Reversible				
Physostigmine	Eserine	Topical	6–12 hr	Glaucoma
Pyridostigmine	Mestinon Regonol	Oral, iv, im	4 hr	Myasthenia gravis Reversal of neuromuscular blockade
Neostigmine	Prostigmin	Oral, iv	4–6 hr	Myasthenia gravis Reversal of neuromuscular blockade
Edrophonium	Tensilon Enlon	iv	1–2 hr	Reversal of neuromuscular blockade Diagnosis of myasthenia gravis
Demecarium	Humorsol	Topical	3–5 days	Glaucoma
Ambenonium	Mytelase	Oral	4 hr	Myasthenia gravis
Nonreversible				
Echothiophate	Phospholine	Topical	3–14 days	Glaucoma
Isofluorophate		Topical	3–7 days	Glaucoma research
Malathion		Topical		Insecticide—relatively safe for mammals because of rapid hepatic metabolism
Parathion		Topical		Insecticide—highly toxic to higher animals; frequent accidental poisoning
Sarin (GB)	Nerve gas	Topical and gas		
Tabun	Nerve gas	Topical and gas		No indications for the use of nerve gas
Soman	Nerve gas	Topical and gas		

Note: Atropine should always be given prior to or with iv cholinesterase inhibitors and when only nicotinic effects are desired; muscarinic effects are dangerous when excessive.

subdivided. Drugs that inhibit the anionic site are called competitive inhibitors. Their action is a result of competition between the anticholinesterase and ACh for the anionic site. These drugs tend to be short acting. Edrophonium is an example of this type. Drugs that inhibit the esteratic site are called acid-transferring inhibitors. These drugs include the longer-acting neostigmine, pyridostigmine, and physostigmine. Thus, the differences in the mechanism of inhibition produced by prosthetic inhibitors (edrophonium) and acid-transferring inhibitors (neostigmine) account for the longer duration of action associated with the latter agents.

Most of the reversible cholinesterase inhibitors are quaternary ammonium compounds and do not cross the blood-brain barrier. Physostigmine is a tertiary amine that readily passes into the CNS (Fig. 12-18). It produces central muscarinic stimulation and, thus, is not used to reverse neuromuscular blockade but can be used to treat atropine poisoning. Conversely, atropine is used to treat physostigmine poisoning. Physostigmine has also been found to be a specific antidote in the treatment of postoperative delirium (see Central Anticholinergic Syndrome section).[3]

The irreversible cholinesterase inhibitors are mostly organophosphate compounds. In addition, the organophosphate compounds are highly lipid soluble; they readily pass into the CNS and are rapidly absorbed through the skin. They are used as the active ingredient in potent insecticides and chemical warfare agents known as nerve gases. Table 12-9 lists some of these agents. The only therapeutic drug of this group is echothiophate, which is available in the form of topical drops for the treatment of glaucoma. Its primary advantage is its prolonged duration of action. Topical absorption is variable but considerable. Echothiophate can remain effective for 2 or 3 weeks following cessation of therapy.[64] A history of use of echothiophate is important in avoiding prolonged action of succinylcholine, which requires pseudocholinesterase for its hydrolysis.

Organophosphate poisoning manifests all the signs and symptoms of excess ACh.[65] The antidote cartridges dispensed to troops to counter the effects of anticholinesterase nerve gases contain only atropine, which would effectively counter

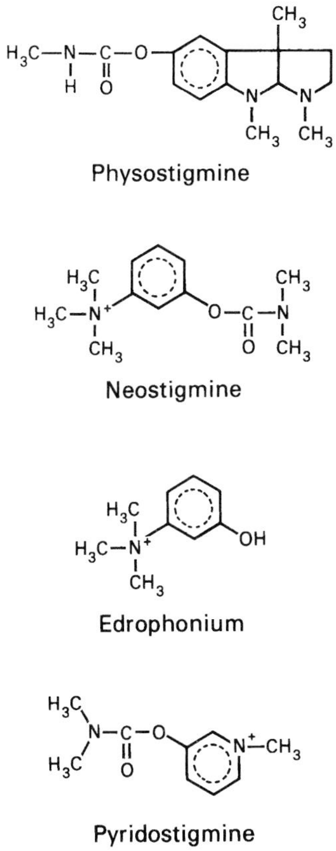

Physostigmine

Neostigmine

Edrophonium

Pyridostigmine

FIGURE 12-18. Structural formulas of clinically useful reversible anticholinesterase drugs. Physostigmine is a tertiary amine and crosses the blood-brain barrier. It is useful in treating the central anticholinergic syndrome.

the muscarinic effects of the gas; however, atropine does little to counter the high-dose nicotinic muscle paralysis or the central ventilation depression that contributes to death from nerve gases. Treatment requires high doses of atropine, 35 to 70 mg/kg IV every 3 to 10 minutes until muscarinic symptoms abate. Lower doses at less frequent intervals may be required for several days. Central ventilatory depression and nicotinic paralysis or weakness require respiratory support and specific therapy of the cholinesterase lesion. Pralidoxime has been reported to reactivate cholinesterase activity by hydrolysis of the phosphate enzyme complex. It is particularly effective with parathion poisoning and is the only cholinesterase reactivator available in the United States.[60]

Muscarinic Antagonists

Muscarinic antagonist refers to a specific drug action for which the term "anticholinergic" is widely used. Any drug that interferes with the action of ACh as a transmitter can be considered an anticholinergic agent. The term anticholinergic refers to a broader classification that would include the nicotinic antagonists.

Atropinic Drugs. Atropine, scopolamine, and glycopyrrolate are the most commonly used muscarinic antagonists used in anesthesia (Fig. 12-19).

The actions of these drugs include inhibition of salivary, bronchial, pancreatic, and gastrointestinal secretions to antagonize the muscarinic side effects of anticholinesterases during reversal of muscle relaxants. Atropine is useful in increasing CO with sinus bradycardia as a result of vagal stimulation if hypoxia is ruled out. It has many uses outside of anesthesia for the treatment of renal colic, gastrointestinal spasm, gastric secretion, and asthma. Historically, atropine was introduced to anesthesia practice to prevent excessive secretions during ether anesthesia and to prevent vagal bradycardia during the administration of chloroform.[66] Atropine and scopolamine also possess antiemetic action. Atropine, however, reduces the opening pressure of the lower esophageal sphincter, which theoretically increases the risk of passive regurgitation. Atropinic drugs also produce dilation of the pupil (mydriasis) and paralysis of accommodation (cycloplegia).

Antimuscarinic agents do not inhibit transmission equally, and there are marked variations in sensitivity at different muscarinic sites owing to differences in penetration and affinities of the various receptors. Differences in relative potency between the different antimuscarinics are outlined in Table 12-10. Glycopyrrolate produces less tachycardia than atropine and is a more potent antisialogogue.

The antimuscarinic effects of the atropinic drugs are the result of competitive inhibition of ACh at the receptors of organs innervated by cholinergic postganglionic nerves. The antagonism can be overcome by sufficient concentrations of cholinomimetic drugs or anticholinesterases that increase ACh levels at the receptor site. This explains most of the therapeutic actions of atropinic drugs; however, they are neither purely antimuscarinic nor purely antagonist.[3]

The belladonna alkaloids (atropine and scopolamine) also block ACh transmission to sweat glands, which, although they are cholinergic, are innervated by the SNS. Antimuscarinic agents produce antinicotinic actions at higher doses and result in important actions on CNS transmission that are pharmacologically similar to the postganglionic cholinergic function.

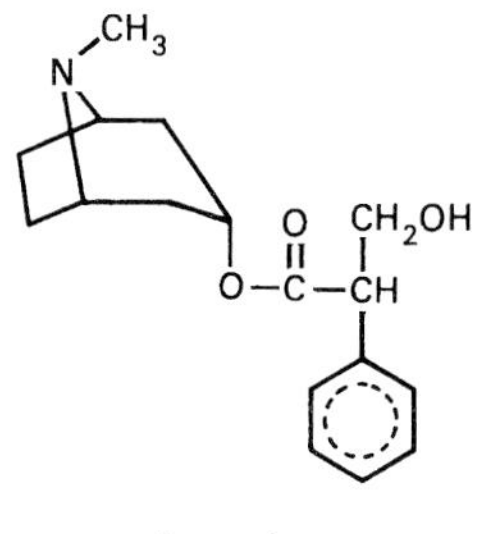

Atropine

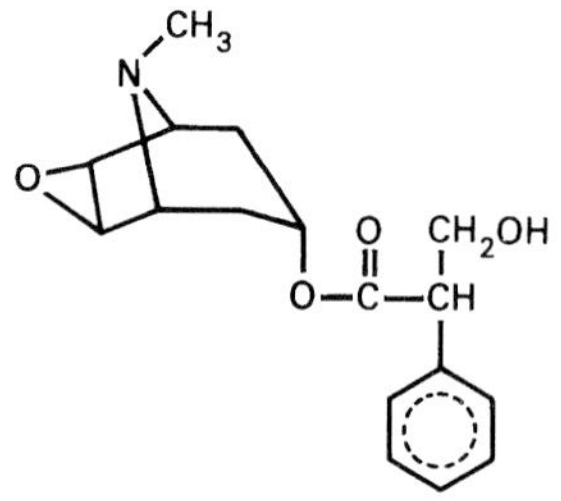

Scopolamine

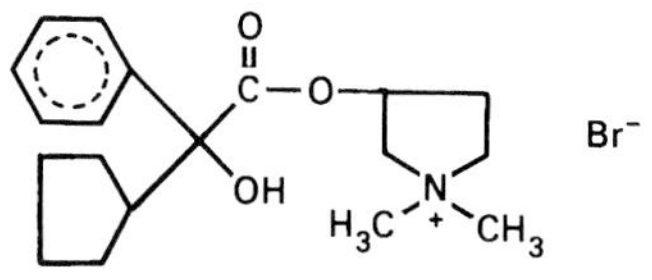

Glycopyrrolate

FIGURE 12-19. Structural formulas of the clinically useful antimuscarinic drugs.

TABLE 12-10

COMPARISON OF ANTIMUSCARINIC DRUGS

	DURATION						
	iv	im	CNS	GI TONE	GASTRIC ACID	AIRWAY SECRETIONS[a]	HEART RATE
Atropine	15–30 min	2–4 hr	++	--	–	–	+++[c]
Scopolamine	30–60 min	4–6 hr	+++[b]	–	–	----	–0[c]
Glycopyrrolate	2–4 hr	6–8 hr	0	---	---	---	+0

[a]Secretions may be reduced by inspissation.
[b]CNS effect often manifest as sedation before stimulation.
[c]May decelerate initially.

Atropine and scopolamine are tertiary amines (see Fig. 12-19) and easily penetrate the blood-brain barrier and placenta. Glycopyrrolate is a quaternary amine that, like the reversible anticholinesterase drugs, does not easily penetrate these barriers. Glycopyrrolate, a synthetic antimuscarinic, has gained popularity because it avoids the central effects of the other two drugs. Atropine and scopolamine have notable CNS effects that are dissimilar. Scopolamine differs from atropine mainly in its central depressant effects, which produce sedation, amnesia, and euphoria. Such properties are widely used for premedication for cardiac patients in combination with morphine and a major tranquilizer. Atropine, as a premedicant, has slight effects on the CNS, including mild stimulation. Higher doses such as those given for reversal of muscle relaxants (1 to 2 mg) may produce restlessness, disorientation, hallucinations, and delirium (see Central Anticholinergic Syndrome section). Excessive stimulation may be followed by depression and paralysis of respiration. Occasionally, scopolamine in low doses may cause restlessness and delirium. This syndrome is more frequently seen in the elderly and patients experiencing pain, for example, in obstetric patients.

Atropine and scopolamine are noted to produce a paradoxical bradycardia when given in low doses. Scopolamine (0.1 to 0.2 mg) usually causes more slowing than atropine but also produces less cardiac acceleration at higher doses. The usual intramuscular premedicant doses of scopolamine causes either a decrease or no change in HR. The paradoxical bradycardia was once thought to be caused by an early central inhibition of the medullary cardioinhibitory center. However, this phenomenon occurs in animals that have had total vagotomy. Atropine may also produce sympathomimetic effects by blocking presynaptic muscarinic receptors found on adrenergic nerve terminals.[6] ACh stimulation of these receptors inhibits NE release, and blockade by atropine releases this inhibition (see Cholinergic Receptors Section).

Atropinic drugs are widely used in ophthalmology as mydriatics and cycloplegics. Atropine is contraindicated in patients with narrow-angle glaucoma. Pupillary dilation thickens the peripheral part of the iris, which narrows the iridocorneal angle. Drainage of aqueous humor is impaired, and intraocular pressure increases. Doses of atropine used for premedication have little effect in this regard, whereas equal doses of scopolamine cause mydriasis. Prudence would dictate avoidance of either agent in patients with narrow-angle glaucoma. The need for antimuscarinic premedication is questionable in this situation.

Atropine is best avoided where tachycardia would be harmful, as may occur in thyrotoxicosis, pheochromocytoma, or obstructive coronary artery disease. Atropine should be avoided in hyperpyrexial patients because it inhibits sweating.

Central Anticholinergic Syndrome. The belladonna alkaloids have long been known to produce undesirable side effects ranging from stupor (scopolamine) to delirium (atropine). This syndrome has otherwise been called postoperative delirium and atropine toxicity. The central anticholinergic syndrome appears to involve the muscarinic receptor.[3] Biochemical studies have demonstrated abundant muscarinic ACh receptors in the brain that can be affected by any drug possessing antimuscarinic activity and capable of crossing the blood-brain barrier. Hundreds of drugs exist that meet these criteria with which this syndrome has been associated. Table 12-11 lists some of those drugs.[3]

High doses of atropinic alkaloids rapidly produce dryness of the mouth, blurred vision with photophobia (mydriasis), hot and dry skin (flushed), and fever. Mental symptoms range from sedation, stupor, and coma to anxiety, restlessness, disorientation, hallucinations, and delirium. Convulsions and ventilatory arrest may occur if lethal poisoning has occurred. Although an alarming reaction may occur, fatalities are rare. Intoxication is usually short lived and followed by amnesia. These reactions can be controlled by the intravenous (iv) injection of physostigmine. Physostigmine is an anticholinesterase that, by virtue of being a tertiary amine, readily passes into the CNS to counter antimuscarinic activity. It should be given slowly in 1-mg doses, not exceeding 3 mg, to avoid producing peripheral cholinergic activity. Neostigmine, pyridostigmine, and edrophonium are not effective because they cannot pass into the CNS. Likewise, atropine is an effective antidote for physostigmine overdose. The duration of physostigmine action may be shorter than that of the offending antimuscarinic agent and require repeated injection if symptoms recur. Physostigmine appears safe when used within dose recommendations and when indications are established. Central disorientation alone does not establish a diagnosis. Peripheral signs of antimuscarinic activity should be present in addition to a central anticholinergic syndrome.

Physostigmine has been reported to reverse the CNS effects of many of the drugs listed in Table 12-11, including antihistamines, tricyclic antidepressants, and tranquilizers. Reversal of the sedative effects of opioids and benzodiazepines has also been reported.[67] However, anticholinesterase agents potentiate cholinergic synaptic transmission and increase neuronal activity, even if no receptor antagonist is present. Thus, arousal may not be a function independent of its cholinesterase activity, and claims that physostigmine is a nonspecific CNS stimulant may not be warranted and could, in fact, be dangerous.[3]

Hemodynamics

Until recently, sympathomimetics were the most common means of treating the hypotension associated with shock. A vasopressor is a drug that is used to elevate arterial blood pressure above the existing level because the pressure is too low. However, elevation of arterial blood pressure alone has repeatedly been demonstrated to be an insufficient goal in the treatment of shock.[68] The goal, instead, is to reestablish blood flow to vital organs. Although blood pressure has been the historical gold standard for estimating perfusion, there is no correlation between blood pressure and flow (Fig. 12-20).[69] In physiologic as well as constructed systems, flow tends to be least when pressure is highest. Flow used in this context refers to CO.

Oxygen transport is the product of the arterial oxygen content (DO_2) and CO:

$$DO_2 = Cao_2 \times CO$$

Therefore, there is a close correlation between oxygen transport and CO. Unfortunately, oxygen transport is not identical to cellular oxygen supply, which can be inadequate despite normal or elevated oxygen transport. Cellular oxygen supply can be inadequate because of maldistribution of blood flow to vital organs or from the inability of the cell to use oxygen.[69] Improving cellular oxygen utilization remains enigmatic, but the catecholamines can be of some assistance in the redistribution of flow.

The physiologic equation that expresses how flow (CO) is generated states that CO is the product of the HR and stroke volume (SV):

$$CO = HR \times SV$$

However, SV is determined by three factors: (1) the contractile or inotropic state of the myocardium, (2) preload, or end-diastolic myocardial fiber length, and (3) afterload, or

TABLE 12-11

ANTIMUSCARINIC COMPOUNDS ASSOCIATED WITH CENTRAL ANTICHOLINERGIC SYNDROME

Belladonna Alkaloids
Atropine sulfate
Scopolamine hydrobromide

Synthetic and Natural Tertiary Amine Compounds
Dicyclomine (Bentyl)—antispasmodic with local anesthetic activity
Thiphenamil (Trocinate)—antispasmodic with local anesthetic activity
Procaine
Cocaine
Cyclopentolate (Cyclogyl) mydriatic

Quaternary Derivatives of Belladonna Alkaloids
Methscopolamine bromide (Pamine)—antispasmodic
Homatropine methylbromide—sedative, antispasmodic
Homatropine hydrobromide—ophthalmic solution—mydriatic

Synthetic Quaternary Compounds
Methantheline bromide (Banthine)
Propantheline bromide (Pro-Banthine)

Antihistamines
Chlorpheniramine (Ornade)
Diphenhydramine (Benadryl)

Plants
Deadly nightshade (atropine)
Bittersweet
Potato leaves and sprouts
Jimson or loco weed
Coca plant (cocaine)

Over-the-Counter
Asthma-Dor—atropine-like
Compoz—scopolamine sedation
Sleep Eze—scopolamine sedation
Sominex—scopolamine sedation

Antiparkinson Drugs
Benztropine (Cogentin)
Trihexphenidyl (Artane)
Biperiden (Akineton)
Ethopropazine (Parsidol)
Procyclidine (Kemadrin)

Antipsychotic Drugs
Chlorpromazine (Thorazine)
Thioriazine (Mellaril)
Haloperidol (Haldol)
Droperidol (Inapsine)
Promethazine (Phenegran)

Tricyclic Antidepressants
Amitriptyline (Elavil)
Imipramine (Tofranil)
Desipramine (Norpramine, Pertofrane)

Synthetic Opioids
Meperidine
Methadone

Note: Trade names are given in parentheses.

resistance to ejection. The physiologic determinants of CO can therefore be expressed as:

$$CO = HR \times (\text{inotropism:preload:afterload})$$

Synchrony of AV contraction is an additional determinant when dysrhythmias develop. This equation is illustrated in Figure 12-21 to emphasize that the biologic mechanisms that produce and regulate flow are interdependent. Terms such as "inotropism," "preload," and "afterload" cannot be defined independently or isolated in the clinical setting. We can now measure, calculate, and manipulate each of the links in the chain of events that determine flow. Note that blood pressure is not among the determinants of flow. It is the product and not the cause. Most catecholamines affect one or more of these factors via the receptors and may cause changes in blood pressure by altering flow, vascular tone, or both. A measured blood pressure does not distinguish changes in flow, resistance, inotropism, or HR; therefore, blood pressure and oxygen transport do not correlate.

Heart Rate

HR becomes an important support of CO when SV is decreased. A change in either HR or SV invariably causes an alteration of the other by reflex activity. Tachycardias can reduce SV by not allowing sufficient diastolic ventricular filling time. Coronary blood flow to the ventricles and especially the subendocardium occurs primarily during diastole. The subepicardial muscle is perfused during systole as well as diastole. However, subendocardial blood flow is totally dependent on diastolic perfusion time, diastolic pressure, and microcirculatory tone.[70]

Diastolic perfusion time becomes even more critical with ventricular hypertrophy. Increases in HR will not only shorten the percent diastolic perfusion time for the endocardium but also increase oxygen demand.[71] Increased HR, alone, has been shown to increase the severity of ischemia and the incidence of reperfusion arrhythmias. Animal studies have shown that myocardial blood flow and contractile function decrease with increased inotropic activity and tachycardia. This does not occur when increased inotropism is not accompanied by tachycardia.

Diastolic perfusion time has a curvilinear relationship with HR, increasing rapidly as rates fall below 75 beats/min (Fig. 12-22). Once HR goes above 90 beats/min in the adult, there is little further decrease in percent diastole. There is an exponential increase in percent diastole below rates of 70 beats/min.[70] Wide swings in percent diastolic time are of little consequence in the patient with normal coronary function but can be critical in those with obstructive coronary artery disease.

Two factors actually determine the duration of systole: HR and electromechanical systole (QS2). HR and QS2 have an inverse relationship (Fig. 12-23).[70] Percent diastolic perfusion time is calculated as the cardiac cycle (R-R) minus QS2. A decrease in HR and/or shortening in QS2 will result in prolongation of the total diastolic period and vice versa. HR is the more

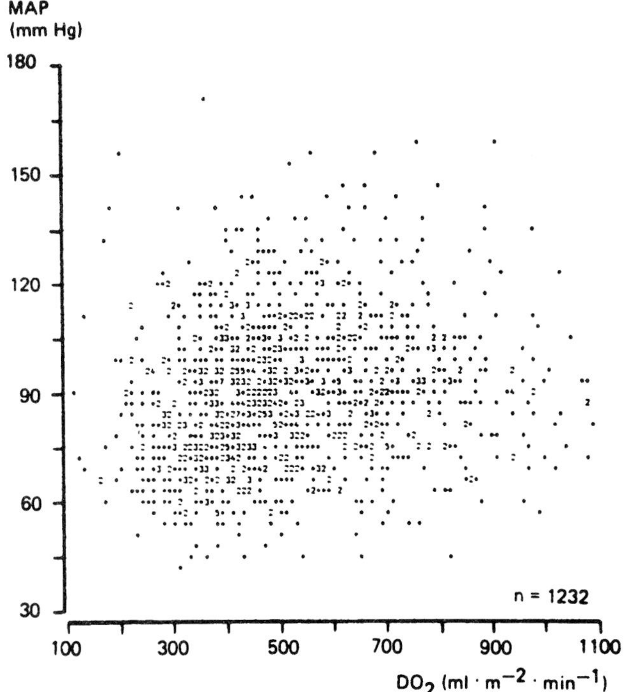

FIGURE 12-20. Correlation between mean arterial pressure (MAP) and O_2 delivery (DO_2) during the perioperative period in patients undergoing aorta bifemoral bypass grafting. (Reprinted with permission from Reinhart K: Principles and Practice of Svo_2 Monitoring, p 121. London, Intensive Care World, King and Worth, Publishers, vol 5, no 4, Dec 1988.)

important factor because small changes in the HR can produce significant changes in percent diastole as a result of the curvilinear relationship between HR and diastolic perfusion time. Changes in HR alone produce movement along that curve, whereas changes in QS2 result in shifts of the curve. Dopamine and dobutamine (DBT) affect diastolic perfusion time by altering HR and QS2. DBT has been shown to increase percent diastole without significantly altering HR. The increase in diastolic perfusion time is because of a shortening of QS2. Isoproterenol reduces percent diastole because it reduces QS2 proportional to the increase in HR. β-blockers, particularly atenolol, will significantly decrease HR and increase percent diastole because it has little effect on QS2 in the usually clinical dose range. The beneficial effects of β-blockers on myocardial oxygen delivery and consumption can be related to a reduced HR alone, although higher doses may reduce inotropism as well. Diastolic perfusion pressure may also increase with β-blockade because of an unopposed relative increase in vascular tone.

Preload

Preload is clinically synonymous with the volume of venous return to the heart, which establishes CO by the purported Frank-Starling mechanism. Preload has repeatedly been demonstrated to be of paramount importance in supporting cardiovascular function in the normal heart. It can be increased by adding volume to the circulation or by acute venous constriction. The catecholamines can be selected for their effect on preload by either increasing (α-1, α-2) or decreasing (β-2, DA1, DA2) venous tone.[72] Positive or negative preloading can be a major unrecognized benefit of some sympathomimetic agents. Although venoconstriction produces little increase in total vascular resistance (afterload), minimal venoconstriction is capable of producing large shifts of blood volume into the central circulation because the capacitance vessels contain 60 to 80% of the total blood volume, an effect that has largely been ignored. The central distributive effect of a catecholamine may be as important as its inotropic action in increasing the CO in the hypovolemic patient. Likewise, a central distribution of capacitance blood may be undesirable if the heart is failing, even though that agent may possess inotropic properties.

Afterload

Afterload is a measure of impedance to ventricular ejection and is the dominant factor in determining CO when inotropism is impaired. In the absence of outlet obstruction, the clinical correlate of afterload to the left ventricle is the systemic vascular resistance reflected by the mean arterial pressure. Afterload is the only factor of the four major determinants of CO that, if increased, will reduce flow. Ohm's law states that blood flow through any organ is directly related to the blood pressure gradient across that organ but is inversely proportional to the resistance (afterload).

Inotropism

Inotropism is defined as the force and velocity of ventricular contraction when preload and afterload are held constant. Vasoactive drugs can be described as having either a positive or negative inotropic effect. Inotropic agents, such as DA and DBT, represent therapeutic agents that altogether increase myocardial contractility. As yet, there are no clinically feasible means to directly measure inotropism at the bedside. We can define failure of inotropism better than we can define what it is. The myocardium permits CO to be regulated at any level below its inotropic state.

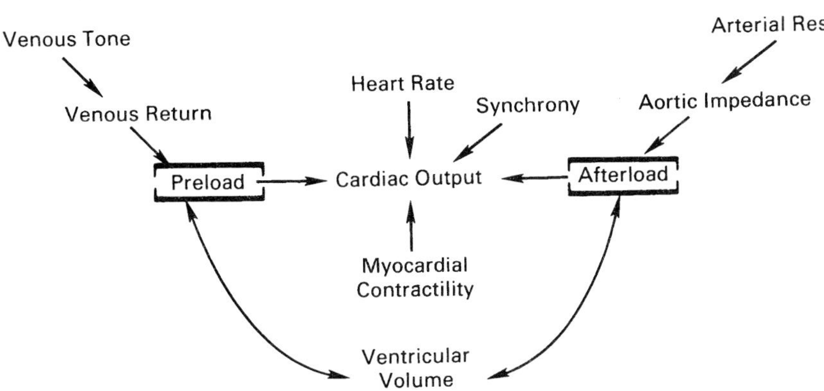

FIGURE 12-21. The four principal factors determining CO are demonstrated. Synchrony of AV contraction is an additional factor becoming important with the development of cardiac dysrhythmias. (Reprinted with permission from Lawson NW, Wallfisch HK: Cardiovascular pharmacology: A new look at the "pressors." In Stoelting RK, Barash PG, Gallagher TJ (eds): Advances in Anesthesia, p 195, Chicago, Year Book Publishers, 1986.)

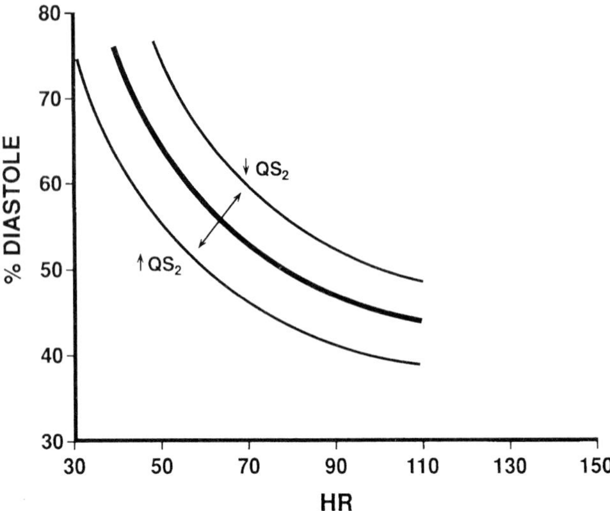

FIGURE 12-22. Small changes in HR produce large changes in percent diastole especially at low HRs because of the curvilinear relationship between rate and diastolic time. Shortening of electromechanical systole (QS_2) produces an upward shift of the curve. Shortening of QS_2 or a decrease in HR, or both, will increase percent diastolic perfusion time. Cardioactive drugs may affect diastolic perfusion time through either or both mechanisms.[70]

Several direct indicators of cardiac inotropism appear useful in lieu of direct force velocity measurements. Pump function can be estimated clinically by work-pressure curves using the Frank-Starling mechanism. When inotropism is normal, CO is more dependent on extracardiac factors such as preload and afterload (see Fig. 12-21).

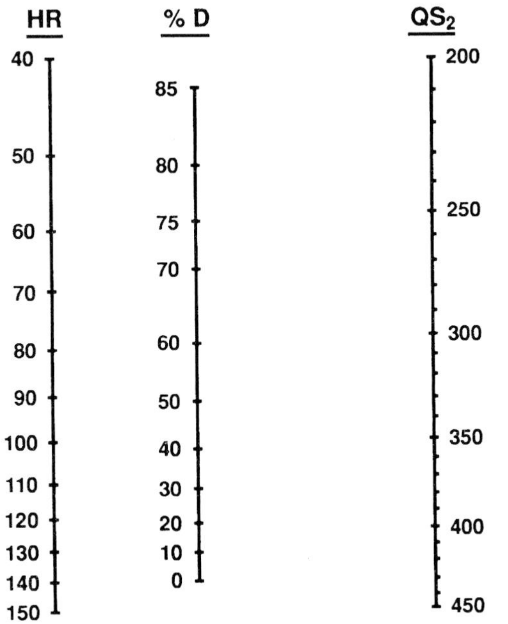

FIGURE 12-23. Nomogram for the relationship between electromechanical systole (QS_2), heart rate (HR), and percent diastole. The percent diastole can be obtained from QS_2 and HR.[70] (Reprinted from Boudoulas H, Rittgers SE, Lewis RP, Leier CV, Weissler AM: Changes in diastolic time with various pharmacologic agents. Circulation 60:164, 1979.)

Lusitropism

Lusitropism is a factor determining CO that is not depicted in Figure 12-21. Lusitropism describes abnormalities of myocardial relaxation, or diastole, as opposed to problems of inotropism. Some vasodilators such as nitroglycerin and some sympathomimetic "inodilators" are thought to improve cardiac function by promoting diastolic relaxation and thus ventricular filling (preloading) and coronary perfusion. Lusitropic dysfunction may play a larger role in chronic heart failure than earlier appreciated because lusitropic dysfunction is now known to play a large role in many myocardial disease processes and may, in fact, precede inotropic dysfunction. Decreased lusitropism is characteristic of the aging myocardium.

Figure 12-21 deliberately emphasizes preload and afterload as balancing forces in producing CO. They are antagonistic and assume differing degrees of dominance depending on whether the myocardium is healthy or failing. Preload is the dominant regulator of CO in the normal cardiovascular system. Afterload dominates flow regulation when the myocardium is failing. Figure 12-24 compares the contrasting effects of preload and afterload on the CO of both the healthy and failing myocardium. Acute increases (in afterload) in the healthy patient are tolerated, up to a fourfold increase. In contrast, even small increases in afterload produce large reductions in CO when the myocardium is depressed by disease or anesthesia. The use of vasodilators for afterload reduction in the patient with a failing myocardium is based on this concept.

The weak links in the chain of cardiovascular events that produce blood flow and oxygen transport can now be selectively detected and manipulated rather than just the mindless increase in blood pressure. The term "vasopressor," once synonymous with vasoconstriction, has now become a generic term for several species of vasoactive drugs that, by whatever means, increase CO that may or may not increase blood pressure. Their uses in anesthesia include (1) maintenance or organ perfusion, (2) treatment of allergic reactions, (3) prolongation of the action of local anesthetics, and (4) for cardiopulmonary resuscitation.

Low-Output Syndrome

Patients with the low CO syndrome have abnormalities of either the heart, blood volume, or blood flow distribution. Those remaining in this state for more than 1 hour usually have dysfunction of all three components. Modern hemodynamic monitoring has pinpointed hypovolemia, relative or absolute, as the most common cause of the low-output syndrome, regardless of the etiology. Initial treatment with adrenergic amines in this setting is likely to delay volume repletion and potentiate the shock state. The proper hemodynamic management of septic shock, the most commonly seen distributive abnormality, remains controversial, but volume repletion is the primary consideration. Likewise, the initial treatment of cardiac dysfunction is optimum volume replacement because hypovolemia is a frequent accompaniment of impaired myocardial performance. Ventricular performance may be improved solely on the basis of increased preload.

The treatment of cardiogenic shock is an example of the low-flow state that requires multiple autonomic interventions common to other forms of the low-output syndrome. An acute reduction of left ventricular contractility (inotropism) produces a cascade of events that worsen in cyclic fashion (Fig. 12-25). One could draw this cascade beginning with any one of the five determinants of CO. Loss of contractility produces a reduction in CO, increased left ventricular end-diastolic pressure, and a host of compensatory reflexes. These compensatory mechanisms include increased sympathetic activity that augments contractility and rate. Chronic dysfunction produces a third compensatory mechanism, hypertrophy.

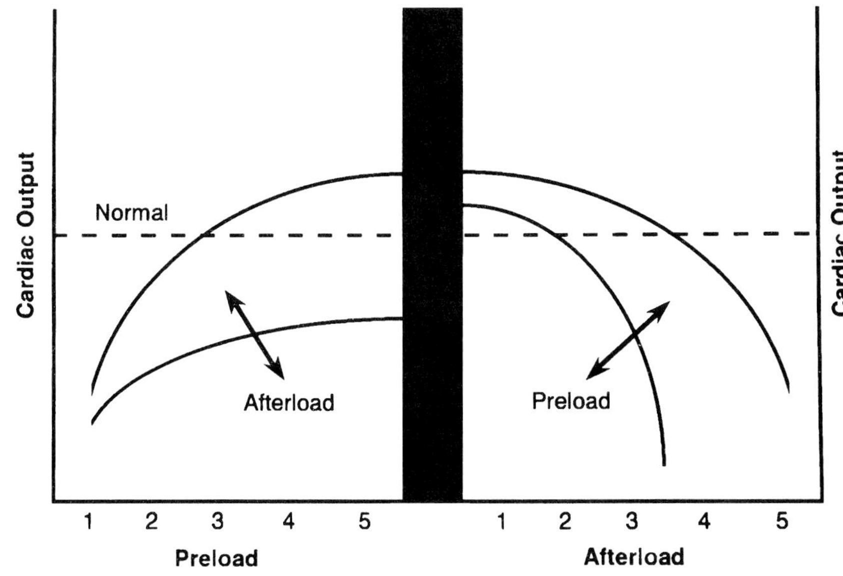

FIGURE 12-24. The contrasting effects of preload and afterload on CO. Increasing preload increases output in the normal myocardium, but to a lesser degree in the failing myocardium. Increased afterload is usually tolerated by the normal myocardium, but even small increases produce large reductions in output in the failing myocardium.

The attributes of the ideal inotropic drug are listed in Table 12-12. The inotropic agent needed for the patient illustrated in Figure 12-25 would be rapid acting and short lived and would not increase HR, preload (unless hypovolemic), afterload, or infarct size. Because the ideal inotropic drug is not available, the peripheral side effects of any inotropic agent become critical to selection because all are multireceptor agonists.

Myocardial failure exists when the heart cannot pump enough blood to meet metabolic needs. The clinical manifestations of heart failure result from peripheral circulatory derangements that are the result of the heart's forward output lagging behind the input. Venous pressure increases and produces congestion. There are marked pathophysiologic differences between chronic heart failure and acute failure from infarction. Patients with chronic heart failure have retention of sodium and water and are typically hypervolemic, whereas patients with acute heart failure are either normovolemic or, commonly, hypovolemic. Cardiomegaly is a common compensatory feature of chronic heart failure (late) but is absent with acute heart failure. Circulating catecholamines and myocardial catecholamine content are decreased in chronic failure but markedly elevated in the acute infarct. Thus, the response to inotropic drugs in chronic heart failure is influenced not only by the lack of myocardial catecholamine stores but also by down-regulation of β receptors. The CO in chronic failure is borderline to decreased, whereas it is usually normal or elevated with acute failure as a result of compensatory mechanisms.

Acute failure is the most common complication of infarction, occurring in 40 to 50% of patients, which reflects a 20 to 25% involvement of the myocardium. In contrast to the patient with chronic heart failure, this dysfunction is usually transient, lasting between 48 to 72 hours. Drugs with a predominant inotropic action are used alone or in combination to acutely improve cardiac contractility. Therefore, one has to be concerned that myocardial damage is not extended during this transient period by inappropriate inotropic or chronotropic support. This is not as major a concern in the patient with hypertrophy, in whom increased inotropism may actually reduce oxygen consumption by reducing ventricular mass.

Table 12-13 presents one approach to the management of cardiogenic shock listed in order of relative importance. The use of sympathomimetic support is placed in proper perspective. It emphasizes the essential role that invasive hemodynamic monitoring and volume management play in confirming a diagnosis of cardiogenic failure. Although volume

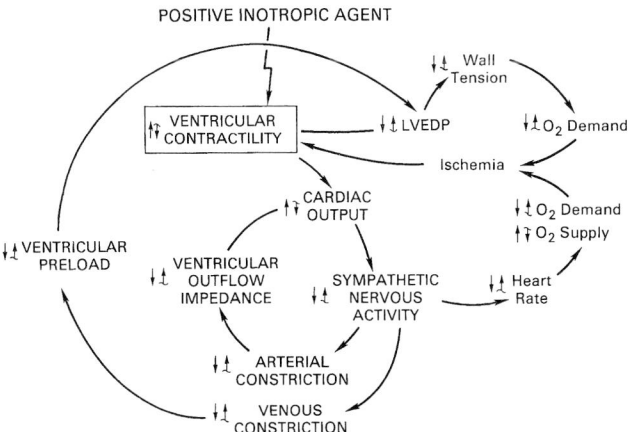

FIGURE 12-25. Reversal of heart failure by intervention (↑) with the ideal positive inotropic agent depicted. (Reprinted with permission from Evans DB, Weishaar RE, Kaplan HR: Strategy for the discovery and development of a positive inotropic agent. Pharmacol Ther 16:303, 1982.)

TABLE 12-12

CHARACTERISTICS OF THE IDEAL POSITIVE INOTROPIC AGENT

Enhances contractile state by increasing velocity and force of myocardial fiber shortening
Lacks tolerance
Does not produce vasoconstriction
No cardiac dysrhythmias
Does not affect heart rate
Controllability—immediate onset and termination of action
Elevates perfusion pressure by raising cardiac output rather than systemic vascular resistance
Redistributes blood flow to vital organs
Direct-acting—not dependent on release of endogenous amines
Compatible with other vasoactive drugs
Effective orally or parenterally

TABLE 12-13

MANAGEMENT OF LOW OUTPUT SYNDROME CAUSED BY MYOCARDIAL DYSFUNCTION

1. Assure adequate ventilation and oxygenation
2. Relieve pain and symptoms of recurrent ischemia
3. Institute hemodynamic monitoring (pulmonary artery, pulmonary capillary wedge, and arterial pressures; urine output; cardiac output)
4. Optimize left ventricular filling pressure
5. Correct metabolic abnormalities
6. Control dysrhythmias (#2 priority if life threatening)
7. Pharmacologic support
   a. Vasodilators
   b. Inotropic drugs
   c. Diuretics—chronic heart failure
8. Rule out "correctable" causes of shock (septal or left ventricle rupture, mitral regurgitation, acute aneurysm)
9. Mechanical support of circulation
10. Surgical correction if possible

Note: Hemodynamic monitoring is essential in confirming a diagnosis, optimizing filling pressures and cardiac output, selecting pharmacologic support, and avoiding complications. Adjustment of left ventricular filling pressure may require additional volume or a relative volume reduction with vasodilators. The diagnostic criteria for cardiogenic shock are not met until step 4 is accomplished.

expansion and reduction of afterload may improve CO, other pharmacologic interventions may still be necessary to optimize CO and its distribution. Invasive monitoring is a prerequisite for the rational use of the vasoactive drugs to (1) establish that a sympathomimetic is necessary, (2) select drugs for the hemodynamic condition, (3) follow resultant hemodynamic changes because many of the beneficial effects of the catecholamines are hidden to the clinical eye, and (4) avoid complications of pressor therapy that are visible to all.

Adrenergic Drugs—Selection

The selection of vasoactive drugs requires a knowledge of both the hemodynamic disturbance and pharmacology of the available drugs. The catecholamines and sympathomimetic drugs continue to be the pharmacologic mainstay of cardiovascular support for the low-flow state. Sustained interest in the catecholamines is related to their predictable pharmacodynamics and favorable pharmacokinetic profiles. Their effects are linearly related to plasma levels, which are directly related to the rate of infusion. There are few clinical surprises within any given dose range and the pharmacokinetics of catecholamines allow rapid titration to the effect. The half-life of most is short, ranging from 2 to 3 minutes. Undesirable side-effects dissipate within minutes of lowering or stopping the infusion. Sympathomimetics, as a group, produce a wide range of hemodynamic effects and can be used in combination to achieve a yet wider spectrum of effects. As a result, one need become familiar with only a few agents to manage most clinical situations.

Table 12-14 is a summary of the hemodynamic effects of some of the currently popular and once popular sympathomimetic drugs. Many of the hemodynamic effects are dose related. The dose ranges are listed and a standard infusion rate cited. Standard rates of infusion are simply guidelines, and the actual dose administered should be determined by patient response.

The goal for managing the low-output or high-output shock syndrome is to establish and maintain adequate tissue perfusion. Aggressive fluid therapy will suffice in most instances. Sympathomimetics are not a substitute for volume. However, once intravascular volume is optimized, a vasoactive drug may be required to sustain CO. The term "inodilator" has entered our lexicon during the early 1990s to supplant the more archaic term vasopressor. This neologism reflects a change in philosophy in managing low-flow states, particularly those characterized by heart failure. The new synthetic sympathomimetics have been chemically engineered to obtain inotropism and vasodilation rather than for pressor effects. The potential for benefit or harm can best be understood in terms of receptor characteristics. For example, activation of the inotropic β-1 and β-2 receptors results in positive inotropism and chronotropism. Selective stimulation of the vascular β-2 receptors causes vasodilatation. Left ventricular outflow may improve as a function of decreased afterload reduction and inotropism. However, chronotropism may not be a desirable feature in a patient with mitral stenosis or coronary artery disease.

Catecholamine Receptor–Effector Coupling

The net physiologic effect of a sympathomimetic is usually defined as the algebraic sum of its relative actions on the α, β, and DA receptors.[73] Most adrenergic drugs activate or block these receptors to varying degrees. Each catecholamine has a distinctive effect, qualitatively and quantitatively, on the myocardium and peripheral vasculature. Table 12-15 demonstrates the relative potency of the adrenergic amines on the various myocardial and vascular receptors. This relative potency is also dose related, adding yet another variable. The use of pluses (+) or zeros (0) is the classical method by which the relative sensitivities of catecholamine-receptor coupling are demonstrated. The use of the (+) is also symbolic of the apparent summation effect of the catecholamines on the receptors. The summation effect further implies a finite number of adrenergic receptor sites to which adrenergic agonists can compete.

For many years, the emphasis on catecholamines was focused almost entirely on their actions on the myocardium and on arteriolar resistance vessels. Changes in venous resistance contribute little to total vascular resistance and blood pressure. However, small changes in venous capacitance result in large changes in venous return because 60 to 70% of the circulating blood volume is the venous circulation.[50] The effect of the sympathomimetic amines on the venous circulation appears to be distributive in that acute venular constriction increases the central blood volume (preload), whereas dilatation decreases venous return by the promotion of peripheral pooling.[74] The distributive effect of a catecholamine may be as important as its inotropic action and more important than its arteriolar effect.[10] Further definition should elucidate some of the complex and confusing data in the literature generated when clinical observations are limited solely to adrenergic effects on the myocardium and arteriolar vasculature.

Intravenous and intra-arterial infusions of EPI in humans have been shown to cause marked constriction of the veins. Arteriolar vasoconstriction may or may not precede venoconstriction; however, SV does not increase until the onset of venoconstriction. The initial increase in CO seen with the infusion of EPI is more an effect of increased preload than an arteriolar or direct cardiac effect. NE produces a similar effect, but the onset of venoconstriction is slower.

A differential ability of the amines to constrict veins has been noted in animals.[75] The data are expressed as the average percentage contribution of venous resistance to total change

DOSE SCHEDULE AND HEMODYNAMIC EFFECTS OF THE ADRENERGIC AGONISTS

DRUG	DOSAGES		SITE OF ACTIVITY					HEMODYNAMICS (↑= INCREASE; ↓= DECREASE; — = NO CHANGE)					
LISTED FROM α TO β	IV PUSH ADULTS	IV INFUSION[a]	α_{1a}	α_{1v}	β_1	β_2	DA	CO	INOTROP	HR	VR	TPR	RBF
										Reflex			
Methoxamine	5–10 mg	N/R	++++	0–+?	0	0	0	–↓	–	↓	–	↑↑	↓↓
Phenylephrine	50–100 μg	a. 10 mg/250 mL											
		b. 40 μg/mL											
		c. 0.15–0.75 μg/kg/min								Reflex			
		d. 0.15 μg/kg/min	++++	+++++	0	0	0	–↓	–	↓	↑↑↑	↑↑	––↓
Norepinephrine	N/R	a. 4 mg/250 mL											
		b. 16 μg/mL											
		c. 0.01–0.1 μg/kg/min								Reflex			
		d. 0.1 μg/kg/min	+++	+++	++++	?+	0	↑–↓	↑	↓	↑↑↑	↑↑↑	↓↓↓
Metaraminol	N/R	a. 100 mg/250 mL											
		b. 400 μg/mL											
		c. 0.5–7 μg/kg/min								Reflex			
		d. 0.5 μg/kg/min	++	++	+++	0	0	–↓	↑	↓	↑	↑↑↑	↓↓↓
Epinephrine	0.3–0.5 mL 1:1000	a. 1 mg/250 mL											
	(0.3–0.5 mg)	b. 4 μg/mL											
	sc—Asthma	0.01–0.03 μg/kg/min	+	+	++++	++++	0	↑↑	↑↑	↑	↑	↑	↑
	iv—Anaphylaxis	c. 0.03–0.15 μg/kg/min	+++	+++	++++	++++		↑–	↑↑	↑↑	↑	↑↑	↓–
		0.15–0.30 μg/kg/min	+++++	+++++				↑–↓	↑↑	↑↑	↑	↑↑↑	↓
	5 mL 1:10,000	d. 0.015 μg/kg/min	+	+	++++	++++	0	↑↑	↑↑	↑	↑	↑	↑
	(0.5 mg) cardiac												
	arrest every 5 min												
Ephedrine	5–10 mg	N/R	++	+++	+++	++	0	↑	↑	↑	↑↑	↑	↑–↓
Mephentermine	15–30 mg	a. 500 mg/250 mL											
		b. 2,000 μg/mL											
		c. 4–8 μg/kg/min											
		d. 4 μg/kg/min	0–++	+?	++++	+?	0	↑	↑↑	↑	↑?	↑	↓–↑
Dopamine[c]	N/R	a. 200 mg/250 mL											
		b. 800 μg/mL											
		0.05–5 μg/kg/min		++++			+++++	↑	–	–	↑	–↓	↑
		c. 2–10 μg/kg/min	+	++++	+++	+++++		↑↑	↑	–↑	↑	–↑	↑
		10 μg/kg/min[b]	+++++	++++	+++++			↑–↓	↑↑	↑↑	↑	↑↑	–↓
		d. 2 μg/kg/min		++++			+++++	↑	–	–	↑	–↓	↑
Dobutamine[c]	N/R	a. 250 mg/250 mL											
		b. 1,000 μg/mL											
		c. 2–30 μg/kg/min											
		d. 5 μg/kg/min	0–+	?	++++	++	0	↑↑	↑↑	–↑	?	–	–↑
Isoproterenol	0.004 mg	a. 1 mg/250 mL											
	(0.2 mL of 0.2	b. 4 μg/mL											
	mg/mL solution)	c. 0.15 μg/kg/min to											
	Third-degree heart	desired effect			+++++	+++++							
	block	d. 0.015 μg/kg/min											
					+++++	+++++		↑–↓	↑↑↑	↑↑↑	↓	↓↓	–↑

[a]a. Mixture
b. Concentration μg/mL
c. Dose range μg/kg/min
d. Standard rate infusion
[b] "Rule of six."
[c]Dopamine and dobutamine employ the same doses. Dosage of either may quickly be calculated by multiplying patient's weight (kg) × 6 = mg added to 100 mL D5%W. The number of drops delivered through a calibrated infusor (60 drops = 1 mL) is the number of μg/kg/min infused into the patient. Example: 70 kg × 6 = 420; 420 mg/100 mL = 4,200 μg/kg or 70 μg gtt; 5 μg/kg/min = 5 gtt/min. N/R, not recommended; CO, cardiac output; Inotrop, contractility; HR, heart rate; VR, venous return (preload); TPR, peripheral resistance (afterload); RBF, renal blood flow.
Reprinted with permission from Lawson NW, Wallfisch HK: Cardiovascular pharmacology: A new look at the "pressors." In Stoelting RK, Barash PG, Gallagher TJ (eds): Advances in Anesthesia, p 195. Chicago, Year Book Medical Publishers, 1986.

TABLE 12-15

ACTIONS OF ADRENERGIC AGONISTS

SYMPATHOMIMETICS	RECEPTORS						DOSE DEPENDENCE	COMMENTS
	α_1	α_2	β_1	β_2	DA_1	DA_2	(α, β, or DA)	
Methoxamine	+++++	?[a]	0	0	0		0	Vasoconstriction only
Phenylephrine	+++++	?	±	0	0		++	Primarily vasoconstriction
Norepinephrine	+++++	+++++	+++	0	0		+++	β_2 effect present but not seen clinically
Metaraminol	+++++	?	+++	0	0		+++	Releases NE
Epinephrine	+++++	+++	++++	++	0		++++	
Ephedrine	++	?	+++	++	0		++	Direct and indirect
Mephentermine	0 to ++	?	++++	+?	0		++	Cerebral stimulation
Dopamine	+ to +++++	?	++++	++	+++	?	+++++	
Dobutamine	0 to +	?	++++	++	0		++	Inotropism greater than chronotropism
Dopexamine	0	0	+	++++	+		++	
Prenalterol	+		++++	++			+	
Isoproterenol	0	0	+++++	+++++	0		0	

[a]The clinical significance of the effects of agonism and antagonism is not yet known.

in vascular resistance (Table 12-16). Methoxamine and NE are considered equipotent α-1 arteriolar vasoconstrictors; however, these effects differ dramatically from their effects on venoconstriction. The lack of venoconstrictor response to methoxamine has been demonstrated in humans.

A similar study in humans found similar results.[76] Table 12-17 demonstrates relative potencies of several catecholamines on resistance versus capacitance vessels. These data represent only the relative potencies of the amines within either resistance or capacitance vessels and are not a comparison of potency ratios between the two. Nevertheless, the data point out the marked differences between the agents. NE is the most potent amine with respect to arteriolar and venous constriction. Metaraminol is 1.5 times more potent than phenylephrine in constricting resistance vessels; however, phenylephrine is 1.5 times more effective in constricting capacitance vessels than metaraminol. NE proved to be 12 times more potent than metaraminol in constricting resistance vessels and 24 times more effective in constricting capacitance vessels.

TABLE 12-16

AVERAGE PERCENTAGES OF CONTRIBUTIONS OF INCREMENTS IN VENOUS RESISTANCE TO INCREMENTS IN TOTAL RESISTANCE ($\Delta VR/\Delta TR \times 100$)

AGENT	$\Delta VR/\Delta TR \times 100$
Norepinephrine	13.8
Tyramine	8.0
Metaraminol	7.2
Ephedrine	3.3
Mephentermine	1.9
Phenylephrine	1.8
Methoxamine	1.4

After Zimmerman BG, Abboud FN, Eckstein JW: Comparison of the effects of sympathomimetic amines upon venous and total vascular resistance in the foreleg of the dog. J Pharmacol Exp Ther 139:290, 1963, with permission.

Brown et al[77] reported the responses of resistance and capacitance vessels to catecholamines in humans on cardiopulmonary bypass. This is a unique method of examining hemodynamic drug response because flow rate (CO) is fixed, excluding the myocardial effects of the drugs. Changes in resistance or capacitance are reflected as either changes in pressure or changes in reservoir volume, respectively. The α agonist phenylephrine produced a marked decrease in venous capacitance (venoconstriction). Arteriolar resistance increased also, but to a lesser degree, confirming the study by Schmid et al.[76] Dopamine produces significant venoconstriction at doses that have no direct arteriolar or cardiac effect, confirming studies of dopamine in animals (Fig. 12-26).[77]

Table 12-18 is a summary of the available data on the relative potencies of the amines on the α receptors of the resistance and capacitance vessels. Scant data permit inaccuracies, but the table is derived from sources that demonstrate remarkable consistency. It is offered as a clinical guide to drug selection. The peripheral receptors of both resistance and capacitance vessels subserve vasoconstriction, but with divergent effects on afterload and preload; therefore, the α-1 receptors have been subdivided into α-1 arterial (α-1a) and α-1 venous (α-1v). Note that methoxamine and phenylephrine, both pure α drugs, are equipotent arterial vasoconstrictors. Phenylephrine, however, is a potent venous constrictor, but methoxamine has virtually no effect on the capacitance vessels. Dopamine has potent venoconstrictor (α-1v) effect at doses at which few α-1a or β-1 effects are noted.

Adverse Effects

The major adverse effects of the sympathomimetic amines are related to excessive α or β activity. The potential for harm can be understood in terms of receptor characteristics. Excessive β-1 activity may increase contractility but increase HR and myocardial oxygen consumption beyond supply. Severe dysrhythmias are a frequent companion of excess β-1 activity as a result of increased conduction velocity, automaticity, and ischemia. The β-2 activity has the potential to increase CO by

TABLE 12-17

RELATIVE POTENCIES OF SEVERAL SYMPATHOMIMETIC AMINES IN HUMANS WITH RESPECT TO CONSTRICTOR EFFECTS ON RESISTANCE VESSELS AND CAPACITANCE VESSELS

RESISTANCE VESSELS		CAPACITANCE VESSELS	
DRUG	RELATIVE POTENCY	DRUG	RELATIVE POTENCY
Norepinephrine	1.0000	Norepinephrine	1.0000
Metaraminol	0.0874	Phenylephrine	0.0570
Phenylephrine	0.0684	Metaraminol	0.0419
Tyramine	0.0148	Methoxamine	0.0068
Mephentermine	0.0049	Ephedrine	0.0025
Ephedrine	0.0020	Tyramine	0.0023
Methoxamine	0.0018	Mephentermine	0.0023

After Schmid PG, Eckstein JW, Abboud FM: Comparison of the effects of several sympathomimetic amines on resistance and capacitance vessels in the forearm of man. Circulation 34:III–209, 1966, with permission.

reducing resistance (afterload) while reducing blood pressure. An excessive decrease in diastolic pressure, however, reduces obstructive coronary perfusion and may further aggravate myocardial ischemia. The β-1 and β-2 effects of adrenergic agonists are more useful clinically than α-1 effects and can be used for longer periods of time. Unfortunately, it is difficult to separate the inotropic, dromotropic, and chronotropic effects in the clinical setting. The characteristics of the ideal positive inotropic agent are listed in Table 12-12 for comparison with each drug as it is discussed.

Drugs with prominent α-1 agonist effects may produce an increase in blood pressure but reduce total flow because of increases in arteriolar resistance (afterload). A more prominent α-1 venous constriction may improve CO by increasing preload or precipitate failure if preload exceeds the contractile limits of the myocardium (see Fig. 12-24).

In general, the α effects of the sympathomimetics are of benefit only when used for specific indications and for the briefest possible time. Other measures are usually more effective in improving flow and are indicated before a pressor should be used. The only time an adrenergic amine should be used as a pressor or in a pressor dose range without consideration of flow is when arterial perfusion pressure must be increased immediately to prevent imminent death or morbidity.[78] Cardiopulmonary resuscitation is the primary example where a pressor effect is necessary to create diastolic coronary perfusion during closed- or open-heart massage. Any drug with strong α agonist properties seems equally effective in this regard. EPI, with its added β properties, has been the first-line agent for this situation. Vasopressin has been added to this first line. Drugs that vasodilate, such as isoproterenol, have little use in this setting even if they possess inotropic properties. Another situation in which a vasoconstrictor may be justified as a temporary measure is acute hypotension when cerebral, coronary, or extracorporeal bypass perfusion pressure is the prime consideration.

The prolonged use of adrenergic agonists with strong α properties commonly results in tachyphylaxis. This phenomenon is probably caused by increasing plasma volume loss through ischemic capillaries and down-regulation of the adrenergic receptors. Precapillary sphincters are under local myogenic control and relax when hypoxic and acidotic, despite strong α stimulation. Postcapillary sphincters are more functional in an hypoxic and acidotic milieu but are under stronger central neurogenic control. Continued postcapillary tone in the face of precapillary relaxation increases hydrostatic pressure with a net loss of intravascular volume. These events are just a few of the explanations for the once mysterious so-called levophed shock, in which patients were unable to be weaned from NE infusions.[79]

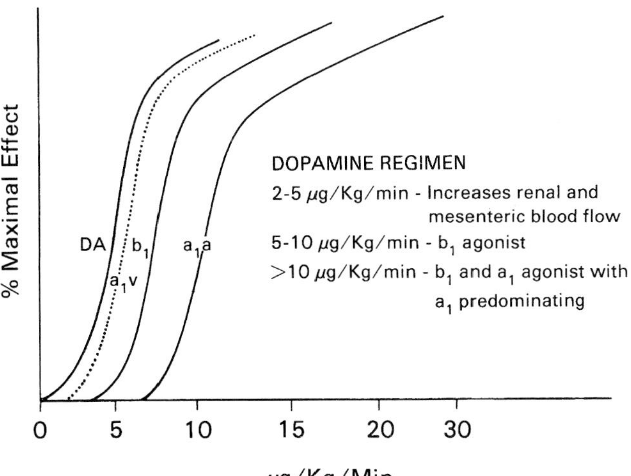

FIGURE 12-26. The spectrum of dose-related adrenergic activity of dopamine is demonstrated. Progressive rates of infusion produce dopaminergic (DA), β, then α activity. Infusion rates of greater than 15 μg/kg/min produce a predominant α effect, like that of NE. Early α-1 venoconstriction may be an important redistributive feature of infused dopamine.

Adrenergie Agonists—α β, DA

Methoxamine and Phenylephrine. Methoxamine is the prototype pure α vasoconstrictor. Phenylephrine produces similar actions, but there are important clinical differences. Methoxamine possesses only α-1 properties and produces almost no venoconstriction. Its only pharmacologic effects are to increase arterial resistance, increase afterload, and reduce flow, even though blood pressure is elevated. Few clinical uses for methoxamine remain. It has been useful for treating paroxysmal atrial tachycardias. A single iv dose of methoxamine can break a paroxysmal atrial tachycardia reflexly through baroreceptor stretch, obviating the need for use of digitalis or countershock. Carotid massage produces similar results by a similar mechanism.

TABLE 12-18

COMPARISON OF RELATIVE α_1 CATECHOLAMINE RESPONSES ON PERIPHERAL RESISTANCE AND CAPACITANCE VESSELS[a]

	VASOCONSTRICTION		
	α_1 ARTERIAL (α_{1a})		α_1 VENOUS (α_{1v})
Norepinephrine	+++++	Norepinephrine	+++++
Metaraminol	+++++	Phenylephrine	+++++
Phenylephrine	++++	Metaraminol	++++
Methoxamine	++++	Dopamine	+++
Epinephrine	0/++++[b]	Epinephrine	0/++++[b]
Dopamine	0/++++[c]	Ephedrine	+++
Ephedrine	++	Mephentermine	+?
Mephentermine	++	Methoxamine	0/+?
Dobutamine	+/0	Dobutamine	?
Isoproterenol	0	Isoproterenol	0

[a]Drugs are listed in descending order of potency within each vascular region.
[b]Dose-dependent; β effects of epinephrine predominate at low doses.
[c]Dose-dependent; DA and β effects predominate at low doses.
Reprinted with permission from Lawson NW, Wallfisch HK: Cardiovascular pharmacology: A new look at the "pressors." In Stoelting RK, Barash PG, Gallagher TJ (eds): Advances in Anesthesia, p 195. Chicago, Year Book Medical Publishers, 1986.

Phenylephrine, also considered a pure α drug, increases venous constriction and arterial constriction in a dose-related manner. Constriction of capacitances vessels precede arteriolar constriction. Venous constriction may be its most redeeming feature when compared with the purely arteriolar effect of methoxamine. One cannot discount the possibility of an inotropic effect now that α-1 receptors are known to exist in the myocardium that improve inotropism. Acutely, venoconstriction favors venous return (preload), even though arterial resistance (afterload) also increases. The net effect may result in an increase in pressure and CO. Phenylephrine, like methoxamine, does not change CO in normal individuals but can cause a decreased output in patients with ischemic heart disease.[80] Phenylephrine has continued to be favored in operating rooms to briefly increase blood pressure during cardiopulmonary bypass as well as during intracranial and peripheral vascular procedures. It does not produce dysrhythmias. Phenylephrine is also useful in reversing right-to-left shunt in tetralogy of Fallot when patients are having "spells" during anesthesia.[81] The arterial vasoconstrictors may reduce the size of an ischemic injury when used in conjunction with intra-aortic balloon pumping or nitroglycerin.[82]

Norepinephrine. NE is the naturally occurring mediator of the SNS and the immediate precursor of EPI. It produces direct-acting hemodynamic effects on the α and β receptors in a dose-related manner when given by infusion. NE produces increased CO and blood pressure when given in low doses (see Table 12-14). Higher doses reduce flow because α arteriolar constriction supersedes the β effects. Reflex baroreceptor bradycardias may occur via active β stimulation.

Increased plasma levels of the endogenous catecholamines NE and EPI are the sympathetic milieu (stress) in which exogenous sympathomimetics are ordinarily given. NE is the catecholamine standard against which other catecholamines are compared. Intravenous NE has received an unseemly reputation over the years that is not merited. Studies indicate that NE was being used in doses that are orders of magnitude greater than that necessary to obtain its best response in producing CO rather than producing a blood pressure. They do not correlate (see Fig 12-20). Complications such as renal failure and tissue necrosis are routine and can be expected when NE is used. If NE is used simply to titrate to blood pressure rather than measured flow, the amount of NE infused is 5 to 10 times more than necessary to obtain the best oxygen delivery and oxygen consumption.[3] Although NE is less commonly used in the critically ill patient than other catecholamines, a resurgence of interest in this agent is noted. It has remained clinically useful because its effects are predictable, prompt, and potent.

Objections to the use of NE for the treatment of cardiogenic shock are based on two considerations: (1) vasoconstriction increases the pressure work of the left ventricle, with an adverse effect on the oxygen economy of the ischemic pump and (2) these drugs cause further vasoconstriction and organ ischemia in a syndrome in which intense constriction may already have occurred.[16] The use of NE requires the use of invasive monitoring; otherwise, complications are to be expected. It is not usually necessary to elevate the systolic blood pressure above 90 to 100 mm Hg. At this level of infusion, the CO will normally be increased as a β effect without excessive peripheral vasoconstriction. NE is also a potent venoconstrictor, which will alter interpretation of venous filling pressures as a guide to adequate volume repletion.

Other undesirable effects associated with NE include renal arteriolar constriction and oliguria. In addition, prolonged therapy may produce a reduction in plasma volume as a result of fluid transudation. Indeed, in some instances, cardiogenic shock requiring continuous NE infusions has been reversed by fluid infusions.[16]

Norepinephrine should only be administered in a centrally placed iv to avoid tissue necrosis from extravasation. It can be used for its intropic effect at low doses and titrated to effect while monitoring cardiac output. Monitoring of blood pressure alone or titrating to a predetermined effect is often detrimental to cardiac output. Blood pressure increases are usually a result of increases in SVR and can diminish forward flow and contribute to cardiac failure. Even moderate doses of norepinephrine may have a detrimental effect on end-organ perfusion, which has given the drug an ill-gotten reputation when used to titrate to pressure rather than flow. However, in those clinical conditions characterized by a low perfusion pressure and high flow (vasodilatation) and maldistribution of flow (sepsis), norepinephrine has been shown to improve renal and splanchnic blood flow by increasing pressure provided the patient has been volume resuscitated.

Epinephrine. EPI is the prototypical endogenous catecholamine. It is synthesized, stored, and released from the adrenal medulla and is the key hormonal element in the fight-or-flight response. It is the most widely used catecholamine in medicine. It is used to treat asthma, anaphylaxis, cardiac arrest, and bleeding and to prolong Regional Anesthesia. The cardiovascular effects of EPI, when given systemically, result from its direct stimulation of both α and β receptors. This is dose dependent and is outlined in Table 12-14.

The effect of EPI on the peripheral vasculature is mixed. It has predominantly α-stimulating effects in some beds (skin, mucosa, and kidney) and β-stimulating actions in others (skeletal muscle). These effects are also dose dependent. At therapeutic doses, β-adrenergic effects predominate in the peripheral vessels, and total resistance may be reduced. Constriction, however, is maintained in the renal and cutaneous areas because of its dominant α effect in these areas. An increase in CO with EPI may be a result of a redistribution of blood to low resistance vessels in the muscle, but with further reduction in flow to vital organs. Cardiac dysrhythmias are a prominent hazard, and the strong chronotropic effects of EPI have limited its use in the treatment of cardiogenic shock.

Epinephrine is commonly used in the perioperative period in anesthesia. It is often used to produce a bloodless field in dentistry, otolaryngology, and skin grafting either topically or in local and field blocks. Anesthesiologists often use it to prolong regional anesthesia. The addition of epinephrine to arthroscopic infusions to attain a bloodless field is another area of increased epinephrine usage with the development of these techniques. These infusions are usually safe in maintaining a dry operative field because the solutions are very dilute at around 1:3,000,000. However, the large volumes infused, the unpredictable absorption of the epinephrine, especially in denuded cancellous bone, offers the opportunity of exposure of the patient to an excessive amount of epinephrine over a short period of time despite the dilution.[83] The unexpected complications are those of epinephrine overdose, that is, acute heart failure, pulmonary edema, or cardiac arrhythmias and arrest in the otherwise young and healthy patient. Impending problems during the infusion of intra-articular fluids will be noted by an increasing blood pressure exceeding that attributable to surgical pain or hypertension that is poorly responsive to deepening of anesthesia. Absent a pulsatile flow or vasoconstriction oximetry may become dysfunctional. The patient will appear pale and cyanotic. Unless alert, one may unintentionally treat an unexpected acute heart failure or cardiac arrest with the very agent that caused the problem. The outcome is universally poor. Vasodilators and β-blockers may save the day instead.

Intravenous and locally infiltrated adrenergic agents should be used cautiously during inhalation anesthesia, especially with halothane. The following schedule has been found to be relatively safe during inhalation anesthesia.[84] (1) EPI concentrations no greater than 1:100,000–1:200,000 (1:200,000 = 5 μg/mL). (2) Adult dose should be no greater than 10 mL of 1:100,000 or 20 mL of 1:200,000 within 10 minutes. (3) Total should not exceed 30 mL of 1:100,000 (60 mL of 1:200,000) within 1 hour.

The dose of submuscosally injected EPI necessary to produce ventricular cardiac dysrhythmia in 50% of patients anesthetized with a 1.25 MAC of a volatile anesthetic was 10.9, 10.9, and 6.7 μg/kg during administration of halothane, enflurane, and isoflurane, respectively.[85] No data are currently available for sevoflurane or desflurane. The incidence of cardiac dysrhythmia is eliminated when this dose is halved in patients anesthetized with halothane or isoflurane. In contrast with adults, children seem to tolerate higher doses of subcutaneous EPI without developing cardiac dysrhythmia.[86]

Ephedrine. Ephedrine is the most commonly used noncatecholamine sympathomimetic agent. It is used extensively for treating hypotension following spinal or epidural anesthesia. Ephedrine stimulates both α and β receptors by direct and indirect actions. It is predominantly an indirect-acting pressor, producing its effects by causing NE release.[16] Tachyphylaxis develops rapidly and is probably related to the depletion of NE stores with repeated injection. The cardiovascular effects of ephedrine (see Table 12-14) are nearly identical to those of EPI but less potent. Its effects are sustained about 10 times longer than those of EPI.

Ephedrine remains the pressor of choice in obstetrics because uterine blood flow improves linearly with blood pressure.[52] This effect is probably not related to its arteriolar vasoconstriction but rather to its venoconstrictive action. Ephedrine is a weak, indirect-acting sympathomimetic agent that produces venoconstriction to a greater degree than arteriolar constriction (see Table 12-18), at the doses ordinarily used.[87] This may be its most important and unappreciated effect. It causes a redistribution of blood centrally, improves venous return (preload), increases CO, and restores uterine perfusion. The mild β action restores HR simultaneously with improved venous return. An increased blood pressure is noted as a result rather than a cause of these events. Mild α-1 arteriolar constriction does occur, but the net effect of improving venous return and HR is increased CO (Fig. 12-27). Uterine blood flow is spared. This response, however, depends on the patient's state of hydration.

Neosynephrine is an attractive alternate vasopressor for obstetrics for similar reasons. It produces strong α-1 venoconstriction and volume redistribution at infusion rates at which α-1a or β effects are minimal (see Table 12-15). Alternatively, the primary disadvantage of the venoconstriction of low doses of dopamine is its lack of immediate availability as an iv push drug. It requires more careful titration than ephedrine. The prophylactic administration of "pressors" before spinal blockade in obstetrics can produce misleading clinical estimates of volume status because of its effects on venous return and arterial pressure.[88]

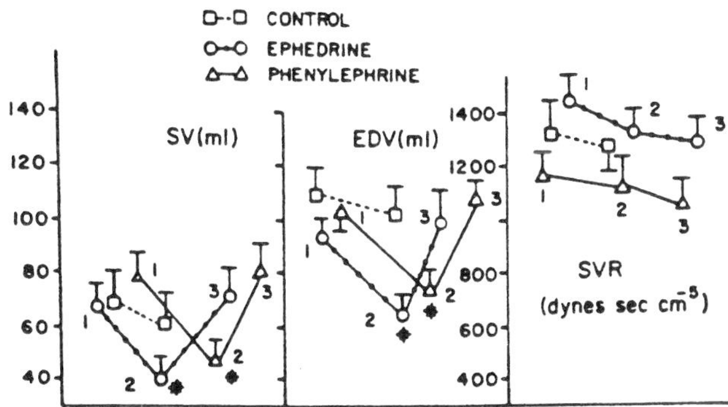

FIGURE 12-27. Stroke volume (SV), end-diastolic volume (EDV), and systemic vascular resistance (SVR) (1) before regional block, (2) during hypotension, and (3) after therapy with ephedrine or phenylephrine. The increase in stroke volume was related entirely to an increased venous return secondary to venoconstriction in these awake, healthy patients. The afterload effects of phenylephrine at higher doses predominate in patients with heart disease or myocardial depression and reduce CO. (Reprinted with permission from Ramanthan S, Grant G: Vasopressor therapy for hypotension due to epidural anesthesia for cesarean section. Acta Anaesthesiol Scand 32:4, 1988.)

Isoproterenol. Isoproterenol is a potent balanced β-1 and β-2 receptor agonist with no vasoconstrictor effects. It increases HR and contractility while decreasing systemic vascular resistance. Although it can increase CO, it is not useful in shock because it redistributes blood to nonessential areas by its preferential effect on the cutaneous and muscular vessels.[89] As a result, it produces variable and unpredictable results on CO and blood pressure. Isoproterenol is a potent dysrhythmogenic drug and extends myocardial ischemic areas. Deleterious effects on an evolving cardiac ischemic process include cardiac dysrhythmias, tachycardia, and reduced diastolic coronary perfusion pressure and time. Increased myocardial oxygen demand makes it an unattractive drug for patients in cardiogenic shock.

Isoproterenol is helpful in managing cardiac failure associated with bradycardia, asthma, and cor pulmonale. It is also a useful chemical pacemaker in third-degree heart block until an artificial pacemaker can be inserted or the cause can be removed. Isoproterenol might be useful in treating both idiopathic and secondary pulmonary hypertension.[15,16] It has also been reported as useful in improving the forward flow in patients with regurgitant aortic valvular disease, but it should not be used if there is an accompanying stenosis.[82]

Dobutamine. Dobutamine is a synthetic catecholamine modified from the classic inodilator isoproterenol. Isoproterenol was, in turn, synthesized from dopamine. Variations and similarities in structure can be seen in Figure 12-7.

DBT has clear advantages over isoproterenol and dopamine in many clinical situations. It acts directly on β-1 receptors but exerts much weaker β-2 stimulation than isoproterenol. It does not cause NE release or stimulate DA receptors. DBT, unlike isoproterenol or DPX, possesses weak α-1 agonism, which can be unmasked by β-blockade as a prompt and dramatic increase in blood pressure.[90] Ordinarily, changes in arterial blood pressure do not occur because the mild α-1 activity is countered by the β-2 activity. DBT produces strong inotropism but with weak chronotropic or vascular effects. Increases in CO are primarily through increased inotropism and secondarily by reduced afterload.

DBT increases automaticity of the SA node and increases conduction through the AV nodes and ventricles. DBT produces less increase in HR per unit gain in CO than dopamine, but it is not devoid of chronotropic activity. Troublesome tachycardias can occur in sensitive individuals and caution should be exercised in patients with established atrial fibrillation or recurrent tachycardias. Early studies found DBT preferable to dopamine, EPI, or isoproterenol because of its reduced chronotropic effects.[91] DBT increases HR more than EPI for a given increase in CO.[92]

DBT may decrease diastolic coronary filling pressure because of its vasodilation in contrast to the constriction produced by dopamine.[71] These studies suggest that dobutamine produces an overall favorable metabolic climate in the ischemic myocardium despite an increase in inotropism. Improvement is rate limited. Dobutamine has been used effectively to improve coronary flow to differentiate, by echocardiography, responsive or unresponsive areas of dyskinesia in patients following myocardial infarction.[93]

Dobutamine is highly controllable with a half-life of 2 minutes. Tachyphylaxis is rare but may be noted if given over 72 hours. The net hemodynamic effects of DBT include an increase in CO, a decrease in left ventricular filling pressure, and a decrease in systemic vascular resistance without a significant increase in chronotropism at lower doses.[94] It has been proven to be as effective as combined dopamine and nitroprusside in treating heart failure with infarction. It is even more effective when summated with the dopaminergic properties of DA. In contrast to dopamine, DBT seems to inhibit hypoxic pulmonary vasoconstriction. Like its parent compound isoproterenol, DBT may prove to be useful in managing right ventricular heart failure.

Dopamine offers some advantages over many sympathomimetics in treating the low-output syndrome.[95] It is a dose-related agonist to all three types of adrenoceptors, and the desired action can be selected by changing the infusion rate. The DA receptors are most sensitive followed by the β, and then α receptors. Dopamine dosage regimens have been traditionally, and arbitrarily, divided into low, medium, and high doses according to its dose-receptor sensitivity (see Table 12-14). Renal and mesenteric vascular dilatation and tubular cell natriuresis are mediated through the DA receptors at low-dose infusion rates of 0.5 to 2.0 μg/kg/min. This is often referred to as "renal dose dopamine" because of the purported enhanced renal blood flow and diuresis. However, the concept of "renal dose" DA may be more imagined than real. The diuresis may also be attributed, in part, to inhibition of aldosterone secretion seen with low-dose DA administration.[96] A general improvement in CO from afterload reduction also contributes to improvements in renal blood flow. These effects have been well demonstrated in patients with heart failure. However, the protective effects of DA on the development of renal failure in the critically ill or injured patient, although an attractive principle, is much less certain. Prevention of renal failure by prophylactic "renal dose" DA (with or without furosemide) in the critically ill[97] or traumatized patient has not been conclusively demonstrated, and no longer tenable. This may be related to the adrenergic milieu into which the DA is given. The vasoconstrictive effects of DA are expected to occur only at relatively high doses. However, even relatively low doses of DA can cause renal vasoconstriction when added into pre-existing high plasma levels of endogenous catecholamines commonly seen in the critically ill or acutely injured patient or those already receiving intravenous sympathomimetics.

The hemodynamic effects of low-dose DA are primarily related to vasodilatation by activation of the DA1 and DA2 receptors. Activation of presynaptic DA2 adrenoceptors add to the vasodilating effect of the DA1 receptors by inhibiting presynaptic NE release in the renal and mesenteric vessels. The reduction of total systemic vascular resistance would be significant when one considers that 25% of the CO goes to the kidneys alone (Fig. 12-28). A reduced diastolic blood pressure is often noted with a slight reflex increase in HR. Increasing the infusion rate of DA to 2 to 5 μg/kg/min begins to activate βreceptors increasing the CO by increasing chronotropism and contractility with early venoconstriction (preload) and systemic vasodilatation (afterload reduction). Blood pressure may not increase despite significant increases in CO. This dose range would appear optimal for managing congestive heart and lung failure because it combines inotropism and afterload reduction with possible diuresis. Further increases in dose activate α receptors, which will increase vascular resistance and blood pressure, but further improvements in CO may be attenuated. Infusion rates of greater than 10 μg/kg/min produce intense a activity, which may override any beneficial DA or β vasodilation effect on total flow. High-dose dopamine behaves much like NE and, in fact, causes NE release at this dose range.[98]

Despite the apparent dose-response divisions of DA, a wide variability of individual responses has been noted. The α-adrenergic effects can be seen in some individuals in doses as low as 5 μg/kg/min, whereas doses as high as 20 μg/kg/min may be required to obtain this effect in shocked patients.[98] This wide variation in dose response has led to a reexamination of DA as a primary adrenergic for patients in cardiogenic shock or failure. Increased venous return may not be desirable in this situation, but dopamine's hemodynamic versatility continues to be useful in cardiogenic shock when

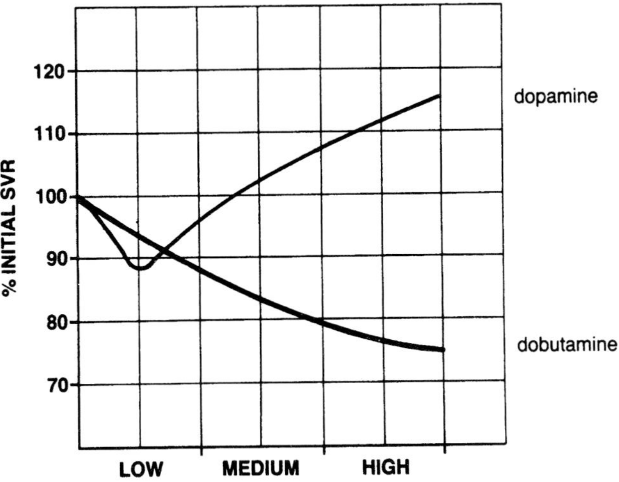

FIGURE 12-28. Dobutamine produces a net reduction in vascular resistance. Its weak α vasoconstrictive effects are balanced by a direct β-2 vasodilation with little change in vascular tone. However, further reflex arterial vasodilation occurs with increased CO. Low-dose dopamine dilates renal and mesentric arterial beds, which reduces afterload but increases resistance at increasing doses as a result of its predominant α effect.

combined with other complementary catecholamines such as dobutamine (Fig. 12-29) (see combinations). The venoconstriction, or distributive effects, of dopamine are useful in surgical patients in whom third-space edema and sepsis are the most common abnormalities. Dopamine increases mean pulmonary arterial pressure and is not recommended for sole support in patients with right heart failure, adult respiratory distress syndrome, or pulmonary hypertension.

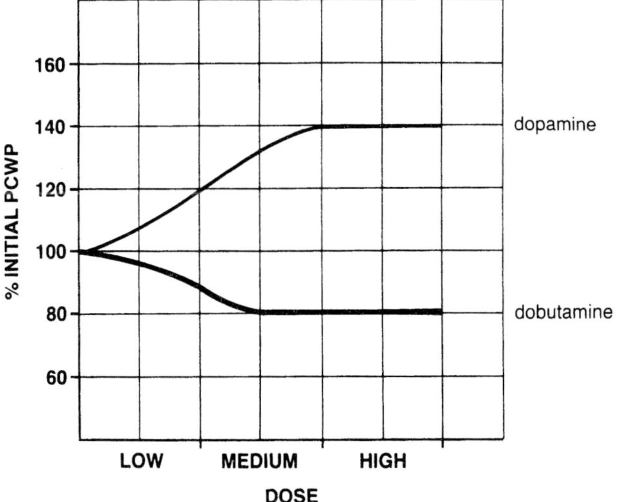

FIGURE 12-29. A decrease in venous capacitance has been demonstrated as an early effect of dopamine. An increase in pulmonary capillary wedge pressure may be noted. Dobutamine may decrease pulmonary capillary wedge pressure by increased inotropism as well as vasodilation with minimal effect on venous capacitance. (Redrawn with permission of Eli Lilly Co., Indianapolis, Indiana.)

Combination Therapy

Dopamine and DBT are two of the most popular inodilators in use today. A comparison of these two drugs will underscore the importance of the extracardiac side effects in selecting a drug either for use alone or in combination.[99] This comparison is particularly appropriate because dopamine and DBT are considered equipotent inotropic agents and are effective in the same dose range of 2 to 15 μg/kg/min. Their differences can be compared at low (0.5 to 4 μg/kg/min), medium (5 to 9 μg/kg/min), and high (10 to 15 μg/kg/min) doses. This comparison will illustrate the divergent effects of two drugs on preload and afterload while sharing the property of inotropism. Although they share several clinical indications, these drugs are pharmacologically distinct and not interchangeable. Their divergent properties, however, make them particularly valuable when used in combination.[100]

DBT is a direct-acting catecholamine that produces a positive inotropic β-1 effect but with minimal changes in β-2 HR or vascular resistance (β-2, α-1 counteraction). Thus, DBT may not alter blood pressure even though CO is markedly improved. Dopamine may do both. Low-dose dopamine can produce hemodynamic changes similar to those of DBT (inotropism and mesenteric vasodilatation) (see Fig. 12-28). Dopamine produces an increase in blood pressure at higher doses related to its direct and indirect α-1 activation. This increased afterload with dopamine may attenuate any further increase in CO comparable to that of an equal dose of DBT. DBT does not have any clinically important venoconstrictor activity in contrast to dopamine in which an increase in ventricular filling pressure can be noted at low doses. This contrasting effect on preload is seen in Figure 12-29. The cardiac response to all vasodilators is dependent on the preexisting preload status. Patients who have acute failure with normal or only slightly elevated end-diastolic volumes may not respond to afterload reduction with an increase in CO. Balanced vasodilators such as nitroprusside or venodilators such as the nitrates may actually reduce CO in these patients. Patients with dilated left ventricles and elevated filling pressures usually have impressive improvement in CO with afterload reduction. This underscores the importance of monitored volume loading before proceeding apace with vasoactive drugs (see Table 12-13). It is possible, and indeed likely, that a portion of the reduced effectiveness of long-term vasodilator therapy results from inadequate preload, which in some circumstances can actually be a consequence of successful drug therapy. Clinical studies suggest that DBT is less likely to increase HR than dopamine for a given dose, a major concern in the patient with coronary artery disease. DBT is a coronary artery dilator, whereas dopamine is not. A dopamine-induced tachycardia, however, may be of less concern in the septic patient who commonly has a maldistribution of volume, low vascular resistance, a preexisting refractory tachycardia, but a previously healthy heart. The empiric preference of dopamine in surgical units and DBT in coronary units has been observed and is perhaps well founded. The surgical patient is more likely to have distributive defects and fluid shifts from major trauma and surgery. The hemodynamics of the septic patient are characterized by low vascular resistance, hypotension, high CO, and some degree of myocardial depression. The mesenteric distribution, inotropic, and pressor effects of dopamine would seem ideal for this condition. However, a shift of blood volume to the central circulation, tachycardia, or an unpredictable increase in afterload may not be appropriate for the patient in congestive heart failure or an acute infarct. DBT, with its dose-related inotropism, afterload reduction, and relative lack of chronotropism, would seem more appropriate for these circumstances.

Dobutamine does not cause NE release or stimulate DA receptors. Dopamine does both, but the effect is dose related.

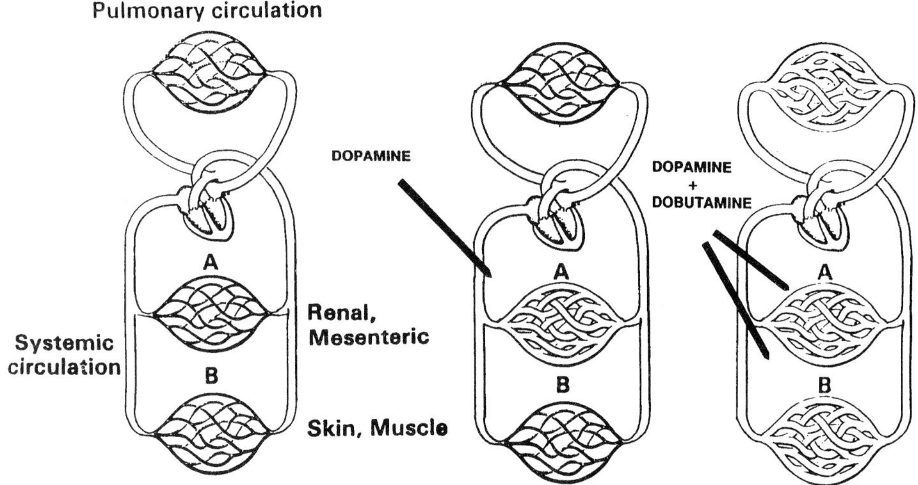

FIGURE 12-30. Combining low doses of dopamine and dobutamine may produce improvements in CO that are greater than can be achieved with either drug alone. This appears to be clinical synergism. However, the vasodilation of different vascular beds likely produces a summed reduction of afterload at the same level of inotropism that only appears to be synergistic. The second law of thermodynamics remains intact.

Dopamine offers possible advantages over many sympathomimetics in managing the low-output syndrome with oliguria. This effect is ablated at higher doses. DBT does not selectively increase renal blood flow but does improve renal blood flow secondarily with improved CO and weak β-2 vasodilation. Much of the reduced afterload observed with the use of DBT may be related more to a reduced sympathetic tone with improved flow than that of active vasodilatation. DBT belongs on the opposite end of the spectrum from amrinone. DBT is a potent inotropic agent but a weak vasodilator, whereas amrinone is a potent vasodilator but weak inotrope.

Dopamine and DBT also have contrasting effects on the pulmonary vasculature. Dopamine has been noted to increase pulmonary artery pressure and does not inhibit the pulmonary hypoxic response. It is not recommended for patients in right heart failure. DBT does vasodilate the pulmonary vasculature and is helpful in treating right heart failure and cor pulmonale.[17] The adrenergic effects of combined sympathomimetics, like the solo drugs, also appear to be additive and competitive for receptor sites. Many combinations of adrenergic drugs have been described as having a synergistic effect. Synergism is the joint action of agents such that their combined effect is greater than the algebraic sum of their individual effects. This synergism may be a clinical interpretation of a summated receptor effect that appears synergistic. For example, infusions of the combination of dopamine and DBT have been noted to produce a greater improvement in CO, at lower doses, than can be achieved by either drug alone. Each drug, although equipotent inotropic agents, dilates different vascular beds. Therefore, the summation of afterload reduction by both drugs could produce a greater improvement in CO than could be achieved by either drug alone, even at the same level of inotropism. Summation is more consistent with current receptor pharmacology and can be used to advantage in avoiding unwanted side effects of one drug while supplementing its desired attributes with another. The summation principle obviates the necessity of knowing a large number of drugs. One need only become familiar with a few agents to manage most clinical situations.

Because of summation, many combinations of vasoactive drugs have been found useful in making fine hemodynamic adjustments in the critically ill. The available sympathomimetic agents provide a wide range of hemodynamic effects, particularly when combined with vasodilators. For example, if a larger positive inotropic action and less vasoconstriction are desired, DBT could be added to dopamine. Also, nitroprusside could be added to dopamine or combined with any other appropriate inodilator.[101] Combinations are also useful in redistributing the CO to vital organs. This is why the combination of DBT and dopamine has been helpful. Dopamine could distribute the CO to the renal and mesenteric vascular bed, whereas DBT could provide additional afterload reduction by opening up the vascular beds of skin and muscle (Fig. 12-30).[102] NE has been successfully used in combination with dopamine to increase vascular resistance in septic patients while distributing a greater portion of the CO to the renal and mesenteric bed.[103]

The studied use of adrenergic combinations in patients with cardiac failure has been proposed because pathophysiology cannot be approached with the attitude that β agonism is all good and a agonism is all bad. The objective is to increase coronary perfusion and CO while decreasing afterload. This is the effect achieved by the intra-aortic balloon pump. No single vasoactive agent can achieve this, but these conditions can be approached with combination therapy. Because of receptor summation during combination therapy, standard rates of infusion (as outlined in Table 12-14) no longer apply. Invasive hemodynamic monitoring is mandatory for success; otherwise, iatrogenic disasters can be expected. Other conditions necessary for success with vasoactive drugs also require that the failing myocardium or vasculature must have functional reserve, the reserve can be stimulated, and perfusion can be maintained.[104,105]

Fenoldopam

Fenoldopam, a benzazepine derivative, is a selective DA1 agonist with no α or β receptor activity compared to dopamine (see Table 12-15).[98,106] Oral bioavailability is poor, but it is an effective antihypertensive when given iv. Intravenous fenoldopam has direct natriuretic and diuretic properties that promote natriuresis, diuresis, and an increase in creatinine clearance. It offers advantages in the acute resolution of severe hypertension compared to sodium nitroprusside, particularly if the patient has preexisting renal impairment.[107] Aronson et al reported a comparative study using SNP and fenoldopam in dogs under general anesthesia. A 30% reduction in mean arterial pressure was produced by either fenoldopam or SNP. Fenoldopam maintained renal blood flow while SNP showed a reduction.[106,108] Preservation or augmentation of renal blood flow during blood pressure reduction presents a potential for use during several situations in the perioperative period. Fenoldopam has an elimination half-life of 5 minutes. This property might well lend itself in producing hypotensive anesthesia while preserving renal function.[108]

Human studies have demonstrated that fenoldopam is a potent direct renal vasodilator. Left ventricular function has been noted to improve with afterload reduction. The study by Kien and colleagues suggests that the improvement in renal function is a direct vasodilator effect of the drug.[108] Intravenous fenoldopam may prove to be ideal for treating conditions in which renal vasoconstriction is an expected complication. Examples are cyclosporine-induced renal vasoconstriction, radiographic dye toxicity, and human kidney recipients.[109–111]

The onset of action with intravenous fenoldopam is about 5 minutes, reaching a steady state in about 20 minutes. The drug is rapidly metabolized in the liver and excreted in the urine. The elimination half-life is about 5 minutes. There has been no evidence of tolerance in reducing blood pressure for up to 24 hours. No rebound on withdrawal has been noted.

The most common adverse effects of fenoldopam are related to vasodilation, which include hypotension, flushing, dizziness, headache, and increases in heart rate, nausea, and hypokalemia. It should be used cautiously in patients with glaucoma as it can increase intraocular pressure. No significant drug interactions have been reported. Concomitant use with β-blockers will reduce the effective dose of fenoldopam.

Fenoldopam is diluted in normal saline or 5% dextrose and is given by continuous infusion without a bolus dose. The effective dosage range is 0.1 to 1.6 μg/kg/min. A reflex tachycardia may be produced. The dosage is titrated upward every 15 minutes according to patient response. Any change in infusion rate should be detectable within 15 minutes.

Clonidine

Clonidine is a centrally acting selective partial α-2 adrenergic agonist (220:1 α-2 to α-1). It is an antihypertensive drug by its ability to decrease central sympathetic outflow. Stimulation of α-2 receptors in the vasomotor centers of the medulla oblongata is thought to produce this effect.[112] It is not clear whether these are pre- or postsynaptic receptors. However, the end result is decreased SNS tone and enhanced vagal tone. Peripherally there is decreased plasma renin activity as well as decreased EPI and NE levels. This drug has been proven to be effective in the treatment of severe hypertension and renin-dependent hypertensive disease.

Clonidine is not available for intravenous use. The usual daily adult oral dose is 0.2 to 0.3 mg. A transdermal clonidine patch is available for use on a weekly basis for surgical patients unable to take oral medication.

Clonidine is clinically useful in anesthesiology in other ways. It has been found to produce dose-dependent analgesia when introduced into the epidural or subarachnoid space in doses of 150 to 450 μgs.[113] The addition of 75 to 150 μg of clonidine to subarachnoid tetracaine or bupivicaine can prolong the duration of sensory and motor blockade of the local anesthetics. Unlike the opioids, clonidine does not depress respiration or cause pruritis, nausea, vomiting, or delayed gastric emptying.[114] Clonidine and morphine do not produce cross-tolerance. Hypotension, sedation, and xerostomia may follow the neuraxial use of clonidine.[115,116]

Oral clonidine (5 μg/kg) when used as a premedicant enhances the postoperative analgesia provided by intrathecal morphine without adding to the side effects of the morphine.[117] Other additional benefits noted from a clonidine premedication include (1) blunted reflex tachycardia for intubation, (2) reduction of vasomotor liability, (3) decreased plasma catecholamines, and (4) dramatic decreases in MAC for inhaled gases or injected drugs.

Other uses of clonidine have been in the diagnosis of pheochromocytoma, treatment of opioid withdrawal, and shivering.[118] Clonidine, 0.3 mg orally, will decrease the plasma concentration of catecholamines in normal patients but not in the presence of a pheochromocytoma. This reflects the ability of clonidine to suppress release of catecholamines from nerve endings but not from the pheochromocytoma. Its usefulness in suppressing opioid withdrawal is likewise attributed to its ability to replace the opioid-mediated inhibition with α-2–mediated inhibition of CNS sympathetic outflow. It may likewise be useful for nicotine withdrawal.

Clonidine is rapidly absorbed by mouth and reaches peak plasma levels within 60 to 90 minutes. The elimination half-life is between 9 to 12 hours. It is equally excreted in the liver and kidneys. The duration of the hypotensive effect after a single dose is about 8 hours. The transdermal administration of clonidine requires about 48 hours to achieve therapeutic levels. The decrease in systolic blood pressure is more prominent than the decrease in diastolic blood pressure. Homeostatic cardiovascular reflexes are maintained, avoiding problems of orthostatic hypotension. There seem to be no effects on glomerular filtration rate.

Side Effects. The most common side effects of clonidine are sedation and a dry mouth. However, skin rashes are frequent with chronic use. Impotence may be seen occasionally and orthostatic hypotension is rare. One of the more worrisome complications of chronic clonidine use is a withdrawal syndrome on acute discontinuation of the drug. This usually occurs about 18 hours after discontinuation. The symptoms are hypertension, tachycardia, insomnia, flushing, headache, apprehension, sweating, and tremulousness. It lasts for 24 to 72 hours and is most likely to occur in patients taking more than 1.2 mg/day of clonidine. The withdrawal syndrome has been noted postoperatively in patients who were withdrawn from clonidine before surgery. It can be confused with anesthesia emergence symptoms particularly in a patient with uncontrolled hypertension. Absent the availability of the oral route in the surgical patient, withdrawal can be treated with clonidine transdermally or more rapidly with rectal clonidine.

Dexmedetomidine

Dexmedetomidine is a more selective α-2 agonist than clonidine.[119] Its potent α-2-agonism is 1620:1 α-2 to α-1. Compared to clonidine, dexmedetomidine is seven times more selective for α-2 receptors and has a shorter half-life of 1.5 hours. It has a more rapid onset of action (less than 5 minutes). The time to peak effect is 15 minutes. It can be given intravenously and has many uses in anesthesiology. It provides excellent sedation, reduces blood pressure and HR, and profoundly decreases plasma catecholamines. Little respiratory depression is evident. Dexmedetomidine has been shown to be an effective anxiolytic and sedative when used as premedication. Pretreatment with dexmedetomidine, like, clonidine, attenuates hemodynamic responses to intubation. Likewise, it decreases the MAC for volatile anesthetics from 35 to 50% but increases the likelihood of hypotension. Dexmedetomidine, like clonidine, increases the range of temperatures not triggering theromoregulator defenses. It is likely to promote perioperative hypothermia but also is effective against shivering.[120]

The following properties of dexmedetomidine seem particularly valuable to the anesthesiologist.[121]

1. Potent analgesia
2. Sedation and anxiolysis
3. Antisialogogue
4. Promotes hemodynaimic stability
5. Homeostatic reflexes remain intact
6. Attenuates opioid rigidity (in animals)

Dexmedetomidine is provided in 2-mL vials (100 mcg/mL) and must be diluted in 48 mL of 0.9% sodium chloride to be used in a controlled infusion device. A loading infusion (1 mcg/kg) must be given over a 10-minute period in a monitored setting. The loading dose should not be bolused. A transient and paradoxical hypertension may be seen during infusion of the loading dose. The HR may be seen to decrease. The increase in BP is attributed to an initial stimulation of α-2 receptors in vascular smooth muscle. The blood pressure usually decreases as the central blockade of central α-2 agonism overrides the peripheral effect.[120,121] The state of sedation must be monitored as episodes of obstructive apnea have occurred with the loading infusion related to the degree of sedation.

Nonadrenergic Sympathomimetic Agents

Table 12-4 classifies the drugs that mimic the SNS into two broad categories, adrenergic or nonadrenergic. Adrenergic agonists exert their action through adrenergic receptors by direct stimulation or indirectly via release of NE. Adrenergic agonists may be catecholamines or noncatecholamines by chemical configuration. Nonadrenergic sympathomimetic drugs also act indirectly by influencing the cAMP-calcium cascade, exclusive of the receptors (see Fig. 12-15). The function of the second messenger (cAMP) and the third messenger (Ca2+) nearly always goes together. This concept reinforces the recent appreciation of the homogeneity of action of a wide variety of drugs previously thought to be unrelated. Sympathomimetics have more pharmacologic similarities than differences.

Vasopressin. Vasopressin and its congener (desmopressin) are exogenous preparations of the endogenous antidiuretic hormone (ADH). ADH and oxytocin are the two principal hormones secreted by the posterior pituitary. Target sites for ADH are the renal-collecting ducts and vascular smooth muscle and cardiac myocytes. Water absorption is passively reabsorbed from renal-collecting ducts into extracellular fluid. Nonrenal actions include inotropism and intense vasoconstriction, accounting for its alternative designation as vasopressin.[122]

Arginine vasopressin (AVP) is the most active form of ADH. Historically, vasopressin has been used for (1) treatment of diabetes insipidus, (2) diagnosis of diabetes insipidus, (3) abdominal distention, (4) and as an adjunct in the treatment of GI hemorrhage and esophageal varices. Recently, three new indications for the use of vasopressin have emerged. These are (1) pressure support for septic shock, (2) cardiac arrest secondary to ventricular fibrillation, and (3) pulseless ventricular tachycardia and heart failure.[123] This discussion is limited to cardiac arrest.

Three AVP receptor subtypes are known. These are V1a, V1b, and V2 receptor subtypes. V1 receptors are found on vascular smooth muscle and cardiac muscle. The V2 receptors regulate renal function. Endogenous ADH is released from the posterior pituitary in response to changes in plasma osmolality or with baroreceptor response to changes in blood volume or pressure. Release is stimulated with a 5 to 10% decrease in blood volume, central blood volume, cardiac output, or blood pressure sensed by the carotid and aortic baroreceptors. Stretch receptors in the left atrium and pulmonary veins may also activate ADH release. It is also released when the osmoreceptors in the hypothalamus sense changes of as little as 1% in osmolality and mediated by the V2 receptors.

Epinephrine is universally the first-line drug applied to pulseless cardiac rhythms such as ventricular fibrillation (VF), ventricular tachycardia, electromechanical dissociation, and asystole. Despite good animal studies, there is little evidence from human data that epinephrine improves outcome from cardiac arrest. Controlled comparative studies in humans between high-dose EPI and standard-dose EPI showed no increase in survival or improved neurologic outcome in survivors receiving high-dose EPI. The search for a more effective vasopressor led to the current advocacy of vasopressin as a replacement for EPI in shock-refractory pulseless rhythms. Survivors of cardiac arrest, compared to nonsurvivors, had demonstrated higher levels of vasopressin both before and after receiving EPI.[124]

Animal studies have shown, both in open- and closed-chest models, vasopressin caused a larger increase in SVR, cerebral perfusion pressure, and coronary perfusion pressure than EPI. Vasopressin is a more effective vasoconstrictor than EPI in the presence of hypoxia and acidosis. In contrast to EPI, vasopressin does not seem to increase MV02 or lactate production.[122] In the 2000 guidelines for advanced cardiac life support (ACLS) of the American Heart Association, vasopressin was updated to a class IIb recommendation (acceptable, possibly helpful, not harmful and supported by fair evidence) for treatment of cardiac arrest secondary to ventricular fibrillation and ventricular tachycardia. EPI was reassigned from a previous class IIb recommendation to "class indeterminate." At the time of this change, there was insufficient evidence to recommend vasopressin for the treatment of asystole or electromechanical dissociation (class indeterminate). However a recent study in out-of-hospital human cardiac arrests has demonstrated that vasopressin is superior to EPI in patients with asystole.[125] Vasopressin followed by EPI may be more effective than EPI alone in the treatment of refractory cardiac arrest. As yet, randomized trials have failed to demonstrate the superiority of vasopressin over EPI in survival of in-hospital cardiac arrest.[126] These data may be skewed by the co-morbid factors requiring hospitalization. Larger trials will be necessary as to whether survival to discharge will be improved by vasopressin.

Vasopressin used for cardiac arrest is known as "vasopressin injection USP" and is available in vials of 20 IU/mL. The dose in cardiac arrest is 40 IU in 40 mL intravenously as a single dose in a peripheral iv line. Extravasation may cause local tissue necrosis. Its use in vasodilated sepsis is by infusion pump starting at 0.04 IU/min.

Adenosine. Adenosine, available for more than 50 years, has been recognized recently as a clinically useful drug. It is a byproduct of ATP and is found in every cell in the body. It is composed of adenine and a pentose sugar. Production can be increased by stimuli such as hypoxia and ischemia. This ubiquitous nucleoside has potent electrophysiologic effects in addition to having a major role in regulation of vasomotor tone. Adenosine is believed to have a cardioprotective effect by regulating oxygen supply and demand. The cardiovascular effects of adenosine depend on which of two receptor sites is activated, α-1 or α-2. The α-1 receptors in the myocardial conduction system are the most sensitive and mediate SA node slowing and AV nodal conduction delay. The α-1 receptor inhibits production of cAMP whose formation is stimulated by β-adrenergic activity (see Table 12-7). The α-2 smooth muscle receptors require higher concentrations of adenosine, which mediate systemic and coronary vasodilatation. The α-2 receptor directly increases the rate of formation of cAMP (see Table 12-7) and functions independently of β activity. Intravenous adenosine, therefore, has significant negative chronotropic effects on the SA node as well as negative dromotropism on the AV node. Thus, adenosine regulates atrial and ventricular rates independently of each other.

Adenosine hyperpolarizes atrial myocytes and decreases their action potential duration via an increase in outward K+ current. These are the acetylcholine-regulated K+ channels. Adenosine mimics the effects of acetylcholine in many ways, including an extremely short plasma half-life of mere seconds. Adenosine also antagonizes the inward Ca2+ current produced by catecholamines. This antidysrhythmic mechanism of Ca2+ channel blockade is thought to be an indirect effect and important only when β stimulation is present. This trait suggests a possible role in countering catecholamine-induced dysrhythmia. Thus, adenosine exhibits some of the traits of a Class IV antidysrhythmic. However, the primary antidysrhythmic effect of adenosine is to interrupt reentrant AV nodal tachycardia, which most likely relates to its K+ current, rather than Ca2+ current effects.

The chief indication for adenosine is paroxysmal supraventricular tachycardia (PSVT), which it may terminate in a matter of seconds. PSVT refers to a broad category of narrow complex tachycardias with acute onset and cessation. The most common forms are AV nodal reentry tachycardia and AV reciprocating tachycardia. PSVT accounts for about one-third of all cases of perioperative dysrhythmia. Clinical studies support the use of adenosine for the treatment of Wolff-Parkinson-White (W-P-W) syndrome and other reentrant tachycardias involving the AV node.[127] The same characteristics that make adenosine an effective therapeutic agent may also make it an ideal agent for diagnosing other types of dysrhythmia. The incidence of incorrect diagnosis of supraventricular dysrhythmia has been reported to be as high as 15% using conventional means.[128] This can lead to utilization of harmful medications. For example, a broad complex tachycardia can either be a VT or an SVT with aberrant conduction. Verapamil can be fatal if the dysrhythmia is VT because the drug is long lasting.[129] However, the fleeting action (9 to 10 seconds) of adenosine assures that no harm will be done if the broad complex is of ventricular origin providing a combined therapeutic and diagnostic test. Adenosine will stop SVT in 90% of cases in which the AV node forms one of the limbs of the reentrant circuit such as AV reciprocating tachycardia and AV nodal reentry; 60% will convert with the first dose. However, adenosine has no effect on ectopic atrial dysrhythmia such as ectopic foci, multifocal SVT, or flutter/fibrillation. Approximately 10% of SVT do not involve AV nodal reentry. Adenosine will nevertheless slow AV nodal conduction in these cases, decrease the ventricular rate, and allow inspection of P waves. Thus, adenosine may be useful in unmasking atrial fibrillation when fast ventricular responses are noted.

A number of side effects have been reported with the use of adenosine, including flushing, headache, dyspnea, bronchospasm, and chest pain. The majority of these are brief (seconds) and not clinically significant. Transient new dysrhythmia (65%) will be noted at the time of cardioversion, but these disappear during the half-life of the drug. Major hemodynamic changes are rare but consist of hypotension and bradycardia. Adenosine should be given by means of a rapid iv bolus with flush because of its extremely short half-life of less than 10 seconds. The initial adult dose is 6 mg (100 to 150 mg/kg pediatrics), which can be followed by 12 mg within 1 to 2 minutes if the initial dose is without effect.[128] The 12-mg dose may be repeated once. The antidysrhythmic effects of adenosine occurs as soon as the drug reaches the AV node.

Phosphodiesterase Inhibitors. Phosphodiesterase inhibitors have pharmacologic properties approaching the characteristics of the ideal inotropic agent (see Table 12-17).[130,131] They do not rely on stimulation of β and/or α receptors. They are the product of a search for a nonglycosidic, noncatecholamine inotropic agent. These drugs combine positive inotropism with vasodilator activity. They selectively inhibit PDE III.[132,133] PDE I and II hydrolyze all cyclic nucleotides, whereas PDE III acts specifically on cAMP. The PDE III inhibitors apparently interact with PDE III at the cell membrane and impede the breakdown of cAMP.[132,134] cAMP levels increase and protein kinase are activated to promote phosphorylation of the SR in a cascade manner similar to the effects of adrenergic drugs. In cardiac muscle, phosphorylation increases the slow inward movement of calcium current, promoting increased intracellular calcium stores. Thus, inotropism increases. In vascular smooth muscle, increased cAMP activity accounts for the vasodilation, decreased peripheral vascular resistance, and lusitropism. Amrinone, like nitroprusside and nitroglycerin, promotes diastolic relaxation, which promotes ventricular filling.[135]

A variety of intravenous PDE inhibitors are undergoing clinical trials. The relative contribution of inotropism and vasodilation differs with each. Amrinone and milrinone are the only PDE inhibitors released for clinical use in the United States. Amrinone is the prototypical PDE III inhibitor. The degree of hemodynamic effect of these drugs depends on the dose, degree of inotropic reserve, and state of cAMP depletion.

Amrinone. Amrinone produces mild inotropic activity and strong vasodilatory effects. The characteristics of amrinone, compared with those of the ideal inotropic agent (see Table 12-12), rank it near the ideal drug. It is the first oral inotrope available since the introduction of digitalis. However, it is not currently prescribed in its oral form. Studies of single-dose and short-term oral and iv amrinone show dose-related improvements at rest in the cardiac index and the left ventricular stroke index (40 to 80% increase); left ventricular end-diastolic pressure (40% decrease); pulmonary capillary wedge pressure (16 to 44% decrease); pulmonary artery pressure (17 to 33% decrease); right atrial pressure (16 to 44% decrease); left ventricular ejection fraction (50% increase); and systemic vascular resistance (23 to 50% decrease). Significantly, HR and mean arterial pressure are not affected.

Peak response with an iv dose occurs after 5 minutes and reveals no evidence of tolerance over short-term trials (24 hours); it is compatible with other adrenergic agonists. It is an effective inotropic agent in patients receiving β-blockers. Its efficacy in the patient who has been digitalized has been demonstrated.

Intravenous amrinone therapy should be initiated with a 0.75-mg/kg bolus given over 2 to 3 minutes. It is continued with a maintenance infusion of 5 to 10 mg/kg/min, adjusted by hemodynamic monitoring. An additional bolus dose of 0.75 mg/kg may be given 30 minutes after initiation of therapy. Care must be taken not to give the bolus too quickly because sudden decreases in peripheral vascular resistance may occur and result in severe hypotension. Hypotension is not a major clinical problem with appropriate monitoring of ventricular filling pressures. The infusion should not exceed a total daily dose of 10 mg/kg, including the bolus doses. Amrinone has the same range of infusion rates as dopamine and DBT, and dose calculation follows the "rule of six" described in Table 12-14.

Amrinone has two uncommon side effects. Dose-related thrombocytopenia occurs in some patients taking long-term oral medication. This usually responds to dose reduction. Acute iv amrinone has not produced thrombocytopenia.[136] Centrilobular hepatic necrosis occurs in dogs given high doses of amrinone for periods exceeding 3 months. There is no evidence of such an effect in humans.

Milrinone. Milrinone is a derivative of amrinone. It has nearly 20 times the inotropic potency of the parent compound. Milrinone is active both intravenously and orally and has beneficial short-term hemodynamic effects in patients with severe refractory congestive heart failure.[137] Improvement of CO appears to result from a combination of enhanced myocardial contractility and peripheral vasodilation. Treatment with oral milrinone for up to 11 months has been effective and well tolerated without evidence of fever, thrombocytopenia, or gastrointestinal effects.[138] Milrinone recently has been approved for short-term iv therapy of congestive heart failure.[139] It is administered with a loading dose of 50 mg/kg over 10 minutes. The maintenance iv infusion rate ranges from a minimum of 0.375 mg/kg/min to a maximum of 0.75 mg/kg/min (not to exceed 1.13 mg/kg/day). Dosage must be adjusted in renal failure patients as milrinone is excreted in the urine primarily in unconjugated form.

Enoximone. Enoximone is a PDE III inhibitor that has proven beneficial in patients suffering from severely impaired myocardial function.[140] Enoximone is structurally unrelated to digitalis, catecholamines, or amrinone. It has not been implicated in platelet compromise. Its hemodynamic effects are similar to those produced by amrinone. It appears to be a more potent inotropic agent than amrinone, whose inotropic effect has been questioned. It produces pulmonary and systemic arteriolar vasodilation and can thus be classified as an inodilator. Any increase in myocardial oxygen consumption (MVO_2) by the increase in inotropism is countered by a decrease in afterload and reduced ventricular size. The drug has been administered by both the bolus technique and infusion. It has been used primarily in patients with cardiogenic shock and for weaning from cardiopulmonary bypass. Its use was instituted in patients who were proven refractory to catecholamine therapy. A definitive dosing therapy has not been established but several studies have given a 1- to 2-mg/kg bolus followed by an infusion of 3 to 10 μg/kg/min. In all cases CI and SV increased with a decrease in ventricular filling pressure, and PVR. No increase in heart rate was noted. The bolus technique alone has been helpful in weaning patients from cardiopulmonary bypass without affecting heart rate or producing arrhythmias.

Glucagon. Glucagon is a single-chain polypeptide of 29 amino acids that is secreted by pancreas a cells in response to hypoglycemia. The liver and kidney are responsible for its degradation. Known effects of this hormone in humans include the following:[82,141] (1) inhibition of gastric motility, (2) enhanced urinary excretion of inorganic electrolytes, (3) increased insulin secretion, (4) hepatic glycogenolysis and gluconeogenesis, (5) anorexia, (6) inotropic and chronotropic cardiac effects, and (7) relaxation of smooth muscle (biliary, i.e., sphincters).

Little attention was given to glucagon until 1968, when it was demonstrated to produce positive inotropic and chronotropic effects in the canine heart. Glucagon enhances the activation of adenyl cyclase in a manner similar to that of NE, EPI, and isoproterenol. These cardiac actions of glucagon are not blocked by β-blockade or catecholamine depletion. Glucagon, in contrast to the xanthines, rarely causes dysrhythmia, even in the face of ischemic heart disease, hypokalemia, and digitalis toxicity. Glucagon may possess antidysrhythmic activity in digitalis toxicity because it has been shown to enhance AV nodal conduction in patients with varying degrees of AV block. Thus, it should be used carefully in patients with atrial fibrillation. An iv dose of 1 to 5 mg of glucagon increases cardiac index, mean arterial pressure, and ventricular contractility, even in the presence of digitalis therapy. After a bolus dose, its action dissipates in approximately 30 minutes. A continuous infusion of 5 μg/kg/min is augmented by an initial bolus of 50 μg/kg. Onset of action occurs in 1 to 3 minutes and peaks at 10 to 15 minutes.

Nausea and vomiting are common side effects in the awake patient, especially following a bolus dose. Hypokalemia, hypoglycemia, and hyperglycemia are also seen. Glucagon is also useful in treating insulin-induced hypoglycemia. Despite the obvious benefits of glucagon in cardiac patients, its use has not become popular. This may be related to its high cost and the multiple metabolic and physiologic effects that are common after its administration. This pancreatic hormone may be of hemodynamic benefit when more conventional approaches have proved refractory in the following settings: (1) low CO syndrome following cardiopulmonary bypass, (2) low CO syndrome with myocardial infarction, (3) chronic congestive heart failure, and (4) excessive β-adrenergic blockade.

Digitalis Glycosides. The most important actions of the digitalis glycosides are those affecting myocardial contractility, conduction, and rhythm. The glycoside most likely to be used by the anesthesiologist is digoxin. The principal uses of digoxin are for the treatment of congestive heart failure and to control supraventricular cardiac dysrhythmia such as atrial fibrillation. Digoxin is one of the few positive inotropes that does not increase HR. Digoxin enhances myocardial inotropism and automaticity but slows impulse propagation through the conduction tissues.[142] Despite nearly two centuries of use, its mechanism of action is only modestly certain. Digitalis reciprocally facilitates calcium entry into the myocardial cell by blocking the Na+, K+ adenosine triphosphatase pump. This calcium influx may account for its positive inotropic action because this inotropic response is not catecholamine- or β-receptor-dependent and is therefore effective in patients taking β-blocking drugs. The inhibition of this enzyme transport mechanism also results in a net K+ loss from the myocardial cell. This contributes to digitalis toxicity with hypokalemia. Calcium potentiates the toxic effects of digitalis. Extreme caution should be observed when calcium is given to a patient taking digitalis or when digitalis administration is contemplated in the patient with hypercalcemia.

Synchrony of the cardiac beat is an important determinant of CO, and digoxin can be beneficial when heart failure is caused by a tachydysrhythmia, even in ischemic myocardial disease. However, the use of β- or calcium channel blockers is increasing in this regard because they both reduce overall myocardial oxygen consumption.

Digitalis has been of no benefit in cardiogenic shock and has proved potentially injurious in patients with uncomplicated myocardial infarction because of its vasoconstrictive properties and effects on myocardial oxygen consumption in the absence of cardiomegaly.

Care must be taken to rule out conditions in which the use of digitalis is of no benefit and is potentially harmful. These include mitral stenosis with normal sinus rhythm and constrictive pericarditis with tamponade. Signs and symptoms of idiopathic hypertrophic subaortic stenosis are often exacerbated by digitalis. With increased strength of contraction, the muscular obstruction can be markedly increased. The same is true for the use of digitalis in patients with infundibular pulmonic stenosis, as occurs with tetralogy of Fallot. Any augmentation of contractility may further reduce an already diminished pulmonary blood flow. Beware of digitalis toxic reactions in the older age group and in patients suffering from arterial hypoxemia, acidosis, renal compromise, hypothyroidism, hypokalemia, or hypomagnesemia as well as in patients receiving quinidine or calcium channel blockers.

The issue of prophylactic digitalization of patients with diminished cardiac reserve who are about to undergo major surgical procedures remains controversial.[142] Indications for preoperative digitalis in which the prophylactic administration of digoxin should be considered include the following: (1) previous heart failure, (2) increased heart size, (3) coronary flow disturbances according to electrocardiogram, (4) age over 60 years, (5) age over 50 years before lung surgery, (6) anticipated massive blood loss, (7) atrial flutter or fibrillation, (8) cardiovascular surgery, and (9) rheumatic valvular lesions.

When entertaining the possibility of perioperative digitalis administration, the following points must be considered. (1) Myocardial oxygen balance is threatened in the nonfailing, nondilated heart. (2) The therapeutic-to-toxic ratio of digitalis is narrow. (3) Inotropic drugs that are less toxic and reversible are readily available. (4) Verapamil or β-blockers are more efficacious for supraventricular tachydysrhythmias not initiated by heart failure. (5) Digitalis may cause serious dysrhythmia in the unstable patient. (6) Serum potassium concentrations may fluctuate in the surgical patient. (7) Any cardiac dysrhythmia that occurs in the presence of digitalis must be considered a toxic phenomenon. (8) Digitalis-induced cardiac dysrhythmias are difficult to treat. (9) Renal compromise will result in toxic effects with standard maintenance doses. (10) Cardioversion may be dangerous after digitalis administration. (11) After initiation of digitalis therapy, the administration of alternative drugs becomes more complicated.

Calcium Salts. Calcium is of great importance in the genesis of the cardiac action potential and is the key to controlling intracellular energy storage and utilization. Movement of extracellular calcium across membranes also governs the function of uterine smooth muscle as well as the smooth muscle of the blood vessels. The sympathomimetic drugs promote the transmembrane influx of calcium, whereas the β-blockers and calcium channel blockers inhibit such movement.

The American Heart Association has recommended against the use of calcium during cardiac arrest except when hyperkalemia, hypocalcemia, or calcium-entry inhibitor toxicity is present.[143]

Traditionally, calcium gluconate has been preferred in pediatric patients and calcium chloride in adult patients. Previous data held that calcium chloride produced consistently higher and more predictable levels of ionized calcium.[144] Studies have shown, however, that ionization of any of the preparations is immediate and equally effective.[145] Intravenous calcium appears effective for the transient reversal of hypotension thought to be the result of myocardial depression from the potent volatile anesthetic drugs.[146] Some clinicians feel that recurrent intraoperative hypotension response to calcium chloride may be an indication for the administration of digoxin. Calcium chloride is also given at the termination of cardiopulmonary bypass to offset the myocardial depression associated with hypothermic potassium cardioplegia and citrate. The use of calcium salts is clearly indicated during rapid or massive transfusions of citrated blood.[147] Citrate binds calcium, and rapid infusion rates of citrated blood result in myocardial depression that is reversible by calcium.

Three forms of calcium salts are available: calcium chloride, calcium gluconate, and calcium gluceptate. Calcium chloride produces only transient (10 to 20 minutes) increases in CO.[142] If inotropic effects are needed for a longer period of time, other inotropic agents should be selected. Bolus doses of 2 to 10 mg/kg (1.5 mg/kg/min) of calcium chloride can produce moderate improvement in contractility. The rapid administration of calcium salts, if the heart is beating, can produce bradycardia and must be used cautiously in the patient who is digitalized because of the hazard of producing toxic effects. Calcium gluceptate can be given in a dose of 5 to 7 mL (4.5 to 6.3 mEq) and calcium gluconate in a dose of 10 to 15 mL (4.8 to 7.2 mEq). These doses are approximately equivalent to that suggested for calcium chloride. Calcium gluconate is unstable and is no longer in frequent use. All of the calcium salts will precipitate as calcium carbonate if mixed with sodium bicarbonate.

Antidepressant Drugs

3 **Monoamine Oxidase Inhibitors.** Monoamine oxidase inhibitors (MAOIs) and the tricyclic antidepressants are used to treat psychotic depression. These drugs are not used in the practice of anesthesia but are a source of potentially serious anesthetics interactions in patients who are taking them chronically. Their use is rapidly declining as the nontricyclic antidepressants such as Prozac are more efficacious and produce fewer side effects. Table 12-19 lists the antidepressants that have been in use and is offered only to be historically complete. Few of the MAO inhibitors or tricyclic antidepressants will be encountered in an anesthesia practice today with the exceptions of phenelzine (Nardil) and amitriptyline (Amitril, Elavil). Their pharmacologic actions and side effects are a direct result of their effect on the cascade of catacholamine metabolism. The nontricyclics also produce their antidepressant effects via this cascade but linked to their inhibition of CNS neuronal uptake of serotonin.

TABLE 12-19

ANTIDEPRESSANT DRUGS

NONPROPRIETARY NAME	TRADE NAME
Monamine Oxidase Inhibitors	
Isocarboxazid	Marplan
Pargyline	Eutonyl
Phenelzine	Nardil
Tranylcypromine	Parnate
Tricyclic Antidepressants	
Imipramine	Imavate, Janimine, Presamine, SK-Pramine, Tofranil
Desipramine	Norpramin, Pertofrane
Amitriptyline	Amitril, Elavil, Endep
Nortriptyline	Aventyl, Pamelor
Doxepin	Adapin, Sinequan
Protriptyline	Vivactil
Amoxapine	Asendin
Maprotiline	Ludiomil
Nontricyclics	
Trazodone	Desyrel
Fluoxetine	Prozac
Buproprion	Wellbutrin

MAOIs (see Table 12-19) block the oxidative deamination of endogenous catecholamines into inactive vanillylmandelic acid (see Fig. 12-12). They do not inhibit synthesis. Thus, blockade of monoamine oxidase would produce an accumulation of NE, EPI, dopamine, and 5-hydroxytryptamine in adrenergically active tissues, including the brain. Alleviation of depression may be related to elevations of the endogenous catecholamines. Overdose with MAOIs is expressed as SNS hyperactivity. They may produce agitation, hallucinations, hyperpyrexia, convulsions, hypertension, and hypotension. Orthostatic hypotension is a common complaint in patients taking MAOIs.[148]

The action of sympathomimetic amines is potentiated in patients taking MAOIs. Indirect-acting sympathomimetics (ephedrine, tyramine) produce an exaggerated response as they trigger the release of accumulated catecholamines. Foods containing a high tyramine content such as cheese, red Italian wine, and pickled herring can also precipitate hypertensive crises.[148] SNS reflex stimulation is also intensified by tyramine. Meperidine has also been reported to produce hypertensive crisis, convulsions, and coma with MAO inhibitors. Hepatotoxicity has been reported that does not seem to be related to dosage or duration of treatment. Its incidence is low but remains a factor in selecting anesthesia.

The anesthetic management of patients taking MAOIs remains controversial, although the need to discontinue them preoperatively is in question. Currently, recommendations for management include discontinuation of the drugs for at least 2 weeks before surgery; however, this recommendation is not based on controlled studies but rather is the result of limited case reports that suggest potent drug interactions.[149] Few adverse effects in humans taking MAOIs given analgesics, opioid anesthesia, or regional blocks have been reported.

However, opioids that cause release of catecholamines (meperidine) should be avoided in these patients. Symptoms of SNS overdose or interactions because of MAOIs can be treated effectively with α- and β-blockers or direct-acting vasodilators.

Tricyclic Antidepressants. This group of antidepressant drugs is referred to as tricyclic antidepressants because of their structure. The important tricyclic antidepressants are listed in Table 12-19. These drugs have almost replaced the MAOIs because of fewer side effects. All of these agents block uptake of NE into adrenergic nerve endings. Just as with the MAOIs, high doses of the tricyclic antidepressants can induce seizure activity that is responsive to diazepam.

Neuroleptic drugs may potentiate the effects of tricyclic antidepressants by competition with metabolism in the liver. Chronic barbiturate use increases metabolism of the tricyclic antidepressants by microsomal enzyme induction. Other sedatives, however, potentiate the tricyclic antidepressants in a manner similar to that occurring with the MAOIs. Atropine also has an exaggerated effect because of the anticholinergic effect of tricyclic antidepressants. Prolonged sedation from thiopental has been reported. Ketamine may also be dangerous in patients taking tricyclic antidepressants by producing acute hypertension and cardiac dysrhythmia.

Despite these serious interactions, discontinuation of these drugs before surgery is probably not necessary. The latency of onset of these drugs is from 2 to 5 weeks; however, the excretion of tricyclic antidepressants is rapid, with approximately 70% of a dose appearing in the urine during the first 72 hours. One might consider a discontinuation of the drug for 72 hours, but the risk of recurrent depression may be greater than that of any untoward drug reaction. The long latency period for resumption of treatment militates against interrupted treatment. A thorough knowledge of the possible drug interactions and autonomic countermeasures now available obviates postponement.

Nontricyclic Antidepressants. The nontricyclic antidepressants are listed in Table 12-19. Their mechanism of action is not fully known but all have in common selective inhibition of neuronal uptake of serotonin. This potentates the behavioral changes induced by the serotonin precursor, 5-hydroxytryptophan.[150] The availability of sympathetic antagonists for possible side effects during anesthesia weighs in favor of continuation of therapy versus the risk of exacerbation of a severe depression.[151]

Prozac (fluoxetine) is a popular oral nontricyclic antidepressant. Unlike desyrel, the elimination half-life of prozac is 1 to 3 days and can lead to significant accumulation of the drug. Prozac's metabolism, like that of other compounds including tricyclic antidepressants, phenobarbital, ethanol, and pentothal, involves the P450IID6 system; concomitant therapy with drugs also metabolized by this enzyme system may lead to drug interactions and prolongation of effect of the benzodiazepines.

Wellbutrin® and Zyban® are the same drug, namely buproprion hydrochloride. Zyban, however, is a sustained-release drug. Wellbutrin® is used as an antidepressant whereas Zyban® is marketed as a nonnicotine aid to smoking cessation. These drugs should not be used concomitantly. Overdose is possible with resultant seizures. Seizure activity is dose related. The neurochemical mechanism of the antidepressant effect of buproprion is not known. It does not inhibit monoamine oxidase and is a weak blocker of the neuronal uptake of serotonin and norepinephrine. It also inhibits the neuronal uptake of dopamine to some extent. No systematic data have been collected on the interactions of buproprion and other drugs. The mechanism by which Zyban® enhances the ability to abstain from smoking is unknown but perhaps it assists the patient through the mental vicissitudes of nicotine withdrawal. High doses higher than 300 mg can result in seizures.[152]

TABLE 12-20

α-ADRENERGIC BLOCKING DRUGS

	TYPE OF ANTAGONISM	SELECTIVITY
Phenoxybenzamine	Noncompetitive	$\alpha_1 > \alpha_2$
Phentolamine	Competitive	$\alpha_1 = \alpha_2$
Tolazoline	Competitive	$\alpha_1 = \alpha_2$
Prazosin	Competitive	$\alpha_1 \gg \alpha_2$
Yohimbine	Competitive	$\alpha_2 \gg \alpha_1$

Adrenergic Antagonists—Sympatholytics

α Antagonists. Drugs that bind selectively to α-adrenergic receptors block the action of endogenous catecholamines or moderate the effects of exogenous adrenergics. The resultant effects may be ascribed together the blockade effect to α-adrenergic agonists or to unopposed β-adrenergic receptor activity. The effect is smooth muscle relaxation. The response to the vasculature may vary over a wide range in a single vascular bed depending on its intrinsic state of constriction. Vessels with higher initial tone have a greater response to α-blockade. Prominent clinical effects of α-blockers include hypotension, orthostatic hypotension, tachycardia and miosis; nasal stuffiness, diarrhea, and inhibition of ejaculation are common side effects.

The α-blockers may be classified according to binding characteristics (Table 12-20). Phenoxybenzmine is an oral α-blocker that produces an irreversible blockade. It is a relatively nonselective α-blocker. Phentolamine, tolazoline, and prazosin are characterized by reversible binding and antagonism.

Phentolamine is 100 times more potent on α-1 receptors than on α-2 receptors. Prazosin is also markedly specific for α-1 receptors, whereas phentolamine has nearly equal blocking activity on both subsets. Phentolamine, by blocking presynaptic inhibitory α-2 receptors, causes greater NE release from the presynaptic terminal.

There are many α-blockers in use today for benign prostatic hypertrophy as well as essential hypertension. When patients are taking these drugs chronically, one should keep in mind that the normal autonomic response to stress, inhalation anesthetics, or extensive regional anesthesia may be blunted. Elevations of catecholamines will not reflexly increase peripheral vascular resistance and may actually decrease if vascular β receptors are unopposed. The effects are similar to the acute sympatholysis seen with spinal or epidural anesthesia. α-blockers are often used in combination with diuretics and other antihypertensives. Volume depletion may not be evident on preoperative examination but unmasked with the induction of anesthesia and the onset of a marked hypotension. This hypotension is usually responsive to volume repletion and the temporary use of a direct acting α-agonist such as neosynephrine. There is no cause for discontinuation of these drugs before surgery but preloading with iv fluids is suggested to ensure adequate central volume.

Phentolamine. Phentolamine is used almost exclusively in the diagnosis and treatment of pheochromocytoma. It is a competitive antagonist at α-1 and α-2 receptors. Phentolamine may also have some antihistaminic and cholinomimetic activity. The cholinomimetic activity may result in abdominal cramping and diarrhea, both of which are blocked by atropine. Tachycardia and hypotension are also common side effects.

Intravenously, phentolamine produces peripheral vasodilatation and a decrease in systemic blood pressure within 2 minutes lasting from 10 to 15 minutes. Blood pressure reduction elicits baroreceptor reflexes and NE release, the result of which is an increased heart rate and cardiac output. Cardiac arrhythmias and angina pectoris may accompany phentolamine administration. It can be given in does of 30 to 70 μg/kg iv to produce a transient decrease in blood pressure. It can also be used as a continuous infusion to maintain blood pressure during resection of a pheochromocytoma.

Phenoxybenzamine (Dibenzyline). Phenoxybenzamine acts as a nonselective α-adrenergic antagonist. α-blockade is 100 times more potent on postsynaptic α-1 receptors than at α-2 receptors. The onset of α-blockade is slow, taking up to 60 minutes to reach peak effect even with iv administration. This is related to the time required for structural modification of the phenoxybenzamine molecule to become active. The elimination half-life is about 24 hours.

Orthostatic hypotension is prominent especially in the presence of preexisting hypertension or hypovolemia. Cardiac output is often increased and renal blood flow is not greatly altered except in preexisting renal vasoconstriction or stenosis. Coronary and cerebral vascular resistance is not changed. In the past it was the drug of choice for treating patients with pheochromocytoma in preparation for surgery. It has been replaced with shorter acting, more specific drugs such as phentolamine.

Prazocin (Minipres). Prazocin is relatively selective for α-1 receptors that leaves the inhibiting effect of α-2 receptor activity on norepinephrine release intact. As a result, it is less likely that nonselective α-antagonists evoke reflex tachycardia. Prazocin dilates both arterioles and veins.

Cardiovascular effects include total body reductions in systemic vascular resistance and venous return. When combined with a diuretic, it is an effective antihypertensive drug. It should not be used with clonidine or α-methylodopa as it appears to decrease their effectiveness. Prazosin may also cause bronchodilation.

Several new oral α-1-blockers are now on the market that have been found useful for benign prostatic hypertrophy (BPH) and hypertension. The anesthesiologist may commonly encounter patients taking these medications on a chronic basis and must be aware of their possible interactions with anesthetics. Doxazosin is a long-acting selective α-1-blocker used for both in treating benign prostatic hypertrophy and hypertension. The most common side effect, as with all α-blockers, is orthostatic hypotension and dizziness. Tamsulosin (flomax) is another α-blocker that is used for BPH. It is not indicated for hypertension but it is capable of producing orthostatic hypotension.

β Antagonists. β-adrenergic-blockers were introduced in the 1960s. Cardiovascular pharmacology has been dominated by the age of these sympatholytic agents that ushered out the age of the pressor. As more indications for their use have been found, more compounds have been developed. They are among the most common drugs used in the treatment of cardiac disease and hypertension. At present, there are β-blocking agents available for oral or intravenous use in the United States. A variety of drugs are available with β-blocking activity that may be distinguished by differing pharmacokinetic and pharmacodynamic properties.Examples of some of the drugs available and their diversity of actions are listed in Table 12-21.

β-blockers can be classified according to whether they are selective or nonselective on the β-1 or β-2 receptor and whether they possess intrinsic sympathomimetric activity (ISA). For example, a β-blocker with selective properties for the β-1 receptor would bind to the cardiac receptors, whereas a nonselective β-blocker would bind to both β-1 (cardiac) and β-2 (vascular, bronchial smooth muscle, and metabolic) receptors. Their biological potency and affinity for β receptor subtypes is determined by their ability to inhibit tachycardia and vasodilatation induced by isoproterenol, a pure nonselective β agonist. Nonselective β antagonists are referred to as first-generation β-blockers. These include propranolol, nadolol, sotalol, and timolol. Second-generation drugs are those considered selective for β-1 adrenergic blockade. These include atenolol, esmolol, and metoprolol.

Those β-blockers possessing ISA exert the partial effect of a partial β agonist while blocking β receptors by more potent β agonists. ISA might be advantageous in patients needing β-blockers but who are troubled by bradycardia or worsening ventricular failure.[153]A distinct advantage to ISA in β-blockers has not been shown in clinical studies.

Over the past decade, and because of their selectivity, the use of β-blockers has expanded to include the treatment of congestive heart failure (CHF).[154] CHF was once a contraindication for the use of β-blockers. This is the result of better understanding of the fluid nature of up- and downregulation of β receptor density once thought to be static.

Selective β-blockade could be of greater benefit in treatment of patients with obstructive airway disease, diabetes, or peripheral vascular disease.However, it must be emphasized that specificity is a relative term and not absolute. Nonselective blocking effects may be seen in all tissues if higher blood levels are reached with "selective" drugs (see Fig. 12-13). For example, the use of β-1 selective blockers in patients with obstructive or reactive airway disease remains controversial. Patients with reactive airway disease may develop serious reductions in ventilatory function even with β-1 selective antagonists.[155] Other drugs are available for treatment of supraventricular arrhythmias and hypertension in asthmatics.

Sympathetic activation generally results in increased circulating glucose levels secondary to enhanced glycogenolysis, lipolysis, and gluconeogensis. Administration of β-2-blockers to insulin-dependent diabetics reduces their ability to recover from hypoglycemic episodes.[156] β-2 antagonists are preferable.

β-blocker therapy should be continued until and after the time of surgery. This issue is no longer controversial for several reasons. Acute withdrawal of β antagonists may produce a hemodynamic withdrawal syndrome similar to thyrotoxicosis.[58] Control of HR and blood pressure perioperatively is easier if chronic medications are continued for the co-morbid factors for which they were prescribed. HR is a major determinant of myocardial oxygen demands. Tachycardia is known to increase the risk of poor outcome in patients with ischemic heart disease,[157] therefore hemodynamic control of HR and BP (work) is important in reducing perioperative risk. In a complete turnabout from a decade ago, several well-founded studies have shown the benefits of prophylactic β-blockade with atenolol in patients at risk for ischemic cardiac disease.[158] The reduction in perioperative morbidity and mortality in these groups of patients was significant.

Several of the β-blockers listed in Table 12-21 also have a local anesthetic-like effect on myocardial membranes at high doses. This effect is similar to that of quinidine in that phase 0 of the cardiac action potential is depressed, slowing conduction. This membrane-stabilizing activity is caused by the D-isomer, whereas the L-isomer is responsible for β-blocking activity. The clinical significance of membrane-stabilizing activity is unclear.

Propranolol. Propranolol is the prototype β-blocking drug against which all others are compared. It is nonselective and has no intrinsic sympathomimetic activity but does have membrane-stabilizing activity at higher doses. It is available in both iv and oral forms. It is highly lipophilic and is metabolized by the liver to more water-soluble metabolites, one of which, 17-OH propranolol, has weak β-blocking activity. There is a significant first-pass effect by the liver after oral administration of the drug. It is highly protein bound, and the free drug level may be altered by other highly bound drugs. The elimination half-life is approximately 4 hours, but the pharmacologic half-life is around 10 hours.

TABLE 12-21

β-ADRENERGIC BLOCKING DRUGS

DRUG	TRADE NAME	RELATIVE β_1 SELECTIVITY	MEMBRANE-STABILIZING ACTIVITY	INTRINSIC SYMPATHOMIMETIC ACTIVITY	PLASMA HALF-LIFE (hr)	ORAL AVAILABILITY (%)	LIPID SOLUBILITY	ELIMINATION	PREPARATIONS
Propranolol	Inderal	0	+	0	3–4	36	+++	Hepatic	Oral, iv
Nadolol	Cogard	0	0	0	14–24	34	0	Renal	Oral
Timolol	Blocadren	0	0	0	4–5	50	+	Hepatic and renal	Oral, eye drops
Pindolol	Visken	0	+	++	3–4	86	+	Hepatic and renal	Oral
Esmolol	Brevibloc	++	0	0	0–16	—	?	RBC esterase	iv
Acebutolol	Sectral	+	+	+	3–4	37[a]	0	Hepatic[a]	Oral
Atenolol	Tenormin	++	0	0	6–9	57	0	Renal	Oral
Metoprolol	Lopressor	++	0	0	3–4	38	+	Hepatic	Oral
Betaxolol	Kerlone	+++	+	0	14–22	89	0	Hepatic[a]	Oral
Penbutolol	Levatol	0	0	+	5	85	0	Hepatic[a]	Oral
Carteolol	Cartrol	0	0	+	6	85	0	Renal	Oral

[a]Primarily hepatic, but active metabolites are formed that must be renally excreted.

4 Hemodynamic effects include decreased HR and contractility. The major factors contributing to the decrease in blood pressure by propranolol are decreased CO and renin release. Systemic vascular resistance may increase on acute administration owing to blockade of β-2 receptors in the peripheral vasculature. With chronic administration, however, peripheral vascular resistance decreases. This is thought to be secondary to decreased renin release and, possibly, decreased central SNS outflow. Complications with the use of propranolol include bradycardia, heart block, worsening of congestive heart failure, bronchospasm, and sedation. During anesthesia with halothane, it may cause severe bradydysrhythmias.

Nadolol. Nadolol is a noncardioselective β-blocker with no membrane-stabilizing activity or intrinsic sympathomimetic activity. It is approximately equipotent to propranolol, but its effects are prolonged owing to slower elimination. It is relatively lipid insoluble and is excreted 70% unchanged in urine and 20% in the feces. The elimination half-life is 24 hours. Because it is lipid insoluble, it does not cross the blood-brain barrier, and sedation is less of a problem than with propranolol. Hemodynamic effects are the same as for propranolol. The main advantage of the drug is the capability for once per day dosing.

Timolol. Timolol is also noncardioselective with little intrinsic sympathomimetic activity and no membrane-stabilizing activity. It is the only β-blocker used as the l-isomer rather than the racemic mixture. It is 5 to 10 times as potent as propranolol. Hepatic metabolism accounts for approximately 66% of its elimination, and another 20% is found unchanged in the urine. The elimination half-life is 5.6 hours, and the pharmacologic half-life is approximately 15 hours. It was first used topically for treatment of glaucoma but is now used in hypertension and has been shown to decrease the risk of reinfarction and death following myocardial infarction.[159] Its hemodynamic effects and side effects are similar to those of other β-blockers. The anesthesiologist should also be aware that timolol eye drops may be absorbed systemically and cause bradycardia and hypotension that are refractory to treatment with atropine.[160]

Pindolol. Pindolol is a nonselective β-blocker with membrane-stabilizing activity and intrinsic sympathomimetic activity. It is 10 to 40 times as potent as propranolol. It is lipid soluble and metabolized by the liver but not as avidly extracted; therefore, its biologic availability after oral administration is more predictable. It is excreted 40% unchanged in the urine. The elimination half-life is 3.5 hours. It is useful in the treatment of angina pectoris, cardiac dysrhythmia, and hypertension. As discussed earlier, the clinical usefulness of the intrinsic sympathomimetic activity property is unclear.

Oxprenolol. Oxprenolol is similar to pindolol except for less intrinsic sympathomimetic activity and lower potency.

Metoprolol. Metoprolol is a relatively selective β-blocking drug with β-blocking effects at moderate and high doses. It has neither intrinsic sympathomimetic activity nor membrane-stabilizing activity. It has a possible advantage in patients with reactive airway disease at oral doses up to 100 mg/day^{-1}. In this case, it should probably be used with a β-2 mimetic drug. It is mostly metabolized in the liver, with only about 5% excreted unchanged in the urine. The elimination half-life is 3.5 hours. It has recently become available in iv as well as oral form; therefore, it may be useful during anesthesia.

Atenolol. Atenolol is similar to metoprolol in that it is relatively cardioselective and has no intrinsic sympathomimetic activity or membrane-stabilizing activity. It is less lipophilic, however, and is eliminated primarily by renal excretion. The elimination half-life is 6 to 7 hours. The lack of first-pass metabolism results in more predictable blood levels after oral dosing.

Acebutolol. Acebutolol is a cardioselective β-blocker with intrinsic sympathomimetic activity and membrane-stabilizing activity. It is metabolized in the liver and is subject to extensive first-pass metabolism. The primary metabolite is diacetolol, which has a pharmacologic profile similar to that of the parent drug and is excreted renally. The pharmacologic effects of the drug, therefore, are dependent on both hepatic transformation and renal excretion. The elimination half-life of acebutolol is 3 to 4 hours and of diacetolol 8 to 13 hours. Elimination is prolonged in the elderly and patients with renal disease. Acebutolol, like pindolol, has intrinsic sympathetic activity that makes it more advantageous than the other β-blockers in patients with bradydysrhythmias or myocardial failure.

Esmolol. Esmolol has several uses in the perioperative period.[161] The most unique feature of the drug is the ester function incorporated into the phenoxypropanolamine structure. This allows for rapid degradation by esterases in the red blood cells and a resultant pharmacologic half-life of 10 to 20 minutes.[161] Esmolol is cardioselective and appears to have little effect on bronchial or vascular tone at doses that decrease HR in humans. It has been used successfully in low doses in patients with asthma[162] but caution is again advised when using β-blockers in these patients.[163] Esmolol is metabolized rapidly in the blood by an esterase located in the red blood cell cytoplasm. It is different from the plasma cholinesterase and is not inhibited to a significant degree by physostigmine or echothiophate but is markedly inhibited by sodium fluoride. There are no apparent important clinical interactions between esmolol and other ester-containing drugs. At the highest infusion rates (500 μg/kg/min), esmolol does not prolong neuromuscular blockade by succinylcholine.

Esmolol has proven to be useful in the perioperative period because of its capability to be administered intravenously and its short half-life.[164] This feature permits a trial of β-blockade in doubtful situations. Esmolol has been shown to blunt the response to intubation of the trachea[161] and is moderately effective in treating postoperative hypertension.[165] Most reported studies in humans have used doses of 50 to 500 μg/kg/min. The most beneficial approach seems to be a loading dose of 500 μg/kg over 30 seconds, followed by continuous infusion of 50 to 300 μg/kg/min. Peak blockade appears to occur within 5 minutes. On discontinuation of the infusion, serum levels decline with an elimination half-life of 9 minutes. The HR response to isoproterenol returns to control in 20 minutes.

Betaxolol. Betaxolol hydrochloride is a β-1 selective (cardioselective) adrenergic receptor antagonist and is freely soluble in water. It has weak membrane-stabilizing activity and no intrinsic sympathomimetic (partial agonist) activity. The preferential effect on β-1 receptors is not absolute. Some β-2 inhibitory activity can be expected in the bronchial and vascular musculature at higher doses. Absorption of an oral dose is complete, with an absolute bioavailability of 90% that is unaffected by ingestion of food or alcohol. The mean elimination half-life is from 11 to 22 hours. It is eliminated primarily by the liver but secondarily through the kidneys. Betaxolol is indicated in the management of hypertension. It may be used alone or concomitantly with other antihypertensive agents.

Penbutolol. Penbutolol is a synthetic β receptor antagonist for oral administration. It is a nonselective β receptor antagonist with some intrinsic sympathomimetic activity. Penbutolol does not appear to have any membrane-stabilizing properties, as does propranolol. Plasma elimination half-life is 5 hours in normal subjects. Ninety percent of radioactive penbutolol was found to be excreted in the urine. There is no change in the effective half-life of penbutolol in healthy patients versus those on renal dialysis. It is indicated primarily for the treatment of hypertension and may be used in combination with other antihypertensives.

Carteolol. Carteolol is a synthetic, nonselective, β-adrenergic–receptor-blocking agent with intrinsic sympathetic activity. It possesses no significant membrane-stabilizing (local anesthetic) activity and is without value in treating intrinsic arrhythmias. Carteolol has equivocal effects on renin secretion because of its intrinsic sympathomimetic activity, in contrast to β-blockers without such activity, which inhibit renin. Carteolol is well absorbed with a half-life of approximately 6 hours. About 50 to 75% of the drug is eliminated by the kidneys; thus, renal impairment increases its half-life in proportion to the reduction in creatinine clearance. Carteolol is primarily indicated for the management of hypertension but may be used in combination with other potent drugs.

Mixed Antagonists

Labetalol. Labetalol is an antihypertensive drug with blocking activity at both α and β receptors. The relative α-/β-blocking effects are dependent on the route of administration. After oral administration, the ratio of α/β effectiveness is 1:3; however, when given intravenously, it is 1:7 (i.e., it is three and seven times more potent on β than on α receptors, respectively). The α effects are primarily on α-1 receptors, whereas the β effects on nonselective.

Hemodynamic effects consist primarily of decreased peripheral resistance and decreased or unchanged HR with little change in CO. Serum renin activity is decreased. Maintenance of lower HRs in the presence of decreased systemic blood pressure is beneficial in controlling the myocardial oxygen supply/demand ratio and is a major benefit of labetalol in patients with coronary artery disease.

Labetalol is eliminated by hepatic glucuronide conjugation. The elimination half-life after iv administration is 5.5 hours and 6 to 8 hours after oral use. Elimination is not markedly prolonged in patients with hepatic or renal failure. Another advantage of the drug is the ability to convert from iv to oral forms of the same drug after the patient is stable. For treatment of hypertension when used as a bolus, the initial dose is 0.25 mg/kg iv over 2 minutes, then repeated every 10 minutes to a total of 300 mg. When used as a continuous infusion, it is usually started at 2 mg/min and titrated to effect. Because there is an enhanced effect by inhalation anesthetics, these doses should be decreased when used intraoperatively.

Complications and contraindications are similar to those for the β-blockers. Labetalol should be used with caution in patients with compromised myocardial function because it may worsen heart failure. Also, owing to β-blocking activity, the drug may induce bronchospasm in asthmatics. As with other β-blockers, abrupt withdrawal is not recommended.

Calcium Entry Blockers

Calcium is regarded as the universal messenger in cells and plays a critical role in a number of biologic processes. It is involved in blood coagulation, a broad array of enzymatic reactions, the metabolism of bone, neuromuscular transmission, the electrical activation of various excitable membranes, as well as endocrine secretion and muscle contraction. Calcium initiates several physiologic events in the specialized automatic and conducting cells in the heart. It is involved in the genesis of the cardiac action potential, and it links excitation to contraction and controls energy stores and utilization. Movement of extracellular calcium across membranes also governs the function of smooth muscle in bronchi and in coronary, pulmonary, and systemic arterioles.

Membrane calcium channels are known to exist that provide a pathway for calcium influx across cell membranes that differs from calcium efflux movements associated with active pumps or exchange. The inward calcium channel exhibits two distinguishing properties: (1) selectivity in that they have the ability to distinguish between ion species and (2) excitability in that they have the property of responding to changes in membrane potential. Separate, ion-specific, channels for sodium and calcium influx are thought to exist. The status of these channels can vary to produce three kinetic states: resting, activated, and inactivated. Sodium channels are referred to as fast channels because the transition among resting, activated, and inactivated states is more rapid than among the calcium channels. Thus, calcium channels are often referred to as membrane "slow channels."[166]

Classification of calcium entry blockers has been difficult since their discovery. They were initially thought to be β-adrenergic-blocking drugs because of their sympatholytic action. Later they were called calcium antagonists. It is clear, however, that these drugs are not true pharmacologic antagonists of calcium. Instead, they interact with the cell membrane to control the intracellular concentration of calcium. The correct terminology for this group of drugs appears to be calcium entry blockers. Slow channel inhibitors or calcium channel blockers are alternate terms. The molecular structures of three clinically useful calcium entry blockers are seen in Figure 12-31. Calcium entry blockers are a heterogeneous group of drugs with dissimilar structures and electrophysiologic and pharmacologic properties. Despite structural dissimilarities, this group shares some important actions that are consistent with the known importance of extracellular calcium and adrenergic function. Any drug that alters slow-channel kinetics could be expected to produce vasodilatation, to depress cardiac conduction velocity (dromotropism), to depress contractility (inotropism), and to decrease HR (chronotropism). All calcium entry blockers

VERAPAMIL

DILTIAZEM

NIFEDIPINE

Bay K 8644

Nitrendipine

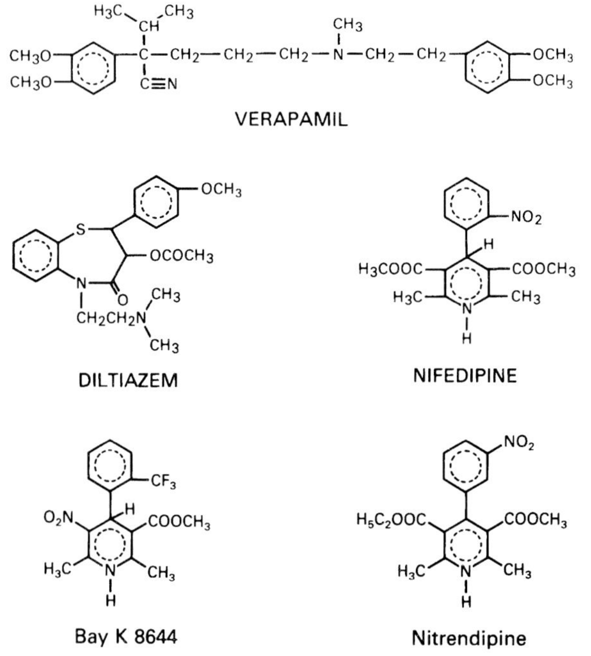

FIGURE 12-31. Structural formulas of the calcium entry blockers demonstrate dissimilar structures consistent with their dissimilar electrophysiologic and pharmacologic properties. They also share some similarities but cannot be considered therapeutically interchangeable. Nifedipine and nitrendipine are structurally similar and are both potent vasodilators; BAY K 8644 is also similar but is a calcium channel agonist.

TABLE 12-22

AUTONOMIC EFFECTS OF CALCIUM ENTRY BLOCKERS IN INTACT HUMANS

	VERAPAMIL	DILTIAZEM	NIFEDIPINE	LIDOFLAZINE
Negative inotropic	+	0/+	0	0
Negative chronotropic	+	0/+	0	0
Negative dromotropic	++++	+++	0	0
Coronary vasodilation	++	+++	++++	++++
Systemic vasodilation	++	++	++++	+++
Bronchodilation	0/+		0/+	

do this, but with varying degrees of potency in the intact human and in vitro (Table 12-22).[167] Thus, despite their similarities, these drugs cannot be considered therapeutically interchangeable. Clinically, nifedipine is a potent coronary artery vasodilator with little direct effect on cardiac conduction. It may reduce dysrhythmia secondarily when increased coronary blood flow is of benefit. Verapamil is valued for its specific antidysrhythmic activity, but it is a myocardial depressant with little vasodilator activity. Verapamil also has slightly greater local anesthetic activity (fast-channel inhibition) than procaine on an equimolar basis.[168] The significance of this observation in humans has not been established. The structural heterogeneity of this group of drugs also suggests more than one site and mechanism of action. Although the molecular basis of the action of these compounds is unknown, they are lipophilic, and it appears likely that they work by producing conformational changes in the cell membranes.

The useful pharmacologic effects of the calcium entry blockers have been confined almost solely to the cardiovascular system, although the list of uses will likely grow.[166] Table 12-23 lists some of the areas of investigation in which they appear to be of clinical benefit. Calcium entry blockers have been described, perhaps erroneously, as selective slow-channel blockers. A review of the literature, however, suggests that these agents are not selective but rather that the slow-channel effects on the cardiovascular system are just more apparent. Their lack of selectivity should not be surprising considering the critical role calcium plays in a wide variety of biologic processes. The sensitivity of a given tissue to the calcium entry blockers is related to that tissue's dependence on extracellular calcium for its function. This would explain the sensitivity of the calcium-dependent myocardium and smooth muscle to these blockers on the one hand and the apparent insensitivity of striated muscle on the other. Extracellular calcium is relatively insignificant in the function of striated muscle, where the SR is the major storage organelle of calcium. Striated muscle can recycle intracellular calcium for prolonged periods, which is in keeping with its function of sustained contraction as opposed to the rhythmic or cyclic contraction of the myocardium and smooth muscle.

TABLE 12-23

USES OF CALCIUM CHANNEL BLOCKERS

Vascular Disorders	**Nonvascular Disorders**
Systemic hypertension	Bronchial asthma
Pulmonary hypertension	Esophageal spasm
Cerebral arterial spasm	Dysmenorrhea
Raynaud's phenomenon	Premature labor
Migraine	

The drugs are all absorbed via the gastrointestinal tract, but the extensive first-pass hepatic extraction of verapamil limits its bioavailability orally (Table 12-24). Onset of action is equivalent for all three drugs and is consistent with rapid membrane transport. All three drugs are extensively protein bound and subject to the effect of changes in plasma protein concentration and competition from other protein-bound drugs and metabolites, but final elimination of verapamil and nifedipine is primarily renal.

Verapamil

Verapamil is a calcium entry blocker that is administered intravenously for terminating supraventricular tachydysrhythmias. Nearly all forms of supraventricular tachydysrhythmias are caused by reentry using either the sinoatrial or the AV node as part of the circuit. Verapamil terminates these cardiac dysrhythmias by decreasing nodal conductivity, converting the unidirectional block of reentry to a bi-directional block. In this regard, its action on supraventricular dysrhythmia is similar to that of quinidine on ventricular reentry cardiac dysrhythmia.

Verapamil does not alter the action potential upstroke in fibers whose resting membrane potential is more negative than −60 mV (i.e., fast-action potentials).[169] It does slow or prevent depolarization in cardiac tissue with a resting membrane potential that is less negative than −50 mV (i.e., calcium-dependent upstroke). Verapamil, therefore, has profound effects on pacemaker cells, which depend on the calcium current for depolarization.[170] It depresses the rate of sinus discharge, reduces conduction velocity, and increases refractoriness of the AV node. A dose-dependent increase in the PR interval and AV interval is produced on the electrocardiogram. This has been described as a quinidine-like effect similar to that produced by Class IA antidysrhythmic drugs (e.g., procainamide), which are also effective for supraventricular dysrhythmia. In contrast to the procainamide, verapamil does not increase the QRS or Q-T interval because it lacks activity on the sodium-dependent action potentials.

Verapamil is a first-line drug for treatment of supraventricular tachydysrhythmias (Table 12-25). The incidence of successful termination of paroxysmal atrial tachycardia with verapamil in adults has approached 90%.[171] It is also effective in treating atrial fibrillation and atrial flutter by either converting to a sinus rhythm or slowing the ventricular response. The ventricular rate will slow as a result of decreased conduction velocity through the AV node even when conversion is not produced. Caution must be exercised in treating patients when the underlying cause of the atrial tachycardia, atrial fibrillation, or atrial flutter is the Wolff-Parkinson-White syndrome. An

TABLE 12-24

COMPARATIVE PHARMACOLOGY OF CALCIUM ENTRY BLOCKERS

	VERAPAMIL	DILTIAZEM	NIFEDIPINE
Dose			
Oral	80–160 mg tid	60–90 mg tid	10–20 mg tid
iv	75–150 μg/kg	75–150 μg/kg	5–15 μg/kg
Absorption			
Oral (%)	>90%	>90%	>90%
Bioavailability			
Oral (%)	<20%	?<20%	60–70%[a]
Onset			
Oral	15–20 min	20–30 min	15–20 min
iv	1 min	?	1 min
Sublingual	—	—	3 min
Peak Effect			
Oral	5 hr	30 min	1–2 hr
iv	5–30 min	?	1–3 hr
Elimination half-life	2–7 hr	4 hr	4–5 hr
Plasma protein binding	90%	80%	90%
Metabolism	70% First-pass hepatic	Deacetylated	80% to lactone
Elimination			
Renal	75%	35%	70%
Gastrointestinal (liver)	15%	75%	<15%
Side effects	Constipation, headache, vertigo, hypotension, atrioventricular conduction disturbances	Headache, dizziness, flushing, atrioventricular conduction disturbances, constipation	Headache, hypotension, flushing, digital dysesthesias, leg edema

[a]Light sensitive.

TABLE 12-25

ACTIONS OF CALCIUM ENTRY BLOCKERS

Verapamil
Vasodilator
↓ systemic vascular resistance → ↑ heart rate → ↑ ejection fraction and cardiac output
Small decrease in left ventricular dP/dt
Little or no change in coronary resistance
↓ conduction through atrioventricular node (↑ P-R interval)
Should not be given with digitalis or β blockers

Diltiazem
More like verapamil than nifedipine
Dilates coronary more than systemic vessels and has less marked hemodynamic effects than nifedipine or verapamil
Little effect on cardiac output
Does not cause tachycardia
Effects on conduction system similar to those of verapamil
Less inotropic effect than verapamil

Nifedipine
Rapid onset of action, may be used sublingually
Potent peripheral vasodilator, may be useful in treatment of hypertension
Has little clinically important negative inotropic activity
Less tendency to produce cardiac decompensation than verapamil
Little effect on nodal activity and no antiarrhythmic activity; therefore causes no electrocardiographic changes
Increased coronary blood flow in normal and ischemic myocardium

accessory bypass tract lies near the AV node that participates in the re-entry of these tachydysrhythmias. Verapamil may terminate the tachydysrhythmia by its specific depressant effects on the AV node, which is one limb of the re-entrant pathway. It may also increase conduction velocity in the accessory tract, in which case the HR may actually increase.

Verapamil has no adverse effects on bronchial asthma or obstructive lung disease and may be selected over propranolol in patients with these conditions. It should be avoided in patients with sick sinus syndrome, AV block, and the presence of heart failure, unless the heart failure is the result of a supraventricular tachycardia.

Studies further support the hypothesis that Ca^{2+} participates directly in the genesis of ventricular dysrhythmia.[172] When sodium channels are inactivated by hypoxia, stretch, or hyperkalemia, the remaining Ca^{2+} can produce a depolarizing current in these abnormal cells, especially in the presence of catecholamines. The conversion of a fast response cell to a cell with slow response characteristics presents all the necessary ingredients for the reentry phenomenon: slow depolarization and delayed conduction. The resulting ventricular dysrhythmia can usually be terminated with one of the Class I drugs as long as the resting membrane potential of the slow response is between –80 and –60 mV. Verapamil has been effective in terminating ventricular tachycardias and premature depolarizations in about two-thirds of the treatment trials when other drugs have failed. The resting membrane potential of these abnormal "slow response" foci has been postulated to be less negative than –60 mV, a range in which lidocaine would be ineffective on the calcium current conduction and depolarization. More information is needed before recommendations can be made for verapamil in treating dysrhythmia other than supraventricular tachydysrhythmias. Other drugs are significantly more effective for the initial treatment of ventricular dysrhythmia.

The important side effects of verapamil are directly related to its predominant pharmacologic action (see Table 12-25). It may produce unwanted AV conduction delays and bradycardia, resulting in cardiovascular collapse. Verapamil must be used carefully, if at all, in the presence of propranolol. The combined effect has produced complete heart block in animals and humans. It must be used carefully in digitalized patients for the same reason. No such interactions exist with nifedipine. The combination of β-blockade and nifedipine may be beneficial in patients with ischemic heart disease because the reflex tachycardia seen with nifedipine can be countered with β-blockade.

Nifedipine

Nifedipine is the most potent calcium entry blocker when tested in isolated tissue preparations. It is an equipotent cardiac depressant and vasodilator. Depression of inotropism and cardiac conduction, however, is not evident in the intact human. It does not affect baroreflex mechanisms and, as a result, the marked vasodilation is accompanied by increased SNS tone and afterload reduction (see Table 12-25).[166] A compensatory tachycardia may result, and CO may actually increase as a result of the afterload reduction.

The most specific therapeutic application for nifedipine is coronary vasospasm (variant of Prinzmetal's angina). It has been more successful than nitroglycerin for this purpose because it produces a more profound and predictable coronary vasodilation. It has also been extremely useful in other types of ischemic heart disease, ranging from unstable angina to myocardial infarction. The decrease in myocardial oxygen demand that results from the reduced afterload and reduced left ventricular volume appears to be the mechanism for the relief of angina. Coronary vasodilation is another factor, but it is not known if this is the antianginal effect in patients with coronary artery disease. The dilating effect may last only 5 minutes, but the antianginal effect may last more than 1 hour.

Diltiazem

The hemodynamic effects of diltiazem lie somewhere between those of verapamil and nifedipine.[166] It is less potent than either of these two agents. Diltiazem is a good coronary artery dilator but a poor peripheral vasodilator. It often produces bradycardia and delayed conduction, and reflex tachycardia is not a problem. It appears to be an effective oral drug for the treatment of coronary disease in which cardiac dysrhythmias are troublesome. Cardiac dysrhythmias are noticeably a part of the clinical picture in patients suffering from coronary spasm. Intravenous administration of diltiazem is effective therapy for supraventricular tachycardias including PSVT, atrial fibrillation, atrial flutter, and reentrant tachycardias such as Wolff-Parkinson-White syndrome.[173] Like verapamil, diltiazem acts by prolonging AV nodal conduction. The peripheral vascular effects of diltiazem, though, are less severe, making it a more desirable therapeutic choice in most cases. A bolus dose of 0.25 mg/kg is administered over 2 minutes and may be repeated at 0.35 mg/kg if necessary after 15 minutes. An infusion of 5 to 15 mg/hr may be necessary to maintain the reduction of HR.

Nicardipine

Nicardipine hydrochloride is a calcium channel blocker that can be administered orally and intravenously. It is the only calcium channel blocker that can be titrated intravenously to achieve blood pressure response. Nicardipine is a smooth muscle relaxant producing vasodilation of peripheral and coronary arteries. It has a rapid onset of action, and the major effects last 10 to 15 minutes. Toxic metabolic products are not produced. It has minimal cardiodepressant effects and does not decrease the rate of the sinus node pacemaker or slow conduction through the AV node. Renal failure does not affect the dosage, but the dosage should be reduced in the elderly and those with hepatic dysfunction. It is compatible with most crystalloid solutions. Side effects of nicardipine include headache, lightheadedness, flushing, and hypotension. Reflex tachycardia is not a frequent finding with nicardipine, as is the case with nitroprusside, hydralazine, or nifedipine.

Nimodipine

Nimodipine is highly lipophilic. It has a greater vasodilating effect on cerebral arteries than on vessels elsewhere because of its lipophilism, which promotes crossing the blood-brain barrier. Clinical studies demonstrate a favorable effect on the severity of neurologic deficits caused by cerebral vasospasm following subarachnoid hemorrhage. However, no radiographic evidence has been presented that nimodipine either prevents or relieves spasm of these arteries. The mechanism for clinical improvement is not known. It is primarily an oral drug that is rapidly absorbed, with a T-terminal half-life of approximately 8 to 9 hours. Earlier elimination rates are much more rapid, which results in a need to redose every 4 hours. The bioavailability of an oral dose is only 13%. Dosage should be reduced in patients with hepatic dysfunction. The primary indication for nimodipine is for the improvement of neurologic deficits caused by spasm following subarachnoid hemorrhage from a ruptured aneurysm.

Felodipine

Felodipine is a second-generation calcium channel inhibitor. Nimodipine and felodipine have demonstrated selectivity for vascular tissue beds. Whereas nimodipine preferentially dilates cerebral vessels, felodipine preferentially dilates peripheral resistance vessels. Neither has significant effects on cardiac muscle. This has important clinical implications in the treatment of hypertension. Early studies indicate that 10 to 20 mg of felodipine daily will reduce blood pressure without reducing CO or HR. Coronary blood flow increases, but no effect on ventricular contraction or relaxation has been reported. This would make the drug appropriate for the active hypertensive patient.

Calcium Entry Blockers and Anesthesia

Evidence indicates that halothane depresses slow-channel kinetics. All of the potent inhalation anesthetics behave in a similar fashion in that they depress myocardial contractility and vascular tone in a dose-related manner. Most studies indicate that the calcium entry blockers and inhalation anesthetics exert additive effects on the inward calcium current.[167] Opioid anesthetics do not appear to add anything to the effects of the calcium entry blockers. Several recent studies indicate an interaction between the calcium entry blockers and the neuromuscular blocking drugs similar to that seen with the mycin antibiotics.[166] This interaction is not well defined, but in vitro and in vivo studies indicate a reduced margin of safety with these drug combinations. Calcium entry blockers appear to augment the effects of both depolarizing and nondepolarizing muscle relaxants.[174] These observations serve as a word of caution because their clinical significance has not been defined. Prolonged apnea and relaxation have been reported when verapamil was used to treat a supraventricular tachycardia in a patient with Duchenne's muscular dystrophy.[175]

Calcium entry blockers should be continued until the time of surgery to maintain control of angina pectoris, hypertension, or cardiac dysrhythmia.[166] It could be anticipated that sudden discontinuation of these drugs theoretically could produce a rebound of symptoms, although this phenomenon has not been reported. Up-regulation of calcium receptors would probably occur during periods of entry blockade.

Verapamil may increase the toxicity of digoxin, the benzodiazepines, carbamazepine, oral hypoglycemics, and possibly quinidine and theophylline.[176] Cardiac failure, AV conduction disturbances, and sinus bradycardia may be more frequent with concurrent use of β-blockers, and severe hypotension and bradycardia may occur with bupivacaine. Decreased lithium effect and lithium neurotoxicity have both been reported with the concurrent use of verapamil.[177] The effects of verapamil may also be increased by cimetidine.

Vasodilators

Increased awareness and treatment of hypertension over the last 20 years has resulted in increasing numbers of patients presenting for anesthesia and surgery who are taking one or more antihypertensive medications. These drugs are numerous, affect multiple organ systems, and have the potential for many deleterious interactions in the perioperative period. Most antihypertensive drugs blunt the ANS or its effector organs or cause reflex increases in ANS outflow. Most anesthetic agents also inhibit ANS tone to some degree and may therefore have additive effects with antihypertensive drugs. In addition, patients with hypertension may exhibit greater lability in blood pressure intraoperatively and rebound hypertension in the postoperative period. The anesthesiologist should therefore maintain a thorough understanding of the commonly used antihypertensive drugs. A rational approach to their perioperative use includes decisions as to holding or continuing them preoperatively, possible interactions with anesthetic drugs, and resumption of treatment postoperatively. The commonly used antihypertensive drugs are grouped below according to their primary mechanism of action and discussed briefly with emphasis on consideration for the anesthesiologist.

Diuretics

Diuretics are the most common prescribed drugs for hypertension. Their basic mechanisms of action are decreased plasma and extracellular volumes. Although the thiazides and furosemide have been shown to have vasodilating properties, the clinical significance of this effect is unclear. Chronic diuretic therapy results in decreased intravascular volume. The cardiovascular response to induction of anesthesia may therefore be accentuated, resulting in hypotension and tachycardia. Other problems associated with diuretic use include hypokalemia, hyponatremia, hypocalcemia, and hyperglycemia. Chronic hypokalemia is common with diuretic therapy and may predispose the patient to cardiac arrhythmias.[178] The clinical relevance of perioperative hypokalemia is unclear and has stirred considerable debate among anesthesiologists as to whether surgery should be postponed until plasma potassium levels are treated.[179]

Sympatholytics

Sympatholytic drugs include those that block central SNS outflow or NE release from the presynaptic neuron at the effector site. Currently included in this group are α-methyldopa and clonidine.

α-Methyldopa. α-methyldopa is a catechol derivative that is enzymatically converted to active compounds by enzymes in the catecholamine synthesis chain (see Fig. 12-9). α-methyldopamine and α-methlynorepinephrine are the primary metabolites. The precise mechanism responsible for decreased SNS tone is unclear, but it is thought that α-methylnorepinephrine, which is stored in presynaptic vesicles, is released and stimulates presynaptic α-2 receptors, thereby inhibiting NE release. Because of the unique metabolism of α-methyldopa to the active compound and the storage of the metabolite in presynaptic vesicles, both the time to onset and duration of action are long. Even after iv administration, the peak effect may not be seen for several hours. Although the elimination half-life is 2 hours, the effect of an oral dose may last up to 24 hours.

Clonidine

Clonidine stimulates presynaptic α-2 receptors and inhibits NE release from both central and peripheral adrenergic terminals. It also has some α-1 agonist activity and in high oral doses may cause paradoxical hypertension by stimulating vascular α-1 receptors. Under normal circumstances, the α-2 effects predominate. The prominent antihypertensive effect is thought to be secondary to stimulation of α-2 receptors in the vasomotor centers of the medulla oblongata.[112] Whether these are presynaptic or postsynaptic receptors remains controversial; however, the end result is decreased SNS and enhanced vagal tone. Peripherally, there is decreased plasma renin activity as well as decreased EPI and NE levels.[180]

Cardiovascular effects of clonidine include decreased peripheral vascular resistance and HR. The cardiovascular response to exercise is usually maintained. Prominent side effects include hypotension, sedation, and dry mouth. One of the more worrisome complications of clonidine use is the occurrence of a withdrawal syndrome on acute discontinuation of the drug. This usually occurs about 18 hours after discontinuation and consists of hypertension, tachycardia, insomnia, flushing, headache, apprehension, sweating, and tremulousness. It lasts for 24 to 72 hours and is most likely to occur in patients taking more than 1.2 mg/day of clonidine. The withdrawal syndrome has been noted postoperatively in patients who were taken off clonidine for surgery. It can be confused with anesthesia emergence symptoms, particularly in a patient with uncontrolled hypertension. Clonidine is not available for iv use, but symptoms of the withdrawal syndrome as well as routine postoperative hypertension can be treated with clonidine administered transdermally or rectally.[181] Withholding clonidine prior to surgery is not recommended.

Dexmedetomidine

Dexmedetomidine is a more selective α-2 agonist than clonidine.[119] It has a much shorter half-life (about 1.5 hours) and a more rapid onset of action (5 minutes). The time to peak effect is 15 minutes. Intravenous dexmedetomidine provides excellent sedation, lowering of blood pressure and HR, and profound decreases in plasma catecholamines. Little respiratory depression is evident. Other studies have shown it to be an effective anxiolytic and sedative when used as premedication for anesthesia for minor gynecologic surgery. In an animal model, dexmedetomidine produces stereospecific and dose-dependent decreases in MAC.[182]

Flacke listed the potential uses of sympatholytic drugs in the future. In addition to the reducing effect of MAC and the absent respiratory depression, the following properties seem particularly valuable to the anesthesiologist:[182] (1) They are potent analgesics. (2) They are sedatives and anxiolytics. (3) They are antisialogogues. (4) They may promote hemodynamic stability. (5) Homeostatic reflexes remain intact. (6) They attenuate opioid rigidity (in animals). (7) Their circulatory actions can be reversed. Clonidine has also been used successfully as a substitute for opiates and nicotine during withdrawal. It reduces sympathetic hyperactivity with head injury and can be used as an analgesic in the subarachnoid and epidural spaces for the treatment of pain.

Converting Enzyme Inhibitors

The renin–angiotensin system is integrally related to the ANS in controlling blood pressure (see Fig. 12-16). The central role of the renin-angiotensin-aldosterone system in the regulation of fluid balance and hemodynamics was not fully appreciated until the discovery and clinical application of inhibitors of the ACE. Captopril, enalapril, and lisinopril inhibit converting enzyme and thereby prevent the conversion of angiotensin I to the active angiotensin II. These drugs have been highly effective in the treatment of all levels of essential hypertension as well as renovascular and malignant hypertension. The cardiovascular effects normally involve only decreased peripheral vascular resistance. CO may remain normal or increase while the filling pressure remains unchanged. Thus, these drugs have been effective in the management of congestive heart failure as well.[183] There is usually no increase in SNS tone in response to the lowered blood pressure. ACE inhibition generally results in reductions in angiotensin–aldosterone, NE, and plasma antidiuretic hormone. This suppression is accompanied by a decrease in aldosterone and an improvement in cumulative plasma potassium levels, which are beneficial in both congestive heart failure and hypertension. It can be concluded that the major humoral responses to chronic congestive heart failure, even overlooking the effects of the diuretics, are affected by the release of angiotensin, aldosterone, and increased SNS tone.

Captopril, the first orally active compound, has proven highly effective in the treatment of all levels of hypertension and congestive heart failure (Table 12-26). Enalapril is a second-generation (nonsulfhydryl) ACE inhibitor. The omission of the sulfhydryl group possibly diminishes side effects. Both captopril and enalapril combine a high degree of clinical efficacy with a low rate of side effects. Both are eliminated via renal excretion and should be given in reduced doses in patients with renal dysfunction. Captopril has a shorter half-life and requires more frequent dosing than enalapril. Enalapril has to be converted by esterase in the liver and other tissues into the active compound enalaprilat. Many new ACE inhibitors are being developed that are eliminated via hepatic routes and may prove advantageous in renal failure. Lisinopril is one of these ACE inhibitors that is absorbed as the active form and is very long-acting.

5 The ACE inhibitors are associated with few side effects and are increasingly popular in treating hypertension. Captopril may produce reversible neutropenia, dermatitis, and angioedema. Enalapril produces syncope, headache, and dizziness in about 1% of elderly patients. All ACE inhibitors may cause hypotension in patients who are hypovolemic and taking diuretic therapy. Diuretic therapy should be discontinued 1 week before starting ACE inhibitor therapy. The hypotensive effects are also enhanced by the concomitant use of calcium channel blockers. The ACE inhibitors blunt the hypokalemic effects of thiazide diuretics and may magnify the potassium-sparing effects of spironolactone, triamterene, and amiloride. In addition, nonsteroidal anti-inflammatory drugs, including aspirin, may magnify the potassium-retaining effects of ACE inhibitors.

Vasodilators

The drugs that directly relax smooth muscle to cause vasodilation reflexively increase ANS tone and are included here for the sake of a complete discussion of antihypertensive drugs.[59] These are discussed with emphasis on perioperative use.

Hydralazine. Hydralazine is the most commonly used vasodilator and can be given by the im, iv, and oral routes. It relaxes smooth muscle tone directly, without interacting with adrenergic or cholinergic receptors. The mechanism of action is unknown. It is most potent in coronary, splanchnic, renal, and cerebral vessels, causing increased blood flow in each of these organs. The decrease in cardiac afterload is beneficial, but, unfortunately, there is usually a concomitant reflex tachycardia that may be severe. It is commonly combined with a β blocker such as propranolol. It may also cause fluid retention and is usually given chronically with a diuretic.[112] Hydralazine

TABLE 12-26

THE ANGIOTENSIN-CONVERTING ENZYME (ACE)

AGENT	MAJOR STUDIES	CHARACTERISTICS
Captopril	Quality of life; SAVE; diabetic nephropathy; ISIS-IV (early Stage AMI, trial negative)	The first ACE inhibitor; overall the best studied
Enalapril	CONSENSUS; SOLVD (prevention and treatment arms); V-HeFT I and II	Longer acting; the best-studied in heart failure
Benazepril	None	Long plasma half-life (22 hr)
Cilazepril	None	Long tissue half-life
Fosinopril	None	Renal and hepatic elimination may allow safer use in renal or hepatic failure
Perindopril	None	Long plasma half-life (35 hr), less initial hypotension
Quinapril	QUIET (Quinapril Ischemic Event Trial: postangioplasty, end-points AMI, sudden death; ready 1995)	Potent binding to tissue ACE prolongs effective half-life
Ramipril	AIRE (acute infarction ramipril efficacy)	Long plasma half-life (>33 hr), proven use in postinfarct CHF
Trandolapril	TRACE Study (Trandolapril Cardiac Evaluation Study) on high-risk AMI patients; ready 1995	Long plasma half-life (20 hr); highly lipid soluble with potential for tissue binding
Lisinopril	GISSI-III: early-stage AMI, mortality reduced by 11%	Active as is; water soluble; long acting

CHF, congestive heart failure.

is metabolized by hepatic acetylation, and oral bioavailability may be low owing to first-pass metabolism. The elimination half-life is about 4 hours, but the pharmacologic half-life is much longer as a result of avid binding of the drug to smooth muscle. The effective half-life is approximately 100 hours. Side effects include a lupus-like syndrome, drug fever, skin rash, pancytopenia, and peripheral neuropathy. The iv dose we recommend for perioperative use is 5 to 10 mg in an iv bolus every 15 to 20 minutes until blood pressure control is achieved. It may also be given 10 to 40 mg im, but the response is slower.

Sodium Nitroprusside. Sodium nitroprusside is an extremely potent vasodilator that is available only for iv administration. It acts directly on smooth muscle, causing both arterial and venous dilation.[59] The mechanism of action is not entirely clear but appears to involve binding to α receptor on the surface of the myocyte, followed by activation of an intracellular vasodilator intermediate. The action of sodium nitroprusside on both venous and arterial sides of the circulation causes decreases in cardiac preload as well as afterload. This results in decreased cardiac work; however, it has been suggested that sodium nitroprusside may further compromise ischemic myocardium in the presence of occlusive coronary artery disease by shunting blood away from the ischemic zone.[184]

Sodium nitroprusside is useful during the perioperative period. It lowers blood pressure within 1 to 2 minutes, with the effect dissipating within 2 minutes after infusion is stopped. It is extremely potent and should be administered through a central venous line by infusion pump while continuously monitoring arterial pressure. The starting dose is 0.25 to 0.5 μg/kg/min. It can be increased slowly as needed to control blood pressure, but chances for toxicity are greater if the dose of 10 μg/kg/min is exceeded. The dose required for steady-state–induced hypotension is variable.

Chemically, sodium nitroprusside consists of a ferrous iron atom bound with five cyanide molecules and one nitric group. The ferrous iron reacts with sulfhydryl groups in red blood cells and releases cyanide. Cyanide is reduced to thiocyanate in the liver and excreted in the urine. The half-life of thiocyanate is 4 days, and it accumulates in the presence of renal failure. There is no evidence, however, that preexisting hepatic or renal failure increases the likelihood of cyanide toxicity. Administration of high doses of sodium nitroprusside can result in cyanide toxicity. The cyanide molecule binds to cytochrome oxidase, interfering with electron transport and causing cellular hypoxia. This can be recognized by increasing tolerance to the drug, elevated mixed venous Pao_2, and metabolic acidosis. The treatment of cyanide toxicity consists of (1) administration of amyl nitrate (by inhalation or directly into the anesthesia circuit), (2) infusion of sodium nitrite 5 mg/kg over 4 to 5 minutes, and (3) administration of sodium thiosulfate 150 mg/kg in 50 mL water over 15 minutes.

The hypotensive effects of sodium nitroprusside may be potentiated by inhalation anesthetics and blood loss; therefore, close perioperative monitoring is essential. It is commonly used to induce hypotension for decreasing blood loss in patients predisposed to major hemorrhage. Administration of sodium nitroprusside causes a reflex increase in sympathetic tone and renin release.[185] Drugs that blunt these reflexes markedly enhance its effects. Preoperative treatment with propranolol or captopril decreases the amount of sodium nitroprusside required for producing hypotension and thus decreases the potential for toxicity.[186]

Glyceril Trinitrate. Glyceril trinitrate, or nitroglycerin, is a venodilator used to treat myocardial ischemia. Its predominant action is on venules, causing increased venous capacitance and decreased cardiac preload. Effects on the arterial side are minimal except at very high doses. Upon iv administration effects can be seen within 2 minutes, and they usually resolve within 5 minutes of discontinuing the drug. Side effects are minimal, and there is no potential for cyanide toxicity as with nitroprusside. Use of nitroglycerin for control of perioperative hypertension has been reported[187] but because of its relatively weak arteriolar action, it is not as useful as other drugs as an antihypertensive agent. In obstetric patients with preeclampsia, however, it may be chosen over nitroprusside to circumvent potential cyanide toxicity to the fetus.[188]

Diazoxide. Diazoxide is a direct-acting vasodilator that may be given iv and is useful in hypertensive emergencies. It has a greater effect on resistance than capacitance vessels, thus decreasing cardiac afterload with little effect on preload. It also causes fluid retention and induces a reflex sympathetic response.[112] The hypotensive effect is potentiated by diuretics, sympatholytics, and hypovolemia. Diazoxide is usually administered as an iv bolus of 300 mg for a 70-kg adult. It is 90% bound to serum albumin; therefore, a substantial portion of the initial bolus may not reach the site of action. Rapid boluses (30 seconds) of 100 mg every 5 minutes are often recommended as an alternative to allow more free drug to reach the arterioles.[112] The hypotensive effect is usually obtained in 5 to 10 minutes and lasts 5 to 12 hours.

Calcium Entry Inhibitors

The calcium entry blockers verapamil, nifedipine, and nitrendipine may also be useful for treating hypertension in the perioperative period (see Adrenergic Antagonists: Calcium Channel Blockers section).

Treatment of Postoperative Hypertension

The wide variety of antihypertensive agents discussed previously makes the treatment of hypertension in the recovery room easier because we can now choose from among multiple routes of administration and variable onsets and durations of action of the different agents.[189] However, treatment may become confusing unless the basic pharmacology of each drug is understood. Those drugs available for only oral administration are not routinely used because of unreliable gastrointestinal function during this period. The etiology of postoperative hypertension in each case should be considered. A determination should be made if this requires emergency therapy or is just urgent. Pain should be eliminated by assurance of adequate analgesia prior to therapy with antihypertensive agents. Also, because of the complex pathophysiology of hypertension, a thorough knowledge of each patient and his or her condition is mandatory in choosing a treatment regimen. The medications required for preoperative control may provide the most information in determining what will be necessary postoperatively. In particular, the use of drugs that may have an associated withdrawal syndrome such as clonidine or β-blockers should be noted as well as if they were withheld prior to surgery. The volume status of the patient is also important. Fluid overload may require diuretic therapy. Volume depletion or hemorrhage may predispose to severe hypotension in response to routine doses of sympatholytics or vasodilators.

For severe elevations of blood pressure that require immediate treatment, sodium nitroprusside is the drug of choice. Intravenous nicardipine can be given and effective before a sodium nitroprusside infusion can be prepared. Labetalol, metoprolol, and esmolol may also be used intravenously. Esmolol has the advantage of being rapidly titratable.[190] α-methyldopa may be used intravenously but takes much longer to work than clonidine. Clonidine can be given per rectum and begins to act in 10 to 20 minutes.[181] If conditions permit, it is helpful to use the drugs the patient was taking preoperatively to ease the transition in the postoperative period. Caution must be exercised if the hypertension is the result of excessive exogenous catecholamines, pheochromocytoma, or thyrotoxicosis. α-blockade should be started before β-blockade. The hypertension may, in fact, worsen if β receptors are blocked first, leaving the α receptors unopposed.

References

1. Guyton AC: The autonomic nervous system: The adrenal medulla. In Guyton AC (ed): Textbook of Medical Physiology, p 686. Philadelphia, WB Saunders, 1986
2. Axelrod J, Weinshilboum R: Catecholamines. N Engl J Med 287:237, 1972
3. Flacke WE, Flacke JW: Cholinergic and anticholinergic agents. In Smith NT, Corbascio AN (eds): Drug Interaction in Anesthesia, p 160. Philadelphia, Lea & Febiger, 1986
4. Berne RM, Levy MN: Control of the heart. In: Berne RM, Levy MN (eds): Cardiovascular Physiology, p 221. St. Louis, Mosby, 1977
5. Bexton RS, Milne JR, Cory-Pearce R, English TA, Camm AJ: Effect of beta blockade on exercise response after cardiac transplantation. Br Heart J 49:584, 1983
6. Shepherd JT, Vanhoutte PM: Spasm of the coronary arteries: Causes and consequences (the scientist's viewpoint). Mayo Clin Proc 60:33, 1985
7. Koizumi K, Brooks CC: The autonomic nervous system and its role in controlling visceral activities. In Mountcastle VB (ed): Medical Physiology, p 783. St. Louis, CV Mosby, 1974
8. O'Rourke ST, Vanhoutte PM: Adrenergic and cholinergic regulation of bronchial vascular tone. Am Rev Respir Dis 146:S11, 1992
9. Comroe JH: Reflexes from the lungs. In Comroe JH (ed): Physiology of Respiration, p 72. Chicago, Year Book, 1979
10. Pearl RG, Maze M, Rosenthal MH: Pulmonary and systemic hemodynamic effects of central venous and left atrial sympathomimetic drug administration in the dog. J Cardiothorac Anesth 1:29, 1987
11. Bevan JA: Some bases of differences in vascular response to sympathetic activity. Circ Res 45:161, 1979
12. Thomas J, Fouad FM, Tarazi RC, Bravo EL: Evaluation of plasma catecholamines in humans. Correlation of resting levels with cardiac responses to beta-blocking and sympatholytic drugs. Hypertension 5:858, 1983
13. Stoelting RK: Sympathomimetics. In Stoelting RK (ed): Pharmacology and Physiology in Anesthetic Practice, p 251. Philadelphia, JB Lippincott, 1987
14. Lawson N: Catecholamines: The first messengers. In Bailliere's Clinical Anesthesiology. London, Bailliere Tindall, 1994
15. Shepherd JT, Vanhoutte PM: Neurohumoral regulation. In The Human Cardiovascular System, p 368. New York, Raven Press, 1984
16. Zaritsky AL, Chernow B: Catecholamines, sympathomimetics. In Ziegler MG, Lake CR (eds): Frontiers of Clinical Neuroscience, p 481. Baltimore, Williams & Wilkins, 1984
17. Chernow B, Rainey TG, Lake CR: Catecholamines in critical care medicine. In Ziegler MG, Lake CR (eds): Frontiers of Clinical Neuroscience, p 368. Baltimore, Williams & Wilkins, 1984
18. Fuder H: Selected aspects of presynaptic modulation of noradrenaline release from the heart. J Cardiovasc Pharmacol 7 (suppl 5):S2, 1985
19. Maze M: Clinical implications of membrane receptor function in anesthesia. Anesthesiology 55:160, 1981
20. Wood M: Cholinergic and parasympathomimetic drugs: Cholinesterases and anticholinesterases. In Wood M, Wood AJJ (eds): Drugs and Anesthesia, p 111. Baltimore, Williams & Wilkins, 1982
21. Goldberg LI: The role of dopamine receptors in the treatment of congestive heart failure. J Cardiovasc Pharmacol 14 (suppl 5):S19, 1989
22. Vanhoutte PM, Flavahan NA: The heterogenicity of adrenergic receptors. In Szabadi E, Bradshaw CM, Nohovski SR (eds): Pharmacology of Adrenoreceptors, p 43. VCH: VCH Verlagsgesellschaft, Germany, 1985
23. Van Zwieten PA: The role of adrenoceptors in circulatory and metabolic regulation. Am Heart J 116:1384, 1988
24. Davey MJ: Alpha adrenoceptors—an overview. J Mole Cell Cardiol 18 (suppl 5):1, 1986
25. Terzic A, Puceat M, Vassort G, Vogel SM: Cardiac alpha 1-adrenoceptors: An overview. Pharmacol Rev 45:147, 1993
26. Aubry ML, Davey MJ, Petch B: Cardioprotective and antidysrhythmic effects of alpha 1-adrenoceptor blockade during myocardial ischaemia and reperfusion in the dog. J Cardiovasc Pharmacol 7 (suppl 6):S93, 1985
27. Hoffman BB, Lefkowitz RJ: Alpha-adrenergic receptor subtypes. N Engl J Med 302:1390, 1980
28. Langer SZ: Presynaptic regulation of catecholamine release. Biochem Pharmacol 23:1793, 1974
29. Cohen RA, Shepherd JT, Vanhoutte PM: Effects of the adrenergic transmitter on epicardial coronary arteries. Fed Proc 43:2862, 1984
30. Griggs DMJ, Chilian WM, Boatwright RB, Shoji T, Williams DO: Evidence against significant resting alpha-adrenergic coronary vasoconstrictor tone. Fed Proc 43:2873, 1984
31. Timmermans PB, Van Zwieten PA: alpha 2 adrenoceptors: Classification, localization, mechanisms, and targets for drugs. J Med Chem 25:1389, 1982
32. Schmitz W, Kohl C, Neumann J, Scholz H, Scholz J: On the mechanism of positive inotropic effects of alpha-adrenoceptor agonists. Basic Res Cardiol 84 (suppl 1):23, 1989
33. Bohm M, Diet F, Feiler G, Kemkes B, Erdmann E: Alpha-adrenoceptors and alpha-adrenoceptor-mediated positive inotropic effects in failing human myocardium. J Cardiovasc Pharmacol 12:357, 1988
34. Maze M, Tranquilli W: Alpha-2 adrenoceptor agonists: Defining the role in clinical anesthesia. Anesthesiology 74:581, 1991
35. Summers RJ, Mohnaar P, Russell F *et al*: Coexistence and localization of beta 1- and beta 2-adrenoceptors in the human heart. Eur Heart J 10 (suppl B):11, 1989
36. Goldberg LI: Dopamine receptors and hypertension. Physiologic and pharmacologic implications. Am J Med 77:37, 1984
37. Kuchel OG, Kuchel GA: Peripheral dopamine in pathophysiology of hypertension. Interaction with aging and lifestyle. Hypertension 18:709, 1991
38. Burns AM: Dopamine: Past, present and future (editorial). Clin Intensive Care 1:148, 1990
39. Miller R: Metoclopramide and dopamine receptor blockade. Neuropharmacology 15:463, 1976
40. Hilberman M, Maseda J, Stinson EB *et al*: The diuretic properties of dopamine in patients after open-heart operation. Anesthesiology 61:489, 1984
41. Keeton TK, Campbell WB: The pharmacologic alteration of renin release. Pharmacol Rev 32:81, 1980
42. Owall A, Gordon E, Lagerkranser M, Lindquist C, Rudehill A, Sollevi A: Clinical experience with adenosine for controlled hypotension during cerebral aneurysm surgery. Anesth Analg 66:229, 1987
43. Lineberger AS, Sprague DH, Battaglini JW: Sinus arrest associated with cimetidine. Anesth Analg 64:554, 1985
44. Prichard BN, Owens CW, Smith CC, Walden RJ: Heart and catecholamines. Acta Cardiol 46:309, 1991
45. Prys-Roberts C: The changing face of adrenergic pharmacology. Curr Opin Anesth 5:113, 1992
46. Brodde OE: Beta-adrenoceptors in cardiac disease. Pharmacol Ther 60:405, 1993
47. Williams LT, Lefkowitz RJ: Receptor binding studies in adrenergic pharmacology. New York, Raven Press, 1979
48. Hoefke W: Clonidine. In Scriabine A (ed): Pharmacology of Antihypertensive Drugs, p 55. New York, Raven Press, 1980
49. Berne RM, Levy MN: Coronary circulation and cardiac metabolism. In Berne RM, Levy MN (eds): Cardiovascular Physiology, p 221. St. Louis, CV Mosby, 1977
50. Guyton AC: Cardiac output, venous return, and their regulation. In Guyton AC (ed): Textbook of Medical Physiology, p 272. Philadelphia, WB Saunders, 1986
51. Baron JF, Decaux-Jacolot A, Edouard A, Berdeaux A, Samii K: Influence of venous return on baroreflex control of heart rate during lumbar epidural anesthesia in humans. Anesthesiology 64:188, 1986
52. Greene NM: Perspectives in spinal anesthesia. Reg Anesth 7:55, 1982
53. Bailey PL, Stanley TH: Anesthesia for patients with a prior cardiac transplant. J Cardiothorac Anesth 4:38, 1990
54. Vatner SF: Regulation of coronary resistance vessels and large coronary arteries. Am J Cardiol 56:16E, 1985
55. Levy MN, Blattberg B: Effect of vagal stimulation on the overflow of norepinephrine into the coronary sinus during cardiac sympathetic nerve stimulation in the dog. Circ Res 38:81, 1976
56. Yasue H, Touyama M, Shimamoto M, Kato H, Tanaka S: Role of autonomic nervous system in the pathogenesis of Prinzmetal's variant form of angina. Circulation 50:534, 1974
57. Torretti J, Gerson JI, Oates RP, Lange JS: Beta-adrenoceptor blockade and tolerance to potassium. Anesthesiology 64:846, 1986
58. Stoelting RK: Antihypertensive drugs. In Stoelting RK (ed): Pharmacology and Physiology in Anesthetic Practice, p 294. Philadelphia, JB Lippincott, 1987
59. Stoelting RK: Peripheral vasodilators. In Stoelting RK (ed): Pharmacology and Physiology in Anesthetic Practice, p 307. Philadelphia, JB Lippincott, 1987
60. Stoelting RK: Anticholinesterase drugs and cholinergic agonists. In Stoelting RK (ed): Pharmacology and Physiology in Anesthetic Practice, p 217. Philadelphia, JB Lippincott, 1987
61. Westfall TC: Muscarinic agents. In Bevan JA (ed): Essentials of Pharmacology, p 116. New York, Harper & Row, 1976
62. Wilkins JL, Hardcastle JD, Mann CV, Kaufman L: Effects of neostigmine and atropine on motor activity of ileum, colon, and rectum of anaesthetized subjects. Br Med J 1:793, 1970
63. Child CS: Prevention of neostigmine-induced colonic activity. A comparison of atropine and glycopyrronium. Anaesthesia 39:1083, 1984
64. De Roetth AJ, Wong A, Dettbarn W, Rosenberg P, Wilensky JG: Blood cholinesterase activity of glaucoma patients treated with phospholine iodide. Am J Ophthalmol 62:834, 1966
65. Milby TH: Prevention and management of organophosphate poisoning. JAMA 216:2131, 1971
66. Stoelting RK: Anticholinergic drugs. In Stoelting RK (ed): Pharmacology and Physiology in Anesthetic Practice, p 232. Philadelphia, JB Lippincott, 1987
67. Spaulding BC, Choi SD, Gross JB, Apfelbaum JL, Broderson H: The effect of physostigmine on diazepam-induced ventilatory depression: A double-blind study. Anesthesiology 61:551, 1984

68. Shoemaker WC, Patil R, Appel PL, Kram HB: Hemodynamic and oxygen transport patterns for outcome prediction, therapeutic goals, and clinical algorithms to improve outcome. Feasibility of artificial intelligence to customize algorithms. Chest 102:617S, 1992
69. Reinart K: Principles and Practice of SV02 Monitoring. In King, Worth (eds): Intensive Care World, p 121. London, vol. 5, 1988.
70. Boudoulas H, Rittgers SE, Lewis RP, Leier CV, Weissler AM: Changes in diastolic time with various pharmacologic agents: Implication for myocardial perfusion. Circulation 60:164, 1979
71. Royster RL: Intraoperative administration of inotropes in cardiac surgery patients. J Cardiothorac Anesth 4(suppl 5):17, 1990
72. De Mey J, Vanhoutte PM: Uneven distribution of postjunctional alpha 1- and alpha 2-like adrenoceptors in canine arterial and venous smooth muscle. Circ Res 48:875, 1981
73. Smith NT, Corbascio AN: The use and misuse of pressor agents. Anesthesiology 33:58, 1970
74. Lundberg J, Norgren L, Thomson D, Werner O: Hemodynamic effects of dopamine during thoracic epidural analgesia in man. Anesthesiology 66:641, 1987
75. Zimmerman BG, Abboud FM, Eckstein JW: Comparison of the effects of sympathomimetic amines upon venous and total vascular resistance in the foreleg of the dog. J Pharmacol Exp Ther 139:290, 1966
76. Schmid PG, Eckstein JW, Abboud FM: Comparison of the effects of several sympathomimetic amines on resistance and capacitance vessels in the forearm of man. Circulation 34:209, 1966
77. Brown BR Jr: Selective venoconstriction by dopamine in comparison with isoproterenol and phenylephrine. Anesthesiology 43:570, 1975
78. Rajfer SI, Goldberg LI: Sympathetic amines in the treatment of shock. In Shoemaker WC, Thompson WL, Holbrook PR (eds); Textbook of Critical Care, p 490. Philadelphia, WB Saunders, 1984
79. Kopin IJ: Metabolic degradation of catecholamines and relative importance of different pathways under physiological conditions and after the administration of drugs. In Blaschko H, Muscholl E (eds): Catecholamines: Handbook of Experimental Pharmacology, p 270. New York, Springer Verlag, 1972
80. Rooke GA, Freund PR, Jacobson AF: Hemodynamic response and change in organ blood volume during spinal anesthesia in elderly men with cardiac disease. Anesth Analg 85:99, 1997
81. Junod AF: Metabolism of vasoactive agents in lung. Am Rev Respir Dis 115:51, 1977
82. Hug CC, Kaplan JA: Pharmacology-cardiac drugs. In Kaplan JA (ed): Cardiac Anesthesia, p 39. New York, Grune & Stratton, 1979
83. Karns JL: Epinephrine-induced potentially lethal arrhythmia during orthoscopic shoulder surgery: A case report. AANA J 67:419, 1999
84. Wood M: Drugs and the sympathetic nervous system. In Wood M, Alistair JJ (eds): Drugs and Anesthesia. p. 407. Baltimore, Williams & Wilkins, 1982
85. Johnston RR, Eger EI, II, Wilson C. A comparative interaction of epinephrine with enflurane, isoflurane, and halothane in man. Anesth Analg 55:709, 1976
86. Karl HW, Swedlow DB, Lee KW, Downes JJ: Epinephrine-halothane interactions in children. Anesthesiology 58:142, 1983
87. Ramanathan S, Grant GJ: Vasopressor therapy for hypotension due to epidural anesthesia for cesarean section. Acta Anaesthesiol Scan 32:559, 1988
88. Tsen LC, Boosalis P, Segal S, Datta S, Bader AM: Hemodynamic effects of simultaneous administration of intravenous ephedrine and spinal anesthesia for cesarean delivery. J Clin Anesth 12:378, 2000
89. Houston MC, Thompson WL, Robertson D: Shock. Diagnosis and management. Arch Intern Med 144:1433, 1984
90. Tarnow J, Komar K: Altered hemodynamic response to dobutamine in relation to the degree of preoperative beta-adrenoceptor blockade. Anesthesiology 68:912, 1988
91. Maekawa K, Liang CS, Hood WB Jr: Comparison of dobutamine and dopamine in acute myocardial infarction. Effects of systemic hemodynamics, plasma catecholamines, blood flows and infarct size. Circulation 67:750, 1983
92. Butterworth JF, Prielipp RC, Royster AL *et al:* Dobutamine increases heart rate more than epinephrine in patients recovering from aortocoronary bypass surgery. J Cardiothorac Vasc Anesth 6:535, 1992
93. Pierard LA, De Landsheere CM, Berthe C, Rigo P, Kulbertus HE: Identification of viable myocardium by echocardiography during dobutamine infusion in patients with myocardial infarction after thrombolytic therapy: comparison with positron emission tomography. J Am Coll Cardiol 15:1021, 1990
94. McGhie AI, Golstein RA: Pathogenesis and management of acute heart failure and cardiogenic shock: Role of inotropic therapy. Chest 102:626S, 1992
95. Goldberg LI: Pharmacological bases for the use of dopamine and related drugs in the treatment of congestive heart failure. J Cardiovasc Pharmacol 14 (suppl 8):S21, 1989
96. Olsen NV, Lund P, Jensen PF *et al:* Dopamine, dobutamine, and dopexamine. A comparison of renal effects in unanesthetized human volunteers. Anesthesiology 79:685, 1993
97. Debaveye YA, Van den Berghe GH: Is there still a place for dopamine in the modern intensive care unit? Anesth Analg 98:461, 2004
98. Murphy MB, Elliott WJ: Dopamine and dopamine receptor agonists in cardiovascular therapy. Crit Care Med 18:S14, 1990
99. Harkine CP, Farber NE: New cardia inotropic drugs, p 461. In Advances in Anesthesiology. St. Louis, Mosby, 1996
100. Lawson N: Therapeutic combinations of vasopressors and inotropic agents. Semin Anesthesiol 9:270, 1990
101. Banic A, Krejci V, Erni D *et al*: Effects of sodium nitroprusside and phenylephrine on blood flow in free musculocutaneous flaps during general anesthesia. Anesthesiology 90:147, 1999
102. Royster RL, Butlerworth JF, Priclipp RC *et al*: Combined inotropic effects of amrinone and epinephrine after cardiopulmonary bypass in humans. Anesth Analg 77:662, 1993
103. el Allaf D, Cremers S, D'Orio V, Carlier J: Combined haemodynamic effects of low doses of dopamine and dobutamine in patients with acute infarction and cardiac failure. Arch Int Physiol Biochim 92:S49, 1984
104. Richard C, Ricome JL, Rimailho A, Bottineau G, Auzepy P: Combined hemodynamic effects of dopamine and dobutamine in cardiogenic shock. Circulation 67:620, 1983
105. Tinker JH: Perioperative myocardial infarction. Semin Anesthesiol 253, 1982
106. Aronson S, Goldberg LI, Roth S *et al*: Preservation of renal blood flow during hypotension induced with fenoldopam in dogs. Can J Anaesth 37:380, 1990
107. Post JB 4th, Frishman WH: Fenoldopam: A new dopamine agonist for the treatment of hypertensive urgencies and emergencies. J Clin Pharmacol 38:2, 1998
108. Kien ND, Moore PG, Jaffe RS: Cardiovascular function during induced hypotension by fenoldopam or sodium nitroprusside in anesthetized dogs. Anesth Analg 74:72, 1992
109. Brooks DP, Drutz DJ, Ruffolo RR Jr: Prevention and complete reversal of cyclosporine A-induced renal vasoconstriction and nephrotoxicity in the rat by fenoldopam. J Pharmacol Exp Ther 254:375, 1990
110. White WB, Radford MJ, Gonzalez FE *et al*: Selective dopamine-1 agonist therapy in severe hypertension: Effects of intravenous fenoldopam. Am J Med 95:161, 1988
111. Lepor NE: A review of pharmacologic interventions to prevent contrast-induced nephropathy. Rev Cardiovasc Med 4 (suppl):S34, 2003
112. Ziegler MG: Antihypertensives. In Chernow B, Lake CR (eds) The Pharmacologic Approach to the Critically Ill Patient, p 303. Baltimore, Williams & Wilkins, 1983
113. Filos KS, Goudas LC, Patroni O, Polyzou V: Hemodynamic and analgesic profile after intrathecal clonidine in humans. A dose-response study. Anesthesiology 81:591, 1994
114. Eisenach JC, De Kock M, Klimscha W: alpha (2)-adrenergic agonists for regional anesthesia. A clinical review of clonidine (1984–1995). Anesthesiology 3:655, 1996
115. Heidemann SM, Sarnaik AP: Clonidine poisoning in children. Crit Care Med 18:618, 1990
116. Payen D, Quintin L, Plaisance P, Chiron B, Lhoste F: Head injury: Clonidine decreases plasma catecholamines. Crit Care Med 18:392, 1990
117. Goyagi T, Nishikawa T: Oral clonidine premedication enhances the quality of postoperative analgesia by intrathecal morphine. Anesth Analg 82:1192, 1996
118. Gold MS, Pottash AC, Sweeney DR, Kleber HD: Opiate withdrawal using clonidine. A safe, effective, and rapid nonopiate treatment. JAMA 243:343, 1980
119. Aantaa R, Kanto J, Scheinin M, Kallio A, Scheinin H: Dexmedetomidine, an alpha 2-adrenoceptor agonist, reduces anesthetic requirements for patients undergoing minor gynecologic surgery. Anesthesiology 73:230, 1990
120. Dyck JB, Maze M, Haack C, Vuorilehto L, Shafer SL: The pharmacokinetics and hemodynamic effects of intravenous and intramuscular dexmedetomidine hydrochloride in adult human volunteers. Anesthesiology 78:813, 1993
121. Hall JE, Uhrich TD, Barney JA, Arain SR, Ebert TJ: Sedative, amnestic and analgesic properties of small-dose dexmedetomidine infusions. Anesth Analg 90:699, 2000
122. Lee CR, Watkins ML, Patterson JH *et al*: Vasopressin: A new target for the treatment of heart failure. Am Heart J 146:9, 2003
123. Wenzel V, Lindner KH: Employing vasopressin during cardiopulmonary resuscitation and vasodilatory shock as a lifesaving vasopressor. Cardiovasc Res 51:529, 2001
124. Lindner KH, Haak T, Keller A, Bothner U, Lurie KG: Release of endogenous vasopressors during and after cardiopulmonary resuscitation. Heart 75:145, 1996
125. Wenzel A, Krismer AC, Amtz HR *et al*: A comparison of vasopressin and epinephrine for out-of-hospital cardiopulmonary resuscitation. N Engl J Med 350:105, 2004
126. Stiell IG, Hebert PC, Wells GA *et al*: Vasopressin versus epinephrine for inhospital cardiac arrest: A randomised controlled trial. Lancet 358:105, 2001
127. Dreifus LS, Hessen SE: Supraventricular tachycardia: Diagnosis and treatment. Cardiology 77:259, 1990
128. Rossi AF, Steinberg LG, Kipel G, Golinko RJ, Griepp RB: Use of adenosine in the management of perioperative arrhythmias in the pediatric cardiac intensive care unit. Crit Care Med 20:1107, 1992

129. Freilich A, Tepper D: Adenosine and its cardiovascular effects. Am Heart J 123:1324, 1992
130. Makabali C, Weil MH, Henning RJ: Dobutamine and other sympathomimetic drugs for the treatment of low cardiac output failure. Seminars in Anesthesia 1:63, 1982
131. Boldt J, Hempelmann G: Phosphodiesteras inhibitors. In Clinical Pharmacology, p 59. London, Baillière Tindall, 1994
132. Conti M, Jin SL, Monaco L, Repaske DR, Swinnen JV: Hormonal regulation of cyclic nucleotide phosphodiesterases. Endocr Rev 12:218, 1991
133. Rutman HI, LeJemtel TH, Sonnenblick EH: Newer cardiotonic agents: Implications for patients with heart failure and ischemic heart disease. J Cardiothorac Anesth 1:59, 1987
134. Levy JH, Bailey JM: Amrinone: pharmacokinetics and pharmacodynamics. J Cardiothorac Anesth 3:10, 1989
135. Pagel PS, Grossman W, Haering JM, Warltier DC: Left ventricular diastolic function in the normal and diseased heart. Perspectives for the anesthesiologist (2). Anesthesiology 79:1104, 1993
136. Pagel PS, Hettrick DA, Warltier DC: Amrinone enhances myocardial contractility and improves left ventricular diastolic function in conscious and anesthetized chronically instrumented dogs. Anesthesiology 79:753, 1993
137. Jhaveri R, Kim S, White AR, Burke S, Berkowitz DE, Nyhan D: Enhanced vasodilatory responses to milrinone in catecholamine-precontracted small pulmonary arteries. Anesth Analg 98:1618, 2004
138. Mollhoff T, Loick HM, Van Aken H *et al*: Milrinone modulates endotoxemia, systemic inflammation, and subsequent acute phase response after cardiopulmonary bypass (CPB). Anesthesiology 90:72, 1999
139. Doolan LA, Jones EF, Kalman J, Buxton BF, Tonkin AM: A placebo-controlled trial verifying the efficacy of milrinone in weaning high-risk patients from cardiopulmonary bypass. J Cardiothorac Vasc Anesth 11:37, 1997
140. Boldt J, Kling D, Moosdorf R, Hempelmann G: Enoximone treatment of impaired myocardial function during cardiac surgery: combined effects with epinephrine. J Cardiothorac Anesth 4:462, 1990
141. Zaloga GP, Chernow B; Insulin, glucagon and growth hormone. In Chernow B, Lake CR (eds): The Pharmacologic Approach to the Critically Ill Patient, p 562. Baltimore, Williams & Wilkins, 1983
142. Stoelting RK: Digitalis and related drugs. In Stoelting RK (ed): Pharmacology and Physiology in Anesthetic Practice, p 269. Philadelphia, JB Lippincott, 1987
143. Montgomery WH, Donegan J, McIntyre K: Standards and guidelines for cardiopulmonary resuscitation and emergency cardiac care. Circulation 74:IV1, 1986
144. White RD, Goldsmith RS, Rodriguez R, Moffitt EA, Pluth JR: Plasma ionic calcium levels following injection of chloride, gluconate, and gluceptate salts of calcium. J Thorac Cardiovasc Surg 71:609, 1976
145. Oshida J, Goto H, Benson KT, Arakawa K: Effects of calcium chloride on verapamil- and diltiazem-pretreated isolated rat hearts. J Cardiothorac Vasc Anesth 7:717, 1993
146. Desai TK, Carlson RW, Thill-Baharozian M, Geheb MA: A direct relationship between ionized calcium and arterial pressure among patients in an intensive care unit. Crit Care Med 16:578, 1988
147. Marquez J, Martin D, Virji MA *et al*: Cardiovascular depression secondary to ionic hypocalcemia during hepatic transplantation in humans. Anesthesiology 65:457, 1986
148. Stoelting RK: Drugs used in treatment of psychiatric disease. In Stoelting RK (ed): Pharmacology and Physiology in Anesthetic Practice, p 347. Philadelphia, JB Lippincott, 1987
149. Wong KC, Ashburn MA: Monoamine oxidase inhibitors and anesthesia. In Literature Scan: Anesthesiology Current Insights, Cedar Knoll, New Jersey, Word Medical Communication, 1990.
150. Bhatara VS, Magnus RD, Paul KL, Preskorn SH: Serotonin syndrome induced by venlafaxine and fluoxetine: A case study in polypharmacy and potential pharmacodynamic and pharmacokinetic mechanisms. Ann Pharmaco 32:432, 1998
151. Catterson ML, Preskorn SH, Martin RL: Pharmacodynamic and pharmoacoinetic considerations in geriatric psychopharmacology. Psychiatric Clinic North America 20:205, 1997
152. Zacny JP, Galinkin JL: Psychotropic drugs used in anesthesia practice. Anesthesiology 90:269, 1999
153. Silke B, Verma SP, Ahuja RC *et al*: Is the intrinsic sympathomimetic activity (ISA) of beta-blocking compounds relevant in acute myocardial infarction? Eur J Clin Pharmacol 27:509, 1984
154. Smith NL, Chan JD, Rea TD, Wiggins KL, Gottdiener JS, Lumley T: Time trends in the use of beta-blockers and other pharmacotherapies in older adults with congestive heart failure. Am Heart J 148:710, 2004
155. Chang LC; Use of practolol in asthmatics: A plea for caution. Lancet 2:321, 1971
156. Woods KL, Wright AD, Kendall MJ, Black E: Lack of effect of propranolol and metoprolol on glucose tolerance in maturity-onset diabetics. Br Med J 281:1321, 1980
157. Slogoff S, Keats AS: Does perioperative myocardial ischemia lead to postoperative myocardial infarction? Anesthesiology 62:107, 1985
158. Wallace A, Layug B, Tateo I *et al*: Prophylactic atenolol reduces postoperative myocardial ischemia. McSPI Research Group. Anesthesiology 88:7, 1998
159. Pratt CM, Young JB, Roberts R: The role of beta-blockers in the treatment of patients after infarction. Cardiol Clin 2:13, 1984
160. Frishman WH: Drug therapy: atenolol and timolol, two new systemic beta-adrenoceptor antagonists. N Engl J Med 306:1456, 1982
161. Menkhaus PG, Reves JG, Kissin I *et al*: Cardiovascular effects of esmolol in anesthetized humans. Anesth Analg 64:327, 1985
162. Steck J, Sheppard D, Byrd R *et al*: Pulmonary effects of esmolol. Clin Res 33:472A, 1985
163. McDevitt DG: Clinical significance of cardioselectivity. Prim Cardio 165:165, 1983
164. de Bruijn NP, Reves JG, Croughwell N, Clements F, Drissel DA: Pharmacokinetics of esmolol in anesthetized patients receiving chronic beta blocker therapy. Anesthesiology 66:323, 1987
165. Jordan D, Shulman SM, Miller ED Jr: Esmolol hydrochloride, sodium nitroprusside, and isoflurane differ in their ability to alter peripheral sympathetic responses. Anesth Analg 77:281, 1993
166. Stoelting RK: Calcium entry blockers. In Stoelting RK (ed): Pharmacology and Physiology in Anesthetic Practice, p 355. Philadelphia, JB Lippincott, 1987
167. Reves JG: The relative hemodynamic effects of Ca++ entry blockers. Anesthesiology 61:3, 1984
168. Kraynack BJ, Lawson NW, Gintautas J: Local anesthetic effect of verapamil in vitro. Reg Anaesth 7:114, 1982
169. Stone PH, Antman EM, Muller JE, Braunwald E: Calcium channel blocking agents in the treatment of cardiovascular disorders. Part II: Hemodynamic effects and clinical applications. Ann Intern Med 93:886, 1980
170. Morad M, Tung L: Ionic events responsible for the cardiac resting and action potential. Am J Cardiol 49:584, 1982
171. Klein HO, Kaplinsky E: Digitalis and verapamil in atrial fibrillation and flutter. Is verapamil now the preferred agent? Drugs 31:185, 1986
172. Clusin WT, Bristow MR, Karagueuzian HS, Katzung BG, Schroeder JS: Do calcium-dependent ionic currents mediate ischemic ventricular fibrillation? Am J Cardiol 49:606, 1982
173. Merin RG: Calcium (slow) channel blocking drugs. American Society of Anesthesiology Annual Refresher Course Lecture 101: 1982
174. Carpenter RL, Mulroy MF: Edrophonium antagonizes combined lidocaine-pancuronium and verapamil-pancuronium neuromuscular blockade in cats. Anesthesiology 65:506, 1986
175. Zalman F, Perloff JK, Durant NN, Campion DS: Acute respiratory failure following intravenous verapamil in Duchenne's muscular dystrophy. Am Heart J 105:510, 1983
176. Roizen MF, Moss J, Muldoon SM: The effects of anesthesia, anesthetic adjuvant drugs, and surgery on plasma norepinephrine. In Ziegler MG, Lake CR (eds): Frontiers of Clinical Neuroscience, p 227. Baltimore: Williams & Wilkins, 1984
177. Price WA, Giannini AJ: Neurotoxicity caused by lithium-verapamil synergism. J Clin Pharmacol 26:717, 1986
178. Holland OB: Diuretic-induced hypokalaemia and ventricular arrhythmias. Drugs 28 (suppl 1):86, 1984
179. McGovern B: Hypokalemia and cardiac arrhythmias. Anesthesiology 63: 127, 1985
180. Maze M, Segal IS, Bloor BC: Clonidine and other alpha2 adrenergic agonists: Strategies for the rational use of these novel anesthetic agents. J Clin Anesth 1:146, 1988
181. Johnston RV, Nicholas DA, Lawson NW, Wallfisch HK, Arens JF: The use of rectal clonidine in the perioperative period. Anesthesiology 64:288, 1986
182. Muzi M, Goff DR, Kampine JP, Roerig DL, Ebert TJ: Clonidine reduces sympathetic activity but maintains baroreflex responses in normotensive humans. Anesthesiology 77:864, 1992
183. Mets B, Miller ED: Angiotensin and angiotensin-converting enzyme inhibitors. In Clinical Pharmacology, p 151. London, Baillière Tindall, 1994
184. Chiariello M, Gold HK, Leinbach RC, Davis MA, Maroko PR: Comparison between the effects of nitroprusside and nitroglycerin on ischemic injury during acute myocardial infarction. Circulation 54:766, 1976
185. Miller EDJ, Ackerly JA, Vaughan EDJ, Peach MJ, Epstein RM: The renin-angiotensin system during controlled hypotension with sodium nitroprusside. Anesthesiology 47:257, 1977
186. Woodside JJ, Garner L, Bedford RF *et al*: Captopril reduces the dose requirement for sodium nitroprusside induced hypotension. Anesthesiology 60:413, 1984
187. Fremes SE, Weisel RD, Mickle DA *et al*: A comparison of nitroglycerin and nitroprusside: II. The effects of volume loading. Ann Thorac Surg 39:61, 1985
188. Hood DD, Dewan DM, James FM, Floyd HM, Bogard TD: The use of nitroglycerin in preventing the hypertensive response to tracheal intubation in severe preeclampsia. Anesthesiology 63:329, 1985
189. Ferguson RK, Vlasses PH: Hypertensive emergencies and urgencies. JAMA 255:1607, 1986
190. Reves JG, Flezzani P: Perioperative use of esmolol. Am J Cardiol 56:57F, 1985

CHAPTER 13 ■ NONOPIOID INTRAVENOUS ANESTHESIA

PAUL F. WHITE AND GLADYS ROMERO

KEY POINTS

1. With the exception of ketamine, intravenous (IV) anesthetics lack analgesic properties.
2. Dexmedetomidine is an α-2 agonist with sedative and opioid-sparing effects.
3. Low doses of IV anesthetics produce sedation, while high doses produce hypnosis (or unconsciousness).
4. All nonopioid IV anesthetics produce dose-dependent central nervous system (CNS) depression.
5. Compared to thiopental and propofol, methohexital produces less CNS depression.
6. Propofol possesses unique antiemetic and appetite-stimulating properties.
7. Etomidate produces less cardiovascular depression than the barbiturates and propofol.
8. Ketamine possesses analgesic and psychomimetic properties.
9. Midazolam possesses amnestic and anxiolytic properties.
10. IV anesthetics in combination with potent opioid analgesics and/or local anesthetics can be used to produce total intravenous anesthesia (TIVA).

The concept of intravenous (IV) anesthesia has evolved from primarily induction of anesthesia to total IV anesthesia (TIVA). TIVA has assumed increasing importance for therapeutic, as well as diagnostic, procedures in both adults and children. This change has been a result of the development of rapid, short-acting IV hypnotic, analgesic, and muscle relaxant drugs; the availability of pharmacokinetic and dynamic-based IV delivery systems; and the development of the electroencephalogram (EEG) base cerebral monitor, which measures the hypnotic component of the anesthetic state. This chapter focuses on the pharmacologic properties and clinical uses of the currently available nonopioid IV anesthetics.

Following its introduction into clinical practice, thiopental quickly became the gold standard of IV anesthetics against which all the newer IV drugs were compared. Many different hypnotic drugs are currently available for use during IV anesthesia (Fig. 13-1). However, the "ideal" IV anesthetic has not yet been developed. The physical and pharmacologic properties that an ideal IV anesthetic would possess include the following:

1. Drug compatibility and stability in solution.
2. Lack of pain on injection, venoirritation, or local tissue damage from extravasation.
3. Low potential to release histamine or precipitate hypersensitivity reactions.
4. Rapid and smooth onset of hypnotic action without excitatory activity.
5. Rapid metabolism to pharmacologically inactive metabolites.
6. A steep dose-response relationship to enhance titratability and minimize accumulation.
7. Lack of acute cardiovascular and respiratory depression.
8. Decreases in cerebral metabolism and intracranial pressure.
9. Rapid and smooth return of consciousness and cognitive skills with residual analgesia.
10. Absence of postoperative nausea and vomiting, amnesia, psychomimetic reactions, dizziness, headache, or prolonged sedation ("hangover").

Despite thiopental's proven clinical usefulness, safety, and widespread acceptance over many decades, it is not the ideal IV anesthetic. The sedative–hypnotic drugs that have been more recently introduced into clinical practice (e.g., midazolam, ketamine, etomidate, propofol) have proven to be extremely valuable in specific clinical situations. These newer compounds combine many of the characteristics of the ideal IV anesthetic but fail in aspects where the other drugs succeed. For some of these IV sedative–hypnotics, disadvantages have led to "restricted" indications (e.g., ketamine, etomidate) or withdrawal

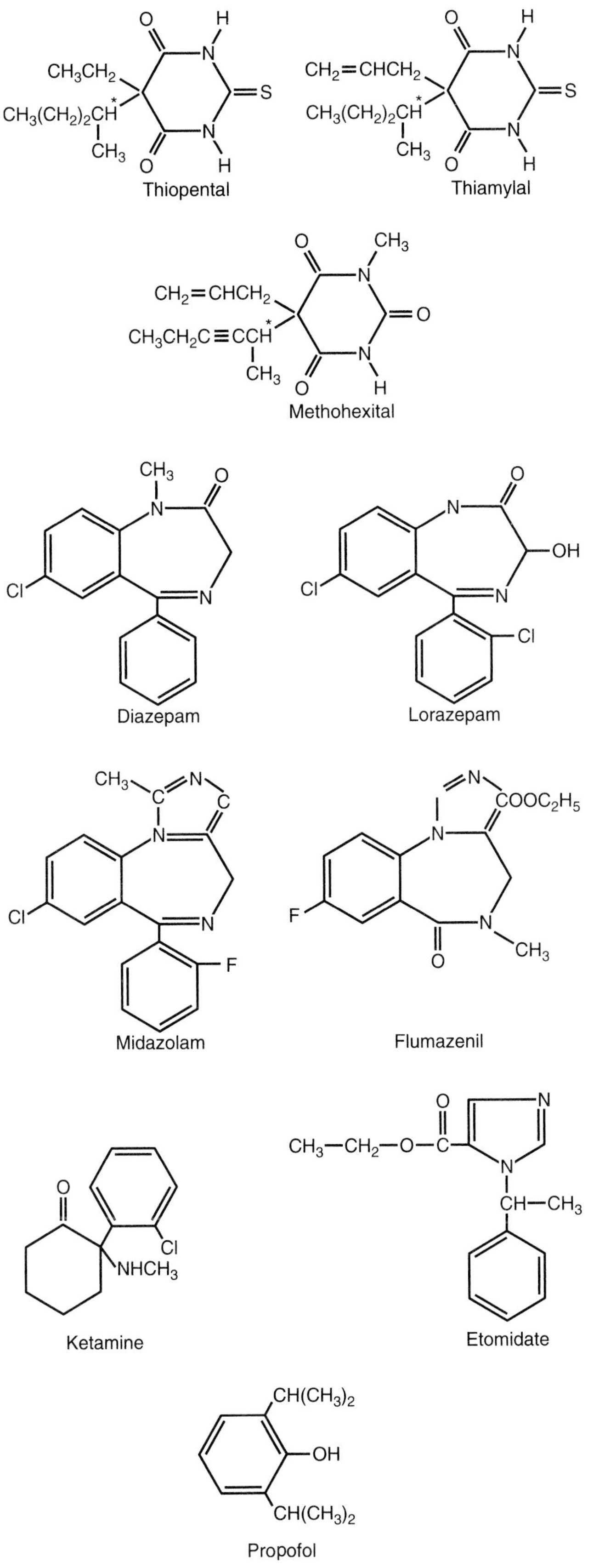

Thiopental

Thiamylal

Methohexital

Diazepam

Lorazepam

Midazolam

Flumazenil

Ketamine

Etomidate

Propofol

FIGURE 13-1. Chemical structures of currently available nonopioid IV anesthetics.

from clinical use (e.g., Althesin, propanidid, eltanolone). Because the optimal pharmacologic properties are not equally important in every clinical situation, the anesthesiologist must make the choice that best fits the needs of the individual patient and the operative procedure.

GENERAL PHARMACOLOGY OF INTRAVENOUS HYPNOTICS

Mechanism of Action

A widely accepted theory of anesthetic action is that both IV and inhalational anesthetics exert their primary sedative and hypnotic effects through an interaction with the inhibitory γ-aminobutyric acid (GABA) neurotransmitter system.[1] GABA is the principal inhibitory neurotransmitter within the CNS. The GABA and adrenergic neurotransmitter systems counterbalance the action of excitatory neurotransmitters. The GABA type A ($GABA_A$) receptor is a receptor complex consisting of up to five glycoprotein subunits. When the $GABA_A$ receptor is activated, transmembrane chloride conductance increases, resulting in hyperpolarization of the postsynaptic cell membrane and functional inhibition of the postsynaptic neuron. Sedative–hypnotic drugs interact with different components of the GABA-receptor complex (Fig. 13-2). However, the allosteric (structural) requirements for activation of the receptor are different for IV and volatile anesthetics.[2]

Benzodiazepines bind to specific receptor sites that are part of the $GABA_A$-receptor complex. The binding of benzodiazepines to their receptor site increases the efficiency of the coupling between the GABA receptor and the chloride ion channel. The degree of modulation of the GABA-receptor function is limited, which explains the "ceiling effect" produced by benzodiazepines with respect to CNS depression. The CNS properties of benzodiazepines (e.g., hypnosis, sedation, anxiolysis, and anticonvulsant effects) are presumed to be associated with stimulation of different receptor subtypes and/or concentration-dependent receptor occupancy. It has been suggested that a benzodiazepine receptor occupancy of 20% provides anxiolysis, while 30 to 50% receptor occupancy is associated with sedation, and 60% receptor occupancy is required for hypnosis (or unconsciousness).

The interaction of barbiturates and propofol with specific membrane structures appears to decrease the rate of dissociation of GABA from its receptor, thereby increasing the duration of the GABA-activated opening of the chloride ion channel (Fig. 13-2). Barbiturates can also mimic the action of GABA by directly activating the chloride channels. The proposed mechanism of action of thiopental relates to its ability to function as a competitive inhibitor at the nicotic acetytcholine receptors (AChRs) in the CNS.[3] Etomidate augments GABA-gated chloride currents (i.e., indirect modulation) and at higher concentrations evokes chloride currents in the absence of GABA (i.e., direct activation). Although the mechanism of action of propofol is similar to that of the barbiturates (i.e., enhancing the activity of the GABA-activated chloride channel), it also possesses ion channel–blocking effects in cerebral cortex tissue and nicotinic acetylcholine receptors, as well as an inhibitory effect on lysophosphatidate signaling in lipid mediator receptors.[4]

Ketamine produces a functional dissociation between the thalamocortical and limbic systems, a state that has been termed "dissociative" anesthesia. Ketamine depresses neuronal function in the cerebral cortex and thalamus, while simultane-
1 ously activating the limbic system. Ketamine's effect on the medial medullary reticular formation may be involved in the affective component of its nociceptive activity. The CNS effects of ketamine appear to be primarily related to its antagonistic

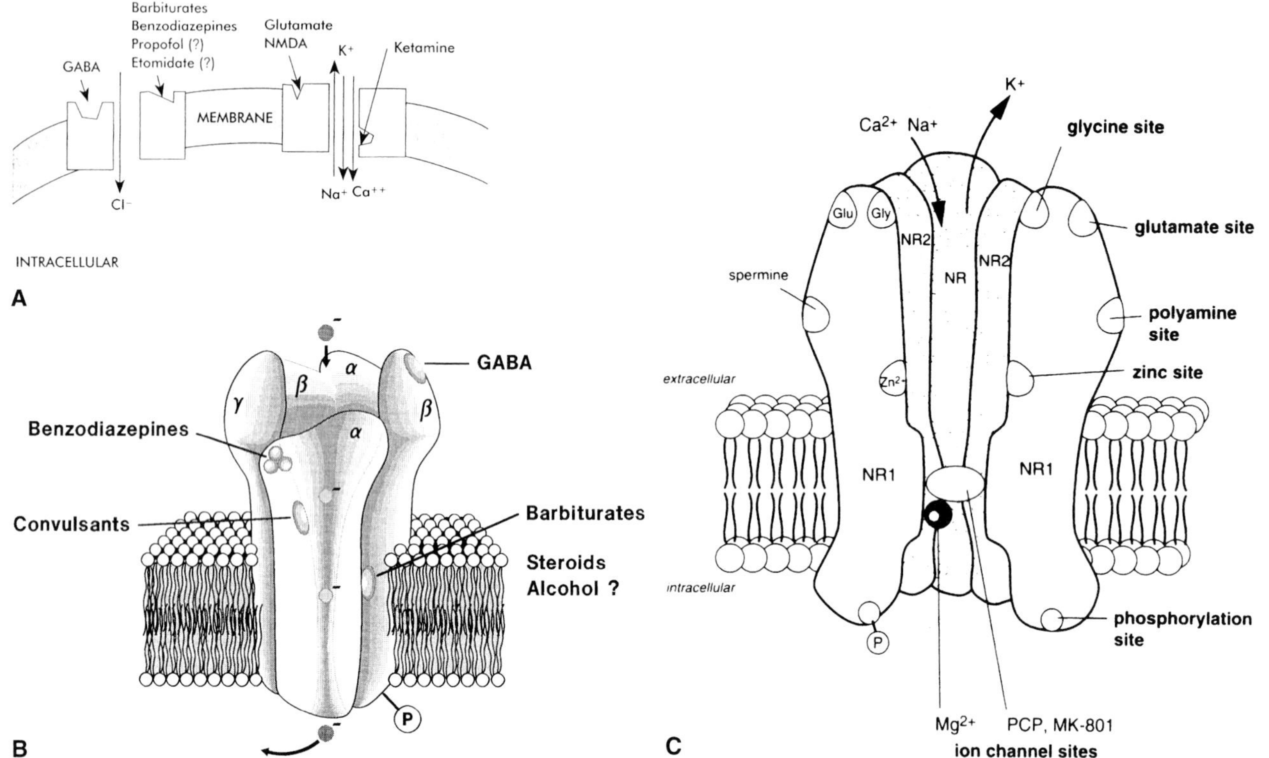

FIGURE 13-2. A. This model depicts the postsynaptic site of GABA and glutamate within the CNS. GABA decreases the excitability of neurons by its action at the $GABA_A$-receptor complex. When GABA occupies the binding site of this complex, it allows inward flux of chloride ion, resulting in hyperpolarizing of the cell and subsequent resistance of the neuron to stimulation by excitatory transmitters. Barbiturates, benzodiazepines, propofol, and etomidate decrease neuronal excitability by enhancing the effect of GABA at this complex, facilitating this inhibitory effect on the postsynaptic cell. Glutamate and its analog N-methyl-D-aspartate (NMDA) are excitatory amino acids. When glutamate occupies the binding site on the NMDA subtype of the glutamate receptor, the channel opens and allows Na^+, K^+, and Ca^{2+} to either enter or leave the cell. Flux of these ions leads to depolarization of the postsynaptic neuron and initiation of an action potential and activation of other pathways. Ketamine blocks this open channel and prevents further ion flux, thus inhibiting the excitatory response to glutamate. (Reprinted with permission from Van Hemelrijck J, Gonzales JM, White PF: Use of intravenous sedative agents. In Rogers MC, Tinker JH, Covino BG, Longnecker DE (eds): Principles and Practice of Anesthesiology, p 1131. St. Louis, Mosby, 1992.) B. Schematic model of the $GABA_A$-receptor complex illustrating recognition sites for many of the substances that bind to the receptor. C. Model of the NMDA receptor showing sites for antagonist action. Ketamine binds to the site labeled PCP (phencyclidine). The pentameric structure of the receptor, composed of a combination of the subunits NR 1 and NR 2, is illustrated. (Altered with permission from Leeson TD, Iversen LL. The glycine site on the NMDA receptor: Structure-activity relationships and therapeutic potential. J Med Chem 37:4054, 1994.)

activity at the *N*-methyl-D-aspartate (NMDA) receptor (Fig. 13-2). Unlike the other IV anesthetics, ketamine does not interact with GABA receptors; however, it binds to non-NMDA glutamate receptors and nicotinic, muscarinic, monoaminergic, and opioid receptors. In addition, it also inhibits neuronal sodium channels (producing a modest local anesthetic action) and calcium channels (causing cerebral vasodilatation).

2 The centrally active α-2 adrenergic receptor agonist, dexmedetomidine, has potent sedative and analgesic-sparing properties. The drug also has effects on the perioperal α-2 receptors involved in regulating the cardiovascular system by inhibiting norepinephrine release. This class of anesthetic drugs can also reduce the tonic levels of sympathetic outflow from the CNS and augment cardiac vagal activity.[5,6]

Pharmacokinetics and Metabolism

An understanding of basic pharmacokinetic principles is integral to the understanding the pharmacologic actions and interactions of IV anesthetic and adjunctive drugs and will allow the anesthesiologist to develop more optimal dosing strategies when using IV techniques. Although lipid solubility facilitates diffusion of IV anesthetics across cellular membranes including the blood–brain barrier, only the nonionized form is able to readily cross neuronal membranes. The ratio of the un-ionized-to-ionized fraction depends on the pKa of the drug and the pH of the body fluids.

The rapid onset of the CNS effect of most IV anesthetics can be explained by their high lipid solubility and the relatively high proportion of the cardiac output (20%) perfusing the brain. However, a variable degree of hysteresis exists between the blood concentration of the hypnotic drug and its onset of action on the CNS. The hysteresis is related in part to diffusion of these drugs into brain tissue and nonspecific CNS receptor binding. However, the number of CNS binding sites is usually saturable and only a small fraction of the available binding sites needs to be occupied to produce clinical effects. Although the total amount of drug in the blood is available for diffusion, the diffusion rate will be more limited for IV anesthetics with

TABLE 13-1

PHARMACOKINETIC VALUES FOR THE CURRENTLY AVAILABLE INTRAVENOUS SEDATIVE–HYPNOTIC DRUGS

■ DRUG NAME	■ DISTRIBUTION HALF-LIFE (min)	■ PROTEIN BINDING (%)	■ DISTRIBUTION VOLUME AT STEADY STATE (L/kg)	■ CLEARANCE (mL/kg/min)	■ ELIMINATION HALF-LIFE (h)
Thiopental	2–4	85	2.5	3.4	11
Methohexital	5–6	85	2.2	11	4
Propofol	2–4	98	2–10	20–30	4–23
Midazolam	7–15	94	1.1–1.7	6.4–11	1.7–2.6
Diazepam	10–15	98	0.7–1.7	0.2–0.5	20–50
Lorazepam	3–10	98	0.8–1.3	0.8–1.8	11–22
Etomidate	2–4	75	2.5–4.5	18–25	2.9–5.3
Ketamine	11–16	12	2.5–3.5	12–17	2–4

a high degree of plasma protein binding (90%) because only the "free" unbound drug can diffuse across membranes and exert central effects. When several drugs compete for the same binding sites, or when the protein concentration in the blood is decreased by preexisting disease (e.g., hepatic failure), a higher fraction of the unbound drug will be available to exert an effect on the CNS. Since only unbound drug is available for uptake and metabolism in the liver, highly protein-bound drugs may have a lower rate of hepatic metabolism as a result of their decreased hepatic extraction ratio (i.e., the fraction of the hepatic blood flow that is cleared of the drug).

The pharmacokinetics of IV hypnotics are characterized by rapid distribution and subsequent redistribution into several hypothetical compartments, followed by elimination (Table 13-1). The initial pharmacologic effects are related to the activity of the drug in the central compartment. The primary mechanism for terminating the central effects of IV anesthetics administered for induction of anesthesia is redistribution from the central highly perfused compartment (brain) to the larger but less well perfused "peripheral" compartments (muscle, fat). Even for drugs with a high hepatic extraction ratio, elimination does not usually play a major role in terminating the drug's CNS effects because elimination of the drug can only occur from the central compartment. The rate of elimination from the central compartment, the amount of drug present in the peripheral compartments, and the rate of redistribution from the peripheral compartments "back" into the central compartment determine the time necessary to eliminate the drug from the body.

Most IV anesthetic agents are eliminated via hepatic metabolism followed by renal excretion of more water-soluble metabolites. Some metabolites have pharmacologic activity and can produce prolonged drug effects (e.g., oxazepam, desmethyldiazepam, norketamine). Moreover, there is considerable interpatient variability in the clearance rates for commonly used IV anesthetic drugs. The elimination clearance is the distribution volume cleared of drug over time and is a measure of the efficacy of the elimination process. The slow elimination of some anesthetics is due in part to their high degree of protein binding that reduces their hepatic extraction ratio. Other drugs may have a high hepatic extraction ratio and elimination clearance despite extensive plasma protein binding (e.g., propofol), indicating that protein binding is not always a rate limiting factor.

For most drugs, the hepatic enzyme systems are not saturated at clinically relevant drug concentrations, and the rate of drug elimination will decrease as an exponential function of the drug's plasma concentration (first-order kinetics). However, when high steady-state plasma concentrations are achieved with prolonged infusions, hepatic enzyme systems can become saturated and the elimination rate becomes independent of the drug concentration (zero-order kinetics). The elimination half-life ($t_{1/2}\beta$) is the time required for the anesthetic concentration to decrease by 50% during the terminal phase of the plasma decay curve. The $t_{1/2}\beta$ is dependent on the volume to be cleared (the distribution volume) and the efficiency of the metabolic clearance system. Because their volumes of distribution are similar, the wide variation in elimination half-life values for the IV anesthetics is a reflection of differences in their clearance values.

When a drug infusion is administered without a loading dose, 3 to 5 times the $t_{1/2}\beta$ value may be required to reach a "steady-state" plasma concentration. The steady-state concentration obtained during an anesthetic infusion depends on the rate of drug administration and its clearance rate. When an infusion is discontinued, the rate at which the plasma concentration decreases is largely dependent on the clearance rate (as reflected by the terminal elimination half-life value). For drugs with shorter elimination half-lives, plasma concentration will decrease at a rate that allows for a more rapid recovery (e.g., propofol). Drugs with long elimination half-life values (e.g., thiopental and diazepam) are usually only administered by continuous IV infusion when the medical condition requires long-term treatment (e.g., elevated intracranial pressure [ICP] as a result of brain injury or prolonged sedation in the ICU because of respiratory failure).

3 Careful titration of an anesthetic drug to achieve the desired clinical effect is necessary to avoid drug accumulation and the resultant prolonged CNS effects after the infusion has been discontinued. Although the value of the terminal half-life indicates how fast a drug is eliminated from the body, a more useful indicator of the acceptability of a hypnotic infusion for maintenance of anesthesia or sedation is the context-sensitive half-time, a value derived from computer simulations of drug infusions.[7] The context-sensitive half-time is defined as the time necessary for the effect-compartment (i.e., effect site) concentration to decrease by 50% in relation to the duration of the infusion. The context-sensitive half-time becomes particularly important in determining recovery after prolonged infusions of sedative–hypnotic drugs. Drugs (e.g., propofol) may have a relatively short context-sensitive half-time despite the fact that a large amount of drug remains present in the "deep" (less well perfused) compartment. The slow return of the anesthetic from the deep compartment contributes little to the concentration of drug in the central compartment from which it is rapidly cleared. Therefore, the concentration in the central compartment rapidly declines below the hypnotic threshold after discontinuation of the infusion, contributing to short emergence times despite the fact that a substantial quantity of anesthetic drug may remain in the body.

Marked interpatient variability exists in the pharmacokinetics of IV sedative–hypnotic drugs. Factors that can influence anesthetic drug disposition include the degree of protein binding, the efficiency of hepatic and renal elimination processes, physiologic changes with aging, preexisting disease states, the operative site, body temperature, and drug interactions (e.g., coadministration of volatile anesthetics). For example, increased age, lean body (muscle) mass and total body water decrease, results in an increase in the steady-state volume of distribution of most IV anesthetics. The increased distribution volume and decreased hepatic clearance leads to a prolongation of their $t_{1/2}\beta$ values. Moreover, a decrease of the volume of the central compartment may result in higher initial drug concentrations and can at least partially explain the decreased induction requirement in the elderly. Additionally, the slower redistribution from the vessel-rich tissues to intermediate compartments (muscles) also contributes to the age-related decrease in the induction dose requirements.[7] Although prolongation of the elimination half-time does not provide an explanation for the decreased induction dose requirement, it is responsible for producing higher steady-state plasma concentrations at any given infusion rate.

The hepatic clearance of IV anesthetics with a high (e.g., etomidate, propofol, ketamine) or intermediate (e.g., methohexital, midazolam) extraction ratio is largely dependent on hepatic blood flow, with most of the drug being removed from the blood as it flows through the liver (so-called perfusion-limited clearance). The elimination rate of drugs with low hepatic extraction ratios (e.g., thiopental, diazepam, lorazepam) is dependent on the enzymatic activity of the liver and is less dependent of hepatic blood flow (so-called capacity-limited clearance). Hepatic blood flow decreases during upper abdominal surgery and, as a result, higher blood levels of drugs with perfusion-limited clearance are achieved at any given infusion rate. With aging, a decreased cardiac output and a redistribution of blood flow can partly explain the lower clearance rate for drugs with perfusion-limited clearance. While concomitant administration of volatile anesthetics (which are known to decrease liver blood flow) has little influence on the elimination of thiopental, they can decrease the clearance of etomidate, ketamine, methohexital, and propofol. Other factors that decrease hepatic blood flow include hypocapnia, congestive heart failure, intravascular volume depletion, circulatory collapse, β-adrenergic blockade, and norepinephrine administration.

Hepatic disease can influence the pharmacokinetics of drugs by: (1) altering the plasma protein content and changing the degree of protein binding, (2) decreasing hepatic blood flow and producing intrahepatic shunting, and (3) depressing the metabolic enzymatic activity of the liver. Therefore, the influence of hepatic disease on pharmacokinetics and dynamics of IV anesthetics is difficult to predict. Renal disease can also alter the concentration of plasma and tissue proteins, as well as the degree of protein binding, thereby producing changes in free drug concentrations. Because IV anesthetic agents are primarily metabolized by the liver, renal insufficiency has little influence on their rate of metabolic inactivation or elimination of the primary compound.

Pharmacodynamic Effects

4 The principal pharmacologic effect of IV anesthetics is to produce progressively increasing sedation and ultimately hypnosis as a result of dose-dependent CNS depression. However, all sedative–hypnotics also directly or indirectly affect other major organ systems. The relationship between the dose of a sedative–hypnotic and its CNS effects can be defined by dose-response curves. Although most IV anesthetics are characterized by steep dose-response curves, they are not always parallel (Fig. 13-3). The characteristics of a dose-response curve can only be interpreted in relation to the specific response for which it was constructed.

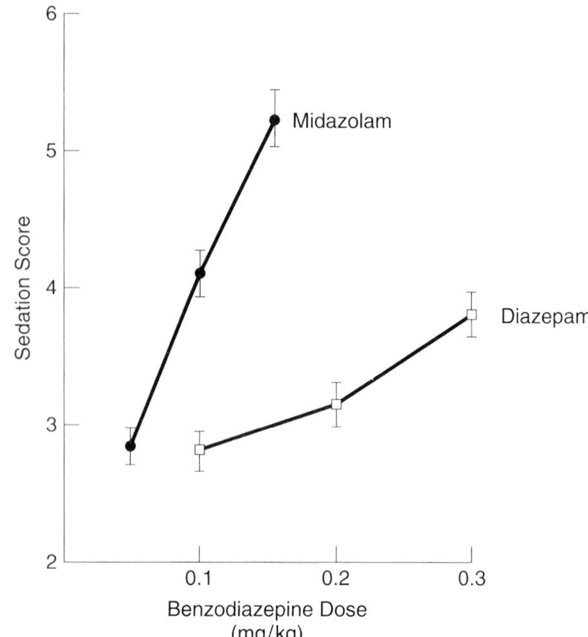

FIGURE 13-3. Dose-response relationships for sedation with midazolam (•) and diazepam (□). The level of sedation (2 = awake and alert to 6 = asleep and unarousable) was assessed 5 minutes after bolus doses of midazolam (0.05, 0.1, or 0.15 mg/kg) or diazepam (0.1, 0.2, or 0.3 mg/kg). Values represent mean values ± SEM. (Reprinted with permission from White PF, Vascones LO, Mathes SA, et al: Comparison of midazolam and diazepam for sedation during plastic surgery. J Plast Reconstruct Surg 81:703, 1988.)

When steady-state plasma concentrations are achieved, it can be presumed that the plasma concentration is in quasi-equilibrium with the effect-site concentration. Under these circumstances, it is possible to describe the relationship between drug and effect using a concentration-effect curve (Fig. 13-4). Because of the pharmacodynamic variability that exists among individuals, the plasma drug concentration necessary to obtain a particular effect is often described in terms of an effective concentration range, the so-called therapeutic window. Efficacy of an IV anesthetic relates to the maximum effect that can be achieved with respect to some measure of CNS function. Depending on the drug effect under consideration, the efficacy of sedative–hypnotics may appear to be less than 100%. For example, it is virtually impossible to produce a burst-suppressive EEG pattern with a benzodiazepine. Potency, on the other hand, relates to the quantity of drug necessary to obtain the maximum CNS effect. The relative potency of sedative–hypnotics also varies depending on the end point chosen. In the presence of an antagonist drug (e.g., flumazenil), the maximal response that can be obtained with a benzodiazepine agonist is further reduced because of competition for the same CNS receptor binding sites.

The influence of sedative–hypnotics on cerebral metabolism, cerebral hemodynamics, and ICP is of particular importance during neuroanesthesia. In patients with reduced cerebral compliance, a small increase in cerebral blood volume can cause a life-threatening increase in ICP. Most sedative–hypnotic drugs cause a proportional reduction in cerebral metabolism ($CMRO_2$) and cerebral blood flow (CBF), resulting in a decrease in ICP. Although a decrease in $CMRO_2$ probably provides only a modest degree of protection against

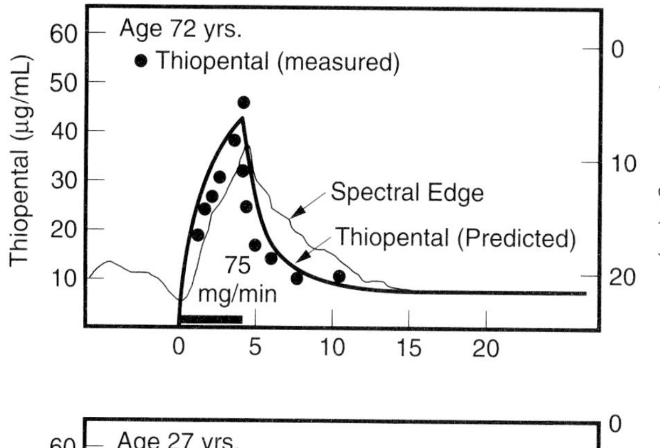

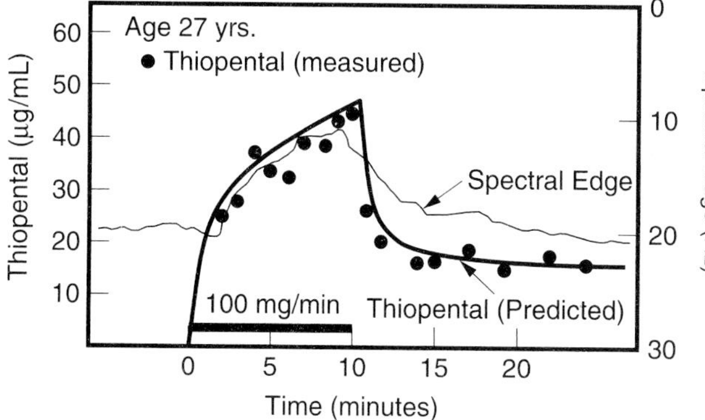

FIGURE 13-4. The concentration of thiopental versus time and spectral edge in an elderly patient (**top**) and in a younger patient (**bottom**). Solid horizontal bars represent the length of thiopental infusion. Filled circles represent the measured thiopental concentration (linear scale), and the solid line next to them represents the fitted data from the pharmacokinetic model. The axis for spectral edge has been inverted for visual clarity. (Reprinted with permission from Homer TD, Stanski DR: The effect of increasing age on thiopental disposition and anesthetic requirement. Anesthesiology 62:714, 1985.)

CNS ischemia or hypoxia, some hypnotics appear to possess cerebroprotective potential. Explanations for the alleged neuroprotective effects of these compounds include a biochemical role as free-radical scavengers and membrane stabilizers (barbiturates and propofol) or NMDA-receptor antagonists (ketamine). With the exception of ketamine, all sedative–hypnotics also lower intraocular pressure (IOP). The changes in IOP generally reflect the effects of the IV agent on systemic arterial pressure and intracranial hemodynamics. However, none of the available sedative–hypnotic drugs protect against the transient increase in IOP that occurs with laryngoscopy and intubation.

Most IV hypnotics have similar EEG effects. Activation of high-frequency EEG activity (15 to 30 Hz) is characteristic of low concentrations (so-called sedative doses) of IV anesthetics. At higher concentrations, an increase in the relative contribution of the lower frequency higher amplitude waves is observed. At high concentrations, a burst-suppressive pattern develops with an increase in the isoelectric periods. Most sedative–hypnotic drugs have been reported to cause occasional EEG seizure-like activity. Interestingly, the same drugs also possess anticonvulsant properties.[8] When considering possible epileptogenic properties of CNS-depressant drugs, it is important to differentiate between true epileptogenic activity (e.g., methohexital) and myoclonic-like phenomena (e.g., etomidate). Myoclonic activity is generally considered to be the result of an imbalance between excitatory and inhibitory subcortical centers, produced by an unequal degree of suppression of these brain centers by low concentrations of hypnotic drugs. Epileptic activity refers to a sudden alteration in CNS seizure-like activity resulting from a high voltage electrical discharge at either cortical or subcortical sites, with subsequent spreading to the thalamic and brainstem centers. As a result of its vasoconstrictive effects on the cerebral vasculature, propofol may be useful for treatment of intractable migraine headaches.[9]

Although some induction drugs can increase airway sensitivity, coughing and airway irritation (e.g., bronchospasm) are usually a result of manipulation of the airway during "light" levels of anesthesia rather than to a direct drug effect. With the exception of ketamine (and to a lesser extent etomidate), IV anesthetics produce dose-dependent respiratory depression, which is enhanced in patients with chronic obstructive pulmonary disease. The respiratory depression is characterized by a decrease in tidal volume and minute ventilation, as well as a transient rightward shift in the CO_2 response curve. Following the rapid injection of a large bolus dose of an IV anesthetic, transient apnea lasting 30 to 90 seconds is usually produced. Ketamine causes minimal respiratory depression when administered in the usual induction doses, while etomidate is associated with less respiratory depressant effects than the barbiturate compounds or propofol. Preliminary experience has demonstrated that dexmedetomidine has minimal depressant effects on respiratory function.[10]

Many different factors contribute to the hemodynamic changes associated with IV induction of anesthesia, including the patient's preexisting cardiovascular and fluid status, resting sympathetic nervous system tone, chronic cardiovascular drugs, preanesthetic medication, the speed of drug injection, and the onset of unconsciousness. In addition, cardiovascular changes can be attributed to the direct pharmacologic actions of anesthetic and analgesic drugs on the heart and peripheral vasculature. Intravenous anesthetics can depress the CNS and peripheral nervous system responses, blunt the compensatory baroreceptor reflex mechanisms, produce direct myocardial depression, and lower peripheral vascular resistance (and/or dilate venous capacitance vessels), thereby decreasing venous return. Profound hemodynamic effects occur at induction in the presence of hypovolemia because a higher than expected drug concentration is achieved in the central compartment. Not surprisingly, the acute cardiocirculatory depressant effects of all IV anesthetics are accentuated in the elderly, as well as in the presence of preexisting cardiovascular disease (e.g., hypertension).

The sympatholytic effects of dexmedetomidine may be useful for producing controlled hypotension.[10] The effects of IV anesthetics on neuroendocrine function are also influenced by the surgical stimuli. Although IV anesthetics are alleged to increase antidiuretic hormone (vasopressin) secretion, it is probably secondary to the surgical stress. Increases in this stress hormone can result in increased peripheral vascular resistance and a reduction of urine output. Similarly, glucose tolerance appears to be decreased by surgical stress, resulting in elevations in the glucose concentration. Most IV sedative–hypnotic drugs lack intrinsic analgesic activity. In fact, thiopental has been alleged to possess so-called antianalgesic activity (i.e., appearing to lower the pain threshold). In contrast to the other drugs in this class, ketamine, and dexmedetomidine, appears to possess analgesic-like activity.

Hypersensitivity (Allergic) Reactions

Allergic reactions to IV anesthetics are rare but can be severe and even life threatening. Intravenous drug administration bypasses the normal "protective barriers" against entrance of foreign molecules into the body. With the exception of etomidate, all IV induction agents have been alleged to cause some histamine release. However, the incidence of severe anaphylactic reactions is extremely low with the currently available IV induction agents. The high frequency of allergic reactions to the cremophor EL–containing formulations led to the early withdrawal of several IV anesthetics containing this solubilizing agent (e.g., propofol EL, propanidid, Althesin). The possible mechanisms for immunologic reactions include: (1) direct action on mast cells, (2) classic complement activation after previous exposure and antibody formation, (3) complement activation through the alternative pathway without previous antigen exposure, (4) antigen–antibody reactions, and (5) the "mixed type" of anaphylactoid reactions.

Severe anaphylactic reactions to IV anesthetics are extremely uncommon; however, profound hypotension attributed to nonimmunologically mediated histamine release has been reported with thiopental use. Although anaphylactic reactions to etomidate have been reported, it does not appear to release histamine and is considered to be the most "immunologically safe" IV anesthetic. While propofol does not normally trigger histamine release, life-threatening anaphylactoid reactions have been reported in patients with a previous history of multiple drug allergies. Barbiturates can also precipitate episodes of acute intermittent porphyria (AIP) and their use is contraindicated in patients who are predisposed to AIP. Although benzodiazepines, ketamine, and etomidate are reported to be safe in humans, these drugs have been shown to be porphyrogenic in animal models.

COMPARATIVE PHYSICO-CHEMICAL AND CLINICAL PHARMACOLOGIC PROPERTIES

Barbiturates

The most commonly used barbiturates are thiopental (5-ethyl-5-[1-methylbutyl]-2-thiobarbituric acid), methohexital (1-methyl-5-allyl-5-[1-methyl-2-pentynyl] barbituric acid), and thiamylal (5-allyl-5-[1-methylbutyl]-2-thiobarbituric acid). Thiopental (Pentothal) and thiamylal (Surital) are thiobarbiturates, while methohexital (Brevital) is an oxybarbiturate. Thiamylal is slightly more potent than thiopental but has a similar pharmacologic profile. Although the l-isomers of thiopental and thyamylal are twice as potent as the D-isomers, both hypnotics are commercially available as racemic mixtures. Because methohexital has two asymmetric centers, it has four stereoisomers. The β-l-isomer is 4 to 5 times more potent than the α-l-isomer, but it produces excessive motor responses. Therefore, methohexital is marketed as the racemic mixture of the two α-isomers.

All three barbiturates are available as sodium salts and must be dissolved in isotonic sodium chloride (0.9%) or water to prepare solutions of 2.5% thiopental, 1 to 2% methohexital, and 2% thiamylal. If refrigerated, solutions of the thiobarbiturates are stable for up to 2 weeks. Solutions of methohexital are stable for up to 6 weeks. When barbiturates are added to Ringer's lactate or an acidic solution containing other water-soluble drugs, precipitation will occur and can occlude the IV catheter. Although the typical solution of thiopental (2.5%) is highly alkaline (pH 9) and can be irritating to the tissues if injected extravenously, it does not cause pain on injection and venoirritation is rare. In contrast, a 1% methohexital solution frequently causes discomfort when injected into small veins. Intra-arterial injection of thiobarbiturates is a serious complication as crystals can form in the arterioles and capillaries, causing intense vasoconstriction, thrombosis, and even tissue necrosis. Accidental intra-arterial injections should be treated promptly with intra-arterial administration of papaverine and lidocaine (or procaine), as well as a regional anesthesia-induced sympathectomy (stellate ganglion block, brachial plexus block) and heparinization.

Thiopental is metabolized in the liver to hydroxythiopental and the carboxylic acid derivative, which are more water soluble and have little CNS activity. When high doses of thiopental are administered, a desulfuration reaction can occur with the production of pentobarbital, which has long-lasting CNS-depressant activity. The low elimination clearance of thiopental (3.4 mL/kg/min) contributes to a long elimination half-life ($t_{1/2}\beta$ of 12 h). Preexisting hepatic and renal disease results in decreased plasma protein binding, thereby increasing the free fraction of thiopental and enhancing its CNS and cardiovascular-depressant properties. During prolonged continuous administration of thiopental, the concentration in the tissues approaches the concentration in the central compartment, with termination of its CNS effects be-
5 coming solely dependent on elimination by nonlinear hepatic metabolism. Methohexital is metabolized in the liver to inactive hydroxyderivatives. The clearance of methohexital (11 mL/kg/min) is higher and more dependent on hepatic blood flow than thiopental, resulting in a shorter elimination half-life ($t_{1/2}\beta$ 3–6 h).

The usual induction dose of thiopental is 3 to 5 mg/kg in adults, 5 to 6 mg/kg in children, and 6 to 8 mg/kg in infants. Because methohexital is approximately 2.7 times more potent than thiopental, a dose of 1.5 mg/kg is equivalent to 4 mg/kg of thiopental in adults. The dose of barbiturates necessary to induce anesthesia is reduced in premedicated patients, patients in early pregnancy (7 to 13 weeks' gestation), and those of more advanced ASA (American Society of Anesthesiologists) physical status (III or IV). Geriatric patients require a 30 to 40% reduction in the usual adult dose because of a decrease of the volume of the central compartment and slowed redistribution of thiopental from the vessel-rich tissues to lean muscle.[11] When the calculation of the induction dose is based on the lean body mass rather than total body weight, dosage adjustments for age, sex, or obesity are not necessary. Thiopental infusion is seldom used to maintain anesthesia because of the long context-sensitive half-time and prolonged recovery period. Plasma thiopental levels necessary to maintain a hypnotic state range between 10 and 20 mg/mL. A typical infusion rate necessary to treat intracranial hypertension or intractable convulsions is 2 to 4 mg/kg/h. The plasma concentration of methohexital needed to maintain hypnosis during anesthesia ranges between 3 and 5 mg/mL and can be achieved with an infusion rate of 50 to 120 mg/kg/min.

Barbiturates produce a proportional decrease in $CMRO_2$ and CBF, thereby lowering ICP. The maximal decrease in $CMRO_2$ (55%) occurs when the EEG becomes isoelectric (burst-suppressive pattern). An isoelectric EEG can be maintained with a thiopental infusion rate of 4 to 6 mg/kg/h (resulting in plasma concentrations of 30 to 50 mg/mL). Because the decrease in systemic arterial pressure is usually less than the reduction in ICP, thiopental should improve cerebral perfusion and compliance. Therefore, thiopental is widely used to improve brain relaxation during neurosurgery and to improve cerebral perfusion pressure (CPP) after acute brain injury. Although barbiturate therapy is widely used to control ICP after brain injury, the results of outcome studies are no better than with other aggressive forms of cerebral antihypertensive therapy.

It has been suggested that barbiturates also possess "neuroprotective" properties secondary to their ability to decrease oxygen demand. Alternative explanations have been suggested, including a reverse steal ("Robin Hood effect") on CBF, free-radical scavenging, stabilization of liposomal membranes, as well as excitatory amino acid (EAA) receptor blockade. Based on evidence from experimental studies and a large randomized prospective multiinstitutional study,[12] it has been concluded that barbiturates have no place in the therapy following resuscitation of a cardiac arrest patient. In contrast, barbiturates are frequently used for cerebroprotection during incomplete brain ischemia (e.g., carotid endarterectomy, temporary occlusion of cerebral arteries, profound hypotension, and cardiopulmonary bypass). By improving the brain's tolerance of incomplete ischemia in patients undergoing open heart surgery with cardiopulmonary bypass, barbiturates are alleged to decrease the incidence of postbypass neuropsychiatric disorders.[13] However, during valvular open heart cardiac surgery, a protective effect of barbiturate loading could not be demonstrated.[14] The routine use of barbiturates during cardiac surgery is not recommended because recent evidence would suggest that the use of moderate degrees of hypothermia (33 to 34°C) may provide superior neuroprotection without prolonging recovery.

Barbiturates cause predictable, dose-dependent EEG changes and possess potent anticonvulsant activity. Continuous infusions of thiopental have been used to treat refractory status epilepticus. However, low doses of thiopental may induce spike wave activity in epileptic patients. Methohexital has well-established epileptogenic effects in patients with psychomotor epilepsy. Low-dose methohexital infusions are frequently used to activate cortical EEG seizure discharges in patients with temporal lobe epilepsy. It is also the IV anesthetic of choice for electroconvulsive therapy.[15] Since the frequency of epileptiform EEG activity during induction of anesthesia with methohexital is significantly less than that which occurs during normal periods of sleep in epileptic patients, this suggests that higher doses of methohexital produces anticonvulsant activity. Methohexital also causes myoclonic-like muscle tremors and other signs of excitatory activity (e.g., hiccoughing).

Barbiturates cause dose-dependent respiratory depression.[16] However, bronchospasm or laryngospasm following induction with thiopental is usually the result of airway manipulation in "lightly" anesthetized patients. Laryngeal reflexes appear to be more active after induction with thiopental than with propofol. The cardiovascular effects of thiopental and methohexital include decreases in cardiac output, systemic arterial pressure, and peripheral vascular resistance. The depressant effects of thiopental on cardiac output are primarily a result of a decrease in venous return caused by peripheral pooling, as well as a result of a direct myocardial depressant effect, which assumes increasing importance in the presence of hypovolemia and myocardial disease.[17] Use of appropriate doses can minimize the cardiodepressant effects of thiopental, even in infants. Bhutada et al demonstrated that thiopental could be used for induction in infants without important changes in heart rate and blood pressure during the intubation period.[18] An equipotent dose of methohexital produces even less hypotension than thiopental because of a greater tachycardic response to the blood pressure lowering effects of the drug. If the blood pressure remains stable, the myocardial oxygen demand–supply ratio remains normal despite the increase in heart rate because of a concurrent decrease in coronary vascular resistance.

Propofol

Propofol (2,6-disopropylphenol), an alkylphenol compound, is virtually insoluble in aqueous solution. The initial cremophor EL formulation of propofol was withdrawn from clinical testing because of the high incidence of anaphylactic reactions. Subsequently, propofol (10 mg/mL) was reintroduced as an egg lecithin emulsion formulation (Diprivan), consisting of 10% soybean oil, 2.25% glycerol, and 1.2% egg phosphatide. Pain on injection occurs in 32 to 67% of patients when injected into small hand veins but can be minimized by injection into larger veins and by prior administration of either lidocaine or a potent opioid analgesic (e.g., fentanyl or remifentanil). A wide variety of drugs have been used for reducing pain on injection of propofol (e.g., metoprolol,[19] granisetron,[20] dolasetron,[21] and even thiopental[22]). Diluting the formulation with additional solvent (Intralipid) or changing the lipid carrier (Lipofundin) also reduced propofol-induced injection pain, probably because of a decrease in the concentration of free propofol in the acqueous phase of the emulsion. A new propofol formulation with sodium metabisulphite (instead of disodium edetate) as an antimicrobial has recently been shown to be associated with less severe pain on injection. Although the presence of the metabisulphite has raised concerns regarding its use in sulphite-allergic patients, this does not appear to be a clinically important problem. Of interest, a 2% formulation is available for long-term sedation to decrease the fluid volume infused as well as the lipid load. Recently, a lower-lipid formulation of propofol (Ampofol) has been introduced into clinical practice for both general anesthesia[23] and sedation.[24] The increased "free" fraction of propofol leads to increased pain when it is injected into small veins. Therefore, it is important to add lidocaine to the Ampofol formulation to minimize the pain on injection. A new water-soluble prodrug of propofol (Aquavan) is rapidly hydrolized in the circulation to release propofol.[25] It has a slower onset than propofol but a similar recovery profile. Although Aquavan does not produce injection site discomfort, a burning perineal sensation has been reported.

Propofol's pharmacokinetics has been studied using single bolus dosing and continuous infusions.[26] In studies using a two-compartment kinetic model, the initial distribution half-life is 2 to 8 minutes and the elimination half-life is 1 to 3 hours. Using a three-compartment model, the initial and slow distribution half-life values are 1 to 8 minutes and 30 to 70 minutes, respectively. The elimination half-life depends largely on the sampling time after discontinuing the administration of propofol and ranges from 2 to 24 hours. This long elimination half-life is indicative of the existence of a poorly perfused compartment from which propofol slowly diffuses back into the central compartment. Propofol is rapidly cleared from the central compartment by hepatic metabolism and the context-sensitive half-life for propofol infusions up to 8 hours is less than 40 minutes. Propofol is rapidly and extensively metabolized to inactive, water-soluble sulphate and glucuronic acid metabolites, which are eliminated by the kidneys. Propofol's clearance rate (1.5 to 2.2 l/min) exceeds hepatic blood flow, suggesting that an extrahepatic route of elimination (lungs) also contributes to its clearance. Nevertheless, changes in liver blood flow would be expected to produce marked alterations in propofol's clearance rate. Surprisingly, few changes in propofol's pharmacokinetics have been reported in the presence of hepatic or renal disease.

The induction dose of propofol in healthy adults is 1.5 to 2.5 mg/kg, with blood levels of 2 to 6 μg/mL producing unconsciousness depending on the concomitant medications (e.g., opioid analgesics), the patient's age and physical status, and the extent of the surgical stimulation.[27] In one of the first reports describing the use of propofol for induction and maintenance of anesthesia with nitrous oxide, an average infusion rate of 120 μg/kg/min was required.[28] The recommended maintenance infusion rate of propofol varies between 100 and 200 μg/kg/min for hypnosis and 25 to 75 μg/kg/min for sedation. Awakening typically occurs at plasma propofol concentrations of 1 to 1.5 μg/mL.[29] Because a 50% decrease in the plasma propofol concentration is usually required for awakening, emergence following anesthesia is rapid even following prolonged infusions.

Analogous to the barbiturates, children require higher induction and maintenance doses of propofol on a mg/kg basis as a result of their larger central distribution volume and higher clearance rate. Elderly and patients in poor health require lower induction and maintenance doses of propofol as a result of their smaller central distribution volume and decreased clearance rate. Although subhypnotic doses of propofol produce sedation and amnesia,[29] awareness has been reported even at higher infusion rates when propofol is used as the sole anesthetic.[30] Propofol often produces a subjective feeling of well-being and even euphoria, and may have some abuse potential as a result of these effects.[31] Propofol possesses dose-dependent effects on thalamocortical transfer of nociceptive information. However, pain-evoked cortical activity remains intact after loss of consciousness.[32]

Propofol decreases $CMRO_2$ and CBF, as well as ICP.[33] However, when larger doses are administered, the marked depressant effect on systemic arterial pressure can significantly decrease CPP. Cerebrovascular autoregulation in response to changes in systemic arterial pressure and reactivity of the cerebral blood flow to changes in carbon dioxide tension are not affected by propofol. Evidence for a possible neuroprotective effect has been reported in in vitro preparations, and the use of propofol to produce EEG burst suppression has been proposed as a method for providing neuroprotection during aneurysm surgery. Its neuroprotective effect may at least partially be related to the antioxidant potential of propofol's phenol ring structure, which may act as a free-radical scavenger, decreasing free-radical induced lipid peroxidation. A recent study reported that this antioxidant activity may offer many advantages in preventing the hypoperfusion/reperfusion phenomenon that can occur during major laproscopic surgery.[34] Although TIVA with propofol and an opioid analgesic is a safe and effective alternative to standard inhalation techniques (i.e., volatile anesthetic with nitrous oxide) for maintenance of anesthesia, concerns have been raised regarding the cost-effectiveness of this technique.[35]

Propofol produces cortical EEG changes that are similar to thiopental. However, sedative doses of propofol increase β-wave activity analogous to the benzodiazepines. Induction of anesthesia with propofol is occasionally accompanied by excitatory motor activity (so-called nonepileptic myoclonia). In a study involving patients without a history of seizure disorders, excitatory movements following propofol were not associated with EEG seizure activity.[36] Propofol appears to possess profound anticonvulsant properties.[37] Propofol has been reported to decrease spike activity in patients with cortical electrodes implanted for resection of epileptogenic foci and has been used successfully to terminate status epilepticus. The duration of motor and EEG seizure activity following electroconvulsive therapy is significantly shorter with propofol than with other IV anesthetics. Propofol produces a decrease in the early components of somatosensory and motor-evoked potentials but does not influence the early components of the auditory evoked potentials.

Propofol produces dose-dependent respiratory depression, with apnea occurring in 25 to 35% of patients after a typical induction dose. A maintenance infusion of propofol decreases tidal volume and increases respiratory rate. The ventilatory response to carbon dioxide and hypoxia is also significantly decreased by propofol. Propofol can produce bronchodilation in patients with chronic obstructive pulmonary disease and does not inhibit hypoxic pulmonary vasoconstriction.

Propofol's cardiovascular depressant effects are generally considered to be more profound than those of thiopental. Both direct myocardial depressant effects and decreased systemic vascular resistance have been implemented as important factors in producing cardiovascular depression. Direct myocardial depression and peripheral vasodilation are dose and concentration dependent. In addition to arterial vasodilation, propofol produces venodilation (due both to a reduction in sympathetic activity and to a direct effect on the vascular smooth muscle), which further contributes to its hypotensive effect. The relaxation of the vascular smooth muscle may be because of an effect on intracellular calcium mobilization or because of an increase in the production of nitric oxide. Experiments in isolated myocardium suggest that the negative inotropic effect of propofol results from a decrease in intracellular calcium availability secondary to inhibition of transsarcolemmal calcium influx.

Propofol also alters the baroreflex mechanism, resulting in a smaller increase in heart rate for a given decrease in arterial pressure.[38] The smaller increase in heart rate with propofol may account for the larger decrease in arterial pressure than with an equipotent dose of thiopental. Recent studies suggest that induction of anesthesia with propofol attenuates desflurane-mediated sympathetic activation.[39] Age enhances the cardiodepressant response to propofol and a reduced dosage is required in the elderly. Patients with limited cardiac reserve seem to tolerate the cardiac depression and systemic vasodilation produced by carefully titrated doses of propofol and maintenance infusions are increasingly used at the end of cardiac surgery when early extubation is desired.

6 Propofol appears to possess antiemetic properties that contribute to a lower incidence of emetic sequelae after general anesthesia. In fact, subanesthetic doses of propofol (10 to 20 mg) have also been successfully used to treat nausea and emesis in the early postoperative period.[40] The postulated mechanisms include antidopaminergic activity, depressant effect on the chemoreceptor trigger zone and vagal nuclei, decreased release of glutamate and aspartate in the olfactory cortex, and reduction of serotonin concentrations in the area postrema. Interestingly, propofol also decreases the pruritus produced by spinal opioids.

Propofol does not trigger malignant hyperthermia (MH) and may be considered the induction agent of choice in MH-susceptible patients. The use of propofol infusions for sedation in the pediatric intensive care unit has been linked to several deaths following prolonged administration because of lipid accumulation and hypotension. Although clinical doses of propofol do not affect cortisol synthesis or the response to adrenocorticotropic hormone (ACTH) stimulation, propofol has been reported to inhibit phagocytosis and killing of bacteria in vitro and to reduce proliferative responses when added to lymphocytes from critically ill patients.[41] Because fat emulsions are known to support the growth of microorganisms, contamination can occur as a result of dilution or fractionated use.[42]

Benzodiazepines

The parenteral benzodiazepines include diazepam (Valium), lorazepam (Ativan), and midazolam (Versed), as well as the antagonist flumazenil (Romazicon). Diazepam and lorazepam are insoluble in water and their formulation contains propylene glycol, a tissue irritant that causes pain on injection and venous irritation. Diazepam is available in a lipid emulsion formulation, which does not cause pain or thrombophlebitis but is associated with a slightly lower bioavailability. Midazolam is a water-soluble benzodiazepine that is available in an acidified (pH 3.5) aqueous formulation that produces minimal local irritation after IV or intramuscular (IM) injection.[43] At physiologic pH, an intramolecular rearrangement occurs that changes the physicochemical properties of midazolam such that it becomes more lipid soluble.

Benzodiazepines undergo hepatic metabolism via oxidation and glucuronide conjugation. Oxidation reactions are susceptible to hepatic dysfunction and coadministration of other anesthetic drugs. Diazepam is metabolized to active metabolites (desmethyldiazepam, 3-hydroxydiazepam), which can prolong diazepam's residual sedative effects because of their long $t_{1/2}\ \beta$ values. These metabolites undergo secondary conjugation to form inactive water-soluble glucuronide conjugates. Drugs that inhibit the oxidative metabolism of diazepam include the H_2-receptor blocking drug cimetidine. Severe liver disease reduces diazepam's protein-binding and hepatic clearance rate, increases its volume of distribution, and thereby further prolongs the $t_{1/2}\beta$ value. Chronic renal disease decreases protein binding and increases the free drug fraction, resulting in enhanced hepatic metabolism and a shorter $t_{1/2}\beta$ value. In elderly patients, the clearance rate of diazepam is significantly decreased, prolonging its $t_{1/2}\beta$ to 75 to 150 hours.

Lorazepam is directly conjugated to glucuronic acid to form pharmacologically inactive metabolites. Age and renal disease have little influence on the kinetics of lorazepam; however, severe hepatic disease decreases its clearance rate.

Midazolam undergoes extensive oxidation by hepatic enzymes to form water-soluble hydroxylated metabolites, which are excreted in the urine. However, the primary metabolite, 1-hydroxymethylmidazolam, has mild CNS-depressant activity. The hepatic clearance rate of midazolam is five times greater than lorazepam and 10 times greater than diazepam. Although changes in liver blood flow can affect the clearance of midazolam, age has relatively little influence on midazolam's elimination half-life.

The benzodiazepines used in anesthesia are classified as either short- (midazolam, flumazenil), intermediate- (diazepam), or long-acting (lorazepam). Because the distribution volumes are similar, the large difference in the elimination half-times is because of differences in their differing clearance rates (see Table 13-1). The context-sensitive half-times for diazepam and lorazepam are very long; therefore, only midazolam should be used by continuous infusion to avoid excessive accumulation.

All benzodiazepines have anxiolytic, amnestic, sedative, hypnotic, anticonvulsant, and spinally mediated muscle relaxant properties. Benzodiazepines differ in potency and efficacy with regard to their distinctive pharmacologic properties.[43] The dose-dependent pharmacologic activity implies that the CNS effects of various benzodiazepine compounds depend on the affinity for receptor subtypes and their degree of receptor binding. Although benzodiazepines can be used as hypnotics, they are primarily used as premedicants and adjuvant drugs because of their anxiolytic, sedative, and amnestic properties. For example, midazolam (0.04 to 0.08 mg/kg IV/IM) is the most commonly used premedicant. In addition, midazolam, 0.4 to 0.8 mg/kg administered orally 10 to 15 minutes before parental separation, is an excellent premedicant in children. In contrast to lorazepam, both diazepam and midazolam can be used to induce anesthesia because they have a relatively short onset time after IV administration. The half-life of equilibration between the plasma concentration of midazolam and its maximal EEG effect is only 2 to 3 minutes. The therapeutic window to maintain unconsciousness with midazolam is reported to be 100 to 200 ng/mL, with awakening occurring at plasma concentrations below 50 ng/mL. However, significant hypnotic synergism occurs when midazolam and opioid analgesics are administered in combination.

The usual induction dose of midazolam in premedicated patients is 0.1 to 0.2 mg/kg IV, with infusion rates of 0.25 to 1 mg/kg/min required to maintain hypnosis and amnesia in combination with inhalational agents and/or opioid analgesics. Higher maintenance infusion rates and prolonged administration will result in accumulation and prolonged recovery times. Lower infusion rates are sufficient to provide sedation and amnesia during local and regional anesthesia.[44] Patient-controlled administration of midazolam during procedures under local anesthesia is well accepted by patients and associated with few perioperative complications.[45]

Benzodiazepines decrease both $CMRO_2$ and CBF analogous to the barbiturates and propofol. However, in contrast to these compounds, midazolam is unable to produce a burst-suppressive (isoelectric) pattern on the EEG. Accordingly, there is a "ceiling" effect with respect to the decrease in $CMRO_2$ produced by increasing doses of midazolam. Midazolam induces dose-dependent changes in regional cerebral perfusion in the parts of the brain that subserve arousal, attention, and memory. Cerebral vasomotor responsiveness to carbon dioxide is preserved during midazolam anesthesia. In patients with severe head injury, a bolus dose of midazolam may decrease CPP with little effect on ICP. Although midazolam may improve neurologic outcome after incomplete ischemia in animal experiments, benzodiazepines have not been shown to possess neuroprotective activity in humans. Like the other sedative–hypnotic drugs, the benzodiazepines are potent anticonvulsants that are commonly used to treat status epilepticus.

Benzodiazepines produce dose-dependent respiratory depression. In healthy patients, the respiratory depression associated with benzodiazepine premedication is insignificant. However, the depressant effect is enhanced in patients with chronic respiratory disease, and synergistic depressant effects occur when benzodiazepines are coadministered with opioid analgesics. Benzodiazepines also depress the swallowing reflex and decrease upper airway reflex activity.

Both midazolam and diazepam produce decreases in systemic vascular resistance and blood pressure when large doses are administered for induction of anesthesia. However, the cardiovascular depressant effects of benzodiazepines are frequently "masked" by the stimulus of laryngoscopy and intubation. The cardiovascular depressant effects are directly related to the plasma concentration; however, a plateau plasma concentration appears to exist above which little further change in arterial blood pressure occurs. In the presence of heart failure, the decrease in preload and afterload produced by benzodiazepines may be beneficial in improving cardiac output. However, the cardiodepressant effect of benzodiazepines may be more marked in hypovolemic patients.

Ro 48-6791, a so-called short-acting intravenous sedative (SAIVS), is a new water-soluble benzodiazepine that has full agonistic activity at CNS benzodiazepine receptors. Compared with midazolam, it is 2- to 2.5-fold more potent, has a higher plasma clearance rate, and has a similar onset and duration of action.[46] In a recent study involving outpatients undergoing endoscopy procedures, the times to ambulation and to recovery from psychomotor impairment were decreased compared to midazolam, although the later recovery end points (e.g., "fitness-for-discharge") were similar.[47]

In contrast to all other sedative–hypnotic drugs, there is a specific antagonist for benzodiazepines. Flumazenil, a 1,4-imidazobenzodiazepine derivative, has a high affinity for the benzodiazepine receptor but minimal intrinsic activity.[48] Flumazenil's molecular structure is similar to other benzodiazepines except for the absence of a phenyl group, which is replaced by a carbonyl group. It is water soluble and possesses moderate lipid solubility at physiologic pH. Flumazenil is rapidly metabolized in the liver, and its metabolites are excreted in the urine as glucuronide conjugates. Flumazenil acts as a competitive antagonist in the presence of benzodiazepine agonist compounds. The residual activity of the benzodiazepines in the presence of flumazenil depends on the relative concentrations of the agonist and antagonist drugs. As a result, it is possible to reverse benzodiazepine-induced anesthesia (or deep sedation) either completely or partially depending on the dose of flumazenil. Flumazenil is short acting, with an elimination half-life of ~1 hour.

Recurrence of the central effects of benzodiazepines (resedation) may occur after a single dose of flumazenil because of residual effects of the more slowly eliminated agonist drug.[49] If sustained antagonism is desired, it may be necessary to administer flumazenil as repeated bolus doses or a continuous infusion. In general, 45 to 90 minutes of antagonism can be expected following flumazenil 1 to 3 mg IV. However, the respiratory depression produced by benzodiazepines is not completely reversed by flumazenil.[50] Reversal of benzodiazepine sedation with flumazenil is not associated with adverse cardiovascular effects or evidence of an acute stress response.[51] Although flumazenil does not appear to change CBF or $CMRO_2$ following midazolam anesthesia for craniotomy, acute increases in ICP have been reported in head-injured patients receiving flumazenil.

Etomidate

Etomidate is a carboxylated imidazole-containing anesthetic compound (R-1-ethyl-1-[a-methylbenzyl] imidazole-5-carboxylate) that is structurally unrelated to any other IV anesthetic. Only the D-isomer of etomidate possesses anesthetic activity. Analogous to midazolam (which also contains an imidazole nucleus), etomidate undergoes an intramolecular rearrangement at physiologic pH, resulting in a closed-ring structure with enhanced lipid solubility. The aqueous solution of etomidate (Amidate) is unstable at physiologic pH and is formulated in a 0.2% solution with 35% propylene glycol (pH 6.9), contributing to a high incidence of pain on injection, venoirritation, and hemolysis. A new lipid emulsion formulation (Etomidate-Lipuro) has recently been introduced in Europe and appears to be associated with a lower incidence of side effects compared to the original propylene glycol formulation.

The standard induction dose of etomidate (0.2 to 0.4 mg/kg IV) produces a rapid onset of anesthesia. Involuntary myoclonic movements are common during the induction period as a result of subcortical disinhibition and are unrelated to cortical seizure activity. The frequency of this myoclonic-like activity can be attenuated by prior administration of opioid analgesics, benzodiazepines, or small sedative doses (0.03 to 0.05 mg/kg) prior to induction of anesthesia.[52] Emergence time after etomidate anesthesia is dose dependent but remains short even after administration of repeated bolus doses or continuous infusions. For maintenance of hypnosis, the target concentration is 300 to 500 $ng \cdot mL^{-1}$ and can be rapidly achieved by administering a two- or three-stage infusion (e.g., 100 mg/kg/min for 10 min followed by 10 mg/kg/min or 100 mg/kg/min for 3 to 5 minutes, followed by 20 mg/kg/min for 20 to 30 minutes, and then 10 mg/kg/min). The pharmacokinetics of etomidate are optimally described by a three-compartment open model.[53] The high clearance rate of etomidate (18 to 25 mL/kg/min) is a result of extensive ester hydrolysis in the liver (forming inactive water-soluble metabolites). A significant decrease in plasma protein binding has been reported in the presence of uremia and hepatic cirrhosis. Severe hepatic disease causes a prolongation of the elimination half-life secondary to an increased volume of distribution and a decreased plasma clearance rate.

Analogous to the barbiturates, etomidate decreases $CMRO_2$, CBF, and ICP. However, the hemodynamic stability associated with etomidate will maintain adequate CPP. Etomidate has been used successfully for both induction and maintenance of anesthesia for neurosurgery. Etomidate's well-known inhibitory effect on adrenocortical synthetic function[54] limits its clinical usefulness for long-term treatment of elevated ICP. Although clear evidence for a neuroprotective effect in humans is lacking, etomidate is frequently used during temporary arterial occlusion and intraoperative angiography (for the treatment of cerebral aneurysms). Etomidate produces an EEG pattern that is similar to thiopental except for the absence of increased β activity at lower doses. Etomidate can induce convulsion-like EEG potentials in epileptic patients without the appearance of myoclonic or convulsant-like motor activity, a property that has been proven useful for intraoperative mapping of seizure foci. Etomidate also possesses anticonvulsant properties and it has been used to terminate status epilepticus. Etomidate produces a significant increase of the amplitude of somatosensory evoked potentials while only minimally increasing their latency. Consequently, etomidate can be used to facilitate the interpretation of somatosensory evoked potentials when the signal quality is poor.

7 Etomidate causes minimal cardiorespiratory depression even in the presence of cardiovascular and pulmonary disease.[55] The drug does not induce histamine release and can be safely used in patients with reactive airway disease. Consequently, etomidate is considered to be the induction agent of choice for poor-risk patients with cardiorespiratory disease, as well as in those situations in which preservation of a normal blood pressure is crucial (e.g., cerebrovascular disease). However, etomidate does not effectively blunt the sympathetic response to laryngoscopy and intubation unless combined with a potent opioid analgesic.

Etomidate is associated with a high incidence of postoperative nausea and emesis when used in combination with opioids for short outpatient procedures. In addition, the increased mortality in critically ill patients sedated with an etomidate infusion has been attributed to its inhibitory effect on cortisol synthesis.[56] Etomidate inhibits the activity of 11-β-hydroxylase, an enzyme necessary for the synthesis of cortisol, aldosterone, 17-hydroxyprogesterone, and corticosterone. Even after a single induction dose of etomidate,[56] adrenal suppression persists for 5 to 8 hours. Although the clinical significance of short-term blockade of cortisol synthesis is not known, the use of etomidate for maintenance of anesthesia has been questioned. Recently, etomidate has been reported to inhibit platelet function, resulting in prolongation of the bleeding time.[57] In spite of its side effect profile, etomidate remains a valuable induction drug still for specific indications (in patients with severe cardiovascular and cerebrovascular disease).

Ketamine

Ketamine (Ketalar or Ketaject) is an arylcyclohexylamine that is structurally related to phencyclidine.[58] Ketamine is a water-soluble compound with a pKa of 7.5 and is available in 1%, 5%, and 10% aqueous solutions. The ketamine molecule contains a chiral center producing two optical isomers. The S(+) isomer of ketamine possesses more potent anesthetic and analgesic properties despite having a similar pharmacokinetic and pharmacodynamic profile as the racemic mixture (or the R[−] isomer).[59,60] Although the S(+)-ketamine is approved for clinical use in Europe, the commonly used solution is a racemic mixture of the two isomers. Ketamine is extensively metabolized by hepatic microsomal cytochrome P-450 enzymes and its primary metabolite, norketamine, is one third to one fifth as potent as the parent compound. The metabolites of norketamine are excreted by the kidney as water-soluble hydroxylated and glucuronidated conjugates. Analogous to the barbiturates and propofol, ketamine has relatively short distribution and redistribution half-life values. Ketamine also has a high hepatic clearance rate (1 L/min) and a large distribution volume (3 L/kg), resulting in an elimination half-life of 2 to 3 hours. The high hepatic extraction ratio suggests that alterations in hepatic blood flow can significantly influence ketamine's clearance rate.

Ketamine produces dose-dependent CNS depression lead-
8 ing to a so-called dissociative anesthetic state characterized by profound analgesia and amnesia, even though patients may be conscious and maintain protective reflexes. The proposed mechanism for this cataleptic state includes electrophysiologic

inhibition of thalamocortical pathways and stimulation of the limbic system. Although it is most commonly administered parenterally, oral and intranasal administration of ketamine (6 mg/kg) has been used for premedication of pediatric patients. Following benzodiazepine premedication, ketamine 1 to 2 mg/kg IV (or 4 to 8 mg/kg IM) can be used for induction of anesthesia. The duration of ketamine-induced anesthesia is in the range of 10 to 20 minutes after a single induction dose; however, recovery to full orientation may require an additional 60 to 90 minutes. Emergence times are even longer following repeated bolus injections or a continuous infusion. S(+)-ketamine has a shorter recovery time compared with the racemic mixture. The therapeutic window for maintenance of unconsciousness with ketamine is between 0.6 and 2 mg/mL in adults and between 0.8 and 4 mg/mL in children. Analgesic effects are evident at subanesthetic doses of 0.1 to 0.5 mg/kg IV and plasma concentrations of between 85 and 160 ng/mL. A low-dose infusion of 4 μg/kg/min IV was reported to result in equivalent postoperative analgesia as an IV morphine infusion of 2 mg/h.

As a result of its NMDA-receptor blocking activity, it has been suggested that ketamine should be highly effective for preemptive analgesia and opioid-resistant chronic pain states.[61] Unfortunately, a well-controlled study failed to demonstrate a preemptive effect when ketamine was administered prior to the surgical incision.[62]

An important consideration in the use of ketamine anesthesia relates to the high incidence of psychomimetic reactions (namely, hallucinations, nightmares, altered short-term memory and cognition) during the early recovery period. The incidence of these reactions is dose dependent and can be reduced by coadministration of benzodiazepines, barbiturates, or propofol. Ketamine has been traditionally contraindicated for patients with increased ICP or reduced cerebral compliance because it increases $CMRO_2$, CBF, and ICP. However, there is recent evidence that IV induction doses of ketamine actually increases ICP in traumatic–brain-injury patients during controlled ventilation with propofol sedation.[63] Prior administration of thiopental or benzodiazepines can blunt ketamine-induced increases in CBF. Since ketamine has antagonistic activity at the NMDA receptor, it has been suggested that it possesses some inherent protective effects against brain ischemia. Nevertheless, ketamine can adversely affect neurologic outcome in the presence of brain ischemia despite its NMDA-receptor blocking activity. Cortical EEG recordings following ketamine induction are characterized by the appearance of fast β activity (30 to 40 Hz) followed by moderate-voltage θ activity, mixed with high-voltage δ waves recurring at 3 to 4 second intervals. At higher dosages, ketamine produces a unique EEG burst-suppression pattern (Fig. 13-5). Although ketamine-induced myoclonic and seizure-like activity has been observed in normal (nonepileptic) patients, ketamine appears to possess anticonvulsant activity.[8] Recently, several have demonstrated the opioid-sparing effects of low-dose Ketamine (75 to 200 mcg/kg) when administered as an adjuvant during anesthesia.[64,65] Interestingly, small-dose ketamine has also been used in the treatment of severe depression in patients with chronic pain syndromes.[66] However, ketamine can produce adverse effects when administered in the presence of triciclyic antidepressants because both drugs inhibit norepinephrine reuptake and could produce severe hypotension, heart failure, and/or myocardial ischemia.[67,68]

Ketamine has well-characterized bronchodilatory activity. In the presence of active bronchospasm, ketamine is considered to be the IV induction agent of choice. Ketamine has been used in subanesthetic dosages to treat persistent bronchospasm in the operating room and ICU. It is also used in combination with midazolam to provide sedation and analgesia for asthmatic patients. In contrast to the other IV anesthetics, protective airway reflexes are more likely to be preserved with ketamine. However, it must be emphasized that the use of ketamine does not obviate the need for tracheal intubation in the patient with a full stomach (because tracheal soiling has been reported in this situation). Ketamine causes minimal respiratory depression in clinically relevant doses and can facilitate the transition from mechanical to spontaneous ventilation after anesthesia. However, its ability to increase oral secretions can lead to laryngospasm during "light" anesthesia.

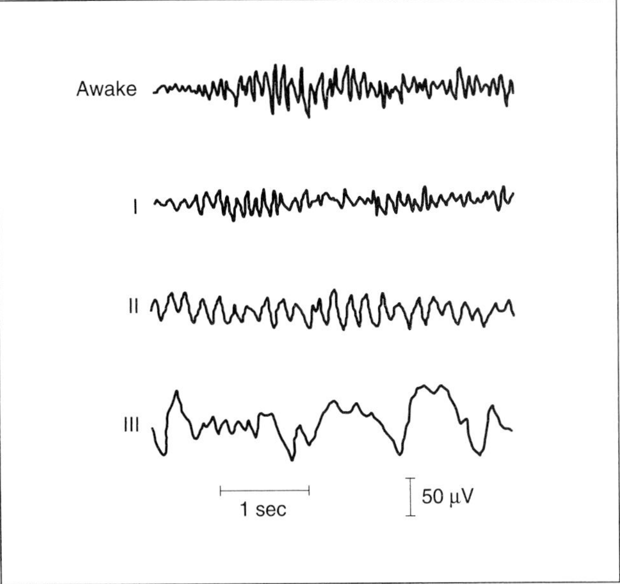

FIGURE 13-5. Progressive changes in the EEG produced by ketamine. Stages I through III are achieved with racemic ketamine and its S(+)isomer. With R(−)ketamine, Stage II was the maximal EEG depression produced. (Reprinted with permission from Shüttler J, Stanski DR, White PF, et al: Pharmacodynamic modeling of the EEG effect of ketamine and its enantiomers in man. J Pharmacokinet Biopharm 15:241, 1987.)

Ketamine has prominent cardiovascular stimulating effects secondary to direct stimulation of the sympathetic nervous system. Ketamine is the only anesthetic that actually increases peripheral arteriolar resistance. As a result of its vasoconstrictive properties, ketamine can reduce the magnitude of redistribution hypothermia.[69] Induction of anesthesia with ketamine often produces significant increases in arterial blood pressure and heart rate. Although the mechanism of the cardiovascular stimulation is not entirely clear, it appears to be centrally mediated. There is evidence to suggest that ketamine attenuates baroreceptor activity via an effect on NMDA receptors in the nucleus tractus solitarius. Because of the increased cardiac work and myocardial oxygen consumption, ketamine negatively affects the balance between myocardial oxygen supply and demand. Consequently, its use is not recommended in patients with severe coronary artery disease. In contrast to the secondary cardiovascular stimulation, ketamine has intrinsic myocardial depressant properties that only become apparent in the seriously ill patient with depleted catecholamine reserves. Because ketamine can also increase pulmonary artery pressure, its use is contraindicated in adult patients with poor right ventricular reserve. Interestingly, the effect on the pulmonary vasculature seems to be attenuated in children.

The anesthetic and analgesic potency of S(+)-ketamine is three times greater than R(−)-ketamine and twice that of the racemic mixture (Fig. 13-6), reflecting its fourfold greater affinity at the phencyclidine binding site on the NMDA receptor compared with the R(−) isomer.[70] The therapeutic index of S(+)-ketamine is 2.5 times greater than both the R(−)

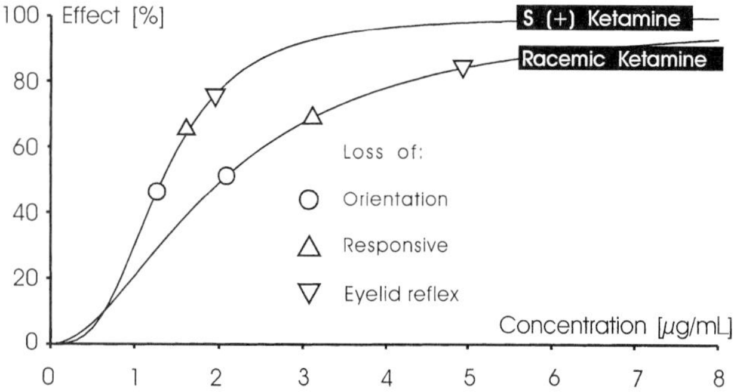

FIGURE 13-6. Concentration-response relationship for racemic ketamine and S(+)ketamine in relation to specific clinical end points. The slowing of the median EEG frequency was used as the effect (end point) and was related to the arterial blood concentrations of ketamine. (Reprinted with permission from Schüttler J, Kloos S, Ihmsen H, et al: Pharmacokinetic-pharmacodynamic properties of S(+)-ketamine versus racemic ketamine: A randomized double-blind study in volunteers. Anesthesiology 77:A330, 1992.)

and the racemic forms. In addition, hepatic biotransformation of S(+)-ketamine occurs 20% faster than that of the R(−) enantiomer, contributing to shorter emergence times and a faster return of cognitive function. Both isomers produce similar cardiovascular stimulating effects and hormonal responses during surgery. Although the incidence of dreaming is similar with S(+)-ketamine and the racemic mixture, subjective mood and patient acceptance are higher with the S(+) isomer.

CLINICAL USES OF INTRAVENOUS ANESTHETICS

Use of Intravenous Anesthetics As Induction Agents

The induction characteristics and recommended dosages of the available IV anesthetic agents are summarized in Table 13-2. As a result of differences in pharmacokinetic (e.g., altered clearance and distribution volumes) and pharmacodynamic (altered brain sensitivity) variables, the induction dosages of all IV anesthetics need to be adjusted to meet the needs of individual patients. For example, advanced age, preexisting diseases (e.g., hypothyroidism, hypovolemia), premedication (e.g., benzodiazepines), and coadministration of adjuvant drugs (e.g., opioids, (α-2 agonists) decrease the induction dose requirements.

When there is concern regarding a possible abnormal response, assessing the effect of a small "test dose" (equal to 10 to 20% of the usual induction dose) will often identify those patients for whom a dosage adjustment is required. Before administering additional medication, adequate time should be allowed for the anesthetic to exert its effect, especially when using drugs with a slow onset of action (midazolam) or in the presence of a "slow" circulation time in elderly patients and those with congestive heart failure.

The clinical uses of propofol have expanded greatly since its introduction into clinical practice in 1989.[71] Intravenous administration of propofol results in a rapid loss of consciousness (usually within one arm-to-brain circulation) that is comparable to the barbiturates. Although an induction dose of 2.5 mg/kg was initially recommended, the use of smaller induction doses of propofol (1 to 2 mg/kg) has minimized its acute cardiovascular and respiratory depressant effects. Recovery from propofol's sedative–hypnotic effects is rapid with less residual sedation, fatigue ("hangover"), and cognitive impairment than with other available sedative–hypnotic drugs after short surgical procedures. Consequently, propofol has become the IV drug of choice for outpatients undergoing ambulatory surgery.

With benzodiazepines, there is wide variation in the dose-response relationships in unpremedicated elective surgery patients. Compared to midazolam, diazepam and lorazepam have slower onset times to achieve a peak effect and their dose-effect relationship is less predictable. As a result, diazepam and lorazepam are rarely used for induction of general anesthesia. In addition, the slow hepatic clearance of diazepam and lorazepam may contribute to prolonged residual effects (sedation, amnesia, fatigue) when they are used for premedication. Midazolam has a slightly more rapid onset and may be a useful induction agent for special indications (when nitrous oxide is contraindicated, or as part of a total IV anesthetic technique). However, when midazolam is used for induction and/or maintenance of anesthesia, return of consciousness takes substantially longer than with other sedative–hypnotic drugs. In spite of its extensive hepatic metabolism, recovery of cognitive function is still slower after midazolam compared with thiopental, methohexital, etomidate, or propofol.

In an effort to optimize the clinical use of midazolam during the induction period, it is utilized increasingly as a coinduction agent with other sedative–hypnotic drugs (propofol,
9 ketamine). Midazolam 2 to 5 mg IV can provide for increased sedation, amnesia, and anxiolysis during the preinduction period. When midazolam is used in combination with propofol, 1.5 to 2 mg/kg IV, or ketamine, 0.75 to 1 mg/kg IV, it facilitates the onset of anesthesia without delaying emergence times.[72]

TABLE 13-2

INDUCTION CHARACTERISTICS AND DOSAGE REQUIREMENTS FOR THE CURRENTLY AVAILABLE SEDATIVE–HYPNOTIC DRUGS

DRUG NAME	INDUCTION DOSE (mg/kg)	ONSET (sec)	DURATION (min)	EXCITATORY ACTIVITY*	PAIN ON INJECTION*	HEART RATE†	BLOOD PRESSURE†
Thiopental	3–6	<30	5–10	+	0–+	↑	↓
Methohexital	1–3	<30	5–10	++	+	↑↑	↓
Propofol	1.5–2.5	15–45	5–10	+	++	0–↓	↓↓
Midazolam	0.2–0.4	30–90	10–30	0	0	0	0/↓
Diazepam	0.3–0.6	45–90	15–30	0	+/+++	0	0/↓
Lorazepam	0.03–0.06	60–120	60–120	0	++	0	0/↓
Etomidate	0.2–0.3	15–45	3–12	+++	+++	0	0
Ketamine	1–2	45–60	10–20	+	0	↑↑	↑↑

*0 = none; + = minimal; ++ = moderate; +++ = severe.
†↓ = decrease; ↑ = increase.

Midazolam attenuates the cardiostimulatory response to ketamine, as well as its psychomimetic emergence reactions. Use of midazolam, 2 to 3 mg IV with propofol reduces recall during the induction period; however, larger doses of midazolam (5 mg IV) will delay emergence after brief surgical procedures.

As a result of their side effect profiles, the clinical use of etomidate and ketamine for induction of anesthesia is restricted to specific situations where their unique pharmacologic profiles offer advantages over other available IV anesthetics. For example, etomidate can facilitate maintenance of a stable blood pressure in high-risk patients with critical stenosis of the cerebral vasculature and in patients with severe cardiac impairment or unstable angina. Ketamine is a useful induction agent for hypovolemic patients, as well as in patients with reactive airway disease or a compromised upper airway.

Use of Intravenous Drugs for Maintenance of Anesthesia

The continued popularity of volatile anesthetics for maintenance of anesthesia is due primarily to their rapid reversibility and ease of administration when using conventional vaporizer delivery system for titrating to the desired end point. The availability of IV drugs with more rapid onset and shorter recovery profiles, as well as user-friendly infusion delivery systems, has facilitated the maintenance of anesthesia with continuous infusions of IV drugs, producing an anesthetic state (namely, TIVA) that compares favorably with the volatile anesthetics. In a comparison of the requirement of postoperative analgesics after inhalation and TIVA techniques, not surprisingly, the postoperative pain was reduced after TIVA.[73] For example, in morbidly obese patients undergoing bariatric surgery, the use of TIVA technique was associated with a superior recovery profile compared to a sevoflurane-based inhalation technique.[74] However, TIVA techniques are more expensive than inhalation or "balanced" anesthetic techniques.[35]

The traditional intermittent bolus administration of IV drugs results in a "depth" of anesthesia (and analgesia) that oscillates above and below the desired level.[75] Because of rapid distribution and redistribution of the IV anesthetics, the high peak blood concentration after each bolus is followed by a rapid decrease, producing fluctuating drug levels in the blood and hence the brain. The magnitude of the drug level fluctuation is dependent on the size of the bolus dose and the frequency of its administration. Wide variation in the plasma drug concentrations can result in hemodynamic and respiratory instability as a result of changes in the depth of anesthesia or sedation. By providing more stable blood (and brain) concentrations with a continuous IV infusion, it might be possible to improve anesthetic conditions and hemodynamic stability, as well as decreasing side effects and recovery times with IV anesthetics.[76] Administration of IV anesthetics by a variable-rate infusion is a logical extension of the incremental bolus method of drug titration, as a continuous infusion is equivalent to the sequential administration of infinitely small bolus doses.

Although an IV anesthetic can be titrated to achieve and maintain the desired clinical effect, a knowledge of basic pharmacokinetic principles is helpful in more accurately predicting the optimal dosage requirements. The required plasma concentration depends on the desired pharmacological effect (hypnosis, sedation), the concomitant use of other adjunctive drugs (opioid analgesics, muscle relaxants, cardiovascular drugs), the type of operation (superficial, intra-abdominal, intracranial), and the patient's sensitivity to the drug (age, drug history, preexisting diseases). Preexisting diseases (cirrhosis, congestive heart failure, renal failure) can markedly alter the pharmacokinetic variables of the highly protein-bound, lipophilic IV anesthetic drugs. In general, children have higher clearance rates, while the elderly have reduced clearance values. Various intraoperative interventions (laryngoscopy, tracheal intubation, skin incision, entry into body cavities) transiently increase the anesthetic and/or analgesic requirements. Therefore, the infusion scheme should be tailored to provide peak drug concentrations during the periods of most intense stimulation. For specific surgical interventions, the so-called therapeutic window of an IV anesthetic is defined as the blood concentration range required to produce a given effect (Table 13-3). It must be emphasized that the therapeutic window for Sedative–hypnotics is markedly influenced by the presence of adjunctive drugs (opioids, α_2 agonists, nitrous oxide).

The use of IV anesthetic techniques requires continuous titration of the drug infusion rate to the desired pharmacodynamic end point.[72] Most anesthesiologists rely on somatic and autonomic signs for assessing depth of IV anesthesia, analogous to the manner in which they titrate the volatile anesthetics. The most sensitive clinical signs of depth of anesthesia appear to be changes in muscle tone (i.e., electromyography [EMG]) and ventilatory rate and pattern.[77] However, if the patient has been given muscle relaxants, the anesthesiologist must rely on signs of autonomic hyperactivity (tachycardia, hypertension, lacrimation, diaphoresis). Unfortunately, the anesthetic drugs (ketamine), as well as adjunctive agents (α_2 agonists, β blockers, adenosine, calcium-channel blockers), can directly influence the cardiovascular response to surgical stimulation. Although the cardiovascular signs of autonomic nervous system hyperactivity may be masked, other autonomic signs (e.g., diaphoresis) and purposeful movements may be more reliable indicators of depth of anesthesia than blood pressure because the latter depends on the ability of the heart to maintain the cardiac output in the face of acute changes in afterload. The heart rate response to surgical stimulation appears to be more useful than the blood pressure response in determining the need for additional analgesic medication. Moreover, it

TABLE 13-3

THERAPEUTIC BLOOD CONCENTRATIONS WHEN INTRAVENOUS ANESTHETICS ARE INFUSED FOR HYPNOSIS OR SEDATION

DRUG NAME	MAJOR SURGERY PROCEDURES	MINOR SURGERY PROCEDURES	SEDATIVE CONCENTRATION	AWAKENING CONCENTRATION
Thiopental	10–20 μg/mL	10–20 μg/mL	4–8 μg/mL	4–8 μg/mL
Methohexital	6–15 μg/mL	5–10 μg/mL	1–3 μg/mL	1–3 μg/mL
Propofol	4–6 μg/mL	2–4 μg/mL	1–2 μg/mL	1–1.5 μg/mL
Midazolam	100–200 ng/mL	50–200 ng/mL	40–100 ng/mL	50–150 ng/mL
Etomidate	500–1000 ng/mL	300–600 ng/mL	100–300 ng/mL	200–350 ng/mL
Ketamine	1–4 μg/mL	0.6–2 μg/mL	0.1–1 μg/mL	NA

NA = not available.

would appear that blood pressure and heart rate responses to surgical stimulation are a less useful guide with IV techniques than with volatile anesthetics.

The clinical assessment of anesthetic depth has become more challenging because IV anesthetic techniques involve a combination of hypnotics, opioids, muscle relaxants, and adjuvant drugs. The interactions between these drugs can result in additive, supra-additive, infra-additive, or even antagonistic effects. An ideal "depth of anesthesia" indicator would integrate the physiologic and neurologic information from all aspects of the anesthetic state. In the absence of a global cerebral function monitor, the "depth of anesthesia" device should provide an indication of one or more of the key components of general anesthesia (e.g., hypnosis, analgesia, amnesia, suppression of the stress response, or muscle relaxation). A simple, noninvasive monitor of the depth of anesthesia, which would reliably predict a patient's response to surgical stimulation, would be extremely valuable when utilizing IV anesthetic techniques.

The EMG activity of the frontalis muscles increases significantly in patients who move in response to specific surgical stimuli.[77] However, EMG changes occur late and their interpretation is obscured by muscle relaxant drugs. The EEG changes depend largely on the type of anesthetic drugs used. Although a common EEG pattern can be recognized with increasing depression of CNS function by sedative–hypnotics and opioid analgesics, there is no characteristic EEG pattern associated with unconscious and amnestic states.[78] Univariate descriptors of EEG activity appear to be of limited clinical usefulness, and no meaningful correlation could be found between EEG spectral edge frequency and hemodynamic response to surgical stimuli during propofol anesthesia.[79] Although EEG variables (spectral edge frequency, median frequency) appear to be useful indicators of the CNS effects of anesthetic and analgesic drugs in the experimental setting, their usefulness in clinical practice is limited because the many confounding factors during the operation (changing drug levels and surgical stimulation). The EEG-based bispectral index (BIS), patient state index (PSI), state entropy (SE), and response entropy (RE) monitors represent newer approaches to the analysis of the spontaneous EEG, have proved to be a useful indicator of anesthetic (hypnotic) depth.[80] Recent studies have demonstrated that the BIS index can improve filtration of both IV and volatile anesthetics during surgery, thereby facilitating the recovery process. Using EEG-based monitoring can reduce the time required to achieve fast-track eligibility after ambulatory surgery.[81,82]

An attractive alternative to the spontaneous EEG is the evoked response of the EEG to sensory stimuli (e.g., auditory evoked potential [AEP] monitors). The ability to quantitatively assess the response of the body to varying levels of stimulation (sensory or auditory evoked responses) may be useful in improving the assessment of depth of anesthesia.[83] Although all sedative–hypnotic drugs affect the brainstem evoked potentials, uncertainty still exists regarding the most useful evoked response(s) to measure. The complexity associated with recording evoked responses is much greater than recording the spontaneous EEG because the value is critically dependent on technical factors (e.g., stimulus intensity, stimulus rate, electrode position), body temperature, as well as the anesthetic drugs. Although most IV anesthetics produce dose-dependent changes in the somatosensory evoked potentials, the correlation between the acute hemodynamic changes to surgical stimuli and the early auditory evoked responses is poor. However, the early cortical (mid-latency) auditory evoked response might be useful in detecting awareness under anesthesia. Furthermore, the auditory evoked potential index (AEPi) may be more discriminatory than BIS in characterizing the transition from wakefulness to unresponsiveness.[84]

As a result of the availability of more rapid and shorter acting sedative–hypnotics, sophisticated computer technology, and new insights into pharmacokinetic–dynamic interactions, use of TIVA techniques has been steadily increasing during the last decade. When utilizing constant rate IV infusions, 4 to 5 half-lives may be required to achieve a steady state anesthetic concentration (Fig. 13-7). To more rapidly achieve a therapeutic blood concentration, it is necessary to administer a loading (priming) dose and to maintain the desired drug concentration using a maintenance infusion. The loading dose (LD) and initial maintenance infusion rate (MIR) can be calculated from previously determined population kinetic values using the following equations:

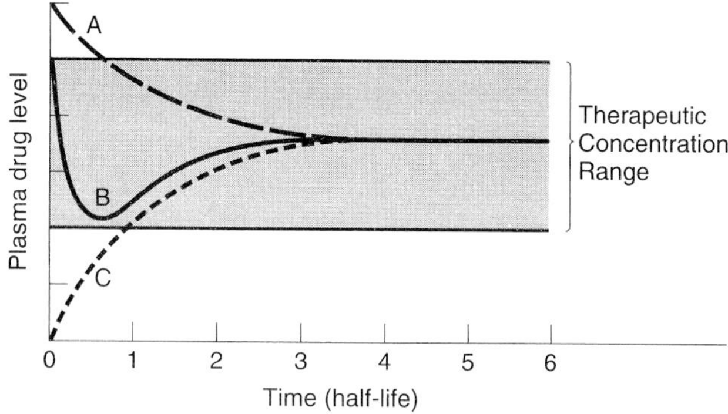

FIGURE 13-7. Simulated drug level curves when a constant infusion is administered following a "full" loading dose equal to [Cp] × Vd_{ss} (*Curve A*), a smaller loading dose equal to [Cp] × Vc (*Curve B*), or in the absence of a loading (*Curve C*). (Reprinted with permission from White PF: Clinical uses of intravenous anesthetic and analgesic infusions. Anesth Analg 68:161, 1989.)

$$\text{LD} = \text{Cp (mg/mL)} \cdot \text{Vd (mL/kg)}$$
$$\text{MIR} = \text{Cp (mL/kg)} \cdot \text{Cl (mL/kg/min)}$$

where Cp = plasma drug concentration; Vd = distribution volume; Cl = drug clearance.

The use of the smaller central volume of distribution (Vc) for the Vd component of the LD equation will underestimate the LD, whereas use of the larger steady-state volume of distribution (Vd_{ss}) will result in drug levels that transiently exceed those that are desired. If a smaller LD is administered, a higher initial MIR will be required to compensate for the drug that is removed from the brain by both redistribution and elimination processes. As the redistribution phase assumes less importance, the MIR will decrease because it becomes solely dependent on the drug's elimination and the desired plasma concentration.

An alternative approach is to begin with a rapid loading infusion with a bolus-elimination transfer (BET) scheme that combines three functions, as shown in the following equation:

$$\text{Input} = \text{V1} \cdot C_{ss} + \text{Cl} \cdot C_{ss} + \text{V1} \cdot C_{ss}\,(k_{21} \cdot e^{-k_{21}t})$$

where V1 = distribution volume of the central compartment; C_{ss} = steady-state plasma concentration; Cl = drug clearance; k_{21} = redistribution constant from the central to the peripheral compartment; k_{21} = redistribution constant from the peripheral to the central compartment. Implementation of the BET infusion scheme requires the use of a microprocessor-controlled pump. If a continuous infusion is to be used in an optimal manner to suppress responses to surgical stimuli, the MIR should be varied according to the individual patient responses (Fig. 13-8). Using an MIR large enough to suppress responses to the most intense surgical stimuli will lead to excessive drug accumulation, postoperative side effects, and delayed recovery. More gradual signs of inadequate or excessive anesthesia can be treated by making 50 to 100% changes in the MIR. Abrupt increases in autonomic activity can be treated by giving a small

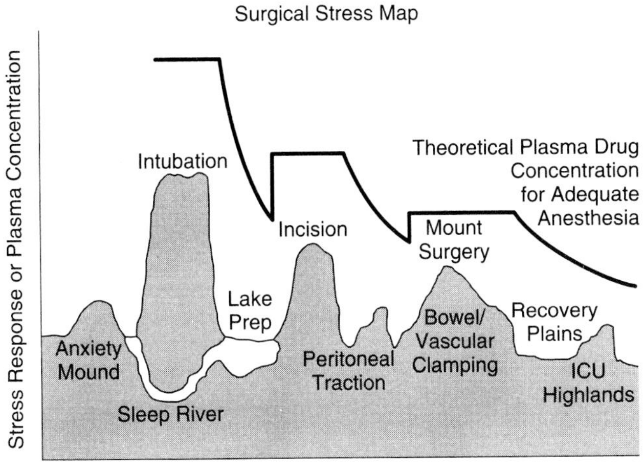

FIGURE 13-8. The "landscape" of surgical anesthesia. The surgical stimuli are not constant during an operation; therefore, the plasma concentration of an IV anesthetic should be titrated to match the needs of the individual patient. (Reprinted with permission from Glass PSA, Shafer SL, Jacobs JR, et al: Intravenous drug delivery systems. In Miller's Anesthesia, 4th ed, p 391. New York, Churchill Livingstone, 1994.)

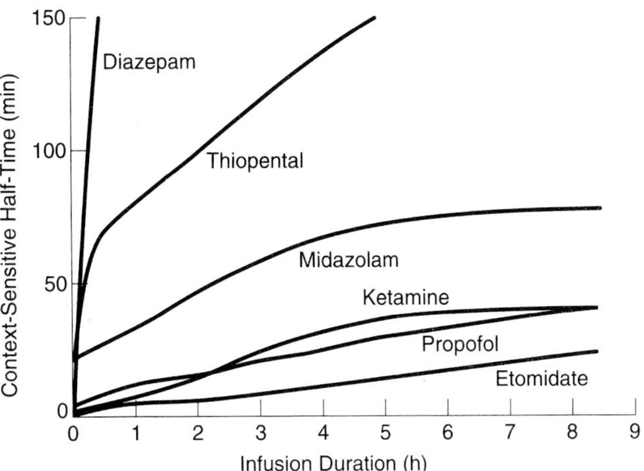

FIGURE 13-9. Context-sensitive half-time values as a function of infusion duration for IV anesthetics, including thiopental, midazolam, diazepam, ketamine, etomidate, and propofol. The context-sensitive half-time for thiopental and diazepam is significantly longer compared with etomidate, propofol, and midazolam with an increasing infusion duration increase. (Reprinted with permission from Hughes MA, Jacobs JR, Glass PSA: Context-sensitive half-time in multicompartment pharmacokinetic models for intravenous anesthesia. Anesthesiology 76: 334, 1992.)

bolus dose equal to 10 to 25% of the initial loading dose and increasing the MIR.

Despite the marked pharmacokinetic and pharmacodynamic variability that exists among surgical patients, computer programs have been developed that allow reasonable predictions of concentration-time profiles for IV anesthetics and analgesics. This new technology has led to the development of target-controlled infusions (TCI), whereby the anesthesiologist chooses a "target" blood or brain (effective site) drug concentration and the micropressor-controlled infusion pump infuses the drug at the rate needed to rapidly achieve and maintain the desired concentration based on population pharmacokinetic-dynamic data.[84] It is obvious that the target concentration must be altered depending on the observed pharmacodynamic effect and the anticipated changes in surgical stimulation.

Closed-loop control based on plasma drug concentrations is not possible because there is no available methodology to obtain frequent measurements of drug concentrations in real time. A more advanced form of TCI uses a feedback signal generated by simulating a mathematical model of the control process. Clearly, the precision of control achievable with a model-based system is only as accurate as the model. An example of a model-based drug delivery system is the computer-assisted continuous infusion (CACI) system. An ideal automatic anesthesia delivery device would titrate anesthetic to meet the needs of the individual patient using an acquired feedback signal which accurately reflects the effect site concentration of the drug. The most successful efforts at feedback control of anesthesia have utilized the BIS and cortical auditory evoked responses to assess the pharmacodynamic end point.[83]

The rapid, short-acting, sedative–hypnotics (e.g., methohexital, propofol) and opioids (e.g., alfentanil, remifentanil) are better suited for continuous administration techniques than the more traditional anesthetic and analgesic agents because they can be more precisely titrated to meet the unique and changing needs of the individual patient. Traditionally, the elimination half-life of a particular drug has been used in attempting to predict the duration of drug action and the time to awakening after discontinuation of the anesthetic infusion. Using conceptual modeling techniques, it has been shown that the concept of context-sensitive half-time is more appropriate in choosing drugs for continuous IV administration (Fig. 13-9). Because none of the currently available IV drugs can provide for a complete anesthetic state without producing prolonged recovery times and undesirable side effects, it is necessary to administer a combination of IV drugs that provide for hypnosis, amnesia, hemodynamic stability, analgesia, and muscle relaxation. Selecting a combination of drugs with similar pharmacokinetics and compatible pharmacodynamic profiles should improve the anesthetic and surgical conditions. Sedative–hypnotics (methohexital, midazolam, propofol, etomidate, ketamine), opioids (fentanyl, alfentanil, sufentanil, remifentanil), and muscle relaxants (cis-atracurium, mivacurium, rocuronium) can be successfully administered using continuous infusion TIVA techniques as alternatives to the volatile anesthetics and nitrous oxide.

Use of Intravenous Anesthetics for Sedation

The use of sedative–hypnotic drugs as part of a monitored anesthesia care (MAC) technique in combination with local anesthetics is becoming increasingly popular.[85–87] During local or regional anesthesia, subhypnotic dosages of IV anesthetics can be infused to produce sedation, anxiolysis, and amnesia and enhance patient comfort. The optimum sedation technique achieves the desired clinical end points without producing perioperative side effects (respiratory depression, nausea, and vomiting). In addition, it should provide for ease of titration to the desired level of sedation while providing for a rapid return to a "clear headed" state on completion of the surgical procedure. Sedation also constitutes an essential element in the management of patients in the ICU. The ideal sedative agent for critically ill patients would have minimal depressant effects on the respiratory and cardiovascular systems, would not influence biodegradation of other drugs, and would be independent of renal and hepatic function for its elimination. Recently, the BIS monitor has been used to monitor the depth of sedation in the ICU. For patients undergoing cardiac surgery, rapid reversibility of the sedative state may result in earlier extubation and lead to a shorter stay in the ICU. Although intermittent bolus injections of sedative–hypnotic drugs (e.g., diazepam 2.5 to

5 mg, lorazepam 0.5 to 1 mg, midazolam 1.25 to 2.5 mg) have been administered during local anesthesia, continuous infusion techniques with propofol are becoming increasingly popular for maintaining a stable level of sedation in the OR and ICU settings.

Benzodiazepines, particularly midazolam, are still the most widely used for sedation in the ICU and for relief of acute situational anxiety during local and regional anesthesia. Midazolam has a steeper dose-response curve than diazepam (Fig. 13-3), and therefore, careful titration is necessary to avoid oversedation and respiratory depression. Midazolam infusion, 0.05 to 5 mg/kg/min, can be highly effective in providing sedation for hemodynamically unstable patients in the ICU.[88] Use of a midazolam infusion has been shown to control agitation and decrease analgesic requirements without producing cardiovascular or respiratory instability. However, marked variability exists for midazolam in the individual patient dose-effect relationships.[88] In addition, marked tolerance may develop to the CNS effects of midazolam with prolonged administration.

Propofol sedation offers advantages over the other sedative–hypnotics (including midazolam) because of its rapid recovery and favorable side effect profile. In addition, the degree of sedation is readily changeable from "light" to "deep" levels by varying the MIR. Following a propofol LD of 0.25 to 0.5 mg/kg, a carefully titrated subhypnotic infusion of 25 to 75 mg/kg/min produces a stable level of sedation with minimal cardiorespiratory depression and a short recovery period. Because even low concentrations of propofol can depress the ventilatory response to hypoxia, supplemental oxygen should always be provided. Sedative infusions of propofol produce less perioperative amnesia than midazolam, and propofol-induced amnesia appears to be directly related to the infusion rate.

A small dose of midazolam (2 mg IV) administered immediately before a variable-rate infusion of propofol has also been shown to significantly decrease intraoperative anxiety and recall of uncomfortable events without compromising the rapid recovery from propofol sedation.[89] Propofol sedation can also be supplemented with potent opioid and nonopioid analgesics to provide sedation analgesia. In comparing propofol and midazolam for patient-controlled sedation, midazolam was associated with less intraoperative recall and pain on injection than propofol, while propofol was associated with less residual impairment of cognitive function. Compared with midazolam in the ICU setting, use of propofol sedation allowed for more rapid weaning of critically ill patients from artificial ventilation.[90] It has been suggested that the more rapid weaning after propofol sedation may be cost-saving compared with midazolam when only a limited period of sedation (<48 hour) is required.[91] Although a pharmacokinetic study yielded no evidence of a change in receptor sensitivity or drug accumulation over a 4-day study period, preliminary data suggest that tolerance to the CNS effects of propofol may develop with more prolonged administration (>1 week).

Concerns have been raised about elevated lipid plasma levels in patients sedated with propofol for several days, especially when high infusion rates (>6 mg/kg/h) are utilized. However, the availability of a propofol formulation with reduced lipid content (Ampofol) should decrease the risk of this problem in the future. Because of conflicting evidence regarding increased mortality as a result of myocardial failure when propofol was used for sedation in the neonatal ICU,[92–94] more safety data are needed to define the indications for the use of prolonged propofol infusions, especially in the pediatric population. Low-dose ketamine infusions (5 to 25 mg/kg/min) can also be used for sedation and analgesia during local or regional anesthetic procedures, as well as in the ICU setting.[59] Midazolam, 0.07 to 0.15 mg/kg infused over 3 to 5 min, followed by ketamine, 0.25 to 0.5 mg/kg IV over 1 to 3 min, produced excellent sedation, amnesia, and analgesia without significant cardiorespiratory depression.

CONCLUSION

It is obvious that many of the goals desirable in an ideal IV anesthetic have not been achieved with the currently available drugs. Nevertheless, each of these sedative–hypnotic drugs possesses characteristics that may be useful in specific clinical situations. For example, thiopental remains a widely used IV anesthetic even though it is unstable in solution and produces a high incidence of postoperative drowsiness and sedation. In situations where a rapid recovery is not essential (e.g., inpatient procedures), the barbiturates may be the most cost-effective IV anesthetics. Although recovery from anesthesia with methohexital is more rapid than with thiopental (and compares favorably with propofol), excitatory side effects (e.g., myoclonus, hiccoughing) are more prominent than with the other barbiturates or propofol. Importantly, methohexital remains the anesthetic of choice for ECT procedures.

Propofol is the IV drug of choice when a rapid and smooth recovery is required (e.g., outpatient [ambulatory] anesthesia). Recovery from propofol anesthesia is characterized by the absence of a "hangover effect" and less PONV. The cardiovascular depressant effects produced by propofol appear to be more pronounced than those of thiopental, but can be minimized by careful titration and the use of a variable-rate infusion during the maintenance period. The ability to combine propofol with potent, rapid and short-acting opioid analgesics (e.g., remifen-
10 tanil) has facilitated the use of TIVA techniques. Improvements in the ability to deliver IV anesthetics (propofol) and analgesics (remifentanil) will lead to a greater acceptance of these techniques in the future.[95]

When administered alone for induction of anesthesia, benzodiazepines are associated with a prolonged recovery profile. In the usual induction doses, benzodiazepines are associated with minimal cardiorespiratory depression and the reliable amnestic effect may be valuable during TIVA (e.g., for acute sedation prior to induction of anesthesia, for maintenance in the absence of nitrous oxide). When administered in smaller doses, midazolam can also be a valuable adjunct as part of a coinduction and/or maintenance technique. Other short-acting benzodiazepines may be developed in the future (e.g., Ro 48-6791).

Etomidate has minimal cardiovascular and respiratory depressant effects and is therefore, an extremely useful induction agent in high-risk patients. It is also used as an alternative to methohexital for ECT procedures. Unfortunately, pain on injection, excitatory phenomena, adrenocortical suppression, and a high incidence of PONV have limited the use of etomidate to special situations in which it offers significant advantages over other available IV anesthetics. The new lipid formulation of etomidate is associated with its fewer side effects and may allow this IV anesthetic to gain wider clinical acceptance in the future.

Ketamine is a unique IV anesthetic that produces a wide spectrum of pharmacologic effects (including sedation, hypnosis, somatic analgesia, bronchodilation, and sympathetic nervous system stimulation). Induction of anesthesia can be rapidly achieved following parenteral injection, making it the drug of choice when IV access is difficult to establish in an emergency situation. Ketamine is also indicated for induction of anesthesia in the presence of hypovolemic shock, acute bronchospastic states, right-to-left intracardiac shunts, and cardiac tamponade. The adverse cardiovascular, cerebrodynamic, and psychomimetic effects of ketamine can be minimized by prior administration of a benzodiazepine (e.g., midazolam) or sedative–hypnotic drugs (e.g., thiopental, propofol), making it useful as part of coinduction and maintenance anesthetic techniques. The introduction of the more potent S(+)-ketamine may increase use of ketamine in small-doses (75 to 250 μg/kg) or by continuous infusion (10 to 25 μg/kg/min) as an IV adjuvant during general anesthesia because of its anesthetic and analgesic-sparing activity.

Intravenous anesthesia has evolved from being used mainly for induction of anesthesia to providing unconsciousness and amnesia for surgical procedures performed under local, regional, and general anesthesia. New insights into the pharmacokinetics and dynamics of IV anesthetics, as well as the development of computer technology to facilitate IV drug delivery (e.g., TCI), have greatly enhanced the use of TIVA techniques. The shorter context-sensitive half-life values of the newer sedative–hypnotic drugs make these compounds more useful as continuous infusions for maintenance of anesthesia or sedation. While the search for the ideal IV anesthetic continues, the challenge for the anesthesiologist is to choose the most cost-effective sedative–hypnotic that most closely matches the needs of a specific clinical situation.

References

1. Franks NP, Lieb WR: Molecular and cellular mechanisms of general anaesthesia. Nature 367:607, 1994
2. Krasowski MD, Koltchine VV, Rick CE *et al*: Propofol and other intravenous anesthetics have sites of action on the gamma-aminobutyric acid type A receptor distinct from that for isoflurane. Mol Pharmacol 53:530, 1998
3. Coates KM, Mather LE, Johnson R, Flood P: Thiopental is a competitive inhibitor at the human alpha7 nicotinic acetylcholine receptor. Anesth Anal 92:930, 2001
4. Rossi MA, Chan CK, Christensen JD *et al*: Interactions between propofol and lipid mediator receptors: inhibition of lysophosphatidate signaling. Anesth Analg 83:1090, 1996
5. Shelly MP: Dexmedetomidine: a real innovation or more of the same? Br. J. Anaesth 87:677, 2001
6. Thomas JE, Judith E, Hall, MA *et al*: The effects of increasing plasma concentrations of Dexmedetomidine in humans. Anesthesiology 93:382, 2000
7. Hughes MA, Jacobs JR, Glass PSA: Context-sensitive half-time in multicompartment pharmacokinetic models for intravenous anesthesia. Anesthesiology 76:334, 1992
8. Modica PA, Tempelhoff R, White PF: Pro- and anticonvulsant effects of anesthetics (Part II). Anesth Analg 70:433, 1990
9. Drummond-Lewis J, Scher C: Propofol: A new treatment strategy for refractory migraine headache. Pain Med 3:366, 2002
10. Hall JE, Uhrich TD, Barney JA *et al*: Sedative, amnestic, and analgesic properties of small-dose dexmedetomidine infusions. Anesth Analg 90:699, 1995
11. Avram J, Krejcie TC, Henthorn TK: The relationship of age to pharmacokinetics of early drug distribution: The concurrent disposition of thiopental and indocyanine green. Anesthesiology 72:403, 1990
12. Abramson N: Randomized clinical study of thiopental loading in comatose survivors of cardiac arrest. N Engl J Med 314:397, 1986
13. Gunaydin B, Babacan A: Cerebral hypoperfusion after cardiac surgery and anesthetic strategies: A comparative study with high-dose fentanyl and barbiturate anesthesia. Ann Thorac Cardiovasc Surg 4:12, 1998
14. Newman MF, Croughwell ND, White WD *et al*: Pharmacologic electroencephalograhic suppression during cardiopulmonary bypass: A comparison of thiopental and isoflurane. Anesth Analg 86:246, 1998
15. Ding Z, White PF: Anesthesia for electroconvulsive therapy. Anesth Analg 94:1351, 2002
16. Blouin RT, Conard PF, Gross JB: Time course of ventilatory depression following induction doses of propofol and thiopental. Anesthesiology 75:940, 1991
17. Vohra A, Thomas AN, Harper NJN, Pollard BJ: Non-invasive measurement of cardiac output during induction of anaesthesia and tracheal intubation: Thiopentone and propofol compared. Br J Anaesth 67:64, 1991
18. Bhutada A, Shani R, Rastogi S, Wung JT: Randomised controlled trial of thiopental for intubation in neonates. Arch Dis Child Fetal Neonatal Ed 82:F34, 2000
19. Asik I, Yorukoglu D, Gulay I, Tulunay M: Pain on injection of propofol: Comparison of metoprolol with lidocaine. Eur J Anaesthesiol 20:487, 2003
20. Dubey PK, Prasad SS: Pain on injection of propofol: The effect of granisetron pretreatment. Clini J Pain 19:121, 2003
21. Piper SN, Rohm KD, Papsdorf M *et al*: Dolasetron reduces pain on injection of propofol. Anaesthesiol Intensivmed Notfallmed Schmerzther 37:528, 2002
22. Agarwal A, Ansari MF, Gupta D *et al*: Pretreatment with thiopental for prevention of pain associated with propofol injection. Anaesth Analg 98:683, 2004
23. Song D, Hamza M, White PF *et al*: The pharmacodynamic effects of a lower-lipid emulsion of propofol: A comparison with the standard propofol emulsion. Anesth Analg 98:687, 2004
24. Song D, Hamza M, White PF *et al*: Comparison of a lower-lipid propofol emulsion with the standard emulsion for sedation during monitored anesthesia care. Anesthesiology, 100:1072, 2004
25. Fechner J, Ihmsen H, Hatterscheid D *et al*: Pharmacokinetics and clinical pharmacodynamics of the new propofol prodrug PGI 15715 in volunteers. Anesthesiology 99:303, 2003
26. Shafer A, Doze VA, Shafer SL, White PF: Pharmacokinetics and pharmacodynamics of propofol infusions during general anesthesia. Anesthesiology 69:348, 1988
27. Sebel PS, Lowdon JD: Propofol: A new intravenous anesthetic. Anesthesiology 71:260, 1989
28. Doze VA, Westphal LM, White PF: Comparison of propofol with methohexital for outpatient anesthesia. Anesth Analg 65:1189, 1986
29. Smith I, White PF, Nathanson M, Gouldson R: Propofol: An update on its clinical use. Anesthesiology 81:1005, 1994
30. Glass PSA: Prevention of awareness during total intravenous anesthesia. Anesthesiology 78:399, 1993
31. Oxorn D, Orser B, Ferris LE, Harrington E: Propofol and thiopental anesthesia: A comparison of the incidence of dreams and perioperative mood alterations. Anesth Analg 79:553, 1994
32. Hofbauer RK, Fiset P, Plourde G *et al*: Dose-dependent effects of propofol on the central processing of thermal pain. Anesthesiology 100:386, 2004
33. Pinaud M, Lelausque JN, Chetanneau A *et al*: Effects of propofol on cerebral hemodynamics and metabolism in patients with brain trauma. Anesthesiology 73:404, 1990
34. Yagmurdur H, Cakan T, Bayrak A *et al*: The effects of etomidate, thiopental, and propofol in induction on hypoperfusion-reperfusion phenomenon during laparoscopic cholecystectomy. Acta Anaesthesiol Scand 48:772, 2004
35. Dolk A, Cannerfelt R, Anderson RE, Jakobsson J: Inhalation anaesthesia is cost-effective for ambulatory surgery clinical comparison with propofol during elective knee arthroscopy. Eur J Anaesthesiol 19:88–92, 2002
36. Reddy RV, Moorthy SS, Dierdorf SF *et al*: Excitatory effects and electroencephalographic correlation of etomidate, thiopental, methohexital, and propofol. Anesth Analg 77:1008, 1993
37. Ebrahim ZY, Schubert A, Van Ness P *et al*: The effect of propofol on the electroencephalogram of patients with epilepsy. Anesth Analg 78:275, 1994
38. Sellgren J, Ejnell H, Elam M *et al*: Sympathetic muscle nerve activity, peripheral blood flows, and baroreceptor reflexes in humans during propofol anesthesia and surgery. Anesthesiology 80:534, 1994
39. Lopatka CW, Muzi M, Ebert TJ: Propofol, but not etomidate, reduces desflurane-mediated sympathetic activation in humans. Can J Anaesth 46:342, 1999
40. Gan TJ, Glass PSA, Howell ST *et al*: Determination of plasma concentrations associated with 50% reduction in postoperative nausea. Anesthesiology 87:779, 1997
41. Krumholz W, Endrass J, Hempelmann G: Propofol inhibits phagocytosis and killing of Staphylococcus aureus and Escherichia coli by polymorphonuclear leukocytes in vitro. Can J Anaesth 41:446, 1994
42. Crowther J, Hrazdil J, Jolly DT *et al*: Growth of microorganisms in propofol, thiopental, and a 1:1 mixture of propofol and thiopental. Anesth Analg 82:475, 1996
43. Reves JG, Fragen RJ, Vinik HR, Greenblatt DJ: Midazolam—Pharmacology and uses. Anesthesiology 62:310, 1985
44. Urquhart ML, White PF: Comparison of sedative infusions during regional anesthesia: Methohexital, etomidate, and midazolam. Anesth Analg 68:249, 1988
45. Ghouri A, Taylor E, White PF: Patient-controlled drug administration during local anesthesia: A comparison of midazolam, propofol, and alfentanil. J Clin Anesth 4:476, 1992
46. Dingemanse J, van Gerven JMA, Schoemaker RC *et al*: Integrated pharmacokinetics and pharmacodynamics of Ro 48-6791, a new benzodiazepine, in comparison with midazolam during first administration to healthy male subjects. Br J Clin Pharmacol 44:477, 1997
47. Tang J, Wang B, White PF *et al*: Comparison of the sedation and recovery profiles of Ro 48-6791, a new benzodiazepine, and midazolam in combination with meperidine for outpatient endoscopic procedures. Anesth Analg 89:893, 1999
48. Brodgen RN, Goa KL: Flumazenil. Drugs 42:1061, 1991
49. Ghouri AF, Ramirez Ruiz MA, White PF: Effect of flumazenil on recovery after midazolam and propofol sedation. Anesthesiology 81:333, 1994
50. Flogel CM, Ward DS, Wada DR, Ritter JW: The effects of large-dose flumazenil on midazolam-induced ventilatory depression. Anesth Analg 77:1207, 1993
51. White PF, Shafer A, Boyle WA *et al*: Benzodiazepine antagonism does not provoke a stress response. Anesthesiology 70:636, 1989
52. Doenicke AW, Roizen MF, Kugler J *et al*: Reducing myoclonus after etomidate. Anesthesiology 90:113, 1999
53. Van Hamme MJ, Ghoneim MM, Amber JJ: Pharmacokinetics of etomidate, a new intravenous anesthetic. Anesthesiology 49:274, 1978
54. Wagner RL, White PF, Kan PB *et al*: Inhibition of adrenal steroidogenesis by the anesthetic etomidate. N Engl J Med 310:1415, 1984

55. Gooding JM, Weng JT, Smith RA *et al*: Cardiovascular and pulmonary response following etomidate induction of anesthesia in patients with demonstrated cardiac disease. Anesth Analg 50:40, 1979
56. Wagner RL, White PF: Etomidate inhibits adrenocortical function in surgical patients. Anesthesiology 61:647, 1984
57. Gries A, Weis S, Herr A *et al*: Etomidate and thiopental inhibit platelet function in patients undergoing infrainguinal vascular surgery. Acta Anaesthesiol Scand 45:44957, 2001
58. White PF, Way WL, Trevor AJ: Ketamine—Its pharmacology and therapeutic uses. Anesthesiology 56:119, 1982
59. White PF, Ham J, Way WL, Trevor AJ: Pharmacology of ketamine isomers in surgical patients. Anesthesiology 52:231, 1980
60. White PF, Schuttler J, Shafer A, Stanski DR et al: Comparative pharmacology of the ketamine isomers. Studies in volunteers. Br J Anaesth 57:197, 1985
61. Rabben T, Skjelbred P, Oye I: Prolonged analgesia effect of ketamine, an N-methyl-D-aspartate receptor inhibitor, in patients with chronic pain. J Pharmocol Ther 289:1060, 1999
62. Dahl V, Ernoe PE, Steen T, Raeder JC, White PF: Does ketamine have preemptive effects in women undergoing abdominal hysterectomy procedures? Anesth Analg 90:1419, 2000
63. Albanese J, Arnaud S, Rey M *et al*: Ketamine decreases intracranial pressure and electroencephalographic activity in traumatic brain injury patients during propofol sedation. Anesthesiology 87:1328, 1997
64. Susuki M, Tsueda K, Lansing PS *et al*: Small-dose ketamine enhances morphine-induced analgesia after outpatient surgery. Anesth Analg 89:98, 1999
65. Menigaux C, Fletcher D, Dupont X, Guinard B, Guirimand F, Chauvin M: The benefits of intraoperative small-dose ketamine on postoperative pain after anterior cruciate ligament repair. Anesth Analg 90:129, 2000
66. Berman RM, Capiello A, Anand A *et al*: Antidepressant effects of ketamine in depressed patients. Biol Psychiatry 47:351, 2000
67. Kudoh A, Takahira Y, Katagai H, Takazawa T: Small-dose ketamine improves the postoperative state of depressed patients. Anesth Analg 95:114, 2002
68. Mortero RF, Clark LD, Tolan MM, Metz RJ, Tsueda K, Sheppard RA: The effects of small-dose ketamine on propofol sedation: Respiration, postoperative mood, perception, cognition and pain. Anesth Analg 92:1465, 2001
69. Ikeda T, Kazama T, Sessler DI *et al*: Induction of anesthesia with ketamine reduces the magnitude of redistribution hyportermia. Anesth Analg 93:934, 2001
70. Khos R, Duriex ME: Ketamine: Teaching an old drug new tricks. Anesth Analg 87:1186, 1998
71. Smith I, White PF, Nathanson M, Gouldson R: Propofol: An update on its clinical use. Anesthesiology 81:1005, 1994
72. White PF: Comparative evaluation of intravenous agents for rapid sequence induction: Thiopental, ketamine, and midazolam. Anesthesiology 57:279, 1982
73. Kamata K, Nagata O, Iwakiri H, Ozaki M: Comparison of requirement for postoperative analgesics after inhalation and total intravenous anesthesia. Masui 52:1200, 2003
74. Salihoglu Z, Karaca S, Kose Y *et al*: Total intravenous anesthesia versus single breath technique and anesthesia maintenance with sevoflurane for bariatric operations. Obes Surg 11:496, 2001
75. White PF: Use of continuous infusion versus intermittent bolus administration of fentanyl or ketamine during outpatient anesthesia. Anesthesiology 59:294, 1983
76. White PF: Clinical uses of intravenous anesthetic and analgesic infusions. Anesth Analg 68:161, 1989
77. Chang T, Dworsky WA, White PF: Continuous electromyography for monitoring depth of anesthesia. Anesth Analg 53:315, 1980
78. Plourde G: Depth of anaesthesia. Can J Anaesth 31:270, 1991
79. White PF, Boyle WA: Relationship between hemodynamic and electroencephalographic changes during general anesthesia. Anesth Analg 68:177, 1989
80. Chen X, Tang J, White PF, Wender RH, Sloninsky A, Kariger R: A comparison of patient state index and bispectral index values during the perioperative period. Anesth Analg 95:1669, 2002
81. Song D, van Vlymen J, White PF: Is the bispectral index useful in predicting fast-track eligibility after ambulatory anesthesia with propofol and desflurane? Anesth Analg 87:1245, 1998
82. White PF, Ma H, Tang J, Wender R, Sloninsky A, Kariger R: Does the use of electroencephalographic bispectral index or auditory evoked potential index monitoring facilitate recovery after desflurane anesthesia in the ambulatory setting? Anesthesiology 100:811, 2004
83. Struys M, Versichelen L, Mortier E *et al*: Comparison of spontaneous frontal EMG, EEG power spectrum and bispectral index to monitor propofol drug effect and emergence. Acta Anaesthesiol Scand 42:628, 1998
84. Schraag S, Bothner U, Gajraj R *et al*: The performance of electroencephalogram bispectral index and auditory evoked potential index to predict loss of consciousness during propofol infusion. Anesth Analg 89:1311, 1999
85. Milne SE, Kenny GN: Future applications for TCI systems. Anaesthesia 53 (suppl 1):56, 1998
86. White PF, Vascones LO, Mathes SA *et al*: Comparison of midazolam and diazepam for sedaetion during plastic surgery. J Plast Reconstruct Surg 81:703, 1988
87. Taylor E, Ghouri AF, White PF: Midazolam in combination with propofol for seadation during local anesthesia. J Clin Anesth 4:213, 1992
88. Sá Rêgo MM, Watcha, MF, White PF: The changing role of monitored anesthesia care in the ambulatory setting. Anesth Analg 85:1020, 1997
89. Shafer A, Doze VA, White PF: Pharmacokinetic variability of midazolam infusions in critically ill patients. Crit Care Med 18:1039, 1990
90. White PF, Negus JB: Sedative infusions during local or regional anesthesia: A comparison of midazolam and propofol. J Clin Anesth 3:32, 1991
91. Aitkenhead AR, Pepperman ML, Willatts SM *et al*: Comparison of propofol and midazolam for long-term sedation in critically ill patients. Lancet 2:704, 1989
92. Carrasco G, Molina R, Costa J *et al*: Propofol vs. midazolam in short-, medium-, and long-term sedation of critically ill patients: A cost-benefit analysis. Chest 103:557, 1993
93. McFarlan CS, Anderson BJ, Short TG. The use of propofol infusions in paediatric anaesthesia: A practical guide. Paediatr Anaesth 9:209, 1999
94. Parke TJ, Steven JE, Rice ASC *et al*: Metabolic acidosis and fatal myocardial failure after propofol infusion in children: five case reports. BMJ 305:613, 1992
95. Martin PH, Murphy BVS, Petros AJ: Metabolic, biochemical and haemodynamic effects of infusion of propofol for long-term sedation of children undergoing intensive care. Br J Anaesth 79:276, 1997
96. Egan T, Shafer SL: Target-controlled infusions for intravenous anesthetics. Anesthesiology 2003:99, 1039

CHAPTER 14 ■ OPIOIDS

BARBARA A. CODA

KEY POINTS

1. The term "opioid" designates all drugs, both natural and synthetic, including endogenous peptides, which have morphine-like properties. In its broadest sense, it refers to agonists, partial agonists, and mixed agonist–antagonists at one or more of the opioid receptors.
2. Opioid receptor classification is based on binding activity of specific ligands: morphine at mu (μ), ketocyclazocine at kappa (κ), enkephalins at delta (δ), and endorphin at epsilon (ϵ) receptors, and specific opioid receptors are responsible for different opioid effects. Most opioids used in clinical anesthesia today (e.g., fentanyl and morphine and their derivatives) are highly selective for μ opioid receptors. Naloxone, the most commonly used opioid antagonist, is not selective for opioid receptor type. Very few endogenous opioids exhibit great selectivity for a single receptor type.
3. Opioids are administered primarily for their analgesic effect, which results from complex interactions at discrete sites in the brain, spinal cord, and under certain conditions, peripheral tissues, and involves both μ_1 and μ_2 opioid effects. For the mixed agonist–antagonist opioids, analgesic effects are also mediated at κ receptors. Opioids act selectively on neurons that transmit and modulate nociception, leaving other sensory modalities and motor functions intact.
4. Opioids are used in combination with volatile anesthetics with or without nitrous oxide to produce balanced anesthesia. Fentanyl and its derivatives reduce the minimum alveolar concentration (MAC) of volatile agents in a dose-dependent fashion. An apparent ceiling effect is seen at 70% MAC reduction, although reduction of up to 90% has been reported for sufentanil and remifentanil.
5. Fentanyl and its derivatives can be combined with a sedative–hypnotic agent to provide total intravenous anesthesia (TIVA). Alfentanil and remifentanil are particularly suited for TIVA because of their rapid onset and short duration of action.
6. Fentanyl and its derivatives can be given in very high doses for "opioid anesthesia," but even at extremely high doses, i.e., those that produce profound analgesia as well as apnea, unconsciousness is not assured.
7. Muscle hypertonus occurs with high-dose opioid administration, and severe chest wall rigidity can interfere with ventilation. It is seen most often on induction with rapid-acting opioids. Opioid-induced muscle rigidity is increased in the presence of nitrous oxide and can be prevented or treated with sedative–hypnotics or low-dose muscle relaxants.
8. All opioids depress respiratory drive in a dose-dependent manner, and ventilatory depression is seen even at doses associated with mild analgesia. Equianalgesic opioid doses produce equivalent magnitudes of respiratory depression. When given in combination with benzodiazepines, opioids can blunt hypoxic drive to a greater extent than the hypercarbic drive and produce profound respiratory depression.
9. Fentanyl or one of its derivatives is often used as a component of anesthetic induction. Small opioid doses reduce the dosage requirements of sedative–hypnotics, and blunt airway reflexes (sympathetic activity in response to laryngoscopy).
10. In low doses, opioids have minimal cardiovascular effects, but bradycardia and hypotension are seen with higher doses. A prominent feature of fentanyl and its derivatives is their remarkable hemodynamic stability. Morphine and meperidine cause histamine release, and high doses of these opioids can produce greater hypotension than fentanyl and its derivatives.
11. All opioids can produce nausea and vomiting through complex interactions at nausea and vomiting centers in the medulla. In general, equianalgesic doses of opioids produce similar magnitude of nausea. Opioid-induced nausea can be exacerbated by vestibular input, and is particularly problematic in ambulatory patients.
12. Opioids produce smooth muscle spasm throughout the gastrointestinal tract. They decrease gastric secretions and delay gastric emptying. Opioids increase the tone of the common bile duct and sphincter of Oddi, although meperidine and the mixed agonist-antagonists cause less biliary spasm than morphine and fentanyl.

HISTORY

Opioids have been used in the treatment of pain for thousands of years. The drug opium, which contains more than 20 alkaloids, is obtained from the exudate of *Papaver somniferum* seed pods, and the word "opium" is derived from *opos*, the Greek word for juice. The first undisputed reference to poppy juice is found in the third century (BCE) writings of Theophrastus.[1] The German pharmacist Sertuener isolated what he called the "soporific principle" in opium in 1806, and in 1817 named it morphine, after the Greek god of dreams, Morpheus.[2] Isolation of other opium alkaloids followed, and by the mid 1800s, the medical use of pure alkaloids rather than crude opium preparations began to spread.[1] Morphine was used widely to treat wounded soldiers during the American Civil War, and in 1869, its use as a premedication was described by Claude Bernard. However, in the absence of muscle relaxants and controlled ventilation, opioids were associated with a significant risk of severe respiratory depression and death. Thus their use in anesthesia was limited at that time.

With the advent of cardiac surgery in the late 1950s came the development of "opioid anesthesia." A decade later, Lowenstein reported the use of progressively higher doses of morphine (0.5 to 3 mg/kg), but found limitations including incomplete suppression of the stress response, hypotension, awareness during anesthesia, and increased fluid and blood requirements.[3]

Fentanyl, a 4-anilinopiperidine derivative of phenoperidine, was synthesized in 1960. The completely synthetic opioids were more potent and had a better safety margin (ratio of median lethal dose to lowest effective dose for surgery) than meperidine. Advances in surgical techniques created the need for potent opioids with a rapid onset, a brief, predictable duration, and a maximal safety margin for use in clinical anesthesia, and led to development of sufentanil, alfentanil, and other fentanyl derivatives between 1974 and 1976. The newest potent opioid, remifentanil, has an ultrashort duration of action because of rapid metabolism by ester hydrolysis and offers an advantage in specific clinical settings.

The search for opioid analgesics without potential for dependence was stimulated by concerns about opioid addiction and led to the identification of multiple opioid receptor types. In the mid 1960s, nalorphine, a morphine antagonist, was also found to have analgesic properties. Two other compounds, pentazocine and cyclazocine, antagonized some of morphine's effects. Pentazocine also produced analgesia, and both produced some psychotropic effects that morphine did not. These and other observations led Martin to propose the theory of receptor dualism. Intrinsic to this theory were two key concepts: (1) the existence of multiple opioid receptors (originally only two were proposed); and (2) the idea of pharmacologic redundancy (i.e., more than one receptor could mediate a physiologic function, such as analgesia).[4] Thus, a drug could be a strong agonist, a partial agonist, or a competitive antagonist at one or more of the different receptor types. Subsequent research has revealed three distinct families of opioid peptides and multiple categories of opioid receptors. Future research may identify compounds that provide potent analgesia but fewer side effects or propensity for abuse based on receptor selectivity.

TERMINOLOGY

The term "opiate" was originally used to refer to drugs derived
1 from opium, including morphine, its semisynthetic derivatives, and codeine. The more general term "opioid" was introduced to designate all drugs, both natural and synthetic, with morphine-like properties, including endogenous peptides. The nonspecific term "narcotic" has been used to refer to morphine and morphine-like analgesics. However, because of its use in a legal context, referring to any drug (including nonopioids, such as cocaine) that can produce dependence, the term narcotic is not useful in a pharmacologic or clinical context.

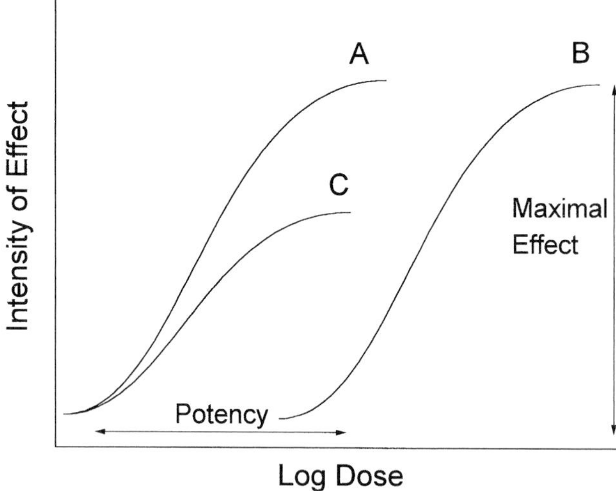

FIGURE 14-1. Log dose-effect curves for two agonists (*A* and *B*) with equal efficacy but different potency, and a partial agonist (*C*). Note that the potencies of A and C are similar, but the efficacy is less and the slope of the dose-response curve is shallower for the partial agonist. Note also that at lower doses, the partial agonist C is more potent than the full agonist B.

In its broadest sense, the term opioid can refer to agonists, partial agonists, mixed agonist–antagonists, and competitive antagonists. Differentiation of these terms requires understanding of receptor–ligand interactions. Receptor theory states that drugs have two independent characteristics at receptor sites: *affinity*, the ability to bind a receptor to produce a stable complex, and intrinsic activity or *efficacy*, which is described by the dose-effect curve resulting from the drug–receptor combination. Efficacy can range from zero (i.e., no effect) to the maximum possible effect, depicted graphically as the plateau of the dose-effect curve (Fig. 14-1). Given a high enough dose, an *agonist* will produce the maximum possible effect of binding with the receptor, whereas an *antagonist* produces no direct effect when it binds the receptor. A *partial agonist* has a dose-effect ceiling that is lower than the maximum possible effect produced by a full agonist, as well as a dose-effect curve that is less steep than that of a full agonist. A *mixed agonist–antagonist* acts as an agonist (or partial agonist) at one receptor and an antagonist at another. It is important to differentiate the term "potency" from "efficacy." Whereas efficacy defines the range in magnitude of an effect produced by a drug–receptor combination relative to the maximum possible effect, potency refers to the relative dose required to achieve an effect, and is related to receptor affinity. Thus, at the lower end of the effect range, a partial agonist may be more potent than a full agonist (see Fig. 14-1). However, even at very large doses the efficacy, or maximum effect achieved by the partial agonist, will be less than the maximum possible effect of a full agonist.

ENDOGENOUS OPIOIDS AND OPIOID RECEPTORS

All of the endogenous opioids are derived from three prohormones: proenkephalin, prodynorphin, and pro-opiomelanocortin (POMC). Each of these precursors is encoded by a separate gene. The three families of peptides differ in their distribution, receptor selectivity, and neurochemical role,[5] but

TABLE 14-1

TENTATIVE CLASSIFICATION OF OPIOID RECEPTOR SUBTYPES AND THEIR ACTIONS

■ RECEPTOR	■ ANALGESIA	■ RESPIRATORY	■ GASTROINTESTINAL	■ ENDOCRINE	■ OTHER
μ	Peripheral		↓ Gastric secretion ↓ GI transit—supraspinal and peripheral Antidiarrheal	Skeletal muscle rigidity	Pruritus ?Urinary retention (and/or δ) Biliary spasm (probably >1 receptor type)
μ_1	Supraspinal			Prolactin release	Acetylcholine turnover Catalepsy
μ_2	Spinal Supraspinal (synergism with spinal)	Respiratory depression	↓ GI transit—spinal and supraspinal		Most cardiovascular effects
κ	Peripheral			↓ ADH release	Sedation
κ_1	Spinal				
κ_2	?				(Pharmacology unknown)
κ_3	Supraspinal				
δ	Peripheral	?Respiratory depression	↓ GI transit—spinal Antidiarrheal—spinal and supraspinal	?Growth hormone release	?Urinary retention (and /or μ)
δ_1	Spinal				Dopamine turnover
δ_2	Supraspinal				
Unknown (receptor type not identified)	Supraspinal				Pupillary constriction Nausea and vomiting

Adapted from Pasternak GW: Pharmacological mechanisms of opioid analgesics. Clin Neuropharmacol 16:1, 1993.

share some features. For example, all begin with the pentapeptide sequences of [Leu]- or [Met]-enkephalin. Proenkephalin includes the pentapeptide sequences for [Met]- and [Leu]-enkephalin, and cells that synthesize proenkephalin are widely distributed throughout the brain, spinal cord, and peripheral sites, particularly the adrenal medulla.[6] Pro-opiomelanocortin is the common precursor of β-endorphin, adrenocorticotropic hormone (ACTH), and melanocyte-stimulating hormone (MSH). The term *endorphin* is reserved for peptides of the POMC family. The major site of POMC synthesis is the pituitary, but it is also found in the pancreas and placenta. The dynorphin peptides all begin with the [Leu]-enkephalin sequence and are widely distributed throughout the brain, spinal cord, and peripheral sites.

Endogenous opioids bind to a number of opioid receptors
2 to produce their effects. Martin's initial classification of opioid receptors into the three types was based on binding activity of the exogenous ligands morphine, ketocyclazocine, and SKF10,047 at mu (μ), kappa (κ), and sigma (σ) receptors, respectively. Other opioid receptors identified since that time are delta (δ) receptors, bound by enkephalins, and epsilon (ϵ) receptors, bound by endorphin.[5,6] There is also evidence supporting the existence of two μ, two δ, and three κ receptor subtypes.[8] While it appears that specific opioid receptors are responsible for different opioid effects and that synthetic opioids may be highly selective for a receptor type or subtype, it is important to note that very few endogenous opioids exhibit great selectivity for a single receptor type.[7] Remember also, that the theory of receptor dualism includes the concept of pharmacologic redundancy of receptor function. Thus, observed opioid effects typically involve complex interactions among the different receptor systems at supraspinal, spinal, and peripheral sites. Table 14-1 summarizes our current understanding of which opioid receptors are responsible for mediating opioid analgesic and side effects. One caveat in interpreting this summary is that species differences in opioid receptor systems exist, so the results of animal studies, from which most of this information is derived,
3 may not always be directly applicable to humans. Most opioids used in clinical anesthesia today (e.g., fentanyl and morphine and their derivatives) are highly selective for μ opioid receptors. Naloxone, the most commonly used opioid antagonist, is not selective for opioid receptor type. In fact, current identification of an opioid-receptor–mediated drug effect requires demonstration of naloxone reversibility. Development of selective opioid receptor subtype antagonists will be helpful tools in improving our understanding of which receptor subtypes mediate specific opioid effects.

At the cellular level, endogenous and exogenous opioids produce their effects by altering patterns of interneuronal communication. Receptor binding initiates a series of physiologic functions resulting in cellular hyperpolarization and inhibition of neurotransmitter release, effects that are mediated by second messengers. All opioid receptors appear to be coupled to G-proteins,[5] which regulate the activity of adenylate cyclase among other functions. G-protein interactions, in turn, affect ion channels; different ion conductances may be involved at different opioid receptor types.[7]

STRUCTURE–ACTIVITY RELATIONSHIPS

The wide array of different molecules that produce morphine-like analgesia and side effects, including endogenous opioids, all share some common structural characteristics. Horn and

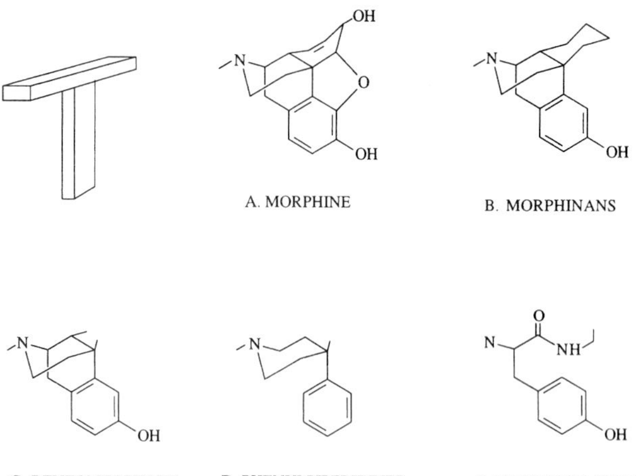

FIGURE 14-2. "T"-shape conformation of opioid molecules. **A.** Morphine, one of the phenanthrene alkaloids, has a rigid five-ring structure, with a phenylpiperidine ring forming a crossbar and a hydroxylated aromatic ring in the vertical axis. **B.** Reducing the number of fused rings to four yields the morphinan class of opium alkaloids. **C.** Benzomorphans have three fused rings. **D.** Phenylpiperidines and the 4-anilinopiperidines such as fentanyl have a flexible two-ring structure. **E.** Finally, the tyramine moiety, which is the amino terminal peptide of both [Leu]- and [Met]-enkephalin, is shown, with a single aromatic ring. Another key feature is the positively charged basic nitrogen equidistant (4.55Å) from the aromatic ring. (Adapted with permission from Thorpe DH: Opiate structures and activity: A guide to understanding the receptor. Anesth Analg 63:143, 1984.)

Rodgers[8] suggested that the tyrosine moiety at the amino terminal of the enkephalins formed the basis of a significant conformational relationship between the enkephalins and opiates. The structure of the phenanthrene class of opium alkaloids is complex and consists of five or six fused rings. Morphine, one of three phenanthrenes, has a rigid five-ring structure that conforms to a "T" shape (Fig. 14-2).[9] The other phenanthrenes are codeine, a derivative of morphine, and thebaine, a precursor of oxycodone and naloxone. Progressively reducing the number of fused rings from the phenanthrenes yields the morphinans, with four rings; the benzomorphans, with three rings; the phenylpiperidines, with two rings; and finally, the tyramine moiety of the endogenous opioid peptides, with a single hydroxylated ring. All of these distinct classes of drugs possess morphine-like activity. Thorpe's[9] opiate receptor model is based on these structural similarities with two aromatic binding sites and one anionic site responsible for binding the positively charged nitrogen. In this model, differences in binding at the aromatic or anionic sites could account for receptor specificity or for agonist versus antagonist activity. Structural modifications alter such important properties as opioid receptor affinity, agonist versus antagonist activity, resistance to metabolic breakdown, lipid solubility, and pharmacokinetics.[1]

PHARMACOKINETICS AND PHARMACODYNAMICS

Basic Considerations

Opioid effects are initiated by the combination of an opioid with one or more receptors at specific tissue sites. The relationship between opioid dose and effects depends on both pharmacokinetic and pharmacodynamic variables. *Pharmacokinetics* determines the relationship between drug dose and its concentration at the effect site(s). *Pharmacodynamic* variables relate the concentration of a drug at its site of action, in this case opioid receptors in the brain and other tissues, and the intensity of its effects. Pharmacokinetics generally refers to the study of blood or plasma drug concentration versus time because blood is easy to sample, bears a definable relationship to tissue concentration, and is the medium by which drugs are distributed throughout the body. Changes in drug concentration over time in the blood, at the effect site and at other sites, are determined by physicochemical properties of the drug as well as the processes of absorption, redistribution, biotransformation, and elimination.

In clinical anesthesia practice, opioids are typically administered intravenously. After an intravenous bolus dose or brief infusion, peak plasma opioid concentrations occur within minutes. Plasma drug concentrations then fall rapidly as the drug is distributed to extravascular sites, including sites of action, noneliminating tissues, and eliminating organs. Compartmental models describe the time course of change in plasma concentration; typically, opioids used in anesthesia are characterized by two- or three-compartment models (see Chapter 11: Basic Principles of Clinical Pharmacology). The early rapid decline in plasma concentration after the peak is called the *distribution phase*, and the subsequent slower decline is the *elimination phase*. From a mathematical curve fitted to measured plasma concentration versus time data, distribution and elimination half-lives, systemic clearance, compartment volumes, and intercompartmental transfer rate constants can be calculated. Table 14-2 summarizes the estimates of key pharmacokinetic parameters and physicochemical characteristics for the most commonly used opioids in clinical anesthesia.

It is important to note that there is tremendous variability in the values published for opioid pharmacokinetic parameters. This is due, in part, to real population differences (e.g., age, diseases), and in part to differences in study design (e.g., sampling site, duration, concomitant events such as surgery, or other drugs that may affect differential flow to sites of metabolism or elimination). In addition, the distributional and elimination half-lives are of limited use in predicting the onset and duration of opioid action in clinical anesthesia. Contributions of distribution processes between physiologic compartments vary with time. In an effort to relate pharmacokinetics to the time of onset and duration of action, concepts such as *effect compartment* in pharmacodynamic modeling[10] and *context-sensitive half-times*[11] have been developed. The application of these concepts are considered later in this chapter.

Physicochemical properties of opioids influence both pharmacokinetics and pharmacodynamics. To reach its effector sites in the central nervous system (CNS), an opioid must cross biologic membranes from the blood to receptors on neuronal cell membranes. The ability of opioids to cross this blood-brain barrier depends on such properties as molecular size, ionization, lipid solubility, and protein binding (see Table 14-2). Of these characteristics, lipid solubility and ionization assume major importance in determining the rate of penetration to the CNS. In the laboratory, lipid solubility is measured as an octanol:water or octanol:buffer partition coefficient. Drug ionization is also an important determinant of lipid solubility; nonionized drugs are 1,000 to 10,000 times more lipid-soluble than the ionized form.[12] The degree of ionization depends on the pK_a of the opioid and the pH of the environment. An opioid with a pK_a much lower than 7.4 will have a much greater nonionized fraction in plasma than one with a pK_a close to or greater than physiologic pH. While greater lipid solubility correlates with membrane permeability, the relationship is not simply a linear one. Hansch[13] has shown that there is an optimal hydrophobicity for blood-brain barrier penetration, and Bernards[14] has demonstrated a similar biphasic relationship between the octanol:buffer distribution coefficient and spinal meningeal

TABLE 14-2

PHYSICOCHEMICAL CHARACTERISTICS AND PHARMACOKINETICS OF COMMONLY USED OPIOID AGONISTS IN ADULTS

PARAMETER	MORPHINE	MEPERIDINE	FENTANYL	SUFENTANIL	ALFENTANIL	REMIFENTANIL
pK_a	7.9	8.5	8.4	8.0	6.5	7.26[a]
% nonionized (pH 7.4)	23	7	8.5	20	89	58[a]
λ_{ow}	1.4	39	816	1757	128	17.9[b]
Protein binding (%)	35	70	84	93	92	66–93[a]
Clearance (mL/min)	1050	1020	1530	900	238	4000
Vd_{ss} (L)	224	305	335	123	27	30
Rapid distribution half-life ($T_{1/2}\pi$, min)			1.2–1.9	1.4	1.0–3.5	0.4–0.5
Slow redistribution half-life ($T_{1/2\alpha}$, min)	1.5–4.4	4–16	9.2–19	17.7	9.5–17	2.0–3.7
Elimination half-life ($T_{1/2}\beta$, h)	1.7–3.3	3–5	3.1–6.6	2.2–4.6	1.4–1.5	0.17–0.33

λ_{ow}, octanol:water partition coefficient, Vd_{ss}, steady-state volume of distribution.
[a] Unpublished information from Glaxo. JG Bovill, personal communication.
[b] Glass PSA *et al*: Anesth Analg 89:S7, 1999.
Adapted from Bovill JG: Pharmacokinetics and pharmacodynamics of opioid agonists. Anaesth Pharmacol Rev 1:122, 1993.

permeability. Plasma protein binding also affects opioid redistribution because only the unbound fraction is free to diffuse across cell membranes. The major plasma proteins to which opioids bind are albumin and α_1-acid glycoprotein (AAG). Alterations in AAG concentration occur in a variety of conditions and disease states and result in acute or chronic changes in opioid requirements.

Two main mechanisms are responsible for drug elimination: *biotransformation* and *excretion*. Opioids are biotransformed in the liver by two types of metabolic processes. Phase I reactions include oxidative and reductive reactions, such as those catalyzed by cytochrome P-450 system, and hydrolytic reactions. Phase II reactions involve conjugation of a drug or its metabolite to an endogenous substrate, such as D-glucuronic acid.[12] Remifentanil is metabolized via ester hydrolysis, which is unique for an opioid. With the exceptions of the *N*-deallylated metabolite of meperidine and the 6- and possibly 3-glucuronides of morphine, opioid metabolites are generally inactive. Opioid metabolites and, to a lesser extent, their parent compounds are excreted primarily by the kidneys. The biliary system and gut are other routes of opioid excretion.

MORPHINE

Morphine produces its major effects in the CNS and the gastrointestinal system, but other systems are also affected. CNS effects include analgesia, sedation, changes in affect, respiratory depression, nausea and vomiting, pruritus, and changes in pupil size. Morphine also affects gastric secretions and gut motility, and has endocrine, urinary, and autonomic effects. It mimics the effects of endogenous opioids by acting as an agonist at μ_1 and μ_2 opioid receptors throughout the body and is considered the standard agonist to which other μ agonists are compared.

Analgesia

Opioids are administered primarily for their analgesic effect. Morphine analgesia results from complex interactions at a number of discrete sites in the brain, spinal cord, and under certain conditions, peripheral tissues, and involves both μ_1 and μ_2 opioid effects. Morphine and related opioids act selectively on neurons that transmit and modulate nociception, leaving other sensory modalities and motor functions intact. At the spinal cord level, morphine acts presynaptically on primary afferent nociceptors to decrease the release of substance P and also hyperpolarizes postsynaptic neurons in the substantia gelatinosa of the dorsal spinal cord to decrease afferent transmission of nociceptive impulses.[15] Spinal morphine analgesia is mediated by μ_2 opioid receptors. Supraspinal opioid analgesia originates in the periaqueductal gray matter (PAG), the locus ceruleus (LC), and nuclei within the medulla, notably the nucleus raphe magnus (NRM), and primarily involves μ_1 opioid receptors. Microinjections of morphine into any of these regions activates the respective descending modulatory systems to produce profound analgesia.[6,15] A more detailed description of the endogenous pain transmission and modulation pathways is given in Chapter 54. Morphine can act at a number of these discrete regions in the CNS to produce synergistic analgesic effects. For example, co-administration at the level of the brain and spinal cord increases morphine's analgesic potency nearly 10-fold,[16] an effect mediated by μ_2 opioid receptors.[6] There are also synergistic interactions between supraspinal sites of opioid action (e.g., between the PAG and the NRM).[6] When inflammation is present, morphine may also produce analgesia by activating opioid receptors on primary afferent neurons.[17]

Although rapidly changing plasma morphine concentrations, such as those that follow bolus dosing, do not correlate well with analgesic effects, constant or very slowly changing (i.e., steady-state) plasma concentrations do correlate with effect intensities. Dahlström measured the minimum effective analgesic concentration (MEAC) of morphine for postoperative pain relief at 10 to 15 ng/mL.[18] For more severe pain, plasma morphine concentrations of 30 to 50 ng/mL are needed to achieve adequate analgesia.[19]

Effect on Minimum Alveolar Concentration of Volatile Anesthetics

μ-agonists are used extensively in conjunction with nitrous oxide (N_2O) with or without volatile anesthetics to provide "balanced anesthesia." In animals, morphine decreases the minimum alveolar concentration (MAC) of volatile anesthetics in a dose-dependent manner,[20,21] but there appears to be a ceiling effect to the anesthetic-sparing ability of morphine, with a plateau at 65% MAC.[20] Measurement of the maximum effect of very high morphine doses on MAC is limited by undesirable side effects such as hypotension and abdominal wall rigidity. Morphine 1 mg/kg administered with 60% N_2O blocked the adrenergic response to skin incision in 50% of patients, a characteristic called MAC-BAR.[22] Neuraxial morphine may also reduce MAC. Epidural morphine 4 mg given 90 minutes prior to incision reduced halothane MAC by nearly 30%.[23] The effect of intrathecal morphine on MAC is unclear. In one study, a relatively large dose of intrathecal morphine (750 μg) reduced halothane MAC approximately 40%,[24] but an equally large dose (15 μg/kg) failed to reduce halothane MAC in another.[25]

Other Central Nervous System Effects

Morphine can produce sedation, as well as cognitive and fine motor impairment, even at plasma concentrations commonly achieved during management of moderate to severe pain.[26] Other subjective side effects include euphoria, dysphoria, and sleep disturbances. High doses of morphine and similar opioids produce a slowing of electroencephalogram (EEG) activity associated with a marked shift toward increased voltage and decreased frequency.[1,27] In routine analgesic doses, morphine can produce sleep disturbances, including reduction in REM and slow wave sleep,[1] as well as vivid dreams. In extremely high doses, morphine can produce seizure activity in animals, but this toxic effect is not seen with doses used clinically in humans.

Morphine produces dose-dependent pupillary constriction (miosis) in humans. A near maximal degree of miosis is seen with 0.5 mg/kg of morphine.[28] In the absence of other drugs, miosis appears to correlate with opioid-induced ventilatory depression. However, hypoxemia from severe opioid-induced respiratory depression will cause pupillary dilation.

Systemic and neuraxial administration of morphine can produce pruritus, although this symptom is more common with spinal administration.[1] Pruritus appears to be a μ receptor–mediated effect produced at the level of the medullary dorsal horn (MDH).[29] Antihistamines are often used to treat this side effect, but pruritus induced by morphine microinjection into the MDH is not histamine mediated.[29] Thus, their effectiveness is probably related to nonspecific sedative effects.

Morphine can also affect the release of several pituitary hormones, both directly and indirectly. Inhibition of corticotropin-releasing factor and gonadotropin-releasing hormone decreases circulating concentrations of ACTH, β-endorphin, follicle-stimulating hormone, and luteinizing hormone. Prolactin and growth hormone concentrations may be increased by opioids, and antidiuretic hormone release is inhibited by opioids.[1]

Respiratory Depression

Morphine and other μ agonists produce dose-dependent ventilatory depression primarily by decreasing the responsivity of the medullary respiratory center to CO_2.[28] Standard therapeutic doses of morphine produces a shift to the right and a decrease in slope of the ventilatory response to CO_2 curve, as well as abnormal breathing patterns.[30,31] The respiratory depressant effects of morphine are similar for young and elderly patients,[30,31] but normal sleep markedly potentiates morphine-induced ventilatory depression.[32] Frequent periods of oxygen desaturation associated with obstructive apnea, paradoxic breathing, and slow respiratory rate have been reported in patients receiving morphine infusions for postoperative analgesia, but occurred only when the patients were asleep.[33] Such reports emphasize the need to consider both the expected severity of postoperative pain as well as diurnal variations in pain and opioid sensitivity when including long-acting opioids such as morphine in an anesthetic. Sleep apnea, seen with ever-increasing frequency in association with obesity, increases the risk of morphine-induced respiratory depression. With increasing morphine doses, periodic breathing resembling Cheyne-Stokes breathing, decreased hypoxic ventilatory drive, and apnea can occur.[34] However, even with severe ventilatory depression, patients are usually arousable and will breathe on command.

Cough Reflex

Morphine and related opioids depress the cough reflex, at least in part by a direct effect on the medullary cough center. Doses required to attenuate the cough reflex are smaller than the usual analgesic dosage, and receptors mediating this effect appear to be less stereospecific and less sensitive to naloxone than those responsible for analgesia.[1] Dextroisomers of opioids, which do not produce analgesia, are also effective cough suppressants.[1]

Muscle Rigidity

Large doses of intravenous morphine (2 mg/kg infused at 10 mg/min) can produce abdominal muscle rigidity and decrease thoracic compliance; this effect plateaus 10 minutes after morphine administration is complete.[35] Subjects receiving smaller doses of intravenous morphine (10 to 15 mg) also report feelings of muscle tension, most frequently in the neck or legs, but occasionally in the chest wall (unpublished observations). Muscle rigidity is drastically increased by the addition of 70% N_2O.[35] Opioid-induced muscle rigidity appears to be mediated by μ receptors at supraspinal sites.[36] Myoclonus, sometimes resembling seizures, but without EEG evidence of seizure activity, has also been observed with high-dose opioids.[37] In clinical practice, opioid-induced muscle rigidity and myoclonus are most often observed on induction of anesthesia, but have been observed postoperatively[38] and can be severe enough to interfere with manual or mechanical ventilation. These effects are reduced or eliminated by naloxone,[38] drugs that facilitate GABA agonist activity (such as thiopental[35] and diazepam), and muscle relaxants.[38]

Nausea and Vomiting

Nausea and vomiting are among the most distressing side effects of morphine and its derivatives. Increased postoperative vomiting is seen with morphine premedication as well as with the use of intraoperative opioids.[39] The incidence of opioid-induced nausea appears to be similar irrespective of the route of administration, including oral, intravenous, intramuscular, subcutaneous, transmucosal, transdermal, intrathecal, and epidural.[39] Furthermore, laboratory and clinical studies comparing the incidence or severity of nausea and vomiting have found no differences among opioids in equianalgesic doses, including morphine, hydromorphone, meperidine, fentanyl, sufentanil, alfentanil, and remifentanil.[39–42] The physiology and neuropharmacology of opioid-induced nausea and vomiting are complex (Fig. 14-3). The vomiting center receives input from the chemotactic trigger zone (CTZ) in the area postrema of the medulla, the pharynx, gastrointestinal tract, mediastinum, and visual center.[39,43] The CTZ is rich in opioid, dopamine (D_2), serotonin (5-HT_3), histamine, and (muscarinic) acetylcholine receptors, and also receives input from the vestibular portion of the eighth cranial nerve. Morphine and related opioids induce nausea by direct stimulation of the CTZ and can also produce increased vestibular sensitivity.[1] Therefore, vestibular stimulation such as ambulation markedly increases the nauseant and emetic effects of morphine. This can be especially problematic in outpatient surgery, when early ambulation is a clinical priority. High doses of morphine and other opioids also have naloxone-reversible antiemetic effects at the level of the vomiting center.[44] In volunteer studies, morphine-induced nausea and vomiting increase after a morphine infusion is stopped,[45] which suggests that antiemetic effects are more short-lived than emetic effects. Another possible explanation for this observation is that the active metabolite morphine-6-glucuronide accumulates and worsens nausea. Prophylaxis and treatment of opioid-induced nausea and vomiting includes the use of drugs that act as antagonists at the various receptor

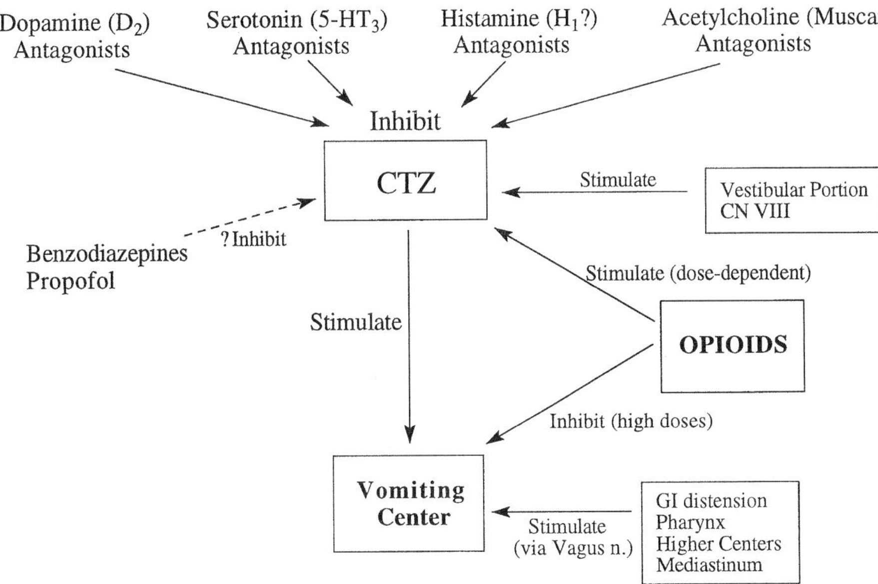

FIGURE 14-3. Pharmacology of nausea and vomiting. The chemotactic trigger zone (CTZ), located in the area postrema of the brainstem, contains dopamine, serotonin, histamine, and muscarinic acetylcholine as well as opioid receptors. The vomiting center receives input from the CTZ as well as peripheral sites via the vagus nerve. As illustrated, the role of opioids is complex, and they appear to have both emetic and antiemetic effects.

sites in the CTZ as well agents such as propofol and benzodiazepines, whose antiemetic mechanisms are unknown.[39]

Gastrointestinal Motility and Secretion

Morphine and other opioids affect gastrointestinal motility and propulsion, as well as gastric and pancreatic secretions via stimulation of opioid receptors in the brain, spinal cord, enteric muscle, and smooth muscle,[34,46] and are mediated by μ, κ, and δ opioid receptors at different anatomic sites.[46] In rodents, μ agonists inhibit gastric secretion, decrease gastrointestinal motility and propulsion, and suppress diarrhea when administered by intracerebroventricular, intrathecal, and peripheral injection.[46] A study in human volunteers demonstrated that methylnaltrexone, an opioid antagonist that does not cross the blood-brain barrier, attenuated morphine-induced delay in gastric emptying,[47] suggesting that this effect is mediated primarily by a peripheral opioid mechanism. Morphine decreases lower esophageal sphincter tone and produces symptoms of gastroesophageal reflux,[34] and diamorphine significantly slows gastric emptying. Thus, preoperative opioid administration should be considered when evaluating the risk of regurgitation and aspiration of gastric contents in patients who will be anesthetized or sedated. Like other opioid effects, gastrointestinal effects are probably dose related. Tone in both the small and large bowel is increased, but propulsive activity is decreased, leading to constipation. Epidurally administered morphine can also delay gastric emptying. A single epidural dose (4 mg) of morphine slowed gastric emptying, while an intramuscular dose did not.[48] How the effects of equianalgesic or repeated doses would compare is unknown.

Biliary Tract

Morphine and other opioids increase the tone of the common bile duct and sphincter of Oddi. Symptoms accompanying increases in biliary pressure can vary from epigastric distress to typical biliary colic, and may even mimic angina. When produced, biliary spasm can elevate plasma amylase and lipase for up to 24 hours.[1] Morphine and other μ agonists such as fentanyl are used in provocative tests to evaluate sphincter of Oddi dysfunction and biliary-type pain. In volunteers, morphine caused a greater delay in gallbladder emptying[49] and an increase in contractions of the sphincter of Oddi[50] than meperidine. Nitroglycerine, atropine, and naloxone can reverse opioid-induced increases in biliary pressure.[1] It has been suggested that morphine causes biliary tract contraction via histamine release, and antagonism of morphine's biliary effects by diphenhydramine supports this hypothesis.[51]

Genitourinary Effects

Urinary retention, seen after both systemic and spinal morphine administration, is because of complex effects on central and peripheral neurogenic mechanisms. It results in dyssynergia between the bladder detrusor muscle and the urethral sphincter because of a failure of sphincter relaxation.[1,52] Estimates of the incidence of this bothersome side effect vary widely and are confounded by the effects of anesthesia and surgery on urinary retention, but it is probably more common after spinal administration. Spinal morphine appears to cause naloxone-reversible urinary retention via μ and/or δ, but not κ opioid receptors.[52] In an animal study, cholinomimetic agents and α-adrenergic agonists aggravated morphine-induced high intravesical pressures, and therefore may be harmful agents to use for treatment of morphine-induced urinary retention.[53]

Histamine Release

Opioids stimulate the release of histamine from circulating basophils and from tissue mast cells in skin and lung.[54,55] Morphine-mediated histamine release is dose dependent; intradermal injection of morphine in a concentration of 1 mg/mL induces an urticarial wheal and flare.[55] Morphine-induced histamine release is not prevented by pretreatment with naloxone,[55] suggesting that histamine release is not mediated by opioid receptors. Morphine-induced histamine release has clinical relevance. The decrease in peripheral vascular resistance seen with high-dose morphine (1 mg/kg) correlates well with elevated plasma histamine concentration.[56] Furthermore, differences in the release of histamine could account for most of the hemodynamic differences between morphine and fentanyl (Fig. 14-4).[56]

Cardiovascular Effects

Opioids are popular in clinical anesthesia because they reliably produce analgesia with minimal changes in cardiovascular parameters. In doses typically used for pain management or as part of balanced anesthesia, morphine has little effect on blood pressure or heart rate and rhythm in the supine,

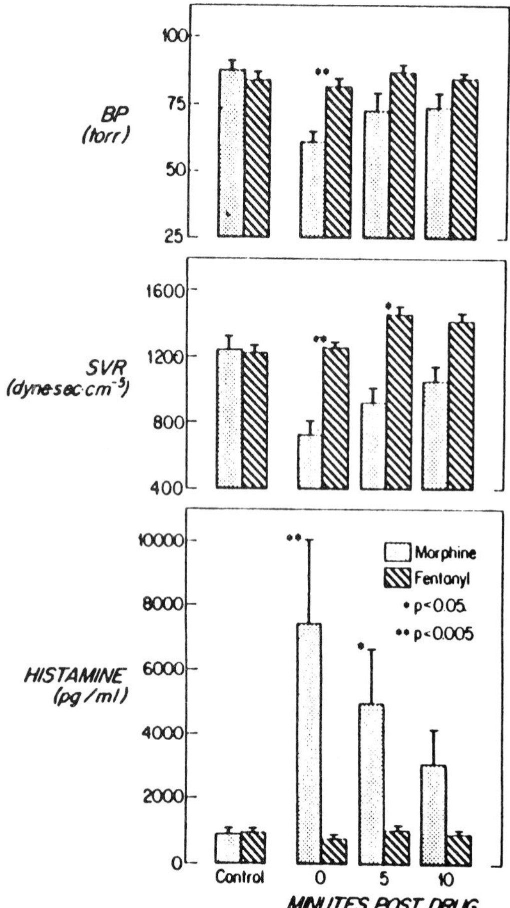

FIGURE 14-4. Mean arterial pressure (BP), systemic vascular resistance (SVR), and plasma histamine concentration (mean ± SE) before and after morphine 1 mg/kg and fentanyl 50 μg/kg (both infused over 10 minutes). Morphine, but not fentanyl, causes significant decrements in BP and SVR, which parallel the increase in plasma histamine concentration. (Reprinted with permission from Rosow CE, Moss J, Philbin DM *et al*: Histamine release during morphine and fentanyl anesthesia. Anesthesiology 56:93, 1982.)

normovolemic patient. However, therapeutic doses of morphine can produce arteriolar and venous dilation, decreased peripheral resistance, and inhibition of baroreceptor reflexes,[1] which can lead to postural hypotension. In addition to histamine release, morphine-mediated central sympatholytic activity and direct action on vascular smooth muscle may also contribute to peripheral vasodilation.[57] Thus, morphine's effect on vascular resistance is greater under conditions of high sympathetic tone.[57] The clinical implications of this finding are important. Patients who are critically ill (e.g., patients with severe trauma or cardiac disease) can be expected to have high sympathetic tone, and thus may experience hypotension in response to doses of morphine that would not normally produce hemodynamic instability. At clinically relevant doses, morphine does not suppress myocardial contractility.[1] However, opioids do produce dose-dependent bradycardia, probably by both sympatholytic and parasympathomimetic mechanisms.[58] In clinical anesthesia practice, opioids are often used to prevent tachycardia and reduce myocardial oxygen demand. Patients undergoing cardiovascular surgery who received morphine 1 to 2 mg/kg experienced minimal changes in heart rate, mean arterial pressure, cardiac index, and systemic vascular resistance. However, outcome was no different from that achieved with carefully administered inhalation-based anesthesia.[58]

Morphine does not directly affect cerebral circulation, but with morphine-induced respiratory depression, CO_2 retention causes cerebral vasodilation and an elevation in cerebrospinal fluid pressure. This effect is not seen when mechanical ventilation is used to prevent hypercarbia.[1] Thus, morphine and other μ agonists must be used cautiously in spontaneously breathing patients with head injury or other conditions associated with elevated intracranial pressure.

Disposition Kinetics

Morphine is rapidly absorbed after intramuscular, subcutaneous, and oral administration. Following intramuscular administration, peak plasma concentration is seen at 20 minutes and absorption half-life is estimated at 7.7 minutes (range 2 to 15 minutes).[59] After intravenous administration morphine undergoes rapid redistribution, with a mean redistribution half-time between 1.5 and 4.4 minutes in awake and anesthetized adults.[59–61] Morphine has a terminal elimination half-life between 1.7 and 3.3 hours.[60–62] Age affects morphine pharmacokinetics. The average elimination half-life of morphine is 7 to 8 hours in neonates less than 1 week of age, and 3 to 5 hours in older infants.[74] In patients between 61 and 80 years old, morphine's terminal elimination half-life was 4.5 hours compared to 2.9 hours in younger patients.[63]

Morphine is about 35% protein bound, mostly to albumin.[12] Its steady-state volume of distribution is large, with estimates in the range of 3 to 4 L/kg in normal adults.[59–61] Morphine's major metabolic pathway is hepatic phase II conjugation, to form morphine-3-glucuronide (M3G) and morphine-6β-glucuronide (M6G). 3-Glucuronidation is the predominant pathway, and following a single intravenous dose, 40% and 10% of the dose are excreted in the urine as M3G and M6G, respectively.[64] Unchanged morphine in the urine accounts for only about 10% of the dose. The rate of hepatic clearance of morphine is high, with a hepatic extraction ratio of 0.7.[59] Thus, morphine elimination may be slowed by processes that decrease hepatic blood flow.[61] Extrahepatic sites, such as kidney, intestine, and lung, have been suggested for morphine glucuronidation, but their importance in humans is unknown.

Active Metabolites

M6G possesses significant μ receptor affinity and potent antinociceptive activity. Appreciable plasma concentrations of M6G and M3G have been measured in cancer patients receiving high doses of oral morphine. During chronic oral morphine therapy, plasma M6G concentrations can be higher than those of the parent morphine compound.[65] Because morphine glucuronides are eliminated by the kidney, it is not surprising that very high M6G:morphine ratios have been reported in patients with renal dysfunction. This accumulation of the active metabolite is thought to be responsible for the unusual sensitivity of renal failure patients to morphine. While common wisdom suggests that glucuronide conjugates do not penetrate the blood-brain barrier, M6G concentration in cerebrospinal fluid (CSF) is 20 to 80% that of morphine.[66] Despite a mounting volume of animal literature demonstrating the analgesic potency of M6G, there is little information in humans concerning the magnitude of analgesia and side effects of M6G relative to morphine. Portenoy et al[66] demonstrated that in cancer patients receiving chronic morphine therapy, pain relief correlated positively with the M6G:morphine ratio, suggesting a contributing role of M6G to overall morphine analgesia. In a study of cancer patients who received synthetic M6G (up to 60 μg/kg), 17 of 19 patients experienced effective analgesia and no adverse effects.[67] However, dizziness, nausea, sedation, muscle aches, and respiratory depression have been reported in volunteers who received M6G.[65] While the contribution of M6G to morphine-induced analgesia and side effects remains to be determined, morphine should be administered cautiously to patients with renal failure.

Dosage and Administration of Morphine

In current clinical practice morphine is used mainly as a premedicant and for postoperative analgesia, and less often as a component of balanced or high-dose opioid anesthesia. Intravenous analgesic doses of morphine for adults typically range from 0.01 to 0.20 mg/kg. When used in a balanced anesthetic technique with N_2O, morphine can be given in total doses of up to 3 mg/kg with remarkable hemodynamic stability, but awareness under anesthesia is a risk. When combined with other inhalation agents, it is unlikely that more than 1 to 2 mg/kg of morphine is necessary. Because of its hydrophilicity, morphine crosses the blood-brain barrier relatively slowly; and while its onset can be observed within 5 minutes, peak effects may be delayed for 10 to 40 minutes. This delay makes morphine more difficult to titrate as an anesthetic supplement than the more rapidly acting opioids.

MEPERIDINE

Meperidine, a phenylpiperidine derivative (Fig. 14-5), was the first totally synthetic opioid. It was initially studied as an anticholinergic agent, but was found to have significant analgesic activity.[1]

Analgesia and Effect on Minimum Alveolar Concentration of Volatile Anesthetics

Meperidine's analgesic potency is about one-tenth that of morphine's and is most likely mediated by μ opioid receptor activation. However, meperidine also has moderate affinity for κ and δ opioid receptors.[1,68] Unlike morphine, meperidine plasma concentrations correlate reasonably well with analgesic effects.[69] While there is considerable interpatient variability, the minimum effective analgesia concentration of meperidine is approximately 200 ng/mL. There is very little information available on the effect of meperidine on the MAC of inhaled anesthetics, but a study in dogs demonstrated a dose-dependent reduction in the MAC of halothane.[70]

Meperidine also has well recognized weak local anesthetic properties. Compared to morphine, fentanyl, and buprenorphine injected perineurally, only meperidine alters nerve conduction and produces analgesia.[71] This has led to some popularity for epidural and subarachnoid administration, particularly in obstetric anesthesia. But because of its local anesthetic effects, neuraxial meperidine may also produce sensory and motor blockade as well as sympatholytic effects that are not seen with other opioids.

Side Effects

Like morphine, therapeutic doses of meperidine can produce sedation, pupillary constriction, and euphoria, and very high doses are associated with CNS excitement and seizures (see later). In equianalgesic doses, meperidine produces respiratory depression equal to that of morphine, as well as nausea, vomiting, and dizziness, particularly in ambulatory patients.[1]

Like other opioids, meperidine causes significant delay in gastric emptying. While meperidine does increase common bile duct pressure, this occurs to a lesser extent than with equianalgesic doses of morphine and fentanyl (Fig. 14-6).[49,72]

Analgesic doses of meperidine in awake patients are not associated with hemodynamic instability, but 1 mg/kg in patients with cardiac disease decreased heart rate, cardiac index, and rate–pressure product.[73] In an isolated papillary muscle preparation, high concentrations of meperidine depressed contractility. This effect was not naloxone reversible and is consistent with a nonspecific, local anesthetic effect.[74] In higher doses, meperidine causes significantly more hemodynamic instability than morphine or fentanyl and its derivatives,[75] an effect at least partially related to histamine release. In a comparison of opioids administered as part of balanced anesthesia, Flacke et al[75] found that 25% patients in the meperidine group experienced severe hypotension and had abnormally elevated plasma histamine concentrations. Interestingly, only one patient in the morphine group (0.6 mg/kg morphine given) had a similar histamine plasma concentration. Thus, meperidine is not recommended in high doses for clinical anesthesia.

Shivering

Meperidine is effective in reducing shivering from diverse causes, including general and epidural anesthesia, fever, hypothermia, transfusion reactions, and administration of amphotericin B. Meperidine reduces or eliminates visible shivering as well as the accompanying increase in oxygen consumption[76] following general and epidural anesthesia. Equianalgesic doses of fentanyl (25 μg) and morphine (2.5 mg) did not reduce postoperative shivering, suggesting that the antishivering effect of meperidine is not mediated by μ-opioid receptors. This effect

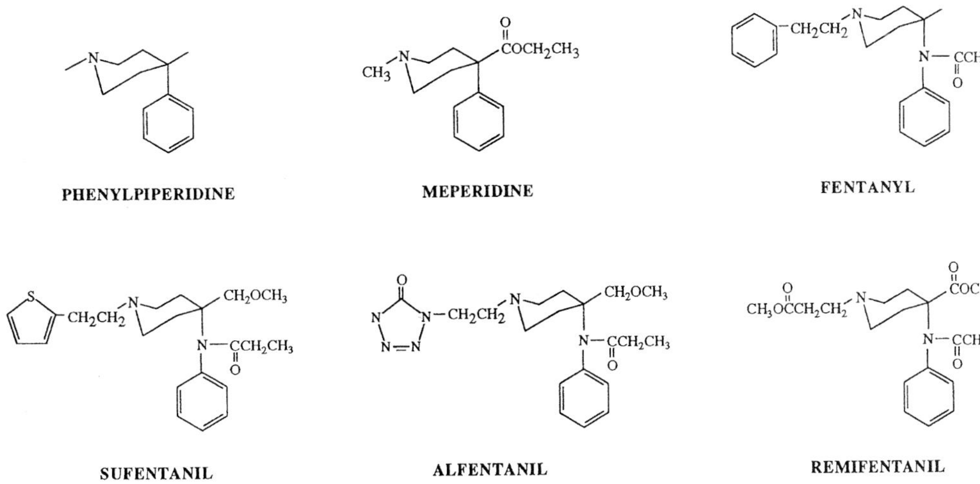

PHENYLPIPERIDINE MEPERIDINE FENTANYL

SUFENTANIL ALFENTANIL REMIFENTANIL

FIGURE 14-5. Chemical structures of phenylpiperidine, meperidine, and the 4-anilinopiperidine derivatives fentanyl, sufentanil, alfentanil, and remifentanil.

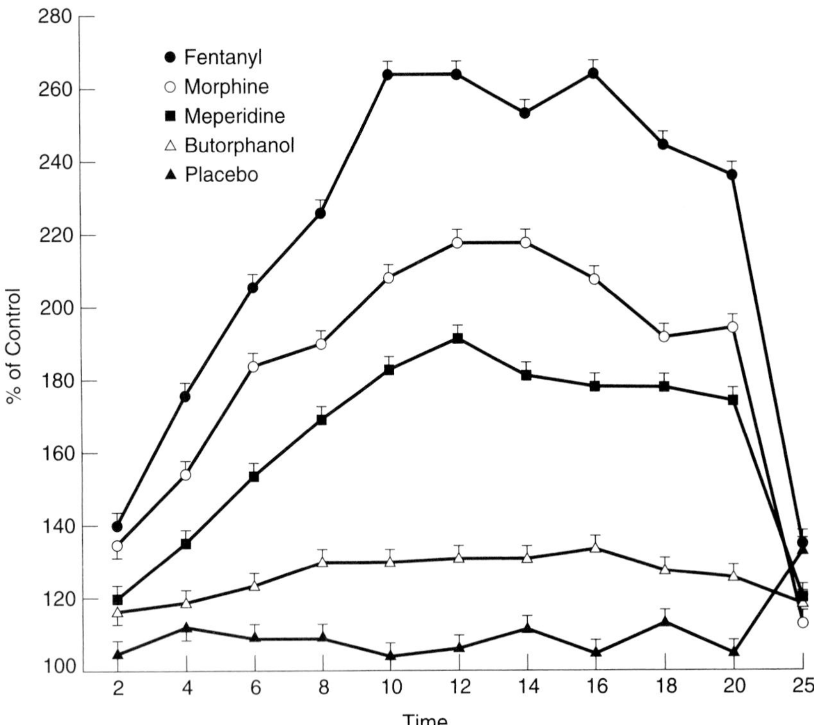

FIGURE 14-6. The effect of several opioids on common bile duct pressures in patients anesthetized with enflurane and N_2O–O_2. Patients received either fentanyl 100 μg/70 kg, morphine 10 mg/70 kg, meperidine 75 mg/70 kg, or butorphanol 2 mg/70 kg. After 20 minutes, the effects were reversed with naloxone. (Reprinted with permission from Radnay PA, Duncalf D, Novakovik M, Lesser ML: Common bile duct pressure changes after fentanyl, morphine, meperidine, butorphanol, and naloxone. Anesth Analg 63:441, 1984.)

may be mediated by κ-opioid receptors. Butorphanol, a drug with significant κ agonist activity, effectively reduces postoperative shivering in a dose of 1 mg.[77] Furthermore, low doses of naloxone, sufficient to block μ receptors, did not reverse meperidine's antishivering effect, but high-dose naloxone, designed to block both μ and κ receptors, did reverse the antishivering effect.[68] The observation that other types of drugs, such as α_1-adrenergic agonists (clonidine 1.5 μg/kg), serotonin (5-HT_2) antagonists,[78] and propofol,[79] can reduce postoperative shivering suggests that a nonopioid mechanism may be involved. Physostigmine 0.04 mg/kg can also prevent postoperative shivering, suggesting a role for the cholinergic system. Perhaps meperidine's greater antishivering effect, relative to other opioids, is because of additive thermoregulatory impairment by more than one mechanism.

Disposition Kinetics

Following intravenous administration, meperidine plasma concentration falls rapidly. Meperidine's redistribution half-life is 4 to 16 minutes, and its terminal elimination half-life is between 3 and 5 hours.[81,82] The elimination half-life is not prolonged in patients 60 to 80 years old. However, in neonates and infants, a median elimination half-life, 8 to 10 hours, with greater individual variability (three- to fivefold) compared to adults. Absorption after intramuscular administration was complete in normal volunteers, with peak plasma concentration at 5 to 15 minutes after injection; but in postoperative patients, intramuscular meperidine absorption is quite variable, with time to reach peak concentration between 5 and 110 minutes.

Meperidine is moderately lipid soluble, and is 40 to 70% protein bound, mostly to albumin and α_1-acid glycoprotein (see Table 14-2).[83] Meperidine has a large steady-state volume of distribution, with estimates in the range of 3.5 to 5 L/kg in adults.[81,82] The high clearance rate (10 mL/kg/min) reflects a high hepatic extraction ratio; it is *N*-demethylated in the liver to form normeperidine, the principal metabolite, and also hydrolyzed to meperidinic acid. Both metabolites may then be conjugated[1] and excreted renally. Normeperidine is pharmacologically active and potentially toxic (see later).

Active Metabolites

Normeperidine has appreciable pharmacologic activity and can produce signs of central nervous system excitation. In humans, mood alterations such as apprehension and restlessness, as well as neurotoxic effects such as tremors, myoclonus, and seizures, have been reported.[84] The elimination half-life of the metabolite normeperidine (14 to 21 hours) is considerably longer than the parent compound, and therefore is likely to accumulate with repeated or prolonged administration, particularly in patients with renal dysfunction.[84] Myoclonus and seizures have been reported in patients receiving meperidine for postoperative or chronic pain. Patients who developed seizures had a mean plasma normeperidine concentration of 0.81 μg/mL,[84] and it appears that a total daily dosage of 1,000 mg is associated with an increased risk of seizures, even in patients without renal dysfunction.

Dosage and Administration of Meperidine

A single dose of meperidine is approximately one-tenth as potent as morphine when given parenterally, but has a shorter duration of action. Intravenous analgesic doses of meperidine for adults typically range from 0.1 to 1 mg/kg. Intravenous doses of 12.5 to 50 mg are effective in reducing postoperative shivering. As discussed earlier, high doses of meperidine for intraoperative use are not recommended because of hemodynamic instability. In addition, very high single doses or prolonged administration may produce seizures because of the metabolite normeperidine; thus, the total daily dose should not exceed 1,000 mg/24 hours.

METHADONE

Methadone, a synthetic opioid introduced in the 1940s, is primarily a μ agonist with pharmacologic properties that are similar to morphine. While its chemical structure is very different from that of morphine, steric factors force the molecule to simulate the pseudopiperidine ring conformation that appears to be required for opioid activity.[1] Because of its long elimination half-life, methadone is most often used for long-term pain management and in treatment of opioid abstinence syndromes.

Analgesia and Use in Anesthesia

Following parenteral administration, the onset of analgesia is rapid, within 10 to 20 minutes. After single doses of up to 10 mg, the duration of analgesia is similar to morphine,[1] but with large or repeated parenteral doses, prolonged analgesia can be obtained. Several investigators have administered methadone intra- and postoperatively with the aim of providing prolonged postoperative analgesia. Patients who received 20 mg methadone intraoperatively and up to 20 mg additional methadone in the immediate postoperative period had a median duration of postoperative analgesia of over 20 hours.[85,86] The effect of methadone on the MAC of volatile anesthetics has not been reported.

Side Effects

Side effects of methadone are similar in magnitude and frequency to those of morphine.[1,85] Patients who received 20 mg methadone at the beginning of surgery were sedated in the immediate postoperative period but did not appear to have clinically significant respiratory depression. About 50% experienced nausea or vomiting, which was easily treated with standard antiemetic therapy.[85] Methadone produces typical opioid effects on smooth muscle. Like morphine, it markedly decreases intestinal propulsive activity and can cause constipation as well as biliary spasm.[1]

Disposition Kinetics

Following an intravenous dose, the plasma concentration–time data for methadone are described by a biexponential equation. The mean redistribution half-time is 6 minutes (range 1 to 24 minutes), and the mean terminal elimination half-time is 34 hours (range 9 to 87 hours).[86] Methadone is well absorbed after an oral dose, with bioavailability approximately 90%, and reaches peak plasma concentration at 4 hours after oral administration.[1] It is nearly 90% plasma protein bound and undergoes extensive metabolism in the liver, mostly *N*-demethylation and cyclization to form pyrrolidines and pyrroline.[1]

Dosage and Administration of Methadone

The use of methadone in clinical anesthesia has focused on attempts to achieve prolonged postoperative analgesia, providing that an adequate initial dose is administered. Because adverse effects can also be prolonged, careful titration of the dose is necessary. In opioid-naïve patients, an initial single dose of 20 mg can provide analgesia without significant postoperative respiratory depression.[85] Wangler and Rosenblatt[87] described a technique to avoid respiratory depression in which 8 to 12 mg methadone is administered to the awake patient until the threshold of respiratory depression (respiratory rate of 6 to 8/min) is reached. Immediately prior to incision, an additional dose equal to half the initial dose is given. For administering supplemental analgesic doses in the immediate postoperative period, it is essential to confirm that patients with ongoing significant pain have no depression of respiration or level of consciousness, and that a 30- to 40-minute interval should elapse between 5-mg doses to allow full assessment of adverse effects. It may be easier and safer to use a sustained release opioid preparation (containing oxycodone or morphine) with a shorter time to peak effect if a long-acting analgesic is desired. This is most easily accomplished by administering the oral medication preoperatively, but it is also important to note that these long-acting opioids are not currently approved for prophylaxis of postoperative pain.

FENTANYL

Fentanyl and its analogs sufentanil and alfentanil are the most frequently used opioids in clinical anesthesia today. Fentanyl, first synthesized in 1960, is structurally related to the phenylpiperidines (see Fig. 14-5) and has a clinical potency ratio 50 to 100 times that of morphine. Clear plasma concentration-effect relationships have been demonstrated for fentanyl (Table 14-3). Scott et al[88] demonstrated progressive EEG changes with increasing serum fentanyl concentration (Fig. 14-7). During a 5-minute fentanyl infusion, the time lag between increasing serum fentanyl concentration and EEG slowing was 3 to 5 minutes. After the infusion was stopped,

TABLE 14-3

PLASMA CONCENTRATION RANGES (ng/mL) FOR VARIOUS THERAPEUTIC AND NONTHERAPEUTIC OPIOID EFFECTS

EFFECT	MORPHINE	MEPERIDINE	FENTANYL	SUFENTANIL	ALFENTANIL	REMIFENTANIL
MEAC	10–15	200	0.6	0.03	15	
Moderate to strong analgesia	20–50	400–600	1.5–5	0.05–0.10	40–80	
50% MAC reduction	NA	>500	0.5–2	0.145	200	1.3
Surgical analgesia with ~70% N_2O	NA	NA	15–25	NA	300–500	
Respiratory depression threshold	25	200	1	0.02–0.04	50–100	
50% ↓ ventilatory response to CO_2	50	NA	1.5–3	0.04	120–350	2.07–2.97
Apnea	NA	NA	7–22	NA	300–600	
Unconsciousness (not reliably achieved with opioids alone)		(Seizures)	15–20	NA	500–1500	

Effects were generally achieved during continuous infusions or patient-controlled analgesia systems. Note that plasma concentrations associated with measurable depression of ventilatory drive are similar to those associated with analgesia for all opioids.
MEAC, minimum effective analgesic concentration, defined in most studies as the plasma opioid concentration associated with just perceptible analgesia; NA, information not available.

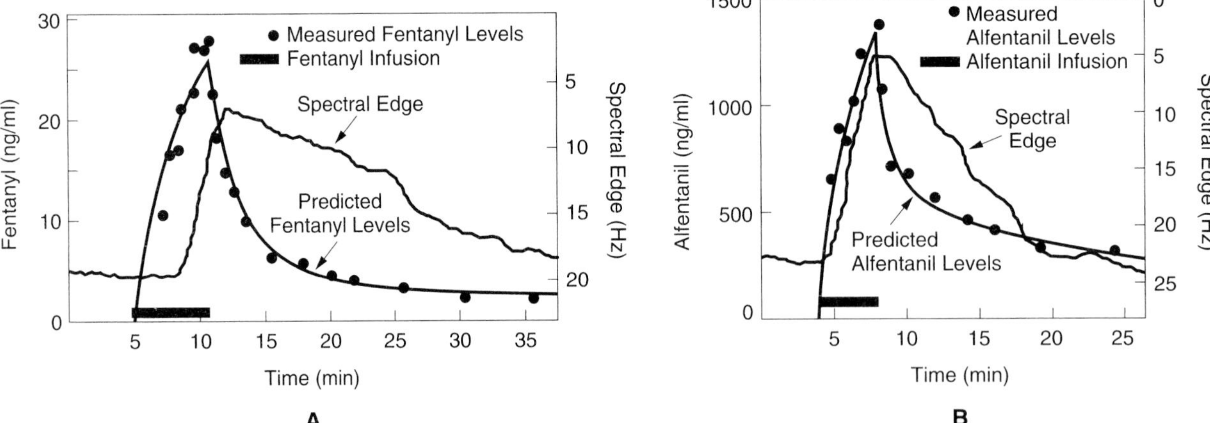

FIGURE 14-7. The time course of EEG spectral edge and serum concentrations of fentanyl (A) and alfentanil (B). Infusion rates were 150 μg/min fentanyl and 1,500 μg/min alfentanil. Increasing opioid effect is seen as a decrease in spectral edge. Changes in spectral edge follow serum concentrations more closely with alfentanil than with fentanyl. (Reprinted with permission from Scott JC, Ponganis KV, Stanski DR: EEG quantitation of narcotic effect: The comparative pharmacodynamics of fentanyl and alfentanil. Anesthesiology 62:234, 1985.)

the resolution of EEG changes lagged behind decreasing serum fentanyl concentration by 10 to 20 minutes.

Analgesia

Fentanyl, a μ-opioid receptor agonist, produces profound dose-dependent analgesia, ventilatory depression, and sedation, and at high doses it can produce unconsciousness. In postoperative patients receiving fentanyl by a patient-controlled analgesia system, the mean fentanyl dose requirement was 55.8 μg/h, and mean minimum effective analgesic concentration (MEAC) in blood was 0.63 ng/mL.[89] A large interpatient variability in MEAC (0.23 to 1.18 ng/mL) typical of opioids was observed, but over the 2-day study period, the MEAC for any individual patient remained relatively constant. In a volunteer study, a mean plasma fentanyl concentration of 1.3 ng/mL reduced experimental pain intensity ratings by 50%.[40] This is consistent with other estimates of plasma fentanyl concentrations associated with moderate to strong analgesia.[90]

Effect on Minimum Alveolar Concentration of Volatile Anesthetics and Use in Anesthesia

4 Fentanyl reduces the MAC of volatile anesthetics in a concentration- or dose-dependent fashion. A single iv bolus dose of fentanyl 3 μg/kg, given 25 to 30 minutes prior to incision, reduced both isoflurane and desflurane MAC by approximately 50%.[91] Fentanyl 1.5 μg/kg administered 5 minutes prior to skin incision reduces the minimum alveolar concentration that blocks adrenergic responses to stimuli (MAC-BAR) of isoflurane or desflurane in 60% N_2O by 60 to 70%.[92] No further drop is seen with an increase in fentanyl dose to 3 μg/kg. During constant plasma concentration of 0.5 to 1.7 ng/mL, fentanyl reduced isoflurane MAC by 50%.[93] Fentanyl produces a steep plasma concentration-related reduction in sevoflurane MAC[94]; (3 ng/mL provides a 59% reduction), but a ceiling effect is reached, such that a threefold increase to 10 ng/mL reduced MAC by only an additional 17%.

Epidural fentanyl also reduces halothane MAC.[95] Epidural fentanyl 1, 2, and 4 μg/kg reduced halothane MAC by 45, 58, and 71%, respectively, while the same doses of fentanyl given iv reduced halothane MAC by 8, 40, and 49%, respectively.

5 Combining opioids with propofol rather than an inhalation agent is another common technique for providing general anesthesia, referred to as *total intravenous anesthesia* or TIVA. For an intravenous anesthetic, the potency index is described as the plasma concentration required to prevent a response in 50% (CP_{50}) or 95% (CP_{95}) of patients to various surgical stimuli. Plasma concentrations of fentanyl and propofol that reduce hemodynamic or somatic responses to various surgical stimuli in 50% of patients have been determined using computer-assisted infusion.[96] Fentanyl plasma concentrations of 1.2, 1.8, and 2.8 ng/mL were required for 50% reductions in propofol's CP_{50}s for skin incision, peritoneal incision, and abdominal retraction, respectively. Greater fentanyl concentrations were required to suppress hemodynamic responses to these same stimuli. Thus, fentanyl reduces requirements for both volatile agents and propofol by a similar proportion.

Several other investigators have also used computer-assisted infusion to administer fentanyl as a component of a balanced anesthetic technique.[97,98] In combination with 50 to 70% N_2O in oxygen, loss of consciousness, and absence of response to skin incision are achieved at plasma fentanyl concentrations of 15 to 25 ng/mL and greater than 3.7 ng/mL, respectively. Intraoperative concentration requirements varied between 1 and 9 ng/mL. Finally, spontaneous ventilation was seen when the fentanyl concentration dropped to 1.5 to 2 ng/mL.[97,98]

6 Fentanyl has been used as the sole agent for anesthesia, a technique that requires a large initial dose of 50 to 150 μg/kg or stable plasma fentanyl concentrations in the range of 20 to 30 ng/mL.[90] The major advantage of this technique is reliable hemodynamic stability. High doses of fentanyl significantly blunt the "stress response"—that is, hemodynamic and hormonal responses to surgical stimuli—while producing only minimal cardiovascular depression. Thus, the technique is sometimes referred to as "stress-free anesthesia." There are also disadvantages to using high-dose fentanyl as the sole anesthetic agent. It appears that no dose of fentanyl will completely block hemodynamic or hormonal responses in all patients.[99] Furthermore, although high doses generally result in unconsciousness, there have been reports of intraoperative awareness and recall in patients who received very high doses (>50 μg/kg) of fentanyl. Because opioids do not produce muscle relaxation, and high-dose fentanyl can produce muscle rigidity, a muscle relaxant is generally required to achieve adequate surgical conditions. This can potentially increase the difficulty in detecting signs of intraoperative awareness. Direct and processed EEG monitoring have been used to assess the depth of anesthesia achieved with high-dose opioids.

Other Central Nervous System Effects

The effects of fentanyl on cerebral blood flow (CBF) and intracranial pressure (ICP) have been studied in normal patients and in those with neurologic disease. An induction dose of 16 μg/kg increased middle cerebral artery flow by 25% in normal patients having noncranial neurosurgery.[100] A smaller dose (3 μg/kg) resulted in an elevation in ICP in ventilated patients with head trauma.[101] However, in brain tumor patients anesthetized with N_2O–O_2, a dose of 5 μg/kg of fentanyl did not result in elevated ICP.[102] In all cases of elevation in ICP and CBF, there were decreases in mean arterial pressure, which may have contributed to these changes.

Muscle rigidity is often seen on induction with high-dose fentanyl and its derivatives. When rigidity is intense, it may
7 be difficult or impossible to ventilate the patient. In a study in normal volunteers, 1,500 μg fentanyl infused over 10 minutes produced rigidity in 50% of subjects.[103] A similar incidence, 35%, was seen in patients receiving 750 to 1,000 μg fentanyl during induction of general anesthesia, and up to 80% of patients receiving 30 μg/kg developed moderate to severe rigidity.[104] Muscle rigidity seen with high doses of fentanyl increases with age[104] and is accompanied by unconsciousness and apnea,[103,104] but lower doses, 7 to 8 μg/kg, have produced chest wall rigidity without unconsciousness or apnea. Streisand et al[103] hypothesized that hypercarbia from fentanyl-induced respiratory depression may have influenced fentanyl ionization and cerebral blood flow and hence the delivery of fentanyl to brain tissue. It would follow that patients instructed to deep-breathe during fentanyl induction may experience less rigidity during induction of anesthesia. This is consistent with observations by Lunn et al.[105] During high-dose fentanyl induction (75 μg/kg), $PaCO_2$ was maintained at 35 to 40 torr by assisting and then controlling respirations. Although chest wall compliance was reduced in 4 of 18 patients, no patient developed rigidity sufficient to impair ventilation.

Fentanyl has been associated with seizure-like movements during anesthetic induction, which are not associated with seizure activity on the EEG.[106] Whereas fentanyl can induce seizures in other animals, the doses required to produce EEG-documented seizures is generally higher than that used in humans. Such activity may represent myoclonus, a result of opioid-mediated blockade of inhibitory motor pathways of cortical origin, or may represent exaggerations of opioid-induced muscle rigidity.[106] However, fentanyl can activate epileptiform EEG activity in patients having surgery for intractable temporal lobe epilepsy.[107]

Fentanyl-induced pruritus often presents as facial itching, but can be generalized. Equianalgesic plasma concentrations of fentanyl, morphine, and alfentanil produce equivalent intensity of pruritus.[40] Fentanyl has also been reported to have a tussive effect. Twenty-eight percent of patients coughed within 1 minute after receiving a bolus dose of fentanyl (1.5 μg/kg). The mechanism is unclear, and it was not attenuated by pretreatment with atropine or midazolam.[108]

Respiratory Depression

Fentanyl produces approximately the same degree of ventila-
8 tory depression as equianalgesic doses of morphine.[40] Respiratory depression—expressed as an elevation in end-tidal CO_2, a decrease in the slope of the CO_2 response curve, or the minute ventilation at an end-tidal CO_2 of 50 mmHg (V_E50)—develops rapidly, reaching a peak in ~5 minutes,[88,109,110] and the time course closely follows plasma fentanyl concentration.[109,111] Even at plasma concentrations associated with mild analgesia, ventilatory depression can be detected, and the magnitude of respiratory depression is linearly related to intensity of analgesia (see Table 14-3).[40,112] In postoperative patients, plasma fentanyl concentrations of 1.5 to 3.0 ng/mL were associated with a 50% reduction in CO_2 responsiveness.[113]

The magnitude of respiratory depression can be greatly increased when fentanyl is given in combination with another respiratory depressant such as midazolam. Bailey et al[110] determined that midazolam alone (0.05 mg/kg) did not depress ventilation or cause hypoxemia. Fentanyl alone (2 μg/kg) reduced the slope of the CO_2 response curve and the V_E50 by 50%, and 6 of 12 subjects became hypoxemic. Fentanyl and midazolam produced no greater depression of the ventilatory response to CO_2 than fentanyl alone, but 11 of 12 subjects became hypoxemic and 6 of 12 became apneic within 5 minutes. These observations suggest that this frequently used combination blunts the hypoxic ventilatory drive to a greater extent than the hypercarbic ventilatory drive. Precautions such as supplemental oxygen and pulse oximetry monitoring are recommended when such drug combinations are used.

Airway Reflexes

9 Although obtundation of airway reflexes by general inhalation anesthetics is well described, little is known about the direct effects of opioids on these protective reflexes. Tagaito et al examined the dose-related effects of fentanyl on airway responses to laryngeal irritation during propofol anesthesia in humans.[114] All patients had laryngeal mask airways; half breathed spontaneously, and half had ventilation controlled to maintain an end-tidal CO_2 of 38 mm Hg. In both groups, stimulation of the larynx (application of water to mucosa) elicited a forced expiration, followed by spasmodic panting mingled with cough reflexes and brief laryngospasm. With three cumulative fentanyl doses (50, 50, and 100 μg), expiration, panting, and coughing decreased in a dose-dependent fashion. After the first dose of fentanyl, apnea with laryngospasm replaced the other reflexes, and with cumulative fentanyl dosing, the duration of laryngospasm shortened. These investigators also noted that cough was the airway reflex most vulnerable to depression by fentanyl. While attenuation of airway reflexes is desirable during general anesthesia, it is equally desirable that these protective reflexes return to baseline rapidly after emergence, and remain intact throughout conscious sedation. Doses required to suppress cough and other reflexes in awake or sedated individuals have not been characterized.

Cardiovascular and Endocrine Effects

Isolated heart muscle models have shown concentration-dependent negative inotropic effects of opioids, including mor-
10 phine, meperidine, and fentanyl.[58] A fentanyl concentration of 10 μg/mL reduced contractility by 50%, but 1 μg/mL had no significant effects on papillary muscle mechanics. In clinical practice, high-dose fentanyl administration (up to 75 μg/kg) produces much lower plasma concentrations, that is, in the range of 50 ng/mL,[105] and is associated with remarkable hemodynamic stability. Patients who received 7 μg/kg fentanyl at induction of anesthesia had a slight decrease in heart rate, but no change in mean arterial pressure compared to control.[75] Fentanyl-induced bradycardia is more marked in anesthetized than conscious subjects, and usually resolves with atropine. With higher fentanyl doses, in the range of 20 to 25 μg/kg, decreases in heart rate, mean arterial pressure, systemic and pulmonary vascular resistance, and pulmonary capillary wedge pressure of approximately 15% were seen in patients with coronary artery disease.[105,115] Very high fentanyl doses, up to 75 μg/kg, produced no further hemodynamic changes. All of these patients had been premedicated with a diazepam or pentobarbital, and scopolamine or atropine. In unpremedicated patients undergoing noncardiac surgery, induction with fentanyl 30 μg/kg produced no changes in heart rate or systolic blood pressure.[104] Hypertension in

response to sternotomy is the most common hemodynamic disturbance during high-dose fentanyl anesthesia and occurs in 40 and 100% in patients receiving 50 to 100 μg/kg.[116] Unlike morphine and meperidine, which induce hypotension, at least in part because of histamine release,[57,117] high-dose fentanyl (50 μg/kg) is not associated with significant histamine release (see Fig. 14-4).

While high doses of fentanyl are associated with minimal cardiovascular changes, combining fentanyl with other drugs can compromise hemodynamic stability. The combination of fentanyl and diazepam produces significant cardiovascular depression.[104,115] Diazepam 10 mg given after 20 to 50 μg/kg of fentanyl decreased stroke volume, cardiac output, systemic vascular resistance, and mean arterial pressure, and increased central venous pressure significantly.[115] Adding 60% N_2O to high-dose fentanyl produced a significant decrease in cardiac output and increases in systemic and pulmonary vascular resistance.[105]

High-dose fentanyl (100 μg/kg) prevented increases in plasma epinephrine, cortisol, glucose, free fatty acids, and growth hormone (the "stress response") during surgery, but lower dose fentanyl (5 μg/kg followed by an infusion of 3 μg/kg/h) did not.[118]

Smooth Muscle and Gastrointestinal Effects

11 Fentanyl, like morphine and meperidine, significantly increases common bile duct pressure (see Fig. 14-6).[72] Like other opioids,
12 fentanyl can cause nausea and vomiting, particularly in ambulatory patients, and can delay gastric emptying and intestinal transit.

Disposition Kinetics

Fentanyl's extreme lipid solubility (see Table 14-2) allows rapid crossing of biologic membranes uptake by highly perfused tissue groups, including the brain, heart, and lung. Thus, after a single bolus dose, the onset of effects is rapid and the duration brief. Hug and Murphy[119] determined the relationships between fentanyl effects and its concentration over time in plasma and various tissues in rats given fentanyl 50 μg/kg (Fig. 14-8). The onset of opioid effects occurred within 10 seconds, and correlated with a rapid increase in brain tissue fentanyl concentration, which equilibrated with plasma by 1.5 minutes. Recovery from fentanyl effects started within 5 minutes and was complete by 60 minutes. Elimination from the "central tissues" (brain, heart, and lung) was also rapid, as fentanyl was redistributed to other tissues, particularly muscle and fat. Peak muscle concentration was seen at 5 minutes, while fat concentration reached a maximum approximately 30 minutes after the dose. The delay in fat uptake despite fentanyl's high lipid solubility is because of the limited blood supply to that tissue. Thus, redistribution to muscle and fat limits the duration of a bolus dose of fentanyl, and accumulation in peripheral tissue compartments can be extensive because of the large mass of muscle and high affinity of fentanyl for fat. With prolonged administration of fentanyl, fat can act as a reservoir of drug.

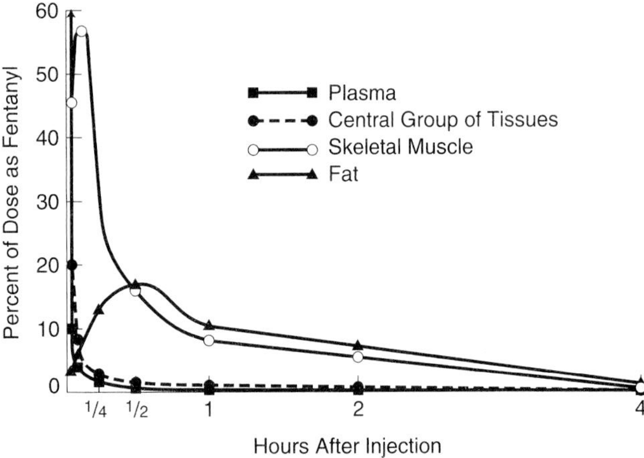

FIGURE 14-8. Fentanyl uptake and elimination in various tissues of the rat following intravenous injection. Unchanged fentanyl tissue concentrations (means for 6 rats) are expressed as percentage of dose. "Central" represents the combined content of brain, heart, and lung tissues. The large mass of muscle (50% body weight of the rat) and high affinity of fat for fentanyl (despite slow equilibration) serve as a drain on the central compartment. (Reprinted with permission from Hug CC, Murphy MR: Tissue redistribution of fentanyl in terms of its effects in rats. Anesthesiology 55:369, 1981.)

Fentanyl pharmacokinetics have been studied in normal volunteers as well as patients under general anesthesia. After an iv dose, plasma fentanyl concentration falls rapidly, and the concentration–time curve has been described by both two- and three-compartment models.[120] McClain and Hug[109] administered fentanyl 3.2 or 6.4 μg/kg to healthy male volunteers and found that nearly 99% of the dose was eliminated from plasma by 60 minutes. These investigators found both rapid and slower distribution phases, with half-times of 1.2 to 1.9 minutes and 9.2 to 19 minutes, respectively. The terminal elimination half-time ranged from 3.1 to 6.6 hours, somewhat longer than that for morphine. Similar values were noted in surgical patients less than 50 years old,[102,121] including morbidly obese patients.[102] Reports of age effects on fentanyl kinetics are conflicting. While fentanyl requirement decreases with increasing age (20 to 89 years), pharmacokinetic parameters do not change.[122] In contrast, Bentley et al[121] observed a marked decrease in clearance and an increase in terminal elimination half-time to approximately 15 hours in patients over 60 years old compared to 4.4 hours in patients less than 50 years old.

Unlike its derivatives, fentanyl is significantly bound to red blood cells, approximately 40%, and has a blood:plasma partition coefficient of approximately 1.[120] Plasma fentanyl is highly protein bound, with estimates in the range of 79 to 87%. It binds avidly to α_1-acid glycoprotein but also binds to albumin.[120,123] Fentanyl protein binding is pH dependent, such that a decrease in pH will increase the proportion of fentanyl that is unbound.[120] Thus, a patient with respiratory acidosis will have a higher proportion of unbound (active) fentanyl, which could exacerbate respiratory depression. Clearance of fentanyl is primarily by rapid and extensive metabolism in the liver. Clearance estimates[109,122] of 8 to 21 mL/kg/min approach liver blood flow and indicate a high hepatic extraction ratio. Thus, hepatic metabolism of fentanyl is expected to be dependent on liver blood flow. Metabolism is primarily by *N*-dealkylation to norfentanyl and by hydroxylation of both the parent and norfentanyl.[120] Only about 6% of the dose of fentanyl is excreted unchanged in the urine.[109]

Dosage and Administration of Fentanyl

From administration as a single bolus dose, fentanyl developed an early reputation as a short-acting opioid, but experience with very large doses and multiple doses revealed that prolonged respiratory depression and delayed recovery could occur. These observations demonstrate that fentanyl's clinical duration is limited by redistribution, and that with prolonged administration, accumulation can occur as discussed later in this chapter.

Fentanyl can be useful as a sedative/analgesic premedication when given a short time prior to induction. For this use, incremental doses of 25 to 50 μg iv can be used and titrated until the desired effect is achieved. It is important to note that although the onset of fentanyl's effects is rapid, peak effect lags behind peak plasma concentration by up to 5 minutes.[88] A transmucosal delivery system for fentanyl is also available and has been shown to be an effective premedicant for pediatric and adult patients as well as an effective treatment for "breakthrough" pain in chronic pain patients. In children, doses of 10 to 20 μg/kg, and in adults, 400 to 800 μg, administered 30 minutes prior to induction or a painful procedure are safe and effective, but dose-dependent side effects typical of opioids are reported.[124,125] Because respiratory depression and hypoxemia can occur, transmucosal fentanyl should usually be administered in a monitored environment.

When fentanyl was administered with 50% N_2O in oxygen for induction, the effective dose for loss of consciousness was 8 to 23 μg/kg.[98] Remember, however, that the combination of N_2O and a moderate to high dose of opioid may cause significant muscle rigidity, which can be attenuated by a variety of adjuvants, including benzodiazepines, barbiturates, and muscle relaxants.

Fentanyl is also used frequently as an adjunct to induction agents, such as thiopental and propofol, to blunt the hemodynamic response to laryngoscopy and tracheal intubation, which can be particularly severe in patients with hypertension or cardiovascular disease. Common clinical practice involves titration of fentanyl in doses of 1.5 to 5 μg/kg prior to administration of a barbiturate or other induction agent. Because fentanyl's peak effect lags behind peak plasma concentration by 3 to 5 minutes, fentanyl titration should be complete approximately 3 minutes prior to laryngoscopy to maximally blunt hemodynamic responses to tracheal intubation. Perhaps the most common clinical use of fentanyl and its derivatives is as an analgesic component of balanced general anesthesia. With this technique, incremental doses of fentanyl 0.5 to 2.5 μg/kg are administered intermittently as dictated by the intensity of the surgical stimulus and may be repeated approximately every 30 minutes. Generally, administration of up to 3 to 5 μg/kg/h will allow recovery of spontaneous ventilation at the end of surgery. As an alternative to intermittent dosing, a loading dose of 5 to 10 μg/kg and continuous fentanyl infusion at a rate between 2 and 10 μg/kg/h are recommended.[98] It is important to remember, however, that anesthetic requirements vary with age, concurrent diseases, and the surgical procedure. For example, fentanyl requirements decrease by 50% as age increases from 20 to 89 years.[122] Fentanyl requirements can also be expected to decrease with the duration of infusion (see discussion of context-specific half-times at the end of this chapter).

Fentanyl combined with high-dose droperidol, and nitrous oxide, is a technique called *neuroleptanesthesia*.[126] Although used for many years, this technique has largely been replaced by the balanced anesthetic technique of fentanyl combined with low-dose inhaled anesthetics. Neuroleptanesthesia is not likely to regain popular use in the United States because of concerns about prolongation of the QT interval of the ECG by high dose droperidol.[127] High-dose (e.g., 50 to 150 μg/kg) fentanyl "anesthesia" has been used extensively for cardiac surgery. With this technique, a mean plasma fentanyl concentration of 15 ng/mL, which prevents hemodynamic changes in response to noxious stimuli,[128] can be achieved with a loading dose of 50 μg/kg, followed by a continuous infusion of 30 μg/kg/h. With high-dose fentanyl, muscle relaxants and mechanical ventilation are required. Whether opioids alone are suitable as the sole "anesthetic" agent continues to be debated.

Finally, fentanyl has been used as an analgesic in management of acute and chronic pain (see Chapters 54 and 55).

Dosage recommendations are summarized in Table 14-5.

SUFENTANIL

Sufentanil, a thienyl derivative of fentanyl (see Fig. 14-5) first described in the mid 1970s, has a clinical potency ratio 2,000 to 4,000 times that of morphine and 10 to 15 times that of fentanyl.[129,130] Like fentanyl, sufentanil equilibrates rapidly between blood and brain, and demonstrates clear plasma concentration-effect relationships. In a study comparing sufentanil and fentanyl effects on the EEG, Scott et al[130] noted similar pharmacodynamic profiles. During a 4-minute sufentanil infusion, the change in spectral edge lagged behind the rising sufentanil concentration by approximately 2 to 3 minutes, while resolution of the EEG changes lagged behind plasma concentration changes by 20 to 30 minutes.

Analgesia

Sufentanil is a highly selective μ-opioid receptor agonist and exerts potent analgesic effects in animals when given by either systemic or spinal routes. While the literature describing clinical experience with sufentanil as a component of general anesthesia is extensive, available information regarding the analgesic potency of systemically administered sufentanil in humans is limited. Geller et al[131] titrated an iv infusion rate to adequate postoperative analgesia, and noted that a mean rate of 8 to 17 μg/h was required during the first 48 hours. This was associated with a fivefold range in plasma sufentanil concentrations, between 0.02 and 0.1 ng/mL. Similar sufentanil requirements (including a wide interpatient variability) are noted in other studies of postoperative and cancer patients,[41,132] and Lehman estimated that the minimum effective analgesic concentration of sufentanil is near 0.03 ng/mL,[132] and the analgesic EC_{50} of sufentanil concentration is approximately 0.05 ng/mL.[133]

Effect on Minimum Alveolar Concentration of Volatile Anesthetics and Use in Anesthesia

In animal studies, sufentanil decreases the MAC of volatile anesthetics in a dose-dependent manner, with the maximum MAC reduction between 70 and 90%.[134] In humans, a plasma sufentanil concentration of 0.145 ng/mL is associated with a 50% reduction in isoflurane MAC.[135] Increasing the plasma sufentanil concentration to 0.5 ng/mL reduced isoflurane MAC by 78%, and a ceiling effect was approached with greater plasma sufentanil concentrations. The maximum MAC reduction seen in humans was 89%, at a sufentanil concentration of 1.4 ng/mL.

In clinical anesthesia practice, sufentanil is used as a component of balanced anesthesia and has been employed extensively in high doses (10 to 30 μg/kg) with oxygen and muscle relaxants for cardiac surgery. In this dose range, sufentanil is at least as effective as fentanyl in its ability to produce and maintain hypnosis. In addition, hemodynamic stability appears to be as good as or better than that achieved with fentanyl.[75,129] Bailey et al[136] used a computer-assisted continuous infusion system to determine the sufentanil plasma concentration response to various noxious stimuli during high-dose sufentanil anesthesia for cardiac surgery. They estimated the plasma concentration associated with a 50% probability of no response (movement, hemodynamic, or sympathetic) to intubation, incision, sternotomy, and mediastinal dissection (CP_{50}). The CP_{50} for intubation, incision, and sternotomy (pooled data) was 7.06 ng/mL, and for mediastinal dissection CP_{50} was 12.1 ng/mL. As is typical of opioids, a wide intersubject variability (3- to 10-fold) was noted in sufentanil concentration requirements. However, when used as the sole anesthetic agent, even high doses may not completely block the hemodyamic responses to noxious stimuli.[99]

Other Central Nervous System Effects

Equianalgesic doses of sufentanil and fentanyl produce similar changes in the EEG.[129,130] In patients who received sufentanil 15 μg/kg, α activity became prominent within a few seconds, and within 3 minutes, the EEG consisted almost entirely of slow δ activity.[129] Rigidity and myoclonic activity resembling seizures have been reported during induction of, and on emergence from, anesthesia with sufentanil in doses of approximately 1 to 2 μg/kg.[37,38]

There has been considerable investigation of the effects of sufentanil on cerebral hemodynamics and intracranial pressure. In patients with intracranial tumors, sufentanil 1 μg/kg was associated with an elevation in spinal cerebrospinal pressure and a decrease in cerebral perfusion pressure.[137] As seen with fentanyl, mean arterial pressure had dropped significantly in these patients. In normal volunteers, a smaller dose of sufentanil (0.5 μg/kg) was not associated with changes in cerebral blood flow.[138] Very large doses of sufentanil (20 μg/kg) in dogs decreased cerebral blood flow in proportion to cerebral metabolism, and intracranial pressure did not change.[139]

Respiratory Depression

Like other μ-opioid agonists, sufentanil causes respiratory depression in doses associated with clinical analgesia.[111,112] Respiratory depression can be especially marked in the presence of inhalation anesthetics. In spontaneously breathing patients anesthetized with 1.5% halothane and N_2O, a small dose of sufentanil (approximately 2.5 μg) reduced mean minute ventilation by 50%, and 4 μg reduced mean respiratory rate by 50%.[140] Postoperative respiratory depression after apparent recovery from anesthesia has been reported for both fentanyl and sufentanil.[141] The lack of exogenous stimulation in the early postoperative period may be an important a factor during early recovery from anesthesia.

In normal volunteers who received bolus doses of fentanyl and sufentanil, changes in end-tidal CO_2 were the same for fentanyl and sufentanil, but the slope of the ventilatory response to CO_2 was depressed to a greater extent by fentanyl.[111] In another volunteer study, a fourfold range of equianalgesic plasma concentrations of morphine and sufentanil produced equivalent respiratory depression, measured as both increased end-tidal CO_2 and a decreased ventilatory response to CO_2.[133]

Cardiovascular and Endocrine Effects

In animal studies, sufentanil produces vasodilation by a sympatholytic mechanism but may also have a direct smooth muscle effect.[142] Clinically, a prominent feature of many trials involving sufentanil is the remarkable hemodynamic stability achieved during balanced and high-dose (up to 30 μg/kg) opioid anesthesia. Only a modest decrease in mean arterial pressure is observed when sufentanil (approximately 15 μg/kg) is used for induction of anesthesia.[75,143] In general, sufentanil and fentanyl have been found to be equivalent for use in balanced and high-dose opioid anesthesia,[99,144] but clinical comparisons between fentanyl and sufentanil suggest that sufentanil may be associated with less respiratory depression and better analgesia in the immediate postoperative period.[145]

The choice of premedication and muscle relaxant may significantly affect hemodynamics during induction and maintenance of anesthesia with sufentanil. Combining vecuronium and sufentanil can cause a decrease in mean arterial pressure during induction,[146] and significant bradycardia and sinus arrest[147] have been reported. Bradycardia is not seen when pancuronium is used during anesthesia with sufentanil.

Sufentanil, like fentanyl, reduces the endocrine and metabolic responses to surgery.[129] However, even a large induction dose (20 μg/kg) did not prevent increases in cortisol, catecholamines, glucose, and free fatty acids during and after cardiopulmonary bypass.[148]

Disposition Kinetics

Sufentanil is extremely lipophilic and has pharmacokinetic properties similar to that of fentanyl. Because of a smaller degree of ionization at physiologic pH and higher degree of plasma protein binding, its volume of distribution is somewhat smaller and its elimination half-life shorter than that of fentanyl (see Table 14-2). Sufentanil pharmacokinetics has been studied in anesthetized patients who had received methohexital for anesthetic induction, followed by the sufentanil dose of 5 μg/kg, and N_2O in oxygen 33%.[149] Plasma sufentanil concentration drops very rapidly after an iv bolus dose, and 98% of the drug is cleared from plasma within 30 minutes. Plasma concentration–time data in this study were best fitted to a three-compartment model, with rapid and slower distribution half-times of 1.4 and 17.7 minutes, respectively, and an elimination half-life of 2.7 hours. In other pharmacokinetic studies with anesthetized patients, reported mean elimination half-lives were in the range of 2.2 to 4.6 hours.[150–152] Obese patients have a larger total volume of distribution and a longer elimination half-life (3.5 vs. 2.2 hours) compared to nonobese patients.[150]

Sufentanil is less red cell bound than fentanyl (22 compared to 40%) and has a whole blood:plasma concentration ratio of 0.741.[120] Plasma sufentanil is approximately 92% protein bound at pH 7.4, mostly to α_1-acid glycoprotein. Clearance of sufentanil is rapid, and like fentanyl has a high hepatic extraction ratio.[120] Metabolism in the liver is by *N*-dealkylation and *O*-demethylation. However, sufentanil clearance and elimination half-life in patients with cirrhosis are similar to controls.[151]

Dosage and Administration of Sufentanil

Like fentanyl, sufentanil is most often used as a component of balanced anesthesia, or as a single agent in high doses, particularly for cardiac surgery (Table 14-5). Several investigations have found similar sufentanil dose requirements for induction of anesthesia.[136,153,175] When sufentanil is titrated during induction, loss of consciousness is seen with total doses between 1.3 to 2.8 μg/kg. Doses in the range of 0.3 to 1.0 μg/kg given 1 to 3 minutes prior to laryngoscopy can be expected to blunt hemodynamic responses to intubation, but muscle rigidity can occur, particularly in the elderly, even at these lower doses.

Balanced anesthesia is maintained with intermittent bolus doses or a continuous infusion. With bolus doses of 0.1 to 0.5 μg/kg, mean maintenance requirements of 0.35 μg/kg/h have been reported.[75] Cork et al[152] administered an initial bolus of 0.5 μg/kg followed by an infusion of 0.5 μg/kg/h, titrated to patient need. This regimen of sufentanil in combination with N_2O 70% in oxygen, with or without isoflurane, provided satisfactory anesthesia with good hemodynamic stability. Thus, for balanced anesthesia, sufentanil-expected dose requirements for bolus administration and continuous infusion are similar, in the range of 0.3 to 1 μg/kg/h. Much higher bolus doses (10 μg/kg) and/or infusion rates (0.15 μg/kg/min) are required to achieve the plasma sufentanil concentration range of 6 to 60 ng/mL required during cardiac anesthesia using sufentanil as the sole agent.

ALFENTANIL

Alfentanil, a tetrazole derivative of fentanyl (see Fig. 14-5), was synthesized 2 years after sufentanil and introduced into clinical practice in the early 1980s. On a milligram basis, its clinical potency is approximately ten times that of morphine and one-fourth to one-tenth that of fentanyl when given in single doses. Alfentanil differs from fentanyl in its pharmacokinetics as well as in its speed of equilibration between plasma and effect site in the brain. In a comparison using EEG spectral edge effects to quantify fentanyl and alfentanil pharmacodynamics, Scott et al[88] demonstrated that alfentanil's effect followed serum drug concentration more closely than fentanyl (see Fig. 14-8). Peak effect lagged behind peak plasma concentration by less than 1 minute, and resolution of effect followed decreasing serum alfentanil concentration by no more than 10 minutes. Alfentanil is a μ-opioid receptor agonist and produces typical naloxone-reversible analgesia and side effects such as sedation, nausea, and respiratory depression.

Analgesia

Alfentanil has been administered intravenously for treatment of postoperative and cancer-related pain, as well as in laboratory pain models with normal volunteers. Clear concentration and dose-related analgesic effects have been demonstrated for alfentanil, but individual requirements in terms of dosage or plasma concentrations vary widely. For postoperative analgesia, the MEAC is approximately 10 ng/mL, with a range of 2 to >40 ng/mL.[154] In a laboratory investigation, 80 ng/mL was associated with a 50% reduction in pain intensity.[40] In clinical studies of patients receiving continuous iv infusion of alfentanil, mean plasma concentrations required for relief of moderate to severe pain are approximately 40 to 80 ng/mL (see Table 14-3).[155] Following an adequate loading dose, average alfentanil requirements for postoperative analgesia are approximately 10 to 20 μg/kg/h.[156,157]

Effect on Minimum Alveolar Concentration of Volatile Anesthetics and Use in Anesthesia

Like other opioids, alfentanil decreases the MAC of enflurane in a curvilinear fashion up to a plateau.[21,158] In dogs, an infusion rate of 8 μg/kg/min (plasma concentration 223 ng/mL) reduced enflurane MAC by 69%, but increasing the infusion rate fourfold did not reduce enflurane MAC further.[158]

In humans, alfentanil plasma concentrations required to supplement N_2O anesthesia for various noxious stimuli have been determined.[159] Patients received a loading dose of 150 μg/kg, followed by an infusion that was titrated between 25 and 150 μg/kg/h according to the patients' responses to surgical stimuli, and steep concentration-effect curves were demonstrated. Plasma concentrations required along with 66% N_2O to obtund somatic, autonomic, and hemodynamic responses to stimuli in 50% of patients were 475, 279, and 150 ng/mL for tracheal intubation, skin incision, and skin closure, respectively. The plasma alfentanil concentration associated with spontaneous ventilation after discontinuation of N_2O was 223 ng/mL. Nearly identical results were obtained in a similar study using computer-controlled infusions to deliver alfentanil (Fig. 14-9).[160] Plasma alfentanil concentrations required in combination with propofol to obtund responses to intubation and surgical stimuli have also been determined.[161] In contrast to combining alfentanil and N_2O, much lower alfentanil plasma concentrations (55 to 92 ng/mL) were required to prevent responses in 50% of patients when alfentanil was combined with propofol at a plasma concentration of 3 μg/mL (Fig. 14-10).

High-dose alfentanil has been used as an induction agent for patients with and without cardiac disease[162] and for induction and maintenance of cardiac anesthesia.[116,163] Patients with cardiac valvular or coronary artery disease required half as much alfentanil to induce unconsciousness.[162] When used as the sole anesthetic agent, mean plasma alfentanil concentrations required to significantly blunt hemodynamic responses to intubation and sternotomy were 700 to 830 ng/mL and 1,200 to 1,800 ng/mL, respectively.[164] These values are approximately twice those reported for alfentanil in combination with 66% nitrous oxide.[159,160] However, even doses that produced very high plasma alfentanil concentrations (1,200 to >2,000 ng/mL) did not eliminate responses to intubation and intraoperative stimuli in all patients.[199] In contrast to fentanyl and sufentanil, the duration of even very large doses of alfentanil is short, so repeated doses or a continuous infusion of alfentanil is required.

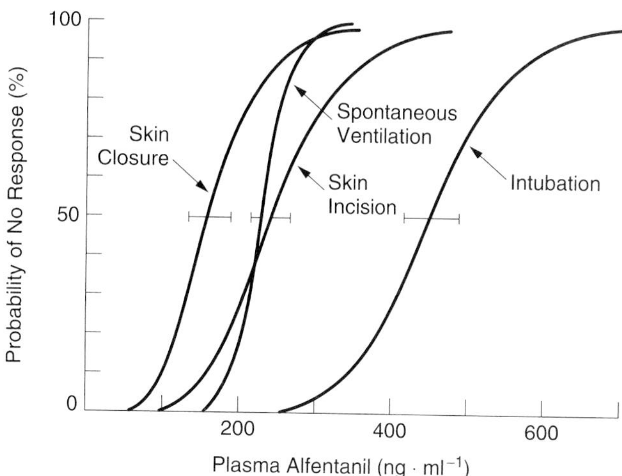

FIGURE 14-9. The relationship between alfentanil plasma concentration (with 66% N_2O) and the probability of no response for intubation, skin incision, and skin closure; and the relationship of plasma alfentanil concentration (without N_2O) and the recovery of adequate spontaneous ventilation. (Reprinted with permission from Ausems ME, Vuyk J, Hug CC *et al:* Comparison of a computer-assisted infusion *versus* intermittent bolus administration of alfentanil as a supplement to nitrous oxide for lower abdominal surgery. Anesthesiology 68:851, 1988.)

Other Central Nervous System Effects

Alfentanil produces the typical generalized slowing of the EEG;[88,165] a plasma concentration of approximately 1,400 ng/mL is associated with the onset of δ-wave activity. Like fentanyl, alfentanil can increase epileptiform EEG activity in patients with intractable temporal lope epilepsy having surgery under general anesthesia.[132] Like fentanyl and sufentanil, alfentanil can produce intense muscle rigidity accompanied by loss of consciousness. In 90 to 100% of patients, induction doses of 150 to 175 μg/kg were associated with muscle rigidity, which was not limited to the chest wall or trunk. Rather, electromyography has shown increased activity of comparable magnitude in muscles of the neck, extremities, chest wall, and abdomen.[137,166]

Alfentanil has been reported to increase cerebrospinal fluid pressure in patients with brain tumors, whereas fentanyl does not.[102] However, Mayberg et al[167] examined the effect of 25 and 50 μg/kg of alfentanil on cerebral blood flow velocity and intracranial pressure in neurosurgical and orthopaedic patients anesthetized with isoflurane and 50% N_2O. Ventilation was controlled to maintain normocapnea, and blood pressure was maintained at baseline for neurosurgical patients. No clinically significant changes in ICP and no evidence of cerebral vasodilation or vasoconstriction were seen.

Respiratory Depression

In animal and human studies, antinociceptive effects could not be separated from respiratory depression in volunteers; mild ventilatory depression (increased end-tidal CO_2; decreased

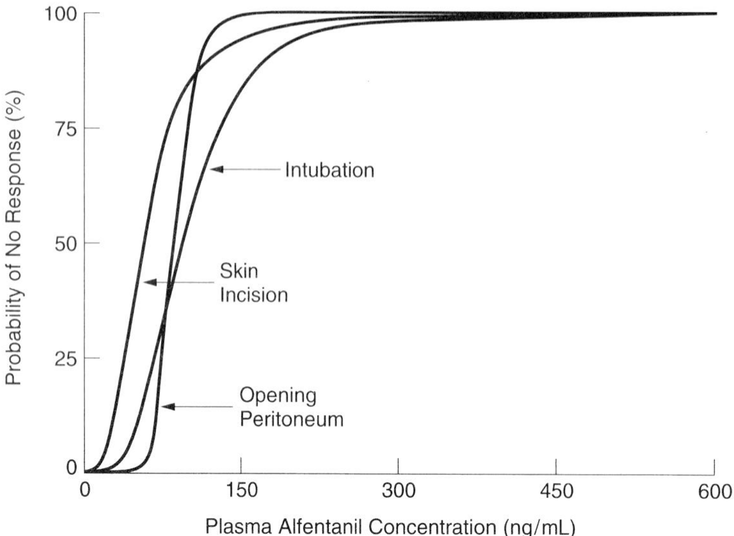

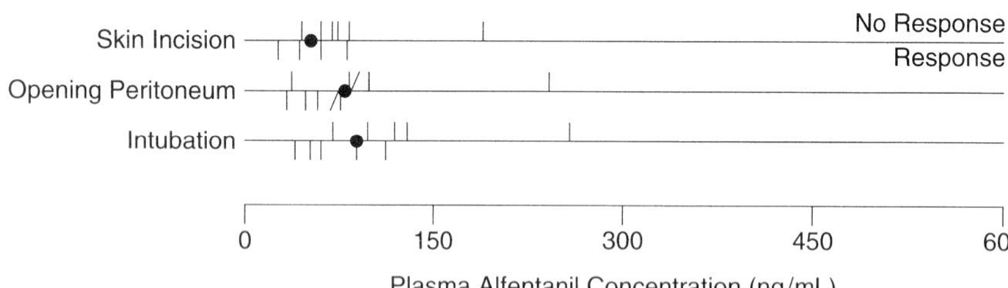

FIGURE 14-10. The alfentanil plasma concentration-effect relationships for intubation, skin incision, and the opening of the peritoneum when given as a supplement to propofol. (Reprinted with permission from Vuyk J, Lim T, Engbers FHM *et al:* Pharmacodynamics of alfentanil as a supplement to propofol or nitrous oxide for lower abdominal surgery in female patients. Anesthesiology 78:1036, 1993.)

slope of the CO_2 response curve) was seen at plasma concentrations as low as 20 ng/mL. At plasma concentrations associated with 50% reduction in pain intensity, respiratory depression was equivalent for alfentanil, fentanyl, and morphine.[10] A clinical study examined postoperative analgesia and respiratory effects of alfentanil administered by a patient-controlled analgesia system.[168] In patients who received a continuous alfentanil infusion at 900 μg/h plus 100- to 200-μg doses as needed, 3 of 10 patients developed respiratory depression (respiratory rate <8/min). Mean alfentanil blood concentration in this group of patients was 80 ng/mL.

Two clinical studies examined the intensity and duration of respiratory depressant effects of alfentanil in the immediate postoperative period.[169,170] Patients received balanced anesthesia 67% N_2O with or without 0.5% halothane and alfentanil 20 to 100 μg/kg/h. At the end of surgery the infusion was decreased to 20 μg/kg/h, which produced plasma alfentanil concentrations between 106 and 120 ng/mL, and good analgesia. Ventilatory response to CO_2 was decreased to 50% of the baseline value, but $PaCO_2$ was only moderately elevated (42 to 48 torr). By 2 hours after alfentanil was discontinued, respiratory function was near baseline. Recovery of ventilatory function was faster with alfentanil compared to fentanyl.[170] Another comparison found that for anesthetics of 1.5 to 2 hours duration, recovery of respiratory function was similar with alfentanil and fentanyl.[171] Like its congeners, alfentanil has been associated with apnea and unconsciousness after apparent recovery from anesthesia.[172]

Cardiovascular Effects

The cardiovascular effects of alfentanil are influenced by preoperative medication, muscle relaxant used, method of administration, and the degree of surgical stimulation. In general, heart rate and mean arterial pressure are unchanged or slightly decreased during induction with alfentanil 40 to 120 μg/kg,[162] but rapid induction with 150 to 175 μg/kg alfentanil can decrease mean arterial pressure by 15 to 20 torr. After induction with etomidate, alfentanil 120 μg/kg decreased mean arterial pressure by approximately 30 torr,[173] and following thiopental (3 to 5 mg/kg) induction, a smaller dose of alfentanil (40 μg/kg) decreased mean arterial pressure by approximately 40 torr.[174] Alfentanil does not appear to have negative inotropic effects,[173] but severe hypotension has been observed when alfentanil is given after 0.125 mg/kg diazepam.[175] In combination with lorazepam premedication or thiopental induction, moderate doses (10 to 50 μg/kg) of alfentanil blunt the cardiovascular and catecholamine responses to laryngoscopy and intubation,[164,174] but for patients over 70 years old, doses in this range given with thiopental can produce significant hypotension after induction.[176] Alfentanil can also cause bradycardia, but this effect is minimized by premedication with atropine and by the vagolytic effect of pancuronium. Alfentanil 50 μg/kg combined with propofol 1 mg/kg for induction of anesthesia can produce significant bradycardia and hypotension after intubation, but premedication with glycopyrrolate prevents these effects.[177]

Nausea and Vomiting

Early clinical reports noted frequent nausea during recovery from balanced anesthesia using alfentanil, but clinical comparisons between alfentanil and sufentanil[178] or fentanyl[179] and N_2O revealed the same incidence of nausea and vomiting. In normal volunteers receiving computer-controlled opioid infusions, the severity of nausea at equianalgesic plasma concentrations was equivalent for alfentanil, fentanyl, and morphine,[40] but alfentanil-induced nausea and vomiting resolved more quickly (Coda BA, unpublished observations).

Disposition Kinetics

Alfentanil pharmacokinetics differs from fentanyl and sufentanil in several respects (see Table 14-3). A unique characteristic is that alfentanil is a weaker base than other opioids. Whereas other opioids have pK_a above 7.4, the pK_a of alfentanil is 6.8; consequently, nearly 90% of unbound plasma alfentanil is nonionized at pH 7.4.[120] This property, together with its moderate lipid solubility, enables alfentanil to cross the blood-brain barrier rapidly and accounts for its rapid onset of action. Compared to fentanyl and sufentanil, which have mean plasma-brain equilibration half-times of 6.4 and 6.2 minutes, respectively,[88,130] alfentanil has a blood-brain equilibration half-time of 1.1 minutes.[110] Alfentanil also has a smaller volume of distribution than fentanyl, which is a result of lower lipid solubility and high protein binding.[180] Approximately 92% of alfentanil is protein bound, mostly to α_1-acid glycoprotein.[120,123]

After iv administration, plasma alfentanil concentration falls rapidly; 90% of the administered dose has left the plasma by 30 minutes,[181] mostly because of distribution to highly perfused tissues. Plasma concentration decay curves in patients most often fit a three-compartment model.[19,181] Like fentanyl, alfentanil is quickly distributed, with rapid and slow distribution half-times of 1.0 to 3.5 minutes and 9.5 to 17 minutes, respectively. However, alfentanil has a terminal elimination half-life of 84 to 90 minutes, which is considerably shorter than those of fentanyl and sufentanil. Clearance of alfentanil, 6.4 mL/kg/min, is just half that of fentanyl, but because alfentanil's volume of distribution is 4 times smaller than fentanyl's, relatively more of the dose is available to the liver for metabolism.[182] Chauvin et al[183] found that alfentanil has an intermediate hepatic extraction coefficient (32 to 53%) in humans, and that its elimination is dependent on hepatic plasma flow.

In animals, alfentanil undergoes *N*-dealkylation and *O*-demethylation in the liver to form inactive metabolites.[120] Liver disease can significantly prolong the elimination half-life of alfentanil. Patients with moderate hepatic insufficiency as a result of cirrhosis have reduced binding to α_1-acid glycoprotein and a plasma clearance one-half that of control patients. These changes result in a marked increase in the elimination half-life, 219 minutes versus 90 minutes in controls.[184] Renal disease also decreases alfentanil protein binding, but does not result in decreased plasma clearance or a prolonged terminal elimination half-life.[185] Alfentanil's elimination half-life is prolonged by about 30% in the elderly and appears to be much shorter (about 40 minutes) in children 5 to 8 years old.[186] Obesity is also associated with a 50% decrease in alfentanil clearance and a prolonged (172 minutes) elimination half-life.[186]

The combination of moderate lipid solubility and short elimination half-life suggests that both redistribution and elimination are important in the termination of alfentanil's effects.[182] After a single bolus dose, redistribution will be the most important mechanism, but after a very large dose, repeated small doses, or a continuous infusion, elimination will be a more important determinant of the duration of alfentanil's effects.

Dosage and Administration of Alfentanil

Because of its rapid onset, alfentanil has been used as an induction agent alone or in combination with other drugs. In healthy patients, doses of about 120 μg/kg produce unconsciousness in 2 to 2.5 minutes, but may also produce muscle rigidity. Premedication with a benzodiazepine (e.g., lorazepam 0.08 mg/kg) is associated with a lower dose requirement, 40 to 50 μg/kg, and a faster onset of unconsciousness, within 1.5 minutes,[162] but may also produce hypotension.

Because of its brief duration of action, alfentanil can be a useful component of general anesthesia in short surgical procedures, especially those associated with minimal postoperative pain, particularly in the outpatient surgery. In this setting, loading doses of 5 to 10 μg/kg provide good analgesia with rapid recovery.[180] For longer procedures, alfentanil can be administered as needed in repeated small bolus doses, but its pharmacokinetic properties make it ideal for administration as a continuous infusion. After induction of anesthesia, a loading dose of alfentanil 10 to 50 μg/kg is followed with supplemental bolus doses of 3 to 5 μg/kg as needed or a continuous infusion starting at 0.4 to 1.7 μg/kg/min with 60 to 70% N_2O or a propofol infusion.[159,160,180,187,188] A pediatric study reported use of similar doses of alfentanil and propofol,[189] while another used higher alfentanil doses (100 μg/kg loading dose followed by 2.5 μg/kg/min) combined with 70% N_2O without propofol.[190]

When high-dose alfentanil is used as the sole anesthetic agent, a continuous infusion of up to 150 to 600 μg/kg/h is adjusted according to the patient's responses to stimuli, but much lower doses can be effective for cardiac surgery if adequate premedication is given.[163] See Table 14-5 for a summary of dosage recommendations.

REMIFENTANIL

Remifentanil, a 4-anilidopiperidine with a methyl ester side chain (see Fig. 14-5) first described in 1990 and approved for clinical use in 1996, was developed to meet the need for an ultrashort-acting opioid. Because its ester side chain is susceptible to metabolism by blood and tissue esterases, remifentanil is rapidly metabolized to a substantially less active compound. Thus, because its ultrashort action is due to metabolism rather than to redistribution, it does not accumulate with repeated dosing or prolonged infusion. Remifentanil demonstrates potent, naloxone-reversible μ-selective opioid agonist activity in animal assays.[191]

Analgesia

In animals and humans, remifentanil produces dose-dependent analgesic effects. Human laboratory studies have examined analgesic effects of bolus iv doses (0.0625 to 2.0 μg/kg)[192] as well as computer-controlled infusions with targeted plasma concentrations (0.75 to 3.0 ng/mL).[193] Bolus doses produced a peak analgesic effect between 1 and 3 minutes and a duration of approximately 10 minutes. In volunteers, MEAC is approximately 0.75 ng/mL, and analgesic EC_{50} is approximately 3 ng/mL.[193] Both studies found remifentanil to be about 40 times as potent as alfentanil.

Clinical investigations have evaluated early postoperative analgesia. One study reported that after remifentanil–propofol anesthesia, nearly 80% of patients were titrated to satisfactory analgesia with remifentanil infusion of 0.05 to 0.15 μg/kg/min.[194] Another early postoperative evaluation demonstrated effective analgesia with patient-controlled infusion of remifentanil to a mean target blood concentration of 2 ng/mL, but noted a fairly high incidence of nausea (26%) with this regimen.[195] Clinical evaluations of remifentanil for labor analgesia have produced conflicting results, and some have found prohibitive rates of unacceptable side effects such as nausea and respiratory depression. However, a dose-ranging study that used remifentanil via PCA reported a median effective bolus dose of 0.4 μg/kg (range 0.2 to 0.8 μg/kg) and consumption of 0.066 μg/kg/min (range 0.027 to 0.207 μg/kg/min).[196]

Effect on Minimum Alveolar Concentration of Volatile Anesthetics and Use in Anesthesia

The effect of remifentanil on the MAC of volatile anesthetics is characterized by steep dose-effect or concentration-effect curves typical of other μ-opioid agonists. In animals, remifentanil decreases enflurane and isoflurane MAC in a dose-dependent fashion up to a maximum near 65%, similar to fentanyl.[197,198] In humans, remifentanil reduces isoflurane MAC logarithmically in a blood concentration–dependent fashion.[199] A whole blood remifentanil concentration of 1.3 ng/mL reduced isoflurane MAC by 50%, with a maximum MAC reduction (91%) at 32 ng/mL. Remifentanil's effect on the MAC-BAR (requirement for blunting the sympathetic response to skin incision) of sevoflurane in 60% N_2O is similar.[200] A remifentanil plasma concentration of 1ng/mL sevoflurane reduced MAC-BAR by 60%, while 3 ng/mL decreased MAC-BAR another 30%.

The rapid onset and brief duration of remifentanil suggest that it is suitable for induction of anesthesia. Although a median ED_{50} of 12 μg/kg for loss of consciousness has been reported, clinical investigations have also found that, as with other opioids, loss of consciousness is not reliably achieved with remifentanil alone, even in doses of 20 μg/kg or more.[201,202] Furthermore, a high incidence of muscle rigidity and purposeless movement was seen. Even at 2 μg/kg remifentanil, moderate muscle rigidity was seen in 40% of patients, and at the 20 μg/kg, 60% of patients had severe muscle rigidity.[201]

Drover and Lemmens[203] used computer-assisted infusions to determine the blood concentrations of remifentanil required to supplement 66% N_2O in patients having abdominal surgery. A range of 0.5 to 7.8 ng/mL target remifentanil concentrations was used, and other than premedication with 1 to 2 mg midazolam, no sedatives or hypnotics were given. During surgery, the remifentanil blood concentration associated with a 50% probability of adequate anesthesia (EC_{50}) was 4.1 ng/mL for men and 7.5 ng/mL for women. The reason for gender differences in these results was not clear, but could have been related to different types of surgeries. A pediatric study of remifentanil and N_2O in O_2 reported an infusion rate twice that used for adults, and quality of anesthesia similar to alfentanil, propofol, and isoflurane, but noted that this regimen may have been an overestimate of remifentanil requirement.[190]

Investigations of remifentanil for balanced anesthesia, including combination with isoflurane,[204,205] sevoflurane,[206] and desflurane,[207] report similar findings of hemodynamic stability and easy titratability. A clinical trial of remifentanil and desflurane–N_2O identified blood remifentanil concentrations that provide an optimal balance between hemodynamic stability and blunting responses to noxious stimulation while permitting rapid recovery.[207] In the presence of 2.2 to 2.7% end-tidal desflurane and N_2O, optimal remifentanil plasma concentrations were 5 to 7 ng/mL for laryngoscopy and skin closure and 10 ng/mL during abdominal surgery. It is interesting to note that adjustments in remifentanil blunted the sympathetic response to noxious stimulation but did not alter desflurane's effect on the bispectral index analysis of the EEG.

Remifentanil is frequently administered with propofol, to provide *total intravenous anesthesia* (TIVA). Both can be administered at fixed infusion rates or by computer-controlled systems that provide target plasma concentrations, commonly referred to as *target-controlled infusions* or TCI. The combination of remifentanil and propofol for TIVA has been used successfully for a variety of inpatient procedures, including coronary artery bypass graft (CABG); other major thoracic, neurosurgical, abdominal, and orthopaedic procedures; as well as ambulatory surgery and other painful procedures in adults and children. Two studies demonstrated that a fairly low plasma concentration of remifentanil, TCI at 3.4 to 4 ng/mL, reduces propofol EC_{50} for intubation by 66%, from approximately 6 ng/mL to 2 ng/mL.[202,208] However, further increases in remifentanil dosage only modestly reduced propofol dose requirements, an apparent ceiling effect.[208] An early clinical study[209] evaluated various combinations of remifentanil and propofol concentrations (EC_{50}) to prevent responses to laryngoscopy and surgical stimuli in 50% of patients. Remifentanil EC_{50} for laryngoscopy was 14.3 ng/mL and 1.4 ng/mL with propofol infusions of 44 and 200 μg/kg/min, respectively. Response to intubation was prevented in 80% of patients by approximately doubling the remifentanil.

Barvais and Sutcliffe reviewed the use of remifentanil for cardiac anesthesia.[210] While high-dose remifentanil (1 to 2 μg/kg/min) has been used as a single agent, it is more commonly administered with propofol or isoflurane for "fast-track cardiac anesthesia." Target remifentanil and propofol concentrations for cardiac surgery[210,211] are very similar to those for other procedures with low-dose propofol. In a study comparing remifentanil, sufentanil, and fentanyl for fast-track cardiac anesthesia, Engoren[212] found that remifentanil patients were more likely to require treatment for blood pressure fluctuations during and after surgery, but otherwise, the three regimens produced similar outcomes with respect to extubation, ICU stay, and cost.

One drawback of remifentanil use for general anesthesia is that patients require analgesics very soon after an infusion is stopped. A continuation of remifentanil to transition to postoperative analgesia can avoid early pain and accompanying detrimental sympatho-adrenal stimulation and is essential for patients undergoing cardiac or other major surgery.

Remifentanil administered by infusion also appears to be useful during monitored anesthesia care (MAC) for conscious sedation in procedures such as extracorporeal shock wave lithotripsy and colonoscopy,[213,214] or in conjunction with regional anesthesia.[215–217] When compared to propofol, remifentanil provides better analgesia, but more nausea and respiratory depression, whereas propofol causes more oversedation. Times required for readiness for discharge are clinically similar. For MAC, the ideal administration regimen appears to be small bolus doses of remifentanil with a continuous infusion combined with low-dose propofol or midazolam.

Other Central Nervous System Effects

Remifentanil produces classic μ-opioid agonist effects on the EEG, that is, a concentration-dependent slowing. The plasma concentration associated with 50% maximal EEG changes (EC_{50}) is 15 to 20 ng/mL.[218,219] Remifentanil's rapid onset and very short duration results in extremely close tracking of changes in EEG spectral edge with plasma remifentanil concentration.[218,219] Like other opioids, remifentanil can produce muscle rigidity, especially with bolus doses. This can be avoided with using smaller doses and injecting over 60 seconds or more.

Several clinical reports have described cerebral hemodynamics in humans. When bolus doses of remifentanil (0.5 or 1.0 μg/kg) or alfentanil (10 or 20 μg/kg) were given during isoflurane/N_2O anesthesia with controlled ventilation, neither opioid affected intracranial pressure and both produced modest, dose-dependent decreases in mean arterial pressure.[220] In another study, patients received higher remifentanil doses, followed by continuous infusion, while isocapnea and mean arterial pressure were maintained. Cerebral blood flow velocity decreased significantly in patients receiving 5 μg/kg, followed by 3 μg/kg/min, but not in those with 2 μg/kg, followed by 1 μg/kg/min remifentanil. A multicenter clinical trial comparing remifentanil/N_2O to fentanyl/N_2O anesthesia found that intracranial pressure (remifentanil 13 ± 10; fentanyl 14 ±

13 mm Hg) and cerebral perfusion pressure (remifentanil 78 ± 14; fentanyl 76 ± 19 mm Hg) were similar with the two regimens.[221] In a study comparing cerebrovascular autoregulation in the awake and anesthetized states, remifentanil 0.5μg/kg/min plus propofol preserved cerebral autoregulation, whereas isoflurane 1.8% did not.[222]

In many cranial and spinal neurosurgical procedures, the ability to monitor motor evoked potentials (MEPs) is important; opioids, sedative hypnotic drugs, and inhalation agents used in general anesthesia are known to suppress MEPs. A human and animal study compared the effects of phenylpiperadine opioids and hypnotics including thiopental, midazolam, and propofol on MEPs.[223] While all opioids and propofol suppressed MEPs in a dose-dependent fashion, remifentanil exerted less suppression than the other opioids and propofol. A target plasma concentration of 9 ng/mL reduced amplitude by 50%, but the quality and reproducibility of MEPs was preserved even at plasma concentration of 15 ng/mL, well within the plasma concentration range that provides surgical anesthesia.

Although remifentanil has not been shown to produce seizure activity, it can be used to reduce methohexital requirement in patients having electroconvulsive therapy. Remifentanil 1 μg/kg allowed a 50% reduction in methohexital dose, which results in seizure prolongation by 50%.[224]

Respiratory Depression

Remifentanil produces dose-dependent respiratory depression as measured by increases in end-tidal CO_2 and decreased oxygen saturation. In a dose-escalation study in normal volunteers, the respiratory depressant effects of remifentanil and alfentanil were compared.[192] Peak respiratory depression occurred at 5 minutes after each dose of remifentanil and alfentanil, and the maximal respiratory depressant effect seen after 2 μg/kg remifentanil was similar to that caused by 32 μg/kg alfentanil. The duration of respiratory depression, measured as time to return of blood gases to within 10% of baseline values, was 10 minutes after 1.5 μg/kg and 20 minutes after 2 μg/kg remifentanil compared to 30 minutes after 32 μg/kg alfentanil. During continuous opioid infusion, the ventilatory response to CO_2 decreased by approximately 30, 45, and 60% in response to 4-hour remifentanil infusions of 0.025, 0.050, and 0.075 μg/kg/min, respectively.[225] Recovery from remifentanil-induced respiratory depression was rapid, and minute ventilation returned to baseline by 8 (range 5 to 15) minutes after the infusion was stopped for all infusion rates. In contrast, a 50% decrease in minute ventilation produced by a 4-hour infusion of alfentanil at 0.5 μg/kg/min required 61 (range 5 to 90) minutes to return to baseline.[225] In a volunteer study, Glass et al reported that the blood remifentanil concentration needed to depress ventilatory response to inspired 8% CO_2 by 50% (EC_{50}) was 1.17 ng/mL.[226] Bouillon et al[227] reported a similar EC_{50} (0.92 ng/mL) determined by an indirect response model and also noted that remifentanil concentrations well tolerated at steady state will produce clinically significant respiratory depression when achieved with bolus dosing. In general, clinical comparisons report that respiratory parameters (respiratory rate, O_2 saturation and end-tidal CO_2) recover more rapidly after remifentanil compared to other opioids given in equipotent dosage.

An animal model suggested that in combination with sevoflurane, remifentanil depressed ventilation more than responses to noxious stimulation. Therefore, maintenance of spontaneous respiration during general anesthesia with remifentanil and volatile agents or propofol may not be feasible unless low doses of remifentanil are used.[228] Clinical experience in spontaneously breathing humans receiving remifentanil combined with either isoflurane or propofol demonstrates respiratory depression in 10 to 35% of patients receiving remifentanil at 0.025 μg/kg/min. It increases to nearly 50% in patients receiving 0.05 μg/kg/min and to >90% in patients receiving remifentanil at 0.075 μg/kg/min.[229] A similar rate of respiratory depression (20%) with need for assisted ventilation is seen in pediatric patients receiving remifentanil/propofol infusions for general anesthesia during bone marrow aspiration.[230] As discussed earlier, remifentanil alone or combined with low-dose propofol or midazolam can be used for conscious sedation and to supplement regional or local anesthesia during monitored anesthesia care. Clinical reports describing these regimens report respiratory depression (respiratory rate <8 or SpO2 <90%) in 2 to 30% of patients; but in all cases, recovery from respiratory depression with remifentanil is more rapid than other agents.[213–216] As with other opioids, higher rates of respiratory depression are seen when propofol is combined with remifentanil (15 to 50% of patients) and careful monitoring and titration are required to minimize this side effect.

Hemodynamic Effects

In healthy volunteers, remifentanil in bolus doses greater than 1.0 μg/kg produces brief increases in systolic blood pressure (5 to 20 torr) and heart rate (10 to 25 beats/min).[192] In patients anesthetized with isoflurane and 66% N_2O in oxygen, remifentanil (up to 5 μg/kg) produces dose-dependent decreases in systolic blood pressure and heart rate. These effects are attenuated by premedication with glycopyrrolate 0.3 to 0.4 mg and are readily reversed with ephedrine or phenylephrine.[231] Sebel et al[232] evaluated hemodynamic responses in patients receiving remifentanil 2 to 30 μg/kg (escalating doses) given during general anesthesia and found that systolic heart rate decreased more than 20% for doses greater than 2 μg/kg. These hemodynamic effects were not mediated by histamine release. Clinical reports of experience with patients receiving opioid-based anesthetics have characterized hemodynamic changes during balanced anesthesia with remifentanil combined with isoflurane ± N_2O/O_2 or propofol. During a comparison of remifentanil- versus alfentanil-based TIVA, a 20% drop in mean arterial pressure, with minimal change in heart rate, was noted after induction, with 35 to 50% of patients experiencing at least one episode of mean arterial pressure less than 70 mmHg.[188] Decreases in blood pressure were transient and easily treated with fluids and downward titration of propofol. In a comparison of remifentanil- and fentanyl-based general anesthetics in more than 2,400 patients (80% ASA I and II), hypotension (systolic BP <80 or treated pharmacologically) occurred in 12% of patients receiving remifentanil compared to 4% with fentanyl.[204] Bradycardia was less common, 2% and 1% of patients in the remifentanil and fentanyl groups, respectively.

Greater hemodynamic changes can be seen in patients with coronary disease. In a comparison of high-dose remifentanil (2 μg/kg/min) and remifentanil 0.5 μg/kg/min plus propofol targeted to 2 μg/mL plasma concentration, both techniques produced similar changes: 30% drop in mean arterial pressure, and 25% drop in cardiac index. Myocardial blood flow and oxygen consumption decreased by about 30 and 40%, respectively. More moderate hemodynamic changes were reported with lower doses (remifentanil target-controlled infusion [TCI] 4 to −8 ng/mL and propofol 1.2 ng/mL).[211] Heart rate and cardiac index dropped 20 and 6%, respectively, and no hypotension was seen. In an early clinical report, DeSouza reported a series of six cases[233] of severe bradycardia (HR <30 beats/min) and hypotension (systolic BP <80 mmHg) in six patients who received a rapid injection of remifentanil 1 μg/kg followed by a continuous infusion at 0.1 to 0.2 μg/kg/min on induction for cardiac surgery.

Hypotension was effectively treated by ephedrine and temporary discontinuation of remifentanil. These severe effects can often be avoided by slower administration (more than 60 seconds or longer) of the loading dose, as smaller bolus doses of remifentanil (0.3 to 0.5 μg/kg) are apparently not associated with severe bradycardia and hypotension.

Gastrointestinal Effects

Like other μ agonists, remifentanil can cause nausea and vomiting, but the occurrence of these adverse effects is influenced to a large extent by surgery, adjuvant anesthetic agents, and antiemetic prophylaxis. In a volunteer study, high infusion rates (1 to 8 μg/kg/min) produced nausea in 70% of subjects.[218] However, much lower doses are typically used for general anesthesia. Philip et al[187] compared nausea and vomiting at multiple time points in outpatient adults for laparoscopic surgery who received remifentanil or alfentanil combined with N_2O and propofol. In this study remifentanil was infused at 0.25 to 0.5 μg/kg/min and alfentanil was infused at 1 to 2 μg/kg/min after induction. Overall, the incidence of nausea was 44 and 53% for remifentanil and alfentanil, respectively; the incidence of vomiting was 21 and 29% for remifentanil and alfentanil, respectively. In outpatients with similar opioid infusions combined with 0.8% isoflurane, nausea occurred in 18 and 20% of patients with remifentanil and alfentanil, respectively.[234] In contrast, a report summarizing adverse events in over 2,400 patients who received remifentanil (range 0.25 to 2 μg/kg/min) or fentanyl with isoflurane or propofol for a variety of surgeries, nausea and vomiting were rare.[204] Another comparison of low-dose remifentanil (0.5 μg/kg and 0.1 μg/kg/min) plus propofol to alfentanil plus propofol reported very low incidence of nausea and vomiting (6 to 12%, mostly at home).[235] A study in 100 otorhinolaryngeal surgery patients who received either remifentanil or alfentanil and propofol reported an intermediate incidence that was equivalent for both opioids.[42] Nausea occurred in 16 and 22% of patients with remifentanil and alfentanil, respectively, and vomiting in 14 and 12% of patients receiving remifentanil and alfentanil, respectively. In a pediatric study, the addition of remifentanil 0.2 μg/kg/min to desflurane anesthesia produced no increase in the incidence of postoperative nausea or vomiting after dental surgery; nausea and vomiting occurred in <5% of patients who received remifentanil. For strabismus surgery in children, vomiting occurred with equal frequency (26 to 31%) with remifentanil, alfentanil, isoflurane, and propofol.[236] Thus, remifentanil appears to produce dose-dependent nausea and vomiting similar to other short-acting μ-agonist opioids that can be attenuated by propofol. Taken together, remifentanil studies confirm the wide variability in occurrence of nausea and vomiting in the clinical setting.

Like other opioids, remifentanil delays gastric emptying[237] and biliary drainage.[238] As expected, biliary effects resolve more quickly than biliary drainage delay from morphine of meperidine.

Other Side Effects

Postoperative shivering occurred in about 40% of patients undergoing otorhinolaryngeal surgery despite active warming, and independent of temperature,[42] while another noted shivering in 10% of outpatients.[234] In both of these studies, shivering was less common with alfentanil. One pediatric investigation reported pruritus in 12% of patients.[236]

In volunteers, remifentanil produced concentration-related subjective and psychomotor side effects typical of μ-opioids.[193] Subjective side effects induced by remifentanil included dry mouth, itching, flushing, sweating, and "turning of the stomach." Remifentanil also impaired performance of psychomotor tests and caused miosis and respiratory depression. Some of these effects lasted an hour or more after remifentanil administration was stopped.

Disposition Kinetics

The key structural feature of remifentanil is an ester functional group that is susceptible to hydrolysis by blood and tissue nonspecific esterases and results in very rapid metabolism. Because butyrocholinesterase (pseudocholinesterase) does not appear to metabolize remifentanil, plasma cholinesterase deficiency and anticholinergic administration do not affect remifentanil clearance.[237] Unlike other opioids, remifentanil clearance is mainly because of enzymatic hydrolysis, with redistribution playing only a minor role. This property reduces its pharmacokinetic variability compared to other opioids. Remifentanil has a small volume of distribution, approximately 0.3 to 0.5 L/kg,[192,240] or about 25 liters in an average adult.[241] Remifentanil's clearance, 3 to 5 L /min, is approximately 3 to 4 times normal hepatic blood flow.[192,240,241] Both two- and three-compartment models have been used to describe the plasma concentration decay curve of remifentanil. A rapid distribution phase of 0.9 minutes and a very short terminal elimination half-life of 9.5 minutes characterized a two-compartment model in adults.[192] In pediatrics, elimination half-life is about 3.5 to 6 minutes.[242] In the three-compartment model, rapid and slow distribution half-times were 0.4 to 0.9 and 2 to 6 minutes, respectively, and the elimination half-time was about 10 to 30 minutes.[219,240]

As for other fentanyl congeners, gender does not affect remifentanil pharmacokinetics, but advanced age is associated with a decrease in clearance and volume of distribution, as well as an apparent increase in potency.[243] Remifentanil pharmacokinetics are similar in lean (within 20% ideal body weight) and obese (at least 80% over ideal body weight) patients, indicating that remifentanil dosing should be based on lean body mass.[244] Although pharmacokinetic parameters of remifentanil are unchanged in patients with severe liver disease[245] or renal failure,[246] patients with hepatic disease appear to be more sensitive to remifentanil-induced respiratory depression.

Dosage and Administration of Remifentanil

Because of its extremely short duration of action, remifentanil is best administered as a continuous infusion, although administration as repeated bolus doses has also been reported to be effective. Outside the United States, remifentanil is often administered by TCI, a pump system designed to infuse the drug based on population kinetics to achieve desired target plasma concentrations. Theoretically, this makes sense especially for remifentanil, because its pharmacodynamic effects track plasma concentrations very closely. However, two studies have found that simple manually controlled infusion is as effective[247,248] and is more economical than computer-controlled infusions.

Numerous reports have described dosing regimens for remifentanil alone or in combination with intravenous and inhaled agents for induction and maintenance of general anesthesia, and as a component of sedation and monitored anesthesia care.

Induction Dosage, Intubation, LMA Placement. As described earlier, remifentanil alone has not been found to be a satisfactory single agent for induction of anesthesia because of unreliability in loss of consciousness as well as significant muscle rigidity.[201] However, induction of anesthesia with high-dose remifentanil 4 to 5 μg/kg, or an infusion of 2 μg/kg/min has been reported.[210] It is important to note that bolus doses of >2 μg/kg can drop arterial pressure 20 to 30%, while hemodynamic changes in cardiac patients receiving high-dose infusion are similar to remifentanil plus propofol.[249] Combined with a potent inhalation agent, a loading dose of 1 μg/kg given over 60 seconds can provide adequate intubating conditions with hemodynamic stability. By far the most commonly reported remifentanil-based regimen for anesthetic induction and laryngoscopy consists of remifentanil 0.5 to 1 μg/kg given over 60 seconds plus propofol 1 to 2 mg/kg, followed by remifentanil infusion of 0.25 to 0.5 μg/kg/min.[204,205,250,251] This may be given with or without a midazolam 1- to 2-mg iv premedication. Similar regimens are recommended for pediatric patients, with substitution of oral midazolam premedication 0.5 mg/kg. In the elderly, dose reduction is indicated, with remifentanil 0.05 μg/kg over 60 seconds plus propofol titrated to loss of consciousness in 10-mg increments, followed by remifentanil infusion of 0.1 μg/kg/min. If TCI is used for induction of anesthesia, an initial remifentanil target of 5 to 7 ng/mL accompanied by 0.5 to 1 MAC inhaled anesthetic or propofol TCI of 2 ng/mL is recommended.[203,241]

Maintenance of General Anesthesia. In combination with 70% N_2O in O_2, remifentanil 0.6 μg/kg/min is generally adequate, but at least one study reported a wide range of infusion rates (0.025 to 2 μg/kg/min).[252] A similar infusion rate for remifentanil with N_2O is recommended for pediatric patients. A lower infusion rate (0.2 to 0.25 μg/kg/min) is needed when remifentanil is combined with sevoflurane (1 to 2%),[206] desflurane (3 to 3.6%),[207,253] or isoflurane (0.2 to 0.8%).[204,205,234] For TIVA, maintenance infusion rates for remifentanil and propofol are 0.25 to 0.5 μg/kg/min and 75 to 100 μg/kg/min, respectively.[188,204,250,254,255] If N_2O is added, remifentanil infusion rates as low as 0.125 μg/kg/min and propofol infusion of 50 to 75 μg/kg/min can be used.[254] For elderly patients or those with cardiac disease, a reduction in propofol by about 25% is recommended. For pediatric patients, reported infusion rates are similar to adults, with remifentanil at 0.25 μg/kg/min and propofol about 100 μg/kg/min. For high-dose opioid anesthesia for cardiac surgery, the remifentanil infusion is maintained at 1 to 3 μg/kg/min and should be adjusted downward for hypothermia as discussed earlier.[210] Adding a low-dose propofol infusion of 50 μg/kg/min to this high-infusion rate effectively suppressed responses to skin incision, sternotomy, and aortic cannulation.[256]

If TCI is used, a target range for remifentanil is 4 to 10 ng/mL for balanced anesthesia and TIVA, and a starting rate of 25 to 30 ng/mL is recommended for high-dose opioid anesthesia.[210,241]

A disadvantage of remifentanil, related to its short duration of action, is that patients may experience substantial pain on emergence from anesthesia. Thus, if moderate to severe postoperative pain is anticipated, continuing the remifentanil infusion between 0.05 and 0.15 μg/kg/min ensures adequate analgesia in most patients.[194] The use of local and regional anesthetic techniques are also effective. When only mild postoperative pain is anticipated, intraoperative administration of a nonsteroidal anti-inflammatory drug 30 to 60 minutes before the end of surgery may provide effective analgesia without additional opioids.

Monitored Anesthesia Care (MAC). Remifentanil can also be used for conscious sedation/analgesia and as an adjunct for sedation or analgesia during regional anesthesia, or for block placement, as part of MAC. When local or regional anesthesia is not used, and the procedure is expected to be painful, remifentanil and propofol can be beneficial. During colonoscopy, a continuous remifentanil infusion of 0.2 to 0.25 μg/kg/min, supplemented with small (10-mg) doses of propofol, provided good analgesia but mild respiratory depression was common.[214] In another clinical evaluation, patients having extracorporeal shock wave lithotripsy received low-dose propofol (50 μg/kg/min) as well as remifentanil. Patients who received low-dose (12.5 to 25 μg) intermittent bolus injection of remifentanil with or without infusion at 0.05μg/kg/min reported better analgesia than continuous infusion of 0.1 μg/kg/min alone.[213] Remifentanil 1 μg/kg with or without a subsequent infusion of 0.2 μg/kg/min administered 90 seconds prior to placement of ophthalmologic block resulted in excellent analgesia,[257] but 14% of patients who received an infusion experienced respiratory depression.

When used as an adjunct to local or regional anesthesia, a much lower maintenance infusion rate, 0.05 to 0.1 μg/kg/min, provides adequate sedation and analgesia.[216,217] Finally, the dose requirement of remifentanil for sedation/analgesia is reduced approximately 50% when combined with midazolam or propofol. When 1 to 2 mg of midazolam premedication is given, 0.01 to 0.07 μg/kg/min remifentanil provides good sedation/analgesia for procedures performed under local or regional anesthesia.[215,216]

Dosage recommendations are summarized in Table 14-5.

PARTIAL AGONISTS AND MIXED AGONIST–ANTAGONISTS

The partial agonist and mixed agonist–antagonist opioids are synthetic or semisynthetic compounds that are structurally related to morphine. They are characterized by binding activity at multiple opioid receptors and their differential effects (agonist, partial agonist, or antagonist) at each receptor type. The clinical effect of a partial agonist at the μ-opioid receptor is complex (Fig. 14-11). Administered alone, a partial agonist has a flatter dose-response curve and a lower maximal effect than a full agonist (see Fig. 14-1 and the lowermost curve in Fig. 14-11). Combined with a low concentration (compare the curve indicated by [Ag] = 0.25 in Fig. 14-11) of a full agonist, the effects of the partial agonist are additive up to the maximum effect of the partial agonist. Combined with increasing concentrations ([Ag] = 0.67 to 256) of full agonist, the partial

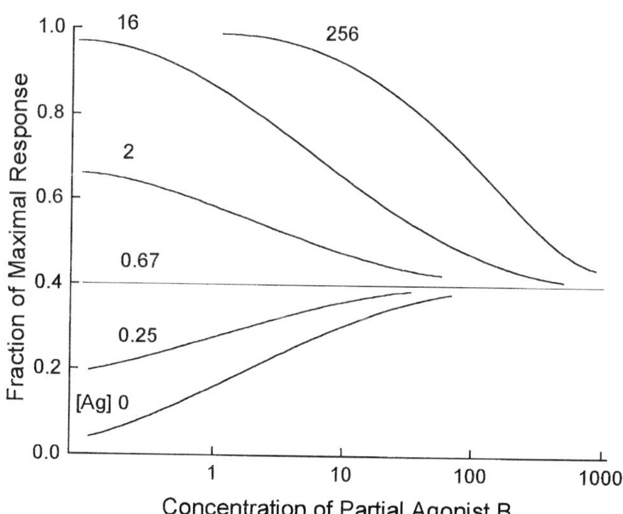

FIGURE 14-11. Hypothetical log dose-effect curves for the combination of a partial agonist, B (intrinsic efficacy of 0.4), with a range of concentrations of a full agonist, A. The observed effect of the combination of A and B is expressed as a fraction of the maximal effect of the full agonist. As the concentration of the partial agonist increases, the effect of the combination converges on the maximum effect of the partial agonist. When added to a low concentration (e.g., [A] = 0.25) of agonist, the partial agonist increases the response; but when added to a large concentration of the agonist, the response decreases—that is, B acts like an antagonist. (Modified with permission from Bowdle TA: Partial agonist and agonist–antagonist opioids: Basic pharmacology and clinical applications. Anaesth Pharmacol Rev 1:135, 1993.)

TABLE 14-4

ACTIONS OF THE NALBUPHINE, BUTORPHANOL, AND BUPRENORPHINE AT OPIOID RECEPTORS

DRUG	μ RECEPTOR	κ RECEPTOR
Nalbuphine	Partial agonist	Partial agonist
Butorphanol	Partial agonist	Partial agonist
Buprenorphine	Partial agonist	?Antagonist

Although nalbuphine and butorphanol have been reported to be antagonists at the μ-opioid receptor, they do cause respiratory depression, which is not a function of κ agonists. Thus, they appear to have at least partial agonist activity at the μ-opioid receptor.
Adapted from Bowdle TA: Partial agonist and agonist–antagonist opioids: Basic pharmacology and clinical applications. Anesth Pharmacol Rev 1:135, 1993.

agonist will act as an antagonist. These drugs mediate their clinical effects via μ- and κ-opioid receptors, as summarized in Table 14-4. The classification scheme presented may change as our understanding of these drugs and of opioid receptors continues to grow. Bowdle extensively reviewed the pharmacology and clinical uses of these and other drugs in this class.[258] Only nalbuphine, butorphanol, and buprenorphine are considered in this chapter.

The major role of the opioid agonist–antagonist and partial agonist drugs continues to be in the provision of postoperative analgesia, but they have also been used for intraoperative sedation, as adjuncts during general anesthesia, and to antagonize some effects of full μ-opioid agonists.

Nalbuphine

Nalbuphine is a phenanthrene opioid derivative. Although it is often classified as a κ agonist and μ antagonist, it is more accurately described as a partial agonist at both κ and μ receptors.[258] While MAC reduction studies have not been done in humans, Murphy and Hug[20] reported that a 0.5 mg/kg dose reduced enflurane MAC by 8% in dogs. However, increasing the dose eightfold produced no further reduction in enflurane MAC. This modest MAC reduction, compared to 65% for morphine, suggests that nalbuphine may not be a useful adjunct for general anesthesia. However, several investigators have examined its effectiveness as a component of balanced anesthesia for cardiac[259] and lower abdominal surgery.[20,260] Combined with diazepam 0.4 mg/kg and 50% N_2O in oxygen, a loading dose of 3 mg/kg was followed by additional doses of 0.25 mg/kg as needed throughout surgery. No significant increases in blood pressure, stress hormones, or histamine were seen, and emergence from anesthesia was uncomplicated.[259] Nalbuphine 0.2 mg/kg was compared to meperidine 0.5 mg/kg as an adjuvant to general anesthesia with 1% halothane and 70% N_2O in oxygen in spontaneously breathing patients undergoing inguinal hernia repair.[261] Both drugs produced a similar degree of respiratory depression, postoperative analgesia, and side effects. The most common side effect was drowsiness. In a double-blind comparison with fentanyl for gynecologic surgery, fentanyl was found to better attenuate hypertensive responses to intubation and surgical stimulation.[260] However, significant respiratory depression was seen in 8 of 30 patients who received fentanyl, and 4 required naloxone, compared to no respiratory depression in the nalbuphine group. Analgesia was similar, and as in other studies, postoperative sedation was common in the nalbuphine group.

The respiratory depression produced by nalbuphine, most likely mediated by μ-opioid receptors, has a ceiling effect equivalent to that produced by ~0.4 mg/kg morphine.[258] Analgesia is mediated by both κ and μ receptors. Because of these effects, nalbuphine has been used to antagonize the respiratory depressant effects of full agonists while still providing analgesic effects. In a double-blind comparison, nalbuphine and naloxone both effectively antagonized fentanyl-induced postoperative respiratory depression, but patients who received nalbuphine had less reversal of analgesia.[262] Nalbuphine has also been effective in antagonizing fentanyl-induced respiratory depression following high-dose (100 to 120 μg/kg) fentanyl anesthesia for cardiac surgery.[263] Only 3 of 21 patients experienced pain after nalbuphine administration, and this was adequately treated with additional nalbuphine. However, in a volunteer study, nalbuphine 0.21 mg/kg did not antagonize the respiratory depressant effects of 0.21 mg/kg morphine.[264] While nalbuphine and other agonist–antagonists have ceiling

TABLE 14-5

DOSAGE FOR FENTANYL, SUFENTANIL, ALFENTANIL, AND REMIFENTANIL DURING ELECTIVE SURGERY IN ADULTS

Doses are guidelines for hemodynamically stable adults. They should be adjusted downward for elderly patients and those with cardiac dysfunction and hemodynamic instability

ANESTHETIC PHASE	FENTANYL	SUFENTANIL	ALFENTANIL	REMIFENTANIL
Premedication (μg)	25–50	2–5	250–500	
Induction				
With hypnotic (μg/kg)	1.5–5	0.1–1	10–50	0.5–1.0 +/or 0.25–0.5 μg/kg/min
With 60–70% N_2O (μg/kg)	8–23	1.3–2.8		
High dose opioid (μg/kg)	50	10–30	120	2–5 +/or 2 μg/kg/min
Maintenance				
Balanced anesthesia				
Intermittent bolus (μg)	25–100	5–20	250–500	25–50
Infusion (μg/kg/min)	0.033	0.005–0.015	0.5–1.5	0.25–0.05
High dose opioid (μg/kg/min)	0.5		2.5–10	1.0–3.0
Transiotion to PACU (μg/kg/min)				0.05–0.15
Monitored Anesthesia Care				
Intermittent bolus (μg)	12.5–50	2.5–10	125–250	12.5–25
Infusion (μg/kg/min)				0.01–0.2

analgesic and respiratory depressant effects, they can be as effective as full μ agonists in providing postoperative analgesia. Nalbuphine 5 to 10 mg has also been used to antagonize pruritus induced by epidural and intrathecal morphine. The usual adult dose of nalbuphine is 10 mg as often as every 3 hours. It is important to be aware that nalbuphine can precipitate withdrawal symptoms in patients who are physically dependent on opioids.

Butorphanol

Butorphanol, a morphinan congener, has partial agonist activity at κ and μ opioid receptors, similar to those of nalbuphine. Compared to nalbuphine and similar drugs, however, butorphanol has a pronounced sedative effect, which is probably mediated by κ receptors. In a laboratory study as well as in clinical use as a premedicant, butorphanol produced dose-dependent sedation comparable to that of midazolam.[265] Like nalbuphine, butorphanol decreases enflurane MAC, in dogs, by a modest amount, 11%, at 0.1 mg/kg.[25] Increasing the butorphanol dose 40-fold does not produce a further reduction. However, like nalbuphine, butorphanol has also been reported to be an effective component of balanced general anesthesia. Combined with diazepam and nitrous oxide, butorphanol and morphine provided equally satisfactory anesthesia.[258]

Given alone, butorphanol produces respiratory depression with a ceiling effect below that of full μ agonists. In postoperative patients a parenteral dose of 3 mg produces respiratory depression approximately equal to that of 10 mg morphine. In a clinical study examining its effectiveness in reversing fentanyl-induced respiratory depression,[266] patients anesthetized with isoflurane, nitrous oxide, and fentanyl 5 μg/kg followed by an infusion of 3 μg/kg/h received three sequential doses of butorphanol 1 mg at 10- to 15-minute intervals. After the first 1-mg dose, respiratory rate and ventilatory response to CO_2 increased, while end-tidal CO_2 decreased significantly. Further progressive changes were not significantly different from the initial response to butorphanol, and analgesia was not significantly affected in 21 of 22 patients.

In contrast to morphine, fentanyl, and even meperidine, butorphanol does not produce significant elevation in intrabiliary pressure[72] (see Fig. 14-6). Butorphanol has also been effective in the treatment of postoperative shivering,[77] but the mechanism for this effect is unknown.

Butorphanol is indicated for use as a sedative and in treatment of moderate postoperative pain. Preliminary clinical experience suggests that butorphanol administered as patient-controlled analgesia is associated with a lower incidence of opioid-induced ileus compared to μ-selective opioids (Dunbar PJ, personal communication). A dose as low as 0.5 mg can provide clinically useful sedation, while single analgesic doses range from 0.5 to 2 mg. Butorphanol has also been administered epidurally and transnasally.

Buprenorphine

Buprenorphine is a highly lipophilic thebaine derivative, which at small to moderate doses is 25 to 50 times more potent than morphine.[1] Unlike nalbuphine and butorphanol, buprenorphine does not appear to have agonist, and may have antagonist, activity at the κ-opioid receptor (see Table 14-4).[258] Another unique characteristic of buprenorphine is its slow dissociation from μ receptors, which can lead to prolonged effects not easily antagonized by naloxone. Buprenorphine also appears to have an unusual bell-shaped dose-response curve such that, at very high doses, it produces progressively less analgesia.[258] In a clinical study, patients who received 10 or 20 μg/kg buprenorphine during surgery were pain-free postoperatively, but half of the patients who received 30 or 40 μg/kg had significant postoperative pain.[267] This observation is consistent with buprenorphine's bell-shaped dose-effect curve, and patients who received very high buprenorphine doses probably had plasma drug concentrations in the range at which declining analgesia is seen.

Buprenorphine also appears to have a ceiling effect to its respiratory depressant dose-response curve. However, although buprenorphine-induced respiratory depression can be prevented by prior naloxone administration, it is not easily reversed by naloxone once the effects have been produced.[1] A dose of 0.3 mg buprenorphine reduces CO_2 responsiveness to about 50% of control values.[268] Large doses of naloxone (5 to 10 mg) were required to antagonize buprenorphine respiratory depression in volunteers, while 1-mg doses were not effective. In addition, the maximum antagonist effect did not occur until 3 hours after naloxone administration, an observation consistent with buprenorphine's slow dissociation from μ receptors. Buprenorphine has been compared to naloxone in its ability to antagonize fentanyl-induced respiratory depression, and appears to increase respiratory rate without antagonizing analgesic effects in slowly administered doses up to 0.5 mg.[269]

Buprenorphine can be effective in treatment of moderate to severe pain. Its onset can be slow, but analgesic duration can be more than 6 hours. A single dose of 0.3 to 0.4 mg appears to produce analgesia equivalent to 10 mg morphine.[1]

Opioid Antagonists (Naloxone and Naltrexone)

Under normal conditions, opioid antagonists produce few effects. They are competitive inhibitors of the opioid agonists, so the effect profile depends on the type and dose of agonist administered as well as the degree to which physical dependence on the opioid agonist has developed. The most widely used opioid antagonist is naloxone, which is structurally related to morphine and oxymorphone, and is a pure antagonist at μ-, κ-, and δ-opioid receptors.[1] Naltrexone is a long-acting oral agent, which also has relatively pure antagonist activity. In some circumstances, naloxone can antagonize effects that appear to be mediated by endogenous opioids. For example, naloxone can reverse "stress analgesia" in animals and man, it can antagonize analgesia produced by low-frequency stimulation with acupuncture needles, and it can also reverse analgesia produced by placebo medications.[1]

In clinical anesthesia practice, naloxone is administered to antagonize opioid-induced respiratory depression and sedation. Because opioid antagonists will reverse all opioid effects, including analgesia, naloxone should be carefully titrated to avoid producing sudden, severe pain in postoperative patients. Sudden, complete antagonism of opioid effects with naloxone has been reported to cause severe hypertension, tachycardia, ventricular dysrhythmias, and acute, sometimes fatal, pulmonary edema.[270] Naloxone-induced pulmonary edema can occur even in healthy young patients who have received relatively small doses (80 to 500 μg) of naloxone.[271,272] The mechanism for this phenomenon is thought to be centrally mediated catecholamine release, which causes acute pulmonary hypertension. Because most patients with opioid-induced respiratory depression will often breathe on command, it is important to stimulate them in addition to administering carefully titrated naloxone doses in the immediate postoperative period. It is also essential to monitor vital signs and oxygenation closely after naloxone is administered to detect occurrence of any of these potentially serious complications.

Naloxone will precipitate opioid withdrawal symptoms in opioid-dependent individuals. Clinicians tend to be aware of this risk when treating patients with known opioid addiction, but it is important to consider the potential for opioid withdrawal syndrome when treating nonaddicts who use opioids chronically, such as cancer patients and severe burn and trauma patients with protracted recovery courses.

Naloxone has a very fast onset of action, and thus is easily titrated. Peak effects occur within 1 to 2 minutes, and duration is dose dependent, but total doses of 0.4 to 0.8 mg generally last 1 to 4 hours.[1] Suggested incremental doses for intravenous titration are 20 to 40 μg given every few minutes until the patient's ventilation improves, but analgesia is not completely reversed. Because naloxone has a short duration of action, respiratory depression may recur if large doses and/or long-acting opioid agonists have been administered. When prolonged ventilatory depression is anticipated, an initial loading dose followed by a naloxone infusion can be used. Infusion rates between 3 and 10 μg/h have been effective in antagonizing respiratory depression from systemic as well as epidural opioids.[273]

USE OF OPIOIDS IN CLINICAL ANESTHESIA

Opioids are used alone or in combination with other agents, such as sedatives or anticholinergic agents, as "premedications." For this purpose, longer acting opioids such as morphine are administered as single doses that are generally within the "analgesic" range. The goal of opioid premedication is to provide moderate sedation, anxiolysis, and analgesia while maintaining hemodynamic stability. Potential risks of opioid premedication include oversedation, respiratory depression, and nausea and vomiting. For induction of anesthesia, opioids are often used to blunt or prevent the hemodynamic responses to tracheal intubation. Opioids with rapid onset of action, such as fentanyl and its derivatives, are appropriate for this use.

Intraoperatively, opioids are administered as components of balanced anesthesia, or alone in high-dose opioid anesthesia. During maintenance of general anesthesia, opioid dosage is titrated to the desired effect based on the surgical stimulus as well as individual patient characteristics, such as age, volume status, neurologic status, liver dysfunction, or other systemic disease states. Plasma opioid concentrations required to blunt hemodynamic responses to laryngoscopy, tracheal intubation, and various surgical stimuli, as well as plasma opioid concentration associated with awakening from anesthesia, have been determined for several opioids. Titration to achieve these plasma concentrations (see Table 14-3), which reflect brain (effect site) concentrations, can be accomplished by administering repeated small bolus doses or by manual- or target-controlled infusion. Fentanyl and its derivatives sufentanil and alfentanil are the opioids most widely used as supplements to general anesthesia; remifentanil is a useful alternative when ultrashort duration is desirable. All of these opioids are more easily titrated than morphine because of their rapid onset of action. However, Shafer and Varvel[10] have emphasized that making a rational choice among these opioids requires an understanding of the relationships between their pharmacokinetics and pharmacodynamics. They have used elegant computer models to simulate the rate of decrease in plasma and effect site (brain) concentrations after various administration methods, including bolus doses, brief infusion, and prolonged infusion. Decreases in effect site concentration will determine time to recovery from various opioid effects. Comparable simulations have also been done for the newer opioid remifentanil.[218] Important pharmacokinetic differences among these opioids include volumes of distribution and intercompartmental (distributional) and central (elimination) clearances. A smaller distribution volume tends to shorten recovery time, and a reduction in clearance tends to increase recovery time.[10] The major pharmacodynamic differences among these opioids are potency and the equilibration times between the plasma and the site of drug effect. Equilibration half-times between plasma and effect site are 5 to 6 minutes for fentanyl and sufentanil and 1.3 to 1.5 minutes for alfentanil and remifentanil.[10,192] Computer simulations demonstrate that simply comparing elimination half-lives will not predict the relative rate of decline in drug concentration at the effect site after either bolus doses or continuous infusion of fentanyl, sufentanil, and alfentanil. The rate of recovery after a continuous infusion will depend on the duration of the infusion as well as the magnitude of decline that is required. Figure 14-12 demonstrates how the times required for 20, 50, and 80% decrements in effect site (i.e., brain)

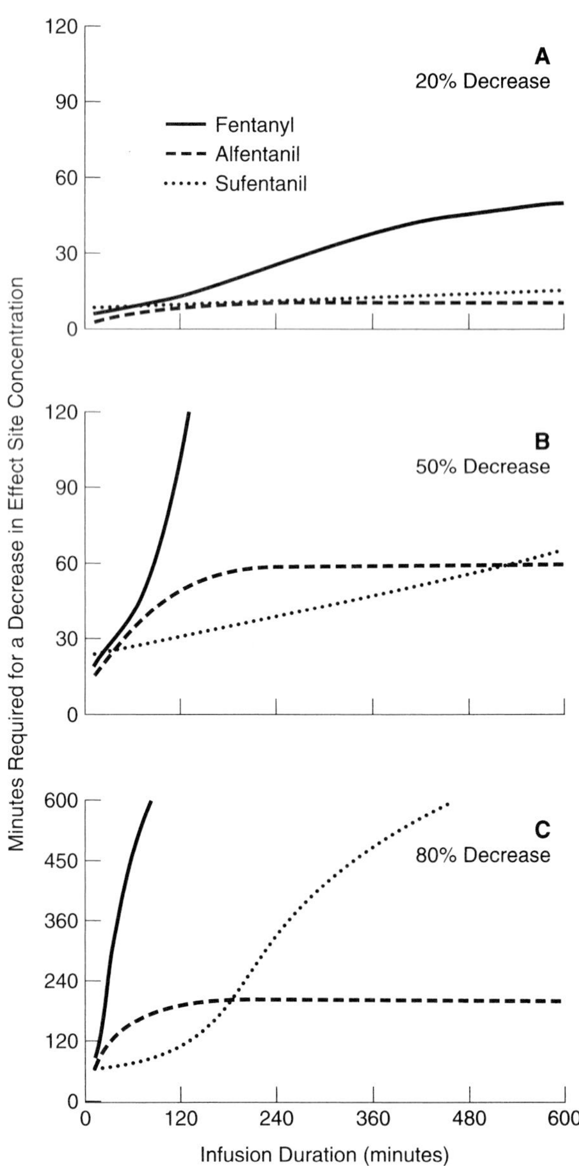

FIGURE 14-12. Recovery curves for fentanyl, sufentanil, and alfentanil showing the time required for decreases of 20% (A), 50% (B), and 80% (C) from maintained intraoperative effect site (brain) concentrations after termination of the infusion. (Reprinted with permission from Shafer SL, Varvel JR: Pharmacokinetics, pharmacodynamics, and rational opioid selection. Anesthesiology 74:53, 1991.)

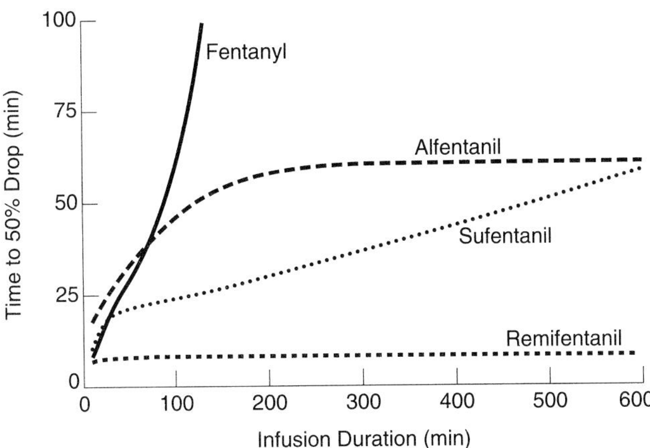

FIGURE 14-13. Context-sensitive half-times for fentanyl, sufentanil, alfentanil, and remifentanil. This computer simulation depicts the time necessary to achieve a 50% reduction in plasma opioid concentration as a function of infusion duration. (Reprinted with permission from Egan TD, Lemmens HJM, Fiset P *et al:* The pharmacokinetics of the new short-acting opioid remifentanil (GI87084B) in healthy adult male volunteers. Anesthesiology 79:881, 1993.)

concentrations vary with each opioid depending on infusion duration. If only a 20% drop in effect site concentration is required (upper panel), recovery from all three opioids will be rapid, although recovery time increases for fentanyl after 3 hours of drug infusion. However, if a 50% decrease is required, recovery from sufentanil will be fastest for infusions less than 6 to 8 hours in duration, but more rapid for alfentanil if infusions are continued for more than 8 hours.

Context-Sensitive Half-Time

Hughes et al[11] expanded the concepts of Shafer and Varvel to define the relative contributions of distribution compartments to central compartment (plasma) drug distribution. These relative contributions vary according to infusion duration. Hughes devised the concept of "context-sensitive half-time," which is defined as the time required for the drug concentration in the central compartment to decrease by 50%, and demonstrated how this half-time changes as drug infusion duration increases. During an infusion, the peripheral (fast and slow) compartments begin to "fill up." After the infusion is stopped, drug will be eliminated, but will also continue to be redistributed as long as the concentration in a peripheral compartment is lower than that in the central compartment. This leads to a rapid drop in central compartment drug concentration. When central compartment (plasma) concentration drops below that of the peripheral compartment(s), the direction of drug redistribution will reverse and will slow the decline in plasma concentration. The degree to which redistribution will affect the rate of drug elimination depends on the ratio of the distributional to elimination time constants. Thus, a drug that can rapidly redistribute will have a correspondingly larger contribution from the peripheral compartment(s), and plasma concentration will drop progressively more slowly as infusion duration continues. Figure 14-13 illustrates the context-sensitive half-times for fentanyl, alfentanil, sufentanil, and remifentanil. This model predicts the time to a 50% concentration decrease in the plasma, which will reflect, but not be equal to, effect site concentrations depicted in Figure 14-12.

Some testing of these computer models in humans has been done. Kapila et al[274] compared modeled context-sensitive half-times with measured decreases in drug concentration and drug effect (respiratory depression) in volunteers receiving remifentanil and alfentanil. After 3-hour opioid infusions, measured whole blood opioid concentrations and recovery of ventilatory drive corresponded closely to modeled values for both drugs. Although the concept of a context-sensitive half-time appears to be useful, Hughes et al[11] noted that it is unknown whether a decrement of 50% provides the most clinically useful description of the rate of offset of opioid effects. If one closely titrates infusions so that minimum effective concentrations are achieved, perhaps much smaller decrements will be necessary. For example, it can be seen in the upper panel of Figure 14-12 that if only a 20% decline in effect site concentration is needed, fentanyl, sufentanil, and alfentanil concentrations all drop rapidly if the infusion duration is 2 hours or less. This rapid resolution is seen for sufentanil and alfentanil even with prolonged (5- to 10-hour) administration if only a 20% decrement is required. In practice, it is relatively easy to administer higher than necessary doses of opioids, particularly to mechanically ventilated patients, because hemodynamic consequences are minimal. Titrating against a quantifiable parameter, such as minute ventilation in a spontaneously breathing patient, may allow a tighter dose titration, but this may not be practical for many surgeries, for example, those requiring the use of muscle relaxants. It does seem clear, however, that some context-sensitive index is more useful than the elimination half-life. Understanding these concepts can be useful when deciding which opioid to use, as well as in adapting guidelines for opioid dosage and infusion rates depending on the duration of anesthesia.

References

1. Jaffe JH, Martin WR: Opioid analgesics and antagonists. In Gilman AG, Goodman LS, Rall TW, et al (eds): The Pharmacological Basis of Therapeutics, p 491. New York, Macmillan, 1985
2. Rey A: L'Examen Clinique en Psychologie. Paris, Presses Universitaires de France, 1964
3. Lowenstein E: "Morphine anesthesia": A perspective. Anesthesiology 35:563, 1971
4. Martin WR: Multiple opioid receptors. Life Sci 128:1547, 1981
5. Pleuvry BJ: The endogenous opioid system. Anaesth Pharmacol Rev 1:114, 1993
6. Pasternak GW: Pharmacologic mechanisms of opioid analgesics. Clin Neuropharmacol 16:1, 1993
7. McFadzean I: The ionic mechanisms underlying opioid mechanisms. Neuropeptides 11:173, 1988
8. Horn AS, Rodgers JR: Structural and conformational relationships between the enkephalins and the opiates. Nature 260:795, 1976
9. Thorpe DH: Opiate structures and activity: A guide to underlying opioid actions. Anesth Analg 63:143, 1984
10. Shafer SL, Varvel JR: Pharmacokinetics, pharmacodynamics, and rational opioid selection. Anesthesiology 74:53, 1991
11. Hughes MA, Glass PSA, Jacobs JR: Context-sensitive half-time in multicompartment pharmacokinetic models for intravenous anesthetic drugs. Anesthesiology 76:334, 1992
12. Bovill JG: Pharmacokinetics and pharmacodynamics of opioid agonists. Anaesth Pharmacol Rev 1:122, 1993
13. Hansch C, Dunn WJ: Linear relationships between lipophilic character and biological activity of drugs. J Pharm Sci 61:1, 1972
14. Bernards CM, Hill HF: Physical and chemical properties of drug molecules governing their diffusion through the spinal meninges. Anesthesiology 77:750, 1992
15. Lipp J: Possible mechanisms of morphine analgesia. Clin Neuropharmacol 14:31, 1991
16. Yeung JC, Rudy TA: Multiplicative interaction between narcotic agonisms expressed at spinal and supraspinal sites of antinociceptive action as revealed by concurrent intrathecal and intracerebroventricular injections of morphine. J Pharmacol Exp Ther 215:633, 1980
17. Stein C, Millan MJ, Shippenberg TS *et al:* Peripheral opioid receptors mediating antinociception in inflammation: Evidence for involvement of μ, δ and κ receptors. J Pharmacol Exp Ther 248:1269, 1989
18. Dahlstrom B, Tamsen A, Psalzow I, Hartvig P: Patient-controlled analgesia therapy. Part IV: Pharmacokinetics and analgesic plasma concentrations of morphine. Clin Pharmacokinetics 7:266, 1982
19. Hill HF, Coda BA, Mackie AM, Iverson K: Patient-controlled analgesic infusions: Alfentanil versus morphine. Pain 49:301, 1992

20. Murphy MR, Hug CC: The enflurane-sparing effect of morphine, butorphanol, and nalbuphine. Anesthesiology 57:489, 1982
21. Lake CL, DiFazio CA, Moscicki JC *et al:* Reduction in halothane MAC: Comparison of morphine and alfentanil. Anesth Analg 64:807, 1985
22. Roizen MF, Horrigan RW, Frazer BM: Anesthetic doses blocking adrenergic (stress) and cardiovascular responses to incision-MAC BAR. Anesthesiology 54:390, 1981
23. Schweiger IM, Klopfenstein CE, Forster A: Epidural morphine reduces halothane MAC in humans. Can J Anaesth 39:911, 1992
24. Drasner K, Bernards CM, Ozanne GM: Intrathecal morphine reduces the minimum alveolar concentration of halothane in humans. Anesthesiology 69:310, 1988
25. Licina MG, Schubert A, Tobin JE *et al:* Intrathecal morphine dose not reduce minimum alveolar concentration of halothane in humans: Results of a double-blind study. Anesthesiology 74:660, 1991
26. Coda BA, Hill HF, Hunt EB *et al:* Cognitive and motor function impairments during continuous opioid analgesic infusions. Hum Psychopharmacol 8:383, 1993
27. Smith NT, Dee-Silver H, Sanford TJ *et al:* EEGs during high-dose fentanyl–, sufentanil–, or morphine–oxygen anesthesia. Anesth Analg 63:386, 1984
28. Martin WR: Pharmacology of opioids. Pharmacol Rev 35:283, 1984
29. Thomas DA, Williams GM, Iwata K *et al:* The medullary dorsal horn: A site of action of morphine in producing facial scratching in monkeys. Anesthesiology 79:548, 1993
30. Arunasalam K, Davenport HT, Painter S *et al:* Ventilatory response to morphine in young and old subjects. Anaesthesia 38:529, 1983
31. Daykin AP, Bowen DJ, Saunders DA, Norman J: Respiratory depression after morphine in the elderly. Anaesthesia 41:910, 1986
32. Forrest WH, Bellville JW: The effect of sleep plus morphine on the respiratory response to carbon dioxide. Anesthesiology 25:137, 1964
33. Catley DM, Thornton C, Jordan C *et al:* Pronounced episodes of oxygen desaturation on the postoperative period: Its association with ventilatory pattern and analgesic regimen. Anesthesiology 63:20, 1985
34. Duthie DJR, Nimmo WS: Adverse effects of opioid analgesic drugs. Br J Anaesth 59:61, 1987
35. Freund FG, Martin WE, Wong KC *et al:* Abdominal-muscle rigidity induced by morphine and nitrous oxide. Anesthesiology 38:358, 1973
36. Weinger MB, Cline EJ, Smith NT *et al:* Localization of brainstem sites which mediate alfentanil-induced muscle rigidity in the rat. Pharmacol Biochem Behav 29:573, 1988
37. Smith NT, Benthuysen JL, Bickford RG *et al:* Seizures during opioid anesthetic induction: Are they opioid-induced rigidity? Anesthesiology 71:852, 1989
38. Bowdle TA, Rooke GA: Postoperative myoclonus and rigidity after anesthesia with opioids. Anesth Analg 78:783, 1994
39. Watcha MF, White PF: Postoperative nausea and vomiting. Anesthesiology 77:162, 1992
40. Hill HF, Chapman CR, Saeger LS *et al:* Steady-state infusions of opioids in human. II. Concentration–effect relationships and therapeutic margins. Pain 43:69, 1990
41. Coda BA, O'Sullivan B, Donaldson G *et al*: Comparative efficacy of patient-controlled administration of morphine, hydromorphone, or sufentanil for the treatment of oral mucositis pain following bone marrow transplantation. Pain 72:333, 1997
42. Crozier TA, Kietzmann D, Dobermeier B: Mood change after anaesthesia with remifentanil or alfentanil. Eur J Anaesthesiol 21:20, 2004
43. Peroutka SJ, Snyder SH: Antiemetics: Neurotransmitter receptor binding predicts therapeutic actions. Lancet 20:659, 1982
44. Costello DJ, Borison HL: Naloxone antagonizes narcotic self blockade of emesis in the cat (abs). J Pharmacol Exp Ther 203:222, 1977
45. Coda BA, Mackie A, Hill HF: Influence of alprazolam on opioid analgesia and side effects during steady-state morphine infusions. Pain 50:309, 1992
46. Burks TF, Fox DA, Hirning LD *et al:* Regulation of gastrointestinal function by multiple opioid receptors. Life Sci 43:2177, 1988
47. Murphy DB, Sutton JA, Prescott LF, Murphy MB: Opioid-induced delay in gastric emptying: A peripheral mechanism in humans. Anesthesiology 87(4):765, 1997
48. Thorén T, Wattwil M: Effects on gastric emptying of thoracic epidural analgesia with morphine or bupivicaine. Anesth Analg 67:687, 1988
49. Hahn M, Baker R, Sullivan S: The effect of four narcotics on cholecystokinin octapeptide stimulated gallbladder contraction. Aliment Pharmacol Ther 2:129, 1988
50. Thune A, Baker RA, Saccone GT *et al:* Differing effects of pethidine and morphine on human sphincter of Oddi motility. Br J Surg 77:992, 1990
51. Ehrenpreis S, Kimura I, Kobayashi T *et al:* Histamine release as the basis for morphine action on bile duct and sphincter of Oddi. Life Sci 40:1695, 1987
52. Dray A: Epidural opiates and urinary retention: New models provide new insights. Anesthesiology 68:323, 1988
53. Durant PAC, Yaksh TL: Drug effects on urinary bladder tone during spinal morphine-induced inhibition of the micturition reflex in unanesthetized rats. Anesthesiology 68:325, 1988
54. Stellato C, Cirillo R, de Paulis A *et al:* Human basophil/mast cell releasability: IX. Heterogeneity of the effects of opioids on mediator release. Anesthesiology 77:32, 1992
55. Hermens JM, Ebertz JM, Hanifin JM, Hirshman CA: Comparison of histamine release in human skin mast cells induced by morphine, fentanyl, and oxymorphone. Anesthesiology 62:124, 1985
56. Rosow CE, Moss J, Philbin DM *et al:* Histamine release during morphine and fentanyl anesthesia. Anesthesiology 56:93, 1982
57. Lowenstein E, Whiting RB, Bittar DA *et al:* Local and neurally mediated effects of morphine on skeletal muscle vascular resistance. J Pharmacol Exp Ther 180:359, 1972
58. Roizen MF: Does the choice of anesthetic (narcotic *versus* inhalational) significantly affect cardiovascular outcome after cardiovascular surgery? In Estafanous FG (ed): Opioids in Anesthesia, p 180. Boston, Butterworth, 1984
59. Stanski DR, Greenblatt DJ, Lowenstein E: Kinetics of intravenous and intramuscular morphine. Clin Pharmacol Ther 24:52, 1978
60. Murphy MR, Hug CC: Pharmacokinetics of intravenous morphine in patients anesthetized with enflurane–nitrous oxide. Anesthesiology 54:187, 1981
61. Mazoit JX, Sandouk P, Zetlaoui P: Pharmacokinetics of unchanged morphine in normal volunteers. Anesth Analg 66:293, 1987
62. Sear JW, Hand CW, Moore RA, McQuay HJ: Studies on morphine disposition: influence of general anesthesia on plasma concentrations of morphine and its metabolites. Br J Aneasth 662:22, 1989
63. Lynn AM, Slattery JT: Morphine pharmacokinetics in early infancy. Anesthesiology 66:136, 1987
64. Osborne R, Joel S, Trew D *et al:* Morphine and metabolite behavior after different routes of morphine administration: Demonstration of the importance of the active metabolite morphine-6-glucuronide. Clin Pharmacol Ther 47:12, 1990
65. Lehmann KA, Zech D: Morphine-6-glucuronide, a pharmacologically active morphine metabolite: A review of the literature. Eur J Pain 14:28, 1993
66. Portenoy RK, Thaler HT, Inturrisi CE *et al:* The metabolite morphine-6-glucuronide contributes to the analgesia produced by morphine infusion in patients with pain and normal renal function. Clin Pharmacol Ther 51:422, 1992
67. Osborne R, Thompson P, Joel S *et al:* The analgesic activity of morphine-6-glucuronide. Br J Clin Pharmacol 34:130, 1992
68. Kurz M, Belani KG, Sessler DI *et al:* Naloxone, meperidine, and shivering. Anesthesiology 79:1193, 1993
69. Tamsen A, Hartvig P, Fagerlund C *et al:* Patient-controlled analgesic therapy, part II: Individual analgesic demand and analgesic plasma concentrations of pethidine in postoperative pain. Clin Pharmacokinet 7:164, 1982
70. Steffey EP, Martucci R, Howland D *et al:* Meperidine–halothane interaction in dogs. Can Anaesth Soc J 24:459, 1977
71. Kaya K, Babacan A, Beyazova M *et al:* Effects of perineural opioids on nerve conduction of N. suralis in man. Acta Neurol Scand 85:337, 1992
72. Radnay PA, Duncalf D, Novakovic M *et al:* Common bile duct pressure changes after fentanyl, morphine, meperidine, butorphanol, and naloxone. Anesth Analg 63:441, 1984
73. Yrjola H, Heinonen J, Tuominen M *et al:* Comparison of haemodynamic effects of pethidine and anileridine in anaesthetised patients. Acta Anaesthesiol Scand 25:412, 1981
74. Rendig SV, Amsterdam EA, Henderson GL, Mason DT: Comparative cardiac contractile actions of six narcotic analgesics: Morphine, meperidine, pentazocine, fentanyl, methadone and L-α-acetylmethadol (LAAM). J Pharmacol Exp Ther 215:259, 1980
75. Flacke JW, Bloor BC, Kripke BJ *et al:* Comparison of morphine, meperidine, fentanyl, and sufentanil in balanced anesthesia: A double-blind study. Anesth Analg 64:897, 1985
76. Macintyre PE, Pavlin EG, Dwersteg JF: Effect of meperidine on oxygen consumption, carbon dioxide production, and respiratory gas exchange in postanesthesia shivering. Anesth Analg 66:751,1987.
77. Vogelsang J, Hayes SR: Butorphanol tartrate (Stadol) relieves postanesthesia shaking more effectively than meperidine (Demerol) or morphine. J Post Anesth Nurs 7:94, 1992
78. Joris J, Banache M, Bonnet F *et al:* Clonidine and ketanserin both are effective treatment for postanesthetic shivering. Anesthesiology 79:532, 1993
79. Matsukawa T, Kurz A, Sessler DI *et al:* Propofol linearly reduces the vasoconstriction and shivering thresholds. Anesthesiology 82:1169, 1995
80. Horn E-P, Standl T, Sessler DI *et al:* Physostigmine prevents postanesthetic shivering as does meperidine or clonidine. Anesthesiology 88:108, 1998
81. Mather LE, Tucker GT, Pflug AE *et al:* Meperidine kinetics in man: Intravenous injection in surgical patients and volunteers. Clin Pharmacol Ther 17:27, 1975
82. Koska AJ, Kramer WG, Romagnoli A *et al:* Pharmacokinetics of high-dose meperidine in surgical patients. Anesth Analg 60:8, 1981
83. Wong YC, Chan K, Lau OW *et al:* Protein binding characterization of pethidine and norpethidine and lack of interethnic variability. Methods Find Exp Clin Pharmacol 13:273, 1991
84. Kaiko RF, Foley KM, Grabinski PY *et al:* Central nervous system excitatory effects of meperidine in cancer patients. Ann Neurol 13:180, 1983
85. Gourlay GK, Wilson PR, Glynn CJ: Pharmacodynamics and pharmacokinetics of methadone during the perioperative period. Anesthesiology 57:458, 1982
86. Gourlay GK, Willis RJ, Wilson PR: Postoperative pain control with methadone: Influence of supplementary methadone doses and blood concentration–response relationships. Anesthesiology 61:19, 1984

87. Wangler MA, Rosenblatt RM: Methadone titration to avoid excessive respiratory depression. Anesthesiology 59:363, 1983
88. Scott JC, Ponganis KV, Stanski DR: EEG quantitation of narcotic effect: The comparative pharmacodynamics of fentanyl and alfentanil. Anesthesiology 62:234, 1985
89. Gourlay GK, Kowalski SR, Plummer JL *et al:* Fentanyl blood concentration–analgesic response relationship in the treatment of postoperative pain. Anesth Analg 67:329, 1988
90. Hug CC: Pharmacokinetics of new synthetic narcotic analgesics. In Estafanous FG (ed): Opioids in Anesthesia, p 50. Boston, Butterworth, 1984
91. Sebel PS, Glass PSA, Fletcher JE *et al:* Reduction of the MAC of desflurane with fentanyl. Anesthesiology 76:52, 1992
92. Daniel M, Weiskopf RB, Noorani M, Eger EI: Fentanyl augments the blockade of the sympathetic response to incision (MAC-BAR) produced by desflurane and isoflurane. Anesthesiology 88:43, 1998
93. Westmoreland CL, Sebel PS, Gropper A: Fentanyl or alfentanil decreases the minimum alveolar anesthetic concentration of isoflurane in surgical patients. Anesth Analg 78:23, 1994
94. Katoh T, Ikeda K: The effects of fentanyl on sevoflurane requirements for loss of consciousness and skin incision. Anesthesiology 88:18, 1998
95. Inagaki Y, Mashimo T, Yoshiya I: Segmental analgesic effect and reduction of halothane MAC from epidural fentanyl in humans. Anesth Analg 74:856, 1992
96. Kazama T, Ikeda K, Morita K: The pharmacodynamic interaction between propofol and fentanyl with respect to the suppression of somatic or hemodynamic responses to skin incision, peritoneum incision, and abdominal wall retraction. Anesthesiology 89:894, 1998
97. Shafer SL, Varvel JR, Aziz N *et al:* Pharmacokinetics of fentanyl administered by computer-controlled infusion pump. Anesthesiology 73:1091, 1990
98. Glass PSA, Jacobs JR, Smith LR *et al:* Pharmacokinetic model-driven infusion of fentanyl: Assessment of accuracy. Anesthesiology 73:1082, 1990
99. Philbin DM, Rosow CE, Schneider RC *et al:* Fentanyl and sufentanil anesthesia revisited: How much is enough? Anesthesiology 73:5, 1990
100. Trindle MR, Dodson BA, Rampil IJ: Effects of fentanyl *versus* sufentanil in equianesthetic doses on middle cerebral artery blood flow volume. Anesthesiology 78:454, 1993
101. Sperry RJ, Bailey PL, Reichman MV *et al:* Fentanyl and sufentanil increase intracranial pressure in head trauma patients. Anesthesiology 77:416, 1992
102. Jung R, Shah N, Reinsel R *et al:* Cerebrospinal fluid pressure in patients with brain tumors: Impact of fentanyl *versus* alfentanil during nitrous oxide–oxygen anesthesia. Anesth Analg 71:419, 1990
103. Streisand JB, Bailey PL, LeMaire L *et al:* Fentanyl-induced rigidity and unconsciousness in human volunteers. Anesthesiology 78:629, 1993
104. Bailey PL, Wilbrink J, Zwanikken P *et al:* Anesthetic induction with fentanyl. Anesth Analg 64:48, 1985
105. Lunn JK, Stanley TH, Eisele J *et al:* High dose fentanyl anesthesia for coronary artery surgery: Plasma fentanyl concentrations and influence of nitrous oxide on cardiovascular responses. Anesth Analg 58:390, 1979
106. Scott JC, Sarnquist FH: Seizure-like movements during a fentanyl infusion with absence of seizure activity in a simultaneous EEG recording. Anesthesiology 62:812, 1985
107. Manninen PH, Burke SJ, Wennberg R *et al:* Intraoperative localization of epileptogenic focus with alfentanil and fentanyl. Anesth Analg 88:1101, 1999
108. Phua WT, Teh BT, Jong W *et al:* Tussive effect of a fentanyl bolus. Can J Anaesth 38:330, 1991
109. McClain DA, Hug CC: Intravenous fentanyl kinetics. Clin Pharmacol Ther 28:106, 1980
110. Bailey PL, Pace NL, Ashburn MA *et al:* Frequent hypoxemia and apnea after sedation with midazolam and fentanyl. Anesthesiology 73:826, 1990
111. Bailey PL, Streisand JB, East KA *et al:* Differences in magnitude and duration of opioid-induced respiratory depression and analgesia with fentanyl and sufentanil. Anesth Analg 70:8, 1990
112. Knill RL: Does sufentanil produce less ventilatory depression than fentanyl? Anesth Analg 71:564, 1990
113. Cartwright P, Prys-Roberts C, Gill K *et al:* Ventilatory depression related to plasma fentanyl concentrations during and after anesthesia in humans. Anesth Analg 62:966, 1983
114. Tagaito Y, Isono S, Nishino T: Upper airway reflexes during a combination of propofol and fentanyl anesthesia. Anesthesiology 88:1459, 1998
115. Stanley TH, Webster LR: Anesthetic requirements and cardiovascular effects of fentanyl–oxygen and fentanyl–diazepam–oxygen anesthesia in man. Anesth Analg 57:411, 1978
116. Bovill JG, Sebel PS, Stanley TH: Opioid analgesics in anesthesia: With special reference to their use in cardiovascular anesthesia. Anesthesiology 61:731, 1984
117. Flacke JW, Flacke WE, Bloor BC *et al:* Histamine release by four narcotics: A double-blind study in humans. Anesth Analg 66:723, 1987
118. Giesecke K, Hamberger B, Järnberg PO *et al:* High- and low-dose fentanyl anaesthesia: Hormonal and metabolic responses during cholecystectomy. Br J Anaesth 61:575, 1988
119. Hug CC, Murphy MR: Tissue redistribution of fentanyl and termination of its effects in rats. Anesthesiology 55:369, 1981
120. Mather LE: Clinical pharmacokinetics of fentanyl and its newer derivatives. Clin Pharmacokinetics 8:422, 1983
121. Bentley JB, Borel JD, Nenad RE *et al:* Age and fentanyl pharmacokinetics. Anesth Analg 61:968, 1982
122. Scott JC, Stanski DR: Decreased fentanyl and alfentanil dose requirements with age: A simultaneous pharmacokinetic and pharmacodynamic evaluation. J Pharmacol Exp Ther 240:159, 1987
123. Meuldermans WEG, Hurkmans RMA, Heykants JJP: Plasma protein binding and distribution of fentanyl, sufentanil, alfentanil and lofentanil in blood. Arch Int Pharmacodyn 257:4, 1982
124. Streisand JB, Stanski DR, Hague B *et al:* Oral transmucosal fentanyl citrate premedication in children. Anesth Analg 69:28, 1989
125. Gerwels JW, Bezzant JL, Le Maire L *et al:* Oral transmucosal fentanyl citrate for painful procedures in patients undergoing outpatient dermatologic procedures. J Dermatol Surg Oncol 20:823, 1994
126. Foldes FF: Neuroleptanesthesia for general surgery. In Oyama T (ed): International Anesthesiology Clinics, p 1. Boston, Little, Brown, 1973
127. White P: Droperidol: A cost-effective antiemetic for over thirty years. Anesth Analg 95:789, 2002
128. Sprigge JS, Wynands JE, Whalley DG *et al:* Fentanyl infusion anesthesia for aortocoronary bypass surgery: Plasma levels and hemodynamic response. Anesth Analg 61:972, 1982
129. Monk JP, Beresford R, Ward A: Sufentanil: A review of its pharmacological properties and therapeutic use. Drugs 36:286, 1988
130. Scott JC, Cooke JE, Stanski DR: Electroencephalographic quantitation of opioid effect: Comparative pharmacodynamics of fentanyl and sufentanil. Anesthesiology 74:34, 1991
131. Geller E, Chrubasik J, Graf R *et al:* A randomized double-blind comparison of epidural sufentanil *versus* intravenous sufentanil or epidural fentanyl analgesia after major abdominal surgery. Anesth Analg 76:1243, 1993
132. Lehmann KA, Gerhard A, Horrichs-Haermeyer G *et al:* Postoperative patient-controlled analgesia with sufentanil: Analgesic efficacy and minimum effective concentrations. Acta Anaesthesiol Scand 35:221, 1991
133. Coda BA, Hill HF, Bernards C *et al:* Comparison of therapeutic margins of sufentanil and morphine during steady-state infusions in volunteers. Anesthesiology
134. Hall RI, Murphy MR, Hug CC: The enflurane sparing effect of sufentanil in dogs. Anesthesiology 67:518, 1987
135. Brunner MD, Braithwaite P, Jhaveri R *et al:* MAC reduction of isoflurane by sufentanil. Br J Anaesth 72:42, 1994
136. Bailey JM, Schweiger IM, Hug CC: Evaluation of sufentanil anesthesia obtained by a computer-controlled infusion for cardiac surgery. Anesth Analg 76:247, 1993
137. Marx W, Shah N, Long C *et al:* Sufentanil, alfentanil, and fentanyl: Impact on cerebrospinal fluid pressure in patients with brain tumors. J Neurosurg Anesth 1:3, 1989
138. Mayer N, Weinstabl C, Podreka I *et al:* Sufentanil does not increase cerebral blood flow in healthy human volunteers. Anesthesiology 73:240, 1990
139. Werner C, Hoffman WE, Baughman VL *et al:* Effects of sufentanil on cerebral blood flow, cerebral blood flow velocity, and metabolism in dogs. Anesth Analg 72:177, 1991
140. Welchew EA, Herbert P: Effects of sufentanil on respiration and heart rate during nitrous oxide and halothane anaesthesia. Br J Anaesth 58:120P, 1986
141. Robinson D: Respiratory arrest after recovery from anaesthesia supplemented with sufentanil. Can J Anaesth 35:101, 1988
142. Karasawa F, Iwanov V, Moulds RF: Sufentanil and alfentanil cause vasorelaxation by mechanisms independent of the endothelium. Clin Exp Pharmacol Physiol 20:705, 1993
143. Sebel PS, Bovil JG: Cardiovascular effects of sufentanil. Anesth Analg 61:115, 1982
144. Rosow CE: Cardiovascular effects of opioid analgesia. Mt Sinai J Med 54:273, 1987
145. Clark NJ, Meuleman T, Liu W *et al:* Comparison of sufentanil–N_2O and fentanyl–N_2O in patients without cardiac disease undergoing general surgery. Anesthesiology 66:130, 1987
146. Thomson IR, MacAdams CL, Hudson RJ *et al:* Drug interactions with sufentanil. Anesthesiology 76:922, 1992
147. Schmeling WT, Bernstein JS, Vucins EJ *et al:* Persistent bradycardia with episodic sinus arrest after sufentanil and vecuronium administration: Successful treatment with isoproterenol. J Cardiothorac Anesth 4:89, 1990
148. Bovill JG, Sebel PS, Fiolet JWT *et al:* The influence of sufentanil on endocrine and metabolic responses to cardiac surgery. Anesth Analg 62:391, 1983
149. Bovill JG, Sebel PS, Blackburn CL *et al:* The pharmacokinetics of sufentanil in surgical patients. Anesthesiology 61:502, 1984
150. Schwartz AE, Matteo RS, Ornstein E *et al:* Pharmacokinetics of sufentanil in obese patients. Anesth Analg 73:790, 1991
151. Chauvin M, Ferrier C, Haberer JP *et al:* Sufentanil pharmacokinetics in patients with cirrhosis. Anesth Analg 68:1, 1989
152. Cork RC, Gallo JA, Weiss LB *et al:* Sufentanil infusion: Pharmacokinetics compared to bolus. Anesth Analg 67:S1, 1988
153. Bowdle TA, Ward RJ: Induction of anesthesia with small doses of sufentanil or fentanyl: Dose *versus* EEG response, speed of onset, and thiopental requirement. Anesthesiology 70:26, 1989
154. Lehmann KA: The pharmacokinetics of opioid analgesics with special

reference to patient-controlled administration. In Harmer M, Rosen M, Vickers MD (eds): Patient-Controlled Analgesia, p 18. Oxford, Blackwell Scientific, 1985
155. van den Nieuwenhuyzen MCO, Engbers FHM, Burm AGL *et al:* Computer-controlled infusion of alfentanil for postoperative analgesia: A pharmacokinetic and pharmacodynamic evaluation. Anesthesiology 79:481, 1993
156. Welchew EA, Hosking J: Patient-controlled postoperative analgesia with alfentanil. Anaesthesia 40:1172, 1985
157. Chauvin M, Hongnat JM, Mourgeon E *et al:* Equivalence of postoperative analgesia with patient-controlled intravenous or epidural alfentanil. Anesth Analg 76:1251, 1993
158. Hall RI, Szlam F, Hug CC: The enflurane-sparing effect of alfentanil in dogs. Anesth Analg 66:1287, 1987
159. Ausems ME, Hug CC, Stanski DR *et al:* Plasma concentrations of alfentanil required to supplement nitrous oxide anesthesia for general surgery. Anesthesiology 65:362, 1986
160. Ausems ME, Vuyk J, Hug CC *et al:* Comparison of a computer-assisted infusion *versus* intermittent bolus administration of alfentanil as a supplement to nitrous oxide for lower abdominal surgery. Anesthesiology 68:851, 1988
161. Vuyk J, Lim T, Engbers FHM *et al:* Pharmacodynamics of alfentanil as a supplement to propofol or nitrous oxide for lower abdominal surgery in female patients. Anesthesiology 78:1036, 1993
162. Nauta J, de Lange S, Koopman D *et al:* Anesthetic induction with alfentanil: A new short-acting narcotic analgesic. Anesth Analg 61:267, 1982
163. Hug CC, Hall RI, Angert KC *et al:* Alfentanil plasma concentration vs. effect relationships in cardiac surgical patients. Br J Anaesth 61:435, 1988
164. Hynynen M, Takkunen O, Salmenperä M *et al:* Continuous infusion of fentanyl or alfentanil for coronary artery surgery. Br J Anaesth 58:1252, 1986
165. Bovill JG, Sebel PS, Wauquier A *et al:* Influence of high-dose alfentanil anaesthesia on the electroencephalogram: Correlation with plasma concentrations. Br J Anaesth 55:199, 1983
166. Benthuysen JL, Smith NT, Sanford TJ *et al:* Physiology of alfentanil-induced rigidity. Anesthesiology 64:440, 1986
167. Mayberg TS, Lam AM, Eng CC *et al:* The effect of alfentanil on cerebral blood flow velocity and intracranial pressure during isoflurane–nitrous oxide anesthesia in humans. Anesthesiology 78:288, 1993
168. Owen H, Currie JC, Plummer JL: Variation in the blood concentration/analgesic response relationship during patient-controlled analgesia with alfentanil. Anaesth Intens Care 19:555, 1991
169. O'Connor M, Escarpa A, Prys-Roberts C: Ventilatory depression during and after infusion of alfentanil in man. Br J Anaesth 55:217S, 1983
170. Andrews CJH, Sinclair M, Prys-Roberts C *et al:* Ventilatory effects during and after continuous infusion of fentanyl or alfentanil. Br J Anaesth 55:211S, 1983
171. Stanley TH, Pace NL, Liu WS *et al:* Alfentanil–N_2O vs fentanyl–N_2O balanced anesthesia: Comparison of plasma hormonal changes, early postoperative respiratory function, and speed of postoperative recovery. Anesth Analg 62:245, 1983
172. Hudson RJ: Apnoea and unconsciousness after apparent recovery from alfentanil-supplemented anaesthesia. Can J Anaesth 37:255, 1990
173. Rucquoi M, Camu F: Cardiovascular responses to large doses of alfentanil and fentanyl. Br J Anaesth 55:223S, 1983
174. Crawford DC, Fell D, Achola KJ *et al:* Effects of alfentanil on the pressor and catecholamine responses to tracheal intubation. Br J Anaesth 59:707, 1987
175. Silbert BS, Rosow CE, Keegan CR *et al:* The effect of diazepam on induction of anesthesia with alfentanil. Anesth Analg 65:71, 1986
176. Kirby IJ, Northwood D, Dodson ME: Modification by alfentanil of the haemodynamic response to tracheal intubation in elderly patients. Br J Anaesth 60:384, 1988
177. Skues MA, Richards MJ, Jarvis A, Prys-Roberts C: Preinduction atropine or glycopyrrolate and hemodynamic changes associated with induction and maintenance of anesthesia with propofol and alfentanil. Anesth Analg 69:386, 1989
178. Bloomfield EL: The incidence of postoperative nausea and vomiting: A retrospective comparison of alfentanil *versus* sufentanil. Mil Med 157:59, 1992
179. Sfez M, Mapihan YL, Gaillard JL *et al:* Analgesia for appendectomy: A comparison of fentanyl and alfentanil in children. Acta Anaesthesiol Scand 34:30, 1990
180. Bovill JG: Which potent opioid? Important criteria for selection. Drugs 33:520, 1987
181. Bovill JG, Sebel PS, Blackburn CL *et al:* The pharmacokinetics of alfentanil (R39209): A new opioid analgesic. Anesthesiology 57:439, 1982
182. Stanski DR, Hug CC: Alfentanil: A kinetically predictable narcotic analgesic. Anesthesiology 57:435, 1982
183. Chauvin M, Bonnet F, Montembault C *et al:* The influence of hepatic plasma flow on alfentanil plasma concentration plateaus achieved with an infusion model in humans: Measurement of alfentanil hepatic extraction coefficient. Anesth Analg 65:999, 1986
184. Ferrier C, Marty J, Bouffard Y *et al:* Alfentanil pharmacokinetics in patients with cirrhosis. Anesthesiology 62:480, 1985
185. Chauvin M, Lebrault C, Levron JC *et al:* Pharmacokinetics of alfentanil in chronic renal failure. Anesth Analg 66:53, 1987
186. Larijani GE, Goldberg ME: Alfentanil hydrochloride: A new short-acting narcotic analgesic for surgical procedures. Clin Pharm 6:275, 1987
187. Philip BK, Scuderi PE, Chung F *et al:* Remifentanil compared with alfentanil for ambulatory surgery using total intravenous anesthesia. The Remifentanil/Alfentanil Outpatient TIVA Group. Anesth Analg 84(3):515, 1997
188. Ozkose Z, Cok OY, Tuncer B, *et al:* Comparison of hemodynamics, recovery profile, early postoperative pain, and costs of remifentnail *versus* alfentanil-based total intravenous anesthesia (TIVA). J Clin Anesthesia 14:161–6, 2002
189. Ganidagli S, Cengiz M, Baysal Z: Remifentanil *vs.* alfentanil in the total intravenous anaesthesia for pediatric surgery. Paediatric Anaesthesia 13:695, 2003
190. Davis PJ, Lerman J, Suresh S *et al*: A randomized multicenter study of remifentanil compared with alfentanil, isoflurane, or propofol in anesthetized pediatric patients undergoing elective strabismus surgery. Anesth Analg 84:282, 1997
191. James MK, Feldman PL, Schuster SV *et al:* Opioid receptor activity of GI87084B, a novel ultra-short acting analgesic, in isolated tissues. J Pharmacol Exp Ther 259:712, 1991
192. Glass PSA, Hardman D, Kamiyama Y *et al:* Preliminary pharmacokinetics and pharmacodynamics of an ultra-short-acting opioid: Remifentanil (GI87084B). Anesth Analg 77:1031, 1993
193. Black ML, Hill JL, Zacny JP: Behavioral and physiological effects of remifentanil and alfentanil in human volunteers. Anesthesiology 90:718, 1999
194. Bowdle TA, Camporesi EM, Maysick L *et al:* A multicenter evaluation of remifentanil for early postoperative analgesia. Anesth Analg 83(6):1292, 1996
195. Schraag S, Kenny GN, Mohl U, Georgieff M: Patient-maintained remifentanil target-controlled infusion for the transition to early postoperative analgesia. Br J Anaesth 81:365, 1998
196. Volmanen P, Akural EI, Raudaskoski T, Alahuhta S: Remifentanil in obstetric analgesia: A dose-finding study. Anesth Analg 94:913, 2002
197. Michlesen LG, Salmenpera M, Hug CC *et al:* Anesthetic potency of remifentanil in dogs. Anesthesiology 84:865, 1996
198. Criado AB, Gómez de Segura IA: Reduction in isoflurane MAC by fentanyl or remifentanil in rats. Veterinary Anesthesia and Analgesia 30:250, 2003
199. Lang E, Kapila A, Shlugman D *et al:* Reduction of isoflurane minimal alveolar concentration by remifentanil. Anesthesiology 85:721, 1996
200. Albertin A, Casati A, Bergonzi P *et al*: Effects of two target-controlled concentrations (1 and 3 ng/ml) of remifentanil on MAC(BAR) of sevoflurane. Anesthesiology 100:255, 2004
201. Jhaveri R, Joshi P, Batenhorst R *et al:* Dose comparison of remifentanil and alfentanil for loss of consciousness. Anesthesiology 87:253, 1997
202. Bouillon TW, Bruhn J, Radulescu L *et al*: Pharmacodynamic interaction between remifentanil and propofol regarding hypnosis, tolerance of laryngoscopy, bispectral index, and electroencephalographic approximate entropy. Anesthesiology 100:1353, 2004
203. Drover DR, Lemmens HJ: Population pharmacodynamics and pharmacokinetics of remifentanil as a supplement to nitrous oxide anesthesia for elective abdominal surgery. Anesthesiology 89(4):869, 1998
204. Joshi GP, Warner DS, Twersky RS *et al*: A comparison of the remifentanil and fentanyl adverse effect profile in a multicenter phase IV study. J Clin Anesth 14:494, 2002
205. Snyed JR, Camu F, Doenicke A *et al*: Remifentanil during anaesthesia for major abdominal and gynaecological surgery. An open, comparative study of safety and efficacy. Eur J Anaesthesiol 18:605, 2110, 2001
206. Van Delden PG, Houweling PL, Bencini AF *et al*: Remifentanil-sevoflurane anaesthesia for laparoscopic cholecystectomy: comparison of three dose regimens. Anaesthesia 57:212, 2002
207. Billard V, Servin F, Guignard B *et al*: Desflurane-remifantnail-nitrous oxide anesthesia for abdominal surgery: Optimal concentrations and recovery features. Acta Anaesthesiol Scand 48:355, 2004
208. Mertens MJ, Olofsen E, Engbers FH *et al*: Propofol reduces perioperative remifentanil requirements in a synergistic manner. Response surface modeling of perioperative remifentanil-propofol interactions. Anesthesiology 99:347, 2003
209. Fragen RJ, Randel GI, Librojo ES *et al:* The interaction of remifentanil and propofol to prevent response to tracheal intubation and the start of surgery for outpatient knee arthroscopy. Anesthesiology 81:A376, 1994
210. Barvais L, Sutcliffe N: Remifentanil for cardiac anesthesia. Adv Exp Med Biol 523:171, 2003
211. Guarracino F, Penzo D, De Cosmo D *et al*: Pharmacokinetic-based total intravenous anesthesia using remifentanil and propofol for surgical myocardial revascularization. Eur J Anaesthesiol 20:385, 2003
212. Engoren M, Luther G, Fenn-Buderer N: A comparison of fentanyl, sufentanil, and remifentanil for fast-track cardiac anesthesia. Anesth Analg 93:859, 2001
213. Sá Rêgo MM, Inagaki Y, White PF: Remifentanil administration during monitored anesthesia care: Are intermittent boluses an effective alternative to a continuous infusion? Anesth Analg 88:518, 1999
214. Rudner R, Przemyslaw J, Kawecki P *et al*: Conscious analgesia/sedation with remifentanil and propofol versus total intravenous anesthesia with fentanyl, midazolam, and propofol for outpatient colonoscopy, Gastrointest Endosc 57:657, 2003

215. Gold MI, Watkins WD, Sung YF *et al:* Remifentanil *versus* remifentanil/midazolam for ambulatory surgery during monitored anesthesia care. Anesthesiology 87(1):51, 1997
216. Lauwers M, Camu F, Breivik H *et al*: The safety and effectiveness of remifentanil as an adjunct sedative for regional anesthesia. Anesth Analg 88:134, 1999
217. Servin FS, Raeder JC, Merle JC *et al*: Remifentanil sedation compared with propofol during regional anaesthesia. Acta Anaesthesiol Scand 46:309, 2002
218. Egan TD, Lemmens HJM, Fiset P *et al:* The pharmacokinetics of the new short-acting opioid remifentanil (GI87084B) in healthy adult male volunteers. Anesthesiology 79:881, 1993
219. Egan TD, Minto CF, Hermann DJ *et al:* Remifentanil *versus* alfentanil: Comparative pharmacokinetics and pharmacodynamics in healthy adult male volunteers [published erratum appears in Anesthesiology 85(3):695, 1996]. Anesthesiology 84(4):821, 1996
220. Warner DS, Hindman BJ, Todd MM *et al:* Intracranial pressure and hemodynamic effects of remifentanil *versus* alfentanil in patients undergoing supratentorial craniotomy. Anesth Analg 83(2):348, 1996
221. Guy J, Hindman BJ, Baker KZ *et al:* Comparison of remifentanil and fentanyl in patients undergoing craniotomy for supratentorial space-occupying lesions [see comments]. Anesthesiology 86(3):514, 1997
222. Engelhard K, Waser C, Mollenaz O, Kochs E: Effects of remifentanil/propofol in comparison with isoflurane on dynamic cerebrovascular autoregulation in humans. Acta Anaesthesiol Scand 45:971, 2001
223. Scheufler KM, Zentner J: Total intravenous anesthesia for intraoperative monitoring of the motor pathways: An integral view combining clinical and experimental data. J Neurosurg 96:571, 2002
224. Smith DL, Angst MS, Brock-Utne JG, DeBattista C: Seizure duration with remifentanil/methohexital vs. methohexital alone in middle-aged patients undergoing electroconvulsive therapy. Acta Anaesthesiol Scand 47:1064, 2003
225. Glass PSA, Hardman HD, Kamiyama Y *et al:* Pharmacodynamic comparison of GI87084B (GI), a novel ultra-short acting opioid, and alfentanil. Anesth Analg 74:S113, 1992
226. Glass PS, Iselin Chaves IA, Goodman D *et al*: Determination of the potency of remifentanil compared with alfentanil using ventilatory depression as the measure of opioid effect. Anesthesiology 90:1556, 1999
227. Bouillon T, Bruhn J, Radu-Radulescu L *et al:* Model of the ventilatory depressant potency of remifentanil in the non-steady state. Anesthesiology 99:779–87, 2003
228. Ma D, Chakrabarti MK, Whitwam JG: The combined effects of sevoflurane and remifentanil on central respiratory activity and nociceptive cardiovascular responses in anesthetized rabbits. Anesth Analg 89:453, 1999
229. Peacock JE, Phillip BK: Ambulatory anesthesia experience with remifentanil. Anesth Analg 89:S22, 1999
230. Keidan I, Berkenstadt H, Sidi A, Perel A: Propofol/remifentanil versus propofol alone for bone marrow aspiration in paediatric haemato-oncological patients. Paediatric Anaesthesia 11:297, 2001
231. Pitts MC, Palmore MM, Salmenpera MT *et al:* Pilot study: Hemodynamic effects of intravenous GI87084B (GI) in patients undergoing elective surgery. Anesthesiology 77:A101, 1992
232. Sebel PS, Hoke JF, Westmoreland C *et al:* Histamine concentrations and hemodynamic responses after remifentanil. Anesth Analg 80:990, 1995
233. DeSouza G, Lewis MC, TerRiet MF: Severe bradycardia after remifentanil [letter]. Anesthesiology 87(4):1019, 1997
234. Cartwright DP, Kvalsvik O, Cassuto J *et al:* A randomized, blind comparison of remifentanil and alfentanil during anesthesia for outpatient surgery. Anesth Analg 85(5):1014, 1997
235. Dershwitz M, Michalowski P, Chang Y *et al*: Postoperative nausea and vomiting after total intravenous anesthesia with propofol and remifentanil or alfentanil: How important is the opioid? J Clin Anesth 14:275, 2002
236. Davis PJ, Lerman J, Suresh S *et al*: A randomized multicenter study of remifentanil compared with alfentanil. Isoflurane or propofol; in anesthetized pediatric patients undergoing elective strabismus surgery. Anesth Analg 84:982, 1997
237. Walldén J, Thörn SE, Wattwil M: The delay of gastric emptying induced by remifentanil is not influenced by posture. Anesth Analg 99:429, 2004
238. Fragen RJ, Vilich F, Spies SM, Erwin WD: The effect of remifentanil on biliary tract drainage into the duodenum. Anesth Analg 89:1561, 1999
239. Manullang J, Egan TD: Remifentanil's effect is not prolonged in a patient with pseudocholinesterase deficiency. Anesth Analg 89(2):529, 1999
240. Westmoreland CL, Hoke JF, Sebel PS *et al:* Pharmacokinetics of remifentanil (GI87084B) and its major metabolite (GI90291) in patients undergoing elective inpatient surgery. Anesthesiology 79:893, 1993
241. Servin F: Remifentanil; from pharmacological properties to clinical practice. Adv Exp Med Biol 523:245, 2003
242. Ross AK, Davis PJ, Dear G deL *et al*: Pharmacokinetics of remifentanil in aesthetized pediatric patients undergoing elective surgery or diagnostic procedures. Anesth Analg 93:1393, 2001
243. Minto CF, Schnider TW, Egan TD *et al:* Influence of age and gender on the pharmacokinetics and pharmacodynamics of remifentanil. I. Model development. Anesthesiology 86(1):10, 1997
244. Egan TD, Huizinga B, Gupta SK *et al:* Remifentanil pharmacokinetics in obese *versus* lean patients [see comments]. Anesthesiology 89(3):562, 1998
245. Dershwitz M, Hoke JF, Rosow CE *et al:* Pharmacokinetics and pharmacodynamics of remifentanil in volunteer subjects with severe liver disease. Anesthesiology 84(4):812, 1996
246. Hoke JF, Shlugman D, Dershwitz M *et al:* Pharmacokinetics and pharmacodynamics of remifentanil in persons with renal failure compared with healthy volunteers. Anesthesiology 87(3):533, 1997
247. Lehmann A, Boldt J, Rompert R *et al*: Target-controlled or manually controlled infusion of propofol in high-risk patients with severely reduced left ventricular function. J Cardiothorac Vasc Anesth 15:445, 2001
248. Fragen RJ, Fitzgerald PC. Is an infusion pump necessary to safely administer remfentanil? Anesth Analg 90:713, 2000
249. Kazmaier S, Hanekop GG, Buhre W *et al:* Myocardial consequences of remifentanil in patients with coronary artery disease. Br J Anaesth 84(5):578, 2000
250. Hogue CW Jr, Bowdle TA, O'Leary C *et al:* A multicenter evaluation of total intravenous anesthesia with remifentanil and propofol for elective inpatient surgery. Anesth Analg 83(2):279, 1996
251. Song D, Whitten CW, White PF: Use of remifentanil during anesthetic induction: A comparison with fentanyl in the ambulatory setting. Anesth Analg 88(4):734, 1999
252. Dershwitz M, Randel GI, Rosow CE *et al:* Initial clinical experience with remifentanil, a new opioid metabolized by estersases. Anesth Analg 81:619, 1995
253. Pinsker MC, Carroll NV: Quality of emergence from anesthesia and incidence of vomiting with remifentanil in a pediatric population. Anesth Analg 89(1):71, 1999
254. Jellish WS, Sheikh T, Baker W *et al*: Hemodynamic stability, myocardial ischemia, and perioperative outcome after carotid surgery with remifentanil/propofol or isoflurane/fentanyl anesthesia. J Neurosurgical Anesthesiology 3:176, 2003
255. Phillip BK, Scuderi PE, Chung F *et al*: Remifentanil compared to alfentanil for ambulatory surgery using total intravenous anesthesia. Anesth Analg 84:515, 1997
256. Randel GI, Fragen RJ, Librojo ES *et al:* Remifentanil blood concentration effect relationship at intubation and skin incision in surgical patients compared to alfentanil. Anesthesiology 81:A375, 1994
257. Ahmad S, Leavell ME, Fragen RJ *et al:* Remifentanil *versus* alfentanil as analgesic adjuncts during placement of ophthalmologic nerve blocks. Reg Anesth Pain Med 24(4):331, 1999
258. Bowdle TA: Partial agonist and agonist–antagonist opioids: Basic pharmacology and clinical applications. Anaesth Pharmacol Rev 1:135, 1993
259. Zsigmond EK, Winnie AP, Raza SMA *et al:* Nalbuphine as an analgesic component in balanced anesthesia for cardiac surgery. Anesth Analg 66:1155, 1987
260. Rawal N, Wennhager M: Influence of perioperative nalbuphine and fentanyl on postoperative respiration and analgesia. Acta Anaesthesiol Scand 34:197, 1990
261. O'Connor SA, Wilkinson DJ: A double-blind study of the respiratory effects of nalbuphine hydrochloride in spontaneously breathing anesthetized patients. Anesth Analg 67:324, 1988
262. Bailey PL, Clark NJ, Pace NL *et al:* Antagonism of postoperative opioid-induced respiratory depression: Nalbuphine *versus* naloxone. Anesth Analg 66:1109, 1987
263. Moldenhauer CC, Roach GW, Finlayson DC *et al:* Nalbuphine antagonism of ventilatory depression following high-dose fentanyl anesthesia. Anesthesiology 62:647, 1985
264. Bailey PL, Clark NJ, Pace NL *et al:* Failure of nalbuphine to antagonize morphine: A double-blind comparison with naloxone. Anesth Analg 65:605, 1986
265. Dershwitz M, Rosow CE, DiBiase PM *et al:* Comparison of the sedative effects of butorphanol and midazolam. Anesthesiology 74:717, 1991
266. Bowdle TA, Greichen SL, Bjurstrom RI *et al:* Butorphanol improves CO_2 response and ventilation after fentanyl anesthesia. Anesth Analg 66:517, 1987
267. Pedersen JE: Perioperative buprenorphine: Do high doses shorten analgesia postoperatively? Acta Anaesthesiol Scand 30:660, 1986
268. Gal TL: Naloxone reversal of buprenorphine-induced respiratory depression. Clin Pharmacol Ther 45:66, 1989
269. Boysen K, Hertel S, Chraemmer-Jorgansen B *et al:* Buprenorphine antagonism of ventilatory depression following fentanyl anaesthesia. Acta Anesthesiol Scand 32:490, 1988
270. Pallasch TJ, Gill CJ: Naloxone-associated morbidity and mortality. Oral Surg Oral Med Oral Pathol 52:602, 1981
271. Partridge BL, Ward CF: Pulmonary edema following low-dose naloxone administration. Anesthesiology 65:709, 1986
272. Prough DS, Roy R, Bumgarner J *et al:* Acute pulmonary edema in healthy teenagers following conservative doses of intravenous naloxone. Anesthesiology 60:485, 1984
273. Rawal N, Schött U, Dahlström B *et al:* Influence of naloxone infusion on analgesia and respiratory depression following epidural morphine. Anesthesiology 64:194, 1986
274. Kapila A, Glass PSA, Jacobs JR *et al:* Measured context-sensitive half-times of remifentanil and alfentanil. Anesthesiology 83:968, 1995

CHAPTER 15 ■ INHALATION ANESTHESIA

THOMAS J. EBERT

KEY POINTS

1. Volatile anesthetics are relatively inexpensive, easily administered via inhalation, readily titrated, and have a high safety ratio in terms of preventing recall. Depth of anesthesia can be quickly adjusted in a predictable way while monitoring tissue levels via end-tidal concentrations. In addition they cause relaxation of skeletal muscle.
2. The inhaled anesthetics are among the most rapidly acting drugs in existence, and their pharmacokinetics are described in four phases: absorption, distribution, metabolism, and excretion. Anesthetic uptake is assessed with the ratio of the fractional concentration of alveolar anesthetic to inspired anesthetic (F_A/F_I), followed over time. The most important factor in the rate of rise of F_A/F_I is F_A because of the avid uptake of anesthetic from the alveoli into the bloodstream. The inhaled anesthetics with the lowest solubilities in blood show the fastest rise in F_A/F_I, and are eliminated most rapidly.
3. The pharmacodynamic effects of inhaled anesthetics is related to dose, described as the *minimum alveolar concentration* or *MAC*. MAC is the alveolar concentration of an anesthetic at one atmosphere that prevents movement in response to a surgical stimulus in 50% of patients.
4. All of the potent, volatile anesthetics depress cerebral metabolic rate and increase cerebral blood flow, varying as a function of dose. Increases in intracerebral pressure with sevoflurane, isoflurane, and possibly desflurane are minimal and far less than with halothane.
5. Sevoflurane has been associated with a lower heart rate compared to desflurane and does not increase sympathetic nervous system activity as does desflurane. Cardiac output is well preserved with sevoflurane, desflurane, and isoflurane, and all three have been associated with cellular protection from ischemia-induced myocardial injury.
6. In dehydrated carbon dioxide absorbents, degradation of desflurane, enflurane, isoflurane, and sevoflurane results in carbon monoxide formation. In rare instances, sevoflurane destruction has led to high heat and fires.
7. Halothane is 20% metabolized and an immune response to the metabolite trifluoroacetyl (TFA) has resulted in hepatitis. Based on % metabolized, halothane>enflurane>

isoflurane>desflurane in antigenic potential. Sevoflurane is not metabolized to a TFA halide; rather it is metabolized to hexafluoroisopropanol that does not serve as a neoantigen. Immunologic memory resulting in hepatitis has been reported years after an initial halothane exposure. In addition, cross-sensitivity has been reported in which exposure to one anesthetic can sensitize patients to a second but different anesthetic.

INTRODUCTION

Inhalation anesthetics are the most common drugs used for the provision of general anesthesia. Adding as little as 1% of a volatile anesthetic to the inspired oxygen results in a state of unconsciousness and amnesia, which are essential components of general anesthesia. When combined with intravenous adjuvants, such as opioids or benzodiazepines, a balanced technique is achieved that results in further sedation/hypnosis and analgesia. The popularity of the inhaled anesthetics for establishing general anesthesia is based on their ease of administration (i.e., via inhalation) and the ability to reliably monitor their effects with both clinical signs and end-tidal concentrations. In addition, the volatile anesthetic gases are relatively inexpensive in terms of the overall cost of the anesthesia care of the patient.

The most popular potent inhaled anesthetics used in adult surgical procedures are sevoflurane, desflurane, and isoflurane (Fig. 15-1). In pediatric cases, halothane and sevoflurane are most commonly employed. Although there are many similarities in terms of the overall effects of the volatile anesthetics (e.g., they all have a dose-dependent effect to decrease blood pressure), there are some unique differences that affect the clinician's selection for use. These differences are weighted against the patient's health and with the particular effects of the planned surgical procedure. Discussion of the four most popular inhaled anesthetics provides the major emphasis of this chapter. For the sake of completeness and for historical purposes related to metabolism and renal toxicity, comments on both enflurane and methoxyflurane also are included.

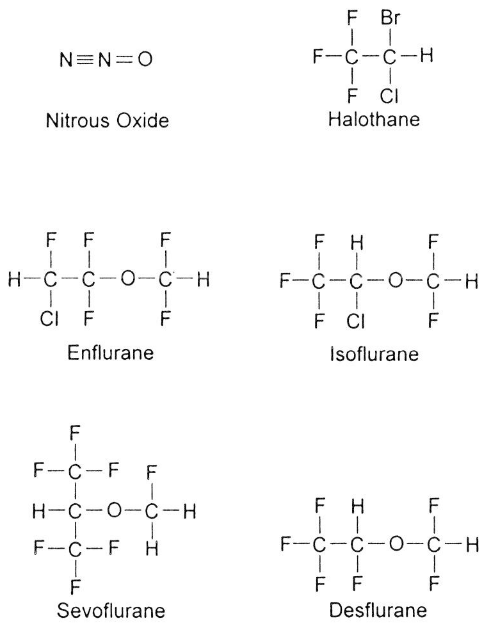

N≡N=O

Nitrous Oxide

Halothane

Enflurane

Isoflurane

Sevoflurane

Desflurane

FIGURE 15-1. Chemical structure of inhaled anesthetics. Halothane is an alkane, a halogen-substituted ethane derivative. Isoflurane and enflurane are isomers that are methyl ethyl ethers. Desflurane differs from isoflurane in the substitution of a fluorine for a chlorine atom and sevoflurane is a methyl isopropyl ether.

HISTORY

The volatile anesthetics in early clinical use consisted of flammable gases, including diethyl ether, cyclopropane, and divinyl ether. Several nonflammable compounds were available, including chloroform and trichloroethylene, but these were associated with hepatic toxicity and neurotoxicity, and were only briefly in clinical use. In the early 1930s, studies on derivatives of the halogenated compound, chloroform, indicated that noncombustible anesthetic gases might be derived using organic fluoride compounds. Advances in fluorine chemistry in the 1940s allowed safe incorporation of fluorine into molecules at a reasonable expense. These advances proved to be pivotal to the development of modern-day anesthetics. Fluorine is the halogen with the lowest atomic weight (18.998; chlorine = 35.45; bromine = 79.90; iodine = 126.9). Fluorine substitutions for other halogens on the ether molecule lowered the boiling point, increased stability, and generally decreased toxicity. The fluoride ion also dampened the flammable hydrocarbon of the ether anesthetic framework.

In 1951, halothane was synthesized and extensively tested in animals by Suckling, working at ICI Laboratory in England. Halothane was introduced into clinical practice in 1956 and was rapidly embraced, owing in part to its nonflammability and in part to its lower tissue solubility. Halothane also had a relatively low pungency and a high potency; thus, it could be administered in high-inspired concentrations (relative to its potency) to induce anesthesia via inhalation. Halothane was associated with a lower incidence of nausea and vomiting.

Despite these desirable properties of halothane, some concerns and drawbacks remained. Most notable were the effects of halothane on sensitizing the myocardium to catecholamines and the later described role of its intermediate metabolite in hepatic necrosis. Thus, the search for better agents continued. Between the years of 1959 and 1966, Terrell and colleagues at Ohio Medical Products (subsequently called Anaquest, Ohmeda, and most currently, Baxter) synthesized more than 700 compounds. The 347th and 469th compounds in the series were methyl ethyl ethers, enflurane and isoflurane, which were halogenated with fluorine and chlorine. Clinical trials of enflurane and isoflurane proceeded nearly in parallel, involving both human volunteer and patient studies. Years later, several compounds in Terrell's series were reexamined. One of these (the 653rd) was problematic because the compound had a vapor pressure close to 1 atmosphere, making it impossible to deliver with a standard wicked vaporizer. However, this particular compound was completely halogenated with fluorine and hence was predicted to have a very low solubility in blood. As synthesis and delivery problems were resolved, this compound, now known as desflurane, was introduced into clinical practice in 1993.

Wallin and colleagues at Travenol Laboratories described other new compounds in the early 1970s, during the course of evaluating fluorinated isopropyl ethers. One of these proved to be a potent anesthetic agent and became known as sevoflurane. Like desflurane, it had a low solubility owing to fluorination of the ether molecule. It was noted that sevoflurane released organic and inorganic fluorides in both animals and humans; thus, the drug was not aggressively developed and marketed. When the patent rights were transferred to Ohio Medical Products, further testing revealed significant

TABLE 15-1

PHYSIOCHEMICAL PROPERTIES OF VOLATILE ANESTHETICS

	SEVO	DES	ISO	ENFLUR	HALO	N_2O
Boiling point (°C)	59	24	49	57	50	−88
Vapor pressure at 20°C (mm Hg)	157	669	238	172	243	38,770
Molecular weight (g)	200	168	184	184	197	44
Oil:gas partition coefficient	47	19	91	97	224	1.4
Blood:gas partition coefficient	0.65	0.42	1.46	1.9	2.50	0.46
Brain:blood solubility	1.7	1.3	1.6	1.4	1.9	1.1
Fat:blood solubility	47.5	27.2	44.9	36	51.1	2.3
Muscle:blood solubility	3.1	2.0	2.9	1.7	3.4	1.2
MAC in O_2 30–60 yr, at 37°C P_B760 (%)	1.8	6.6	1.17	1.63	0.75	104
MAC in 60–70% N_2O (%)	0.66	2.38	0.56	0.57	0.29	
MAC, >65 yr (%)	1.45	5.17	1.0	1.55	0.64	–
Preservative	No	No	No	No	Thymol	No
Stable in moist CO_2 absorber	No	Yes	Yes	Yes	No	Yes
Flammability (%) (in 70% N_2O/30% O_2)	10	17	7	5.8	4.8	
Recovered as metabolites (%)	2–5	0.02	0.2	2.4	20	

breakdown of sevoflurane in the presence of soda lime, raising safety concerns that limited further evaluation. Maruishi Pharmaceutical in Japan undertook testing and development of sevoflurane, releasing the drug for general use in Japan in July 1990. Because of the rapid acceptance and safety record of sevoflurane in Japan, Abbott Laboratories began pursuing laboratory and clinical trials with sevoflurane in the United States. After its safety was established, sevoflurane was introduced in U.S. clinical practice in 1995.

The new inhaled anesthetics sevoflurane and desflurane differ from isoflurane most importantly in their kinetic behavior. They both have significantly lower solubility in blood, which increases their speed for washin and washout and their speed in adjustment of anesthetic depth (Table 15-1). These characteristics mesh well with the ambulatory anesthesia environment of modern day practice.

PHARMACOKINETIC PRINCIPLES

Pharmacokinetics as a discipline began with the study of noninhaled drugs before the concepts were applied to the inhaled anesthetics. Kety in 1950 was the first to examine the pharmacokinetics of inhaled agents in a systematic fashion.[1] Eger and colleagues accomplished much of the early research in the field leading to his landmark text on the subject in 1974.[2] The inhaled anesthetics differ substantially from nearly all other drugs because they are gases given via inhalation. This makes their pharmacokinetics unique as well, and most major textbooks of anesthesia continue to devote considerable space to pharmacokinetic principles of currently used agents.

Drug pharmacology is classically divided into two disciplines, pharmacodynamics and pharmacokinetics. *Pharmacodynamics* can be defined as what drugs do to the body. It describes the desired and undesired effects of drugs, as well as the cellular and molecular changes leading to these effects. *Pharmacokinetics* can be defined as what the body does to drugs. It describes where drugs go, how they are transformed, and the cellular and molecular mechanisms underlying these processes.

Systemic drug pharmacokinetics have four phases: absorption, distribution, metabolism, and excretion. *Absorption* is the phase in which drug is transferred from the administration site (e.g., digestive tract, lung, muscle) into the bloodstream. Intravenous drugs have no absorption phase because they are delivered directly into the bloodstream. *Distribution* is the phase in which drug is transferred to tissue sites throughout the body. *Metabolism* refers to the physiochemical processes by which substances in a living organism are synthesized (anabolism) or altered (catabolism); but in the context of anesthetic drugs only drug alteration is pertinent. Finally, *excretion* is the phase in which changed or unchanged drug is transferred from tissues or blood into some vehicle (e.g., bile, exhaled air, urine) for removal from the body.

Tissues are often grouped into hypothetical *compartments* based on perfusion. An important implication of different compartments and perfusion rates is the concept of *redistribution*. After a given amount of drug is administered, it reaches highly perfused tissue compartments first where it can equilibrate rapidly and exert its effects. With time, however, compartments with lower perfusion rates receive the drug and additional equilibria are established between blood and these tissues. As the tissues with lower perfusion absorb drug, maintenance of equilibria throughout the body requires drug transfer from highly perfused compartments back into the bloodstream. This lowering of drug concentration in one compartment by delivery into another compartment is called redistribution.

In discussions of the inhaled anesthetics, the terminology just described is subject to some minor differences. The absorption phase is usually called *uptake*, the metabolic phase is usually called *biotransformation*, and the excretion phase is usually called *elimination*. The terms are completely interchangeable.

Unique Features of Inhaled Anesthetics

Speed, Gas State, and Route of Administration

2 The inhaled anesthetics are among the most rapidly acting drugs in existence, and when administering a general anesthetic, this speed provides a margin of safety. The ability to quickly increase or decrease anesthetic levels as necessary can mean the difference between an anesthetic state and an anesthetic misadventure. Speed also means efficiency. Rapid induction and recovery may lead to faster operating room turnover

times, shorter recovery room stays, and earlier discharges to home.

Technically, nitrous oxide is the only true gas, while the potent anesthetics are the vapors of volatile liquids. But for simplicity, all of them are called gases because they are all in the gas phase when administered via the lungs. As gases, none deviate significantly from ideal gas behavior. These agents are all nonionized and have low molecular weights. This allows them to diffuse rapidly without the need for facilitated diffusion or active transport from bloodstream to tissues. The other advantage of gases is that they can be delivered to the bloodstream via a unique route available in all patients: the lungs.

The lung route of administration is unique to the inhaled anesthetics, except for bronchodilators or endotracheal administration of cardiac resuscitation drugs. These exceptions are, however, a "one-way street" because their route of delivery is different from their elimination route. Inhaled anesthetics have a "two-way street" in the lungs; they are delivered and primarily eliminated via this route.

Speed, gaseous state, and the lung route of administration combine to form the major beneficial feature of the inhaled anesthetics—the ability to decrease plasma concentrations as easily and as rapidly as they are increased.

Physical Characteristics of Inhaled Anesthetics

The goal of delivering inhaled anesthetics is to produce the anesthetic state by establishing a specific concentration of anesthetic molecules in the central nervous system (CNS). This is done by establishing the specific partial pressure of the agent in the lungs, which ultimately equilibrates with the brain and spinal cord. Equilibration is a result of three factors:

1. Inhaled anesthetics are gases rapidly transferred bidirectionally via the lungs to and from the bloodstream and subsequently to and from CNS tissues as partial pressures equilibrate.
2. Plasma and tissues have a low capacity to absorb the inhaled anesthetics relative to the amount we can deliver to the lungs, allowing us to quickly establish or abolish anesthetizing concentrations of anesthetic in the bloodstream and ultimately the CNS.
3. Metabolism, excretion, and redistribution of the inhaled anesthetics are minimal relative to the rate at which they are delivered or removed from the lungs. This permits easy maintenance of blood and CNS concentrations.

At equilibrium, CNS partial pressure equals blood partial pressure, which in turn equals alveolar partial pressure:

$$P_{\text{CNS}} = P_{\text{blood}} = P_{\text{alveoli}} \tag{15-1}$$

where P is partial pressure. The physical characteristics of inhaled anesthetics are shown in Table 15-1.

Inhaled anesthetics are delivered to the lung as gases and follow the ideal gas law, $PV = nRT$, where P is pressure, V is volume, n is number of moles of gas, R is the gas constant, and T is absolute temperature. If a gas is heated in a fixed volume, pressure will increase. If a gas is heated or if molecules of gas are added while keeping its pressure constant, its volume must increase. If the number of molecules of gas is increased into a fixed volume, pressure will increase.

The so-called *permanent gases*, such as oxygen and nitrogen, exist only as gases at ambient temperatures. Gases such as nitrous oxide can be compressed into liquids under high pressure at ambient temperature. Most *potent volatile anesthetics* are liquids at ambient temperature and pressure. Some molecules with sufficient energy escape the liquid and enter a gas phase above the surface of the liquid as a vapor. Pure gases always diffuse from an area of high pressure to an area of low pressure, because of their *chemical potential*, μ. Chemical potential, also called the escaping tendency, is a thermodynamic concept. It is similar to an electrical potential. In this case, however, it is gases that continue to seek equilibration until μ is equal throughout the system. Chemical potential depends on the substance and characteristics of the system in which it exists, such as temperature, pressure, and presence of other substances.

If the system in which the volatile liquid resides is a closed container, molecules of the substance will equilibrate between the liquid and gas phases (to equalize μ). At equilibrium the pressure exerted by molecular collisions of the gas against the container walls is the *vapor pressure*. One important property of vapor pressure is that as long as *any* liquid remains in the container, the vapor pressure is independent of the volume of that liquid. As with any gas, however, vapor pressure is proportional to temperature.

For all of the potent agents at 20°C the vapor pressure is below atmospheric pressure. If the temperature is raised the vapor pressure increases. The *boiling point* of a liquid is the temperature at which its vapor pressure exceeds atmospheric pressure in an open container. Desflurane is bottled in a special container because its boiling point of 23.5°C makes it boil at typical room temperatures. Boiling does not occur within the bottle because it is countered by buildup of vapor pressure within the bottle; but once opened to air, the desflurane would quickly boil away. The bottle is designed to allow transfer of desflurane from bottle to vaporizer without exposure to the atmosphere.

Gases in Mixtures

For any mixture of gases in a closed container, each gas exerts a pressure proportional to its *fractional mass* (or fractional *volume* according to $PV = nRT$, since "volume" is a more familiar term when dealing with gases). This is its *partial pressure*. The sum of the partial pressures of each gas in a mixture of gases equals the total pressure of the entire mixture (Dalton's law).

$$P_{\text{total}} = P_{\text{gas1}} + P_{\text{gas2}} + \cdots + P_{\text{gasN}} \tag{15-2}$$

The entire mixture behaves just as if it were a single gas according to the ideal gas law.

Gases in Solution

Partial pressures of gases in solution are more complicated. Any gas/vapor dissolved in a liquid exerts a force to drive molecules out of solution and into the gas phase. Molecules in the gas phase counter this by exerting a force that drives them into the liquid phase. Only at a given concentration of molecules in the gas phase will the forces (hence chemical potentials) be equal and the system in equilibrium. This force is called the *tension*, and the concentration of molecules in the gas phase at equilibrium will determine the pressure of that phase according to the ideal gas law. Tension is conveniently described by the partial pressure of the gas in equilibrium with the liquid phase. The terms "tension" and "partial pressure" are used synonymously in this chapter.

The *concentration* of gas molecules in solution is more complicated still, owing to intermolecular interaction. Gas molecules within a liquid interact with solvent molecules to a much larger extent than do molecules in the gas phase. The gas molecules will be present in the liquid only to the extent that this equalizes the chemical potential between the liquid and gas phases. The chemical potential of the gas in a liquid depends dramatically on the liquid itself and the energy-state of that liquid. "Solubility" is the term used to describe the tendency of a gas to equilibrate with a solution, hence determining its concentration in solution. The solubility coefficient, λ is an expression of this tendency:

$$\lambda = V_{dissolved\ gas}/V_{liquid} \text{ at } 37^\circ C \tag{15-3}$$

where V = volume.

The principles of partial pressures and solubility apply in mixtures of gases in solution. That is, the concentration of any one gas in a mixture of gases in solution depends on two factors: (1) its partial pressure in the gas phase in equilibrium with the solution, and (2) its solubility within that solution. Thus, the partial pressure of a particular gas is proportional to its fractional volume in the gas phase, not the liquid phase.

The implications of these properties are that anesthetic gases administered via the lungs diffuse into blood until the partial pressures in alveoli and blood are equal. The concentration of anesthetic in the blood depends on the partial pressure at equilibrium and the blood solubility. Likewise, transfer of anesthetic from blood to target tissues also proceeds toward equalizing partial pressures. The concentration of anesthetic in target tissue depends on the partial pressure at equilibrium and the target tissue solubility. Because inhaled anesthetics are gases, and because partial pressures of gases equilibrate throughout a system, monitoring the alveolar concentration of inhaled anesthetics provides an index of their effects in the brain.

In summary:

1. Inhaled anesthetics equilibrate based on their partial pressures in each tissue (or tissue compartment), *not* based on their concentrations.
2. The partial pressure of a gas in solution is always defined by the partial pressure in the gas phase with which it is in equilibrium.
3. The concentration of anesthetic in a tissue depends on its partial pressure and tissue solubility.

Finally, the particular terminology used when referring to gases in the gas phase or absorbed in plasma or tissues is important. Inspired concentrations or fractional volumes of inhaled anesthetic are typically used rather than partial pressure. For most drugs, concentration is expressed as mass (mg) per volume (mL), but it can also be expressed in percent by weight or volume. Since volume of a gas in the gas phase is directly proportional to mass according to the ideal gas law, it is easier to express this fractional concentration as a percent by volume. Tension and partial pressure, on the other hand, are expressed in mmHg, or torr (1 torr = 1 mmHg), or kPa (kilopascals). In the gas phase, fractional concentration is equal to the partial pressure (or tension) divided by ambient pressure, usually atmospheric, or:

$$\text{Fractional volume} = P_{anesthetic}/P_{barometric} \tag{15-4}$$

Anesthetic Transfer: Machine to Central Nervous System

Anesthetics follow a multistep route from anesthesia machine to patient (and back). Each of these steps represents a transfer point or interface between hypothetical compartments. The compartments are organized by location or pharmacokinetic properties in an effort to simplify the concept of anesthetic flow. For example, one-way flow occurs from the fresh gas outlet to the anesthesia circuit and to the waste gas scavenging system. Equilibrium flow occurs between the anesthesia circuit and the airways (and alveoli) and between the alveoli and pulmonary blood. Bulk flow of blood accounts for anesthetic transfer to systemic blood and equilibrium flow occurs between systemic blood and tissues. The flow of anesthetic from compartment to compartment can be characterized by pharmacokinetics. Technically, the flow from fresh gas outlet (FGO) to circuit is not a pharmacokinetic concern because it does not characterize what the body does to the drug. But it is typically discussed as a pharmacokinetic parameter because it has important clinical implications.

When the fresh gas flow and the vaporizer are turned on, fresh gas with a fixed fractional concentration of anesthetic leaves the FGO and mixes with the gas in the circuit—the bag, tubing, absorbent canister, and piping. It is immediately diluted to a lower fractional concentration, then slowly rises as this compartment equilibrates with the fresh gas flow. With spontaneous patient ventilation by mask, the anesthetic gas passes from circuit to airways. The fractional concentration of anesthetic leaving the circuit is designated as F_I (fraction inspired). In the lungs the gas comprising the dead space in the airways (trachea, bronchi) and the alveoli further dilutes the circuit gas. The fractional concentration of anesthetic present in the alveoli is F_A (fraction alveolar). The anesthetic then passes across the alveolar–capillary membrane and dissolves in pulmonary blood according to the partial pressure of the gas and its solubility. It is further diluted and travels via bulk blood flow throughout the vascular tree. The anesthetic then passes via simple diffusion from blood to tissues as well as between tissues.

The vascular system delivers blood to three physiologic tissue groups; the vessel-rich group (VRG), the muscle group, and the fat group. The VRG includes the brain, heart, kidney, liver, digestive tract, and glandular tissues. The percent body mass and perfusion of each are shown in Table 15-2. The CNS tissues of the VRG are referred to as *tissues of desired effect*. The other tissues of the VRG comprise the compartment frequently referred to as *tissues of undesired effects*. The tissues of the muscle and fat groups comprise the *tissues of accumulation*.

Anesthetic is delivered most rapidly to the VRG because of high blood flow. Here it diffuses according to partial pressure gradients. CNS tissue takes in the anesthetic according to the tissue solubility, and at a high enough tissue concentration unconsciousness is achieved. Increasing CNS tissue concentrations causes progressively deeper stages of anesthesia. As this is occurring, anesthetic is also distributing to other VRG tissues. Also coincident with delivery to the CNS, anesthetic is being delivered—albeit more slowly because of lower perfusion—to muscle and fat where it accumulates and may affect the speed of emergence from the anesthetic. In reality, the fat solubilities provide little influence on emergence in cases lasting <4 hours since the delivery of anesthetic to fat tissue is extremely slow as a result of low blood flow. The concentration of inhaled anesthetic in a given tissue at a particular time during the

TABLE 15-2

GROUP	% BODY MASS	% CARDIAC OUTPUT	PERFUSION mL/min/100 g
Vessel rich	10	75	75
Muscle	50	19	3
Fat	20	6	3

administration depends not only on tissue blood flow, but also on tissue solubility, which governs how the inhaled anesthetics partition themselves between blood and tissue. Partitioning depends on the relative solubilities of the anesthetic for each compartment. These relative solubilities are expressed by a partition coefficient, δ, which is the ratio of dissolved gas (by volume) in two-tissue compartments at equilibrium. Alternatively it is the ratio of tissue:gas solubilities in the two compartments. For a pure gas in the gas phase, λ equals 1, that is, $V_{\text{"dissolved"gas}}/V_{gas} = 1$. Thus blood:gas partition coefficient is the same as blood solubility:

$$\delta_{b/g} = \lambda_{blood}/\lambda_{gas} = \lambda_{blood}/1 = \lambda_{blood} \quad (15\text{-}5)$$

where $\delta_{b/g}$ is the blood:gas partition coefficient.

For other partition coefficients such as brain:blood ($\delta_{br/bl}$), the volume of anesthetic dissolved in brain is divided by the volume of anesthetic dissolved in blood:

$$\delta_{br/bl} = \lambda_{brain}/\lambda_{blood} \quad (15\text{-}6)$$

Some of the partition coefficients for the inhaled anesthetics are shown in Table 15-1.

As explained earlier, one of the reasons why inhaled anesthetics are rapidly titratable is that their tissue solubilities are low relative to delivery rate; thus delivery of a desired partial pressure to the CNS is possible despite redistribution and accumulation of anesthetic in other tissues.

Uptake and Distribution

F_A/F_I

A simple, common way to assess anesthetic uptake is to follow the ratio of fractional concentration of alveolar anesthetic to inspired anesthetic (F_A/F_I) over time. Experimentally derived data for F_A/F_I versus time during induction are shown in Figure 15-2.

The inhaled anesthetics with the lowest solubilities in blood show the fastest rise in F_A/F_I. The shape of these curves has several regions with different origins. As fresh gas carrying anesthetic begins to flow into the air-filled circuit (assuming complete mixing), the concentration in the circuit (F_I) will rise according to first-order kinetics:

$$F_I = F_{FGO}(1 - e^{-T/\tau}) \quad (15\text{-}7)$$

F_{FGO} is the fraction of inspired anesthetic in the gas leaving the fresh gas outlet (i.e., the vaporizer setting), T is time, and τ is a time constant. Because all anesthetics in the circuit are in the gas phase, F (fractional volume or concentration) is also P (partial pressure) divided by P_B (barometric pressure), and inspired anesthetic can be expressed as either F_I or P_I. The time constant is simply the volume or "capacity" of the circuit (V_C) divided by the fresh gas flow (FGF) or $\tau = V_C$ /FGF. For example, if the bag, tubing, absorbent canister, and piping comprise 8 L, and the fresh gas flow is 2 L, the time constant $\tau = 8/2 = 4$. One of the characteristics of first-order kinetics is that 95% of maximum is reached after 3 time constants—in this case, $3 \times 4 = 12$ minutes.

Because 12 minutes is relatively long, starting with a higher F_{FGO} can increase the rate of rise of F_I. Using the earlier example with $\tau = 4$, by first-order kinetics 63% of maximum is reached after one time constant, or 4 minutes. To attain an F_I of 2% at 4 instead of 12 minutes, the F_{FGO} can be set to 3.2% (2% divided by 0.63) and then lowered to 2% at the 4-minute mark.

Other ways to speed the increase in F_I include increasing the fresh gas flow, thus decreasing τ. Furthermore, the rebreathing bag can be collapsed prior to starting the fresh gas flow, such

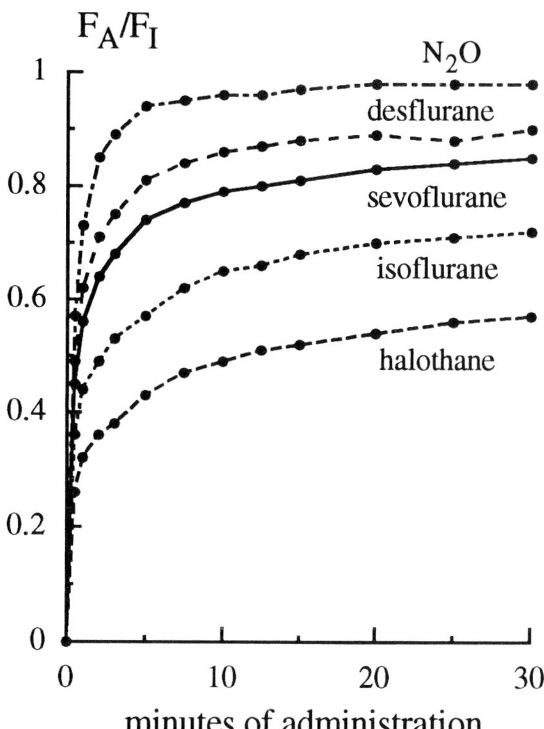

FIGURE 15-2. The rise in alveolar (F_A) anesthetic concentration toward the inspired (F_I) concentration is most rapid with the least soluble anesthetics, nitrous oxide, desflurane, and sevoflurane. It rises most slowly with the more soluble anesthetics, for example, halothane. All data are from human studies. (Adapted from Yasuda N, Lockhart SH, Eger EI II *et al*: Comparison of kinetics of sevoflurane and isoflurane in humans. Anesth Analg 72:316, 1991; and Yasuda N, Lockhart SH, Eger EI II *et al*: Kinetics of desflurane, isoflurane, and halothane in humans. Anesthesiology 74:489, 1991.)

that the capacity in the circuit (V_C) is less, which also decreases τ. Finally, at high flows (>4 L/min) there is far less mixing because fresh gas pushes "old" gas out of the circuit via the pop-off valve before complete mixing occurs, causing F_I to increase at a greater rate.

One factor that delays the rate of rise of F_I arises from the fact that CO_2 absorbent can adsorb and decompose the inhaled anesthetics. From a practical standpoint, this does not affect the rate of rise in F_I to a significant extent compared to other factors. Another factor that delays the rate of rise of F_I is solubility of the inhaled anesthetics in some of the plastic and rubber parts of the anesthesia circuit. This absorption has been quantified, but plays only a small role in decreasing the rate of rise of F_I.

Rise in F_A in the Absence of Uptake

The rate of rise in F_I discussed earlier assumes that no anesthetic is mixing with gas in the patient's lungs. In reality, circuit gas mixes with exhaled gases from the lung with each breath. If extremely high fresh gas flows (producing a high volume of gas at the desired concentration) are used, little mixing with exhaled air occurs and F_I is relatively fixed. In this situation, circuit gas enters the lungs where it mixes with alveolar gas. If there were no blood flow to the lungs, F_A would rise in a fashion analogous to F_I; that is:

$$F_A = F_I(1 - e^{-T/\tau}) \quad (15\text{-}8)$$

In this equation, τ is the time constant for alveolar rise in anesthetic concentration and equals the functional residual capacity (FRC) of the patient's lungs divided by minute ventilation, $\dot{V}_A$. There are two ways to speed the equilibration of F_A with F_I, that is, to decrease τ. One way is to increase minute ventilation, and the other is to decrease FRC. Both of these methods can be used to speed induction by mask: the patient can exhale deeply before applying the mask (to decrease the initial FRC), and the patient can breathe deeply and rapidly (to increase $\dot{V}_A$) after the mask is applied. One of the reasons that pediatric inductions by spontaneous breathing of inhaled anesthetics are so much quicker than adult inductions is that the low FRC relative to $\dot{V}_A$ of children makes for a low time constant, and hence a rapid increase in F_A/F_I. One important caveat about the relationship of F_A to FRC is that FRC includes airway dead space; thus, in reality, F_A by Equation 15-8 is not just the concentration of inhaled anesthetic in the alveoli but also the concentration in the entire lung. However, it is simply called the alveolar concentration because the dead space in the airways is relatively insignificant and only the alveolar gas is exchanging anesthetic with the blood.

Rise in F_A in the Presence of Uptake

Because in reality there *is* pulmonary blood flow, the most important factor in the rate of rise of F_A/F_I is uptake of anesthetic from the alveoli into the bloodstream. The rate of rise of F_A/F_I (the slope of the curves seen in Fig. 15-2) reflects the speed at which alveolar anesthetic (F_A) equilibrates with that being delivered to the lungs (F_I). F_A is not solely a function of F_I and time. Inhaled anesthetics so avidly transfer into and are diluted by the bloodstream that uptake into blood is a primary determinant of F_A; that is, the greater the uptake, the slower the rate of rise of F_A/F_I. Uptake is proportional to tissue solubility. The less soluble the anesthetic (such as desflurane), the lesser its uptake and the faster it reaches equilibrium.

Consider a hypothetical example. Suppose that halothane and desflurane are soluble in blood, but insoluble in all other tissues. Suppose further that total lung capacity and blood volume were both 5 liters. If a fixed volume of anesthetic is delivered to the lungs (by asking the patient to take one deep breath and hold it), according to partition coefficients, 70.6% of the delivered halothane will be transferred to the blood while 29.4% remains in the alveoli (70.6/29.4 = 2.4). In contrast 29.6% of the desflurane will be transferred to the blood while 70.4% remains in the alveoli (29.6/70.4 = 0.42). Therefore, 2.4 times (70.6/29.6) more halothane than desflurane (by volume or number of molecules) will be transferred from alveoli to bloodstream before partial pressures equilibrate. At equilibrium, the partial pressures of halothane and desflurane are 29.4% and 70.4% of their inhaled values, respectively.

But anesthetics *are* soluble in tissues, and they are delivered *continuously* rather than in a "one-shot" fashion; thus they are again characterized by first-order kinetics:

$$P_{bl}(\text{blood}) = P_A(\text{alveoli}) \times (1 - e^{-T/\tau}),$$
$$\text{where } P_A = F_A \times P_B\,(\text{barometric}) \qquad (15\text{-}9)$$

Here, P_B is the barometric pressure, and the time constant, τ, equals "capacity" (volume of anesthetic dissolved in blood at the desired alveolar partial pressure) divided by flow (volume of anesthetic delivered per unit time). For any given flow of anesthetic into the system, this capacity for the more soluble halothane is greater than the capacity for the less soluble desflurane; thus, τ for halothane is greater than that for desflurane. The more soluble an inhaled anesthetic, the larger the capacity of the blood and tissues for that anesthetic, and the longer it takes to saturate at any given delivery rate.

Anesthetic flow can be described by a series of first-order rate equations: F_I as a function of F_{FGO}, F_A as a function of F_I, blood uptake as a function of F_A, and so on. These differential equations can then be solved to determine any value as a function of time. Relatively straightforward equations help describe which parameters determine the rate of rise of F_A/F_I.

During any given period of time, the alveolar anesthetic fraction, F_A, as a proportion of the inspired anesthetic fraction, F_I, will equal the ratio of $\dot{V}_{expired}$ to $\dot{V}_{inspired}$; that is:

$$F_A/F_I = \dot{V}_{expired}/\dot{V}_{inspired} \qquad (15\text{-}10)$$

If F_A/F_I is zero and starts to increase as inhaled anesthetic reaches the alveoli from the circuit but uptake of anesthetic in the pulmonary blood nearly equals its delivery to the alveoli, then F_A/F_I will not rise. All of the anesthetic arriving at the alveoli is transferred immediately to the blood. Since blood capacity to absorb anesthetic is finite, F_A will eventually begin to rise relative to F_I. If, on the other hand, blood uptake is very small, F_A and F_I quickly become nearly equal.

Blood uptake of anesthetic is expressed by the equation:

$$\dot{V}_B = \delta_{b/g}{}^{*} Q \times ((P_A - P_v)/P_B) \qquad (15\text{-}11)$$

Where $\dot{V}_B$ is blood uptake, $\delta_{b/g}$ is the blood:gas partition coefficient, Q is cardiac output, P_A is alveolar partial pressure of anesthetic, P_v is mixed venous partial pressure of anesthetic, and P_B is barometric pressure. This is the Fick equation applied to blood uptake of inhaled anesthetics. The parameters that increase or decrease the rate of rise in F_A/F_I during induction can be clearly defined and these important factors have been substantiated in experimental models (Table 15-3).

TABLE 15-3

FACTORS THAT INCREASE OR DECREASE THE RATE OF RISE OF F_A/F_I

■ INCREASE	■ DECREASE	
Low λ_B	High λ_B	The lower the blood:gas solubility, the faster the rise in F_A/F_I
Low Q	High Q	The lower the cardiac output, the faster the rise in F_A/F_I
High $\dot{V}_A$	Low $\dot{V}_A$	The higher the minute ventilation, the faster the rise in F_A/F_I
High (P_A-P_v)	Low (P_A-P_v)	At the beginning of induction, P_v is zero but rises rapidly (thus $[P_A-P_v]$ falls rapidly) and F_A/F_I increases rapidly. Later, during induction and maintenance, P_v rises more slowly so F_A/F_I rises more slowly.

Parameters as described in Equation 15–16: λ_B, blood solubility; Q, cardiac output; $\dot{V}$, minute ventilation; P_A, P_v, pulmonary arterial and venous blood partial pressure.

Before induction, P_v is zero because no anesthetic is present in the bloodstream. P_A is established with the first inspiration of anesthetic, and the alveolar to pulmonary blood partial pressure gradient, P_A-P_v, determines the rate of increase in F_A/F_I. Initially, P_A climbs at a much greater rate than P_v because circulation and dilution as well as tissue uptake together keep P_v low. As significant tissue concentrations of anesthetic start to accumulate, P_v rapidly climbs as the pulmonary blood, originally carrying no anesthetic, becomes saturated with anesthetic. This early rapid rise in F_A/F_I followed by slowing is seen in Figure 15-2.

Distribution (Tissue Uptake)

Until P_v starts to increase, the maximum F_A/F_I at a given inspired concentration of anesthetic, cardiac output, and minute ventilation are entirely dependent on the solubility of that drug in the blood as characterized by the blood:gas partition coefficient $\delta_{b/g}$. This can be seen in the time curves for the rise in F_A/F_I during induction for the various inhalation anesthetics shown in Figure 15-2. The first "knee" in each curve in Figure 15-2 represents the point at which the rapid rise in P_v begins to taper off, that is, when significant inhaled anesthetic concentrations begin to build up in the bloodstream because of distribution to and equilibration with the various tissue compartments.

Each of the three perfusion compartments—VRG, muscle, and fat—takes up anesthetic based on the Fick equation:

$$\dot{V}_{\text{Compart.}} = \lambda_{\text{Compart.}} \times Q_{\text{Compart.}} \times ((P_{a\text{Compart.}} - P_{v\text{Compart.}})/P_B) \quad (15\text{-}12)$$

where $P_{a\text{Compart.}}$ and $P_{v\text{Compart.}}$ are arterial and venous partial pressures in the tissue compartment. Mixed venous partial pressure of anesthetic in the pulmonary outflow, P_v, depends on the relative uptake in each of these perfusion compartments. To the extent that the mass and blood flow to each of these compartments differs, anesthetic uptake will differ.

As blood is equilibrating with alveolar gas, it also begins to equilibrate with the VRG, muscle, and, more gradually, the fat compartments based on perfusion. Muscle is not that different from the VRG, having partition coefficients that range from 1.2 (nitrous oxide) to 3.4 (halothane), just under a 3-fold difference; and for each anesthetic except nitrous oxide, the muscle partition coefficient is approximately double that for the VRG. Although both VRG and muscle are lean tissues, the muscle compartment equilibrates far more slowly than the VRG. The explanation comes from Equation 15-12 and the mass of the compartments relative to perfusion. The perfusion of the VRG is about 75 mL/min/100 g of tissue, whereas it is only 3 mL/min/100 g of tissue in the muscle (see Table 15-2). This 25-fold difference in perfusion between VRG (especially brain) and muscle means that even if the partition coefficients were equal, the muscle would still take 25 times longer to equilibrate with blood.

Fat is perfused to a lesser extent than muscle and its time for equilibration with blood is considerably slower because the partition coefficients are so much greater. All of the potent agents are highly lipid soluble. Partition coefficients range from 27 (desflurane) to 51 (halothane). On average, the solubility for these agents is about 25 times greater in fat than in the VRG group. Thus, fat equilibrates far more slowly with the blood and does not play a significant role in determining speed of induction. After long anesthetic exposures (>4 hours), the high saturation of fat tissue may play a role in delaying emergence.

Nitrous oxide represents an exception. Its partition coefficients are fairly similar in each tissue, it does not accumulate to any great extent and is not a very potent anesthetic. Its utility lies as an adjunct to the potent agents, and as a vehicle to speed induction.

Metabolism

Data suggest that enzymes responsible for biotransformation of inhaled anesthetics become saturated at less than anesthetizing doses of these drugs, such that metabolism plays little role in opposing induction. It may, however, have some significance to recovery from anesthesia as discussed later.

Overpressurization and the Concentration Effect

There are several ways to speed uptake and induction of anesthesia with the inhaled anesthetics. The first is *overpressurization*, which is analogous to an intravenous (IV) bolus. This is the administration of a higher partial pressure of anesthetic (F_I) than the alveolar concentration (F_A) actually desired for the patient.

Inspired anesthetic concentration (F_I) can influence both F_A and the *rate of rise* of F_A/F_I. The greater the inspired concentration of an inhaled anesthetic, the greater the rate of rise. This concentration effect has two components. The first is a concentrating effect, and the second is an augmented gas inflow effect.

For example, consider the administration of 10% anesthetic (10 parts anesthetic and 90 parts other gas) to a patient in which 50% of the anesthetic in the alveoli is absorbed by the blood. In this case 5 parts (0.5×10) anesthetic remain in the alveoli, 5 parts enter the blood, and 90 parts remain as other alveolar gas. The alveolar concentration is now $5/(90 + 5) = 5.3\%$. Consider next administering 50% anesthetic with the same 50% uptake. Now 25 parts anesthetic remain in alveoli, 25 parts pass into blood, and 50 parts remain as other alveolar gas. The alveolar concentration becomes $25/(50 + 25) = 33\%$. Giving five times as much anesthetic has led to a $33\%/5.3\% = 6.2$ times greater alveolar concentration. The higher the F_I, the greater the effect. Thus nitrous oxide, typically given in concentrations of 50 to 70%, has the greatest concentrating effect. This is why the F_A/F_I versus time curve in Figure 15-2 rises the most quickly with nitrous oxide, even though desflurane has a slightly lower blood:gas solubility. The concentrating effect becomes most prominent with the most soluble anesthetic. Therefore, halothane and isoflurane *should* benefit most at any particular concentration of anesthetic, F_I. But because equipotent concentrations for halothane and isoflurane are lower than those of the less soluble anesthetics, sevoflurane and desflurane, these agents benefit from the concentration effect less than expected—that is, *concentration outweighs solubility*. The typical inspired concentrations of N_2O are so much greater than the potent anesthetics that its low tissue solubility is of no consequence.

This isn't the complete picture; there is yet another factor to consider. As gas is leaving the alveoli for the blood, new gas at the original F_I is entering to replace that which is lost. This other aspect of the concentration effect has been called *augmented gas inflow*. Again, take the example of 10% anesthetic delivered with 50% uptake into the bloodstream. The 5 parts anesthetic absorbed by the bloodstream are replaced by gas in the circuit that is still 10% anesthetic. The 5 parts anesthetic and 90 parts other gas left in the lungs mix with 5 parts replacement gas, or $5 \times 0.10 = 0.5$ parts anesthetic. Now the alveolar concentration is $(5 + 0.5)/(100\%) = 5.5\%$ (as compared to 5.6% without augmented inflow). For 50%

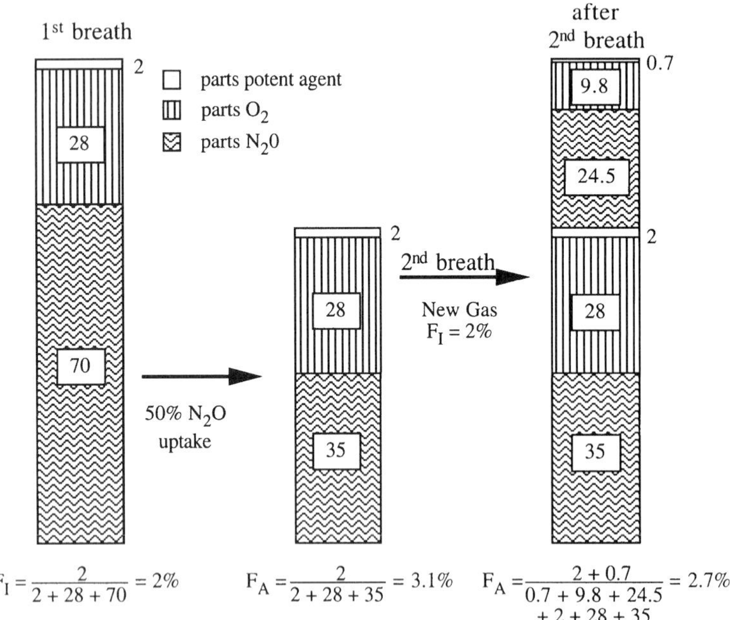

FIGURE 15-3. A graphic and the equations to demonstrate the second gas effect. In this hypothetical example, the second gas is set at 2% of a potent anesthetic and the model is set for 50% uptake of the first gas (nitrous oxide) in the first inspired breath. The second gas is concentrated because of the uptake of N_2O (**middle panel**). On replenishing the inspired second gas ($F_I = 2\%$) in the next breath, the second gas has been concentrated to be 2.7% because of the uptake of N_2O in the previous breath.

anesthetic and 50% uptake, 25 parts of anesthetic removed from the alveoli are replaced with 25 parts of 50% anesthetic, giving a new alveolar concentration of $(25 + 12.5)/(100\%) = 37.5\%$ (as compared to 50% without augmented inflow). Thus five times the F_I leads to $37.5/5.5 = 6.8$ times greater F_A (compared to 6.2 times without augmented gas inflow). Of course, this cycle of absorbed gas being replaced by fresh gas inflow is continuous and has a finite rate so our example is a simplification.

Second Gas Effect

A special case of concentration effect applies to administration of a potent anesthetic with nitrous oxide—that is, two gases simultaneously. Along with the concentration of potent agent in the alveoli via its uptake, there is further concentration via the uptake of nitrous oxide, a process called the *second gas effect*. The second gas is the potent agent. The principle is simple (Figs. 15-3 and 15-4). Consider, for example, administering 2% of a potent anesthetic in 70% nitrous oxide and 28% oxygen. In this case, nitrous oxide, with its extremely high vapor pressure (despite low solubility), partitions into the blood more rapidly than the potent anesthetic, decreasing the alveolar N_2O concentration by some amount (e.g., by 50%). Ignoring uptake of the potent anesthetic, the uptake of N_2O is 35 parts, leaving 35 parts N_2O, 28 parts O_2, and 2 parts potent agent in the alveoli. The second gas is now present in the alveoli at a concentration of $2/(2 + 35 + 28) = 3.1\%$. The second gas has been concentrated.

Ventilation Effects

As indicated by Figure 15-2 and Equation 15-3, inhaled anesthetics with very low tissue solubility have an extremely rapid rise in F_A/F_I with induction. This suggests that there is very little room to improve this rate by increasing or decreasing ventilation. This is consistent with the experimental evidence shown in Figure 15-5. The greater the solubility of an inhaled anesthetic, the more rapidly it is absorbed by the bloodstream, such that anesthetic delivery to the lungs may be rate limiting. Therefore, for more soluble anesthetics, augmentation of anesthetic delivery by increasing minute ventilation also increases the rate of rise in F_A/F_I.

Spontaneous minute ventilation is not static, however, and to the extent that the inhaled anesthetics depress spontaneous ventilation with increasing inspired concentration, V_A will decrease and so will the rate of rise of F_A/F_I. This is demonstrated in Figure 15-5. This negative feedback should not be considered

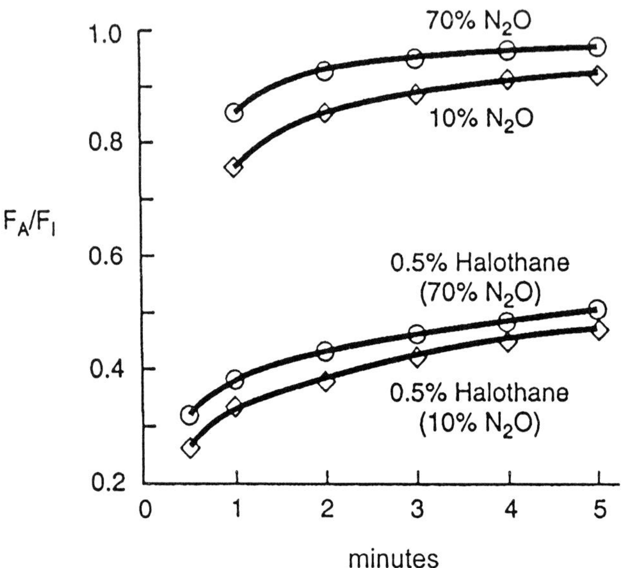

FIGURE 15-4. The concentration effect is demonstrated in the top half of the graph from dogs receiving nitrous oxide. Administration of 70% nitrous oxide produces a more rapid rise in the F_A/F_I ratio of nitrous oxide than administration of 10% nitrous oxide. The second gas effect is demonstrated in the lower graphs. The F_A/F_I ratio for 0.5% halothane rises more rapidly when given with 70% nitrous oxide than when given with 10% nitrous oxide. (Adapted from Epstein R, Rackow H, Salanitre E *et al*: Influence of the concentration effect on the uptake of anesthetic mixtures: The second gas effect. Anesthesiology 25:364, 1964.)

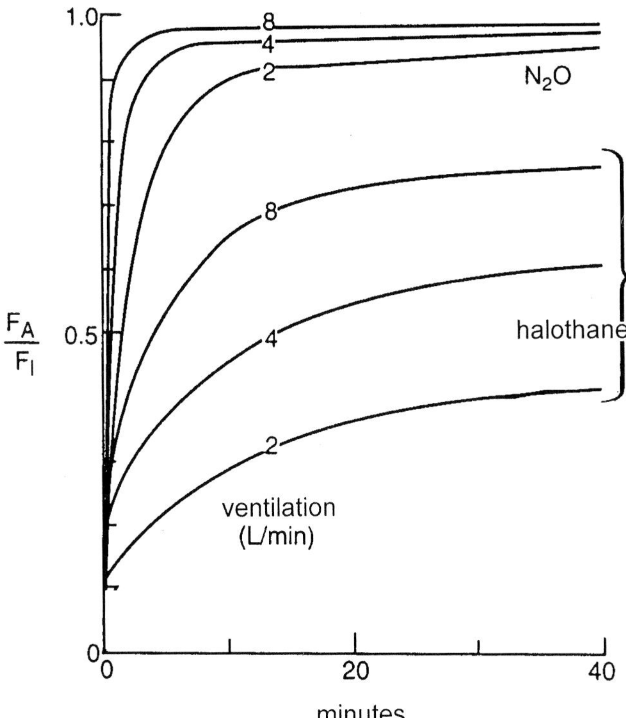

FIGURE 15-5. The F_A/F_I ratio rises more rapidly if ventilation is increased from 2 to 8 L/min. Solubility modifies this impact of ventilation; for example, the effect is greatest with the least soluble anesthetic, nitrous oxide (top 3 lines), and least with the more-soluble anesthetic, halothane. (Adapted from Eger EI II: Ventilation, circulation and uptake. In Eger EI II (ed): Anesthetic Uptake and Action, p 122. Baltimore, Williams & Wilkins, 1974.)

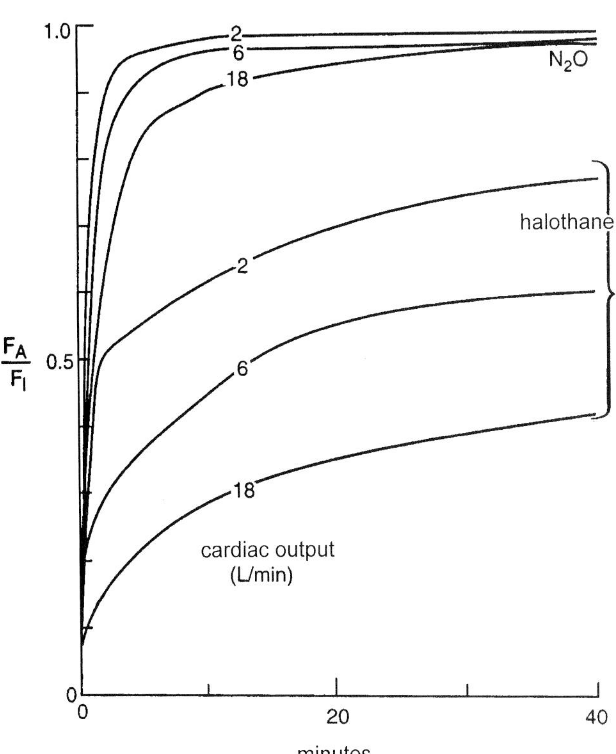

FIGURE 15-6. If ventilation is fixed, an increase in cardiac output from 2 to 18 L/min will decrease the alveolar anesthetic concentration by augmenting uptake, thereby slowing the rise of the F_A/F_I ratio. This effect is most prominent with the more-soluble anesthetics (halothane) than with the less-soluble anesthetics (nitrous oxide). (Adapted from Eger EI II: Ventilation, circulation and uptake. In Eger EI II (ed): Anesthetic Uptake and Action, p 131. Baltimore, Williams & Wilkins, 1974.)

a drawback of the inhaled anesthetics, because the respiratory depression produced at high anesthetic concentrations essentially slows the rise in F_A/F_I. This might arguably add a margin of safety in preventing an overdose.

Perfusion Effects

As with ventilation, cardiac output is not static during the course of induction. For the insoluble agents, changes in cardiac output do not affect the rate of rise of F_A/F_I to a great extent, but for the more soluble agents the effect is noticeable, as seen in Figure 15-6. However, as inspired concentration increases, greater cardiovascular depression reduces anesthetic uptake and actually increases the rate of rise of F_A/F_I. This positive feedback can rapidly lead to profound cardiovascular depression. Figure 15-6 presents experimental data in which lower cardiac outputs lead to a much more rapid rise in F_A/F_I when $\dot{V}_A$ is held constant. This more rapid rise is greater than can be accounted for just by concentration effect.

Ventilation–Perfusion Mismatching

Ventilation and perfusion are normally fairly well matched in healthy patients such that P_A (alveolar partial pressure)/ P_I and P_a (arterial partial pressure)/ P_I are the same curve. If significant intrapulmonary shunt occurs, however, as in the case of inadvertent bronchial intubation, the rate of rise of alveolar and arterial anesthetic partial pressures can be affected. The effects, however, depend on the solubility of the anesthetic, as seen in Figure 15-7. Ventilation of the intubated lung is dramatically increased while perfusion increases slightly. The nonintubated lung receives no ventilation, while perfusion decreases slightly. For the less-soluble anesthetics, increased ventilation of the intubated lung cannot appreciably increase alveolar partial pressure relative to inspired concentration on that side, but alveolar partial pressure on the nonintubated side is essentially zero. Pulmonary mixed venous blood, therefore, comprises nearly equal parts blood containing normal amounts of anesthetic and blood containing no anesthetic, that is, diluted relative to normal. Thus the rate of rise in P_a relative to P_I is significantly reduced. There is less total anesthetic uptake, so the rate of rise of P_A relative to P_I increases even though induction of anesthesia is slowed because CNS partial pressure equilibrates with P_a. For the more soluble anesthetics, increased ventilation of the intubated lung *does* increase the alveolar partial pressure relative to inspired concentration on that side. Pulmonary venous blood from the intubated side contains a higher concentration of anesthetic that lessens the dilution by blood from the nonintubated side. Thus the rate of rise of P_a/P_I is not as depressed as that for the less soluble anesthetics, and induction of anesthesia is less delayed.

Elimination

Percutaneous and Visceral Loss

Although the loss of inhaled anesthetics via the skin is very small, it does occur and is the greatest for nitrous oxide. These anesthetics also pass across gastrointestinal viscera and the

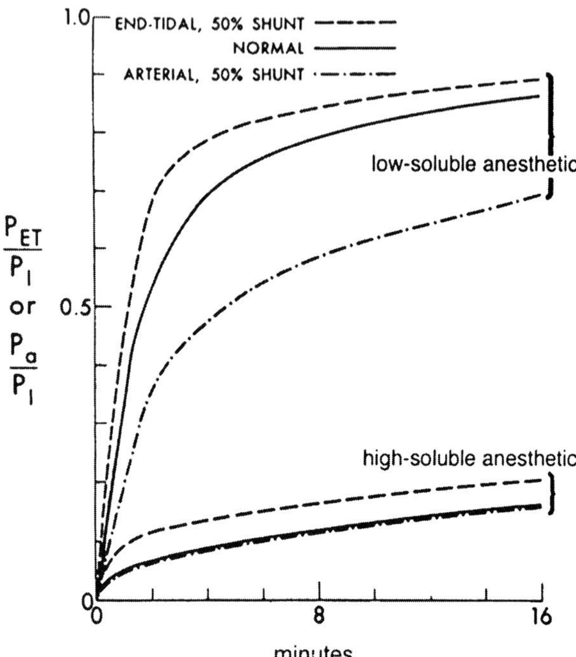

FIGURE 15-7. When no ventilation/perfusion abnormalities exist, the alveolar (P_A) or end-tidal (P_{ET}) and arterial (P_a) anesthetic partial pressures rise together (*continuous lines*) toward the inspired partial pressure (P_I). When 50% of the cardiac output is shunted through the lungs, the rate of rise of the end-tidal partial pressure (*dashed line*) is accelerated while the rate of rise of the arterial partial pressure (*dot-dashed line*) is slowed. The greatest effect of shunting is found with the least soluble anesthetics. (Adapted from Eger EI II, Severinghaus JW: Effect of uneven pulmonary distribution of blood and gas on induction with inhalation anesthetics. Anesthesiology 25:620, 1964.)

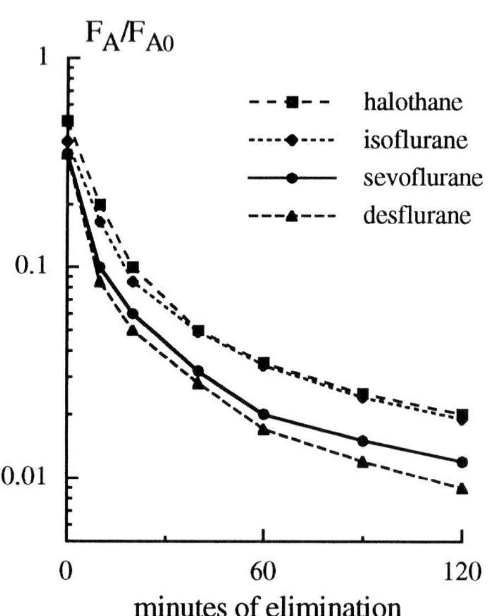

FIGURE 15-8. Elimination of anesthetic gases is defined as the ratio of end-tidal anesthetic concentration (F_A) to the last F_A during administration and immediately before the beginning of elimination (F_{AO}). During the 120-minute period after ending the anesthetic delivery, the elimination of sevoflurane and desflurane is 2 to 2.5 times faster than isoflurane or halothane (note logarithmic scale for the ordinate). (Adapted from Yasuda N, Lockhart SH, Eger EI II *et al*: Comparison of kinetics of sevoflurane and isoflurane in humans. Anesth Analg 72:316, 1991; and Yasuda N, Lockhart SH, Eger EI II *et al*: Kinetics of desflurane, isoflurane, and halothane in humans. Anesthesiology 74:489, 1991.)

pleura. During open abdominal or thoracic surgery there is some anesthetic loss via these routes. Relative to losses by all other routes, losses via percutaneous and visceral routes are insignificant.

Diffusion between Tissues

Using more elaborate mathematical modeling of inhaled anesthetic pharmacokinetics than presented here, several laboratories have derived a five-compartment model that best describes tissue compartments. These compartments are the alveoli, the VRG, the muscle, the fat, and one additional compartment. Current opinion is that this fifth compartment represents adipose tissue adjacent to lean tissue that receives anesthetic via intertissue diffusion. This transfer of anesthetic is not insignificant, and may account for up to one-third of uptake during long administration.

Metabolism

Inhaled anesthetic biotransformation is discussed in more depth elsewhere in this chapter. Metabolism is greatest for halothane, up to 50% of loss. In fact, there is evidence that decreases in the alveolar concentrations of halothane during emergence outpace those for isoflurane, presumably because of this significant metabolism. Experimentally, it has been determined that metabolism does not significantly affect recovery from isoflurane.

Exhalation and Recovery

Recovery from anesthesia, like induction, depends on anesthetic solubility, cardiac output, and minute ventilation. Solubility is the primary determinant of the rate of fall of F_A (Fig. 15-8). The greater the solubility of inhaled anesthetic, the larger the capacity for absorption in the bloodstream and tissues. The "reservoir" of anesthetic in the body at the end of administration depends on tissue solubility (which determines the capacity) and the dose and duration of anesthetic (which determine how much of that capacity is filled). Recovery from anesthesia, or "washout," is usually expressed as the ratio of expired fractional concentration of anesthetic (F_E) to the expired concentration at time zero (F_{E0}) when the anesthetic was discontinued (or F_A/F_{A0}). Elimination curves of low and high soluble anesthetics are shown in Figure 15-9. The longer the duration of a highly soluble anesthetic, the greater the reservoir of anesthetic in the body, and the higher the curve seen in the right half of Figure 15-9. This effect is nearly absent with low soluble agents such as nitrous oxide, desflurane, and sevoflurane.[3]

There are two major pharmacokinetic differences between recovery and induction. First, whereas overpressurization can increase the speed of induction, there is no "under pressurization." Both induction and recovery rates depend on the P_A to P_v gradient, and P_A can never fall below zero. Second, whereas all tissues begin induction with zero anesthetic, each begins recovery with quite different anesthetic concentrations. The VRG tissues begin recovery with the same anesthetic partial pressure as that in alveoli, since $P_{CNS} = P_{blood} = P_{alveoli}$. The partial pressures in muscle and fat depend on the inspired concentration during anesthesia, the duration of administration, and the anesthetic tissue solubilities. As long as an arterial-to-tissue partial pressure gradient exists, these tissues will absorb anesthetic—especially fat, since it is a huge potential reservoir whose anesthetic partial pressures are typically low after hours of anesthesia. After discontinuation of anesthesia, muscle and fat may continue to absorb anesthetic, even hours later. The redistribution continues until blood/alveolar anesthetic partial

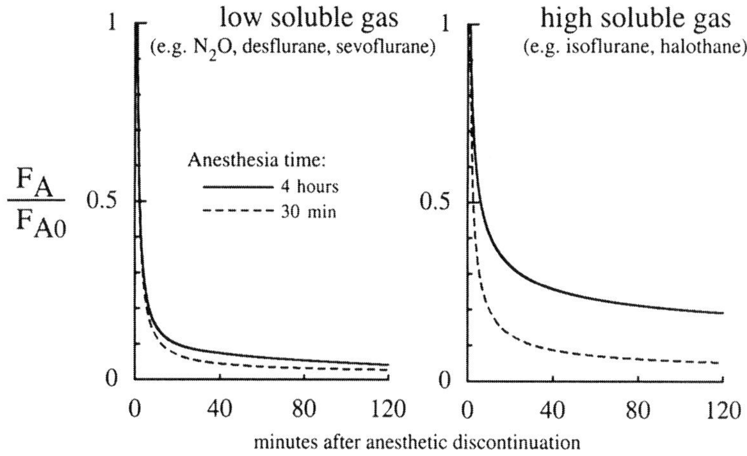

FIGURE 15-9. Both solubility and duration of anesthesia affect the decrease of the alveolar concentration (F_A) from its value immediately preceding the cessation of anesthetic administration (F_{AO}). A longer anesthetic time (from 15 minutes to 240 minutes) only slightly slows the decrease with low soluble anesthetics (**left graph**). An agent with a higher blood and tissue solubility (**right graph**) slows the elimination of the anesthetic and enhances the effect of duration. (Adapted from Stoelting RK, Eger EI II: The effects of ventilation and anesthetic solubility on recovery from anesthesia: An in vivo and analog analysis before and after equilibrium. Anesthesiology 30:290, 1969.)

pressure falls below tissue partial pressure. This redistribution causes the early rate of decline in alveolar anesthetic concentration during recovery to exceed its increase during induction.

Because VRG tissues are highly perfused and washout of anesthetic is mostly via elimination from these tissues early in recovery, all anesthetics regardless of duration of administration, have approximately the same rate of elimination to 50% of F_{E0}. Unfortunately, halving the CNS concentration of anesthetic is rarely sufficient for waking the patient. More commonly, 80 to 90% of inhaled anesthetic must be eliminated before emergence. At these amounts of washout, the more soluble anesthetics are eliminated more slowly than less soluble agents.

Diffusion Hypoxia

During recovery from anesthesia, washout of high concentrations of nitrous oxide can lower alveolar concentrations of oxygen and carbon dioxide, a phenomenon called *diffusion hypoxia*. The resulting alveolar hypoxia can cause hypoxemia, and alveolar hypocarbia can depress respiratory drive, which may exacerbate hypoxemia. It is therefore appropriate to initiate recovery from nitrous oxide anesthesia with 100% oxygen rather than less concentrated O_2/air mixtures.

CLINICAL OVERVIEW OF CURRENT INHALED ANESTHETICS

Halothane

Halothane, a relatively nonflammable liquid, is the most potent of the currently used volatile anesthetics. It is an alkane—a halogen-substituted ethane derivative (see Fig. 15-1)—that was placed into clinical use in 1956. The halogenated structure provided nonflammability. It has an intermediate blood solubility and is relatively nonpungent; hence, it can be inhaled via the face mask. The carbon–fluorine bond is important in providing nonflammability of halothane at room temperature and the trifluorocarbon group contributes to its molecular stability. Despite its chemical stability, halothane oxidizes spontaneously and is broken down by ultraviolet light. It decomposes to hydrochloric acid (HCL), hydrobromic acid (Hbr), chloride (CL^-), bromide (Br^-), and phosgene ($COCl_2$). To prevent this decomposition, halothane is stored in amber-colored bottles and 0.01% thymol is added as a preservative to prevent spontaneous oxidative decomposition. The thymol preservative can "gum up" vaporizers, mandating a more difficult and more frequent cleaning schedule than that for vaporizers specific to other volatile anesthetics. Halothane also is adsorbed by contact with dry soda lime and broken down to BCDFE (2-bromo-2-chloro-1,1-difluoroethene), which has organ toxicity in animal models. In humans, halothane has been associated with an immune-mediated hepatitis and a sensitization to epinephrine resulting in arrhythmias. It also has been associated with bradycardia when used in the pediatric population.

Enflurane

Enflurane, a halogenated methyl ethyl ether, is an isomer of isoflurane (see Fig. 15-1). It is a nonflammable liquid at room temperature and is pungent. Its use in high concentrations has been associated with seizure-like activity on the EEG. Its metabolism has resulted in an increase in blood fluoride concentration and, rarely, with a renal concentrating deficiency. Its popularity has generally been reserved owing to competition from isoflurane—the near-simultaneously introduced volatile anesthetic, which has few side effects—and more recently, the introduction of new anesthetics with lower solubilities.

Isoflurane

Isoflurane, a halogenated methyl ethyl ether, is a clear, nonflammable liquid at room temperature and has a high degree of pungency (see Fig. 15-1). The second most potent of the volatile anesthetics in clinical use, isoflurane has great physical stability and undergoes essentially no deterioration during storage for up to 5 years or on exposure to sunlight. It has become the gold standard anesthetic since its introduction in the 1970s. There has been a brief period of controversy concerning the use of isoflurane in patients with coronary disease because of the possibility for coronary "steal," arising from the potent effects of isoflurane on coronary vasodilation. In clinical use, however, this has been, at most, a rare occurrence.

Desflurane

Desflurane is a fluorinated methyl ethyl ether that differs from isoflurane by just one atom: a fluorine atom is substituted for a chlorine atom on the α-ethyl component of isoflurane (see Fig. 15-1). The process of completely fluorinating the ether molecule has several effects. It decreases blood and tissue solubility (the blood:gas solubility of desflurane equals that of nitrous oxide), and it results in a loss of potency (the MAC of desflurane is five times higher than isoflurane). Moreover, the complete fluorination of the methyl ether molecule results in a high vapor pressure (owing to decreased intermolecular attraction). Thus, a new vaporizer technology has been developed to deliver a regulated concentration of desflurane as a gas. A heated, pressurized vaporizer requiring electrical power and more frequent servicing is required. One of the advantages of desflurane is the near-absent metabolism to serum trifluoroacetate. This makes immune-mediated hepatitis extremely unlikely. Desflurane is the most pungent of the volatile anesthetics and cannot be administered via the face mask as it results in coughing, salivation, breath holding, and laryngospasm. In extremely dry CO_2 absorbers, desflurane (and to a lesser extent isoflurane, enflurane, and sevoflurane) degrades to form carbon monoxide. Desflurane has the lowest blood:gas solubility of the potent volatile anesthetics; moreover, its fat solubility is roughly half of that of the other volatile anesthetics. Thus, desflurane offers a theoretical advantage in long surgical procedures by virtue of decreased tissue saturation. Desflurane has been associated with tachycardia, hypertension, and, in select cases, myocardial ischemia when used in high concentrations or rapidly increasing the inspired concentration (without using opioid adjuvants to prevent such a response).

Sevoflurane

Sevoflurane is a sweet-smelling, completely fluorinated methyl isopropyl ether (see Fig. 15-1). Its vapor pressure is most similar to that of enflurane and it can be used in a conventional vaporizer. The blood:gas solubility of sevoflurane is second only to desflurane in terms of potent volatile anesthetics. Sevoflurane is approximately half as potent as isoflurane, and some of the preservation of potency, despite fluorination, is because of the bulky propyl side chain on the ether molecule. Sevoflurane has minimal odor, no pungency, and is a potent bronchodilator. These attributes make sevoflurane an excellent candidate for administration via the face mask on induction of anesthesia in both children and adults. Sevoflurane is half as potent a coronary vasodilator as isoflurane, but is 10 to 20 times more vulnerable to metabolism than isoflurane. Like that of enflurane and methoxyflurane, the metabolism of sevoflurane results in inorganic fluoride; the increase in plasma fluoride after sevoflurane administration has not been associated with renal concentrating defects, as is the case with methoxyflurane. Unlike other potent volatile anesthetics, sevoflurane is not metabolized to trifluoroacetate; rather, it is metabolized to an acyl halide (hexafluoroisopropanol). This does not stimulate formation of antibodies, and immune-mediated hepatitis has not been reported with sevoflurane. Sevoflurane can form carbon monoxide during exposure to dry CO_2 absorbents and an exothermic reaction in dry absorbent has resulted in canister fires. Sevoflurane breaks down in the presence of the carbon dioxide absorber to form a vinyl halide called compound A. Compound A has been shown to be a dose-dependent nephrotoxin in rats, but has not been associated with renal injury in human volunteers or patients, with or without renal impairment, even when fresh gas flows are 1 L/min or less.

Xenon

Xenon is an inert gas. Difficult to obtain, and hence extremely expensive, it has received considerable interest in the last few years because it has many characteristics approaching those of an "ideal" inhaled anesthetic.[5,6] Its blood:gas partition coefficient is 0.14, and unlike the other potent volatile anesthetics (except methoxyflurane), xenon provides some degree of analgesia. Unfortunately, the MAC in humans is 71%, which might prove to be a limitation. It is nonexplosive, nonpungent, and odorless, and thus can be inhaled with ease. In addition, it does not produce significant myocardial depression.[5] Because of its scarcity and high cost, new anesthetic systems need to be developed to provide for recycling of xenon. If this proves to be too difficult from either a technical or patient safety standpoint, it may be necessary to use it in a very low, or closed, fresh gas flow system to reduce wastage.

Nitrous Oxide

Nitrous oxide is a sweet-smelling, nonflammable gas of low potency (MAC = 104%) and is relatively insoluble in blood. It is most commonly administered as an anesthetic adjuvant in combination with opioids or volatile anesthetics during the conduct of general anesthesia. Although not flammable, nitrous oxide will support combustion. Unlike the potent volatile anesthetics in clinical use, nitrous oxide does not produce significant skeletal muscle relaxation, but it does have documented analgesic effects. Despite a long track record of use, controversy has surrounded nitrous oxide in four areas: its role in postoperative nausea and vomiting, its potential toxic effects on cell function via inactivation of vitamin B_{12}, its adverse effects related to absorption and expansion into air-filled structures and bubbles, and last, its effect on embryonic development. The one concern that seems most valid and most clinically relevant is the ability of nitrous oxide to expand air-filled spaces because of its greater solubility in blood compared to nitrogen. Several closed gas spaces such as the bowel and middle ear exist in the body and other spaces may occur as a result of disease or surgery such as a pneumothorax. The nitrogen cannot be removed readily via the bloodstream. Unfortunately, nitrous oxide delivered to a patient diffuses from the blood into these closed gas spaces quite easily such that the spaces must increase pressure and potentially expand. Movement of nitrous oxide into these spaces continues until the partial pressure equals that of the blood and alveoli. Compliant spaces will continue to expand until sufficient pressure is generated to oppose further N_2O flow into the space. The higher the inspired concentration of nitrous oxide, the higher the partial pressure required for equilibration.

Seventy-five percent N_2O can expand a pneumothorax to double or triple its size in 10 and 30 minutes, respectively. Air-filled cuffs of pulmonary artery catheters and endotracheal tubes also expand with the use of N_2O, possibly causing tissue damage via increased pressure in the pulmonary artery or trachea, respectively.[6,7] In a rabbit model, the volume of an air embolus resulting in cardiovascular compromise is less during coadministration of nitrous oxide.[8] Accumulation of nitrous oxide in the middle ear can diminish hearing postoperatively[9] and is relatively contraindicated for tympanoplasty because the increased pressure can dislodge a tympanic graft.

NEUROPHARMACOLOGY OF INHALED ANESTHETICS

The inhaled anesthetics establish the anesthetic state by effects on spontaneous neuronal activity and metabolism. The exact anesthetic mechanisms of inhaled agents remain poorly understood and the associated nervous system effects may in part be mediated by these undetermined mechanisms. Therefore as a whole, the current understanding of inhaled anesthetic neuropharmacology tends to be more descriptive than mechanistic in nature.

The mechanisms of anesthesia are elusive partly because there is no uniform definition of when the brain is anesthetized;

however, a useful definition may be a brain that is incapable of self-awareness or subsequent recall. This definition is helpful conceptually, but from a practical standpoint it is difficult to know when the brain is no longer self-aware or will have no recall, and to know the dose of inhaled anesthetic at that point. The ability to determine, establish, and maintain this level of anesthesia is part of the art of anesthesia. It depends on the integration of knowledge of inhaled anesthetic pharmacokinetics and pharmacodynamics, direct observation of the patient, and interpretation of data from a complex array of monitors. With the recent advent of the processed electroencephalogram (EEG) monitor, the first, albeit crude, index of anesthetic "depth" via continuous real-time analysis of the patient's EEG might provide relevant information. The utility of this device remains controversial, and it is likely that relevant information might need tailoring to each anesthetic regimen.

Minimum Alveolar Concentration

The pharmacodynamic effects of inhaled anesthetics must be
3 based on a dose, and this dose is the *minimum alveolar concentration* or *MAC*. MAC is the alveolar concentration of an anesthetic at one atmosphere that prevents movement in response to a surgical stimulus in 50% of patients. It is analogous to the ED_{50} expressed for intravenous drugs. A variety of surgical stimuli have been used to establish the MAC for each inhaled anesthetic, but the classic, defining, noxious stimulus is incision of the abdomen. Likewise, skeletal muscle movement is the defining patient response, but other responses have been used to establish MAC as well. Experimentally determined MAC values for humans for the inhaled anesthetics are shown in Table 15-1.

The 95% confidence ranges for MAC are approximately ± 25% of the listed MAC values. Manufacturer's recommendations and clinical experience establish 1.2 to 1.3 times MAC as a dose that consistently prevents patient movement during surgical stimuli. Loss of consciousness typically precedes the absence of stimulus-induced movement by a wide margin. While 1.2 to 1.3 MAC values do not *absolutely* ensure the defining criteria for brain anesthesia (the absence of self-awareness and recall), vast clinical experience suggests it is extremely unlikely for a patient to be aware of, or to recall the surgical incision at these anesthetic concentrations unless other conditions exist such that MAC is increased in that patient (Table 15-4).

Concentrations of inhaled anesthetics that provide loss of self-awareness and recall are about 0.4 to 0.5 MAC. Several lines of reasoning lead to this conclusion. First, most patients receiving only 50% nitrous oxide (approximately 0.4 to 0.5 MAC) as in a typical dentist's office will have no recall of their procedure during N_2O administration. Second, various studies have shown that a shift in EEG dominance to the anterior leads, that is, the shift from self-aware to nonself-aware, accompanies loss of consciousness, and in primates, the EEG

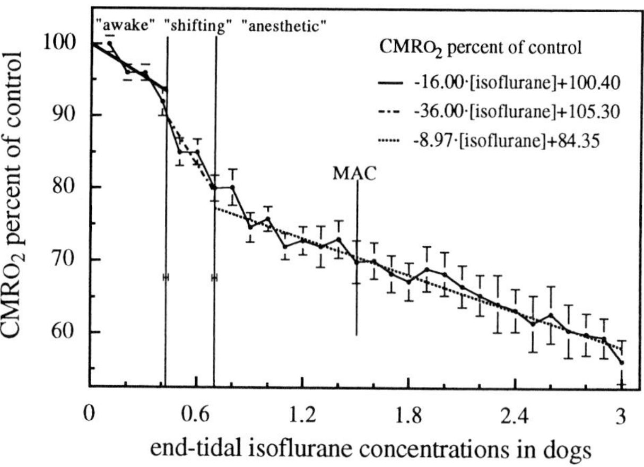

FIGURE 15-10. The effects of halothane on $CMRO_2$ as a percentage of control ("awake"). $CMRO_2$ is plotted versus end-tidal isoflurane concentration. Regression lines for changes in $CMRO_2$ are drawn for each EEG determined area. The pattern depicted here is characteristic of all of the anesthetics examined (enflurane, halothane, and isoflurane). (Adapted from Stullken EH Jr, Milde JH, Michenfelder JD *et al*: The non-linear responses of cerebral metabolism to low concentrations of halothane, enflurane, isoflurane and thiopental. Anesthesiology 46:28, 1977.)

shift and loss of consciousness occur at 0.5 MAC.[10] Third, in dogs, loss of consciousness accompanies a sudden nonlinear fall in cerebral metabolic rate (CMR) at approximately 0.5 MAC (Fig. 15-10).

MAC values can be established for any measurable response. MAC-awake, or the alveolar concentration of anesthetic at which a patient opens his or her eyes to command, varies from 0.15 to 0.5 MAC.[11] Interestingly, transition from awake to unconscious and back typically shows some hysteresis, in that it quite consistently takes 0.4 to 0.5 MAC to lose consciousness, but less than that (as low as 0.15 MAC) to regain consciousness. This may be because of the speed of alveolar washin versus washout.[12] MAC-BAR, or the alveolar concentration of anesthetic that blunts adrenergic responses to noxious stimuli, has likewise been established and is approximately 50% higher than standard MAC.[13] MAC also has been established for discreet levels of EEG activity, such as onset of burst suppression or isoelectricity.

Standard MAC values are roughly additive. Administering 0.5 MAC of a potent agent and 0.5 MAC of nitrous oxide is equivalent to 1 MAC of potent agent in terms of preventing *patient movement*, although this does not hold over the entire range of N_2O doses. MAC effects for other response parameters are not necessarily additive. Because MAC-movement probably differs from MAC for various secondary side effects (such hypothetical situations as "MAC-dysrhythmia," "MAC-hypotension," or "MAC-tachycardia," etc.), combinations of a potent agent and nitrous oxide may decrease or increase these secondary effects relative to potent agent alone. For example, combining 0.6 MAC of nitrous oxide with 0.6 MAC of isoflurane produces less hypotension than 1.2 MAC of isoflurane alone because isoflurane is a more potent vasodilator and myocardial depressant at equivalent MAC than N_2O.

Various factors increase (Table 15-4) or decrease (Table 15-5) MAC. Unfortunately, no single mechanism explains these alterations in MAC, supporting the view that anesthesia is the net result of numerous and widely varying physiologic alterations. In general, those factors that increase CNS metabolic activity and neurotransmission, increase CNS neurotransmitter levels, and upregulation of CNS responses to chronically depressed neurotransmitter levels (as in chronic alcoholism) also seem to increase MAC. Conversely, those factors that

TABLE 15-4

FACTORS THAT INCREASE MAC

- Increased central neurotransmitter levels (monoamine oxidase inhibitors, acute dextroamphetamine administration, cocaine, ephedrine, levodopa)
- Hyperthermia
- Chronic ethanol abuse (determined in humans)
- Hypernatremia

TABLE 15-5

FACTORS THAT DECREASE MAC

- Increasing age
- Metabolic acidosis
- Hypoxia (PaO_2, 38 mm Hg)
- Induced hypotension (MAP <50 mmHg)
- Decreased central neurotransmitter levels (alpha-methyldopa, reserpine, chronic dextroamphetamine administration, levodopa)
- Alpha-2 agonists
- Hypothermia
- Hyponatremia
- Lithium
- Hypoosmolality
- Pregnancy
- Acute ethanol administration[a]
- Ketamine
- Pancuronium[a]
- Physostigmine (10 times clinical dose)
- Neostigmine (10 times clinical dose)
- Lidocaine
- Opioids
- Opioid agonist–antagonist analgesics
- Barbiturates[a]
- Chlorpromazine[a]
- Diazepam[a]
- Hydroxyzine[a]
- Δ-9-Tetrahydrocannabinol
- Verapamil
- Anemia (<4.3 mL O_2/dL blood)

[a]Determined in humans.

decrease CNS metabolic activity and neurotransmission, decrease CNS neurotransmitter levels, and downregulation of CNS responses to chronically elevated neurotransmitter levels seem to decrease MAC. Many notable factors do not alter MAC, including duration of inhaled anesthetic administration, gender, type of surgical stimulation, thyroid function, hypo- or hypercarbia, metabolic alkalosis, hyperkalemia, and magnesium levels. However, there may be a genetic component influencing MAC. Redheaded females have a 19% increase in MAC compared to dark-haired females.[14] These data suggest involvement of mutations of the *MCIR* allele. Variants of the *MCIR* allele also have been implicated in altering analgesic responses to a κ opioid.[15] MAC also can vary in relationship to genotype and chromosomal substitutions as shown in rats.[16]

The Effect of Age on MAC

The MAC for each of the potent anesthetic gases shows a clear, age-related change (Fig. 15-11). MAC decreases with age and there are similarities between agents in the decline in MAC and age. Excluding data in patients less than 1 year of age (where MAC can be lower[17]), there is a linear model that describes the decrease in MAC with increasing age.[18] The slope of this model is: MAC = $a(10^{bx})$, where "x" is the difference in age in years from 40, "b" is –.00269, and "a" is the MAC at age 40. This equation defines a change in MAC of approximately 6% per decade, a 22% decrease in MAC from age 40 to age 80, and a 27% decrease in MAC from age 1 to 40 years. MAC is typically expressed for an intermediate age (40 years), and these are:

- Halothane 0.75%
- Isoflurane 1.17%
- Enflurane 1.63%
- Sevoflurane 1.80%

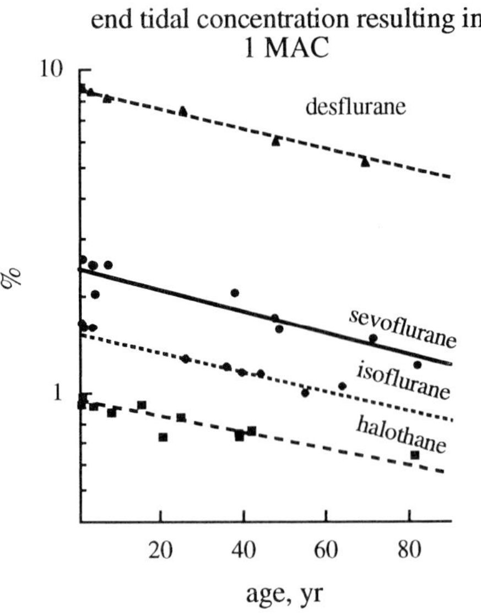

FIGURE 15-11. Effect of age on MAC. Regression lines are fitted to published values from separate studies. Data are from patients ages 1 to 80 years. (Adapted from Mapleson WW: Effect of age on MAC in humans: A meta-analysis. Br J Anaesth 76:179, 1996.)

- Desflurane 6.60%
- Nitrous Oxide 104.00%

Other Alterations in Neurophysiology

The four, current, widely used, potent agents, halothane, isoflurane, desflurane, and sevoflurane, all have reasonably similar effects on a wide range of parameters including cerebral metabolic rate, the EEG, cerebral blood flow (CBF), and flow–metabolism coupling. There are notable differences in effects on intracerebral pressure, cerebrospinal fluid production and resorption, CO_2 vasoreactivity, CBF autoregulation, and cerebral protection. Nitrous oxide departs from the potent agents in several important respects, and is therefore discussed separately.

Cerebral Metabolic Rate and Electroencephalogram

All of the potent agents depress cerebral metabolic rate (CMR) to varying degrees in a nonlinear fashion. In isoflurane-anesthetized dogs, there is a sudden decrease in $CMRO_2$ paralleling a change in the EEG from an awake to anesthetized pattern at about 0.4 to 0.6 MAC as seen in Figure 15-10.[19] For most of the potent agents, CMR is decreased only to the extent that spontaneous cortical neuronal activity (as reflected in the EEG) is decreased. Once spontaneous cortical neuronal activity is absent (an isoelectric EEG), no further decreases in CMR are generated. Halothane is the exception. Halothane causes a 20 to 30% decrease in CMR at normal clinical concentrations, and at 4.5% produces an isoelectric EEG. Further increases in inspired concentration cause further decreases in $CMRO_2$. This further depression of $CMRO_2$ is because of toxic effects on oxidative phosphorylation. Toxic effects begin at concentrations as low as 2.3%, at which point brain lactate concentrations increase, but this dose is typically well above those used clinically for halothane.

Isoflurane causes a larger MAC-dependent depression of CMR than halothane, and does not depress $CMRO_2$ once an isoelectric EEG is produced.[20] Because of this greater depression in neuronal activity, isoflurane abolishes EEG activity at doses used clinically and can usually be tolerated from a hemodynamic standpoint.[38] Desflurane and sevoflurane both cause decreases in CMR similar to isoflurane.[21,22] Interestingly, while both desflurane and sevoflurane depress the EEG and abolish activity at clinically tolerated doses of approximately 2 MAC,[21,22] in *dogs* desflurane-induced isoelectric EEG reverts to continuous activity with time despite an unchanging MAC, a property unique to desflurane.[21] Sevoflurane at isoelectric EEG concentrations in *cats* is not associated with a reversion to continuous EEG activity, although species differences could account for the differing results.[23] The reversion from an isoelectric to a continuous EEG does not occur in desflurane anesthetized swine[24] and there are no case reports of this phenomenon in humans.

Potential for cerebral toxicity has been studied for sevoflurane as compared to halothane. At normal CO_2 and blood pressure no evidence of sevoflurane toxicity exists.[25] With extreme hyperventilation to decrease cerebral blood flow by half, brain lactate levels increase, but significantly less than with halothane. There are conflicting data as to whether sevoflurane has a proconvulsant effect.[22,23,26] High, long-lasting concentrations of sevoflurane (1.5 to 2.0 MAC), a sudden increase in cerebral sevoflurane concentrations, and hypocapnia can trigger EEG abnormalities that often are associated with increases in heart rate in both adults and children.[27,28] This has raised the question as to the appropriateness of sevoflurane in patients with epilepsy.[29]

Cerebral Blood Flow, Flow–Metabolism Coupling, and Autoregulation

4 All of the potent agents increase CBF in a dose-dependent manner. Halothane is a very potent cerebral vasodilator[30] and causes the greatest increase in CBF per MAC-multiple. Because of this, halothane is rarely used in neurosurgery today, even though it was the dominant anesthetic for these cases until the early 1970s. Despite causing the greatest increase in CBF, the vasodilating effects of halothane are blunted by hyperventilating subjects to a $PaCO_2$ of 25 mm Hg prior to or simultaneous to the administration of halothane.[31]

Isoflurane, sevoflurane, and desflurane cause far less cerebral vasodilation per MAC-multiple than halothane (Fig. 15-12).[30,32,33] In human studies, isoflurane produces insignificant or no changes in CBF.[34] Desflurane and sevoflurane both influence CBF in a fashion similar to isoflurane.[21,22] All of these inhaled anesthetic agents affect CBF in a time-dependent as well as dose-dependent manner. In animals, an initial dose-dependent increase in CBF with halothane and isoflurane administration recovers to preinduction levels approximately 2 to 5 hours after induction. The mechanism of this recovery is unclear.

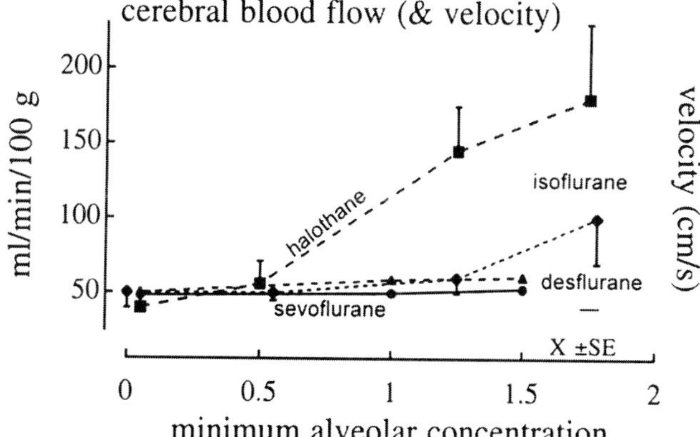

FIGURE 15-12. Cerebral blood flow (and velocity) measured in the presence of normocapnia and in the absence of surgical stimulation in volunteers receiving halothane or isoflurane. At light levels of anesthesia, halothane (but not isoflurane) increased cerebral blood flow. At 1.6 MAC isoflurane also increased cerebral blood flow. (Adapted from Eger, E. I. II. Isoflurane (Forane): A compendium and reference. Madison, Ohio Medical Products.) Cerebral blood flow velocity measured before and during sevoflurane and desflurane anesthesia up to 1.5 MAC showed no change in CBFV. (Adapted from Bedforth NM, Hardman JG, Nathanson MH: Cerebral hemodynamic response to the introduction of desflurane: A comparison with sevoflurane. Anesth Analg 91:152, 2000.)

The increase in CBF with increasing dose caused by the potent agents occurs despite decreases in CMR. This phenomenon has been called "uncoupling," but from a mechanistic standpoint, true uncoupling of flow from metabolism may not occur. That is, as CMR is depressed by the volatile anesthetics there still is a coupled decline in CBF opposed by a coincident direct vasodilatory effect on the cerebral blood vessels. The net effect on the cerebral vessels depends on the sum of indirect vasoconstricting and direct vasodilating influences.

This view is supported by several facts. First, at low doses, both halothane (<0.375%) and isoflurane (0.5%) can actually decrease CBF.[35,36] This likely reflects intact coupling of CBF to CMR with the depression in neuronal activity and metabolism causing a coupled decline in perfusion. At higher doses, increases in CBF occur presumably because direct vasodilation at these doses outweighs indirect vasoconstriction. Second, if CMR is maximally or near maximally depressed with a barbiturate, halothane and isoflurane produce similar increases in CBF.[37] This is consistent with the greater depression of CMR seen with isoflurane. From a starting point of normal CMR, isoflurane causes a greater dose-dependent decrease in CMR resulting in greater indirect vasoconstriction and less vasodilation. When CMR is maximally depressed prior to isoflurane or halothane administration, no further indirect vasoconstriction is possible, and the two agents dilate cerebral vessels to a similar extent. Third, CBF to $CMRO_2$ ratios are the same for many volatile anesthetics at equivalent MAC, and increase with increasing dose in a similar fashion.[38] Finally, regional CBF–CMR relationships are arguably a better indicator of coupling than the global CBF to CMR ratio, and both isoflurane and halothane show strong coupling between decreases in CMR and CBF in individual brain regions.[39]

Autoregulation is the intrinsic myogenic regulation of vascular tone. In normal brain, the mechanisms of autoregulation of CBF over a range of mean arterial pressures from 50 to 150 mm Hg are incompletely understood. Because the volatile anesthetics are direct vasodilators, all are considered to diminish autoregulation in a dose-dependent fashion such that at high anesthetic doses CBF is essentially pressure-passive. Sevoflurane preserves autoregulation up to approximately 1 MAC.[22] At 1.5 MAC, the dynamic rate of autoregulation (change in middle cerebral artery blood flow to a rapid change in blood pressure [BP]) is better preserved with sevoflurane than isoflurane (Fig. 15-13). This may be a result of less of a direct vasodilator effect of sevoflurane, preserving the ability of the vessel to respond to changes in BP at 1.5 MAC. Based on a similar model but a separate study of dynamic autoregulation of cerebral blood flow, 0.5 MAC desflurane reduced autoregulation and isoflurane did not. At 1.5 MAC, both anesthetics substantially reduced autoregulation (see Fig. 15-13).

Intracerebral Pressure

Probably the area of greatest clinical interest to the anesthesiologist is the effect of volatile anesthesia on intracerebral pressure (ICP). In general, ICP will increase or decrease in proportion to changes in CBF. Halothane increases ICP to the greatest extent, reflecting its effects on CBF that are the largest of the potent agents.[52] In fact, brain protrusion during craniotomy is greater with halothane than isoflurane, consistent with the greater increase in ICP by halothane.[40] At concentrations above 0.5 MAC, halothane has the propensity to increase

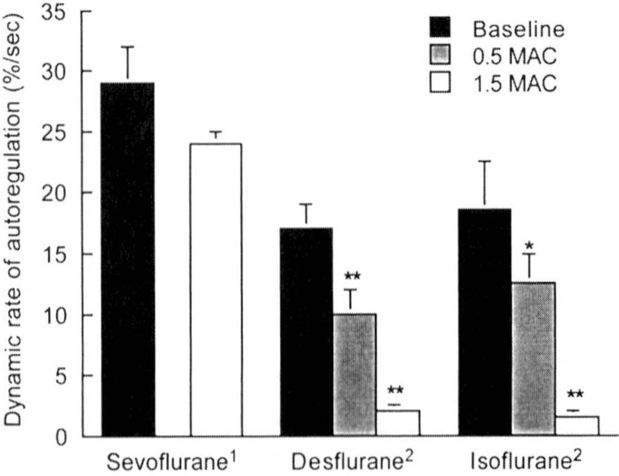

FIGURE 15-13. Dynamic rate of autoregulation (dRoR) during awake (or fentanyl and N_2O baseline), 0.5, and 1.5 minimum alveolar anesthetic concentration (MAC) anesthesia. Values are mean ± SD (SE for iso/des). * $p<0.05$ versus baseline, ** $p<0.001$ versus baseline and sevoflurane. (Data from Summors AC, Gupta AK, Matta BF: Dynamic cerebral autoregulation during sevoflurane anesthesia: A comparison with isoflurane. Anesth Analg 88:341, 1999; and Strebel S, Lam A, Matta B *et al*: Dynamic and static cerebral autoregulation during isoflurane, desflurane, and propofol anesthesia. Anesthesiology 83:66, 1995.)

CBF and ICP. This effect, in association with a blood pressure decrease, may cause profound decreases in cerebral perfusion pressure. Preinduction hyperventilation and hyperventilation with induction blunt the increases in ICP seen with halothane administration.[52] Barbiturate coadministration likewise blunts or prevents halothane-induced increases in ICP.

In contrast to halothane, isoflurane increases ICP minimally in animals both with and without brain pathology, including those with an already elevated ICP.[51] In human studies there usually are mild increases in ICP with isoflurane administration that, as with halothane, are blocked or blunted by hyperventilation or barbiturate coadministration.[41] There are some contradictory data, however. In one human study, hypocapnia did not prevent elevations in ICP with isoflurane administration in patients with space-occupying brain lesions.[42] Nonetheless, the increase in ICP is far less for isoflurane than for halothane. Furthermore, any isoflurane-induced increases in ICP tend to be of short duration, in one study only 30 minutes,[43] as opposed to halothane in which ICP increases may last for hours.

Like isoflurane, both sevoflurane and desflurane above 1 MAC produce mild increases in ICP, paralleling their mild increases in CBF.[21,22,44,45] One potential advantage of sevoflurane is that its lower pungency and airway irritation may lessen the risk of coughing and bucking and the associated rise in ICP as compared to desflurane or isoflurane. In fact, introduction of desflurane after propofol induction of anesthesia has led to significant increases in HR, MAP, and middle cerebral artery blood flow velocity that were not noted in patients given sevoflurane.[54] This may relate to the airway irritant effects of desflurane rather than a specific alteration in neurophysiology. However, several studies in both children and adults suggest that increases in ICP from desflurane are slightly greater than from either isoflurane or sevoflurane.[46,47] The bottom line is that all four potent agents may be used at appropriate doses, especially with adjunctive and compensatory therapies, in just about any neurosurgical procedure. However, patients with traumatic head injuries, elevated ICP, or space-occupying brain lesions are probably better served with isoflurane, sevoflurane, and possibly desflurane than halothane.

Cerebrospinal Fluid Production and Resorption

Studies indicate that 1 MAC halothane decreases cerebrospinal fluid (CSF) production but increases resistance to resorption, the net effect being an increase in CSF volume.[63] Isoflurane does not appear to alter CSF production,[43] but may increase, decrease, or leave unchanged the resistance to resorption depending on dose. Sevoflurane at 1 MAC depresses CSF production up to 40%.[48] Desflurane at 1 MAC leaves CSF production unchanged or increased.[47,49] In general, anesthetic effects on ICP via changes in CSF dynamics are clinically far less important than anesthetic effects on CBF.

Cerebral Blood Flow Response to Hyper- and Hypocarbia

Significant hypercapnia is associated with dramatic increases in CBF whether volatile anesthetics are administered or not. As discussed earlier, hypocapnia can blunt or abolish volatile anesthetic-induced increases in CBF depending on when the hypocapnia is produced. This vasoreactivity to CO_2 may be somewhat altered by the volatile anesthetics as compared to normal. Neither isoflurane nor halothane abolish hypocapnic vasoconstriction, and at least two studies suggest that halothane actually enhances CO_2 reactivity.[32,50] CO_2 vasoreactivity under desflurane anesthesia is normal up to 1.5 MAC,[51] and CO_2 vasoreactivity for sevoflurane is preserved at 1 MAC.[52]

Cerebral Protection

Because all of the potent agents significantly depress CMR, one might reason that they all could offer some degree of neuroprotection. Unfortunately, this is not the case. In halothane anesthetized dogs, focal ischemia caused by middle cerebral artery occlusion led to larger infarct size and worse neurological outcome than for awake animals.[53] Fortunately the well-known neuroprotective effects of pentobarbital are preserved with halothane since pentobarbital coadministration minimized the pathological and functional damage.[54]

In comparison, isoflurane may provide neuroprotective effects in both mice and dogs during hypoxemia or ischemia.[55,56] In one study, cerebral hypoperfusion secondary to hypotension from isoflurane was associated with better tissue oxygen content than during hypotension by other means, consistent with the profound decrease in $CMRO_2$ seen with isoflurane.[57] The most compelling evidence for an advantage of isoflurane over halothane for neuroprotection was shown in two studies of human carotid endarterectomy surgery. In these patients, not only was the incidence of ischemic EEG changes less using isoflurane than halothane,[58] but ischemic EEG changes occurred at a lower CBF with isoflurane than with halothane.[59]

Both sevoflurane and desflurane have been shown to improve neurological outcome in comparison to N_2O-fentanyl after incomplete cerebral ischemia in a rat model.[60,61] In piglets undergoing low-flow cardiopulmonary bypass, desflurane improved neurologic outcome compared to a fentanyl/droperidol-based anesthetic.[62] In humans, desflurane has been shown to increase brain tissue PO_2 during administration, and to maintain PO_2 to a greater extent than thiopental during temporary cerebral artery occlusion during cerebrovascular surgery.[63] Human neuroprotection outcome studies for sevoflurane and desflurane have not been published. Interpretation of the published data suggests that surgical cases in which temporary cerebral arterial occlusion is planned or probable would benefit more from isoflurane, sevoflurane, or desflurane than halothane anesthesia, but further studies are necessary.

Nitrous Oxide

The effects of nitrous oxide on cerebral physiology are not clear. Both the MAC for N_2O and its effects on CMR vary widely depending on species. The difference in CMR effects may in part be accounted for by differences in MAC, but MAC-equivalent effects on CMR also differ. In several studies in dogs, goats, and swine N_2O causes an increase in $CMRO_2$ and CBF, while in rodents no such increases or only slight increases occur. In human studies, N_2O administration preserved CBF but decreased $CMRO_2$.[38]

Another problem is the fact that N_2O is a coanesthetic used to supplement potent agents, not a complete anesthetic in itself, and CMR effects may differ depending on presence or absence of potent agent as well as the particular agent and dose. N_2O causes a greater increase in CBF and CMR in dogs at 0.2% halothane than at 0.8% halothane. In contrast, addition of N_2O to 1 or 2.2 MAC isoflurane does not alter $CMRO_2$, but does increase CBF at 1 MAC and not 2.2 MAC.

Barbiturates, narcotics, or a combination of the two appear to decrease or eliminate the increases in CMR and CBF produced by N_2O. The effect of pentobarbital/N_2O is dose dependent, with preserved increases in CMR by N_2O at low-dose pentobarbital, and no changes in CMR at high-dose pentobarbital.[64] N_2O and benzodiazepine coadministration is particularly confusing. Midazolam/N_2O in dogs increased CBF but did not alter $CMRO_2$[65] while the opposite was true in rats,[66] and both CBF and $CMRO_2$ declined in rats given diazepam/N_2O. N_2O administration increases ICP, but as is the case for CMR and CBF, changes in ICP are decreased or eliminated by a variety of co-anesthetics and more importantly by hypocapnia.

N_2O appears to have an antineuroprotective effect, as addition of N_2O to isoflurane during temporary ischemia is associated with greater tissue damage and worsened neurologic outcome.[66] In a study in mice, survival time after a hypoxic event was decreased by addition of N_2O.[68] Given the conflicting data on the effects of N_2O on CMR, CBF, ICP, and the apparent antineuroprotective effect of this agent, avoidance or discontinuation of its use should be considered in surgical cases with a high likelihood of elevated ICP or significant cerebral ischemia.

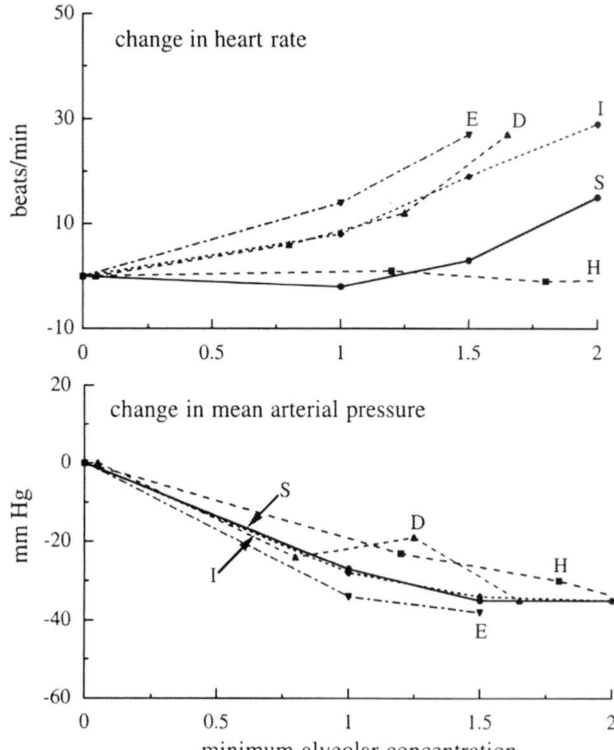

FIGURE 15-14. Heart rate and blood pressure changes (from awake baseline) in volunteers receiving general anesthesia with a potent anesthetic. Halothane and sevoflurane produced little change in heart rate at less than 1.5 MAC. All anesthetics caused similar decreases in blood pressure. (Adapted from Malan TP Jr, DiNardo JA, Isner RJ *et al*: Cardiovascular effects of sevoflurane compared with those of isoflurane in volunteers. Anesthesiology 83:918, 1995; Weiskopf RB, Cahalan MK, Eger EI II *et al*: Cardiovascular actions of desflurane in normocarbic volunteers. Anesth Analg 73:143, 1991; and Calverley RK, Smith NT, Prys-Roberts C *et al*: Cardiovascular effects of enflurane anesthesia during controlled ventilation in man. Anesth Analg 57:619, 1978.)

THE CIRCULATORY SYSTEM

Hemodynamics

The cardiac, vascular and autonomic effects of the volatile anesthetics have been carefully defined by a number of studies carried out in human volunteers not undergoing surgery.[69–75] In general, the information from these volunteer studies has translated well to the patient population commonly exposed to these anesthetics during elective and emergent surgeries. There are clearly factors such as interactions with anesthetic adjuvants and altered responses because of underlying disease that modify the circulatory effects of the volatile anesthetics.

A common effect of the potent volatile anesthetics has been a dose-related decrease in arterial blood pressure, with essentially no differences between the volatile anesthetics at steady-state, equi-anesthetic concentrations (Fig. 15-14). However, the mechanism by which they decrease arterial blood pressure is somewhat more specific for each anesthetic. Halothane is most noted for its decrease in cardiac output and this contributes importantly to its blood pressure lowering effect (Fig. 15-15).[76] The mechanism by which halothane decreases cardiac output is primarily a result of a profound depression of myocardial contractility and has been associated with an increase in right atrial pressure (see Fig. 15-15).[77] This contrasts to the newer volatile anesthetics, desflurane, sevoflurane, and isoflurane, which are known to maintain cardiac output.[73,78] Their primary mechanism to decrease blood pressure with increasing dose is related to their potent effects on regional and systemic vascular resistance (see Fig. 15-15). Enflurane falls somewhere between halothane and the newer volatile anesthetics in terms of its effects on cardiac output and peripheral resistance.

In terms of the effects of the volatile anesthetics on heart rate, data from animal studies indicate that desflurane consistently increases heart rate,[79,80] whereas sevoflurane provides
5 a relatively stable heart rate.[81] In volunteers, sevoflurane and halothane up to about 1 MAC result in minimal, if any, changes in steady-state heart rate (see Fig. 15-14). This contrasts to both enflurane and isoflurane, which have been associated with an increase in heart rate of 10 to 20% at 1 MAC. At anesthetic levels greater than 1 MAC, desflurane has been associated with an increase in heart rate to equal that of isoflurane.[82] This is generally reflected as a 10 to 15 beats/min increase in heart rate. Both desflurane and, to a lesser extent, isoflurane have been associated with transient and significant increases in heart rate during rapid increases in the inspired concentration of either anesthetic.[82] Although the mechanism(s) underlying these transient heart rate surges are not known, it is conjectured that the relative pungency of these anesthetics activates airway receptors leading to a reflex tachycardia.[83] This tachycardia can be lessened with fentanyl, alfentanil or clonidine pretreatment.[84–86]

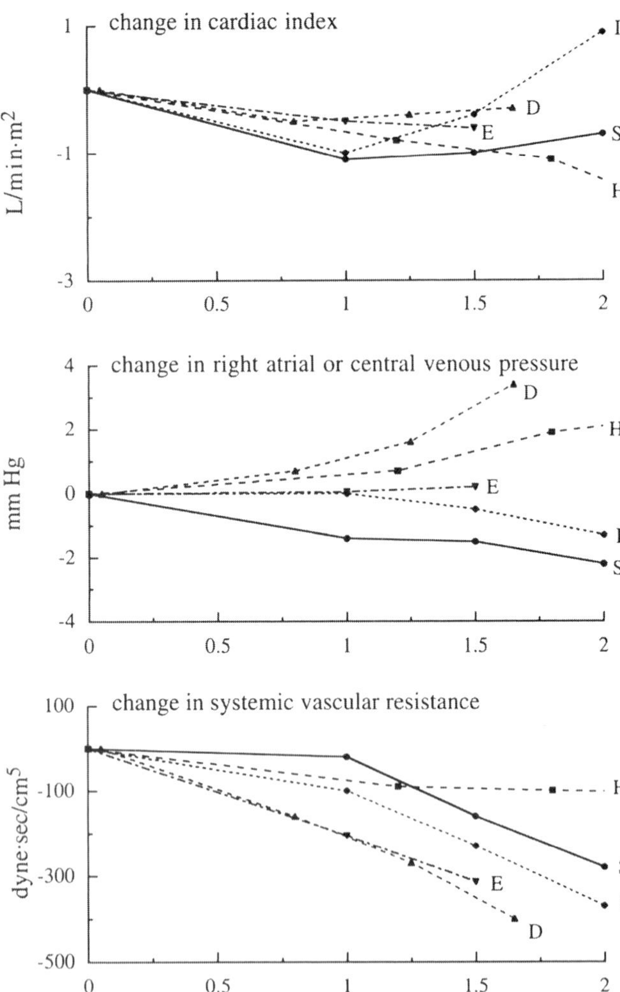

FIGURE 15-15. Cardiac index, systemic vascular resistance, and central venous pressure (or right atrial pressure) changes (from awake baseline) in volunteers receiving general anesthesia with a potent anesthetic. Increases in central venous pressure from halothane and desflurane might be because of different mechanisms. With halothane, the increase might be because of myocardial depression, whereas with desflurane, the increase is more likely because of venoconstriction. (Adapted from Malan TP Jr, DiNardo JA, Isner RJ, et al: Cardiovascular effects of sevoflurane compared with those of isoflurane in volunteers. Anesthesiology 83:918, 1995; Weiskopf RB, Cahalan MK, Eger EI II, et al: Cardiovascular actions of desflurane in nonmocarbic volunteers. Anesth Analg 73:143, 1991; and Calverley RK, Smith NT, Prys-Roberts C, et al: Cardiovascular effects of enflurane anesthesia during controlled ventilation in man. Anesth Analg 57:619, 1978.).

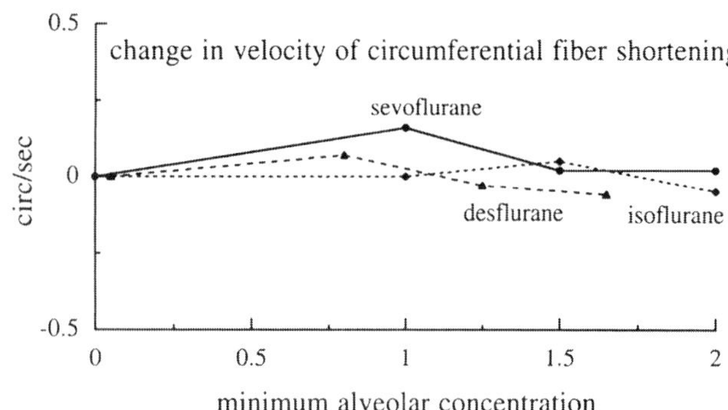

FIGURE 15-16. Noninvasive assessment of myocardial contractility with echocardiography during anesthesia in volunteers. Sevoflurane, desflurane, and isoflurane did not cause changes suggestive of myocardial depression. (Adapted from Malan TP Jr, DiNardo JA, Isner RJ, et al: Cardiovascular effects of sevoflurane compared with those of isoflurane in volunteers. Anesthesiology 83:918, 1995; Weiskopf RB, Cahalan MK, Eger EI II, et al: Cardiovascular actions of desflurane in normocarbic volunteers. Anesth Analg 73:143, 1991; and Calverley RK, Smith NT, Prys-Roberts C, et al: Cardiovascular effects of enflurane anesthesia during controlled ventilation in man. Anesth Analg 57:619, 1978.)

Myocardial Contractility

Myocardial contractility indices have been directly evaluated in animals and indirectly evaluated in humans during the administration of each of the volatile anesthetics.[87] The older anesthetics, halothane and enflurane, have been studied in humans using a relatively imprecise technique called ballistocardiography, which permits an indirect measure of contractility (IJ amplitude). At 1 MAC, enflurane caused a 40% decrease in IJ amplitude, whereas halothane caused a 30% decrease in IJ amplitude.[69,70] At 1.5 MAC, greater depression of myocardial contractility was noted for both volatile anesthetics. These changes were noted in conjunction with approximately 20% decreases in cardiac output at 1 MAC halothane and enflurane. Animal and human studies indicate that the myocardial depression from halothane is greater than isoflurane and enflurane. In contrast, human studies with the newer volatile anesthetics, isoflurane, sevoflurane, and desflurane, have not demonstrated significant changes in echocardiographic-determined indices of myocardial function, including the more noteworthy measurement of the velocity of circumferential fiber shortening (Fig. 15-16). More precise indices of myocardial contractility have been obtained for sevoflurane, isoflurane, and desflurane in chronically instrumented dogs after autonomic innervation of the heart was pharmacologically blocked. These studies of the direct myocardial effects of the volatile anesthetics demonstrate that isoflurane, desflurane, and sevoflurane cause dose-dependent depression of myocardial function with no differences between the three anesthetics (Fig. 15-17). Thus, the direct effect of volatile anesthetics is a dose-dependent myocardial depression; however, halothane and enflurane have greater effects on myocardial contractility than do isoflurane, sevoflurane, and desflurane.

Other Circulatory Effects

The majority of the volatile anesthetics have been studied during both controlled and spontaneous ventilation.[71,73,88] The process of spontaneous ventilation reduces the high intrathoracic pressures from positive pressure ventilation. The negative intrathoracic pressure during the inspiratory phase of spontaneous ventilation augments venous return and cardiac filling and improves cardiac output and, hence, blood pressure. A second result of spontaneous ventilation is higher $PaCO_2$, and this change causes cerebral and systemic vascular relaxation and further contributes to an improved cardiac output via afterload reduction. Thus, spontaneous ventilation decreases systemic vascular resistance and increases heart rate, cardiac output, and stroke volume as contrasted to positive pressure ventilation. It has been suggested that spontaneous ventilation might improve the safety of inhaled anesthetic administration, because the concentration of a volatile anesthetic that produces cardiovascular collapse exceeds the concentration resulting in apnea.

A curious observation with the potent volatile anesthetics has been an alteration in the cardiovascular effects during prolonged anesthetic exposures, noted as a small increase in heart rate and cardiac index, a gradual decrease in systemic vascular resistance, and no change in myocardial indices.[72,73] Activation

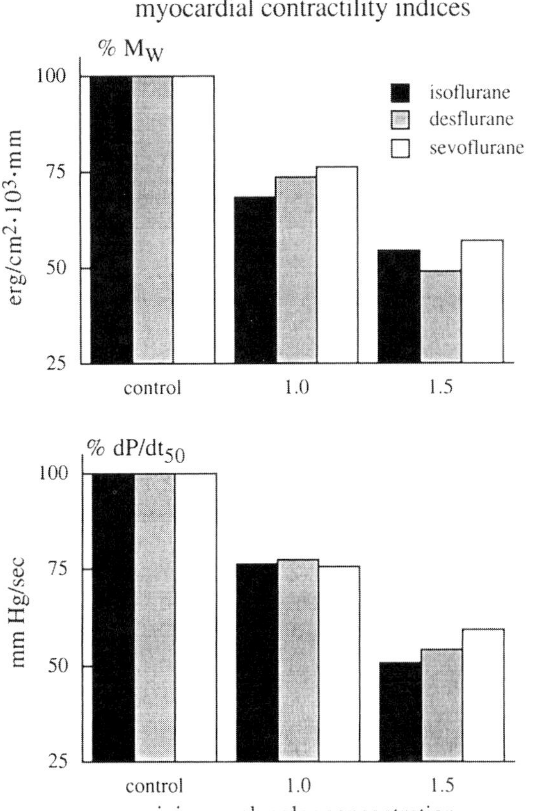

FIGURE 15-17. Myocardial contractility indices from chronically instrumented dogs. For these measurements, pharmacologic blockade of the autonomic nervous system was established to eliminate neural or circulating humoral influences on the inotropic state of the heart. The conscious control data were assigned 100%, and subsequent reductions in the inotropic state are depicted for both 1 and 1.5 minimum alveolar anesthetic concentrations of sevoflurane, desflurane, and isoflurane. There were no differences between these three volatile anesthetics. M_W, slope of the regional preload recruitable stroke work relationship; dP/dt_{50}, change in pressure per unit of time. (Adapted from Pagel PS, Kampine JP, Schmeling WT *et al*: Influence of volatile anesthetics on myocardial contractility in vivo: Desflurane versus isoflurane. Anesthesiology 74:900, 1991; and Harkin CP, Pagel PS, Kersten JR *et al*: Direct negative inotropic and lusitropic effects of sevoflurane. Anesthesiology 81:156, 1994.)

of beta-sympathetic receptors has been suggested as a mechanism contributing to the increased heart rate and cardiac output from prolonged anesthesia with halothane; however, this possibility has been questioned based on recent studies with prolonged exposure to desflurane anesthesia.[72]

Nitrous oxide is commonly combined with potent volatile anesthetics to maintain general anesthesia. Nitrous oxide has unique cardiovascular actions.[75,89] It increases sympathetic nervous system activity and vascular resistance when given in a 40% concentration.[89] When nitrous oxide is combined with volatile anesthetics and compared to equipotent concentrations of the volatile anesthetic without nitrous oxide, there still is evidence of sympathetic nervous system activation, with an increased systemic vascular resistance and an improved arterial pressure with little effect on cardiac output.[73] Part of these effects might not be because of the nitrous oxide per se, but may simply be attributed to a decrease in the concentration of the co-administered potent volatile anesthetic to achieve a MAC equivalent when using nitrous oxide.

Oxygen consumption is decreased approximately 10 to 15% during general anesthesia. The distribution of cardiac output also is altered by anesthesia. Blood flow to liver, kidneys,

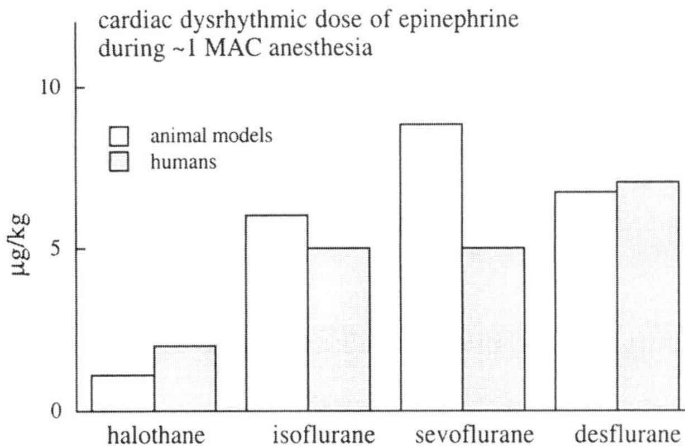

FIGURE 15-18. The dose of epinephrine associated with cardiac arrhythmias in animal and human models was least with halothane. The ether anesthetics, isoflurane, desflurane, and sevoflurane, required 3- to 6-fold greater doses of epinephrine to cause arrhythmias. (Adapted from Navarro R, Weiskopf RB, Moore MA, et al: Humans anesthetized with sevoflurane or isoflurane have similar arrhythmic response to epinephrine. Anesthesiology 80:545, 1994; Weiskopf RB, Eger EI II, Holmes MA, et al: Epinephrine-induced premature ventricular contractions and changes in arterial blood pressure and heart rate during I-653, isoflurane, and halothane anesthesia in swine. Anesthesiology 70:293, 1989; Hayashi Y, Sumikawa K, Tashiro C, et al: Arrhythmogenic threshold of epinephrine during sevoflurane, enflurane, and isoflurane anesthesia in dogs. Anesthesiology 69:145, 1988; and Moore MA, Weiskopf RB, Eger EI II, et al: Arrhythmogenic doses of epinephrine are similar during desflurane or isoflurane anesthesia in humans. Anesthesiology 79:943, 1993.)

and gut is decreased, particularly at deep levels of anesthesia. In contrast, blood flow to the brain, muscle, and skin is increased or not changed during general anesthesia.[79,90] In humans, increases in muscle blood flow are noted with isoflurane, desflurane, and sevoflurane with very small differences between anesthetics at equipotent concentrations.[91]

In contrast to halothane, the ether-based anesthetics (isoflurane, enflurane, sevoflurane, and desflurane) have not predisposed patients to ventricular arrhythmias, nor sensitized the heart to the arrhythmogenic effects of epinephrine (Fig. 15-18). The use of IV lidocaine can lessen the epinephrine effect during halothane anesthesia. Some of the differences between volatile anesthetics in their ability to promote arrhythmias can be attributed to their direct effects on cardiac pacemaker cells and conduction pathways.[92] SA node discharge rate is slowed by the volatile anesthetics and conduction in the His-Purkinje system and conduction pathways in the ventricle are also prolonged by the volatile anesthetics.[92] A greater slowing by halothane over isoflurane in the His-Purkinje system might promote dysrhythmias via a reentry phenomena.

Coronary Steal

Because the potent volatile anesthetics relax vascular smooth muscle and lead to vasodilation, there has been a concern related to abnormal distribution of blood flow in coronary blood vessels of patients with ischemic heart disease. This effect has been called coronary steal and became a concern with the introduction of isoflurane to clinical practice. Isoflurane (and most other potent volatile anesthetics) increases coronary blood flow many times beyond that of the myocardial oxygen demand, thereby creating potential for "steal." Steal is the diversion of blood from a myocardial bed with limited or inadequate perfusion to a bed with more adequate perfusion, especially one that has a remaining element of autoregulation. In instrumented animal models, the pronounced coronary vasodilation produced by isoflurane was shown to cause steal[93] and early patient studies provided additional support.[94] However, more recent work in a chronically instrumented, canine model of multivessel coronary artery obstruction has shown that neither isoflurane, sevoflurane, nor desflurane at concentrations up to 1.5 MAC resulted in abnormal collateral coronary blood flow redistribution (steal), whereas adenosine, a potent coronary vasodilator, clearly resulted in abnormal flow distribution.[95–97] Interestingly, sevoflurane favorably increased (rather than decreased) collateral coronary blood flow in this instrumented animal model when aortic pressure was held constant (similar to what might be seen with systemic blood pressure support).[95]

Myocardial Ischemia and Cardiac Outcome

Not surprisingly, the clinical relevance of coronary steal with isoflurane has been debated and is generally thought to be minimal.[98] Outcome studies have failed to associate the use of isoflurane in patients undergoing coronary artery bypass operations with an increased incidence of myocardial infarction or perioperative death.[98,99] Most studies would suggest that determinants of myocardial oxygen supply and demand, rather than the anesthetic, are of far greater importance to patient outcomes.

Several studies have evaluated the two new anesthetics, sevoflurane and desflurane, to comparator anesthetics, in terms of myocardial ischemia and outcome in patients with coronary artery disease either undergoing noncardiac or coronary artery bypass graft (CABG) surgery.[100,101] In both populations, sevoflurane appears to be essentially equivalent to isoflurane in terms of the incidence of myocardial ischemia and adverse cardiac outcomes. Desflurane appears to result in similar outcome effects as isoflurane in cardiac patients having coronary artery bypass grafting,[102] with one exception. In a study where desflurane was given without opioids to patients with coronary artery disease requiring CABG surgery, significant ischemia mandating the use of beta-blockers was noted.[103] Desflurane has not been evaluated in terms of ischemia and outcome in a patient population with coronary disease undergoing noncardiac surgery.

Cardioprotection from Volatile Anesthetics

There is a new body of literature describing the potential for organ protective effects (particularly cardioprotective effects) of the potent inhaled agents.[104,105] Organ protection would be defined as "reducing tissue damage after hypoxic ischemia or toxic insult." A preconditioning stimulus of brief coronary occlusion and ischemia initiates a signaling cascade of intracellular events that reduces ischemia and reperfusion myocardial injury. There is a memory effect from an ischemic stimulus that offers 2 to 3 hours of protection. The volatile anesthetics mimic ischemic preconditioning and trigger a similar cascade of intracellular events resulting in myocardial protection that lasts beyond the elimination of the anesthetic. Numerous factors may be involved in preconditioning, including the sodium:hydrogen exchanger, the adenosine receptor (particularly a1 and a2 subtypes), inhibitory g proteins, protein kinase c, tyrosine kinase, and potassium (K_{ATP}) channel opening. Pharmacologic blockade of these factors, for example, with adenosine blockers, delta-1 opioids, pertussis toxin, or glibenclamide, reduces or eliminates the cardioprotective effect of ischemic preconditioning and of the volatile anesthetics.[106,107] Alternatively, administration of certain drugs can mimic ischemic or volatile anesthetic preconditioning. These include adenosine, opioid agonists, and K_{ATP} channel openers. In contrast to the inhalation of volatile anesthetics, these cardioprotective drugs must be given into a coronary artery because systemic administration has serious side effects.

Lipophilic volatile anesthetics diffuse through myocardial cell membranes and alter mitochondrial electron transport leading to reactive oxygen species formation.[107] This may be the trigger for preconditioning via protein kinase C activation of K_{ATP} channel opening.[108] Approximately 30 to 40% of the cardioprotection from the volatile anesthetics appears to be related to a reduced loading of calcium into the myocardial cells during ischemia.[105] Preconditioned hearts may tolerate ischemia for 10 minutes longer than nonconditioned hearts.[109] While these evolving data generally derive from animal models, there now is increasing evidence in cardiac patient populations that anesthetic cardioprotection lessens myocardial damage (based on troponin levels) during "on and off pump" cardiac surgery.[110] This effect seems to be common to all current-day potent volatile anesthetics and may favorably influence ICU length of stay after coronary surgery.[111]

Sulfonylurea oral hyperglycemic drugs close K_{ATP} channels abolishing anesthetic preconditioning. They should be discontinued 24 to 48 hours prior to elective surgery in high-risk patients.[106] But hyperglycemia also prevents preconditioning, so insulin therapy should be started when holding oral agents.[112]

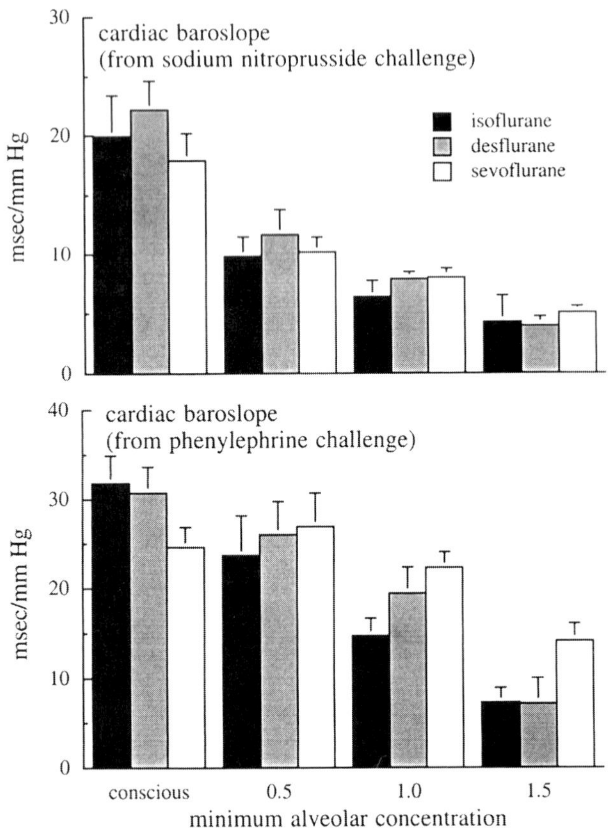

FIGURE 15-19. Summary data of the baroreflex regulation of heart rate (R-R interval) in response to a decreasing pressure stimulus (sodium nitroprusside) or in response to an increasing pressure stimulus (phenylephrine). These data were acquired in healthy volunteers who were randomized to receive isoflurane, desflurane, or sevoflurane. With increasing minimum alveolar anesthetic concentration (MAC), each of the volatile anesthetics led to a progressive reduction in the cardiac baroslope (an index of baroreflex sensitivity derived by relating changes in mean pressure to changes in R-R interval). There were no statistical differences between anesthetics. (Adapted from Ebert TJ, Harkin CP, Muzi M: Cardiovascular responses to sevoflurane: A review. Anesth Analg 81:S11, 1995.)

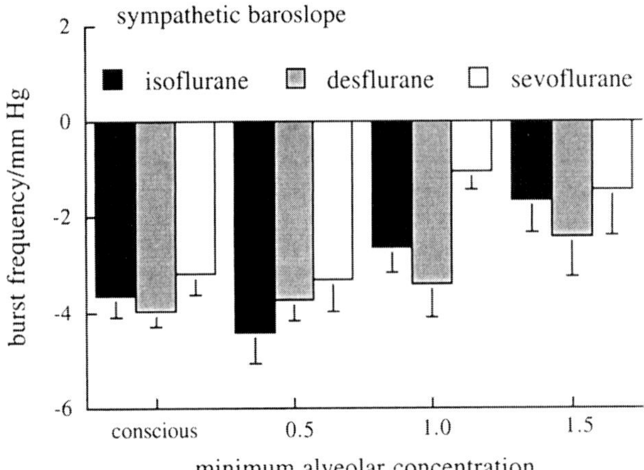

FIGURE 15-20. The sympathetic baroreflex function of healthy volunteers randomized to receive isoflurane, desflurane, or sevoflurane. The slope (sensitivity) is the relationship between decreasing diastolic pressure and increasing efferent sympathetic nerve activity. The reflex regulation of sympathetic outflow was fairly well preserved at 0.5 and 1.0 minimum alveolar anesthetic concentration (MAC) of anesthetic. At 1.5 MAC, there was a 50% decrease in the slope with all anesthetics. (Adapted from Ebert TJ, Harkin CP, Muzi M: Cardiovascular responses to sevoflurane: A review. Anesth Analg 81:S11, 1995.)

Autonomic Nervous System

Studies that have focused on the efferent activity of the parasympathetic and sympathetic nervous systems indicate that the volatile anesthetics depress their activity in a dose-dependent fashion.[113,114] However, because the autonomic nervous system (ANS) is importantly modulated by baroreceptor reflex mechanisms, the effects of the anesthetic on the efferent system cannot be reported without taking into account their effects on different components of the baroreflex arc. Thus, although both limbs of the autonomic nervous system have been shown to be attenuated by the anesthetics, the afferent activity from the arterial baroreceptors has been found to be increased with some of the anesthetics, including halothane and isoflurane.[113,115,116] This increased discharge of the baroreceptors actually contributes to the depression of the entire baroreflex arc by tonically lowering the overall level of the outflow of the sympathetic nervous system. From the perspective of clinical relevance, studies have examined the behavior of arterial baroreflex system during a hypotensive or hypertensive stimulus by evaluating changes in heart rate and sympathetic nerve activity. The arterial baroreflex is the most rapid system responding to blood pressure perturbations. Early investigations focused primarily on the regulation of heart rate (and this reflects primarily a vagally mediated end point). Halothane, enflurane, and isoflurane[117,118] all depress, in a dose-dependent fashion, the arterial baroreflex control of heart rate, although there was a suggestion that isoflurane had less of a prominent effect than halothane or enflurane.[117] Similar effects on the reflex control of heart rate have recently been demonstrated with sevoflurane and desflurane (Fig. 15-19).[119–121]

There is greater difficulty in evaluating the sympathetic component of the baroreflex arc in humans, but a technique called sympathetic microneurography has been utilized to directly record vasoconstrictor impulses directed to blood vessels in humans.[74,82] There is a dose-dependent depression of the reflex control of sympathetic outflow that appears to be relatively equivalent for isoflurane, sevoflurane, and desflurane (Fig. 15-20). Importantly, at low levels of anesthesia, for example, 0.5 MAC, there is little if any depression of reflex function and this might have important implications in the compromised patient population. Opioid and benzodiazepine adjuvants have only minimal effects on reflex function and combining these with low levels of potent anesthetics might preserve reflex function.[122,123] Another important observation has been the more rapid return of baroreflex function with the less-soluble anesthetic sevoflurane versus isoflurane.[124] This might add to hemodynamic stability in the postoperative period when tissue concentrations of the volatile anesthetics are declining.

Desflurane has a unique and prominent effect on sympathetic outflow in humans, which is not apparent in animal models. With increasing steady-state concentrations of desflurane, there is a progressive increase in resting sympathetic nervous system activity and plasma norepinephrine levels.[74,82,125] Despite this increase in tonic sympathetic outflow, blood pressure decreases similarly to sevoflurane and isoflurane. This raises the question as to whether desflurane has the ability to uncouple neuroeffector responses. In addition, desflurane can cause marked activation of the sympathetic nervous system when the inspired concentration is increased, especially to concentrations above 5 to 6% (Fig. 15-21).[74,82,125] There is a transient surge in sympathetic outflow leading to both hypertension and tachycardia. In addition, the endocrine axis is activated as evidenced by 15- to 20-fold increases in plasma antidiuretic hormone and epinephrine (Fig. 15-22). The hemodynamic response persists for 4 to 5 minutes and the endocrine response persists for 15 to 25 minutes. Adequate concentrations of opioids or clonidine given prior to increasing the concentration of desflurane have been shown to attenuate these responses.[84–86] The source of the neuroendocrine activation has been actively sought, and it would appear that there are receptors in both the upper and the lower airways, and/or perhaps in a highly perfused tissue near the airways, that initiates the sympathetic activation.[83] The possibility that desflurane activates airway

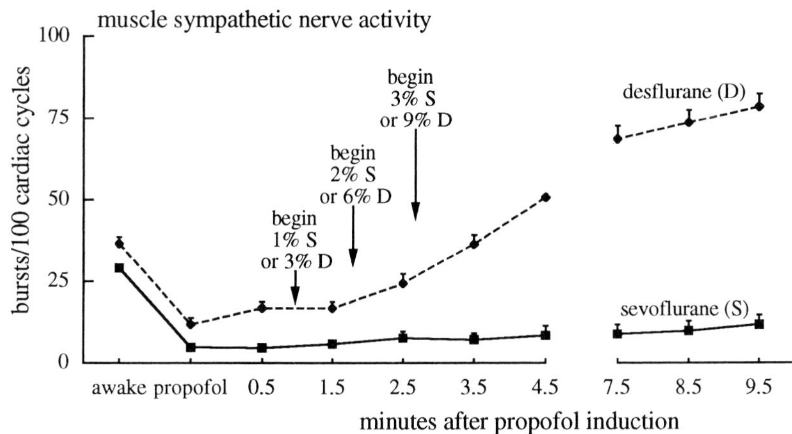

FIGURE 15-21. Consecutive measurements of sympathetic nerve activity (SNA)(mean ± SE) from human volunteers during induction of anesthesia with propofol and the subsequent mask administration of sevoflurane or desflurane for a 10-minute period. The inspired concentration of these anesthetics was increased at 1-minute intervals beginning precisely 2 minutes after propofol administration (0.41 MAC of sevoflurane and desflurane). In both groups, propofol reduced SNA and MAP. Desflurane resulted in significant increases in sympathetic nerve activity that persisted throughout the 10-minute mask administration period. (Adapted from Ebert TJ, Muzi M, Lopatka CW: Neurocirculatory responses to sevoflurane in humans. A comparison to desflurane. Anesthesiology 83:88, 1995.)

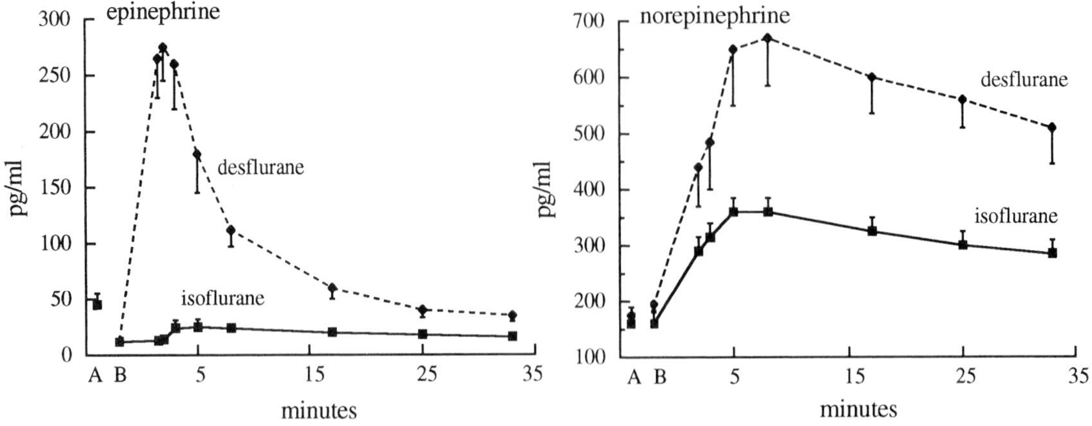

FIGURE 15-22. Stress hormone responses to a rapid increase in anesthetic concentration, from 4 to 12% inspired. Volunteers given desflurane showed a larger increase in plasma epinephrine and norepinephrine concentrations than when given isoflurane. Data are mean ± SE. A, awake value; B, value after 32 minutes of 0.55 MAC; time represents minutes after the first breath of increased anesthetic concentration. (Adapted from Weiskopf RB, Moore MA, Eger EI II *et al*: Rapid increase in desflurane concentration is associated with greater transient cardiovascular stimulation than with rapid increase in isoflurane concentration in humans. Anesthesiology 80:1035, 1994.)

irritant receptors is quite strong, since desflurane is the most pungent of the anesthetics available for clinical use.[126]

THE PULMONARY SYSTEM

The volatile anesthetics have multiple and important effects on many aspects of pulmonary physiology, including respiratory rate and tidal volume, responses to CO_2 and hypoxia, effects on bronchiolar smooth muscle tone, and mucociliary function. Less pronounced, but still important effects of the volatile anesthetics have been observed on pulmonary vascular resistance and pulmonary blood flow.

General Ventilatory Effects

All volatile anesthetics decrease tidal volume but have lesser effects on decreasing minute ventilation because of an offsetting

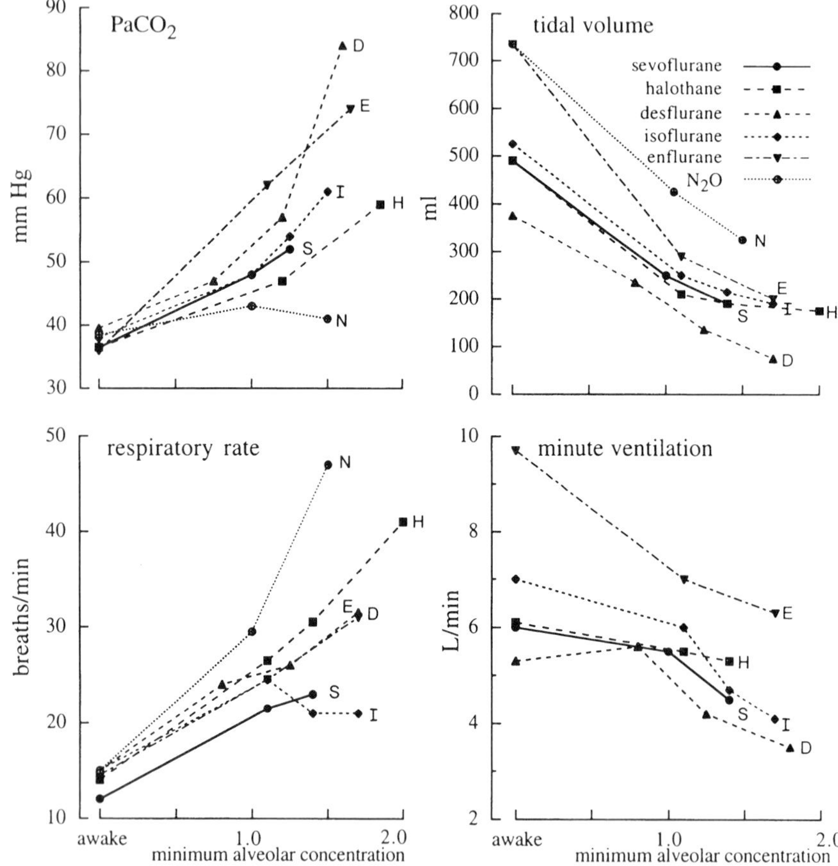

FIGURE 15-23. Comparison of mean changes in resting $PaCO_2$, tidal volume, respiratory rate, and minute ventilation in patients anesthetized with either halothane, isoflurane, enflurane, sevoflurane, desflurane, or nitrous oxide. Anesthetic-induced tachypnea compensates in part for the ventilatory depression caused by all volatile anesthetics (decrease in minute ventilation and tidal volume and concomitant increase in $PaCO_2$). Desflurane results in the greatest increase in $PaCO_2$ with corresponding reductions in tidal volume and minute ventilation. Isoflurane, like all other inhaled agents, increases respiratory rate, but does not result in dose-dependent tachypnea. (Adapted from Lockhart SH, Rampil IJ, Yasuda N, et al: Depression of ventilation by desflurane in humans. Anesthesiology 74:484, 1991; Doi M, Ikeda K: Respiratory effects of sevoflurane. Anesth Analg 66:241, 1987; Fourcade HE, Stevens WC, Larson CP Jr, et al: The ventilatory effects of Forane, a new inhaled anesthetic. Anesthesiology 35:26, 1971; and Calverley RK, Smith NT, Jones CW, et al: Ventilatory and cardiovascular effects of enflurane anesthesia during spontaneous ventilation in man. Anesth Analg 57:610, 1978.)

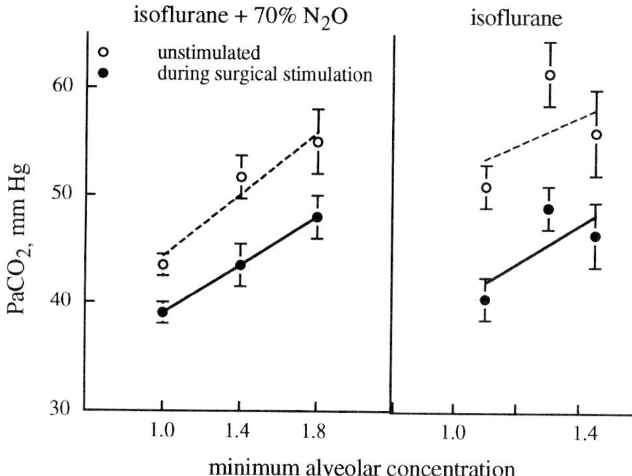

FIGURE 15-24. The effect of surgical stimulation on the ventilatory depression of inhaled anesthesia with isoflurane in the presence and absence of nitrous oxide. Surgical stimulation increased alveolar ventilation and decreased $PaCO_2$ at all depths of anesthesia examined. (Adapted from Eger EI II, Dolan WM, Stevens WC *et al*: Surgical stimulation antagonizes the respiratory depression produced by forane. Anesthesiology 36:544, 1972.)

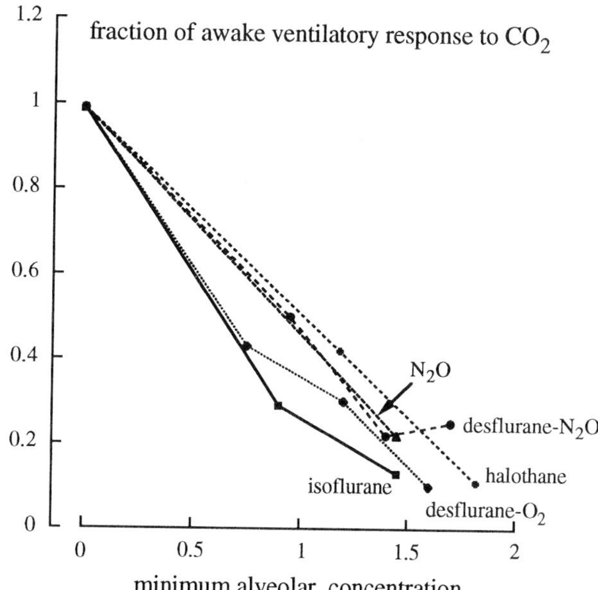

FIGURE 15-25. All inhaled anesthetics produce similar dose-dependent decreases in the ventilatory response to carbon dioxide. (Adapted from Eger EI II: Desflurane. Anesth Rev 20:87, 1993.)

response to increase respiratory rate (Fig. 15-23). These effects are dose dependent, with higher concentrations of volatile anesthetics, resulting in greater decreases in tidal volume and greater increases in respiratory rate. Their net effect of a gradual decrease in minute ventilation has been associated with increasing resting $PaCO_2$. The relative increases in $PaCO_2$ as an index of respiratory depression with volatile anesthetics evaluated at less than 1.24 MAC are as follows: enflurane > desflurane = isoflurane > sevoflurane = halothane. The respiratory depression can be partially antagonized during surgical stimulation where respiratory rate has been shown to increase, resulting in a decrease in the $PaCO_2$ (Fig. 15-24). In addition, resting $PaCO_2$ during desflurane or sevoflurane anesthesia is significantly decreased (returned toward normal) with the addition of nitrous oxide. This comparison (with and without nitrous oxide) requires a lessening of the potent volatile anesthetic to maintain an equi-MAC concentration when adding nitrous oxide to the inspired gas and this probably contributes to the return of $PaCO_2$ toward normal. The degree of respiratory depression from inhaled anesthetics may be lessened during prolonged administration of the anesthetic.[127]

Ventilatory Mechanics

Functional residual capacity is decreased during general anesthesia and this has been explained by a number of mechanisms, including a decrease in the intercostal muscle tone, alteration in diaphragm position, changes in thoracic blood volume, and the onset of phasic expiratory activity of respiratory muscles.[128–130] About 40% of the muscular work of breathing is via intercostal muscles and about 60% is from the diaphragm. The diaphragmatic muscle function is relatively spared when contrasted to the parasternal intercostal muscles.[128] However, inspiratory rib cage expansion is reasonably well maintained during anesthesia because of preserved activity of the scalene muscles.[128] Expiration is generally considered a passive function mediated by the elastic recoil of the lung. The process of applying a resistance or load to expiration typically results in a slowing of respiration but under anesthesia additional noted responses included a substantial asynchrony of the thoracic movements with respiration.[131] This suggests that in patients with pulmonary disease associated with increased expiratory resistance, the act of spontaneous ventilation during general anesthesia might be associated with increased risk.

Response to Carbon Dioxide and Hypoxemia

In awake subjects a high sensitivity to CO_2 has been noted by increases in minute ventilation of approximately 3 L/min per 1 mm Hg increase in $PaCO_2$. It is mediated by central chemoreceptors and has been used as an index of ventilatory drive. All of the inhaled anesthetics produce a dose-dependent depression of the ventilatory response to hypercarbia (Fig. 15-25). Early studies suggested that the addition of nitrous oxide to halothane depressed ventilation less than an equi-MAC dose of halothane alone;[132] however, this does not appear to be the case for desflurane (see Fig. 15-25). During anesthesia with spontaneous ventilation, an apneic threshold can be determined that is generally 4 to 5 mm Hg below the prevailing resting $PaCO_2$, and this threshold is not related to the slope of the CO_2 response curves or to the level of the resting $PaCO_2$. The clinical relevance of this threshold may be important when assisting ventilation in an anesthetized patient who is breathing spontaneously. This only serves to lower the $PaCO_2$ to approach that of the apneic threshold, therefore mandating more control of ventilation.

Inhaled anesthetics, including nitrous oxide, also produce dose-dependent attenuation of the ventilatory response to hypoxia.[133,134] This action appears to be dependent on the peripheral chemoreceptors. In fact, even subanesthetic concentrations of volatile anesthetics (0.1 MAC) elicit anywhere from a 15 to 75% depression of the ventilatory drive to hypoxia (Fig. 15-26).[135] The mechanism of this depression still remains poorly understood. Studies have suggested that hypoxia may decrease the probability that potassium channels are open, thus causing membrane depolarization, influx of calcium ions, and release of neurotransmitters.[136] One theory is that the potassium channels are responding to reactive oxygen species, such as those formed as a result of halothane administration. In one study, the administration of antioxidants prior to the administration of halothane prevented the depression of the hypoxic

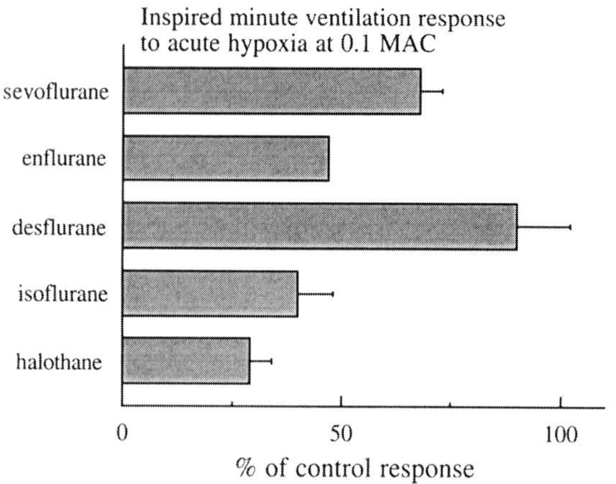

FIGURE 15-26. Influence of 0.1 MAC of five volatile anesthetic agents on the ventilatory response to a step decrease in end-tidal oxygen concentration. Values are mean ± SD. Subanesthetic concentrations of the volatile anesthetics, except desflurane and sevoflurane, profoundly depress the response to hypoxia. (Adapted from Sarton E, Dahan A, Teppema L *et al*: Acute pain and central nervous system arousal do not restore impaired hypoxic ventilatory responses during sevoflurane sedation. Anesthesiology 85:295, 1996.)

response.[137] The extreme sensitivity of the volatile anesthetics in terms of inhibiting hypoxic responsiveness has important clinical implications. Residual effects of volatile anesthetics may impair the ventilatory drive of patients in the recovery room. In this regard, the short-acting anesthetics (sevoflurane and desflurane) may prove advantageous because of their more rapid washout and their minimal effect on hypoxic sensitivity at subanesthetic concentrations (see Fig. 15-26). The effects of the volatile anesthetics on hypoxic drive may play an even more important role in patients who rely on hypoxic drive to set their level of ventilation, such as those with chronic respiratory failure.

Bronchiolar Smooth Muscle Tone

Bronchoconstriction under anesthesia occurs because of direct stimulation of the laryngeal and tracheal areas and the administration of adjuvant drugs that cause histamine release, and from noxious stimuli especially in lightly anesthetized patients.[138] These responses are enhanced in patients with known reactive airway disease, (including those requiring bronchodilator therapy or those with chronic smoking histories). Airway smooth muscle, which extends as far distally as the terminal bronchioles, is under the influence of both parasympathetic and sympathetic nerves. The parasympathetic nerves mediate baseline airway tone and reflex bronchoconstriction, via an M3 muscarinic receptor on the airway smooth muscle that increases intracellular cyclic GMP. Adrenergic receptors also are located on bronchial smooth muscle with the beta-2 receptor subtype playing an important role in promoting bronchiolar muscle relaxation through an increase in intracellular cyclic-AMP. The volatile anesthetics relax airway smooth muscle by directly depressing smooth muscle contractility and indirectly by inhibiting the reflex neural pathways.[139] They also may have protective effects by acting on the bronchial epithelium via a nonadrenergic, noncholinergic mechanism, possibly involving the nitric oxide pathway.[140] A recent study in patients comparing isoflurane, halothane, and sevoflurane to a control group receiving thiopental indicated that sevoflurane may have a more rapid onset of bronchodilation than isoflurane or halothane.[141] Studies from our laboratory suggest that desflurane administration shortly after thiopental induction and tracheal intubation results in a transient increase in respiratory system resistance (bronchoconstriction), and we have attributed this to a direct effect from the pungency and airway irritability of desflurane (Fig. 15-27). This effect is worsened in patients with an active smoking history. Volatile anesthetics have been used effectively to treat status asthmaticus when other conventional treatments have failed.[142] Although halothane has been successfully used in these situations, sevoflurane may be a better choice because of its quick onset, lack of pungency, lack of cardiovascular depression, and lower risk of cardiac arrhythmias compared to halothane.

Mucociliary Function

Adequate mucociliary function may be important in preventing postoperative atelectasis and hypoxemia. There are a number of factors involved in diminished mucociliary function, particularly in the mechanically ventilated patient. Anesthesia plays an as yet poorly defined role. Halothane, enflurane, and nitrous oxide with halothane have been shown to decrease, in a dose-dependent fashion, mucociliary movement. It also is known that smokers have impaired mucociliary function compared to nonsmokers, and the combination of a volatile anesthetic in a smoker who is mechanically ventilated sets up a scenario for inadequate clearing of secretions, mucous plugging, atelectasis, and hypoxemia.

Pulmonary Vascular Resistance

Although vascular smooth muscle is clearly affected by the volatile anesthetics, the pulmonary vasodilator action of the clinically relevant concentrations of inhaled anesthetics, including halothane, isoflurane, enflurane, sevoflurane, and desflurane, is minimal. In addition, any decrease in cardiac output that might occur from a volatile anesthetic tends to offset the direct vasodilator action of the anesthetic, resulting in little or no change in pulmonary artery pressures and pulmonary blood

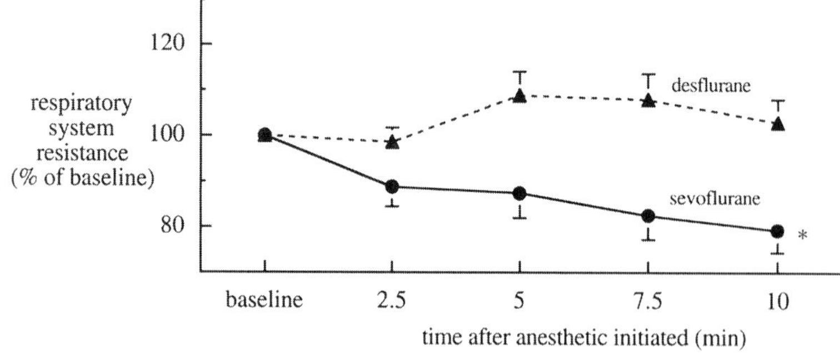

FIGURE 15-27. Changes in respiratory system resistance (*Rrs*) expressed as a percentage of the "thiopental" baseline recorded after tracheal intubation but prior to administration of sevoflurane or desflurane to the inspired gas mixture. Airway resistance responses to sevoflurane were significantly different from desflurane (*$p<0.05$). (Adapted from Goff MJ, Arain SR, Ficke DJ *et al*: Absence of bronchodilation during desflurane anesthesia: A comparison to sevoflurane and thiopental. Anesthesiology 93:404, 2000.)

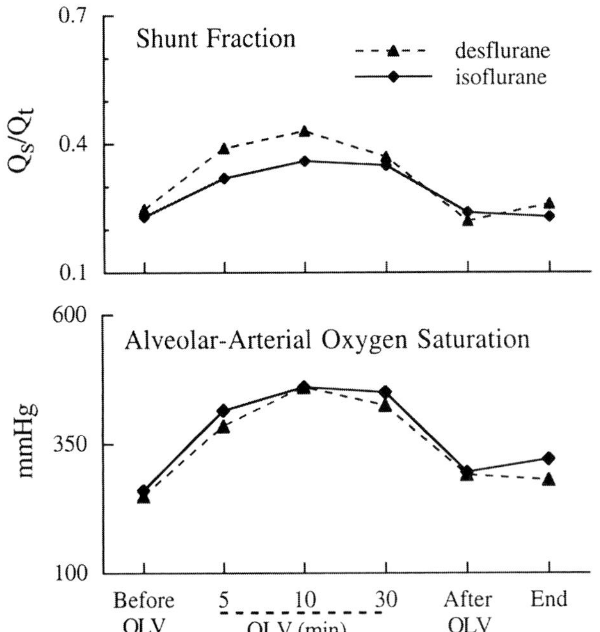

FIGURE 15-28. Shunt fraction (**top panel**) and the alveolar–arterial oxygen gradient (**bottom panel**) immediately before, during, and after one-lung ventilation (OLV) in patients anesthetized with desflurane or isoflurane. Data are means. (Adapted from Pagel PS, Fu JL, Damask MC *et al*: Desflurane and isoflurane produce similar alterations in systemic and pulmonary hemodynamics and arterial oxygenation in patients undergoing one-lung ventilation during thoracotomy. Anesth Analg 87:800, 1998.)

flow. Even nitrous oxide, which has little effect on cardiac output and pulmonary blood flow, has at best a small effect to increase pulmonary vascular resistance. However, the effect of nitrous oxide may be magnified in patients with resting pulmonary hypertension.[143] Perhaps more important in terms of volatile anesthetics and pulmonary blood flow is their potential to attenuate hypoxic pulmonary vasoconstriction (HPV). During periods of hypoxemia, HPV reduces blood flow to underventilated areas of the lung, thereby diverting blood flow to areas of the lung with greater ventilation. The net effect is to improve the V/Q matching, resulting in a reduced amount of venous admixture and improved arterial oxygenation. Although all of the inhaled anesthetics in high concentrations have been shown to attenuate HPV in animal models, the situation is less clear in patient studies. This may reflect the multifactorial effects of the volatile anesthetics on factors involved in pulmonary blood flow, including their cardiovascular, autonomic and humoral actions. Furthermore, nonpharmacologic variables impair HPV, including surgical trauma, temperature, pH, $PaCO_2$, size of the hypoxic segment, and intensity of the hypoxic stimulus. In patients undergoing one lung ventilation during thoracic surgery, PaO_2 and intrapulmonary shunt fraction (Qs/Qt) have been minimally affected when changing from two-lung to one-lung ventilation (OLV) during either halothane, isoflurane, enflurane, desflurane anesthesia (Fig. 15-28).[144] Isoflurane appears to be less inhibitory on HPV than halothane and, although this effect is subtle,[144] it might be attributed to the greater maintenance of cardiac output known to occur with isoflurane. Both sevoflurane and desflurane preserve cardiac output and should also help lessen shunt fraction during OLV. Propofol appears to be no more beneficial on shunt fraction during OLV compared to sevoflurane.[145] Finally, the addition of 4 cm positive end-expiratory pressure (PEEP) to the dependent lung may not impair cardiac output but reduces shunt fraction during OLV.[146]

HEPATIC EFFECTS

Although postoperative liver dysfunction has been associated with many of the volatile anesthetics in current use, the most concern has been focused on halothane. There appears to be two distinct mechanisms by which halothane can cause hepatitis. One is more common but relatively mild, does not require a previous exposure, and has a low morbidity. The second is associated with repeat exposure and probably represents an immune reaction to oxidatively derived metabolites of halothane and has been associated with severe liver damage and fulminant hepatic failure.

The liver has two blood supplies. One is the well-oxygenated blood from the hepatic artery and the second is the poorly oxygenated blood supply from the portal vein. Hepatocyte hypoxia is a significant contributor to postoperative hepatic injury. A pleasant attribute of the ether-based anesthetics (isoflurane, sevoflurane, and desflurane) is their ability to maintain or increase hepatic artery blood flow while decreasing (or not changing) portal vein blood flow.[79,147] This contrasts to halothane where decreases in portal vein blood flow are not compensated by increases in hepatic artery blood flow (Fig. 15-29). Rather, halothane causes selective hepatic artery vasoconstriction. It is estimated in animal models that there is a 65% reduction in oxygen availability during halothane anesthesia, while during isoflurane the reduction in availability is only 35%.[148]

Situations that decrease hepatic blood flow or increase hepatic oxygen demand make patients vulnerable to the unwanted effects of halothane on hepatic blood flow. For example, surgery in the area of the liver (or elsewhere in the abdominal cavity) that might compromise hepatic blood flow puts patients at risk for hepatic cell injury. In addition, enzyme induction, which increases oxygen demand, enhances the vulnerability of patients to the effects of halothane. Furthermore, patients who are critically dependent on oxygen supply for

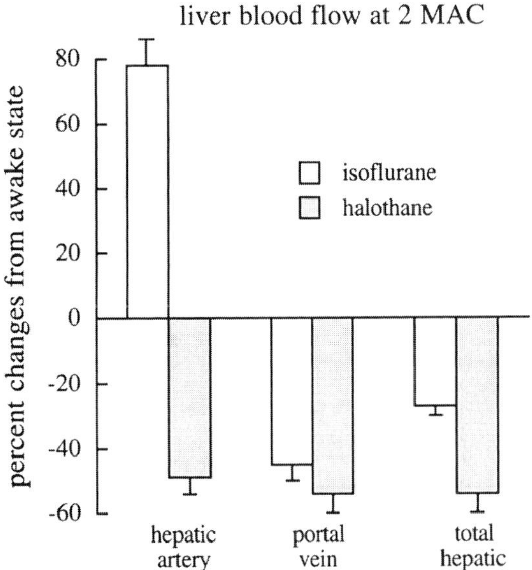

FIGURE 15-29. Changes (%, mean ± SE) in hepatic blood flow during administration of isoflurane or halothane. Decreases in portal vein blood flow produced by 2 MAC isoflurane are offset by increases in hepatic artery blood flow (autoregulation). Halothane resulted in decreases in both portal vein and hepatic artery blood flow, thereby significantly compromising total hepatic artery blood flow. (Adapted from Gelman, S, Fowler, KC, Smith, LR: Liver circulation and function during isoflurane and halothane anesthesia. Anesthesiology 61:726, 1984.)

survival of remaining liver tissue, such as the cirrhotic patient, are at a higher risk for further hepatic injury than noncirrhotic individuals.[149] Whether this injury can simply be explained by a direct effect of halothane during hypoxic conditions or be attributed to reductive metabolism of halothane that is enhanced under hypoxic conditions is not entirely clear.[150]

Changes in liver function tests have been used as an index of hepatic injury during anesthesia. Transient increases in plasma alanine aminotransferase (ALT) activity followed the administration of enflurane, but not desflurane, isoflurane, or sevoflurane in human volunteers.[147,151,152] Although changes in the ALT or aspartate aminotransferase (AST) is an accepted index of liver cell damage, these measures may not accurately reflect the extent of hepatic injury and are not uniquely specific to the liver. Most cases of halothane hepatitis demonstrate lesions in the centrilobular area of the liver and not coincidentally, this area is most susceptible to hypoxia. Therefore, a more sensitive measure of injury may be glutathione-S-transferase (GST) since it is distributed primarily in the centrilobular hepatocytes. In patient studies comparing halothane anesthesia to isoflurane and enflurane,[153] significant increases in GST occurred after halothane (increases of 24 to 50%) and enflurane (20%), but not after isoflurane. There were two peaks in the GST responses; the first was 3 to 6 hours after halothane and the other was approximately 24 hours after halothane. It has been suggested that the early peak reflects direct damage or impaired liver blood flow and the second peak may be caused by metabolites or an immune response. The immune mechanism of hepatitis is considered later in this chapter in the section labeled "Anesthetic Metabolism."

NEUROMUSCULAR SYSTEM AND MALIGNANT HYPERTHERMIA

Compared to the alkane halothane, the ether-derived, fluorinated, volatile anesthetics produce about 2-fold greater skeletal muscle relaxation. Nitrous oxide does not relax skeletal muscles and in doses greater than 1 MAC may, in fact, result in skeletal muscle rigidity. Interestingly, the inhaled anesthetics, in addition to the direct effects of relaxing skeletal muscle, also potentiate the action of neuromuscular blocking drugs.[154,155] Although the mechanism of this potentiation is not entirely clear, it appears to be largely because of a postsynaptic effect at the nicotinic acetylcholine receptor located at the neuromuscular junction.[156] Specifically, at the receptor level, the volatile anesthetics act synergistically with the neuromuscular blocking drugs to enhance their action.[157] The degree of enhancement is related to their aqueous concentration so that at equi-MAC concentrations, the less potent anesthetics (e.g., desflurane and sevoflurane versus isoflurane) should have a greater inhibitory effect on neuromuscular transmission. Support for this concept comes from a clinical study demonstrating 20% lower requirement for vecuronium to maintain a stable twitch depression during 1.25% desflurane compared to 1.25% isoflurane.[158] In contrast, equipotent concentrations of desflurane, isoflurane, and sevoflurane acted similarly to enhance the effect of cisatracurium on neuromuscular function.[154] This may relate to major structural differences between neuromuscular blocking drugs.

All of the potent volatile anesthetics serve as triggers for malignant hyperthermia in genetically susceptible patients.[159–161] In contrast, nitrous oxide is only a weak trigger for malignant hyperthermia.[161] Studies evaluating the caffeine-induced contractures indicate the augmentation of the contractures by nitrous oxide is 1.3, whereas that for isoflurane is 3-fold, enflurane 4-fold, and halothane 11-fold.[161] Thus, halothane may be the most potent trigger of the volatile anesthetics for malignant hyperthermia. Although desflurane is a weak trigger for malignant hyperthermia, it has been associated with an unusual delayed onset of symptoms if succinylcholine was not used for neuromuscular blockade.[159,162]

GENETIC/CELLULAR EFFECTS

In tests employed to identify chemicals that cause a mutagenic or carcinogenic response, all of the volatile anesthetics, including nitrous oxide, have proven to be negative. The Ames test identifies chemicals that act as mutagens and carcinogens and has been shown to be negative for enflurane, isoflurane, desflurane, sevoflurane, and nitrous oxide.[149] Although halothane results in a negative Ames test, metabolites may be positive.

Virtually every volatile anesthetic agent has been shown to be teratogenic in animal studies, but none has been shown to be teratogenic in humans. Animal studies have indicated that nitrous oxide exposure in the early periods of gestation may result in adverse effects, including an increased incidence of fetal resorption.[163] The same vulnerability does not exist during the administration of the potent volatile anesthetics.[164]

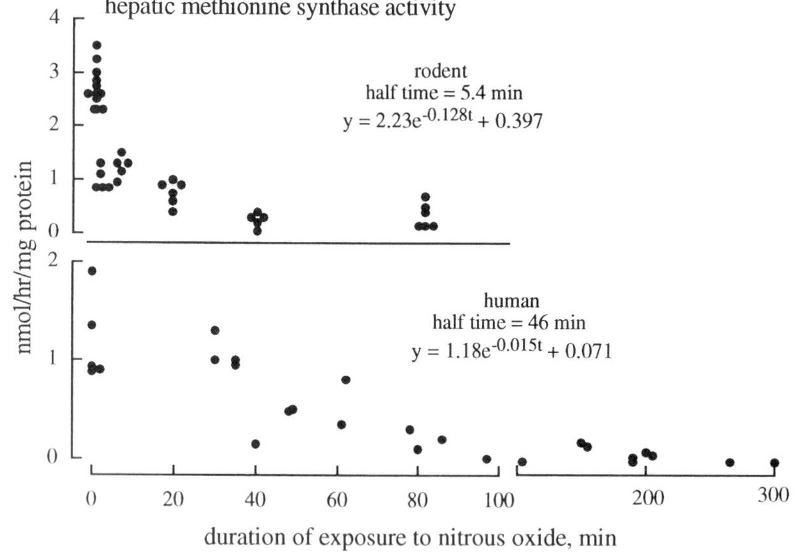

FIGURE 15-30. Time course of inactivation of hepatic methionine synthase (synthetase) activity during administration of 50% nitrous oxide to rats or 70% nitrous oxide to humans. The half-life was substantially less in rats. (Adapted from Royston BD, Nunn JF, Weinbren HK *et al*: Rate of inactivation of human and rodent hepatic methionine synthase by nitrous oxide. Anesthesiology 68:213, 1988.)

However, learning function may be impaired in newborn animals exposed in utero to inhaled anesthetics.[165]

There has been an ongoing concern about the incidence of spontaneous abortions in operating room personnel chronically exposed to trace concentrations of inhaled anesthetics, especially nitrous oxide.[163] Animal studies using intermittent exposure to trace concentrations of nitrous oxide, halothane, enflurane, and isoflurane have not revealed harmful reproductive effects.[166] Methionine synthetase and thymidylate synthetase are vitamin B12–dependent enzymes that have been shown to decrease in activity during nitrous oxide exposure. The mechanism appears to be an irreversible oxidation of the cobalt atom of vitamin B12 by nitrous oxide. The half-time for inactivation of methionine synthetase is 46 minutes when 70% nitrous oxide is administered to patients (Fig. 15-30). Methionine synthetase and thymidylate synthetase are involved in the formation of myelin and the formation of DNA, respectively. Thus, the concern that these changes might have an effect on a rapidly developing embryo/fetus seems appropriate. Inhibition of these enzymes could also manifest as depression of bone marrow function and neurologic disturbances. In fact, megaloblastic changes in bone marrow are consistently observed in patients exposed to nitrous oxide for 24 hours,[239] and four days of exposure to nitrous oxide has resulted in agranulocytosis. Furthermore, animals exposed to 15% nitrous oxide for up to 15 days developed a neuropathy presented as ataxia and spinal cord and peripheral nerve degeneration. A sensory motor polyneuropathy that is often combined with signs of posterior lateral spinal cord degeneration resembling pernicious anemia has been described in humans who chronically inhale nitrous oxide for recreational use.[167] These effects have been attributed to reduced activity of the vitamin B12–dependent enzymes.

Despite the unproven influence of trace concentrations of the volatile anesthetics on congenital development and spontaneous abortions, these concerns have resulted in the use of scavenging systems to remove anesthetic gases from the operating room and the establishment of Occupational Saftey and Health Administration standards for waste gas exposure. The National Institute for Occupational Safety and Health recommended exposure levels for nitrous oxide is 25 parts per million (ppm) as a time-weighted average over the time of exposure. The exposure limit for halogenated anesthetics (without nitrous oxide exposure) is 2 ppm.

OBSTETRIC EFFECTS

Similar to the effects of volatile anesthetics on vascular smooth muscle, a dose-dependent decrease in uterine smooth muscle contractility and blood flow occurs, and the response appears to be similar among the volatile anesthetics.[168,169] Consequently, a common technique used to provide general anesthesia for urgent Caesarean sections is to administer low concentrations of the volatile anesthetic, such as 0.5 MAC, combined with nitrous oxide. This decreases the likelihood of uterine atony and blood loss, especially at a time after delivery when uterine contraction is essential.[170] Uterine relaxation can become troubling at concentrations of volatile anesthesia greater than 1 MAC, and higher concentrations might delay the onset time of newborn respiration.[170] In some situations, uterine relaxation may be desirable, such as to remove a retained placenta. In this case, a brief, high concentration of a volatile anesthetic may be advantageous. In terms of neonatal effects of general anesthesia, APGAR scores and acid-base balance are not affected by anesthetic technique, such as spinal versus general.[171] More sensitive measures of neurologic and behavioral function, such as the Scanlon Early Neonatal Neurobehavioral Scale (ENNS) and the neurological and adaptive capacities score (NACS) indicate some transient depression of scores following general anesthesia that did not persist at 24 hours postdelivery measurements.[171,172] Fetal loss seems to increase following surgery in the first or second trimester, but the majority of these findings have been in patients following acute abdomen or trauma in emergency settings. Generally, elective surgeries are delayed until at least 6 weeks postpartum, or until the late second or early third trimester. Perhaps the most important factor in promoting good fetal outcome is maintaining good uterine blood flow during anesthesia and surgery.

ANESTHETIC DEGRADATION BY CARBON DIOXIDE ABSORBERS

The majority of adult general anesthesia is given through closed or semiclosed breathing circuits. This mandates the use of a carbon dioxide absorbent in the circuit. One of the problems with the CO_2 absorbents in use today is their chemical makeup, which consists of monovalent hydroxide bases (KOH and NaOH). These strong bases result in breakdown or degradation of all modern-day, potent anesthetics.[173] Degradation of the anesthetics is slightly greater with potassium hydroxide. Barium hydroxide lime, which contains potassium but not sodium hydroxide, causes more anesthetic degradation than soda lime (which contains less potassium hydroxide and more sodium hydroxide).[174] In the case of halothane and sevoflurane, the reaction with carbon dioxide absorbents results in degradation of these anesthetics to haloalkenes.[5] Halothane degrades to form trace amounts of BCDFE (2-bromo-2-chloro-1,1-difluoroethene) and sevoflurane degrades to form trace amounts of compound A (2,2-difluoro-1-[trifluoromethyl] vinyl ether). These haloalkenes have been shown to be nephrotoxic in rats,[175] although clinically significant renal effects of haloalkene formation in surgical patients have not been reported. In dehydrated carbon dioxide absorbents, degradation of desflurane, enflurane, isoflurane, and sevoflurane results in carbon monoxide formation [176,177,248]

Special mention of several novel carbon dioxide absorbents that have reduced or eliminated sodium and potassium hydroxide content is warranted prior to delving into the discussion of compound A, carbon monoxide, and fires. The new absorbents, called Amsorb Plus and DrägerSorb® Free, contain primarily calcium hydroxide. These new absorbents are chemically unreactive with sevoflurane, enflurane, isoflurane, and desflurane, and thus, they essentially eliminate the degradation of these anesthetics to carbon monoxide and compound A (Fig. 15-31).[178–180]

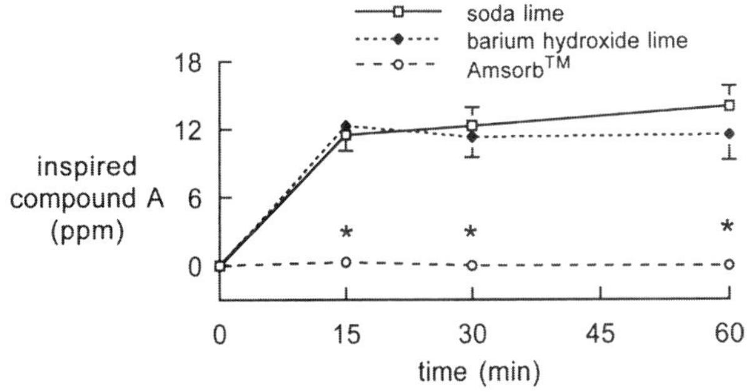

FIGURE 15-31. Compound A levels produced from three carbon dioxide absorbents during 1 MAC sevoflurane anesthesia delivered to volunteers at 1 lpm fresh gas flow (mean ± SE). Gas samples were taken from the inspired limb of the anesthesia circuit. *different from Baralyme® or soda lime ($p<0.05$). (Adapted from Mchaourab A, Arain SR, Ebert TJ: Lack of degradation of sevoflurane by a new carbon dioxide absorbent in humans. Anesthesiology 94:1007, 2001.)

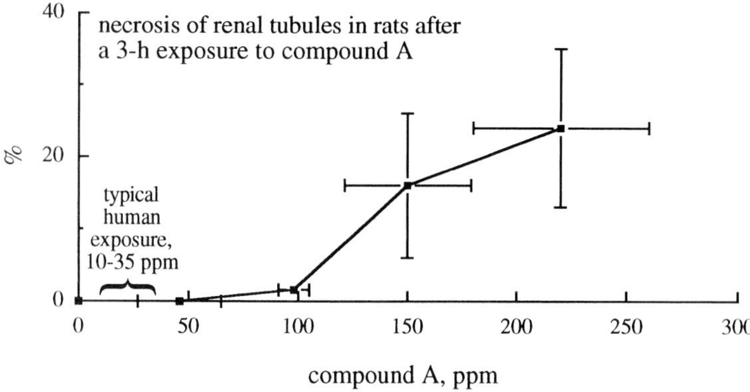

FIGURE 15-32. Renal biopsy results from rats inhaling different concentrations of compound A for 3 hours. The derived threshold to cause renal necrosis is around 100 ppm (300 ppm · hr). The typical human exposure during the administration of sevoflurane in a semiclosed circuit is between 10 and 35 ppm of compound A, which falls well below the threshold to cause renal injury in rats. (Adapted from Kharasch ED, Hoffman GM, Thorning D *et al*: Role of the renal cysteine conjugate β-lyase pathway in inhaled compound A nephrotoxicity in rats. Anesthesiology 88:1624, 1998.)

Compound A

Sevoflurane undergoes base-catalyzed degradation in carbon dioxide absorbents to form a vinyl ether called "compound A." The production of compound A is enhanced in low-flow or closed-circuit breathing systems and by warm or very dry CO_2 absorbents. Barium hydroxide lime produces more compound A than soda lime and this can be attributed to slightly higher absorbent temperature during CO_2 extraction.[174]

Studies in rats where compound A has been administered in the inspired gas have identified a threshold for renal tubular necrosis between 290 and 340 parts per million (ppm) × hour (e.g., 50 ppm × 6 hr = 300 ppm·hr) (Fig. 15-32).[181,182] The nephrotoxicity is characterized by cell necrosis of the cortical medullary tubules located in the proximal tubules.[175] The associated biochemical markers include elevations of serum BUN and creatinine, glucosuria, and proteinuria.[175,181] In addition, several enzymes from the tubule cells have been used as markers of cell injury including increases in urinary excretion of n-acetyl-beta-D-glucosaminidase (NAG) and alpha-glutathione-S-transferase (αGST).[175,181]

There are well-defined species differences in the threshold for compound A–induced nephrotoxicity. The threshold is approximately 300 ppm · hr in 250-gm rats,[181,262] greater than 612 ppm · hr in pigs,[183] and between 600 and 800 ppm · hr in monkeys.[184] In patients and volunteers receiving sevoflurane in closed-circuit or low-flow delivery systems, inspired compound A concentrations averaged 8 to 24 and 20 to 32 ppm with soda lime and barium hydroxide lime, respectively.[185–187] Total exposures as high as 320 to 400 ppm · hr have had no clear effect on clinical markers of renal function.[188,189] In randomized and prospective volunteer and patient studies, no adverse renal effects from low-flow (0.5 to 1.0 L/min) or closed-circuit sevoflurane anesthesia were detected using both standard clinical markers of renal function (serum creatinine and BUN concentrations) and experimental markers of renal function and structural integrity (proteinuria, glucosuria, and enzymuria).[185,186,189,190–192] In fact, several new studies evaluated the renal effects of long duration, low-flow sevoflurane in patients with preexisting renal disease (plasma creatinine >1.5 mg/dL).[193,194] The fresh gas flow was 1 LPM, barium hydroxide absorbent was employed, and minimal anesthetic adjuvants were given to maximize the dose of sevoflurane and production of compound A. There were no adverse effects from sevoflurane determined with both standard clinical markers and biochemical markers of renal function. Recent evidence from patients undergoing elective surgery indicates that transient proteinuria, glucosuria, and enzymuria also occur after desflurane, isoflurane, and propofol anesthesia, without changes in serum BUN and creatinine.[186,187] Despite solid evidence for the renal safety of low-flow sevoflurane from randomized prospective studies, the renal safety of sevoflurane has been questioned and debated.[195,196]

Aside from the high probability that the absence of renal injury in patients is because of low compound A levels during the clinical use of sevoflurane in a low-flow system, another probable explanation must be considered. Compound A is not itself toxic to organs. Rather it is the biodegradation of compound A to cysteine conjugates and the further action of a renal enzyme called beta-lyase on the conjugates that can result in formation of a potentially toxic thiol (Fig. 15-33).[182,197] There is clear evidence for species differences in the biotransformation of compound A to cysteine-s conjugates.[198] Recent evidence suggests that the cysteine conjugates can be handled in one (or both) of two ways.[199] They can be acetylated to mercapturic acid through a detoxication pathway, which results in no organ toxicity, or acted on by an enzyme in the kidneys

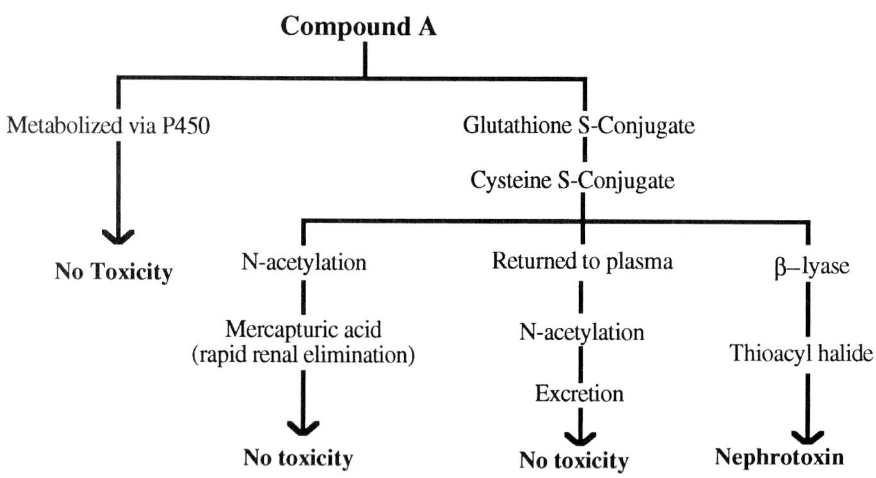

FIGURE 15-33. Known pathways for metabolism and elimination of compound A in humans. A potential toxin results only from the action of renal beta-lyase on cysteine-S-conjugates. The activity of this enzyme in humans is 8- to 30-fold less than in rats. Considerable handling of the cysteine-S-conjugates in humans is via N-acetylation to mercapturic acid. (Adapted from Kharasch ED, Jubert C: Compound A uptake and metabolism to mercapturic acids and 3,3,3-trifluoro-2-fluoromethoxypropanoic acid during low-flow sevoflurane anesthesia. Anesthesiology 91:1267, 1999.)

called renal beta-lyase, to form reactive intermediates (toxification pathway). These reactive intermediates are responsible for the renal cell necrosis seen in rats. The beta-lyase-dependent metabolism pathway in humans is far less extensive than the beta-lyase pathway in rats (8 to 30 times less active).[198] Thus, compared with rats, humans receive markedly lower doses of compound A and metabolize a lower fraction of compound A via the renal beta-lyase pathway. This may account for the safety of sevoflurane in both human volunteers and patients when compared to rat models. Finally, pharmacovigilance suggests sevoflurane is not nephrotoxic. The anesthetic has been in clinical use for nearly a decade, and many countries outside the United States have no flow restrictions on sevoflurane, yet not a single case report of renal harm from sevoflurane has been presented in the literature.

Carbon Monoxide and Heat

CO_2 absorbents degrade sevoflurane, desflurane, enflurane, and isoflurane to carbon monoxide when the normal water content of the absorbent (13 to 15%) is markedly decreased below 5%.[176,177,200] The degradation is the result of an exothermic reaction of the anesthetics with the absorbent. The anesthetic molecular structure and the presence of a strong base in the carbon dioxide absorbent are involved in the formation
6 of CO. Desflurane, enflurane, and isoflurane contain a difluoromethoxy moiety that is essential for the formation of CO. When studies are conducted with CO_2 absorbents maintained at or just above room temperature, desflurane and enflurane given at just under 1 MAC produced up to 8,000 and 4,000 ppm of CO, respectively, versus 79 ppm with nearly 2 MAC sevoflurane.[176] In dehydrated barium hydroxide, CO production from desflurane was nearly 3-fold higher than with soda lime but was trivial with sevoflurane. In normal clinical use, CO_2 canister temperatures are 25 to 45°C, but can be higher when employing a very low fresh gas flow. In a laboratory setting, when CO_2 canister temperature is not controlled and sevoflurane is administered to desiccated barium hydroxide, the exothermic reaction can increase canister temperatures. If CO_2 canister temperature exceeds 80°C, significant CO production is noted with sevoflurane.[177] Instances of CO poisoning have been reported in situations where the CO_2 absorbent has been presumably dried (desiccated) because an anesthetic machine has been left on with a high fresh gas flow passing through the CO_2 absorbent over an extended period of time.[201–204] In an experimental setting, overnight drying of barium hydroxide for 14 hours at 10L/min fresh gas flow did not result in significant CO production from desflurane, whereas 24 to 66 hours of fresh gas flow drying produced significant CO production.[205]

Although desflurane produces the most CO with anhydrous CO_2 absorbers, the reaction with sevoflurane produces the most heat. The strong exothermic reaction has caused significant heat production, fires, and patient injuries.[206,207] Although sevoflurane is not flammable at less than 11%, formaldehyde, methanol, and formate have been identified and these alone or in combination with oxygen might be flammable at high canister temperatures. In experimental settings, long exposure of 1 MAC sevoflurane to desiccated absorbents resulted in canister temperatures in excess of 300°C and can be associated with smoldering, melting of plastic components, explosions, and fires.[177]

There are newer CO_2 absorbents that do not degrade anesthetics (to either compound A or carbon monoxide) and they should reduce exothermic reactions. "From a patient safety perspective, widespread adoption of a nondestructive CO_2 absorbent should be axiomatic."[173] Although the cost of these new CO_2 absorbents (Amsorb® Plus and DrägerSorb® Free) is higher and the absorptive capacity may be lower than either barium hydroxide lime or soda lime, their benefit may be substantial. The use of a nondestructive absorbent eliminates all of the potential complications related to anesthetic breakdown and therefore minimizes the possibility of additional costs as a result of those complications, including additional lab tests, hospital days and medical/legal expenses. Adoption of these new absorbents into routine clinical practice is consistent with the patient safety goals of our anesthesia societies.

ANESTHETIC METABOLISM

Fluoride-Induced Nephrotoxicity

Metabolism (biotransformation) of halogenated anesthetics to free inorganic fluoride, resulting in nephrotoxicity, is now an accepted fact for the anesthetic methoxyflurane. The metabolism of methoxyflurane and, to a lesser extent, enflurane has resulted in a well-described injury to renal collecting tubules.[208,209] The nephrotoxicity associated with these anesthetics presents as a high output renal insufficiency that is unresponsive to vasopressin and is characterized by dilute polyuria, dehydration, serum hypernatremia, hyperosmolality, elevated BUN, and creatinine. An association between increased plasma fluoride concentrations and metabolism of these anesthetics led to a "fluoride hypothesis."[208] Nephrotoxicity is caused by metabolism of the volatile anesthetics to fluoride, and the inorganic fluoride is the ultimate substance producing the renal injury. This hypothesis has been reexamined recently in part because sevoflurane undergoes 5% metabolism that results in transient increases in serum fluoride concentrations but has not been associated with a renal concentrating defect.[209] The traditional hypothesis stated that both the duration of the high systemic fluoride concentrations (area under the fluoride time curve) and the peak fluoride concentration (peaks above 50 μM appear to represent the toxic threshold) were related to nephrotoxicity (Fig. 15-34).[208] The safety of sevoflurane and the relative safety of enflurane with regard to fluoride concentrations may be because of a rapid decline in plasma fluoride concentrations as a result of less availability of the anesthetic for metabolism from a faster washout compared to methoxyflurane.[210]

A recent report further clarifies this issue and has led to a modification of the traditional fluoride hypothesis for renal toxicity.[211] That is, the site of metabolism is an important factor in toxicity (i.e., intrarenal metabolism contributes to nephrotoxicity). The metabolism of methoxyflurane to fluoride in the kidney is significantly greater than that of sevoflurane and enflurane. This may be related to the multiple cytochrome P450 enzymes in the kidney responsible for metabolism of methoxyflurane (P450-2A6, P450-3A, P450-2E1).[211] In contrast, sevoflurane and enflurane are primarily metabolized by the cytochrome P450-2E1. Thus, intrarenal fluoride generated from methoxyflurane metabolism and/or the multiple P450 isoenzymes involved in methoxyflurane metabolism may account for the nephrotoxicity from this anesthetic. Therefore, the potential for toxicity from relatively high plasma levels of fluoride following long exposure to sevoflurane and enflurane is offset by the minimal amount of renal defluorination and this may explain the relative absence of renal concentrating defects with these anesthetics.[209,211,273]

Factors such as total dose of anesthetic, enzyme induction, and obesity have been proven to enhance biotransformation. The activity of hepatic cytochrome P450 enzymes is increased by a variety of drugs, including phenobarbital, phenytoin, and isoniazid.[212] Obesity causes increased metabolism (defluorination) in halothane, enflurane, and isoflurane. However, the effects of obesity on the defluorination of sevoflurane are less clear.[213]

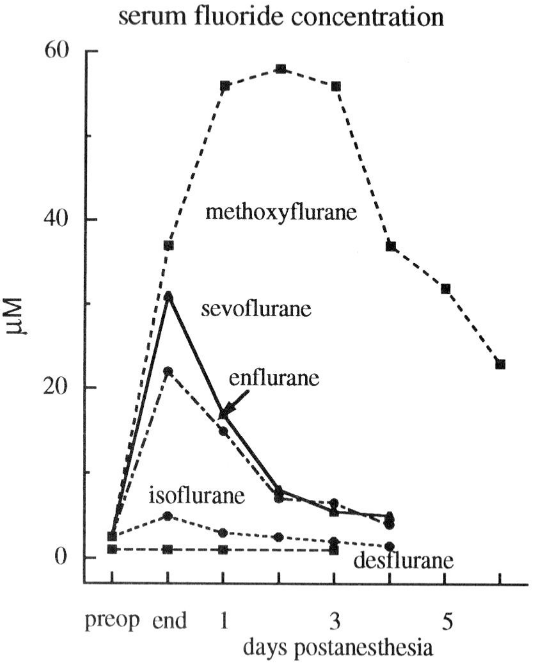

FIGURE 15-34. Plasma inorganic fluoride concentrations (mean ± SE) before and after 2 to 4 hours of methoxyflurane, enflurane, sevoflurane, isoflurane, and desflurane anesthesia. (Adapted from Kharasch ED, Armstrong AS, Gunn K, et al: Clinical sevoflurane metabolism and disposition. II. The role of cytochrome P450 2E1 in fluoride and hexafluoroisopropanol formation. Anesthesiology 82:1379, 1995; Mazze RI: Metabolism of the inhaled anaesthetics: Implications of enzyme induction. Br J Anaesth 56:27S, 1984; and Sutton TS, Koblin DD, Gruenke LD, et al: Fluoride metabolites after prolonged exposure of volunteers and patients to desflurane. Anesth Analg 73:180, 1991.)

Hepatic Injury from Metabolism: Halothane Hepatitis

Although postoperative liver dysfunction has been associated with most of the volatile anesthetics in current use, the most focused attention has been directed to halothane. This is in part because of the relatively recent demonstration of binding of an oxidatively derived metabolite of halothane to liver cytochromes, which could then act as haptens and induce an immune reaction. This hypersensitivity reaction has been as-
7 sociated with severe liver damage and fulminant hepatic failure. There are many causes of postoperative jaundice and abnormal liver function tests, including viral hepatitis, coexisting liver disease (such as Gilbert's disease), blood transfusions, septicemia, drug reactions, intra- and postoperative hypoxia and hypotension, and direct tissue trauma as a result of the surgical procedure.[150] The diagnosis of halothane hepatitis is generally made based on "incomplete exclusion," defined as the appearance of liver damage within 28 days of halothane exposure in a person in whom other known causes of liver disease have been excluded.

Halothane was introduced into clinical practice in 1956, and case reports of unexplained jaundice following anesthesia with halothane began to appear in 1958. By 1963, at least 350 putative cases of "halothane hepatitis" had been reported. In 1967, it was identified that approximately 18% of halothane was metabolized in man.[214] The metabolites were oxidatively derived. It is now known that oxidative metabolism of halothane, catalyzed by hepatic cytochrome P450 2E1, produces a reactive intermediate, trifluoroacetyl (TFA) that can covalently modify liver microsomal proteins. This complex can produce an immune response in some individuals that is characterized by immunoglobulin G antibodies. However, halothane-associated hepatitis can present as one of two clinical syndromes and it is likely that only one syndrome can be explained by an immune mechanism.[150,215] Each syndrome may develop after an uneventful anesthesia and surgery with no apparent time-to-dose relationship. The most common syndrome, which occurs in close to 20% of the adult patients receiving halothane, is a mild, self-limited postoperative illness that has been attributed to *reductive* metabolism of halothane and this route of metabolism is enhanced under low oxygen or hypoxic conditions. Reductive metabolism of isoflurane, desflurane, sevoflurane, and enflurane does not occur. This may relate to the fact that halothane uniquely reduces hepatic blood flow (both portal vein and hepatic artery blood flow).[216,217] The typical presentation of hepatitis from reductive metabolism is a rapid (1 to 3 days) but mild, unprogressing pattern of liver injury characterized by nausea, lethargy, fever, moderately increased concentrations of liver transaminases, and, rarely, transient jaundice. It does not require a repeat exposure, as does the immune mechanism of hepatitis; it can occur on the first exposure to halothane.

Several more recent observations suggest that reductive metabolism is not an important mechanism in the evolution of the immune-mediated halothane hepatitis.[150] The possibility existed that binding of a metabolite of halothane to liver cytochromes could act as haptens and induce a hypersensitivity response.[218] Supporting this possibility were the clinical manifestations of hepatitis, including eosinophilia, fever, rash, arthralgia, and prior exposure to halothane. The possibility of a genetic susceptibility factor is suggested by case reports of halothane hepatitis in closely related patients.[215] The most compelling evidence for an immune-mediated mechanism is the presence of circulating immunoglobulin G (IgG) antibodies in up to 70% of patients with diagnosis of halothane hepatitis.[150,218] This antibody is not directed against the reductive metabolite of halothane, but against an oxidative compound, TFA halide, which is incorporated onto the surface of the hepatocyte (Fig. 15-35).[219] TFA proteins have been identified from the liver of rats after halothane exposure with enzyme-linked immunosorbent assays and immunoblotting techniques. These altered proteins can be seen by the immune

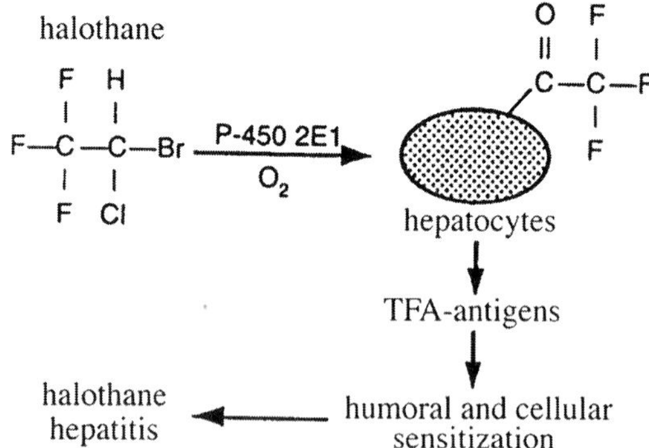

FIGURE 15-35. Halothane is metabolized to a trifluoroacetylated (TFA) adduct that binds to liver proteins. In susceptible patients, this adduct (altered protein) is seen as nonself (neoantigen), generating an immune response (production of antibodies). Subsequent exposure to halothane may result in hepatotoxicity. A similar process may occur in genetically susceptible individuals after anesthetic exposure to other fluorinated volatile anesthetics (enflurane, isoflurane, desflurane) that also generate a TFA adduct. (Adapted from Njoku D, Laster MJ, Gong DH *et al*: Biotransformation of halothane, enflurane, isoflurane, and desflurane to trifluoroacetylated liver proteins: Association between protein acylation and hepatic injury. Anesth Analg 84:173, 1997.)

system as nonself (neoantigen), generating production of antibodies. These can now be identified from serum samples of humans by identifying anti-TFA albumin activity on an ELISA screening evaluation.[220]

This metabolic pathway involving the cytochrome P450 2E1 system during halothane exposure is identical to the metabolic pathway noted with enflurane, isoflurane, and desflurane. However, the expression of the neoantigens should be related to the amount of metabolism of each agent. This would suggest that halothane is > enflurane > isoflurane > desflurane in terms of antigenic load.[221] Indeed, case reports have appeared in the literature linking each of these anesthetics with immune-mediated hepatitis.[220,222,223,311] If the incidence of fulminant hepatic failure after halothane is 1 in 35,000,[224] hepatic failure caused by isoflurane may occur in only 1 in 3,500,000 isoflurane anesthetics, and a lower incidence would be expected with desflurane. There are no reports of fulminant hepatic necrosis associated with sevoflurane in humans. Sevoflurane is not metabolized to a TFA halide; rather it is metabolized to hexafluoroisopropanol, which does not serve as a neoantigen (Fig. 15-36).[147] Desflurane is the least metabolized of the volatile anesthetics, resulting in very small amounts of adduct, and only one case report of hepatotoxicity from desflurane has been described.[220] Sensitization of this patient by two exposures to halothane (18 years and 12 years previously) precipitated massive hepatotoxicity. Anti-TFA antibodies were identified in the serum.

Herein lies another problem. Immunologic memory resulting in hepatitis has been reported 28 years after an initial halothane exposure.[225] In addition, cross-sensitivity has been reported in which exposure to one anesthetic can sensitize patients to a second but different anesthetic.[220,226] Recently these autoantibodies have been identified in 10% of health care workers (PACU nurses, nurse anesthetists, and anesthesiologists) chronically exposed to low levels of anesthetics.[221,227] Although this finding is intriguing if not alarming, the implication that anesthetics with the highest rates of metabolism (halothane, enflurane, and perhaps even isoflurane) should be removed from the OR setting requires further validation. It is worth recalling that despite case reports of hepatic damage associated with halothane, which appeared in the literature within 2 years of its introduction, it has taken some 35 years of research and debate to reach the current consensus on the mechanism of halothane-associated hepatitis and fulminant hepatic failure. It is the opinion of these authors that halothane should not be used in adult surgical cases and should be strongly discouraged in the pediatric population. Although the incidence of hepatitis appears to be much lower in the pediatric population, our concern is related to immunologic memory resulting in hepatitis later in life during a repeat exposure to anesthesia; additional concerns relate to health care workers who are chronically exposed to trace amounts of halothane. The new volatile anesthetics have an extremely low potential for hepatotoxicity and the possibility of avoiding even one case of fulminant hepatic failure from a volatile anesthetic is sufficiently compelling to discourage use of the older, more metabolized anesthetics including halothane and enflurane.

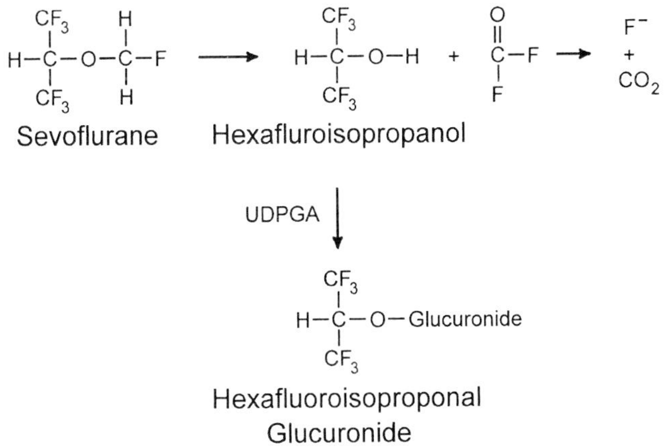

$$\underset{\text{Sevoflurane}}{(CF_3)_2CH{-}O{-}CH_2F} \longrightarrow \underset{\text{Hexafluroisopropanol}}{(CF_3)_2CH{-}OH} + O{=}CF_2 \longrightarrow F^- + CO_2$$

$$\text{Hexafluroisopropanol} \xrightarrow{\text{UDPGA}} \underset{\text{Hexafluoroisoproponal Glucuronide}}{(CF_3)_2CH{-}O{-}\text{Glucuronide}}$$

FIGURE 15-36. Pathway for oxidative metabolism of sevoflurane (UDPGA, uridine diphosphate glucuronic acid). Trifluoroacetylated (TFA) adducts are not formed from the metabolism of sevoflurane. (Adapted from Frink EJ Jr, Ghantous H, Malan TP *et al*: Plasma inorganic fluoride with sevoflurane anesthesia: Correlation with indices of hepatic and renal function. Anesth Analg 74:231, 1992.)

CLINICAL UTILITY OF VOLATILE ANESTHETICS

For Induction of Anesthesia

Although current-day practices for establishing the anesthetic state consist of initial administration of an IV sedative–hypnotic, there is an increasing interest in the use of volatile anesthetics via the face mask. This is commonplace in pediatric anesthesia but relatively rare in adult anesthesia. Historically, in the days of ether and cyclopropane, the standard induction technique was a mask induction. The renewed interest in this technique is attributed primarily to the newer potent and poorly soluble anesthetic, sevoflurane, which is nonpungent and, therefore, can easily be inhaled.[228] An important attribute of the gaseous induction technique is the ability to take the patient "deep" in a rapid fashion, thereby avoiding some of the unwanted side effects of stage 2 of anesthesia (excitation, salivation, coughing, movement), noted historically with the use of the highly soluble anesthetic, ether. Induction of anesthesia with halothane in the pediatric population is quite common. The resurgence of interest in mask induction in the adult population centers on the potential safety and utility of this technique when using sevoflurane.[229–232] The safety issues consist primarily of the fact that spontaneous ventilation is preserved with a gas induction, and patients essentially regulate their own depth of anesthesia, as excessive sevoflurane would, in fact, suppress ventilation. Safety would be compromised if stage 2 excitation was problematic; however, clinical studies indicate that this is not the case. It is likely that the low blood:gas solubility of sevoflurane makes for a rapid induction. Typical times to loss of consciousness average approximately 1 minute when delivering 8% sevoflurane via the face mask. Sevoflurane also has been used in the approach to the difficult adult airway because of the preservation of spontaneous ventilation and absence of salivation with this technique.[233] The traditional "awake look" in the suspected difficult airway (where IV drugs are titrated to a level that allows direct laryngoscopy in the awake patient) has been modified to consist of spontaneous ventilation of high concentrations of sevoflurane until laryngoscopic evaluation is tolerated. Laryngeal mask placement can be successfully achieved 2 minutes after administering 7% sevoflurane via the face mask.[230] The addition of nitrous oxide to the inspired gas mixture does not add significantly to the induction sequence. The gas induction technique is promoted by pretreatment with benzodiazepines but complicated by apnea with opioid pretreatment.[231] Of course the utility of this technique is that clinicians simply need to pay attention to the airway during the induction sequence, rather than reaching for drugs and injecting them through an IV port. Importantly, patient acceptance of this technique has been relatively high, exceeding 90% of the cases.[232] There have been a number of techniques described to use sevoflurane for induction of anesthesia via face mask. These include priming the circuit (emptying the rebreathing bag, opening the "pop-off" valve, dialing the vaporizer to 8% while using a fresh gas flow of 8 L/min, and maintaining this for 60 seconds prior to applying the face mask to the patient); a single-breath induction from end-expiratory volume to maximum inspired volume; and simply deep breathing. All seem to have the successful end result of loss of consciousness, generally within 1 minute.

For Maintenance of Anesthesia

The volatile anesthetics are clearly the most popular drug used to maintain anesthesia. They are easily administered via inhalation, they are readily titrated, they have a high safety ratio in terms of preventing recall, and the depth of anesthesia can be quickly adjusted in a predictable way while monitoring tissue levels via end-tidal concentrations. They are effective regardless of age or body habitus. They have some properties that prove beneficial in the operating room, including relaxation of skeletal muscle, in most cases preservation of cardiac output and cerebral blood flow, and relatively predictable recovery profiles. Some of the drawbacks to the use of the current volatile anesthetics are the absence of analgesic effects, their association with postoperative nausea and vomiting, and their potential for carbon monoxide poisoning and hepatitis.

PHARMACOECONOMICS AND VALUE-BASED DECISIONS

In the current environment of cost containment, clinicians are constantly being pressured to use less-expensive anesthetic agents, including antiemetics, neuromuscular blocking drugs, and volatile anesthetics. If succumbing to these pressures, the clinician must focus on providing value-based anesthesia. That is, to obtain the best results at the most practical cost. Factors involved in the value-based decision include the efficacy of the drug, the side effects, its direct costs, and its indirect effects. In terms of efficacy, all of the volatile anesthetics are reasonably similar, that is, they can be used to establish state of anesthesia for surgical interventions and can be easily reversed. In terms of side effects, the things to consider are serious side effects or toxicities versus manageable side effects, and to what extent these manageable side effects increase the cost. Regarding serious side effects, although halothane is the least expensive of the volatile anesthetics, it has definite life-threatening potential in terms of sensitization of the heart to arrhythmias and the development of an immune response that can cause fulminant hepatic necrosis. One can make a strong argument that halothane does not belong in the operating room. A common side effect of the volatile anesthetics is nausea and vomiting. The need for rescue medications to treat nausea and vomiting after volatile anesthesia needs to be weighed into any legitimate cost analysis. Direct costs are not simply the cost/mL of liquid or cost/bottle of anesthetic. Rather, they reflect the combination of the potency of the drug to establish a MAC level, the fresh gas flow, and the cost of the anesthetic. At 2 L/min fresh gas flow, delivering 1 MAC, both desflurane and sevoflurane cost about $13.00 to $15.00/hr. This contrasts to generically priced isoflurane, which costs $1.00 to $2.00/MAC⁻hr when delivered at 2 L/min.[234] Simply reducing the fresh gas flow of sevoflurane and desflurane can halve the cost/MAC⁻hr of these more expensive anesthetics without compromising their speed and effectiveness. The indirect costs are probably the most difficult to pinpoint, but may be the most important to evaluating the cost of using the new volatile anesthetics. Examples of indirect costs include costs associated with OR time, time in the PACU versus bypassing the PACU to a step-down unit, and labor costs and outcome related costs, such as litigation to defend a bad outcome from an anesthetic drug.

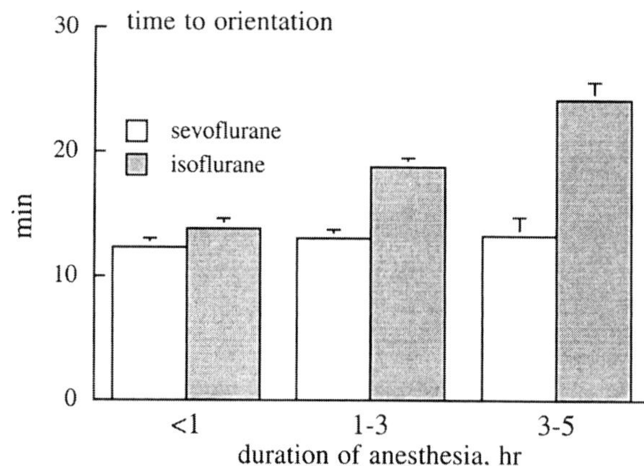

FIGURE 15-37. The recovery times to orientation after anesthesia of varying durations. With the less-soluble anesthetic sevoflurane, the time to orientation was independent of the anesthetic duration. In contrast, long anesthetic durations with isoflurane were associated with delayed times to orientation. (Adapted from Ebert TJ, Robinson BJ, Uhrich TD *et al*: Recovery from sevoflurane anesthesia: A comparison to isoflurane and propofol anesthesia. Anesthesiology 89:1524, 1998.)

One of the arguments for using the newer, more expensive volatile anesthetics, sevoflurane and desflurane, has been their relative speed in terms of emergence from anesthesia. It seems that this speed matches the ambulatory anesthesia environment in which we practice and the "move 'em in, move 'em out" approach to surgical patients. This argument has been tempered somewhat by the basic knowledge that one of the skills of the clinician is the titration of the volatile anesthetics. Even the more soluble drugs can be titrated based on clinical experience or with the aid of processed EEG monitors (such as the bispectral index system), permitting fast wake-ups regardless of the choice of anesthetic agent. However, there is strong evidence to support the use of the less-soluble (but most expensive) drugs in the longest surgical cases (Fig. 15-37).[3] In these cases the high direct cost of the anesthetic is balanced by the much improved recovery profile, including a more rapid time to emergence and a more rapid discharge from the recovery room. Curiously, the discharge advantage with the low soluble anesthetics has been difficult to show after shorter surgical procedures.

ACKNOWLEDGMENTS

The author wishes to acknowledge the contribution of Dr. Philip Schmid, Department of Anesthesiology, University of Iowa, for his work on the section entitled Pharmacokinetic Principles in the previous edition of this chapter.

References

1. Kety SS: The physiological and physical factors governing the uptake of anesthetic gases by the body. Anesthesiology 11:517, 1950
2. Eger EI II: Anesthetic Uptake and Action. Baltimore, Williams & Wilkins, 1974
3. Ebert TJ, Robinson BJ, Uhrich TD, Mackenthun A, Pichotta PJ: Recovery from sevoflurane anesthesia: A comparison to isoflurane and propofol anesthesia. Anesthesiology 89:1524, 1998
4. Nakata Y, Goto T, Morita S: Comparison of inhalation inductions with xenon and sevoflurane. Acta Anaesthesiol Scand 41:1157, 1997
5. Hettrick DA, Pagel PS, Kersten JR *et al*: Cardiovascular effects of xenon in isoflurane-anesthetized dogs with dilated cardiomyopathy. Anesthesiology 89:1166, 1998

6. Stanley TH, Kawamura R, Graves C: Effects of nitrous oxide on volume and pressure of endotracheal tube cuffs. Anesthesiology 41:256, 1974
7. Kaplan R, Abramowitz MD, Epstein BS: Nitrous oxide and air-filled balloon-tipped catheters. Anesthesiology 55:71, 1981
8. Munson ES, Merrick HC: Effect of nitrous oxide on venous air embolism. Anesthesiology 27:783, 1966
9. Waun JE, Sweitzer RS, Hamilton WK: Effect of nitrous oxide on middle ear mechanics and hearing acuity. Anesthesiology 28:846, 1987
10. Tinker JH, Sharbrough FW, Michenfelder JD: Anterior shift of the dominant EEG rhythm during anesthesia in the Java monkey: Correlation with anesthetic potency. Anesthesiology 46:252, 1977
11. Gross JB, Alexander CM: Awakening concentrations of isoflurane are not affected by analgesic doses of morphine. Anesth Analg 67:27, 1988
12. Katoh T, Suguro Y, Kimura T, Ikeda K: Cerebral awakening concentration of sevoflurane and isoflurane predicted during slow and fast alveolar washout. Anesth Analg 77:1012, 1993
13. Roizen MF, Horrigan RW, Frazer BM: Anesthetic doses blocking adrenergic (Stress) and cardiovascular responses to incision—MAC BAR. Anesthesiology 54:390, 1981
14. Liem EB, Lin C-M, Suleman M-I *et al*: Anesthetic requirement is increased in redheads. Anesthesiology 101:279, 2004
15. Mogil JS, Wilson SG, Chesler EJ *et al*: The nelanocortin-1 receptor gene mediates female-specific mechanisms of analgesia in mice and humans. Proc Natl Acad Sci U S A 100:4867, 2003
16. Stekiel TA, Contney SJ, Bosnjak ZJ, Kampine JP, Roman RJ, Stekiel WJ: Reversal of minimum alveolar concentrations of volatile anesthetics by chromosomal substitution. Anesthesiology 101:796, 2004
17. LeDez, KM, Lerman J: The minimum alveolar concentration (MAC) of isoflurane in preterm neonates. Anesthesiology 67(3):301, 1987
18. Mapleson WW: Effect of age on MAC in humans: A meta-analysis. Br J Anaesth 76:179, 1996
19. Stullken EH Jr, Milde JH, Michenfelder JD, Tinker JH: The non-linear responses of cerebral metabolism to low concentrations of halothane, enflurane, isoflurane and thiopental. Anesthesiology 46:28–34, 1977
20. Michenfelder JD: The in vivo effects of massive concentrations of anesthetics on canine cerebral metabolism. In Halsey MJ, Kent DW (eds): Molecular Mechanisms of Anesthesia, p 537. New York, Raven Press, 1975
21. Lutz LJ, Milde JH, Milde LN: The cerebral functional, metabolic, and hemodynamic effects of desflurane in dogs. Anesthesiology 73:125, 1990
22. Scheller MS, Nakakimura K, Fleischer JE, Zornow MH: Cerebral effects of sevoflurane in the dog: Comparison with isoflurane and enflurane. Br J Anaesth 65(3):388, 1990
23. Osawa M, Shingu K, Murakawa M *et al*: Effects of sevoflurane on central nervous system electrical activity in cats. Anesth Analg 79:52, 1994
24. Rampil IJ, Laster M, Dwyer RC, Taheri S, Eger EI II: No EEG evidence of acute tolerance to desflurane in swine. Anesthesiology 74:889, 1991
25. Fujibayashi T, Sugiura Y, Yanagimoto M, Harada J, Goto Y: Brain energy metabolism and blood flow during sevoflurane and halothane anesthesia: Effects of hypocapnia and blood pressure fluctuations. Acta Anaesthesiol Scand 38:413, 1994
26. Yli-Hankala A, Vakkuri A, Särkelä M, Lindgren L, Korttila K, Jäntti V: Epileptiform electroencephalogram during mask induction of anesthesia with sevoflurane. Anesthesiology 91:1596, 1999
27. Julliac B, Guehl D, Chopin F, Burbaud P, Cros AM: Sharp increase in cerebral sevoflurane concentration during mask induction in adults is a major risk factor of spike wave occurrence. Anesthesiology A-132, 2004
28. Jääskeläinen SK, Kaisti K, Suni L, Hinkka S, Scheinin H: Sevoflurane is epileptogenic in healthy subjects at surgical levels of anesthesia. Neurology 61:1073, 2003
29. Hisada K, Morioka T, Fukui K *et al*: Effects of sevoflurane and isoflurane on electrocorticographic activities in patients with temporal lobe epilepsy. J Neurosurg Anesthesiol 13:333, 2001
30. Todd MM, Drummond JC: A comparison of the cerebrovascular and metabolic effects of halothane and isoflurane in the cat. Anesthesiology 60:276, 1984
31. Adams RW, Gronert GA, Sundt TM Jr, Michenfelder JD: Halothane, hypocapnia, and cerebrospinal fluid pressure in neurosurgery. Anesthesiology 37:510, 1972
32. Drummond JC, Todd MM: The response of the feline cerebral circulation to Pa_{CO2} during anesthesia with isoflurane and halothane and during sedation with nitrous oxide. Anesthesiology 62:268, 1985
33. Bedforth NM, Hardman JG, Nathanson MH: Cerebral hemodynamic response to the introduction of desflurane: A comparison with sevoflurane. Anesth Analg 91:152, 2000
34. Algotsson L, Messeter K, Nordström CH, Ryding E: Cerebral blood flow and oxygen consumption during isoflurane and halothane anesthesia in man. Acta Anaesthesiol Scand 32:15, 1988
35. Brüssel T, Fitch W, Brodner G, Arendt I, Van Aken H: Effects of halothane in low concentrations on cerebral blood flow, cerebral metabolism, and cerebrovascular autoregulation in the baboon. Anesth Analg 73:758, 1991
36. Van Aken H, Fitch W, Graham DI, Brüssel T, Themann H: Cardiovascular and cerebrovascular effects of isoflurane-induced hypotension in the baboon. Anesth Analg 65:565, 1986
37. Drummond JC, Todd MM, Scheller MS, Shapiro HM: A comparison of the direct cerebral vasodilating potencies of halothane and isoflurane in the New Zealand white rabbit. Anesthesiology 65:462, 1986
38. Smith AL, Wollman H: Cerebral blood flow and metabolism: Effects of anesthetic drugs and techniques. Anesthesiology 36:378, 1972
39. Hansen TD, Warner DS, Todd MM, Vust LJ: The role of cerebral metabolism in determining the local cerebral blood flow effects of volatile anesthetics: Evidence for persistent flow-metabolism coupling. J Cereb Blood Flow Metab 9:323, 1989
40. Drummond JC, Todd MM, Toutant SM, Shapiro HM: Brain surface protrusion during enflurane, halothane, and isoflurane anesthesia in cats. Anesthesiology 59:288, 1983
41. Adams RW, Cucchiara RF, Gronert GA, Messick JM Jr, Michenfelder JD: Isoflurane and cerebrospinal fluid pressure in neurosurgical patients. Anesthesiology 54:97, 1981
42. Grosslight K, Foster R, Colohan AR, Bedford RF: Isoflurane for neuroanesthesia: risk factors for increases in intracranial pressure. Anesthesiology 63:533, 1985
43. Artru A: A. Isoflurane does not increase the rate of CSF production in the dog. Anesthesiology 60(3):193, 1984
44. Talke P, Caldwell J, Dodsont B, Richardson CA: Desflurane and isoflurane increases lumbar cerebrospinal fluid pressure in normocapnic patients undergoing transsphenoidal hypophysectomy. Anesthesiology 85:999, 1996
45. Talke P, Caldwell JE, Richardson CA: Sevoflurane increases lumbar cerebrospinal fluid pressure in normocapnic patients undergoing transsphenoidal hypophysectomy. Anesthesiology 91:127, 1999
46. Sponheim S, Skraastad Ø, Helseth E, Due-Tønnesen B, Aamodt G, Breivik H: Effects of 0.5 and 1.0 MAC isoflurane, sevoflurane and desflurane on intracranial and cerebral perfusion pressures in children. Acta Anaesthesiol Scand 47:932, 2003
47. Muzzi DA, Losasso TJ, Dietz NM, Faust RJ, Cucchiara RF, Milde LN: The effect of desflurane and isoflurane on cerebrospinal fluid pressure in humans with supratentorial mass lesions. Anesthesiology 76:720, 1992
48. Sugioka S: Effects of sevoflurane on intracranial pressure and formation and absorption of cerebrospinal fluid in cats. [Japanese]. Masui 41:1434, 1992
49. Artru AA: Rate of cerebrospinal fluid formation, resistance to reabsorption of cerebrospinal fluid, brain tissue water content, and electroencephalogram during desflurane anesthesia in dogs. J Neurosurg Anesthesiol 5:178, 1993
50. Wollman H, Alexander C, Cohen PJ, Smith TC, Chase PE, van der Molen RA: Cerebral circulation during general anesthesia and hyperventilation in man. Thiopental induction to nitrous oxide and d-Tubocurarine. Anesthesiology 26:329, 1998
51. Lutz LJ, Milde JH, Milde LN: The response of the canine cerebral circulation to hyperventilation during anesthesia with desflurane. Anesthesiology 74:504, 1991
52. Bundgaard H, von Oettingen G, Larsen KM *et al*: Effects of sevoflurane on intracranial pressure, cerebral blood flow and cerebral metabolism. Acta Anaesthesiol Scand 42:621, 1998
53. Hoff J, Schmith A, Nielsen S, et al: Effects of barbiturate and halothane anaesthesia on focal cerebral infarction in the dog. Surg Forum 24:449, 1973
54. Michenfelder JD, Milde JH, Sundt JM Jr: Cerebral protection by barbiturate anesthesia. Use after middle cerebral artery occlusion in Java monkeys. Arch Neurol 33, 1976
55. Newberg, LA, Michenfelder JD: Cerebral protection by isoflurane during hypoxemia or ischemia. Anesthesiology 59(1):23–28, 1983
56. Newberg LA, Milde JH, Michenfelder JD: Systemic and cerebral effects of isoflurane-induced hypotension in dogs. Anesthesiology 60:541, 1984
57. Seyde WC, Longnecker DE: Cerebral oxygen tension in rats during deliberate hypotension with sodium nitroprusside, 2-chloroadenosine, or deep isoflurane anesthesia. Anesthesiology 64:480, 1986
58. Michenfelder JD, Sundt TM, Fode N, Sharbrough FW: Isoflurane when compared to enflurane and halothane decreases the frequency of cerebral ischemia during carotid endarterectomy. Anesthesiology 67:336, 1987
59. Messick JM Jr, Casement B, Sharbrough FW, Milde LN, Michenfelder JD, Sundt TM Jr: Correlation of regional cerebral blood flow (rCBF) with EEG changes during isoflurane anesthesia for carotid endarterectomy: Critical rCBF. Anesthesiology 66:344, 1987
60. Werner C, Möllenberg O, Kochs E, Schulte am Esch J: Sevoflurane improves neurological outcome after incomplete cerebral ischaemia in rats. Br J Anaesth 75:756, 1995
61. Engelhard K, Werner C, Reeker W *et al*: Desflurane and isoflurane improve neurological outcome after incomplete cerebral ischaemia in rats. Br J Anaesth 83:415, 1999
62. Loepke AW, Priestley MA, Schultz SEMJ, Golden J, Kurth CD: Desflurane improves neurologic outcome after low-flow cardiopulmonary bypass in newborn pigs. Anesthesiology 97:1521, 2002
63. Hoffman WE, Charbel FT, Edelman G, Ausman JI: Thiopental and desflurane treatment for brain protection. Neurosurgery 43:1050, 1998
64. Sakabe T, Tsutsui T, Maekawa T, Ishikawa T, Takeshita H: Local cerebral glucose utilization during nitrous oxide and pentobarbital anesthesia in rats. Anesthesiology 63:262, 1985
65. Fleischer JE, Milde JH, Moyer TP, Michenfelder JD: Cerebral effects of high-dose midazolam and subsequent reversal with Ro 15-1788 in dogs. Anesthesiology 68:234, 1988

66. Hoffman WE, Miletich DJ, Albrecht RF: The effects of midazolam on cerebral blood flow and oxygen consumption and its interaction with nitrous oxide. Anesth Analg 65:729, 1986
67. Baughman VL, Hoffman WE, Thomas C, Albrecht RF, Miletich DJ: The interaction of nitrous oxide and isoflurane with incomplete cerebral ischemia in the rat. Anesthesiology 70:767, 1989
68. Hartung J, Cottrell JE: Nitrous oxide reduces thiopental-induced prolongation of survival in hypoxic and anoxic mice. Anesth Analg 66:47–52, 1987
69. Eger EI II, Smith NT, Stoelting RK, Cullen DJ, Kadis LB, Whitcher CE: Cardiovascular effects of halothane in man. Anesthesiology 32:396, 1970
70. Calverley RK, Smith NT, Prys-Roberts C, Eger EI II, Jones CW: Cardiovascular effects of enflurane anesthesia during controlled ventilation in man. Anesth Analg 57:619, 1978
71. Stevens WC, Cromwell TH, Halsey MJ, Eger EI II, Shakespeare TF, Bahlman SH: The cardiovascular effects of a new inhalation anesthetic, Forane, in human volunteers at a constant arterial carbon dioxide tension. Anesthesiology 35:8, 1971
72. Weiskopf RB, Cahalan MK, Eger EI II *et al:* Cardiovascular actions of desflurane in normocarbic volunteers. Anesth Analg 73:143, 1991
73. Malan TP Jr, DiNardo JA, Isner RJ *et al:* Cardiovascular effects of sevoflurane compared with those of isoflurane in volunteers. Anesthesiology 83:918, 1995
74. Ebert TJ, Muzi M, Lopatka CW: Neurocirculatory responses to sevoflurane in humans. A comparison to desflurane. Anesthesiology 83:88, 1995
75. Ebert TJ, Kampine JP: Nitrous oxide augments sympathetic outflow: Direct evidence from human peroneal nerve recordings. Anesth Analg 69:444, 1989
76. Bastard OG, Carter JG, Moyers JR, Bross BA: Circulatory effects of isoflurane in patients with ischemic heart disease: A comparison with halothane. Anesth Analg 63:635, 1984
77. Pagel PS, Kampine JP, Schmeling WT, Warltier DC: Alteration of left ventricular diastolic function by desflurane, isoflurane, and halothane in the chronically instrumented dog with autonomic nervous system blockade. Anesthesiology 74:1103, 1991
78. Eger EI II: Isoflurane: A review. Anesthesiology 55:559, 1981
79. Merin RG, Bernard J, Doursout M, Cohen M, Chelly JE: Comparison of the effects of isoflurane and desflurane on cardiovascular dynamics and regional blood flow in the chronically instrumented dog. Anesthesiology 74:568, 1991
80. Pagel PS, Kampine JP, Schmeling WT, Warltier DC: Evaluation of myocardial contractility in the chronically instrumented dog with intact autonomic nervous system function: Effects of desflurane and isoflurane. Acta Anaesthesiol Scand 37:203, 1993
81. Bernard J-M, Wouters PF, Doursout M-F, Florence B, Chelly JE, Merin RG: Effects of sevoflurane and isoflurane on cardiac and coronary dynamics in chronically instrumented dogs. Anesthesiology 72:659, 1990
82. Ebert TJ, Muzi M: Sympathetic hyperactivity during desflurane anesthesia in healthy volunteers. A comparison with isoflurane. Anesthesiology 79:444, 1993
83. Muzi M, Ebert TJ, Hope WG, Bell LB: Site(s) mediating sympathetic activation with desflurane. Anesthesiology 85:737, 1996
84. Pacentine GG, Muzi M, Ebert TJ: Effects of fentanyl on sympathetic activation associated with the administration of desflurane. Anesthesiology 82:823, 1995
85. Weiskopf RB, Eger EI II, Noorani M, Daniel M: Fentanyl, esmolol, and clonidine blunt the transient cardiovascular stimulation induced by desflurane in humans. Anesthesiology 81:1350, 1994
86. Yonker-Sell AE, Muzi M, Hope WG, Ebert TJ: Alfentanil modifies the neurocirculatory responses to desflurane. Anesth Analg 82:162, 1996
87. Housmans PR, Murat I: Comparative effects of halothane, enflurane, and isoflurane at equipotent anesthetic concentrations on isolated ventricular myocardium of the ferret. II. Relaxation. Anesthesiology 69:464, 1988
88. Weiskopf RB, Cahalan MK, Ionescu P *et al*: Cardiovascular actions of desflurane with and without nitrous oxide during spontaneous ventilation in humans. Anesth Analg 73:165, 1991
89. Ebert TJ: Differential effects of nitrous oxide on baroreflex control of heart rate and peripheral sympathetic nerve activity in humans. Anesthesiology 72:16, 1990
90. Crawford MW, Lerman J, Saldivia V, Carmichael FJ: Hemodynamic and organ blood flow responses to halothane and sevoflurane anesthesia during spontaneous ventilation. Anesth Analg 75:1000, 1992
91. Ebert TJ, Harkin CP, Muzi M: Cardiovascular responses to sevoflurane: A review. Anesth Analg 81:S11, 1995
92. Atlee JL III, Bosnjak ZJ: Mechanisms for cardiac dysrhythmias during anesthesia. Anesthesiology 72(2):347, 1990
93. Buffington CW, Romson JL, Levine A, Duttlinger NC, Huang AH: Isoflurane induces coronary steal in a canine model of chronic coronary occlusion. Anesthesiology 66:280, 1987
94. Reiz S, Balfors E, Sorensen MB, Ariola S Jr, Friedman A, Truedsson H: Isoflurane—a powerful coronary vasodilator in patients with coronary artery disease. Anesthesiology 59:91, 1983
95. Kersten JR, Brayer AP, Pagel PS, Tessmer JP, Warltier DC: Perfusion of ischemic myocardium during anesthesia with sevoflurane. Anesthesiology 81:995, 1994
96. Hartman JC, Kampine JP, Schmeling WT, Warltier DC: Steal-prone coronary circulation in chronically instrumented dogs: Isoflurane versus adenosine. Anesthesiology 74:744, 1991
97. Hartman JC, Pagel PS, Kampine JP, Schmeling WT, Warltier DC: Influence of desflurane on regional distribution of coronary blood flow in a chronically instrumented canine model of multivessel coronary artery obstruction. Anesth Analg 72:289, 1991
98. Slogoff S, Keats AS, Dear WE *et al*: Steal-prone coronary anatomy and myocardial ischemia associated with four primary anesthetic agents in humans. Anesth Analg 72:22, 1991
99. Tuman KJ, McCarthy RJ, Spiess BD, DaValle M, Dabir R, Ivankovich AD: Does choice of anesthetic agent significantly affect outcome after coronary artery surgery? Anesthesiology 70:189, 1989
100. Searle NR, Martineau RJ, Conzen P *et al*: Comparison of sevoflurane/fentanyl and isoflurane/fentanyl during elective coronary artery bypass surgery. Can J Anaesth 43:890, 1996
101. Ebert TJ, Kharasch ED, Rooke GA, Shroff A, Muzi M. Sevoflurane Ischemia Group: Myocardial ischemia and adverse cardiac outcomes in cardiac patients undergoing noncardiac surgery with sevoflurane and isoflurane. Anesth Analg 85:993, 1997
102. Thomson IR, Bowering JB, Hudson RJ, Frais MA, Rosenbloom M: A comparison of desflurane and isoflurane in patients undergoing coronary artery surgery. Anesthesiology 75:776, 1991
103. Helman JD, Leung JM, Bellows WH *et al*: The risk of myocardial ischemia in patients receiving desflurane versus sufentanil anesthesia for coronary artery bypass graft surgery. Anesthesiology 77:47, 1992
104. Kersten JR, Schmeling TJ, Pagel PS, Gross GJ, Warltier DC: Isoflurane mimics ischemic preconditioning via activation of KATP channels. Anesthesiology 87:361, 1997
105. Novalija E, Fujita S, Kampine JP, Stowe DF: Sevoflurane mimics ischemic preconditioning effects on coronary flow and nitric oxide release in isolated hearts. Anesthesiology 91:701, 1999
106. Riess ML, Stowe DF, Warltier DC: Cardiac pharmacolocial preconditioning with volatile anesthetics: From bench to bedside? Am J Physiol 286:H1603, 2004
107. Stowe DF, Kevin LG: Cardiac preconditioning by volatile anesthetic agents: A defining role for altered mitochondrial bioenergetics. Antioxid Redox Signal 6:439, 2004
108. Novalija E, Kevin LG, Camara AK, Bosnjak ZJ, Kampine JP, Stowe DF: Reactive oxygen species precede the epsilon isoform of protein kinase C in the anesthetic preconditioning signaling cascade. Anesthesiology 99:421, 2003
109. Kevin LG, Katz P, Camara AK, Novalija E, Riess ML, Stowe DF: Anesthetic preconditioning: effects on latency to ischemic injury in isolated hearts. Anesthesiology 99:385, 2003
110. Conzen PF, Fischer S, Detter C, Peter K: Sevoflurane provides greater protection of the myocardium than propofol in patients undergoing off-pump coronary artery bypass surgery. Anesthesiology 99:826, 2003
111. De Hert SG, Van der Linden PJ, Cromheecke S *et al*: Choice of primary anesthetic regimen can influence intensive care unit length of stay after coronary surgery with cardiopulmonary bypass. Anesthesiology 101:9, 2004
112. Gu W, Pagel PS, Warltier DC, Kersten JR: Modifying cardiovascular risk in diabetes mellitus. Anesthesiology 98:774, 2003
113. Seagard JL, Hopp FA, Donegan JH, Kalbfleisch JH, Kampine JP: Halothane and the carotid sinus reflex: evidence for multiple sites of action. Anesthesiology 57:191, 1982
114. Seagard JL, Hopp FA, Bosnjak ZJ, Osborn JL, Kampine JP: Sympathetic efferent nerve activity in conscious and isoflurane-anesthetized dogs. Anesthesiology 61:266, 1984
115. Seagard JL, Hopp FA, Bosnjak ZJ, Elegebe EO, Kampine JP: Extent and mechanism of halothane sensitization of the carotid sinus baroreceptors. Anesthesiology 58:432, 1983
116. Seagard JL, Elegbe EO, Hopp FA *et al*: Effects of isoflurane on the baroreceptor reflex. Anesthesiology 59:511, 1983
117. Kotrly KJ, Ebert TJ, Vucins EJ, Igler FO, Kampine JP: Human baroreceptor control of heart rate under isoflurane anesthesia. Anesthesiology 60:173, 1984
118. Muzi M, Ebert TJ: A randomized, prospective comparison of halothane, isoflurane and enflurane on baroreflex control of heart rate in humans. In: Bosnjak Z, Kampine JP (eds). Advances in Pharmacology, Vol. 31: Anesthesia and Cardiovascular Disease, p 379. San Diego, Academic Press, 1994
119. Tanaka M, Nishikawa T: Arterial baroreflex function in humans anaesthetized with sevoflurane. Br J Anaesth 82:350, 1999
120. Muzi M, Ebert TJ: A comparison of baroreflex sensitivity during isoflurane and desflurane anesthesia in humans. Anesthesiology 82:919, 1995
121. Ebert TJ, Perez F, Uhrich TD, Deshur MA: Desflurane-mediated sympathetic activation occurs in humans despite preventing hypotension and baroreceptor unloading. Anesthesiology 88:1227, 1998
122. Kotrly KJ, Ebert TJ, Vucins EJ, Roerig DL, Stadnicka A, Kampine JP: Effects of fentanyl-diazepam-nitrous oxide anaesthesia on arterial baroreflex control of heart rate in man. Br J Anaesth 58:406, 1986
123. Ebert TJ, Kotrly KJ, Madsen KS, Bernstein JS, Kampine JP: Fentanyl-diazepam anesthesia with or without N_2O does not attenuate cardiopulmonary baroreflex-mediated vasoconstrictor responses to controlled hypovolemia in humans. Anesth Analg 67:548, 1988

124. Tanaka M, Nishikawa T: Sevoflurane speeds recovery of baroreflex control of heart rate after minor surgical procedures compared with isoflurane. Anesth Analg 89:284, 1999
125. Muzi M, Lopatka CW, Ebert TJ: Desflurane-mediated neurocirculatory activation in humans: Effects of concentration and rate of change on responses. Anesthesiology 84:1035, 1996
126. Bunting HE, Kelly MC, Milligan KR: Effect of nebulized lignocaine on airway irritation and haemodynamic changes during induction of anaesthesia with desflurane. Br J Anaesth 75:631, 1995
127. Calverley RK, Smith NT, Jones CW, Prys-Roberts C, Eger EI II: Ventilatory and cardiovascular effects of enflurane anesthesia during spontaneous ventilation in man. Anesth Analg 57:610, 1978
128. Warner DO, Warner MA, Ritman EL: Mechanical significance of changing rib cage-diaphragm interactions to the ventilatory depression of halothane anesthesia. Anesthesiology 84:309, 1996
129. Warner DO, Warner MA, Ritman EL: Human chest wall function while awake and during halothane anesthesia. I: Quiet breathing. Anesthesiology 82:6, 1995
130. Warner DO, Warner MA, Ritman EL: Atelectasis and chest wall shape during halothane anesthesia. Anesthesiology 85:49, 1996
131. Kochi T, Ide T, Isono S, Mizuguchi T, Nishino T: Different effects of halothane and enflurane on diaphragmatic contractility in vivo. Anesth Analg 70:362, 1990
132. Hornbein TF, Martin WE, Bonica JJ *et al*: Nitrous oxide effects on the circulatory and ventilatory responses to halothane. Anesthesiology 31:250, 1969
133. Hirshman CA, McCullough RE, Cohen PJ, Weil JV: Depression of hypoxic ventilatory response by halothane, enflurane and isoflurane in dogs. Br J Anaesth 49:957, 1977
134. Yacoub O, Doell D, Kryger MH, Anthonisen NR: Depression of hypoxic ventilatory response by nitrous oxide. Anesthesiology 45:385, 1976
135. van den Elsen M, Sarton E, Teppema L, Berkenbosch A, Dahan A: Influence of 0.1minimum alveolar concentration of sevoflurane, desflurane and isoflurane on dynamic ventilatory response to hypercapnia in humans. Br J Anaesth 80:174, 1998
136. Lopez-Barneo J, Pardal R, Ortega-Saenz P: Cellular mechanisms of oxygen sensing. Annu Rev Physiol 63:259, 2001
137. Dahan A, Teppema LJ: Influence of anaesthesia and analgesia on the control of breathing. Br J Anaesth 91:40, 2003
138. Hirshman CA, Bergman NA: Factors influencing intrapulmonary airway calibre during anaesthesia. Br J Anaesth 65:30, 1990
139. Hirshman CA, Edelstein G, Peetz S, Wayne R, Downes H: Mechanism of action of inhalational anesthesia on airways. Anesthesiology 56:107, 1982
140. Lindeman KS, Baker SG, Hirshman CA: Interaction between halothane and the nonadrenergic, noncholinergic inhibitory system in porcine trachealis muscle. Anesthesiology 81:641, 1994
141. Rooke GA, Choi J-H, Bishop MJ: The effect of isoflurane, halothane, sevoflurane, and thiopental/nitrous oxide on respiratory system resistance after tracheal intubation. Anesthesiology 86:1294, 1997
142. Mori N, Nagata H, Ohta S, Suzuki M: Prolonged sevoflurane inhalation was not nephrotoxic in two patients with refractory status asthmaticus. Anesth Analg 83:189, 1996
143. Reiz S: Nitrous oxide augments the systemic and coronary haemodynamic effects of isoflurane in patients with ischaemic heart disease. Acta Anaesthesiol Scand 27:464, 1983
144. Benumof JL, Augustine SD, Gibbons JA: Halothane and isoflurane only slightly impair arterial oxygenation during one-lung ventilation in patients undergoing thoracotomy. Anesthesiology 67:910, 1987
145. Beck DH, Doepfmer UR, Sinemus C, Bloch A, Schenk MR, Kox WJ: Effects of sevoflurane and propofol on pulmonary shunt fraction during one-lung ventilation for thoracic surgery. Br J Anaesth 86:38, 2001
146. Abe K, Mashimo T, Yoshiya I: Arterial oxygenation and shunt fraction during one-lung ventilation: A comparison of isoflurane and sevoflurane. Anesth Analg 86:1266, 1998
147. Frink EJ Jr, Ghantous H, Malan TP *et al*: Plasma inorganic fluoride with sevoflurane anesthesia: Correlation with indices of hepatic and renal function. Anesth Analg 74:231, 1992
148. Hursh D, Gelman S, Bradley EL: Hepatic oxygen supply during halothane or isoflurane anesthesia in guinea pigs. Anesthesiology 67:701, 1987
149. Baden JM, Serra M, Fujinaga M, Mazze RI: Halothane metabolism in cirrhotic rats. Anesthesiology 67:660, 1987
150. Elliott RH, Strunin L: Hepatotoxicity of volatile anaesthetics. Br J Anaesth 70:339, 1993
151. Weiskopf RB, Eger EI II, Ionescu P *et al*: Desflurane does not produce hepatic or renal injury in human volunteers. Anesth Analg 74:570, 1992
152. Eger EI II. Isoflurane (Forane): A compendium and reference. Madison, Ohio, Medical Products, 1985
153. Hussey AJ, Aldridge LM, Paul D, Ray DC, Beckett GJ, Allan LG: Plasma glutathione-S-transferase concentration as a measure of hepatocellular integrity following a single general anaesthetic with halothane, enflurane or isoflurane. Br J Anaesth 60:130, 1988
154. Wulf H, Kahl M, Ledowski T: Augmentation of the neuromuscular blocking effects of cisatracurium during desflurane, sevoflurane, isoflurane or total i.v. anaesthesia. Br J Anaesth 80:308, 1998
155. Kurahashi K, Maruta H: The effect of sevoflurane and isoflurane on the neuromuscular block produced by vecuronium continuous infusion. Anesth Analg 82:942, 1996
156. Dilger JP, Vidal AM, Mody HI, Liu Y: Evidence for direct actions of general anesthetics on an ion channel protein. Anesthesiology 81:431, 1994
157. Paul M, Fokt RM, Kindler CH, Dipp NCJ, Yost CS: Characterization of the interactions between volatile anesthetics and neuromuscular blockers at the muscle nicotinic acetylcholine receptor. Anesth Analg 95:362, 2002
158. Wright PMC, Hart P, Lau M *et al*: The magnitude and time course of vecuronium potentiation by desflurane versus isoflurane. Anesthesiology 82:404, 1995
159. Allen GC, Brubaker CL: Human malignant hyperthermia associated with desflurane anesthesia. Anesth Analg 86:1328, 1998
160. Ducart A, Adnet P, Renaud B, Riou B, Krivosic-Horber R: Malignant hyperthermia during sevoflurane administration. Anesth Analg 80:609, 1995
161. Reed SB, Strobel GE: An in vitro model of malignant hyperthermia: differential effects of inhalation anesthetics on caffeine-induced muscle contractures. Anesthesiology 48:254, 1978
162. Papadimos TJ, Almasri M, Padgett JS, Rush JE: A suspected case of delayed onset malignant hyperthermia with desflurane anesthesia. Anesth Analg 98:548, 2004
163. Lane GA, Nahrwold ML, Tait AR: Anesthetics as teratogens: Nitrous oxide is fetotoxic, xenon is not. Science 210:899, 1980
164. Mazze RI, Fujinaga M, Rice SA, Harris SB, Baden JM: Reproductive and teratogenic effects of nitrous oxide, halothane, isoflurane, and enflurane in Sprague-Dawley rats. Anesthesiology 64:339, 1986
165. Mazze RI, Wilson AI, Rice SA *et al*: Effects of isoflurane on reproduction and fetal development in mice. Anesth Analg 63:249, 1984
166. Mazze RI: Fertility, reproduction, and postnatal survival in mice chronically exposed to isoflurane. Anesthesiology 63:663, 1985
167. Layzer RB, Fishman RA, Schafer JA: Neuropathy following use of nitrous oxide. Neurology 28:504, 1978
168. Munson ES, Embro WJ: Enflurane, isoflurane and halothane and isolated human uterine muscle. Anesthesiology 46:11, 1977
169. Palahniuk RJ, Shnider SM: Maternal and fetal cardiovascular and acid-base changes during halothane and isoflurane anesthesia in the pregnant ewe. Anesthesiology 41:462, 1974
170. Abboud TK, Zhu J, Richardson M, Peres Da Silva E, Donovan M: Desflurane: A new volatile anesthetic for cesarean section. Maternal and neonatal effects. Acta Anaesthesiol Scand 39:723, 1995
171. Abboud TK, Nagappala S, Murakawa K *et al*: Comparison of the effects of general and regional anesthesia for cesarean section on neonatal neurologic and adaptive capacity scores. Anesth Analg 64:996, 1985
172. Warren TM, Datta S, Ostheimer GW, Naulty JS, Weiss JB, Morrison JA: Comparisons of the maternal and neonatal effects of halothane, enflurane and isoflurane for cesarean delivery. Anesth Analg 62:516, 1983
173. Kharasch ED: Putting the brakes on anesthetic breakdown. Anesthesiology 91:1192, 1999
174. Frink EJ Jr, Malan TP, Morgan SE, Brown EA, Malcomson M, Brown BR Jr: Quantification of the degradation products of sevoflurane in two CO_2 absorbents during low-flow anesthesia in surgical patients. Anesthesiology 77:1064, 1992
175. Jin L, Baillie TA, Davis MR, Kharasch ED: Nephrotoxicity of sevoflurane compound A [fluoromethyl-2,2-difluoro-1-(trifluoromethyl)vinyl ether] in rats: Evidence for glutathione and cysteine conjugate formation and the role of renal cysteine conjugate beta-lyase. Biochem Biophys Res Commun 210:498, 1995
176. Fang ZX, Eger EI II, Laster MJ, Chortkoff BS, Kandel L, Ionescu P: Carbon monoxide production from degradation of desflurane, enflurane, isoflurane, halothane, and sevoflurane by soda lime and baralyme. Anesth Analg 80:1187, 1995
177. Holak EJ, Mei DA, Dunning MBI *et al*: Carbon monoxide production from sevoflurane breakdown: Modeling of exposures under clinical conditions. Anesth Analg 96:757, 2003
178. Murray JM, Renfrew CW, Bedi A, McCrystal CB, Jones DS, Fee JPH: Amsorb. A new carbon dioxide absorbent for use in anesthetic breathing systems. Anesthesiology 91:1342, 1999
179. Kobayashi S, Bito H, Obata Y, Katoh T, Sato S: Compound A concentration in the circle absorber system during low-flow sevoflurane anesthesia: Comparison of Dragersorb Free, Amsorb, and Sodasorb II. J Clin Anesth 15:33, 2003
180. Kharasch ED, Powers KM, Artru AA: Comparison of Amsorb, sodalime, and Baralyme degradation of volatile anesthetics and formation of carbon monoxide and compound a in swine in vivo. Anesthesiology 96:173, 2002
181. Kharasch ED, Hoffman GM, Thorning D, Hankins DC, Kilty CG: Role of the renal cysteine conjugate β-lyase pathway in inhaled compound A nephrotoxicity in rats. Anesthesiology 88:1624, 1998
182. Kharasch ED, Thorning DT, Garton K, Hankins DC, Kilty CG: Role of renal cysteine conjugate β-lyase in the mechanism of compound A nephrotoxicity in rats. Anesthesiology 86:160, 1997
183. Steffey EP, Laster MJ, Ionescu P, Eger EI II, Gong D, Weiskopf RB: Dehydration of Baralyme increases compound A resulting from sevoflurane degradation in a standard anesthetic circuit used to anesthetize swine. Anesth Analg 85:1382, 1997

184. Mazze RI, Friedman M, Delgado-Herrara L, Galvez S, Mayer DB: Renal toxicity of compound A plus sevoflurane compared with isoflurane in nonhuman primates. Anesthesiology 89:A490, 1998
185. Bito H, Ikeda K: Closed-circuit anesthesia with sevoflurane in humans. Effects on renal and hepatic function and concentrations of breakdown products with soda lime in the circuit. Anesthesiology 80:71, 1994
186. Kharasch ED, Frink EJ Jr, Zager R, Bowdle TA, Artru A, Nogami WM: Assessment of low-flow sevoflurane and isoflurane effects on renal function using sensitive markers of tubular toxicity. Anesthesiology 86:1238, 1997
187. Ebert TJ, Arain SR: Renal effects of low-flow anesthesia with desflurane and sevoflurane in patients. Anesthesiology 91:A404, 1999
188. Eger EI II, Gong D, Koblin DD *et al*: Dose-related biochemical markers of renal injury after sevoflurane versus desflurane anesthesia in volunteers. Anesth Analg 85:1154, 1997
189. Ebert TJ, Frink EJ Jr, Kharasch ED: Absence of biochemical evidence for renal and hepatic dysfunction after 8 hours of 1.25 minimum alveolar concentration sevoflurane anesthesia in volunteers. Anesthesiology 88:601, 1998
190. Ebert TJ, Messana LD, Uhrich TD, Staacke TS: Absence of renal and hepatic toxicity after four hours of 1.25 minimum alveolar concentration sevoflurane anesthesia in volunteers. Anesth Analg 86:662, 1998
191. Bito H, Ikeda K: Renal and hepatic function in surgical patients after low-flow sevoflurane or isoflurane anesthesia. Anesth Analg 82:173, 1996
192. Groudine SB, Fragen RJ, Kharasch ED, Eisenman TS, Frink EJ, McConnell S: Comparison of renal function following anesthesia with low-flow sevoflurane and isoflurane. J Clin Anesth 11:201, 1999
193. Litz RJ, Hübler M, Lorenz W, Meier VK, Albrecht DM: Renal responses to desflurane and isoflurane in patients with renal insufficiency. Anesthesiology 97:1133, 2002
194. Conzen PF, Kharasch ED, Czerner SFA *et al*: Low-flow sevoflurane compared with low-flow isoflurane anesthesia in patients with stable renal insufficiency. Anesthesiology 97:578, 2002
195. Mazze RI, Jamison RL: Low-flow (1 l/min) sevoflurane: Is it safe? Anesthesiology 86:1225, 1997
196. Bedford RF, Ives HE: The renal safety of sevoflurane. Editorial. Anesth Analg 90:505, 2000
197. Spracklin D, Kharasch ED: Evidence for the metabolism of fluoromethyl-1,1-difluoro-1-(trifluoromethyl)vinyl ether (Compound A), a sevoflurane degradation product, by cysteine conjugate β-lyase. Chem Res Toxicol 9:696, 1996
198. Iyer RA, Anders MW: Cysteine conjugate β-lyase-dependent biotransformation of the cysteine S-conjugates of the sevoflurane degradation product compound A in human, nonhuman, nonhuman primate, and rat kidney cytosol and mitochondria. Anesthesiology 85:1454, 1996
199. Kharasch ED, Jubert C: Compound A uptake and metabolism to mercapturic acids and 3,3,3-trifluoro-2-fluoromethoxypropanoic acid during low-flow sevoflurane anesthesia. Anesthesiology 91:1267, 1999
200. Fang ZX, Eger EI II: Source of toxic CO explained: $-CHF_2$ anesthetic + dry absorbent. UCSF research shows CO comes from CO_2 absorbent. APSF Newsletter 9:25, 1994
201. Woehlck HJ, Dunning MI, Gandhi S, Chang D, Milosavljevic D: Indirect detection of intraoperative carbon monoxide exposure by mass spectrometry during isoflurane anesthesia. Anesthesiology 83:213, 1995
202. Lentz RE: CO poisoning during anesthesia poses puzzle. APSF Newsletter 9:13, 1994
203. Woehlck HJ: Severe intraoperative CO poisoning. Anesthesiology 90:353, 1999
204. Berry PD, Sessler DI, Larson MD: Severe carbon monoxide poisoning during desflurane anesthesia. Anesthesiology 90:613, 1999
205. Woehlck HJ, Dunning MI, Raza T, Ruiz F, Bolla B, Zink W: Physical factors affecting the production of carbon monoxide from anesthetic breakdown. Anesthesiology 94:453, 2001
206. Fatheree RS, Leighton BL: Acute respiratory distress syndrome after an exothermic Baralyme®-sevoflurane reaction. Anesthesiology 101:531, 2004
207. Castro BA, Freedman LA, Craig WL, Lynch CI: Explosion within an anesthesia machine: Baralyme®, high fresh gas flows and sevoflurane concentration. Anesthesiology 101:537, 2004
208. Cousins MJ, Mazze RI: Methoxyflurane nephrotoxicity: A study of dose-response in man. JAMA 225:1611, 1973
209. Frink EJ Jr, Malan TP Jr, Isner RJ, Brown EA, Morgan SE, Brown BR Jr: Renal concentrating function with prolonged sevoflurane or enflurane anesthesia in volunteers. Anesthesiology 80:1019, 1994
210. Mazze RI: The safety of sevoflurane in humans. Anesthesiology 77:1062, 1992
211. Kharasch ED, Hankins DC, Thummel KE: Human kidney methoxyflurane and sevoflurane metabolism. Intrarenal fluoride production as a possible mechanism of methoxyflurane nephrotoxicity. Anesthesiology 82:689, 1995
212. Kharasch ED: Biotransformation of sevoflurane. Anesth Analg 81:S27, 1995
213. Frink EJ Jr, Malan TP Jr, Brown EA, Morgan S, Brown BR Jr: Plasma inorganic fluoride levels with sevoflurane anesthesia in morbidly obese and nonobese patients. Anesth Analg 76:1333, 1993
214. Rehder K, Forbes J, Alter H, Hessler O, Stier A: Halothane biotransformation in man: A quantitative study. Anesthesiology 28:711, 1967
215. Brown BR Jr, Gandolfi AJ: Adverse effects of volatile anaesthetics. Br J Anaesth 59:14, 1987
216. Frink EJ Jr, Morgan SE, Coetzee A, Conzen PF, Brown BR Jr: The effects of sevoflurane, halothane, enflurane, and isoflurane on hepatic blood flow and oxygenation in chronically instrumented greyhound dogs. Anesthesiology 76:85, 1992
217. Gatecel C, Losser M-R, Payen D: The postoperative effects of halothane versus isoflurane on hepatic artery and portal vein blood flow in humans. Anesth Analg 96:740, 2003
218. Kenna G, Satoh H, Christ DD, Pohl LR: Metabolic basis for drug hypersensitivity; antibodies in sera from patients with halothane hepatisis recognise liver neo-antigens that contain the tri-fluoroacetyl group derived from halothane. J Pharmacol Exp Ther 245:1103, 1988
219. Kenna JG, Martin JL, Satoh H, Pohl LR: Factors affecting the expression of trifluoroacetylated liver microsomal protein neoantigens in rats treated with halothane. Drug Metab Dispos 18:188, 1990
220. Martin JL, Plevak DJ, Flannery KD *et al*: Hepatotoxicity after desflurane anesthesia. Anesthesiology 83:1125, 1995
221. Njoku D, Laster MJ, Gong DH, Eger EII, Reed GF, Martin JL: Biotransformation of halothane, enflurane, isoflurane, and desflurane to trifluoroacetylated liver proteins: Association between protein acylation and hepatic injury. Anesth Analg 84:173, 1997
222. Lewis JH, Zimmerman HJ, Ishak KG, Mullick FG: Enflurane hepatotoxicity. A clinicopathologic study of 24 cases. Ann Intern Med 98:984, 1983
223. Stoelting RK, Blitt CD, Cohen PF, Menn RG: Hepatic dysfunction after isoflurane anesthesia. Anesth Analg 66:147, 1987
224. Ray DC, Drummond GB: Halothane hepatitis. Br J Anaesth 67:84, 1991
225. Martin JL, Dubbink DA, Plevak DJ *et al*: Halothane hepatitis 28 years after primary exposure. Anesth Analg 74:605, 1992
226. Sigurdsen J, Hreidarsson AB, Thiodleifsson B: Enflurane hepatitis. A report of a case with a previous history of halothane hepatitis. Acta Anaesthesiol Scand 29:495, 1985
227. Njoku DB, Greenberg RS, Bourdi M *et al*: Autoantibodies associated with volatile anesthetic hepatitis found in the sera of a large cohort of pediatric anesthesiologists. Anesth Analg 94:243, 2002
228. Doi M, Ikeda K: Airway irritation produced by volatile anaesthetics during brief inhalation: Comparison of halothane, enflurane, isoflurane and sevoflurane. Can J Anaesth 40:122, 1993
229. Tanaka S, Tsuchida H, Nakabayashi K, Seki S, Namiki A: The effects of sevoflurane, isoflurane, halothane, and enflurane on hemodynamic responses during an inhaled induction of anesthesia via a mask in humans. Anesth Analg 82:821, 1996
230. Muzi M, Robinson BJ, Ebert TJ, O'Brien TJ: Induction of anesthesia and tracheal intubation with sevoflurane in adults. Anesthesiology 85:536, 1996
231. Muzi M, Colinco MD, Robinson BJ, Ebert TJ: The effects of premedication on inhaled induction of anesthesia with sevoflurane. Anesth Analg 85:1143, 1997
232. Thwaites A, Edmends S, Smith I: Inhalation induction with sevoflurane: A double-blind comparison with propofol. Br J Anaesth 78:356, 1997
233. Mostafa SM, Atherton AMJ: Sevoflurane for difficult tracheal intubation. Br J Anaesth 79:392, 1997
234. Dion P: The cost of anesthetic vapors. Can J Anaesth 39:633, 1992

CHAPTER 16 ■ NEUROMUSCULAR BLOCKING AGENTS

FRANÇOIS DONATI AND DAVID R. BEVAN

KEY POINTS

1. Neuromuscular blocking agents are used to improve conditions for tracheal intubation, to provide immobility during surgery, and to facilitate mechanical ventilation.
2. The main site of action of neuromuscular blocking agents (muscle relaxants) is on the nicotinic cholinergic receptor at the endplate of muscle. They also have effects at presynaptic receptors located on the nerve terminal.
3. Succinylcholine is a blocking agent that produces depolarization at the endplate and binds to extrajunctional receptors. In spite of many side effects, such as hyperkalemia, its rapid offset makes it the drug of choice for rapid sequence induction.
4. All other drugs available are nondepolarizing. They compete with acetylcholine for the same binding sites.
5. Fade-in response to high frequency stimulation (e.g. train-of-four, 2 Hz for 2 sec) is a characteristic of nondepolarizing blockade. Train-of-four fade is difficult to evaluate manually or visually during recovery when ratio is >0.4.
6. The upper airway is particularly sensitive to the effects of nondepolarizing blockade. Complete recovery does not occur until train-of-four ratio at the adductor pollicis >0.9.
7. Residual paralysis is more frequent with long-duration than intermediate-duration agents.
8. Reversal with anticholinesterases should be attempted when a certain degree of spontaneous recovery is manifest. Ideally, all four twitches in response to train-of-four stimulation should be visible before reversal is given.

It appears paradoxical that drugs having peripheral effects on neuromuscular transmission might have a role in anesthesia. If the patient is anesthetized, why provide agents to prevent movement? Yet, the introduction of muscle relaxants, more appropriately called neuromuscular blocking agents, into clinical practice more than 60 years ago is an important milestone in the history of anesthesia.[1] However, in 1954, in a paper on anesthetic mortality, Beecher and Todd claimed that mortality increased by sixfold when muscle relaxants were used.[2] This situation was probably because of the suboptimal use of mechanical ventilation and reversal drugs, but other controversies arose in recent years, for a variety of reasons.

For example, the incidence of awareness is greater when neuromuscular blocking agents are used,[3] and some authors recommend restricting the use of these drugs whenever possible, as patient movement might be an indicator of

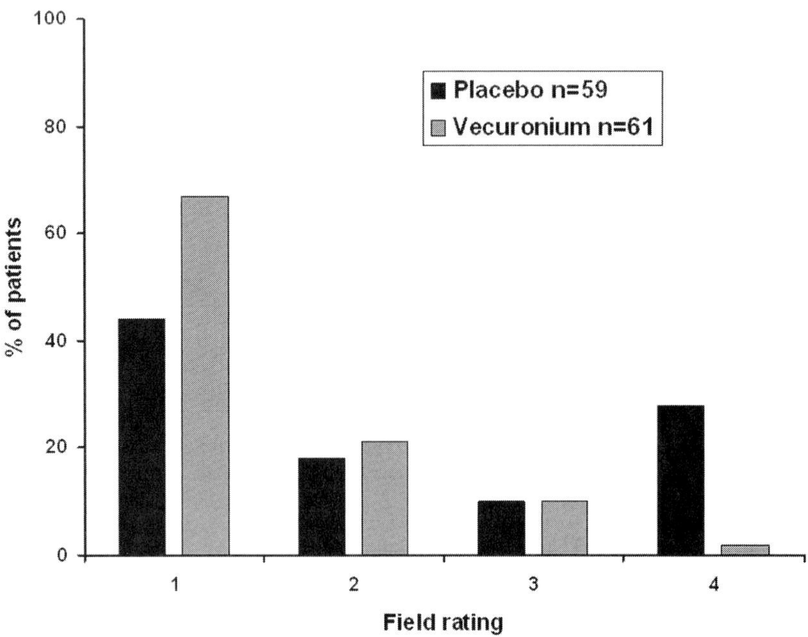

FIGURE 16-1. Surgeon's assessment of muscle relaxation during lower abdominal surgery. Rating goes from 1 (excellent) to 4 (poor). The incidence of poor rating was greater in patients not given vecuronium (29%) compared with those who received the drug (2%). Redrawn from King et al.[5]

consciousness. However, anesthetics act at the spinal cord level to produce immobility, and movement in response to a noxious stimulus indicates inadequate analgesia, not insufficient unconsciousness.[4] Therefore, awareness does not occur because too much of a neuromuscular blocking agent has been given, but because too little anesthetic is administered. This seems to be supported by an incident report review where an inadequate dose of anesthetic drugs was suspected in 68 of 81 cases of awareness.[3]

1 Complete paralysis is not required all the time for all surgical procedures. For example, anesthesiologists might tend to inject more mivacurium than really needed by surgeons. However, neuromuscular blocking agents were found to make a difference in lower abdominal surgery, where, in spite of generous doses of isoflurane, surgical conditions were better in patients receiving vecuronium (Fig. 16-1).[5] In addition to providing immobility and better surgical conditions, neuromuscular blocking agents improve intubating conditions. The doses of narcotics required for acceptable intubating conditions in the absence of muscle paralysis produce significant hypotension (Fig. 16-2).[6] Providing optimal intubating conditions is not a trivial objective. It has been demonstrated that poor intubating conditions are associated with an increased incidence of voice hoarseness and vocal cord damage (Fig. 16-3).[7] Furthermore, giving neuromuscular blocking agents improved the quality of intubating conditions.

As it is important to provide adequate anesthesia while a patient is totally or partially paralyzed, it is also essential to make sure that the effects of neuromuscular blocking drugs have worn off or are reversed before the patient regains consciousness. With the introduction of shorter acting neuromuscular blocking agents, it was thought that reversal of blockade could be omitted. However, residual paralysis is still a problem, even 25 years after if was first described (Table 16-1).[8] In addition, the threshold for complete neuromuscular recovery is now considered to be a train-of-four (TOF) ratio of 0.9, instead of the traditional 0.7 (Fig. 16-4).[9] Thus, an understanding of the pharmacology of neuromuscular blocking agents and reversal drugs is essential.

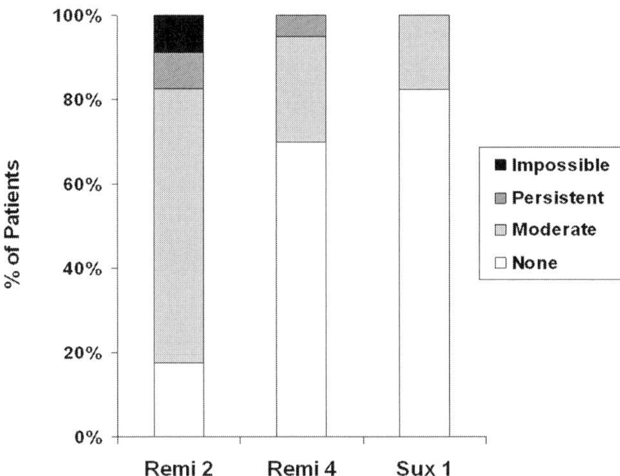

FIGURE 16-2. Neuromuscular blocking agents provide better intubating conditions than high doses of narcotics, without hypotension. In the study mentioned earlier, patients were randomized to remifentanil, 2 μg/kg (Remi 2), or 4 μg/kg (Remi 4), or succinylcholine 1 mg/kg (Sux 1). Mean arterial pressure decreased by a mean value of 21, 28, and 8%, respectively. Intubating conditions were rated as impossible or according to the degree of coughing produced (persistent, moderate, or none). Data from McNeil et al.[6]

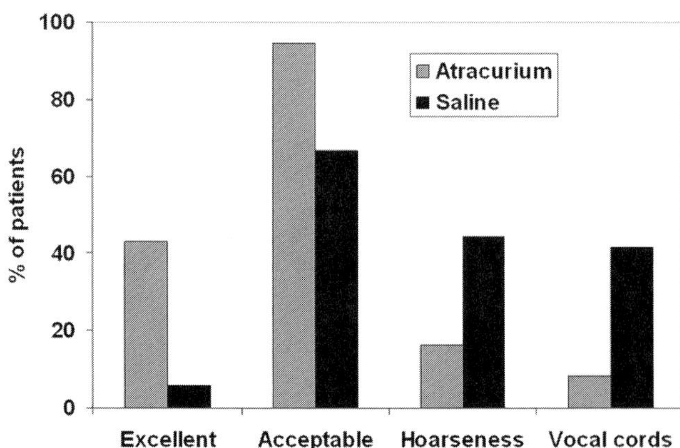

FIGURE 16-3. Neuromuscular blocking agents improve intubating conditions and reduce vocal cord sequelae. The graph depicts the incidence of excellent and acceptable (defined as good or excellent) intubating conditions after atracurium or saline. The percentage of patients who reported hoarseness and those with vocal cord lesions documented by stroboscopy is also shown. Data from Mencke et al.[7]

TABLE 16-1

REPORTS OF RESIDUAL PARALYSIS 1979–2004

STUDY	LONG-ACTING DRUGS USED	INTERMEDIATE-ACTING DRUGS USED	REVERSAL	TOF THRESHOLD	RESIDUAL PARALYSIS (% OF PATIENTS)	COMMENTS
Viby-Mogensen et al 1979[8]	*d*-tubocurarine Pancuronium Gallamine		Yes	0.7	42	
Bevan et al 1988[169]	Pancuronium		Yes	0.7	36	Less paralysis with atracurium and vecuronium
		Atracurium	Yes	0.7	4	
		Vecuronium	Yes	0.7	9	
Fawcett et al 1995[99]		Atracurium/ vecuronium bolus	Yes	0.7	12	More paralysis with infusions
		Atracurium/ vecuronium infusion	Yes	0.7	24	
Berg et al 1997[155]	Pancuronium		Yes	0.7	26	More atelectasis when residual paralysis present
		Atracurium/ vecuronium	Yes	0.7	5	
Bissinger et al 2000[170]	Pancuronium		Yes	0.7	20	More hypoxia with TOF <0.7
		Vecuronium	Yes	0.7	8	
Baillard et al 2001[154]		Vecuronium	No	0.7	42	
Hayes et al 2001[171]		Atracurium/ vecuronium/ rocuronium	Optional	0.7 0.8	41 52	
Gatke et al 2002[135]		Rocuronium without AMG monitoring	Yes	0.8	17	Less paralysis when AMG used
		Rocuronium with AMG monitoring	Yes	0.8	3	
Debaene et al 2003[134]		Atracurium/vecuro-nium/rocuronium	No	0.7 0.9	16 45	Paralysis could be present even 4 h after injection
Murphy et al 2004[156]	Pancuronium		Yes	0.7 0.9	47 97	More hypoxia and discharge delayed with pancuronium
		Rocuronium	Yes	0.7 0.9	7 33	

AMG, acceleromyography; TOF, train-of-four ratio.

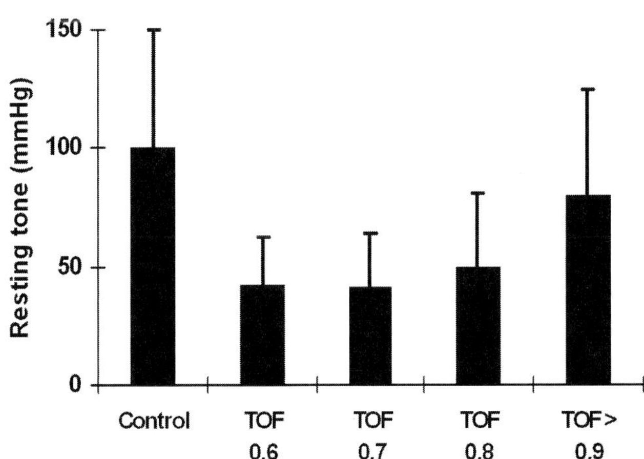

FIGURE 16-4. Upper esophageal resting tone in volunteers given vecuronium. Train-of-four ratio was measured at the adductor pollicis. Statistically significant decreases compared with control were found at all levels of paralysis until TOF >0.9. Redrawn from Eriksson et al.[146]

PHYSIOLOGY AND PHARMACOLOGY

Structure

The cell bodies of motor neurons supplying skeletal muscle lie in the spinal cord. They receive and integrate information from the central nervous system. This information is carried via an elongated structure, the axon, to distant parts of the body. Each nerve cell supplies many muscle cells (or fibers) a short distance after branching into nerve terminals. The terminal portion of the axon is a specialized structure, the synapse, designed for the production and release of acetylcholine. The synapse is separated from the endplate of the muscle fiber by a narrow gap, called the synaptic cleft, which is approximately 50 nm in width (0.05 μm) (Fig. 16-5).[10] The nerve terminal is surrounded by a Schwann cell, and the synaptic cleft has a basement membrane and contains filaments that anchor the nerve terminal to the muscle.

The endplate is a specialized portion of the membrane of the muscle fiber where nicotinic acetylcholine receptors are concentrated. During development, multiple connections are made

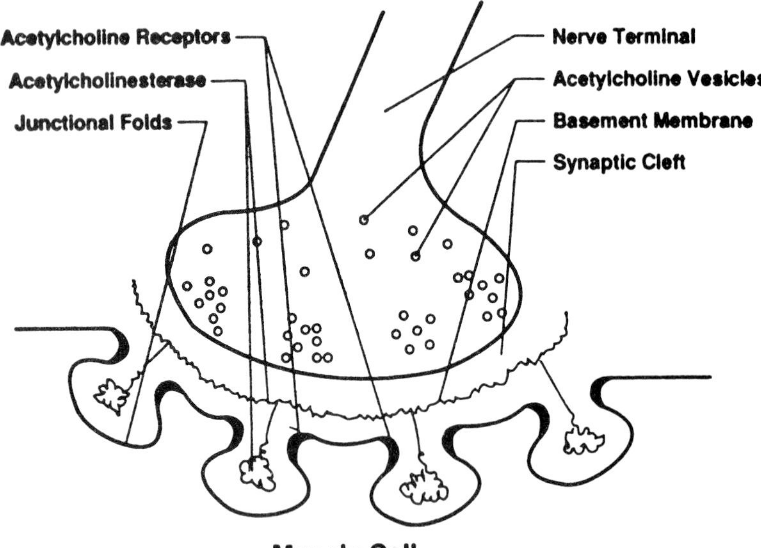

FIGURE 16-5. Schematic representation of the neuromuscular junction (not drawn to scale).

between nerve terminals and a single muscle fiber. However, as maturation continues, most of these connections atrophy and disappear, usually leaving only one connection per muscle fiber. This endplate continues to differentiate from the rest of the muscle fiber. The nerve terminal enlarges, and folds appear. The acetylcholine receptors cluster at the endplate, especially at the crests of the folds and their density decreases to almost zero in extrajunctional areas.[11,12] Mammalian endplates usually have an oval shape with the short axis perpendicular to the fiber. The width of the endplate is sometimes as large as the diameter of the fiber, but is usually smaller. However, its length is only a small fraction of that of the fiber.

Nerve Stimulation

Under resting conditions, the electrical potential of the inside of a nerve cell is negative with respect to the outside (typically –90 mV). If this potential is made less negative (depolarization), sodium channels open and allow sodium ions to enter the cell. This influx of positive ions makes the potential inside the membrane positive with respect to the outside. This potential change in turn causes depolarization of the next segment of membrane, causing more sodium channels to open, and an electrical impulse, or action potential, propagates. The duration of the action potential is brief (<1 msec), because of rapid inactivation of sodium channels and activation of potassium channels. An action potential also triggers the opening of calcium channels, allowing calcium ions to penetrate the cell. This entry of calcium facilitates release of the neurotransmitter at the nerve terminal.

The sodium channels in the axon may be activated in response to electrical depolarization provided by a nerve stimulator. A peripheral nerve is made up of a large number of axons, each of which axon responds in an all-or-none fashion to the stimulus applied. Thus, in the absence of neuromuscular blocking agents, the relationship between the amplitude of the muscle contraction and current applied is sigmoid.[13] At low currents, the depolarization is insufficient in all axons. As current increases, more and more axons are depolarized to threshold and the strength of the muscle contraction increases. When the stimulating current reaches a certain level, all axons are depolarized to threshold and propagate an action potential. Increasing current beyond this point does not increase the amplitude of muscle contraction: the stimulation is supramaximal (Fig. 16-6). Most commercially available stimulators deliver impulses lasting 0.1 to 0.2 msec.

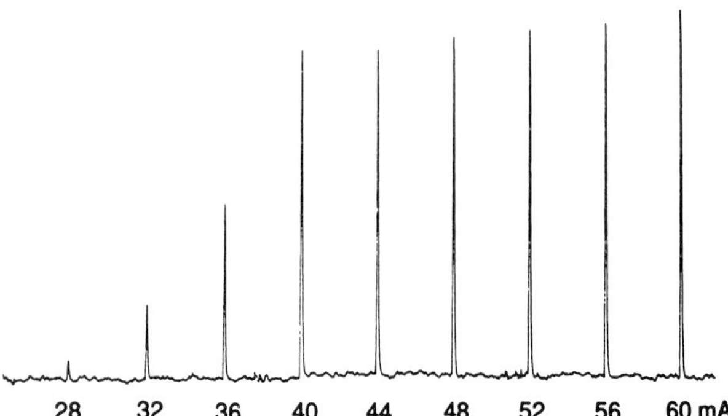

FIGURE 16-6. Example of increasing stimulating current in one patient. Current pulses, 0.2-msec duration, were delivered to the ulnar nerve at the wrist every 10 seconds. The force of contraction of the adductor pollicis was measured and appears as spikes. No twitch was seen if the current was <28 mA. At current strengths of ≥40 mA, the current became supramaximal, increasing the current produced little change in force.

Release of Acetylcholine

Acetylcholine is synthesized from choline and acetate and packaged into 45-nm vesicles. Each vesicle contains 5,000 to 10,000 acetylcholine molecules. Some of these vesicles cluster near the cell membrane opposite the crests of the junctional folds of the endplate, in areas called active zones (see Fig. 16-5).[12]

Although there have been doubts regarding the vesicular hypothesis, it is now widely accepted that acetylcholine is released in packets, or quanta, and that a quantum represents the contents of one vesicle.[14] In the absence of nerve stimulation, quanta are released spontaneously, at random, and this is seen as small depolarizations of the endplate (miniature endplate potential; MEPP). When an action potential invades the nerve terminal, ~200 to 400 quanta are released simultaneously, unloading ~1 to 4 million acetylcholine molecules into the synaptic cleft.[10,14] Calcium, which enters the nerve terminal through channels that open in response to depolarization, is required for vesicle fusion and release. Calcium channels are located near docking proteins, and this special geometric arrangement provides high intracellular concentrations of calcium to allow binding of specialized proteins on the vesicle membrane with docking proteins.[12] Binding produces fusion of the membranes and release of acetylcholine ensues. When the calcium concentration is decreased, or if the action of calcium is antagonized by magnesium, the release process is inhibited and transmission failure may occur. Other proteins regulate storage and mobilization of acetylcholine vesicles. It appears that a small proportion of vesicles is immediately releasable, while a much larger reserve pool can be mobilized more slowly. Each impulse releases 0.2 to 0.5% of the 75,000 to 100,000 vesicles in the nerve terminal.[14] With repetitive stimulation, the amount of acetylcholine released decreases rapidly because only a small fraction of the vesicles is in a position to be released immediately. To sustain release during high-frequency stimulation, vesicles must be mobilized from the reserve pool, and this process requires calcium.[14]

Postsynaptic Events

The 1 to 10 million receptors located at the endplate are made up of five glycoprotein subunits arranged in the form of a rosette and lying across the whole cell membrane (Fig. 16-7). Two of these noncontiguous subunits, designated α, are identical. The other three units are called β, δ and γ or ϵ There are two acetylcholine binding sites, each located on the outside part of the α subunit. When two acetylcholine molecules bind simultaneously to each binding site, an opening is created in the center of the rosette, allowing sodium ions to enter the cell.[10,15] This depolarizes the endplate, that is, its inside becomes less negative. There is a high density of sodium channels in the folds of synaptic clefts and in the perijunctional area.[15] These channels open when the membrane is depolarized beyond a critical point, allowing more sodium to enter the cell, and producing further depolarization. This depolarization generates an action potential, which propagates by activation of sodium channels along the whole length of the muscle fiber. The

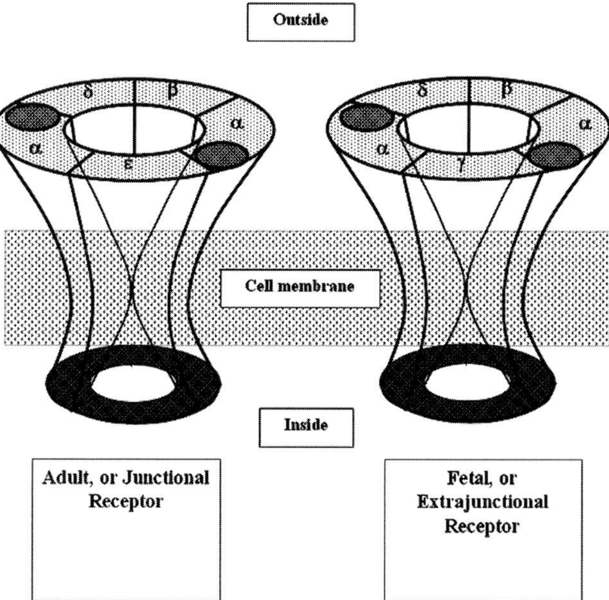

FIGURE 16-7. Two types of nicotinic receptors in muscle. Both have the same five subunits, except for a substitution of the ε for the γ subunits. The acetylcholine binding sites are represented by a shaded oval area. They are on the α subunit, at the δ and ε or γ interface, respectively. According to some authors, the order of the β and δ is inverted.

muscle action potential has a duration 5 to 15 milliseconds and can be recorded as a electromyogram (EMG). It precedes the onset of contraction, or twitch, which lasts 100 to 200 milliseconds. With high-frequency (>10 Hz) stimulation, the muscle fiber does not have time to relax before the next impulse, so contractions fuse and add up, and a tetanus is obtained.

There are two types of nicotinic acetylcholine receptors. Early in development, receptors are evenly distributed along the whole length of the muscle fiber. These receptors, called fetal receptors, have a γ subunit (see Fig. 16-7). When the endplate develops, receptors tend to cluster at the neuromuscular junction and leave only few receptors in the extrajunctional areas. As maturation continues, the γ subunit is substituted by an ε subunit, which is characteristic of the adult-type, junctional receptor.[11,12] In humans, the switch occurs in the last weeks of pregnancy. Maintenance of adult receptors at the endplate depends on the integrity of nerve supply. A few γ-type, extrajunctional receptors still persist in adults, but can proliferate in cases of denervation. Both types of receptor have slightly different sensitivities to agonist and antagonist drugs.[12] Both have two binding sites for acetylcholine, located on the subunit, at the interface between the δ and the ϵ or γ or subunits, respectively.[16]

2 The main action of nondepolarizing neuromuscular blocking drugs is to block the postsynaptic acetylcholine receptor by binding to at least one of the two α subunits, thus preventing access by acetylcholine. Under normal circumstances, only a small fraction of available receptors must bind to acetylcholine to produce sufficient depolarization to trigger a muscle contraction. In other words, there is a wide "margin of safety." This implies that neuromuscular blocking drugs must be bound to a large number of receptors before any blockade is detectable. Animal studies suggest that 75% of receptors must be occupied before twitch height decreases in the presence of *d*-tubocurarine, and blockade is complete when 92% of receptors are occupied.[17] The actual number depends on species and type of muscle, and humans might have a reduced margin of safety compared with other species.[18] So, it is futile to correlate receptor occupancy data obtained in cats with certain clinical tests in humans, such as hand grip and head lift, which involve different muscle groups. However, the general concept that a large proportion of receptors must be occupied before blockade becomes detectable, and that measurable blockade occurs over a narrow range of receptor occupancy, remains applicable to clinical practice. Because it must overcome the margin of safety, the initial dose of neuromuscular blocking agent is greater than maintenance doses.

Acetylcholine is hydrolyzed rapidly by the enzyme acetyl cholinesterase, which is present in the folds of the endplate as well as embedded in the basement membrane of the synaptic cleft. The presence of the enzyme in the synaptic cleft suggests that not all the acetylcholine released reaches the endplate; some is hydrolyzed en route.[14]

Presynaptic Events

The release of acetylcholine normally decreases during high-frequency stimulation because the pool of readily releasable acetylcholine becomes depleted faster than it can be replenished. Under normal circumstances, the reduced amount released is well above what is required to produce muscle contraction because of the high margin of safety at the neuromuscular junction. However, during partial nondepolarizing blockade this decrease in transmitter output produces fade—a progressive decrease in muscle response with each stimulus. Nondepolarizing neuromuscular blocking drugs probably accentuate the fade by blocking presynaptic nicotinic receptors, which differ structurally from postsynaptic receptors.[19] The function of the presynaptic receptors is to sustain acetylcholine mobilization in the face of continuing stimulation, in other words to provide positive feedback. Nondepolarizing agents have a greater affinity for presynaptic than postsynaptic receptors. Only small doses of nondepolarizing relaxants are needed to block presynaptic receptors.[20] Whatever the exact mechanism of fade, it remains a key property of nondepolarizing neuromuscular blocking drugs and is useful for monitoring purposes.

NEUROMUSCULAR BLOCKING AGENTS

Neuromuscular blocking drugs interact with the acetylcholine receptor either by depolarizing the endplate or by competing with acetylcholine for binding sites. The former mechanism is characteristic of depolarizing drugs and the latter of nondepolarizing agents. The only depolarizing agent still in use is succinylcholine. All others are of the nondepolarizing type.

Pharmacological Characteristics of Neuromuscular Blocking Agents

The effect of neuromuscular blocking drugs is measured as the depression of adductor muscle contraction (twitch) following electrical stimulation of the ulnar nerve. The value is compared with a control value, obtained before injection of the drug. Each drug has onset, potency, and recovery characteristics.

Potency of each drug is determined by constructing dose-response curves, which describe the relationship between twitch depression and dose (Fig. 16-8). Then, the effective dose 50, or ED_{50}, which is the median dose corresponding to 50% twitch depression, is obtained. A more clinically relevant value, the ED_{95}, corresponding to 95% block, is more commonly used. For example, the ED_{95} for vecuronium is 0.05 mg/kg, which means that half the patients will achieve at least 95% block of single twitch (compared with the prevecuronium value) with that dose, and half the subjects will reach less than 95% block. Rocuronium has an ED_{95} of 0.3 mg/kg. Therefore, it has one-sixth the potency of vecuronium because 6 times as much rocuronium has to be given to produce the same effect. The ED_{95} of known neuromuscular blocking agents vary over two orders of magnitude (Table 16-2).

Onset time, or time to maximum blockade, can be shortened if the dose is increased. When two or more drugs are compared, it is meaningful to compare only equipotent doses, and usually, clinically relevant doses ($2 \times ED_{95}$) are considered.

Duration of action is the time from injection of the neuromuscular blocking agent to return of 25% twitch height (compared with control). Duration increases with dose, so comparisons are normally made with $2 \times ED_{95}$ doses. The 25% twitch height figure was chosen because rapid reversal can normally be achieved at that level. Categories were proposed for neuromuscular blocking drugs according to their duration of action (see Table 16-2).[21] Same duration agents may have markedly different onsets.

Recovery index is the time interval between 25% and 75% twitch height. It provides information about the speed of recovery once return of twitch is manifest. It is sometimes preferred to duration of action, because it does not depend heavily on the dose given. The values for ED_{95}, onset time, duration of action, and recovery index depend on which muscle is used to make measurements. For consistency's sake, the adductor pollicis has been retained as the gold standard, not because of its physiological significance, but because it is most commonly monitored and data on it are most abundant.

The pharmacological characteristics of neuromuscular blocking agents are completed by an assessment of intubating conditions, which do not always parallel twitch height at the adductor pollicis. Intubating conditions depend on paralysis of centrally located muscles, but also on type and quantity of narcotic and hypnotic drug given for induction of anesthesia. To decrease variability between studies, criteria to grade intubating conditions as excellent, good, poor, or impossible in a scoring system were adopted by a group of experts who met in Copenhagen in 1994.[22]

DEPOLARIZING DRUGS: SUCCINYLCHOLINE

Among drugs that depolarize the endplate, only succinylcholine
3 is still used clinically. Decamethonium, a depolarizing drug with a slow onset and intermediate duration, has been replaced by nondepolarizing alternatives. However, succinylcholine still

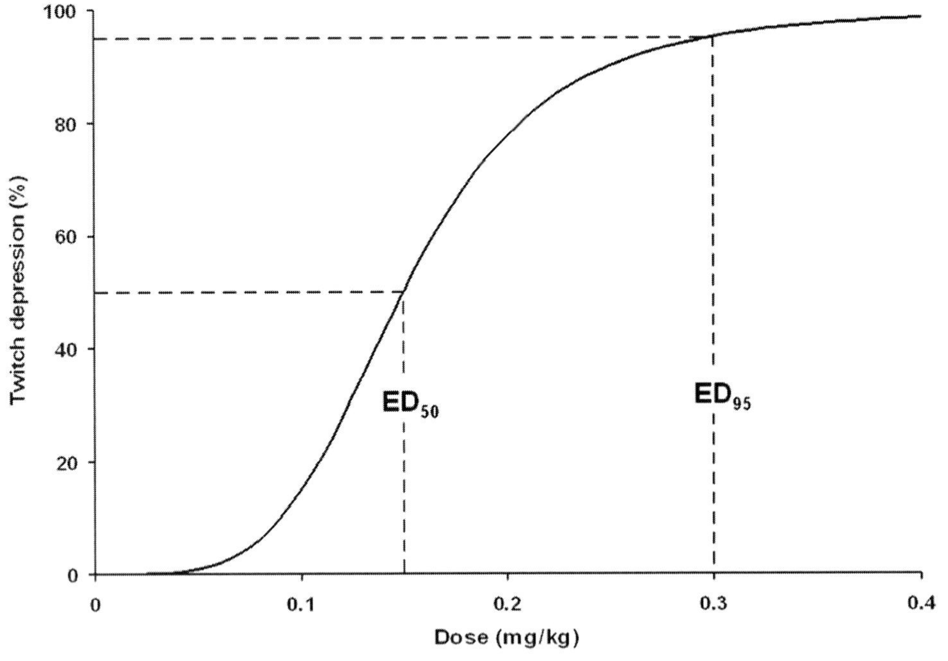

FIGURE 16-8. Example of a dose-response relationship. The actual numbers are approximately those for rocuronium. The ED_{50} is the dose corresponding to 50% blockade and ED_{95} the dose corresponding to 95% blockade.

TABLE 16-2

POTENCY, ONSET TIME, DURATION, AND RECOVERY INDEX OF NEUROMUSCULAR BLOCKING AGENTS

AGENT	ED_{95} (mg/kg)	ONSET TIME (min)	DURATION TO 25% RECOVERY (min)	RECOVERY INDEX (25–75% RECOVERY) (min)
ULTRASHORT-DURATION AGENTS				
Succinylcholine	0.3	1–1.5	6–8	2–4
GW280430A[a]	0.19	1.7	6–8	2.5
SHORT-DURATION AGENTS				
Mivacurium	0.08	3–4	15–20	7–10
Rapacuronium[b]	0.75	1–1.5	15–25	5–7
INTERMEDIATE-DURATION AGENTS				
Atracurium	0.2–0.25	3–4	35–45	10–15
Cisatracurium	0.05	5–7	35–45	12–15
Rocuronium	0.3	1.5–3	30–40	8–12
Vecuronium	0.05	3–4	35–45	10–15
LONG-DURATION AGENTS				
Alcuronium[b]	0.25	3–5	60–90	30–40
Doxacurium	0.025	5–10	40–120	30–40
d-Tubocurarine[b]	0.5	2–4	60–120	30–45
Gallamine[b]	2	1.5–3	60–120	30–60
Metocurine[b]	0.3	3–5	60–150	40–60
Pancuronium	0.07	2–4	60–120	30–40
Pipecuronium[b]	0.05	3–5	90–130	35–45

Typical values for the average young adult patient. Onset and duration data depend on dose. The values presented are the best estimates available for twice the ED_{95} and are measured at the adductor pollicis. Actual values may vary markedly from one individual to the next, and may be affected by age, other medications, and/or disease states. The categories under which the drugs are classified are somewhat arbitrary.
[a]Being investigated at the time of writing.
[b]No longer used or very limited use in North America.

enjoys some popularity, despite a long list of undesired effects, because it is the only ultrarapid onset, ultrashort duration neuromuscular blocking drug available.

Neuromuscular Effects

The effects of succinylcholine at the neuromuscular junction are not completely understood. The drug depolarizes presynaptic, postsynaptic, and extrajunctional receptors. However, when the receptor is in contact with any agonist, including acetylcholine, for a prolonged time, it ceases to respond to the agonist. Normally, this desensitization process does not take place because of the rapid breakdown of acetylcholine (<1 msec). However, succinylcholine remains at the endplate for much longer, and desensitization can develop. Another possible mechanism is the inactivation of sodium channels in the junctional and perijunctional area, which occurs when the membrane remains depolarized. This inactivation prevents the propagation of the action potential.

Within 1 minute after succinylcholine injection and before paralysis is manifest, some disorganized muscular activity is observed frequently. This phenomenon is called "fasciculations" and is probably a result of depolarization of the nerve terminal produced by activation of presynaptic receptors. The effectiveness of small doses of nondepolarizing drugs in reducing the incidence of fasciculations suggests that the presynaptic receptors are relatively sensitive to these drugs.[20]

Succinylcholine has yet another neuromuscular effect. In some muscles, like the masseter and to a lesser extent the adductor pollicis, a sustained increase in tension that may last for several minutes can be observed. The mechanism of action of this tension change is uncertain but is most likely mediated by acetylcholine receptors because it is blocked by large amounts of nondepolarizing drugs.[23] The increase in masseteric tone, which is probably always present to some degree but greater in some susceptive individuals, may lead to imperfect intubating conditions in a small proportion of patients. Masseter spasm may be an exaggerated form of this response.

Characteristics of Depolarizing Blockade

After injection of succinylcholine, single-twitch height is decreased. However, the response to high-frequency stimulation is sustained: minimal train-of-four and tetanic fade is observed. The block is antagonized by nondepolarizing agents so that the ED_{95} is increased by a factor two if a small dose of nondepolarizing drug is given before.[24] Succinylcholine blockade is potentiated by inhibitors of acetyl cholinesterase, such as neostigmine and edrophonium.[25]

Phase II Block

After administration of 7 to 10 mg/kg, or 30 to 60 minutes of exposure to succinylcholine, train-of-four and tetanic fade become apparent. Neostigmine or edrophonium can antagonize this block, which has been termed "nondepolarizing," "dual," or "Phase II block." The onset of Phase II block coincides with tachyphylaxis, as more succinylcholine is required for the same effect.[26]

Pharmacology of Succinylcholine

Succinylcholine is rapidly hydrolyzed by plasma cholinesterase (also called pseudocholinesterase), with an elimination half-life of <1 minute in patients.[27] Because of the rapid disappearance of succinylcholine from plasma, the maximum effect is reached quickly. Subparalyzing doses (up to 0.3 to 0.5 mg/kg) reach their maximal effect within ~1.5 to 2 minutes at the adductor pollicis,[24] and within 1 minute at more central muscles, such as the masseter and the larynx. With larger doses (1 to 2 mg/kg), abolition of twitch response can be reached even more rapidly.

The mean dose producing 95% blockade (ED_{95}) at the adductor pollicis is 0.30 to 0.35 mg/kg with opioid–nitrous oxide anesthesia.[28] In the absence of nitrous oxide, the ED_{95} is increased to 0.5 mg/kg.[29] These values are doubled if *d*-tubocurarine, 0.05 mg/kg, is given as a defasciculating agent.[24] The time until full recovery is dose dependent and reaches 10 to 12 minutes after a dose of 1 mg/kg.[28]

Side Effects

Cardiovascular

Sinus bradycardia with nodal or ventricular escape beats (or both) may occur, especially in children, and asystole has been described after a second dose of succinylcholine in both pediatric and adult patients. These parasympathetic effects can be attenuated with atropine or glycopyrrolate.[30] Succinylcholine increases catecholamine release, and this effect may explain, in part, why bradycardia does not occur more frequently. The mechanism for the enhanced bradycardic effect of a second dose is not known.

Anaphylaxis

Succinylcholine has been incriminated as the trigger of allergic reactions more often than any other drug used in anesthesia. Successive studies conducted in France indicate that the number of reported events is decreasing, corresponding to the gradual replacement of succinylcholine by nondepolarizing drugs.[31] The incidence of anaphylactic reactions to succinylcholine is difficult to establish, but is probably of the order of 1:5,000 to 1:10,000.

Fasciculations

The prevalence of fasciculations is high (60 to 90%) after the rapid injection of succinylcholine, especially in muscular adults. Although this is a benign side effect of the drug, most clinicians prefer to prevent fasciculations. In this respect, a small dose of a nondepolarizing neuromuscular blocking drug is given 3 to 5 minutes before succinylcholine is effective. When the drug was available, *d*-tubocurarine 0.05 mg/kg was used for this purpose. Rocuronium is an acceptable alternative, as long as appropriate doses (0.03 to 0.04 mg/kg, that is, 10% of the ED_{95}) are given.[32] In one study, rocuronium, 0.03 mg/kg, decreased the incidence of fasciculations from 90 to 10%.[33] A dose of 0.06 mg/kg leads to an unacceptably high incidence of symptoms of neuromuscular weakness, such as blurred vision, heavy eyelids, voice changes, difficulty swallowing, or even dyspnea, in the awake patient.[34] Atracurium 0.02 mg/kg is also effective. Pancuronium, vecuronium, cisatracurium, and mivacurium are not as effective as defasciculants. After these nondepolarizing drugs, the dose of succinylcholine must be increased from 1 mg/kg to 1.5 or even 2 mg/kg because of the antagonism between depolarizing and nondepolarizing drugs.[24] Other drugs, such as diazepam, lidocaine, fentanyl, calcium, vitamin C, magnesium, and dantrolene, have all been used to prevent fasciculations. The results are no better than with nondepolarizing relaxants, and they may have undesirable effects of their own. "Self-taming," the administration of small (10-mg) doses of succinylcholine 1 minute before the intubating dose, does not appear to be effective[33] and has largely been abandoned.

Muscle Pains

Generalized aches and pains, similar to the myalgia that follows violent exercise, are common 24 to 48 hours after succinylcholine administration. They occur in 1.5 to 89% of patients receiving succinylcholine and are more common in young, ambulatory patients.[35] The intensity of muscle pains is not always correlated with the intensity of fasciculations, but the methods that have been shown effective to prevent fasciculations usually prevent muscle pains. For example, a precurarization dose of a nondepolarizing neuromuscular blocking agent is effective. Lidocaine (1 to 1.5 mg/kg), especially in conjunction with precurarization, has also been shown to be of value.[35] Calcium, vitamin C, benzodiazepines, magnesium, and dantrolene have been tried with inconclusive results.[35]

Intragastric Pressure

Succinylcholine increases intragastric pressure, and this effect is blocked by precurarization. However, succinylcholine causes even greater increases in lower esophageal sphincter pressure. Thus, succinylcholine does not appear to increase the risk of aspiration of gastric contents unless the lower esophageal sphincter is incompetent.

Intraocular Pressure

Intraocular pressure increases by 5 to 15 mm Hg after injection of succinylcholine. The mechanism is unknown but occurs after detachment of extraocular muscle, suggesting an intraocular etiology. Precurarization with a nondepolarizing blocker has little or no effect on this increase. This background information has led to the widespread recommendation to avoid succinylcholine in open eye injuries. However, it must be appreciated that other factors, such as inadequate anesthesia, elevated systemic blood pressure, and insufficient neuromuscular blockade during laryngoscopy and tracheal intubation, might increase intraocular pressure more than succinylcholine. In addition, there is little evidence that the use of succinylcholine has led to blindness or extrusion of eye content.[36]

Intracranial Pressure

Succinylcholine may increase intracranial pressure (ICP), and this response is probably diminished by precurarization.[37] Most of this change may be a result of an increase in PCO_2 produced by fasciculations. Again, laryngoscopy and tracheal intubation with inadequate anesthesia or muscle relaxation are likely to increase ICP even more than succinylcholine.

Hyperkalemia

Serum potassium increases by 0.5 to 1.0 mEq/L after injection of succinylcholine. This increase is not prevented completely by precurarization. In fact, only large doses of nondepolarizing blockers reliably abolish this effect.[38] Subjects with preexisting hyperkalemia, such as patients in renal failure, do not have a greater increase in potassium levels, but the absolute level might reach the toxic range. Succinylcholine is safe in normokalemic renal failure patients.[39] However, severe hyperkalemia, occasionally leading to cardiac arrest, has been described in patients after major denervation injuries, spinal cord transection, peripheral denervation, stroke, trauma, extensive burns, and prolonged immobility with disease, and may be related to potassium loss via a proliferation of extrajunctional receptors.[38] Hyperkalemia has been reported with myotonia and muscle dystrophies, and cardiac arrests have been reported in children before the diagnosis of the disease was made.[38]

Severe hyperkalemia after succinylcholine resulting in cardiac arrest has also been observed in acidotic hypovolemic patients.

Abnormal Plasma Cholinesterase

Plasma cholinesterase activity can be reduced by a number of endogenous and exogenous causes, such as pregnancy, liver disease, uremia, malnutrition, burns, plasmapheresis, and oral contraceptives. These conditions usually lead to a slight, clinically unimportant increase in the duration of action of succinylcholine.[40] Plasma cholinesterase activity is reduced by some anticholinesterases (e.g., neostigmine) so that the duration of succinylcholine given after neostigmine, but not after edrophonium, is increased.[25]

A small proportion of patients have a genetically determined inability to metabolize succinylcholine. Either plasma cholinesterase is absent or an abnormal form of the enzyme is present. Only patients homozygous for the condition (approximately 1:2,000 individuals) have prolonged paralysis (3 to 6 hours) after usual doses of succinylcholine (1 to 1.5 mg/kg). In heterozygous patients (1:30 cases), the duration of action is only slightly prolonged compared with normal individuals. Traditional methods for identifying plasma cholinesterase phenotype involve measurement of enzyme activity with a substrate and inhibition with dibucaine, fluoride, and chloride. These tests are only capable of identifying some enzyme variants. The complete amino acid sequence of plasma cholinesterase has now been determined using molecular genetics techniques. The cholinesterase gene is located on chromosome 3 at q26,[40] and 20 mutations in the coding region of the plasma cholinergic gene have been identified. Although whole blood or fresh frozen plasma (FFP) can be given to accelerate succinylcholine metabolism in patients with low or absent plasma cholinesterase, the best course of action is probably mechanical ventilation of the lungs until full recovery of neuromuscular function can be demonstrated. Neostigmine and edrophonium are unpredictable in the reversal of abnormally prolonged succinylcholine blockade and are best avoided.

Clinical Uses

The main indication for succinylcholine is to facilitate tracheal intubation. In adults, a dose of 1.0 mg/kg yields 75 to 80% excellent intubation conditions within 1 to 1.5 minutes after an induction sequence that includes a hypnotic (propofol or thiopental) and a moderate dose narcotic.[41] The dose must be increased to 1.5 to 2.0 mg/kg if a precurarizing dose of nondepolarizing blocker has been used.

Succinylcholine is especially indicated for the "rapid sequence induction," when a patient presents with a full stomach and the possibility of aspiration of gastric contents. In this situation, manual ventilation of the lung is avoided if possible to reduce the probability of aspiration because of excessive pressure in the stomach. Thus, the ideal neuromuscular blocking agent has both a fast onset, to reduce the time between induction and intubation of the airway, and a rapid recovery, to allow return of normal breathing before the patient becomes hypoxic. The duration of action of succinylcholine, given at a dose of 1 mg/kg, is short enough so that in the majority of properly preoxygenated patients resume respiratory efforts (5 to 6 minutes) before hypoxia can be detected.[42] It has been argued that this is valid only in relatively healthy subjects and not in all cases. As a result, a lower dose has been suggested. However, a dose of 0.6 mg/kg results in substantially fewer patients with excellent intubating conditions, and the decrease in duration is modest.[41] For maintenance of relaxation, typical infusion rates are ~50 to 100 μg/kg/min.[26] However, the availability of short and intermediate nondepolarizing drugs makes succinylcholine infusions obsolete.

Children are slightly more resistant to succinylcholine than adults,[43] and doses of 1 to 2 mg/kg are required to facilitate intubation. In infants, 2 to 3 mg/kg may be required. Precurarization is not necessary in patients younger than 10 years because fasciculations are uncommon in this age group. Bradycardia is common in children unless atropine or glycopyrrolate is given.[30] Succinylcholine, at a dose of 4 mg/kg, is the only effective intramuscular neuromuscular blocking agent in children with difficult intravenous access and provides adequate intubating conditions in about 4 minutes. However, this route of administration should not be the method of choice.[44]

NONDEPOLARIZING DRUGS

4 Nondepolarizing neuromuscular blocking drugs bind to the postsynaptic receptor in a competitive fashion, by binding to one of the α subunits of the receptor (see Fig. 16-7).[12]

Characteristics of Nondepolarizing Blockade

The fade observed in response to high-frequency stimulation (>0.1 to 0.15 Hz) is characteristic of nondepolarizing blockade. With EMG recordings, fade is relatively constant in the range 2 to 50 Hz.[45] Mechanical fade is greater with 100 Hz than with 50 Hz.[46] Tetanic stimulation is followed by posttetanic facilitation, which is an increased response to any stimulation applied soon after the tetanus. The intensity and duration of this effect depend on the frequency and duration of the tetanic stimulation. With a 50-Hz tetanus of 5-second duration, twitch responses have been found to fall within 10% of their pretetanic values in 1 to 2 minutes, and in most cases in 1 minute (Fig. 16-9).

Finally, nondepolarizing blockade can be antagonized with anticholinesterase agents such as edrophonium, neostigmine, or pyridostigmine. It is also antagonized by depolarizing agents, such as succinylcholine, provided that the nondepolarizing blockade is intense and that the succinylcholine dose is too small to produce a block of its own.

Pharmacokinetics

As is the case for other drugs used in anesthesia, the elimination half-life of neuromuscular blocking agents does not always correlate with duration of action because termination of action sometimes depends on redistribution instead of elimination. However, knowledge of the kinetics of the drug helps us understand the behavior of the drug in special situations (prolonged administration, disease of the organs of elimination, and so on).

Several mechanisms can explain the various categories of durations of action listed in Table 16-3:

1. All long-acting drugs all have a long (1 to 2 hours) elimination half-life and depend on liver and/or kidney function for termination of action.
2. Intermediate-duration drugs either have an intermediate elimination half-life (atracurium and cisatracurium); or they have long elimination half-lives (1 to 2 hours) but depend on redistribution rather than elimination for termination of effect (vecuronium and rocuronium) (Fig. 16-10).
3. Short-duration drugs have either short elimination half-lives (the active isomers of mivacurium) or long

TABLE 16-3

TYPICAL PHARMACOKINETIC DATA FOR NEUROMUSCULAR BLOCKING AGENTS IN ADULTS, EXCEPT WHERE STATED

DRUG	VOLUME OF DISTRIBUTION (L/kg)	CLEARANCE (mL/kg/min)	ELIMINATION HALF-LIFE (min)
ULTRASHORT-DURATION AGENTS			
Succinylcholine	0.04	37	0.65
SHORT-DURATION AGENTS			
Mivacurium			
Trans–trans	0.05	29	2.4
Cis–trans	0.05	46	2.0
Cis–cis	0.18	7	30
Rapacuronium	0.2	7	100
INTERMEDIATE-DURATION AGENTS			
Atracurium	0.14	5.5	20
Cisatracurium			
Adults	0.12	5	23
Intensive care	0.26	6.5	25
Rocuronium			
Adults	0.3	3	90
Intensive care	0.7	3	330
Vecuronium	0.4	5	70
LONG-DURATION AGENTS			
Doxacurium	0.2	2.5	95
d-Tubocurarine			
Adults	0.3	1–3	90
Elderly	0.3	0.8	270
Neonates	0.7	1.1	300
Infants	0.5	1.0	300
Children	0.3	1.5	90
Pancuronium	0.3	1.8	140

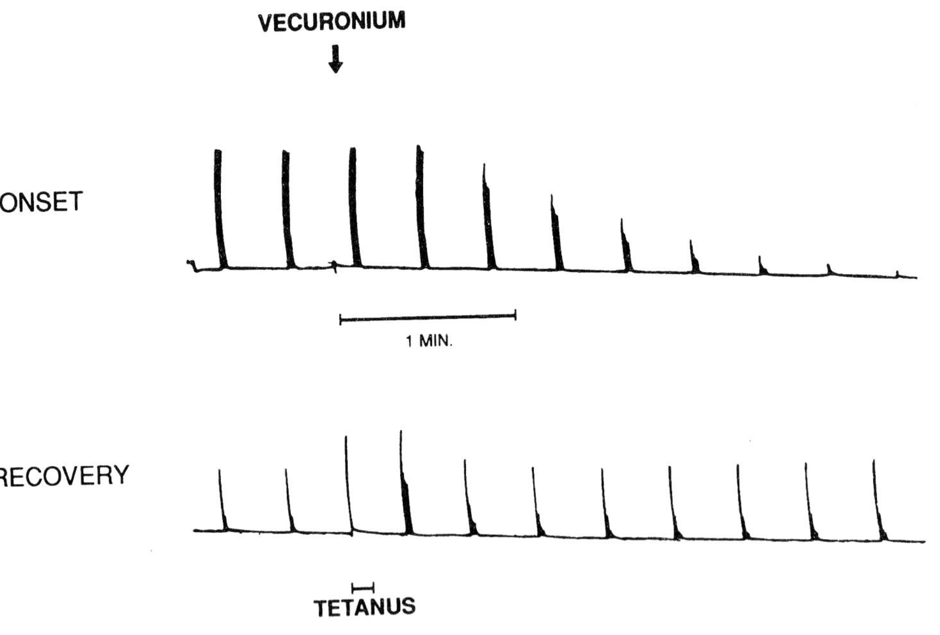

FIGURE 16-9. Characteristics of nondepolarizing blockade. Train-of-four responses are equal before administration of vecuronium (*arrow*). For a given twitch depression, fade is less during onset (*top trace*) than recovery (*bottom trace*). A 50 Hz- tetanus was applied during recovery. Tetanic fade is seen, with posttetanic facilitation, that is a greater train-of-four response after than before the train.

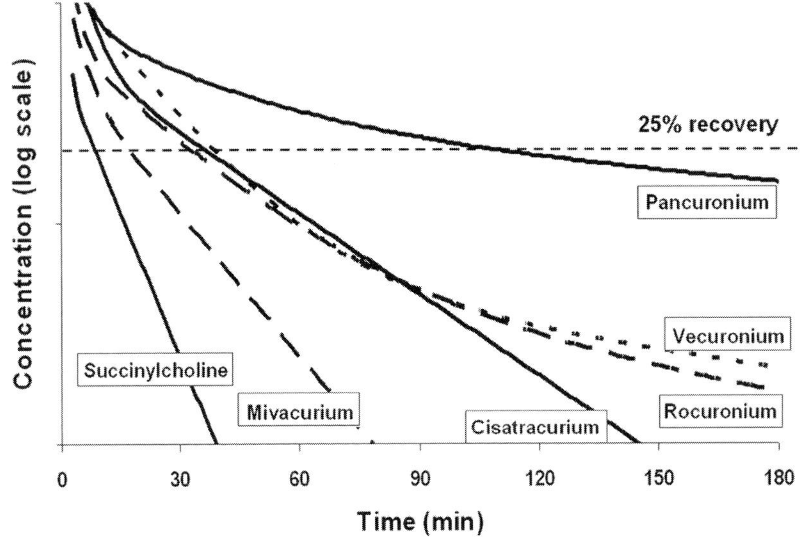

FIGURE 16-10. Representative concentrations at the neuromuscular junction for six representative drugs, after bolus doses of 2 × ED_{95}. Concentrations at the neuromuscular junction lag somewhat behind plasma concentrations. The level corresponding to 25% recovery is indicated. The curves were moved up or down so that the 25% level matched. Succinylcholine and the active mivacurium isomers have a rapid elimination. Pancuronium has a long half-life and recovery occurs during the elimination phase. Cisatracurium has an intermediate terminal half-life, and recovery also occurs during the elimination phase. Rocuronium and vecuronium have an elimation half-life comparable to that of pancuronium. However, an important redistribution occurs before, and 25% recovery occurs during that redistribution process. As a result, both rocuronium and vecuronium have a duration of action comparable to that of cisatracurium.

elimination half-life but extensive redistribution (rapacuronium).

4. Ultrashort-duration drugs have a very short elimination half-life (succinylcholine).

The volume of distribution of all these agents is approximately equal to extracellular fluid (ECF) volume (0.2 to 0.4 L/kg) (see Table 16-3). Drugs with short elimination half-lives (succinylcholine and mivacurium) have even smaller volumes of distribution because they are degraded before distribution is complete. In infants, in whom the ECF volume, as a proportion of body weight, is increased, the volume of distribution parallels ECF volume closely.

Onset and Duration of Action

Onset and duration of action of neuromuscular blocking drugs are determined by the time required for drug concentrations at the site of action to reach, and return below, a critical level, respectively. For duration, this level is determined chiefly by plasma concentrations, at least for intermediate- and long-duration drugs. However, onset time (2 to 7 minutes) lags behind peak plasma concentrations (<1 minute). This delay reflects the time required for drug transfer between plasma and neuromuscular junction and is represented quantitatively by a rate constant (k_{eo}). This rate constant corresponds to half-times of 5 to 10 minutes for most nondepolarizing drugs and is determined by all the factors that modify access of the drug to, and its removal from, the neuromuscular junction. These include cardiac output, distance of the muscle from the heart, and muscle blood flow. Thus, onset times are not the same in all muscles because of different blood flows. If metabolism or redistribution is very rapid, the onset time is accelerated. This probably plays a role only for succinylcholine and mivacurium. Finally, potent drugs have a slower onset of action than less potent agents (Fig. 16-11).[47] This is because a large proportion of receptors must be occupied before blockade can be observed. Blockade of these receptors will occur faster, and onset will be more rapid, if more drug molecules are available, that is, if

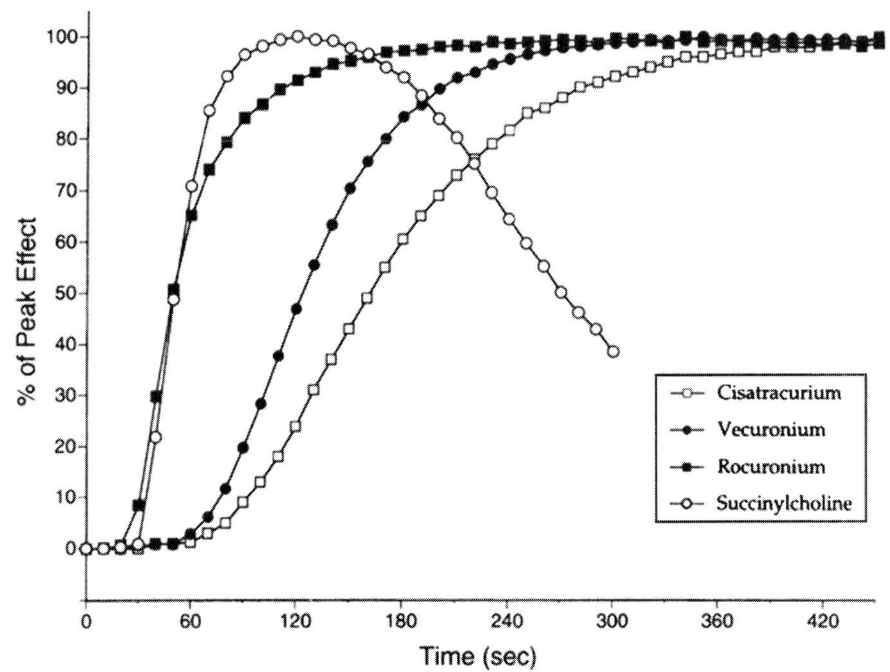

FIGURE 16-11. Neuromuscular blockade as a function of time for four neuromuscular blocking agents. Onset is faster for the less potent succinycholine and rocuronium than for the more potent vecuronium and cisatracurium. Reproduced from Kopman et al.[47]

potency is low. Table 16-2 shows that onset tends to be slower if a drug is potent, that is if ED_{95} is small.

Individual Nondepolarizing Agents

Since 1942, nearly 50 nondepolarizing neuromuscular blocking agents have been introduced into clinical anesthesia. This section covers only those drugs currently available in North America and Europe, plus a few others of historical interest. The first agent to undergo clinical investigation was Intocostrin, or *d*-tubocurarine, the purified and standardized product of curare obtained from the plant *Chondodendrum tomentosum*.[1] *d*-Tubocurarine has been almost completely replaced by more modern synthetic analogues.

d-Tubocurarine

The ED_{95} of *d*-tubocurarine is 0.5 mg/kg. At that dose, the duration of action is typical of a long-duration agent (see Table 16-2).[48]

Pharmacology. The molecule undergoes minimal metabolism so that 24 hours after its administration about 10% of the compound is found in the urine and 45% in the bile. Like most other neuromuscular blocking drugs, it is not extensively (30 to 50%) protein bound. Excretion is impaired in renal failure with an increase in elimination half-life.[49]

Cardiovascular Effects. Hypotension frequently accompanies the administration of *d*-tubocurarine even at doses less than ED_{95}. The mechanism involved is mainly histamine release, and skin flushing is frequently observed. Autonomic ganglionic blockade may also play a minor role in the production of hypotension.

Age. Pharmacokinetic studies have been performed in all age groups, and the results are helpful in understanding the behavior of all nondepolarizing agents in patients at the extremes of age. The potency of *d*-tubocurarine on a mg/kg basis does not vary greatly with age. Infants demonstrate greater blockade than older children or adults if the same concentration of *d*-tubocurarine is applied. However, this increased sensitivity of the neuromuscular junction in infants is concealed by the increased volume of distribution (see Table 16-3),[50] and this phenomenon has also been observed with other neuromuscular blocking agents. The onset of action is more rapid in the young as a result of a more rapid circulation time. However, the decreased glomerular filtration rate (GFR) in the very young and the very old results in an increase in $T_{1/2}\beta$ and prolonged duration of action.[50]

Burns. Patients with massive burns demonstrate resistance to *d*-tubocurarine and other nondepolarizing drugs that is dependent on the size of the burn and the time since injury.[51] Resistance is associated with higher concentrations of the free drug to produce a given degree of twitch depression compared with nonthermally injured patients. As in denervation injury, there is an increase in the number of acetylcholine receptors in muscles close to the site of injury, and less so in more distant muscles.[52]

Clinical Use. The long duration and cardiovascular effects of *d*-tubocurarine have restricted its use and constituted a stimulus for the production of alternative agents. Initially, this led to the introduction of pancuronium, which replaced the hypotension of *d*-tubocurarine with hypertension and tachycardia. More recently, drugs of intermediate duration (atracurium, cisatracurium, vecuronium, and rocuronium) with virtually no cardiovascular effects have almost eliminated the use of *d*-tubocurarine. When available, *d*-tubocurarine has been mainly confined to be used as a "precurarization" (3 mg/70 kg) before succinylcholine to reduce fasciculations and muscle pains. Rocuronium has largely replaced *d*-tubocurarine for this indication.

Alcuronium

Although it has never been available in North America, alcuronium still enjoys limited use in some countries. The ED_{95} is approximately 0.2 to 0.25 mg/kg. Intubating doses are usually limited to 0.3 mg/kg because of the long duration of action. Although it was introduced as an intermediate-duration drug, its recovery index (37 minutes) makes it a long-acting neuromuscular blocking agent.[53]

Atracurium

Atracurium is a bisquaternary ammonium benzylisoquinoline compound. It was developed in an attempt to produce a short-acting muscle relaxant that was independent of the liver and the kidney for termination of its action. It is a mixture of 10 isomers of different potencies. In humans, atracurium is degraded via two metabolic pathways. One of these pathways is the Hofmann reaction, a nonenzymatic degradation the rate of which increases as temperature and/or pH increases. The second pathway is nonspecific ester hydrolysis. The enzymes involved in this metabolic pathway are a group of tissue esterases, which are distinct from plasma or acetyl cholinesterases. The same group of enzymes is involved in the degradation of esmolol and remifentanil. It has been estimated that two-thirds of atracurium is degraded by ester hydrolysis and one-third by Hofmann reaction.[54] Subjects with abnormal plasma cholinesterase have a normal response to atracurium.

The end products of the degradation of atracurium are laudanosine and acrylate fragments. Laudanosine has been reported as causing seizures in animals, but at doses largely exceeding the clinical range. No deleterious effect of laudanosine has been demonstrated conclusively in humans.[55] Laudanosine is excreted by the kidney. Acrylates have the potential to inhibit cell growth, and this has been demonstrated in vitro.[56] However, the concentrations and exposure times required to obtain this effect are much greater than what is obtained normally in clinical practice.

Pharmacology. Atracurium is an intermediate-duration drug, with a terminal half-life of approximately 20 minutes. Termination of effect occurs during the elimination phase of the drug. Because degradation does not depend on an end-organ function, duration of action is not dependent on renal or hepatic function. It does not increase with age.

The ED_{95} of atracurium is 0.2 to 0.25 mg/kg. The onset of action of equipotent doses is similar for atracurium, pancuronium, *d*-tubocurarine, and vecuronium. It is slower than succinylcholine. As with any neuromuscular blocking agent, onset time can be reduced if the dose is increased, but it is not recommended to exceed 0.5 mg/kg, because of hypotension and histamine release. The duration of action is also dose related. The time to 25% first twitch recovery after 0.5 mg/kg is approximately 30 to 40 minutes.

Cardiovascular Effects. Atracurium releases histamine if large doses ($2 \times ED_{95}$ or greater) are administered, with hypotension and tachycardia as frequent manifestations. Similar changes occur after the use of *d*-tubocurarine or metocurine but at lower equipotent doses. The most obvious clinical manifestation of histamine release is skin flushing. Bronchospasm may also occur. These responses can be avoided by slow injection over 1 to 3 minutes or by pretreatment with H_1 and H_2 receptor blockade. Anaphylactic reactions to atracurium have been described, but they do not appear to be more frequent than after other neuromuscular blocking drugs.[31]

Special Situations. Dosage requirements are similar in the elderly, younger adults, and children, presumably reflecting the organ independence of atracurium's elimination. Similarly, no dosage adjustment is required in individuals with renal or hepatic failure. As with other nondepolarizing agents, the dose must be increased in burn patients, partly because of increased protein binding, partly because of up-regulation of receptors, causing resistance at the endplate. In the obese patient, the dose of atracurium, as for all neuromuscular blocking agents, should be calculated based on lean body mass.

Clinical Uses. To obtain adequate intubating conditions, relatively large doses must be used (0.5 mg/kg), and laryngoscopy should be attempted only after 2 to 3 minutes. Cardiovascular manifestations of histamine release are often seen at that dose, and perfect intubating conditions are seen in only half the patients (see Fig. 16-3).[7] Increasing the dose may improve intubating conditions, but at the expense of greater cardiovascular effects. For intubation, there has been a tendency to replace atracurium by agents, such as rocuronium, with a shorter onset time and more cardiovascular stability. Atracurium is, however, convenient and versatile for maintenance of relaxation, either as a continuous infusion (5 to 10 μg/kg/min) or as intermittent injections (0.05 to 0.1 mg/kg every 10 to 15 minutes).

Cisatracurium

In an attempt to increase the margin of safety between the neuromuscular blocking dose and the histamine-releasing dose, a potent isomer of atracurium, cisatracurium, was identified. Like atracurium, its cardiovascular effects are manifest at doses exceeding 0.4 mg/kg, but its ED_{95} (0.05 mg/kg) is much lower. As a result, manifestations of histamine release are not seen in practice. The metabolism of cisatracurium is similar to that of atracurium, but it seems that the relative importance of Hofmann elimination is somewhat greater than for atracurium, and the role of ester hydrolysis is correspondingly less.[57] The end products of metabolism, laudanosine and acrylate fragments are the same as for atracurium.

Pharmacology. Because cisatracurium is a potent drug, its onset time is longer than that of atracurium and longer still than that of rocuronium. For example, equipotent doses of cisatracurium (0.092 mg/kg) and rocuronium (0.72 mg/kg) had onset times of 4 minutes and 1.7 minutes, respectively.[58] The elimination half-life (22 to 25 minutes) is similar to that of atracurium,[59] so that the duration of action for 2 × ED_{95} doses (0.1 mg/kg) is 30 to 45 minutes. However, in an attempt to accelerate onset, the recommended dose was increased to 0.15 mg/kg. This is well below the threshold for histamine release, but the duration of action is prolonged to 45 to 60 minutes.

Because the doses required to obtain paralysis are considerably less for cisatracurium than for atracurium, less laudanosine and less acrylate byproducts are produced.[56] Peak concentrations of laudanosine have been found to be five times less with equipotent doses of cisatracurium. Thus, the concerns raised by the potential toxic effects of these metabolites are virtually eliminated.

Special Situations. As for atracurium, there is no need to adjust dosage in the elderly, children, or infants, when compared with young adults. The experience in burn and obese patients is limited, but the same principles that are valid for atracurium are expected to apply.

Side Effects. In contrast to atracurium, cisatracurium is devoid of histamine-releasing properties even at high doses (8 × ED_{95}). It is also devoid of cardiovascular effects. However, anaphylactic reactions have been described.[31]

Clinical Use. Cisatracurium may be used to facilitate tracheal intubation at doses equivalent to 3 to 4 times the ED_{95} (0.15 to 0.2 mg/kg) when manual ventilation is possible after induction of anesthesia and when the duration of the procedure is expected to exceed 1 hour. Duration is shorter with lower doses, but onset time is prolonged and intubating conditions are less ideal. Neuromuscular blockade is easily maintained at a stable level by continuous intravenous infusion of cisatracurium (1 to 2 μg/kg/min) at a constant rate and does not change with time, suggesting the lack of a significant cumulative drug effect and lack of dependence on renal and/or hepatic clearance mechanisms.[60] The rate of recovery is independent of the dose of cisatracurium and the duration of the administration.

Because cisatracurium does not depend on end-organ function for its elimination, the drug appears suitable for administration in the intensive care unit (ICU). The infusion rates to keep patients paralyzed is greater than in the operating room (typically 5 μg/kg/min), with wide interindividual variability.[61] It is likely that prolonged exposure of the receptors to a neuromuscular blocking agent causes some up-regulation, with a corresponding requirement for a higher dose.

Doxacurium

Doxacurium is a long-acting bisquaternary ammonium compound that is devoid of histamine-releasing or cardiovascular side effects. It has a prolonged elimination half-life (1 to 2 hours) and depends on the kidney and the liver for its disposition. Thus, duration of action is prolonged in the elderly and in subjects with impaired renal or hepatic function. Doxacurium is also a weak substrate for plasma cholinesterase. The ED_{95} for doxacurium is 25 μg/kg (see Table 16-2).[62] Doxacurium has a limited place in clinical practice because of its very slow onset and long duration of action. Nevertheless, it may be useful in patients with ischemic heart disease who are undergoing prolonged anesthesia or long-term mechanical ventilation of the lungs. The slow onset time, prolonged duration of action, and slow recovery make doxacurium unsuitable for facilitating tracheal intubation or for providing skeletal muscle relaxation during brief surgical procedures. When infused for several days to patients in the ICU, recovery after stopping the infusion exceeded 10 hours.

Gallamine

Gallamine was introduced in 1948 and has only historical interest. It is a low potency nondepolarizing drug (ED_{95} = 2 mg/kg) and it has a long duration of action. Gallamine produces significant tachycardia because of a vagolytic effect, even at doses associated with incomplete blockade at the adductor pollicis. It is effective when used to prevent succinylcholine-induced fasciculations.

GW280430A

The new compound called GW280430A is a nondepolarizing drug and belongs to the class of asymmetric mixed-onium chlorofumarates. Its main degradation pathway involves cysteine in the plasma and is independent of plasma cholinesterase. The ED_{95} in humans is 0.19 mg/kg.[63] Cardiovascular effects are observed at doses exceeding 3 × ED_{95}, and are most probably related to histamine release. At doses anticipated to be required for tracheal intubation (0.4 to 0.6 mg/kg), onset at the adductor pollicis is 1.5 minutes and duration to 25% T1 recovery is 8 to 10 minutes, making this drug comparable to succinylcholine in duration of action. At the time of writing, this compound was still an investigational drug.

Metocurine

Metocurine, produced by methylation of two hydroxy groups of *d*-tubocurarine, is twice as potent as the parent compound and produces less histamine release. Its ED_{95} is approximately 0.3 mg/kg.[48] Its duration of action is comparable to that of *d*-tubocurarine, making it a long-acting agent.

Metocurine causes less histamine release and cardiovascular effects than equipotent doses of *d*-tubocurarine. Because of this, metocurine enjoyed a brief period of popularity before the introduction of atracurium and vecuronium. Metocurine and pancuronium combined were found to be synergistic with opposing cardiovascular effects, and the mixture was recommended for use in patients with severe cardiovascular disease.[64] However, the introduction of shorter duration alternatives without cardiovascular effects has made metocurine obsolete.

Mivacurium

Mivacurium is a benzylisoquinoline derivative with an intermediate onset and short duration of action that is hydrolyzed by plasma cholinesterase, like succinylcholine.[65] Contrary to succinylcholine, however, mivacurium produces nondepolarizing blockade. The drug is presented as a mixture of three isomers. Two, the cis–trans and trans–trans, have short half-lives, but the cis–cis isomer has a much longer half-life (see Table 16-3). The cis–cis isomer accounts for only 6% of the mixture, has less than one-tenth the potency of the other isomers and thus contributes little if anything to neuromuscular block during anesthesia. The pharmacology of mivacurium is governed largely by the behavior of the trans–trans and cis–trans isomers.

Pharmacology. Under steady-state nitrous oxide–narcotic anesthesia, the ED_{95} of mivacurium is 0.08 mg/kg (see Table 16-2). However, there is evidence that mivacurium is less effective when given at induction of anesthesia than during stable anesthesia.[66] This might be because cardiac output is decreased and/or peripheral blood flow might be increased after induction of anesthesia. Decreasing cardiac output tends to increase the effect of short-acting drugs because a bolus dose is diluted in a smaller volume, producing greater plasma concentrations. In any event, doses that are twice the ED_{95} mg/kg determined under steady-state anesthesia are associated with poor intubating conditions. In 9 out of 9 patients, a dose of 0.15 mg/kg provided unacceptable conditions.[67] These conditions are markedly improved if the dose is increased to 0.2 or 0.25 mg/kg but were not as good as with succinylcholine.[67] Onset time is surprisingly long for a drug whose active isomers have a terminal half-life of less than 2 minutes. At 2 to 3 × ED_{95}, twitch disappears in 2.5 to 4 minutes.[65] This long onset time is probably the result of the high potency of mivacurium. For all neuromuscular blocking agents, a direct relationship between onset time and potency has been demonstrated. Drugs with a low ED_{95}, expressed in μmoles/kg, have a longer onset time.[47] On the other hand, recovery to 25% does not depend heavily on dose, being in the range of 15 to 25 minutes for doses of 0.15 to 0.25 mg/kg. The infusion rate to maintain blockade constant does not vary with time, and recovery is as rapid after many hours of infusion than after a bolus dose, suggesting that the slowly eliminated cis–cis metabolite contributes very little to the overall neuromuscular effect.

Side Effects. Like atracurium, mivacurium releases histamine in a dose-related fashion. At doses of 0.15 mg/kg or less, the drug has virtually no cardiovascular effects. Hypotension and tachycardia are seen frequently when doses are increased to 0.2 mg/kg or more. Cutaneous signs, such as erythema and flushing, are also observed frequently with large doses. They can be seen in isolation or be accompanied by cardiovascular changes. These histamine-related effects are short lived (2 to 3 minutes) and should not normally be considered a manifestation of anaphylaxis, which is a rare event. Bronchospasm is rare, but may be seen more frequently with mivacurium than with other neuromuscular blocking agents.[68] Manifestations of histamine release may be decreased if the drug is either given slowly (in more than 30 seconds) or in divided doses (0.15 mg/kg followed 30 seconds later by 0.1 mg/kg).

Special Situations. In infants and children the ED_{95} is approximately the same as in adults, but onset of block and recovery are more rapid.[69] Cardiovascular effects are not as important as in adults, so doses up to 0.3 mg/kg have been used. Duration to 25% recovery is shorter (10 minutes) in infants and children than in adults.[69] The infusion rate required to maintain blockade is greater in children than in adults.[70] In the elderly, the ED_{95} is the same as in younger adults. However, duration of action is prolonged by a few minutes and the infusion rate to maintain neuromuscular blockade is decreased.[71]

Burns. In burn patients, upregulation of the receptors, and to a lesser extent increased protein binding, causes a resistance to all nondepolarizing neuromuscular blocking agents. Thus, a larger dose of the drug is normally required. However, for mivacurium, the situation is different because plasma cholinesterase activity is decreased in burn patients. The net effect is either a normal or even an enhanced effect of usual doses.[72]

Reversal. Administration of anticholinesterase agents after mivacurium has been controversial for two main reasons. First, neostigmine, but not edrophonium, inhibits plasma cholinesterase. Therefore, the breakdown of mivacurium may be slower in the presence of neostigmine. In fact, neostigmine has been shown to delay recovery if given during intense neuromuscular block, presumably when high concentrations of mivacurium are still present.[73] However, if neostigmine is given when signs of spontaneous recovery are present (two twitches or more present), the rate of recovery is accelerated. Edrophonium does not interfere with plasma cholinesterase activity and was found to accelerate recovery, even when given when blockade is profound (one twitch in the train-of-four).[73] Also, mivacurium reversal has been suggested to be unnecessary because spontaneous recovery is rapid and its avoidance may reduce the incidence of side effects such as postoperative nausea and vomiting. However, this may result in residual block on arrival in the recovery room, particularly if large doses of mivacurium are used up to the end of anesthesia.

Plasma Cholinesterase. Mivacurium is metabolized by plasma cholinesterase somewhat more slowly than succinylcholine. The conditions associated with a decrease plasma cholinesterase activity known to affect succinylcholine metabolism also alter mivacurium duration of action. For example, a moderate increase in the duration of action of mivacurium can be seen in postpartum patients. Patients homozygous for atypical plasma cholinesterase may show very prolonged block.

Clinical Use. Mivacurium is well suited to surgical procedures requiring brief muscle relaxation, particularly those in which rapid recovery is required, such as ambulatory and laparoscopic surgery. However, it is not recommended for rapid sequence induction. Because of its slow onset, conditions for tracheal intubation are unsatisfactory unless large bolus doses, at least 0.2 mg/kg, are given and a delay of at least 2 minutes is allowed before intubation is attempted.[67] However, by using two doses of 0.15 and 0.1 mg/kg separated by 30 seconds, good to excellent intubating conditions have been achieved in almost 90% of patients, an onset similar to that of succinylcholine.[74] Small doses of mivacurium (0.04 to 0.08 mg/kg) have been suggested to facilitate insertion of a laryngeal mask airway.[75] Conditions and success rate are usually better than in the absence of neuromuscular blocking agent. The rapid recovery makes it necessary to monitor neuromuscular activity continuously during its administration, which is accomplished more easily by constant infusion (5 to 7 μg/kg/min in young and middle-aged adults) than by intermittent bolus injection. This infusion rate has to be increased in children and reduced in the elderly.[76] In children, mivacurium has a faster onset of action and more rapid recovery than in adults, so the drug can be used for intubation and maintenance of relaxation for short procedures.[69,70]

Pancuronium

Pancuronium belongs to a series of bisquaternary aminosteroid compounds. It is metabolized to a 3-OH compound, which has one-half the neuromuscular blocking activity of the parent compound. The ED_{95} of pancuronium is 0.07 mg/kg. The duration of action is long, being 1.5 to 2 hours after a 0.15 mg/kg dose. Clearance is decreased in renal and hepatic failure, demonstrating that excretion is dependent on both organs. The onset of action is more rapid in infants and children than in adults and recovery is slower in the elderly.

Cardiovascular Effects. Pancuronium is associated with increases in heart rate, blood pressure, and cardiac output, particularly after large doses ($2 \times ED_{95}$). The cause is uncertain but includes a vagolytic effect at the postganglionic nerve terminal, a sympathomimetic effect as a result of blocking of muscarinic receptors that normally exert some braking on ganglionic transmission, and an increase in catecholamine release. Pancuronium does not release histamine.

Clinical Use. The slow onset of action of pancuronium limits its usefulness in facilitating tracheal intubation. Administration in divided doses, with a small dose given 3 minutes before induction of anesthesia (priming principle), produces a small but measurable acceleration, but the intermediate- and short-acting compounds are more suitable when succinylcholine is contraindicated. In patients with myocardial ischemia, tachycardia should be avoided. However, pancuronium has enjoyed popularity in cardiac anesthesia because it counteracts the bradycardic effect of high doses of opioids. With the increased tendency toward early extubation in cardiac surgery, the appropriateness of pancuronium in this setting must be reevaluated. The use of pancuronium instead of rocuronium is associated with a greater incidence of muscular weakness in the recovery room after cardiac surgery,[77] and reversal should be considered seriously. The continued popularity of pancuronium is dependent on cost: generic pancuronium is cheaper than other nondepolarizing relaxants. Its use is associated with a high incidence of residual block in the postanesthesia care unit (PACU), at least in adults (see Table 16-1).[8,78] Pancuronium neuromuscular block is more difficult to reverse than that of the intermediate duration agents.[79]

Pipecuronium

In an effort to obtain a pancuronium without cardiovascular side effects, pipecuronium was developed. Its ED_{95} is slightly less (0.05 mg/kg) than that of pancuronium, and it is virtually without any cardiovascular effects. However, pipecuronium soon became obsolete because it had the drawbacks of long-acting agents (difficulty to reverse, residual paralysis, lack of versatility), and the absence of cardiovascular effects was also seen with the shorter acting vecuronium and rocuronium.

Rapacuronium

Rapacuronium is also an aminosteroid compound that was introduced for clinical use in 1999. It was withdrawn in 2001 because of rare, but severe cases of bronchospasm after intubation. Being less potent than rocuronium, it had a more rapid onset of action. Following 1.5 mg/kg, good to excellent intubation conditions were produced at 60 seconds, clinical duration (25% T_1 recovery) occurs in 17 minutes and spontaneous recovery to train-of-four ratio of 0.7 occurs in 35 minutes.[80] The intubating conditions were not as good as with succinylcholine and the duration of action was longer. Rapacuronium is metabolized to a 17-OH derivative (ORG 9488) that has twice the neuromuscular blocking activity of the parent compound and is excreted slowly via the kidneys.

Rapacuronium produces mild dose-related tachycardia and hypotension, and these cardiovascular changes do not appear to be because of histamine release. Mild to moderate increases in airway pressure and bronchospasm were observed in more patients given rapacuronium than succinylcholine.[80] The mechanism for this effect is not a hypersensitivity or allergic reaction, but is most likely related to the effect of rapacuronium on M2 and M3 muscarinic receptors in the lung. Activation of the postsynaptic M3 receptors by acetylcholine produces brochosconstriction in the lungs, and the effect is terminated by presynaptic M2 receptors that counteract this effect. Rapacuronium has the potential to block both receptors, but it has a greater affinity for the M2 receptor. The concentrations required for M2 blockade are well within the clinical range, while much more is required for M3 inhibition. The net effect is that if M2 receptors are blocked selectively, for example, in susceptible individuals, bronchoconstriction by activation of the M3 receptors is unopposed.[81] Other neuromuscular blocking agents, such as vecuronium and cisatracurium, have similar differential effects on the M2 and M3 receptors, but at concentrations higher than encountered clinically.[81]

Rocuronium

Rocuronium is an aminosteroid compound with structural similarity with vecuronium and pancuronium. Its duration of action is comparable to that of vecuronium, but onset is shorter.

Pharmacology. Plasma concentrations of rocuronium decrease rapidly after bolus injection because of hepatic uptake.[82] Thus, the duration of action of the drug is determined chiefly by redistribution, rather than by its rather long terminal elimination half-life (1 to 2 hours) (see Fig. 16-10). Metabolism to 17-deacetylrocuronium is a very minor elimination pathway. Most of the drug is excreted unchanged in the urine, bile, or feces.[82]

With an ED_{95} of 0.3 mg/kg, rocuronium has one-sixth the potency of vecuronium, a more rapid onset, but a similar duration of action and similar pharmacokinetic behavior. With equipotent doses, rocuronium onset at the adductor pollicis was much faster than that of cisatracurium, atracurium, and vecuronium (see Fig. 16-11).[47] After doses of 0.6 mg/kg ($2 \times ED_{95}$) maximal block occurs in 1.5 to 2 minutes. In a multicenter study of 349 patients, intubating conditions at 60 seconds after 0.6 mg/kg rocuronium were good to excellent in 77% of cases. To obtain results similar to those after 1 mg/kg succinylcholine, the dose of rocuronium had to be increased to 1.0 mg/kg, which provided 92% good or excellent conditions.[83] However, the duration of action is longer than for succinylcholine, ranging between 30 to 40 minutes for a 0.6 mg/kg dose to approximately 60 minutes after 1 mg/kg in adults. Thus, rocuronium is an intermediate-duration drug.

As for other nondepolarizing agents the onset of action of rocuronium is more rapid at the diaphragm and adductor laryngeal muscles than at the adductor pollicis,[84] probably a result of a greater blood flow to centrally located muscles. Laryngeal adductor muscles are important in anesthesia because they close the vocal cords and insufficient relaxation prevents easy passage of the tracheal tube. Laryngeal adductor muscles are resistant to the effect of rocuronium, and the plasma concentration required for equivalent blockade is greater at the larynx than at the adductor pollicis.[85] The same is true of the diaphragm, which is resistant to the effect of rocuronium and other neuromuscular blocking agents. Recovery is faster at the diaphragm and larynx than at the adductor pollicis.[84]

Cardiovascular Effects. No hemodynamic changes (blood pressure, heart rate, or ECG) were seen in humans, and there were no increases in plasma histamine concentrations after doses of up to $4 \times ED_{95}$ (1.2 mg/kg).[86] Only slight hemodynamic changes are observed during coronary artery bypass surgery. Anaphylactic reactions have been described, and it has been claimed that these events occur more frequently with rocuronium than with other neuromuscular blocking agents.[31] However, it now appears that many of these reports might not be a true anaphylactic reaction to rocuronium, because up to 50% of the general population show a positive intradermal or pick test to the drug.[87] Clearly, many patients who were investigated for a possible anaphylactic reaction were falsely labeled allergic to the drug, because of the high rate of false-positive tests. It is possible that overdiagnosis has played a role in the relatively high incidence of rocuronium anaphylaxis reported in Norway (29 cases in 150,000 administrations, or 1:5,000)[88] or in France,[31] while reports from other Nordic countries suggest a much lower incidence (7 cases in 800,000 administrations or less than 1:100,000).[88] Current evidence suggests that withholding rocuronium because of the fear of anaphylactic reactions is unjustified.

Special Situations. The potency of rocuronium has been reported to be slightly greater in women than in men, the ED_{95} being 0.27 and 0.39 mg/kg, respectively, with an increased duration in women.[89] Some ethnic groups are more sensitive to the drug. Chinese subjects living in Vancouver were found to be more sensitive than Caucasians.[90] Children (2 to 12 years old) require more rocuronium and duration of action is less. Onset of action is shorter in the pediatric than in the adult population. For example, a dose of 1.2 mg/kg provides an onset time (39 seconds) comparable to that of succinylcholine, 2 mg/kg, and mean duration of action is 41 minutes.[91] Thus, the recommended doses are 0.9 to 1.2 mg/kg in this age group. Rocuronium is more potent in infants than in older children.[92] Doses of 0.6 mg/kg have a longer duration in neonates (<1 month) than in infants (5 to 12 months), so a reduced dosage (0.45 mg/kg) is recommended.[93] Rocuronium may be used for rapid-sequence induction as succinylcholine is relatively contraindicated because of the possible presence of undiagnosed muscle dystrophy in pediatric patients, especially in boys.[38]

In elderly patients, the ED_{95} is similar to that found in younger adults, but the duration of action is prolonged slightly.[94] Rocuronium has an increased terminal half-life in renal failure patients, probably because of its partial renal elimination, but this translates into very minor, if any, prolongation of block.[95] In hepatic disease, the slower uptake and elimination of rocuronium by the liver tends to prolong the duration of action of the drug, but this is compensated to some extent by the larger volume of distribution.[96]

Clinical Use. The rapid onset and intermediate duration of action makes this agent a potential replacement for succinylcholine in conditions where rapid tracheal intubation is indicated. However, large doses (>1 mg/kg) are required with a prolonged duration of action. Contrary to succinylcholine, the option to wait for spontaneous breathing to resume before hypoxia is manifest does not exist with rocuronium. To shorten the onset time, the "priming principle," which involves the administration of a small dose of rocuronium usually 3 minutes before induction, has been advocated. Unfortunately, the optimal priming dose, that is the largest dose that will not produce symptoms of weakness in the awake patient, is rather small. As with defasciculating doses before succinylcholine, it is not recommended to administer more than $0.1 \times ED_{95}$,[32] which, in the case of rocuronium, amounts to 0.03 mg/kg. Such a small dose has minimal effects on onset times provided by much larger doses (0.6 to 1.0 mg/kg). However, priming might have an effect if the intubating dose is small (0.45 mg/kg). A "timing principle" has been described in which 0.6 mg/kg rocuronium is given *before* the induction agent, which is administered at the onset of ptosis. Considering that loss of consciousness does not occur immediately after injection of the induction agent, this technique is not recommended. Rocuronium and thiopental do not mix. They form a precipitate when they are in the same intravenous line. If thiopental is used for induction of anesthesia, the line must be flushed carefully before rocuronium is given.

Except in countries where it is not available, rocuronium has replaced vecuronium as an intermediate-duration relaxant because of its more rapid onset. Initial doses of 0.6 mg/kg iv will usually produce good intubating conditions within 90 seconds. Duration of action is 30 to 40 minutes. Smaller doses (typically 0.45 mg/kg) have a shorter duration of action, but time to intubation must be increased. Subsequent doses of 0.1 to 0.2 mg/kg will provide clinical relaxation for 10 to 20 minutes. Alternatively, rocuronium might be given by continued infusion, titrated with the help of a nerve stimulator. Infusion rates are in the range 5 to 10 μg/kg/min.[60] Recovery after infusions is slower than after bolus doses.[97]

Vecuronium

Vecuronium is an intermediate-duration aminosteroid neuromuscular relaxant without cardiovascular effects. Its ED_{95} is 0.04 to 0.05 mg/kg. Its duration and recovery characteristics are comparable to those of rocuronium. However, its onset of action is slower.

Pharmacology. Vecuronium is a monoquaternary ammonium compound produced by demethylation of the pancuronium molecule. The demethylation reduces the acetylcholine-like characteristics of the molecule and increases its lipophilicity, which encourages hepatic uptake. Vecuronium undergoes spontaneous deacetylation to produce 3-OH, 17-OH, and 3,17-$(OH)_2$ metabolites. The most potent of these metabolites, 3-OH vecuronium, about 60% of the activity of vecuronium, is excreted by the kidney, and may be responsible, in part, for prolonged paralysis in patients in the intensive care unit.[98] Like rocuronium, vecuronium has been found less potent and with a shorter duration of action in men than in women, probably because of a greater volume of distribution in men.

Duration of action of vecuronium, like that of rocuronium, is governed by redistribution, not by elimination (see Fig. 16-10). Attempts have been made to speed the onset of action by using the priming principle, that is by administering a small, subparalyzing dose several minutes before the principal dose is given. For vecuronium, the best results have been obtained with a priming dose of 0.01 mg/kg, followed 3 to 4 minutes later by 0.1 mg/kg. However, the introduction of rocuronium, which has a more rapid onset of action, is likely to make this practice obsolete.

Cardiovascular Effects. Vecuronium usually produces no cardiovascular effects with clinical doses. It does not induce histamine release. Bradycardia has been described with high-dose opioid anesthesia, and this might be the reflection of the opioid effect. Allergic reactions have been described, but no more frequently than after the use of other neuromuscular blocking drugs.[31]

Clinical Use. The cardiovascular neutrality and intermediate duration of action make vecuronium a suitable agent for use in patients with ischemic heart disease or those undergoing short, ambulatory surgery. Care should be taken when vecuronium is administered immediately after thiopental because a precipitate of barbituric acid may be formed that may obstruct the intravenous cannula.

Large doses, 0.1 to 0.2 mg/kg, with or without priming, can be used to facilitate tracheal intubation instead of succinylcholine. For maintenance of relaxation, vecuronium may be given using intermittent boluses, 0.01 to 0.02 mg/kg, or by continuous infusion at a rate of 1 to 2 μg/kg/min. However, the rate of spontaneous recovery of neuromuscular function is slower after administration by infusion than by intermittent boluses.[99] Vecuronium has now largely been replaced by the more rapid rocuronium.

DRUG INTERACTIONS

Interactions between neuromuscular blocking drugs and several anesthetic and nonanesthetic drugs have been suggested. Although some interactions have been confirmed, many remain as isolated case reports or theoretical possibilities. Only some of these interactions will be discussed here.

Anesthetic Agents

Inhalational Agents

The anesthetic vapors potentiate neuromuscular blockade in a dose-related fashion. Studies attempting to quantify the magnitude of this effect have led to conflicting results, because the time factor is also important. The older halogenated agents halothane, enflurane, and isoflurane may take 2 hours or more to equilibrate with muscle, so in practice the potentiating effect of these vapors might not be immediately apparent. At similar MAC, enflurane appears to potentiate nondepolarizing blockade more than does isoflurane, which in turn potentiates to a greater extent than halothane. The newer agents sevoflurane and desflurane equilibrate more rapidly with muscle, but the effect may be measurable only after 30 minutes or more. For example, the duration of action of a bolus dose of mivacurium given at induction of anesthesia is not altered by the presence of sevoflurane (1 MAC). However, the infusion rate required to maintain block decreases by 75% over the next 1.5 hours, compared with no change under propofol anesthesia.[100] The degree of potentiation increases with the concentration of sevoflurane.[70] Recovery rate is longer in the presence of sevoflurane, even if the infusion rate of mivacurium was less.[70] There is evidence that desflurane might have a greater potentiating effect on the neuromuscular junction than sevoflurane.[101]

The mechanism of action of potentiation by halogenated agents is uncertain, but it appears that they produce their effects at the neuromuscular junction. Isoflurane and sevoflurane inhibit current through the nicotinic receptor at the neuromuscular junction, and this inhibition is dose dependent.[102]

Intravenous Anesthetics

Although some slight potentiation of neuromuscular blockade has been demonstrated with high doses of most iv induction agents in animals, clinical doses of drugs such as midazolam, thiopental, propofol, fentanyl, and ketamine have little or no neuromuscular effect in humans.

Local Anesthetics

Lidocaine, procaine, and other local anesthetic agents produce neuromuscular blockade in their own right as well as potentiating the effects of depolarizing and nondepolarizing neuromuscular blocking drugs. However, these data were obtained in vitro, with concentrations of local anesthetics rarely obtained systemically in practice.

Interactions between Nondepolarizing Blocking Drugs

Combinations of two nondepolarizing neuromuscular blocking drugs are either additive or synergistic, depending on which two drugs are involved. Addition occurs when the total effect equals that of equipotent doses of each drug. For instance, pancuronium and vecuronium have an additive interaction.[103] An ED_{95} of either pancuronium (0.07 mg/kg) or vecuronium (0.05 mg/kg) yields 95% blockade. Half the ED_{95} of pancuronium (0.035 mg/kg) administered with half the ED_{95} of vecuronium (0.025 mg/kg) will also produce 95% block. However, some combinations are synergistic, that is their combined effect is greater than if an equipotent dose of either one of the constituents is given alone. For example, cisatracurium (ED_{95} = 0.05 mg/kg) and rocuronium (ED_{95} = 0.3 mg/kg) will produce a greater blockade than equipotent amounts of each drug given alone. To get 95% block, not one-half but approximately one-fourth the ED_{95} of each drug needs to be given together, that is cisatracurium, 0.0125 mg/kg with rocuronium, 0.075 mg/kg.[104] Generally, combinations of chemically similar drugs—for example, pancuronium–vecuronium, *d*-tubocurarine–metocurine, and atracurium–mivacurium—have additive effects. Combinations of dissimilar agents tend to show potentiation, but the rule is not always followed. For example, mivacurium and cisatracurium show synergism,[104] while vecuronium and atracurium show very little, if any. The first such synergism was demonstrated for pancuronium–metocurine combinations, and the mixture has less cardiovascular effects than either drug alone for the same neuromuscular block.[64] The use of combinations may be recommended to reduce cost, and this might be advocated for cisatracurium–rocuronium mixtures, which show synergism. Another reason to use mixtures of drugs is to take advantage of the properties of two drugs. For example, synergism occurs between mivacurium and rocuronium, and the mixture retains the fast onset of rocuronium, while having the short duration of action of mivacurium.[105]

The mechanism by which two drugs produce a greater effect than either one alone is unknown, except in rare cases. For example, synergism is expected between mivacurium and pancuronium, because of the inhibition of plasma cholinesterase that pancuronium produces, thus accentuating the effect of mivacurium. However, such a simple mechanism is absent in most cases. Administration of a combination of relaxants does not affect the degree of protein binding of either drug. Surprisingly, when drug mixtures are applied to receptors in vitro, no potentiation is observed.[106] Perhaps the interaction occurs via presynaptic receptors or some other, unknown, mechanism.

Interactions of a different nature occur when administration of a nondepolarizing agent is followed by injection of another nondepolarizing agent. Usually, the duration of action of the second agent is that of the first drug given. For example, if mivacurium, a short-acting agent, is given after mivacurium, it has a duration of action of 12 minutes. However, if the same dose of mivacurium, 0.05 mg/kg, is given after rocuronium, its duration of action is prolonged to 42 minutes.[107] On the contrary, if mivacurium is the first drug, rocuronium has a short duration of action. Thus, switching from a long- or intermediate-duration agent to a shorter duration drug to obtain paralysis of short duration at the end of a case will not provide paralysis of short duration. The reason why the characteristics of the first agent given are determinant is that the size of the loading dose is greater than that of the maintenance dose, so that even when the second dose is given, the majority of receptors is still occupied by the first drug.

Nondepolarizing–Depolarizing Interactions

Depolarizing and nondepolarizing relaxants are mutually antagonistic. When *d*-tubocurarine or other nondepolarizing agents are given before succinylcholine to prevent fasciculations and muscle pain, the succinylcholine is less potent and has a shorter duration of action.[24] The exception is with pancuronium, because it inhibits plasma cholinesterase. Mixtures of succinylcholine with mivacurium or atracurium demonstrate antagonism.[108] However, nondepolarizing drugs are somewhat more effective when administered after the effect of succinylcholine has worn off, compared with no prior succinylcholine. Finally, the response to a small dose of succinylcholine at the end of an anesthetic in which a nondepolarizing agent has been used is difficult to predict. It may either antagonize or potentiate the blockade, depending on the degree of nondepolarizing block. Antagonism is more likely if blockade is deep and potentiation if blockade is shallow. If an anticholinesterase agent has been given, then the effect of the succinylcholine is potentiated because of inhibition of plasma cholinesterase.

Antibiotics

Neomycin and streptomycin are the most potent of the aminoglycosides in depressing neuromuscular function.[109] The polymixins also depress neuromuscular transmission.[109] These antibiotics are not used frequently any more. Other aminoglycosides (e.g., gentamicin, netilmicin, tobramycin) also potentiate nondepolarizing neuromuscular blockade. They prolong the action of steroidal neuromuscular agents, but their effect on benzylisoquinoline compounds is less apparent.[110] The lincosamines clindamycin and lincomycin have prejunctional and postjunctional effects, but prolongation of blockade by clindamycin is unlikely to occur clinically unless large doses are used.[111] The penicillins, cephalosporins, tetracyclines, and erythromycin are devoid of neuromuscular effects at clinically relevant doses.[111] Metronidazole does not appear to have clinically significant effects at the neuromuscular junction.

Anticonvulsants

Acute administration of phenytoin produces augmentation of neuromuscular block.[112] Resistance to pancuronium, metocurine, vecuronium, and rocuronium, but not to atracurium or mivacurium, has been demonstrated in patients receiving chronic anticonvulsant therapy with carbamazepine or phenytoin.[113,114] A least part of the phenomenon has a pharmacokinetic origin. In patients with chronic carbamazepine therapy, the clearance of vecuronium was found to be increased and its terminal half-life decreased.[114]

Cardiovascular Drugs

Beta-blocking drugs and calcium channel antagonists have been found to have neuromuscular effects in vitro, but in practice, the duration of action of neuromuscular blocking agents is not altered in patients taking these drugs chronically.[115] Ephedrine given at induction of anesthesia has been found to accelerate onset of action of rocuronium while esmolol prolongs onset time.[116] The mechanism for this effect is probably by alteration of drug delivery to the site of action by changes in cardiac output. The acceleration of onset by ephedrine has not been found in all studies.

Miscellaneous

Metoclopramide inhibits plasma cholinesterase and thus prolongs the action of succinylcholine and mivacurium. Inconsistent interactions have been described for diuretics, digoxin, and corticosteroids, probably because these drugs induce chronic fluid and electrolyte shifts, the magnitude of which depends on the condition being treated. Magnesium at doses used for antiarrhythmic treatment or preeclampsia has profound potentiation effects on depolarizing and nondepolarizing blockade.[117]

ALTERED RESPONSES TO NEUROMUSCULAR BLOCKING AGENTS

Intensive Care Unit

Neuromuscular blocking agents are useful in the ICU to facilitate mechanical ventilation. It is essential to provide sedation to patients who receive paralyzing agents, to prevent discomfort associated with the inability to move. Enthusiasm for the liberal use of neuromuscular blocking agents in the ICU has waned considerably over the past decade or so, because of several reports of critically ill patients who demonstrated residual weakness for unexpectedly long periods after discontinuation of a neuromuscular blocking agent. In some, recovery took several months. Pancuronium and vecuronium have been used most frequently, but recent descriptions of similar syndromes after atracurium and cisatracurium[118] suggest that the frequency of reports of weakness reflects the popularity of the drugs rather than a particular association with steroid-based compounds. Electromyographic (EMG) studies have shown variable lesions from myopathy to axonal degeneration of motor and sensory fibers. The picture is complicated by the syndrome of "critical illness neuropathy," which occurs in patients with sepsis and multiorgan failure, even in individuals not given neuromuscular blocking agents. Administration of corticosteroids is also considered a risk factor.[119] Symptoms include failure to wean from mechanical ventilation, limb weakness, and impaired deep tendon reflexes, but sensory function is usually not affected. There are no controlled clinical studies to allow the several initiating factors to be identified and matched with particular syndromes. In the absence of more definitive studies, it is recommended to administer neuromuscular blocking agents only to patients who cannot be managed otherwise, to limit the duration of administration to a few days or less, and to use only the dose that is necessary.[120]

Studies in ICU patients in whom the administration of relaxant was adjusted according to strict neuromuscular monitoring criteria have shown considerable variation in the requirement for neuromuscular blocking agent to maintain the same effect among patients and a wide within-patient pharmacokinetic variability.[121,122] Vecuronium and rocuronium have been associated with prolonged recovery times. For example, a mean of 3 hours was found between the end of rocuronium infusion and a train-of-four ratio of 0.7.[122] With cisatracurium, this interval was shorter (approximately 1 hour) and less variable.[121] Drug requirement is variable from patient to patient, is usually greater than in the operating room, and tends to increase with time. These reports suggest the need for more careful monitoring of neuromuscular block in ICU patients, although the optimal method and level of block to be achieved are uncertain. It is suggested to titrate neuromuscular blocking agents to the minimum infusion rate that will optimize oxygenation.

Myasthenia Gravis

Myasthenia gravis is an autoimmune disease in which circulating antibodies produce a functional reduction in the number of acetylcholine receptors.[10,16] The lesion is postsynaptic: the number of acetylcholine quanta is normal and their content is either normal or increased.

Diagnosis and Management

The hallmark of myasthenia gravis is fatigue. Presentation is extremely varied, but typically, ocular symptoms, such as diplopia and ptosis, occur first. Bulbar involvement is usually seen next. Patients may go on to have extremity weakness and respiratory difficulties.[10] The characteristic EMG finding in myasthenia gravis is a voltage decrement to repeated stimulation at 2 to 5 Hz. This finding is also characteristic of nondepolarizing blockade in nonmyasthenic individuals. Edrophonium, 2 to 8 mg, produces brief recovery from myasthenia gravis and can be used as a diagnostic test. Finally, up to 80% of patients have an increased titer of the acetylcholine receptor antibody.[10]

Treatment is largely symptomatic. Anticholinesterase agents such as pyridostigmine are used to increase neurotransmission at the neuromuscular junction. Corticosteroids and immunotherapy, with azathioprine, might produce long-term improvement. Plasmapharesis might be effective by eliminating the circulating antibody. Finally, many myasthenics have an associated thymoma, and surgical removal of the thymus may be indicated.[10]

Response to Neuromuscular Blocking Agents

Patients with myasthenia gravis are usually resistant to succinylcholine, with larger than usual doses required to produce complete blockade. This effect might be offset by the inhibition of plasma cholinesterase activity provided by pyridostigmine. Sensitivity to nondepolarizing neuromuscular blocking drugs is increased to a variable extent, depending on the severity of the disease. The ED_{95} of vecuronium was found to be decreased by more than half in myasthenic patients, and the response of the orbicularis oculi is depressed even more than that of the adductor pollicis, reflecting some degree of ocular involvement.[123]

Management of Anesthesia

Traditionally, neuromuscular blocking drugs have been avoided in the patient with myasthenia gravis by the use of inhalational vapors with or without local anesthesia. More recently, there have been several reports of the successful use of small, titrated doses of atracurium, mivacurium, vecuronium, or rocuronium, administered under careful neuromuscular monitoring. Mivacurium might have a prolonged duration in myasthenic patients, especially those who have been treated with an anticholinesterase agent preoperatively, as plasma cholinesterase is inhibited by pyridostigmine. In addition, the effect of reversal drugs might be less than expected because myasthenic patients already receive drugs that produce cholinesterase inhibition. Thus, it is preferable to continue mechanical ventilation until spontaneous recovery is manifest.

Two problems remain after thymectomy: postoperative anticholinesterase therapy and predicting the need for mechanical support of ventilation. In most patients, the dose of anticholinesterases is reduced for 1 to 2 days after surgery. The need for mechanical ventilation of the lungs usually correlates with preoperative lung function tests.

Myotonia

Myotonia is characterized by an abnormal delay in muscle relaxation after contraction. Several forms have been described: myotonic dystrophy (dystrophia myotonica, myotonia atrophica, Steinert's disease), myotonia congenita (Thomsen's disease), hyperkalemic periodic paralysis, and paramyotonia congenita.

Diagnosis

Repeated nerve stimulation leads to a gradual but persistent increase in muscle tension. The EMG is pathognomonic; myotonic after-discharges are seen in peripheral muscle, consisting of rapid bursts of potential produced by tapping the muscle or moving the needle. They produce typical "dive-bomber" sounds on the loudspeaker.

Response to Neuromuscular Blocking Agents

The characteristic response to succinylcholine is a sustained, dose-related contracture that may make ventilation difficult for several minutes. Muscle membrane fragility may be responsible for the exaggerated hyperkalemia that is produced after succinylcholine.[38] Most case reports suggest that the response to nondepolarizing drugs is normal. However, myotonic responses have been observed after reversal with neostigmine.

Anesthesia

Succinylcholine is best avoided. Short- or intermediate-duration nondepolarizing agents may be used in usual doses with careful neuromuscular monitoring. Reversal agents are best avoided.

Muscular Dystrophy

The muscular dystrophies are a group of many diseases, with variability in presentation and typical age at onset of symptoms. The most common of these is the Duchenne-type muscular dystrophy (DMD), an X-linked hereditary disease that usually becomes apparent in childhood. Other types of muscular dystrophy include Becker, limb-girdle, fasciohumeral, Emery-Dreifuss, nemaline rod, and oculopharyngeal dystrophy. There have been several reports of cardiac arrest after administration of succinylcholine in children, often associated with hyperkalemia. Resuscitation was found to be difficult, and several of these cases were fatal.[38] The most likely explanation for these adverse events is previously undiagnosed, latent, muscular dystrophy. In 1993, the number of such reports encouraged Burroughs Wellcome, the manufacturer of Anectine (succinylcholine), to state that "succinylcholine [is] contraindicated in children and adolescents except when used for emergency tracheal intubation." After further discussion the recommendation was modified to a warning.

Response to Neuromuscular Blocking Agents

Most case reports describe a normal response to nondepolarizing agents, such as vecuronium, atracurium, and mivacurium, although there have been sporadic instances of increased sensitivity. There are little data on the response to anticholinesterases. There is considerable controversy over whether DMD patients are susceptible to malignant hyperthermia (MH).

Anesthesia

Succinylcholine should be avoided in patients with muscular dystrophy, especially if onset of symptoms occurred in childhood or adolescence. The possibility of latent or unrecognized DMD in young males (less than 10 years old) may be a reason to avoid succinylcholine in this patient population. Careful titration of short- or intermediate-duration nondepolarizing agents should be done. Reversal agents do not appear to be contraindicated.

Upper Motor Neuron Lesions

Patients with hemiplegia or quadriplegia as a result of central nervous system lesions show an abnormal response to both depolarizing and nondepolarizing agents. Hyperkalemia and cardiac arrest have been described after succinylcholine, probably as a result of extrajunctional receptor spread. Hyperkalemia is typically seen if the drug is given between from 1 week to 6 months after the lesion, but may be seen before and after that time period.[38] There is resistance to nondepolarizing neuromuscular blocking drugs below the level of the lesion. In hemiplegic patients, monitoring of the affected side shows that the block is less intense and recovery is more rapid than on the unaffected side. However, the apparently normal side also demonstrates some resistance to nondepolarizing drugs.

Similar findings have been reported after a stroke, with a greater resistance on the affected side.

Burns

As a result of the proliferation of extrajunctional receptors, succinylcholine produces severe hyperkalemia in patients with burns, and this may lead to cardiac arrest. The magnitude of the problem depends on the extent of the injury. It may appear as early as 24 to 48 hours after the burn injury and usually ends with healing.[38] Resistance to the effects of nondepolarizing neuromuscular blocking agents is manifest, even in muscles that are apparently not affected by the burn.[51,52] Mivacurium requirements may be decreased in burn patients, because of the lower plasma cholinesterase activity.[124]

Miscellaneous

Denervated muscle demonstrates potassium release after succinylcholine and resistance to nondepolarizing relaxants. Contractures in response to succinylcholine have also been observed in amyotrophic lateral sclerosis and multiple sclerosis. Succinylcholine is usually avoided in several neurologic diseases, including Friedrich's ataxia, polyneuritis, and Parkinson's disease, because of isolated reports of hyperkalemia.

MONITORING NEUROMUSCULAR BLOCKADE

Why Monitor?

Deep levels of paralysis are usually desired during anesthesia to facilitate tracheal intubation and to obtain an immobile surgical field. However, complete return of respiratory function must be attained before the trachea is extubated. Administration of neuromuscular blocking drug must be individualized because blockade occurs over a narrow range of receptor occupancy,[18] and because there is considerable interindividual variability in response. Thus, it is important for the clinician to assess the effect of neuromuscular blocking drugs without the confounding influence of volatile agents, intravenous anesthetics, and opioids. To test the function of the neuromuscular junction, a peripheral nerve is stimulated electrically, and the response of the muscle is assessed.

Stimulator Characteristics

The response of the nerve to electrical stimulation depends on three factors: the current applied, the duration of the current, and the position of the electrodes. Stimulators should deliver a maximum current in the range of 60 to 80 mA. Most stimulators available for clinical use are designed to provide constant current, irrespective of impedance changes because of drying of the electrode gel, cooling, decreased sweat gland function, and so forth. However, this constant current feature does not hold for high impedances (>5 kΩ). Thus, electrodes should be firmly applied to the skin. A current display monitor on the stimulator is an asset, because accidental disconnection can be identified easily by a current approaching 0 mA. The duration of the current pulse should be long enough for all axons in the nerve to depolarize but short enough to avoid the possibility of exceeding the refractory period of the nerve. In practice, pulse durations of 0.1 to 0.2 msec are acceptable. At least one electrode should be on the skin overlying the nerve to be stimulated. If the negative electrode is used for this purpose, the threshold to supramaximal stimulation is less than for the positive electrode.[13] However, the difference is not large in practice. The position of the other electrode is not critical, but it should not be placed in the vicinity of other nerves. There is no need to use needle electrodes. Silver–silver chloride surface electrodes, used to monitor the electrocardiogram, are adequate for peripheral nerve stimulation, without the risk of bleeding, infection, and burns. In practice, applying these electrodes along the course of a nerve gives the best results (Fig. 16-12).

Monitoring Modalities

Different stimulation modalities were introduced into clinical practice to take advantage of the characteristic features of nondepolarizing neuromuscular blockade: fade and posttetanic facilitation with high-frequency stimulation. Thus, the following discussion refers mostly to nondepolarizing block.

Single Twitch

The simplest way to stimulate a nerve is to apply a single stimulus, at intervals of >10 seconds. The amplitude of

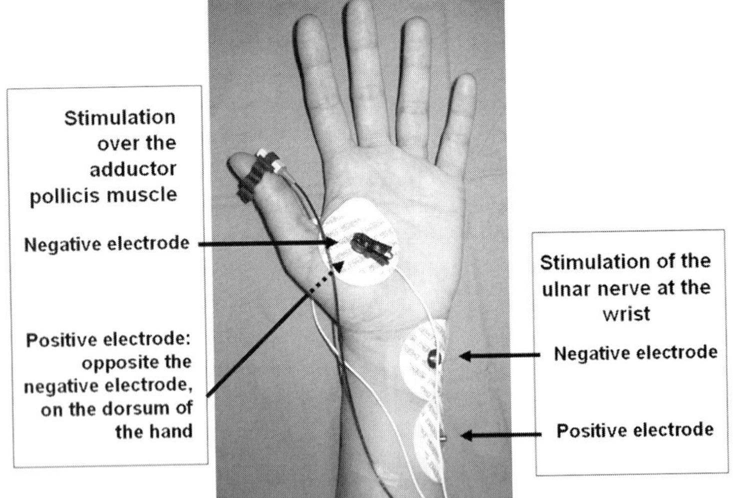

FIGURE 16-12. Electrode placement to obtain contraction of the adductor pollicis muscle. The traditional method is to stick the electrodes over the course of the ulnar nerve at the wrist, with the negative electrode distal (*right*). An alternate method is to position the electrodes over the adductor pollicis (*left*), the negative electrode on the palm of the hand, the positive in the same location, but on the dorsum of the hand. The device fixed to the thumb is an accelerometer.

response is compared with a control, preblockade twitch height. The single-twitch modality is useful to construct dose-response curves and to evaluate onset time. However, because a control value is required, the clinical usefulness of this mode of stimulation is limited.

Tetanus

When stimulation is applied at a frequency of ≥30 Hz, the mechanical response of the muscle is fusion of individual twitch responses. In the absence of neuromuscular blocking drugs, no fade is present and the response is sustained. During nondepolarizing blockade, the mechanical response appears as a peak, followed by a fade (see Fig. 16-9). The sensitivity of tetanic stimulation in the detection of residual neuromuscular blockade is greater than that of single twitch, that is, tetanic fade might be present while twitch height is normal. Most nerve stimulators provide a 5-second train at a frequency of 50 Hz. This frequency was adopted because at >100 Hz, some fade may be seen even in the absence of neuromuscular blocking drugs. However, more fade is seen with 100-Hz than 50-Hz frequencies, and 100-Hz, 5-second trains are most useful in the detection of residual block.[46] With tetanic stimulation, no control prerelaxant response is required, as the degree of muscle paralysis can be assessed by the degree of fade following tetanic stimulation. However, the main disadvantage of this mode of stimulation is posttetanic facilitation (see Fig. 16-9), the extent of which depends on the frequency and duration of the tetanic stimulation. For a 50-Hz tetanus applied for 5 seconds, the duration of this interval appears to be at least 1 to 2 minutes.[125] If single-twitch stimulation is performed during that time, the response is spuriously exaggerated.

Train-of-Four

With 2-Hz stimulation, the mechanical or electrical response decreases little after the fourth stimulus, and the degree of fade is similar to that found at 50 Hz.[45] Thus, applying train-of-four stimulation at 2 Hz provides more sensitivity than single twitch and approximately the same sensitivity as tetanic stimulation at 50 Hz. In addition, this relatively low frequency allows the response to be evaluated manually or visually. Moreover, the presence of a small number of impulses (4) eliminates the problem of posttetanic facilitation. Train-of-four stimulation can be repeated every 12 to 15 seconds. There is a fairly close relationship between single-twitch depression and train-of-four response, and no control is required for the latter.[126] During recovery, the second twitch reappears at 80 to 90% single-twitch block, the third at 70 to 80%, and when blockade is 65 to 75%, all four twitches become visible.[127] Then, the train-of-four ratio, the height of the fourth twitch to that of the first twitch, is linearly related to first twitch height when blockade is <70%. When single-twitch height has recovered to 100%, the train-of-four ratio is ~70%.

Posttetanic Count

During profound neuromuscular blockade, there is no response to single-twitch, tetanic, or train-of-four stimulation. To estimate the time required before the return of a response, one may use a technique that depends on the principle of posttetanic facilitation. A 50-Hz tetanus is applied for 5 seconds, followed by a 3-second pause and by stimulation at 1 Hz. The train-of-four and tetanic responses are undetectable, but facilitation produces a certain number of visible posttetanic twitches (Fig. 16-13). The number of visible twitches correlates inversely with the time required for a return of single-twitch or train-of-four responses.[128] For intermediate-duration drugs, the time from a posttetanic count of 1 to reappareance of twitch is 10 to 20 minutes.

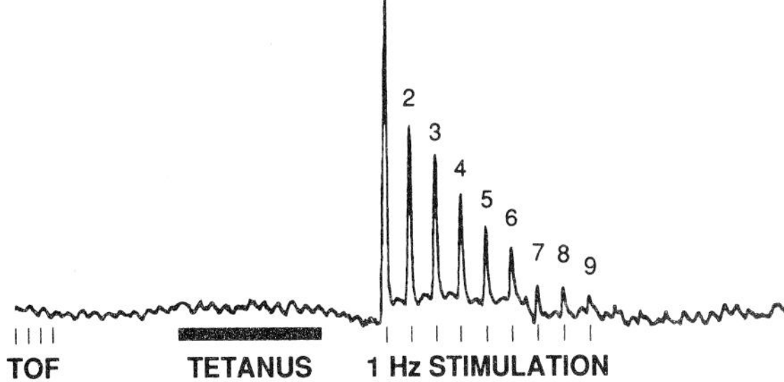

FIGURE 16-13. Posttetanic count (PTC). During profound blockade, no response is seen to train-of-four (TOF) or tetanus. However, because there is posttetanic facilitation, some twitches (in the case earlier, 9) can be seen after tetanic stimulation. In the example above, the PTC is 9.

Double-Burst Stimulation

Train-of-four fade may be difficult to evaluate by visual or tactile means during recovery from neuromuscular blockade. Irrespective of experience, it is difficult for anesthesiologists to detect train-of-four fade when actual train-of-four ratio is 0.4 or greater, meaning that residual paralysis can go undetected.[129] This shortcoming can be overcome, to a certain extent, by applying two short tetanic stimulations (three impulses at 50 Hz, separated by 750 msec), and by evaluating the ratio of the second to the first response. The double-burst stimulation ratio correlates closely with the train-of-four ratio, but is easier to detect manually.[129] At least 12 to 15 seconds must elapse between two consecutive double-burst stimulations.

Recording the Response

Visual and Tactile Evaluation

5 When electrical stimulation is applied to a nerve, the easiest and least expensive way to assess the response is to observe or feel the response of the muscle. This method is easily adaptable to any superficial muscle. However, serious errors in assessment can be made. In the case of evaluating the response of the adductor pollicis to ulnar nerve stimulation, the train-of-four count can be made reliably during a surgical procedure,[127] but the quantitative assessment of train-of-four ratio is difficult to make during recovery. Several investigations suggest that train-of-four ratios as low as 0.3[129] can remain undetected. The detection rate for tetanic fade (50 Hz) is no better.[130] With double-burst stimulation, fade can be detected reliably up to train-of-four ratios in the range of 0.5 to 0.6.[129] With 100-Hz tetanic stimulation, fade might be detected at train-of-four ratios of 0.8 to 1.0[46] and may be seen in individuals with no neuromuscular block.

Measurement of Force

A force transducer can overcome the shortcomings of one's senses. If applied correctly, the device provides accurate and reliable responses, displayed as either a digital or an analog signal on a monitor. Force measurement can be measured after single-twitch, tetanus, train-of-four, double-burst, or posttetanic stimulation. However, the availability of tetanus and double-burst stimulation is superfluous if accurate recording of the train-of-four response can be made. Unfortunately, transducers are expensive, bulky, cumbersome, and can be applied to only one muscle, usually the adductor pollicis.

Electromyography

It is possible to measure the electrical instead of the mechanical response of the muscle. One electrode should be positioned over the neuromuscular junction, which is usually close to the midportion of the muscle, and the other near the insertion of the muscle. A third, neutral electrode can be located anywhere else. Theoretically, any superficial muscle can be used for EMG recordings. In practice, such recordings are limited to the hypothenar eminence, the first dorsal interosseous, and the adductor pollicis muscles, which are supplied by the ulnar nerve. Most EMG recording devices compute the area under the EMG curve during a specified time window (usually 3 to 18 msec) after the stimulus is applied.[131] This integrated EMG response is considered a better representation of the overall muscular activity than the measurement of peak response. There is usually good correlation between EMG and force of the adductor pollicis if the EMG signal is taken from the thenar eminence. The signal obtained from the hypothenar eminence is larger and less subject to movement artifacts, but it can underestimate the degree of paralysis when compared with the adductor pollicis.[132]

Accelerometry

According to Newton's law, acceleration is proportional to force if mass remains unchanged. The device is usually attached to the tip of the thumb (see Fig. 16-12) and a digital readout is obtained. The setup is sensitive to inadvertent displacement of the thumb and, in the absence of neuromuscular blocking drugs, train-of-four ratios >100% can be obtained.[133] In spite of these shortcomings, accelerometers have become increasingly popular because they are easy to use, are less cumbersome, can be used on muscles other than the adductor pollicis, and are relatively inexpensive. The use of accelerometry is helpful in the diagnosis of residual paralysis[134] and can reduce the incidence of the condition.[135]

Displacement

A variety of devices have been proposed that include a piezoelectric wafer that responds to motion or displacement. They are designed for the adductor pollicis. A thorough evaluation of these devices has not been made, but data indicate that there are slight, but clinically insignificant differences between the results such displacement trasnducers and mechanomyography provide.[136]

Phonomyography

A contracting muscle emits low frequency sounds. Train-of-four response and fade can be heard with a stethoscope placed over the adductor pollicis muscle. A quantitative response can be obtained with special microphones sensitive to frequencies (2 Hz) below the threshold of the human ear. An excellent correlation between phonomyography and force measurement has been found at several muscles, including the adductor pollicis and the corrugator supercilii.[84] At the time of writing, no commercial devices using phonomyography were available.

Choice of Muscle

Muscles do not respond in a uniform fashion to neuromuscular blocking drugs. After administration of a neuromuscular blocking agent, differences can be measured with respect to onset time, maximum blockade, and duration of action. It is not practical to monitor the muscles of physiological importance, for example, the abdominal muscles during surgery, or the respiratory and upper airway muscles postoperatively. A better approach is to choose a monitoring site that has a response similar to the muscle of interest. For example, monitoring the response of the facial nerve around the eye is a good indicator of intubating conditions, and the use of the adductor pollicis during recovery reflects upper airway muscle function. Another strategy is to stick to one monitoring site, such as the adductor pollicis, and interpret the information provided from knowledge of the different responses between muscles (Fig. 16-14).

Adductor Pollicis

The adductor pollicis is accessible during most surgical procedures. It is supplied by the ulnar nerve, which becomes superficial at the wrist where a negative electrode can be positioned. The positive electrode is applied a few centimeters proximally (see Fig. 16-12). The force of contraction of the adductor pollicis can be measured easily, and it has become a standard in research. After injection of a dose that produces less than 100% blockade, the time to maximal blockade is longer than in centrally located muscles.[137,138] The adductor pollicis is relatively sensitive to nondepolarizing neuromuscular blocking drugs, and during recovery it is blocked more than some respiratory muscles such as the diaphragm,[137] laryngeal adductors,[138] and abdominal muscles (see Fig. 16-14).[139] There

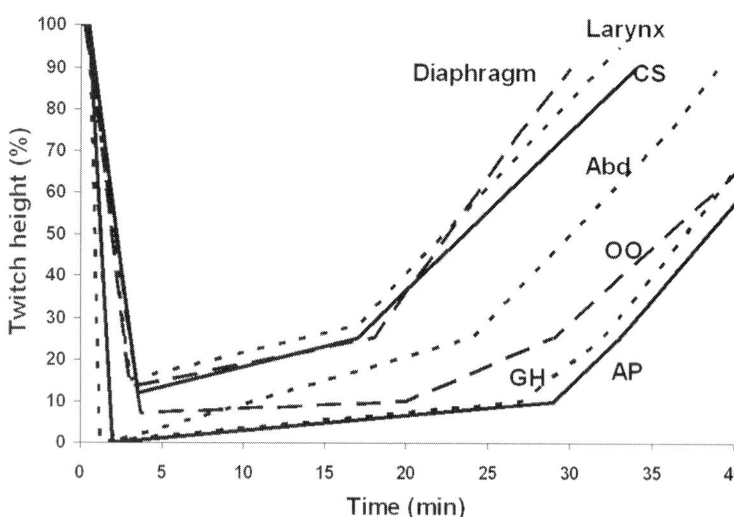

FIGURE 16-14. Approximate time course of twitch height after rocuronium, 0.6 mg/kg, at different muscles. Diaphragm: diaphragm; larynx: laryngeal adductors (vocal cords); CS: corrugator supercilii (eyebrow); abd: abdominal muscles; OO: orbicularis oculi (eyelid); GH: geniohyoid (upper airway); AP: adductor pollicis (thumb). The data are taken or inferred from Plaud et al,[142] Dhonneur et al,[166] Kirov et al,[139] and d'Honneur et al.[140]

is evidence that recovery of the adductor pollicis and of upper airway muscles occurs more or less simultaneously (see Fig. 16-14).[140]

The adductor pollicis can also be stimulated by applying electrodes directly over it. This can be accomplished by placing the two electrodes in the space lying between the base of the first and second metacarpals, on the palmar and dorsal aspects on the hand, respectively (see Fig. 16-12). Such a stimulation avoids the confounding movement of hypothenar muscles. Direct muscle stimulation with this electrode position does not normally occur, because neuromuscular blocking agents abolish the response completely.[141]

Other Muscles of the Hand

Ulnar nerve stimulation also produces flexion and abduction of the fifth finger, which usually recovers before the adductor pollicis, the discrepancy in first twitch or train-of-four ratio being of the order of 15 to 20%.[132] Relying on the response of the fifth finger might overestimate recovery from blockade. Abduction of the index finger also results from stimulation of the ulnar nerve because of contraction of the first dorsal interosseous, the sensitivity of which is comparable to that of the adductor pollicis. The hypothenar eminence (near the fifth finger) and the first dorsal interosseous are particularly well suited for EMG recordings.[132] Stimulation in the hand (see Fig 16-12) eliminates contraction of the hypothenar muscles, but may evoke movement of the first dorsal interosseous.

Muscles Surrounding the Eye

There seem to be major differences in the response of muscles innervated by the facial nerve and located around the eye, and these differences have introduced some confusion in the literature. The orbicularis oculi essentially covers the eyelid, and its response to neuromuscular blocking agents is similar to that of the adductor pollicis.[142] However, it is customary to observe the movement of the eyebrow, and recordings at that site are similar to that of the laryngeal adductors (see Fig 16-14).[142] Onset of blockade is more rapid and recovery occurs sooner than at the adductor pollicis. Thus, facial nerve stimulation with inspection of the response of the eyebrow (which most likely represents the effect of the corrugator supercilii, not the orbicularis oculi) is indicated to predict intubating conditions and to monitor profound blockade. The facial nerve can be stimulated 2 to 3 cm posterior to the lateral border of the orbit. There is no need to use stimulating currents greater than 20 to 30 mA.

Muscles of the Foot

The posterior tibial nerve can be stimulated behind the internal malleolus to produce flexion of the big toe by contraction of the flexor hallucis. The response of this muscle is comparable to that of the adductor pollicis. Stimulation of the external peroneal nerve produces dorsiflexion, but the sensitivity of the muscles involved has not been measured.

Clinical Applications

Monitoring Onset

The quality of intubating conditions depends chiefly on the state of relaxation of muscles of the jaw, pharynx, larynx, and respiratory system. Onset of action is faster in all these muscles than in the hand or foot because they are closer to the central circulation and they receive a greater blood flow. Among these central muscles, the diaphragm and especially the laryngeal adductors are the most resistant to nondepolarizing agents. Data on laryngeal muscles are important not only because easy passage of the tracheal tube can be performed if vocal cords are relaxed, but also because all other muscles can be presumed to be blocked if the resistant laryngeal muscles are blocked. The relationship between onset time in laryngeal and hand muscles depends on dose. At relatively low doses (e.g., rocuronium, 0.3 to 0.4 mg/kg), onset time is slower at the adductor pollicis than at the laryngeal muscles. If the dose is increased (e.g., rocuronium, 0.6 to 1.0 mg/kg), onset is faster at the adductor pollicis because these doses produce 100% blockade at the adductor pollicis without blocking laryngeal muscles completely (see Fig. 16-14).[143] Onset time decreases considerably in any muscle if the dose given is sufficient to reach 100%. Finally, if the dose is large enough to block the laryngeal muscles completely, onset time again becomes shorter at the larynx. It is not surprising that monitoring the adductor pollicis muscle predicts intubating conditions poorly. Facial nerve stimulation with visual observation of the response over the eyebrow gives better results because the response of the corrugator supercilii is close to that of the vocal cords. Train-of-four fade takes longer to develop than single-twitch depression (see Fig. 16-9), and during onset, train-of-four stimulation does not have any advantages over single-twitch stimulation at 0.1 Hz.

Monitoring Surgical Relaxation

Adequate surgical relaxation is usually obtained when fewer than two or three visible twitches are observed at the adductor pollicis. However, this criterion might prove inadequate in certain circumstances when profound relaxation is required owing to the discrepancy between the adductor pollicis and other muscles. In this case, the posttetanic count can be used at the adductor pollicis,[128] provided that this type of stimulation is not repeated more often than every 2 to 3 minutes. A suitable alternative is stimulation of the facial nerve with observation of the response over the eyebrow, which recovers at the same rate as such resistant muscles as the diaphragm.[137,142]

Monitoring Recovery

Complete return of neuromuscular function should be achieved at the conclusion of surgery unless mechanical ventilation is planned. Thus, monitoring is useful in determining whether spontaneous recovery has progressed to a degree that allows reversal agents to be given and to assess the effect of these agents.

The effectiveness of anticholinesterase agents depends directly on the degree of recovery present when they are administered. Preferably, reversal agents should be given only when four twitches are visible,[144] which corresponds to a first-twitch recovery of >25%. For this assessment, using the adductor pollicis is preferable. The presence of spontaneous respiration is not a sign of adequate neuromuscular recovery. The diaphragm recovers earlier than the much more sensitive upper airway muscles, such as the geniohyoid, which recovers, on average, at the same time as the adductor pollicis.[140] To prevent upper airway obstruction after extubation, it is preferable to use the adductor pollicis to monitor recovery, instead of the more resistant muscles of the hypothenar eminence or those around the eye.

Finally, the adequacy of recovery should be assessed. Traditionally, a train-of-four ratio of 0.7 was considered to be the threshold below which residual weakness of the respiratory muscles could be present. There is abundant evidence that significant weakness may occur up to train-of-four values of 0.9. Awake volunteers given mivacurium failed to perform the head-lift test when the train-of-four ratio at the adductor pollicis decreased below 0.62, but needed a train-of-four ratio of

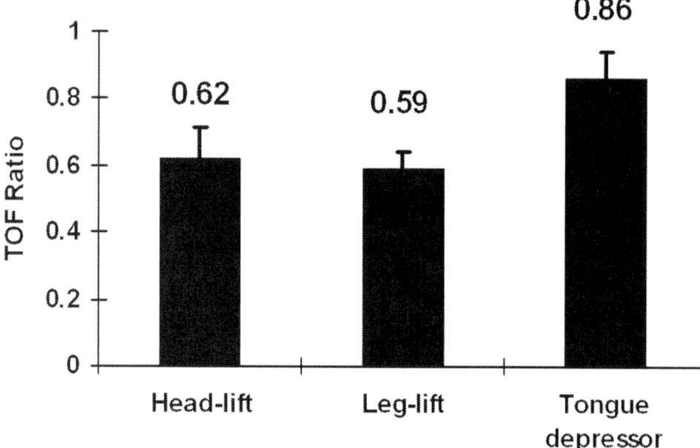

FIGURE 16-15. Correlation between train-of-four responses at the adductor pollicis and certain clinical tests of neuromuscular recovery. Volunteers were given mivacurium and were asked to lift their head for 5 seconds (head lift), lift their leg for 5 seconds (leg lift), or hold a tongue depressor between their teeth against force (tongue depressor). The minimum train-of-four ratio (and SD) when each of these tests was passed is indicated. Data from Kopman et al.[145]

at least 0.86 to hold a tongue depressor between their teeth (Fig. 16-15).[145] This suggests that the head-lift test does not 6 guarantee full recovery, and that the upper airway muscles used to retain a tongue depressor are very sensitive to the residual effects of neuromuscular blocking drugs. Furthermore, impairment in swallowing and laryngeal aspiration of a pharyngeal fluid was observed at train-of-four ratios as high as 0.9 in volunteers given vecuronium (see Fig. 16-4).[146]

Anesthetized patients appear considerably more sensitive to the ventilatory effects of neuromuscular blocking drugs than are awake patients. Whereas tidal volume and end-tidal CO_2 are preserved in awake patients receiving relatively high doses of neuromuscular blocking drugs,[147] anesthetized adults have a decreased tidal volume and increased PCO_2 with doses of pancuronium as low as 0.5 mg.[148] In conscious volunteers, administration of small doses of vecuronium to maintain train-of-four at less than 0.9 leads to severe impairment of the ventilatory response to hypoxia (Fig. 16-16).[149] The response to hypercapnia is maintained, and this indicates that the response to hypoxia is not a result of respiratory muscle weakness.[149]

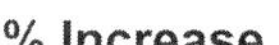

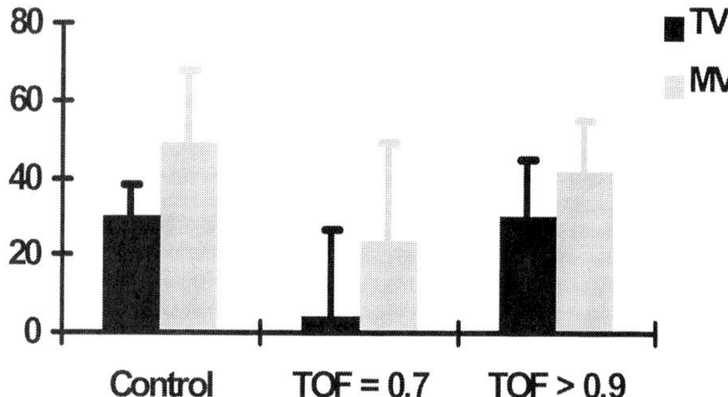

FIGURE 16-16. Response to hypoxia is impaired during recovery from vecuronium blockade. Normal response is an increase in minute volume (MV) or tidal volume (TV) (control). These increases are decreased significantly when vecuronium produces a train-of-four ratio of 0.7 at the adductor pollicis. They return to near normal values at a train-of-four ratio >0.9. Data from Eriksson et al.[149]

Taken together, the results of these investigations indicate that normal respiratory and upper airway function does not return to normal unless the train-of-four ratio at the adductor pollicis is 0.9 or more. However, it has become apparent that human senses fail to detect either a train-of-four or 50-Hz tetanic fade when the train-of-four ratio is as low as 0.3.[129,130] With double-burst stimulation, detection failures may occur at train-of-four ratios of 0.5 to 0.6.[129] Compared with the train-of-four, the ability to detect fade is not improved by using tetanic stimulation at 50 Hz for 5 seconds. However, in one study fade could be detected visually at train-of-four ratios of 0.8 to 0.9 by using 100-Hz tetanic stimulation.[46] It is unclear, however, whether fade induced by inhalational agents alone can be seen. Because of the presence of posttetanic facilitation, 50- or 100-Hz stimuli should not be applied more often than every 2 minutes. Because of the limitations of one's senses, it has been advocated that quantitative assessment of the train-of-four ratio be made routinely.[9] Mechanographic and EMG equipment give reliable values of train-of-four ratio, but the use of this equipment is limited by size, cost, and convenience. Accelerometers are less bulky and cheaper, but they can overestimate the value of train-of-four ratio during recovery.[133] It has been suggested that a train-of-four ratio of 1.0 obtained by accelerometry must be obtained before neuromuscular function can be considered complete.[150] Monitoring devices based on the measurement of displacement or sound may prove to have more reliable train-of-four ratios than accelerometry. In one study, a transmission module sensitive to bending and deformation was found to yield train-of-four ratio values comparable to mechanomyography during the recovery period.[136]

In response to the shortcomings of visual or tactile evaluations, another approach to recovery is to wait until sufficient spontaneous recovery is present and give reversal agents systematically. Kopman et al[151] suggested that neostigmine be given at a train-of-four count of 2 or greater if the neuromuscular blocking agent is cisatracurium or rocuronim. Complete recovery took longer than expected, as some patients still had train-of-four ratios less than 0.9 after 30 minutes. In any event, clinicians must be aware of the limitations of the tests they are using and complete their evaluations with clinical tests.

Factors Affecting the Monitoring of Neuromuscular Blockade

Many drugs interfere with neuromuscular function and these are dealt with elsewhere. However, certain situations make the interpretation of data on neuromuscular function difficult. Central hypothermia may slow the metabolism of neuromuscular blocking agents and prolong blockade. If the extremity where monitoring is performed is cold, the degree of block will be accentuated. Thus, if only the monitored hand is cold, without central hypothermia, the degree of paralysis will appear to be increased. Resistance to nondepolarizing neuromuscular blocking drugs occurs with nerve damage, including peripheral nerve trauma, cord transection, and stroke. In this case, monitoring of the involved limb would tend to underestimate the degree of muscle paralysis. The level of paralysis should also be adjusted for the type of patient, as well as the type of surgery. For example, it is not necessary to paralyze frail individuals or patients at the extremes of age to the same extent as young muscular adults. The same applies to patients with debilitating muscular diseases.

Neuromuscular monitoring by itself does not guarantee adequate relaxation during surgery and complete recovery postoperatively. The surgical field may be poor in spite of full paralysis of the hand, because of difference in response between muscles.

Residual paralysis might occur because of excess neuromuscular blocking agents given, early administration of reversal, or an abnormal response of the patient. The effect of the neuromuscular blocking drug is the same whether or not monitoring is used. Neuromuscular monitoring can help in the diagnosis of inadequate skeletal muscle relaxation during surgery or insufficient recovery after surgery, but does not, in itself, treat these conditions.

ANTAGONISM OF NEUROMUSCULAR BLOCK

In most circumstances, all efforts should be made to ensure that the patient leaves the operating room with unimpaired muscle strength. Specifically, respiratory and upper airway muscles must function normally, so the patient can breathe, cough, swallow secretions, and keep his or her airway patent. Two strategies can be adopted to achieve this goal. The first is to titrate neuromuscular blocking agents carefully, so that no residual effect is manifest at the end of surgery. The second is to accelerate recovery by giving a reversal drug. This second option is probably safer, but both strategies require careful assessment of blockade.

Assessment of Neuromuscular Blockade

Spontaneous breathing can resume even if relatively deep degrees of paralysis are still present. Spontaneous ventilation, adequate to prevent hypercapnia, can be maintained despite considerable measurable skeletal muscle weakness if a patent airway is ensured. The ability to perform maneuvers such as vital capacity, maximum voluntary ventilation, and forced expiratory flow rate recovers at less intense levels of paralysis because it requires a greater strength.[147] Such tests are, however, difficult to perform in everyday practice, particularly when the patient is recovering from general anesthesia. Moreover, the weakest point in the respiratory system is the upper airway. When given vecuronium, swallowing was impaired and laryngeal aspiration occurred when the TOF ratio was 0.9 or less.[146] These problems are difficult to diagnose when a tracheal tube is in place. Consequently, several indirect indices, which are easier to measure, have been correlated with the more specific tests of lung and upper airway function.

Clinical Evaluation

Several crude tests have been suggested, including head lift for 5 seconds, tongue protrusion, and the ability to lift the legs off the bed to determine recovery of neuromuscular function. Pavlin et al[147] correlated the maximum inspiratory pressure (MIP) with tests of skeletal muscle strength and of airway musculature in conscious volunteers receiving *d*-tubocurarine. As the dose was increased, head lift and leg raising were affected first. Then, the ability to swallow, touch teeth, and maintain a patent airway was impaired. Hand grip strength was decreased markedly by then. Nevertheless, as long as the mandible was elevated by an observer, the $PETCO_2$ was normal even when all the tests were failed. From these data, it was concluded that ability to maintain head lift for 5 seconds usually indicates sufficient strength to protect the airway and support ventilation.[147] However, Kopman et al have shown, in volunteers, that the most sensitive test is the ability to clamp the jaws shut and prevent removal of a wooden spatula.[145] This correlated with a TOF ratio measured at the adductor pollicis of >0.86, whereas head lift and leg lift could be performed at more intense levels of paralysis (TOF approximately 0.6) (see Fig. 16-15). All subjects complained of visual symptoms until TOF >0.9. Pressure measurements in the upper esophagus have been shown to be decreased (see Fig. 16-4) and laryngeal aspiration detected at a TOF ratio <0.9.[146,152] Thus, it appears that a normal head lift or leg lift is insufficient to guarantee normal upper airway function. The ability to resist removal of an object (such as a tongue depressor or a tracheal tube) from the mouth by closing the teeth probably correlates better with adequate upper airway function.

Evoked Responses to Nerve Stimulation

The clinical tests described above are usually unobtainable in the patient recovering from anesthesia. Furthermore, it is preferable to assess the degree of recovery before emergence. Evoked responses to nerve stimulation are then appropriate. The target is a TOF >0.9, considering that upper airway function does not recover completely until the train-of-four ratio at the adductor pollicis is at least 0.9. Even at that level, some subjects show some signs of weakness.[134]

With the introduction of short- and intermediate-duration nondepolarizing agents into clinical practice, the use of reversal agents has been considered by some as optional. The decision to omit pharmacological reversal of neuromuscular blockade must be made carefully, because the presence of residual paralysis may be missed. As mentioned earlier, manual and tactile evaluation of neuromuscular blockade by train-of-four or 50-Hz tetanic stimulation may fail to detect fade.[129,130] Double-burst stimulation is more sensitive, but becomes unreliable at train-of-four ratios in the 0.6 to 0.9.[129] The most sensitive test is the ability to maintain sustained contraction to 100-Hz tetanus for 5 seconds. Fade is detected when TOF ratio is as high as 0.8 to 0.9.[46] Tetanic stimulation at 100 Hz is painful and must be performed only in adequately anesthetized patients.

Because of the limitations of the visual and tactile estimate of the train-of-four response during recovery, objective measurement has been advocated.[9] Acceleromyographic recordings might be the most practical, because accelerometers are cheap and easy to use. However, it must be appreciated that the TOF ratio obtained with accelerometry is greater than that measured with mechanomyography and may exceed 1.0. An accelerographic TOF ratio of 1.0 has been proposed as the equivalent of a mechanomyographic TOF of 0.9.[150]

Residual Paralysis

7 Several studies have demonstrated that residual neuromuscular blockade is frequent in patients in the recovery room after surgery. Viby-Mogensen et al found in 72 adult patients given long-acting agents that the train-of-four ratio was 0.7 in 30 (42%) patients, and that 16 of the 68 patients (24%) who were awake were unable to sustain head lift for 5 seconds.[8] In that study, the patients received appropriate doses of neostigmine. Similar results have been obtained in Sweden, Australia, Canada, and the United States (see Table 16-1).[153] The incidence of train-of-four ratio 0.7 is reduced from about 30% to less than 10% if the intermediate agents atracurium or vecuronium are substituted for the long-acting drugs and if reversal is given.[153] Recovery from mivacurium is even more rapid. However, the actual incidence of residual paralysis was certainly underestimated in these studies because of the criterion used (train-of-four ratio of 0.7). Recently, there has been a trend for a greater incidence of residual paralysis, even with intermediate-duration drugs. This can be explained by two factors. The threshold for residual paralysis has been raised from a train-of-four ratio of 0.7 to 0.8 and then to 0.9.[134] However, the most important reason for high incidence of residual paralysis seems to be omission of reversal. In one study, this incidence was 42% after vecuronium, using the 0.7 criterion.[154]

Clinical Importance

Residual paralysis in the recovery room has been shown to be associated with significant morbidity. In 1997, Berg et al studied nearly 700 general surgical patients who randomly received pancuronium, vecuronium, or atracurium to produce surgical relaxation.[155] In patients who had received pancuronium, the incidence of postoperative partial paralysis, defined by a train-of-four ratio <0.7, was five times that in patients receiving either of the two intermediate-acting drugs (26 versus 5%). In addition, the incidence of atelectasis demonstrated on chest radiographs taken 2 days later was greater in patients who had received pancuronium and who had not attained a train-of-four ratio of 0.7 (16%) than in those who exceeded this threshold (4.8%).[155] Intense residual block has been demonstrated in patients after cardiac surgery, and choosing rocuronium over pancuronium has been associated with fewer symptoms of weakness and a shorter time to extubation.[156]

Reversal Agents

So far, the only compounds that have been widely used to reverse the effect of neuromuscular blocking agents are the anticholinesterase drugs. The pharmacologic principle involved is inhibition of acetylcholine breakdown to increase its concentration of acetylcholine at the neuromuscular junction, thus tilting the competition for receptors in favor of the neurotransmitter. Other drugs such as suramin and 3–4 aminopyridine are not as effective, or more toxic, or both. At the time of writing, a chelating agent, ORG25696, designed to rid the organism of rocuronium, was investigated for its ability to reverse neuromuscular blockade.

Anticholinesterases: Mechanism of Action

Neostigmine, edrophonium, and pyridostigmine inhibit acetylcholinesterase, but this may not be the only mechanism by which blockade is antagonized. This inhibition is present at all cholinergic synapses in the peripheral nervous system. Thus, the anticholinesterases have potent parasympathomimetic activity, which is attenuated or abolished by the administration of an antimuscarinic agent, atropine or glycopyrrolate. Neostigmine, edrophonium, and pyridostigmine are quaternary ammonium compounds, which do not penetrate the blood-brain barrier well. Thus, although these agents have the ability to affect cholinergic function in the central nervous system, the concentrations in the brain are usually too small for such an effect. Physostigmine is an anticholinesterase that can cross the blood-brain barrier easily. For this reason, it is not used to reverse neuromuscular blockade. Neostigmine injected intrathecally is a good analgesic, but produces nausea and vomiting.

Neostigmine and pyridostigmine are attached to the anionic and esteratic sites of the acetylcholinesterase molecule and produce longer lasting inhibition than edrophonium. Neostigmine and pyridostigmine are inactivated by the interaction with the enzyme, whereas edrophonium is unaffected.[153]

Inhibition of acetylcholinesterase results in an increased amount of acetylcholine reaching the receptor and in a longer time for acetylcholine to remain in the synaptic cleft. This causes an increase in the size and duration of the end plate potentials.[157] There is evidence that some of the effects of neostigmine are not the result of cholinesterase inhibition.[157] Anticholinesterases also have presynaptic effects. In the absence of neuromuscular blocking drugs, they potentiate the normal twitch response in a way similar to succinylcholine, probably as a result of the generation of action potentials that spread antidromically.[20] A ceiling effect, that is, the inability for large doses to produce an increasing effect, has been demonstrated in vitro.

Neostigmine Block

Large doses of anticholinesterases, greater than those used clinically, may produce neuromuscular blockade. Fade of both EMG and mechanical responses has been observed during tetanic stimulation after clinical doses of neostigmine but not edrophonium were given to reverse neuromuscular blockade.[158] Paradoxically, this neostigmine effect is antagonized with small doses of nondepolarizing blocking agents. The mechanism involved is uncertain. There are no clinical reports of postoperative weakness attributed to reversal agents, and this may be because all patients who received the anticholinesterase also had been given some neuromuscular blocking agent.

Potency

Dose-response curves have been constructed for edrophonium, neostigmine, and pyridostigmine. During a constant infusion of neuromuscular blocking drugs, the curves are obtained by plotting the peak effect versus the dose of reversal agent. In this situation, neostigmine was found to be approximately 12 times as potent as edrophonium.[159] However, the curves are not parallel, that of edrophonium being flatter. This indicates that edrophonium is effective over a narrower range of blockade and less effective against deep blockade. This was verified when neostigmine and edrophonium were used to reverse atracurium blockade. More neostigmine and edrophonium were required to reverse deep (99%) than moderate (90%) block, but the difference was greater for edrophonium.[160] There is no difference in the dose-response relationship of anticholinesterases if vecuronium is infused instead of pancuronium, but there is a marked shift to the left for the curves obtained during vecuronium block if the reversal agent is given during spontaneous recovery.[161] This indicates that anticholinesterase-assisted recovery is the sum of two components: (1) spontaneous recovery from the neuromuscular blocking agent itself, which depends on the pharmacokinetic characteristics of the drug, and (2) assisted recovery, which is a function of the dose and type of anticholinesterase agent given.

Pharmacokinetics

Following bolus iv injection, the plasma concentration of the anticholinesterases decreases rapidly during the first 5 to 10 minutes and then more slowly.[153] Volumes of distribution are in the range of 0.7 to 1.4 L/kg and the elimination half-life is 60 to 120 minutes. The drugs are water-soluble, ionized compounds so that their principal route of excretion is the kidney. Their clearances are in the range of 8 to 16 mL/kg/min, which is much greater than the GFR because they are actively secreted into the tubular lumen. Their clearance is reduced markedly in patients in renal failure.

Pharmacodynamics

The onset of action of edrophonium (1 to 2 minutes) to peak effect is much more rapid than that of neostigmine (7 to 11 minutes) or pyridostigmine (15 to 20 minutes) (Fig. 16-17).[159] The reason for the differences is uncertain, but may be related to the different rates of binding to the enzyme. The duration of action (1 to 2 hours) is similar to their elimination half-life. Even when used to reverse blockade produced by long-acting agents, duration of action of anticholinesterase agents is comparable to or most often exceeds that of the neuromuscular blocking drug. Well-documented recurarization has not been reported. In practice, cases of apparent reparalysis in the recovery room are incomplete reversal that was initially thought to be complete. Either manual or visual assessment is performed using the train-of-four or tetanus mode, which can yield to gross underevaluation of residual paralysis, or respiratory function

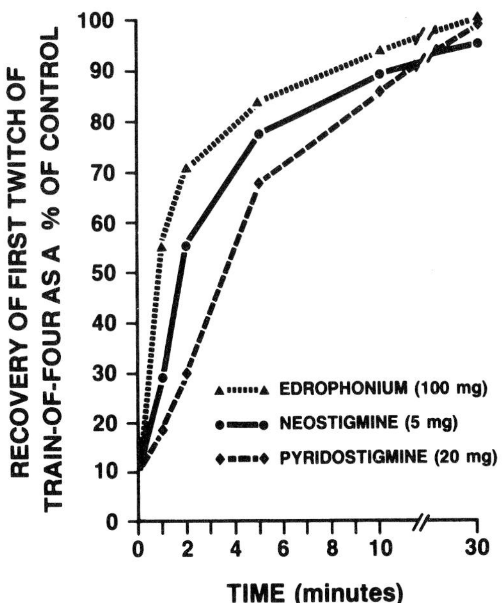

FIGURE 16-17. Reversal of pancuronium blockade at 10% twitch recovery. Reversal is given at time zero. Edrophonium is faster then neostigmine, which is faster than pyrodostigmine. Redrawn from Ferguson et al.[167]

appeared adequate when the tracheal tube was in place, but once extubated, the patient cannot maintain a patent airway.

Factors Affecting Reversal

Several factors modify the rate of recovery of neuromuscular activity after reversal.

Intensity of Block

The more intense the block at the time of reversal, the longer the recovery of neuromuscular activity (Fig. 16-18).[160] In addition, neostigmine is more effective than edrophonium or pyridostigmine in antagonizing intense (90%) blockade.[160] When reversal is administered after spontaneous recovery to $\geq$25% T_1 has occurred, recovery is rapid and the time from reversal to TOF 0.9 is usually only a few minutes, although recovery after pancuronium may not be complete.[79] Thus, it has been recommended that reversal should not be attempted until $T_1 \geq 25\%$
8 when four twitches to TOF stimulation are visible. Attempted reversal at only two twitches may take 30 minutes or more to reach TOF = 0.9.[151]

It is sometimes argued that reversal can be attempted earlier, for instance when there is only one or no twitch visible following train-of-four stimulation, because time has to be spent anyway waiting for all four twitches to reappear. Several studies dealt with the problem of total time between injection of the neuromuscular blocking agent until complete recovery, with the reversal agent given at different levels of spontaneous recovery. Bevan et al[162] administered large doses of neostigmine (0.07 mg/kg) after rocuronium and vecuronium and measured time until train-of-four ratio was 0.9. Neostigmine decreased the time to recovery, no matter when it was given. However, time from injection to full reversal was not less when neostigmine was given 5 minutes after rocuronium (42.1 minutes) than at 25% recovery (28.2 minutes) (Fig. 16-19).[162] In addition, giving the reversal agent too early leads to a period of "blind paralysis," because neostigmine-assisted recovery is characterized by an early, rapid phase, followed by slower recovery. As a result, the interval between a train-of-four ratio of 0.4 to 0.9, that is, the time when fade is difficult to detect, is likely to be much longer with early neostigmine administration. Thus, there is little advantage in attempting early reversal.

Dose

Over a certain dose range, the degree and rate of reversal depends directly on dose.[163] However, all anticholinesterase agents demonstrate a ceiling effect (see Fig. 16-18). Usually, there is no added benefit in giving doses exceeding 0.07 mg/kg neostigmine, or 1.0 mg/kg edrophonium.

Choice of Neuromuscular Blocking Agent

Recovery of neuromuscular activity after reversal is dependent on the rate of spontaneous recovery as well as the acceleration induced by the reversal agent. Consequently, the overall recovery of intermediate-acting agents (atracurium, vecuronium, mivacurium, rocuronium) following the same dose of anticholinesterase is more rapid and more complete than after pancuronium, *d*-tubocurarine, or gallamine.[79] This is probably why residual paralysis is more frequent with longer acting neuromuscular blocking agents. After prolonged infusions, recovery is slower than after intermittent bolus administration.[97] This is especially true of drugs that depend on redistribution for termination of action, such as rocuronium and vecuronium.

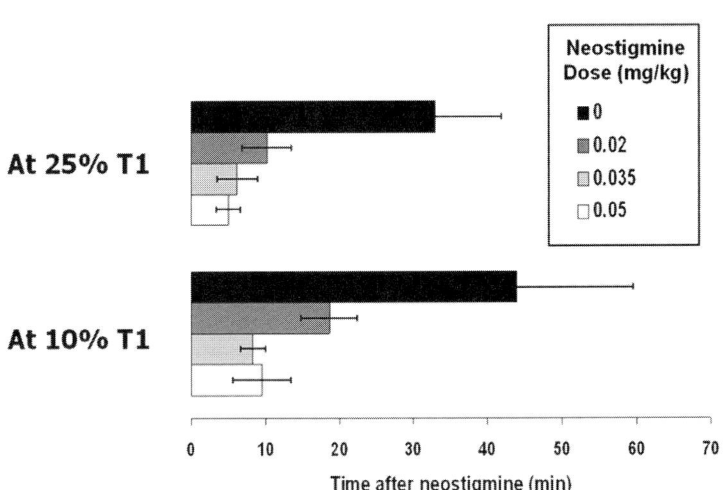

FIGURE 16-18. Neostigmine is more effective at greater degree of recovery from rocuronium blockade. Time to reach a train-of-four ratio of 0.8 after various doses of neostigmine. This time is less if neostigmine is given at 25% than at 10% first-twitch recovery. Notice a ceiling effect for neostigmine at doses greater than 0.035 mg/kg. A dose of 0 indicates no reversal given. Data from McCourt et al.[168]

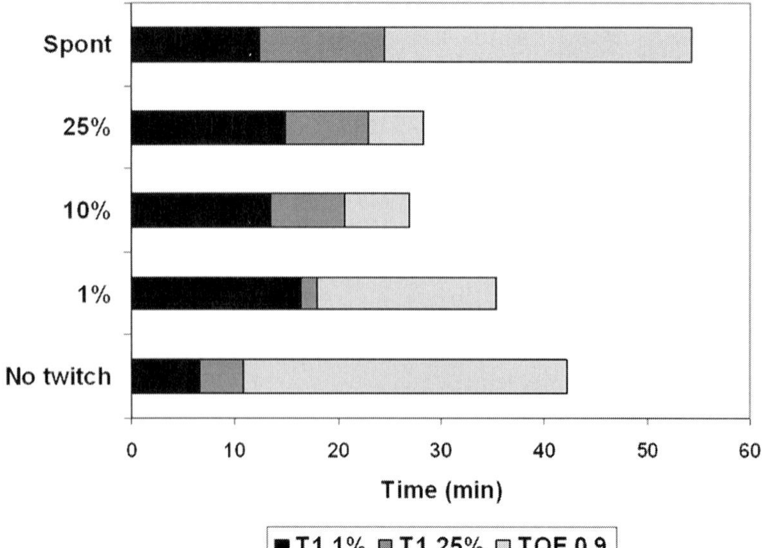

FIGURE 16-19. Time from injection of rocuronium until recovery to train-of-four ratio of 0.9 in adults. Reversal with neostigmine was either not given (spont), or given at 25, 10, or 1% twitch recovery, or given 5 minutes after rocuronium, when there was no twitch. Times from rocuronium injection to 1% first twitch, 25% first twitch and train-of-four ratio of 0.9 are indicated. Neostigmine was optimal when given at 10 to 25%. Giving it early had no advantage. Data from Bevan et al.[162]

Age

Recovery of neuromuscular activity occurs more rapidly with smaller doses of anticholinesterases in infants and children than in adults (Fig. 16-20).[162] Residual weakness in the recovery room is found less frequently in children than in adults. The effectiveness of reversal has not been studied extensively in the elderly. Although the elimination of anticholinesterases is reduced in this age group, this is counterbalanced by the tendency for neuromuscular blockade to wear off more slowly. This is especially true of steroid neuromuscular blocking agents, such as vecuronium and rocuronium, which have a slower recovery index in the elderly.

Drug Interactions

Drugs that potentiate neuromuscular blockade can slow reversal or produce recurarization if given after anticholinesterase administration. Halogenated agents, when continued after neostigmine administration, prolong time to full reversal. Even when they are discontinued at the time of anticholinesterase drug administration, reversal time is not reduced significantly, probably because wash out of the vapor from muscle tissue takes time. Care must be taken if aminoglycoside antibiotics or magnesium must be given shortly after reversal agents.[117]

Renal Failure

Anticholinesterases are actively secreted into the tubular lumen so that their clearance is reduced in renal failure.[153] Thus, duration of action of neostigmine and edrophonium is increased in renal failure, at least to a comparable extent as duration of action of the neuromuscular blocking agent. No cases of recurarization have been reported.

Anticholinesterases: Other Effects

Cardiovascular

Anticholinesterases provoke profound vagal stimulation. The time course of the vagal effects parallels the reversal of block: rapid for edrophonium and slower for neostigmine. However, the bradycardia and bradyarrhythmias can be prevented with anticholinergic agents. Atropine has a rapid onset of action (1 minute), duration of 30 to 60 minutes, and crosses the

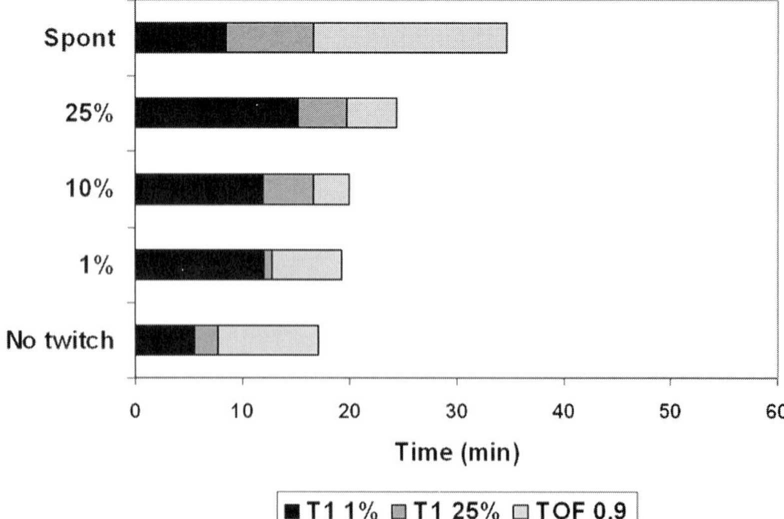

FIGURE 16-20. Same graph as in Figure 16-19, but in children 2 to 12 years old. Spontaneous recovery from rocuronium blockade is more rapid, as well as neostigmine-assisted recovery. Data from Bevan et al.[162]

blood-brain barrier. Its time course makes it appropriate for use in combination with edrophonium,[159] whereas glycopyrrolate (onset 2 to 3 minutes) is more suitable with neostigmine or pyridostigmine. Because glycopyrrolate does not cross the blood-brain barrier, it is believed that the incidence of memory deficits after anesthesia is less than that after atropine. If atropine is given with neostigmine, the dose is approximately half that of neostigmine (atropine 20 μg/kg for neostigmine 40 μg/kg). Such a combination leads to an initial tachycardia followed by a slight bradycardia. With glycopyrrolate, the dose is one-fourth to one-fifth that of neostigmine. Atropine requirements are less with edrophonium than with nesotigmine (atropine 7 to 10 μg/kg versus edrophonium 0.5 mg/kg).

Other Cholinergic Effects

Anticholinesterases produce increased salivation and bowel motility. Although atropine blocks the former, it appears to have little effect on peristalsis. Some reports claim an increase in bowel anastomotic leakage after the reversal of neuromuscular blockade. Others have held the use of anticholinesterases to be responsible for an increased incidence of vomiting after ambulatory surgery. In a recent meta-analysis, it was concluded that neostigmine (2.5 mg or more in adults) was associated with a higher incidence of nausea and vomiting than no reversal.[164] This conclusion is heavily affected by two studies showing a large effect, while all other studies showed no effect. The meta-analysis suggested that lower doses (1.5 mg or less) were not associated with a greater incidence of nausea and vomiting. Since then, two more studies failed to show any relationship between administration of neostigmine and an increased incidence of postoperative nausea and vomiting. This emetic effect has not been found for edrophonium. At any rate, possible nausea and vomiting is preferable to signs and symptoms of respiratory paralysis.

Respiratory Effects

Anticholinesterases may cause an increase in airway resistance, but anticholinergics reduce this effect. Several other factors, such as pain, the presence of an endotracheal tube, or light anesthesia, may predispose to bronchoconstriction at the end of surgery so that it is difficult to incriminate the reversal agents.

Clinical Use

Several reversal regimens have been proposed and are effective. In general, the more intense the block, the greater the dose of anticholinesterase that is required. However, there does not seem to be any advantage in giving more than the equivalent of neostigmine 0.07 mg/kg. Neostigmine is preferred to edrophonium for intense block, but the rapid action of edrophonium has the advantage of allowing the extent of reversal to be assessed in the operating room. Pyridostigmine has a slow onset of action, and does not appear to accelerate reversal of short- and intermediate-duration drugs to a great extent.

ORG 25969

A new method of reversing neuromuscular blockade has been advocated recently by the introduction of a cyclodextrin, ORG 25969, which, at the time of writing, was still in the investigational stage in humans.[165] The compound is made up of eight sugars arranged in a ring. It has a high affinity for rocuronium, with which it forms a complex, and the complex is excreted. ORG 25969 has less affinity for other steroidal neuromuscular blocking agents like vecuronium and pancuronium, and apparently no affinity for other endogenous steroidal compounds. It does not bind benzylisoquinoline-type neuromuscular blocking agents. The ability to produce a rapid return of twitch height even at deep levels of paralysis and the lack of side effects make this compound a promising new development in anesthesia.

References

1. Griffith HR, Johnson GE: The use of curare in general anesthesia. Anesthesiology 3:418, 1942
2. Beecher TK, Todd DP: Study of deaths associated with anesthesia and surgery based on a study of 599,458 anesthesias in 10 institutions 1948–1952 inclusive. Ann Surg 140:2, 1954
3. Bergman IJ, Kluger MT, Short TG: Awareness during general anaesthesia: A review of 81 cases from the Anaesthetic Incident Monitoring Study. Anaesthesia 57:549, 1954
4. Sonner JM, Antognini JF, Dutton RC *et al*: Inhaled anesthetics and immobility: Mechanisms, mysteries, and minimum alveolar anesthetic concentration. Anesthesia Analgesia 97:718, 2003
5. King M, Sujirattanawimol N, Danielson DR, Hall BA, Schroeder DR, Warner DO: Requirements for muscle relaxants during radical retropubic prostatectomy. Anesthesiology 93:1392, 2000
6. McNeil IA, Culbert B, Russell I: Comparison of intubating conditions following propofol and succinylcholine with propofol and remifentanil 2 micrograms kg-1 or 4 micrograms kg-1. Br J Anaesth 85:623, 2000
7. Mencke T, Echternach M, Kleinschmidt S *et al*: Laryngeal morbidity and quality of tracheal intubation: A randomized controlled trial. Anesthesiology 98:1049, 2003
8. Viby-Mogensen J, Jorgensen BC, Ording H: Residual curarization in the recovery room. Anesthesiology 50:539, 1979
9. Eriksson LI: Evidence-based practice and neuromuscular monitoring: It's time for routine quantitative assessment. Anesthesiology 98:1037, 2003
10. Boonyapisit K, Kaminski HJ, Ruff RL: Disorders of neuromuscular junction ion channels. Am J Med 106:97, 1999
11. Sanes JR, Lichtman JW: Development of the vertebrate neuromuscular junction. Annu Rev Neurosci 22:389, 1999
12. Naguib M, Flood P, McArdle JJ, Brenner HR: Advances in neurobiology of the neuromuscular junction: Implications for the anesthesiologist. Anesthesiology 96:202, 2002
13. Brull SJ, Silverman DG: Pulse width, stimulus intensity, electrode placement, and polarity during assessment of neuromuscular block. Anesthesiology 83:702, 1995
14. Van der Kloot W, Molgo J: Quantal acetylcholine release at the vertebrate neuromuscular junction. Physiol Rev 74:899, 1994
15. Wood SJ, Slater CR: The contribution of postsynaptic folds to the safety factor for neuromuscular transmission in rat fast- and slow-twitch muscles. J Physiol (Lond) 500(Pt 1):165, 1997
16. Lindstrom JM: Acetylcholine receptors and myasthenia. Muscle Nerve 23:453, 2000
17. Waud BE, Waud DR: The relation between the response to "train-of-four" stimulation and receptor occlusion during competitive neuromuscular block. Anesthesiology 37:413, 1972
18. Wood SJ, Slater CR: Safety factor at the neuromuscular junction. Prog Neurobiol 64:393, 2001
19. MacDermott AB, Role LW, Siegelbaum SA: Presynaptic ionotropic receptors and the control of transmitter release. Annu Rev Neurosci 22:443, 1999
20. Baker T, Stanec A: Drug actions at mammalian motor nerve endings: The suppression of neostigmine-induced fasciculations by vecuronium and isoflurane. Anesthesiology 67:942, 1987
21. Donati F: Neuromuscular blocking drugs for the new millennium: Current practice, future trends—comparative pharmacology of neuromuscular blocking drugs. Anesth Analg 90:S2, 2000
22. Viby-Mogensen J, Engbaek J, Eriksson LI *et al*: Good clinical research practice (GCRP) in pharmacodynamic studies of neuromuscular blocking agents. Acta Anaesthesiol Scand 1996;40:59, 2000
23. Smith CE, Saddler JM, Bevan JC, Donati F, Bevan DR: Pretreatment with non-depolarizing neuromuscular blocking agents and suxamethonium-induced increases in resting jaw tension in children. Br J Anaesth 64:577, 1990
24. Szalados JE, Donati F, Bevan DR: Effect of d-tubocurarine pretreatment on succinylcholine twitch augmentation and neuromuscular blockade. Anesth Analg 71:55, 1990
25. McCoy EP, Mirakhur RK: Comparison of the effects of neostigmine and edrophonium on the duration of action of suxamethonium. Acta Anaesthesiol Scand 39:744, 1995
26. Donati F, Bevan DR: Long-term succinylcholine infusion during isoflurane anesthesia. Anesthesiology 58:6, 1983
27. Roy JJ, Donati F, Boismenu D, Varin F: Concentration-effect relation of succinylcholine chloride during propofol anesthesia. Anesthesiology 97:1082, 2002

28. Vanlinthout LE, van Egmond J, de Boo T, Lerou JG, Wevers RA, Booij LH: Factors affecting magnitude and time course of neuromuscular block produced by suxamethonium. Br J Anaesth 69:29, 1992
29. Szalados JE, Donati F, Bevan DR: Nitrous oxide potentiates succinylcholine neuromuscular blockade in humans. Anesth Analg 72:18, 1991
30. Lerman J, Chinyanga HM: The heart rate response to succinylcholine in children: A comparison of atropine and glycopyrrolate. Can Anaesth Soc J 30:377, 1983
31. Mertes PM, Laxenaire MC, Alla F: Anaphylactic and anaphylactoid reactions occurring during anesthesia in France in 1999–2000. Anesthesiology 99:536, 2003
32. Kopman AF, Khan NA, Neuman GG: Precurarization and priming: A theoretical analysis of safety and timing. Anesth Analg 93:1253, 2001
33. Harvey SC, Roland P, Bailey MK, Tomlin MK, Williams A: A randomized, double-blind comparison of rocuronium, d-tubocurarine, and "mini-dose" succinylcholine for preventing succinylcholine-induced muscle fasciculations. Anesth Analg 87:719, 1998
34. Mencke T, Schreiber JU, Becker C, Bolte M, Fuchs-Buder T: Pretreatment before succinylcholine for outpatient anesthesia? Anesth Analg 94:573, 2002
35. Wong SF, Chung F: Succinylcholine-associated postoperative myalgia. Anaesthesia 55:144, 2000
36. Vachon CA, Warner DO, Bacon DR: Succinylcholine and the open globe. Tracing the teaching. Anesthesiology 99:220, 2003
37. Minton MD, Grosslight K, Stirt JA, Bedford RF: Increases in intracranial pressure from succinylcholine: Prevention by prior nondepolarizing blockade. Anesthesiology 65:165, 1986
38. Gronert GA: Cardiac arrest after succinylcholine: Mortality greater with rhabdomyolysis than receptor upregulation. Anesthesiology 94:523, 2001
39. Thapa S, Brull SJ: Succinylcholine-induced hyperkalemia in patients with renal failure: An old question revisited. Anesth Analg 91:237, 2000
40. Davis L, Britten JJ, Morgan M: Cholinesterase. Its significance in anaesthetic practice. Anaesthesia 52:244, 1997
41. Donati F: The right dose of succinylcholine. Anesthesiology 99:1037, 2003
42. Hayes AH, Breslin DS, Mirakhur RK, Reid JE, O'Hare RA: Frequency of haemoglobin desaturation with the use of succinylcholine during rapid sequence induction of anaesthesia. Acta Anaesthesiol Scand 45:746, 2001
43. Meakin G, McKiernan EP, Morris P, Baker RD: Dose-response curves for suxamethonium in neonates, infants and children. Br J Anaesth 62:655, 1989
44. Donati F, Guay J: No substitute for the intravenous route. Anesthesiology 94:1, 2001
45. Lee C, Katz RL: Fade of neurally evoked compound electromyogram during neuromuscular block by d-tubocurarine. Anesth Analg 56:271, 1977
46. Baurain MJ, Hennart DA, Godschalx A *et al*: Visual evaluation of residual curarization in anesthetized patients using one hundred-hertz, five-second tetanic stimulation at the adductor pollicis muscle. Anesth Analg 87:185, 1998
47. Kopman AF, Klewicka MM, Kopman DJ, Neuman GG: Molar potency is predictive of the speed of onset of neuromuscular block for agents of intermediate, short, and ultrashort duration. Anesthesiology 90:425, 1999
48. Savarese JJ, Ali HH, Antonio RP: The clinical pharmacology of metocurine: Dimethyltubocurarine revisited. Anesthesiology 47:277, 1977
49. Miller RD, Matteo RS, Benet LZ, Sohn YJ: The pharmacokinetics of d-tubocurarine in man with and without renal failure. J Pharmacol Exp Ther 202:1, 1977
50. Fisher DM, O'Keeffe C, Stanski DR, Cronnelly R, Miller RD, Gregory GA: Pharmacokinetics and pharmacodynamics of d-tubocurarine in infants, children, and adults. Anesthesiology 57:203, 1982
51. Martyn JA, White DA, Gronert GA, Jaffe RS, Ward JM: Up-and-down regulation of skeletal muscle acetylcholine receptors. Effects on neuromuscular blockers. Anesthesiology 76:822, 1992
52. Ibebunjo C, Martyn JA: Thermal injury induces greater resistance to d-tubocurarine in local rather than in distant muscles in the rat. Anesth Analg 91:1243, 2000
53. Diefenbach C, Kunzer T, Buzello W, Theisohn M: Alcuronium: A pharmacodynamic and pharmacokinetic update. Anesth Analg 80:373, 1995
54. Stiller RL, Cook DR, Chakravorti S: In vitro degradation of atracurium in human plasma. Br J Anaesth 57:1085, 1985
55. Fodale V, Santamaria LB: Laudanosine, an atracurium and cisatracurium metabolite. Eur J Anaesthesiol 19:466, 2002
56. Amann A, Rieder J, Fleischer M *et al*: The influence of atracurium, cisatracurium, and mivacurium on the proliferation of two human cell lines in vitro. Anesth Analg 93:690, 2001
57. Kisor DF, Schmith VD, Wargin WA, Lien CA, Ornstein E, Cook DR: Importance of the organ-independent elimination of cisatracurium. Anesth Analg 83:1065, 1996
58. Eikermann M, Peters J: Nerve stimulation at 0.15 Hz when compared to 0.1 Hz speeds the onset of action of cisatracurium and rocuronium. Acta Anaesthesiol Scand 44:170, 2000
59. Lien CA, Schmith VD, Belmont MR, Abalos A, Kisor DF, Savarese JJ: Pharmacokinetics of cisatracurium in patients receiving nitrous oxide/opioid/barbiturate anesthesia. Anesthesiology 84:300, 1996
60. Miller DR, Wherrett C, Hull K, Watson J, Legault S: Cumulation characteristics of cisatracurium and rocuronium during continuous infusion. Can J Anaesth 47:943, 2000
61. Dhonneur G, Cerf C, Lagneau F, Mantz J, Gillotin C, Duvaldestin P: The pharmacokinetics of cisatracurium in patients with acute respiratory distress syndrome. Anesth Analg 93:400, 2001
62. Basta SJ, Savarese JJ, Ali HH *et al*: Clinical pharmacology of doxacurium chloride. A new long-acting nondepolarizing muscle relaxant. Anesthesiology 69:478, 1988
63. Belmont MR, Lien CA, Tjan J *et al*: Clinical pharmacology of GW280430A in humans. Anesthesiology 100:768, 2004
64. Lebowitz PW, Ramsey FM, Savarese JJ, Ali HH: Potentiation of neuromuscular blockade in man produced by combinations of pancuronium and metocurine or pancuronium and d-tubocurarine. Anesth Analg 59:604, 1980
65. Savarese JJ, Ali HH, Basta SJ *et al*: The clinical neuromuscular pharmacology of mivacurium chloride (BW B1090U). A short-acting nondepolarizing ester neuromuscular blocking drug. Anesthesiology 68:723, 1988
66. Plaud B, Debaene B, Donati F: Duration of anesthesia before muscle relaxant injection influences level of paralysis. Anesthesiology 97:616, 2002
67. Maddineni VR, Mirakhur RK, McCoy EP, Fee JP, Clarke RS: Neuromuscular effects and intubating conditions following mivacurium: A comparison with suxamethonium. Anaesthesia 48:940, 1993
68. Bishop MJ, O'Donnell JT, Salemi JR: Mivacurium and bronchospasm. Anesth Analg 97:484, 2003
69. Brandom BW, Meretoja OA, Simhi E *et al*: Age related variability in the effects of mivacurium in paediatric surgical patients. Can J Anaesth 45:410, 1998
70. Bevan JC, Reimer EJ, Smith MF *et al*: Decreased mivacurium requirements and delayed neuromuscular recovery during sevoflurane anesthesia in children and adults. Anesth Analg 87:772, 1998
71. Goudsouzian N, Chakravorti S, Denman W, Schwartz A, Yang HS, Cook DR: Prolonged mivacurium infusion in young and elderly adults. Can J Anaesth 44:955, 1997
72. Martyn JA, Goudsouzian NG, Chang Y, Szyfelbein SK, Schwartz AE, Patel SS: Neuromuscular effects of mivacurium in 2- to 12-yr-old children with burn injury. Anesthesiology 92:31, 2000
73. Kao YJ, Le ND: The reversal of profound mivacurium-induced neuromuscular blockade. Can J Anaesth 43:1128, 1996
74. Ali HH, Lien CA, Witkowski T *et al*: Efficacy and safety of divided dose administration of mivacurium for a 90-second tracheal intubation. J Clin Anesth 8:276, 1996
75. Chui PT, Cheam EW: The use of low-dose mivacurium to facilitate insertion of the laryngeal mask airway. Anaesthesia 53:491, 1998
76. Goudsouzian N, Chakravorti S, Denman W, Schwartz A, Yang HS, Cook DR: Prolonged mivacurium infusion in young and elderly adults. Can J Anaesth 44:955, 1997
77. Murphy GS, Szokol JW, Marymont JH *et al*: Recovery of neuromuscular function after cardiac surgery: Pancuronium versus rocuronium. Anesth Analg 96:1301, 2003
78. Murphy GS, Szokol JW, Franklin M, Marymont JH, Avram MJ, Vender JS: Postanesthesia care unit recovery times and neuromuscular blocking drugs: A prospective study of orthopedic surgical patients randomized to receive pancuronium or rocuronium. Anesth Analg 98:193, 2004
79. Baurain MJ, Hoton F, D'Hollander AA, Cantraine FR: Is recovery of neuromuscular transmission complete after the use of neostigmine to antagonize block produced by rocuronium, vecuronium, atracurium and pancuronium? Br J Anaesth 77:496, 1996
80. Sparr HJ, Mellinghoff H, Blobner M, Nolge-Schomburg G: Comparison of intubating conditions after rapacuronium (Org 9487) and succinylcholine following rapid sequence induction in adult patients. Br J Anaesth 82:537, 1999
81. Jooste E, Klafter F, Hirshman CA, Emala CW: A mechanism for rapacuronium-induced bronchospasm: M2 muscarinic receptor antagonism. Anesthesiology 98:906, 2003
82. Proost JH, Eriksson LI, Mirakhur RK, Roest G, Wierda JM: Urinary, biliary and faecal excretion of rocuronium in humans. Br J Anaesth 85:717, 2000
83. Andrews JI, Kumar N, van den Brom RH, Olkkola KT, Roest GJ, Wright PM: A large simple randomized trial of rocuronium versus succinylcholine in rapid-sequence induction of anaesthesia along with propofol. Acta Anaesthesiol Scand 43:4, 1999
84. Hemmerling TM, Donati F: Neuromuscular blockade at the larynx, the diaphragm and the corrugator supercilii muscle: A review: Can J Anaesth 50:779, 2003
85. Plaud B, Proost JH, Wierda JM, Barre J, Debaene B, Meistelman C: Pharmacokinetics and pharmacodynamics of rocuronium at the vocal cords and the adductor pollicis in humans. Clin Pharmacol Ther 58:185, 1995
86. Levy JH, Davis GK, Duggan J, Szlam F: Determination of the hemodynamics and histamine release of rocuronium (Org 9426) when administered in increased doses under N2O/O2-sufentanil anesthesia. Anesth Analg 78:318, 1994
87. Dhonneur G, Combes X, Chassard D, Merle JC: Skin sensitivity to rocuronium and vecuronium: A randomized controlled prick-testing study in healthy volunteers. Anesth Analg 98:986, 2004
88. Laake JH, Rottingen JA: Rocuronium and anaphylaxis—a statistical challenge. Acta Anaesthesiol Scand 45:1196, 2001
89. Xue FS, Tong SY, Liao X, Liu JH, An G, Luo LK: Dose-response and time course of effect of rocuronium in male and female anesthetized patients. Anesth Analg 85:667, 1997

90. Collins LM, Bevan JC, Bevan DR *et al*: The prolonged duration of rocuronium in Chinese patients. Anesth Analg 91:1526, 2000
91. Woolf RL, Crawford MW, Choo SM: Dose-response of rocuronium bromide in children anesthetized with propofol: A comparison with succinylcholine. Anesthesiology 87:1368, 1997
92. Taivainen T, Meretoja OA, Erkola O, Rautoma P, Juvakoski M: Rocuronium in infants, children and adults during balanced anaesthesia. Paediatr Anaesth 6:271, 1996
93. Rapp HJ, Altenmueller CA, Waschke C: Neuromuscular recovery following rocuronium bromide single dose in infants. Paediatr Anaesth 14:329, 2004
94. Bevan DR, Fiset P, Balendran P, Law-Min JC, Ratcliffe A, Donati F: Pharmacodynamic behaviour of rocuronium in the elderly. Can J Anaesth 40:127, 1993
95. Szenohradszky J, Fisher DM, Segredo V *et al*: Pharmacokinetics of rocuronium bromide (ORG 9426) in patients with normal renal function or patients undergoing cadaver renal transplantation. Anesthesiology 77:899, 1992
96. Khalil M, d'Honneur G, Duvaldestin P, Slavov V, De Hys C, Gomeni R: Pharmacokinetics and pharmacodynamics of rocuronium in patients with cirrhosis. Anesthesiology 80:1241, 1994
97. Jellish WS, Brody M, Sawicki K, Slogoff S: Recovery from neuromuscular blockade after either bolus and prolonged infusions of cisatracurium or rocuronium using either isoflurane or propofol-based anesthetics. Anesth Analg 91:1250, 2000
98. Segredo V, Caldwell JE, Matthay MA, Sharma ML, Gruenke LD, Miller RD: Persistent paralysis in critically ill patients after long-term administration of vecuronium. N Engl J Med 327:524, 1992
99. Fawcett WJ, Dash A, Francis GA, Liban JB, Cashman JN: Recovery from neuromuscular blockade: Residual curarisation following atracurium or vecuronium by bolus dosing or infusions. Acta Anaesthesiol Scand 39:288, 1995
100. Motamed C, Donati F: Sevoflurane and isoflurane, but not propofol, decrease mivacurium requirements over time. Can J Anaesth 49:907, 2002
101. Hemmerling TM, Schuettler J, Schwilden H: Desflurane reduces the effective therapeutic infusion rate (ETI) of cisatracurium more than isoflurane, sevoflurane, or propofol. Can J Anaesth 48:532, 2001
102. Paul M, Fokt RM, Kindler CH, Dipp NC, Yost CS: Characterization of the interactions between volatile anesthetics and neuromuscular blockers at the muscle nicotinic acetylcholine receptor. Anesth Analg 95:362, table, 2002
103. Ferres CJ, Mirakhur RK, Pandit SK, Clarke RS, Gibson FM: Dose-response studies with pancuronium, vecuronium and their combination. Br J Clin Pharmacol 18:947, 1984
104. Kim KS, Chun YS, Chon SU, Suh JK: Neuromuscular interaction between cisatracurium and mivacurium, atracurium, vecuronium or rocuronium administered in combination. Anaesthesia 53:872, 1998
105. Motamed C, Donati F: Intubating conditions and blockade after mivacurium, rocuronium and their combination in young and elderly adults. Can J Anaesth 47:225, 2000
106. Paul M, Kindler CH, Fokt RM, Dipp NC, Yost CS: Isobolographic analysis of non-depolarising muscle relaxant interactions at their receptor site. Eur J Pharmacol 438:35, 2002
107. Kim DW, Joshi GP, White PF, Johnson ER: Interactions between mivacurium, rocuronium, and vecuronium during general anesthesia. Anesth Analg 83:818, 1996
108. Kim KS, Na DJ, Chon SU: Interactions between suxamethonium and mivacurium or atracurium. Br J Anaesth 77:612, 1996
109. Sokoll MD, Gergis SD: Antibiotics and neuromuscular function. Anesthesiology 55:148, 1981
110. Dupuis JY, Martin R, Tetrault JP: Atracurium and vecuronium interaction with gentamicin and tobramycin. Can J Anaesth 36:407, 1989
111. Sloan PA, Rasul M: Prolongation of rapacuronium neuromuscular blockade by clindamycin and magnesium. Anesth Analg 94:123, 2002
112. Spacek A, Nickl S, Neiger FX *et al*: Augmentation of the rocuronium-induced neuromuscular block by the acutely administered phenytoin. Anesthesiology 90:1551, 1999
113. Spacek A, Neiger FX, Spiss CK, Kress HG: Atracurium-induced neuromuscular block is not affected by chronic anticonvulsant therapy with carbamazepine. Acta Anaesthesiol Scand 41:1308, 1997
114. Alloul K, Whalley DG, Shutway F, Ebrahim Z, Varin F: Pharmacokinetic origin of carbamazepine-induced resistance to vecuronium neuromuscular blockade in anesthetized patients. Anesthesiology 84:330, 1996
115. Loan PB, Connolly FM, Mirakhur RK, Kumar N, Farling P: Neuromuscular effects of rocuronium in patients receiving beta-adrenoreceptor blocking, calcium entry blocking and anticonvulsant drugs. Br J Anaesth 78:90, 1997
116. Szmuk P, Ezri T, Chelly JE, Katz J: The onset time of rocuronium is slowed by esmolol and accelerated by ephedrine. Anesth Analg 90:1217, 2000
117. Fawcett WJ, Stone JP: Recurarization in the recovery room following the use of magnesium sulphate. Br J Anaesth 91:435, 2003
118. Fodale V, Pratico C, Girlanda P *et al*: Acute motor axonal polyneuropathy after a cisatracurium infusion and concomitant corticosteroid therapy. Br J Anaesth 92:289, 2004
119. Fletcher SN, Kennedy DD, Ghosh IR *et al*: Persistent neuromuscular and neurophysiologic abnormalities in long-term survivors of prolonged critical illness. Crit Care Med 31:1012, 2003
120. Hund E: Neurological complications of sepsis: critical illness polyneuropathy and myopathy. J Neurol 248:929, 2001
121. Lagneau F, d'Honneur G, Plaud B *et al*: A comparison of two depths of prolonged neuromuscular blockade induced by cisatracurium in mechanically ventilated critically ill patients. Intensive Care Med 28:1735, 2002
122. Sparr HJ, Wierda JM, Proost JH, Keller C, Khuenl-Brady KS: Pharmacodynamics and pharmacokinetics of rocuronium in intensive care patients. Br J Anaesth 78:267, 1997
123. Itoh H, Shibata K, Yoshida M, Yamamoto K: Neuromuscular monitoring at the orbicularis oculi may overestimate the blockade in myasthenic patients. Anesthesiology 93:1194, 2000
124. Martyn JA, Chang Y, Goudsouzian NG, Patel SS: Pharmacodynamics of mivacurium chloride in 13- to 18-yr-old adolescents with thermal injury. Br J Anaesth 89:580, 2002
125. Brull SJ, Connelly NR, O'Connor TZ, Silverman DG: Effect of tetanus on subsequent neuromuscular monitoring in patients receiving vecuronium. Anesthesiology 74:64, 1991
126. Ali HH, Utting JE, Gray TC: Quantitative assessment of residual antidepolarizing block. II. Br J Anaesth 43:478, 1971
127. O'Hara DA, Fragen RJ, Shanks CA: Comparison of visual and measured train-of-four recovery after vecuronium-induced neuromuscular blockade using two anaesthetic techniques. Br J Anaesth 58:1300, 1986
128. Viby-Mogensen J, Howardy-Hansen P, Chraemmer-Jorgensen B, Ording H, Engbaek J, Nielsen A: Posttetanic count (PTC): A new method of evaluating an intense nondepolarizing neuromuscular blockade. Anesthesiology 55:458, 1981
129. Drenck NE, Ueda N, Olsen NV *et al*: Manual evaluation of residual curarization using double burst stimulation: A comparison with train-of-four. Anesthesiology 70:578, 1989
130. Dupuis JY, Martin R, Tessonnier JM, Tetrault JP: Clinical assessment of the muscular response to tetanic nerve stimulation. Can J Anaesth 37:397, 1990
131. Kalli I: Effect of surface electrode position on the compound action potential evoked by ulnar nerve stimulation during isoflurane anaesthesia. Br J Anaesth 65:494, 1990
132. Kopman AF: The relationship of evoked electromyographic and mechanical responses following atracurium in humans. Anesthesiology 63:208, 1985
133. Kopman AF, Klewicka MM, Neuman GG: The relationship between acceleromyographic train-of-four fade and single twitch depression. Anesthesiology 96:583, 2002
134. Debaene B, Plaud B, Dilly MP, Donati F: Residual paralysis in the PACU after a single intubating dose of nondepolarizing muscle relaxant with an intermediate duration of action. Anesthesiology 98:1042, 2003
135. Gatke MR, Viby-Mogensen J, Rosenstock C, Jensen FS, Skovgaard LT: Postoperative muscle paralysis after rocuronium: Less residual block when acceleromyography is used. Acta Anaesthesiol Scand 46:207, 2002
136. Dahaba AA, Von Klobucar F, Rehak PH, List WF: The neuromuscular transmission module versus the relaxometer mechanomyograph for neuromuscular block monitoring. Anesth Analg 94:591, 2002
137. Donati F, Meistelman C, Plaud B: Vecuronium neuromuscular blockade at the diaphragm, the orbicularis oculi, and adductor pollicis muscles. Anesthesiology 73:870, 1990
138. Donati F, Meistelman C, Plaud B: Vecuronium neuromuscular blockade at the adductor muscles of the larynx and adductor pollicis. Anesthesiology 74:833, 1991
139. Kirov K, Motamed C, Dhonneur G: Differential sensitivity of abdominal muscles and the diaphragm to mivacurium: An electromyographic study. Anesthesiology 95:1323, 2001
140. d'Honneur G, Guignard B, Slavov V, Ruggier R, Duvaldestin P: Comparison of the neuromuscular blocking effect of atracurium and vecuronium on the adductor pollicis and the geniohyoid muscle in humans. Anesthesiology 82:649, 1995
141. Nepveu ME, Donati F, Fortier LP: Train-of-four stimulation for adductor pollicis neuromuscular monitoring can be applied at the wrist or over the hand. Anesth Analg 100:149, 2005
142. Plaud B, Debaene B, Donati F: The corrugator supercilii, not the orbicularis oculi, reflects rocuronium neuromuscular blockade at the laryngeal adductor muscles. Anesthesiology 95:96, 2001
143. Wright PM, Caldwell JE, Miller RD: Onset and duration of rocuronium and succinylcholine at the adductor pollicis and laryngeal adductor muscles in anesthetized humans. Anesthesiology 81:1110, 1994
144. Kirkegaard H, Heier T, Caldwell JE: Efficacy of tactile-guided reversal from cisatracurium-induced neuromuscular block. Anesthesiology 96:45, 2002
145. Kopman AF, Yee PS, Neuman GG: Relationship of the train-of-four fade ratio to clinical signs and symptoms of residual paralysis in awake volunteers. Anesthesiology 86:765, 1997
146. Eriksson LI, Sundman E, Olsson R *et al*: Functional assessment of the pharynx at rest and during swallowing in partially paralyzed humans: Simultaneous videomanometry and mechanomyography of awake human volunteers. Anesthesiology 87:1035, 1997
147. Pavlin EG, Holle RH, Schoene RB: Recovery of airway protection compared with ventilation in humans after paralysis with curare. Anesthesiology 70:381, 1989
148. Nishino T, Yokokawa N, Hiraga K, Honda Y, Mizuguchi T: Breathing pattern of anesthetized humans during pancuronium-induced partial paralysis. J Appl Physiol 64:78, 1988

149. Eriksson LI, Lennmarken C, Wyon N, Johnson A: Attenuated ventilatory response to hypoxaemia at vecuronium-induced partial neuromuscular block. Acta Anaesthesiol Scand 36:710, 1992
150. Capron F, Alla F, Hottier C, Meistelman C, Fuchs-Buder T: Can acceleromyography detect low levels of residual paralysis? A probability approach to detect a mechanomyographic train-of-four ratio of 0.9. Anesthesiology 100:1119, 2004
151. Kopman AF, Zank LM, Ng J, Neuman GG: Antagonism of cisatracurium and rocuronium block at a tactile train-of-four count of 2: Should quantitative assessment of neuromuscular function be mandatory? Anesth Analg 98:102, 2004
152. Sundman E, Witt H, Olsson R, Ekberg O, Kuylenstierna R, Eriksson LI: The incidence and mechanisms of pharyngeal and upper esophageal dysfunction in partially paralyzed humans: Pharyngeal videoradiography and simultaneous manometry after atracurium. Anesthesiology 92:977, 2000
153. Bevan DR, Donati F, Kopman AF: Reversal of neuromuscular blockade. Anesthesiology 77:785, 1992
154. Baillard C, Gehan G, Reboul-Marty J, Larmignat P, Samama CM, Cupa M: Residual curarization in the recovery room after vecuronium. Br J Anaesth 84:394, 2000
155. Berg H, Roed J, Viby-Mogensen J *et al*: Residual neuromuscular block is a risk factor for postoperative pulmonary complications. A prospective, randomised, and blinded study of postoperative pulmonary complications after atracurium, vecuronium and pancuronium. Acta Anaesthesiol Scand 41:1095, 1997
156. Murphy GS, Szokol JW, Marymont JH, Avram MJ, Vender JS, Rosengart TK: Impact of shorter-acting neuromuscular blocking agents on fast-track recovery of the cardiac surgical patient. Anesthesiology 96:600, 2002
157. Fiekers JF: Concentration-dependent effects of neostigmine on the endplate acetylcholine receptor channel complex. J Neurosci 5:502, 1985
158. Astley BA, Katz RL, Payne JP: Electrical and mechanical responses after neuromuscular blockade with vecuronium, and subsequent antagonism with neostigmine or edrophonium. Br J Anaesth 59:983, 1987
159. Cronnelly R, Morris RB, Miller RD: Edrophonium: duration of action and atropine requirement in humans during halothane anesthesia. Anesthesiology 57:261, 1982
160. Donati F, Smith CE, Bevan DR: Dose-response relationships for edrophonium and neostigmine as antagonists of moderate and profound atracurium blockade. Anesth Analg 68:13, 1989
161. Smith CE, Donati F, Bevan DR: Dose-response relationships for edrophonium and neostigmine as antagonists of atracurium and vecuronium neuromuscular blockade. Anesthesiology 71:37, 1989
162. Bevan JC, Collins L, Fowler C *et al*: Early and late reversal of rocuronium and vecuronium with neostigmine in adults and children. Anesth Analg 89:333, 1999
163. Breen PJ, Doherty WG, Donati F, Bevan DR: The potencies of edrophonium and neostigmine as antagonists of pancuronium. Anaesthesia 40:844, 1985
164. Tramer MR, Fuchs-Buder T: Omitting antagonism of neuromuscular block: Effect on postoperative nausea and vomiting and risk of residual paralysis. A systematic review. Br J Anaesth 82:379, 1999
165. Epemolu O, Bom A, Hope F, Mason R: Reversal of neuromuscular blockade and simultaneous increase in plasma rocuronium concentration after the intravenous infusion of the novel reversal agent Org 25969. Anesthesiology 99:632, 2003
166. Dhonneur G, Kirov K, Slavov V, Duvaldestin P: Effects of an intubating dose of succinylcholine and rocuronium on the larynx and diaphragm: An electromyographic study in humans. Anesthesiology 90:951, 1999
167. Ferguson A, Egerszegi P, Bevan DR: Neostigmine, pyridostigmine, and edrophonium as antagonists of pancuronium. Anesthesiology 53:390, 1980
168. McCourt KC, Mirakhur RK, Kerr CM: Dosage of neostigmine for reversal of rocuronium block from two levels of spontaneous recovery. Anaesthesia 54:651, 1999
169. Bevan DR, Smith CE, Donati F: Postoperative neuromuscular blockade: A comparison between atracurium, vecuronium, and pancuronium. Anesthesiology 69:272, 1988
170. Bissinger U, Schimek F, Lenz G: Postoperative residual paralysis and respiratory status: A comparative study of pancuronium and vecuronium. Physiol Res 49:455, 2000
171. Hayes AH, Mirakhur RK, Breslin DS, Reid JE, McCourt KC: Postoperative residual block after intermediate-acting neuromuscular blocking drugs. Anaesthesia 56:312, 2001

CHAPTER 17 ■ LOCAL ANESTHETICS

SPENCER S. LIU AND RAYMOND S. JOSEPH, Jr.

KEY POINTS

1. Local anesthetics block the generation, propagation, and oscillations of electrical impulses in electrically excitable tissue.
2. Molecular and genetic studies indicate that local anesthetics primarily work by binding to a modulated receptor located on the interior of the sodium channel.
3. In addition to sodium channel block, mechanisms of action of both peripheral and central neural block may involve decremental conduction, partial block of information carrying electrical oscillations, and interactions with other neurotransmitters such as GABA.
4. In general, the more potent and longer acting agents are more lipid soluble, have increased protein binding, less systemic absorption, but more potential for systemic toxicity.
5. All currently available local anesthetics are racemic mixtures with the exception of lidocaine (achiral), levobupivacaine (l = S), and ropivacaine (S). It appears that S isomers have nearly equal efficacy but less potential for systemic toxicity.
6. Efficacy for clinical use of local anesthetics may be increased by addition of epinephrine, opioids, and alpha-2 adrenergic agonists. The value of alkalinization of local anesthetics appears to be debatable as a clinically useful tool to improve anesthesia.
7. Systemic toxicity from the clinical use of local anesthetics for regional anesthesia appears to be an uncommon occurrence. Surveys from France and the United States approximate the seizure rate to be 1/10,000 for epidural injection and 7/10,000 for peripheral nerve block.
8. Nonetheless, systemic toxicity from local anesthetics should be promptly treated. Patients with cardiovascular collapse from bupivacaine, ropivacaine, and levobupivacaine may be especially difficult to resuscitate.

INTRODUCTION

Local anesthetics block the generation, propagation, and oscillations of electrical impulses in electrically excitable tissue. Use of local anesthetics in clinical anesthesia is varied and includes direct injection into tissues, topical application, and intravenous administration to produce clinical effects at varied locations including the central neuraxis, peripheral nerves, mucosa, skin, heart, and airway. Detailed knowledge of pertinent anatomy and pharmacology will aid in optimal therapeutic use of local anesthetics. Care should be taken to avoid potential central nervous system (CNS) and cardiovascular toxicity from local anesthetics.

MECHANISMS OF ACTION OF LOCAL ANESTHETICS

Anatomy of Nerves

Local anesthetics are often used to block nerves either peripherally or centrally. Peripheral nerves are mixed nerves containing afferent and efferent fibers that may be myelinated or unmyelinated. Each axon within the nerve fiber is surrounded by endoneurium composed of nonneural glial cells. Individual nerve fibers are gathered into fascicles and surrounded by perineurium composed of connective tissue. Finally, the entire

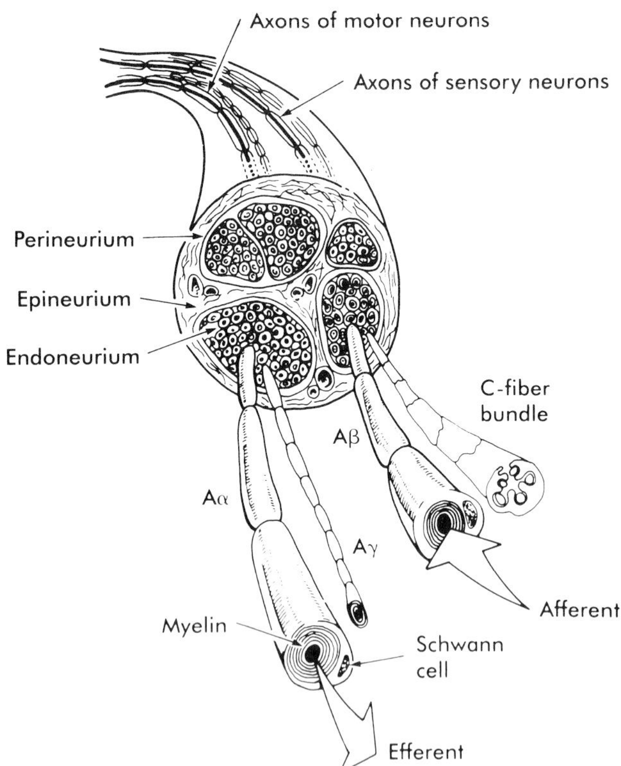

FIGURE 17-1. Schematic cross section of typical peripheral nerve. The epineurium, consisting of collagen fibers, is oriented along the long axis of the nerve. The perineurim is a discrete cell layer, whereas the endoneurium is a matrix of connective tissue. Both afferent and efferent axons are shown. Sympathetic axons (not shown) are also present in mixed peripheral nerves. (Adapted with permission from Strichartz GR: Neural physiology and local anesthetic action. In Cousins MJ, Bridenbaugh PO [eds]: Neural Blockade in Clinical Anesthesia and Management of Pain, p 35. Philadelphia, Lippincott–Raven, 1998.)

peripheral nerve is encased by epineurium composed of dense connective tissue (Fig. 17-1). Thus, several layers of protective tissue surround individual axons, and these layers act as barriers to the penetration of local anesthetics.[1] In addition to the enveloping connective tissue, all mammalian nerves with a diameter greater than 1 μm are myelinated. Myelinated nerve fibers are segmentally enclosed by Schwann cells forming a bilayer lipid membrane that is wrapped several hundred times around each axon.[2] Thus, myelin accounts for over half the thickness of nerve fibers >1 μm (Fig. 17-2). Separating the myelinated regions are the nodes of Ranvier where structural elements for neuronal excitation are concentrated (Fig. 17-3).[3] The nodes are covered by interdigitations from nonmyelinating Schwann cells[4] and by negatively charged glycoproteins. Although axonal membranes are not freely in contact with their environment at the nodes, these areas do allow passage of drugs and ions.[5] Furthermore, the negatively charged proteins may bind basic local anesthetics and thus act as a depot. Unmyelinated nerve fibers (diameter <1 μm) are encased by a Schwann cell that simultaneously insulates several (5 to 10) axons (Fig. 17-2). These fibers are continuously encased by Schwann cells and do not possess interruptions (nodes of Ranvier). The existence of multiple protective layers around both myelinated and unmyelinated nerve fibers presents a substantial barrier to the entry of clinically used local anesthetics. For example, animal models suggest that only 1.6% of an injected dose of local anesthetic penetrates into the nerve following performance of peripheral nerve blocks.[6]

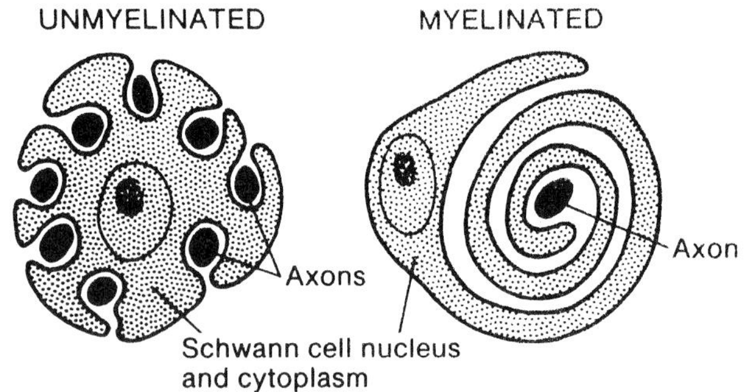

FIGURE 17-2. Schwann cells form myelin around one myelinated axon or encompass several unmyelinated axons. (Adapted with permission from Carpenter RL, Mackey DC: Local anesthetics. In Barash PG, Cullen BF, Stoelting RF [eds]: Clinical Anesthesia, p 413. Philadelphia, Lippincott–Raven, 1996.)

Nerve fibers are commonly classified by size, conduction velocity, and function (Table 17-1). In general, increasing myelination and nerve diameter lead to increased conduction velocity. The presence of myelin accelerates conduction velocity because of increased electrical insulation of nerve fibers and saltatory conduction. Increased nerve diameter accelerates conduction velocity both by increased myelination and by improved electrical cable conduction properties of the nerve. Myelinated and unmyelinated nerves carry out both afferent and efferent functions.

Electrophysiology of Neural Conduction

Ionic disequilibria across semipermeable membranes form the basis for neuronal resting potentials and for the potential energy needed to initiate and maintain electrical impulses. The resting potential of neural membranes averages −60 to −70 mV, with the cell interior being negative to the cell exterior. This resting potential is predominantly maintained by a potassium gradient with a 10 times greater concentration of potassium within the cell. This gradient is maintained by an active protein pump that transports potassium into the cell and sodium out of the cell through voltage-gated potassium channels that are open at resting potentials.[7] Potassium equilibrium is not the only factor in resting potential, as a resting potential of approximately −90 mV is predicted by the Nernst equation if only potassium is considered. In addition to

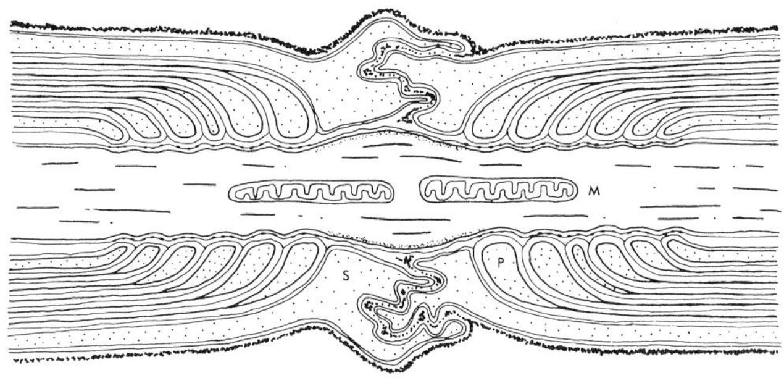

FIGURE 17-3. Diagram of node of Ranvier displaying mitochondria (M), tight junctions in paranodal area (P), and Schwann cell (S) surrounding node. (Adapted with permission from Strichartz GR: Mechanisms of action of local anesthetic agents. In Rogers MC, Tinker JH, Covino BG, et al [eds]: Principles and Practice of Anesthesiology, p 1197. St. Louis, Mosby Year Book, 1993.)

TABLE 17-1

CLASSIFICATION OF NERVE FIBERS

CLASSIFICATION	DIAMETER (μ)	MYELIN	CONDUCTION (m/sec)	LOCATION	FUNCTION
A-alpha A-beta	6–22	+	30–120	Afferents/efferents for muscles and joints	Motor and proprioception
A-gamma	3–6	+	15–35	Efferent to muscle spindle	Muscle tone
A-delta	1–4	+	5–25	Afferent sensory nerve	Pain Touch Temperature
B	<3	+	3–15	Preganglionic sympathetic	Autonomic function
C	0.3–1.3	–	0.7–1.3	Postganglionic sympathetic Afferent sensory nerve	Autonomic function Pain Temperature

potassium channels, voltage-independent channels that allow "leak" currents of sodium, chloride, and other ions affect the resting potential.

In contrast to the dependence of resting membrane potential on potassium disequilibria, generation of action potentials is primarily a result of activation of voltage-gated sodium channels.[7] These channels are protein structures spanning the bilayer lipid membrane composed of structural elements, an aqueous pore, and voltage-sensing elements that control passage of ions through the pore (Fig. 17-4).[8] Sodium channels exist in several conformations depending on membrane potential and time. At resting membrane potential, sodium channels predominantly exist in a resting (closed) conformation.[7,9] During membrane depolarization, channels open within a few hundred microseconds and allow passage of 10^7 ions/sec^{-1}. Sodium channels are relatively selective, but other monovalent ions can also gain passage through the channel. For example, lithium traverses about as well as sodium, whereas potassium only about one-tenth as well. Following activation (opening) of the sodium channel and depolarization, the channel will spontaneously close into an inactivated state in a time-dependent fashion to allow repolarization and then revert to a resting conformation.[10] Thus, a three-state kinetic scheme (Fig. 17-5) conceptualizes the changes in sodium channel conformation that account for changes in sodium conductance during depolarization and repolarization.

An action potential will be generated by depolarization when the impulse-firing threshold of the axon is reached. That is the point at which no further depolarization is required for local processes to generate a complete action potential. This threshold is not an absolute voltage, but rather depends on the dynamics of the sodium and potassium channels. For example, a brief maximally depolarizing stimulus will not generate an

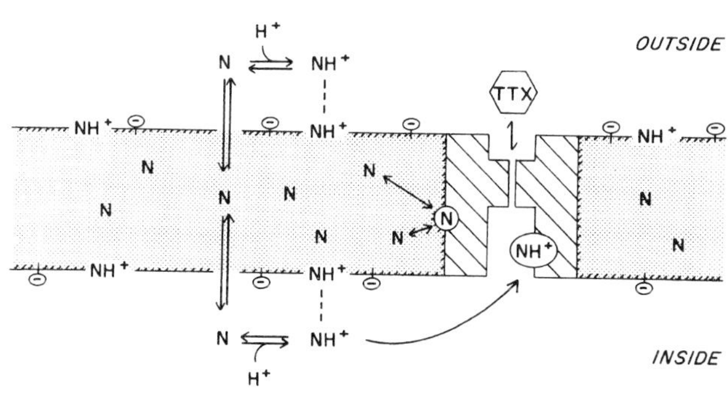

FIGURE 17-4. Diagram of bilayer lipid membrane of conductive tissue with sodium channel (*cross-hatching*) spanning the membrane. Tertiary amine local anesthetics exist as neutral base (N) and protonated, charged form (NH^+) in equilibrium. The neutral base (N) is more lipid soluble, preferentially partitions into the lipophilic membrane interior, and easily passes through the membrane. The charged form (NH^+) is more water soluble and binds to the sodium channel at the negatively charged membrane surface. Both forms can affect function of the sodium channel. The N form can cause membrane expansion and closure of the sodium channel. The NH^+ form will directly inhibit the sodium channel by binding with a local anesthetic receptor. The natural "local anesthetic" tetrodotoxin (TTX) binds at the external surface of the sodium channel and has no interaction with clinically used local anesthetics. (Adapted with permission from Strichartz GR: Neural physiology and local anesthetic action. In Cousins MJ, Bridenbaugh PO [eds]: Neural Blockade in Clinical Anesthesia and Management of Pain, p 35. Philadelphia, Lippincott–Raven, 1998.)

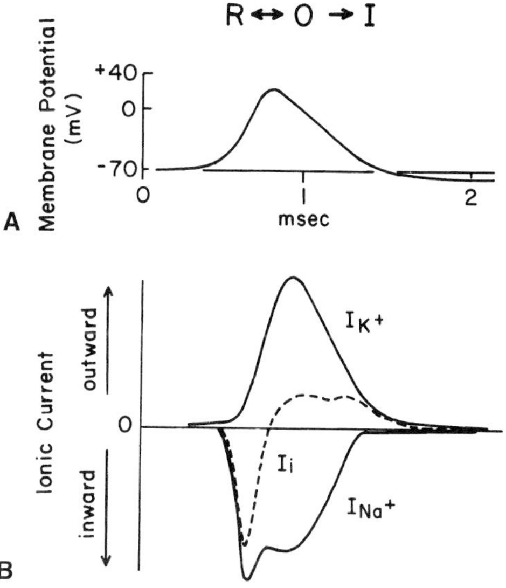

FIGURE 17-5. Illustration of dominant form of sodium channel during generation of an action potential. R = resting form, O = open form, I = inactive form. **Figure A** demonstrates the concurrent generation of an action potential, as the membrane depolarizes from resting potential. **Figure B** demonstrates concurrent changes in ion flux, as inward sodium current (I_{Na^+}) and outward potassium current (I_{K^+}) together yield the net ionic current across the membrane (I_i). (Adapted with permission from Strichartz GR: Neural physiology and local anesthetic action. In Cousins MJ, Bridenbaugh PO [eds]: Neural Blockade in Clinical Anesthesia and Management of Pain, p 35. Philadelphia, Lippincott–Raven, 1998.)

action potential because there is insufficient time for sodium channels to open. Nor will a depolarizing stimulus that increases too slowly create an action potential. As the stimulus slowly increases, initially activated sodium channels will spontaneously inactivate, so there will never be enough open channels at one time to generate an action potential. Furthermore, voltage-sensitive potassium channels would begin to increase potassium conductance that would further inhibit generation of an action potential. Thus, successful generation of an action potential requires a depolarizing stimulus of correct intensity and duration.

Once an action potential is generated, propagation of the potential along the nerve fiber is required for information to be transmitted. Both impulse generation and propagation are "all or nothing" phenomena. In the case of impulse propagation, either the locally generated action potential reaches the threshold potential of adjacent segments and causes propagation along the nerve, or the local depolarization ends. Nonmyelinated fibers require achievement of threshold potential at the immediately adjacent membrane, whereas myelinated fibers require generation of threshold potential at a subsequent node of Ranvier.

Repolarization after action potential generation and propagation rapidly follows owing to increasing equilibria of internal and external sodium ions, a time-controlled decrease in sodium conductance, and a voltage-controlled increase in potassium conductance.[11] In addition, active internal concentration of potassium occurs via the membrane-bound enzyme Na^+/K^+/ATPase that extrudes three sodium ions for every two potassium ions absorbed. Although many mammalian nonmyelinated nerve fibers develop a period of hyperpolarization after the action potential, myelinated nerve fibers return directly to resting membrane potential.[11]

Molecular Mechanisms of Action of Local Anesthetics

2 The sodium channel is the key target of local anesthetic activity. The wide variety of compounds that exhibit local anesthetic activity combined with the different effects of neutral and charged local anesthetics suggest that local anesthetics may act on the sodium channel either by modification of the lipid membrane surrounding it or by direct interaction with its protein structure.

Previous studies have demonstrated that anesthetics can reduce sodium conductance through sodium channels by interacting with the surrounding lipid membrane.[12] Alterations in neuronal membranes by local anesthetics can occur by altering the fluidity of the membrane that causes membrane expansion and subsequent closure of the sodium channel. Furthermore, alterations in membrane composition may lower the probability of occurrence of the open sodium channel state. Such observations can account for local anesthetic actions of neutral and lipophilic local anesthetics, but do not explain the different activity of clinically used, tertiary amine local anesthetics (e.g., lidocaine).

Instead, the mechanisms of action of these local anesthetics are best explained by direct interaction with the sodium channel (modulated receptor theory).[13] The commonly used tertiary amine local anesthetics exist in free equilibrium as both a lipid-soluble neutral form and a hydrophilic, charged form depending on pK_a and environmental pH. Although the neutral form may exert anesthetic actions as described earlier, the cationic species is clearly the more potent form (see Fig. 17-4).[13] These tertiary amine local anesthetics also demonstrate greater sodium channel blockade when the neural membrane is repetitively depolarized (1 to 100 Hz),[14,15] whereas neutral local anesthetics exhibit little change in activity with increased frequency of stimulation (use-dependent block). Increasing frequency of stimulation increases the probability that sodium channels will exist in the open and inactive forms as compared to the unstimulated state. Thus, differences in activity of tertiary amine local anesthetics between use-dependent (repetitive stimulation) and tonic (unstimulated) block are well explained by the existence of a single local anesthetic receptor within the sodium channel that possesses different affinities during different channel conformations (resting, open, inactive). Specifically, higher affinities occur during the open and inactive phases. In support of this theory, when the affinity of inactive channels for local anesthetics is decreased through genetic manipulation, use-dependent block is reduced.[16,17]

Molecular manipulation of the sodium channel has revealed specifics of the local anesthetic receptor.[8] Binding sites to local anesthetics are located on the intracellular side of the sodium channel, may have different binding areas during the open and inactivated conformations of the sodium channel, and possess stereoselectivity with preference for the *R* isomers.[9,17,18]

Mechanism of Blockade of Peripheral Nerves

3 Local anesthetics may block function of peripheral nerves through several mechanisms. As discussed earlier, sodium channel blockade leads to attenuation of neural action potential formation and propagation. Although it remains unknown in humans by what percent the neural action potential must be decreased before functional block occurs, animal studies suggest that the action potential must be decreased by at least 50% before measurable loss of function is observed.[6] Previous studies have examined the differences in susceptibility of nerve fiber to local anesthetic blockade based on size, myelination, and length of fiber exposed to local anesthetic. Clinically, one can often discern a differential pattern of sensory block after application of local anesthetic to a peripheral nerve.[19] Classically, the sensation of temperature is lost, followed by sharp pain, then light touch. Thus, an initial assumption was that small, unmyelinated (C) fibers conducting temperature sensation were inherently more susceptible to local anesthetic blockade than large, myelinated (A) fibers conducting touch. However, experimental studies reveal a more complex picture. In vivo studies of sciatic nerve block in rats with lidocaine indicate that larger A fibers are more susceptible to tonic and phasic block than smaller C fibers.[15] Differential block of large and small nerve fibers is also affected by choice of local anesthetic. Those with an amide group, high pK_a, and lower lipid solubility are more potent blockers of C fibers. Thus, experimental studies indicate that local anesthetic block of nerve fibers will intrinsically depend on type (size) of fiber, frequency of membrane stimulation, and choice of local anesthetic.[14,20]

During clinical applications, the exposure length of the nerve fiber may explain differential block,[21,22] as small nerve fibers require a shorter length of fiber exposed to local anesthetic for block to occur than do large fibers. It is theorized that this observation is because of decremental conduction block of a "critical length" of nerve.[22] Decremental conduction describes the decreased ability of successive nodes of Ranvier to propagate an impulse in the presence of local anesthetic (Fig. 17-6). As internodal distances become greater with increasing nerve fiber size,[23] larger nerve fibers will demonstrate increasing resistance to local anesthetic block. Evidence for this mechanism is conflicting. Sciatic nerve blocks in rats demonstrate greater length of spread along the nerve and greater intraneural content of radiolabeled lidocaine with injections of high volume and low concentrations of lidocaine. However, the use of small volumes and greater concentrations of lidocaine produced more effective sensory and motor block despite lesser spread and intraneural penetration of lidocaine.[24] Further clinical studies on decremental conduction and role of "critical

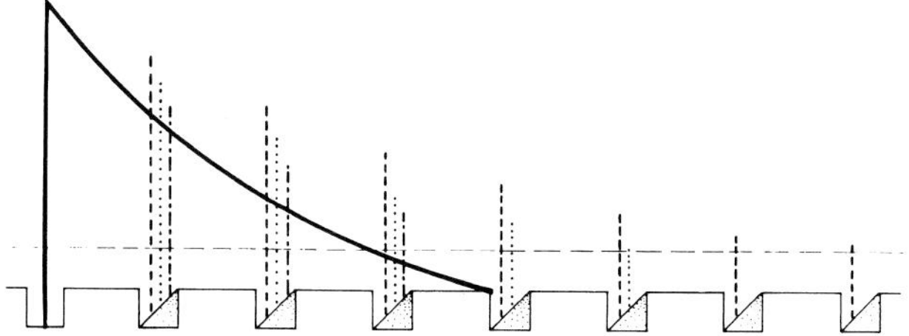

FIGURE 17-6. Diagram illustrating the principle of decremental conduction block by local anesthetic at a myelinated axon. The first node of Ranvier at left contains no local anesthetic and gives rise to a normal action potential (*solid curve*). If the nodes succeeding the first are occupied by a concentration of local anesthetic high enough to block 74 to 84% of the sodium conductance, then the action potential amplitudes decrease at successive nodes (amplitudes are indicated by interrupted bars representing three increasing concentration of local anesthetic). Eventually, the impulse decays to below threshold amplitude if the series of local anesthetic containing nodes is long enough. Propagation of the impulse has then been blocked by decremental conduction, even though none of the nodes are completely blocked. Concentrations of local anesthetic that block more than 84% of the sodium conductance at three successive nodes prevent any impulse propagation at all. (Adapted with permission from Fink BR: Mechanisms of differential axial blockade in epidural and spinal anesthesia. Anesthesiology 70:851, 1989.)

length" will be needed, especially as nerve blocks in humans typically involve much greater lengths of affected nerve than animal models. For example, sciatic nerve blocks in humans probably result in 5 to 10 cm of affected nerve length.[6]

A final mechanism whereby local anesthetics may block peripheral nerve function is via degradation of transmitted electrical patterns. It is theorized that a large part of the sensory information transmitted via peripheral nerves is carried via coding of electrical signals in after-potentials and after-oscillations.[25] Evidence for this theory is found in studies demonstrating loss of sensory nerve function after incomplete local anesthetic blockade. For example, sensation of temperature of the skin can be lost despite unimpeded conduction of small fibers.[26] Furthermore, a surgical depth of epidural and peripheral nerve block anesthesia can be obtained with only minor changes in somatosensory evoked potentials from the anesthetized area.[27,28] Previous studies have demonstrated that application of sub-blocking concentrations of local anesthetic will suppress normally occurring after-potentials and after-oscillations without significantly affecting action potential conduction.[29] Thus, disruption of coding of electrical information by local anesthetics may be another mechanism for block of peripheral nerves.

Mechanism of Blockade of Central Neuraxis

Central neuraxial block via spinal or epidural administration of local anesthetics involves the same mechanisms at the level of spinal nerve roots, either intra- or extradural, as discussed earlier. In addition, central neuraxial administration of local anesthetics allows multiple potential actions of local anesthetics within the spinal cord at different sites. For example, within the dorsal horn, local anesthetics can exert familiar ion channel block of sodium and potassium channels in dorsal horn neurons and inhibit generation and propagation of nociceptive electrical activity.[30] Other spinal cord neuronal ion channels, such as calcium channels, are also important for afferent and efferent electrical activity. Administration of calcium channel blockers to spinal cord N (neuronal) calcium channels results in hyperpolarization of cell membranes, resistance to electrical stimulation from nociceptive afferents, and intense analgesia.[31] Local anesthetics appear to have similar actions on calcium channels, which may contribute to analgesic actions of central neuraxially administered local anesthetics.[32]

In addition to ion channels, multiple neurotransmitters are involved in nociceptive transmission in the dorsal horn of the spinal cord.[33] For example, tachykinins (substance P) are important neurotransmitters modulating nociception from C fibers.[34] Administration of local anesthetics in concentrations that occur after spinal and epidural anesthesia inhibits postsynaptic depolarizations driven by substance P and may decrease nociception via this inhibitory mechanism.[35] Other neurotransmitters that are important for nociceptive processing in the spinal cord, such as acetylcholine, γ-aminobutyric acid (GABA), and N-methyl-D-aspartate (NMDA), can all be affected by local anesthetics either pre- or postsynaptically.[8,35] These studies suggest that antinociceptive effects of central neuraxial local anesthetic block may be mediated via complex interactions at neural synapses in addition to ion channel blockade.

PHARMACOLOGY AND PHARMACODYNAMICS

Chemical Properties and Relationship to Activity and Potency

The clinically used local anesthetics consist of a lipid-soluble, substituted benzene ring linked to an amine group (tertiary or quaternary depending on pK_a and pH) via an alkyl chain containing either an amide or ester linkage (Fig. 17-7). The type of linkage separates the local anesthetics into either *aminoamides*, metabolized in the liver, or *aminoesters*, metabolized by plasma cholinesterases. Several chemical properties of local anesthetics will affect their efficacy and potency.

All clinically used local anesthetics are weak bases that can exist as either the lipid-soluble, neutral form or as the charged, hydrophilic form. The combination of pH of the environment and pK_a, or dissociation constant, of a local anesthetic determines how much of the compound exists in each form (Table 17-2). As previously discussed, the primary site of action of local anesthetics appears to exist on the intracellular side of the sodium channel, and the charged form appears to be the predominantly active form.[13] Penetration of the lipid-soluble form through the lipid neural membrane appears to be the primary form of access of local anesthetic molecules, although some access by the charged form can be gained via the aqueous sodium channel pore (see Fig. 17-4).[39] Thus, decreasing pK_a for a given environmental pH will increase the percentage of lipid-soluble forms in existence, hastening penetration of neural membranes and onset of action.

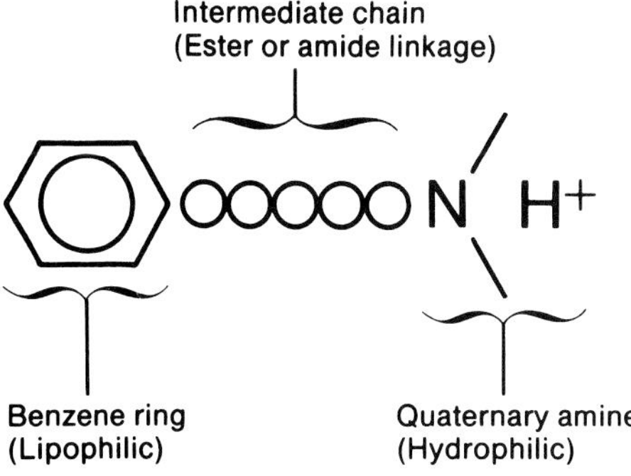

FIGURE 17-7. General struture of clinically used local anesthetics. (Adapted with permission from Carpenter RL, Mackey DC: Local anesthetics. In Barash PG, Cullen BF, Stoelting RF [eds]: Clinical Anesthesia, p 413. Philadelphia, Lippincott–Raven, 1996.)

TABLE 17-2

PHYSICOCHEMICAL PROPERTIES OF CLINICALLY USED LOCAL ANESTHETICS

LOCAL ANESTHETIC	pKa	% IONIZED (AT pH 7.4)	PARTITION COEFFICIENT (LIPID SOLUBILITY)	% PROTEIN BINDING
AMIDES				
Bupivacaine[a]	8.1	83	3,420	95
Etidocaine	7.7	66	7,317	94
Lidocaine	7.9	76	366	64
Mepivacaine	7.6	61	130	77
Prilocaine	7.9	76	129	55
Ropivacaine	8.1	83	775	94
ESTERS				
Chloroprocaine	8.7	95	810	N/A
Procaine	8.9	97	100	6
Tetracaine	8.5	93	5,822	94

N/A, not available.
[a] Levo-bupivacaine has same physicochemical properties as racemate.
Data from Liu SS. Local anesthetics and analgesia. In Ashburn MA, Rice LJ (eds): The Management of Pain, pp 141–170. New York, Churchill Livingstone Inc., 1997.

Lipid solubility is another important determinant of activity. Although increasing lipid solubility may hasten penetration of neural membranes, increasing solubility may also result in increased sequestration of local anesthetic in myelin and other lipid-soluble compartments. Thus, increasing lipid solubility usually slows the rate of onset of action.[40] Similarly, duration of action is increased as absorption of local anesthetic molecules into myelin and surrounding neural compartments creates a
4 depot for slow release of local anesthetics.[40] Finally, increased lipid solubility increases potency of the local anesthetic.[12,13] This observation may be explained by a correlation between lipid solubility and both sodium channel receptor affinity and ability to alter sodium channel conformation by direct effects on lipid cell membranes.

Degree of protein binding also affects activity of local anesthetics, as only the unbound form is free for pharmacologic activity. In general, the more lipid soluble and longer acting agents have increased protein binding.[41] Although the sodium channel is a protein structure, it does not appear that degree of local anesthetic protein binding correlates with binding to the local anesthetic receptor. Studies suggest that dissociation of local anesthetic molecules from the sodium channel occurs in a matter of seconds regardless of degree of protein binding of the local anesthetic.[42] Thus, prolongation in duration of action associated with an increased degree of protein binding must involve other extracellular or membranous proteins.

A final physical property of interest is stereoisomeric mixture of the commercially available local anesthetics. All currently available local anesthetics are racemic mixtures with the exception of lidocaine (achiral), ropivacaine (*S*), and
5 levo-bupivacaine ($l = S$).[43,44] Stereoisomers of local anesthetics appear to have potentially different effects on anesthetic potency, pharmacokinetics, and systemic toxicity.[19,43,44] For example, *R* isomers appear to have greater in vitro potency for block of both neural and cardiac sodium channels and may thus have greater therapeutic efficacy and potential systemic toxicity.[18,43–45]

Relative in vitro potencies of the clinically used local anesthetics have been identified and vary depending on individual nerve fibers and frequency of stimulation, and overall increasing lipid solubility of local anesthetic correlates with increasing anesthetic potency (see Table 17-2).[46] However, clinical use of local anesthetics is complex and in vivo potencies often do not correlate with in vitro determinants.[47] Local factors affecting diffusion and spread of anesthetic will have great impact on clinical effects and will vary with different applications (e.g., peripheral nerve block vs. spinal injection). Furthermore, clinical use may not require absolute suppression of the compound action potential, but rather a disruption of information coding in the pattern of discharges. Few rigorous studies have been performed to evaluate relative clinical potencies of local anesthetics, and commonly accepted values are listed in Table 17-3.

Tachyphylaxis to Local Anesthetics

Tachyphylaxis to local anesthetics is a clinical phenomenon whereby repeated injection of the same dose of local anesthetic leads to decreasing efficacy. Tachyphylaxis has been described after central neuraxial blocks, peripheral nerve blocks, and for different local anesthetics.[48,49] An interesting clinical feature of tachyphylaxis to local anesthetics is dependence on dosing interval. If dosing intervals are short enough such that pain does not occur, tachyphylaxis does not develop. Conversely, longer periods of patient discomfort before redosing hasten development of tachyphylaxis.[48] Both pharmacokinetic and dynamic mechanisms may be involved. A study examining repeated sciatic nerve blocks and infiltration analgesia in rats noted tachyphylaxis accompanied by increased clearance of radiolabeled lidocaine out of nerves and skin.[50] Not all studies support a pharmacokinetic mechanism for tachyphylaxis. For example, with the development of clinical tachyphylaxis, there is no difference in local anesthetic spread within or clearance from the epidural space.[51]

The observation that pain is important for the development of tachyphylaxis has led to speculation that there is a pharmacodynamic mechanism for tachyphylaxis via spinal cord sensitization.[52] Rats receiving repeated sciatic nerve blocks failed to develop tachyphylaxis in the absence of noxious stimulation. Exposure of the rats to increasingly noxious degrees of thermal stimulation increasingly hastened development of tachyphylaxis, whereas pretreatment with an NMDA antagonist (MK-801) that prevents spinal cord sensitization also prevented development of tachyphylaxis. Second-messenger effects of nitric oxide for NMDA pathways may be especially important, as administration of nitric oxide synthetase inhibitors prevented development of tachyphylaxis in a

TABLE 17-3

RELATIVE POTENCY OF LOCAL ANESTHETICS FOR DIFFERENT CLINICAL APPLICATIONS

	BUPIVACAINE	CHLOROPROCAINE	LIDOCAINE	MEPIVACAINE	PRILOCAINE	ROPIVACAINE
Peripheral nerve	3.6	N/A	1	2.6	0.8	3.6
Spinal	9.6	1	1	1	1	N/A
Epidural	4	0.5	1	1	1	4

N/A, not available.
Data from Camorcia M. Minimum local analgesic doses of ropivacaine, levobupivacaine, and bupivacaine for intrathecal labor analgesia. Anesthesiology 2005:102:646. Faccenda KA. A comparison of levobupivacaine 0.5% and racemic bupivacaine 0.5% for extradural anesthesia for caesarean section. Reg Anesth Pain Med 2003;28:394. McDonald SB. Hyperbaric spinal ropivacaine: a comparison to bupivacaine in volunteers. Anesthesiology 1999:90:971. Marsan A. Prilocaine or mepivacaine for combined sciatic-femoral nerve block in patients receiving elective knee arthroscopy. Minerva Anestesiol 2004;70:763. Casati A. Lidocaine versus ropivacaine for continuous interscalene brachial plexus blockafter open shoulder surgery. Acta Anaesthesiol Scand 2003;47:35. Casati A. A double-blind study of axillary brachial plexus block by 0.75% ropivacaine or 2% mepivacaine. Eur J Anaesthesiol 1998;15:549. Fanelli G. A double-blind comparison of ropivacaine, bupivacaine, and mepivacaine during sciatic and femoral nerve blockade. Anesth Analg, 1998;87:597. Yoos JR. Spinal 2-chloroprocaine: a comparison with small-dose bupivacaine in volunteers. Anesth Analg 2005 Feb;100:566. Kouri ME. Spinal 2-chloroprocaine: a comparison with lidocaine in volunteers. Anesth Analg 2004 Jan:98:75.

dose-dependent manner in the same model.[53] The clinical relevance of these findings needs to be explored, but the development of a mechanism for tachyphylaxis may lead to clinical means for its prevention.

Additives to Increase Local Anesthetic Activity

Epinephrine

3 Epinephrine has been added to local anesthetics since the early 1890s. Reported benefits of epinephrine include prolongation of local anesthetic block, increased intensity of block, and decreased systemic absorption of local anesthetic.[54] Epinephrine's vasoconstrictive effects augment local anesthetics by antagonizing inherent vasodilating effects of local anesthetics, decreasing systemic absorption and intraneural clearance, and perhaps by redistributing intraneural local anesthetic.[54,55]

Direct analgesic effects from epinephrine may also occur via interaction with α-2 adrenergic receptors in the brain and spinal cord,[56] especially because local anesthetics increase the vascular uptake of epinephrine.[57] Clinical use of epinephrine is listed in Table 17-4. The smallest dose is suggested, as epinephrine combined with local anesthetics may have toxic effects on tissue,[58] the cardiovascular system,[59] peripheral nerves, and the spinal cord.[33,54]

Alkalinization of Local Anesthetic Solution

Since the late 1800s, local anesthetic solutions have been alkalinized in order to hasten onset of neural block.[60] The pH of commercial preparations of local anesthetics ranges from 3.9 to 6.47 and is especially acidic if prepackaged with epinephrine.[61]

TABLE 17-4

EFFECTS OF ADDITION OF EPINEPHRINE TO LOCAL ANESTHETICS

	INCREASE DURATION	DECREASE BLOOD LEVELS (%)	DOSE/CONCENTRATION OF EPINEPHRINE
NERVE BLOCK			
Bupivacaine	+−	10–20	1:200,000
Lidocaine	++	20–30	1:200,000
Mepivacaine	++	20–30	1:200,000
Ropivacaine	−−	0	1:200,000
EPIDURAL			
Bupivacaine	+−	10–20	1:300,000–1:200,000
L-bupivacaine	+−	10	1:200,000–400,000
Chloroprocaine	++		1:200,000
Lidocaine	++	20–30	1,600,000–1:200,000
Mepivacaine	++	20–30	1:200,000
Ropivacaine	−−	0	1:200,000
SPINAL			
Bupivacaine	+−		0.2 mg
Lidocaine	++		0.2 mg
Tetracaine	++		0.2 mg

++, overall supported; −−, overall not supported; +−, inconsistent.
Data from Liu SS. Local Anesthetics and Analgesia. In, Ashburn MA, Rice LJ (eds): The Management of Pain. New York: Churchill Livingstone Inc., 1997:141–170 and Kopacz DJ. A comparison of epidural levobupivacaine 0.5% with or without epinephrine for lumbar spine surgery. Anesth Analg 2001;93:755.

As the pK_a of commonly used local anesthetics ranges from 7.6 to 8.9 (see Table 17-2), less than 3% of the commercially prepared local anesthetic exists as the lipid-soluble neutral form. As previously discussed, the neutral form is believed to be the most important for penetration into the neural cytoplasm, whereas the charged form primarily interacts with the local anesthetic receptor within the sodium channel. Therefore, the rationale for alkalinization was to increase the percentage of local anesthetic existing as the lipid-soluble neutral form. However, clinically used local anesthetics cannot be alkalinized beyond a pH of 6.05 to 8 before precipitation occurs,[61] and such pHs will only increase the neutral form to about 10%.

Clinical studies that have shown an association between alkalinization of local anesthetics and hastening of block onset have shown a decrease of less than 5 minutes when compared to commercial preparations.[60,62] In addition, a recent animal study suggests that alkalinization of lidocaine decreases the duration of peripheral nerve blocks if the solution does not also contain epinephrine.[63] Overall, the value of alkalinization of local anesthetics appears debatable as a clinically useful tool to improve anesthesia.

Opioids

Addition of opioids to local anesthetics has gained popularity. Opioids have multiple central neuraxial and peripheral mechanisms of analgesic action. Supraspinal administration of opioids results in analgesia via opiate receptors in multiple sites,[64] via activation of descending spinal pathways[65] and via activation of nonopioid analgesic pathways.[66] Spinal administration of opioids provides analgesia primarily by attenuating C fiber nociception[67] and is independent of supraspinal mechanisms.[68] Coadministration of opioids with central neuraxial local anesthetics results in synergistic analgesia.[69] An exception to this analgesic synergy is 2-chloroprocaine, which appears to decrease the effectiveness of epidural opioids when used for epidural anesthesia.[70] The mechanism for this action is unclear but does not appear to involve direct antagonism of opioid receptors.[71] Overall, clinical studies support the practice of central neuraxial coadministration of local anesthetics and opioids in humans for prolongation and intensification of analgesia and anesthesia.[69]

The discovery of peripheral opioid receptors offers yet another circumstance in which the coadministration of local anesthetics and opioids may be useful.[72] The most promising clinical results have been from intra-articular administration of local anesthetic and opioid for postoperative analgesia,[73] whereas combining local anesthetics and opioids for nerve blocks appears to be ineffective.[74] There are several reasons for a predicted lack of effect of coadministration of local anesthetic and opioid for peripheral nerve blocks. Anatomically, peripheral opioid receptors are found primarily at the end terminals of afferent fibers.[75] However, peripheral nerves are commonly blocked by deposition of anesthetic proximal to the end terminals of nerve fibers. In addition, common sites for peripheral nerve blocks are encased in multiple layers of connective tissue that the anesthetics must traverse before gaining access to peripheral opioid receptors. Finally, previous studies have demonstrated the importance of concomitant local tissue inflammation for analgesic effectiveness of peripheral opioid receptors.[72] The mechanism for the underlying dependence on local inflammation is speculative and may involve upregulation or activation of peripheral opioid receptors or "loosening" of intercellular junctions to allow passage of opioids to receptors. Lack of inflammation at the site of a peripheral nerve block may also reduce the effects of coadministration of local anesthetic and opioid. All of these factors combine to decrease the theoretical effectiveness of combinations of local anesthetics and opioids for peripheral nerve blocks. In summary, coadministration of opioids and local anesthetic in the central neuraxis appears to be an effective, nontoxic[33] means to improve activity of local anesthetic, whereas there is little theoretical reason to expect the mixture to enhance peripheral nerve block.

α-2 Adrenergic Agonists

α-2 adrenergic agonists can be a useful adjuvant to local anesthetics. α-2 agonists, such as clonidine, produce analgesia via supraspinal and spinal adrenergic receptors.[76] Clonidine also has direct inhibitory effects on peripheral nerve conduction (A and C nerve fibers).[77] Thus, addition of clonidine may have multiple routes of action depending on type of application. Preliminary evidence suggests that coadministration of an α-2 agonist and local anesthetic results in central neuraxial and peripheral nerve analgesic synergy,[78] whereas systemic (supraspinal) effects are additive.[79] Overall, clinical trials indicate that clonidine enhances intrathecal and epidural anesthesia, peripheral nerve blocks,[80] and intravenous regional anesthesia[81] without evidence for neurotoxicity.[33]

PHARMACOKINETICS OF LOCAL ANESTHETICS

Clearance of local anesthetic from neural tissue and from the body governs both duration of effect and potential toxicity. Clinical effects of neural block from local anesthetics are primarily dependent on local factors as discussed in the Pharmacology section. However, systemic toxicity is primarily dependent on blood levels of local anesthetics. Resultant blood levels after administration of local anesthetics for neural blockade depend on absorption, distribution, and elimination of local anesthetics.

Systemic Absorption

In general, local anesthetics with decreased systemic absorption will have a greater margin of safety in clinical use. The rate and extent of absorption will depend on numerous factors, of which the most important are the site of injection, the dose of local anesthetic, the physicochemical properties of the local anesthetic, and the addition of epinephrine.

The relative amounts of fat and vasculature surrounding the site of local anesthetic injection will interact with the physicochemical properties of the local anesthetic to affect rate of systemic uptake. In general, areas with greater vascularity will have more rapid and complete uptake as compared to those with more fat, regardless of type of local anesthetic. Thus, rates of absorption from injection of local anesthetic into various sites generally decrease in the following order: intercostal > caudal > epidural > brachial plexus > sciatic/femoral (Table 17-5).[82,83]

The greater the total dose of local anesthetic injected, the greater the systemic absorption and peak blood levels (C_{max}). This relationship is nearly linear (Fig. 17-8) and is relatively unaffected by anesthetic concentration[84] and speed of injection.[82,83]

Physicochemical properties of local anesthetics will affect systemic absorption. In general, the more potent agents with greater lipid solubility and protein binding will result in lower systemic absorption and C_{max} (Fig. 17-9).[83] Increased binding to neural and nonneural tissue probably explains this observation.

The effects of epinephrine have been previously discussed. In brief, epinephrine can counteract the inherent vasodilating characteristics of most local anesthetics. The reduction in C_{max} with epinephrine is most effective for the less lipid-soluble,

TABLE 17-5

TYPICAL C_{max} AFTER REGIONAL ANESTHETICS WITH COMMONLY USED LOCAL ANESTHETICS

LOCAL ANESTHETIC	TECHNIQUE	DOSE (mg)	C_{max} (mcg/mL)	T_{max} (min)	TOXIC PLASMA CONCENTRATION (mcg/mL)
Bupivacaine	Brachial plexus	150	1.0	20	3
	Celiac plexus	100	1.50	17	
	Epidural	150	1.26	20	
	Intercostal	140	0.90	30	
	Lumbar sympathetic	52.5	0.49	24	
	Sciatic femoral	400	1.89	15	
L-bupivacaine	Epidural	75	0.36	50	4
	Brachial plexus	250	1.2	55	
Lidocaine	Brachial plexus	400	4.00	25	5
	Epidural	400	4.27	20	
	Intercostal	400	6.8	15	
Mepivacaine	Brachial plexus	500	3.68	24	5
	Epidural	500	4.95	16	
	Intercostal	500	8.06	9	
	Sciatic femoral	500	3.59	31	
Ropivacaine	Brachial plexus	190	1.3	53	4
	Epidural	150	1.07	40	
	Intercostal	140	1.10	21	

C_{max}, peak plasma levels; T_{max}, time until C_{max}.
Data from Liu SS. Local Anesthetics and Analgesia. In Ashburn MA, Rice LJ (eds): The Management of Pain. New York: Churchill Livingstone Inc., 1997:141–170, Berrisford RG. Plasma concentrations of bupivacaine and its enantiomers during continuous extrapleural intercostal nerve block. British Journal of Anaesthesia 70:201, 1993. Kopacz DJ. A comparison of epidural levobupivacaine 0.5% with or without epinephrine forlumbar spine surgery. Anesth Analg 2001 Sep:93:755, and Crews JC. Levobupivacaine for axillary brachial plexus block: a pharmacokinetic and clinical comparison in patients with normal renal function or renal disease. Anesth Analg 2002;95:219.

less potent, shorter acting agents (see Table 17-4), as increased tissue binding rather than local blood flow may be a greater determinant of absorption for the long-acting agents.

Distribution

After systemic absorption, local anesthetics are rapidly distributed to the body. Regional distribution of local anesthetic will depend on organ blood flow, the partition coefficient of local anesthetic between compartments, and plasma protein binding. The end organs of main concern for toxicity are within the cardiovascular and the central nervous systems. Both are considered members of the "vessel-rich group" and will have local anesthetic rapidly distributed to them. Despite the high blood perfusion, regional blood and tissue levels of local anesthetics within these organs will not initially correlate with systemic blood levels because of hysteresis.[85] As regional, rather than systemic, pharmacokinetics govern subsequent pharmacodynamic effects, systemic blood levels may not correlate with effects of local anesthetics on end organs.[86] Regional pharmacokinetics of local anesthetics for the heart and brain have not been fully delineated; thus the volume of distribution at steady state (VDss) is often used to describe local anesthetic distribution (Table 17-6). However, VDss describes the extent of total body distribution and may be inaccurate for specific organ systems.

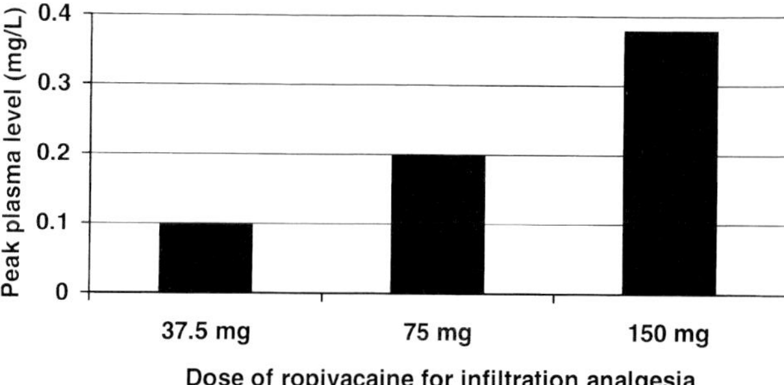

FIGURE 17-8. Increasing doses of ropivacaine used for wound infiltration result in linearly increasing maximal plasma concentrations (C_{max}). (Data from from Mulroy MF, Burgess FW, Emanuelsson B-M: Ropivacaine 0.25% and 0.5%, but not 0.125%, provide effective wound infiltration analgesia after outpatient hernia repair, but with sustained plasma drug levels. Reg Anesth Pain Med 24:136, 1999.)

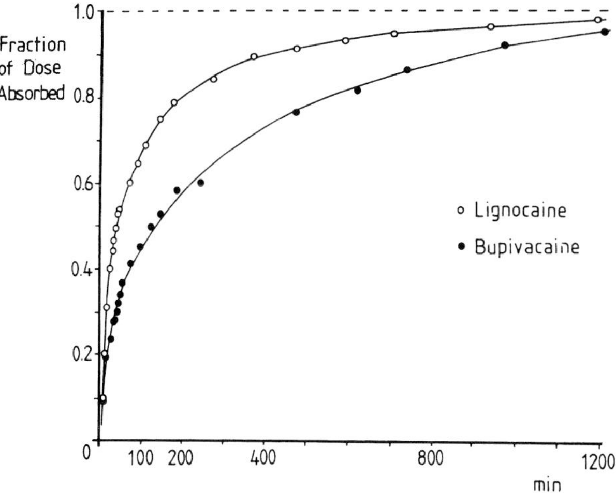

FIGURE 17-9. Fraction of dose absorbed into the systemic circulation over time from epidural injection of lidocaine or bupivacaine. Bupivacaine is a more lipid soluble, more potent agent with less systemic absorption over time. (Adapted with permission from Tucker GT, Mather LE: Properties, absorption, and disposition of local anesthetic agents. In Cousins MJ, Bridenbaugh PO [eds]: Neural Blockade in Clinical Anesthesia and Management of Pain, p 55. Philadelphia, Lippincott–Raven, 1998.)

TABLE 17-6

PHARMACOKINETIC PARAMETERS OF CLINICALLY USED LOCAL ANESTHETICS

■ LOCAL ANESTHETIC	■ VDss (L/kg)	■ CL (L/kg/hr)	■ T1/2 (hr)
Bupivacaine	1.02	0.41	3.5
Levo-bupivacaine	0.78	0.32	2.6
Chloroprocaine	0.50	2.96	0.11
Etidocaine	1.9	1.05	2.6
Lidocaine	1.3	0.85	1.6
Mepivacaine	1.2	0.67	1.9
Prilocaine	2.73	2.03	1.6
Procaine	0.93	5.62	0.14
Ropivacaine	0.84	0.63	1.9

Data from Denson DD: Physiology and pharmacology of local anesthetics. In Sinatra RS, Hord AH, Ginsberg B, et al (eds): Acute Pain. Mechanisms and Management, p 124. St. Louis, Mosby Year Book, 1992 and Burm AG, van der Meer AD, van Kleef JW, et al: Pharmacokinetics of the enantiomers of bupivacaine following intravenous administration of the racemate. Br J Clin Pharmacol 38:125–129, 1994.

TABLE 17-7

RELATIVE POTENCY FOR SYSTEMIC CENTRAL NERVOUS SYSTEM TOXICITY BY LOCAL ANESTHETICS AND RATIO OF DOSAGE NEEDED FOR CARDIOVASCULAR SYSTEM: CENTRAL NERVOUS SYSTEM (CVS:CNS) TOXICITY

■ AGENT	■ RELATIVE POTENCY FOR CNS TOXICITY	■ CVS:CNS
Bupivacaine	4.0	2.0
Levo-bupivacaine	2.9	2.0
Chloroprocaine	0.3	3.7
Etidocaine	2.0	4.4
Lidocaine	1.0	7.1
Mepivacaine	1.4	7.1
Prilocaine	1.2	3.1
Procaine	0.3	3.7
Ropivacaine	2.9	2.0
Tetracaine	2.0	

Data from Liu SS. Local Anesthetics and Analgesia. In Ashburn MA, Rice LJ, (eds): The Management of Pain. New York: Churchill Livingstone Inc., 1997:141–170. Groban L. Central nervous system and cardiac effects from long-acting amide local anesthetic toxicity in the intact animal model. Reg Anesth Pain Med 2003 Jan–Feb; 28(1):3–11.

Elimination

Clearance (CL) of aminoester local anesthetics is primarily dependent on plasma clearance by cholinesterases,[87] whereas aminoamide local anesthetic clearance is dependent on clearance by the liver.[88] Thus, hepatic extraction, hepatic perfusion, hepatic metabolism, and protein binding (Table 17-2) will primarily determine the rate of clearance of aminoamide local anesthetics. In general, local anesthetics with higher rates of clearance will have a greater margin of safety.[83]

Clinical Pharmacokinetics

The primary benefit of knowledge of the systemic pharmacokinetics of local anesthetics is the ability to predict C_{max} after the agents are administered, thereby avoiding the administration of toxic doses (Tables 17-5, 17-7, and 17-8). However, pharmacokinetics are difficult to predict in any given circumstance as both physical and pathophysiologic characteristics will affect the individual pharmacokinetics. There is some evidence for increased systemic levels of local anesthetics in the very young and in the elderly owing to decreased clearance and increased absorption,[83] whereas correlation of resultant systemic blood levels between dose of local anesthetic and patient weight is often inconsistent (Figure 17-10).[89] Effects of gender on clinical pharmacokinetics of local anesthetics have not been well defined,[90] although pregnancy may decrease clearance.[83] Pathophysiologic states such as cardiac and hepatic disease will alter expected pharmacokinetic parameters (Table 17-9), and lower doses of local anesthetics should be used for these patients. As expected, renal disease has little effect on pharmacokinetic parameters of local anesthetics (Table 17-9). Finally, the skill of the anesthesiologist should be considered, as a large dose of local anesthetic placed in the correct location may have much less potential for systemic toxicity than a small dose incorrectly injected intravascularly. All of these factors should be considered when utilizing local anesthetics and minimizing systemic toxicity, the commonly accepted maximal dosages (Table 17-8) notwithstanding.

CLINICAL USE OF LOCAL ANESTHETICS

Local anesthetics are used in a variety of ways in clinical anesthesia practice. Probably the most common clinical use of local anesthetics for anesthesiologists is for regional anesthesia and analgesia. Central neuraxial anesthesia and analgesia can be accomplished by epidural or spinal injections of local anesthetics. Placement of epidural and spinal catheters can allow continuous infusion of local anesthetics and other analgesics for extended durations. Intravenous regional anesthesia and peripheral nerve blocks allow for anesthesia of the head and neck including the airway, upper extremities, trunk, and lower extremities. Newly developed catheters for continuous peripheral nerve blocks can also be placed to allow continuous infusions of local anesthetics and other analgesics for prolonged analgesia in a fashion similar to continuous epidural analgesia. Topical application of local anesthetics to the airway, eye, and skin provides sufficient anesthesia for painless performance of minor anesthetic and surgical procedures such as tracheal intubation, intravenous catheter placement, or dural puncture.[91] Typical applications for each local anesthetic are listed in Table 17-8.[92]

Other common clinical uses for local anesthetics include administration of lidocaine to blunt responses to tracheal instrumentation and to suppress cardiac dysrhythmias. Intravenous or topical administrations of lidocaine have been used with variable success to blunt hemodynamic response to tracheal intubation and extubation.[93,94] In addition to hemodynamic responses, instrumentation of the airway can result in coughing, bronchoconstriction, and other airway responses. Intravenous lidocaine can be effective for decreasing airway sensitivity to instrumentation by depressing airway reflexes and decreasing calcium flux in airway smooth muscle.[95,96] Doses of intravenous lidocaine from 2 to 2.5 mg/kg are needed to consistently blunt hemodynamic and airway responses to tracheal instrumentation.[95–97] Intravenous lidocaine is also effective for attenuating increases in intra-ocular pressure, intracranial pressure, and intra-abdominal pressure during

TABLE 17-8

CLINICAL PROFILE OF LOCAL ANESTHETICS

LOCAL ANESTHETIC	CONCENTRATION (%)	CLINICAL USE	ONSET	DURATION (h)	RECOMMENDED MAXIMUM SINGLE DOSE (mg)
AMIDES					
Bupivacaine	0.25	Infiltration	Fast	2–8	175/225 + epinephrine
L-bupivacaine*	0.25–0.5	Peripheral nerve block*	Slow	4–12	150
	0.5–0.75	Epidural anesthesia*	Moderate	2–5	150
	0.03–0.25	Epidural analgesia	NA	NA	NA
	0.5–0.75	Spinal anesthesia	Fast	1–4	20
Etidocaine	0.5	Infiltration	Fast	2–8	300/400 + epinephrine
	0.5–1	Peripheral nerve block	Fast	3–12	300/400 + epinephrine
	1–1.5	Epidural anesthesia	Fast	2–4	300/400 + epinephrine
Lidocaine	0.5–1	Infiltration	Fast	1–4	300/500 + epinephrine
	0.25–0.5	IV regional anesthesia	Fast	0.5–1	300
	1–1.5	Peripheral nerve block	Fast	1–3	300/500 + epinephrine
	1.5–2	Epidural anesthesia	Fast	1–2	300/500 + epinephrine
	1.5–5	Spinal anesthesia	Fast	0.5–1	100
	4	Topical	Fast	0.5–1	300
Mepivacaine	0.5–1	Infiltration	Fast	1–4	400/500 + epinephrine
	1–1.5	Peripheral nerve block	Fast	2–4	400/500 + epinephrine
	1.5–2	Epidural anesthesia	Fast	1–3	400/500 + epinephrine
	2–4	Spinal anesthesia	Fast	1–2	100
Prilocaine	0.5–1	Infiltration	Fast	1–2	600
	0.25–0.5	IV regional anesthesia	Fast	0.5–1	600
	1.5–2	Peripheral nerve block	Fast	1.5–3	600
	2–3	Epidural	Fast	1–3	600
Ropivacaine	0.2–0.5	Infiltration	Fast	2–6	200
	0.5–1	Peripheral nerve block	Slow	5–8	250
	0.5–1	Epidural anesthesia	Moderate	2–6	200
	0.05–0.2	Epidural analgesia	NA	NA	NA
MIXTURE					
Lidocaine + prilocaine	2.5/2.5	Skin topical	Slow	3–5	20 gm
ESTERS					
Benzocaine	Up to 20	Topical	Fast	0.5–1	200
Chloroprocaine	1	Infiltration	Fast	0.5–1	800/1,000 + epinephrine
	2	Peripheral nerve block	Fast	0.5–1	800/1,000 + epinephrine
	2–3	Epidural anesthesia	Fast	0.5–1	800/1,000 + epinephrine
Cocaine	4–10	Topical	Fast	0.5–1	150
Procaine	10	Spinal anesthesia	Fast	0.5–1	1,000
Tetracaine	2	Topical	Fast	0.5–1	20
	0.5	Spinal anesthesia	Fast	2–6	20

Adapted with permission from Covino BG, Wildsmith JAW: Clinical pharmacology of local anesthetic agents. In Cousins MJ, Bridenbaugh PO (eds): Neural blockade in clinical anesthesia and management of pain, pp 97–128. Philadephia, Lippincott–Raven, 1998.

airway instrumentation.[98] Attenuation of all these responses may be beneficial in selected clinical situations (e.g., corneal laceration or increased intracranial pressure). Intravenous lidocaine has well-recognized cardiac antidysrhythmic effects.[99]

Finally, intravenous lidocaine (1 to 5 mg/kg) is an effective analgesic and has been used to treat postoperative[100] and chronic neuropathic pain.[101] Peripheral and central inhibition of generation and propagation of spontaneous electrical activity in injured C nerve fibers and Aδ nerve fibers are thought to be primary mechanisms as opposed to typical conduction block.[102–104] Positron emission tomography in patients with neuropathic pain suggests that altered activity in cerebral blood flow to the thalamus[105] may also contribute to systemic analgesic effects of local anesthetics. The ability of local anesthetics to provide systemic analgesic effects at central and peripheral sites may in part explain the ability of a single neural block to provide long-lasting analgesia from neuropathic pain. In addition, orally administered mexiletine (a Class I antidysrhythmic agent similar to lidocaine) has been successfully used to treat chronic pain conditions.[101]

TOXICITY OF LOCAL ANESTHETICS

Systemic Toxicity of Local Anesthetics

Central Nervous System Toxicity

Local anesthetics readily cross the blood-brain barrier, and generalized CNS toxicity may occur from systemic absorption or

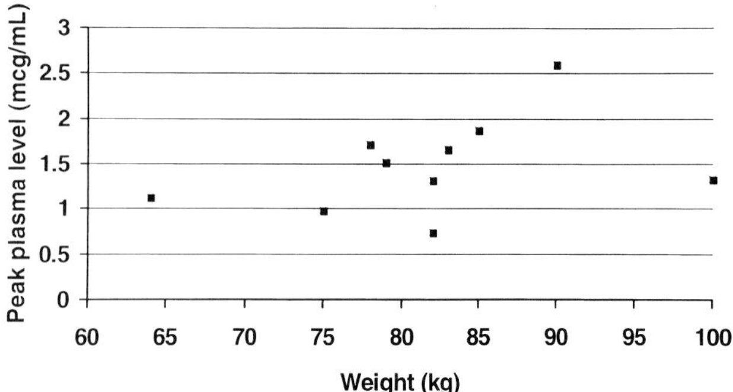

FIGURE 17-10. Lack of correlation between patient weight and peak plasma concentration after epidural administration of 150 mg of bupivacaine. (Data from Sharrock NE, Mather LE, Go G, et al: Arterial and pulmonary concentrations of the enatiomers of bupivacaine after epidural injection in elderly patients. Anesth Analg 86:812, 1998.)

TABLE 17-10

DOSE-DEPENDENT SYSTEMIC EFFECTS OF LIDOCAINE

PLASMA CONCENTRATION (mcg/mL)	EFFECT
1–5	Analgesia
5–10	Lightheadedness Tinnitus Numbness of tongue
10–15	Seizures Unconsciousness
15–25	Coma Respiratory arrest
>25	Cardiovascular depression

direct vascular injection. Signs of generalized CNS toxicity because of local anesthetics are dose dependent (Table 17-10). Low doses produce CNS depression, and higher doses result in CNS excitation and seizures.[106] The rate of intravenous administration of local anesthetic will also affect signs of CNS toxicity, as higher rates of infusion of the same dose will lessen the appearance of CNS depression while leaving excitation intact.[107] This dichotomous reaction to local anesthetics may be a result of a greater sensitivity of cortical inhibitory neurons to the impulse blocking effects of local anesthetics.[106,108,109]

Local anesthetic potency for generalized CNS toxicity approximately parallels action potential blocking potency (Tables 17-3 and 17-7).[106] In general, decreased local anesthetic protein binding and clearance will increase potential CNS toxicity. External factors can increase potency for CNS toxicity, such as acidosis and increased P_{CO_2}, perhaps via increased cerebral perfusion or decreased protein binding of local anesthetic.[106] There are also external factors that can decrease local anesthetic potency for generalized CNS toxicity. For example, seizure thresholds of local anesthetics are increased by administration of barbiturates and benzodiazepines.[110]

Addition of vasoconstrictors such as epinephrine may reduce or promote the potential for generalized local anesthetic CNS toxicity. Addition of epinephrine to local anesthetics will decrease systemic absorption and peak blood levels and increase the safety margin. On the other hand, the convulsive threshold for intravenous administration of lidocaine in the rat is decreased by about 42% when epinephrine (1:100,000), norepinephrine, or phenylephrine is added to the plain solution.[111] The mechanisms of increased toxicity with addition of epinephrine are unclear but appear to depend on the development of hypertension from vasoconstriction. A hyperdynamic circulatory system may enhance the toxic effects of local anesthetics by causing increased cerebral blood flow and delivery of lidocaine to the brain[112,113] or through disruption of the blood-brain barrier.[114] In addition to enhancing distribution of local anesthetic to the brain, hyperdynamic circulatory changes can also decrease clearance of local anesthetic from the body because of changes in distribution of blood flow away from the liver. Changes in total body clearance from hyperdynamic circulatory changes induced by local anesthetic seizures have been studied in dogs.[115] Seizures significantly increased heart rate, blood pressure, and cardiac output while significantly decreasing total body clearance (29 to 68%) of lidocaine, mepivacaine, bupivacaine, and etidocaine.

Clinical reports suggest toxicity from local anesthetics used for regional anesthesia is uncommon. Surveys from France and
7 the United States of over 280,000 cases of regional anesthesia report an incidence of seizures with epidural injection approximating 1/10,000 and an incidence of 7/10,000 with peripheral nerve blocks.[108,109] There appears to be a higher incidence of local anesthetic toxicity during peripheral nerve blocks, perhaps because of differences in practice or less clinical awareness. Nonetheless, epidural anesthesia (primarily obstetrical) constituted all the cases of death or brain damage resulting from unintentional intravenous injection of local anesthetic in an analysis of closed malpractice claims in the United States from 1980 to 1999.[116]

TABLE 17-9

EFFECTS OF CARDIAC, HEPATIC, AND RENAL DISEASE ON LIDOCAINE PHARMACOKINETICS

	VDss (L/Kg)	CL (mL/kg/min)	T1/2(hr)
Normal	1.32	10.0	1.8
Cardiac failure	0.88	6.3	1.9
Hepatic disease	2.31	6.0	4.9
Renal disease	1.2	13.7	1.3

VDss, volume of distribution at steady state; CL, total body clearance; T1/2, terminal elimination half-life.
Data from Thomson PD. Lidocaine pharmacokinetics in advanced heart failure, liver disease, and renal failure in humans. Ann Intern Med 1973;78:499.

Cardiovascular Toxicity of Local Anesthetics

In general, much greater doses of local anesthetics are required to produce cardiovascular (CV) toxicity than CNS toxicity. Similar to CNS toxicity, potency for CV toxicity reflects the anesthetic potency of the agent (Tables 17-3 and 17-7). Attention has focused on the apparently exceptional cardiotoxicity of the more potent, more lipid-soluble agents (bupivacaine, levo-bupivacaine, ropivacaine). These agents appear to have a different sequence of CV toxicity than less potent agents, with bupivacaine being the most cardiotoxic. For example, increasingly toxic doses of lidocaine lead to hypotension, bradycardia, and hypoxia, whereas toxic doses of bupivacaine, levo-bupivacaine, and ropivacaine often result in sudden cardiovascular collapse as a result of ventricular dysrhythmias that are resistant to resuscitation (Fig. 17-11).[106,110,117]

Use of the single–optical isomer (*S*/*L*) preparations of ropivacaine and levo-bupivacaine may improve the safety profile for long-lasting regional anesthesia. Both ropivacaine and

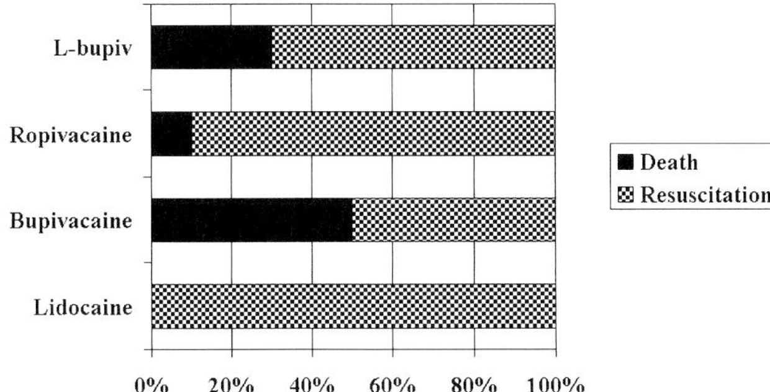

FIGURE 17-11. Success of resuscitation of dogs after cardiovascular collapse from intravenous infusions of lidocaine, bupivacaine, levo-bupivacaine, and ropivacaine. Success rates were greater for lidocaine (100%), than ropivacaine (90%), than levo-bupivacaine (70%), and than bupivacaine (50%). Required doses to induce cardiovascular collapse were greater for lidocaine (127 mg/kg), than ropivacaine (42 mg/kg), than levo-bupivacaine (27 mg/kg), and than bupivacaine (22 mg/kg). (Data from Groban L, Deal DD, Vernon JC, et al: Cardiac resuscitation after incremental overdosage with lidocaine, bupivacaine, levobupivacaine, and ropivacaine in anesthetized dogs. Anesth Analg 92:37, 2001.)

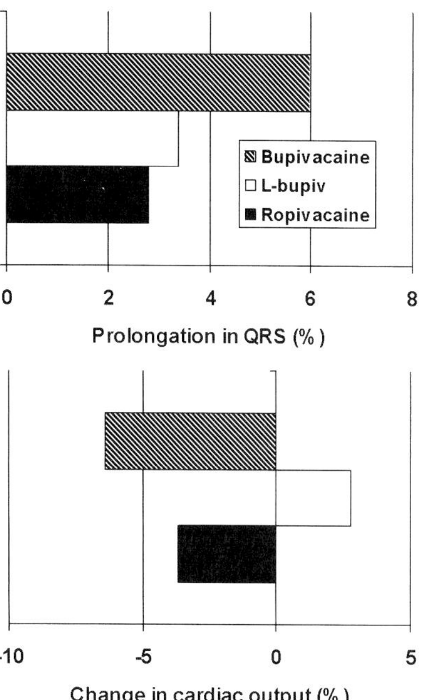

FIGURE 17-13. Mild prolongation in QRS interval and reduction in cardiac output are observed after intravenous infusions of bupivacaine (103 mg), levobupivacaine (37 mg), and ropivacaine (115 mg) in healthy volunteers. Data from: Knudsen K, Beckman Suurkula M, et al. Central nervous and cardiovascular effects of i.v. infusions of ropivacaine, bupivacaine and placebo in volunteers. Br Anaesth 1997:78:507. Stewart J, Kellett N, Castro D. The central nervous system and cardiovascular effects of levobupivacaine and ropivacaine in healthy volunteers. Anesth Analg 2003:97:412.

levo-bupivacaine appear to be approximately equipotent to racemic bupivacaine for epidural and plexus anesthesia (see Table 17-3).[118,119] Both ropivacaine and levo-bupivacaine have approximately 30 to 40% less systemic toxicity than bupivacaine on a mg:mg basis in animal studies[46,106] (Fig. 17-12), although human studies are less dramatic (Fig. 17-13).[120,121] Reduced potential for cardiotoxicity is likely because of reduced affinity for brain and myocardial tissue from their single isomer preparation.[18,45,106] In addition to stereoselectivity, the larger butyl side chain in bupivacaine may also have more of a cardiodepressant effect as opposed to the propyl-side chain of ropivacaine.[122]

Cardiovascular Toxicity Mediated at the CNS. It has been demonstrated that the central and peripheral nervous systems may be involved in the increased cardiotoxicity with bupivacaine. The nucleus tractus solitarii in the medulla is an important region for autonomic control of the cardiovascular system. Neural activity in the nucleus tractus solitarii of rats is markedly diminished by intravenous doses of bupivacaine immediately prior to development of hypotension. Furthermore, direct intracerebral injection of bupivacaine can elicit sudden dysrhythmias and cardiovascular collapse.[123]

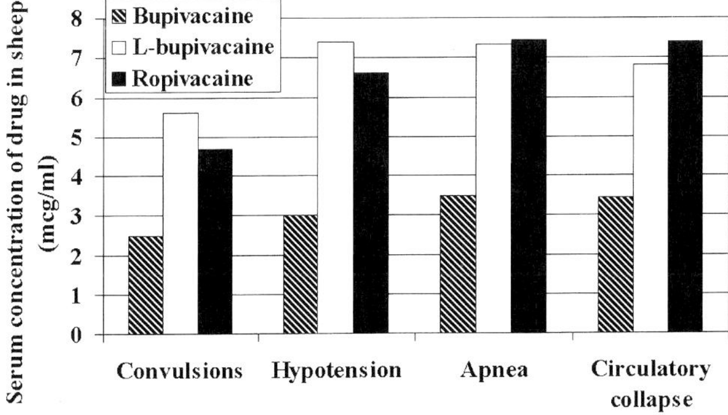

FIGURE 17-12. Serum concentrations in sheep at each toxic manifestation for bupivacaine, levo-bupivacaine, and ropivacaine in sheep. Both levo-bupivacaine and ropivacaine required significantly greater serum concentrations than bupivacaine. (Data from Santos AC, DeArmas PI: Systemic toxicity of levobupivacaine, bupivacaine, and ropivacaine during continuous intravenous infusion to nonpregnant and pregnant ewes. Anesthesiology 95:1256, 2001.)

Peripheral effects of bupivacaine on the autonomic and vasomotor systems may also augment its CV toxicity. Bupivacaine possesses a potent peripheral inhibitory effect on sympathetic reflexes[123] that has been observed even at blood concentrations similar to those measured after uncomplicated regional anesthesia.[124] Finally, bupivacaine also has potent direct vasodilating properties, which may exacerbate cardiovascular collapse.[125]

Cardiovascular Toxicity Mediated at the Heart. The more potent local anesthetics appear to possess greater potential for direct cardiac electrophysiologic toxicity.[45,106] Although all local anesthetics block the cardiac conduction system via a dose-dependent block of sodium channels, two features of bupivacaine's sodium channel blocking abilities may enhance its cardiotoxicity. First, bupivacaine exhibits a much stronger binding affinity to resting and inactivated sodium channels than lidocaine.[126] Second, local anesthetics bind to sodium channels during systole and dissociate during diastole (Fig. 17-14). Bupivacaine dissociates from sodium channels during cardiac diastole much more slowly than lidocaine. Indeed, bupivacaine dissociates so slowly that the duration of diastole at physiologic heart rates (60 to 180 bpm) does not allow enough time for complete recovery of sodium channels and bupivacaine conduction block accumulates. In contrast, lidocaine fully dissociates from sodium channels during diastole and little accumulation of conduction block occurs (Fig. 17-15).[126,127] Thus, enhanced electrophysiologic effects of more potent local anesthetics on the cardiac conduction system may explain their increased potential to produce sudden cardiovascular collapse via cardiac dysrhythmias.

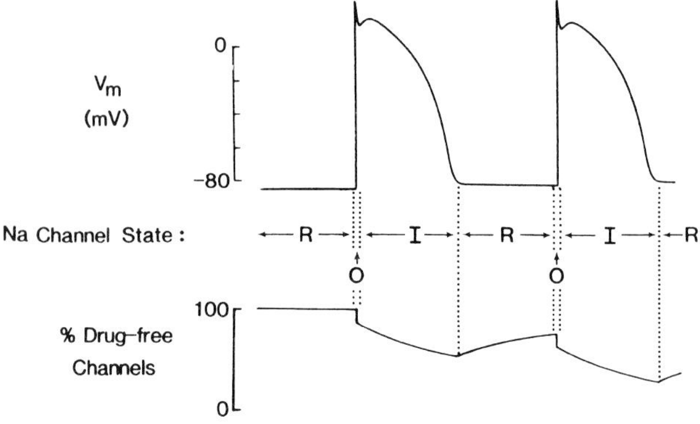

FIGURE 17-14. Diagram illustrating relationship between cardiac action potential (**top**), sodium channel state (**middle**), and block of sodium channels by bupivacaine (**bottom**). R = resting, O = open, and I = inactive forms of the sodium channel. Sodium channels are predominantly in the resting form during diastole, open transiently during the action potential upstroke, and are in the inactive form during the action potential plateau. Block of sodium channels by bupivacaine accumulates during the action potential (systole) with recovery occurring during diastole. Recovery of sodium channels is from dissociation of bupivacaine and is time dependent. Recovery during each diastolic interval is incomplete and results in accumulation of sodium channel block with successive heartbeats. (Adapted with permission from Clarkson CW, Hondegham LM: Mechanisms for bupivacaine depression of cardiac conduction: Fast block of sodium channels during the action potential with slow recovery from block during diastole. Anesthesiology 62:396, 1985.)

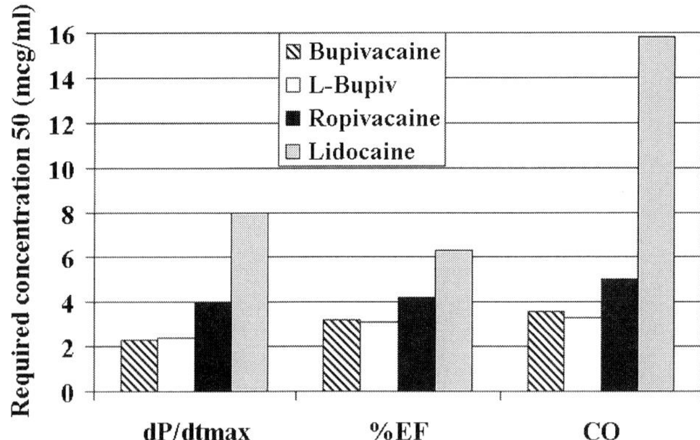

FIGURE 17-16. Plasma concentrations required to induce myocardial depression in dogs administered bupivacaine, levo-bupivacaine, ropivacaine, and lidocaine. dP/dtmax = 35% reduction of inotropy from baseline measure. %EF = 35% reduction in ejection fraction from baseline measure. CO = 25% reduction in cardiac output from baseline measure. (Data from Groban L, Deal DD, Vernon JC, et al: Does local anesthetic stereoselectivity or structure predict myocardial depression in anesthetized canines? Reg Anesth Pain Med 27:460, 2002.)

Increased potency for direct myocardial depression from the more potent local anesthetics is another contributing factor to increased cardiotoxicity (Fig. 17-16).[106,122] Again, multiple mechanisms may account for the increased potency for myocardial depression from more potent local anesthetics. Bupivacaine, the most completely studied potent local anesthetic, possesses a high affinity for sodium channels in the cardiac myocyte.[18,45,106] Furthermore, bupivacaine inhibits myocyte release and utilization of calcium[128] and reduces mitochondrial energy metabolism, especially during hypoxia.[129] Thus, multiple direct effects of bupivacaine on activity of the cardiac myocyte may explain the cardiotoxicity of bupivacaine and other potent local anesthetics.

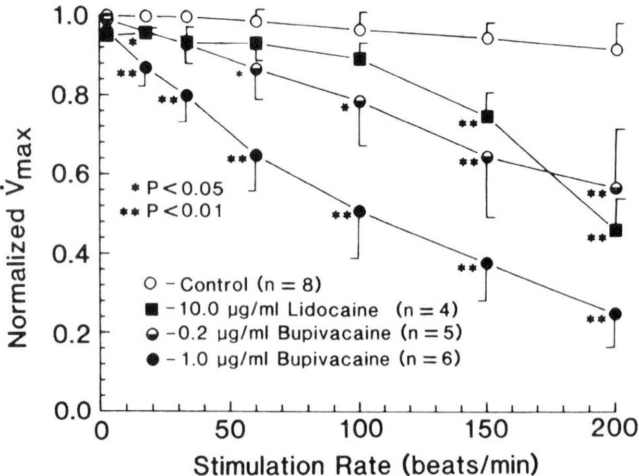

FIGURE 17-15. Heart rate dependent effects of lidocaine and bupivacaine on velocity of the cardiac action potential (V_{max}). Bupivacaine progressively decreases V_{max} at heart rates above 10 bpm because of accumulation of sodium channel block, whereas lidocaine does not decrease V_{max} until heart rate exceeds 150 bpm. (Adapted with permission from Clarkson CW, Hondegham LM: Mechanisms for bupivacaine depression of cardiac conduction: Fast block of sodium channels during the action potential with slow recovery from block during diastole. Anesthesiology 62: 396, 1985.)

Treatment of Systemic Toxicity from Local Anesthetics

8 The best method for avoiding systemic toxicity from local anesthetics is through prevention. Toxic systemic levels can occur by unintentional intravenous or intra-arterial injection or by systemic absorption of excessive doses placed in the correct area. Unintentional intravascular and intra-arterial injections can be minimized by frequent syringe aspiration for blood, use of a small test dose of local anesthetic (~3 mL) to test for subjective systemic effects from the patient (e.g., tinnitus, circumoral numbness), and either slow injection or fractionation of the rest of the dose of local anesthetic.[110] Detailed knowledge of local anesthetic pharmacokinetics will also aid in reducing the administration of excessive doses of local anesthetics. Ideally, heart rate, blood pressure, and the electrocardiogram should be monitored during administration of large doses local anesthetics. Pretreatment with a benzodiazepine may also lower the probablility of seizure by raising the seizure threshhold.

Treatment of systemic toxicity is primarily supportive. Injection of local anesthetic should be stopped. Oxygenation and ventilation should be maintained, as systemic toxicity of local anesthetics is enhanced by hypoxemia, hypercarbia, and acidosis.[110] If needed, the patient's trachea should be intubated and positive pressure ventilation instituted. As previously discussed, signs of CNS toxicity will typically occur prior to CV events. Seizures can increase body metabolism and cause hypoxemia, hypercarbia, and acidosis. Pharmacologic treatment to terminate seizures may be needed if oxygenation and ventilation cannot be maintained. Intravenous administration of thiopental (50 to 100 mg), midazolam (2 to 5 mg), and propofol (1 mg/kg) can terminate seizures from systemic local anesthetic toxicity. Succinylcholine (50 mg) can terminate muscular activity from seizures and facilitate ventilation and oxygenation. However, succinylcholine will not terminate seizure activity in the CNS, and increased cerebral metabolic demands will continue unabated.

Cardiovascular depression from less potent local anesthetics (e.g., lidocaine) is usually mild and caused by mild myocardial depression and vasodilation. Hypotension and bradycardia can usually be treated with ephedrine (10 to 30 mg) and atropine (0.4 mg). As previously discussed, potent local anesthetics (e.g., bupivacaine) can produce profound CV depression and malignant dysrhythmias that should be promptly treated. Oxygenation and ventilation must be immediately instituted, with cardiopulmonary resuscitation if needed. Ventricular dysrhythmias may be difficult to treat and may need large and multiple doses of electrical cardioversion, epinephrine, vasopressin, and amiodarone. The use of calcium channel blockers in this setting is not recommended, as its cardiodepressant effect is exaggerated.[110] A novel and promising treatment for cardiac toxicity is the administration of intravenous lipid to theoretically remove bupivacaine from sites of action. Administration of a 20% lipid solution at a dose of 4 mL/kg followed by a 0.5 mL/kg/min infusion for 10 minutes allowed for the resuscitation of 100% of dogs with induced bupivacaine cardiotoxicity at a dose of 10mg/kg.[130] None of the dogs given an equivalent volume of crystalloid were rescuscitated in this study. These findings raise the question of whether propofol in a 10% lipid solution would be a preferred treatment for cardiac toxicity. Propofol has been reported to terminate bupivacaine-induced seizures and cardiac depression in patients.[130] However, the dose of lipid in a standard induction dose of propofol (2 mg/kg) would be only 3% of the dose used in the aforementioned animal experiment. As effects of lipid on cardiac toxicity are dose related, further information is needed prior to reaching conclusions on clinical use of propofol for local anesthetic–induced cardiac toxicity.

Neural Toxicity of Local Anesthetics

In addition to systemic toxicity, local anesthetics can cause injury to the central and peripheral nervous system from direct exposure. Mechanisms for local anesthetic neurotoxicity remain speculative, but previous studies have demonstrated local anesthetic–induced injury to Schwann cells, inhibition of fast axonal transport, disruption of the blood-nerve barrier, decreased neural blood flow with associated ischemia, and disruption of cell membrane integrity via a detergent property of local anesthetics.[131,132] Although all clinically used local anesthetics can cause concentration-dependent nerve fiber damage in peripheral nerves when used in high enough concentrations, previous studies have demonstrated that local anesthetics in clinically used concentrations are generally safe for peripheral nerves.[133] The spinal cord and the nerve roots, on the other hand, are more prone to injury.

Spinal cord toxicity of local anesthetics has been assessed by administration of local anesthetics to rabbits via intrathecal catheters. These studies suggest that bupivacaine (2%), lidocaine (8%), and tetracaine (1%) cause histopathologic changes and neurologic deficits. On the other hand, clinically relevant concentrations of these agents, chloroprocaine and ropivacaine (2%), did not disrupt spinal cord histology or cause nerurological deficits.[134] Desheathed peripheral nerve models, designed to mimic unprotected nerve roots in the cauda equina, have been used to further assess electrophysiologic neurotoxicity of local anesthetics.[135–137] Lidocaine 5% and tetracaine 0.5% caused irreversible conduction block in these models, whereas lidocaine 1.5%, bupivacaine 0.75%, and tetracaine 0.06% did not. Electrophysiologic toxicity of lidocaine in isolated nerve preparations represented by incomplete recovery of neuromuscular function occurs at 40 m*M* (~1%) (Fig. 17-17), with irreversible ablation of the compound action potential seen at

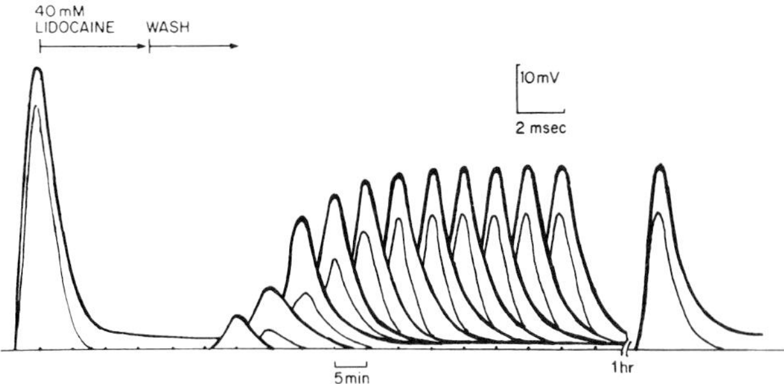

FIGURE 17-17. The nonreversible effect of 40 mM lidocaine on the compound action potential (CAP) of frog sciatic nerve. Lidocaine was applied to a stable nerve preparation for 15 minutes and then washed with frog Ringer's solution for 2 hours. Tracings represent CAPs in response to stimulus (1-Hz stimulus = heavy line; 40-Hz stimulus = thin line). 40 mM lidocaine completely ablated the CAP when applied to the nerve. The 1-Hz CAP response began to return after 10 to 15 minutes of washing and reached a new level in 45 minutes, where it was stable for the subsequent 2 hours of observation. The recovered 1-Hz CAP is only 65% of the original. (Adapted with permission from Bainton C: Concentration dependence of lidocaine-induced irreversible conduction loss frog nerve. Anesthesiology 81:657, 1994.)

80 m*M* (~2%). Although such studies do not reflect in vivo conditions, they suggest that lidocaine and tetracaine may be especially neurotoxic in a concentration-dependent fashion and that neurotoxicity could theoretically occur with clinically used solutions. Local anesthetic effects on spinal cord blood flow, another possible etiology of neurotoxicity from direct drug exposure, appear benign. Spinal administration of bupivacaine, lidocaine, mepivacaine, and tetracaine cause vasodilation and increase spinal cord blood flow, whereas ropivacaine causes vasoconstriction and reduction in spinal cord blood flow in a concentration-dependent fashion.[138]

Neurohistopathologic data in humans after intrathecal exposure to local anesthetics is not available. Electrophysiologic parameters such as somatosensory evoked potentials, monosynaptic H-reflex,[139] and cutaneous current perception thresholds[140] have been used to evaluate recovery after spinal anesthesia. These measurements have shown complete return to baseline activity after 5% lidocaine spinal anesthesia in very small study populations. Prospective surveys of over 80,000 spinal anesthetics report an incidence of 0 to 0.02% long-term neurologic injury in patients undergoing spinal anesthesia.[109] Thus, spinally administered local anesthetics have not notably manifested clinical neurotoxicity.

Transient Neurologic Symptoms after Spinal Anesthesia

Prospective, randomized studies reveal a 4 to 40% incidence of transient neurologic symptoms (TNS), including pain or sensory abnormalities in the lower back, buttocks, or lower extremities, after lidocaine spinal anesthesia.[139] These symptoms have been reported with other local anesthetics as well (Table17-11). Increased risk of TNS is associated with lidocaine, the lithotomy position, and ambulatory anesthesia, but not with baricity of solution or dose of local anesthetic.[139] The potential neurological etiology of this syndrome coupled with known concentration-dependent toxicity of lidocaine led to concerns over a neurotoxic etiology for TNS from spinal lidocaine.

As previously discussed, laboratory work in both intrathecal and desheathed peripheral nerve models has proved that

TABLE 17-11

INCIDENCES OF TRANSIENT NEUROLOGICAL SYMPTOMS (TNS) VARY WITH TYPE OF SPINAL LOCAL ANESTHETIC AND SURGERY

LOCAL ANESTHETIC	CONCENTRATION (%)	TYPE OF SURGERY	APPROXIMATE INCIDENCE OF TNS (%)
Lidocaine	2–5	Lithotomy position	30–36
	2–5	Knee arthroscopy	18–22
	0.5	Knee arthroscopy	17
	2–5	Mixed supine position	4–8
Mepivacaine	1.5–4	Mixed	23
Procaine	10	Knee arthroscopy	6
Bupivacaine	0.5–0.75	Mixed	1
Levo-bupivacaine	0.5	Mixed	1
Prilocaine	2–5	Mixed	1
Ropivacaine	0.5–0.75	Mixed	1

Data from: Pollock JE. Transient neurologic symptoms: etiology, risk factors, and management. Reg Anesth Pain Med 2002;27:581 and Breebaart MB. Urinary bladder scanning after day-case arthroscopy under spinal anaesthesia: comparison between lidocaine, ripovacaine, and levobupivacaine. Br J Anaesth 2003;90:309.

the concentration of lidocaine is a critical factor in neurotoxicity. As concentrations of lidocaine below 40 m*M* (~1.0%) are not neurotoxic to desheathed peripheral nerve, such dilute concentrations of spinal lidocaine should not cause TNS if the syndrome is a result of subclinical concentration-dependent neurotoxicity. The dilution of lidocaine to as low as 0.5%, however, does not decrease the incidence of TNS.[141] The high incidence of TNS observed with lidocaine concentrations <1% despite further dilution in cerebrospinal fluid lessens the plausibility of a concentration-dependent neurotoxic etiology. Furthermore, a volunteer study comparing individuals with and without TNS symptoms after lidocaine spinal anesthesia showed no difference detected by electromyography, nerve conduction studies, or somatosensory evoked potentials. Overall, there is little evidence to support a neurotoxic etiology for TNS.[139] Other potential etiologies for TNS include patient positioning, sciatic nerve stretch, muscle spasm, and myofascial strain.[139]

Interest in finding a short-acting spinal anesthetic with a lesser incidence of TNS has served as an impetus for investigations into the use of 2-chloroprocaine as a spinal anesthetic. Preliminary studies show that preservative-free 2-chloroprocaine provides an anesthetic profile similar to lidocaine without report of TNS, which would make 2-chloroprocaine potentially useful for outpatient procedures (Table 17-12). Enthusiasm for spinal 2-chloroprocaine should be tempered by the potential for neurotoxicity. In a laboratory study, 2-chloroprocaine (14 mg/kg) administered to rats via intrathecal catheter was noted to be histologically neurotoxic to the spinal cord to the same degree as 2.5% lidocaine. This finding calls into question the long held belief that the antioxidant sodium bisulfite is to blame for 2-chloroprocaine's clinical neurotoxicity.[142] The clinical applicability of this finding is uncertain, as the dose of chloroprocaine is far greater than the dose used for spinals in humans (0.6 mg/kg).

Myotoxicity of Local Anesthetics

Toxicity to skeletal muscle is an uncommon side effect of local anesthetic injection. Experimental data suggests, however, that local anesthetics have the potential for myotoxicity in clinically applicable concentrations (Fig. 17-18). Histopathologic evidence shows that the injection of these agents causes diffuse myonecrosis, which is both reversible and clinically imperceptible. The reversible nature of this injury is possibly because of the relative resilience of myoblasts, which regenerate damaged tissue. Theoretical mechanisms of injury are numerous but dysregulation of intracellular calcium concentrations is the most likely culprit. One study shows that ropivacaine is less myotoxic than bupivacaine primarily because of the latter causing

TABLE 17-12

DOSE RANGE OF SPINAL 2-CHLOROPROCAINE AND COMPARISON TO LIDOCAINE

2-CHLOROPROCAINE	30 mg	45 mg	60 mg	LIDOCAINE 40 mg
Sensory Block Height				
Peak	T7	T5	T2	T8
Time to L1 regression (mins)	53 ± 30	75 ± 14	92 ± 13	84 ± 35
Thigh tourniquet tolerance (mins)	37 ± 11	42 ± 11	62 ± 10	38 ± 24
Complete regression (mins)	98 ± 20	116 ± 15	132 ± 23	126 ± 16
Time to ambulation (mins)	**100 ± 20**	**119 ± 15**	**133 ± 20**	**134 ± 14**
Time to bladder void (mins)	100 ± 21	132 ± 19	141 ± 21	134 ± 14

Data from Kouri ME, Kopacz DJ: Spinal 2-chloroprocaine: A comparison with lidocaine in volunteers. Anesth Analg 98(1):75–80, Jan 2004, and Smith KN, Kopacz DJ, McDonald SB: Spinal 2-chloroprocaine: A dose-ranging study and the effect of added epinephrine. Anesth Analg 98(1): 81–88, Jan 2004.

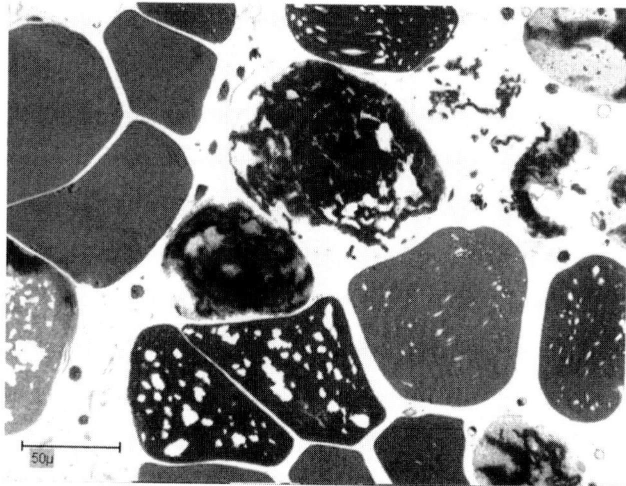

FIGURE 17-18. Skeletal muscle cross section with characteristic histologic changes after continuous exposure to bupivacaine for 6 hours. A whole spectrum of necrobiotic changes can be encountered, ranging from slightly damaged vacuolated fibers and fibers with condensed myofibrils to entirely disintegrated and necrotic cells. The majority of the myocytes are morphologically affected. Additionally, a marked interstitial and myoseptal edema appears within the sections. However, scattered fibers remain intact. (Reprinted with permission from Zink W, Graf B: Local anesthetic myotoxicity. Reg Anesth Pain Med 29(4):333–40, Jul–Aug 2004.)

apoptosis (programmed cell death).[143] Further investigation is needed to determine the clinical relevance of local or systemic myotoxicity following single injection or continuous infusion of local anesthetics.

Allergic Reactions to Local Anesthetics (see also Chapter 49)

True allergic reactions to local anesthetics are rare and usually involve Type I (IgE) or Type IV (cellular immunity) reactions.[144,145] Type I reactions are worrisome, as anaphylaxis may occur, and are more common with ester than amide local anesthetics. True Type I allergy to aminoamide agents is extremely rare.[145] Increased allergenic potential with esters may be a result of hydrolytic metabolism to para-aminobenzoic acid, which is a documented allergen. Added preservatives such as methylparaben and metabisulfite can also provoke an allergic response. Skin testing with intradermal injections of preservative-free local anesthetics has been advocated as a means to determine tolerance to local anesthetic. These tests should be undertaken with caution, as potentially severe and even fatal reactions can occur in truly allergic patients.[145]

References

1. Ritchie JM, Ritchie B, Greengard P: The effect of the nerve sheath on the action of local anesthetics. J Pharmacol Exp Ther 150:160, 1965
2. Coggeshall RE: A fine structured analysis of the myelin sheath in rat spinal roots. Anat Rec 194:201, 1979
3. Waxman SG, Ritchie JM: Molecular dissection of the myelinated axon. Ann Neurol 33:121, 1993
4. Landon N, Williams PL: Ultrastructure of the node of Ranvier. Nature 199:575, 1963
5. London DN, Langely OK: The local chemical environment of nodes of Ranvier: A study of cation binding. J Anat 108:419, 1971
6. Popitz-Berger FA, Leeson S, Strichartz GR, et al: Relation between functional deficit and intraneural local anesthetic during peripheral nerve block. Anesthesiology 83:583, 1995
7. Wann KT: Neuronal sodium and potassium channels: Structure and function. Br J Anaesth 71:2, 1993
8. Ogata N, Ohishi Y: Molecular diversity of structure and function of the voltage-gated Na+ channels. Jpn J Pharmacol 88:365, 2002
9. French RJ, Zamponi GW, Sierralta IE: Molecular and kinetic determinants of local anaesthetic action on sodium channels. Toxicol Lett 100:247, 1998
10. Caterall WA: The molecular basis of neuronal excitability. Science 223:653, 1984
11. Chiu SY, Ritchie JM, Rogart RB: A quantitative description of membrane current in rabbit myelinated nerve. J Physiol (Lond) 292:149, 1979
12. Yun I, Cho ES, Jang HO, et al: Amphiphilic effects of local anesthetics on rotational mobility in neuronal and model membranes. Biochim Biophys Acta 1564:123, 2002
13. Butterworth JF, Strichartz GR: Molecular mechanisms of local anesthesia: A review. Anesthesiology 72:711, 1990
14. Huang JH, Thalhammer JG, Raymond SA, et al: Susceptibility to lidocaine of impulses in different somatosensory afferent fibers of rat sciatic nerve. J Pharmacol Exp Ther 282:802, 1997
15. Gokin AP, Philip B, Strichartz GR: Preferential block of small myelinated sensory and motor fibers by lidocaine: In vivo electrophysiology in the rat sciatic nerve. Anesthesiology 95:1441, 2001
16. Yarov-Yarovoy V, McPhee JC, Idsvoog D, et al: Role of amino acid residues in transmembrane segments IS6 and IIS6 of the Na+ channel alpha subunit in voltage-dependent gating and drug block. J Biol Chem 277:35393, 2002
17. Li HL, Galue A, Meadows L, et al: A molecular basis for the different local anesthetic affinities of resting versus open and inactivated states of the sodium channel. Mol Pharmacol 55:134, 1999
18. Nau C, Strichartz GR: Drug chirality in anesthesia. Anesthesiology 97:497, 2002
19. Butterworth J, Ririe DG, Thompson RB, et al: Differential onset of median nerve block: Randomized, double-blind comparison of mepivacaine and bupivacaine in healthy volunteers. Br J Anaesth 81:515, 1998
20. Jaffe RA, Rowe MA: Differential nerve block: Direct measurements on individual myelinated and unmyelinated dorsal root axons. Anesthesiology 84:1455, 1996
21. Raymond SA, Steffensen SC, Gugino LD, et al: The role of length of nerve exposed to local anesthetics in impulse blocking action. Anesth Analg 68:563, 1989
22. Fink BR: Mechanisms of differential axial blockade in epidural and spinal anesthesia. Anesthesiology 70:851, 1989
23. Ritchie JM: On the relation between fiber diameter and conduction velocity in myelinated nerve fibers. Proc R Soc Lond 29:B217, 1982
24. Nakamura T, Popitz-Bergez F, Birknes J, et al: The critical role of concentration for lidocaine block of peripheral nerve in vivo: studies of function and drug uptake in the rat. Anesthesiology 99:1189, 2003
25. Waikar SS, Thalhammer JG, Raymond SA, et al: Mechanoreceptive afferents exhibit functionally-specific activity dependent changes in conduction velocity. Brain Res 721:91, 1996
26. Mackenzie RA, Burke D, Skuse NF: Fibre function and perception during cutaneous nerve block. J Neurol Neurosurg Psychiatry 38:865, 1975
27. Narita Y, Nagai M, Kuzuhara S: Trigeminal somatosensory evoked potentials before, during and after an inferior alveolar nerve block in normal subjects. Psych Clin Neurosci 51:241, 1997
28. Zaric D, Hallgren S, Leissner L, et al: Evaluation of epidural sensory block by thermal stimulation, laser stimulation, and recording of somatosensory evoked potentials. Reg Anesth 21:124, 1996
29. Raymond SA: Subblocking concentrations of local anesthetics: Effects on impulse generation and conduction in single myelinated sciatic nerve axons in frog. Anesth Analg 75:906, 1992
30. Olschewski A, Wolff M, Brau ME, et al: Enhancement of delayed-rectifier potassium conductance by low concentrations of local anaesthetics in spinal sensory neurones. Br J Pharmacol 136:540, 2002
31. Bowersox SS, Luther R: Pharmacotherapeutic potential of omega-conotoxin MVIIA (SNX-111), an N-type neuronal calcium channel blocker found in the venom of *Conus magus*. Toxicon 36:1651, 1998
32. Xiong Z, Bukusoglu C, Strichartz GR: Local anesthetics inhibit the G protein-mediated modulation of K+ and Ca++ currents in anterior pituitary cells. Mol Pharmacol 55:150, 1999
33. Hodgson PS, Neal JM, Pollock JE, et al: The neurotoxicity of drugs given intrathecally (spinal). Anesth Analg 88:797, 1999
34. Too HP, Maggio JE: Immunocytochemical localization of neuromedin K (neurokinin B) in rat spinal ganglia and cord. Peptides 12:431, 1991
35. Nagy I, Woolf CJ: Lignocaine selectively reduces C fibre-evoked neuronal activity in rat spinal cord in vitro by decreasing N-methyl-D-aspartate and neurokinin receptor-mediated post-synaptic depolarizations; implications for the development of novel centrally acting analgesics. Pain 64:59, 1996
36. Nordmark J, Rydqvist B: Local anaesthetics potentiate GABA-mediated Cl^- currents by inhibiting GABA uptake. Neuroreport 8:465, 1997
37. Pascual JM, Karlin A: Delimiting the binding site for quaternary ammonium lidocaine derivatives in the acetylcholine receptor channel. J Gen Physiol 112:611, 1998
38. Sugimoto M, Uchida I, Mashimo T: Local anaesthetics have different mechanisms and sites of action at the recombinant N-methyl-D-aspartate (NMDA) receptors. Br J Pharmacol 138:876, 2003
39. Frazier DY, Narahashi T, Yamada M: The site of action and active form of local anesthetic. II. Experiments with quaternary compounds. J Pharmacol Exp Ther 171:45, 1970
40. Gissen AJ, Covino BG, Gregus J: Differential sensitivity of fast and slow

fibers in mammalian nerve. II. Margin of safety for nerve transmission. Anesth Analg 61:561, 1982
41. Taheri S, Cogswell LP 3rd, Gent A, et al: Hydrophobic and ionic factors in the binding of local anesthetics to the major variant of human alpha1-acid glycoprotein. J Pharmacol Exp Ther 304:71, 2003
42. Ulbricht W: Kinetics of drug action and equilibrium results at the node of Ranvier. Physiol Rev 61:785, 1981
43. Foster RH, Markham A: Levobupivacaine: A review of its pharmacology and use as a local anaesthetic. Drugs 59:551, 2000
44. Wang RD, Dangler LA, Greengrass RA: Update on ropivacaine. Expert Opin Pharmacother 2:2051, 2001
45. Heavner JE: Cardiac toxicity of local anesthetics in the intact isolated heart model: A review. Reg Anesth Pain Med 27:545, 2002
46. Strichartz GR, Sanchez V, Arthur GR: Fundamental properties of local anesthetics. II. Measured octanol:buffer partition coefficients and pK_a values of clinically used drugs. Anesth Analg 71:158, 1990
47. Pateromichelakis S, Prokopiou AA: Local anaesthesia efficacy: Discrepancies between in vitro and in vivo studies. Acta Anaesthesiol Scand 32:672, 1988
48. Bromage PR, Pettigrew RT, Crowell DE: Tachyphylaxis in epidural analgesia: I. Augmentation and decay of local anesthetic. J Clin Pharmacol 9:30, 1969
49. Baker CE, Berry RL, Elston RC: Effects of pH of bupivacaine on duration of repeated sciatic nerve blocks in the albino rat: Local anesthetics for neuralgia study group. Anesth Analg 72:773, 1991
50. Choi RH, Birknes JK, Popitz-Bergez FA, et al: Pharmacokinetic nature of tachyphylaxis to lidocaine: Peripheral nerve blocks and infiltration anesthesia in rats. Life Sci 61:PL177, 1997
51. Mogensen T, Simonsen L, Scott NB: Tachyphylaxis associated with repeated epidural injections of lidocaine is not related to changes in distribution or the rate of elimination of the epidural space. Anesth Analg 69:71, 1989
52. Lee K-C, Wilder RT, Smith RL et al: Thermal hyperalgesia accelerates and MK-801 prevents the development of tachyphylaxis to rat sciatic nerve blockade. Anesthesiology 81:1284, 1994
53. Wilder RT, Sholas MG, Berde CB: NG-nitro-L-arginine methyl ester (L-NAME) prevents tachyphylaxis to local anesthetics in a dose-dependent manner. Anesth Analg 83:1251, 1996
54. Neal JM: Effects of epinephrine in local anesthetics on the central and peripheral nervous systems: Neurotoxicity and neural blood flow. Reg Anesth Pain Med 28:124, 2003
55. Sinnott CJ, Cogswell III LP, Johnson A et al: On the mechanism by which epinephrine potentiates lidocaine's peripheral nerve block. Anesthesiology 98:181, 2003
56. Curatolo M, Petersen-Felix S, Arendt-Nielsen L et al: Epidural epinephrine and clonidine: Segmental analgesia and effects on different pain modalities. Anesthesiology 87:785, 1997
57. Ueda W, Hirakawa M, Mori K: Acceleration of epinephrine absorption by lidocaine. Anesthesiology 63:717, 1985
58. Magee C, Rodeheaver GT, Edgerton MT, et al: Studies of the mechanisms by which epinephrine damages tissue defenses. J Surg Res 23:126, 1977
59. Hall JA, Ferro A: Myocardial ischaemia and ventricular arrhythmias precipitated by physiological concentrations of adrenaline in patients with coronary artery disease. Br Heart J 67:419, 1992
60. Lambert DH: Clinical value of adding sodium bicarbonate to local anesthetics. Reg Anesth Pain Med 27:328, 2002
61. Ikuta PT, Raza SM, Durrani Z: pH adjustment schedule for the amide local anesthetics. Reg Anesth 14:229, 1989
62. Neal JM, Hebl JR, Gerancher JC, et al: Brachial plexus anesthesia: essentials of our current understanding. Reg Anesth Pain Med 27:402, 2002
63. Sinnott CJ, Garfield JM, Thalhammer JG: Addition of sodium bicarbonate to lidocaine decreases the duration of peripheral nerve block in the rat. Anesthesiology 93:1045, 2000
64. Fields HL: Pain modulation: Expectation, opioid analgesia and virtual pain. Prog Brain Res 122:245, 2000
65. Matos FF, Rollema H, Brown JL, et al: Do opioids evoke the release of serotonin in the spinal cord? An in vivo microdialysis study of the regulation of extracellular serotonin in the rat. Pain 48:439, 1992
66. Barke KE, Hough LB: Simultaneous measurement of opiate-induced histamine release in the periaqueductal gray and opiate antinociception: An in vivo microdialysis study. J Pharmacol Exp Ther 266:934, 1993
67. Wang C, Chakrabarti MK, Galletly DC, et al: Relative effects of intrathecal administration of fentanyl and midazolam on A delta and C fibre reflexes. Neuropharmacology 31:439, 1992
68. Niv D, Nemirovsky A, Rudick V: Antinociception induced by simultaneous intrathecal and intraperitoneal administration of low doses of morphine. Anesth Analg 80:886, 1995
69. Walker SM, Goudas LC, Cousins MJ, et al: Combination spinal analgesic chemotherapy: a systematic review. Anesth Analg 95:674, 2002
70. Karambelkar DJ, Ramanathan S: 2-Chloroprocaine antagonism of epidural morphine analgesia. Acta Anaesth Scand 41:774, 1997
71. Coda B, Bausch S, Haas M, et al: The hypothesis that antagonism of fentanyl analgesia by 2-chloroprocaine is mediated by direct action on opioid receptors. Reg Anesth 22:43, 1997
72. Janson W, Stein C: Peripheral opioid analgesia. Curr Pharm Biotechnol 4:270, 2003
73. Kalso E, Smith L, McQuay HJ, et al: No pain, no gain: Clinical excellence and scientific rigour—lessons learned from IA morphine. Pain 98:269, 2002
74. Picard PR, Tramer MR, McQuay HJ, et al: Analgesic efficacy of peripheral opioids (all except intra-articular): A qualitative systematic review of randomised controlled trials. Pain 72:309, 1997
75. Fields HL, Emson PC, Leigh BK: Multiple opiate receptor sites on primary afferent fibres. Nature 284:351, 1980
76. Eisenach JC, De Kock M, Klimscha W: Alpha(2)-adrenergic agonists for regional anesthesia: A clinical review of clonidine (1984–1995). Anesthesiology 85:655, 1996
77. Butterworth JF, Strichartz GR: The α_2-adrenergic agonists clonidine and guanfacine produce tonic and phasic block of conduction in rat sciatic nerve fibers. Anesth Analg 76:295, 1993
78. Gaumann DM, Brunet PC, Jirounek P: Clonidine enhances the effects of lidocaine on C fiber action potential. Anesth Analg 74:719, 1992
79. Pertovaara A, Hamalainen MM: Spinal potentiation and supraspinal additivity in the antinociceptive interaction between systemically administered α_2-adrenoreceptor agonist and cocaine in the rat. Anesth Analg 79:261, 1994
80. Bernard JM, Macaire P: Dose–range effects of clonidine added to lidocaine for brachial plexus block. Anesthesiology 87:277, 1997
81. Reuben SS, Steinberg RB, Klatt JL, et al: Intravenous regional anesthesia using lidocaine and clonidine. Anesthesiology 91:654, 1999
82. Tucker GT, Moore DC, Bridenbaugh PO: Systemic absorption of mepivacaine in commonly used regional block procedures. Anesthesiology 37:277, 1972
83. Tucker GT, Mather LE: Properties, absorption, and disposition of local anesthetic agents. In Cousins MJ, Bridenbaugh PO (eds): Neural Blockade in Clinical Anesthesia and Management of Pain, 3d ed, p 55. Philadelphia, Lippincott–Raven, 1998
84. Morrison LM, Emanuelsson BM, McClure JH: Efficacy and kinetics of extradural ropivacaine: Comparison with bupivacaine. Br J Anaesth 72:164, 1994
85. Huang YF, Upton RN, Runciman WB: I.V. bolus administration of subconvulsive doses of lignocaine to conscious sheep: Myocardial pharmacokinetics. Br J Anaesth 70:326, 1993
86. Huang YF, Upton RN, Runciman WB: I.V. bolus administration of subconvulsive doses of lidocaine to conscious sheep: Relationships between myocardial pharmacokinetics and pharmacodynamics. Br J Anaesth 70:556, 1993
87. Kuhnert BR, Kuhnert PM, Philipson EH: The half-life of 2-chloroprocaine. Anesth Analg 65:273, 1986
88. Rutten AJ, Mather LE, Nancarrow C: Cardiovascular effects and regional clearances of intravenous ropivacaine in sheep. Anesth Analg 70:577, 1990
89. Braid DP, Scott DB: Dosage of lignocaine in epidural block in relation to toxicity. Br J Anaesth 38:596, 1966
90. Adinoff B, Devous MD Sr, Best SE, et al: Gender differences in limbic responsiveness, by SPECT, following pharmacologic challenge in healthy subjects. Neuroimage 18:697, 2003
91. Chen BK, Cunningham BB: Topical anesthetics in children: Agents and techniques that equally comfort patients, parents, and clinicians. Curr Opin Pediatr 13:324, 2001
92. Covino BG, Wildsmith JAW: Clinical pharmacology of local anesthetic agents. In Cousins MJ, Bridenbaugh PO (eds): Neural Blockade in Clinical Anesthesia and Management of Pain, 3rd ed, p 97. Philadelphia, Lippincott–Raven, 1998
93. Paulissian R, Salem MR, Joseph NJ, et al: Hemodynamic responses to endotracheal extubation after coronary artery bypass grafting. Anesth Analg 73:10, 1991
94. Kindler CH, Schumacher PG, Schneider MC, et al: Effects of intravenous lidocaine and/or esmolol on hemodynamic responses to laryngoscopy and intubation: A double-blind, controlled clinical trial. J Clin Anesth 8:491, 1996
95. Gonzalez RM, Bjerke RJ, Drobycki T, et al: Prevention of endotracheal tube-induced coughing during emergence from general anesthesia. Anesth Analg 79:792, 1994
96. Yukioka H, Hayashi M, Terai T, et al: Intravenous lidocaine as a suppressant of coughing during tracheal intubation in elderly patients. Anesth Analg 77:309, 1993
97. Helfman SM, Gold MI, DeLisser EA, et al: Which drug prevents tachycardia and hypertension associated with tracheal intubation: Lidocaine, fentanyl, or esmolol? Anesth Analg 72:482, 1991
98. Nakayama M, Fujita S, Kanaya N, et al: Effect of intravenous lidocaine on intraabdominal pressure response to airway stimulation. Anesth Analg 78:1149, 1994
99. Chamberlain DA: Antiarrhythmic drugs in resuscitation. Heart 80:408, 1998
100. Koppert W, Weigand M, Neumann F, et al: Perioperative intravenous lidocaine has preventive effects on postoperative pain and morphine consumption after major abdominal surgery. Anesth Analg 98:1050, 2004
101. Kingery WS: A critical review of controlled clinical trials for peripheral neuropathic pain and complex regional pain syndromes. Pain 73:123, 1997
102. Devor M, Wall PD, Catalan N: Systemic lidocaine silences neuroma and DRG discharge without blocking nerve conduction. Pain 48:261, 1992

103. Tanelian DL, MacIver MB: Analgesic concentrations of lidocaine suppress tonic A-delta and C fiber discharges produced by acute injury. Anesthesiology 74:934, 1991
104. Persaud N, Strichartz GR: Micromolar lidocaine selectively blocks propagating ectopic impulses at a distance from their site of origin. Pain 99:333, 2002
105. Cahana A, Carota A, Montadon ML, et al: The long-term effect of repeated intravenous lidocaine on central pain and possible correlation in positron emission tomography measurements. Anesth Analg 98:1581, 2004
106. Groban L: Central nervous system and cardiac effects from long-acting amide local anesthetic toxicity in the intact animal model. Reg Anesth Pain Med 28:3, 2003
107. Shibata M, Shingu K, Murakawa M: Tetraphasic actions of local anesthetics on central nervous system electrical activity in cats. Reg Anesth 19:255, 1994
108. Brown DL, Ransom DM, Hall JA, et al: Regional anesthesia and local anesthetic-induced systemic toxicity: Seizure frequency and accompanying cardiovascular changes. Anesth Analg 81:321, 1995
109. Auroy Y, Benhamou D, Bargues L, et al: Major complications of regional anesthesia in France: The SOS Regional Anesthesia Hotline Service. Anesthesiology 97:1274, 2002
110. Weinberg GL: Current concepts in resuscitation of patients with local anesthetic cardiac toxicity. Reg Anesth Pain Med 27:568, 2002
111. Yokoyama M, Hirakawa M, Goto H: Effect of vasoconstrictive agents added to lidocaine on intravenous lidocaine-induced convulsions in rats. Anesthesiology 82:574, 1995
112. Yamauchi Y, Kotani J, Ueda Y: The effects of exogenous epinephrine on a convulsive dose of lidocaine: Relationship with cerebral circulation. J Neurosurg Anesth 10:178, 1998
113. Sokrab TEO, Johansson BB: Regional cerebral bloodflow in acute hypertension induced by adrenaline, noradrenaline, and phenylephrine in the conscious rat. Acta Physiol Scand 137:101, 1989
114. Mayhan WG, Faraci FM, Siems JL: Role of molecular charge in disruption of the blood–brain barrier during acute hypertension. Circ Res 64:658, 1989
115. Arthur GR, Feldman HS, Covino BG: Alterations in the pharmacokinetic properties of amide local anaesthetics following local anaesthetic induced convulsions. Acta Anaesthesiol Scand 32:522, 1988
116. Lee LA, Posner KL, Domino KB, et al: Injuries associated with regional anesthesia in the 1980s and 1990s: A closed claim analysis. Anesthesiology 101:143, 2004
117. Klein SM, Pierce T, Rubin Y, et al: Successful resuscitation after ropivacaine induced ventricular fibrillation. Anesth Analg 97:901, 2003
118. McClellan KJ, Faulds D: Ropivacaine: An update of its use in regional anaesthesia. Drugs 60:1065, 2000
119. McLeod GA, Burke D: Levobupivacaine. Anaesthesia 56:331, 2001
120. Knudsen K, Beckman Suurkula M, Blomberg S, et al: Central nervous and cardiovascular effects of i.v. infusions of ropivacaine, bupivacaine and placebo in volunteers. Br J Anaesth 78:507, 1997
121. Stewart J, Kellett N, Castro D: The central nervous system and cardiovascular effects of levobupivacaine and ropivacaine in healthy volunteers. Anesth Analg 97:412, 2003
122. Groban L, Deal DD, Vernon JC, et al: Does local anesthetic stereoselectivity or structure predict myocardial depression in anesthetized canines? Reg Anesth Pain Med 27:460, 2002
123. Pickering AE, Waki H, Headley PM, et al: Investigation of systemic bupivacaine toxicity using the in situ perfused working heart-brainstem preparation of the rat. Anesthesiology 97:1550, 2002
124. Chang KSK, Yang M, Andresen MC: Clinically relevant concentrations of bupivacaine inhibit rat aortic baroreceptors. Anesth Analg 78:501, 1994
125. Hogan QH, Stadnicka A, Bosnjak ZJ, et al: Effects of lidocaine and bupivacaine on isolated rabbit mesenteric capacitance veins. Reg Anesth Pain Med 23:409, 1998
126. Guo XT, Castle NA, Chernoff DM, et al: Comparative inhibition of voltage-gated cation channels by local anesthetics. Ann N Y Acad Sci 625:181, 1991
127. Clarkson CW, Hondegham LM: Mechanisms for bupivacaine depression of cardiac conduction: Fast block of sodium channels during the action potential with slow recovery from block during diastole. Anesthesiology 62:396, 1985
128. Mio Y, Fukuda N, Kusakari Y, et al: Bupivacaine attenuates contractility by decreasing sensitivity of myofilaments to $Ca2+$ in rat ventricular muscle. Anesthesiology 97:1168, 2002
129. Nouette-Gaulain K, Forestier F, Malgat M, et al: Effects of bupivacaine on mitochondrial energy metabolism in heart of rats following exposure to chronic hypoxia. Anesthesiology 97:1507, 2002
130. Weinberg G, Ripper R, Feinstein DL, et al: Lipid emulsion infusion rescues dogs from bupivacaine-induced cardiac toxicity. Reg Anesth Pain Med 28:198, 2003
131. Kitagawa N, Oda M, Totoki T: Possible mechanism of irreversible nerve injury caused by local anesthetics and membrane disruption. Anesthesiology 100:962, 2004
132. Kalichman MW: Physiologic mechanisms by which local anesthetics may cause injury to nerve and spinal cord. Reg Anesth 18:448, 1993
133. Selander D: Neurotoxicity of local anesthetics: Animal data. Reg Anesth 18:461, 1993
134. Yamashita A, Matsumoto M, Matsumoto S, et al: A comparison of the neurotoxic effects on the spinal cord of tetracaine, lidocaine, bupivacaine, and ropivacaine administered intrathecally in rabbits. Anesth Analg 97:512, 2003
135. Bainton C, Strichartz G: Concentration dependence of lidocaine-induced irreversible conduction loss in frog nerve. Anesthesiology 81:657, 1994
136. Kanai T, Katsuki H, Takasake M: Graded, irreversible changes in crayfish giant axon as manifestations of lidocaine neurotoxicity in vitro. Anesth Analg 86:569, 1998
137. Lambert L, Lambert D, Strichartz G: Irreversible conduction block in isolated nerve by high concentrations of local anesthetics. Anesthesiology 80:1082, 1994
138. Iida H, Watanabe Y, Dohi S, et al: Direct effects of ropivacaine and bupivacaine on spinal pial vessels in canine. Anesthesiology 87:75, 1997
139. Pollock JE: Transient neurologic symptoms: Etiology, risk factors, and management. Reg Anesth Pain Med 27:581, 2002
140. Liu S, Kopacz D, Carpenter R: Quantitative assessment of differential sensory nerve block after lidocaine spinal anesthesia. Anesthesiology 82:60, 1995
141. Pollock JE, Liu SS, Neal JM, et al: Dilution of lidocaine does not decrease the incidence of transient neurologic symptoms. Anesthesiology 90:445, 1999
142. Taniguchi M, Bollen AW, Drasner K: Sodium bisulfite: Scapegoat for chloroprocaine neurotoxicity? Anesthesiology 100:85, 2004
143. Zink W, Graf B: Local anesthetic myotoxicity. Reg Anesth Pain Med 29:333, 2004
144. Chen AH: Toxicity and allergy to local anesthesia. J California Dent Assoc 26:683, 1998
145. Finder RL, Moore PA: Adverse drug reactions to local anesthesia. Dent Clin North Am 46:747, 2002

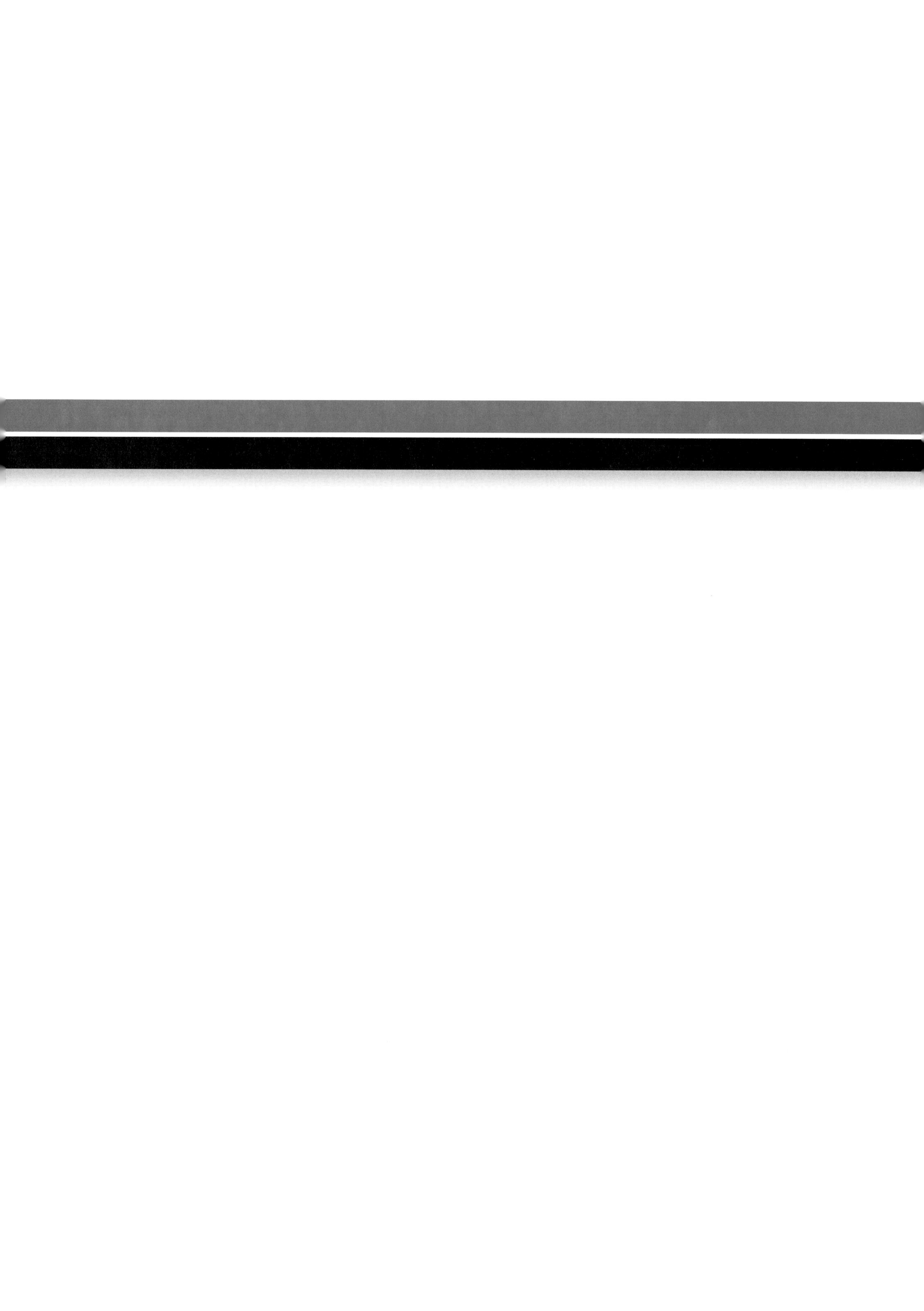

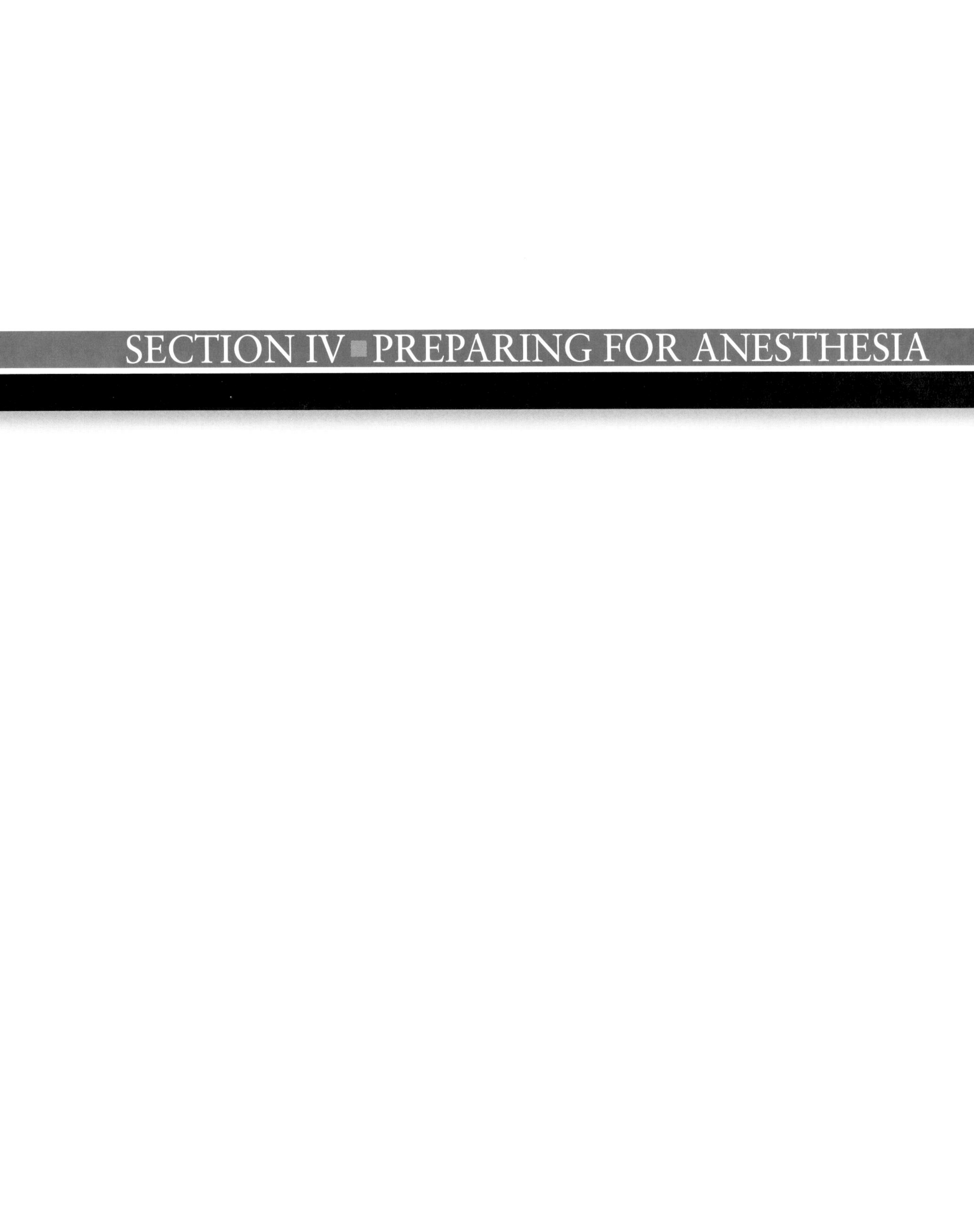

SECTION IV ▪ PREPARING FOR ANESTHESIA

CHAPTER 18 ■ PREOPERATIVE EVALUATION AND MANAGEMENT

TARA M. HATA AND JOHN R. MOYERS

KEY POINTS

1. The Joint Commission for the Accreditation of Healthcare Organizations (JCAHO) requires that all patients receive a preoperative anesthetic evaluation and the American Society of Anesthesiologists (ASA) has approved Basic Standards for Preoperative Care.
2. When evaluating the patient with hypertension, it is important to determine the presence of end-organ damage (heart, lung, and cerebrovascular systems).
3. Exercise tolerance is a major determinant of cardiac risk and need for further testing.
4. The algorithm for preoperative evaluation of cardiac patients undergoing noncardiac surgery is very useful in guiding further testing and evaluation.
5. Preoperative laboratory tests should be ordered only based on defined indications such as positive findings on history and physical exam.
6. No best drug or combination of drugs exists for preoperative medication.
7. Psychological preparation is as important as pharmacologic preparation for anesthesia and surgery.
8. Timing of delivery is as important as drug selection with preoperative medication.
9. Age of the child is a major determinant of the approach to preoperative medication.

The goals of preoperative evaluation are to reduce patient risk and the morbidity of surgery, as well as to promote efficiency and reduce costs. 1 The Joint Commission for the Accreditation of Healthcare Organizations (JCAHO) requires that all patients receive a preoperative anesthetic evaluation. The American Society of Anesthesiologists (ASA) has approved Basic Standards for Preanesthetic Care, which outlines the minimum requirements for a preoperative evaluation. Conducting a preoperative evaluation is based on the premise that it will modify patient care and improve outcome. There is evidence, although not entirely convincing in all instances, that the preoperative evaluation will increase patient safety. That is, armed with knowledge preoperatively the anesthesiologist can formulate and conduct an anesthetic plan that avoids dangers inherent in patient disease states. Furthermore, preoperative evaluations may very well reduce costs and cancellation rates, increasing resource utilization in the operating room. This assumes that evaluations are done by anesthesiologists and others familiar with anesthetics, surgery, and perioperative events.

The preoperative evaluation has several components and goals. One should obtain a history and perform a physical exam pertinent to the patient and surgery contemplated. Based on the history and physical, the appropriate laboratory tests and preoperative consultations should be obtained. Through these one needs to determine whether the patient's preoperative condition may be improved prior to surgery. Guided by the above, the anesthesiologist should choose the appropriate anesthetic and care plan. Finally, the process should be used to educate the patient about anesthesia and the perioperative period, answer all questions, and obtain informed consent.

The first part of this chapter outlines clinical risk factors pertinent to patients scheduled for anesthesia and surgery and the use of tests to confirm diagnoses. The second part discusses preoperative medication. The chapter provides only an overview of the preoperative management process; for more details, the reader is referred to chapters focusing on specific organ systems.

CHANGING CONCEPTS IN PREOPERATIVE EVALUATION

In the past, patients were admitted to the hospital at least a day prior to surgery. Currently, more and more patients are admitted to the hospital on the day of surgery. Older patients are scheduled for more complex procedures, and there is more pressure on the anesthesiologist to reduce the time between cases. The first time the anesthesiologist performing the anesthetic sees the patient may be just prior to anesthesia and surgery. The patient has been seen previously by others in a preoperative evaluation clinic. Only a short time exists to engender trust and answer last-minute questions. It is often impossible to alter medical therapy at this juncture immediately preoperatively. However, preoperative screening clinics are becoming more effective and clinical practice guidelines becoming more prevalent. Information technology has helped the anesthesiologist in previewing the upcoming patients that will be anesthetized. Preoperative questionnaires and computer-driven programs have become alternatives to traditional information gathering. Finally, when anesthesiologists are responsible for ordering preoperative laboratory tests, cost saving occurs and cancellations of planned surgical procedures become less likely. In this setting it is important that communication between the preoperative evaluation clinic and the anesthesiologist performing the anesthetic occur through the patient record and in person.

APPROACH TO THE HEALTHY PATIENT

The preoperative evaluation form is the basis for formulating the best anesthetic plan tailored to the patient. It should aid the anesthesiologist in identifying potential complications, as well as serve as a medicolegal document. The importance of the design has increased because of the fact that it is more common today for the evaluation to be completed in a preop clinic by another physician or health professional who will not personally be performing the anesthetic, but also because regulatory agencies such as JCAHO demand better documentation. Therefore, the information obtained needs to be complete, concise, and legible. In those hospitals that have computerized patient forms, legibility is no longer an issue. A group from University of California, San Diego (UCSD) studied the quality of preoperative evaluation forms across the United States and rated them in three categories: informational content, ease of use, and ease of reading.[1] Their results revealed that a surprisingly high percentage of forms are missing important information. Figure 18-1 is an example of the preoperative evaluation form in use at the University of Iowa Hospitals, which attempts to document all pertinent information.

The approach to the patient should always begin with a thorough history and physical exam. This alone may be sufficient (without additional routine laboratory tests) prior to noninvasive procedures.

The indication for the surgical procedure is part of the preoperative history, because it will help determine the urgency of the surgery. True emergent procedures, which are associated with an accepted higher anesthetic morbidity and mortality, require a more abbreviated evaluation. A less-defined area is the approach to urgent procedures. For example, ischemic limbs require surgery soon after presentation, but can usually be delayed for 24 hours for further evaluation. The indication for the surgical procedure may also have implications on other aspects of perioperative management. For example, the presence of a small bowel obstruction has implications regarding the risk of aspiration and the need for a rapid sequence induction. The extent of a lung resection will dictate the need for further pulmonary testing and perioperative monitoring. Patients undergoing carotid endarterectomy may require a more extensive neurologic examination, as well as testing to rule out coronary artery disease (CAD). Frequently, further information will be required that necessitates contacting the surgeon. Perioperative care of the patient, as well as efficiency in the operating room, is always enhanced by close communication with the surgeons.

The ability to review previous anesthetic records is helpful in detecting the presence of a difficult airway, a history of malignant hyperthermia, and the individual's response to surgical stress and specific anesthetics. The patient should be questioned regarding any previous difficulty with anesthesia or other family members having difficulty with anesthesia. A patient history relating an "allergy" to anesthesia should make one suspicious for malignant hyperthermia.

The history should include a complete list of medications, including over-the-counter and herbal products, to define a preoperative medication regimen, anticipate potential drug interactions, and provide clues to underlying disease. A complete list of drug allergies, including previous reactions, should also be obtained.

The anesthesiologist should determine when the patient last ate, as well as note the sites of preexisting intravenous cannulae and invasive monitors. Once the general issues are completed, the preoperative history and physical exam can focus on specific systems.

Systems Approach

Airway

A basic concern of the anesthesiologist is always the patient's airway. The ability to review previous anesthetic records is especially useful in uncovering unsuspected "difficult airways" or to confirm previous uneventful intubations, assuming the patient's body habitus has not changed in the interim. Evaluation of the airway involves determination of the thyromental distance, the ability to flex the base of the neck and extend the head, and examination of the oral cavity including dentition. The Mallampati classification has become the standard for assessing the relationship of the tongue size relative to the oral cavity (Table 18-1),[2] although **by itself** the Mallampati classification has a low positive predictive value in identifying patients who are difficult to intubate.[3,4] In trauma patients, as well as those with severe rheumatoid arthritis or Down

PRE-ANESTHETIC EVALUATION
Operation Proposed
Surgical Diagnosis
Age ______ Gender ______ Wt ______ Ht ______
BP P rr T
Allergies ☐ Latex allergy
Medications (Include Drugs, OTC and Herbals):
Anesthetic History ☐ Malignant hyperthermia
HEENT ☐ Hx of difficult airway
Teeth:
Class: I II III IV
Chin:
Neck:
Respiratory System ☐ WNL
☐ Asthma ☐ Bronchitis ☐ COPD ☐ Pneumonia
☐ TB ☐ Penumothorax ☐ Recent URI ☐ Dyspnea
☐ Cough ☐ RequiresO_2 ☐ Steroids ☐ Snoring/Sleep Apnea
Tobacco: ____ppd ____ YR
Chest Exam:
CxR:
Anesthetic options / risks discussed ______________
☐ Risks discussed and patient/guardian understands
Print Name/Signature Time Date

Patient Name
Cardiovascular System ☐ WNL
☐ CHD ☐ HTN ☐ CAD ☐ MI ☐ Valve disease
☐ Cardiomyopathy ☐ CHF ☐ RF ☐ Pacer ☐ Dysrrhythmia
☐ PVD ☐ Angina ☐ DOE ☐ Orthopnea ☐ Murmur
Exercise tolerance:
CV Exam:
EKG:
Echo/Cath:
Central Nervous System ☐ WNL
☐ CVA ☐ TIA ☐ LOC ☐ Seizures ☐ ↑ ICP
☐ HA ☐ NM disease ☐ Weakness ☐ Parethesias ☐ Psych disorder
☐ Altered MS/GCS ☐ Spinal cord injury
Renal ☐ WNL
☐ Insufficiency ☐ Failure ☐ Dialysis: last date______
GI, Hepatic ☐ WNL
☐ Liver disease ☐ Hepatitis ☐ Bowel obstruction ☐ N/V ☐ Reflux
ETOH_drinks / ______
Endocrine, Metabolic, Infections, Other ☐ WNL
☐ Diabetes ☐ Thyroid disease ☐ RA ☐ Steroids
☐ Coagulopathy ☐ Chemotherapy ☐ Sickle Cell ☐ Pregnant
☐ Anemia ☐ HIV ☐ MRSA ☐ VRE
Additional Information / Interval History
☐ Advance directive(s) documented elsewhere
NPO Status:
Invasive monitors:
IV Access:
Pt Instructions:
Print Staff Name/Signature Time Date

Hospital Number
Lab Data
☐ Patient examined and chart reviewed. Patient approved for anesthesia.
☐ Potential post-op ICU admission
A/P:
Attending Signature Time Date
POSTANESTHETIC EVALUATION
PACU / ICU / Ward
☐ Extubated O_2 sat ____
☐ Satisfactory spont vent P____
☐ Protective reflexes BP____
☐ Follows commands IT ____
☐ Report given T____
Signature Time Date
POSTANESTHETIC PROGRESS NOTE
☐ No anesthesia related adverse events
Signature Time Date

FIGURE 18-1. Example of pre-anesthetic evaluation form.

syndrome, assessment of the cervical spine is critical. In appropriate patients, the presence of pain or symptoms of cervical cord compression on movement should be assessed. In other instances, radiographic examination may be required.

Pulmonary

A screening evaluation should include questions regarding the history of tobacco use, shortness of breath, cough, wheezing, stridor, and snoring or sleep apnea. The patient should also be questioned regarding the presence or recent history of an upper respiratory tract infection. Physical exam should assess the respiratory rate as well as the chest excursion, use of accessory muscles, nail color, and the patient's ability to carry on a conversation or to walk without dyspnea. Auscultation should be used to detect decreased breath sounds, wheezing, stridor, or rales. For the patient with positive findings, see preoperative evaluation of the pulmonary patient.

TABLE 18-1

AIRWAY CLASSIFICATION SYSTEM

■ CLASS	■ DIRECT VISUALIZATION, PATIENT SEATED	■ LARYNGOSCOPIC VIEW
I	Soft palate, fauces, uvula, pillars	Entire glottic
II	Soft palate, fauces, uvula	Posterior commissure
III	Soft palate, uvular base	Tip of epiglottis
IV	Hard palate only	No glottal structures

Modified with permission from Mallampati RS, Gatt SP, Gugino LD *et al*: A clinical sign to predict difficult tracheal intubation: A prospective study. Can Anaesth Soc J 32:429, 1985.

Cardiovascular System

When screening a patient for cardiovascular disease prior to surgery, the anesthesiologist is most interested in recognizing signs and symptoms of uncontrolled hypertension and unstable cardiac disease such as myocardial ischemia, congestive heart failure, valvular heart disease, and significant cardiac dysrhythmias. Symptoms of cardiovascular disease should be carefully determined, especially the characteristics of chest pain, if present. Certain populations of patients, such as the elderly, women, or diabetics, may present with more atypical features. The presence of unstable angina has been associated with a high perioperative risk of myocardial infarction (MI).[5] The perioperative period is associated with a hypercoagulable state and surges in endogenous catecholamines, both of which may exacerbate the underlying process in unstable angina, increasing the risk of acute infarction.[6] The preoperative evaluation can affect both a patient's short- and long-term health by instituting treatment of unstable angina. Symptoms of clinically important valvular disease should be sought, such as angina, syncope, or congestive heart failure from aortic stenosis that would require further evaluation. A history of other valvular disease such as mitral valve prolapse may simply dictate the need for SBE prophylaxis.

The exam of the cardiovascular system should include blood pressure, measuring both arms when appropriate. The anesthesiologist should take into account the effects of preoperative anxiety and may want a record of resting blood pressure measurements. However, Bedford and Feinstein reported that the admission blood pressure was the best predictor of response to laryngoscopy.[7] Auscultation of the heart is performed, specifically listening for a murmur radiating to the carotids suggestive of aortic stenosis or abnormal rhythms, or a gallop suggestive of heart failure. The presence of bruits over the carotid arteries would warrant further work-up to determine the risk of stroke. The extremities should also be examined for the presence of peripheral pulses to exclude peripheral vascular disease or congenital cardiovascular disease.

Neurologic System

A screening of the neurological system in the apparently healthy patient can mostly be accomplished through simple observation. The patient's ability to answer health history questions practically ensures a normal mental status. Questions can be directed to exclude the presence of increased intracranial pressure, cerebrovascular disease, seizure history, preexisting neuromuscular disease, or nerve injuries. The neurologic examination may be cursory in healthy patients, or extensive in patients with coexisting disease. Testing of strength, reflexes, and sensation may be important in patients if the anesthetic plan or surgical procedure may result in a change in the condition.

Endocrine System

Each patient should be screened for endocrine diseases that may affect the perioperative course: diabetes, thyroid disease, parathyroid disease, endocrine-secreting tumors, and adrenal cortical suppression.

Evaluation of the Patient with Known Systemic Disease

Cardiac Disease

The preoperative evaluation of the patient with suspected cardiovascular disease has been approached in two ways: clinical risk indices and preoperative cardiac testing. The goals are to define risk, determine which patients will benefit from further testing, form an appropriate anesthetic plan, and identify patients who will benefit from perioperative beta-blockade, intervention therapy, or even surgery. Clinical risk indices range from the physical status index of the American Society of Anesthesiologists (Table 18-2) to the Goldman Cardiac Risk Index, which has recently been updated.

TABLE 18-2

AMERICAN SOCIETY OF ANESTHESIOLOGISTS PHYSICAL STATUS CLASSIFICATION

■ STATUS	■ DISEASE STATE
ASA Class 1	No organic, physiologic, biochemical, or psychiatric disturbance
ASA Class 2	Mild to moderate systemic disturbance that may not be related to the reason for surgery
ASA Class 3	Severe systemic disturbance that may or may not be related to the reason for surgery
ASA Class 4	Severe systemic disturbance that is life threatening with or without surgery
ASA Class 5	Moribund patient who has little chance of survival but is submitted to surgery as a last resort (resuscitative effort)
Emergency operation (E)	Any patient in whom an emergency operation is required

From information in American Society of Anesthesiologists: New classification of physical status. Anesthesiology 24:111, 1963.

In an update of the Goldman Cardiac Risk Index, the investigators studied 4,315 patients aged 50 years and older who were undergoing elective, major noncardiac procedures.[8] Six independent predictors of complications were identified and included in a revised risk index: high-risk type of surgery, history of ischemic heart disease, history of congestive heart failure, history of cerebrovascular disease, preoperative treatment with insulin, and preoperative serum creatinine >2.0 mg/dL. Cardiac complications rose with an increase in the number of risk factors present. Rates of major cardiac complications with 0, 1, 2, or 3 of these factors were 0.5, 1.3, 4, and 9%, respectively, in the derivation cohort and 0.4, 0.9, 7, and 11%, respectively, among 1,422 patients in the validation cohort (Fig. 18-2).

While all of these indices provide information to assess the probability of complications and provide an estimate of risk, they do not prescribe perioperative management. In contrast,

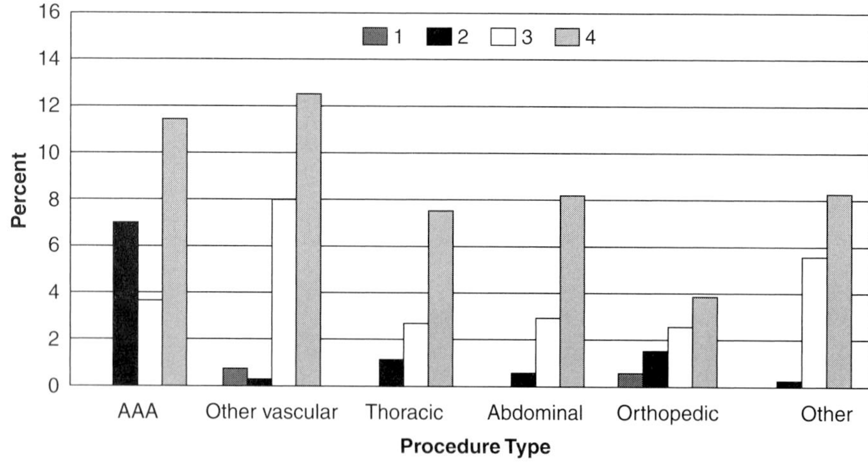

FIGURE 18-2. CRI cardiac risk index. Bars represent rate of major cardiac complications in entire patient population (both derivation and validation cohorts combined) for patients in revised CRI classes according to type of procedure performed. AAA, abdominal aortic aneurysm. Note that, by definition, patients undergoing AAA, thoracic, and abdominal procedures were excluded from Class I. In all subsets except patients undergoing AAA, there was a statistically significant trend toward greater risk with higher-risk class. See text for details. (Reproduced with permission from Lee TH, Marcantonio ER, Mangione CM *et al*: Derivation and prospective validation of a simple index for prediction of cardiac risk of major noncardiac surgery. Circulation 100:1043, 1999.)

the anesthesiologist is most concerned with forming an anesthetic plan after defining the cardiovascular risk factors.

In patients with symptomatic coronary disease, the preoperative evaluation may lead to the recognition of a change in the frequency or pattern of anginal symptoms. Certain populations of patients—for example, the elderly, women, or diabetics—may present with more atypical features. The presence of unstable angina has been associated with a high perioperative risk of MI.[5]

In virtually all studies, the presence of active congestive heart failure preoperatively has been associated with an increased incidence of perioperative cardiac morbidity.[9,10] Stabilization of ventricular function and treatment for pulmonary congestion are important prior to elective surgery. Because the type of perioperative monitoring and treatments would be different, clarifying the cause of heart failure is important. Congestive symptoms may be a result of nonischemic cardiomyopathy or cardiac valvular insufficiency and/or stenosis.

Adults with a prior MI almost always have coronary artery disease. Traditionally, risk assessment for noncardiac surgery was based on the time interval between the MI and surgery. Multiple studies have demonstrated an increased incidence of reinfarction if the MI was within 6 months of surgery.[11–13] With improvements in perioperative care, this difference has decreased. Therefore, the importance of the intervening time interval may no longer be valid in the current era of interventional therapy and risk stratification after an acute MI. Although many patients with an MI may continue to have myocardium at risk for subsequent ischemia and infarction, other patients may have their critical coronary stenoses either totally occluded or widely patent. For example, the use of percutaneous transluminal coronary angioplasty, thrombolysis, and early coronary artery bypass grafting (CABG) has changed the natural history of the disease.[14,15] Therefore, patients should be evaluated from the perspective of their risk for ongoing ischemia. The American Heart Association/American College of Cardiology Task Force on Perioperative Evaluation of the Cardiac Patient Undergoing Noncardiac Surgery has defined three risk groups—major, intermediate, and minor (Table 18-3). They indicate that recent MI (MI <30 days) places patients in the group at highest risk; after that period, a prior MI places the patient at intermediate risk.[16]

TABLE 18-3

CLINICAL PREDICTORS OF INCREASED PERIOPERATIVE CARDIOVASCULAR RISK (MYOCARDIAL INFARCTION, CONGESTIVE HEART FAILURE, DEATH)

Major
Unstable coronary syndromes
- Recent myocardial infarction[a] with evidence of important ischemic risk by clinical symptoms or noninvasive study
- Unstable or severe[b] angina (Canadian Class III or IV)[c]

Decompensated congestive heart failure
Significant arrhythmias
- High-grade atrioventricular block
- Symptomatic ventricular arrhythmias in the presence of underlying heart disease
- Supraventricular arrhythmias with uncontrolled ventricular rate

Severe valvular disease

Intermediate
Mild angina pectoris (Canadian Class I or II)
Prior myocardial infarction by history or pathological Q waves
Compensated or prior congestive heart failure
Diabetes mellitus

Minor
Advanced age
Abnormal ECG (left ventricular hypertrophy, left bundle-branch block, ST-T abnormalities)
Rhythm other than sinus (e.g., atrial fibrillation)
Low functional capacity (e.g., inability to climb one flight of stairs with a bag of groceries)
History of stroke
Uncontrolled systemic hypertension

[a]The American College of Cardiology National Database Library defines recent MI as greater than 7 days but less than or equal to 1 month (30 days).
[b]May include "stable" angina in patients who are unusually sedentary.
[c]Campeau L: Grading of angina pectoris. Circulation 54:522, 1976.
Reproduced with permission from Eagle K, Brundage B, Chaitman B *et al*: Guidelines for perioperative cardiovascular evaluation of the noncardiac surgery. A report of the American Heart Association/American College of Cardiology Task Force on Assessment of Diagnostic and Therapeutic Cardiovascular Procedures. Circulation 93:1278, 1996.

Patients with Coronary Artery Disease

For those patients without overt symptoms or history, the probability of CAD varies with the type and number of atherosclerotic risk factors present. Peripheral arterial disease has been shown to be associated with CAD in multiple studies.[17] Diabetes mellitus is a common disease in the elderly and represents a process that affects multiple organ systems. Complications of diabetes mellitus are frequently the cause of urgent or emergent surgery, especially in the elderly. Diabetes accelerates the progression of atherosclerosis, so it is not surprising that diabetics have a higher incidence of CAD than nondiabetics do. There is a high incidence of both silent myocardial infarction and myocardial ischemia.[18] Eagle et al demonstrated that diabetes is an independent risk factor for perioperative cardiac morbidity.[19] In attempting to determine the degree of this increased probability, the length of the disease and other associated end-organ dysfunction should be taken into account. Autonomic neuropathy has been found to be the best predictor of silent coronary artery disease.[20] Because these patients are at very high risk for a silent MI, an electrocardiogram (ECG) should be obtained to examine for the presence of Q waves.

Hypertension has also been associated with an increased incidence of silent myocardial ischemia and infarction.[18] Hypertensive patients who have left ventricular hypertrophy and are undergoing noncardiac surgery are at a higher perioperative risk than nonhypertensive patients.[21] Investigators have suggested that the presence of a strain pattern on ECG suggests a chronic ischemic state.[22] Therefore, these patients should also be considered to have an increased probability of CAD and for perioperative morbidity.

There is controversy regarding a trigger to delay or cancel a surgical procedure in a patient with untreated or inadequately treated hypertension. Hypertension has been divided into three stages, with Stage 3 denoting that which might be used as a cutoff (Table 18-4).[23] Aggressive treatment of blood pressure is associated with increased reduction in long-term risk, although the effect diminishes in all but diabetic patients
2 as diastolic blood pressure is reduced below 90 mmHg. Although there has been a suggestion in the literature that a case should be delayed if the diastolic pressure is greater than 110 mm Hg, the study often quoted as the basis for this determination demonstrated no major morbidity in that small group of patients.[24] Other authors state that there is little association between blood pressures of less than 180 mmHg systolic or 110 mm Hg diastolic and postoperative outcomes. However, such patients are prone to perioperative myocardial ischemia, ventricular dysrhythmias, and lability in blood pressure. It is less clear in patients with blood pressures above

TABLE 18-4

BLOOD PRESSURE (mmHg)

CATEGORY	SYSTOLIC		DIASTOLIC
Optimal	<120	and	<80
Normal	<130	and	<85
High-normal	130–139	or	85–89
Hypertension			
Stage 1	140–159	or	90–99
Stage 2	160–179	or	100–109
Stage 3	≥180	or	≥110

Reproduced with permission from Sixth report of the Joint National Committee on Prevention, Detection, Evaluation, and Treatment of High Blood Pressure. Arch Intern Med 157:2413, 1997.

TABLE 18-5

CARDIAC RISK[a] STRATIFICATION FOR NONCARDIAC SURGICAL PROCEDURES

HIGH	(Reported cardiac risk often >5%) • Emergent major operations, particularly in the elderly • Aortic and other major vascular • Peripheral vascular • Anticipated prolonged surgical procedures associated with large fluid shifts and/or blood loss
INTERMEDIATE	(Reported cardiac risk generally <5%) • Carotid endarterectomy • Head and neck • Intraperitoneal and intrathoracic • Orthopaedic • Prostate
LOW[b]	(Reported cardiac risk generally <1%) • Endoscopic procedures • Superficial procedures • Cataract • Breast

[a]Combined incidence of cardiac death and nonfatal myocardial infarction.
[b]Do not generally require further preoperative cardiac testing.
Reproduced with permission from Eagle K, Brundage B, Chaitman B *et al*: Guidelines for perioperative cardiovascular evaluation of the noncardiac surgery. A report of the American Heart Association/American College of Cardiology Task Force on Assessment of Diagnostic and Therapeutic Cardiovascular Procedures. Circulation 93:1278, 1996.

180/100 mmHg, although no absolute evidence exists that postponing surgery will reduce risk.[25] In the absence of end-organ changes, such as renal insufficiency or left ventricular hypertrophy with strain, it would seem appropriate to proceed with surgery. In contrast, a patient with a markedly elevated blood pressure and new onset of a headache should have surgery delayed for further treatment.

Several other risk factors have been used to suggest an increased probability of CAD. These include the atherosclerotic processes associated with tobacco use and hypercholesterolemia. Although these risk factors increase the probability of developing coronary artery disease, they have not been shown to increase perioperative risk. When attempting to determine the overall probability of disease, the number of risk factors and severity of each are important.

Importance of Surgical Procedure

The surgical procedure influences the scope of preoperative evaluation required by determining the potential range of physiologic flux during the perioperative period. Few hard data exist defining the surgery-specific incidence of complications. It is known that peripheral procedures, such as those included in a study of ambulatory surgery completed at the Mayo Clinic, are associated with an extremely low incidence of morbidity and mortality,[26] while major vascular procedures are associated with the highest incidence of complications. Eagle et al published data on the incidence of perioperative myocardial infarction and mortality by procedure for patients enrolled in the Coronary Artery Surgery Study (CASS).[27] They determined the overall risk of perioperative morbidity in patients with known coronary artery disease treated medically compared to those patients who had prior coronary artery bypass grafting. High-risk procedures include major vascular, abdominal, thoracic, and orthopaedic surgery. The American Heart Association/American College of Cardiology Guidelines described a risk stratification for noncardiac surgery that is shown in Table 18-5.[16]

Importance of Exercise Tolerance

3 Exercise tolerance is one of the most important determinants of perioperative risk and the need for further testing and invasive monitoring. An excellent exercise tolerance, even in patients with stable angina, suggests that the myocardium can be stressed without failing. If a patient can walk a mile without becoming short of breath, the probability of extensive coronary artery disease is small. Alternatively, if patients experience dyspnea associated with chest pain during minimal exertion, the probability of extensive coronary artery disease is high, which has been associated with greater perioperative risk. Additionally, these patients are at risk for developing hypotension with ischemia, and therefore may benefit from more extensive monitoring, coronary intervention therapy, or revascularization. Exercise tolerance can be assessed with formal treadmill testing or with a questionnaire that assesses activities of daily living (Table 18-6).[16]

Reilly et al have evaluated the predictive value of self-reported exercise tolerance for serious perioperative complications and demonstrated that a poor exercise tolerance (could not walk four blocks and climb two flights of stairs) independently predicted a complication with an odds ratio of 1.94.[28] The likelihood of a serious adverse event was inversely related to the number of blocks that could be walked. Therefore, there is good evidence to suggest that minimal additional testing is necessary if the patient is able to describe a good exercise tolerance.

INDICATIONS FOR FURTHER CARDIAC TESTING

Multiple algorithms have been proposed to determine which patients require further testing. As described previously, the risk associated with the proposed surgical procedure influences the decision to perform further diagnostic testing and interventions. Guidelines must be tempered by recent studies in which perioperative cardiac morbidity was greatly reduced by perioperative β-adrenergic blockade administration.[29] With the reduction in perioperative morbidity, it has been suggested that extensive cardiovascular testing is not necessary. However,

TABLE 18-6

ESTIMATED ENERGY REQUIREMENT FOR VARIOUS ACTIVITIES[a]

1 MET	Can you take care of yourself? Eat, dress, or use the toilet? Walk indoors around the house? Walk a block or two on level ground at 2–3 mph or 3.2–4.8 km/hr? Do light work around the house like dusting or washing dishes?	4METs	Walk on level ground at 4 mph or 6.4 km/hr? Run a short distance Do heavy work around the house like scrubbing floors or lifting or moving heavy furniture? Participate in moderate recreational activities like golf, bowling, dancing, doubles tennis, or throwing a baseball or football?
4 METs	Climb a flight of stairs or walk up a hill?	>10 METs	Participate in strenuous sports like swimming, singles tennis, football, basketball, or skiing?

MET= metabolic equivalent.
[a]Adapted from the Duke Activity Status Index and AHA Exercise Standards.
Reproduced with permission from Eagle K, Brundage B, Chitman B *et al*: Guidelines for perioperative cardiovascular evaluation of the noncardiac surgery. A report of the American Heart Association/American College of Cardiology Task Force on Assessment of Diagnostic and Therapeutic Cardiovascular Procedures. Circulation 93:1278, 1996.

until these findings can be confirmed, further testing may be warranted.

4 The algorithm to determine the need for testing proposed by the American College of Cardiology/American Heart Association Task Force and an update in 2002,[30] is based on the available evidence and expert opinion that integrates clinical history, surgery-specific risk, and exercise tolerance (Fig. 18-3).[16] In step one, the clinician evaluates the urgency of the surgery and the appropriateness of a formal preoperative assessment. Next, determine if the patient has undergone a recent revascularization procedure or coronary evaluation. Those patients with unstable coronary syndromes should be identified, and appropriate treatment instituted. Finally, the decision to undergo further testing depends on the interaction of the clinical risk factors, surgery-specific risk, and functional capacity. For patients at intermediate clinical risk, both exercise tolerance and the extent of the surgery are taken into account to determine the need for further testing. Importantly, no preoperative cardiovascular testing should be performed if the results will not change perioperative management.

Cardiovascular Tests

Electrocardiogram

Preoperative 12-lead electrocardiogram can provide important information on the state of the patient's myocardium and coronary circulation. Abnormal Q waves in high-risk patients are highly suggestive of a past myocardial infarction. Confirmation of active ischemia usually requires changes in at least two leads. It has been estimated that approximately 30% of myocardial infarctions occur without symptoms ("silent infarctions") and can only be detected on routine electrocardiograms, with the highest incidence occurring in patients with either diabetes or hypertension. The Framingham study showed that long-term prognosis is not improved by lack of symptoms.[18] The absence of Q waves on the electrocardiogram does not exclude the occurrence of a Q-wave myocardial infarction in the past. It has been shown that 5 to 27% of Q waves disappear over the 10-year period following an infarction.[32] Those patients in whom the electrocardiogram reverts to normal have improved survival compared with those with consistent abnormalities, with or without Q waves. The presence of Q waves on a preoperative electrocardiogram in a high-risk patient, regardless of symptoms, should alert the anesthesiologist to the increased perioperative risk and the possibility of active ischemia.

It has not been established that information obtained from the preoperative electrocardiogram affects clinical care. A review of clinical studies on the matter is inconclusive. In a retrospective review of adult patients undergoing ambulatory surgery, the preoperative electrocardiogram was not predictive of perioperative risk.[33] Although controversy exists, current recommendations include the need for a preoperative electrocardiogram in the presence of systemic vascular disease (for example, those patients with hypertension or peripheral vascular disease), for males over 40 years of age and for females over 50.

Noninvasive Cardiovascular Testing

The exercise electrocardiogram has been the traditional method in the past for evaluating patients with suspected coronary artery disease. It represents the most cost-effective and least invasive method for detecting ischemia, with a sensitivity of 70 to 80% and a specificity of 60 to 75% for identifying coronary artery disease. A positive exercise stress test alerts the anesthesiologist that the patient is at risk for ischemia over a wide range of heart rates, with the greatest risk in those who develop ischemia only after mild exercise. However, as discussed previously, the ability to exercise suggests that no further testing is necessary, and therefore stress electrocardiography is infrequently indicated.

A number of high-risk patients are either unable to exercise or have contraindications to exercise, for example, those with claudication. Therefore, pharmacologic stress testing and ambulatory electrocardiography have come into vogue, particularly as preoperative cardiovascular tests in patients scheduled for vascular surgery. Pharmacologic stress thallium imaging is useful in those patients who are unable to exercise. Dipyridamole or adenosine is administered as a coronary vasodilator to assess flow heterogeneity. The presence of a redistribution defect is predictive of postoperative cardiac events, especially in patients undergoing peripheral vascular surgery (Fig. 18-4). Similarly, dopamine can be used to increase myocardial oxygen demand, by increasing heart rate and blood pressure, in those patients who cannot exercise.

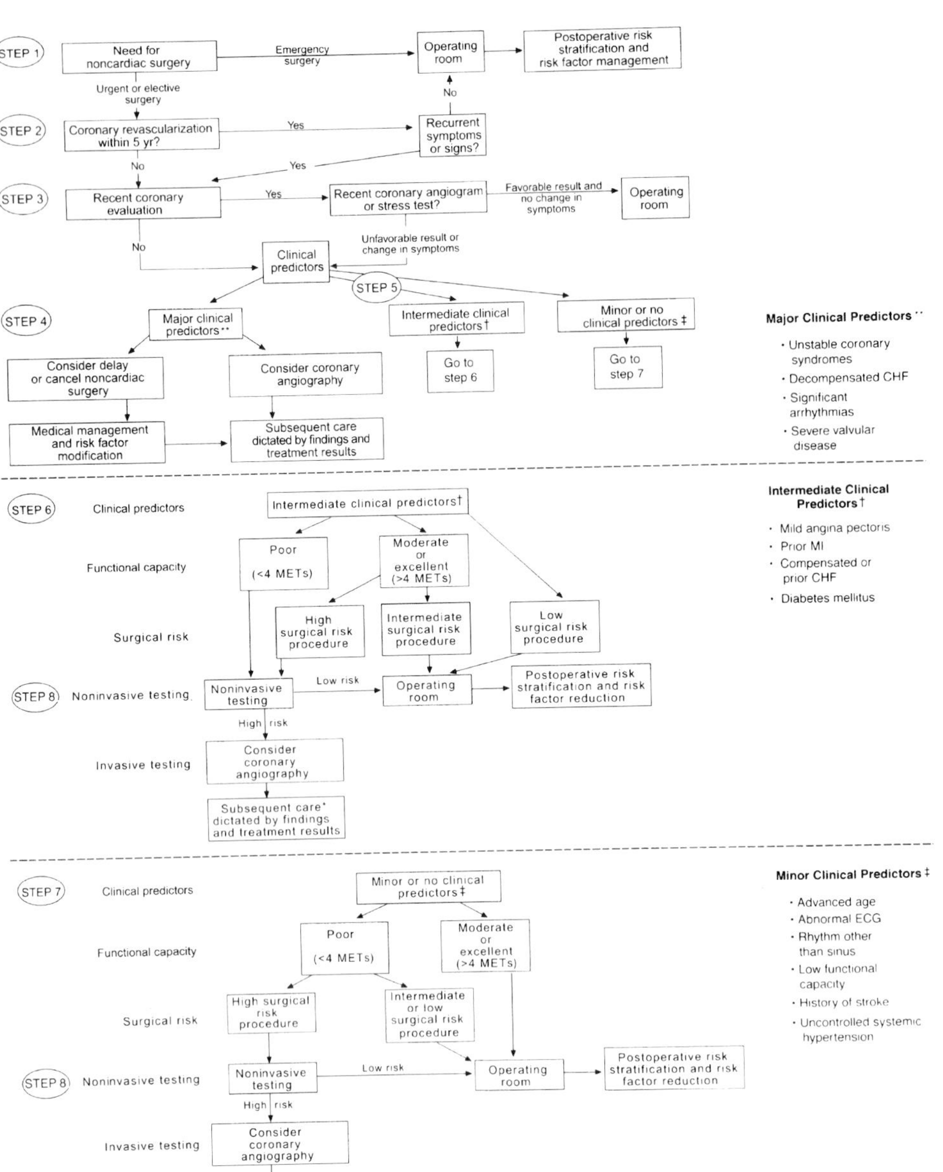

FIGURE 18-3. The American Heart Association/American College of Cardiology Task Force on Perioperative Evaluation of Cardiac Patients Undergoing Noncardiac Surgery has proposed an algorithm for decisions regarding the need for further evaluation. This represents one of multiple algorithms proposed in the literature. It is based on expert opinion and incorporates six steps. First, the clinician must evaluate the urgency of the surgery and the appropriateness of a formal preoperative assessment. Next, he or she must determine whether the patient has had a previous revascularization procedure or coronary evaluation. Those patients with unstable coronary syndromes should be identified, and appropriate treatment should be instituted. The decision to have further testing depends on the interaction of the clinical risk factors, surgery-specific risk, and functional capacity. (Adapted with permission from Eagle K, Brundage B, Chaitman B *et al*: Guidelines for perioperative cardiovascular evaluation of noncardiac surgery. A report of the American Heart Association/American College of Cardiology Task Force on Assessment of Diagnostic and Therapeutic Cardiovascular Procedures. Circulation 93: 1278, 1996.)

The ambulatory ECG (Holter monitoring) provides a means of continuously monitoring the electrocardiogram for significant ST segment changes preoperatively. One study demonstrated that the presence of silent ischemia is a strong predictor of outcome, while its absence is associated with a favorable outcome in 99% of the patients studied.[34] Other investigators have demonstrated the value of ambulatory ECG monitoring, although the negative predictive values have not been as high as reported by some.

Stress echocardiography is another preoperative test that may be of value in evaluating patients with suspected coronary artery disease. The appearance of either new or more severe regional wall motion abnormalities with exercise is considered a positive test. Either represents areas at risk for myocardial ischemia. The advantage of the stress echocardiogram is that it is a dynamic assessment of ventricular function. Dobutamine echocardiography has also been studied and found to have among the best predictive values. It is generally accepted that the group at risk is comprised by those who demonstrate regional wall motion abnormalities at low heart rates.

Several groups have published meta-analyses of preoperative diagnostic tests. One group of investigators demonstrated good predictive values using ambulatory ECG monitoring, radionuclide angiography, dipyridamole thallium imaging, or dobutamine stress echocardiography.[35] Shaw et al also demonstrated good predictive values of dipyridamole thallium imaging and dobutamine stress echocardiography.[36] Both of these studies demonstrated the superior value of dobutamine stress echocardiography; however, there was significant overlap of the confidence intervals with other tests. The most important determinant with respect to the choice of preoperative testing is the expertise of the local institution. The decision to perform further invasive testing should be based on the knowledge that the intervention will affect both short- and long-term outcomes.

Assessment of Ventricular and Valvular Function

Both echo and radionuclide angiography can assess cardiac ejection fraction at rest and under stress, but echo is less invasive and is also able to assess regional wall motion abnormalities, wall thickness, valvular function, and valve area. Pulse-wave Doppler can be used to determine the velocity time integral. Ejection fraction can then be calculated by determining the cross-sectional area of the ventricle. Conflicting results exist with regard to the predictive value of ejection fraction

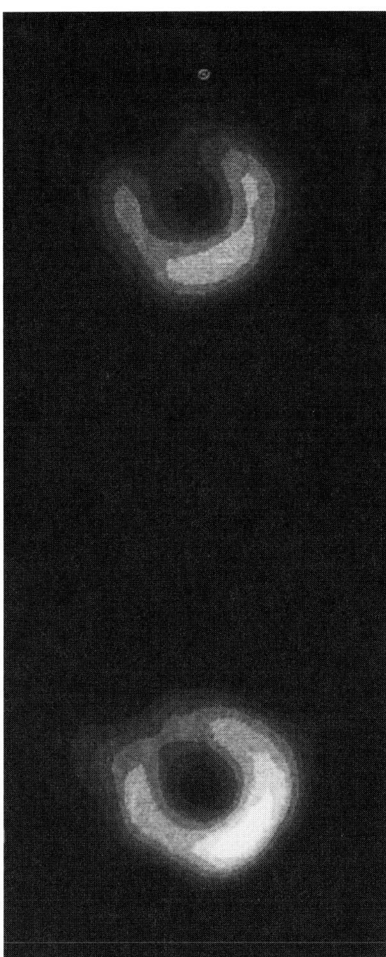

FIGURE 18-4. A dipyridamole-thallium SPECT image demonstrating a reversible defect. The top image demonstrates defects consistent with areas of low perfusion or ischemia, which fills in on subsequent imaging (*bottom*). (See upper left portion of image.)

using either echocardiographic or radionuclide measurements. Echocardiography can provide important information regarding valvular function, which may have important implications for either cardiac or noncardiac surgery, and is discussed more fully later in this text. Aortic stenosis has been associated with a poor prognosis in noncardiac surgical patients, and knowledge of valvular lesions may modify perioperative hemodynamic therapy.[9]

Coronary Angiography

Coronary angiography is currently the best method for defining coronary anatomy. In addition, information regarding ventricular and valvular function can also be assessed. Hemodynamic indices can be determined such as ventricular pressures and pressure gradients across valves. This information is routinely available in patients scheduled for coronary bypass grafting. Narrowing of the left main coronary artery and certain other lesions may be associated with a greater perioperative risk. Diffuse atherosclerosis in small vessels, as seen in diabetics, may lead to incomplete revascularization and a risk of developing ischemia despite coronary bypass grafting. Coronary angiography is used by cardiologists to determine whether coronary vascularization is an option.

Unlike the exercise or pharmacologic stress tests discussed earlier, coronary angiography provides anatomic, not functional, information. Although a critical coronary stenosis delineates an area of risk for developing myocardial ischemia, the functional response of that ischemia cannot be assessed by angiography alone. A critical stenosis may or may not be the underlying cause for a perioperative myocardial infarction that occurs. In the ambulatory population, many infarctions are the result of acute thrombosis of a noncritical stenosis. Therefore, the value of routine angiography prior to noncardiac surgery depends on the identification of lesions that will cause morbidity and mortality.

The American College of Physician Guidelines attempt to apply the evidence-based approach.[37] The initial decision point is the assessment of risk using the Detsky modification of the CRI.[10] If patients are Class II or III, they are considered high risk. If they are Class I, the presence of other clinical factors can be used to further stratify risk. Those who exhibit multiple markers for cardiovascular disease according to these risk indices and who are undergoing major vascular surgery are considered appropriate for further diagnostic testing, either by dipyridamole imaging or by dobutamine stress echocardiography. The Guidelines suggest that there is insufficient evidence to recommend diagnostic testing for nonvascular surgery patients.

Perioperative Coronary Interventions

The strategies to reduce the perioperative risk of noncardiac surgery have recently been studied. There are several large studies that suggest that in patients who survive CABG, the risk of subsequent noncardiac surgery is low.[5,8] While there is little data to support the notion of coronary revascularization solely for the purpose of improving perioperative outcome, it is true that for some patients scheduled for high-risk surgery long-term survival may be enhanced by revascularization. Two studies utilized the Coronary Artery Surgery Study database and found that CABG significantly improved survival in those patients with both peripheral vascular disease and triple-vessel coronary disease, especially the group with depressed ventricular function.[6] After reviewing all available data, most clinicians believe the indication for CABG prior to noncardiac surgery remains the same as in other settings and is independent of the proposed noncardiac surgery.

The value of percutaneous translumimal coronary angioplasty (PTCA) is less well established. The current evidence does not support the use of PTCA beyond established indications for nonoperative patients.

Coronary stent placement may be a unique issue. In a case series of 39 patients who had undergone coronary stent placement within 1 month of noncardiac surgery there was a significant incidence of perioperative death and hemorrhage for patients who had surgery within 14 days of stent placement.[31] The authors of the ACC/AHA Guideline recommended waiting a minimum of 2 weeks, and preferably 4 weeks.

PULMONARY DISEASE

Introduction

Pulmonary complications remain a major cause of morbidity and mortality for patients undergoing surgery and anesthesia. They occur more frequently than cardiac complications, with an incidence of 5 to 10% in those having major noncardiac procedures. Perioperative pulmonary complications include atelectasis, pneumonia, bronchitis, bronchospasm, hypoxemia, and respiratory failure requiring mechanical ventilation.[38]

The site and type of surgery are the strongest predictors of complications. With regard to the surgical *site*, thoracic or upper abdominal surgery is associated with the highest risk for postoperative pulmonary problems. Risk increases as the incision approaches the diaphragm.[38–40] Decreases in postoperative vital capacity and functional residual capacity, as well as diaphragmatic dysfunction, contribute to hypoxemia and atelectasis.[41] Functional residual capacity may take up to 2 weeks to return to baseline. Diaphragmatic dysfunction occurs despite adequate analgesia and is theorized to be because of phrenic nerve inhibition.[42] The *types* of surgery carrying the highest risks were AAA repair, thoracic, and upper abdominal surgery, followed by neck, peripheral vascular, and neurosurgery. Neurosurgery and neck surgery may be associated with perioperative aspiration pneumonia.

The need for emergency surgery and the need for general anesthesia are also associated with a slightly increased risk. Not only can the surgery affect pulmonary function, but general anesthesia also results in mechanical changes such as a decrease in the FRC and altered diaphragmatic motion leading to $\dot{V}/\dot{Q}$ mismatch with shunting and dead space ventilation. General anesthesia also aggravates these changes by its effects at the microscopic level: inhibition of mucociliary clearance, increased alveolar-capillary permeability, inhibition of surfactant release, increased nitric oxide synthetase, and increased sensitivity of the pulmonary vasculature to neurohumoral mediators. Subanesthetic levels of intravenous or volatile agents have the ability to blunt the ventilatory response to hypoxemia and hypercarbia. Duration of anesthesia is a well-established risk factor for postoperative pulmonary complications, with morbidity rates increasing after 2 to 3 hours.[43] However, although laparoscopic surgery is often longer in duration, the decreased pulmonary complications postoperatively compared to an open procedure usually outweigh the risks of increased anesthesia time.[44]

Patient-Related Factors (Table 18-7)

Preoperative evaluation of patients with preexisting pulmonary disease should include assessment of the type and severity of disease, as well as its reversibility. Because clinical observations are often the best predictors for the development of postoperative pulmonary complications, a careful history and physical examination is imperative. The anesthesiologist should inquire about exercise intolerance, chronic cough, or unexplained dyspnea. On physical exam, findings of wheezing, rhonchi, decreased breath sounds, dullness to percussion, and a prolonged expiratory phase are important. Preoperative pulmonary function testing is usually reserved for those scheduled for lung resection, or for those scheduled for major surgery who have unexplained pulmonary signs and symptoms after a careful history and physical examination. Early intervention helps to ensure that the patient's medical status is optimal prior to surgery.

TABLE 18-7

POTENTIAL PATIENT-RELATED RISK FACTORS FOR POSTOPERATIVE PULMONARY COMPLICATIONS

POTENTIAL RISK FACTOR	TYPE OF SURGERY	UNADJUSTED RELATIVE RISK ASSOCIATED WITH FACTOR
Smoking	Coronary bypass	3.4
	Abdominal	1.4–4.3
ASA Class > II	Unselected	1.7
	Thoracic or abdominal	1.5–3.2
Age > 70 yr	Unselected	1.9–2.4
	Thoracic or abdominal	0.9–1.9
Obesity	Unselected	1.3
	Thoracic or abdominal	0.8–1.7
COPD	Unselected	2.7–3.6
	Thoracic or abdominal	4.7

ASA, American Society of Anesthesiologists; COPD, chronic obstructive pulmonary disease.
Adapted from Smetana GW: Preoperative pulmonary evaluation. N Engl J Med 340(12):942, 1999.

Tobacco

The use of tobacco is an important risk factor, but one that usually cannot be influenced. Even among smokers who have not developed chronic lung disease, smoking is known to increase carboxyhemoglobin levels, decrease ciliary function and increase sputum production, as well as cause stimulation of the cardiovascular system secondary to the nicotine. While cessation of smoking for 2 days can decrease carboxyhemoglobin levels, abolish the nicotine effects, and improve mucous clearance, a prospective study by Warner showed that smoking cessation for at least 8 weeks was necessary to reduce the rate of postoperative pulmonary complications.[45] Because smokers often show increased airway reactivity under general anesthesia, it is useful to administer a bronchodilator such as albuterol preoperatively.

Asthma

Asthma is one of the most common coexisting diseases that confronts the anesthesiologist. During the patient interview it is important to elicit information regarding inciting factors, severity, reversibility, and current status. Frequent use of bronchodilators, hospitalizations for asthma, and the requirement for systemic steroids are all indicators of the severity of the disease. After an episode of asthma, airway hyperreactivity may persist for several weeks.[46] In addition to bronchodilators, perioperative steroids are worth considering as prophylaxis for the severe asthmatic; for example, hydrocortisone 100 mg intravenously every 8 hours on the day of surgery. The possibility of adrenal insufficiency is also a concern in those patients who have received more than a "burst and taper" of steroids in the previous 6 months. This group of patients should be administered "stress doses" of steroids perioperatively. Kabalin et al found there was a low complication rate for asthmatics treated with short-term steroids undergoing surgery.[47] Significantly, they found no association with impaired wound healing or infections. For patients using inhaled steroids, they should be administered regularly starting at least 48 hours prior to surgery for optimal effectiveness.

Endocrine Disease

Diabetes mellitus is the most common endocrinopathy and has acute and chronic disease manifestations. Because of this and other factors, diabetics are more likely to require surgery. Some recent studies in the critical care literature have sparked a trend toward tighter perioperative glucose control, especially in diabetics. Because the majority of diabetics develop disease in one or more systems, end-organ disease must be identified and managed carefully in the perioperative period. While long-term, close control of glucose may limit some of the microvascular effects of diabetes (retinopathy, neuropathy, and nephropathy), macrovascular events, such as myocardial infarctions or

TABLE 18-8

CLINICAL MANIFESTATIONS OF THYROID AND PARATHYROID DISEASES

	HYPERTHYROIDISM	HYPOTHYROIDISM	HYPERPARATHYROIDISM
General	Weight loss; heat intolerance; warm, moist skin	Cold intolerance	Weight loss, polydipsia
Cardiovascular	Tachycardia, atrial fibrillation, congestive heart failure	Bradycardia, congestive heart failure, cardiomegaly, pericardial or pleural effusion	Hypertension, heart block
Neurologic	Nervousness, tremor, hyperactive reflexes	Slow mental function, minimal reflexes	Weakness, lethargy, headache, insomnia, apathy, depression
Musculoskeletal	Muscle weakness, bone resorption	Large tongue, amyloidosis	Bone pains, arthritis, pathologic fractures
Gastrointestinal	Diarrhea	Delayed gastric emptying	Anorexia, nausea, vomiting, constipation, epigastric pain
Hematologic	Anemia, thrombocytopenia		
Renal		Impaired free water clearance	Polyuria, hematuria

Adapted from Roizen MF: Anesthesia for the patient with endocrine disease, Part 1. Curr Rev Clin Anesth 6:43, 1987.

stroke, may not be altered in incidence. Diabetics have an increased risk of coronary artery disease, perioperative myocardial infarction, hypertension, and congestive heart failure. In addition, they are more likely than the general population to have cerebral vascular, peripheral vascular, and renal vascular disease. Myocardial infarction or ischemia may be "silent" if diabetic autonomic neuropathy is present. A high index of suspicion for myocardial ischemia or past infarction should be maintained throughout the preoperative period. Administration of perioperative beta-blockers should be considered in diabetic patients with coronary artery disease to help limit perioperative myocardial ischemia. Some may have concerns regarding the use of beta-blockade in diabetics as a result of the fears of worsening glucose intolerance and masking hypoglycemic symptoms. Despite the controversy, many clinicians believe diabetics benefit at least as much as the general population in receiving perioperative beta-blockers. Significant renal disease develops commonly in diabetics, many times necessitating chronic dialysis. Peripheral and autonomic neuropathies are common in diabetics. These deficits should be documented prior to anesthesia and surgery with the anesthetic plan adjusted accordingly. Joint rigidity (stiff joint syndrome) may significantly affect the temporomandibular, atlantooccipital, and cervical spine joints in patients with long-standing type 1 diabetes. The joint limitation may result in difficulty with intubation and should be identified prior to anesthesia and airway manipulation.

Thyroid and parathyroid disease have clinical manifestations that are important to the preoperative evaluation (Table 18-8). Thyroid disease is usually adequately evaluated by clinical history, although of course, the thyroid function tests are more sensitive. The preoperative evaluation should focus on evaluating the signs and symptoms of hyperthyroidism and hypothyroidism. Hypothyroidism can lead to the development of hypothermia, hypoglycemia, hypoventilation and hyponatremia, as well as a susceptibility to depressant drugs. Anesthesiologists should be alerted to the possibility of the hypermetabolic state of thyroid storm in patients with hyperthyroidism. A large thyroid mass may distort the upper airway, producing wheezing, especially evident in the supine position. In these cases, a chest x-ray should be obtained looking for evidence of tracheal deviation or narrowing. A computed tomography (CT) scan of the upper airway and trachea will provide better detail of any airway compromise. Patients with hyperparathyroidism often have hypercalcemia, indicating preoperative determination of a serum calcium level. The classic findings for pheochromocytoma include intermittent hypertension, headache, diaphoresis, and tachychardia. In patients with other endocrine tumors, a pheochromocytoma should be ruled out as the cause of unexplained hypertension as part of a multiple endocrine neoplasia syndrome. The preoperative preparation of a patient with a pheochromocytoma is fully discussed in Chapter 41. Over time the mortality for surgical resection of a pheochromocytoma has decreased because of improvements in perioperative therapy for patients with the syndrome. The important issue is to identify patients with a pheochromocytoma preoperatively before they are scheduled for other types of surgery. In patients on long-term corticosteroids, one should have a high index of suspicion for adrenal-cortical suppression and Cushing's syndrome. The hallmark symptoms found in Cushing's syndrome include moon facies, striations of the skin, trunk obesity, hypertension, easy bruisability, and hypovolemia. The preoperative preparation includes correction of the fluid and electrolyte abnormalities. There is consensus that for patients taking corticosteroids for long periods that perioperative steroid supplementation is indicated to cover the stresses of anesthesia and surgery. However, in patients who have had only a short course of steroids within the 12 months prior to surgery, the use of steroid supplementation is controversial, although most clinicians would favor their use preoperatively (Table 18-9).

Other Organ Systems

Renal disease has important implications for fluid and electrolyte management, as well as metabolism of drugs (see Chapter 35). Liver disease is associated with altered protein binding and volume of distribution of drugs, as well as coagulation abnormalities (see Chapter 39). Coagulation disorders may influence the choice of regional anesthesia. The anesthesiologist should inquire about bruising, bleeding, and the use of medications that influence platelet function such as aspirin, other nonsteroidal anti-inflammatory drugs, and anticoagulants. The perioperative management of hemoglobinopathies is reviewed in Chapter 19. Musculoskeletal disorders have been associated with an increased risk of malignant hyperthermia. Osteoarthritis may result in difficulty exposing the glottic opening for tracheal intubation or difficulty in positioning for regional anesthetic. Because rheumatoid arthritis is a multisystem disease, it is important in such patients to perform a thorough review of systems. These patients may have restrictive lung disease, pleural effusions, pericarditis, anemia, and atlantooccipital instability. Finally, the anesthesiologist should inquire about

TABLE 18-9

PERIOPERATIVE CORTICOSTEROID COVERAGE

For minor surgery	The patient should take 1.5–2 times his or her usual prednisone dosage on the morning of surgery. The following day the patient should take his or her normal prednisone dose (or parenteral equivalent if gut cannot be used). The surgeon and anesthesiologist should be aware that the patient is glucocorticoid dependent and should be prepared to administer more "steroids" if the surgery becomes prolonged or more extensive.
For moderate surgery	The patient should be given 2 times his or her usual glucocorticoid dosage orally (if possible) on the morning of surgery and/or 25 mg hydrocortisone iv before the operation, then 75 mg hydrocortisone iv during the operation, and 50 mg hydrocortisone iv after the operation; then the dose should be rapidly tapered over 48 hr to the usual dose—if the postoperative course is uncomplicated.
For major surgery	The patient should be given 2 times his or her usual glucocorticoid dosage orally (if possible) on the morning of surgery and/or 50 mg hydrocortisone iv before the operation, then 100 mg hydrocortisone iv during the operation. After the operation, 100 mg iv q 8 hr × 24 hr should be administered and then rapidly tapered (over 48–72 hr) to the patient's usual glucocorticoid dosage—if the postoperative course is uncomplicated.

Adapted from Brussel T, Chernow B: Perioperative management of endocrine problems: Thyroid, adrenal cortex, pituitary. Am Soc Anesthesiol 3:48, 1990.

infectious diseases such as HIV or antibiotic-resistant infections.

PREOPERATIVE LABORATORY TESTING

The Value of Preoperative Testing: Normal Values

In attempting to determine the optimal choice of preoperative tests, it is important to understand the interpretation of the results. Ideally, tests would either confirm or exclude the presence of a disease; however, the vast majority of tests only increase or decrease the probability of disease. In determining reference ranges for diagnostic tests, values that fall outside of
5 the 95% confidence intervals for normal individuals are considered abnormal. Therefore, up to 5% of normal individuals can have "abnormal" test results. To determine its clinical relevance, a test must be interpreted within the context of the clinical situation. Performing tests in patients with no risk for having the pathophysiologic process of interest can yield a high number of false-positive results. For example, a low potassium (3.0 mg/dL) in an otherwise healthy individual is most likely a normal result. Interpreting this test as abnormal, and initiating treatment, could lead to harm without any benefit.

The Value of Preoperative Testing: Bayesian Analysis

The use of noninvasive testing is another area in which the clinical situation significantly affects the interpretation. It is rare for a test result to be pathognomonic for a disease state; that is, no test is 100% sensitive and specific. For example, exercise or pharmacologic stress testing has sensitivities ranging from 60 to 90% and specificities ranging from 60 to 80% for a significant coronary artery stenosis. To interpret the results of a noninvasive test, it is important to know the prevalence of disease in the population as well as the sensitivity and specificity of the test. If a test is used in a population with a very low prevalence of disease, a positive result is frequently a false-positive. Similarly, a negative result in a population with a very high prevalence of disease may be a false-negative. Bayes' theorem suggests a test is most useful in a population with a moderate probability of disease.[75]

Risks and Costs Versus Benefits

The use of medical testing is associated with significant cost, both in real dollars and in potential harm. Routine preoperative testing has been estimated to cost $3 billion annually. An "abnormal" test that is later determined to be a false result can lead to significant cost and real harm. For example, a positive exercise electrocardiographic stress test in a healthy 40-year-old female may lead to coronary angiography. Coronary angiography is not a benign procedure, and can lead to vascular injuries. Based on Bayesian analysis, a positive test result in this patient is most likely a false-positive, and the test was inappropriately used. Therefore, the woman and her physician would gain no additional information, thousands of dollars in medical costs would accrue, and she would sustain morbidity.

Several studies have evaluated the implications of reduced testing. Golub et al retrospectively reviewed the records of 325 patients who had undergone pre-admission testing prior to ambulatory surgery.[48] Of these, 272 (84%) had at least one abnormal screening test result, while only 28 surgeries were delayed or canceled. The authors estimated that only three patients potentially benefited from pre-admission testing, including a new diagnosis of diabetes in one and nonspecific ECG changes in two, one of which had known ischemic heart disease.

In a study published in 1991, Narr and colleagues at the Mayo Clinic demonstrated minimal benefits from routine testing and proposed that routine laboratory screening tests were not required in healthy patients.[49] In a follow-up study published in 1997, a cohort of patients who had no preoperative testing during 1994 was reviewed and found to include no deaths or major perioperative morbidity.[50] They concluded that current anesthetic and medical practices rapidly identify indications for laboratory evaluation when necessary and therefore routine testing was not indicated in this healthy cohort.

Even if testing better defines a disease state, the risks of any intervention based upon the results may outweigh the benefit. Cardiovascular testing is a classic example (Fig. 18-5). If a noninvasive test is positive, coronary angiography may be performed. A positive angiogram may then result in coronary artery bypass grafting prior to the planned noncardiac surgery. Although cardiovascular morbidity and mortality may be reduced in patients with significant coronary artery disease who have undergone coronary revascularization, the morbidity associated with both the testing and revascularization procedure may be greater than any potential benefit.

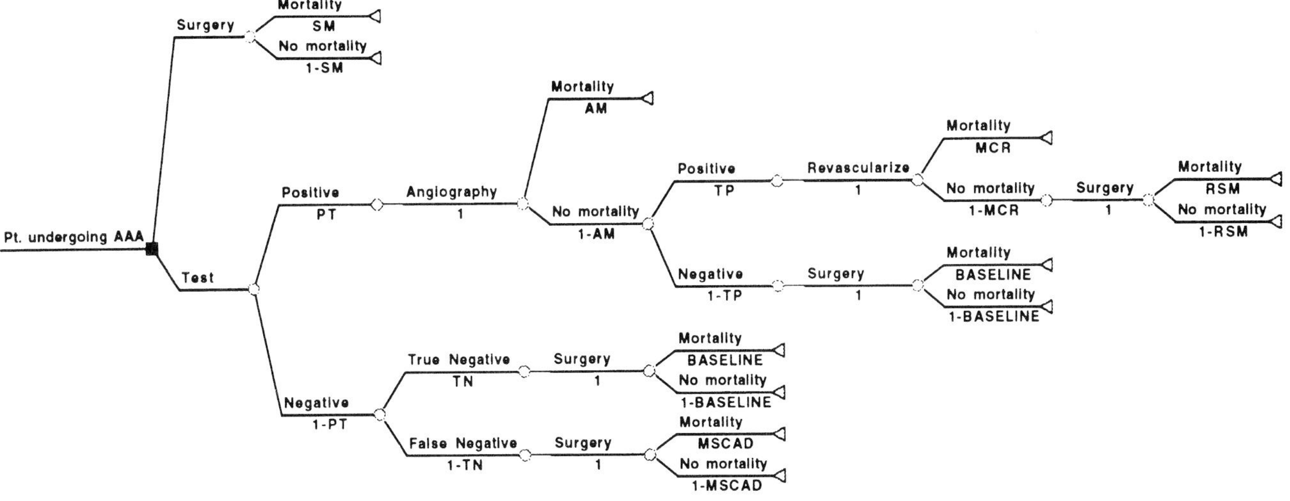

FIGURE 18-5. A decision algorithm evaluating the decision between vascular surgery alone or coronary artery revascularization before vascular surgery. There are currently no randomized trials to address the optimal strategy. By outlining the multiple decision points at which a patient can sustain mortality by choosing to undergo coronary revascularization first, the optimal strategy for preoperative evaluation can be demonstrated. Specifically, variation in mortalities at each decision point can change the optimal strategy. (Reproduced with permission from Fleisher LA, Skolnick ED, Holroyd KJ, Lehmann HP: Coronary artery revascularization before abdominal aortic aneurysm surgery: A decision analytic approach. Anesth Analg 79:661, 1994.)

Roizen and Cohn have suggested a protocol for screening tests based on the preoperative evaluation using a benefit–risk analysis.[51]

Recommended Laboratory Testing

Blood Count
Neonates
Physiologic age ≥75 yr
Class C procedure
Malignancy
Renal disease
Tobacco use
Anticoagulant use

Coagulation Studies
Chemotherapy
Hepatic disease
Bleeding disorder
Anticoagulants

Electrolytes
Renal disease
Diabetes
Diuretic, digoxin, or steroid use
CNS disease

BUN/Creatinine
Physiologic age ≥75 yr
Class C procedure
Cardiovascular disease
Renal disease
Diabetes
Diuretic or digoxin use
CNS disease

Blood Glucose
Physiologic age ≥75 yr
Class C procedure
Diabetes
Steroid use
CNS disease

Liver Function Tests
Hepatic disease
Hepatitis exposure
Malnutrition

Chest X-Ray
Physiologic age ≥75 yr
Cardiovascular disease
Pulmonary disease
Malignancy
Radiation Therapy
Tobacco ≥20 p-y

ECG
Physiologic age ≥75 yr
Class C procedure
Cardiovascular disease
Pulmonary disease
Radiation therapy
Diabetes
Digoxin use
CNS disease

Pregnancy Test
Possible pregnancy

Albumin
Physiologic age ≥75 yr
Class C procedure
Malnutrition

T/S
Physiologic age ≥75 yr
Class C procedure

Complete Blood Count and Hemoglobin Concentration

The use of a preoperative hemoglobin has been suggested as the only test necessary in many patients prior to elective surgery; however, even this minimal standard has been questioned. Baron et al reviewed the records of 1,863 pediatric patients scheduled for elective outpatient procedures.[52] In only 1.1% of patients was the hematocrit abnormal, and in none of these patients was the procedure canceled or anesthetic plan modified. However, a baseline hematocrit is still indicated in any procedure with a risk of blood loss.

The standard regarding the lowest acceptable perioperative hematocrit and indication for a preoperative transfusion has changed during the past decade. The current recommendations of the National Blood Resource Education Committee is that a hemoglobin of 7 g/dL is acceptable in patients without systemic disease. In patients with systemic disease, signs of inadequate systemic oxygen delivery (tachycardia, tachypnea) are an indication for transfusion.

Electrolytes

In the past, patients routinely received a chemistry panel prior to surgery. Because of technology issues, it may be cheaper to obtain a standard battery than to determine one particular test. However, testing rarely leads to any change in perioperative management.

There are numerous guidelines regarding the need for preoperative electrolytes. The only consensus is the lack of routine testing in asymptomatic adults, although a creatinine and glucose has been recommended in older patients. In patients with systemic diseases or on medications that affect the kidneys, a BUN and creatinine are indicated.

Coagulation Studies

Coagulation disorders can have significant impact on the surgical procedure and perioperative management. However, abnormal laboratory studies in the absence of clinical abnormalities will rarely lead to perioperative problems. Patients with known inherited coagulopathies, such as hemophilia or von Willebrand's disease, require preoperative preparation of the patient. It is important to identify such disorders from or history of bleeding problems. A prothrombin, partial thromboplastin time analysis is indicated in the presence of previous bleeding disorders such as following injuries; after tooth extraction or surgical procedures; and in patients with known or suspected liver disease, malabsorption or malnutrition, and on certain medications such as antibiotics and chemotherapeutic agents.

Bleeding time previously was advocated as a means of determining the presence of a qualitative platelet defect. However, recently clinicians have questioned the value of this test in clinical practice. The test is extremely operator dependent, and some authors have suggested that the test should be abandoned in favor of clinical history. In the absence of a clinical bleeding diathesis, complications are extremely rare. If such a history exists, it may be prudent to avoid regional anesthesia.

Pregnancy Testing

Routine pregnancy testing in women of child-bearing potential is a subject of considerable debate. The rationale is that specific agents may be avoided, or surgery may be delayed. Information regarding the last menstrual period can help define the potential, but does not eliminate the possibility. Roizen and Cohn suggest that pregnancy testing should be limited to females who believe they are pregnant or cannot tell if they are pregnant.[51] However, a number of studies have evaluated the validity of history as a means of assessing pregnancy status in adolescents with conflicting results. Current practice varies dramatically among centers and anesthesiologists and may be a function of the population served with regard to the need to routinely test those women with a negative pregnancy history.

Chest X-Rays

A preoperative chest x-ray can identify abnormalities that may lead to either delay or cancellation of the planned surgical procedure or modification of perioperative care. For example, identification of pneumonia, pulmonary edema, pulmonary nodules, or a mediastinal mass could all lead to modification of care. However, routine testing in the population without risk factors can lead to more harm than benefit. Roizen and Cohn have demonstrated substantial harm from additional procedures based on shadows performed solely as a routine preoperative chest x-ray.[51]

The American College of Physicians suggests that a chest x-ray is indicated in the presence of active chest disease or an intrathoracic procedure, but not solely on the basis of advanced age alone.[53] Other guidelines suggest that a preoperative chest x-ray is reasonable in patients over the age of 60 years. In a meta-analysis, Archer et al reviewed the published reports from 1966 to 1992 in the English, French, and Spanish literature.[54] Twenty-one reports were identified with sufficient data to evaluate the use of testing. On average, abnormalities were reported in 10% of routine preoperative chest x-rays, of which only 1.3% were unexpected. These findings result in modification in management in only 0.1% of patients, with unknown influence on outcome. The authors estimated that each finding that influenced management would cost $23,000, concluding that routine chest x-rays without a clinical indication were not justified. Therefore, a preoperative chest x-ray is indicated in patients with a history or clinical evidence of active pulmonary disease, and *may* be indicated routinely only in patients with advanced age.

Pulmonary Function Tests

Pulmonary function tests can be generally divided into two categories, spirometry and an arterial blood gas. Spirometry can provide information on forced vital capacity (FVC), forced expiratory volume in 1 sec (FEV_1), ratio of FEV_1/FVC, and average forced expiratory flow from 25 to 75%. Although each of these measures has a sound physiologic basis, their practical assessment can vary greatly among healthy persons. Objective measures defining high risk for pulmonary resection have been proposed. For nonpulmonary surgery, they rarely provide additional information beyond that obtained from history. The one possible indication is the use of pulmonary function testing with bronchodilator therapy to assess responsiveness in a patient who is wheezing.

With the advent of the pulse oximeter, the use of preoperative arterial blood gas sampling has become less important. It may still be indicated, since determining the baseline CO_2 is useful in managing postoperative ventilation settings and resting hypercapnia is associated with increased perioperative risk. However, the physical act of obtaining an arterial blood gas can lead to hyperventilation and change the $PaCO_2$. One method of assessing the probability of CO_2 retention is evaluation of the serum bicarbonate. A normal serum bicarbonate will virtually exclude the diagnosis of CO_2 retention. If the serum bicarbonate is elevated, then an arterial blood gas either preoperatively or immediately prior to induction may be indicated.

Another indication for an arterial blood gas has been determination of oxygen concentration. With the advent and availability of pulse oximetry in the preoperative screening clinic, this is rarely an indication.

SUMMARY

The preoperative evaluation of the surgical patient continues to be an important component of the anesthesiologist's role. A thorough history and physical examination can be used to identify those medical conditions that might affect perioperative management and direct further laboratory testing. In the current era of capitated care and the desire to reduce inappropriate utilization of medical technology, the anesthesiologist can have a significant impact on health resource utilization by performing appropriate laboratory tests. By combining data from the history, physical examination, exercise tolerance, and the stress of the surgical procedure, inappropriate testing can be reduced; but more importantly, appropriate screening tests will be performed.

TABLE 18-10

COMPARISON OF PREOPERATIVE VISIT AND PENTOBARBITAL (2 mg/kg im) (PERCENTAGE OF PATIENTS)

	■ FELT DROWSY	■ FELT NERVOUS	■ ADEQUATE PREPARATION
Control group	18	58	35
Pentobarbital group	30	61	48
Preoperative visit	26	40	65
Preoperative visit and pentobarbital	38	38	71

Data from Egbert LD, Battit GE, Turndorf H *et al*: The value of the preoperative visit by an anesthetist. JAMA 185:553, 1963.

PREOPERATIVE MEDICATION

Anesthetic management for patients begins with preoperative psychological preparation and, if necessary, preoperative medication. Specific pharmacologic actions should be kept in mind
6 when these drugs are administered before operation, and they should be tailored to the needs of each patient. The anesthesiologist should assess the patient's mental and physical condition during the preoperative visit. Because it is part of and the beginning of the anesthetic, choice of preoperative medication is based on the same considerations as the choice of anesthesia, including the patient's medical problems, requirements of the surgery, and the anesthesiologist's skills. Satisfactory preoperative preparation and medication facilitate an uneventful perioperative course. Poor preparation may begin a series of problems and misadventures.

No consensus exists on the choice of preoperative medications. Their use has been dominated by tradition, which has been modified somewhat by the change in anesthetic agents and techniques over the years. Beecher stated that "empirical procedures firmly established in the habits of good doctors have a life, not to say, immortality of their own."[55] Similarly, "the emotional attachment of an anesthesiologist to his own regimen is often more obvious than his objective assessment of its effects."[56] Another reason for lack of consensus may be that several different drugs or combinations of drugs can accomplish the same goals. However, there is general agreement that most patients should enter the operating room after anxiety has been relieved and other specific goals have been met through preoperative preparation and medication. This should be accomplished without undue sedation, which can interfere with patient safety or, given the dramatic increase in the number of outpatient surgical procedures, prolong length of stay in the operating room.

PSYCHOLOGICAL PREPARATION

Psychological preparation of the patient involves the preoperative visit and interview with the patient and family members. The anesthesiologist should explain anticipated events and the
7 proposed anesthetic management in an effort to reduce anxiety and allay apprehension. Patients may perceive the day of surgery as the biggest, most threatening day in their lives; they do not wish to be treated impersonally in the operating room. The anesthesiologist's first direct encounter with the patient may be in the immediate preoperative period. A growing number of patients receive their pre-anesthetic evaluations by others in preoperative evaluation clinics or just prior to surgery. Preoperative visits must be conducted efficiently, but they must also be informative and reassuring, answering all questions. Most of the anesthesiologist's time is spent with an unconscious or sedated patient; therefore, he or she must take time before the operation to earn the trust and confidence of that patient.

Most patients are anxious before surgery. Studies show that, depending on the intensity of inquiry, from 40 to 85% of patients are apprehensive before surgery. Preoperative anxiety states are at a high level, and most patients expect apprehension to be relieved before they arrive in the operating room. The classic study by Egbert et al showed that an average of 57% of patients felt anxious before operation.[57] An informative and comforting preoperative visit may replace many milligrams of depressant medication. For example, the study by Egbert and colleagues showed that more patients were adequately prepared for surgery after a preoperative interview than after 2 mg/kg of pentobarbital given intramuscularly 1 hour before surgery (see Table 18-10).[57] However, psychological preparation cannot accomplish everything and will not relieve all anxiety. Besides psychological preparation, there are other goals of preoperative medication. Control of pain and satisfactory levels of amnesia or sedation cannot be achieved with consistent success at the preoperative visit alone. In addition, emergency situations may provide little or no time for a preoperative interview. More seriously ill or elderly patients, conversely, may not tolerate the physiologic effects of sedative medications. Always remember that the substitution of preoperative depressant drugs for a comforting and tactful preoperative visit may compromise patient safety.

PHARMACOLOGIC PREPARATION

The ideal drug or combination of drugs for preoperative pharmacologic preparation is as elusive as is the ideal anesthetic techniques and is not based on a large body of data that is either definitive or persuasive. Routine administration of the same drugs to all patients has fallen into disfavor as a selective approach has emerged. In selecting the appropriate drugs for preoperative medication, the patient's psychological condition, physical status, and age must be considered. The surgical procedure and its duration are important factors, as well. Is this an outpatient procedure? Is it elective surgery or emergency surgery? The anesthesiologist must know the patient's weight, prior response to depressant drugs, including unwanted side effects, and allergies. Finally, the anesthesiologist's experience and familiarity with certain preoperative medications more than others are determinants.

The goals to be achieved for each patient with preoperative medication are intimately involved in the selection process (Table 18-11). The desired goals may be multiple and should

TABLE 18-11

VARIOUS GOALS FOR PREOPERATIVE MEDICINE

1. Relief of anxiety
2. Sedation
3. Amnesia
4. Analgesia
5. Drying of airway secretions
6. Prevention of autonomic reflex responses
7. Reduction of gastric fluid volume and increased pH
8. Antiemetic effects
9. Reduction of anesthetic requirements
10. Facilitation of smooth induction of anesthesia
11. Prophylaxis against allergic reactions

Modified from Stoelting RK: Psychological preparation and preoperative medication. In Miller RD (ed): Anesthesia. New York, Churchill Livingstone, 1981.

TABLE 18-12

COMMON PREOPERATIVE MEDICATIONS, DOSES, AND ADMINISTRATION ROUTES

MEDICATION	ADMINISTRATION ROUTE	DOSE (mg)
Diazepam	Oral	5–20
Lorazepam	Oral, im	1–4
Midazolam	im	3–7
	iv	Titration of 1.0–2.5-mg doses
Secobarbital	Oral, im	50–200
Pentobarbital	Oral, im	50–200
Morphine	im	5–15
Meperidine	im	50–150
Cymetidine	Oral, im, iv	150–300
Ranitidine	Oral	50–200
Metoclopramide	Oral, im, iv	5–20
Atropine	im, iv	0.3–0.6
Glycopyrrolate	im, iv	0.1–0.3
Scopolamine	im, iv	0.3–0.6

im, intramuscular; iv, intravenous.
Modified from Stoelting RK, Miller RD (eds): Basics of Anesthesia. New York, Churchill Livingstone, 1984.

be tailored to the needs of each patient. Some of the goals, such as relief of anxiety and production of sedation, apply to almost every patient, whereas others are important only occasionally. Prophylaxis against allergic reactions applies in just a few instances. Prevention of autonomic reflexes mediated through the vagus nerve or an antiemetic effect may be better attempted immediately before the anticipated need rather than achieved at the time of preoperative medication. Preoperative medication regimens do not produce sufficient obtundation to be clinically significant in reducing anesthetic requirement. Some patients should not receive depressant drugs before surgery. Patients with little physiologic reserve, at the extremes of age, with a head injury, or with hypovolemia may be harmed more than helped by many of the medications normally used before operation. In contrast, the conditions of others demand that attempts be made pharmacologically to reduce anxiety, provide analgesia, or dry secretions in the airway to produce a safer perioperative course. For elective surgery, the anesthesiologist will, in most instances, want the patient to enter the operating room free of anxiety and sedated, yet easily arousable and cooperative. The patient should not be overly obtunded or display other unwanted side effects of the preoperative drugs. The pa-
8 tient who asks to be "asleep" before leaving the hospital room should be told that apprehension and sedation may be reduced but it would be unsafe to produce a comatose state. The time and route of administration of the preoperative medications are important. As a general rule, oral medications should be given to the patient 60 to 90 minutes before arrival in the operating room. It is acceptable to administer oral drugs with up to 150 mL of water.[58] Intravenous agents produce effects after a few circulation times, while for full effect, intramuscular medications should be given at least 20 minutes and preferably 30 to 60 minutes before the patient's arrival in the operating room. Every attempt should be made to have the preoperative medications achieve their full effect before the patient's arrival in the operating room rather than after induction of anesthesia. The drug(s), doses, route of administration, and effects should be recorded on the anesthetic record. A list of common preoperative medications is presented in Table 18-12.

Sedative–Hypnotics and Tranquilizers

Benzodiazepines

Benzodiazepines are among the most popular drugs used for preoperative medication (Table 18-13). They are used to produce anxiolysis, amnesia, and sedation. Because the site of action of benzodiazepines is on specific receptors in the central nervous system (Fig. 18-6) there is relatively little depression of ventilation or of the cardiovascular system with premedicant doses. Benzodiazepines have a wide therapeutic index and a low incidence of toxicity. Other than central nervous

TABLE 18-13

COMPARISON OF PHARMACOLOGIC VARIABLES OF BENZODIAZEPINES

	DIAZEPAM	LORAZEPAM	MIDAZOLAM
Dose equivalent (mg)	10	1–2	3–5
Time to peak effect after oral dose (hr)	1–1.5	2–4	0.5–1
Elimination half-time (hr)	20–40	10–20	1–4
Clearance (mL/kg/min)	0.2–0.5	0.7–1.0	6.4–11.1
Volume of distribution (L/kg)	0.7–1.7	0.8–1.3	1.1–1.7

Adapted from Reves JG, Fragen RJ, Vinick HR *et al*: Midazolam: Pharmacology and uses. Anesthesiology 62:310, 1985; and Stoelting RK: Pharmacology and Physiology in Anesthetic Practice. Philadelphia, JB Lippincott, 1987.

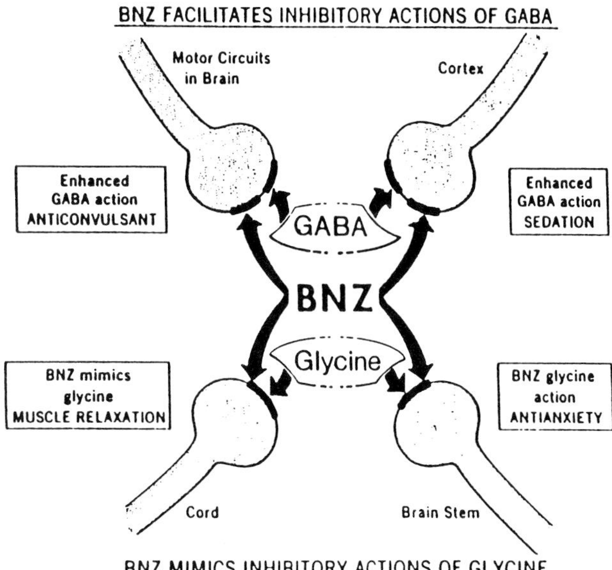

FIGURE 18-6. Schematic diagram of possible mechanisms for pharmacologic effects of benzodiazepines (BNZs). GABA, γ-aminobutyric acid. (Reprinted from Richter JJ: Current theories about the mechanisms of benzodiazepines and neuroleptic drugs. Anesthesiology 54:66, 1981.)

system depression, there are few side effects of this group of drugs. Specifically, nausea and vomiting are not usually associated with administration of benzodiazepines for preoperative medication.

There are some hazards and unwanted side effects of the benzodiazepines. The central nervous system depression they cause is sometimes long and excessive, especially with use of lorazepam. There may be pain at the intramuscular or intravenous injection site with diazepam, as well as the possibility of phlebitis. These drugs are not analgesic agents. Benzodiazepines may not always produce a calming effect but may cause agitation, as evidenced by restlessness and delirium.

Diazepam. While diazepam is often the standard against which other benzodiazepines are compared, it has largely been replaced. Because it is insoluble in water and must be dissolved in organic solvents, pain may occur on intramuscular or intravenous injection. Phlebitis is often a sequela of intravenous injection.

Lorazepam. Lorazepam resembles oxazepam structurally and is 5 to 10 times as potent as diazepam. Lorazepam can produce profound amnesia, relief of anxiety, and sedation (Fig. 18-7).[59] When lorazepam is compared with diazepam, their effects are very similar. Although it is insoluble in water and requires a solvent such as polyethylene glycol or propylene glycol, administration of lorazepam, unlike diazepam, is not associated with pain on injection or phlebitis. Prolonged sedation is more likely after lorazepam administration. Even though the elimination half-life of diazepam is longer than that of lorazepam (20 to 40 hours versus 10 to 20 hours), the effect of diazepam may be shorter because it more rapidly dissociates from the benzodiazepine receptor.[60]

Lorazepam is reliably absorbed both orally and intramuscularly. Maximal effect occurs 30 to 40 minutes after intravenous injection. Bradshaw et al demonstrated clinical effects 30 to 60 minutes after oral administration of lorazepam.[61] A study by Blitt et al demonstrated that lack of recall was not produced until 2 hours after intramuscular injection.[62] Peak plasma concentrations may not occur until 2 to 4 hours after oral administration. Therefore, lorazepam must be ordered well before surgery so that the drug has time to be effective before the patient arrives in the operating room. Lorazepam also may be given sublingually. As stated previously, the elimination half-life is 10 to 20 hours. The usual dose is about 25 to 50 μg/kg. The dose for an adult should usually not exceed 4.0 mg.[59,60] With recommended doses, anterograde amnesia may be produced for as long as 4 to 6 hours without excessive sedation. Higher doses lead to prolonged and excessive sedation without more amnesia. Because of its slow onset and length of action, lorazepam is not useful in instances in which rapid awakening is necessary, such as with outpatient anesthesia. There are no active metabolites of lorazepam; and because its metabolism is not dependent on microsomal enzymes, there is less influence on its effect from age or liver disease. As with diazepam, little cardiorespiratory depression occurs with lorazepam. However, there is the danger of unwanted respiratory depression in those with lung disease.

Midazolam. Midazolam has predominantly replaced the use of diazepam for preoperative medication and conscious sedation. It is common to administer sedative doses intravenously just prior to the trip to the operating room. The physicochemical properties of the drug allow for its water solubility and rapid metabolism. As with other benzodiazepines, midazolam produces anxiolysis, sedation, and amnesia. It is two to three times as potent as diazepam because of its increased affinity for the benzodiazepine receptor. The usual intramuscular dose is 0.05 to 0.1 mg/kg and titration of 1.0 to 2.5 mg at a time intravenously. There is no irritation or phlebitis with injection of midazolam. The incidence of side effects after administration is low, although depression of ventilation and sedation may be greater than expected, especially in elderly patients or when the drug is combined with other central nervous system

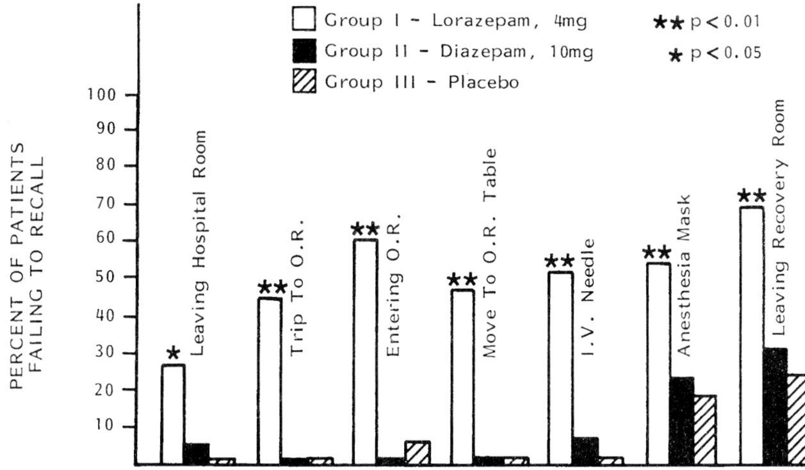

FIGURE 18-7. Percentage of patients in each group failing to recall specific events of the operative day. Medications were administered intramuscularly. (Reprinted with permission from Fragen RJ, Caldwell N: Lorazepam premedication: Lack of recall and relief of anxiety. Anesth Analg 55:792, 1976.)

depressants. There is more rapid onset of action and predictable absorption after intramuscular injection of midazolam than after diazepam. The time of onset after intramuscular injection is 5 to 10 minutes, with peak effect occurring after 30 to 60 minutes. The onset after intravenous administration of 5 mg would be expected to occur after 1 to 2 minutes. In addition to quicker onset, more rapid recovery occurs after midazolam administration compared with diazepam. This is probably the result of the lipid solubility of midazolam and its rapid distribution in the peripheral tissues and metabolic biotransformation. For these reasons, midazolam usually should be given within an hour of induction.[63] Midazolam is metabolized by hepatic microsomal enzymes to essentially inactive hydroxylated metabolites. H_2 receptor antagonists do not interfere with its metabolism. The elimination half-life of midazolam is approximately 1 to 4 hours and may be extended in the elderly. Tests show that mental function usually returns to normal within 4 hours of administration.[63] After administration of 5 mg, amnesia lasts from 20 to 30 minutes. Intramuscular administration may produce longer periods of amnesia. The lack of recall may be augmented by concomitant administration of scopolamine. The properties of midazolam make it ideal for shorter procedures.

Other Benzodiazepines. Oxazepam, another benzodiazepine that has been used for preoperative medication, is one of the pharmacologically active metabolites of diazepam. It is absorbed slowly after oral administration and has an elimination half-life of 5 to 15 hours. Temazepam has been given in oral doses of 20 to 30 mg before surgery. It must be given well before surgery because peak plasma levels do not occur until approximately 2 to 2.5 hours after administration. Triazolam is a short-acting benzodiazepine. The adult oral dose of the drug is 0.25 to 0.5 mg. Peak plasma concentrations occur in about 1 hour and its elimination half-life is 1.7 to 5.2 hours. The drug may become long-acting in the elderly. Similarly, a study by Pinnock et al did not show triazolam to be of short duration when compared with diazepam for premedication for minor gynecologic surgery.[64] Alprazolam (1 mg) given to adults has been shown to produce a modest reduction in anxiety before surgery.

Barbiturates

Use of barbiturates for preoperative medication is a time-tested practice with a long record of safety. These drugs are used primarily for their sedative effects. While barbiturate administration for pharmacologic preparation before surgery has been replaced in many instances by the use of benzodiazepines, they may be useful in certain settings. There is little cardiorespiratory depression associated with the usual preoperative doses. The barbiturates may be given orally as well as parenterally, and the drugs are relatively inexpensive. Barbiturates, however, are unlikely to produce sedation in the presence of pain. In fact, disorientation and paradoxical excitation may result. Low doses of barbiturates have been said to lower the pain threshold and be antianalgesic. The agents lack specificity of action on the central nervous system and have a lower therapeutic index than the benzodiazepines. Barbiturates should not be used in patients with certain kinds of porphyria.

Secobarbital. Secobarbital usually is administered to adults in oral doses of 50 to 200 mg when used for preoperative medication. Onset usually occurs 60 to 90 minutes after administration, and sedative effects last 4 hours or longer. Indeed, even though secobarbital traditionally has been considered a "short-acting" barbiturate, it may impair performance for as long as 10 to 22 hours.[65]

Other Sedative Drugs

Hydroxyzine. Hydroxyzine is a nonphenothiazine tranquilizer. It is often given for its proposed additive effects to opioids and does not cause an increase in side effects. Hydroxyzine has sedative action and anxiolytic properties. It has limited analgesic properties and does not produce amnesia. It is an antihistamine and an antiemetic.

Diphenhydramine. Diphenhydramine is a histamine receptor antagonist with sedative and anticholinergic activity. It is also an antiemetic. A dose of 50 mg will last 3 to 6 hours in an adult. Diphenhydramine has been used recently in combination with cimetidine, steroids, and other drugs for prophylaxis in patients with chronic atopy and for prophylaxis before chemonucleolysis and dye studies. Diphenhydramine blocks the histamine receptor to prevent effects of histamine peripherally.

Phenothiazines. Promethazine, promazine, and perphenazine are often used in combination with opioids. Phenothiazines have sedative, anticholinergic, and antiemetic properties. These effects, added to the analgesic effects of the opioids, have been used for preoperative medication.

Opioids

Morphine and meperidine were historically the most frequently used opioids for intramuscular preoperative medication. Recently, the use of intravenous fentanyl just before surgery has become more popular. Opioids are used when analgesia is needed before operation. It has been stated in the strict sense that "unless there is pain, there is no need for narcotic in preanesthetic medication."[66] For the patient experiencing pain before operation, the opioids can produce good analgesia and even euphoria. Opioids have been ordered for patients before operation to ameliorate the discomfort that may occur during regional anesthesia or the insertion of invasive monitoring catheters or large intravenous lines. The dose of opioid may need to be reduced in the debilitated or elderly patient. The elderly patient often exhibits a reduced sensitivity to pain. Furthermore, elderly patients can have an increased analgesic response to opioids. Opioids also have been used before operation in the opioid-dependent patient.

Preoperative administration of opioids in other settings has been controversial. They have been given before surgery prior to a nitrous oxide–opioid anesthetic. This is done in an attempt to have a basal state of anesthesia on board when the patient arrives in the operating room and to get a preview of the patient's response to opioids. Opioids have been given to patients before operation to provide analgesia on their awakening in the recovery room. The other approach is to titrate the opioid intravenously during emergence or on the patient's arrival in the recovery room. Preoperative administration of opioids can lower anesthetic requirements. This may or may not be clinically significant for a specific patient receiving a particular anesthetic technique. Some anesthesiologists use opioids in combination with other drugs before operation to facilitate anesthetic induction by mask. It must be remembered that opioids decrease ventilation during spontaneous breathing and therefore decrease uptake of inhalation drugs. If necessary, the anesthesiologist may want to use assisted or controlled ventilation of the lungs to overcome the respiratory depressant effects of the opioids. Finally, opioids are not the best drugs to relieve apprehension, produce sedation, or prevent recall.

Administration of opioids has the potential for causing several side effects. Preoperatively, they usually exhibit no direct myocardial effects. However, opioids do interfere with the compensatory constriction of smooth muscles of the peripheral vasculature. This may lead to orthostatic hypotension. Histamine release after injection of morphine may compound these circulatory effects. As with most preoperative medications, it is probably safest to have the patient remain at bed rest after opioid premedication. The analgesic properties and respiratory depressant effects of opioids usually go hand in hand. The decrease in the carbon dioxide drive at the medullary respiratory center may be prolonged. Furthermore, there is a decrease in the responsiveness to hypoxia at the carotid body after injection of only low doses of opioids.[67] The anesthesiologist may wish to consider supplemental oxygen for the patient receiving opioid premedication. In general, the opioid agonist–antagonists produce less respiratory depression, but they also produce less analgesia. Rather than euphoria, the opioids may produce dysphoria. When this side effect does occur, it is most commonly seen in a patient who does not have pain before operation and has received the opioid premedication. Nausea and vomiting may result from opioid administration. The effect of opioids on the vestibular apparatus leading to motion sickness or stimulation of the medullary chemoreceptor trigger zone is a postulated reason for nausea and vomiting. Choledochoduodenal sphincter (sphincter of Oddi) spasm has occasionally been noted subsequent to injection of opioids. The opioid produces smooth muscle constriction, which leads to right upper quadrant pain. Pain relief may be achieved with naloxone or possibly glucagon. Occasionally, the pain from biliary tract spasm is difficult to differentiate from the pain of angina pectoris. The administration of nitroglycerin should relieve angina pectoris and pain resulting from biliary tract spasm; an opioid antagonist should relieve only pain resulting from biliary tract spasm. Some question the use of opioid premedication in patients with biliary tract disease. All opioids have the potential to induce choledochoduodenal sphincter spasm. Meperidine is less likely than morphine to produce this side effect. Opioids may produce pruritus. Morphine, possibly through histamine release, often produces itching, especially around the nose. Opioids also may cause flushing, dizziness, and miosis.

Other drugs are often combined with opioids for their additive effects or to overcome the disadvantages of opioid side effects. The sedative–hypnotics and scopolamine are often used with opioids to produce sedation, anxiolysis, and amnesia in addition to analgesia. In selected patients, the combination of morphine and a benzodiazepine or scopolamine may be useful for pharmacologic preoperative preparation.

Morphine

Morphine is well absorbed after intramuscular injection. The onset of effect should occur within 15 to 30 minutes. The peak effect occurs in 45 to 90 minutes and lasts as long as 4 hours. After intravenous administration, the peak effect usually occurs within 20 minutes. Morphine is not reliably absorbed after oral administration. As with the other opioids, depression of ventilation and orthostatic hypotension may occur after injection of morphine. The effect of morphine on the chemoreceptive trigger zone may produce nausea and vomiting. Nausea and vomiting may also occur owing to a vestibular component.

Meperidine

Meperidine is about one-tenth as potent as morphine. It may be given orally or parenterally. A single dose of meperidine usually lasts 2 to 4 hours. The onset after intramuscular injection is unpredictable, and a great deal of variability in time to peak effect exists.

Fentanyl

Fentanyl is a synthetic opioid agonist structurally similar to meperidine. It is 75 to 125 times more potent than morphine in its analgesic characteristics. The lipid solubility of fentanyl is greater than that of morphine, which contributes to its rapid onset of action. Peak plasma concentrations occur within 6 to 7 minutes following intravenous administration and its elimination half-time is 3 to 6 hours. The drug's short duration of action is attributed to redistribution to inactive tissues, such as the lungs, fat, and skeletal muscle. Metabolism occurs primarily by *N*-demethylation to norfentanyl, which is a less potent analgesic. A decreased clearance rate in the elderly may prolong elimination.

In doses of 1 to 2 μg/kg intravenously, fentanyl may be used to provide preoperative analgesia. Oral transmucosal fentanyl preparations of fentanyl are available, delivering 5 to 20 μg/kg of the drug. This form has been examined as a premedicant in both adults and children to relieve anxiety and pain. Because of a high incidence of preoperative nausea and vomiting, oral transmucosal fentanyl (in doses greater than 15 μg/kg) is not recommended in children younger than six years of age.[68] Fentanyl causes neither myocardial depression nor histamine release, but may be associated with ventilatory depression and profound bradycardia. Synergistic effects with benzodiazepines warrant close observation when this combination is given in the preoperative period.

Opioid Agonist–Antagonists

Opioid agonist-antagonists have been chosen for preoperative medication in an attempt to reduce the ventilatory side effects of pure opioid agonists. However, there is a ceiling on the analgesia that can be produced by agonist–antagonist drugs. They are similar to the pure opioids with regard to side effects. In addition, dysphoria may be even more likely to occur after their administration. Another issue to remember is that the agonist–antagonist drug can reduce the effectiveness of a pure opioid agonist needed to control postoperative pain. The most commonly used opioid agonist–antagonists are pentazocine, butorphanol, and nalbuphine.

Gastric Fluid pH and Volume

Many patients who come to the operating room are at risk for aspiration pneumonitis. The classic example is the patient with acute pain and a "full stomach" who must have emergency surgery. The pregnant patient, the obese patient, the diabetic, the patient with hiatal hernia or gastroesophageal reflux, all may be at risk for aspiration of gastric contents and subsequent chemical pneumonitis. Although it is not certain, it is believed that in adults aspiration of more than 25 mL of gastric fluid with a pH lower than 2.5 will cause pulmonary sequelae. This has not been, and probably never will be, proved in humans. However, using these guidelines, some have estimated that 40 to 80% of patients scheduled for elective surgery may be at risk.[69,70] However, clinically significant pulmonary aspiration of gastric contents is very rare in healthy patients having elective surgical procedures, and few anesthesiologists advocate routine prophylaxis.[71]

The necessity of prolonged fasting (nothing by mouth after midnight) before induction of anesthesia for elective surgery has been challenged.[72] Some institutions allow ingestion of clear liquids until 3 or even 2 hours before surgery in selected patients. Indeed, gastric fluid volume immediately after induction of anesthesia is not increased by ingestion of 150 mL of water, coffee, or orange juice 2 to 3 hours earlier. A study by Shevde and Trivedi described the administration of 240 mL of water, coffee, or pulp-free orange juice to healthy volunteers. All had gastric volumes of less than 25 mL with a slight decrease in pH within 2 hours of taking one of the three liquids.[73] There is concern about comfort, hypovolemia, and hypoglycemia in the pediatric age group perioperatively after prolonged fasting. An investigation by Splinter and associates concluded that drinking clear fluid up to 3 hours before scheduled surgery does not have a measurable effect on gastric volume and pH of healthy children aged 2 to 12 years.[74] Other studies in infants,

TABLE 18-14

SUMMARY OF FASTING RECOMMENDATIONS TO REDUCE THE RISK OF PULMONARY ASPIRATION[a]

INGESTED MATERIAL	MINIMUM FASTING PERIOD (APPLIED TO ALL AGES)
Clear liquids[b]	2 hours
Breast milk	4 hours
Infant formula	6 hours
Nonhuman milk	6 hours
Light meal (toast and clear liquids)	6 hours

[a]Applies only to healthy patients who are undergoing elective procedures and are not intended for women in labor. Following the guidelines does not guarantee complete gastric emptying.
[b]Examples of clear liquids include water, fruit juices without pulp, carbonated beverages, clear tea, and black coffee.
Adapted from Practice Guidelines for Preoperative Fasting and the Use of Pharmacologic Agents to Reduce the Risk of Pulmonary Aspiration: Application to Healthy Patients Undergoing Elective Procedures. A Report by the American Society of Anesthesiologists Task Force on Preoperative Fasting. Anesthesiology 90:896, 1999.

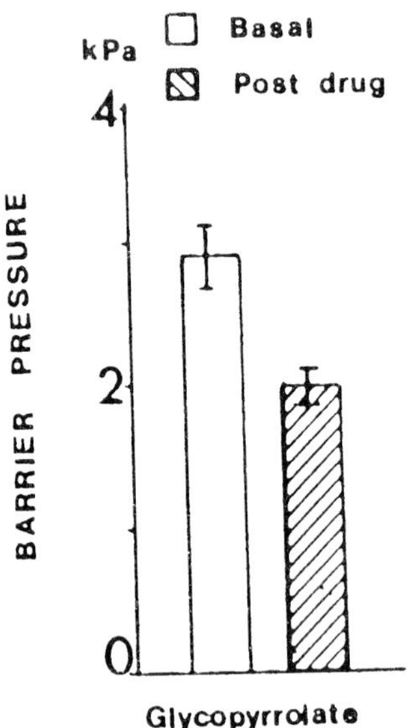

FIGURE 18-8. Barrier pressure (esophageal sphincter pressure minus gastric pressure) before and after intravenous administration of glycopyrrolate, 0.3 mg, to adult patients. Mean ± SE. (Reprinted with permission from Brock-Utne JG, Welman RS, Moshal MG *et al*: The effect of glycopyrrolate [Robinul] on the lower esophageal sphincter. Can Anaesth Soc J 25:144, 1978.)

children, and healthy adults scheduled for elective surgery have found similar results. Therefore, fears that ingestion of oral fluid on the morning of surgery will invariably result in a predictable increase in gastric fluid volume are unfounded. It must be appreciated, however, that these data are from healthy patients not "at risk" for aspiration and apply only to ingestion of clear liquids. The American Society of Anesthesiologists has defined and summarized preoperative fasting practices through guidelines adapted in 1998 (Table 18-14).[71]

Many different kinds of drugs have been used to alter gastric fluid volume and increase the pH of gastric fluid. Anticholinergics, H_2 receptor antagonists, antacids, and gastrokinetic agents have all been used to reduce the possibility of aspiration pneumonitis.

Anticholinergics

Neither atropine nor glycopyrrolate has been shown to be very effective in increasing gastric fluid pH or reducing gastric fluid volume.[69,70] Furthermore, intravenous doses of anticholinergics may cause relaxation of the gastroesophageal junction (Fig. 18-8). Therefore, the risk of aspiration pneumonitis may be increased, but this specific effect of intramuscular administration of anticholinergics for preoperative use has not been proved.

Histamine Receptor Antagonists

The H_2 receptor antagonists cimetidine, ranitidine, famotidine, and nizatidine reduce gastric acid secretion. They block the ability of histamine to induce secretion of gastric fluid with a high hydrogen ion concentration. Therefore, the H_2 receptor antagonists increase gastric fluid pH. Their antagonism of the histamine receptor occurs in a selective and competitive manner. It is important to remember that these drugs cannot be expected reliably to affect gastric fluid volume or gastric emptying time. Compared with other premedicants, they have relatively few side effects. Because there are few side effects, many anesthesiologists have advocated the liberal preoperative use of H_2 receptor antagonists. Multiple-dose regimens may be more effective in increasing gastric pH than a single dose before operation on the day of surgery. An H_2 antagonist also may be used for the allergic patient or in preparing a patient for exposure to a trigger of the allergic response, such as radiologic dye.

Cimetidine. Cimetidine usually is administered in 150 to 300 mg doses orally or parenterally. Administration of 300 mg of cimetidine orally 1 to 1.5 hours before surgery has been shown to increase the gastric fluid pH above 2.5 in 80% of patients.[75,76] Cimetidine can be given intravenously for those unable to take oral medications. Cimetidine can cross the placenta, but adverse fetal effects are unproved. The gastric effects of cimetidine last as long as 3 or 4 hours, and therefore this drug is suitable for operations of that duration.

Cimetidine has few side effects, but there are some of note. It inhibits the hepatic mixed-function oxidase enzyme system; therefore, it can prolong the half-life of many drugs, including diazepam, chlordiazepoxide, theophylline, propranolol, and lidocaine. The clinical significance of this after one or two preoperative doses of cimetidine is uncertain. Life-threatening cardiac dysrhythmias, hypotension, cardiac arrest, and central nervous system depression have been reported after cimetidine administration. These side effects may be especially likely to occur in critically ill patients after rapid intravenous administration. As discussed previously, cimetidine does not affect gastric fluid already present.

Ranitidine. Ranitidine is more potent, specific, and longer acting than cimetidine. The usual oral dose is 50 to 200 mg. Ranitidine, 50 to 100 mg, given parenterally will decrease gastric fluid pH within 1 hour. It is as effective in reducing the number of patients at risk for gastric aspiration as cimetidine and produces fewer cardiovascular or central nervous system side effects. The effects of ranitidine last up to 9 hours. Thus, it may be superior to cimetidine at the conclusion of lengthy procedures in reducing the risk of aspiration pneumonitis during emergence from anesthesia and extubation of the trachea.

Other Histamine Receptor Antagonists. Famotidine is a third H_2 receptor blocker that has been given preoperatively to raise gastric fluid pH. Its pharmacokinetics are similar to those of cimetidine and ranitidine, with the exception of having a longer serum elimination half-life than the other two drugs. Famotidine in a dose of 40 mg orally 1.5 to 3 hours preoperatively has been shown to be effective in increasing gastric pH. Nizatidine 150 to 300 mg orally 2 hours before surgery will similarly decrease preoperative gastric acidity.[77–79]

Antacids

Antacids are used to neutralize the acid in gastric contents. A single dose of antacid given 15 to 30 minutes before induction of anesthesia is almost 100% effective in increasing gastric fluid pH above 2.5. The nonparticulate antacid, 0.3 *M* sodium citrate, is commonly given before operation when an increase in gastric fluid pH is desired. The nonparticulate antacids do not produce pulmonary damage themselves if aspiration of gastric fluid containing these antacids should occur. Colloid antacid suspension may be more effective than the nonparticulate antacids in increasing gastric fluid pH. However, aspiration of gastric fluid containing particulate antacids may cause significant and persistent pulmonary damage, despite the increase in gastric fluid pH. The serious pulmonary sequelae have been manifested in the form of pulmonary edema and arterial hypoxemia.

Antacids work at the time given. There is no "lag time," as with the H_2 receptor blockers. Antacids are effective on the fluid already present in the stomach. This makes them especially attractive in emergency situations for those patients who are able to take medications orally.

However, antacids do increase gastric fluid volume, unlike H_2 receptor blockers.[75] The risk of aspiration depends on both the pH and the volume of gastric content. The increase in gastric fluid volume from antacid administration may become readily apparent after repeated doses, such as during labor, during which opioid administration may also contribute to delayed gastric emptying. Withholding antacids because of concern about increasing gastric volume is not warranted, considering animal evidence documenting increased mortality after aspiration of low volumes of acidic gastric fluid (0.3 mL/kg, pH 1) compared with aspiration of large volumes of buffered gastric fluid (1 to 2 mL/kg, pH 1.8).[80] Antacids may slow gastric emptying, and complete mixing with all gastric contents may be questionable in the immobile patient. The effect of antacids on food particles within the stomach is unknown.

Omeprazole

Omeprazole suppresses gastric acid secretion in a dose-dependent manner by binding to the proton pump of the parietal cell. For an adult patient intravenous doses of 40 mg 30 minutes before induction have been used. Oral doses of 40 to 80 mg must be given 2 to 4 hours before surgery to be effective. Effect on gastric pH may last as long as 24 hours. Much like the other H_2 receptor antagonists, investigators have found increases in gastric pH and inconsistent effects on gastric volume with administration of omeprazole.[81–83]

Gastrokinetic Agents

Gastrokinetic agents are useful because of their effectiveness in reducing gastric fluid volume. Metoclopramide is an example of a gastrokinetic agent that may be administered before operation.

Metoclopramide. Metoclopramide is a dopamine antagonist that stimulates upper gastrointestinal motility, increases gastroesophageal sphincter tone, and relaxes the pylorus and duodenum. It also has antiemetic properties. Metoclopramide speeds gastric emptying but has no known effect on acid secretion and gastric fluid pH. It may be administered orally or parenterally. A parenteral dose of 5 to 20 mg is usually given 15 to 30 minutes before induction. When the drug is administered intravenously over 3 to 5 minutes, it usually prevents the abdominal cramping that can occur from more rapid administration. An oral dose of 10 mg achieves onset within 30 to 60 minutes. The elimination half-life of metoclopramide is approximately 2 to 4 hours.

The clinical usefulness of the gastrokinetic agents is found in those patients who are likely to have large gastric fluid volumes, such as parturients, patients scheduled for emergency surgery who have just eaten, obese patients, patients with trauma, outpatients, and those with gastroparesis secondary to diabetes mellitus.

However, the administration of metoclopramide does not guarantee gastric emptying. Significant gastric fluid volume may still be present despite its administration. The effect of metoclopramide on the upper gastrointestinal tract may be offset by concomitant atropine administration or prior injection of opioids. It will not further reduce gastric volume in patients undergoing elective surgery with already small gastric volumes. It may not be effective after administration of sodium citrate. In contrast, metoclopramide may be especially effective in reducing the risk of aspiration pneumonitis when combined with an H_2 receptor antagonist (for example, ranitidine) before elective surgery.

As mentioned previously, the drugs used to alter gastric fluid pH and volume are relatively free of side effects. The risk–benefit ratio for these drugs in reducing the risk of pulmonary sequelae from aspiration is often very favorable. Indeed, the drugs do decrease the number of patients at risk. However, none of the drugs or combinations of drugs is absolutely reliable in preventing the risk of aspiration pneumonitis in all patients all of the time. Therefore, their use does not eliminate the need for careful anesthetic techniques to protect the airway during induction, maintenance, and emergence from anesthesia.

Antiemetics

There are several groups of patients in whom the antiemetic effects of drugs may be helpful in reducing nausea and vomiting. Droperidol, metoclopramide, ondansetron, and dexamethasone, singly or in combination, are agents in common usage.[84] These are patients scheduled for ophthalmologic surgery, patients with a prior history of nausea and vomiting or motion sickness, patients scheduled for laparoscopic surgery or gynecologic procedures, and patients who are obese. A risk score for predicting postoperative nausea and vomiting after inhalation anesthesia identified four risk factors: female gender, prior history of motion sickness or postoperative nausea, nonsmoking, and the use of postoperative opioids. The investigators suggested prophylactic antiemetic therapy when two or more of the risk factors were present when using volatile anesthetics.[85] Many anesthesiologists prefer not to administer antiemetics as part of a preoperative regimen, but believe that antiemetics should be administered intravenously just before they are needed at the conclusion of surgery.

Anticholinergics

Previously, anticholinergic drugs were widely used when inhalation anesthetics produced copious respiratory tract secretions and intraoperative bradycardia was a frequent danger. The advent of newer inhalation agents has almost completely dispelled the routine use of anticholinergic drugs for preoperative medication. Their routine use has been questioned by several authors, who believe that the same care in selection of anticholinergics should be exhibited as in the choice of other drugs. Specific indications for an anticholinergic before surgery are (1) antisialagogue effect and (2) sedation and amnesia (Table 18-15). Uses that are less firmly established and not universally agreed on include the preoperative prescription of

TABLE 18-15

COMPARISON OF SOME OF THE EFFECTS OF ANTICHOLINERGIC DRUGS

	ATROPINE	GLYCOPYRROLATE	SCOPOLAMINE
Increased heart rate	+++	++	+
Antisialagogue	+	++	+++
Sedation	+	0	+++

0, no effect; +, small effect; ++, moderate effect; +++, large effect.
Adapted from Stoelting RK: Pharmacology and Physiology in Anesthetic Practice. Philadelphia, JB Lippincott, 1991.

anticholinergics for their vagolytic action or in an attempt to decrease gastric acid secretion.

Antisialagogue Effect

Anticholinergics have been prescribed in a selective fashion when drying of the upper airway is desirable. For example, when endotracheal intubation is contemplated, an anesthesiologist may want to reduce secretions. In the study by Falick and Smiler, conditions were more often rated as satisfactory after endotracheal intubation when an anticholinergic drug had been administered.[86] The antisialagogue effect may be important for intraoral operations and instrumentations of the airway such as bronchoscopic examination. Administration of anticholinergics may be desirable before the use of topical anesthesia for the airway to prevent a dilutional effect of secretions and to allow contact of the local anesthetic with the mucosa.

Scopolamine is a more potent drying agent than atropine. It is less likely to increase heart rate and more likely to produce sedation and amnesia. Glycopyrrolate is a more potent and longer acting antisialagogue than atropine, with less likelihood of increasing heart rate. Because glycopyrrolate is a quaternary amine, it does not easily cross the blood-brain barrier and does not produce sedation. Anticholinergics are not the only drugs that can dry secretions. As demonstrated by the study of Forrest et al, several other drugs and placebo (presumably a reflection of apprehension) can cause a patient to have a dry mouth before operation[87] (Table 18-16).

Sedation and Amnesia

When sedation and amnesia are desired before operation, scopolamine is frequently the anticholinergic chosen, especially in combination with morphine. Scopolamine and atropine both cross the blood-brain barrier. Scopolamine is a much more potent sedative and amnestic drug than atropine. In a study of patient acceptance of preoperative medication, the combination of morphine and scopolamine was superior to that of morphine and atropine.[88] Scopolamine does not produce amnesia in all patients. It may not be as effective as lorazepam or diazepam in preventing recall. Scopolamine has an additive amnestic effect when combined with benzodiazepines. The study by Frumin et al showed that the combination of diazepam and scopolamine produced amnesia more often than did diazepam alone.[89]

Vagolytic Action

Vagolytic action of the anticholinergic drugs is produced through the blockade of effects of acetylcholine on the sinoatrial node. Atropine given intravenously is more potent than glycopyrrolate and scopolamine in increasing heart rate. The vagolytic action of the anticholinergic drugs is useful in the prevention of reflex bradycardia during surgery. Bradycardia may result from traction on extraocular muscles or abdominal viscera, from carotid sinus stimulation, or after the administration of repeated doses of intravenous succinylcholine. The prevention of reflex bradycardia with intramuscular doses of the anticholinergics is unreliable, given the drug dosages and timing usually involved with preoperative medication administered on the unit. Many anesthesiologists prefer to give atropine or glycopyrrolate intravenously just before surgery and the anticipated bradycardic stimulus. Atropine and glycopyrrolate given intravenously immediately before surgery have been equally effective in preventing bradycardia resulting from repeated doses of succinylcholine.

Elevation of Gastric Fluid pH Level

High doses of anticholinergics often are needed to alter gastric fluid pH. Even then, when given in the preoperative setting, anticholinergics cannot be relied on consistently to decrease

TABLE 18-16

INCIDENCE OF SIDE-EFFECTS 1 HOUR AFTER PREOPERATIVE MEDICATION (PERCENTAGE OF PATIENTS)

MEDICATION	DRY MOUTH	SLURRED SPEECH	DIZZY	NAUSEATED	RELAXED
Pentobarbital (50–150 mg)	29	27	10	7	2
Secobarbital (50–150 mg)	41	32	8	9	4
Diazepam (5–15 mg)	35	20	10	3	12
Hydroxyzine (50–150 mg)	45	31	6	2	9
Morphine (5–10 mg)	80	33	15	7	20
Meperidine (50–100 mg)	85	45	20	12	25
Placebo	34	21	7	12	4

Modified from Forrest WH, Brown CR, Brown BW *et al*: Subjective responses to six common preoperative medications. Anesthesiology 47:241, 1977.

gastric hydrogen ion secretion.[70] This function has largely been replaced by the use of H_2 receptor antagonists (see Gastric Fluid pH and Volume section).

Side Effects in Anticholinergic Drugs

Scopolamine and atropine may cause central nervous system toxicity, the so-called central anticholinergic syndrome. This is most likely to occur after the administration of scopolamine, but can be seen after high doses of atropine. The symptoms of central nervous system toxicity resulting from anticholinergic drugs include delirium, restlessness, confusion, and obtundation. Elderly patients and patients with pain appear to be particularly susceptible. The central nervous system toxic effect of anticholinergics has been noted to be potentiated by inhalation anesthetics. Some clinicians have successfully treated the syndrome after it occurred with 1 to 2 mg of physostigmine intravenously.

The anticholinergics relax the lower esophageal sphincter. In theory, after parenteral administration of an anticholinergic drug, the risk of pulmonary aspiration of gastric contents is increased. This has yet to be proved as an important clinical issue.

Mydriasis and cycloplegia from anticholinergic drugs could be unwanted in patients with glaucoma because of resulting increased intraocular pressure. This seems unlikely with the doses used for preoperative medication. Atropine and glycopyrrolate may be less likely to increase intraocular pressure than scopolamine. In patients with glaucoma, most anesthesiologists feel safe in continuing medications for glaucoma up until the time of surgery and using atropine or glycopyrrolate when necessary (see Chapter 33).

Because anticholinergic drugs block vagal activity, relaxation of bronchial smooth muscle occurs and respiratory dead space increases. The magnitude of the increase in dead space depends on prior bronchomotor tone, but increases as large as 25 to 33% have been reported. Anticholinergic drugs cause secretions to dry and thicken. In theory, a dose of anticholinergic drug given before operation could lead to inspissation of secretions and an increase in airway resistance. This may develop into more than a theoretical issue when patients with diseases such as cystic fibrosis are being considered.

Sweat glands of the body are innervated by the sympathetic nervous system and use cholinergic transmission. Therefore, administration of anticholinergic agents interferes with the sweating mechanism, which may cause body temperature to increase. This side effect of anticholinergic medication must be considered carefully in a child with a fever.

Atropine is more likely than glycopyrrolate or scopolamine to cause an increase in heart rate. Unwanted increases in heart rate are much more likely after intravenous administration than after intramuscular administration. In fact, heart rate may transiently decrease after intramuscular administration as a result of a peripheral agonist effect of the anticholinergic agent.

Adrenergic Agonists

Alpha-2 adrenergic agonists have been used as premedicants.[90,91] Clonidine in doses of 2.5 to 5 μg/kg has been administered preoperatively to produce sedation, reduce maximum allowable concentration, and prevent hypertension and tachycardia from endotracheal intubation and surgical stimulation. It has even been used as part of anesthetic technique to produce induced hypotension. Dexmedetomidine is another alpha-2 adrenergic agonist studied for preoperative use to attenuate intraoperative sympathoadrenal responses.[90] After the administration of clonidine preoperatively, one is more likely to see episodes of hypotension and bradycardia during anesthesia when there are periods of little surgical stimulation. Furthermore, some anesthesiologists ask if preoperative alpha-2 adrenergic agonists are a substitute for a properly conducted anesthetic if appropriate attention is given to depth of anesthesia.

Other Drugs Given with Preoperative Medications

Although they are not preoperative medications in the strict sense, other drugs are often given at the time of preoperative medication. Examples of such drugs are insulin, steroids, antibiotics, and methadone for patients who are addicted to opioids. They may be prescribed by either the anesthesiologist or the surgeon to be given on the ward or in the operating room immediately prior to surgery. Regardless of these factors, their actions may affect the anesthetic, and the anesthesiologist must be knowledgeable about their administration and actions.

Beta-Blockers

For patients with known or suspected coronary artery disease, preoperative beta-blockers may add to safety in the perioperative period. Clinical studies have shown that beta-blockers in this setting have reduced mortality and the incidence of nonfatal myocardial infarction after surgery. Because benefit has been shown with several different beta-blockers, it is probably a drug class effect or hemodynamic effect rather than the result of employing a specific beta-blocker. Contraindications to preoperative beta-blocker therapy include known allergy to beta-blockers, second- or third-degree heart block, congestive heart failure, acute bronchospasm, low systolic blood pressure (less than 100 mm Hg), slow heart rate (less than 60 beats per minute), and other hemodynamic instability. Many clinicians use either atenolol (50 to 100 milligrams po daily) or metoprolol (25 to 50 milligrams po twice daily). They are chosen because of their long action and relative beta-1 selectivity. The goals are to achieve a heart rate near 50 to 70 beats per minute, while maintaining a systolic blood pressure greater than 110 mm Hg. The beta-blockade is usually maintained throughout the perioperative period to achieve maximum effect. Intravenous metoprolol may be given just prior to surgery if inadequate blockade has been achieved with the oral medications. The oral beta-blockers may be started several days prior to surgery.

Antibiotics

Antibiotics are often administered immediately before operation for contaminated, potentially contaminated, or dirty surgical wounds. Prophylactic antibiotics may be warranted for "clean" surgical procedures when infection would be catastrophic. Other instances for the use of prophylactic antibiotics include in the immunosuppressed patient, in the aged, or in patients taking steroids. Antibiotics given immediately before surgery are also used for the prevention of endocarditis.[92] Antibiotic administration comes under the anesthesiologist's purview because of the desire to have such agents given immediately before exposure to pathogens, which is just before the beginning of surgery.

It has been estimated that 60 to 70% of surgical patients receive antibiotics just before surgery or intraoperatively. Cephalosporins are the most popular. However, no drug or combination of drugs may be relied on to protect against all potential pathogens in all patients for all types of surgery. As with any other medication, the anesthesiologist must know the side effects and complications of the antibiotics to be administered. Some are associated with allergic reactions, hypotension, and bronchospasm (e.g., penicillin and vancomycin). Allergic reactions from cephalosporin administration have been estimated to occur in about 5% of patients. Cross-reactivity of the cephalosporins in patients with a known penicillin allergy has been estimated at anywhere from 5 to 20%. The aminoglycosides, vancomycin, and the polymyxins have been implicated in nephrotoxicity. In addition, ototoxicity has resulted from aminoglycoside and vancomycin administration. Pseudomembranous colitis is a known complication of clindamycin administration. Finally, the aminoglycosides are known to extend the neuromuscular blocking effects of muscle relaxants.

Steroids

Steroid administration may be necessary immediately before surgery in the patient treated for hypoadrenocorticism or in the patient with suppression of the pituitary-adrenal axis owing to present or previous administration of corticosteroids. It is impossible to identify the specific duration of therapy or dose of steroids that produces pituitary and adrenal suppression. Marked variability among patients exists. Certainly, more suppression may be expected the higher the dose and the longer the duration of therapy. A conservative estimate is to consider treatment in any patient who has received corticosteroid therapy for at least 1 month in the past 6 to 12 months.

Because of disease states of the pituitary-adrenal axis or its suppression from steroid therapy, patients may not be able to respond to the stress of surgery. The dose and duration of supplemental steroid administration depend on an estimate of the stress of the surgical procedure in the perioperative period. One regimen is to administer 25 mg of cortisol preoperatively and then give an intravenous infusion of 100 mg of cortisol over the next 12 to 24 hours for adult patients. Another method is to administer 100 mg of hydrocortisone intravenously before, during, and after surgery. This dose is meant to equal the estimated maximum amount of steroid that stress could produce in patients perioperatively. When considering whether to administer steroids or a higher dose of steroids, the anesthesiologist should keep in mind that the risk–benefit ratio is usually very small.

Insulin

Anesthesia and surgery may interrupt the regular meal schedule and insulin administration of diabetics (see Chapter 41). Perioperative stress may increase serum glucose concentrations. A plan for perioperative insulin and glucose management must be agreed on among the anesthesiologist, the surgeon, and the endocrinologist involved in the diabetic patient's care. There are several methods of doing this, none of which has proved superior to the others. One method is to administer one-fourth to one-half of the usual daily dose of intermediate-acting insulin preoperatively in the morning of surgery and begin an infusion of glucose-containing fluid. A second way is to administer no insulin or no glucose preoperatively and to measure serum glucose levels frequently during anesthesia. Regular insulin or glucose is then administered intraoperatively and postoperatively as needed. A third method is to begin an infusion of insulin and glucose immediately preoperatively and to check serum glucose levels frequently.

Opioid Dependency

Withdrawal produced by drug cessation is a preoperative issue in the patient who is taking methadone or is dependent on other opioids. There should be an attempt to maintain opioid use at the usual level by continuing methadone or substituting other appropriate agents for methodone. The anesthesiologist should be cautioned about using agonist-antagonist drugs in these patients in the preoperative period for fear of producing withdrawal.

DIFFERENCES IN PREOPERATIVE MEDICATION BETWEEN PEDIATRIC AND ADULT PATIENTS

Differences between children and adults with regard to preoperative medication include aspects of psychological preparation, the emphasis on oral medications when pharmacologic preparation is desired, and more frequent use of anticholinergics for their vagolytic activity. What remains the same is the need to assess the needs of each child individually and to tailor the psychological preparation and preoperative medication accordingly (see Chapter 44).

Psychological Factors in Pediatric Patients

Hospital admission and major surgery can produce long-lasting psychological effects in some children. The hospital stay is stressful and full of apprehension over the short term for almost all children. The demeanor and communicative efforts of the anesthesiologist can make a difference to the child and family who are getting ready for a trip to the operating room, anesthesia, and surgery.

Age is probably the most important aspect when psychological preparation of the pediatric patient is considered.[93] A baby younger than 6 to 8 months of age is not emotionally upset when separated from his or her mother. Others in the health care team can substitute very easily. Preoperative preparation in this age group is often directed toward other goals, for example, obtundation of vagal reflex responses. However, preschool children are upset when separated from their mothers and fear the operating room. This is an age when hospitalization may be the most upsetting. It is difficult to explain the forthcoming events to children in this age group. It is easier to communicate with patients from age 5 years to adolescence. The anesthesiologist can explain and offer reassurance about such issues as separation from parents and the home, operating room events, and any of the patient's perceived fears of surgery and anesthesia. Adolescent patients may already be anxious and apprehensive. They may also be worried about loss of consciousness, have a fear of death, or be apprehensive about what they will do or say after preoperative sedation or during anesthesia. The more fearful child may be difficult to identify. This is usually the child who is quiet during the preoperative interview and appears nonchalant or even detached. If these patients can be identified before operation, they are often candidates for heavy pharmacologic preparation.

Psychological Preparation

For the above reasons, a good preoperative visit and proper psychological preparation may be even more important in children than adults. This is an art that is acquired by the anesthesiologist. The preoperative visit is a time of reassurance and explanation. It is an opportunity to gain the child's trust. Most anesthesiologists will want to involve the parents when possible. Some hospitals have found brochures, motion pictures, and slide shows to be helpful in preparing pediatric patients for the operating room. The child may want to bring a personal belonging, such as a stuffed animal or blanket, to the operating room for security. Some children wish to take an active role by doing such things as holding the face mask during inhalation induction of anesthesia. It may be helpful in a case with supportive parents to have them accompany the child to the operating room suite after an explanation of events that may occur during induction. It is common in many hospitals for a parent to go into the operating room and stay until induction is complete.

Differences in Pharmacologic Preparation

The discussion of pharmacologic preparation for the pediatric patient presumes proper psychological preparation, a satisfactory operating room environment, and preparation for an efficient and timely induction of anesthesia (see Chapter 44).

Sedative–Hypnotics

As in adults, the sedative–hypnotic medications are used to reduce apprehension, produce sedation and amnesia, and to facilitate smooth induction of anesthesia when an inhalation method is to be used. The use of preoperative medication is controversial in pediatric patients and may not be completely successful in as many as 20% of instances. It has not been proved to reduce unwanted psychological outcome after surgery and anesthesia. Neither has it been shown that the uneventful induction of anesthesia is less likely to produce long-lasting psychological problems in children. After 6 months to 1 year of age, the child scheduled for a surgical procedure may benefit from a sedative–hypnotic drug before surgery. There is some emphasis on avoiding intramuscular injections in children. The oral route is often used for preoperative medication in the older child, whereas in preschool children drugs may also be given rectally. Many different sedative–hypnotic drugs via different routes (oral, intranasal, and rectal) have been prescribed for children before operation. Midazolam can be given intramuscularly (0.05 to 0.2 mg/kg). However, the most effective and acceptable route for midazolam is the oral route, achieved by mixing 0.5 to 0.75 mg/kg with flavored syrup, apple juice, or cola because of its bitter taste.[94] It is effective in producing sedation and compliance, but not usually sleep, in about 15 minutes and lasts for 30 to 60 minutes. Oral ketamine 5 to 10 mg has been prescribed 20 to 30 minutes before induction. Although often allowing smooth separation from parents, oral secretions and preoperative or postoperative delirium can be problems. Both ketamine (3 to 8 mg/kg) and midazolam (0.2 mg/kg) can be given using a nasal atomizer, with the caveat that nasal drug administration and bitter aftertaste are disadvantageous. Ketamine (5 mg/kg) and midazolam (0.3 to 1.0 mg/kg) have also been given rectally before induction of anesthesia. A further option in the pharmacologic preparation of children is the rectal administration of methohexital (Fig. 18-9). Methohexital (20 to 30 mg/kg) may be given immediately before operation, using pulse oximetry and while the child is still in the parent's arms. The intramuscular route is also possible.

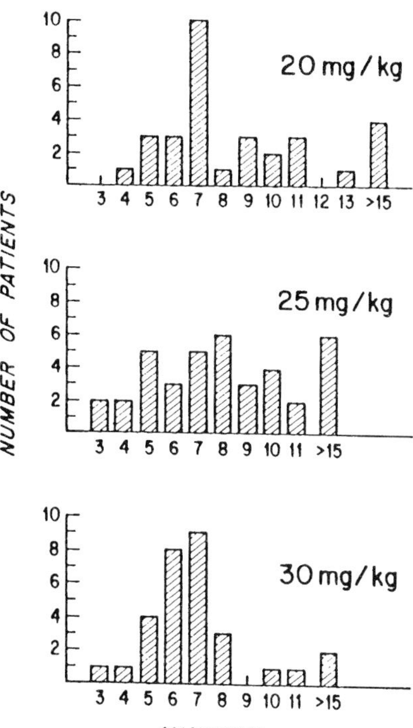

FIGURE 18-9. Frequency distribution of sleep induction times after rectal instillation of methohexital. Patients averaged 3.3 years in age and 15 kg in body weight. (Reprinted from Liu LMP, Goudsouzian NG, Liu PL: Rectal methohexital premedication in children, a dose-comparison study. Anesthesiology 53:343, 1980.)

Opioids

There is the occasional need for opioid premedication in children. Methadone has the advantage of oral administration, usually prescribed in the 0.1 to 0.2 mg/kg dose range. Intramuscular morphine and meperidine are used, often in combination with other premedications. Intramuscular morphine is often seen as part of the pharmacologic preparation for the child with congenital heart disease. In many hospitals, opioids have been combined with sedative–hypnotic and anticholinergic drugs to make a "cocktail" that may be given orally for preoperative medication. Transmucosal administration of fentanyl (5 to 20 μg/kg) appears to be effective in producing sedation preoperatively. However, transmucosal fentanyl may increase gastric fluid volume and also increase the incidence of rigidity, respiratory depression, pruritus, nausea, and vomiting.[68] Fentanyl (2 μg/kg) and sufentanil (3.0 μg/kg) given by the intranasal route have been shown to calm pediatric patients preoperatively. Again, postoperative nausea and vomiting, in addition to respiratory complications, have resulted in lack of enthusiasm for this technique.

Anticholinergics

Easily induced vagal reflexes make anticholinergics especially important in children. Bradycardia may result from airway manipulation, surgical manipulation, or anesthetic drugs such as halothane or succinylcholine. Also, the child's cardiac output is more dependent on heart rate than is the adult's. If no contraindication exists, most pediatric patients receive atropine intravenously immediately after induction of anesthesia and placement of an intravenous catheter. If the intramuscular route has been used for atropine, it will often be administered immediately after the patient becomes unconscious during induction of anesthesia. Glycopyrrolate also has been used in children in this setting. Scopolamine has a place in premedication of the pediatric patient to produce sedation, amnesia, and drying of the airways. One must be aware of the hazards of administering an anticholinergic to a child with a fever or when inspissation of secretions is not wanted. Finally, it has been noted that patients with Down syndrome appear to be sensitive to atropine. This is especially evident with the effect on heart rate and mydriasis.

(For information on Anesthesia for Ambulatory Surgery, see Chapter 46.)

References

1. Takata MN, Benumof JL, Mazzei WJ: The preoperative evaluation form: Assessment of quality from one hundred thirty-eight institutions and recommendations for a high-quality form. J Clin Anes 13(5):345, 2001
2. Mallampati RS, Gatt SP, Gugino LD *et al:* A clinical sign to predict difficult tracheal intubation: A prospective study. Can Anaesth Soc 32:429, 1985

3. Frerk CM: Predicting difficult intubation. Anaesthesia 46:1005, 1991
4. Savva D: Prediction of difficult tracheal intubation. Br J Anaesth 73:149, 1994
5. Shah KB, Kleinman BS, Rao T *et al*: Angina and other risk factors in patients with cardiac diseases undergoing noncardiac operations. Anesth Analg 70:240, 1990
6. Tuman KJ, McCarthy RJ, March RJ *et al*: Effects of epidural anesthesia and analgesia on coagulation and outcome after major vascular surgery. Anesth Analg 73:696, 1991
7. Bedford R, Feinstein B: Hospital admission blood pressure, a predictor for hypertension following endotracheal intubation. Anesth Analg 59:367, 1980
8. Lee TH, Marcantonio ER, Mangione CM *et al*: Derivation and prospective validation of a simple index for prediction of cardiac risk of major noncardiac surgery. Circulation 100:1043, 1999
9. Goldman L, Caldera DL, Nussbaum SR *et al*: Multifactorial index of cardiac risk in noncardiac surgical procedures. N Engl J Med 297:845, 1977
10. Detsky A, Abrams H, McLaughlin J *et al*: Predicting cardiac complications in patients undergoing non-cardiac surgery. J Gen Intern Med 1:211, 1986
11. Tarhan S, Moffitt EA, Taylor WF, Giuliani ER: Myocardial infarction after general anesthesia. JAMA 220:1451, 1972
12. Rao TL, Jacobs KH, El-Etr AA: Reinfarction following anesthesia in patients with myocardial infarction. Anesthesiology 59:499, 1983
13. Shah KB, Kleinman BS, Sami H *et al*: Reevaluation of perioperative myocardial infarction in patients with prior myocardial infarction undergoing noncardiac operations. Anesth Analg 71:231, 1990
14. Califf RM, Topol EJ, George BS *et al*: One-year outcome after therapy with tissue plasminogen activator: Report from the Thrombolysis and Angioplasty in Myocardial Infarction trial. Am Heart J 119:777, 1990
15. Rouleau JL, Talajic M, Sussex B *et al*: Myocardial infarction patients in the 1990s—their risk factors, stratification and survival in Canada: The Canadian Assessment of Myocardial Infarction (CAMI) study. J Am Coll Cardiol 27:1119, 1996
16. Eagle K, Brundage B, Chaitman B *et al*: Guidelines for perioperative cardiovascular evaluation of the noncardiac surgery. A report of the American Heart Association/American College of Cardiology Task Force on Assessment of Diagnostic and Therapeutic Cardiovascular Procedures. Circulation 93:1278, 1996
17. Hertzer NR, Bevan EG, Young JR *et al*: Coronary artery disease in peripheral vascular patients: A classification of 1000 coronary angiograms and results of surgical management. Ann Surg 199:223, 1984
18. Kannel W, Abbott R: Incidence and prognosis of unrecognized myocardial infarction: An update on the Framingham study. N Engl J Med 311:1144, 1984
19. Eagle KA, Coley CM, Newell JB *et al*: Combining clinical and thallium data optimizes preoperative assessment of cardiac risk before major vascular surgery. Ann Int Med 110:859, 1989
20. Acharya DU, Shekhar YC, Aggarwal A, Anand IS: Lack of pain during myocardial infarction in diabetics: Is autonomic dysfunction responsible? Am J Cardiol 68:793, 1991
21. Hollenberg M, Mangano DT, Browner WS *et al*: Predictors of postoperative myocardial ischemia in patients undergoing noncardiac surgery. The Study of Perioperative Ischemia Research. JAMA 268:205, 1992
22. Pringle SD, MacFarlane PW, McKillop JH *et al*: Pathophysiologic assessment of left ventricular hypertrophy and strain in asymptomatic patients with essential hypertension. J Am Coll Cardiol 13:1377, 1989
23. Sixth report of the Joint National Committee on Prevention, Detection, Evaluation, and Treatment of High Blood Pressure. Arch Intern Med 157:2413, 1997
24. Goldman L, Caldera DL: Risks of general anesthesia and elective operation in the hypertensive patient. Anesthesiology 50:285, 1979
25. Howell SJ, Sear JW, Foex P: Hypertension, hypertensive heart disease and perioperative cardiac risk. British Journal of Anaesthesia 92:570, 2004
26. Warner MA, Shields SE, Chute CG: Major morbidity and mortality within 1 month of ambulatory surgery and anesthesia. JAMA 270:1437, 1993
27. Eagle KA, Rihal CS, Mickel MC *et al*: Cardiac risk of noncardiac surgery: Influence of coronary disease and type of surgery in 3368 operations. CASS Investigators and University of Michigan Heart Care Program. Circulation 96:1882, 1997
28. Reilly DF, McNeely MJ, Doerner D *et al*: Self-reported exercise tolerance and the risk of serious perioperative complications. Arch Intern Med 159:2185, 1999
29. Poldermans D, Boersma E, Bax JJ *et al*: The effect of bisoprolol on perioperative mortality and myocardial infarction in high-risk patients undergoing vascular surgery. N Engl J Med 341:1789, 1999
30. American College of Cardiology and the American Heart Association: ACC/AHA Guideline Update on Perioperative Cardiovascular Evaluation for Noncardiac Surgery. ACC/AHA Practice Guidelines 2002
31. Rihal C, Gersh B, Whisnant J *et al*: Influence of coronary heart disease on morbidity and mortality after carotid endarterectomy: A population-based study in Olmsted County, Minnesota (1970–1988). J Am Coll Cardiol 19:1254, 1992
32. Kalbfleisch JM, Shudaksharappa KS, Conrad LL, Sarkar NK: Disappearance of the Q deflection following myocardial infarction. Am Heart J 76:193, 1968
33. Gold BS, Young ML, Kinman JL *et al*: The utility of preoperative electrocardiograms in the ambulatory surgical patient. Arch Intern Med 152:301, 1992
34. Raby KE, Goldman L, Creager MA *et al*: Correlation between perioperative ischemia and major cardiac events after peripheral vascular surgery. N Engl J Med 321:1296, 1989
35. Mantha S, Roizen MF, Barnard J *et al*: Relative effectiveness of four preoperative tests for predicting adverse cardiac outcomes after vascular surgery: A meta-analysis. Anesth Analg 79:422, 1994
36. Shaw LJ, Eagle KA, Gersh BJ, Miller DD: Meta-analysis of intravenous dipyridamole–thallium-201 imaging (1985 to 1994) and dobutamine echocardiography (1991 to 1994) for risk stratification before vascular surgery. J Am Coll Cardiol 27:787, 1996
37. Anonymous: Guidelines for assessing and managing the perioperative risk from coronary artery disease associated with major noncardiac surgery. Ann Intern Med 127:313, 1997
38. Arozullah AM, *et al*: Multifactorial risk index for predicting postoperative respiratory failure in men after major noncardiac surgery. The National Veterans Administration Surgical Quality Improvement Program. Ann Surg 232:242, 2000
39. Smetana GW: Preoperative pulmonary evaluation. N Engl J Med 340:937, 1999
40. Arozullah AM, Khuri SF, Henderson WG *et al*: Development and validation of a multifactorial risk index for predicting postoperative pneumonia after major noncardiac surgery. Ann Intern Med 135:847, 2001
41. Meyers JR, Lembeck L, O'Kane H *et al*: Changes in functional residual capacity of the lung after operation. Arch Surg 110:576, 1975
42. Dureuil B, Viires N, Cantineau JP *et al*: Diaphragmatic contractility after upper abdominal surgery. J Appl Physiol 61:1775, 1986
43. Fisher BW, Majumdar SR, McAlistar FA: Predicting pulmonary complications after nonthoracic surgery: a systematic review of blinded studies. Am J Med 112:219, 2002
44. Hall JC, Tarala RA, Hall JL: A case-control study of postoperative pulmonary complications after laparoscopic and open cholecystectomy. J Laparoendosc Surg 6:87, 1996
45. Warner MA, Divertie MB, Tinker JH: Preoperative cessation of smoking and pulmonary complications in coronary artery bypass patients. Anesth 60:609, 1984
46. Whyte MK, Choudry NB, Ind PW: Bronchial hyperresponsiveness in patients recovering from acute severe asthma. Respir Med 87:29, 1993
47. Kabalin CS, Yarnold PR, Grammer LC: Low complication rate of corticosteroid-treated asthmatics undergoing surgical procedures. Arch Intern Med 155:1379, 1995
48. Golub R, Cantu R, Sorrento JJ, Stein HD: Efficacy of preadmission testing in ambulatory surgical patients. Am J Surg 163:565(discussion 571), 1992
49. Narr BJ, Hansen TR, Warner MA: Preoperative laboratory screening in healthy Mayo patients: Cost-effective elimination of tests and unchanged outcomes. Mayo Clin Proc 66:155, 1991
50. Narr BJ, Warner ME, Schroeder DR, Warner MA: Outcomes of patients with no laboratory assessment before anesthesia and a surgical procedure. Mayo Clin Proc 72:505, 1997
51. Roizen MF, Cohn S: Preoperative evaluation for elective surgery: What laboratory tests are needed? In Advances in Anesthesia, p 25. St Louis, Mosby–Year Book, 1993
52. Baron MJ, Gunter J, White P: Is the pediatric preoperative hematocrit determination necessary? South Med J 85:1187, 1992
53. Sox HCJ: Common Diagnostic Tests: Use and Interpretation. Philadelphia, American College of Physicians, 1990
54. Archer C, Levy AR, McGregor M: Value of routine preoperative chest x-rays: A meta-analysis. Can J Anaesth 40:1022, 1993
55. Beecher HK: Preanesthetic medication. JAMA 157:242, 1955
56. Lyons SM, Clarke RSJ, Vulgaraki K: The premedication of cardiac surgical patients. Anaesthesia 30:459, 1975
57. Egbert LD, Battit GE, Turndorf H *et al*: The value of the preoperative visit by the anesthetist. JAMA 185:553, 1963
58. Soreide E, Holst-Larsen K, Reite K *et al*: Effects of giving water 20–450 ml with oral diazepam premedication 1–2 h before operation. Br J Anaesth 71:503, 1993
59. Fragen RJ, Caldwell N: Lorazepam premedication: Lack of recall and relief of anxiety. Anesth Analg 55:792, 1976
60. White PF: Pharmacologic and clinical aspects of preoperative medication. Anesth Analg 65:963, 1986
61. Bradshaw EG, Ali AA, Mulley BA *et al*: Plasma concentrations and clinical effects of lorazepam after oral administration. Br J Anaesth 53:517, 1981
62. Blitt CD, Petty WC, Wright WA *et al*: Clinical evaluation of injectable lorazepam as a premedicant: The effect on recall. Anesth Analg 55:522, 1976
63. Reves JG, Fragen RJ, Vinick HR et al: Midazolam: Pharmacology and uses. Anesthesiology 62:310, 1985
64. Pinnock CA, Fell D, Hunt PCW *et al*: A comparison of triazolam and diazepam as premedication for minor gynaecologic surgery. Anaesthesia 40:324, 1985
65. Koch-Weser J, Greenblatt DJ: The archaic barbiturate hypnotics. N Engl J Med 291:790, 1974

66. Cohen EN, Beecher HK: Narcotics in preanesthetic medication: A controlled study. JAMA 147:1664, 1951
67. Weil JV, McCullough RE, Kline JS: Diminished ventilatory response to hypoxia and hypercapnia after morphine in man. N Engl J Med 292:1103, 1975
68. Epstein RH, Mendel HG, Witkowski TA *et al*: The safety and efficacy of oral transmucosal fentanyl citrate for preoperative sedation in young children. Anesth Analg 83:1220, 1996
69. Stoelting RK: Responses to atropine, glycopyrrolate and Riopan on gastric fluid pH and volume in adult patients. Anesthesiology 48:367, 1978
70. Manchikanti L, Roush JR: The effect of preanesthetic glycopyrrolate and cimetidine in gastric fluid pH and volume in outpatients. Anesth Analg 63:40, 1984
71. A Report by the American Society of Anesthesiologists Task Force on Preoperative Fasting: Practice guidelines for preoperative fasting and the use of pharmacologic agents to reduce the risk of pulmonary aspiration: Application to healthy patients undergoing elective procedures. Anesthesiology 90:896, 1999
72. Kallar SK, Everett LL: Potential risks and preventive measures for pulmonary aspiration: New concepts in preoperative fasting guidelines. Anesth Analg 77:171, 1993
73. Shevde K, Trivedi N: Effects of clear liquids on gastric volume and pH in healthy volunteers. Anesth Analg 72:528, 1991
74. Splinter WM, Schaefer SE, Zunder IH: Clear fluids three hours before surgery do not affect the gastric fluid contents of children. Can J Anaesth 37:498, 1990
75. Stoelting RK: Gastric fluid pH in patients receiving cimetidine. Anesth Analg 57:675, 1978
76. Maliniak K, Vahil AH: Pre-anesthetic cimetidine and gastric pH. Anesth Analg 58:309, 1979
77. Feldman M, Burton ME: Histamine-2 receptor antagonists. N Engl J Med 323:1672, 1990
78. Escolano F, Castaño J, Lopez R *et al*: Effects of omeprazole, ranitidine, famotidine and placebo on gastric secretion in patients undergoing elective surgery. Br J Anaesth 69:404, 1992
79. Mikawa K, Nishina K, Maekawa N *et al*: Gastric fluid volume and pH after nizatidine in adults undergoing elective surgery: Influence of timing and dose. Can J Anaesth 42:730, 1995
80. James CF, Modell JH, Gibbs CP *et al*: Pulmonary aspiration: Effects of volume and pH in the rat. Anesth Analg 63:665, 1984
81. Rocke DA, Rout CC, Gouws E: Intravenous administration of the proton pump inhibitor omeprazole reduces the risk of acid aspiration at emergency cesarean section. Anesth Analg 78:1093, 1994
82. Haskins DA, Jahr JS, Texidor M *et al*: Single-dose oral omeprazole for reduction of gastric residual acidity in adults for outpatient surgery. Acta Anaesthesiol Scand 36:513, 1992
83. Atanassoff PG, Alon E, Pasch T: Effects of single-dose intravenous omeprazole and ranitidine on gastric pH during general anesthesia. Anesth Analg 75:95, 1992
84. Apfel CC, Korttila K, Abdalla M *et al*: A factorial trial of six interventions for the prevention of postoperative nausea and vomiting. N Engl J Med 350:2441, 2004
85. Apfel CC, Läärä E, Koivuranta M *et al*: A simplified risk score for predicting postoperative nausea and vomiting. Anesthesiology 91:693, 1999
86. Falick YS, Smiler BG: Is anticholinergic premedication necessary? Anesthesiology 43:472, 1975
87. Forrest WH, Brown CR, Brown BW: Subjective responses to six common preoperative medications. Anesthesiology 47:241, 1977
88. Conner JT, Bellville JW, Wender R *et al*: Morphine, scopolamine and atropine as intravenous surgical premedicants. Anesth Analg 56:606, 1977
89. Frumin MJ, Herekar VR, Jarvik ME: Amnesic actions of diazepam and scopolamine in man. Anesthesiology 45:406, 1976
90. Abi-Jaoude F, Brusset A, Ceddaha A *et al*: Clonidine premedication for coronary artery bypass grafting under high-dose alfentanil anesthesia: Intraoperative and postoperative hemodynamic study. J Cardiothorac Vasc Anesth 7:35, 1993
91. Jaakola ML, Kanto J, Scheinin H *et al*: Intramuscular dexmedetomidine premedication: An alternative to midazolam–fentanyl combination in elective hysterectomy? Acta Anaesthesiol Scand 38:238, 1994
92. Dajani AS, Taubert KA, Wilson W *et al*: Prevention of bacterial endocarditis Recommendations by the American Heart Association. JAMA 277:1794, 1997
93. Vetter TR: The epidemiology and selective identification of children at risk for preoperative anxiety reactions. Anesth Analg 77:96, 1993
94. Weldon BC, Watcha MF, White PF: Oral midazolam in children: Effect of time and adjunctive therapy. Anesth Analg 75:51, 1992

CHAPTER 19 ■ ANESTHESIA FOR PATIENTS WITH RARE AND COEXISTING DISEASES

STEPHEN F. DIERDORF AND J. SCOTT WALTON

KEY POINTS

1. The muscle membrane in patients with muscular dystrophy has an abnormal structure and is susceptible to damage from succinylcholine. Massive release of intracellular contents, especially potassium, may occur.
2. Myotonic dystrophy produces cardiac conduction delay that can manifest as first-, second-, or third-degree atrioventricular heart block.
3. Patients with myasthenia gravis are exquisitely sensitive to nondepolarizing muscle relaxants. Short-acting muscle relaxants and careful objective and clinical monitoring of neuromuscular function are indicated.
4. Many types of cancer in addition to small cell lung carcinoma can produce myasthenic syndrome.
5. Patients with multiple sclerosis should be advised that they may have an exacerbation of neurologic symptoms during the perioperative period.
6. Repeated episodes of sickling in patients with sickle cell disease cause pulmonary hypertension. Pulmonary hypertension in sickle cell patients is associated with increased mortality.
7. Rheumatoid arthritis is a multisystem disease that causes subclinical cardiac and pulmonary dysfunction.
8. Many patients with rheumatoid arthritis have significant degeneration of the cervical spine with few neurologic symptoms. Cervical manipulation during laryngoscopy and intubation requires special precautions.
9. Esophageal dysfunction in patients with scleroderma or dermatomyositis increases the risk of aspiration pneumonitis.
10. Patients with epidermolysis bullosa can have undiagnosed myocardial dysfunction.

Knowledge of the pathophysiology of coexisting diseases and an understanding of the implications of concomitant drug therapy are essential for the optimal management of anesthesia for an individual patient. In many instances, the nature of the coexisting disease has more impact on the management of anesthesia than does the actual surgical procedure. A variety of rare disorders may influence the selection and conduct of anesthesia (Table 19-1). Recent advances in molecular genetics and biology have clarified the pathophysiology of many uncommon diseases. These discoveries have radically altered the treatment of some disorders. Consequently, anesthesiologists must periodically update their diagnostic skills and clinical knowledge to recognize when additional evaluation or treatment may be required.

MUSCULOSKELETAL DISEASES

Muscular Dystrophy

The cytoskeleton of the muscle cell is composed of different proteins such as dystrophin, merosin, utrophin, syntrophin, dystrobrevin, and sarcoglycans. Abnormal muscle proteins or

TABLE 19-1

COEXISTING DISEASES THAT INFLUENCE ANESTHESIA MANAGEMENT

■ MUSCULOSKELETAL
Muscular dystrophy
Myotonic dystrophy
Familial periodic paralysis
Myasthenia gravis
Lambert-Eaton (myasthenic) syndrome
Guillain-Barré syndrome
■ CENTRAL NERVOUS SYSTEM
Multiple sclerosis
Epilepsy
Parkinson's disease
Huntington's disease
Alzheimer's disease
Amyotrophic lateral sclerosis
Creutzfeldt-Jakob disease
■ ANEMIAS
Nutritional deficiency
Hemolytic
Hemoglobinopathies
Thalassemias
■ COLLAGEN VASCULAR
Rheumatoid arthritis
Systemic lupus erythematosus
Scleroderma
Polymyositis
■ SKIN
Epidermolysis bullosa
Pemphigus

insufficient quantities of normal proteins diminish the integrity of the muscle membrane, making it more susceptible to damage (Fig. 19-1). The muscular dystrophies are diseases associated with abnormalities of the muscle membrane (Table 19-2).[1]

Muscular dystrophies are characterized by a progressive, but variable loss of skeletal muscle function. Although many of the presenting signs and symptoms of muscular dystrophy are a result of skeletal muscle weakness, cardiac and smooth

TABLE 19-2

TYPES OF MUSCULAR DYSTROPHY

Duchenne
Becker
Emery-Dreifuss
Limb-girdle
Oculopharyngeal
Fascioscapulohumeral
Congenital muscular dystrophy

muscle are also affected. In many types of muscular dystrophy, cardiac muscle dysfunction may be more significant than skeletal muscle dysfunction, and preoperative evaluation of cardiac function can influence perioperative management.

Recent research has revealed a wide variety of unrelated genetic defects that produce clinically similar muscle diseases. It is still, however, more clinically useful to classify muscle diseases by clinical expression rather than genetic origin (Fig. 19-2).

Duchenne's Muscular Dystrophy

Duchenne's muscular dystrophy is produced by a genetic abnormality resulting in a lack of production of dystrophin, a major component of the skeleton of the muscle membrane. Duchenne's dystrophy is characterized by painless degeneration and atrophy of skeletal muscle. This disorder is a sex-linked recessive trait clinically evident in boys, although sensitive testing may reveal subclinical abnormalities in carrier females. Progressive muscle weakness produces symptoms between the ages of 2 and 5 years and limitation of movement usually confines the patient to a wheelchair by 12 years of age. Axial skeletal muscle imbalance produces kyphoscoliosis that often requires operative instrumentation for stabilization. Death is usually secondary to congestive heart failure or pneumonia. Aggressive treatment of cardiopulmonary dysfunction has improved survival for many patients until the age of 30 years. Serum creatine kinase levels reflect the progression of the disease. Early in the patient's life the creatine kinase level is increased. Later, as significant amounts of muscle have degenerated, the creatine kinase level decreases.

Involvement of cardiac muscle is reflected by a progressive loss of R-wave amplitude in the lateral precordial leads of the

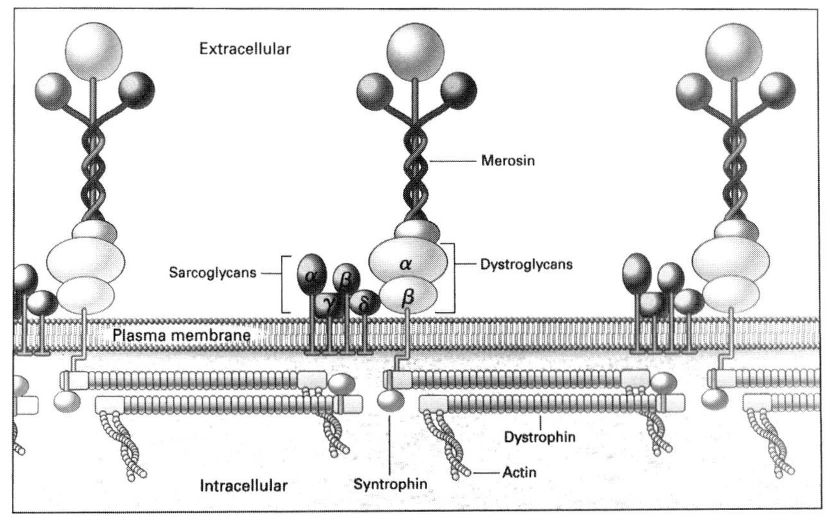

FIGURE 19-1. Muscle cell cytoskeleton. (Reprinted with permission from Duggan DJ, Gorospe JR, Fanin M *et al*: Mutations in the sarcoglycan genes in patients with myopathy. N Engl J Med 336:618, 1997.)

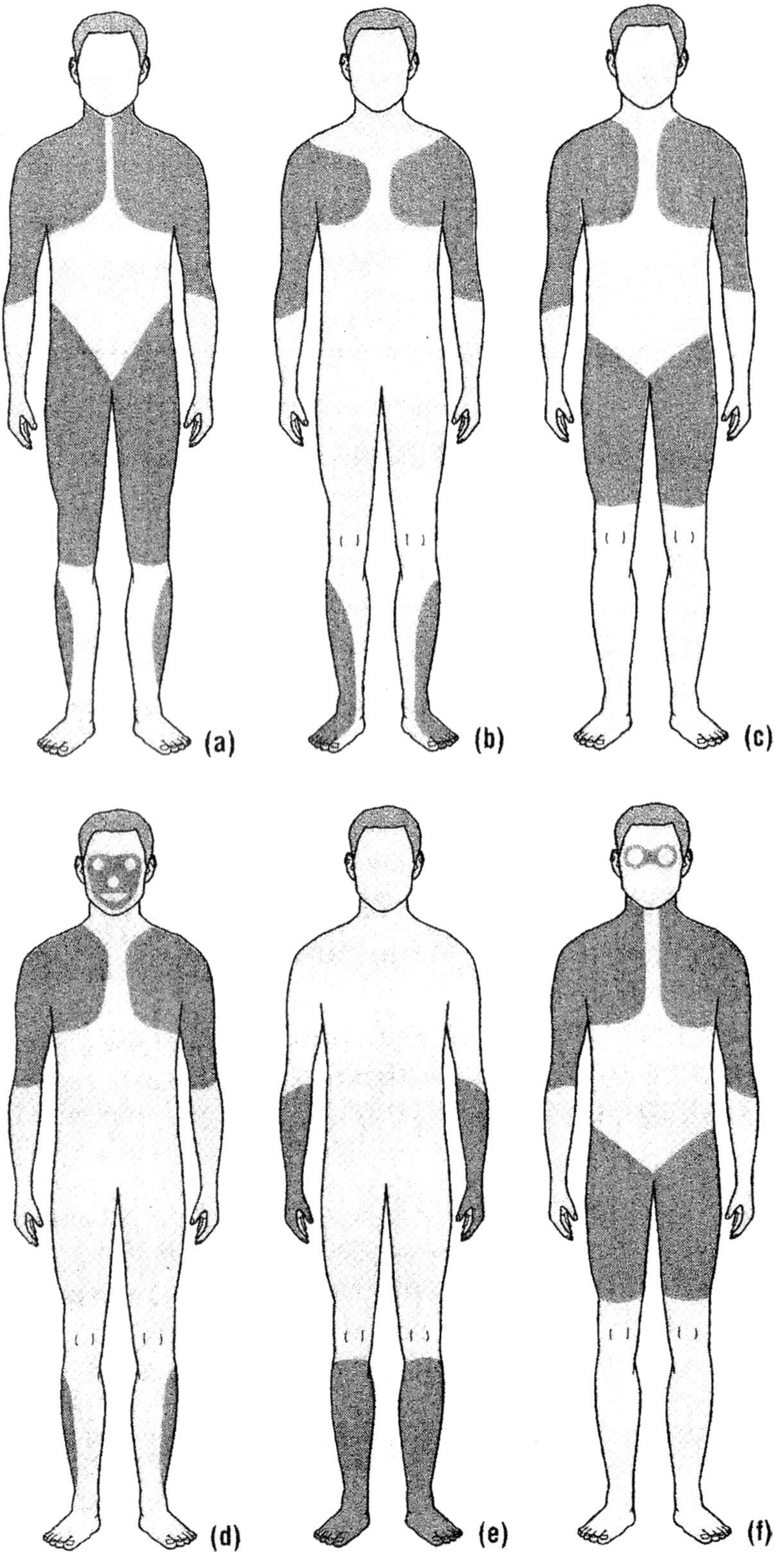

FIGURE 19-2. Distribution of predominant muscle weakness in different types of muscular dystrophy. A. Duchenne-type and Becker-type. B. Emery-Dreifuss. C. Limb-girdle. D. Fascioscapulohumeral. E. Distal. F. Oculopharyngeal. (Reproduced with permission from the BMJ Publishing Group Emery AEH: BMJ 317:991, 1998.)

electrocardiogram as the patient ages. Routine echocardiography can provide important information about cardiac function and is indicated at regular intervals. Progressive loss of myocardial tissue results in cardiomyopathy, ventricular dysrhythmias, and mitral regurgitation. Treatment of cardiac dysfunction may include angiotensin-converting enzyme (ACE) inhibitors and beta-adrenergic blockers.[2]

Degeneration of respiratory muscles can be measured with pulmonary function testing (spirometry), which reveals a restrictive pulmonary disease pattern. Diminished muscle strength produces an ineffective cough resulting in retention of pulmonary secretions, pneumonia, and death. Smooth muscle involvement causes intestinal tract hypomotility, delayed gastric emptying, and gastroparesis.

Although the genetic defect that causes Duchenne's dystrophy is known, specific genetic therapy remains elusive. Current treatment is supportive and directed at better nutrition and improvement of cardiorespiratory function.

Emery-Dreifuss Muscular Dystrophy

Emery-Dreifuss muscular dystrophy is characterized by contractures of the elbows, ankles, and spine as well as humeropectoral muscle weakness. There are two types of Emery-Dreifuss dystrophy. The autosomal dominant type is caused by a defect in the cell nuclear protein lamin, while the X-linked recessive type is caused by a defect in the nuclear protein emerin. The skeletal muscle manifestations are usually mild, whereas cardiac conduction defects can be fatal.[3] Implantable defibrillating pacemakers are often indicated for patients with Emery-Dreifuss muscular dystrophy.

Limb-Girdle Muscular Dystrophy

Patients with limb-girdle dystrophy exhibit weakness of the muscles of the shoulder and pelvic girdles. Cardiomyopathy and atrioventricular conduction defects can occur in patients with limb-girdle dystrophy. Although most cases of limb-girdle dystrophy are inherited as an autosomal recessive trait, some forms are inherited as autosomal dominant traits. Fifteen different genetic defects have been discovered and most cause an abnormality in the sarcoglycan proteins.

Fascioscapulohumeral Muscular Dystrophy

Fascioscapulohumeral muscular dystrophy is inherited as an autosomal dominant trait. Patients with this disease have diverse clinical manifestations. Weakness of the facial, scapulohumeral, anterior tibial, and pelvic-girdle muscles is prominent. Other abnormalities include retinal vascular disease, deafness, and neurologic dysfunction. Cardiac conduction defects and dysrhythmias may occur.

Oculopharyngeal Muscular Dystrophy

Oculopharyngeal muscular dystrophy typically presents in late adulthood. The primary clinical manifestations are ptosis and dysphagia. Dysphagia is secondary to pharyngeal skeletal muscle weakness and esophageal smooth muscle dysfunction. Weakness of the muscles of the head, neck and arms may also develop.

Congenital Muscular Dystrophy

Congenital muscular dystrophy is characterized by early onset (infancy, in utero) of muscle weakness, mental retardation, feeding difficulties, and respiratory dysfunction. Included in this group of muscular dystrophies are merosin-deficient muscular dystrophy, Fukuyama muscular dystrophy, Walker-Warburg syndrome, Ulrich's disease, muscle-eye-brain (MEB) disease, rigid spine muscular dystrophy, central core disease, myotubular myopathy, and nemaline myopathy.[4]

Management of Anesthesia

Most of the significant complications from anesthesia in patients with muscular dystrophy are secondary to the effects of anesthetic drugs on myocardial and skeletal muscle. Myocardial dysfunction makes patients with muscular dystrophy more susceptible to the myocardial depressant effects of potent inhaled anesthetics. There are numerous case reports of cardiac arrest occurring during the induction of anesthesia. These reports are associated with rhabdomyolysis and hyperkalemia and have occurred with volatile anesthetics alone or in combination with succinylcholine. In view of the weakened muscle structure of patients with muscular dystrophy, succinylcholine may damage the muscle membrane and release intracellular
1 contents. Succinylcholine is best avoided in patients with muscular dystrophy. The effect of volatile anesthetics on abnormal skeletal muscle is not known. It could be speculated that volatile anesthetics, by releasing calcium from the sarcoplasmic reticulum, could damage the muscle membrane and cause rhabdomyolysis. Sevoflurane is a less-potent stimulus for release of calcium from the sarcoplasmic reticulum and may be the preferred volatile agent for patients with muscular dystrophy.[5] Some patients with muscular dystrophy may be susceptible to malignant hyperthermia, but this is unpredictable.

Nondepolarizing muscle relaxants can be used although patients with Duchenne's muscular dystrophy may have prolonged recovery. The response to mivacurium is, however, normal.[6] The response of patients with other forms of muscular dystrophy to nondepolarizing muscle relaxants is variable and close monitoring of neuromuscular function is indicated.

Degeneration of gastrointestinal smooth muscle with hypomotility of the intestinal tract and delayed gastric emptying in conjunction with impaired swallowing increases the risk of perioperative aspiration of gastric contents. After surgery, the patient with muscular dystrophy must be closely monitored for evidence of pulmonary dysfunction and retention of pulmonary secretions. Vigorous respiratory therapy and mechanical ventilation may be required.

The Myotonias

The myotonias are a diverse group of diseases that share a common pathologic feature: myotonia. Myotonia is the delayed relaxation of skeletal muscle after voluntary contraction. Typically, muscle relaxants and regional anesthesia will not prevent or treat myotonia. Drugs that alter ion channel activity and skeletal muscle membrane excitability such as mexilitene, tocainide, and quinine may relax a myotonic contracture. Recent research has identified a wide variety of genetic defects that produce abnormalities in ion channels in the muscle membrane (Table 19-3). These defects can occur in the sodium, chloride, and calcium ion channels.

Myotonic Dystrophy (Steinert's Disease)

Myotonic dystrophy is the most common of the myotonic disorders. Myotonic dystrophy is an autosomally dominant inherited disorder with symptoms occurring during the second and third decades of life. In addition to myotonia, other clinical features of myotonic dystrophy include muscle degeneration, cataracts, premature balding, diabetes mellitus, thyroid dysfunction, adrenal insufficiency, gonadal dystrophy, and

TABLE 19-3

CLASSIFICATION OF MYOTONIC DYSTROPHY

- Protein kinase deficiency
  - Myotonic dystrophy
- Sodium channel diseases
  - Hyperkalemic periodic paralysis
  - Paramyotonic congenita
- Calcium channel diseases
  - Hypokalemic periodic paralysis
- Chloride channel diseases
  - Myotonia congenita (Thomsen)
  - Recessive myotonia
- Unknown defect
  - Proximal myotonic dystrophy

cardiac conduction abnormalities. Myotonic dystrophy is the result of an enlarged trinucleotide repeat of cytosine, thymine, and guanine (CTG) on chromosome 19. This defect produces a decrease in protein kinase that causes a degeneration of the sarcoplasmic reticulum.

Cardiac abnormalities have been well described in patients
2 with myotonic dystrophy. The most prominent cardiac disorders include atrioventricualr conduction delays (A-V block), atrial flutter and fibrillation, and ventricular dysrhythmias. First-degree A-V block may actually precede the onset of skeletal muscle symptoms. Sudden death may be a result of the abrupt onset of third-degree A-V block. Other cardiac abnormalities associated with myotonic dystrophy include mitral valve prolapse, left ventricular diastolic dysfunction, and cardiac failure.[7]

Pulmonary function studies demonstrate a restrictive lung disease pattern, mild arterial hypoxemia, and diminished ventilatory responses to hypoxia and hypercapnia. Brainstem respiratory control mechanisms may also be defective. Weakness of the respiratory muscles diminishes the effectiveness of cough and may lead to pneumonia. Myotonia of the respiratory muscles can produce intense dyspnea requiring treatment with procainamide. Alteration of smooth muscle function produces gastric atony and intestinal hypomotility. Pharyngeal muscle weakness in conjunction with delayed gastric emptying increases the risk of aspiration of gastric contents.

Pregnancy often produces an exacerbation of myotonic dystrophy that may be secondary to increased levels of progesterone. Congestive heart failure is also more likely to occur during pregnancy. Cesarean section must often be performed because of uterine smooth muscle dysfunction. Some infants of mothers with myotonic dystrophy may develop congenital myotonic dystrophy. Congenital myotonic dystrophy is characterized by hypotonia, respiratory insufficiency, and difficulty with feeding. Mental retardation is common in patients with the congenital form of myotonic dystrophy.

Therapy for myotonic dystrophy is directed at treatment of cardiac dysrhythmias (pacemaker implantation) and surgical therapy for cataracts and gallbladder disease. Mexilitene is effective for the treatment of myotonia. Treatment with growth hormone, selenium, vitamin E, coenzyme Q, and dehydroepiandrosterone may be effective but are as yet unproven.

Other Myotonias

Other forms of myotonic dystrophy include proximal myotonic myopathy, myotonic dystrophy type 2, and proximal myotonic dystrophy.

Patients with proximal myotonic myopathy have myotonia, proximal muscle weakness, and cataracts, but no facial muscle weakness. Cardiac dysrhythmias occur less frequently than in patients with myotonic dystrophy.

Myotonic dystrophy type 2 patients have clinical manifestations similar to myotonic type 1 patients but have a different mode of inheritance.

Proximal myotonic dystrophy produces clinical manifestations similar to proximal myotonic myopathy but with more severe muscle degeneration.[8]

Management of Anesthesia

Considerations for anesthesia for patients with myotonic dystrophy include the presence of cardiac and respiratory muscle disease and the abnormal responses to drugs used during anesthesia. Succinylcholine produces an exaggerated contracture and its use should be avoided (Fig. 19-3). The myotonic response to succinylcholine can be so severe that ventilation and tracheal intubation are difficult or impossible. Most patients with myotonic dystrophy develop a chronic myopathy

Succinylcholine (mg/kg)

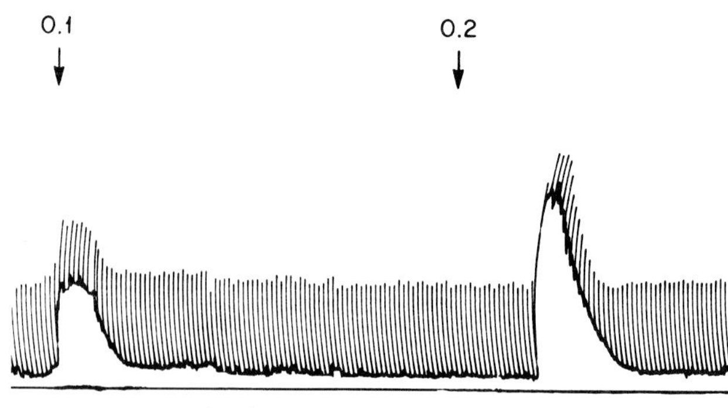

FIGURE 19-3. Administration of low does of succinylcholine to a patient with myotonic dystrophy produces an exaggerated contraction of skeletal muscle. (Reprinted with permission from Mitchell MM, Ali HH, Savarese JJ: Myotonia and neuromuscular blocking drugs. Anesthesia 49:44, 1978.)

and the response to nondepolarizing muscle relaxants may be enhanced. It would be prudent to use short-acting muscle relaxants such as mivacurium or cis-atracurium with close monitoring of the response. Reversal with neostigmine may provoke myotonia. The response to the peripheral nerve stimulator must be carefully interpreted because muscle stimulation may produce myotonia. The myotonic response may be misinterpreted as sustained tetanus when significant neuromuscular blockade still exists.

Patients with myotonic dystrophy are sensitive to the respiratory depressant effects of opioids (systemic and neuraxial), barbiturates, benzodiazepines, and inhaled anesthetics. The severity of the respiratory depression parallels the progression of the disease and may be the result of depression of central respiratory centers as well as peripheral muscle effects. In a study of more than 200 patients with myotonic dystrophy undergoing surgery, respiratory complications were more likely to occur in the early postoperative period after upper abdominal surgery or in those patients in whom preoperative upper extremity weakness was clinically evident.[9]

No specific anesthetic technique has been shown to be superior for patients with myotonic dystrophy. Higher doses of propofol have been associated with prolonged recovery. Carefully controlled propofol infusions have been successfully used for patients with myotonic dystrophy. Inhaled anesthetics may be used but close monitoring of cardiac rhythm and cardiovascular function is indicated. Postoperative mechanical ventilation should be employed until muscle strength and function return.[10] Successful regional anesthesia has been described for both children and adults with myotonic dystrophy.[11]

Skeletal muscle weakness and myotonia are exacerbated during pregnancy. Labor is typically prolonged and there is an increased incidence of postpartum hemorrhage (placenta accreta). Spinal and epidural anesthesia have been successfully used for pregnant patients.

Familial Periodic Paralysis

Genetic research required a reclassification of the periodic paralyses and some types of myotonias. These diseases have been reclassified as the skeletal muscle channelopathies.[12] The skeletal muscle channelopathies include hyperkalemic and hypokalemic periodic paralysis, paramyotonia congenita, and potassium aggravated myotonia.

TABLE 19-4

CLINICAL FEATURES OF FAMILIAL PERIODIC PARALYSIS

■ HYPOKALEMIC

Calcium channel defect
Potassium level <3 mEq/L during symptoms
Precipitating factors
- High glucose meals
- Strenuous exercise
- Glucose-insulin infusions
- Stress
- Hypothermia

Other features
- Chronic myopathy with aging

■ HYPERKALEMIC

Sodium channel defect
Potassium level normal or >5.5 mEq/L during symptoms
Precipitating factors
- Rest after exercise
- Potassium infusions
- Metabolic acidosis
- Hypothermia

Other features
- Skeletal muscle weakness may be localized to tongue and eyelids

Hyperkalemic Periodic Paralysis

Hyperkalemic periodic paralysis is inherited as an autosomal dominant trait that causes a mutation in the sodium ion channel. Hyperkalemic periodic paralysis is characterized by episodes of myotonia and muscle weakness that may last several hours after exposure to a trigger. Weakness can occur during rest after strenuous exercise, infusions of potassium, metabolic acidosis, or hypothermia. The weakness may be so severe that ventilatory support is required. The hyperkalemia is often transient, occurring only at the onset of weakness and potassium levels measured during the attack may be normal or decreased. Treatment consists of a low-potassium diet and the administration of thiazide diuretics (Table 19-4).

Hypokalemic Periodic Paralysis

Hypokalemic periodic paralysis is inherited as an autosomal dominant trait that produces a defect in the calcium ion channel. Paralysis may be produced by the ingestion of carbohydrates, strenuous exercise, and the infusion of glucose and insulin. Paralysis is usually incomplete, affecting the limbs and trunk, but sparing the diaphragm. Vocal cord paralysis can cause respiratory distress. Low potassium levels during acute episodes can cause cardiac dysrhythmias. Treatment consists of potassium infusion and the administration of acetazolamide and dichlorphenamide. Chronic muscle weakness occurs in most patients with hypokalemic periodic paralysis as they age.

Management of Anesthesia

The primary goal of the perioperative management of patients with both forms of periodic paralysis is the maintenance of normal potassium levels and avoidance of events that precipitate weakness. If possible, any electrolyte abnormality should be corrected prior to surgery. These patients may be sensitive to nondepolarizing muscle relaxants. Short-acting muscle relaxants are preferred and the response should be monitored with a peripheral nerve stimulator. Succinylcholine is best avoided as its administration may alter serum potassium levels. Metabolic changes (acidosis and alkalosis) or medications (glucose and insulin, diuretics) that reduce potassium levels may initiate an episode of paralysis. Since changes in the potassium level may precede the onset of weakness, serial measurement of potassium levels during prolonged surgical procedures and the early postoperative period should be considered. The electrocardiogram (ECG) should be continuously monitored for evidence of potassium-related dysrhythmias. Other recommendations include the avoidance of carbohydrate loads, hypothermia, and excessive hyperventilation. Any cause of potassium depletion can produce muscle weakness in patients with hypokalemic periodic paralysis. Halogenated inhaled anesthetics have been administered without complication. Regional anesthesia has also been successfully used.[13] Malignant hyperthermia has been associated with both forms of periodic paralysis.

After surgery, adequate muscle strength must be assured before mechanical ventilation of the lungs is discontinued.

Myasthenia Gravis

Myasthenia gravis is an autoimmune disease with antibodies directed against the nicotinic acetylcholine receptor or other muscle membrane proteins. Eighty-five percent of patients with myasthenia gravis have identifiable antiacetylcholine receptor antibodies. The majority of previously described "seronegative" patients have been found to have antibodies to muscle-specific receptor tyrosine kinase (MuSK).[14] Antiacetylcholine receptor antibodies damage the postsynaptic muscle membrane via a complement-mediated reaction causing an increased degradation and decreased formation of acetylcholine receptors. The thymus may play a central role in the pathogenesis of myasthenia gravis as 90% of patients have histologic abnormalities such as thymoma, thymic hyperplasia, or thymic atrophy. Many myasthenic patients also have antinuclear and antithyroid antibodies and other autoimmune diseases such as systemic lupus erythematosus, rheumatoid arthritis, pernicious anemia, and thyroiditis is associated with myasthenia gravis.

The clinical hallmark of myasthenia gravis is skeletal muscle weakness. Typically, the weakness is aggravated by repetitive muscle use and there are periods of exacerbation alternating with remission. Any skeletal muscle may be affected, although there is a predilection for muscles innervated by cranial nerves. Initial symptoms include diplopia, dysarthria, dysphagia, or limb-muscle weakness. Although respiratory insufficiency is not a common presenting symptom, undiagnosed myasthenia gravis should be included in the differential diagnosis of respiratory failure.[15] A myasthenic crisis will occur in 15 to 20% of patients during the course of their disease. Myasthenic crises are often precipitated by pulmonary infections and result in respiratory failure requiring mechanical ventilation. Potential cardiac manifestations of myasthenia gravis include focal myocarditis, atrial fibrillation, atrioventricular conduction delay, and left ventricular diastolic dysfunction.

Many conditions such as viral infection, pregnancy, extreme heat, stress, and surgery may initiate or exacerbate the symptoms of myasthenia, but the response to such stressors is unpredictable. Some pregnant patients have a remission during pregnancy while others (20 to 40%) have increased symptoms during gestation. Postpartum respiratory failure can occur. Fifteen to 20% of neonates born to myasthenic mothers have transient myasthenia from passive placental transfer of antiacetylcholine receptor antibodies. Signs and symptoms of neonatal myasthenia begin 12 to 48 hours after birth and may persist for several weeks.

There are several types of myasthenia gravis. Disease classification is based on skeletal muscle groups affected as well as the age of onset (Table 19-5). The Osserman staging system is based on the severity of the disease. Type I: ocular signs and symptoms only; type IIA: generalized muscle weakness;

TABLE 19-5

DIFFERENT PRESENTATIONS OF MYASTHENIA GRAVIS

	ETIOLOGY	ONSET	SEX	THYMUS	COURSE
Neonatal myasthenia	Passage of antibodies from myasthenic mothers across the placenta	Neonatal	Both sexes	Normal	Transient
Congenital myasthenia	Congenital end-plate pathology, genetic, autosomal recessive pattern of inheritance	0–2 yr	Male > female	Normal	Nonfluctuating, compatible with long survival
Juvenile myasthenia	Autoimmune disorder	2–20 yr	Female > male (4:1)	Hyperplasia	Slowly progressive, tendency to relapse and remission
Adult myasthenia	Autoimmune disorder	20–40 yr	Female > male	Hyperplasia > thymoma	Maximum severity within 3–5 yr
Elderly myasthenia	Autoimmune disorder	>40 yr	Male > Female	Thymoma (benign or locally invasive)	Rapid progress, higher mortality

Reproduced with permission from Barka A: Anesthesia and myasthenia gravis. Can J Anaesth 39:476, 1992.

type IIB: generalized moderate weakness and/or bulbar dysfunction; type III: acute fulminant presentation and/or respiratory dysfunction; and type IV: severe, generalized myasthenia.

The diagnosis of myasthenia gravis is based on the clinical history, the edrophonium test, electromyography, and the detection of circulating antiacetylcholine receptor antibodies. No single test, however, is definitive. The administration of edrophonium, for example, can improve muscle strength in myasthenic patients and in patients with other neuromuscular disorders.

Treatment modalities include the administration of cholinesterase inhibitors, corticosteroids, immunosuppressants, plasmapharesis, and thymectomy. The mainstay of medical therapy is the cholinesterase inhibitor pyridostigmine. Cholinesterase inhibitors function by effectively increasing the concentration of acetylcholine at the nicotinic postsynaptic membrane. Consistent control of myasthenia with cholinesterase inhibitors can be quite challenging. Underdosing will result in increased muscle weakness, whereas overdosing will produce a "cholinergic crisis." Excessive amounts of cholinesterase inhibitors produce abdominal cramping, salivation, bradycardia, and skeletal muscle weakness that mimics the weakness of myasthenia.

The immunosuppressive effects of corticosteroids produce an improvement in muscle strength in myasthenic patients although the precise mechanism is unknown. High-dose corticosteroids may, however, cause a transient increase in muscle weakness. Other immunosuppresants used for the treatment of myasthenia include azathioprine, cyclosporine, cyclophosphamide, tacrolimus, rituximab, and mycophenolate mofetil. Plasmapharesis removes antiacetylcholine receptor antibodies from the circulation and is effective treatment for patients in myasthenic crisis. Intravenous immunoglobulin may also be effective for the treatment of myasthenic crisis.

The association between the thymus and myasthenia gravis has been known for decades. The role of thymectomy for the treatment of myasthenia gravis is, however, not clearly established. Although a thymoma is a clear indication for thymectomy, thymectomy for other myasthenic patients is controversial. Thymectomy may be more effective if performed in the early stages of the disease. Should thymectomy be recommended, the surgical approach is also controversial. It is not clear whether wide surgical exposure through a sternal splitting approach is better than a transcervical or a video-assisted thorascopic (VATS) approach. The less-invasive approaches offer fewer postoperative complications, but may result in an incomplete resection of the thymus.[16]

Management of Anesthesia

The primary concern in anesthesia for the patient with myasthenia gravis is the potential interaction between the disease, treatment of the disease, and neuromuscular blocking drugs. The uncontrolled or poorly controlled myasthenic pa-
3 tient is exquisitely sensitive to nondepolarizing muscle relaxants. Small defasiculating doses of nondepolarizers can produce significant respiratory muscle weakness and respiratory distress. It should be anticipated that any patient with myasthenia, no matter how localized, will have increased sensitivity to nondepolarizing muscle relaxants (Fig. 19-4). An anesthetic technique that avoids the use of a muscle relaxant may be

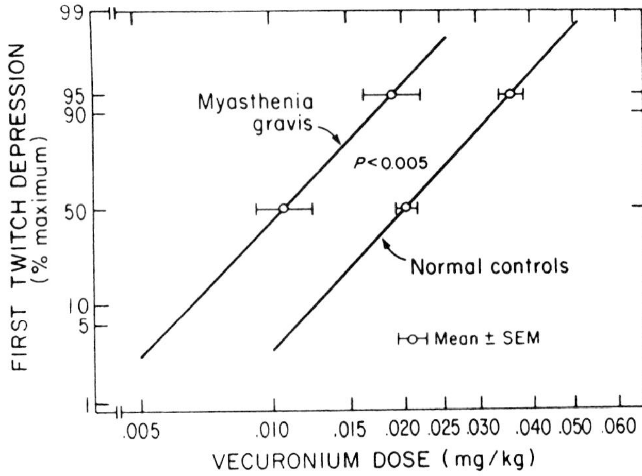

FIGURE 19-4. Dose-response for vecuronium in normal patients and patients with myasthenia gravis. (Reprinted with permission from Eisenkraft JB, Book WJ, Paparestas AE: Sensitivity to vecuronium in myasthenia gravis: A dose-responsive study. Can J Anaesth 37;301, 1990.)

preferred for patients with myasthenia gravis.[17] Conditions suitable for tracheal intubation can be obtained with a standard induction technique (thiopental, propofol) and the inhalation of volatile halogenated agents. Isoflurane, sevoflurane, and desflurane depress neuromuscular transmission and may provide enough muscle relaxation so that tracheal intubation can be performed without neuromuscular blocking drugs after an adequate depth of anesthesia has been attained. Adjuvant drugs such as propofol, opioids, and lidocaine that blunt responses to laryngosocpy may be useful.

Myasthenia and the cholinesterase inhibitor drugs used to treat myasthenia will influence the response to both depolarizing and nondepolarizing muscle relaxants. Certain recommendations are indicated. Pretreatment doses of nondepolarizers and long-acting nondepolarizing muscle relaxants (pancuronium) should not be used in myasthenic patients. If additional muscle relaxation is required for the procedure, short-acting nondepolarizers in small doses should be used for myasthenic patients. Close, objective monitoring of neuromuscular transmission and clinical effect is necessary. Atracurium, cisatracurium, mivacurium, vecuronium, and rocuronium have been used. The response of the myasthenic patients to these drugs varies greatly. Although patients with myasthenia have a resistance to succinylcholine, a dose of 1.5 to 2 mg/kg will be adequate for rapid tracheal intubation. Preoperative administration of pyridostigmine, however, may prolong the action of succinylcholine and mivacurium.[18]

Adjuvant drugs that may exacerbate muscle weakness in myasthenic patients include aminoglycoside antibiotics, polymyxins, beta-adrenergic blockers, procainamide, corticosteroids, and phenytoin. Patients with myasthenia gravis may have central respiratory depression and the respiratory depressant effects of barbiturates, benzodiazepines, opioids, and propofol may be accentuated. Vigilant monitoring of respiratory function is required.

Most modern anesthetic techniques permit weaning from mechanical ventilation and tracheal extubation of myasthenic patients soon after surgery.[19] Less-invasive surgical techniques for thymectomy, such as a transcervical approach or video-assisted thoracoscopic thymectomy, produce less disruption of respiratory function than transsternal thymectomy. Because of the unpredictability of postoperative recovery, however, it would be prudent to make preoperative arrangements for postoperative ventilation. Risk factors that increase the likelihood of postoperative insufficiency include a long duration of myasthenia, chronic respiratory disease, and treatment requiring high doses of pyridostigmine. The patient with myasthenia gravis can be quite challenging to wean from ventilatory support. Skeletal muscle strength can vary greatly during a short period of time.

Epidural analgesia and anesthesia can be used for labor and delivery. Muscle relaxation induced by regional anesthesia may, however, compound the weakness caused by myasthenia. This potential synergism necessitates careful monitoring of the patient's muscle strength. Amide local anesthetics may be better than ester local anesthetics as the metabolism of amides is not affected by cholinesterase activity. Exacerbations of myasthenia must be anticipated during pregnancy.

Myasthenic Syndrome (Lambert-Eaton Syndrome)

The Lambert-Eaton myasthenic syndrome (LEMS) is a disorder of neuromuscular transmission associated with carcinomas, particularly small cell carcinoma of the lung and lymphoproliferative diseases (Table 19-6). The onset of the myasthenic syndrome may actually precede the discovery of the malignancy by as much as 5 years. LEMS is an autoimmune disease in which immunoglobulin G (IgG) antibodies against voltage-gated calcium channels (presynaptic) are produced. In those cases associated with carcinoma, the autoantibodies are directed at calcium channels in the tumor. These autoantibodies, however, cross-react with calcium channels at the neuromuscular junction. The result is a decreased release of acetylcholine in response to nerve stimulation. Typically, the patient is a man, 50 to 70 years of age, complaining of proximal extremity weakness (hip, shoulder) that markedly affects gait and the ability to stand and climb stairs. Rarely, the clinical presentation may be respiratory failure. Autonomic dysfunction, such as xerostomia, impotence, orthostatic hypotension, constipation, and altered sweating responses may also develop.[20]

Treatment of the underlying neoplasm may improve the neurologic condition. The most effective drug for the treatment of myasthenic syndrome is 3,4-diaminopyridine. 3,4-diaminopyridine improves synaptic transmission by opening voltage-gated potassium channels, which prolongs the action potential and increases release of acetylcholine. Side effects of 3,4-diaminopyridine include perioral and digital paresthesias and seizures. Immunosuppression with corticosteroids, azathioprine, and cyclosporine may also be effective.

TABLE 19-6

COMPARISON OF MYASTHENIC SYNDROME AND MYASTHENIA GRAVIS

	MYASTHENIC SYNDROME	MYASTHENIA GRAVIS
Manifestations	Proximal limb weakness (arms > legs)	Extraocular, bulbar, and facial muscle weakness
	Exercise improves with strength	Fatigue with exercise
	Muscle pain common	Muscle pain uncommon
	Reflexes absent or decreased	Reflexes normal
Gender	Male > female	Female > male
Coexisting pathology	Small cell carcinoma of the lung	Thymoma
Response to muscle relaxants	Sensitive to succinylcholine and nondepolarizing muscle relaxants	Resistant to succinylcholine Sensitive to nondepolarizing muscle relaxants
	Poor response to anticholinesterases	Poor response to anticholinesterases

Reprinted with permission from Stoelting RK, Dierdorf SF (eds): Anesthesia and Co-existing Disease, 3rd ed. New York, Churchill Livingstone.

Plasmapharesis and intravenous immunoglobulin may produce short-term improvement.[21]

Management of Anesthesia

Patients with myasthenic syndrome are sensitive to the effects of both depolarizing and nondepolarizing muscle relaxants. Consequently, doses of these drugs should be reduced and neuromuscular function should be monitored carefully. The administration of 3,4-diaminopyridine should be continued up to the time of surgery.

Because the myasthenic syndrome is difficult to diagnose, a high index of suspicion should be maintained if unexpected muscle weakness occurs in patients with malignant tumors. Although myasthenic syndrome is most frequently associated with small cell carcinoma of the lung, muscle weakness can
4 occur with other malignancies as well.

Guillain-Barré Syndrome (Polyradiculoneuritis)

Guillain-Barré syndrome is the most common cause of acute, flaccid paralysis. Guillain-Barré syndrome is an autoimmune disease triggered by a bacterial or viral infection. The list of infectious triggers is long and includes Epstein-Barr virus, hemophilus parainfluenza, influenza, adenovirus, herpes simplex, varicella, human immunodeficiency virus, mycoplasma, and campylobacter. The infection triggers an immune response that produces antibodies to an antigen of the infectious agent. The antigen mimics an epitope of the Schwann cell and the antibodies damage myelin nerve sheaths.

Most patients have a history of a respiratory or gastrointestinal infection within 4 weeks of the onset of neurologic symptoms. Guillain-Barré syndrome is characterized by the acute or subacute onset of skeletal muscle weakness or paralysis of the legs. Sensory disturbances such as paresthesias often precede the paralysis. The paralysis typically progresses cephalad to include the muscles of the trunk and arms. Difficulty in swallowing and impaired ventilation secondary to intercostal muscle paralysis can occur. Progression occurs over 10 to 12 days, followed by gradual recovery. The most serious immediate problem is ventilatory insufficiency. The vital capacity should be measured frequently. If the vital capacity decreases to less than 15 to 20 mL/kg, mechanical ventilation of the lungs is indicated. The more rapid the onset of quadriplegia, the more likely the need for ventilatory support. Although 85% of patients with this syndrome achieve a good or full recovery, chronic recurrent neuropathy develops in 3 to 5% of patients. Subtypes of Guillain-Barré syndrome include acute inflammatory demyelinating polyneuropathy (AIDP), acute motor axonal neuropathy (AMAN), acute motor-sensory axonal neuropathy (AMSAN), and Miller-Fisher syndrome (MFS).

The primary therapy for Guillain-Barré syndrome is intensive respiratory care and management of autonomic dysfunction. Intensive critical care has reduced mortality from Guillain-Barré syndrome to less than 5%. Plasmapharesis and the administration of intravenous immunoglobulin may help alleviate the harmful effects of the disordered immune response.[22]

Autonomic nervous system dysfunction occurs in many patients with Guillain-Barré syndrome. This dysfunction can produce wide fluctuations in cardiovascular parameters. In a manner similar to autonomic hyperreflexia, physical stimulation can precipitate hypertension, tachycardia, and cardiac dysrhythmias. Appropriate alpha- and beta-adrenergic blockade may be required. Mild hepatic dysfunction may also develop in patients with Guillain-Barré syndrome.

Management of Anesthesia

Autonomic nervous system dysfunction indicates that compensatory cardiovascular responses may be absent, resulting in significant hypotension secondary to postural changes, blood loss, or positive airway pressure. On the other hand, noxious stimuli such as laryngoscopy and tracheal intubation may produce exaggerated increases in heart rate and blood pressure. Direct-acting vasopressors may be required to control blood pressure. Cardiovascular function should be carefully monitored in the perioperative period.

The administration of succinylcholine should be avoided because of the danger of drug-induced potassium release and hyperkalemia. This risk may actually persist after clinical recovery from the disorder.[23] A nondepolarizing muscle relaxant with minimal cardiovascular effects such as cisatracurium, vecuronium, or rocuronium would be a useful choice. The sensitivity of patients with Guillain-Barré syndrome to nondepolarizing muscle relaxants, however, may vary from extreme sensitivity to resistance, depending on the phase of the disease.[24] It is likely that mechanical ventilation will be required during the immediate postoperative period. Patients with Guillain-Barré syndrome that have pronounced sensory disturbances may benefit from the administration of epidural opioids.

It should be remembered that it can be very difficult to differentiate Guillain-Barré syndrome from other neurologic disorders such as anterior spinal syndrome or chronic inflammatory demyelinating polyneuropathy. Guillain-Barré syndrome can occur after surgery.

CENTRAL NERVOUS SYSTEM DISEASES

Multiple Sclerosis

Multiple sclerosis is an acquired disease of the central nervous system (CNS) characterized by central nervous system inflammation and multiple sites of demyelination in the brain and spinal cord. The cause of multiple sclerosis is multifactorial and involves a complex series of immunologic events occurring in genetically susceptible individuals. Initially, a virus or other agent (? ischemia) triggers an inflammatory reaction that causes a T-cell–mediated autoimmune response to myelin. Demyelination exposes the axon to harmful factors and interferes with neural transmission. The nerve's ability to repair itself during the early phases of the process explains the relapsing nature of the disease.[25]

The symptoms of multiple sclerosis depend on the sites of demyelination in the brain and spinal cord. Demyelination of the optic tracts produces visual disturbances, whereas demyelination of the oculomotor pathways results in nystagmus. Lesions of the spinal cord produce limb weakness and paresthesias. The legs are affected more than the arms. Bowel retention and urinary incontinence are frequent complaints. Brainstem involvement can produce diplopia, trigeminal neuralgia, cardiac dysrhythmias, and autonomic dysfunction, while alterations in ventilation can lead to hypoxemia, apnea, and respiratory failure. The course of multiple sclerosis is characterized by exacerbation of symptoms at unpredictable intervals over a period of years. Residual symptoms eventually persist and may lead to severe disability. Three clinical courses are recognized: relapsing-remitting MS (RR-MS), primary-progressive MS (PP-MS), and secondary-progressive MS (SP-MS). Ten to 20% of patients with multiple sclerosis have a relatively benign course with little disability. Pregnancy is associated with an improvement in symptoms, but relapse frequently occurs in the first three postpartum months.

The diagnosis of multiple sclerosis is based primarily on clinical determinants. Clinical criteria include age of onset between 10 and 50 years, neurologic signs and symptoms of CNS white matter disease, two or more attacks separated by a month or more, and involvement of two or more noncontiguous anatomic areas. Laboratory confirmation of the diagnosis can be made by chemical analysis of the cerebrospinal fluid and cranial magnetic resonance imaging (MRI). Seventy percent of patients with multiple sclerosis have elevated levels of IgG in the CSF. An elevated level of albumin in the CSF is indicative of blood-brain barrier dysfunction. MRI is a sensitive diagnostic tool for multiple sclerosis and provides direct evidence of the location of demyelinated plaques in the central nervous system. MRI can also be used as a measure of the effectiveness of treatment.

Current therapy for multiple sclerosis is directed at modulating the immunologic and inflammatory responses that damage myelin. Corticosteroids (methylprednisolone) are the primary agents for treatment of an acute exacerbation of multiple sclerosis. Corticosteroids have diverse effects that suppress cellular immune responses. Interferon (IFN) alters the inflammatory response and augments natural disease suppression and has been shown to reduce the relapse rate. Side effects of interferon therapy include aggravation of spasticity, development of autoantibodies, and flu-like symptoms. Glatiramer is a mixture of polypeptides that mimics the structure of myelin and serves as a decoy for autoantibodies. A number of immunosuppressants have been studied but patient response has been variable. Mitoxantrone can be used to treat aggressive multiple sclerosis. Mitoxantrone, however, is cardiotoxic. Currently under investigation are therapies directed at remyelination such as Schwann cell transplantation.[26] Symptomatic therapy for some of the complications of multiple sclerosis include diazepam, dantrolene, and baclofen for spasticity. Painful dysesthesias, tonic seizures, dysarthria, and ataxia may be treated with carbamazepine. Nonspecific measures include the avoidance of excessive fatigue, emotional stress, and hyperthermia. Demyelinated nerve fibers are extremely sensitive to increases in temperature. A temperature increase of 0.5 degrees C can block impulse conduction in demyelinated fibers.

Management of Anesthesia

The effect of surgery and anesthesia on the course of multiple sclerosis is controversial. Regional and general anesthesia have been reported to exacerbate multiple sclerosis, while other reports have found no correlation between anesthesia and the course of the disease. Factors other than anesthesia such as infection, emotional stress, and hyperpyrexia may contribute to an increased risk of a perioperative exacerbation. Preoperatively, the patient should be advised that surgery and anesthesia could produce a relapse despite a well-managed
5 anesthetic. Ideally, the patient should have a thorough neurologic examination before the operation to document coexisting neurologic deficits. After surgery, the examination can be repeated so that pre- and postoperative findings can be compared.

Although the mechanism is not known, spinal anesthesia has been associated with an exacerbation of the disease. It could be speculated that demyelinated areas of the spinal cord are more sensitive to the effects of the local anesthetic causing a relative neurotoxicity. Further evidence for this theory is found by the observation that higher concentrations of bupivacaine (0.25%) used for labor epidural analgesia were more likely to produce relapse than lower concentrations.[27] With such a precaution in mind, epidural analgesia can be safely provided for women during labor. Neuraxial local anesthetics and opioids may also be indicated for the treatment of chronic, refractory pain syndromes in patients with multiple sclerosis.

Selection of agents for general anesthesia should take into consideration potential interactions with medications the patient is receiving. Patients being treated with corticosteroids may require intravenous corticosteroid supplementation during the perioperative period. Immunosuppressants can produce cardiotoxicity and subclinical cardiac dysfunction. Baclofen can produce an increase sensitivity to nondepolarizing muscle relaxants, while anticonvulsants produce resistance to nondepolarizers. In theory, succinylcholine could produce an exaggerated release of potassium, although this has not been reported. Autonomic dysfunction caused by multiple sclerosis may exaggerate the hypotensive effects of volatile anesthetics. Careful monitoring of cardiovascular function is indicated. Respiratory muscle weakness and respiratory control dysfunction increase the likelihood of the need for supplemental oxygen and/or mechanical ventilation during the immediate postoperative period.[28]

Epilepsy

A seizure is a common manifestation of many types of CNS diseases. A seizure results from an excessive discharge of large numbers of neurons that become depolarized in a synchronous fashion. Idiopathic seizures usually begin during childhood. The sudden onset of seizures in a young or middle-aged adult should arouse suspicion of focal brain disease, particularly a tumor. The onset of seizures after 60 years of age is usually secondary to cerebrovascular disease but can be a result of head injury, tumor, metabolic disturbances, or central nervous system infection. The onset of seizures mandates a thorough neurologic evaluation to determine the etiology. Advanced neuroimaging techniques provide powerful diagnostic tools for the determination of structural causes of epilepsy. Research in molecular biology and genetics has revealed that some forms of epilepsy are caused by mutations in ion channels. The availability of new antiseizure drugs has increased the therapeutic options for patients with epilepsy. Selecting the right drug or drugs for the treatment of epilepsy may require trial and error to balance efficacy with side effects.[29]

There are more than 40 types of epilepsy based on several clinical features. The most common classification is the International Classification of Epileptic Seizures (Table 19-7). A description of the most frequently encountered types of seizures follows.

1. Grand Mal Seizures
   A grand mal seizure is characterized by generalized tonic-clonic activity. All respiratory activity is arrested and a period of arterial hypoxemia ensues. The tonic phase lasts for 20 to 40 seconds and is followed by the clonic phase. In the postictal period, the patient is lethargic and confused. Initial therapy is directed toward maintaining arterial oxygenation and stopping the seizure activity. Diazepam and thiopental are effective for the treatment of acute, generalized seizures. Antiseizure drugs effective for seizure control and prevention are valproate, phenytoin, felbamate, carbamazepine, and lamotrigine (Table 19-8). Epileptic patients resistant to drug therapy may benefit from surgical resection of a seizure focus or vagal nerve stimulator implantation.[30]
2. Focal Cortical Seizure
   Focal cortical seizure, also known as Jacksonian epilepsy, may be sensory or motor, depending on the site of neuronal discharge. There is usually no loss of consciousness, although the seizure activity may spread to produce a grand mal seizure.

TABLE 19-7

CLASSIFICATION OF SEIZURES

■ LOCALIZATION-RELATED EPILEPSIES AND SEIZURES
Idiopathic
Benign childhood epilepsy
Childhood epilepsy with occipital paroxysms
■ GENERALIZED EPILEPSIES
Idiopathic
Absence epilepsy
Childhood
Juvenile
Benign neonatal convulsions
Myoclonic epilepsy
Neonatal
Juvenile
Grand mal seizures on awakening
Idiopathic and/or symptomatic
West's syndrome
Lennox-Gestaut syndrome
Myoclonic–astatic seizures
Myoclonic absences
Symptomatic
Nonspecific etiology
■ UNDETERMINED EPILEPSIES AND SYNDROMES
With both generalized and focal seizures
Neonatal seizures
Severe myoclonic epilepsy of infancy
Acquired epileptic aphasia
■ SPECIAL SYNDROMES
Febrile seizures
Alcohol-related seizures

Modified with permission from Riela AR: Management of seizures. Crit Care Clin 5:863, 1989.

3. Absence Seizure (Petit Mal)
   Absence seizures, previously called petit mal seizures, are characterized by a brief loss of awareness lasting 30 seconds. Additional manifestations include staring, blinking, and rolling of the eyes. There is an immediate resumption of consciousness. Absence seizures typically occur in children and young adults. Absence seizures without other seizure activity are best treated with ethosuximide. Valproate is the drug of choice for absence seizures associated with other seizure activity.
4. Akinetic Seizure
   Akinetic seizures are characterized by a sudden, brief loss of consciousness and loss of postural tone. These types of seizures usually occur in children and can produce severe head injury from a fall.
5. Myoclonic Seizure
   Myoclonic seizures occur as isolated clonic jerks in response to a sensory stimulus. In most cases a single group of muscles is involved. Myoclonic seizures are often associated with degenerative and metabolic brain diseases.
6. Psychomotor Seizure
   Psychomotor seizures are seen as an impairment of consciousness, inappropriate motor acts, hallucinations, amnesia, and unusual visceral symptoms. This type of seizure is preceded by an aura.
7. Status Epilepticus
   Status epilepticus is defined as two consecutive tonic-clonic seizures without regaining consciousness, or seizure activity that is unabated for 30 minutes or more. Status epilepticus can include all types of seizure activity. Grand mal status epilepticus is of the greatest concern because mortality can be as high as 20%. Grand mal status epilepticus typically lasts for 48 hours with a seizure frequency of four to five per hour. As the seizure progresses, skeletal muscle activity diminishes and seizure activity may be evident only on the electroencephalogram (EEG). Respiratory effects of status epilepticus include inhibition of the respiratory centers, uncoordinated skeletal muscle activity that impairs ventilation, and abnormal autonomic activity that produces bronchoconstriction. In addition to the danger of arterial hypoxemia, there is a high likelihood of permanent neuronal damage from continued seizures. Diazepam or lorazepam are considered the drugs of choice for treatment of status epilepticus. Because the effects of the benzodiazepines are transient, a longer acting anticonvulsant such as phenytoin or phenobarbital must also be administered. Thiopental is quite effective for the initial treatment of status epilepticus, but the effect is transient. Muscle relaxants may be required to facilitate tracheal intubation if a secured airway is necessary. Although muscle relaxants will terminate the skeletal muscle manifestations of a seizure, there is no effect on seizure activity in the brain. On rare occasions, general anesthesia with isoflurane or barbiturates may be required for treatment of status epilepticus.

Management of Anesthesia

Patients receiving antiseizure medications should be maintained on their normal medication regimen until the time of surgery. After surgery, medications should be given parenterally until oral intake can be resumed. A decline in blood levels of anticonvulsant drugs will increase the likelihood of postoperative seizures.

In the management of anesthesia for the patient with a seizure disorder, the potential influence of anticonvulsants on the response to anesthesia must be considered. Conversely, an anesthesia technique should be used that will not increase the likelihood of seizure activity. Because anticonvulsant drugs affect the liver and neuromuscular systems, the potential for significant drug interactions certainly exists. Stimulation of the hepatic microsomal enzymes by anticonvulsants may increase the magnitude of biotransformation of anesthetic drugs. Increased biotransformation of volatile halogenated anesthetics may increase the risk of organ toxicity. Other known side effects of anticonvulsants include leukopenia, anemia, and hepatitis from phenytoin; pancreatitis, hepatic failure, and coagulopathy from valproate; aplastic anemia, cardiotoxicity, and hypothyroidism from carbamazepine; leukopenia from felbamate; and rash and hypersensitivity from lamotrigine.[31]

Although most inhaled anesthetics, including nitrous oxide, have been reported to produce seizure activity, such activity during the administration of isoflurane, sevoflurane, and desflurane is extremely rare. In general, these anesthetics produce a dose-dependent depression of EEG activity. The use of ketamine is controversial. Ketamine has been shown to produce seizure activity in patients with known seizure disorders. Similarly, methohexital may produce seizure activity. It would seem reasonable to avoid the use of ketamine and methohexital for patients with seizure disorders when alternative drugs such as thiopental, propofol, and benzodiazepines are available. Propofol has a more depressant effect on the EEG than thiopental and has been shown to increase the seizure threshold in patients receiving electroconvulsive therapy.

Potent opioids such as fentanyl, sufentanil, and alfentanil may produce myoclonic activity or chest wall rigidity that can be confused with seizure activity. In clinical doses, opioid induced seizures are unlikely. Prolonged administration of

TABLE 19-8

ANTICONVULSANT DRUGS

DRUG	SEIZURE TYPE	THERAPEUTIC BLOOD LEVELS (μg/mL)	SIDE EFFECTS
Phenobarbital	Generalized	15–35	Sedation, increased drug metabolism
Valproate	Generalized Absence	50–100	Pancreatitis, hepatic dysfunction
Felbamate	Generalized Partial	20–140	Insomnia, ataxia, nausea
Phenytoin	Generalized Partial	10–20	Gingival hyperplasia Dermatitis Resistance to NM blockers
Fosphenytoin	Generalized Partial		Paresthesias Hypotension
Carbamazepine	Generalized Partial	6–12	Cardiotoxic, hepatitis Resistance to NM blockers
Lamotrigine	Generalized Partial	2–16	Rash Stevens-Johnson syndrome
Topiramate	Generalized Partial	4–10	
Gabapentin	Generalized Partial	4–16	Fatigue, somnolence
Primidone	Generalized Partial	6–12	Nausea, ataxia
Clonazepam	Absence	0.01–0.07	Ataxia
Ethosuximide	Absence	40–100	Leuopenia Erythema multiforme
Levetiracetam	Generalized Partial	5–45	Dizziness, headache Somnolence
Oxycarbazepine	Partial	10–35	Hyponatremia, diplopia Somnolence
Tiagabine	Partial		Tremor, depression
Zonisamide	Generalized Partial	10–40	Anorexia Decreased cognition

large doses of fentanyl (200 to 400 μg/kg) or sufentanil (40 to 160 μg/kg) may produce seizures and should be used with caution in patients with seizure disorders.

Patients receiving phenytoin or carbamazepine exhibit resistance to nondepolarizing muscle relaxants.

Parkinson's Disease

Parkinson's disease, one of the most common disabling neurologic diseases, affects 1% of the population over 60 years of age. Parkinson's disease is a degenerative disease of the central nervous system caused by loss of dopaminergic fibers in the basal ganglia of the brain. The characteristic pathologic feature is destruction of dopamine-containing nerve cells in the substantia nigra of the basal ganglia. Lewy bodies, a hallmark of the pathology of Parkinson's disease, are proteinaceous cytoplasmic cell inclusions. Theories of the etiology of Parkinson's disease include mitochondrial dysfunction with disordered oxidative metabolism, excitotoxicity (persistent activation of glutamatergic receptors), inadequate neurotrophic support, and exposure to toxins (pesticides, herbicides, industrial chemicals, or viral infection).[32] Other than the well-known postencephalitic Parkinson's disease, however, there is little evidence that Parkinson's disease is caused by a virus.

The clinical effects of Parkinson's disease are caused by dopamine deficiency. Dopamine deficiency increases activity of gamma-aminobutyric acid (GABA). GABA inhibits thalamic and brainstem nuclei, which suppress cortical motor activity, thereby causing tremor, akinesia, and gait and posture abnormalities. The most characteristic clinical features of Parkinson's disease are resting tremor, cogwheel rigidity of the extremities, bradykinesia, shuffling gait, stooped posture, and facial immobility. These features are all secondary to diminished inhibition of the extrapyramidal motor system as a result of depletion of dopamine from the basal ganglia. Other features that occur in patients with Parkinson's disease are seborrhea, sialorrhea, orthostatic hypotension, bladder dysfunction, pupillary abnormalities, diaphragmatic spasm, oculogyric crises, dementia, and mental depression.

The treatment of Parkinson's disease is directed toward increasing dopamine levels in the brain but preventing the adverse peripheral effects of dopamine. Levodopa is the single most effective therapy for patients with Parkinson's disease. When administered orally, however, levodopa is converted to dopamine and causes side effects such as nausea, vomiting, and hypotension. To avoid such side effects, levodopa is administered in combination with a peripheral decarboxylase inhibitor (carbidopa). Cardiovascular side effects of levodopa include depletion of myocardial norepinephrine stores, peripheral vasoconstriction, hypovolemia, and orthostatic hypotension. Although levodopa has significantly reduced morbidity and mortality from Parkinson's disease, motor fluctuations causing significant disability occur in levodopa treated patients. There is also some evidence that levodopa may accelerate the pathologic process that causes Parkinson's disease. In an effort to delay the use of levodopa, other drugs such as selegiline, dopamine agonists, amantadine, COMT inhibitors, and apomorphine have been used as initial treatment drugs.[33] Anticholinergic drugs (trihexyphenidyl, benztropine) are effective because they counteract loss of inhibition of cholinergic neurons. Anticholinergics can worsen dementia and are reserved for younger patients in the early phases of Parkinson's disease. Amantadine is a glutamate receptor antagonist and may exert a neuroprotective effect on neurons in the basal ganglia. Dopamine receptor agonists (bromocriptine, pergolide, pramipexole, ropinirole) exert their effect on dopamine receptors in the brain. Side effects of dopamine agonists include pulmonary and retroperitoneal fibrosis, erythromelalgia, and Raynaud's phenomenon. Selegiline is a selective MAO-B inhibitor that decreases the metabolism of dopamine. COMT inhibitors (entacapone, tolcapone) prevent the degradation of levodopa. Many of the aforementioned types of drugs, although not entirely successful as sole agents for the treatment of Parkinson's disease, are effective in combination with levodopa. Therapies directed at neuroprotection with a variety of agents (coenzyme Q10, creatine, vitamin E) are under study. Patients with advanced drug-resistant Parkinson's disease may benefit from surgical implantation of deep brain stimulators.[34]

Management of Anesthesia

Management of anesthesia is usually determined by potential interaction between anesthesia drugs and anti-Parkinson medications and the severity of neurologic impairment. The patient's medications should be administered on the morning of surgery. The half-life of levodopa is short and interruption of therapy for more than 6 to 12 hours can result in severe skeletal muscle rigidity that interferes with ventilation. Dopamine antagonists such as phenothiazines, droperidol, and metoclopramide should be avoided. Alfentanil and fentanyl may produce acute dystonic reactions in patients with Parkinson' disease. Although ketamine could produce an exaggerated sympathetic nervous system response with resultant tachycardia and hypertension, it has been used without difficulty in patients with Parkinson's disease. The likelihood of coexisting heart disease in elderly patients with Parkinson's disease, however, makes the use of ketamine less attractive. There are no reports of adverse responses to isoflurane, sevoflurane, or desflurane in patients with Parkinson's disease. Although definitive studies of anesthesia for patients receiving selegiline have not been performed, clinical experience indicates that anesthesia is usually uneventful. There have been reports of agitation, muscle rigidity, and hyperthermia in patients receiving meperidine and selegiline. Patients with Parkinson's disease who are being treated with dopamine agonists may be at risk for neuroleptic malignant syndrome. Apomorphine is a dopamine agonist that can be administered subcutaneously or intravenously in the perioperative period if oral levodopa cannot be administered.

Autonomic dysfunction is common in patients with Parkinson's disease. Gastrointestinal dysfunction is manifested by excessive salivation, dysphagia, and esophageal dysfunction. Consequently, the patient with Parkinson's disease should be considered to be at risk for aspiration pneumonitis. The most consistent cardiovascular abnormality is orthostatic hypotension. The disease process undoubtedly contributes to hypotension, which is further compounded by the tendency for anti-Parkinson drugs to cause peripheral vasodilation. Patients with Parkinson's disease would be more likely to develop exaggerated decreases in blood pressure in response to inhaled halogenated anesthetics.

Perioperative respiratory complications are common in patients with Parkinson's disease.[35] Upper airway obstruction may occur as a result of poor coordination of upper airway muscles secondary to neurotransmitter imbalance caused by the disease process or induced by the administration of antidopaminergic drugs. Some Parkinson's patients with upper airway obstruction may respond to the administration of anti-Parkinson drugs.

In the postoperative period, patients with Parkinson's disease are susceptible to mental confusion and even hallucinations. These alterations in mental function may not appear until the day after surgery. The patient and the patient's caregiver should be advised of this possibility.

Huntington's Disease

Huntington's disease is a neurodegenerative disease caused by severe neuronal atrophy in the corpus striatum and later the cortex. Huntington's disease is one of the trinucleotide repeat disorders. An increase in cytosine, adenine, and guanine (CAG) repeat sequences on chromosome 4 causes the genetic defect that causes Huntington's disease. This gene encodes for the huntingtin protein. Although the function of the huntingtin protein is not known, intranuclear inclusions of huntingtin and ubiquitin are found in neurons that eventually die. Huntington's disease is a heritable disorder that is transmitted as an autosomal dominant trait. Identification of the Huntington's gene provides a reliable technique for predictive testing; however, the delayed nature of the clinical manifestations of the disease presents legal and ethical concerns about early predictive testing.[36]

The hallmark clinical features are choreiform movements and dementia. Onset is typically between the ages of 35 and 40 years, although a juvenile form may develop as early as 5 years of age. Although chorea is the most common movement disorder, athetosis and dystonia also occur. Movement abnormalities can involve the extremities, trunk, face, eyes, oropharynx, and respiratory muscles. The disease progresses for several years and mental depression makes suicide a frequent occurrence. Death usually results from malnutrition and aspiration pneumonitis. The duration of Huntington's disease averages 17 years from the time of diagnosis to death.

There is no specific therapy for Huntington's disease. Pharmacotherapy is directed at relief of mental depression and control of movement disorders. Drugs that reduce dopaminergic transmission such as phenothiazines, butyrophenones, and thioxanthines or drugs that deplete dopamine such as tetrabenzamine and reserpine reduce the severity of chorea. Selective serotonin reuptake inhibitors (SSRIs) such as fluoxitene, sertraline, and paroxitene are the primary drugs for treatment of depression.[37]

Management of Anesthesia

Many of the manifestations of Huntington's disease are typical of patients with neurodegenerative disorders. As the disease progresses, the pharyngeal muscles become dysfunctional and the risk of aspiration pneumonitis increases. Appropriate anti-aspiration maneuvers should be used.

If preoperative and postoperative sedation are necessary, the butyrophenones or phenothiazines are logical choices. Cases of neuroleptic malignant syndrome in patients with Huntington's disease are most likely secondary to the administration of neuroleptic drugs rather than intrinsic effects of Huntington's disease. Although there are no specific contraindications to the use of inhaled or intravenous anesthetics, recovery from propofol may be faster than from other intravenous hypnotics. Short-acting neuromuscular blocking drugs would be preferable to longer acting relaxants. Decreased plasma cholinesterase activity may prolong the relaxant effects of succinylcholine and mivacurium. Although reported experience with regional anesthesia is sparse, spinal anesthesia has been successfully administered.

As for any patient with a progressive neurologic disease, delayed emergence and an increased likelihood of respiratory complications must be anticipated in the immediate postoperative period.

Alzheimer's Disease

Alzheimer's disease is the major cause of dementia in the United States and the major reason that patients are admitted to nursing homes. The incidence of Alzheimer's disease is 1% in 60 year olds and 30% in 85 year olds. Although dementia is caused by more than 60 disorders, Alzheimer's disease is responsible for 50 to 60% of the cases. Dementia is characterized by intellectual and cognitive deterioration that impairs social function. Memory impairment and language deterioration occur early in the disease process. Motor and sensory abnormalities, gait disturbances, seizures, agitation, and psychosis are later features of the disease. Any systemic cause of dementia must be eliminated before the diagnosis of Alzheimer's is made. Laboratory testing for thyroid dysfunction, infection, and heavy metal exposure may be indicated. Computed tomography (CT), MRI, and positron emission tomography (PET) are helpful in differentiating Alzheimer's from other causes of dementia.

The deposition of beta-amyloid peptide appears to be central to the process of degeneration and neuronal death. The pathologic features of Alzheimer's such as neurofibrillary tangles and neuritic plaques are secondary to beta-amyloid deposition. Different genetic patterns may explain variations in clinical presentation and age of onset. To date, no effective antiamyloid therapies are available.

Treatment of Alzheimer's disease is directed in four areas: neuroprotection, cholinesterase inhibitors, psychopharmacologic agents to improve behavior, and health maintenance.[38] Neuroprotective therapies under investigation include vitamin E, selegiline, memantine, and anti-inflammatory agents. The administration of cholinesterase inhibitors is now considered standard of care treatment for patients with Alzheimer's disease. The three most commonly used cholinesterase inhibitors are donepezil, rivastigmine, and galantamine. Cholinesterase inhibitors improve the patient's ability to perform daily living activities and may improve cognition. Side effects of cholinesterase inhibitors include nausea, vomiting, bradycardia, syncope, and fatigue. Appropriate psychotropic drugs can be used to treat psychosis and depression. Treatment of the medical and nutritional problems of a neurodegenerative disease and the elderly patient are indicated to reduce morbidity and mortality.

Management of Anesthesia

Selection of anesthetic drugs and techniques for patients with Alzheimer's disease is guided by the patient's general physiologic condition, the degree of neurologic deterioration, and the potential for interaction between anesthetics and medications the patient is receiving. Because of dementia, these patients are likely to be disoriented and uncooperative preoperatively. Sedative preoperative drugs are rarely indicated as further mental confusion could result. Anesthetics known to result in rapid recovery, such as propofol, desflurane, and sevoflurane are advantageous because they permit a rapid return to the patient's preoperative state. If an anticholinergic is required, glycopyrrolate, which does not cross the blood-brain barrier, is preferable to atropine or scopolamine. An anticholinergic drug that crosses the blood-brain barrier could exacerbate the dementia. Patients receiving cholinesterase inhibitors may have a prolonged response to succinylcholine and mivacurium. The patient's preoperative drug list should be reviewed for the possibility of interactions with anesthetics.

Amyotrophic Lateral Sclerosis

Amyotrophic lateral sclerosis (ALS) is a degenerative disease of motor cells (anterior horn cells) throughout the central nervous system. Progression of the disease is relentless and death usually follows within 3 to 5 years of diagnosis. Ten percent of ALS patients, however, survive for 10 years. Upper and lower motor neurons are involved, although lower motor neurons are affected first. The cause of ALS is unknown, but proposed causes include glutamate excitotoxicity, free radical stress, impaired neural protein repair, viral or prion infections, heavy metal exposures, or an autoimmune response. Although the similarity between ALS and poliomyelitis is striking, there is no increase in the incidence of ALS in postpolio patients. Five to 10% of the cases of ALS are hereditary.[39]

The signs and symptoms of ALS reflect the upper and lower motor neuron dysfunction. Initial symptoms are weakness, atrophy, and skeletal muscle fasciculation, often beginning in the intrinsic muscles of the hand. Deep tendon reflexes are inappropriately brisk. As the disease progresses, the atrophy and weakness involve most skeletal muscles, including those of the tongue, pharynx, larynx, and chest. Dysarthria and dysphagia are a result of bulbar involvement. Pulmonary function tests demonstrate a decrease in vital capacity, maximal voluntary ventilation, and diminished expiratory muscle function. In rare instances, the initial presentation of ALS may be respiratory failure. Eventually, respiratory failure develops in all patients with ALS and ventilatory support is required. Although mechanical ventilation can prolong life, many patients with ALS do not opt for aggressive ventilatory management because of the futility of life-prolonging measures. Intellectual and cognitive function is preserved.[40] Patients with ALS have evidence of autonomic dysfunction as evidenced by an increased resting heart rate, orthostatic hypotension, and elevated levels of epinephrine and norepinephrine. There may be a decreased R-R interval variation on the ECG and a decreased heart rate response to atropine. The cause of death for patients with ALS is usually respiratory failure. Sudden death from circulatory collapse frequently occurs in ventilator-dependent patients with ALS.

Riluzole, an antiglutamate drug, is the only specific drug approved for the treatment of ALS. Although not curative, riluzole may modestly prolong survival and delay the need for tracheostomy. Side effects of riluzole include dizziness and hepatic dysfunction. Investigations of other drug therapies have been unproductive.[41] Creatine therapy has been shown to produce some benefit in a mouse model of ALS. Although similar efficacy has not yet been shown in humans, many ALS patients take creatine supplements. Palliative care may include ventilatory and nutritional support and medications for the relief of muscle cramps and fasiculations.

Management of Anesthesia

Neuromuscular transmission is markedly abnormal in patients with ALS and these patients can be very sensitive to nondepolarizing muscle relaxants. As with other patients with lower motor neuron disease, ALS patients should be considered vulnerable to hyperkalemia in response to succinylcholine. Bulbar involvement with dysfunction of pharyngeal muscles predisposes patients with ALS to pulmonary aspiration. The need for postoperative ventilatory support is highly likely for these patients. There is no evidence that a specific anesthetic drug or combination of drugs is best for patients with ALS. Subclinical autonomic dysfunction can produce very exaggerated decreases in cardiovascular function in response to anesthesia.[42]

Creutzfeldt-Jakob Disease

Creutzfeldt-Jakob disease (CJD) is one of three disorders that constitute the class of diseases known as the human spongiform encephalopathies. The other two diseases in this group are kuru and Gerstmann-Straussler syndrome. Pathologically these diseases are characterized by vacuolation of brain tissue and neuronal loss. Creutzfeldt-Jakob disease is caused by a prion. A prion is a small proteinaceous infectious agent that modifies nucleic acids. Most cases of CJD are sporadic although some are hereditary. Iatrogenic transmission of CJD has been linked to contaminated dural graft material, the use of contaminated surgical instruments, corneal transplants, and pooled human growth hormone. Although CJD was previously considered to be a rare form of dementia, the discovery of transmission of another prion disease (bovine spongiform encephalopathy, mad cow disease) from cows to humans in the mid 1990s catapulted CJD to media prominence. This disease is termed variant CJD (vCJD) and it differs clinically from classic CJD.[43] The typical clinical characteristics of classic CJD are subacute dementia, myoclonus, and EEG changes. The EEG pattern is relatively characteristic with diffuse, slow activity, and periodic complexes. Progressive loss of cognitive and neurologic function occurs. Patients with vCJD present at an earlier age with psychiatric features such as dysphoria, withdrawal, anxiety, and insomnia. Neurologic features develop 1 to 2 months after the psychiatric changes commence.[44] Presumably, transmission of vCJD is by the ingestion of contaminated animal products. Accurate epidemiologic studies are difficult because the incubation period is several years. Scrapie and chronic wasting disease (mule and elk) are other animal forms of spongiform encephalopathy. The risk of transmission of these diseases to humans is unknown.

Management of Anesthesia

Creutzfeldt-Jakob is a transmissible disease and appropriate precautions must be observed when administering anesthesia. High-risk patient tissues include brain, spinal cord, cerebrospinal fluid, and lymphoid tissue. Human to human transmission via blood transfusion has occurred. Single-use anesthesia supplies, including facemasks, breathing circuits, laryngoscopes, and tracheal tubes, should be employed.[45]

Patients with degenerative neurologic diseases are prone to aspirate gastric contents because they have impaired swallowing function and decreased activity of laryngeal reflexes. Appropriate anti-aspiration precautions are indicated during anesthesia. Because lower motor neuron dysfunction occurs in CJD patients, the use of succinylcholine should be avoided. The autonomic and peripheral nervous systems may be adversely affected, which may result in abnormal cardiovascular responses to anesthesia and vasoactive drugs.

ANEMIAS

Anemia is defined as an absolute or relative deficiency in the concentration of circulating functional red blood cells. Anemias can be classified as nutritional, hemolytic, and genetic (hemoglobinopathies, thalassemias) (Table 19-9).

Regardless of the cause of the anemia, compensatory physiologic mechanisms develop to offset the decreased oxygen carrying capacity of the blood. In a healthy person, symptoms do not develop until the hemoglobin level decreases below 7 g/dL. Symptoms are variable and depend on other concurrent disease processes. Physiologic compensation includes increased plasma volume, increased cardiac output, and increased levels of red blood cell 2,3-diphosphoglycerate (Table 19-10). Because elderly patients with chronic anemia have an increased plasma volume, transfusion of whole blood in these patients may result in congestive heart failure. Similarly, the myocardial depressant effects of anesthetics may be exaggerated for patients with increased cardiac output at rest as compensation for anemia.

Concern about the transmission of blood-borne infections has greatly influenced the perioperative use of blood products. Traditional hematocrit levels that have triggered the need for blood transfusion have been radically altered and there is no universally accepted hematocrit level that demands transfusion. The patient's physiologic status and coexisting diseases must be factored into a subjective decision.

TABLE 19-9

TYPES OF ANEMIA

Types of anemia
NUTRITIONAL
Iron deficiency
Vitamin B12 deficiency
Folic acid deficiency
Chronic illness
HEMOLYTIC
Spherocytosis
Glucose-6-phosphate dehydrogenase deficiency
Immune-mediated
Drug-induced ABO incompatibility
GENETIC
Hemoglobin S (sickle cell)
THALASSEMIAS
Thalassemia major (Cooley's anemia)
Thalassemia intermedia
Thalassemia minor

Nutritional Deficiency Anemias

The three primary causes of nutritional deficiency anemia are iron deficiency, vitamin B_{12} deficiency, and folic acid deficiency. Chronic illness, as well as poor dietary intake, can result in nutritional deficiency anemia.

Iron deficiency anemia produces the typical microcytic, hypochromic red blood cell. Iron deficiency anemia may be an absolute deficiency secondary to decreased oral intake or a relative deficiency caused by a rapid turnover of red

TABLE 19-10

COMPENSATORY MECHANISMS TO INCREASE OXYGEN DELIVERY WITH CHRONIC ANEMIA

Compensatory mechanisms
Increased cardiac output
Increased red blood cell 2,3-diphosphoglycerate
Increased P-50
Increased plasma volume
Decreased blood viscosity

blood cells (e.g., chronic blood loss, hemolysis). Measuring the hemoglobin and serum ferritin levels is a rapid and effective method for differentiating true iron deficiency anemia from other causes. Severe iron deficiency anemia can result in respiratory distress, congestive heart failure, thrombocytopenia, and neurologic abnormalities.

Megaloblastic anemia can be caused by vitamin B_{12} (cobalamin) deficiency, folate deficiency, or refractory bone marrow disease. Absorption of vitamin B_{12} by the gastrointestinal tract depends on production of intrinsic factor, a glycoprotein produced by gastric parietal cells. Atrophy of the gastric mucosa causes vitamin B_{12} deficiency and megaloblastic anemia. Chronic gastritis and gastric atrophy may be caused by autoantibodies to gastric parietal cells. In addition to megaloblastic anemia, vitamin B_{12} deficiency can interfere with myelination and produce nervous system dysfunction. In adults, this is manifested by a peripheral neuropathy secondary to degeneration of the lateral and posterior spinal cord columns. The neuropathy is evidenced by symmetric loss of proprioception and vibratory sensation, especially in the lower extremities. Administration of parenteral vitamin B_{12} reverses both the hematologic and neurologic changes in adults. Congenital vitamin B_{12} deficiency, however, produces severe neurologic changes that can only be partially reversed with therapy. The coexisting neuropathy of vitamin B_{12} deficiency must be considered when regional anesthesia or peripheral nerve blocks might be used. The clinical significance of the effects of nitrous oxide on vitamin B_{12} metabolism is controversial. Nitrous oxide inactivates the vitamin B_{12} component of methionine synthetase and prolonged exposure to nitrous oxide results in megaloblastic anemia and neurologic changes similar to those that occur with pernicious anemia. Relatively short exposures to nitrous oxide have also been reported to produce megaloblastic changes. Whether the duration of exposure to nitrous oxide obtained during the course of a normal anesthetic produces such changes in humans has not been established. The issue of nitrous oxide causing postoperative neurologic dysfunction is very controversial and case reports of neuropathy linked to intraoperative nitrous oxide exposure have increased. Whether these reports influence the future use of nitrous oxide is not clear.

Folic acid deficiency also produces megaloblastic anemia. Although peripheral neuropathy may occur, it is not as common as with vitamin B_{12} deficiency. The administration of folic acid during early pregnancy markedly reduces the risk of neural tube defects in infants. Causes of folic acid deficiency include alcoholism, pregnancy, and malabsorption syndromes. Methotrexate, phenytoin, and ethanol are among the drugs known to interfere with folic acid absorption.

Hemolytic Anemias

The normal life span of an erythrocyte is 120 days. Abnormalities in the erythrocyte may result in the premature destruction of the cell (hemolysis). Causes of hemolytic anemia include structural erythrocyte abnormalities, enzyme deficiencies, and immune hemolytic anemias.

Hereditary Spherocytosis

Spherocytosis, elliptocytosis, pyropoikilocytosis, and stomatocytosis are the four types of hereditary red cell membrane defects resulting in abnormally shaped red blood cells.

Hereditary spherocytosis is the most common of the red blood cell membrane defects producing hemolysis. Spherocytosis is a disorder of the proteins (spectrin) of the red blood cell cytoskeleton in which the red blood cell is more rounded, more fragile, and more susceptible to hemolysis than the normal, biconcave red blood cell. As a result of this increased fragility, the spleen destroys the abnormal red blood cells and a chronic anemia ensues. Cholelithiasis from chronic hemolysis and elevation of the serum bilirubin occur frequently in patients with hereditary spherocytosis. Patients with hereditary spherocytosis may have hemolytic crises accompanied by anemia, vomiting, and abdominal pain. These crises may be triggered by infection or folic acid deficiency.

Hereditary spherocytosis is treated by splenectomy, which is usually delayed until the patient is 6 years of age or older. Splenectomy before that age is associated with a high incidence of bacterial infections, especially those secondary to pneumococcus. Before splenectomy, most patients require a folic acid supplement owing to excessive utilization of folic acid for red blood cell production. Transfusion is rarely necessary because adequate compensatory mechanisms for chronic anemia have developed in these patients.

Glucose-6-Phosphate Dehydrogenase Deficiency

Glucose-6-phosphate dehydrogenase (G6PD) deficiency is the most common enzymopathy in humans and afflicts 400 million people worldwide. G6PD deficiency may confer malarial resistance and the distribution of this variant parallels the geographic distribution of malaria. African Americans, Africans, Asians, and Mediterranean populations are susceptible to the abnormality. In patients with G6PD deficiency, G6PD activity decreases by 50% during the 120 day life span of the red blood cell. G6PD initiates the hexose monophosphate shunt. This shunt produces nicotinamide-adenine dinucleotide phosphate (NADPH). Without NADPH, the red blood cell is susceptible to damage by oxidation. A deficiency of G6PD results in decreased levels of glutathione when the red blood cell is exposed to oxidants. This increases the rigidity of the red blood cell membrane and accelerates clearance of the cell from the circulation. In severe forms of G6PD deficiency, oxidation produces denaturation of globin chains and causes intravascular hemolysis. Glutathione synthetase is another enzyme of the hexose monophosphate shunt, and deficiency of this enzyme may also produce anemia.

There are a number of drugs that accentuate the destruction of erythrocytes in patients with G6PD deficiency, including analgesics, antibiotics, sulfonamides, and antimalarials (Table 19-11). There is considerable variability in the hemolytic response to drugs; many drugs (e.g., aspirin) cause hemolysis only in very high doses. Patients with G6PD deficiency are unable to reduce the methemoglobin produced by sodium nitrate; therefore sodium nitroprusside and prilocaine should not be administered. Characteristically, the crisis begins 2 to 5 days

TABLE 19-11

DRUGS THAT PRODUCE HEMOLYSIS IN PATIENTS WITH GLUCOSE-6-PHOSPHATE DEHYDROGENASE DEFICIENCY

Phenacetin	Nalidixic acid
Aspirin (high doses)	Isoniazid
Penicillin	Primaquine
Streptomycin	Quinine
Chloramphenical	Quinidine
Sulfacetamide	Doxorubicin
Sulfanilimide	Methylene blue
Sulfapyridine	Nitrofurantoin

after drug administration. The hemolytic episode is usually self-limited because only the older red blood cells are affected. Bacterial infections can also trigger hemolytic episodes. Presumably, the oxidants produced by active white blood cells may hemolyze susceptible red blood cells. Anesthetic drugs have not been implicated as hemolytic agents; however, early postoperative evidence of hemolysis might indicate a G6PD deficiency.

Pyruvate Kinase Deficiency

Pyruvate kinase is a glycolytic enzyme of the Embden-Meyerhof pathway. This pathway converts glucose to lactate and is the primary pathway for adenosine triphosphate synthesis in the red blood cell. A deficiency of pyruvate kinase produces a potassium leak from red blood cells, increasing their rigidity and accelerating destruction in the spleen. Pyruvate kinase deficiency is responsible for 95% of the deficiency syndromes in the Embden-Meyerhof pathway, whereas deficiency of glucose phosphate isomerase accounts for 4%.

Clinically, these patients exhibit anemia, premature cholelithiasis, and splenomegaly. The degree of anemia varies from a very mild anemia to a severe, transfusion dependent anemia. The clinical features resemble those for patients with spherocytosis. There are no special considerations for anesthesia other than those for any patient with chronic anemia.

Immune Hemolytic Anemia

The immune hemolytic anemias are characterized by immunologic alterations in the red blood cell membrane and are caused by drugs, disease, or erythrocyte sensitization. There are three types of immune hemolytic anemia: autoimmune hemolysis, drug-induced immune hemolysis, and alloimmune hemolysis (erythrocyte sensitization).[46] Autoimmune hemolytic anemia includes warm and cold antibody hemolytic anemia. Cold autoimmune hemolytic anemia is of special concern to the anesthesiologist because of the likelihood that the cold operating room environment and hypothermia during cardiopulmonary bypass may initiate a hemolytic crisis. Cold hemagglutinin disease is caused by IgM autoantibodies that react with the I antigen of red blood cells. Maintaining a warm environment is essential for prevention of hemolysis. Plasmapheresis to reduce the titer of cold antibody is recommended before hypothermic procedures such as cardiopulmonary bypass. Collagen vascular diseases, neoplasia, and infections produce immune hemolytic anemias by a variety of mechanisms including warm and cold antibody-mediated hemolysis.

There are three types of drug-induced immune hemolysis: autoantibody type, hapten-induced type, and immune complex type. Hemolysis induced by alpha-methyldopa is of the autoimmune type mediated by an IgG antibody that does not fix complement. The hapten-induced type is characteristic of the response to penicillin and other antibiotics. The immune complex type of reaction can occur after the administration of quinidine, quinine, sulfonamides, isoniazid, phenacetin, acetaminophen, cephalosporins, tetracycline, hydralazine, and hydrochlorothiazide.

The classic example of alloimmune hemolysis (erythrocyte sensitization) is hemolytic disease of the newborn produced by Rh sensitization. An Rh-negative mother with Rh antibodies produces hemolysis in an Rh-positive fetus. Differences in fetal and maternal ABO groups may also cause hemolysis. This is, however, unusual because A and B antibodies are of the IgM class and do not readily cross the placenta.

Hemoglobinopathies

There are more than 300 different hemoglobinopthies described in the literature. Most are quite rare and may never be encountered by an anesthesiologist during his or her career. Sickle cell diseases are the most common hemoglobinopathies in the United States. An estimated 8 to 10% of African Americans have the sickle cell trait, and 1 in 400 has sickle cell anemia.

Sickle Cell Disease

Normal hemoglobin is composed of four globin polypeptide units arranged in a tetramer. There are four globin proteins in normal human hemoglobin designated: alpha (α), beta (β), delta (δ), gamma (γ). In adult hemoglobin the tetramer $\alpha_2\beta_2$ predominates and is called hemoglobin A. Hemoglobin F (tetramer $\alpha_2\gamma_2$) predominates in fetal and neonatal life. In sickle cell disease an abnormal globin is produced and is designated β^s and the tetramer $\alpha_2\beta_2{}^s$ is hemoglobin S. The β^s globin is abnormal in that valine is substituted for glutamic acid in the sixth amino acid position. This abnormality causes the hemoglobin to aggregate and form a polymer when exposed to low concentrations of oxygen. The formation of polymeric hemoglobin strands within the erythrocyte causes the red blood cell to sickle. As the sickle prone cell passes through the microcirculation, the cell is exposed to progressively lower oxygen tensions. The deformed sickle cells can occlude small vessels causing reduced blood flow and stasis. The sickled erythrocyte may return to a normal shape when reexposed to higher oxygen tensions. Permanent alterations to the cell membrane do occur and worsen with each cycle of sickling, resulting in early removal of the red blood cell from the circulation. Erythrocyte life span is only 12 to 17 days in sickle cell disease compared to the normal 120 days. The altered red blood cell membrane increases the adhesion of sickle cells to the vascular endothelium. This adhesion activates coagulation and releases inflammatory mediators. Hemolysis of altered erythrocytes with release of free hemoglobin causes oxidant injury to tissues and decreases nitric oxide levels. The basis of multiple organ system damage in sickle cell disease is vascular occlusion, tissue ischemia, infarction, hypercoagulability, thrombosis, and inflammation.

The definitive diagnosis of sickle cell disease is made with hemoglobin electrophoresis. This test not only detects hemoglobin S but also reveals any other types of hemoglobin present.

Clinical Manifestations. The clinical manifestations of sickle cell disease can develop in any organ system (Table 19-12). The most frequent manifestation is pain. A "painful episode" is thought to be because of tissue ischemia and usually affects the back, chest, extremities, and abdomen. The severity of painful events may range from annoying to severe and disabling. Parenteral narcotic analgesics are the mainstay of therapy but may be supplemented with nonsteroidal anti-inflammatory drugs (NSAIDs). Supplemental oxygen and intravenous fluids are administered to maximize tissue oxygenation. The term "crisis" is used to describe painful episodes that coincide with life-threatening events. Crises that may be seen in sickle cell disease are: splenic sequestration, aplastic anemia, right upper quadrant syndrome, and acute chest syndrome. The concentration of hemoglobin F may be predictive of clinical manifestations as increased levels of hemoglobin F decrease the likelihood of clinical events.

Splenic sequestration occurs when there is a dramatic acceleration of erythrocyte trapping in an enlarged spleen. The removal of large numbers of erythrocytes causes the hematocrit to fall precipitously. Hypovolemia and shock may develop. Left upper quadrant pain is a prominent symptom. Infusion of fluids and red blood cells must be performed to restore the intravascular volume and hematocrit. Splenectomy is often performed following the acute episode to prevent recurrence.

TABLE 19-12

CLINICAL MANIFESTATIONS OF SICKLE CELL DISEASE

■ HEMATOLOGIC	■ PULMONARY
Hemolytic anemia Aplastic anemia	Acute chest syndrome Pulmonary infarction Fibrosis Asthma Pulmonary hypertension Thromboembolism Pneumonia
■ SPLEEN	**■ GENITOURINARY**
Infarction Hyposplenism Splenic sequestration	Priapism Infection
■ CENTRAL NERVOUS SYSTEM	**■ HEPATOBILIARY**
Stroke Hemorrhage Aneurysm Meningitis	Right upper quadrant syndrome Hepatitis Cirrhosis Cholelithiasis Cholestasis Jaundice
■ MUSCULOSKELETAL	**■ IMMUNE SYSTEM**
Painful episodes Bone marrow hyperplasia Avascular necrosis (hip and shoulder) Osteomyelitis Bone infarcts	Immunosuppression
■ CARDIAC	**■ PSYCHOSOCIAL**
Cardiomegaly	Depression Anxiety Substance abuse
■ RENAL	
Papillary necrosis Glomerular sclerosis Renal failure	

An *aplastic crisis* occurs when there is a failure of reticulocyte formation. The high turnover rate of erythrocytes in sickle cell disease results in a rapid worsening of anemia when erythrocyte formation is interrupted. Symptoms of an aplastic crisis are nonspecific and are related to severe anemia. Transfusion is performed to maintain an adequate hematocrit until reticulocyte formation returns to normal.

Right upper quadrant syndrome is heralded by pain in the right upper quadrant. Fever, jaundice, and liver failure follow. The right upper quadrant pain may represent hepatic ischemia, cholecystitis, cholangitis, or ischemia of other visceral organs. Transfusion will reduce the concentration of hemoglobin S and optimize the hematocrit. Intravenous fluids, analgesics, antibiotics, and supplemental oxygen are usually required.

Acute chest syndrome (ACS) is characterized by chest pain, dyspnea, fever, and acute pulmonary hypertension. ACS may be fatal. Transfusion or exchange transfusion is performed to maintain the hematocrit at 30%. Supplemental oxygen, antibiotics, and inhaled bronchodilators are administered as required.

Sickle cell disease also produces chronic cardiac, pulmonary,
6 and renal dysfunction. Cor pulmonale may result from chronic hypoxemia, pulmonary fibrosis, and pulmonary hypertension. Cardiac dysfunction is characterized by systolic and diastolic dysfunction. The renal medulla is vulnerable to infarction and there may be an inability to concentrate the urine. Other systemic effects of sickle cell disease include cholelithiasis (chronic hemolysis), cerebral infarction, and priapism.[47,48]

There are at least 40 variants of S hemoglobinopathy. Patients with SA hemoglobin (sickle cell trait) usually have a normal life expectancy and few complications. Hemoglobin levels are normal and sickling occurs only under extreme physiologic conditions. Although the risk of anesthesia is small, there have been some reports of death in the perioperative period in patients with sickle cell trait. Hemoglobin C also results from a mutation of the β globin at the 6th amino acid position. Lysine is substituted for glutamic acid. Some patients have both the sickle cell gene and the hemoglobin C gene (hemoglobin SC). Hemoglobin S may also be combined with thalassemia trait resulting in hemoglobin S-thalassemia trait. The severity of sickle cell disease from worst to least is: SS > S-thalassemia > SC > CC > SA (Table 19-13).

Treatment. Although the exact molecular defect of S hemoglobin has been known for over 50 years, there is no specific corrective therapy. Supportive therapy has improved, increasing survival, so that many patients with SS disease live more than 50 years. In some cases bone marrow transplantation may be curative, especially when performed in early childhood. Because of the risks of bone marrow transplantation, this therapy is reserved for very severe cases.[49] An unaffected sibling is usually required for donor matching.

Preventive treatment is begun as soon as the diagnosis is made. Patients should be referred to centers that provide a multidisciplinary approach for routine and urgent care. Daily oral penicillin is begun in infancy as prophylaxis against pneumococcal sepsis. Patients receiving frequent transfusions should be monitored for iron overload. Liver biopsy is the most common method of monitoring the effects of excessive iron. If iron overload occurs, chelation therapy must be instituted to prevent cardiomyopathy and cirrhosis. Hydroxyurea is often administered to increase production of hemoglobin F and reduce the likelihood of sickling.

Management of Anesthesia. Surgery is frequently required for patients with sickle cell disease. Operations commonly performed on these patients include cholecystectomy, liver biopsy, splenectomy, tonsillectomy, hip replacement, and obstetric procedures. It is ideal for the anesthesiologist, hematologist, and

TABLE 19-13

COMMON HEMOGLOBIN S VARIANTS

	■ HEMOGLOBIN SS	■ HEMOGLOBIN SC	■ HEMOGLOBIN SA
Hemoglobin level (g/dL)	7–8	9–12	13–15
Life expectancy (years)	30	Slightly reduced	Normal
Propensity for sickling	++++	++	+
Clinical features	Vaso-occlusive crises Splenic infarction Hepatomegaly Skin ulceration	Vaso-occlusive crises Retinal thrombosis Femoral head necrosis	Few, under physiologic conditions

TABLE 19-14

SYMPTOM-BASED PREOPERATIVE EVALUATION IN SICKLE CELL DISEASE PATIENTS FOR MAJOR SURGERY

All patients
Hemoglobin and hematocrit

Hemoglobin > 9 gm/dL *or* hematocrit > 28% *or* exchange transfusion planned
Hemoglobin electrophoresis

Cardiac symptoms *or* History of acute chest syndrome *or* Dyspnea on exertion
Electrocardiogram
Echocardiogram
Chest radiograph

Renal Dysfunction
Serum electrolytes
BUN
Creatinine

Hepatic Dysfunction
Platelet count
PT/PTT, INR
Fibrinogen

Change in Neurologic Status
Cranial MRI

Transcranial Doppler

surgeon to interact closely when sickle cell patients require surgery. Prevention of conditions that favor sickling is the basis for recommendations regarding perioperative management. Adequate oxygenation, avoidance of excessive oxygen consumption, assurance of adequate oxygen-carrying capacity, and avoidance of vascular stasis are imperative. Normothermia should be achieved as this minimizes oxygen consumption. Hypothermia may cause peripheral vasoconstriction and vascular stasis; whereas hyperthermia accelerates hemoglobin S polymerization. A warm ambient temperature supplemented with forced air warming is desired. Vascular stasis is minimized with adequate hydration and anticipation of intraoperative volume loss. Use of the tourniquet should be reserved for those operations where its use is essential for the success of the surgery.

The hemoglobin and hematocrit should be measured preoperatively. Adequate oxygen carrying capacity is maintained by transfusion to keep the hematocrit at 30%. Exchange transfusion may be used to keep the hematocrit at 30% and reduce the concentration of hemoglobin S to 30 to 40%. Exchange transfusion is the preferred method for patient preparation for cardiopulmonary bypass (Table 19-14).

Drugs commonly used for anesthesia do not have any significant direct effects on the sickling process. The anesthetic technique may influence outcome if it produces hypoxemia, vascular stasis, and reduced cardiac output. Regional anesthesia has been successfully employed for surgery, labor and delivery, and pain management. Pain management of patients with sickle cell disease in the postoperative period can be quite challenging. A variety of techniques, including opioids (morphine), nonnarcotic analgesics, and regional anesthesia have been used.

Close monitoring of the sickle cell patient during the postoperative period for pulmonary complications and aggressive treatment with supplemental oxygen is necessary as hypoxemia may be the primary trigger of acute chest syndrome. Acute chest syndrome during the early postoperative period produces significant morbidity and mortality.[50,51]

Thalassemia

The thalassemias are a group of genetically transmitted (autosomal recessive) anemias caused by insufficient production of one of the globin polypeptide components of hemoglobin. Although there are four globin chains (α, β, γ, δ), α and β thalassemias are the most common. Thalassemia genes are most prevalent in the Mediterranean region, the Middle East, India, Southeast Asia, and malarial zones. The carrier incidence in these areas is 2.4 to 15%.

There are three prominent clinical features of thalassemia: anemia, hemolysis, and marked hyperplasia of the bone marrow. The anemia is microcytic and hypochromic and can be profound. In addition to anemia, there is unbalanced production of globin pairs. In β thalassemia, there is inadequate production of β globin, but normal production of α globin. The excess α globins are poorly soluble and precipitate to form inclusion bodies in erythroid precursor cells. The excess globins are highly reactive and cause free radical cellular injury. Many erythrocytes fail to mature and others are destroyed by the spleen and reticuloendothelial system. Splenomegaly, hepatomegaly, cholelithiasis, and jaundice are common. Anemia causes a vigorous secretion of erythropoietin that produces bone marrow hyperplasia. Bone marrow hyperplasia causes skeletal abnormalities such as retarded growth, fractures, and facial dysmorphism. Extramedullary marrow develops in the pleura, sinuses, epidural space, and pleural cavities. Spontaneous bleeding from extramedullary marrow is common and can cause hemothorax, epidural hematoma, and epistaxis.[52]

A wide variety of clinical phenotypes are manifest, from very mild anemia to very severe anemia. The anemia in thalassemia major (Cooley's anemia) is severe and often life threatening. β thalassemia minor produces a mild anemia of iron deficiency. β thalassemia intermedia is an intermediate form of thalassemia that usually does not require transfusion. α thalassemia produces a mild hemolytic anemia (Table 19-15).

Treatment of thalassemia is based on the severity of the anemia. Thalassemia major must be treated aggressively to reduce

TABLE 19-15

THALASSEMIC SYNDROMES

■ HEMOGLOBIN BART'S HYDROPS FETALIS (FATAL IN UTERO)

Thalassemia hemoglobin Bart's is a γ^4 globin tetramer that is produced because of complete lack of α globin production

Thalassemia Major
Homozygous
β^0-thalassemia
Severe β^+-thalassemia

Heterozygous
β^0-thalassemia
Severe β^+-thalassemia

Thalassemia Intermedia
Homozygous
Known as hemoglobin H disease. Hgb H is a β4 globin tetramer produced because of a relative lack of α globin

Heterozygous
Severe β^+-thalassemia
Mild β^+-thalassemia

Thalassemia Minor
Mild reductions in α and β globin production

Note: ^{0} indicates none of that type of globin is produced.
$^+$ indicates a subnormal amount of that globin is produced.

complications and prolong life. Bone marrow transplantation may cure thalassemia and can be undertaken after 2 years of age if the illness is likely to be severe. Thalassemia major patients who do not qualify for or fail bone marrow transplantation will require transfusion therapy. Three transfusion protocols are employed: palliative transfusion, hypertransfusion, and supertransfusion. Palliative transfusion is used to treat only severe complications of anemia. Extramedullary erythropoiesis is not suppressed by palliative transfusion. Palliative transfusion is generally practiced in areas where there is poor access to medical care. The goal of hypertransfusion is to maintain a hemoglobin level of 9 to 10 grams/dL. Transfusion is required every 3 to 4 weeks. Extramedullary erythropoiesis is substantially reduced. Supertransfusion is used to maintain a hemoglobin level greater that 12 grams/dL in an effort to suppress all erythropoiesis. Frequent blood transfusion predictably causes hemosiderosis. Chelation therapy with deferoxamine or deferiprone is required to reduce the likelihood of cardiac and hepatic iron toxicity (cirrhosis).

Management of Anesthesia. Anesthetic considerations depend on the severity of the anemia. Hemosiderosis is likely in patients receiving regular transfusion therapy. A preoperative echocardiogram may be indicated if there is any suggestion of cardiac dysfunction. Extramedullary erythropoiesis can produce hyperplasia of the facial bones and narrowing of the nasal passages and make direct laryngoscopy and tracheal intubation difficult. Epidural, spinal, and intrapleural anesthesia are relatively contraindicated as the presence of extramedullary bone marrow in these sites increases the likelihood of bleeding and hematoma formation. Massive bleeding into the epidural and pleural spaces can occur. Patients receiving palliative transfusion therapy are at greater risk for extramedullary erythropoiesis than those receiving hypertransfusion therapy.

COLLAGEN VASCULAR DISEASES

A number of diseases are classified as the collagen vascular diseases or connective tissue diseases (Table 19-16). The four most common disorders of this group are rheumatoid arthritis, systemic lupus erythematosus, scleroderma, and dermatomyositis/polymyositis. Although many such patients can be categorized as having discrete disease syndromes, many others with collagen vascular diseases are considered to have overlap syndromes (also termed mixed connective tissue diseases) with features of different collagen vascular diseases, and cannot be conveniently classified. The etiology of the collagen vascular diseases is unknown, although the immune system is clearly involved in the cascade of pathologic events that cause clinical manifestations of the diseases. Although all of these diseases have effects on joints, each has diffuse systemic effects as well. The alterations in joint function and systemic effects will both have significant impact on the management of anesthesia.

TABLE 19-16

COLLAGEN VASCULAR DISEASES

- Rheumatoid arthritis
- Lupus
  - Systemic lupus erythematosus
  - Drug-induced lupus
  - Discoid lupus
- Scleroderma
  - Progressive systemic sclerosis
  - CREST syndrome (calcinosis cutis, Raynaud's phenomenon, esophageal dysfunction, sclerodactyly, telangectasia)
  - Focal scleroderma
- Polymyositis/dermatomyositis
- Overlap syndromes

Rheumatoid Arthritis

Rheumatoid arthritis is a chronic inflammatory disease characterized by a symmetric polyarthropathy and significant systemic involvement. Although the etiology of rheumatoid arthritis is not known, the pathogenesis has been delineated. An as yet unknown antigen provokes a cellular immune response in which monocytes, macrophages, and fibroblasts release cytokines (TNF-tumor necrosis factor and interleukin-1). These cytokines initiate an inflammatory cascade that damages synovial and joint tissue. B lymphocyte dysregulation causes additional damage via complement fixation.[53] The presence of rheumatoid factor (IgM) in 75% of patients with rheumatoid arthritis supports the concept of rheumatoid arthritis as an autoimmune disease. The pathologic changes of rheumatoid arthritis begin with cellular hyperplasia of the synovium followed by invasion of the synovium by lymphocytes, plasma cells, and fibroblasts. Ultimately, the cartilage and articular surfaces are destroyed.

The hands and wrists are involved first, particularly the metacarpophalangeal and interphalangeal joints. In the lower extremity, the knee is involved most frequently. Compression of lower extremity peripheral nerves by the deformed knee can produce paresis and sensory loss over the lower leg. The upper cervical spine is affected in nearly 80% of patients with rheumatoid arthritis. Instability of the upper cervical spine can manifest as atlantoaxial instability, cranial settling, and subaxial instability. Plain radiography and CT of the cervical spine will demonstrate the bony changes of rheumatoid arthritis. MRI is better suited to the study of the bony and soft tissue changes on the spinal cord. The degree of cord compression, however, may not correlate with the patient's symptoms. Although a very rare event, spinal cord damage after laryngoscopy and tracheal intubation has been reported.[54] Intradural cord compression secondary to rheumatoid nodules or pannus formation can also occur. Rheumatoid arthritis commonly affects the joints of the larynx, resulting in limitation of vocal cord movement and generalized erythema and edema of the laryngeal mucosa that may progress to airway obstruction. Arthritic changes in the temporomandibular joints also occur. All of these abnormalities can complicate laryngoscopy and tracheal intubation.

Extra-articular and systemic manifestations of rheumatoid arthritis are diverse (Table 19-17). Pericarditis occurs in nearly one-third of patients with rheumatoid arthritis and can produce constrictive pericarditis or cardiac tamponade. Although cardiac tamponade develops in only a small proportion of patients with rheumatoid arthritis, rheumatoid arthritis is more likely to cause tamponade than systemic lupus erythematosus. Cardiovascular disease is a common cause of mortality in patients with rheumatoid arthritis and there is a high incidence of subclinical cardiac dysfunction.[55] Cardiovascular effects include myocarditis, coronary arteritis, pulmonary hypertension, diastolic dysfunction, dysrhythmias, and aortitis (aortic root dilation, aortic insufficiency). Pulmonary changes are common and include pleural effusions, pulmonary nodules, interstitial lung disease, obstructive lung disease, and restrictive lung disease. Several of the antirheumatic drugs can cause or accentuate pulmonary dysfunction. Renal failure is a common cause of death in patients with rheumatoid arthritis. Renal dysfunction may be secondary to vasculitis, amyloidosis, and anti-rheumatic drugs.

TABLE 19-17

EXTRA-ARTICULAR MANIFESTATIONS OF RHEUMATOID ARTHRITIS

Skin
- Raynaud's phenomenon
- Digital necrosis

Eyes
- Scleritis
- Corneal ulceration

Lung
- Pleural effusion
- Pulmonary fibrosis

Heart
- Pericarditis
- Cardiac tamponade
- Coronary arteritis
- Aortic insufficiency

Kidney
- Interstitial fibrosis
- Glomerulonephritis
- Amyloid deposition

Peripheral Nervous System
- Compression syndromes
- Mononeuritis

Central Nervous System
- Dural nodules
- Necrotizing vasculitis

Liver
- Hepatitis

Blood
- Anemia
- Leukopenia

Mild anemia is present in almost all patients with rheumatoid arthritis. The anemia may be secondary to a cytokine-induced decrease in erythropoiesis or may result from side effects of drug therapy. Felty's syndrome is the clinical complex of rheumatoid arthritis, leukopenia, and hepatosplenomegaly.

Neurologic complications of rheumatoid arthritis include peripheral nerve compression (carpal tunnel syndrome) and cervical nerve root compression. Mononeuritis multiplex is presumed to be caused by deposition of immune complexes in blood vessels supplying the affected nerves. Rheumatoid vasculitis may affect cerebral blood vessels, producing a cerebral necrotizing vasculitis.

There is no treatment that cures rheumatoid arthritis. The goals for therapy are induction of a remission, improved function, and maintenance of a remission. There are three groups of drugs used to treat rheumatoid arthritis: NSAIDs, corticosteroids, and disease-modifying antirheumatic drugs (DMARDs). Since NSAIDs do not affect the course of the disease, they are used in conjunction with DMARDs. Corticosteroids are potent anti-inflammatory and anti-immune drugs, but the side effects associated with long-term treatment limit their usefulness. DMARDS are now the first line of therapy for the early treatment of rheumatoid arthritis. Methotrexate has proven to be very effective and is often the initial drug of choice. Other synthetic DMARDs include leflunomide, cyclosporine, azathioprine, gold, sulfasalazine, minocycline, and hydroxychloroquine. Biologic DMARDs that inhibit TNF-alpha include infliximab, etanercept, and adalimumab. Anakinra inhibits interleukin-1. The primary side effect of the biologic DMARDs is an increased susceptibility to infection.[56] Most of the drugs used for the treatment of rheumatoid arthritis have significant side effects that may limit their use (Table 19-18). Surgical procedures such as synovectomy, tenolysis, and joint replacement are performed to relieve pain and restore joint function.

Management of Anesthesia

Because rheumatoid arthritis is a multisystem disease and the clinical manifestations are so diverse, individualized preoper-
7 ative evaluation is important in the identification of systemic effects.

TABLE 19-18

ADVERSE EFFECTS OF DRUGS USED TO TREAT COLLAGEN VASCULAR DISEASES

DRUG	EFFECT
Immunosuppressants	
Methotrexate	Hepatotoxicity, anemia, leukopenia
Azathioprine	Biliary stasis, leukopenia
Cyclosporine	Renal dysfunction, hypertension Hypomagnesemia
Cyclophosphamide	Leukopenia, hemorrhagic cystitis Inhibition of pseudocholinesterase
Leflunomide	Hepatoxicity, weight loss, hypertension
TNF Antagonists	
Etanercept	Bacterial infections, tuberculosis
Infliximab	Lymphoma, heart failure
Adalimumab	
Interleukin-1 Antagonists	
Anakinra	Infection, skin irritation
Corticosteroids	Hypertension, fluid retention Osteoporosis, infection
Aspirin	Platelet dysfunction, peptic ulcer Hepatic dysfunction, hypersensitivity
NSAIDs	Peptic ulcer, hypertension, hyperglycemia, leukopenia
COX-2 inhibitors	Renal dysfunction
Gold	Aplastic anemia, dermatitis, nephritis
Antimalarials	Myopathy, retinopathy
Penicillamine	Glomerulonephritis, myasthenia, aplastic anemia

The joint effects of rheumatoid arthritis, including arthritic changes in the temporomandibular joints, cricoarytenoid joints, and cervical spine, can render rigid, direct laryngoscopy and tracheal intubation very difficult. The mobility of these joints should be evaluated before surgery so that a plan for airway management can be formulated. If atlantoaxial instability exists, flexion of the neck may compress the spinal cord. Neck pain radiating to the occiput may be the first sign of cervical spine involvement. Patients with symptoms or evidence of cervical cord compression can be fitted with a cervical collar preoperatively to minimize the risk of overmanipulation of the neck during surgery. Many patients with rheumatoid arthritis, however, are asymptomatic with respect to cervical spine disease (Fig. 19-5). Preoperative imaging (radiography, CT, MRI) may be indicated if the degree of cervical involvement is unknown. Although there have been no documented reports of spinal cord damage in patients with rheumatoid arthritis undergoing tracheal intubation for elective surgery, alleged neurologic damage after laryngoscopy has been the source of liti-
8 gation against anesthesiologists. Any preoperative evidence of neurologic function should be documented before surgery. To minimize the risk of neurologic damage during tracheal intubation, awake, fiberoptic laryngoscopy may be the best means of performing tracheal intubation in patients with significant cervical spine involvement. Because patients with rheumatoid arthritis undergo repeated anesthetics, it is quite helpful if the technique of airway management is clearly documented in the patient's medical record. Progression of the rheumatoid

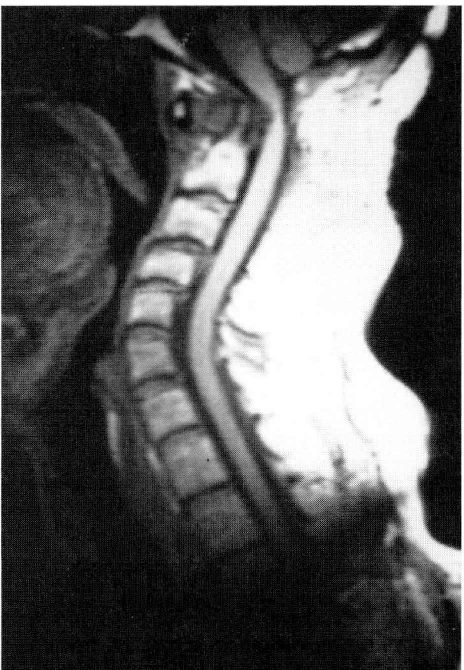

FIGURE 19-5. Magnetic resonance imaging of a cervical spine in a patient with rheumatoid arthritis. Although the patient had no neurologic symptoms, there is severe spinal stenosis in the upper cervical spine.

process may, however, alter joint function to the extent that neck motion may diminish with time and render a previously successful intubation technique useless. Criocoarytenoid arthritis produces erythema and edema of the vocal cords. Involvement of the cricoarytenoid joints reduces the size of the glottic inlet and necessitates the use of a smaller than predicted tracheal tube. Exaggerated postextubation edema and stridor may occur.

The degree of cardiopulmonary involvement by the rheumatoid process influences the selection of the type of anesthesia. Functional evaluation of the heart and lungs is necessary if the clinical history suggests dysfunction. It may be difficult to determine if the dysfunction is secondary to rheumatoid arthritis or other common causes of cardiopulmonary disease such as arteriosclerosis or smoking. The need for postoperative ventilatory support should be anticipated if severe pulmonary disease is present.

Medications that the patient is receiving influence the management of anesthesia. Corticosteroid supplementation may be necessary during the perioperative period. Aspirin and other anti-inflammatory drugs interfere with platelet function and clotting may be abnormal. Many rheumatoid medications suppress red blood cell formation and anemia is common. Drug induced hepatic and renal dysfunction may be present.

Restriction of joint mobility necessitates careful positioning of the patient during the operation. The extremities should be positioned to minimize the risk of neurovascular compression and further joint injury. Preoperative evaluation of joint motion will help determine how the extremities should be positioned.

Rheumatoid arthritis is a multisystem disease. Potential joint disabilities have been well documented in the medical literature and are often obvious. More significant and less evident are the effects on the spinal cord, heart, lungs, kidneys, and liver. The type and severity of systemic dysfunction must be considered when planning an anesthetic for patients with rheumatoid arthritis.[57,58]

Systemic Lupus Erythematosus

Systemic lupus erythematosus (SLE) is an autoimmune disease with diverse clinical and immunologic manifestations. The etiology of SLE is unknown, but appears to be a complex interaction between genetic susceptibility and hormonal and environmental factors. Patients with SLE produce autoantibodies primarily to DNA, but also RNA polymerase, cardiolipin, and ribosomal phosphoproteins. Some of the clinical manifestations of SLE may be the result of the production of an autoantibody highly specific for a single protein within an organ.[59]

The clinical manifestations of SLE are diverse. The most common presenting features are polyarthritis and dermatitis. The arthritis is oligoarticular and migratory. Any joint may be involved including the cervical spine. The classic malar rash is present in only one-third of SLE patients. Renal disease is a common cause of morbidity and mortality in patients with SLE. Proteinuria, hypertension, and decreased creatinine clearance are the usual manifestations of SLE nephritis. Of patients with SLE, 10 to 20% develop end-stage renal disease and require dialysis or transplantation. Central nervous system involvement occurs in 50% of patients with SLE and is a result of vasculopathy. CNS manifestations include seizures, stroke, dementia, psychosis, myelitis, and peripheral neuropathy. The cranial MRI may demonstrate vascular lesions, but is not adequate for patients with diffuse cerebral disease.[60]

SLE produces a diffuse serositis that manifests as pleuritis and pericarditis. Although 60% of SLE patients have a pericardial effusion, cardiac tamponade is uncommon. In rare cases, cardiac tamponade may be the presenting sign of SLE. Myocarditis, cardiac conduction abnormalities, ventricular dysfunction, and coronary arteritis can occur in patients with SLE.[61] A noninfectious endocarditis (Libman-Sacks endocarditis) often affects the mitral valve and can produce mitral insufficiency. Effective treatment of SLE has improved survival, but has increased the likelihood of ischemic heart disease. Pulmonary effects of SLE include pleural effusion, pneumonitis, pulmonary hypertension, and alveolar hemorrhage. There is a high incidence of pulmonary hypertension in SLE patients who have Raynaud's phenomenon. Patients with SLE are susceptible to infection that may present as pneumonia or adult respiratory distress syndrome. Pulmonary function studies typically demonstrate a restrictive lung disease pattern and a decreased diffusing capacity. Patients with SLE may have cricoarytenoid arthritis that can manifest as hoarseness, stridor, or airway obstruction.

Nearly one-third of patients with SLE have detectable antiphospholipid antibodies and may have thromboembolic complications. Lupoid hepatitis typically occurs in young women with SLE. Other potentially serious manifestations of SLE include peritonitis, pancreatitis, bowel ischemia, and protein-losing enteropathy.

There is no specific etiologic therapy for SLE. Despite the diverse effects of SLE and the lack of specific therapy, current regimens have improved survival. NSAIDs are used for mild arthritis. Antimalarials (hydroxychloroquine) control arthritis and exert antithrombotic effects. Corticosteroids are effective for moderate and severe SLE, but toxicity limits the dose. Immunosuppressants such as methotrexate, azathioprine, cyclophosphamide, and mycophenolate mofetil are effective and permit lower dosages of corticosteroids. The potential for side effects from any of the drugs used to treat SLE is significant and can result in morbidity.[62]

Drug-induced lupus may be caused by procainamide, quinidine, hydralazine, methyldopa, enalapril, captopril, clonidine, isoniazid, or minocycline. Drug-induced lupus may be caused by reactive drug metabolites and reactive T cells. The clinical manifestations of drug-induced lupus are generally mild and include arthralgia, fever, anemia, and leukopenia. These effects typically resolve within 4 weeks of discontinuation of the drug.

Management of Anesthesia

Careful preoperative evaluation of the patient with SLE is necessary because of the diverse systemic effects of the disease. Preoperative chest radiography, echocardiography, or pulmonary function testing may be necessary if the clinical history suggests dysfunction. Anesthesia management is influenced not only by the degree of organ dysfunction, but also by the drugs used to treat SLE. Although there are no specific contraindications to a particular type of anesthetic, myocardial dysfunction will certainly influence the choice of anesthetic and the type of intraoperative monitors. Because renal dysfunction is so common, renal function should be quantified preoperatively if there is any suggestion of a recent change in renal function. Although minor abnormalities in hepatic function are present in many patients with SLE, these changes are not usually significant. Patients with SLE are at increased risk for postoperative infections.

Arthritic involvement of the cervical spine is unusual in patients with SLE and tracheal intubation is not generally difficult. The potential for laryngeal involvement and upper airway obstruction does, however, require clinical evaluation of laryngeal function. Should postextubation laryngeal edema or stridor occur, intravenous administration of corticosteroids is effective for alleviation of symptoms.

Drugs administered to the patient for treatment of SLE may also influence the management of anesthesia. Patients receiving corticosteroids may require intraoperative administration of corticosteroids. Cyclophosphamide inhibits plasma cholinesterase and may prolong the response to succinylcholine and mivacurium.

Scleroderma

Scleroderma (systemic sclerosis) is characterized by excessive deposition of collagen and fibrosis in the skin and internal organs. The etiology of scleroderma is unknown. Infectious or environmental trigger agents have been proposed. Alterations in the function of fibroblasts, endothelial cells, and T and B lymphocytes result in exaggerated deposition of collagen, inflammation, obliteration of small arteries and arterioles, and ultimately fibrosis and atrophy of organs. Endothelial cell injury may be the earliest manifestation of scleroderma. The endothelial cells appear to be deficient in intrinsic vasodilators while having increased levels of the potent vasoconstrictor endothelin-1. Increased activity of connective tissue growth factor (CTGF) and transforming growth factor-beta (TGF-β) may be responsible for the deposition of large amounts of collagen.[63]

The manifestations of scleroderma are most evident in the skin, which becomes thickened and swollen. Eventually, the skin becomes atrophic and small arteries are obliterated. The skin becomes fibrotic and taut and produces severe restriction of joint mobility. Raynaud's phenomenon is present in 85% of patients with scleroderma and is often the presenting symptom.

The same pathologic process that affects the vascular system in the skin affects small blood vessels in other organs as well. Lung involvement occurs in 80% of patients with scleroderma and is characterized by interstitial fibrosis, pulmonary hypertension, and an impaired diffusing capacity. These changes in conjunction with the effects of chronic aspiration pneumonitis produce a restrictive lung disease. The onset of pulmonary hypertension is an ominous prognostic sign.[64] Myocardial fibrosis occurs in 70 to 80% of patients with scleroderma, although only 25% have clinical symptoms. Echocardiography may reveal a decreased ejection fraction and impaired left ventricular filling. Degeneration of cardiac conducting tissue may cause conduction defects and cardiac dysrhythmias. Pericarditis with effusion is very common.

Renal dysfunction is relatively common in patients with scleroderma. This dysfunction is secondary to pathologic changes in the renal vasculature similar to the changes in the digital arteries that produce Raynaud's phenomenon. Renal dysfunction can be so severe that a scleroderma renal crisis develops with hypertension, retinopathy, and a rapid deterioration in renal function.

Gastrointestinal motility is decreased and is very pronounced in the esophagus. The frequent episodes of gastroesophageal reflux and aspiration pneumonitis exacerbate pulmonary dysfunction. Involvement of the colon and small
9 intestine may result in pseudoobstruction.

Currently, the therapy for scleroderma is limited to the treatment of specific organ dysfunction, immunosuppressants (corticosteroids, methotrexate, cyclophosphamide, antithymocyte globulin), and decreasing collagen production (penicillamine). Vasodilators such as calcium channel blockers, ACE inhibitors, and prostacyclin analogs are frequently used for the treatment of cardiac dysfunction, pulmonary hypertension, and Raynaud's phenomenon.[65]

Management of Anesthesia

Scleroderma, like other collagen vascular diseases, is a multiorgan disease with many systemic manifestations. The altered organ systems must be thoroughly evaluated so that a logical plan for anesthesia can be selected. There are no specific contraindications to the use of any type of anesthesia, although the selection must be guided by the degree of organ dysfunction.

Tracheal intubation can be quite difficult. Fibrotic and taut facial skin can markedly hinder active and passive mobility of the temporomandibular joints. Awake fiberoptic-assisted laryngoscopy and tracheal intubation may be required; tracheostomy may be necessary in severely affected patients. Orotracheal intubation is preferred as the fragility of the nasal mucosa increases the risk of severe nasal hemorrhage from nasotracheal intubation.

The patient with scleroderma is at risk for aspiration pneumonitis during the induction of anesthesia owing to the high incidence of esophageal dysmotility and gastroesophageal reflux. Appropriate measures to minimize the risk of acid aspiration, such as the use of histamine-2 blockers and oral antacids, may be indicated.

Chronic arterial hypoxemia is often present because of restriction of lung expansion and impaired oxygen diffusion. Controlled ventilation with an increased oxygen concentration is usually necessary. Compromised myocardial function and decreased coronary vascular reserve often necessitate the use of invasive cardiovascular monitoring because the response to inhaled anesthetics may be exaggerated. Transesophageal echocardiography can provide valuable information about cardiac function, although passage of the probe may be difficult because of esophageal stricture. Venous access can be difficult and a venous cutdown or central venous catheterization may be required. Muscle involvement may increase the sensitivity to muscle relaxants and short-acting neuromuscular blockers should be used.

Regional anesthesia may be administered to patients with scleroderma, although the response to local anesthetics may be prolonged. The anesthesiologist is often consulted as to the efficacy of sympathetic blockade for the treatment of vasospasm secondary to Raynaud's phenomenon. Stellate ganglion blockade, however, may produce deleterious effects on contralateral blood flow in patients with scleroderma. Intractable ischemic limb pain may necessitate long-term pain management.

Polymyositis/Dermatomyositis

Three diseases comprise the inflammatory myopathies: polymyositis, dermatomyositis, and inclusion-body myositis. Clinical features common to these three diseases are severe muscle weakness, and noninfectious muscle inflammation. The etiology of these diseases is unknown; however, many of the processes that cause the inflammation have been delineated. Dermatomyositis is the result of an antibody induced complement activation that lyses muscle capillaries and causes muscle necrosis. Muscle fiber necrosis in polymyositis and inclusion-body myositis is caused by cytotoxic T cells.[66]

Common presenting symptoms of polymyositis are muscle pain, tenderness, and proximal muscle weakness. Patients with dermatomyosisits have skin manifestations that may precede the muscle weakness. The skin rash of dermatomyositis is characterized by a purplish discoloration of the eyelids (heliotrope rash), periorbital edema, erythematous lesions on the knuckles and a sun-sensitive rash on the face, neck, and chest. Inclusion-body myositis typically presents with weakness of the quadriceps and ankle dorsiflexors in men over 50 years of age. Although the pathogenic processes of these diseases are different, the effects on the heart and lungs are similar. Of patients with polymyositis and dermatomyositis, 50% have evidence of pulmonary disease. Pulmonary manifestations include interstitial lung disease, bronchopneumonia, and alveolitis. Aspiration is one of the most common complications of polymyositis. Intrinsic lung disease and thoracic muscle weakness produce a restrictive lung disease and decreased diffusing capacity. Myocardial fibrosis can result in congestive heart failure and cardiac dysrhythmias.

The most effective treatment for the inflammatory myopathies are corticosteroids (prednisone). Patients that do not respond to corticosteroids are treated with immunosuppressants such as azathioprine, methotrexate, cyclophosphamide, cyclosporine, and mycophenolate mofetil. Intravenous immunoglobulin and total body lymphocyte irradiation have been recommended for patients resistant to other forms of therapy.[67]

Management of Anesthesia

Mobility of the temporomandibular joints and cervical spine is usually adequate in patients with polymyositis. Some patients, however, have restricted mobility that can make direct laryngoscopy difficult. Adequate mouth and neck mobility must be ascertained before induction of anesthesia. Awake flexible fiberoptic laryngoscopy and tracheal intubation may be required for those patients with restricted neck mobility and inadequate mouth opening.

Dysphagia and gastroesophageal reflux are very common and there is an increased likelihood of aspiration pneumonitis. Appropriate precautions to minimize the risk of aspiration of gastric contents should be taken during the perioperative period. Gastrointestinal perforations that necessitate surgical intervention are relatively common in patients with polymyositis.

Although the typical electromyographic changes of polymyositis suggest the potential for hyperkalemia after succinylcholine, succinylcholine has been administered to patients with polymyositis without complication.[68] Prolonged neuromuscular blockade may occur after the administration of nondepolarizing muscle relaxants. This prolonged response may be secondary to the myopathy or an interaction between the muscle relaxant and immunosuppressants. The reported experience with anesthesia for patients with inflammatory myopathies is very limited and generalizations from a few case reports must be interpreted with caution. It should be anticipated that considerable variation in response to muscle relaxants will occur. It would seem to be prudent to avoid the administration of succinylcholine and to use short-acting nondepolarizing muscle relaxants such as mivacurium, cisatracurium, and rocuronium.

The degree of cardiopulmonary dysfunction influences the choice of anesthesia and selection of intraoperative monitors. Further preoperative evaluation of cardiopulmonary function may be required if the clinical history suggests deterioration in cardiac or pulmonary function. Because of the preoperative muscle weakness, postoperative ventilatory support may be necessary.

SKIN DISORDERS

Most primary diseases of the skin are localized and cause few systemic effects or complications during the administration of anesthesia. Two blistering skin disorders, however, can result in complications during anesthesia: epidermolysis bullosa and pemphigus.

Epidermolysis Bullosa

Epidermolysis is a rare skin disorder that can be inherited or acquired. Patients with heritable forms have abnormalities that cause defects in the anchoring systems of skin layers. The acquired forms are autoimmune disorders in which autoantibodies are produced that destroy the basement membrane of the skin and mucosa. The end result is the loss or absence of normal intercellular bridges and separation of skin layers (Fig. 19-6). The separation of the skin layers results in intradermal fluid accumulation and bullae formation. Even minor skin trauma produces skin blisters. Lateral shearing forces applied to the skin are especially damaging. Pressure applied perpendicular to the skin is not as hazardous. Although there are 25 subtypes of epidermolysis bullosa, these disorders can be categorized into three groups depending on where the actual skin separation occurs: epidermolytic (epidermolysis simplex), junctional, and dermolytic (epidermolysis bullosa dystrophica). Although serious complications from skin and mucosal loss can occur with any form of epidermolysis, the simplex form is generally benign. Patients with the junctional form rarely survive beyond early childhood. Laryngeal involvement is unusual, but is most likely to occur with the junctional type.

Epidermolysis dystrophica is caused by a defect in type VII collagen. This form produces severe scarring of the fingers and toes with pseudosyndactyly formation and ankylosis of the interphalangeal joints and resorption of the metacarpals and metatarsals (Fig. 19-7). Malignant degeneration of the skin is common. Involvement of the esophageal mucosa is present in most patients, resulting in dysphagia and esophageal strictures that contribute to poor nutrition.[69] Secondary infection of bullae with staphylococcus aureus or beta hemolytic streptococcus is frequent. Glomerulonephritis may be secondary to streptococcal infection. Hypoalbuminemia, secondary to nephritis, protein loss into bullae, and poor nutrition, is usual.
10 Other consequences of chronic infection and malnutrition are anemia and cardiomyopathy. Mitral valve prolapse may occur. Hypoplasia of tooth enamel results in carious degeneration of the teeth and the need for extensive dental restorations. Diseases associated with epidermolysis bullosa include porphyria

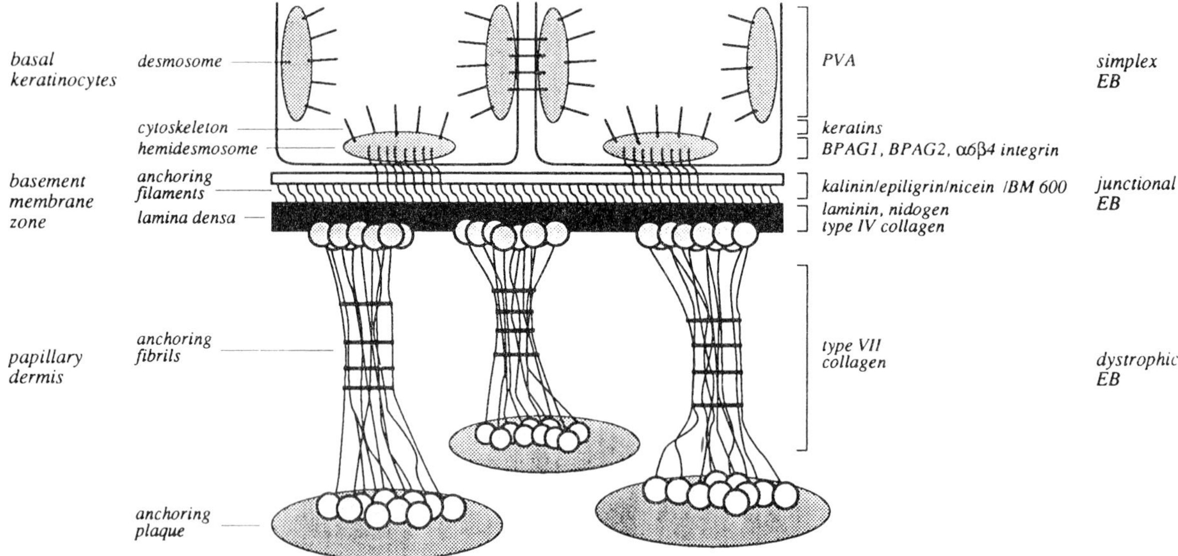

FIGURE 19-6. The ultrastructure for the zones of the skin. The diagram demonstrates where skin separation occurs in the different types of epidermolysis bullosa. (Reproduced with permission from Uitto J, Christiano AM: Molecular genetics of the cutaneous basement membrane zone. J Clin Invest 90;687, 1992; copyright of the American Society for Clinical Investigation.)

cutanea tarda, amyloidosis, multiple myeloma, diabetes mellitus, and hypercoagulation. Patients with epidermolysis bullosa dystrophica rarely survive beyond the third decade of life.

Medical therapy for epidermolysis bullosa has not been very successful. Phenytoin, a collagenase inhibitor, may produce short-term improvement. Corticosteroids are not effective. Coverage of denuded skin with cultured human skin preparations may be effective. Surgical therapy is directed at preservation and improvement of hand function.

Management of Anesthesia

It is critical that trauma to the skin and mucous membranes be avoided or minimized during the intraoperative period. Trauma from adhesive tape, blood pressure cuffs, and adhesive ECG electrodes can cause bullae formation. The blood pressure cuff should be padded with loose cotton dressing. Intravascular catheters should be anchored with sutures or a gauze dressing rather than adhesive tape. Trauma from a facemask may be reduced by lubrication of the mask and the patient's face. Use of upper airway instruments, including oropharyngeal and nasopharyngeal airways, should be kept to a minimum because the squamous epithelial lining of the oropharynx and esophagus is susceptible to bullous formation. Frictional trauma to the oropharynx may result in the formation of large intraoral bullae, airway obstruction, and extensive hemorrhage from denuded mucosa. For similar reasons, insertion of an esophageal stethoscope should be avoided. Laryngeal involvement in patients with epidermolysis bullosa dystrophica is rare. If tracheal intubation is required, the laryngoscope and tracheal tube should be well lubricated to reduce friction against the oropharyngeal mucosa. Scarring of the oral cavity can cause microstomia and immobility of the tongue, which increases the difficulty of tracheal intubation. Fiberoptic-assisted tracheal intubation may be required. Although the safety of tracheal intubation has been established for patients with epidermolysis bullosa dystrophica, similar safety has not been established for patients with the junctional form. The junctional form affects all mucosa, including the respiratory epithelium. The types of surgical procedures (intra-abdominal) required in infants with the junctional type, however, usually mandate tracheal intubation.

Surgical procedures for patients with epidermolysis are usually peripheral and involve the hands. Ketamine is very useful for such superficial procedures because it provides good analgesia and usually does not require supplemental inhalation anesthesia. There are, however, no contraindications to inhaled anesthetics. Porphyria cutanea tarda, often associated with epidermolysis bullosa, does not have the same implications for anesthesia as acute intermittent porphyria. Regional anesthesia, including spinal, epidural, and brachial plexus anesthesia, has been used successfully for patients with epidermolysis bullosa.

Despite all the potential complications with anesthesia for patients with epidermolysis bullosa, appropriate intraoperative management is associated with surprisingly few complications. This is especially true when care is provided at a center experienced with the management of patients with epidermolysis bullosa.[70,71]

Pemphigus

Pemphigus is a vesiculobullous disease that may involve extensive areas of the skin and mucous membranes. Pemphigus is an autoimmune disease in which IgG antibodies attack the desmosomal proteins desmoglein 3 and desmoglein 1, leading to disruption of cell adhesion and separation of epithelial layers. A growing number of drugs have been implicated in the cause or exacerbation of pemphigus. These drugs include penicillamine, cephalosporins, ACE inhibitors, phenobarbital, propranolol, levodopa, piroxicam, and nifedipine.

There are several types of pemphigus including pemphigus vulgaris, pemphigus foliaceus, pemphigus vegetans, pemphigus erythematosus, and paraneoplastic pemphigus.[72] Pemphigus vulgaris is the most common type and the most clinically significant for the anesthesiologist because of the occurrence of oral lesions. Oral lesions develop in 50 to 70% of patients with pemphigus vulgaris and usually precede the cutaneous lesions. Lesions of the pharynx, larynx, esophagus, conjunctiva, urethra, cervix, and anus can develop. Extensive

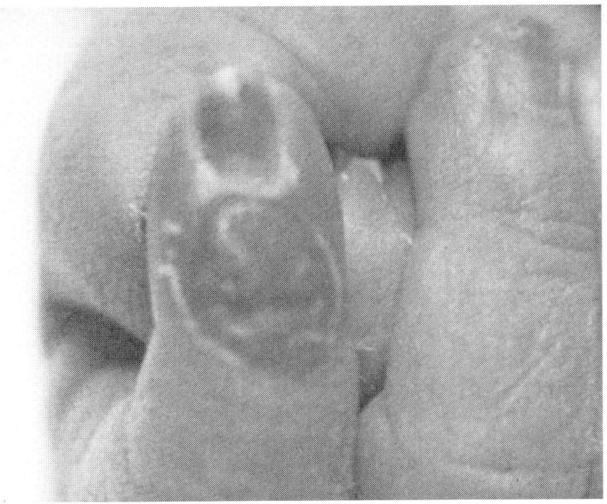

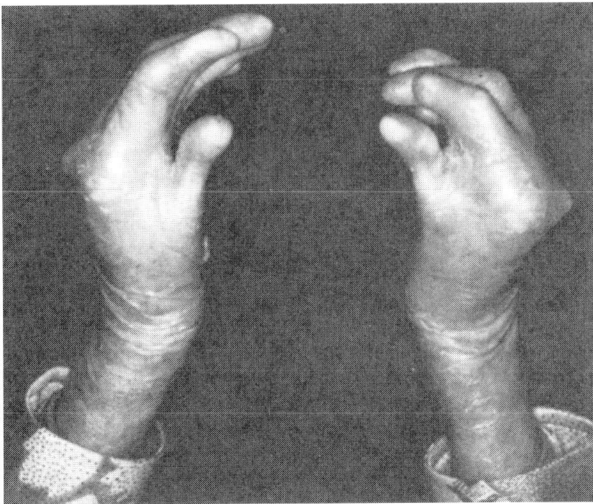

FIGURE 19-7. Epidermolysis bullosa. A. Bullous lesion of the finger of a neonate with epidermolysis. B. Hands of an older child with epidermolysis progression to produce severe scarring and pseudosyndactyly. (Courtesy of James E. Bennett, MD, Division of Plastic Surgery, Indiana University School of Medicine, Indianapolis, IN.)

oropharyngeal lesions may make eating painful to the extent that malnutrition occurs. Skin denudation and bullae formation can result in significant fluid and protein losses and the risk of secondary bacterial infection is great. As with epidermolysis bullosa, lateral shearing force is more likely to produce bullae than pressure exerted perpendicular to the skin surface. Systemic corticosteroids are the most effective therapy for pemphigus vulgaris. Improvement may be seen within days of corticosteroid therapy with full healing in 6 to 8 weeks. Adjuvant immunosuppressants such as azathioprine, cyclophosphamide, methotrexate, and mycophenolate mofetil can be used to reduce corticosteroid doses and side effects.[73]

Paraneoplastic pemphigus is an autoimmune disease associated with a number of malignant tumors, especially lymphomas and leukemias. IgG antibodies are produced that react to desmoglein 3 and 1. Oral and cutaneous lesions occur in most patients. Obstructive respiratory failure may result from inflammation and sloughing of the tracheobronchial mucosa.[74]

Pemphigus foliaceus (superficial pemphigus) is a less-severe form of pemphigus in which skin separation occurs near the epithelial surface; the oral mucosa is not affected. Pemphigus foliaceus can, however, be fatal if not treated. Pemphigus erythematosus (Senear-Usher syndrome) is a superficial form of pemphigus with erythematous hyperkeratotic lesions over the nose and malar areas; the oral cavity is not involved.

Management of Anesthesia

Preoperative drug therapy and the extreme fragility of the mucous membranes are the primary concerns for the management of anesthesia for patients with pemphigus. Corticosteroid supplementation will be necessary during the perioperative period. Management of the airway and tracheal intubation should be performed as described for patients with epidermolysis bullosa. Ketamine and regional anesthesia have been used successfully for patients with pemphigus.[75]

There are no specific contraindications to the use of any inhaled or intravenous anesthetics; however, potential side effects of treatment drugs and interactions with anesthetics must be considered. Methotrexate produces hepatorenal dysfunction and bone marrow suppression, and cyclophosphamide may prolong the action of succinylcholine and mivacurium by inhibiting cholinesterase activity.

References

1. Emery AEH: The muscular dystrophies. Lancet 359: 687, 2002
2. Muntoni F: Cardiomyopathy in muscular dystrophies. Curr Opin Neurol 16: 577, 2003
3. Boriani G, Gallina M, Merlini L *et al*: Clinical relevance of atrial fibrillation/flutter, stroke, pacemaker implant, and heart failure in Emery-Dreifuss muscular dystrophy: A long term longitudinal study. Stroke 34: 901, 2003
4. Wagner KR: Genetic diseases of muscle. Neurol Clin N Am 20: 645, 2002
5. Kunst G, Graf BM, Schreiner R *et al*: Differential effects of sevoflurane, isoflurane, and halothane on Ca release from the sarcoplasmic reticulum of skeletal muscle. Anesthesiology 91: 179, 1999
6. Uslu M, Mellinghoff H, Diefenbach C: Mivacurium for muscle relaxation in a child with Duchenne's muscular dystrophy. Anesth Analg 89: 340, 1999
7. Bhakta D, Lowe M, Groh W: Prevalence of structural abnormalities in patients with myotonic dystrophy type 1. Am Heart J 147: 224, 2004
8. Nagamitsu S, Ashizawa T: Myotonic dystophies. Adv Neurol 88: 293, 2002
9. Mathieu J, Allard P, Gobeil G *et al*: Anesthetic and surgical complications in 219 cases of myotonic dystrophy. Neurology 49: 1646, 1997
10. Rosenbaum HK, Miller JD: Malignant hyperthermia and myotonic disorders. Anes Clin N Am 20: 623, 2002
11. Aquilina A, Groves J: A combined technique utilising regional anesthesia and target-controlled sedation in a patient with myotonic dystrophy. Anaesthesia 57: 385, 2002
12. Davies NP, Hanna MG: The skeletal muscle channelopathies: Distinct entities and overlapping syndromes. Curr Opin Neurol 16: 559, 2003
13. Weller JF, Elliott RA, Pronovost PJ: Spinal anesthesia for a patient with familial hyperkalemic periodic paralysis. Anesthesiology 97: 259, 2002
14. Palace J, Vincent A, Beeson D: Myasthenia gravis: Diagnostic and management dilemmas. Curr Opin Neurol 14: 583, 2001
15. Vincent A, Palace J, Hilton-Jones D: Myasthenia gravis. Lancet 357: 2122, 2001
16. Saperstein DS, Barohn RJ: Management of myasthenia gravis. Semin Neurol 24: 41, 2004
17. Rocca GD, Coccia C, Diana L *et al*: Propofol or sevoflurane anesthesia without muscle relaxants allow early extubation of myasthenic patients. Can J Anaesth 50: 547, 2003
18. Abel M, Eisenkraft JB: Anesthetic implications of myasthenia gravis. Mount Sinai J Med 69: 31, 2002
19. Dillon FX: Anesthesia issues in the perioperative management of myasthenia gravis. Semin Neurol 24: 83, 2004
20. Sanders DB: The Lambert-Eaton myasthenic syndrome. Adv Neurol 88: 189, 2002
21. Newsom-Davis J: Therapy in myasthenia gravis and Lambert-Eaton myasthenic syndrome. Semin Neurol 23: 191, 2003
22. Kieseier BC, Hartung H-P: Therapeutic strategies in the Guillain-Barré syndrome. Semin Neurol 23: 159, 2003
23. Feldman JM: Cardiac arrest after succinylcholine administration in a pregnant patient recovered from Guillain-Barré syndrome. Anesthesiology 72: 942, 1990
24. Fiacchino F, Gemma M, Bricchi M *et al*: Hypo- and hypersensitivity to vecuronium in a patient with Guillain-Barré syndrome. Anesth Analg 78: 187, 1994

25. Kornek B, Lassmann H: Neuropathology of multiple sclerosis—new concepts. Brain Res Bull 61: 321, 2003
26. Noseworthy JH: Treatment of multiple sclerosis and related disorders: What's new in the past 2 years? Clin Neuropharm 26: 28, 2003
27. Bader AM, Hunt CO, Datta S *et al*: Anesthesia for the patient with multiple sclerosis. J Clin Anesth 1: 21, 1988
28. Dorotta IR, Schubert A: Multiple sclerosis and anesthetic implications. Curr Opin Anaesthesiol 15: 365, 2002
29. Blume WT: Diagnosis and management of epilepsy. CMAJ 168: 441, 2003
30. Nguyen DK, Spencer SS: Recent advances in the treatment of epilepsy. Arch Neurol 26: 38, 2003
31. Bazil CW, Pedley TA: Clinical pharmacology of antiepileptic drugs. Clin Neuropharm 26: 38, 2003
32. Chung KKK, Dawson VL, Dawson TM: New insights into Parkinson's disease. J Neurol 250(suppl 3): 15, 2003
33. Dewey RB: Management of motor complications in Parkinson's disease. Neurology 62(suppl 4): S3, 2004
34. Olanow CW: The scientific basis for the current treatment of Parkinson's disease. Annu Rev Med 55: 41, 2004
35. Galvez-Jimenez N, Lang AE: The perioperative management of Parkinson's disease revisited. Neurol Clin N Am 22: 367, 2004
36. Sutton-Brown M, Suchowersky O: Clinical and research advances in Huntington's disease. Can J Neurol Sci 30(suppl 1): S45, 2003
37. Sharma N, Satandaert DG: Inherited movement disorders. Neurol Clin N Am 20: 759, 2002
38. Cummings JL: Drug therapy: Alzheimer's disease. N Engl J Med 351: 56, 2004
39. Rowland LP, Shneider NA: Amyotrophic lateral sclerosis. N Engl J Med 344: 1688, 2001
40. Borasio GD, Miller RG: Clinical characteristics and management of ALS. Semin Neurol 21: 155, 2001
41. Dib M: Amyotrophic lateral sclerosis: progress and prospects for treatment. Drugs 63: 289, 2003
42. Jacka MJ, Sanderson F: Amyotrophic lateral sclerosis presenting during pregnancy. Anesth Anal 86: 542, 1998
43. Irani DN, Johnson RT: Diagnosis and prevention of bovine encephalopathy and variant Creutzfeldt-Jakob disease. Annu Rev Med 54: 305, 2003
44. Spencer MD, Knight RSG, Will RG: First hundred cases of variant Creutzfeldt-Jakob disease: Retrospective case review of early psychiatric and neurological features. BMJ 324: 1479, 2002
45. Farling P, Smith G: Anaesthesia for patients with Creutzfeldt-Jakob disease. A practical guide. Anaesthesia 58: 627, 2003
46. Gehrs BC, Friedberg RC: Autoimmune hemolytic anemia. Am J Hematol 69: 258, 2002
47. Claster S, Vichinsky EP: Managing sickle cell disease. BMJ 327: 1151, 2003
48. Gladwin MT, Sachdev V, Jison ML *et al*: Pulmonary hypertension as a risk factor for death in patients with sickle cell disease. N Engl J Med 350: 886, 2004
49. Vermylen C: Hematopoietic stem cell transplantation in sickle cell disease. Blood Rev 17: 163, 2003
50. Firth PG, Head CA: Sickle cell disease and anesthesia. Anesthesiology 101: 766, 2004
51. Danzer BI, Birnbach DJ, Thys DM: Anesthesia for the parturient with sickle cell disease. J Clin Anesth 8: 598, 1996
52. Lo L, Singer ST: Thalassemia: current approach to an old disease. Pediatr Clin N Am 49: 1165, 2002
53. Olsen NJ, Stein CM: New drugs for rheumatoid arthritis. N Engl J Med 350: 2167, 2004
54. Yaszemski MJ, Shepler TR: Sudden death from cord compression associated with atlantoaxial instability in rheumatoid arthritis. Spine 15: 338, 1990
55. Gonzalez-Juanatey C, Testa A, Garcia-Castelo A *et al*: Echocardiographic and doppler findings in long term treated rheumatoid arthritis patients without clinically evident cardiovascular disease. Semin Arthritis Rheum 33: 231, 2004
56. O'Dell JR: Therapeutic strategies for rheumatoid arthritis. N Engl J Med 350: 2591, 2004
57. Petrozza PH: Major spine surgery. Anes Clin N Am 20: 405, 2002
58. Matti MV, Sharrock NE: Anesthesia on the rheumatoid patient. Rheum Dis Clin N Am 24: 19, 1998
59. Mok CC, Lau CS: Pathogenesis of systemic lupus erythematosus. J Clin Pathol 56: 481, 2003
60. Nadeau SE: Neurologic manifestations of connective tissue disease. Neurol Clin N Am 20: 151, 2002
61. Wijetunga M, Rockson S: Myocarditis in systemic lupus erythematosus. Am J Med 113: 419, 2002
62. Dall'era M, Davis JC: Systemic lupus erythematosus. Postsgraduate Med 114: 31, 2003
63. Jimenez SA, Derk CT: Following the molecular pathways toward an understanding of the pathogenesis of systemic sclerosis. Ann Intern Med 140: 37, 2004
64. Fagan KA, Badesch DB: Pulmonary hypertension associated with connective tissue disease. Prog Cardiovasc Dis 45: 225, 2002
65. Leighton C: Drug treatment of scleroderma. Drugs 61: 419, 2001
66. Dalakas MC, Hohlfeld R: Polymyositis and dermatomyositis. Lancet 362: 971, 2003
67. Dalakas MC: Therapeutic approaches in patients with inflammatory myopathies. Semin Neurol 23: 199, 2003
68. Brown S, Shupack RC, Patel C *et al*: Neuromuscular blockade in a patient with active dermatomyositis. Anesthesiology 77: 1031, 1992
69. Anderson SHC, Meenan J, Williams KN *et al*: Efficacy and safety of endoscopic dilation of esophageal stricture in epidermolysis bullosa. Gastrointest Endosc 59: 28, 2004
70. Lin AN, Lateef F, Kelly R *et al*: Anesthetic management of epidermolysis bullosa: Review of 129 anesthetic episodes in 32 patients. J Am Acad Dermatol 30: 412, 1994
71. Herod J, Denyer J, Goldman A, Howard R: Epidermolysis bullosa in children: Pathophysiology, anaesthesia and pain management. Paediatr Anaesth 12: 388, 1994
72. Cotell S, Robinson ND, Chan LS: Autoimmune blistering skin diseases. Am J Emerg Med 18: 288, 2000
73. Harman KE, Albert S, Black MM: Guidelines for management of pemphigus vulgaris. Br J Dermatol 149: 926, 2003
74. Kimyai-Asadi A, Jih MH: Paraneoplastic pemphigus. Int J Dermatol 40: 367, 2001
75. Mahalingam TG, Kathirvel S, Sodhi P: Anaesthetic management of a patient with pemphigus vulgaris for emergency laparotomy. Anaesthesia 55: 155, 2000

CHAPTER 20 ■ MALIGNANT HYPERTHERMIA AND OTHER PHARMACOGENETIC DISORDERS

HENRY ROSENBERG, BARBARA W. BRANDOM, NYAMKHISHIG SAMBUUGHIN, AND JEFFREY E. FLETCHER

KEY POINTS

1. Malignant hyperthermia syndrome (MH) is an uncommon pharmacogenetic disorder of skeletal muscle. This means several things: (a) MH is inherited. (b) The syndrome is induced by pharmacologic agents in almost all cases. A few cases have been documented to result from exercise and heat exposure. (c) The pathophysiology involves biochemical changes in skeletal muscle physiology resulting in hypermetabolism. (d) The incidence is approximately one in 10,000 general anesthetics in the general population.
2. Unexpected elevation of end-tidal carbon dioxide in the absence of equipment malfunction is the most sensitive and specific sign of MH. Other signs of MH include tachycardia, tachypnea, acidosis, muscle rigidity, and rhabdomyolysis. MH may occur at any time in the course of an anesthetic from induction to emergence.
3. Masseter muscle rigidity after succinylcholine is more common in children than adults. It is predictive of MH susceptibility in up to 25% of cases and is associated with myoglobinuria. Trigger agents should be discontinued after masseter muscle rigidity.
4. Sudden cardiac arrest in a young male during general anesthesia, with or without succinylcholine, is likely a result of hyperkalemia in a patient with an occult myopathy, especially Duchenne muscular dystrophy.
5. Disorders that predispose patients to MH include central core disease and rarer forms of myotonia (e.g., hypokalemic periodic paralysis).
6. Trigger agents for MH include all potent inhalation agents and succinylcholine.
7. The gold standard test for diagnostic testing is the caffeine halothane contracture test (of freshly biopsied muscle) wherein muscle is exposed to incremental doses of caffeine or to halothane.
8. The essential points in treatment are the immediate discontinuation of trigger agents, hyperventilation, administration of dantrolene in doses of 2.5 mg/kg, repeated prn to signs of MH, and cooling by all routes available (especially nasogastric lavage, treatment of hyperkalemia in a standard fashion). Following an MH episode the patient should be treated with dantrolene for at least 36 hours.
9. Prevention of MH and avoidance of medicolegal action consists of obtaining a thorough history related to anesthetic complications, avoiding MH trigger agents in susceptibles and their relatives, having dantrolene immediately

available, and monitoring body temperature during general anesthesia.

10 MH susceptibility is inherited in an autosomal dominant pattern in humans. Administration of triggering agents such as all halogenated an aesthetic agents and/or succinylcholine leads to an uncontrolled release of free calcium from the sarcoplasmic reticulum of skeletal muscle. Several genes have been linked to MH, with mutations found in three, the ryanodine receptor gene, the dihydropyridine receptor gene, and the gene that elaborates the sodium channel of muscle. In humans, over 18 mutations have been found to be causal for MH. Mutations in these genes alter the function of the calcium channel leading to increased calcium release from the sarcoplasmic reticulum. There are many other DNA variants whose significance is yet to be determined.

Many inherited disorders have significant implications for anesthetic management. In this chapter we discuss those disorders that are precipitated by drugs often administered by anesthesiologists. In some cases, such as the porphyrias, the illness may be induced by agents other than anesthetics. In other enzymatic disorders, such as pseudocholinesterase abnormalities, it would be unlikely for a patient to have any problems until he or she is exposed to the depolarizing neuromuscular blocking agent succinylcholine. Malignant hyperthermia (MH) or malignant hyperpyrexia is perhaps the most significant inherited disorder triggered by exposure to anesthetic drugs.

MALIGNANT HYPERTHERMIA

Malignant hyperthermia was first formally described in 1960 in Lancet[1] by Denborough and Lovell and subsequently in *The British Journal of Anaesthesia*.[2] That first case report laid the foundation for much of our understanding of the clinical presentations of MH. The patient was a young man who claimed that several of his relatives died without apparent cause during anesthesia. He was anesthetized with halothane and developed tachycardia, hot sweaty skin, peripheral mottling, and cyanosis. Early recognition and symptomatic treatment saved him. It became apparent that this new syndrome had the following elements: patients were otherwise healthy unless exposed to an anesthetic agent, temperature elevation was a hallmark, a heritable or genetic component was present, and a high mortality rate was likely. In addition, with early recognition and treatment it was possible to abort the malignant effects of the syndrome.

The association between porcine stress syndrome (PSS) or "pale soft exudative porksyndrome" and MH was described in the early 1970s, thus providing an animal model for MH.[3] Porcine breeds such as the Landrace, Poland China, and Pietrain show the classic presentations of MH when potent inhalation agents and/or succinylcholine are administered. During the 1970s, many more clinical presentations of MH were reported. The development of an in vitro diagnostic test was suggested by Kalow et al based on exposure of a skeletal muscle biopsy specimen to caffeine and then halothane.[4] In 1975, Harrison reported that dantrolene could be effective in treating and preventing MH in pigs.[5] By 1979, a sufficient number of cases were described showing that intravenous dantrolene could successfully reverse the human form of MH, and the drug was approved for use by the U.S. Food and Drug Administration (FDA). In the 1980s, lay organizations in the United States, Canada, and Great Britain were formed to disseminate information to patients affected by MH as well as to enhance awareness of the syndrome among physicians. Application of the muscle biopsy diagnostic halothane–caffeine contracture test was standardized and a registry for MH was created in the United States in the late 1980s. In addition, a variety of other tests for diagnosing MH were introduced, many of which subsequently were found to be of little or no validity.

A major step forward occurred in 1985, when Lopez and colleagues directly demonstrated an increased intracellular concentration of calcium ion in muscle from MH-susceptible pigs and humans.[6] The intracellular calcium concentration dramatically increased during an MH crisis and was reversed by the administration of dantrolene.

In the 1990s molecular biologic techniques were applied to identify the genes associated with MH susceptibility. It is anticipated that better understanding of the genetic substrate of the pathophysiology of MH will result in a less invasive diagnostic test than the contracture tests used at present. In the 1990s epidemiologic information helped to differentiate MH from other life-threatening anesthetic complications. It was appreciated that some deaths in children formerly attributed to MH were really the result of destruction of muscle cells that occurred during anesthesia with volatile agents and succinylcholine in patients with unrecognized myopathies, specifically the dystrophinopathies, Duchenne and Becker muscular dystrophy.[7]

Clinical Presentations

As our knowledge of MH has grown, the definition of MH has changed. At first, MH was thought in all cases to be a heritable syndrome consisting of an extremely elevated body temperature, skeletal muscle rigidity, and acidosis associated with a high mortality rate. However, MH should be thought of in terms of its underlying pathophysiologic characteristics. MH is a hypermetabolic disorder of skeletal muscle with varied pre-
1 sentations, depending on species, breed, and triggering agents. An important pathophysiologic process in this disorder is intracellular hypercalcemia in skeletal muscle. Intracellular hypercalcemia activates metabolic pathways that result in adenosine triphosphate depletion, acidosis, membrane destruction, and cell death. Although a heritable component is present in many cases, it is not invariably apparent from patient family history. In addition, disorders that may have symptoms and signs similar to those of MH, such as neuroleptic malignant syndrome (NMS), and heat stroke may not have an inherited basis.

Classic Malignant Hyperthermia

Malignant hyperthermia may present in several ways. In almost all cases, the first manifestations of the syndrome occur in the operating room. However, MH also may occur in the recovery room or (rarely) even later. In the classic case, the initial signs of tachycardia and tachypnea result from sympathetic nervous system stimulation secondary to underlying hypermetabolism and hypercarbia derived primarily from the skeletal muscle. Because many patients receive neuromuscular blockers and controlled ventilation during general anesthesia, tachypnea usually is not recognized. Shortly after the increase in heart rate, an increase in blood pressure occurs, often associated with ventricular dysrhythmias induced by sympathetic nervous system stimulation resulting from hypercarbia or caused by hyperkalemia or catecholamine release. Thereafter, muscle rigidity or an increase in muscle tone may become apparent. Increase in body temperature, at a rate of 1 to 2°C every 5 minutes, follows. With the increase in metabolism, the patient may "break through" the neuromuscular blockade. At the same time, the CO_2

absorbent becomes activated and warm to the touch (because the reaction with CO_2 is exothermic). The patient will display peripheral mottling and, on occasion, sweating and cyanosis. Blood gas analysis usually reveals hypercarbia with respiratory and metabolic acidosis without marked oxygen desaturation. Elevation of end-tidal CO_2 is one of the earliest most sensitive
2 and specific signs of MH. However, vigorous hyperventilation may mask such hypercarbia and delay the diagnosis.[8] A mixed venous blood sample will show even more dramatic evidence of CO_2 retention and metabolic acidosis.[9] Hyperkalemia, hypercalcemia, lactacidemia, and myoglobinuria are characteristic. An increase in creatine kinase (CK) levels is dramatic, often exceeding 20,000 units in the first 12 to 24 hours. Death results unless the syndrome is promptly treated. Even with treatment and survival, the patient is at risk for life-threatening myoglobinuric renal failure and disseminated intravascular coagulation. Another significant clinical problem is recrudescence of the syndrome within the first 24 to 36 hours.[10,11] If succinylcholine is used during induction of anesthesia, an acceleration of the manifestations of MH may occur such that tachycardia, hypertension, marked temperature elevation, and dysrhythmias are seen over the course of 5 to 10 minutes. However, a completely normal response to succinylcholine does not rule out the subsequent development of MH when potent volatile agents are used.

Masseter Muscle Rigidity

3 Rigidity of the jaw muscles after administration of succinylcholine is referred to as *masseter muscle rigidity* (MMR) or *masseter spasm*. The association of this phenomenon with MH was underlined by many case reports of MMR preceding MH.[12,13] Although MMR probably occurs in patients of all ages, it is distinctly most common in children and young adults. MMR occurs in about 1% of children induced with halothane prior to administration of succinylcholine. Several studies have shown a peak age incidence at 8 to 12 years of age. Characteristically, anesthesia is induced by inhalation of halothane or sevoflurane, after which succinylcholine is administered. Snapping of the jaw or rigidity on opening of the jaw is seen. Although less common MMR may follow induction with thiopental or propofol prior to succinylcholine administration. However, this rigidity can be overcome with effort and usually abates within 2 to 3 minutes. Repeat doses of succinylcholine do not relieve the problem nor do nondepolarizing relaxants. A peripheral nerve stimulator usually reveals flaccid paralysis. However, increased tone of other muscles also may be noted. Tachycardia and dysrhythmias are not infrequent. Only in rare cases does frank MH supervene immediately after MMR. More commonly (if the anesthetic is continued with a triggering agent), the initial signs of MH appear in 20 minutes or more. If the anesthetic is discontinued, the patient usually recovers uneventfully. However, within 4 to 12 hours, myoglobinuria occurs and CK elevation is detected.

Muscle biopsy with caffeine–halothane contracture testing has shown that approximately 25% of patients who experience MMR are also susceptible to MH.[14,15] Therefore, one may elect to discontinue anesthesia and postpone surgery after an episode of MMR. If surgery must be continued, it should be with nontriggering anesthetics and the use of end-tidal CO_2 and core temperature monitoring. The issue of whether to give dantrolene after an episode of MMR is unresolved. Dantrolene is most useful only when there is a clear diagnosis of MH. When MMR is accompanied by rigidity of chest or limb, MH is more likely to follow than after isolated jaw rigidity.[16,17]

The differential diagnosis of MMR consists of the following: (1) myotonic syndrome, (2) temporomandibular joint dysfunction, (3) underdosing with succinylcholine, (4) not allowing sufficient time for succinylcholine to act before intubation, (5) increased resting tension after succinylcholine in the presence of fever or elevated plasma epinephrine. A variety of reports have shown that succinylcholine increases jaw muscle tone in patients with normal muscle.[18] This normal agonistic effect of succinylcholine, further increased by temperature[19] and epinephrine in the presence of halothane, may account for some cases of MMR. Signs of temporomandibular dysfunction as well as myotonia should be sought following the MMR episode. If rigidity precluding laryngoscopy occurred without temporomandibular joint dysfunction, the patient should be evaluated by a neurologist for the presence of occult myopathy and counseled regarding the need for a muscle biopsy and diagnostic contracture test to evaluate MH susceptibility. It is incumbent on the anesthesiologist to alert the patient to the possibility that MH may follow in subsequent procedures.

MMR has been shown in both retrospective as well as prospective studies to occur in as many as 1 in 100 children anesthetized with halothane and given succinylcholine. A retrospective study based on the information supplied to the Danish Malignant Hyperthermia Registry found that the incidence of MMR was 1 in 12,000 (including adults and children).[20] A prospective study found MMR in 1 of 500 children who received halothane and then intravenous succinylcholine.[21]

Our advice regarding MMR is as follows:

1. When it occurs, the anesthesiologist should, if at all possible, discontinue the anesthetic and postpone surgery. If end-tidal CO_2 monitoring and dantrolene are available and the anesthesiologist is experienced in managing MH, he or she may elect to continue with a nontriggering anesthetic.
2. After episodes of MMR, the patient should be observed carefully for a period of 12 to 24 hours for myoglobinuria and signs of MH. Administration of 1 to 2 mg/kg of dantrolene should be considered.
3. The family should be informed of the episode of MMR and its implications.
4. Creatine kinase levels should be checked 6, 12, and 24 hours after the episode. If the CK level is still grossly elevated at 12 hours, additional samples should be drawn until it begins to return to normal.
5. If the CK level is greater than 20,000 IU in the perioperative period and a concomitant myopathy is not present, the diagnosis of MH is very likely.[22] If contracture test results are within normal limits after an episode of MMR, we currently do not recommend that other family members undergo testing, but advise that succinylcholine be avoided in future anesthetics for that patient.

A study by Littleford et al[23] has shown that acidosis and rhabdomyolysis occur when anesthesia is continued with a volatile inhalation agent after MMR, although fulminant MH may not occur. MMR has been documented most frequently in association with succinylcholine, although it may occur after induction with any anesthetic agent, intravenous or inhalation, before succinylcholine administration.[24] Hence, pediatric anesthesiologists avoid the use of succinylcholine except on specific indication. (See also Myodystrophies Exacerbated by Anesthesia section.)

Late Onset of MH and Myoglobinuria

Malignant hyperthermia may occur in the postoperative period, usually within the first few hours of recovery from anesthesia. The characteristic tachycardia, tachypnea, hypertension, and dysrhythmias indicate that an episode of MH may be about to follow. Myoglobinuria may occur without an obvious increase in metabolism.[25] Succinylcholine may cause rhabdomyolysis in patients who have other muscle disorders that may not be clinically obvious on cursory examination.[7,26,27] Myoglobinuria may result from interactions with other drugs such as inhibitors of cholesterol formation.[28] The presence of myoglobinuria mandates that the patient be referred to a neurologist for further investigation.

Myodystrophies Exacerbated by Anesthesia: Relation to Malignant Hyperthermia

Patients suffering from *muscular dystrophy,* Duchenne or Becker's, are at risk to develop hyperkalemic cardiac arrest after administration of succinylcholine. The same may occur following administration of volatile anesthetic agents only. These adverse events were first believed to represent a form of MH.[29,30] It now appears that the pathophysiology of the hyperkalemic episodes and MH is different. Case reports collected by the Malignant Hyperthermia Association of the United States (MHAUS) and the North American MH Registry indicate that when an apparently healthy child experiences a sudden unexpected cardiac arrest on induction of anesthesia, once hypoxemia and ventilatory problems are ruled out, hyperkalemia should be considered. Of 29 patients with such a presentation, 60% died. In 50% there was evidence of undiagnosed myopathy (usually muscular dystrophy).[7] The treatment of hyperkalemic arrests includes administration of calcium chloride,
4 glucose, insulin, bicarbonate, and hyperventilation.

In 1993 and in 1994 the package insert for succinylcholine was modified to warn against routine use of succinylcholine in children. Of course, in special circumstances, such as airway emergencies and the presence of a "full stomach," succinylcholine may still be appropriate. However, administration of rapid-acting nondepolarizing neuromuscular blockers in these situations may be an appropriate alternative to use of succinylcholine.

5 *Central core disease* (CCD) is a congenital myopathy characterized by muscle weakness. CCD is generally inherited in an autosomal dominant manner, although a few families with autosomal recessive inheritance and many sporadic cases have been reported.[31] Mutations that predispose to central core disease, similar to MH, are usually associated with the ryanodine receptor gene. Many cases of MH have been reported in patients with CCD. Therefore, precautions regarding MH must be taken for all patients with central core disease.[32]

The *myotonias* are a varied set of disorders resulting from abnormalities in either the sodium or chloride channel of muscle. The common pathophysiologic process is prolonged depolarization of the muscle membrane following activation. Patients with any of these disorders will display muscle contractures after succinylcholine. Hypokalemic periodic paralysis and a rare form of myotonia, myotonia fluctuans, have been linked to MH susceptibility by the halothane–caffeine contracture test.[33,34]

King or *King-Denborough* syndrome is a rare myopathy characterized by cryptorchidism, markedly slanted eyes, low-set ears, pectus deformity, scoliosis, small stature, and hypotonia. Several patients with this disorder have been diagnosed as MH susceptible both clinically and by muscle biopsy.[35,36] Skeletal abnormalities such as osteogenesis imperfecta[37] and the Schwartz-Jampel[38] syndrome *myotonia* have been associated with signs of MH. Metabolism is increased in patients with osteogenesis imperfecta because of the bone disease. Fever during anesthesia is common in these patients. The Schwartz-Jampel syndrome is an autosomal recessive myotonic-like condition with osteoarticular deformities. Fever is common in these patients because of continuous muscle activity. In both these conditions, association with MH is sporadic. Despite a few well-documented cases of MH in patients with osteogenesis imperfecta, we (and others[39]) have not confirmed MH susceptibility in three cases of osteogenesis imperfecta tested with the halothane–caffeine contracture test. Inhalation anesthetics have been administered without complication to many patients with osteogenesis imperfecta. But we have found typical contractures in one other muscle biopsy from a patient with osteogenesis imperfecta.

Syndromes with a Clinical Resemblance to MH

Pheochromocytoma may be mistaken for MH because it presents with tachycardia, hypertension, and fever during anesthesia. However, pheochromocytoma does not predispose to MH.[40] Thyrotoxicosis could also be mistaken for MH. Carbon dioxide production is lower in these endocrine disorders than in MH. Hypertension is greater in pheochromocytoma than in thyrotoxicosis, and even less in MH. Neither endocrine crisis is associated with muscle rigidity as in MH. Metabolic acidosis is generally not present during thyrotoxicosis and not as great during pheochromocytoma as during MH. Thyroid crisis did not trigger MH even in susceptible pigs.[41]

Sepsis is most often confused with MH. Patients undergoing urinary tract surgery; ear, nose, and throat surgery; or appendectomy for appendicitis can and will develop fever and sometimes acidosis in the PACU. Hyperkalemia may also appear during episodes of sepsis. Unlike MH, however, muscle rigidity is uncommon, although rigors may be mistaken for rigidity. In addition, signs of sepsis are treated effectively with nonsteroidal anti-inflammatory agents and antibiotics. MH will not respond to such nonspecific therapy. Dantrolene may often be associated with acute reduction of fever. This, however, is also nonspecific. Differentiating sepsis from MH is often not possible clinically.

Hypoxic encephalopathy is characterized by failure to awaken from anesthesia, posturing and opisthotonus, and hyperthermia. It has been mistaken for MH. The diagnosis is based on the clinical presentation.

Mitochondrial myopathies resemble MH. Defects within the mitochondrial genome affect oxidative phosphorylation and result in impaired production of ATP. These disorders have many manifestations, usually presenting at an early age with central nervous system (CNS) and muscle pathology. Failure to thrive, developmental delays, muscle weakness, and cardiomyopathy may be present. Elevated serum lactate and pyruvate are found on laboratory examination. There does not appear to be a relation between the mitochondrial myopathies and MH. However, respiratory depression is often seen following anesthesia. Succinylcholine is best avoided in these patients because of the potential for hyperkalemia. There is insufficient evidence in the literature to characterize the response to potent volatile agents.[42]

Periodic paralyses are inherited disorders characterized by marked muscle weakness and paralysis resulting from small deviations in potassium concentrations. The disorders are inherited and result from mutations in the gene that elaborates the sodium channel or the calcium channel of skeletal muscle.

In *hypokalemic periodic paralysis*, the patient is exquisitely sensitive to lowered potassium as may occur with administration of a glucose load or fasting. As mentioned earlier, there has been a relation to MH described in some patients.[33]

In *hyperkalemic periodic paralysis* small increases in potassium will lead to muscle weakness and paralysis. A relation to MH susceptibility has not been described. In almost all cases the patient will relate a family history of muscle weakness and paralysis under conditions where there is a change in serum potassium.

Malignant Hyperthermia Outside the Operating Room

The often-repeated observation that an MH-like syndrome can occur in certain pig breeds in response to stressful situations supports the suggestion that MH may occur outside the operating room in humans. Gronert et al have described a patient who had episodic fevers and whose muscle produced a contracture consistent with MH susceptibility.[43] The fevers were controlled by dantrolene. A minority of exercise-induced rhabdomyolysis and heat stroke cases are also related to MH. Mutations in the RYR1 receptor gene, known to be causative of MH, have been found in a patient who died of heat stroke[44] and in some patients with exercise-induced rhabdomyolysis.[45]

In 1997 Tobin and associates documented an apparent awake episode of fatal MH in a 12-year-old-boy. The child had recovered from an episode of clinical MH during anesthesia several months prior to the episode. Following soccer practice on a day that was not overly hot and humid, he complained of muscle discomfort and rapidly developed ventricular fibrillation. His CK rose to 9,000 IU. Genetic investigation revealed the presence of a ryanodine receptor mutation known to be causal for MH. Other family members also harbor the mutation.

A few other cases of apparent awake episodes of fatal MH have been reported from other countries.

Neuroleptic Malignant Syndrome and Other Drug-Induced Hyperthermic Reactions

The symptoms and signs of the NMS include fever, rhabdomyolysis, tachycardia, hypertension, agitation, muscle rigidity, and acidosis.[46] The mortality rate is unknown, but is significant. Dantrolene is an effective therapeutic modality in many cases of NMS. Therefore, it is not unusual for an anesthesiologist to be consulted in the management of patients with this disorder.

Although the resemblance of NMS to MH is striking, there are significant differences between the two. MH is acute, whereas NMS often occurs after longer term drug exposure. Phenothiazines and haloperidol or any of the newer potent antipsychotic agents alone or in combination are usually triggering agents for NMS. Sudden withdrawal of drugs used to treat Parkinson's disease may also trigger NMS. Electroconvulsive therapy (ECT) with succinylcholine does not appear to trigger the syndrome.[47] Also, NMS does not seem to be inherited, and there are no case reports of it in family members who have had an episode of MH.

Many believe that the changes in NMS are a reflection of dopamine depletion in the central nervous system by psychoactive agents. In support of this theory, therapy with bromocriptine, a dopamine agonist, is often useful in treatment of NMS. Therefore, although there appear to be similarities between MH and NMS,[46] a common pathophysiology is not readily apparent. From an anesthesiologist's viewpoint, it is best to monitor patients with NMS as though they were susceptible to MH. However, drugs such as succinylcholine have been used for ECT without problems in MH patients.

A similar set of signs may be observed in some patients taking serotonin uptake inhibitors. Much less is known regarding this syndrome.

Other drugs known to induce a hypermetabolic syndrome and rhabdomyolysis, probably through mechanisms not related to those of MH, are cocaine, amphetamines, and MDMA. Dantrolene has been used sporadically as an adjunct to treatment of marked hyperthermia with promising results. Treatment, however, is usually symptomatic.

TABLE 20-1

SAFE VERSUS UNSAFE DRUGS IN MALIGNANT HYPERTHERMIA

■ SAFE DRUGS	■ UNSAFE DRUGS
Antibiotics	All inhalation agents (except nitrous oxide)
Antithistamines	Succinylcholine
Barbiturates	
Benzodiazepines	
Droperidol	
Ketamine	
Local anesthetics	
Nitrous oxide	
Nondepolarizing neuromuscular blockers	
Opioids	
Propofol	
Propranolol	
Vasoactive drugs	

Drugs That Trigger Malignant Hyperthermia

It is clearly established that the potent inhalation agents, includ-
6 ing sevoflurane, desflurane, isoflurane, halothane, methoxyflurane, cyclopropane, and ether, may trigger MH. Succinylcholine and decamethonium are also triggers. Other anesthetic drugs and adjuvants are not MH triggers. Table 20-1 indicates the drugs believed to be safe and those that are unsafe.

Local Anesthetics

All local anesthetics are safe for MH-susceptible patients.[48] Preliminary studies of local anesthetics during an MH crisis (e.g., for dysrhythmia control) do not show an exacerbation of MH by amide local anesthetics.

Catecholamines

Although plasma catecholamines increase during an MH crisis, such an elevation is usually secondary to metabolic and cardiovascular changes. Vasopressors and other catecholamines are not involved in triggering MH.[49] Therefore, these drugs should be used as necessary but only with simultaneous treatment of the MH crisis.

Nondepolarizing Relaxants and Anticholinesterases

Vecuronium, rocuronium, atracurium, pancuronium, and all other nondepolarizing drugs are considered safe to use in patients with MH. Clinical studies have shown that anticholinesterase–anticholinergic combinations are safe for reversal of nondepolarizing relaxants in MH-susceptible patients.[50]

Phenothiazines and Drugs Used to Treat Psychoses

Phenothiazines increase intracellular calcium ion concentration and may cause contractures in vitro in muscle from MH-susceptible patients.[51] Phenothiazines also induce the related neuroleptic malignant syndrome. Therefore, although there have been several reports that phenothiazines are effective in managing temperature fluctuations during recovery from MH, these compounds should be used cautiously in MH-susceptible patients. Medications used in the treatment of psychiatric conditions such as haloperidol, atypical antipsychotics may induce NMS. Since NMS and MH are dissimilar, there is no evidence that these agents are precipitants of MH.

Other Drugs

Digoxin, quinidine, and calcium salts do not induce MH in the swine.[52] Therefore, it is reasonable to assume that they are safe to use in clinical situations. Neither ketamine nor propofol are MH triggers.[53]

Incidence and Epidemiology

Although the incidence of reported episodes of MH has increased, the mortality rate from MH has declined. In part, these two trends reflect a greater awareness of the syndrome, earlier diagnosis, and better therapy. The incidence of MH varies from country to country, based on differences in gene pools. In the upper midwest of the United States, for example, there are many families containing large numbers of MH-susceptible people. In contrast, other areas of the country and parts of the world have rarely reported MH. For example, Bachand and colleagues examined the incidence of MH in the province of Quebec, Canada, where many families had been biopsied. They traced the pedigrees of the patients to the original immigrants from France and found an incidence of MH susceptibility of 0.2% in this province. However, that represented only five extended families.[54] A study in Great Britain revealed 3 cases of MH in 100,000 administered anesthetics.[55] The best epidemiologic study of MH was done in the mid 1980s by Ording.[20] Based on information supplied to the Danish Malignant Hyperthermia Registry comprising the reported incidence of MH in Denmark (population approximately 5 million), this study revealed fulminant MH in approximately 1 in 250,000 administered anesthetics. However, if the definition of MH is expanded to include abortive cases of MH and is further refined to include only cases in which inhalation anesthetics and succinylcholine were used, the incidence was as high as 1 in 4,000 anesthetic administrations![20]

A better understanding of the prevalence of MH is likely to emerge from the widespread use of molecular genetics for the diagnosis of MH susceptibility. For example, Monnier and colleagues estimate that one in 2,000 to 3,000 persons in France harbor one of the known MH causative mutations.[56] Currently, the consensus is that mortality from MH is under 5% in Western countries. However, the epidemiologic characteristics of MH are very difficult to define for the following reasons:

1. Widespread diagnostic testing for MH is difficult to apply.
2. The clinical diagnosis of MH is often questionable.
3. Triggering of MH even in susceptible patients may not occur on each anesthetic exposure. In some cases, susceptible patients have received triggering agents for up to 13 anesthetics without any problems, only to have MH triggered on the subsequent anesthetic. Investigation of the Danish Malignant Hyperthermia Registry found the MH genotype to be expressed in only 34 to 54% of anesthetic exposures.[57]
4. Registries of MH cases do not capture all data. There is a paucity of data concerning the frequency of use of anesthesia in the general population.

Inheritance of Malignant Hyperthermia

Many of the difficulties that limit an understanding of the epidemiologic characteristics of MH also limit accurate assessment of its inheritance. The animal model does not clarify the issue of inheritance in humans. MH in most pig breeds is inherited in an autosomal recessive fashion.[58] Variability in clinical presentation and the fact that MH is not regularly apparent on exposure to triggering agents, even in those who are susceptible, result in great difficulty in assessing the inheritance of MH in affected families. Nevertheless, it is generally accepted that MH in humans is inherited as an autosomal dominant trait with variable penetrance.[59] This implies that children of MHS patients have a 50% chance of being MHS themselves.

Diagnostic Tests for Malignant Hyperthermia

Development of the In Vitro Contracture Test

In 1970, Kalow et al demonstrated that isolated muscle from MH-susceptible patients was unusually sensitive to caffeine when exposed in vitro.[4] Shortly thereafter, Ellis and coinvestigators demonstrated that muscle from MH-susceptible patients also had a more sensitive than normal contracture response to halothane. The European MH Group (EMHG)[60,61] and North American MH Group (NAMHG)[62–64] separately have standardized protocols for contracture testing. Treatment of muscle biopsy specimens in a tissue bath with either halothane or caffeine has come to be the standard test for diagnosing MH susceptibility.

Other tests have been proposed to differentiate patients with MH from those who are normal. None of these tests distinguished MHS patients from normals with accuracy. However, several newer approaches suggest that nonmuscle biopsy tests might be valuable as an initial estimation of likelihood of MH susceptibility and are discussed later in the chapter.

Halothane–Caffeine Contracture Test

Although some procedures and interpretations differ between
7 the EMHG and NAMHG protocols, the following steps are similar. Skeletal muscle (1 to 3 g) is usually biopsied from the vastus lateralis muscle. Strips of muscle weighing 100 to 200 mg and measuring 15 to 30 mm ($\geq$25 mm preferred) in length by 2 to 3 mm in width by 2 to 3 mm in thickness are carefully isolated and mounted in a standard muscle bath apparatus (Fig. 20-1). The tissue bath contains a modified Krebs solution at 37°C bubbled with O_2 and CO_2 (95%/5%), and the resting tension is adjusted to the optimum length for maximal twitch tension (usually about 2 g). The bundles are stimulated supramaximally with pulses of frequency 0.1 to 0.2 Hz with 2 msec pulses to verify viability. After a 15- to 60-minute equilibration in which the preparation is oxygenated with O_2/CO_2 (95/5%), halothane is added to the gas phase, either as a bolus dose or in incrementally increasing concentrations (Fig. 20-2). The concentration of halothane is verified by gas chromatography. A second set of muscle strips is equilibrated and subsequently exposed to incrementally increasing concentrations of caffeine-free base (see Fig. 20-2). It is recommended that the caffeine strips be tested early in the procedure because they tend to be more sensitive to instability over time. Testing is usually completed within about 5 hours of biopsy to ensure adequate viability of the muscle preparations. Owing to time constraints, it is essential that the biopsy be performed at or within about 1 hour of the testing laboratory. Usually, a histologic evaluation accompanies the contracture test to examine whether the subject has a muscle disorder other than MH.

Interpretation of the Halothane–Caffeine Contracture Test. Two protocols have been adopted for use over the past decade. These protocols were initiated to standardize procedures so that the results from groups of laboratories could be pooled for analysis. A uniform approach was necessary to standardize the phenotype derived from the contracture test for use in genetic analysis.

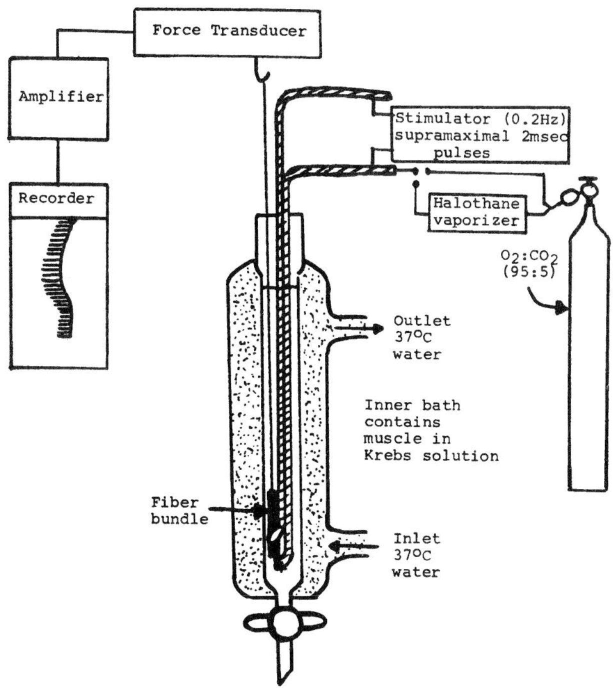

FIGURE 20-1. Diagram of the muscle bath apparatus used for contracture testing for diagnosing MH susceptibility.

In the EMHG protocol, also known as the IVCT for In Vitro Contracture Test,[60,61] halothane is added incrementally (0.5, 1.0, 2.0%) with the preparation exposed to each concentration for 3 minutes. A response indicative of MH susceptibility is based on a contracture threshold (>0.2 g) at a halothane concentration ≤2% in either of the two muscle strips tested. Caffeine is also added incrementally in concentrations of 0.25, 0.5, 1.0, 1.5, 2.0, 3.0, and 4.0 m*M*. Each caffeine concentration is maintained until the contracture plateau is reached, or for 3 minutes, whichever is sooner. A positive response is a contracture threshold (>0.2 g) at a concentration of caffeine of 2 m*M* or less in either of two strips tested.

In the NAMHG protocol,[62] also known as the Caffeine Halothane Contracture Test (CHCT), a bolus dose of halothane 3% is added to the gas phase for each of three muscle strips and the maximum contracture within 10 minutes is recorded. A positive response is a contracture >0.7 g tension to halothane 3% and a negative response is <0.5 g. An equivocal response to halothane (MH-equivocal, or MHE) is between 0.5 and 0.7 g.[63] As in the EMHG protocol, caffeine is added incrementally, but the concentrations are 0.5, 1.0, 2.0, 4.0, 8.0, and 32 m*M*. A positive response is a contracture >0.3 g (determined by the specific laboratory) to 2 m*M* caffeine. The interpretations of the outcomes of the halothane and caffeine tests differ between the EMHG and NAMHG protocols. The EMHG protocol requires a positive response to halothane and a positive response to caffeine for a diagnosis of MH-susceptible (MHS). If the outcomes of both tests are negative, then the subject is diagnosed as MH-normal (MHN). If only the caffeine test is abnormal, the patient is considered MHE to caffeine (MHEc). If only the halothane test is abnormal, the patient is considered MHE to halothane (MHEh). The NAMHG protocol differs in that the subject is considered MH positive (MH+ or MHS) if either the response to halothane or the response to caffeine is abnormal. The patient is diagnosed as normal (MH− or MHN) if neither test is positive. As in the EMHG protocol, MHE subjects are treated clinically as MH susceptible.

Sensitivity and Specificity of the Halothane–Caffeine Contracture Test. The sensitivity of the NAMHG protocol (CHCT) is 100% with specificity 78% (false-negatives are to be avoided).[64] The EMHG test (IVCT) has sensitivity of 98% with specificity of 93%. It is difficult to be certain of the sensitivity and specificity of the contracture test because although one can be fairly certain of the clinical phenotype of MHS based on anesthetic exposures, it is almost impossible to be assured that control subjects do not harbor a causative mutation. Determination of the sensitivity and specificity is based on contracture studies of patients with no known MH history undergoing routine surgery (controls) compared to contracture studies from patients who experienced a clinical episode of MH. When the genetic characterization of MH is more complete, the sensitivity and specificity of the contracture test may be clarified.

Other Contracture Tests

In an attempt to further improve the specificity and sensitivity of the contracture test, other agents have been tested for their effect on skeletal muscle.

Ryanodine. An additional contracture test using the plant alkaloid ryanodine was proposed for inclusion in the EMHG protocol. Ryanodine binds to and activates the calcium release channel of the sarcoplasmic reticulum. It was reasoned that this test would afford maximum specificity for MH, and early studies supported this concept.[65–68]

The basic testing conditions for ryanodine are similar to those described for halothane and caffeine testing. High-purity ryanodine is employed. A bolus of ryanodine (1 μM) is added to the bath and the time to onset of contracture, time to 0.2-g contracture, time to 1-g contracture, and the time and amplitude of maximum contracture are recorded. Discrimination was improved by using the time to initial contracture and time to development of a 10-m*N* (1 g) contracture.[69]

4-Chloro-*m*-cresol. 4-Chloro-*m*-cresol (4-CmC) is a potent activator of ryanodine receptor–mediated Ca^{2+} release. Cumulative administration of 25, 50, 75, 100, 150, and 200 μmol/L 4-CmC produced concentration-dependent contractures. Contractures developed earlier and to a greater magnitude in muscle from patients identified as MHS by the EMHG protocol than in normal muscle.[70] The addition of testing with this compound has been approved by the EMHG.

Pitfalls in the Contracture Test

Ideally, each laboratory should derive specimens from patients who are clearly and unequivocally normal and those who are clearly and unequivocally MH susceptible to verify that cut-points for MH susceptibility are diagnostic within the laboratory. Unfortunately, because of the variation in presentation of MH and the confusion with signs associated with non-MH causes, it is not always possible to have complete agreement on the MH status of a patient based on a clinical history, even among experts in the field. This problem has made estimates of sensitivity and specificity difficult.

A clinical grading scale has been developed to address concerns for objectively evaluating the clinical episode.[71] This scale lacks sensitivity, because incomplete recording of necessary data or early termination of the crisis would not yield scores indicative of MH, even if an episode had occurred. The scoring system also is designed to avoid overweighting duplicative indicators representing the same processes. The value of the grading scale is mainly in identifying those subjects with the most convincing episodes of MH for subsequent evaluation of the sensitivity and specificity of the diagnostic tests. The clinical grading scale (Table 20-2) is useful in evaluating clinical episodes in those cases in which the subject is rated a D6 (Diagnostic rank 6, almost certainly MH), but lower scores should not be considered for actual diagnosis. We would even encourage the practice of sending patients rated D6 for diagnostic muscle contracture testing, because these individuals are rare

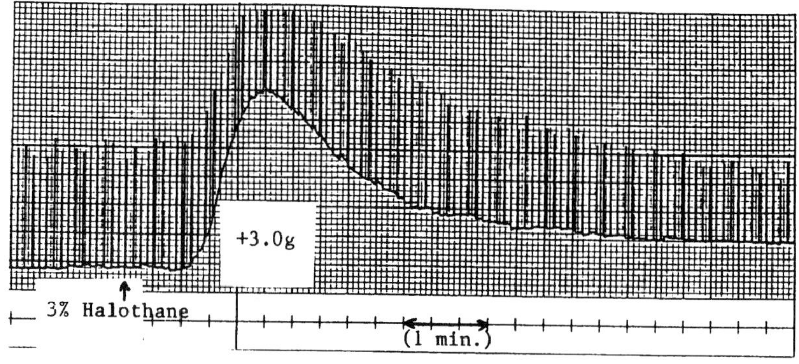

Abnormal Halothane Contracture

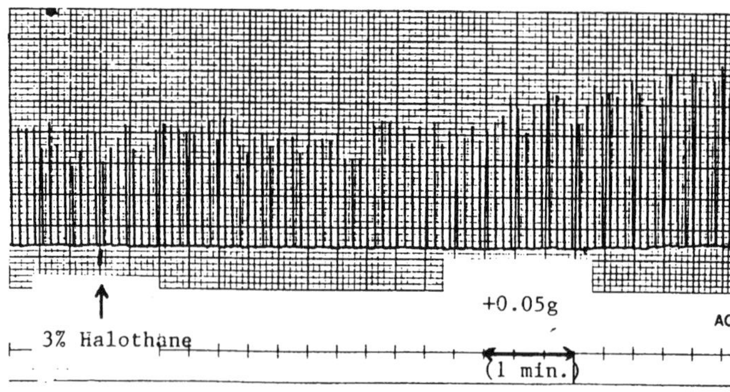

A Normal Halothane Contracture

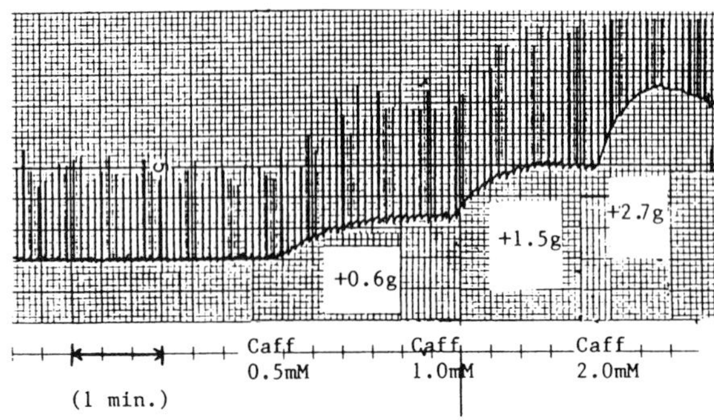

Abnormal Caffeine Dose Response

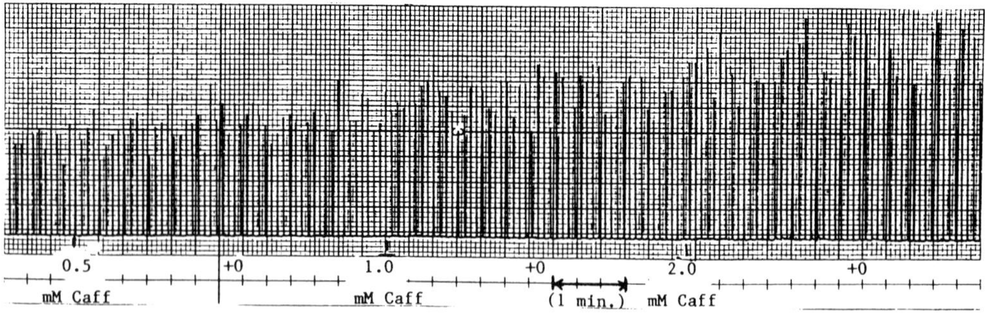

B Normal Caffeine Dose Response

FIGURE 20-2. Muscle strips weighing approximately 150 mg and stimulated supramaximally are exposed to 3% halothane or incremental doses of caffeine. **A.** A 3-g contracture is recorded from this strip from an MHS patient after exposure of the muscle to 3% halothane (*top*); a normal response to 3% halothane (*bottom*). **B.** Contractures noted after exposure to 0.5, 1, and 2 m*M* caffeine in MHS muscle (*top*); no contracture response to the same caffeine concentrations. Twitch height augmentation is normal following caffeine addition (*bottom*).

TABLE 20-2

CRITERIA USED IN THE MH CLINICAL GRADING SCALE

Process I: Muscle Rigidity	
Generalized Rigidity	15
Masseter Rigidity	15
Process II: Myonecrosis	
Elevated CK>20,000 (+Succ.)	15
Elevated CK>10,000 (No Succ.)	15
Cola Colored Urine	10
Myoglobin in urine >60 ug/L	5
Blood/plasma/serum K>6 mEg/L	3
Process III: Respiratory Acidosis	
$PetCO_2$>55 with CV	15
$PaCO_2$>60 with CV	15
$PetCO_2$>60 with SV	15
Inappropriate hypercarbia	15
Inappropriate tachypnea	10
Process IV: Temperature Increase	
Rapid increase in temperature	15
Inappropriate temperature >38.8 in perioperative period	10
Process V: Cardiac Involvement	
Inappropriate tachycardia	3
V. tach or V. fib	3

See Larach et al[71] for full details of this scoring system. Briefly, a case may receive 15 points for the worst presentation in five of the first six categories. A sum of more than 50 points is termed "D6," almost certainly a case of MH. A sum of 35 to 49 points is "D5," very likely to be a case of MH.

and essential for the continuing evaluation of the sensitivity and specificity of the contracture test and for study of the genetics of MH.

There have been a few reports describing patients who were diagnosed as nonsusceptible by contracture testing subsequently experiencing clinical episodes highly suggestive of MH; and in one case, the estimated false-negative rate was 4 out of 171 subjects (2%).[72,73] MH experts are not convinced that these are valid cases of MH. A mimic of MH such as sepsis may explain the clinical problem.[73] In contrast, studies have reported 16 MHN patients receiving triggering agents on 23 occasions[74] and 13 MHN patients receiving triggering agents on 26 occasions,[75] all without complications. Unfortunately, studies like these are difficult to conduct because they require large patient populations and tracking of subjects diagnosed several years before the actual study. Until more data are gathered, it is difficult to put the occasional false-negative diagnosis into proper perspective.

Variability seems to exist between families in the magnitude of contracture.[76] This may be because of the inheritance of different genetic defects. Until such time as all the basic biochemical defects of MH are uncovered, the contracture test will be subject to some differences in interpretation. However, the halothane–caffeine contracture test is currently the only method of MH diagnosis that has been standardized and has had sensitivity and specificity confirmed in any manner by multiple centers throughout the world. When a patient is diagnosed as MHS by the contracture test, then MH trigger agents are to be avoided. IF the patient is MHN, then volatile agents may be used.

Tests with More Limited Usefulness in Malignant Hyperthermia Diagnosis

Alternative tests that have not gained acceptance within the EMHG or NAMHG have been reviewed elsewhere.[77,78] These tests include lymphocyte tests, platelet aggregation, skinned fiber tests, adenosine triphosphate depletion, erythrocyte osmotic fragility, and others. The tests discussed later have at least some usefulness in some cases of MH.

Elevated resting CK values are associated with MH susceptibility in a few families. However, many subjects susceptible to MH do not have elevated CK values, making this method of diagnosis relatively insensitive.[78] Also, several muscle disorders are associated with elevated resting CK values, making this test nonspecific.[78] We caution that this method of diagnosis is only tentative and should be confirmed by contracture testing. Elevated CK values also may be useful in preliminarily identifying key family members to be referred for contracture testing and in identifying MH in children too young to undergo contracture testing.

The use of resting CK values for general screening for MH is neither sensitive nor specific, but there is a relationship between high postoperative CK values associated with masseter muscle rigidity (MMR) and the probability for diagnosis as MH susceptible by the contracture test.[15,22] Although it is not a perfect indicator of MH susceptibility,[79] the chances are about 80% that a CK value >20,000 after MMR will yield a positive diagnosis by contracture testing.[15,22] A relatively normal CK postoperatively does not rule out the possibility of an acute MH reaction during that anesthetic.[80]

A variety of minimally invasive diagnostic tests are in development at present. One utilizes nuclear magnetic resonance spectroscopy to evaluate ATP depletion during graded exercise in vivo. MH patients have a greater breakdown of ATP and creatine phosphate as well as an increase in acid content compared to normals.[81] Utilizing cultured muscle cells[82] or B lymphocytes,[83] it has been shown that agents such as caffeine and chlorocresol will raise intracellular calcium ion concentrations to a greater extent in tissue derived from MHS individuals than normals. Injection of a small amount of caffeine through a microdialysis catheter inserted into muscle will elicit an enhanced release of carbon dioxide locally. Metabolic changes are measured through the catheter.[84,85] Repetitive nerve stimulation produces a different pattern of contraction and relaxation in MHS muscle than in normal muscle.[86,87] All of these tests are still in the developmental stage.

Molecular Genetic Testing for MH Susceptibility

The discovery of multiple MH causing mutations in the RYR1 gene[31,59] has led to the introduction of genetic testing of MH susceptibility on a limited basis in Europe and the US. The guidelines published by the European Malignant Hyperthermia Group suggest that for clinical diagnosis a panel of 23 of the more common RYR1 mutations should be examined. <www.emhg.org> A limitation of genetic testing in the United States is the sensitivity of about 23% when testing for 21 mutations.[87a] Screening of the entire coding region of the RYR1 identifies sequence variants in more than 50% of patients.[87b] Therefore sensitivity of genetic tests will improve as more mutations are identified as causative of MH.

Patients should consider genetic testing if:

1. They have had a positive contracture test.
2. A family member has had a positive contracture test.
3. They have suffered a very likely MH episode but have not had a contracture test.
4. A family member has been found to have a causal mutation.

When a mutation known to be causative for MH is identified in a family member who has had an abnormal contracture response to halothane or caffeine, it is possible to determine MH susceptibility in other members of that family by examination of their RYR1 DNA for that mutation. Those with the mutation are MH susceptible (with high specificity) but those without the mutation cannot be considered MH negative as they may harbor another mutation. The patient cannot be presumed to be MH-negative without negative results on muscle contracture testing.[88] The decision to undergo genetic testing is complex. The pros and cons of testing should be discussed with either an MH expert or a genetic counselor.

Treatment of Malignant Hyperthermia

Malignant hyperthermia is a treatable disorder. All institu-
8 tions in which anesthetic agents are administered should have dantrolene available (36 ampules [720 mg] is recommended) and a management plan.

The Acute Episode

The following steps should be taken immediately when MH is diagnosed:

1. Administration of all inhalation agents and succinylcholine should be discontinued and assistance should be secured. (It is helpful to have a dedicated cart available containing the agents for treatment of MH.)
2. Hyperventilation with 100% oxygen should be instituted at >10 L/min. Oxygen flow should be 10 L/min to hasten purging of residual anesthetic gases. Time should not be wasted in securing another anesthetic machine, but an ambu bag and E-cylinder of oxygen can be used.
3. Assistance should be obtained in mixing dantrolene. The present preparation of dantrolene is poorly soluble. Each vial containing 20 mg should be mixed with 50 mL of bacteriostatic sterile distilled water (not saline solution). It is important to store sterile water in clearly labeled containers of a different size from that used for routine intravenous solutions. It may be helpful to keep a mixing system adjacent. Dantrolene will dissolve faster as temperature of the diluent increases from 20 to 40°C.[89] Intravenous therapy should be started with 2.5 mg/kg with repeat doses as needed. More than 10 mg/kg of dantrolene may be given as dictated by clinical circumstances, however many acute episodes are controlled with 2 to 3 mg/kg. There is 300 mg mannitol with each 20 mg dantrolene. Therefore a bladder catheter should be inserted to facilitate monitoring urine output.
4. Titration of dantrolene and bicarbonate to heart rate, body temperature, and $PaCO_2$ is the best clinical guideline of therapy.
5. In fulminant cases in which significant metabolic acidosis is present, 2 to 4 mEq/kg bicarbonate should be given. Large volumes of fluid may be needed to replace loss into edematous tissues and into the urine.
6. If it is not already available, a capnometer should be obtained so that CO_2 excretion can be documented.
7. Dysrhythmia control usually follows hyperventilation, dantrolene therapy, and correction of acidosis. Calcium channel blockers should not be used in the acute treatment of MH. Verapamil can interact with dantrolene to produce hyperkalemia and myocardial depression.[90,91] Lidocaine can be given safely during an MH crisis.
8. Body temperature elevation should be managed by placing ice packs on the groin and in the axillae and by use of gastric, wound, and rectal lavage. Gastric lavage is the quickest, most practical means for rapid temperature control. Some have recommended peritoneal dialysis and others, cardiopulmonary bypass. Cooling should be stopped when core temperature reaches 38°C to avoid hypothermia.
9. Although arterial blood is useful for assessing acidosis, central mixed venous blood gas determinations (or, if not available, femoral venous blood gas readings) serve as a better guideline for therapy.
10. Hyperkalemia should be managed in the usual fashion with glucose, insulin, bicarbonate, and hyperventilation. If hyperkalemia is associated with significant cardiac effects, calcium chloride, one gram or 10 mg/kg, should be given. During therapy of MH, hypokalemia frequently results. However, potassium replacement should be undertaken very cautiously, if at all, because potassium may retrigger an MH episode.
11. Baseline laboratory tests should include creatinine, coagulation profile, and creatine kinase (CK). CK elevations may not occur for 6 to 12 hours after an MH episode and should be followed as a rough guide to therapy. These tests will serve as a baseline for management of subsequent complications.

Management After the Acute Episode

After the acute episode, the clinician should be concerned about three complications of MH:

1. Recrudescence of MH. As many as 25% of patients may experience acute recrudescence, a relapse, within hours of the first episode.[92,93–95]
2. Disseminated intravascular coagulation (DIC).[94] DIC has often been described in cases of MH, probably resulting from release of thromboplastins secondary to shock and core temperature >41°C[95] and/or release of cellular contents on membrane destruction. The usual regimen for treatment of DIC should be followed.
3. Myoglobinuric renal failure. Myoglobinuria may occur within hours after the episode begins. If analysis shows that there is blood in the urine, urine should be sent to measure RBCs and myoglobin. If there are no RBCs, myoglobinuria is presumed present. If the urine is acid, bicarbonate should be given to decrease the chance that myoglobin will injure renal tubules.

The guidelines for the dose and duration of dantrolene therapy after resolution of acute MH are empirical. It would seem prudent to continue dantrolene, 1 mg/kg every 6 hours intravenously (iv), for at least 24 to 36 hours but more may be given if signs of MH reappear. Some recommend conversion of dantrolene therapy from iv to oral form (4 mg/kg per day or more) with continuation for several days.

Significant muscle weakness and pain may follow MH, resulting from muscle destruction along with dantrolene administration; this should be managed symptomatically. Recovery of strength may require weeks to months.

A variety of other electrolyte changes may occur, such as hypocalcemia and hyperphosphatemia. Sodium and chloride changes may occur secondary to fluid shifts during the acute episode. All these changes usually respond to control of the acute episode.

Dantrolene

Dantrolene sodium is a hydantoin derivative (1-[[[5-(4-nitrophenyl)-2-furanyl]methylene]imino]-2,4-imidazolidinedione). In 1979, iv dantrolene was approved for treatment of MH. Until that time, the primary use of dantrolene was in the management of spasticity. Dantrolene is a unique muscle relaxant. Unlike neuromuscular blocking agents (whose site of action is at the nicotinic receptor of the neuromuscular junction) or the nonspecific relaxants (which modulate spinal cord synaptic reflexes), dantrolene acts within the muscle cell itself by reducing calcium release by the sarcoplasmic reticulum. $[^3H]$azidodantrolene, a pharmacologically active, photoaffinity analog of dantrolene, specifically binds to a site on the ryandodine receptor.[96,97] During an MH episode, dantrolene reduces intracellular calcium levels. Therefore, dantrolene is a specific and effective agent in the treatment of MH. In the usual clinical doses, dantrolene has little effect on myocardial contractility.[98]

Studies have also indicated that doses of neuromuscular blocking agents need not be changed significantly after dantrolene administration. However, the drug should be used cautiously in patients with neuromuscular disease.[99]

The serum level of dantrolene required for prophylaxis against MH is about 2.5 μg/mL. The half-life of iv dantrolene, the only form recommended, is approximately 12 hours. However, the therapeutic level of dantrolene usually persists for 4 to 6 hours after a usual iv dose of 2.5 mg/kg.[100] Therefore, dantrolene should be supplemented at least every 6 hours after a clinical episode. Muscle weakness may persist for 24 hours after dantrolene therapy is discontinued. Nausea and phlebitis are other complications of acute dantrolene administration. Hepatotoxicity has been demonstrated only with long-term use of oral dantrolene. Prophylaxis for MH should be carried out with iv or oral dantrolene (5 mg/kg per 24 hours) in those *rare* situations where prophylaxis is desired.[101]

Management of the Patient Susceptible to Malignant Hyperthermia

Because of an increasing awareness of MH and more widespread use of diagnostic tests, it is not unusual for an anesthesiologist to be confronted with a MH-susceptible patient or a patient who has a family history of MH. The management of such patients should be carefully planned.

In the preoperative interview, the anesthesiologist should try to obtain sufficient information regarding previous episodes of MH and their documentation. If the family has participated in the North American Malignant Hyperthermia Registry, the Registry may be able to give details to the anesthesia provider. The anesthesiologist should allow adequate time to reassure patients and their families that he or she is familiar with MH and its implications and that appropriate monitoring and therapy will be instituted as necessary. It may be worth mentioning that there have been no deaths from MH in previously diagnosed MH-susceptible patients when the anesthesia team was aware of the problem. Anesthesia and premedication should be designed to produce a low normal heart rate. Standard premedicant drugs such as opioids, benzodiazepines, ataractics, barbiturates, antihistamines, and anticholinergics do not cause problems in MH-susceptible patients when administered in appropriate doses; however, phenothiazines are not recommended. Dantrolene need not be given preoperatively if nontriggering agents are used and end-tidal CO_2 and core temperature are monitored. Dantrolene must be immediately available in the operating room, and equipment for rapid measurement of blood gases and electrolytes should be available.

The anesthesia machine is prepared by draining, removing, or disabling anesthetic vaporizers, and changing tubing and CO_2 absorbent and flowing oxygen at 10 L/min for 20 minutes.[102] The modern anesthesia workstation is larger than older anesthesia machines and requires 30 minutes to flush out with 10 L/min at 1 L tidal volume, if new breathing hoses, bag, and soda lime cartridge have been placed.[103] Obviously, iced solutions and adequate supplies of dantrolene must be available in the vicinity of the operating room when MH-susceptible patients are anesthetized.

Exhaled CO_2 should be monitored because the earliest sign of MH is an increase in CO_2 production and excretion.[104] Arterial and central venous monitoring is recommended for MH-susceptible patients, as dictated by the surgical procedure. Body core temperature should be monitored by nasopharyngeal, rectal, or esophageal routes in all patients for all surgical procedures. Skin temperature, although acceptable, is not as desirable because it may not reflect core temperature.[105]

If possible, a regional, local, or major conduction anesthetic should be used with either amide or ester local anesthetics. If not possible, iv induction of anesthesia followed by nitrous oxide, oxygen, and a nondepolarizing relaxant with opioid supplementation is recommended. Induction agents that have not been implicated in MH are midazolam, diazepam, droperidol, and propofol.

Neuromuscular blocking agents such as pancuronium, vecuronium, atracurium, cisatracurium, rocuronium, and mivacurium are safe. Routine reversal of nondepolarizing relaxants with anticholinesterase and anticholinergic agents is recommended.

Many thousands of safe anesthetics have been administered with nitrous oxide in MH-susceptible patients. Two cases have been reported in which early signs of MH have been documented despite the use of a safe anesthetic technique.[106] Therefore, even under the most controlled circumstances, the anesthesiologist should be alert to the early signs of MH.

Administration of dantrolene after surgery is not recommended if there are no signs of MH. However, the patient must be observed closely for 4 to 6 hours. If there is no sign of MH in the first hour postoperatively after safe anesthetic techniques were used, it is very unlikely that MH will occur later. The patient may be discharged on the same day as surgery.[107,108] Complete rehydration with iv fluid and adequate oral intake decreases the chance that fever will occur postdischarge as a result of dehydration.

The same precautions should be taken for the obstetric patient as for the routine surgical patient. Evidence that the stress of labor may precipitate MH is not convincing, and well-conducted epidural anesthesia for labor and delivery without dantrolene pretreatment but with careful monitoring of vital signs is recommended. If an emergency cesarean section with general anesthesia is necessary, alternatives to succinylcholine should be used. The maternal:fetal partition ratio for dantrolene is probably 0.4.[109] Dantrolene has not been reported to produce significant problems for the fetus or newborn, but existing data are very scanty.

Malignant Hyperthermia in Species Other Than Pigs and People

Malignant hyperthermia has been reported sporadically in many species. Clinical episodes have been documented in cats, dogs, and horses.[110] Capture myopathy is a syndrome characterized by temperature elevation, rhabdomyolysis, acidosis, and death in wild animals (e.g., zebra, elk).[111] This also has been suggested to be an MH variant.

Medicolegal Aspects

In this era of malpractice actions, it is not surprising that MH cases have been the subject of malpractice suits. Because MH may be considered an inborn genetic problem with a relatively fixed associated mortality that may go unrecognized before a patient's exposure to triggering agents, it may be used as a "cover" for other problems.

Fever, opisthotonic posturing, and neurologic abnormalities may accompany hypoxic brain injury, and because of their similarity to MH, MH may be incorrectly implicated in the differential diagnosis. Furthermore, after cardiac arrest from any cause, CK and potassium levels may be significantly elevated. The incidence of litigation after the occurrence of MH is unknown.

Some have stated that, with the advent of dantrolene, there should be no deaths from MH. This is unrealistic because the syndrome may be truly explosive in some cases and impossible to control with current therapy. Also, all the factors that lead to MH are not known. The dose of dantrolene needed to prevent recrudescence cannot be determined with certainty. Nevertheless, certain common themes underlie the basis for litigation in MH:

9
1. Failure to obtain a thorough personal history in regard to anesthetic problems and a family history of any unexplained perioperative problems.
2. Failure to monitor core temperature continuously with an electronic temperature monitoring device. Several jury trial cases have been lost by the defense because the patient's temperature was not monitored. Intraoperative temperature monitoring is now considered a "standard of care" in the United States by the legal profession, despite the failure of the American Society of Anesthesiologists to recommend routine temperature monitoring during administration of all general anesthetics.
3. Failure to have adequate supplies of dantrolene on hand with a plan of management of MH.
4. Failure to investigate unexplained increases in body temperature and increased skeletal muscle tone (especially after succinylcholine administration) when associated with increased heart rate and dysrhythmias.

Several examples of medicolegal cases involving these principles are described below:

1. A young female patient had shoulder surgery with isoflurane–nitrous oxide–oxygen. Temperature was not monitored continuously. At the end of the procedure, premature ventricular beats and increasing end-tidal carbon dioxide were noted. The patient had a cardiac arrest as the dysrhythmia was being treated. As the drapes were being removed, the patient felt warm. A temperature probe revealed a reading of nearly 42°C. The patient was diagnosed as having an acute episode of MH. Dantrolene was administered an hour later. The patient developed DIC over the next day and died. The case was settled out of court.
2. A 26-year-old woman was undergoing a breast augmentation in a plastic surgeon's office using general anesthesia with isoflurane. Toward the end of the procedure, her heart rate increased as did end-tidal carbon dioxide and skin temperature. Dantrolene was not available and the patient was sent to a nearby emergency room. By the time dantrolene was given, her temperature was about 43°C. She developed DIC and died. The case was settled without jury trial. The company providing insurance for the physician now mandates that dantrolene be immediately available wherever general anesthesia is administered.
3. Symptoms of bowel obstruction developed in a middle-aged man. He was taken to a local hospital, and anesthesia was administered with nitrous oxide–oxygen–halothane and succinylcholine. His temperature was not monitored, but an unexplained tachycardia (140 to 160 beats/min) was present throughout the 2-hour procedure. On arrival in the intensive care unit after the operation, the patient was slightly hypotensive. Invasive monitoring was started. Despite marked metabolic and respiratory acidosis, a Pa_{CO_2} of 100 mm Hg, and a recorded temperature of nearly 42°C, MH was not diagnosed. A cooling blanket and antibiotics failed to arrest the decrease in the patient's blood pressure, which eventually led to cardiac arrest. A judgment against the physicians and hospital of $4.5 million was reached.

There have been several malpractice cases filed against anesthesiologists in which cardiac arrest and death occurred after succinylcholine was used in patients with an undiagnosed myopathy. The usual outcome is an out-of-court settlement.

The message is clear. All facilities where general anesthesia is administered (including hospitals, outpatient surgery centers, physician offices, and dental offices) should have a full supply of dantrolene available. All patients undergoing general anesthesia should have standard monitoring, including end-tidal carbon dioxide and, except for brief cases, body temperature.

Patient Support Services

To answer the needs of patients and families who wished to learn more about MH and of those families whose relatives have died from MH, support groups were founded in several countries (e.g., the Malignant Hyperthermia Association [of Canada] and the Malignant Hyperthermia Association of the United States [MHAUS]). Both groups serve as a repository of information about MH, provide names of physicians knowledgeable about MH and the location of MH diagnostic centers, and simply lend an ear to those with MH who have questions. Both organizations have an advisory committee of physicians. The Malignant Hyperthermia Association of the United States publishes a quarterly newsletter, *The Communicator,* with excerpts from the medical literature, explanatory articles, questions and answers, and related information. In addition MHAUS organized two hotlines so that a health care provider with an urgent question about MH or NMS can be placed in contact with a knowledgeable volunteer specialist. Approximately 30 to 40 calls a month are handled by the MH Hotline, 1-800-644-9737, and a smaller number by the Neurolept Malignant Syndrome Information Service (NMSIS).

The address of the Malignant Hyperthermia Association of the United States is 11E State Street, Box 1069, Sherburne, New York, 13460-1069, FAX 607-674-7910. The phone number is 1-800-98MHAUS. The hotline number is 1-800-MHHyper. The Web site address is http://www.mhaus.org.

In 1989, the North American MH Registry was formed. Now based in Pittsburgh, Pennsylvania (Children's Hospital of Pittsburgh, 412-692-5464), the Registry is the repository for patient and family specific information for MH-susceptible patients. MH susceptible patients are invited to contact the Registry. If an MHS individual wishes to join the Registry, he or she must complete a questionnaire and sign a consent form. The Registry was merged with MHAUS in 1995. A description of the Registry is available at www.anesth.upmc.edu. The forms used in the Registry can be reviewed at www.mhreg.org.

Pathogenesis and Etiology

Several major developments have contributed to the present
10 understanding of the complex pathophysiology of MH. The first was the recognition that the syndrome is genetically transmitted.[2] This finding is significant because it suggests that a rigorous application of modern molecular genetics will lead to the identification of mutations in specific proteins causing the disorder. A second finding was a greater sensitivity of biopsied skeletal muscle from MH-susceptible patients to halothane or caffeine. This was the basis for an in vitro diagnostic test and studies of the mechanisms underlying MH. The third was the recognition of similarities between human MH and porcine stress syndrome. This animal model was used to elucidate the role of altered Ca^{2+} regulation in MH and led to the finding that a mutation in the ryanodine receptor may be a causative factor in many families with MH.[112] Fourth, MH has

been identified as a heterogeneous disorder.[31,59] Heterogeneity may account for some variability in presentation and forces investigators to consider the role of a final common pathway resulting from a mutation in any one of several different proteins. Fifth, the finding that pigs or human subjects with MH do not always trigger in response to adequate triggering agents, has suggested that modulators influence the expression of the syndrome.[113,114]

Experimental Models for Malignant Hyperthermia

Although MH is rare in humans, breeding pigs for leaner meat and better musculature has resulted in the appearance of the MH gene in a relatively high frequency in a number of herds (e.g., Poland, China, Landrace, Pietrain). A syndrome in pigs undergoing anesthesia is similar to the MH syndrome in humans. However, the porcine syndrome can also be elicited in the absence of anesthetics, by factors such as heat and stress. Although pigs administered MH-triggering anesthetics have provided a model for human MH, there is little evidence that a human stress syndrome analogous to PSS exists in the majority of patients. However, there is a weak association between exertional heat stroke and MH.[115–117] A single genetic defect in the ryanodine receptor has been associated with porcine MH, and this specific mutation is found in some humans with MH. The mode of inheritance in swine (autosomal recessive) is different from that in humans (autosomal dominant). The porcine model has been extensively exploited in studies of MH. Reports of MH exist, but are rare, in horses, dogs, and cats. Of these, only the dog has been proposed as a model of human MH.[118] The pattern of inheritance in the dog appears to be autosomal dominant, yet there are some differences between the anesthesia-elicited canine and human MH syndromes.

Understanding the Malignant Hyperthermia Defect: Necessary Concepts

A hypothesis explaining MH must account for the puzzling clinical observations surrounding this disorder. Most importantly, the large majority of these patients function normally in the absence of anesthetics. Therefore, the defect should not significantly interfere with normal muscle physiology. The defect, at least in humans, appears to be expressed significantly only in skeletal muscle. The expression of the syndrome shows a large variability among individuals. For example, 30% of patients have had up to three uneventful anesthetics.[57,119] A spectrum of presentations can occur, ranging from relatively minor intraoperative complications to rapid temperature rise, muscle rigidity, acidosis, dysrhythmias, and death. Some cases have a greater latency to onset and are not made manifest until several hours postoperatively. MH does not always occur in response to triggering agents. This is a well-established observation in human MH and similar observations have been reported in swine. Also, while most investigators would agree that PSS is a more consistently triggered syndrome than the human MH syndrome, even adult swine occasionally do not respond to adequate triggering agents in either a barnyard challenge with halothane alone[120] or prolonged halothane,[121] or halothane and succinylcholine challenge.[11] The term "MH" may, in fact, be a misnomer, as sometimes patients show no signs of temperature elevation. Finally, many cases do not exhibit rigidity. The large variability among individuals may be explained by different genes causing MH in different families or by other predisposing factors being expressed differently in different patients or families.[76] The function of many different proteins has been reported to be altered in MH skeletal muscle. Thus, it is reasonable to assume that systems other than those directly involved in Ca^{2+} regulation are secondarily altered in MH and these may play a crucial role in modifying the response to triggering agents. The involvement of secondary systems would explain the high variability in the phenotype.

Skeletal Muscle: Site of the Malignant Hyperthermia Defect

The MH and PSS defects are expressed in skeletal muscle, as evidenced by the in vitro contracture test for MH susceptibility. Results regarding other tissues are more controversial, especially in humans, and are not considered in detail in this chapter. The defects are expressed in type I and type II fibers.[122] While the distributions and amounts of protein in whole skeletal muscle and in isolated sarcoplasmic reticulum appear to be normal by electrophoretic analysis, downregulation of specific proteins, including the ryanodine receptor[123] and dihydropyridine receptor,[124] has been reported. Additionally, the expression of subtypes of the sodium channel is altered in MH muscle.[125–127]

Altered Calcium Regulation: The Common Final Pathway

Ultimately, the main problem in skeletal muscle is a lack of control of myoplasmic Ca^{2+} concentration during anesthesia,[6,128] which may be manifest clinically as muscle rigidity. Ca^{2+} levels are controlled by a complex interaction of Ca^{2+} release from the terminal cisternae, the adenosine triphosphate–driven Ca^{2+} pumps at the sarcoplasmic reticulum and sarcolemma, Na^+/Ca^{2+} exchange, several Ca^{2+} buffering proteins (calsequestrin, parvalbumin), and mitochondrial Ca^{2+} regulation (Fig. 20-3). Although several of these systems may become involved as the MH syndrome progresses, the difficulty in Ca^{2+} regulation appears to originate in the Ca^{2+} release mechanism in the terminal cisternae. The Ca^{2+} release mechanism could be made sensitive to anesthetics by any of several possibilities, including a mutation in the skeletal muscle calcium release channel, termed the ryanodine receptor (*RYR*1); a protein directly coupled to *RYR*1 (e.g., dihydropyridine receptor); or an altered modulator of *RYR*1 function (e.g., fatty acids). Succinylcholine opens the acetylcholine receptor and depolarizes the muscle membrane by opening the voltage dependent sodium channels, which may have altered function in MH. Depolarization leads to Ca^{2+} release from the sarcoplasmic reticulum. Dantrolene antagonizes Ca^{2+} release from the sarcoplasmic reticulum, lowers elevated intracellular Ca^{2+} levels, and reverses an episode of MH.[6]

Presence or Absence of a Malignant Hyperthermia-Associated Defect Within Skeletal Muscle Organelles: Sarcolemma

The sarcolemma (see Fig. 20-3) maintains the membrane potential of the muscle cell and acts as a permeability barrier to ions, including Na^+, K^+, Cl^-, and Ca^{2+}. Skeletal muscle, in most cases, does not require extracellular Ca^{2+} for nerve or electrically evoked contractility. In contrast, halothane-induced contractures[128,129] and, to a lesser extent (depending on the species), caffeine-induced contractures[128] require extracellular Ca^{2+}. A loss of integrity in the sarcolemma could cause a large influx of Ca^{2+} from the extracellular medium. Also, opening specific Ca^{2+} channels (e.g., dihydropyridine receptors) in the sarcolemma would allow the entry of extracellular Ca^{2+}.

Terminal Cisternae: Ca^{2+} Release. The terminal cisternae of the sarcoplasmic reticulum are the sites of Ca^{2+} sequestration. They are coupled to the t-tubules through the ryanodine receptor and the dihydropyridine receptor (Fig. 20-4; see Fig. 20-3). Several investigators have reported a hypersensitive Ca^{2+}-induced Ca^{2+} release in terminal cisternae preparations from porcine MH muscle.[130–132] Also observed for PSS

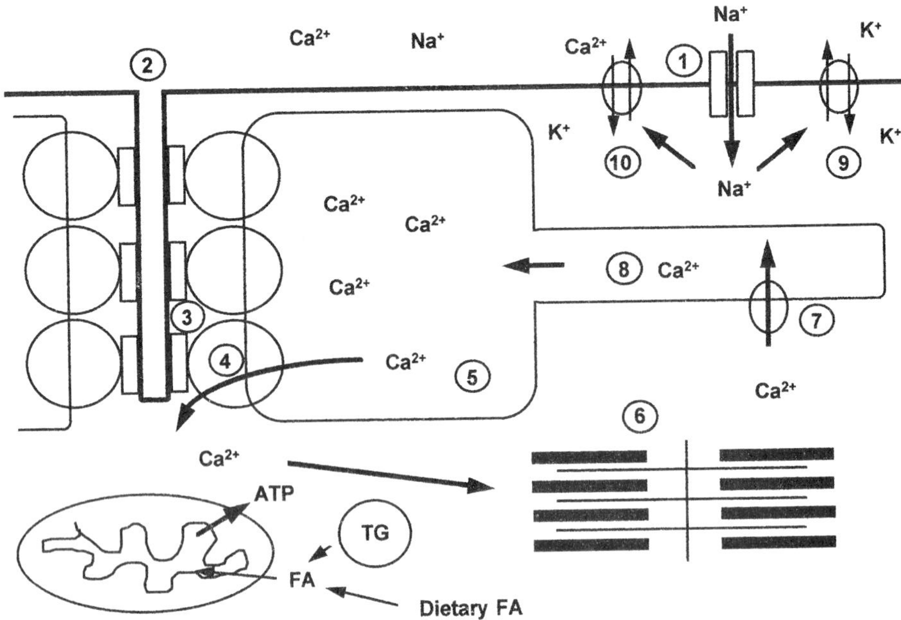

FIGURE 20-3. Excitation–contraction coupling and MH. The action potential generated at the endplate region of the neuromuscular junction is propagated down the sarcolemma (muscle plasma membrane) by the opening of voltage-dependent Na^+ channels (*1*). The action potential continues down into the t-tubules (*2*) to the dihydropyridine receptors (*3*). The dihydropyridine receptors in skeletal muscle function as voltage sensors and are coupled to the Ca^{2+} release channels (*4*). Through this coupled signaling process, the Ca^{2+} release channels are opened, some of the available terminal cisternae Ca^{2+} stores (*5*) are released, and the levels of myoplasmic Ca^{2+} are elevated. The Ca^{2+} then diffuses to the myofibrils (*6*) and interacts with the troponin/tropomyosin complex associated with actin (*thin lines*) and allows interaction of actin with myosin (*thick lines*) for mechanical movement. The Ca^{2+} diffuses away from the myofibrils and this Ca^{2+} signal is terminated by an ATP-driven Ca^{2+} pump (*7*), which pumps Ca^{2+} into the longitudinal sarcoplasmic reticulum (*8*). The Ca^{2+} diffuses from the longitudinal sarcoplasmic reticulum to the terminal cisternae, where it is concentrated for release by Ca^{2+} binding proteins. Na^+ entering during the action potential is subsequently extruded from the cell by the Na^+/K^+-ATPase (*9*) and possibly through Na^+/Ca^{2+} exchange (*10*). This latter process would elevate intracellular Ca^{2+} and could result from delayed inactivation of Na^+ currents. A major form of energy for supplying cellular ATP for the ion pumps and numerous other energy consuming processes is fatty acids (FA) derived from the serum (dietary FA), or from intramuscular triglyceride (TG) stores. Therefore, a defect in the intracellular Ca^{2+} regulating processes (increased Ca^{2+} release or decreased Ca^{2+} uptake), or a defect in the sarcolemma could account for an increase in myoplasmic Ca^{2+}.

Ca^{2+}-induced Ca^{2+} release are an enhanced rate of release from skinned fibers[133] and terminal cisternae preparations.[134,135]

The maximum amount of Ca^{2+} released is normal for PSS vesicles.[136] In the human MH population, the Ca^{2+} release process appears to be less dramatically affected than that in PSS muscle. For example, the threshold of Ca^{2+}-induced Ca^{2+} release in terminal cisternae–containing fractions is not altered in a human MH population.[131,137] Although the alterations in Ca^{2+} release reported in swine cannot be observed in isolated heavy sarcoplasmic reticulum preparations from humans, abnormalities in Ca^{2+} release are observed when preparations containing additional cellular components are examined, such as skinned fiber preparations (Fig. 20-5). MH subjects have a greater than normal rate and hypersensitivity of Ca^{2+}-induced Ca^{2+} release[138] and Ca^{2+} release is hypersensitive to caffeine using the skinned fiber preparation.[139]

With respect to anesthetic action, the rate of halothane induced Ca^{2+} release is abnormally high in PSS susceptibles.[132,140] In contrast, in human MH muscle[141] and PSS muscle,[142] the dose-response curves for halothane-induced Ca^{2+} release are normal when the amount of Ca^{2+} release is monitored. Free calcium was determined (with fura-2) in voltage-clamped human muscle fibers.[143] The kinetics and voltage dependence of calcium release for MH muscle was normal; however, the maximal peak rate of Ca^{2+} release increased about 3-fold. Although resting Ca^{2+} concentrations are normal, human skeletal muscle cell cultures have a 2-fold greater than normal sensitivity to halothane.[144] There is no effect of temperature on the rate of halothane-induced Ca^{2+} release.[140,145]

In heavy sarcoplasmic reticulum preparations (containing triads and sarcoplasmic reticulum), halothane at clinically relevant concentrations cannot induce a sustained net Ca^{2+} release if physiologic levels of adenosine triphosphate and Mg^{2+} are included. This ability to overcome the effects of halothane under approximate physiologic conditions is because of the enormous capacity of the Ca^{2+} pumping system.[137] The addition of fatty acids, even to vesicles isolated from normal muscle, markedly (~20- to 30-fold) decreases the concentration of halothane required for the sustained opening of the Ca^{2+} release channel in the presence of adenosine triphosphate and Mg^{2+}.[137] Under these conditions, fatty acids can cause a sustained Ca^{2+} release at clinical concentrations of halothane. Unlike studies of Ca^{2+} release in the absence of fatty acids,[145] there is an absolute temperature dependence (occurs at 37°C, not at 25°C) of the fatty acid enhancement of halothane-induced Ca^{2+} release, which is consistent with the temperature dependence of halothane-induced contractures of MH muscle.[146]

Mitochondria. Mitochondria oxidize a variety of substrates to generate the form of energy (adenosine triphosphate) most useful for driving cellular reactions. Defects in mitochondrial function do not appear to initiate the MH syndrome. The uncoupling of Ca^{2+}-stimulated, but not adenosine diphosphate-stimulated, mitochondrial succinate

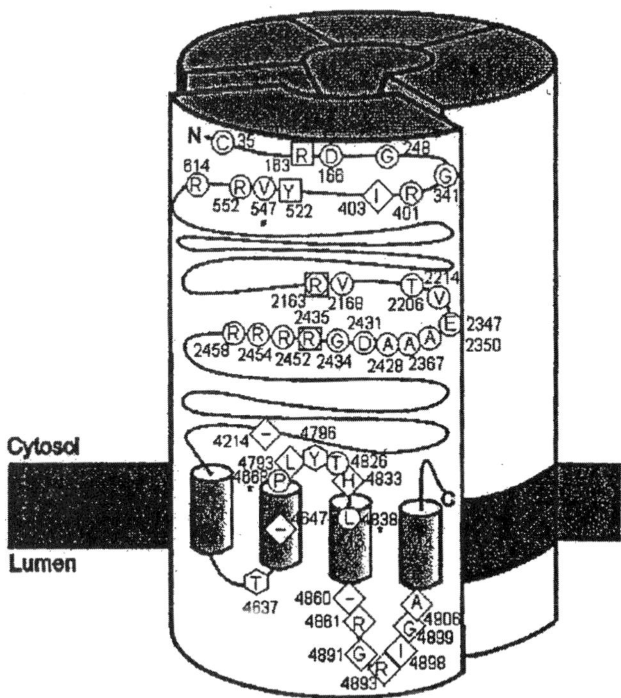

FIGURE 20-4. Schematic illustration of the homotetrameric ryanodine receptor, the calcium release channel situated in the membrane of the sarcoplasmic reticulum (SR). The cytosolic part of the protein complex, the so-called foot, bridges the gap between the transverse tubular system and the SR. Mutations have been described for the skeletal muscle ryanodine receptor (RYR1), which cause susceptibility to malignant hyperthermia (MHS) and central core disease (CCD). (From Lehmann-Horn F, Lerche H, Jurkat-Rott K: Skeletal muscle channelopathies: Myotonias, periodic paralyses and malignant hyperthermia. In Stahlberg E (ed): Clinical Neurophyisology of Disorders of Muscle and Neuromuscular Junction. Handbook of Clinical Neurophysiology, vol 2. Elsevier BV, 2003:476.)

oxidation has been demonstrated in muscle from pigs and humans[147] susceptible to MH.

Longitudinal Sarcoplasmic Reticulum: Ca^{2+} Uptake. The longitudinal sarcoplasmic reticulum (see Fig. 20-3) is primarily involved in removing Ca^{2+} from the myoplasm through the adenosine triphosphate–driven Ca^{2+} pump. While earlier studies had suggested a defect in Ca^{2+} uptake might cause the loss of Ca^{2+} regulation associated with MH, subsequent studies have ruled out a role for the Ca^{2+} pump in causing MH.[140]

Myofibrils. Relatively few studies have been conducted on myofibrils in MH. However, there is apparently no defect in the Ca^{2+} sensitivity of the fast or slow fibers of the contractile system from MH skeletal muscle.

Proteins or Systems Reported Altered in Malignant Hyperthermia Muscle

Calcium Release Channel of Skeletal Muscle

The human skeletal muscle calcium release channel is encoded by a ryanodine receptor type 1 (*RYR*1) gene located on chromosome 19q13.1.[148] There are other types of RYR that exist in cardiac muscle (type 2) and brain (type 3) tissues, respectively. *RYR*1 is the primary conduit through which the sarcoplasmic reticulum stores of Ca^{2+} are released to the sarcoplasm.[112] *RYR*1 is an extremely large homotetramer, having subunits of about 560,000 MW each. *RYR*1 has binding sites for the contracture-inducing plant alkaloid ryanodine[149] and the preservative 4-chloro-*m*-cresol.[150]

In about 50% of MH susceptible families, susceptibility to MH is linked to chromosome 19 and a mutation in *ryr*1.[31,59,151] The hypothesis that mutation in *RYR*1 causes MH susceptibility is supported by physiologic studies showing subtle effects of halothane on isolated *RYR*1 currents in human MH muscle.[152] Halothane can open a hypersensitive *RYR*1, leading to an uncontrolled release of Ca^{2+} into the myoplasm and the MH syndrome. However, the buffering capacity of the Ca^{2+} pump in the presence of adenosine triphosphate is able to sustain normal Ca^{2+} regulation in the presence of halothane in terminal cisternae preparations isolated from MH muscle.[114] These observations are consistent with the observed interindividual variability in human MH and the occurrence of nonrigid MH. When ATP is low the syndrome occurs and the lower the energy stores are, the worse the MH sysndrome is. Unlike the hypersensitive Ca^{2+} release in porcine muscle,[130] Ca^{2+} regulation in human MH heavy sarcoplasmic reticulum fractions appeared to be normal.[131] However, using planar bilayer approaches capable of monitoring single *RYR*1 channels, subtle changes in the function of *RYR*1 have been observed in human MH muscle,[152,153] similar in some respects to those in PSS muscle in planar bilayers.[154] These differences relate primarily to an increased probability of the MH *RYR*1 being in an open state. While differences between normal and PSS susceptibles have been reported in the absence of halothane or caffeine,[154] human MH muscle requires the presence of caffeine[153] or halothane[152] to detect differences in *RYR*1 function. In human MH muscle two populations of ion channels appear to be present: one halothane-insensitive and the other halothane-sensitive.[152] The halothane-sensitive channels have an increased probability of opening in the presence of clinically relevant concentrations of halothane. The halothane-sensitive channels do not occur in muscle from all MH patients, and both types (or states) of channels can coexist in the same muscle biopsy. Whether these subtle differences in *RYR*1 function in planar bilayers, or the differences in K_d of ryanodine binding,[149] in human muscle reflect a different acylation or phosphorylation state of *RYR*1 is not known. Consistent with the altered function of the PSS *RYR*1, there has been a specific mutation identified (Arg^{615} to Cys^{615}) in *RYR*1 in PSS.[155] The mutation is on the cytoplasmic surface of *RYR*1.[156] This mutation accounts for the altered functional states of *RYR*1 and ryanodine binding in PSS swine. However, the porcine mutation does not appear to account directly for the caffeine sensitivity of PSS muscle.[157] In between 2 and 11% of MH families the human equivalent (Arg^{614} to Cys^{614}) to the PSS *RYR*1 mutation has been identified. However, there may be discordance between the presence of this mutation and the outcome of the diagnostic contracture test.[158–160] A major reason for the attenuated effects of the *RYR*1 mutation in human muscle is likely the dominant mode of inheritance with reduced penetrance and genetic heterogeneity of MH versus recessive mutation in the pig. Thus, normal copies of *RYR*1 are expressed in human MH muscle, but not PSS muscle. The number of sequence variants in *RYR*1 reported at scientific meetings to date is more than 200, including Arg614Cys, and this number is constantly rising. The majority of these are usually found in only one or two families.

There is a 2-fold greater than normal sensitivity to halothane in cell cultures from MH muscle.[144] However, a 2-fold increase in sensitivity to triggering agents in cell culture does not equate to the much greater sensitivity of MH muscle to halothane observed in vivo. Transfection of human MH skeletal

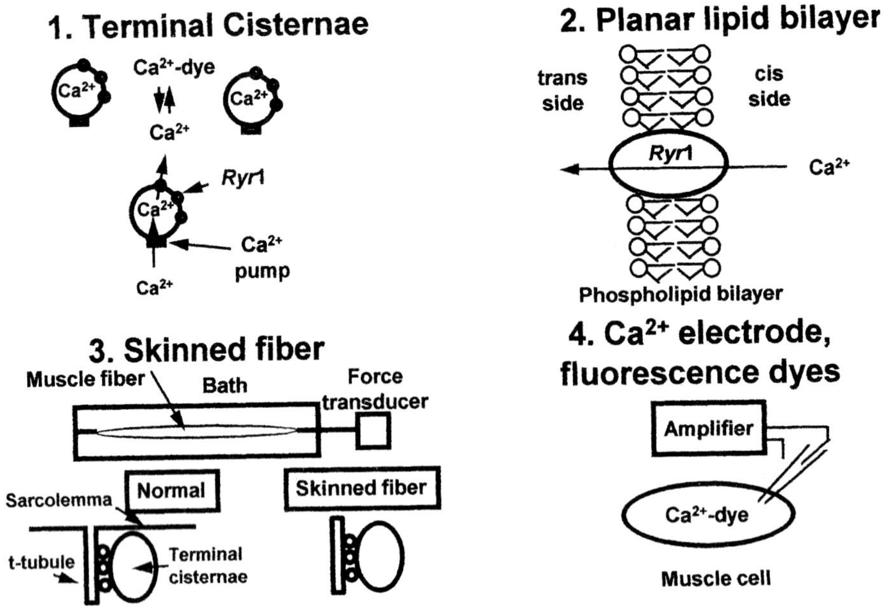

FIGURE 20-5. Methods to examine Ca^{2+} regulation. (*1*) *Terminal cisternae.* Skeletal muscle can be homogenized and resealed portions of the terminal cisternae containing the Ca^{2+} release channel (*RYR*1) can be recovered by a series of centrifugation steps. These vesicles can take up Ca^{2+} from the bathing medium by means of the ATP-driven Ca^{2+} pump and can subsequently release Ca^{2+} by opening of *RYR*1. Ca^{2+} levels in the extravesicular medium can be monitored spectrophotometrically by a number of dyes (usually metalochrome indicators such as arsenazo III or antipyrylazo III). Alternatively, $^{45}Ca^{2+}$ and filtration of the vesicles can be used. The amount of calcium released is usually determined by the decrease in radioactivity retained on the filters that contain the vesicles. Both the spectrophotometric and radioisotopic approaches allow monitoring of Ca^{2+} uptake and Ca^{2+} release, and these processes can be dissociated pharmacologically with the *RYR*1 blocker, ruthenium red. The terminal cisternae method allows the overall response of a large population of channels to be examined and may best reflect the overall responsiveness of the muscle. (*2*) *Planar lipid bilayers.* It is possible to incorporate *RYR*1 into artificial lipid bilayers (i.e., planar lipid bilayer) and monitor the Ca^{2+} current as electrical charge movement through one to several channels at a time. Although this method can provide very useful, detailed information on the opening and closing of individual *RYR*1s, it does not provide an indication of the overall responsiveness of the muscle in which both Ca^{2+} uptake and Ca^{2+} release are participating and in which many modulating substances are present. (*3*) *Skinned fibers.* A third approach involves skinned fiber preparations in which the sarcolemma is either removed mechanically or made permeable chemically, and the function of the sarcoplasmic reticulum (Ca^{2+} uptake and release) and myofibrils (actin and myosin) monitored by the contractile response of the fiber. This preparation has an interesting advantage in that type I and type II fibers can be distinguished. Also, the t-tubules seal completely, allowing the function of the dihydropyridine receptors and Na^+ channels to be examined. This method only examines one muscle fiber at a time, which might be a slight disadvantage in MH or PSS skeletal muscle, because the defect is not uniformly expressed throughout the tissue. (*4*) Ca^{2+} *electrodes and fluorescence dyes.* The cytoplasmic Ca^{2+} levels can be monitored in intact muscle either with fluorescence dyes or Ca^{2+} electrodes. The former can monitor a muscle mass, while the latter examines individual fibers. Both approaches can be used with muscle fibers or cell culture systems.

muscle cell cultures with normal (wild-type) *RYR*1 does not result in the MH-negative phenotype (judged by sensitivity of Ca^{2+} transients to halothane), whereas expression of a mutated *ryr*1 (Arg^{163} to Cys^{163}) in normal muscle cells causes hypersensitivity to halothane.[144] Transfection of nonmuscle cell lines with any one of 19 *RYR*1 mutations increased the sensitivity of the cells to relatively high concentrations of halothane and caffeine.[161,162] Therefore, cell cultures can be useful models for elucidating the mechanisms by which MH mutations enhance the sensitivity of muscle to triggering agents.

In summary, there are physiologic, biochemical, pharmacologic, and molecular genetic data supporting a mutation in *RYR*1 as an important factor, and perhaps an initiating factor, in about 50% of the families with MH. The effects of the altered *RYR*1 function on Ca^{2+} regulation determined in vitro are not as pronounced in humans as in swine, possibly owing to the dominant mode of inheritance and genetic heterogeneity of MH in humans. It is highly probable that other systems come into play as modulators of the MH response. This may better explain the extreme intra- and interindividual variability in the human MH syndrome, which is in contrast to the more consistent response in MH swine.

Sodium Channel

Skeletal and cardiac muscle sodium channels are composed of two subunits (α, 220,000 MW; β, 40,000 MW). The α subunit forms the ion pore, allowing Na^+ to enter the cell, and the smaller β subunit can modify the kinetics of the ion flux.[163,164] Sodium channels in skeletal muscle are of two, and possibly three,[127] subtypes. These subtypes can be differentiated by their sensitivity to tetrodotoxin (TTX), a toxin from the puffer fish that blocks the channel pore. The adult sodium channel (SKM1) is 90% blocked by a 100 n*M* concentration of TTX. The "embryonic" sodium channel (SKM2) in skeletal muscle is identical to the cardiac sodium channel, and is blocked by a 10-μM concentration of TTX in cell culture. A third channel is expressed following denervation, and this subtype is not antagonized by TTX, even at a 100-μM concentration. The adult sodium channel α subunit, encoded on chromosome 17,[163,164] was formerly believed to be the only subtype expressed in normal, mature skeletal muscle. The embryonic sodium channel α subunit appears early in muscle differentiation and is encoded on chromosome 3. Each of the α subunits interacts with the same β subunit (β_1), encoded on chromosome 19.[165] The sodium channels of normal human skeletal muscle (vastus lateralis) are composed of approximately 50% SkM1 and 50% SkM2.[127] Specific mutations in the α subunit of SkM1 have been implicated as the cause of other disorders of skeletal muscle, including the myotonic form of hyperkalemic periodic paralysis,[164,166] paramyotonia congenita,[167] and myotonia fluctuans.[168] These disorders are well known to exhibit masseter muscle rigidity and whole body rigidity to agents associated with the MH syndrome,[169] although they lack the signs of acidosis characteristic of MH.

Altered sodium channel function may play a role in the expression of MH. The function of the sodium channel is abnormal in primary cultures of human MH skeletal muscle.[170] There are two populations of sodium currents separated by their kinetics of inactivation (i.e., closing of the channel). These are the normally inactivating and delayed inactivating fast sodium currents. There is a greater proportion of the slow inactivation of the Na^+ current in cultured human MH muscle[125] that would keep the sodium current active for a longer time (delayed inactivation). The consequence of this prolonged sodium current in MH muscle is a longer membrane depolarization and increased period of Ca^{2+} release from the terminal cisternae. A toxin from the sea anemone (ATX II) causing delayed inactivation of the sodium current, as found in human MH muscle cultures, enhances the response of normal muscle to halothane, caffeine, and ryanodine.[171] This finding supports a role for altered Na^+ channel currents in the response of MH muscle to triggering agents. Veratridine, also a sodium channel inhibitor, enhances the response of MH muscle to halothane.[173] Therefore, altered Na^+ currents may be important for at least some of the signs associated with MH. Those patients expressing sodium channel abnormalities may be more likely to exhibit certain signs, such as muscle rigidity.

The expression of sodium channel subtypes is also altered in MH skeletal muscle. SkM2 (embryonic form) appears to be downregulated in MH, in cell culture systems, or in biopsies of vastus lateralis muscle.[126] This would lead to a predominance of SkM1 in MH muscle. SkM1 is more sensitive to halothane than SkM2.[173] There also is evidence for linkage of MH to chromosome 17[174,175] at or near the locus encoding the Na^+ channel α subunit.[176] In one family, a Gly1306Ala mutation in the sodium channel known to cause myotonia fluctuans cosegregated with MH susceptibility, as determined by contracture testing.[34] Two of these patients had whole body rigidity and/or masseter muscle rigidity to succinylcholine, although without metabolic acidosis. As with *RYR*1, it is not clear in most cases if the altered function reflects a primary defect in the Na^+ channel protein, or if the function is altered indirectly by processes such as phosphorylation or acylation.[177]

In summary, changes in sodium channel expression or function could be the result of mutations within a sodium channel subtype, or a secondary effect of a primary mutation in another protein (e.g., *RYR*1). Also, second-messenger systems, such as fatty acids, may play a role in altered sodium channel function and expression. These changes in sodium channel function may be essential for the phenotypic expression of certain aspects of the MH syndrome, such as muscle rigidity.

Elevated Fatty Acid Production

Lipids are an important component of a cell, as they provide energy and structure (e.g., membranes) and participate in function. Several lipid metabolites, including fatty acids, serve second-messenger functions.[178] Fatty acids are the major source of energy in the resting state of skeletal muscle and can also contribute up to 65% of the energy during exercise.[179] Fatty acids provide about 70% of the energy in resting muscle. Therefore, fatty acid utilization is likely upregulated in MH muscle to compensate for the energy consumed by the adenosine triphosphatases attempting to maintain Na^+ and Ca^{2+} homeostasis.

In addition to existing in a free form, fatty acids are esterified to phospholipids, triacylglycerides, diacylglycerides, monoacylglycerides, cholesterol esters, and many proteins. Free fatty acids are maintained at very low levels in a cell (since they are not only essential, but very toxic) and most of the "free" fatty acids actually are bound to fatty acid–binding proteins.[180]

Fatty acid production is elevated in mitochondrial fractions[147] and whole muscle homogenates from PSS and MH susceptibles. There is an age-related increase in fatty acid production in skeletal muscle that parallels an age-related increase in susceptibility to the PSS.[181] When only static levels of free fatty acids are examined, they are at normal levels in human MH and PSS muscle. However, the flux of fatty acids through β-oxidation can still be increased to a large extent in MH muscle without increasing the levels of free fatty acids. The fatty acid flux is derived from triacylglycerides, and this likely accounts for the low levels of triacylglycerides (or total neutral lipid) in biopsied MH or PSS skeletal muscle.[138] The effects of fatty acids on Ca^{2+} release from skeletal muscle sarcoplasmic reticulum are significant, but not dramatic, in the absence of anesthetics,[182,183] and they are not mediated through *RYR*1.[184] However, the fatty acids act in synergy with halothane and decrease the amount of halothane required for sustained Ca^{2+} release by 20- to 30-fold![114,131] This fatty acid enhancement of halothane-induced Ca^{2+} release, in contrast with all other studies of Ca^{2+} release, exhibits the same temperature dependence (i.e., it occurs only at 37°C, not at 25°C) as halothane-induced contractures of skeletal muscle and is mediated through *RYR*1.[114] While the concentration of fatty acid required for this effect exceeds that of the normal unbound form, halothane can displace fatty acids from fatty acid–binding proteins.[185] Therefore, it is highly likely that sufficient concentrations of fatty acids could be achieved at the site of halothane action. If the production of free fatty acids is sustained by accelerated triacylglyceride breakdown and the fatty acids are shunted toward acylation of *RYR*1 and the sodium channel, then this could lead to greatly elevated myoplasmic Ca^{2+} levels. In the case of *RYR*1, this would lead to a greater sensitivity to halothane.

Phospholipase C and Inositol 1,4,5-Trisphosphate

One specific metabolite of phospholipase C action, IP_3, has been demonstrated to be elevated in human MH[186] and PSS[187] muscle, but not in MH human blood specimens.[186] This product of the hydrolysis of the phospholipid, phosphatidylinositol 4,5-bisphosphate, causes Ca^{2+} release from intracellular stores.[188] The elevation of all products of phosphatidylinositol hydrolysis is observed,[188] and this suggests that phospholipase C activity may be elevated in MH. Activation of phospholipase C in skeletal muscle also elevates diacylglycerol and indirectly elevates free fatty acids by deacylation of the diacylglycerol. Diacylglycerol and fatty acids have diverse cell signaling effects.[178,189] In addition to elevated IP_3 production, MH muscle is also hypersensitive to IP_3.[190] Therefore, secondary involvement of this system could have multiple effects that together increase the sensitivity of Ca^{2+} release.

Molecular Biology of Malignant Hyperthermia

The identification of the porcine mutation causing PSS and the location of the human RYR1 gene on chromosome 19q13.1 has helped to establish a direct link of this gene to MH.[148,191] RYR1 was proposed as a candidate gene for MH and the "pig" mutation Arg614Cys was identified in an MH family subsequently.[155] Further genetic linkage studies and research on mutations in RYR1 have revealed that MH is characterized by genetic heterogeneity. About 50% of MH families are linked to RYR1. RYR1 is one of the largest human genes. It contains 106 exons that are transcribed into a 15,364 nucleotide mRNA. Transcription occurs practically only in skeletal muscle level. More than 200 different sequence variants have been identified in the RYR1 gene. The majority are clustered in three regions: the N-terminal region between codons 34 and 614, the central region between codons 2163 and 2458 and the C-terminal region between codons 4136 and 4973.[31,59,192,193] This preferential localization raised speculations concerning the specific role of these regions. The central region is close to the region where the protein would interact with the regulatory protein, FKBP12, and the dihydropyridine receptor, a voltage sensor of RYR1. The C-terminal region that corresponds to the transmembrane domain of the protein.[192] The pathogenic character of many RYR1 gene mutations has been studied by kinetic measures of intracellular calcium release in response to caffeine or halothane with use of different cell lines.[161,162,194,195] Sei and colleagues have demonstrated the presence of calcium channels similar to those found in skeletal muscle in the B lymphocyte. Enhanced intracellular calcium levels are found in lymphocytes from cell lines with mutated ryanodine genes upon exposure to caffeine or chlorocresol.[196,197]

The phenotype and genotype correlation studies are very limited in MH because it is difficult to establish correlation between the mutation and contractile data because of variables among diagnostic laboratories and because of the fact that clinical episodes of MHS that fulfill all criteria are rare as a result of successful intervention during anesthetic complications. Nevertheless, the most severe phenotype as a result of RYR1 mutation is central core disease (CCD), characterized by marked hypotonia and muscle weakness. Interestingly, the majority of RYR1 mutations causing CCD are located in the transmembrane region of the protein, suggesting a critical role of this region in Ca^+ regulation. In addition, the mutations causing both MH and CCD (R163C, R2163H, and R2435H) exhibit more severe caffeine and halothane responses than those associated with MH alone.[198]

Genetic studies have identified linkage of five other chromosomal regions to MH, suggesting genetic heterogeneity of the disorder. However, only a single gene has been identified to date. The Arg1086His mutation was identified in the CACNL1A3 gene of a large French MH family. CACNL1A3 codes for the skeletal muscle L-type calcium channel's alpha1 subunit.[199] This voltage-dependant channel is also called the dihydropyridine receptor (DHPR) and serves as a voltage sensor for RYR1. Mutational screening studies, however, indicate that only 1% of MHS families exhibit mutations in the DHPR.

There have been several reports of discordance between segregation of mutations identified in *RYR*1 and the outcome of the in vitro contracture test for MH.[158,159,200] This discordance is relatively rare and the reason for it is unknown. However, a study in swine has demonstrated that there is an excellent correlation between the contracture test outcome and the genetic susceptibility for MH. In human families, specific ryanodine mutations usually correlate extremely well with the in vitro contracture test result. Hence, in a particular family the presence of the familial MH mutation predicts MH susceptibility.[201]

The Future of Research in Malignant Hyperthermia

While molecular genetics has dominated the research in MH in recent years, a deeper understanding of the physiology and biochemistry of the interplay among *RYR*1, the Na^+ channel, and fatty acid metabolism still is needed. DNA-based linkage analyses are no longer pursued to the same extent as in the early 1990s. Instead, the focus of recent molecular genetic studies has been on identifying new mutations in *RYR*1. Further linkage studies are necessary to identify other chromosomes linked to MH. Molecular genetic approaches may be the only hope for a diagnostic blood test. However, at present molecular genetic testing will be most useful for the 50% of MH susceptible families in which a specific proven causative mutation is known to exist.

Summary

Mutations associated with skeletal muscle control of intracellular calcium concentration are causal for most cases of classic MH. Any one of at least six different genes may cause MH, although the exact proteins remain to be identified in some cases. Mutations have been identified in *RYR*1 and in the dihydropyridine receptor gene. A variety of poorly understood biochemical and/or gene expression factors influence the clinical manifestations of MH. For example, mutations in a sodium channel subunit may be associated with some signs of MH, but this clinical MH requires the expression of other factors also. A disturbance in fatty acid metabolism, as a secondary effect, alters the function of several organelles and can lead to a hypersensitive *RYR*1 response to halothane and altered Na^+ channel subunit expression in skeletal muscle. The MH syndrome is the result of a complex and poorly understood interaction among several systems in skeletal muscle.

OTHER INHERITED DISORDERS

Inherited diseases affect every bodily organ and every physiologic and biochemical process. Some are mild and allow a relatively normal life span, whereas others are incompatible with extrauterine existence even for a few days. Adding to the complexity is a natural variability of genetic penetrance and expressivity even in a single family. All of these disorders have as a common feature an abnormality in one or more genes that affects the function of one or more enzymes. The metabolic basis of inherited diseases is the subject of several well-known books,[202] which may be consulted for an in-depth appreciation of our state of knowledge of many of these disorders.

DISORDERS OF PLASMA CHOLINESTERASE

Plasma cholinesterase, pseudocholinesterase, or nonspecific cholinesterase is an enzyme with a molecular weight of 320,000 and a tetrahedral structure. It is found in plasma and most tissue but not in red blood cells. Pseudocholinesterase degrades acetylcholine released at the neuromuscular junction, as well as other choline and aliphatic esters.[203] The half-life of pseudocholinesterase has been estimated to be 8 to

16 hours. It is very stable in serum samples and can be stored for long periods of time at –20°C with little or no activity loss. Cholinesterase is synthesized in the liver. Therefore, decreased plasma cholinesterase activity occurs in advanced cases of hepatocellular dysfunction.

Inherited variants of pseudocholinesterase are of interest to the anesthesiologist because the duration of action of succinylcholine, mivacurium, and (in some cases) ester-linked local anesthetics, as well as the toxicity of cocaine,[204] is a function of the activity of this enzyme system. Prolonged apnea after succinylcholine, or mivacurium, administration occurs in patients who have very low absolute activity of pseudocholinesterase or have enzyme variants.[205,206] These patients otherwise have no symptoms.

Many physiologic, pharmacologic, and pathologic factors can either increase or decrease the activity of this enzyme to a significant extent. However, it is only when there is a >75% decrease in the levels of the normal pseudocholinesterase that there is clinically evident prolongation of succinylcholine activity (see later). Table 20-3 lists some of the causes for variation in plasma cholinesterase activity.

TABLE 20-3

SOME CAUSES OF CHANGES IN CHOLINESTERASE ACTIVITY

INHERITED
Cholinesterase variants that may lead to decreased or increased activity (e.g., silent gene or C5 variant)
PHYSIOLOGIC
Decreases in last trimester of pregnancy
Reduced activity of the newborn
ACQUIRED DECREASES
Liver diseases
Carcinoma
Debilitating diseases
Collagen diseases
Uremia
Malnutrition
Myxedema
ACQUIRED INCREASES
Obesity
Alcoholism
Thyrotoxicosis
Nephrosis
Psoriasis
Electroshock therapy
DRUGS RELATED TO DISEASES
Neostigmine
Pyridostigmine
Chlorpromazine
Echothiophate iodide
Cyclophosphamide
Monoamine oxidase inhibitors
Pancuronium
Contraceptives
Organophosphorus insecticides
Hexaflurenium
OTHER CAUSES OF DECREASED ACTIVITY
Plasmapheresis
Extracorporeal circulation
Tetanus
Radiation therapy
Burns

The significance of these factors depends on the severity of disease, drug dosage, and individual variation.
Adapted from Whittaker M: Plasma cholinesterase variants and the anesthetist. *Anaesthesia* 35:174, 1980.

Succinylcholine-Related Apnea

Succinylcholine is hydrolyzed by a two-step process, first to succinylmonocholine and then to succinic acid. It has been estimated that only about 5% of the injected drug reaches the end-plate region because of a combination of both hydrolysis and diffusion from the plasma. Urinary excretion and protein binding play unimportant roles in the disposition of the drug when plasma cholinesterase activity is normal. The rate of metabolism determines the duration of action of succinylcholine.

A variety of assay procedures are available for pseudocholinesterase activity. However, most involve the reaction of a thiocholine (e.g., butyrylthiocholine) with serum or plasma containing cholinesterase. The reaction product is coupled with 5,5′-dithiobis(2-nitrobenzoic acid) and forms a colored product that can be followed spectrophotometrically. The use of benzoylcholine, a specific substrate for plasma cholinesterase, avoids contamination of the assay for plasma cholinesterase by the esterase in red blood cells that is released when hemolysis occurs.

Kalow and Genest were the first to show that qualitative as well as quantitative differences in the pseudocholinesterase enzyme determine the duration of succinylcholine apnea.[207] Kalow found that in certain persons displaying succinylcholine sensitivity, the local anesthetic dibucaine (Nupercaine) inhibited the hydrolysis of a benzylcholine substrate less than it inhibited the reaction in those displaying a normal response to succinylcholine. Thus, this atypical phenotype may be referred to as dibucaine-resistant. The percentage inhibition of the reaction was termed the *dibucaine number.* It was found to be constant for a person and did not depend on the concentration of the enzyme.

A discontinuous distribution of dibucaine numbers suggested an inheritance pattern based on alteration at a single gene locus (Table 20-4). Those with dibucaine numbers in the range of 80 would be homozygous normal with a normal response to succinylcholine, those with dibucaine numbers of 20 would be homozygous atypical with a marked prolongation of succinylcholine activity, and those with dibucaine numbers in the 60 range would be heterozygous and, in general, have a normal response to succinylcholine.

Over the years, two other major allelic variants were discovered. In one case, the silent gene, the enzyme is not produced. In the other, there is a differential inhibition of cholinesterase activity by fluoride.[208] In those with prolonged duration of succinylcholine activity with this genotype, fluoride ion inhibits the in vitro hydrolysis of substrate by the enzyme less than it does in normals. Thus the phenotype may be referred to as fluoride resistant. A *fluoride number,* similar to a dibucaine number, is thereby created. Other variants exist, including the K variant, which can be identified only by genetic analysis, not by the current tests of substrate degradation.

When there is a question of succinylcholine sensitivity, the absolute activity of pseudocholinesterase should be determined as well as the dibucaine and fluoride numbers. In some cases, because of biologic variability or unusual combinations of genotype (e.g., combination of atypical and fluoride genes), it is helpful to use other inhibitors of the cholinesterase reaction in genotyping the patient. Bromide, urea, sodium chloride, and succinylcholine have been used to distinguish the various genotypes (see Table 20-4).

Molecular genetic techniques have been successfully applied to pseudocholinesterase variants. La Du's laboratory

TABLE 20-4

BIOCHEMICAL CHARACTERISTICS OF SOME CHOLINESTERASE VARIANTS

GENOTYPE	ACTIVITY	DIBUCAINE #	FLUORIDE#	CHLORIDE#	SUCCINYLCHOLINE#
EuEu	677–1860	78–86	55–65	1–12	89–98
EaEa	140–525	18–26	16–32	46–58	4–19
EuEa	285–1008	51–70	38–55	15–34	51–78
EuEf	579–900	74–80	47–48	14–30	87–91
EfEa	475–661	49–59	25–33	31–36	56–59
EfEs	351	63	26	25	81

Eu = normal enzyme gene; Ea = atypical enzyme gene; Ef = fluoride-resistant gene; Es = silent gene.
Reproduced with permission from Viby-Mogensen J: Succinylcholine neuromuscular blockade in subjects homozygous for atypical plasma cholinesterase. Anesthesiology 55:429, 1981.

has identified a point mutation in the gene for human serum cholinesterase in which a nucleotide change leads to an alteration of a single amino acid (adenine to guanine) in the protein.[209] This change apparently alters the affinity of atypical cholinesterase for choline esters. Other base pair alterations account for other atypical variants, including the K and J silent gene variants, which, while common, produce little to no clinical prolongation of succinylcholine action (Table 20-5).[210]

The identification of causative mutations offers the prospect that more accurate and precise diagnostic tests for atypical pseudocholinesterase variants will exist in the future.

The frequencies of occurrence of the various genes vary to some extent with ethnic background. For example, South African blacks[211] and Eskimo populations have the silent gene much more frequently, patients with Huntington's chorea are more likely to have an Ef gene (fluoride-resistant) than are normal controls, and Israelis have a higher chance of having an atypical genotype than Americans. In European studies, the approximate percentages in the population of the genotypes are as follows: EuEu (96%), EuEa (2.5%), EuEf or EuEs (0.3%), EaEf (0.005%), EaEa (0.05%), and EfEf or EfEs (0.006%).[212]

Patients homozygous for atypical, fluoride, or silent genes as well as those with the combination of atypical with fluoride, atypical with silent genes, or fluoride with silent genes should wear safety identification bracelets indicating that succinylcholine administration will lead to prolonged apnea. Relatives should be tested as well. There are only a few cholinesterase research units that investigate families and interpret results: Whittaker's in Great Britain, Hanel and Viby-Mogensen's in Denmark, and La Du's in the United States (University of Michigan, Department of Anesthesiology).

Clinical Implications of Pseudocholinesterase Abnormalities

Important questions for the anesthesiologist are: Which patients are at risk for development of an abnormal response to succinylcholine? What are the clinical characteristics of this response? and What are the treatment options?

TABLE 20-5

STRUCTURAL CHANGES OF BCHE VARIANTS

Fluoride-2	117 GLY→Frame shift
Atypical	70ASP→GLY
Silent	117 GLY→Frame shift
Fluoride-1	243 THR→MET
Fluoride-2	390 GLY→VAL
K Variant	539 ALA→THR
H Variant	142 VAL→MET
J Variant	497 GLU→VAL

Significant prolongation of succinylcholine's effects occurs in the following genotypes: EaEa, EfEf, EaEs, EfEa, and EsEs. The more common situations in which homozygote normals and heterozygotes are at risk are as follows: patients who have been receiving echothiophate eyedrops (up to 2 weeks after therapy is discontinued), patients who are undergoing plasmapheresis patients with severe liver disease, and patients (particularly heterozygotes) who have received succinylcholine after reversal of nondepolarizing blockade with neostigmine.

Viby-Mogensen[205,206] has studied the question of plasma cholinesterase apnea in detail. His cholinesterase unit found that 6.2% of patients who displayed apnea for 50 to 250 minutes after a "usual" dose of succinylcholine had an acquired deficiency of plasma cholinesterase. He then studied 70 patients who were genotypically normal for pseudocholinesterase and administered 1.0 mg/kg of succinylcholine during a 50% nitrous oxide–oxygen–1% halothane anesthetic and followed the depression and return of thumb twitch. He found that there was indeed a relationship between the duration of apnea, the return of a full twitch response, and plasma cholinesterase activity. However, only moderate prolongation of apnea was found when cholinesterase was depressed by as much as 70%. Apnea is significantly prolonged only with extreme depression of cholinesterase activity.

In a second study with a similar protocol, he found that heterozygotes having one normal gene (e.g., EuEa, EuEf) had a normal response to succinylcholine, including typical fasciculations and a depolarizing type of block with train-of-four stimulations.[205] However, heterozygotes without the usual gene (e.g., EaEf) had a prolonged response to succinylcholine, with apnea lasting as long as 24 minutes. Most showed typical fasciculations. Fade with train-of-four stimulations was the rule. It should be noted that others have found that heterozygotes with one normal gene display a prolonged response to succinylcholine under certain conditions. About 1 in 500 heterozygotes is prone to such a response.

Apnea lasts from 120 minutes to more than 300 minutes in homozygous atypical patients (EaEa) when they are given succinylcholine.[206] The other class of patients who regularly display prolonged apnea after succinylcholine administration comprises patients who are homozygous for the silent gene.

Treatment of Succinylcholine Apnea

The safest course of treatment after the patient fails to breathe within 10 to 15 minutes after succinylcholine administration is to continue mechanical ventilation until adequate muscle tone has returned. Two units of blood may contain adequate amounts of pseudocholinesterase to hydrolyze the succinylcholine,[213] although blood transfusion is not recommended for routine treatment of succinylcholine-induced apnea.

The use of cholinesterase inhibitors in treating succinylcholine apnea is controversial. When given along with blood or plasma, the improvement is rapid and lasting. If they are administered alone before there is evidence of fade with train-of-four stimulation, there may be a transient improvement followed by intensification of the neuromuscular block. Remember that neostigmine inhibits the degradation of succinylcholine by plasma cholinesterase. The best chance for reversal of succinylcholine-related apnea in these situations occurs when no more than 0.03 mg/kg of neostigmine is given 90 to 120 minutes after succinylcholine when a nondepolarizing type of blockade is present.

C5 Variant

An isoenzyme of pseudocholinesterase has been demonstrated whereby the hydrolysis of succinylcholine is increased, and therefore the duration of apnea is decreased after succinylcholine administration. The gene does not appear to be an allele of the Eu and Ea gene and is found infrequently in the population.[214]

Plasma Cholinesterase Abnormalities and the Metabolism of Local Anesthetics

Although the ester-linked local anesthetics (e.g., procaine, tetracaine, 2-chloroprocaine) are metabolized by pseudocholinesterase, prolongation of block and/or clinical toxicity of these local anesthetics in homozygous atypical patients has rarely been documented.[215,216] Jatlow et al have shown delayed hydrolysis of cocaine in vitro with plasma from homozygote atypicals.[217] They theorized that such persons may be at risk for toxic reaction from normal doses of cocaine.

Mivacurium Disposition and Plasma Cholinesterase. The short duration of action of mivacurium is because of its degradation by pseudocholinesterase. Although it is theoretically possible to reverse neuromuscular block in patients with atypical pseudocholinesterase who receive mivacurium, the few cases so far reported indicate that anticholinesterase agents may not be effective under such situations. These individuals should be managed in a manner similar to patients with the atypical enzyme who received succinylcholine.[218] When abnormal plasma cholinesterase does not metabolize mivacurium as rapidly as expected, the neuromuscular blocker is cleared by the kidneys as is curare. The most rapid adequate recovery from mivacurium-induced block will be obtained when the plasma concentration of mivacurium has decreased to the level at which three to four responses to a train-of-four stimulation to the ulnar nerve are palpable. Then neostigmine should induce recovery as it would from blocker that was expected to be long acting.

THE PORPHYRIAS

All the porphyrias result from a defect in heme synthesis. The heme pigments are tetrapyrroles that are the essential elements in hemoglobin, myoglobin, and the cytochromes, that is, compounds that are involved in the transport of oxygen, activation of oxygen, and the electron transport chain. Cytochrome P-450 is a hemoprotein intimately involved in the conversion of lipid-soluble nonpolar drugs to soluble polar compounds that may be excreted in the urine.

A complete deficiency of enzymes that are involved in heme synthesis is incompatible with life. However, a partial deficiency may lead to the accumulation of one or more of the molecular intermediates in heme production. Such an accumulation of precursors is responsible for the clinical manifestations of the porphyrias (in an as-yet unexplained manner).

The rate-limiting step in heme synthesis is the conjugation of succinyl-CoA with glycine to form D-aminolevulinic acid (the enzyme is aminolevulinic acid synthetase). In the porphyrias, there is a partial deficiency of enzymes subsequent to this initial step, which results in a stimulation of this reaction to form aminolevulinic acid. The result is overproduction of intermediate products before the deficient step (Figs. 20-6 and 20-7).

The porphyrias generally manifest after puberty. Inheritance is through an autosomal dominant pattern, but congenital erythropoietic porphyria is inherited as an autosomal recessive pattern.

A functional classification for the anesthesiologist is based on a division of the porphyrias into inducible and noninducible forms. The inducible porphyrias are those in which the acute symptoms are precipitated on drug exposure (Table 20-6).[219] These forms are acute intermittent porphyria, variegate porphyria, and hereditary coproporphyria. These porphyrias cause an acute neurologic syndrome and are therefore of interest to the anesthesiologist. Cutaneous manifestations, with particular sensitivity to ultraviolet light exhibited by skin fragility and bleeding, are the chief features of the other porphyrias. About 80% of patients with variegate porphyria are photosensitive. Some patients with hereditary coproporphyria also may have skin lesions. The porphyrias are very difficult to diagnose in the latent phase of the disorder. Direct assay of the intermediates themselves may be used in the acute state to measure the elevated levels of the heme intermediates. The inducible porphyrias are seen as a neurologic syndrome with a variety of presentations.

The central, peripheral, and autonomic nervous systems may be involved in the porphyrias. A frequent manifestation

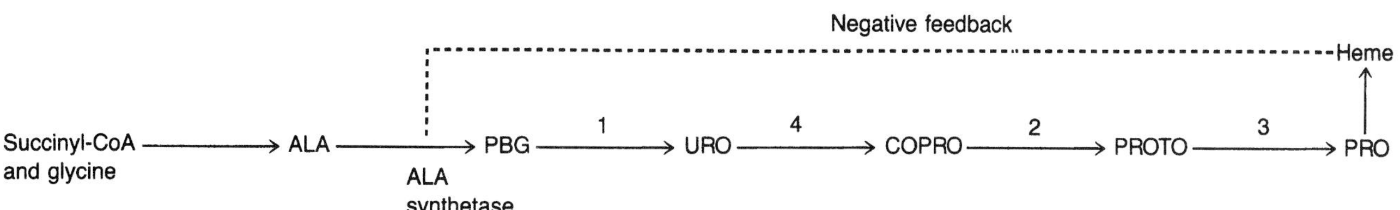

FIGURE 20-6. Biosynthesis of heme and sites of defects in certain porphyrias. (ALA = aminolevulinic acid; PBG = porphobilinogen; URO = uroporphyrinogen; COPRO = coproporphyrinogen; PROTO = protoporphyrinogen; PRO = protoporphyrin.) In intermittent acute porphyria, there is a partial deficiency of the enzyme at site 1. In hereditary coproporphyria, there is an enzyme deficiency at site 2. In variegate porphyria, the enzyme problem is at site 3. In porphyria cutanea tarda, there is a deficiency at site 4. (Reprinted with permission from Mees DL, Frederickson EL: Anesthesia and the porphyrias. South Med J 68:29, 1975.)

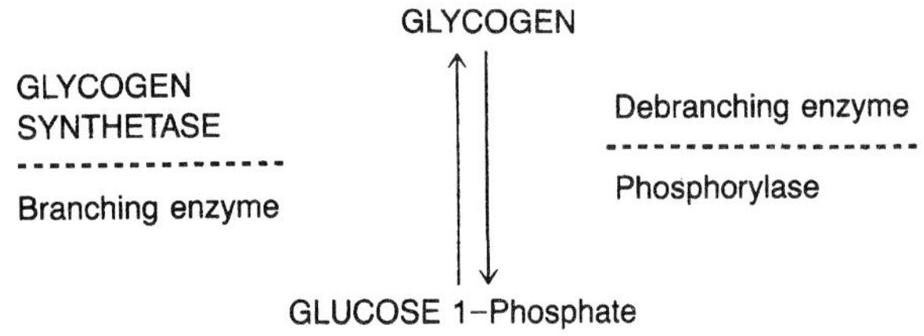

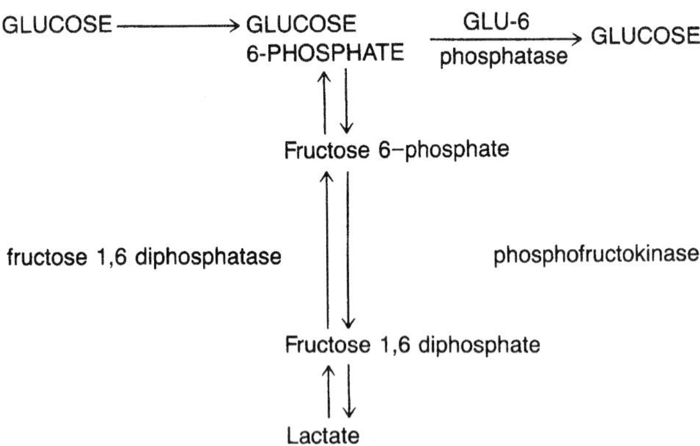

FIGURE 20-7. The glycogen–glucose–lactate pathway.

is colicky abdominal pain, often with nausea and vomiting, which may suggest the diagnosis of acute abdomen, leading to exploratory laparotomy. Other symptoms are psychiatric disturbance, quadriplegia, hemiplegia, alterations of consciousness, and pain. Hyponatremia and hypokalemia may result from vomiting during the acute attack or may be related to hypothalamic disturbance. Death may result from paralysis of the respiratory muscles. The cause of these changes is unknown; they may be related to metabolites of the intermediates or result from deficiency of the heme pigment in the nerve cell itself.

Because the porphyrias are unusual disorders, there is limited experience with the clinical use of many anesthetic drugs. In vitro studies suggest that certain anesthetics or anesthetic adjuvants may be contraindicated, but sufficient clinical experience is lacking (see later).[220]

TABLE 20-6

DRUGS KNOWN TO PRECIPITATE PORPHYRIA

SEDATIVES	Barbiturates Hypnotics such as chlordiazepoxide, glutethimide, diazepam
ANALGESICS	Pentazocaine, antipyrine, aminopyridine Lidocaine
ANTICONVULSANTS	Phenytoin, methsuximide
ANTIBIOTICS	Sulfonamides, chloramphenicol
STEROIDS	Estrogens, progesterones
HYPOGLYCEMIC SULFONYLUREAS	Tolbutamide, chlorpropramide
TOXINS	Lead, ethanol
MISCELLANEOUS	Ergot preparations Amphetamines Methyldopa

Management of Patients with Porphyria

It is important to recognize porphyria in patients who are scheduled for surgery. It may become apparent through a careful family history and personal history related to anesthesia. A careful history in the patient with porphyria should concentrate on neurologic background. Laboratory work should include electrolyte and blood urea nitrogen levels. Physical examination includes inspection of cutaneous lesions over the body.

In the anesthetic management of patients with porphyria, the chief concern is to avoid the administration of drugs that can induce a crisis; the drugs that induce cytochrome enzyme production can trigger the syndrome. Chief among those are the barbiturates; therefore, all barbiturates are contraindicated in porphyria. Ethyl alcohol, nonbarbiturate sedatives, hydantoin anticonvulsants, and a variety of other drugs also can induce a crisis (see Table 20-5). Other factors, such as fasting, infection, and estrogens, may also precipitate porphyria. Diagnosis can be especially difficult because attacks may occur at a variable time period after drug administration or they may not occur at all despite administration of inducing drugs.

Propofol appears to be a safe induction agent.[221] Nitrous oxide, muscle relaxants, and opioids are unequivocally safe drugs. Experience with other inhalation agents and reversal agents has been favorable, but in vitro studies suggest that they might exacerbate a crisis.

Most experts have advised that regional techniques be avoided to prevent confusion should neurologic signs develop after operation. However, reports of uneventful epidural anesthesia in the parturient with acute intermittent porphyria may indicate that this technique can be safely performed in these patients.[222] Blistered or fragile skin areas should be padded and given special attention. Glucose infusion should be started because starvation may induce an attack.

The acute attack should be treated with glucose infusion, and correction of hyponatremia, hypokalemia, and hypomagnesemia. Pyridoxine and hematin also have been valuable in some cases. Supportive therapy for respiratory insufficiency and treatment of pain is also suggested.

GLYCOGEN STORAGE DISEASES

The metabolic pathways involving glucose degradation to lactate, glucose conversion to glycogen, and the breakdown of glycogen to glucose are important to the whole body biochemistry as well as to cellular physiology in general. The enzymatic steps involved in glucose metabolism have been studied intensively since the earliest days of modern biochemistry. The glycogen storage diseases are inherited and are characterized by dysfunction of one of the many enzymes involved in glucose metabolism. To date, several different glycogen storage disorders, each based on the deficiency of an enzyme involved in glucose metabolism, have been identified. Some of the glycogen storage diseases are incompatible with life past infancy, whereas others are not. Anesthetic experience with these diseases is limited, but several particular problems have been identified.[223]

Hypoglycemia. Hypoglycemia is a constant risk in these patients. It results from failure to metabolize stored glycogen to glucose.

Acidosis. This is related to fat and protein metabolism because glycogen stores are not metabolically available.

Cardiac and Hepatic Dysfunction. This is secondary to destruction and displacement of normal tissue by the accumulated glycogen.

Detailed descriptions of glucose metabolism are given elsewhere. Figure 20-7 outlines the glycogen–glucose–lactate pathway. There are, of course, multiple enzymatic steps to reach each of the end points.

Defects in Glucose Metabolism

Type I (Von Gierke's Disease; Glucose-6-phosphate Deficiency). Inheritance is autosomal recessive. The prognosis is moderately good, with many patients surviving into adulthood. Short stature and liver enlargement are characteristic. These patients tolerate fasting very poorly. Hypoglycemia, acidosis, and convulsions may be a problem. Prolonged bleeding has been described. Often, preoperative hyperalimentation is used to reduce liver glycogen stores. Portacaval shunt has been performed with limited success in these patients.

Type II (Pompe's Disease). Inheritance of this disease is considered to be autosomal recessive. This is a devastating disease with a very poor prognosis. There is a deficiency of lysosomal acid maltase with an accumulation of glycogen in the lysosomes, especially in the heart, liver, muscle, and central nervous system. Cardiac compromise resulting from outflow obstruction of hypertrophied muscle occurs, as does congestive heart failure secondary to myocardial disruption by glycogen stores. A case report has been described in which halothane was used without incident.[224] In another case, halothane led to prompt hypotension and intractable cardiac failure.[225] A late-onset form with a better prognosis has been described as well.

Type III (Forbes' Disease; Debranching Enzyme Deficiency). Inheritance of this disease is autosomal recessive.

Type IV (Andersen's Disease; Branching Enzyme Deficiency). This is a very rare disorder, characterized by a defect in the synthesis of normal glycogen. Cirrhosis of the liver and death are characteristic before a patient reaches age 2 years.

Type V (McArdle's Disease; Muscle Phosphorylase Deficiency). An autosomal recessive inheritance pattern and cramping with exercise are characteristic of this disorder. Skeletal muscle is not able to mobilize glycogen stores, the usual fuel in muscle, for sustained exercise. Myoglobinuria occurs with overexertion in these patients and may occur after succinylcholine administration as well. Muscle atrophy occurs in adulthood. Tourniquets should not be used in these patients, and frequent automated blood pressure readings should be done with caution. Severe rhabdomyolysis has been observed after bypass for cardiac surgery.[226]

Type VI (Hers' Disease; Reduced Hepatic Phosphorylase). A decreased ability to mobilize hepatic glycogen occurs in this disorder, with normal muscle and cardiac physiology.

Type VII (Muscle Phosphofructokinase Deficiency). This disorder is similar to McArdle's disease and is characterized by muscle cramping. The same enzymatic defect in erythrocytes leads to chronic hemolysis.

Type VIII (Deficient Hepatic Phosphorylase Kinase). This results from a deficiency in the regulatory enzyme controlling the phosphorylase enzyme. A case report has described fever and acidosis during succinylcholine, halothane, and ketamine anesthesia.[227] Liver transplantation has been used with success in the more severe forms of the glycogen storage diseases.

Defects of Fructose Metabolism

Fructose-6-phosphate is converted to fructose-1,6-diphosphate during glucose breakdown to lactate. Conversely, fructose-1,6-diphosphate is converted to fructose-6-phosphate by the enzyme fructose-1,6-diphosphatase during gluconeogenesis.

In fructose-1,6-diphosphatase deficiency, there is an inability to produce glycogen from lactate. Hypoglycemia may result. Acidosis has been reported because lactate is formed preferentially. In errors of fructose metabolism, like those of glucose metabolism, hypoglycemia and acidosis pose the greatest threats to the patient.[228]

THE MUCOPOLYSACCHARIDOSES

The mucopolysaccharides are polysaccharides that yield mixtures of monosaccharides and derived products after hydrolysis. The mucopolysaccharides contain *N*-acetylated hexosamine in a characteristic repeating unit. For example, chondroitin sulfate A is a monosaccharide of *d*-glucuronic acid and *N*-acetyl *d*-galactosamine 4-sulfate. Monopolysaccharides are found in all cells.

The mucopolysaccharidoses are genetically determined diseases in which mucopolysaccharides are stored in tissues in abnormal quantities and excreted in large amounts in the urine. The disorders result from a deficiency of a specific lysosomal enzyme that is required to break down these compounds. As a result, mucopolysaccharides accumulate in tissues, producing specific clinical manifestations. There are seven basic forms of mucopolysaccharidoses and several subgroups. Most of the mucopolysaccharidoses are inherited as autosomal recessive traits. All the mucopolysaccharidoses are progressive, and patients characteristically are marked by coarse facial features (gargoylism); associated skeletal abnormalities such as lumbar lordosis, stiff joints, chest deformity, dwarfing, and hypoplasia of the odontoid process (Morquio's syndrome); corneal opacities; limitation of joint motion; and heart, liver, and spleen enlargement resulting from mucopolysaccharide accumulation. Mental deterioration also occurs frequently. Some cases have been successfully treated by bone marrow transplantation at a young age.

The Hunter and Hurler syndromes are the best known variants of the mucopolysaccharidoses. The Hunter syndrome is an X-linked recessive disease.[229] Respiratory infection and heart disease, both valvular and ischemic, often lead to death when patients are young. Patients may commonly present for repair of inguinal hernia or ear, nose, and throat or orthopaedic procedures. The thick, soft tissues and the copious, thick secretions make perioperative and intraoperative airway management a particular problem. In Leroy and Crocker's series, minor difficulties occurred with anesthesia in patients in more than one-third of 60 operations.[229] The use of a laryngeal mask airway may not be successful.[230] Postoperative respiratory obstruction was noted in several cases. Because of the underlying heart disease, these patients should have electrocardiograms and echocardiographic tests performed before surgery.

Mucopolysaccharidosis IV (Morquio's syndrome) is associated with perhaps the most significant skeletal deformities. In addition to cardiovascular disorders and respiratory insufficiency from marked chest wall deformity, acute, subacute, or chronic myelopathy is extremely common. This is secondary to severe hypoplasia or absence of the odontoid process of the second cervical vertebra. In anesthesia care, the head should be positioned carefully and precautions, such as avoidance of succinylcholine, should be taken with patients with spinal cord compromise.

OSTEOGENESIS IMPERFECTA

Osteogenesis imperfecta is seen in approximately 1 of 50,000 births. Most cases are autosomal dominant; some are autosomal recessive. The pathophysiologic characteristics include decreased collagen synthesis, which leads to osteoporosis, joint laxity, and tendon weakness. The manifestations of osteogenesis imperfecta are small bowed limbs, large head, short neck, blue sclerae, otosclerosis, joint laxity, brittle teeth, and a tendency to fractures. An increased bleeding tendency is also seen resulting from abnormal platelet function, and aortic and mitral valve dysfunction resulting from dilation of the valve ring. Temperature elevation is common, possibly because of elevated basal metabolic rate.

The patient should be handled carefully because minor trauma may lead to fractures. Airway management may also be difficult because of cervical spine involvement with this disorder. Patients have short necks, and mandibular fractures frequently occur. The patient's cardiovascular status should be evaluated, especially mitral and aortic valve function. Kyphoscoliosis may also occur, with pulmonary compromise. Care should be taken to pad the pressure areas, particularly for long procedures. One should be prepared to obtain platelet transfusions. The patient's core temperature should be monitored because hyperthermia (possibly resulting from central nervous system dysfunction or excessive metabolism in bone) has been reported.[231] Signs consistent with MH have been observed, but contracture tests for MH susceptibility have not confirmed a constant association between osteogenesis imperfecta and MH.[39]

RILEY-DAY SYNDROME (FAMILIAL DYSAUTONOMIA)

A deficiency of dopamine β-hydroxylase that leads to decreased norepinephrine at the nerve endings is thought to be the cause of Riley-Day syndrome.[232] This syndrome is inherited in an autosomal recessive fashion. Patients with Riley-Day syndrome exhibit copious pulmonary secretions, dysphagia, denervation supersensitivity, no sensitivity to pain, no response to histamine, and impairment of temperature control. The impairment of temperature control leads to intermittent fevers.

There are numerous problems related to anesthesia. These include corneal abrasions, excess secretions, pneumonia, labile blood pressure secondary to baroreceptor insensitivity, a decreased vascular volume, possible decreased response to hypoxia and hypercarbia, increased potential for aspiration because of swallowing problems, postural hypotension, and sensitivity to vasopressors.

Anesthesia management is well summarized by Axelrod et al.[233] Perioperative management should include diazepam (0.1 to 0.2 mg/kg po) without an opioid. Antacid may be given on call. Intraoperative management should include temperature monitoring and careful blood pressure monitoring. Application of regional techniques may result in more stable cardiovascular function. Fresh gases should be humidified. Vasopressors need to be titrated carefully because of the hypersensitivity response. After operation secretions can be managed with chest percussion therapy. Postoperatively, opioids should be used only with great care to minimize the risk of apnea.[234]

References

1. Denborough MA, Lovell RRH: Anaesthetic deaths in a family. Lancet 2:45, 1960
2. Denborough MA, Forster JFA, Lovell RRH *et al*: Anaesthetic deaths in a family. Br J Anaesth 34:395, 1962
3. Nelson TE: Porcine stress syndromes. In Gordon RA, Britt BA, Kalow W (eds): International Symposium on Malignant Hyperthermia, p 191. Springfield, IL, Charles C Thomas, 1973
4. Kalow W, Britt BA, Terreau ME, Haist C: Metabolic error of muscle metabolism after recovery from malignant hyperthermia. Lancet 2:895, 1970
5. Harrison GG: Control of the malignant hyperpyrexic syndrome in MHS swine by dantrolene sodium. Br J Anaesth 47:62, 1975
6. Lopez JR, Allen PD, Alamo L *et al*: Myoplasmic free [Ca^{2+}] during a malignant hyperthermia episode in swine. Muscle Nerve 11:82, 1988
7. Larach MG, Rosenberg H, Gronert GA, Allen GC: Hyperkalemic cardiac arrest during anesthesia in infants and children with occult myopathies. Clin Pediatr 36:9, 1997
8. Karan SM, Crowl F, Muldoon SM: Malignant hyperthermia masked by capnographic monitoring. Anesth Analg 78:590, 1994
9. Gronert GA, Ahern CP, Milde JH: Treatment of porcine malignant hyperthermia: Lactate gradient from muscle to blood. Can Anaesth Soc J 33:729, 1986
10. Mathieu A, Bogosian AJ, Ryan JF *et al*: Recrudescence after survival of an initial episode of malignant hyperthermia. Anesthesiology 51:454, 1979
11. Short JA, Cooper CM: Suspected recurrence of malignant hyperthermia after post-extubation shivering in the intensive care unit, 18 h after tonsillectomy. Br J Anaesth 82:945, 1999
12. Donlon JV, Newfield P, Sreter I, Ryan JF: Implications of masseter spasm after succinylcholine. Anesthesiology 49:298, 1978
13. Relton JES, Creighton RE, Conn AW, Nabeta S: Generalized muscular hypertonicity associated with general anaesthesia: A suggested anaesthetic management. Can Anaesth Soc J 14:22, 1967
14. Ellis FR, Halsall PJ: Suxamethonium spasm. A differential diagnostic conundrum. Br J Anaesth 56:381, 1984
15. O'Flynn RP, Shutack JG, Rosenberg H, Fletcher JE: Masseter muscle rigidity and malignant hyperthermia susceptibility in pediatric patients: An update on management and diagnosis. Anesthesiology 80:1228, 1994
16. Larach MG, Rosenberg H, Larach DG, Broennle AM: Prediction of malignant hyperthermia susceptibility by clinical signs. Anesthesiology 66:57, 1987
17. Hackl W, Mauritz W, Schemper M *et al*: Prediction of malignant hyperthermia susceptibility: Statistical evaluation of clinical signs. Br J Anaesth 64:425, 1990
18. Van Der Speck AFL, Fang WB, Ashton-Miller JA *et al*: The effects of succinylcholine on mouth opening. Anesthesiology 67:459, 1987
19. Storella RJ, Keykhah MM, Rosenberg H: Halothane and temperature interact to increase succinylcholine-induced jaw contracture in the rat. Anesthesiology 79:1261, 1993
20. Ording H: Incidence of malignant hyperthermia in Denmark. Anesth Analg 64:700, 1985
21. Hannallah RS, Kaplan RF: Jaw relaxation after a halothane/succinylcholine sequence in children. Anesthesiology 81:99, 1994
22. Rosenberg H, Fletcher JE: Masseter muscle rigidity and malignant hyperthermia susceptibility. Anesth Analg 65:161, 1986
23. Littleford JA, Patel LR, Bose D *et al*: Masseter muscle spasm in children: Implications of continuing the triggering anesthetic. Anesth Analg 72:151, 1991
24. Albrecht A, Wedel DJ, Gronert GA: Masseter muscle rigidity and nondepolarizing neuromuscular blocking agents. Mayo Clin Proc 72:329, 1997
25. Friedman S, Baker T, Gatti M *et al*: Probable succinylcholine-induced rhabdomyolysis in a male athlete. Anesth Analg 81:422, 1995
26. Miller ED, Sanders DB, Rowlingson JC *et al*: Anesthesia-induced rhabdomyolysis in a patient with Duchenne's muscular dystrophy. Anesthesiology 48:146, 1978
27. Sullivan M, Thompson WK, Gill GD: Succinylcholine-induced cardiac arrest in children with undiagnosed myopathy. Can J Anaesth 41:497, 1994
28. Rosenberg AD, Neuwirth MG, Kagen LJ *et al*: Intraoperative rhabdomyolysis in a patient receiving pravastatin, a 3-hydroxy-3-methylgutaryl coenzyme A (HMG CoA) reductase inhibitor. Anesth Analg 81:1089, 1995
29. Kelfer HM, Singer WD, Reynolds RN: Malignant hyperthermia in a child with Duchenne muscular dystrophy. Pediatrics 71:118, 1983
30. Smith CL, Bush GH: Anaesthesia and progressive muscular dystrophy. Br J Anaesth 57:1113, 1985
31. McCarthy TV, Quane KA, Lynch PJ: Ryanodine receptor mutations in malignant hyperthermia and central core disease. Hum Mut 15:410, 2000
32. Frank JP, Harati Y, Butler IJ *et al*: Central core disease and malignant hyperthermia syndrome. Ann Neurol 7:11, 1980
33. Lambert C, Blanloeil Y, Krivosic-Horber R *et al*: Malignant hyperthermia in a patient with hypokalemic periodic paralysis. Anesth Analg 79:1012, 1994
34. Vita GM, Olckers A, Jedlicka AE *et al*: Masseter muscle rigidity associated with glycine1306-to-alanine mutation in the adult muscle sodium channel α-subunit gene. Anesthesiology 82:1097, 1995

35. McPherson EW, Taylor CA Jr: The King syndrome: Malignant hyperthermia, myopathy, and multiple anomalies. Am J Med Genet 8:159, 1981
36. Isaacs H, Badenhorst ME: Dominantly inherited malignant hyperthermia (MH) in the King-Denborough syndrome. Muscle Nerve 15:740, 1992
37. Rampton AJ, Kelly DA, Shanahan EC, Ingram GS: Occurrence of malignant hyperpyrexia in a patient with osteogenesis imperfecta. Br J Anaesth 56:1443, 1984
38. Viljoen D, Beighton P: Schwartz-Jampel syndrome (chondrodystrophic myotonia). J Med Gen 29:58, 1992
39. Porsborg P, Astrup G, Bendixen D *et al*: Osteogenesis imperfecta and malignant hyperthermia. Is there a relationship? Anaesthesia 61:863, 1996
40. Allen GC, Rosenberg H: Phaeochromocytoma presenting as acute malignant hyperthermia—a diagnostic challenge. Can J Anaesth 37:593, 1990
41. Kumar MV, Carr RJ, Komanduri V *et al*: Differential diagnosis of thyroid crisis and malignant hyperthermia in an anesthetized porcine model. Endocr Res 25:87, 1999
42. Shear T, Tobias JT. Anesthetic implications of Leigh's syndrome. Pediatric Anesthesia 14:792, 2004
43. Gronert GA, Thompson RL, Onofrio BM: Human malignant hyperthermia: Awake episodes and correction by dantrolene. Anesth Analg 59:377, 1980
44. Tobin JR, Jason DR, Challa VR, Nelson TE, Sambuughin N: Malignant hyperthermia and apparent heat stroke. JAMA 286:168, 2001
45. Wappler F, Fiege M, Steinfath M *et al*: Evidence for susceptibility to malignant hyperthermia in patients with exercise-induced rhabdomyolysis. Anesthesiology 94:95, 2001
46. Caroff SN: The neuroleptic malignant syndrome. J Clin Psych 41:79, 1980
47. Addonizio G, Susman VL: ECT as a treatment alternative for patients with symptoms of neuroleptic malignant syndrome. J Clin Psych 48:102, 1987
48. Berkowitz A, Rosenberg H: Femoral block with mepivacaine for muscle biopsy in malignant hyperthermia patients. Anesthesiology 62:651, 1985
49. Gronert GA, Milde JH, Taylor SR: Porcine muscle responses to carbachol, α and β adrenoreceptor agonist, halothane or hyperthermia. J Physiol 307:319, 1980
50. Ording H, Nielsen VG: Atracurium and its antagonism by neostigmine (plus glycopyrrolate) in patients susceptible to malignant hyperthermia. Br J Anaesth 58:1001, 1986
51. Hon CA, Landers DF, Platts AA: Effects of neuroleptic agents on rat skeletal muscle contracture in vitro. Anesth Analg 72:194, 1991
52. Gronert GA, Ahern CP, Milde JH *et al*: Effect of CO_2, calcium, digoxin, and potassium on cardiac and skeletal muscle metabolism in malignant hyperthermia susceptible swine. Anesthesiology 64:24, 1986
53. Raff M, Harrison GG: The screening of propofol in MHS swine. Anesth Analg 68:750, 1989
54. Bachand M, Vachond N, Boisvert M *et al*: Clinical reassessment of malignant hyperthermia in Abitibi-Temiscamingue. Can J Anaesth 44:696, 1997
55. Lunn JN, Farrow SC, Fowkes FGR *et al*: Epidemiology in anaesthesia. Br J Anaesth 54:803, 1982
56. Monnier N, Krivosic-Horber R, Payen J-F *et al:* Presence of two different genetic traits in malignant hyperthermia families: implications for genetics analysis, diagnosis, and incidence of malignant hyperthermia susceptibility. Anesthesiology 97:1067, 2002
57. Bendixen D, Skovgaard LT, Ording H: Analysis of anaesthesia in patients suspected to be susceptible to malignant hyperthermia before diagnostic in vitro contracture test. Acta Anaesthesiol Scand 41:480, 1997
58. Seewald MJ, Eichinger HM, Lehmann-Horn F, Iaizzo PA: Characterization of swine susceptible to malignant hyperthermia by in vivo, in vitro and postmortem techniques. Acta Anaesthesiol Scand 35:345, 1991
59. Jurkat-Rott K, McCarthy T, Lehmann-Horn F: Genetics and pathogenesis of malignant hyperthermia. Muscle Nerve 23:4, 2000
60. European Malignant Hyperpyrexia Group: A protocol for the investigation of malignant hyperpyrexia. Br J Anaesth 56:1267, 1984
61. European MH Group: Laboratory diagnosis of malignant hyperpyrexia susceptibility (MHS). Br J Anaesth 57:1038, 1985
62. Larach MG: Standardization of the caffeine–halothane muscle contracture test. Anesth Analg 69:511, 1989
63. Allen GC, Larach MG, Kunselman AR: The sensitivity and specificity of the caffeine–halothane contracture test: A report from the North American Malignant Hyperthermia Registry. The North American Malignant Hyperthermia Registry of MHAUS. Anesthesiology 88:570, 1998
64. Larach MG, Landis JR, Bunn JS *et al*: Prediction of malignant hyperthermia susceptibility in low-risk subjects. An epidemiologic investigation of caffeine–halothane contracture responses. Anesthesiology 76:16, 1992
65. Hopkins PM, Ellis FR, Halsall PJ: Ryanodine contracture: A potentially specific in vitro diagnostic test for malignant hyperthermia. Br J Anaesth 66:611, 1991
66. Lenzen C, Roewer N, Wappler F *et al*: Accelerated contractures after administration of ryanodine to skeletal muscle of malignant hyperthermia susceptible patients. Br J Anaesth 71:242, 1993
67. Wappler F, Roewer N, Lenzen C *et al*: High-purity ryanodine and 9,21-dehydroryanodine for in vitro diagnosis of malignant hyperthermia in man. Br J Anaesth 72:240, 1994
68. Hopkins PM, Ellis FR, Halsall PJ: Comparison of in vitro contracture testing with ryanodine, halothane and caffeine in malignant hyperthermia and other neuromuscular disorders. Br J Anaesth 70:397, 1993
69. Hopkins PM, Hartung E, Wappler F: Multicentre evaluation of ryanodine contracture testing in malignant hyperthermia. The European Malignant Hyperthermia Group. Br J Anaesth 80:389, 1998
70. Wappler F, Scholz J, von Richthofen *et al*: 4-Chloro-m-cresol-induced contractures of skeletal muscle specimen from patients at risk for malignant hyperthermia. Anaesthesiol Intensivmed Notfallmed Schmerzther 32:541, 1997
71. Larach MG, Localio AR, Allen GC *et al*: A clinical grading scale to predict malignant hyperthermia susceptibility. Anesthesiology 80:771, 1994
72. Isaacs H, Badenhorst M: False-negative results with muscle caffeine–halothane contracture testing for malignant hyperthermia. Anesthesiology 79:5, 1993
73. Wedel DJ, Nelson TE: Malignant hyperthermia—diagnostic dilemma: False-negative contracture responses with halothane and caffeine alone. Anesth Analg 78:787, 1994
74. Allen GC, Rosenberg P, Fletcher JE: Safety of general anesthesia in patients previously tested negative for malignant hyperthermia susceptibility. Anesthesiology 72:619, 1990
75. Ording H, Hedengran AM, Skovgaard LT: Evaluation of 119 anaesthetics received after investigation for susceptibility to malignant hyperthermia. Acta Anaesthesiol Scand 35:711, 1991
76. Urwyler A, Censier K, Kaufmann MA, Drewe J: Genetic effects on the variability of the halothane and caffeine muscle contracture tests. Anesthesiology 80:1287, 1994
77. Fletcher JE: Current laboratory methods for the diagnosis of malignant hyperthermia susceptibility. In Levitt RC (ed): Anesthesia Clinics of North America, Temperature Regulation in Anesthesia, p 553, Philadelphia, WB Saunders, 1994
78. Ording H: Diagnosis of susceptibility to malignant hyperthermia in man. Br J Anaesth 60:287, 1988
79. Kaplan RF, Rushing E: Isolated masseter muscle spasm and increased creatine kinase without malignant hyperthermia susceptibility or other myopathies. Anesthesiology 77:820, 1992
80. Antognini JF: Creatine kinase alterations after acute malignant hyperthermia episodes and common surgical procedures. Anesth Analg 81:1039, 1995
81. Bendahan D, Kozak-Ribbens G, Rodet L *et al*. [3]Phosphorus magnetic resonance spectroscopy characterization of muscular metabolic anomalies in patients with malignant hyperthermia: application to diagnosis. Anesthesiology 88:96, 1998
82. Treves S, Larini F, Menegazzi P *et al*: Alteration of intracellular Ca^{2+} transients in COS-7 cells transfected with the cDNA encoding skeletal-muscle ryanodine receptor carrying a mutation associated with malignant hyperthermia. Biochem J 301:661, 1994
83. Sei Y, Brandom BW, Bina S, Hosoi E *et al*: Patients with malignant hyperthermia demonstrate an altered calcium control mechanism in B lymphocytes. Anesthesiology 97:1052, 2002
84. Anetseder M, Hager M, Muller C, Roewer N: Regional lactate and carbondioxide concentrations in a metabolic test for malignant hyperthermia. Lancet 359:1579, 2002
85. Anetseder M, Hager M, Muller-Reible C, Roewer N. Diagnosis of susceptibility to malignant hyperthermia by use of a metabolic test. Lancet 362:494, 2003
86. Hoyer A, Veeser M, Schaupp F, Albrecht Y, Roewer N: Compound muscle action potentials (CMAP) of malignant hyperthermia susceptible (MHS) and non-susceptible human skeletal muscles (MHN) differ under repetitive stimulation (RS) in vivo. ASA Meeting, abstract 997, 2002
87. Hoyer A, Veeser M, Schaupp F, Albrecht Y, Roewer N: The initially higher contraction velocity of malignant hyperthermia susceptible (MH)-susceptible human muscles (MHS) decreases earlier and more distinctly under the influence of repetive stimulation (RS) than in non-susceptibles (MHN). ASA Meeting, abstract 1014, 2002
87a. Sei Y, Sambuughin NN, Davis EJ, *et al:* Malignant hyperthermia in North America genetic screening of the three hot spots in the type 1 ryanodine receptor gene. Anesthesiology 101:824–30, 2004
87b. Sambuughin N, Holley H, Muldoon S, *et al:* Screening of the entire ryanodine receptor type 1 coding region for sequence variants associated with malignant hyperthermia susceptibility in the North American population. Anesthesiology 102:515–21, 2005
88. Urwyler A, Deufel T, McCarthy T, West S: Guidelines for molecular genetic detection of susceptibility to malignant hyperthermia. Br J Anaesth 86: 283, 2001
89. Mitchell LW, Leighton BL: Warmed diluent speeds dantrolene reconstitution. Can J Anaesth 50:127, 2003
90. Rubin AS, Zablocki AD: Hyperkalemia, verapamil, and dantrolene. Anesthesiology 66:246, 1987
91. Saltzman LS, Kates RA, Corke BC *et al*: Hyperkalemia and cardiovascular collapse after verapamil and dantrolene administration in swine. Anesth Analg 63:473, 1984
92. Brandom BW, Larach MG. the North American MH Registry: Reassessment of the safety and efficacy of dantrolene. Anesthesiology 97:A1199, 2002

93. Fletcher R, Blennow G, Olsson AK *et al*: Malignant hyperthermia in a myopathic child: Prolonged postoperative course requiring dantrolene. Acta Anaesthesiol Scand 26:435, 1982
94. Jensen AG, Bach V, Werner MU *et al*: A fatal case of malignant hyperthermia following isoflurane anaesthesia. Acta Anaesthesiol Scand 30:293, 1986
95. Bouchama A, Knochel JP: Heat stroke. N Engl J Med 346:1978, 2002
96. Paul-Pletzer K, Palnitkar SS, Jimenez LS *et al*: The skeletal muscle ryanodine receptor identified as a molecular target of [^{3}H]azidodantrolene by photoaffinity labeling. Biochemistry 40:531, 2001
97. Paul-Pletzer K, Yamamoto T, Bhat MB *et al*: Identification of a dantrolene-binding sequence on the skeletal muscle ryanodine receptor. J Biol Chem 277:34918, 2002
98. Britt BA: Dantrolene. Can Anaesth Soc J 31:61, 1984
99. Watson CB, Reierson N, Norfleet EA: Clinically significant muscle weakness induced by oral dantrolene sodium prophylaxis for malignant hyperthermia. Anesthesiology 65:312, 1986
100. Lerman J, McLeod ME, Strong HA: Pharmacokinetics of intravenous dantrolene in children. Anesthesiology 70:625, 1989
101. Allen GC, Cattran CB, Peterson RG, Lalande M: Plasma levels of dantrolene following oral administration in malignant hyperthermia-susceptible patients. Anesthesiology 69:900, 1988
102. Beebe JJ, Sessler DI: Preparation of anesthesia machines for patients susceptible to malignant hyperthermia. Anesthesiology 69:395, 1988
103. Schonell LH, Sims C, Bulsara M: Preparing a new generation anaesthetic machine for patients susceptible to malignant hyperthermia. Anaesth Intensive Care 31:58, 2003
104. Neubauer KR, Kaufman RD: Another use for mass spectrometry: Detection and monitoring of malignant hyperthermia. Anesth Analg 64:837, 1985
105. Vaughan MS, Cork RC, Vaughan RW: Inaccuracy of liquid crystal thermometry to identify core temperature trends in postoperative adults. Anesth Analg 61:284, 1982
106. Ruhland G, Hinkle AJ: Malignant hyperthermia after oral and intravenous pretreatment with dantrolene in a patient susceptible to malignant hyperthermia. Anesthesiology 60:159, 1984
107. Pollock N, Langton E, Stowell K, Simpson C, McDonnell N: Safe Duration of Postoperative Monitoring for Malignant Hyperthermia Susceptible Patients. Anaesthesia Intensive Care 32:502, 2004
108. Yentis SM, Levine MF, Hartley EJ: Should all children with suspected or confirmed malignant hyperthermia susceptibility be admitted after surgery? A 10-year review, Anesth Analg 75:345, 1992
109. Shime J, Gare D, Andrews J, Britt B: Dantrolene in pregnancy: Lack of adverse effects on the fetus and newborn infant. Am J Obstet Gynecol 159:831, 1988
110. Aleman M, Riehl J, Aldridge BM, Lecouteur RA, Stot JL, Pessah IN: Association of a mutation in the ryanodine receptor 1 gene with equine malignant hyperthermia. Muscle Nerve 30:356, 2004
111. Harthoorn AM, Young E: A relationship between acid-base balance and capture myopathy in zebra (*Equus burchelli*) and apparent therapy. Vet Rec 95:337, 1974
112. MacLennan DH, Phillips MS: Malignant hyperthermia. Science 256:789, 1992
113. Fletcher JE, Calvo PA, Rosenberg H: Phenotypes associated with malignant hyperthermia susceptibility in swine genotyped as homozygous or heterozygous for the ryanodine receptor mutation. Br J Anaesth 71:410, 1993
114. Fletcher JE, Tripolitis L, Rosenberg H, Beech J: Malignant hyperthermia: Halothane- and calcium-induced calcium release in skeletal muscle. Biochem Mol Biol Int 29:763, 1993
115. Figarella-Branger D, Kozak-Ribbens G, Rodet L *et al*: Pathological findings in 165 patients explored for malignant hyperthermia susceptibility. Neuromuscul Disord 3:553, 1993
116. Hopkins PM, Ellis FR, Halsall PJ: Evidence for related myopathies in exertional heat stroke and malignant hyperthermia. Lancet 338:1491, 1991
117. Kochling A, Wappler F, Winkler G, Schulte am Esch JS: Rhabdomyolysis following severe physical exercise in a patient with predisposition to malignant hyperthermia. Anaesth Intensive Care 26:315, 1998
118. Nelson TE: Malignant hyperthermia in dogs. J Am Vet Med Assoc 198:989, 1991
119. Halsall PJ, Cain PA, Ellis FR: Retrospective analysis of anaesthetics received by patients before susceptibility to malignant hyperpyrexia was recognized. Br J Anaesth 51:949, 1979
120. Gallant EM, Rempel WE: Porcine malignant hyperthermia: False negatives in the halothane test. Am J Vet Res 48:488, 1987
121. Haggendal J, Jonsson L, Carlsten J: The role of sympathetic activity in initiating malignant hyperthermia. Acta Anaesthesiol Scand 34:677, 1990
122. Ervasti JM, Strand MA, Hanson TP *et al*: Ryanodine receptor in different malignant hyperthermia-susceptible porcine muscles. Am J Physiol 260:C58, 1991
123. Mickelson JR, Ervasti JM, Litterer LA *et al*: Skeletal muscle junctional membrane protein content in pigs with different ryanodine receptor genotypes. Am J Physiol 267:C282, 1994
124. Ervasti JM, Claessens MT, Mickelson JR, Louis CF: Altered transverse tubule dihydropyridine receptor binding in malignant hyperthermia. J Biol Chem 264:2711, 1989
125. Wieland SJ, Fletcher JE, Rosenberg H, Gong QH: Malignant hyperthermia: Slow sodium current in cultured human muscle cells. Am J Physiol 257:C759, 1989
126. Wieland SJ, Gong QH, Fletcher JE, Rosenberg H: Altered sodium current response to intracellular fatty acids in halothane-hypersensitive skeletal muscle. Am J Physiol 271:C347, 1996
127. Fletcher JE, Wieland SJ, Karan SM *et al*: Sodium channel in human malignant hyperthermia. Anesthesiology 86:1023, 1997
128. Iaizzo PA, Klein W, Lehmann-Horn F: Fura-2 detected myoplasmic calcium and its correlation with contracture force in skeletal muscle from normal and malignant hyperthermia susceptible pigs. Pflugers Arch 411:648, 1988
129. Fletcher JE, Huggins FJ, Rosenberg H: The importance of calcium ions for in vitro malignant hyperthermia testing. Can J Anaesth 37:695, 1990
130. Nelson TE: Abnormality in calcium release from skeletal sarcoplasmic reticulum of pigs susceptible to malignant hyperthermia. J Clin Invest 72:862, 1983
131. Fletcher JE, Mayerberger S, Tripolitis L *et al:* Fatty acids markedly lower the threshold for halothane-induced calcium release from the terminal cisternae in human and porcine normal and malignant hyperthermia susceptible skeletal muscle. Life Sci 49:1651, 1991
132. Mickelson JR, Ross JA, Reed BK, Louis CF: Enhanced Ca^{2+}-induced calcium release by isolated sarcoplasmic reticulum vesicles from malignant hyperthermia susceptible pig muscle. Biochim Biophys Acta 862:318, 1986
133. Carrier L, Villaz M, Dupont Y: Abnormal rapid Ca^{2+} release from sarcoplasmic reticulum of malignant hyperthermia susceptible pigs. Biochim Biophys Acta 1064:175, 1991
134. Mickelson JR, Gallant EM, Litterer LA *et al*: Abnormal sarcoplasmic reticulum ryanodine receptor in malignant hyperthermia. J Biol Chem 263:9310, 1988
135. Mickelson JR, Gallant EM, Rempel WE *et al*: Effects of the halothane-sensitivity gene on sarcoplasmic reticulum function. Am J Physiol 257:C787, 1989
136. Foster PS, White MD, Denborough MA: Characterization of the terminal cisternae and longitudinal tubules of sarcoplasmic reticulum from malignant hyperpyrexia susceptible porcine skeletal muscle. Int J Biochem 21:1119, 1989
137. Fletcher JE, Tripolitis L, Erwin K *et al*: Fatty acids modulate calcium-induced calcium release from skeletal muscle heavy sarcoplasmic reticulum fractions: Implications for malignant hyperthermia. Biochem Cell Biol 68:1195, 1990
138. Endo M, Yagi S, Ishizuka T *et al*: Changes in the Ca-induced Ca release mechanism in the sarcoplasmic reticulum of the muscle from a patient with malignant hyperthermia. Biomed Res 4:83, 1983
139. Takagi A, Sunohara N, Ishihara T *et al*: Malignant hyperthermia and related neuromuscular diseases: Caffeine contracture of the skinned muscle fibers. Muscle Nerve 6:510, 1983
140. Louis CF, Zualkernan K, Roghair T, Mickelson JR: The effects of volatile anesthetics on calcium regulation by malignant hyperthermia-susceptible sarcoplasmic reticulum. Anesthesiology 77:114, 1992
141. McSweeney DM, Heffron JJ: Uptake and release of calcium ions by heavy sarcoplasmic reticulum fraction of normal and malignant hyperthermia-susceptible human skeletal muscle. Int J Biochem 22:329, 1990
142. O'Brien PJ: Porcine malignant hyperthermia susceptibility: Hypersensitive calcium-release mechanism of skeletal muscle sarcoplasmic reticulum. Can J Vet Res 50:318, 1986
143. Struk A, Lehmann-Horn F, Melzer W: Voltage-dependent calcium release in human malignant hyperthermia muscle fibers. Biophys J 75:2402, 1998
144. Censier K, Urwyler A, Zorzato F, Treves S: Intracellular calcium homeostasis in human primary muscle cells from malignant hyperthermia-susceptible and normal individuals. Effect of overexpression of recombinant wild-type and Arg163Cys mutated ryanodine receptors. J Clin Invest 101:1233, 1998
145. Nelson TE: Porcine malignant hyperthermia: Critical temperatures for in vivo and in vitro responses. Anesthesiology 73:449, 1990
146. Sullivan JS, Denborough MA: Temperature dependence of muscle function in malignant hyperpyrexia-susceptible swine. Br J Anaesth 53:1217, 1981
147. Cheah KS, Cheah AM, Fletcher JE, Rosenberg H: Skeletal muscle mitochondrial respiration of malignant hyperthermia-susceptible patients: Ca^{2+}-induced uncoupling and free fatty acids. Int J Biochem 21:913, 1989
148. McCarthy TV, Healy JM, Heffron JJ *et al*: Localization of the malignant hyperthermia susceptibility locus to human chromosome 19q12-13.2. Nature 343:562, 1990
149. Hawkes MJ, Nelson TE, Hamilton SL: [3H]ryanodine as a probe of changes in the functional state of the Ca^{2+}-release channel in malignant hyperthermia. J Biol Chem 267:6702, 1992
150. Herrmann-Frank A, Richter M, Sarkozi S *et al*: 4-Chloro-m-cresol, a potent and specific activator of the skeletal muscle ryanodine receptor. Biochim Biophys Acta 1289:31, 1996
151. Robinson R, Curran JL, Hall WJ *et al*: Genetic heterogeneity and HOMOG analysis in British malignant hyperthermia families. J Med Genet 35:196, 1998
152. Nelson TE: Halothane effects on human malignant hyperthermia skeletal muscle single calcium-release channels in planar lipid bilayers. Anesthesiology 76:588, 1992
153. Fill M, Stefani E, Nelson TE: Abnormal human sarcoplasmic reticulum Ca^{2+} release channels in malignant hyperthermic skeletal muscle. Biophys J 59:1085, 1991

154. Fill M, Coronado R, Mickelson JR *et al*: Abnormal ryanodine receptor channels in malignant hyperthermia. Biophys J 57:471, 1990
155. Fujii J, Otsu K, Zorzato F *et al*: Identification of a mutation in porcine ryanodine receptor associated with malignant hyperthermia. Science 253:448, 1991
156. Mickelson JR, Knudson CM, Kennedy CF *et al*: Structural and functional correlates of a mutation in the malignant hyperthermia-susceptible pig ryanodine receptor. FEBS Lett 301:49, 1992
157. Shomer NH, Mickelson JR, Louis CF: Caffeine stimulation of malignant hyperthermia-susceptible sarcoplasmic reticulum Ca^{2+} release channel. Am J Physiol 267:C1253, 1994
158. Deufel T, Sudbrak R, Feist Y *et al*: Discordance, in a malignant hyperthermia pedigree, between in vitro contracture-test phenotypes and haplotypes for the MHS1 region on chromosome 19q12-13.2, comprising the C1840T transition in the RYR1 gene. Am J Hum Genet 56:1334, 1995 [erratum: Am J Hum Genet 57(2):520, 1995]
159. Fagerlund TH, Ording H, Bendixen D *et al*: Discordance between malignant hyperthermia susceptibility and RYR1 mutation C1840T in two Scandinavian MH families exhibiting this mutation. Clin Genet 52:416, 1997
160. Robinson RL, Anetseder MJ, Brancadoro V *et al*: Recent advances in the diagnosis of malignant hyperthermia susceptibility: how confident can we be of genetic testing? Eur J Hum Genet 11:342, 2003
161. Tong J, Oyamada H, Demaurex N *et al*: Caffeine and halothane sensitivity of intracellular Ca^{2+} release is altered by 15 calcium release channel (ryanodine receptor) mutations associated with malignant hyperthermia and/or central core disease. J Biol Chem 272:26332, 1997
162. Tong J, McCarthy TV, MacLennan DH: Measurement of resting cytosolic Ca^{2+} concentrations and Ca^{2+} store size in HEK-293 cells transfected with malignant hyperthermia or central core disease mutant Ca^{2+} release channels. J Biol Chem 274:693, 1999
163. Lehmann-Horn F, Rudel R: Molecular pathophysiology of voltage-gated ion channels. In: Reviews of Physiology, Biochemistry and Pharmacology, p 195. Berlin, Springer, 1996
164. Cannon SC: Sodium channel defects in myotonia and periodic paralysis. Ann Rev Neurosci 19:141, 1996
165. Kallen RG, Cohen SA, Barchi RL: Structure, function and expression of voltage-dependent sodium channels. Mol Neurobiol 7:383, 1993
166. Rojas CV, Wang JZ, Schwartz LS *et al*: A Met-to-Val mutation in the skeletal muscle Na^+ channel α-subunit in hyperkalaemic periodic paralysis. Nature 354:387, 1991
167. Ptacek LJ, George AL Jr, Barchi RL *et al*: Mutations in an S4 segment of the adult skeletal muscle sodium channel cause paramyotonia congenita. Neuron 8:891, 1992
168. Ricker K, Moxley RT 3rd, Heine R, Lehmann-Horn F: Myotonia fluctuans. A third type of muscle sodium channel disease. Arch Neurol 51:1095, 1994
169. Russell SH, Hirsch NP: Anaesthesia and myotonia. Br J Anaesth 72:210, 1994
170. Wieland SJ, Fletcher JE, Gong QH, Rosenberg H: Effects of lipid-soluble agents on sodium channel function in normal and MH-susceptible skeletal muscle cultures. Adv Exp Med Biol 301:9, 1991
171. Fletcher JE, Adnet PJ, Reyford H *et al*: ATX II, a sodium channel toxin, sensitizes skeletal muscle to halothane, caffeine, and ryanodine. Anesthesiology 90:1294, 1999
172. Adnet PJ, Etchrivi TS, Halle I *et al*: Effects of veratridine on mechanical responses of human malignant hyperthermic muscle fibers. Acta Anaesthesiol Scand 42:246, 1998
173. Ruppersberg JP, Rudel R: Differential effects of halothane on adult and juvenile sodium channels in human muscle. Pflugers Arch 412:17, 1988
174. Moslehi R, Langlois S, Yam I, Friedman JM: Linkage of malignant hyperthermia and hyperkalemic periodic paralysis to the adult skeletal muscle sodium channel (SCN4A) gene in a large pedigree. Am J Med Genet 76:21, 1998
175. Levitt RC, Olckers A, Meyers S *et al*: Evidence for the localization of a malignant hyperthermia susceptibility locus (MHS2) to human chromosome 17q. Genomics 14:562, 1992
176. Olckers A, Meyers DA, Meyers S *et al*: Adult sodium channel α-subunit is a gene candidate for malignant hyperthermia susceptibility. Genomics 14:829, 1992
177. Schmidt JW, Catterall WA: Palmitylation, sulfation, and glycosylation of the α subunit of the sodium channel. Role of post-translational modifications in channel assembly. J Biol Chem 262:13713, 1987
178. Graber R, Sumida C, Nunez EA: Fatty acids and cell signal transduction. J Lipid Mediat Cell Signal 9:91, 1994
179. Carroll JE: Myopathies caused by disorders of lipid metabolism. Neurol Clin 6:563, 1988
180. Glatz JF, Vork MM, Cistola DP, van der Vusse GJ: Cytoplasmic fatty acid binding protein: Significance for intracellular transport of fatty acids and putative role on signal transduction pathways. Prostaglandins Leukot Essent Fatty Acids 48:33, 1993
181. Cheah KS, Cheah AM, Waring JC: Phospholipase A2 activity, calmodulin, $Ca^{2+}$and meat quality in young and adult halothane sensitive and halothaner insensitive British Landrace pigs. Meat Sci 17:37, 1986
182. Cheah AM: Effect of long chain unsaturated fatty acids on the calcium transport of sarcoplasmic reticulum. Biochim Biophys Acta 648:113, 1981
183. Messineo FC, Rathier M, Favreau C *et al*: Mechanisms of fatty acid effects on sarcoplasmic reticulum. III. The effects of palmitic and oleic acids on sarcoplasmic reticulum function—a model for fatty acid membrane interactions. J Biol Chem 259:1336, 1984
184. Dettbarn C, Palade P: Arachidonic acid-induced Ca^{2+} release from isolated sarcoplasmic reticulum. Biochem Pharmacol 45:1301, 1993
185. Dubois BW, Evers AS: ^{9}F-NMR spin-spin relaxation (T2) method for characterizing volatile anesthetic binding to proteins. Analysis of isoflurane binding to serum albumin. Biochemistry 31:7069, 1992
186. Wappler F, Scholz J, Kochling A *et al*: Inositol 1,4,5-trisphosphate in blood and skeletal muscle in human malignant hyperthermia. Br J Anaesth 78:541, 1997
187. Foster PS, Gesini E, Claudianos C *et al*: Inositol 1,4,5-trisphosphate phosphatase deficiency and malignant hyperpyrexia in swine. Lancet 2:124, 1989
188. Henzi V, MacDermott AB: Characteristics and function of Ca^{2+}- and inositol 1,4,5-trisphosphate-releasable stores of Ca^{2+} in neurons. Neuroscience 46:251, 1992
189. Nishizuka Y: Intracellular signaling by hydrolysis of phospholipids and activation of protein kinase C. Science 258:607, 1992
190. Lopez JR, Perez C, Linares N *et al*: Hypersensitive response of malignant hyperthermia-susceptible skeletal musculae to inositol 1,4,5-triphosphate induced release of calcium. Naunyn Schmiedebergs Arch Pharmacol 352:4423, 1995
191. MacLennan DH, Duff C, Zorzato F *et al*: Ryanodine receptor gene is a candidate for predisposition to malignant hyperthermia. Nature 343:559, 1990
192. Nelson TE: A pharmacogenetic disease of Ca^{++}-regulating proteins. Curr Mol Med 2:347, 2002
193. Davis MR, Haan E, Jungbluth H *et al*: Principal mutation hotspot for central core disease and related myopathies in the C-terminal transmembrane region of the RYR1 gene. Neuromuscul Disord 13:151, 2003
194. Tilgen N, Zorzato F, Halliger-Keller B *et al*: Identification of four novel mutations in the C-terminal membrane spanning domain of the ryanodine receptor 1: association with central core disease and alteration of calcium homeostasis. Hum Mol Genet 10:2879, 2001
195. Wehner M, Rueffert H, Koenig F, Olthoff D: Functional characterization of malignant hyperthermia-associated RyR1 mutations in exon 44, using the human myotube model. Neuromuscul Disord 14:429, 2004
196. Sei Y, Gallagher KL, Basile AS: Skeletal muscle type ryanodine receptor is involved in calcium signaling in human B lympoctyes. J Biol Chem 274:5995, 1999
197. Girard T, Cavagna D, Padocan E *et al*: B-lymphocytes from malignant hyperthermia susceptible patients have an increased sensitivity to skeletal muscle ryanodine receptor activators. J Biol Chem 276:48077, 2001
198. Robinson RL, Brooks C, Brown SL *et al*: RYR1 mutations causing central core disease are associated with more severe malignant hyperthermia in vitro contracture test phenotypes. Hum Mutat 20:88, 2002
199. Monnier N, Procaccio V, Stieglitz P, Lunardi J: Malignant-hyperthermia susceptibility is associated with a mutation of the alpha 1-subunit of the human dihydropyridine-sensitive L-type voltage-dependent calcium-channel receptor in skeletal muscle. Am J Hum Genet 60:1316, 1997
200. Serfas KD, Bose D, Patel L *et al*: Comparison of the segregation of the RYR1 C1840T mutation with segregation of the caffeine/halothane contracture test results for malignant hyperthermia susceptibility in a large Manitoba Mennonite family. Anesthesiology 84:322, 1996
201. Girard T, Treves S, Voronkov E, Siegemund M, Urwyler A: Molecular genetic testing for malignant hyperthermia susceptibility. Anesthesiology 100:1076, 2004
202. Stanbury JB, Wyngaarden JB, Frederickson DS: The Metabolic Basis of Inherited Disease, 6th ed. New York, McGraw-Hill, 1989
203. Whittaker M: Chemical and Biochemical Properties In Monographs in Human Genetics, Vol. 11. New York, Karger, 1986
204. Xie W, Altamirano CV, Bartels CF *et al*: An improved cocaine hydrolase: The A328Y mutant of human butyrylcholinesterase is 4-fold more efficient. Mol Pharmacol 55:83, 1999
205. Viby-Mogensen J: Correlation of succinylcholine duration of action with plasma cholinesterase activity in subjects with normal enzyme. Anesthesiology 53:517, 1980
206. Viby-Mogensen J: Succinylcholine neuromuscular blockade in subjects heterozygous for abnormal plasma cholinesterase. Anesthesiology 55:231, 1981
207. Kalow W, Genest K: A method for the detection of atypical forms of human serum cholinesterase: Determination of dibucaine numbers. Can J Biochem 35:339, 1957
208. Harris H, Whittaker M: Differential inhibition of serum cholinesterase with fluoride: Recognition of two new phenotypes. Nature (Lond) 191:496, 1961
209. Primo-Parma SL, Bartels CF, Wiersema B *et al*: Characterization of 12 silent alleles of the human butyrylcholinesterase (BCHE) gene. Am J Hum Genet 58:52, 1996
210. McGuire M, Noguiera CG, Bartels CF *et al*: Identification of the structured mutation responsible for the dibucaine-resistant (atypical) variant form of human cholinesterase. Proc Natl Acad Sci USA 86:953, 1989
211. Krause A, Lane AB, Jenkins T: Pseudocholinesterase variation in southern Africa populations. South African Med J 71:298, 1987

212. Hanel HK, Viby-Mogensen J, Schaffalitzky de Muckadell OB: Serum cholinesterase variants in the Danish population. Acta Anaesthesiol Scand 22:505, 1978
213. Lovely MJ, Patteson SK, Beuerlein FJ, Chesney JT: Perioperative blood transfusion may conceal atypical pseudocholinesterase. Anesth Analg 70:326, 1990
214. Harris H, Hopkinson DA, Robson EB *et al*: Genetic studies on a new variant of serum cholinesterase detected by electrophoresis. Ann Hum Genet 26:359, 1963
215. Brodsky JB, Campos FA: Chloroprocaine analgesia in a patient receiving echothiophate iodide eye drops. Anesthesiology 48:288, 1978
216. Raj PP, Rosenblatt R, Miller J *et al*: Dynamics of local anesthetic compounds in regional anesthesia. Anesth Analg 56:110, 1977
217. Jatlow P, Barash PG, Van Dyke C *et al*: Cocaine and succinylcholine sensitivity: A new caution. Anesth Analg 58:235, 1979
218. Petersen RS, Bailey PL, Kalameghan R, Ashwood ER: Prolonged neuromuscular block after mivacurium. Anesth Analg 76:194, 1993
219. Murphy PC: Acute intermittent porphyria: The anaesthetic problem and its background. Br J Anaesth 36:801, 1964
220. James MFM, Hift RJ: Porphyrias. Br J Anaesth 85:143, 2000
221. McLoughlin C: Use of propofol in a patient with porphyria. Br J Anaesth 62:114, 1989
222. McNeill MJ, Bennet A: Use of regional anaesthesia in a patient with acute porphyria. Br J Anaesth 64:371, 1990
223. Cox JM: Anesthesia and glycogen storage disease. Anesthesiology 29:1221, 1963
224. McFarlane HJ, Soni N: Pompe's disease and anesthesia. Anaesthesia 41:1219, 1986
225. Ellis FR: Inherited muscle disease. Br J Anaesth 52:153, 1980
226. Lobato EB, Janelle GM, Urdaneta F, Malias MA: Noncardiogenic pulmonary edema and rhabdomyolysis after protamine administration in a patient with unrecognized McArdle's disease. Anesthesiology 91:303, 1999
227. Edelstein G, Hirshman CA: Hyperthermia and ketoacidosis during anesthesia in a child with glycogen-storage disease. Anesthesiology 52:90, 1980
228. Hashimoto Y, Watanabe H, Satou M: Anesthetic management of a patient with hereditary fructose 1,6-diphosphate deficiency. Anesth Analg 57:503, 1978
229. Leroy JG, Crocker AC: Clinical definition of the Hurler-Hunter phenotypes. Am J Dis Child 112:518, 1966
230. Busoni P, Cognani G: Failure of laryngeal mask to secure the airway in a patient with Hunter's syndrome (mucopolysaccharidosis type II). Paediatr Anaesth 9:153, 1999
231. Oliverio RM: Anesthetic management of intramedullary nailing in osteogenesis imperfecta: Report of a case. Anesth Analg 52:232, 1973
232. Brown BR, Watson PD, Taussig LM: Congenital metabolic diseases of pediatric patients. Anesthesiology 43:197, 1975
233. Axelrod FB, Donenfeld RF, Danzinger F, Turndorf M: Anesthesia in familial dysautonomia. Anesthesiology 68:631, 1988
234. Stubbig K, Schmidt H, Schreckenberger R *et al*: Anaesthesia and intensive therapy in autonomic dysfunction. Anaesthetist 42:316, 1993

CHAPTER 21 ■ DELIVERY SYSTEMS FOR INHALED ANESTHETICS

RUSSELL C. BROCKWELL AND J. JEFFREY ANDREWS

KEY POINTS

1. The low-pressure circuit (LPC) is the "vulnerable area" of the anesthesia workstation because it is most subject to breakage and leaks. The LPC is located downstream from all anesthesia machine safety features except the oxygen analyzer, and it is the portion of the machine that is missed if an inappropriate LPC leak test is performed. Leaks in the LPC can cause delivery of a hypoxic mixture and/or patient awareness during anesthesia.
2. Because most Ohmeda anesthesia machines have a one-way check valve in the LPC, a negative leak test is required to detect leaks in the LPC. A positive pressure leak test will not detect leaks in the LPC of most Datex-Ohmeda products.
3. Internal vaporizer leaks can only be detected with the vaporizer turned "on."
4. Prior to an anesthetic, the circle system must be checked for leaks and for flow. To test for leaks, the circle system is pressurized to 30-cm water pressure, and the circle system airway pressure gauge is observed (static test). To check for appropriate flow to rule out obstructions and faulty valves, the ventilator and a test lung (breathing bag) are used (dynamic test).
5. Some new anesthesia workstation self-tests do not detect internal vaporizer leaks unless each vaporizer is individually turned on during the self-test.
6. In the event of a pipeline crossover, two actions must be taken. The backup oxygen cylinder must be "on," and the wall supply sources must be disconnected.
7. Fail-safe valves and proportioning systems help minimize delivery of a hypoxic mixture, but they are not foolproof. Delivery of a hypoxic mixture can result from (1) the wrong supply gas, (2) a defective or broken safety device, (3) leaks downstream from the safety devices, (4) inert gas administration, and (5) dilution of the inspired oxygen concentration by high concentrations of inhaled anesthetics.
8. Because of desflurane's low boiling point and high vapor pressure, controlled vaporization of desflurane requires special sophisticated vaporizers such as the Datex-Ohmeda Tec 6 and the Aladin cassette vaporizer.
9. Misfiling an empty variable bypass vaporizer with desflurane could theoretically be catastrophic, resulting in delivery of a hypoxic mixture and a massive overdose of inhaled desflurane anesthetic.
10. Inhaled anesthetics can interact with CO_2 absorbents and produce toxic compounds. During sevoflurane anesthesia, compound A can be formed, particularly at low fresh gas flow rates, and during desflurane anesthesia, carbon monoxide can be produced, particularly with desiccated absorbents.

11 Desiccated strong base absorbents (particularly Baralyme) can react with sevoflurane, producing extremely high absorber temperatures and combustible decomposition products. These in combination with the oxygen or nitrous oxide–enriched environment of the circle system can produce fires within the breathing system.

12 Anesthesia ventilators with ascending bellows (bellows that ascend during the expiratory phase) are safer than descending bellows because disconnections will readily manifest with ascending bellows.

13 Use of the oxygen flush valve during the inspiratory phase of mechanical ventilation can cause barotrauma, particularly in pediatric patients.

14 Ventilators that use fresh gas decoupling technology virtually eliminate the possibility of barotrauma by oxygen flushing during the inspiratory phase because fresh gas flow and oxygen flush flow is diverted to the reservoir breathing bag. However, if the breathing bag has a leak or is absent, patient awareness under anesthesia and delivery of a lower than expected oxygen concentration could occur because of entrainment of room air.

15 With newer Ohmeda anesthetic ventilators such as the 7100 and 7900 Smart Vent, both the patient gas and the drive gas are scavenged resulting in substantially increased volumes of scavenged gas. Thus, the scavenging systems must be set appropriately to accommodate the increased volume or pollution of the operating room environment could result.

INTRODUCTION

The anesthesia delivery system has evolved from a simple pneumatic device to a complex integrated computer-controlled multisystem workstation (Figs. 21-1 and 21-2). The subsystems within the anesthesia workstation function in harmony to safely deliver the inhaled anesthetic to the patient. These component systems include what was formerly referred to as the anesthesia machine-proper (i.e., the pressure-regulating and gas-mixing components), the vaporizers, the anesthesia breathing circuit, the ventilator, the scavenging system, and respiratory and physiologic monitoring systems.

For anesthesia providers to safely use the many features of the anesthesia workstation, a thorough understanding of its operation is essential. Because of large-scale education efforts, in addition to improvements in the engineering and design of the anesthesia workstation, malpractice claims associated with gas-delivery equipment are becoming less frequent. On the other hand, because of the continual development of new volatile anesthetics, aftermarket add-on devices, and even new anesthesia workstation features, claims are not likely to go away completely. In fact, in a review of the American Society of Anesthesiologists (ASA) "Closed Claim" database, Caplan found that although claims related to the medical gas-delivery system were rare, when they occurred, they were usually severe, often resulting in death or permanent brain injury.[1]

In this chapter the anesthesia workstation is examined piece by piece. The normal operation, function, and integration of major anesthesia workstation subsystems are described. More importantly, the potential problems and hazards associated with the various components of the anesthesia delivery system, and the appropriate preoperative checks that may help to detect and prevent such problems, are illustrated.

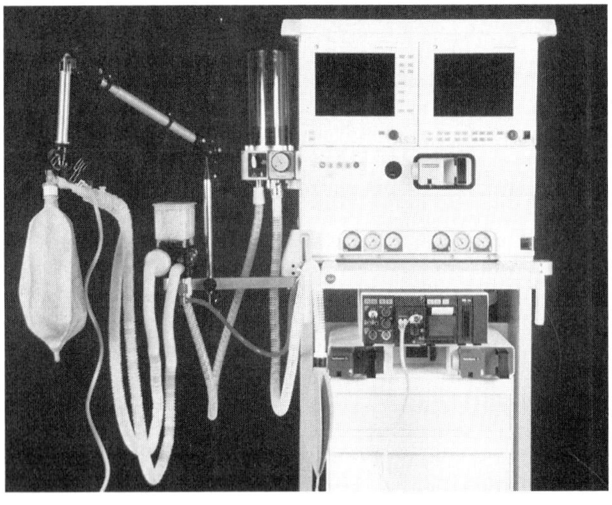

ANESTHESIA WORKSTATION STANDARDS AND PRE-USE PROCEDURES

A few years ago, a fundamental knowledge of the basic anesthesia machine pneumatics would suffice for most anesthesia providers. Today, a detailed understanding of pneumatics, electronics, and even computer science is necessary to fully understand the capabilities and complexities of the anesthesia workstation. Along with the changes in the composition of the anesthesia workstation to include more complex ventilation systems and integrated monitoring, recently there has also been increasing divergence between anesthesia workstation designs from different manufacturers. In 1993, a joint effort between the ASA and the U.S. Food and Drug Administration (FDA) produced the 1993 FDA Anesthesia Apparatus Pre-use Checkout Recommendations (Appendix A). This pre-use checklist was versatile and could be applied to most commonly available anesthesia machines equally well and did not require users to vary the pre-use procedure significantly from machine to machine.

Today, because of increasing fundamental anesthesia workstation design variations, the 1993 FDA pre-use checklist may

FIGURE 21-1. GE/Datex-Ohmeda S/5 Anesthesia Delivery Unit (ADU) workstation. Courtesy GE Medical.

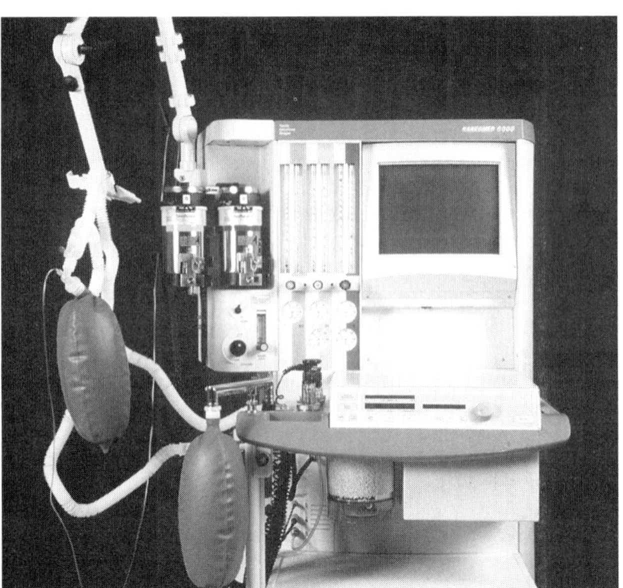

FIGURE 21-2. Dräger Narkomed 6000 anesthesia workstation.

no longer be applicable to certain anesthesia workstations. In such cases, anesthesia providers must be aware of this, and the original equipment manufacturer's recommended pre-use checklist should be followed. Some of the newer workstations even have computer-assisted self-tests that automatically perform all or a part of the pre-use machine checkout procedure. The availability of such automated checkout features further adds to the complexity of constructing a standardized pre-use anesthesia machine checklist such as the one utilized in the recent past. Ultimately, the responsibility of performing adequate pre-use testing of the anesthesia workstation falls to the individual user. That anesthesia provider of record must be aware of which anesthesia workstation components are tested by these automated self-tests and which ones are not. Because of the number of machines available and the variability among their self-testing procedures, the following discussion will be limited to general topics related to these systems.

STANDARDS FOR ANESTHESIA MACHINES AND WORKSTATIONS

Standards for anesthesia machines and workstations provide guidelines to manufacturers regarding their minimum performance, design characteristics, and safety requirements. During the past two decades, the progression of anesthesia machine standards has been as follows:

1979: American National Standards Institute (ANSI) Z79.8-1979,[2]

1988: American Society for Testing and Materials (ASTM) F1161-88,[3]

1994: ASTM F1161-94[4] (reapproved in 1994 and discontinued in 2000),

2000: ASTM F1850-00[5]

To comply with the 2000 ASTM F1850-00 standard, newly manufactured workstations must have monitors that measure the following parameters: continuous breathing system pressure, exhaled tidal volume, ventilatory CO_2 concentration, anesthetic vapor concentration, inspired oxygen concentration, oxygen supply pressure, arterial hemoglobin oxygen saturation, arterial blood pressure, and continuous electrocardiogram. The anesthesia workstation must have a prioritized alarm system that groups the alarms into three categories: high, medium, and low priority. These monitors and alarms may be automatically enabled and made to function by turning on the anesthesia workstation, or the monitors and alarms can be manually enabled and made functional by following a pre-use checklist.[5]

CHECKING THE ANESTHESIA WORKSTATION

A complete anesthesia apparatus checkout procedure must be performed each day prior to the first use of the anesthesia workstation. An abbreviated version should be performed before each subsequent case. Several checkout procedures exist, but the 1993 FDA Anesthesia Apparatus Checkout Recommendations reproduced in Appendix A are the most popular and remain applicable to the majority of anesthesia machines in use worldwide.[6–10] It should be noted that many machines have been modified in the field. The addition of aftermarket products may mandate modification of the pre-use checklist. The user must refer to the operator's manual for special procedures or precautions.

The three most important preoperative checks are (1) oxygen analyzer calibration, (2) the low-pressure circuit leak test, and (3) the circle system test. Each is discussed in the following sections. Additional details regarding these systems will be presented in subsequent sections describing the anatomy of the anesthesia workstation. For a simplified diagram of a two-gas anesthesia machine and the components described in the following discussion, please refer to Figure 21-3. A comprehensive discussion of Figure 21-3 can also be found in the Anesthesia Workstation Pneumatics section.

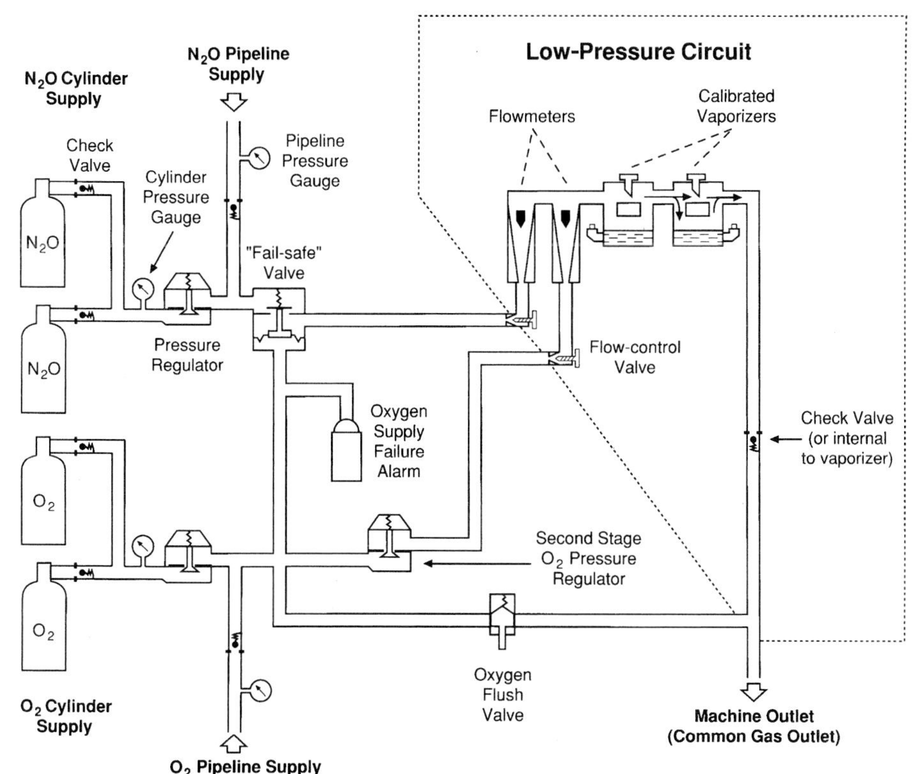

FIGURE 21-3. Diagram of a generic two-gas anesthesia machine. (Modified with permission from Check-Out, A Guide for Preoperative Inspection of an Anesthesia Machine. Park Ridge, Illinois, American Society of Anesthesiologists, 1987.)

TABLE 21-1

CHECK VALVES AND MANUFACTURER-RECOMMENDED LEAK TEST

■ ANESTHESIA MACHINE	■ MACHINE OUTLET CHECK VALVE	■ VAPORIZER OUTLET CHECK VALVE	■ LEAK TEST RECOMMENDED BY MANUFACTURER	
			■ POSITIVE PRESSURE	■ NEGATIVE PRESSURE (SUCTION BULB)
Dräger Narkomed 2A, 2B, 2C, 3, 4, GS	No	No	X	
Fabius GS	No	No		Self-Test
Narkomed 6000	No	No		Self-Test
Ohmeda Unitrol	Yes	Variable		X
Ohmeda 30/70	Yes	Variable		X
Ohmeda Modulus I	Yes	Variable		X
Ohmeda Modulus II	Yes	No		X
Ohmeda Excel series	Yes	No		X
Ohmeda Modulus II Plus	No	No		X
Ohmeda CD	No	No		X
Datex-Ohmeda Aestiva	Yes	No		X
Datex-Ohmeda S5/ADU	No	No		Self-Test

Data from Ohio Medical Products, Ohmeda, Datex-Ohmeda, North American Dräger, Dräger Medical.

Oxygen Analyzer Calibration

The oxygen analyzer is one of the most important monitors on the anesthesia workstation. It is the only machine safety device that evaluates the integrity of the low-pressure circuit in an ongoing fashion. Other machine safety devices, such as the fail-safe valve, the oxygen supply failure alarm, and the proportioning system, are all upstream from the flow control valves. The only machine monitor that detects problems downstream from the flow control valves is the oxygen analyzer. Calibration of this monitor is described in Appendix A (Anesthesia Apparatus Checkout Recommendations, 1993, #9). The actual procedure for calibrating the oxygen analyzer has remained reasonably similar over the recent generations of the anesthesia workstations. Generally, the oxygen concentration sensing element must be exposed to room air for calibration to 21%. This may require manually setting a dial on older machines, but on newer ones, it usually only involves temporary removal of the sensor, selecting and then confirming that the oxygen calibration is to be performed from a set of menus on the workstation's display screen, and finally reinstalling the sensor.

Low-Pressure Circuit Leak Test

1 The low-pressure leak test checks the integrity of the anesthesia machine from the flow control valves to the common outlet. It evaluates the portion of the machine that is downstream from all safety devices except the oxygen analyzer. The components located within this area are *precisely* the ones most subject to breakage and leaks. Leaks in the low-pressure circuit can cause hypoxia or patient awareness.[11,12] Flow tubes, the most delicate pneumatic component of the machine, can crack or break. A typical three-gas anesthesia machine has 16 O-rings in the low-pressure circuit. Leaks can occur at the interface between the glass flow tubes and the manifold, and at the O-ring junctions between the vaporizer and its manifold. Loose filler caps on vaporizers are a common source of leaks, and these leaks can cause patient awareness under anesthesia.[11,13]

Several different methods have been used to check the low-pressure circuit for leaks. They include the oxygen flush test, the common gas outlet occlusion test, the traditional positive pressure leak test, the North American Dräger positive pressure leak test, the Ohmeda 8000 internal positive pressure leak test, the Ohmeda negative pressure leak test, the 1993 FDA universal negative pressure leak test, and others. One reason for the large number of methods is that the internal design of various machines differs considerably. The most notable example is that most GE Healthcare/Datex-Ohmeda (hereafter referred to as Datex-Ohmeda) workstations have a check valve near the common gas outlet, whereas Dräger medical workstations do not. The presence or absence of the check valve profoundly influences which preoperative check is indicated.

Several mishaps have resulted from application of the wrong leak test to the wrong machine.[14–17] Therefore, it is mandatory to perform the appropriate low-pressure leak test each day. To do this, it is essential to understand the exact location and operating principles of the Datex-Ohmeda check valve. Many Datex-Ohmeda anesthesia workstations have a machine outlet check valve located in the low-pressure circuit (Table 21-1). The check valve is located downstream from the vaporizers and upstream from the oxygen flush valve (see Fig. 21-3). It is open (Fig. 21-4, left) in the absence of back pressure. Gas flow from the manifold moves the rubber flapper valve off its seat and allows gas to proceed freely to the common outlet. The

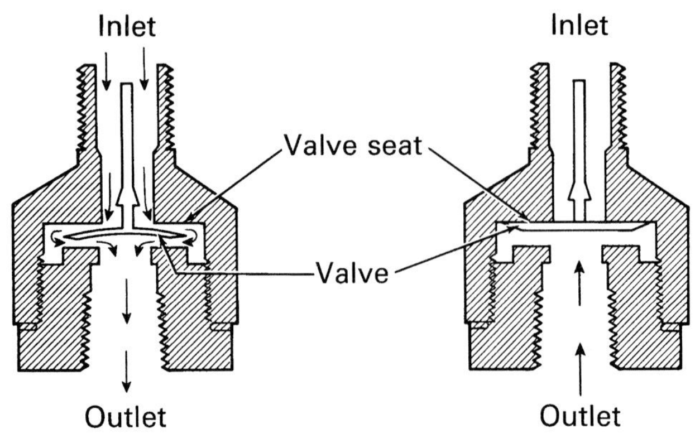

FIGURE 21-4. Machine outlet check valve. See text for details. (Reproduced with permission from Bowie E, Huffman LM: The Anesthesia Machine: Essentials for Understanding. Madison, Ohmeda, Inc., a Division of BOC Health Care, 1985.)

valve closes (Fig. 21-4, right) when back pressure is exerted on it.[8] Back pressure sufficient to close the check valve may occur with the following conditions: oxygen flushing, peak breathing circuit pressures generated during positive pressure ventilation, or use of a positive pressure leak test.

Generally speaking, the low-pressure circuit of anesthesia workstations without an outlet check valve can be tested using a positive pressure leak test, and machines with check valves must be tested using a negative pressure leak test. When performing a positive pressure leak test, the operator generates positive pressure in the low-pressure circuit using flow from the anesthesia machine or from a positive pressure bulb to detect a leak. When performing a negative pressure leak test, the operator creates negative pressure in the low-pressure circuit using a suction bulb to detect leaks. Two different low-pressure circuit leak tests are described below.

Oxygen Flush Positive-Pressure Leak Test

Historically, older anesthesia machines did not have check valves in the low-pressure circuit. Therefore, it was common practice to pressurize the breathing circuit and the low-pressure circuit with the oxygen flush valve to test for internal anesthesia machine leaks. Because many modern Datex-Ohmeda machines now have check valves in the low-pressure circuit, application of a positive-pressure leak test to these machines can be misleading or even dangerous (Fig. 21-5). Inappropriate use of the oxygen flush valve or the presence of a leaking flush valve may lead to inadequate evaluation of the low-pressure circuit for leaks. In turn, this can lead the workstation user into a false sense of security despite the presence of large leaks.[15–19] Positive pressure from the breathing circuit results in closure of the outlet check valve, and the value on the airway pressure gauge will fail to decline. The system appears to be tight, but in actuality, only the circuitry downstream from the check valve is leak free.[20] Thus, a vulnerable area exists from the check valve back to the flow control valves because this area is not tested by a positive pressure leak test.

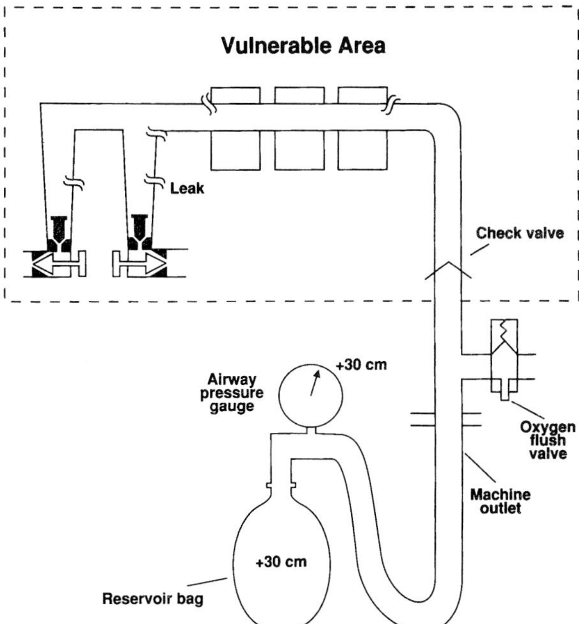

FIGURE 21-5. Inappropriate use of the oxygen flush valve to check the low-pressure circuit of an Ohmeda machine equipped with a check valve. The area within the rectangle is not checked by the inappropriate use of the oxygen flush valve. The components located within this area are *precisely* the ones most subject to breakage and leaks. Positive pressure within the patient circuit closes the check valve, and the value on the airway pressure gauge does not decline despite leaks in the low-pressure circuit.

1993 FDA Negative-Pressure Leak Test

The 1993 FDA Universal negative pressure leak test[10] (Appendix A, #5) was so named "universal" because at that time it could be used to check all contemporary anesthesia machines regardless of the presence or absence of check valves in the low-pressure circuit. It remains effective for many anesthesia workstations and can be applied to many Datex-Ohmeda machines, Dräger Medical machines, and others. Unfortunately, some newer machines are no longer compatible with this test. The ASA Committee on Equipment and Facilities in conjunction with the FDA is expected to update the 1993 Anesthesia Apparatus Pre-Use Checkout Recommendations as this chapter comes to press. Until the new recommendations become available, the 1993 guidelines should continue to be followed as closely as possible, since they remain applicable to the vast majority of anesthesia workstations in use worldwide.

The 1993 FDA check is based on the Datex-Ohmeda negative-pressure leak test (Fig. 21-6). It is performed using a negative-pressure leak testing device, which is a simple suction bulb. The machine master switch, the flow control valves, and vaporizers are turned off. The suction bulb is attached to the common fresh gas outlet and squeezed repeatedly until it is fully collapsed. This action creates a vacuum in the low-pressure circuitry. The machine is leak free if the hand bulb remains collapsed for at least 10 seconds. A leak is present if the bulb reinflates during this period. The test is repeated with each vaporizer individually turned to the on position because internal vaporizer leaks can be detected only with the vaporizer turned on.

3 The FDA "universal" negative-pressure low-pressure circuit leak test has several advantages.[21] The universal test is quick and simple to perform. It has an obvious end point, and it may help isolate the problem. For example, if the bulb reinflates in less than 10 seconds, a leak is present somewhere in the low-pressure circuit. Therefore, it differentiates between breathing-circuit leaks and leaks in the low-pressure circuit. The universal negative-pressure leak test is the most sensitive of all contemporary leak tests because it is not volume dependent. That is, it does not involve the use of a breathing bag or corrugated hoses whose compliance could mask a significant leak. It can detect leaks as small as 30 mL/min. Finally, the operator does not need a detailed or in-depth knowledge of proprietary design differences. If the operator performs the universal test correctly, the leak will be detected.

Circle System Tests

The circle system tests (Appendix A, #11–12) evaluate the integrity of the circle breathing system, which spans from the common gas outlet to the Y-piece (Fig. 21-7). It has two parts—the *leak test* and the *flow test.* To thoroughly check the circle
4 system for leaks, valve integrity, and obstruction, both tests must be performed preoperatively. The *leak test* is performed by closing the pop-off valve, occluding the Y-piece, and pressurizing the circuit to 30 cm water pressure using the oxygen flush valve. The value on the pressure gauge will not decline if the circle system is leak free, but this does not assure valve integrity. The value on the gauge will read 30 cm water even if the unidirectional valves are stuck shut or if the valves are incompetent.

The *flow test* checks the integrity of the unidirectional valves, and it detects obstruction in the circle system. It can be performed by removing the Y-piece from the circle system and breathing through the two corrugated hoses individually. The valves should be present, and they should move appropriately.

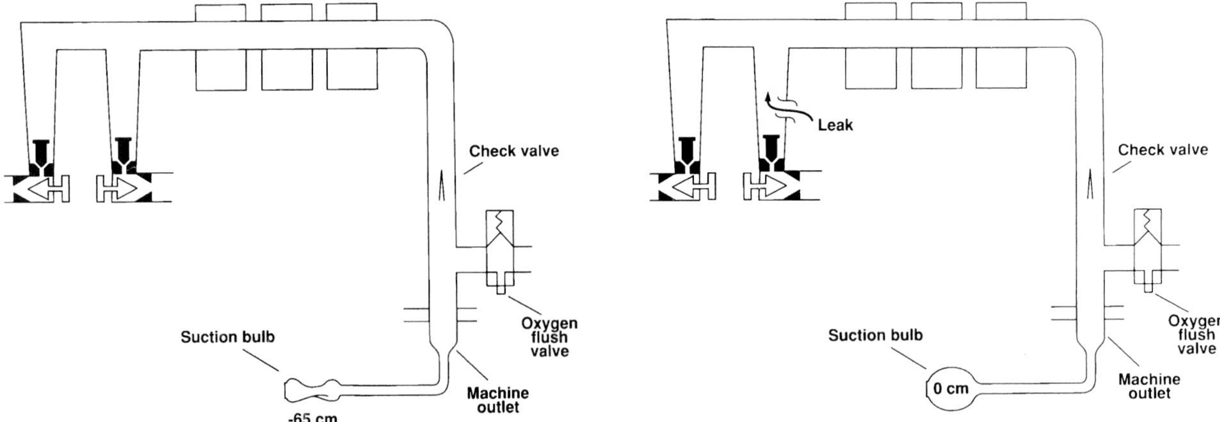

FIGURE 21-6. FDA negative pressure leak test. (*Left*) A negative-pressure leak testing device is attached directly to the machine outlet. Squeezing the bulb creates a vacuum in the low-pressure circuit and opens the check valve. (*Right*) When a leak is present in the low-pressure circuit, room air is entrained through the leak and the suction bulb inflates. (Reprinted with permission from Andrews JJ: Understanding anesthesia machines. In 1988 Review Course Lectures, p 78. Cleveland, International Anesthesia Research Society, 1988.)

The operator should be able to inhale but not be able to exhale through the inspiratory limb. The operator should be able to exhale but not inhale through the expiratory limb. The flow test can also be performed by using the ventilator and a breathing bag attached to the "Y" piece as described in the 1993 FDA Anesthesia Apparatus Checkout Recommendations (Appendix A, #12).[10]

Workstation Self-Tests

As previously mentioned, many new anesthesia workstations now incorporate technology that allows the machine to either automatically or manually walk the user through a series of self-tests to check for functionality of electronic, mechanical, and pneumatic components. Tested components commonly include the gas supply system, flow control valves, the circle system, ventilator, and in the case of the Datex-Ohmeda ADU, even the Aladin cassette vaporizer. The comprehensiveness of these self-diagnostic tests varies from one model and manufacturer to another. If these tests are to be employed, users must be sure to read and strictly follow all manufacturer recommendations. Although a thorough understanding what the particular workstation's self-tests include is very helpful, this information is often difficult to obtain and may vary greatly between devices.

One particularly important point of caution with self-tests should be noted on systems with manifold mounted vaporizers 5 such as the Dräger Medical Fabius GS and Narkomed 6000 series. A manifold mounted vaporizer does not become a part of an anesthesia workstation's gas flow stream until its concentration control dial is turned to the on position. Therefore, to detect internal vaporizer leaks on this type of a system, the "leak test" portion of the self-diagnostic must be repeated separately with each individual vaporizer turned to the on position. If this precaution is not taken, large leaks that could potentially result in patient awareness, such those from a loose filler cap or cracked fill indicator, could go undetected.

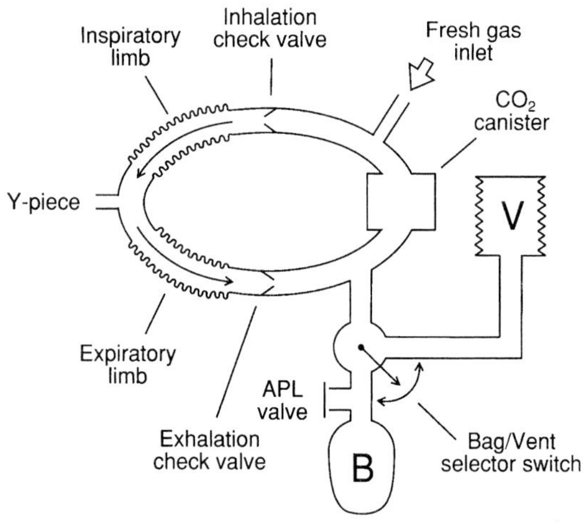

FIGURE 21-7. Components of the circle system. *B* = Reservoir Bag; *V* = ventilator; APL = Adjustable Pressure Limiting. (Reproduced with permission from Brockwell RC: Inhaled Anesthetic Delivery Systems. In Miller RD (ed): Anesthesia, 6th ed, p 295. Philadelphia, Churchill Livingstone, 2004.)

Anesthesia Workstation Pneumatics

The Anatomy of an Anesthesia Workstation

A simplified diagram of a generic two-gas anesthesia machine is shown in Figure 21-3. The pressures within the anesthesia workstation can be divided into three circuits: a high-pressure, an intermediate-pressure, and a low-pressure circuit (see Fig. 21-3). The ***high-pressure circuit*** is confined to the cylinders and the cylinder primary pressure regulators. For oxygen, the pressure range of the high-pressure circuit extends from a high of 2,200 pounds per square inch gauge (psig) to 45 psig, which is the regulated cylinder pressure. For nitrous oxide in the high-pressure circuit, pressures range from a high of 750 psig in the cylinder to a low of 45 psig. The ***intermediate-pressure circuit*** begins at the regulated cylinder supply sources at 45 psig and it includes the pipeline sources at 50 to 55 psig and extends to the flow control valves. Depending on the manufacturer and specific machine design, second-stage pressure regulators may be used to decrease the pipeline supply pressures to the flow control valves to even lower pressures such as 14 psig or 26 psig within the intermediate pressure circuit.[22,23] Finally, the ***low-pressure circuit*** extends from the flow control valves to the common gas outlet. Therefore, the low-pressure circuit includes the flow tubes, vaporizer manifold, vaporizers, and the one-way check valve on most Datex-Ohmeda machines.[22]

Both oxygen and nitrous oxide have two supply sources. These consist of a pipeline supply source and a cylinder supply source. The pipeline supply source is the primary gas source for the anesthesia machine. The hospital pipeline supply system provides gases to the machine at approximately 50 psig, which is the normal working pressure of most machines. The cylinder supply source serves as a back-up if the pipeline supply fails or the primary supply if the anesthesia workstation is being used in a location without the availability of pipeline supplied gases. As previously described, the oxygen cylinder source is regulated from 2,200 to approximately 45 psig, and the nitrous oxide cylinder source is regulated from 745 to approximately 45 psig.[22–24]

A safety device traditionally referred to as the **fail-safe** valve is located downstream from the nitrous oxide supply source. It serves as an interface between the oxygen and nitrous oxide supply sources. This valve shuts off or proportionally decreases the supply of nitrous oxide (and other gases) if the oxygen supply pressure decreases. To meet ASTM standards, contemporary machines have an alarm device to monitor the oxygen supply pressure. A high-priority alarm is actuated as declining oxygen supply pressure reaches a predetermined threshold, such as 30 psig.[22–24]

Many Datex-Ohmeda machines have a second-stage oxygen regulator located downstream from the oxygen supply source in the intermediate pressure circuit. It is adjusted to a precise pressure level, such as 14 psig.[23] This regulator supplies a constant pressure to the oxygen flow control valve regardless of fluctuating oxygen pipeline pressures. For example, the flow from the oxygen flow control valve will be constant if the oxygen supply pressure is greater than 14 psig.

The flow control valves represent an important anatomic landmark within the anesthesia workstation because they separate the intermediate-pressure circuit from the low-pressure circuit. The low-pressure circuit is that part of the machine that lies downstream from the flow control valves. The operator regulates flow entering the low-pressure circuit by adjusting the flow control valves. The oxygen and nitrous oxide flow control valves are linked mechanically or pneumatically by a proportioning system to help prevent inadvertent delivery of a hypoxic mixture. After leaving the flow tubes, the mixture of gases travels through a common manifold and may be directed to a calibrated vaporizer. Precise amounts of inhaled anesthetic can be added, depending on vaporizer control dial setting. The total fresh gas flow plus the anesthetic vapor then travel toward the common gas outlet.[22,23]

Many Datex-Ohmeda anesthesia machines have a one-way check valve located between the vaporizers and the common gas outlet in the mixed-gas pipeline. Its purpose is to prevent back flow into the vaporizer during positive pressure ventilation, therefore minimizing the effects of downstream intermittent pressure fluctuations on inhaled anesthetic concentration (see Vaporizers: Intermittent Back Pressure section). The presence or absence of this check valve ***profoundly*** influences which preoperative leak test is indicated (see Checking Your Anesthesia Workstation). The oxygen flush connection joins the mixed-gas pipeline between the one-way check valve (when present) and the machine outlet. Thus, when oxygen flush valve is activated the pipeline oxygen pressure has a "straight shot" to the common gas outlet.[22,23]

Pipeline Supply Source

Under normal conditions, the pipeline supply serves as the primary gas source for the anesthesia machine. Most hospitals today have a central piping system to deliver medical gases such as oxygen, nitrous oxide, and air to the operating room. The central piping system must supply the correct gases at the appropriate pressure for the anesthesia workstation to function properly. Unfortunately, this does not always occur. Proven as recently as 2002, even large medical centers with huge cryogenic bulk oxygen storage systems are not immune to component failures that may contribute to critical oxygen pipeline supply failures.[25] In this case, a faulty joint ruptured at the bottom of the primary cryogenic oxygen storage tank, releasing 8,000 gallons of liquid oxygen to flood the streets in the surrounding area. This mishap suddenly compromised the oxygen delivery to a major medical center.

In a survey of approximately 200 hospitals in 1976, 31% reported difficulties with pipeline systems.[26] The most common problem was inadequate oxygen pressure, followed by excessive pipeline pressures. The most devastating reported hazard, however, was accidental crossing of oxygen and nitrous oxide pipelines, which has led to many deaths. This problem caused 23 deaths in a newly constructed wing of a general hospital in Sudbury, Ontario, during a 5-month period.[26,27] More recently, in 2002, two additional hypoxic deaths were reported in New Haven, Connecticut. These resulted from a medical gas system failure in which an altered oxygen flowmeter was inadvertently connected to a wall supply source for nitrous oxide.[28]

In the event a pipeline crossover is ever suspected, the work-
6 station user must immediately make **two** corrective actions. First, the back-up oxygen cylinder should be turned on. Then, the pipeline supply must be disconnected. This second step is mandatory because the machine will preferentially use the inappropriate 50 psig pipeline supply source instead of the lower-pressure (45 psig) oxygen cylinder source if the wall supply is not disconnected.

Gas enters the anesthesia machine through the pipeline inlet connections (see Fig. 21-3; see arrows). The pipeline inlet fittings are gas-specific Diameter Index Safety (DISS) threaded body fittings. The DISS provides threaded noninterchangeable connections for medical gas lines, which minimize the risk of misconnection. A check valve is located downstream from the inlet. It prevents reverse flow of gases from the machine to the pipeline or the atmosphere.

Cylinder Supply Source

Anesthesia workstations have E cylinders for use when a pipeline supply source is not available or if the pipeline system fails. Anesthesia providers can easily become complacent and falsely assume that back-up gas cylinders are in fact present on the back of the anesthesia workstation, and further, that if they are present, that they contain an adequate supply of compressed gas. The pre-use checklist should contain steps that confirm both.

Medical gases supplied in E cylinders are attached to the anesthesia machine via the hanger yoke assembly. The hanger yoke assembly orients and supports the cylinder, provides a gas-tight seal, and ensures a unidirectional flow of gases into the machine.[30] Each hanger yoke is equipped with the Pin Index Safety System (PISS). The PISS is a safeguard introduced to eliminate cylinder interchanging and the possibility of accidentally placing the incorrect gas on a yoke designed to accommodate another gas. Two metal pins on the yoke assembly are arranged so that that they project into corresponding holes on the cylinder valve. Each gas or combination of gases has a specific pin arrangement.[31]

Once the cylinders are turned on, compressed gases may pass from their respective high-pressure cylinder sources into the anesthesia machine (see Fig. 21-3). A check valve is located downstream from each cylinder if a double-yoke assembly is used. This check valve serves several functions. First, it minimizes gas transfer from a cylinder at high pressure to one with lower pressure. Second, it allows an empty cylinder to be exchanged for a full one while gas flow continues from the other cylinder into the machine with minimal loss of gas or supply pressure. Third, it minimizes leakage from an open cylinder to the atmosphere if one cylinder is absent.[23,30] A cylinder supply pressure gauge is located downstream from the check valves. The gauge will indicate the pressure in the cylinder having the higher pressure when two reserve cylinders of the same gas are opened at the same time.

Each cylinder supply source has a pressure-reducing valve known as the cylinder pressure regulator. It reduces the high and variable storage pressure present in a cylinder to a lower, more constant pressure suitable for use in the anesthesia machine. The oxygen cylinder pressure regulator reduces the oxygen cylinder pressure from a high of 2,200 psig to approximately 45 psig. The nitrous oxide cylinder pressure regulator receives pressure of up to 745 psig and reduces it to approximately 45 psig.[22,23]

The gas supply cylinder valves should be turned off when not in use, except during the preoperative machine checking period. If the cylinder supply valves are left on, the reserve cylinder supply can be silently depleted whenever the pressure inside the machine decreases to a value lower than the regulated cylinder pressure. For example, oxygen pressure within the machine can decrease below 45 psig with oxygen flushing or possibly even during use of a pneumatically driven ventilator, particularly at high inspiratory flow rates. Additionally, the pipeline supply pressures of all gases can fall to less than 45 psig if problems exist in the central piping system. If the cylinders are left on when this occurs, they will eventually become depleted and no reserve supply may be available if a pipeline failure occurs.[20,23]

The amount of time that an anesthesia machine can operate from the E-cylinder supplies is important knowledge. This is particularly true now that anesthesia is being provided more frequently in office-based and in remote (outside the OR) hospital settings. For oxygen, the volume of gas remaining in the cylinder is proportional to the cylinder pressure. One author has proposed the following equation to help estimate the remaining time.[32]

$$\text{Approx. Remaining Time (Hrs)} \approx \frac{\text{Oxygen cylinder pressure (psig)}}{200 \times \text{oxygen flow rate (L/Min)}}$$

It should be noted that this calculation will provide only a gross estimate of remaining time and may not be exact. Furthermore, users should be cautioned that use of a pneumatically driven mechanical ventilator will dramatically increase oxygen utilization rates and decrease the remaining time until cylinder depletion. Hand ventilating with low fresh gas flow rates may consume <5% the amount of oxygen as compared to intermediate flowmeter settings coupled with the use of pneumatically powered mechanical ventilation.[25] Because piston type anesthesia ventilators such as found in the Dräger Medical Fabius GS and Narkomed 6000 series do not impact oxygen consumption rates, they may be preferable to conventional gas-driven ventilators in practice settings that are dependent on the use of compressed gas cylinders as the primary gas sources.

Oxygen Supply Pressure Failure Safety Devices

Oxygen and nitrous oxide supply sources existed as independent entities in older models of anesthesia machines, and they were not pneumatically or mechanically interfaced. Therefore, abrupt or insidious oxygen pressure failure had the potential to lead to the delivery of a hypoxic mixture. The 2000 ASTM F1850-00 standard states that, "The anesthesia gas supply device shall be designed so that whenever oxygen supply pressure is reduced to below the manufacturer specified minimum, the delivered oxygen concentration shall not decrease below 19% at the common gas outlet."[5] Contemporary anesthesia machines have a number of safety devices that act together in a cascade manner to minimize the risk of delivery of a hypoxic gas mixture as oxygen pressure decreases. Several of these devices are described in the following sections.

Pneumatic and Electronic Alarm Devices

Many older anesthesia machines have a pneumatic alarm device that sounds a warning when the oxygen supply pressure decreases to a predetermined threshold value such as 30 psig. The 2000 ASTM F1850-00 standard mandates that a medium priority alarm shall be activated within 5 seconds when the oxygen pressure decreases below a manufacturer-specific pressure threshold.[5] Electronic alarm devices are now used to meet this guideline.

Fail-Safe Valves

A fail-safe valve is present in the gas line supplying each of the flowmeters except oxygen. Controlled by oxygen supply pressure, the valve shuts off or proportionally decreases the supply pressure of all other gases (nitrous oxide, air, CO_2, helium, nitrogen) as the oxygen supply pressure decreases. Unfortunately,
7 the misnomer "fail-safe" has led to the misconception that the valve prevents administration of a hypoxic mixture. This is not the case. Machines that are either not equipped with a flow proportioning system (see Proportioning Systems section) or ones whose system may be disabled by the user can deliver a hypoxic mixture under normal working conditions. On such a system, the oxygen flow control valve can be closed intentionally or accidentally. Normal oxygen pressure will keep other gas lines open so that a hypoxic mixture can result.[22,23]

Many Datex-Ohmeda machines are equipped with a fail-safe valve known as the pressure-sensor shutoff valve (Fig. 21-8). This valve operates in a threshold manner and is either open or closed. Oxygen supply pressure opens the valve, and the valve return spring closes the valve. Figure 21-8 shows a nitrous oxide pressure-sensor shutoff valve with a threshold pressure of 20 psig. In Figure 21-8A, an oxygen supply pressure greater than 20 psig is exerted on the mobile diaphragm. This pressure moves the piston and pin upward and the valve opens. Nitrous oxide flows freely to the nitrous oxide flow control valve. In Figure 21-8B, the oxygen supply pressure is less than 20 psig, and the force of the valve return spring completely closes the valve.[23] Nitrous oxide flow stops at the closed

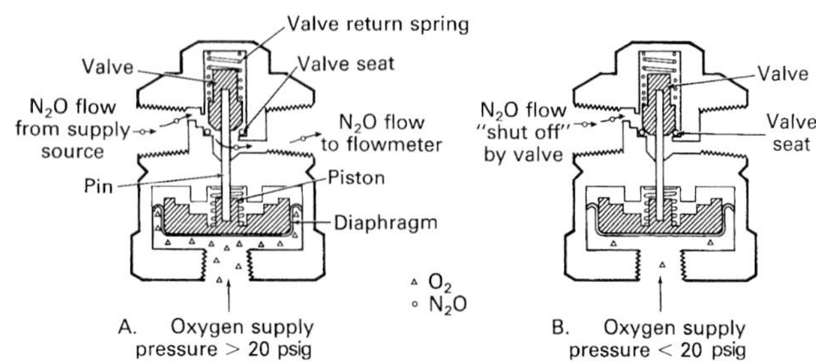

FIGURE 21-8. Pressure-sensor shutoff valve. The valve is open in *A* because the oxygen supply pressure is greater than the threshold value of 20 psig. The valve is closed in *B* because of inadequate oxygen pressure. (Redrawn with permission from Bowie E, Huffman LM: The Anesthesia Machine: Essentials for Understanding. Madison, Wisconsin, Ohmeda, a Division of BOC Health Care, Inc, 1985.)

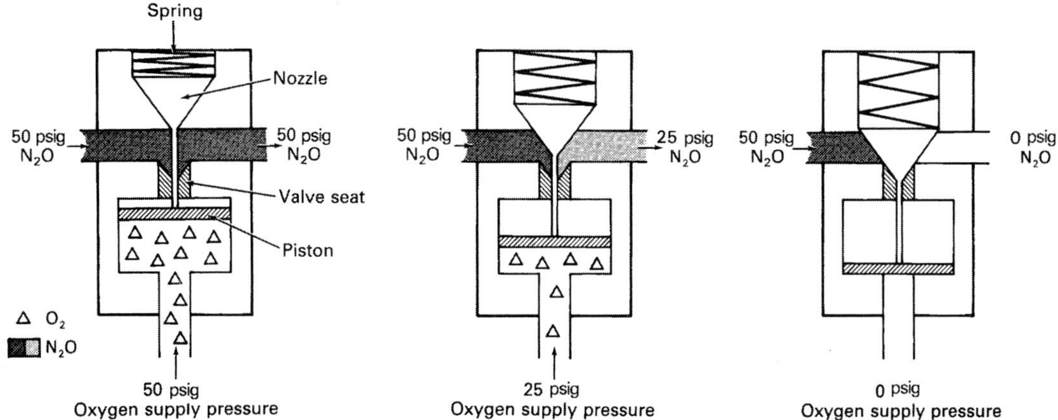

FIGURE 21-9. Oxygen Failure Protection Device/Sensitive Oxygen Ratio Controller (OFPD/S-ORC), which responds proportionally to changes in oxygen supply pressure. (Redrawn with permission from Narkomed 2A Anesthesia System: Technical Service Manual, 6th ed. Telford, PA, North American Dräger, June 1985.)

fail-safe valve, and it does not advance to the nitrous oxide flow control valve.

North American Dräger uses a different fail-safe valve known as the Oxygen Failure Protection Device (OFPD) to interface the oxygen pressure with that of other gases, such as nitrous oxide or other inert gases. This is in contrast to Datex-Ohmeda's oxygen pressure-sensor shutoff valve, because the OFPD is based on a proportioning principle rather than a threshold principle. The pressure of all gases controlled by the OFPD will decrease proportionally with the oxygen pressure. The OFPD consists of a seat-nozzle assembly connected to a spring-loaded piston (Fig. 21-9). The oxygen supply pressure in the left panel of Figure 21-9 is 50 psig. This pressure pushes the piston upward, forcing the nozzle away from the valve seat. Nitrous oxide and/or other gases advance toward the flow control valve at 50 psig. The oxygen pressure in the right panel is zero psig. The spring is expanded and forces the nozzle against the seat, preventing flow through the device. Finally, the center panel shows an intermediate oxygen pressure of 25 psig. The force of the spring partially closes the valve. The nitrous oxide pressure delivered to the flow control valve is 25 psig. There is a continuum of intermediate configurations between the extremes (0 to 50 psig) of oxygen supply pressure. These intermediate valve configurations are responsible for the proportional nature of the OFPD. An important concept to be understood with these particular fail-safe devices is that the Datex-Ohmeda Pressure Sensor Shutoff Valve is threshold in nature (all-or-nothing), whereas the Dräger Oxygen Failure Protection Device is a variable flow type proportioning system.

Second-Stage Oxygen Pressure Regulator

Most contemporary Datex-Ohmeda workstations have a second-stage oxygen pressure regulator set at a specific value ranging from 12 to 19 psig. Output from the oxygen flowmeter is constant when the oxygen supply pressure exceeds the threshold (minimal) value. The pressure-sensor shutoff valve of Datex-Ohmeda is set at a higher threshold value (20 to 30 psig) to ensure that oxygen is the last gas flowing if oxygen pressure failure occurs.

Flowmeter Assemblies

The flowmeter assembly (Fig. 21-10) precisely controls and measures gas flow to the common gas outlet. With traditional glass flowmeter assemblies, the flow control valve regulates the amount of flow that enters a tapered, transparent flow tube known as a Thorpe tube. A mobile indicator float inside the flow tube indicates the amount of flow passing through the associated flow control valve. The quantity of flow is indicated on a scale associated with the flow tube.[22,23] Some newer

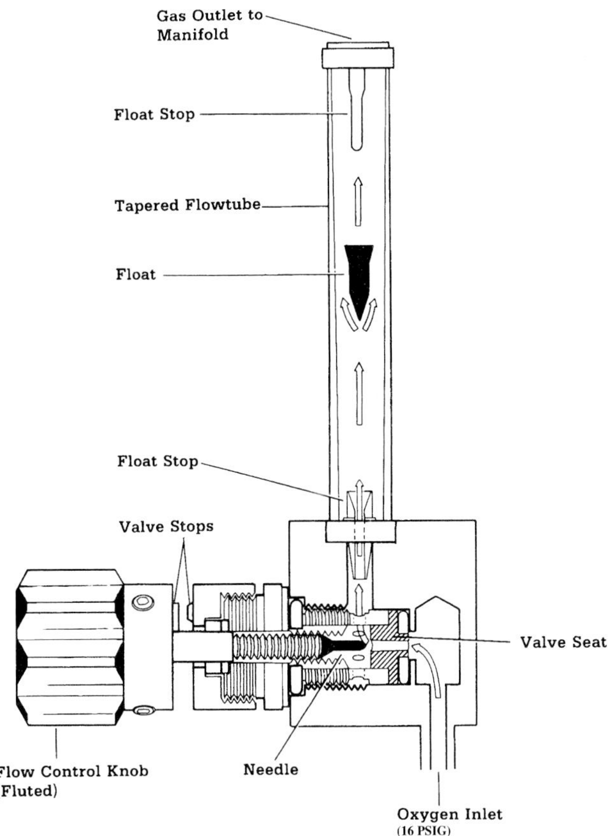

FIGURE 21-10. Oxygen flowmeter assembly. The oxygen flowmeter assembly is composed of the flow control valve assembly plus the flowmeter subassembly. (Reproduced with permission from Bowie E, Huffman LM: The Anesthesia Machine: Essentials for Understanding. Madison, Wisconsin, Ohmeda, a Division of BOC Health Care, Inc, 1985.)

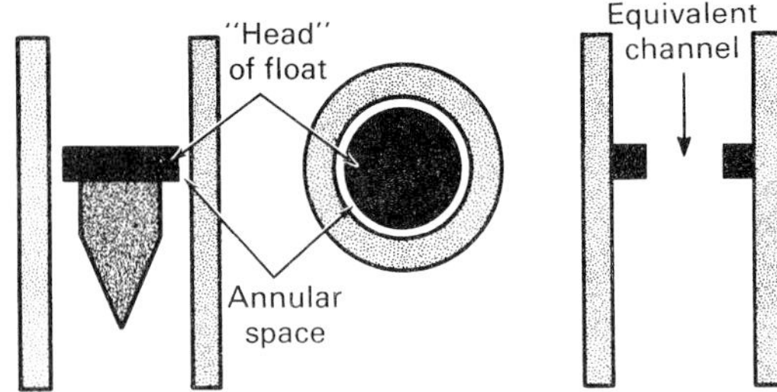

FIGURE 21-11. The annular space. The clearance between the head of the float and the flow tube is known as the annular space. It can be considered an equivalent to a circular channel of the same cross-sectional area. (Redrawn with permission from Macintosh R, Mushin WW, Epstein HG: Physics for the Anaesthetist, 3rd ed. Oxford, England, Blackwell Scientific Publications, 1963.)

anesthesia workstations have now replaced the conventional glass flow tubes with electronic flow sensors that measure the flows of the individual gases. These flow rate data are then presented in either numerical format, graphical format, or a combination of the two. The integration of these "electronic flowmeters" is an essential step in the evolution of the anesthesia workstation if it is to become fully integrated with anesthesia data-capturing systems such as computerized anesthesia record keepers.

Operating Principles of Conventional Flowmeters

Opening the flow control valve allows gas to travel through the space between the float and the flow tube. This space is known as the annular space (Fig. 21-11). The indicator float hovers freely in an equilibrium position where the upward force resulting from gas flow equals the downward force on the float resulting from gravity at a given flow rate. The float moves to a new equilibrium position in the tube when flow is changed.

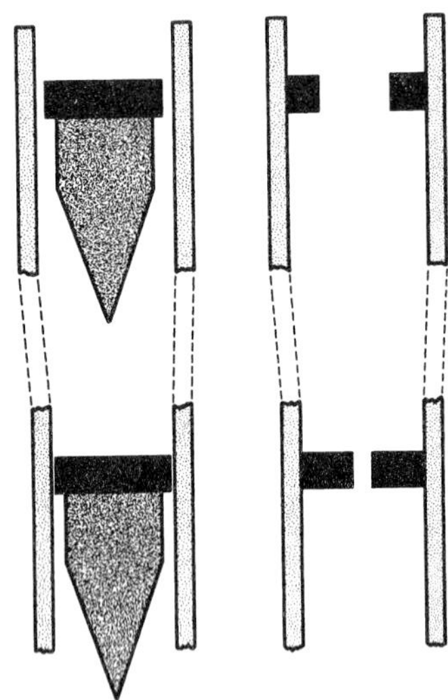

FIGURE 21-12. Flow tube constriction. The lower pair of illustrations represents the lower portion of a flow tube. The clearance between the head of the float and the flow tube is narrow. The equivalent channel is tubular because its diameter is less than its length. Viscosity is dominant in determining gas flow rate through this tubular constriction. The upper pair of illustrations represents the upper portion of a flow tube. The equivalent channel is orificial because its length is less than its width. Density is dominant in determining gas flow rate through this orificial constriction. (Redrawn with permission from Macintosh R, Mushin WW, Epstein HG: Physics for the Anaesthetist, 3rd ed. Oxford, England, Blackwell Scientific Publications, 1963.)

These flowmeters are commonly referred to as *constant pressure* flowmeters because the pressure decrease across the float remains constant for all positions in the tube.[22,31,33]

Flow tubes are tapered, with the smallest diameter at the bottom of the tube and the largest diameter at the top. The term *variable orifice* designates this type of unit because the annular space between the float and the inner wall of the flow tube varies with the position of the float. Flow through the constriction created by the float can be laminar or turbulent, depending on the flow rate (Fig. 21-12). The characteristics of a gas that influence its flow rate through a given constriction are viscosity (laminar flow) and density (turbulent flow). Because the annular space is tubular, at low flow rates laminar flow is present and *viscosity* determines the gas flow rate. The annular space simulates an orifice at high flow rates, and turbulent gas flow then depends predominantly on the *density* of the gas.[22,33]

Components of the Flowmeter Assembly

Flow Control Valve Assembly. The flow control valve (see Fig. 21-10) assembly is composed of a flow control knob, a needle valve, a valve seat, and a pair of valve stops.[22] The assembly can receive its pneumatic input either directly from the pipeline source (50 psig) or from a second-stage pressure regulator. The location of the needle valve in the valve seat changes to establish different orifices when the flow control valve is adjusted. Gas flow increases when the flow control valve is turned counterclockwise, and it decreases when the valve is turned clockwise. Extreme clockwise rotation may result in damage to the needle valve and valve seat. Therefore, flow control valves are equipped with valve "stops" to prevent this occurrence.[23]

Safety features. Contemporary flow control valve assemblies have numerous safety features. The oxygen flow control knob is physically distinguishable from other gas knobs. It is distinctively fluted, projects beyond the control knobs of the other gases, and is larger in diameter than the flow control knobs of other gases. All knobs are color-coded for the appropriate gas, and the chemical formula or name of the gas is permanently marked on each. Flow control knobs are recessed or protected with a shield or barrier to minimize inadvertent change from a preset position. If a single gas has two flow tubes, the tubes are arranged in series and are controlled by a single flow control valve.[5]

Flowmeter Subassembly. The flowmeter subassembly (see Fig. 21-10) consists of the flow tube, the indicator float with float stops, and the indicator scale.[22]

Flow tubes. Contemporary flow tubes are made of glass. Most have a single taper in which the inner diameter of the flow tube increases uniformly from bottom to top. Manufacturers provide double flow tubes for oxygen and nitrous oxide to provide better visual discrimination at low flow rates. A fine flow tube indicates flow from approximately 200 mL/min to 1 mL/min, and a coarse flow tube indicates flow from approximately 1 mL/min to 10 to 12 mL/min. The two tubes are connected in series and supplied by a single flow control valve. The total gas flow is that shown on the higher flowmeter.

Indicator floats and float stops. Contemporary anesthesia machines use several different types of bobbins or floats, including plumb-bob floats, rotating skirted floats, and ball floats. Flow is read at the top of plumb-bob and skirted floats and at the center of the ball on the ball-type floats.[22] Flow tubes are equipped with float stops at the top and bottom of the tube. The upper stop prevents the float from ascending to the top of the tube and plugging the outlet. It also ensures that the float will be visible at maximum flows instead of being hidden in the manifold. The bottom float stop provides a central foundation for the indicator when the flow control valve is turned off.[22,23]

Scale. The flowmeter scale can be marked directly on the flow tube or located to the right of the tube.[5] Gradations corresponding to equal increments in flow rate are closer together at the top of the scale because the annular space increases more rapidly than does the internal diameter from bottom to top of the tube. Rib guides are used in some flow tubes with ball-type indicators to minimize this compression effect. They are tapered glass ridges that run the length of the tube. There are usually three rib guides that are equally spaced around the inner circumference of the tube. In the presence of rib guides, the annular space from the bottom to the top of the tube increases almost proportionally with the internal diameter. This results in a nearly linear scale.[22] Rib guides are employed on many Dräger Medical flow tubes.

Safety features. The flowmeter subassemblies for each gas on the Datex-Ohmeda Modulus I, Modulus II, Modulus II Plus, CD, and Aestiva are housed in independent, color-coded, pin-specific modules. The flow tubes are adjacent to a gas-specific, color-coded backing. The flow scale and the chemical formula (or name of the gas) are permanently etched on the backing to the right of the flow tube. Flowmeter scales are individually hand-calibrated using the specific float to provide a high degree of accuracy. The tube, float, and scale make an inseparable unit. The entire set must be replaced if any component is damaged.

Dräger Medical does not use a modular system for the flowmeter subassembly. The flow scale, the chemical symbol, and the gas-specific color codes are etched directly onto the flow tube. The scale in use is obvious when two flow tubes for the same gas are used.

Problems with Flowmeters

Leaks. Flowmeter leaks are a substantial hazard because the flowmeters are located downstream from all machine safety devices except the oxygen analyzer.[34] Leaks can occur at the O-ring junctions between the glass flow tubes and the metal manifold or in cracked or broken glass flow tubes, the most fragile pneumatic component of the anesthesia machine. Even though gross damage to conventional glass flow tubes is usually apparent, subtle cracks and chips may be overlooked, resulting in errors of delivered flows.[35] The use of electronic flowmeters and the removal of conventional glass flow tubes from some newer anesthesia workstations (Datex-Ohmeda S/5 ADU and the Dräger Fabius) may help to eliminate these potential sources of leaks (see Electronic Flowmeters section).

Eger et al in 1963[36] demonstrated that, in the presence of a flowmeter leak, a hypoxic mixture is less likely to occur if

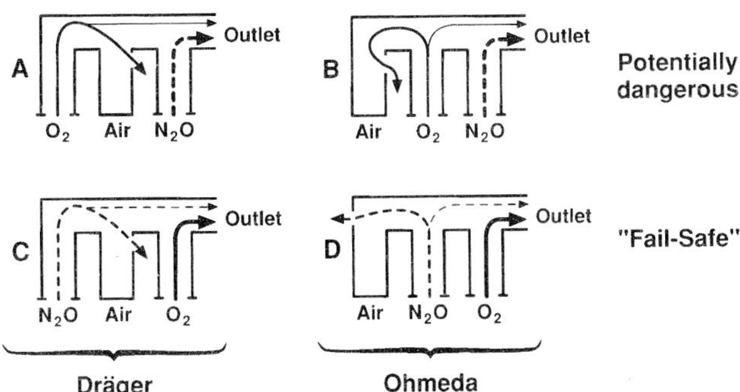

FIGURE 21-13. Flowmeter sequence—a potential cause of hypoxia. In the event of a flowmeter leak, a potentially dangerous arrangement exists when nitrous oxide is located in the downstream position (*A* and *B*). The safest configuration exists when oxygen is located in the downstream position (C and *D*). See text for details. (Modified with permission from Eger EI II, Hylton RR, Irwin RH *et al*: Anesthetic flowmeter sequence—a cause for hypoxia. Anesthesiology 24:396, 1963.)

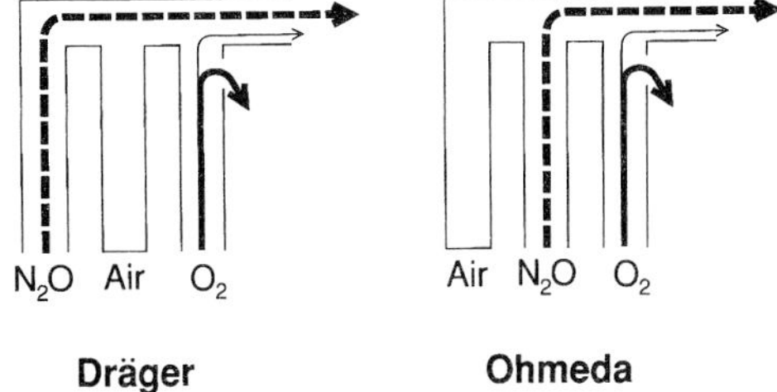

FIGURE 21-14. Oxygen flow tube leak. An oxygen flow tube leak can produce a hypoxic mixture regardless of flow tube arrangement. (Reproduced with permission from Brockwell RC: Inhaled Anesthetic Delivery Systems. In Miller RD (ed): Anesthesia, 6th ed, p 281. Philadelphia, Churchill Livingstone, 2004.)

the oxygen flowmeter is located downstream from all other flowmeters. Figure 21-13 is a more contemporary version of the figure in Eger's original publication. The unused air flow tube has a large leak. Nitrous oxide and oxygen flow rates are set at a ratio of 3:1. A potentially dangerous arrangement is shown in Figure 21-13A and 21-13B because the nitrous oxide flowmeter is located in the downstream position. A hypoxic mixture can result because a substantial portion of oxygen flow passes through the leak, and all nitrous oxide is directed to the common gas outlet. A safer configuration is shown in Figure 21-13C and 21-13D. The oxygen flowmeter is located in the downstream position. A portion of the nitrous oxide flow escapes through the leak, and the remainder goes toward the common gas outlet. A hypoxic mixture is less likely because all the oxygen flow is advanced by the nitrous oxide.[36] North American Dräger flowmeters are arranged as in Figure 21-13C, and Datex-Ohmeda flowmeters are as in Figure 21-13D.

A leak in the oxygen flow tube may result in creation of a hypoxic mixture even when oxygen is located in the downstream position (Fig. 21-14).[34,35] Oxygen escapes through the leak and nitrous oxide continues to flow toward the common outlet, particularly at high ratios of nitrous oxide to oxygen flow.

Inaccuracy. Flow measurement error can occur even when flowmeters are assembled properly with appropriate components. Dirt or static electricity can cause a float to stick, and the actual flow may be higher or lower than that indicated. Sticking of indicator float is more common in the low flow ranges because the annular space is smaller. A damaged float can cause inaccurate readings because the precise relationship between the float and the flow tube is altered. Back pressure from the breathing circuit can cause a float to drop so that it reads less than the actual flow. Finally, if flowmeters are not aligned properly in the vertical position (plumb), readings can be inaccurate because tilting distorts the annular space.[17,22,35]

Ambiguous Scale. Before the standardization of flowmeter scales and the widespread use of oxygen analyzers, at least two deaths resulted from confusion created by ambiguous scales.[17,35,37] The operator read the float position beside an adjacent but erroneous scale in both cases. Today this error is less likely to occur because contemporary flowmeter scales are marked either directly onto the flow tube or immediately to the right of it.[5] The possibility of confusion is minimized when the scale is etched directly onto the tube.

Electronic Flowmeters

As mentioned earlier, some newer anesthesia workstations such as the Datex-Ohmeda S/5 ADU and the North American Dräger Fabius GS among others have conventional control knobs and flow control valves, but have electronic flow sensors and digital displays rather than glass flow tubes. The output from the flow control valve is represented graphically and/or numerically in liters per minute on the workstation's integrated user interface. These systems are dependent on electrical power to provide a precise display of gas flow. However, even when electrical power is totally interrupted, since the flow control valves themselves are nonelectronic, oxygen should continue to flow. Since these machines do not have individual flow tubes that physically quantitate flow of each gas, electronic flow sensors and often a small conventional pneumatic "fresh gas" or "total flow" indicators are provided that give the user an estimate of the total quantity fresh gas flowing from all flow control valves. This miniature flow tube indicator serves to inform the user of the approximate quantity of gas that is leaving the anesthesia workstation's common gas outlet, and is functional even in the event of a total power failure.

Proportioning Systems

Manufacturers equip anesthesia workstations with proportioning systems in an attempt to prevent creation and delivery of a hypoxic mixture. Nitrous oxide and oxygen are interfaced mechanically and/or pneumatically so that the minimum oxygen concentration at the common gas outlet is between 23 to 25% depending on manufacturer.

Datex-Ohmeda Link-25 Proportion Limiting Control System

Conventional Datex-Ohmeda machines use the Link-25 System. The heart of the system is the mechanical integration of the nitrous oxide and oxygen flow control valves. It allows independent adjustment of either valve, yet automatically intercedes to maintain a minimum 25% oxygen concentration with a maximum nitrous oxide–oxygen flow ratio of 3:1. The Link-25 automatically increases oxygen flow to prevent delivery of a hypoxic mixture.

Figure 21-15 illustrates the Datex-Ohmeda Link-25 System. The nitrous oxide and oxygen flow control valves are identical. A 14-tooth sprocket is attached to the nitrous oxide flow control valve, and a 28-tooth sprocket is attached to the oxygen flow control valve. A chain physically links the sprockets. When the nitrous oxide flow control valve is turned through two revolutions, or 28 teeth, the oxygen flow control valve will revolve once because of the 2:1 gear ratio. The final 3:1 flow ratio results because the nitrous oxide flow control valve is supplied by approximately 26 psig, whereas the oxygen flow control valve is supplied by 14 psig. Thus, the combination of the mechanical and pneumatic aspects of the system yields the final oxygen concentration. The Datex-Ohmeda Link-25 proportioning system can be thought of as a system which *increases oxygen flow* when necessary to prevent delivery of a fresh gas mixture with oxygen concentration of less than 25%.

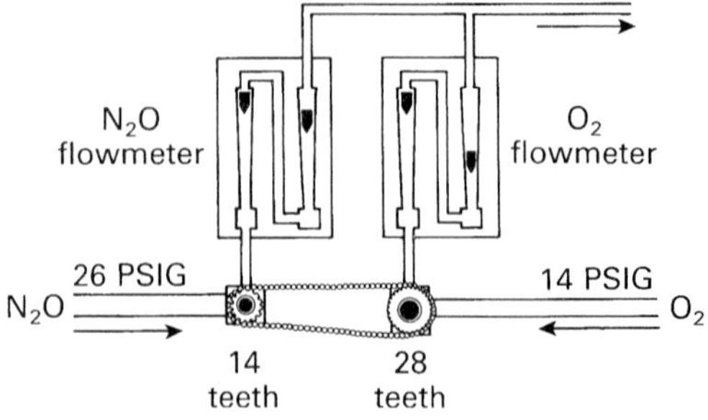

FIGURE 21-15. Ohmeda Link-25 Proportion Limiting Control system. See text for details.

A few reports have described failures of the Datex-Ohmeda Link-25 system.[37–41] The authors of these reports describe failures that resulted in either inability to administer oxygen without nitrous oxide or that allowed creation of a hypoxic mixture.

North American Dräger Oxygen Ratio Monitor Controller/Sensitive Oxygen Ratio Controller System

North American Dräger's proportioning system, the Oxygen Ratio Monitor Controller (ORMC), is used on the North American Dräger Narkomed 2A, 2B, 3, and 4. An equivalent system is known as the Sensitive Oxygen Ratio Controller (S-ORC) on some newer Dräger anesthesia workstations such as the Dräger Fabius GS and Narkomed 6000 series. The ORMC and the S-ORC are pneumatic oxygen–nitrous oxide interlock systems designed to maintain a fresh gas oxygen concentration of at least 25 ± 3%. They control the fresh gas oxygen concentration to levels substantially higher than 25% at oxygen flow rates less than 1 L/min. The ORMC and S-ORC limit nitrous oxide flow to prevent delivery of a hypoxic mixture. This is unlike the Datex-Ohmeda Link-25, which actively increases oxygen flow.

A schematic of the ORMC is shown in Figure 21-16. It is composed of an oxygen chamber, a nitrous oxide chamber, and a nitrous oxide slave control valve. All are interconnected by a mobile horizontal shaft. The pneumatic input into the device is from the oxygen and the nitrous oxide flowmeters. These flowmeters are unique because they have specific resistors located downstream from the flow control valves. These resistors create back pressures directed to the oxygen and nitrous oxide chambers. The value of the oxygen flow tube resistor is three to four times that of the nitrous oxide flow tube resistor, and the relative value of these resistors determines the value of the controlled fresh gas oxygen concentration. The back pressure in the oxygen and nitrous oxide chambers pushes against rubber diaphragms attached to the mobile horizontal shaft. Movement of the shaft regulates the nitrous oxide slave control valve, which feeds the nitrous oxide flow control valve.

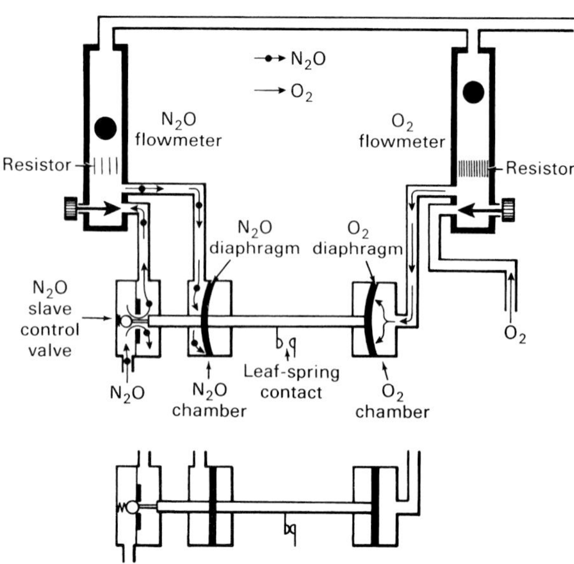

FIGURE 21-16. North American Dräger Oxygen Ratio Monitor Controller. See text for details. (Redrawn with permission from Schreiber P: Safety Guidelines for Anesthesia Systems. Telford, Pennsylvania, North American Dräger, 1984.)

If the oxygen pressure is proportionally higher than the nitrous oxide pressure, the nitrous oxide slave control valve opens more widely, allowing more nitrous oxide to flow. As the nitrous oxide flow is increased manually, the nitrous oxide pressure forces the shaft toward the oxygen chamber. The valve opening becomes more restrictive and limits the nitrous oxide flow to the flowmeter.

Figure 21-16 illustrates the action of a single ORMC/S-ORC under different sets of circumstances. The back pressure exerted on the oxygen diaphragm, in the upper configuration is greater than that exerted on the nitrous oxide diaphragm. This causes the horizontal shaft to move to the left, opening the nitrous oxide slave control valve. Nitrous oxide is then able to proceed to its flow control valve and out through the flowmeter. In the bottom configuration, the nitrous oxide slave control valve is closed because of inadequate oxygen back pressure.[24] To summarize, in contrast to the Datex-Ohmeda Link-25 system that actively increases oxygen flow to maintain a fresh gas oxygen concentration greater than 25%, the Dräger ORMC and S-ORC are systems that limit nitrous oxide flow to prevent delivery of a fresh gas mixture with an oxygen concentration of less than 25%.

Limitations

Proportioning systems are not foolproof. Workstations equipped with proportioning systems can still deliver a hypoxic mixture under certain conditions. Following is a description of some of the situations in which this may occur.

Wrong Supply Gas. Both the Datex-Ohmeda Link-25 and the Dräger ORMC/S-ORC will be fooled if a gas other than oxygen is present in the oxygen pipeline. In the Link-25 System, the nitrous oxide and oxygen flow control valves will continue to be mechanically linked. Nevertheless, a hypoxic mixture can proceed to the common gas outlet. In the case of the Dräger ORMC or S-ORC, the rubber diaphragm for oxygen will reflect adequate supply pressure on the oxygen side even though the incorrect gas is present, and flow of both the wrong gas plus nitrous oxide will result. The oxygen analyzer is the only workstation monitor besides an integrated multigas analyzer that would detect this condition in either system.

Defective Pneumatics or Mechanics. Normal operation of the Datex-Ohmeda Link-25 and the North American Dräger ORMC/S-ORC is contingent on pneumatic and mechanical integrity.[42] Pneumatic integrity in the Datex-Ohmeda System requires properly functioning second-stage regulators. A nitrous oxide–oxygen ratio other than 3:1 will result if the regulators are not precise. The chain connecting the two sprockets must be intact. A 97% nitrous oxide concentration can occur if the chain is cut or broken.[43] In the North American Dräger System, a functional Oxygen Failure Protection Device (OFPD) is necessary to supply appropriate pressure to the ORMC. The mechanical aspects of the ORMC/S-ORC, such as the rubber diaphragms, the flow tube resistors, and the nitrous oxide slave control valve, must likewise be intact.

Leaks Downstream. The ORMC/S-ORC and the Link-25 function at the level of the flow control valves. A leak downstream from these devices, such as a broken oxygen flow tube (see Fig. 21-14), can result in delivery of a hypoxic mixture to the common gas outlet. In this situation, oxygen escapes through the leak, and the predominant gas delivered is nitrous oxide. The oxygen monitor and/or integrated multigas analyzer are the only machine safety devices that can detect this problem.[34] For the majority of its products, Dräger Medical recommends a preoperative positive pressure leak test to detect such a leak. However, in addition to this test, for many North American Dräger products, application of the negative-pressure leak test as well may provide a more sensitive way to detect such a leak. Datex-Ohmeda almost universally recommends a preoperative negative pressure leak test for its workstations, because of the frequently present check valve located at the common gas outlet (see Checking Your Anesthesia Workstation section).

Inert Gas Administration. Administration of a third inert gas, such as helium, nitrogen, or CO_2, can cause a hypoxic mixture because contemporary proportioning systems link only nitrous oxide and oxygen.[44] Use of an oxygen analyzer is mandatory (or preferentially a multigas analyzer when available) if the operator uses a third gas.

Dilution of Inspired Oxygen Concentration by Volatile Inhaled Anesthetics. Volatile inhaled anesthetics, like inert gases, are added to the mixed gases downstream from both the flowmeters and the proportioning system. Concentrations of less-potent inhaled anesthetics such as desflurane may account for a larger percentage of the total fresh gas composition than more potent agents. This can be seen when the maximum vaporizer dial settings of the various volatile agents are examined (e.g., desflurane maximum dial setting 18% versus isoflurane maximum dial setting of 5%). Since significant percentages of these inhaled anesthetics may be added downstream of the proportioning system, the resulting gas/vapor mixture may contain an inspired oxygen concentration that is less than 21% oxygen despite a functional proportioning system. The anesthesia provider must be aware of this possibility, particularly when high concentrations of less potent volatile inhaled anesthetics are used.

Oxygen Flush Valve

The oxygen flush valve allows direct communication between the oxygen high-pressure circuit and the low-pressure circuit (see Fig. 21-3). Flow from the oxygen flush valve enters the low-pressure circuit downstream from the vaporizers and most importantly downstream from the Datex-Ohmeda machine outlet check valve. The spring-loaded oxygen flush valve stays closed until the operator opens it by depressing the oxygen flush button. Actuation of the valve delivers 100% oxygen at 35 to 75 L/min to the breathing circuit.[23]

The oxygen flush valve can provide a high pressure oxygen source suitable for jet ventilation under the following circumstances: (1) the anesthesia machine is equipped with a one-way check valve positioned between the vaporizers and the oxygen flush valve; and (2) when a positive pressure relief valve exists downstream of the vaporizers, this pressure relief valve must be upstream of the outlet check valve. Because the Ohmeda Modulus II has such a one-way check valve and its positive pressure relief valve is upstream from the check valve, the entire oxygen flow of 35 to 75 L/min is delivered to the common gas outlet at a high pressure of 50 psig. On the other hand, the Ohmeda Modulus II Plus and some Ohmeda Excel machines are not capable of functioning as an appropriate oxygen source for jet ventilation. The Ohmeda Modulus II plus, which does not have the check valve, provides only 7 psig at the common gas outlet because some oxygen flow travels retrograde through an internal relief valve located upstream from the oxygen flush valve. The Ohmeda Excel 210, which does have a one-way check valve, also has a positive pressure relief valve downstream from the check valve and therefore is unsuitable for jet ventilation. Older North American Dräger machines such as the Narkomed 2A (which also does not have the outlet check valve) provide an intermediate pressure of 18 psig to the common gas outlet because some pressure is vented retrograde through a pressure relief valve located in the vaporizers.[45]

Several hazards have been reported with the oxygen flush valve. A defective or damaged valve can stick in the fully open position, resulting in barotrauma.[46] A valve sticking in a partially open position can result in patient awareness because the oxygen flow from the incompetent valve dilutes the inhaled anesthetic.[19,47] Improper use of normally functioning oxygen flush valves also can result in problems. Overzealous intraoperative oxygen flushing can dilute inhaled anesthetics. Oxygen flushing during the inspiratory phase of positive pressure ventilation can produce barotrauma in patients if the anesthesia machine does not incorporate fresh gas decoupling or an appropriately adjusted inspiratory pressure limiter. Anesthesia systems (Dräger Narkomed 6000 series, Julian, Fabius GS and Datascope Anestar) with fresh gas decoupling are inherently safer from the standpoint of minimizing the chance of producing barotrauma from inappropriate oxygen flush valve use. These systems physically divorce the fresh gas inflow from either the flowmeters or the oxygen flush valve from the delivered tidal volume presented to the patient's lungs (see Fresh Gas Decoupling section). With traditional anesthesia breathing circuits, excess volume cannot be vented during the inspiratory phase of mechanical ventilation because the ventilator relief valve is closed and the Adjustable Pressure Limiting (APL) valve is either out-of-circuit or closed.[48] An alternative way to manage this problem can be seen on the Datex-Ohmeda S/5 ADU and Aestiva. These circle systems utilize an integrated adjustable pressure limiter. If this device is properly adjusted, it functions like the APL valve to limit the maximum airway pressure to a safe level, thereby reducing the possibility of barotrauma.

Some very old anesthesia systems made use of a freestanding vaporizer downstream from the common gas outlet; on these systems, oxygen flushing could rapidly deliver large quantities of inhaled anesthetic to the patient. Finally, inappropriate preoperative use of the oxygen flush to evaluate the low-pressure circuit for leaks can be misleading, particularly on Datex-Ohmeda machines with a one-way check valve at the common outlet.[18] Since back pressure from the breathing circuit closes the one-way check valve air-tight, major low-pressure circuit leaks can go undetected with this leak test (see Checking Your Anesthesia Workstation section).

VAPORIZERS

As dramatically as the evolution of the anesthesia workstation has been in recent years, vaporizers have also changed from rudimentary ether inhalers and copper kettles to the present temperature compensated, computer-controlled, and flow-sensing devices we use today. In 1993, with the introduction of desflurane to the clinical setting, an even more sophisticated vaporizer was introduced to handle the unique physical properties of this agent. Now, a new generation of anesthesia vaporizers blending both "old" copper kettle-like technology and "new" computerized control technology has emerged in the Datex-Ohmeda Aladin cassette vaporizer system. Before the discussion of variable bypass vaporizers, the Datex-Ohmeda Tec 6 desflurane vaporizer, and the Datex-Ohmeda Aladin cassette vaporizer, certain physical principles will be reviewed briefly to facilitate understanding of the operating principles, construction, and design of contemporary volatile anesthetic vaporizers.

Physics

Vapor Pressure

Contemporary inhaled volatile anesthetics exist in the liquid state at temperatures below 20°C. When a volatile liquid is in a closed container, molecules escape from the liquid phase to the vapor phase until the number of molecules in the vapor phase is constant. These molecules in the vapor phase bombard

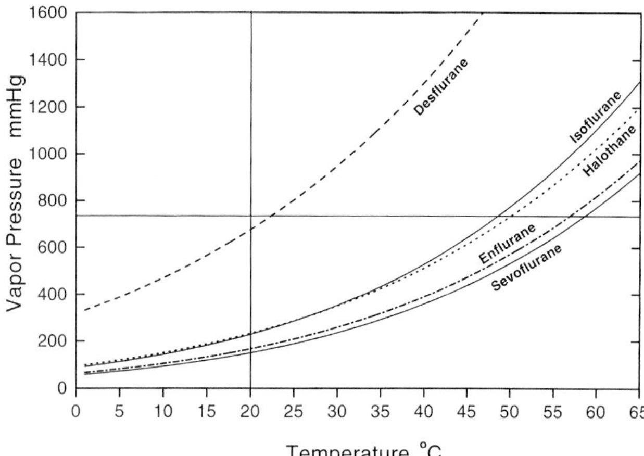

FIGURE 21-17. Vapor pressure versus temperature curves for desflurane, isoflurane, halothane, enflurane, and sevoflurane. The vapor pressure curve for desflurane is both steeper and shifted to higher vapor pressures when compared with the curves for other contemporary inhaled anesthetics. (From inhaled anesthetic package insert equations and from Susay SR, Smith MA, Lockwood GG: The saturated vapor pressure of desflurane at various temperatures. Anesth Analg 83:864, 1996.)

the wall of the container and create a pressure known as the *saturated vapor pressure*. As the temperature increases, more molecules enter the vapor phase, and the vapor pressure increases (Fig. 21-17). Vapor pressure is independent of atmospheric pressure and is contingent only on the temperature and physical characteristics of the liquid. The *boiling point* of a liquid is defined as that temperature at which the vapor pressure equals atmospheric pressure.[49–51] At 760 mm Hg, the boiling points for desflurane, isoflurane, halothane, enflurane, and sevoflurane are approximately 22.8, 48.5, 50.2, 56.5, and 58.5°C, respectively. Unlike other contemporary inhaled anesthetics, desflurane boils at temperatures that may be encountered in clinical settings such as pediatric and burn operating rooms. This unique physical characteristic alone mandates a special vaporizer design to control the delivery of desflurane. If agent-specific vaporizers are inadvertently misfilled with incorrect liquid anesthetic agents, the resulting mixtures of volatile agents may demonstrate unique properties from those of the individual component agents. The altered vapor pressure and other physical properties of the resulting azeotropic mixtures that result from the mixing of various agents may alter the output of the anesthetic vaporizer (see Variable Bypass Vaporizers: Misfilling section).[52]

Latent Heat of Vaporization

When a molecule is converted from a liquid to the gaseous phase, energy is consumed because the molecules of a liquid tend to cohere. The amount of energy that is consumed for a given liquid as it is converted to a vapor is referred to as the *latent heat of vaporization*. It is more precisely defined as the number of calories required to change 1 g of liquid into vapor without a temperature change. The energy for vaporization must either come from the liquid itself or from an outside source. The temperature of the liquid itself will decrease during vaporization in the absence of an outside energy source. This energy loss can lead to significant decreases in temperature of the remaining liquid, and can greatly decrease subsequent vaporization.[49,51,53]

Specific Heat

The *specific heat* of a substance is the number of calories required to increase the temperature of 1 g of a substance by

1°C.[21,49,51] The substance can be a solid, liquid, or gas. The concept of specific heat is important to the design, operation, and construction of vaporizers because it is applicable in two ways. First, the specific heat value for an inhaled anesthetic is important because it indicates how much heat must be supplied to the liquid to maintain a constant temperature when heat is being lost during vaporization. Second, manufacturers select vaporizer component materials that have a high specific heat to minimize temperature changes associated with vaporization.

Thermal Conductivity

Thermal conductivity is a measure of the speed with which heat flows through a substance. The higher the thermal conductivity, the better the substance conducts heat.[49] Vaporizers are constructed of metals that have relatively high thermal conductivity, these help to maintain a uniform internal temperature.

Ambient Pressure Effects

See Datex-Ohmeda Tec-6 Vaporizer for Desflurane: Factors that Influence Vaporizer Output: Varied Altitudes.

Variable Bypass Vaporizers

The Datex-Ohmeda Tec 4, Tec 5, and Tec 7, as well as the North American Dräger Vapor 19.n and 20.n vaporizers are classified as variable bypass, flow-over, temperature-compensated, agent-specific, out of breathing circuit vaporizers.[49] *Variable bypass* refers to the method for regulating the anesthetic agent concentration output from the vaporizer. The concentration control dial setting determines the ratio of flow that goes through the bypass chamber and through the vaporizing chamber as fresh gas from the flowmeters enters the vaporizer inlet. The gas channeled through the vaporizing chamber flows over a wick system saturated with the liquid anesthetic and subsequently also becomes saturated with vapor. Thus, *flow-over* refers to the method of vaporization and is in contrast to a bubble-through system that may be seen in some copper kettle type vaporizers of old. The Tec 4, Tec 5, and Tec 7, and the DrägerVapor 19.n and 20.n are further classified as *temperature compensated*. Each of these is equipped with an automatic temperature-compensating device that helps maintain a constant vaporizer output over a wide range of operating temperatures. These vaporizers are *agent specific* and *out-of-circuit* because each is designed to accommodate a single anesthetic agent and to be physically located outside of the breathing circuit. Variable bypass vaporizers are used to deliver halothane, enflurane, isoflurane, and sevoflurane, but not desflurane.

Basic Operating Principles

A diagram of a generic, variable bypass vaporizer is shown in Figure 21-18. Vaporizer components include the concentration control dial, the bypass chamber, the vaporizing chamber, the filler port, and the filler cap. Using the filler port, the operator fills the vaporizing chamber with liquid anesthetic. The maximum safe fill level is predetermined by the position of the filler port, which is positioned to minimize the chance of overfilling. If a vaporizer is overfilled or tilted, liquid anesthetic can spill into the bypass chamber. If this were to happen, both the vaporizing chamber flow and the bypass chamber flow could potentially be carrying saturated anesthetic vapor, and an overdose would result. The concentration control dial is a variable restrictor, and it can be located either in the bypass chamber or the outlet of the vaporizing chamber. The function of the concentration control dial is to regulate the relative flow rates through the bypass and vaporizing chambers.

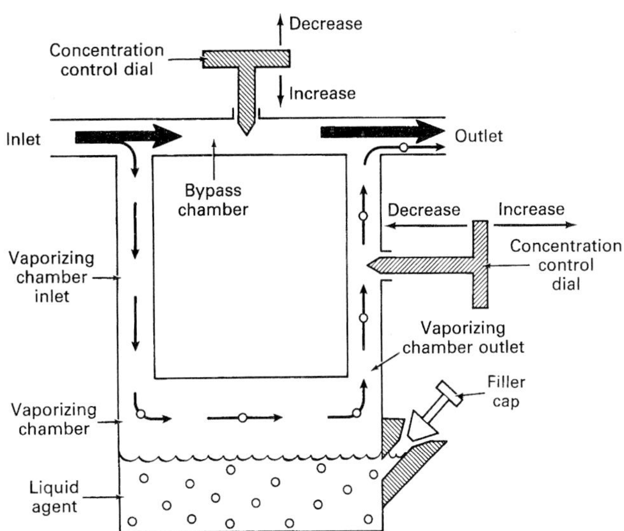

FIGURE 21-18. Generic variable bypass vaporizer. See text for details.

Flow from the flowmeters enters the inlet of the vaporizer. More than 80% of the flow passes straight through the bypass chamber to the vaporizer outlet, and this accounts for the name "bypass chamber." Less than 20% of the flow from the flowmeters is diverted through the vaporizing chamber. Depending on the temperature and vapor pressure of the particular inhaled anesthetic, the fresh gases entering the vaporizing chamber entrain a specific flow of the inhaled anesthetic agent. The mixture that exits the vaporizer is the combination of flow through the bypass chamber, flow through the vaporizing chamber, and flow of entrained anesthetic vapor. The final concentration of inhaled anesthetic is the ratio of the flow of the inhaled anesthetic to the total gas flow.[49,54]

The vapor pressure of an inhaled anesthetic depends on the ambient temperature (see Fig. 21-17). For example, at 20°C the vapor pressure of isoflurane is 238 mm Hg, whereas at 35°C the vapor pressure almost doubles (450 mm Hg). Variable bypass vaporizers have an internal mechanism to compensate for variations in ambient temperature. The temperature-compensating valve of the Datex-Ohmeda Tec 4 is shown in Figure 21-19. At relatively high ambient temperatures, such as those commonly seen in operating rooms designated for the care of pediatric or burn patients, the vapor pressure inside

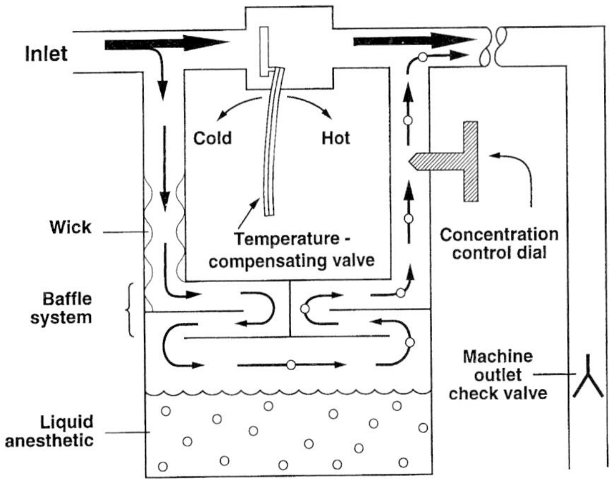

FIGURE 21-19. Simplified schematic of the Ohmeda Tec Type Vaporizer. See text for details.

the vaporizing chamber is high. To compensate for this increased vapor pressure, the bimetallic strip of the temperature-compensating valve leans to the right, decreasing the resistance to flow through the bypass chamber. This allows more flow to pass through the bypass chamber and less flow to pass through the vaporizing chamber. In contrast, in a cold operating room environment, the vapor pressure inside the vaporizing chamber is reduced. To compensate for this decrease in vapor pressure, the bimetallic strip leans to the left. This increases the resistance to flow through the bypass chamber, causing more flow to pass through the vaporizing chamber and less to pass through the bypass chamber. The net effect in both situations is maintenance of relatively constant vaporizer output.

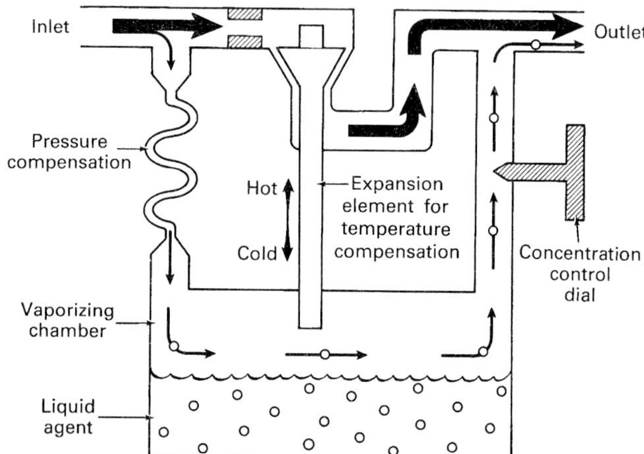

FIGURE 21-20. Simplified schematic of the North American Dräger Vapor 19.1 vaporizer. See text for details.

Factors That Influence Vaporizer Output

If an ideal vaporizer existed, with a fixed dial setting, its output would be constant regardless of varied flow rates, temperatures, back pressures, and carrier gases. Designing such a vaporizer is difficult because as ambient conditions change, the physical properties of gases and of vaporizers themselves can change.[54] Contemporary vaporizers approach ideal but still have some limitations. Even though some of the most sophisticated vaporizer systems now available use computer-controlled components and multiple sensors, they have yet to become significantly more accurate than conventional vaporizers. Several factors that affect vaporizer performance in general are described below.

Flow Rate. With a fixed dial setting, vaporizer output can vary with the rate of gas flowing through the vaporizer. This variation is particularly notable at extremes of flow rates. The output of all variable bypass vaporizers is less than the dial setting at low flow rates (less than 250 mL/min). This results from the relatively high density of volatile inhaled anesthetics. Insufficient turbulence is generated at low flow rates in the vaporizing chamber to upwardly advance the vapor molecules. At extremely high flow rates, such as 15 L/min, the output of most variable bypass vaporizers is less than the dial setting. This discrepancy is attributed to incomplete mixing and failure to saturate the carrier gas in the vaporizing chamber. Also, the resistance characteristics of the bypass chamber and the vaporizing chamber can vary as flow increases. These variations can result in decreased output concentration.[54]

Temperature. Because of improvements in design, the output of contemporary temperature-compensated vaporizers is almost linear over a wide range of temperatures. Automatic temperature-compensating mechanisms in the bypass chamber maintain a constant vaporizer output with varying temperatures.[23] As previously described, a bimetallic strip (see Fig. 21-19) or an expansion element (Fig. 21-20) directs a greater proportion of gas flow through the bypass chamber as temperatures increase.[54] Additionally, the wick systems are placed in direct contact with the metal wall of the vaporizer to help replace energy (heat) consumed during vaporization. The materials vaporizers are constructed from are chosen because they have a relatively high specific heat and high thermal conductivity. These factors help minimize the effect of cooling during vaporization.

Intermittent Back Pressure. Intermittent back pressure that results from either positive pressure ventilation or use of the oxygen flush valve may result in higher than expected vaporizer output. This phenomenon, known as the *pumping effect*, is more pronounced at low flow rates, low dial settings, and low levels of liquid anesthetic in the vaporizing chamber.[49,54–57] Additionally, the pumping effect is increased by rapid respiratory rates, high peak inspired pressures, and rapid drops in pressure during expiration.[47–51] Newer variable bypass vaporizers such as the Datex-Ohmeda Tec 4, Tec 5, and Tec 7, and North American Dräger Vapor 19.n and 20.n are relatively immune from the pumping effect. One proposed mechanism for the pumping effect is dependent on retrograde pressure transmission from the patient circuit to the vaporizer during the inspiratory phase of positive pressure ventilation. Gas molecules are compressed in both the bypass and vaporizing chambers. When the back pressure is suddenly released during the expiratory phase of positive-pressure ventilation, vapor exits the vaporizing chamber via both the vaporizing chamber outlet and retrograde through the vaporizing chamber inlet. This occurs because the output resistance of the bypass chamber is lower than that of the vaporizing chamber, particularly at low dial settings. The enhanced output concentration results from the increment of vapor that travels in the retrograde direction to the bypass chamber.[54–57]

To decrease the pumping effect, the vaporizing chambers of newer systems are smaller than those of early variable bypass vaporizers such as the Fluotec Mark II (750 mL).[56] Therefore, no substantial volumes of vapor can be discharged from the vaporizing chamber into the bypass chamber during the expiratory phase. The North American Dräger Vapor 19.1 and 20.n (see Fig. 21-20) have a long spiral tube that serves as the inlet to the vaporizing chamber.[56] When the pressure in the vaporizing chamber is released, some of the vapor enters this tube but does not enter the bypass chamber because of tube length.[50] The Tec 4 (see Fig. 21-19) has an extensive baffle system in the vaporizing chamber, and a one-way check valve has been inserted at the common gas outlet to minimize the pumping effect. This check valve attenuates but does not eliminate the pressure increase because gas still flows from the flowmeters to the vaporizer during the inspiratory phase of positive pressure ventilation.[49,58]

Carrier Gas Composition. Vaporizer output is influenced by the composition of the carrier gas that flows through the vaporizer.[59–66] During experimental conditions, when the carrier gas is rapidly changed from 100% oxygen to 100% nitrous oxide, a sudden transient decrease in vaporizer output occurs, followed by a slow increase to a new steady-state value (Fig. 21-21B).[64,65] Because nitrous oxide is more soluble than oxygen in the halogenated liquid within the vaporizer sump, when this switch occurs the output from the vaporizing chamber is transiently reduced.[64] Once the anesthetic liquid is totally saturated with nitrous oxide, vaporizing chamber output increases somewhat, and a new steady state is established.

The explanation for the new steady-state output value is less well understood.[66] With contemporary vaporizers such as the North American Dräger Vapor 19.n and 20.n and the Ohmeda Tec–type conventional vaporizers, the steady-state output value

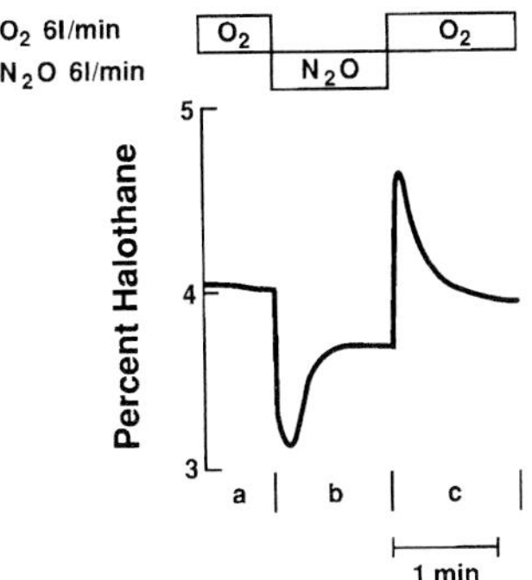

FIGURE 21-21. Halothane output of a North American Dräger Vapor 19.1 vaporizer with different carrier gases. The initial output concentration is approximately 4% halothane when oxygen is the carrier gas at flows of 6 L/min (A). When the carrier gas is quickly switched to 100% nitrous oxide (B), the halothane concentration decreases to 3% within 8 to 10 seconds. Then, a new steady-state concentration of approximately 3.5% is attained within 1 minute. See text for details. (Modified with permission from Gould DB, Lampert BA, MacKrell TN: Effect of nitrous oxide solubility on vaporizer aberrance. Anesth Analg 61:939, 1982.)

is less when nitrous oxide rather than oxygen is the carrier gas (see Fig. 21-21B). Conversely, the output of some older vaporizers is enhanced when nitrous oxide is the carrier gas instead of oxygen.[59,61] The steady-state plateau is achieved more rapidly with increased flow rates, regardless of the ultimate output value.[65] Factors that contribute to the characteristic steady-state response resulting when various carrier gases are used include the viscosity and density of the carrier gas, the relative solubilities of the carrier gas in the anesthetic liquid, the flow-splitting characteristics of the specific vaporizer, and the concentration control dial setting.[61,64–66]

Safety Features

Newer generations of anesthesia vaporizers including the North American Dräger 19.n and 20.n, and the Datex-Ohmeda Tec 4, Tec 5, and Tec 7 now have built-in safety features that have minimized or eliminated many hazards once associated with variable bypass vaporizers. Agent-specific, keyed filling devices help prevent filling a vaporizer with the wrong agent. Overfilling of these vaporizers is minimized because the filler port is located at the maximum safe liquid level. Finally, today's vaporizers are firmly secured to a vaporizer manifold on the anesthesia workstation. Thus, problems associated with vaporizer tipping have become much less frequent. Contemporary interlock systems prevent administration of more than one inhaled anesthetic.

Hazards

Despite many safety features, some hazards are still associated with contemporary variable bypass vaporizers.

Misfilling. Vaporizers not equipped with keyed fillers have been occasionally misfilled with the wrong anesthetic liquid.[67] A potential for misfilling exists even on contemporary vaporizers equipped with keyed fillers.[68–70] When a vaporizer misfilling occurs, patients can inadvertently be rendered inadequately, or excessively, anesthetized depending on which drug is placed in the vaporizer. The use of a multigas analyzer may alert the user to such a problem.

Contamination. Contamination of anesthetic vaporizer contents has occurred by filling an isoflurane vaporizer with a contaminated bottle of isoflurane. A potentially serious incident was avoided because the operator detected an abnormal acrid odor.[71]

Tipping. Tipping of a vaporizer can occur when they are incorrectly "switched out" or moved. However, tipping is unlikely when a vaporizer is attached to the anesthesia workstation manifold short of the entire machine being turned over. Excessive tipping can cause the liquid agent to enter the bypass chamber and can cause output with extremely high agent concentration.[72] The Tec 4 is slightly more immune to tipping than the North American Dräger Vapor 19.n because of its extensive baffle system. However, if either vaporizer is tipped, it should not be used until it has been flushed for 20 to 30 minutes at high fresh gas flow rates. During this procedure, having the vaporizer concentration control dial set at a low concentration maximizes bypass chamber flow and will aid in removal of any residual liquid anesthetic in that area.[49] After following this procedure, the use of a multigas analyzer is strongly recommended. The Dräger Vapor 20.n series vaporizers now have a transport ("T") dial setting that helps prevent tipping-related problems. When the dial is placed in this position, the vaporizer sump is isolated from the bypass chamber, thereby reducing the likelihood of tipping and a resulting accidental overdose. Therefore, any time one of these vaporizers is moved separate from the anesthesia workstation, the control dial should be placed in the "T" position.

The design of the Tec-6 and the Aladin cassette vaporizer systems, both from Datex-Ohmeda, has practically eliminated the possibility of tipping from these products. Since the Aladin cassette vaporizer's bypass chamber is physically separated from the "cassette," and permanently resides in the anesthesia workstation, the possibility of tipping is virtually eliminated. Tipping of the Aladin cassettes themselves when they are not installed in the vaporizer is not problematic.

Overfilling. Improper filling procedures combined with failure of the vaporizer sight glass can cause overfilling and patient overdose. Liquid anesthetic enters the bypass chamber, and up to 10 times the intended vapor concentration can be delivered to the common gas outlet.[73] Most modern vaporizers are now relatively immune to overfilling because of side-fill rather than top-fill designs. Side-fill systems largely prevent overfilling.

Underfilling. Just as with overfilling, underfilling of anesthetic vaporizers may also be problematic. When a Tec 5 sevoflurane vaporizer is in a low-fill state and used under conditions of high fresh gas flow rates (>7.5 L/min) and high dial setting (such as seen during inhalational inductions), the vaporizer output may abruptly decrease to less than 2%. The causes of this problem are most likely multifactorial. However, the combination of low vaporizer fill state (<25% full) in combination with the high vaporizing chamber flow, can result in a clinically significant and reproducible fall in vaporizer output.[74]

Simultaneous Inhaled Anesthetic Administration. On some older anesthesia machines from Datex-Ohmeda that are equipped with the Select-a-Tec® three-vaporizer manifold that does not utilize a vapor-interlock system, two inhaled anesthetics can be administered simultaneously when the center vaporizer is removed. On such machines, the left or right vaporizer should be moved to the central position if the central vaporizer is removed (as indicated by the manifold warning label). Once this is done, the vaporizer's interlock system will allow only one agent to be administered at a time. More contemporary Select-a-Tec vaporizer manifolds have a built-in vapor-interlock or vapor-exclusion device that prevents this problem. On these newer three-vaporizer systems, a U-shaped plastic device links the vaporizer extension rods even when the vaporizers are not adjacent to one another on the manifold. On such a system, the manifold plus the vaporizers themselves comprise the vapor-interlock or vapor-exclusion system.

Leaks. Vaporizer leaks occur frequently, and can potentially result in patient awareness during anesthesia.[11,15,55,75] A loose filler cap is the most common source of vaporizer leaks. With some key-filled Penlon and Dräger vaporizers, a loose filler screw clamp allows escape of saturated anesthetic vapor.[11] Leaks can occur at the O-ring junctions between the vaporizer and its manifold. To detect a leak within a vaporizer, the concentration control dial must be in the on position. Even though vaporizer leaks in Dräger Systems can potentially be detected with a conventional positive-pressure leak test (because of the absence of an outlet check valve), a negative-pressure leak test is more sensitive and allows the user to detect even small leaks. Datex-Ohmeda recommends a negative-pressure leak testing device (suction bulb) to detect vaporizer leaks in the Modulus I, Modulus II, Excel, and the Aestiva workstations because of the check valve located just upstream of each machine's fresh gas outlet (see Checking Your Anesthesia Workstation section).

Many newer anesthesia workstations are capable of performing self-testing procedures that, in some cases, may eliminate the need for the conventional negative-pressure leak testing. However, it is of vital importance that anesthesia providers understand that these self-tests may not detect internal vaporizer leaks on systems with add-on vaporizers. For the self-tests to determine if an internal vaporizer leak is present, the leak test must be repeated with each vaporizer sequentially while its concentration control dial is turned to the on position. Recall that when a vaporizer's concentration control dial is set in the off position, it may not be possible to detect even major internal leaks such as an absent or loose filler cap.

Anesthesia Vaporizers and Environmental Considerations. Today, more than ever, anesthetics are being administered to patients outside the operating room. One such location that has proved sometimes difficult to work in is the MRI suite. The presence of a powerful magnet field, the significant noise pollution, and limited access to the patient during the procedure all complicate care in this setting. It is imperative that only nonferrous (MRI compatible) equipment be used in these settings. Some anesthesia vaporizers, although they may appear nonferrous by testing with a horseshoe magnet, may indeed contain substantial internal ferrous components. Inappropriate use of such a device in an MRI suite may potentially turn them into a dangerous missile if left unsecured.[76]

The Datex-Ohmeda Tec 6 Vaporizer for Desflurane

Because of its unique physical characteristics, the controlled vaporization of desflurane required a novel approach to vaporizer design. Datex-Ohmeda developed the Tec 6 vaporizer, the first
8 such system, and released it into clinical use in the early 1990s. The Tec 6 vaporizer is an electrically heated, pressurized device specifically designed to deliver desflurane.[77,78] The vapor pressure of desflurane is three to four times that of other contemporary inhaled anesthetics, and it boils at 22.8°C,[79] which is near room temperature (see Fig. 21-17). Desflurane has a minimum alveolar anesthetic concentration (MAC) value of 6 to 7%.[79] Desflurane is valuable because it has a low blood gas solubility coefficient of 0.45 at 37°C, and recovery from anesthesia is more rapid than with many other potent inhaled anesthetics.[79] In 2004, Dräger Medical received FDA approval for its own version of the Tec 6 desflurane vaporizer. The operating principles described in the following discussion are applicable to either system, even though we refer to the Tec 6 specifically.

Unsuitability of Contemporary Variable Bypass Vaporizers for Controlled Vaporization of Desflurane

Desflurane's high volatility and moderate potency preclude
9 its use with contemporary variable bypass vaporizers such as Datex-Ohmeda Tec 4, Tec 5, and Tec 7, or the North American Dräger Vapor 19.n or 20.n for two primary reasons:[77]

1. At 20°C the vapor pressure of desflurane is near one atmosphere.

   The vapor pressures of enflurane, isoflurane, halothane, and desflurane at 20°C are 172, 240, 244, and 669 mm Hg, respectively (see Fig. 21-17).[79] Equal amounts of flow through a traditional vaporizer would vaporize many more volumes of desflurane than any other of these agents. For example, at one atmosphere and 20°C, 100 mL/min passing through the vaporizing chamber would entrain 735 mL/min desflurane versus 29, 46, and 47 mL/min of enflurane, isoflurane, and halothane, respectively.[77] Under these same conditions, to produce 1% desflurane output the amount of bypass flow necessary to achieve sufficient dilution of the large volume of desflurane saturated anesthetic vapor would be approximately 73 L/min, compared to 5 L/min or less for the other three anesthetics. Additionally, above 22.8°C at one atmosphere, desflurane will boil. The amount of vapor produced would be limited only by the heat energy available from the vaporizer owing to its specific heat.[77]
2. Contemporary vaporizers lack an external heat source.

   The latent heat of vaporization for desflurane is approximately equal to that of enflurane, isoflurane, and halothane; however its MAC is 4 to 9 times higher than those of the other three inhaled anesthetics. Thus, the absolute amount of desflurane vaporized over a given time period is considerably greater than the other anesthetic drugs. Supplying desflurane via a conventional vaporizer in higher (equivalent MAC) concentrations would lead to excessive cooling of the vaporizer and would significantly reduce its output. In the absence of an external heat source, temperature compensation using traditional mechanical devices would be almost impossible. Because of the broad range of temperatures seen in the clinical setting, and because of desflurane's steep vapor pressure versus temperature curve (see Fig. 21-17), the delivery of desflurane in a conventional anesthetic vaporizer would be at best unpredictable.[77]

Operating Principles of the Tec 6 and Tec 6 Plus

To achieve controlled vaporization of desflurane, Datex-Ohmeda introduced the Tec 6 vaporizer to widespread clinical practice in 1993. This was the first clinically available vaporizer ever to be electrically heated and pressurized. The physical appearance and operation of the Tec 6 are similar to contemporary vaporizers, but some aspects of the internal design and operating principles are radically different. The Tec 6 Plus represents a later version of the original Tec 6. The Tec 6 Plus has the same basic Tec 6 design, but also incorporates an enhanced audible alarm system not previously available on the Tec 6.

Functionally, the Tec 6's operation is more accurately described as a dual-gas blender than as a vaporizer. A simplified schematic of the Tec 6 is shown in Figure 21-22. The vaporizer has two independent gas circuits arranged in parallel. The fresh gas circuit is shown in gray, and the vapor circuit is shown in white. The fresh gas from the flowmeters enters at the fresh gas inlet, passes through a fixed restrictor (R1), and exits at the vaporizer gas outlet. The vapor circuit originates at the desflurane sump, which is electrically heated and thermostatically controlled to 39°C, a temperature well above desflurane's boiling point. The heated sump assembly serves as a reservoir of desflurane vapor. At 39°C, the vapor pressure in the sump is approximately 1,300 mm Hg absolute,[80] or approximately 2 atmospheres absolute (see Fig. 21-17). Just downstream from the sump is the shutoff valve. After the vaporizer warms up, the shutoff valve fully opens when the concentration control valve is turned to the on position. A pressure-regulating valve located

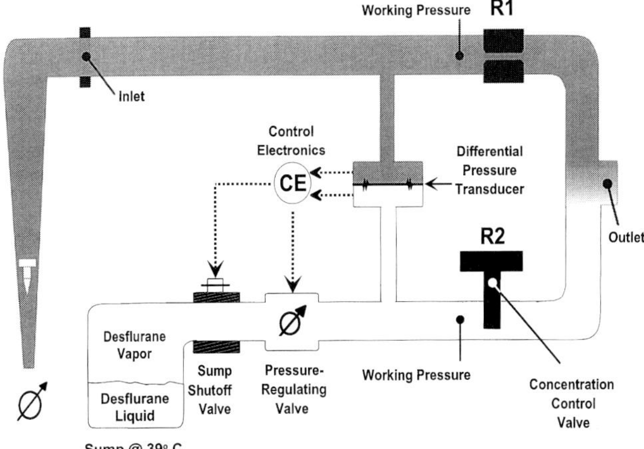

FIGURE 21-22. Simplified schematic of the Tec 6 desflurane vaporizer. (From Andrews JJ: Operating Principles of the Ohmeda Tec 6 Desflurane Vaporizer: A Collection of Twelve Color Illustrations. Washington, DC, Library of Congress, Copyright 1996, with permission.)

downstream from the shutoff valve downregulates the pressure to approximately 1.1 atmospheres absolute (74 mm Hg gauge) at a fresh gas flow rate of 10 L/min. The operator controls desflurane output by adjusting the concentration control valve (R2), which is a variable restrictor.[77]

The vapor flow through R2 joins the fresh gas flow through R1 at a point downstream from the restrictors. Until this point, the two circuits are physically divorced. They are interfaced pneumatically and electronically, however, through differential pressure transducers, a control electronics system, and a pressure-regulating valve. When a constant fresh gas flow rate encounters the fixed restrictor, R1, a specific back pressure, proportional to the fresh gas flow rate, pushes against the diaphragm of the control differential pressure transducer. The differential pressure transducer conveys the pressure difference between the fresh gas circuit and the vapor circuit to the control electronics system. The control electronics system regulates the pressure-regulating valve so that the pressure in the vapor circuit equals the pressure in the fresh gas circuit. This equalized pressure supplying R1 and R2 is the working pressure, and the working pressure is constant at a fixed fresh gas flow rate. If the operator increases the fresh gas flow rate, more back pressure is exerted upon the diaphragm of the control pressure transducer, and the working pressure of the vaporizer increases.[77]

Table 21-2 shows the approximate correlation between fresh gas flow rate and working pressure for a typical vaporizer. At a fresh gas flow rate of 1 L/min, the working pressure is 10 millibars, or 7.4 mm Hg gauge. At a fresh gas flow rate of 10 L/min, the working pressure is 100 millibars, or 74 mm Hg gauge. Therefore, there is a linear relationship between fresh gas flow rate and working pressure. When the fresh gas flow rate is increased 10-fold, the working pressure increases 10-fold.[77]

Listed below are two specific examples to demonstrate the operating principles of the Tec 6.[77]

Example A: Constant fresh gas flow rate of 1 L/min, with an increase in the dial setting.

With a fresh gas flow rate of 1 L/min, the working pressure of the vaporizer is 7.4 mm Hg. That is, the pressure supplying R1 and R2 is 7.4 mm Hg. As the operator increases the dial setting, the opening at R2 becomes larger, allowing more vapor to pass through R2. Specific vapor flow values at different dial settings are shown in Table 21-3.

Example B: Constant dial setting with an increase in fresh gas flow from 1 to 10 L/min.

At a fresh gas flow rate of 1 L/min, the working pressure is 7.4 mm Hg, and at a dial setting of 6% the vapor flow rate through R2 is 64 mL/min (see Tables 21-2 and 21-3). With a 10-fold increase in the fresh gas flow rate, there is a concomitant 10-fold increase in the working pressure to 74 mm Hg. The ratio of resistances of R2 to R1 is constant at a fixed dial setting of 6%. Because R2 is supplied by 10 times more pressure, the vapor flow rate through R2 increases 10-fold to 640 mL/min. Vaporizer output is constant because both the fresh gas flow and the vapor flow increase proportionally.

Factors that Influence Vaporizer Output

Varied altitude and carrier gas composition influence Tec 6 output. Each is discussed in the following sections.

Varied Altitudes. Although ambient pressure changes affect conventional vaporizer output significantly in terms of volumes percent (%v/v, i.e. concentration), their effect on anesthetic potency (i.e. partial pressure) is minimal. This effect is illustrated using the example of isoflurane shown in Table 21-4. With a constant dial setting of 0.89%, at 1 atm (760 mm Hg), if perfectly calibrated, the %v/v delivered would be 0.89% and the partial pressure of isoflurane would be 6.8 mm Hg. Maintaining the same dial setting and lowering ambient pressure to 0.66 atm or 502 mm Hg (roughly equivalent to 10,000 ft elevation) would result in an increase in the concentration output to 1.75% (almost double), but the partial pressure only increases to 8.77 mm Hg (only a 29% increase) because of the proportionate decline in ambient pressure.

It is generally considered that the partial pressure of the anesthetic agent in the central nervous system, not its concentration, is responsible for the anesthetic effect. To obtain a consistent depth of anesthesia when gross changes in barometric pressure occur, the %v/v must be changed in inverse

TABLE 21-2

FRESH GAS FLOW RATE VERSUS WORKING PRESSURE

FRESH GAS FLOW RATE (L/min)	WORKING PRESSURE AT R1 AND R2 (GAUGE) (GAS INLET PRESSURE)		
	mbar	cm WATER	mmHG
1	10	10.2	7.4
5	50	51.0	37.0
10	100	102.0	74.0

Reprinted with permission from Andrews JJ, Johnston RV Jr: The new Tec 6 desflurane vaporizer. Anesth Analg 76:1338, 1993.

TABLE 21-3

DIAL SETTING VERSUS FLOW THROUGH RESTRICTOR R2

DIAL SETTING (VOL%)[a]	FRESH GAS FLOW RATE (L/min)	APPROXIMATE VAPOR FLOW RATE THROUGH R2 (mL/min)
1	1	10
6	1	64
12	1	136
18	1	220

[a] Volume percent = [(vapor flow rate)/(fresh gas flow rate) + (vapor flow rate)] × 100%.
Reprinted with permission from Andrews JJ, Johnston RV Jr: The new Tec 6 desflurane vaporizer. Anesth Analg 76:1338, 1993.

proportion to the barometric pressure. For the most part, traditional variable bypass vaporizers automatically compensate for this change and for practical purposes the effect of barometric pressure can generally be ignored.

This should be considered in stark contrast to the response of the Tec-6 desflurane vaporizer at varied altitudes (Table 21-4). One must remember this device is more accurately described as a dual gas "blender" than a vaporizer. Regardless of the ambient pressure, the Tec-6 will maintain a constant concentration of vapor output (%v/v), not a constant partial pressure. This means that at high altitudes, the partial pressure of desflurane for any given dial setting will be decreased in proportion to the atmospheric pressure divided by the calibration pressure (normally 760 mm Hg) per the following formula.

$$\text{Required Dial Setting} = \frac{\text{Normal Dial Setting (\%v/v)} \times 760 \text{ mm Hg}}{\text{Ambient Pressure (mm Hg)}}$$

For example at an altitude of 2000 m (6564 ft) where the ambient pressure is 608 mm Hg, the Tec-6 dial setting must be advanced from 10%v/v to 12.5%v/v to avoid underdosing that could potentially result in patient awareness. Conversely, the Tec-6's maintenance of a constant %v/v in hyperbaric conditions could produce significant increases in partial pressure output, and if not accounted for, the potential for anesthetic overdose. Therefore, in hyperbaric settings the Tec-6 dial setting would need to be reduced to maintain the desired partial pressure output of desflurane.

Carrier Gas Composition. Vaporizer output approximates the dial setting when oxygen is the carrier gas because the Tec 6 vaporizer is calibrated using 100% oxygen. At low flow rates when a carrier gas other than 100% oxygen is used, however, a clear trend toward reduction in vaporizer output emerges. This reduction parallels the proportional decrease in viscosity of the carrier gas. Nitrous oxide has a lower viscosity than oxygen, so the back pressure generated by resistor R1 (see Fig. 21-22) is less when nitrous oxide is the carrier gas, and the working pressure is reduced. At low flow rates using nitrous oxide as the carrier gas, vaporizer output is approximately 20% less than the dial setting. This suggests that, at clinically useful fresh gas flow rates, the gas flow across resistor R1 is laminar, and the working pressure is proportional to both the fresh gas flow rate and the viscosity of the carrier gas.[81]

Safety Features

Because desflurane's vapor pressure is near one atmosphere, misfilling contemporary vaporizers with desflurane could theoretically result in both desflurane overdose and creation

TABLE 21-4

PERFORMANCE OF TEC TYPE VAPORIZERS VS. THE TEC 6 DESFLURANE VAPORIZER AT VARYING AMBIENT PRESSURES

		ISOFLURANE VAPORIZER WITH A DIAL SETTING OF 0.89%			TEC 6 DESFLURANE VAPORIZER WITH A DIAL SETTING OF 6%
ATMOSPHERES	AMBIENT PRESSURE (mm Hg)	cc ISOFLURANE VAPOR ENTRAINED BY 100 cc O_2	OUTPUT CONCENTRATION IN PERCENT	PARTIAL PRESSURE OUTPUT (mm Hg)	PARTIAL PRESSURE OUTPUT OF DESFLURANE (mm Hg)
0.66 (2/3)	500 (10,000 feet)	91	1.753%	8.77	30
0.74	560	74	1.429%	8.0	33.6
0.80	608 (6,564 feet)	64.32	1.25%	7.6	36.5
1.0	760	46	0.89%	6.8	45.6
1.5	1,140	26.4	0.515%	5.87	68.4
2	1,520	19	0.36%	5.5	91.2
3	2,280	11.65	0.228%	5.198	136

(The following were assumed: 5,000 cc bypass chamber flow, 100 cc vaporizing chamber flow - Equivalent to an isoflurane dial setting of 0.89%)

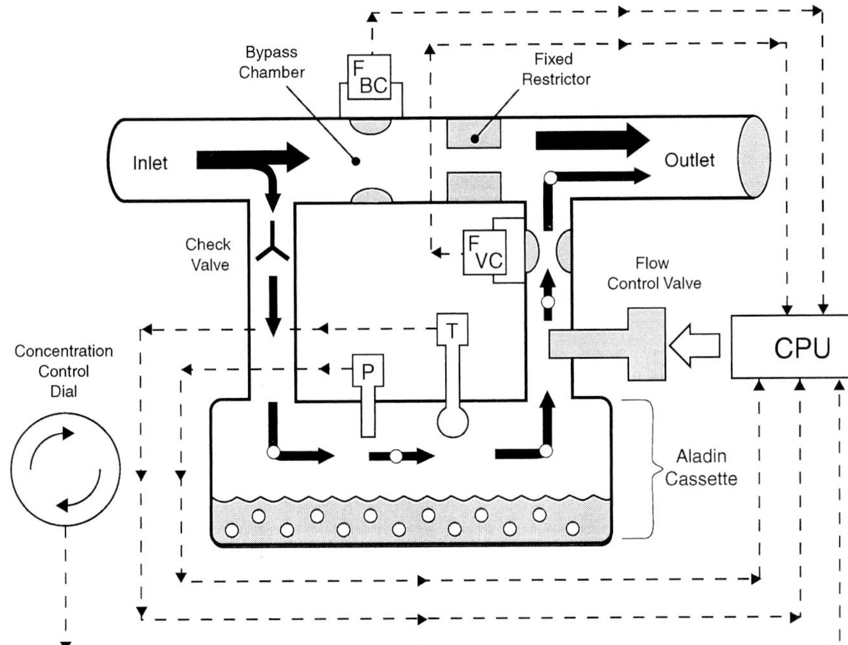

FIGURE 21-23. Simplified schematic of Datex-Ohmeda Aladin Cassette Vaporizer. The *black arrows* represent flow from the flowmeters, and the *white circles* represent anesthetic vapor. The heart of the vaporizer is the electronically controlled flow control valve located in the outlet of the vaporizing chamber. CPU, central processing unit; F_{BC}, flow measurement unit, which measures flow through the bypass chamber; F_{VC} = flow measurement unit, which measures flow through the vaporizing chamber; P, pressure sensor; T, temperature sensor. (Modified from Andrews, JJ: Operating Principles of the Datex-Ohmeda Aladin Cassette Vaporizer: A Collection of Color Illustrations. Washington, DC, Library of Congress, 2000.)

of a hypoxic gas mixture.[82] Datex-Ohmeda has introduced a unique, anesthetic-specific filling system to minimize occurrence of this potential hazard. The agent-specific filler of the desflurane bottle known as the "Saf-T-Fill" adapter is intended to prevent its use with traditional vaporizers. The filling system also minimizes spillage of liquid or vapor anesthetic by maintaining a "closed system" during the filling process. Each desflurane bottle has a spring-loaded filler cap with an O-ring on the tip. The spring seals the bottle until it is engaged in the filler port of the vaporizer. Thus, this anesthetic-specific filling system interlocks the vaporizer and the dispensing bottle, preventing loss of anesthetic to the atmosphere. A case report described the misfilling of a Tec 6 desflurane vaporizer with sevoflurane. This error was possible because of similarities between a new type of keyed filler for sevoflurane and the desflurane Saf-T-fill adapter. In this case, the desflurane vaporizer detected this error and automatically shut itself off.[70]

Major vaporizer faults cause the shutoff valve located just downstream from the desflurane sump (see Fig. 21-22) to close, producing a no-output situation. The valve is closed and a "no-output" alarm is activated immediately if any of the following conditions occur: (1) the anesthetic level decreases to below 20 mL; (2) the vaporizer is tilted; (3) a power failure occurs; or (4) there is a disparity between the pressure in the vapor circuit versus the pressure in the fresh gas circuit exceeding a specified tolerance.

Summary

The Tec 6 vaporizer is an electrically heated, thermostatically controlled, constant-temperature, pressurized, electromechanically coupled dual circuit, gas-vapor blender. The pressure in the vapor circuit is electronically regulated to equal the pressure in the fresh gas circuit. At a constant fresh gas flow rate, the operator regulates vapor flow using a conventional concentration control dial. When the fresh gas flow rate increases, the working pressure increases proportionally. For a given concentration setting even when varying the fresh gas flow rate, the vaporizer output is constant because the amount of flow through each circuit remains proportional.[77]

The Datex-Ohmeda Aladin Cassette Vaporizer

The vaporizer system used in the Datex-Ohmeda S5/Anesthesia Delivery Unit (ADU) is unique in that the single electronically controlled vaporizer is designed to deliver five different inhaled anesthetics including halothane, isoflurane, enflurane, sevoflurane, and desflurane. The vaporizer consists of a permanent internal control unit housed within the ADU and an interchangeable Aladin agent cassette that contains anesthetic liquid. The Aladin agent cassettes are color coded for each anesthetic agent, and they are also magnetically coded so that the Datex-Ohmeda ADU can identify which anesthetic cassette has been inserted. The cassettes are filled using agent-specific fillers.[49]

Though very different in external appearance, the functional anatomy of the S/5 ADU cassette vaporizer (Fig. 21-23) is very similar to that of the Dräger vapor 19.1 and 20.n and the Datex-Ohmeda Tec 4, Tec 5, and Tec 7 vaporizers. The Aladin system is functionally similar to these conventional vaporizers because it is also made up of a bypass chamber and vaporizing chamber. A fixed restrictor is located in the bypass chamber, and flow measurement sensors are located both in the bypass chamber and in the outlet of the vaporizing chamber. The heart of the S/5 ADU cassette vaporizer is the electronically regulated flow control valve located in the vaporizing chamber outlet. This valve is controlled by a central processing unit (CPU). The CPU receives input from multiple sources including the concentration control dial, a pressure sensor located inside the vaporizing chamber, a temperature sensor located inside the vaporizing chamber, a flow measurement unit located in the bypass chamber, and a flow measurement unit located in the outlet of the vaporizing chamber. The CPU also receives input from the flowmeters regarding the composition of the carrier gas. Using data from these multiple sources, the CPU is able to precisely regulate the flow control valve to attain the desired vapor concentration output. Appropriate electronic control of the flow control valve is essential to the proper function of this vaporizer.[49,84]

A fixed restrictor is located in the bypass chamber, and it causes flow from the vaporizer inlet to split into two flow streams (see Fig. 21-23). One stream passes through the bypass chamber, and the other portion enters the inlet of the vaporizing chamber and passes through a one-way check valve. The presence of this check valve is unique to the Aladin system. This one-way valve prevents retrograde flow of the anesthetic vapor back into the bypass chamber, and its presence is crucial when delivering desflurane if the room temperature is greater than the boiling point for Desflurane (22.8°C).[49] A precise amount of vapor-saturated carrier gas passes through the flow control valve, which is regulated by the CPU. This flow then joins the bypass flow and is directed to the outlet of the vaporizer.[49]

As mentioned during the discussion of the Tec 6, the controlled vaporization of desflurane presents a unique challenge, particularly when the room temperature is greater than the boiling point of desflurane (22.8°C). At higher temperatures, the pressure inside the vaporizer sump increases, and the sump becomes pressurized. When the sump pressure exceeds the pressure in the bypass chamber, the one-way check valve located in the vaporizing chamber inlet closes preventing carrier gas from entering the vaporizing chamber. At this point, the carrier gas passes straight through the bypass chamber and its flow sensor. Under these conditions, the electronically regulated flow control valve simply meters in the appropriate flow of pure desflurane vapor needed to achieve the desired final concentration selected by the user. At least one case report has described a failure of the vaporizing chamber inlet check valve to function as designed. In this case, an anesthetic overdose occurred as a result of regurgitation of desflurane from the vaporizing chamber in a retrograde fashion back into the bypass chamber. This report merits ADU users to be cautious of this potential problem, especially when desflurane is used.[84]

During operating conditions in which high fresh gas flow rates and/or high dial settings are used, large quantities of anesthetic liquid are rapidly vaporized. As a result, the temperature of the remaining liquid anesthetic and the vaporizer itself decrease as a result of energy consumption of the latent heat of vaporization. To offset this cooling effect, the S/5 ADU is equipped with a fan that forces warmed air from an "agent heating resistor" across the cassette (vaporizer sump) to raise its temperature when necessary. The fan is activated during two common clinical scenarios: (1) desflurane induction and maintenance, and (2) sevoflurane induction.

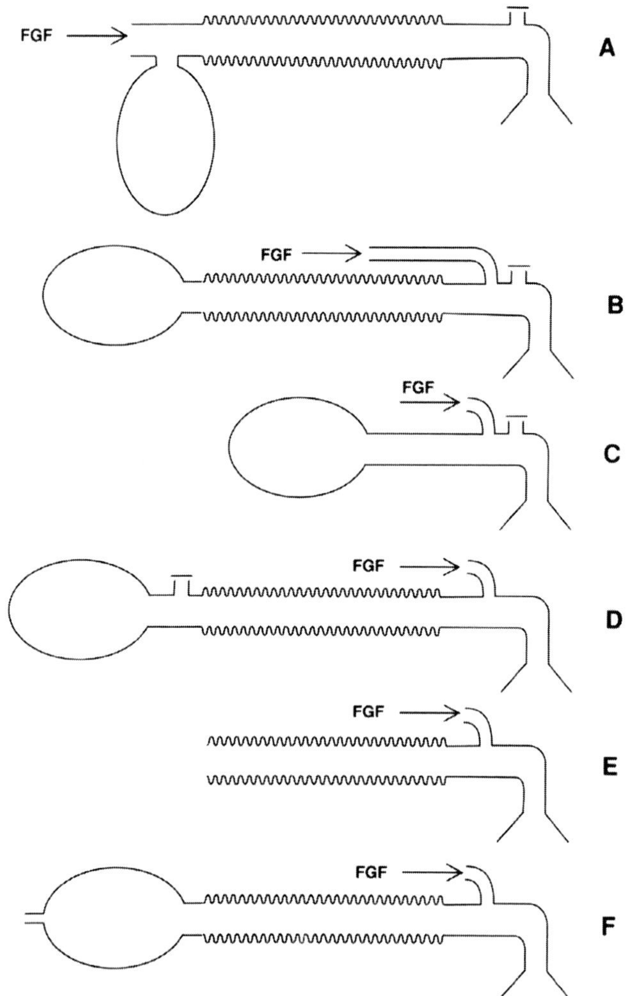

FIGURE 21-24. Mapleson Breathing Systems A-F. (Redrawn with permission. Willis BA, Pender JW, Mapleson WW: Rebreathing in a T-piece: Volunteer and Theoretical Studies of the Jackson-Rees Modification of Ayre's T-piece during spontaneous respiration. Br J Anaesth 47:1239, 1975.)

ANESTHETIC BREATHING CIRCUITS

As the prescribed mixture of gases from the flowmeters and vaporizer exits the anesthesia workstation at the common gas outlet, it then enters an anesthetic breathing circuit. The function of the anesthesia breathing circuit is not only to deliver oxygen and anesthetic gases to the patient, but also to eliminate CO_2. CO_2 can be removed either by washout with adequate fresh gas inflow or by the use of CO_2 absorbent media (e.g., soda lime absorption). The following discussion focuses on the semiclosed rebreathing circuits and the circle system.

Mapleson Systems

In 1954 Mapleson described and analyzed five different semiclosed anesthetic systems, and they are now classically referred to as the Mapleson Systems and are designated with letters A through E (Fig. 21-24).[85] Subsequently in 1975, Willis et al described the F system that was added to the original five.[86] The Mapleson Systems consist of several common components. Theses components commonly include a facemask, a spring-loaded pop-off valve, reservoir tubing, fresh gas inflow tubing, and a reservoir bag. Within the Mapleson Systems, three distinct functional groups can be seen. They include the A, the BC, and DEF groups. The Mapleson A, also known as the Magill Circuit, has a spring-loaded pop-off valve located near the facemask, and the fresh gas flow enters the opposite end of the circuit near the reservoir bag. In the B and C systems, the spring-loaded pop-off valve is located near the facemask, but the fresh gas inlet tubing is located near the patient. The reservoir tubing and breathing bag serve as a blind limb where fresh gas, dead space gas, and alveolar gas can collect. Finally, in the Mapleson D, E, F group or "T-piece" group, the fresh gas enters near the patient, and excess gas is popped off at the opposite end of the circuit.

Even though the components and component arrangement are simple, functional analysis of the Mapleson Systems can be complex.[87,88] The amount of CO_2 rebreathing associated with each system is multifactorial, and variables which dictate the ultimate CO_2 concentration include the following: (1) the fresh gas inflow rate, (2) the minute ventilation, (3) the mode of ventilation (spontaneous or controlled), (4) the tidal volume, (5) the respiratory rate, (6) the I:E ratio, (7) the duration of the expiratory pause, (8) the peak inspiratory flow rate, (9) the volume of the reservoir tube, (10) the volume of the breathing bag, (11) ventilation by mask, (12) ventilation through an endotracheal tube, and (13) the CO_2 sampling site.

The performance of the Mapleson Systems is best understood by studying the expiratory phase of the respiratory cycle.[89] Illustrations of the various Mapleson System component arrangements may be found in Figure 21-24. During spontaneous ventilation, the Mapleson A has the best efficiency of the six systems requiring a fresh gas inflow rate of only one times the minute ventilation to prevent rebreathing of CO_2. But it has the worst efficiency during controlled ventilation, requiring a minute ventilation as high as 20 L/min to prevent rebreathing. Systems DEF are slightly more efficient than systems BC. To prevent rebreathing CO_2, the DEF systems require a fresh gas inflow rate of approximately 2.5 times the minute ventilation, whereas the fresh gas inflow rates required for BC systems are somewhat higher.[88]

The following summarizes the relative efficiency of different Mapleson Systems with respect to prevention of rebreathing, during spontaneous ventilation: A > DFE > CB. During controlled ventilation, DFE > BC > A.[85,88] The Mapleson A, B, and C systems are rarely used today, but the D, E, F systems are commonly employed. In the United States, the most popular representative from the D, E, F group is the Bain Circuit, and it will be discussed in the next section.

Bain Circuit

The Bain circuit is a coaxial circuit and a modification of the Mapleson D system. The fresh gas flows through a narrow inner tube within the outer corrugated tubing.[91] The central fresh gas tubing enters the outer corrugated hose near the reservoir bag, but the fresh gas actually empties into the circuit at the patient end (Fig. 21-25). Exhaled gases enter the corrugated tubing and are vented through the expiratory valve near the reservoir bag. The Bain circuit may be used for both spontaneous and controlled ventilation. The fresh gas inflow rate necessary to prevent rebreathing is 2.5 the minute ventilation.

The Bain circuit has many advantages over other systems. It is lightweight, convenient, easily sterilized, and may be reusable. Scavenging of the gases from the expiratory valve is facilitated because the valve is located away from the patient. Exhaled gases in the outer reservoir tubing add warmth by countercurrent heat exchange to inspired fresh gases. The main hazards related to the use of the Bain circuit are either an unrecognized disconnection or kinking of the inner fresh gas hose. These problems can cause hypercarbia from inadequate gas flow or increased respiratory resistance. As with other circuits, an obstructed antimicrobial filter positioned between the Bain circuit and the endotracheal tube can result in increased resistance in the circuit. This may produce hypoventilation and hypoxemia, and may even mimic the signs and symptoms of severe bronchospasm.[92]

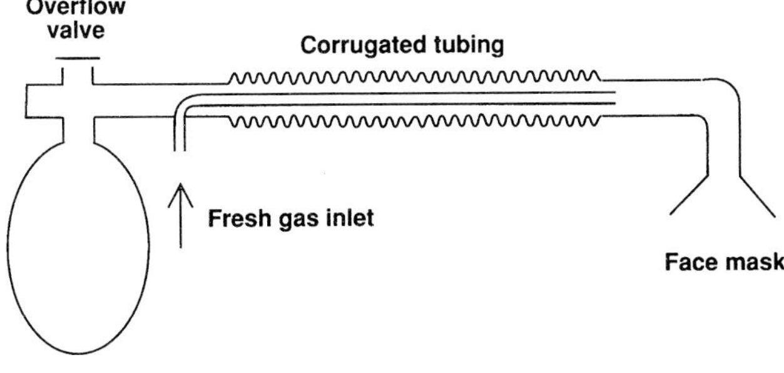

FIGURE 21-25. The Bain Circuit. (Redrawn with permission from Bain JA, Spoerel WE: A streamlined anaesthetic system. Can Anaesth Soc J 19:426, 1972.)

The outer corrugated tube should be transparent to allow ongoing inspection of the inner tube. The integrity of the inner tube can be assessed as described by Pethick.[93] With his technique, high-flow oxygen is fed into the circuit while the patient end is occluded until the reservoir bag is filled. The patient end is opened, and oxygen is flushed into the circuit. If the inner tube is intact, the venturi effect occurs at the patient end. This causes a decrease in pressure within the circuit, and as a result, the reservoir bag deflates. Conversely, a leak in the inner tube allows the fresh gas to escape into the expiratory limb, and the reservoir bag will remain inflated. This test is recommended as a part of the pre-anesthesia check if a Bain circuit is used.

Circle Breathing Systems

For many years, the overall design of the circle breathing system has changed very little from one anesthesia workstation manufacturer to the next. Both the individual components and the order in which they appeared in the circle system were consistent across major platforms. More recently, however, with the increasing technological complexity of the anesthesia workstation, the circle system has gone through some major changes as well. These changes have resulted in part from an effort to improve patient safety (as in the integration of Fresh Gas Decoupling and Inspiratory Pressure Limiters), but have also allowed the deployment of new technological advances. Examples of major new technologies include (1) a return to the application of single-circuit piston-type ventilators and (2) use of new spirometry devices that are located at the Y-connector instead of at the traditional location on the expiratory circuit limb. The following discussion first focuses on the traditional circle breathing system, and then is followed by a brief discussion of some variations in the designs of newer circle systems.

The Traditional Circle Breathing System

The circle system remains the most popular breathing system in the United States. It is so named because its components are arranged in a circular manner (see Fig. 21-7). One version of the traditional circle system, referred to as either a "Universal F" or "single limb circuit," has increased in popularity over recent years. Though these systems appear very different externally, they have the same overall functional layout as the traditional circle system and the following discussion is applicable to both the traditional circle system and the "Universal F" system.

The circle system prevents rebreathing of CO_2 by use of CO_2 absorbents but allows partial rebreathing of other exhaled gases. The extent of rebreathing of the other exhaled gases depends on breathing circuit component arrangement and the fresh gas flow rate. A circle system can be semiopen, semiclosed, or closed, depending on the amount of fresh gas inflow.[94] A semiopen system has no rebreathing and requires a very high flow of fresh gas. A semiclosed system is associated with some rebreathing of exhaled gases and is the most commonly used application in the United States. A closed system is one in which the inflow gas exactly matches that being taken up, or consumed, by the patient. In a closed system, there is complete rebreathing of exhaled gases after absorption of CO_2, and the overflow (pop-off or APL) valve or ventilator relief valve remains closed.

The circle system (see Fig. 21-7) consists of seven primary components, including the following: (1) a fresh gas inflow source; (2) inspiratory and expiratory unidirectional valves; (3) inspiratory and expiratory corrugated tubes; (4) a Y-piece connector; (5) an overflow or pop-off valve, referred to as the Adjustable Pressure-Limiting (APL) valve; (6) a reservoir bag;

and (7) a canister containing a CO_2 absorbent. The inspiratory and expiratory valves are placed in the system to ensure gas flow through the corrugated hoses remains unidirectional. The fresh gas inflow enters the circle by a connection from the common gas outlet of the anesthesia machine.

Numerous variations of the circle arrangement are possible, depending on the relative positions of the unidirectional valves, the pop-off valve, the reservoir bag, the CO_2 absorber, and the site of fresh gas entry. However, to prevent rebreathing of CO_2 *in a traditional circle system*, three rules must be followed: (1) a unidirectional valve must be located between the patient and the reservoir bag on both the inspiratory and expiratory limbs of the circuit; (2) the fresh gas inflow cannot enter the circuit between the expiratory valve and the patient; and (3) the overflow (pop-off) valve cannot be located between the patient and the inspiratory valve. If these rules are followed, any arrangement of the other components will prevent rebreathing of CO_2.[90] Some newer anesthesia workstations now employ less traditional circle breathing systems. Two of these systems are discussed in detail below (see Anesthesia Workstation Variations section).

The most efficient circle system arrangement with the highest conservation of fresh gases is one in which the unidirectional valves are near the patient and the pop-off valve is located just downstream from the expiratory valve. This arrangement minimizes dead space gas and preferentially eliminates exhaled alveolar gases. A more practical arrangement, the one used on most conventional anesthesia machines (see Fig. 21-7), is somewhat less efficient because it allows alveolar and dead space gases to mix before they are vented.[95,96]

The main advantages of the circle system over other breathing systems include its (1) maintenance of relatively stabil inspired gas concentrations, (2) conservation of respiratory moisture and heat, and (3) prevention of operating room pollution. Additionally, the circle system can be used for closed system anesthesia or semiclosed with very low fresh gas flows. The major disadvantage of the circle system stems from its complex design. Commonly, the circle system may have 10 or more different connections. These multiple connection sites set the stage for misconnections, disconnections, obstructions, and leaks. In an ASA "closed claim" analysis of adverse anesthetic outcomes arising from gas delivery equipment, over one-third (25/72) of malpractice claims resulted from breathing circuit misconnections or disconnections.[1] Malfunction of the circle system's unidirectional valves can result in life-threatening problems. Rebreathing can occur if the valves stick in the open position, and total occlusion of the circuit can occur if they are stuck shut. If the expiratory valve is stuck in the closed position, breath-stacking and barotrauma or volutrauma can result. Obstructed filters located in the expiratory limb of the circle breathing system have caused increased airway pressures, hemodynamic collapse, and bilateral tension pneumothorax. Causes of circle system obstruction and failure include manufacturing defects, debris, patient secretions, and particulate obstruction from other odd sources such as albuterol nebulization.[97–100] Some systems, such as the Datex-Ohmeda 7900 SmartVent, use flow transducers located on both the inspiratory and expiratory limbs of the circle system. In one report cracks in the flow transducer tubing used by this system produced a leak in the circle system that was difficult to detect.[101]

CO_2 ABSORBENTS

In the early 2000s, there were several reports of adverse chemical reactions between CO_2 absorbent materials and anesthetic agents. Some of these undesirable interactions are quite dramatic such as sevoflurane interacting with desiccated Baralyme®, resulting in fires within the breathing system and severe patient injury.[102,103] Although other sources of ignition and fire in the breathing system continue to be described,[104] the Baralyme®-sevoflurane problem is somewhat unique in that nothing "unusual" is added to or removed from the breathing system for this to occur. Other reactions such as desflurane or sevoflurane with desiccated strong base absorbents can produce more insidious patient morbidity and even death from the release of byproducts such as carbon monoxide or compound A.[105] Although absorbent materials may be problematic, they still represent an important component of the circle breathing system. Different anesthesia breathing systems eliminate CO_2 with varying degrees of efficiency. The closed and semiclosed circle system both **require** that CO_2 be absorbed from the exhaled gases to avoid hypercapnea. If one could design an ideal CO_2 absorbent, its characteristics would include lack of reactivity with common anesthetics, lack of toxicity, low resistance to air flow, low cost, ease of handling, and efficiency in CO_2 absorption.

The Absorber Canister

On modern anesthesia machines, the absorber canister (see Fig. 21-7) is composed of two clear plastic canisters arranged in series. The canisters can be filled with either loose bulk absorbent or with absorbent supplied by the factory in prefilled plastic disposable cartridges called prepacks. Free granules from bulk absorbent can create a clinically significant leak if they lodge between the clear plastic canister and the O-ring gasket of the absorber. Leaks have also been caused by defective prepacks, which were larger than factory specifications.[106] Prepacks can also cause total obstruction of the circle system if the clear plastic shipping wrapper is not removed prior to use.[107]

Chemistry of Absorbents

Three formulations of CO_2 absorbents are commonly available today: soda lime, Baralyme®, and calcium hydroxide lime (Amsorb®). Of these agents, the most commonly used is soda lime. All serve to eliminate CO_2 from the breathing circuit with varying degrees of efficiency.

By weight the approximate composition of "high moisture" soda lime is 80% calcium hydroxide, 15% water, 4% sodium hydroxide, and 1% potassium hydroxide (an activator). Small amounts of silica are added to produce calcium and sodium silicate. This addition produces a harder more stable pellet and thereby reduces dust formation. The efficiency of the soda lime absorption varies inversely with the hardness; therefore, little silicate is used in contemporary soda lime. Sodium hydroxide is the catalyst for the CO_2 absorptive properties of soda lime.[108,109] Baralyme® is a mixture of approximately 20% barium hydroxide and 80% calcium hydroxide. It may also contain some potassium hydroxide. Baralyme® is the primary CO_2 absorbent implicated as an agent that may produce fires in the breathing system when used with sevoflurane. Calcium hydroxide lime is one of the newest clinically available CO_2 absorbents. It consists primarily of calcium hydroxide and calcium chloride and contains two setting agents: calcium sulfate and polyvinylpyrrolidine. The latter two agents serve to enhance the hardness and porosity of the agent.[110] The most significant advantage of calcium hydroxide lime over other agents is its lack of the strong bases, sodium and potassium hydroxide. The absence of these chemicals eliminates the undesirable production of carbon monoxide, the nephrotoxic substance known as compound A, and may reduce or eliminate the possibility of a fire in the breathing circuit.[111] The most significant disadvantages of calcium hydroxide lime are (1) less absorptive capacity—about 50% less than strong-base containing absorbents, and (2) generally higher cost per unit than other absorbents.[112,113]

The size of the actual absorptive granules has been determined over time by trial and error. The current size particles represent a compromise between resistance to air flow and absorptive efficiency.[114] The smaller the granule size, the greater the surface area that is available for absorption. However, as particle size decreases, air flow resistance increases. The granular size of soda lime and Baralyme® used in clinical practice is between 4 and 8 mesh, a size at which absorptive surface area and resistance to flow are optimized. Mesh size refers to the number of openings per linear inch in a sieve through which the granular particles can pass. A 4-mesh screen means that there are four quarter-inch openings per linear inch. Likewise, an 8-mesh screen has eight per linear inch.[108]

The absorption of CO_2 by absorbents such as soda lime occurs by a series of chemical reactions; it is not a physical process like soaking water into a sponge. CO_2 combines with water to form carbonic acid. Carbonic acid reacts with the hydroxides to form sodium (or potassium) carbonate and water. Calcium hydroxide accepts the carbonate to form calcium carbonate and sodium (or potassium) hydroxide. The equations are as follows:

1. $CO_2 + H_2O \Longleftrightarrow H_2CO_3$
2. $H_2CO_3 + 2NaOH\ (KOH) \Longleftrightarrow Na_2CO_3\ (K_2CO_3) + 2H_2O + \text{Heat}$
3. $Na_2CO_3\ (K_2CO_3) + Ca(OH)_2 \Longleftrightarrow CaCO_3 + 2NaOH\ (KOH)$

Some CO_2 may react directly with $Ca(OH)_2$, but this reaction is much slower.

The reaction with Baralyme® differs from that of soda lime because more water is liberated by a direct reaction of barium hydroxide and CO_2.

1. $Ba(OH)_2 + 8H_2O + CO_2 \Longleftrightarrow BaCO_3 + 9H_2O + \text{Heat}$
2. $9H_2O + 9CO_2 \Longleftrightarrow 9H_2CO_3$
   Then by direct reactions and by KOH and NaOH,
3. $9H_2CO_3 + 9Ca(OH)_2 \Longleftrightarrow CaCO_3 + 18H_2O + \text{Heat}$

Absorptive Capacity

The maximum amount of CO_2 that can be absorbed by soda lime is 26 L of CO_2 per 100 g of absorbent. The absorptive capacity of calcium hydroxide lime is significantly less, and has been reported at 10.2 L per 100 g of absorbent.[110,113] However, as previously mentioned, absorptive capacity is the product of both available chemical reactivity and physical (granule) availability. As the absorbent granules stack up in the absorber canisters, small passageways inevitably form. These small passages channel gases preferentially through low resistance areas. Because of this phenomenon, functional absorptive capacity of either soda lime or calcium hydroxide lime may be substantially decreased. In practice, because of channeling, the efficiency of soda lime may be reduced to allow only 10 to 20 L or less of CO_2 to actually be absorbed per 100 g of absorbent.[115]

Indicators

Ethyl violet is the pH indicator added to both soda lime and Baralyme to help assess the functional integrity of the absorbent. This compound is a substituted triphenylmethane dye with a critical pH of 10.3.[109] Ethyl violet changes from colorless to violet in color when the pH of the absorbent decreases as a result of CO_2 absorption. When the absorbent is fresh, the pH exceeds the critical pH of the indicator dye, and it exists in its colorless form (Fig. 21-26, A). However, as absorbent becomes exhausted, the pH decreases below 10.3, and ethyl violet changes to its violet form (Fig. 21-26, B) because of alcohol dehydration. This change in color indicates the absorptive capacity of the material has been consumed. Unfortunately, in some circumstances ethyl violet may not always be a reliable indicator of the functional status of absorbent. For example, prolonged exposure of ethyl violet to fluorescent lights can produce photodeactivation of this dye. When this occurs, the absorbent appears white even though it may have a reduced pH and its absorptive capacity has been exhausted.[116]

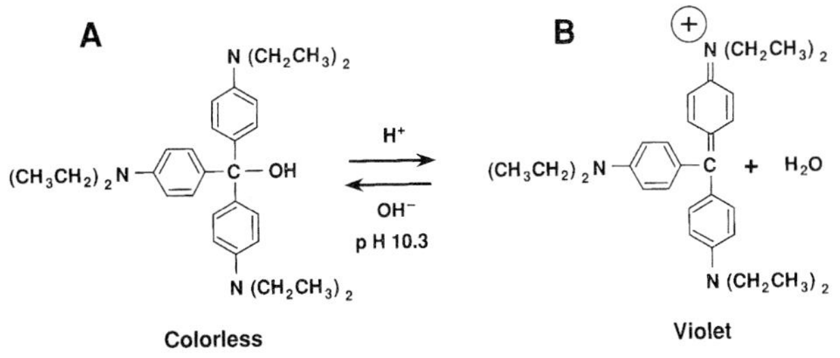

FIGURE 21-26 A and B. Ethyl Violet. See text for details. (Reprinted with permission from Andrews JJ, Johnston RV Jr, Bee DE, Arens JF: Photodeactivation of ethyl violet: A potential hazard of sodasorb. Anesthesiology 72:59, 1990.)

Interactions of Inhaled Anesthetics with Absorbents

It is important and desirable to have CO_2 absorbents that neither release toxic particles or fumes nor produce toxic compounds when exposed to common anesthetics. Soda lime and Baralyme generally fit this description, but inhaled anesthetics do interact with absorbents to some extent. Historically speaking, an uncommon anesthetic, trichloroethylene, reacts with soda lime to produce toxic compounds. In the presence of alkali and heat, trichloroethylene degrades into the cerebral neurotoxin dichloroacetylene, which can cause cranial nerve lesions and encephalitis. Phosgene, a potent pulmonary irritant, is also produced and phosgene can cause adult respiratory distress syndrome (ARDS).[117]

Sevoflurane has been shown to produce degradation products upon interaction with CO_2 absorbents.[105,118,119] The major degradation product produced is an olefin compound known as fluoromethyl-2, 2-difluoro-1-(trifluoromethyl) vinyl ether, or compound A. During sevoflurane anesthesia, factors apparently leading to an increase in the concentration of compound A include: (1) low flow or closed circuit anesthetic techniques; (2) the use of Baralyme® rather than soda lime; (3) higher concentrations of sevoflurane in the anesthetic circuit; (4) higher absorbent temperatures; and (5) fresh absorbent.[118–121] Interestingly, the dehydration of Baralyme increases the concentration of compound A, but the dehydration of soda lime decreases the concentration of compound A.[122,123] Apparently, the degradation products released during clinical conditions do not commonly result in adverse effects in humans even during low flow anesthesia,[120] but further studies are needed to verify this.[124–126]

10 Desiccated strong-base absorbents can also degrade contemporary inhaled anesthetics to clinically significant concentrations of carbon monoxide (CO) as well as trifluoromethane, which can interfere with anesthetic gas monitoring.[105] Under certain conditions, this process can produce very high carboxyhemoglobin concentrations, reaching 35% or more.[127] Higher levels of carbon monoxide are more likely after prolonged contact between absorbent and anesthetics, and

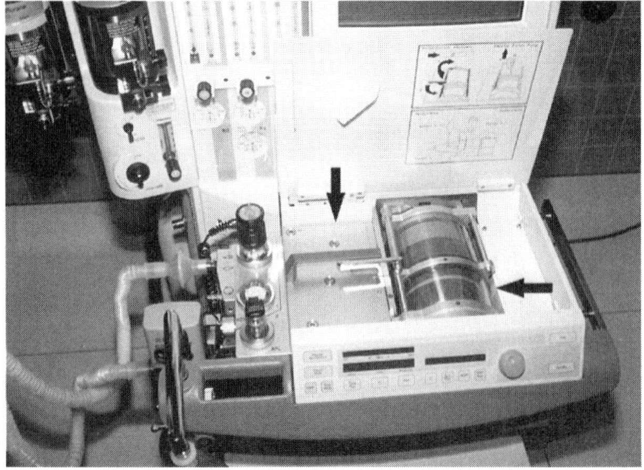

FIGURE 21-27. The Dräger Medical Narkomed 6000 with its single-circuit ventilator. The *horizontal arrow* indicates the piston cylinder unit of the Divan Ventilator. The *vertical arrow* indicates the rectangular valve manifold for fresh gas decoupling.

after disuse of an absorber for at least 2 days, especially over a weekend. Thus, case reports describing carbon monoxide poisoning have been most common in patients anesthetized on Monday morning, presumably because continuous flow from the anesthesia machine dehydrated the absorbents over the weekend.[128,129] Fresh gas flow rates of 5 liters per minute or more through the breathing system and absorbent (without a patient connected) are sufficient to cause critical drying of the absorbent material. This is even worse when the breathing bag is left off the breathing circuit. Absence of the reservoir bag facilitates retrograde flow through the circle system (Fig. 21-27).[127] Because the inspiratory valve leaflet produces some resistance to flow, the fresh gas flow takes the retrograde path of least resistance through the absorbent and out the 22 mm breathing bag mount.

Several factors appear to increase the production of carbon monoxide and resulting elevated carboxyhemoglobin levels. Those factors include (1) the inhaled anesthetic used (for a given MAC multiple, the magnitude of CO production from greatest to least is desflurane $\geq$ enflurane $>$isoflurane $>>$ halothane $=$ sevoflurane); (2) the absorbent dryness (completely dry absorbent produces more CO than hydrated absorbent); (3) the type of absorbent (at a given water content, Baralyme® produces more CO than does soda lime); (4) the temperature (an increased temperature increases CO production); (5) the anesthetic concentration (more CO is produced from higher anesthetic concentrations);[130] (6) low fresh gas flow rates; and (7) reduced experimental animal (patient) size[105,131] per 100 g of absorbent.

Several interventions have been suggested to reduce the incidence of carbon monoxide exposure in humans undergoing general anesthesia.[129] These interventions include (1) educating anesthesia personnel regarding the etiology of CO production; (2) turning off the anesthesia machine at the conclusion of the last case of the day to eliminate fresh gas flow that dries the absorbent; (3) changing CO_2 absorbent if fresh gas was found flowing during the morning machine check; (4) rehydrating desiccated absorbent by adding water to the absorbent;[113] (5) changing the chemical composition of soda lime to reduce or eliminate potassium hydroxide (such products now available include Dragersorb® 800 plus, Sofnolime®, and Spherasorb®); and (6) using absorbent materials such as calcium hydroxide lime that are free of both sodium and postassium hydroxides. The elimination of sodium and potassium hydroxides from desiccated soda lime diminishes or eliminates degradation of desflurane to carbon monoxide and sevoflurane to compound A, but does not compromise CO_2 absorption.[111,132]

One extremely rare, but potentially life-threatening complication related to CO_2 absorbent use is the development of fires within the breathing system. Specifically, this can occur as the
11 result of interactions between the strong-base absorbents (particularly Baralyme®) and the inhaled anesthetic, sevoflurane. In August 2003, Abbott Laboratories changed the package insert for sevoflurane to describe this rare phenomenon and the conditions under which it could occur. Almost 1 year later, in the fall of 2004, several case reports describing patient injuries related to this problem were published (all involving Baralyme®). It seems that when desiccated strong-base absorbents are exposed to sevoflurane, absorber temperatures of several hundred degrees may result from their interaction.[103] The build-up of very high temperatures, the formation of combustible degradation byproducts (formaldehyde, methanol, and formic acid), plus the oxygen- or nitrous oxide–enriched environment provide all the substrates necessary for a fire to occur.[105] Avoidance of the use of the combination of sevoflurane with strong-base absorbents, particularly Baralyme®, especially if it has become desiccated is the best way to prevent this unusual potentially life-threatening complication.

ANESTHESIA VENTILATORS

The ventilator on the modern anesthesia workstation serves as a mechanized substitute for the manual squeezing of the reservoir bag of the circle system, the Bain circuit, or another breathing system. As recently as the late 1980s, anesthesia ventilators were mere adjuncts to the anesthesia machine. Today, in newer anesthesia workstations, they have attained a prominent central role. In addition to the near ubiquitous role of the anesthesia ventilator in today's anesthesia workstation, many advanced ICU-style ventilation features have also been integrated into anesthesia ventilators (see Fig. 21-27). Although many similarities exist between today's anesthesia ventilator and ICU ventilator, some fundamental differences in ventilation parameters and control systems still remain. This discussion focuses on the classification, operating principles, and hazards associated with contemporary anesthesia ventilators.

Classification

Ventilators can be classified according to their power source, drive mechanism, cycling mechanism, and bellows type.[133,134]

Power Source

The power source required to operate a mechanical ventilator is provided by compressed gas, electricity, or both. Older pneumatic ventilators required only a pneumatic power source to function properly. Contemporary electronic ventilators from Dräger Medical, Datex-Ohmeda, and others require either an electrical only or both an electrical and a pneumatic power source.

Drive Mechanism and Circuit Designation

Double-circuit ventilators are most commonly used on modern anesthesia workstations. Generally, these conventional ventilators are pneumatically driven. In a double-circuit ventilator, a driving force such as pressurized gas compresses a component analogous to the reservoir bag known as the ventilator bellows. The bellows then in turn delivers ventilation to the patient. The driving gas in the Datex-Ohmeda 7000, 7810, 7100, and 7900 is 100% oxygen. In the North American Dräger AV-E and AV-2 +, a venturi device mixes oxygen and air. Some newer pneumatic anesthesia workstations have the ability for the user to select whether compressed air or oxygen is used as the driving gas.

In recent years, with the introduction of circle breathing systems that integrate fresh gas decoupling, resurgence has been seen in the utilization of mechanically driven anesthesia ventilators. These "piston"-type ventilators utilize a computer-controlled stepper motor instead of compressed drive gas to actuate gas movement in the breathing system. In these systems, rather than having dual circuits with patient gas in one and drive gas in another, a single patient gas circuit is present. Thus, they are classified as piston-driven single-circuit ventilators. The piston operates much like the plunger of a syringe to deliver the desired tidal volume or airway pressure to the patient. Sophisticated computerized controls are able to provide advanced types of ventilatory support such as synchronized intermittent mandatory ventilation (S-IMV), pressure-controlled ventilation (PCV), and pressure support–assisted ventilation, in addition to the conventional control mode ventilation. Since the patient's mechanical breath is delivered without the use of compressed gas to actuate a bellows, these systems consume dramatically less compressed gas during ventilator operation than traditional pneumatic ventilators. This improvement in efficiency may have clinical significance when the anesthesia workstation is used in a setting where no pipeline gas supply is available (e.g., remote locations or office-based anesthesia practices).

Cycling Mechanism

Most anesthesia machine ventilators are time cycled and provide ventilator support in the control mode. Inspiratory phase is initiated by a timing device. Older pneumatic ventilators use a fluidic timing device. Contemporary electronic ventilators use a solid-state electronic timing device and are thus classified as time cycled and electronically controlled. More advanced ventilation modes such as S-IMV, PCV, and modes that utilize a pressure-support option may have an adjustable threshold pressure trigger as well. In these modes, pressure sensors provide feedback to the ventilator control system to allow it to determine when to initiate and/or terminate the respiratory cycle.

Bellows Classification

The direction of bellows movement during the expiratory phase determines the bellows classification. *Ascending (standing) bellows* ascend during the expiratory phase (Fig. 21-28B, right), whereas *descending (hanging) bellows* descend during the expiratory phase. Older pneumatic ventilators and some new anesthesia workstations use weighted descending bellows, while most contemporary electronic ventilators have an ascending bellows design. Of the two configurations, the ascending bel-
12 lows is generally safer. An ascending bellows will not fill if a total disconnection occurs. However, the bellows of a descending bellows ventilator will continue its upward and downward movement despite a patient disconnection. The driving gas pushes the bellows upward during the inspiratory phase. During the expiratory phase, room air is entrained into the breathing system at the site of the disconnection because gravity acts on the weighted bellows. The disconnection pressure monitor and the volume monitor may be fooled even if a disconnection is complete (see Breathing Circuit Problems section).[34] Some contemporary anesthesia workstation designs have returned to the descending bellows to integrate fresh gas decoupling (Dräger Medical Julian and Datascope Anestar). An essential safety feature on any anesthesia workstation that utilizes a descending bellows is an integrated CO_2 apnea alarm that cannot be disabled while the ventilator is in use.

Operating Principles of Ascending Bellows Ventilators

Contemporary examples of ascending bellows, double-circuit, electronic ventilators include the Dräger Medical AV-E, AV-2+, the Datex-Ohmeda 7000, 7800, and 7900 series. A generic ascending bellows ventilator is illustrated in Figure 21-26. It may be viewed as a breathing bag (bellows) located within a clear plastic box. The bellows physically separates the driving gas circuit from the patient gas circuit. The driving gas circuit is located outside the bellows, and the patient gas circuit is inside the bellows. During the inspiratory phase (Fig. 21-28A, left) the driving gas enters the bellows chamber, causing the pressure within it to increase. This increase in pressure is responsible for two events. First, the ventilator relief valve closes, preventing anesthetic gas from escaping into the scavenging system. Second, the bellows is compressed, and the anesthetic gas within the bellows is delivered to the patient's lungs. This compression action is analogous to the hand of the anesthesiologist squeezing the breathing bag.[48]

During the expiratory phase (see Fig. 21-28B), the driving gas exits the bellows housing. This produces a drop to atmospheric pressure within both the bellows housing and the pilot line to the ventilator relief valve. The decrease in pressure to the ventilator relief valve causes the "mushroom valve" portion of the assembly to open. Exhaled patient gases refill the bellows before any scavenging can begin. The bellows refill first because a weighted ball [like those used in ball-type positive end-expiratory pressure (PEEP) valves] or similar device is incorporated into the base of the ventilator relief valve. This ball produces 2 to 3 cm water of back pressure; therefore, scavenging occurs only after the bellows fills completely and the pressure inside the bellows exceeds the pressure threshold of the "ball valve." This design causes all ascending bellows ventilators to produce 2 to 3 cm water pressure of PEEP within the breathing circuit when the ventilator is in use. Scavenging occurs only during the expiratory phase, as the ventilator relief valve is open only during expiration.[48]

It is important to understand that on most anesthesia workstations, gas flow from the anesthesia machine into the breathing circuit is continuous and independent of ventilator activity. During the inspiratory phase of mechanical ventilation, the ventilator relief valve is closed (see Fig. 21-28A), and the breathing system's Adjustable Pressure Limiting Valve ("pop-off" valve) is most commonly out of circuit. Therefore, the patient's lungs receive the volume from the bellows plus that from the flowmeters during the inspiratory phase. Factors that influence the correlation between set tidal volume and exhaled tidal volume include the flowmeter settings, the inspiratory time, the compliance of the breathing circuit, external leakage, and the location of the tidal volume sensor. Usually, the volume gained from the flowmeters during inspiration is counteracted by the volume lost to compliance of the breathing circuit, and set tidal volume generally approximates the exhaled tidal volume. However, certain conditions such as inappropriate activation of the oxygen flush valve during the inspiratory phase can result in barotrauma and/or volutrauma because excess pressure and volume may not be able to be vented from the circle system.[48]

Problems and Hazards

Numerous hazards are associated with anesthesia ventilators. These include problems with the breathing circuit, the bellows assembly, and the control assembly.

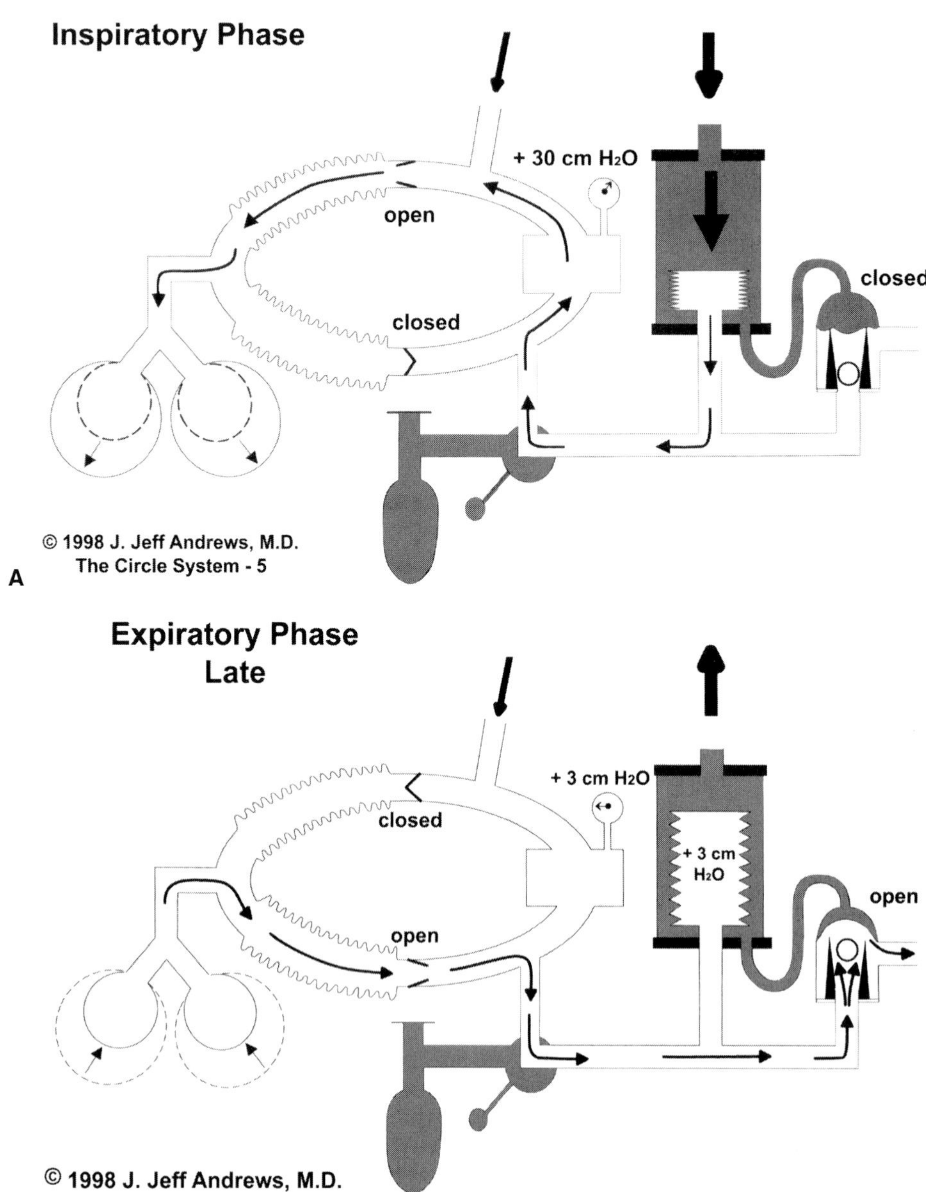

FIGURE 21-28A and B. Inspiratory (A) and expiratory (B) phases of gas flow in a traditional circle system with an ascending bellows ventilator. The bellows physically separates the driving-gas circuit from the patient gas circuit. The driving-gas circuit is located outside the bellows, and the patient gas circuit is inside the bellows. During inspiratory phase (A), the driving gas enters the bellows chamber, causing the pressure within it to increase. This causes the ventilator relief valve to close, preventing anesthetic gas from escaping into the scavenging system, and the bellows to compress, delivering anesthetic gas within the bellows to the patient's lungs. During expiratory phase (B), pressure within the bellows chamber and the pilot line decreases to zero, causing the mushroom portion of the ventilator relief valve to open. Gas exhaled by the patient refills the bellows before any scavenging occurs, because a weighted ball is incorporated into the base of the ventilator relief valve. Scavenging occurs only during the expiratory phase, because the ventilator relief valve is only open during expiration. (Reprinted with permission from Andrews JJ: The Circle System. A Collection of 30 Color Illustrations. Washington, DC, Library of Congress, 1998.)

Traditional Circle System Problems

Breathing circuit misconnections and disconnection are a leading cause of critical incidents in anesthesia.[1,135] The most common disconnection site is at the Y-piece. Disconnections can be complete or partial (leaks). In the past, a common source of leaks with older absorbers was failure to close the Adjustable Pressure Limiting Valve (APL or pop-off valve) upon initiation of mechanical ventilation. On today's anesthesia workstations, the bag/ventilator selector switch has virtually eliminated this problem, as the APL valve is usually out of circuit when the ventilator mode is selected. Preexisting undetected leaks can exist in compressed, corrugated, disposable anesthetic circuits. To detect such a leak preoperatively, the circuit must be fully expanded before the circuit is checked for leaks.[136] As previously mentioned, disconnections and leaks manifest more readily with the ascending bellows ventilator systems because they result in a situation in which the bellows will not refill.[34]

Several disconnection monitors exist, although none should replace vigilance. Monitoring of breath sounds and observation of chest wall excursion should continue despite use of both mechanical (spirometers and pressure sensors) and physiologic monitors.

Pneumatic and electronic pressure monitors are helpful in diagnosing disconnections. Factors that influence monitor effectiveness include the disconnection site, the pressure sensor location, the threshold pressure alarm limit, the inspiratory flow rate, and the resistance of the disconnected breathing circuit.[137,138] Various anesthesia workstations and ventilators have different locations for the airway pressure sensor and different values for the threshold pressure alarm limit. The threshold pressure alarm limit may be preset at the factory or adjustable. An audible or visual alarm is actuated if the peak inspiratory pressure of the breathing circuit does not exceed the threshold pressure alarm limit. When an adjustable threshold pressure alarm limit is available, such as on many workstations from Dräger Medical, the operator should set the pressure alarm limit to within 5 cm water of the peak inspiratory pressure. On systems that have an "autoset" feature, when activated, the threshold limit is automatically set at 3 to 5 cm water

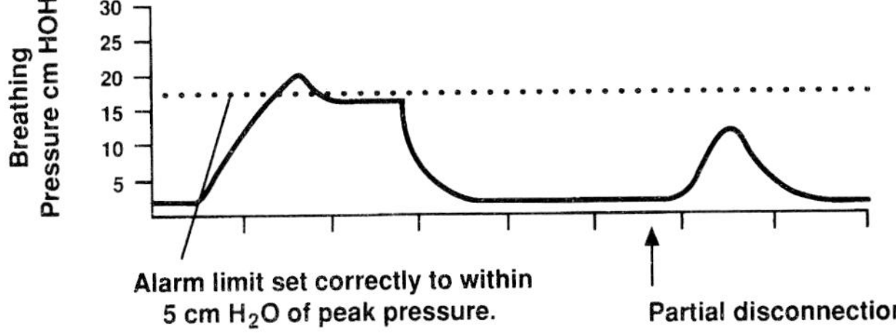

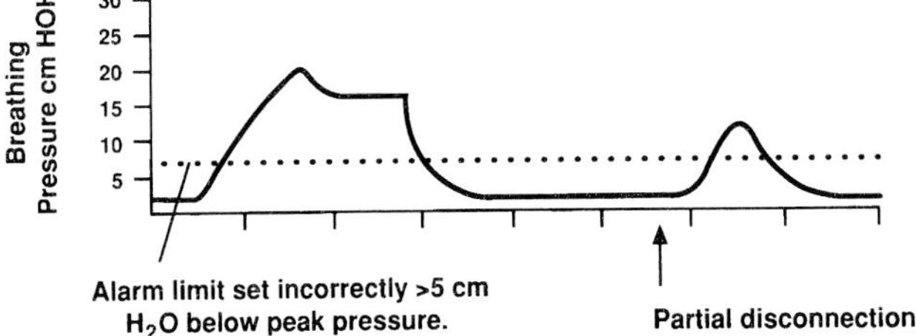

FIGURE 21-29. Threshold pressure alarm limit. (*Top*) The threshold pressure alarm limit (*dotted line*) has been set appropriately. An alarm is actuated when a partial disconnection occurs (*arrow*) because the threshold pressure alarm limit is not exceeded by the breathing circuit pressure. (*Bottom*) A partial disconnection is unrecognized by the pressure monitor because the threshold pressure alarm limit has been set too low. (Redrawn with permission from Baromed Breathing Pressure Monitor: Operator's Instruction Manual. Telford, Pennsylvania, North American Dräger, August 1986.)

pressure below the current peak inspiratory pressure. On such systems, failure to reset the threshold pressure alarm limit may result in either an "Apnea Pressure" or "Threshold Low" alert. Figure 21-29 illustrates how a partial disconnection (leak) may be unrecognized by the low-pressure monitor if the threshold pressure alarm limit is set too low or if the factory preset value is relatively low.

Respiratory volume monitors are useful in detecting disconnections. Volume monitors may sense exhaled tidal volume, inhaled tidal volume, minute volume, or all three. The user should bracket the high and low threshold volumes slightly above and below the exhaled volumes. For example, if the exhaled minute volume of a patient is 10 L/min, reasonable alarm limits would be 8 to 12 L/min. Many Datex-Ohmeda ventilators are equipped with volume monitor sensors that use infrared light/turbine technology. These volume sensors are usually located in the expiratory limb of the breathing circuit and thus measure exhaled tidal volume. In the case of the Datex-Ohmeda S/5 ADU, a special attachment known as the D-Lite® spirometry connector is placed in the breathing circuit. This device is actually placed at or near the level of the patient connection and permits measurement of both inhaled and exhaled volumes and pressures (see Anesthesia Workstation Variations section). With the older infrared type sensors, exposure to a direct beam of light from the overhead surgical lighting could cause erroneous volume readings as the surgical beam interfered with the infrared sensor.[139] Other types of expiratory volume sensors can be seen in systems such as the Datex-Ohmeda Aestiva, Aespire, and other workstations that incorporate the 7100 ventilator or 7900 SmartVent. These systems generally utilize differential pressure transduction technology to determine inhaled and exhaled volumes as well as to measure airway pressures. The Dräger Medical Narkomed 6000 series, 2B and GS workstations commonly use an ultrasonic flow sensor located on the expiratory limb. Still other systems from Dräger measure exhaled volume using "hot wire" sensor technology. With this type of sensor, a tiny array of two platinum wires is electrically heated to a high temperature. As gas flows past the heated wires, they tend to be cooled. The amount of energy required to maintain the temperature of the wire is proportional to the volume of gas flowing past it. This system has been associated in at least one report with accidental development of a fire in the breathing circuit.[104]

CO_2 monitors are probably the best devices for revealing patient disconnections. CO_2 concentration is measured near the Y-piece either directly (mainstream) or by aspiration of a gas sample to the instrument (sidestream). Either a sudden change in the differences between the inspiratory and end-tidal CO_2 concentrations or the acute absence of measured CO_2 indicates a disconnection, a nonventilated patient, or other problems.[34] Importantly, an absence of exhaled CO_2 can be an indication of absent cardiac output rather than a mechanical equipment problem.

Misconnections of the breathing system are unfortunately, relatively common. Despite the efforts of standards committees to eliminate this problem by assigning different diameters to various hoses and hose terminals, they continue to occur. Anesthesia workstations, breathing systems, ventilators, and scavenging systems incorporate many of these diameter-specific connections. The "ability" of anesthesia providers to outwit these "fool-proof" systems has led to various hoses being cleverly adapted or forcefully fitted to inappropriate terminals and even to various other solid cylindrically shaped protrusions of the anesthesia machine.[34]

Occlusion (obstruction) of the breathing circuit may occur. Tracheal tubes can become kinked. Hoses throughout the breathing circuit are subject to occlusion by internal obstruction or external mechanical forces, which can impinge on flow and have severe consequences. For example, blockage of a bacterial filter in the expiratory limb of the circle system has resulted in bilateral tension pneumothorax.[98] Incorrect insertion of flow direction–sensitive components can result in a no-flow state.[34] Examples of these components include some PEEP valves and cascade humidifiers. Depending on the location of the occlusion relative to the pressure sensor, a high-pressure alarm may alert practitioners to the problem.

Excess inflow to the breathing circuit from the anesthesia machine during the inspiratory phase can cause barotrauma. The best example of this phenomenon is oxygen flushing. Excess volume cannot be vented from the system during inspiration because the ventilator relief valve is closed and the APL valve is out of circuit.[48] A high-pressure alarm, if present, may be activated when the pressure becomes excessive. With many Dräger Medical systems, both audible and visual alarms are actuated when the high-pressure threshold is exceeded. In the Modulus II Plus System, the Datex-Ohmeda 7810 ventilator automatically switches from the inspiratory to the expiratory phase when the adjustable peak pressure threshold is exceeded.

On workstations equipped with adjustable inspiratory pressure limiters such as the Datex-Ohmeda S/5 ADU, Aestiva, Dräger Medical's Narkomed 6000 series, 2B, 2C, GS and Fabius GS, maximal inspiratory pressure may be set by the user to a desired peak airway pressure. An adjustable pressure relief valve will open when the predetermined user-selected pressure is reached. This theoretically prevents generation of excessive airway pressure. Unfortunately, this feature is dependent on the user having preset the appropriate "pop-off" pressure. If the setting is too low, insufficient pressure for ventilation may be generated, resulting in inadequate minute ventilation; if set too high, the excessive airway pressure may still occur, resulting in barotrauma. The piston-driven Fabius GS, as well as others may also include a factory preset inspiratory pressure safety valve that opens at a preset airway pressure such as 75 cm of water pressure to minimize the risk of barotrauma. These strategies may reduce the risk of barotrauma and volutrauma; however, they are no substitute for vigilance.

Bellows Assembly Problems

Leaks can occur in the bellows assembly. Improper seating of the plastic bellows housing can result in inadequate ventilation because a portion of the driving gas is vented to the atmosphere. A hole in the bellows can lead to alveolar hyperinflation and possibly barotrauma in some ventilators because high-pressure driving gas can enter the patient circuit. The oxygen concentration of the patient gas may increase when the driving gas is 100% oxygen, or it may decrease if the driving gas is composed of an air–oxygen mixture.[140]

The ventilator relief valve can cause problems. Hypoventilation occurs if the valve is incompetent because anesthetic gas is delivered to the scavenging system during the inspiratory phase instead of to the patient. Gas molecules preferentially exit into the scavenging system because it represents the path of least resistance, and the pressure within the scavenging system can be subatmospheric. Ventilator relief valve incompetency can result from a disconnected pilot line, a ruptured valve, or from a damaged flapper valve.[141,142] A ventilator relief valve stuck in the closed or partially closed position can produce either barotrauma or undesired PEEP.[143] Excessive suction from the scavenging system can draw the ventilator relief valve to its seat and close the valve during both the inspiratory and expiratory phases.[34] In this case, breathing circuit pressure escalates because excess anesthetic gas cannot be vented. It is worthwhile to note that during expiratory phase, some newer machines from Datex-Ohmeda (S/5 ADU, 7100 and 7900 SmartVent) scavenge both excess patient gases and the exhausted ventilator drive gas. That is, when the ventilator relief valve opens, and waste anesthetic gases are vented from the breathing circuit, the drive gas from the bellows housing joins with it to enter the scavenging system. Under certain conditions, the large volume of exhausted gases could overwhelm the scavenging system, resulting in pollution of the operating room with waste anesthetic gases (see Scavenging Systems section). Other mechanical problems that can occur include leaks within the system, faulty pressure regulators, and faulty valves. Unlikely problems such as an occluded muffler on the Dräger AV-E ventilator can result in barotrauma. In this case, obstruction of driving gas outflow closes the ventilator relief valve, and excess patient gas cannot be vented.[144]

Control Assembly and Power Supply Problems

The control assembly can be the source of both electrical and mechanical problems. Electrical failure can be total or partial; the former is the more obvious. As anesthesia workstations are becoming more dependent on integrated computer-controlled systems, power interruptions become more significant. Battery back-up systems are designed to continue operation of essential electronics during brief (up to several hours') outages. However, even with these systems, in the event of a failure, some time may be required to reboot after an electrical outage has occurred. During this time the availability of certain workstation features such as manual or mechanical ventilation can be variable. One cluster of electrical failures that could have potentially resulted in operating room fires was reported early on after the release of the Dräger Medical Narkomed 6000. Problems with the workstation's power supply printed circuit boards prompted a corrective recall action in November 2002.[145]

ANESTHESIA WORKSTATION VARIATIONS

With the introduction of new technology, often comes the need for adaptation of current technology to successfully allow its integration into existing systems. Otherwise, a more comprehensive redesign of an entire anesthesia system "from the ground up" could be necessary. One such example of adaptation in the anesthesia workstation can be seen with two new design variations of the circle breathing system. The first of these is found on the Datex-Ohmeda S/5 ADU (Fig. 21-1), and the second is incorporated into the Dräger Narkomed 6000 series (Fig. 21-2) and Fabius GS workstations. Since use of the circle system is fundamental to the day-to-day practice for most anesthesiologists, a comprehensive understanding of these new systems is crucial for their safe use.

The Datex-Ohmeda S/5 ADU (Fig. 21-1)

The Datex-Ohmeda S/5 ADU debuted as the AS/3 ADU in 1998. Along with its more comprehensive safety features and integrated design that eliminated glass flow tubes and conventional anesthesia vaporizers in exchange for a computer screen with digital fresh gas flow scales and the built-in Aladin Cassette vaporizer system, the machine had a radically different appearance in general. It is not until closer inspection that the other unique properties of the ADU begin to stand out. The principal difference in the ADU's circle system lies in the incorporation of the specialized "D-lite" flow and pressure transducer fitting into the circle at the level of the Y-connector. On most traditional circle systems, exhaled tidal volume is measured by a spirometry sensor located in proximity to the expiratory valve. The placement of the D-lite fitting at the Y-connector provides a better location to perform exhaled volume measurement; allows airway gas composition and pressure monitoring to be done with a single adapter instead of with multiple fittings added to the breathing circuit; and it provides the ability to assess both inspiratory and expiratory gas flow and therefore generation of complete flow-volume spirometry. The relocation of the spirometer sensor to the Y-connector also makes it possible to move the location of the fresh gas inlet to the "patient" side of the inspiratory valve without adversely affecting accuracy of exhaled tidal volume measurement.

This atypical circle system arrangement with the fresh gas entering on the patient side of the inspiratory valve is advantageous for several reasons. It is likely to be more efficient in delivering fresh gas to the patient, while preferentially eliminating exhaled gases. Importantly, it is also less likely to cause desiccation of the CO_2 absorbent (see Interactions of Inhaled Anesthetics with Absorbents section). Other notable changes on the S/5 ADU circle system include a compact proprietary CO_2 absorbent canister design that can be changed during ventilation without loss of circle system integrity, and the relocation of the inspiratory and expiratory unidirectional valves from a horizontal position to a vertical position on the "compact block" assembly just below the absorbent canister. The reorientation of the unidirectional valves reduces the breathing circuit resistance encountered by a spontaneously ventilated patient. The vertically oriented unidirectional valves only have to be tipped away from the vertical position to be opened, unlike conventional horizontal valve discs, which have to be physically lifted off of the valve seat against gravity to be opened.

The Dräger Medical Narkomed 6000 Series (Fig. 21-2) and Fabius GS

Several important differences exist between the traditional circle breathing systems of the newest Dräger products. At first glance, the most notable difference lies in the appearance and design of the ventilators used with these systems. From the inconspicuous horizontally mounted Divan piston ventilator

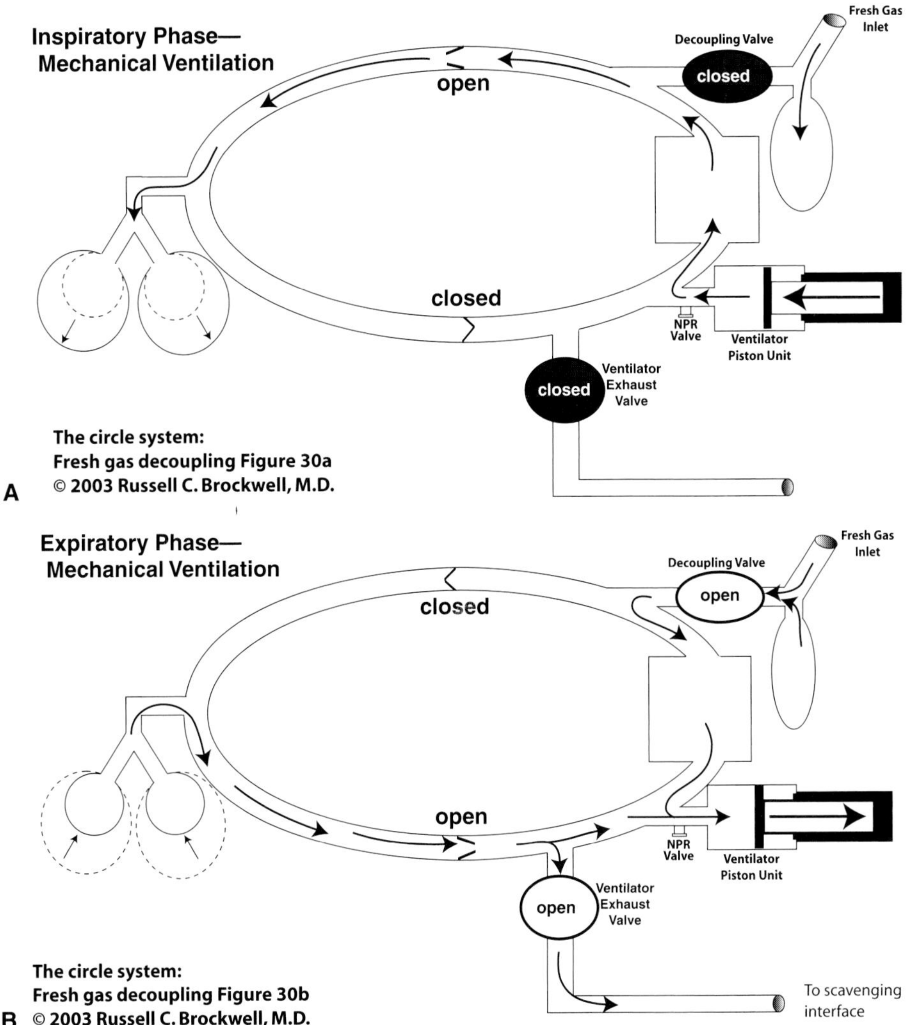

FIGURE 21-30A and B. Inspiratory and expiratory phase gas flows of a Dräger Narkomed 6000–type circle system with piston ventilator and fresh gas decoupling. NPR valve = Negative Pressure Relief Valve. See text for details. (Reprinted with permission from Brockwell RC: New Circle System Designs: A Collection of figures privately published in Birmingham, AL 2003.)

of the Narkomed 6000 to the vertically mounted and visible piston ventilator of the Fabius GS with its absent flow tubes and glowing electronic fresh gas flow indicators, these systems appear drastically different from traditional anesthesia systems. The piston ventilators of the Dräger Narkomed 6000 and Fabius Series anesthesia systems are classified as electrically powered, piston driven, single circuit, electronically controlled with fresh gas decoupling."

The circle breathing systems utilized by these Dräger workstations incorporate a feature known as Fresh Gas Decoupling (FGD). The incorporation of this patient safety enhancing technology has required a significant redesign of the traditional circle system. A functional schematic of a circle system similar to the one used by the Dräger Narkomed 6000 series during both inspiratory and expiratory phase of mechanical ventilation can be seen in Figure 21-30A and 21-30B. To understand the operating principles of FGD, it is important to have a good understanding of gas flows in a traditional circle system both during inspiratory and expiratory phases of mechanical ventilation. A complete discussion of this was presented earlier in the section entitled Operating Principles of Ascending Bellows Ventilators.

The key concept of the fresh gas decoupled breathing system can be illustrated during the inspiratory phase of mechanical ventilation. With the traditional circle system, several events are occurring (see Fig. 21-28A): (1) continuous fresh gas flow from the flowmeters and/or the oxygen flush valve is entering the circle system at the fresh gas inlet; (2) the ventilator is delivering the prescribed tidal volume to the patient's lungs; and (3) the ventilator relief valve (ventilator exhaust valve) is closed, so no gas is escaping the circle system except into the patient's lungs.[146] In a traditional circle system, when these events coincide and fresh gas inflow is coupled directly into the circle system, the total volume delivered to the patient's lungs is the sum of the volume from the ventilator plus the volume of gas that enters the circle via the fresh gas inlet. In contrast, when FGD is used, during the inspiratory phase (see Fig. 21-30A) the fresh gas coming from the anesthesia workstation via the fresh gas inlet is diverted into the reservoir bag by a decoupling valve that is located between the fresh gas source and the ventilator circuit. The reservoir (breathing) bag serves as an accumulator for fresh gas until the expiratory phase begins. During expiratory phase (see Fig. 21-30B), the decoupling valve opens, allowing the accumulated fresh gas in the reservoir bag to be drawn into the circle system to refill the piston ventilator chamber or descending bellows. Since the ventilator exhaust valve also opens during expiratory phase, excess fresh gas and exhaled patient gases are allowed to escape to the scavenging system.

Current fresh gas decoupled systems are designed with either piston-type or descending bellows–type ventilators. Since the bellows in either of these type of systems refills under slight negative pressure, it allows the accumulated fresh gas from the reservoir bag to be drawn into the ventilator for delivery to the patient during the next ventilator cycle. Because of this design requirement, it is unlikely that fresh gas decoupling, as described here, can be used with conventional ascending bellows ventilators, which refill under slight positive pressure.

The most significant advantage of circle systems using
14 FGD is decreased risk of barotrauma and volutrauma. With a traditional circle system, increases in fresh gas flow from the flowmeters or from inappropriate use of the oxygen flush valve may contribute directly to tidal volume, which if excessive, may result in pneumothorax or other injury. Since systems with FGD isolate fresh gas coming into the system from the patient while the ventilator exhaust valve is closed, the risk of barotrauma is greatly reduced.

Possibly the greatest disadvantage to the new anesthesia circle systems that utilize FGD is the possibility of entraining room air into the patient gas circuit. As previously discussed, in a fresh gas decoupled system the bellows or piston refills under slight negative pressure. If the volume of gas contained in the reservoir bag volume plus the returning volume of gas exhaled from the patient's lungs is inadequate to refill the bellows or piston, negative patient airway pressures could develop. To prevent this, a negative pressure relief valve is placed in the breathing system (see Fig. 21-30A and 21-30B). If breathing system pressure falls below a preset value such as -2 cm H_2O pressure, then the relief valve opens and ambient air is entrained into the patient gas circuit. If this goes undetected, the entrained atmospheric gases could lead to dilution of either or both the inhaled anesthetic agents or an enriched oxygen mixture (lowering an enriched oxygen concentration toward 21%). If unchecked, this could lead to either intraoperative awareness or hypoxia. High-priority alarms with both audible and visual alerts should notify the user that fresh gas flow is inadequate and room air is being entrained.

Another potential problem with an FGD system such as seen on the Narkomed 6000 series lies in its reliance on the reservoir bag to accumulate the incoming fresh gas. If the reservoir bag is removed during mechanical ventilation, or if it has a significant leak from poor fit on the bag mount or a perforation, room air may enter the breathing circuit as the ventilator piston unit refills during expiratory phase. This may also result in dilution of either or both the inhaled anesthetic agents or an enriched oxygen mixture, potentially resulting in awareness during anesthesia or hypoxia. Furthermore, this type of a disruption could lead to significant pollution of the operating room with anesthetic gases as fresh gases would be allowed to escape into the atmosphere. Other FGD designs, such as those seen in the Dräger Medical Fabius GS and the recently released Apollo anesthesia systems do not use the breathing bag as the fresh gas reservoir, but instead have an alternate location for fresh gas accumulation during inspiratory phase.

SCAVENGING SYSTEMS

Scavenging is the collection and the subsequent removal of waste anesthetic gases from the operating room.[147] In most cases, the amount of gas used to anesthetize a patient for a given anesthetic far exceeds the minimal amount needed. Therefore, scavenging minimizes operating room pollution by removing this excess of gases. In 1977, the National Institute for Occupational Safety and Health (NIOSH) prepared a document entitled "Criteria for a Recommended Standard: Occupational Exposure to Waste Anesthetic Gases and Vapors."[148] Although it was maintained that a minimal safe level of exposure could not be defined, the NIOSH proceeded to issue the recommendations shown in Table 21-5.[148] In 1991 the American Society for Testing and Materials (ASTM) released the ASTM F1343-91 standard entitled "Standard Specification for Anesthetic Equipment—Scavenging Systems for Anesthetic Gases."[149] The document provided guidelines for devices that safely and effectively scavenge waste anesthetic gases to reduce contamination in anesthetizing areas.[149] In 1999, the ASA Task Force on Trace Anesthetic Gases developed a booklet entitled "Waste Anesthetic Gases: Information for Management in Anesthetizing Areas and the Postanesthesia Care Unit." This publication addresses analysis of the literature, the role of regulatory agencies, scavenging and monitoring equipment, and recommendations.[150]

TABLE 21-5

NIOSH RECOMMENDATIONS FOR TRACE GAS LEVEL

ANESTHETIC GAS	MAXIMUM TWA[a] CONCENTRATION (ppm)
Halogenated agent alone	2
Nitrous oxide	25
Combination of halogenated agent plus nitrous oxide:	
Halogenated agent	0.5
Nitrous oxide	25
Dental facilities (nitrous oxide alone)	50

[a] TWA, time-weighted average. Time-weighted average sampling, also known as time-integrated sampling, is a sampling method that evaluates the average concentration of anesthetic gas over a prolonged period of time, such as 1 to 8 hours.

Reprinted with permission from US Department of Health, Education, and Welfare: Criteria for a recommended standard: Occupational exposure to waste anesthetic gases and vapors. March ed, Washington DC, 1977.

The two major causes of waste gas contamination in the operating room are the anesthetic technique employed and equipment issues.[150,151] Regarding the anesthetic technique, the following factors cause operating room contamination: (1) failure to turn off gas flow control valves at the end of an anesthetic, (2) poorly fitting masks, flushing the circuit, (3) filling anesthetic vaporizers, (4) use of uncuffed endotracheal tubes, and (5) use of breathing circuits such as the Jackson-Rees, which are difficult to scavenge. Equipment failure or lack of understanding of proper equipment use can also contribute to operating room contamination. Leaks can occur in the high-pressure hoses, the nitrous oxide tank mounting, the high-pressure circuit and low-pressure circuit of the anesthesia machine, or in the circle system, particularly at the CO_2 absorber assembly. The anesthesia provider must be certain that the scavenging system is operational and adjusted properly to ensure adequate scavenging. If side stream CO_2 or multigas analyzers are used, the analyzed gas (50 to 250 cc/min) must be directed to the scavenging system or returned to the breathing system to prevent pollution of the operating room.[150,151]

Components

Scavenging systems generally have five components (Fig. 21-31): (1) the gas-collecting assembly, (2) the transfer means, (3) the scavenging interface, (4) the gas-disposal assembly tubing, and (5) an active or passive gas-disposal assembly.[149] An "active system" uses a central evacuation system to eliminate waste gases. The "weight" or pressure of the waste gas itself produces flow through a "passive system."

Gas-Collecting Assembly

The gas-collecting assembly captures excess anesthetic gas and delivers it to the transfer tubing.[134] Waste anesthetic gases are

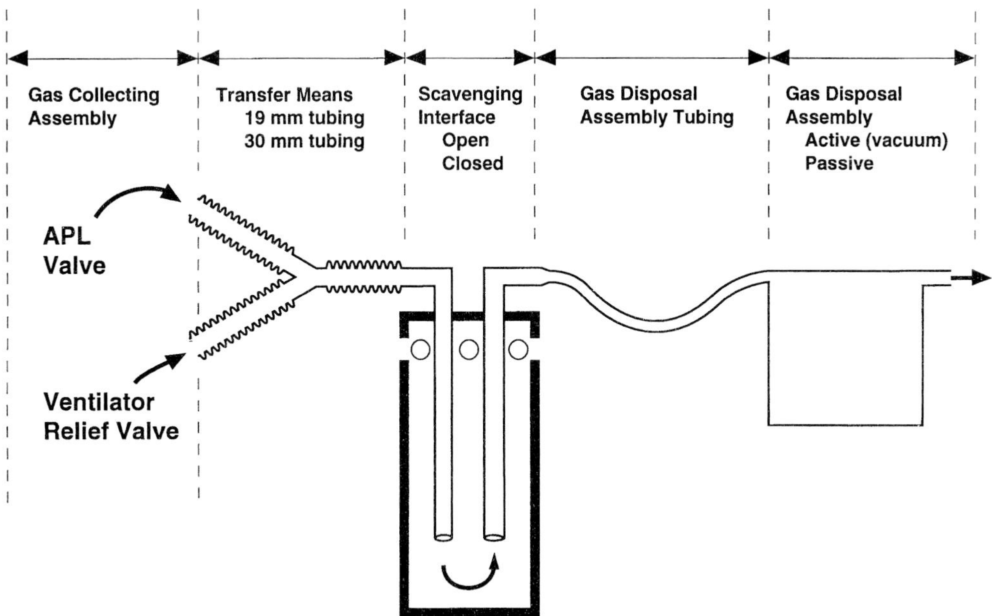

FIGURE 21-31. Components of a scavenging system. APL = adjustable pressure limiting valve.

vented from the anesthesia system either through the APL valve or through the ventilator relief valve. All excess patient gas is either vented into the room (e.g., from a poor facemask fit or endotracheal tube leak) or exits the breathing system through one of these valves. Gas passing through these valves accumulates in the gas-collecting assembly, and is directed to the transfer means. In some newer Datex-Ohmeda systems such as the S5/ADU and others that incorporate either the 7100 or 7900 ventilators, the ventilator drive gas is also exhausted into the scavenging system. This is significant, because under conditions of high fresh gas flows and high minute ventilation, the gases flowing into the scavenging interface may overwhelm the evacuation system. If this occurs, waste anesthetic gases may overflow the system via the positive-pressure relief valve (closed systems) or through the atmospheric vents (open systems) polluting the operating room. In contrast, most other pneumatic ventilators from both Datex-Ohmeda and Dräger exhaust their drive gas (100% oxygen or oxygen/air mixture) into the operating room through a small vent on the back of the ventilator control housing.

Transfer Means

The transfer means carries excess gas from the gas-collecting assembly to the scavenging interface. The tubing must be either 19 or 30 mm, as specified by the ASTM F1343-91 standard.[149] The tubing should be sufficiently rigid to prevent kinking, and as short as possible to minimize the chance of occlusion. Some manufacturers color code the transfer tubing with yellow bands to distinguish it from 22-mm breathing system tubing. Many machines have separate transfer tubes for the APL valve and for the ventilator relief valve. The two tubes frequently merge into a single hose before they enter the scavenging interface. Occlusion of the transfer means can be particularly problematic since it is upstream from the pressure-buffering features of the scavenging interface. If the transfer means is occluded, baseline breathing circuit pressure will increase, and barotrauma can occur.

Scavenging Interface

The scavenging interface is the most important component of the system because it protects the breathing circuit or ventilator from excessive positive or negative pressure.[147] The interface should limit the pressures immediately downstream from the gas collecting assembly to between −0.5 and +10 cm water with normal working conditions.[149] Positive pressure relief is mandatory, irrespective of the type of disposal system used, to vent excess gas in case of occlusion downstream from the interface. If the disposal system is an "active system," negative pressure relief is necessary to protect the breathing circuit or ventilator from excessive subatmospheric pressure. A reservoir is highly desirable with active systems, since it stores waste gases until the evacuation system can remove them. Interfaces can be open or closed, depending on the method used to provide positive and negative pressure relief.[147]

Open Interfaces. An open interface contains no valves and is open to the atmosphere, allowing both positive and negative pressure relief. Open interfaces should be used only with active disposal systems that use a central evacuation system. Open interfaces require a reservoir because waste gases are intermittently discharged in surges, whereas flow from the evacuation system is continuous.[147]

Many contemporary anesthesia machines are equipped with open interfaces like those in Figure 21-32A and 21-32B.[152] An open canister provides reservoir capacity. The canister volume should be large enough to accommodate a variety of waste gas flow rates. Gas enters the system at the top of the canister and travels through a narrow inner tube to the canister base. Gases are stored in the reservoir between breaths. Positive and negative pressure relief is provided by holes in the top of the canister. The open interface shown in Figure 21-32A differs somewhat from the one shown in Figure 21-32B. The operator can regulate the vacuum by adjusting the vacuum control valve shown in Figure 21-32B.[152]

The efficiency of an open interface depends on several factors. The vacuum flow rate per minute must equal or exceed the minute volume of excess gases to prevent spillage. The volume of the reservoir and the flow characteristics within the interface are important. Spillage will occur if the volume of a single exhaled breath exceeds the capacity of the reservoir. The flow characteristics of the system are important because gas leakage can occur long before the volume of waste gas equals the reservoir volume if significant turbulence occurs within the interface.[153]

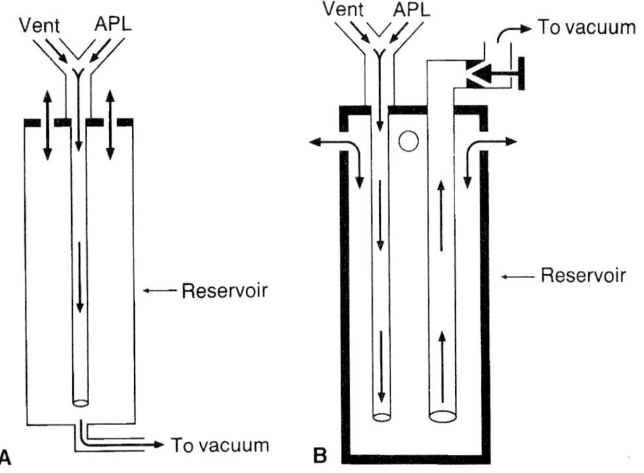

FIGURE 21-32 A and B. Two open scavenging interfaces. Each requires an active disposal system. APL, adjustable pressure limiting valve. See text for details. (Modified with permission from Dorsch JA, Dorsch SE: Controlling trace gas levels. In Dorsch JA, Dorsch SE (eds): Understanding Anesthesia Equipment, 4th ed, p 355. Baltimore, Williams & Wilkins, 1999.)

Closed Interfaces. A closed interface communicates with the atmosphere through valves. All closed interfaces must have a positive-pressure relief valve to vent excess system pressure if obstruction occurs downstream from the interface. A negative-pressure relief valve is mandatory to protect the breathing system from subatmospheric pressure if an active disposal system is used.[147] Two types of closed interfaces are commercially available. One has positive pressure relief only; the other has both positive and negative pressure relief. Each type is discussed in the following sections.

Positive pressure relief only. This interface (Fig. 21-33, left) has a single positive-pressure relief valve and is designed to be used only with passive disposal systems. Waste gas enters the interface at the waste gas inlets. Transfer of the waste gas from the interface to the disposal system relies on the "weight" or pressure of the waste gas itself since a negative pressure evacuation system is not used. The positive-pressure relief valve opens at a preset value such as 5 cm water if an obstruction between the interface and the disposal system occurs.[154] On this type of system, a reservoir bag is not required.

Positive and negative pressure relief. This interface has a positive-pressure relief valve, and at least one negative-pressure relief valve, in addition to a reservoir bag. It is used with active disposal systems. Figure 21-33 (right) is a schematic of Dräger Medical's closed interface for suction systems. A variable volume of waste gas intermittently enters the interface through the waste gas inlets. The reservoir intermittently accumulates excess gas until the evacuation system eliminates it. The operator should adjust the vacuum control valve so that the reservoir bag is properly inflated (**A**), not over distended (**B**), or completely deflated (**C**). Gas is vented to the atmosphere through the positive-pressure relief valve if the system pressure exceeds +5 cm water. Room air is entrained through the negative-pressure relief valve if the system pressure is more negative than −0.5 cm water. On some systems, a back-up negative-pressure relief valve opens at −1.8 cm water if the primary negative-pressure relief valve becomes occluded.

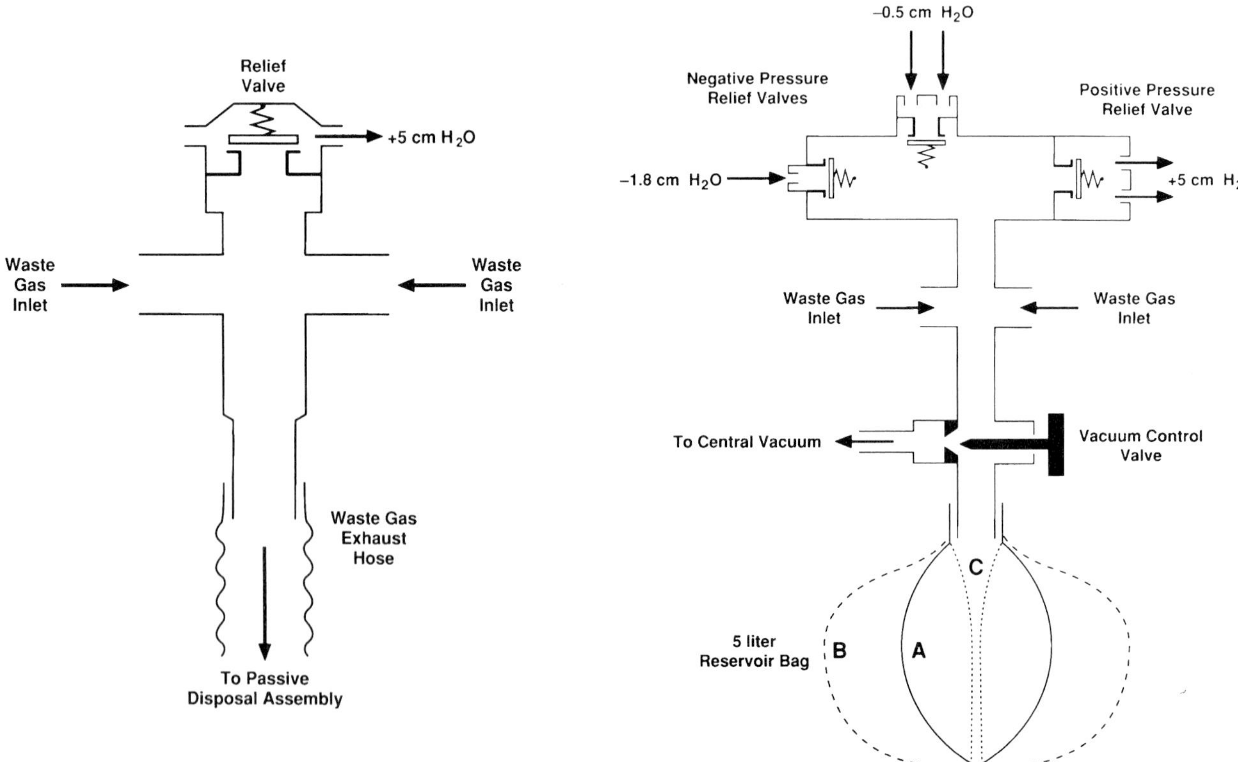

FIGURE 21-33. Closed scavenging interfaces. (*Left*) Interface used with a passive disposal system. (*Right*) Interface used with an active system. See text for details. (Modified with permission (*left*) from Scavenger Interface for Air Conditioning: Instruction Manual. Telford, Pennsylvania, North American Dräger, October 1984; (*right*) from Narkomed 2A Anesthesia System: Technical Service Manual. Telford, Pennsylvania. North American Dräger, 1985.)

The effectiveness of a closed system in preventing spillage depends on the rate of waste gas inflow, the evacuation flow rate, and the size of the reservoir. Leakage of waste gases into
5 the atmosphere occurs only when the reservoir bag becomes fully inflated and the pressure increases sufficiently to open the positive pressure relief valve. In contrast, the effectiveness of an open system to prevent spillage depends not only on the volume of the reservoir but also on the flow characteristics within the interface.[153]

Gas-Disposal Assembly Conduit

The gas-disposal assembly conduit (see Fig. 21-31) conducts waste gas from the scavenging interface to the gas-disposal assembly. It should be collapse proof and should run overhead, if possible, to minimize the chances of accidental occlusion.[149]

Gas-Disposal Assembly

The gas-disposal assembly ultimately eliminates excess waste gas (see Fig. 21-31). There are two types of disposal systems: active and passive.

The most common method of gas disposal is the active assembly, which uses a central evacuation system. A vacuum pump serves as the mechanical flow-inducing device that removes the waste gases usually to the outside of the building. An interface with a negative-pressure relief valve is mandatory because the pressure within the system is negative. A reservoir is very desirable, and the larger the reservoir, the lower the suction flow rate needed.[147,153]

A passive disposal system does not use a mechanical flow-inducing device. Instead, the "weight" or pressure from the heavier-than-air anesthetic gases produces flow through the system. Positive pressure relief is mandatory, but negative pressure relief and a reservoir are unnecessary. Excess waste gases can be eliminated from the surgical suite in a number of ways. Some include venting through the wall, ceiling, floor, or to the room exhaust grill of a nonrecirculating air conditioning system.[147,153]

Hazards

Scavenging systems minimize operating room pollution, yet they add complexity to the anesthesia system. A scavenging system functionally extends the anesthesia circuit all the way from the anesthesia machine to the ultimate disposal site. This extension increases the potential for problems. Obstruction of scavenging pathways can cause excessive positive pressure in the breathing circuit, and barotrauma can occur. Excessive vacuum applied to a scavenging system can result in undesirable negative pressures within the breathing system. Finally, in 2004, another unusual problem that resulted from waste gas scavenging was reported by Lees et al.[155] They reported cases of fires in engineering equipment rooms that house the vacuum pumps used for waste anesthetic gas evacuation. It seems that in some hospitals, waste gases are not directly vented outside, but may be vented into machine rooms that have vents that open to the outside. Since some new anesthesia machines such as the Datex-Ohmeda S5/ADU and Aestiva, among others, now also scavenge ventilator drive gas (which is 100% oxygen in most cases) in addition to gas from the breathing system, the environments in these machine rooms may become highly enriched with oxygen gas. The result of this has been the production of fires in these spaces outside the operating room. These sites may contain equipment or materials such as petroleum distillates (pumps/oil/grease) that in the presence of an oxygen-enriched atmosphere could be excessively combustible and a severe fire hazard.

References

1. Caplan RA, Vistica MF, Posner KL *et al*: Adverse anesthetic outcomes arising from gas delivery equipment. Anesthesiology 87:741, 1997
2. American National Standards Institute: Minimum Performance and Safety Requirements for Components and Systems of Continuous Flow Anesthesia Machines for Human Use (ANSI Z79.8-1979). New York, American National Standards Institute, 1979
3. American Society for Testing and Materials: Standard specification for minimum performance and safety requirements for components and systems of anesthesia gas machines. (ASTM F1161-88). Philadelphia, American Society for Testing and Materials, 1988
4. American Society for Testing and Materials: Standard Specification for Minimum Performance and Safety Requirements for Components and Systems of Anesthetic Gas Machines (ASTM 1161-94). Philadelphia, American Society for Testing and Materials, 1994
5. American Society for Testing and Materials: Standard specification for particular requirements for anesthesia workstations and their components (ASTM F1850-00). Philadelphia, American Society for Testing and Materials, West Conshohoken, 2000
6. Cooper JB: Toward prevention of anesthetic mishaps. Int Anesthesiol Clin 22:167, 1984
7. Spooner RB, Kirby RR: Equipment related anesthetic incidents. Int Anesthesiol Clin 22:133, 1984
8. Emergency Care Research Institute: Avoiding anesthetic mishaps through pre-use checks. Health Devices 11:201, 1982
9. Food and Drug Administration: Anesthesia Apparatus Checkout Recommendations, FDA. 8th ed. Rockville, Maryland, Food and Drug Administration, 1986
10. Food and Drug Administration: Anesthesia Apparatus Checkout Recommendations. Rockville, Maryland, Food and Drug Administration, 1993
11. Lewis SE, Andrews JJ, Long GW: An unexpected Penlon sigma elite vaporizer leak. Anesthesiology 90:1221, 1999
12. Myers JA, Good ML, Andrews JJ: Comparison of tests for detecting leaks in the low-pressure system of anesthesia gas machines. Anesth Analg 84:179, 1997
13. Dorsch JA, Dorsch SE: Hazards of anesthesia machines and breathing systems. In Dorsch JA, Dorsch SE (eds): Understanding Anesthesia Equipment, 4th ed, p 399. Baltimore, Williams and Wilkins, 1999
14. Yasukawa M, Yasukawa K: Hypoventilation due to disconnection of the vaporizer and negative-pressure leak test to find disconnection. Masui–Japanese Journal of Anesthesiology 41(8):1345, 1992
15. Peters KR, Wingard DW: Anesthesia machine leakage due to misaligned vaporizers. Anesth Rev 14:36, 1987
16. Comm G, Rendell-Baker L: Back pressure check valves a hazard. Anesthesiology 56:227, 1982
17. Rendell-Baker L: Problems with anesthetic and respiratory therapy equipment. Int Anesthesiol Clin 20:1, 1982
18. Dodgson BG: Inappropriate use of the oxygen flush to check an anaesthetic machine. Can J Anaesth 35:336, 1988
19. Mann D, Ananian J, Alston T: Oxygen flush valve booby trap. Anesthesiology 101:558, 2004
20. Dorsch JA, Dorsch SE: Equipment checking and maintenance. In Dorsch JA, Dorsch SE (eds): Understanding Anesthesia Equipment, 4th ed, p 937. Baltimore, Williams & Wilkins, 1999
21. Myers JA, Good ML, Andrews JJ: Comparison of tests for detecting leaks in the low-pressure system of anesthesia gas machines. Anesth Analg 84:179, 1997
22. Dorsch JA, Dorsch SE: The anesthesia machine. In Dorsch JA, Dorsch SE (eds): Understanding Anesthesia Equipment, 4th ed, p 75. Baltimore, Williams & Wilkins, 1999
23. Bowie E, Huffman LM: The Anesthesia Machine: Essentials for Understanding. Madison, Ohmeda, The BOC Group, Inc, 1985
24. Cicman JH, Jacoby MI, Skibo VF *et al*: Anesthesia systems. Part 1: Operating principles of fundamental components. J Clin Monit 8:295, 1992
25. Schumacher SD, Brockwell RC, Andrews JJ *et al*: Bulk liquid oxygen supply failure: Anesthesiology 100:186, 2004
26. Feeley TW, Hedley-Whyte J: Bulk oxygen and nitrous oxide delivery systems: Design and dangers. Anesthesiology 44:301, 1976
27. Pelton DA: Non-flammable medical gas pipeline systems. In Wyant GM (ed): Mechanical Misadventures in Anesthesia, p 8. Toronto, University of Toronto Press, 1978
28. Stassou A. (1/16/2002 1105pm). Two die in Hospital Mix-up. WTHN News, New Haven CT, 1992. http://www.wtnh.com/Global/story.asp?S=624589. Last retrieved 11/6/2004.
29. Serlin S: Check your tanks (Letter to the Editor). Anesth Analg 98:870, 2004
30. Dorsch JA, Dorsch SE: The anesthesia machine. In Dorsch JA, Dorsch SE (eds): Understanding Anesthesia Equipment, 4th ed, p 75. Baltimore, Williams & Wilkins, 1999
31. Adriani J: Clinical application of physical principles concerning gases and vapor to anesthesiology. In Adriani J (ed): The Chemistry and Physics of Anesthesia, 2nd ed, p58. Springfield, Illinois, Charles C Thomas, 1962

32. Atlas G: A method to quickly estimate remaining time for an oxygen E-cylinder. Anesth Analg 98:1190, 2004
33. Macintosh R, Mushin WW, Epstein HG: Flowmeters. In Macintosh R, Mushin WW, Epstein HG (eds): Physics for the Anaesthetist, 3rd ed, p 196. Oxford, Blackwell Scientific Publications, 1963
34. Schreiber P: Safety guidelines for anesthesia systems. Telford, Pennsylvania, North American Dräger, 1984
35. Eger EI II, Epstein RM: Hazards of anesthetic equipment. Anesthesiology 24:490, 1964
36. Eger EI II, Hylton RR, Irwin RH *et al*: Anesthetic flowmeter sequence—a cause for hypoxia. Anesthesiology 24:396, 1963
37. Mazze RI: Therapeutic misadventures with oxygen delivery systems. The need for continuous in-line oxygen monitors. Anesth Analg 51:787, 1972
38. Cheng CJ, Garewal DS: A failure of the chain link mechanism of the Ohmeda Excel 210 anesthetic Machine. Anesth Analg 92:913, 2001
39. Lohman G: Fault with an Ohmeda Excel 410 Machine (Letter and Response). Anaesthesia 46:695, 1991
40. Kidd AG, Hall I: Fault with an Ohmeda Excel 210 Anesthetic Machine (Letter and response). Anaesthesia 49:83, 1994
41. Paine GF, Kochan JJ: Failure of the chain link mechanism of the Ohmeda Excel 210 anesthesia machine (Letter to the Editor). Anesth Analg 94:1374, 2002
42. Richards C: Failure of a nitrous oxide-oxygen proportioning device. Anesthesiology 71:997, 1989
43. Abraham ZA, Basagoitia B: A potentially lethal anesthesia machine failure. Anesthesiology 66:589, 1987
44. Neubarth J: Another hazardous gas supply misconnection (Letter). Anesth Analg 80:206, 1995
45. Gaughan SD, Benumof JL, Ozaki GT: Can an anesthesia machine flush valve provide for effective jet ventilation? Anesth Analg 76:800, 1993
46. Anderson CE, Rendell-Baker L: Exposed O_2 flush hazard. Anesthesiology 56:328, 1982
47. Anonymous. Internal leakage from anesthesia unit flush valves. Health Devices 10:172, 1981
48. Andrews JJ: Understanding your anesthesia machine and ventilator. *Review Course Lectures IARS 63rd Congress Lake Buena Vista, Florida, March 4–8, 1989*. International Anesthesia Research Society, p 59. Cleveland 1989
49. Dorsch JA, Dorsch SE; Vaporizers (anesthetic agent delivery devices). In Dorsch JA, Dorsch SE (eds): Understanding Anesthesia Machines, 4th ed, p 121. Baltimore, Williams and Wilkins, 1999
50. Macintosh R, Mushin WW, Epstein HG: Vapor pressure. In Macintosh R, Mushin WW, Epstein HG (eds): Physics for the Anaesthetist, 3rd ed, p 68. Oxford, Blackwell Scientific Publications, 1963
51. Adriani J: Principles of physics and chemistry of solids and fluids applicable to anesthesiology. In Adriani J (ed): The Chemistry and Physics of Anesthesia, 2nd ed, p 7. Springfield, Illinois, Charles C. Thomas, 1962
52. Korman B, Richie IM: Chemistry of halothane-enflurane mixtures applied to anesthesia. Anesthesiology 63:152, 1985
53. Macintosh R, Mushin WW, Epstein HG: Vaporization. In Macintosh R, Mushin WW, Epstein HG (eds): Physics for the Anaesthetist, 3rd ed, p 26. Oxford, Blackwell Scientific Publication, 1963
54. Schreiber P: Anaesthetic equipment: Performance, classification, and safety. New York, Springer-Verlag, 1972
55. Hill DW, Lowe HJ: Comparison of concentration of halothane in closed and semi-closed circuits during controlled ventilation. Anesthesiology 23:291, 1962
56. Hill DW: The design and calibration of vaporizers for volatile anaesthesia agents. In Scurr C, Feldman S (eds): Scientific Foundations of Anaesthesia, 3rd ed, p 544. London, William Heineman Medical Books, 1982
57. Hill DW: The design and calibration of vaporizers for volatile anaesthetic agents. Br J Anaesth 40:648, 1968
58. Morris LE: Problems in the performance of anesthesia vaporizers. Int Anesthesiol Clin 12:199, 1974
59. Stoelting RK: The effects of nitrous oxide on halothane output from Fluotec Mark 2 vaporizers. Anesthesiology 35:215, 1971
60. Diaz PD: The influence of carrier gas on the output of automatic vaporizers. Br J Anaesth 48:387, 1976
61. Nawaf K, Stoelting RK: Nitrous oxide increases enflurane concentrations delivered by ethrane vaporizers. Anesth Analg 58:30, 1979
62. Prins L, Strupat J, Clement J: An evaluation of gas density dependence of anaesthetic vaporizers. Can Anaesth Soc J 27:106, 1980
63. Lin CY: Assessment of vaporizer performance in low-flow and closed-circuit anesthesia. Anesth Analg 59:359, 1980
64. Gould DB, Lampert BA, MacKrell TN: Effect of nitrous oxide solubility on vaporizer aberrance. Anesth Analg 61:938, 1982
65. Palayiwa E, Sanderson MH, Hahn CEW: Effects of carrier gas composition on the output of six anaesthetic vaporizers. Br J Anaesth 55:1025, 1983
66. Scheller MS, Drummond JC: Solubility of N_2O in volatile anesthetics contributes to vaporizer aberrancy when changing carrier gases. Anesth Analg 65:88, 1986
67. Karis JH, Menzel DB: Inadvertent change of volatile anesthetics in anesthesia machines. Anesth Analg 61:53, 1982
68. Riegle EV, Desertspring D: Failure of the agent-specific filling device (Letter). Anesthesiology 73:353, 1990
69. George TM: Failure of keyed agent-specific filling devices. Anesthesiology 61:228, 1984
70. Broka SM, Gourdange PA, Joucken KL: Sevoflurane and desflurane confusion. Anesth Analg 88:1194, 1999
71. Lippmann M, Foran W, Ginsburg R *et al*: Contamination of anesthetic vaporizer contents. Anesthesiology 78:1175, 1993
72. Munson WM: Cardiac arrest: A hazard of tipping a vaporizer. Anesthesiology 26:235, 1965
73. Sinclair A: Vaporizer overfilling. Can J Anaesth 40:77, 1993
74. Seropian MA, Robins B: Smaller than expected sevoflurane concentrations using the SevoTec 5 vaporizer at low fill states and high fresh gas glows. Anesth Analg 91:834, 2000
75. Meister GC, Becker KE Jr: Potential fresh gas flow leak through Dräger vapor 19.1vaporizer with key-index fill port. Anesthesiology 78:211, 1993
76. Zimmer C, Janssen M, Treschan T, Peters J: Near-miss accident during magnetic resonance imaging. Anesthesiology 100:1329, 2004
77. Andrews JJ, Johnston RV Jr: The new Tec 6 desflurane vaporizer. Anesth Analg 76:1338, 1993
78. Weiskopf RB, Sampson D, Moore MA: The desflurane (Tec 6) vaporizer: Design, design considerations and performance evaluation. Br J Anaesth 72:474, 1994
79. Eger EI: New inhaled anesthetics. Anesthesiology 80:906, 1994
80. Susay SR, Smith MA, Lockwood GG: The saturated vapor pressure of desflurane at various temperatures. Anesth Analg 83:864, 1996
81. Johnston RV Jr, Andrews JJ: The effects of carrier gas composition on the performance of the Tec 6 desflurane vaporizer. Anesth Analg 79:548, 1994
82. Andrews JJ, Johnston RV Jr, Kramer GC: Consequences of misfilling contemporary vaporizers with desflurane. Can J Anaesth 40:71, 1993
83. Rupani G: Refilling a Tec 6 desflurane vaporizer (Letter to the Editor). Anesth Analg 96:1526, 2003
84. Hendrickx JF, Carette RM, Deloof T *et al*: Severe ADU desflurane vaporizing unit malfunction. Anesthesiology 99:1459, 2003
85. Mapleson WW: The elimination of rebreathing in various semiclosed anaesthetic systems. Br J Anaesth 26:323, 1954
86. Willis BA, Pender JW, Mapleson WW: Rebreathing in a T-piece: Volunteer and theoretical studies of the Jackson-Rees modification of Ayre's T-piece during spontaneous respiration. Br J Anaesth 47:1239, 1975
87. Rose DK, Froese AB: The regulation of $PaCO_2$ during controlled ventilation of children with a T-piece. Canad Anaesth Soc J 26(2):104, 1979
88. Froese AB, Rose DK: A detailed analysis of T-piece systems. In Steward (ed): Some Aspects of Paediatric Anaesthesia, p 101. Elsevier North-Holland Biomedical Press, 101, 1982
89. Sykes MK: Rebreathing circuits: A review. Br J Anaesth 40:666, 1968
90. Dorsch JA, Dorsch SE: The breathing system II. The Mapleson systems. In Dorsch JA, Dorsch SE (eds): Understanding Anesthesia Equipment, 2nd ed, p 182. Baltimore, Williams and Wilkins, 1984
91. Bain JA, Spoerel WE: A streamlined anaesthetic system. Can Anaesth Soc J 19:426, 1972
92. Aarhus D, Holst-Larsen E, Holst-Larsen H: Mechanical obstruction in the anaesthesia delivery-system mimicking severe bronchospasm. Anaesthesia 52:992, 1997
93. Pethick SL: Letter to the Editor. Can Anaesth Soc J 22:115, 1975
94. Moyers J: A nomenclature for methods of inhalation anesthesia. Anesthesiology 14:609, 1953
95. Eger EI II: Anesthetic systems: Construction and function. In Eger EI II (ed): Anesthetic Uptake and Action. p 206. Baltimore, Williams & Wilkins, 1974
96. Eger EI II, Ethans CT: The effects of inflow, overflow and valve placement on economy of the circle system. Anesthesiology 29:93, 1968
97. Smith CR, Otworth JR, Kaluszyk GSW: Bilateral tension pneumothorax due to a defective anesthesia breathing circuit filter. J Clin Anesth 3:229, 1991
98. McEwan AI, Dowell L, Karis JH: Bilateral tension pneumothorax caused by a blocked bacterial filter in an anesthesia breathing circuit. Anesth Analg 76:440, 1993
99. Walton JS, Fears R, Burt N, Dorman BH: Intraoperative breathing circuit obstruction caused by albuterol nebulization. Anesth Analg 89:650, 1999
100. Chacon A, Kuczkowski K, Sanchez R: Unusual case of breathing circuit obstruction: Plastic packaging revisited (Letter to the Editor). Anesthesiology 100:753, 2004
101. Dhar P, George I, Sloan P: Flow transducer gas leak detected after induction. Anesth Analg 89:1587, 1999
102. Kanno T, Aso C, Saito S *et al*: A combustive destruction of expiration valve in an anesthetic circuit. Anesthesiology 98:577, 2003
103. Laster M, Roth P, Eger E II: Fires from the interaction of anesthetics with desiccated absorbent. Anesth Analg 99:769, 2004
104. Fatheree R, Leighton B: Acute respiratory distress syndrome after an exothermic baralyme-sevoflurane reaction. Anesthesiology 101:531, 2004
105. Holak E, Mei D, Dunning M III *et al*: Carbon monoxide production from sevoflurane breakdown. Anesth Analg 96:757, 2003
106. Kshatri AM, Kingsley CP: Defective carbon dioxide absorber as a cause for a leak in a breathing circuit. Anes 84:475, 1996
107. Norman PH, Daley MD, Walker JR *et al*: Obstruction due to retained carbon dioxide absorber canister wrapping. Anesth Analg 83:425, 1996

108. Adriani J: Carbon dioxide absorption. In Adriani J (ed): The Chemistry and Physics of Anesthesia, 2nd ed, p 151. Springfield, Illinois, Charles C. Thomas, 1962
109. Dewey & Almy Chemical Division: The Sodasorb Manual of CO_2 Absorption. New York, W.R. Grace and Company, 1962
110. Murray MM, Renfrew CW, Bedi A *et al*: A new carbon dioxide absorbent for use in anesthetic breathing systems. Anesthesiology 91:1342, 1999
111. Versichelen LF, Bouche MP, Rolly G *et al*: Only carbon dioxide absorbents free of both NaOH and KOH do not generate compound-A during *in vitro* closed system sevoflurane. Anesthesiology 95:750, 2001
112. Sosis M: Why not use Amsorb alone as the CO_2 absorbent and avoid any risk of CO production? (Letter to the Editor). Anesthesiology 98:1299, 2003
113. Higuchi H, Adachi Y, Arimura S *et al*: The carbon dioxide absorption capacity of Amsorb is half that of soda lime. Anesth Analg 93:221, 2001
114. Hunt HE: Resistance in respiratory valves and canisters. Anesthesiology 16:190, 1955
115. Brown ES: Performance of absorbents: Continuous flow. Anesthesiology 20:41, 1959
116. Andrews JJ, Johnston RV Jr, Bee DE *et al*: Photodeactivation of ethyl violet: A potential hazard of sodasorb. Anesthesiology 72:59, 1990
117. Case History 39: Accidental use of trichloroethylene (Trilene, Trimar) in a closed system. Anesth Analg 43:740, 1964
118. Morio M, Fujii K, Satoh N *et al*: Reaction of sevoflurane and its degradation products with soda lime. Anesthesiology 77:1155, 1992
119. Kharasch ED, Powers KM *et al*: Comparison of Amsorb, Sodalime, Baralyme® degradation of volatile anesthetics and formation of carbon monoxide and compound A in swine in vivo. Anesthesiology 96:173, 2002
120. Frink EJ Jr, Malan TP, Morgan SE *et al*: Quantification of the degradation products of sevoflurane in two CO_2 absorbents during low-flow anesthesia in surgical patients. Anesthesiology 77:1064, 1992
121. Fang ZX, Kandel L, Laster MJ *et al*: Factors affecting production of compound-A from the interaction of sevoflurane with Baralyme® and soda lime. Anesth Analg 82:775, 1996
122. Eger EI II, Ion P, Laster MJ *et al*: Baralyme dehydration increases and soda lime dehydration decreases the concentration of compound A resulting from sevoflurane degradation in a standard anesthetic circuit. Anesth Analg 85:892, 1997
123. Steffey EP, Laster MJ, Ionescu P *et al*: Dehydration of baralyme® increases compound A resulting from sevoflurane degradation in a standard anesthetic circuit used to anesthetize swine. Anesth Analg 85:1382, 1997
124. Eger EL II, Koblin DD, Bowland T *et al*: Nephrotoxicity of sevoflurane versus desflurane anesthesia in volunteers. Anesth Analg 84:160, 1997
125. Kharasch ED, Frink Jr EJ, Zager R *et al*: Assessment of low-flow sevoflurane and isoflurane effects on renal function using sensitive markers of tubular toxicity. Anesthesiology 86:1238, 1997
126. Bito H, Ikeuchi Y, Ikeda K: Effects of low-flow sevoflurane anesthesia on renal function: Comparison with high-flow sevoflurane anesthesia and low-flow isoflurane anesthesia. Anesthesiology 86:1231, 1997
127. Berry PD, Sessler DI, Larson MD: Severe carbon monoxide poisoning during desflurane anesthesia. Anesthesiology 90:613, 1999
128. Baxter PJ, Kharasch ED: Rehydration of desiccated baralyme prevents carbon monoxide formation from desflurane in an anesthesia machine. Anesthesiology 86:1061, 1997
129. Woehlick HJ, Dunning M, Connolly LA: Reduction in the incidence of carbon monoxide exposures in humans undergoing general anesthesia. Anesthesiology 87:228, 1997
130. Fang ZX, Eger EI, Laster MJ *et al*: Carbon monoxide production from degradation of desflurane, enflurane, isoflurane, halothane, and sevoflurane by soda lime and baralyme®. Anesth Analg 80:1187, 1995
131. Bonome C, Belda J, Alavarez-Refojo F *et al*: Low-flow anesthesia and reduced animal size increase carboxyhemoglobin levels in swine during desflurane and isoflurane breakdown in dried soda lime. Anesth Analg 89:909, 1999
132. Neumann MA, Laster MJ, Weiskopf RB *et al*: The elimination of sodium and potassium hydroxides from desiccated soda lime diminishes degradation of desflurane to carbon monoxide and sevoflurane to compound A but does not compromise carbon dioxide absorption. Anesth Analg 89:768, 1999
133. Spearman CB, Sanders HG: Physical principles and functional designs of ventilators. In Kirby RR, Smith RA, Desautels DA (eds): Mechanical Ventilation, p 59. New York, Churchill Livingstone, 1985
134. McPherson SP, Spearman CB: Introduction to ventilators. In McPherson SP, Spearman CB (eds): Respiratory Therapy Equipment, 3rd ed, p 230. St. Louis, C.V. Mosby, 1985
135. Cooper JB, Newbower RS, Kitz RJ: An analysis of major errors and equipment failures in anesthesia management. Consideration for prevention and detection. Anesthesiology 60:34, 1984
136. Reinhart DJ, Friz R: Undetected leak in corrugated circuit tubing in compressed configuration. Anesthesiology 78:218, 1993
137. Raphael DT, Weller RS, Doran DJ: A response algorithm for the low-pressure alarm condition. Anesth Analg 67:876, 1988
138. Slee TA, Pavlin EG: Failure of low pressure alarm associated with use of a humidifier. Anesthesiology 69:791, 1988
139. Sattari R, Reichard PS, Riddle RT: Temporary malfunction of the Ohmeda modulus CD series volume monitor caused by the overhead surgical lighting. Anesthesiology 91:894, 1999
140. Feeley TW, Bancroft ML: Problems with mechanical ventilators. Int Anesthesiol Clin 20:83, 1982
141. Khalil SN, Gholston TK, Binderman J: Flapper valve malfunction in an Ohio closed scavenging system. Anaesth Analg 66:1334, 1987
142. Sommer RM, Bhalla GS, Jackson JM: Hypoventilation caused by ventilator valve rupture. Anesth Analg 67:999, 1988
143. Bourke D, Tolentino D: Inadvertent positive end-expiratory caused by a malfunctioning ventilator relief valve. Anesth Analg 97:492, 2003
144. Roth S, Tweedie E, Sommer RM: Excessive airway pressure due to a malfunctioning anesthesia ventilator. Anesthesiology 65:532, 1986
145. Usher A, Cave D, Finegan B: Critical incident with Narkomed 6000 anesthesia system (Letter to the Editor). Anesthesiology 99:762, 2003
146. Dorsch JA, Dorsch SE: Anesthesia ventilators. In Dorsch JA, Dorsch SE (eds): Understanding Anesthesia Equipment, 4th ed, p 309. Baltimore, Williams and Wilkins, 1999
147. Dorsch JA, Dorsch SE: Controlling trace gas levels. In Dorsch JA, Dorsch SE (eds): Understanding Anesthesia Equipment, 4th ed, p 355. Baltimore, Williams and Wilkins, 1999
148. US Department of Health, Education, and Welfare: Criteria for a Recommended Standard: Occupational Exposure to Waste Anesthetic Gases and Vapors. March ed. Washington, DC, US Department of Health, Education, and Welfare, 1977
149. American Society for Testing and Materials: Standard Specification for Anesthetic Equipment-Scavenging Systems for Anesthetic Gases (ASTM F1343-91). Philadelphia, American Society for Testing and Materials, 1991
150. ASA Task Force on Trace Anesthetic Gases: McGregor DG, Chair: Waste Anesthetic Gases; Information for Management in Anesthetizing Areas and the Postanesthesia Care Unit (PACU), p 3. Park Ridge, Illinois, American Society of Anesthesiologists, 1999
151. Kanmura Y, Sakai J, Yoshinaka H *et al*: Causes of nitrous oxide contamination in operating rooms. Anesthesiology 90:693, 1999
152. Open Reservoir Scavenger: Operator's Instruction Manual. Telford, Pennsylvania, North American Dräger, 1986
153. Gray WM: Scavenging equipment. Br J Anaesth 57:685, 1985
154. Scavenger Interface for Air Conditioning: Instruction Manual. Telford, Pennsylvania, North American Dräger, 1984
155. Allen M, Lees DE. Fires in Medical Vacuum Pumps: Do you need to be concerned? ASA Newsletter 68(10):22, 2004

APPENDIX A

Anesthesia Apparatus Checkout Recommendations

This checkout, or a reasonable equivalent, should be conducted before administration of anesthesia. These recommendations are only valid for an anesthesia system that conforms to current and relevant standards and includes an ascending bellows ventilator and at least the following monitors: Capnograph, pulse oximeter, oxygen analyzer, respiratory volume monitor (spirometer), and breathing system pressure monitor with high- and low-pressure alarms. This is a guideline that users are encouraged to modify to accommodate differences in equipment design and variations in local clinical practice. Such local modifications should have appropriate peer review. Users should refer to the operator's manual for the manufacturer's specific procedures and precautions, especially the manufacturer's low-pressure leak test (step #5).

Emergency Ventilation Equipment

*1. **Verify Back-up Ventilation Equipment is Available & Functioning**

High-Pressure System

*2. **Check Oxygen Cylinder Supply**
   a. Open O_2 cylinder and verify at least half full (about 1,000 psi).
   b. Close cylinder.

*3. **Check Central Pipeline Supplies**
   a. Check that hoses are connected and pipeline gauges read about 50 psi.

Low-Pressure System

*4. Check Initial Status of Low-Pressure System
   a. Close flow control valves and turn vaporizers off.
   b. Check fill level and tighten vaporizers' filler caps.

*5. Perform Leak Check of Machine Low-Pressure System
   a. Verify that the machine master switch and flow control valves are OFF.
   b. Attach "Suction Bulb" to common (fresh) gas outlet.
   c. Squeeze bulb repeatedly until fully collapsed.
   d. Verify bulb stays *fully* collapsed for at least 10 seconds.
   e. Open one vaporizer at a time and repeat "c" and "d" as above.
   f. Remove suction bulb, and reconnect fresh gas hose.

*6. **Turn on Machine Master Switch** and all other necessary electrical equipment.

*7. **Test Flowmeters**
   a. Adjust flow of all gases through their full range, checking for smooth operation of floats and undamaged flow tubes.
   b. Attempt to create a hypoxic O_2/N_2O mixture and verify correct changes in flow and/or alarm.

Scavenging System

*8. **Adjust and Check Scavenging System**
   a. Ensure proper connections between the scavenging system and both APL (pop-off) valve and ventilator relief valve.
   b. Adjust waste gas vacuum (if possible).
   c. Fully open APL valve and occlude Y-piece.
   d. With minimum O_2 flow, allow scavenger reservoir bag to collapse completely and verify that absorber pressure gauge reads about zero.
   e. With the O_2 flush activated, allow the scavenger reservoir bag to distend fully, and then verify that absorber pressure gauge reads < 10 cm H_2O.

Breathing System

*9. **Calibrate O_2 Monitor**
   a. Ensure monitor reads 21% in room air.
   b. Verify low O_2 alarm is enabled and functioning.
   c. Reinstall sensor in circuit and flush breathing system with O_2.
   d. Verify that monitor now reads greater than 90%.

10. **Check Initial Status of Breathing System**
   A. Set selector switch to "Bag" mode.
   B. Check that breathing circuit is complete, undamaged, and unobstructed.
   C. Verify that CO_2 absorbent is adequate.
   D. Install breathing circuit accessory equipment (e.g., humidifier, PEEP valve) to be used during the case.

11. **Perform Leak Check of the Breathing System**
   A. Set all gas flows to zero (or minimum).
   B. Close APL (pop-off) valve and occlude Y-piece.
   C. Pressurize breathing system to about 30 cm H_2O with O_2 flush.
   D. Ensure that pressure remains fixed for at least 10 seconds.
   E. Open APL (pop-off) valve and ensure that pressure decreases.

Manual and Automatic Ventilation Systems

12. **Test Ventilation Systems and Unidirectional Valves**
   A. Place a second breathing bag on Y-piece.
   B. Set appropriate ventilator parameters for next patient.
   C. Switch to automatic ventilation (Ventilator) mode.
   D. Turn ventilator ON and fill bellows and breathing bag with O_2 flush.
   E. Set O_2 flow to minimum, other gas flows to zero.
   F. Verify that during inspiration bellows delivers appropriate tidal volume and that during expiration bellows fills completely.
   G. Set fresh gas flow to about 5 L/min.
   H. Verify that the ventilator bellows and simulated lungs fill *and empty* appropriately without sustained pressure at end expiration.
   I. *Check for proper action of unidirectional valves.*
   J. Exercise breathing circuit accessories to ensure proper function.
   K. Turn ventilator OFF and switch to manual ventilation (bag/APL) mode.
   L. Ventilate manually and assure inflation and deflation of artificial lungs and appropriate feel of system resistance and compliance.
   M. Remove second breathing bag from Y-piece.

Monitors

13. **Check, Calibrate, and/or Set Alarm Limits of all Monitors**
   Capnometer
   Oxygen Analyzer
   Pressure monitor with High- and Low-Airway Pressure Alarms
   Pulse Oximeter
   Respiratory Volume Monitor (Spirometer)

Final Position

14. **Check Final Status of Machine**
   A. Vaporizers off.
   B. APL valve open.
   C. Selector switch to "Bag."
   D. All flowmeters to zero (or minimum).
   E. Patient suction level adequate.
   F. Breathing system ready to use.

**If an anesthesia provider uses the same machine in successive cases, these steps need not be repeated or may be abbreviated after the initial checkout.*

ACKNOWLEDGMENT

Portions of this chapter have appeared with permission in Andrews JJ, Brockwell RC: Inhaled anesthesia delivery systems. In Miller (ed): Anesthesia, 6th ed., p 273. Philadelphia, Churchill Livingstone, 2004.

CHAPTER 22 ■ AIRWAY MANAGEMENT

WILLIAM H. ROSENBLATT

KEY POINTS

1. Three mechanisms account for 75% of airway management injuries: inadequate ventilation, esophageal intubation, and difficult tracheal intubation.
2. Several physical evaluation measures of the difficult airway have become popularized, though their reproducibility and predictability are disputed.
3. Multivariate composite indexes of airway exam findings have improved positive predicted value and specificity.
4. Tracheal intubation should be considered nonroutine under the following conditions: (1) the presence of equally important priorities to the management of the airway ("full stomach," "open globe," etc.), (2) abnormal airway anatomy, (3) an emergency, or (4) direct injury to the larynx and/or trachea.
5. It must be noted that the patient with normal lung compliance should require no more than 20 to 25 cm H_2O pressure to inflate the lungs.
6. Laryngeal mask airway (LMA) size selection is critical to its successful use, and to the avoidance of minor as well as more significant complications.
7. Timing of the removal of the LMA at the end of surgery is critical to avoid complications.
8. It is important to assure that the first attempt at laryngoscopy is a "best attempt."
9. The Functional Airway Assessment (FAA) places an emphasis on the interdependence of anatomic characteristics rather than on their individual size or functional integrity.
10. If, during the laryngoscopy, a satisfactory laryngeal view is not achieved, the backward-upward-rightward pressure (BURP) maneuver may aid in improving the view.
11. Extubation of the trachea must not be considered a benign procedure. Most adult patients are extubated after the return of consciousness and spontaneous respiration, the resolution of neuromuscular block, and the ability to follow simple commands.
12. The LMA had been "repositioned" from the emergency to the routine management pathway of the American Society of Anesthesiologists (ASA) Difficult Airway Algorithm.
13. The ASA defines the difficult airway as the situation in which the conventionally trained anesthesiologist experiences difficulty with mask ventilation or both. Entry into the algorithm begins with the evaluation of the airway.
14. Awake airway management remains a mainstay of the ASA's Difficult Airway Algorithm.
15. There is no true or firm indication for fiberoptic bronchoscope (FOB)–aided intubation, as there might be with direct laryngoscopy.
16. Retrograde wire intubation (RWI) can be a primary intubation technique (elective or urgent) and also employed after failed attempts at direct laryngoscopy, fiberoptic-aided intubation, and LMA-guided intubation.
17. The ASA Difficult Airway Algorithm lists transtracheal jet ventilation as an option in the cannot-mask ventilate, cannot-intubate situation.

PERSPECTIVES ON AIRWAY MANAGEMENT

The airway manager of the twenty-first century is faced with a mind-boggling choice of devices and techniques. The penultimate decade of the last century reintroduced the concept of supralaryngeal ventilation for a large number of surgical procedures. This was followed in the late 1990s by a proliferation of capable supraglottic airways (SGA). Two prominent movements in medicine fueled this movement: evidence-based analysis of medical therapies and a trend toward reduced invasiveness in instrumentation. Techniques of difficult airway management are influenced by both the expanded clinical applications and clinician comfort with SGA ventilation, and new, nonirritating inhalation agents.

Techniques and practices in airway management have long been an important concern of the American Society of Anesthesiologists (ASA). In 1991, Caplan et al reported that 24% of 1,541 liability claims in the ASA closed claims database
1 were related to adverse respiratory events.[1] Three mechanisms accounted for 75% of these injuries: inadequate ventilation, esophageal intubation, and difficult tracheal intubation. A more recent analysis of the closed claims data examined

airway injuries (6% of 4,460 claims as of 1996). Interestingly, most injuries to the larynx occurred during routine tracheal intubations.[2]

Airway management remains as much art as science. "Experience matters" holds as much truth for airway management as "vigilance" does for the entire field of anesthesiology. In part, this is because of the lack of adequate means of preoperatively detecting the patient who is difficult to tracheally intubate by direct laryngoscopy (DL). More information has surfaced showing that routine patient evaluation fails to detect a major source of these failures.[3] Fortunately, this has become a less significant problem as SGA use proliferates and new means of intubation are adopted.[4] Still DL remains the fastest means of achieving tracheal intubation across all operators.

It is clear that management of the airway is paramount to safe perioperative care and the following steps become necessary to favorably affect outcome: (1) a thorough airway history and physical examination; (2) consideration of management plans for use of a supraglottic means of ventilation (e.g., facemask, Laryngeal Mask Airway [LMA]); (3) a management plan for intubation and extubation techniques; and (4) an alternative plan of action should difficulties arise.

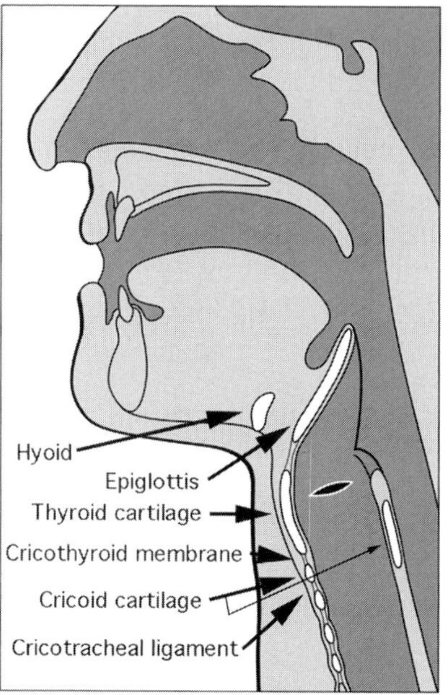

FIGURE 22-1. The major landmarks of the airway mechanism. Note that the cricoid cartilage is less than 1 cm in height in its anterior aspect, but may be 2 cm in height posteriorly (*small arrow*).

Review of Airway Anatomy

The term "airway," refers to the upper airway—consisting of the nasal and oral cavities, pharynx, larynx, trachea, and principal bronchi. The airway in humans is primarily a conducting pathway. Because the oroesophageal and nasotracheal passages cross each other, anatomic and functional complexities have evolved for protection of the sublaryngeal airway against aspiration of food that passes through the pharynx. Anatomically complex, the airway undergoes growth and development and significant changes in its size, shape, and relation to cervical spine between infancy and childhood.[5] Similar to other systems in the body, it is not immune from the influence of genetic, nutritional, and hormonal factors. Table 22-1 illustrates the anatomic differences in the larynx between the infant and adult.

The laryngeal skeleton consists of nine cartilages (three paired and three unpaired); together, these house the vocal folds, which extend in an anterior–posterior plane from the thyroid cartilage to the arytenoid cartilages. The shield-shaped thyroid cartilage acts as the anterior "protective housing" of the vocal mechanism (Fig. 22-1). Movements of the laryngeal structures are controlled by two groups of muscles: the extrinsic muscles, which move the larynx as a whole, and the intrinsic muscles, which move the various cartilages in relation to one another. The larynx is innervated bilaterally by two branches of each vagus nerve: the superior laryngeal nerve and the recurrent laryngeal nerve. Because the recurrent laryngeal nerves supply all of the intrinsic muscles of the larynx (with the exception of cricothyroid), trauma to these nerves can result in vocal cord dysfunction. As a result of unilateral nerve injury, airway function is usually unimpaired, but the protective role of larynx in preventing aspiration may be compromised.

TABLE 22-1

ANATOMIC DIFFERENCES BETWEEN THE PEDIATRIC AND ADULT AIRWAYS

Proportionately smaller infant/child larynx
Narrowest portion: cricoid cartilage in infant/child; vocal folds in adult
Relative vertical location: C3, C4, C5 in infant/child; C4, C5, C6 in adult
Epiglottis: longer, narrower, and stiffer in infant/child
Aryepiglottic folds closer to midline in infant/child
Vocal folds: anterior angle with respect to perpendicular axis of larynx in infant/child
Pliable laryngeal cartilage in infant/child
Mucosa more vulnerable to trauma in infant/child

The cricothyroid membrane (CTM) provides coverage to the cricothyroid space. The membrane, which is typically 9 mm in height and 3 cm in width, is composed of a yellow elastic tissue that lies directly beneath to the skin and a thin facial layer. It is located in the anterior neck between the thyroid cartilage superiorly and the cricoid cartilage inferiorly. It can be identified 1 to 1.5 fingerbreadths below the laryngeal prominence (thyroid notch, or Adam's apple). It is often crossed horizontally in its upper third by the anastomosis of the left and right superior cricothyroid arteries. The membrane has a central portion known as the conus elasticus and two lateral portions, which are thinner and located directly over the laryngeal mucosa. Because of anatomic variability in the course of veins and arteries and its proximity to the vocal folds (which are 0.9 cm above the ligaments' upper border), it is suggested that any incisions or needle punctures to the cricothyroid membrane be made in its inferior third and be directed posteriorly.

At the base of the larynx, suspended by the underside of the cricothyroid membrane, is the signet ring–shaped cricoid cartilage. This cartilage is approximately 1 cm in height anteriorly, but almost 2 cm in height in its posterior aspect as it extends in a cephalad direction, behind the cricothyroid membrane and the thyroid cartilage (see Fig. 22-1). The trachea is suspended from the cricoid cartilage by the cricotracheal ligament (CTL). The trachea measures ~15 cm in adults and is circumferentially supported by 17 to 18 C-shaped cartilages, with a posterior membranous aspect overlying the esophagus (Fig. 22-2).

The first tracheal ring is anterior to the sixth cervical vertebrae. The tracheal cartilages are interconnected by fibroelastic tissue, which allows for expansion of the trachea both in length

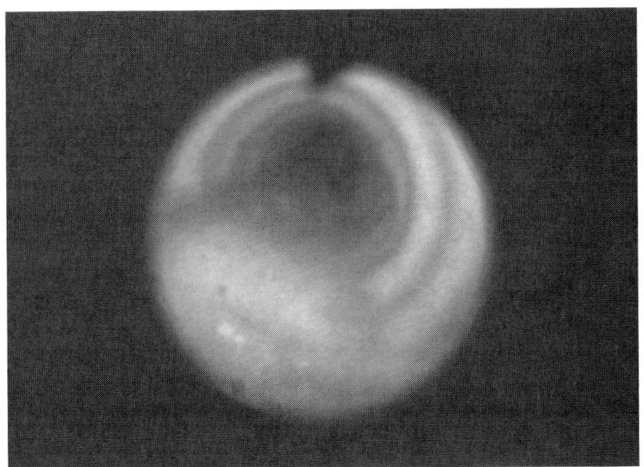

FIGURE 22-2. Bronchoscopic view of the adult trachea. The cartilaginous, C-shaped tracheal rings are seen anteriorly, and the membranous portion, overlying the esophagus, is posterior.

and diameter with inspiration/expiration and flexion/extension of the thoracocervical spine. The trachea ends at the carina at the level of the fifth thoracic vertebra, where it bifurcates into the principal bronchi (Fig. 22-3). The right principal bronchus is larger in diameter than the left, and deviates from the plane of the trachea at a less acute angle. Aspirated materials, as well as a deeply inserted tracheal tube, tend to gain entry into the right principal bronchus though left sided position should be excluded. Cartilaginous rings support the first seven generations of the bronchi.

Patient History and Physical Exam

Preoperative evaluation of the patient should elicit a thorough history of airway-related untoward events as well as related symptoms. A search for documentation to confirm or elucidate these problems should be conducted. Signs and symptoms related to the airway should be elicited, such as snoring (e.g., obstructive sleep apnea), chipped teeth, changes in voice, dysphagia, stridor, bleeding, cervical spine pain or limited range of motion, upper extremity neuropathy, temporomandibular joint pain or dysfunction, and significant or prolonged sore throat/mandible after a previous anesthetic. Many congenital and acquired syndromes are associated with difficult airway management (Table 22-2).

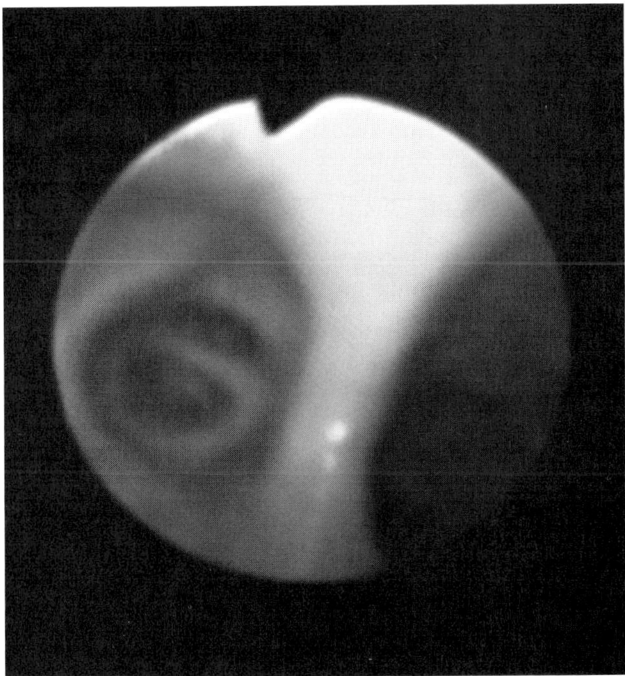

FIGURE 22-3. The adult tracheal carina. The cartilaginous rings of the principal bronchi are easily visualized beyond the carina.

2 Over the last two decades, several physical evaluation measures have become popularized, though their reproducibility and predictability are disputed.[6] The difficulty in developing the perfect airway evaluation tool lies in two interrelated areas: simplicity and interdependency. Though simple bedside evaluation tools are useful, adequate evaluation may require endoscopic, radiologic, or other uncommon examinations.[3] Interdependency refers to the predictive value of one airway exam measure based on the findings of another. This is discussed under the topic of functional airway assessment (FAA) in a later section.

El-Ganzouri et al designed a model for stratifying risk of difficult direct laryngoscopy using a large population.[7] This group examined five common indices individually and in a multivariate model to assess predictive power. As can be seen in Table 22-3, no individual measure proved both sensitive and specific. Though the Mallampati classification (Fig. 22-4) was the most sensitive index, it had low specificity (many false-positives), and low-positive predictive value (4% for a grade IV laryngeal view).[8] Positive predictive values were low for all the commonly used indices.

This multivariate index (MI) assigned relative weights to each exam finding based on the odds of a high-grade laryngeal view on DL with increasing exam score. The scoring of each of these physical exams is listed in Table 22-4. The authors noted that at increasing MI scores, positive predictive value increased, but sensitivity decreased (i.e., higher MI scores occur when there are more positive physical findings, but not all difficult laryngoscopy patients will manifest multiple findings). Com-
3 pared to the Mallampati classification alone, the multivariate composite index had an improved positive predictive and specificity value at equal sensitivity. Of course, some pathology will only present on the induction of anesthesia and/or attempts at laryngoscopy (Fig. 22-5).[10]

Few studies have objectively determined those findings that identify the difficult-to-mask ventilate patient. This basic airway maneuver was examined in a control study by Langeron et al.[11] Of 1,502 patients (excluding planned rapid-sequence induction or emergency cases), 5% were characterized as difficult mask ventilation (DMV). Only one patient in the series was impossible to ventilate by face mask. Table 22-5 describes the criteria for defining a DMV and the five independent clinical predictors. The presence of two predictors indicted a high likelihood of DMV.

4 In general, tracheal intubation should be considered nonroutine under the following conditions: (1) the presence of equally important priorities to the management of the airway ("full stomach," "open globe," etc.), (2) abnormal airway anatomy, (3) an emergency, or (4) direct injury to the larynx and/or trachea. Although the finding of abnormal anatomy is not necessarily synonymous with the difficult airway, it should kindle a heightened level of suspicion. Several investigators have identified anatomic features as having unfavorable influences on the mechanics of direct laryngoscopy; these are explainable on the basis of inability to create a line of sight from the operator's eye to the aperture of the larynx. In the earliest attempt to describe anatomic correlates of difficult intubation, Cass et al placed emphasis on a short muscular neck with a

TABLE 22-2

SYNDROMES ASSOCIATED WITH DIFFICULT AIRWAY MANAGEMENT

PATHOLOGIC CONDITION	PRINCIPAL PATHOLOGIC CLINICAL FEATURES PERTAINING TO AIRWAY
CONGENITAL	
Pierre Robin syndrome	Micrognathia, macroglossia, glossoptosis, cleft soft palate
Treacher Collins syndrome (mandibulofacial dysostosis)	Auricular and ocular defects; malar and mandibular hypoplasia, microstomia, choanal atresia
Goldenhar's syndrome (oculo–auriculo–vertebral syndrome)	Auricular and ocular defects; malar and mandibular hypoplasia; occipitalization of atlas
Down's syndrome (mongolism)	Poorly developed or absent bridge of the nose; macroglossia, microcephaly, cervical spine abnormalities
Klippel-Feil syndrome	Congenital fusion of a variable number of cervical vertebrae; restriction of neck movement
Alpert's syndrome (acrocephalosyndactyly)	Maxillary hypoplasia, prognathism, cleft soft palate, tracheobronchial cartilaginous anomalies
Beckwith's syndrome (infantile gigantism)	Macroglossia
Cherubism	Tumorous lesion of mandibles and maxillae with intraoral masses
Cretinism (congenital hypothyroidism)	Absent thyroid tissue or defective synthesis of thyroxine; macroglossia, goiter, compression of trachea, deviation of larynx/trachea
Cri du chat syndrome	Chromosome 5-P abnormal; microcephaly, micrognathia, laryngomalacia, stridor
Meckel's syndrome	Microcephaly, micrognathia, cleft epiglottis
von Recklinghausen disease (neurofibromatosis)	Increased incidence of pheochromocytoma; tumors may occur in the larynx and right ventricle outflow tract
Hurler's syndrome (mucopolysaccharidosis I)	Stiff joints, upper airway obstruction because of infiltration of lymphoid tissue; abnormal tracheobronchial cartilages
Hunter's syndrome (mucopolysaccharidosis II)	Same as in Hurler's syndrome, but less severe; pneumonias
Pompe's disease (glycogen storage II)	Muscle deposits, macroglossia
ACQUIRED	
Infections	
Supraglottitis	Laryngeal edema
Croup	Laryngeal edema
Abscess (intraoral, retropharyngeal)	Distortion and stenosis of the airway and trismus
Papillomatosis	Chronic viral infection forming obstructive papillomas, primarily supraglottic
Ludwig's angina	Distortion and stenosis of the airway and trismus
Arthritis	
Rheumatoid arthritis	Temporomandibular joint ankylosis, cricoarytenoid arthritis, deviation of larynx, restricted mobility of cervical spine
Ankylosing spondylitis	Ankylosis of cervical spine; less commonly ankylosis of temporomandibular joints; lack of mobility of cervical spine
Benign Tumors	
Cystic hygroma, lipoma, adenoma, goiter	
Stenosis or distortion of the airway	
Malignant Tumors	
Carcinoma of tongue, carcinoma of larynx, carcinoma of thyroid	Stenosis or distortion of the airway; fixation of larynx or adjacent tissues (e.g., infiltration or fibrosis from irradiation)
Trauma	
Head injury, facial injury, cervical spine injury	Cerebrospinal rhinorrhea, edema of the airway; hemorrhage; unstable fracture(s) of the maxillae and mandible; intralaryngeal damage
Miscellaneous Conditions	
Morbid obesity	Short, thick neck and large tongue are likely to be present
Acromegaly	Macroglossia; prognathism
Acute burns	Edema of airway

full dentition, a receding mandible with obtuse mandibular angles, protruding maxillary incisor teeth, decreased mobility at temporomandibular joints, a long high arched palate, and increased alveolar–mental distance.[12] Early radiographic studies showed that the posterior depth of the mandible (the distance between the bony alveolus immediately behind the third molar tooth and the lower border of mandible) was an important factor in determining the ease or difficulty of laryngoscopy.[13] As is discussed later, this anatomic feature is receiving renewed interest.

TABLE 22-3

STATISTICAL ACCURACY OF COMMONLY APPLIED PHYSICAL AIRWAY INDEXES[7–9]

	SENSITIVITY[a] %	SPECIFICITY[a] %	POSITIVE PREDICTIVE VALUE[a]
Mouth opening (<4 cm)	26.3	94.8	25
Thyromental distance (<6 cm)	7	99.2	38.5
Mallampati Class III	44.7	89.0	21
Neck movement <80	10.4	98.4	29.5
Inability to prognath	16.5	95.8	20.6
Body weight >110	11.1	94.6	11.8
History of difficult intubation	4.5	99.8	69.0

[a]For finding of grade III/IV view on direct laryngoscopy.

CLINICAL MANAGEMENT OF THE AIRWAY

Preoxygenation

Preoxygenation (also commonly termed "denitrogenation") should be practiced in all cases when time permits.[14] This procedure entails the replacement of the nitrogen volume of the lung (upwards of 69% of the functional residual capacity [FRC]) with oxygen to provide a reservoir for diffusion into the alveolar capillary blood after the onset of apnea.[15] Preoxygenation with 100% O_2 via a tight-fitting facemask for 5 minutes in a spontaneously breathing patient can furnish up to 10 minutes of oxygen reserve following apnea (in a patient without significant cardiopulmonary disease and a normal oxygen consumption).[16] In one study of healthy, nonobese patients who were allowed to breathe 100% O_2 preoperatively, subjects sustained an oxygen saturation of greater than 90% for 6 ± 0.5 min, whereas obese patients experienced oxyhemoglobin desaturation to under 90% in 2.7 ± 0.25 min.[17] The patient breathing room air (21% O_2) will experience oxyhemoglobin desaturation to a level of under 90% after approximately 2 minutes under ideal conditions. Patients in respiratory failure, or with conditions affecting metabolism or lung volumes, frequently evidence desaturation sooner owing to increased O_2 extraction, decreased FRC, or right-to-left transpulmonary shunting. The most common reason for not achieving a maximum alveolar FIO_2 during preoxygenation is a loose-fitting mask, allowing the entrainment of room air.[14] Less time-consuming methods of preoxygenation have also been described. Using a series of four vital capacity breaths of 100% O_2 over a 30-second period, a high arterial PaO_2 (339 mm Hg) can be achieved, but the time to desaturation is consistently shorter as compared to techniques of breathing 100% O_2 for 5 minutes.[18] A modified vital capacity technique, wherein the patient is asked to take eight deep breaths in a 60-second period, shows promise in terms of prolonging the time to desaturation.[14,19] I prefer the technique of applying a tight-fitting mask for 5 minutes or more of tidal volume breathing; the mask is placed immediately after the patient has been made comfortable on the operating room table and remains in place during intravenous catheter insertion and application of monitors. Pharyngeal insufflation of oxygen is a technique that has been described to prolong the duration that an apneic patient sustains an oxyhemoglobin saturation of >90%. In this technique, oxygen is insufflated at a rate of 3 L/min via a catheter passed through the nares. This technique relies on the phenomenon of apneic oxygenation, a process by which gases are entrained into the alveolar space during apnea, as long as there is a patent airway.[20] This entrainment can provide enough oxygen to sustain hemoglobin saturation for prolonged periods. It is based on the decrease in intrathoracic pressure, relative to atmospheric pressure, produced as approximately 210 cm^3 of oxygen diffuses into the alveolar capillary bed each minute while as little as 12 cm^3 of carbon dioxide diffuses into

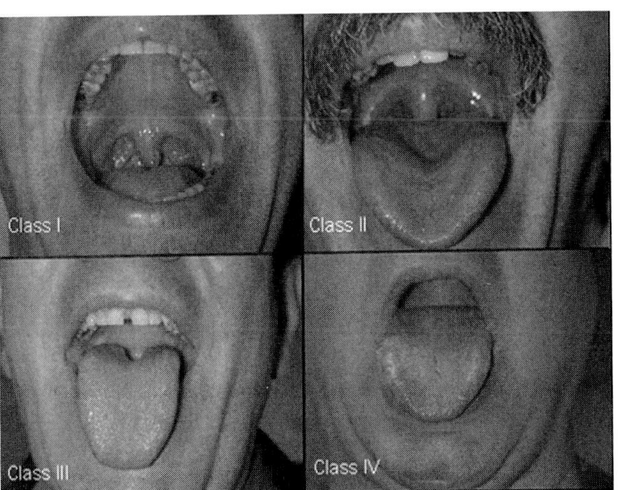

FIGURE 22-4. Mallampati/Samsoon–Young classification of the oropharyngeal view.[10] *Class I:* uvula, faucial pillars, soft palate visible; *Class II:* faucial pillars, soft palate visible; *Class III:* soft and hard palate visible; *Class IV:* hard palate visible only (added by Samsoon and Young).

TABLE 22-4

TECHNIQUES OF COMMON AIRWAY INDEXES MEASUREMENT

Thyromental distance: measured along a straight line from tip of mentum to thyroid notch in neck-extended position
Mouth opening: interincisor distance (or inter-alveolus distance when edentulous) with the mouth fully opened[7]
Mallampati score (see legend, Fig. 22-4)
Head and neck movement: the range of motion from full extension to full flexion[9]
Ability to prognath: capacity to bring the lower incisors in front of the upper incisors[7]

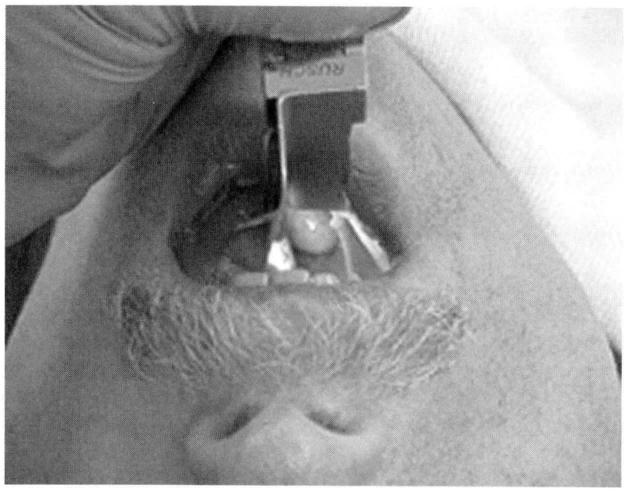

FIGURE 22-5. A 40-year-old male whose epiglottic cyst was discovered at laryngoscopy.

the alveolar space (the remainder of the carbon dioxide being buffered in the blood or tissues). The alveolar carbon dioxide is not removed in this situation, limiting the duration of this technique of oxygenation.

Support of the Airway with the Induction of Anesthesia

With the induction of anesthesia and the onset of apnea, ventilation and oxygenation are supported by the anesthesiologist. Traditional methods include the anesthesia facemask and the tracheal tube. During the last decade several SGA devices have been introduced into worldwide clinical practice. Of these, the LMA has gained significant acceptance among anesthesiologists in the United States, with use rates as high as 35% of all general anesthesia cases, in some settings.[21] The use of the LMA in routine surgery, including cases traditionally managed with tracheal intubation, has been previously discussed.[58]

TABLE 22-5

ASSESSMENT AND PREDICTABILITY OF DIFFICULT MASK VENTILATION[11]

	Odds ratio
Criteria for difficult mask ventilation	
Inability for one anesthesiologist to maintain oxygen saturation >92%	
Significant gas leak around face mask	
Need for ≥IS 4 min gas flow (or use of fresh gas flow button more than twice)	
No chest movement	
Two-handed mask ventilation needed	
Change of operator required	
Independent risk factors for difficult mask ventilation	
Presence of a beard	3.18
Body mass index >26 ng/m^2	2.75
Lack of teeth	2.28
Age >55	2.26
History of snoring	1.84

The Anesthesia FaceMask

The anesthesia facemask is the device most commonly used to deliver anesthetic gases and oxygen, as well as to ventilate the patient who has been made apneic.

The skillful use of a facemask may be challenging and, despite the many advances in airway management, remains a mainstay in the delivery of anesthesia and resuscitation. When the induction of anesthesia is initiated, the patient's level of consciousness changes from the awake state, with a competent and protected airway, to the unconscious state, with an unprotected and potentially obstructed airway. This drug-induced central ventilatory drive depression with a relaxation of the musculature of the upper airway can rapidly lead to hypercapnea and hypoxia. Facemask ventilation is minimally invasive and virtually universal and requires the least sophisticated equipment, thus making it critical to management of the airway.

Appropriate positioning of the patient is paramount to successful mask ventilation. With the patient in the supine position, the head and neck are placed in the *sniffing* position, which is discussed extensively later in the chapter. This position improves mask ventilation by anteriorizing the base of the tongue and the epiglottis.

The mask is gently held over the patient's face with the left hand, leaving the right hand free for other uses (Fig. 22-6).

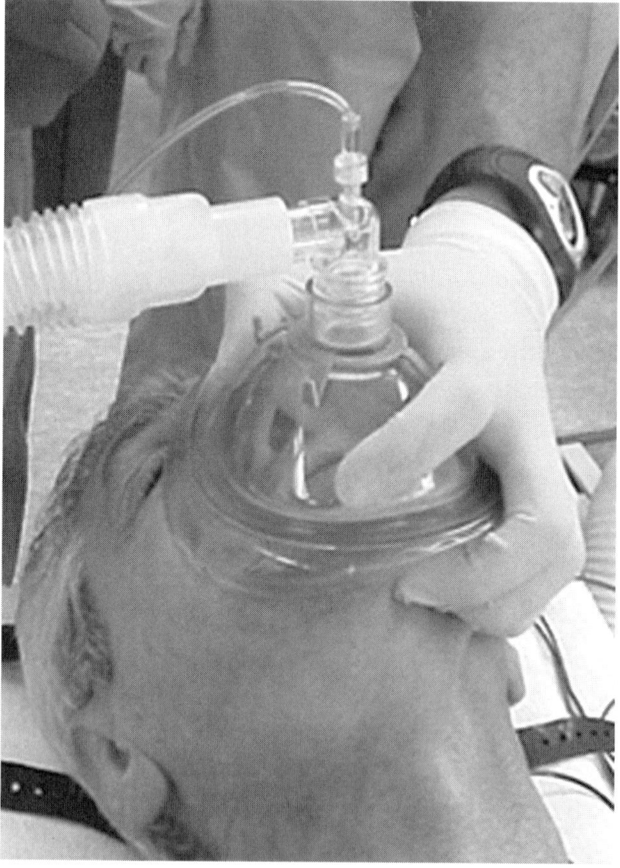

FIGURE 22-6. Holding the anesthesia mask on the face. The thumb and the first finger grip the mask in such a fashion that the anesthesia circuit (or ambu bag) connection abuts the web between these digits. This allows the palm of the hand to apply pressure to the left side of the mask, while the tips of these three digits apply pressure over the right. The third finger helps to secure under the mentum, while the fourth finger is under the angle of the mandible or along the lower mandibular ridge. Mask straps (on pillow) may be used to complement the hand grip by securing the right side of the mask.

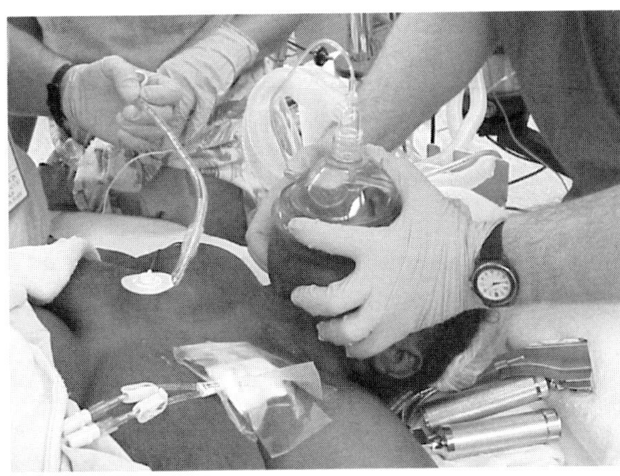

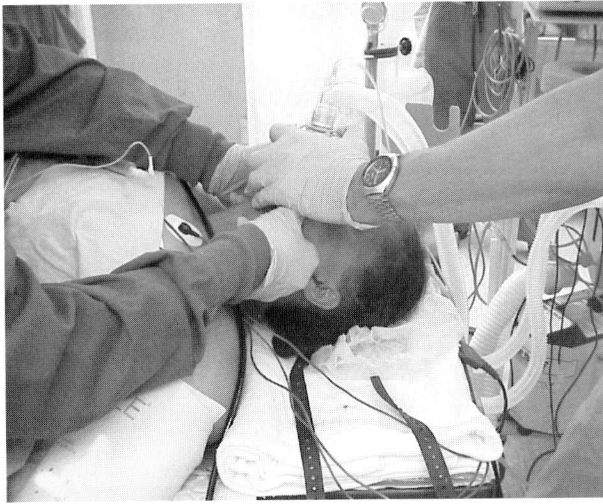

FIGURE 22-7. When mask ventilation is difficult owing to upper airway obstruction, a second operator may be required so that (A) two or (B) three hands can be used in a jaw-thrust maneuver.

Elastic "mask straps" may be used to help secure the mask in the awake or anesthetized patient who is breathing spontaneously and without obstruction, or to complement the left-hand grip. The mask straps can be particularly helpful for the clinician with short fingers. However, prolonged use of tight-fitting mask straps has been associated with motor and sensory neuropraxias.

After induction of anesthesia, a tight fit of the facemask is achieved by downward displacement of the mask between the thumb and first/second fingers with concurrent upward displacement of the mandible with the remaining fingers. This latter maneuver, commonly known as a *jaw thrust,* raises the soft tissues of the anterior airway off of the pharyngeal wall and allows for improved ventilation. In those patients who are obese, edentulous, or bearded, two hands or a mask strap may be required to ensure a tight-fitting mask seal. When two hands are required for holding the facemask, a second operator will obviously be required to ventilate the patient (Fig. 22-7). If need be, the second operator can lend a third hand to the mask fitting, providing for both jaw thrust and chin lift.

5 It must be noted that the patient with normal lung compliance should require no more than 20 to 25 cm H_2O pressure to inflate the lungs. If more pressure than this is required, the clinician should reevaluate the adequacy of the airway, then adjust the mask fit, seek the aid of a second operator to perform two- or three-handed mask holds, and/or consider other devices that aid in the creation of an open passage for airflow through the upper airway. Both rigid oral airways and soft nasal airways create an artificial passage between the roof of the mouth, tongue, and the posterior pharyngeal wall (Fig. 22-8).

Oral airways, which come in a wide variety of sizes, can stimulate the semiconscious patient and provoke coughing, vomiting, and/or laryngospasm. The level of anesthesia must be assessed before they are inserted. Likewise, an SGA may be used at this juncture if the anesthetic is adequate. Nasal airways, less stimulating to the patient, can cause significant nasal trauma

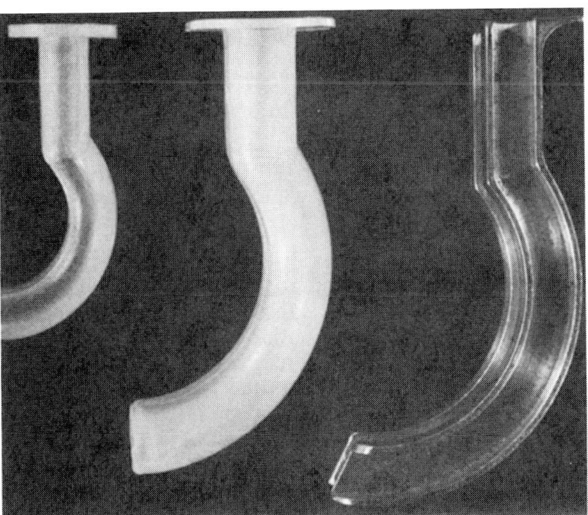

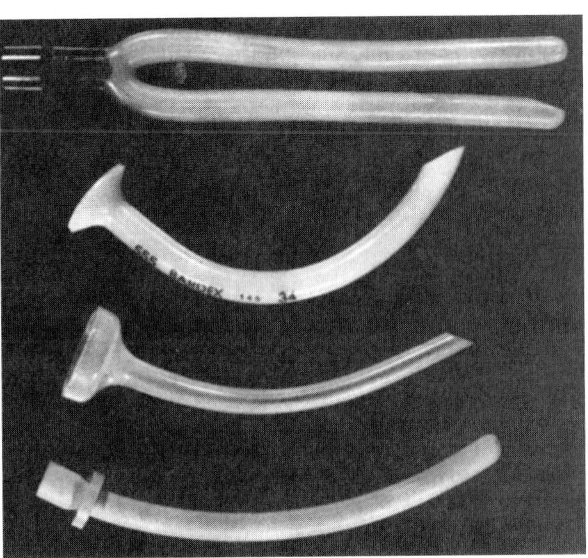

FIGURE 22-8. A variety of oral (A) and nasal (B) airways are available. The goal of these devices is to hold the base of the tongue forward to create an air passage.

and bleeding and should be used with extreme caution in patients with known coagulopathy or nasal deformities. These devices are contraindicated in the patient with a basilar skull fracture.

Obstruction to mask ventilation may be caused by laryngospasm, a reflex closure of the vocal folds. Laryngospasm occurs as a result of foreign body (e.g., oral or nasal airway); saliva, blood, or vomitus touching the glottis; or even a light plane of anesthesia. Hypoxia as well as noncardiogenic pulmonary edema can result if there is continued spontaneous ventilation against closed vocal cords. Treatment of laryngospasm includes removal of an offending stimulus (if it can be identified), continuous positive airway pressure, deepening of the anesthetic state, and the use of a rapid-acting muscle relaxant.

If there are no contraindications (e.g., a "full stomach" or other aspiration risk), mask ventilation can be the technique employed for the duration of anesthesia maintenance. Otherwise, it is commonly used to administer anesthetic gases until the anesthetic state is adequate for use of another means of airway support (e.g., SGA, tracheal tube). This decision is made after careful consideration of the patient's coexisting diseases and surgical requirements.

Supraglottic Airways

The LMA ushered in the first major use of SGAs in the United States. But, by the time of its initial introduction in 1989 and approval by the U.S. Federal Drug Administration (FDA) in 1991, it was being used in more than 500 hospitals in the United Kingdom. Though initially approved for use as a substitute for facemask ventilation and when tracheal intubation was not achievable, it soon enjoyed wide use in surgical cases traditionally managed with tracheal intubation.[21]

Though other SGAs were available in the early 1990s (e.g., COPA J. Mallinkroft Medical, Athlone, Ireland), it was not until the patent of original LMA design, the LMA-Classic®, expired in 2002 that there was a proliferation of similar devices. A wealth of information exists on the LMA and its subsequent iterations (all by the original inventor, Dr. Archie Brain). Much of this knowledge may apply to newer SGAs but studies on those devices are few at the time of this writing. This chapter devotes considerable text to the family of LMAs. This is not meant to infer preference, but rather a relative availability of information.

The advent of the LMA as well as other supralaryngeal airways have led some to question the relative safety of tracheal intubation.[22] A recent study by Tanaka et al demonstrated vocal cord edema and increased airflow resistance in patients undergoing minor surgery with a tracheal tube.[23] These changes

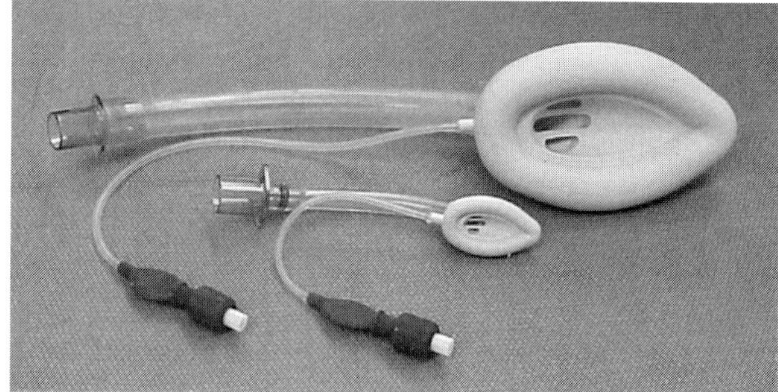

FIGURE 22-9. The original LMA design: a size 1 and size 6 LMA-Classic. The two bars over the airway aperture prevent the epiglottis from obstructing the LMA barrel.

were not seen with LMA use. This, along with ASA closed claim database information, lends support to the search for safe alternatives to tracheal intubation whenever possible.[24]

LMA Design. The LMA is composed of a small "mask" designed to sit in the hypopharynx, with an anterior surface aperture overlying the laryngeal inlet (Fig. 22-9). The rim of the mask is composed of an inflatable silicone cuff that fills the hypopharyngeal space, creating a seal that allows positive-pressure ventilation with up to 20 cm H_2O pressure.[25] The adequacy of the seal is dependent on correct placement and appropriate size. It is less dependent on the cuff filling pressure or volume. Attached to the posterior surface of the mask is a barrel (airway tube) that extends from the mask's central aperture through the mouth and can be connected to an ambu bag or anesthesia circuit.

6 LMA size selection is critical to its successful use, and to the avoidance of minor as well as more significant complications. Neonatal to large adult sizes are available. Table 22-6 gives the recommended size for patient weight and the maximum inflation volumes. The manufacturer recommends that the clinician choose the largest size that will comfortably fit in the oral cavity, then inflate to the minimum pressure that allows ventilation to 20 cm H_2O without an air leak. The intracuff pressure should never exceed 60 cm H_2O (and should be periodically monitored if nitrous oxide is used as part of the anesthetic). When an adequate seal cannot be obtained with 60 cm H_2O cuff pressure, the LMA may be malpositioned and/or sizing should be reevaluated. Light anesthesia may also contribute to poor seal or partial or complete laryngospasm.

LMA Insertion. The insertion of the LMA as described by its inventor, Dr. Archie J. I. Brain, has been modified by a number of writers. Discussion of these various alternatives is beyond the scope of this text. Dr. Brain's initial contemplations

TABLE 22-6

LMA SIZING AND INFLATION VOLUMES

LMA SIZE	PATIENT WEIGHT	INCREASE IN SIZE (%)	MAXIMUM INFLATION VOLUME (mL)	TEST INFLATION VOLUME (mL)
1	Neonates/infants up to 5 kg	—	4	6
1.5	5–10 kg	21	7	10
2	10–20 kg	21	10	15
2.5	20–30 kg	18	14	21
3	>30 kg	15.7	20	30
4	Small adults	14.4	30	45
5	Normal adults	13.8	40	60
6	Large adults	8.1	50	80

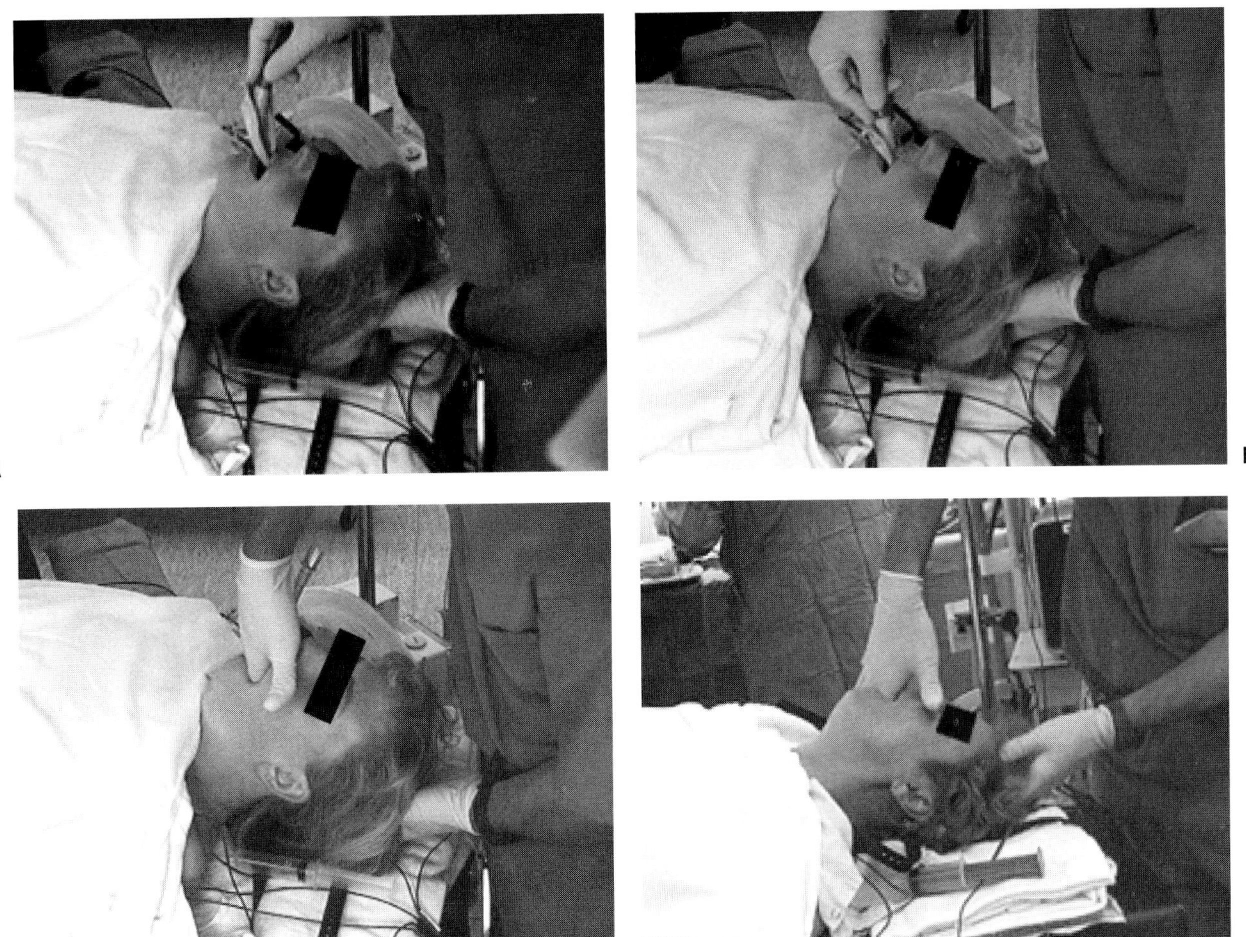

FIGURE 22-10. Insertion of the LMA. The LMA is inserted with the index finger of the dominant hand pressing with a force vector against the hard palate (A and B). The outward force vector is continued from the hard palate to the pharynx and hypopharynx (C) until the index finger meets resistance against the upper esophageal sphincter (D).

of this unique airway considered routine and natural placement of a "foreign body" in the hypopharynx—food. It was Dr. Brain's intent to mimic the placement of food into the hypopharynx and thereby establish the placement of a device, which could then serve as an airway. All varieties of the LMA (with the exception of the LMA-Fastrach) follow the same insertion technique.

To understand the insertion technique, we must therefore review the processes of deglutination: lubrication with saliva; formation of a flat oval food bolus by the tongue; initiation of the swallowing reflex by stimulation of the palate; upward pressure by the tongue flattening the food bolus against the palate; directing of the food bolus toward the posterior pharyngeal wall and into the hypopharynx by the shape of the palate and pharyngeal wall; head extension and neck flexion opening the space behind the larynx to allow passage of the food bolus into the hypopharynx; and finally, opening of the upper esophageal sphincter to allow esophageal entry of the food bolus. These functions allow the food bolus to reach its mark blindly, while avoiding the anterior pharyngeal structures and avoiding reflex responses meant to protect the airway.

Prototype insertion methods involved rotation through 180° and the early use of an introducer to prevent down-folding of the epiglottis. The currently recommended technique, illustrated in Figure 22-10, has been found to be less traumatic and has a 98% success rate. In this technique the mask is lubricated with a nonsilicone, nonlocal anesthetic–containing lubricant (simulating the saliva) and is fully deflated to form a thin, flat wedge shape (masticated food bolus). The operator's nondominant hand is placed under the occiput to flex the neck on the thorax and extend the head at the atlanto-occipital joint (creating a space behind the larynx; this action also tends to open the mouth).[26] The index finger of the dominant hand is placed in the cleft between the mask and barrel. The hard palate is visualized and the superior (nonaperture) surface of the mask is placed against it. Force is applied by the index finger in an upward direction toward the top of the patient's head. This will cause the mask to flatten out against the palate and follow the shape of the palate as it slides into the pharynx and hypopharynx. The index finger continues along this arc, always applying an outward pressure until the resistance of the upper esophageal sphincter is met. The most common error made by clinicians is applying pressure with a posterior vector. This tends to catch the tip of the LMA on the posterior pharyngeal wall, causing folding with resultant misplacement and trauma.

Once insertion is complete, removal of the inserting hand is facilitated by gentle stabilization of the LMA barrel with the nondominant hand. Prior to attachment of the anesthesia circuit, the LMA is inflated with the minimum amount of gas to form an effective seal. Though it is difficult to suggest a particular volume of gas to be used, the operator should be accustomed to the feel of the pilot bulb when it is inflated to 60 cm H_2O pressure, the maximum suggested seal pressure. Accompanying the inflation, one should be able to observe a rising of the cricoid and thyroid cartilage and lifting of the barrel out of the mouth by approximately 1 cm as the mask is lifted off the upper esophageal sphincter. The mask is fixed in position by bringing the barrel down against the chin and taping in the midline while a gentle upward pressure is exerted against the hard palate. If a midline position is not possible owing to the nature of the patient position or surgical procedure, a flexible LMA (discussed later) should be considered. A bite block is recommend to prevent biting and occlusion of the LMA barrel.

The LMA and Gastroesophageal Reflux. Although the distal tip of the LMA's mask sits in the esophageal inlet, it does not reliably seal it. A predominant clinical perception is that the LMA does not protect the trachea from regurgitated gastric contents. As of 2004, just 23 cases of suspected pulmonary aspiration have been reported (with an estimated 200,000,000 uses of the LMA worldwide). Of these, only 13 were verified as true aspiration events and none resulted in death, though five patients required positive-pressure ventilation. There were predisposing factors in most of the cases, including obesity, dementia, emergency surgery, upper abdominal surgery, Trendelenburg position, intraperitoneal insufflation, or a difficult airway.[27–40] Indeed, when used in patients at low risk for regurgitation, the rate of aspiration during LMA use is similar to that in all non-LMA general anesthetics (~2 in 10,000 cases), though the incidence of gastroesophageal reflux may be increased when compared to use of the facemask.[41–45]

Some evidence suggests that there may be more gastroesophageal reflux during LMA use with a patient in the Trendelenburg or lithotomy position.[43,45] If regurgitated gastric contents are noted in the LMA barrel, maneuvers similar to those applied when using an ETT should be instituted: Trendelenburg position, administer 100% oxygen, leave the LMA in place and use a flexible suction device down the barrel, deepen anesthetic if necessary.

When populations of patients considered to have a full stomach are studied (in controlled trials, prospective series, or anecdotally), there is a very low incidence of aspiration noted with elective or emergency LMA use. Reports have included patients who are morbidly obese or experience frequent gastroesophageal reflux and those undergoing elective cesarean section or airway rescue during labor and those presenting to emergency departments or paramedic crews.[46–56] During cardiopulmonary resuscitation, the incidence of gastroesophageal regurgitation is four times greater with a bag-valve mask than with the LMA.[57]

Unconventional Use of the LMA. Since its introduction, a wealth of clinical data has indicated that the LMA can be safely used in the operating room in a variety of clinical situations. A large number of clinical situations traditionally managed with tracheal intubation and mechanical ventilation have been performed with the LMA.[58]

LMA and Positive-Pressure Ventilation. Though first introduced for use with spontaneous ventilation, the LMA has proved useful for cases in which positive-pressure ventilation is either desired or preferred.[59,60] Contrary to initial impression, positive-pressure ventilation can be safely accomplished with the LMA.[61–64] There is no difference found in gastric inflation with positive pressure (<17 cm H_2O) when comparing the LMA and the ETT.[65,66] When using the LMA, one should limit tidal volumes to 8 mL/kg and airway pressure to 20 cm H_2O since this is the sealing pressure of the device under normal circumstances. LMA use has been described with the supine, prone, lateral, oblique, Trendelenburg, and lithotomy positions.[67] Though the manufacturer recommends use for a maximum of 2 to 3 hours, reports of use lasting more than 24 hours can be found.[68]

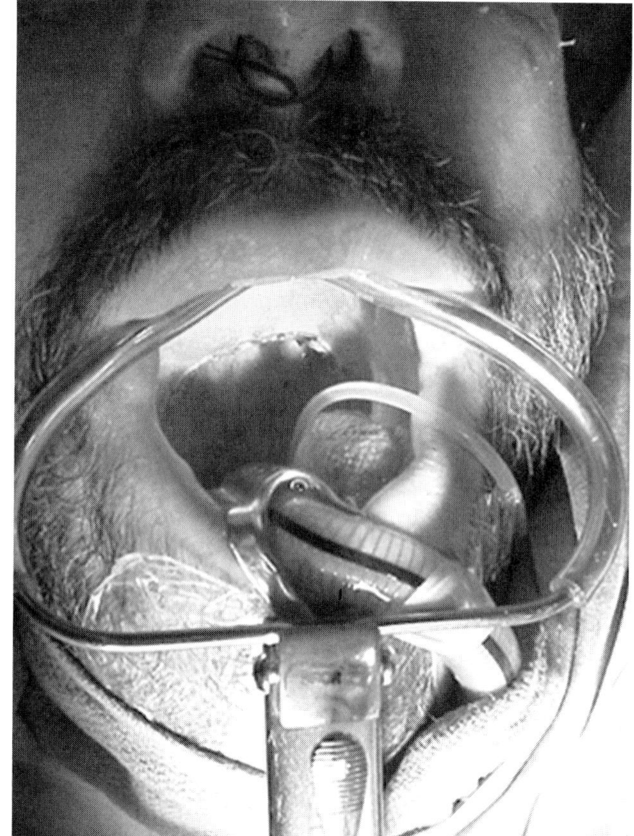

FIGURE 22-11. An LMA-flexible in place with a Crow-Davis mouth gag during a tonsillectomy and uvulopharyngopalatoplasty. The uvula has been removed. The LMA mask is not visible to the surgeon when correctly placed.

The LMA-Flexible. The advent of the LMA-flexible (Fig. 22-11) has permitted extension of LMA use to a variety of cases in which the airway is shared with the surgical team (e.g., otolaryngologic surgery).[69] The LMA-flexible differs from the original design by virtue of a thin-walled, small-diameter, wire-reinforced (kink-resistant) barrel, which can be positioned out of the midline without affecting the hypopharyngeal position of the mask. It was designed to be used with a tonsillar mouth gag, as employed in surgery on the mouth and pharynx.[70,71] The LMA-flexible has also proved useful when heavy drapes are placed over the head and airway (e.g., mastoidectomy), when there is movement of the head position during surgery (e.g., typanostomy tubes), or when the LMA barrel cannot be secured in the midline (e.g., mid or lateral facial surgery). The use of this mask in surgery above the level of the hypopharynx, including tonsillectomy, affords a number of clinically important advantages over tracheal intubation (Table 22-7).

When correctly placed, the LMA mask serves to block the airway from blood, secretions, and surgical debris above the level of the mask, as compared to the tracheal tube, which is known not to protect the trachea from liquids instilled into the pharynx[72–75] (Fig. 22-12).

The LMA and Bronchospasm. As a supraglottic airway, the LMA appears to be well suited to the patient with a history of extrinsic asthma. The LMA presents a unique opportunity for the clinician to conveniently and effectively control the airway without having to introduce a foreign body into the trachea. Thus, it may be an ideal airway tool in the asthmatic patient who is not at risk for reflux and aspiration.[76–78] Because the halogenated inhaled anesthetics are potent bronchodilators, it is at the time of emergence (when the anesthetic is discontinued)

TABLE 22-7

ADVANTAGES OF THE LMA IN SUPRAGLOTTIC SURGERY

Improved protection of the airway from blood and surgical debris
Reduced cardiovascular responses
Reduced coughing on emergence
Reduced laryngospasm after airway device removal
Improved oxygen saturation after airway device removal
Ability to administer oxygen until complete restoration of airway reflexes

that the patient at risk for bronchospasm is most likely to wheeze. In the patient managed with the LMA, there is no foreign body in the sensitive bronchorespiratory tree and the patient can be fully emerged prior to removal of the device. In the event that uncontrollable bronchospasm does occur intraoperatively (e.g., from vagal stimuli such as traction on the peritoneum), intubation can be performed through the LMA or after its removal.[79]

7 **LMA Removal.** Timing of the removal of the LMA at the end of surgery is critical.[80,81] The LMA should be removed either when the patient is deeply anesthetized or after protective reflexes have returned and the patient is able to open the mouth on command. Removal during excitation stages of emergence can be accompanied by coughing and/or laryngospasm. Many clinicians remove the LMA fully inflated; thus, it acts as a "scoop" for secretions above the mask, bringing them out of the airway.[82] This has been particularly useful in otolaryngologic surgery (see Fig. 22-12).

Contraindications to LMA Use. The primary contraindication to elective use of the LMA is a risk of gastric-contents aspiration (e.g., full stomach, hiatus hernia with significant gastroesophageal reflux, morbid obesity, intestinal obstruction, delayed gastric emptying, poor history). Other contraindications include poor lung compliance or high airway resistance, glottic or subglottic airway obstruction, and limited mouth opening (<1.5 mm).[67]

LMA Use Complications. Apart from gastroesophageal reflux and aspiration, reported complications have included laryngospasm, coughing, gagging, retching, bronchospasm, and other events characteristic of airway manipulation. The incidence of sore throat is approximately 10%, as compared to 30% with tracheal intubation, but has been reported as 0 to 70%.[67] Also reported are hoarseness (4 to 47%) and dysphagia (4 to 24%). The LMA may cause transient changes in vocal cord function.[80] This is possibly related to cuff overinflation during prolonged procedures.

There have been few reports of nerve injury associated with LMA use. As of March 2004, 14 cases of nerve palsy have been reported: recurrent (7), hypoglossal (5), and lingual (2).[84,85] All but one of these resolved spontaneously. In all cases, size 3 and 4 LMAs were in use and, in all but one case, nitrous oxide was one of the inhalation agents (which can increase cuff pressures by 9 to 38%).[86] Cuff pressures were not monitored in any of the cases. It is hypothesized that lingual nerve injuries occur as the nerve is trapped between the mandible and the LMA barrel lying lateral to the tongue. The hypoglossal nerve runs rostral and lateral to the hyoid bone and may be trapped against it. The recurrent nerve may be compressed between the LMA cuff and the cricoid or thyroid cartilage. Unmonitored increases in pressure as a result of N_2O diffusion, light anesthesia with constriction of pharyngeal musculature, tissue edema and venous engorgement from a head-down position, and lidocaine gel lubricant have been blamed for nerve injury.[87] To prevent such injury, the cuff of the LMA should be inflated to no more than 60 cm H_2O and should be monitored if N_2O is in use. The use of a larger LMA, with less pressure, has also been recommended.[88] Lidocaine should not be present in cuff lubricants.

One death has been associated with an LMA device. An elderly woman suffered a tear of her esophagus after use of the intubating LMA (LMA-Fastrach®), dying 9 weeks later from septic shock after a series of related complications.[89] Interestingly, the actual complication was most likely a small esophageal tear from an inadvertent esophageal intubation. Therefore, this complication was more of a misadventure of "blind intubation" not inherently attributable to the LMA-Fastrach itself. No other deaths because of complication of LMA use have been reported in the literature. It has been estimated, though, that 600 deaths occur each year in the developed world because of complications of difficult tracheal intubation.[90]

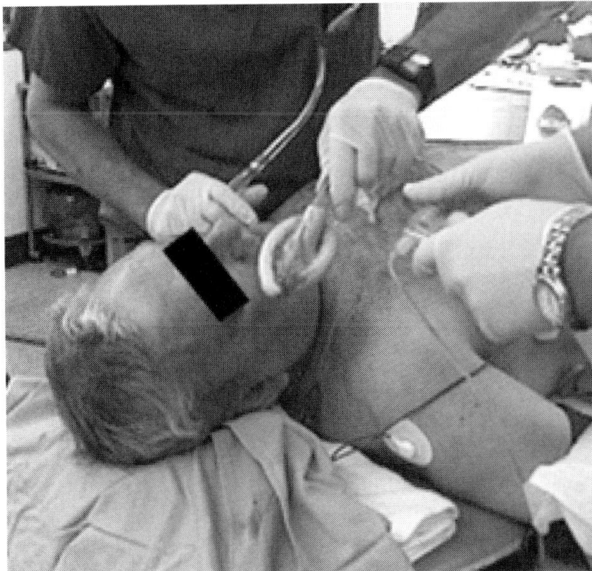

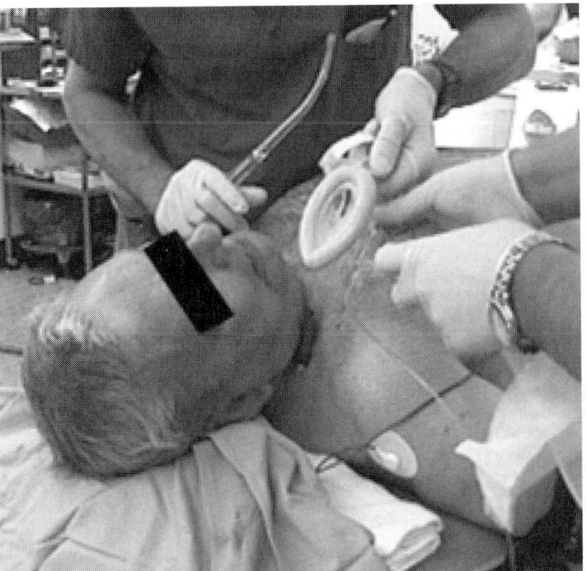

FIGURE 22-12. Following endoscopic sinus surgery, (**A**) the superior, pharyngeal surface of the LMA is blood-stained, whereas (**B**) the laryngeal surface remains clean.

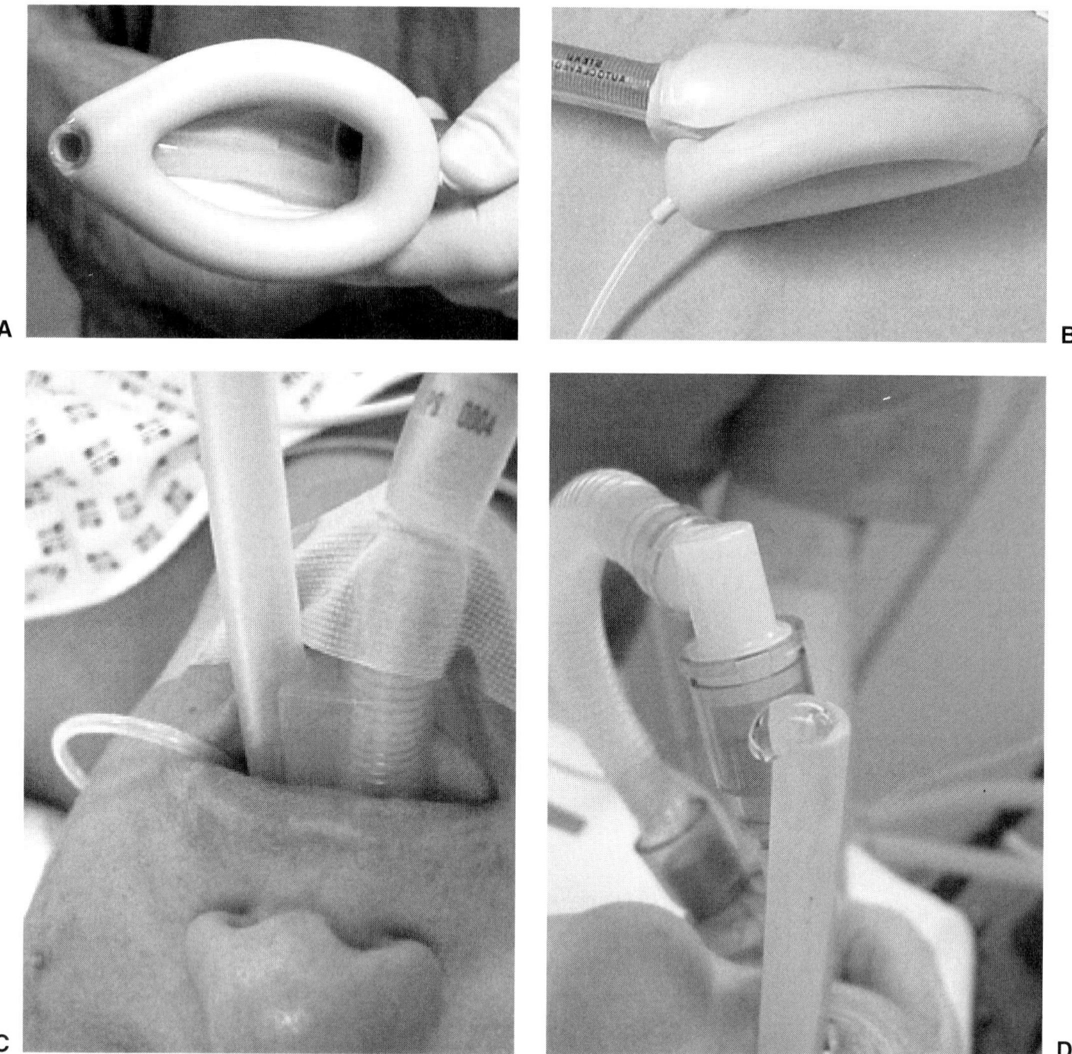

FIGURE 22-13. The LMA-Proseal: A. Anterior view showing gastric drain passing through the bowl. B. Lateral view showing the circumferential and posterior mask cuffs. (In the photograph, the view of the esophageal lumen is obscured by the airway lumen.) C. The airway lumen and gastric drain, separated by an integral bite block, emerge from the patient. D. A drop of water-soluble lubricant has been placed in the proximal aperture of the esophageal lumen to monitor for gas leak, which should not be present.

The LMA-Proseal®. Although the original LMA and the LMA-flexible have been used successfully for positive-pressure ventilation, they are not ideally suited to this task for two reasons: first, if poorly seated in the hypopharynx, gastric inflation may occur; second, the seal pressure is limited to approximately 20 cm H_2O. In 1994, an LMA prototype that included a gastric drain was described.[91] The LMA-Proseal® was introduced to clinical practice in 2001 (Fig. 22-13). It was believed that such a design would reduce both the risk of gastric inflation (by providing a low-resistance pathway for pressure transmitted to the esophagus) and the risk of aspiration of refluxed gastric contents. Subsequently, it was found that the design, which also incorporates a second, posterior cuff, could reliably allow positive-pressure ventilation with 40 cm H_2O pressure. It is inserted in an identical manner as describe previously for the LMA-classic. A metallic insertion device is available from the manufacturer. Table 22-8 lists the unique features of the LMA-Proseal and the resultant clinical advantage.

The LMA-Proseal has been shown to achieve a higher effective seal than the LMA-classic (40 to 45 cm H_2O) and allow easier and quicker gastric tube placement.[93,94] A wide variety of surgical cases have been performed with the LMA-Proseal. Many of these have previously been considered contraindicated for supraglottic airway use.[93] Maltby et al have pioneered the use of the LMA-Proseal laparoscopic cholecystectomy in obsess patients.[93] This surgical procedure has long been considered the prototypical case for contraindicated LMA use because of high intraperitoneal pressures, as well as intraoperative stomach manipulation. Laparoscopic cholecystectomy was performed in 46 patients, 12 of whom had a body mass index of greater than 30 kg/m^2. The median airway pressure at which a gas leak occurred was 34 cm H_2O (range 18 to 45). Four obese patients crossed over to a control, tracheal tube group. Stomach size (e.g., distension) was equal between groups.

Apart from being successfully used as a positive pressure as well as spontaneous ventilation airway, the LMA-Proseal has a distinct advantage over all currently available supraglottic airways. The presence of the gastric drain allows position diagnosis.[95] This facility, originally intended by Dr. Brain, has been extensively researched by Drs. M. Stix and C. O'Connor. These authors have developed a protocol for

TABLE 22-8

FEATURES OF THE LMA-PROSEAL

FEATURE	CLINICAL IMPACT
Gastric drain	• Position confirmation • Active gastric emptying • Passive gastric emptying • Protection from gastric content aspiration[92]
Posterior cuff	• Increased seal pressure
Bite block	• Prevents patient biting obstruction
Wire-reinforced airway barrel	• Reduced overall size • Decreased ability to tracheally intubate
Large barrel/bite block configuration	• First attempt insertion less successful than LMA-classic • Confers rotational stability • Size choice—size down from LMA-classic

judging LMA-Proseal position, a task typically difficult for the less experienced LMA user. The protocol of Stix and O'Connor follows a simple logic based on the observations of Dr. Brain and their own observations.

Bite block depth. Based on the successful use of the LMA-Proseal in 147 women and 127 men, a first approximation of insertion adequacy can be made from observation of the integral bite block. The midway point of the bite block was found to be proximal to the incisors (e.g., within the oral cavity) in 78% of women and 92% of men.[96] Though mid (or greater) bite block advancement into the esophagus indicated good placement, a normal distribution of depths indicate that the bite block test affords a "first approximation" of LMA-Proseal position adequacy.

Suprasternal notch test (SSN). When correctly positioned, the proximal orifice of the gastric drain tube should be within the boundaries of the upper esophagus, making it contiguous with the esophageal lumen.[95] Gentle percussion over the suprasternal notch results in a brief pressure increase in the lumen of the gastric drain. This can be demonstrated with the placement of a seal of surgical jelly, or preferably, nontoxic soap (e.g., children's bubble-making soap) over the distal end of gastric drain (Fig. 22-13D).[97] Inadequate insertion depth and glottic or folded positions will result in a negative SSN test.[98]

Airway seal test. Once the insertion depth and esophageal position of the proximal gastric drain orifice is assured, positive-pressure breaths are given. If an adequate separation of the alimentary and airway tracks has been achieved, no insufflated gas should emerge from the distal gastric drain.[95] The surgical jelly-soap or bubble seal of the distal gastric drain will aid in detection of escaping gas.[99]

Gastric drain patency. Posterior folding of the distal aspect of the LMA-Proseal mask has been described.[100] Folding of the mask in the hypopharynx may not be detected during routine ventilation. Dr. Brimacombe and colleagues have stated that one or more of the above-mentioned tests may give a false-positive results.[101] These authors suggest supplementing the LMA-Proseal position testing with the insertion of a gastric tube, thereby assuring gastric drain patency.

The importance of position testing was highlighted in a report of pulmonary aspiration of gastric contents during a cholecystectomy with an LMA-Proseal.[102] No position testing had been performed, and though adequate ventilation was achieved and with airway pressures of 27 cm H_2O, the LMA-Proseal had been unknowingly placed in a folded position. This case illustrates the importance of the LMA-Proseal in modern clinical practice: as of this writing more than 10 supraglottic airways are in use in clinical practice. Because many are recent arrivals to the clinical arena, there is little or no information available regarding gastric insufflation with positive-pressure ventilation and protection from gastric content aspiration. The LMA-Proseal remains the only device where these questions have been repeatedly investigated, and position testing is a possibility.

Similarly, little is known of the resuscitation utility of new SGAs. The LMA-Proseal would be expected to function similarly to the LMA-Classic in a cannot intubate/cannot ventilate situation, and adds gastric emptying as a resuscitative maneuver.[103,104]

Esophageal and gastric insufflation have been noted with some proseal LMA placements.[105] The incidence and clinical signature of this air trapping are unknown.

The LMA and the Difficult Airway. Apart from its role as a routine anesthetic airway device, the LMA has a history of being a valuable tool in the care of the patient with the anticipated, or the unanticipated, difficult airway. This will be considered later in this chapter.

The Laryngeal Tube. The laryngeal tube (LT) (VBM Modizintechnile, GmbH, Sulz aN, Germany) consists of a single lumen tube with an approximately 130 degree midshaft angle and two (distal and proximal) low pressure cuffs (Fig. 22-14A). An oval aperture between the cuffs serves as a ventilation artifice. The distal end of the tube is scaled around the distal cuff. When inserted correctly, the distal cuff seals the oral and nasal pharynx. Ventilation (spontaneous or positive pressure) occurs via the midcuff orifice. The cuffs are inflated via a common pilot valve. The LT is reusable, requires a mouth opening of at least 2.3 cm and is inserted either blindly or with the aid of a laryngoscope. Six sizes (0 through 5) are suitable for neonates to large adults. Several studies have examined the use of the LT in spontaneous and controlled ventilation, and in comparison to the LMA classic and the LMA-proseal. Gaitini et al used the LT in 175 patients presenting for elective surgery.[106] Positive-pressure ventilation was successful in 96.6% of cases.

Ocker et al compared the LT to the LMA classic in 50 patients undergoing routine surgery. Time of insertion and adequacy of ventilation were similar for both devices.[107] Peak airway pressure and airway leak pressure were higher with the LT (leak pressures LT 36 $\pm$ 3 cm H_2O, LMA 22 $\pm$ 3 cm H_2O).

The Cobra Pharyngeal. Laryngeal Airway (Engineered Medical Systems, Indianapolis, IN, USA) is a disposable supralaryngeal airway device. It has a single lumen that terminates in a widened distal end (Fig. 22-14B). A pharyngeal cuff serves to occlude the upper airway from the oral cavity. A series of

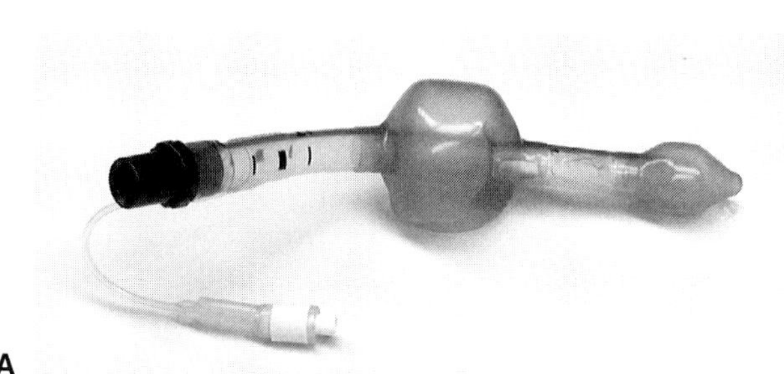
A

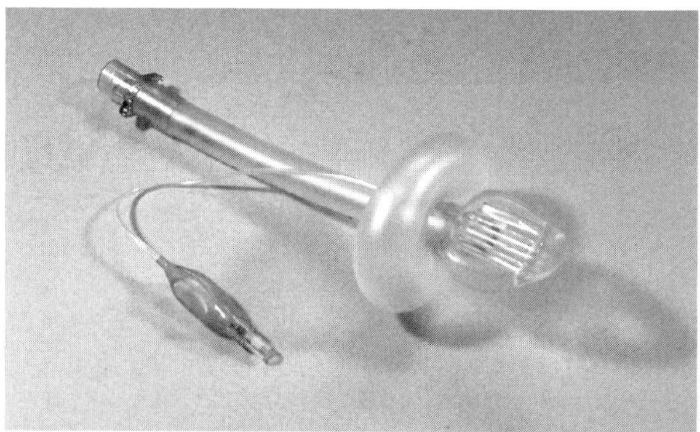
B

FIGURE 22-14. **A.** The Laryngeal Tube. **B.** The Cobra Pharyngeal Laryngeal Airway.

slots in the widened end serve to hold the epiglottis out of the barrel. A fiberscope and/or ETT may be passed through the barrel and the slots. Reports have demonstrated the use of the cobra in airway rescue, as well as routine anesthetic care with spontaneous as well as positive-pressure ventilation.[108,109]

Tracheal Intubation

Routine Laryngoscopy

Preparing for laryngoscopy and the "best attempt." Whether laryngoscopy is undertaken with the patient in an awake or unconscious state, repeated attempts often result in edema and bleeding of the anterior upper airway structures (e.g., tongue, vallecula, epiglottis, laryngeal structures), hindering subsequent attempts at visualization and causing increased
8 airway obstruction. It is therefore important to assure that the first attempt at laryngoscopy is a "best attempt."

First, when faced with the critically ill patient, the most skilled laryngoscopist available should be positioned to perform the laryngoscopy. In less acute situations, it is not inappropriate for a trainee, clinician extender, or other skilled personnel to assume this role. Second, the availability of all the materials needed to perform laryngoscopy and intubation should be assured, as should the availability of materials needed to manage a failed intubation. When devices are available in a variety of sizes (e.g., tracheal tubes, LMAs), the operator should have at hand the presumed correct size, as well as one size smaller and one size larger of each item (Table 22-9).

Other devices that complete the equipment list, but may not be uniformly available, include: end-tidal CO_2 monitoring (e.g., capnography or colorimetric device [e.g., Easy Cap II, Mallinckrodt]), pulse oximetry, transtracheal jet ventilation catheter, and a high-pressure oxygen source.

The height of the supine patient surface should be at the level of the laryngoscopist's xyphoid cartilage, with the bed or operating room table in a non-movable mode (e.g., wheels locked). The clinician performing the intubation must have unobstructed access to the head.

Direct laryngoscopy. Successful laryngoscopy involves the distortion of the normal anatomic planes of the supralaryngeal airway to produce a line of direct visualization from the operator's eye to the larynx: this requires the creation of a new (nonintrinsic) visual axis, through maximal alignment of the axes of the oral and pharyngeal cavities, and displacement of the tongue. Unanticipated failure of direct laryngoscopy is primarily a problem of tongue displacement (inability to align the axes can be anticipated by physical exam).[3] Some investigators have focused the search for the cause of difficult direct laryngoscopy on the relative position of the tongue. Chow et al have found that a hypopharyngeal tongue (e.g., the greater mass of the tongue is within the hypopharynx) is accompanied by a caudad larynx, which is in turn determined by measurement of the mandibular hyoid distance (a measure of the cephalocaudad separation of the mandible and hyoid during fetal development).[110]

Benumof eloquently explains this finding in terms of ontogeny and the descent of the larynx to create the phonics of the human pharyngeal space (antagony recapitulates phylongony). A long descent of the larynx results in a large part of the tongue to be in the hypopharynx.[111] Poor descent of the larynx results in a small thyromental distance (TMD) and can indicate a difficult intubation. Chow et al also noted that the long mandibularhyoid distance can be in part because of a shortened mandibular ranus. A short ranus results in the floor of the mouth being more rostrad and less compliant, and therefore displacement of the tongue is more difficult.[112] If both a small TMD as well as a large TMD can both predict difficult laryngoscopy, then how can this measure be useful to the airway evaluator? As pointed out by the ASA Difficult Airway Algorithm, no one measure may be adequate to determine difficulty of DL, and multiple measures must be integrated to make sensible airway management decisions.[113]

Another mandibular dimension that has been examined is the mandibular depth index (the posterior depth of the mandible/mandibular length).[114] Kikkawa et al have noted that a deep or short mandible (higher index) indicates a large hypopharyngeal tongue and difficulty with displacement. Though

TABLE 22-9

EQUIPMENT FOR LARYNGOSCOPY[a]

Oxygen source and self-inflating ventilation bag (e.g., ambu bag)
Face mask[b]
Oropharyngeal and nasopharyngeal airways[b]
Tracheal tubes[b]
Tracheal tube stylet
Syringe for tracheal tube cuff inflation
Suction apparatus
Laryngoscope handle (2), tested for working order and battery freshness
Laryngoscope blades: Common blades include the curved (Macintosh) and straight (Miller)[b]
Pillow, towel, blanket, or foam for head positioning
Stethoscope

[a]Equipment that should be immediately available in the ideal clinical setting.
[b]Presumed size as well as one larger and one smaller should be immediately available.

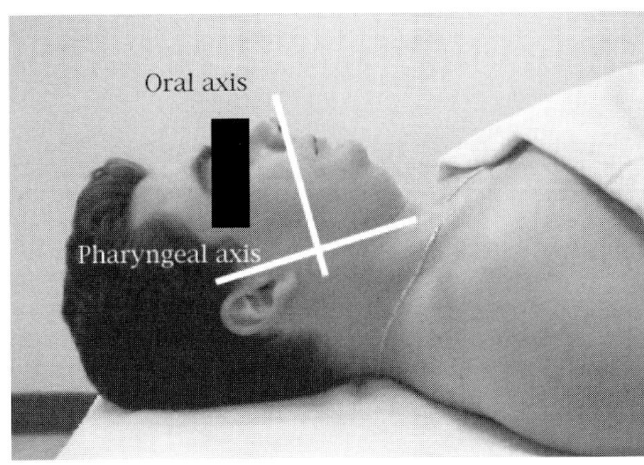

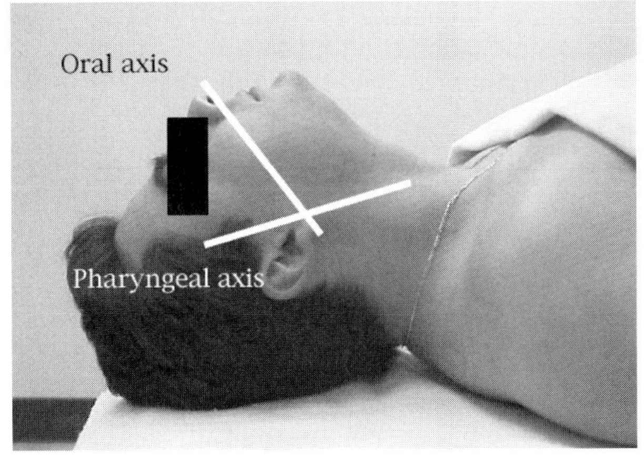

FIGURE 22-15. A. With the patient supine, the oral and pharyngeal axes do not overlap. B. Extenstion at the atlanto-occipital joint maximally overlaps the oral and pharyngeal axes.

the mandibular hyoid distance and the mandibular depth index are distinct measures, they approach the problem of difficulty with DL similarly: anatomic relationships of the mandible may predict a difficult to displace hypopharyngeal tongue. They also highlight that a single measure (e.g., thyromental distance) does not yield enough information to be predictive.

Though congenital, anatomic variation may occur, pathologic variations may mimic the same problem of hypopharyngeal tongue mass: Ovassapian et al have identified hyperplasia of the lymphoid tissue at the base of the tongue as the principle cause of unanticipated difficult laryngoscopy.[3] Visualization of this tissue is currently the only method of diagnosis. It is therefore typically discovered during a failed DL.

Direct laryngoscopy requires the creation of a line of sight from the operator's eye to the aperture of the larynx. Bannister and MacBeth proposed a three-axis model to explain the anatomic relationships involved in this operation.[115] Recently, this explanation has been challenged.[116] Work by Adnet et al noted that whereas extension at the atlanto-occipital joint maximally facilitated an oral cavity/pharyngeal alignment, no significant improvement was achieved with flexion of the cervical spine on the thorax. Chow and Wu refined this approach by noting that laryngeal axis alignment is unnecessary.[117] The end point of the effort to create an in-line space for tracheal intubation is the glottic aperture: alignment of the entire larynx is therefore unnecessary. These authors propose a two-axes/tongue-displacement model. This model does not depend on the alignment of all axes to create an in-line view of the larynx, but rather maximizes the spaces between the alveolar ridge and laryngeal aperture through oral-pharyngeal alignment and tongue displacement. This concept can be used to understand not only the problems that may hinder direct laryngoscopy, but also why common indexes of airway assessment fail in their predictive power. This concept has been described previously and can be viewed as functional airway assessment
9 (FAA).[118] FAA is a method of examining the functional nature of each of the anatomic correlates of the commonly used assessment indices. FAA places an emphasis on the interdependence of these anatomic characteristics rather than on their individual size or functional integrity. As explained by Chow and Wu, when the head and neck are in the neutral position, the oral and pharyngeal axis are perpendicular to each other.[117] With maximal extension of a normal atlanto-occipital joint, 35 degree of motion is attained Fig. 22-15. This brings the angle between the oral and pharyngeal axis to 125 degree. Though an improvement, certainly not the 180 degree required for creation of a line of sight to the glottis. A different space must be created. This space is created by displacement of the tongue with the laryngoscope. Though atlanto-occipital extension cannot by itself allow direct laryngeal vision, it does provide anterior displacement of the mass of the tongue and brings upper the alveolar ridge into improved position relative to the tongue and larynx. The extension of the atlanto-occipital point also provides an advantage in mouth opening.[26] Calder et al has shown that the maximal mouth opening is 50% greater in full atlanto-occipital extension as compared to the neutral head position. Temporal-mandibular jaw (TMJ) function also contributes to the displacement of the tongue away from the required visual axis. Rotation and translation of the TMJ result in a relaxation of the tongue insertion, as well as creation of the aperture width needed for instrumentation.

Using the FAA approach to airway evaluation also helps to explain the value of the popular yet highly criticized Mallampati and Thyromental distance indices. These two measures have historically been considered important because they approximate the relative mass of the tongue (Mallampati) and the anterior-posterior borders of space in which it will be displaced (TMD) by the laryngoscope. As noted elsewhere, these indices have shown to have poor and/or variable predictive power. Two groups have considered the interrelated nature of these measures in a way which reveals why they perform poorly when considered individually: Ayoub et al found a high Mallampati score to be predictive of a difficult DL when the TMD was less than 4 cm.[119] When the TMD was greater than 4 cm, relative tongue size (as determined by the Mallampati) was not predictive: Iohon et al found similar results using a TMD cutoff of 6 cm.[120] The finding that the predictive power of the Mallampati improves when the mandible is short is consistent with the concept of FAA: When the mandibular space is restricted, tongue size is important. When the space is large, a tongue of any nonpathologic size should be accommodated. An exception to this may be hypopharyngeal tongue as described by Chow and Wu, though according to those authors, measurement of the mandibular hyoid distance should help in diagnosing this.[110]

An unforeseen cause of difficulty in direct laryngoscopy is a pathologic increase in tongue size. Ovassapian et al have identified lingual tonsil hyperplasia (LTH) as the most commonly undiagnosed cause of unanticipated difficult direct laryngoscopy.[3,121] Ovassapian et al reviewed the cases of unanticipated difficult direct laryngoscopy in their institution from 1989 to 2000. Thirty-three patients were identified. All patients were found to have LTH on fiberoptic exam.

Devices that aid in positioning the patient in a sniff position pillow have become available. These include the Sniff position pillow (AliMed, Inc. of Dedham, MA) developed by Michael

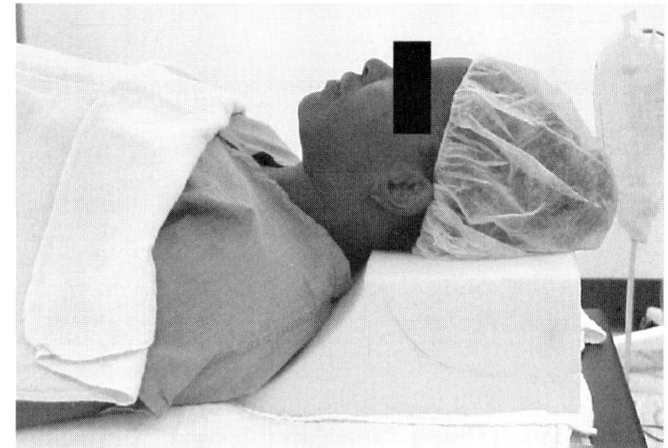

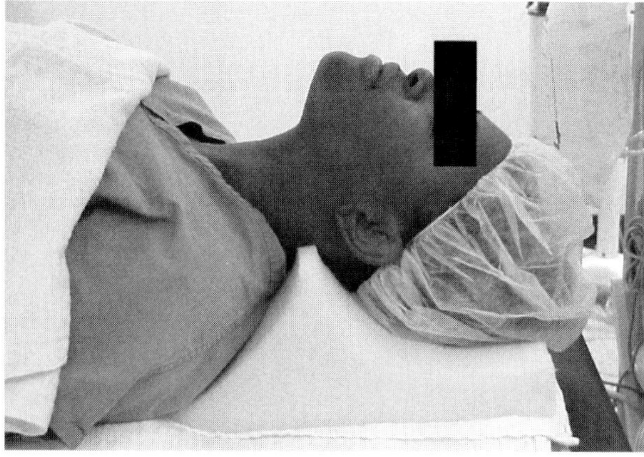

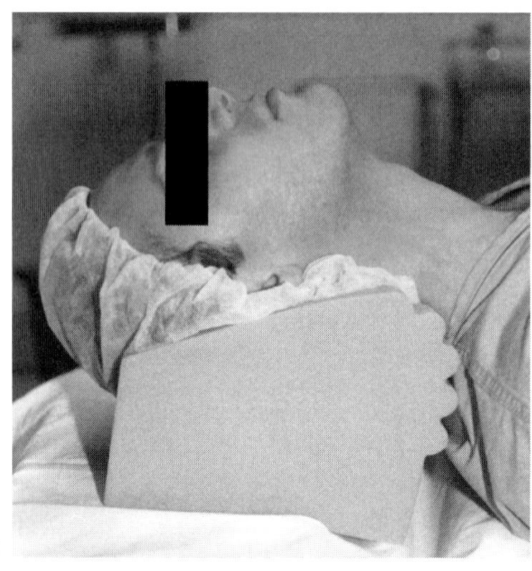

FIGURE 22-16. **A** Pi's pillow (Dupaco, Oceanside, CA) places the patient in a comfortable position prior to the induction of anesthesia and (**B**) in an ideal "sniff" position during airway management. **C** The Popitz sniff position pillow.

Popitz, and Pi's pillow (Dupaco, Oceanside, CA), which is comfortable for the awake patient but easily reconfigured after anesthetic induction to provide an ideal position, has been developed by Dr. Kaiduan Pi (Fig. 22-16).

The obese patient may need further positioning to move the mass of the chest away from the plane across which the laryngoscope handle will sweep as it is manipulated into the mouth. This may require placing a wedge-shaped lift (e.g., blankets, pillows) under the scapula, shoulders, and nape of neck, raising the head and neck above the thorax and providing a grade to allow gravity to take the mass away from the airway (Fig. 22-17).

10 If, during the laryngoscopy, a satisfactory laryngeal view is not achieved, the backward-upward-rightward pressure (BURP) maneuver may aid in improving the view. In this maneuver, a second operator displaces the larynx (*B*) backward against the cervical vertebrae, (*U*) superiorly as possible, and (*R*) slightly laterally to the right, using external pressure over the cricoid cartilage. The BURP maneuver has been shown to improve the laryngeal view, decreasing the rate of difficult intubation in 1,993 patients from 4.7 to 1.8%.[122,123] When a left-handed operator is using a left-handed laryngoscope blade, the lateral external pressure should displace the larynx to the left. Similarly, Benumof describes "optimal external laryngeal manipulation," which consists of pressing posteriorly and cephalad over the thyroid, hyoid, and cricoid, as improving laryngeal view by at least one Cormack and Lehane grade.[124,125]

Once alignment has been achieved, the mouth is opened by one of two techniques (Fig. 22-18). The first accomplishes hyperextension of the atlanto-occipital joint by the use of the dominant hand under the occiput. This maneuver tends to open the mouth, and can be accentuated by using the fifth finger of the nondominant hand (holding the laryngoscope) to apply pressure over the chin in a caudad direction (Fig. 22-18A). In the second technique, which tends to be more effective but requires contact of the (gloved) hand with the teeth and/or gum, caudad pressure is applied with the thumb of the dominant hand on the mandibular molars on the patient's same side while the first finger, crossed above or below the thumb, applies cephalad pressure to the ipsilateral maxillary molars (Fig. 22-18B). The ultimate goal of both techniques is rotation and translation of the temporomandibular joint to achieve the widest interincisor gap. The patient, whether conscious or not, is now ready for laryngoscopy.

Though direct laryngoscopy remains the most utilized method for tracheal intubation,[126] it is far from successful in all cases nor always benign when successful. DL may be difficult or impossible 8.5% and 1.8%, respectively, of the time.[126] Domino et al's analysis of the ASA closed claims database reveals that laryngeal injury during DL occurs more often in "easy" as opposed to difficult laryngoscopies.[24] Among the 4,460 cases in the ASA closed claim database, 87 instances of laryngeal trauma were recorded. Of these, 80% occurred during routine (non-difficult) tracheal intubation, where no injury was suspected. This has led some to question whether routine tracheal intubation is as safe as assumed.[22]

Use of the laryngoscope blade. Proper use of the laryngoscope blade is vital to the success of this basic airway management technique. Two blade types are commonly available and each is applied in a unique manner (Fig. 22-19). The curved (Macintosh) blade is used to pull the epiglottis out of the line of sight by tensing the glossoepiglottic ligament, whereas the straight blade (Miller) compresses the epiglottis against the base of the tongue. Both blades include a flange along the left

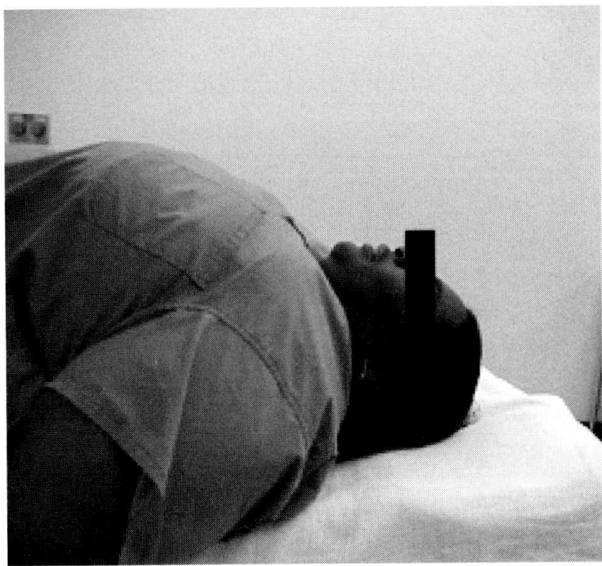
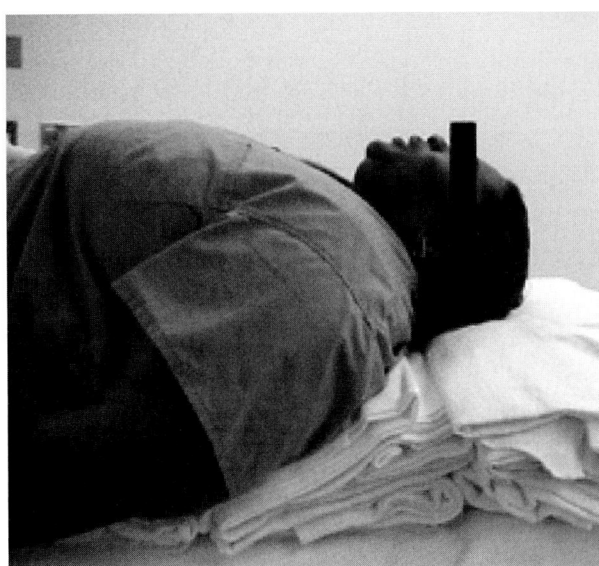

FIGURE 22-17. A. With the morbidly obese patient, a 10-cm pillow may not provide a position adequate for laryngoscopy. B. A wedge-shaped lift is used to move the mass of the morbidly obese patient's chest away from the area of laryngoscopy and to improve the compliance of the thoracic cavity.

side of their length, which is used to sweep the tongue to the left side of the mouth. Blades with a right-side flange are available for the left-handed practitioner, but they are not commonly found in practice.

Historically, choice of laryngoscopic blade had a theoretical bases in airway innervation. The internal branch of the superior laryngeal nerve (a branch of the vagus) provides sensory innervation from the level of the vocal cords to the underside of the epiglottis. Stimulation of these structures (with the Miller blade) was believed to cause more vagally related reactions (laryngospasm, bradycardia, hypertension.) The vallecula, stimulated by the curved, Macintosh blade, is innervated by the glossopharyngeal nerve.

In most available systems the flange incorporates the light source, either a bulb placed near the distal blade aspect or a rigid fiberoptic cable that transmits light produced within the handle. In either case, these blades must be long enough to achieve their respective applications. Therefore, blade size needs to be chosen appropriately and, on occasion, exchanged after a failed attempt. As a generalization, the Macintosh blade is regarded as advantageous whenever there is little room to pass an endotracheal tube (e.g., small mouth), whereas the Miller blade is considered better in the patient who has a small mandibular space, large incisor teeth or a large epiglottis.[127] The straight-against-the tongue nature of the Miller blade affords maximal transfer of effort from the operator's elbow and shoulder to the displacement of the tongue into a small mandibular space.

With the left hand holding the laryngoscope handle, the blade is inserted into the right side of the mouth, with care taken not to compress the upper lip against the teeth. As the blade is advanced toward the epiglottis, it is swept leftward, using the flange to displace the tongue to the left as the blade compresses it into the mandibular space. Once reaching the base of the tongue (the Macintosh blade tip in the vallecula, or the Miller blade compressing the epiglottis against the base of

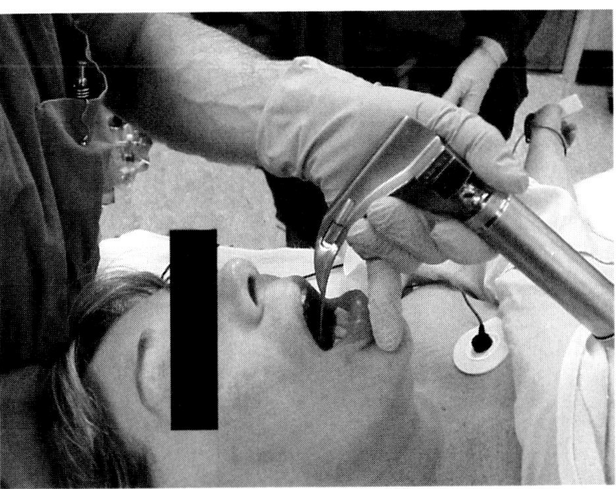
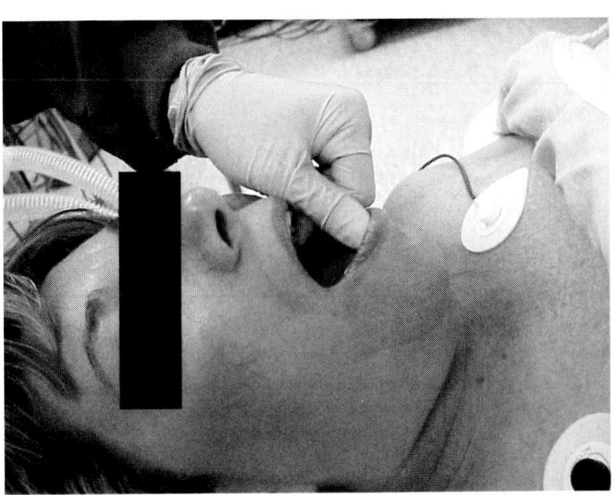

FIGURE 22-18. Techniques of opening the mouth in preparation for laryngoscopy. A. Hyperextension of the atlanto-occipital joint and use of the fifth finger of the dominant hand. B. The thumb–first finger "scissors" technique.

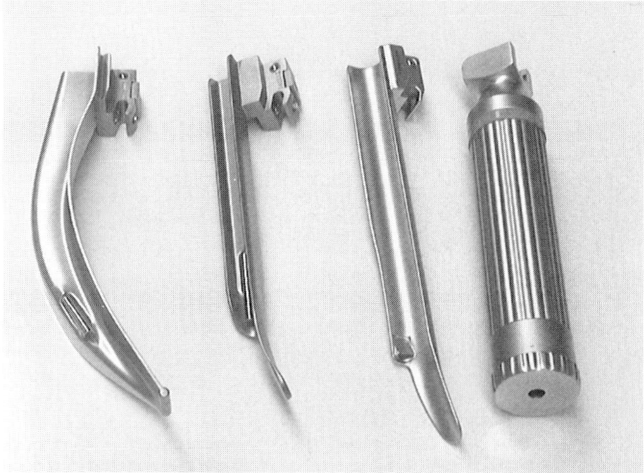

FIGURE 22-19. Macintosh, Miller, and Henderson laryngoscope blades with small and regular-sized handles.

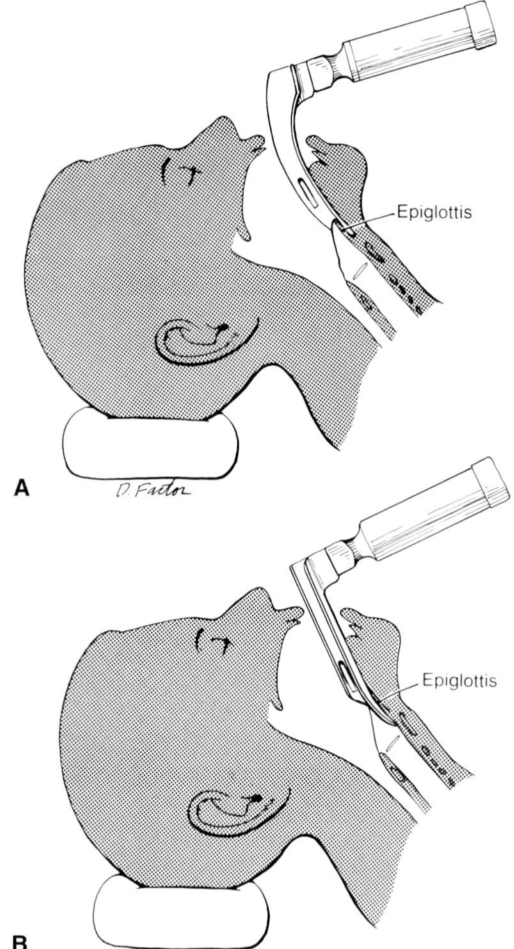

FIGURE 22-20. A. When a curved laryngoscope blade is used, the tip of the blade is placed in the vallecula, the space between the base of the tongue and the pharyngeal surface of the epiglottis. B. The tip of a straight blade is advanced beneath the epiglottis.

the tongue), the operator's arm and shoulder lift in an anterior and caudad direction (Fig. 22-20).

Importantly, the laryngoscopist must strive to avoid rotating the wrist and laryngoscope handle in a cephalad direction, bringing the blade against the upper incisor teeth. Extending either blade style too deeply can bring the tip of the blade to rest under the larynx itself, so that forward pressure lifts the entire airway from view (Fig. 22-21).

Special considerations apply to the technique of laryngoscopy and intubation in the infant and child. Because of the relatively larger size of the occiput in children, producing an anatomic sniffing position, elevation of the head (as done in the adult) is not needed.[128] On occasion, one may need to elevate the thorax instead. The relatively short neck gives the impression of an anterior position of the larynx. Posterior cricoid pressure is often required to place the laryngeal inlet into view. A straight blade is more helpful in displacing the stiff, omega-shaped, and high epiglottis. Since the cricoid cartilage is the narrowest aspect of the airway until 6 to 8 years of age, the intubator must be sensitive to resistance to advancement of the ETT that has easily passed the vocal folds. Hyperextension at the atlanto-occipital joint, as done in adult, may cause airway obstruction because of the relative pliability of the trachea. In the child, there is a higher risk of endobronchial intubation or extubation with head movement owing to the short length of the trachea.

With laryngoscopy, the view of the larynx may be complete, partial, or impossible. A laryngeal view scoring system that has won general acceptance was developed by Cormack and Lehane, who described four grades of laryngeal view.[125] Grade 1 includes visualization of the entire glottic aperture; Grade 2 includes visualization of only the posterior aspects of the glottic aperture; Grade 3 is visualization of the tip of the epiglottis; Grade 4 is visualization of no more than the soft palate (Fig. 22-22). A Cormach–Lehane Grade 3 or 4 is expected in 1.5 to 8.5% of adult laryngoscopies.[129]

This system has proved useful not only as a means of recording the laryngeal view on individual patients, but also as a clinical end point in the evaluation of preoperative airway assessment tools. A modification of the Cormack and Lehane score (MCLS) has been proposed by Koh et al, who noted that partial vocal cord view (MCLS 2A) was significantly easier to intubate than when only the artynoids and epiglottis were seen (MCLS 2B).[130]

Once the larynx is visualized with a left side–flanged blade, the tracheal tube is inserted from the right-hand side, care being taken not to obstruct the view of the vocal folds. Whenever possible, the action of the endotracheal tube passing through the vocal folds should be witnessed by the laryngoscopist. The tracheal tube should be inserted to a depth of at least 2 cm after the disappearance of the tracheal tube cuff past the vocal folds to approximate placement in the midtrachea. This should present the 21-cm and 23-cm external markings at the teeth for the typical adult female and male, respectively.[131] Choice of adult tracheal tube size may be made by the generalization that for women, size 7 to 8 id (internal diameter) may be used, and for a man, size 8 to 9 id. The larger tracheal tubes may be desirable if pulmonary toilet or diagnostic or therapeutic bronchoscopy is to be part of the clinical course. Pediatric laryngoscope blades and tracheal tube sizes are discussed in detail elsewhere in this chapter (Table 22-10).

An alternative approach to direct laryngoscopy has been described by Henderson.[132] In this approach to tongue displacement, a straight-bladed laryngoscope is introduced into the right side of the mouth. The blade is advanced between the tongue and palastine tonsil. The blade passes below the epiglottis, which is then elevated. This approach subjects the tongue to less compressive forces. It has been suggested that this technique may improve the view of the larynx in the presence of linguar tonsil hyperplasia (see Fig. 22-19).

Verification of successful tracheal tube placement is made by a variety of methods. The gold standard for confirmation

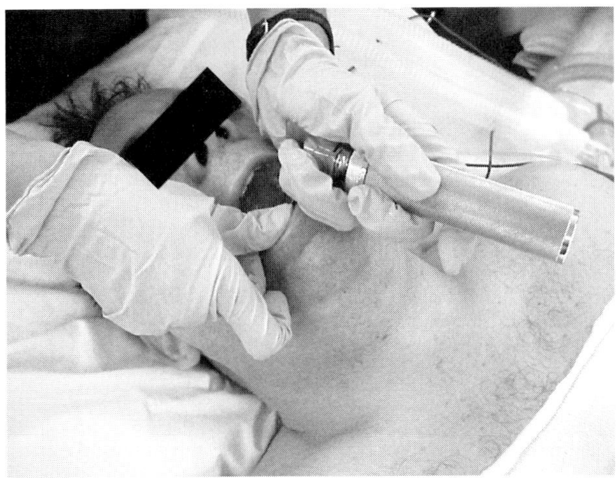

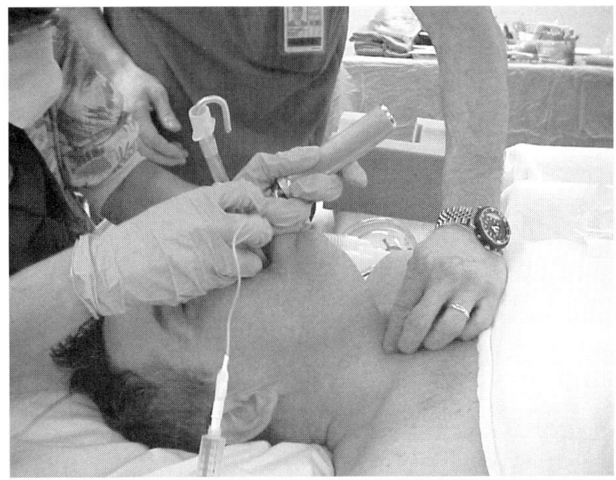

A B

FIGURE 22-21. The sequence of routine laryngoscopy. **A.** With the mouth maximally opened, the laryngoscope is held in the left hand and the blade inserted on the right side of the mouth. Using the blade flange, the tongue is swept to the left as the wrist pulls in a caudad direction. **B.** While visualizing the laryngeal inlet, the tracheal tube is inserted.

of placement includes visualization of placement through the vocal folds and sustained detection of exhaled carbon dioxide as measured with capnography or a disposable chemical colorimetric device such as the Easy Cap II (Mallinckrodt). Other portable techniques include auscultation over the chest and abdomen, visualization of the chest excursion, observation of condensation in the ETT, use of a self-inflating bulb (Tubechek-B, Ambu, Linthicum, MD), lighted stylets (Trachlight, Laerdal Medical, Armonk, NY; SURCH-LITE, Aaron Medical Industries, St. Petersburg, FL), fiberoptic bronchoscope (FOB) identification of the tracheal rings, or chest x-ray.[132,133]

NPO Status and the Rapid-Sequence Induction. Induction of anesthesia in patients who have "full stomachs" or incompetent gastroesophageal sphincters can result in regurgitation and pulmonary aspiration. Individuals at risk include the morbidly obese, pregnant women, diabetics with gastroparesis, those who require emergency operations, patients with gastroesophageal reflux disease, and patients who have recently eaten. Individuals experiencing emotional stress have increased gastric acid secretions and are also at an increased risk for aspiration.[134] A complete discussion of the pharmacologic therapy for aspiration prophylaxis is available elsewhere in this text.

The technique of rapid-sequence induction is performed to gain control of the airway in the least amount of time after the ablation of protective airway reflexes with the induction of anesthesia. In the rapid-sequence technique, the administration of an intravenous anesthetic induction agent is immediately followed by a rapidly acting neuromuscular blocking drug. Direct laryngoscopy and intubation are performed as soon as muscle relaxation is confirmed. Cricoid pressure (Sellick's maneuver) is applied by an assistant from the beginning of induction until confirmation of endotracheal tube placement. Cricoid pressure entails the downward displacement of the cricoid cartilage against the vertebral bodies (Fig. 22-22). In this manner, the lumen of the esophagus is ablated, while the completely circular nature of the cricoid cartilage maintains the tracheal lumen. Early cadaveric studies showed that correctly applied cricoid pressure was effective in preventing gastric fluids, under 100 cm H_2O pressure, from leaking into the pharynx. Unfortunately, the esophagus is laterally displaced in a majority of normal patients.[135] Because cricoid pressure further lateralizes the esophagus, the adequacy of esophageal abalation has been questioned. Cricoid pressure is contraindicated with active vomiting (risk of esophageal rupture), cervical spine fracture, and laryngeal fracture. Historically, facemask ventilation is not undertaken for the 40 to 90 seconds of time required to achieve adequate neuromuscular relaxation. This practice is based on minimal data and has recently been questioned.

If during rapid-sequence induction there are difficulties in securing the airway and oxyhemoglobin desaturation occurs, gentle positive-pressure ventilation may be used while maintaining cricoid pressure. This positive pressure should require <25 cm H_2O pressure. If more positive pressure is used, there is a risk of gastric distention and regurgitation.

The Intubating Laryngeal Mask Airway (LMA-Fastrach). Blind, fiberoptic aided, stylet-guided, and laryngoscopy-directed intubation via the LMA has been widely reported in adults and children.[79,136–142] There are several limitations to this procedure including the maximal size ETT that can be used, the minimal length of the ETT required to ensure that its cuff is within the larynx and not wedged between or above the vocal folds, and the difficulty in removing the LMA after intubation.[79,143] In an effort to overcome these limitations, Brain introduced a version of the LMA with a large-diameter (13 mm id), short-length (14 cm) rigid stainless steel barrel curved to align the mask aperture to the glottic vestibule (Fig. 22-24).[144–146]

The mask incorporates a vertically oriented semirigid bar, fixed at the proximal end of the bowl aperture and positioned to sit beneath the epiglottis in the average adult. A handle at the proximal end of the barrel is used for insertion, repositioning, and removal. A secondary advantage of the handle is that the operator need never place fingers into the patient's mouth. This device, the LMA-Fastrach, can accommodate up to an 8.0-mm id cuffed ETT, which can be inserted blindly or over a fiberscope or other stylet device. The LMA-Fastrach is designed to be used with a straight, armored, silicone tracheal tube (Euromedics, Malaysia), although standard or Parker Flex-tip (Parker Medical, Englewood, Colorado) polyvinyl chloride tracheal tubes have been used.[147] To date, the LMA-Fastrach has been distributed in adult sizes with cuffs equivalent to the size 3, 4, and 5 LMAs. Experience has suggested that most adults between 40 and 70 kg are best managed with a size 4 LMA-Fastrach, larger persons requiring the size 5. Pediatric sizes are not yet available.

The LMA-Fastrach is indicated for routine, elective intubation and for anticipated and unanticipated difficult intubation.

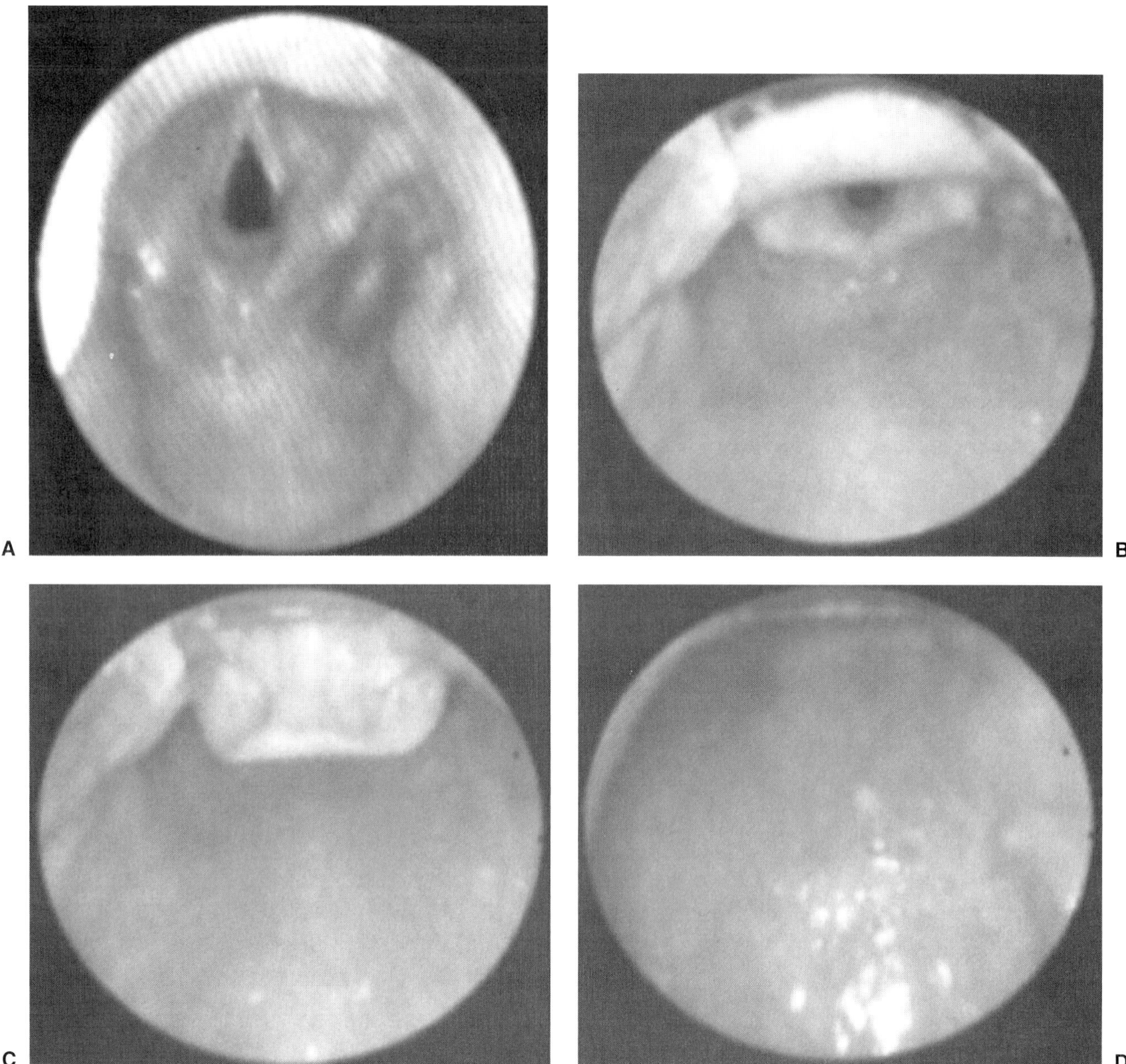

FIGURE 22-22. The Cormack–Lehane laryngeal view scoring system: (A) Grade 1, (B) Grade 2, (C) Grade 3, (D) Grade 4.

Since it was designed to facilitate blind tracheal intubation, the presence of airway secretions, blood, or edema (e.g., from previous intubation attempts or trauma) does not interfere with its use. Because the design of the barrel is based on the normal adult palate-to-glottis relationship, patients who are evaluated as being manageable with tracheal intubation based on external exam, but subsequently are found to have a high Cormack–Lehane score (because of lingual tonsil hyperplasia or cervical spine immobility, for example) should be successfully managed with the LMA-Fastrach.[125] In the largest trial of the LMA-Fastrach to date, ventilation was satisfactory in 95% and unsatisfactory in 1% of 500 uses, and 96% were intubated within three attempts (79.8% on first, 12.4% on second, 4% on third).[148] Patients who are assessed as grossly abnormal on preoperative airway exam may often still be managed with the LMA-Fastrach.[149] The LMA-Fastrach has been demonstrated to be useful as a ventilatory and intubating device after failed rapid sequence intubation.[147]

A large study has shown the utility of the LMA-Fastrach in anticipated as well as unanticipated difficult to intubate patients. Ferson et al successfully intubated 234 patients over a 3-year period using the LMA-Fastrach.[150] Studied patients included those with normal-appearing airways on routine exam who were unexpectedly difficult to manage, patients with a Cormack and Lehane laryngeal view grade 4 on laryngoscopy, patients with immobilized or traumatized cervical spines and patients with airway tumors, prior airway surgery, or radiation. Successful blind intubation via the LMA-Fastrach occurred in 96.99%, the remaining ones facilitated with supplemental use of a fiberoptic intubation scope. [A new design of the LMA-Fastrach, the C-Trach, introduced in 2004 incorporates a fiberoptic cable and miniaturized monitor into the LMA-Fastrach design (Fig 22-24C)].

Notably in this series all patients who presented with a cannot intubate/cannot ventilate situation were successfully ventilated and intubated with the LMA-Fastrach, emphasizing its

TABLE 22-10

SIZE AND LENGTH OF TRACHEAL TUBES RELATIVE TO AIRWAY ANATOMY

AGE	INTERNAL DIAMETER (mm)	DISTANCE FROM LIPS TO MIDTRACHEA[a] (cm)	DIAMETER OF TRACHEA (mm)	LENGTH OF TRACHEA (cm)	DISTANCE FROM LIPS TO CARINA (cm)
Premature	2.5	8			
Full term	3.0	10			
1–6 mo	3.5	11	5	6	13
6–12 mo	4.0	12			
2 yr	4.5	13			
4 yr	5.0	14			
6 yr	5.5	15			
8 yr	6.5	16	8	8	18
10 yr	7.0	17–18			
12 yr	7.5	18–20			
14 yr	8.0–9.0	20–22	20[b] 15[c]	14[b] 12[c]	28[b] 24[c]

[a]Add 2–3 cm for nasal tubes.
[b]Males.
[c]Females.

importance in the cannot intubate/cannot mask ventilate and emergency pathways of the ASA Difficult Airway Algorithm.[113]

Contraindications to the LMA-Fastrach are similar to those of the LMA. Since the end point of LMA-Fastrach procedure is tracheal intubation, it may prove useful for the management of patients at moderate risk for gastroesophageal regurgitation and aspiration, or for high-risk patients on whom other techniques have failed.

The LMA-Fastrach is inserted with the head in a neutral position. It can be used in the unconscious or awake patient (with the use of topical anesthetics). The mask of the LMA-Fastrach is tested, deflated, and lubricated as described for the LMA. It is inserted into the mouth, with the handle held parallel to the chest, so the mask lies flat against the palate. Gentle pressure on the handle and barrel, toward the chin, reproduces the palatal pressure described for insertion of the LMA. A smooth backward rotation of the handle toward the top of the head seats the tip of the mask in the hypopharynx, posterior to the cricoid cartilage. Once seated, the LMA-Fastrach's mask is inflated via the pilot cuff. An ambu bag or anesthesia circuit is attached to the proximal end of the LMA-Fastrach barrel

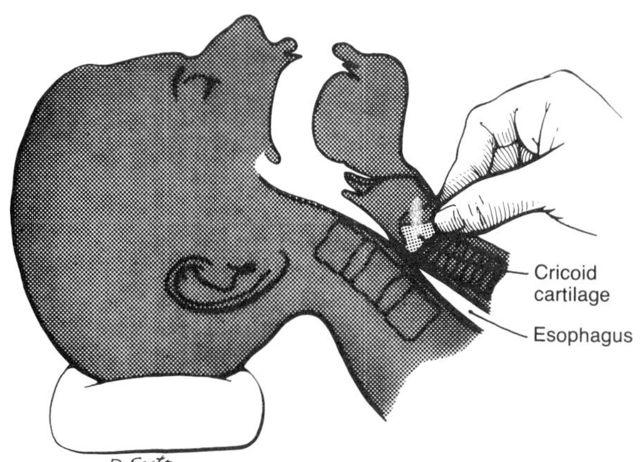

FIGURE 22-23. Cricoid pressure (Sellick's maneuver) is applied to occlude the esophagus and prevent aspiration of gastric contents.

and ventilation is attempted. By using the LMA-Fastrach handle, the position of the device can be optimized by lateral and anterior–posterior manipulation. This is termed the Chandy Maneuver (after Dr. Chandy Verghese, United Kingdom). A seemingly common cause of airway obstruction is the down-folding of the epiglottis. This can be relieved with a smooth rotational movement of the inflated LMA-Fastrach out of the airway (6 cm along the axis of the insertion) while the cuff remains inflated, and immediate re-placement (the "up-down" maneuver).

After adequate ventilation is achieved, the ETT is advanced through the barrel. As the ETT exits the bowl aperture of the LMA-Fastrach, the semirigid elevating bar is pushed anteriorly, carrying the epiglottis out of the way of the airway. If positioned correctly, the ETT can freely enter the glottis.

The second part of the Chandy Maneuver may facilitate blind tracheal intubation. In this maneuver the handle is used to gently lift (without rotation) the LMA-Fastrach anteriorly, sealing the bowl against the larynx.

When blind intubation fails (esophageal insertion or obstruction) several maneuvers are undertaken.[150] Early obstruction is typically a result of a down-folded epiglottis. An up-down maneuver, as described earlier, can be employed and tracheal intubation attempts repeated. Early resistance (within 1 cm of the Euromedics ETT exit mark) may also signify vallecular entrapment secondary to too large an LMA-Fastrach. The operator may remove the LMA-Fastrach and place a smaller size. Obstruction at 3 cm past the exit mark may signify entrapment or too small a device, and again, a change is indicated.

When intubation fails despite the Chandy or up-down maneuvers, or a change in the ILM size, the clinician should recall that the LMA-Fastrach is a ventilation device first! Typically ventilation will be adequate despite failure to intubate. At this juncture the clinician can (1) continue with short surgical procedures using the LMA-Fastrach as a simple SGA (procedures longer than 15 minutes may be ill advised because of the pressure excited by the LMA-Fastrach on tissues), (2) change to another LMA device, (3) diagnose the intubation impediment with the aid of another device (e.g., fiberoptic bronchoscope or FAST (Clarus Medical), (4) remove the LMA-Fastrach and continue with DL, or an another technique of tracheal intubation, or (5) in the resuscitative situation, perform a surgical airway while continuing ventilation with the LMA-Fastrach.

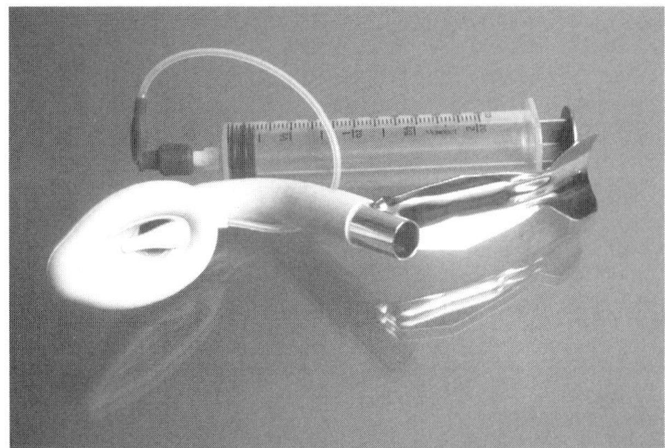

A

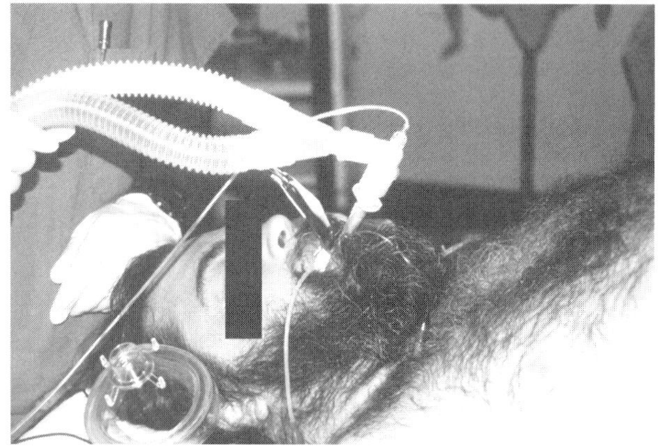

B

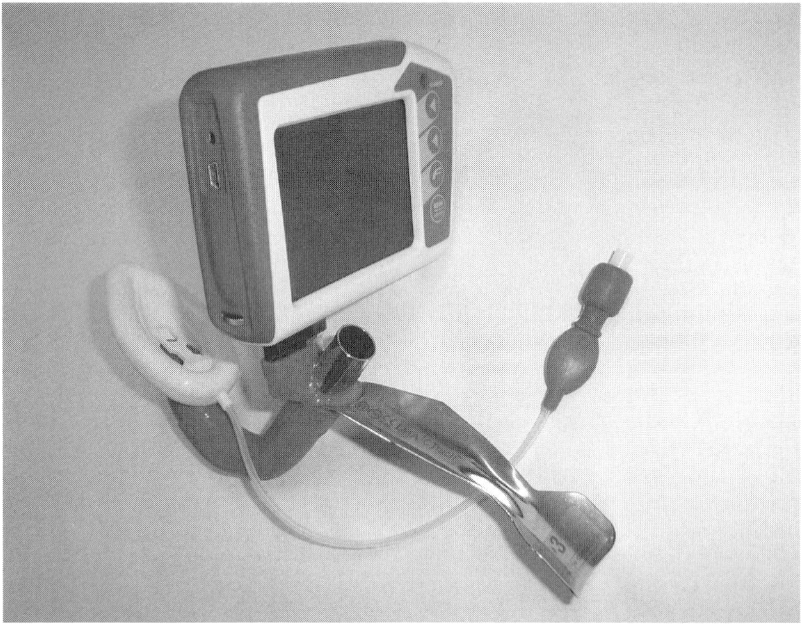

C

FIGURE 22-24. A. The LMA-Fastrach. B. The LMA-Fastrach used for intubation in a patient outside the operating room. C. The LMA C-Trach.

This last procedure may be an underappreciated facility of all LMAs and the SGAs. These devices may serve as a bridge while invasive airway procedures are performed.

Once intubation is achieved and confirmed (e.g., by auscultation or capnography), the ETT circuit adapter is removed and the LMA-Fastrach is withdrawn over the ETT. During this removal procedure, the ETT is stabilized by one of two methods. A silicone stabilizing rod (supplied by the manufacturer) can be held against the ETT as the LMA-Fastrach is retreated out of the mouth. The advantage of this technique is that the operator's hands do not have to enter the oral cavity. The disadvantage is that in the midremoval position, the operator loses direct contact with the ETT. In the second technique, described by Rosenblatt and Murphy, a Magill forceps is used to hold the proximal tip of the ETT while the LMA-Fastrach is removed.[147] In the midremoval position, a finger is placed in the mouth to identify and stabilize the ETT, while the Magill forceps is removed and the LMA-Fastrach is fully retreated. This technique requires the hand to be placed in the mouth, but allows improved control of the ETT.

Extubation of the Trachea

Though a wealth of literature is focused on the field of tracheal intubation, few reviews have well contemplated the area of extubation after completion of surgery, or prolonged ventilatory support.[151] Indeed, the period of extubation may be far more treacherous than that of intubation (Table 22-11 [see section A]).

11 **Routine Extubation.** Extubation of the trachea must not be considered a benign procedure. It is not simply the elimination or reversal of tracheal intubation. Extubation is fraught with its own set of potential complications (Table 22-11 [see section B]). Appropriately trained personnel and equipment should be immediately available at the time of extubation. This may range from a postanesthetic care unit nurse or respiratory therapist with a set of laryngoscopes to a surgeon prepared to perform an emergency tracheostomy.

Most adult patients are extubated after the return of consciousness and spontaneous respiration, the resolution of neuromuscular block, and the ability to follow simple commands (Table 22-12). The patient is asked to open the mouth and a suction catheter is used to remove excessive secretions and/or blood. The airway pressure is allowed to rise to 5 to 15 cm of H_2O to allow for a "passive cough," and the endotracheal tube is removed after the cuff (if present) is deflated.[151] If coughing or straining is contraindicated or hazardous (e.g., increased intracranial pressure), extubation may be performed while the patient is in a surgical plane of anesthesia. In patients at risk for gastric contents aspiration (e.g., full stomach) or upper

TABLE 22-11

TRACHEAL EXTUBATION

A. Causes of Ventilatory Compromise during Tracheal Extubation
- Residual anesthetic
- Poor central respiratory effort
- Decreased respiratory rate
- Decreased respiratory drive in response to CO_2
- Decreased respiratory drive in response to O_2
- Reduced tone of upper airway musculature
- Reduced gag and swallow reflex
- Decreased threshold to laryngospasm
- Surgical airway compromise
- Surgical airway edema
- Vocal cord paralysis
- Arytenoid cartilage dislocation
- Supraglottic edema with airway obstruction by the epiglottis
- Retroarytenoid edema with limited vocal fold abduction
- Subglottic edema
- Tracheomalacia (from long-standing tracheal intubation)
- Bronchospasm

B. Complications of Tracheal Extubation
- Respiratory drive failure
- Hypoxia (e.g., atelectasis)
- Upper airway obstruction (e.g., edema, residual anesthetic)
- Vocal fold–related obstruction (e.g., vocal cord paralysis)
- Tracheal obstruction (e.g., subglottic edema)
- Bronchospasm
- Aspiration
- Hypertension
- Increased intracranial pressure
- Increased pulmonary artery pressure
- Increased bronchial stump pressure (e.g., after pulmonary resection)
- Increased ocular pressure
- Increased abdominal wall pressure (e.g., risk of wound dehiscence)

TABLE 22-12

CRITERIA FOR ROUTINE "AWAKE" EXTUBATION

Subjective Clinical Criteria:
- Follows commands
- Clear oropharynx/hypopharynx (e.g., no active bleeding, secretions cleared)
- Intact gag reflex
- Sustained head lift for 5 seconds, sustained hand grasp
- Adequate pain control
- Minimal end-expiratory concentration of inhaled anesthetics

Objective Criteria:
- Vital capacity: $\geq$10 mL/kg
- Peak voluntary negative inspiratory pressure: >20 cm H_2O
- Tidal volume >6 cc/kg
- Sustained tetanic contraction (5 sec)
- T_1/T_4 ratio >0.7
- Alveolar-Arterial PaO_2 gradient (on FIO_2 of 1.0): <350 mm Hg[a]
- Dead space to tidal volume ratio: $\leq$0.6[a]

[a]Used during weaning from mechanical ventilation in the intensive care setting.

airway obstruction, the clinician needs to assess the relative risk of each potential morbidity. For the latter risk, and possibly the former, a maneuver has been described in which an LMA is placed posterior to the ETT, which is then removed. This obviates the problem of upper airway obstruction, and may offer some protection against regurgitation and aspiration.[152–154] Because of the risks of atelectasis and diffusion hypoxia, the ability to administer oxygen should be available at the time of extubation.

Difficult Extubation. The patient who presented as a difficult airway at the time of anesthetic induction must be considered a difficult airway at the time of extubation, even when corrective surgery was performed in the interim (e.g., uvulopharyngoplasty in the obstructive sleep apnea patient).

As a cause of ventilatory compromise, laryngospasm deserves special attention because of it prevalence in children and because it accounts for 23% of all critical postoperative respiratory events in adults.[151] Laryngospasm may be triggered by respiratory secretions, vomitus, or blood in the airway; pain in any part of the body; and pelvic or abdominal visceral stimulation. The cause of airway obstruction during laryngospasm is the contraction of the lateral cricoarytenoids, the thyroarytenoid, and the cricothyroid muscles. Management of laryngospasm consists of the immediate removal of the offending stimulus (if identifiable), administration of oxygen with continuous positive airway pressure, and, if other maneuvers are unsuccessful, the use of a small dose of short-acting muscle relaxants.[151]

Negative-pressure pulmonary edema may result from any airway obstruction in a patient who continues to have a voluntary respiratory effort. Negative intrathoracic pressure is transmitted to the alveoli, which are unable to expand owing to the more proximal obstruction. Fluid is entrained from the pulmonary capillary bed. Negative-pressure pulmonary edema is treated as any other form of noncardiogenic edema.

Identification of patients at risk at extubation. A number of well known clinical situations may place patients at increased risk for complication at the time of extubation. Table 22-13 lists the risk factors for extubation complications. However, the clinician should evaluate every patient in terms of potential problems, in the same manner that they are prepared for the unanticipated difficult intubation.

Approach to the difficult extubation. When there is a suspicion that a patient may have difficulty with oxygenation or ventilation after tracheal extubation, the clinician may choose from a number of management strategies. These may range from the preparation of standby reintubation equipment to the active establishment of a route or guide for reintubation and/or oxygenation. When the patient's intubation is without difficulty and there is no substantial reason to believe that an interim insult to the airway has occurred, extubation may be accomplished in a routine fashion, with a heightened state of readiness for reintubation. When there has been difficulty with intubation or there is a clinical suspicion that reintubation will be difficult, extubation over a guiding stylet may be a successful technique. Any number of devices can be used as a stylet (Table 22-14).

A popular test to predict airway patency after extubation is the detection of a leak on deflation of the ETT cuff. A recent investigation has cast doubt on the reliability of this test as a predictor of airway incompetence: though the absence of an airway leak on cuff deflation was not predictive of subsequent ventilatory failure after extubation, no patient with a positive leak test (leak around the ETT cuff) developed problems after extubation.[155]

Another technique may be the use of an FOB to view the tracheal structures during the removal of the ETT. If extubation is tolerated, the FOB can be slowly withdrawn into the subglottic region. If secretions do not obstruct the objective lens, the vocal folds and other structures may be visualized and evaluated.

A number of obturators are available for use in trial extubation (where they may be left in place in the airway for extended periods) or endotracheal tube exchange (e.g., failure of the ETT cuff).[156] It is beyond the scope of this text to

TABLE 22-13

CLINICAL SITUATIONS PRESENTING INCREASED RISK FOR COMPLICATIONS AT EXTUBATION[151]

Paradoxical vocal cord motion (preexisting)	Poorly understood mechanism
Thyroid surgery	4.3% recurrent laryngeal nerve injury Local edema Tracheomalacia (from long-standing goiter)
Laryngoscopy (diagnostic)	Edema, laryngospasm, especially with biopsy
Uvulopalatoplasty	Palatal and oropharyngeal edema
Obstructive sleep apnea syndrome (uncorrected)	
Carotid endarterectomy	Wound hematoma, glottic edema, nerve palsies
Maxillofacial trauma	Laryngeal fracture Reduced level of consciousness Requirements for mandibular/maxillary wires
Cervical vertebrae decompression	Supraglottic and hypopharyngeal edema
Parkinson's disease	
Rheumatoid arthritis	
Generalized edema	Laryngotracheal narrowing
Angioneurotic edema	Laryngotracheal narrowing
Anaphylaxis	Laryngotracheal narrowing
Hypopharyngeal infections	Laryngotracheal narrowing
Hypoventilation syndromes[a]	
Hypoxemic syndromes[b]	
Inadequate airway protective reflexes	Aspiration risk

[a]Residual anesthetic or preoperative medications (including alcohol and illicit drugs), central sleep apnea, carotid endarterectomy, poliomyelitis, Guillain-Barré syndrome, myasthenia gravis, botulism, thoracic skeletal deformity, severe pain (with diaphragmatic splinting), morbid obesity, severe chronic obstructive pulmonary disease.
[b]Hypoventilation, ventilation–perfusion mismatch, intracardiac or intrapulmonary shunting, increased oxygen consumption, severe anemia, impaired alveolar oxygen diffusion.

describe all the commercially available catheters. The Cook Airway Exchange Catheters (Cook Critical Care, Bloomington, IN) are manufactured with external diameters of 2.7, 3.7, 4.7, and 6.33 mm (Fig. 22-25A). The smallest diameter catheter (which can fit within a 3.0-mm id ETT) is 45 cm long, whereas the others are 83 cm in length. They all have a central lumen and rounded, atraumatic ends. The catheters are graduated from the distal end. The proximal end is fitted with either a 15-mm or a Luer-lock Rapi-Fit adapter, which can be quickly removed and replaced for ETT removal or change. With these adapters an oxygen source can be used to provide insufflated or jet-ventilated oxygen if the patient fails extubation and/or if reintubation over the catheter fails.

The Cardiomed endotracheal ventilation catheter (Gromley, Ontario, Canada) designed by Richard Cooper, MD, a Canadian anesthesiologist, is 85 cm in length, and has inner and outer diameters of 3 and 4 mm, respectively. An integral Luer-lock fitting adapter is found at the proximal end, whereas the blunted distal end incorporates eight helically arranged side holes in addition to the distal end hole (Fig. 22-25B). The arrangement of these holes is meant to center the catheter during oxygen insufflation, and prevent traumatic "whipping" within the trachea. The use of this catheter for ETT exchange, tracheal reintubation, oxygen insufflation, jet ventilation, and end-tidal CO_2 detection after extubation has been documented by the inventor.[151]

THE DIFFICULT AIRWAY

The Difficult Airway Algorithm

In 1993, the ASA's Task Force on the Difficult Airway first published an algorithm that has become a staple of management for clinicians. This algorithm was reissued in 2003.[113,157] The

TABLE 22-14

DEVICES USED AS EXTUBATING STYLETS

DEVICE	ADVANTAGE	DISADVANTAGE
Fiberoptic bronchoscope	Visualize structures Oxygen can be insufflated through working channel	ETT cannot be exchanged
Eschmann catheter or similar device	Inexpensive, semirigid	Cannot visualize or oxygenate
Exchange/ventilatory catheter	Oxygen can be insufflated through central lumen	Cannot visualize, may be too flexible

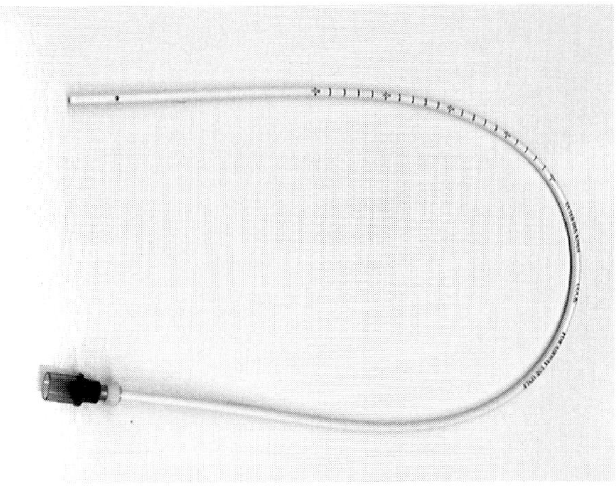

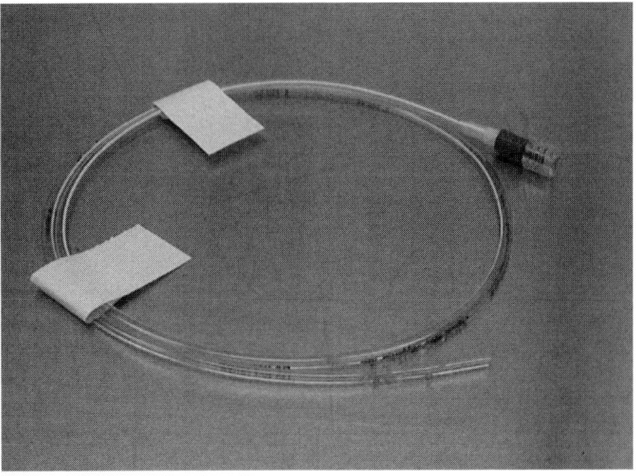

FIGURE 22-25. **A.** The Cook airway exchange catheter fitted with a Rapifit Luer-lock adapter (Cook Critical Care, Bloomington, IN). A 15-mm Rapifit adapter for attachment to an anesthesia circuit or ambu bag is also available. **B.** The Cardiomed endotracheal ventilation catheter.

most dramatic change in the ASA Difficult Airway Algorithm
2 (ASA-DAA) was the repositioning of the LMA from the emer-
3 gency to the routine management pathway (Fig. 22-26). The ASA defines the difficult airway as the situation in which the "conventionally trained anesthesiologist experiences difficulty with mask ventilation or both." Based on available data, the incidence of failed intubation is 0.05 to 0.35%, whereas the incidence of failed intubation/inability to perform mask ventilation is 0.01 to 0.03%.[158,159]

The ASA algorithm stands as a model for the approach to the difficult airway for nurse anesthetists, emergency medicine physicians, and prehospital personnel, as well as for anesthesiologists. Although the algorithm largely speaks for itself, its salient features are discussed here. One statement in this document summarizes the difficulty of writing and recommending practices in the difficult airway management: "The difficult airway represents a complex interaction between patient factors, the clinical setting and the skills of the practitioner."[113]

Entry into the algorithm begins with the evaluation of the airway. Although there is some debate as to the value of particular evaluation methods and indices, clinicians must use all available data and their own clinical experience to reach a general impression as to the difficulty of the patient's airway in terms of laryngoscopy and intubation, supraglottic ventilation techniques, aspiration risk, or apnea tolerance.

This evaluation should direct the clinician to enter the ASA algorithm at one of its two root points: A—awake intubation, or B—intubation attempts after the induction of general anesthesia (see Fig. 22-26). This highlights the misnomer of the algorithm: it is not only for difficult airways, but is relevant to

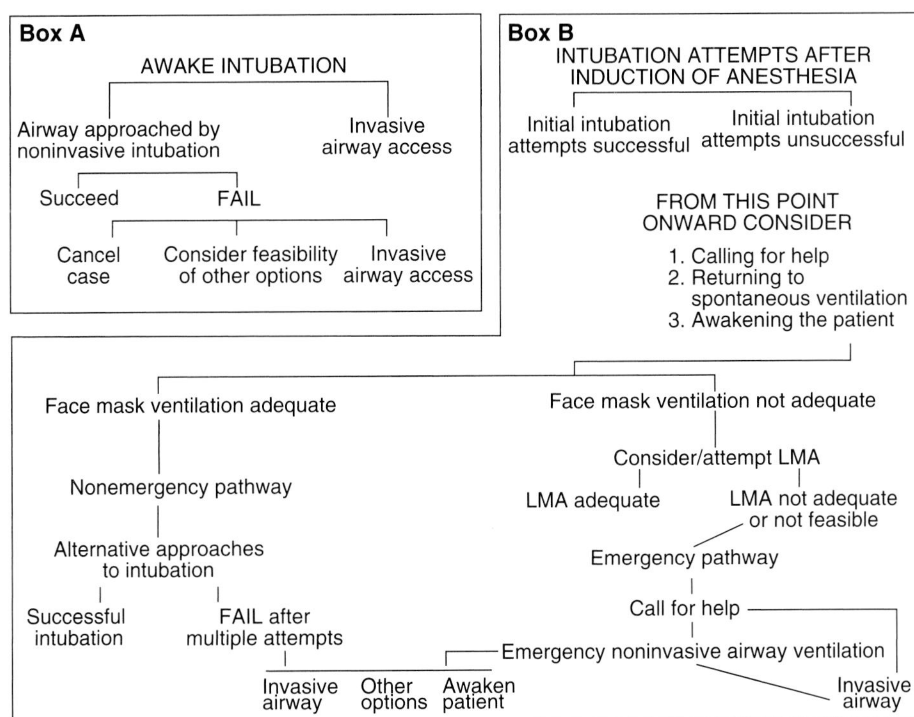

FIGURE 22-26. The American Society of Anesthesiologists Difficult Airway Algorithm. (Adapted from Practice guidelines for the management of the difficult airway: An updated report by the American Society of Anesthesiologists Task Force on Management of the Difficult Airway. Anesthesiology 98:1269, 2003.)

TABLE 22-15

FACTORS TO CONSIDER IN PROCEEDING WITH REGIONAL ANESTHESIA (RA) AFTER THE PATIENT HAS BEEN JUDGED TO HAVE A DIFFICULT AIRWAY

■ MAY CONSIDER RA	■ SHOULD NOT CONSIDER RA
Superficial surgery	Cavity-invading surgery
Minimal sedation needed	Significant sedation needed
Anesthetic may be provided with local infiltration	Extensive neuroaxial local anesthetic administration will be required, or risk of intravascular injection/absorption is high
Access to the airway is good	Access to the airway is poor
Surgery can be halted at any time	Surgery cannot be stopped once started

all instances where the airway is managed. Box B describes the approach taken in the majority of tracheal intubations (and is applicable to facemask– and SGA-managed patients). The decision to enter the algorithm via box A or B is a premanagement one. Box A is chosen when difficulty is anticipated, while box B is for the situation when no difficulty is anticipated. This decision can be refined in light of the proliferation of SGAs. Takenaka et al, have questioned the need to enter the ASA-DAA box A when SGAs are deemed usable despite an anticipated difficult tracheal intubation by DL.[160] This has been further delineated into a preoperative decision tree by Rosenblatt.[161] Figure 22-27 outlines the Airway Approach Algorithm (AAA), which is a simple, one-pathway algorithm for entering into the ASA-DAA. Branch choice, like the earlier-noted statement from the ASA practice guidelines, is highly dependent on the clinician's skill and experience. Details of the AAA can be found elsewhere and are summarized here:[161]

1. Is airway control necessary? No matter how routine sedation or general anesthesia become to potentially make a patient apneic, should always be considered seriously and alternatives should be considered.
2. Will DL be (at all) difficult? If there is no indication that DL will be difficult (based on physical exam and history), the clinician may proceed with any technique (induction, DL, LMA, etc.) as clinically appropriate. This is the essence of box B of the ASA-DAA.
3. Can SGA ventilation be used? If the clinician feels that there is a physical reason that SGA ventilation (by facemask, LMA, or other device) will be difficult, the juncture of possible "cannot intubate/cannot ventilate" (CNI/CNV) has been reached. Because this is a preoperative algorithm, box A of the ASA-DAA may be the root entry point.
4. Is there an aspiration risk? As discussed earlier, the patient at risk for aspiration is not a candidate for elective SGA use. A juncture of "cannot intubate/should not ventilate" has been reached and box A of the ASA-DAA is chosen.
5. Will the patient tolerate an apneic period? Question 3 from this list is difficult to answer and is highly dependent on the skills and experience of the clinician. Should intubation fail, and SGA ventilation not be adequate, the patient's ability to sustain oxygen saturation will dictate their ability to tolerate an apneic period. Factors such as age, obesity, pulmonary status, abnormal oxygen consumption (e.g., fever), and choice of induction agents will influence this. These factors have been discussed in detail elsewhere.[161] To illustrate the clinical application of the AAA, the path through this algorithm will be traced for the clinical scenarios at the end of this chapter.

The exception to the AAA is the patient who is unable to cooperate owing to mental retardation, intoxication, anxiety, depressed level of consciousness, or age. This patient may still enter box A, but awake intubation may need to be modified in favor of techniques which maintain spontaneous ventilation (e.g., inhalation induction).

Preparation of the patient for awake intubation is discussed later. In most instances, awake intubation is successful if approached with care and patience. When awake intubation fails, the clinician has a number of options. First, one can consider cancellation of the surgical case. In this situation, specialized equipment or personnel can be assembled for a return to the operating room. Where cancellation is not an option, regional anesthetic techniques can be considered, or, if demanded by the situation, a surgical airway (e.g., tracheostomy) may be called for.

The decision to proceed with regional anesthesia because the airway has been assessed or proven to be difficult to manage must be considered in terms of risks and benefits (Table 22-15). The ASA-DAA truly becomes useful in the unanticipated difficult airway (box B, unable to intubate by DL after the induction of anesthesia). When induction agents (with or without muscle relaxants) have been administered and the airway cannot be controlled, vital management decisions must be made rapidly. Typically, the clinician has attempted direct laryngoscopy and intubation after successful or failed anesthesia mask ventilation (unless a rapid-sequence induction is being performed). Even if the patient's oxygen saturation remains adequate throughout these efforts, the number of laryngoscopy attempts should be limited to three. As discussed earlier, significant soft tissue trauma can result from multiple laryngoscopies, thereby worsening the situation. First, mask ventilation should be instituted. If facemask ventilation is adequate, the ASA-DAA nonemergency pathway is entered. The clinician may then turn to the most convenient and/or appropriate technique for establishing tracheal intubation, if needed. This might include, but is not limited to, blind oral or nasal intubation; intubation facilitated by a fiberoptic bronchoscope, LMA, LMA-Fastrach, bougie, lighted stylet, or a retrograde wire; or a surgical airway. (The most widely applied of these procedures, as well as new techniques, is discussed within the clinical scenarios in a later section of this chapter.) When mask ventilation fails, the algorithm suggests supraglottic ventilation via any LMA. If successful, the nonemergency pathway of the ASA-DAA has again been entered and alternative techniques of tracheal intubation may be utilized, if needed (e.g., perhaps LMA ventilation is adequate for the clinical situation).

Should LMA ventilation fail to sustain the patient, the emergency pathway is entered. The ASA-DAA suggests use of an Esophageal-Tracheal Combitube, rigid bronchoscopy, transtracheal oxygenation, or a surgical airway.

At any juncture, the decision to awaken the patient should be considered based on the adequacy of ventilation, the risk of aspiration, and the risk of proceeding with intubation attempts or the surgical procedure.

The repositioning of the LMA within the algorithm (in its 2003 republication) was based on more than 12 years of clinical use in the United States (and more than 20 years' experience worldwide). Relatively few cases of LMA failure in the face of the CNI/CNV situation have been reported.[10,162–168] Three broad categories account for these failures: acute oral–pharyngeal angle, obstruction at the level of the hypopharynx, obstruction below the vocal folds. Conversely many cases of LMA rescue of the failed airway have been reported. Though control studies are lacking, Parmet et al noted that all cases of CNI/CNV (with the exception of an iatrogenic subglottic obstruction) occurring in a 2-year period in a single hospital were rescued with an LMA.[162]

Awake Airway Management

14 Awake airway management remains a mainstay of the ASA's Difficult Airway Algorithm. Awake intubation provides many advantages over the anesthetic state, including maintenance of spontaneous ventilation in the event that the airway cannot be secured rapidly, increased size and patency of the pharynx, relative forward placement of the base of the tongue, posterior placement of the larynx, and patency of the retropalatal space.[169,170] The effect of sedatives and general anesthetics on airway patency may be secondary to direct effects on motoneurons and on the reticular activating system.[171] The sleep apnea patient may be particularly prone to obstruction with minimal sedation. Additionally, the awake state confers some maintenance of upper and lower esophageal sphincter tone, thus reducing the risk of reflux. In the event that reflux occurs, the patient can close the glottis and/or expel aspirated foreign bodies by cough to the extent that these reflexes have not been obtunded by local anesthesia.[172] Lastly, patients at risk for neurologic sequelae (e.g., patients with unstable cervical spine pathology) may undergo sensory-motor monitoring after tracheal intubation. In an emergent situation, there may be cautions (e.g., cardiovascular stimulation in the presence of cardiac ischemia or ischemic risk, bronchospasm, increased intraocular pressure, increased intracranial pressure) but no absolute contraindications to awake intubation.[173] Contraindications to elective awake intubation include patient refusal or inability to cooperate (e.g., child, profound mental retardation, dementia, intoxication) or allergy to local anesthetics.

Once the clinician has decided to proceed with awake airway management, the patient must be prepared both physically and psychologically. Most adult patients will appreciate an explanation of the need for an awake airway exam and will be more cooperative once they realize the importance of, and rationale for any uncomfortable procedures. Once the airway has been prepared, patients will realize that they should experience no further discomfort during the intubation.

Apart from appropriate explanation, medication can also be used to allay anxiety. If sedatives are to be used, the clinician must keep in mind that producing obstruction or apnea in the difficult airway patient can be devastating and an overly sedated patient may not be able to protect the airway from regurgitated gastric contents, or cooperate with procedures. Small doses of benzodiazepines (diazepam, midazolam, lorazapam) are commonly used to alleviate anxiety without producing significant respiratory depression. These drugs may be given in iv or oral forms (when available) and may be reversed with specific antagonists (e.g., flumazenil). Opioid receptor agonists (e.g., fentanyl, alfentanil, remifentanil) can also be used in small, titrated doses for their sedative and antitussive effects, although caution must be exercised. A specific antagonist (e.g., naloxone) should always be immediately available. Ketamine and droperidol and the new agent, dexmetomodine, have also been popular among clinicians.

Administration of antisialagogues is important to the success of awake intubation techniques. As will be discussed below, clearing of airway secretions is essential to the use of indirect optical instruments (e.g., fiberoptic bronchoscope, rigid fiberoptic laryngoscope) because small amounts of any liquid can obscure the objective lens. The commonly used drugs atropine (0.5 to 1 mg im or iv) and glycopyrrolate (0.2 to 0.4 mg im or iv) have other significant effects: by reducing saliva production, these drugs increase the effectiveness of topically applied local anesthetics by removing a barrier to mucosal contact and reducing drug dilution. Vasoconstriction of the nasal passages is needed if there is to be instrumentation of this part of the airway. If the patient is at risk for gastric regurgitation and aspiration, prophylactic measures should be undertaken. It is also prudent to supply supplemental oxygen to the patient by nasal cannula (which can be placed over the nose or mouth).

Local anesthetics are a cornerstone of awake airway control techniques. The airway, from the base of the tongue to the bronchi, comprises an undeniably sensitive series of tissues. Topical anesthesia and injected nerve block techniques have been developed to blunt the protective airway reflexes as well as to provide analgesia. As is well known to the anesthetic practitioner, local anesthetics are both effective and potentially dangerous drugs. The clinician should have a thorough understanding of the mechanism of action, metabolism, toxicities, and acceptable cumulative doses of the drugs that he or she chooses to employ in the airway. Because much of the agent used will be within the tracheal–bronchial tree and will travel to the alveoli, there will be significant and rapid intravascular absorption.

Despite the availability of myriad local anesthetics, only those most commonly used in airway preparation will be discussed here.

Among otolaryngologists, cocaine is a popular topical agent. Not only is it a highly effective local anesthetic, but also it is the only local anesthetic that is a potent vasoconstrictor. It is commonly available in a 4% solution. The total dose applied to the mucosa should not exceed 200 mg in the adult. Cocaine should not be used in patients with a known cocaine hypersensitivity, hypertension, ischemic heart disease, preeclampsia, or those taking monoamine oxidase inhibitors.[174] Since cocaine is metabolized by pseudocholinesterase, it is contraindicated in patients deficient in this enzyme.

Lidocaine, an amide local anesthetic, is available in a wide variety of preparations and doses (Table 22-16). Topically applied, peak onset is within 15 minutes. Toxic plasma levels are not impossible to achieve but are not commonly reported in airway management.

Tetracaine is an amide local anesthetic with a longer duration of action than either cocaine or lidocaine. Solutions of 0.5%, 1%, and 2% are available. Absorption of this drug from the respiratory and GI tracts is rapid, and toxicity after nebulized application has been reported with doses as low as 40 mg, although the acceptable safe dose in adults is 100 mg.[175]

TABLE 22-16

AVAILABLE LIDOCAINE PREPARATIONS

PREPARATION	DOSES
Injectable/topical solution	1%, 2%, 4%
Viscous solution	1%, 2%
Ointment	1%, 5%
Aerosol	10%

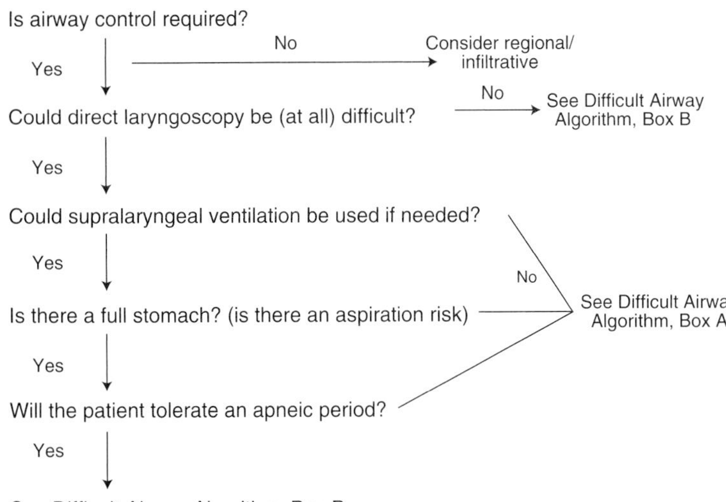
AIRWAY APPROACH ALGORITHM
Is airway control required?
Yes
No
Consider regional/ infiltrative
Could direct laryngoscopy be (at all) difficult?
No
See Difficult Airway Algorithm, Box B
Yes
Could supralaryngeal ventilation be used if needed?
Yes
No
Is there a full stomach? (is there an aspiration risk)
See Difficult Airway Algorithm, Box A
Yes
Will the patient tolerate an apneic period?
Yes
See Difficult Airway Algorithm, Box B

FIGURE 22-27. The Airway Approach Algorithm: A decision tree approach to entry into the American Society of Anesthesiologists Difficult Airway Algorithm (see Fig. 22-26). (From Rosenblatt W. The airway approach algorithm. J Clin Anesthesia 16:312, 2004.)

Benzocaine is popular among some clinicians because of its very rapid onset (<1 minute) and short duration (~10 minutes). It is available in 10%, 15%, and 20% solutions. It has been combined with tetracaine (Hurricaine®, Beutlich Pharmaceuticals) to prolong the duration of action. A 0.5-second aerosol administration of Hurricaine delivers 30 mg of benzocaine, the toxic dose being 100 mg. Another common preparation is Cetacaine spray, which combines benzocaine with tetracaine, butyl aminobenzoate, benzalkonium chloride, and cetyldimethylethyl ammonium bromide. Benzocaine may produce methemoglobinemia, which is treated by the administration of methylene blue.

There are three anatomic areas to which the clinician directs local anesthetic therapy: the nasal cavity/nasopharynx, the pharynx/base of tongue, and the hypopharynx/larynx/trachea. The nasal cavity is innervated by the greater and lesser palantine nerves (innervating the nasal turbinates and most of the nasal septum) and the anterior ethmoid nerve (innervating the nares and anterior third of the nasal septum). The two palantine nerves arise from the sphenopalantine ganglion, located posterior to the middle turbinate. Two techniques for nerve block have been described. The ganglion can be approached through a noninvasive nasal approach: cotton-tipped applicators soaked in local anesthetic are passed along the upper border of the middle turbinate until the posterior wall of the nasopharynx is reached. They are left in place for 5 to 10 minutes. In the oral approach, a needle is introduced into the greater palantine foramen, which can be palpated in the posterior lateral aspect of the hard palate, 1 cm medial to the second and third maxillary molars. Anesthetic solution (1 to 2 mL) is injected with a spinal needle inserted in a superior/posterior direction at a depth of 2 to 3 cm. Care must be taken not to inject into the sphenopalantine artery. The anterior ethmoid nerve can be blocked by cotton-tipped applicators soaked in local anesthetic placed along the dorsal surface of the nose until the anterior cribriform plate is reached. The applicator is left in place for 5 to 10 minutes.

The oropharynx is innervated by branches of the vagus, facial, and glossopharyngeal nerves. The glossopharyngeal nerve (GPN) travels anteriorly along the lateral surface of the pharynx, its three branches supplying sensory innervation to the posterior third of the tongue, the vallecula, the anterior surface of the epiglottis (lingual branch), the walls of the pharynx (pharyngeal branch), and the tonsils (tonsillar branch). A wide variety of techniques may be used to anesthetize this part of the airway. The simplest techniques involve aerosolized local anesthetic solution, or a voluntary "swish and swallow." As long as the clinician has developed a plan to anesthetize all relevant structures, has allowed enough time for drying agents to work, and remains continually cognizant of the total dose of local anesthetics administered, most patients will be adequately anesthetized in this way.

Some patients may require a GPN block, especially when topical techniques do not adequately block the gag reflex. The branches of this nerve are most easily accessed as they transverse the palatoglossal folds. These folds are seen as soft tissue ridges, which extend from the posterior aspect of the soft palate to the base of the tongue, bilaterally (Fig. 22-28).

A noninvasive technique employs anesthetic-soaked cotton-tip applicators, which are positioned against the inferior-most aspect of the folds and left in place for 5 to 10 minutes. When the noninvasive technique proves inadequate, local anesthetic can be injected. Standing on the side contralateral to the nerve to be blocked, the operator displaces the extended tongue to

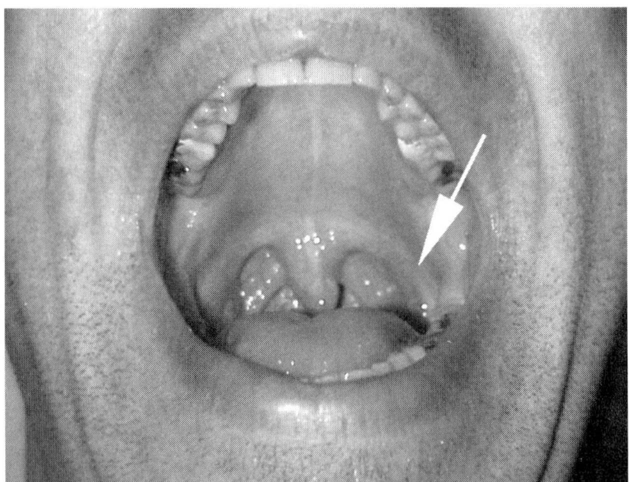

FIGURE 22-28. The palatoglossal arch (*arrow*) is a soft tissue fold that is a continuation of the posterior edge of the soft palate to the base of the tongue. A local anesthetic–soaked swab placed in the gutter along the base of the tongue is left in contact with the fold for 5 to 10 minutes.

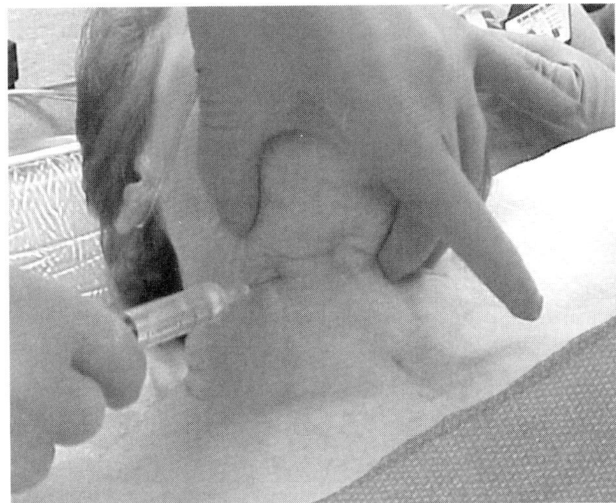

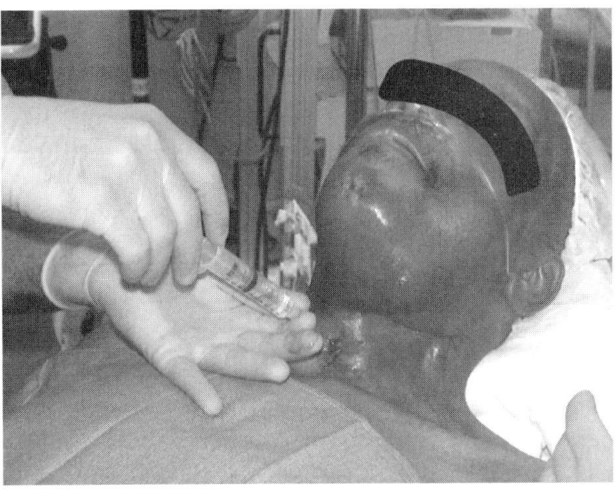

FIGURE 22-29. When a superior laryngeal nerve block is performed, pressure is applied to the contralateral greater cornu of the hyoid to facilitate identification of anatomic landmarks. The needle is inserted at the level of the thyrohyoid membrane just inferior to the greater cornu of the thyroid cartilage. **A.** Superior laryngeal nerve block. **B.** Transtracheal aspiration and injection of local anesthetic (note bubble of aspirated tracheal air).

the contralateral side and a 25-G spinal needle is inserted into the membrane near the floor of the mouth. An aspiration test is performed. If air is aspirated, the needle has passed through-and-through the membrane. If blood is aspirated, the needle is redirected more medially. The lingual branch is most readily blocked in this manner, but retrograde tracking of the injectate has also been demonstrated.[172] Though providing a reliable block, this technique is reported to be painful and may result in a bothersome and persistent hematoma.[176] A posterior approach to the GPN has been described in the otolaryngologic literature (for tonsillectomy). It may be difficult to visualize the site of needle insertion, which is behind the palatopharyngeal arch where the nerve is in close proximity to the carotid artery. Because of the risk for arterial injection and bleeding, the technique will not be described here; however, the reader is referred to a more authoritative text.[177]

The internal branch of the superior laryngeal nerve (SLN), which is a branch of the vagus nerve, provides sensory innervation to the base of the tongue, epiglottis, aryepiglottic folds, and arytenoids. The branch originates from the SLN lateral to the cornu of the hyoid bone. It then pierces the thyrohyoid membrane and travels under the mucosa in the pyriform recess. The remaining portion of the SLN, the external branch, supplies motor innervation to the cricothyroid muscle. Several blocks of this nerve have been described. In many instances topical application of anesthetics in the oral cavity will provide adequate analgesia. An external block is performed with the patient supine with the head extended and the clinician standing on the side ipsilateral to the nerve to be blocked. Beneath the angle of the mandible the clinician identifies the superior cornu of the hyoid bone (Fig. 22-29). Using one hand, medially directed pressure is applied to the contralateral hyoid cornu, displacing the ipsilateral hyoid cornu toward the clinician. Caution must be taken to locate the carotid artery and displace it if necessary. The needle can be inserted directly over the hyoid cornu and then "walked" off the cartilage in an anterior-caudad direction until it can be passed through the membrane to a depth of 1 to 2 cm (Fig. 22-29A). Before the injection of local anesthetic, an aspiration test should be performed to ensure that one has not entered the pharynx or a vascular structure. Local anesthetic with epinephrine (1.5 to 2 mL) is injected in the space between the thyrohyoid membrane and the pharyngeal mucosa. The superior laryngeal nerve can also be blocked with a noninvasive block internal technique. The patient is asked to open the mouth widely, and the tongue is grasped using a gauze pad or tongue blade. A right-angle forceps (e.g., Jackson-Krause forceps) with anesthetic-soaked cotton swabs is slid over the lateral tongue and into the pyriform sinuses bilaterally. The cotton swabs are held in place for 5 minutes.

Sensory innervation of the vocal folds and the trachea is provided by the recurrent laryngeal nerve. Transtracheal injection of local anesthetic can easily be performed to produce adequate analgesia, and the technique is described in detail below (see Retrograde Intubation section, Case 2) (Fig. 22-29B). Lidocaine, 4 mL of 2% or 4% solution, is injected.

An effective and noninvasive technique of tracheal and vocal cord topical analgesia utilizes the working channel of the fiberoptic bronchoscope. A disadvantage of this technique is that solutions leaving the working channel can obscure the objective lens. This can be overcome by use of an epidural catheter, inserted through the working channel, as described by Ovassapian.[178] Not only does this prevent the obscuring of the view, but also it allows specific "aiming" of the anesthetic stream.

Clinical Difficult Airway Scenarios

The clinician approaching the patient with a difficult airway has a vast armamentarium of techniques and instruments that can be applied to securing and maintaining oxygenation and ventilation.[179] Although this array can be confusing, textbook authors cannot dictate specific approaches in every situation; moreover, the variability of patient presentation makes specific recommendations difficult. Thus, to discuss management, the following section presents a number of brief clinical scenarios and the author's own approach. The major alternative airway management techniques are discussed in this manner. All of the clinical cases described herein have been managed by the author or a colleague. Other techniques that might be applied in each situation are also discussed, together with the author's own "decision tree" regarding their applicability. In these cases, as in actual practice, the first technique applied may not have

TABLE 22-17

THE AIRWAY APPROACH ALGORITHM AS APPLIED TO THE CLINICAL CASES PRESENTED IN THIS CHAPTER

■ CASE[a]	■ REQUIRE CONTROL?[b]	■ DL DIFFICULT?[b]	■ SGA POSSIBLE?[b]	■ ASPIRATION RISK?[b]	■ APNEA[b]	■ BOX[b]
1	Yes	Yes	Yes	Yes		A
2	Yes	Yes	?	—		A
3	Yes	No	—	—		B
4	Yes	No	—	—		B
5	Yes	Yes	Yes	No		B

[a]Refer to clinical cases.
[b]Refer to Figure 22-7.

been the best one. The principle of flexibility (and a keen eye to the need to change course quickly) is emphasized repeatedly. In view of the critical importance of the act of airway control, the clinician must be prepared to alter his or her approach as the situation demands. Table 22-17 shows the author's route through the AAA (Figure 22-27) with each case.

When DL and tracheal intubation fail, the clinician has a large armamentarium of tools to turn to. Because successful DL is dependent on sufficient tissue distortion (to create a line of sight), techniques that do not require similar anatomic alignment may be successful after failed DL. Fiberoptic, SGA, stylet-assisted (e.g., lighted stylet) and retrograde techniques may provide a successful alternative. But these techniques also call on alternative skill sets. In a difficult or even critical situation it is unlikely that turning to an unpracticed technique will be helpful.[180]

Unfortunately, clinicians rarely employ alternative techniques until a difficult situation arises. Heidegger et al introduced a simple algorithm for incorporating flexible fiberoptic-aided tracheal intubation into daily practice as a routine alternative to DL.[180] Their incidence of difficult intubation was 6 in 1,324 cases, or 0.049%, markedly lower than the 0.3% reported previously.[181]

Case 1: Flexible Fiberoptic-Aided Intubation

A 50-year-old man with symptomatic cervical vertebrae disk herniation presents for disk resection and spinal fixation. He has a history of tobacco use, alcohol consumption, and gastroesophageal reflux. In the preoperative holding area 0.4 mg of glycopyrrolate is administered. Fifteen minutes later, when the patient states that his oral secretions are minimized, topical anesthesia is administered to the airway. The patient receives 4 mg of intravenous midazolam. An intubating oral airway is placed without eliciting a gag reflex and a flexible fiberoptic bronchoscope is advanced into the airway. The vocal ligaments are visualized, and 4 mL of 4% lidocaine solution are injected through the fiberscope's working channel, being seen to bathe the laryngeal and sublaryngeal structures. The distal end of the fiberscope is advanced into the larynx, and a 7.0-id endotracheal tube, which had been threaded onto the fiberscope's insertion shaft, is advanced into the trachea. The fiberscope is removed while the structures of the carina, trachea, and, finally, the tracheal tube are observed. The anesthesia circuit is attached to the tracheal tube and a steady output of carbon dioxide is detected by capnography. A brief sensory and motor neurologic exam is performed by the attending surgeon and general anesthesia is induced.

Use of the Fiberoptic Bronchoscope in Airway Management. The FOB is a ubiquitous instrument in anesthesia, being available to 99% of surveyed active ASA members.[179] The technique of fiberoptic-aided intubation was first performed using a choledochoscope in a patient with Still's disease (idiopathic, adult onset arthritis).[182] By the late 1980s it was recognized that the use of the flexible FOB represented such a significant advancement in the management of the patient with a difficult airway that experts stated that no anesthesiologist could afford not to be facile with this technique.[183] It is now generally accepted that for a variety of clinical situations, the FOB is a critical tool in the armamentarium of the anesthesiologist dealing with the awake or unconscious patient who is, or appears to be, difficult to intubate.[184] The FOB has proven to be the most versatile tool available in this regard.[178]

15 There is no true or firm indication for FOB-aided intubation, as there might be with direct laryngoscopy (e.g., rapid-sequence induction for the full-stomach patient). There are, however, many clinical situations where the FOB can be of unparalleled aid in securing the airway, especially if the clinician has made an effort to master the necessary skills by using it in routine intubations.[178,180] These include anticipated difficult intubation because of historical or physical exam findings, unanticipated difficult intubation (where other techniques have failed), lower and upper airway obstruction, unstable or fixed cervical spine disease, mass effect in the upper or lower airways, dental risk or damage, and awake intubation.[178] Unlike the other devices used to intubate the trachea, the FOB can also serve to visualize structures below the level of the vocal folds. For example, it can identify the placement of the tracheal tube or aid in placement of a double lumen tracheal tube. It may be helpful in diagnosis within the trachea and bronchial tree, or in pulmonary toilet (Fig. 22-30).

Contraindications to FOB-aided intubation are relative and revolve about the limitations of the device (Table 22-18).

Because the optical elements are small (the objective lens is typically 2 mm in diameter or smaller), minute amounts of airway secretions, blood, or traumatic debris can hinder visualization. Care must be taken to remove these obstacles from the airway beforehand: application of intramuscular or intravenous antisialagogues (e.g., glycopyrrolate, 0.2 to 0.4 mg; atropine, 0.5 to 1 mg) will produce a drying effect within 15 minutes, but caution should be taken in patients who may not be able to tolerate an increase in heart rate. Vasoconstriction of the nose using topical oxymetazoline, phenylephrine, or cocaine reduces the chances of bleeding should this route be chosen. If an awake intubation is planned using the FOB, the patient must be able to cooperate—a "quiet" airway, with little motion of the head, neck, tongue, and larynx, is vital to success. Finally, because FOB-aided intubation of the trachea can require significant time, especially if the clinician is not facile with the device, hypoxia or impending hypoxia is a contraindication, and a more rapid method of securing an airway (e.g., LMA or surgical airway) should be considered.

Elements of the Fiberoptic Bronchoscope. The FOB is a fragile device with optical and nonoptical elements. The

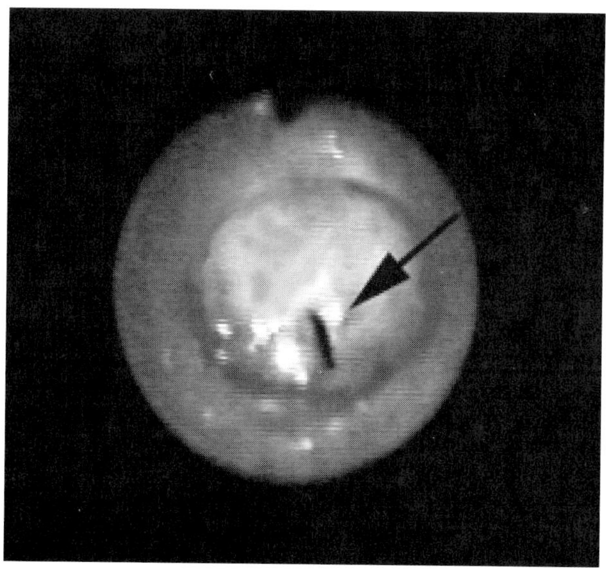

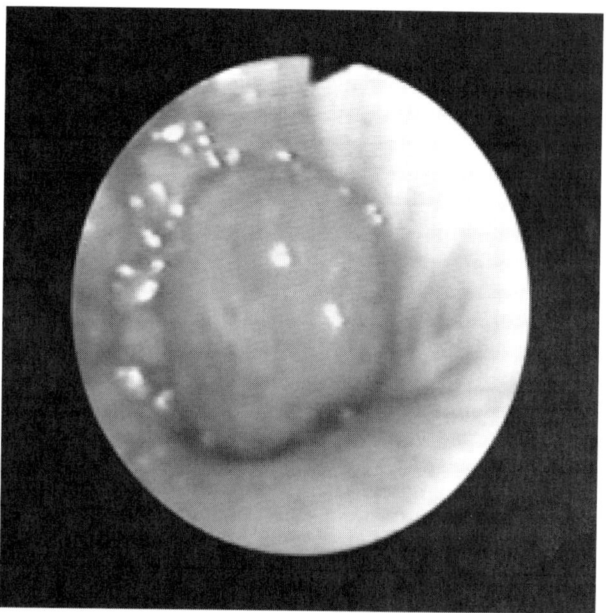

FIGURE 22-30. The fiberoptic bronchoscope may be useful for diagnosis and therapy below the level of the vocal ligaments including bronchial segments exam and toilet (see Fig. 22-30). **A.** Laryngeal web. **B.** Bronchial tumor.

fundamental element consists of a glass-fiber bundle. Each fiber is 8 to 12 microns in diameter and is coated with a secondary glass layer, turned the cladding. The cladding aids in maintaining the image within each fiber as the light is reflected off the sidewall 10,000 times per meter as it moves from the objective lens to the eyepiece lens in the operator's handle. The typical intubating FOB has 10,000 to 30,000 such fibers encased in a 60-cm, water-impermeable insertion cord, with graduation marks every 10 cm. Though the fibers are allowed to rotate over each other throughout the length of the cord, they are fused together at the two ends in a coherent pattern; that is, the arrangement of the fibers at the eyepiece end is identical to the arrangement at the objective lens, where a diopter ring allows focusing. Therefore, one might envision that the image before the objective lens (i.e., the objective) is divided into 10,000 individual and unique pictures, which independently travel down an unwieldy cord, to be reassembled in front of the eyepiece lens. Broken fibers, which may occur because of bending of the insertion cord, entrapping the cord in other equipment, and dropping the FOB, are readily apparent and are generally no more than a nuisance until the number of broken fibers interferes with the visual field.

The insertion cord also contains a *working channel*: a lumen, up to 2 mm in diameter, which travels from the distal tip to the handle. It can be used for applying suction, or oxygen, and instilling lavaging fluids or drugs (e.g., local anesthetics). There is one report of gastric rupture attributed to the insufflation of oxygen through the working channel when the FOB was within the esophagus.[185] In general, FOBs <2 mm in external diameter (e.g., pediatric) do not have a working channel.

Two wires traveling from a lever in the handle down the length of the insertion cord control movement of the distal tip in the sagittal plane. The entire insertion cord is protected by a metal "wrap" until the level of the distal tip, which is hinged for movement. Coronal plane movement is accomplished by a combined use of the control lever and rotation of the entire FOB from handle to distal end. Because the fibers are able to move over one another, except for where they are fused at the extreme ends of the optic cord, rotational control is maximized by reducing any curves in the FOB shaft (Fig. 22-31).

The final element of the FOB is the light source. Illumination of the objective is provided by one or two noncoherent bundles of glass fibers that transmit light from the handle to the distal tip. The light is provided either by a "universal" cord that emerges from the handle and is inserted into a medical-grade endoscopic light source, or may be provided by a battery-operated light source on the handle.

Preparation of the Fiberoptic Bronchoscope. When approaching the FOB-aided intubation, one must ensure that the device is in working order. A series of inspections are made, as listed in Table 22-19.

Use of the Fiberoptic Bronchoscope. The FOB is held in the nondominant hand, the thumb over the control lever and the index finger poised over the working channel valve (see Fig. 22-31). The dominant hand will be used to steady and hold the insertion cord as it is manipulated in the patient. Many operators are tempted to "switch" hands, but the thumb of the nondominant hand should be capable of controlling the gross movement of the control lever. Any experienced endoscopist will recognize that the fine control required to hold the shaft of the endoscope steady, advance the objective end into the airway, and make directional adjustments is where the art of endoscopy lies.

TABLE 22-18

CONTRAINDICATIONS TO FIBEROPTIC BRONCHOSCOPY

- Hypoxia
- Heavy airway secretions not relieved with suction or antisialagogues
- Bleeding from the upper or lower airway not relieved with suction
- Local anesthetic allergy (for awake attempts)
- Inability to cooperate (for awake attempts)

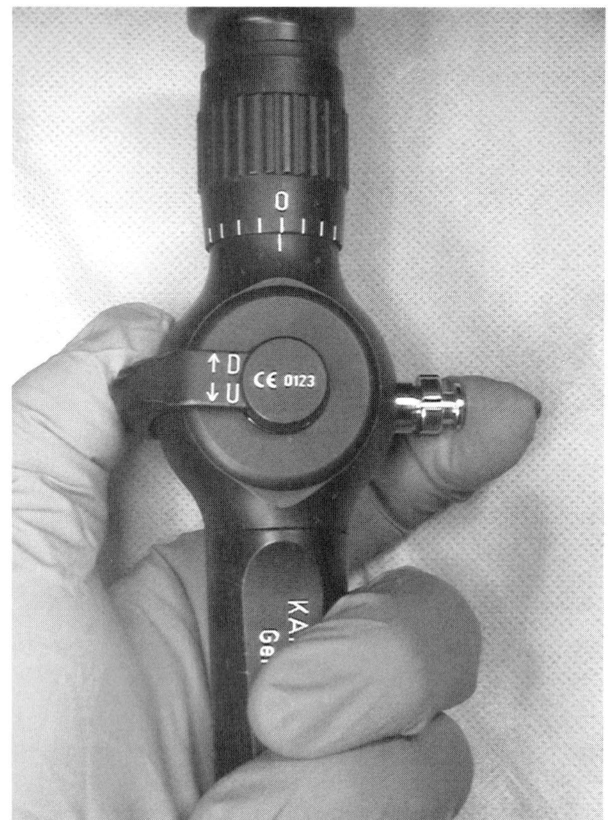

A

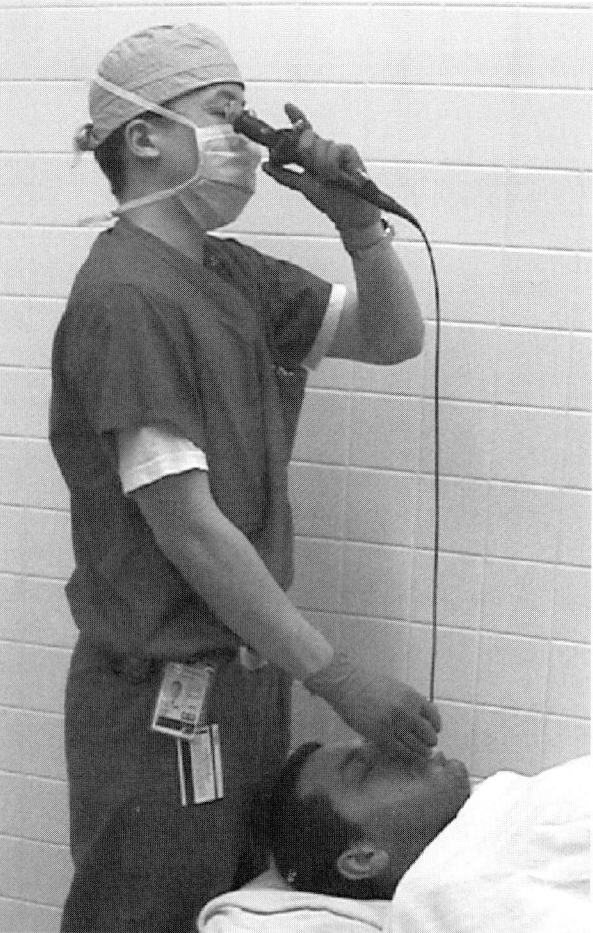

B

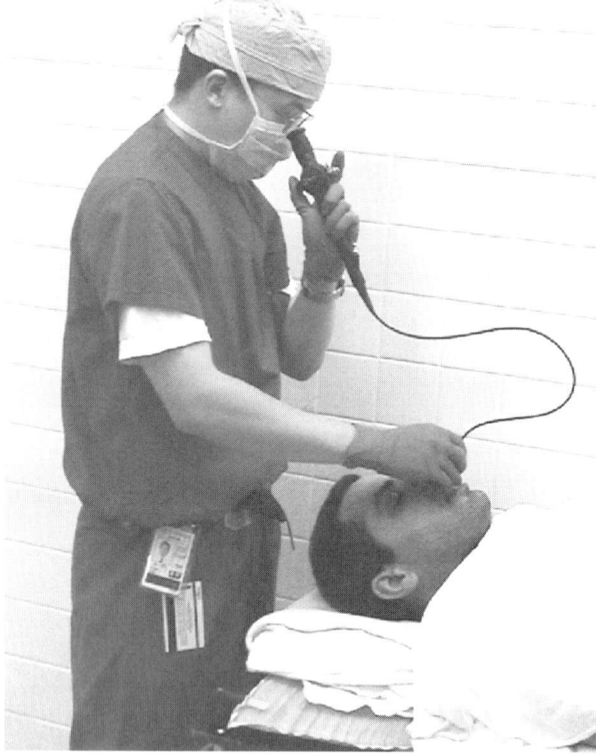

C

FIGURE 22-31. Handling of the fiberoptic bronchoscope. **A.** The handle is held in the nondominant hand with the tip of thumb over the sagittal plane control lever. The index finger can be used to control the working channel (e.g., suction, oxygen insufflation). The dominant hand is used for fine manipulation at the distal end. **B.** The operator's two hands should be kept maximally apart so as to keep the insertion shaft as straight as possible, maximizing coronal plane rotational control. **C.** Curves introduced along the shaft reduce coronal plane rotational control.

TABLE 22-19

PREPARATION OF THE FIBEROPTIC BRONCHOSCOPE

■ PROCEDURE	■ FINDING	■ SIGNIFICANCE AND ACTION
Inspect passive angulation: Allow FOB to hang from the hand.	Observer deviations from "plum."	Angulation may signify damage to the insertion shaft. If lever controls are operative, the FOB may be usable. Excessive angulation or curvature may make manipulation difficult, disorienting the operator, so the scope should not be used.
Active angulation: The control lever is used to manipulate the distal tip	Does the lever control move the tip in the sagittal plane smoothly and to the extent stated by the manufacturer?	There may be a damaged or entrapped control wire. The device should be repaired by the manufacturer.
Apply suction to the working channel.	No or minimal suction at distal aperture.	Caking of secretions within channel may require cleaning by the manufacturer. Crimping of insertion cord requires repair.
Picture clarity: Observe printed writing a few millimeters in front of the objective lens.	Foggy or dirty picture.	The objective lens and eyepiece lens can be cleaned with a lint-free cloth. Use a commercial defogger. Prior to placing in the patient, warm water may prevent further fogging by equalizing the lens and patient temperatures. Suction or oxygen insufflation. If these are unsuccessful, the FOB may need cleaning by the manufacturer.

The insertion shaft is lubricated with a water-soluble lubricant, and it is threaded through the lumen of an ETT, the objective end emerging from the main ETT orifice. A clinically appropriate ETT should be chosen, but the larger the ratio between the internal diameter of the ETT and the external diameter of the insertion shaft, the greater the risk of "hangup" on airway structures, as occurs in 20 to 30% of attempts (Fig. 22-32).[178]

Hangup occurs when a cleft exists between these two devices because of the differential sizes. Hangup may involve entrapment of the epiglottis, corniculate/arytenoid cartilages, the aryepiglottic folds, or the vocal folds, and can occur with any number of stylet-guided techniques (e.g., fiberoptic, retrograde wire, lighted stylet) though it is most thoroughly described with fiberoptic aided intubation.[186,187] The orientation of the tracheal tube bevel is important in this regard. In orotracheal intubation, the bevel cleft is likely to entrap the right arytenoid cartilage when the ETT is in its typical concavity anterior position. Rotation of the ETT counterclockwise 90° places the bevel facing positively and improves passage. During nasotraceheal intubation, the epiglottis may be entrapped, and a bevel-up position (rotation of the ETT 90° clockwise) may facilitate passage. [188]

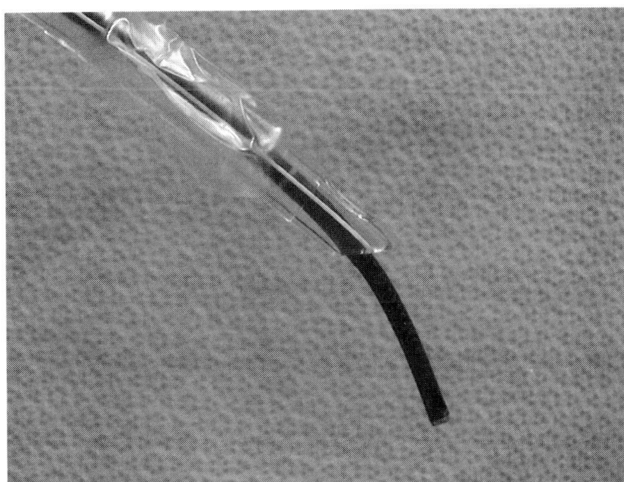

FIGURE 22-32. The size discrepancy between the fiberoptic bronchoscope and the tracheal tube that has been threaded onto it can create a cleft that can entrap anterior anatomic structures, hindering advancement of the tracheal tube into the larynx (hangup).

The type of tracheal tube may also affect passage. It has been suggested that the Parker Flex-tip (Parker Medical, Cincinnati, OH) may pass the airway structures more easily than a standard ETT bevel.[189] The use of soft-tipped ETTs, asking the patient to inspire deeply during the ETT advancement, and the "double setup" ETT, which uses a small ETT (e.g., 5.0 id) within a clinically adequate ETT (e.g., 7.5 id) to overcome the clefts caused by size differentials have been described.[186,190]

The clinician chooses the route of intubation, either oral or nasal, based on clinical requirements, surgical needs, operator experience, and other intubation techniques available should FOB-aided intubation fail. This last factor is important because should an attempt at nasal intubation fail, there may be significant bleeding hindering other indirect visualization techniques. The nasal route is considered easier by many clinicians. The differences between oral and nasal FOB-aided intubation are discussed in Table 22-20.

A variety of intubating oral airways (IOA) are commercially available. Their chief function is to provide a clear visual path from the oral aperture to the pharynx, keep the bronchoscope in the midline, prevent the patient from biting the insertion cord, and provide a clear airway for the spontaneously or mask-ventilated patient. The common characteristic of all IOAs is a channel along the length of the airway large enough to allow the passage of the endotracheal tube. The Ovassapian airway (Fig. 22-33) provides two sets of semicircular, incomplete flexible flanges that stabilize the ETT (up to size 9.0 id) in the midline but allow its removal from the airway after intubation has been accomplished so that the IOA can be removed from

TABLE 22-20

TECHNIQUES OF NASAL AND ORAL FOB-AIDED INTUBATION

	■ NASAL	■ ORAL
Preparation	Antisialagogues, topical decongestant, serial dilations with soft and lubricated nasal trumpets[a]	Antisialagogue, intubating oral airway (IOA)
ETT	Softened by placing in warm water. May be kept either on proximal insertion cord (near handle) or inserted[b] into the nose so that it is felt to turn the bend from the nasal cavity into the nasopharynx	Kept either on proximal insertion cord (near handle) or inserted 4-5 cm into the IOA
Structures seen	Floor of nose, nasal turbinates, superior aspect of the soft palate, nasopharyngeal posterior wall, base of tongue, epiglottis (distal tip),[c] arytenoid cartilages, vocal folds, tracheal rings, carina	IOA (anterior or anterior/posterior depending on IOA) Soft palate/uvula Epiglottis (distal tip),[c] arytenoid cartilages, vocal folds, tracheal rings, carina

[a]Although phenylephrine and cocaine have been used to decongest the nose, evidence suggests that oxymetazoline may be the best agent.
[b]The bevel of the ETT should follow along the nasal septum, away from the turbinates. If the ETT will not turn into the nasopharynx, it may be rotated 90° in a clockwise or counterclockwise direction and readvanced.
[c]An obstructing base of tongue or epiglottis can be moved by extension at the atlanto-occipital joint, jaw thrust, chin lift, or having an assistant pull the tongue forward.

the mouth. The flat lingual surface of the airway gives it good lateral and rotational stability. The Patil-Syracuse endoscopic airway and the Luomanen oral airway (see Fig. 22-33) were also designed for fiberoptic-aided intubation. Each has a central groove, open at the lingual (Patil-Syracuse) or palatal (Luomanen) aspect, which allows easy removal of the ETT. The flat lingual surface provides good stability. Though this style of IOA provides superb access to the pharynx, it is larger than other airways and is often uncomfortable for the patient. The Williams airway (see Fig. 22-33) and the Berman airway were both designed for blind oral intubation. It is often difficult to manipulate the tip of the fiberscope when it is within these narrow airways. Both are molded plastic with a complete circular internal lumen which guides the ETT toward the larynx. These airways have a small profile and are often better tolerated by the awake patient, but tend to be less stable on the tongue. Because the internal lumen is a complete circle, the Williams airway must be retreated off the ETT if it is going to be removed after intubation. This may pose difficulty if the ETT in use has a fused circuit adapter. The Berman airway solves this problem by being split along the length of one side. The plastic of the opposite side is thin and malleable. If the interincisor gap is adequate, the airway can be opened laterally to allow removal from the ETT.

After successful navigation through the supraglottic airway, the endoscopist visualizes the vocal folds. If glottic closure,

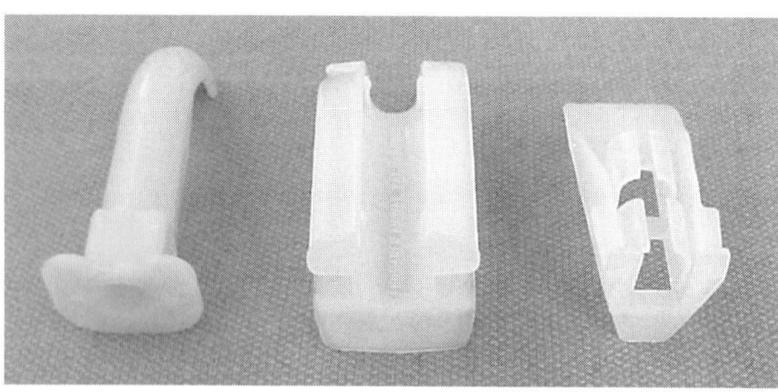

FIGURE 22-33. **Left.** Williams airway. **Middle.** Luomanen airway. **Right.** Ovassapian fiberoptic intubating airway.

gag, or coughing occur as the FOB distal tip stimulates the structures of the larynx, the operator can choose to apply local anesthetic through the working channel, administer more sedation, or withdraw the scope and reinforce preparatory procedures. The clinician might also decide to advance the FOB into the larynx without further preparation. The actions taken must be dictated by the individual clinical situation; in the elective scenario, for example, there may be time for reinforced airway analgesia, whereas in the face of impending respiratory arrest patient discomfort may need to be tolerated. Once the larynx is entered, the operator may choose a structure, such as the tracheal carina, to serve as an identifying landmark as the ETT is advanced. Simply because the FOB has entered the trachea, there is no guarantee that the intubation will be successful. As noted earlier, 20 to 30% of ETT advancements are accompanied by hangup. Therefore, a patient with a critical airway should not be induced with a general anesthetic with the assumption that the ETT will be easy to pass.

Once the ETT enters the trachea, the clinician may choose to view the ETT and a chosen anatomic landmark simultaneously (e.g., the tracheal carina) to assure correct ETT placement before the FOB is withdrawn.

There have been a number of variations and adjuncts to FOB-aided intubation. The reader is referred to the primary literature listed in Table 22-21, which is not meant to be exhaustive.

Although FOB-aided intubation is a versatile and vital technique, there are several pitfalls, most of which have been discussed. Table 22-22 lists the most common reasons for failure of FOB-aided intubation.

Flexible fiberoptic-aided intubation is a technology-intense technique. Apart from the delicate fiberoptic device, there are cameras, recorders, light sources, and a variety of disposable adjuncts that are typically required. Dedicated wheeled carts, designed carry required as well as optional equipment in a functional arrangement, are available (Fig. 22-34). The clinician called to manage the patient outside the operating theater may benefit from portable arrangements (Fig. 22-35).

Rigid Fiberoptic Intubation Devices. Rigid fiberoptic devices allow indirect views of the larynx and act as an ETT guide for intubation. More than one-third of all anesthesiologists have access to these devices.[179] The most commonly available of these devices include the Bullard (ACMI, Santa

TABLE 22-21

AIDS TO FIBEROPTIC-AIDED INTUBATION

■ TECHNIQUE	■ ADVANTAGE
Endoscopy mask	Control ventilation maintained during or between attempts at FOB-aided intubation
Laryngeal mask	Excellent view of the larynx and ability to ventilate during or between attempts at FOB-aided intubation
Fiberoptic-aided retrograde intubation	Guiding of the FOB with a wire known to be entering the trachea
Retrograde fiberoptic intubation	Changing a tracheostomy to an oral or nasal tracheal tube when antegrade intubation is difficult or impossible
FOB-aided intubation with the aid of a rigid laryngoscope	Helpful with an obstructing mass or large epiglottis

Barbara, CA, USA) and WuScope (Pentax Precision Instruments, Orangeburg, NY) laryngoscopes (Fig. 22-36). Although these laryngoscopes may be used in routine clinical situations, they are particularly useful when movement of the patient's head and neck is impossible or contraindicated (e.g., atlanto-occipital joint disease and the spine-injured patient). They are also applicable when there is a limited oral aperture (0.64 cm in the case of the Bullard). These devices consist of a rigid, stainless-steel laryngoscope-like blade that encases a fiberoptic cable with a proximal eyepiece and distal objective lens. The blades have an anatomic curve to match the neutral position of the human oral cavity-pharynx-hypopharynx relationship. Alignment of the oral, pharyngeal, and tracheal axes is not required. Illumination is provided by a second fiberoptic cable transmitting light from a battery or free-standing light source.

The Bullard scope, which comes in adult and pediatric sizes, has been the best investigated. It features a fixed fiberoptic cable located on the posterior aspect of the blade. The eyepiece lens has an adjustable diopter. A working channel also runs the length of the blade. Once the larynx is visualized, the ETT is advanced using a detachable stylet, although other techniques have been described.[191] The advantages of the Bullard scope over traditional laryngoscope blades in managing the spine-injured patient and the obese patient have been investigated.[192–194]

Adequate exposure with the Bullard laryngoscope may be achieved after failed DL.[195]

The Upsher scope is available in an adult size as of this writing. Instead of a stylet, the ETT is held and advanced through a C-shaped lumen in the blade. There is no working channel in this scope. The eyepiece is focusable.

The Wu scope differs from the other devices in that a flexible fiberoptic endoscope is fitted into a passage within a three-part stainless steel handle and blade. A second, larger lumen accepts the ETT. A working channel is positioned alongside the endoscope lumen. Two adult sizes are manufactured. Once the larynx is visualized and the ETT advanced into the trachea, the two stainless-steel pieces of the laryngoscope blade are disassembled and removed from the mouth. Unlike the other two devices, the Wu scope can also be used for nasal intubation by assembling only the anterior blade portion and the handle. An ETT, previously placed in the pharynx via the nares, can be fitted into the anterior portion of the blade.

A new generation of fiberoptic devices is focused on simplicity and portability, by incorporating optical and light source elements into a single stylet-like stainless steel sheath. The lack of a tongue displacing blade and a suction/oxygen channel are potential disadvantages. The Bonfils Intubation Fiberscope (Karl Storz Endoscopy, Tuttingen, Germany) (Fig. 22-37A) is a long, rigid tubular device with conventional optical and light transmitting fiberoptic elements.[196] A proximal end eyepiece (with adjustable diopter) can be used with the naked eye or fitted with a standard endoscopy camera. A cable (or battery powered attachment) brings illumination from an external light source. The distal end has a 40° angulation. Suction may be applied through a working channel. The technique of use replicates the paraglossal approach of laryngoscopy discussed previously in this chapter. The Shikani Seeing Optical Stylet (Clarus Medical, LLC, Minneapolis, MN) (SOS) has a similar configuration to the Bonfils with the exception that the distal one-half of the stylet is malleable (Fig. 22-37B). The light source may be self-contained (a proprietary powered handle or a green line

TABLE 22-22

COMMON REASONS FOR FAILURE DURING FIBEROPTIC-AIDED INTUBATION

Lack of experience: Not practicing on routine intubations
Failure to adequately dry the airway: Underdose or rushed technique
Failure to adequately anesthetize the airway of the awake patient: Secretions not dried; rushed technique
Nasal cavity bleeding: Inadequate vasoconstriction; rushed technique; forcible ETT insertion
Obstructing base of tongue or epiglottis: Poor choice of intubating airway; require chin lift/jaw thrust
Inadequate sedation of the awake patient
Hangup: ETT too large
Fogging of the FOB: Suction or oxygen not attached to working channel; cold bronchoscope

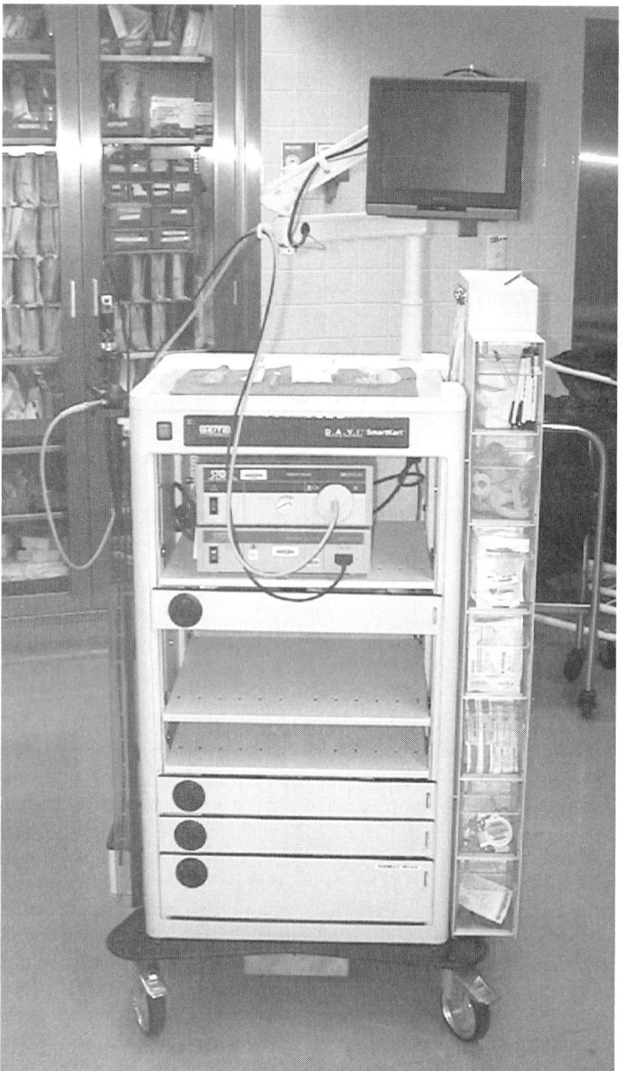

FIGURE 22-34. The Difficult Airway SmartKart (Seitz Technical Products, Avondale, PA) is designed to transport several fiberscopes as well as other difficult airway equipment, accessories, and the electronics required for video viewing through indirect optical devices.

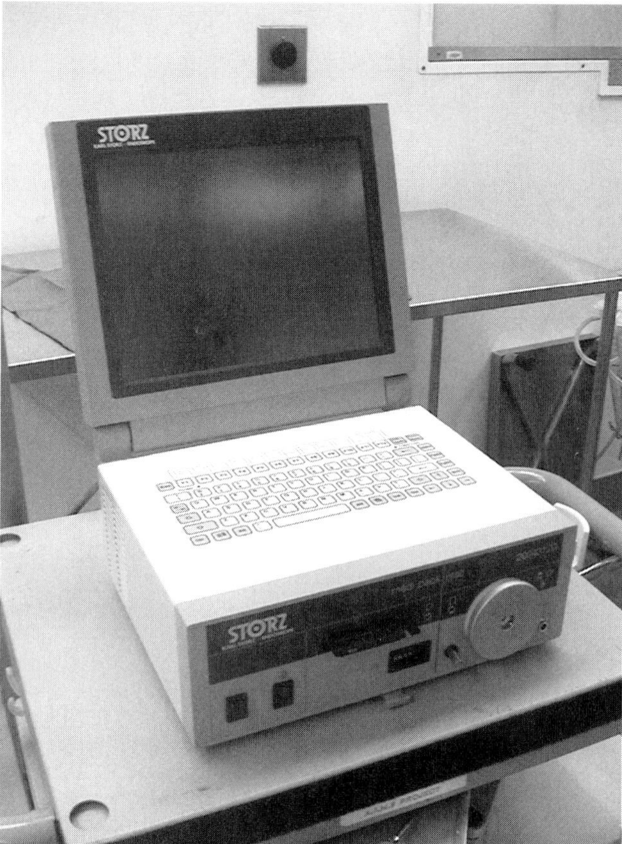

FIGURE 22-35. The Medipack (Karl Storz Endoscopy, Culver City, CA) incorporates a light source, fiberscope camera receiver, and video screen in one package.

[Rusch Medical, Duluth, Georgia] laryngoscope handle) or cabled. Unlike the Bofils, a midline approach is recommended. Studies have investigated the use of the SOS as a substitute for the laryngoscope in routine anesthetic cases.[197] The hypothetical benefit of this practice is the reduction of unanticipated difficult intubations and the maintenance of alternative technique skills by incorporating this or similar devices into daily practice.[180]

Glidescope© (Fig. 22-38)

New innovations in video delivery have given rise to the next generation of video-assisted laryngoscopy tools. The Glidescope (Saturn Biomedical Systems, Burnaby, BC, Canada) provides an electronically projected image on a video monitor emanating from a video chip set at the distal end of a conventional-like laryngoscope blade, but with a more acute (60°) angulation.[198] Illumination is likewise generated at the distal aspect. This configuration affords several advantages: (1) It may be handled with a skill set similar to that used with conventional DL. (2) The operator's point of sight (e.g., the video apparatus) is positioned close to the distal blade aspect (thereby eliminating fragile fiberoptic elements). The operator therefore "sees" at a position behind the tongue, and displacement as with conventional DL, is not necessary in most cases. Similarly, lingual tonsil hyperplasia should not affect the visual axis as it does with conventional DL.[3] (3) The video image of the airway is displayed on a lightweight portable screen. The video display allows for visualization by more than one individual (e.g., aid, mentor, student). (4) Less stress is imposed on the airway by virtue of reduced compressive force directed to the tongue. (5) An external light source is not needed. At the time of this writing, no controlled trial information is available on this device.

Video-Macintosh Laryngoscope (Fig. 22-39)

The Video-Macintosh (VM) (Karl-Storz Endovision, Culver City, California) consists of a conventional-appearing laryngoscope handle and blade. A stainless-steel shaft built into the blade flange accepts a short, fiberoptic cable containing both light source and optical cables. This fiberoptic cable enters the handle where the camera elements are housed. Two larger (and less fragile) cables exit proximal handle and connect to standard light- and video-processing devices from the same manufacturer. The video image is displayed on a standard NTSC monitor. Though the image projected from the VM closely resembles that seen with the naked eye (1) ETT placement is facilitated because the operator need not maintain an unobstructed line of sight (his eye using the video monitor), (2) external laryngeal manipulation can be observed by a second operator, and (3) use of the VM is identical standard DL, making the

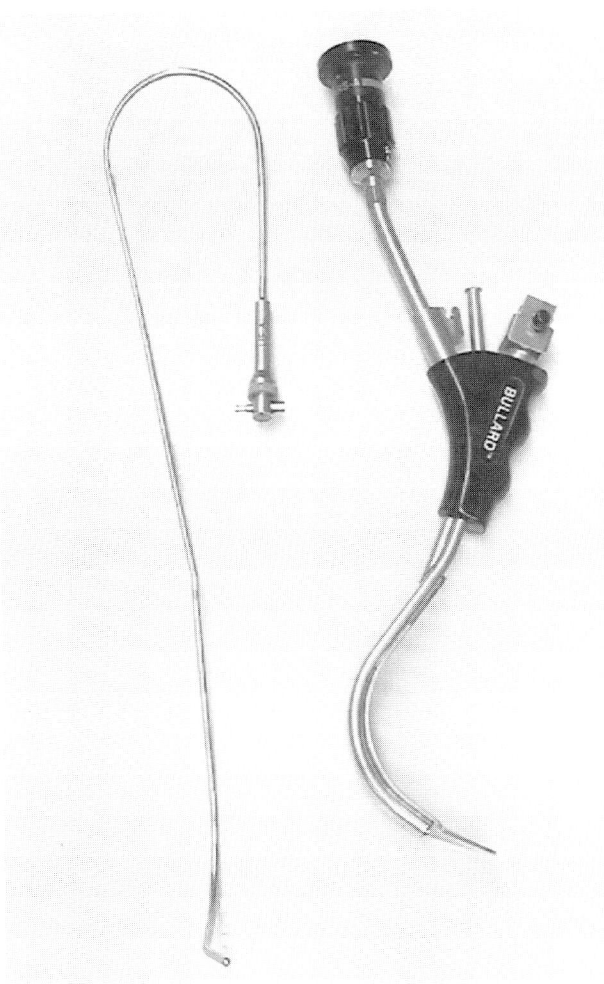

FIGURE 22-36. The Bullard laryngoscope, battery handle, and stylet.

video facility uniquely valuable during supervised instruction. Though large controlled trials have not been published at the time of this writing, the VM will likely have a significant advantage in teaching and some difficult laryngoscopies.

Case 2: Retrograde Wire Intubation

A 65-year-old female with a 60-pack/year history of smoking and advanced rheumatoid arthritis presents to the emergency department (ED) in respiratory distress. Her oxygen saturation with a nonrebreather oxygen mask is 85%. She has a limited oral aperture (~2.5 cm) and a thyromental distance of 6 cm. Although the cricothyroid membrane can be palpated, there is limited access to it and the tracheal rings owing to a significant cervical kyphosis. The sputum is noted to be blood-tinged and contains thickened bronchial secretions. Awake blind nasal intubation is attempted twice by the emergency medicine physicians, is unsuccessful, and results in epistaxis. Retrograde intubation of the airway is performed with the patient in a sitting position. After initial local anesthetic infiltration of the skin over the membrane, on 18 G angiocatheter is advanced over the mid-cricothyroid membrane at an angle of 45° to the chest. After the free aspiration of air is noted, the Teflon sheath of the catheter is advanced into the trachea. A 0.035-inch radiologic guidewire 110 inches in length is advanced via the catheter until the proximal end emerges from the mouth. A 7.0 ETT is placed over the wire and is guided into the trachea. The wire is removed by pushing it into the percutaneous puncture site and retrieving it from the proximal end of the tracheal tube. Breath sounds are auscultated over the lung fields as ventilation is assisted with positive pressure. Once improved oxygen saturation is noted, the patient receives sedation with intravenous midazolam (in divided doses, titrating to the sedative effect).

Use of the Retrograde Wire Intubation in Airway Management. Retrograde wire intubation (RWI) involves the antegrade pulling or guiding of an ETT into the trachea using a wire or catheter, which has been passed into the trachea via a percutaneous puncture through the cricothyroid membrane or the cricotracheal membrane and blindly passed retrograde into the larynx, hypopharynx, pharynx and out of the mouth or nose. Retrograde intubation was first described in 1960 by Butler and Cirillo, with the placement a red rubber urethral catheter via a previous tracheostomy up through the larynx and out of the mouth.[199] The percutaneous technique used today was first described by Waters in 1963, using an epidural catheter.[200] In 1993 the technique was included in the ASA's Difficult Airway Algorithm.[157] The basic equipment used in the retrograde intubation technique is listed in Table 22-23.

16 Retrograde wire intubation has been described in a number of clinical situations as a primary intubation technique (elective or urgent) and after failed attempts at direct laryngoscopy, fiberoptic-aided intubation, and LMA-guided intubation.[201] The most common indications are inability to visualize the vocal folds owing to blood, secretions, or anatomic variations; unstable cervical spine, upper airway malignancy; and mandibular fracture. Contraindications include lack of access to the cricothyroid membrane or the cricotracheal ligament

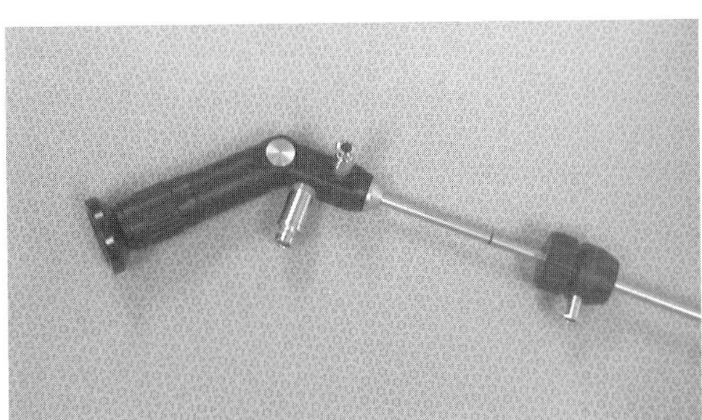

A

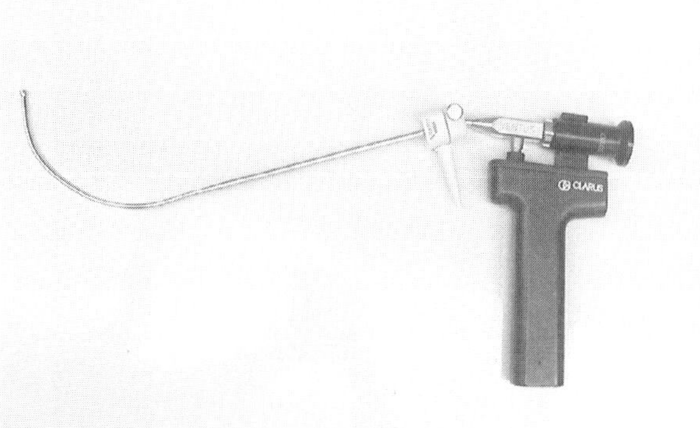

B

FIGURE 22-37. Optical stylets. **A.** The objective end of the Bonfils (Karl Storz Endoscopy, Culver City, CA). **B.** The Shikani Seeing Optical Stylet (Clarus Medical, Minneapolis, MN).

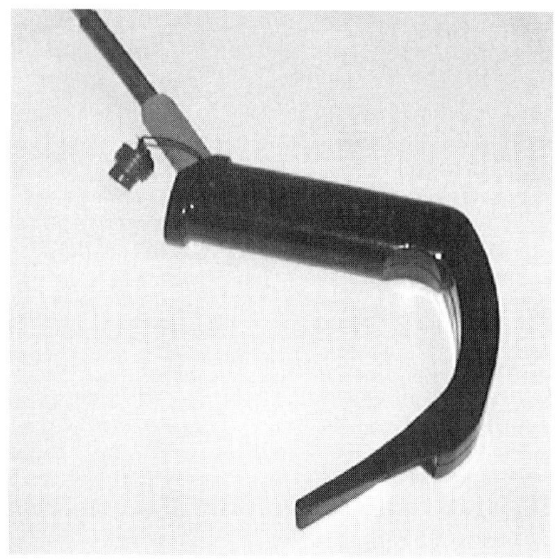

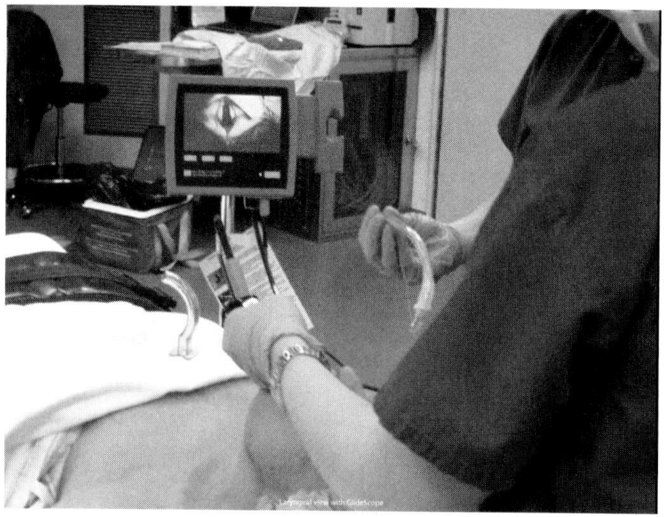

FIGURE 22-38. A. The Glide Scope. B. Glide Scope screen in use during laryngoscopy (photograph courtesy of Dr. Richard Cooper).

(because of severe neck deformity, obesity, mass), laryngotracheal disease (stenosis, malignancy, infection), coagulopathy, and skin infection.

The anatomic relationships to be considered in RWI have been described elsewhere in this chapter. Typically, the procedure requires 5 minutes to perform.[202] Because most clinicians are not facile with the technique, it may take several minutes in inexperienced hands; therefore, RWI is relatively contraindicated in the hypoxic patient. RWI has been used in elective and emergent situations, in adults and infants, in the operating room, ED, and the prehospital environment. Complications reported with RWI are listed in Table 22-24.

In the current patient (as in Case 1), RWI was chosen in a setting where the patient was not apneic and was therefore supporting her own ventilation and oxygenation, albeit poorly. The two cases differ in impending respiratory failure (Case 2) versus FOB-aided intubation undertaken in an stable situation (Case 1). In many situations, where awake intubation is an obvious initial approach to securing the airway, there is little time for patient preparation (e.g., the administration of antisialagogues, topical anesthetics, and/or sedation). In this regard, RWI does not require a clear visual field or significant patient cooperation and can often be performed with little analgesia of the airway. The technique of RWI differs greatly from other methods of tracheal intubation familiar to the anesthesiologist. Preferably RWI should be learned on a simulator/mannequin model before being attempted in a patient. In addition, unless RWI is practiced often, it may be time-consuming. For this reason, RWI may be a poor choice for rescue of an acutely compromised airway.

Performing Retrograde Wire Intubation (Fig. 22-40). RWI is generally performed with the patient in a supine position, although the sitting position is often used for patients in respiratory distress. Extension of the head or the neck displaces the cricoid and tracheal cartilages anteriorly and displaces the sternocleidomastoid muscles laterally, though, as in Case 2, this may not always be possible. The skin should be prepared. If the patient is conscious, a local anesthetic skin wheel is made over the puncture site. Local anesthesia of the airway should be administered to prevent discomfort and airway reflexes as time permits. In general, topical anesthesia of the trachea, larynx, pharynx, and nasal passages is desirable. Translaryngeal anesthesia is a particularly convenient technique since a percutaneous entry of the trachea is required during the RWI. Structures above and below the vocal folds are anesthetized during the ensuing patient cough if a local anesthetic–filled syringe is used to facilitate the recognition of appropriate placement

FIGURE 22-39. The Video Macintosh (Karl Storz Endoscopy, Culver City, CA).

TABLE 22-23

EQUIPMENT FOR RETROGRADE WIRE INTUBATION

18 G or larger angiocatheter
Luer-lock syringe, 3 mL or larger
Guidewire:

- Preferably J-type end
- Length: at least 2.5 times the length of a standard ETT (typically 110 to 120 cm)
- Diameter: capable of passing via angiocatheter being chosen

Other: Scalpel blade, nerve hook, Magill forceps, 30″ silk suture, epidural catheter

TABLE 22-24

COMPLICATIONS ASSOCIATED WITH RETROGRADE WIRE INTUBATION[201]

Bleeding (11)
Subcutaneous emphysema (4)
Pneumomediastinum (1)
Breath-holding (1)
Catheter traveling caudad (2)
Trigeminal nerve trauma (1)
Pneumothorax (1)

(with tracheal air bubbles) and then is injected to provide airway anesthesia (see Fig. 22-29B).[203]

As noted earlier, the CTM and CTL are both potential sites for translaryngeal puncture. Although the CTM has the advantage of being directly anterior to the large posterior surface of the cricoid cartilage, thereby protecting the esophagus from a puncturing needle, it places the needle in close proximity (0.9 to 1.5 cm) to the vocal folds and hence allows for a somewhat smaller margin of error at the time of the intubation.

Although classically performed with a Tuohy needle and epidural catheter, the advent of smaller diameter, stiffer wires with atraumatic "J" tips has made the guidewire modification popular. These guidewires are typically 0.032 to 0.038 inches in diameter, being able to pass through an 18-G intravenous catheter. The typical length is between 110 and 120 cm. The only requirement for length is that the wire be more than twice as long as the tracheal tube to be used, so that no matter where in its course along the wire the tracheal tube should be, both ends of the wire are always accessible to the operator. Kits that conveniently incorporate all the necessary equipment are available (Cook Critical Care, Bloomington, IN).

The needle/catheter approaches the trachea at 90° to the coronal and sagittal planes if possible (as it was not in Case 2). In this orientation, the needle is likely to impact the posterior aspect of the cricoid cartilage if advanced too far, and not puncture the esophagus. Additionally, this angle will help to avoid trauma to the near-lying vocal folds.

After the percutaneous puncture is made and the trachea identified by free air aspiration, the catheter is angled cephalad and the wire is advanced (J-tip) into the trachea until it emerges from the mouth or nose. The wire may need to be retrieved from the mouth with a "sweeping" finger, Magill forceps, or nerve hook. Any obstruction to advancement of the wire should prompt re-evaluation of the angle of the catheter

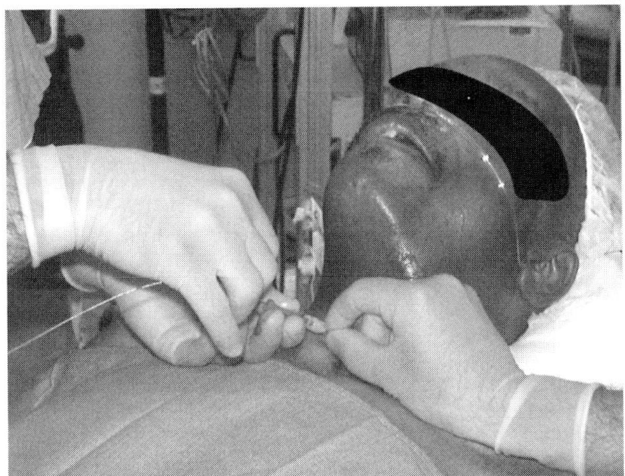
A

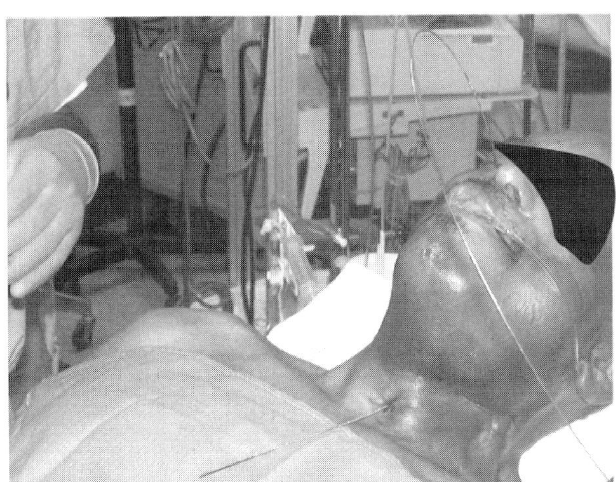
B

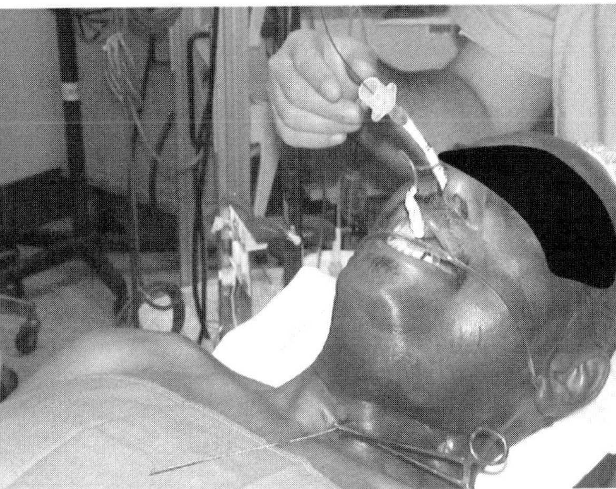
C

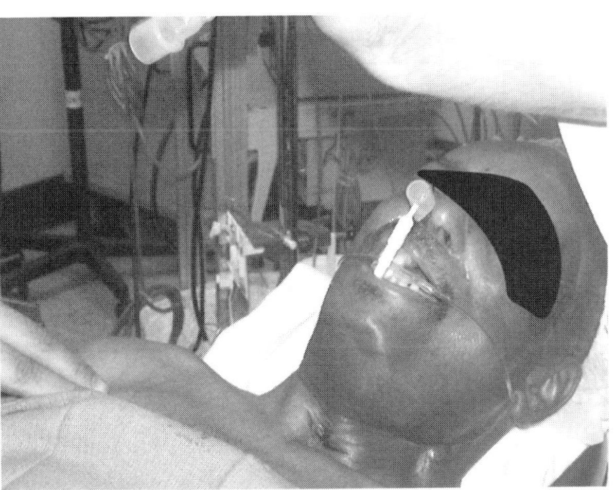
D

FIGURE 22-40. The sequence of retrograde wire intubation after the cricothyroid or cricotracheal ligament is identified and a percutaneous puncture is performed with air aspiration (see Fig. 22-29B). (**A**) The retrograde device (twisted wire, Cook Critical Care) is advanced until (**B**) it emerges from the mouth or nose. (**C**) The wire is clamped at the entrance site and the endotracheal tube is advanced over the wire in an antegrade fashion. (**D**) The wire is removed, leaving the tracheal tube in place.

TABLE 22-25

TECHNIQUES OF ETT ADVANCEMENT OVER A RETROGRADE WIRE

TECHNIQUE	ADVANTAGE	DISADVANTAGE
Wire travels through entire main lumen of the ETT	Standard technique	Margin of error[a] equals distance from vocal folds to puncture site No stylet after removal of wire "Railroading"[b] can occur
Wire placed into ETT lumen via Murphy eye	Increased margin of error Decreased railroading	Cannot use stylet (below)
Wire enters distal end of ETT and exits via Murphy eye	Decreased railroading	Margin of error equals distance from vocal folds to puncture site Cannot use stylet (below)
ETT "exchange" stylet is placed over wire, prior to placement of ETT	Decreased railroading Can use stylet to vastly increase margin of error once wire is removed	Cost
Fiberoptic bronchoscope is placed over wire prior to placement of ETT	Decreased railroading Can use stylet to vastly increase margin of error once wire is removed Visualization	Cost
Silk suture	No railroading Margin of error issues reduced	May be difficult to place silk suture
Small ETT	Reduced railroading	May not be clinically adequate

[a]*Margin of error* refers to the distance below the vocal folds that the endotracheal tube extends at the time that the guidewire is removed. If this distance is not adequate, there is a risk of immediate extubation.
[b]*Railroading* refers to the differential size of the guidewire and the tracheal tube. A large discrepancy in size allows for a cleft, which may entrap the epiglottis, arytenoid cartilages, aryepiglottic folds, or vocal folds, hindering intubation attempts.

and the position of the head and neck (e.g., catheter directed posterior and/or caudad, neck flexed). Coughing typically heralds caudad traveling of the wire. If the wire is retracted and found to be bent, it is prudent to procure a new one. When complaints of pain are encountered above the level of the larynx, it is typically a result of the wire passing into an inadequately prepared nasal cavity. Options include retracting the wire modestly and asking the patient to open the mouth and maximally protrude the tongue during the readvancement, reaching into the oropharynx to retrieve the wire, or patiently repreparing the nasal passages. Once the wire is satisfactorily retrieved, placement of the tracheal tube may be performed using the wire in a number of fashions, depending on the operator's preference and previous experience. Table 22-25 lists common techniques, together with their advantages and disadvantages. Details of these techniques have been described elsewhere.[204]

In the case reported, other techniques may have been considered. Although indirect visual devices (flexible fiberoptic bronchoscope, rigid fiberoptic laryngoscope) may have also been helpful in this case, three elements worked against their use: (1) tissue trauma from repeated attempts at blind nasal intubation produced a bloody airway, frustrating the use of these devices; (2) the patient was unable to cooperate owing to her respiratory distress; (3) because of the impending respiratory failure, there was little time for adequate airway analgesia. A coughing, gagging, conscious patient makes fiberoptic techniques nearly impossible. Straining and coughing during fiberoptic intubation attempts have resulted in Mallory-Weiss tears of the esophagus, resulting in significant hemorrhage.

Blind nasal intubation was the first technique attempted in this patient. Until recently, blind nasal intubation has been a staple of airway control, especially in the emergency department, where it has been largely supplanted by rapid-sequence intubation.[205] This technique requires significant analgesia of the nasal passages in the awake patient. Success is far more likely in the spontaneously breathing patient. With the head in the Magill position, the ETT is advanced into the nares, nasal passage (keeping the ETT bevel alongside the nasal septum), and into the pharynx. Breath sounds are auscultated from the ETT, and its position adjusted to keep them maximized. The patient's head and larynx can be manipulated externally as necessary.

Case 3: Esophageal Tracheal Combitube

A 55-year-old male with a history of cirrhosis and esophageal varices requires airway control as a result of acute, recurrent upper gastrointestinal bleeding. Apart from fresh blood in the airway, physical exam of his external airway is consistent with a routine laryngoscopy. Furthermore, he had been intubated for similar events in the past. After a rapid-sequence induction, the larynx cannot be visualized on three laryngoscopies owing to fresh blood emanating from the esophagus. On all three attempts, the ETT is advanced blindly, and the absence of breath sounds over the thorax together with the presence of copious blood in the ETT leads to the diagnosis of esophageal intubation. A large adult-sized esophageal tracheal Combitube (Tyco Healthcare, Mansfield, NY) is requested, blindly inserted into the airway, and the pharyngeal and distal cuffs are inflated. Ventilation through the pharyngeal perforations lumen (blue) produces bilateral breath sounds to auscultation, and the oxygen saturation increases to >90%. Copious blood is suctioned from the esophageal lumen. The patient is transported to the angiography suite where his esophageal varices are embolized. The esophageal tracheal Combitube is removed and the patient is intubated with direct laryngoscopy.

History of the Tracheal Esophageal Combitube. The tracheal esophageal Combitube was developed from the concept of the esophageal obturator (ESO) airway, which was introduced in 1968.[206] The ESO consisted of a tracheal-like tube,

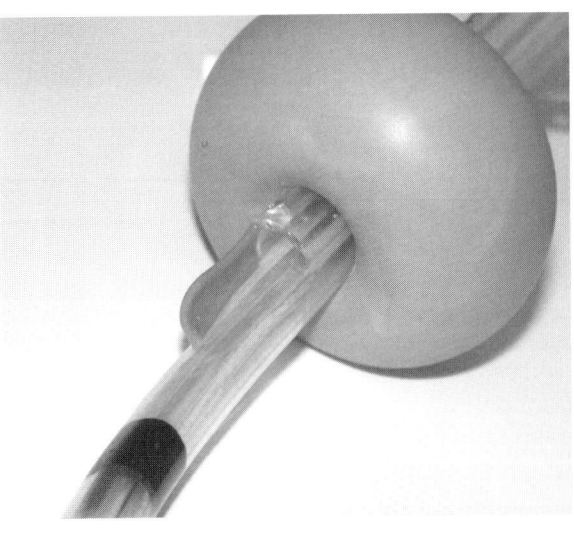

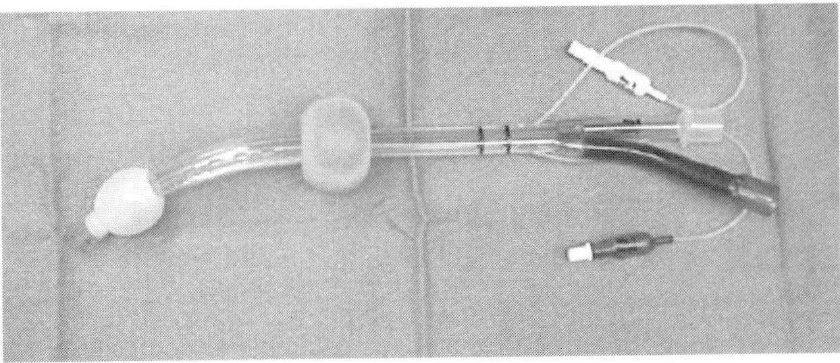
A

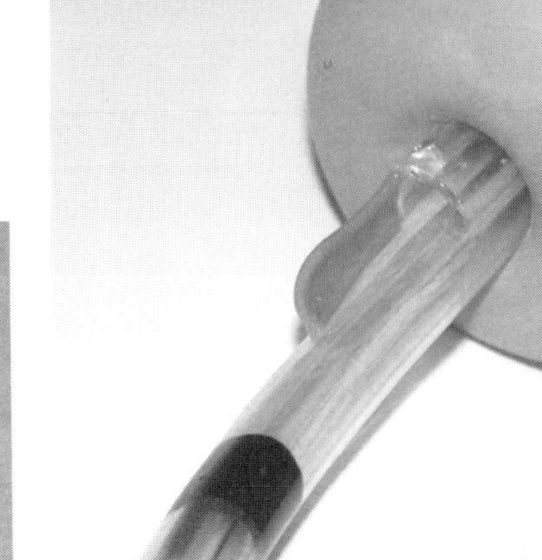
B

FIGURE 22-41. A. The esophageal tracheal Combitube. B. The fiberoptic port of the Easy Tube.

34 cm in length, with an inflatable cuff at its sealed, distal end. It was inserted blindly into the esophagus, so that the cuff lay at a level caudad and posterior to the tracheal carina. Sixteen holes communicating with the central lumen were positioned so as to be in the hypopharynx when inserted to the proper depth. A facemask at the proximal end was used to "seal" the airway. Ventilation was achieved by applying positive pressure to the proximal open aperture, where it emerged from the facemask. Unfortunately, significant problems/complications became apparent as the ESO came into common practice.

These shortcomings of the ESO were addressed by Dr. Michael Frass, a critical care physician in Vienna, Austria, in 1986.[207] The facemask of the ESO was replaced by an oropharyngeal balloon, sealing the upper airway and anchoring the device against the hard palate. As with the ESO, perforations at the hypopharyngeal level allowed egress of air near the level of the larynx. A second lumen, patent from proximal to distal end, without perforations was substituted for the blind esophageal tube of the ESO. As with the ESO, a cuff at the distal aspect of the esophageal lumen occludes the esophagus. This design, named the Tracheal Esophageal Combitube, is functional if introduced into the esophagus (ventilation being achieved through the esophageal lumen, via the hypopharyngeal perforations) or in the trachea (ventilation being achieved through the tracheal lumen, via the distal aperture). In either case, the proximal balloon seals both the oral and nasal passages, and the distal conventional tracheal tube cuff isolates the respiratory system from the gastrointestinal system. The device is available in two sizes: the 41Fr size is used for larger adults (height >5.5 feet) and the 37Fr size is used for adults 4 to 6 feet tall (Fig. 22-41). Though a single-use device, Combitube reprocessing and reuse has been reported.[208]

Use of the Esophageal Tracheal Combitube. The esophageal tracheal Combitube is inserted "blindly." The operator lifts the lower jaw and tongue anteriorly with one hand, and the esophageal tracheal Combitube is inserted with a downward, caudad-curved motion until the proximal depth indicator (two black rings printed on the double lumen tube) come to rest at the level of the teeth. The oropharyngeal balloon is inflated with 100 mL of air through a blue plastic pilot balloon (85 mL in the small adult size) while the distal cuff is inflated with 5 to 15 mL (via a white pilot balloon). An ambu bag or anesthesia circuit is attached to the proximal end of the esophageal lumen (constructed of blue polyvinyl chloride), and ventilation is confirmed by auscultation or other means. Because 90% of esophageal tracheal Combitube placements result in an esophageal position, ventilation occurs via this lumen's hypopharyngeal perforations. If no breath sounds are auscultated and/or gastric inflation is noted, the esophageal tracheal Combitube has been positioned in the trachea. Without repositioning, ventilation is changed to the distal end of tracheal lumen (clear polyvinyl chloride). If no maneuver improves ventilation, the device is most likely in the esophagus, but has been advanced too deeply, with the oropharyngeal cuff obstructing the airway.[209] In this case, the cuffs should be deflated, the device withdrawn 2 cm, and the ventilation sequence repeated.

Advantages of the esophageal tracheal Combitube include rapid airway control, airway protection from regurgitation, ease of use by the inexperienced operator, no requirement to visualize the larynx, and being able to maintain the neck in a neutral position, though cervical spine movement may be greater than that seen with the LMA, LMA-Fastrach, and flexible fiberscope.[210] It has been shown to be useful in the patient with massive upper gastrointestinal bleeding or vomiting, and as a rescue device in failed rapid-sequence induction or unanticipated difficult intubation. It is also useful in the morbidly obese, in acute bronchospasm, during cardiopulmonary resuscitation, and for prolonged ventilation after airway rescue.[129,163–174,211–217] Several series have demonstrated the effectiveness esophageal tracheal Combitube in prehospital management of the airway.[218–220] Urtubia et al have used the esophageal tracheal Combitube for elective surgery with a high success and low complication rate.[221]

Techniques for exchange of the esophageal tracheal Combitube (after patient stabilization) for an endotracheal tube have been described.[222]

Contraindications to use of the esophageal tracheal Combitube use include esophageal obstruction or other abnormality, ingestion of caustic agents, upper airway foreign body or mass, lower airway obstruction, height less than 4 feet, and an intact gag reflex. Since the esophageal tracheal Combitube includes latex in its construction, it should not be used in patients with latex allergy.

Complications associated with the esophageal tracheal Combitube have included lacerations to the pyriform sinus and esophageal wall resulting in subcutaneous emphysema, pneumomediastinum, pneumoperitoneum, and esophageal rupture.[223–225]

A device similar to the esophageal tracheal Combitube has been available in many parts of the world since 2003.[226] The Easy Tube (EzT) (Rusch International, Kernen, German) is distributed in two sizes, 41ch for patients above 130 cm in height and 28ch for patients 90 to 130 cm in height. Unlike the Combitube, the distal lumen of the EzT is designed to resemble an ETT (including a Murphy eye). The pharyngeal aperture is designed to allow easy passage of a fiberscope (or suction catheter) (Fig. 22-41B). The EzT was designed for routine anesthetics as well as emergency and cannot intubate/cannot ventilate situations. Contraindications to EzT use are identical to those for the Combitube. Though it may be inserted blindly, it is designed to be used with a laryngoscope (much like a standard ETT). Unlike the Combitube, it is latex free.

Case 4: Failed Rapid-Sequence Induction and the LMA

A 39-year-old male presents for elective uvulopharyngopalatoplasty. He has no previous surgical history. His maximal incisor gap is 5 cm, thyromental distance is 7 cm, and his oropharyngeal view is a Samsoon–Young Class 2. There is no limitation in head and neck flexion and extension. During a sleep apnea study, he had 15 apneic events each hour. The patient has a significant history of gastroesophageal reflux, and rapid-sequence induction is planned. After the administration of pentothal, succinylcholine, and cricoid pressure (Sellick maneuver), direct laryngoscopy with a Macintosh number 3 laryngoscope blade reveals a large epiglottis obscuring the view of the vocal folds (Cormack–Lehane Grade 3).[125] Significant hyperplasia of the base of the tongue, which prevents its full displacement, is also noted. The BURP maneuver does not improve the view.[122] A Macintosh 4 and Miller 3 blades are used and do not improve the view. Oxygen saturation, which was 100% prior to induction, is now 92%, and facemask ventilation is initiated with the Sellick maneuver in place. Complete obstruction to ventilation is encountered, despite chin and/or jaw lift, two-person ventilation, and a reduction in the degree of cricoid pressure. The oxygen saturation falls to 85% and a size 5 LMA (which had been prepared prior to the induction of anesthesia) is inserted with the technique as described by the inventor. Immediately, a clear airway is established, and the Sellick pressure remains in place. A second dose of pentothal is administered, and the patient is intubated by the blind passage of a 7.0-id ETT via the LMA. The LMA is then removed using a Cook airway exchange catheter (Cook Critical Care, Bloomington, IN) as a stylet, and the surgical case proceeds.

The LMA in the Failed Airway. One clear advantage of LMA use is in the failed airway. There have been many reported (and unreported) cases of failed intubation and failure to ventilate by facemask in which the airway was rescued with an LMA.[227,228] Parmet et al estimate that 1:800,000 failed airway patients cannot be managed with an LMA, providing an 80-fold increase in margin of safety over the oft-noted 1:10,000 patients who cannot be ventilated by mask nor intubated by traditional means.[162] Likewise, a wealth of literature describes the use of the LMA in elective difficult airway management in awake and unconscious patients, in anticipated and unanticipated situations, in cervical spine injury, and in pediatric dysmorphic syndromes.[103,104,162,229,230] The characteristics of the LMA that underlie its superiority as a tool in the difficult airway armamentarium are that it is well tolerated by the patient, simulating the natural distension of the hypopharyngeal tissues by food, and that its insertion follows an intrinsic pathway, requiring no tissue distortion (as with laryngoscopy), which may not be possible in all patients. Finally, it is a blind technique not hindered by blood, secretions, debris, and edema from previous attempts at laryngoscopy.[229] Because the LMA's ease of insertion is not dependent on anatomy that can be assessed on routine physical exam, typical airway assessment measures do not apply to its application.[230] The major disadvantage of the LMA in resuscitation is the lack of mechanical protection from regurgitation and aspiration. Lower rates of regurgitation during CPR (3.5%) than with the bag-valve mask ventilation (12.4%) have been shown.[52,231–233] Even in the face of regurgitation, pulmonary aspiration is a rare event with the LMA.[234] Unfortunately, the use of the Sellick maneuver may prevent proper seating of the LMA in a minority of instances.[235–237] This may require the brief removal of the cricoid pressure until the LMA has been properly seated. Cricoid pressure is effective with an LMA in situ. Had it been available, the Fastrack-LMA would also have been an ideal device in this case scenario.

Case 5: Deviation from the Difficult Airway Algorithm

Thirteen hours after admission to the intensive care unit, a 76-year-old female who had sustained trauma to the face, head, and neck in a motor vehicle accident is noted to have progressive decline in her level of consciousness and respiratory effort. On examination, there appears to be an adequate interincisor gap and thyromental distance. The oropharyngeal view and range of motion of the head and neck cannot be evaluated. Owing to the inability to fully evaluate the airway with respect to ease of intubation, an awake procedure is chosen. Fiberoptic devices are not considered usable because of the presence of fresh and clotted blood in the mouth as a result of continued epistaxis. Other airway techniques that require significant patient preparation are not considered because of the rapid progression of the patient's respiratory failure. Additionally, the presence of fresh blood in the oral and pharyngeal cavities will hinder adequate drying and analgesia. Blind nasal intubation is considered contraindicated based upon the obvious facial trauma and the risk of cribriform plate disruption. Neither equipment for retrograde intubation nor the tracheal esophageal Combitube is readily available. A lighted stylet intubation guide is available, but no clinician present is experienced with this technique. Although the mental status change is believed to reflect an intracranial process (e.g., intracranial hypertension), the risk of complete loss of the airway is judged to be the primary clinical hazard. Awake direct laryngoscopy is attempted with manual in-line stabilization of the neck. After clearing fresh blood from the pharynx with a Yankauer suction catheter, a Cormack–Lehane Grade 3 laryngeal view is obtained; but because of patient resistance (biting on the laryngoscope and movement), tracheal intubation is not achieved. The decision is made to proceed with rapid-sequence induction and intubation, with preparations made for an emergency tracheostomy. After surgical preparation of the neck and preoxygenation, intravenous succinylcholine and etomidate are administered, direct laryngoscopy is undertaken, the larynx is easily visualized, and the trachea is intubated.

Muscle Relaxants and Direct Laryngoscopy. In the case described, the use of muscle relaxants significantly improved the ability to visualize the larynx.[238–240] In a recent study, the use of muscle relaxants during a direct laryngoscopy increased the success rate of intubation and was associated with fewer incidents of airway trauma, intubation attempts, esophageal intubations, aspiration, and even death.[241] Intubating conditions with and without muscle relaxation have been investigated in few well-controlled trials because the superior intubating conditions achieved with muscle relaxants has discouraged inclusion of control groups.[242] The effects of muscle relaxation actions that improve laryngoscopic view include allowing complete temporomandibular joint relaxation and opening, anterior movement of the epiglottis, and widening of the laryngeal vestibule and laryngeal sinus.[243,244] In addition, the finding that laryngoscopic stimulation of the pharyngeal musculature causes the upper airway lumen to appear small is offset by the use of relaxants.

Leaving the Algorithm. The situation described in Case 5 is unusual in that rapid-sequence induction was attempted because the clinical situation had deviated from the ASA Difficult Airway Algorithm owing to the progressive nature of the airway compromise. The situation was more akin to the "crash" airway described by Walls et al.[205] In this case, the institution of muscle relaxation, which might be considered contraindicated in the apparently difficult-to-intubate patient, allowed for full visualization of the larynx. Knowing that failure to intubate in this case would result in probable loss of the airway, the clinician was prepared for cricothyroidotomy. Although the ASA's Difficult Airway Algorithm is a valuable tool in the process of approaching the difficult airway, the clinician must always be prepared for the case that does not fit the mold. As stated earlier, adaptability in a rapidly changing clinical situation is critical to the success of airway management. Also of interest in this case was the availability of a lighted stylet for use in similar difficult airway scenarios. Although this device may have been useful in the current case, no clinician present was familiar with its operation. A critical situation is not an occasion for trying an unfamiliar technology.

Other Devices

An ever-increasing number of airway management devices are commercially available. Although encyclopedic coverage of these tools is beyond the scope of this chapter, a review of the more established equipment follows.

Lighted Stylets

These devices rely on transillumination of the airway. A light source introduced into the trachea will produce a well-circumscribed glow of the tissues over the larynx and trachea. The same light placed in the esophagus will produce no or a diffuse light. A number of devices have become available, including disposable, partly disposable, and fully reusable systems. Although there are many reports of successful intubation using these devices, some common problems have been noted: In general, the operating theater lights must be dimmed to best appreciate the circumscribed glow; a stylet tip successfully placed in the trachea, but not pointing in an anterior direction, may give a false-negative impression; it is often difficult to remove the semirigid stylet from the ETT after intubation.

Airway Bougie

These encompass a series of solid or hollow, semimalleable stylets that may be blindly manipulated in to the trachea. An ETT is then "threaded" over the bougie and into the trachea. These bougies are generally low in cost and highly portable. The Eschmann introducer (Eschmann Health Care, Kent, England) was introduced in 1949. It is 60 cm long, 15Fr-gauge, and angled 40 degrees 3.5 cm from its distal end (Fig. 22-42). It is constructed from a woven polyester base, which is malleable. It can be very helpful when the larynx cannot be visualized with laryngoscopy. The introducer (also known as the gum elastic bougie) can be manipulated under the epiglottis, its angled segment directed anteriorly toward the larynx. Once it has entered the larynx and trachea, a distinctive "clicking" feel is elicited as the tip passes over the cartilaginous structures. A similar device, the Frova Intubating Introducer (Cook Critical Care, Bloomington, IN), is a disposable device, with an optional "stiffening" stylet and a hollow bore. The internal lumen allows for the insufflation of oxygen, the detection of carbon dioxide, and the use of a self-inflating bulb to detect inadvertent esophageal placement.[245]

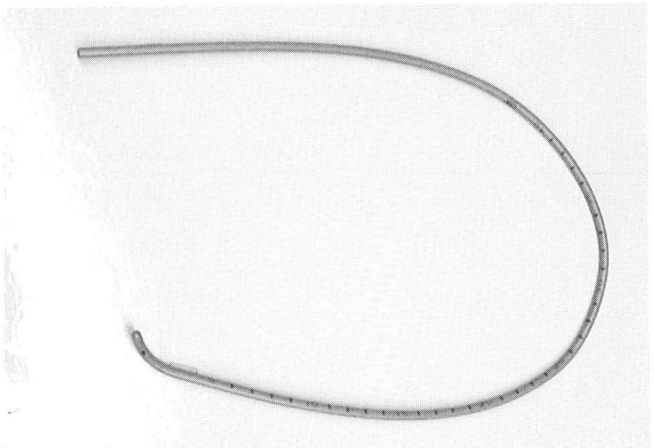

FIGURE 22-42. Frova Intubating Introducer (Cook Critical Care, Bloomington, IN)

Minimally Invasive Transtracheal Procedures

When access to the airway from the mouth or nose fails or is unavailable (e.g., maxillofacial, pharyngeal, or laryngeal trauma, pathology, or deformity), emergency access via the extrathoracic trachea is a feasible route to the airway. The clinician must be familiar with these alternative techniques of oxygenation and ventilation. The decision to proceed with an invasive procedure can be difficult, and most clinicians will hesitate at potentially grave risk to the patient. One should consider becoming facile with at least one of these techniques in elective situations (such as transtracheal aspiration for airway analgesia or elective retrograde intubation or, consider, for example, assisting a surgical colleague on a tracheostomy). Although tracheostomy and cricothyroidotomy are beyond the scope of this chapter, percutaneous techniques will be considered.

Cricothyroidotomy, cricothyrotomy, coniotomy, and minitracheostomy are synonyms for establishing an air passage through the cricothyroid membrane. The anatomy of this structure and those surrounding it was discussed earlier in this chapter. Although cricothyrotomy is the procedure of choice in an emergency situation, it may also apply to an elective situation when there is limited access to the trachea (e.g., severe cervical kyphoscoliosis). Cricothyrotomy is contraindicated in neonates and children under 6 years of age, and in patients with laryngeal fractures.

Percutaneous Transtracheal Jet Ventilation

Percutaneous transtracheal jet ventilation (TTJV), as a form of cricothyroidotomy, is the most familiar to anesthesiologists.[246]
17 The ASA Difficult Airway Algorithm lists transtracheal jet ventilation as an option in the cannot mask ventilate/cannot intubate situation. TTJV is a simple and relatively safe means to sustain the patient's life in this critical situation.[247] An intravenous catheter of 12-, 14-, or 16-gauge, attached to a 5-mL or larger empty or partially fluid-filled (saline or local anesthetic) syringe should be used to enter the airway. The patient is positioned supine, with the head midline or extended on the neck and thorax (if not contraindicated by the clinical situation). After aseptic preparation, local anesthetic is injected over the cricothyroid membrane (if the patient is awake and time permits). The right-handed clinician stands on the right side of the patient, facing the head. The clinician can use his or her nondominant hand to stabilize the larynx. The catheter-needle is advanced at right angles to all planes in the caudad third of the membrane. From the moment of skin puncture there should be constant aspiration on the syringe plunger. Free aspiration of

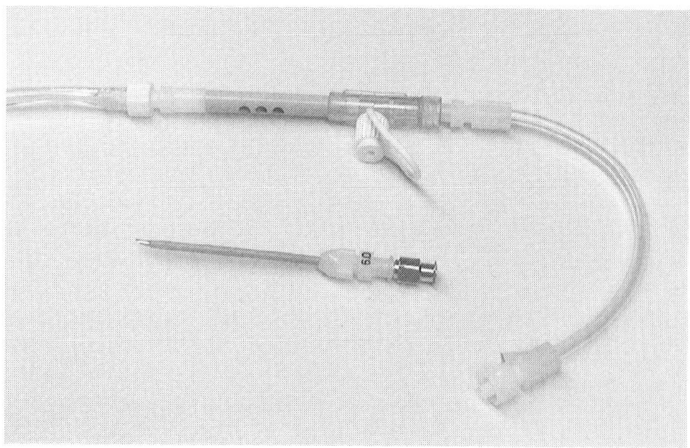

FIGURE 22-43. The Cook Critical Care transtracheal ventilation catheter and Enk Flow Modulator (Cook Critical Care, Bloomington, IN).

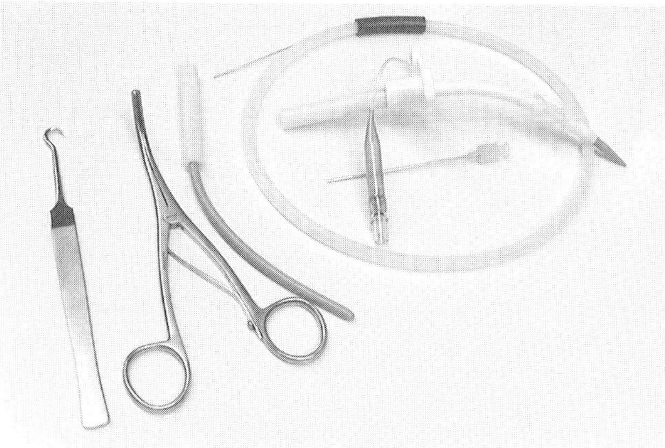

FIGURE 22-45. The Melker cricothyroidotomy cannula and curved dialator (Cook Critical Care, Bloomington, IN). The guidewire is not shown.

air confirms entrance into the trachea. Unless there is significant pulmonary fluid (e.g., blood, aspirated gastric contents, or water from drowning), the aspiration of tracheal air should be incontrovertible. The needle-catheter assembly should be advanced slightly, and subsequently the catheter advanced fully into the airway alone. Although this technique has been described with common angiocatheters, dedicated devices made of kink-resistant materials and with accessory ports are available (Fig. 22-43).

Once the catheter has been successfully placed in the airway, an oxygen source is attached. The clinician may have several options in this regard. If a high-pressure system is available—for example, a metered and adjustable oxygen source with a hand-controlled valve (Fig. 22-44) and a Luer-lock connector—25 to 30 psi of oxygen (central hospital supply or regulated cylinder) can be delivered directly through the catheter, with insufflations of 1 to 1.5 seconds at a rate of 12 insufflations per minute. If a 16-gauge catheter has been placed, this system will deliver a tidal volume of 400 to 700 mL. Low-pressure systems cannot provide enough flow to expand the chest adequately for oxygenation and ventilation (e.g., ambu bag: 6 psi, common gas outlet: 20 psi).

Low-pressure oxygen flow meters can be used for TTJV. These systems are capable of delivering a brief (0.5 second) 30 psi burst pressure, which quickly decays to 5 psi or less.[248] If this oxygen source is to be used an I:E ratio of 1:1 with a

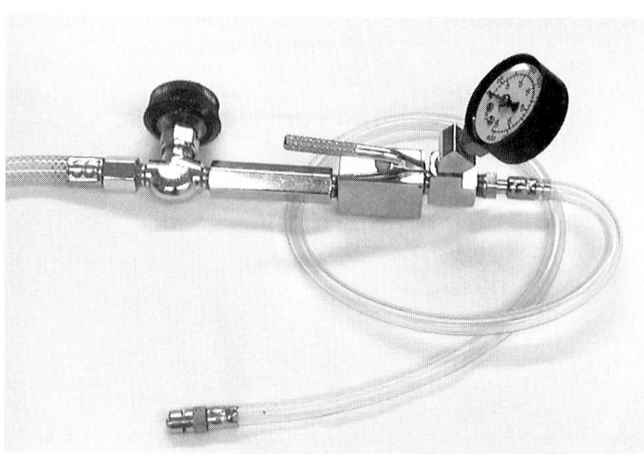

FIGURE 22-44. System for regulation of a high-pressure oxygen source for transtracheal jet ventilation.

rate of 30 to 60 breaths per minute should be used to assure adequate burst pressures.

The Muallem Jet Ventilator (Dr. Muallem Lebanon) automates respiratory cycles during jet ventilation. This device was developed primarily for use during bronchoscopy but could be applicable to TTJV.[249]

Specialized percutaneous cricothyroidotomy systems have been developed that improve the ease of this technique. These devices generally provide a large-bore access that is adequate for oxygenation and ventilation with low-pressure systems. The Melker emergency cricothyroidotomy catheter set (Cook Critical Care, Bloomington, IN) uses a Seldinger—catheter-over-a-wire—technique familiar to most anesthesia practitioners (Fig. 22-45). The set comes in a variety of cannula sizes (3.5-, 4-, and 6-mm internal diameter cuffed and uncuffed). Preparation and positioning of the patient are the same as with needle cricothyroidotomy. A 1- to 1.5-cm vertical incision of the skin only is made over the lower third of the cricothyroid membrane. Aiming 45° caudad, a percutaneous puncture of the subcutaneous tissue and cricothyroid membrane is made with the provided 18-gauge needle-catheter assembly and syringe. After air is aspirated, the catheter is advanced into the trachea. The provided guidewire is inserted through the catheter and into the trachea. The catheter is removed and the tracheal cannula, fitted internally with a curved dilator, is threaded onto the wire. The dilator is advanced through the membrane using firm pressure. Significant resistance to its advancement may indicate that the skin incision needs to be extended. Once the cannula-dilator has been fully inserted, the dilator and wire are removed. The 15-mm circuit adapter end of the cannula is now attached to an ambu bag or anesthesia circuit.

Other percutaneous systems include Nu-Trake (Weiss Emergency Airway System; International Medical Devices) and the QuickTrach® transtracheal catheter (VBM Medizintechnik GMBH). Nonneedle puncture techniques are beyond the current discussion.

CONCLUSION

Apart from monitoring, the management of the "routine" patient airway is the most common task of the anesthesiologist—even during the administration of regional anesthesia, the airway must be monitored and possibly supported. Unfortunately, routine tasks often become neglected tasks in terms of the care and vigilance that is afforded each event. But the consequences of a lost airway are so devastating that the clinician can never afford a lackadaisical approach.

Although the ASA's Task Force on the Difficult Airway has given the medical community an immensely valuable tool in the approach to the patient with the difficult airway, the Task Force's algorithm must be viewed as a starting point only. Judgment, experience, the clinical situation, and available resources all affect the appropriateness of the chosen pathway through, or divergence from, the algorithm. The clinician need not be expert in all the equipment and techniques currently available. Rather, a broad range of approaches should be mastered, so that the failure of one does not present a road block to success.

Similarly, the medical manufacturing community, and the far-sighted clinicians who supply it with concepts for airway management products, has supplied a vast array of devices. Many represent redundancy in concept, and each has its supporters and detractors. No one device can be considered superior to another when considered in isolation. It is the clinician and his or her resources (both equipment and personnel) and judgment that determine the effectiveness of any technique. In the management of the difficult airway, flexibility, and not rigidity, prevails.[250,251]

References

1. Caplan RA, Posner KL, Ward RJ *et al:* Adverse respiratory events in anesthesia: A closed claims analysis. Anesthesiology 72:828, 1990
2. Domino KB, Posner KL, Caplan RA, Cheney FW: Airway Injury during Anesthesia: A Closed Claims Analysis. Anesthesiology 91:1703, 1999
3. Ovassapian A, Glassenberg R, Randel GI, Klock A, Mesnick PS, Klafta JM: The unexpected difficult airway and lingual tonsil hyperplasia. A case series and a review of the literature. Anesthesiology 97:124, 2002
4. Takenaka I, Kadoya T, Aoyama K: Is awake intubation necessary when the laryngeal mask is feasible? Anesth Analg 91:246, 2000
5. Westhorpe RN: The position of the larynx in children and its relationship to the ease of intubation. Anaesth Intens Care 15:384, 1987
6. Karkouti K, Rose DK, Ferris LE, Wigglesworth DF, Meisami-Fard T, Lee H: Inter-observer reliability of ten tests used for predicting difficult tracheal intubation. Can J Anesth 43:554, 1996
7. el-Ganzouri AR, McCarthy RJ, Tuman KJ, Tanck EN, Ivankovich AD: Preoperative airway assessment: Predictive value of a multivariate risk index. Anesth Analg 82:1197, 1996
8. Mallampati SR, Gatt SP, Gugino LD *et al:* A clinical sign to predict difficult tracheal intubation: A prospective study. Can Anaesth Soc J 32:429, 1985
9. Wilson ME, Spiegelhalter D, Robertson J, Lesser P. Predicting difficult intubation Br J Anaesth 61:211, 1988
10. Patel SK, Whitten CW, Ivy R 3rd *et al:* Failure of the laryngeal mask airway: An undiagnosed laryngeal carcinoma. Anesth Analg 86:438, 1998
11. Langeron O, Masso E, Huraux C *et al:* Prediction of difficult mask ventilation. Anesthesiology 92:1229, 2000
12. Cass NM, James NR, Lines V: Difficult direct laryngoscopy complicating intubation for anesthesia. Br Med J 1:488, 1956
13. White A, Kander: Anatomical factors in difficult direct laryngoscopy. Br J Anaesth 47:468, 1975
14. Benumof JL: Preoxygenation: Best method for both efficacy and efficiency (editorial). Anesthesiology 91:603, 1999
15. Wilson WC: Emergency airway management on the ward. In Hannowell LA, Waldron RJ (eds): Airway Management, p 443, Lippincott-Raven Publishers, 1996
16. Gambee AM, Hertzka RE, Fisher DM: Preoxygenation techniques: Comparison of three minutes and four breaths. Anesth Analg 66:468, 1987
17. Jense HG, Dubin SA, Silverstein PI, O'Leary-Escolas U: Effect of obesity on safe duration of apnea in anesthetized humans. Anesth Analg 72:89, 1991
18. Gold MI, Duarte I, Muravchick S: Arterial oxygenation in conscious patients after 5 minutes and after 30 seconds of oxygen breathing. Anesth Analg 60:313, 1981
19. Baraka AS, Taha SK, Aouad MT *et al:* Preoxygenation: Comparison of maximal breathing and tidal volume breathing techniques. Anesthesiology 91:612, 1999
20. Frumin MJ, Epstein RM, Cohen G: Apneic oxygenation in man. Anesthesiology 20:789, 1959
21. Rosenblatt WH, Ovassappian A, Eige S: Use of the laryngeal mask airway in the United States: A randomized survey of ASA members. ASA Annual Meeting, Orlando, Florida, 1998
22. Maktabi MA, Smith RB, Todd MM: Is routine endotracheal intubation as safe as we think or wish (Editorial). Anesthesiology 99:247, 2003
23. Tanaka A, Isono S, Ishikawa T, Soto J, Nishio T: Laryngeal resistance before and after minor surgery: Endotracheal tube versus laryngeal mask airway. Anesthesiology 99:252, 2003
24. Domino KB, Posner KL, Caplan PA, Cheney FW: Airway injury during anesthesia: A closed claims analysis. Anesthesiology 91:1703, 1999
25. Keller C, Brimacombe J: Mucosal pressure, mechanism of seal, airway sealing pressure, and anatomic position for the disposable versus reusable laryngeal mask airways. Anesth Analg 88:1418, 1999
26. Calder I, Picard J, Chapman M, O'Sullivan C, Crockard HA. Mouth opening: A new angle. Anesthesiology 99:799, 2003
27. Brain AIJ: The laryngeal mask and the oesophagus. Anaesthesia 46:701, 1991
28. Wilkinson PA, Cyna AM, MacLeod DM *et al:* The laryngeal mask: Cautionary tales. Anaesthesia 45:167, 1990
29. Nanji GM, Maltby JR: Vomiting and aspiration pneumonitis with the laryngeal mask airway. Can J Anaesth 38:69, 1992
30. Brimacombe J, Berry A: Aspiration and the laryngeal mask airway—a survey of Australian intensive care units. Anaesth Intens Care 20:534, 1992
31. Griffin RM, Hatcher IS: Aspiration pneumonia and the laryngeal mask airway. Anaesthesia 45:1039, 1990
32. Koehli N: Aspiration and laryngeal mask airway. Anaesthesia 46:419, 1991
33. Alexander R, Arrowsmith JE, Frossard JR: The layrngeal mask airway: Safe in the x-ray department. Anaesthesia 48:734, 1993
34. Maroof M, Khan RM, Siddique MS: Intraoperative aspiration pneumonitis and the laryngeal mask airway. Anesth Analg 77:405, 1993
35. Langer A, Hempel V, Ahlhelm T *et al:* Die Kehlkopfmaske bei 1900 allgeneinanasthesien—Erfahrungsbericht. Anaesthesiol Intensivmed Notfalmed Schmerzther, 28:156, 1993
36. Lussman RF, Gerber HR: Severe aspiration pneumonia with the laryngeal mask. Anaesthesiol Intensivmed Notfalmed Schmerzther 32:194, 1997
37. Ismail-Zade IA, Vanner RG: Regurgitation and aspiration of gastric contents in a child during general anaesthesia using the laryngeal mask airway. Paediatr Anaesth 6:325, 1996
38. Koay CK. A case of aspiration using the proseal LMA [Case Reports. Letter]. Anaesth Intensive Care 31(1):123, 2003, Feb
39. Cassinello F, Rodrigo FJ, Munoz-Alameda L, Perez-Tejerizo G, Vallejo D: Postoperative pulmonary aspiration of gastric contents in an infant after general anesthesia with laryngeal mask airway (LMA) [Case Reports. Letter]. Anesth Analg 90(6):1457, 2000
40. Brimacombe J, Keller C. Aspiration of gastric contents during use of a ProSeal laryngeal mask airway secondary to unidentified foldover malposition [Case Reports. Journal Article]. Anesth Analg 97(4):1192, table of contents, 2003 Oct.
41. Brimacombe JR, Berry A: The incidence of aspiration associated with the laryngeal mask airway: A meta-analysis of published literature. J Clin Anesth 7:297, 1995
42. Owens TM, Robertson P, Twomey C *et al:* The incidence of gastroesophageal reflux with the laryngeal mask: A comparison with the face mask using esophageal lumen pH electrodes. Anesth Analg 80:980, 1995
43. McCrory CR, McShane AJ: Gastroesophageal reflux during spontaneous respiration with the laryngeal mask airway. Can J Anaesth 46:268, 1999
44. Joshi GP, Morrison SG, Okonkwo NA, White PF: Continuous hypopharyngeal pH measurements in spontaneously breathing anesthetized outpatients: Laryngeal mask airway versus tracheal intubation. Anesth Analg 82:254, 1996
45. el Mikatti N, Luthra AD, Healy TE, Mortimer AJ: Gastric regurgitation during general anaesthesia in different positions with the laryngeal mask airway. Anaesthesia 50:1053, 1995
46. Hong S-Y, Byung-Te S: Laryngeal Mask Airway for Cesarean Section. World Congress of Anaesthesiologists D770, 1996
47. Liew E, Chan-Liao M: Experience of Using Laryngeal Mask Anesthesia for Cesarean Section. World Congress of Anaesthesiologists D771. 14, 1996
48. Dysart R: The Laryngeal Mask Airway in Pregnancy and Postpartum (Abstract). New Zealand Society of Anaesthetists & Australia College of Anaesthetists, 1993
49. Pennant JH, Walker MB: Comparison of the endotracheal tube and laryngeal mask in airway management by paramedical personnel. Anesth Analg 74:531, 1992
50. Hayes A, McCarrol SM: Airway management in unskilled personnel—a comparison of laryngeal mask airway, pocket mask and bag valve mask techniques. Anesthesiology 83:A223, 1995
51. Grantham H, Phillips G: The laryngeal mask in prehospital emergency care. Emerg Med 7:57, 1995
52. Tanigawa K, Shigematsu A: Choice of airway devices for 12,020 cases of nontraumatic cardiac arrest in Japan. Prehosp Emerg Care 2:96, 1998
53. Atherton GL, Johnson JC: Ability of paramedics to use the Combitube in prehospital cardiac arrest. Ann Emerg Med 22:1263, 1993
54. Haden RM, Pinnock CA, Scott PV: Incidence of aspiration with the laryngeal mask airway. Br J Anaesth 72:496, 1994
55. Yardy N, Hancox D, Strang TSO: A comparison of two airway aids for emergency use by unskilled personnel: The Combitube and laryngeal mask. Anaesthesia 54:181, 1999
56. Han TH, Brimacombe J, Lee EJ, Yang HS: The laryngeal mask airway is effective (and probably safe) in selected healthy parturients for elective Cesarean section: A prospective study of 1067 cases. Can J Anaesth 48:1117, 2001

57. Stone BJ, Chantler PJ: The incidence of regurgitation during cardiopulmonary resuscitation: A comparison between the bag valve mask and laryngeal mask airway. Resuscitation 38:3, 1998
58. Rosenblatt WH. Airway Management. In Barash PG, Cullen BF, Stoelting RK (eds): Clinical Anesthesia, p 595. Philadelphia, Lippincott Williams and Wilkins, 2000
59. Verghese C, Brimacombe J: Survey of laryngeal mask airway usage in 11,910 patients: Safety and efficacy for conventional and nonconventional usage. Anesth Analg 82:129, 1996
60. Graziotti PJ: Intermittent positive pressure ventilation through a laryngeal mask airway. Is a nasogastric tube useful? Anaesthesia 47:1088, 1992
61. Ho BY, Skinner HJ, Mahajan RP: Gastro-oesophageal reflux during day case gynaecological laparoscopy under positive pressure ventilation: Laryngeal mask vs. tracheal intubation. Anaesthesia 54:93, 1999
62. Voyagis GS, Papakalou EP: A comparison of the laryngeal mask and tracheal tube for controlled ventilation. Acta Anaesthesiol Belg 47:81, 1996
63. André E, Capdevila X, Vialles N *et al:* Pressure-controlled ventilation with a laryngeal mask airway during general anaesthesia. Br J Anaesth 80 (suppl 1):244, 1998
64. Gursoy F, Algren JT, Skjonsby BS: Positive pressure ventilation with the laryngeal mask airway in children. Anesth Analg 82:33, 1996
65. Latorre F, Eberle B, Weiler N *et al:* Laryngeal mask airway position and the risk of gastric insufflation. Anesth Analg 86:867, 1998
66. Brimacombe JR, Brain AI, Berry AM *et al:* Gastric insufflation and the laryngeal mask. Anesth Analg 86:914, 1998
67. Brimacombe JR, Brain AIJ: The laryngeal mask airway. A Review and Practical Guide, 2nd ed. London, WB Saunders, 2004
68. Brimacombe J, Shorney N: The laryngeal mask airway and prolonged balanced regional anaesthesia. Can J Anaesth 40:360, 1993
69. Brimacombe J, Keller C: Comparison of the flexible and standard laryngeal mask airways. Can J Anaesth 46:558, 1999
70. Williams PJ, Bailey PM: Comparison of the reinforced laryngeal mask airway and tracheal intubation for adenotonsillectomy. Br J Anaesth 70:30, 1993
71. Brimacombe JR, Keller C, Gunkel AR *et al:* The influence of the tonsillar gag on efficacy of seal, anatomic position, airway patency, and airway protection with the flexible laryngeal mask airway: A randomized, cross-over study of fresh adult cadavers. Anesth Analg 89:181, 1999
72. John RE, Hill S, Hughes TJ: Airway protection by the laryngeal mask: A barrier to dye placed in the pharynx. Anaesthesia 46:366, 1991
73. Cork RC, Depa RM, Standen JR: Prospective comparison of use of the laryngeal mask and endotracheal tube for ambulatory surgery. Anesth Analg 79:719, 1994
74. Kaplan A, Crosby GJ, Bhattacharyya N: Airway protection and the laryngeal Mask Airway. Laryngoscope 114:652, 2004
75. Young PJ, Basson C, Hamilton D *et al:* Prevention of tracheal aspiration using the pressure-limited tracheal tube cuff. Anaesthesia 54:559, 1999
76. Kim ES, Bishop MJ: Endotracheal intubation, but not laryngeal mask airway insertion, produces reversible bronchoconstriction. Anesthesiology 90:391, 1999
77. Berry A, Brimacombe J, Keller C *et al:* Pulmonary airway resistance with the endotracheal tube versus laryngeal mask airway in paralyzed anesthetized adult patients. Anesthesiology 90:395, 1999
78. Groudine SB, Lumb PD, Sandison MR: Pressure support ventilation with the laryngeal mask airway: A method to manage severe reactive airway disease post-operatively. Can J Anaesth 42:341, 1995
79. Benumof JL: Laryngeal mask airway and the ASA difficult airway algorithm. Anesthesiology 84:686, 1996
80. Erskine RJ, Rabey PG: The laryngeal mask airway in recovery. Anaesthesia 47:354, 1992
81. Kitching AJ, Walpole AR, Blogg CE: Removal of the laryngeal mask airway in children: Anaesthetized compared with awake (Abstract). Br J Anaesth 76:874, 1996
82. Deakin CD, Diprose P, Majumdar R, Pulletz M: An investigation into the quantity of secretions removed by inflated and deflated laryngeal mask airways. Anaesthesia 55:478, 2000
83. Beckford NS, Mayo R, Wilkinson A 3d *et al:* Effects of short-term endotracheal intubation on vocal function. Laryngoscope 100:331, 1990
84. Lowinger D, Benjamin B, Gadd L: Recurrent laryngeal nerve injury caused by a laryngeal mask airway. Anaesth Intens Care 27:202, 1999
85. Sommer M, Shuldt M, Runge U, Gielen-Wijffels S, Marcus MAE: Bilateral hypoglossal nerve injury following the use of the laryngeal mask airway without the use of nitrous oxide. Acta Anesthesiology Scand 48:377, 2004
86. Lumb AB, Wrigley MW: The effect of nitrous oxide on laryngeal mask cuff pressure: *In vitro* and *in vivo* studies. Anaesthesia 47:320, 1992
87. Lowinger D, Benjamin B, Gadd L: Recurrent laryngeal nerve injury caused by a laryngeal mask airway. Anaesth Intens Care 27:202, 1999
88. Brain AI: Pressure in laryngeal mask airway. Anaesthesia 51:603, 1996
89. Branthwaite MA: An unexpected complication of the intubating laryngeal mask. Anaesthesia 54:166, 1999
90. Bellhouse CP, Dore C: Criteria for estimating likelihood of difficulty of endotracheal intubation with the Macintosh laryngoscope. Anaesth Intens Care 16:329, 1988
91. Brain AI: The oesophageal vent-laryngeal. Br J Anaesth 72:727, 1994
92. Keller C, Brimacombe J, Dleinsosser A, Loeckinger A. Does the proseal laryngeal mask prevent aspiration of regurgitated fluid. Anesth Analg 91:1017, 2000
93. Maltby JR, Beriault MT, Watson NC, Liepert D, Gordon HF. The LMA-proseal is an effective alternative to tracheal intubation for laparoscopic cholecystectomy. Can J Anaesth 49:857, 2002
94. Brimacombe J, Keller C, Fullkrug B *et al:* A multicenter study comparing the proseal and classic laryngeal mask airway in anesthetized, non-paralyzed patients. Anesthesiology 96:289, 2002
95. Brain AIJ, Verghese C, Strube PJ: The LMA Proseal—a laryngeal mask with an oesophageal vent. Br J Anaesth 84:650, 2000
96. Stix MS, O'Connor: Depth of insertion of the proseal laryngeal mask airway. Br J Anesth 90:235, 2003
97. O'Connor CJ, Borromeo CJ, Stix MS: Assessing proseal laryngeal mask position: The suprasternal notch test (Letter). Anesth Analg 94:1374, 2002
98. Brimacombe J, Keller C, Berg A: Gastric insufflation with the proseal laryngeal mask. Anesth Analg 92:1614, 2001
99. O'Connor CJ, Davies SR, Stix MS: Soap bubbles and gauze thread drain tube tests. Anesth Analg 93:1078, 2001
100. Brimacombe J, Keller C, Berg A: Gastric insufflation with the proseal laryngeal mask. Anesth Analg 92:1614, 2001
101. Brimacombe J, Keller C, Berg A, Mitchell S: Assessing proseal laryngeal mask positioning: The suprasternal notch test. Anesth Analg 94:1375, 2002
102. Brimacombe J, Keller C: Aspiration of gastric contents during use of a proseal laryngeal mask airway secondary to unidentified folded malpositions. Anesth Analg 97:1192, 2003
103. Rosenblatt WH: The use of the LMA-proseal in airway resuscitation. Anesth Analg 97:1773, 2004
104. Awan R, Nolan JP, Cook TM: Use of the proseal laryngeal mask for airway maintenance during emergency cesarean section of the failed tracheal intubation. Br J Anaesth 92:144, 2004
105. Stix MS, Borromeo CJ, O'Connor CJ: Esophageal insufflation with normal fiber optic position of the proseal laryngeal mesh airway. Anesth Analog 94:1036, 2002
106. Gaitini LA, Vaida SJ, Samri M *et al:* An evaluation of the laryngeal tube during general aesthesia using mechanical ventilation. Anesth Analog 96:1750, 2003
107. Ocker H, Volker W, Schmucker P, Steinfath M, Volker D: A comparison of the laryngeal tube with the laryngeal mask airway during routine surgical procedures. Anesth Analg 95:1094, 2002
108. Agro' F, Carassitti M, Barzoi 6, Millozzi F, Galli B: A first report on the diagnosis and treatment of acute postoperative airway obstruction with the cobra PLA. Can J Anesth 51:640, 2004
109. Gaitini LA, Samri MJ, Mesh K, Yanovski B, Vaida S: A comparison of the laryngeal mask airway unique, pharyngeal X press and per laryngeal airway cobra in paralyzed anesthetized adult patients. Anesthesiology A-1494, 2003
110. Chow HC, Wu TL: Thyromental distance and anterior larynx: misconceptional and misname? Anesth Analg 96:1526, 2003
111. Benumof JL: Both a large and small thyromental distance can predict difficult intubation. Anesth Analg 97:1543, 2003
112. Chow HC, Wu TL: Br J Anaes 71:335, 1993
113. Practice guidelines for the management of the difficult airway: An updated report by the American Society of Anesthesiologists Task Force on Management of the Difficult Airway. Anesthesiology 98:1269, 2003
114. Kikkawa YS, Koichi T, Nimi S: Prediction and surgical management of difficult laryngoscopy. Laryngoscopy 114:776, 2003
115. Bannister FB, MacBeth RG: Direct laryngoscopy and tracheal intubation. Lancet ii:651, 1944
116. Adnet F, Borran SW, Lapostalle F, Lapandry C: The three axis alignment theory and the sniffing position: Perpetuation of an anatomic myth? Anesthesiology 91:1964, 1999
117. Chow HC, Wu TL: Rethinking the three axis alignment theory for direct laryngoscopy. Acta Anaesthesiol Scand 45:261, 2001
118. Rosenblatt WH: Preoperative planning of airway management in critical care patients. Critical Care Medicine 32(suppl 4):186, 2004
119. Ayoub C, Baraka A, el-Khatib M, Muallem M, Kawkabani N, Soueide A: A new cut-off point of thyromental distance for prediction of difficult airway. Middle East J Anesthesiol 15(6):619. 2000 Oct
120. Iohom G, Ronayne M, Cunningham AJ: Prediction of difficult tracheal intubation. Eur J Anaesthesiol 20:31, 2003
121. Ovassapian A: Case reports. In Ovassapian A (ed): Fiberoptic Airway Endoscopy in Anesthesia and Critical Care, p 149. New York, Raven Press 1990
122. Ulrich B, Listyo R, Gerig HJ *et al:* The difficult intubation: The value of BURP and 3 predictive tests of difficult intubation. Anaesthesist 47:45, 1998
123. Takahata O, Kubota M, Mamiya K et al: The efficacy of the "BURP" maneuver during a difficult laryngoscopy. Anesth Analg 84:419, 1997
124. Benumof JL, Cooper SD: Quantitative improvement in laryngoscopic view by optimal external laryngeal manipulation. J Clin Anesth 8:136, 1996
125. Cormack RS, Lehane J: Difficult tracheal intubation in obstetrics. Anaesthesia 39:1105, 1984
126. Rose DK, Cohen MM. The airway: Problems and predictions in 18,500 patients. Canadian J of Anaesth 41:372, 1994

127. Benumof JL: The American Society of Anesthesiologists' management of the difficult airway algorithm and explanation-analysis of the algorithm. In Benumof JL (ed): Airway Management: Principles and Practice. St Louis, Mosby, 1996
128. Wheeler M: The difficult pediatric airway. In Hagberg C (ed): Handbook of Difficult Airway Management. Philadelphia, Churchill Livingston, 2000
129. Crosby ET, Cooper RM, Douglas MJ *et al*: The unanticipated difficult airway with recommendations for management. Can J Anaesth 45:757, 1998
130. Koh LK, Kong CE, Ip-Yam PC: The modified Cormack-Lehane score for the grading of direct laryngoscopy: Evaluation in the Asian population. Anaesth Intensive Care 30:48, 2002
132. Henderson JJ: The use of the paraglossal straight blade laryngoscopy in difficult tracheal intubation. Anaesthesia 52:552, 1997
131. Benumof JBL: Conventional (laryngoscopic) orotracheal and nasotracheal intubation (single-lumen tube). In Benumof JBL (ed): Airway Management: Principles and Practice, p 261. St Louis, Mosby, 1996
132. Salem MR, Wafai Y, Joseph NJ *et al:* Efficacy of the self-inflating bulb in detecting esophageal intubation. Does the presence of a nasogastric tube or cuff deflation make a difference? Anesthesiology 80:42, 1994
133. Cardoso MM, Banner MJ, Melker RJ *et al:* Portable devices used to detect endotracheal intubation during emergency situations: A review. Crit Care Med 26:957, 1998
134. Bresnick WH, Rask-Madsen C, Hogan DL *et al:* The effect of acute emotional stress on gastric acid secretion in normal subjects and duodenal ulcer patients. J Clin Gastroenterol 17:117, 1993
135. Smith KJ, Dombranowski J, Yip G, Dauphin A, Choi PTL: Cricoid pressure displaces the esophagus: An observational study using magnetic resonance imaging. Anesthesiology 99:60, 2003
136. Rabb MF, Minkowitz HS, Hagberg CA: Blind intubation through the laryngeal mask airway for management of the difficult airway in infants. Anesthesiology 84:1510, 1996
137. Heard CMB, Caldicott LD, Fletcher JE *et al:* Fiberoptic-guided endotracheal intubation via the laryngeal mask airway in pediatric patients: A report of a series of cases. Anesth Analg 82:1287, 1996
138. Brimacombe J, Agro F, Carassiti M *et al:* Use of a lighted stylet for intubation via the laryngeal mask airway (abstract). Can J Anaesth 45:556, 1998
139. Atherton DP, O'Sullivan E, Lowe D *et al:* A ventilation-exchange bougie for fibreoptic intubations with the laryngeal mask airway. Anaesthesia 51:1123, 1996
140. Gajraj NM: Tracheal intubation through the laryngeal mask using a gum elastic bougie. Anaesthesia 51:796, 1996
141. Gabbott DA, Sasada MP: Tracheal intubation through the laryngeal mask using a gum elastic bougie in the presence of cricoid pressure and manual in-line stabilisation of the neck. Anaesthesia 51:389, 1996
142. Elwood T, Cox RG: Laryngeal mask insertion with a laryngoscope in paediatric patients. Can J Anaesth 43:435, 1996
143. Bahk JH, Kim CS: A method for removing the laryngeal mask airway after using it as an intubation guide. Anesthesiology 86:1218, 1997
144. Brain AIJ, Verghese C, Addy EV *et al:* The intubating laryngeal mask. I: Development of a new device for intubation of the trachea. Br J Anaesth 79:699, 1997
145. Kapila A, Addy EV, Verghese C *et al:* The intubating laryngeal mask airway: An initial assessment of performance. Br J Anaesth 79:710, 1997
146. Brain AIJ, Verghese C, Addy EV *et al:* The intubating laryngeal mask. II: A preliminary clinical report of a new means of intubating the trachea. Br J Anaesth 79:704, 1997
147. Rosenblatt WH, Murphy M: The intubating laryngeal mask: Use of a new ventilating intubating device in the emergency department. Ann Emerg Med 33:234, 1999
148. Baskett PJ, Parr MJ, Nolan JP: The intubating laryngeal mask: Results of a multicentre trial with experience of 500 cases. Anaesthesia 53:1174, 1998
149. Monrigal JP, Tesson B, Granry JC: Evaluation of the efficiency of the LMA Fastrach in case of difficult intubation. Anesthesiology 9:A1359, 1999
150. Ferson DZ, Rosenblatt WH, Johansen MJ, Osborne I, Ovassapian A: Use of the Intubating LMA-Fastrach in 254 Patients with Difficult-to-manage Airways. Anesthesiology 95:1175, 2001
151. Cooper RM: Extubation and changing the endotracheal tube. In Benumof JL (ed): Airway Management: Principles and Practice, p 864. St Louis, Mosby, 1996
152. Asai T: Use of the laryngeal mask during emergence from anaesthesia. Eur J Anaesthesiol 15:379, 1998
153. Asai T, Shingu K: Use of the laryngeal mask during emergence from anesthesia in a patient with an unstable neck. Anesth Analg 88:469, 1999
154. Nair I, Bailey PM: Use of the laryngeal mask for airway maintenance following trachea extubation (Letter). Anaesthesia 50:174, 1995
155. Engoren M: Evaluation of the cuff-leak test in a cardiac surgery population. Chest 116:1029, 1999
156. Loudermilk EP, Hartmannsgruber M, Stoltzfus DP *et al:* A prospective study of the safety of tracheal extubation using a pediatric airway exchange catheter for patients with a known difficult airway. Chest 111:1660, 1997
157. Practice guidelines for management of the difficult airway: A report by the American Society of Anesthesiologists Task Force on Management of the Difficult Airway. Anesthesiology 78:597, 1993
158. Rocke DA, Murry WB, Rout CC *et al:* Relative risk analysis factors associated with difficult intubation in obstetric anesthesia. Anesthesiology 77:597, 1993
159. Lyons G: Failed intubation. Anaesthesia 40:759, 1985
160. Takenaka I, Kadoya T, Aoyama K: Is awake intubation necessary when the laryngeal mask is feasible? (Letter). Anesth Analg 91:247, 2000
161. Rosenblatt W: The airway Approach Algorithm. J Clin Anesth 16:312, 2004
162. Parmet JL, Colonna-Romano P, Horrow JC *et al:* The laryngeal mask airway reliably provides rescue ventilation in cases of unanticipated difficult tracheal intubation along with difficult mask ventilation. Anesth Analg 87:661, 1998
163. Christian AS: Failed obstetric intubation (Case Reports). Anaesthesia 45:995, 1990
164. Browning ST, Whittet HB, Williams A: Failure of insertion of a laryngeal mask airway caused by a variation in the anatomy of the thyroid cartilage. Anaesthesia 54:884, 1999
165. Ishimura H, Minami K, Sata T, Shigematsu A, Kadoya T: Impossible insertion of the laryngeal mask airway and oropharyngeal axes. Anesthesiology 83:867, 1995
166. Gataure PS, Hughes JA: The laryngeal mask airway in obstetrical anaesthesia. Can J Anaesth 42:130, 1995
167. Kokkinis K, Papageorgiou E: Failure of the laryngeal mask airway (LMA) to ventilate patients with severe tracheal stenosis. Resuscitation 30:21, 1995
168. Busoni P, Fognani G: Failure of the laryngeal mask to secure the airway in a patient with Hunter's syndrome (mucopolysaccharidosis type II). Paediatr Anaesth 9:153, 1999
169. Nandi PR, Charlesworth CH, Taylor SJ *et al:* Effect of general anaesthesia on the pharynx. Br J Anaesth 66:157, 1991
170. Hudgel DW, Hendricks C: Palate and hypopharynx—sites of inspiratory narrowing of the upper airway during sleep. Am Rev Resp Dis 138:1542, 1988
171. Iscoe SD: Central control of the upper airway. In Mathew OP, Sant'Ambrogio G (eds): Respiratory function of the upper airway. New York, Marcel Dekker, 1988
172. Benumof JL: Management of the difficult adult airway: With special emphasis on awake tracheal intubation. Anesthesiology 75:1087, 1991
173. McLeskey CH, Cullen BF, Kennedy RD *et al:* Control of cerebral perfusion pressure during induction of anesthesia in high-risk neurosurgical patients. Anesth Analg 53:985, 1974
174. Fleming JA, Byck R, Barash P: Pharmacology and therapeutic application of cocaine. Anesthesiology 73:518, 1990
175. Weisel W, Tella RA: Reaction to tetracaine used as topical anesthetic in bronchoscopy: A study of 1000 cases. JAMA 147:218, 1951
176. Sitzman BT, Rich GF, Rockwell JJ *et al:* Local anesthetic administration for awake direct laryngoscopy. Are glossopharyngeal nerve blocks superior? Anesthesiology 86:34, 1997
177. Sanchez A, Trivedi NS, Morrison DE: Preparation of the patient for awake intubation. In Benumof JL (ed): Airway Management: Principles and Practice, p 159. St Louis, Mosby, 1996
178. Ovassapian A: Fiberoptic Endoscopy and the Difficult Airway, 2nd ed. Philadelphia, Lippincott-Raven, 1996
179. Rosenblatt WH, Wagner PJ, Ovassapian A *et al:* Practice patterns in managing the difficult airway by anesthesiologists in the United States. Anesth Analg 87:153, 1998
180. Heidegger T, Gerig HJ, Ulrich B, Kreinenbul. Validation of a simple algorithm for tracheal intubation: Daily practice is the key to success in emergencies and analysis of 13,248 intubations. Anesth Anal 92:517, 2001
181. Rose, DK, Cohen MM: The airway. Problems and predictions in 18,300 patients. Canad J Anaesth 41:372, 1994
182. Murphy P: A fibre-optic endoscope used for nasal intubation. Anaesthesia 22:489, 1967
183. Ovassapian A, Yelich SJ, Dykes MH *et al:* Learning fibreoptic intubation: Use of simulators v. traditional teaching. Br J Anaesth 61:217, 1988
184. Benumof JL: Management of the difficult airway. Anesthesiology 75:1087, 1991
185. Hershey MD, Hannenberg AA: Gastric distention and rupture from oxygen insufflation during fiberoptic intubation. Anesthesiology 85:1479, 1996
186. Rosenblatt WH: Overcoming obstruction during bronchoscope-guided intubation of the trachea with the double setup endotracheal tube. Anesth Analg 83:175, 1996
187. Ovassapian A, Yellich J, Dykes MHM, Brunner EE: Fiberoptic nasotracheal intubation: Incidence and causes of failure. Anesth Analg 62:692, 1983
188. Jones He, Pearce AC, Moore P: Fiberoptic intubation: influence of tracheal tube tip design. Anaesthesia 48:672, 1993
189. Kristensen MS: The Parker flex-tip tube versus a standard tube for fiberoptic orotracehal intubation: randomized double blind study. Anesthesiology 98:334, 2003
190. Brull SJ, Wiklund R, Ferris C *et al:* Facilitation of fiberoptic orotracheal intubation with a flexible tracheal tube. Anesth Analg 78:746, 1994
191. Gorback MS: Management of the challenging airway with the Bullard laryngoscope. J Clin Anesth 3:473, 1991
192. Hastings RH, Vigil AC, Hanna R *et al:* Cervical spine movement during laryngoscopy with the Bullard, Macintosh, and Miller laryngoscopes. Anesthesiology 82:859, 1995

193. Cohn AI, McGraw SR, King WH: Awake intubation of the adult trachea using the Bullard laryngoscope. Can J Anaesth 42:246, 1995
194. Cohn AI, Hart RT, McGraw SR *et al:* The Bullard laryngoscope for emergency airway management in a morbidly obese parturient. Anesth Analg 81:872, 1995
195. Cooper SD, Benumof JL, Ozaki ST. Evaluation of the Bullard laryngoscope using the new intubating stylet: Comparison with conventional laryngoscopy. Anesth Analg 79:965, 1994
196. Halligan M, Charters P: A clinical evaluation of the Bonfils intubation fiberscope. Anaesthesia 58:1087, 2003
197. Young CF, Rosenblatt WH. Comparison of the Shikani Optical Stylet to direct laryngoscopy for orotracheal intubation by a first year anesthesiology resident (Abstract). Anesthesiology, 2004
198. Cooper RM. Use of a new video laryngoscope (Glidescope®) in the management of a difficult airway. Can J of Anaesth 50:611, 2003
199. Butler FS, Cirillo AA: Retrograde tracheal intubation. Anesth Analg 39:333, 1960
200. Waters DJ: Guided blind endotracheal intubation. Anaesthesia 18:158, 1963
201. Sanchez A, Pallares V: Retrograde intubation technique. In Benumof JL (ed): Airway Management: Principles and Practice. St Louis, Mosby, 1996
202. Barriot P, Riou B: Retrograde technique for tracheal intubation in trauma patients. Crit Care Med 16:712, 1988
203. Reynaud J, Lacour M, Diop L *et al:* Intubation tracheale guidee a bouche fermee (technic de D.J. Waters). Bull Soc Med Afr Noire Lang Fr 12774, 1967
204. Sanchez A, Pallares V: Retrograde intubation technique. In Benumof JL (ed): Airway Management: Principles and Practice. St Louis, Mosby, 1996
205. Walls RM: Management of the difficult airway in the trauma patient. Emerg Med Clin North Am 16:45, 1998
206. Don Michael TL, Lambert EH, Mehran A: Mouth to lung airway for cardiac resuscitation. Lancet 2:1329, 1968
207. Frass M, Frenzer R, Zahler J: Respiratory tube or airway. U.S. Patent 1987, no. 4, 688,568
208. Lipp MDW, Jaehnichen G, Golecki N, Fecht G, Reichl R, Heeg P: Microbiological, microstructure, and material science examinations of reprocessed combitubes after multiple reuse. Anesth Analg 91:693, 2000
209. Green-KS, Beger-TH SO: Proper use of the Combitube (Letter). Anesthesiology 81:513, 1994
210. Brimacombe J, Keller C, Kunzel KH, Gaber O, Boehler M, Puhringer F: Cervical spine motion during airway management: A cinefluoroscopic study of the posteriorly destabilized third cervical vertebrae in human cadavers. Anesth Analg 91:1274, 2000
211. Kulozik U, Georgi R, Krier C: Intubation with the Combitube-TM in massive hemorrhage from the locus Kieselbachii. Anasthesiol Intensivmed Notfallmed Schmerzther 31:191, 1996
212. Hofbauer R, Roggla M, Staudinger T *et al:* Emergency intubation with the Combitube in a patient with persistent vomiting. Anasthesiol Intensivmed Notfallmed Schmerzther 29:306, 1994
213. Deroy R, Ghoris M: The Combitube elective anesthetic airway management in a patient with cervical spine fracture. Anesth Analg 87:1441, 1998
214. Banyai M, Falger S, Roggla M *et al:* Emergency intubation with the Combitube in a grossly obese patient with bull neck. Resuscitation 26:271, 1993
215. Liao D, Shalit M: Successful intubation with the Combitube in acute asthmatic respiratory distress by a paramedic. J Emerg Med 14:561, 1996
216. Blostein PA, Koestner AJ, Hoak S: Failed rapid sequence intubation in trauma patients: Esophageal tracheal Combitube is a useful adjunct. J Trauma 44:534, 1998
217. Frass M, Frenzer R, Mayer G *et al:* Mechanical ventilation with the esophageal tracheal combitube (ETC) in the intensive care unit. Arch Emerg Med 4:219, 1987
218. Rumball CJ, MacDonald D: The PTL, Combitube, laryngeal mask, and oral airway: A randomized prehospital comparative study of ventilatory device effectiveness and cost-effectiveness in 470 cases of cardiorespiratory arrest. Prehosp Emerg Care 1:1, 1997
219. Tanigawa K, Shigematsu A: Choice of airway devices for 12,020 cases of nontraumatic cardiac arrest in Japan. Prehosp Emerg Care 2:96, 1998
220. Lefrancios DP, Dufour DG: Use of the esophageal tracheal Combitube by basic emergency medical technicians. Resuscitation 52:77, 2002
221. Urtubia R, Medina J, Alzamora R *et al:* Insertion of the Esophageal-Tracheal Combitube using inhalational induction of anesthesia with sevoflurane as single agent. Difficult Airway 3:51, 2002
222. Gaitini LA, Vaida SJ, Somri M *et al:* Fiberoptic-guided airway exchange of the esophageal-tracheal Combitube in spontaneously breathing versus mechanically ventilated patients. Anesth Analg 88:193, 1999
223. Richards CF: The pyriform sinus perforation during Esophageal Tracheal Combitube. J Emerg Med 16:37, 1998
224. Vezina D, Lessard MR, Bussieres J *et al:* Complications associated with the use of the Esophageal Tracheal Combitube. Can J Anaesth 45:76, 1998
225. Klein H, Williamson M, Sue Ling HM *et al:* Esophageal rupture associated with the use of the Combitube. Anesth Analg 85:937, 1997
226. Thierbach AR: A new device for emergency airway management. The easy tube resuscitation. 61(3):347, 2004
227. Martin SE, Ochsner MG, Jarman RH *et al:* Laryngeal mask airway in air transport when intubation fails: Case report. J Trauma Injury Infect Crit Care 42:333, 1997
228. Brimacombe JR, De Maio B: Emergency use of the laryngeal mask airway during helicopter transfer of a neonate. J Clin Anesth 7:689, 1995
229. Asai T, Latto P: Role of the laryngeal mask in patients with difficult tracheal intubation and difficult ventilation. In Latto IP, Vaughan RS (eds): Difficulties in Tracheal Intubation, p 177. London, WB Saunders, 1997
230. Brimacombe JR, Berry AM: Mallampati grade and laryngeal mask placement. Anesth Analg 82:1112, 1996
231. Baskett PJF: The use of the laryngeal mask airway by nurses during cardiopulmonary resuscitation: Results of a multicentre trial. Anaesthesia 49:3, 1994
232. Verghese C, Prior Willeard PFS: Immediate management of the airway during cardiopulmonary resuscitation in a hospital without a resident anaesthesiologist. Eur J Emerg Med 1:123, 1994
233. Samarkandi AH, Seraj MA: The role of the laryngeal mask airway in cardiopulmonary resuscitation. Resuscitation 2:103, 1994
234. Keller C, Brimacombe J, Bittersohl J., Lirk P, von Goedecke A. Aspiration and Laryngeal mask airway: three cases and a review of the literature. British Journal of Anaesthesia 93:579–582, 2004
235. Brimacombe J: Does the laryngeal mask airway have a role outside the operating theatre? Can Anaesth J 42:258, 1995
236. Aoyama K, Takenaka I: Cricoid pressure impedes positioning and ventilation through the laryngeal mask. Can J Anaesth 43:1035, 1996
237. Strang TI: Does the laryngeal mask airway compromise cricoid pressure? Anaesthesia 47:829, 1992
238. Asai T, Barcklay K: Cricoid pressure impedes placement of the laryngeal mask airway and subsequent tracheal intubation through the mask. Br J Anaesth 72:47, 1994
239. Baumgarten RK, Carter CE, Reynolds WJ *et al:* Priming with nondepolarizing relaxants for rapid tracheal intubation: A double-blind evaluation. Can J Anaesth 35:5, 1988
240. Cicala R, Westbrook L: An alternative method of paralysis for rapid-sequence induction. Anesthesiology 69:983, 1988
241. Gnauck K, Lungo JB, Scalzo A *et al:* Emergency intubation of the pediatric medical patient: Use of anesthetic agents in the emergency department. Ann Emerg Med 23:1242, 1994
242. Li J, Murphy-Lavoie H, Bugas C *et al:* Complications of emergency intubation with and without paralysis. Am J Emerg Med 17:141, 1999
243. Sosis M: Modified rapid sequence induction I. Anesthesiology 70:1031, 1989
244. Sivarajan M, Joy JV: Effects of general anesthesia and paralysis on upper airway changes due to head position in humans. Anesthesiology 85:787, 1996
245. Tuzzo DM, Frova G. Application of the self-inflating bulb to a hollow intubating introducer. Minerva Anestesiologica 67:127, 2001
246. Benumof JL, Gaughan SD: Concerns regarding barotrauma during jet ventilation (letter). Anesthesiology 76:1072, 1992
247. Benumof JL: Transtracheal jet ventilation via percutaneous catheter and high-pressure source. In Benumof JL (ed): Airway Management: Principles and Practice. St Louis, Mosby—Year Book, 1996
248. Gaughn SD, Gzaki GT, Benumof JL: Comparison in a lung model of low and high flow regulators for transtracheal jet ventilation. Anesthesiology 77:189, 1992
249. Muallem MK: Muallem Jet Ventilator. Middle East J Anesth 15:575, 2000
250. Dunn SM, Robbins L, Connelly NR: The LMA ProSeal™ may not be the best option for difficult to intubate/ventilate patients. Anesth Analg 99:310, 2004
251. Rosenblatt WH: In response. Anesth Analg 99:311, 2004

CHAPTER 23 ■ PATIENT POSITIONING

MARK A. WARNER

KEY POINTS

1. Sedated or anesthetized patients should not be placed in positions that are not comfortable while they are awake.
2. Elevated lower-extremity positions (e.g., lithotomy) may reduce perfusion pressure in the elevated extremities and increase the opportunity for developing compartment syndromes, especially when the extremities are elevated for prolonged periods.
3. Padding provided by any number of different materials (e.g., gel or foam pads, blankets) should be used to widely disperse point pressure on body parts or tissues.
4. Brachial plexus neuropathy associated with sternotomy in anesthetized patients undergoing cardiac procedures may mimic as peripheral ulnar neuropathy.
5. The etiology of ulnar neuropathy is not always clear. Most commonly it develops postoperatively in men 40 to 70 years of age who undergo abdominal or pelvic procedures. There are anatomic and neurophysiologic reasons for men compared to women to develop this problem.
6. Excessive flexion or extension of the spine in anesthetized patients who are placed in unique surgical positions may contribute to spinal cord ischemia and catastrophic neurologic damage.
7. Perioperative vision loss occurs most frequently in anesthetized patients undergoing cardiac surgical procedures. Patients undergoing extensive spine procedures while positioned prone also have a high frequency of vision loss, primarily from posterior ischemic optic neuropathy.
8. Neuropathies that result in motor function loss as well as sensory loss compared to those with isolated sensory loss generally are associated with more prolonged or permanent nerve dysfunction.

Positioning a patient for a surgical procedure is frequently (1) a compromise between what the anesthetized patient can tolerate, both structurally and physiologically, and what the surgical team requires for access to their anatomic targets.[1,2] Physiologic instability resulting from disease or injury may be magnified by rapidly moving a seriously ill patient from bed to transport cart, through corridors and elevators, and onto the operating table. Induction of anesthesia and positioning may need to be delayed until that patient is hemodynamically stable, or establishment of the intended surgical posture may need to be modified to match the patient's tolerance. This chapter presents the physiologic significance of various positions in which a patient may be placed during an operation, briefly describes the techniques of establishing the positions, and discusses the potential complications of each posture.

It is very important for clinicians to understand the physiologic and potential pathologic consequences of patient positioning. Although considerable information is available on the physiologic effects of various positions, there is a paucity of information on the complications of positioning. Until recently, there have been few studies, either retrospective or prospective, that provided epidemiologic evidence of the frequency and natural history of many of the perioperative positioning complications. Why? In decades preceding the 1990s, catastrophic perioperative outcomes, such as death or hypoxic brain injury from either the delivery of inadequate oxygen or failure adequately to ventilate patients, were infrequent but potentially avoidable consequences of the delivery of anesthesia. The development of pulse oximetry and end-tidal respiratory monitoring in the 1980s, the subsequent acceptance of monitoring standards of care by the anesthesia community, the introduction of improved drugs, and improved physician education contributed to a dramatic decline in the frequency of these major events. Less catastrophic, yet still disabling, perioperative complications, such as those possibly related to positioning, consequently became a higher priority for study.

In the 1990s and more recently, a number of studies of large surgical populations provided new information on the frequency and natural history of rare perioperative events such as neuropathies and vision loss. These studies occasionally provided sufficient data to allow speculation on potential mechanisms of injury. Based on the findings of these studies, investigators are seeking to confirm mechanisms of injury and the efficacy of novel interventions to decrease the frequency of, or to prevent, these perioperative events. For now, however, the mechanism and even the onset of many potential positioning-related complications often are unknown.

The lack of solid scientific information on basic mechanisms of positioning-related complications often leads to medicolegal entanglements. Attempts to determine the etiology of complications alleged to be caused by patient positioning are often unconscionably biased. Notations on anesthesia and operating room records may be absent or uninformative. On some occasions, medicolegal conclusions have been shaped by assumptions and assertions made by people having no understanding of the case in question and no personal familiarity with proceedings in an operating room. Careful, but laconic, descriptive notations about positions used during anesthesia and surgery, as well as brief comments about special protective measures such as eye care and pressure-point padding, are useful information to include on the anesthesia record. In potentially complicated or contentious circumstances, a brief resume in the progress notes is advisable. Only in this manner can subsequent inquiries be properly answered on behalf of either the patient or the anesthesiologist. When credible, expanded knowledge that further delineates mechanisms of positioning-related complications is available, these issues and the care of patients will be improved.

DORSAL DECUBITUS POSITIONS

Physiology

Circulatory

In the horizontal supine position (Fig. 23-1A), the influence of gravity on the vascular system is minimal. Intravascular pressures from head to foot vary little from mean pressures at the level of the heart; therefore, almost no perfusion gradient exists between the heart and arteries in either the head or the lower extremities. Similarly, venous gradients from the periphery to the right atrium consist principally of the cyclic intrathoracic pressure changes that occur with respiration.

If the patient in the dorsal decubitus position is tilted head high or head low, the effects of gravity on blood flow in the head or the feet can become quite significant as the gradient to or from the heart increases. Pressures have been shown to change by 2 mm Hg for each 2.5 cm that a given point varies in vertical height above or below the reference point at the heart.[3]

When the lower extremities are below the level of the heart, blood pools in distensible dependent vessels, causing a reduction in effective circulating volume, cardiac output, and systemic perfusion. If the head is high and blood pressure measured at the level of the heart is low, the blood pressure in the brain is decreased further according to the magnitude of the head elevation.

If the head is tilted down (Fig. 23-1B), pressure in the cerebral veins increases in proportion to the gradient upward to the heart. Many alert patients so positioned complain of a rapidly occurring, pounding vascular headache. Congestion develops in the nasal mucosa and conjunctivae. In the presence of an intracranial pathologic process, such as a head injury or a stroke, elevations of cerebral venous pressure resulting from head-down tilt can provoke or intensify cerebral edema and dangerously raise intracranial pressure. Head-down tilt also increases cerebrospinal fluid pressure in the cranial vault, adding its effect to the total intracranial pressure elevation. Finally, venous congestion and resultant edema may cause a "compartment syndrome" in areas within the head as vessels and nerves are squeezed as they traverse small bony spaces.

West et al[4] have identified three separate perfusion zones in the pulmonary circulation, based on the interrelationship among pressures in the alveoli, arterioles, and venules.

In zone 1, alveolar pressure exceeds either arterial or venous pressure and perfusion of the lung unit is prevented. Although it is rarely present in a normal lung, zone 1 can be produced by pulmonary hypotension, excessive positive end-expiratory pressure (PEEP), or overdistention of alveolar units from large tidal volumes during positive-pressure ventilation.

In zone 2, arterial pressure exceeds alveolar pressure, whereas alveolar pressure remains higher than venous pressure. This relationship is found in nondependent portions of the lung, and perfusion is the result of a fluctuating balance between arterial and alveolar pressures.

In zone 3, hydrostatic forces in the dependent portion of the lung produce venous congestion, and perfusion is determined by the difference between arterial pressure and venous pressure.

In the dorsal recumbent positions, the pulmonary circulation tends to be most congested along the dorsal body wall and least congested substernally. When the patient is tilted head high, zone 3 moves toward the lung bases as better ventilatory mechanics improve gas exchange. If the tilt is head down, zone 3 shifts cephalad into the poorly ventilated lung apices, and abnormal ventilation–perfusion ratios can be expected to intensify.

Respiratory

In the supine position, mobile abdominal viscera gravitate toward the dorsal body wall and press the dorsal parts of the diaphragm cephalad. The displacement lengthens muscle fibers in that portion of the diaphragm and increases the strength and effectiveness of its contractions during spontaneous ventilation. The benefit is improved aeration of the congested, compacted, and less compliant lung bases. With head-up tilt (Fig. 23-1C), the visceral weight shifts away from the diaphragm and ventilation is enhanced. In the head-down position, the visceral mass, its weight potentially increased by the presence of abdominal fat, fluid, or tumors, can cause significant respiratory embarrassment by impeding caudad excursions of the contracting diaphragm and preventing adequate expansion of the lung bases.

In the supine position, gravity-induced vascular congestion forces the dorsal portions of the lung to function as a zone 3.[4] Consequently, the compliance of the area is reduced, and passive ventilation tends to distribute gas preferentially to more easily distensible substernal units where pulmonary blood volume is less. To prevent development of a clinically significant ventilation–perfusion imbalance during use of controlled ventilation, tidal volumes must be used that are greater than the average amount that is sufficient for the spontaneously breathing, conscious patient.[5]

Variations of the Dorsal Decubitus Position

Supine

Horizontal. In the traditional horizontal supine position (dubbed "lying at attention"), the patient lies on his or her back with a small pillow beneath the head (see Fig. 23-1A). The arms are either comfortably padded and restrained

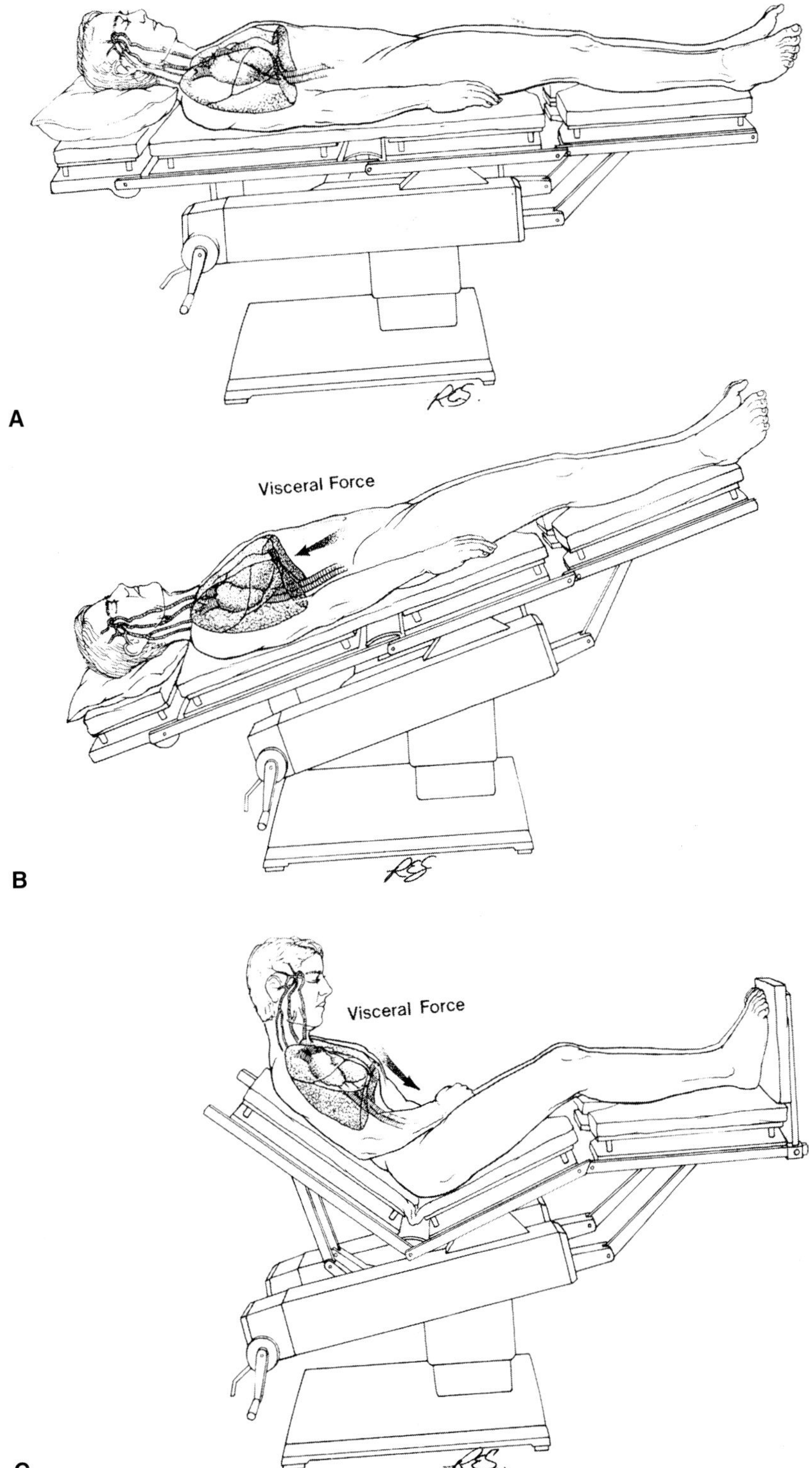

FIGURE 23-1. **A.** Supine adult with minimal gradients in the horizontal vascular axis. Pulmonary blood volume is greatest dorsally. Viscera displace the dorsal diaphragm cephalad. Cerebral circulation is slightly above heart level if the head is on a small pillow. **B.** Head-down tilt aids blood return from lower extremities but encourages reflex vasodilation, congests vessels in the poorly ventilated lung apices, and increases intracranial blood volume. **C.** Elevation of the head shifts abdominal viscera away from the diaphragm and improves ventilation of the lung bases. According to the gradient above the heart, pressure in arteries of the head and neck decreases; pressure in accompanying veins may become subatmospheric.

alongside the trunk or abducted on well padded arm boards. Either arm (or both) may be extended ventrally and the flexed forearm secured to an elevated frame in such a way that perfusion of the hand is not compromised, no skin-to-metal contact exists to cause electrical burns if a cautery is used, and the brachial neurovascular bundle is neither stretched nor compressed at the axilla (see the left arm arrangement in Fig. 23-13). The lumbar spine may need padded support to prevent a postoperative backache (see Complications of the Dorsal Decubitus Positions section). Bony contact points at the occiput, elbows, and heels should be padded.

Although the horizontal supine posture has a long history of widespread use, it does not place hip and knee joints in neutral positions and is poorly tolerated for any length of time by an immobilized, awake patient.

Contoured. A contoured supine posture (Fig. 23-2C) has been termed the *lawn chair position*.[6] It is established by arranging the surface of the operating table so that the

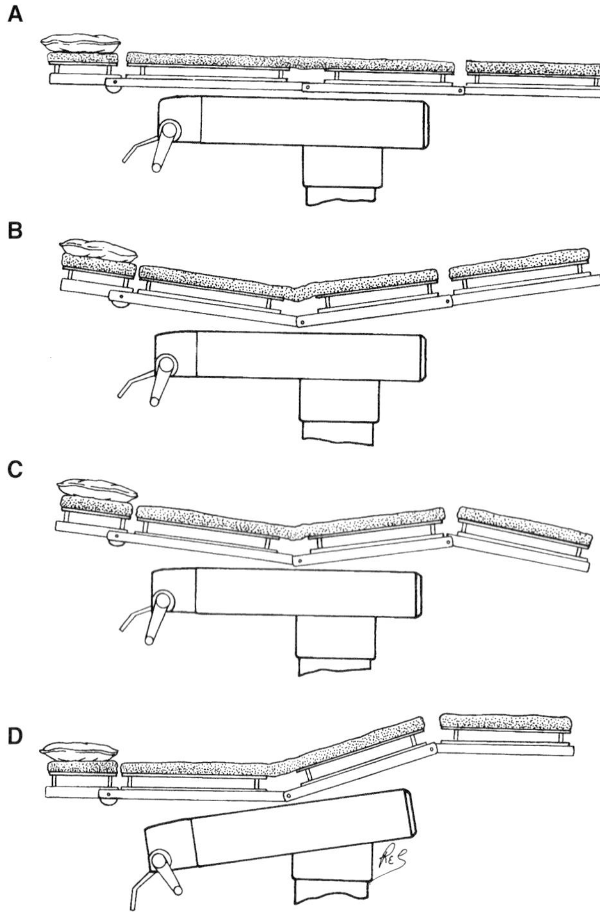

FIGURE 23-2. Establishment of the contoured supine ("lawn chair") position. A. Traditional flat supine table top. B. Thighs flexed on trunk. C. Knees gently flexed in final body position. D. Trunk section leveled to stabilize floor-supported arm board. (Reproduced with permission from Figure 5-3 (p. 42) of Martin JT, Warner MA [eds]: Positioning in Anesthesia and Surgery, 3rd ed. Philadelphia, WB Saunders, 1997.)

trunk–thigh hinge is angulated approximately 15 degrees and the thigh–knee hinge is angulated a similar amount in the opposite direction. Alternatively, a rolled towel or blanket can be placed beneath the patient's knees to keep them flexed. The patient of average height then lies comfortably with hips and knees flexed gently. Quite often a person who has been required to lie motionless on a rigid horizontal table and then is changed to the contoured supine position offers an almost involuntary expression of relief and appreciation.

As in the horizontal supine position, the patient should have a pad or pillow beneath the occiput, elbows, and heels. Arms can be positioned as described for the horizontal supine posture.

Frog-Leg. On occasion, a surgeon may wish to have access to the perineum. Placing the patient supine with the knees bent and the soles of the feet together separates the thighs sufficiently to permit access to the perineum and vagina for the surgeon standing at the patient's flank. If the patient's skeleton is stiff, lateral spread of the knees may seriously stress the hips or stretch branches of the obturator nerves;[7] a pad of sufficient size should be used to support each knee (1) to minimize the opportunity for postoperative hip and back pain and (2) to prevent a dislocated hip or fracture of an osteoporotic femur during the operation.

Lateral Uterine or Abdominal Mass Displacement. With a patient in the supine position, a mobile abdominal mass, such as a very large tumor or a pregnant uterus, can rest on the great vessels of the abdomen and compromise circulation. This is known as the *aortocaval syndrome* or the *supine hypotensive syndrome.* A significant degree of perfusion can be restored if the compressive mass is rolled toward the left hemiabdomen by leftward tilt of the table top or by a wedge under the right hip.[8]

Lithotomy

Standard. In the standard lithotomy position (Fig. 23-3), the patient lies supine with arms crossed on the trunk or with one or both arms extended laterally to less than 90 degrees on arm boards. Each lower extremity is flexed at the hip and knee, and both limbs are simultaneously elevated and separated so that the perineum becomes accessible to the surgeon. For many gynecologic and urologic procedures, the patient's thighs are flexed approximately 90 degrees on the trunk and the knees are bent sufficiently to maintain the lower legs nearly parallel to the floor. More acute flexion of the knees or hips can threaten to angulate and compress major vessels at either joint. In addition, hip flexion to greater than 90 degrees on the trunk has been shown to increase stretch of the inguinal ligaments.[7] Branches of the lateral femoral cutaneous nerves often pass directly through these ligaments and can be impinged and become ischemic within the stretched ligament.

Numerous devices are available to hold legs that are elevated during delivery or operation. Each should be fitted to the stature of the individual patient. Care should be taken to ensure that angulations or edges of the padded holder do not compress the popliteal space or the upper dorsal thigh. Compartment syndromes of one or both lower extremities have resulted from prolonged use of the lithotomy position with some types of support devices.[9]

When the legs are to be lowered to the original supine position at the end of the procedure, they should first be brought together at the knees and ankles in the sagittal plane and then lowered slowly together to the table top. This minimizes torsion stress on the lumbar spine that would occur if each leg were lowered independently. It also permits gradual accommodation to the increase in circulatory capacitance, thereby avoiding sudden hypotension.[10]

Low. For most urologic procedures and for many procedures that require simultaneous access to the abdomen and perineum, the degree of thigh elevation in the lithotomy position is only approximately 30 to 45 degrees (Fig. 23-4). This reduces perfusion gradients to and from the lower extremities and improves access to a perineal surgical site for members of the operating team who may need to stand at the lateral aspect of either leg.

High. Some surgeons prefer to improve access to the perineum by suspending the patient's feet from high poles. The effect is to have the patient's legs almost fully extended on the thighs (Fig. 23-5) and the thighs flexed 90 degrees or more on the trunk. The posture produces a significant uphill gradient for arterial perfusion into the feet, requiring careful avoidance of systemic hypotension. Less mobile patients may tolerate this posture poorly because of angulation and compression of the contents of the femoral canal by the inguinal ligament (see Fig. 23-5A), or stretch of the sciatic nerve (see Fig. 23-5B), or both.

Exaggerated. Transperineal access to the retropubic area requires that the patient's pelvis be flexed ventrally on the spine, the thighs almost forcibly flexed on the trunk, and the lower legs aimed skyward so as to be out of the way (Fig. 23-6). The result places the long axis of the symphysis pubis almost parallel to the floor. This exaggerated lithotomy position stresses the lumbar spine, produces a significant uphill gradient for perfusion of the feet, and may restrict ventilation because of abdominal compression by bulky thighs. It can be tolerated under anesthesia but can rarely be assumed by an awake patient.

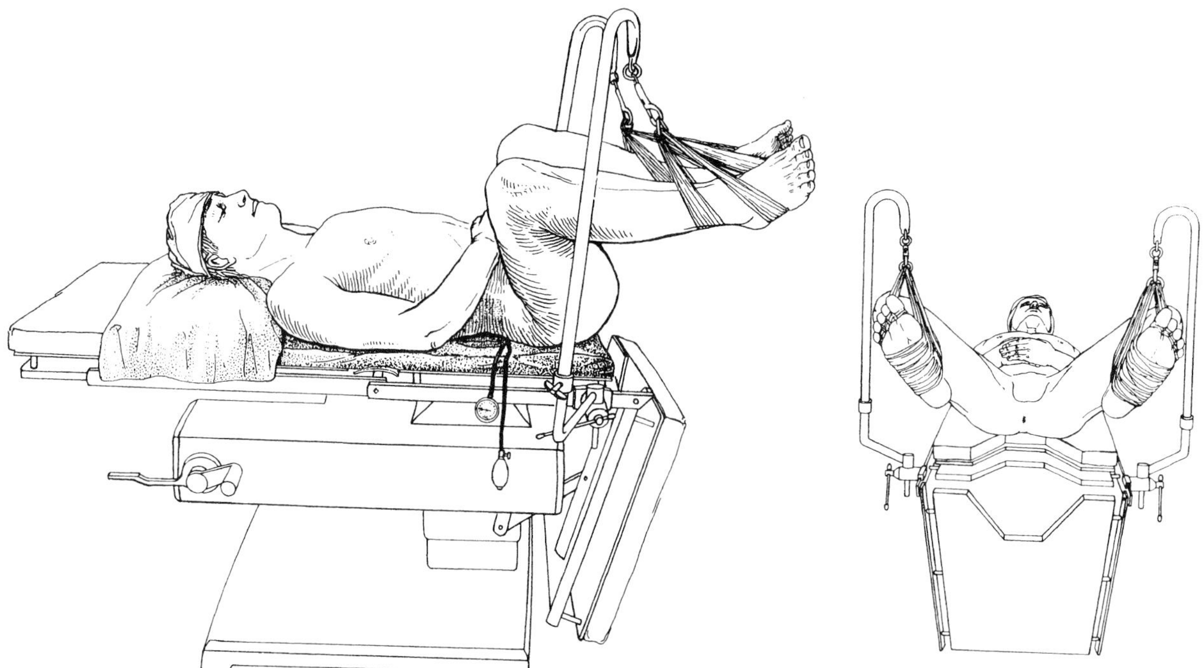

FIGURE 23-3. Standard lithotomy position with "candy cane" extremity support. Thighs are flexed approximately 90 degrees on abdomen; knees are flexed enough to bring lower legs grossly parallel to the torso section of the table top. Arms are retained on boards, crossed on the abdomen, or snugged at the sides of patient. (Modified with permission from Figures 6-5 and 6-14 of Martin JT, Warner MA [eds]: Positioning in Anesthesia and Surgery, 3rd ed. Philadelphia, WB Saunders, 1997.)

Control of ventilation is usually necessary. If painful lumbar spine disease exists, an alternative surgical position may need to be chosen beforehand to avoid severely accentuating the lumbar distress after surgery. This position has been associated
2 with a very high frequency of lower extremity compartment syndrome.[11] Maintenance of adequate perfusion pressure in the legs is important.

Tilted. Frequently, some degree of head-down tilt is added to one of the lithotomy positions. If the tilt is great enough, and particularly in the instance of the exaggerated lithotomy position, the patient may slide cephalad. Care must be taken to avoid this situation; there are several anecdotes from medicolegal actions involving patients who slid off operating tables with resulting head injuries.

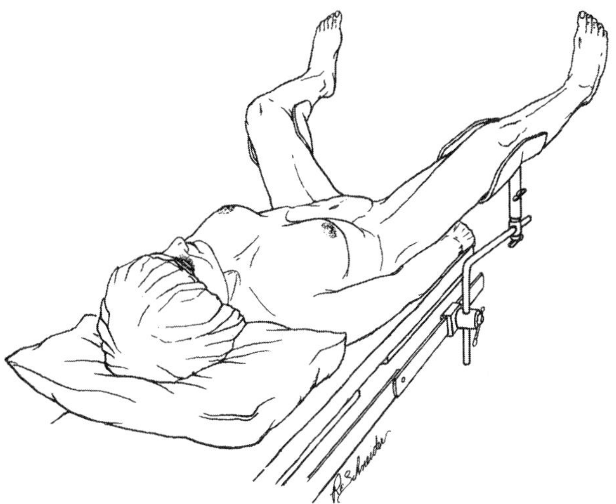

FIGURE 23-4. Low lithotomy position for perineal access, transurethral instrumentation, or combined abdominoperineal procedures. (Modified with permission from Figure 8-4, (p. 99) of Martin JT, Warner MA [eds]: Positioning in Anesthesia and Surgery, 3rd ed. Philadelphia, WB Saunders, 1997.)

Depending on the degree of head depression, the addition of tilt to the lithotomy position combines the worst features of both the lithotomy and the head-down postures. The weight of abdominal viscera on the diaphragm adds to whatever abdominal compression is produced by the flexed thighs of an obese patient or of one placed in an exaggerated lithotomy position. Ventilation should be assisted or controlled. Because elevation of the lower extremities above the heart produces an uphill perfusion gradient, systemic hypotension and compressive leg wrapping may limit perfusion to the periphery, a factor in the development of compartment syndromes in the legs of lithotomized patients.[9] This perfusion gradient often is unpredictable and exaggerated, potentially increasing the risk of compartment syndrome.[12,13]

Head-Down Tilt. Sometime during the mid 1800s, Bardenhauer, an innovative German surgeon in Cologne, began to elevate the hips of patients to gravitate the viscera cephalad and help expose lesions deep within the pelvis.[14] Others may have used the posture at about the same time. That unique maneuver, tilting a patient 30 to 45 degrees head down (Fig. 23-7), was adopted and popularized by Friedrich Trendelenburg of Bonn and Leipzig before 1870 (thus the often-used term "Trendelenburg position"). However, its publication apparently awaited an article by Meyer, an American pupil of Trendelenburg, in 1885.[15]

Reich and associates,[16] studying well-instrumented, anesthetized patients, have compared circulatory variables in the level supine position with those recorded after 3 minutes of marked (60-degree) elevation of the lower extremities or after 3 minutes of 20 degrees of head-down tilt. They found that head-down tilt only minimally increased cardiac output and mean arterial pressure, whereas leg raising slightly increased

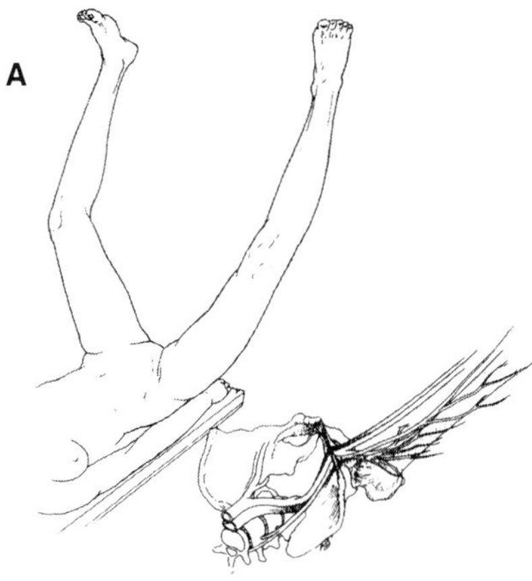

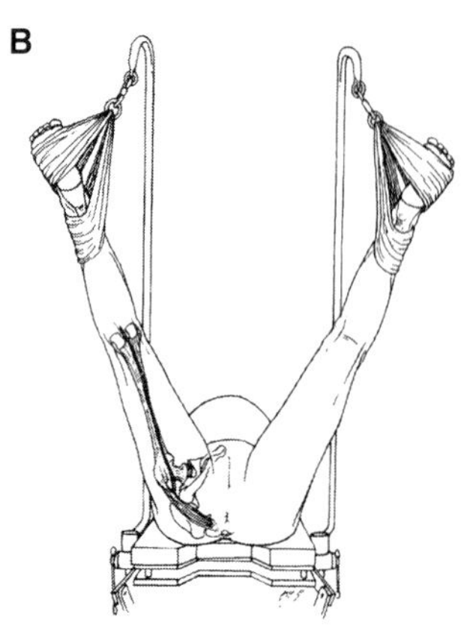

FIGURE 23-5. High lithotomy position. Note potential for angulation and compression/obstruction of contents of femoral canal (**A**, *insert*) or stretch of sciatic nerve (**B**). (**A** reproduced with permission from McLeskey CH [ed]: Geriatric Anesthesiology. Baltimore, Williams & Wilkins, 1997. **B** reproduced with permission from Figure 6-11 and 6-12, (pp. 61 & 63) of Martin JT, Warner MA [eds]: Positioning in Anesthesia and Surgery, 3rd ed. Philadelphia, WB Saunders, 1997.)

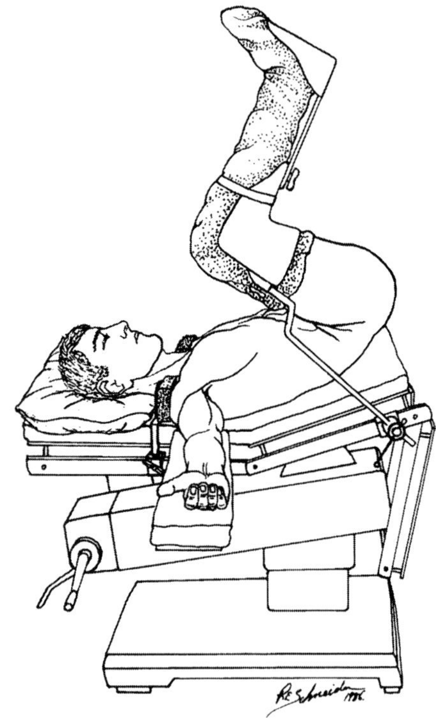

FIGURE 23-6. The exaggerated lithotomy position. Shoulder braces, usually needed to stabilize the torso, are placed over the acromioclavicular area to minimize compression of the brachial plexus and adjacent vessels. (Reprinted with permission from Figure 6-7 (p. 54) of Martin JT, Warner MA [eds]: Positioning in Anesthesia and Surgery, 3rd ed. Philadelphia, WB Saunders, 1997.)

mean arterial pressure without affecting cardiac output. In each posture, there was evidence of deteriorating pulmonary function and right ventricular stress. They urged caution in the use of either maneuver in patients with pulmonary disease or right ventricular compromise.

Cephalad displacement of the diaphragm and obstruction of its caudad inspiratory stroke accompany a head-down position because of gravity-shifted abdominal viscera. Consequently, the work of spontaneous ventilation is increased for an anesthetized patient in a posture that already worsens the ventilation–perfusion ratio by gravitational accumulation of blood in the poorly ventilated lung apices. During controlled ventilation, higher inspiratory pressures are needed to expand the lung.

Intracranial vascular congestion and increased intracranial pressure can be expected to result from head-down tilt. For patients with known or suspected intracranial disease, the position should be used only in those rare instances in which a surgically useful alternate posture cannot be found. Maintenance of the position should then be as brief as possible, and the need for postoperative neurologic intensive care should be anticipated.

Steep head-down tilt positions (e.g., 30 to 45 degrees of head-down tilt) may require some means of preventing the patient from sliding cephalad out of position. The use of anklets and bent knees is a satisfactory method of retaining the tilted patient in position (see Fig. 23-7) if the anklets are not excessively tight and if the flexed knee joints are placed sufficiently caudad of the leg–thigh hinge of the table top so that the adjacent firm edge of the depressed leg section of the table cannot indent either proximal calf. Should indentation occur, compressive ischemia and phlebitis or a compartment syndrome may result.

Historically, shoulder braces also have been used to prevent cephalad sliding in steep head-down tilt positions. These braces are best tolerated if placed over the acromioclavicular joints, but care must be taken to see that the shoulder is not forced sufficiently caudad to trap and compress the subclavian neurovascular bundle between the clavicle and the first rib. If the braces are placed medially against the root of the neck, they may easily compress neurovascular structures that emerge from the area of the scalene musculature. For these and other reasons, the use of shoulder braces has waned in popularity.

Complications of the Dorsal Decubitus Positions

Postural Hypotension

Depending on the resilience of the patient's vasocompensatory mechanisms, postural hypotension may be seen when a head-elevated position is being established. If mean arterial pressure at the circle of Willis remains within the range of cerebral blood flow autoregulation in a patient who is not hypertensive, the postural hypotension may require little treatment other than

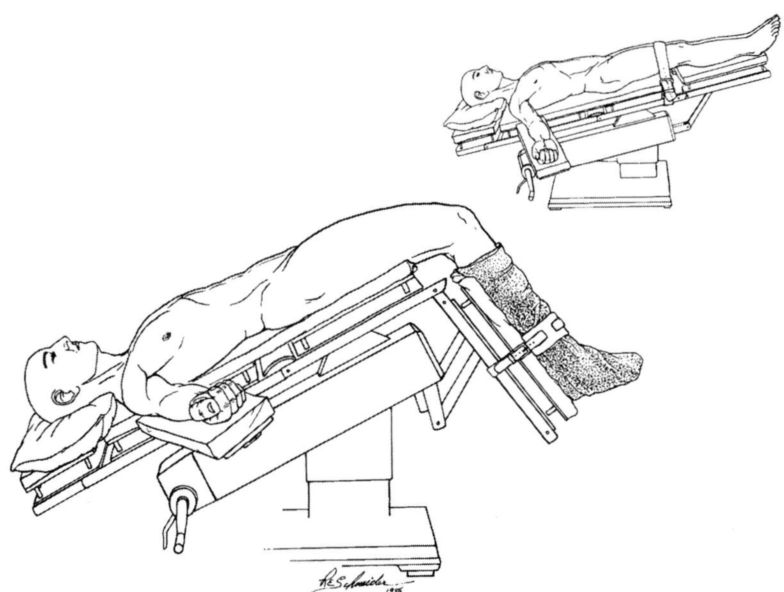

FIGURE 23-7. Head-down tilt. *Foreground figure* shows traditional steep (30- to 45-degree) tilt described by Trendelenburg. Leg restraints and knee flexion stabilize the patient, avoiding the need for wristlets or shoulder braces that threaten the brachial plexus. *Upper figure* shows 10 to 15 degrees of head-down tilt, which is more common in modern surgical procedures. (Reprinted with permission from Martin JT, Warner MA [eds]: Positioning in Anesthesia and Surgery, 3rd ed. Philadelphia, WB Saunders, 1997.)

to appropriately decrease the concentration of anesthetic drugs to preserve compensatory reflexes. If the degree of hypotension encountered is more severe, further head elevation should be delayed until the level of anesthetic is decreased; in addition, judicious use of fluids and vasopressors can reestablish effective perfusion.

Postural hypotension may also appear in the presence of inadequately replaced blood loss when the intravascular space has been functionally increased either by lowering the legs to horizontal at the termination of the lithotomy position or by returning a head-down tilt to horizontal. Volume repletion is the indicated therapy, although judiciously small doses of vasopressors may sometimes be needed initially.

Pressure Alopecia

Prolonged compression of hair follicles can produce hair loss. Abel and Lewis[17] described patients who had pain, swelling, and exudation where the occiput had been supporting the weight of the head for long periods in the Trendelenburg position. Alopecia occurred between the 3rd and 28th postoperative day; regrowth was complete within 3 months. Use of tight head straps to hold anesthetic face masks and prolonged hypotension and hypothermia have also been associated with compression alopecia.[18] Frequently turning the patient's head during long operations[19] and use of padded, soft head supports are recommended to reduce the risks of this complication.

Pressure-Point Reactions

Weight-bearing bony prominences can produce ischemic necro-
3 sis of overlying tissue unless proper padding is applied. Hypothermia and vasoconstrictive hypotension may enhance the process. The heels, the elbows, and the sacrum are particularly vulnerable. The use of a variety of pads (e.g., foam or gel) may disperse point pressure if used for protection. While their use may protect against skin and soft tissue compression and ischemia, there are no studies that have proven their use to be beneficial in reducing peripheral neuropathies in the perioperative period.

BRACHIAL PLEXUS AND UPPER EXTREMITY INJURIES

Brachial Plexus Neuropathy

Root Injuries

Shoulder braces placed tight against the base of the neck can compress and injure the roots of the brachial plexus. Braces, if needed at all, are considered less harmful when placed more laterally over the acromioclavicular joint.

The dorsal decubitus positions do not usually threaten structures in the patient's neck unless considerable lateral displacement of the head occurs. In that position, the roots of the brachial plexus on the side of the obtuse head–shoulder angle can be stretched and damaged. If the upper extremity is fixed at the wrist, the stretch injury of the plexus can be accentuated as the head moves laterally away from the anchoring point of the wrist. Similarly, exaggerated rotation of the head away from an extended arm can be associated with a brachial plexus injury.

Sternal Retraction

Frequently, the patient undergoing a median sternotomy has both arms padded and secured alongside the torso. An alternative is to have both arms abducted.[20] Vander Salm et al[21,22]
4 described first rib fractures and brachial plexus injuries associated with median sternotomies. They related the extent of the injury to the amount of retractor displacement of the rib, with the most severe injury being caused by displacement sufficient to produce a first rib fracture. Roy and associates,[23] in a study of 200 consecutive adults scheduled for cardiac surgery via a median sternotomy, positioned the left arm either abducted and padded on an arm board with the palm supinated or secured by a draw sheet alongside the trunk; the right arm was always placed alongside the trunk. They found a 10% incidence of upper extremity nerve injury that was not influenced by internal mammary artery harvest, internal jugular vein catheterization, or left arm position. Surgical manipulation was more contributory than extremity positioning in producing trauma to the

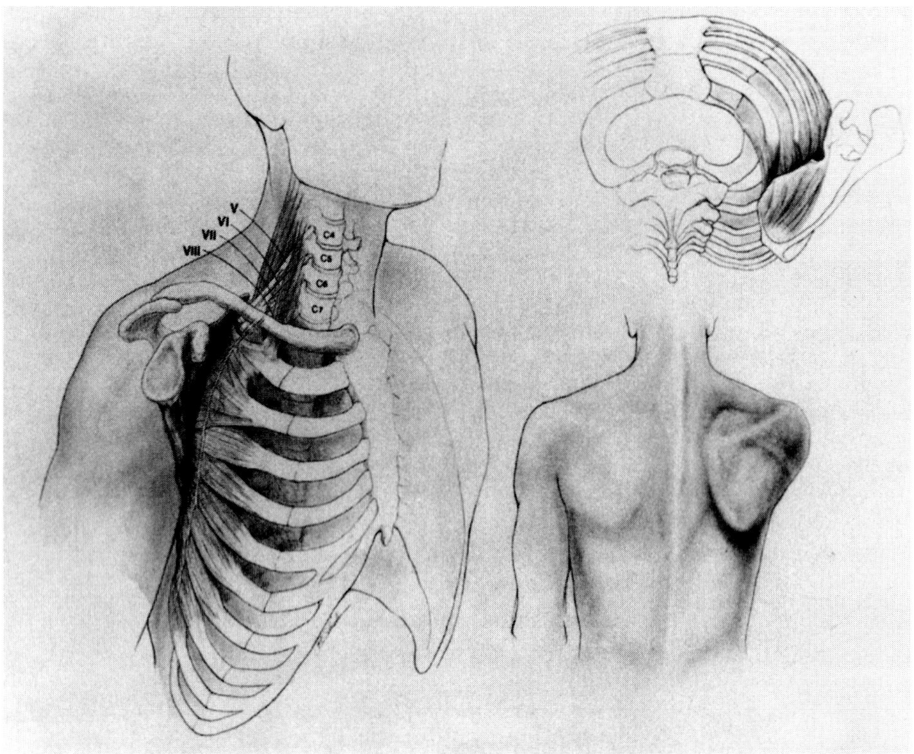

FIGURE 23-8. Scapular winging. The serratus anterior muscle (*upper right*) is supplied solely by the long thoracic nerve that branches immediately from C5, C6, C7, and sometimes C8 (*left figure*). Arising on the lateral ribs and inserting on the deep surface of the scapula, the muscle keeps the shoulder girdle approximated to the dorsal rib cage. Long thoracic nerve palsy allows dorsal protrusion of the scapula (*lower right*). See text. (Reproduced with permission from Martin JT: Postoperative isolated dysfunction of the long thoracic nerve: A rare entity of uncertain etiology. Anesth Analg 69:614, 1989.)

brachial plexus. Jellish et al[20] reported that there is less slowing of somatosensory evoked potentials (SSEPs) of the ulnar nerve during sternotomy when both arms are abducted instead of tucked at the sides. However, they found no differences in perioperative symptoms between patients in the arm-abducted versus arm-at-side groups.

Long Thoracic Nerve Dysfunction

Several lawsuits have centered on postoperative serratus anterior muscle dysfunction and winging of the scapula (Fig. 23-8) alleged to be the result of position-related injuries to the long thoracic nerve of Bell, which arises from nerve roots C5, C6, and C7. Because C5 and C6 fibers of the nerve course through the middle scalene muscle and emerge from its lateral border to join the fibers from C7, it has been proposed that neuropathies of the long thoracic nerve are traumatic in origin.[24] Johnson and Kendall[25] described the widely variable etiology of serratus anterior muscle paralysis in a review of 111 cases and found only 13% occurring after either a surgical procedure or an obstetric delivery. Because the nerve is not routinely involved in a stretch injury of the brachial plexus and because the plexus is not routinely involved when long thoracic nerve dysfunction occurs, the relationship between postoperative long thoracic nerve palsy and patient positioning remains speculative. Based on evidence of Foo and Swann[26] plus data from litigations, Martin[27] concluded that in the absence of demonstrable trauma, postoperative dysfunctions of the long thoracic nerve were quite likely the result of coincidental neuropathies, possibly of viral origin.

Axillary Trauma from the Humeral Head

Excessive abduction of the arm on an arm board may thrust the head of the humerus into the axillary neurovascular bundle. The bundle is stretched at that point and its neural structures may be damaged. In the same manner, vessels can be compressed or occluded and perfusion of the extremity can be jeopardized.

Radial Nerve Compression

The radial nerve, arising from roots C6-8 and T1, passes dorsolaterally around the middle and lower portions of the humerus in its musculospiral groove. At a point on the lateral aspect of the arm, approximately three fingerbreadths proximal to the lateral epicondyle of the humerus, the nerve can be compressed against the underlying bone and injured. Pressure from the vertical bar of an anesthesia screen or a similar device against the lateral aspect of the arm[28] and excessive cycling of an automatic blood pressure cuff[29] have been implicated in causing damage to the radial nerve. Postoperative radial nerve dysfunction is a relatively rare reason for malpractice litigation.[30,31]

Clinical manifestations of a radial nerve lesion include wrist drop, weakness of abduction of the thumb, inability to extend the metacarpophalangeal joints, and loss of sensation in the web space between the thumb and index finger.[32] Radial nerve function can be rapidly assessed by noting the patient's ability actively to extend the distal phalanx of the thumb.

Median Nerve Dysfunction

Isolated perioperative injuries to the median nerve are uncommon and the mechanism is obscure.[30,31] A potential source of injury is iatrogenic trauma to the nerve during access to vessels in the antecubital fossa, as might occur during venipuncture. Anecdotally, this problem appears to occur primarily in men 20 to 40 years of age who cannot easily extend their elbows completely. Forced elbow extension after administration of muscle relaxants and while positioning the arms, with resultant stretch of the median nerve, has been suggested as one potential mechanism for this problem. A quick check of sensation over the dorsal and palmar surfaces of the distal phalanges of the first and second fingers identifies an acute injury.

Ulnar Neuropathy

Improper anesthetic care and patient malpositioning have been implicated as causative factors in the development of ulnar neuropathies since reports by Büdinger[33] and Garriques[34] in the 1890s. These factors likely play an etiologic role for this problem in some surgical patients. Other factors, however, may contribute to the development of postoperative ulnar neuropathies. In a series of 12 inpatients with newly acquired ulnar neuropathy, Wadsworth and Williams[35] determined that external compression of an ulnar nerve during surgery was a factor in only two patients. Ulnar neuropathies develop in medical as well as surgical patients.[36] The mechanisms of ulnar neuropathy are unclear.

5 Typically, anesthesia-related ulnar nerve injury is thought to be associated with external nerve compression or stretch caused by malpositioning during the intraoperative period. Although this implication may be true for some patients, three findings suggest that other factors may contribute. First, patient characteristics (e.g., male sex, high body mass index [≥38], and prolonged postoperative bed rest) are associated with these ulnar neuropathies.[37] Various reports suggest that 70 to 90% of patients who have this problem are men.[30,31,35–37] Second, many patients with perioperative ulnar neuropathies have a high frequency of contralateral ulnar nerve conduction dysfunction.[38] This finding suggests that many of these patients likely have asymptomatic but abnormal ulnar nerves before their anesthetics, and these abnormal nerves may become symptomatic during the perioperative period. Finally, many patients do not notice or complain of ulnar nerve symptoms until more than 48 hours after their surgical procedures.[37,38] A prospective study of ulnar neuropathy in 1,502 surgical patients found that none of the patients had symptoms of the neuropathy during the first 2 postoperative days.[39] It is not clear whether onset of symptoms indicates the time that an injury has occurred to the nerve. Prielipp et al[40] found that 8 of 15 awake volunteers who had notable alterations in their ulnar nerve SSEP signals from direct ulnar nerve pressure did not perceive a paresthesia, even when the SSEP waveforms decreased as much as 72%.

Elbow flexion can cause ulnar nerve damage by several mechanisms. In some patients, the ulnar nerve is compressed by the aponeurosis of the flexor carpi ulnaris muscle and cubital tunnel retinaculum when the elbow is flexed by more than 110 degrees[41,42] (Fig. 23-9). In other patients, this fibrotendinous roof of the cubital tunnel is poorly formed and can lead to anterior subluxation or dislocation of the ulnar nerve over the medial epicondyle of the humerus during elbow flexion. This displacement has been observed in approximately 16% of cadavers in whom the flexor muscle aponeurosis and supporting tissues have not been dissected.[43,44] Ashenhurst[44] has speculated that the ulnar nerve may be chronically damaged by recurrent mechanical trauma as the nerve subluxates over the medial epicondyle.

External compression in the absence of elbow flexion also may damage the ulnar nerve.[45,46] Although compression within the medial epicondylar groove may be possible if the groove is shallower than normal, the bony groove usually is deep and the nerve is well protected from external compression.[47] External compression may occur distal to the medial epicondyle, where the nerve and its associated artery are relatively superficial. In an anatomic study, Contreras et al[48] observed that the ulnar nerve and posterior recurrent ulnar artery pass posteromedially to the tubercle of the coronoid process, where they are covered only by skin, subcutaneous fat, and a thin distal band of the aponeurosis of the flexor carpi ulnaris.

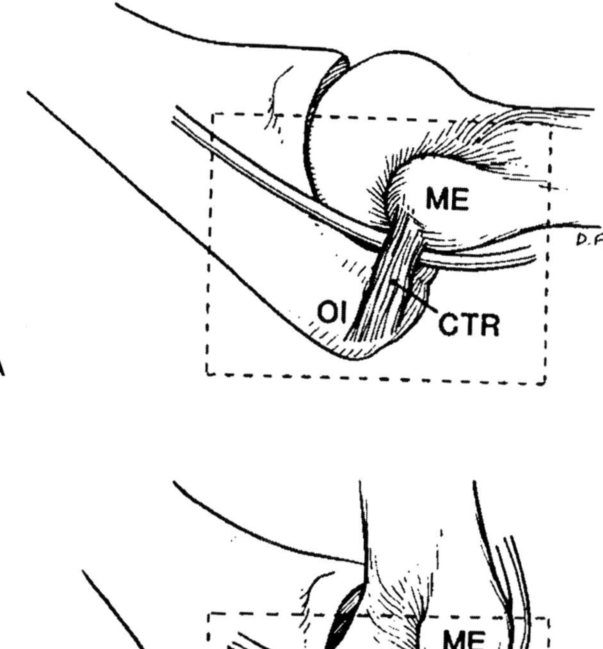

FIGURE 23-9. Medial-to-lateral view of right elbow. The cubital tunnel retinaculum (CTR) is lax in extension (**A**) as it stretches from the medial epicondyle (ME) to the olecranon (Ol). The retinaculum tightens in flexion (**B**) and can compress the ulnar nerve (*arrow*). (Reprinted with permission from O'Driscoll SW, Horii E, Carmichael SW *et al:* The cubital tunnel and ulnar neuropathy. J Bone Joint Surg Am 73:613, 1991.)

Why are men more likely to have this complication? There are several anatomic differences between men and women that may increase the likelihood of perioperative ulnar neuropathy developing in men. First, two anatomic differences may increase the chance of ulnar nerve compression in the region of the elbow. The tubercle of the coronoid process is approximately 1.5 times larger in men than women.[48] In addition, there is less adipose tissue over the medial aspect of the elbow of men compared with women of similar body fat composition.[48–50] Second, men may be more likely to have a well-developed cubital tunnel retinaculum than women, and the retinaculum, if present, is thicker. A thicker cubital tunnel retinaculum may increase the risk of ulnar nerve compression in the cubital tunnel when the elbow is flexed.

Clinical manifestations of ulnar nerve dysfunction vary with the location and extent of the lesion.[51] Nearly all patients have numbness, tingling, or pain in the sensory distribution of the ulnar nerves once they become symptomatic. However, there can be considerable ulnar nerve dysfunction before symptoms appear. Prielipp et al[40] found that only 8 of 15 male volunteers with significant ulnar nerve conduction slowing noted any symptoms. More studies are needed to understand better the mechanism and natural history of ulnar neuropathy.

Ulnar nerve injury is relatively common.[30,31,39] Also, a significant proportion of patients have symptoms of bilateral ulnar nerve dysfunctions both before and after surgery.[38] Therefore, some have speculated it might be helpful during the preanesthetic interview to inquire about a history of ulnar neuropathies ("crazy bone" problems) or previous surgery at the elbow. If such a history is indicated, the finding must be recorded and a discussion with the patient or family should present the possibility of a postoperative recurrence despite special precautions of padding and positioning.

The time of recognition of digital anesthesia associated with ulnar nerve dysfunction may be quite important in establishing the origin of the postoperative syndrome. If ulnar hypesthesia or anesthesia is noted promptly after the end of anesthesia, as in the recovery facility, the condition is likely to be associated with events that occurred during anesthesia or surgery. If the recognition is delayed for many hours, the likelihood of cause shifts from the intra-anesthetic period to postoperative events. In a review of closed claims, Kroll and associates[30] commented that postoperative ulnar dysfunction can occur as a result of events in the postanesthetic period and that nerve injury may develop in certain susceptible patients "despite conventionally accepted methods of positioning and padding."

Opioids may mask postoperative dysesthesias and pain, but even strong analgesics cannot mask a loss of sensation as a result of nerve dysfunction. It may be helpful to assess ulnar nerve function and record these observations before discharging the patient from the recovery room.

Arm Complications

An arm that is hyperabducted can force the head of the humerus into the axillary neurovascular bundle and damage nerves and vessels to the arm. Abduction of the arm to more than 90 degrees from the trunk should be avoided. An arm board should be securely attached to the operating table to prevent its accidental release. An arm that is not properly secured can slip over the edge of the table or arm board, resulting in injury to the capsule of the shoulder joint by excessive dorsal extension of the humerus, fracture of the neck of an osteoporotic humerus, or injury to the ulnar nerve at the elbow. Conversely, in the unlikely event that the retaining strap is excessively tight across the supinated forearm (Fig. 23-10), the potential exists for pressure to compress the anterior interosseous nerve, a branch of the median nerve in the upper forearm that courses with its artery along the volar surface of the tough interosseous membrane. The result is an ischemic injury to the distribution of the nerve and artery that resembles a compartment syndrome in the lower extremity and may require prompt surgical decompression.[52–54]

Backache

Lumbar backache can be worsened by the ligamentous relaxation that occurs with general, spinal, or epidural anesthesia. Loss of normal lumbar curvature in the supine position is apparently the issue. Padding (see Fig. 23-3) placed under the lumbar spine before the induction of anesthesia may help retain lordosis and make a patient with known lumbar distress more comfortable. Hyperlordosis should be

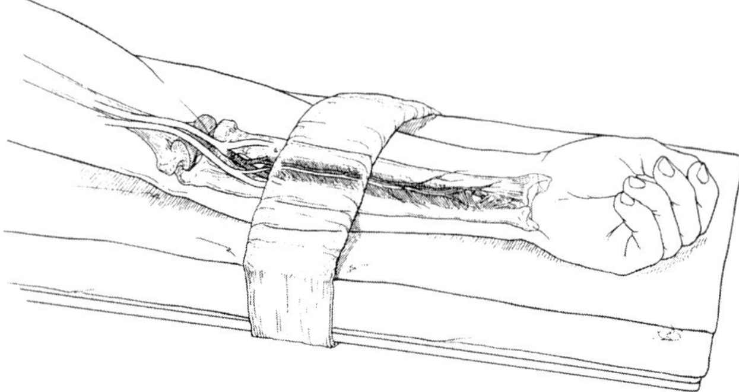

FIGURE 23-10. Arm restraint, if excessively tight, can compress the anterior interosseous nerve and vessel against the interosseous membrane in the volar forearm to produce an ischemic neuropathy. (Reproduced with permission from McLeskey CH [ed]: Geriatric Anesthesiology. Baltimore, Williams & Wilkins, 1997.)

avoided, however. Hyperextension of the lumbar spine, especially to an angulation of more than 10 degrees at the L2-3 apex of the lumbar spine, may result in ischemia of the spinal nerves.[55]

Elevation of the legs can worsen the pain of a herniated nucleus pulposus. When the lithotomy position is contemplated for a patient with a history of low back pain or a herniated lumbar disk, gentle passive attempts to have the patient assume the posture before anesthesia may be helpful in determining whether the position can be tolerated.

Perineal Crush Injury

The supine patient who is placed on a fracture table for repair of a fractured femur usually has the pelvis retained in place by a vertical pole at the perineum (Fig. 23-11), with the foot of the injured extremity fixed to a mobile rest. A worm gear on the rest lengthens the distance between the foot and the pelvis so that the bone fragments can be distracted and realigned. Unless the pole is well padded, severe pressure can be exerted on the pelvis, and damage can occur to the genitalia and the pudendal nerves. Complete loss of penile sensation has been reported after use of the fracture table.[56,57] The correct position for the pole is against the pelvis between the genitalia and the uninjured limb.[56]

Compartment Syndrome

If, for whatever reason, perfusion to an extremity is inadequate, a compartment syndrome may develop. Characterized by ischemia, hypoxic edema, elevated tissue pressure within fascial compartments of the leg, and extensive rhabdomyolysis, the syndrome produces extensive and potentially lasting damage to the muscles and nerves in the compartment. Because the pathologic process is at tissue level, distal pulses and capillary refill may remain intact while a compartment syndrome is developing in an extremity; thus, they are not useful indicators of the ongoing process. Ferrihemate, resulting from myoglobin destruction, exerts a direct toxic effect on renal tubular epithelium, and renal failure is likely.[58] Circulating debris from infections in the involved extremities is apt to be filtered by pulmonary microvasculature with injurious consequences for the lung.

Causes of a compartment syndrome while a patient is in any of the dorsal decubitus positions include (1) systemic hypotension and loss of driving pressure to the extremity (augmented by elevation of the extremity); (2) vascular obstruction of major leg vessels by intrapelvic retractors, by excessive flexion

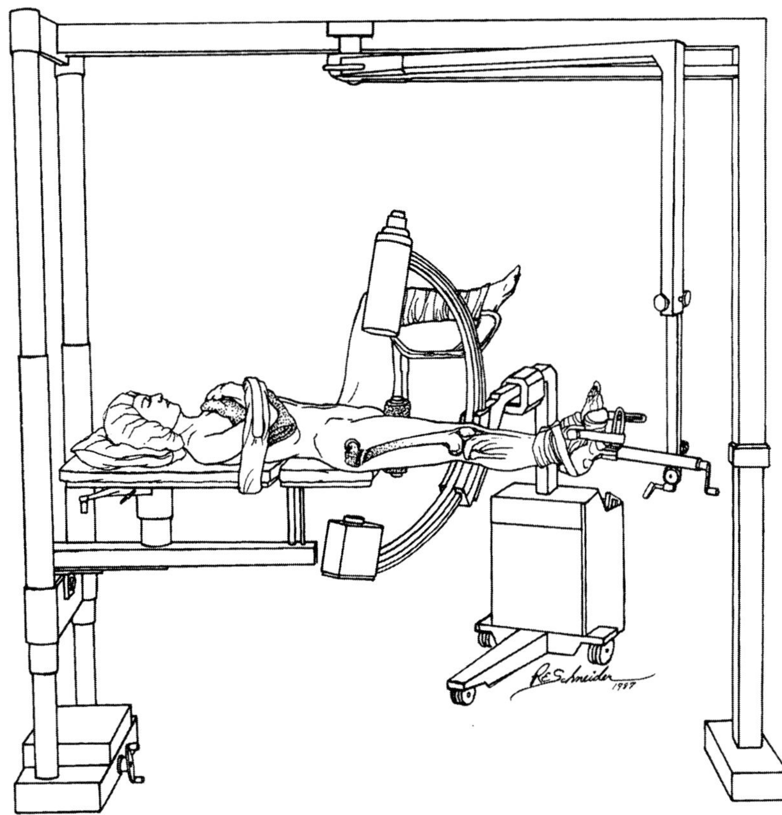

FIGURE 23-11. Traction table with perineal post stabilizing patient while leg is elongated to reposition bone ends. Elevated leg risks hypoperfusion; pelvic post threatens genitalia. (Reproduced with permission from Figure 6-6, (p. 54) of Martin JT, Warner MA [eds]: Positioning in Anesthesia and Surgery, 3rd ed. Philadelphia, WB Saunders, 1997.)

of knees or hips, or by undue popliteal pressure from a knee crutch; and (3) external compression of the elevated extremity by straps or leg wrappings that are too tight, by the inadvertent pressure of the arm of a surgical assistant, or by the weight of the extremity against a poorly supportive leg holder.[9,59] A tight strap on an arm as well as tight "drawsheets" for maintaining arms at the patient's sides may compress the anterior interosseous neurovascular bundle and may be associated with an anterior interosseous neuropathy or a forearm or a hand compartment syndrome.[53,54]

Several clinical characteristics seem to be associated with perioperative compartment syndrome. Prolonged lithotomy posture in excess of 5 hours has been a common factor in literature anecdotes of postlithotomy compartment syndromes. For lengthy procedures in the lithotomy position, well-padded holders that immobilize the limb by supporting the foot without compressing the calf or popliteal fossa seem to be the least threatening choice. There is considerable variability in the perfusion pressure of the lower extremity in elevated legs. Halliwill et al[12] and Pfeffer et al[13] found significant blood pressure variation at the ankle in volunteers placed in various lithotomy positions. Several volunteers had mean pressures of less than 20 mm Hg when positioned in the high lithotomy position. This pressure is less than intracompartment pressures commonly measured in many lithotomy positions.

Warner et al[60] have shown that perioperative compartment syndromes occur in patients in positions other than lithotomy. In fact, the frequency of this problem occurs as often (approximately 1:9,000 patients) in anesthetized patients who are positioned laterally as in similar patients who are positioned in lithotomy. The difference between compartment syndromes in these two groups is that patients in a lateral decubitus position tend to have compartment syndromes of either arm, while those in a lithotomy position have compartment syndromes of the lower extremities.[60]

Finger Injury

In 1968, Courington and Little[61] described the amputation of a young woman's fingers that were caught between the leg and thigh sections of the operating table as the leg section was returned to the horizontal position at the termination of an operation during which the patient was in the lithotomy position. A towel used to create a boxing glove–like wrap on the hands of lithotomized patients or carefully removing the patient's hands from the risk position before raising the foot of the table may prevent such a tragic misadventure.[62]

LATERAL DECUBITUS POSITIONS

Physiology

Circulatory

In the lateral decubitus position, the patient is turned onto one side of the trunk and stabilized to prevent accidental rolling toward either the supine or the prone posture. It is of practical and legal importance to note that the side of the body that rests on the table is the side that determines the name of the position (left side down = left lateral decubitus position).

If the legs are maintained in the long axis of the body, almost no pressure gradients exist along the great vessels from head to foot. Small hydrostatic differences are detected between the values when blood pressure is recorded simultaneously on the two arms.

If the lower extremities are positioned below the level of the heart, blood pools in the distensible vessels of the dangling legs because of gravity-induced increases in venous pressure and resultant venous stasis. Wrapping the legs and thighs in compressive bandages has been commonly used to combat venous pooling. Marked flexion of the lower extremities at knees and hips can partially or completely obstruct venous return to the inferior vena cava either by angulation of vessels at the popliteal space and inguinal ligament or by thigh compression against an obese abdomen. A small support placed just caudad of the down-side axilla can be used to lift the thorax enough to relieve pressure on the axillary neurovascular bundle and prevent disturbed blood flow to the arm and hand. However, this chest support (inappropriately called an *axillary roll* by some) has not been proven to reduce the frequency of ischemia, nerve damage, or compartment syndrome to the down-side upper extremity. It may, however, decrease shoulder discomfort postoperatively. Any padding should support only the chest wall and it should be periodically observed to ensure that it doesn't impinge on the neurovascular structures of the axilla.

In the low-pressure pulmonary circuit, hydrostatic gradients occur between the two hemithoraces. Although the degree of gravity-induced lateral displacement of the heart is different in the two lateral decubitus positions, it is generally true that most of the down-side lung lies below the level of the atrium and that the up-side lung lies above it. Vascular congestion of the down-side lung resembles a zone 3 of West et al,[4] whereas the relative hypoperfusion of the up-side lung resembles a zone 2. Kaneko et al[63] found that the transition between zone 3 and zone 2 occurred at approximately 18 cm above the most dependent part of the lung.

If the cervical spine of the patient who is placed in a horizontal lateral decubitus position is carefully maintained in alignment with the thoracolumbar spine, almost no gradient occurs between pressures in the mediastinum and those in the head. However, if the head is not supported and sufficient lateral angulation of the neck occurs in either direction, obstruction of jugular flow may occur.

Respiratory

In the presence of a supple chest, the lateral decubitus position can decrease the volume of the down-side hemithorax. The weight of the chest may force the down-side rib cage into a less expanded conformation. Gravity-induced shifts of mediastinal structures toward the down-side chest wall tend further to reduce the volume of the dependent lung. Abdominal viscera force the down-side diaphragm cephalad if the long axis of the trunk is horizontal or head down.

Spontaneous ventilation can partially compensate for the diaphragmatic stretching in the dependent hemithorax because the contractile efficiency of the elongated diaphragmatic muscle fibers is increased. The compacted lung base and zone 3 vascular congestion decrease compliance and interfere with the distribution of gas during positive-pressure ventilation. An elevated kidney rest placed against either the down-side rib margin or flank, or that migrates into that position as the patient shifts on it, further interferes with movement of the down-side hemidiaphragm and passive ventilation of the dependent lung.

The up-side hemithorax is much less compressed than the dependent side, and because the lung lies above the level of the atria, it has less vascular congestion than the down-side lung. As a result, unless contralateral flexion has stretched the up-side flank muscles to the point of rigidity and limited excursions of the costal margin, positive-pressure ventilation is directed preferentially to the more compliant up-side lung. The result can easily be excessive ventilation of the underperfused up-side lung and hypoventilation of the congested down-side lung. The potential for a clinically significant ventilation–perfusion mismatch is obvious, particularly in the presence of pulmonary disease.

Variations of the Lateral Decubitus Positions

Standard (Horizontal) Lateral Position

In the horizontal lateral decubitus position (Fig. 23-12), the patient is rolled onto one side on a flat table surface and stabilized in that posture by flexing the down-side thigh. The down-side knee is bent to retain the leg on the table and improve stabilization of the trunk. The common peroneal nerve of that side is padded to minimize compression damage caused by the weight of the legs. The up-side thigh and leg are extended comfortably, and pillows are placed between the lower extremities. The head is supported by pillows or a head rest so that the cervical and thoracic spines are properly aligned. A small pad, thick enough to raise the chest wall and prevent excessive compression of the shoulder or entrapment/compression of the neurovasclar structures of the axilla, is placed just caudad to the down-side axilla. This padding may support adequate perfusion of the down-side hand and minimize circumduction of the dependent shoulder, which might stretch its suprascapular nerve.

Arms may be extended ventrally and retained on a single arm board with suitable padding between them, or they may be individually retained on a padded two-level arm support that can also help to stabilize the thorax. An alternate method of arm arrangement is to flex each elbow and place the arms on suitable padding on the table in front of the patient's face.

The patient is stabilized in the lateral position by the use of one or more retaining tapes or straps stretched across the hip and fixed to the underside of the table top. Care must be taken to see that the hip tapes or straps lie safely between the iliac crest and the head of the femur rather than over the head of the femur. An additional restraining tape or strap may be used across the thorax or shoulders if needed.

Semisupine and Semiprone

The semilateral postures are designed to allow the surgeon to reach anterolateral (semisupine) and posterolateral (semiprone) structures of the trunk. In the semisupine position, the up-side arm must be carefully supported so that it

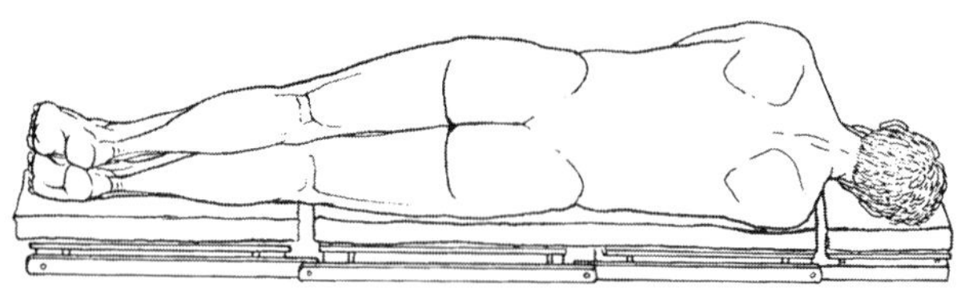

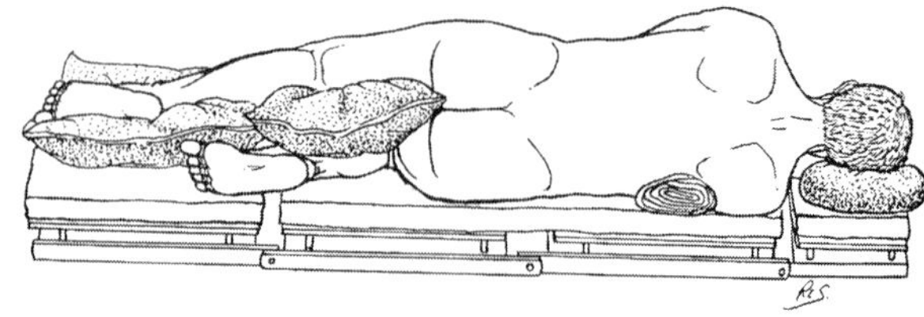

FIGURE 23-12. The standard lateral decubitus position. Proper head support, axillary roll, and leg pillow arrangement are shown on *lower figure*. Down-side leg is flexed at hip and knee to stabilize torso. Retaining straps and pad for down-side peroneal nerve are not shown. (Reproduced with permission from Figure 9-1, (p. 127) of Martin JT, Warner MA [eds]: Positioning in Anesthesia and Surgery, 3rd ed. Philadelphia, WB Saunders, 1997.)

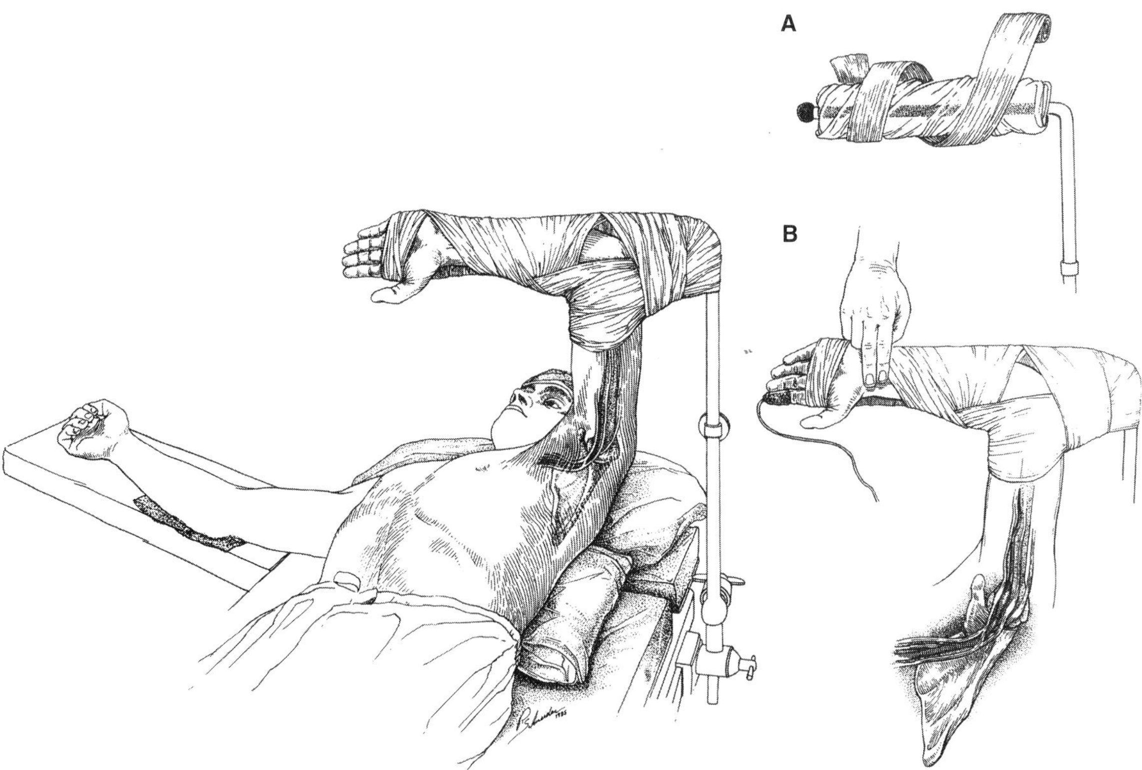

FIGURE 23-13. The semisupine position with dorsal pads supporting the torso, the extended arm padded at the elbow, and the elevated arm restrained on a well cushioned, adjustable overhead bar (**A**). Axillary contents (**B**) are not under tension and are not compressed by the head of the humerus, and a pulse oximeter ensures that the digital circulation is not compromised. The position is safe only if the arm does not become a hanging mechanism to support the torso. (Reproduced with permission from Figure 7-2, (p. 176) of Collins VJ [ed]: Principles of Anesthesiology, 3rd ed. Philadelphia, Lea & Febiger, 1993.)

is not hyperextended and no traction or compression is applied to the brachial and axillary neurovascular bundles (Fig. 23-13). The supporting bar should be well wrapped to prevent electrical grounding contact (see Fig. 23-13A). Sufficient noncompressible padding should be placed under the dorsal torso (see Fig. 23-13, *large figure*) and hip to prevent the patient from rolling supine and stretching the anchored extremity. The pulse of the restrained wrist should be checked to ensure adequate circulation in the elevated arm and hand (Fig. 23-13B).

Flexed Lateral Positions

Lateral Jackknife. The lateral jackknife position places the down-side iliac crest over the hinge between the back and thigh sections of the table (Fig. 23-14). The table top is angulated at that point to flex the thighs on the trunk laterally. After the patient has been suitably positioned and restrained, the chassis of the table is tipped so that the uppermost surface of the patient's flank and thorax becomes essentially horizontal. As a result, the feet are below the level of the atria, and significant amounts of blood may pool in distensible vessels in each leg.

The lateral jackknife position is usually intended to stretch the up-side flank and widen intercostal spaces as an asset to a thoracotomy incision. However, in terms of lumbar stress, restriction by the taut flank of up-side costal margin motion, and pooling of blood in depressed lower extremities, the position imposes a significant physiologic insult. Actually, its usefulness to the surgeon is brief, and its use should be limited. Once the rib-spreading retractor is placed in the incision, the position has reduced value for the rest of the operation.[64]

Kidney. The kidney position (Fig. 23-15) resembles the lateral jackknife position, but it adds the use of an elevated rest (the *kidney rest*) under the down-side iliac crest to increase the amount of lateral flexion and improve access to the up-side kidney under the overhanging costal margin. Unlike the lateral jackknife position, the kidney position does not have a useful alternative for a flank approach to the kidney. Thus, the physiologic insults associated with the posture need to be limited by vigilant anesthesia and rapid surgery. Strict stabilizing precautions should be taken to prevent the patient from subsequently shifting caudad on the table in such a manner that the elevated rest relocates into the down-side flank and becomes a severe impediment to ventilation of the dependent lung.

Complications of the Lateral Decubitus Positions

Eyes and Ears

Injuries to the dependent eye are unlikely if the head is properly supported during and after the turn from the supine to the lateral position. If the patient's face turns toward the mattress, however, and the lids are not closed or the eyes otherwise protected, abrasions of the ocular surface can occur. Direct pressure on the globe can displace the crystalline lens, increase intraocular pressure or, particularly if systemic hypotension is present, cause ischemia.

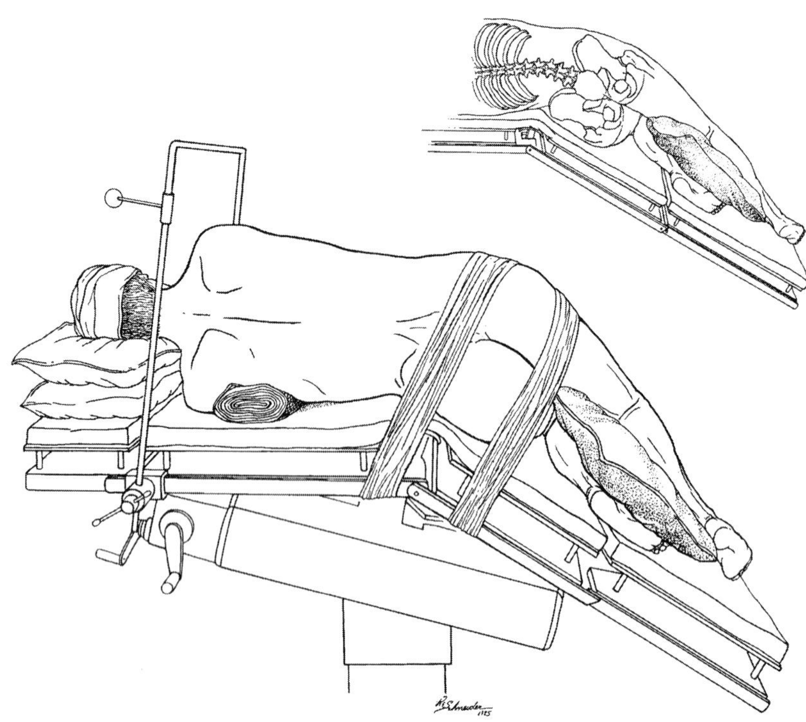

FIGURE 23-14. The lateral jackknife position, intended to open intercostal spaces. Note the properly placed restraining tapes (*large figure*) thrusting cephalad to retain the iliac crest at the flexion point of the table and prevent caudad slippage, which compresses the down-side flank (*insert*). (Reproduced with permission from Figure 9-4, (p. 130) of Martin JT, Warner MA [eds]: Positioning in Anesthesia and Surgery, 3rd ed. Philadelphia, WB Saunders, 1997.)

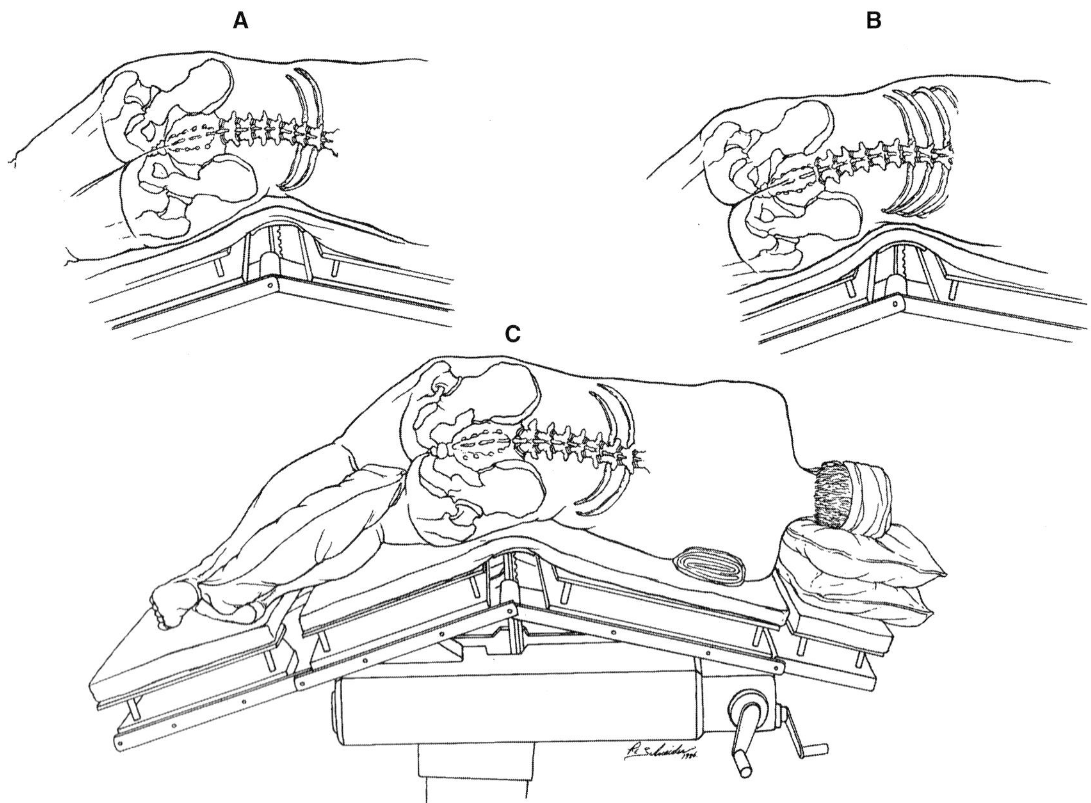

FIGURE 23-15. The flexed lateral (kidney) position. Upper panels show improper locations of the elevated transverse rest, the flexion point of the table, in the flank (**A**) or at the lower costal margin (**B**) to impede ventilation of the down-side lung. The iliac crest at the proper flexion point (**C**), allowing the best possible expansion of the down-side lung. Restraining tapes deleted for clarity. (Reproduced with permission from Figure 9-6, (p. 132) of Martin JT, Warner MA [eds]: Positioning in Anesthesia and Surgery, 3rd ed. Philadelphia, WB Saunders, 1997.)

In the lateral position, the weight of the head can press the down-side ear against a rough or wrinkled supporting surface. Careful padding with a pillow or a foam sponge is usually sufficient protection against contusion of the ear. The external ear should also be palpated to ensure that it has not been folded over in the process of placing support beneath the head.

Neck

Lateral flexion of the neck is possible when the head of a patient in the lateral position is inadequately supported. If the cervical spine is arthritic, postoperative neck pain can be troublesome. Pain from a symptomatic protrusion of a cervical disk can be intensified unless the head is carefully positioned so that lateral or ventral flexion, extension, or rotation is avoided. Patients with unstable cervical spines can be intubated while awake and turned gently into the operative position while repeated neurologic checks, with which the patient cooperates and responds, are accomplished to detect the development of a positioning injury.[65]

Suprascapular Nerve

Ventral circumduction of the dependent shoulder can rotate the suprascapular notch away from the root of the neck (Fig. 23-16). Because the suprascapular nerve is fixed both paravertebrally and at the notch, circumduction can stretch the nerve and produce troublesome, diffuse, dull shoulder pain. The diagnosis is established by blocking the nerve at the notch and producing pain relief. Treatment may require resecting the ligament over the notch to decompress the nerve. A supporting pad placed under the thorax just caudad of the axilla and thick enough to raise the chest off the shoulder should prevent a circumduction stretch injury to the nerve.

Long Thoracic Nerve

Instances of postoperative winging of the scapula (see Fig. 23-8) have followed use of the lateral decubitus position.[27] Although coincidental viral neuropathies of the long thoracic nerve may play a major etiologic role in postoperative appearances of scapular winging in patients for whom only a dorsal decubitus position was used, the possibility of trauma to the nerve while establishing the lateral position is difficult to refute. Lateral flexion of the neck may stretch the long thoracic nerve in the obtuse angle of the neck.

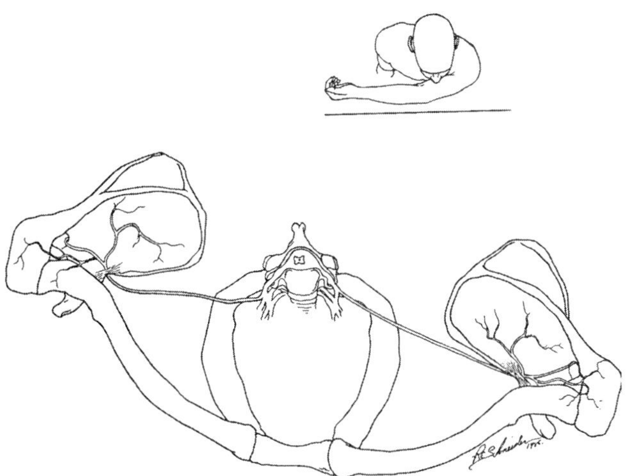

FIGURE 23-16. Circumduction of the arm displacing the scapula and stretching the suprascapular nerve between its anchoring points at the cervical spine and the suprascapular notch. (Reproduced with permission from Figure 9-14, (p. 147) of Martin JT, Warner MA [eds]: Positioning in Anesthesia and Surgery, 3rd ed. Philadelphia, WB Saunders, 1997.)

VENTRAL DECUBITUS (PRONE) POSITIONS

Physiology

Circulatory

In the *prone position*, the circulatory dynamics vary according to the postural modification in use. If the legs remain essentially horizontal, pressure gradients in the blood vessels are minimal. If the patient is kneeling, or if the table chassis is rotated head high, significant pooling of venous blood in distensible dependent vessels is likely to occur.

With the patient lying on the soft abdominal wall, pressure of compressed viscera is transmitted to the dorsal surface of the abdominal cavity. Mesenteric and paravertebral vessels are compressed, causing engorgement of veins within the spinal canal. Obstruction of the inferior vena cava can produce immediate, visible distention of vertebral veins. Because bleeding from incised vessels about the spine is increased under these circumstances, numerous modifications of the prone position have been created to free the abdomen from pressure, reduce the congestion of intraspinal veins, and facilitate surgical hemostasis.[66]

If the head of a prone patient is below the level of the heart, venous congestion of the face and neck becomes evident. Turning the patient's head can alter arterial perfusion and venous drainage in both extracranial and intracranial vessels. Conjunctival edema is usual and reflects the influence of gravity on accumulation of extravascular fluid (see Complications of the Ventral Decubitus Positions: Blindness section).

If the head is above the level of the heart, mean vascular pressures are decreased according to the distance above the heart and conjunctival edema is less evident or absent, but air entrainment in open veins is possible.

Kaneko et al[63] described the perfusion of the entire lung of prone subjects in terms that subsequently fit the zone 3 of West et al.[4] Backofen and Schauble[67] found that even the carefully established and supported prone position caused a significant fall in stroke volume and cardiac index, despite the development of increased vascular resistance in both the systemic and pulmonary circuits. No significant changes were detected in mean arterial pressure, right atrial pressure, or pulmonary artery occlusion pressure. On the basis of these observations, they recommend that, in patients whose cardiovascular status is precarious, invasive hemodynamic monitors be introduced to detect otherwise unrecognizable deterioration of cardiac function caused by positioning.

Respiratory

Using computed tomography, Gattinoni's group[68] found a dramatic redistribution of densities from the dorsal (paravertebral supine) to the ventral (substernal) portions of the lungs when subjects in respiratory failure were turned from the supine to the prone position. The original areas of compression atelectasis reopened when those parts of the lung became nondependent, whereas fresh areas of compression atelectasis formed rather promptly in newly dependent areas of the lung. In their study group, they found no change in oxygenation or shunting when pronation occurred.

If the thorax is supple or compliant, the body weight of an anesthetized, prone patient compresses the anteroposterior diameter of the relaxed chest to a degree that is real but poorly defined. If the particular prone posture in use allows the pressure of the abdominal viscera to be sufficient to force the diaphragm cephalad, the lung is shortened along its long axis. With both the dorsoventral and the cephalocaudad dimensions of the lung decreased, and in the presence of the relative vascular congestion of a zone 3 of West et al,[4] the compliance of the compacted prone lung can be anticipated to decrease. The result of decreased pulmonary compliance in a poorly positioned, prone, anesthetized patient is either an increased work of spontaneous ventilation or the need for higher inflation pressures during positive-pressure ventilation.

Proper positioning can retain more nearly normal pulmonary compliance by minimizing the cephalad shift of the diaphragm caused by compressed abdominal viscera. If the patient is arranged so that the abdomen hangs free, the loss of functional residual capacity is less in the prone position than in either the supine or the lateral position.[69] Rehder et al[70] noted that the weight of the freed abdominal contents had an "inspiratory effect on the diaphragm" when the pronated patient was properly supported by pads under the shoulder girdle and pelvis.

Variations of the Ventral Decubitus Position

Full (Horizontal) Prone

In the so-called *full* or *horizontal prone position* (Fig. 23-17), the requirement to elevate the trunk off the supporting surface so that the ventral abdominal wall is freed of compression almost always results in the head and lower extremities being below the level of the spine. If the table top is angulated at the trunk–thigh hinge to remove the lumbar lordosis and separate the lumbar spinous processes, and if the chassis is then rotated head-up sufficiently to level the patient's back, a significant perfusion gradient may develop between the legs and the heart. Wrapping the legs in compressive bandages, or the use of full-length elastic hosiery, minimizes pooling of blood in distensible vessels and supports venous return.

Various ventral supports, including parallel rolls of tightly packed sheets, padded and adjustable metal frames, and four-pillar frames, have been devised to free the abdomen from compression.[66,71] Each has merit, and no specific unit has been shown to be better than the others for hemodynamic or respiratory maintenance or patient safety. The choice is based on the physique of the patient, the requirements of the surgical procedure, and the available equipment.

Pronated patients with limited mobility of the neck, a history of postural neck pain, or a history suggesting a symptomatic cervical disk should have their heads retained in the sagittal plane, either with a skull-pin head clamp[72] or with a face rest. If the neck is pain free and its mobility is satisfactory, the head can be turned laterally and supported to prevent pressure on the down-side eye and ear.[73] However, forced rotation of the pronated head should be carefully avoided lest it induce postoperative neck pain or cervical nerve root or vascular compression.

When a patient is scheduled to be pronated after induction of anesthesia, it is worthwhile during the preanesthetic interview to obtain and record information about any limitations that may exist in his or her ability to raise the arms overhead during work or sleep.[66] If the patient is symptomatic, it may be prudent to place the arms alongside the torso after pronation (see the discussion of the Thoracic Outlet Syndrome, later). If the arms are placed alongside the head (i.e., extended ventrally at the shoulder, flexed at the elbow, and abducted onto arm boards; the "surrender" position), the musculature about the shoulders should be under no tension, neither humeral head should stretch or compress its axillary neurovascular bundle (i.e., shoulders should be abducted less than 90 degrees), ulnar nerves at the elbow should be padded, and the pulses at the wrists should remain full. Anterior (forward) flexion of the shoulders may reduce tension on the neurovascular structures of the axilla.

Prone Jackknife

The prone jackknife posture is used to provide access to the sacral, perianal, and perineal areas as well as to the lower alimentary canal (Fig. 23-18). The thighs are flexed on the trunk more than is usual in the full prone position, with the table surface hinges determining the degree of flexion achievable.[66]

Prone Kneeling

Kneeling positions have been used to improve operative conditions in the lumbar and cervicooccipital areas (Fig. 23-19).

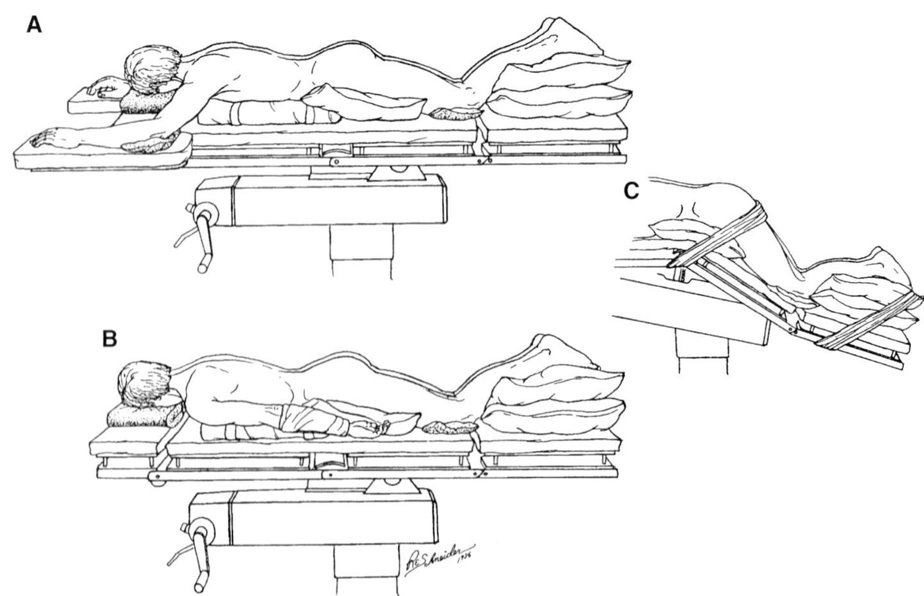

FIGURE 23-17. The classic prone position. **A.** Flat table with relaxed arms extended alongside patient's head. Parallel chest rolls extended from just caudad of clavicle to just beyond inguinal area, with pillow over pelvic end. Elbows and knees are padded, and legs are bent at the knees. Head is turned onto a C-shaped foam sponge that frees the down-side eye and ear from compression. **B.** Same posture with arms snugly retained alongside torso. **C.** Table flexed to reduce lumbar lordosis; subgluteal area straps placed after the legs are lowered to provide cephalad thrust and prevent caudad slippage. (Reproduced with permission from Figure 10-1, (p. 156) of Martin JT, Warner MA [eds]: Positioning in Anesthesia and Surgery, 3rd ed. Philadelphia, WB Saunders, 1997.)

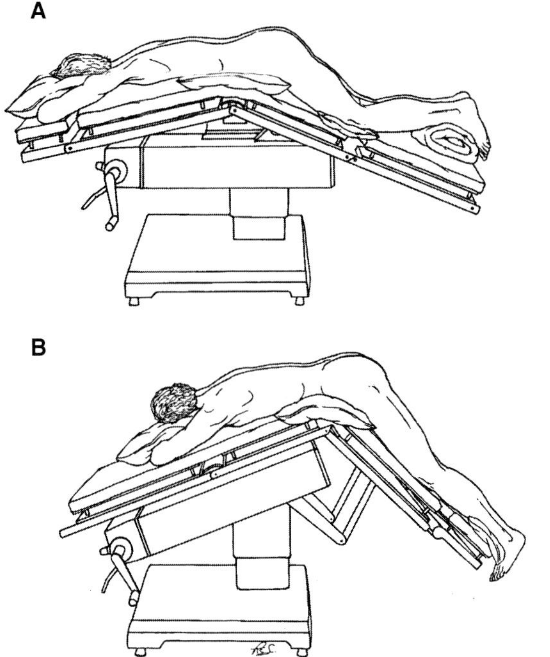

FIGURE 23-18. The prone jackknife positions. **A.** Low jackknife position with the trunk–thigh hinge of the table used as the flexion position and augmented by a pillow under the pelvis. **B.** Full jackknife position with the thigh–leg hinge of the table used as the flexion point to achieve more acute angulation of the hips on the torso. (Reproduced with permission from Figure 10-14 & 10-15, (p. 163 & 164) of Martin JT, Warner MA [eds]: Positioning in Anesthesia and Surgery, 3rd ed. Philadelphia, WB Saunders, 1997.)

Numerous frames have been constructed to support the weight of a kneeling patient, and their usefulness again depends on local use and the physique of the patient. If the vertebral column is unstable, kneeling frames are not as useful as parallel longitudinal supports because kneeling risks application of shearing forces at the fracture site, with the potential for damage of the contents of the spinal canal. In massively obese patients who must be operated on in the prone position, kneeling frames tend to prevent pressure on the abdomen more successfully than longitudinal frames.

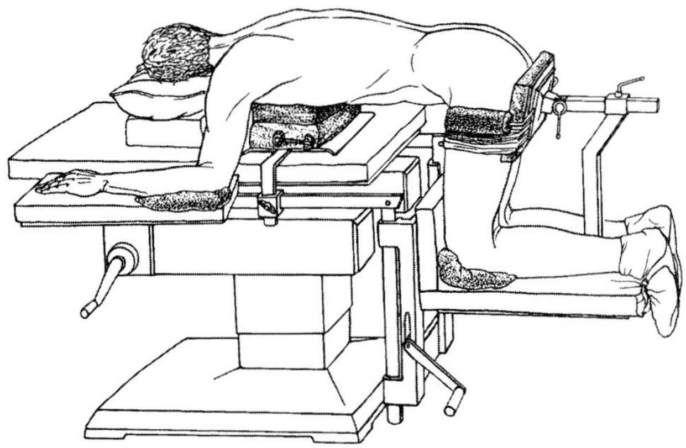

FIGURE 23-19. The Andrews kneeling frame with Wiltse's thoracic jack in use. (Reproduced with permission from Figure 10-9, (p. 161) of Martin JT, Warner MA [eds]: Positioning in Anesthesia and Surgery, 3rd ed. Philadelphia, WB Saunders, 1997.)

Complications of the Ventral Decubitus Positions

Eyes and Ears

The eyes and ears may sustain injury in the prone position. The eyelids should be closed, and each eye should be protected in some manner so that the lids cannot be accidentally separated and the cornea scratched. Instillation of lubrication in the eyes should be considered, although the value of this treatment is debated. The eyes should also be protected against the head turning medially after positioning as well as against pressure being exerted on the globe. Monitoring wires and intravenous tubing should be checked after pronation to see that none has migrated beneath the head. If the head is retained in the sagittal plane, the eyes should be checked after positioning to ensure that they are safe from compression by any head rest.

Conjunctival edema usually occurs in the eyes of the pronated patient if the head is at or below the level of the heart. It is usually transient, inconsequential, and requires only reestablishment of the normal tissue perfusion gradients of the supine position, or of a slight amount of head-up tilt, to be redistributed.

7 **Blindness.** Permanent loss of vision can occur after nonocular surgical procedures, especially those performed in a ventral decubitus position.[74–89] The occurrence of this devastating complication is particularly associated with extensive surgical procedures done in the prone position, such as reconstructive spine surgery, where there is associated blood loss, anemia, and hypotension. Visual loss after neurovascular and cardiopulmonary bypass procedures is well recognized and may be related to embolic events produced by the surgical intervention itself, hypoperfusion, or other nonpositioning causes.[90–93] Visual loss after noncardiac, nonneurovascular procedures may initially be noticed by a loss of acuity, a loss of visual field, or both.

Speculated causes of significant permanent postoperative visual loss usually involve compromise of oxygen delivery to elements of the visual pathway and include ischemic optic neuropathy (anterior or posterior), retinal artery occlusion (central or branch), and cortical blindness.[94] No case series exist to provide information regarding the frequency of these events after nonocular, noncardiac surgery in a general surgical population. Roth et al[76] surveyed approximately 61,000 patients undergoing nonocular surgery (including cardiac surgery) over a 4-year period and identified 34 ocular injuries (mostly corneal abrasions), including one case of permanent postoperative visual loss from ischemic optic neuropathy after lumbar spinal fusion. In a review of 3,450 spinal surgeries, Stevens et al[82] identified three patients who had permanent postoperative visual loss. Brown et al[95] identified three patients in whom postoperative ischemic optic neuropathy developed after noncardiac surgery over a 10-year period in one institution. Warner et al[96] noted none of nearly 11,000 prone-positioned patients developed perioperative vision loss. However, these authors subsequently have experienced several patients who have developed complete blindness after spinal surgery performed with patients positioned prone. Reflecting concern about the apparent increased incidence of perioperative blindness, the American Society of Anesthesiologists, Committee on Professional Liability, has created a formal registry to monitor and document the incidence of this complication (see http://www.asahq.org).

Positioning appears to be a risk factor for some of these events. Studies noting a relative high frequency of postoperative visual loss in spinal surgery patients have implicated positioning as one causative factor.[77–80,83,92] Use of the knee–chest position,[77] the prone position,[78,83,97] and the horseshoe head rest[79] have been cited as potential causes of visual loss, perhaps

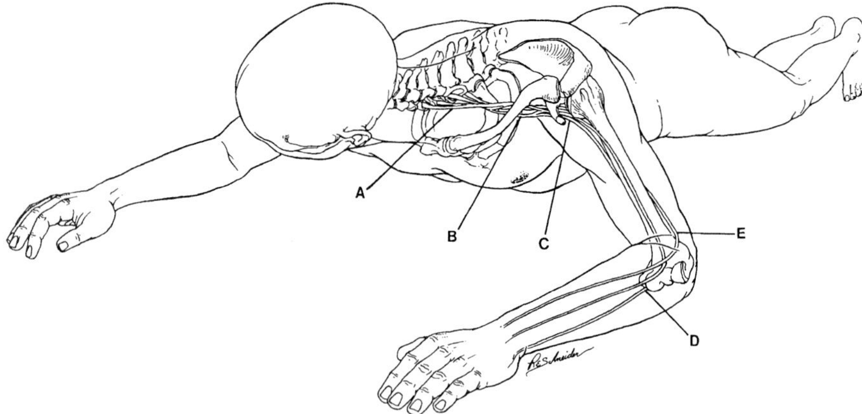

FIGURE 23-20. Sources of potential injury to the brachial plexus and its peripheral components when the patient is in the prone position. **A.** Neck rotation, stretching roots of the plexus. **B.** Compression of the plexus and vessels between the clavicle and first rib. **C.** Injury to the axillary neurovascular bundle from the head of the humerus. **D.** Compression of the ulnar nerve before, beyond, and within the cubital tunnel. **E.** Area of vulnerability of the radial nerve to lateral compression proximal to the elbow. (Reproduced with permission from Figure 10-29, (p. 185) of Martin JT, Warner MA [eds]: Positioning in Anesthesia and Surgery, 3rd ed. Philadelphia, WB Saunders, 1997.)

by direct pressure on the globe increasing the intraocular pressure beyond the perfusion pressure of the retina. Other reports, including those of spinal surgery patients, describe visual loss after prolonged procedures, intraoperative hypotension, and massive blood loss,[74–76,81,82] which may prevent adequate oxygen delivery to the visual apparatus. For example, all patients with ischemic optic neuropathy in the series of Brown et al[95] experienced periods of significant anemia (hemoglobin concentration <8 g/dL) and intraoperative hypotension. It is possible that venous congestion and edema in the head associated with the prone position may be a contributing factor.

Neck Problems

Anesthesia impairs reflex muscle spasm that protects the skeleton against motion that would be painful if the patient were alert. Lateral rotation of the head and neck of an anesthetized, pronated patient, particularly one with an arthritic cervical spine, can stretch relaxed skeletal muscles and ligaments and injure articulations of cervical vertebrae. Postoperative neck pain and limitation of motion can result. The arthritic neck is usually best managed by keeping the head in the sagittal plane when the patient is prone.

Extremes of head and neck rotation can also interfere with flow in either the ipsilateral or contralateral vessels to and from the head. Excessive head rotation can reduce flow in both the carotid[98] and vertebral systems.[99] Impaired cerebral perfusion is the obvious consequence.

Brachial Plexus Injuries

Stretch injuries to the roots of the brachial plexus (Fig. 23-20A) on the side contralateral to the turned face are possible if the contralateral shoulder is held firmly caudad by a wrist restraint. If an arm is placed on an arm board alongside the head, care must be taken to ensure that the head of the humerus is not stretching and compressing the axillary neurovascular bundle (see Fig. 23-20B,C).

When an arm is placed on an arm board alongside the head, the forearm naturally pronates. As a result, the ulnar nerve, lying in the cubital tunnel (the groove between the olecranon process and the medial epicondyle of the humerus), is vulnerable to being compressed by the weight of the elbow (see Fig. 23-20D). Consequently, the medial aspect of the elbow must be well padded and its weight borne principally on the medial epicondyle.

Asking patients about their ability to work or sleep with arms elevated overhead may identify patients with *thoracic outlet obstruction*.[66] A useful preoperative test if the history is in question is to have the patient clasp hands behind the occiput during the interview (Fig. 23-21). If the patient describes dysesthesias, it may be prudent to keep the arms alongside the trunk in the prone position. Agonizing, debilitating, and unremitting postoperative pain has been known to follow overhead arm placement in pronated patients who have had prior discomfort in their arms in that position.[66]

Breast Injuries

The breasts of a pronated woman, if forced laterally by ventral chest supports, can be stretched and injured along their sternal borders. Medial and cephalad displacement seems better

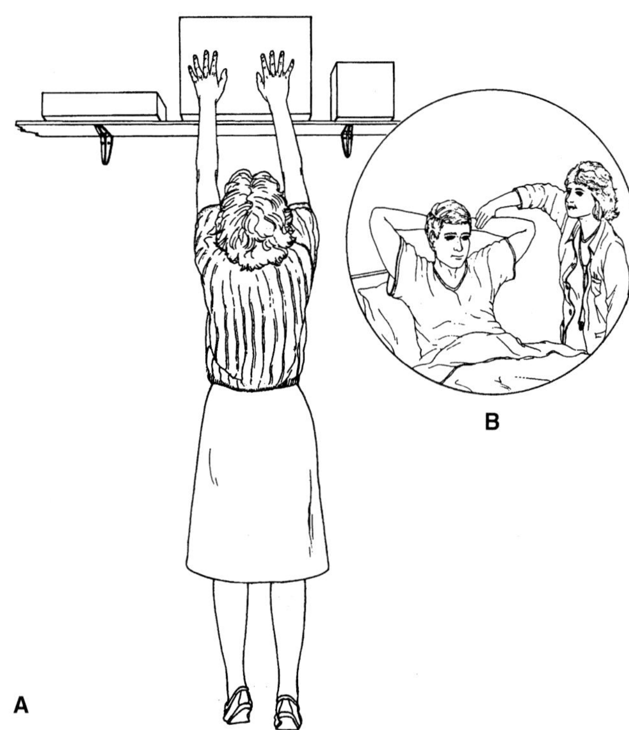

FIGURE 23-21. Assessment of a potential thoracic outlet syndrome. **A.** The patient has a history of distress when trying to work or sleep with arms over head. **B.** Interview was carried out with patient's hands clasped on occiput and radial pulses checked for damping. (Reproduced with permission from Figure 10-30, (p. 186) of McLeskey CH [ed]: Geriatric Anesthesiology. Baltimore, Williams & Wilkins, 1997.)

tolerated. Direct pressure on breasts (particularly if breast prostheses are present) can cause ischemia to breast tissue and should be avoided.

Abdominal Compression

Compression of the abdomen by the weight of the prone patient's trunk can cause viscera to force the diaphragm cephalad enough to impair ventilation. If intra-abdominal pressure approaches or exceeds venous pressure, return of blood from the pelvis and lower extremities is reduced or obstructed. Because the vertebral venous plexuses communicate directly with the abdominal veins, increased intra-abdominal pressure is transmitted to the perivertebral and intraspinal surgical field in the form of venous distention and increased difficulty with hemostasis. All of the various supportive pads and frames, when properly used, are designed to remove pressure from the abdomen and avoid these problems.[66]

Viscerocutaneous Stomata

Stomata that drain visceral contents into containers affixed to the abdominal wall are at risk in the prone position if they lie against a part of the ventral supporting frame or pad (Fig. 23-22). Compressive ischemia of the stomal orifice can cause it to slough.

Knee Injuries

Obese patients, or those who have pathologic conditions of the knees, can have their knee joints injured in the kneeling position if the supportive ledges are not heavily padded (see Fig. 23-19). Often there is no suitable alternative position for these patients, and the possibility of postoperative knee problems caused by the kneeling prone position should be carefully discussed in the preanesthetic interview.

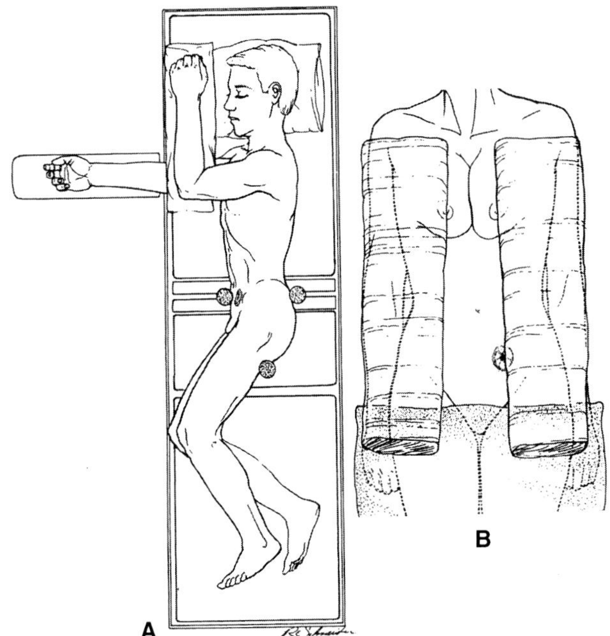

FIGURE 23-22. Postural supports compromising visceral stoma. Both the vertical abdominal support of a device designed to maintain a patient in the lateral position (A) and the longitudinal chest rolls supporting a pronated patient (B) can cause ischemic compression of a viscerocutaneous anastomosis and subsequent necrosis. Surgical repair of the stoma may be needed. (Modified with permission from Figure 22-18, (p. 340) of McLeskey CH [ed]: Geriatric Anesthesiology. Baltimore, Williams & Wilkins, 1997.)

HEAD-ELEVATED POSITIONS

Physiology

Circulatory

Coonan and Hope[100] have reviewed circulatory changes that occur in alert humans with the change from the supine to the erect position. As the head is raised above the level of the heart, pressure gradients develop and increase with the degree of elevation. Blood shifts from the upper body toward the feet. Atrial filling pressures decrease, sympathetic tone increases, parasympathetic tone decreases, the renin-angiotensin-aldosterone system is activated, and fluid and electrolytes are retained by the kidneys.[101,102] Albin et al[103,104] and Dalrymple[105] noted similar alterations in cardiovascular parameters when the head-elevated position was established after patients were anesthetized. Although significant changes were not encountered with less than 60 degrees of head-up tilt, the magnitude of changes in anesthetized patients was often greater than in the awake patients.

The presence of an intracranial pathologic process can be expected to exacerbate potentially harmful reductions in cerebral blood flow associated with head elevation.[106] In the anesthetized, seated patient, mean arterial pressure should be measured at the level of the circle of Willis because that site is more reliable as an indicator of cerebral perfusion pressure in the head-elevated posture than is measurement at the level of the arm or wrist.[100] Additional information regarding the neurosurgical implications of the head-elevated (sitting) position appear in Chapter 27.

Respiratory

As the patient becomes more upright in the head-elevated dorsal decubitus position, the inspiratory stroke of the diaphragm becomes less impeded by the bulk of abdominal viscera. Spontaneous chest wall motion requires less effort, and less pressure is needed to inflate the lungs during passive inspiration. Functional residual capacity increases in the head-elevated positions.[107]

Variations of the Head-Elevated Positions

Sitting

The classic *sitting position* for surgery places the patient in a semireclining posture on an operating table, with the legs elevated to approximately the level of the heart and the head flexed ventrally on the neck (Fig. 23-23). Head flexion should not be sufficient to force the chin into the suprasternal notch (see Midcervical Tetraplegia section). Elastic stockings or compressive wraps around the legs reduce pooling of blood in the lower extremities. The head often is held in place by some type of a face rest or by a three-pin skull fixation frame.

Supine—Tilted Head Up

A dorsal recumbent position with the head of the patient elevated is used for many operations involving the ventral and lateral aspects of the head (Fig. 23-24) and neck, and occasionally with the neck flexed, for transcranial access to the top of the brain. Its purpose is to improve access to the surgical target

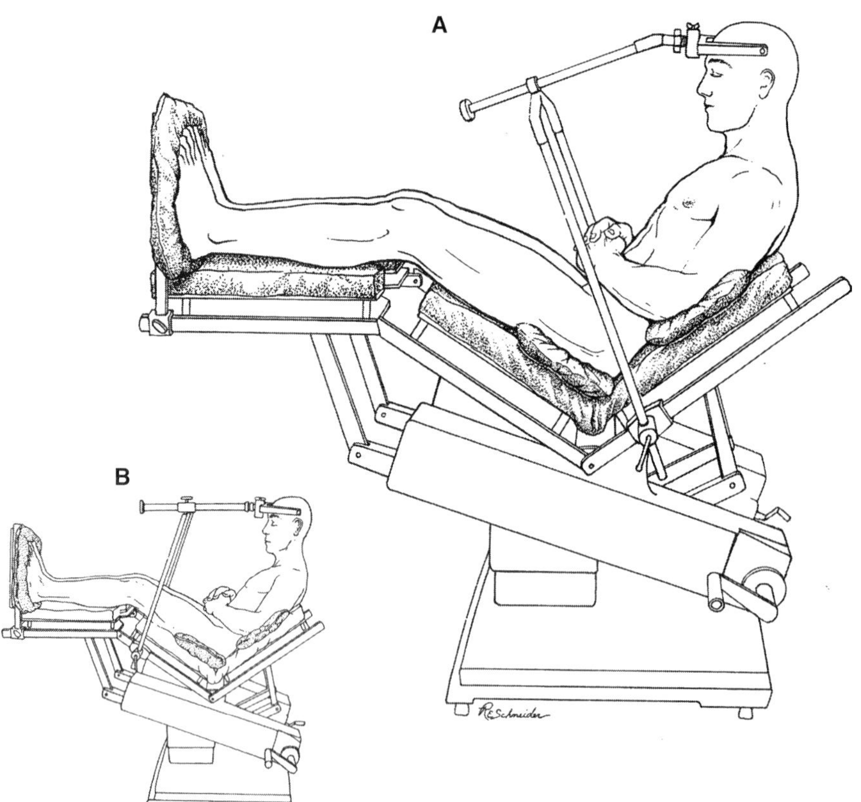

FIGURE 23-23. **A.** Conventional neurosurgical sitting position. The legs are at approximately the level of the heart and gently flexed on the thighs; the feet are supported at right angles to the legs; subgluteal padding protects the sciatic nerve. The frame of the head holder is *properly* clamped to the side rails of the back section in the event of hemodynamically significant air embolism. **B.** *Improper* attachment of the head frame to the table side rails at the thigh section. In this position, the patient's head could not be quickly lowered because it would require disengaging the skull clamp. (Reproduced with permission from Figure 7-1, (p. 72) of Martin JT, Warner MA [eds]: Positioning in Anesthesia and Surgery, 3rd ed. Philadelphia, WB Saunders, 1997.)

for the operating team as well as to drain blood and irrigation solutions away from the wound. The back section of the surgical table can be elevated as needed to produce a low sitting position (see Fig. 23-24A), or the entire table can be rotated head-high with the patient's extended legs supported by a foot rest (see Fig. 23-24B). Although the degree of tilt typically is not great, small pressure gradients are created along the vascular axis that can pool blood in the lower extremities or entrain air in patulous vessels that are incised above the level of the heart.

For operations around the shoulder joint, the patient may be placed in a head-elevated semisupine position, with the upper torso rotated toward the nonsurgical shoulder and supported by a firm roll or pad (Fig. 23-25). The upper trunk is moved laterally until the raised surgical shoulder extends beyond the edge of the operating table. The torso is supported so that the hips are on the table, the surgical shoulder is off and above the table edge, and the head rests on either a pillow (see Fig. 23-25A) or a horseshoe head rest (see Fig. 23-25B). Access is thereby provided to both the dorsal and ventral aspects of the shoulder girdle. The surgical arm remains on the ventral torso and is prepared and draped to be mobile in the surgical field.

Lateral—Tilted Head Up

The lateral decubitus position with the head somewhat elevated, a means of access to occipitocervical lesions, has also been referred to as the *park bench position*.[108] All the stabilizing requirements needed for the usual lateral decubitus position apply. The head may be held firmly in a three-pin skull fixation holder, which can be readjusted as needed during surgery, or supported by pillows or padding. Although the degree of head elevation used typically is less than 15 degrees, the position does not completely remove the threat of air embolization. The anesthesiologist has good access to the patient's face and ventral thorax for purposes of monitoring, manipulation,

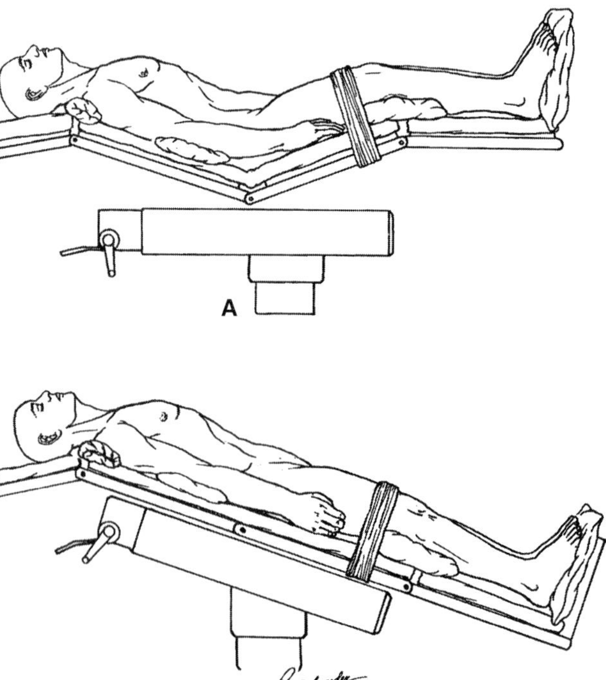

FIGURE 23-24. Head-elevated positions often used for operations about the ventral and ventrolateral aspects of the head, face, neck, and cervical spine. **A.** The legs are at approximately heart level and the gradient into the head is appreciable but slight. **B.** The flat table and foot rest are useful when a thyroidectomy is planned under regional anesthesia. (Reproduced with permission from Figure 7-7, (p. 89) of Martin JT, Warner MA [eds]: Positioning in Anesthesia and Surgery, 3rd ed. Philadelphia, WB Saunders, 1997.)

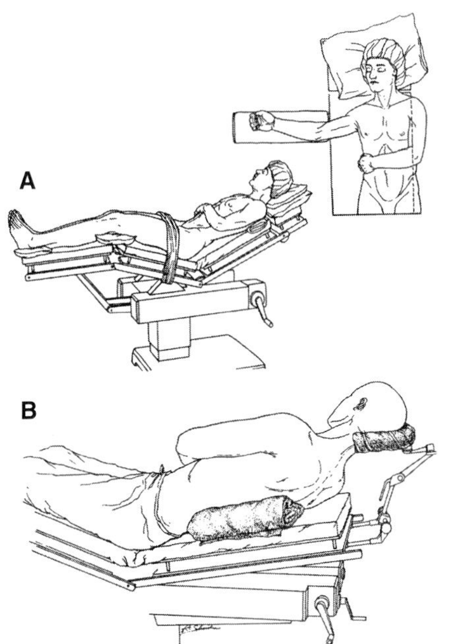

FIGURE 23-25. A. The barber chair position for surgery around the shoulder joint. B. The upper torso is rotated toward the nonsurgical shoulder and supported with a firm roll or pad.

and resuscitation. Considerable attention should be directed to avoiding compression of neck veins, which can lead to an increase in intracranial pressure and to edema of the tongue.

Prone—Tilted Head Up

The ventral decubitus posture with the table rotated head high (Fig. 23-26) can be used to access dorsal structures of the head and neck. Usually the perceived advantage of this position compared to a sitting position is the avoidance of air embolization.

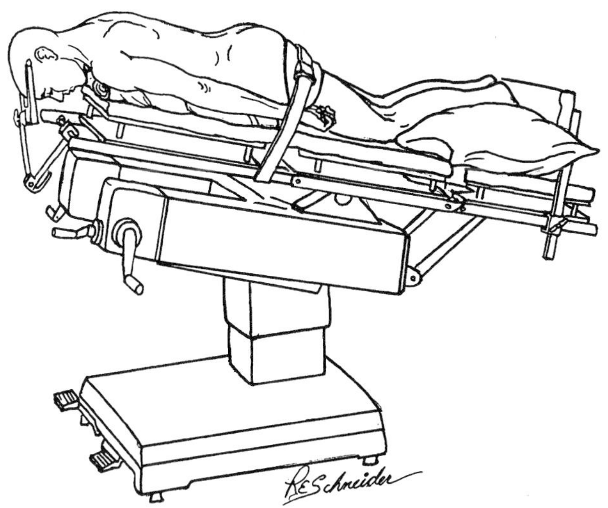

FIGURE 23-26. The skull-pin head rest used to stabilize a patient in the head-elevated prone position. Note the chest rolls used to free the abdomen from compression and the gluteal strap to minimize caudad slippage after head-up tilt. (Reproduced with permission from Figure 7-6, (p. 88) of Martin JT, Warner MA [eds]: Positioning in Anesthesia and Surgery, 3rd ed. Philadelphia, WB Saunders, 1997.)

Although the pressure gradients for air entrainment into patulous veins are less than in the full sitting position, the hazard is not eliminated. As a result of the positive-pressure inflation cycle of passive ventilation, a bothersome recurrent flux of cerebrospinal fluid into and out of the exposed wound may be encountered. The posture also restricts resuscitative access to the ventral thorax.

Complications of the Head-Elevated Positions

Postural Hypotension

In the anesthetized patient, establishing any of the head-elevated positions is frequently accompanied by some degree of reduction in systemic blood pressure. The normal protective reflexes are inhibited by drugs used during anesthesia. Measuring mean arterial pressures at the level of the circle of Willis is recommended to assess cerebral perfusion pressures more accurately.

Air Embolus

Air embolization is potentially lethal. In the bloodstream, air migrates to the heart, where it creates a compressible foam that destroys the propulsive efficiency of ventricular contraction and irritates the conduction system. Air can also move into the pulmonary vasculature, where bubbles obstruct small vessels and compromise gas exchange, or it can cross through a patent foramen ovale to the left side of the heart and the systemic circulation.

The potential for venous air embolization increases with the degree of elevation of the operative site above the heart. Although the occurrence of air emboli is a relatively frequent phenomenon in head-elevated positions, most of the emboli are small in volume, clinically silent, and recognizable only by sophisticated Doppler detection techniques. Nevertheless, the potential for continuing, dangerous accumulations of entrained air requires immediate detection of the embolization, a careful search for its portal of entry, and prompt treatment of its clinical effects.

Pneumocephalus

In the usual craniotomy, most of the brain lies subjacent to the incision. After the dura is incised, cerebrospinal fluid is removed to improve working conditions, and the surgical field is open to the air. During closure of the craniotomy, most of the intracranial air escapes from the wound and any residual pneumocephalus is of little consequence. However, when an incision is made through the dura in the posterior fossa or cervical spine of a seated patient, the bulk of the brain lies above the incision. Cerebrospinal fluid drains downward out of the wound, and tissue retraction can allow air to bubble up over the surfaces of the brain to become trapped in the upper reaches of the cranium.[109] When brain mass is decreased by ventricular drainage, steroids, and diuresis, the space available to a pneumocephalus is enlarged. Diffusion of nitrous oxide into the accumulated air, or the warming of trapped gas, can produce a tension pneumocephalus with signs of increased intracranial pressure and delayed awakening from anesthesia.

Toung et al[110] found postoperative pneumocephalus in all of a group of seated patients and in most of those who had been in the prone or the park bench position. Intraventricular air was present in most of the seated patients and was rare in those in the other positions. None of their group of 100 patients had neurologic changes attributable to the trapped intracranial air. Standefer et al[111] reported a 3% incidence of symptomatic (tension) pneumocephalus in seated, anesthetized patients whose duras were opened.

Ocular Compression

Pressure from a padded head rest on the eyes of a patient who has been placed in a head-elevated position can dislocate a crystalline lens or render the globe ischemic. Unilateral blindness has been reported as a result (see Blindness section).[112] Modern skull-pin head clamps that grip firmly when properly applied have made ocular compression in the sitting position a rarity. In the head-elevated lateral decubitus or prone position, the threats to the eyes are those described in the preceding discussions of those nonelevated postures.

Edema of the Face, Tongue, and Neck

Severe postoperative macroglossia, apparently because of venous and lymphatic obstruction, can be caused by prolonged, marked neck flexion.[113] Try to avoid placing the patient's chin firmly against the chest and use of an oral airway to protect the endotracheal tube. Ellis et al[114] reported a patient who needed a tracheostomy because of massive swelling of the tongue, lips, pharynx, and epiglottis occurring shortly after extubation at the end of a lengthy anesthetic in the sitting position that involved deliberate hypotension. Extremes of neck flexion, with or without head rotation, have been widely used to gain access to structures in the posterior fossa and cervical spine, but their potential for damage should be understood and excessive flexion–rotation avoided if possible. Moore and associates[115] have described five cases of macroglossia in patients with posterior fossa disease and have suggested that the primary mechanism is neurologically determined rather than being the result of either vascular obstruction or local trauma. This problem also has been described with the use of transesophogeal echocardiography probes.

Midcervical Tetraplegia

This devastating injury occurs after hyperflexion of the neck, with or without rotation of the head, and is attributed to stretching of the spinal cord with resulting compromise of its vasculature in the midcervical area. An element of spondylosis or a spondylotic bar may be involved.[116,117] The result is paralysis below the general level of the fifth cervical vertebra. Although most reports in the literature have described the condition as occurring after the use of the sitting position, midcervical tetraplegia has also occurred after prolonged, nonforced head flexion for intracranial surgery in the supine position.

Sciatic Nerve

Stretch injuries of the sciatic nerve can occur in some seated patients if the hips are markedly flexed without bending the knees. Prolonged compression of the sciatic nerve as it emerges from the pelvis is possible in a thin, seated patient if the buttocks are not suitably padded. Foot drop may be the result of injuries to either the sciatic nerve or the common peroneal nerve and can be bilateral.

PERIOPERATIVE PERIPHERAL NEUROPATHIES

Prevention

The American Society of Anesthesiologists approved an advisory on peripheral neuropathies in 1999.[118] This advisory includes pertinent literature and a summary of the opinions of anesthesia providers on a variety of positioning and

TABLE 23-1

SUMMARY OF TASK FORCE CONSENSUS

Preoperative assessment: When judged appropriate, it is helpful to ascertain that patients can comfortably tolerate the anticipated operative position.

Upper Extremity Positioning:
- Arm abduction should be limited to 90 degrees or less in supine patients. Patients who are positioned prone may comfortably tolerate arm abduction of 90 degrees or more.
- Arms should be positioned to decrease pressure on the postcondylar groove of the humerus (ulnar groove). When arms are tucked at the side, a neutral forearm position is recommended. When arms are abducted on arm boards, either supination or a neutral forearm position is acceptable.
- Prolonged pressure on the radial nerve in the spiral groove of the humerus should be avoided.
- Extension of the elbow beyond a comfortable range may stretch the median nerve.

Lower Extremity Positioning:
- Lithotomy positions that stretch the hamstring muscle group beyond a comfortable range may stretch the sciatic nerve.
- Prolonged pressure on the peroneal nerve at the fibular head should be avoided.
- Neither extension nor flexion of the hip increases the risk of femoral neuropathy.

Protective Padding:
- Padded armboards may decrease the risk of upper extremity neuropathy.
- The use of chest rolls in laterally positioned patients may decrease the risk of upper extremity neuropathies.
- Padding at the elbow and at the fibular head may decrease the risk of upper and lower extremity neuropathies, respectively.

Equipment:
- Properly functioning automated blood pressure cuffs on the upper arms do not affect the risk of upper extremity neuropathies.
- Shoulder braces in steep head-down positions may increase the risk of brachial plexus neuropathies.

Postoperative Assessment: A simple postoperative assessment of extremity nerve function may lead to early recognition of peripheral neuropathies.

Documentation: Charting specific positioning actions during the care of patients may result in improvements of care by (1) helping practitioners focus attention on relevant aspects of patient positioning and (2) providing information that continuous improvement processes can use to lead to refinements in patient care.

peripheral neuropathy issues. The paucity of literature related to these issues limited the advisory to recommendations based on opinions and current practices of a broadly representative group of anesthesia providers from around the United States. Additional input and opinions were obtained from consultants from around the world. A summary of the findings of the advisory is shown in Table 23-1.

Practical Considerations

Efforts to prevent perioperative neuropathies are frequently debated, and there often is confusion over how to manage a neuropathy once it has occurred. In general, there are no data to support recommendations on any of these issues. Therefore, the following opinions have been formulated by personal experience, guided by advice from neurologists who primarily care for patients with peripheral neuropathies, and seasoned or supported by speculation derived from anecdotal case reports.

Padding-Exposed Peripheral Nerves

Many types of padding materials are advocated to protect exposed peripheral nerves. They often consist of cloth (e.g., blankets and towels), foam sponges (e.g., "eggcrate" foam), and gel pads. There are no data to suggest that any of these materials is more effective than any other, or that any is better than no padding at all. A good rule of thumb would be to position and pad exposed peripheral nerves to (1) prevent their stretch beyond normally tolerated limits while awake; (2) avoid their direct compression, if possible; and (3) distribute over as large an area as possible any compressive forces that must be placed on them.

Prolonged Duration in One Position

Prolonged duration in one position appears to increase the risk of neuropathy and other integumentary damage. For example, prolonged duration in lithotomy positions greatly increases the risk of lower extremity neuropathy.[119,120] When possible, it would appear prudent to limit as much as practical the time any patient spends in one position. However, intermittent movement of the limbs or head during the intraoperative period may increase the opportunity for a number of different problems, including but not limited to dislodging an endotracheal tube, abrading a cornea, or moving an extremity into a suboptimal position. Practitioners must judge the benefits versus risks of any intraoperative changes in a patient's position.

Course of Action for the Patient with a Neuropathy

Although each situation is unique and requires careful assessment, the following guidelines may suggest a basic course of action that will lead to appropriate care:[121]

- Is the neuropathy sensory or motor? Sensory lesions are
8 more frequently transient than motor lesions. If the symptoms are numbness or tingling only, it may be appropriate to inform the patient that many of these neuropathies can be expected to resolve during the first 5 days.[39] The patient should be instructed to avoid postures that might compress or stretch the involved nerve. Arrangements should be made for frequent contact with the patient. A call to alert a neurologist is appropriate, and if the symptoms still persist on postoperative day 5, the neurologist should be consulted.
- If the neuropathy has a motor component, a neurologist should be consulted immediately. Electromyographic studies may be needed to assess the location of any acute lesion. This knowledge may direct an appropriate treatment plan. The studies may also demonstrate chronic abnormalities of the nerve or, if applicable, the contralateral nerve.

References

1. Martin JT, Warner MA (eds): Positioning in Anesthesia and Surgery, 3rd ed. Philadelphia, WB Saunders, 1997
2. Anderton JM, Keen RI, Neave R (eds): Positioning the Surgical Patient. London, Butterworths, 1988
3. Enderby GEH: Postural ischemia and blood pressure. Lancet 1:185, 1954
4. West JB, Dollery CT, Naimark A: Distribution of blood flow in isolated lung: Relations to vascular and alveolar pressures. J Appl Physiol 19:713, 1964
5. Froese AB, Bryan AC: Effects of anesthesia and paralysis on diaphragmatic mechanics in man. Anesthesiology 41:242, 1974
6. Warner MA: Supine positions. In Martin JT, Warner MA (eds): Positioning in Anesthesia and Surgery, 3rd ed, p 39. Philadelphia, WB Saunders, 1977
7. Litwiller JP, Wells RE, Halliwill JR *et al*: Effect of lithotomy positions on strain of the obturator and lateral femoral cutaneous nerves. Clin Anat 17:45, 2004
8. Smith BE: Obstetrics. In Martin JT, Warner MA (eds): Positioning in Anesthesia and Surgery, 3rd ed, p 267. Philadelphia, WB Saunders, 1997
9. Martin JT: 1992–Compartment syndromes: Concepts and perspectives for the anesthesiologist. Anesth Analg 75:275, 1992
10. Little DM: Posture and anesthesia. Can Anaesth Soc J 7:2, 1960
11. Angermeier KW, Jordan GH: Complications of the exaggerated lithotomy position: A review of 177 cases. J Urol 151:866, 1994
12. Halliwill JR, Hewitt SA, Joyner MJ *et al:* Effects of various lithotomy positions on lower extremity blood pressures. Anesthesiology 89:1373, 1999
13. Pfeffer SD, Halliwill JR, Warner MA: Effects of lithotomy position and external compression on lower leg muscle compartment pressure. Anesthesiology 95:632, 2001
14. Wilcox S, Vandam LD: Alas, poor Trendelenburg and his position! A critique of its uses and effectiveness. Anesth Analg 67:574, 1988
15. Meyer W: Ueber die Nachbehandlung des hohen Steinschnittes sowie ueber Verwenbarkeit desselben zur Operation von Blasenscheidenfisteln. Archiv für Klinische Chiruque 31:494, 1885
16. Reich DL, Konstadt SN, Hubbard M, Thys DM: Do Trendelenburg and passive leg raising improve cardiac performance? Anesth Analg 67:S184, 1988
17. Abel RR, Lewis GM: Postoperative alopecia. Arch Dermatol 81:72, 1960
18. Gormley T, Sokoll MD: Permanent alopecia from pressure of a headstrap. JAMA 199:157, 1967
19. Lawson NW, Mills NL, Ochsner JL: Occipital alopecia following cardiopulmonary bypass. J Thorac Cardiovasc Surg 71:342, 1976
20. Jellish WS, Blakeman B, Warf P, Slogoff S: Hands-up positioning during asymmetric sternal retraction for internal mammary artery harvest: A possible method to reduce brachial plexus injury. Anesth Analg 84:260, 1997
21. Vander Salm TJ, Cereda J-M, Cutler BS: Brachial plexus injury following median sternotomy. J Thorac Cardiovasc Surg 80:447, 1980
22. Vander Salm TJ, Cutler BS, Okike ON: Brachial plexus injury following median sternotomy: Part II. J Thorac Cardiovasc Surg 83:914, 1982
23. Roy RC, Stafford MA, Charlton JE: Nerve injury and musculoskeletal complaints after cardiac surgery: Influence of internal mammary artery dissection and left arm position. Anesth Analg 67:277, 1988
24. Gregg JR, Labosky D, Harty M *et al:* Serratus anterior paralysis in the young athlete. J Bone Joint Surg Am 61:825, 1979
25. Johnson JTH, Kendall HO: Isolated paralysis of the serratus anterior muscle. J Bone Joint Surg Am 37:567, 1955
26. Foo CL, Swann M: Isolated paralysis of the serratus anterior. J Bone Joint Surg Br 65:552, 1983
27. Martin JT: Postoperative isolated dysfunction of the long thoracic nerve: A rare entity of uncertain etiology. Anesth Analg 69:614, 1989
28. Britt BA, Gordon RA: Peripheral nerve injuries associated with anesthesia. Can Anaesth Soc J 11:514, 1964
29. Bickler PE, Schapera A, Bainton CR: Acute radial nerve injury from use of an automatic blood pressure monitor. Anesthesiology 73:186, 1990
30. Kroll DA, Caplan RA, Posner K *et al:* Nerve injury associated with anesthesia. Anesthesiology 73:202, 1990
31. Cheney FW, Domino KB, Caplan RA *et al:* Nerve injury associated with anesthesia. Anesthesiology 90:1062, 1999
32. Chusid JG: Correlative Neuroanatomy and Functional Neurology, p 145. Los Altos, CA: Lange Medical Publications, 1985
33. Büdinger K: Ueber Lähmungen nach Chloroform-Narkosen. Archiv für Klinische Chiruque 47:121, 1894
34. Garriques HJ: Anaesthesia-paralysis. Am J Med Sci 133:81, 1897

35. Wadsworth TG, Williams JR: Cubital tunnel external compression syndrome. BMJ 1:662, 1973
36. Warner MA, Warner DO, Harper CM *et al:* Ulnar neuropathy in medical patients. Anesthesiology 92:613, 2000
37. Warner MA, Warner ME, Martin JT: Ulnar neuropathy: Incidence, outcome, and risk factors in sedated or anesthetized patients. Anesthesiology 81:1332, 1994
38. Alvine FG, Schurrer ME: Postoperative ulnar-nerve palsy: Are there predisposing factors? J Bone Joint Surg Am 69:255, 1987
39. Warner MA, Warner DO, Matsumoto JY *et al:* Ulnar neuropathy in surgical patients. Anesthesiology 90:54, 1999
40. Prielipp RC, Morell RC, Walker FO *et al:* Ulnar nerve pressure: Influence of arm position and relationship to somatosensory evoked potentials. Anesthesiology 91:345, 1999
41. Campbell WW, Pridgeon RM, Riaz G *et al:* Variations in anatomy of the ulnar nerve at the cubital tunnel: Pitfalls in the diagnosis of ulnar neuropathy at the elbow. Muscle Nerve 14:733, 1991
42. O'Driscoll SW, Horii E, Carmichael SW *et al:* The cubital tunnel and ulnar neuropathy. J Bone Joint Surg Am 73:613, 1991
43. Childress HM: Recurrent ulnar nerve dislocation at the elbow. J Bone Joint Surg 38:978, 1956
44. Ashenhurst EM: Anatomical factors in the etiology of ulnar neuropathy. CMAJ 87:159, 1962
45. Macnicol MF: Extraneural pressures affecting the ulnar nerve at the elbow. Hand 14:5, 1982
46. Morell RC, Prielipp RC, Harwood TN *et al:* Men are more susceptible than women to direct pressure on unmyelinated ulnar nerve fibers. Anesth Analg 97:1183, 2003
47. Pechan J, Julis I: The pressure measurement in the ulnar nerve: A contribution to the pathophysiology of the cubital tunnel syndrome. J Biomech 8:75, 1975
48. Contreras MG, Warner MA, Charboneau WJ *et al:* The anatomy of the ulnar nerve at the elbow: Potential relationship of acute ulnar neuropathy to gender differences. Clin Anat 11:372, 1998
49. Shimokata H, Tobin JD, Muller DC *et al:* Studies in the distribution of body fat: I. Effects of age, sex, and obesity. J Gerontol 44:66, 1989
50. Hattori K, Numata N, Ikoma M *et al:* Sex differences in the distribution of subcutaneous and internal fat. Hum Biol 63:53, 1991
51. Chusid JG: Correlative Neuroanatomy and Functional Neurology, p 149. Los Altos, CA: Lange Medical Publications, 1985
52. Hill NA, Howard FM, Huffer BR: The incomplete anterior interosseous nerve syndrome. J Hand Surg [Am] 10:4, 1985
53. Kies SJ, Danielson DR, Dennison DJ *et al:* Perioperative compartment syndrome of the hand. Anesthesiology 2004; 101:1232–4
54. Contreras MG, Warner MA, Carmichael SW *et al:* Perioperative anterior interosseous neuropathy. Anesthesiology 96:243, 2002
55. Amoiridis G, Wöhrle JC, Langkafel M *et al:* Spinal cord infarction after surgery in a patient in the hyperlordotic position. Anesthesiology 84:228, 1996
56. Hofmann A, Jones RE, Schoenvogel R: Pudendal nerve neuropraxia as a result of traction on the fracture table. J Bone Joint Surg Am 64:136, 1982
57. Lindenbaum SD, Fleming LL, Smith DW: Pudendal nerve palsies associated with closed intramedullary femoral fixation. J Bone Joint Surg Am 64:934, 1982
58. Orken DE: Modern concepts of the role of nephrotoxic agents in the pathogenesis of acute renal failure. Prog Biochem Pharmacol 7:219, 1972
59. Matsen FA III: Compartmental syndrome: A unified concept. Clin Orthop 113:8, 1975
60. Warner ME, LaMaster LM, Thoeming AK *et al:* Compartment syndrome in surgical patients. Anesthesiology 94:705, 2001
61. Courington FW, Little DM Jr: The role of posture in anesthesia. Clin Anesth 3:24, 1968
62. Martin JT: Lithotomy positions. In Martin JT, Warner MA (eds): Positioning in Anesthesia and Surgery, 3rd ed, p 47. Philadelphia, WB Saunders, 1997
63. Kaneko K, Milic-Emily J, Dolovich MB *et al:* Regional distribution of ventilation and perfusion as a function of body position. J Appl Physiol 21:767, 1966
64. Lawson NW, Meyer DJ Jr: The lateral decubitus position: Anesthesiologic considerations. In Martin JT, Warner MA (eds): Positioning in Anesthesia and Surgery, 3rd ed, p 127. Philadelphia, WB Saunders, 1997
65. Lee C, Barnes A, Nagel EL: Neuroleptanalgesia for awake pronation of surgical patients. Anesth Analg 56:276, 1977
66. Martin JT: The ventral decubitus (prone) positions. In Martin JT, Warner MA (eds): Positioning in Anesthesia and Surgery, 3rd ed, p 155. Philadelphia, WB Saunders, 1997
67. Backofen JE, Schauble JR: Hemodynamic changes with prone positioning during general anesthesia. Anesth Analg 64:194, 1985
68. Gattinoni L, Pelosi P, Vitale G *et al:* Body position changes redistribute lung computed-tomographic density in patients with acute respiratory failure. Anesthesiology 74:15, 1991
69. Douglas WW, Rehder K, Beynen FM *et al:* Improved oxygenation in patients with acute respiratory failure: The prone position. Am Rev Respir Dis 115:559, 1977
70. Rehder K, Knopp TJ, Sessler AD: Regional intrapulmonary gas distribution in awake and anesthetized-paralysed prone man. J Appl Physiol 45:528, 1978
71. Chusid JG: Correlative Neuroanatomy and Functional Neurology, p 157. Los Altos, CA: Lange Medical Publications, 1985
72. Reid SA, Grundy BL: The head-elevated positions: Surgical aspects: The neurosurgical skull clamp. In Martin JT, Warner MA (eds): Positioning in Anesthesia and Surgery, 3rd ed, p 71. Philadelphia, WB Saunders, 1997
73. Gravenstein N, Grundy BL, Lobato EB: The central nervous system. In Martin JT, Warner MA (eds): Positioning in Anesthesia and Surgery, 3rd ed, p 291. Philadelphia, WB Saunders, 1997
74. Johnson MW, Kincaid MC, Trobe JD: Bilateral retrobulbar optic nerve infarctions after blood loss and hypotension. Ophthalmology 94:1577, 1987
75. Rizzo JF, Lessell L: Posterior ischemic optic neuropathy during general surgery. Am J Ophthalmol 103:808, 1987
76. Roth S, Thisted RA, Erickson JP *et al:* Eye injuries after nonocular surgery. Anesthesiology 85:1020, 1996
77. Stambough JL, Cheeks ML: Central retinal artery occlusion: a complication of the knee-chest position. J Spinal Disord 5:363, 1992
78. Bekar A, Türeyen K, Aksoy K: Unilateral blindness due to patient positioning during cervical syringomyelia surgery: Unilateral blindness after prone position. J Neurosurg Anesthesiol 8:227, 1996
79. Myers MA, Hamilton SR, Bogosian AJ *et al:* Visual loss as a complication of spinal surgery. Spine 22:1325, 1997
80. Katz DM, Trobe JD, Cornblath WT *et al:* Ischemic optic neuropathy after lumbar spine surgery. Arch Ophthalmol 112:925, 1994
81. Katzman SS, Moschonas CG, Dzioba RB: Amaurosis secondary to massive blood loss after lumbar spine surgery. Spine 19:468, 1994
82. Stevens WR, Glazer PA, Kelley SD *et al:* Ophthalmic complications after spinal surgery. Spine 22:1319, 1997
83. Levin H, Ben-David B: Transient blindness during hysteroscopy: A rare complication. Anesth Analg 81:880, 1995
84. Cheng MA, Sigurdson W, Tempelhoff R *et al:* Visual loss after spine surgery: A survey. Neurosurgery 46:625, 2000
85. Cheng MA, Todorov A, Tempelhoff R *et al:* The effect of prone positioning on intraocular pressure in anesthetized patients. Anesthesiology 95:1351, 2001
86. Tsamparlakis J, Casey TA, Howell W *et al:* Dependence of intraocular pressure on induced hypotension and posture during surgical anesthesia. Trans Ophthalmol Soc UK 100:521, 1980
87. Roth S, Nunez R, Schreider BD: Unexplained visual loss after lumbar spinal fusion. J Neurosurg Anesth 9:346, 1997
88. Lee LA, Lam AM: Unilateral blindess after prone lumbar spine surgery. Anesthesiology 95:793, 2001
89. Roth S: Postoperative visual loss: Still no answers—yet. Anesthesiology 95:575, 2001
90. Sweeny PJ, Breuer AC, Selshorst JB *et al:* Ischemic optic neuropathy: A complication of cardiopulmonary bypass surgery. Neurology 32:560, 1982
91. Shaw PJ, Bates D, Cartlidge NEF *et al:* Neurologic and neuropsychologic morbidity following major surgery: Comparison of coronary artery bypass and peripheral vascular surgery. Stroke 18:700, 1987
92. Shapira OM, Kimmel WA, Lindsey PS *et al:* Anterior ischemic optic neuropathy after open heart operations. Ann Thorac Surg 61:660, 1996
93. Nuttall GA, Garrity JA, Dearani JA *et al:* Risk factors for ischemic optic neuropathy after cardiopulmonary bypass: A matched case/control study. Anesth Analg 93:1410, 2001
94. Roth S, Gillesberg I: Injuries to the visual system and other sense organs. In Benumof JL, Saidman LJ (eds): Anesthesia and Perioperative Complications, 2nd ed. St. Louis, Mosby, 1999
95. Brown RH, Schauble JF, Miller NR: Anemia and hypotension as contributors to perioperative vision loss. Anesthesiology 80:222, 1994
96. Warner ME, Warner MA, Garrity JA *et al:* The frequency of perioperative vision loss. Anesth Analg 93:1417, 2001
97. Connolly SE, Gordon KB, Horton JC: Salvage of vision after hypotension-induced ischemic optic neuropathy. Am J Ophthalmol 117:235, 1994
98. Sherman DD, Hart RG, Easton JD: Abrupt change in head position and cerebral infarction. Stroke 12:2, 1981
99. Toole JF: Effects of change of head, limb and body position on cephalic circulation. N Engl J Med 279:307, 1968
100. Coonan TJ, Hope CE: Cardio-respiratory effects of change of body position. Can Anaesth Soc J 30:424, 1983
101. Sonkodi S, Agabiti-Rosei E, Fraser R *et al:* Response of the renin-angiotensin-aldosterone system to upright tilting and to intravenous furosemide: Effect of prior metoprolol and propranolol. Br J Clin Pharmacol 13:341, 1982
102. Williams GH, Cain JP, Dluly RG *et al:* Studies on the control of plasma aldosterone concentration in normal man: 1. Response to posture, acute and chronic volume depletion and sodium loading. J Clin Invest 51:1731, 1972
103. Albin MS, Janetta PJ, Maroon JC *et al:* Anaesthesia in the sitting position. In Recent Progress in Anesthesiology and Resuscitation. Amsterdam, Excerpta Medica International Congress Series No. 347:775, 1975
104. Albin MS, Babinski M, Wolf S: Cardiovascular response to the sitting position (Letter). Br J Anaesth 52:961, 1980
105. Dalrymple DG: Cardiorespiratory effects of the sitting position in neurosurgery. Br J Anaesth 51:1079, 1979

106. Shenkin HA, Scheuerman EB, Spitz EB *et al:* Effect of change of posture upon cerebral circulation of man. J Appl Physiol 2:317, 1949
107. Don HF: The measurement of trapped gas in the lungs at functional residual capacity and the effects of posture. Anesthesiology 35:582, 1971
108. Gilbert RGB, Brindle F, Galindo A: Anesthesia for Neurosurgery, p 126. Boston, Little, Brown, 1966
109. Kitahata LM, Katz JD: Tension pneumocephalus after posterior fossa craniotomy, a complication of the sitting position. Anesthesiology 44:448, 1976
110. Toung TKJ, McPherson RW, Ahn H: Pneumocephalus: Effects of patient position on incidence of aerocele after posterior fossa and upper cervical cord surgery. Anesth Analg 65:65, 1986
111. Standefer M, Bay JW, Trusso R: The sitting position in neurosurgery: A retrospective analysis of 488 cases. Neurosurgery 14:649, 1984
112. Hollenhorst RW, Svein HJ, Benoit CF: Unilateral blindness occurring during anesthesia for neurosurgical operations. Arch Ophthalmol 52:819, 1954
113. McAllister RG: Macroglossia: A positional complication. Anesthesiology 40:199, 1974
114. Ellis SC, Bryan-Brown CW, Hyderally H: Massive swelling of the head and neck. Anesthesiology 42:102, 1975
115. Moore JK, Chaudhri S, Moore AP, Easton J: Macroglossia and posterior fossa disease. Anaesthesia 43:382, 1988
116. Hitselberger WE, House WF: A warning regarding the sitting position for acoustic tumor surgery. Archives of Otolaryngology 106:69, 1980
117. Wilder BL: Hypothesis: The etiology of midcervical quadriplegia after operation with the patient in the sitting position. Neurosurgery 11:530, 1982
118. American Society of Anesthesiologists Task Force on Prevention of Perioperative Peripheral Neuropathies: Practice advisory for the prevention of perioperative peripheral neuropathies. Anesthesiology 92:1168, 2000
119. Warner MA, Martin JT, Schroeder DR *et al:* Lower extremity motor neuropathy associated with surgery performed on patients in a lithotomy position. Anesthesiology 81:6, 1994
120. Warner MA, Warner DO, Harper CM *et al:* Lower extremity neuropathies associated with the lithotomy position. Anesthesiology 93:938, 2000
121. Warner MA: Perioperative neuropathies. Mayo Clin Proc 73:567, 1998

CHAPTER 24 ■ MONITORING THE ANESTHETIZED PATIENT

GLENN S. MURPHY AND JEFFERY S. VENDER

KEY POINTS

1. Effective monitoring reduces the potential for adverse outcomes in the perioperative setting by identifying derangements before they result in serious injury.
2. Alterations in ventilation, cardiac output, distribution of pulmonary blood flow, and metabolic activity can all influence the capnograph display during carbon dioxide gas analysis.
3. During direct invasive arterial pressure monitoring, systemic fidelity is optimized when the catheter and tubing are stiff, the mass of the fluid is small, and the length of the connecting tubing is not excessive.
4. On the basis of available evidence, it is difficult to draw meaningful conclusions regarding the effectiveness of pulmonary artery catheter monitoring in reducing morbidity and mortality in critically ill patients. Expert opinion suggests that perioperative complications may be reduced if pulmonary artery catheters (PACs) are used in the appropriate patients and settings, and if clinicians interpret and apply the data provided by the PAC correctly.
5. Transesophageal echocardiography provides a more accurate estimation of ventricular preload than pulmonary artery catheterization. Transesophageal echocardiography also allows the clinician to rapidly assess patients for evidence of myocardial ischemia, cardiac valvular dysfunction, and causes of perioperative hemodynamic instability.

Monitoring represents the process by which anesthesiologists recognize and evaluate potential physiologic problems in a timely manner. The term is derived from *monere*, which in Latin means to warn, remind, or admonish. In perioperative care, monitoring implies the following four essential features: observation and vigilance, instrumentation, interpretation of data, and initiation of corrective therapy when indicated.

Monitoring is an essential aspect of anesthesia care. Patient safety is enhanced when appropriate monitoring is operational and clinical judgments are proper. Effective monitoring reduces the potential for poor outcomes that may follow anesthesia by
1 identifying derangements before they result in serious or irreversible injury. Electronic monitors improve a physician's ability to respond because they are able to make repetitive measurements at higher frequencies than humans and do not fatigue or become distracted. Monitoring devices increase the specificity and precision of clinical judgments. At no time in the history of anesthesia have practitioners had the capability routinely to monitor so many diverse physiologic variables in real time, often noninvasively, as they do today. Our understanding of the physiologic effects of anesthesia and its inherent risks is enhanced by using appropriate intraoperative physiologic monitoring.

This chapter discusses the methods by which anesthesiologists monitor organ function during anesthesia care. The descriptions of the technologic and scientific principles used in monitoring devices have been simplified for clarity.

Cost containment has been raised as a reason to discourage the use of expensive, technologically advanced monitoring systems. The value of a given monitor depends on the clinical expertise of the anesthesiologist, the clinical setting, the anesthetic technique, and the performance of the specific equipment in question. Monitoring devices should not be denied solely on the basis of expense.[1] Although it is appropriate for society to demand cost containment, anesthesiologists have a responsibility to assess how monitoring should be used. Professional societies, regulatory agencies, and the legal profession have played important roles in establishing current monitoring practices.

Standards for basic anesthetic monitoring have been established by the American Society of Anesthesiologists (ASA).

Since 1986, these standards have emphasized the evolution of technology and practice. Today's standards (last affirmed on October 15, 2003) emphasize the importance of regular and frequent measurements, integration of clinical judgment and experience, and the potential for extenuating circumstances that can influence the applicability or accuracy of monitoring systems.[2]

Standard I requires qualified personnel to be present in the operating room, to monitor the patient continuously and modify anesthesia care based on clinical observations and the responses of the patient to dynamic changes resulting from surgery or drug therapy. Standard II focuses attention on continually evaluating the patient's oxygenation, ventilation, circulation, and temperature. Standard II specifically mandates the following:

1. Using an oxygen analyzer with a low concentration limit alarm during general anesthesia.
2. Quantitatively assessing blood oxygenation during any anesthesia care.
3. Continuously ensuring the adequacy of ventilation by physical diagnostic techniques during all anesthesia care. Quantitative monitoring of tidal volume and capnography are encouraged in patients undergoing general anesthesia.
4. Ensuring the adequacy of circulation by the continuous display of the electrocardiogram (ECG), and determining the arterial blood pressure at least at 5-minute intervals. During general anesthesia, circulatory function is to be continually evaluated by assessing the quality of the pulse, either electronically or by palpation or auscultation.
5. Endotracheal intubation or laryngeal mask airway insertion requires qualitative identification of carbon dioxide in the expired gas. During general anesthesia, capnography and end-tidal carbon dioxide analysis are encouraged.
6. During all anesthetics, the means for continuously measuring the patient's temperature must be available. When changes in body temperature are intended or anticipated, temperature should be continuously measured and recorded on the anesthesia record.

The ASA standards emphasize the melding of physical signs with instrumentation. Electronic monitoring, no matter how sophisticated or comprehensive, does not necessarily reduce the need for clinical skills such as inspection, palpation, and auscultation. Although the authors believe that electronic monitors augment clinical judgments when properly used, there is little evidence that electronic monitors, by themselves, reduce mortality or morbidity. Moreover, there is considerable controversy regarding the need to apply specific monitors in unique clinical situations, particularly those that may add significant cost. Monitoring can be classified as invasive, minimally invasive, or noninvasive. Invasive monitors place patients at risk for complications related to their application and use. Anesthesiologists must balance the potential risk of instituting invasive monitoring with the presumed benefits derived from its application.

The variety of devices available for patient monitoring is expansive and changing as advances in biomedical engineering find their way into the marketplace. The Association for the Advancement of Medical Instrumentation has been effective in promoting design guidelines to ensure patient and operator safety and reduce stress and distractions often associated with medical monitoring.[3]

The proliferation of alarm tones during anesthesia care can be disturbing and may paradoxically impair clinical vigilance. Monitoring systems may be insufficiently sensitive to reject errors. During routine anesthesia care, a minimum of five alarms (inspired oxygen, airway pressure, oximetry, blood pressure, and heart rate) should be operational. Unfortunately, spurious warnings occur with high frequency during routine anesthesia monitoring. The integration of alarm signals is an important area in need of continuing evaluation. Loeb[4] reported that anesthesia providers have difficulty in accurately recognizing the source of an alarm tone. Alarm annunciators using unique sound and visual prompts are incorporated into anesthesia equipment. Warning signals for ventilation, oxygenation, drug administration, temperature, and cardiovascular parameters need to be designed so that problem identification is fast, simple, and relevant.

INSPIRATORY AND EXPIRED GAS MONITORING: OXYGEN

The concentration of oxygen in the anesthetic circuit must be measured. Measuring inspired oxygen does not guarantee the adequacy of arterial oxygenation.[5] Gas machine manufacturers place oxygen sensors on the inspired limb of the anesthesia circuit to ensure that hypoxic gas mixtures are never delivered to patients. Oxygen monitors require a fast response time (2 to 10 seconds), accuracy (± pm2%), and stability when exposed to humidity and inhalation agents.

Paramagnetic Oxygen Analysis

Oxygen is a highly paramagnetic gas. Paramagnetic gases are attracted to magnetic energy because of unpaired electrons in their outer shell orbits. Differential paramagnetic oximetry has been incorporated into a variety of operating room monitors. These instruments detect the change in sample line pressure resulting from the attraction of oxygen by switched magnetic fields. Signal changes during electromagnetic switching correlate with the oxygen concentration in the sample line.

Galvanic Cell Analyzers

Galvanic cell analyzers meet the performance criteria necessary for operative monitoring. These analyzers measure the current produced when oxygen diffuses across a membrane and is reduced to molecular oxygen at the anode of an electrical circuit. The electron flow (current) is proportional to the partial pressure of oxygen in the fuel cell. Galvanic cell analyzers require regular replacement of the galvanic sensor capsule. In the sensor, the electric potential for the reduction of oxygen results from a chemical reaction. Over time, the reactants require replenishment.[6]

Polarographic Oxygen Analyzers

Polarographic oxygen analyzers are commonly used in anesthesia monitoring. In this electrochemical system, oxygen diffuses through an oxygen-permeable polymeric membrane and participates in the following reaction: $O_2 + 2H_2O + 4e \rightarrow 4\ OH^-$. The current change is proportional to the number of oxygen molecules surrounding the electrode. Polarographic oxygen sensors are versatile and are important components of gas machine oxygen analyzers, blood gas analyzers, and transcutaneous oxygen analyzers.

MONITORING OF EXPIRED GASES

Carbon Dioxide

Expiratory CO_2 monitoring ($PECO_2$) has evolved as an important physiologic and safety monitor. CO_2 is usually sampled near the endotracheal–gas delivery interface. Alterations
2 in ventilation, cardiac output (CO), distribution of pulmonary blood flow, and metabolic activity influence $PECO_2$ and the capnograph display obtained during quantitative expired gas analysis.

Capnometry is the measurement and numeric representation of the CO_2 concentration during inspiration and expiration. A *capnogram* is a continuous concentration–time display of the CO_2 concentration sampled at a patient's airway during ventilation. *Capnography* is the continuous monitoring of a patient's capnogram. The capnogram is divided into four distinct phases (Fig. 24-1). The first phase (A–B) represents the initial stage of expiration. Gas sampled during this phase occupies the anatomic dead space and is normally devoid of CO_2. At point B, CO_2-containing gas presents itself at the sampling site, and a sharp upstroke (B–C) is seen in the capnogram. The slope of this upstroke is determined by the evenness of ventilation and alveolar emptying. Phase C–D represents the alveolar or expiratory plateau. At this phase of the capnogram, alveolar gas is being sampled. Normally, this part of the waveform is almost horizontal. Point D is the highest CO_2 value and is called the *end-tidal* CO_2 ($ETCO_2$). $ETCO_2$ is the best reflection of the alveolar CO_2 ($PACO_2$). As the patient begins to inspire, fresh gas is entrained and there is a steep downstroke (D–E) back to baseline. Unless rebreathing of CO_2 occurs, the baseline approaches zero.

The utility of capnography depends on an understanding of the relationship between arterial CO_2 ($PaCO_2$), alveolar CO_2 ($PACO_2$), and $ETCO_2$. This concept assumes that ventilation and perfusion are appropriately matched, that CO_2 is easily diffusible across the capillary–alveolar membrane, and that no sampling errors occur during measurement. If these conditions are met, changes in $ETCO_2$ reflect changes in $PaCO_2$ even if it is assumed that all alveoli do not empty at the same time. If one assumes an idealized mathematical model of ventilation–perfusion, $ETCO_2 \approx PACO_2 \approx PaCO_2$. If the $PaCO_2$–$PACO_2$ gradient is constant and small, capnography provides a noninvasive, continuous, real-time reflection of ventilation. During general anesthesia, the $ETCO_2$–$PaCO_2$ gradient typically is 5 to 10 mm Hg. A maldistribution of ventilation and perfusion ($\dot{V}/\dot{Q}$) or problems in gas sampling may result in a widening of the $ETCO_2$–$PaCO_2$ gradient. $\dot{V}/\dot{Q}$ maldistribution is a common cause of an increased $PaCO_2$–$PACO_2$ gradient. Other patient factors that may influence the accuracy of $ETCO_2$ monitoring by widening the $PaCO_2$–$ETCO_2$ gradient include shallow tidal breaths, prolongation of the expiratory phase of ventilation, or uneven alveolar emptying.

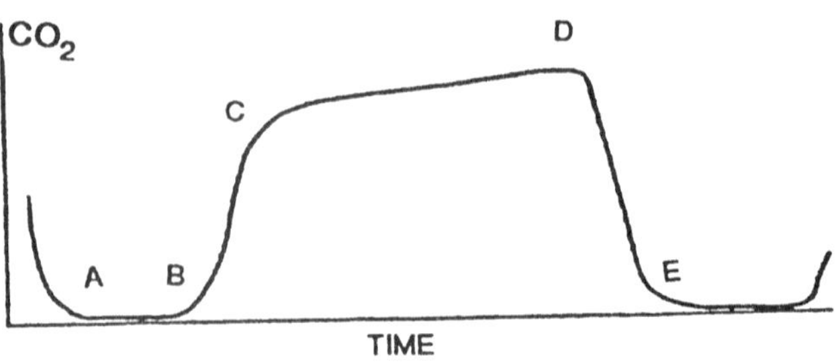

FIGURE 24-1. The normal capnogram. *Point D* delineates the end-tidal CO_2. $ETCO_2$ is the best reflection of the alveolar CO_2 tension.

Dead space (wasted) ventilation is the extreme example of $\dot{V}/\dot{Q}$ mismatch, where a complete absence of perfusion in the presence of adequate alveolar ventilation occurs. Because only perfused alveoli can participate in gas exchange, the nonperfused alveoli have a $PaCO_2$ of zero. The ventilation-weighted average of the perfused and nonperfused alveoli determines the $ETCO_2$. Therefore, conditions resulting in an increase of dead space ventilation lower the $ETCO_2$ measurement and increase the $PaCO_2$–$ETCO_2$ gradient. The common clinical causes associated with a widened $PaCO_2$–$ETCO_2$ gradient include embolic phenomena (thrombus, fat, air, amniotic fluid), hypoperfusion states with reduced pulmonary blood flow, and chronic obstructive pulmonary disease. In contrast, conditions that increase pulmonary shunt (perfusion in the absence of ventilation) result in minimal changes in the $PaCO_2$–$ETCO_2$ gradient.

Capnography is an essential element in determining the appropriate placement of endotracheal tubes. The presence of a stable $ETCO_2$ for three successive breaths indicates that the tube is not in the esophagus. A continuous, stable CO_2 waveform ensures the presence of alveolar ventilation but does not necessarily indicate that the endotracheal tube is properly positioned in the trachea. For example, the tip of the tube could be located in a main-stem bronchus. Capnography is also a monitor of potential changes in perfusion or dead space, is a very sensitive indicator of anesthetic circuit disconnects and gas circuit leaks, and is a method to detect the quality of CO_2 absorption. Increases in $ETCO_2$ can be expected when CO_2 production exceeds ventilation, such as in hyperthermia or when an exogenous source of CO_2 is present. Table 24-1 summarizes the common elements that may be reflected by changes in $ETCO_2$ during anesthesia care.

A sudden drop in $ETCO_2$ to near zero followed by the absence of a CO_2 waveform is a potentially life-threatening problem that could indicate malposition of an endotracheal tube into the pharynx or esophagus, sudden severe hypotension, pulmonary embolism, a cardiac arrest, or an artifact resulting from disruption of sampling lines. When a sudden drop of the $ETCO_2$ occurs, it is essential to quickly verify that there is pulmonary ventilation and to identify physiologic and mechanical factors that might account for a zero-line capnogram. During life-saving cardiopulmonary resuscitation, the generation of adequate perfusion can be assessed by the restoration of the CO_2 waveform.

Whereas abrupt decreases in the $ETCO_2$ are often associated with an altered cardiopulmonary status (e.g., embolism or hypoperfusion), gradual reductions in $ETCO_2$ more often

TABLE 24-1

FACTORS THAT MAY CHANGE END-TIDAL CO_2 ($ETCO_2$) DURING ANESTHESIA

Increases in $ETCO_2$	Decreases in $ETCO_2$
ELEMENTS THAT CHANGE CO_2 PRODUCTION	
Increases in metabolic rate	**Decreases in metabolic rate**
Hyperthermia	Hypothermia
Sepsis	Hypothyroidism
Malignant hyperthermia	
Shivering	
Hyperthyroidism	
ELEMENTS THAT CHANGE CO_2 ELIMINATION	
Hypoventilation	Hyperventilation
Rebreathing	Hypoperfusion
	Pulmonary embolism

reflect decreases in $Pa{CO_2}$ that occur after increases in minute ventilation where ventilation overmatches CO_2 production.

The size and shape of the capnogram waveform can be informative.[7] A slow rate of rise of the second phase (B–C, see Fig. 24-1) is suggestive of either chronic obstructive pulmonary disease or acute airway obstruction as from bronchoconstriction (asthma). A normally shaped capnogram with an increase in $ET{CO_2}$ suggests alveolar hypoventilation or an increase in CO_2 production. Transient increases in $ET{CO_2}$ are often observed during tourniquet release, aortic unclamping, or the administration of bicarbonate.

Several methods for the quantification of CO_2 have been applied to patient monitoring systems. One of the most commonly used methods is based on infrared absorption spectrophotometry (IRAS).

Infrared Absorption Spectrophotometry

Asymmetric, polyatomic molecules like CO_2 absorb infrared light at specific wavelengths. Operating room IRAS devices can detect CO_2, N_2O, and the potent inhaled anesthetic agents. Operating room instruments are designed to measure the unique energy absorbed by the gases and vapors of interest when a sample of the inspired and expired gas is placed into the optical path of an infrared beam.[8] The mixtures complicate the analysis because of interactions between the gases and vapors and the closeness of absorption spectra for the gases of interest. All anesthetic vapors absorb infrared light at 3.6 μm. Therefore, manufacturers using this signature cannot display with certainty the concentration of a specific anesthetic agent of interest. Optical filters and unique detection systems enhance the sensitivity of IRAS monitoring and permit estimation of CO_2, N_2O, and the specific potent inhalational agent present in the measurement chamber. IRAS devices have five components: an infrared light source, a gas sampler, an optical path, a detection system, and a signal processor. The light source produces the infrared energy. The light is focused and filtered so that the quality of the photons with respect to the energy and frequency is stable over time. Narrow wavelengths are then presented to the gas stream. Once the sample has entered the measurement chamber, a detection system calibrated to determine the concentration of a specific gas or agent over time is activated. Changes in temperature, pressure, and acoustic characteristics in the detection chamber can be used to determine the concentration of the gas or agents of interest. Signal detectors create electrical currents analyzed by the signal processor, which transforms the current change to a measurement. The capnogram or agent waveform is an oscilloscopic representation of the electrical current changes over time. The signal-processing section of an IRAS instrument has a memory section that correlates the absorbed energy with a concentration as predicted by the Lambert-Beer law.

Multiple Expired Gas Analysis

Most operating room gas analyzers incorporate methods so that they can monitor concentrations of at least O_2, CO_2, and the inhaled anesthetic agents. *Mass spectrometry systems* bombard the gas mixture with electrons, creating ion fragments of a predictable mass and charge. These fragments are accelerated in a vacuum. A sample of this mixture enters a measurement chamber, where the fragment stream is subjected to a high magnetic field. The magnetic field separates the fragments by their mass and charge. The fragments are deflected onto a detector plate, and each gas has a specific landing site on the detector plate. The ion impacts are proportional to the concentration of the parent gas or vapor. The processor section of the mass spectrometer system calculates the concentration of the gases of interest.

Another unique approach to monitor respiratory gases is based on *Raman scattering.* Raman scattering results when photons generated by a high-intensity argon laser collide with gas molecules. After impact, the gases are momentarily excited to unstable vibrational and rotatory states. When the gases return to their normal state, photons of a characteristic frequency are emitted. The scattered photons are measured as peaks in a spectrum that determine the concentration and composition of respiratory gases and inhaled vapors. Advances in laser technology have made Raman spectroscopic monitors available for clinical use. The instrument is fast and easy to calibrate. O_2, N_2, N_2O, CO_2, and H_2O vapor are all measurable using Raman scattering technology.

The clinical indications for routine CO_2 and O_2 gas monitoring are well documented. Monitors equipped to measure anesthetic gases are also prevalent and desirable. Nitrogen monitoring provides quantification of washout during preoxygenation. A sudden rise in N_2 in the exhaled gas indicates either introduction of air from leaks in the anesthesia delivery system or venous air embolism. Critical events that can be detected by the analysis of respiratory gases and anesthetic vapors are listed in Table 24-2.

TABLE 24-2

DETECTION OF CRITICAL EVENTS BY IMPLEMENTING GAS ANALYSIS

EVENT	MONITORING MODALITY
Error in gas delivery	O_2, N_2, CO_2, agent analysis
Anesthesia machine malfunction	O_2, N_2, CO_2, agent
Disconnection	CO_2, O_2, agent analysis
Vaporizer malfunction or contamination	Agent analysis
Anesthesia circuit leaks	N_2, CO_2 analysis
Endotracheal cuff leaks	N_2, CO_2
Poor mask or LMA fit	N_2, CO_2
Hypoventilation	CO_2 analysis
Malignant hyperthermia	CO_2
Airway obstruction	CO_2
Air embolism	CO_2, N_2
Circuit hypoxia	O_2 analysis
Vaporizer overdose	Agent analysis

LMA, laryngeal mask airway.
Modified with permission from Knopes KD, Hecker BR: Monitoring anesthetic gases. In Lake CL (ed): Clinical Monitoring, p 24. Philadelphia, WB Saunders, 1990.

OXYGENATION MONITORING

The assessment of oxygenation is an integral part of anesthesia practice. Early detection and prompt intervention may limit serious sequelae of hypoxemia. The clinical signs associated with hypoxemia (e.g., tachycardia, altered mental status, cyanosis) are often masked or difficult to appreciate during anesthesia. The mechanisms responsible for hypoxemia are multifactorial. Oxygen analyzers assess oxygen delivery to the patient. Other noninvasive technologies detect the presence of arterial hypoxemia. Arterial oxygen monitors do not ensure adequacy of oxygen delivery to, or utilization by, the tissues and should not be considered a replacement for arterial blood gas measurements when more definitive information regarding oxygenation is desired.

Pulse Oximetry

Pulse oximetry is the standard of care for monitoring oxygenation during anesthesia. Pulse oximeters measure pulse rate and oxygen saturation of hemoglobin (Hb) (Spo_2) on a noninvasive, continuous basis. Figure 24-2 displays the oxyhemoglobin dissociation curve that defines the relationship of hemoglobin saturation and oxygen tension. On the steep part of the curve, a predictable correlation exists between Sao_2 and Po_2. In this range, the Sao_2 is a good reflection of the extent of hypoxemia and the changing status of arterial oxygenation. Shifts in the oxyhemoglobin dissociation curve to the right or to the left define changes in the affinity of Hb for oxygen. At a Po_2 of >75 mm Hg, the Sao_2 plateaus and loses its ability to reflect changes in Pao_2.

Pulse oximetry is based on several premises:

1. The color of blood is a function of oxygen saturation.
2. The change in color results from the optical properties of Hb and its interaction with oxygen.
3. The ratio of O_2Hb and reduced Hb can be determined by absorption spectrophotometry.

Pulse oximetry combines the technology of plethysmography and spectrophotometry. Plethysmography produces a pulse trace that is helpful in tracking circulation. Oxygen saturation is determined by spectrophotometry, which is based on the Beer-Lambert law. At a constant light intensity and Hb concentration, the intensity of light transmitted through a tissue is a logarithmic function of the oxygen saturation of Hb. Two wavelengths of light are required to distinguish O_2Hb from reduced Hb. Light-emitting diodes in the pulse sensor emit red (660 nm) and near infrared (940 nm) light. The percentage of O_2Hb and reduced Hb is determined by measuring the ratio of infrared and red light sensed by a photodetector. Pulse oximeters perform a plethysmographic analysis to differentiate the pulsatile "arterial" Hb saturation from the nonpulsatile signal resulting from "venous" absorption and other tissues such as skin, muscle, and bone. The absence of a pulsatile waveform during extreme hypothermia or hypoperfusion limits the ability of a pulse oximeter to calculate the Spo_2.

The Spo_2 measured by pulse oximetry is not the same as the arterial saturation (Sao_2) measured by a laboratory co-oximeter. Pulse oximetry measures the "functional" saturation,

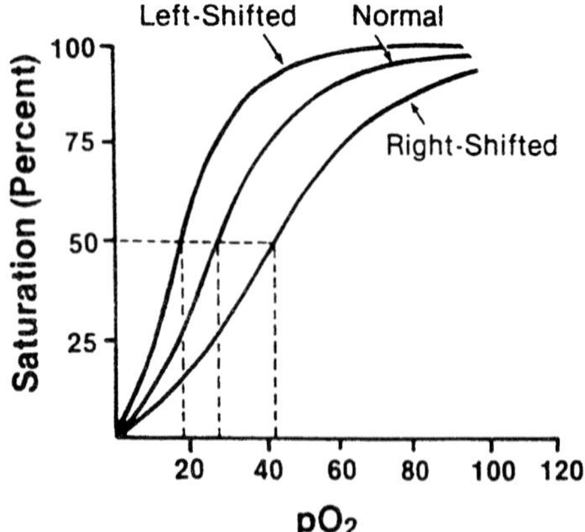

FIGURE 24-2. The oxyhemoglobin dissociation curve. The relationship between arterial saturation of hemoglobin and oxygen tension is represented by the sigmoid-shaped oxyhemoglobin dissociation curve. When the curve is left-shifted, the hemoglobin molecule binds oxygen more tightly. (Reproduced with permission from Brown M, Vender JS: Non-invasive oxygen monitoring. Crit Care Clin 4:493, 1988.)

which is defined by the following equation:

$$\text{Functional } Sao_2 = O_2Hb/(O_2Hb + \text{reduced Hb}) \times 100$$

Laboratory co-oximeters use multiple wavelengths to distinguish other types of Hb by their characteristic absorption. Co-oximeters measure the "fractional" saturation, which is defined by the following equation:

$$\text{Fractional } Sao_2 = O_2Hb/(O_2Hb + \text{reduced Hb} + COHb + MetHb) \times 100$$

In clinical circumstances where other Hb moieties are present, the Spo_2 measurement is higher than the Sao_2 reported by the blood gas laboratory. In most patients, MetHb and COHb are present in low concentrations so that the functional saturation approximates the fractional value.

Pulse oximetry has been used in all patient age groups to detect and prevent hypoxemia. The clinical benefits of pulse oximetry are enhanced by its simplicity. Modern pulse oximeters are noninvasive, continuous, and autocalibrating. They have quick response times and their battery backup provides monitoring during transport. The clinical accuracy is typically reported to be ±pm 2 to 3% at 70 to 100% saturation and ± 3% at 50 to 70% saturation. Published data from numerous investigations support accuracy and precision reported by instrument manufacturers.

The appropriate use of pulse oximetry necessitates an appreciation of both physiologic and technical limitations. Despite the numerous clinical benefits of pulse oximetry, other factors affect its accuracy and reliability. Factors that may be present during anesthesia care and that affect the accuracy and reliability of pulse oximetry include dyshemoglobins, vital dyes, nail polish, ambient light, light-emitting diode variability, motion artifact, and background noise. Electrocautery can interfere with pulse oximetry if the radiofrequency emissions are sensed by the photodetector. Reports of burns or pressure necrosis exist but are infrequent. These complications can be reduced by inspecting the digits during monitoring.

Recent developments in pulse oximetry technology permit more accurate measurements of Spo_2 during patient movement or low-perfusion conditions. These instruments use complex signal processing of the two wavelengths of light to improve the signal-to-noise ratio and reject artifact. Studies in volunteers suggest that the performance of pulse oximeters incorporating this technology is superior to conventional oximetry during motion of the hand.[9]

There is overwhelming evidence supporting the capability of pulse oximetry for detecting desaturation before it is clinically apparent. Pulse oximetry has wide applicability in many hospital and nonhospital settings. However, there are no definitive data demonstrating a reduction in morbidity or mortality associated with the advent of pulse oximetry. An older large, randomized trial did not detect a significant difference in postoperative complications when routine pulse oximetry was used.[10] However, there was a sense that use of Spo_2 provided early warning of hypoxemia, and anesthesiologists using Spo_2 felt a greater level of comfort than those who did not use Spo_2. A reduction of anesthesia mortality, as well as fewer malpractice claims for respiratory events, coincident with the introduction of pulse oximeters suggests that the routine use of these devices may have been a contributing factor. Pulse oximetry is an inexpensive, essential tool for anesthesia care.

BLOOD PRESSURE MONITORING

Perioperative measurement of arterial blood pressure is an important indicator of the adequacy of circulation. Systemic blood pressure monitoring is commonly performed indirectly

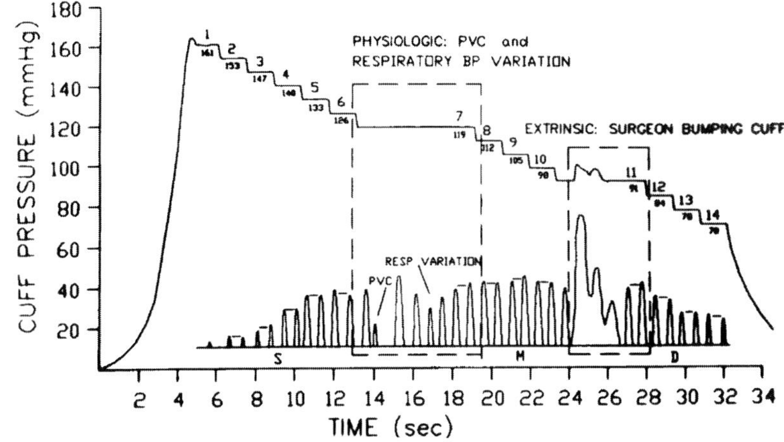

FIGURE 24-3. Diagram illustrating motion artifact, a premature ventricular contraction, and respiratory artifact as sensed by a Dinamap noninvasive blood pressure monitor. (Reproduced with permission from Ramsey M: Blood pressure monitoring: Automated oscillometric devices. J Clin Monit 7:56, 1991.)

using extremity-encircling cuffs or directly by inserting a catheter into an artery and transducing the arterial pressure trace. Today, anesthesiologists have a variety of techniques available for measuring changes in systolic, diastolic, and mean arterial pressure (MAP).

Indirect Measurement of Arterial Blood Pressure

The simplest method of blood pressure determination estimates systolic blood pressure by palpating the return of the arterial pulse while an occluding cuff is deflated. Modifications of this technique include the observance of the return of Doppler sounds, the transduced arterial pressure trace, or a photoplethysmographic pulse wave as produced by a pulse oximeter.

Auscultation of the Korotkoff sounds permit estimation of both systolic (SP) and diastolic (DP) blood pressures. MAP can be calculated using an estimating equation (MAP = DP + 1/3 [SP – DP]). Korotkoff sounds result from turbulent flow within an artery created by the mechanical deformation from the blood pressure cuff. Systolic blood pressure is signaled by the appearance of the first Korotkoff sound. Disappearance of the sound or a muffled tone signals the diastolic blood pressure.

The detection of sound changes is subjective and prone to errors based on deficiencies in sound transmission or hearing. Cuff deflation rate also influences accuracy. Quick deflations underestimate blood pressure. Palpation and auscultatory techniques require pulsatile blood flow and are unreliable during conditions of low flow. These techniques are reasonably accurate when aneroid gauges are within calibration, the encircling cuff is appropriately sized and positioned, the inflation is above the true systolic pressure, and the Korotkoff sounds or pulse is properly identified.

The American Heart Association recommends that the bladder width for indirect blood pressure monitoring should approximate 40% of the circumference of the extremity. Bladder length should be sufficient to encircle at least 60% of the extremity. Falsely high estimates result when cuffs are too small, when cuffs are applied too loosely, or when the extremity is below heart level. Falsely low estimates result when cuffs are too large, when the extremity is above heart level, or after quick deflations.

Since 1976, microprocessor-controlled oscillotonometers have replaced auscultatory and palpatory techniques for routine perioperative blood pressure monitoring. Standard oscillometry measures mean blood pressure by sensing the point of maximal fluctuations in cuff pressure produced while deflating a blood pressure cuff. Most current instruments use oscillometric techniques to measure systolic, diastolic, and mean blood pressures by determining parameter identification points during cuff deflation.

In a generic noninvasive oscillometric monitor (*noninvasive blood pressure,* or NIBP), cuff pressure is sensed by a pressure transducer whose output is digitized for processing. After the cuff is inflated by an air pump, cuff pressure is held constant while oscillations are sampled. If no oscillations are sensed by the pressure transducer, the microprocessor switches open a deflation valve, and the next lower pressure level is sampled for the presence of oscillations. The microprocessor controlling the operation of the NIBP compares the amplitude of oscillation pairs and numerically displays the blood pressure estimate. Figure 24-3 depicts how a typical NIBP is obtained. In this example, the effect of respiratory variation, a premature ventricular complex, and cuff movement are demonstrated.

Automated oscillometry has been demonstrated to correlate well with direct intra-arterial measurement of MAP and diastolic blood pressure. Automated oscillometry may underestimate systolic blood pressure, with mean errors reported from –6.9 to –8.6 mm Hg compared with direct radial artery pressure measurements.

Oscillometry requires the careful evaluation of several cardiac cycles at each increment of deflation to smooth out pronounced respiratory variations or motion artifacts. Cuff movement or erratic pulse transmission influences accuracy. In the anesthetized patient, automated oscillometry is usually accurate and versatile. A variety of cuff sizes makes it possible to use oscillometry in all age groups.

Problems With Noninvasive Blood Pressure Monitoring

Cuff-based pressure monitoring continues to be the standard method used in the perioperative period. When clinical circumstances require frequent blood pressure readings for a prolonged period, it is advisable periodically to move the cuff to alternative sites. Failure to deflate the cuff increases venous pressure. Hematomas have been described both beneath and distal to the cuff. Tremors or shivering can delay cuff deflation and prolong the deflation cycle. A compartment syndrome attributed to a prolonged inflation cycle has been described. Ulnar neuropathy has been reported after the use of automated cycled blood pressure cuffs. Compression of the ulnar nerve can be avoided by applying the encircling cuff proximal to the ulnar groove. Automated sequencing may alter the timing of intravenous drug administration when the access site is located in the same extremity. Hydrostatic errors result when blood pressure cuffs are placed on extremities that are above or below the level of the right atrium. The hydrostatic offset can be mathematically corrected by adding or subtracting 0.7 mm Hg for each centimeter that the cuff is off the horizontal plane of the heart.

Indirect Continuous Noninvasive Techniques

Several methods for monitoring blood pressure continuously and noninvasively have been designed and evaluated for intraoperative blood pressure surveillance. These techniques provide clinicians with a continuous blood pressure estimate and an accurate display of the arterial blood pressure trace. *Indirect continuous noninvasive techniques* (ICNTs) continue to be evaluated because it is desirable to enhance beat-to-beat blood pressure monitoring while reducing the inherent risks and costs of direct intra-arterial monitoring. Clinical studies suggest that accuracy and precision of ICNTs are satisfactory, even under conditions of rapidly changing hemodynamics.[11–13] At present, however, ICNTs are not considered substitutes for direct arterial pressure monitoring in critically ill patients in the operating room.

Invasive Measurement of Vascular (Arterial Blood) Pressure

Indwelling arterial cannulation permits the opportunity to monitor arterial blood pressure continuously and to have vascular access for arterial blood sampling. Intra-arterial blood pressure monitoring uses saline-filled tubing to transmit the force of the pressure pulse wave to a pressure transducer that converts the displacement of a silicon crystal into voltage changes. These electrical signals are amplified, filtered, and displayed as the arterial pressure trace. Intra-arterial pressure transducing systems are subject to many potential errors based on the physical properties of fluid motion and the performance of the catheter-transducer-amplification system used to sense, process, and display the pressure pulse wave.

The behavior of transducers, fluid couplings, signal amplification, and display systems can be described by a complex second-order differential equation. Solving the equation predicts the output and characterizes the fidelity of the system's ability faithfully to display and estimate the arterial pressure over time. The fidelity of fluid-coupled transducing systems is
3 constrained by two properties: *damping* (ζ) and *natural frequency* (Fo). Zeta (ζ) describes the tendency for saline in the measuring system to extinguish motion. Fo describes the tendency for the measuring system to resonate. The fidelity of the transduced pressure depends on optimizing ζ and Fo so that the system can respond appropriately to the range of frequencies contained in the pressure pulse wave. Analysis of high-fidelity recordings of arterial blood pressure indicates that the pressure trace contains frequencies from 1 to 30 Hz.

The performance of a transducing system is often described by its *bandwidth*. The bandwidth contains the frequencies in which the transducing system faithfully reproduces the frequencies contained in the pulse pressure wave. Conventional disposable, saline-coupled transducers with 60 in of pressure tubing have an acceptable bandwidth and commonly have frequency responses approaching 30 Hz. If the system begins to resonate (ringing) or becomes damp (inertia), the fidelity of the system is impaired and estimates of blood pressure become less accurate. Measuring the bandwidth of transducer systems requires complicated equipment. Estimates of ζ and Fo can be obtained at the bedside.

Studies have demonstrated that system fidelity is optimized when catheters and tubing are stiff, the mass of the fluid is small, the number of stopcocks is limited, and the connecting tubing is not excessive. Damping lowers the effective bandwidth of the transducer system, which promotes the potential for resonance. Figure 24-4 demonstrates the effect of damping on the character of the arterial pressure trace. In clinical practice, underdamped catheter–transducer systems tend to overestimate systolic pressure by 15 to 30 mm Hg and amplify artifact (catheter whip). Likewise, excessive increases in ζ reduce fidelity and underestimate systolic pressure. The presence of air bubbles in the coupling fluid reduces the natural frequency of the transducing system. For clinical use, it is sufficient to place the transducer at the level of the right atrium, open the stopcock to atmosphere, and balance the electronic amplifying system to display "zero." Periodic checks of the zero reference point ensures that transducer drift is eliminated.

Gardner[14] suggested using the "fast flush" test to determine the natural frequency and damping characteristics of the transducing system. This test examines the characteristics of the resonant waves recorded after the release of a flush. Damping is estimated by the amplitude ratio of the first pair of resonant waves and the natural frequency is estimated by dividing the paper speed by the interval cycle. Kleinman et al[15] have confirmed the utility of the fast flush test. Because many therapeutic decisions are based on changes in arterial blood pressure, it is imperative that anesthesiologists understand the physical limitation imposed by fluid-filled pressure transducer systems. Significant exaggeration of pressure measurements occur when the transducer system has a resonant frequency in the range of the pressure wave frequencies. Systolic pressure is underestimated when measured with overdamping systems and overestimated by underdamping or resonating systems. Mean pressure estimates are typically less affected even when damping and resonance are not optimal.

Arterial Cannulation

Multiple arteries can be used for direct measurement of blood pressure, including the radial, brachial, axillary, femoral, and dorsalis pedis arteries. The radial artery remains the most popular site for cannulation because of its accessibility and the presence of a collateral blood supply. In the past, assessment of the patency of the ulnar circulation by performance of an *Allen's test* has been recommended before cannulation. Allen's test is performed by compressing both radial and ulnar arteries while the patient tightens his or her fist. Releasing pressure on each respective artery determines the dominant vessel supplying blood to the hand. The prognostic value of the Allen's test in assessing the adequacy of the collateral circulation has not been confirmed.[16,17]

Radial artery cannulation and blood pressure monitoring have been associated with several problems. The radial artery pulse pressure wave is subject to inaccuracies inherent to its distal location. After separation from cardiopulmonary bypass, large pressure gradients between aortic and radial arteries have been described.

Complications of Invasive Arterial Monitoring

Traumatic cannulation has been associated with hematoma formation, thrombosis, and damage to adjacent nerves. Abnormal radial artery blood flow after catheter removal occurs frequently. Studies suggest that blood flow normalizes in 3 to 70 days. Radial artery thrombosis can be minimized by using small catheters, avoiding polypropylene-tapered catheters, and reducing the duration of arterial cannulation. Flexible guidewires may reduce the potential trauma associated with catheters negotiating tortuous vessels. During cannula removal, the potential for thromboembolism may be diminished by compressing the proximal and distal arterial segment while aspirating the cannula during withdrawal.

Many cannulation sites have been used for direct arterial blood pressure monitoring (Table 24-3). Three techniques for cannulation are common: direct arterial puncture,

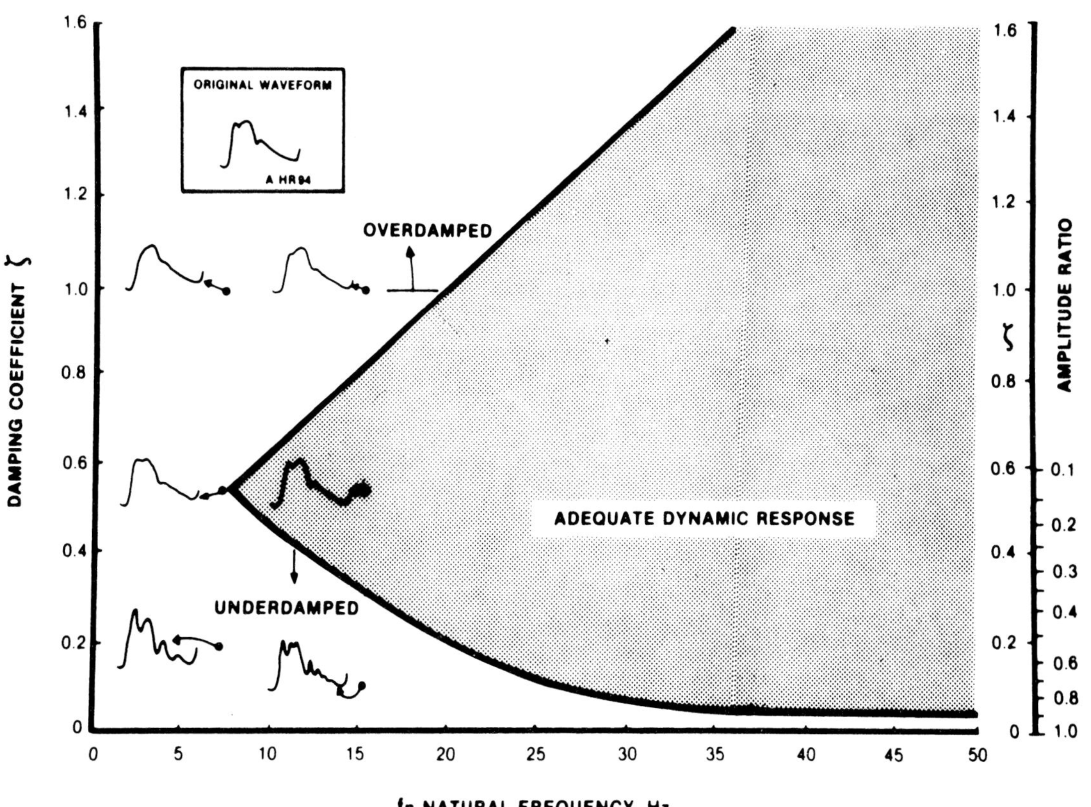

FIGURE 24-4. The relationship between the frequency of fluid-filled transducing systems and damping. The *shaded area* represents the appropriate range of damping for a given natural frequency (Fn). The size of the wedge also depends on the steepness of the arterial pressure trace and heart rate. (Reproduced with permission from Gardner RM: Direct blood pressure measurement: Dynamic response requirements. Anesthesiology 54:231, 1981.)

guidewire-assisted cannulation (Seldinger's technique), and the transfixion–withdrawal method. A necessary condition for percutaneous placement is identification of the arterial pulse, which may require a Doppler flow detection device in patients with poor peripheral pulses.

Arterial cannulation is regarded as an invasive procedure with a documented morbidity. Ischemia after radial artery cannulation resulting from thrombosis, proximal emboli, or prolonged shock has been described.[18] Contributing factors include severe atherosclerosis, diabetes, low cardiac output, and intense peripheral vasoconstriction. Ischemia, hemorrhage, thrombosis, embolism, cerebral air embolism (retrograde flow associated with flushing), aneurysm formation, arteriovenous fistula formation, skin necrosis, and infection have occurred as the direct result of arterial cannulation, arterial blood sampling, or high-pressure flushing.

Continuous-flush devices are incorporated into disposable transducer kits and infuse at 3 to 6 mL/h. In neonates, the infusion volume may contribute to fluid overload. Continuous-flush devices have little effect on the blood pressure measurement. However, pressurized flush systems may serve as a source of an air embolism. Removing air from the pressurized infusion bag, stopcocks, and tubing minimizes the potential for air embolism.

Direct arterial pressure monitoring requires constant vigilance. The data displayed must correlate with clinical conditions before therapeutic interventions are initiated. Sudden increases in the transduced blood pressure may represent a hydrostatic error because the position of the transducer was not adjusted after change in the operating room table's height. Sudden decreases often result from kinking of the catheter or

TABLE 24-3

ARTERIAL CANNULATION AND DIRECT BLOOD PRESSURE MONITORING

■ ARTERIAL CANNULATION SITE	■ CLINICAL POINTS OF INTEREST
Radial artery	Preferred site for monitoring Nontapered catheters preferred
Ulnar artery	Complication similar to radial Primary source of hand blood flow
Brachial artery	Insertion site medial to biceps tendon Median nerve damage is potential hazard Can accommodate 18-gauge cannula
Axillary artery	Insertion site at junction of pectoralis and deltoid muscle Specialized kits available
Femoral artery	Easy access in low flow states Potential for local and retroperitoneal hemorrhage Longer catheters preferred
Dorsalis pedis artery	Collateral circulation = posterior tibial artery Higher systolic pressure estimates

tubing. Before initiating therapy, the transducer system should be "rezeroed" and the patency of the arterial cannula verified. This ensures the accuracy of the measurement and avoids a potentially dangerous medication error.

Central Venous and Pulmonary Artery Monitoring

Central venous cannulas are important portals for intraoperative vascular access and for the assessment of changes in vascular volume. Central venous cannulas permit the rapid administration of fluids, insertion of PACs, insertion of transvenous electrodes, monitoring of central venous pressure (CVP), and a site for observation and treatment of venous air embolism.

The right internal jugular vein is the preferred site for cannulation because it is accessible from the head of the operating table, has a predictable anatomy, and has a high success rate in both adults and children.[19] The left-sided internal jugular vein is also available but is less desirable because of the potential for damaging the thoracic duct or difficulty in maneuvering catheters through the jugular–subclavian junction. Accidental carotid artery puncture is a potential problem with either location.

Three techniques (posterior, central, and anterior) have been described for internal jugular cannulation. Each insertion point is referenced to the triangle formed by the sternal and clavicular heads of the sternocleidomastoid muscle and the clavicle. Venipuncture using a 22-gauge "seeker" needle minimizes trauma to adjacent structures. When the location of the internal jugular vein is difficult to ascertain, ultrasonography can assist in identifying the proximity of internal jugular vein and the carotid artery. Alternatives to the internal jugular vein include the external jugular, subclavian, antecubital, and femoral veins.

Central Venous Pressure Monitoring

The benefit of CVP monitoring has been the subject of considerable debate. Proponents of CVP monitoring believe that CVP pressures are essentially equivalent to right atrial pressures and serve as a reflection of right ventricular preload.[20] Conditions that affect right atrial pressure also influence the CVP pressure trace. The normal CVP waveform consists of three peaks (a, c, and v waves) and two descents (x, y), each resulting from the ebb and flow of blood in the right atrium (Fig. 24-5). Corresponding events occur in the left atrium and similar pressure contours are observed during monitoring of pulmonary artery pressure when the PAC is placed in the occluded position.

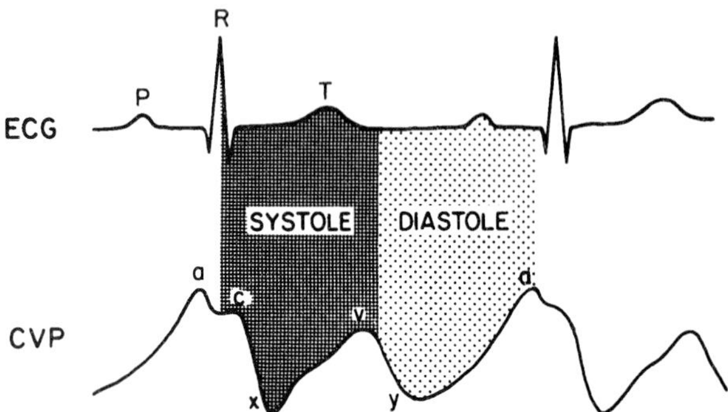

FIGURE 24-5. The normal central venous pressure trace. (Redrawn with permission from Mark JB: Central venous pressure monitoring: Clinical insights beyond the numbers. J Cardiothorac Vasc Anesth 5:163, 1991.)

The character of the CVP trace depends on many factors, including heart rate, conduction disturbances, tricuspid valve function, normal or abnormal intrathoracic pressure changes, and changes in right ventricular compliance. In patients with atrial fibrillation, a waves are absent. When resistance to the emptying of the right atrium is present, large a waves are often observed. Examples include tricuspid stenosis, right ventricular hypertrophy as a result of pulmonic stenosis, or acute or chronic lung disease associated with pulmonary hypertension. Large a waves may also be observed when right ventricular compliance is impaired.

Tricuspid regurgitation typically produces giant v waves that begin immediately after the QRS complex. Large v waves are often observed when right ventricular ischemia or failure is present or when ventricular compliance is impaired by constrictive pericarditis or cardiac tamponade. A prominent v wave during CVP monitoring may suggest right ventricular papillary muscle ischemia and tricuspid regurgitation. When right ventricular compliance decreases, the CVP often increases with prominent a and v waves fusing to form an *m* or *w* configuration.

Central venous pressure monitoring is often unreliable for estimating left ventricular filling pressures, especially when cardiopulmonary disease processes alter the normal cardiovascular pressure–volume relationships. CVP monitoring is less invasive and less costly than pulmonary artery monitoring and offers unique understanding of right-sided hemodynamic events and the status of vascular volume.

Pulmonary Artery Monitoring

The development of the flow-directed, balloon flotation PAC was a major advance in hemodynamic monitoring, and it has become an important tool in the quantitative assessment of cardiopulmonary function. Numerous articles have reviewed the various applications and benefits of pulmonary artery monitoring.[21] Use should be guided by the information needed for enhanced diagnosis and therapy.[22] Today, PAC monitoring is commonly used in surgical patients to help evaluate and treat hemodynamic alterations, which contribute significantly to the morbidity and mortality inherent to the surgical care of high-risk patients.

In 1993, the ASA published practice guidelines that examined the evidence supporting the clinical effectiveness of PAC
4 monitoring. These guidelines were updated in 2003.[23] Issues such as the timing of PAC monitoring, its effect on treatment decisions, patient selection and case mix, and evidence regarding PAC monitoring contribution to positive or negative outcomes were evaluated using stringent evidence-based methodology. This effort identified many flaws in the body of evidence, which made it difficult to draw meaningful conclusions regarding the effectiveness of PAC monitoring to reduce morbidity or mortality. The consensus opinion implies that PAC monitoring may reduce perioperative complications if critical hemodynamic data obtained during appropriate PAC monitoring are accurately interpreted and appropriate treatment is tailored to the conditions as they change over time.[23] Monitoring the hemodynamic status of high-risk patients may reduce cardiac complications (e.g., myocardial ischemia, congestive heart failure, dysrhythmias), renal insufficiency, brain injury, and pulmonary complications.

Pulmonary artery catheters permit the measurement of intracardiac pressures, thermodilution CO (TCO), mixed venous oxygen saturation, intracavitary electrograms, and lung water. This information can help define clinical problems, monitor the progression of hemodynamic dysfunctions, and guide the response of corrective therapy.

TABLE 24-4

DERIVED HEMODYNAMIC VARIABLES

NAME	ABBREVIATION	CALCULATION	UNITS
Cardiac index	CI	CO/BSA	1 liters/min/m^2
Systemic vascular resistance	SVR	(MAP-CVP/CO) × 80	dyne-cm/s
Pulmonary vascular resistance	PVR	(MPAP-PCWP/CO) × 80	dyne-cm/s
Stroke index	SI	CI/heart rate	mL/beat/m^2
Left ventricular stroke work index	LVSWI	SI × (MAP-PCWP) × 0.0136	gm/beat/m^2
Right ventricular stroke work index	RVSWI	SI × (MPAP-CVP) × 0.0136	gm/beat/m^2

BSA, body surface area; MAP, mean arterial pressure; CVP, central venous pressure; MPAP, mean pulmonary arterial pressure; PCWP, pulmonary capillary wedge pressure.

The measurement of intracardiac pressures can indirectly assess left ventricular preload, diagnose the existence of pulmonary hypertension, or differentiate cardiac and noncardiac causes of pulmonary edema. PACs allow for the rapid and reproducible measurements of TCO, calculation of oxygen delivery (CO × arterial O_2 content), and assessment of cardiac work. Hemodynamic measurements are often predicated on the manipulation of preload, afterload, and contractility. Several derived indices of hemodynamic function necessitate measurements commonly obtained from PAC monitoring (Table 24-4).

Access to mixed venous blood from the pulmonary artery port provides an indirect assessment of the balance between O_2 delivery and O_2 utilization. Mixed venous oxygen saturation ($S\bar{v}O_2$) measurements are needed to calculate mixed venous oxygen content ($C\bar{v}O_2$). $C\bar{v}O_2$ is an important variable used for calculating intrapulmonary (Eq. 24-1) or intracardiac shunts (Eq. 24-2).

$$\frac{Cco_2 - Cao_2}{Cco_2 - C\bar{v}o_2} = \frac{\dot{Q}s}{\dot{Q}t} \tag{24-1}$$

$$\frac{Sao_2 - SRAo_2}{Sao_2 - S\bar{v}o_2} = \frac{\dot{Q}p}{\dot{Q}s} \tag{24-2}$$

Where Cco_2 = capillary O_2 content, Cao_2 = arterial O_2 content, $C\bar{v}o_2$ = mixed venous O_2 content, $\dot{Q}s/\dot{Q}t$ = shunt fraction, Sao_2 = arterial O_2 saturation, $SRAo_2$ = right atrial O_2 saturation, $S\bar{v}o_2$ = mixed venous O_2 saturation, and $\dot{Q}p/\dot{Q}s$ = pulmonary-to-systemic shunt.

The validity of PAC monitoring depends on a properly functioning pressure monitoring system, correctly identifying the "true" *pulmonary capillary wedge pressure* (PCWP), and integration of the various factors that affect the relationship of PCWP, and the other cardiac pressures and volumes that are determinants of ventricular function. Figure 24-6 depicts the transduced pressure waves observed as a PAC is floated to the wedged position. Catheter placement is most commonly performed by observing the pressure waves as the catheter is floated from the CVP position through the right heart chambers into the pulmonary artery.

Pulmonary artery catheter monitoring necessitates an appreciation of the various physiologic determinants of CO and oxygen delivery. The PAC is used to continuously monitor the pulmonary artery pressure and intermittently monitor pulmonary wedge pressure. PCWP is used to assess left ventricular preload indirectly by reflecting changes in left ventricular end-diastolic pressure (LVEDP). Figure 24-7 depicts the relationship between the various pressures in the cardiopulmonary system.

It has been well demonstrated that right-sided pressures in the heart often are poor indicators of left ventricular filling, either as absolute numbers or in terms of the direction of change in response to therapy. The correlation of these pressures as estimates of LVEDP (or left ventricular end-diastolic volume [LVEDV]) is directly related to their proximity to the left ventricle and the status of ventricular compliance. Assuming an open conduit from the catheter tip to the left ventricle, when the PAC is occluded ("wedged"), the right-sided heart chambers and valves are bypassed. During end-diastole, there is cessation of forward blood flow, and a static fluid column is presumed to exist from the left ventricle to the PAC tip. Ideally, changes in LVEDP are reflected by all proximal pressures (left atrial, pulmonary venous, pulmonary artery end-diastolic pressure [PAEDP], and PCWP). Alterations of internal or external forces applied to the open conduit during PCWP measurements may invalidate the PCWP-LVEDP-LVEDV relationship.

Factors Affecting the Accuracy of Pulmonary Artery Catheter Data

Pulmonary Vascular Resistance. Any disease process or condition that increases pulmonary vascular resistance has the

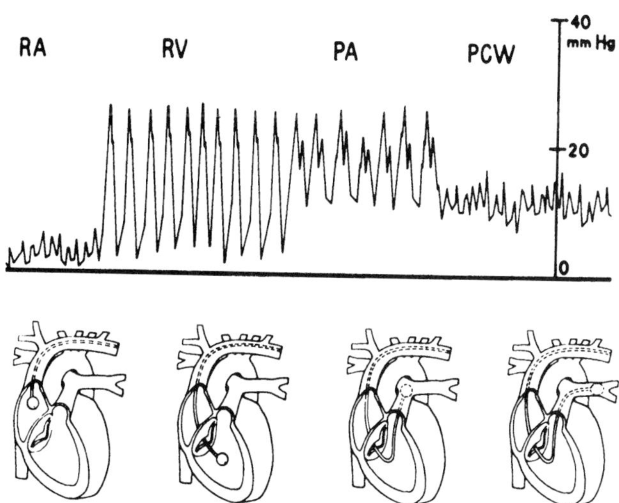

FIGURE 24-6. Pressure tracing observed during the flotation of a pulmonary artery catheter. (Reproduced with permission from Dizon CT, Barash PG: The value of monitoring pulmonary artery pressure in clinical practice. Conn Med 41:622, 1979.)

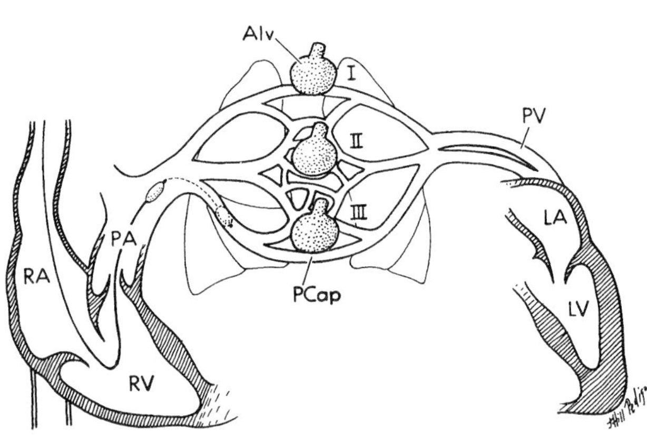

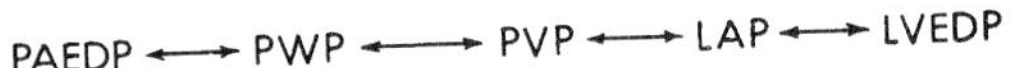

FIGURE 24-7. The anatomic position of a pulmonary artery catheter in the pulmonary artery. The *dashed line* positions the inflated balloon in the "wedged" position. (RA, right atrium; RV, right ventricle; PA, pulmonary artery; Alv, alveolus; Pcap, pulmonary capillary; PV, pulmonary vein; LA, left atrium; LV, left ventricle.) I, II, and III characterize the relationship of $P_{aveolar}$, $P_{arterial}$, and P_{venous} as described by West. The bottom of the figure shows a progressive correlation of vascular pressures. (Reproduced with permission from Vender JS: Invasive cardiac monitoring. Crit Care Clin 4:455, 1988.)

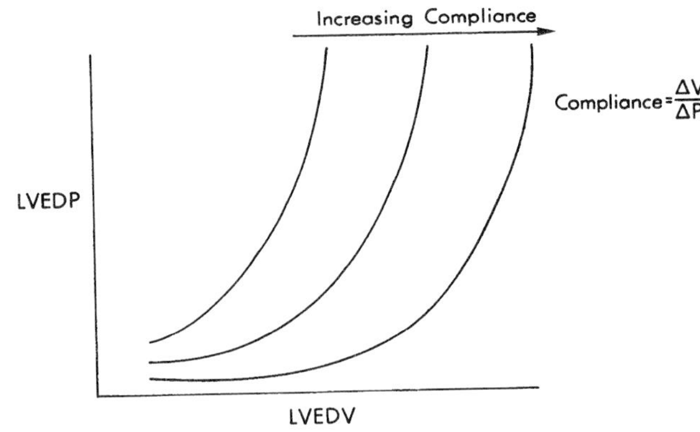

FIGURE 24-8. Typical ventricular compliance curve. (Reproduced with permission from Vender JS: Invasive cardiac monitoring. Crit Care Clin 4:455, 1988.)

potential to reduce pulmonary blood flow and alter the relationship between PCWP and PAEDP. Pathologic conditions such as acute or chronic lung disease, pulmonary emboli, alveolar hypoxia, acidosis, and hypoxemia, and many vasoactive drugs increase pulmonary vascular resistance and have the potential to modify the PCWP–PAEDP relationship. Tachycardia shortens ventricular diastole and also increases pulmonary vascular resistance.

Alveolar–Pulmonary Artery Pressure Relationships. West et al[25] described a gravity-dependent difference between ventilation and perfusion in the lung. The variability in pulmonary blood flow is a result of differences in pulmonary artery (PA), alveolar (Palv), and venous pressures (PV) and is categorized into three distinct zones. Only Zone III (PA > PV > Palv) meets the criteria for uninterrupted blood flow and a continuous communication with distal intracardiac pressures. Increases in alveolar pressure, decreases in perfusion, or changes in positioning can convert areas of Zone III into either Zone II or I. Flow-directed PACs usually advance to gravity-dependent areas of highest blood flow.

The location of a PAC can be confirmed by a lateral chest film to ascertain that the catheter tip is below the level of the left atrium. The following characteristics suggest that the PAC tip is not in Zone III: PCWP > PAEDP, nonphasic PCWP tracing, and inability to aspirate blood from the distal port when the catheter is wedged.

Respiratory Pattern and Airway Pressure. Changes in intrathoracic and intrapleural pressure affect transmural cardiac pressures. Transmural pressure is defined as the net distending pressure of the left ventricle. Changes in intrathoracic pressure affect the PCWP–LVEDP relationship. Positive end–expiratory pressure (PEEP) therapy can induce changes in both intravascular and intrapleural pressures. PEEP increases alveolar pressure, potentially converting Zone III areas to Zone II. If PEEP is transmitted across the alveoli, intrapleural pressure increases. Pulmonary compliance determines the extent of this effect. PEEP alters ventricular distensibility and decreases venous return. This causes a disproportionate increase in PCWP (and LVEDP) compared with changes in LVEDV.

The effect of PEEP therapy is minimal if the levels of PEEP are low (≤10 cm) and the PAC is located in Zone III. Higher levels of PEEP influence the PCWP–LVEDP relationship. During high PEEP therapy, esophageal pressure measurements can be made to determine intrapleural pressure. Alternatively, subtracting 1 to 2 mm Hg from the displayed "wedge" pressure for each 5 cm H_2O of PEEP therapy gives an estimate when PEEP is above 10 cm H_2O.

Intracardiac Factors. Pathologic obstruction at the mitral valve secondary to mitral stenosis, atrial myxoma, or clot can interfere with the ability of left atrial pressure to reflect LVEDP. Similarly, mitral regurgitation, a noncompliant left atrium, or left-to-right intracardiac shunting often is associated with large v waves.

Decreases in left ventricular compliance, aortic regurgitation, or premature closure of the mitral valve may reverse the left atrial pressure–LVEDP pressure gradient. When this occurs, PCWP is not a valid reflection of LVEDV.

Figure 24-8 graphically depicts the relationship between LVEDP and LVEDV. The LVEDP–LVEDV relationship is not linear. A family of LVEDP–LVEDV compliance curves characterizes the effect of changing the stiffness of the left ventricle. Ventricular compliance is a dynamic factor influenced by many physiologic and pathologic variables. The LVEDP–LVEDV compliance curves suggest that at low preloads, larger increases in LVEDV produce smaller changes in LVEDP. Conversely, at higher preloads, a similar change in LVEDV produces a greater pressure change. For a given LVEDV, any decrease in ventricular compliance results in an increase in LVEDP. This explains the development of hydrostatic pulmonary edema at normal LVEDV. Factors that are associated with changes in ventricular compliance are listed in Table 24-5.

Complications of Pulmonary Catheter Monitoring

Adverse effects from PAC monitoring can result during central venous access, the catheterization procedure, or any time after

TABLE 24-5

DECREASED LEFT VENTRICULAR COMPLIANCE: COMMON ETIOLOGIES

Myocardial ischemia	Cardiac tamponade
Restrictive myopathies	Myocardial fibrosis
Right-to-left intraventricular shunts	Inotropic drugs
Aortic stenosis	Hypertension

TABLE 24-6

ADVERSE EFFECTS ASSOCIATED WITH PULMONARY ARTERY MONITORING

■ COMPLICATION	■ REPORTED INCIDENCE (%)
Central venous access	
Arterial puncture	1.1–13
Postoperative neuropathy	5.3
Pneumothorax	0.3–1.1
Air embolism	0.3–4.5
Flotation of pulmonary artery catheter	
Minor dysrhythmias	4–68.9
Ventricular tachycardia or fibrillation	0.3–62.7
Right bundle-branch block	0.1–4.3
Complete heart block (prior left bundle-branch block)	0–8.5
Complications associated with catheter residence	
Pulmonary artery rupture	0.1–1.5
Positive cultures from catheter tip	1.4–34.8
Sepsis secondary to catheter resistance	0.7–11.4
Thrombophlebitis	6.5
Venous thrombosis	0.5–66.7
Pulmonary infarction	0.1–5.6
Mural thrombus	28–61
Valvular or endocardial vegetations	2.2–100
Deaths attributed to pulmonary artery catheter	0.02–1.5

ASA Task Force on Pulmonary Artery Catheterization.
Practice Guidelines for Pulmonary Artery Catheterization: an updated report by The American Society of Anesthesiologists Task Force on Pulmonary Catheterization. Anesthesiology 99:988–1014, 2003.

PAC placement. Central venous access represents an invasive process with inherent risks, some of which are potentially life threatening.

Unintentional puncture of nearby arteries, bleeding, neuropathy, and pneumothorax may result from needle insertion into adjacent structures. Air embolism may occur if a cannula is open to the atmosphere and air is entrained during or after CVP placement. Dysrhythmias are common during the catheterization procedure, with a reported incidence of 4.7 to 68.9%. Ventricular tachycardia or fibrillation may be induced during catheter advancement. Catheter advancement has been associated with right bundle-branch block and, in patients with preexisting left bundle-branch block, may precipitate complete heart block. Table 24-6 summarizes the adverse effects as reported by the ASA task force on pulmonary artery catheterization.[23]

The rate of iatrogenic deaths associated with PAC monitoring is uncertain. The most dreaded complication associated with PAC monitoring is pulmonary artery rupture. Pulmonary hypertension, coagulopathy, and heparinization are often present in patients who have died of pulmonary artery rupture. Perforations and subsequent hemorrhage can be avoided by restricting "overwedging," minimizing the number of balloon inflations, and using proper technique during balloon inflations.

Infection is a potential complication of the continued use of CVP and PAC catheters. Guidelines for the prevention of intravascular catheter-related infections have recently been published by the Centers for Disease Control and Prevention (CDC).[24] Methods recommended to reduce the incidence of local and bloodstream infections include (1) education and training of clinicians who insert and maintain central catheters; (2) use of maximal sterile barrier precautions (mask, cap, sterile gloves and gown, and large sterile drape); (3) use of 2% chlorhexidine for skin preparation; and (4) avoidance of routine replacement of CVP and PAC catheters solely for the purpose of reducing the risk of infection.

Since the advent of PACs, several modifications have been integrated into the design that enhance their monitoring capabilities. The first significant design modification incorporated a thermistor at the tip, permitting the measurement of CO. Other features have been introduced for clinical use or evaluation. These include mixed venous oximetry, measurement of right ventricular ejection fraction, pacing options, and continuous CO monitoring (CCOM).

Mixed Venous Oximetry

Continuous estimates of $S\bar{v}O_2$ provide a reflection of total tissue oxygen balance. Oxygen delivery ($\dot{D}O_2$) equals the arterial oxygen content multiplied by the CO ($\dot{D}O_2 = [Hb \times 13.8] \times CO$), where 13.8 represents the volume of oxygen carried by Hb converted to grams per liter. Oxygen consumption ($\dot{V}O_2$) is determined by the difference between arterial and venous oxygen delivery. The relationship between $S\bar{v}O_2$, $\dot{V}O_2$, and $\dot{D}O_2$ is demonstrated in the following equation derived from the Fick relationship:

$$S\bar{v}O_2 = SaO_2 - \frac{\dot{V}O_2}{Hb \times 13.8} \times CO$$

This equation indicates that changes in $S\bar{v}O_2$ vary directly with changes in CO, Hb, and SaO_2 and inversely with $\dot{V}O_2$. The normal $S\bar{v}O_2$ is 75%, which denotes tissue oxygen extraction = 25%.

The oximetric PAC uses reflectance spectrophotometry and technology similar to pulse oximetry. Several wavelengths are transmitted through optical fibers embedded in the pulmonary artery. The reflected intensity of light identifies the saturation of blood surrounding the tip of the PAC. Three-wavelength in vivo systems correlate well with simultaneous samples measured by co-oximetry.[26,27] An example of the utility of mixed venous oximetry is depicted in Figure 24-9.

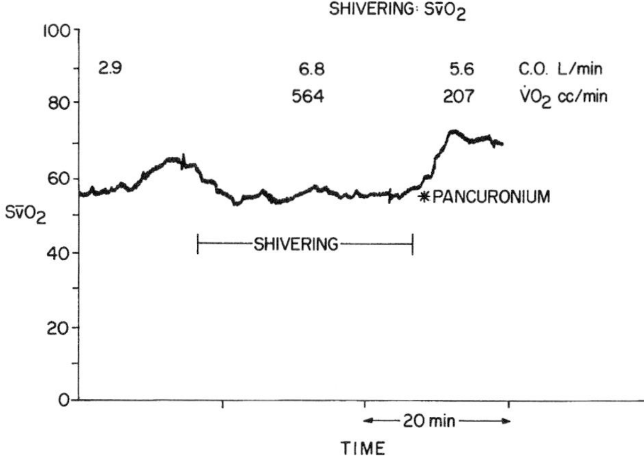

FIGURE 24-9. This $S\bar{v}O_2$ recording in a postcoronary artery bypass patient demonstrates the effects of shivering and its treatment, and the relationship between $S\bar{v}O_2$, cardiac output (CO), and metabolic rate ($\dot{V}O_2$). (Reproduced with permission from Vender JS: Invasive cardiac monitoring. Crit Care Clin 4:455, 1988.)

Indicator Dilution Applications

Indicator dilution determination of CO is based on a concept proposed by Stewart and tested by Hamilton and colleagues. TCO determination is the most widely used adaptation of the indicator dilution principle, which was first described by Fegler in 1954.[28] Today, 5% dextrose or 0.9% saline is used as the indicator. A thermistor located at the PAC tip records the decrease in temperature as the bolus of cooled injectate passes through the pulmonary artery. Computers contend with the complexity of the TCO equation, which includes the following factors: specific heat of the blood and the indicator fluid, the volume of injectate, catheter size, specific gravity of the blood and indicator, the volume of the injectate, and the area of the blood temperature curve. Comparison studies suggest that using either room-temperature or iced injectates provides accurate estimates of CO. Iced injectate is preferred because it produces a more exacting curve with a better signal-to-noise ratio.[29]

When properly performed, TCO measurements correlate well with direct Fick or dye dilution estimates of CO. In clinical practice, triplicate determinations are averaged to increase precision. Differences in values of 12 to 15% are not of clinical significance. TCO estimates vary with the respiratory cycle. This variability can be reduced by performing measurements at peak inspiration or end expiration. Precision is enhanced by ensuring that the rate of injection and the volume are constant. Most CO computers delay the repeat measurement 30 to 90 seconds to stabilize the thermal environment of the pulmonary thermistor.

Adaptations for Continuous Cardiac Output Monitoring

Continuous CO monitoring offers the potential to identify acute changes in ventricular performance as they occur. A properly positioned PAC provides access to the right atrium, right ventricle, and pulmonary artery outflow tract. These locations provide many options for assessment of CCOM. Several thermal techniques are currently used. Pulsed thermodilution uses a coiled right ventricular filament that is randomly heated. A thermistor at the tip of the PAC detects changes in blood temperature and sends the temperature information to a microcomputer that uses stochastic analysis to create a thermodilution curve. CO is computed continuously from a conservation of heat equation.[30]

Another technique applies heat to a thermistor located at the tip of a PAC. The right ventricular outflow subsequently cools the tip. The temperature changes registered are proportional to the decreased temperature produced by right ventricular blood flow. Both of these systems require calibration using standard thermodilution before initiating the CCOM mode. CCOM compares favorably with bolus CO measurements, even under conditions of varying patient temperature and CO.[31]

Right Ventricular Ejection Fraction

Calculation of right ventricular ejection fraction and end-diastolic volume may be performed with a special PAC that uses a rapid response thermistor and a sophisticated computer system. This system analyzes the exponential decay of the pulmonary artery temperature over several cardiac cycles and calculates the ejection fraction by subtracting the mean residual fraction from the CO. Studies have demonstrated good correlation with in vitro techniques and clinical utility for detecting intraoperative right ventricular ischemia.[32–34] Right ventricular ejection fraction monitoring has been recommended when impairment of right ventricular function is suspect. Accuracy requires proper placement. Atrial fibrillation and tricuspid regurgitation can affect the accuracy of the thermal decay methodology.

Clinical Benefits of Pulmonary Artery Monitoring

The debate regarding the clinical benefit of PAC monitoring has persisted since the mid 1980s. Perioperative outcomes have been reported to be improved, worsened, or unchanged by PAC use. At the present time, assessment of the benefits of PAC monitoring is hampered by the lack of well-designed outcome trials. Interpretation of most clinical trials is significantly limited by important flaws in study design, which include inadequate sample size to detect meaningful outcomes, lack of randomization, and lack of standardization of treatments based on PAC data.[24] A study by Sandham et al. was designed to address many of the methodologic limitations present in previous PAC outcome trials.[35] This large-scale, randomized, controlled, single-blind study examined the impact of PAC monitoring in high-risk patients undergoing major surgical procedures. Patients were randomized to a protocol group (PACs used to achieve specific targeted hemodynamic treatment goals) or a standard care group (no PAC use). No differences in major morbidity or mortality were observed between the two groups. Additional well-designed studies are needed to determine the benefits and risks of invasive right-heart catheterization.

Inadequate understanding and application by physician users have been implicated as conditions that limit the benefit of PAC monitoring. To optimize clinical outcome and reduce complications, the care provider must be able to interpret and use the data provided by the PAC. A questionnaire that measured physician knowledge of the technical and theoretical aspects of PAC monitoring was administered to critical care specialists in the United States and Europe. These surveys revealed knowledge of pulmonary artery catheterization is not uniformly good among intensive care unit physicians, with only half of respondents able to read the PCWP correctly from a clearly marked tracking.[36,37] Changes in training and credentialing have been proposed to improve these deficiencies in knowledge.[38,39] In experienced and knowledgeable hands, the PAC can add valuable information with limited risk.

NONINVASIVE TECHNIQUES FOR CARDIAC OUTPUT

The quest for technically simple, noninvasive methods for accurately estimating CO continues. Three methods are available for clinical use.

Impedance Plethysmography

Impedance plethysmography is based on determining the pulsatile changes in resistance occurring during ventricular ejection. Four electrodes are applied to the neck and thorax and a small electric current is applied. Impedance measurements (dZ/dT) are made using two thoracic electrode pairs. Changes in impedance correlate with stroke volume. CO is estimated by determining stroke volume and ventricular ejection time.[40] Electrode placement is an important source of error. Other factors influencing bioimpedance measurements include intrathoracic fluid shifts and changes in hematocrit. More than 150 validation studies have been published, and both poor and good correlations between impedance plethysmography and a reference method have been reported.[41] Although impedance plethysmography has not gained wide acceptance, the technique offers clinicians a simple, quick method to determine CO with minimal direct patient risk.

Doppler Ultrasonography

Doppler ultrasonography can measure the velocity of blood in the ascending or descending aorta or outflow tract of the pulmonary artery. CO is calculated by multiplying the time-weighted average velocity of blood flow by an estimate of aortic or pulmonary artery cross-sectional area that can be directly measured or predicted from a nomogram. Accuracy and precision depend on the estimate of the vessel diameter and the alignment of the Doppler probe. Velocity measurements are most accurate when the Doppler probe and the blood flow are parallel. If the alignment exceeds 25 degrees, velocity measurements lose precision. Suprasternal, transtracheal, and transesophageal probes have been designed for clinical use.[42,43] The development of esophageal Doppler probes allows for continuous, minimally invasive estimation of CO, and may allow for optimization of intravascular volume status without the use of a CVP or PAC.[44]

Arterial Pulse Contour Analysis

Pulse contour analysis of the arterial pressure waveform allows clinicians to determine beat-to-beat measurements of left ventricular output. Computer algorithms are used to calculate the area under the systolic portion of the arterial pulse waveform (from the end of diastole to the end of the ejection phase). Stroke volume is determined by dividing the resulting area by the aortic impedance. A limitation of arterial pulse contour analysis is that the technique requires calibration with another method of measuring cardiac output. Reference cardiac output determinations for calibration can be obtained using moderately invasive (thermodilution CO using a PAC or transpulmonary themodilution using a central venous and arterial line) or minimally invasive (lithium dilution using a peripheral venous and arterial catheter) technology. A number of clinical studies have demonstrated that the precision and accuracy of arterial pulse contour analysis is acceptable when compared with thermodilution CO measurements obtained by PACs.[45,46]

TRANSESOPHAGEAL ECHOCARDIOGRAPHY

The use of transesophageal echocardiography (TEE) in the perioperative period has increased significantly since its first application in humans was reported by Frazen in 1976. (See also Chapter 3) Rapid technological advances have occurred since then, including a reduction in transducer size, the development of multiplane probes, and the use of pulsed-wave, continuous-wave, and color flow Doppler. Improvements in computer design and image acquisition have allowed for a more comprehensive examination of the heart and surrounding structures. TEE appears to offer distinct advantages over other monitors of cardiovascular function and can provide the anesthesiologist with unique diagnostic information in the operating room.

Modern TEE machines offer a number of imaging techniques. In *M-mode,* or motion mode, all of the structures along a narrow ultrasound beam are plotted on the x-axis versus time on the y-axis. M-mode allows only a few millimeters of the heart to be visualized at any one time. *Two-dimensional (2-D) mode* uses multiple scanning lines to create a two-dimensional image of a cross section of the heart. This image is updated 30 to 60 times per second, which produces a real-time display of cardiac motion.

Doppler technology provides information about blood flow in the heart and major vessels. The *Doppler effect* is based on the principle that moving objects (red blood cells) change the frequency of the emitted ultrasound beam. If an object is moving toward the transducer, the ultrasound beam is compressed, which increases the frequency of the transmitted signal. An object moving away from the transducer lowers the frequency of the transmitted ultrasound beam. This information allows the calculation of blood flow velocity within the cardiovascular system. Current TEE machines use three Doppler systems: pulsed-wave, continuous-wave, and color flow Doppler. *Pulsed-wave Doppler* uses a single crystal to emit and receive short bursts of ultrasound at a known frequency (pulse repetition frequency). By measuring the time required for the transmitted ultrasound bursts to return to the transducer, the velocity of blood flow at precise locations in the heart can be measured. A major limitation of pulsed-wave Doppler is that high-velocity flows cannot be accurately quantified. The maximal velocity that can be measured is limited to one half of the pulse repetition frequency; this is known as the Nyquist limit. *Continuous-wave Doppler* uses two crystals (one to transmit, one to receive) to measure blood flow velocity continuously. This allows for accurate measurement of high-velocity flows, but does not permit precise localization. *Color flow Doppler* uses pulsed-wave technology to measure blood flow velocity at multiple sites. Blood flow toward the transducer is coded red and flow away from the transducer is coded blue. Rapidly accelerating or turbulent flow is coded green. By superimposing this color map on a 2-D image of the heart, the direction and velocity of blood flow in the heart can be easily imaged.

Monitoring Applications

There are a number of important monitoring applications for TEE in the perioperative period. In 1996, the ASA and the Society of Cardiovascular Anesthesiologists published practice guidelines to define the proper indications for performing TEE in the operative setting.[47] Indications were divided into three categories.

Category I indications are supported by the strongest evidence or expert opinion; TEE frequently is useful in improving clinical outcomes and is often indicated, depending on patient risk and practice setting. Category II indications are supported by weaker evidence and expert consensus; TEE may be useful in improving clinical outcomes, depending on individual circumstances. Category III indications have little current scientific or expert support, and TEE is infrequently useful in improving clinical outcomes. These indications are summarized in Table 24-7.

Transesophageal echocardiography is used extensively as a monitor of ventricular function. TEE appears to provide more accurate estimates of left ventricular preload than pulmonary artery catheterization. In echocardiography, preload is determined by measuring end-diastolic area. Studies in patients undergoing cardiac or vascular surgery revealed that end-diastolic
5 area calculated by TEE correlated well with left ventricular preload, whereas pulmonary artery diastolic pressure correlated poorly with left ventricular preload.[48,49] Left atrial and left ventricular pressures may also be calculated using Doppler measurements of flow across the mitral valve, or from the pulmonary veins into the left atrium. TEE estimates of intracardiac filling pressures correlate well with data obtained from PACs.[50] Left ventricular contractility can be estimated using a variety of techniques. Ejection fraction can be determined by measuring left ventricular end-diastolic area (EDA) and end-systolic area (ESA):

$$\text{ejection fraction area} = \frac{\text{EDA} - \text{ESA}}{\text{EDA}} \times 100$$

TABLE 24-7

INDICATIONS FOR PERIOPERATIVE TRANSESOPHAGEAL ECHOCARDIOGRAPHY

Category I indications: Supported by the strongest evidence or expert opinion; TEE is frequently useful in improving clinical outcomes in these settings and is often indicated, depending on individual circumstances (e.g., patient risk and practice setting).
- Intraoperative evaluation of acute, persistent, and life-threatening hemodynamic disturbances in which ventricular function and its determinants are uncertain and have not responded to treatment
- Intraoperative use in valve repair
- Intraoperative use in congenital heart surgery for most lesions requiring cardiopulmonary bypass
- Intraoperative use in repair of hypertrophic obstructive cardiomyopathy
- Intraoperative use for endocarditis when preoperative testing was inadequate or extension of infection to perivalvular tissue is suspected
- Preoperative use in unstable patients with suspected thoracic aortic aneurysms, dissection, or disruption who need to be evaluated quickly
- Intraoperative assessment of aortic valve function in repair of aortic dissections with possible aortic valve involvement
- Intraoperative evaluation of pericardial window procedures
- Use in intensive care unit for unstable patients with unexplained hemodynamic disturbances, suspected valve disease, or thromboembolic problems (if other tests or monitoring techniques have not confirmed the diagnosis or patients are too unstable to undergo other tests)

Category II indications: Supported by weaker evidence and expert consensus; TEE may be useful in improving clinical outcomes in these settings, depending on individual circumstances, but appropriate indications are less certain.
- Perioperative use in patients with increased risk of myocardial ischemia or infarction
- Perioperative use in patients with increased risk of hemodynamic disturbances
- Intraoperative assessment of valve replacement
- Intraoperative assessment of repair of cardiac aneurysms
- Intraoperative evaluation of removal of cardiac tumors
- Intraoperative detection of foreign bodies
- Intraoperative detection of air emboli during cardiotomy, heart transplantation operations, and upright neurosurgical procedures
- Intraoperative use during intracardiac thrombectomy
- Intraoperative use during pulmonary embolectomy
- Intraoperative use for suspected cardiac trauma
- Preoperative assessment of patients with suspected acute thoracic aortic dissections, aneurysms, or disruption
- Intraoperative use during repair of thoracic aortic dissections without suspected aortic valve involvement
- Intraoperative detection of aortic atheromatous disease or other sources of aortic emboli
- Intraoperative evaluation of pericardectomy or pericardial effusions, or evaluation of pericardial surgery
- Intraoperative evaluation of anastomotic sites during heart or lung transplantation
- Monitoring placement and function of assist devices

Category III indications: Little current scientific or expert support; TEE is infrequently useful in improving clinical outcomes in these settings, and appropriate indications are uncertain.
- Intraoperative evaluation of myocardial perfusion, coronary artery anatomy, or graft patency
- Intraoperative use during repair of cardiomyopathies other than hypertrophic obstructive cardiomyopathy
- Intraoperative use for uncomplicated endocarditis during noncardiac surgery
- Intraoperative monitoring for emboli during orthopaedic procedures
- Intraoperative assessment of repair of thoracic aortic injuries
- Intraoperative use for uncomplicated pericarditis
- Intraoperative evaluation of pleuropulmonary diseases
- Monitoring placement of intra-aortic balloon pumps, automatic implantable cardiac defibrillators, or pulmonary artery catheters
- Intraoperative monitoring of cardioplegia administration

TEE, transesophageal echocardiography.
Reproduced with permission from American Society of Anesthesiologists and Society of Cardiovascular Anesthesiologists Task Force on Transesophageal Echocardiography: Practice guidelines for perioperative transesophageal echocardiography. Anesthesiology 84:96, 1996.

Stroke volume can be calculated by measuring the Doppler velocity of flow across an area of the heart (aortic valve, pulmonary artery, left ventricular outflow tract) and multiplying this value times the area through which the flow occurs. The stroke volume times heart rate yields CO. The use of biplane or multiplane probes appears to increase the accuracy of CO measurements.[51]

Transesophageal echocardiography may provide a more meaningful reference standard for myocardial ischemia than ECG. Within seconds of the onset of myocardial ischemia, abnormal inward motion and thickening of the affected myocardial segment occurs. Wall motion abnormalities precede changes in the ECG or PAC. Clinical studies suggest that many episodes of ischemia detected by TEE are missed by standard intraoperative ECG monitoring.[52,53] However, not all wall motion abnormalities are because of ischemia. Ventricular pacing, conduction abnormalities, translational motion of the heart, stunned myocardium, and changes in loading conditions can all mimic myocardial ischemia on TEE.

Transesophageal echocardiography is the only intraoperative monitor that provides information on the structure and function of the mitral, aortic, tricuspid, and pulmonic valves. The severity of stenotic or regurgitant valvular disease can be determined using Doppler studies. One of the most important indications for TEE in the operating room is in the assessment of patients requiring valvular surgery. The use of TEE before cardiopulmonary bypass provides new information or prompts changes in valve surgery in 9 to 13% of cases.[47] In patients undergoing mitral valve repair, postcardiopulmonary bypass TEE revealed persistent valvular dysfunction in 6 to 11% of patients, leading to second pump runs in 3 to 10% of cases.[47]

Transesophageal echocardiography may be used to determine the etiology of acute hypotension in the perioperative period. Left ventricular failure or dysfunction can be differentiated from other common causes of severe hypotension, such as hypovolemia or decreased systemic vascular resistance. Unusual causes of acute hypotension, including pericardial tamponade, pulmonary embolism, and aortic dissection, can be rapidly diagnosed with TEE. The early detection of the cause of hemodynamic instability allows for the appropriate therapy to be instituted (volume expansion, inotropes, vasopressors).

Transesophageal echocardiography is moderately invasive and is associated with major and minor complications. Major complications (esophageal trauma, dysrhythmias, hemodynamic instability) occur in 0.2 to 0.5% of examinations.[47] Minor complications (lip injuries, dental injuries, hoarseness, dysphagia) occur in 0.1 to 13% of cases and may be related to endotracheal intubation rather than TEE.[47] Complication rates may be reduced when examinations are performed by experienced practitioners. Most complication rates have been reported from studies in awake patients; some complications may be less frequent in anesthetized surgical patients.

MONITORING NEUROLOGIC FUNCTION

The best assessment of neurologic function is a thorough neurologic examination that evaluates the integration of brain and spinal cord function. However, anesthesia, sedation, and muscle relaxants, as well as existing neuropathology or trauma, may significantly impair the sensitivity or even the ability to perform a standard neurologic examination in the operating room. Therefore, monitoring neurologic function has become an important component of anesthesia care. Intraoperative neurologic monitoring often guides anesthesia and surgical decision making. Many intraoperative factors have the potential to influence spontaneous or evoked neural activity. General anesthesia can influence synaptic transmission and neural activity directly or by altering physiologic factors such as blood flow or blood pressure.

Intracranial Pressure Monitoring

Intracranial pressure (ICP) monitoring was initially used in trauma, where the relationship between uncontrolled ICP elevation and fatality has been firmly established.[54] ICP can be monitored by insertion of a subarachnoid bolt, a ventricular catheter, or an epidural transducer, or by insertion of a fiberoptic sensor in the cranial cavity. Each of these techniques requires a burr hole for intracranial access.

The cerebrospinal fluid (CSF) pressure wave is pulsatile and oscillates with the cardiac and respiratory cycle. Normal ICP is less than 15 mm Hg. Continuous recordings of the ICP in neurotrauma victims demonstrate three distinct pathologic waveforms. *A waves* (plateau waves) are found in patients with elevated baseline ICP and consist of a further elevation of ICP for periods from 5 to 20 minutes; A waves result from abrupt increases in regional cerebral blood volume where cerebral blood flow is decreased because of brain swelling, venous obstruction, or obstruction of CSF flow. *B* and *C waves* are of lesser magnitude and are related to respiratory pattern and blood pressure. Unlike A waves, they are not thought to be useful in guiding therapy or predicting outcome.

Intracranial pressure monitoring assumes that *cerebral perfusion pressure* (CPP = MAP − ICP) is uniformly distributed and that intracranial hypertension results in ischemia, displacement, compression, or herniation of the brain. ICP monitoring does not measure neural function or neural recovery.

Electroencephalogram

The electroencephalogram (EEG) represents the spontaneous electrical activity of the superficial cerebral cortex as recorded from either the scalp or surface electrodes. The EEG signal originates from postsynaptic excitatory and inhibitory potentials produced by the pyramidal cells located in the outer cerebral cortex. In the operating room, the EEG signal can often be recorded to assess cortical activity. Signal processing requires the amplification of small voltages (10 to 100 mV), which are 1,000 times smaller than ECG signals. Conventional EEG analysis uses scalp electrodes positioned at standardized points referenced to cranial dimensions. The voltage difference between a pair of EEG electrodes is amplified and compared with measurements using a reference electrode. This method, differential amplification, reduces artifacts. The resulting signal is then passed through electronic filters, which reduce or remove unwanted frequencies, and is then displayed as voltage over time. The EEG is usually characterized by activity in four frequency bands: *beta* (>112 Hz), *alpha* (8–12 Hz), *theta* (4–8 Hz), and *delta* (<4 Hz).

In unanesthetized patients, the EEG trace demonstrates background rhythms regulated by "pacemaker neurons" of the lower brain structures and the local electrical activity resulting from cortical neurons underlying the active electrode. During anesthesia, the background alpha rhythm predominates. With deeper anesthesia or during ischemia, EEG activity generally decreases in both amplitude and frequency. A total of 50% of the brain's oxygen consumption has been attributed to the energy requirement for the generation of EEG activity.

Electroencephalographic monitoring has been advocated for the intraoperative detection of cerebral ischemia during carotid endarterectomy, during deliberate hypotension, for the intraoperative or perioperative assessment of pharmacologic interventions, for identification of epileptic foci, or for the assessment of coma or brain death.[55]

Deep anesthesia, cerebral ischemia, or other pathologic states abolish or reduce normal neural EEG activity (alpha and beta rhythms), and slower frequencies (delta and theta) predominate. Sleep or surgical anesthesia typically increases amplitude (synchronization), whereas arousal characteristically decreases amplitude (desynchronization). High concentrations of isoflurane or desflurane can cause periods of electrical silence interspersed with brief episodes of activity. This pattern is termed *burst suppression.* Similar effects are seen by many intravenous sedative drugs such as barbiturates. Increasing depth of anesthesia often results in EEG slowing with increases in amplitude, leading to burst suppression. At the highest levels of anesthesia, the EEG can become *isoelectric*, mimicking the effect of hypothermia or brain hypoxia. EEG interpretation requires experienced observers and the ability to integrate the changes with anesthetic, physiologic, and surgical events.

Processing Electroencephalographic Data

Several signal-processing techniques have been used to improve the ability of clinicians to interpret changes in the EEG and evaluate trends. The EEG signal is usually digitized, processed, and then graphically displayed for interpretation. Real-time analysis using Fourier transformation to identify amplitudes and frequencies of interest or a periodic analysis are often performed to convert voltage/time data to power spectral information, where power versus frequency information is graphically displayed over epochs (e.g., the *compressed spectral array*).

The *spectral edge frequency* is often calculated and displayed to summarize the changes in the power spectrum. The spectral edge is the frequency that is just above 95% of the power contained in the raw EEG. Monitoring the spectral edge has been considered useful in detection of cerebral ischemia and anesthetic depth.[56] Other descriptors such as the peak power frequency or the median power frequency have been used to describe EEG data under anesthesia.[57]

The *bispectral index* (BIS) is a variable derived from the EEG that is a measure of the hypnotic effect of anesthetic agents. The BIS is the first processed EEG descriptor that purports to predict depth of consciousness. Previous EEG parameters, such as the spectral edge frequency, do not change in a linear manner with increasing depth of anesthesia. Furthermore, different anesthetic agents have differing effects on the processed EEG.

The calculation of the BIS integrates four different processed EEG descriptors into a single variable. These four parameters were selected on the basis of EEG data collected from thousands of anesthetics. The EEG data were correlated with the clinical state of the patient (level of consciousness, response to surgical incision). Each parameter has a particular stage of anesthesia where it performs most accurately. The Beta-Ratio parameter reflects light sedation, the SynchFastSlow detects surgical levels of anesthesia, and the burst suppression ratio (BSR) and QUAZI predominate during deep levels of anesthesia.[58] The parameters are then ranked and combined to yield a single number, the BIS. The range of valves for the BIS is from 0 to 100, with decreasing numbers indicating deeper levels of sedation or anesthesia. BIS valves of less than 60 appear to predict absence of consciousness.

Clinical studies have demonstrated that the BIS can reliably predict the level of sedation, loss of consciousness, and the probability of recall using a variety of anesthetic agents.[59–62] The BIS does not appear to be as reliable in predicting movement in response to a noxious stimulation. Motor responses to painful stimuli may be mediated by subcortical structures, which are not measured by the BIS monitor. The use of the BIS can facilitate faster emergence and improved recovery from general anesthesia by allowing more precise titration of anesthetic effect.[63]

Other monitoring systems have been developed for clinical use that process EEG data in order to quantify depth of anesthesia. The *Patient State Index* (PSI) monitor records the EEG from anterior and posterior scalp sites. The EEG is analyzed using a multivariate algorithm that quantifies the most probable level of sedation or anesthesia. PSI values range from 0 to 100, with lower numbers indicating deeper states of hypnosis. These PSI values correlate well with level of consciousness and anesthesia, and use of PSI monitoring may allow for faster emergence and recovery from anesthesia.[64] The *Narcotrend* monitor classifies the EEG into 14 distinct stages from stage A (awake) to stage F1 (isoelectric EEG). Decreasing Narcotrend stages during anesthesia have been associated with decreasing BIS values.[65] Clinical studies suggest that the Narcotrend monitor is able to distinguish all states of anesthesia accurately.[66]

Evoked Potential Monitoring

Stimulation of neural structures to evoke responses is useful for monitoring the functional integrity of brainstem, visual, auditory, or peripheral neural pathways. Evoked potentials (EPs) represent small electrical signals generated in neural pathways after periodic stimulation. In the cortex and subcortex, EPs are smaller than the background EEG, and it is necessary to remove the random background electrical activity to record EP data. Computer signal averaging and filtering permits display of the EP voltages over time. EPs are usually quantitated by the time from stimulation (*latency*) and the *amplitude* of the peaks generated by the neural structures of interest. Three sensory pathways are available for intraoperative monitoring.[67]

Brainstem auditory evoked responses (BAERs) are monitored by stimulation of the cochlea using pulsed sound waves in the ear. Three to five waves are usually recorded using electrodes placed near the ear and cortex. BAERs are useful in assessing brainstem function in comatose patients and during surgical procedures of the cerebellopontine angle, floor of the fourth ventricle, or procedures in proximity to the fifth, seventh, or eighth cranial nerves.[68] Unlike other EPs, the BAERs are relatively resistant to the effects of anesthesia. A commercially available auditory evoked potential monitor has been developed that allows clinicians to accurately determine the depth of anesthesia in the perioperative setting.[69]

Visual evoked potentials (VEPs) are produced by flashing light to stimulate the retina and recording the EPs over the occipital cortex. VEPs assess the integrity of the visual pathway and have been used during resection of pituitary tumors, craniopharyngiomas, or surgery in the vicinity of the optic tracts. Unlike BAERs, VEPs are technically difficult to obtain during anesthesia, and questions have arisen about their usefulness in surgery.

Somatosensory evoked potentials (SSEPs) are produced by stimulating peripheral nerves and recording responses from electrodes monitoring the transmission of the EPs through the sensory pathway. The nerves usually stimulated are the median, ulnar, peroneal, or posterior tibial. Surface electrodes are placed to record the signal from peripheral nerves, plexuses, nerve roots, the dorsal columns, the brainstem lemniscal pathways to the thalamus, and the sensory cortex.

Median nerve SSEPs have been used to monitor cerebral function in patients undergoing neurosurgical procedures or those with cerebral ischemia. In these patients, examination of the timing and amplitude of the response measured over the contralateral scalp at 20 milliseconds (N20) represents the cortical response to stimulation. Similarly, examination of the negative waves occurring 11 to 14 milliseconds interrogates spinal roots, spinal cord, and brainstem.

Monitoring the responses of upper or lower extremity nerves may assist in evaluating spinal cord function during instrumentation of the spine or during thoracoabdominal surgery, where spinal cord ischemia is a possible risk factor. Deterioration of spinal cord function decreases the amplitude and increases the latency of the SSEP waveform. Monitoring of SSEPs is thought to be a sensitive indicator of the spinal cord's functional integrity. Despite the fact that SSEP monitoring does not evaluate the function of the motor pathway, it appears to be useful during spinal surgery, notably for correction of scoliosis.[70] Intraoperative SSEPs should be regarded as an extension of the sensory neurologic examination during anesthesia care, but may not totally replace the "wake-up" test. During anesthesia, monitoring both the area of risk and the contralateral pathways helps identify changes resulting from surgery as opposed to those as a result of other global variables, such as the effect of anesthesia.

Motor evoked potentials (MEPs) provide a means of assessing descending motor pathways during neurosurgical, orthopaedic, or vascular procedures. MEPs can be obtained by transcranial electrical stimulation, transcranial magnetic stimulation, or direct spinal cord stimulation.[71] Attenuation of transcranially elicited MEPs by commonly used anesthetic techniques has limited their usefulness during surgery. Further investigation with MEPs is needed to define fully their use during surgery.[72]

Facial nerve stimulation is commonly performed during procedures in the posterior fossa. Intentional stimulation or surgical irritation of the facial nerve can be evaluated visually or by evaluating the electromyogram. Although facial nerve function is rather insensitive to anesthetic influences, muscle relaxants need to be limited to provide adequate monitoring conditions.

TEMPERATURE MONITORING

The ability to monitor body temperature is a standard of anesthesia care. The continual observation of temperature changes in anesthetized patients allows for the detection of accidental heat loss or malignant hyperthermia. Humans maintain their core temperature by balancing heat production from metabolism and the many environmental factors that supply heat or cool the body. Regional temperature information from skin, muscle, the body cavities, spinal cord, and brain are integrated in the central nervous system. Conceptually, thermoregulation involves the integration of "set points," which, when exceeded, trigger temperature-dissipating, temperature-conserving, or heat-producing mechanisms. Both general and regional anesthesia inhibit afferent and efferent control of thermoregulation.[73,74] In addition, the operating room environment and surgical exposure often contribute to excessive heat losses. Heat loss is common during surgery because the surgical environment transfers heat from the patient and anesthesia reduces heat production and diminishes the capability of patients to monitor and maintain thermoregulation.

Heat is produced as a consequence of cellular metabolism. In adults, thermoregulation involves the control of basal metabolic rate, muscular activity, sympathetic arousal, vascular tone, and hormone activation balanced against exogenous factors that determine the need for the body to create heat or to adjust the transfer of heat to the environment.

Heat losses may result from radiation, conduction, convection, and evaporation. Radiation refers to the infrared rays emanating from all objects above absolute temperature. Conduction refers to the transfer of heat from contact with objects. Convection refers to the transfer of heat from air passing by objects. Evaporation represents the heat loss resulting when water vaporizes. For every gram of water evaporated, 0.58 kcal of heat is lost.

Perioperative hypothermia predisposes patients to increases in metabolic rate (shivering) and cardiac work, decreases in drug metabolism and cutaneous blood flow, and impairments of coagulation. Clinical studies have demonstrated that patients in whom intraoperative hypothermia develops are at a higher risk for development of postoperative myocardial ischemia and wound infection compared with patients who are normothermic in the perioperative period.[75,76] Anesthesiologists frequently monitor temperature and attempt to maintain central core temperature at near-normal values in all patients undergoing anesthesia.

Central core temperatures can be estimated using probes that can be placed into the bladder, distal esophagus, ear canal, trachea, nasopharynx, or rectum.[77] Pulmonary artery blood temperature is also a good estimate of central core temperature.

Temperature is usually measured using electrical probes containing calibrated thermistors or thermocouples that serve as temperature transducers. Thermistors respond to temperature changes by changing their electrical resistance. Thermocouples are constructed by passing current through a circuit where the electrodes are made of two dissimilar metals. The current measured is directly proportional to the temperature difference between the two metal junctions. Thermocouple temperature probes maintain one junction at a known temperature and place the second junction on the temperature probe tip. Skin temperature can also be monitored using liquid crystal thermometry. Although convenient, temperature strips do not correlate with core temperature measurements.[78]

Thermoregulatory responses are based on a physiologically weighted average reflecting changes in the mean body temperature. Mean body temperature is estimated by the following equation:

$$\text{Mean temperature} = 0.85\ \text{T core} + 0.15\ \text{T skin}$$

Skin temperature monitoring has been advocated to identify peripheral vasoconstriction but is not adequate to determine alterations in mean body temperature that may occur during surgery. Core temperature sites have been established as reliable indicators of changes in mean temperature. During routine noncardiac surgery, temperature differences between these sites are small. When anesthetized patients are being cooled, changes in rectal temperature often lag behind those of other probe locations, and the adequacy of rewarming is best judged by measuring temperature at several locations.

FUTURE TRENDS IN MONITORING

Diagnostic and therapeutic advances in medicine have had a great impact on the strategies and techniques available for intraoperative monitoring. Today's anesthesia practice has narrowed the distinction between laboratory medicine and patient monitoring. Technologic advances in instrument design, computerization, and engineering have made it possible to have ready access to serum chemistries, hematologic profiles, assessment of coagulation, and arterial blood gas measurements. Modern monitoring systems have the potential to transfer processed and raw data from the operating room to information management systems, which offer the potential for creating meaningful paperless anesthesia records and enhanced archiving of the conduct of anesthesia care as depicted by real-time monitoring trends.

The U.S. Department of Health and Human Services proposed implementation of patient record systems in 1996.[79] Proprietary systems for automated anesthesia records are now in the marketplace. These offer file sharing so that information that is traditionally viewed as patient monitoring can also be used for billing, ordering supplies, and quality improvement. Although computerization of the hospital environment has direct and indirect costs, the benefits to physicians, patients, insurers, and hospital administrators indicate that, like in other business environments, information management is coming to operating room monitoring and anesthesiology.[80,81] The clinical and administrative data that can be obtained from anesthesia work stations integrated with hospital information systems should enhance the quality of care and improve the intraoperative monitoring of anesthetized patients.

References

1. Roizen MF, Schreider B, Austin W *et al*: Pulse oximetry, capnography, and blood gas measurements: Reducing cost and improving the quality of care with technology. J Clin Monit 9:237, 1993
2. American Society of Anesthesiologists: Standards for Basic Anesthetic Monitoring. Park Ridge, Illinois, 2003. http://www.asahq.org/publicationsAndServices/standards/02.pdf#2 (last viewed 24 August 2004)
3. Association for the Advancement of Medical Instrumentation: Human Factors, Engineering Guidelines and Preferred Practices for the Design of Medical Devices. Arlington, Virginia, Association for the Advancement of Medical Instrumentation, 1988 http://www.aami.org/ (last viewed 24 August 2004)
4. Loeb RG: A measure of intraoperative attention to monitor displays. Anesth Analg 76:337, 1993
5. Barker L, Webb RK, Runiciman EB *et al*: The Australian Incident Monitoring Study. The oxygen analyzer: Applications and limitations—an analysis of 200 incident reports. Anaesth Intensive Care 21:570, 1993
6. Mayer RM: Oxygen analyzers: Failure rates and life-spans of galvanic cells. Journal of Clinical Monitoring 6:196, 1990
7. Williamson JA, Webb RK, Cockings J *et al*: The Australian Incident Monitoring Study: The capnograph applications and limitations—an analysis of 2000 incident reports. Anaesth Intensive Care 21:551, 1993
8. Walder B, Lauber R, Zbinden AM: Accuracy and cross-sensitivity of 10 different anesthetic gas monitors. J Clin Monit 9:364, 1993
9. Barker SH, Shah WK: The effects of motion on the performance of pulse oximeters in volunteers. Anesthesiology 86:101, 1997

10. Moller JT, Pederson T, Rasmussen LS *et al*: Randomized evaluation of pulse oximetry in 20,802 patients: II. Perioperative events and postoperative complications. Anesthesiology 78:445, 1993
11. Langewouters GJ, Settels JJ, Roelandt R *et al*: Why use Finapres or Pertapres rather than intra-arterial or intermittent non-invasive techniques of blood pressure measurement? J Med Eng Technol 22:37, 1998
12. Vogel AJ, Van Montfrans GA: Reproducibility of twenty-four hour finger arterial blood pressure, variability and systemic hemodynamics. J Hypertens 15:1761, 1997
13. Hirschl MM, Binder M, Harken H *et al*: Accuracy and reliability of noninvasive continuous finger blood pressure measurement in critically ill patients. Crit Care Med 24:1684, 1996
14. Gardner RM: Direct blood pressure measurement: Dynamic response requirements. Anesthesiology 54:227, 1981
15. Kleinman B, Powell S, Kumar P, Gardner RM: The fast flush test measures the dynamic response for the entire pressure monitoring system. Anesthesiology 77:1215, 1992
16. Slogoff S, Keats AS, Arlund C: On the safety of radial artery cannulation. Anesthesiology 59:42, 1983
17. McGregor AD: The Allen test: An investigation of its accuracy by fluorescein angiography dye. J Hand Surg Br 12:82, 1987
18. Vender JS, Watts RD: Differential diagnosis of hand ischemia in the presence of an arterial cannula. Anesth Analg 61:465, 1982
19. Sanford TJ: Internal jugular vein cannulation versus subclavian vein cannulation. An anesthesiologist's view: The right internal jugular vein. J Clin Monit 1:58, 1985
20. Mark JB: Central venous pressure monitoring: Clinical insights beyond the numbers. J Cardiothorac Anesth 5:163, 1991
21. Vender JS: Pulmonary artery catheter monitoring. Anesthesiol Clin North America 6:743, 1988
22. Tuman KJ, Carroll GC, Ivankovich AD: Pitfalls of interpretation of pulmonary artery catheter data. J Cardiothorac Anesth 3:625, 1989
23. Practice guidelines for pulmonary artery catheterization: An updated report by the American Society of Anesthesiologists Task Force on pulmonary artery catheterization. Anesthesiology 99(4):988, 2003
24. Guidelines for the prevention of intravascular catheter-related infections. Centers for Disease Control and Prevention. Recommendations and Reports. August 9, 2002/51(RR 10); 1–26
25. West JB, Dollery CT, Naimark A: Distribution of blood flow in isolated lung: Relation to vascular and alveolar pressures. J Appl Physiol 19:713, 1984
26. Gettinger A, Glass D: In vivo comparison of two mixed venous saturation catheters. Anesthesiology 66:373, 1987
27. Scuderi PE, MacGregor DA, Bowton DL *et al*: A laboratory comparison of three pulmonary artery oximetry catheters. Anesthesiology 81:245, 1994
28. Fegler G: Measurement of cardiac output in anesthetized animals by thermodilution method. Q J Exp Physiol 39:153, 1954
29. Pearl RGB, Rosenthal MH, Mielson L *et al*: Effect of injectate volume and temperature on thermodilution cardiac output determination. Anesthesiology 64:798, 1986
30. Yelderman ML, Ramsey MA, Quinn MD *et al*: Continuous thermodilution cardiac output measurement in intensive care unit patients. J Cardiothorac Vasc Anesth 6:270, 1992
31. Mihm FG, Gettinger A, Hanson CW *et al*: A multicenter evaluation of a new continuous cardiac output pulmonary artery catheter system. Crit Care Med 26:1346, 1998
32. Hines R, Barash PG: Intraoperative right ventricular dysfunction detected with a right ventricular ejection fraction catheter. J Clin Monit 2:206, 1986
33. Mukherjee R, Spinale FG, VonRecum AF *et al*: In vitro validation of right ventricular thermodilution ejection fraction system. Ann Biomed Eng 19:165, 1991
34. Dennis JW, Menawat S, Sobowale O *et al*: Superiority of end-diastolic volume and ejection fraction measurements over wedge pressure in evaluating cardiac function during aortic reconstruction. J Vasc Surg 16:372, 1992
35. Sandham JD, Hull RD, Brant RF *et al*: A randomized, controlled trial of the use of pulmonary artery catheters in high-risk surgical patients. N Engl J Med 348(1):5, 2003
36. Iberti TJ, Fischer EP, Leibowitz AB *et al*: A multicenter study of physician's knowledge of pulmonary artery catheter. JAMA 264:2928, 1990
37. Gnaegi A, Feihl F, Perret C: Intensive care physicians insufficient knowledge of right-heart catheterization at the bedside: Time to act? Crit Care Med 25:213, 1997
38. Papadakos PJ, Vender JS: Training requirement for pulmonary artery catheter utilization in adult patients. New Horiz 5:287, 1997
39. Ginosar Y, Thijs LG, Sprung CL: Raising the standard of hemodynamic monitoring: Targeting the practice or practitioner? Crit Care Med 25:209, 1997
40. Young JD, McQuillan P: Comparison of thoracic electrical bioimpedance and thermodilution for the measurement of cardiac index in patients with severe sepsis. Br J Anaesth 70:58, 1993
41. Raaijmakers E, Faes TJ, Scholten RJ *et al*: A meta-analysis of three decades of validating thoracic impedance cardiography. Crit Care Med 27:1203, 1999
42. Perrino AC, Fleming J, LaMantia KR: Transesophageal Doppler cardiac output monitoring: Performance during aortic reconstructive surgery. Anesth Analg 73:705, 1991
43. Perrino AC, O'Connor T, Luther M: Transtracheal Doppler cardiac output monitoring: Comparison to thermodilution during noncardiac surgery. Anesth Analg 78:1060, 1994
44. Sinclair S, James S, Singer M: Intraoperative intravascular volume optimization and length of hospital stay after repair of proximal femoral fracture: Randomized controlled trial. BMJ 315:909, 1997
45. Della Rocca G, Costa MG, Coccia C *et al*: Cardiac output monitoring: aortic transpulmonary thermodilution and pulse contour analysis agree with standard thermodilution methods in patients undergoing lung transplantation. Can J Anaesth 50(7):707, 2003
46. Buhre W, Weyland A, Kazmaier S *et al*: Comparison of cardiac output assessed by pulse-contour analysis and thermodilution in patients undergoing minimally invasive direct coronary artery bypass grafting. J Cardiothorac Vasc Anesth 13(4):437, 1999
47. American Society of Anesthesiologists and Society of Cardiovascular Anesthesiologists Task Force on Transesophageal Echocardiography: Practice guidelines for perioperative transesophageal echocardiography. Anesthesiology 84:96, 1996
48. Harpole DH, Clements FM, Quill T *et al*: Right and left ventricular performance during and after abdominal aortic aneurysm repair. Ann Surg 209:356, 1989
49. Cheung AT, Savino JS, Weiss SJ *et al*: Echocardiographic and hemodynamic indexes of left ventricular preload in patients with normal and abnormal ventricular function. Anesthesiology 81:376, 1994
50. Kuecherer HF, Muhiuden IA, Kusumoto FM: Estimation of mean left atrial pressure from transesophageal pulsed Doppler echocardiography of pulmonary venous flow. Circulation 81:1488, 1990
51. Hozumi T, Shakudo M, Applegate R *et al*: Accuracy of cardiac output estimation with biplane transesophageal echocardiography. J Am Soc Echocardiogr 6:62, 1993
52. Hauser AM, Gangadharen F, Ramos RG *et al*: Sequence of mechanical, electrocardiographic, and clinical effects of repeated coronary artery occlusion in human beings: Echocardiographic observations during coronary angioplasty. J Am Coll Cardiol 5:193, 1980
53. Smith JS, Cahalan MK, Benefiel DJ *et al*: Intraoperative detection of myocardial ischemia in high-risk patients: Electrocardiography versus two-dimensional transesophageal echocardiography. Circulation 72:1015, 1985
54. Saul TG, Druker TB: Effect of intracranial pressure monitoring and aggressive treatment on mortality in severe head injury. J Neurosurg 56:498, 1982
55. Nuwer MR: Intraoperative electroencephalography. J Clin Neurophysiol 10:437, 1993
56. Rampil I, Correll JW, Rosenbaum SH *et al*: Computerized electroencephalogram monitoring and carotid artery shunting. Neurosurgery 13:276, 1983
57. Sidi A, Halimi P, Cotev S: Estimating anesthetic depth by electroencephalography during anesthetic induction and intubation in patients undergoing cardiac surgery. J Clin Anesth 2:101, 1990
58. Rampil IJ: A primer for EEG signal processing in anesthesia. Anesthesiology 89:980, 1998
59. Lui J, Singh H, White PF: Electroencephalographic bispectral index correlates with intraoperative recall and depth of propofol-induced sedation. Anesth Analg 84:185, 1997
60. Myles PS, Lesli K, McNeil J *et al*: Bispectral index monitoring to prevent awareness during anaesthesia: The B-Aware randomised controlled trial. Lancet 363:1757, 2004
61. Sebel PS, Lang E, Rampil IJ *et al*: A multicenter study of bispectral electroencephalogram analysis for monitoring anesthetic effect. Anesth Analg 84:891, 1997
62. Kearse LA, Rosow C, Zaslavski A *et al*: Bispectral analysis of the electroencephalogram predicts conscious processing of information during propofol sedation and hypnosis. Anesthesiology 88:25, 1998
63. Song D, Joshi GP, White PF: Titration of volatile anesthetics using bispectral index facilitates recovery after ambulatory anesthesia. Anesthesiology 87:847, 1997
64. Drover DR, Lemmens HJ, Pierce ET *et al*: Patient state index: Titration of delivery and recovery from propofol, alfentanil, and nitrous oxide anesthesia. Anesthesiology 97(1):82, 2002
65. Kreuer S, Biedler A, Larsen R *et al*: The Narcotrend: A new EEG monitor designed to measure the depth of anesthesia-a comparison with Bispectral Index monitoring during propofol-remifentanil anesthesia. Anaesthesist 50:921, 2001
66. Schmidt GN, Bischoff P, Standl T *et al*: Comparative evaluation of Narcotrend, Bispectral Index, and classical electroencephalographic variables during induction, maintenance, and emergence of a propofol/remifentanil anesthesia. Anesth Analg 98:1346, 2004
67. American Electroencephalographic Society: Guidelines on evoked potentials. J Clin Neurophysiol 11:40, 1994
68. Nagao S, Roccaforte P, Moody RA: Acute intracranial hypertension and auditory brain-stem responses: II. The effect of posterior fossa mass lesions on brain-stem function. J Neurosurg 52:351, 1980
69. Nishiyama T, Matsukawa T, Hanaoka K: A comparison of the clinical usefulness of three different electroencephalogram monitors: Bispectral Index, processed electroencephalogram, and Alaris Auditory Evoked Potentials. Anesth Analg 98:1341, 2004

70. Forbes HJ, Allen PW, Waller CS *et al*: Spinal cord monitoring in scoliosis surgery: Experience with 1168 cases. J Bone Joint Surg Br 73:487, 1991
71. Adams DC, Emerson RG, Heyer EJ *et al*: Monitoring of intraoperative motor-evoked potentials under conditions of controlled neuromuscular blockade. Anesth Analg 77:913, 1993
72. Zentner J, Albrech T, Heuser D: Influence of halothane, enflurane, and isoflurane on motor evoked potentials. Neurosurgery 31:298, 1992
73. Sessler DI: Central thermoregulatory inhibition by general anesthesia. Anesthesiology 75:557, 1991
74. Ozaki M, Kurz A, Sessler DI *et al*: Thermoregulatory thresholds during epidural and spinal anesthesia. Anesthesiology 81:282, 1994
75. Kurz A, Sessler DJ, Lenhardt R: Perioperative normothermia to reduce the incidence of surgical wound infection and shorten hospitalization. N Engl J Med 334:1209, 1996
76. Frank SM, Fleisher LA, Breslow MJ *et al*: Perioperative maintenance of normothermic reduces the incidence of morbid cardiac events: A randomized clinical trial. JAMA 277:1127, 1997
77. Yamakage M, Kawanna S, Watanabe H *et al*: The utility of tracheal temperature monitoring. Anesth Analg 76:795, 1993
78. Vaughan MS, Cork RD, Vaughan RW: Inaccuracy of liquid crystal thermometry to identify core temperature trends in postoperative adults. Anesth Analg 61:284, 1982
79. U.S. Department of Health and Human Services: Initiatives Toward the Electronic Health Care System of the Future. Washington, DC, U.S. Department of Health and Human Services, 1992
80. Smith NT: The M-15: A truly different workstation. J Clin Monit 10:352, 1994
81. Gibby GL: Anesthesia information-management systems: Their role in risk-versus cost assessment and outcomes research. J Cardiothorac Vasc Anesth 11(2 suppl 1):2, 1997

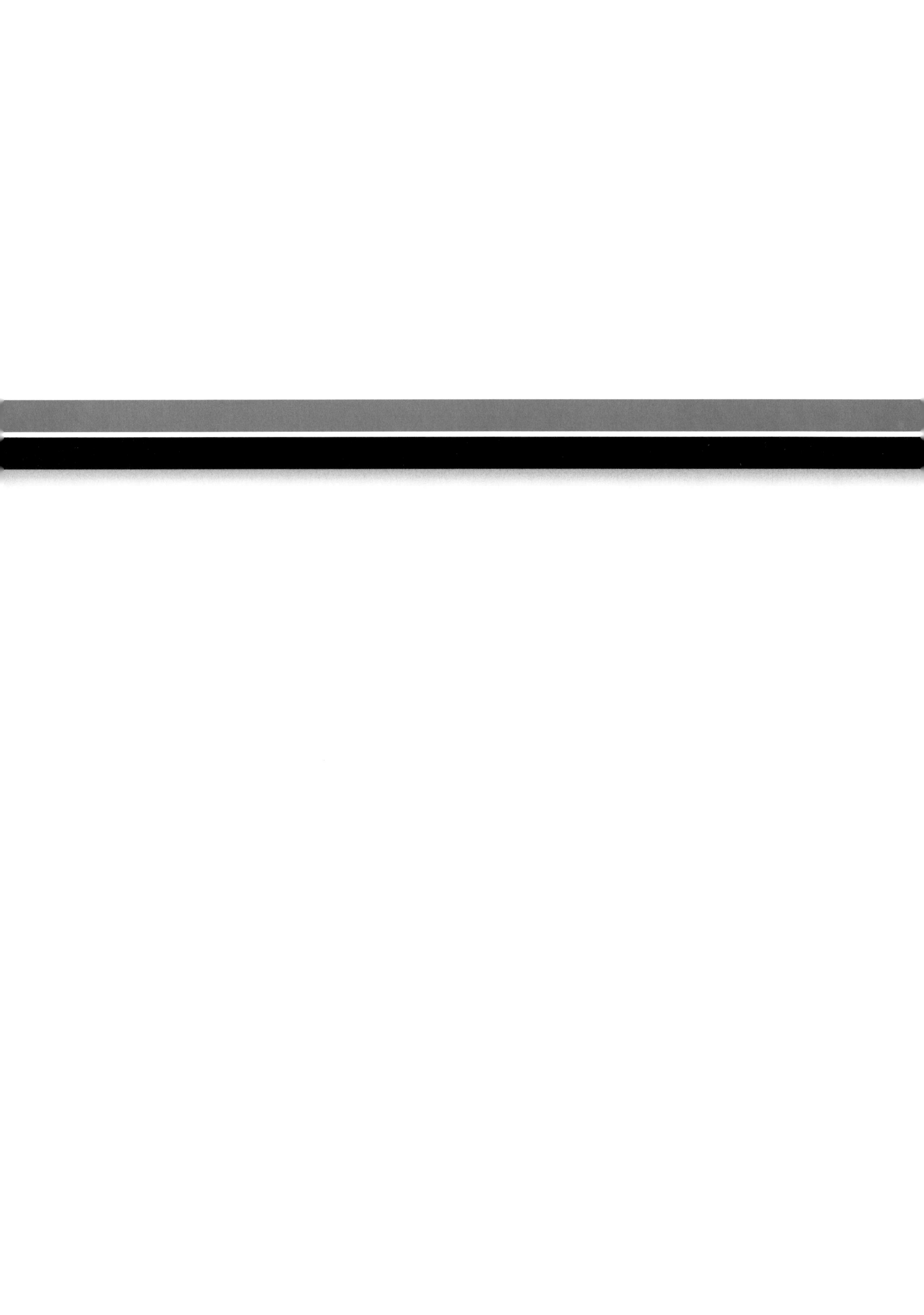

SECTION V MANAGEMENT OF ANESTHESIA

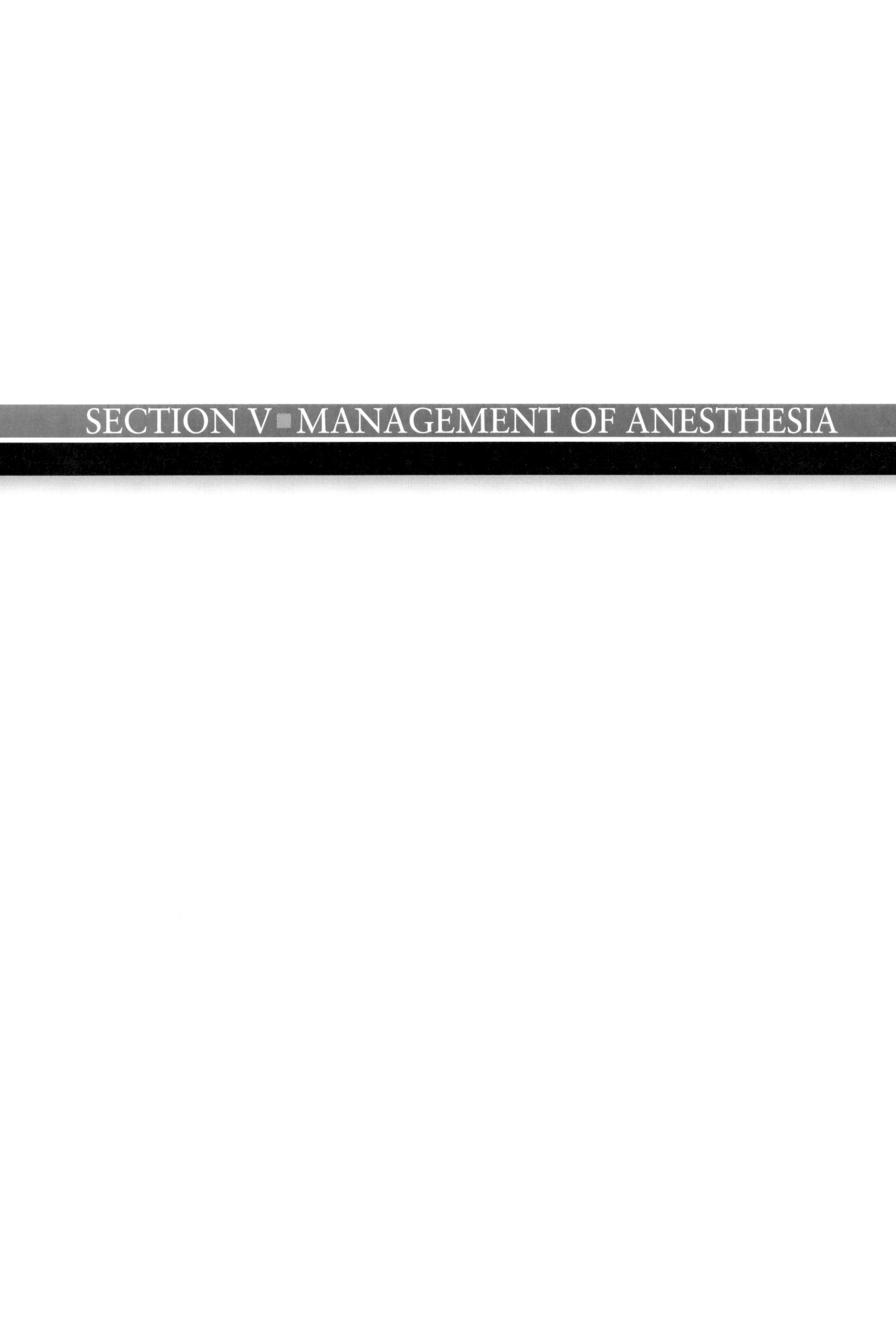

CHAPTER 25 ■ EPIDURAL AND SPINAL ANESTHESIA

CHRISTOPHER M. BERNARDS

KEY POINTS

1. The epidural fat and the epidural venous plexus do not form a continuous "sheet" surrounding the spinal cord as is often depicted. Rather, the epidural fat lies in discrete pockets in the posterior and lateral epidural space and the epidural veins travel primarily in the anterior and lateral epidural space and are normally absent in the posterior epidural space.
2. Clinicians must develop a three-dimensional mental picture of the spinal anatomy so that when they contact boney structures during attempted epidural or spinal needle placement they can redirect the needle in a reasoned and systematic manner and not subject the patient to random needle "pokes" in an effort to place the block.
3. Serious systemic toxicity during attempted epidural block is almost always the result of inadvertent local anesthetic injection directly into the vasculature. Consequently, an appropriate test dose designed to identify intravascular injection is critical.
4. Physical characteristics (e.g., height, weight, cerebrospinal fluid [CSF] volume) and age do have an effect on spinal and epidural block characteristics. However, the magnitude of the effects are relatively small and of such low predictive power that these characteristics are not useful predictors of local anesthetic dose in any individual patient.
5. The risk of hemodynamic complications of epidural and spinal anesthesia increases with increasing block height.
6. Lidocaine appears to be worse than other local anesthetics in terms of the risk of neurological toxicity (i.e., cauda equina syndrome and transient radicular irritation).
7. Recent human studies suggest that the new preservative free formulation of chloroprocaine is safe for spinal anesthesia. This drug may offer a viable alternative to lidocaine for short duration spinal anesthesia.
8. Administration of drugs that impair coagulation can put patients at increased risk of spinal hematoma. Our understanding of the relative risk of different classes of drugs affecting the clotting system is constantly evolving. Clinicians are directed to the consensus statement from the American Society for Regional Anesthesia and Pain Medicine for the most recent recommendations (*www.asra.com/items of interest/consensus statements/*)

There are no absolute indications for spinal or epidural anesthesia. However, there are clinical situations in which patient preference, patient physiology, or the surgical procedure makes central neuraxial block the technique of choice. There is also growing evidence that these techniques may improve outcome in selected situations. Spinal and epidural anesthesia have been shown to blunt the "stress response" to surgery,[1] to decrease intraoperative blood loss,[2,3] to lower the incidence of postoperative thromboembolic events,[2–5] and to decrease morbidity and mortality in high-risk surgical patients.[6,7] In addition, both spinal and epidural techniques can be used to extend analgesia into the postoperative period, where their use has been shown to provide better analgesia than can be achieved with parenteral opioids.[8] In addition, central neuraxial analgesia has become an indispensable technique to provide analgesia to nonsurgical patients. Thus, these techniques are an indispensable part of modern anesthetic practice, and every anesthesiologist should be adept at performing them.

ANATOMY

Proficiency in spinal and epidural anesthesia requires a thorough understanding of the anatomy of the spine and spinal cord. The anesthesiologist must be familiar with the surface anatomy of the spine but must also develop a mental picture of the three-dimensional anatomy of deeper structures. In addition, one must appreciate the relationship between the cutaneous dermatomes, the spinal nerves, the vertebrae, and the spinal segment from which each spinal nerve arises.

Vertebrae

The *spine* consists of 33 *vertebrae* (7 cervical, 12 thoracic, 5 lumbar, 5 fused sacral, and 4 fused coccygeal) (Fig. 25-1). With the exception of C1, the cervical, thoracic, and lumbar vertebrae consist of a *body* anteriorly, two *pedicles* that project posteriorly from the body, and two *laminae* that connect the pedicles (Fig. 25-2). These structures form the *vertebral canal*, which contains the spinal cord, spinal nerves, and epidural space. The laminae give rise to the *transverse processes* that project laterally and the *spinous process* that projects posteriorly. These bony projections serve as sites for muscle and ligament attachments. The pedicles contain a superior and inferior *vertebral notch* through which the spinal nerves exit the vertebral canal. The superior and inferior *articular processes* arise at the junction of the lamina and pedicles and form joints with the adjoining vertebrae. The first cervical vertebra differs from this typical structure in that it does not have a body or a spinous process.

The five sacral vertebrae are fused together to form the wedge-shaped *sacrum*, which connects the spine with the iliac wings of the pelvis (see Fig. 25-1). The 5th sacral vertebra is not fused posteriorly, giving rise to a variably shaped opening known as the *sacral hiatus*. Occasionally other sacral vertebrae do not fuse posteriorly, giving rise to a much larger sacral hiatus. The *sacral cornu* are bony prominences on either side of the hiatus and aid in identifying it. The sacral hiatus provides an opening into the sacral canal, which is the caudal termination of the epidural space. The four rudimentary coccygeal vertebrae are fused together to form the *coccyx*, a narrow triangular bone that abuts the sacral hiatus and can be helpful in identifying it. The tip of the coccyx can often be palpated in the proximal gluteal cleft and by running one's finger cephalad along its smooth surface, the sacral cornu can be identified as the first bony prominence encountered.

Identifying individual vertebrae is important for correctly locating the desired interspace for epidural and spinal blockade. The spine of C7 is the first prominent spinous process encountered while running the hand down the back of the neck. The spine of T1 is the most prominent spinous process and immediately follows C7. The 12th thoracic vertebra can be identified by palpating the 12th rib and tracing it back to its attachment to T12. A line drawn between the iliac crests crosses the body of L5 or the 4-5 interspace.

Ligaments

The vertebral bodies are stabilized by five ligaments that increase in size between the cervical and lumbar vertebrae (see Fig. 25-2). From the sacrum to T7, the *supraspinous ligament* runs between the tips of the spinous processes. Above T7 this ligament continues as the *ligamentum nuchae* and attaches to the occipital protuberance at the base of the skull. The *interspinous ligament* attaches between the spinous processes and blends posteriorly with the supraspinous ligament and anteriorly with the ligamentum flavum. The *ligamentum flavum* is a tough, wedge-shaped ligament composed of elastin. It consists of right and left portions that span adjacent vertebral laminae and fuse in the midline to varying degrees.[7,8] The ligamentum flavum is thickest in the midline, measuring 3 to 5 mm at the L2–3 interspace of adults. This ligament is also farthest from the spinal meninges in the midline, measuring 4 to 6 mm at the L2–3 interspace.[9] As a result, midline insertion of an epidural needle is least likely to result in unintended meningeal puncture. The anterior and posterior *longitudinal ligaments* run along the anterior and posterior surfaces of the vertebral bodies.

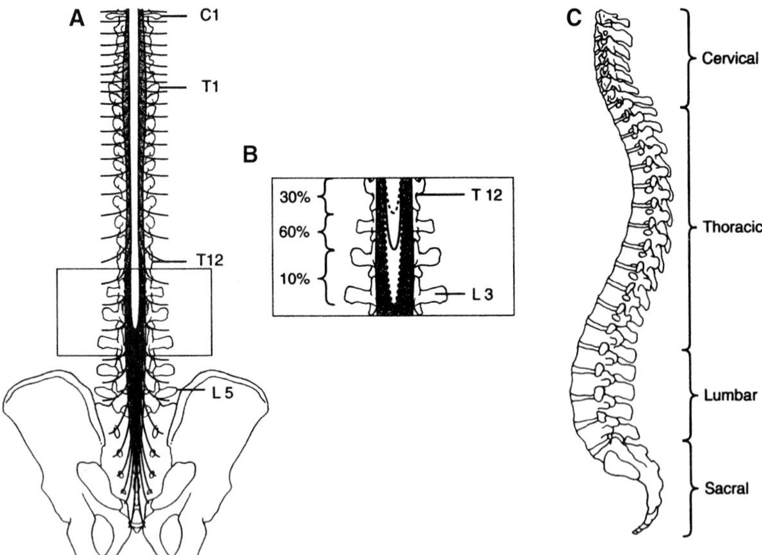

FIGURE 25-1. Posterior (**A**) and lateral (**C**) views of the human spinal column. Note the inset (**B**), which depicts the variability in vertebral level at which the spinal cord terminates.

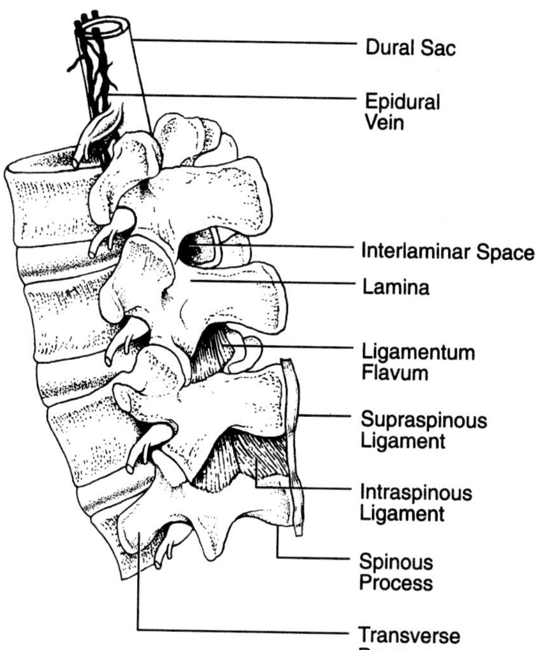

FIGURE 25-2. Detail of the lumbar spinal column and epidural space. Note that the epidural veins are largely restricted to the anterior and lateral epidural space.

Epidural Space

The epidural space is the space that lies between the spinal meninges and the sides of the vertebral canal (Fig. 25-3). It is bounded cranially by the foramen magnum, caudally by the sacrococcygeal ligament covering the sacral hiatus, anteriorly by the posterior longitudinal ligament, laterally by the vertebral pedicles, and posteriorly by both the ligamentum flavum and vertebral lamina. The epidural space is not a closed space but communicates with the paravertebral space by way of the intervertebral foramina.[10] The epidural space is shallowest anteriorly where the dura may in some places fuse with the posterior longitudinal ligament. The space is deepest posteriorly,

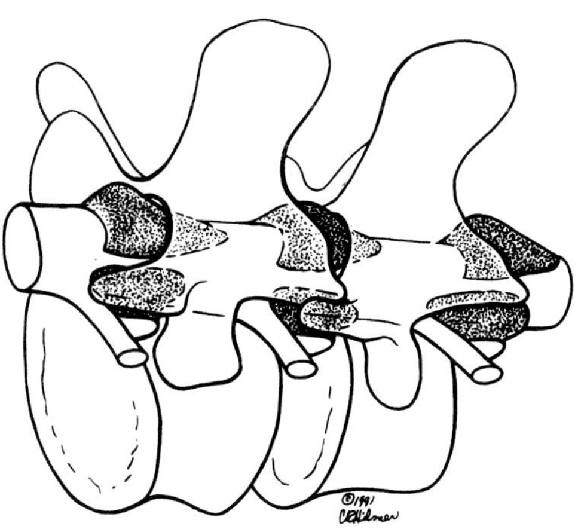

FIGURE 25-3. The compartments of the epidural space (*stippled areas*) are discontinuous. Areas where no compartments are indicated represent a potential space where the dura mater normally abuts the sides of the vertebral canal. (Reprinted with permission from Hogan Q: Lumbar epidural anatomy: A new look by cryomicrotome section. Anesthesiology 75:767, 1991.)

although the depth varies because the space is intermittently obliterated by contact between the dura mater and the ligamentum flavum or vertebral lamina. Contact between the dura mater and the pedicles also interrupts the epidural space laterally. Thus, the epidural space is composed of a series of discontinuous compartments that become continuous when the
1 potential space separating the compartments is opened up by injection of air or liquid. A rich network of valveless veins (Batson's plexus) courses through the anterior and lateral portions of the epidural space with few if any veins present in the posterior epidural space (see Fig. 25-2).[11] The epidural veins anastomose freely with extradural veins, including the pelvic veins, the azygous system, and the intracranial veins. The epidural space also contains lymphatics and segmental arteries running between the aorta and the spinal cord.

Epidural Fat

The most ubiquitous material in the epidural space is fat, which is principally located in the posterior and lateral epidural space (see Fig. 25-3).[10] Interestingly, the epidural fat appears to have clinically important effects on the pharmacology of epidurally and intrathecally administered drugs. For example, using a pig model, Bernards et al showed that there is a linear relationship between an opioid's lipid solubility and its terminal elimination half-time in the epidural space, its mean residence time in the epidural space, and its concentration in epidural fat.[12] In addition, net transfer of opioid from the epidural space to the intrathecal space was greatest for the least lipid soluble opioid (morphine) and least for highly lipid soluble opioids (fentanyl, sufentanil). In effect, increasing lipid solubility resulted in opioid "sequestration" in epidural fat, thereby, reducing the bioavailability of drug in the underlying subarachnoid space and spinal tissue.

Epidural fat also appears to play a role in the pharmacokinetics of epidurally administered local anesthetics. Specifically, sequestration in epidural fat likely explains why a highly lipid soluble local anesthetic like etidocaine is only approximately equipotent with lidocaine in the epidural space despite the fact that etidocaine is roughly seven times more potent than lidocaine in vitro. Because of its much greater lipid solubility, etidocaine is more likely than lidocaine to be sequestered in epidural fat, thereby reducing the amount of drug available to produce block in the spinal nerve roots and spinal cord. Consistent with this hypothesis, Lebeaux and Tucker showed that after administering 80 mg etidocaine and 50 mg lidocaine into the epidural space of sheep, the amount of etidocaine still present in epidural fat 12 hours later was more than 100 times greater than the amount of lidocaine.[13] Thus, sequestration in epidural fat appears to play an important role in the pharmacokinetics of local anesthetics just as it does for epidural opioids.

Meninges

The spinal meninges consist of three protective membranes (dura mater, arachnoid mater, and pia mater), which are continuous with the cranial meninges (Fig. 25-4).

Dura Mater

The dura mater is the outermost and thickest meningeal tissue. The spinal dura mater begins at the foramen magnum where it fuses with the periosteum of the skull, forming the cephalad border of the epidural space. Caudally, the dura mater ends at approximately S2 where it fuses with the filum terminale. The dura mater extends laterally along the spinal nerve roots and becomes continuous with the connective tissue of the epineurium at approximately the level of the intervertebral foramina. The dura mater is composed of randomly arranged

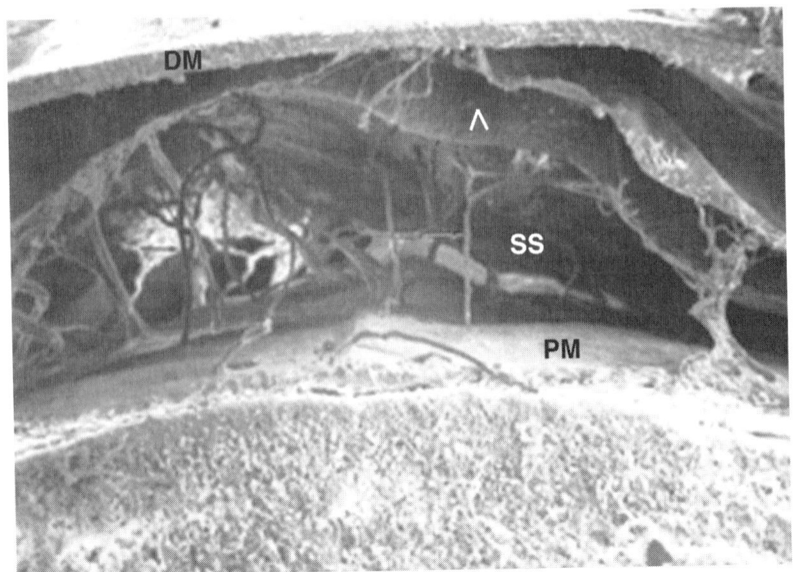

FIGURE 25-4. The spinal meninges of the dog, demonstrating the pia mater (*PM*) in apposition to the spinal cord, the subarachnoid space (*SS*), the arachnoid mater (*AM*), trabeculae (*arrow*), and the dura mater (*DM*). The separation between the arachnoid mater and the dura mater demonstrates the subdural space. The subdural space is only a potential space in vivo but is created here as an artifact of preparation. (Reprinted with permission from Peters A, Palay SL, Webster H (eds): The Fine Structure of the Nervous System: The Neurons and Supporting Cells. Philadelphia, WB Saunders, 1976.)

collagen fibers and elastin fibers arranged longitudinally and circumferentially.[14] The dura mater is largely acellular except for a layer of cells that forms the border between the dura and arachnoid mater.

There is controversy regarding the existence and clinical significance of a midline connective tissue band, the *plica medianis dorsalis*, running from the dura mater to the ligamentum flavum. Anatomic studies using epiduroscopy[15] and epidurography[16] have demonstrated the presence of the *plica medianis dorsalis* and have led to speculation that this tissue band may on occasion be responsible for difficulty in inserting epidural catheters and for unilateral epidural block. However, using cryomicrotome sections to investigate the epidural space, Hogan failed to find evidence of a substantial connection between the dura mater and the ligamentum flavum.[10] He speculated that the injection of either air or contrast required for the earlier studies may have compressed epidural contents (e.g., fat) and produced an artifact mimicking a connective tissue band. In addition, Hogan has shown in a clinical study that there is no significant impediment to spread of injectate across the midline.[17] Thus, the *plica medianis dorsalis* does not appear to be clinically relevant with respect to clinical epidural anesthesia.

The inner surface of the dura mater abuts the arachnoid mater. There is a potential space between these two membranes called the *subdural space* (see Fig. 25-4). Occasionally a drug intended for either the epidural space or the subarachnoid space is injected into the subdural space.[18] Subdural injection has been estimated to occur in 0.82% of intended epidural injections.[19] The radiology literature suggests that the incidence of subdural injection during intended subarachnoid injection may be as high as 10%.[20]

Arachnoid Mater

The arachnoid mater is a delicate, avascular membrane composed of overlapping layers of flattened cells with connective tissue fibers running between the cellular layers. The arachnoid cells are interconnected by frequent tight junctions and occluding junctions. These specialized cellular connections likely account for the fact that the arachnoid mater is the principal physiologic barrier for drugs moving between the epidural space and the spinal cord.[21]

In the region where the spinal nerve roots traverse the dura and arachnoid membranes, the arachnoid mater herniates through the dura mater into the epidural space to form arachnoid granulations. As with the cranial arachnoid granulations, the spinal arachnoid granulations serve as a site for material in the subarachnoid space to exit the central nervous system (CNS). Although some have postulated that the arachnoid granulations are a preferred route for drugs to move from the epidural space to the spinal cord, the available experimental data suggest that this is not the case.[22]

The *subarachnoid space* lies between the arachnoid mater and the pia mater and contains the CSF. The spinal CSF is in continuity with the cranial CSF and provides an avenue for drugs in the spinal CSF to reach the brain. In addition, the spinal nerve roots and rootlets run in the subarachnoid space.

Pia Mater

The spinal pia mater is adherent to the spinal cord and is composed of a thin layer of connective tissue cells interspersed with collagen. Trabeculae connect the pia mater with the arachnoid mater and the cells of these two meninges blend together along the trabeculae. Unlike the arachnoid mater, the pia mater is fenestrated in places so that the spinal cord is in direct communication with the subarachnoid space. The pia mater extends to the tip of the spinal cord where it becomes the *filum terminale*, which anchors the spinal cord to the sacrum. The pia mater also gives rise to the dentate ligaments, which are thin connective tissue bands extending from the side of the spinal cord through the arachnoid mater to dura mater. These ligaments serve to suspend the spinal cord within the meninges.

Spinal Cord

In the first-trimester fetus, the spinal cord extends from the foramen magnum to the end of the spinal column. Thereafter, the vertebral column lengthens more than the spinal cord so that at birth the spinal cord ends at about the level of the third lumbar vertebra. In the adult, the caudad tip of the spinal cord typically lies at the level of the first lumbar vertebra. However, in 30% of individuals the spinal cord may end at T12, while in 10% it may extend to L3 (see Fig. 25-1).[23] A sacral spinal cord has been reported in an adult.[23] Flexion of the vertebral column causes the tip of the spinal cord to move slightly cephalad.

The spinal cord gives rise to 31 pairs of *spinal nerves*, each composed of an *anterior motor root* and a *posterior sensory root*. The nerve roots are in turn composed of multiple rootlets.

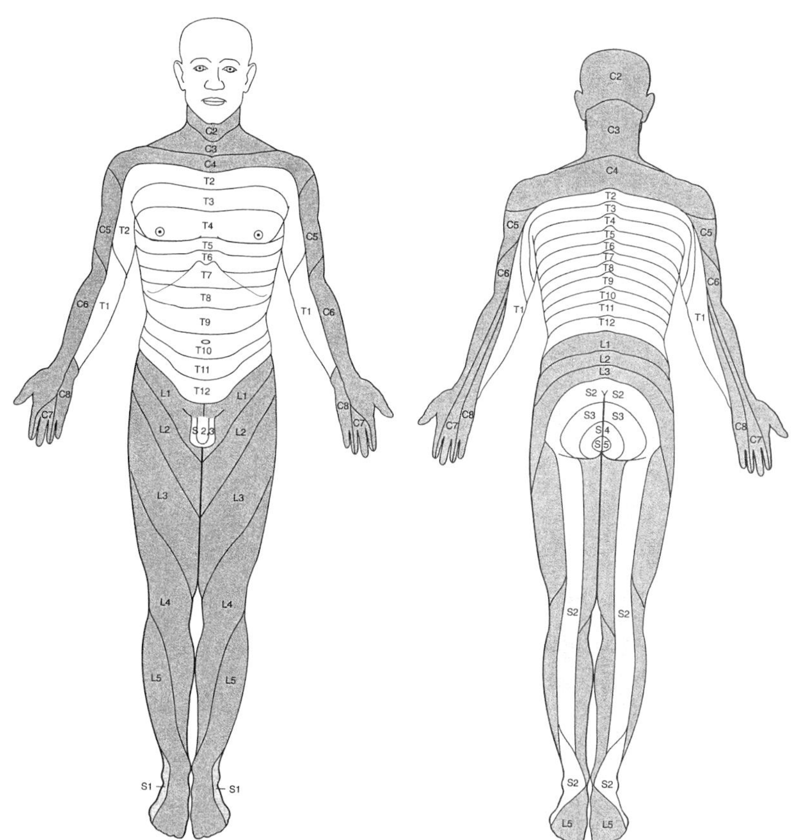

FIGURE 25-5. Human sensory dermatomes.

The portion of the spinal cord that gives rise to all of the rootlets of a single spinal nerve is called a cord segment. The skin area innervated by a given spinal nerve and its corresponding cord segment is called a *dermatome* (Fig. 25-5). The intermediolateral gray matter of the T1 through L2 spinal cord segments contains the cell bodies of the *preganglionic sympathetic neurons*. These sympathetic neurons run with the corresponding spinal nerve to a point just beyond the intervertebral foramen where they exit to join the sympathetic chain ganglia.

The spinal nerves and their corresponding cord segments are named for the intervertebral foramen through which they run. In the cervical region, the spinal nerves are named for the vertebra forming the caudad half of the intervertebral foramen; for example, C4 emerges through an intervertebral foramen formed by C3 and C4. In the thoracic and lumbar region, the nerve roots are named for the vertebrae forming the cephalad half of the intervertebral foramen; for example, L4 emerges through an intervertebral foramen formed by L4 and L5. Because the spinal cord ends between L1 and L2, the thoracic, lumbar, and sacral nerve roots run increasingly longer distances in the subarachnoid space to get from their spinal cord segment of origin to the intervertebral foramen through which they exit. Those nerves that extend beyond the end of the spinal cord to their exit site are collectively known as the cauda equina (see Fig. 25-1).

TECHNIQUE

Spinal and epidural anesthesia should be performed only after appropriate monitors are applied and in a setting where equipment for airway management and resuscitation are immediately available. Before positioning the patient, all equipment for spinal block should be ready for use, for example, local anesthetics mixed and drawn up, needles uncapped, prep solution available, and so on. Preparing all equipment ahead of time will minimize the time required to perform the block and thereby enhance patient comfort.

Needles

Spinal and epidural needles are named for the design of their tips (Fig. 25-6). The Whitacre and Sprotte spinal needles have a "pencil-point" tip with the needle hole on the side of the shaft. The Greene and Quincke needles have beveled tips with cutting edges. The pencil-point needles require more force to insert than the bevel-tip needles but provide a better tactile "feel" of the various tissues encountered as the needle is inserted. In addition, the bevel has been shown to cause the needle to be deflected from the intended path as it passes through tissues while the pencil-point needles are not deflected.[24] Epidural needles have a larger diameter than spinal needles to facilitate the injection of fluid or air when using the "loss-of-resistance" technique to identify the epidural space. In addition, the larger diameter allows for easier insertion of catheters into the epidural space. The Tuohy epidural needle has a curved tip to help control the direction that the catheter moves in the epidural space. The Hustead needle tip is also curved, although somewhat less than the Tuohy needle. The Crawford needle tip is straight, making it less suitable for catheter insertion. The outside diameter of both epidural and spinal needles is used to determine their gauge. Larger gauge (i.e., smaller diameter) spinal needles are less likely to cause postdural puncture headaches (PDPH), but are more readily deflected than smaller gauge needles. Epidural needles are typically sized 16 to 19 gauge and spinal needles 22 to 29 gauge. Spinal needles smaller than 22 gauge are often easier to insert if an introducer needle is used. The introducer is inserted into the interspinous ligament in the intended direction of the spinal needle and the spinal needle is then

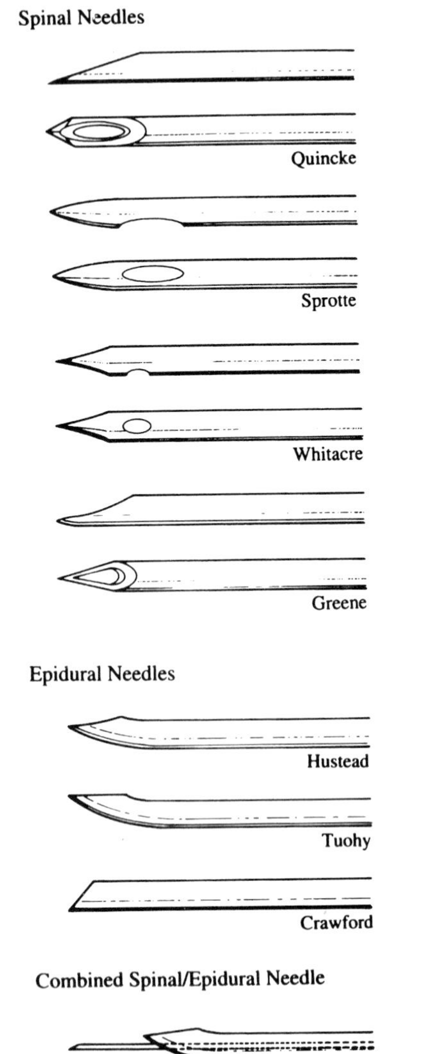

FIGURE 25-6. Some of the commercially available needles for spinal and epidural anesthesia. Needles are distinguished by the design of their tips.

inserted through the shaft of the introducer. The introducer prevents the spinal needle from being deflected or bent as it passes through the interspinous ligament.[24] Needles of the same outside diameter may have different inside diameters. This is important because inside diameter determines how large a catheter can be inserted through the needle and determines how rapidly CSF will appear at the needle hub during spinal needle insertion. All spinal and epidural needles come with a tight-fitting stylet. The stylet prevents the needle from being plugged with skin or fat and importantly prevents dragging skin into the epidural or subarachnoid spaces, where the skin may grow and form dermoid tumors.

Sedation

If the patient desires, light sedation is appropriate before placement of spinal or epidural block. Generally, the patient should not be heavily sedated because successful spinal and epidural anesthesia requires patient participation to maintain good position, evaluate block height, and indicate to the anesthesiologist about paresthesias if the needle contacts neural elements. In addition, patient cooperation is required to properly evaluate an epidural test dose; and sedation with as little as 1.5 mg midazolam plus 75 μg fentanyl has been shown to reduce the reliability of patient reports of subjective symptoms of intravenous local anesthetic injection.[25] Once the block is placed and adequate block height assured, the patient can be sedated as deemed appropriate.

Spinal Anesthesia

Position

Careful attention to patient positioning is critical to successful spinal puncture. Poor positioning can turn an otherwise easy spinal anesthetic into a challenge for both the anesthesiologist and the patient. Spinal needles are most often inserted with the patient in the lateral decubitus position and this technique is described in detail later. However, both the prone jackknife and sitting positions offer advantages under specific circumstances. The sitting position is sometimes used in obese patients because it is often easier to identify the midline with the patient sitting. In addition, the sitting position allows one to restrict spinal block to the sacral dermatomes (saddle block) when using hyperbaric local anesthetic solutions. Spinal block is generally performed in the prone jackknife position only when this is the position to be used for surgery. The use of hypobaric local anesthetic solutions with the patient in the prone jackknife position produces sacral block for perirectal surgery.

In the lateral decubitus position, the patient lies with the operative side down when using hyperbaric local anesthetic solutions and with the operative side up when using hypobaric solutions, thus assuring that the earliest and most dense block occurs on the operative side. The back should be at the edge of the table so that the patient is within easy reach. The patient's shoulders and hips are both positioned perpendicular to the bed to help prevent rotation of the spine. The knees are drawn to the chest, the neck is flexed, and the patient is instructed to actively curve the back outward. This will spread the spinous processes apart and maximize the size of the interlaminar foramen. It is useful to have an assistant who can help the patient maintain this position. Using the iliac crests as a landmark, the L2–3, L3–4, and L4–5 interspaces are identified and the desired interspace chosen for needle insertion. Interspaces above L2-3 are avoided to decrease the risk of hitting the spinal cord with the needle. Some find it helpful to mark the spinous processes flanking the desired interspace with a skin marker. This obviates the need to reidentify the intended interspace after the patient is prepped and draped.

The patient is prepped with an appropriate antiseptic solution and draped. All antiseptic solutions are neurotoxic, and care must be taken not to contaminate spinal needles or local anesthetics with the prep solution. How one drapes is a matter of personal preference, but the author finds that prepping and draping out a large area (e.g., T12-S1) with towels is preferable to using a commercial one-piece drape with a limited center hole. Draping a large area permits easier identification of a rotated or inadequately flexed back and allows one to readily move to another interspace if this becomes necessary.

Midline Approach

For the midline approach to the subarachnoid space, the skin overlying the desired interspace is infiltrated with a small amount of local anesthetic to prevent pain when inserting the spinal needle. One should avoid raising too large a skin wheal because this can obscure palpation of the interspace, especially in obese patients. Additional local anesthetic (1 to 2 mL) is then deposited along the intended path of the spinal

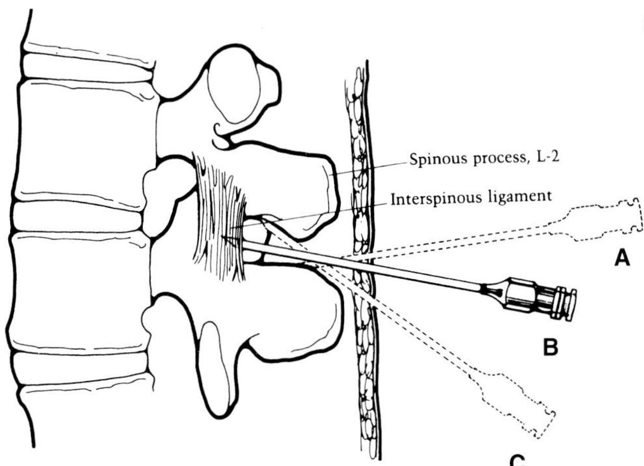

FIGURE 25-7. Midline approach to the subarachnoid space. The spinal needle is inserted with a slight cephalad angulation and should advance in the midline without contacting bone (**B**). If bone is contacted, it may be either the caudad (**A**) or the cephalad spinous process (**C**). The needle should be redirected slightly cephalad and reinserted. If bone is encountered at a shallower depth, then the needle is likely walking up the cephalad spinous process. If bone is encountered at a deeper depth, then the needle is likely walking down the inferior spinous process. If bone is repeatedly contacted at the same depth, then the needle is likely off the midline and walking along the lamina. (Reprinted with permission from Mulroy MF: Regional Anesthesia: An Illustrated Procedural Guide. Boston, Little Brown, 1989.)

needle to a depth of 1 to 2 inches. This deeper infiltration provides additional anesthesia for spinal needle insertion and helps identify the correct path for the spinal needle.

The spinal needle or introducer needle is inserted in the middle of the interspace with a slight cephalad angulation of 10 to 15 degrees (Fig. 25-7). The needle is then advanced, in order, through the subcutaneous tissue, supraspinous ligament, interspinous ligament, ligamentum flavum, epidural space, dura mater, and finally arachnoid mater. The ligaments produce a characteristic "feel" as the needle is advanced through them, and the anesthesiologist should develop the ability to distinguish a needle that is advancing through the high-resistance ligaments from one that is advancing through lower-resistance paraspinous muscle. This will allow early detection and correction of needles that are not advancing in the midline. Penetration of the dura mater produces a subtle "pop" that is most easily detected with the pencil-point needles. Detection of dural penetration will prevent inserting the needle all the way through the subarachnoid space and contacting the vertebral body. In addition, learning to detect dural penetration will allow one to insert the spinal needle quickly without having to stop every few millimeters and remove the stylet to look for CSF at the needle hub.

Once the needle tip is believed to be in the subarachnoid space, the stylet is removed to see if CSF appears at the needle hub. With small diameter needles (26 to 29 gauge) this generally requires 5 to 10 seconds, but may require $\geq$1 minute in some patients. Gentle aspiration may speed the appearance of CSF. If CSF does not appear, the needle orifice may be obstructed by a nerve root and rotating the needle 90 degrees may result in CSF flow. Alternatively, the needle orifice may not be completely in the subarachnoid space and advancing an additional 1 to 2 mm may result in brisk CSF flow. This is particularly true of pencil-point needles, which have their orifice on the side of the needle shaft proximal to the needle tip. Finally, failure to obtain CSF suggests that the needle orifice is not in the subarachnoid space and the needle should be reinserted.

2 If bone is encountered during needle insertion, the anesthesiologist must develop a reasoned, systematic approach to redirecting the needle. Simply withdrawing the needle and repeatedly reinserting it in different directions is not appropriate. When contacting bone, the depth should be immediately noted and the needle redirected slightly cephalad. If bone is again encountered at a greater depth, then the needle is most likely walking down the inferior spinous process and it should be redirected more cephalad until the subarachnoid space is reached. If bone is encountered again at a shallower depth, then the needle is most likely walking up the superior spinous process and it should be redirected more caudad. If bone is repeatedly encountered at the same depth, then the needle is likely off the midline and walking along the vertebral lamina (see Fig. 25-7).

When redirecting a needle it is important to withdraw the tip into the subcutaneous tissue. If the tip remains embedded in one of the vertebral ligaments, then attempts at redirecting the needle will simply bend the shaft and not reliably change needle direction. When using an introducer needle, it must also be withdrawn into the subcutaneous tissue before being redirected. Changes in needle direction should be made in small increments because even small changes in needle angle at the skin may result in fairly large changes in position of the needle tip when it reaches the spinal meninges at a depth of 4 to 6 cm. Care should be exercised when gripping the needle to ensure that it does not bow. Insertion of a curved needle will cause it to veer off course.

If the patient experiences a paresthesia, it is important to determine whether the needle tip has encountered a nerve root in the epidural space or in the subarachnoid space. When the paresthesia occurs, immediately stop advancing the needle, remove the stylet, and look for CSF at the needle hub. The presence of CSF confirms that the needle encountered a cauda equina nerve root in the subarachnoid space and the needle tip is in good position. Given how tightly packed the cauda equina nerve roots are, it is surprising that all spinal punctures do not produce paresthesias. If CSF is not visible at the hub, then the paresthesia probably resulted from contact with a spinal nerve root traversing the epidural space. This is especially true if the paresthesia occurs in the dermatome corresponding to the nerve root that exits the vertebral canal at the same level that the spinal needle is inserted. In this case the needle has most likely deviated from the midline and should be redirected toward the side opposite the paresthesia. Occasionally, pain experienced when the needle contacts bone may be misinterpreted by the patient as a paresthesia and the anesthesiologist should be alert to this possibility.

Once the needle is correctly inserted into the subarachnoid space, it is fixed in position and the syringe containing local anesthetic is attached. CSF is gently aspirated to confirm that the needle is still in the subarachnoid space and the local anesthetic slowly injected ($\leq$0.5 ml/s-1). After completing the injection, a small volume of CSF is again aspirated to confirm that the needle tip remained in the subarachnoid space while the local anesthetic was deposited. This CSF is then reinjected and the needle, syringe, and any introducer removed together as a unit. If the surgical procedure is to be performed in the supine position, the patient is helped onto his back. To prevent excessive cephalad spread of hyperbaric local anesthetic, care should be taken to ensure that the patient's hips are not raised off the bed as they turn.

Once the block is placed, strict attention must be paid to the patient's hemodynamic status with blood pressure and/or heart rate supported as necessary. Block height should also be assessed early by pin prick or temperature sensation. Temperature sensation is tested by wiping the skin with alcohol and may be preferable to pin prick because it is not painful. If, after a few minutes, the block is not rising high enough or is rising too high, the table may be tilted as appropriate to influence further spread of hypobaric or hyperbaric local anesthetics.

Paramedian Approach

The paramedian approach to the epidural and subarachnoid spaces is useful in situations where the patient's anatomy does not favor the midline approach, e.g., inability to flex the spine or heavily calcified interspinous ligaments. This approach can be used with the patient in any position and is probably the best approach for the patient in the prone jackknife position.

The spinous process forming the lower border of the desired interspace is identified. The needle is inserted ~1 cm lateral to this point and is directed toward the middle of the interspace by angling it ~45 degrees cephalad with just enough medial angulation (~15 degrees) to compensate for the lateral insertion point. The first significant resistance encountered should be the ligamentum flavum. Bone encountered prior to the ligamentum flavum is usually the vertebral lamina of the cephalad vertebra and the needle should be redirected accordingly. An alternative method is to insert the needle perpendicular to the skin in all planes until the lamina is contacted. The needle is then walked off the superior edge of the lamina and into the subarachnoid space. The lamina provides a valuable landmark that facilitates correct needle placement; however, repeated needle contact with the periosteum can be painful.

Lumbosacral Approach

The lumbosacral (or Taylor) approach to the subarachnoid and epidural spaces is simply a paramedian approach directed at the L5-S1 interspace, which is the largest interlaminar space. This approach may be useful when anatomic constraints make other approaches unfeasible. The patient may be positioned laterally, prone or sitting, and the needle inserted at a point 1 cm medial and 1 cm inferior to the posterior superior iliac spine. The needle is angled cephalad 45 to 55 degrees and just medial enough to reach the midline at the level of the L5 spinous process. As with the paramedian approach, the interspinous ligament is bypassed and the first significant resistance felt should be the ligamentum flavum.

Continuous Spinal Anesthesia

Inserting a catheter into the subarachnoid space increases the utility of spinal anesthesia by permitting repeated drug administration as often as necessary to extend the level or duration of spinal block. A common and reasonable recommendation for subsequent dosing or "topping up" of continuous spinal blocks is to administer half the original dose of local anesthetic when the block has reached two thirds of its expected duration.

The technique is similar to that described for "single shot" spinal anesthesia except that a needle large enough to accommodate the desired catheter must be used. After inserting the needle and obtaining free-flowing CSF, the catheter is simply threaded into the subarachnoid space a distance of 2 to 3 cm. It is often easier to insert the catheter if it is directed cephalad or caudad instead of lateral. If the catheter does not easily pass beyond the needle tip, rotating the needle 180 degrees may be helpful or another interspace may be used. The catheter should never be withdrawn back into the needle shaft because of the risk of shearing the catheter off into the subarachnoid space.

A variety of catheters and needles are available for continuous spinal anesthesia. Commonly, 18-gauge epidural needles and 20-gauge catheters are used. However, needles and catheters this size carry a higher risk of PDPH, especially in young patients. Because of this risk, smaller needle and catheter combinations have been developed with catheters ranging in size from 24 to 32 gauge. Although smaller catheters decrease the risk of PDPH, they have also been associated with multiple reports of neurologic injury, specifically, cauda equina syndrome (see Complications). For this reason, the United States Food and Drug Administration has advised against using any catheter smaller than 24 gauge for continuous spinal anesthesia.

Epidural Anesthesia

For the novice, correct placement of an epidural needle can be technically more challenging than spinal needle placement because there is less room for error. However, with experience, epidural needle placement is often easier than spinal needle placement because the larger gauge needles used for epidural anesthesia are less likely to be deflected from their intended path and they produce much better tactile feel of the interspinous and flaval ligaments. In addition, the loss of resistance technique provides a much clearer end point when entering the epidural space than does the subtle pop of a spinal needle piercing the dura mater.

Patient preparation, positioning, monitors, and needle approaches for epidural anesthesia are the same as for spinal anesthesia. Unlike spinal anesthesia, epidural anesthesia may be performed at any intervertebral space. However, at vertebral levels above the termination of the spinal cord, the epidural needle may accidentally puncture the spinal meninges and damage the underlying spinal cord. To prevent accidental meningeal puncture, the anesthesiologist must learn to identify the interspinous ligaments and the ligamentum flavum by their feel. In addition, epidural needles must be advanced slowly and, most importantly, under control.

After proper positioning, sterile skin preparation, and draping, the desired interspace is identified and a local anesthetic skin wheal is raised at the point of needle insertion. Because epidural needles are relatively blunt, it is sometimes helpful to pierce the skin with a ≥18-gauge hypodermic needle before inserting the epidural needle. For epidural anesthesia using the midline approach, the epidural needle is inserted through the subcutaneous tissue and into the interspinous ligament. The interspinous ligament has a characteristic "gritty" feel, much like inserting a needle into a bag of sand. This is especially true of younger patients. If the interspinous ligament is not clearly identified, then one should be suspicious that the needle is not in the midline. After engaging the interspinous ligament, the needle is advanced slowly through it until an increase in resistance is felt. This increased resistance represents the ligamentum flavum.

The epidural needle must now traverse the ligamentum flavum and stop within the epidural space before puncturing the spinal meninges. Numerous techniques for identifying the epidural space have been used successfully; however, the loss of resistance to fluid has the advantage of simplicity, reliability, and, most importantly, a higher success rate when compared to the use of air for loss of resistance.[26] In addition, use of fluid instead of air for loss of resistance decreases the risk of postdural puncture headache in the event of accidental meningeal puncture.[27]

A glass syringe or a specially designed low resistance plastic syringe is filled with 2 to 3 mL of saline and a small (0.1 to 0.3 mL) air bubble. The syringe is attached to the epidural needle and the plunger pressed until the air bubble is visibly compressed. If the needle tip is properly embedded within the ligamentum flavum, it should be possible to compress the air bubble without injecting fluid. In this way the air bubble serves as a gauge of the appropriate amount of pressure to exert on the syringe plunger. If the air bubble cannot be compressed without injecting fluid, then the needle tip is most likely not in the ligamentum flavum. In this case, the needle tip may still be in the

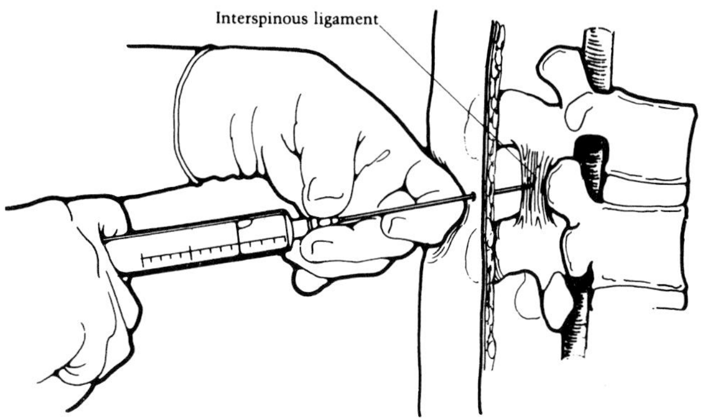

FIGURE 25-8. Proper hand position when using the loss-of-resistance technique to locate the epidural space. After embedding the needle tip in the ligamentum flavum, a syringe with 2 to 3 mL saline and an air bubble is attached. The left hand rests securely on the back and the fingers of the left hand grasp the needle firmly. The left hand advances the needle slowly and under control by rotating at the wrist. The fingers of the right hand maintain constant pressure on the syringe plunger but do not aid in advancing the needle. If the needle tip is properly engaged in the ligamentum flavum, it should be possible to compress the air bubble without injecting the saline. As the needle tip enters the epidural space, there will be a sudden loss of resistance and the saline will be suddenly injected. (Reprinted with permission from Mulroy MF: Regional Anesthesia: An Illustrated Procedural Guide. Boston, Little Brown, 1989.)

interspinous ligament, or it may be off the midline in the paraspinous muscles. To differentiate between these possibilities, one can carefully advance the needle and syringe a few millimeters in an effort to engage the ligamentum flavum. If it is still not possible to compress the air bubble, withdraw the needle into the subcutaneous tissue, and reinsert it.

Once the ligamentum flavum is identified, the needle is slowly advanced with the nondominant hand while the dominant hand maintains constant pressure on the syringe plunger (Fig. 25-8). As the needle tip enters the epidural space, there will be a sudden and dramatic loss of resistance as the saline is rapidly injected. Saline injection into the epidural space can be moderately painful and patients should be forewarned. If the needle is advancing obliquely through the ligamentum flavum, it is possible to enter into the paraspinous muscles instead of the epidural space. In this case the loss of resistance will be less dramatic. To help verify that the needle has entered the epidural space, 0.5 mL of air can be drawn into the syringe and injected. In the epidural space there will be virtually no resistance to air injection, while in the paraspinous muscles air injection will encounter demonstrable resistance.

After entering the epidural space, stop advancing the needle. Because the dura mater abuts the ligamentum flavum in many places, the dura may now be tented over the needle tip and advancing the needle any farther than necessary heightens the risk of accidental meningeal puncture, i.e., "wet tap." When the syringe is disconnected from the needle, it is common to have a small amount of fluid flow from the needle hub. This is usually the saline flowing back out of the epidural space but could be CSF if the needle accidentally entered the subarachnoid space. CSF can often be distinguished by the fact that CSF will usually flow out in a volume greatly exceeding that used for the loss of resistance, CSF will be warm compared to saline, and CSF will test positive for glucose.

If a "single shot" technique is to be used, then a local anesthetic test dose should be administered to help rule out undetected subarachnoid or intravenous (iv) needle placement. After a negative test dose, the desired volume of local anesthetic should be administered in small increments (e.g., 5 mL) at a rate of 0.5 to 1 mL/s-1. Slow, incremental injection decreases the risk of pain during injection and allows detection of adverse reactions to accidental iv or subarachnoid placement before the entire dose is administered.

Continuous Epidural Anesthesia

Use of a catheter for epidural anesthesia affords much greater flexibility than the "single shot" technique because the catheter can be used to prolong a block that is too short, to extend a block that is too low, or to provide postoperative analgesia. On the downside, catheters may migrate into an epidural vein, into the subarachnoid space, or out an intervertebral foramen. Catheter use is also more likely to result in unilateral epidural block, a clinical fact shown to result from catheter tips that end up in the anterior epidural space or migrate out an intervertebral foramina.[17,28] An ever-changing selection of epidural catheters is commercially available. They differ in diameter, stiffness, location of injection holes, presence or absence of a stylet, construction material, and the like. Whichever catheter is chosen, it is important to verify that it passes easily through the epidural needle before the needle is placed in the epidural space. Epidural catheters are usually inserted through either Tuohy or Hustead needles because their curved tips help direct the catheter away from the dura mater. The needle bevel should be directed either cephalad or caudad, although the direction of the bevel does not guarantee that the catheter will travel in that direction. The catheter will typically encounter resistance as it reaches the curve at the tip of the needle, but steady pressure will usually result in passage into the epidural space. If the catheter will not pass beyond the needle tip, it is possible that the needle opening is not completely in the epidural space or that some structure in the epidural space is preventing catheter insertion (e.g., epidural fat). In this instance, the needle can be carefully advanced 1 to 2 mm more or rotated 180 degrees and the catheter reinserted. Although either of these maneuvers may result in successful catheter placement, they also increase the risk of accidental meningeal puncture. Alternatively, the procedure can be repeated at another interspace or with a different needle approach, for example, paramedian. Occasionally a catheter will advance only a short distance past the needle tip. This raises the possibility that the needle tip is not in the epidural space and needs to be repositioned. In this case, the catheter should not be withdrawn back into the epidural needle because of the risk that the catheter tip will be sheared off by the bevel's sharp edge. Rather, the needle and catheter should be pulled out in tandem and the procedure repeated.

The catheter should be advanced only 3 to 5 cm into the epidural space. Placing a longer length of catheter in the epidural space increases the risk that it will enter an epidural vein, puncture the spinal meninges, exit an intervertebral foramen, wrap around a nerve root, or wind up in some other disadvantageous location. Once the catheter is appropriately positioned in the epidural space, the needle is slowly withdrawn with one hand as the catheter is stabilized with the other. After the needle is removed, the length of catheter in the epidural space is confirmed by subtracting the distance between the skin and the epidural space from the length of catheter below the skin. Documenting this distance is important when trying to determine if catheters used in the postoperative period have been dislodged.

An epidural test dose must be administered through the catheter to test for iv or subarachnoid placement before incrementally delivering the entire epidural drug dose. In addition, because of the risk of undetected iv or subarachnoid migration of the catheter over time, additional test doses must be administered before each top-up dose is given through the catheter. As with continuous spinal anesthesia, a reasonable guideline for top-up doses is to administer half the initial local anesthetic dose at an interval equal to two thirds the expected duration of the block.

Epidural Test Dose

The epidural test dose is designed to identify epidural needles
3 or catheters that have entered an epidural vein or the subarachnoid space. Failure to perform the test may result in intravascular injection of toxic doses of local anesthetic or total spinal block. Aspirating the catheter or needle to check for blood or CSF is helpful if positive, but the incidence of false-negative aspirations is too high to rely on this technique alone.[29]

The most common test dose is 3 mL of local anesthetic containing 5 mg/mL-1 epinephrine (1:200,000). The dose of local anesthetic should be sufficient that subarachnoid injection will result in clear evidence of spinal anesthesia. Intravenous injection of this dose of epinephrine typically produces an average 30 beats per minute—one heart rate increase between 20 and 40 seconds after injection.[30,31] Heart rate increases may not be as evident in some patients taking β-blocking drugs; reflex bradycardia usually occurs in these patients.[30,32] In β-blocked patients, a systolic blood pressure increase of $\geq$20 mm Hg may be a more reliable indicator of intravascular injection.[30,32]

Importantly, the sensitivity of the standard 15 μg epinephrine test dose has been shown to be markedly diminished by preexisting high thoracic epidural anesthesia and/or concurrent general anesthesia.[33] Larger epinephrine doses may be effective at detecting intravenous injection in these settings, but that has not been shown experimentally.

Isoproterenol has also been used to detect intravascular injection.[34] In addition, air injection combined with a precordial doppler to detect the characteristic murmur has been used successfully to test for iv placement of epidural catheters.[29] These techniques have been developed for use in laboring women where the sensitivity of epinephrine as a test dose is disturbingly low because maternal heart rate increases during contractions are often as large as those produced by epinephrine.[35] The clinical indications for these alternative tests of intravascular injection await additional larger studies.

Combined Spinal–Epidural Anesthesia

Combined spinal–epidural anesthesia (CSEA) is a useful technique by which a spinal block and an epidural catheter are placed simultaneously. This technique is popular because it combines the rapid onset, dense block of spinal anesthesia with the flexibility afforded by an epidural catheter. There are special epidural needles with a separate lumen to accommodate a spinal needle available for CSEA (see Fig. 25-6). However, the technique is easily performed by first placing a standard epidural needle in the epidural space and then inserting an appropriately sized spinal needle through the shaft of the epidural needle and into the subarachnoid space. The desired local anesthetic is injected into the subarachnoid space, the spinal needle removed, and a catheter placed in the epidural space via the epidural needle. The catheter can then be used to extend the height or duration of intraoperative block or can be used to provide postoperative epidural analgesia.

An interesting pharmacologic aspect of CSEA is the observation that after the peak spinal block height is established, both saline and local anesthetic injected into the epidural space are effective at pushing the block level higher.[36–38] This observation has been interpreted to indicate that the mechanism by which the epidural "top-up" increases block height is by a volume effect (i.e., compression of the spinal meninges forcing CSF cephalad) as well as a local anesthetic effect.

A potential risk of this technique is that the meningeal hole made by the spinal needle may allow dangerously high concentrations of subsequently administered epidural drugs to reach the subarachnoid space. Anecdotal case reports and in vitro animal studies suggest that this may be a legitimate concern.[35,39–41] Although CSEA shows great promise, additional prospective studies are necessary to identify the relative risks and limitations of the technique.

PHARMACOLOGY

Successful spinal or epidural anesthesia requires a block that is high enough to block sensation at the surgical site and lasts for the duration of the planned procedure. However, because variability between patients is considerable (Figs. 25-9 and 25-10), reliably predicting the height and duration of central neuraxial block that will result from a particular local anesthetic dose is difficult. Thus, recommendations regarding local anesthetic choice and dose must be viewed as approximate guidelines. The clinician must understand the factors governing spinal and epidural block height and duration to individualize local anesthetic choice and dose for each patient and procedure.

Spinal Anesthesia

Block Height

Table 25-1 lists some common surgical procedures that are readily performed under spinal anesthesia and the block height that is usually sufficient to ensure patient comfort. Also listed are techniques that are appropriate to achieve the desired block height. The rationale for these recommendations is explained in the following section.

Baricity and Patient Position. The height of spinal block is thought to be determined by the cephalad spread of local anesthetic within the CSF. Table 25-2 lists some of the many

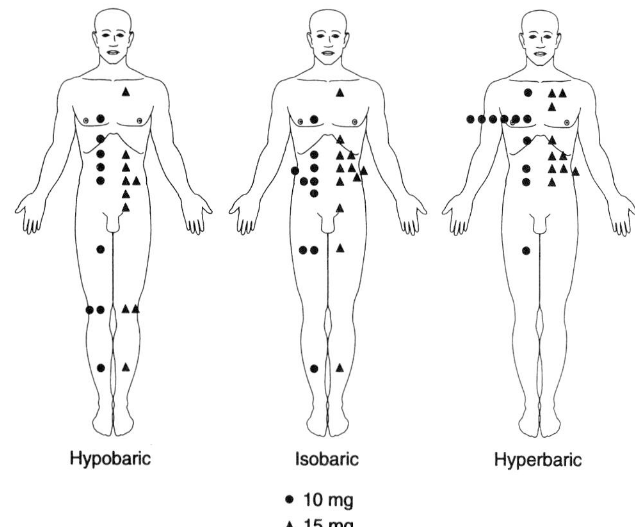

FIGURE 25-9. Peak spinal block height following 10- and 15-mg doses of hypobaric, isobaric, and hyperbaric tetracaine solutions injected at L3-4 with patients in the lateral horizontal position. Note that dose has no influence on block height and that there is considerable interindividual variability in peak block height, especially with the hypobaric solution. (Adapted with permission from Brown DT, Wildsmith JA, Covino BG, Scott DB: Effect of baricity on spinal anaesthesia with amethocaine. Br J Anaesth 52:589, 1980.)

TABLE 25-1

REPRESENTATIVE SURGICAL PROCEDURES APPROPRIATE FOR SPINAL ANESTHESIA

■ SURGICAL PROCEDURE	■ SUGGESTED BLOCK HEIGHT	■ TECHNIQUE	■ COMMENTS
Perianal Perirectal	L1-2	Hyperbaric solution/sitting position Hypobaric solution/jackknife position Isobaric solution/horizontal position	Patients must remain in relative head-up or head-down position when using hypobaric and hyperbaric solutions to maintain restricted spread during the procedure
Lower extremity Hip Transurethral resection of the prostate Vaginal/cervical	T10	Isobaric solution	Hypobaric and hyperbaric solutions are also suitable but may produce higher blocks than necessary
Herniorraphy Pelvic procedures Appendectomy	T6-8	Hyperbaric solution/horizontal position	Isobaric solutions injected at L2-3 interspace may also be suitable
Abdominal Cesasean section	T4-6	Hyperbaric solution/horizontal position	Upper abdominal procedures usually require concomitant general anesthesia to prevent vagal reflexes and pain from traction on diaphragm, esophagus, and the like

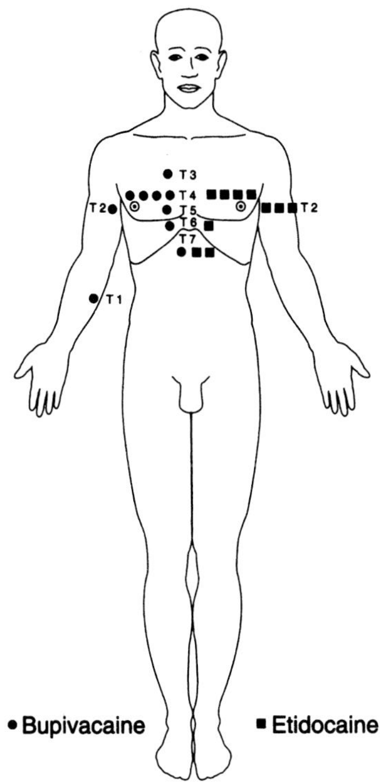

FIGURE 25-10. Peak epidural block height following 20 mL of 0.75% bupivacaine and 1.5% etidocaine injected via a catheter at the L1-2 interspace. Note that despite a well-controlled technique, the interindividual variability in block height is considerable and demonstrates the difficulty in accurately predicting block height in an individual patient. (Adapted with permission from Sinclair CJ, Scott DB: Comparison of bupivacaine and etidocaine in extradural blockade. Br J Anaesth 56:147, 1984.)

variables that have been proposed to influence the spread of local anesthetics within the subarachnoid space. Many of these variables have been shown to be of negligible clinical importance. Of those factors that do exert significant influence on local anesthetic spread, the baricity of the local anesthetic solution relative to patient position is probably the most important. Baricity is defined as the ratio of the density (mass/volume) of the local anesthetic solution divided by the

TABLE 25-2

FACTORS THAT HAVE BEEN SUGGESTED AS POSSIBLE DETERMINANTS OF SPREAD OF LOCAL ANESTHETIC SOLUTIONS WITHIN THE SUBARACHNOID SPACE

■ CHARACTERISTICS OF THE LOCAL ANESTHETIC SOLUTION
Baricity Local anesthetic dose Local anesthetic concentration Volume injected
■ PATIENT CHARACTERISTICS
Age Weight Height Gender Pregnancy Patient position
■ TECHNIQUE
Site of injection Speed of injection Barbotage Direction of needle bevel Addition of vasoconstrictors
■ DIFFUSION

Adapted with permission from Greene NM: Distribution of local anesthetic solutions within the subarachnoid space. Anesth Analg 64:715, 1985.

TABLE 25-3

BARICITY OF SOLUTIONS COMMONLY USED FOR SPINAL ANESTHESIA

	BARICITY[a]
HYPERBARIC	
Tetracaine: 0.5% in 5% dextrose	1.0133
Bupivacaine: 0.75% in 8.25% dextrose	1.0227
Lidocaine: 5% in 7.5% dextrose	1.0265
Procaine: 10% in water	1.0104
ISOBARIC[b]	
Tetracaine: 0.5% in normal saline	0.9997
Bupivacaine: 0.75% in saline	0.9988
Bupivacaine: 0.5% in saline	0.9983
Lidocaine: 2% in saline	0.9986
HYPOBARIC	
Tetracaine: 0.2% in water	0.9922
Bupivacaine: 0.3% in water	0.9946
Lidocaine: 0.5% in water	0.9985

[a]Measured at 37°C, except for hypobaric 0.5% lidocaine measured at 25°C. At 37°C, this solution's baricity is less.
[b]These solutions are slightly hypobaric but are used clinically as if they were isobaric.
Data from Horlocker TT, Wedel DJ: Density, specific gravity, and baricity of spinal anesthetic solutions at body temperature. Anesth Analg 76:1015, 1993; Lambert D, Covino B: Hyperbaric, hypobaric and isobaric spinal anesthesia. Resident Staff Physician 33:79, 1987; Greene NM: Distribution of local anesthetic solutions within the subarachnoid space. Anesth Analg 64:715, 1985; and Bodily N, Carpenter R, Owens B: Lidocaine 0.5% spinal anaesthesia: A hypobaric solution for short-stay perirectal surgery. Can J Anaesth 39:770, 1992.

density of CSF, which averages 1.0003 ± 0.0003 g/mL-1 at 37°C. Solutions that have the same density as CSF have a baricity of 1.0000 and are termed isobaric. Solutions that are more dense than CSF are termed hyperbaric, whereas solutions that are less dense than CSF are termed hypobaric.

Table 25-3 lists the baricity of local anesthetic solutions commonly used for spinal anesthesia. For practical purposes, solutions with a baricity <0.9990 can be expected to reliably behave hypobarically in all patients. Hypobaric solutions are typically prepared by mixing the local anesthetic solution in distilled water. Solutions with a baricity of ≥1.0015 can be expected to reliably behave hyperbarically. Hyperbaric solutions are typically prepared by mixing the local anesthetic in 5% to 8% dextrose. The baricity of the resultant solution depends on the amount of dextrose added; however, dextrose concentrations between 1.25 and 8% result in equivalent block heights.[42,43] Lower dextrose concentrations have been shown to have a concentration-dependent effect on block height, with 0.33% producing a block to T9.5 on average, 0.83% producing a block to T7.2, and 8% producing a block to T3.6.[44]

Baricity is important in determining local anesthetic spread and thus block height because gravity causes hyperbaric solutions to flow downward in CSF to the most dependent regions of the spinal column, whereas hypobaric solutions tend to rise in CSF. In contrast, gravity has no effect on the distribution of truly isobaric solutions. Thus, the anesthesiologist can exert considerable influence on block height by choice of anesthetic solution and proper patient positioning. Spinal block can be restricted to the sacral and low lumbar dermatomes ("saddle block") by administering a hyperbaric local anesthetic solution with the patient in the sitting position[45] or by administering a hypobaric solution with the patient in the prone jackknife position. Similarly, high thoracic to midcervical levels of anesthesia can be reached by administering hyperbaric solutions with the patient in the horizontal and Trendelenburg positions[46,47] or by administering hypobaric solutions with the patient in a semisitting position. However, this use of hypobaric solutions is not recommended because the high block achieved and the diminished venous return associated with the upright posture can lead to significant cardiovascular compromise.

The sitting, Trendelenberg, and jackknife positions have marked influences on the distribution of hypobaric and hyperbaric solutions because these positions accentuate the effect of gravity. However, most spinal anesthetics are administered as hyperbaric solutions injected while patients are in the horizontal lateral position after which they are turned to the horizontal supine position. In this situation the influence of gravity is more subtle because the dependent areas of the spinal column do not deviate as much from the horizontal. While the patient is turned laterally, gravity has a small but measurable effect on local anesthetic distribution in that hyperbaric solutions will produce a denser, longer lasting block on the dependent side, while hypobaric solutions will have the opposite effect.[48] This makes hypobaric solutions ideal for unilateral procedures performed in the lateral position (e.g., hip surgery). Hyperbaric solutions can be used to advantage for unilateral procedures performed in the supine position if the operative side is dependent during drug injection and the patient is left in the lateral position for at least 6 minutes.[48] Despite differences in block density and duration, peak block height will be comparable between the dependent and nondependent sides.

When the patient is turned supine following hyperbaric drug injection in the lateral position, the normal spinal curvature will influence subsequent movement of the injected solution. Hyperbaric solutions injected at the height of the lumbar lordosis will tend to flow cephalad to pool in the thoracic kyphosis and caudad to pool in the sacrum (Fig. 25-11). Pooling of hyperbaric local anesthetic solutions in the thoracic kyphosis has been evoked to explain the clinical observation that hyperbaric solutions tend to produce blocks with an average height in the midthoracic region (see Fig. 25-9). In addition, hyperbaric solutions have also been observed to produce blocks with a bimodal distribution, that is, one group of patients with blocks centered in the low thoracic region and a second group of patients with

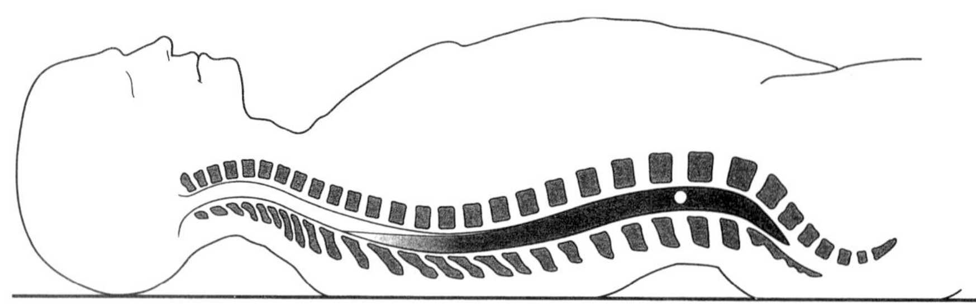

FIGURE 25-11. In the horizontal supine position, hyperbaric local anesthetic solutions injected at the height of the lumbar lordosis (*circle*) flow down the lumbar lordosis to pool in the sacrum and in the thoracic kyphosis. Pooling in the thoracic kyphosis is thought to explain the fact that hyperbaric solutions produce blocks with an average height of T4-6.

blocks centered in the high thoracic region.[49,50] The presumed explanation for this observation is that the lumbar lordosis produces "splitting" of the local anesthetic solution with some portion flowing caudad toward the sacrum and the remainder flowing cephalad into the thoracic kyphosis. The cephalad extent of the block then depends on what fraction of the injected drug flows cephalad. Consistent with this hypothesis is the fact that eliminating the lumbar lordosis by maintaining the hips flexed has been shown to significantly reduce[50] or eliminate[49] the bimodal distribution of blocks without affecting maximal block height.

Obviously, gravity influences the distribution of hyperbaric and hypobaric solutions only until they are sufficiently diluted in CSF so that they become isobaric. At this point, the local anesthetic solution no longer moves in response to changes in patient position and the block is said to be "fixed." Interestingly, the time required for a local anesthetic solution to become fixed may be considerable. Povey et al showed that hyperbaric bupivacaine injected in the sitting position produces a saddle block that is restricted to the lumbar segments for as long as the subjects remained sitting.[45,46] However, even 60 minutes after bupivacaine injection the block spread to midthoracic levels after turning the patients supine. Similarly, Bodily et al[51] found that hypobaric lidocaine administered in the jackknife position rose as many as 6 dermatomes when patients were allowed to sit upright in the recovery room as long as 60 minutes after lidocaine injection. Whether it is also possible to affect spread so long after injecting hyperbaric or hypobaric solutions in the horizontal position is unclear. Nonetheless, these findings demonstrate that in some situations it may be possible to exert influence on block height by adjusting patient position for at least 60 minutes after local anesthetic injection.

In contrast to the situation with hyperbaric solutions, patient position has no effect on the distribution of isobaric solutions because these solutions are not influenced by gravity. Consequently, isobaric solutions tend not to spread as far from the site of injection and produce blocks with an average height in the low thoracic region (see Fig. 25-9).[43,52] The obvious caveat is that the local anesthetic solution must be truly isobaric in the patient in whom it is used. Because of the variability in CSF density among patients, it is difficult to produce reliably isobaric local anesthetic solutions. Nonetheless, as indicated in Table 25-3, several local anesthetic solutions are used as if they were isobaric. It is noteworthy that while isobaric solutions produce an average block height that is lower than comparable hyperbaric solutions,[43,52–54] the "isobaric" solutions produce blocks with a much greater variability in height.[55–57] Logan et al have termed plain bupivacaine "an unpredictable spinal anesthetic agent."[55] The greater variability in spread may stem in part from the fact that these solutions are actually slightly hypobaric and their spread has been shown to be affected by patient position.[58,59] Temperature-related changes in baricity may also play a role in the variability in distribution of these nearly isobaric solutions. For example, Steinstra and van Poorten[60] have shown that the distribution of plain bupivacaine is significantly altered by changes in temperature of the injected solution. In addition, McClure et al[61] have shown that increasing the volume and decreasing the concentration of isobaric tetracaine also increases the variability in block height. These and other unknown factors may play a role in the unpredictability of these nearly isobaric solutions. Although unpredictability is cause for concern, it should be pointed out that the lower average block height achieved offers potential advantages for surgical procedures below the umbilicus because of the decreased incidence of cardiovascular side effects associated with lower blocks. The isobaric solution that has been shown to most reliably produce a low thoracic block is 10 mg of tetracaine crystals diluted in 1- or 2-mL room temperature saline and injected in the horizontal position.[61]

Dose, Volume, and Concentration. Studies aimed at determining the effect of these three interdependent variables on block height are difficult to conduct and interpret because it is not possible to change one variable without simultaneously changing another. Nonetheless, it is possible to draw some conclusions regarding the effect of these variables on block height. Several studies with isobaric tetracaine and bupivacaine solutions have found that neither injected volume nor drug concentration affects block height when dose is held constant.[61–65] Drug dose does appear to play a small role in determining block height with isobaric bupivacaine. Two studies have found that 10 mg of isobaric bupivacaine results in significantly lower blocks than does 15 or 20 mg, but there is no difference in block height between the two higher doses.[66,67] In contrast, two studies that examined the effect of different doses of isobaric tetracaine found that doses between 5 and 15 mg had no effect on block height, producing blocks with an average height of T9-T10.[52,68]

Drug dose and volume appear to be relatively unimportant in predicting the spread of hyperbaric local anesthetic solutions injected in the horizontal position. Increasing the dose and volume of hyperbaric tetracaine, while holding concentration constant, does not affect block height when doses between 7.5 and 15 mg are used.[52,68,69] Similarly, increasing the dose and volume of hyperbaric 0.5% bupivacaine does not increase block height when doses between 10 and 20 mg are used.[70,71] However, doses of hyperbaric 0.5% bupivacaine <10 mg have been shown to result in blocks that are ~2.5 dermatomes lower than those achieved with doses >10 mg.[70] The fact that bupivacaine dose affects block height only at the extreme low end of the usual dose range is consistent with the experience with isobaric bupivacaine reported earlier. The fact that drug dose is relatively unimportant in determining block height with hyperbaric solutions likely results from an overwhelming effect of baricity and patient position in determining spread of these solutions.

Injection Site. The site of injection can have an important effect on block height in some situations. In particular, sensory block height resulting from isobaric 0.5% bupivacaine is reduced by 2 dermatomes per interspace when comparing different groups of patients who received injections at the L2-3, L3-4, or L4-5 interspaces.[72,73] In an even more convincing study, this group of investigators performed repeated blocks in the same patient and found that by moving from the L3-4 to the L4-5 interspace means block height could be reduced from T6 to T10 when using isobaric 0.5% bupivacaine.[74] In contrast, Sundnes et al[70] found no relationship between injection site and block height when using a hyperbaric bupivacaine solution, presumably because of the overwhelming effect of gravity and patient position on distribution of hyperbaric local anesthetics. Whether isobaric and hyperbaric solutions of other local anesthetics will behave similarly is not clear.

Patient Characteristics. In young adults, it was determined that the most important variable governing block height with hyperbaric local anesthetic solutions may be lumbosacral CSF volume.[75] However, it is unclear if these findings can be extrapolated to other local anesthetics or patient ages.

Higuchi and colleagues performed a detailed examination of the effect of lumbar CSF volume, CSF density, lumbar CSF motion, patient age, patient weight, patient height, and patient body mass index (BMI) on spinal block with isobaric bupivacaine.[76] Multiple linear regression demonstrated that neither patient age nor height correlated with any clinical characteristic of spinal block. However, CSF volume and weight were correlated with peak block height. CSF volume was the only variable to correlate with time to voiding. BMI was the only significant predictor of time to onset of complete sensory block.

Although these variables were statistically significant predictors of several important aspects of spinal block, the

TABLE 25-4

DOSE AND DURATION OF LOCAL ANESTHETICS USED FOR SPINAL ANESTHESIA

		DURATION OF SENSORY BLOCK (MIN)[b]		
DRUG	DOSE (MG)[a]	2-DERMATOME REGRESSION	COMPLETE RESOLUTION	PROLONGATION BY ADRENERGIC AGONISTS (%)[c]
Procaine	50–200	30–50	90–120	30–50
Chloroprocaine	30–100	30–50	70–150	NR
Lidocaine	25–100	40–100	140–240	20–50
Bupivacaine	5–20	90–140	240–380	20–50
Tetracaine	5–20	90–140	240–380	50–100

[a]The lowest doses are used primarily for very restricted blocks, e.g., saddle block, lest they become too dilute to be effective.
[b]Duration is influenced by dose and block height. The duration of surgical anesthesia will obviously depend upon the surgical site.
[c]The effect of adrenergic agonists depends on the dose and choice of agonist. Prolongation is greatest at lumbar and sacral dermatomes and least at thoracic dermatomes.
NR: Not Recommended; see text for explanation.

coefficients of determination (R^2) were generally small (average: 0.23; range: 0.08 to 0.46), indicating that these variables account for a relatively small amount of the variability in each of the block outcomes examined. Clearly, other factors contribute significantly to the clinical characteristics of spinal block with isobaric bupivacaine.

4 While these studies are mechanistically important, their clinical application is necessarily limited by the difficulty in determining an individual patient's CSF volume, CSF density, and velocity of CSF movement.

Importantly, several investigators have found that patient age, weight, BMI, and height are either not predictive of clinical characteristics of spinal block[77,78,80–82] or are of such low predictive power as to be unreliable predictors in any individual patient.[57,72,79,83,84]

Onset

Most patients can sense the onset of spinal block within a very few minutes after drug injection regardless of the local anesthetic used. However, there is a significant difference among drugs in the time to reach peak block height. Lidocaine and mepivacaine tend to reach peak block height between 10 and 15 minutes, whereas tetracaine and bupivacaine may require >20 minutes before peak block height is reached.

Duration

Spinal blocks do not end abruptly after a fixed period of time. Rather, they recede gradually from the most cephalad dermatome to the most caudad. As a result, surgical anesthesia lasts significantly longer at sacral levels than at thoracic levels. Therefore, when discussing the duration of spinal block it is necessary to distinguish between duration at the surgical site and the time required for the block to completely resolve. The former is important for providing adequate surgical anesthesia, and the latter is important for assuring a timely recovery. A thorough understanding of the factors that govern block duration is necessary if the clinician is to choose techniques that result in an appropriate duration of spinal blockade.

Local Anesthetic. The principal determinant of spinal block duration is the local anesthetic drug employed. Procaine is the shortest acting local anesthetic for subarachnoid use, lidocaine and mepivacaine are agents of intermediate duration, while bupivacaine and tetracaine are the longest acting drugs available for use in the United States. Table 25-4 lists the range of times required for sensory block to regress 2 dermatomes and to completely resolve with the local anesthetics most commonly used for spinal anesthesia. Although drug choice is the principal determinant of block duration, other variables are responsible for the wide range of block duration found in Table 25-4.

Drug Dose. Increasing local anesthetic dose clearly increases the duration of spinal block.[66,67,69,85,86] For example, Brown et al[52] demonstrated that duration of sensory block at L1 following 15 mg tetracaine was ~20% greater than following 10 mg. Sheskey et al[67] demonstrated an ~40% increase in block duration at L2 when comparing 10 mg bupivacaine with 15 mg. Similarly, Axelsson et al.[85] found that duration of sensory block at L2 was nearly doubled when comparing 10 mg bupivacaine with 20 mg.

Block Height. If drug dose is held constant, higher blocks tend to regress faster than lower blocks.[86] Consequently, isobaric local anesthetic solutions will generally produce longer blocks than hyperbaric solutions using the same dose. The conventional wisdom is that greater cephalad spread results in relatively lower drug concentration in the CSF and spinal nerve roots. As a result, it takes less time for local anesthetic concentration to decrease below the minimally effective concentration.

Adrenergic Agonists. Adrenergic agonists, such as epinephrine, phenylephrine, and more recently clonidine, are added to local anesthetics in an effort to prolong the duration of spinal anesthesia. Their effectiveness depends on the local anesthetic with which they are combined. In addition, they are more effective at prolonging block in the lumbar and sacral dermatomes than in thoracic dermatomes.

Epinephrine is typically administered in doses of 0.2 to 0.3 mg and phenylephrine in doses of 2 to 5 mg. There is evidence to suggest a relationship between the dose of vasoconstrictor added and the duration of spinal anesthesia; however, the relationship is not strong.[87–90] At the maximal doses used clinically, phenylephrine (5 mg) prolongs spinal block to a greater degree than epinephrine (0.5 mg).[91,92] At lower doses, epinephrine (0.2 to 0.3 mg) and phenylephrine (2 to 3 mg) appear to be equally effective in prolonging spinal block.[90,93] Thus, both choice of adrenergic agonist and dose administered appear to play a role in determining block duration.Clonidine has most commonly been added to intrathecal local anesthetics in a dose of 75 to 150 milligram to prolong spinal block.[94,95] At these doses, it is at least as effective as moderate doses of phenylephrine and epinephrine at prolonging sensory block but has been associated with greater decreases in blood pressure in some[94] but not all studies.[95] Interestingly, clonidine also prolongs spinal block when administered orally.[96–98]

Tetracaine is the local anesthetic that is most dramatically prolonged by addition of adrenergic agonists. The duration of tetracaine spinal block may be increased 70% to 100% at

TABLE 25-5

LOCAL ANESTHETICS USED FOR SURGICAL EPIDURAL BLOCK

DRUG[a]	DURATION OF SENSORY BLOCK		
	TWO-DERMATOME REGRESSION (MIN)	COMPLETE RESOLUTION (MIN)	PROLONGATION BY EPINEPHRINE (%)
Chloroprocaine 3%	45–60	100–160	40–60
Lidocaine 2%	60–100	160–200	40–80
Mepivacaine 2%	60–100	160–200	40–80
Ropivacaine 0.5–1.0%	90–180	240–420	No
Etidocaine 1–1.5%	120–240	300–460	No
Bupivacaine 0.5–0.75%	120–240	300–460	No

[a]These concentrations are recommended for surgical anesthesia; more dilute concentrations are appropriate for epidural analgesia.

lumbar and sacral dermatomes by addition of phenylephrine. Epinephrine may prolong tetracaine spinal anesthesia by 40% to 60%. Clonidine prolongs tetracaine spinal block by 50% to 70%, with the larger effect occurring at lumbar dermatomes.

Bupivacaine spinal block is also prolonged by adrenergic agonists, although the effect is somewhat less than that seen with tetracaine (see Table 25-4). Epinephrine in doses of 0.2 mg prolongs bupivacaine spinal block by 20% to 30%, but only in lumbar dermatomes. Larger doses of epinephrine (0.3 to 0.5 mg) prolong sensory block in thoracic dermatomes as well by 30% to 50%. Clonidine prolongs bupivacaine spinal block by 30% to 50% as well.

The effect of adrenergic agonists on the duration of lidocaine spinal block is controversial. Some clinical studies have demonstrated that adrenergic agonists clearly prolong lidocaine spinal block,[88,99–101] whereas others have concluded that adrenergic agonists do not produce clinically useful prolongation.[102,103] This discrepancy may be explained, in part, by the fact that spinal block duration is so variable that studies using small numbers of patients may lack sufficient statistical power to detect real differences in mean block duration between groups. This problem was obviated in an interesting study by Chiu et al[104] who used a crossover study design to demonstrate that 0.2 mg of epinephrine significantly prolonged lidocaine sensory block in lumbar and sacral dermatomes. Thus, the available data suggest that adding epinephrine to lidocaine will result in a somewhat longer block, at least in lumbar and sacral dermatomes, than would be achieved if epinephrine were not added.

The mechanism by which adrenergic agonists prolong spinal block is not clear. Originally, epinephrine and phenylephrine were added to local anesthetics with the intent of reducing local spinal cord blood flow and thereby slowing the rate of drug elimination from the spinal cord and CSF. There are animal studies that support this mechanism[105,106] and others that do not.[107,108] Animal studies with clonidine indicate that it does reduce regional spinal cord blood flow.[109] There are no human studies that have investigated the effect of intrathecal adrenergic agonists on spinal cord blood flow. However, there are human studies that demonstrate that epinephrine decreases the rate of local anesthetic clearance from the CSF[110,111] and also slows the rate at which subarachnoid local anesthetic appears in the plasma.[99] These findings are consistent with a vasoconstrictor-mediated decrease in drug clearance from the spinal cord; however, they are not proof that this is the only or even the principal mechanism by which adrenergic agonists prolong spinal anesthesia.

Adrenergic agonists are potent analgesic agents in their own right when administered into the subarachnoid space.[112] Analgesia results from inhibition of nociceptive afferents, an effect that is mediated by stimulation of α-adrenergic receptors in the spinal cord dorsal horn. In addition, large intrathecal doses of α-adrenergic agonists have been shown to produce flaccidity in animal models by hyperpolarizing motor neurons.[113] Thus, prolongation of motor and sensory block by adrenergic agonists may be due, in part, to direct inhibitory effects of these drugs on sensory and motor neurons.

Epidural Anesthesia

Any procedure that can be performed under spinal anesthesia can also be performed under epidural block and requires the same block height (see Table 25-1). As with spinal anesthesia, there is a great deal of variability among patients in spread (see Fig. 25-10) and duration of epidural block (Table 25-5). Therefore, to choose the most appropriate local anesthetic and dose for a particular clinical situation, the anesthesiologist must be familiar with the variables that affect spread and duration of epidural anesthesia.

Block Spread

Injection Site. Unlike spinal anesthesia, epidural anesthesia produces a segmental block that spreads both caudally and cranially from the site of injection (Fig. 25-12). Thus, injection site is arguably the most important determinant of the spread of epidural block.*Caudal* epidural blocks are largely restricted to sacral and low lumbar dermatomes. Low thoracic levels can be reached with caudal injections if large volumes are used (e.g., 30 mL). However, the block at thoracic dermatomes tends to be patchy and short lived following caudal injection.[114] *Lumbar* local anesthetic injections with volumes of 10 mL often extend caudad to include all sacral dermatomes, although the onset of block in the L5 and S1 roots is often delayed and may be patchy.[115] Twenty-milliliter volumes produce better quality sacral anesthesia following lumbar injection. The slow onset at L5 and S1 is thought to result from their larger diameter and consequent slower drug penetration. Lumbar injections can be extended to midthoracic levels (T4-6) when 20-mL volumes of local anesthetic are used. *Thoracic* injections produce a symmetric segmental band of anesthesia, the width of which depends on the dose of local anesthetic administered. When using a mid to upper thoracic injection site, it is prudent to reduce the local anesthetic doses by ~30% to 50% relative to lumbar doses to prevent excessive cephalad spread. It is generally not feasible to produce surgical anesthesia in low lumbar and sacral dermatomes with midthoracic or higher injection sites. Thoracic epidural block is ideally suited for anesthesia of the chest and abdomen.

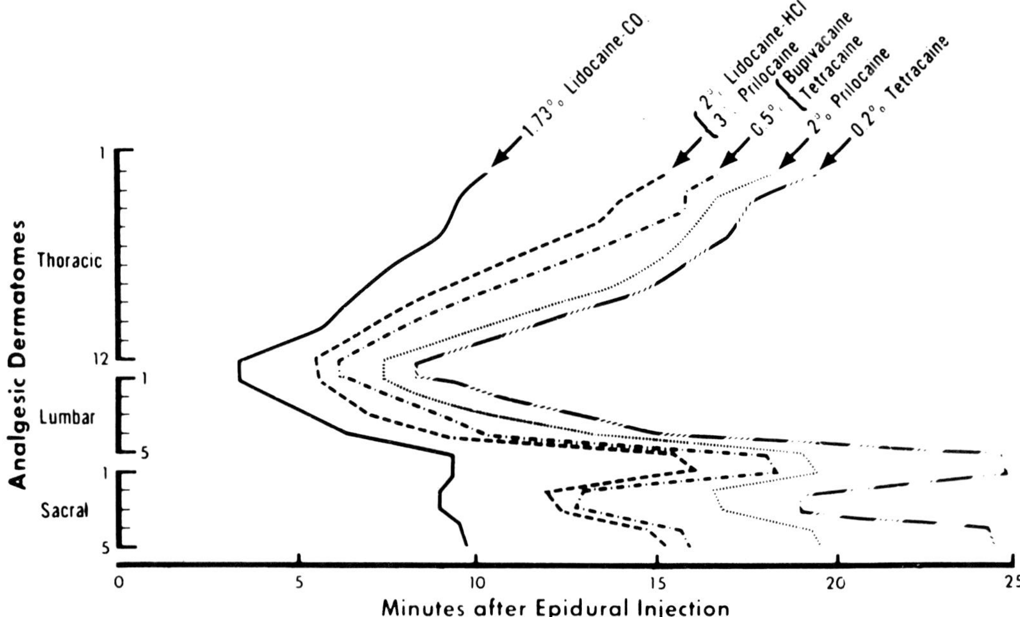

FIGURE 25-12. Spread of epidural sensory block over time following injection of various local anesthetic solutions at the L2-3 interspace. All solutions contained epinephrine 1:200,000. Sensory block spreads both cephalad and caudad from the site of injection with time. Note the delay in onset of block at the L5 and S1 dermatomes with all solutions tested. (Reprinted with permission from Bromage PR: Epidural Analgesia. Philadelphia, WB Saunders, 1978.)

Dose, Volume, and Concentration. Within the range typically used for surgical anesthesia, drug concentration is relatively unimportant in determining block spread. However, drug dose and volume are important variables determining both spread and quality of epidural block. If drug concentration is held constant, increasing the volume of local anesthetic (and thereby the dose) will result in significantly greater average spread and greater block density. However, the relationship is nonlinear. For example, doubling the volume and dose of 1.5% lidocaine or 0.75% bupivacaine from 10 mL to 20 mL has been shown to increase spread by only three to four spinal segments.[115,116] Volume appears to be important in determining block spread independent of drug dose, but again the relationship is nonlinear. Erdemir et al showed that tripling the injected volume of lidocaine from 10 mL to 30 mL while holding the dose constant (300 mg) increased the cephalad extent of block by only 4.3 dermatomes.[117] This tendency toward greater spread is thought to be explained by the observation that increasing the volume of solution injected into the epidural space increases cephalad distribution.[118]

Position. When using a single-shot technique, maintaining patients in the lateral position during and after epidural injection of surgical doses of local anesthetics does not seem to have a clinically important effect on spread of the block from side to side.[119] Similarly, studies examining the effect of patient position on cephalad spread of epidural block have generally found that the effect of posture on spread is not clinically important.[120] Interestingly, Ponhold et al[121] demonstrated that maintaining a 30 degree head-up position significantly increased the frequency of adequate block at the L5 and S1 nerve roots even though there was no effect on the cephalad extent of anesthesia.

Patient Characteristics

Age. Most,[115,116,122–125] but not all,[126] studies that have examined the effect of age on epidural block have demonstrated greater spread in older patients. However, the effect of age is probably clinically significant only when comparing adults whose ages differ by three or more decades. Even so, the difference in block height is not likely to be more than 3 or 4 dermatomes. Greater spread in older patients is thought to be related to a less-compliant epidural space and diminished ability for epidural solutions to leak out of intervertebral foramina.[118,127] Both of these age-related changes would be expected to result in more extensive spread of solutions within the epidural space.

Height and Weight. The correlation between patient height[115,116,125,126] or weight[125,126] and spread of epidural block is weak and of little clinical significance except perhaps in patients who are extremely tall, extremely short, or morbidly obese.

Pregnancy. Studies examining the effect of pregnancy on spread of epidural block are conflicting. Some studies have demonstrated greater spread at term[128] and during early pregnancy,[129] suggesting that greater spread during pregnancy is not simply the result of anatomic changes associated with pregnancy. However, other studies have not found a significant difference in spread of epidural block between pregnant and nonpregnant women.[130,131]

Atherosclerosis. Atherosclerosis has been suggested as an important determinant of the spread of epidural block.[128] However, subsequent studies have failed to find any relationship between block spread and atherosclerosis.[116,122,132]

Given the myriad factors that have some effect on spread of epidural anesthesia, how should anesthesiologists choose an appropriate local anesthetic dose for a single-shot epidural block? A useful recommendation is to assume that a 20-mL volume of all local anesthetics intended for surgical anesthesia will produce a midthoracic block on average after lumbar injection. If there are multiple reasons to expect that the block may spread excessively in an individual patient (e.g., advanced age, obesity, very short stature, high injection site) or if the procedure does not require a high block, then reduce the dose accordingly. If there are multiple reasons to expect that the spread may be reduced from the average, then increase the volume accordingly. Obviously, choice of the appropriate local anesthetic dose is obviated if an epidural catheter is used. In this situation, begin with a lower dose than one anticipates will be needed and administer additional local anesthetic as necessary to extend the block to the desired level.

Onset

The onset of epidural block with all local anesthetics can usually be detected within 5 minutes in the dermatomes immediately surrounding the injection site. The time to peak effect differs somewhat among local anesthetics. Shorter acting drugs generally reach their maximum spread in 15 to 20 minutes, whereas longer acting drugs require 20 to 25 minutes. Increasing the dose of local anesthetic speeds the onset of both motor and sensory block.

Duration

Local Anesthetic. As with spinal anesthesia, choice of local anesthetic is the most important determinant of the duration of epidural block. Chloroprocaine is the shortest duration drug used for epidural anesthesia, lidocaine and mepivacaine provide blocks of intermediate duration, and bupivacaine, ropivacaine, and etidocaine produce the longest lasting epidural block. Table 25-5 lists local anesthetics commonly used for epidural block and approximate duration of surgical anesthesia. Of note, tetracaine and procaine are not generally used for epidural block because of the poor quality block that these drugs produce.

Importantly, when used epidurally some local anesthetics exhibit considerable separation in both the intensity and duration of sensory and motor block. Etidocaine produces the most intense motor block and is unusual among local anesthetics in that motor block may considerably outlast sensory block.[133] The phenomenon of the postoperative patient who is in pain yet still unable to move his or her legs has led some anesthesiologists to abandon etidocaine for epidural use. This is unfortunate because etidocaine's superior muscle relaxation is sometimes beneficial intraoperatively. Bupivacaine has the opposite sensorimotor profile in that low concentrations of bupivacaine produce sensory block that is relatively more intense than motor block. This separation of sensory and motor block underlies the common practice of using dilute bupivacaine solutions for epidural analgesia.

Dose. Increasing the dose of local anesthetic administered results in increased duration[115,134–136] and density[115,135,136] of epidural block.

Age. Studies that have evaluated the effect of age on epidural block duration are inconclusive. Veering et al.[124] found that duration of epidural block with plain bupivacaine was not significantly affected by age. Nydahl et al.[123] found that epidural block using bupivacaine with epinephrine was actually shorter in older patients. In contrast, Park et al.[122] found that epidural block using lidocaine with epinephrine was slightly but significantly longer in older patients. Additional studies are necessary to clarify the effect of age on duration of epidural block.

Adrenergic Agonists. Epinephrine, in a concentration of 5 mcg/mL (1:200,000), is the most common adrenergic agonist added to epidural local anesthetics. It has been shown to prolong the duration of lidocaine and mepivacaine epidural block by as much as 80%.[137] The mechanism by which epinephrine prolongs epidural block is not clear. Vasoconstrictors have been assumed to prolong block by producing local vasoconstriction and thus decreased local anesthetic clearance from the epidural space. The fact that epinephrine reduces peak plasma concentrations of some local anesthetics following epidural injection is considered to be supportive evidence of this mechanism. However, iv infusion of epinephrine also decreases peak plasma concentration of epidurally administered local anesthetics, presumably by increasing their volume of distribution.[138] Thus, it is unclear what role local vasoconstriction plays in epinephrine's ability to prolong epidural block. As discussed earlier for spinal anesthesia, prolongation of motor and sensory block may be due, in part, to direct inhibitory effects of epinephrine on sensory and motor neurons.

Epinephrine does not significantly prolong the duration of anesthesia when added to concentrated solutions of bupivacaine,[139,140] etidocaine,[135,140] or ropivacaine[141] that are generally used for surgical anesthesia. However, epinephrine does appear to prolong analgesia and improve the quality of block when added to more dilute solutions of these local anesthetics, such as those used for labor analgesia.[142–144]

Summary

The extent and duration of both spinal and epidural block are influenced by a number of variables, some of which are under the control of the anesthesiologist. Understanding the impact of these variables will allow the anesthesiologist to rationally select the most appropriate drug and dose for any clinical situation. However, even the most experienced anesthesiologist will still have blocks that are not adequate for the planned procedure. The frequency of failed blocks can be kept to a minimum if the clinician aims to produce blocks that are a little higher and a little longer than seems necessary. It is often easier to deal with a block that is too high or too long than to cover up for a block that is too low or too brief.

PHYSIOLOGY

Neurophysiology

The physiology of local anesthetic neural blockade is discussed in detail in Chapter 17. This section briefly presents aspects of the physiology of neural blockade that are unique to spinal and epidural anesthesia.

Site of Action

The site of action of spinal and epidural anesthesia is not precisely known. Following epidural administration, local anesthetic is found in the spinal nerves within the epidural space, in spinal nerve rootlets within the CSF, and in the spinal cord. Similarly, following intrathecal administration in animals, local anesthetic is found in all sites between the spinal nerve rootlets and the interior of the spinal cord.[145,146] Thus, neural blockade can potentially occur at any or all points along the neural pathways extending from the site of drug administration to the interior of the spinal cord.

In an interesting study in humans, Boswell et al demonstrated that patients are able to feel paresthesias during direct electrical stimulation of the spinal cord under spinal anesthesia.[147] Cortical evoked potentials from direct spinal cord stimulation were also maintained under spinal anesthesia, although amplitudes were decreased. In contrast, paresthesias and cortical evoked potentials from tibial nerve stimulation were abolished by spinal anesthesia. These investigators concluded that neural pathways within the spinal cord were largely intact during spinal anesthesia and that the spinal nerve rootlets were the principal site of neural blockade.

The site of epidural block is less well localized. Monkey studies suggest that epidural block occurs largely at sites within the spinal meninges, including the cauda equina nerve roots, dorsal root entry zone, and the long tracts of spinal cord white matter.[148] However, these findings are not entirely consistent with the segmental onset of epidural anesthesia (see Fig. 25-12) or with the limited segmental blocks that can be produced with small doses of lumbar epidural local anesthetics in humans. These clinical observations are most readily explained by block of the segmental spinal nerves as they traverse the epidural or paravertebral spaces. In reality, epidural block likely occurs at both extradural and subdural sites with extradural radicular block predominating early and subdural spinal block predominating later. This supposition is consistent with human studies by Urban who rigorously examined the anatomic pattern of analgesia that occurred during onset and regression of epidural block.[149] He concluded that local anesthetics initially acted on radicular structures followed later by actions within the spinal cord.

Interestingly, human studies demonstrate that somatosensory evoked potentials are maintained during epidural anesthesia, although amplitudes are decreased and latencies increased. This contrasts with spinal block in which evoked potentials are completely eliminated and supports the clinical impression that epidural block is generally less dense than that achieved with spinal anesthesia.

Differential Nerve Block

Differential block refers to a clinically important phenomenon in which nerve fibers subserving different functions display varying sensitivity to local anesthetic blockade. In vivo sympathetic nerve fibers appear to be blocked by the lowest concentration of local anesthetic followed in order by fibers responsible for pain, touch, and motor function. This observation has led to the widely held belief that differences in sensitivity to local anesthetic blockade is explained solely by differences in fiber diameter, with smaller diameter neurons exhibiting greater sensitivity than larger diameter neurons. While the mechanism for differential block in spinal and epidural anesthesia is not known, it is clear that fiber diameter is not the only, or perhaps not even the most important, factor contributing to differential block.[150,151] Differential block is also discussed in Chapter 17.

Differential block occurs with both peripheral nerve blocks and central neuraxial blocks. In the peripheral nervous system, differential block is a temporal phenomenon with sympathetic block occurring first followed in time by sensory and motor block. In contrast, with spinal and epidural anesthesia differential block is manifest as a spatial separation in the modalities blocked. This is seen most clearly with spinal anesthesia where sympathetic block may extend as many as 2 to 6 dermatomes higher than pin-prick sensation,[152] which in turn extends 2 to 3 dermatomes higher than motor block. This spatial separation is believed to result from a gradual decrease in local anesthetic concentration within the CSF as a function of distance from the site of injection. With epidural anesthesia, similar zones of differential sensory and sympathetic block are found.[153]

Perhaps the most troublesome consequence of differential block is the occasional patient who has intact touch and proprioception at the surgical site despite adequate blockade of pain sensation. Even the most stoic patients are likely to find this unpleasant and may lie in fear that the procedure will soon become painful. In no instance should the anesthesiologist downplay the distress this may cause patients. Reassurance and judicious sedation as necessary are usually sufficient to overcome this problem.

Another important neurophysiologic aspect of central neuroaxial block is that it produces sedation,[154] potentiates the effect of sedative hypnotic drugs,[155–157] and markedly decreases minimum alveolar concentration (MAC).[158] The mechanism(s) underlying these effects is not known but "deafferentation," that is, the loss of ascending sensory input to the brain, is commonly invoked as causative.

Cardiovascular Physiology

Cardiovascular side effects, principally hypotension and bradycardia, are arguably the most important and most common physiologic changes during spinal and epidural anesthesia. Understanding the homeostatic mechanisms responsible for control of blood pressure and heart rate is essential for understanding and treating the cardiovascular changes associated with spinal and epidural anesthesia.

Spinal Anesthesia

Blockade of sympathetic efferents is the principal mecha-
5 nism by which spinal anesthesia produces cardiovascular derangements. As would be expected, the incidence of significant hypotension or bradycardia is generally related to the extent of sympathetic blockade, which in turn parallels block height.[159,160] However, the severity of cardiovascular changes has been shown not to correlate with peak block height in one study[161] and to correlate poorly in another (Fig. 25-13).[159] Additional risk factors associated with hypotension include age >40 to 50 years, concurrent general anesthesia, obesity, hypovolemia, and addition of phenylephrine to the local anesthetic.[159,162]

Hypotension during spinal anesthesia is the result of both arterial and venodilation. Venodilation increases volume in capacitance vessels, thereby decreasing venous return and right-sided filling pressures.[161,163–165] This fall in preload is thought to be the principal cause of decreased cardiac output during high spinal anesthesia. Arterial dilation during spinal anesthesia results in significant decreases in total peripheral resistance (Fig. 25-14).[164,166] Thus, the hypotension that accompanies 30% to 40% of spinal anesthetics may be the result of reductions in afterload, reductions in cardiac output, or both (see Fig. 25-14).

Heart rate does not change significantly during spinal anesthesia in most patients (see Fig. 25-14). However, clinically significant bradycardia occasionally occurs with a reported incidence of 10% to 15%. As with hypotension, the risk of bradycardia increases with increasing block height.[159] Additional

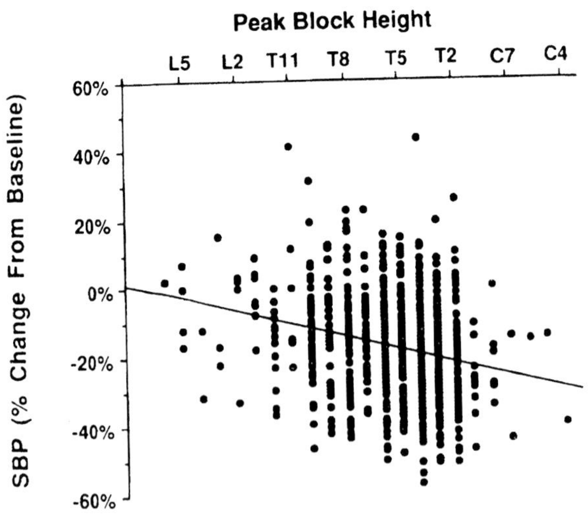

FIGURE 25-13. The relationship between peak block height and change in systolic blood pressure (SBP) during spinal anesthesia. Although there is a statistically significant correlation between block height and decrease in systolic blood pressure, the interindividual variability is so great that the relationship has little predictive value. This is reflected in the R^2 of 0.07 for the linear regression line. (From Carpenter RL, Caplan RA, Brown DL *et al*: Incidence and risk factors for side effects of spinal anesthesia. Anesthesiology 76:906, 1992.)

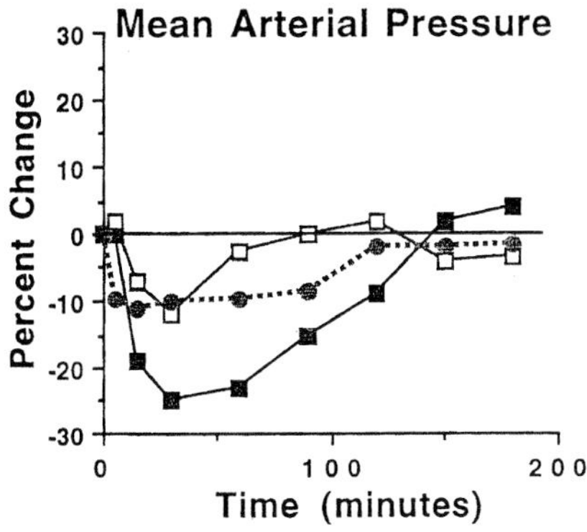

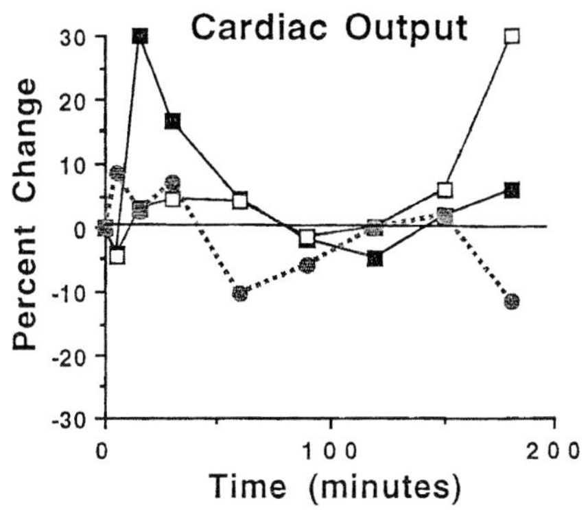

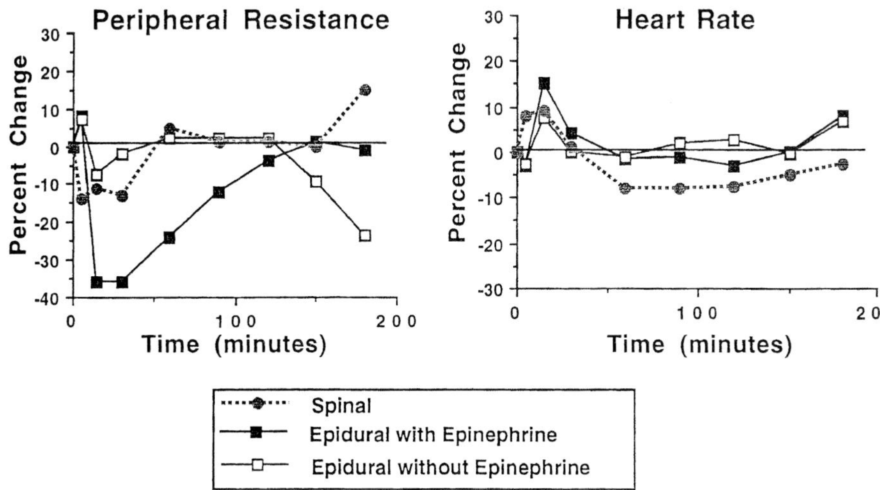

FIGURE 25-14. The cardiovascular effects of spinal and epidural anesthesia in volunteers with T5 blocks. The effects of spinal anesthesia and epidural anesthesia without epinephrine were generally comparable and are both qualitatively and quantitatively different from the effects of epidural anesthesia with epinephrine. (Modified from Bonica JJ, Kennedu WF Jr, Ward RJ, Tolas AG: A comparison of the effects of high subarachnoid and epidural anesthesia. Acta Anaesthesiol Scand [Suppl] 23:429, 1966.)

risk factors associated with bradycardia include age younger than 50 years, ASA 1 physical status, and concurrent use of βblockers.[159,162] The mechanism responsible for bradycardia is not clear. Blockade of the sympathetic cardioaccelerator fibers originating from T1-4 spinal segments is often suggested as the cause. The fact that bradycardia is more common with high blocks supports this mechanism. However, significant bradycardia sometimes occurs with blocks that are seemingly too low to block cardioaccelerator fibers. Diminished venous return has also been proposed as a cause of bradycardia during spinal anesthesia. Intracardiac stretch receptors have been shown to reflexively decrease heart rate when filling pressures fall.[167] Consistent with this mechanism, Jacobsen et al demonstrated a significant reduction in left ventricular volumes and heart rate during hypotensive episodes in two patients during epidural anesthesia.[168] They concluded that central volume depletion elicited a vagally mediated reflex slowing of heart rate. Similarly, Baron et al demonstrated that vagal activity is enhanced by decreased venous return during epidural anesthesia.[169] However, this mechanism does not operate at all times in all patients. Anzai and Nishikawa demonstrated significant heart rate increases in 40 patients who had their filling pressures suddenly decreased by body tilt during spinal anesthesia.[165] In reality, both blockade of cardioaccelerator fibers and decreased filling pressures as well as other unrecognized factors likely contribute to bradycardia during spinal anesthesia.

Although bradycardia is usually of moderate severity and well tolerated, there have been reports of sudden, unexplained, severe bradycardia and asystole during both spinal and epidural anesthesia.[170,171] In addition, multiple case reports document that spinal anesthesia can also produce second- and third-degree heart block[172–174] and that preexisting first-degree block may be a risk factor for progression to higher grade blocks during spinal anesthesia.[172] These reports document the need for continued vigilance with prompt and, if needed, aggressive treatment of the cardiovascular changes that accompany central neuraxial blockade.

Epidural Anesthesia

The hemodynamic changes produced by epidural anesthesia are largely dependent on whether or not epinephrine is added to the local anesthetic solution (see Fig. 25-14).[175] High epidural block with nonepinephrine-containing solutions results in decreased stroke volume, cardiac output, total peripheral resistance, and arterial pressure. The magnitude of these changes is generally less than that seen with comparable levels of spinal block.[175] As with spinal anesthesia, these hemodynamic changes are believed to result from venous and arterial dilation induced by sympathetic blockade. In contrast, when epinephrine-containing solutions are used for epidural anesthesia, stroke volume and cardiac output increase significantly (see Fig. 25-14).[175] However, peripheral resistance falls dramatically, resulting in a decrease in arterial pressure greater than that seen with nonepinephrine-containing solutions. β-2–adrenergic-mediated vasodilatation produced by low doses of absorbed epinephrine accounts for the greater decrease in peripheral vascular resistance and blood pressure. Decreased peripheral resistance may also contribute to the marked increase in cardiac output. However, epinephrine-induced venoconstriction with a resultant increase in venous return may also play an important role in increasing cardiac output.[176]

Treating Hemodynamic Changes

Treatment of hypotension secondary to spinal and epidural block must be aimed at the root causes: decreased cardiac output and/or decreased peripheral resistance. Bolus crystalloid administration has often been advocated as a means of restoring venous return and thus cardiac output during central neuraxial blockade. However, the effectiveness of this therapy in normovolemic patients is controversial. Prehydrating patients with 500 to 1,500 mL of crystalloid does not reliably prevent hypotension, but it has been shown to decrease the incidence of hypotension during spinal anesthesia in some,[177,178] but not all, studies.[160] Similarly, prehydration with crystalloid has been shown not to be effective in preventing hypotension during spinal anesthesia for cesarean section.[179] Thus, although judicious crystalloid preloading of patients before central neuraxial blocks may benefit some patients, this practice cannot be relied on to prevent clinically significant hypotension in all or even most patients. The reason for this is that increasing preload can only increase stroke volume, which has limited ability to restore blood pressure if heart rate or systemic vascular resistance remains low. In this regard colloids offer an interesting alternative to crystalloids for preloading before central neuraxial blocks. Marhofer and colleagues have shown that 500 mL 6% hetastarch actually increases systemic vascular resistance index (SVRI) in elderly patients having spinal anesthesia, while 1,500 mL crystalloid significantly decreases SVRI.[180]

Vasopressors are a more reliable approach to treating hypotension secondary to central neuraxial blockade. Drugs with both α- and β-adrenergic activity have been shown to be superior to pure α-agonists for correcting the cardiovascular derangements produced by spinal and epidural anesthesia.[181,182] Ephedrine is the drug most commonly used to treat hypotension. Ephedrine boluses of 5 to 10 mg increase blood pressure by restoring cardiac output and peripheral vascular resistance. Dopamine, in low to moderate doses, has also been shown to correct the hemodynamic changes induced by central neuraxial block.[183,184] Dopamine may be preferable to ephedrine for long-term infusion because tachyphylaxis can develop to repeated ephedrine boluses. Pure α-adrenergic agonists, most commonly phenylephrine, are also used to correct hypotension during spinal anesthesia. However, α-agonists increase blood pressure largely by increasing systemic vascular resistance, sometimes at the expense of further decreasing cardiac output.[182] In addition, phenylephrine boluses have been shown to produce transient left ventricular dysfunction during epidural anesthesia with nonepinephrine-containing local anesthetics.[185] A potential, but as yet unstudied, role for α-agonists may be to treat hypotension that occurs during epidural anesthesia with epinephrine-containing local anesthetics. Because the principal derangement in this situation is a marked decrease in systemic vascular resistance, α-agonists may be an appropriate choice for treating hypotension in this setting.

Deciding when to treat hemodynamic derangements during spinal and epidural anesthesia is perhaps more difficult than deciding how to treat them. There are currently no studies that clearly define the lower limit of acceptable blood pressure or heart rate for any group of patients. In the absence of such data, several authors have recommended treating blood pressure if it decreases more than 25% to 30% below baseline or in normotensive patients, if systolic pressure falls below 90 mm Hg. Recommendations regarding bradycardia suggest initiating treatment if heart rate falls below 50 to 60 beats/minutes-1. These recommendations are reasonable, although not universally applicable. Ultimately, anesthesiologists must decide what is an acceptable blood pressure and heart rate for an individual patient based on that patient's underlying medical condition.

Respiratory Physiology

Spinal and epidural blocks to midthoracic levels have little effect on pulmonary function in patients without preexisting lung disease. Drugs used perioperatively for sedation during spinal or epidural block likely have a larger impact on pulmonary function than the block per se. In particular, lung volumes, resting minute ventilation, dead space, arterial blood gas tensions, and shunt fraction show little or no change during spinal or epidural anesthesia. Interestingly, the ventilatory response to hypercapnia is actually increased by spinal and epidural block.[186,187]

High blocks associated with abdominal and intercostal muscle paralysis can impair ventilatory functions requiring active exhalation. For example, expiratory reserve volume, peak expiratory flow, and maximum minute ventilation may be significantly reduced by high spinal and epidural blocks. The negative impact of high blocks on active exhalation suggests caution when using spinal or epidural anesthesia in patients with obstructive pulmonary disease who may rely on their accessory muscles of respiration to maintain adequate ventilation.

Patients with high spinal or epidural blocks may complain of dyspnea despite normal or elevated minute ventilation. This likely results from the patient's inability to feel the chest wall move while breathing. This is understandably frightening to the patient, but reassurance is usually effective in alleviating their fear. The anesthesiologist must be alert to the possibility that the complaint of dyspnea stems from incipient respiratory failure secondary to respiratory muscle paralysis. A normal speaking voice, as opposed to a faint gasping voice, suggests ventilation is normal.

Gastrointestinal Physiology

The gastrointestinal effects of spinal and epidural anesthesia are largely the result of sympathetic blockade. The abdominal organs derive their sympathetic innervation from T6-L2. Blockade of these fibers results in unopposed parasympathetic activity by way of the vagus nerve. Consequently, secretions increase, sphincters relax, and the bowel becomes constricted. Some surgeons believe this improves surgical exposure. Nausea is a common complication of spinal and epidural anesthesia. The etiology is unknown but an increased incidence of nausea during spinal anesthesia is associated with blocks higher than T5, hypotension, opioid premedication, and a history of motion sickness.[159,162]

Endocrine-Metabolic Physiology

Surgery produces numerous endocrine and metabolic changes, including increased protein catabolism and oxygen consumption as well as increases in circulating concentrations of catecholamines, growth hormone, renin, angiotensin, thyroid-stimulating hormone, β-endorphin, glucose, and free fatty acids, among others.[1] These endocrine–metabolic changes have collectively been termed the "surgical stress response."

The mechanisms responsible for the stress response are complex and incompletely understood. However, afferent sensory information from the surgical site plays an important role in initiating and maintaining these changes.[1] Not surprisingly, spinal and epidural anesthesia have been shown to inhibit many of the endocrine–metabolic changes associated with the stress response. The inhibitory effect is greatest with lower abdominal and lower extremity procedures and least with upper abdominal and thoracic procedures.[1] The salutary effect of spinal and epidural anesthesia is believed to result from blockade of the afferent sensory information that helps initiate the stress response.

Although some aspects of the surgical stress response may be beneficial, it is generally viewed as maladaptive and possibly a contributor to postoperative morbidity and mortality.[1] Despite the ability of central neuraxial block to decrease the stress response, there is as yet no clear evidence that this results in decreased morbidity or mortality.

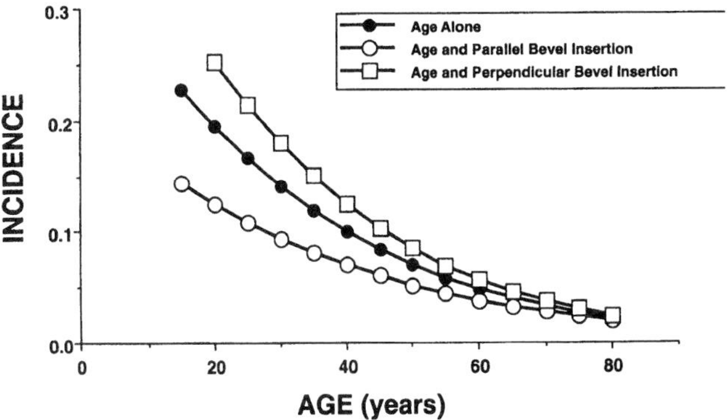

FIGURE 25-15. The incidence of postdural puncture headache decreases as patient age increases. When using beveled needles, the incidence is higher than average at any given age if the needle is inserted perpendicular to the spinal meninges and lower if inserted parallel to the spinal meninges. (Modified from Lybecker H, Møller JT, May O, Nielsen HK: Incidence and prediction of post-dural puncture headache: A prospective study of 1021 spinal anesthesias. Anesth Analg 70:389, 1990.)

COMPLICATIONS

Backache

Although postoperative backache occurs following general anesthesia, it is more common following epidural and spinal anesthesia.[188] Compared with spinal anesthesia, back pain following epidural anesthesia is more common (11% versus 30%) and of longer duration.[189] Importantly, back pain has been cited in one study as the most common reason for patients to refuse future epidural block.[189] The etiology of backache is not clear, although needle trauma, local anesthetic irritation, and ligamentous strain secondary to muscle relaxation have been offered as explanations.

Postdural Puncture Headache

Postdural puncture headache is a common complication of spinal anesthesia with a reported incidence as high as 25% in some studies. The risk of PDPH is less with epidural anesthesia, but it occurs in up to 50% of young patients following accidental meningeal puncture with large diameter epidural needles. The headache is characteristically mild or absent when the patient is supine, but head elevation rapidly leads to a severe fronto-occipital headache, which again improves on returning to the supine position. Occasionally cranial nerve symptoms (e.g., diploplia, tinnitis) and nausea and vomiting are also present. The headache is believed to result from the loss of CSF through the meningeal needle hole resulting in decreased buoyant support for the brain. In the upright position the brain sags in the cranial vault putting traction on pain-sensitive structures. Traction on cranial nerves is believed to cause the cranial nerve palsies occasionally seen.

The incidence of PDPH decreases with increasing age (Fig. 25-15) and with the use of small diameter spinal needles with noncutting tips.[190,191] Inserting cutting needles with the bevel aligned parallel to the long axis of the meninges has also been shown to decrease the incidence of PDPH.[191,192] Some authors have suggested that parallel insertion spreads dural fibers, whereas perpendicular insertion cuts the fibers resulting in a larger meningeal hole. However, the collagen fibers of the dura mater are arranged randomly; therefore, as many fibers will be cut with parallel insertion as with perpendicular insertion. A more likely explanation arises from the fact that the dura mater is under longitudinal tension. Thus, a slit-like hole oriented perpendicular to this longitudinal tension will tend to be pulled open while a hole oriented parallel to this tension will be pulled closed. Some studies have suggested that women are at greater risk of developing PDPH. However, if age differences are accounted for, there does not appear to be a gender difference in the incidence of PDPH.[191] Folklore aside, remaining supine following meningeal puncture does not decrease the incidence of PDPH. Finally, use of fluid, instead of air, for loss of resistance during attempted epidural anesthesia does not alter the risk of accidental meningeal puncture, but does markedly decrease the risk of subsequently developing PDPH.[27] PDPH usually resolves spontaneously in a few days to a week for most patients. However, there are reports of PDPH persisting for months following meningeal puncture. Initial treatment is appropriately conservative if this meets the patient's needs. Bed rest and analgesics as necessary are the mainstay of conservative treatment. Caffeine has also been shown to produce short-term symptomatic relief.[193]

Epidural Blood Patch. Patients who are unable or unwilling to await spontaneous resolution should be offered epidural blood patch. Epidural blood patch is believed to form a clot over the meningeal hole, thereby preventing further CSF leak while the meningeal rent heals. Ten to 20 mL of autologous blood is aseptically injected into epidural space at or near the interspace at which the meningeal puncture occurred. This is effective in relieving symptoms within 1 to 24 hours in 85% to 95% of patients; ~90% of patients who fail an initial blood patch will respond to a second patch. The most common side effects of blood patch are backache and radicular pain, although transient bradycardia and cranial nerve palsies have also been reported.

The timing of epidural blood patch has been controversial. Early studies suggested that prophylactic blood patch in patients at high risk for PDPH was ineffective. This led several authors to suggest that blood patch should not be performed before patients develop symptoms of PDPH. Subsequent studies, which used larger volumes of blood in the epidural space (15 to 20 mL), have shown that prophylactic blood patch is effective in preventing PDPH in patients in whom the meninges were accidentally punctured during attempted epidural anesthesia.[194,195] Prophylactic blood patch is not appropriate for most patients but is worth considering in high-risk outpatients for whom a return trip to the hospital for epidural blood patch would be difficult.

Epidurally administered fibrin glue has been shown to be an effective alternative to blood administration for treatment of PDPH.[196] Whether it is superior to blood requires further study but it may be an attractive alternative for some patients. In the future it may be necessary to drop the term "blood patch" in favor of "meningeal patch."

Hearing Loss

Lamberg et al demonstrated that a transient (1 to 3 days) mild decrease in hearing acuity (greater than 10 dB) is common after spinal anesthesia with an incidence of roughly 40% and a 3:1 female:male predominance.[197] Similarly, Gültekin et al[198] demonstrated a 45% incidence of hearing impairment in subjects undergoing prilocaine spinal anesthesia but a much lower incidence (18%) in patients having bupivacaine spinal anesthesia. The mechanism of hearing loss in these studies is unclear, but the marked female predominance, the absence of PDPH, and the difference in incidence between prilocaine and bupivacaine suggest that CSF leak is not the cause.

Systemic Toxicity

Systemic toxicity of local anesthetics is discussed in detail in Chapter 17. Systemic toxicity does not occur with spinal anesthesia because the drug doses used are too low to cause toxic reactions even if injected intravenously. Both CNS and cardiovascular toxicity may occur during epidural anesthesia. CNS toxicity may result from local anesthetic absorption from the epidural space but more commonly occurs following accidental intravascular injection of local anesthetic. In contrast, cardiovascular toxicity from epidural local anesthetics can only occur unintended intravascular injection because the plasma concentrations of local anesthetics required to produce serious cardiovascular toxicity are very high. An adequate IV test dose and incremental injection of local anesthetics are the most important methods to prevent both CNS and cardiovascular toxicity during epidural anesthesia.

Total Spinal

Total spinal anesthesia occurs when local anesthetic spreads high enough to block the entire spinal cord and occasionally the brainstem during either spinal or epidural anesthesia. Profound hypotension and bradycardia are common secondary to complete sympathetic blockade. Respiratory arrest may occur as a result of respiratory muscle paralysis or dysfunction of brainstem respiratory control centers. Management includes vasopressors, atropine, and fluids as necessary to support the cardiovascular system, plus oxygen and controlled ventilation. If the cardiovascular and respiratory consequences are managed appropriately, total spinal block will resolve without sequelae.

Neurologic Injury

Serious neurologic injury is a rare but widely feared complication of epidural and spinal anesthesia. Multiple large series of spinal and epidural anesthesia report that neurologic injury occurs in ~0.03% to 0.1% of all central neuraxial blocks, although in most of these series the block was not clearly proven to be causative.[199] Persistent paresthesias and limited motor weakness are the most common injuries, although paraplegia and diffuse injury to cauda equina roots (*cauda equina syndrome*) do occur rarely. Injury may result from direct needle trauma to the spinal cord or spinal nerves, from spinal cord ischemia, from accidental injection of neurotoxic drugs or chemicals, from introduction of bacteria into the subarachnoid or epidural space, or very rarely from epidural hematoma.[199]

Importantly, local anesthetics intended for epidural and intrathecal use can themselves be neurotoxic in concentrations used clinically.[200] In particular, hyperbaric 5% lidocaine has been implicated as a cause of multiple cases of cauda equina syndrome following subarachnoid injection through
6 small-bore ("microspinal") catheters during continuous spinal anesthesia.[201] Hyperbaric solutions injected through these high-resistance catheters have been shown to produce very little turbulence and thus poor mixing of the local anesthetic within CSF.[202] Nerve injury is believed to result from pooling of toxic concentrations of undiluted lidocaine around dependent cauda equina nerve roots. Consequently, the U.S. Food and Drug Administration has banned the use of these small-gauge catheters for continuous spinal anesthesia. Although the combination of microspinal catheters and high concentrations of lidocaine have clearly been implicated in causing cauda equina syndrome, this complication has also occurred when using larger (20 gauge) catheters,[201] 2% lidocaine,[203] and 0.5% tetracaine.[201] A common thread in all of these reports has been the apparent maldistribution of the local anesthetic within the CSF. Maldistribution should be suspected whenever spinal block is unexpectedly restricted and maneuvers, such as altering patient position or drug baricity, should be employed to improve drug distribution before additional drug is injected through a continuous spinal catheter. If these maneuvers fail to improve drug distribution, an alternative anesthetic technique should be employed.

The mechanism by which local anesthetics produce cauda equina syndrome is not yet clear; however, in vitro evidence suggests that local anesthetics produce excitotoxic damage by depolarizing neurons and increasing intracellular calcium concentrations.[204] It is also unclear as yet whether adjuncts added to local anesthetics, for example, epinephrine, contribute to cauda equina syndrome. However, based on animal studies, it has been argued that epinephrine should not be added to intrathecal lidocaine.[205] Rather, if a prolonged duration of spinal anesthesia is necessary, then a longer acting drug like bupivacaine should be used.

Transient Neurologic Symptoms (TNS). In addition to cauda equina syndrome, the occurrence of *transient neurologic symptoms* (TNS) or *transient radicular irritation* (TRI) has also emerged as a concern following central neuraxial blockade. TRI is defined as pain, dysesthesia, or both in the legs or buttocks after spinal anesthesia and was first proposed as a recognizable entity by Schneider.[206] All local anesthetics have been shown to cause TRI although the risk appears to be greater with lidocaine than other local anesthetics.[207–213]

In a large epidemiologic study of nearly 2,000 patients, Freedman et al characterized the clinical picture of TRI.[214] They found that patients receiving lidocaine were significantly more likely to develop TRI than were patients receiving spinal tetracaine or bupivacaine although TRI did occur with these latter two drugs as well. Additional risk factors for TRI included surgery in the lithotomy position when lidocaine, but not when bupivacaine or tetracaine, was used, and outpatient status; obesity was a borderline risk factor. Variables shown not to increase the risk of TRI included lidocaine dose, type of spinal needle, addition of epinephrine to lidocaine, paresthesia, hypotension, and blood tinged CSF among others. In a separate study, Sakura has shown that the addition of phenylephrine is a risk factor for TRI when using 0.5% tetracaine for spinal anesthesia.[215]

Pain from TRI was not trivial, with the majority of patients rating it as moderate (VAS = 4 to 7/10). The pain usually resolved spontaneously within 72 hours but a very few patients required 6 months.[214]

The mechanism responsible for TRI is unknown; however, it would be inappropriate to conclude that TRI is simply a milder manifestation of cauda equina syndrome. Differences in clinical presentation, risk factors, and so on suggest that these are not simply two points along a continuum of the same process.

Chloroprocaine

Chloroprocaine was introduced into clinical practice in 1951 and was used for spinal anesthesia beginning in that year. In the early 1980s, however, clinicians reported multiple cases of neurological injury following intrathecal injection of chloroprocaine. Importantly, the chloroprocaine solution available at the time contained either methylparaben as an antimicrobial or bisulfite as an antioxidant. Subsequent animal studies demonstrated that bisulfite and metabisulfite at low pH were capable of causing neurological injury, but that plain chloroprocaine was not. Nonetheless, concern about the potential for chloroprocaine-mediated neurotoxicity led to its nearly complete abandonment as a spinal anesthetic. This occurred despite the fact that the U.S. Food and Drug Administration had concluded that chloroprocaine was not more neurotoxic than lidocaine, bupivacaine, or mepivacaine. This abandonment of chloroprocaine for spinal use was facilitated by the clinical impression that lidocaine was a safer alternative for short duration spinal anesthetics.

However, we now recognize that lidocaine is not without risk of neurological toxicity. This observation, coupled with the fact that a preservative-free chloroprocaine formulation is now available, has led to a reevaluation of chloroprocaine as a short-acting spinal anesthetic. In 2004, Kouri and Kopacz compared the block characteristics of 40 mg plain 2% lidocaine with
7 40 mg plain 2% preservative-free chloroprocaine in humans using a double-blind, randomized crossover study design.[216] They found that both drugs produced identical average block heights (T8), but that chloroprocaine resulted in more rapid resolution of sensory block (103 ± 13 minutes versus 126 ± 16 minutes.) and faster attainment of discharge criteria (104 ± 12 minutes versus 134 ± 14 minutes). In addition, seven of eight volunteers experienced TNS following intrathecal lidocaine while none experienced TNS following 2% chloroprocaine. In other studies from the same research group, chloroprocaine spinal block height and duration were shown to be positively correlated with chloroprocaine dose[217] and addition of dextrose was shown not to alter spinal block characteristics except that it increased postvoid bladder volume.[218] This group also performed studies to determine the effect of epinephrine and fentanyl as block-prolonging adjuvants to spinal chloroprocaine. Vath and Kopacz found that the addition of 20 μg fentanyl to 40 mg chloroprocaine increased average peak block height (T5 versus T9), prolonged the time for sensory block regression to L1 (78 ± 7 minutes versus 53 ± 19), and modestly increased the time to complete regression (104 ± 7 minutes versus 95 ± 9 minutes).[219] Interestingly, Smith et al. found that epinephrine (0.2 mg) increased chloroprocaine block duration but that it's use was associated with a high incidence of myalgia, arthralgia, malaise, and anorexia that lasted up to 48 hours.[217] The authors had no explanation for the epinephrine-associated side effects, but recommended against its use with intrathecal chloroprocaine.

Thus, these studies, coupled with concerns about the potential for lidocaine-mediated neurotoxicity, raise the possibility that chloroprocaine will reenter the mainstream as a spinal anesthetic, especially for ambulatory anesthesia. Additional, larger studies demonstrating chloroprocaine's safety will help to clarify this drug's role in spinal anesthesia.

Importantly, as of this writing, chloroprocaine is not specifically indicated for spinal anesthesia, therefore, its use is "off-label." But then so to is the use of multiple drugs that are routinely administered intrathecally, including plain bupivacaine, fentanyl, and sufentanil.

Spinal Hematoma

Spinal hematoma is a rare but potentially devastating complication of spinal and epidural anesthesia, with an incidence estimated to be less than 1 in 150,000. Patients most commonly present with numbness or lower extremity weakness, a fact that can make early detection difficult in patients receiving perioperative spinal local anesthetics for pain control. Early detection is critical because a delay of more than 8 hours in decompressing the spine reduces the odds of good recovery.[220]

Coagulation defects are the principal risk factor for epidural hematoma. This raises the legitimate question as to how
8 to treat patients who are or who will be anticoagulated. This issue has been addressed in a Consensus Statement from the American Society for Regional Anesthesia and Pain Medicine[221] and the recommendations presented here are taken from this consensus statement. In brief, patients taking nonsteroidal anti-inflammatory drugs with antiplatelet effects (e.g., cyclooxygenase-1 inhibitors) or receiving subcutaneous unfractionated heparin for DVT prophylaxis are not viewed as being at increased risk of spinal hematoma.

In contrast, other classes of antiplatelet drugs, like thienopryidine derivatives (e.g., ticlopidine, clopidogrel) and GP IIb/IIIa antagonists (e.g., abciximab, eptifibitide, tirofiban) have a more potent effect on platelet aggregation and neuraxial block should generally not be performed in patients taking these or similar medications. Further, the consensus statement recommends that ticlopidine be discontinued for 2 weeks and clopidogrel for 1 week before performing central neuraxial blocks. The GP IIb/IIIa antagonists have a shorter duration of action, thus it is recommended that abciximab should be discontinued 24 to 48 hours before central neuraxial block and eptifibitide, and tirofiban 4 to 8 hours beforehand.

Patients receiving fractionated low-molecular weight heparin (e.g., enoxaprin, dalteparin, tinzaparin) are considered to be at increased risk of spinal hematoma. Patients receiving these drugs preoperatively at thromboprophylactic doses should have the drug held for 10 to 12 hours before central neuraxial block. At higher doses, such as those used to treat established DVT, central neuraxial block should be delayed for 24 hours after the last dose. For patients in whom low-molecular-weight heparin is begun after surgery, single-shot central neuraxial blocks are not contraindicated provided that the first low-molecular-weight heparin dose is not administered until 24 hours postoperatively if using a twice daily dosing regimen and 6 to 8 hours if using a once-daily dosing regimen. If an indwelling central neuraxial catheter is in place, it should not be removed until 10 to 12 hours after the last low-molecular-weight heparin dose and the subsequent doses should not begin until at least 2 hours after catheter removal.

Patients who are "fully anticoagulated" (i.e., have elevated PT or PTT) or who are receiving thrombolytic or fibrinolytic therapy are considered to be at increased risk of spinal hematoma. These patients should not receive central neuraxial block except in very unusual circumstances where other options are not viable.

Importantly for those patients who may have an epidural or intrathecal catheter placed, its removal is nearly as great a risk for spinal hematoma as its insertion and the timing of removal and anticoagulation should be coordinated. Also, drugs/regimens not considered to put patients at increased risk of neuraxial bleeding when used alone (e.g., minidose unfractionated heparin and NSAIDS) may in fact increase risk when combined. This discussion is necessarily abbreviated and the reader who confronts these issues clinically should review the complete consensus statement.

CONTRAINDICATIONS

The only absolute contraindication to spinal or epidural anesthesia is patient refusal. However, several preexisting conditions increase the relative risk of these techniques and the anesthesiologist must carefully weigh the expected benefits before proceeding. Some conditions that increase the apparent risk of central neuraxial block include the following:

1. Hypovolemia or shock increase the risk of hypotension.
2. Increased intracranial pressure increases the risk of brain herniation when CSF is lost through the needle, or if a further increase in intracranial pressure follows injection of large volumes of solution into the epidural or subarachnoid spaces.
3. Coagulopathy or thrombocytopenia increase the risk of epidural hematoma.
4. Sepsis increases the risk of meningitis.
5. Infection at the puncture site increases the risk of meningitis.

Preexisting neurologic disease, particularly diseases that wax and wane (e.g., multiple sclerosis), have been considered a contraindication to central-neuraxial block by some authors. However, there is no evidence to suggest that spinal or epidural anesthesia alters the course of any preexisting neurologic disease. Recommendations to avoid regional anesthesia in these patients stem largely from a medicolegal concern that the anesthetic may be incorrectly blamed for any subsequent worsening of the patient's preexisting condition. Although this is a legitimate concern, it is not a reason to avoid central-neuraxial block if this is an otherwise appropriate choice.

SPINAL OR EPIDURAL ANESTHESIA?

Spinal and epidural anesthesia each have advantages and disadvantages that may make one or the other technique better suited to a particular patient or procedure. Controlled studies comparing both techniques for surgical anesthesia have consistently found that spinal anesthesia takes less time to perform, produces more rapid onset of better quality sensorimotor block, and is associated with less pain during surgery. Despite these important advantages of spinal anesthesia, epidural anesthesia offers advantages, too. Chief among them are the lower risk of PDPH, less hypotension if epinephrine is not added to the local anesthetic, the ability to prolong or extend the block via an indwelling catheter, and the option of using an epidural catheter to provide postoperative analgesia.

References

1. Kehlet H: The stress response to surgery: Release mechanisms and the modifying effect of pain relief. Acta Chir Scand Suppl 550:22, 1988
2. Modig J, Borg T, Karlström G, Maripuu E, Sahlstedt B: Thromboembolism after total hip replacement: Role of epidural and general anesthesia. Anesth Analg 62:174, 1983
3. Thornburn J, Louden J, Vallance R: Spinal and general anesthesia in total hip replacement: Frequency of deep vein thrombosis. Br J Anaesth 52:1117, 1980
4. Christopherson R, Beattie C *et al:* Perioperative morbidity in patients randomized to epidural or general anesthesia for lower extremity vascular surgery. Anesthesiology 79:422, 1993
5. Rosenfeld B, Beattie C, Christopherson R *et al:* The effects of different anesthetic regimens on fibrinolysis and the development of postoperative arterial thrombosis. Anesthesiology 79:435, 1993
6. Yeager M, Glass D, Neff R, Brinck-Johnsen T: Epidural anesthesia and analgesia in high-risk surgical patients. Anesthesiology 66:729, 1987
7. Moraca RJ, Sheldon DG, Thirlby RC: The role of epidural anesthesia and analgesia in surgical practice. Ann Surg 238:663, 2003
8. Block BM, Liu SS, Rowlingson AJ, Cowan AR, Cowan JA, Jr., Wu CL: Efficacy of postoperative epidural analgesia: A meta-analysis. J Am Med Assoc 290:2455, 2003
9. Zarzur E: Anatomic studies of the human lumbar ligamentum flavum. Anesth Analg 63:499, 1984
10. Hogan Q: Lumbar epidural anatomy. A new look by cryomicrotome section. Anesthesiology 75:767, 1991
11. Meijenhorst GC: Computed tomography of the lumbar epidural veins. Radiology 145:687, 1982
12. Bernards CM, Shen DD, Sterling ES *et al:* Epidural, cerebrospinal fluid, and plasma pharmacokinetics of epidural opioids (part 1): Differences among opioids. Anesthesiology 99(2):455, 2003
13. Tucker G, Mather L: Properties, absorption, and disposition of local anesthetic agents. In Cousins M, Bridenbaugh P (eds): Neural Blockade in Clinical Anesthesia and Management of Pain, 2nd ed, pp 47–110. Philadelphia, JB Lippincott,1988
14. Fink BR, Walker S: Orientation of fibers in human dorsal lumbar dura mater in relation to lumbar puncture. Anesth Analg 69:768, 1989
15. Blomberg R: The dorsomedian connective tissue band in the lumbar epidural space of humans: An anatomical study using epiduroscopy in autopsy cases. Anesth Analg 65:747, 1986
16. Savolaine ER, Pandya JB, Greenblatt SH, Conover SR: Anatomy of the human lumbar epidural space: New insights using CT-epidurography. Anesthesiology 68:217, 1988
17. Hogan Q: Epidural catheter tip position and distribution of injectate evaluated by computed tomography. Anesthesiology 90:964, 1999
18. Manchada V, Murad S, Shilyansky G, Mehringer M: Unusual clinical course of accidental subdural local anesthetic injection. Anesth Analg 62:1124, 1983
19. Lubenow T, Keh-Wong E, Kristof K, Ivankovich O, Ivankovich A: Inadvertant subdural injection: A complication of epidural block. Anesth Analg 67:175, 1988
20. Jones M, Newton T: Inadvertent extra-arachnoid injections in myelography. Radiology 80:818, 1983
21. Bernards C, Hill H: Morphine and alfentanil permeability through the spinal dura, arachnoid and pia mater of dogs and monkeys. Anesthesiology 73:1214, 1990
22. Bernards C, Hill H: The spinal nerve root sleeve is not a preferred route for redistribution of drugs from the epidural space to the spinal cord. Anesthesiology 75:827, 1991
23. Reiman A, Anson B: Vertebral level of termination of the spinal cord with report of a case of sacral cord. Anat Rec 88:127, 1944
24. Drummond G, Scott D: Deflection of spinal needles by the bevel. Anaesthesia 35:854, 1980
25. Moore JM, Liu SS, Neal JM: Premedication with fentanyl and midazolam decreases the reliability of intravenous lidocaine test dose. Anesth Analg 86:1015, 1998
26. Evron S, Sessler D, Sadan O, Boaz M, Glezerman M, Ezri T: Identification of the epidural space: Loss of resistance with air, lidocaine, or the combination of air and lidocaine. Anesth Analg 99:245, 1999
27. Aida S, Taga K, Yamakura T, Endoh H, Shimoji K: Headache after attempted epidural block: The role of intrathecal air. Anesthesiology 88:76, 1998
28. Asato F, Goto F: Radiographic findings of unilateral epidural block. Anesth Analg 83:519, 1996
29. Leighton BL, Norris MC, DeSinome CA, Rosko T, Gross JB: The air test as a clinically useful indicator of intravenously placed epidural catheters. Anesthesiology 73:610, 1990
30. Mackie K, Lam A: Epinephrine-containing test dose during beta-blockade. J Clin Monit 7:213, 1991
31. Moore D, Batra M: The components of an effective test dose prior to epidural block. Anesthesiology 55:693, 1981
32. Guinard J, Mulroy M, Carpenter R, Knopes K: Test doses: Optimal epinephrine content with and without acute beta-adrenergic blockade. Anesthesiology 73:386, 1990
33. Liu SS: Hemodynamic responses to an epinephrine test dose in adults during epidural or combined epidural-general anesthesia. Anesth Analg 83:97, 1996
34. Leighton B, DeSimone C, Norris M, Chayen B: Isoproterenol is an effective marker of intravenous injection in laboring women. Anesthesiology 71:206, 1989
35. Leighton BL, Norris MC, Sosis M, Epstein R, Chayen B, Larijani GE: Limitations of epinephrine as a marker of intravascular injection in laboring women. Anesthesiology 66:688, 1987
36. Takiguchi T, Okano T, Egawa H, Okubo Y, Saito K, Kitajima T: The effect of epidural saline injection on analgesic level during combined spinal and epidural anesthesia assessed clinically and myelographically [see comments]. Anesth Analg 85:1097, 1997

37. Stienstra R, Dahan A, Alhadi BZ, van Kleef JW, Burm AG: Mechanism of action of an epidural top-up in combined spinal epidural anesthesia. Anesth Analg 83:382, 1996
38. Stienstra R, Dilrosun-Alhadi BZ, Dahan A, van Kleef JW, Veering BT, Burm AG: The epidural "top-up" in combined spinal-epidural anesthesia: The effect of volume versus dose. Anesth Analg 88:810, 1999
39. Myint Y, Bailey P, Milne B: Cardiorespiratory arrest following combined spinal epidural anaesthesia. Anaesthesia 48:684, 1993
40. Bernards C, Kopacz D, Michel M: Effect of needle puncture on morphine and lidocaine flux through the spinal meninges of the monkey. Anesthesiology 80:853, 1994
41. Hodgkinson R, Husain FJ: Obesity, gravity, and spread of epidural anesthesia. Anesth Analg 60:421, 1981
42. Lee A, Ray D, Littlewood D, Wildsmith J: Effect of dextrose concentration on the intrathecal spread of amethocaine. Br J Anaesth 61:135, 1988
43. Chambers WA, Edstrom HH, Scott DB: Effect of baricity on spinal anaesthesia with bupivacaine. Br J Anaesth 53:279, 1981
44. Bannister J, McClure JH, Wildsmith JA: Effect of glucose concentration on the intrathecal spread of 0.5% bupivacaine. Br J Anaesth 64:232, 1990
45. Povey HM, Jacobsen J, Westergaard-Nielsen J: Subarachnoid analgesia with hyperbaric 0.5% bupivacaine: Effect of a 60-min period of sitting. Acta Anaesthesiol Scand 33:295, 1989
46. Povey HM, Olsen PA, Pihl H: Spinal analgesia with hyperbaric 0.5% bupivacaine: Effects of different patient positions. Acta Anaesthesiol Scand 31:616, 1987
47. Sinclair CJ, Scott DB, Edström H: Effect of the Trendelenberg position on spinal anaesthesia with hyperbaric bupivacaine. Br J Anaesth 54:497, 1982
48. Martin-Salvaj G, Van Gessel E, Forster A, Schweizer A, Iselin-Chaves I, Gamulin Z: Influence of duration of lateral decubitus on the spread of hyperbaric tetracaine during spinal anesthesia: A prospective time-response study. Anesth Analg 79:1107, 1994
49. Smith T: The lumbar spine and subarachnoid block. Anesthesiology 29:60, 1968
50. Logan MR, Drummond GB: Spinal anesthesia and lumbar lordosis. Anesth Analg 67:338, 1988
51. Bodily M, Carpenter R, Owens B: Lidocaine 0.5% spinal anaesthesia: A hypobaric solution for short-stay perirectal surgery. Can J Anaesth 39:770, 1992
52. Brown DT, Wildsmith JA, Covino BG, Scott DB: Effect of baricity on spinal anesthesia with amethocaine. Br J Anaesth 52:589, 1980
53. Cummings GC, Bamber DB, Edstrom HH, Rubin AP: Subarachnoid blockade with bupivacaine. A comparison with cinchocaine. Br J Anaesth 56:573, 1984
54. Møller IW, Fernandes A, Edström HH: Subarachnoid anaesthesia with 0.5% bupivacaine: Effects of density. Br J Anaesth 56:1191, 1984
55. Logan MR, McClure JH, Wildsmith JA: Plain bupivacaine: An unpredictable spinal anaesthetic agent. Br J Anaesth 58:292, 1986
56. McKeown DW, Stewart K, Littlewood DG, Wildsmith JA: Spinal anesthesia with plain solutions of lidocaine (2%) and bupivacaine (0.5%). Regional Anesth 11:68, 1986
57. Cameron AE, Arnold RW, Ghorisa MW, Jamieson V: Spinal analgesia using bupivacaine 0.5% plain. Variation in the extent of the block with patient age. Anaesthesia 36:318, 1981
58. Kalso E, Tuominen M, Rosenberg PH: Effect of posture and some c.s.f. characteristics on spinal anaesthesia with isobaric 0.5% bupivacaine. Br J Anaesth 54:1179, 1982
59. Tuominen M, Kalso E, Rosenberg P: Effects of posture on the spread of spinal anaesthesia with isobaric 0.75% or 0.5% bupivacaine. Br J Anaesth 54:313, 1982
60. Stienstra R, van Poorten JF: The temperature of bupivacaine 0.5% affects the sensory level of spinal anesthesia. Anesth Analg 67:272, 1988
61. McClure JH, Brown DT, Wildsmith JA: Effect of injected volume and speed of injection on the spread of spinal anaesthesia with isobaric amethocaine. Br J Anaesth 54:917, 1982
62. Van Zundert AA, De Wolf AM: Extent of anesthesia and hemodynamic effects after subarachnoid administration of bupivacaine with epinephrine. Anesth Analg 67:784, 1988
63. Nielsen TH, Kristoffersen E, Olsen KH, Larsen HV, Husegaard HC, Wernberg M: Plain bupivacaine: 0.5% or 0.25% for spinal analgesia? Br J Anaesth 62:164, 1989
64. Bengtsson M, Malmqvist LA, Edström HH: Spinal analgesia with glucose-free bupivacaine—Effects of volume and concentration. Acta Anaesthesiol Scand 28:583, 1984
65. Blomqvist H, Nilsson A, Arweström E: Spinal anaesthesia with 15 mg bupivacaine 0.25% and 0.5%. Regional Anesth 13:165, 1988
66. Mukkada TA, Bridenbaugh PO, Singh P, Edström HH: Effects of dose, volume, and concentration of glucose-free bupivacaine in spinal anesthesia. Regional Anesth 11:98, 1986
67. Sheskey MC, Rocco AG, Bizzarri-Schmid M, Francis DM, Edstrom H, Covino BG: A dose-response study of bupivacaine for spinal anesthesia. Anesth Analg 62:931, 1983
68. Wildsmith J, McClure J, Brown D, Scott D: Effects of posture on the spread of isobaric and hyperbaric amethocaine. Br J Anaesth 53:273, 1981
69. Pflug AE, Aasheim GM, Beck HA: Spinal anesthesia: Bupivacaine versus tetracaine. Anesth Analg 55:489, 1976
70. Sundnes KO, Vaagenes P, Skretting P, Lind B, Edström HH: Spinal analgesia with hyperbaric bupivacaine: Effects of volume of solution. Br J Anaesth 54:69, 1982
71. Chambers WA, Littlewood DG, Scott DB: Spinal anesthesia with hyperbaric bupivacaine: Effect of added vasoconstrictors. Anesth Analg 61:49, 1982
72. Taivainen T, Tuominen M, Rosenberg PH: Influence of obesity on the spread of spinal analgesia after injection of plain 0.5% bupivacaine at the L3-4 of L4-5 interspace. Br J Anaesth 64:542, 1990
73. Tuominen M, Kuulasmaa K, Taivainen T, Rosenberg PH: Individual predictability of repeated spinal anaesthesia with isobaric bupivacaine. Acta Anaesthesiol Scand 33:13, 1989
74. Tuominen M, Taivainen T, Rosenberg PH: Spread of spinal anaesthesia with plain 0.5% bupivacaine: Influence of the vertebral interspace used for injection. Br J Anaesth 62:358, 1989
75. Carpenter RL, Hogan QH, Liu SS, Crane B, Moore J: Lumbosacral cerebrospinal fluid volume is the primary determinant of sensory block extent and duration during spinal anesthesia [see comments]. Anesthesiology 89:24, 1998
76. Higuchi H, Hirata J, Adachi Y, Kazama T: Influence of lumbosacral cerebrospinal fluid density, velocity, and volume on extent and duration of plain bupivacaine spinal anesthesia. Anesthesiology 100:106, 2004
77. Pargger H, Hampl KF, Aeschbach A, Paganoni R, Schneider MC: Combined effect of patient variables on sensory level after spinal 0.5% plain bupivacaine. Acta Anaesthesiol Scand 42:430, 1998
78. Veering BT, Burm AG, van Kleef JW, Hennis PJ, Spierdijk J: Spinal anesthesia with glucose-free bupivacaine: effects of age on neural blockade and pharmacokinetics. Anesth Analg 66:965, 1987
79. Pitkänen M, Haapaniemi L, Tuominen M, Rosenberg PH: Influence of age on spinal anaesthesia with isobaric 0.5% bupivacaine. Br J Anaesth 56:279, 1984
80. Norris M: Height, weight, and the spread of subarachnoid hyperbaric bupivacaine in the term parturient. Anesth Analg 67:555, 1988
81. Norris MC: Patient variables and the subarachnoid spread of hyperbaric bupivacaine in the term parturient. Anesthesiology 72:478, 1990
82. Wildsmith JA, Rocco AG: Current concepts in spinal anesthesia. Regional Anesth 10:119, 1985
83. McCulloch WJ, Littlewood DG: Influence of obesity on spinal analgesia with isobaric 0.5% bupivacaine. Br J Anaesth 58:610, 1986
84. Pitkänen MT: Body mass and spread of spinal anesthesia with bupivacaine. Anesth Analg 66:127, 1987
85. Axelsson KH, Edström HH, Sundberg AE, Widman GB: Spinal anaesthesia with hyperbaric 0.5% bupivacaine: Effects of volume. Acta Anaesthesiol Scand 26:439, 1982
86. Bengtsson M, Edström HH, Löfström JB: Spinal analgesia with bupivacaine, mepivacaine and tetracaine. Acta Anaesthesiol Scand 27:278, 1983
87. Racle J, Benkhadra A, Poy J, Gleizal B: Effect of increasing amounts of epinephrine during isobaric bupivacaine spinal anesthesia in elderly patients. Anesth Analg 66:882, 1987
88. Vaida GT, Moss P, Capan LM, Turndorf H: Prolongation of lidocaine spinal anesthesia with phenylephrine. Anesth Analg 65:781, 1986
89. Egbert LD, Deas TC: Effect of epinephrine upon the duration of spinal anesthesia. Anesthesiology 21:345, 1960
90. Concepcion M, Maddi R, Francis D, Rocco AG, Murray E, Covino BG: Vasoconstrictors in spinal anesthesia with tetracaine—A comparison of epinephrine and phenylephrine. Anesth Analg 63:134, 1984
91. Meagher RP, Moore DC, DeVries JC: Phenylephrine: The most effective potentiator of tetracaine spinal anesthesia. Anesth Analg 45:134, 1966
92. Caldwell C, Nielsen C, Baltz T, Taylor P, Helton B, Butler P: Comparison of high-dose epinephrine and phenylephrine in spinal anesthesia with tetracaine. Anesthesiology 62:804, 1985
93. Park WY, Balingit PE, Macnamara TE: Effects of patient age, pH of cerebrospinal fluid, and vasopressors on onset and duration of spinal anesthesia. Anesth Analg 54:455, 1975
94. Fukuda T, Dohi S, Naito H: Comparisons of tetracaine spinal anesthesia with clonidine or phenylephrine in normotensive and hypertensive humans. Anesth Analg 78:106, 1994
95. Bonnet F, Brun-Buisson V, Saada M, Boico O, Rostaing S, Touboul C: Dose-related prolongation of hyperbaric tetracaine spinal anesthesia by clonidine in humans. Anesth Analg 68:619, 1989
96. Dobrydnjov I, Samarutel J: Enhancement of intrathecal lidocaine by addition of local and systemic clonidine. Acta Anaesthesiol Scand 43:556, 1999
97. Ota K, Namiki A, Ujike Y, Takahashi I: Prolongation of tetracaine spinal anesthesia by oral clonidine. Anesth Analg 75:262, 1992
98. Ota K, Namiki A, Iwasaki H, Takahashi I: Dosing interval for prolongation of tetracaine spinal anesthesia by oral clonidine in humans. Anesth Analg 79:1117, 1994
99. Axelsson K, Widman B: Blood concentration of lidocaine after spinal anaesthesia using lidocaine and lidocaine with adrenaline. Acta Anaesthesiol Scand 25:240, 1981
100. Leicht CH, Carlson SA: Prolongation of lidocaine spinal anesthesia with epinephrine and phenylephrine. Anesth Analg 65:365, 1986
101. Moore DC, Chadwick HS, Ready LB: Epinephrine prolongs libocaine spinal: Pain in the operative site is the most accurate method of determining local anesthetic duration. Anesthesiology 67:416, 1987

102. Chambers WA, Littlewood DG, Logan MR, Scott DB: Effect of added epinephrine on spinal anesthesia with lidocaine. Anesth Analg 60:417, 1981
103. Spivey DL: Epinephrine does not prolong lidocaine spinal anesthesia in term parturients. Anesth Analg 64:468, 1985
104. Chiu AA, Liu S, Carpenter RL, Kasman GS, Pollock JE, Neal JM: The effects of epinephrine on lidocaine spinal anesthesia: a cross-over study. Anesth Analg 80:735, 1995
105. Kozody R, Swartz J, Palahniuk RJ, Biehl DR, Wade JG: Spinal cord blood flow following subarachnoid lidocaine. Can Anaesth Soc J 32(5):472, 1985
106. Kozody R, Palahniuk RJ, Cumming MO: Spinal cord blood flow following subarachnoid tetracaine. Can Anaesth Soc J 32(1):23, 1985
107. Kozody R, Ong B, Palahniuk RJ, Wade JG, Cumming MO, Pucci WR: Subarachnoid bupivacaine decreases spinal cord blood flow in dogs. Can Anaesth Soc J 32(3):216, 1985
108. Denson DD, Bridenbaugh PO, Turner PA, Phero JC, Raj PP: Neural blockade and pharmacokinetics following subarachnoid lidocaine in the rhesus monkey. I. Effects of epinephrine. Anesth Analg 61:746, 1982
109. Crosby G, Russo M, Szabo M, Davies K: Subarachnoid clonidine reduces spinal cord blood flow and glucose utilization in conscious rats. Anesthesiology 73:1179, 1990
110. Converse JG, Landmesser CM, Harmel MH: The concentration of pontocaine hydrochloride in the cerebrospinal fluid during spinal anesthesia, and the influence of epinephrine in prolonging the sensory anesthetic effect. Anesthesiology 15:1, 1954
111. Mörch ET, Rosenberg MK, Truant AT: Lidocaine for spinal anesthesia. A study of the concentration in the spinal fluid. Acta Anaesthesiol Scand 1:105, 1957
112. Reddy SV, Maderdrut JL, Yaksh TL: Spinal cord pharmacology of adrenergic agonist-mediated antinociception. J Pharmacol Exp Ther 213:525, 1980
113. Phillis J, Tebecis A, York D: Depression of spinal motoneurons by noradrenalin, 5-hydroxytryptamine and histamine. Eur J Pharmacol 4:471, 1968
114. Park W, Massengale M, Macnamara T: Age, height, and speed of injection as factors determining caudal anesthetic level and occurrence of severe hypertension. Anesthesiology 51:81, 1979
115. Park WY, Hagins FM, Rivat EL, Macnamara TE: Age and epidural dose response in adult men. Anesthesiology 56:318, 1982
116. Grundy EM, Ramamurthy S, Patel KP, Mani M, Winnie AP: Extradural analgesia revisited. Br J Anaesth 50:805, 1978
117. Erdemir HA, Soper LE, Sweet RB: Studies of factors affecting peridural anesthesia. Anesth Analg 44:400, 1965
118. Burn JM, Guyer PB, Langdon L: The spread of solutions injected into the epidural space. Br J Anaesth 45:338, 1973
119. Apostolou GA, Zarmakoupis PK, Mastrokostopoulos GT: Spread of epidural anesthesia and the lateral position. Anesth Analg 60:584, 1981
120. Park WY, Hagins FM, Massengale MD, Macnamara TE: The sitting position and anesthetic spread in the epidural space. Anesth Analg 63:863, 1984
121. Ponhold H, Kulier A, Rehak P: 30 degree trunk elevation of the patient and quality of lumbar epidural anesthesia. Effects of elevation in operations on the lower extremities. Anaesthetist 42:788, 1993
122. Park WY, Massengale M, Kim SI, Poon KC, Macnamara TE: Age and the spread of local anesthetic solutions in the epidural space. Anesth Analg 59:768, 1980
123. Nydahl PA, Philipson L, Axelsson K, Johansson JE: Epidural anesthesia with 0.5% bupivacaine: Influence of age on sensory and motor blockade. Anesth Analg 73:780, 1991
124. Veering BT, Burm AG, van Kleef JW, Hennis PJ, Spierdijk J: Epidural anesthesia with bupivacaine: Effects of age on neural blockade and pharmacokinetics. Anesth Analg 66:589, 1987
125. Hirabayashi Y, Saitoh K, Fukuda H, Shimizu R: Effect of age on dose requirement for lumbar epidural anesthesia. Masui 42:808, 1993
126. Duggan J, Bowler GM, McClure JH, Wildsmith JA: Extradural block with bupivacaine: Influence of dose, volume, concentration and patient characteristics. Br J Anaesth 61:324, 1988
127. Hirabayashi Y, Shimizu R, Matsuda I, Inoue S: Effect of extradural compliance and resistance on spread of extradural analgesia. Br J Anaesth 65:508, 1990
128. Bromage P: Spread of analgesic solutions in the epidural space and their site of action: a statistical study. Br J Anaesth 34:161, 1962
129. Fagraeus L, Urban BJ, Bromage PR: Spread of epidural analgesia in early pregnancy. Anesthesiology 58:184, 1983
130. Grundy EM, Zamora AM, Winnie AP: Comparison of spread of epidural anesthesia in pregnant and nonpregnant women. Anesth Analg 57:544, 1978
131. Kalas DB, Senfield RM, Hehre FW: Continuous lumbar peridural anesthesia in obstetrics. IV: Comparison of the number of segments blocked in pregnant and nonpregnant subjects. Anesth Analg 45:848, 1966
132. Sharrock NE: Lack of exaggerated spread of epidural anesthesia in patients with arteriosclerosis. Anesthesiology 47:307, 1977
133. Axelsson K, Nydahl PA, Philipson L, Larsson P: Motor and sensory blockade after epidural injection of mepivacaine, bupivacaine, and etidocaine—A double-blind study. Anesth Analg 69:739, 1989
134. Kerkkamp HE, Gielen MJ, Wattwil M *et al:* An open study comparison of 0.5%, 0.75% and 1.0% ropivacaine, with epinephrine, in epidural anesthesia in patients undergoing urologic surgery. Regional Anesth 15:53, 1990
135. Buckley FP, Littlewood DG, Covino BG, Scott DB: Effects of adrenaline and the concentration of solution on extradural block with etidocaine. Br J Anaesth 50:171, 1978
136. Scott DB, McClure JH, Gaisi RM, Seo J, Covino BG: Effects of concentration of local anaesthetic drugs in extradural block. Br J Anaesth 52:1033, 1980
137. Bromage PR, Burfoot MF, Crowell DE, Pettigrew RT: Quality of epidural blockade. I: Influence of physical factors. Br J Anaesth 36:342, 1964
138. Sharrock NE, Go G, Mineo R: Effect of i.v. low-dose adrenaline and phenylephrine infusions of plasma concentrations of bupivacaine after lumbar extradural anaesthesia in elderly patients. Br J Anaesth 67:694, 1991
139. Kier L: Continuous epidural analgesia in prostatectomy: Comparison of bupivacaine with and without adrenaline. Acta Anaesthesiol Scand 18:1, 1974
140. Sinclair CJ, Scott DB: Comparison of bupivacaine and etidocaine in extradural blockade. Br J Anaesth 56:147, 1984
141. Cederholm I, Anskär S, Bengtsson M: Sensory, motor, and sympathetic block during epidural analgesia with 0.5% and 0.75% ropivacaine with and without epinephrine. Regional Anesth 19:18, 1994
142. Abboud T, Sheik-ol-Eslam A, Yanagi T *et al:* Safety and efficacy of epinephrine added to bupivacaine for lumbar epidural analgesia in obstetrics. Anesth Analg 64:585, 1985
143. Eisenach JC, Grice SC, Dewan DM: Epinephrine enhances analgesia produced by epidural bupivacaine during labor. Anesth Analg 66:447, 1987
144. Finucane B, McCraney J, Bush D: Double-blind comparison of lidocaine and etidocaine during continuous epidural anesthesia for vaginal delivery. South Med J 71:667, 1978
145. Cohen E: Distribution of local anesthetic agents in the neuroaxis of the dog. Anesthesiology 29:1002, 1968
146. Post C, Freedman J, Ramsay C, Bonnevier A: Redistribution of lidocaine and bupivacaine after intrathecal injection in mice. Anesthesiology 63:410, 1985
147. Boswell M, Iacono R, Guthkelch A: Sites of action of subarachnoid lidocaine and tetracaine: Observations with evoked potential monitoring during spinal cord stimulator implantation. Reg Anesth 17:37, 1992
148. Cusick J, Myklebust J, Abram S: Differential neural effects of epidural anesthetics. Anesthesiology 53:299, 1980
149. Urban B: Clinical observations suggesting a changing site of action during induction and recession of spinal and epidural anesthesia. Anesthesiology 39:496, 1973
150. Fink BR: Mechanisms of differential axial blockade in epidural and subarachnoid anesthesia. Anesthesiology 70:851, 1989
151. Fink BR, Cairns AM: Lack of size-related differential sensitivity to equilibrium conduction block among mammalian myelinated axons exposed to lidocaine. Anesth Analg 66:948, 1987
152. Chamberlain D, Chamberlain B: Changes in skin temperature of the trunk and their relationship to sympathetic block during spinal anesthesia. Anesthesiology 65:139, 1986
153. Brull SJ, Greene NM: Zones of differential sensory block during extradural anaesthesia. Br J Anaesth 66:651, 1991
154. Gentili M, Huu PC, Enel D, Hollande J, Bonnet F: Sedation depends on the level of sensory block induced by spinal anaesthesia. Br J Anaesth 81:970, 1998
155. Ben-David B, Vaida S, Gaitini L: The influence of high spinal anesthesia on sensitivity to midazolam sedation [see comments]. Anesth Analg 81:525, 1995
156. Tverskoy M, Shagal M, Finger J, Kissin I: Subarachnoid bupivacaine blockade decreases midazolam and thiopental hypnotic requirements. J Clin Anesth 6:487, 1994
157. Tverskoy M, Shifrin V, Finger J, Fleyshman G, Kissin I: Effect of epidural bupivacaine block on midazolam hypnotic requirements. Reg Anesth 21:209, 1996
158. Hodgson P, Liu S, Gras T: Does epidural anesthesia have general anesthetic effects? A prospective, randomized, double-blind, placebo-controlled trial. Anesthesiology 91:1687, 1999
159. Carpenter RL, Caplan RA, Brown DL, Stephenson C, Wu R: Incidence and risk factors for side effects of spinal anesthesia. Anesthesiology 76:906, 1992
160. Coe AJ, Revanäs B: Is crystalloid preloading useful in spinal anaesthesia in the elderly? Anaesthesia 45:241, 1990
161. Phero JC, Bridenbaugh PO, Edström HH *et al:* Hypotension in spinal anesthesia: A comparison of isobaric tetracaine with epinephrine and isobaric bupivacaine without epinephrine. Anesth Analg 66:549, 1987
162. Tarkkila P, Isola J: A regression model for identifying patients at high risk of hypotension, bradycardia and nausea during spinal anesthesia. Acta Anesthesiol Scand 36:554, 1992
163. Shimosato S, Etsten BE: The role of the venous system in cardiocirculatory dynamics during spinal and epidural anesthesia in man. Anesthesiology 30:619, 1969
164. Kennedy WF, Jr. , Bonica JJ, Akamatsu TJ, Ward RJ, Martin WE, Grinstein A: Cardiovascular and respiratory effects of subarachnoid block in the presence of acute blood loss. Anesthesiology 29:29, 1968

165. Anzai Y, Nishikawa T: Heart rate responses to body tilt during spinal anesthesia. Anesth Analg 73:385, 1991
166. Ward RJ, Bonica JJ, Freund FG, Akamatsu T, Danziger F, Englesson S: Epidural and subarachnoid anesthesia. Cardiovascular and respiratory effects. JAMA 191:275, 1965
167. Pathak CL: Autoregulation of chronotropic response of the heart through pacemaker stretch. Cardiology 58:45, 1973
168. Jacobsen J, Søfelt S, Brocks V, Fernandes A, Warberg J, Secher NH: Reduced left ventricular diameters at onset of bradycardia during epidural anaesthesia. Acta Anaesthesiol Scand 36:831, 1992
169. Baron JF, Decaux-Jacolot A, Edouard A, Berdeaux A, Samii K: Influence of venous return on baroreflex control of heart rate during lumbar epidural anesthesia in humans. Anesthesiology 64:188, 1986
170. Caplan RA, Ward RJ, Posner K, Cheney FW: Unexpected cardiac arrest during spinal anesthesia: A closed claims analysis of predisposing factors. Anesthesiology 68:5, 1988
171. Mackey DC, Carpenter RL, Thompson GE, Brown DL, Bodily MN: Bradycardia and asystole during spinal anesthesia: A report of three cases without morbidity. Anesthesiology 70:866, 1989
172. Bernards CM, Hymas NJ: Progression of first degree heart block to high-grade second degree block during spinal anaesthesia. Can J Anaesth 39:173, 1992
173. Jordi EM, Marsch SC, Strebel S: Third degree heart block and asystole associated with spinal anesthesia. Anesthesiology 89:257, 1998
174. Shen CL, Hung YC, Chen PJ, Tsao CM, Ho YY: Mobitz type II AV block during spinal anesthesia. Anesthesiology 90:1477, 1990
175. Bonica JJ, Kennedy WF, Jr., Ward RJ, Tolas AG: A comparison of the effects of high subarachnoid and epidural anesthesia. Acta Anaesthesiol Scand 23:429, 1966
176. Kerkkamp HE, Gielen MJ: Hemodynamic monitoring in epidural blockade: Cardiovascular effects of 20 ml 0.5% bupivacaine with and without epinephrine. Regional Anesth 15:137, 1990
177. Graves CL, Underwood PS, Klein RL, Kim YI: Intravenous fluid administration as therapy for hypotenstion secondary to spinal anesthesia. Anesth Analg 47:548, 1968
178. Venn PJ, Simpson DA, Rubin AP, Edstrom HH: Effect of fluid preloading on cardiovascular variables after spinal anaesthesia with glucose-free 0.75% bupivacaine. Br J Anaesth 63:682, 1989
179. Rout CC, Rocke DA, Levin J, Gouws E, Reddy D: A reevaluation of the role of crystalloid preload in the prevention of hypotension associated with spinal anesthesia for elective cesarean section. Anesthesiology 79:262, 1993
180. Marhofer P, Faryniak B, Oismuller C, Koinig H, Kapral S, Mayer N: Cardiovascular effects of 6% hetastarch and lactated Ringer's solution during spinal anesthesia. Reg Anesth Pain Med 24:399, 1999
181. Butterworth J, Piccione W, Berrizbeitia L, Dance G, Shemin R, Cohn L: Augmentation of venous return by adrenergic agonists during spinal anesthesia. Anesth Analg 65:612, 1986
182. Ward RJ, Kennedy WF, Bonica JJ, Martin WE, Tolas AG, Akamatsu T: Experimental evaluation of atropine and vasopressors for the treatment of hypotension of high subarachnoid anesthesia. Anesth Analg 45:621, 1966
183. Lundberg J, Norgren L, Thomson D, Werner O: Hemodynamic effects of dopamine during thoracic epidural analgesia in man. Anesthesiology 66:641, 1987
184. Butterworth JF, 4th, Austin JC, Johnson MD *et al:* Effect of total spinal anesthesia on arterial and venous responses to dopamine and dobutamine. Anesth Analg 66:209, 1987
185. Goertz AW, Seeling W, Heinrich H, Lindner KH, Rockemann MG, Georgieff M: Effect of phenylephrine bolus administration of left ventricular function during high thoracic and lumbar epidural anesthesia combined with general anesthesia. Anesth Analg 76:541, 1993
186. Sakura S, Saito Y, Kosaka Y: Effect of lumbar epidural anesthesia on ventilatory response to hypercapnia in young and elderly patients. J Clin Anesth 5:109, 1993
187. Steinbrook R, Concepcion M, Topulos G: Ventilatory responses to hypercapnia during bupivacaine spinal anesthesia. Anesth Analg 67:247, 1988
188. Dahl JB, Schultz P, Anker-Møller E, Christensen EF, Staunstrup HG, Carlsson P: Spinal anaesthesia in young patients using a 29-gauge needle: Technical considerations and an evaluation of postoperative complaints compared with general anaesthesia. Br J Anaesth 64:178, 1990
189. Seeberger MD, Lang ML, Drewe J, Schneider M, Hauser E, Hruby J: Comparison of spinal and epidural anesthesia for patients younger than 50 years of age. Anesth Analg 78:667, 1994
190. Halpern S, Preston R: Postdural puncture headache and spinal needle design. Anesthesiology 81:1376, 1994
191. Lybecker H, Møller JT, May O, Nielsen HK: Incidence and prediction of postdural puncture headache. A prospective study of 1021 spinal anesthesias. Anesth Analg 70:389, 1990
192. Flaatten H, Thorsen T, Askeland B *et al:* Puncture technique and postural postdural puncture headache. A randomised, double-blind study comparing transverse and parallel puncture. Acta Anaesthesiol Scand 42:1209, 1998
193. Camann WR, Murray RS, Mushlin PS, Lambert DH: Effects of oral caffeine on postdural puncture headache. A double-blind, placebo-controlled trial. Anesth Analg 70:181, 1990
194. Cheek TG, Banner R, Sauter J, Gutsche BB: Prophylactic extradural blood patch is effective. Br J Anaesth 61:340, 1988
195. Colonna-Romano P, Shapiro BE: Unintentional dural puncture and prophylactic epidural blood patch in obstetrics. Anesth Analg 69:522, 1989
196. Crul BJ, Gerritse BM, van Dongen RT, Schoonderwaldt HC: Epidural fibrin glue injection stops persistent postdural puncture headache. Anesthesiology 91:576, 1999
197. Lamberg T, Pitkanen MT, Marttila T, Rosenberg PH: Hearing loss after continuous or single-shot spinal anesthesia. Reg Anesth 22:539, 1997
198. Gültekin S, Yilmaz N, Ceyhan A, Karamustafa I, Kilic R, Unal N: The effect of different anesthetic agents in hearing loss following spinal anaesthesia. Eur J Anaesthesiol 15:61, 1998
199. Kane R: Neurologic deficits following epidural or spinal anesthesia. Anesth Analg 60:150, 1981
200. Lambert LA, Lambert DH, Strichartz GR: Irreversible conduction block in isolated nerve by high concentrations of local anesthetics. Anesthesiology 80:1082, 1994
201. Rigler M, Drasner K, Krejcie T *et al:* Cauda equina syndrome after continuous spinal anesthesia. Anesth Analg 72:275, 1991
202. Ross B, Coda B, Heath C: Local anesthetic distribution in a spinal model: A possible mechanism of neurologic injury after continuous spinal anesthesia. Reg Anesth 17:69, 1992
203. Drasner K, Rigler M, Sessler D, Stoller M: Cauda equina syndrome following intended epidural anesthesia. Anesthesiology 77:582, 1992
204. Gold MS, Reichling DB, Hampl KF, Drasner K, Levine JD: Lidocaine toxicity in primary afferent neurons from the rat. J Pharmacol Exp Ther 285:413, 1998
205. Drasner K: Lidocaine spinal anesthesia: A vanishing therapeutic index? [editorial; comment]. Anesthesiology 87:469, 1997
206. Schneider M, Ettlin T, Kaufmann M *et al:* Transient neurologic toxicity after hyperbaric subarachnoid anesthesia with 5% lidocaine [see comments]. Anesth Analg 76:1154, 1993
207. Hiller A, Rosenberg PH: Transient neurological symptoms after spinal anaesthesia with 4% mepivacaine and 0.5% bupivacaine. Br J Anaesth 79:301, 1997
208. Liguori GA, Zayas VM, Chisholm MF: Transient neurologic symptoms after spinal anesthesia with mepivacaine and lidocaine [see comments]. Anesthesiology 88:619, 1998
209. Martinez-Bourio R, Arzuaga M, Quintana JM *et al:* Incidence of transient neurologic symptoms after hyperbaric subarachnoid anesthesia with 5% lidocaine and 5% prilocaine [see comments]. Anesthesiology 88:624, 1998
210. Hampl KF, Heinzmann-Wiedmer S, Luginbuehl I *et al:* Transient neurologic symptoms after spinal anesthesia: A lower incidence with prilocaine and bupivacaine than with lidocaine [see comments]. Anesthesiology 88:629, 1998
211. Salmela L, Aromaa U: Transient radicular irritation after spinal anesthesia induced with hyperbaric solutions of cerebrospinal fluid-diluted lidocaine 50 mg/ml or mepivacaine 40 mg/ml or bupivacaine 5 mg/ml. Acta Anaesthesiol Scand 42:765, 1998
212. Axelrod EH, Alexander GD, Brown M, Schork MA: Procaine spinal anesthesia: A pilot study of the incidence of transient neurologic symptoms. J Clin Anesth 10:404, 1998
213. Bergeron L, Girard M, Drolet P, Grenier Y, Le Truong HH, Boucher C: Spinal procaine with and without epinephrine and its relation to transient radicular irritation. Can J Anaesth 46:846, 1999
214. Freedman JM, Li DK, Drasner K, Jaskela MC, Larsen B, Wi S: Transient neurologic symptoms after spinal anesthesia: An epidemiologic study of 1,863 patients [published erratum appears in Anesthesiology 89(6)1614, 1998]. Anesthesiology 89:633, 1998
215. Sakura S, Sumi M, Sakaguchi Y, Saito Y, Kosaka Y, Drasner K: The addition of phenylephrine contributes to the development of transient neurologic symptoms after spinal anesthesia with 0.5% tetracaine [see comments]. Anesthesiology 87:771, 1997
216. Kouri ME, Kopacz DJ: Spinal 2-chloroprocaine: A comparison with lidocaine in volunteers. Anesth Analg 98:75, 2004
217. Smith KN, Kopacz DJ, McDonald SB: Spinal 2-chloroprocaine: a dose-ranging study and the effect of added epinephrine. Anesth Analg 98:81, 2004
218. Warren DT, Kopacz DJ: Spinal 2-chloroprocaine: The effect of added dextrose. Anesth Analg 98:95, 2004
219. Vath JS, Kopacz DJ: Spinal 2-chloroprocaine: The effect of added fentanyl. Anesth Analg 98:89, 2004
220. Vandermeulen EP, Van Aken H, Vermylen J: Anticoagulants and spinal-epidural anesthesia. Anesth Analg 79:1165, 1994
221. American Society for Regional Anesthesia and Pain Medicine (www.asra.com/items_of_interest/consensus_statements/)

CHAPTER 26 ■ PERIPHERAL NERVE BLOCKADE

MICHAEL F. MULROY

KEY POINTS

1. Peripheral nerve blocks provide longer and more localized pain relief than neuraxial techniques while also avoiding the side effects of systemic medication.
2. Larger volumes of local anesthetic may increase the success potential of peripheral blocks, but the total milligram dosage must be limited to avoid systemic toxicity because of slow absorption. Higher concentrations of local anesthetics on peripheral nerves will increase the degree of motor blockade, but larger volumes of more dilute solutions can be used with less risk of toxicity.
3. Nerve blocks associated with bony or vascular landmarks are more reliable and easy to perform than those that depend on surface landmarks alone.
4. Several peripheral nerve blocks are acceptable alternatives to neuraxial techniques in the anticoagulated patient.
5. Peripheral nerve stimulators are useful tools to facilitate nerve blockade, but they do not eliminate the risk of nerve injury. In the adult patient, responsiveness must be maintained to allow reporting of nerve contact or pain on injection.

GENERAL PRINCIPLES

Regional anesthesia of the extremities and of the trunk is a useful alternative to general anesthesia in many situations. Peripheral nerve blocks have attracted renewed interest because of their salutary role in reducing postoperative pain[1] and shortening outpatient recovery.[2]

Local Anesthetic Drug Selection and Doses

1 The pharmacology of local anesthetics is reviewed at length in Chapter 17. Although high concentrations of drug are needed to produce rapid onset of anesthesia in the epidural space, lower concentrations (e.g., 1% to 1.5% lidocaine, 0.25% to 0.5% bupivacaine) are more appropriate on peripheral nerves because of concerns about local and systemic toxicity. Lo-
2 cal toxicity of these anesthetics appears to be concentration dependent.[3] Lower concentrations are also indicated when larger volumes are required to anesthetize poorly localized peripheral nerves or to block a series of nerves. The use of a high-concentration solution may be useful to increase motor blockade but increases the total milligram dose of local anesthetic.

The absorption of drug and the duration of anesthesia vary with the dose, drug, location injected, and presence of vasoconstrictors. The highest blood levels of local anesthetic occur after intercostal blockade, followed by epidural, caudal, and brachial plexus blockade. Similarly, the duration depends on the blood supply of the area of injection. Equivalent doses of local anesthetic may produce only 3 to 4 hours of anesthesia when placed in the epidural space, but 12 to 14 hours in the arm and 24 to 36 hours when placed on the sciatic nerve. In general, the addition of epinephrine 1:200,000 to 1:400,000 is advantageous in prolonging the duration of blockade and in reducing systemic blood levels of local anesthetic. Its use is not appropriate in the vicinity of "terminal" blood vessels, such as in the digits or penis, or when using an intravenous (IV) regional technique. The recommended doses and drugs in this chapter assume the addition of epinephrine to the solution. In general, the recommendations will be for an effective volume for a sensory block: the final choice of drug, volume, and concentration will be the determinants of the duration of block and the degree of motor blockade.

Nerve Localization

The blockade techniques associated with reliable proximity of nerves to bones or arteries are the easiest technically to perform (e.g., intercostal, axillary). Less reliable landmarks, such as the psoas compartment or obturator foramen, require either large volumes of local anesthetic solution or the establishment of a distinct localization of the desired nerve to provide adequate anesthesia. Paresthesias are the traditional sign of successful localization, but the use of electrical stimulation has gained popularity with the development of improved equipment.[4] A low-current electrical impulse applied to a peripheral nerve produces stimulation of motor fibers and identifies the proximity of the nerve without actual needle contact or patient discomfort. Because the nerve stimulator does not technically contact the nerve, its use may reduce the chance for nerve injury, although it still may occur and paresthesias have been elicited with this technique before motor responses. A familiarity with anatomy and technique is still necessary to bring the needle into proximity to the nerve. The ideal stimulator should have a variable-amperage output. This allows a high current to be delivered in the exploration phase and then a progressively lower current to document proximity of the nerve. The accuracy of the localization can be improved by the use of insulated needles. Current flow can also be improved by using the positive (red) pole of the stimulator as the ground (or reference) electrode and the negative (black) lead as the connection to the needle itself. Whereas 1 to 2 mA can be used to produce the first motor twitch, actual injection of anesthetic should be delayed until stimulation is produced by as little as 0.3 to 0.5 mA. At that point, 2 to 3 mL of local anesthetic should be sufficient to abolish motor twitch, indicating that it is appropriate to inject the remainder of the proposed dose.

Seeking a sensory paresthesia with the needle remains an acceptable alternative, though there is potential for intraneural injection if paresthesias are obtained. This is usually signaled by a complaint from the patient of a "cramping" or "aching" pain during the initial injection. If this occurs, the needle should be immediately withdrawn by a few millimeters and a small test injection repeated. Even without intraneural injection, residual neuropathy of peripheral nerves appears more likely if paresthesias are obtained. A third problem with this technique is the inevitable associated discomfort; patient education and sedation must be handled appropriately.

Another alternative is the use of ultrasound guidance to localize nerves, especially if located near an artery (axillary or femoral). These techniques show promise, but require more complex equipment and experience. The choice of localization technique depends on many factors, especially the experience and training of the operator.

Equipment

Although reusable syringes and needles can be manufactured to a higher standard, their cost and concern about infection generally lead to a preference for disposable equipment. There is a large number of high-quality disposable kits available on the market, and many of the major manufacturers customize their packages at the request of large institutions willing to commit to purchasing a sufficient volume. The use of disposable trays places the burden of sterilization on the manufacturer, although the liability for checking the sterility of contents always remains with the user.

Needles used for regional techniques are often modified from standard injection needles. For peripheral blockade, the "short bevel" or "B bevel" is often used to reduce the potential for injury to nerves. Other modifications, such as the "pencil-point" insulated needle, have been introduced in attempts to reduce nerve injury.

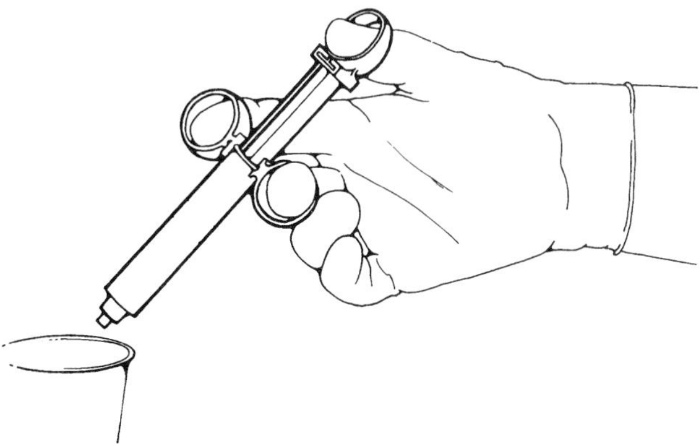

FIGURE 26-1. The three-ring ("control") syringe. Use of this adaptation to the plunger of a standard 10-mL syringe allows greater control of injection, easier aspiration, and the opportunity to refill the syringe with one hand. Plastic adapters are available for disposable syringes as demonstrated. (Reproduced with permission from Mulroy M: Handbook of Regional Anesthesia. Philadelphia, Lippincott Williams & Wilkins, 2002.)

Special syringes are also useful for performing peripheral nerve blockades. Plastic and glass are equally useful. With respect to size, a 10-mL syringe is usually a good compromise. Large volumes are often required for peripheral nerve blockade, so that 3- and 5-mL syringes are rarely adequate. Larger than 10-mL volume often presents such bulk and weight that fine control is hampered. If a larger syringe is used, it is usually advisable to attach it to the needle by a short length of extension tubing. The use of finger rings (the "control syringe") is helpful in controlling injection, facilitating aspiration, and allowing the operator to refill the syringe with one hand (Fig. 26-1). Luer-Lok adapters for the syringe-hub connection are also advantageous. Although friction fittings produce tight seals, the amount of force required for attaching or removing the syringe may displace a needle that has been meticulously maneuvered into the appropriate close contact with a nerve.

Continuous Catheters

A recent addition to the armamentarium of the regional anesthesiologist is continuous-infusion catheters adapted for peripheral nerve blockade. Kits are available that include a standard polyamide catheter, such as previously used for epidural analgesia, combined with a Tuohy needle for insertion that has been modified to include nerve stimulation capability. These kits allow the localization of a peripheral nerve with an electrical current and the threading of a catheter to lie contiguous to that nerve to provide prolonged postoperative analgesia. Further enhancements include the development of stimulating catheters, which include an electrode in the catheter tip that allows more precise localization of the catheter as it is advanced alongside the nerve. Catheter infusions provide prolonged postoperative analgesia following major joint replacement, as well as significant analgesia of an extremity following short-stay orthopedic surgery.[1] Standard precautions are required to preserve the sterility of the catheter and the insertion site, but complications have been rare with these techniques and new devices. There are a number of continuous-infusion devices now available, both in inpatient and outpatient configuration, which allow delivery of dilute local anesthetic concentrations for as long as 72 hours after surgery. These devices range from simple pressure infusion plastic apparatuses that deliver a fixed flow rate to many that can be preprogrammed to variable flow rates and include a patient-controlled supplemental bolus feature. The selection of the ideal catheter and infusion device combination for a specific patient and situation requires individual review of the available options.

The selection of antiseptic solutions is usually a local preference. Chlorhexadine, alcohol, and organic iodine preparations are current standards for skin asepsis. For major deep nerve blockade, a wide area of skin preparation is more desirable, and the borders of the clean area can be extended by draping on four sides with sterile towels. Regional anesthesia does not require the same degree of sterile preparation and gowning as indicated for surgery, but strict attention to asepsis is desirable to reduce the chance of infection.

Common Complications

Systemic toxicity of local anesthetics is not the most common but is the most serious concern.[5] This syndrome and the problems of allergy and other unique toxicities are addressed in Chapter 17. Central nervous system excitation and myocardial depression are the two most common hazards associated with high blood levels of local anesthetics. No peripheral nerve blockade using significant quantities of local anesthetic should be performed without oxygen and appropriate resuscitation equipment immediately available. This includes blockades using small quantities of anesthetic near cerebral vessels, such as stellate ganglion or cervical plexus blockade. With peripheral nerve blockade, careful use of a test dose and small incremental injections are appropriate if intravascular injection is a risk. Toxicity can also occur owing to slow absorption of high doses. Patients should be observed carefully for 20 to 30 minutes following injection because peak levels occur at this time.

While complications of peripheral blockade appear less frequent than after neuraxial blockade, peripheral nerve damage does appear to be a frequent cause for filing of a malpractice claim.[6] Peripheral neuropathy usually results from intraneural local anesthetic injection or needle trauma, although there are other causes.[7] Careful attention should be paid to positioning the patient with numb extremities. Postoperative follow-up is important in confirming that neurologic function has returned to normal. If a deficit is detected, early neurologic assessment is critical in determining whether a preexisting neuropathy was involved. Fortunately, most of these syndromes resolve uneventfully, but full recovery of some peripheral injuries requires several months as a result of slow regeneration of injured peripheral nerves. Sympathetic concern and involvement of the anesthesiologist in arranging physical therapy during recovery help reduce patient dissatisfaction.

Other minor complications such as pain at the site of injection and local hematoma formation are not uncommon but are usually of short duration and respond to reassurance by the anesthesiologist. Hematoma around a peripheral nerve is not of
4 the same significance as that in the epidural or subarachnoid space. Again, expressed concern and help with local therapy and analgesics alleviate patient dissatisfaction.

PATIENT PREPARATION

Patient Selection

In general, all patients scheduled for extremity, thoracic, abdominal, or perineal surgery should be considered candidates for peripheral regional anesthetic techniques. These can be used as the only anesthetic, as a supplement to provide analgesia and muscle relaxation along with general anesthesia, or as the initial step for provision of prolonged postoperative analgesia such as with intercostal blockade or continuous peripheral nerve catheters. Adamant refusal of regional anesthesia by a patient is a contraindication to the procedure. However, patient refusal is frequently a "relative" refusal. If the patient's real objections are to "being awake" or "being aware," this can be managed by the use of sedatives and amnestic drugs. Other contraindications include local infection and severe systemic coagulopathy. The presence of preexisting neurologic disease is often discussed. Some data are available in the case of spinal anesthesia, but the use of peripheral nerve blockade in this situation is unclear. Although some physicians avoid any procedure that may confuse the picture of postoperative neuropathy, others believe that if there is a clear difference in the potential injury and the preexisting disease, regional techniques are appropriate. There are no clear answers in this regard, and full patient education and cooperation are most appropriate. Finally, the level of patient anxiety is an important consideration. Extreme apprehension regarding surgery necessitates heavy sedation, and the advantages of regional anesthesia in providing rapid recovery, alertness, and protection of airway reflexes may be negated. The use of regional anesthesia in these situations is a matter of judgment and experience.

Premedication and Sedation

The best preparation for a regional technique is careful patient education. Supplemental medication is also useful. In addition to the general comments about premedication discussed in earlier chapters, regional anesthesia techniques have special requirements. First, sedation must be adjusted to the required level of patient cooperation. With either the elicitation of a paresthesia or electrical stimulation technique, medication must be light enough to allow the patient to identify and report nerve contact. Although a mild dose of opioid (50 to 100 μg of fentanyl or equivalent) will help ease the discomfort of nerve localization, patient responsiveness must be maintained. This does not preclude the use of an amnestic agent. Small doses of propofol or midazolam may provide excellent amnesia at levels of consciousness that still allow cooperation.

Monitoring

Although current discussions of "monitoring" typically include
5 mechanical and electrical devices, repetitive assessment of the patient's mental status when receiving local anesthetics is of paramount importance. The anesthesiologist must maintain frequent verbal contact with these patients and ideally have an uninvolved assistant available to assess the level of consciousness at all times. There are no electrical or mechanical devices that detect rising blood levels of local anesthetic; close observation for peak levels owing to iv (within 2 minutes) and subcutaneous (~20 minutes) absorption is essential. An electrical or mechanical pulse counter is appropriate to detect the pulse rise seen with epinephrine when it is included in a test dose. Pulse monitoring is also useful as an indicator of systemic toxicity with bupivacaine. A baseline blood pressure should be obtained whenever any sympathetic blockade is performed and at frequent intervals thereafter. Beyond these specific comments, the standards for monitoring and record keeping on any patient undergoing regional anesthesia are the same as for patients undergoing any general anesthetic.

Discharge Criteria

Concern is occasionally expressed about discharging patients from postanesthesia care units when an extremity is still anesthetized. If regional anesthesia is administered to provide prolonged analgesia, numbness may be expected to persist for 10 (with intercostal anesthesia) to 24 (with sciatic blockade) hours after bupivacaine or ropivacaine administration. Patients with numb extremities have been successfully discharged from the postanesthesia care unit to the floors as long as their mental alertness is adequate. Outpatients may be discharged home with numb arms or legs (or even with continuous peripheral nerve infusions) as long as the patient is reliable and adequate instruction about ambulation and care of the insensitive extremity is provided.

SPECIFIC TECHNIQUES

The remainder of this chapter is devoted to the details of the performance of specific types of blockade, arranged by sections of the body. No attempt has been made to describe every regional technique practiced, but to focus on those of clinical usefulness to the anesthesiologist.

Head and Neck

Regional anesthesia of the head and neck has limited surgical application. Concern about control and maintenance of the airway makes many anesthesiologists uncomfortable with regional techniques when intraoperative airway intervention is awkward. Trigeminal nerve blockade and occipital nerve blockade are used for diagnostic or neurolytic blockade for chronic pain syndromes. Cervical plexus blockade is useful for some surgical procedures on the neck, and topical–regional airway anesthesia is effective in reducing the subjective discomfort and hemodynamic responses to tracheal intubation.

Trigeminal Nerve Blockade

Sensory and motor nerve function of the face is provided by the branches of the fifth cranial (trigeminal) nerve. The roots of this nerve arise from the base of the pons and send sensory branches to the large gasserian (or semilunar) ganglion, which lies on the superior margin of the petrous bone just inside the skull above the foramen ovale. A smaller motor fiber nucleus lies behind it and sends motor branches to one terminal nerve, the mandibular. The three major branches of the trigeminal each have a separate exit from the skull (Fig. 26-2). The uppermost ophthalmic branch passes through the sphenoidal fissure into the orbit. The main terminal fibers of this nerve, the frontal nerve, bifurcate into the supratrochlear and supraorbital nerves. These two branches traverse the orbit along the superior border and exit on the front of the face in the easily palpated supraorbital notch for the former and along the medial border of the orbit for the latter.

The two major branches of the trigeminal nerve are the middle (maxillary) and lower (mandibular). The maxillary nerve contains only sensory fibers and exits the skull through the foramen rotundum. It passes beneath the skull anteriorly through the sphenomaxillary fossa. At this point, it lies medial to the lateral pterygoid plate on each side. At the anterior end of this channel, it again moves superiorly to reenter the skull in the infraorbital canal in the floor of the orbit. In the sphenomaxillary fossa, it branches to form the sphenopalatine nerves and to give off the posterior dental branches. The anterior dental nerves arise from the main trunk as it passes through the infraorbital canal. The terminal infraorbital nerve emerges from the foramen of the same name just below the eye and lateral to the nose and gives off the terminal palpebral, nasal, and labial nerves. The mandibular nerve is the third and largest branch of the trigeminal, and the only one to receive motor fibers. It exits the skull posterior to the maxillary nerve through the foramen ovale. At this point, it is just posterior to the lateral pterygoid plate of the sphenoid bone. The motor nerves separate into an anterior branch immediately below the foramen ovale. The main branch continues as the inferior alveolar nerve medial to the ramus of the mandible. This nerve curves anteriorly to follow the mandible and exits as a terminal branch through the mental foramen. The mental nerve provides sensation to the lower lip and jaw.

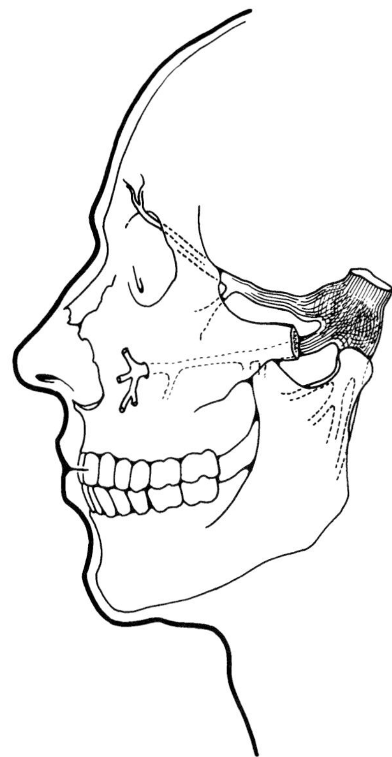

FIGURE 26-2. Lateral view of major branches of the trigeminal nerve. Each major branch exits the skull by a separate foramen. The ophthalmic branch travels in the orbit. The maxillary and mandibular branches emerge from the skull medial to the lateral pterygoid plate, which serves as the landmark for their identification. (Reproduced with permission from Mulroy M: Handbook of Regional Anesthesia. Philadelphia, Lippincott Williams & Wilkins, 2002.)

Gasserian Ganglion Blockade

Ideally, the simplest blockade of the trigeminal nerve is performed in the central ganglion. It is used for treatment of disabling trigeminal neuralgia. This blockade is technically the most difficult and has the most undesirable potential for the complications; it is usually performed by neurosurgeons under fluoroscopic guidance and will not be described in detail here.

Superficial Trigeminal Nerve Branch Blockade

Fortunately, most anesthetic applications of trigeminal blockade can be more easily performed by injection of the individual terminal superficial branches. This is relatively simple because the three superficial branches and their associated foramina all lie in the same sagittal plane on each side of the face (Fig. 26-3). Each of these foramina is readily palpable, and these nerves can be easily blocked with superficial injections of small quantities of local anesthetic. Although the bony landmarks are usually sufficient themselves, paresthesias are desirable before alcohol injection. Each of these blocks can be performed with

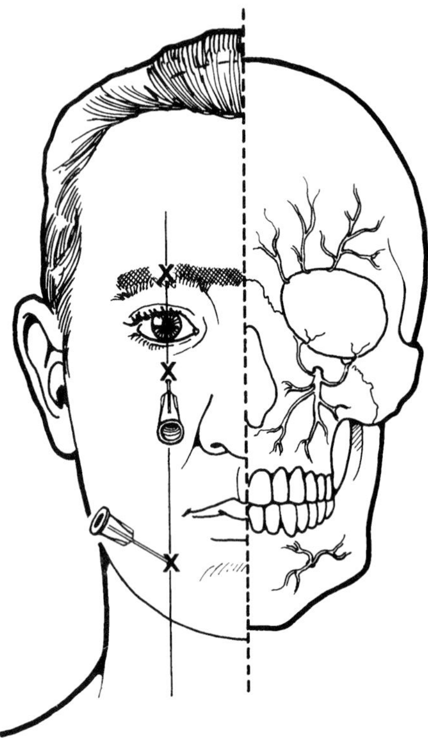

FIGURE 26-3. Terminal branches of the trigeminal nerve. Each of the three terminal branches (the supraorbital, infraorbital, and mental) exits its respective bony canal in the same sagittal plane, approximately 2.5 cm from the midline. The infraorbital canal is angled slightly cephalad, while the mental canal can be entered if the needle is directed medially and slightly caudad. (Reproduced with permission from Mulroy M: Handbook of Regional Anesthesia. Philadelphia, Lippincott Williams & Wilkins, 2002.)

the patient in the supine position. The procedure for blockade follows:

1. The supraorbital notch is easily palpated along the medial superior rim of the orbit, usually 2.5 cm from the midline. Two to 3 mL of local anesthetic injected immediately in the vicinity of the notch produces anesthesia of the ipsilateral forehead. Anesthesia of the supratrochlear nerve by superficial infiltration of the medial aspect of the orbital rim is needed if the band of anesthesia is to cross the midline.
2. The infraorbital foramen lies below the inferior orbital rim in the same plane at approximately the same distance from the midline as the supraorbital notch (usually 2.5 cm). If the foramen cannot be palpated directly, it can be sought by gently probing with a small-gauge needle. This needle should be introduced through a skin wheal approximately 0.5 cm below the expected opening, because the canal angles cephalad from this point toward the orbital floor. Again, injection of a small quantity of local anesthetic immediately in the vicinity of the foramen produces anesthesia of the middle third of the ipsilateral face.
3. The mental nerve also emerges approximately 2.5 cm from the midline, usually midway between the upper and lower borders of the mandible. The mental canal angles medially and inferiorly so that, in this case, needle insertion should start approximately 0.5 cm above and 0.5 cm lateral to the anticipated location of the orifice if it cannot be palpated directly. In older patients, resorption of the superior margin of the mandibular bone will make the foramen appear to lie more superiorly along the ramus. Again, 2 mL of local anesthesia injected into the canal produces anesthesia of the mandibular area.

Maxillary Nerve Blockade

If anesthesia in superior dental nerves is also required or if superficial infraorbital nerve blockade does not produce adequate anesthesia, proximal block of the maxillary nerve is required. This can be performed by a lateral approach to the sphenopalatine fossa. The procedure for blockade follows:

1. The patient lies supine with a small towel under the occiput and the head turned slightly away from the side to be blocked. The zygomatic arch is marked along its course, and the patient is asked to open and close the mouth slowly so that the curved upper border of the mandible can be identified. The lowest point of the mandibular notch is palpated, and an "X" is marked at this spot, which is usually at the midpoint of the zygoma. A skin wheal is raised at the "X" after the appropriate skin preparations.
2. With the patient's jaw in the open position, a 7.5-cm needle is introduced through the "X" and directed 45 degrees cephalad and slightly anterior. This direction should be toward the imagined posterior border of the globe of the eye.
3. The needle should contact the pterygoid plate. It is then withdrawn and redirected slightly anterior until it succeeds in passing beyond the pterygoid plate. At this point, the nerve should lie approximately 1 cm deeper. A paresthesia in the nose or the upper teeth confirms the nerve localization.
4. Anesthesia can be achieved by injecting 5 mL into the fossa, either on obtaining the paresthesia or blindly by advancing 1 cm beyond the plate. The major complication of concern is spread of the anesthetic to adjacent structures, especially to the nerves in the orbit.

Mandibular Nerve Blockade

This nerve can also be blocked for inferior dental pain. It is the only branch where anesthesia carries the risk of loss of motor (mastication) function. The procedure for blockade follows:

1. Head position and landmarks are the same as those described for the maxillary nerve blockade.
2. A 5-cm needle is introduced through the skin wheal and directed medially but slightly posterior and without the cephalad angulation required for maxillary nerve anesthesia. This leaves the needle approximately perpendicular to the skin in all planes.
3. When the pterygoid plate is contacted, the needle is redirected posteriorly until it passes beyond the plate. It should contact the nerve 0.5 to 1 cm deep to this point.
4. Paresthesia of the jaw or cheek confirms identification of the nerve. Five to 10 mL of solution injected incrementally at this point should produce anesthesia of the terminal branches. If paresthesias are essential, exploration should be carried gently cephalad and caudad from the initial point where the needle passes posterior to the plate. As with maxillary blockade, paresthesias can be painful to the patient, and the use of an assistant to secure the head is occasionally necessary. Facial nerve anesthesia can occasionally be seen when large volumes are injected to block the mandibular nerve. This is of little consequence unless neurolytic agents are used. A more serious complication is the possibility of intravascular injection in this highly vascularized area. Injection should be performed incrementally with small quantities and

there should be constant observation for signs of central toxicity.

Cervical Plexus Blockade

Sensory and motor fibers of the neck and posterior scalp arise from the nerve roots of the second, third, and fourth cervical nerves. This cervical plexus is unique in that the sensory fibers separate from the motor fibers early in their course and can be blocked separately. Classic plexus anesthesia along the tubercles of the vertebral body produces both motor and sensory blockade. The transverse processes of the cervical vertebrae form peculiar elongated troughs for the emergence of their nerve roots. These troughs lie immediately lateral to a medial opening for the cephalad passage of the vertebral artery. The trough at the terminal end of the transverse process divides into an anterior and a posterior tubercle, which can often be easily palpated. These tubercles also serve as the attachments for the anterior and middle scalene muscles, which thus form a compartment for the cervical plexus as well as for the brachial plexus immediately below. The compartment at this level is less developed than the one formed around the brachial plexus. The motor branches (including the phrenic nerve) curl anteriorly around the lateral border of the anterior scalene and proceed caudad and medially toward the muscles of the neck. They give anterior branches to the sternocleidomastoid muscle as they pass behind it. The sensory fibers, as mentioned, also emerge behind the anterior scalene muscle but separate from the motor branches and continue laterally to emerge superficially under the posterior border of the sternocleidomastoid muscle. They provide sensory anesthesia to the anterior and posterior skin of the neck and shoulder.

Anesthesia of either the superficial cervical nerves or the cervical plexus itself can be used for operations on the lateral or anterior neck such as thyroidectomy and carotid endarterectomy. In carotid surgery, local infiltration of the carotid bifurcation may be necessary to block reflex hemodynamic changes associated with glossopharyngeal stimulation.

1. The patient is placed supine with a small towel under the head, with the head turned slightly to the side opposite the one to be blocked.
2. The mastoid process is identified and marked. The transverse processes can often be palpated. If not, the most prominent tubercle, that of C6, is marked, and a line is drawn between it and the mastoid process (Fig. 26-4).
3. The cervical processes should be felt approximately 0.5 cm posterior to the line drawn between the mastoid and the sixth cervical tubercle. The second vertebral process should lie approximately 1.5 cm below the mastoid itself. (There is no process for the first vertebra.)

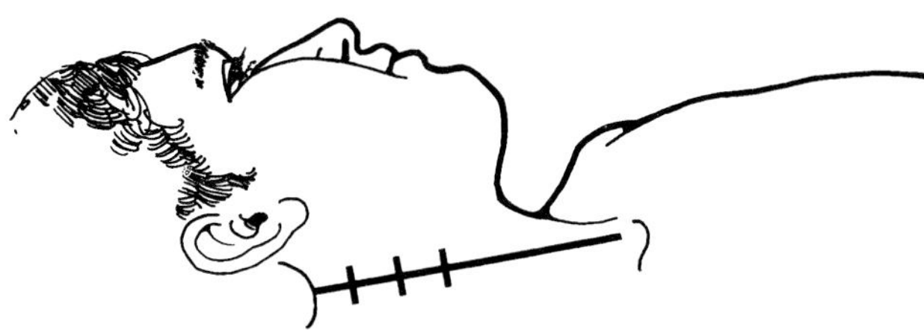

FIGURE 26-4. Superficial landmarks for cervical plexus blockade. A line is drawn from the mastoid process to the prominent tubercle of C6. The transverse processes of C2, C3, and C4 lie 0.5 cm posterior to this line and at 1.5-cm intervals below the mastoid. (Reproduced with permission from Mulroy M: Handbook of Regional Anesthesia. Philadelphia, Lippincott Williams & Wilkins, 2002.)

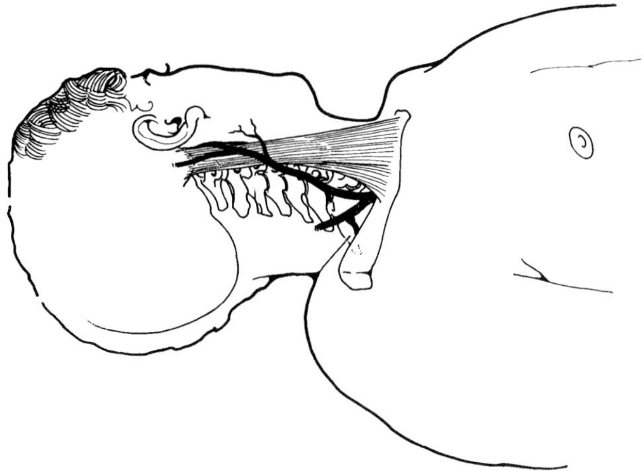

FIGURE 26-5. Anatomy of deep cervical plexus blockade. The transverse processes lie under the lateral border of the sternocleidomastoid muscle, each with a distal trough or sulcus that defines the path of nerve exit. (Reproduced with permission from Mulroy M: Handbook of Regional Anesthesia. Philadelphia, Lippincott Williams & Wilkins, 2002.)

4. The third and fourth processes lie approximately 1.5 cm below their respective superior neighbors.
5. Skin wheals are raised at the three "X" marks that have been placed over the transverse processes.
6. A 3.75-cm needle is introduced perpendicular to the skin and directed posterior and slightly caudad at each "X" until it rests on the transverse process. It is important to maintain a caudad direction to avoid entry directly into the intervertebral foramina. The needle is walked caudad. It should slip off the bone if it is truly on the process rather than continuing to contact bone if it is on the vertebral body. It is important to contact the transverse process as far laterally as possible to avoid any contact of the needle with the vertebral artery (Fig. 26-5).
7. A syringe is connected to the needle, and 5 mL of local anesthetic solution is deposited along the transverse process. Anesthesia in the distribution of the nerve should follow within 5 minutes.

The major potential complication of this procedure is intravascular injection into the vertebral artery. If the needle is advanced too far medially into the vertebral foramen, epidural or even subarachnoid anesthesia may be produced. This is more likely in the cervical region because of longer sleeves of dura that accompany these nerve branches.

Phrenic nerve blockade occurs with deep cervical plexus anesthesia. This blockade is not indicated in any patient who depends on the diaphragm for tidal ventilation, nor is bilateral blockade desirable in most patients. Recurrent laryngeal nerve or vagal blockade can also occur because of diffusion of the local anesthetic. This is a troublesome but not serious complication. It may interfere with the ability to evaluate vocal cord function following thyroid surgery.

Superficial Cervical Plexus Blockade. This is performed in the same position as deep cervical plexus blockade and results in anesthesia only of the sensory fibers of the plexus. The procedure for blockade follows:

1. An "X" is made along the posterior border of the sternocleidomastoid muscle at the level of C4. This usually corresponds with the junction of the external jugular vein as it crosses the posterior border of the muscle (Fig. 26-6).

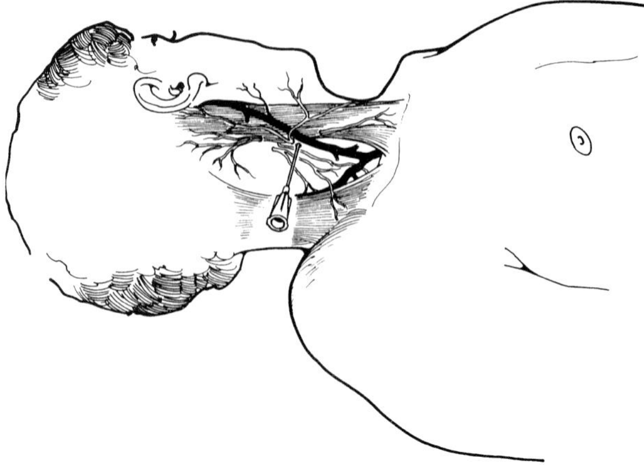

FIGURE 26-6. Superficial cervical plexus blockade. The sensory fibers of the plexus all emerge from behind the lateral border of the sternocleidomastoid muscle. A needle inserted at its midpoint, usually where the external jugular vein crosses the muscle, can be directed superiorly and inferiorly to block all these terminal branches. (Reproduced with permission from Mulroy M: Handbook of Regional Anesthesia. Philadelphia, Lippincott Williams & Wilkins, 2002.)

2. A skin wheal is raised at this mark, and superficial local anesthetic infiltration is performed along the posterior border of the sternocleidomastoid muscle 4 cm above and below the level of the "X." Ten to 12 mL of local anesthetic solution usually provides sensory anesthesia of the anterior neck and shoulder.

Occipital Nerve Blockade

The ophthalmic branch of the trigeminal nerve provides sensory innervation of the forehead and anterior scalp, but the remainder of the scalp is innervated by fibers of the greater and lesser occipital nerves, terminal branches of the cervical plexus. These nerves can be blocked by superficial injection at the point on the posterior skull where they emerge from below the muscles of the neck (Fig. 26-7). Anesthesia is rarely used for surgical procedures; it is more often applied as a diagnostic step in evaluating head and neck pain complaints. The procedure for blockade follows:

1. The block is performed in the sitting position, with the patient leaning the head forward to expose the prominent nuchal ridge of bone at the posterior base of the skull.
2. The external occipital protuberance is identified in the midline, and a mark is placed lateral to this prominence along the nuchal line at the lateral border of the insertion of the erector muscles of the neck, usually 2.5 cm from the midline. The branches of the greater occipital nerve usually pass laterally from behind the muscle to cross the nuchal line at this point.
3. After skin preparation, a small needle is introduced through the mark to the depth of the skull itself. A ridge of 1 to 4 mL of local anesthetic (1% lidocaine or equivalent) is then deposited across the path of the emerging nerves just above the level of the bone. Paresthesias are occasionally encountered but are not essential for obtaining simple skin anesthesia.
4. If more anterior anesthesia of the scalp is required, the lesser occipital nerve branches are also blocked by advancing the needle subcutaneously from this point in an anterior direction toward the mastoid process. A band of anesthetic solution is deposited along the line between the skin entry and the mastoid. A larger volume (6 to 8 mL) is required.

Complications of this technique are rare. Care must be taken not to advance the needle anteriorly under the skull, as the foramen magnum might be entered unintentionally with a long needle. Local hematoma may be produced with the superficial injection, but this is only a temporary problem.

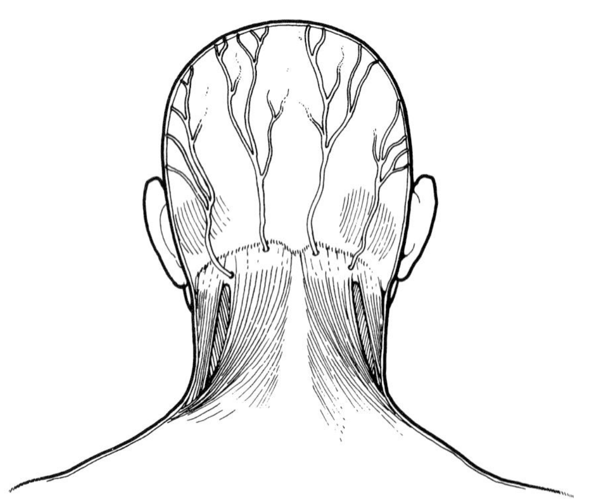

FIGURE 26-7. Occipital nerve blockade. The greater and lesser branches of the occipital nerve emerge from under the muscles at the level of the nuchal ridge on the posterior scalp. They can be easily blocked by a subcutaneous ridge of anesthetic solution. (Reproduced with permission from Mulroy M: Handbook of Regional Anesthesia. Philadelphia, Lippincott Williams & Wilkins, 2002.)

Airway Anesthesia

Manipulation of the airway either during laryngoscopy or during tracheal intubation is often associated with laryngospasm, coughing, and undesirable cardiovascular reflexes (see also Chapter 22). The anesthesiologist can abolish or blunt these reflexes by anesthetizing one or all of the sensory pathways involved. The nasal mucosa is innervated by fibers of the sphenopalatine ganglion, a branch of the middle division of the fifth cranial nerve. These branches lie on the lateral wall of the nasal passages on each side, under the mucosa just posterior to the middle turbinate (Fig. 26-8). The branches of these fibers continue caudad to provide sensory innervation to the superior portion of the pharynx, uvula, and tonsils. Anesthesia of the maxillary branch of the trigeminal nerve is possible but not a practical solution for airway anesthesia. Transmucosal topical application of local anesthetic is more appropriate. Below the sphenopalatine fiber distribution, sensory innervation of the oral pharynx and supraglottic regions is provided by branches of the glossopharyngeal nerve. These nerves lie laterally on each side of the pharynx submucosally in the region of the posterior tonsillar pillar. Direct submucosal injection can be performed but carries the risk of unintentional intravascular injection into several blood vessels in this area. Topical anesthesia of the terminal branches in the mouth and throat is again an easier approach, but deep injection of the glossopharyngeal nerve may be required to block the gag reflex completely. The larynx itself is innervated by the superior laryngeal branch of the vagus nerve in the area above the vocal cords. This branch leaves the main vagal trunk in the carotid sheath and passes anteriorly. Its internal branch penetrates the thyrohyoid membrane and divides to provide the sensory fibers to the cords, epiglottis, and arytenoids.

The recurrent laryngeal nerve provides innervation to the areas below the vocal cords, including motor innervation for all but one of the intrinsic laryngeal muscles. The trachea itself is innervated by the recurrent laryngeal nerve. Topical anesthesia is again the simplest approach to this nerve.

Airway anesthesia can be performed by anesthetizing one or all of these sensory distributions. Full anesthesia facilitates procedures such as nasal intubation or fiberoptic laryngoscopy. Airway anesthesia below the vocal cords is best avoided if there is concern about potential pulmonary aspiration of gastric contents. Topical postpharyngeal anesthesia may also ablate protective laryngeal reflexes.

Many patients find it more comfortable to be semiupright or sitting when topical anesthesia is sprayed into the posterior pharynx. These positions allow them greater ease in swallowing excess solutions and may reduce gagging. In whatever position chosen, there should be a firm support behind the head to reduce involuntary withdrawal motions by the patient, which might dislocate needles being used for injections.

1. For nasal mucosal anesthesia, cotton pledgets soaked with anesthetic solution are introduced through the nares and passed along the turbinates all the way to the posterior end of the nasal passage (see Fig. 26-8). A second set of pledgets is introduced with a cephalad angulation to follow the middle turbinate back to the mucosa overlying the sphenoid bone. This pledget is the more critical because anesthesia in this mucosal area is most likely to anesthetize the branches of the sphenopalatine ganglia as they pass along the lateral wall of the airway. Bilateral anesthesia is preferable, even if a nasal tube is to be inserted only on one side; bilateral blockade of the sphenopalatine fibers also produces posterior pharyngeal anesthesia caudad to this level. The pledgets should be allowed to remain in contact with the nasal mucosa for at least 2 to 3 minutes to allow adequate diffusion of local anesthetic. Cocaine in a 4% solution has been the traditional topical anesthetic for this application because of its unique vasoconstrictive properties. Alternate solutions have been recommended, primarily a mixture of 3% to 4% lidocaine and 0.25% to 0.5% phenylephrine.
2. Topical anesthesia to the posterior pharynx can be performed while the nasal applicators are in place. This can be done with a commercial spray or with an atomizer filled with a 4% solution of lidocaine. (A higher concentration of local anesthetic is required to penetrate mucosal membranes.) For effective anesthesia in the posterior pharyngeal wall, topical application is performed in two stages. First, the tongue itself is sprayed with a local anesthetic, and the patient is encouraged to gargle and swallow the residual liquid in the mouth. The numb tongue is then grasped with a gauze pad with one hand while the spray device is inserted into the mouth with the other. The patient is then encouraged to take rapid deep breaths ("pant like a puppy") while the spray is applied on inspiration. The inspiratory flow of gases should be enough to draw the lidocaine solution into the posterior pharynx and even to the vocal cords themselves. If superior laryngeal nerve blockade has been performed before this, it is likely that the aerosol will be carried into the trachea itself. Again, a few minutes are needed for adequate onset of topical anesthesia in the pharynx. Topical anesthesia is less effective if there are copious secretions. Premedication with an anticholinergic is frequently beneficial.
3. Superior laryngeal nerve blockade can also be performed while the nasal pledgets are in place (Fig. 26-9). This nerve is blocked bilaterally by identifying the superior ala of the thyroid cartilage, which usually lies just inferior to the posterior portion of the hyoid bone on each side. A 5-mL syringe with a 1% lidocaine solution with a 23-gauge, 1.75-cm needle is used. The index finger of one hand retracts the skin of the neck caudad down over the thyroid cartilage; the needle is inserted until it rests on the superior margin of the cartilage. The tension on the skin is then released and the needle is withdrawn slightly and allowed to walk superiorly off the cartilage. The needle is then reinserted and passed through the thyrohyoid membrane, which is perceived as a discernible resistance. After careful aspiration, 2.5 mL of solution is injected into the space below the membrane. This procedure is repeated on the opposite side. This blockade can be

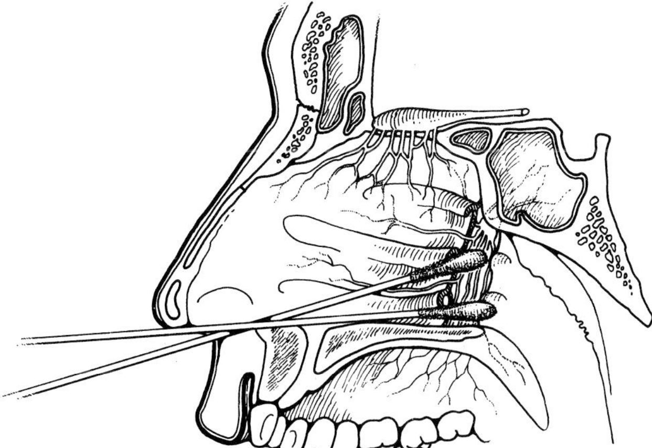

FIGURE 26-8. Nasal airway anesthesia. Cotton pledgets soaked with anesthetic are inserted along the inferior and middle turbinates to produce anesthesia of the underlying sphenopalatine ganglion by transmembrane diffusion of the solution. Wide pledgets also are needed to provide maximal topical anesthesia and vasoconstriction of the nasal mucosa. (Reproduced with permission from Mulroy M: Handbook of Regional Anesthesia. Philadelphia, Lippincott Williams & Wilkins, 2002.)

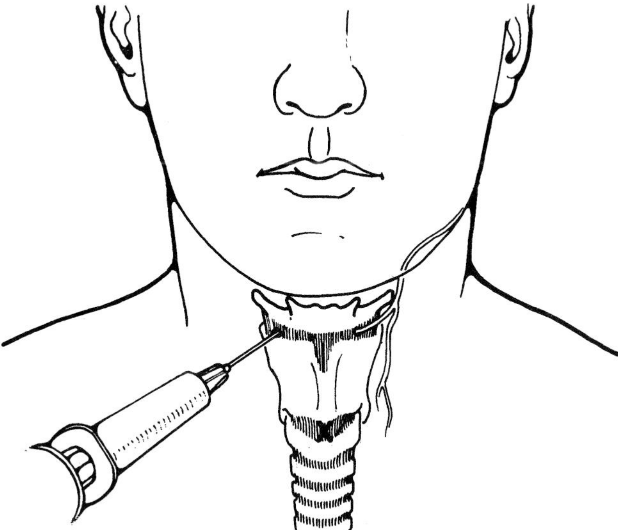

FIGURE 26-9. Superior laryngeal nerve blockade. The needle is advanced superiorly off the lateral wing of the thyroid cartilage to drop through the thyrohyoid membrane. (Reproduced with permission from Mulroy M: Handbook of Regional Anesthesia. Philadelphia, Lippincott Williams & Wilkins, 2002.)

performed as part of total airway anesthesia or it can be used independently to provide increased acceptance of indwelling endotracheal tubes in the intensive care unit.
4. The glossopharyngeal nerve can be blocked by a direct injection into the base of the anterior tonsillar pillar if persistent gagging is a problem. The tongue is retracted medially with a gloved finger or a tongue blade to expose the base of the anterior pillar. A long 25-gauge (spinal) needle is inserted 0.5 cm subcutaneously into the base of the pillar 0.5 cm lateral to the base of the tongue. After careful aspiration, 2 mL of 1.5% lidocaine is injected, and the procedure is repeated on the opposite side. This produces anesthesia of the lingual branch (base of the tongue) and may even anesthetize the pharyngeal and tonsillar branches by diffusion. This allows laryngoscopy with less gagging and hemodynamic response.
5. Tracheal anesthesia can be performed by a direct transcricoid ("transtracheal") injection. This is accomplished by raising a small skin wheal over the cricothyroid membrane. A 20-gauge iv catheter is then inserted gently through this skin wheal and through the membrane. Entry into the trachea can be confirmed by the ability to aspirate air through the catheter. The steel stylet is then removed, and the plastic catheter is left in the trachea. A syringe with 4 mL of 4% lidocaine is attached to the catheter, and the local anesthetic is sprayed into the trachea during inspiration. The flow of air usually carries the local anesthetic distally; the resultant cough continues to spread the anesthetic more proximally up to the underside of the vocal cords and the larynx.
6. After each of these steps has been completed, the pledgets can be removed from the nasal passages and nasal intubation performed. If tracheal or laryngeal anesthesia has been omitted because of concern about aspiration, there should be some pharmacologic intervention to reduce the cardiovascular response to the passage of the tube into the trachea. This can be facilitated by pretreatment with iv β-adrenergic-blocking drugs, by administration of sedation, or by administration of propofol immediately after the airway is secured.

Complications of these techniques are rare. Systemic toxicity from the local anesthetics is a distinct possibility because of the large quantities of drug required to produce sufficient mucosal anesthesia. If all four stages of airway anesthesia are undertaken, the total milligram doses applied usually exceed the maximal recommended dose for peripheral injection. Fortunately, the mucosal absorption is less than the peripheral absorption, but close attention to the patient's mental status and preparation for treatment of toxicity are necessary. Aspiration of gastric contents is also a possibility when the protective reflexes of the airway are interrupted.

Upper Extremity

The innervation of the upper extremity is conveniently derived from five closely approximated nerve roots, extending from C5 to T1 (the brachial plexus). These roots undergo a series of mergers and divisions that produce the terminal nerves of the arm and hand. The plexus branches are close enough to each other to allow reliable anesthesia to be achieved at several points associated with consistent bony or vascular landmarks.

In their proximal course, the nerve roots lie in a well demarcated fascial envelope formed by the anterior fascia of the middle scalene muscle and the posterior fascia of the anterior scalene. These muscles attach to the posterior and anterior tubercles of the transverse processes of the cervical vertebrae from which the nerves emerge. The tubercle can be used as a faithful landmark to guide localization of the nerve, and the fascial planes serve to keep anesthetic solution injected between them close to the nerve bundle. The fascia extends outward for a variable distance from the lateral border of the muscles to enclose the nerves in a "sheath," which can extend below the clavicle. This enclosed bundle passes over the first rib just behind the midpoint of the clavicle (and just posterior to the insertion of the anterior scalene on the rib), where it is joined by the subclavian artery. At the midpoint of the rib, the plexus has consolidated into only three trunks; these rapidly subdivide into the terminal branches. The musculocutaneous nerve is the first major branch to leave the companionship of its partners as it passes into the body of the coracobrachialis muscle high in the axilla. As the individual nerves form, separate compartments in the sheath are formed by developing septa, and blockade of all the nerves with a single injection is not reliable below the clavicle.

Although many approaches to the brachial plexus have been described, there are basically four anatomic locations where anesthetics are placed: (1) the interscalene groove near the transverse processes, (2) the subclavian sheath at the first rib, (3) near the coracoid process in the infraclavicular fossa, and (4) surrounding the axillary artery in the axilla. Because of the specific configuration of the nerves at each of these levels, the anesthesia produced is different with each approach and applicable to different situations.[8] Interscalene injection at the level of the sixth cervical transverse process produces extension of the blockade to the lower fibers of the cervical plexus and is ideally suited for shoulder operations and upper arm procedures. It frequently spares the lowest branches of the plexus, the C8 and T1 fibers, which innervate the caudad (ulnar) border of the forearm. Blockade at the level of the first rib is most reliable in producing anesthesia of all four terminal nerves of the forearm and hand. Injection in the infraclavicular fossa produces excellent anesthesia of the entire arm and hand, although multiple injections may be required. The axillary technique is simpler but carries the risk of missing the musculocutaneous and medial antebrachial cutaneous nerves that depart the sheath high in the axilla, and thus might produce inadequate anesthesia of the forearm. The choice of the appropriate approach depends not only on the patient's anatomy but also on the site of surgery.

The terminal branches can also be anesthetized by local anesthetic injection along their peripheral courses as they cross the joint spaces, or by the injection of a dilute local anesthetic solution intravenously below a pneumatic tourniquet on the upper arm ("intravenous regional," or Bier block).

Brachial Plexus Blockade: Interscalene Approach

Localization of the nerves uses a combination of the muscular and bony landmarks surrounding the nerves.[9] The use of long-acting local anesthetics will provide analgesia for 12 to 14 hours. For longer analgesia, insertion of a continuous catheter is effective for procedures such as shoulder rotator cuff repairs,[10] although securing the catheters in the mobile neck tissues is a challenge.

1. The patient is positioned supine with the head turned to the side opposite that to be blocked. A small towel is placed under the occiput. The arm on the side to be blocked is held at the side, and the patient is asked to hold the shoulder down by pretending to reach for the hip.
2. The lateral border of the sternocleidomastoid muscle is identified and marked, and the patient is then asked to raise the head slightly into a "sniffing" position. This tenses the scalene muscles behind the sternocleidomastoid muscle, and the groove between the anterior and middle scalene is palpated by rolling the fingers posteriorly off the lateral border of the sternocleidomastoid muscle. This groove is marked along its entire extent, as

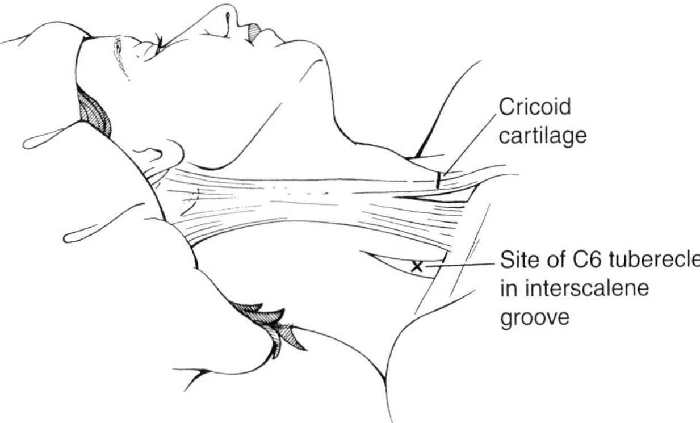

FIGURE 26-10. Superficial landmarks for interscalene brachial plexus blockade. The sternocleidomastoid muscle is identified, and the anterior scalene muscle is found by moving the fingertips over the lateral border of the larger muscle while it is slightly tensed. The groove between the anterior and middle scalene muscles can usually be felt easily, along with the tubercle of the sixth cervical vertebra, which lies at the level of the cricoid cartilage. (Reproduced with permission from Mulroy M: Handbook of Regional Anesthesia. Philadelphia, Lippincott Williams & Wilkins, 2002.)

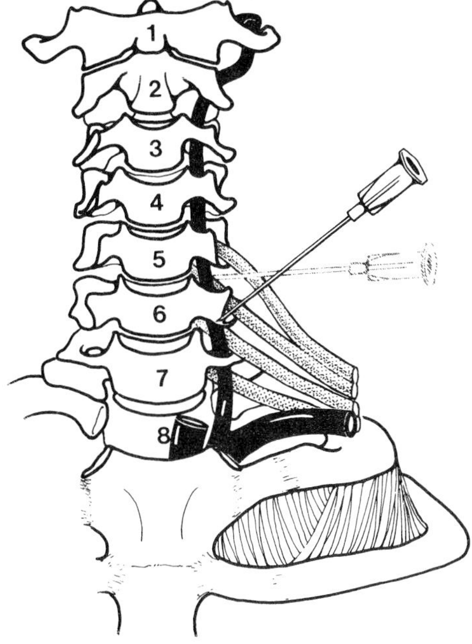

FIGURE 26-12. Needle direction for interscalene blockade. The needle is always kept in a 45-degree caudad direction; medial insertion allows the point to pass into the intervertebral foramen and produces epidural, spinal, or intra-arterial injection of anesthetic. Note the relation of the vertebral artery and the nerve roots to the transverse processes. (Reproduced with permission from Mulroy M: Handbook of Regional Anesthesia. Philadelphia, Lippincott Williams & Wilkins, 2002.)

high up as possible. The patient then relaxes the muscles of the neck, and the level of the cricoid cartilage is marked. The index finger then gently palpates in the groove at the level of the cricoid (Fig. 26-10). The prominent transverse process of C6 can often be felt directly.

3. After aseptic skin preparation, a skin wheal is raised in the groove at the level of the cricoid. A 22-gauge, 3.75-cm needle is introduced through the wheal perpendicular to the skin in all planes so that it is directed medially, caudad, and slightly posteriorly (Fig. 26-11).
4. The needle is advanced until the tubercle is contacted or nerve localization is elicited (Fig. 26-12). If bone is contacted before nerve, the needle is withdrawn and redirected in small steps in an anteroposterior plane until the nerves are identified.
5. Once the nerve is located (usually a motor response in the deltoid or biceps, or a paresthesia to the thumb or upper arm), the needle is fixed in this position with one hand while 25 to 30 mL of local anesthetic solution is injected. Careful aspiration is performed first, and the initial injection is performed in small increments to detect intraneural or intraarterial placement of the needle. A larger volume (30 to 40 mL) is required if greater spread is desired, such as to the cervical plexus or inferiorly to the C8 to T1 fibers.
6. If a catheter is to be inserted, the needle entry point may be moved a centimeter cephalad and the corresponding angle of insertion is a little steeper and more tangential to the course of the plexus. The opening of the tip of the introducing needle should be directed laterally. After the catheter is introduced a few centimeters beyond the tip, the proximal end may be secured more firmly by tunneling 3 to 4 cm below the skin by passing it back through an intravenous catheter that has been introduced subcutaneously near the entry site. Securing catheters in the freely mobile neck is a challenge.
7. If arm surgery requiring a tourniquet is planned, a subcutaneous ring of anesthetic across the axilla is usually required to block the superficial intercostobrachial fibers crossing from the chest wall into the axilla.

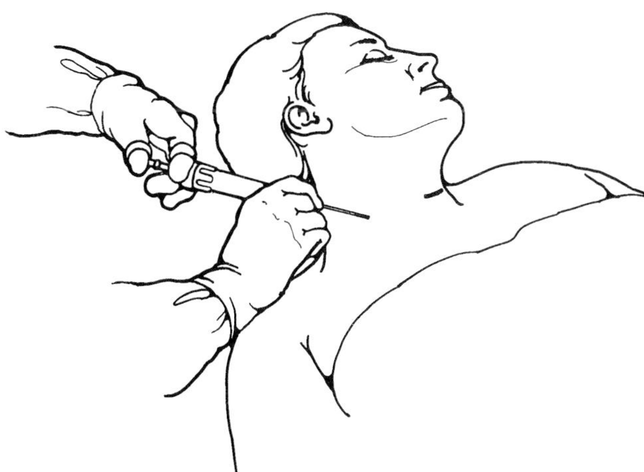

FIGURE 26-11. Hand position for interscalene blockade. The needle is directed medially and caudad into the interscalene groove while one hand exerts constant control of the depth by resting on the clavicle. (Reproduced with permission from Mulroy M: Handbook of Regional Anesthesia. Philadelphia, Lippincott Williams & Wilkins, 2002.)

Complications from this approach are related to the structures located in the vicinity of the tubercle. The cupola of the lung is close and can be contacted if the needle is directed too far caudad. Pneumothorax should be considered if cough or chest pain is produced while exploring for the nerve. If the needle is allowed to pass directly medially, it may enter the intervertebral foramina, and injection of local anesthetic may produce spinal or epidural anesthesia. The vertebral artery passes posteriorly at the level of the sixth vertebra to lie in its canal in the transverse process; direct injection into this vessel can rapidly produce central nervous system toxicity and convulsions.

Careful aspiration and incremental injections are helpful in avoiding both of these potential problems.

Even with appropriate injection, the local anesthetic solution spreads to contiguous nerves. This produces cervical plexus blockade with high volumes, including the motor fibers to the diaphragm, which may be a problem in patients with respiratory insufficiency. A Horner's syndrome is common because of spread to the sympathetic chain on the anterior vertebral body.

Neuropathy of the C6 root is a potential problem because the needle may unintentionally pin the nerve root against the tubercle and predispose to intraneural injection. The needle should be withdrawn slightly if the first injection produces the characteristic "crampy" pain sensation.

Inadequate anesthesia is most likely to occur in the ulnar distribution. As mentioned previously, this may be reduced by the use of higher volumes.

Brachial Plexus Blockade: Supraclavicular Approach

The description of the approach to the brachial plexus at this level is originally attributed to Kulenkampff. Current techniques avoid medial direction of the needle, as originally described, which may contact the pleura.

1. The patient lies in the same position as for interscalene blockade, with the ipsilateral arm held at the side and pulled downward to exaggerate the landmarks of the clavicle and the neck muscles.
2. The outline of the clavicle is drawn on the skin, as well as the interscalene groove (as described previously). The midpoint of the clavicle is marked. An "X" is placed posterior to this midpoint in the interscalene groove, usually 1 cm behind the clavicle. On the thin patient, the pulsation of the subclavian artery can be appreciated in the groove or just anterior to it.
3. After aseptic preparation, a skin wheal is raised at the mark, and a 3.75-cm, 22-gauge needle attached to a 10-mL syringe is introduced in the sagittal plane and advanced caudad until the first rib is contacted (Fig. 26-13). It is important that the direction of the needle remain perpendicular to the rib, which usually requires that the syringe remain parallel to the axis of the head and neck. If the rib is not contacted, careful exploration should be carried out first laterally to the mark and, last of all, medially. The greatest danger of contacting the pleura occurs when probing medially.
4. If a nerve response is not obtained on needle insertion, exploration is continued until the rib is identified. A 5-cm needle may be needed to reach the rib in the heavier patient. Once the rib is contacted, the needle is walked in an anteroposterior plane until a nerve response is found. Again, the needle is kept in the sagittal plane on the dorsal surface of the rib during exploration. If the needle advances beyond the anterior or posterior border of the rib as it curves medially at these two points, it is simply redirected in the opposite direction until the rib is found again. Medial direction is avoided. While exploring along the direction of the rib, the needle should be withdrawn almost to the skin before redirection for each pass. If it is lifted only a few millimeters from the rib, it may simply push the nerve bundle ahead of it without making contact.
5. If no nerve response is obtained, the artery can be used as a landmark. Once it is entered with the needle, a series of injections posterior to it can be used to produce a "wall" of 40 mL of anesthetic solution in this area.
6. An alternate approach is to introduce the needle just above the clavicle from the anterior surface of the body, and advance it directly posterior, following a line that would be traversed by a plumb bob toward the floor (assuming the patient is supine).If no nerve response is encountered, the syringe and needle are withdrawn and rotated caudally in small increments and advanced again. Theoretically, the needle will encounter the nerves before contacting the rib or the pleura. The safety of this approach may be improved by starting with an even greater cephalad angulation, 40 degrees off the vertical.[11]
7. If a nerve response is produced during the course of exploration, the anesthetic solution is injected while the needle is fixed in position. Twenty-five to 40 mL of local anesthetic will produce adequate analgesia. Multiple nerve responses are not required.
8. If a tourniquet is to be used, a ring of subcutaneous anesthesia should be infiltrated along the axilla to block the sensory fibers from the chest wall that cross here to innervate the inner aspect of the upper arm.

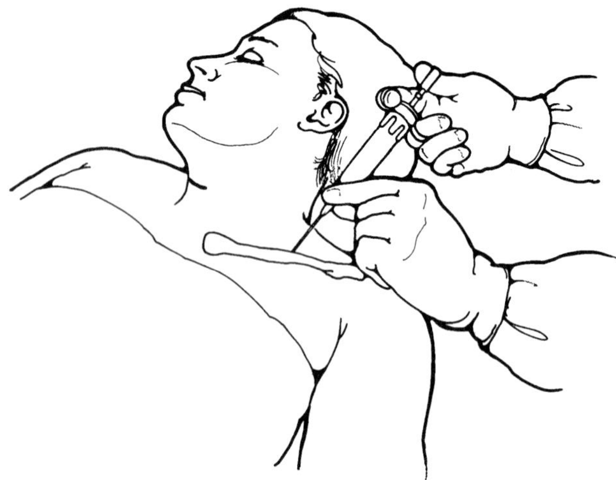

FIGURE 26-13. Hand position for supraclavicular blockade. The needle is directed caudad behind the midpoint of the clavicle in the interscalene groove. Again, control of depth is maintained by the hand resting on the clavicle. The syringe is kept in the sagittal plane parallel to the patient's head to prevent medial angulation, which would increase the chance of pneumothorax. (Reproduced with permission from Mulroy M: Handbook of Regional Anesthesia. Philadelphia, Lippincott Williams & Wilkins, 2002.)

Pneumothorax is the most serious complication of this technique. Although it is rare in experienced hands, it does occur more frequently with this approach to the brachial plexus than with any other approach. This may limit the use of this technique, particularly in outpatients, in whom the insertion of a chest tube would then require hospitalization. Other complications of peripheral blockade of the brachial plexus do not occur with any greater frequency with this blockade than with other methods of blockade.

Brachial Plexus: Infraclavicular Block

Approaching the brachial plexus in the infraclavicular area at the point where the plexus passes below the coracoid process appears to have a lower risk of pneumothorax (Fig. 26-14). Here the plexus consists of three cords, with the musculocutaneous nerve already departed from the bundle. Nerve localization is more challenging than with other techniques because of the depth from the skin, but the approach in the infraclavicular area offers the potential of excellent analgesia of the entire arm with only two separate injections, and also allows for the introduction for continuous catheters to provide prolonged postoperative pain relief. The original description of this

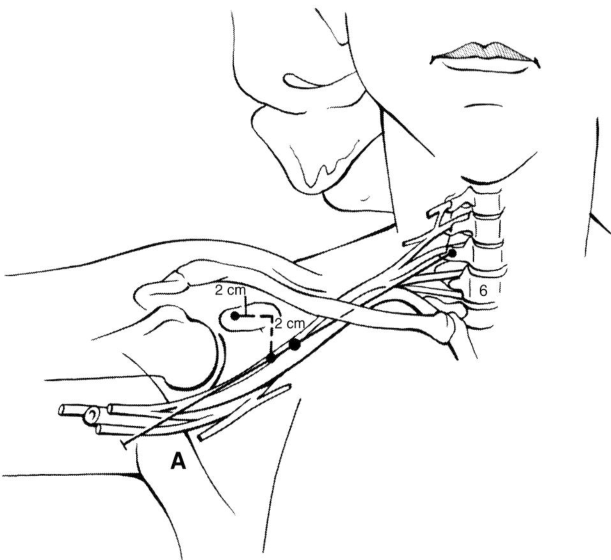

FIGURE 26-14. Infraclavicular approach. The nerves and trunks of the brachial plexus lie basically along a straight line that can be projected from the lateral tubercle of the C6 vertebral body to the axillary artery in the axilla. At the midpoint of this line, the plexus consists of three trunks, with the musculocutaneous nerve potentially having already departed from the neurovascular bundle. This midpoint lies below the clavicle and lateral to the rib cage. The nerves can be identified by drawing a line ending 2 cm medially from the cricoid process and 2 cm inferiorly. A needle inserted directly posterior at this point should contact the nerves at a depth of between 5 and 10 cm. (Reproduced with permission from Mulroy M: Handbook of Regional Anesthesia. Philadelphia, Lippincott Williams & Wilkins, 2002.)

procedure was a complex one that was limited in its accuracy; more recent anatomic and radiographic studies have provided a simpler approach,[12] as follows:

1. Patient is placed in the supine position with the arm at the side. The coracoid process is palpated below the clavicle and marked with a circle. A line is drawn 2 cm medially and then extended 2 cm inferiorly from this point, and an "X" is placed on the skin.
2. After skin preparation and skin wheal, a 10-cm needle is inserted directly perpendicularly through the "X" and advanced through the pectoralis muscle, searching for a nerve response. The first response obtained is usually the musculocutaneous nerve. This nerve can be blocked by an injection of 5 mL of local anesthetic. For complete anesthesia of the hand, a separate response in the hand itself needs to be obtained. When movement or sensation in the hand is elicited, a further 25 mL of local anesthetic can be injected, presumably within the neurovascular sheath at this point. The sheath usually lies just caudad to the musculocutaneous nerve. The artery may be also identified easily at this point, and careful aspiration is required to prevent intravascular injection.
3. If a response is not elicited before contact is made with bone (usually the scapula posteriorly), then the needle is withdrawn to near the skin and reintroduced with a slightly different angulation, usually in a caudad direction. Several passes may be required because the nerves lie at an average depth of 5 cm from the skin. At this point, small changes in needle angulation may produce wide variations in the location of the tip of the needle.
4. If a catheter is to be threaded, it should be only in response to nerve localization in the hand itself. The tip of the Tuohy needle should be directed laterally to allow the catheter to run in the direction of the nerves. It should be advanced only a short distance beyond the tip of the needle because of the risk of puncturing the artery at this level. The catheter can be secured to the skin and remain indwelling for several days.[13]

Complications of this technique include hematoma formation and nerve injury. The risk of pneumothorax is minimized by avoiding any medial deviation of the needle point.

Brachial Plexus: Axillary Technique

The axillary technique carries the least chance of pneumothorax and thus may be a preferred technique for the outpatient. The nerves are anesthetized around the axillary artery, where they have regrouped into their terminal branches. Because of the observation that the single sheath may be broken up into separate compartments by fascial septa surrounding individual nerves in the axilla, local anesthetic should be injected at multiple sites in the axilla in contrast to the single injections possible with proximal approaches. Another obstacle to the single-injection technique at this level is the early departure of the musculocutaneous branch from the sheath high in the axilla.

1. The patient lies supine with the arm extended 90 degrees from the side and flexed at the elbow. Extension beyond 90 degrees potentially compresses the axillary artery because of the pressure from the head of the humerus and may make identification of the landmarks more difficult. A pillow under the forearm also reduces rotation of the shoulder joint, which can obscure the pulse.
2. The axillary artery is marked as high in its course in the axilla as is practical. It is usually felt in the intramuscular groove between the coracobrachialis and the triceps muscles. It also passes between the insertions of the pectoralis major and the latissimus dorsi muscles on the humerus.
3. After aseptic preparation, a skin wheal is raised over the proximal portion of the artery. The index and middle fingers of the nondominant hand straddle the artery just below this point, both localizing the pulsation and compressing the neurovascular bundle below the intended site of injection (Fig. 26-15).

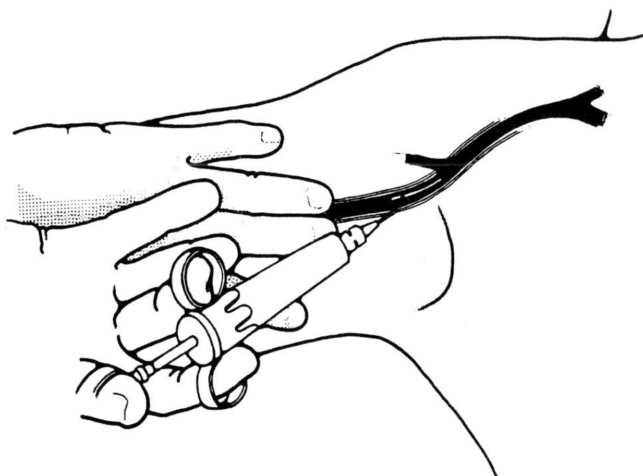

FIGURE 26-15. Hand position for axillary blockade. Two fingers of equal length straddle the artery while the needle is introduced along its long axis with a central angulation. The palpating fingers serve not only to identify the vessel but also to compress the perivascular sheath and encourage the spread of anesthetic solution centrally. (Reproduced with permission from Mulroy M: Handbook of Regional Anesthesia. Philadelphia, Lippincott Williams & Wilkins, 2002.)

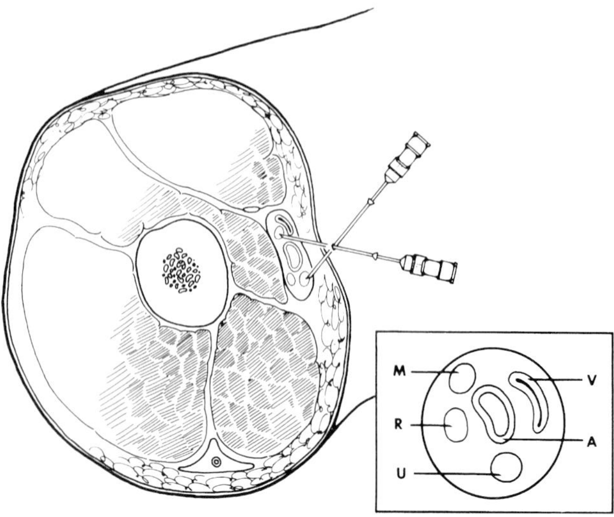

FIGURE 26-16. Needle position for axillary injection. The median (*M*) and musculocutaneous nerves lie on the superior side of the artery (*A*), although the latter may have already departed the axillary sheath at the level of injection. The ulnar nerve (*U*) lies inferior, and the radial nerve (*R*) is inferior and posterior. *V*, vein.

4. Common Approaches

A) *Direct Nerve Localization.* The traditional method is to identify each of the nerves with either a paresthesia or nerve stimulator technique. Ideally, the nerves serving the area of proposed surgery are sought first. The median and the musculocutaneous nerves lie on the superior aspect of the artery (as viewed by the operator), whereas the ulnar and radial nerves lie below and behind the vessel (Fig. 26-16). A three-ring syringe is especially useful in this technique to allow aspiration during the nerve search, to help identify the potential for switching to a transarterial approach if the artery is entered. When a nerve response is obtained, 5 to 10 mL are injected, taking precautions to avoid intraneural injection. Firm pressure is maintained on the distal sheath to encourage the solution to move centrally from the point of injection, hopefully to include the point of origin of the musculocutaneous nerve. With the multiple-injection technique, other nerve responses should be elicited within 5 minutes of the original injection. Beyond this time, spread of the solution may produce hypesthesia of the other nerves, which prevents their identification. The second nerve response should be sought on the side of the artery opposite the original one. While some have had success in patients in simply injecting a large volume on a single-nerve response, most practitioners have found the need to identify at least two or three separate nerves to ensure success.

Alternatively, all four major peripheral nerves may be stimulated and anesthetized lower in the arm, at the junction of the upper and middle third of the humerus (midhumeral approach[14]). At this point, the median nerve is stimulated subcutaneously near the artery, the ulnar nerve is deeper and medial to the artery, the musculocutaneous nerve is under the biceps and 2 to 4 cm away from the artery, and the radial nerve is behind the humerus.

B) *Perivascular infiltration.* Using the same approach with a shorter, smaller gauge needle, 5 to 10 mL of local anesthetic is injected closely on each side of the artery, using multiple passes with a moving needle *not* seeking nerve responses, producing a "wall" of solution that intercepts the paths of each of the branches. After initial infiltration, sensation or motor function is tested in the peripheral nerve distribution within 5 minutes. If anesthesia is not present, reinjection of the area is again performed with multiple passes. This approach is simpler and can be performed rapidly, but requires clear identification of the pulse.

C) *Transarterial.* Another simple alternative is to deliberately enter the artery with the needle. The needle is advanced through the vessel until aspiration confirms that it has passed just posterior; at this point, half the anesthetic solution is injected incrementally with careful attention to avoid intravascular placement. The needle is then withdrawn back through the vessel until aspiration confirms that it is just anterior to the artery. The other half of the solution is injected. This technique is simple and effective and should be kept in mind as an alternative if the vessel is unintentionally entered during either of the aforementioned techniques.

5. If forearm anesthesia is required, supplementary anesthesia of the musculocutaneous nerve may be obtained by injecting an additional 5 to 10 mL of anesthetic solution into the body of the coracobrachialis muscle. This muscle can be easily grasped between the thumb and forefinger, and the entry into its fascial compartment is readily identified. Alternatively a direct nerve response can be elicited with a stimulator. This step may be required even if 40 mL of solution is used in the perivascular injection because the musculocutaneous nerve may be spared as often as 25% of the time even with this or larger volumes. A supplemental subcutaneous injection of 5 mL inferior to the artery is also required to anesthetize the medial antebrachial cutaneous nerve.
6. If a continuous technique is desired, a catheter can be threaded centrally after nerve localization, or simply after identifying the "sheath" by perceiving the characteristic fascial pop on entry that is more easily appreciated with the larger blunter needles used for catheter insertion. Securing the catheter in the axilla is challenging, and may require immobilization of the arm.

The complications of the axillary approaches to the brachial plexus are minimal compared with those of the more proximal approaches. The problem of neuropathy is the foremost consideration, and the relative risk with various techniques remains controversial. Hematoma can occur if the vessel is punctured, but this is rarely a problem. The use of small-gauge needles may reduce this possibility. The advantages of any one technique in reducing complications remains unclear, and the success rate of the various techniques is variable and appears to depend on personal familiarity.

Intravenous Regional Anesthesia (Bier Block)

The simplest technique of arm anesthesia is the injection of local anesthetic into the venous system below an occluding tourniquet.

1. A small-gauge (20 or 22) iv plastic catheter is inserted in the arm to be blocked on the dorsum of the hand. It is taped firmly in place, and a heparin port or small syringe is attached and saline is injected to maintain patency. A pneumatic tourniquet is applied over the upper arm.
2. The arm is elevated to promote venous drainage. An elastic bandage may be applied to produce further exsanguination. After exsanguination, the tourniquet is inflated to 300 mm Hg or 2.5 times the patient's systolic

blood pressure and is tested for adequate occlusion of the radial pulse.

3. The arm is returned to the horizontal position, a 50-mL syringe with 0.5% lidocaine is attached to the previously inserted cannula, and the contents are injected. The forearm discolors, and the patient perceives a transient "pins and needles" sensation as anesthesia ensues over the following 5 minutes. Epinephrine should not be added to the local anesthetic solution.
4. For short procedures, the cannula can be removed at this point. If surgery may extend beyond 1 hour, the cannula can be left in place and reinjected after 90 minutes.
5. Beyond 45 minutes of surgery, many patients experience discomfort at the level of the tourniquet. Special "double-cuff" tourniquets are available for this blockade to alleviate this problem. The proximal cuff is inflated first, allowing anesthesia to be induced in the area under the distal cuff. If discomfort ensues, the distal cuff is inflated over the anesthetized area of skin, and the uncomfortable proximal cuff is released. This step is critical because the major risk of this procedure is premature release of solution into the circulation. If a double cuff is used, both cuffs should be tested before starting and the proper sequence for inflation and deflation meticulously followed. The potential for leakage of anesthetic into the circulation is greater with these narrower cuffs used in the double setup. Because the shifting process also increases the potential for unintentional release of anesthetic, the use of a single, wider cuff may be better for short procedures.
6. If surgery is completed in less than 20 minutes, the tourniquet is left inflated for at least that total period of time. If 40 minutes has elapsed, the tourniquet can be deflated as a single maneuver. Between 20 and 40 minutes, the cuff can be deflated, reinflated immediately, and finally deflated after 1 minute to delay the sudden absorption of anesthetic into the systemic circulation, although this may not lower the eventual peak levels achieved.
7. The duration of anesthesia is minimal beyond the time of tourniquet release. Although bupivacaine may produce a slight prolongation of analgesia, the advantage is short. Furthermore, the cardiotoxicity of systemic levels of bupivacaine makes this drug a less desirable choice for a Bier block.

The simplicity of this technique is offset by the significant risk of systemic local anesthetic toxicity if the tourniquet fails or is released prematurely. Careful testing of the tourniquet and slow injection of solution into a peripheral (not antecubital) vein will reduce the chance of leakage under the tourniquet. Systemic blood levels are time dependent, and careful attention should be paid to the sequence of tourniquet release and to patient monitoring during this period. A separate iv site for injection of resuscitation drugs is needed as well as ready availability of all appropriate resuscitative equipment. With careful attention to these details, this technique is one of the most effective and reliable available to the anesthesiologist.

Distal Upper Extremity Blockade

The nerves to the hand can be blocked at the point where they cross the two major joints, the elbow and the wrist (Fig. 26-17). At these two levels, the overlying muscles are thinned and the bony landmarks are more prominent, allowing easier identification of the nerves. Peripheral blockade is usually not as dense as central blockade but may be useful in anesthetizing one branch that was missed with a central blockade or in providing localized anesthesia on the hand. Because the sensory branches to the forearm from the musculocutaneous nerve and the internal cutaneous nerve have already branched so ex-

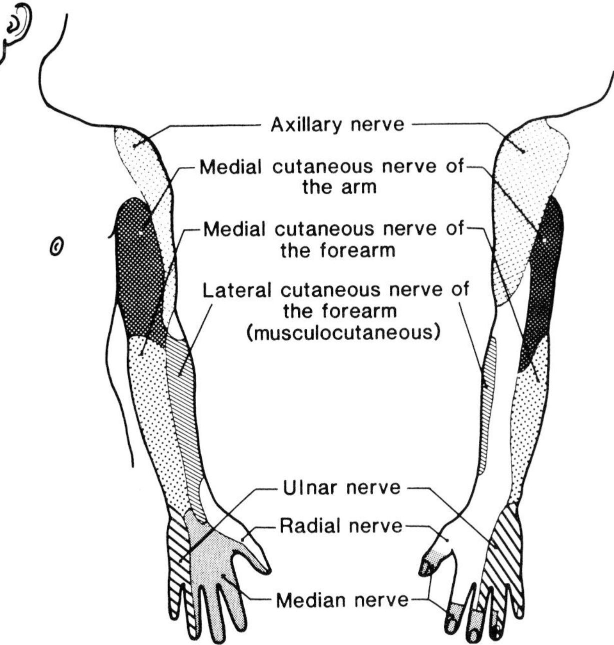

FIGURE 26-17. Sensory dermatomes of the arm. Sensation is provided by the terminal nerves, as identified. This pattern is different from the classic dermatomal distribution of the nerve roots. Different patterns of anesthesia develop if the blockade is performed at the root level (interscalene blockade) versus the terminal nerve level (axillary blockade). (Reproduced with permission from Mulroy M: Handbook of Regional Anesthesia. Philadelphia, Lippincott Williams & Wilkins, 2002.)

tensively that adequate anesthesia of the forearm is not easily obtained, blockade at the elbow really produces no greater anesthesia than blockade at the wrist.

Blockade at the Elbow. Two nerves to the hand cross this joint on the inner aspect. The ulnar travels posteriorly in its well-known superficial groove.

1. The ulnar nerve is blocked by injection of 1 to 4 mL of local anesthetic proximal to the groove formed by the medial condyle of the humerus and the olecranon with the joint flexed at approximately 30 degrees. Further flexion may cause the nerve to roll medially and anterior to the condyle. Paresthesias can usually be readily obtained, but direct injection on an elicitation of a paresthesia or directly into the groove under pressure is not advised because of the risk of damage to the nerve. If the injection is made deep to the fascia, anesthesia should commence within 5 minutes.
2. The median nerve crosses the joint in the company of the brachial artery. A line is drawn between the two condyles on the inner aspect of the joint, and a skin wheal is raised at the point where this line crosses the pulsation of the brachial artery, usually 1 cm to the ulnar side of the biceps tendon. A needle is introduced perpendicularly at this point, and nerve responses are sought immediately adjacent to the artery. Five milliliter of solution is sufficient to produce anesthesia, and, again, intraneural injection is carefully avoided.
3. The radial nerve is identified along the same intracondylar line, approximately 2 cm lateral to the biceps tendon. Another skin wheal is raised here, and, again, a needle is inserted to search for nerve responses in a fan-shaped pattern. If nerve responses are not obtained, a "wall" of anesthetic solution can be deposited here but with less chance of reliable anesthesia.

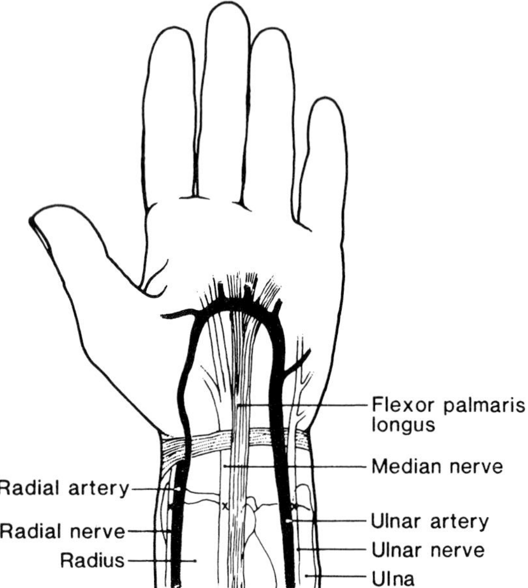

FIGURE 26-18. Terminal nerves at the wrist. The median nerve lies just to the radial side of the flexor palmaris longus. The ulnar and radial nerves lie just "outside" their respective arteries. The radial nerve has already begun branching at this level and must be blocked by a wide subcutaneous ridge of anesthetic. (Reproduced with permission from Mulroy M: Handbook of Regional Anesthesia. Philadelphia, Lippincott Williams & Wilkins, 2002.)

Blockade at the Wrist. The nerves lie more superficially at this joint and are closely associated with easily identified landmarks (Fig. 26-18).

1. The ulnar nerve lies between the ulnar artery and the flexor carpi ulnaris. A skin wheal is raised at the level of the styloid process on the palmar side of the forearm between these two landmarks. A small-gauge needle is inserted, and 3 mL of solution is injected into the area, with or without paresthesias.
2. At the same level on the forearm, the median nerve lies between the tendons of the palmaris longus and the flexor carpi radialis. If only the palmaris longus can be felt, the nerve is just to the radial side of this tendon. A skin wheal is raised, and a needle is inserted until it pierces the deep fascia. Three milliliter of solution produces anesthesia.
3. The radial nerve requires a broader injection because it has already started to ramify as it crosses the wrist. The anatomic "snuffbox" formed by the tendons of the extensor pollicus longus and extensor pollicis brevis tendons is located, and 3 mL of solution is injected here. A subcutaneous wheal is then raised from this point, extending over the dorsum of the wrist 3 to 4 cm onto the back of the hand.

Suprascapular Block

The suprascapular nerve is another terminal branch of the brachial plexus that can be anesthetized by a separate injection. Anesthesia of this nerve provides postoperative pain relief following shoulder arthroscopy or reconstructive surgery. The nerve arises from the superior trunk of the brachial plexus in the neck, courses through the suprascapular notch, and then passes behind the lateral border of the spine of the scapula to the infraspinatus fossa. It has two terminal branches, a sensory articular branch to the shoulder joint and a motor branch to the supraspinatus muscle. The technique for nerve blockade is as follows:

1. The patient is placed in the upright sitting position, leaning forward so that the scapulae are accentuated. The spine of the scapula is identified and marked along its entire length. The inferior tip of the scapula is then identified, and the original line of the spine is bisected at a point immediately superior to this inferior tip.
2. A skin wheal is raised approximately 1 cm superior and 1 cm lateral from this midpoint of the scapular spine, and a 3.75-cm needle is advanced through the skin until contact is made with the superior surface of the scapula. The needle is then withdrawn and redirected cephalad and medially toward the midline until the edge of the suprascapular notch is encountered. At this point, the patient may perceive a paresthesia into the shoulder joint, or the nerve stimulator may produce an internal rotation of the arm itself.
3. Once the nerve is localized, 10 mL of local anesthetic is injected. Even in the absence of nerve localization, this volume of solution injected into the notch should produce adequate anesthesia of the shoulder joint.

Trunk

Anesthesia of the abdomen and chest is most simply obtained with spinal and epidural injections of local anesthetics, as discussed in Chapter 25. In some situations, a narrower band of intercostal or paravertebral anesthesia is preferable, or epidural injection may be hazardous because of the presence of an infection or coagulopathy. In many clinical situations, it may also be desirable to separate the anesthesia of the somatic and sympathetic fibers that occurs in combination when axial blockades are performed. The sympathetic nerves separate from their somatic counterparts early in their course, which makes independent somatic and sympathetic blockade a practical consideration. Sympathetic blockade is most commonly performed at the major ganglia, particularly the stellate, celiac, and lumbar plexus. These blockades often require multiple injections and are technically more difficult than axial anesthesia, but they do offer advantages in certain clinical situations.

The somatic nerves of the chest emerge from their respective intervertebral foramina and pass through the narrow, triangular-shaped paravertebral space. In this triangle, they give off the sympathetic branch and also a small dorsal branch, which provides sensation to the midline of the back. The main trunks then pass into the intercostal groove along the ventral caudad surface of each rib. An artery and vein travel along with each of these nerves in the groove under the protection of the overhanging external edge of the rib. The fasciae of the internal and external intercostal muscles provide interior and external borders of this intercostal groove. As the nerves travel beyond the midaxillary line, they give off a lateral sensory branch while the main trunk continues on to the anterior abdominal wall to provide sensory and motor innervation for the trunk and abdomen down to the level of the pubis. The intercostal groove becomes much less well defined anterior to the midaxillary line, and the nerve begins to move away from its protected position. The lowermost intercostal nerve (the twelfth) is much less closely applied to its accompanying rib and is not as easy to identify and anesthetize using a classic intercostal blockade technique. The upper lumbar roots form the ilioinguinal nerves, which pass laterally within the muscles of the abdominal wall at the level of the iliac crest and eventually move anteriorly to provide innervation of the groin region as the ilioinguinal nerves.

The anatomic basis for separate sympathetic anesthesia is the early separation of sympathetic fibers. The white rami communicantes join the sympathetic ganglia, which lie anteriorly on each side of the vertebral bodies. These preganglionic fibers of the sympathetic system usually arise only from the first thoracic through the second lumbar segments. The spinal ganglia formed by these fibers constitute the sympathetic trunks, which extend upward into the neck and caudad along the lumbar spine. They give terminal sympathetic branches to all the areas of the body. The sympathetic innervation of the head and the lower extremities is derived from fibers that originate from the spinal cord, join sympathetic trunks, and then pass cephalad or caudad along the chain of ganglia before reaching their target organs. Segmental sympathetic innervation of the body from the cervical to the sacral roots is provided by postganglionic nerves departing from the chains (the gray rami communicantes), which rejoin the somatic nerves early in their course. In the head (where motor and sensory innervation is by cranial nerves), the sympathetic fibers reach their end organs by traveling with the arterial vascular supply. The sympathetic ganglia in the neck lie along the lateral border of the relatively flat vertebral bodies. In the chest, the vertebral bodies become more rounded, and the chain of ganglia lies more posteriorly on the lateral side of the vertebral body near the head of each rib. In the abdomen and pelvis, the sympathetic chains begin to move anteriorly and lie on the ventral surface of the vertebral bodies and thus are more widely separated from their respective somatic nerves.

Intercostal Nerve Blockade

Anesthesia of the intercostal nerves provides both motor and sensory anesthesia of the abdominal wall from the xiphoid to the pubis. The sixth to eleventh ribs are usually easily identified, and their accompanying nerves are reliably blocked by injections along the easily palpated sharp posterior angulation of the ribs, which occurs between 5 and 7 cm from the midline in the back. Ribs above the fifth are difficult to palpate because of the overlying scapula and paraspinous muscles and are therefore most easily blocked using the paravertebral technique. Establishing five or six levels of intercostal nerve blockade is a useful anesthetic procedure for providing analgesia and motor relaxation for upper abdominal procedures such as cholecystectomy and gastric surgery. Unilateral blockade of these nerves is a useful treatment for the pain of rib fracture and also serves to reduce postoperative analgesia requirements in patients with subcostal incisions. Several segments must be blocked in each of these applications because of the overlap of the intercostal nerves. This technique is also useful in reducing the pain associated with the insertion of chest tubes or percutaneous biliary drainage procedures.

1. For the performance of intercostal blockade, the patient may be in the lateral, sitting, or prone position. For operative anesthesia, the prone position is most practical. A pillow is placed under the abdomen to provide slight flexion of the thoracic spine. The arms are draped over the edge of the stretcher or operating table so that the scapula falls away laterally from the midline. The anesthesiologist stands at the patient's side. Most anesthesiologists prefer to stand on the side that allows their dominant hand to hold the syringe at the caudad end of the patient.
2. The spinous processes in the midline from T6 through T12 are marked (Fig. 26-19). The ribs are then identified along the line of their most extreme posterior angulation. For the twelfth rib, this is usually 7 cm from the midline. At the level of the sixth rib, this posterior angulation is best appreciated somewhat more medially, usually 5 cm from the midline. These two ribs are marked first at their inferior borders, and a line is drawn between these two points. The rest of the ribs between them are identified, and a mark is placed on the inferior border of each rib along the angled parasagittal plane identified by the first line between the sixth and twelfth ribs.

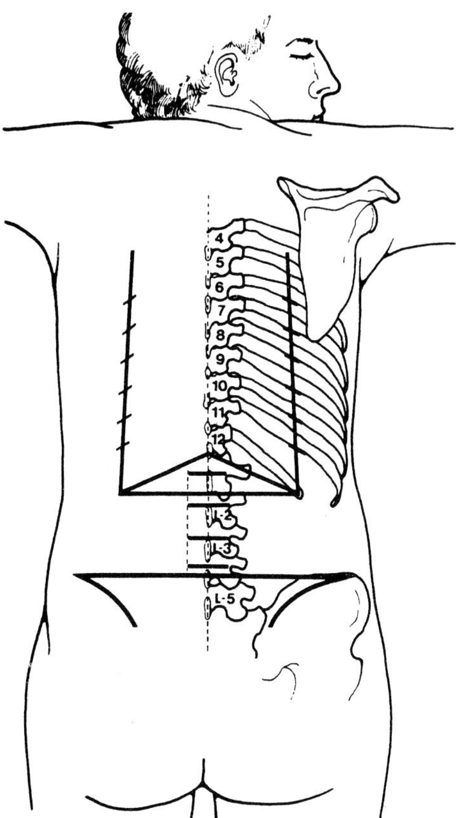

FIGURE 26-19. Landmarks for intercostal blockade. The inferior borders of the ribs are identified at their most prominent points on the back. The marks then usually lie along a line that angles slightly medially from the twelfth to the sixth rib. The triangle drawn between the twelfth ribs and their spinous processes is used for the celiac plexus blockade. (Reproduced with permission from Mulroy M: Handbook of Regional Anesthesia. Philadelphia, Lippincott Williams & Wilkins, 2002.)

3. After aseptic preparation, sedation and analgesia are provided for the patient, and a skin wheal is raised at each mark.
4. The ribs are blocked starting with the lowermost and moving upward.
5. Starting with the lowest rib on the side closest to the anesthesiologist, the index finger of the cephalad hand is placed on the skin above the identifying mark; this finger should lie immediately over the midpoint of the rib. The skin is then retracted in a cephalad direction, so that the previous mark now lies over the rib itself, somewhat toward the inferior side. The anesthesiologist's other hand inserts a 22-gauge, 3.75-cm needle directly onto the rib. This needle is attached to a 10-mL syringe filled with local anesthetic. The syringe and needle are held in such a way that they maintain a constant 10-degree cephalad angulation.
6. Once the needle is safely "parked" on the dorsal surface of the rib, the cephalad hand releases the tension on the skin and takes control of the needle and syringe (Fig. 26-20). This is done by placing the ulnar border of the hand firmly against the skin and grasping the hub of the needle firmly between the thumb and index finger. The middle finger of this hand rests along the shaft of the needle to provide guidance. Once the syringe is firmly gripped by the cephalad hand, the fingers of the

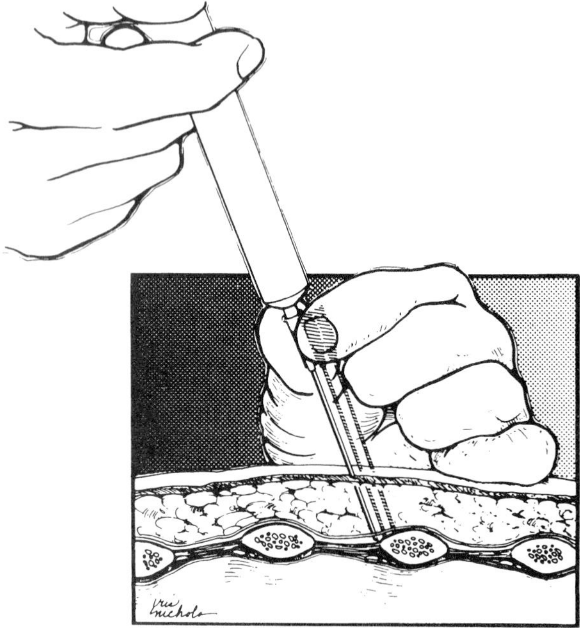

FIGURE 26-20. Hand and needle positions for intercostal blockade. The depth of the needle is controlled by the hand resting on the back. The other hand injects solution when the needle is under the rib, but that is the only function performed while the needle is near the pleura. (Reproduced with permission from Mulroy M: Handbook of Regional Anesthesia. Philadelphia, Lippincott Williams & Wilkins, 2002.)

caudad hand are placed in an "injection" position, either in the rings of a three-ring syringe or on the plunger of a straight syringe.

7. The needle and syringe are then raised slightly off the bone and walked in a caudad direction until they pass below the inferior border of the rib. The entire needle and syringe unit is kept at a 10-degree cephalad angle to the rib at all times. As it passes the inferior border, the needle is advanced 4 to 6 mm under the rib, with the needle actually pointing slightly cephalad into the intercostal groove.
8. Once in the groove, aspiration is performed, and 3 to 5 mL of local anesthetic solution is injected.
9. As soon as the injection is complete, the needle is withdrawn from the groove and moved cephalad and "parked" again on the safe dorsal surface of the rib. The fingers of the caudad hand are then removed from the injection position and assume control of the syringe again. The cephalad hand now relinquishes control and is moved up to the next rib to repeat this cyclic process.
10. The ribs on the opposite side are blocked in a similar manner. This can be done with the anesthesiologist standing on the same side and reaching across the back, or by moving to the opposite side of the patient.
11. Intercostal nerve blockades can be supplemented by a number of somatic paravertebral nerve blockades or sympathetic blockade of the celiac plexus. Care should be taken to adjust the total dose of drug in such combinations of techniques so that the maximal recommended amounts are not exceeded.

Despite frequent concern about the incidence of pneumothorax with intercostal blockade, this complication is rare in experienced hands. This depends primarily on maintaining strict safety features of the described technique. Emphasis should be placed on absolute control of the syringe and needle at all times, particularly during the injection.

A common complication is related to the sedation required to perform this blockade in the prone position. Overdose can lead to airway obstruction and respiratory depression in the prone position. Attention must be paid to the patient's mental status because this blockade produces the highest blood levels of local anesthetics when compared with any other regional anesthetic technique. When the blockade is performed for postoperative pain relief, the dose should be reduced to 0.25% bupivacaine or ropivacaine to minimize the chance for toxicity.

It is possible to produce partial spinal or epidural anesthesia if the injection is made close to the midline and the anesthetic tracks along a dural sleeve to the epidural or subarachnoid space. Respiratory insufficiency can also be seen if the intercostal muscles are blocked in a patient who depends on them for ventilation. Patients with chronic obstructive disease with ineffective diaphragm motion are not good candidates for this technique.

Paravertebral Blockade

The upper five ribs are more difficult to palpate laterally, and blockade of their associated intercostal nerves is best performed with a paravertebral injection. This approach is technically more difficult and has slightly greater potential for complications because of the proximity of the lung and of the intervertebral foramina. Anatomically, the injection is made into the triangle formed by the intervertebral body, the pleura, and the plane of the transverse processes (Fig. 26-21). The intervertebral foramina at each level lie between the transverse processes and approximately 2 cm anterior to the plane formed by the transverse processes in their associated fasciae. At this point, the sympathetic ganglia lie close to the somatic nerves, and coincidental sympathetic blockade is usually attained. This is also related to the injection of larger volumes of local anesthetic, which is required because location of the nerve is less reliable with this technique. Nevertheless, it is a useful technique for segmental anesthesia, particularly of the upper thoracic segments. It is also useful if a more proximal blockade is needed, such as to relieve the pain of herpes zoster or of a proximal rib fracture. Lumbar paravertebral blockade has been used successfully for outpatient hernia operations, providing significant postoperative analgesia.

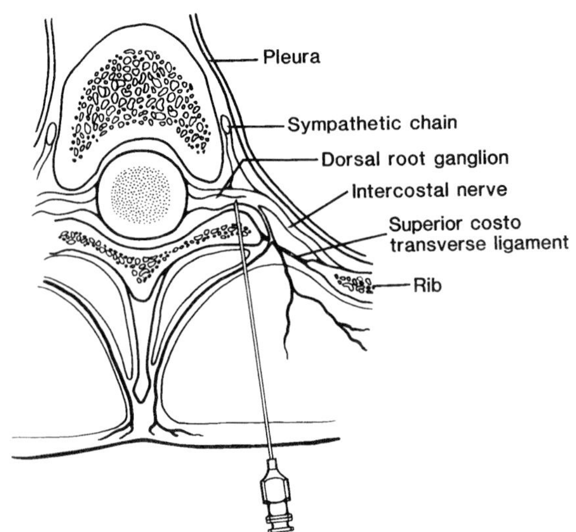

FIGURE 26-21. Paravertebral blockade. As it exits the intervertebral foramen, the thoracic somatic nerve enters a small triangular space formed by the vertebral body, the plane of the transverse process, and the pleura. Medial direction of the needle is obviously important in reducing the chance of a pneumothorax.

The paravertebral approach varies somewhat, depending on the spinal level. In the upper thoracic spine, the transverse process is located lateral to the spinous process of the vertebral body above it. In the lower thoracic spine, the spinous processes are less steeply angled, so that the eleventh and twelfth spinous processes lie between the associated transverse processes. In the lumbar region, the spinous processes are straight, and the transverse processes lie opposite their own respective spinous process. Thus, paravertebral blockade in the upper thoracic region is performed at each level by identifying the spinous process of the vertebra above the level to be blocked; in the lumbar region, the spinous process of the level to be blocked is used to locate the transverse process.

1. This blockade is also performed in the sitting or prone position, with a pillow under the patient's abdomen to produce flexion of the thoracic and lumbar spine. The spinous processes in the region to be blocked are marked. These can be identified by counting upward from the fourth lumbar process (which usually lies just at or above the line joining the two iliac crests) or by counting down from the seventh cervical process (which is the most prominent in the cervical region).
2. Transverse lines are drawn across the cephalad border of the spinous processes and extended laterally to overlie the transverse process (~1 to 4 cm). In the lumbar region, the lines overlie the transverse process of the associated vertebra. In the thoracic region, they indicate the transverse process of the vertebral body immediately below the associated spinous process. Finally, a vertical line is drawn parallel to the spine 3 to 4 cm lateral to it, joining the transverse lines from the spinous processes. For a diagnostic blockade, a single nerve may need to be anesthetized. For pain control, several levels must be identified. The injection of at least three segments (as in intercostal blockade) is required to produce reliable segmental blockade because of sensory overlap.
3. After aseptic skin preparation, skin wheals are raised at the intersections of the vertical and transverse lines.
4. A 22-gauge needle is introduced through the skin wheal in the sagittal plane and directed slightly cephalad to contact the transverse process. A 7.5-cm needle is usually required in the average patient, and the transverse process lies between 3 and 5 cm from the skin. Gentle cephalad or caudad exploration may be required to identify the bone. The depth of the transverse process is carefully noted on the needle shaft.
5. The needle is now withdrawn from the transverse process and walked inferiorly to pass below its caudad edge. This usually requires more perpendicular direction relative to the skin. The needle is advanced 2 cm below the transverse process and angled slightly medial to attempt to contact the vertebral body. Nerve responses are not sought unless a neurolytic injection is planned. When the needle has entered the paravertebral space, 5 to 10 mL of local anesthetic solution is injected after careful aspiration.

The complication of pneumothorax is more likely in the thoracic region with a paravertebral technique than with intercostal blockade. The needle should be directed medially as it passes below the transverse process and never more than 2 cm beyond the transverse process (see Fig. 26-21). If cough or chest pain occurs, a chest radiograph should be performed to rule out pneumothorax. Subarachnoid injection is also more likely in the thoracic area because of the extension of the dural sleeves to the level of the intervertebral foramina. Careful aspiration is important but may not prevent the unintentional injection of local anesthetic into a subdural pocket. Total spinal anesthesia can result with a 5- to 10-mL injection. Systemic toxicity is also a possibility because of the need for relatively large volumes of local anesthetic. Attention must be paid to the total milligram dose injected. The volume required for each level obviously limits the concentrations that can be used and the total number of levels that can be blocked. If lumbar paravertebral injections are combined with intercostals, the concentration and total volume for both blockades may have to be reduced.

Intrapleural Anesthesia

Upper abdominal analgesia can also be obtained by inserting an epidural catheter into the intrapleural space for injection or infusion of local anesthetic. The anesthetic appears to diffuse through the parietal pleura onto the intercostal nerves and produces anesthesia similar to that provided by injection of multiple intercostal nerve blocks. It may also act on the sympathetic nerves by diffusion to the ganglia lying along the anterior vertebral borders.

1. As with intercostal block, the technique can be performed with the patient in the prone, lateral, or sitting position.
2. The seventh or eighth intercostal space is identified 8 to 10 cm from the midline and marked at the upper border of the lower rib.
3. A skin wheal is made at this site, and a blunt-tipped epidural needle (e.g., Touhy) is inserted with the bevel directed cephalad and advanced over the inferior rib in a slightly medial and cephalad angle through the intercostal muscles. Once in the intercostal layers, the stylet is removed, and an air-filled 5-mL glass syringe is attached.
4. The needle is advanced farther until the parietal pleura is punctured, signaled by a negative pressure that moves the plunger of the syringe forward. The syringe is removed, and a standard epidural catheter is threaded 5 to 6 cm beyond the tip. Aspiration is performed to exclude perforation of the lung or a blood vessel.
5. Twenty milliliter of 0.5% bupivacaine or ropivacaine with epinephrine is injected into the pleural space, and the catheter is carefully taped to the skin. Reinjection is required every 3 to 6 hours, or a constant infusion of 0.25% bupivacaine (0.125 mL/kg^{-1}/h^{-1}) or 0.2% ropivacaine can be initiated.

There have been several enthusiastic reports of success with this technique, but limitations have been described. Pain relief is usually reliable, and respiratory depression is not a problem. However, the duration is short enough that large quantities of local anesthetic are required to maintain analgesia, and systemic toxicity has been reported in 1.3% of patients.[15] The incidence of pneumothorax (averaging 2%) is not inconsequential, especially with first attempts. Puncture of the lung also occurs, apparently with a higher incidence if a loss-of-resistance technique is used rather than the passive identification process described earlier. A major limitation is the unilateral analgesia, which limits this technique to procedures such as cholecystectomy and nephrectomy, rib fracture, and treatment of herpetic pain. Loss of local anesthetic solution to thoracostomy drainage makes this technique unreliable for thoracotomy pain.

Ilioinguinal Blockade

The L1 nerve root (occasionally joined by a branch of the T12 root) provides sensory innervation to the lowermost portion of the abdominal wall and the groin by means of its superior iliohypogastric branch and its inferior ilioinguinal branch. These nerves travel in a path similar to that of the intercostal nerves, but without the convenient bony landmark of a rib to identify them. Nevertheless, they can be anesthetized relatively easily in the groin because of their relationship to the anterosuperior iliac spine. Anesthesia of these two nerves is useful in providing lower abdominal wall anesthesia to supplement intercostal blockade. It is more commonly used to produce field anesthesia for inguinal hernia repair surgery. Anesthesia of these nerves alone is not sufficient for hernia repair; subcutaneous infiltration is also necessary.

1. The patient lies in a supine position, and the anterosuperior iliac spine is identified. An "X" is placed on the skin 2.5 cm medial to the spine and slightly cephalad.
2. After aseptic preparation, a skin wheal is raised at the "X."
3. A 2.5-cm, 22-gauge needle is introduced through the "X" and directed perpendicular to the skin until it reaches the fascia of the external oblique muscle. A "wall" of local anesthetic solution is then laid down between this point and the iliac spine and also opposite the mark on an imaginary line extending toward the umbilicus. Injections are made at and below the level of the external oblique, with some solution injected at the level of the internal oblique. A total of 10 to 15 mL of anesthetic is usually required.
4. If field anesthesia for inguinal hernia repair is required, further subcutaneous infiltration of anesthetic is performed along the skin crease of the groin and along the imaginary line extending to the umbilicus. This produces a triangular-shaped area of skin anesthesia. For hernia operations, further anesthesia of the spermatic cord is required. This is usually performed by local injections in the area of the cord and the internal ring. Although epinephrine is useful in the subcutaneous and ilioinguinal blockade, it should be avoided in solutions used to anesthetize the base of the penis or the spermatic cord (see Penile Blockade section). Further anesthesia of the groin area and below can be obtained by blockade of the femoral and lateral femoral cutaneous nerves, but this may result in unwanted weakness of the leg musculature, which may prevent ambulation.

Complications of this procedure are extremely rare. Hematoma formation and unwanted motor blockade of the femoral nerve are possible, but rare. More commonly, anesthesia produced by this technique is inadequate for hernia repair because the patient is still able to perceive the discomfort of peritoneal traction. Administration of local anesthesia by the surgeon or systemic opioids may be required.

Penile Blockade

If surgery is confined to the penis (e.g., circumcision, urethral procedures), the organ should be blocked with simple local infiltration. Two skin wheals are raised at the dorsal base of the penis, one on each side just below and medial to the pubic spine. A 25-gauge, 3.75-cm needle is introduced on each side, and 5 mL of anesthetic is deposited superficially and deep along the lower border of the pubic ramus to anesthetize the dorsal nerve. An additional 5 mL is infiltrated in the subcutaneous tissue around the underside of the shaft to produce a complete ring of anesthetic. A larger needle or a second injection site may be needed to complete the ring. Twenty to 25 mL of 0.75% lidocaine or 0.25% bupivacaine usually suffices. Epinephrine is strictly avoided.

Sympathetic Blockade

Stellate Ganglion

Separate blockade of the sympathetic fibers of the upper extremity and head can be achieved by a single injection of a local anesthetic on the stellate ganglion. The ganglion is the large fusion of the first thoracic sympathetic ganglion with the lower cervical ganglion on each side, and it lies on the generally flat lateral border of the vertebral body of C7. All the fibers to the middle and superior cervical ganglia pass through this lowermost collection and thus can be anesthetized with a single injection. Although technically simple, the location of this ganglion near the carotid artery, the vertebral artery, and the pleura makes this a challenging blockade. It is useful in providing pain relief for sympathetic dystrophies of the upper arm. Stellate ganglion blockade may relieve the pain of acute herpes zoster infection of the head or neck region. It has also been advocated as a means of reducing post-thoracotomy pain by blocking the sympathetic sensory fibers to the pleural cavity. The procedure for blockade follows:

1. The patient is placed in a supine position with a small towel or pillow under the neck, and the arms are held at the side.
2. The medial border of the sternocleidomastoid muscle on the involved side is marked, as is the level of the cricoid cartilage. Gentle palpation approximately 2 cm lateral to the cartilage often reveals the anterior tubercle of the transverse process of the sixth cervical vertebra (*Chassaignac's tubercle*). A circle is marked over this tubercle, and an "X" is placed 1.5 to 2 cm caudad to this mark at the same distance from the midline. This "X" should overlie the tubercle of the seventh cervical vertebra and should fall at the medial border of the sternocleidomastoid muscle body and approximately two fingerbreadths above the clavicle itself.
3. A skin wheal is made at the "X" after aseptic skin preparation.
4. With the index and middle finger of one hand, the sternocleidomastoid muscle and the carotid sheath are retracted laterally (Fig. 26-22). A 22- or 25-gauge, 3.75-cm needle is introduced through the "X" and

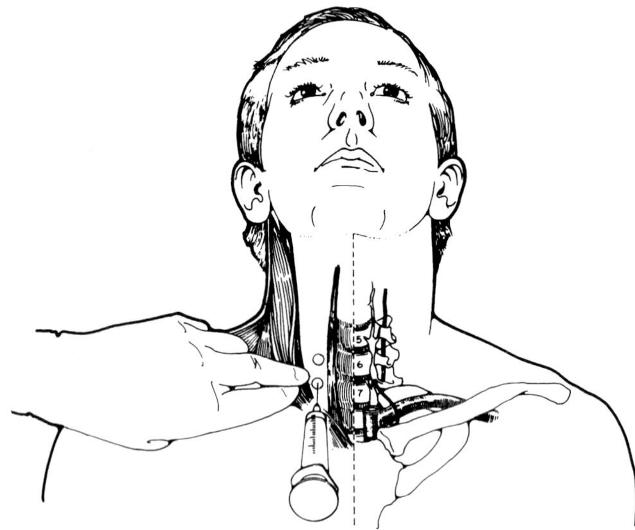

FIGURE 26-22. Stellate ganglion blockade. The sternocleidomastoid muscle and the carotid sheath are retracted laterally with one hand while the needle is introduced directly onto the lateral border of the seventh vertebral body, just medial to the transverse process. The vertebral artery passes posteriorly at this level to enter its canal in the transverse process, but here it lies near the level of intended injection. After contacting bone, the needle is withdrawn slightly and careful aspiration is performed before incremental injection. (Reproduced with permission from Mulroy M: Handbook of Regional Anesthesia. Philadelphia, Lippincott Williams & Wilkins, 2002.)

passed directly posterior until it rests on bone. A paresthesia of the brachial plexus implies that the needle is too far laterally and has passed beyond the transverse process. It may have to be readjusted slightly more medially and perhaps more cephalad or caudad.

5. Once bone is contacted, the needle is withdrawn a few millimeters, and careful aspiration is performed to rule out contact with the vertebral artery. A 2-mL test dose is injected to evaluate further an unrecognized intravascular position. The patient's mental status must be closely observed.
6. If no change occurs, a total of 10 mL of local anesthetic can be injected incrementally with frequent aspiration. One percent lidocaine or 0.25% bupivacaine or their equivalents are more than adequate to produce anesthesia of the sympathetic nerves.
7. Onset of sympathectomy is usually, but not reliably, indicated by the appearance of a *Horner's syndrome* on the ipsilateral side. Ptosis, miosis, and anhydrosis usually develop within 10 minutes, as well as vasodilatation in the arm. Nasal congestion is another common sign usually associated with Horner's syndrome.

There are several potential complications of stellate ganglion blockade. The pleura can be punctured, with resulting pneumothorax. Intravascular injection is the most serious complication because of the proximity of the vertebral artery to the site of injection. Careful aspiration and incremental injections are essential. Only a few milligrams of local anesthetic is required to produce cerebral symptoms when injected directly into the vertebral circulation. Cardiovascular changes are possible with the loss of the cardiac accelerator fibers from the cervical sympathetic ganglia. This is particularly a problem if bilateral blockade is performed, a procedure rarely indicated. Hoarseness from recurrent laryngeal nerve paralysis is a minor but troublesome side effect. Somatic anesthesia of the brachial plexus nerves can be produced by injection behind the level of the tubercle, and phrenic nerve paralysis has also been reported. Subarachnoid injection is also a possibility if the needle is misplaced. The close association of so many vital structures has discouraged the use of neurolytic agents in the region of the stellate ganglion.

Celiac Plexus

The thoracic sympathetic ganglia send branches anteriorly that merge as greater and lesser splanchnic nerves to pass below the diaphragm and around the aorta to coalesce in a diffuse periaortic supplementary sympathetic ganglion known as the celiac plexus. This extensive network is usually located at the level of the first lumbar vertebra in the retroperitoneal space, along the aorta at the level of the origin of the celiac artery. Fibers from this ganglion send postganglionic innervation to all the intraabdominal organs and appear to carry pain sensation from many of the intraperitoneal organs such as the pancreas and liver. Injection into this retroperitoneal space allows anesthetic solution to diffuse around the ganglia and the splanchnic nerves to provide blockade of these fibers. This blockade produces supplementary intraabdominal anesthesia when used in conjunction with intercostal blockade or general anesthesia. It is more commonly applied as a neurolytic sympathetic blockade for the relief of pain from malignancy of the pancreas, liver, or other upper abdominal organs.

1. As with intercostal blockade, the patient is placed in the prone position with the thoracic spine flexed by the use of a pillow under the abdomen.
2. The spinous processes of the twelfth thoracic and the first lumbar vertebral bodies are identified and marked along their entire extent. The twelfth rib is likewise identified and marked 7 cm from the midline. A line is drawn between the twelfth ribs on each side, usually crossing the midline at the level of the spinous process of the L1 vertebra. Lines are also drawn from the spinous process of the twelfth thoracic vertebra to the points on these ribs on both sides. The net result is a shallow triangle, with the spinous process of the twelfth vertebra at its apex (see Fig. 26-19).
3. Skin wheals are raised bilaterally at the marks along the ribs after aseptic skin preparation. Deeper infiltration of local anesthetic with a 22-gauge needle is often helpful in improving patient tolerance of this procedure.
4. On each side, a 12.5-cm, 22- or 20-gauge needle is introduced through the skin wheals and advanced anteriorly and medially and cephalad along the two lines of the triangle that was previously drawn (Fig. 26-23). The needle should be passed at approximately a 45-degree angle anteriorly so that it will contact the lateral border of the vertebral body of L1 at a depth of approximately 5 cm from the skin. (The twelfth spinous process partially overlies the L1 vertebral body.)
5. When contact with a vertebral body is made, the needle is withdrawn several centimeters, and the angle of insertion is steepened so that it advances more anteriorly with subsequent passage, in the hope that it will walk off the anterior border of the vertebral body. The periosteum may be encountered several times during this attempt and should always be palpated gently because of the associated discomfort. Intravenous sedation may be required for tolerance of this blockade, although it must be kept to a minimum if evaluation of a diagnostic pain blockade is desired.
6. Once the anterior border of the vertebral body is reached, the needle is advanced 2 to 3 cm beyond this, and careful aspiration is performed. On the left side, advancement should be halted whenever aortic pulsation is appreciated. If the artery is unintentionally

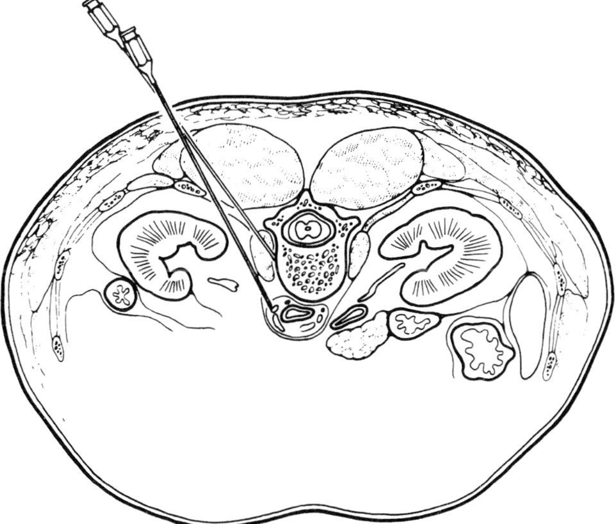

FIGURE 26-23. Celiac plexus blockade. The surface landmarks are described in Figure 26-19. The needles are advanced medially and superiorly to contact the lateral aspect of the vertebral body. They are then advanced more anteriorly to pass beyond the vertebra to the prevertebral space, where the greater and lesser splanchnic nerves and their subsequent celiac plexus lie. No attempt is made to advance the needles to the anterior aspect of the vessels. (Reproduced with permission from Mulroy M: Handbook of Regional Anesthesia. Philadelphia, Lippincott Williams & Wilkins, 2002.)

punctured, the needle should be withdrawn slightly and cleared immediately of blood. On the right side, the needle can often be advanced 1 to 2 cm farther than the needle on the left side.

7. If radiographic confirmation is desired, it is obtained at this point, before injection of the anesthetic. The bony landmarks themselves are usually sufficient to identify the retroperitoneal space anterior to the first lumbar vertebral body. If neurolytic agents are to be used or if the anatomy is difficult, fluroscopic confirmation is desirable.
8. Careful aspiration is performed, and a test dose is injected on each side to rule out subarachnoid or intravascular injection.
9. A large volume of local anesthetic solution is required. Twenty to 25 mL of 0.75% lidocaine or 0.25% bupivacaine is usually adequate.
10. The most reliable sign of successful anesthesia is the disappearance of pain in patients or the appearance of hypotension in normal patients. Patients with pain must remain supine for several hours and should have appropriate iv fluid supplementation to avoid orthostatic hypotension. Gradual ambulation is mandatory.

Hypotension is the most common complication of celiac plexus blockade. It can be reduced by the administration of 1L of balanced salt solution before performing the blockade. The most serious complication is the development of paralysis from unrecognized subarachnoid injection of a neurolytic drug. Radiographic confirmation of needle location is advisable before injection of any neurolytic drug. Even with correct placement of neurolytic drugs, back pain is common and patients may require iv opioids. This pain can be reduced by diluting the alcohol solution with an equal volume of local anesthetic such that a total volume of 50 mL is injected, consisting of 25 mL of alcohol and 25 mL of anesthetic. Even with this approach, diaphragmatic irritation (manifested as shoulder pain) is not uncommon. The duration of pain relief in the patient with chronic pain is unpredictable but is often 2 to 6 months. The blockade can be repeated as often as necessary, although a trial diagnostic blockade with a local anesthetic agent is indicated before each use of neurolytic drugs. One minor side effect of celiac plexus blockade is the increased peristalsis of the gut produced by the shift in the balance of the parasympathetic and sympathetic innervations. This may produce diarrhea within the first 12 hours after the blockade and may be a source of relief to patients on chronic opioid therapy for cancer pain.

Lumbar

As with the sympathetic innervation of the head and arm, the sympathetic nerves to the lower extremities all exit the cord above L2 and all pass through a common "gateway" ganglion in the sympathetic chain at the L2 level. Thus, as in the neck, sympathetic blockade of the lower extremity can be achieved by a single injection of one ganglion. The approach to this ganglion is similar to paravertebral anesthesia, as discussed previously, except that in the lumbar region, the sympathetic chain lies much more anterior from the somatic nerves, and thus a clean separation of sympathetic blockade from somatic blockade can be attained more easily.

As in the upper extremity, lumbar sympathectomy can be used in the treatment of sympathetic dystrophies. It is also occasionally used in patients with severe vascular disease in the lower extremities to give some indication of whether the patient would profit from permanent chemical or surgical sympathectomy.

1. The patient position is similar to that for celiac plexus blockade. The patient lies prone with a pillow under the lumbar spine.
2. The spinous processes of L2 and L3 are identified and marked over their entire course. A horizontal line is drawn through the midpoint of the L2 spinous process and extended 5 cm to either side of the midline. An "X" is placed at this point, which should overlie the space between the transverse process of the second and third vertebrae or the caudad edge of the second transverse process.
3. A skin wheal is raised after aseptic skin preparation at each "X."
4. A 10-cm needle is introduced on each side through the "X," angled 30 to 45 degrees cephalad, and advanced until it contacts the transverse process (Fig. 26-24).
5. The depth of the needle insertion is marked, and the needle is then withdrawn slightly, angled caudad, and walked inferiorly off the transverse process (usually in a direction perpendicular to the skin). A slight medial angulation is used in the hope of contacting the vertebral

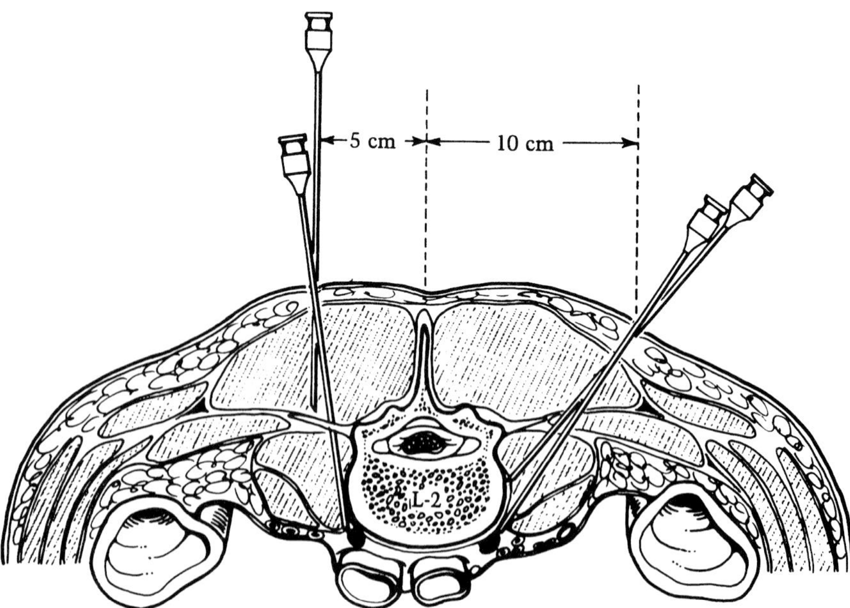

FIGURE 26-24. Lumbar sympathetic blockade. The needle is first placed on the transverse process of L2 and then advanced below it to pass 5 cm deeper. The needle can be angled slightly medially to contact the body of the vertebra; the sympathetic chain lies along the anterior margin of these bodies. (Reproduced with permission from Mulroy M: Handbook of Regional Anesthesia. Philadelphia, Lippincott Williams & Wilkins, 2002.)

body below the transverse process. The needle is advanced 5 cm below the depth of the transverse process. If it encounters a vertebral body, it is angled slightly more anteriorly to walk off that body at the desired depth.

6. Once the needle is in position, careful aspiration is performed, and a test dose is injected on both sides. Ten milliliter of local anesthetic solution injected on each side should produce sympathetic blockade. Again, 1% lidocaine, 0.25% bupivacaine, or an equivalent concentration is more than sufficient to produce sympathetic nerve blockade. If a neurolytic drug such as phenol is used, confirmation of needle position by radiography should be obtained. A slightly more caudad site of injection may be more effective for neurolytic blockade; injection of smaller quantities at several levels may be more appropriate for neurolytic drugs.
7. Care is taken not to inject anesthetic solution as the needle is withdrawn, because this may produce a somatic nerve blockade as the needle passes the course of the L2 nerve root.
8. Vasodilatation and increase in skin temperature should be noted within the leg in 5 to 10 minutes. This can be quantitated objectively if a skin temperature probe is placed on the foot before the start of the blockade.

Complications with this technique are unusual, but, again, intravascular or subarachnoid injection can be a potential problem. The most troublesome and frequent complication is simultaneous blockade of the L2 somatic nerve root. This produces a band of anesthesia across the lateral and anterior thigh, which may confuse the evaluation of a diagnostic sympathetic blockade.

Hypogastric Plexus

At the terminal end of the prevertebral sympathetic chain is the superior hypogastric plexus, which extends from the lower one-third of the fifth lumbar vertebral body to the upper third of the first sacral vertebral body. Fibers passing through this ganglion provide visceral sensation to the pelvic organs. Malignancies in the pelvis often produce chronic pain syndromes that involve transmission of nociception through this ganglion plexus, and significant relief can be obtained by the performance of neurolytic blocks in this area.[16]

1. The patient is placed in the prone position with a pillow under the pelvis to reduce the lumbar lordosis.
2. The L4-5 intervertebral space is identified and marked, and a line drawn at the midline of this space. An "X" is then placed on the skin 5 to 7 cm lateral to this interspace on both sides.
3. Aseptic skin preparation is performed, and a skin wheal raised at the "X" marks at each side.
4. Fifteen-centimeter, 22-gauge needles are then introduced through the skin wheals and directed medially. Both needles are advanced at approximately a 45-degree angle with a 30-degree caudad deflection to approach the anterolateral body of the L5-S1 space. If the L5 vertebral body is encountered, the needle is redirected more anteriorly. The use of fluoroscopy and contrast dye documents the correct placement of the needles just anterior to the L5-S1 intervertebral space.
5. After careful aspiration to exclude intravascular placement, anesthesia can be obtained with 8 mL of 0.25% bupivacaine for a diagnostic block. For neurolytic procedures, an equal volume of 10% phenol can be used on each side.

The major risk of this block is intravascular placement of the drug. The side effects and complications of neurolytic agents apply here if they are used.

Lower Extremity

The nerves to the lower extremity are most easily blocked by the spinal, caudal, or epidural techniques described in Chapter 25. There are occasions when anesthesia by these routes is contraindicated because of systemic sepsis or coagulopathy, or when selective anesthesia of one leg or foot is needed. Peripheral nerve blockade is possible because the motor and sensory fibers to the lower extremities are somewhat similar to those of the upper extremities in that they form a series of intertwined branching roots and divisions that are enclosed in a fascial sheath before they emerge as the terminal nerves to the extremity. They can also be successfully blocked by a single injection in one plane, although the anatomic landmarks identifying this fascial sheath are not as clearly defined as those in the upper extremity. Because of this, the majority of lower extremity blockades are performed more distally, where the nerves have already separated into terminal branches. Thus, in addition to the fascial compartment approach (psoas blockade), there are peripheral approaches described at the hip, knee, and ankle.

The nerves to the legs emerge from the roots of L2 through the third sacral spinal segments (Fig. 26-25). The upper nerve roots from L2 to L4 form the lumbar plexus, which then ramifies eventually to form the lateral femoral cutaneous, femoral, and obturator nerves. These primarily provide sensorimotor innervation of the upper leg, although a branch of the femoral nerve commonly extends along the medial side of the knee as far down as the big toe. A branch of this lumbar plexus, the lumbosacral trunk of L4 and L5, joins the sacral fibers to form the major trunks of the large nerve of the posterior thigh and lower leg, the sciatic. The sciatic nerve is made up of two main trunks, the tibial and the common peroneal, which divide just above the knee. As in the brachial plexus, the upper nerve roots emerge from their foramina into a compartment lined by the fasciae of muscles anterior and posterior to it. In this case, the

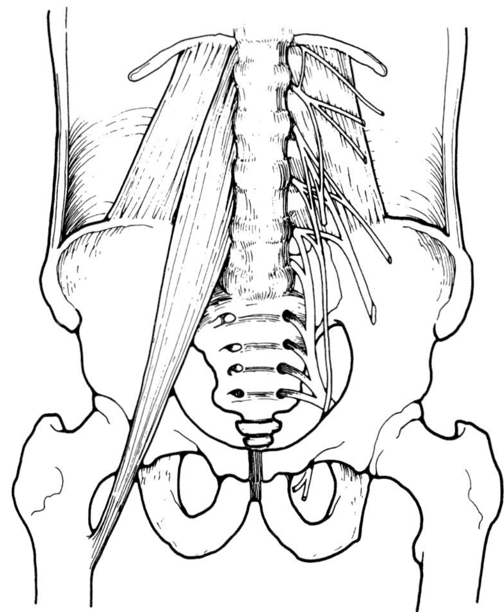

FIGURE 26-25. Psoas compartment anatomy. The roots of the lumbar plexus emerge from their foramina into a fascial plane between the quadratus lumborum muscle posteriorly and the psoas muscle anteriorly. The origin of the lumbosacral plexus is broader than the corresponding brachial plexus in the neck, and the lower sacral roots cannot be easily reached by a single injection. (Reproduced with permission from Mulroy M: Handbook of Regional Anesthesia. Philadelphia, Lippincott Williams & Wilkins, 2002.)

quadratus lumborum is posterior, while the posterior fascia of the psoas muscle provides the anterior border of the compartment before the nerves move into the body of the muscle. The sacral roots have a similar envelope except that the posterior border is the bone of the ilium.

The lumbar plexus branches form their three terminal nerves early. Each of these passes anteriorly and laterally to circle around the pelvis and emerge anteriorly in the groin. The femoral nerve becomes associated with the femoral artery in the area of the groin and passes under the inguinal ligament just lateral to the artery. The lateral femoral cutaneous nerve migrates laterally early and passes under the inguinal ligament near the anterosuperior iliac spine. The third branch of the lumbar plexus, the obturator, remains somewhat medial and posterior in the pelvis and emerges under the superior ramus of the pubis through the obturator foramen to supply motor and sensory fibers to the medial thigh and medial border of the knee.

The branches of the sacral plexus also travel laterally within the pelvis before exiting posteriorly through the sciatic notch as the sciatic nerve. This largest nerve of the body is actually the conjunction of two trunks. The lateral trunk forms from the roots of L4 through S2 and eventually emerges as the common peroneal nerve. Other branches of L4 through S3 form the medial trunk, eventually becoming the tibial nerve. These combined nerves exit through the sciatic notch and pass anteriorly to the piriformis muscle between the ischial tuberosity and the greater trochanter of the femur. They curve caudad and descend the posterior thigh immediately behind the femur. After their bifurcation high in the popliteal fossa, the peroneal nerve provides the motor and sensory fibers to the anterior calf and dorsum of the foot. The tibial nerve remains posterior and provides sensation to the calf and sole of the foot. There are three major branches that cross the knee: the femoral, tibial, and peroneal. By the time these nerves reach the ankle, there are five branches that cross this joint to provide innervation for the skin and muscles of the foot.

Psoas Compartment Blockade

The fascial compartment of the lumbar plexus is more difficult to identify than that of the brachial plexus in the upper extremity and lies much deeper beneath the skin than its equivalent in the neck (see Fig. 26-25). Nevertheless, psoas compartment blockade is useful if single-injection anesthesia of the leg is desired.[17]

1. The patient is placed in the lateral position. The spinous processes of the lumbar vertebrae and the posterior superior iliac spine are identified, and a line drawn parallel to the spine from the top of this iliac spine (Fig. 26-26). Another line is drawn perpendicular to this one intersecting the L4 spine. This line is then trisected, and an "X" is placed on the skin at the junction of the lateral third and medial two-thirds of the line.
2. After aseptic preparation, a skin wheal is raised at the "X." A 10-cm needle is advanced perpendicular to the skin in all planes and passed through the muscles of the back. The transverse process of the vertebral body is sought, which may lie at a depth of between 5 and 8 cm. Once the bone is contacted, the needle is redirected caudally and advanced 2 cm further. Regardless of the depth of the bone from the skin, the nerve roots should lie 2 cm further. Although in some patients the well-demarcated fascial planes can identify the entry into the perineural sheath, anesthesia is more reliable if nerve responses are obtained. If they are not obtained at a 2.5-cm depth beyond the bone, probing with the needle in a fan-like manner should be performed in a cephalad-caudad plane (which is perpendicular to the known paths of the emerging nerves).
3. When a nerve response is obtained, the needle is fixed in position and careful aspiration and administration of a test dose are used to rule out intravascular or subarachnoid placement. Thirty-five to 45 mL of local anesthetic solution is usually required to fill the sheath. Fifteen to 20 minutes may be required for spread of the anesthetic to all the roots of the lumbosacral plexus. It may take longer to produce anesthesia of the caudad branches (the lower sacral fibers that form the tibial nerve), or they may not be anesthetized at all.
4. A catheter may be inserted here, with the direction of the bevel ideally lateral and away from the neuraxial canal. Infusions provide postoperative analgesia for knee and hip replacement surgeries.

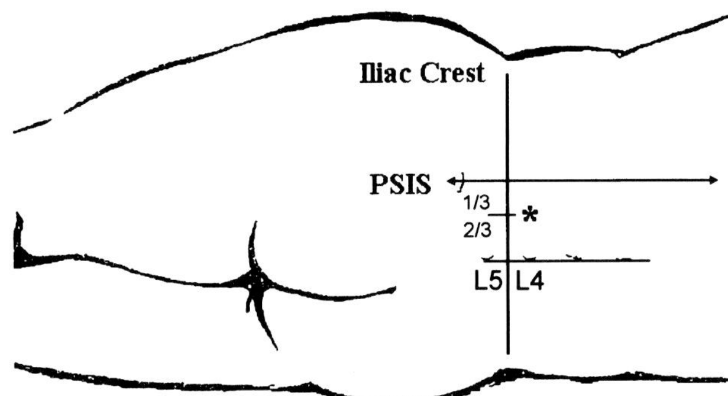

FIGURE 26-26. Psoas block. The nerves of the lumbar plexus can be approached posteriorly by insertion of a needle at a point lying lateral to the L4 spinous process, two thirds of the way between a line drawn along the spinous processes themselves, and a parallel line intersecting the posterior superior iliac spine. (Reprinted with permission from Capdevilla X, Macaire P, Dadure C, *et al*: Anesth Analg 94:1606, 2003.)

Complications of this technique include hematoma in the muscle sheath and retroperitoneal space or the kidney. Neuropathy of the nerves is possible. Unintended spread to the epidural or even subarachnoid space has also been reported. Inadequate anesthesia of some of the branches may occur more frequently than these rare complications.

Anesthesia at the Level of the Hip

Many anesthesiologists feel more confident when administering regional anesthesia in the hip region when nerve responses are sought for each of the major nerves. This technique is cumbersome and usually requires the patient to assume at least two separate positions for the injections. The anesthesia requires a larger volume of anesthetic drug. Each of the four nerves may be blocked selectively on an individual basis. Anesthesia of the lateral femoral cutaneous nerve is occasionally used to provide sensory anesthesia for obtaining a skin graft from the lateral thigh. It can also be blocked as a diagnostic tool to identify cases of meralgia paresthetica. A sciatic nerve blockade alone provides adequate anesthesia for the sole of the foot and lower leg. Procedures on the knee require anesthesia of the femoral and the obturator nerves, although postoperative analgesia of the knee can usually be provided by femoral nerve block alone. Femoral nerve block provides significant postoperative analgesia for the first 18 hours after total knee arthroplasty,and the use of a continuous technique can facilitate rehabilitation.[18]

Sciatic Nerve Blockade, Classic Posterior Approach

1. The patient lies with the side to be blocked uppermost and rolls slightly anterior, flexing the knee so that the

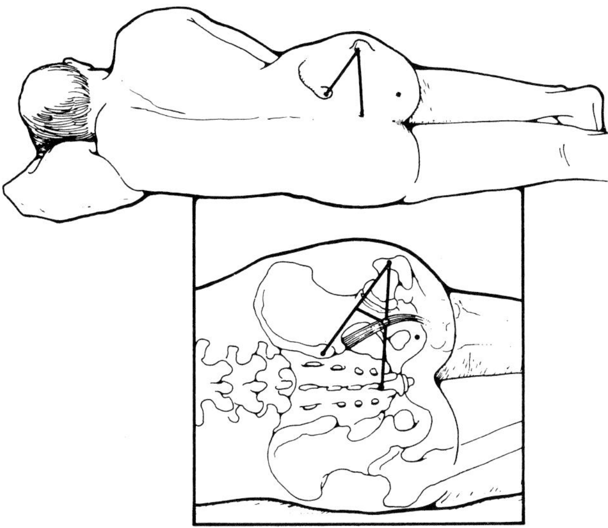

FIGURE 26-27. Sciatic nerve blockade, classic posterior approach. With the patient in the lateral position and the hip and knee flexed, the muscles overlying the sciatic nerve are stretched to allow easier identification. The nerve lies beneath a point 5 cm caudad along the perpendicular line that bisects the line joining the posterosuperior iliac spine and the greater trochanter of the femur. This is also usually the intersection of that perpendicular line with another line joining the greater trochanter and the sacral hiatus. (Reproduced with permission from Mulroy M: Handbook of Regional Anesthesia. Philadelphia, Lippincott Williams & Wilkins, 2002.)

ankle of the involved side rests on top of the knee of the opposite side (Fig. 26-27). This position rotates the femur so that the trochanter is more easily palpated and the muscles overlying the sciatic nerve become stretched.

2. The superior aspect of the greater trochanter of the hip is marked with a circle. A similar circle is placed on the posterosuperior iliac spine, and a line is drawn between these two points.
3. A perpendicular line is drawn from the midpoint of this original line and extended 5 cm in the caudad direction. An "X" is marked at this point. A third line drawn between the greater trochanter and the sacral hiatus should intersect this "X." In the taller patient, the original perpendicular may need to be extended caudad to intersect with the third line, and the nerve may lie closer to the intersection of the second and third lines than to the original "X."
4. A skin wheal is raised at the "X" after aseptic skin preparation.
5. A 10-cm needle is introduced perpendicular to the skin in all planes, and nerve responses of the lower leg and foot are sought. If they are not obtained at the full depth of the needle, the needle is withdrawn to the skin and reintroduced in a fanwise fashion in a path perpendicular to the imagined course of the nerve in the hip. This path can usually be visualized by following the muscular groove on the back of the thigh up and into the imagined position of the sciatic notch. The bony edges of the sciatic notch itself may be encountered. These should be noted, and the search continued. The nerve should lie at approximately this depth as it emerges from inside the pelvis. If localization cannot be obtained in the first 10 minutes, the landmarks should be reassessed.
6. When a nerve response in the foot is obtained, the needle is held immobile, and 25 mL of local anesthetic is injected. A low concentration of local anesthetic may be needed if several nerves are to be blocked, which requires a large total volume of anesthetic in several locations.

Sciatic Nerve Blockade, Supine Approach (Lithotomy). If a patient is uncomfortable in the lateral position or cannot be turned to the side because of a fracture or pain, the nerve can be blocked with the patient in the supine position. An assistant is required to elevate the leg into a lithotomy-type position so that the posterior aspect can be reached.

1. With the patient supine, the hip is flexed by an assistant so that the upper leg is at a 90-degree angle to the torso.
2. The greater trochanter is identified as well as the ischial tuberosity, and a line is drawn between these two. An "X" is marked on the midpoint of this line.
3. A skin wheal is raised at the "X" after aseptic skin preparation. A 10-cm needle is introduced, and nerve responses are sought in a direction along the length of this line (which is perpendicular to the course of the nerve).
4. When a nerve response in the foot is obtained, 25 mL of local anesthetic is injected.

Lateral Femoral Cutaneous Nerve Blockade. The other three nerves of the leg can be blocked at the level of the hip with the patient in the supine position.

1. In the supine position, the anterosuperior iliac spine is identified and marked. An "X" is placed on the skin 2.5 cm below and 2.5 cm medial to the spine.
2. A skin wheal is raised at the "X" after aseptic preparation.
3. A 3.75-cm, 22-gauge needle is introduced through the wheal and directed laterally until a "pop" is felt as it pierces the fascia lata. Three to 5 mL of local anesthetic solution is injected as the needle is withdrawn slowly. The needle is then reinserted slightly medially, and the procedure is repeated until a "wall" of anesthesia has been spread over a 5-cm area above and below the fascia lata extending medially from the level of the anterosuperior spine. A total of 15 to 20 mL of local anesthetic may be required. No nerve responses are sought.

Femoral Nerve Blockade. This blockade can be performed blindly, or nerve responses can be sought for a "three-in-one" blockade (see Lumbar Plexus ["Three-in-One"] Blockade section). The procedure for "blind" blockade follows:

1. In the supine position, a line is drawn from the anterosuperior iliac spine to the pubic tubercle. The femoral artery is identified as it passes below this line, and an "X" is marked on the skin lateral to the artery 2.5 cm below the line.
2. After aseptic preparation, a skin wheal is raised at the mark.
3. A 5-cm, 22-gauge needle is introduced through the "X" and passed perpendicular to the skin until it lies next to the artery and slightly deep to it (Fig. 26-28).
4. Five milliliter of local anesthetic is injected slowly as the needle is withdrawn. The needle is then reinserted slightly more laterally, and the process is repeated twice to create a "wall" of anesthesia lateral to and slightly deep to the femoral artery.
5. Anesthesia of the thigh should ensue within 5 to 10 minutes.

Obturator Nerve Blockade. This nerve is more difficult to locate because of its depth.

1. In the supine position, the pubic tubercle is identified and an "X" is placed 1.5 cm below and 1.5 cm lateral to this structure. This should lie medial to the femoral artery, and a line drawn between the three "Xs" used for these three nerve blockades should be parallel to the line between the superior spine and the pubic tubercle.

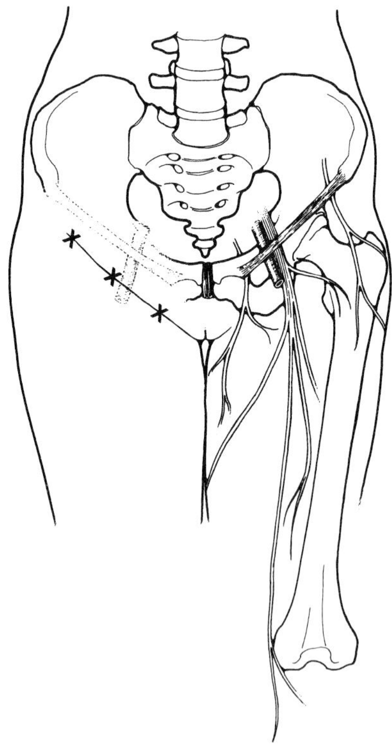

FIGURE 26-28. Blockade of the anterior lumbosacral branches in the groin. The lateral femoral cutaneous nerve emerges approximately 2.5 cm medial to the anterosuperior iliac spine and is best blocked 2.5 cm caudad to this point. The femoral nerve emerges alongside and slightly posterior to the femoral artery and is again easily approached approximately 2.5 cm below the inguinal ligament. On that same line, the obturator nerve emerges from the obturator canal but is deeper and less reliably located. (Reproduced with permission from Mulroy M: Handbook of Regional Anesthesia. Philadelphia, Lippincott Williams & Wilkins, 2002.)

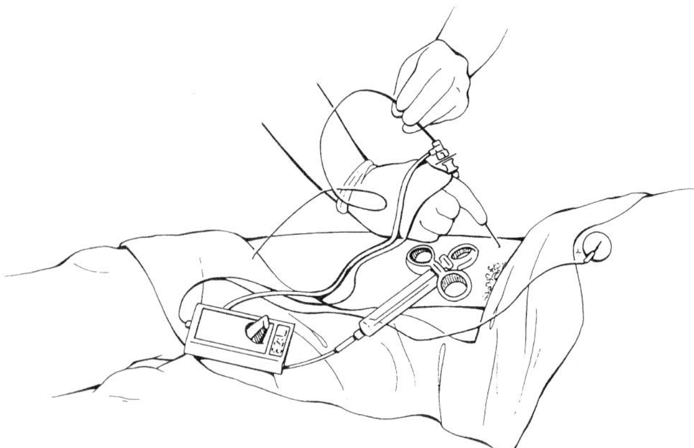

FIGURE 26-29. Continuous femoral catheter. The inguinal approach to the femoral nerve can also be used for the insertion of a continuous catheter. The needle is inserted just lateral to the artery and a motor response is sought in the quadriceps muscle, producing patellar elevation. On identification of the nerve, a continuous catheter is threaded cephalad from this point. A 45-degree angulation of the needle facilitates easy passage of the catheter and encourages spread of the local anesthetic proximally. (Reproduced with permission from Mulroy M: Handbook of Regional Anesthesia. Philadelphia, Lippincott Williams & Wilkins, 2002.)

2. After aseptic skin preparation, a skin wheal is raised at the "X," and a 7.5-cm, 22-gauge needle is introduced through the "X" perpendicular to the skin.
3. The needle is advanced until it contacts bone, which should be the inferior ramus of the pubis. The needle is withdrawn slightly and redirected laterally and slightly caudad to enter the obturator foramen. It is advanced another 2 to 3 cm, and 5 mL of anesthetic is injected as the needle is withdrawn through the presumed depth of the obturator foramen.
4. The needle is then reinserted slightly more laterally, and the process is repeated again until 20 mL of anesthetic solution has been injected to form another "wall" along the presumed path of the obturator nerve (see Fig. 26-28).
5. Alternatively, motor response to a nerve stimulator (adduction of the thigh) can confirm nerve localization.

Lumbar Plexus ("Three-in-One") Blockade. The concept of a single-injection blockade for the lumbar plexus, utilizing the fascial plane that the femoral nerve travels in as it crosses the pelvis, is popular. The premise of this block is that injection of a large quantity of local anesthetic solution in this plane will spread upward into the pelvis and anesthetize the obturator and lateral femoral cutaneous nerves at the point where they still travel in conjunction with the femoral nerve. Unfortunately, the obturator is frequently missed with this technique.[19] Because it is essential to have the needle exactly in the plane of the nerve, eliciting nerve responses is critical for this approach.

1. Preparation for femoral nerve blockade is made as described previously.
2. The needle is inserted in a cephalad manner rather than in a perpendicular angle recommended previously (Fig. 26-29). It is advanced alongside the artery angled at about 45 degrees so that it passes under the inguinal ligament. A nerve response is sought, recognizing that the nerve lies slightly posterior to and occasionally partially under the femoral artery. When the nerve response is obtained, the needle is fixed and the fingers of an assistant are used to compress the femoral artery and the neural sheath below the inguinal ligament while the operator injects 40 mL of anesthetic solution. The injection is performed incrementally after careful aspiration.
3. A continuous perineural catheter can be inserted with this approach, keeping the bevel of the introducing needle directed cephalad to allow the catheter to advance centrally in the fascial plane. Advancement of more than 5 cm of catheter may result in coiling or other misdirection.[20]
4. An alternative to direct localization is identification of the fascial plane by the penetration of the two fascial sheaths by the "pop" sensation of the needle passing through them (the "fascia iliaca block).[21] A needle is introduced 1 cm caudad to the junction of the lateral and middle third of a line marking the inguinal ligament. The needle will first pierce the fascia lata, then the fascia iliaca, and will lie in the nerve compartment. Local anesthetic can be injected directly, or the needle angled 30 degrees cephalad and a catheter threaded. This technique requires little patient cooperation, and is ideal in children, or for repeating a partially successful block (when further stimulation of the femoral nerve may not be successful).

Complications of these techniques are rare. Hematomas can occur in any of the areas of injection and are annoying but rarely serious. The problem of systemic toxicity is significant because of the large volumes of anesthetic solution required. As mentioned previously, careful attention must be paid to the total milligram dose involved when multiple injections are used. Neuropathy is a possibility. Intraneural injection must be avoided by watching for signs of any discomfort at the time of

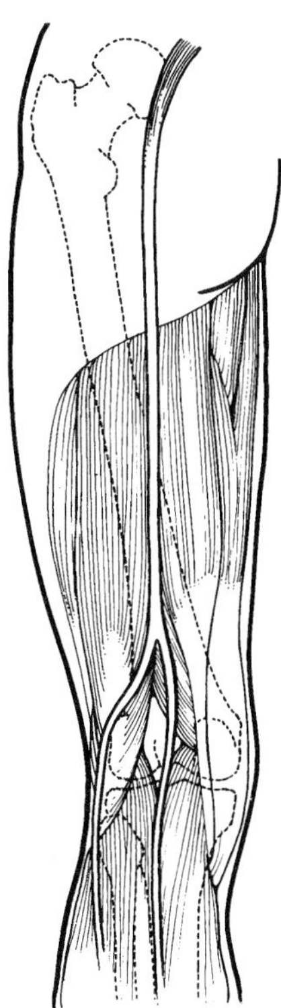

FIGURE 26-30. Popliteal fossa blockade. The two major trunks of the sciatic bifurcate in the popliteal fossa 7 to 10 cm above the knee. A triangle is drawn using the heads of the biceps femoris and the semitendinosus muscles and the skin crease of the knee; a long needle is inserted 1 cm lateral to a point 5 cm cephalad on the line from the skin crease that bisects this triangle. (Reproduced with permission from Mulroy M: Handbook of Regional Anesthesia. Philadelphia, Lippincott Williams & Wilkins, 2002.)

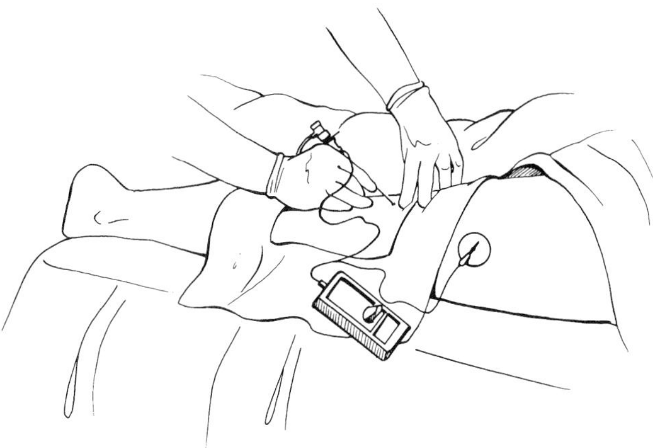

FIGURE 26-31. Popliteal fossa blockade, needle direction. The needle is inserted at the point described in Figure 26-32 and angled 45 degrees cephalad. The nerves usually are contacted halfway between the skin and the femur. This approach is suitable for single injection or catheter insertion. (Reproduced with permission from Mulroy M: Handbook of Regional Anesthesia. Philadelphia, Lippincott Williams & Wilkins, 2002.)

actual injection. If the technique is used for analgesia following outpatient surgery, quadriceps weakness may limit ambulation, and crutches may be needed to enable patient discharge home.

Popliteal Fossa Blockade

The nerves of the lower leg can also be anesthetized by injections at the level of the knee. The success of this technique depends on locating the sciatic nerve near its bifurcation into the tibial and peroneal branches high in the popliteal fossa (Fig. 26-30). Supplemental anesthesia of the femoral nerve is needed to block its terminal saphenous branch, which serves the medial anterior calf and the dorsum of the foot. Insertion of a continuous perineural catheter can provide prolonged analgesia for foot procedures.[22]

Classical Approach.

1. The patient is placed in a prone position. The triangular borders of the popliteal fossa are outlined by drawing the borders of the biceps femoris and the semitendinosus muscles. The base of the triangle is the skin crease behind the knee. The patient can help identify the muscles by slightly flexing the lower leg.
2. After the triangle is drawn, a perpendicular line is drawn from the midpoint of the base to the apex of the triangle. Six centimeters from the base, an "X" is drawn 1 cm lateral to this bisecting line.
3. After aseptic skin preparation, a skin wheal is raised at the "X."
4. A 7.5- or 10-cm needle is introduced through the "X" and directed 45 degrees cephalad along the middle of the triangle (Fig. 26-31). A fanwise search is conducted perpendicular to this line until the nerve is contacted. If the femur is contacted by the needle, the depth is noted. The nerve should lie midway between the skin and the femur.
5. Once a nerve response is obtained, the needle is fixed in position and 30 to 40 mL of local anesthetic solution is injected.
6. A perineural catheter can be inserted here, and advanced 5 cm beyond the needle.
7. The femoral branches can be injected in the same position by raising a subcutaneous wheal of 5 to 10 mL of local anesthetic along the medial tibial head just below the knee.

Lateral Approach. An alternative approach to the block of the popliteal fossa is from the lateral side while the patient is lying supine.

1. On the lateral side of the knee, the groove between the biceps femoris tendon and the vastus lateralis muscle is identified and marked. An "X" is placed 7 cm cephalad to the lateral femoral epicondyle.
2. A 22-gauge, 10-cm needle is inserted at this mark at a horizontal plane. The shaft of the femur is usually contacted within about 5 cm. The needle is then redirected 30 degrees posteriorly to search for the sciatic nerve or its divisions at approximately the same depth of the femur. A response to nerve stimulation in the foot (toe movement is particularly helpful) identifies the nerve, usually the common peroneal nerve that lies laterally. A second nerve response of the tibial nerve may be sought. Ten to 15 mL of anesthesia injected around each nerve provides adequate anesthesia.

Ankle Blockade

All the nerves of the foot can be blocked at the level of the ankle. Although this approach is ideal in producing the least amount of immobility of the lower extremity, it is technically more difficult because at least five nerves must be anesthetized (Fig. 26-32). Several of these nerves can be blocked by simple infiltration of a "wall" of anesthesia, but increased reliability can be produced by seeking paresthesias of the major branches. If paresthesias are not sought, this blockade may actually be

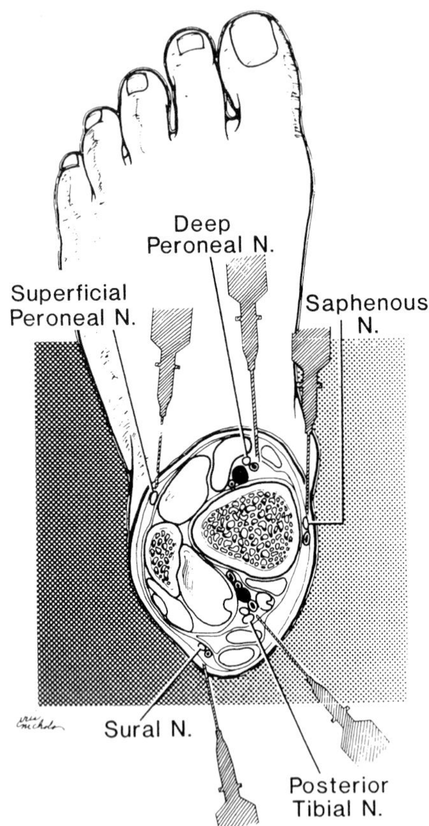

FIGURE 26-32. Ankle blockade. Injections are made at five separate nerve locations. The superficial peroneal nerve, sural nerve, and saphenous nerve are usually blocked simply by subcutaneous infiltration because they may have already generated many superficial branches as they cross the ankle joint. Paresthesias can be sought in the posterior tibial or the deep peroneal nerve, but the bony landmarks usually suffice to provide adequate localization for the deeper injections. (Reproduced with permission from Mulroy M: Handbook of Regional Anesthesia. Philadelphia, Lippincott Williams & Wilkins, 2002.)

less time-consuming than other techniques, even though five separate injections are required. The procedure for blockade follows:

1. Posterior tibial nerve. The posterior tibial nerve is the major nerve to the sole of the foot. It can be approached with the patient either in the prone position or with the hip and knee flexed so that the foot rests on the bed. The medial malleolus is identified, along with the pulsation of the posterior tibial artery behind it. A needle is introduced through the skin just behind the posterior tibial artery and directed 45 degrees anteriorly, seeking a paresthesia in the sole of the foot. Five milliliter of a local anesthetic produce anesthesia if a paresthesia is identified. If not, a fan-shaped injection of 10 mL can be performed in the triangle formed by the artery, the Achilles tendon, and the tibia itself.
2. Sural nerve. With the foot in the same position, the other posterior nerve of the ankle can be blocked by injection on the lateral side. The subcutaneous injection of a ridge of anesthesia behind the lateral malleolus, filling the groove between it and the calcaneus, produces anesthesia of the sural nerve. This will require another 5 mL of local anesthetic.
3. Saphenous nerve. The last three branches of the ankle lie anteriorly. The patient is either turned supine, or the leg can now be extended so that the anesthesiologist's attention is turned to the anterior surface. The saphenous nerve is anesthetized by infiltrating 5 mL of local anesthetic around the saphenous vein at the level where this vein passes anterior to the medial malleolus. A wall of anesthesia between the skin and the bone itself suffices to block the nerve.
4. Deep peroneal nerve. This is the major nerve to the dorsum of the foot and lies in the deep plane of the anterior tibial artery. Pulsation of the artery is sought at the level of the skin crease on the anterior midline surface of the ankle. If it can be felt, 5 mL of local anesthetic is injected just lateral to this. If the artery is not palpable, the tendon of the extensor hallucis longus can be identified by asking the patient to extend the big toe. Injection can be made into the deep planes below the fascia using either one of these landmarks.
5. Superficial peroneal branches. Finally, a subcutaneous ridge of anesthetic solution is laid along the skin crease between the anterior tibial artery and the lateral malleolus. This subcutaneous ridge overlies the previous subfascial injection for the deep peroneal nerve. Another 5 to 10 mL of local anesthetic may be required to cover this area.

Anesthesia of the foot should ensue within 15 minutes after performance of these five injections. Complications of this blockade are rare, although neuropathy can be produced. Care should be taken not to pin any of the deep nerves against the bone at the time of injection, and intraneural injection should be avoided as usual.

References

1. Liu SS, Salinas FV: Continuous plexus and peripheral nerve blocks for postoperative analgesia. Anesth Analg 96:263, 2003
2. Pavlin DJ, Rapp SE, Polissar NL *et al:* Factors affecting discharge time in adult outpatients. Anesth Analg 87:816, 1998
3. Selander D, Brattsand R, Lundborg G *et al:* Local anesthetics: Importance of mode of application, concentration, and adrenaline for the appearance of nerve lesions. Acta Anaesthesiol Scand 23:127, 1979
4. Hadzic A, Vloka J, Hadzic N, Thys DM, Santos AC: Nerve stimulators used for peripheral nerve blocks vary in their electrical characteristics. Anesthesiology 98:969, 2003
5. Brown DL, Ransom DM, Hall JA *et al:* Regional anesthesia and local anesthetic-induced systemic toxicity: Seizure frequency and accompanying cardiovascular changes. Anesth Analg 81:321, 1995
6. Lee LA, Posner KL, Domino KB, Caplan RA, Cheney FW: Injuries associated with regional anesthesia in the 1980s and 1990s: A closed claims analysis. Anesthesiology 101:143, 2004
7. Auroy Y, Benhamou D, Bargues L *et al:* Major complications of regional anesthesia in France: The SOS Regional Anesthesia Hotline Service. Anesthesiology 97:1274, 2002
8. Lanz E, Theiss D, Jankovic D: The extent of blockade following various techniques of brachial plexus block. Anesth Analg 62:55, 1983
9. Winnie AP: Interscalene brachial plexus block. Anesth Analg 49:455, 1970
10. Klein SM, Nielsen KC, Martin A *et al:* Interscalene brachial plexus block with continuous intraarticular infusion of ropivacaine. Anesth Analg 93:601, 2001
11. Klaastad O, VadeBoncouer TR, Tillung T, Smedby O: An evaluation of the supraclavicular plumb-bob technique for brachial plexus block by magnetic resonance imaging. Anesth Analg 96:862, 2003
12. Wilson JL, Brown DL, Wong GY, Ehman RL, Cahill DR: Infraclavicular brachial plexus block: Parasagittal anatomy important to the coracoid technique. Anesth Analg 87:870, 1998
13. Ilfeld BM, Morey TE, Enneking FK: Infraclavicular perineural local anesthetic infusion: A comparison of three dosing regimens for postoperative analgesia. Anesthesiology 100:395, 2004
14. Bouaziz H, Narchi P, Mercier FJ *et al:* Comparison between conventional axillary block and a new approach at the midhumeral level. Anesth Analg 84:1058, 1997
15. Stromskag KE, Minor B, Steen PA: Side effects and complications related to intrapleural analgesia: An update. Acta Anaesthesiol Scand 34:473, 1990
16. Plancarte R, de Leon-Casasola OA, El-Helaly M *et al:* Neurolytic superior hypogastric plexus block for chronic pelvic pain associated with cancer. Regional Anesthesia 22:562, 1997

17. Capdevila X, Macaire P, Dadure C *et al:* Continuous psoas compartment block for postoperative analgesia after total hip arthroplasty: New landmarks, technical guidelines, and clinical evaluation. Anesth Analg 94:1606, 2002
18. Singelyn FJ, Deyaert M, Joris D *et al:* Effects of intravenous patient-controlled analgesia with morphine, continuous epidural analgesia, and continuous three-in-one block on post-operative pain and knee rehabilitation after unilateral total knee arthroplasty. Anesth Analg 87:88, 1998
19. Parkinson SK, Mueller JB, Little WL, Bailey SL: Extent of blockade with various approaches to the lumbar plexus. Anesth Analg 68:243, 1989
20. Ganapathy S, Wasserman RA, Watson JT *et al:* Modified continuous femoral three-in-one block for postoperative pain after total knee arthroplasty. Anesth Analg 89:1197, 1999
21. Capdevila X, Biboulet P, Bouregba M *et al:* Comparison of the three-in-one and fascia iliaca compartment blocks in adults: clinical and radiographic analysis. Anesth Analg 86:1039, 1998
22. Hadzic A, Vloka JD, Singson R, Santos AC, Thys DM: A comparison of intertendinous and classical approaches to popliteal nerve block using magnetic resonance imaging simulation. Anesth Analg 94:1321, 2002

CHAPTER 27 ■ ANESTHESIA FOR NEUROSURGERY

AUDRÉE A. BENDO, IRA S. KASS, JOHN HARTUNG, AND JAMES E. COTTRELL

KEY POINTS

1. The intracranial compartment has a fixed volume. Increases in the volume of the brain, the blood, or the cerebral spinal fluid can lead to an increase in intracranial pressure; this may compromise blood flow or cause the brain to herniate.
2. Hypoxia and ischemia lead to neuronal death. With severe insults the neurons die of necrosis, which leads to inflammation and extensive damage to other neurons in the area; after less severe insults, neurons may be damaged so they cannot function properly and die of a regulated cell death process called apoptosis, which does not injure adjacent neurons.
3. Both intravenous and volatile anesthetic agents reduce brain metabolism. It is the balance of this effect with blood flow, because of flow metabolism coupling, that determines the extent of the increase or decrease in cerebral blood flow with a particular anesthetic agent.
4. Cerebral preconditioning and augmentation of endogenous processes of repair, including both neurogenesis and diaschisis, are promising approaches to cerebral protection.
5. Until and unless the deleterious effects of mild hypothermia can be reduced, or the brain can be cooled without reducing systemic temperature below 35°C, clinical evidence does not support induction of intra-operative mild hypothermia for neurosurgical procedures.
6. Current evidence cautions against the use of prophylactic etomidate prior to temporary vessel occlusion, magnesium loading in ischemic stroke patients, intra-operative nitrous oxide and ketamine, intra-operative moderate hypothermia in subarachnoid hemorrhage (SAH) patients, postoperative nimodipine and tirilazad, and postoperative hypothermia in head trauma patients.
7. Electrophysiologic and cerebral oxygenation/metabolism monitors are used perioperatively to assess cerebral function and pharmacologic interventions and to detect cerebral ischemia.
8. Image-guided neurosurgical procedures are used for diagnosis, three-dimensional localization, and resection of intracranial lesions.
9. The administration of anesthesia to neurosurgical patients requires an understanding of the basic principles of neurophysiology and the effects of anesthetic agents on intracranial dynamics.
10. Neuroanesthetic management of patients with supratentorial disease maximizes therapeutic modalities that reduce intracranial pressure.
11. Because of the relatively confined space within the posterior fossa, the challenge of infratentorial surgery is to prevent further neurologic damage from surgical position and exploration.

12 The anesthetic goals for intracranial aneurysm surgery are to avoid aneurysm rupture, maintain cerebral perfusion pressure and transmural aneurysm pressure, and provide a "slack" brain.

13 With more extensive arteriovenous malformations, hypothermia and high-dose barbiturates have been recommended for brain protection. Induced hypotension may also be required to reduce lesion size and blood flow.

14 Severe intracranial hypertension can precipitate reflex arterial hypertension and bradycardia (Cushing's triad). A reduction in systemic blood pressure in these patients can further aggravate cerebral ischemia by reducing cerebral perfusion pressure.

NEUROPHYSIOLOGY AND NEUROANESTHESIA

To understand how anesthetics act on the nervous system and how these actions may affect the practice of neuroanesthesia, one first needs to understand the basic principles of neurobiology. The following description of cellular neurophysiology provides background information only; greater detail may be sought elsewhere.[1]

Membrane Potentials

Neurons have an electrical potential across their cell membrane owing to different intra- and extracellular ion concentrations. These concentration differences lead to an opposing voltage called the *equilibrium potential*. Sodium (Na) and potassium (K) are the main ions responsible for membrane potentials in neurons. The equilibrium potential for K (E_K) is approximately −90 mV and for Na (E_{Na}) +45 mV. An ion's contribution to the membrane potential of a neuron is determined by its conductance, which is proportional to the membrane's permeability for that ion. Because the conductance to potassium (g_K) is much higher than the sodium conductance (g_{Na}) in an unexcited neuron, the resting membrane potential (approximately −60 mV) is nearer to the potassium equilibrium potential (−90 mV) than the sodium equilibrium potential (+45 mV).

The conductance of ions across the cell membrane is through channels, which are proteins that span the membrane; gates open and close these channels. During rest, most of the sodium channels have their gates closed, whereas more potassium channels have gates in the open position. That is why there is a greater conductance to K in resting neurons.

Neurons transmit signals over long distances by propagating action potentials, which are rapid depolarizations of the membrane, along their axons. The action potential is caused by a rapid increase in the sodium conductance (because of the opening of the sodium activation gate) and a slower increase in the potassium conductance. These conductance changes are triggered by a depolarization of the cell membrane, and therefore the channels that open in response to the depolarization are described as voltage-sensitive channels. When the neuron depolarizes past a threshold voltage level, an action potential is generated. The peak voltage of the action potential is approximately +20 mV; this level is attained because, at the peak, the sodium conductance is much greater than the potassium conductance. The voltage during the action potential returns rapidly to resting levels (repolarizes) because the sodium conductance shuts itself off by closing a second gate (inactivation gate) in the channel, and the potassium conductance increases as a result of the opening of potassium channels.

Synaptic Transmission

Neurons communicate using chemical synapses. The chemical, called a transmitter, is released from the presynaptic neuron, diffuses across the synaptic cleft, and combines with a receptor molecule on the postsynaptic neuron. The release of the neurotransmitter is initiated by an action potential traveling down the axon of the presynaptic neuron, causing the depolarization of the presynaptic terminal. This depolarization leads to the opening of voltage-dependent calcium channels and the entry of calcium from the extracellular fluid into the terminal. Vesicles containing the neurotransmitter then fuse with the terminal membrane, releasing the neurotransmitter into the synaptic cleft. The combination of the neurotransmitter with its receptor located on the postsynaptic cell alters ion channels associated with the receptor. These channels are described as ligand-gated channels. The opening of these ion channels leads to a change in the membrane potential of the postsynaptic neuron. If the transmitter is excitatory, this postsynaptic neuron is depolarized and therefore is more likely to generate an action potential. If the transmitter is inhibitory, the neuron is hyperpolarized and is less likely to generate an action potential.

In addition to opening ion channels, neurotransmitters work through intracellular second messengers. One example of a second messenger is cyclic cAMP, which activates protein kinases to phosphorylate proteins and changes their activity. Ion channels may be phosphorylated, which may change their conductance. A group of proteins that bind guanosine triphosphate, called G proteins, are activated when a transmitter binds to a specific receptor molecule. In some cases these G proteins activate ion channels directly, but in other cases they can either stimulate (G_s) or inhibit (G_i) adenylate cyclase, the enzyme that converts adenosine triphosphate (ATP) into cyclic AMP. G proteins can also activate the phosphatidylinositol second-messenger system; in this case, a transmitter binds to a receptor, which causes another G protein (G_p) to activate phospholipase C. This membrane-bound enzyme breaks down a membrane phospholipid into diacylglycerol and inositol trisphosphate, both of which are second messengers. Diacylglycerol activates protein kinase C, which will then phosphorylate other proteins, whereas inositol trisphosphate increases cytosolic calcium by releasing it from intracellular stores (endoplasmic reticulum).

There are many neurotransmitters in the brain. In this chapter two common neurotransmitters and their receptors are examined.

γ-Aminobutyric acid (GABA) is a major inhibitory amino acid transmitter that is active throughout the brain and reduces the excitability of neurons by hyperpolarizing them. There are two major GABA receptors. Activation of the $GABA_A$ receptor opens chloride channels; this activity is enhanced by benzodiazepines and barbiturates. The $GABA_B$ receptor acts via a second messenger to open potassium channels, but does not affect chloride channels.[2] The response to $GABA_B$ receptor activation has a slower onset and a more prolonged activation than the response to the $GABA_A$ receptor. Both receptors may be present on the same neuron, providing a mechanism for rapid and prolonged inhibition.

Glutamate is the major excitatory transmitter in the brain. Its activation depolarizes neurons, making it more likely that they will fire action potentials. There are three main inotropic glutamate receptors, which have been named for their preferential pharmacologic agonists. Most of the AMPA and kainate receptors allow sodium and potassium but not calcium through their channels.[3] These channels are responsible for the normal excitatory responses seen with glutamate. The third glutamate receptor, the *N*-methyl-D-aspartate receptor (NMDA), is activated when neurons are depolarized; the channels associated with this receptor are not opened by glutamate at normal resting membrane potentials. These channels allow passage of calcium as well as sodium and potassium. NMDA receptor activation is important in changing a neuron's excitability over a period of hours and days (long-term potentiation); this has been correlated with learning in animals.[3] Glutamate receptors have also been associated with neuronal injury after ischemia and anoxia. In addition to inotropic effects, glutamate activates metabotropic receptors, which act via a second messenger. Inositol trisphosphate, a second messenger, releases calcium from intracellular stores; this can affect the excitability of the neuron.

The information here is a simple description of how synapses operate to convey information from one neuron to another. This process is finely controlled; there are neurotransmitters that act on presynaptic terminals to regulate the amount of transmitter the terminal releases. There are compounds called *neuromodulators* that, when applied to a neuron alone, have no observable effect on the excitability of that neuron but alter the effect of other excitatory or inhibitory inputs to that neuron.

Brain Metabolism

The main substance used for energy production in the brain is glucose.[4] When oxygen levels are sufficient, glucose is metabolized to pyruvate in the glycolytic pathway (Fig. 27-1). This biochemical process generates ATP from adenosine diphosphate and inorganic phosphate and produces the reduced form of nicotinamide adeninedinucleotide (NADH) from nicotinamide adenine dinucleotide (NAD). Pyruvate from this reaction then enters the citric acid cycle, which, with regard to energy production, primarily generates NADH from NAD. The mitochondria use oxygen to couple the conversion of NADH back to NAD with the production of ATP from ADP and inorganic phosphate. This process, called *oxidative phosphorylation,* forms

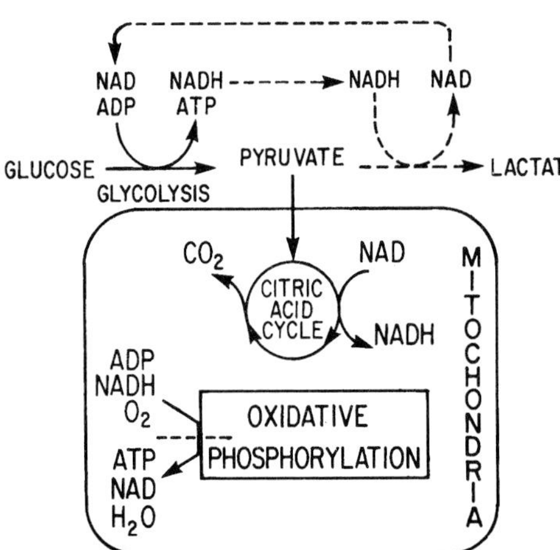

FIGURE 27-1. Energy metabolism in the brain. *Dotted lines* indicate reactions that occur during ischemia. The *dotted line* across the oxidative phosphorylation reaction indicates that this reaction is blocked during ischemia.

TABLE 27-1

CELLULAR PROCESSES THAT REQUIRE ENERGY

Intracellular signaling
Metabolism of DNA, RNA, proteins, lipids, carbohydrates, and other molecules
Transporting of molecules within cells and across the cell membrane
Pumping ions across membranes to maintain ion gradients
Synaptic transmission
Neuronal plasticity (structural and biochemical changes)

three ATP molecules for each NADH converted. The process of aerobic metabolism yields 38 ATP molecules for each glucose molecule metabolized.

This pathway requires oxygen; if oxygen is not present, the mitochondria can neither make ATP nor regenerate NAD from NADH. The metabolism of glucose requires NAD as a cofactor and is blocked in its absence. Thus, in the absence of oxygen, glycolysis proceeds by a modified pathway termed *anaerobic glycolysis*; this modification involves the conversion of pyruvate to lactate, regenerating NAD. There is a net hydrogen ion production, which lowers the intracellular pH. A major problem with anaerobic glycolysis, in addition to lowering pH, is that only two molecules of ATP are formed for each molecule of glucose metabolized. This level of ATP production is insufficient to meet the brain's energy needs.

When the oxygen supply to a neuron is reduced, mechanisms that reduce and/or slow the fall in ATP levels include: (1) the utilization of phosphocreatine stores (a high-energy phosphate that can donate its energy to maintain ATP levels), (2) the production of ATP at low levels by anaerobic glycolysis, and (3) a rapid cessation of spontaneous electrophysiologic activity.

Pumping ions across the cell membrane is the largest energy requirement in the brain (Table 27-1). The sodium, potassium, and calcium concentrations of a neuron are maintained against large electrochemical differences with respect to the outside of the cell. When a neuron is not excited (firing action potentials), there is a slow leak of potassium out of the cells and of sodium into the cells. Neuronal activity markedly increases the flow of potassium, sodium, and calcium; this increases the rate of ion pumping required to maintain the neuron's ion concentration. Because ion pumping uses ATP as an energy source, the ATP requirement of active neurons is greater than that for resting neurons. If energy production does not meet the demand of energy use in the brain, the neurons first become unexcitable and then are irreversibly damaged.[5,6]

Neurons require energy to maintain their structure and internal function. The cell's membranes, internal organelles, and cytoplasm are made of carbohydrates, lipids, and proteins, which require energy for their synthesis. Ion channels, enzymes, and structural components are important protein molecules that are continuously formed, modified, and broken down in the cell. If ATP is not available, protein synthesis cannot continue and the neuron will die. Carbohydrates and lipids are also continuously synthesized and degraded in normally functioning neurons; their metabolism also requires energy. Most cellular synthesis takes place in the cell body; thus, energy is required for the transport of components down the axon to the nerve terminal. The importance of this transport is illustrated by the death of the distal end of an axon when it is severed from its cell body. Thus, energy is required to maintain the integrity of neurons even in the absence of electrophysiologic activity.

The overall metabolic rate for the brain of a young adult man (mean age, 21 years) is 3.5 mL O_2/min/100 g brain tissue or 5.5 mg glucose/min/100 g.[4] This rate is virtually the same in elderly men (mean age, 71 years). Children (mean age, 6 years) have a markedly higher metabolic rate of 5.2 mL O_2/min/100 g brain tissue. Although the reasons for this high metabolic rate are unknown, it may reflect extra energy requirements for the growth and development of the nervous system.[4]

Cerebral Blood Flow

The brain receives approximately 15% of cardiac output, yet makes up only 2% of total body weight.[4] The disproportionately large blood flow is a result of the high metabolic rate of the brain. Global blood flow and metabolic rate remain fairly stable. Regional blood flow and metabolic rate of the brain can change dramatically; when metabolic rate goes up in a region of the brain, the blood flow to that region also increases. The mechanism of this coupling of blood flow and metabolism is not known; however, an increase in either potassium or hydrogen ion concentrations in the extracellular fluid surrounding arterioles may lead to dilatation and increased flow. Other agents that may mediate the coupling are calcium, adenosine, nitric oxide, and the eicosanoids (e.g., prostaglandins).[5] None of these mechanisms need be exclusive, and more than one or all of them may contribute to this exquisite coupling of flow and metabolism.

Increasing carbon dioxide level causes vasodilatation and increased blood flow (Fig. 27-2). Increasing the carbon dioxide tension from 40 to 80 mmHg doubles the flow; reducing the carbon dioxide from 40 to 20 mmHg halves the flow.[7,8] These changes are transient, and blood flow returns to normal in 6 to 8 hours, even if the altered carbon dioxide levels are maintained. These effects may be related to the hydrogen ion concentration. High carbon dioxide levels increase the extracellular hydrogen ion concentration and blood flow, whereas low carbon dioxide levels decrease the extracellular hydrogen ion concentration and reduce blood flow. The bicarbonate concentration in the extracellular fluid of the brain adjusts, bringing the pH back to normal, even though the carbon dioxide levels remain altered.[9] This has important clinical implications in patients hyperventilated for prolonged periods. If normocarbia is rapidly reestablished, brain interstitial fluid pH will decrease and cerebral blood flow (CBF) will increase dramatically, perhaps increasing intracranial pressure (ICP).

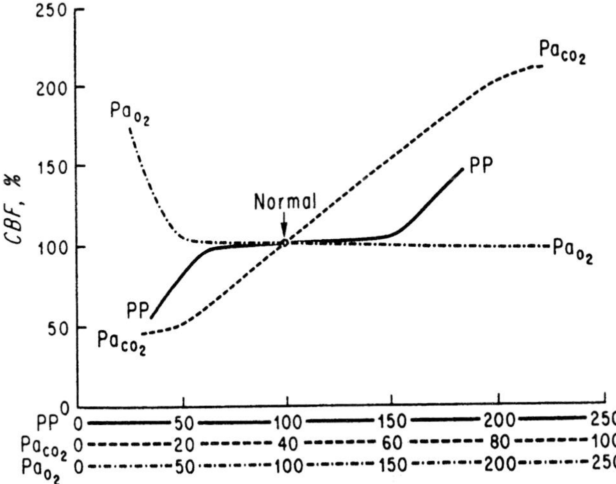

FIGURE 27-2. The effect of perfusion pressure (PP), arterial carbon dioxide pressure ($PaCO_2$), and arterial oxygen pressure (PaO_2) on cerebral blood flow. Each parameter on the abscissa is varied independently while the other parameters are held at their normal levels. (Reprinted with permission from Michenfelder JD: Anesthesia and the Brain, pp 6, 94–113. New York, Churchill Livingstone, 1988.)

If a patient is hypoventilated, carbon dioxide increases, pH decreases, and blood flow increases throughout the brain. The arterioles could become maximally dilated throughout the brain, impeding the ability to direct flow to areas of high metabolic demand. Thus, this luxury flow caused by high carbon dioxide levels throughout the brain could "steal" blood flow from areas that require extra oxygen and produce metabolites. This is particularly important during focal ischemia with the blockage of an intracerebral artery. The vessels supplying collateral flow to the area of the blocked artery would already be maximally dilated because of the metabolic demands of the ischemic tissue, and high Pa_{CO2} would cause blood flow to be shunted away to areas of less demand. The blood flow to the brain can be manipulated to advantage during focal ischemia. Reducing carbon dioxide with hyperventilation or reducing metabolism with agents such as thiopental would reduce blood flow to most areas of the brain, and the vessels in the ischemic area would be maximally dilated because of low pH. These manipulations, which are sometimes called *inverse steal,* could have the effect of maximizing blood flow to compromised areas.[10] The clinical relevance of flow redistribution because of hypocarbia has been questioned.[11]

The CBF autoregulates with respect to pressure changes. In normotensive individuals, mean arterial pressure (MAP) can vary from 50 to 150 mmHg and CBF will be maintained constant because of an adjustment of the cerebral vascular resistance (see Fig. 27-2). This phenomenon is a myogenic response of the arterioles because of their ability to constrict in response to an increased distending pressure. This response takes a few minutes to develop; therefore, after a rapid increase in MAP, there is a short period (about 1 to 3 minutes) of increased blood flow.[12] If mean blood pressure falls below 50 mmHg, CBF is reduced; at a pressure of 40 mmHg, mild symptoms of cerebral ischemia occur.[12] Patients who are hypertensive demonstrate a shift of autoregulation to a higher blood pressure. Their lower limit of autoregulation could be well above 50 mmHg; their upper limit of autoregulation is also increased. This shift, a result of hypertrophy of the vessel wall, takes 1 or 2 months to become established.[13]Autoregulation can be abolished by trauma, hypoxia, and certain anesthetic and adjuvant anesthetic drugs. When blood pressure exceeds the autoregulated range, it can cause a disruption of the blood-brain barrier and cerebral edema.

The cerebral vasculature is also regulated by neurogenic factors that seem to have their greatest influence on the larger cerebral vessels. They control flow to large areas of the brain and play less of a role in the regulation of local CBF.[12] The innervation includes cholinergic, adrenergic, and serotonergic systems. Sympathetic activation leads to increased MAP and shifts the autoregulatory curve to the right, increasing the pressure at which the breakthrough of autoregulation occurs.[13]

Cerebrospinal Fluid

The neurons in the brain are exquisitely sensitive to changes in their environment. Small alterations in extracellular ion levels can profoundly alter neuronal activity. Substances that circulate in the blood, such as catecholamines, if not sequestered from direct contact with the brain, might also disrupt brain function. Thus the composition of the fluid surrounding the

TABLE 27-2

COMPOSITION OF CEREBROSPINAL FLUID AND SERUM IN MAN

	CSF	SERUM
Sodium (mEq/l)	141	140
Potassium (mEq/l)	2.9	4.6
Calcium (mEq/l)	2.5	5.0
Magnesium (mEq/l)	2.4	1.7
Chloride (mEq/l)	124	101
Bicarbonate (mEq/l)	21	23
Glucose (mg/100 mL)	61	92
Protein (mg/100 mL)	28	7,000
pH	7.31	7.41
Osmolality (mOsm/kg H_2O)	289	289

Adapted with permission from Artru AA: Cerebrospinal fluid. In Cottrell JE, Smith DS (eds): Anesthesia and Neurosurgery, p 95. St Louis, CV Mosby, 1994.

brain is tightly regulated and distinct from extracellular fluid in the rest of the body (Table 27-2).[14] There are two barriers, the blood-brain barrier and the blood-cerebrospinal fluid barrier, that maintain the difference between blood and cerebrospinal fluid (CSF) composition.

Brain capillary endothelial cells (the blood-brain barrier) have tight junctions that prevent extracellular passage of substances between the endothelial cells. They also have a low level of pinocytotic activity, which reduces the transport of large molecules across the cells. Processes of astrocyte glial cells are interposed between the neurons of the brain and the capillaries. The functional importance of the astrocytes to the blood-brain barrier is currently unknown; however, they are located wherever the blood-brain barrier is present and appear to be necessary for the development and perhaps the maintenance of the barrier. The blood-brain barrier impedes the flow of ions such as potassium, calcium, magnesium, and sodium; polar molecules such as glucose, amino acids, and mannitol; and macromolecules such as proteins.[14] Lipid-soluble compounds, water, and gases such as carbon dioxide, oxygen, and volatile anesthetics pass rapidly through the blood-brain barrier. Many substances that do not cross the blood-brain barrier are required for brain function; these substances are transported across the capillary endothelial cell by carrier-mediated processes. These processes consist of either active transport, which requires the expenditure of energy, or passive transport, which does not. Passive transport, also referred to as *facilitated diffusion,* can move molecules into the brain only if their concentration in the blood is higher than their concentration in the brain. Glucose is an example of a molecule that enters the brain by passive transport. All of these transport processes have a limited capacity. The blood-brain barrier can become disrupted by acute hypertension, osmotic shock, disease, tumor, trauma, irradiation, and ischemia.

Cerebrospinal fluid is primarily formed in the choroid plexus of the cerebral ventricles. The capillaries of the choroid plexus have fenestrations and intercellular gaps that allow free movement of molecules across the endothelial cells; however, they are surrounded by choroid plexus epithelial cells, which have tight junctions and form the basis of the blood-CSF barrier. It is these cells that secrete the CSF. The CSF volume in the brain is between 100 and 150 mL; it is formed and reabsorbed at a rate of 0.3 to 0.4 mL/min. This allows a complete replacement of the CSF volume three or four times a day. The blood-CSF barrier is similar to the blood-brain barrier in that it allows the free movement of water, gases, and lipid-soluble compounds but requires carrier-mediated active or passive transport processes for glucose, amino acids, and ions. Proteins are largely excluded from the CSF. The CSF is primarily formed by the transport of sodium, chloride, and bicarbonate with the osmotic movement of water. Two clinically used substances that reduce CSF formation are furosemide, which inhibits the combined transport of sodium and chloride, and acetazolamide, which reduces bicarbonate transport by inhibiting carbonic anhydrase.[15] The CSF flows from the lateral ventricles to the third and fourth ventricles and then to the cisterna magna. It then flows around the brain and spinal cord in the cerebral and spinal subarachnoid space. The fluid in the subarachnoid space provides cushioning for the brain, reducing the effect of head trauma. The CSF is absorbed into the venous system of the brain by the villi in the arachnoid membrane. These arachnoid villi allow one-way flow of CSF from the subarachnoid space into the venous sinuses when CSF pressure is greater than the pressure in these sinuses. Owing to the high rate of CSF formation and its absorption into the venous system, proteins and other matter released into the brain extracellular fluid are removed. If the foramina connecting the ventricles or the arachnoid villi are blocked, pressure builds and hydrocephalus develops.

Intracranial Pressure

1 The brain is enclosed in the cranium, which has a fixed volume; therefore, if any of the components located in the cranial vault increase in volume, the ICP will increase (Table 27-3). An increase in volume of one of these components can increase ICP and result in two major deleterious effects on the organism. The first is to reduce blood flow to the brain. The cerebral perfusion pressure (CPP) is determined by the MAP minus the ICP. If ICP increases to a greater extent than MAP, CPP is reduced. If ICP rises sufficiently, the brain can become ischemic. The second important effect of increased ICP is its ability to induce brain herniation. This herniation could be across the meninges, down the spinal canal, or through an opening in the skull. Herniation can rapidly lead to neurologic deterioration and death.

The ICP in humans is normally less than 10 mmHg. Under normal circumstances, a small increase in intracranial volume will not greatly increase ICP because of the elastance of the components located in the cranium (Fig. 27-3). After a certain point, however, the capacity of the system to adjust to increased volume is exceeded and even a small increase in volume will increase ICP.[16] Increases in ICP can be caused by the following: (1) increased CSF volume because of blockage of the circulation or absorption of the CSF, as described earlier; (2) increased blood volume from vasodilatation or hematoma; and (3) increased brain tissue volume caused by a tumor or edema.

Brain edema is typically classified as cytotoxic or vasogenic. The former is because of neuronal damage, which leads to increased sodium and water in the brain cells, and therefore an increase in intracellular volume. Vasogenic edema is caused by a breakdown of the blood-brain barrier and the movement

TABLE 27-3

THE THREE MAJOR COMPONENTS THAT OCCUPY SPACE IN THE SKULL

The brain, which includes neurons and glia
The cerebrospinal fluid and extracellular fluid
The blood perfusing the brain

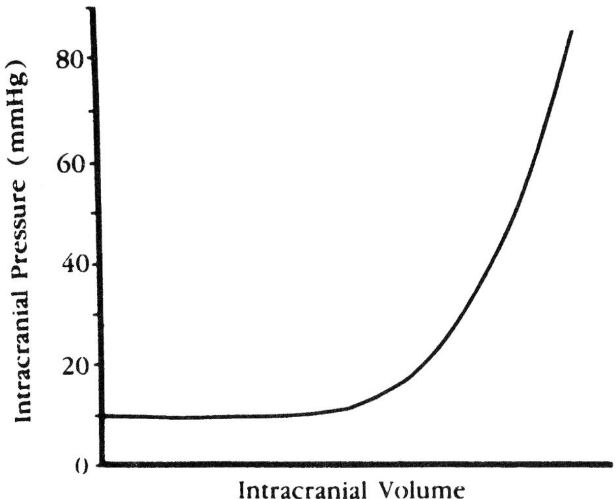

FIGURE 27-3. The effect of increasing volume on intracranial pressure. At first, as volume is increased, pressure does not increase, owing to the elastance of intracranial structures. This elastance is exceeded and then a small increase in volume can cause a large increase in intracranial pressure. (Modified from Miller JD, Garibi J, Pickard JD: The effects of induced changes of cerebrospinal fluid volume during continuous monitoring of ventricular pressure. Arch Neurol 28:265, 1973.)

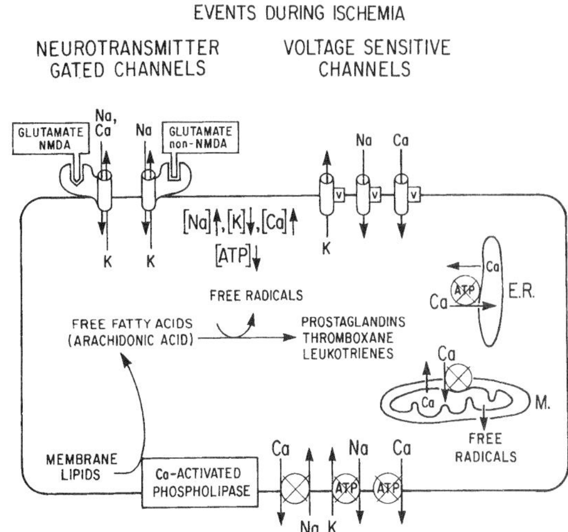

FIGURE 27-4. The effect of hypoxia or ischemia on ion and metabolite levels in neurons. For clarity, ion channels are shown on the top membrane and ion pumps on the bottom membrane; their actual location can be on any membrane surface. *Circles* indicate energy-driven pumps, and a *crossed-through circle* indicates that this pump is blocked or has reduced activity during ischemia. *V* indicates a voltage-dependent channel.

of protein from the blood into the brain's extracellular space. Water moves osmotically with the protein, increasing the extracellular fluid volume in the brain.

Pathophysiology

The brain is the organ most sensitive to ischemia; therefore, when the blood supply to the brain is limited, ischemic damage to neurons can occur.[17] To understand the rationale for treatments used to protect the brain against anoxic and ischemic damage, one needs an appreciation of the pathophysiologic mechanisms that may lead to this damage. The central event precipitating damage is reduced energy production because of blockage of oxidative phosphorylation. This causes ATP production per molecule of glucose to be reduced by 95%. At this rate of production, ATP levels fall, leading to the loss of energy-dependent homeostatic mechanisms. (Complete ischemia would block all ATP production.) The activity of ATP-dependent ion pumps is reduced and the intracellular levels of sodium and calcium increase, while intracellular potassium levels decrease (Fig. 27-4). These ion changes cause the neurons to depolarize and release excitatory amino acids such as glutamate. High levels of glutamate further depolarize the neurons and allow more calcium to enter through the NMDA receptor channel. The high intracellular calcium level is thought to trigger a number of events that could lead to the anoxic or ischemic damage. These include increasing the activity of proteases and phospholipases.[17] The latter would increase the levels of free fatty acids and free radicals. Free radicals are known to damage proteins and lipids, whereas free fatty acids interfere with membrane function. In addition, there is a buildup of lactate and hydrogen ions. All of these processes, coupled with the reduced ability to synthesize proteins and lipids because of the reduced ATP levels, may lead to irreversible damage with ischemia. In addition, phospholipase activation leads to the production of excess arachidonic acid, which, on reoxygenation, can form eicosanoids, including thromboxane, prostaglandins, and leukotrienes. Thromboxane can cause intense vasoconstriction and reduced blood flow in the postischemic period, while leukotrienes can increase edema. Thus, procedures that may protect against ischemia should interfere with these damaging mechanisms (Table 27-4). Specific agents that might accomplish these objectives are detailed in the section on brain protection later in the chapter.

Ischemia can be either global or focal in nature; an example of the former would be cardiac arrest, of the latter, a localized stroke. The mechanisms leading to neuronal damage are probably similar for both, but there are important distinctions between the two. In focal ischemia there are three regions. The first receives no blood flow and responds the same as globally ischemic tissue; the second, called the *penumbra,* receives collateral flow and is partially ischemic; the third is normally perfused. If the insult is maintained for a prolonged period, the neurons in the penumbra will die. More neurons in the penumbra will survive if collateral blood flow is increased. Mechanisms such as inverse steal (described in the Cerebral Blood Flow section) will enhance collateral blood flow, and hence neuron survival, in focal but not global ischemia.

Epileptic activity is sudden, excessive, and synchronous discharges of large numbers of neurons. Aside from those patients with established epilepsy, this massive increase in activity is seen

TABLE 27-4

PROCEDURES THAT MAY PROTECT AGAINST ISCHEMIC DAMAGE

Maintaining blood flow
Maintaining ATP levels by reducing the metabolic rate
Blocking sodium or calcium influx
Scavenging free radicals
Blocking the release of or receptors for excitatory amino acids
Inhibiting proteins that activate or contribute to damage (e.g., proteases, phospholipases, and some kinases)
Activating proteins that induce repair or rescue from apoptosis and necrosis (e.g., some kinases)

in patients with ionic and electrolyte imbalances, disorders of brain metabolism, infection, brain tumor, brain trauma, or elevated body temperature.[18] The electroencephalogram (EEG) shows spikes, which are rapid changes in voltage corresponding to excess activity in many neurons. During the epileptiform activity, sodium and calcium ions enter the cells and potassium leaves. Thus the cells use more energy (ATP) for ion pumping. High extracellular potassium may be responsible for the large and progressive depolarization of the neurons that is commonly found. The mechanisms that lead to permanent neuronal damage with epilepsy may be similar to those that damage cells during ischemia. Intracellular calcium levels rise, which may precipitate the damage. It is clear that during epileptiform activity the energy demand, and hence the cerebral metabolic rate (CMR) and blood flow, increases greatly. Thus, in conditions in which blood flow to the brain may be compromised, it is imperative to avoid excess brain activity. Anticonvulsant medications increase neuronal inhibition or reduce excitatory processes in the brain. Epileptic activity may be accompanied by systemic lactic acidosis, reduced arterial oxygenation, and increased carbon dioxide; therefore, it is important to maintain ventilation, oxygenation, and blood pressure. Prolonged or recurring epileptic activity can lead to profound brain damage.

Brain trauma can directly lead to permanent physical neuronal damage. Primary damage can also be caused by brain herniation or severing of blood vessels in the brain, resulting in direct ischemia. Reversal of the primary damage is not possible; however, much of the brain injury in trauma patients is secondary and occurs following the initial insult.[19] Calcium influx resulting from the trauma has been implicated as a trigger for the damage. It is important to prevent the secondary ischemia that frequently follows brain trauma and is possibly a result of the release of vasoconstrictive substances during reperfusion. In addition, hemorrhage may increase intracranial blood volume and ICP, reducing CPP. The intracranial blood can be damaging by directly promoting free-radical formation using the iron in hemoglobin. Secondary damage may be reduced with proper monitoring and treatment. Treatment includes reducing ICP, maintaining blood flow, reducing vasospasm, removing blood from the subarachnoid space, and perhaps using pharmacologic agents that interfere with the cascade of events that lead to neuron damage.

Brain tumors are expanding, space-occupying lesions that may significantly increase ICP and lead to reduced CPP or brain herniation. Frequently, the blood vessels supplying the tumor have a leaky blood-brain barrier, which may contribute to vasogenic brain edema and elevated ICP.

Thus, for several pathophysiologic events in the brain, ATP depletion; ionic imbalance (particularly high intracellular calcium levels); free-radical formation; and kinase, protease, and phospholipase activation have been implicated as triggers of
2 neuronal damage. A common mechanism of neuronal cell death for various pathophysiologic events may exist. There are two major processes that lead to neuronal death. The first, necrosis, is characterized by a disintegration of the cell and an activation of microglia and the immune response.[20,21] The immune response and inflammation activates and recruits neutrophils and macrophages that produce free radicals and damage adjacent neurons. This expands the lesion in volume and time allowing for continued and expanded neuronal damage.[21] The second process, apoptosis or programmed cell death, involves an active process, which does not damage adjacent neurons.[20] Apoptosis uses a metabolic process that is normally used to kill off unneeded neurons. This process is responsible for the death of many neurons during development and can be reactivated when neurons are damaged subsequent to ischemia.[22] A severe insult, such as would be encountered in the core of an ischemic area, leads predominantly to necrosis, while less-compromised areas undergo a greater degree of apoptosis. The mitochondria, which produce ATP for the cell when oxygen is available, are thought to be central to the initiation of apoptosis (Fig. 27-5). The release of a mitochondrial protein, cytochrome c, can initiate this process by leading to the activation of caspases that then cause the programmed cell death. The pathway of apoptosis is tightly regulated; some molecules, such as *bcl-2*, inhibit this process while other similar molecules, such as *bad* and *bax*, stimulate apoptosis.[23] Neurons can undergo apoptosis in the absence of ischemia. Neurons have receptors for trophic factors such as nerve growth factor, neurotrophins, and brain-derived growth factor. These factors activate receptors that phosphorylate tyrosine residues on certain proteins, thereby inhibiting apoptosis. If these growth factors are not present, the receptors are not activated and the proteins are not phosphorylated; then the neurons will undergo apoptosis. Indeed the loss of growth factors subsequent to neuronal degeneration after ischemia can exacerbate the delayed neuronal loss.

NEUROANESTHESIA

Effects of Anesthetics and Other Adjunctive Drugs on Brain Physiology

Volatile Anesthetics

Halothane, enflurane, sevoflurane, desflurane, and isoflurane have direct vasodilatory effects that increase CBF (Table 27-5). Halothane with nitrous oxide (1.5 minimal alveolar concentrations [MAC]) has been shown to increase blood flow almost 65%, whereas enflurane and isoflurane have a lesser effect at equal anesthetic potency.[24] Enflurane increased blood flow approximately 35%; isoflurane caused an even smaller increase. The increase in CBF returns to baseline levels approximately 3 hours after the initial exposure to 1.3 MAC of anesthetic. Sevoflurane and desflurane appear similar to isoflurane with respect to CBF;[25,26] however, desflurane increases CBF to a greater and sevoflurane to a lesser extent than isoflurane.[27,28] Desflurane has been reported to impair autoregulation.[29] The importance of increased CBF is its influence on ICP. Increasing blood flow would tend to increase the amount of blood in the brain, which could lead to increases in ICP under conditions of abnormal intracranial elastance. In animal studies, sevoflurane demonstrated a smaller increase of ICP than isoflurane, while desflurane showed a larger increase; these differences disappeared with hyperventilation.[30] In any case if high ICP is a potential problem it is better to use an intravenous agent such as
3 propofol since it does not have any direct vasodilatory effect.[31] The volatile anesthetics reduce the CMR; isoflurane reduces the metabolic rate to a greater extent than halothane. Sevoflurane reduces CMR to a similar extent as isoflurane.[32] It is thought that isoflurane's metabolic effect, which reduces CBF, competes with its direct vasodilatory action to limit the net increase in CBF with this agent. Enflurane has been shown to induce seizure-type discharges; this effect is potentiated by hypocapnia. Seizures induced with 1.5 MAC enflurane, hypocapnia, and an auditory stimulus increased CMR and blood flow by 50%.[33] The main advantage of desflurane over isoflurane is a faster onset and recovery from anesthesia. Studies have indicated that it can cause greater ICP increases than isoflurane in patients with altered intracranial elastance.[34] Therefore, it is not recommended for patients with space-occupying lesions. Desflurane has also been shown to cause sympathetic hyperactivity in healthy volunteers.[35] Sevoflurane has the potential for toxicity, since it can be converted to toxic agents; however, the concentration of these agents is normally below the toxic threshold. Sevoflurane has been shown to be a useful alternative to halothane for pediatric induction, however there are

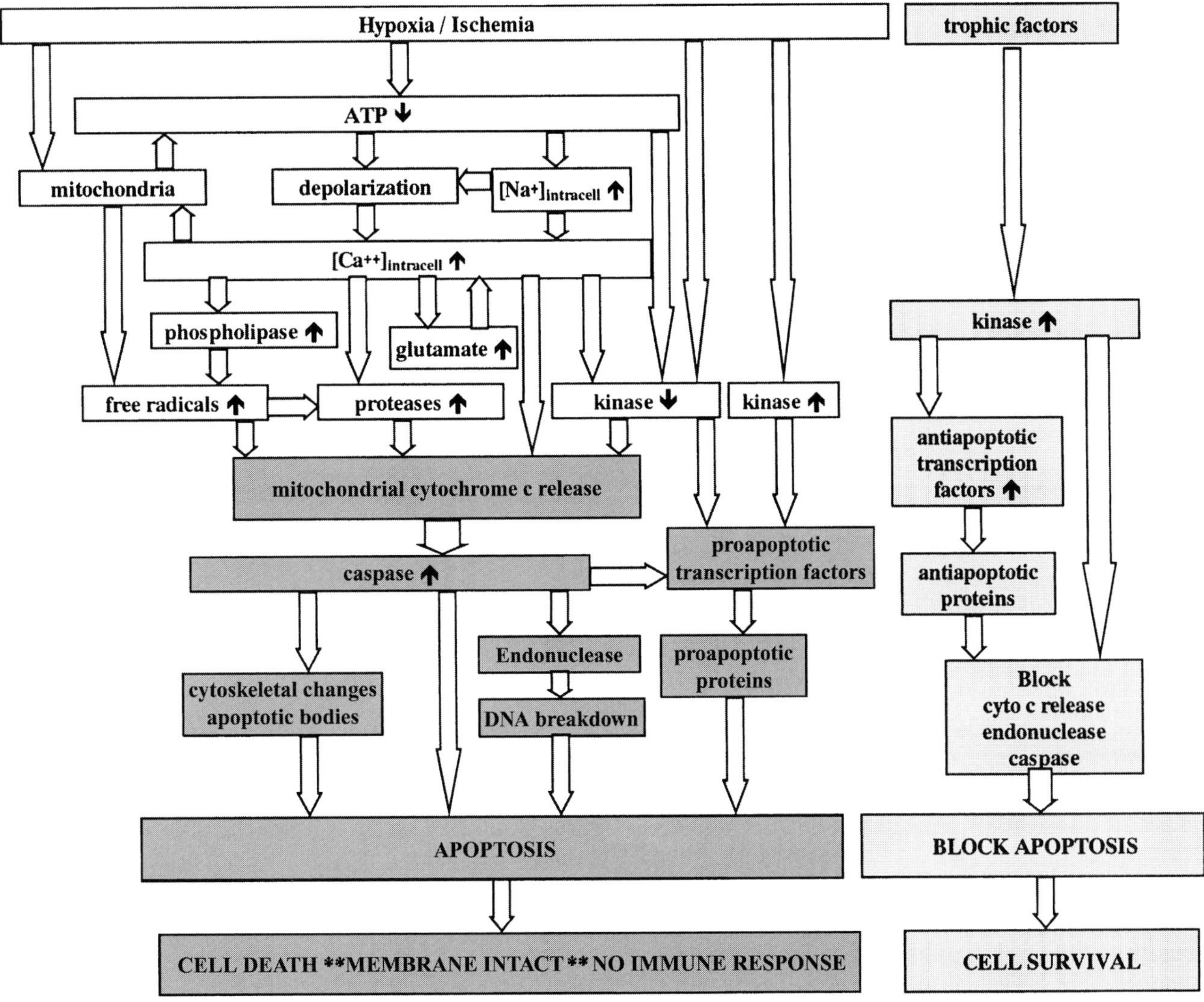

FIGURE 27-5. The effect of hypoxia or ischemia on cellular changes leading to apoptosis. The mitochondria are central to the activation of apoptosis, when hypoxic or ischemic triggers activate mitochondrial release of cytochrome c this leads to the activation of a caspase, which activates other caspases, endonucleases, and other proapoptotic proteins. This causes a cell suicide in which there is little damage to surrounding cells. Trophic factors can activate kinases that activate proteins that arrest apoptosis and can lead to cell survival. This is a complex pathway with control points that can either block or initiate cell death.

reports of epileptiform discharges in patients given sevoflurane at induction doses (1.5 to 2 MAC).[36] Sevoflurane demonstrated cerebral protection during incomplete ischemia in rats when compared to fentanyl with nitrous oxide.[37] These considerations make sevoflurane and isoflurane the volatile anesthetics of choice for neuroanesthesia. However, both of these agents are vasodilators and have the potential to increase ICP under certain circumstances.[24]

Nitrous oxide can increase CBF and ICP.[24,38] Barbiturates and hypocapnia in combination may prevent these increases. There are indications that, even when given independently, barbiturates, benzodiazepines, and morphine are effective in blunting nitrous oxide's effect on CBF and ICP. In contrast, a volatile anesthetic may add to the increases in CBF obtained with nitrous oxide. Although the data on nitrous oxide's effect on brain metabolism are far from unequivocal, the evidence seems to indicate that there can be a substantial increase in CMR if nitrous oxide is administered alone.[38] Although nitrous oxide is commonly used in neuroanesthesia, its use should be carefully considered given its potential effects on CBF, CMR, and ICP.[39]

Intravenous Anesthetics

Barbiturates decrease the CMR and CBF.[24] A major problem with barbiturates is that they can substantially reduce MAP, which, if not controlled, can reduce CPP. At high doses (10 to 55 mg/kg), thiopental can produce an isoelectric EEG and decrease the CMR by 50%.[40] This direct metabolic effect of thiopental leads to constriction of the cerebral vasculature and thereby reduces CBF. Barbiturates are also effective in reducing elevated ICP and controlling epileptiform activity. Methohexital is an exception with regard to epileptiform activity; it can activate some seizure foci in patients with temporal lobe epilepsy.[41]

Etomidate, like the barbiturates, reduces CMR and CBF.[24] In addition to the indirect effect of reduced cerebral metabolism on blood flow, etomidate is also a direct vasoconstrictor even

TABLE 27-5

EFFECTS OF ANESTHETICS ON CBF/$CMRO_2$

	CBF	$CMRO_2$	DIRECT CEREBRAL VASODILATION
Halothane	↑↑↑	↓	Yes
Enflurane	↑↑	↓	Yes
Isoflurane	↑	↓↓	Yes
Desflurane	↑	↓↓	Yes
Sevoflurane	↑	↓↓	Yes
N_2O alone	↑	↑	—
N_2O with volatile anesthetics	↑↑	↑	—
N_2O with intravenous anesthetics	0	0	—
Thiopental	↓↓↓	↓↓↓	No
Etomidate	↓↓	↓↓	No
Propofol	↓↓	↓↓	No
Midazolam	↓	↓	No
Ketamine	↑↑	↑	No
Fentanyl	↓/0	↓/0	No

before metabolism is suppressed.[24] Its advantage over the barbiturates is that it does not produce clinically significant cardiovascular depression. Prolonged use of etomidate may suppress the adrenocortical response to stress.[42]

Propofol is a rapidly acting intravenous anesthetic that, like etomidate and the barbiturates, reduces the CMR and CBF.[24] It reduces the CMR to a similar extent as sevoflurane,[43] but since it does not increase cerebral blood flow it is able to reduce ICP. However, because it also reduces MAP, its effect on CPP must be carefully monitored.[44] Recent studies have shown a lower jugular bulb oxygen saturation during hyperventilation for patients undergoing propofol anesthesia when compared to patients anesthetized with sevoflurane; thus care must be taken when hyperventilating patients anethetized with propofol.[45] Propofol demonstrated longer lasting ventilatory depression when compared with barbiturates.[46]

Benzodiazepines have been shown to reduce CMR and CBF;[24] however, this effect is not as pronounced as that with the barbiturates. As with the barbiturates, the blood flow reduction by benzodiazepines is thought to be secondary to a reduction in CMR. Benzodiazepines may reduce ICP owing to their effect on CBF. Flumazenil is a benzodiazepine antagonist that has been shown to reverse the CMR-, CBF-, and ICP-lowering effects of the benzodiazepine midazolam.[47] Thus, flumazenil should be used cautiously, if at all, in patients with high ICP or abnormal intracranial elastance.

The opioid anesthetics, morphine and fentanyl, cause either a minor reduction or no effect on CBF and CMR when compared with conditions in the unstimulated brain.[24] There is controversy concerning the effects of sufentanil: some studies demonstrate a reduction in CBF and metabolism,[48,49] whereas others report an increase in blood flow and ICP.[50] The duration of the increased blood flow and ICP effects of sufentanil in these earlier cited studies was short and could be overcome by hypocapnia. In animal studies, alfentanil decreased CBF and metabolism after 35 minutes and had no significant effect on ICP.[51] In patients with brain tumors, alfentanil increased CSF pressure.[52] Its effect on CSF pressure was less than that found with sufentanil but greater than that found with fentanyl. Alfentanil had the greatest effect on MAP and CPP.[50] Remifentanil, a rapidly metabolized opioid, had similar effects to fentanyl on CBF; both agents maintained CO_2 reactivity.[53] Remifentanil's main advantage is that it allows a more rapid neurologic assessment of the patient. Aside from the difference in recovery time, there appear to be only minor differences between the different opioid anesthetics.[54] Opioid anesthetics do not substantially suppress metabolism as does propofol; however, there was no difference in cognitive function following coronary artery bypass surgery comparing these two classes of anesthetics.[55]

Dexmedetomidine is an α-2 selective agonist that has analgesic and sedative effects. It is useful since the patient is sedated but cooperative.[56] Dexmedetomidine has been shown to reduce arousal and decrease cerebral blood flow.[57]

Ketamine, a dissociative anesthetic, activates certain areas in the brain and can increase CBF and CMR.[58,59] It is therefore not commonly used in neuroanesthesia.

Barbiturates, propofol, and benzodiazepines are intravenous agents recommended for neuroanesthesia; opioids, particularly fentanyl and remifentanil, have also proved useful.

BRAIN PROTECTION

Morbidity and mortality rates for elective neurosurgery are so low that detecting a decrease in mortality is virtually out of the question and daunting sample sizes would be required to detect less than a 30% improvement in major morbidity. Accordingly, inferences about cerebral protection are limited to those that we can draw from the laboratory, from clinical trials of therapies that are instituted subsequent to ischemic injury—primarily in stroke and head-trauma patients—and from the small number of clinical trials that test for prophylactic neuroprotection in neuro- and cardiac surgery.

Cerebral Preconditioning

Using the retina as a model for the CNS, Barbe and coauthors found that subjecting rats to heat shock (15 minutes at 41°C) protected neurons from high-intensity light damage if the rats were allowed to recover for 18 hours subsequent to heat exposure.[60] This phenomenon was soon replicated in a model of cerebral ischemia[61] and induction of endogenous proteins of repair, and the genes that code for them are now well documented.[62] Among the most intriguing recent genomic discoveries is Stenzel-Poore and colleagues' finding that ischemic preconditioning in a homeothermic mammal elicits "an evolutionarily conserved endogenous response to decreased blood flow and oxygen limitation such as seen during hibernation."[63]

Perhaps preconditioning will bring us closer to a vision articulated by James Cottrell more than a decade ago: "Much research has been directed toward enabling homeothermic mammals to gain the benefits of hypothermia without paying the costs, as do hibernators. If that research succeeds, we may eventually be able to provide brain protection during protracted periods of 'ischemic' CBF and even induce circulatory arrest in neurosurgical patients without going on bypass."[62]

Clinically acceptable means of accomplishing cerebral preconditioning are being sought. Experimental results suggest the possibility of preop hyperbaric oxygen, normobaric 100% oxygen exposure, electroconvulsive shock, and the potassium channel opener diazoxide among other candidates.[62] The first human trial of a cerebral preconditioning agent[64] employs a substance that is endogenously produced in the brain after hypoxic or ischemic insults—erythropoietin (EPO).

Although EPO is well characterized in its systemic role as a cytokine growth hormone that increases the production of erythrocytes by preventing their apoptotic self-destruction during differentiation, EPO's role in the brain has only recently been elucidated. EPO is produced in the adult mammalian brain primarily by astrocytes in the ischemic penumbra. EPO receptors (EPOr) are upregulated by neurons in the ischemic penumbra, and the EPO ->> EPOr interaction in these and other cerebral and cerebrovascular cell types has been reported to stimulate proteins of repair, diminish neuronal excitotoxicity, reduce inflammation, inhibit neuronal apoptosis, and stimulate both neurogenesis and angiogenesis subsequent to experimental ischemic, hypoxic, and toxic injury.[62]

Limiting their study to ischemic stroke patients whose treatment could begin within 8 hours of the onset of symptoms, Ehrenreich and co-authors found that intravenous injection of recombinant EPO once daily for 3 days led to 60- to 100-fold increases of EPO in the CNS, reduced serum concentrations of the glial marker of cerebral injury $S100\beta$, reduced infarct size, and improved recovery.[64] If these results hold up in a multicenter, randomized, controlled trial, there is reason to hope that EPO would be even more effective as a prophylactic protectant—because we might be able to harness EPO's preconditioning effects by initiating administration 24 to 48 hours prior to surgery, deliver EPO during surgery (often intraventricularly, which is particularly effective), and maintain administration in the neuro ICU.

Unfortunately, EPO has the attribute of increasing hematocrit—a potentially deleterious effect in the context of ischemic injury. Fortunately, nonhematopoietic analogues of EPO, such as asialoEPO, have been developed and are showing equivalent potency as neuroprotectants in the laboratory.

Neurogenesis and Diaschisis

4 The old adage that neurogenesis is only for the young has been shown to be wrong.[65] Activated neural stem cells contribute to stroke-induced neurogenesis and neuroblast migration toward the infarct boundary in adult rats[66] and therapy of stroke in rats with a nitric oxide donor and human bone marrow stromal cells enhances angiogenesis and neurogenesis subsequent to 2 hours of middle cerebral artery occlusion. This kind of evidence lends encouragement to the hypothesis that adult neurogenesis is functional and that "neural precursors resident in the brain initiate a compensatory response to stroke that results in the production of new neurons. Moreover, administration of growth factors can enhance this compensatory response . . . [and] we may eventually be able to manipulate these precursors to improve recovery of function in individuals afflicted by this devastating injury."[67]

At the other end of the ladder of repair, "Stroke produces an area of focal damage and distant areas of reduced blood flow and metabolism, termed *diaschisis* . . . diaschisis may be part of a process of structural reorganization after injury."[68] In other words, perhaps the brain is such a tightly integrated circuit that dysfunctional subcircuits add noise to the system and need to be removed to facilitate rewiring. Accordingly, we should be cautious, if not outright skeptical, of proposed therapies that nonselectively impede programmed cell death or *apoptosis*—that is, the prevailing assumption seems to be that all neuron death is bad, but this may be wrong.

Mild Hypothermia and Postoperative Fever

5 Laboratory results have demonstrated since 1956 that the beneficial attributes of mild hypothermia are likely to outweigh its real but manageable untoward effects when neurosurgical procedures are high risk and/or protracted. Berntman et al found that one degree of hypothermia (to 36°C) maintains ATP at normoxic levels during an hypoxic insult that depletes ATP by half at normothermia (37°C), and three degrees of hypothermia (to 34°C) more than doubled preservation of phosphocreatine.[69] These results suggest the possibility that the initial decline of CMR during hypothermia is greater than has been previously assumed.[70,71]

Unfortunately, the most current and definitive clinical trial of mild hypothermia has conclusively shown a failure to improve outcome after surgery for repair of a ruptured cerebral aneurysm. The Intraoperative Hypothermia for Intracranial Aneurysm Surgery Trial (IHAST) was completed in 2003. With 499 patients randomized to undergo aneurysm clipping at 33°C compared to 501 controls at 36.5°C, the study had ample power to detect a 10% increase in the frequency of good outcomes. Mild hypothermia was not beneficial.

Preliminary results for Intention-to-Treat analysis indicate that 66% of patients in the hypothermic group had a good outcome at 90 days versus 63% of patients in the normothermic group. Because people do not easily cool down as scheduled, only 373 of the 499 patients assigned to the hypothermic group actually reached a core temperature below 33.5°C, while 467 of the 501 normothermic patients maintained core temperature above 36°C.[72] In a planned secondary analysis of these patients who were within 0.5°C of their target temperature during aneurysm clipping, 62% of the hypothermic patients had a good outcome versus 63% of the normothermic patients. It is of interest to note that the warmer patients in the entire hypothermic group (>33.5°C, N = 126) had more good outcomes (77%) than the cooler patients (<33.5°C, N = 373) in the hypothermic group (62%) ($p<0.003$, two-way Fisher exact).[73] The only statistically significant intergroup difference in adverse outcomes was a higher incidence of bacteremia in the hypothermic group.

Why has so much laboratory evidence for a therapeutic benefit of mild hypothermia not been born out in aneurysm patients? It should be remembered that almost all of that evidence is from, or is analogous to, models of ischemic stroke, as distinct from hemorrhagic stroke, and the few hemorrhagic stroke models that do exist have applied hypothermia before, during, or within a few hours of the intracranial bleed—as distinct from several days postrupture. If there is any benefit of intraoperative mild hypothermia for hemorrhagic stroke patients, it may not be detectable because it is dwarfed by damage that precedes surgery (the initial bleed) and damage that occurs in the postsurgical ICU (vasospasm, etc.). The initial bleed may also activate functional diaschisis and postinjury repair mechanisms to which intra-operative mild hypothermia is not therapeutically additive.

The multi-institutional study of postoperative mild hypothermia in head-injury patients came to an even more discouraging conclusion—the study was terminated by its

Safety Monitoring Board after enrollment of 392 patients.[74] A decrease in the number of hypothermic patients with ICP >30 mmHg (59% vs. 41%) did not produce a difference in mortality (28% vs. 27% in the normothermic group) and normothermic patients experienced fewer bouts of critical bradycardia and hypotension, and fewer medical complications.

These findings accord well with results from a clinical study of the effect of prolonged mild hypothermia on electrolyte balance. Polderman and co-authors found that serum magnesium, phosphate, and potassium fell to critical levels "despite the fact that moderate and, in some cases, substantial doses of electrolyte supplementation were given."[75] More generally, some of the most competent laboratory studies indicate that hypothermia administered subsequent to an ischemic event only delays neuronal death, and other in vivo work suggests that if there is a window of opportunity for inducing protective postischemic hypothermia, it is very narrow.[62]

Indeed, the narrowness of that window may account for reports of neuroprotective effects from mild hypothermia after cardiac arrest. In both major studies,[76,77] most patients were mildly hypothermic on admission, and it is reasonable to speculate that their brains began to cool as soon as they lost CBF. Patients assigned to the hypothermic groups were cooled further for 12 to 24 hours, while those assigned to the normothermic groups were passively warmed to normothermia or above over a 6- to 8-hour period, such that the hypothermic groups began to cool immediately and were kept cool for a substantial period of time while patients in the normothermic groups began to cool immediately but did not remain hypothermic for a substantial period of time. Put differently, both groups of patients became hypothermic within the window of opportunity, but the opportunity for a protective effect may have been lost too soon thereafter in the normothermic patients.

Evidence that this consideration might be critically important comes from the definitive head-injury study: "Among the patients who had normothermia on admission, the outcomes were similar in the two treatment groups.... [But] among the patients who had hypothermia on admission and were treated with hypothermia, 61 percent had poor outcomes, as compared with 78 percent of those with hypothermia on admission who were in the normothermia group (P = 0.09)... [and] among patients 45 years of age or younger who had hypothermia on admission, 52 percent of those assigned to the hypothermia group had poor outcomes, as compared with 76 percent in the normothermia group (P = 0.02)."[74]

Until and unless the deleterious effects of mild hypothermia can be reduced, or the brain can be cooled without reducing systemic temperature below 35°C, clinical evidence does not support induction of perioperative hypothermia for neurosurgical procedures that do not entail circulatory bypass.

Nevertheless, fever in the neurosurgical or cardiac intensive care unit associates strongly with poor outcome.[62] In vitro results indicate that just as hypothermia preserves ATP, reduces CA^{2+} influx, and improves electrophysiologic recovery from hypoxia, so does hyperthermia deplete ATP, increase CA^{2+} influx, and impair recovery.[78,79] A potentially promising development in ICU temperature control is the concept of low normothermia—keeping nonventilated patients servo-controlled at 36°C in order to provide substantial assurance against bouts of fever.[80]

Anesthetic and Adjuvant Drugs

Clinically verified pharmacological brain protection is even more elusive than the benefits of mild hypothermia. Delayed neuronal necrosis, apoptosis, diaschisis, and neurogenesis can cause protection, which appears to be evident within 1 to 100 hours of experimental infarct, to vanish after 3 to 6 months. Accordingly, decades of laboratory research on the short-term cerebroprotective effects of general anesthetics, both inhalational and intravenous, is called into question by studies that have found no long-term differences.[81,82] Until and unless long-term laboratory studies suggest a difference in the neuroprotective efficacy of general anesthetics that are widely used for neurosurgery, clinical decisions about which anesthetic is most appropriate should be based on considerations other than potential to provide superior cerebral protection per se. Nevertheless, as with hypothermia, the search continues for the optimal anesthetic in subgroups of patients.

Barbiturates

As with mild hypothermia, reduction of CMR is a catch-all term that may or may not indicate cerebral protection. Although an intellectual backlash has challenged the operating hypothesis that lowering CMR has a substantial protective effect,[83] all known means of lowering CMR entail simultaneous negative effects, with the continuum of drugs, techniques, and toxins that reduce CMR ranging, on balance, from protective to damaging. Nakashima and co-authors found that for similar reductions of CMR obtained with hypothermia, pentobarbital, or isoflurane, hypothermia resulted in substantially longer times to depolarization of cerebral cortex subsequent to cardiac arrest.[84] Concomitantly, Verhaegen and co-authors found that hypothermia reduces CMR during ischemia proportionately more than does pentobarbital or isoflurane.[85]

Accordingly, we find mild hypothermia near the protective end of the continuum, followed at some distance by anesthetics (reversible neurotoxins), then moving to the damaging end, we find nonreversible neurotoxins followed at some distance by blunt trauma—all of which lower cerebral metabolism. The point here is that the benefit of reducing CMR remains constant while the cost of doing so varies from minor to lethal. From this perspective it seems rash to challenge the efficacy of reducing CMR in and of itself.

Some of the proximate mechanisms by which barbiturates lower CMR include reduction of calcium influx, sodium channel blockade, inhibition of free-radical formation, potentiation of GABAergic activity, and inhibition of glucose transfer across the blood-brain barrier. All of these mechanisms are consistent with Goodman and co-authors' report that pentobarbital coma markedly reduces lactate, glutamate, and aspartate in the extracellular space of head-injured patients with severely increased ICP.[86] An in vitro investigation suggests that thiopental also delays the loss of transmembrane electrical gradients caused by application of NMDA and AMPA. This stands in marked contrast to the effect of propofol, which can aggravate glutamate excitotoxicity and increase neuronal damage.[87]

Sodium Channel Blockade—Lidocaine

Sodium influx is the first step in the ischemic cascade. Truncating initial steps of the cascade, as distinct from blocking glutamate receptors and scavenging free radicals, reduces damage done by downstream events and lowers the probability of interfering with endogenous mechanisms of repair. In addition to blocking sodium influx, lidocaine may also reduce postnecrotic injury. Recent in vivo data suggest that lidocaine truncates "ischemic damage in the penumbra by blocking the apoptotic cell death pathways that involve cytochrome C release and caspase-3 activation."[88] These appear to be some of the mechanisms by which experimental, prophylactic, low-dose lidocaine has demonstrated neuroprotective properties both in vitro[89,90] and in vivo.[91,92]

Looking for neuroprotection in cardiac valve patients, Mitchell and co-authors found that lidocaine infusion begun at induction of anesthesia and continued for 48 hours with a target plasma concentration between 6 and 12 μmol/L increased scores in 6 of 11 neuropsychological tests and in patients' memory inventory.[93] Similar results were obtained by Wang and co-authors in coronary artery bypass patients,[94] but a third trial of lidocaine in cardiac patients failed to find a protective effect and found an adverse effect in diabetic patients.[95] Nevertheless, initial data presentation indicates a substantial positive effect in nondiabetic lidocaine patients compared to nondiabetic controls. An additional consideration is that these patients were maintained at 30 to 32°C during surgery—which cardiac colleagues tend to think of as not hypothermic—but which may provide a level of neuroprotection to which lidocaine is not additive.

Calcium Channel Blockade—Magnesium

Magnesium blocks both ligand and voltage dependant calcium entry, has shown considerable neuroprotection in animal experiments, and appears to neurologically protect preterm infants if administered to their mothers immediately before birth. The fact that magnesium is also powerfully protective in vitro[96] suggests that it may critically reduce calcium influx in addition to improving CBF subsequent to cerebrovascular dilation. Recent laboratory work indicates that magnesium deficiency exacerbates traumatic brain injury while magnesium loading shortly subsequent to trauma reduces injury. If the same holds for stroke patients, efficacy is most likely to be realized by the FAST-MAG (Field Administration of Stroke Treatment—Magnesium) trial. A preliminary report on the first 20 FAST-MAG patients indicates that paramedics can administer a 4 g loading dose of magnesium sulfate en route to the hospital without substantial complications.[97] In distinction, the long-awaited RCT of not-fast MgSO4 (within 12 hours of stroke) has shown rather conclusively (2,386 patients) that magnesium loading is not neuroprotective and may increase mortality in stroke patients.[98]

For reasons detailed earlier regarding intra-operative hypothermia in stroke patients, cardiac patients are probably a better model for testing the general neuroprotective efficacy of MgSO4. Unfortunately, however, a meta-analysis indicates that the only benefit of prophylactic magnesium in cardiac surgery patients is a reduction in postsurgical atrial fibrillation.

Additional Clinical Trials—Remacemide and High-dose Mannitol

Remacemide reduces glutamate release, and so excitotoxicity, by blocking NMDA channels. Evidence for a prophylactic beneficial effect of this NMDA blocker was gleaned by combining scores from nine neuropsychological tests in coronary artery bypass patients. Those data allow the inference ($p<0.03$) that in exchange for a higher risk of dizziness during 9 days of drug administration, patients in the treatment group retained more of their ability to learn.[99]

"Comatose patients with severe diffuse brain swelling and recent clinical signs of impending brain death"[100] have a justifiably lower threshold for being subjected to experimental treatments. Cruz and colleagues reported dramatic success with administration of high-dose mannitol versus conventional-dose mannitol in such patients randomized in the emergency room to receive either 1.4 g/kg or 0.7 g/kg mannitol. "Ultra-early improvement of bilateral abnormal pupillary widening was significantly more frequent in the high-dose mannitol group than in the conventional-dose group" as was the number of patients with Good or Moderate (GOS) 6-month clinical outcomes (10 in the high-dose group versus 2 in the conventional-dose group, $p<0.02$). These stark results beg to be tested in a multinational randomized controlled trial.[101]

What to Avoid

As with postoperative mild hypothermia in head-injury patients (see earlier), evidence against some anesthetic and adjuvant drugs is stronger than the evidence in their favor.

Calcium Channel Blockers—Postoperative

Several clinical trials and two meta-analyses suggest that calcium channel blockers nimodipine, nicardipine, and AT877 reduce the frequency of vasospasm subsequent to subarachnoid hemorrhage and/or improve outcome.[102] The most favorable finding of the recent meta-analyses suggests that nimodipine improves outcome, on average, by preventing one poor outcome in 1 out of every 13 patients treated.[100] Whether the reduction in blood pressure that accompanies these Ca^{2+} blockers improves outcome relative to hypertensive, hypervolemic, hemodilution remains controversial. Neither meta-analysis was able to detect a statistically significant reduction in mortality. Two subsequently published clinical trials, one that administered nimodipine within 24 hours of acute stroke[103] and one that administered nimodipine within 6 hours of stroke,[104] failed to detect a beneficial effect.

The most disturbing reports yet published about nimodipine, disturbing for medical research in general, are two systematic reviews that reveal a lack of evidence to justify Phase 3 clinical trials. Contrary to conventional assumption, published laboratory experiments found as many negative as positive results, and animal experiments and clinical studies ran simultaneously. Making matters worse, several methodologically sound clinical studies of calcium antagonists in ischemic stroke patients remained unpublished. In each of those unpublished studies, results were significantly worse for patients in the treatment groups.[105]

Etomidate

EEG burst suppression with etomidate prior to temporary vessel occlusion gained prominence eleven years ago on the basis of a clinical trial for which there was no control group, no alternative drug tested, and no historical standard for comparison. Despite the absence of supportive clinical evidence, and the presence of troubling laboratory results,[106] etomidate remains the standard regimen for cerebral protection at several institutions. We now have clinical evidence that the standard propylene glycol formulation of etomidate induces more cerebral tissue hypoxia, tissue acidosis, and neurological deficits than an EEG-equivalent dose of desflurane.[107]

Nitrous Oxide and Ketamine

In 1938 C.D. Courville published "The pathogenesis of necrosis of the cerebral gray matter following nitrous oxide anesthesia"—an article that presents photographs of vacuolated cortical neurons from patients who died subsequent to administration of nitrous oxide (N_2O).[108] Sixty years later, Jevtovic-Todorovic and co-authors published compelling evidence that N_2O causes vacuolation of both the endoplasmic reticulum and mitochondria of neurons in the posterior cingulate and retrosplenial cortices of rats.[109] Are we on our way to where we might have been if Courville's work had received more sustained attention?[110]

Nitrous oxide's mechanism of action is NMDA receptor antagonism, and like other NMDA antagonists, N_2O has been shown to reduce damage from excessive glutamate release. Unfortunately, however, because NMDA also excites inhibitory neurons, NMDA blockade causes inhibition of GABA release, and thus general disinhibition. This is probably a component of the mechanism by which N_2O, like other NMDA antagonists (e.g., ketamine, phencyclidine, dextrorphan, MK-801), can cause neuronal damage.[111]

The question of N_2O's effect on the neuroprotective efficacy of primary anesthetics has been addressed by several investigations. Following Arnfred and Secher's demonstration that thiopental more than doubles survival time in mice subjected to hypoxia while N_2O reduces survival,[112,113] it was found that co-administration of N_2O virtually eliminates the protective effect of thiopental in the same model.[114] Two years later, Baughman and co-authors found that N_2O cut the protective effect of isoflurane in half.[115] More recently, Jevtovic-Tedrovic and co-authors found that N_2O converts a nontoxic dose of ketamine into a substantially toxic dose in rats,[116] and adding N_2O to isoflurane or isoflurane with midazolam substantially exacerbates those agents' pro-apoptotic effect during the brain growth spurt in developing rats.[117]

Evidence that the earlier-mentioned clinical and laboratory findings resulted in part from a direct neurotoxic effect of N_2O is bolstered by our findings in the hippocampal slice model, where nitrous oxide markedly reduced electrophysiological recovery from severe hypoxia without affecting fundamental biochemical parameters like ATP concentration, Ca influx, K efflux, and Na influx.[118] Direct neurotoxicity aside, N_2O has been repeatedly shown to increase CMR, CBF, and ICP when used alone, but these effects are variable when N_2O is used as an adjunct anesthetic, with or without hypocapnia, and with or without EEG burst suppression. Recent evidence indicates that N_2O disturbs CBF/$CMRO_2$ coupling in humans receiving sevoflurane.[43] In patients with folic acid deficiency, a single exposure to N_2O can cause spinal cord degeneration.[119] Less direct, but also less rare, exposure to N_2O causes a substantial increase in plasma homocysteine, which can increase coagulation, decrease flow-mediated vasodilation, and increase postoperative myocardial ischemia—all of which complicate recovery in the neuro ICU. Prolonged hyperhomocysteinemia is also an independent risk factor for cerebrovascular disease.

Perhaps the most pressing question regarding the use of N_2O in neurosurgical patients has been framed by Enlund, Edmark, and Revenas: "It is no consolation for the patient who suffers from an irreversible neurological sequela after nitrous oxide exposure that he happens to be the first one at your clinic for the last five years. For those like us who administer drugs, or for the regulatory authorities, such an incident might nevertheless be acceptable provided that a great number of patients receive indispensable benefits, which outweigh a severe side effect. Are there such pros [benefits] from nitrous oxide?"[120]

Steroids—Tirilazad

Clinical application of the 21-amino steroid tirilazad looked promising.[121] Unfortunately, more substantive results from a North American trial in subarachnoid hemorrhage patients failed to reach statistical significance,[122] and a follow-up study of high-dose tirilazad in women depended on an idiosyncratic grouping of data to reach statistical significance.[123] A detailed commentary on that analysis concluded that "any eventually proven therapeutic efficacy is likely to be modest,"[124] and a systematic review of tirilazad use in 1,757 stroke patients concluded that "Tirilazad mesylate increases death and disability by about one fifth when given to patients with acute ischemic stroke."[125] A recent reanalysis of initially promising results has revealed a failure to adjust for imbalances in baseline characteristics.

Caution and Hope

6 Current evidence cautions against the use of prophylactic etomidate prior to temporary vessel occlusion, magnesium loading in ischemic stroke patients, intra-operative nitrous oxide and ketamine, intra-operative moderate hypothermia in subarachnoid hemorrhage (SAH) patients, postoperative nimodipine and tirilazad, and postoperative hypothermia in head-trauma patients. On the positive side, cerebral preconditioning and augmentation of endogenous processes of repair may deliver standard-of-care brain protection to neurosurgical patients within a decade.

MONITORING

Electroencephalogram

7 The EEG can be used to monitor cerebral function during general anesthesia. The primary use of intraoperative EEG monitoring is the detection of cerebral ischemia during carotid endarterectomy, cerebral aneurysm, and arteriovenous malformation management and cardiopulmonary bypass procedures. EEG monitoring is also used for intraoperative or perioperative assessment of pharmacologic interventions, such as barbiturate-induced burst suppression, during deliberate hypotension, and for the assessment of coma or brain death. Another important intra-operative application of EEG is in the diagnosis and management of intractable epilepsy.

The EEG waves recorded on the surface of the scalp are spontaneous electrical potentials generated by the pyramidal cells of the granular cortex. The EEG signal consists of graded summations of inhibitory and excitatory postsynaptic potentials that create dipole fields in the dendrites of the pyramidal cells. When a number of dipoles develop at once, the summation creates electrical potentials large enough to produce detectable voltage on the scalp.

The EEG waveforms are interpreted by pattern recognition and quantification. Specific complexes are described in terms of morphology, spatial and temporal distribution, and reactivity of the waveforms. Quantification involves measuring frequency and amplitude. Frequency is measured in hertz (Hz) and is defined as the number of times per second the wave crosses the zero voltage line. Amplitude, which is measured in microvolts (μV), is the electrical height of the wave. The frequency bands are divided into delta (0–3 Hz), theta (4–7 Hz), alpha (8–13 Hz), and beta (>13 Hz) rhythms (Table 27-6).

The traditional EEG is a plot of voltage against time. Sixteen channels are usually recorded, allowing analysis of activity of different regions of the brain. EEG waveform changes associated with anesthetic drugs, PaO_2, $PaCO_2$, and temperature are described in Table 27-7.

The EEG response to anesthetic agents can vary from cortical excitation through depression to isoelectricity. Usually,

TABLE 27-6

EEG FREQUENCY RANGES

Delta rhythm (0–3 Hz)	Deep sleep, deep anesthesia, or pathologic states (e.g., brain tumors, hypoxia, metabolic encephalopathy)
Theta rhythm (4–7 Hz)	Sleep and anesthesia in adults, hyperventilation in awake children and young adults
Alpha rhythm (8–13 Hz)	Resting, awake adult with eyes closed; predominantly seen in occipital leads
Beta rhythm (>13 Hz)	Mental activity, light anesthesia

TABLE 27-7

EEG CHANGES ASSOCIATED WITH ANESTHETIC DRUGS, PaO_2, $PaCO_2$, AND TEMPERATURE

■ INCREASED FREQUENCY
Barbiturates (low dose)
Benzodiazepines (low dose)
Etomidate (low dose)
Propofol (low dose)
Ketamine
N_2O (30–70%)
Inhalation agents (<1 MAC)
Hypoxia (initially)
Hypercarbia (mild)
Seizures
■ DECREASED FREQUENCY/INCREASED AMPLITUDE
Barbiturates (moderate dose)
Etomidate (moderate dose)
Propofol (moderate dose)
Opioids
Inhalation agents (>1 MAC)
Hypoxia (mild)
Hypocarbia (moderate to extreme)
Hypothermia
■ DECREASED FREQUENCY/DECREASED AMPLITUDE
Barbiturates (high dose)
Hypoxia (mild)
Hypercarbia (severe)
Hypothermia (<35°C)
■ ELECTRICAL SILENCE
Barbiturates (coma dose)
Etomidate (high dose)
Propofol (high dose)
Desflurane (2 MAC)
Isoflurane (2 MAC)
Sevoflurane (2 MAC)
Hypoxia (severe)
Hypothermia (<15–20°C)
Brain death

anesthetic induction produces a decrease in alpha and an increase in beta activity. As the depth of anesthesia increases, EEG frequency decreases until theta and delta activity predominate. By further increasing the dose of anesthesia, the EEG changes to a burst suppression pattern, which coincides with near-maximal depression of cerebral metabolic activity. Complete electrical silence or isoelectricity follows an additional increase in anesthesia. Anesthesia-induced burst suppression is used to provide cerebral protection by metabolic suppression. EEG monitoring verifies burst suppression and electrical silence and is valuable when determining the dose of drug required to induce and maintain barbiturate coma.

Efforts to use the EEG as a monitor of depth of anesthesia have been problematic because of the variety of agents used to maintain anesthesia and because some anesthetic agents do not follow the general pattern described above.[33] Several different cerebral-monitoring techniques based on EEG-derived algorithms, electromyograms, auditory evoked responses, or combinations of these have been introduced to more precisely determine "depth of anesthesia" during surgery.[126–128] These various techniques are currently under investigation with promising results.[129,130] A recently published multicenter, randomized controlled trial revealed that Bispectral index (BIS) monitoring reduced the risk of awareness in at-risk adult surgical patients (cardiac surgery, cesarean section, and trauma surgery) undergoing relaxant general anesthesia.[130]

Intraoperative EEG monitoring allows early detection of cerebral hypoxia and ischemia. Inadequate PaO_2 or insufficient CBF is reflected within seconds in the EEG.[131] Hypoxia may initially produce EEG activation, which is followed by slowing and eventually electrical silence.

Other physiologic parameters that affect EEG waveforms are $PaCO_2$, temperature, and sensory stimulation. Hypocarbia causes EEG slowing. Mild hypercarbia causes increased frequency, and severe hypercarbia produces a decrease in frequency and amplitude. When body temperature falls below 35°C, hypothermia causes a progressive slowing of activity. Complete electrical silence occurs at 15 to 20°C. Sensory stimulation is associated with EEG activation.

When monitoring an EEG during anesthesia, the changes resulting from hypoxia or ischemia must be distinguished from the drug and physiologic effects that also may influence the EEG. Because of this, the EEG must always be interpreted within the clinical context in which it is observed.

A specific intra-operative application of the EEG, called *electrocorticography* (ECoG), is the localization of epileptic foci during surgery for intractable epilepsy. For these procedures, recording electrodes are applied on or in the brain. The craniotomy can be performed under local anesthesia with conscious sedation (typically using propofol and fentanyl) or under a light general anesthetic using nitrous oxide, narcotic and low dose isoflurane (maximum 0.25% end-tidal concentration). The anesthetic administered must avoid pharmacologic cortical depression, which would prevent provocative seizure activity. Provocative techniques and agents, such as hyperventilation, low-dose barbiturates (methohexital 10 to 50 mg, thiopental 25 to 50 mg), propofol 10 to 20 mg, or etomidate 2 to 4 mg, have been used to activate the foci. Under general anesthesia, alfentanil 20 to 50 μg/kg and fentanyl 10 μg/kg also have been used to successfully produce ECoG activation.

Computerized EEG Processing

The development of the computer-processed EEG has facilitated intraoperative EEG monitoring. The most widely used and best validated technique is *power-spectrum analysis*, which uses a computer to perform a Fourier transformation. A given epoch of EEG (usually 2 to 8 seconds) is converted from a plot of voltage against time to a plot of power (amplitude squared) against frequency. With this technique, data are displayed in one of three formats: the compressed spectral array, the density spectral array, and the band spectral array or power bands. For example, to generate the compressed spectral array format, the Fourier transformation converts the irregular EEG waves to equivalent sine waves of known frequency and power (Fig. 27-6).[131] This display shows time and power as one axis (vertical) and frequencies on the horizontal axis. The Fourier spectral data from successive segments are stacked one on top of the other, creating a pseudo three-dimensional display; that is, the plot is shifted vertically with time and compressed. A major advantage of power-spectrum analysis is that it retains almost all the information in the original EEG. Power-spectrum analysis has documented value as a monitor of cerebral ischemia and possible value in the determination of anesthetic depth.[126] The main disadvantages of this analysis technique are lack of detection of spike activity, inclusion of artifact within frequency bands, and limited review of raw EEG data to determine reliability of the ongoing input.

Several technical matters must be considered to effectively implement intraoperative EEG monitoring. Awake controls should be obtained before induction of general anesthesia. Monitoring should be continuous throughout anesthesia and

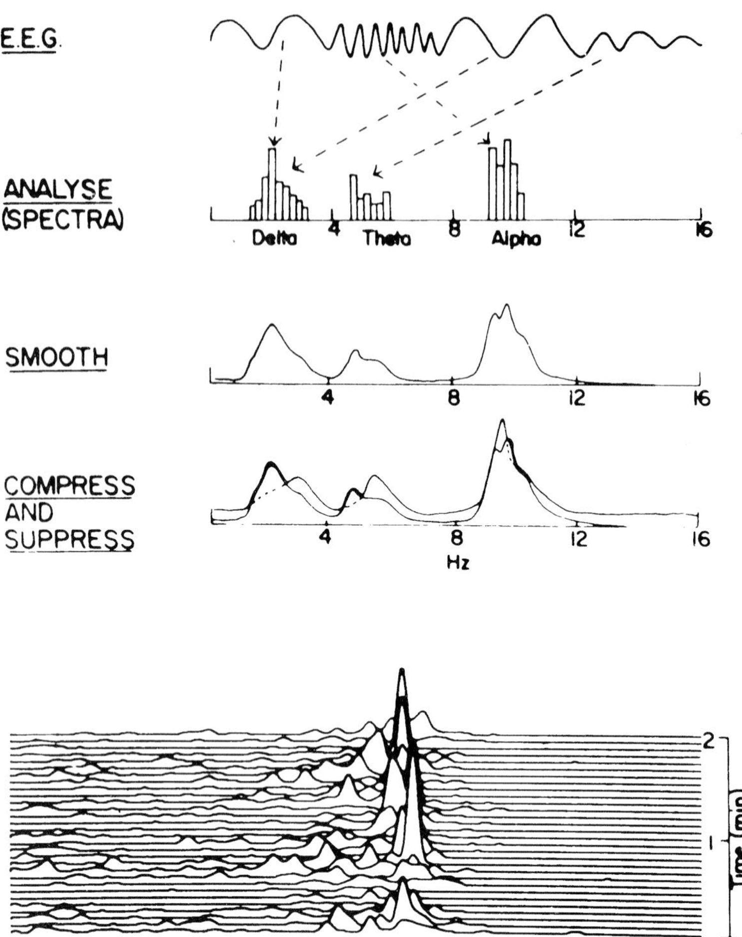

FIGURE 27-6. Schematic diagram of technique used to generate compressed spectral array. Below the diagram is an example of compressed spectra of the alpha rhythm from a normal subject. (Reprinted with permission from Stockard JJ, Bickford RG: The neurophysiology of anesthesia. In Gordon E (ed): A Basis and Practice of Neuroanesthesia, 2nd ed, pp 3-49. Amsterdam, Elsevier, 1981.)

continue until the patient is awake. Bilateral data must be obtained, especially during cerebrovascular procedures. For example, during a carotid endarterectomy, bilateral changes may indicate anesthetic or systemic effects, whereas ipsilateral changes on the operating side are most likely consistent with surgical trauma or ischemia. Marked changes in anesthetic depth, systemic blood pressure, $PaCO_2$, and brain temperature must be avoided in order to distinguish between anesthetic and physiologic effects on the EEG and those resulting from hypoxia or ischemia.

Evoked Potentials

Evoked potentials are used intraoperatively to monitor the integrity of specific sensory and motor pathways. Sensory evoked potentials (SEPs) evaluate the functional integrity of ascending sensory pathways, whereas motor evoked potentials (MEPs) test the functional integrity of descending motor pathways.

There are major differences between evoked potentials and the EEG. The EEG is a recording of spontaneous, random electrical activity that has a nonspecific function and generates a relatively large signal, for example, 50 μV or more. Evoked potentials are comparatively small-amplitude responses (0.1 to 20 μV) to a specific stimulus that are pathway-specific.

Sensory Evoked Potentials

The application of a sensory stimulus—a click, a flash, a shock—results in an afferent nerve impulse that can be detected by appropriately placed surface electrodes as transient potential differences. The amplitude of these evoked potentials is very small and obscured by normal background bioelectric activity from the EEG, electrocardiogram (ECG), muscle activity, and other extraneous electrical activity. Signal averaging is required to extract the evoked responses from this background noise. The background noise is random and is eliminated by the averaging process.

Three SEP modalities are employed clinically: *somatosensory* (SSEP), *auditory* (BAEP), and *visual* (VEP). The waves of the evoked potential are thought to represent potentials from specific neural generators. The individual peaks in the waveform are described in terms of polarity (negative, positive), post-stimulus latency (msec), and peak-to-peak amplitude (μV or nV). They are also described by the distance separating the neural generators and recording electrodes (near-field, far-field).

Anesthetic Considerations for Sensory Evoked Potential Recording. Compromise or injury of a neurologic pathway is manifested as an increase in the latency and/or a decrease in the amplitude of evoked potential waveforms. For SSEPs, a 50% reduction in amplitude from baseline in response to a specific surgical maneuver is considered to be a significant change warranting action to avert potential damage. For BAEPs, an increase in latency of more than 1 millisecond is considered clinically significant. Accordingly, anesthetic, physiologic, and environmental factors capable of producing this pattern of alteration must be controlled when recording evoked potentials. All anesthetics that have been studied influence evoked potentials to some extent. Table 27-8 summarizes the

TABLE 27-8

EFFECTS OF INTRAVENOUS AND INHALED AGENTS ON SENSORY EVOKED POTENTIALS

	BAEPS		CSSEPS		VEPS	
INTRAVENOUS AGENTS	LAT	AMP	LAT	AMP	LAT	AMP
Thiopental						
4–6 mg/kg	0	0	0/↑	↓	↑•	↓•
20 mg/kg	↑	0	↑	↓	↑•	↓•
75 mg/kg	↑	↓	↑	↓	↑•	↓•
Pentobarbital						
9–18 mg/kg	0/↑	0	↑	↓	↑	↓
Propofol						
2–6 mg/kg	0	0	↑	↓/0	0	↓
Etomidate						
0.05–0.3 mg/kg/min	0	0	↑	↑	↑	0
Ketamine	0	0	↑/0	↑	↑	↓
Diazepam						
0.1 mg/kg	0	0	↑/0	↓/0	0	↓
Midazolam	0	0	↑/0	↓/0	—	—
Droperidol						
0.1 mg/kg	—	—	↑	↓	—	—
Lidocaine						
1.5 mg/kg; 3 mg/kg/h	0/↑	0	↑	↓	—	—
Morphine	—	—	0/↑	↓	—	—
Fentanyl	0	0	0/↑	↓/0	↑	↓
Sufentanil	0	0	↑/0	↓	—	—
Alfentanil	0	0	0/↑	↓	—	—
Remifentanil	—	—	—	↓	—	—
Clonidine	0	0	0	0	—	—
Dexmedetomidine	—	—	—	↓	—	—
INHALATION AGENTS						
Desflurane	↑	0	↑	↓	—	—
Enflurane	↑	0	↑	↓[a]	↑	↓
Halothane	↑	0	↑	↓	↑	↓
Isoflurane	↑	0	↑	↓[a]	↑	↓
Sevoflurane	↑	0	↑	↓[b]	↑[a]	↓[a]
Nitrous oxide	0	↓/0	0	↓	↑	↓

BAEPs = brainstem auditory evoked potentials; cSSEPs = cortical somatosensory evoked potentials; VEPs = visual evoked potentials; ↑ = increased; ↓ = decreased; 0 = no change; — = no data; Lat = latency; Amp = amplitude; • = response abolished.

[a] 1.5 MAC will occasionally abolish the response.

[b] At 1.7 to 2.5 MAC, 100% ↑ in amplitude (fusion to a single cortical high-amplitude wave with abolition of all later wave components).

known effects of intravenous and inhaled agents. The sensitivity of evoked potentials to drug effects varies with the sensory modality being monitored. Evoked potentials of cortical origin (i.e., the cortical component of the somatosensory evoked potentials [SSEP] and visual evoked potentials [VEP]) are more vulnerable to anesthetic influences than brainstem potentials (e.g., brainstem auditory evoked potentials [BAEP] and the subcortical components of SSEP). In general, to obtain satisfactory intraoperative SEP recordings, it is important to maintain constant anesthetic drug levels. Specifically, bolus administration of intravenous agents and step changes in inspired inhalation agent concentration must be avoided, especially at times when neurologic injury might occur. When recording cortical evoked potentials (SSEPs or VEPs), one should employ intravenous techniques. High concentrations of volatile agents essentially eliminate cortical evoked potentials. However, end-tidal concentrations of 0.5 MAC of a volatile agent are compatible with satisfactory recordings in patients who are neurologically normal. The newer inhaled agents, desflurane and sevoflurane, may permit the use of higher inhaled concentrations during electrophysiological monitoring.

In general, volatile agents cause a dose-dependent increase in latency and a decrease in amplitude of the cortical SSEP or VEP.[132] As exemplified in a study by Peterson et al (Fig. 27-7), reductions in SSEP amplitude greater than 50% were observed with 1 MAC halothane, 0.5 MAC enflurane, and 0.5 MAC isoflurane, all administered with 60% nitrous oxide in oxygen.[133] The authors concluded that halothane disrupted the SSEP the least, and enflurane disrupted it the most. At doses of 1.5 MAC sevoflurane and desflurane, increases in cortical latency and decreases in amplitude occur. Desflurane up to 1 MAC without nitrous oxide is compatible with cortical median nerve SSEP monitoring during scoliosis surgery. At 1.5 MAC without nitrous oxide, the amplitude of cortical SSEPs is preserved at 60% of baseline with desflurane. Visual evoked potentials tend to be more sensitive than cortical SSEPs to the effects of anesthetics. Nitrous oxide alone has been shown to produce significant decreases in amplitude with minimal latency changes in the cortical SSEP, but it decreases amplitude and increases latency in the VEP. When nitrous oxide is administered in combination with a volatile anesthetic, it produces a profound depressant effect on SSEPs and VEPs.

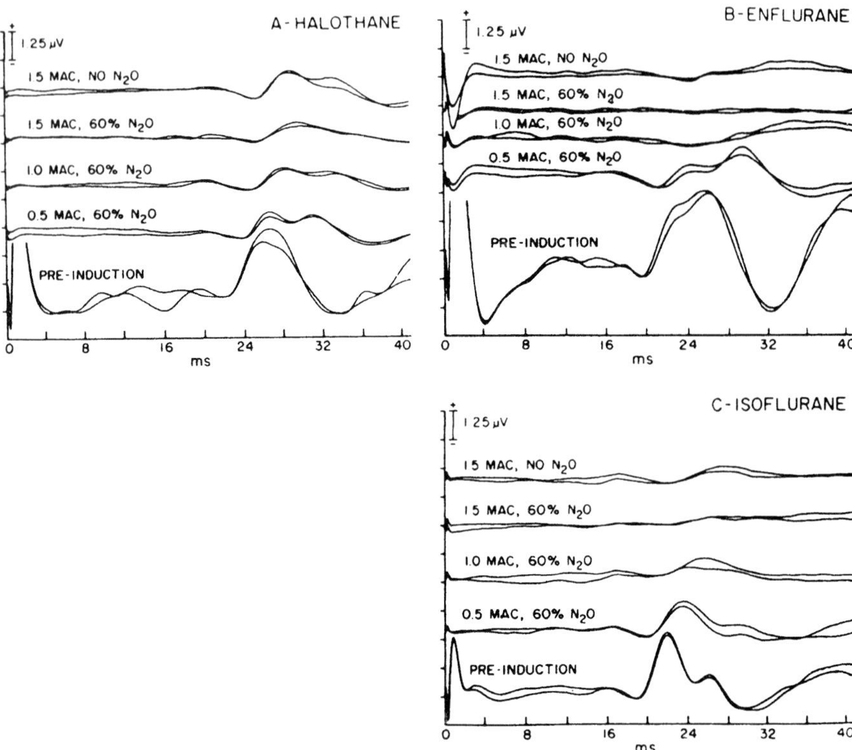

FIGURE 27-7. The responses of cortical somatosensory evoked potentials to various MACs of halothane, enflurane, and isoflurane. A marked alteration of evoked potentials occurs at 1 MAC and higher levels of inhaled agents, and a modest improvement of the response occurs when N_2O is withdrawn. (Reprinted with permission from Peterson DO, Drummond JC, Todd MM: Effects of halothane, enflurane, isoflurane, and nitrous oxide in multilevel somatosensory evoked potentials. Anesthesiology 65:35, 1986.)

Brainstem responses are considerably more resistant to anesthetic influences than are cortical responses. For example, clinically used concentrations of the inhaled agents tend to increase the latencies of early or subcortical peaks of the BAEP with minimal amplitude effects. Most anesthetic regimens are compatible with recording of brainstem responses. However, as with the other evoked potential modalities, large step changes (greater than 0.5 MAC) in inspired inhalation agent concentration should be avoided during critical periods.

Studies on the effects of intravenous agents demonstrate that induction doses of thiopental, etomidate, and fentanyl preserve SSEP recordings. Increasing doses of thiopental result in dose-dependent increases in latency and decreases in amplitude in cortical SSEPs and progressive increases in latency in BAEPs. Very high doses of thiopental, exceeding that which produce an isoelectric EEG, alter SSEPs and BAEPs predictably, but waveforms are preserved. VEPs are more sensitive than the other sensory modalities to the effects of barbiturates with only the early potentials persisting at low doses and increasing in latency at higher doses. Either bolus administration or intravenous infusion of etomidate causes increases in latency and increases in amplitude of cortical SSEPs and slight decreases in amplitude of cervical potentials. Etomidate produces minimal changes in the early or subcortical peaks of the BAEP, but causes a dose-dependent attenuation and prolongation of the middle latency cortical peaks. Etomidate alone does not change VEP amplitudes (P100 or N70), but increases latency (P60, N70, and P100). During fentanyl–nitrous oxide anesthesia, etomidate causes decreases in amplitude and increases in latency of VEPs. The benzodiazepines produce minimal SSEP and VEP changes and no changes in BAEPs. Propofol increases the latency and decreases the amplitude of cortical SSEPs. Propofol (2 mg/kg iv followed by an infusion) increases the BAEP latency of I, III, and V waves without changing the amplitudes. Propofol completely suppresses middle latency auditory potentials.

The opioids produce minimal changes in SEP waveforms. For example, fentanyl causes minimal latency prolongation and amplitude depression of the SSEP waveforms. Compared with the combination of fentanyl and nitrous oxide, the remifentanil/isoflurane technique preserved cortical amplitude better and with less variability in latency and amplitude. High-dose opioid administration also has been shown to be compatible with reproducible recordings of SSEPs. Opioids also produce minimal to no effect on BAEP recordings. Furthermore, low-dose continuous infusions of opioids tend to depress SEPs less than intermittent bolus injections.

Because opioids preserve SEP recordings even in relatively high doses, they are recommended for use as infusions during intra-operative monitoring. As with all intravenous agents used, bolus administration should be avoided during critical times when neurologic injury might occur.

Clonidine and dexmedetomidine are α-2 receptor agonists that are used to decrease anesthetic requirements. Clonidine administered alone or added to 1 MAC isoflurane does not change cortical SSEP latency or amplitude. Dexmedetomidine affects SSEP amplitude minimally and has been shown to blunt isoflurane's effect on SSEP amplitude. Both agents can be used as an anesthetic adjuvant without compromising SSEP monitoring.

Physiologic factors such as temperature, systemic blood pressure, PaO_2, and $PaCO_2$ can alter SEPs and must be controlled during intra-operative recordings.[132] Both hypothermia and hyperthermia alter all SEPs. In addition, fluids used to irrigate the brain or spinal cord can cause marked changes in recordings despite normal core temperature measurement. Therefore, body temperature–irrigating fluids should be used. Systemic hypotension below levels of cerebral autoregulation produces progressive decreases in amplitude of cortical SSEPs until the waveform is lost. During scoliosis surgery, SSEP changes have been observed that resolved with increases in systemic blood pressure, suggesting that spinal cord manipulation during "safe" levels of hypotension may cause significant ischemia. Changes in PaO_2 and $PaCO_2$ also alter SEPs, probably reflecting changes in blood flow or oxygen delivery to neural structures.

Motor Evoked Potentials

A motor evoked potential (MEP) can be produced by direct (epidural) or indirect (transosseous) stimulation of the brain or spinal cord. Following transcranial stimulation, the signal descends through both the dorsolateral and ventral spinal cord. It is primarily localized in the pyramidal tracts, and can be recorded from spinal cord (epidural space), peripheral nerve, and muscle using conventional electromyographic and evoked potential averaging techniques. Stimulation of the motor cortex elicits contralateral peripheral nerve signals, electromyographic signals, or limb movements.

Transosseous activation of motor neurons is accomplished by either electrical or magnetic stimulation. Transcranial electrical stimulation of the motor cortex is a reliable method of eliciting intraoperative MEPs. It is achieved by delivering brief high-voltage pulses through scalp electrodes. Transcranial magnetic stimulation is produced by placing a magnetic coil over the motor cortex. This technique is painless and noninvasive and does not require direct contact with the scalp. Because high-resistance tissues such as bone and skin are transparent to magnetic fields, smaller voltages can be used to stimulate neural elements below the surface.

With either electrical or magnetic stimulation, there is concern that repetitive cortical stimulation can induce epileptic activity, neural damage, and cognitive or memory dysfunction. Guidelines for transcranial MEP stimulation recommend intermittent rather than continuous stimulation over several hours and cautious use in patients with a history of seizures, possible skull fractures, or implanted metallic devices. Disruptions of the calvarium—that is, a skull fracture—could focus the current toward certain regions of the brain and potentially cause neural damage. Other situations of concern are patients with cardiac pacemakers and central venous or pulmonary artery catheterization. Transcranial MEP stimulation should probably be avoided in these patients.

There are several indications for intraoperative monitoring of MEPs. They are especially useful in preserving motor function during procedures in which surgically induced damage may be specific to the motor system. For example, surgical removal of intramedullary tumors can result in selective damage to corticospinal tracts, and MEPs are used to guide surgical resection. During scoliosis surgery, a direct monitor of motor pathway function obviates the need for the intraoperative wake-up test and provides continuous information about motor function throughout the surgical procedure. During cerebrovascular procedures and resection of cerebral tumors involving the motor cortex or subcortical motor pathways, the ability to guide the surgical resection by monitoring motor function prevents postoperative motor deficits. Paralysis is an unpredictable complication that can occur after aortic aneurysm surgery. Myogenic MEP monitoring can detect ventral horn ischemia during aortic reconstruction, thus allowing the surgeon to initiate strategies to improve spinal cord perfusion. In all of these procedures, MEPs should be monitored in conjunction with SSEPs to fully evaluate the functional integrity of both motor and sensory pathways.

Motor evoked potentials are extremely sensitive to depression by anesthetics.[134] The volatile agents are powerful depressants of myogenic MEPs. Nitrous oxide appears to be less suppressive than other inhaled agents. Moderate doses of up to 50% N_20 have been used successfully to supplement other agents during myogenic MEP monitoring. Benzodiazepines, barbiturates, and propofol also produce marked depression of myogenic MEP. However, successful recordings have been obtained during propofol anesthesia by controlling serum propofol concentrations and increasing stimuli rates. Fentanyl, etomidate, and ketamine have little or no effect on myogenic MEP and are compatible with intra-operative recording. Muscle relaxants affect the recorded electromyographic response by depressing myoneural transmission. By adjusting a continuous infusion of muscle relaxant to maintain one or two twitches in a train of four, reliable MEP responses have been recorded.

Although it appears that MEPs are more sensitive to the effects of anesthetic agents, reliable responses have been recorded with a nitrous oxide–narcotic technique and with agents such as ketamine or etomidate. Multistimulus techniques can improve monitoring during anesthesia with more depressive agents such as propofol. As with SEPs, hypothermia, hypoxia, and hypotension will alter MEPs under anesthesia.

Cranial Nerve Monitoring

Potential injury to the cranial nerves can occur during posterior fossa and lower brainstem procedures. The integrity of these cranial nerves can be preserved by monitoring the electromyographic (EMG) potential of cranial nerves with motor components (V, VII, IX, X, XI, XII). Both spontaneous and triggered muscle activity can be recorded. Recordings can be obtained by placing two wire electrodes within the muscle or using surface electrodes. Simultaneous spontaneous EMG and compound muscle action potential (CMAP) recordings can be obtained by using intramuscular wire and surface electrodes. Intramuscular wire electrodes increase the sensitivity for detecting spontaneous EMG activity, while surface electrodes allow for more reliable monitoring of CMAP amplitude and morphology. With accidental surgical trespass, spontaneous neural activity changes into phasic "bursts" or "train" activity, which suggests injury potential. Evoking the nerves with electrical stimulation facilitates identification and hence preservation of the cranial nerve. Although it is possible to record EMG potentials during partial neuromuscular blockade, it is recommended that muscle relaxants not be administered during cranial nerve monitoring.

Intracranial Pressure Monitoring

Since Lundberg's[135] report in 1960, continuous ICP monitoring has been used to guide the perioperative management of patients with head injury, large brain tumor, ruptured intracranial aneurysm, cerebrovascular occlusive disease, and hydrocephalus. With continuous ICP monitoring, it is possible to optimize CPP (MAP-ICP) in critically ill neurosurgical patients. It also allows early detection and prompt treatment of brain hemorrhage, swelling, and herniation. An important intraoperative indication for ICP monitoring is to detect intracranial hypertension in the multiple trauma patients during a nonneurosurgical procedure.

Techniques used to monitor ICP include ventricular catheters, subdural-subarachnoid bolts or catheters, various epidural transducers, and intraparenchymal fiberoptic devices (Fig. 27-8). The intraventricular catheter is the standard method of monitoring ICP. This technique requires a small scalp incision and a burr hole through the skull. A soft, nonreactive plastic catheter is introduced into the lateral ventricle and connected by sterile tubing filled with saline solution to an external transducer. The intraventricular catheter measures CSF pressures reliably. It allows therapeutic CSF drainage and can also be used for compliance testing. There are, however, several potential problems with this technique. This device depends on the transmission of ICP through fluid-filled tubing that can occlude, thus damping or obliterating the recording. In a patient with severe brain swelling or a large mass lesion and small ventricles, it may be technically difficult to locate the lateral ventricle. Besides not being able to pass the catheter into the CSF, there is a possibility of brain tissue damage,

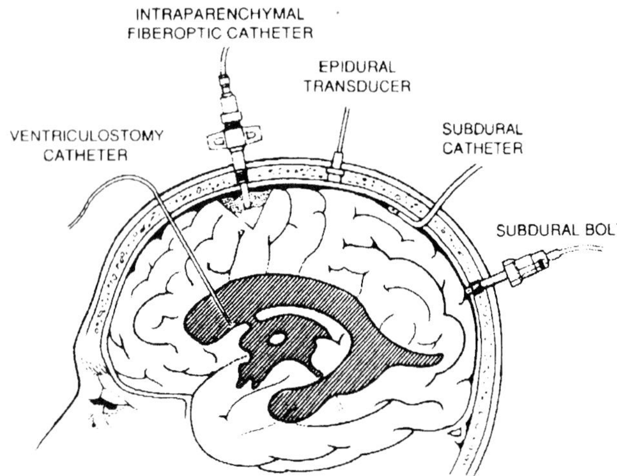

FIGURE 27-8. Techniques used to measure intracranial pressure.

hematoma, and infection. Studies report a low infection rate for the first 4 days after catheter placement. Catheter removal is, therefore, recommended on or before the fifth day, with replacement at a different site if continued ICP monitoring is necessary.

The subdural-subarachnoid bolt usually consists of some type of hollow screw fixed to the calvarium, with the tip passing through the incised dura. The advantages of the bolt are that it does not require brain tissue penetration or knowledge of ventricular position and can be placed in any skull location that avoids major venous sinuses. There are several disadvantages to use of this technique. The bolt cannot be used to lower ICP by CSF drainage or to test compliance reliably. As with the intraventricular catheter, the bolt is connected to a transducer with tubing filled with sterile saline. Not only can the tubing block, but also brain substance can obstruct the tip of the bolt; in either situation, the recording may be damped or lost. Drilling side holes just proximal to the tip of the bolt compensates for this problem to some extent. Subdural devices are easily inserted, but can malfunction if they are not coplanar to the brain surface or if they become loose. The major complication of this procedure is infection, commonly meningitis, osteomyelitis, or a localized infection. Epidural bleeding and focal seizures, if the bolt is inserted too deeply, can also occur.

Two primary types of epidural transducers have been developed. One uses a device that has a pressure-sensitive membrane mounted close to or contacting the dura; the other type, known as the Ladd epidural transducer, is based on the principle of the Numoto pressure switch. Although the risk of infection to the brain is lower because of the extradural placement, there are several disadvantages associated with using these devices. Placement in this potential space is more difficult, and there is a risk of bleeding. Technical problems in positioning and calibrating the transducer in situ can also occur. Another shortcoming of the epidural transducer is that intracranial compliance testing and therapeutic CSF drainage cannot be performed.

Intraparenchymal ICP monitoring techniques allow direct measurement of brain tissue pressure, which may be important in edema formation and regional capillary blood flow. Intraparenchymal devices use a fiberoptic catheter that is inserted within cortical gray matter. In comparison to ventriculostomies, these monitors are easier to insert, have a smaller diameter, and are less disruptive of brain tissue. Because there is no fluid column, the risk of infection is lower.

Cerebral monitoring devices are being developed with miniaturized sensors, transducers, and probes using fiberoptic solid state technology. These devices can be inserted into the subdural, intraparenchymal, or intraventricular compartments. Because these are solid-state monitors, the problems of infection, leaks, catheter occlusion, and drift that attend fluid- or air-filled systems are minimized or avoided. Animal and human studies show that pressure recordings obtained with these devices are accurate and reliable. The main disadvantage of these devices is that they cannot be recalibrated in situ. Another limitation is that they cannot be used for CSF drainage or compliance testing unless inserted in conjunction with a ventriculostomy.

New generations of fiberoptic ICP monitors allow simultaneous measurement of ICP, local CBF using laser Doppler flowmetry, brain tissue oxygen pressure (PO_2), carbon dioxide pressure (PCO_2), pH, and other metabolic markers. By simultaneously monitoring ICP, local CBF, and brain tissue oxygenation, early signs of ischemia can be identified and the effectiveness of therapeutic maneuvers more fully determined. The various ICP monitors are seldom used intra-operatively. They are most valuable in managing critically ill neurosurgical patients in the intensive care unit.

All of the clinically available monitors have recognized advantages and disadvantages. Despite the problems associated with these devices, ICP monitoring provides useful information for evaluating the patient's condition, progress, and need for therapy. Research efforts continue to improve monitoring techniques in terms of reliability, accuracy, and safety.

Transcranial Doppler Ultrasound

Transcranial Doppler (TCD) ultrasound is used for clinical imaging of intracranial vasculature. TCD uses a 2-MHz probe, which is range-gated. The probe is placed over low-density bone regions of the skull, and the beam is focused on the desired vessel. The ultrasonic beam reflects off the blood flowing in the vessel, producing a Doppler shift that is proportional to blood flow velocity. This technique can provide continuous assessment of the systolic, diastolic, and mean flow velocities in the target vessel. Any downstream resistance is proportional to the difference between systolic and diastolic velocities. One commonly used resistance index is the "pulsatility index" defined as:

$$PI = \frac{\text{Systolic Velocity} - \text{Diastolic Velocity}}{\text{Mean Velocity}}$$

TCD does not measure CBF. It determines velocity and direction of the moving column of blood in a major artery. The TCD is used to monitor flow velocity in large vessels in the Circle of Willis and its major branches. The transtemporal approach above the zygomatic arch allows insonating the anterior, middle, and posterior cerebral arteries. The suboccipital route, through the foramen magnum, allows insonating the basilar and vertebral arteries.

TCD has several applications both in critical care and intraoperatively. It can be used to determine the "reserve" of cerebral blood vessels by measuring CO_2 reactivity and autoregulation and to estimate CPP by using the PI. TCD also is used to identify patients with vasospasm, hyperemia, emboli, stenosis, abnormal collateral blood flow, and inadequate CBF. For intraoperative application, the probe is affixed to the temporal bone with a strap. During craniotomy, a skin adhesive is applied to mount the probe.

Limitations of this technique include between-subject variation of TCD velocities, within-subject variation if vessel diameter changes in response to vasoactive agents or conditions, and error from changing the angle of insonation. However, the advantages of TCD are that it is noninvasive and nonradioactive and provides continuous information about the cerebral circulation.

Cerebral Oxygenation/Metabolism Monitors

Brain Tissue Oxygenation

A multiparameter sensor is available for measuring brain tissue PO_2, PCO_2, pH, and temperature using a combined electrode–fiberoptic system. The sensor was originally designed for continuous intra-arterial blood gas monitoring. It is supplied as a sterile, disposable device comprising two modified optical fibers for the measurements of PCO_2 and pH, a miniaturized Clark electrode for PO_2 measurement, and a thermocouple for determining temperature. Coupled with a dialysis catheter, the device permits measurement of other metabolic markers, including lactate, glucose, and excitotoxic amino acids. This sensor is invasive, requiring insertion into the cortex tissue of interest under direct visualization. The measurements obtained are limited to the parenchyma where the electrode is inserted.

Jugular Bulb Venous Oximetry

Continuous or intermittent estimation of the global balance between cerebral oxygen demand and supply can be achieved by jugular bulb venous oximetry. This is done by measuring the oxygen saturation of jugular venous blood ($SjVO_2$) through percutaneous retrograde cannulation of the internal jugular vein with an intravascular catheter with embedded optical fibers. Normal $SjVO_2$ is 60 to 70%. In the absence of anemia and any change in oxygen saturation, increases in $SjVO_2$ to above 75% are indicative of absolute or relative hyperemia; that is, supply is in excess of metabolic requirement. This can occur as a result of reduced metabolic need (e.g., a comatose or brain-dead patient) or from excessive flow (e.g., severe hypercapnia). A value less than 50% reflects increased oxygen extraction and indicates a potential risk of ischemic injury. This may be because of increased metabolic demand (e.g., fever or seizure) not matched by an equivalent increase in flow, or it may be because of an absolute reduction in flow. Changes in the oxygenation of systemic blood also influence the saturation of blood in the jugular bulb.

This monitor is used intraoperatively and postoperatively to diagnose cerebral ischemia from inadequate perfusion pressure or excessive hyperventilation. Its major limitation is that it does not detect focal ischemia.

Transcranial Oximetry

Near-infrared spectroscopy (NIRS) is a noninvasive optical method for monitoring cerebral regional oxygenation. It is based on the principle that light in the near-infrared range (700 to 900 nm) readily penetrates skin and bone, but reflects off certain chromophores in the brain, such as oxy- and deoxyhemoglobin and cytochrome AA[3]. Therefore, by monitoring the absorption of light at several wavelengths in the near-infrared range, brain tissue concentrations of oxy- and deoxyhemoglobin, total hemoglobin, and hemoglobin oxygen saturation can be measured. The tissue field beneath the sensor contains capillaries, arteries, and veins, reflecting a mixed vascular saturation, which NIRS monitors. Cerebral oximetry can be used to monitor ischemia in several clinical neurosurgical conditions, including carotid endarterectomy, head injury, and subarachnoid hemorrhage. Its major limitations include intersubject variability, variable optical path length, potential contamination from extracranial blood, and lack of a definable threshold. At present, it is considered a trend monitor, with each patient acting as his or her own control. In situations of potential regional ischemia, for example, carotid endarterectomy and temporary clip application during intracranial aneurysm surgery, bilateral monitoring should be used.

NEURORADIOLOGY

8 Common neuroradiology procedures are computed tomography (CT), magnetic resonance imaging (MRI), angiography, and a variety of invasive interventional procedures. These require total immobility on the part of the patient. Therefore, uncooperative patients, specifically children, fearful adults, and retarded or obtunded patients, would require general anesthesia. All the standard equipment and monitors required for the administration of a general anesthetic and possible cardiopulmonary resuscitation must be present.

Computed Tomography Scan

The CT scan produces a series of cross-sectional images by computerized processing of x-ray absorption measurements (photon attenuation data as measured by sodium iodide crystals rotating about the patient's head). Performance of a brain scan requires that the patient lie on a table with his or her head inside a rotating gantry that makes a 180° arc, producing one axial slice or cut. Depending on the generation of the scanner, the rotation may take from a few seconds to 4.5 minutes per cut. Eight cuts are usually required for a complete examination of the head. When contrast enhancement is indicated, the dye may be infused intravenously and the scan repeated. The patient must remain supine and immobile throughout the entire scan.

CT scanning is an excellent modality for detecting skull fractures and acute subarachnoid hemorrhage. It is relatively insensitive for viewing structures within the posterior fossa because image degradation results from artifact produced by the interface of bone and brain parenchyma. For trauma patients, spiral acquisition CT is becoming more popular. Larger anatomic regions can be imaged as the patient is moved at a continuous, constant speed through the scanning field with the x-ray tube rotating continuously.

Most CT examinations are performed without an anesthesiologist present. Oral or intravenous sedation is used for many pediatric examinations and is usually administered by radiology personnel. Iodinated contrast medium, which is particularly valuable in studies of vascular malformations, vascularized tumors, and blood-brain defects, may also be administered orally or intravenously. When general anesthesia is requested, the patient's "nothing-by-mouth" status must be determined. Other issues that need to be resolved before the administration of general anesthesia are remote access to the patient and the establishment of monitoring and equipment that meets the same standard of care that exists in the operating room.

The CT scanner uses ionizing radiation. The radiation exposure during CT is similar to that of a conventional skull radiograph (1.0 to 2.5 rad). Exposure values for personnel attending the patient are minimal (e.g., 1 to 2 mrad/hr for the anesthesiologist positioned next to the scan). However, radiation monitoring badges and lead aprons should be worn by personnel who participate in CT scanning on a regular basis.

Magnetic Resonance Imaging

Magnetic resonance imaging is a noninvasive diagnostic technique that is superior to CT in many CNS disorders. This technique employs a strong magnetic field and pulsed radiofrequency energy to generate images. When a biologic specimen is placed within a static magnetic field, certain atomic nuclei

(nuclei with an odd number of protons, such as ^{1}H nuclei) act like magnets and are aligned. The atoms are then subjected to a radiofrequency pulse that deflects their orientation. When the radiofrequency pulse is discontinued, the nuclei rotate back into alignment with the static magnetic field. The energy released as the nuclei "relax" is used to create the MR image. The magnet of the MRI system is in the form of a tube that can accommodate the human body. The patient must remain still during investigation, which may last 1 hour, to prevent imaging artifacts.

The MRI is an extremely valuable diagnostic tool that provides excellent contrast between gray and white brain matter. The images can be displayed in axial, coronal, or sagittal planes. Because there is no dental or bony artifact, the MRI is superior to the CT scan in examining the posterior fossa. Other areas optimally imaged by MRI include the pineal gland region, sella and parasellar structures, the limbic system, cranial nerves, internal auditory canal, the cerebellopontine angle, and leptomeninges. Magnetic resonance angiography (MRA) provides images of arterial and dural sinus blood flow. Magnetic resonance spectroscopy provides noninvasive biochemical measurements of specific brain metabolites and can be helpful in the early detection of stroke.

The intense magnetic field creates unique challenges for the anesthesiologist. The high-static magnetic field (0.12 to 2.00 tesla [T]) and the radiofrequency energy transmitted during image acquisition may damage or cause malfunction of electrical, electronic, or mechanical life support and monitoring equipment. Conversely, the radiofrequency energy generated by these devices can interfere with MR signal detection, producing artifacts that degrade the image. Another problem unique to MRI is that ferromagnetic substances placed within the magnetic field are propelled toward the scanner. A list of MRI-compatible equipment and monitors has been published.[136]

Laryngoscopes are not magnetic, but the batteries are. Therefore, to use a laryngoscope within the scanning room, plastic- or paper-coated batteries must be used. A prebent RAE tube is recommended owing to limited vertical space within the scanner. Very long breathing tubes are required, and either pipeline gases or a remotely placed anesthesia machine can be used. Aluminum cylinders can be used safely within the scanning room. MRI-compatible anesthesia machines and ventilators are available. The anesthesia machine can be bolted to the wall or modified by removal of ferromagnetic components. The ventilators are pneumatically driven and volume-cycled and have fluidic controls. The ventilator is completely powered by high-pressure oxygen delivered by a wall source or from large cylinders placed outside the imaging room, and electronic parts have been replaced with plastic, aluminum, or nonmetallic alloys.

The implementation of monitoring during MRI is difficult because of remote access to the patient and the interactions between various monitoring devices and the MR scanner, as previously described. For example, standard ECG monitors produce problems with image degradation from wire leads acting as antennas and with artifact produced by radiofrequency pulses and static magnetic fields. Burns under ECG electrodes have been reported. MR-compatible ECG monitors, cables, fasteners, and electrodes have been developed. However, this ECG provides only heart rate and rhythm and cannot be used to monitor ischemia. Additional suggestions for improving ECG monitoring include placing electrodes close together near the three-dimensional center of the imager and twisting the leads. Both noninvasive and invasive pressure monitoring have been successfully used during MRI. Blood pressure is easily measured with an ordinary cuff and long pressure tubing without metal connections. The blood pressure dial must be kept away from the magnetic field. Automated blood pressure devices without metal connectors have also been used. Using nonmetallic components, pressure transducers connected to intravascular catheters for central venous, pulmonary artery, and arterial pressure monitoring can function near the magnet. Transducers are affixed along the side of the magnet at its midpoint to minimize artifact. Shielded electric extension cables couple the transducers to the monitors located outside the scanning room. There have been reports of image degradation with the pulse oximeter. Placing the oximeter a distance from the magnet and the probe on the patient's toe, which is usually outside the magnet, and using a fiberoptic cable may improve image quality. Monitoring of heart rate and respiration can be achieved using nonmetallic precordial or esophageal stethoscopes; however, the drum-like noise of the scanner may obscure auscultated heart and breath sounds. A standard vascular Doppler has also been used to monitor heart rate. Capnography is possible with long tubing and high-powered suction. Changes in respiratory rate are easily observed, but the end-tidal CO_2 reading may be less than the actual value. Although temperature monitoring is particularly important in the cold MRI suite, especially in pediatric patients, it has been difficult to implement. The wires conducting the signal from the thermistor may function as an antenna for radiofrequency signals and produce imaging artifact and burns. Nonferromagnetic disposable temperature strips may be used. All efforts to minimize patient heat loss should be implemented: using bags of warmed intravenous fluids, heating pads, and airway humidification and covering the patient.

Guidelines for using the MRI have been issued and are updated by the Institute for Magnetic Resonance Safety, Education and Research.[137] It is recommended that women in the first trimester of pregnancy not be scanned because of possible developmental consequences. Patients with demand pacemakers should not be scanned because the varying magnetic field can induce electric currents in the pacemaker wires, which may be mistaken for the natural electrical activity of the heart, inhibiting pacemaker output. Metallic objects such as vascular clips or shrapnel can move and become displaced when exposed to the magnetic field. Patients who have a large metallic implant or prosthesis can be scanned until the heat at the site of the implant or prosthesis becomes uncomfortable. There is a possibility that induced currents can affect myocardial contractility or produce arrhythmias. Full resuscitation facilities should be available.

Positron Emission Tomography

Biochemical or physiologic processes involved in cerebral metabolism can be imaged with positron emission tomography (PET). After receiving intravenous radionuclide, such as fluorodeoxyglucose (FDG), the patient is scanned in a specialized detector system. This system detects the positron energy emitted from the radionuclide. Computerized reconstruction procedures produce tomographic images. The information from PET can be overlaid on CT or MR images to improve anatomic localization of detected activity. When the MRI is normal in a patient with seizures, PET might provide localizing information prior to focal resection treatment. The injection of FDG renders the patient radioactive for 24 hours. The usual protocol involves two initial scans lasting 15 to 20 minutes followed by another scan in 2 to 3 hours. PET scanners do not require nonferromagnetic monitors and equipment.

Cerebral Angiography

Angiography is used to delineate the vasculature of the brain. Catheters are usually introduced through the common femoral artery, which has replaced direct carotid artery puncture.

Digital subtraction angiography reduces the required volume of intra-arterial contrast and the overall duration of the procedure.

There are several risks and problems associated with angiography, including an incidence of neurologic problems related to angiography itself. In addition, arterial spasm, hematoma, and local infection can occur at the site of needle puncture. Subintimal dissection or occlusion of the vessel may result from injection into the vessel wall. Iodine-containing contrast media produce vasodilation and a burning sensation in the distribution of the injected vessel. Septicemia, cerebral embolism, anaphylactic reactions to the iodinated contrast material, and, rarely, seizures or death are all potential complications of cerebral angiography.

The introduction of low-ionic and nonionic contrast material has reduced both the discomfort and toxicity associated with angiography. Because of this, patients usually do not require general anesthesia and are able to tolerate the procedure with minimal or no sedation. When general anesthesia is requested for children or uncooperative adults, the angiogram quality may be enhanced by hyperventilation. Hypocarbia is thought to improve study quality by slowing the cerebral circulation and improving delineation of tumor blood vessels, perhaps through an inverse steal phenomenon.

Interventional Neuroradiology

Interventional neuroradiology (INR) has developed from traditional neuroradiology and neurosurgery to procedures that treat CNS disease by endovascular access.[138] Procedures such as therapeutic embolization and superselective angiography of vascular malformations, coiling of cerebral aneurysms, balloon angioplasty of occlusive cerebrovascular disease or cerebral vasospasm, therapeutic carotid occlusion for giant aneurysms and brain tumors, and others may be performed. Because these procedures are inherently dangerous, anesthesiologists can help prevent and manage morbidity and mortality.

Most interventional neuroradiology procedures can be accomplished with conscious sedation. The agents chosen for conscious sedation must alleviate pain and discomfort and provide anxiolysis, patient immobility, and a rapid return to consciousness for neurologic testing. A variety of sedation regimens, most often using a combination of midazolam, opioid, and propofol, have been successfully administered. The goal of drug titration is to render the patient well-sedated with a patent airway.

General anesthesia is always administered for small children and uncooperative adult patients. In addition, many neuroradiologists now prefer general anesthesia to reduce motion artifacts and to improve the quality of images during high-risk procedures, even though it prevents awake neurologic testing. The specific choice of anesthesia and airway control via endotracheal tube or laryngeal mask airway may be guided by the condition and physical status of the patient. Cannulation of the femoral artery is the most stimulating portion of the procedure, and the total anesthetic requirement is usually minimal. Total intravenous techniques or combinations of inhalation and intravenous agents with muscle relaxant are chosen with the goal of maintaining adequate systemic and intracranial hemodynamics and immobility throughout the procedure and producing a rapid return to consciousness during emergence.[139]

Before initiating anesthesia, the patient is made comfortable with padding under head, neck, and body, and all pressure points are protected. Two large-bore intravenous catheters are inserted, and standard monitoring is applied. Arterial pressure is monitored for intracranial and spinal cord procedures and whenever blood pressure manipulation is required. Awake neurologic assessment and other CNS monitors (e.g., EEG, evoked potentials, or transcranial Doppler) may be used. During and after these procedures, careful management of coagulation is required to prevent thromboembolic complications. It is important to communicate with the radiologist concerning the degree, timing, and continuation of anticoagulation. A clot with devastating embolic potential can easily develop on a catheter during the procedure, if heparinization is not adequately maintained. At the end of the procedure, protamine may or may not be necessary for heparin reversal. Special techniques such as deliberate hypotension or hypertension and hypercapnia may be requested during certain procedures.

Complications during instrumentation of the cerebral vasculature can be sudden and dramatic. Simultaneous with airway maintenance, it is important to determine whether the problem is hemorrhagic or occlusive. Hemorrhagic disasters require immediate heparin reversal with protamine and low normal blood pressure. Occlusive disasters require deliberate hypertension, titrated to neurologic examination, with or without direct thrombolysis. Other resuscitative measures that might be initiated include rapid fluid infusion, 15° head-up position, hyperventilation, diuretics, anticonvulsants, hypothermia (33 to 34°C), and thiopental infusion titrated to EEG burst suppression.

ANESTHETIC MANAGEMENT OF NEUROSURGICAL PATIENTS

9 The administration of anesthesia to neurosurgical patients requires an understanding of the basic principles of neurophysiology and the effects of anesthetic agents on intracranial dynamics, as reviewed in the previous sections of this chapter.

Preoperative Evaluation

During the preoperative evaluation, the patient's overall medical condition must be considered and integrated into the formulation of an anesthetic management plan. Neurosurgical procedures tend to be lengthy, requiring unusual positioning of the patient and the institution of special techniques such as hyperventilation, cerebral dehydration, and deliberate hypotension. Not all patients can tolerate the position desired by the surgeon; this must be addressed and, if possible, evaluated preoperatively. Furthermore, in patients with cardiac disease, routine institution of osmotherapy or hyperventilation may compromise organ function. Such patients must be medically optimized and, when indicated, cardiac monitoring should be instituted. Except for neurosurgical emergencies (e.g., head trauma or impending herniation), most neurosurgical procedures can be delayed to treat medically unstable conditions.

The preoperative evaluation must include a complete neurologic examination with special attention to the patient's level of consciousness, presence or absence of increased ICP, and extent of focal neurologic deficits. The signs and symptoms frequently associated with intracranial hypertension are headache, nausea, papilledema, unilateral pupillary dilation, and oculomotor or abducens palsy. With advanced stages of intracranial hypertension, the patient exhibits a depressed level of consciousness and irregular respiration. The clinical signs do not reliably indicate the level of ICP. Only a direct CSF pressure measurement can be used to quantitate the pressure; however, indirect evidence of elevated ICP can be determined by evaluating the MRI or CT scan for a mass lesion accompanied by a midline shift of 0.5 cm or greater and/or encroachment of expanding brain on CSF cisterns.

The location of the lesion in the supratentorial or infratentorial compartment will determine the clinical presentation and anesthetic management. Supratentorial disease is usually associated with problems in the management of intracranial hypertension, whereas infratentorial lesions cause problems related to mass effects on vital brainstem structures and elevated ICP as a result of obstructive hydrocephalus.

Fluid and electrolyte abnormalities are common in patients with reduced levels of consciousness. Patients are usually dehydrated and develop electrolyte abnormalities because of decreased fluid intake, iatrogenic water restriction, neuroendocrine abnormalities, and diuresis from diuretics, steroid-related hyperglycemia, and x-ray contrast agents. Fluid and electrolyte abnormalities must be corrected before induction of anesthesia to prevent cardiovascular instability.

COMMON INTRACRANIAL PATHOLOGY

Supratentorial Intracranial Tumors

Supratentorial tumors (meningiomas, gliomas, and metastatic lesions) change intracranial dynamics predictably. Initially, when the lesion is small and slowly expanding, volume-spatial compensation occurs by compression of the CSF compartment and nearby cerebral veins, which prevents increases in ICP. As the lesion grows, compensatory mechanisms become exhausted, and any further increase in tumor mass will cause progressively greater increases in ICP. Primary or metastatic tumors or chronic subdural hematomas can present as chronic mass lesions. Because of the ability of the intracranial compartment to compensate up to a point, patients may exhibit minimal neurologic dysfunction despite the presence of a large mass, elevated ICP, and shifts in the position of brain structures.

Significant changes in ICP can occur with supratentorial tumors if they develop a central area of hemorrhagic necrotic tissue or a wide border of brain edema. As the tumor enlarges, it can outstrip its blood supply, developing a central hemorrhagic area that may expand rapidly, increasing ICP. Brain edema surrounding the tumor increases the effective bulk of the tumor and represents an additional portion of the brain that is not autoregulating. In such situations of compromised intracranial compliance, small increases in arterial pressure may produce large increases in CBF, which can markedly increase intracranial volume and ICP with its attendant complications—cerebral ischemia and herniation. In addition to hypertension, other causes of increased cerebral blood volume, such as hypercarbia, hypoxia, vasodilating agents, and jugular venous obstruction, can adversely affect cerebral hemodynamics and must be avoided perioperatively.

Anesthetic Techniques and Drugs

10 The goal of neuroanesthetic care for patients with supratentorial tumors is to maximize therapeutic modalities that reduce intracranial volume. ICP must be controlled before the cranium is opened, and optimal operating conditions obtained by producing a slack brain that facilitates surgical dissection. Various maneuvers and pharmacologic agents have been used to reduce brain bulk (Table 27-9). For example, administration of diuretics or steroids, hyperventilation, and systemic blood pressure control may be implemented preoperatively to reduce cerebral edema and brain bulk, thereby reducing ICP. The application of these methods selectively or together, when necessary, is often accompanied by marked clinical improvement.

Clinical Control of Intracranial Hypertension. Rapid brain dehydration and ICP reduction can be produced by administering the osmotic diuretic, mannitol, or the loop diuretic, furosemide. Mannitol is given as an intravenous infusion in a dose of 0.25 to 1.0 g/kg. Its action begins within 10 to 15 minutes and is effective for approximately 2 hours. Larger doses produce a longer duration of action but do not necessarily reduce ICP more effectively. Furthermore, larger doses and repeated administration can result in metabolic derangement. Mannitol is effective when the blood-brain barrier is intact. By increasing the osmolality of blood relative to the brain, mannitol pulls water across an intact blood-brain barrier from brain to blood to restore the osmolar balance. When the blood-brain barrier is disrupted, mannitol may enter the brain and increase osmolality. Mannitol could pull water into the brain as the plasma concentration of the agent declines and cause a rebound increase in ICP. This rebound increase in ICP may be prevented by maintaining a mild fluid deficit. Mannitol has been shown to cause vasodilation of vascular smooth muscle, which is dependent on dose and rate of administration. Mannitol-induced vasodilation affects intracranial and extracranial vessels and can transiently increase cerebral blood volume and ICP while simultaneously decreasing systemic blood pressure. Because mannitol may initially increase ICP, it should be given slowly ($\geq$10-minute infusion) and in conjunction with maneuvers that decrease intracranial volume (e.g., steroids or hyperventilation). Prolonged use of mannitol may produce dehydration, electrolyte disturbances, hyperosmolality, and impaired renal function.

Hypertonic saline, another osmotic diuretic, is currently under investigation.[140] Hypertonic saline solutions have been shown to reduce ICP in animal models and in human studies and may be more effective than other diuretics in certain clinical conditions, for example, patients with refractory intracranial hypertension or in those who require brain debulking and maintenance of intravascular volume.[140,141] Hypertonic saline also can be used as an alternative or adjunct to intraoperative use of mannitol. There are several potential adverse effects of hypertonic saline therapy (Table 27-10). Significant complications such as central pontine myelinolysis and intracranial hemorrhage have not been reported in human studies. Different types of hypertonic saline solutions with different methods

TABLE 27-9

CLINICAL CONTROL OF INTRACRANIAL HYPERTENSION

Diuretics: Osmotic: Mannitol (0.25–1 g/kg iv), hypertonic saline (under investigation).
Furosemide: 0.5–1 mg/kg iv alone or 0.15–0.3 mg/kg iv in combination with mannitol.
Corticosteroids: Dexamethasone (effective for localized cerebral edema surrounding tumors; requires 12–36 hours).
Adequate ventilation: $PaO_2 \geq 100$ mmHg, $PaCO_2$ 33–35 mmHg; hyperventilation on demand.
Optimize hemodynamics (MAP, CVP, PCWP, HR): Target normotension and maintain cerebral perfusion pressure (CPP = MAP – ICP) to avoid cerebral ischemia.
Fluid therapy: Target normovolemia before anesthetic induction to prevent hypotension. Use glucose-free isoosmolar crystalloid solutions to prevent increases in brain water content (from hypoosmolality) and ischemic damage (from hyperglycemia).
Position to improve cerebral venous return (neutral, head-up position).
Drug-induced cerebral vasoconstriction (e.g., thiopental, propofol).
Temperature control: Avoid hyperthermia perioperatively. Consider using mild intraoperative hypothermia.
Cerebral spinal fluid drainage—to acutely reduce brain tension.

TABLE 27-10

HYPERTONIC SALINE: POTENTIAL ADVERSE EFFECTS OF INTRAVENOUS ADMINISTRATION

■ CENTRAL NERVOUS SYSTEM	■ SYSTEMIC
Decreased level of consciousness	Hyperosmolality
Seizures	Hypernatremia
Central pontine myelinolysis[a]	Congestive heart failure
Subdural and intraparenchymal hemorrhage[a]	Hypokalemia
Rebound cerebral edema	Hyperchloremic acidosis
	Coagulopathy
	Phlebitis
	Renal failure

[a]Not reported in human studies.

of infusion (bolus and continuous) have been reported in the literature. Published data are encouraging, but more studies are required to determine dose-response curves and the safety and efficacy of these solutions.

Hypertonic agents, either mannitol or hypertonic saline, should be administered cautiously in patients with preexisting cardiovascular disease. In these patients, the transient increase in intravascular volume may precipitate left ventricular failure. Furosemide may be a better agent to reduce ICP in patients with impaired cardiac reserve.

The loop diuretic furosemide reduces ICP by inducing a systemic diuresis, decreasing CSF production, and resolving cerebral edema by improving cellular water transport. Furosemide lowers ICP without increasing cerebral blood volume or blood osmolality; however, it is not as effective as mannitol in reducing ICP. Furosemide can be given alone as a large initial dose (0.5 to 1 mg/kg) or as a lower dose with mannitol (0.15 to 0.30 mg/kg). A combination of mannitol and furosemide diuresis has been shown to be more effective than mannitol alone in reducing ICP and brain bulk but causes more severe dehydration and electrolyte imbalances. With combined therapy, it is necessary to monitor electrolytes intraoperatively and replace potassium as indicated.

Corticosteroids reduce edema around some brain tumors; however, steroids require many hours or days before a reduction in ICP becomes apparent. The administration of steroids preoperatively frequently causes neurologic improvement that can precede the ICP reduction. One explanation for this is that the neurologic improvement is accompanied by partial restoration of the previously abnormal blood-brain barrier. Postulated mechanisms of action for steroidal reduction in brain edema are brain dehydration, blood-brain barrier repair, prevention of lysosomal activity, enhanced cerebral electrolyte transport, improved brain metabolism, promotion of water and electrolyte excretion, and inhibition of phospholipase A_2 activity. The potential complications of continuous perioperative steroid administration are hyperglycemia, glucosuria, gastrointestinal bleeding, electrolyte disturbances, and increased incidence of infection. Therefore, the potential risks and benefits of continuous steroid administration need to be evaluated in these patients.

Hyperventilation reduces brain volume by decreasing CBF through cerebral vasoconstriction. For every 1 mm Hg change in $PaCO_2$, CBF changes by 1–2 mL/100 g/min. The duration of effectiveness of hyperventilation for lowering ICP may be as short as 4 to 6 hours, depending on the pH of the CSF. Hyperventilation is only effective when the CO_2 reactivity of the cerebrovasculature is intact. Impaired responsiveness to changes in CO_2 tension occurs in areas of vasoparalysis, which are associated with extensive intracranial disease such as ischemia, trauma, tumor, and infection.

The typical target $PaCO_2$ is 30 to 35 mmHg. A $PaCO_2$ less than 25 to 30 mmHg in some pathologic conditions may be associated with ischemia caused by extreme cerebral vasoconstriction.[142,143] By monitoring global cerebral oxygenation with, for example, $SjVO_2$, the therapeutic effectiveness of hyperventilation can be determined and more safely applied.

The autoregulation of CBF has been discussed, as has the relationship between blood pressure and ICP when autoregulation is disturbed. The therapeutic goals are to maintain CPP and to control intracranial dynamics so that cerebral ischemia, edema, hemorrhage, and herniation are avoided. Severe hypotension results in cerebral ischemia and should be treated with volume replacement, inotropes, or vasopressors as dictated by clinical need. Severe hypertension, conversely, can worsen cerebral edema and cause intracranial hemorrhage and herniation. The β-adrenergic blockers propranolol and esmolol and the combined α- and β-adrenergic blocker labetalol are effective in reducing systemic blood pressure in patients with raised ICP with minimal or no effect on CBF or ICP.

Restricted fluid intake was a traditional approach to intracranial decompression therapy but is now rarely used to lower ICP. Severe fluid restriction over several days is only modestly effective in reducing brain water and can cause hypovolemia, resulting in hypotension, inadequate renal perfusion, electrolyte and acid-base disturbances, hypoxemia, and reductions in CBF. In patients who are dehydrated preoperatively, intravascular volume must be restored to normal before induction of anesthesia to prevent hypotension in response to anesthetic agents and positive-pressure ventilation. Fluid resuscitation and maintenance fluids in the routine neurosurgical patient are provided with glucose-free isoosmolar crystalloid solutions to prevent increases in brain water content from hypoosmolality. For routine craniotomy, the patient receives hourly maintenance fluids and replacement of urine output. Blood loss is replaced at approximately a 3:1 ratio (crystalloid:blood) down to a hematocrit of approximately 25 to 30%, depending on the patient's physiologic status.

Solutions containing glucose are avoided in all neurosurgical patients with normal glucose metabolism, since these solutions exacerbate ischemic damage and cerebral edema. Hyperglycemia augments ischemic damage by promoting neuronal lactate production, which worsens cellular injury. Intravenous fluids containing glucose and water ($D_5W_{0.45\%}$ NaCl or D_5W) are particularly problematic because the glucose is metabolized and the free water remains in the intracranial fluid compartment, resulting in brain edema. Brain water can interfere with surgical exposure and, after closure of the skull, can compromise cerebral perfusion. In normal patients, both preoperative dexamethasone treatment and general anesthesia–induced gluconeogenesis may elevate resting glucose levels. Therefore, blood glucose levels should be monitored during craniotomy and maintained at near low-normal range. This should be accomplished mainly by withholding glucose.

For most neurosurgical patients, a neutral head position, elevated 15 to 30°, is recommended to decrease ICP by improving venous drainage. Flexing or turning of the head may obstruct cerebral venous outflow, causing a dramatic ICP elevation that has been shown to resolve with resumption of a neutral head position. Lowering the head impairs cerebral venous drainage, which can quickly result in an increase in brain bulk and ICP.

The application of positive end-expiratory pressure (PEEP) to mechanically ventilated patients can potentially increase ICP. This effect occurs when PEEP increases mean intrathoracic pressure, impairing cerebral venous outflow and cardiac output. When PEEP is required to maintain oxygenation, it should be applied cautiously and with appropriate monitoring to minimize decreases in cardiac output and increases in ICP. PEEP levels of 10 cm H_2O or less have been used without significant increases in ICP or decreases in CPP. When higher levels of PEEP are required to optimize the PaO_2-PEEP–CPP relationship, both central venous pressure and ICP monitoring are indicated.

The administration of pharmacologic agents that increase cerebral vascular resistance can acutely reduce ICP. Thiopental and propofol are potent cerebral vasoconstrictors that can be used for this purpose. The effects of these agents on CBF, cerebral metabolic rate for oxygen ($CMRO_2$), ICP, and CPP are reviewed in this chapter. These agents are usually administered during induction of anesthesia but may also be administered in anticipation of noxious stimuli or to treat persistently elevated ICP in the intensive care unit.

Although rarely used to reduce ICP, hypothermia does this by decreasing brain metabolism, CBF, cerebral blood volume, and CSF production.[144] Drugs that centrally suppress shivering, muscle relaxants, and mechanical ventilation are required when hypothermic techniques are employed. Intraoperatively, a modest degree of hypothermia, approximately 34°C, has been recommended as a way to confer neuronal protection during focal ischemia. Hypothermic techniques are also employed to cool febrile neurosurgical patients. Hyperthermia is particularly dangerous in neurosurgical patients because it increases brain metabolism, CBF, and the propensity for cerebral edema.

To acutely reduce brain tension, CSF drainage either by direct surgical puncture of the lateral ventricle or by lumbar spinal catheter can be employed. Lumbar CSF drainage should be used cautiously and only when the dura is open and the patient is at least mildly hyperventilated to prevent acute brain herniation. Brain tension can be effectively reduced by draining 10 to 20 mL of CSF.

Premedication

Lethargic patients do not receive premedication. Patients who are alert and anxious may receive an anxiolytic (e.g., midazolam 5 mg po) before coming to the operating room. If there is any doubt about the patient's level of consciousness, the patient may be given sedation or analgesics in the operating room after an intravenous route is established. For the preinduction insertion of invasive monitoring devices in an awake, conversant patient, premedicants (e.g., small doses of opioids) should be considered to alleviate the discomfort from needle punctures.

Monitoring

In addition to the routine monitors, measurement of intra-arterial blood pressure, arterial blood gases, central venous pressure, and urine output is recommended for all major neurosurgical procedures. An arterial cannula is inserted before induction of anesthesia to continuously monitor blood pressure and to estimate CPP. When the arterial pressure transducer is at midhead level (usually the level of the external auditory meatus), MAP approximates the MAP at the level of the circle of Willis. Cerebral perfusion pressure is calculated as the difference between MAP and central venous pressure in patients without intracranial hypertension or the ICP in those with intracranial hypertension. When the cranium is open, ICP equals atmospheric pressure and CPP equals MAP. With direct arterial pressure monitoring, the hemodynamic consequences of the pharmacologic agents administered during anesthesia are recognized instantly. In addition, the arterial catheter provides ready access for intraoperative measurement of arterial blood gases, hematocrit, serum electrolytes, glucose, and osmolality. Arterial blood gas measurement is necessary to verify the adequacy of hyperventilation. In the elderly and those with ventilation/perfusion mismatch, end-tidal CO_2 may correlate poorly with the $PaCO_2$. Therefore, the difference between $PaCO_2$ and end-tidal CO_2 must be determined for a given patient in a given position. Radial, femoral, or brachial arteries are suitable for short-term cannulation; however, after ulnar artery collateral blood flow is tested, cannulation of the radial artery is preferred.

Because most neurosurgical patients are dehydrated preoperatively and then subjected to intraoperative diuresis, the measurement of cardiac preload and urine output is important. A right atrial catheter reflects cardiac preload and is used to determine the preoperative fluid deficit and rate of intraoperative fluid infusion. When possible, the central venous pressure catheter should be inserted through an antecubital vein instead of the jugular or subclavian veins. This avoids increased ICP from both the head-down position and decreased cerebral venous outflow. The position of the antecubital central venous pressure can be verified by chest radiograph, transducer pressure waveform, or p-wave configuration on the ECG.

Urine output is also measured as an indicator of perioperative fluid balance. During craniotomy, a diuresis occurs initially following the administration of osmotic or loop diuretics. Reduced urine output may reflect either hypovolemia or release of antidiuretic hormone.

Preoperative ICP monitoring is rarely used in patients for elective supratentorial tumor operations. ICP monitoring is an invasive procedure that can cause bleeding or infection. When performed with local anesthesia before induction, the procedure can be uncomfortable to the patient.

Muscle Relaxants

An increase in ICP has been reported after administration of succinylcholine in animals and humans. Intravenous administration of succinylcholine is reported to produce activation of the EEG and increases in CBF and ICP in dogs with normal brains.[145] These cerebral effects have been attributed to succinylcholine-induced increases in muscle afferent activity that produce cerebral stimulation. In many, but not all, patients with compromised intracranial compliance, succinylcholine has been shown to increase ICP. This increase can be blocked with a full, paralyzing dose of vecuronium or a pretreatment (defasciculating) dose of metocurine.[144] The nondepolarizing agent apparently eliminates the massive afferent input to the brain after succinylcholine.

To achieve muscle relaxation for intubation of the trachea, succinylcholine is not recommended for elective neurosurgical cases; however, succinylcholine remains the best agent for achieving total paralysis for the rapid-sequence intubation of the trachea. Therefore, in an emergency room or ICU setting, when there is a risk of aspiration or a need for immediate reassessment of neurologic status, succinylcholine should be used. Simultaneously, an effort should be made to control anesthetic depth to protect against the ICP-elevating effects of such noxious stimuli as laryngoscopy, intubation, or tracheal suctioning. In the hemiplegic (or paraplegic) patient, succinylcholine is avoided because of the risk of hyperkalemia. Succinylcholine-induced hyperkalemia has also been reported after closed head injury and ruptured cerebral aneurysms in patients who were not hemiplegic or paraplegic.

Nondepolarizing muscle relaxants are used during induction and maintenance of anesthesia in neurosurgical patients. Agents that release histamine are avoided, however. Histamine alone may lower blood pressure and increase ICP, thus lowering CPP. When the blood-brain barrier is disrupted, histamine can produce cerebrovasodilation and increases in CBF. Depending on the dose and rate of administration, most of the benzylisoquinolinium compounds (*d*-tubocurarine, metocurine, atracurium, mivacurium) have the potential to release histamine and thus increase ICP. Doxacurium and cisatracurium produce minimal to no histamine release over a wide dose range. Atracurium in intubating doses is reported to have no significant effect on ICP, blood pressure, or CPP in neurosurgical patients. The release of laudanosine by atracurium does not appear to have clinical significance in humans. Laudanosine has been reported to produce seizure activity in animals.

The steroidal compounds (pancuronium, pipecuronium, vecuronium, and rocuronium) may be better relaxants for neurosurgical patients because they do not directly affect ICP. Pancuronium does not produce an increase in CBF, $CMRO_2$, or ICP in dogs.[144] However, pancuronium's vagolytic effects can cause increases in heart rate and blood pressure, which may elevate ICP in patients with disturbed autoregulation. Pipecuronium, another long-acting agent, is reported to have no significant effect on ICP or CPP in patients with intracranial tumors and no hemodynamic side effects. Vecuronium has no effect on ICP, heart rate, or blood pressure in neurosurgical patients. To achieve relatively rapid airway control (within 90 seconds), a priming dose of vecuronium (0.01 mg/kg) can be administered followed by a higher dose (0.10 mg/kg), or high doses of vecuronium (to 0.4 mg/kg) can be safely administered without hemodynamic consequence. Rocuronium also has no effect on ICP in neurosurgical patients, but may have some mild vagolytic activity in higher doses (0.9 mg/kg).

Induction, Maintenance, and Emergence

When the patient is brought into the operating room, a gross neurologic examination should be repeated and documented because changes in the patient's neurologic status can occur overnight. In patients with elevated ICP by clinical exam, CT scan, and/or ICP measurement, osmotherapy may be indicated before induction of anesthesia. After appropriate monitoring devices are applied, the cooperative patient is asked to hyperventilate while preoxygenation is provided. Before laryngoscopy and intubation of the trachea, the patient is smoothly and deeply anesthetized with agents that reduce ICP. In the presence of elevated ICP, thiopental is commonly used to induce anesthesia; however, alternative agents such as propofol or midazolam can be used depending on the patient's medical condition. The following induction sequence is suggested: The intravenous administration of thiopental (3 to 5 mg/kg) or propofol (1.25 to 2.5 mg/kg) is followed by an opioid (fentanyl, 3 to 5 μg/kg) and muscle relaxant. If no airway difficulties are anticipated, a nondepolarizing muscle relaxant is administered while controlled hyperventilation with 100% oxygen is instituted. In patients who have been vomiting because of elevated ICP, cricoid pressure is applied during mask ventilation. To deepen the anesthetic, fentanyl is administered in 50-μg increments to a total dose of 10 μg/kg, depending on the blood pressure response. Lidocaine (1.5 mg/kg) is also administered intravenously 90 seconds before intubation to suppress laryngeal reflexes. When the peripheral muscle twitch response disappears, an additional 2 to 3 mg/kg bolus of thiopental is administered, and endotracheal intubation is performed as rapidly and smoothly as possible. An esmolol infusion or bolus may also be used to reduce the heart rate and blood pressure response to laryngoscopy and intubation. After induction of anesthesia, ventilation of the lung is controlled mechanically. Arterial blood gases are measured after intubation to establish the arterial end-tidal CO_2 gradient.

Routine institution of hyperventilation is no longer recommended in neurosurgical patients because of the risk of cerebral ischemia in some pathologic conditions. In other words, surgical conditions should define the $PaCO_2$ level for each patient. For example, in patients with significant intracranial hypertension or when using volatile agents, $PaCO_2$ is usually adjusted between 30 to 35 mmHg to reduce brain bulk.[146] After direct visualization of the brain and/or discussion with the neurosurgeon, the $PaCO_2$ level should be adjusted as necessary.

Since anesthetics affect the intracranial environment, there continues to be controversy over the best choice of anesthetic technique for neurosurgical patients, that is, intravenous- or volatile-based techniques. In practice, the anesthetics most frequently administered to neurosurgical patients are either propofol-opioid or isoflurane-opioid.[31] The opioids selected are usually fentanyl or remifentanil. There have been no large clinical outcome studies conducted comparing anesthetic techniques. Our choice of anesthetics has been based primarily on information derived from experimental and clinical studies of cerebral hemodynamics (CBF, $CMRO_2$), ICP and recovery characteristics of different agents.

A popular maintenance technique for neurosurgical patients is the continuous infusion of propofol with remifentanil or fentanyl. In brain tumor patients, this technique has been shown to reduce ICP more effectively than either isoflurane or sevoflurane,[31] and in nonneurosurgical patients, propofol with remifentanil produced a quicker emergence than either desflurane or sevoflurane.[147] This technique would seem ideal for neurosurgical patients; however, questions have been raised regarding the risk of cerebral hypoperfusion with propofol anesthesia.[148,149] Studies suggest that propofol anesthesia produces a reduction of CBF larger than a reduction of CMR, resulting in a decrease of the CBF/CMR ratio.[149,150] In susceptible patients, the risk of cerebral hypoperfusion may be even greater when patients are hyperventilated under propofol anesthesia.[149,150]

Nitrous oxide, 50 to 70% in oxygen, is administered by some to decrease the total dose of intravenous agent or the required concentration of volatile agent. The cerebrovascular effects of nitrous oxide are not benign,[38,144] and studies report that at equipotent doses, isoflurane has less adverse effects on ICP and CBF than nitrous oxide. In patients with elevated ICP or low compliance, some clinicians avoid the administration of either nitrous oxide or high concentrations of isoflurane (i.e., greater than 1.0%). Alternatively, an opioid–thiopental or propofol anesthetic technique may be employed with midazolam or low-dose isoflurane added for amnesia. When severe intracranial hypertension exists and the brain is tight despite adequate hyperventilation and the administration of steroids and diuretics, a totally intravenous technique using a thiopental infusion (2 to 3 mg/kg/hr) and fentanyl boluses or infusion (1 to 4 μg/kg/hr) is recommended.

In the usual craniotomy for excision of a supratentorial tumor, the conduct of the anesthetic is aimed at awakening and extubating the patient at the end of the procedure to permit early assessment of surgical results and postoperative neurologic follow-up. The risks and benefits of an early versus delayed recovery in neurosurgical patients have been reviewed.[151] The authors recommend extubation of the neurosurgical patient only when there is complete systemic and brain homeostasis. There are several conditions listed in Table 27-11 that can delay awakening in neurosurgical patients and should be considered prior to developing an extubation plan.

Intracranial hematoma and major cerebral edema are the most feared complications after intracranial surgery. In a retrospective study of 11,214 craniotomy patients, a relationship was demonstrated between perioperative hypertension and the development of postoperative hematomas.[152] Therefore, emergence from anesthesia should be as smooth as possible, avoiding straining or bucking on the endotracheal tube. Bucking can cause arterial hypertension and elevated ICP, which can lead to postoperative hemorrhage and cerebral edema. To avoid bucking, muscle relaxants are not reversed until the head dressing is applied. Intravenous lidocaine (1.5 mg/kg) can be administered 90 seconds before suctioning and extubation to minimize cough, straining, and hypertension. Antihypertensive agents such as labetalol and esmolol also are also administered during emergence to control systemic hypertension.

TABLE 27-11

CAUSES OF DELAYED AWAKENING

Preoperative decreased level of consciousness
Large intracranial tumor
Residual anesthetics
Metabolic or electrolyte disturbances
Residual hypothermia
Surgical complications
- Seizures
- Cerebral edema
- Hematoma
- Pneumocephalus
- Vessel occlusion/ischemia

The patient is extubated only when fully reversed from paralysis, and when he or she is awake and following commands. If the patient is not responsive, the endotracheal tube remains in place until the patient is awake and following commands. A brief neurologic examination is performed before and after extubation of the trachea. The patient is positioned with the head elevated 15 to 30° and transferred to the recovery room with oxygen by mask and oxygen saturation monitoring. Close monitoring and care, including frequent neurologic examinations, are continued in the recovery room.

Awake Craniotomy

Awake craniotomy with functional mapping is recommended for removal of tumors involving the eloquent cortex. Functional mapping is performed by stimulating the brain with a small electrical charge. A neuropsychologist then performs neurocognitive testing and/or monitors motor responses during mapping and later tumor resection. This technique allows maximal tumor resection with minimal postoperative neurological deficits from retraction, edema and/or resection of eloquent tissue. Other advantages include avoidance of general anesthesia and need for more intensive monitoring intra-operatively and postoperatively, a low complication rate, and reduction in resource utilization (e.g., shorter intensive care time and total hospital stay).[153,154]

Preoperative selection, evaluation, and preparation of the patients for awake craniotomy is slightly different than for general anesthesia. The patient must be cooperative and able to participate in neurocognitive testing. In addition, the patient must have an uncomplicated airway and be a candidate for general anesthesia. Most centers provide the patient with detailed information about the procedure and what to expect in verbal, written, and visual form.

In the operating room, there are several challenges for the anesthesiologist. As with any craniotomy, optimal operating conditions providing adequate surgical exposure and brain relaxation are required. For the awake craniotomy, the patient must be positioned very comfortably with bolsters and additional padding. Adequate analgesia and sedation are needed for head frame application, skin incision, craniotomy, and opening of the dura. During cortical mapping and tumor resection, the patient must be fully alert and cooperative, and able to participate in complex neurocognitive testing.

Several different anesthetic protocols have been reported for awake craniotomy.[154] These include neurolept anesthesia, propofol with or without opioid infusions, and asleep, awake, asleep techniques using laryngeal mask airways. Dexmedetomidine, a highly specific α-2 adrenoreceptor agonist, has been recommended for use during awake craniotomy.[155] It has the advantage of providing sedation and analgesia without respiratory depression.

All awake procedures with sedation run the risk of respiratory depression and poor patient cooperation. Complications such as seizures, increased ICP, hypertension, nausea, and vomiting, which are more likely to occur during craniotomy, also require prompt treatment.[153,156] Most anesthetic protocols include prophylaxis with antihypertensives, anticonvulsants and antiemetics to prevent these complications from occurring.

Infratentorial Intracranial Tumors

11 The perioperative management of infratentorial tumors poses significant surgical and anesthetic challenges because of the relatively confined space within the posterior fossa. The posterior fossa contains the medulla, pons, cerebellum, major motor and sensory pathways, primary respiratory and cardiovascular centers, and lower cranial nerve nuclei. Because of the posterior fossa's small size, a localized tumor can significantly compromise these vital brainstem structures and cranial nerves. Consequently, when evaluating patients with infratentorial tumors, the anesthesiologist should be aware that these patients have the potential to develop profound neurologic damage. Patients may exhibit depressed levels of consciousness secondary to increased ICP from obstructive hydrocephalus and/or exhibit signs of brainstem compression with depressed respiration and cranial nerve palsies. Preoperative endotracheal intubation and respiratory support may be required.

Special Anesthetic Considerations

Patient Position. A major challenge of infratentorial surgery is preventing further neurologic damage from the position of the patient and exploration. There is considerable controversy among neurosurgeons as to the best position for infratentorial surgery.[157]

Exploration of the posterior fossa has been traditionally performed in the sitting position because it provides excellent surgical exposure and facilitates venous and CSF drainage. From the standpoint of the anesthesiologist, the sitting position provides better ventilation and easier access to the chest, airway, endotracheal tube, and extremities. Furthermore, facial and conjunctival edema is reduced. However, the sitting position is associated with significant risks. In older or debilitated patients, the sitting position can produce cardiovascular instability, resulting in hypotension with cerebral and cardiovascular compromise. A significant risk of venous air embolism occurs in patients operated on in the sitting position, and an attendant risk of paradoxical air embolism may also occur in patients with a patent foramen ovale or other right-to-left shunt.

Other problems associated with the sitting position are peripheral nerve injury, pneumocephalus, jugular venous obstruction, and quadriplegia. Peripheral nerve injuries to the ulnar, sciatic, or lateral peroneal nerves can result if care is not taken in positioning and padding the respective pressure points. Pneumocephalus occurs frequently in patients who have surgery performed in the sitting position.[157] Pneumocephalus may develop into tension pneumocephalus postoperatively, producing serious neurologic dysfunction. Nitrous oxide has been implicated in the pathogenesis of tension pneumocephalus.[157] Because of this, when used, nitrous oxide should be discontinued before dural and cranial closure and avoided if surgery recurs within 14 days. Jugular venous obstruction causing swelling of the face and tongue may result from hyperflexion of the neck. To avoid this, head flexion should be limited by placing two fingers between the mandible and sternum. Paraplegia, triplegia, and quadriplegia have been reported following surgery in the sitting position. This complication has been attributed to mechanical compression of the cervical spinal cord or vertebrobasilar blood vessels and stretching of spinal cord blood vessels, causing ischemia during head flexion. If hypotension occurs, the brainstem and cervical spinal cord are rendered even more vulnerable to an ischemic insult. During positioning for posterior fossa exploration, cases of position-related brainstem and cervical spinal cord ischemia have been reported. Therefore, flexion of the head on the cervical spine may be hazardous in some patients with large posterior fossa tumors and in elderly or arthritic patients. A preoperative examination of the mobility of the cervical spine, including a review of radiologic studies to determine the width of the cervical canal, should be performed to establish whether the patient can tolerate the position required for surgery. In addition, the application of SEP monitoring during positioning for surgery may be used to detect position-related ischemia.

Other positions used for posterior fossa exploration are the lateral, prone, and "park bench" or three-fourths prone positions. These alternative positions have been advocated because of the lower incidence of air emboli and greater cardiovascular stability associated with them. Potential disadvantages of these positions are malignant cerebellar edema and venous hemorrhage. To date, there is no evidence that operative position affects postoperative outcome. In a study that reviewed 579 posterior fossa craniectomies, patients in the sitting position had less blood loss and postoperative cranial nerve dysfunction than patients operated on in the horizontal position (supine, prone, lateral, and park bench), and there was no difference in the incidence of hypotension and postoperative cardiopulmonary complications between groups.[158] The incidence of venous air embolism in this series of patients was significantly greater in sitting versus horizontal patients (45 vs. 12%), but it was not associated with a significantly increased morbidity or mortality.[158] The authors concluded that there are significant advantages and disadvantages to both sitting and horizontal positions and that these positions can be used safely.

Because of various advantages and disadvantages to both sitting and horizontal positions, no one best position exists for all patients requiring exploration of the posterior fossa. The selection of the most appropriate position for an individual patient should be based on the location of the tumor, surgical exposure, the patient's medical condition, and consideration of the risks and benefits.

Monitoring. During posterior fossa exploration, surgical retraction or manipulation of the brainstem or cranial nerves can cause significant cardiac dysrhythmia or alterations in blood pressure. Adequate warning of brainstem compromise is obtained by monitoring the ECG for alterations in cardiac rate and rhythm. In addition, direct arterial pressure monitoring provides continuous information on sudden changes in systemic blood pressure and an estimate of CPP. (To estimate CPP in the sitting position, the arterial transducer should be zeroed to the highest point on the skull.) The hemodynamic consequences of dysrhythmias or air embolism are also instantly recognized with direct arterial pressure monitoring.

Electrophysiologic monitoring of SEPs is used to detect ischemia and compromise of the brainstem or cranial nerves. For example, BAEPs are monitored during surgery for acoustic neuroma to help preserve function of cranial nerve VIII or during posterior fossa procedures to monitor brainstem ischemia. Depending on the tumor's location, SSEPs may also be used to detect brainstem compromise. Position-related ischemia has been observed during monitoring with either BAEPs or SSEPs. Electromyography is used during resection of acoustic neuromas and microvascular decompression to test seventh nerve function when the face is not accessible to palpation or visual assessment.

Venous Air Embolism. Venous air embolism may occur whenever the operative field is elevated 5 cm or more above the right atrial level. Whereas the incidence of air embolism is on average 40 to 45% in patients operated on in the sitting position, entrainment of air also occurs during operations performed in the lateral, supine, or prone positions. The primary pathophysiologic event in venous air embolism is intense vasoconstriction of the pulmonary circulation, which results in ventilation/perfusion mismatch, interstitial pulmonary edema, and reduced cardiac output as pulmonary vascular resistance increases.

Air may also pass directly through the pulmonary circulation or through right-to-left intracardiac shunts (e.g., probe-patent foramen ovale) to the coronary and cerebral circulation when right atrial pressure exceeds left atrial pressure. A patent foramen ovale exists in 20 to 30% of the population on autopsy study. In the sitting position, a reported 50% of patients develop right atrial pressure greater than left atrial pressure and thus have the potential for paradoxical air embolism. The calculated risk of paradoxical air embolism is 5 to 10%. Preoperative screening with precordial two-dimensional contrast echocardiography during a Valsalva maneuver and cough has been suggested as a method to identify patients with patent foramen ovale. An alternative technique is to perform contrast TEE with a ventilation maneuver after induction of anesthesia, but before surgery.[159] If a patent foramen ovale is detected with either screening method, a position other than sitting is recommended for surgery because of the risk of paradoxical air embolism.

Monitors used for detecting venous air embolism are listed in Table 27-12. The two-dimensional transesophageal echocardiogram detects air bubbles with an echocardiographic probe placed behind the heart. The transesophageal echocardiogram is slightly more sensitive than the precordial Doppler, but is invasive and cumbersome. The transesophageal echocardiogram has the advantage of monitoring air in the right and left cardiac chambers and the aorta, and thus can be used to detect both venous and arterial air embolism.

The precordial Doppler ultrasound transducer is the most sensitive noninvasive monitor of venous air embolism. It detects amounts of air as small as 0.25 mL. The transducer is positioned along the right parasternal border between the third and sixth intercostal spaces to maximize audible signals from the right atrium. Proper placement is confirmed by rapid injection of 5–10 mL of saline into a right atrial catheter. The resultant turbulent flow changes the Doppler sounds to a high-pitched noise similar to the sounds produced by intravascular air.

TABLE 27-12

MONITORS FOR DETECTION OF VENOUS AIR EMBOLISM

Most Sensitive
- Transesophageal echocardiography
- Precordial Doppler
- Pulmonary artery catheter (↑ PAP)
- Capnography (↓ $ETCO_2$)
- Mass spectrometry (↑ ETN_2, most specific and quantitative)

Least Sensitive

PAP = pulmonary artery pressure; $ETCO_2$ = end-tidal carbon dioxide; ETN_2 = end-tidal nitrogen.

Pulmonary artery (PA) catheterization has been advocated for patients who undergo surgery in the sitting position. Passage of air into the pulmonary circulation leads to mechanical obstruction and reflex vasoconstriction from local hypoxemia. The PA catheter detects the resultant hypertension. (The change in pulmonary artery pressure correlates with the hemodynamic significance of the embolus because pulmonary artery pressure increases proportionally with the volume of air entering the pulmonary arteries.) Pulmonary artery pressure measurement is slightly more sensitive than capnography for detecting venous air embolism, but it is invasive. The PA catheter lumen is poorly designed for air aspiration. In addition, the fixed distance between the PA catheter tip and the right atrial port makes it difficult to position for both pulmonary capillary wedge pressure measurement and air aspiration. The catheter can be used to identify patients at risk for paradoxical air embolism, that is, patients who develop right atrial pressure greater than pulmonary capillary wedge pressure. When this occurs, measures to elevate pulmonary capillary wedge pressure, such as volume loading or repositioning, are undertaken.

In the operating room, exhaled gases can be measured by infrared analysis, mass spectrometers, and analyzers based on Raman scattering. The infrared absorption technique is the most popular method of measuring the concentration of CO_2 in the airway. The capnograph is very useful for diagnosing venous air embolism. Small volumes of intravascular air produce a ventilation/perfusion mismatch, which is reflected in a reduced end-tidal CO_2. The capnograph complements the capabilities of the precordial Doppler by differentiating hemodynamically insignificant emboli that are heard with the Doppler from significant emboli. Doppler sounds without reduction in end-tidal CO_2 usually indicate insignificant amounts of air.

End-tidal N_2 monitoring is specific for detecting air but is slightly less sensitive than end-tidal CO_2 in detecting subclinical air embolism. As intravascular air in the pulmonary circulation crosses the capillary–alveolar membrane, it is exhaled, increasing the end-tidal N_2 concentration. The advantage of knowing the value of the end-expired N_2 is the ability to calculate the volume of air entrained. When a patient is ventilated with an air–oxygen mixture, the increase in end-tidal N_2 with venous air embolism may not be evident. In addition, other causes of increases in end-tidal N_2 must be eliminated, such as a leak in the breathing circuit or an incomplete seal around the endotracheal tube cuff.

A central venous pressure catheter is inserted whenever there is a risk for venous air embolism. When the catheter is correctly positioned, entrained air can be aspirated from the right atrium. It is suggested that the optimal position for the tip of a single orifice catheter is 3.0 cm above the superior vena cava and the right atrial junction. The position of the right atrial catheter may be confirmed by a chest film, by using a saline-filled catheter as a unipolar lead and following the configuration of the P waves on the ECG, or by transducing a venous waveform. Multiorifice right atrial catheters are more effective than single-orifice catheters in aspirating air from the circulation.

Early diagnosis of air embolism is essential for successful treatment. The precordial Doppler unit is considered the basic monitoring device for detection of air embolism and is most effective when used in conjunction with end-tidal monitoring. The clinical significance of air embolism detected by Doppler ultrasonography can be assessed by a decrease in end-expired C_2 or an increase in pulmonary artery pressure. A Doppler in conjunction with either a capnograph or a PA catheter usually detects air before physiologic alteration begins. Treatment is directed at preventing further influx of air. Whenever air embolism is suspected, the surgeon is notified immediately. The surgical field is flooded with saline and packed, and bone edges are waxed. Nitrous oxide, if present, is discontinued to prevent further expansion of embolized air. Neck veins are compressed as a means of increasing jugular venous pressure, which prevents further air entry and helps to localize the source of air. Aspiration of air from the right atrial catheter is attempted. With significant air embolism, patient position should be changed to lower the head to heart level when possible. If necessary, vasopressors and volume infusion are administered to treat hypotension. Positive end-expiratory pressure or Valsalva maneuver are avoided because they increase right atrial pressure and the likelihood of paradoxical embolus from venous air embolism.

Anesthetic Management. When selecting an anesthetic technique for patients in the sitting position, conditions of particular concern are cardiovascular stability and risk of air embolism. In changing an anesthetized patient from the supine to sitting position, a mild transient postural hypotension occurs in about one third of cases and marked hypotension in about 2 to 5% of cases.[144,157] General anesthesia with positive-pressure ventilation is associated with a reduction in blood pressure mainly caused by a decrease in cardiac output. As patients are placed into the sitting position, venous return is impeded, causing further reductions in cardiac output and blood pressure. Therefore, efforts are directed at promoting venous return and maintaining cardiac output during the anesthetic management of these patients. An anesthetic technique that causes the least impairment of cardiovascular performance should be administered when patients are placed in the sitting position. Measures to avoid hypotension are also instituted. These include adequate preoperative hydration, wrapping the legs with elastic bandages, and flexing the patient's hips and knees at heart level. The patient's position is slowly changed, titrating position against systemic blood pressure. Administration of fluids (balanced salt solutions) and small amounts of vasopressors may be necessary.

The choice of anesthetic technique must take into account the hemodynamic consequences of the selected surgical position and the requirements of facial or evoked potential monitoring. In sitting position cases, the use of nitrous oxide remains controversial because of the potential to expand embolized air or contribute to tension pneumocephalus.[144,157] Because of these concerns, an anesthetic technique without nitrous oxide is usually administered, for example, air–oxygen, potent inhalation agent with opioids and muscle relaxant. When electrophysiologic monitoring is instituted, a propofol-based intravenous technique with opioid and muscle relaxant is recommended, and for facial nerve monitoring, this technique without supplementary administration of muscle relaxant provides successful monitoring conditions.

Postoperative Concerns. The potential for significant cardiorespiratory and neurologic deterioration exists in the immediate postoperative period following posterior fossa exploration. Therefore, direct arterial pressure and ECG monitoring should be continued for the first 24 to 48 hours postoperatively, and neurologic examinations should be performed frequently.

Central apnea requiring postoperative ventilatory support may result from damage to respiratory centers caused by extensive posterior fossa exploration. If respiratory centers have been manipulated but not destroyed, respiratory impairment is temporary. Postoperative impairment of swallowing and pharyngeal sensation may occur secondary to stretch or manipulation of cranial nerves IX, X, and XII. These patients are at increased risk for aspiration pneumonia or hypoxia and therefore should remain intubated until airway protective reflexes return.

Systemic hypertension frequently occurs after posterior fossa surgery and requires immediate treatment to prevent brain edema and hematoma formation. Postoperative hypertension usually resolves within the first 24 hours. Atrial and ventricular ectopic beats may also occur within the first 24 hours.

Because of the proximity of respiratory and cardiovascular centers, any edema, hematoma, or infarction of the brainstem and cerebellum can produce serious compromise. When a patient fails to awaken satisfactorily from anesthesia, bleeding or acute swelling of the structures in the posterior fossa must be suspected. In addition, patients who are awake and talking may become unresponsive secondary to obstructive hydrocephalus or brainstem compression. Decreased level of consciousness is an early reliable sign of brainstem compression. More serious signs are systemic hypertension, bradycardia, and irregular or absent respirations. Reintubation and prompt surgical intervention to relieve pressure on the brainstem are necessary.

The preoperative level of consciousness and intra-operative conditions will determine whether the patient is extubated at the end of the procedure. A patient with a depressed level of consciousness preoperatively should not be expected to improve immediately after surgery. In general, patients who require preoperative mechanical ventilation usually require postoperative mechanical ventilation. Furthermore, if the surgical procedure is extensive, producing an engorged, swollen brain, postoperative mechanical ventilation is usually necessary.

Pituitary Tumors

The pituitary gland is located at the base of the skull in the sella turcica, a bony cavity within the sphenoid bone, and it is divided into anterior (adenohypophysis) and posterior (neurohypophysis) lobes. A fold of dura (the diaphragma sella) on the superior surface of the sella is pierced by the infundibular stalk, which connects the posterior lobe of the pituitary gland to the hypothalamus. The hypothalamus regulates hormone release from the anterior pituitary through regulatory peptides (hypothalamic releasing and inhibiting factors) that reach the anterior pituitary by a complex portal vascular system. Control of hypothalamic secretion is complex and occurs from neuronal and chemical influences, including feedback from target organ hormones. The larger glandular anterior pituitary secretes at least seven hormones. The smaller posterior pituitary stores and secretes two hormones, antidiuretic hormone and oxytocin, which are synthesized in specialized hypothalamic neurons and transported as granules in axons down the pituitary stalk to the posterior pituitary gland. The anterior and posterior pituitary hormones are listed in Table 27-13.

Pituitary tumors can be divided into two general categories, nonfunctioning and hypersecreting. Nonfunctioning pituitary tumors are usually diagnosed when they become large and produce symptoms related to mass effects by impinging on adjacent structures. Headache, impaired vision, cranial nerve palsies, increased ICP, and hypopituitarism may result. The most common nonfunctioning tumors are chromophobe adenomas, craniopharyngiomas, and meningiomas. As these tumors enlarge, they can cause selective or global impairment of pituitary function by compressing the normal gland. A sudden enlargement of the pituitary caused by spontaneous hemorrhage or infarction into the tumor produces a symptom complex known as pituitary apoplexy, a life-threatening condition characterized by acute neurologic deficits and a rapid decline in pituitary function. Therapy includes rapid administration of corticosteroids and emergency surgical decompression.

Functioning pituitary adenomas produce an excess of one or more of the anterior pituitary hormones, and therefore are usually diagnosed when the tumors are small. The most frequently occurring are prolactinomas followed by growth hormone- and adrenocorticotropin-secreting adenomas. Adenomas secreting thyrotropin or follicle-stimulating hormone and luteinizing hormone are rare. Adenomas secreting both growth hormone and prolactin are common, however. Prolactinomas may produce the amenorrhea-galactorrhea syndrome in females and decreased libido and impotence in males. Excessive production of growth hormone before puberty results in gigantism; after puberty, in acromegaly. Cushing's disease develops from an adrenocorticotropin-secreting adenoma that causes bilateral adrenal hyperplasia.

Special Anesthetic Considerations

Preoperative Evaluation. The preoperative evaluation of patients with pituitary tumors requires an assessment of endocrine function and associated medical disorders. Endocrine tests are performed in the basal state and are supplemented by appropriate provocative tests (Table 27-14). These tests diagnose hyperfunctioning or hypofunctioning tumors, the extent of endocrine disturbance, and the adequacy of treatment.

In Cushing's disease, the increased corticotropin and cortisol can produce multiple systemic effects such as diabetes mellitus with insulin-resistant hyperglycemia, hyperaldosteronism with hypokalemia and metabolic alkalosis, hypertension, mild congestive heart failure, and obesity. These patients require preoperative evaluation and management of hypertension, diabetes, and electrolyte imbalances, as well as a cardiovascular evaluation for ischemic heart disease and congestive heart failure.

TABLE 27-13

PITUITARY GLAND HORMONES

■ ANTERIOR PITUITARY	■ POSTERIOR PITUITARY
Growth hormone	Antidiuretic hormone
Prolactin	Oxytocin
Gonadotropins:	
Follicle-stimulating hormone	
Luteinizing hormone	
Adrenocorticotropin (ACTH)	
β-Lipotropin	
Thyrotropin (TSH)	

TABLE 27-14

PREOPERATIVE ENDOCRINE STUDIES FOR PITUITARY TUMORS

■ ANTERIOR PITUITARY FUNCTION TESTS

Basal levels of pituitary hormones: GH, prolactin, ACTH, TSH, FSH, LH
Serum levels: cortisol (AM and PM), thyroxine, testosterone, estradiol
Urinary levels: 17-ketosteroids, 17-hydroxycorticosteroids, free cortisol, estrogens
Provocative and suppression tests as indicated:
- GH reserve—glucagon stimulation
- GH suppression—glucose suppression (acromegaly)
- Prolactin reserve—chlorpromazine or thyrotropin-releasing hormone provocative testing
- Low- and high-dose dexamethasone suppression (Cushing's syndrome)
- Metyrapone test (Cushing's syndrome)

■ POSTERIOR PITUITARY FUNCTION TESTS

ADH reserve: Serum and urine osmolality before and after 8–12 hours' water deprivation.

Patients with acromegaly exhibit a general overgrowth of skeletal, connective, and soft tissues. Hands and feet become markedly enlarged and facial features become coarse. All major organs increase in size, including the heart, lungs, liver, and kidneys. These patients also require an evaluation for systemic hypertension, diabetes, ischemic heart disease, cardiomegaly, and congestive heart failure, with appropriate medical management instituted before surgery. Significant anatomic airway changes can occur in acromegalics, making airway management difficult. Facial bone hypertrophy, particularly of the mandible and nose, thick tongue and lips, and hypertrophy of nasal turbinates, soft palate, tonsils, epiglottis, and larynx create difficulties with mask fit and visualization of the larynx. Glottic stenosis caused by soft tissue overgrowth may cause preoperative hoarseness and dyspnea. These patients usually require a smaller endotracheal tube than anticipated based on the size of the patient's facial features, and may be predisposed to postextubation edema. Stretching or compression of the recurrent laryngeal nerves from laryngeal soft tissue or thyroid gland enlargement may result in vocal cord paralysis. Because of these anatomic changes, a thorough preoperative airway examination is required. Patients complaining of hoarseness, dyspnea, or inspiratory stridor should undergo indirect laryngoscopy and x-ray examination of the neck to analyze airway conformation and lumen diameter. Based on this evaluation, preparations for difficult airway management and intubation should be anticipated. For patients with difficult airways and glottic abnormalities, an awake fiberoptic intubation is recommended. This obviates the need for a tracheostomy in all but the most severe cases. Patients without upper airway or vocal cord involvement can be managed in the routine manner.

Pressure effects on the normal pituitary gland from parasellar tumors or other lesions can cause panhypopituitarism. Patients who have panhypopituitarism require replacement therapy with appropriate hormones. These patients should be euthyroid before surgery. Glucocorticoid replacement is required when thyroxine replacement is begun to avoid stressing the insufficient adrenocortical axis. Because glucocorticoids are also necessary to facilitate renal excretion of a water load, diabetes insipidus is usually not observed in the patient with pituitary insufficiency until cortisol replacement therapy is instituted. Preoperatively, the patient with panhypopituitarism will be receiving oral steroid and thyroxine therapy and, when indicated, intranasal instillation of synthetic vasopressin.

During the preanesthetic evaluation, the size and location of the tumor and its effect on intracranial dynamics should be determined. Pituitary microadenomas do not produce mass effects. Pituitary tumors with suprasellar extension, craniopharyngiomas, and other suprasellar tumors may exert a mass effect. In these patients, the CT scan or MRI and the neurologic examination are evaluated for signs of increased ICP. All patients scheduled for pituitary surgery are given supplemental short-acting glucocorticoid therapy perioperatively. Because the surgery involves manipulation or removal of the anterior pituitary, transient or permanent deficiency of adrenocorticotropin and cortisol secretion may result. To assess function of the optic nerves and chiasm, a visual examination, including examination of the visual fields, is performed. When transsphenoidal surgery is planned, an otolaryngologic examination of the nasal passages and nasopharynx is also performed, and a nasal culture is obtained to guide antibiotic therapy in the event of postoperative infection.

Surgical Considerations. Since the introduction of the operating microscope, transsphenoidal excision has been recommended for all pituitary tumors that do not have marked suprasellar extension. Advantages of the transsphenoidal approach include the following: lower morbidity and mortality rates with decreased incidence and severity of diabetes insipidus; elimination of frontal lobe retraction and external scars; magnified visualization and removal of small tumors, which spares normal tissue; decreased frequency of blood transfusions; and shorter hospitalization. Relative disadvantages include the possibility of CSF leakage and meningitis (which is rare with the use of antibiotics), inability to visualize neural structures adjacent to a large tumor, inaccessibility of tumors extending into middle and anterior fossae, and the possibility of bleeding from cavernous sinuses or carotid arteries (which can lead to intracranial hemorrhage, brainstem compression, and significant blood loss). The transcranial approach to the sella permits direct visualization of suprasellar structures: the vascular sinus ring, optic chiasm, hypothalamus, and pituitary stalk. This approach is recommended for pituitary tumors of uncertain diagnosis and those that have significant suprasellar extension with optic nerve or hypothalamic involvement. With this approach, there is potential for damage to the olfactory nerves, frontal lobe vasculature, and optic nerves and chiasm. In addition, the incidence of permanent diabetes insipidus and anterior pituitary insufficiency is increased.

Anesthetic Considerations. The anesthetic management of patients undergoing pituitary surgery is not fundamentally different from that of patients undergoing other craniotomies. Basic neuroanesthetic principles apply whether the transsphenoidal or transcranial approach is used. With the transcranial approach, however, intra-operative measures to control ICP are instituted because of pressure effects, the necessity for brain retraction, and the potential for greater blood loss.

During transsphenoidal procedures, central venous pressure is not routinely monitored. When the patient is positioned with a significant head-up tilt, however, air embolism may occur during this procedure. Therefore, precordial Doppler monitoring and right atrial catheterization are recommended for detection and treatment of air embolism when a significant surgical site–cardiac gradient (15° or more) exists.

Evoked potential monitoring of VEPs may be used during pituitary surgery to monitor direct compression or compromise of blood supply to optic nerves and chiasm. Technical difficulties that cause intra-operative recording problems include changes in pupil size, deviation of eyes, goggle size and bulkiness, and stimulus delivery (light flashes). Because VEPs are entirely cortical in origin, they are also more vulnerable to the effects of general anesthetics.

For transsphenoidal procedures, a sublabial incision and dissection through the nasal septum is performed; therefore, oral endotracheal intubation is required. The nasal septum can be prepared with 4% cocaine pledgets placed in the nares, followed by injection of 2% lidocaine with epinephrine 1:200,000 into the submucosa. This combination develops a dissection plane, decreases bleeding, and buffers the hypertensive response to nasal dissection. Initially, the cocaine and epinephrine may cause hypertension, tachycardia, and dysrhythmias, and drugs to treat these responses should be available. After oral endotracheal intubation with a RAE tube, the oropharynx is packed with saline-soaked gauze to minimize blood pooling in the glottis, esophagus, and stomach. Intra-operative C-arm fluoroscopy of the skull (lateral views) is used during this procedure, rendering the patient's head and arms relatively inaccessible once the patient is draped.

Potential intraoperative complications during transsphenoidal procedures relate to the anatomic landmarks surrounding the sella turcica. The cavernous sinuses occupy the lateral walls of the sella and contain venous structures, the internal carotid artery, and cranial nerves III, IV, V, and VI. The optic chiasm, with its associated optic nerves and tracts, lies directly above the diaphragma sella in front of the pituitary stalk. Surgical manipulation in the region surrounding the sella can result in the following: hemorrhage from the venous sinuses or internal carotid artery, arterial spasm or thrombotic occlusion secondary to arterial manipulation, venous air embolism if head-up tilt is excessive, cranial nerve weakness secondary to trauma or stretching, and visual complications secondary to damage of the optic nerve or chiasm.[160]

The chosen anesthetic technique should permit gross visual acuity examination before patient extubation. If vision is the same or improved, extubation can proceed. If acuity is worse, further diagnostic studies and emergent decompressive surgery may be required. After transsphenoidal surgery, the patient will awaken with nasal packing, necessitating mouth breathing postoperatively. Therefore, these patients must be fully awake and following commands before extubation of the trachea.

Postoperative Concerns. In the immediate postoperative period after either transsphenoidal or transcranial procedures, the primary concerns are corticosteroid coverage and fluid balance. Dexamethasone followed by prednisone is given for 5 days after surgery or until postoperative testing shows an intact pituitary–adrenal axis. Fluid balance is assessed by strict attention to hourly fluid intake and output and urine specific gravity. Development of diabetes insipidus is uncommon during surgery but may occur early in the postoperative course. Diabetes insipidus is commonly seen during the first 12 hours postoperatively and usually lasts for 2 to 4 days. Diagnosis is based on the following: polyuria (2 to 15 L/day), hypernatremia, high serum osmolality (≥300 mOsm/kg), decreased urine osmolality (200 mOsm/kg), and decreased urine specific gravity (1.005 or less). Therapy includes replacement of urine losses with intravenous fluids. When urine volumes are excessive, exogenous vasopressin is given, for example, aqueous vasopressin (5 to 10 IU, iv or im, q 6 hr) or the synthetic analog of ADH, desmopressin acetate (0.5 to 2 μg, iv, q 8 hr; 1 to 4 mg, sc q 6 to 12 hr; or nasal inhalation 10 to 20 μg).

Other complications of pituitary tumor surgery include CSF rhinorrhea, hypothalamic injury or stroke, cerebral ischemia, and meningitis. After transsphenoidal surgery, patients must be carefully monitored in the recovery room for airway obstruction caused by bleeding and secretions in the pharynx. Frequent neurologic examinations are performed to note any changes in mental status. Patients who have had an uncomplicated hospital course after transsphenoidal surgery are often discharged within 5 to 6 days.

Cerebrovascular Malformations

Intracranial Aneurysms

SAH from rupture of an intracranial aneurysm is a devastating disease, affecting an estimated 27,000 Americans annually.[161,162] Despite considerable advances in the management of these patients, outcome remains poor with overall mortality rates of 25% and significant morbidity among approximately 50% of survivors. In the most recent studies, the overall incidence of SAH is 8 to 10 per 100,000 people. The peak incidence for rupture is in the fifth and sixth decades of life and is greater for women than men. Several potential risk factors for aneurysm rupture have been identified (Table 27-15).

The management of patients with unruptured intracranial aneurysms (UIAs) remains controversial.[162–165] The International Study of Unruptured Intracranial Aneurysms (ISUIA) was recently published.[165] Four thousand, sixty patients were assessed—1,692 did not undergo aneurysmal repair, 1,917 underwent open surgery, and 451 underwent endovascular procedures. The study revealed that rupture rates were often equaled or exceeded by the risks associated with surgical or endovascular repair of comparable lesions. Patients' age was a strong predictor of surgical outcome; the size and location of an aneurysm predicted both surgical and endovascular outcomes.

TABLE 27-15

POTENTIAL RISK FACTORS FOR ANEURYSM RUPTURE

- Cigarette smoking
- Hypertension
- Alcohol consumption
- Cocaine and amphetamine abuse
- Oral contraceptive use
- Plasma cholesterol >6.3 mmol/l
- Genetic conditions, e.g., ADPKD
- Familial (first-degree relatives)

A patient with aneurysmal SAH is classified according to the Hunt and Hess Classification (Table 27-16) or the World Federation of Neurosurgeons (WFNS) SAH scale (Table 27-17). These classifications are used by neurosurgeons to estimate surgical risk and outcome. Higher grades, or patients who are clinically more impaired, are associated with the presence of cerebral vasospasm, intracranial hypertension, and increased surgical mortality. In general, the poorer the grade on hospital admission, the worse the prognosis.

The presence of blood in the subarachnoid space causes an abrupt, marked rise in ICP, which often results in systemic hypertension and dysrhythmias. The abrupt increase in ICP accounts for the acute onset of a sudden, severe headache. The classic presentation of aneurysmal SAH is that of severe headache associated with stiff neck, photophobia, nausea, vomiting, and often transient loss of consciousness. With this presentation, the diagnosis of SAH is obvious. In about 50% of patients, a small bleed or "warning leak" precedes a major aneurysmal rupture. Warning symptoms and signs tend to be mild and nonspecific (headache, dizziness, orbital pain, slight motor or sensory disturbance) and are generally ignored or misdiagnosed by both patient and physician.

The diagnosis of SAH is made by the combination of clinical findings and a noncontrast CT scan of the head. When performed within a day of aneurysm rupture, CT reveals high-density (white) blood clot in basal subarachnoid cisterns in about 95% of patients. This has traditionally been followed by selected cerebral angiography to document the presence and anatomic features of the aneurysm. More recently, spiral CT angiography (CTA) has been used for detection and evaluation

TABLE 27-16

HUNT AND HESS CLASSIFICATION OF PATIENTS WITH SUBARACHNOID HEMORRHAGE

GRADE	CRITERIA
0	Unruptured aneurysm
I	Asymptomatic, or minimal, headache and slight nuchal rigidity
II	Moderate to severe headache, nuchal rigidity, no neurologic deficit other than cranial nerve palsy
III	Drowsiness, confusion, or mild focal deficit
IV	Stupor, moderate to severe hemiparesis, early decerebration, vegetative disturbance
V	Deep coma, decerebrate rigidity, moribund

(Adapted from Hunt WE, Hess RM: Surgical risk as related to time of intervention in the repair of intracranial aneurysms. J Neurosurg 28:14, 1968.)

TABLE 27-17

WORLD FEDERATION OF NEUROSURGEONS (WFNS) SAH SCALE

WFNS GRADE	GCS SCALE[a]	MOTOR DEFICIT
I	15	Absent
II	13–14	Absent
III	13–14	Present
IV	7–12	Present or absent
V	3–6	Present or absent

SAH = subarachnoid hemorrhage; GCS = Glasgow Coma Scale.
[a] Refer to Table 27-20 for definition of scale.
(Adapted from Drake CG, Hunt WE, Sank K *et al:* Report of World Federation of Neurological Surgeons Committee on a universal subarachnoid hemorrhage grading scale. J Neurosurg 68:985, 1988.)

of intracranial aneurysms. Compared to conventional angiography, the minimally invasive CTA has high specificity, sensitivity and diagnostic accuracy in detecting intracranial aneurysms.

Aneurysms are classified according to location and size. They arise at a branch of bifurcation, usually at a point where a major vessel makes a turn changing the axial flow of blood.

Complications. There are several potential complications of SAH and surgical treatment of aneurysms (Table 27-18). The most important of these are intracranial hypertension, rebleeding, vasospasm, and hydrocephalus.

Rebleeding occurs most commonly during the first 24 hours following initial SAH. The chance of rebleeding is about 4% within the first day; after 48 hours, it is 1.5% per day, with a cumulative rebleeding rate of 19% by the end of 2 weeks.[166] Recurrent aneurysmal hemorrhage is a devastating complication associated with increased morbidity and mortality.

Because of the incidence of rebleeding with conservative management of SAH, early aneurysm clipping (days 0 to 3) is currently recommended for patients who are alert on admission. The debate over "early versus late" surgery was largely resolved following the report of The International Cooperative Study on the Timing of Aneurysm Surgery (ICSTAS).[167,168] In this trial, overall management results demonstrated a similar mortality (20%) and good outcome (60%) for patients with surgery planned for early (0 to 3 days) and late (11 to 14 days) intervals. The least favorable outcome and highest mortality occurred in patients with planned surgery for days 7 to 10 after SAH. Patients who were alert on admission did best with early surgery. When only the North American patients were analyzed, early surgery (days 0 to 3) provided the best results in lower grade patients.[168] There was no difference in the incidence of intra-operative rupture between early and late surgery, and although there was a relationship between "tightness" of the brain during surgery and the interval from SAH to operation, aneurysm dissection was no more difficult in early than in late surgery.[168] The timing of surgery does not influence the risk for cerebral vasospasm.

Cerebral vasospasm is a major cause of morbidity and mortality in SAH patients.[167] Angiographic evidence of vasospasm can be detected in up to 70% of patients. However, clinical vasospasm with ischemic deficits is observed in approximately 30% of patients, most often between days 4 and 12, with a peak at 6 to 7 days following SAH.[167] The clinical syndrome of vasospasm is often heralded by worsening headache and increasing blood pressure. It is characterized by progressive symptoms of confusion and lethargy, followed by focal motor and speech impairments corresponding to the arterial territory involved. The syndrome may resolve gradually or progress to coma and death within a period of hours to days. The diagnosis of vasospasm is confirmed by angiography. The transcranial Doppler (TCD) is a safe, repeatable, noninvasive method to identify and quantify vasospasm and can be used to evaluate the effectiveness of various therapies.

The mechanism responsible for vasospasm is unknown; however, structural and pathologic changes have been demonstrated in the vessel wall. There is also evidence that vasospasm after SAH correlates with the amount of blood in the subarachnoid space, and removal of extravasated blood decreases the occurrence and severity of ischemic deficits. The component in blood implicated in causing cerebral arterial vasospasm is oxyhemoglobin.

Many drugs have been investigated for prevention or treatment of vasospasm but most are ineffective. The calcium channel blocker nimodipine has become standard prophylactic therapy. However, the efficacy of prophylactic nimodipine after SAH has been seriously challenged.[102] A meta-analysis showed a reduction in vasospasm in nimodipine groups, but a corresponding reduction in mortality was slight and not statistically significant compared to control groups.

"Triple-H" therapy—hypervolemia, hypertension, and hemodilution—has become the mainstay of treatment for ischemic neurologic deficits caused by cerebral vasospasm.[170,171] To improve cerebral blood flow to areas of impaired autoregulation, cerebral perfusion pressure is increased by intravascular volume expansion and induced hypertension. Intravascular volume expansion is accomplished with infusion of crystalloid, colloid, or blood to a pulmonary capillary wedge pressure of 12 to 18 mmHg or a central venous pressure of 10–12 mmHg. If this regimen does not reverse the deficit, a vasopressor (e.g., dopamine) is introduced to raise systemic blood pressure until the neurologic deficits subside or reverse. This therapy can worsen cerebral edema, increase ICP, and cause hemorrhagic infarction. Systemic complications include pulmonary edema and cardiac failure in patients at risk. Hemodilution, the last component of triple-H therapy, decreases blood viscosity and improves cerebral blood flow. The optimal hematocrit thought to maximize the oxygen delivery to tissues has been estimated at 33%, but may be higher in ischemic brain. A randomized controlled trial of triple-H therapy has not been undertaken,[170] and there is uncertainty about its efficacy in reducing the occurrence of delayed ischemic deficits and death after SAH.[171]

Another method for treating symptomatic vasospasm is cerebral angioplasty. Transluminal angioplasty can be used to dilate constricted major cerebral vessels in patients who are refractory to conventional treatment.[144] Superselective intra-arterial infusion of papaverine dilates distal vessels not accessible to angioplasty. However, intra-arterial papaverine may be neurotoxic. There is a move away from its use in favor of intra-arterial verapamil.[172] Transluminal angioplasty procedures are usually performed under general anesthesia to minimize movement and permit accurate placement of the intra-arterial balloon used to dilate the cerebral vessels. The risks of angioplasty include aneurysm rupture, intimal dissection, vessel rupture, ischemia, and infarction.

TABLE 27-18

POTENTIAL COMPLICATIONS OF SUBARACHNOID HEMORRHAGE

- Rebleeding
- Vasospasm
- Intracranial hypertension
- Hydrocephalus
- Hyponatremia/volume contraction
- Seizures

Intracranial hypertension is present to some degree in most patients following an SAH. In the uncomplicated case, intracranial hypertension does not require specific treatment. Intracranial pressure gradually returns to normal by the end of the first week. If an intracerebral hemorrhage, intraventricular hemorrhage, vasospasm, or hydrocephalus develops, intracranial hypertension may be severe and require treatment. Patients may require emergency ventriculostomy, steroids, diuretics, or intubation and hyperventilation. Intracranial pressure should be lowered gradually, especially in patients with unclipped aneurysms. Abrupt lowering of ICP by lumbar puncture, ventricular drainage, or rapid infusion of mannitol can induce rebleeding.

Acute (obstructive) *hydrocephalus* after SAH complicates approximately 20% of cases.[173] Although controversial, ventriculostomy has been recommended for treating acute hydrocephalus in patients with diminished level of consciousness after SAH.[173] Ventriculostomy has been associated with increased bleeding and infection.

Endovascular Treatment of Cerebral Aneurysms

Endovascular embolization is a therapeutic alternative to surgical clipping of some cerebral aneurysm. Initially, only patients with high risk or inaccessible aneurysms and/or co-morbid medical conditions were candidates for INR procedures. These procedures are now recommended for treatment of unruptured intracranial aneurysms, depending on aneurysm location, size and age of patient.[165]

A randomized trial comparing clipping and coiling of ruptured aneurysms was recently published [The International Subarachnoid Aneurysm Trial (ISAT)].[174] The study enrolled 2,143 patients treated at 43 centers, mostly in Europe. The study was stopped early by the data safety and monitoring committee. At stopping, 801 patients were treated by endovascular therapy and 793 patients were treated surgically and followed for 1 year. Death or dependency occurred in 23.7% of endovascular cases and 30.6% of surgical cases; a relative risk reduction of 22.6% with endovascular therapy ($p = 0.0019$) was reported.[174] This study has been criticized for not including a representative population, studying only ruptured aneurysms, and poor surgical results and follow-up.[175]

The endovascular technique most commonly performed for occlusion of cerebral aneurysms is insertion of Guglielmi detachable coils (GDC). The field is rapidly evolving and new techniques (microballoons, neurovascular stents) and investigational devices (liquid embolic agents, bioactive coils) are being developed and investigated. An anesthesiologist is present for most of these procedures to monitor the patient, to provide appropriate anesthesia for the procedure, and to manage complications that arise. The reader is referred to an earlier section in this chapter for discussion of anesthetic management during INR procedures.

Special Anesthetic Considerations

Preoperative Evaluation. When the neurologic examination is performed, the patient's clinical grade is noted (see Table 27-17). The patient's CT scan or MR image is evaluated to assess the presence and severity of intracranial hypertension. The severity, acuteness, and stage of the SAH as well as the presence of intracranial hypertension and the timing of surgery will determine the anesthetic management. Because the circle of Willis is proximal to the hypothalamus, an SAH in this area can cause a variety of disturbances related to hypothalamic dysfunction (e.g., ECG changes, temperature instability, various changes in endocrine [pituitary] function, various electrolyte disturbances). Sympathetic overactivity and overstimulation of both adrenal cortex and medulla can contribute to hypertension and diabetes, requiring treatment with insulin.

Electrolyte abnormalities frequently occur secondary to the *syndrome of inappropriate antidiuretic hormone* (SIADH) secretion or diabetes insipidus. Hyponatremia is the most common electrolyte disturbance detected and is often associated with a high urinary sodium and osmolality, which is expected with SIADH. Unlike a patient with SIADH, however, the patient with SAH usually has a contracted intravascular volume despite hyponatremia. This cerebral salt-wasting syndrome may be caused by release of atrial natriuretic factor from damaged brain. The recommended therapy is to maintain normovolemia with isotonic saline solutions. Other factors contributing to intravascular volume contraction in these patients are supine diuresis secondary to increased thoracic blood volume, negative nitrogen balance, decreased erythropoiesis, increased catecholamine levels, and iatrogenic blood loss. Fluid balance and electrolyte abnormalities should be corrected prior to surgery.

Most aneurysm surgery requires significant intravascular volume shifts (diuresis followed by volume loading) and extensive systemic blood pressure manipulations (deliberate hypotension or hypertension). Therefore, patients with a history of hypertension, ischemic heart disease, and/or congestive heart failure must be in optimal condition to tolerate the hemodynamic changes required for this surgery. Depending on the degree of cardiovascular disease, inadvertent or deliberate hypotension may be poorly tolerated. When patients have significant hypertension, the blood pressure should be lowered gradually to normotensive levels to avoid cerebral ischemia. Agents such as propranolol, labetalol, or esmolol are used in neurosurgical patients because these agents do not affect cerebral blood volume or ICP. When the systemic blood pressure is lowered, a critical level below which neurologic deficits occur may be observed. Systemic blood pressure below this level should be avoided intra-operatively.

Electrocardiographic abnormalities are commonly associated with ruptured cerebral aneurysms. The ECG changes include ST-segment depression or elevation, T-wave inversion or flattening, U waves, prolonged Q-T intervals, and dysrhythmia. The ECG changes are not necessarily associated with increased operative morbidity and mortality or consistent increases in serum myoglobin or creatine kinase. They usually resolve within 10 days following SAH and require no special treatment. When indicated, cardiac troponin-I levels should be drawn to determine the clinical significance of these abnormalities. When cardiac dysrhythmia and occasional frank subendocardial ischemia result in cardiac failure, appropriate treatment must be instituted.

12 **Anesthetic Management.** The anesthetic goals for intracranial aneurysm surgery are to avoid aneurysm rupture, maintain cerebral perfusion pressure and transmural aneurysm pressure, and provide a "slack" brain. Patients in WFNS scale I or II who appear anxious should receive premedication. Cerebral perfusion pressure is maintained by using drugs in doses that avoid sudden or profound decreases in systemic blood pressure or increases in ICP. Similarly, transmural pressure, which is defined as the difference between mean arterial pressure and ICP, must be maintained. (The pressure within an aneurysm is equal to the systemic blood pressure.) The relationship between transmural pressure and wall stress or tension of the aneurysm is linear. An increase in mean arterial pressure or fall in ICP will increase transmural pressure, wall stress, and risk of aneurysm rupture. Methods to control brain volume and ICP, such as hyperventilation, diuretics, spinal drainage, and head position, facilitate surgical exposure and minimize the retraction pressure that can cause tissue injury.

Standard monitoring plus an arterial pressure catheter is routinely used. A CVP or PA catheter is recommended in WFNS scale III or higher to provide a more accurate measure of the patient's volume status and cardiac function intraoperatively and postoperatively in the prevention or management of cerebral vasospasm. Electrophysiologic monitoring with the EEG or SSEPs may be used to monitor the adequacy of cerebral perfusion during induced hypotension or temporary/permanent aneurysm clip application. When barbiturates are administered for brain protection, the EEG is used to guide the dose required to achieve a burst suppression pattern.

To minimize the risk of hypertension and aneurysmal rupture during induction of anesthesia, intravenous lidocaine and the β-adrenergic antagonist esmolol or labetalol are recommended. Following induction, ventilation is mechanically controlled to maintain normocarbia if ICP is normal. If intracranial hypertension is present, the $PaCO_2$ can be lowered to 30–35 mmHg. A deep plane of anesthesia must be established prior to insertion of head pins, scalp incision, turning the bone flap, and opening the dura in order to avoid a hypertensive response. When intracranial hypertension is present, anesthesia should be deepened with additional doses of thiopental and fentanyl until the skull is opened. Several techniques can be instituted during aneurysm surgery to provide a "slack" brain and facilitate dissection. These are hyperventilation of the lungs, osmotic diuresis, barbiturate administration, and CSF drainage during the procedure. A lumbar subarachnoid catheter or spinal needle is inserted after induction to allow CSF drainage during the procedure. Excessive loss of CSF must be avoided during insertion of the lumbar drain because it can decrease ICP, thus increasing aneurysmal transmural pressure and the potential for rupture. Removal of CSF after opening the dura is done cautiously with guidance by the surgeons.

The drugs most frequently used to maintain anesthesia during aneurysm surgery are fentanyl or remifentanil and propofol infusions in conjunction with 0.5 MAC of a potent inhalation agent in oxygen and nondepolarizing muscle relaxant. The total dose of fentanyl should not exceed 10 to 12 μg/kg, unless postoperative ventilation is planned. In conditions of poor intracranial compliance, a continuous infusion of thiopental (1 to 3 mg/kg/hr following a bolus dose of 5 mg/kg) may be substituted for propofol as the primary anesthetic. Potential disadvantages to using thiopental are blood pressure instability and prolonged recovery from anesthesia. With this technique, a pulmonary artery catheter should be inserted to monitor and optimize cardiovascular performance and intravascular volume. Following an uneventful aneurysm clip application, the thiopental infusion is discontinued to prevent a delay in recovery.

Prior to aneurysm clipping, isotonic crystalloid solutions without glucose are administered to replace overnight fluid losses and provide hourly maintenance fluid requirements. When the aneurysm is secured, intra-operative fluid deficits are replaced and additional volume is administered. At the time of aneurysm dissection, blood is available for transfusion in case the aneurysm ruptures. A bolus of thiopental (3 to 5 mg/kg) may be given before temporary occlusion of a major intracranial vessel and before aneurysm clipping. If temporary occlusion lasts longer than 10 minutes, recirculation should be established, and additional thiopental administered before reapplying the temporary clip. Following aneurysm clipping, the central venous pressure and pulmonary capillary wedge pressure are raised to 10 to 12 mmHg or 12 to 18 mmHg, respectively, with crystalloid, colloid, or blood. A postoperative hematocrit of 30 to 35% is desirable. As discussed previously, intravascular volume expansion with hemodilution is recommended to reduce the risk of postoperative cerebral vasospasm.

When considering the use of *deliberate hypotension* during aneurysm dissection, the risk–benefit ratio must be assessed for each patient. The potential benefit of deliberate hypotension must be weighed against the risk of causing cerebral ischemia or ischemia to other organs. Patients with a history of cardiovascular disease, occlusive cerebrovascular disease, intracerebral hematoma, fever, anemia, and renal disease are not good candidates for deliberate hypotension. Such patients should only be subjected to moderate reductions in systemic blood pressure (20 to 30 mmHg), if at all. When deliberate hypotension is required, the best choice among the agents listed in Table 27-19 is probably the drug or drug combination with which you have the most experience. Commonly used agents to induce hypotension have been sodium nitroprusside, isoflurane, and esmolol.

Overall, deliberate hypotension has declined in use and has been replaced by temporary clipping. The temporary occlusion of a feeding artery produces an acute reduction in focal blood flow and a slack aneurysm, thus eliminating the need for deliberate hypotension and its systemic effects. Depending on the location of the aneurysm, either somatosensory evoked potentials or brainstem auditory evoked potentials can be used to monitor the safety of temporary occlusion.

The major intraoperative complication of aneurysm surgery is hemorrhage. When an aneurysm ruptures intra-operatively, there is potential for major ischemic damage from hypotension and the surgical efforts to control bleeding. Hemorrhagic death is also possible. When the leak is small and the dissection is complete, it may be possible for the surgeon to gain control with suction and then apply the permanent clip to the neck of the aneurysm. Alternatively, temporary clips can be applied proximal and distal to the aneurysm to gain control. Thiopental may be given to provide some protection prior to the placement of the temporary clip. During temporary occlusion, normotension should be maintained to maximize collateral perfusion. If temporary occlusion is not planned or not possible and blood loss is not significant, the mean arterial pressure may be transiently decreased to 50 mmHg or lower to facilitate surgical control. When bleeding is excessive, aggressive fluid resuscitation and blood transfusion must commence immediately. Administration of cerebroprotective agents may not be possible because of associated hemodynamic effects. Under these conditions, deliberate hypotension is not advised as the intravascular volume must be restored first.

Intraoperative Cerebral Protection. Thiopental has been the drug of choice for intra-operative cerebral protection during aneurysm surgery. In animal models, barbiturates have shown protection during incomplete focal ischemia but not during global ischemia.[144] Barbiturates are the only agents shown to be useful in humans.[144]

Many practitioners institute mild intraoperative hypothermia (32 to 34°C) during aneurysm surgery to enhance the brain's ability to tolerate ischemia. Unfortunately, its value remains unproven. An NIH supported multicenter trial of the use of mild intraoperative hypothermia (IHAST, The International Hypothermia in Aneurysm Trial) was completed in 2003.[72] The investigators found no alteration in outcome, when patients received intraoperative cooling prior to aneurysm clipping.[176]

Emergence. The primary goals at the conclusion of surgery are to avoid coughing, straining, hypercarbia, and hypertension. For patients in Grades I and II who have no intraoperative complications, the endotracheal tube should be removed in the operating room and a neurologic examination performed. Patients who have intraoperative complications or have depressed consciousness preoperatively (Grades III toV) should remain intubated and receive mechanical ventilation until their neurologic status improves.

Postoperative Concerns. Variation in systemic blood pressure is common postoperatively and contributes significantly to morbidity and mortality in patients following aneurysm repair. Causes of hypertension include preexisting hypertension, pain, and CO_2 retention from residual anesthesia. The treatment of postoperative hypertension is critical to prevent the formation of cerebral edema or hematoma. Antihypertensive

TABLE 27-19

DOSAGE, MECHANISM OF ACTION, ADVANTAGES, AND DISADVANTAGES OF COMMONLY USED AGENTS FOR INDUCING HYPOTENSION

■ DRUG	■ DOSAGE	■ MECHANISM OF ACTION	■ ADVANTAGES	■ DISADVANTAGES
Sodium nitroprusside	0.5–10 μg/kg/min	Nitric oxide-mediated direct vasodilatation	Rapid onset/offset titration control	Cyanide toxicity ↑ ICP Rebound hypertension Coagulation abnormalities ↑ Pulmonary shunting
Nitroglycerin	1–10 μg/kg/min	Nitric oxide-mediated direct vasodilatation	Rapid onset/offset titration control	↑ ICP Rebound hypertension Coagulation abnormalities ↑ Pulmonary shunting
Trimethaphan	1–5 mg/min	Ganglionic blockade	Rapid onset/offset	Histamine release Cerebral compromise below MAP 55 mm Hg ↓ Pseudocholinesterase
Esmolol	0.2–0.5 mg/kg/min loading dose 50–200 μg/kg/min	β-adrenergic blockade	Rapid onset/offset	Limited efficacy Cardiac depression Bronchospasm
Labetalol	20 mg test dose 0.5–2 mg/min (total 300 mg)	α- and β-adrenergic blockade	Reduced probability of adverse effects	Limited efficacy Bronchospasm
Prostaglandin E_1	0.1–0.65 μg/kg/min	Direct vasodilatation	Rapid onset ↓ Reflex tachycardia Stable CBF	Slow offset Bradycardia Hyperthermia
Nicardipine	Begin 5 mg/h infusion, max 15 mg/h	Coronary and peripheral vasodilatation	Rapid onset ↓ Reflex tachycardia	Slow offset Resists antihypotensive therapy ↑ Pulmonary shunting
Inhalation anesthetics	Titrate by inspired concentration	Vasodilatation and myocardial depression	Provides surgical anesthesia	↑ ICP ↑ Cerebral edema ↓ Vital organ blood flow

drugs should be administered after respiratory depression and pain are eliminated as causes. The hypertensive response usually subsides within 12 hours. When indicated, preoperative antihypertensive drugs are reinstituted and maintained.

After clipping of the aneurysm, cerebral vasospasm continues to pose a threat to neurologic integrity. Postoperative hypotension must be avoided, and the patient's intravascular volume must be accurately assessed with either a central venous pressure or pulmonary artery catheter. As previously discussed, a higher than normal intravascular fluid volume should be maintained.

Arteriovenous Malformations

An arteriovenous malformation (AVM) of the brain consists of a tangle of congenitally malformed blood vessels that forms an abnormal communication between the arterial and venous systems. The arterial afferents flow directly into venous efferents without the usual resistance of an intervening capillary bed; thus, oxygenated blood is shunted directly into the venous system, leaving surrounding brain tissue transiently or permanently ischemic. These lesions predominate in males over females (2:1), with the onset of complaints between the ages of 10 and 40. The chief clinical features are parenchymal hemorrhage or SAH, focal epilepsy, and progressive focal neurologic sensory-motor deficits occurring in a child or young adult. A vein of Galen AVM in infants may present with hydrocephalus and/or high-output cardiac failure. The natural history of AVMs is not completely understood.[177] The risk of hemorrhage is approximately 1 to 4% per year. The rate of rebleeding is 6% in the first year after a hemorrhage and about 2% per year thereafter.[176] Mortality from initial hemorrhage is high, with reports between 10 and 30%. Recurrence of hemorrhage with a fatal outcome is a constant danger. There are several options for the management of AVMs, including surgical excision, embolization, stereotactic radiosurgery (proton beams, gamma rays, or linear accelerator), a combination of the above, and leaving AVMs alone. Arteriovenous malformations of suitable size and location can be managed successfully with surgical excision. Surgical mortality ranges from 0.6 to 14% and correlates with size, location, and pattern of involvement of the AVM.[177] Early postoperative morbidity ranges from 17 to 23%; however, outcome studies report improvement in morbidity over time.[177] To avoid intraoperative or postoperative massive brain swelling or hemorrhage of large AVMs, operations may be staged or follow preoperative embolization.

Special Anesthetic Considerations

In addition to providing anesthesia for craniotomy and resection of the AVM, anesthesia may be required for radiologic embolization of the AVM. Closed embolization of cerebral AVMs is uncomfortable and invasive. This procedure may be performed under local anesthesia with sedation or under general anesthesia. It has been performed successfully with various combinations of sedative drugs (fentanyl, midazolam, or propofol) that allow neurologic examinations during the procedure and permit immediate diagnoses of complications.[138,177] Children, uncooperative patients, and those with intracranial hypertension or airway problems usually require general anesthesia. General anesthesia does not allow direct neurologic assessment. Potential complications of embolization procedures are embolic or ischemic stroke and hemorrhage from the AVM, either acute or delayed.[178] New onset or preexisting seizures may occur during the embolization procedure, requiring treatment with benzodiazepines or barbiturates.

The anesthetic management of patients with AVMs is similar to the management of patients for aneurysm surgery. Depending on the presentation, the anesthetic approach is modified. For example, a large bleed may present with symptoms relating to mass effects and require maneuvers to reduce ICP. High flow through a large intact AVM may cause a "steal" with resulting cerebral ischemia and require different techniques to improve
13 CPP. With more extensive lesions, hypothermia and high-dose barbiturates have been recommended for brain protection. Induced hypotension may also be required to reduce lesion size and blood flow.

Hyperemic complications, defined as perioperative edema or hemorrhage, may occur after removal of the AVM. Although the mechanism is unclear, one theory proposes that breakthrough cerebral edema and hemorrhage result when blood flow from the surgically obliterated AVM is diverted to the surrounding brain. The smaller vessels in the brain surrounding the AVM are not accustomed to the higher pressure-flow state, and autoregulation is exceeded, resulting in severe brain swelling, edema, and hemorrhage. The clinical syndrome of cerebral hyperperfusion with normal CPP has been called *normal perfusion pressure breakthrough*.[177] Other studies report information that is not consistent with this theory.[177,179] Immediate treatment should include the simultaneous application of high-dose barbiturates, osmotic diuretics, hyperventilation, and maintenance of a low-normal MAP. When marked brain swelling occurs intraoperatively, the patient should remain intubated, hyperventilated, and sedated postoperatively. Hypertension during emergence and postoperatively must be controlled, preferably with β-blockers, to prevent bleeding into the bed of the AVM.

TABLE 27-20

MODIFIED GLASGOW COMA SCALE

■ EYE OPENING	
Spontaneously	4
To verbal command	3
To pain	2
None	1
■ BEST VERBAL RESPONSE	
Oriented, conversing	5
Disoriented, conversing	4
Inappropriate words	3
Incomprehensible sounds	2
No verbal response	1
■ BEST MOTOR RESPONSE	
Obeys verbal commands	6
Localizes to pain	5
Flexion/withdrawal	4
Abnormal flexion (decorticate)	3
Extension (decerebrate)	2
No response (flaccid)	1

Mild head injury = 13–15; moderate = 9–12; severe = ≤8.
(Adapted from Teasdale G, Jennett B: Assessment of coma and impaired consciousness: A practical scale. Lancet 2:81, 1974; and Jennett B: Assessment of the severity of head injury. J Neurol Neurosurg Psychiatry 39:647, 1976.)

HEAD INJURY

Head injury is a leading cause of permanent disability and death, occurring most frequently in adolescents, young adults, and people older than 75 years of age. In all age groups, males are affected two times more often than females and are more likely to sustain severe head injury. The leading causes of traumatic brain injuries (TBI) are motor vehicle crashes, violence, and falls. More than 50% of patients with severe head injury have multiple injuries resulting in significant blood loss, systemic hypotension, and hypoxia.[180]

Classification of severe head injury is based on the Glasgow Coma Scale (Table 27-20), which defines neurologic impairment in terms of eye opening, speech, and motor function. The total score that can be obtained is 15, and severe head injury is determined by a score of 8 or less persisting for 6 hours or more. The Glasgow Coma and Glasgow Outcome Scales permit comparison between series of traumatically head-injured patients based on initial clinical presentation and eventual outcome. The prognosis after head injury depends on the type of lesion sustained, the age of the patient, and the severity of the injury as defined by the Glasgow Coma Scale. In general, mortality is closely related to the initial score on the coma scale. For any given lesion and score, however, the elderly have a poorer outcome than do younger patients.

Following head trauma, the primary injury results from the biomechanical effect of forces applied to the skull and brain at the time of the insult and is manifested within milliseconds. Currently, there is no treatment for the primary injury. Secondary injury occurs minutes to hours after the impact and represents complicating processes initiated by the primary injury, such as ischemia, brain swelling and edema, intracranial hemorrhage, intracranial hypertension, and herniation. Factors that aggravate the initial injury include hypoxia, hypercarbia, hypotension, anemia, and hyperglycemia. These contributing factors to secondary injury are preventable. Seizures, infection, and sepsis that may occur hours to days after injury will further aggravate brain damage and must also be prevented or treated promptly.

Secondary insults complicate the course of more than 50% of head-injured patients.[180,181] An outcome study using data from the Traumatic Coma Data Bank revealed that hypotension occurring after head injury is profoundly detrimental, with more than 70% of patients experiencing significant morbidity and mortality (Table 27-21).[181] Furthermore, the combination of hypoxia and hypotension is significantly more detrimental than that of hypotension alone (>90% of patients with severe outcome or death). These findings confirm the importance of avoiding hypovolemic shock in head-injured patients. The management goal in head-injured patients is to initiate timely and appropriate therapy to prevent secondary brain injury. When the initial injury is not fatal, subsequent neurologic damage and systemic complications should be preventable in most patients.

Primary injury or biomechanical trauma to brain parenchyma includes concussion, contusion, laceration, and hematoma. Not all severely head-injured patients require surgery. Generalized brain injury with edema or contusion is a common finding in patients, whether or not a surgically correctable mass lesion is present. Diffuse cerebral swelling occurs because of sudden intracerebral congestion and hyperemia. Twenty-four hours or more after the initial insult, cerebral edema develops in the extracellular spaces of the white matter. Nonoperative treatment of diffuse cerebral swelling includes hyperventilation, diuresis with mannitol and furosemide, and barbiturates in conjunction with ICP monitoring.

TABLE 27-21

IMPACT OF HYPOXIA AND HYPOTENSION[a] ON OUTCOME AFTER SEVERE HEAD INJURY (GCS ≤ 8)

SECONDARY INSULTS	NUMBER OF PATIENTS	OUTCOME PERCENTAGE: GOOD OR MODERATE	SEVERE OR VEGETATIVE	DEAD
Total cases	699	43	21	37
Neither	456	51	22	27
Hypoxia	78	45	22	33
Hypotension	113	26	14	60
Both	52	6	19	75

Hypoxia = PaO_2 < 60 mmHg; hypotension = SBP < 90 mmHg; GCS = Glasgow Coma Scale.
[a]At time of hospital arrival.
Data adapted from the Traumatic Coma Data Bank[181]

Depressed skull fractures and acute epidural, subdural, and intracerebral hematomas usually require craniotomy. Chronic subdural hematomas are often evacuated through burr holes. Depressed skull fractures under lacerations should be elevated and debrided within 24 hours to minimize the risk of infection. Bony fragments and penetrating objects should not be manipulated in the emergency room, because they may be tamponading a lacerated vessel or dural sinus. Traumatic epidural hematoma is an infrequent complication of head injury, usually the result of a motor vehicle accident. The initial injury tears middle meningeal vessels or dural sinuses and causes unconsciousness. When a spasm and clot occur in the vessel(s), the bleeding stops and the patient recovers, experiencing a lucid interval. Over the next several hours, the vessel bleeds and the patient rapidly deteriorates (especially with arterial bleeding). In rapidly deteriorating conditions, treatment should not be delayed pending radiologic evaluation. Emergency evacuation is necessary. Venous epidural hematomas develop more slowly, and there may be time for diagnostic testing. The clinical presentation of acute subdural hematomas ranges from minimal deficits to unconsciousness and signs of a mass lesion (hemiparesis, unilateral decerebration, and pupillary enlargement). A lucid interval may occur. The most common cause of subdural hematoma is trauma, but it may occur spontaneously and is associated with coagulopathies, aneurysms, and neoplasms. It is considered acute if the patient becomes symptomatic within 72 hours, subacute between 3 and 15 days, and chronic after 2 weeks. Subacute and chronic subdural hematoma are usually observed in patients over age 50 years. There may be no history of head trauma. The clinical presentation in these patients may vary from focal signs of brain dysfunction to a depressed level of consciousness or development of an organic brain syndrome. Intracranial hypertension is usually associated with acute subdural hematoma. Intensive medical therapy to correct elevated ICP and control brain edema and swelling may be required before, during, and after hematoma evacuation. With intracerebral hematomas, the clinical picture may vary from minimal neurologic deficits to deep coma. Large, solitary intracerebral hematomas should be evacuated. Lesions causing delayed neurologic deterioration from fresh hemorrhage are also evacuated but carry a poor prognosis. Depending on the degree of cerebral injury, patients with intracerebral hematomas may require intensive medical therapy to control intracranial hypertension and cerebral edema. Coup and contrecoup injuries usually cause cerebral contusion and intracerebral hemorrhage. In general, contused brain tissue is not removed; occasionally, however, contused tissue over the frontal or temporal poles may be removed to control edema formation and prevent herniation.

Emergency Therapy

Emergency therapy should begin at the site of the accident, in the ambulance, and most certainly, in the emergency room. The first step is to secure an open airway and ensure adequate ventilation to prevent secondary injury from hypoxia and hypercarbia. Before securing the airway in a head-injured patient, a quick assessment of the patient's neurologic status and concomitant injuries should be made.

The incidence of cervical spine injuries in surviving head-injury victims is 1 to 3% in adults and 0.5% in children.[182,183] Victims of head-first falls or high-speed motor vehicle accidents have a 10% or greater chance of cervical spine fractures. X-ray evaluation with a cross-table lateral view can miss 20% of cervical spine fractures.[183] To increase the reliability of radiographic evaluation, anteroposterior and odontoid views, in addition to a lateral view, have been recommended. Reportedly, this combination misses only 7% of fractures.[182] When a cervical spine fracture has not been excluded by x-ray evaluation, cervical alignment with in-line stabilization is recommended during emergent intubation.[184,185] (In-line stabilization requires an assistant to stabilize the patient's head by positioning his or her hands along the side of the head with fingertips on the mastoid holding the occiput down on a backboard.)

When facial fractures and soft tissue edema prevent direct visualization of the larynx, a fiberoptic intubation or intubation with an illuminated stylet or intubating laryngeal mask airway may be attempted. In the presence of severe facial and/or laryngeal injuries, a cricothyrotomy may be required. Nasal intubations are avoided in the presence of a suspected basal skull fracture, severe facial fractures, and bleeding diathesis.

For patients without facial injuries, the simplest and most expeditious approach to intubation is preoxygenation followed by rapid-sequence induction with cricoid pressure and maintenance of in-line stabilization. All head-injured patients are assumed to have a full stomach. Awake, oral intubation without anesthetic agents may be possible in the severely injured patient, but this is difficult in the awake or uncooperative, combative patient. Depending on the patient's cardiovascular status, virtually any of the intravenous induction agents, except ketamine, can be used. The choice of muscle relaxants is controversial. Succinylcholine can increase ICP. In the setting of acute airway compromise, full stomach, and need to perform subsequent neurologic examinations, the benefits of rapid onset and elimination of succinylcholine may outweigh the risk of transiently increasing ICP.

Following control of the airway in the head-injured patient, attention should focus on resuscitation of the cardiovascular system. Transient hypotension after head injury is not uncommon, but sustained hypotension usually results from hemorrhage secondary to other systemic injuries. These injuries must be sought and aggressively treated.

When multiple trauma complicates head injury, there is no ideal crystalloid resuscitation fluid. A major concern during resuscitation is the development of cerebral edema. Animal investigations reveal that total serum osmolality is a key factor in brain edema formation.[186,187] When serum osmolality is reduced, cerebral edema develops in normal and abnormal brain. This occurs because the blood-brain barrier is relatively impermeable to sodium. Solutions containing sodium in concentrations lower than that in serum cause water movement into the brain, increasing brain water. Thus, hypoosmolar solutions (0.45% NaCl and lactated Ringer's solution) are more likely than isoosmolar fluids (0.9% saline) to increase brain water content. Large-volume fluid resuscitation with isoosmolar crystalloids reduces colloid oncotic pressure and increases peripheral tissue edema. However, in animal investigations, the brain behaves differently than other tissues, and profound lowering of colloid oncotic pressure with maintenance of serum osmolality does not result in edema in normal brain[186] and in some head-injury models.[187,188] These results can be explained by the unique structure of the blood-brain barrier and the fact that colloid oncotic pressure gradients generate weak forces in comparison with osmolar gradients.[186] Some doubt has been cast on the applicability of these laboratory findings to clinical practice. The cryogenic-injury model used in these experiments may not be equivalent to head injury in patients. In head-injured patients, brain capillary permeability may be rendered similar to that of peripheral tissues when the blood-brain barrier is damaged. In addition, the time course of these experiments did not allow observation of edema developing 24 to 48 hours after initial resuscitation, which occurs in head-injured patients. An investigation using the percussive head-injury model in rats has shown that reduction in colloid oncotic pressure can aggravate cerebral edema under certain conditions.[189] Therefore, it seems reasonable to avoid a profound reduction in colloid oncotic pressure in clinical practice. Isoosmolar colloid solutions, such as 5% albumin or 6% hetastarch, can be administered to maintain oncotic pressure and intravascular volume. Fresh whole blood, when available, is the ideal colloid resuscitation fluid for hypovolemic patients with ongoing blood loss.

Hypertonic saline solutions (3%, 7.5%) can be very useful for volume resuscitation in head-injured patients because they lower ICP, increase blood pressure, and may improve regional CBF.[190] Hypertonic saline produces an osmotic diuretic effect on the brain that is similar to that of other hyperosmolar solutions (e.g., mannitol). Hypertonic saline therapy may be more effective than other diuretics in certain clinical conditions, for example, in patients with refractory intracranial hypertension[141] or in those who require brain debulking and maintenance of intravascular volume.[140] With long-term use, there is concern over the physiologic implications of elevated serum sodium, such as a depressed level of consciousness and/or seizures. More studies are required to determine dose-response curves and the safety and efficacy of these solutions.

During fluid resuscitation of the head-injured patient, the goals are to maintain serum osmolality, avoid profound reduction in colloid oncotic pressure, and restore circulating blood volume. Immediate therapy is directed at preventing hypotension and maintaining CPP above 60 mmHg.[191] When indicated, an ICP monitor is inserted to guide fluid resuscitation and prevent severe elevations in ICP. Isoosmolar crystalloid solutions, colloid solutions, or both are administered acutely to restore circulating blood volume. Glucose-containing solutions should not be administered because of a significant association between plasma glucose levels and worse neurologic outcome in head-injured patients. Substantial blood loss requires transfusion with crossmatched or fresh whole blood. A minimum hematocrit between 30 and 33% is recommended to maximize oxygen transport.

Hypertension, tachycardia, and increased cardiac output often develop in patients with isolated head trauma, especially young adults.[144] ECG abnormalities and fatal arrhythmias have been reported. The hyperdynamic circulatory responses and ECG changes may result from a surge in epinephrine that accompanies head injury.[144] Either labetalol or esmolol can be used to control hypertension and tachycardia in this situation.

14 In some patients, severe intracranial hypertension precipitates reflex arterial hypertension and bradycardia (Cushing's triad). A reduction in systemic blood pressure in these patients can further aggravate cerebral ischemia by reducing CPP. Systemic blood pressure must be lowered cautiously when intracranial hypertension is severe. In such cases, a reduction of ICP may interrupt this reflex response.

After stabilization of head-injured patients, including control of airway and systemic blood pressure, therapeutic interventions to control intracranial hypertension are instituted. The head is elevated 15° and maintained in a neutral position without rotation or flexion. Mannitol, 0.25 to 1 g/kg, is given to lower ICP acutely, or a combination of furosemide and mannitol may be administered. Hyperventilation and barbiturate therapy may be considered when other measures have failed.[191,192] Appropriate monitoring must be instituted and hypotension avoided.

Mechanical hyperventilation to a $PaCO_2$ 25 to 30 mmHg was routinely employed in head-injured patients based on an assumption that hyperventilation, by reducing CBF, will reduce ICP, thereby preserving CPP and CBF. Clinical investigations suggest that head-injured patients are ischemic within the first 24 hours of injury.[143,194] In these patients hyperventilation may further decrease CBF and aggravate cerebral ischemia.

Recently published guidelines for the management of severe traumatic brain injury no longer recommend hyperventilation to a $PaCO_2$ of 25 to 30 mmHg as a first-tier therapy.[192,193] In fact, the 2000 guidelines recommend avoiding the use of prophylactic hyperventilation ($PaCO_2 \leq 35$ mmHg) therapy during the first 24 hours after severe TBI.[193] When hyperventilation is initiated for control of intracranial hypertension, the $PaCO_2$ should be maintained in the range of 30 to 35 mmHg in order to accomplish ICP control while minimizing the associated risk of ischemia. Hyperventilation to $PaCO_2$ values less than 30 mmHg should be considered only when second-tier therapy of refractory intracranial hypertension is required. Continuous measurement of jugular bulb oxygen saturation or CBF monitoring is recommended during hyperventilation to guide therapy.[192] In emergency situations, we should continue to hyperventilate patients in whom the clinical control of intracranial hypertension is the primary concern. However, when the clinical situation no longer requires it or there is evidence of cerebral ischemia, normocapnic ventilation should be instituted.

Anesthetic Management

The patient is evaluated by CT scan and taken directly to the operating room. There is usually minimal time available for resuscitation and preanesthetic assessment. Information that should be obtained preoperatively is described in Table 27-22.

TABLE 27-22

PRE-ANESTHETIC ASSESSMENT OF THE HEAD-INJURED PATIENT

Airway (cervical spine)
Breathing: ventilation and oxygenation
Circulatory status
Associated injuries
Neurologic status (Glasgow Coma Scale)
Preexisting chronic illness
Circumstances of the injury:
  Time of injury
  Duration of unconsciousness
  Associated alcohol or drug use

The anesthetic management is a continuation of the initial resuscitation, including airway management, fluid and electrolyte balance, and ICP control. The routine monitors for major neurosurgical procedures are applied.

Major goals of anesthetic management are to optimize cerebral perfusion and oxygenation, to avoid secondary damage, and to provide adequate surgical conditions. Cerebral perfusion pressure (CPP = MAP − ICP) should be maintained between 60 and 110 mmHg. If ICP increases to a greater extent than MAP, CPP is reduced, and the brain becomes ischemic. Uncontrolled increases in ICP can result in herniation and death. The choice of anesthetic agents depends on the condition of the patient. In the hemodynamically stable patient with severe intracranial hypertension, narcotics in conjunction with a thiopental infusion (2 to 3 mg/kg/h) and nondepolarizing muscle relaxant can be administered with oxygen and air. In patients with less severe intracranial hypertension, anesthesia can be maintained with various combinations of barbiturates, benzodiazepines, narcotics, and sub-MAC concentration of a potent inhalation agent. Anesthetic management is directed at avoidance of secondary brain injury. Intraoperative hypotension secondary to blood loss or precipitated by anesthetic drugs must be avoided by appropriate volume expansion. Maintenance of ventilation ($PaCO_2$ of 35 mmHg) and oxygenation ($PaO_2 \geq 60$ mmHg) is extremely important.

Intraoperative brain swelling or herniation from the operative site may complicate hematoma decompression. Such causes as improper patient positioning, contralateral intracerebral hematoma, venous drainage obstruction from packing, and acute hydrocephalus from intraventricular hemorrhage must be eliminated. In this setting, the adequacy of hyperventilation must also be verified. A large alveolar-arterial CO_2 gradient may exist, so that end-tidal CO_2 may not reflect arterial CO_2. The respiratory system and equipment should be reviewed to ensure normal peak inspiratory and expiratory pressures. Hemopneumothorax, high intra-abdominal pressures, a kinked endotracheal or expiratory tube, or a stuck expiratory valve can produce marked peak inspiratory or expiratory pressures as well as hypoxemia and hypercarbia. Fluid and electrolyte balance must be reevaluated in patients with cerebral swelling. Mannitol loses its effect after 1 to 3 hours, and it may be necessary to repeat the mannitol bolus to increase osmolarity. Volume overload and hyponatremia may also cause cerebral swelling and must be corrected. If cerebral swelling persists, the anesthetic should be converted to opioid and thiopental infusions with oxygen and air. Thiopental may be given in a series of boluses over 5 to 10 minutes to a total dose of 5 to 25 mg/kg, followed by an infusion of 4 to 10 mg/kg/h. To avoid barbiturate-induced myocardial depression and hypotension, it may be necessary to increase preload and add a vasopressor such as dopamine. Malignant brain swelling may require removal of brain tissue and a temporary scalp closure with a loose dural patch to minimize ICP after closure.

Emergence from anesthesia usually involves transporting an intubated, ventilated, and anesthetized patient to the intensive care unit. Even in an uncomplicated craniotomy for evacuation of hematoma, a period of postoperative ventilation is recommended because brain swelling is maximal 12 to 72 hours after injury. Hypertension and coughing or bucking on the endotracheal tube should be avoided because it can lead to significant intracranial bleeding. Labetalol or esmolol can be used to treat hypertension, and supplemental barbiturates are given to sedate the patient.

Systemic Sequelae

The systemic effects of head injury are diverse and can complicate management.[195] These include cardiopulmonary problems (airway obstruction, hypoxemia, shock, adult respiratory distress syndrome, neurogenic pulmonary edema, ECG changes), hematologic problems (disseminated intravascular coagulation), endocrinologic problems (pituitary dysfunction—i.e., diabetes insipidus, SIADH), metabolic problems (nonketotic hyperosmolar hyperglycemic coma), and gastrointestinal problems (stress ulcers, hemorrhage). Conditions not discussed elsewhere in this chapter are reviewed.

Aspiration, pneumonia, fluid overload, and trauma-related adult respiratory distress syndrome are common causes of pulmonary dysfunction in head-injured patients. A fulminant pulmonary edema may also occur. Neurogenic pulmonary edema is characterized by marked pulmonary vascular congestion, intra-alveolar hemorrhage, and a protein-rich edema fluid. Specific features of this syndrome are its rapid onset, its relationship to hypothalamic lesions, and the ability to prevent or attenuate it by α-blockers and CNS depressants. Neurogenic pulmonary edema is thought to result from massive sympathetic discharge from injured brain secondary to intracranial hypertension. Traditional therapy for pulmonary edema of cardiac origin is ineffective, and the outcome is frequently fatal. Therapy consists of immediate pharmacologic or surgical relief of intracranial hypertension, supportive respiratory care, and careful fluid management.

In head-injured patients, several clotting abnormalities may be present. Disseminated intravascular coagulation has been reported after mild and severe brain trauma and anoxic brain damage, and it presumably develops after release of brain tissue thromboplastin into the systemic circulation. Treatment of the underlying disease process usually results in spontaneous recovery of the coagulation defects. Occasionally, administration of cryoprecipitate, fresh frozen plasma, platelet concentrates, and blood may be required.

Anterior pituitary insufficiency after head injury is a rare occurrence. However, patients exhibiting post-traumatic diabetes insipidus may develop a delayed impairment of anterior pituitary hormones, requiring replacement therapy. Posterior pituitary dysfunction occurs more frequently after head trauma. Diabetes insipidus may occur after craniofacial trauma and basal skull fracture. Its clinical presentation includes polyuria, polydipsia, hypernatremia, high-serum osmolality, and dilute urine. Frequently, post-traumatic diabetes insipidus is transient, and treatment is based on water replacement. If the patient cannot maintain fluid balance, exogenous vasopressin may be administered. The SIADH secretion is associated with hyponatremia, serum and extracellular fluid hypoosmolality, renal excretion of sodium, urine osmolality greater than serum osmolality, and normal renal and adrenal function. The patient develops symptoms and signs of water intoxication (anorexia, nausea, vomiting, irritability, personality changes, and neurologic abnormalities). SIADH secretion usually begins 3 to 15 days after trauma, lasting no more than 10 to 15 days with appropriate therapy. Treatment includes water restriction with or without hypertonic saline.

Many factors in neurosurgical patients predispose to nonketotic hyperosmolar hyperglycemic coma, such as steroids, prolonged mannitol therapy, hyperosmolar tube feedings, phenytoin, and limited water replacement.[195] Diagnostic criteria for nonketotic hyperosmolar hyperglycemic coma are hyperglycemia, glucosuria, absence of ketosis, plasma osmolality >330 mOsm/kg, dehydration, and CNS dysfunction. Hypovolemia and hypertonicity are the immediate threats to life. Serum sodium may be high, normal, or low, depending on the state of hydration. Serum potassium is low. Serial laboratory tests are essential. Once sodium deficits are replaced and blood pressure and urine output are stable, water deficits are replaced with 0.45% saline. Hyperglycemia usually responds to relatively small doses of insulin. Intermittent furosemide therapy may be given for cerebral edema prophylaxis in the elderly, the adult-onset diabetic, or the patient with compromised renal function.

SUMMARY

Guidelines for the management of severe traumatic brain injury were published by The Brain Trauma Foundation in 1996.[192] Revisions to the guidelines were published in 2000 in a document that discusses various management protocols and treatments in light of supporting evidence.[193] Management updates are being published on the Web as new information is made available and the guidelines are revised.[191] Publication of these recommendations, guidelines, and/or standards by The Brain Trauma Foundation reflects on ongoing effort to improve outcome in this high-risk population through evidence-based management and standardized care.

References

1. Kandel ER, Schwartz JH, Jessel TM: Principles of Neural Science. New York, McGraw-Hill, 2000
2. Bormann J: Electrophysiology of $GABA_A$ and $GABA_B$ receptor subtypes. TINS 11:112, 1988
3. McDermott AB, Dale N: Receptors, ion channels and synaptic potentials underlying the integrative actions of excitatory amino acids. TINS 10:280, 1987
4. Clark DD, Sokoloff L: Circulation and energy metabolism of the brain. In Siegel G, Agranoff B, Albers RW *et al* (eds): Basic Neurochemistry, p 645. New York, Raven Press, 1994
5. Siesjo BK: Cell damage in the brain: A speculative synthesis. J Cereb Blood Flow Metab 1:155, 1981
6. Hansen AJ: Effect of anoxia on ion distribution in the brain. Physiol Rev 65:101, 1985
7. Michenfelder JD: Anesthesia and the Brain, p 23. New York, Churchill Livingstone, 1988
8. Smith AL, Wollman H: Cerebral blood flow and metabolism: Effects of anesthetic drugs and techniques. Anesthesiology 36:378, 1972
9. Plum F, Siesjo BK: Recent advances in CSF physiology. Anesthesiology 42:708, 1975
10. Safar P: Resuscitation of the ischemic brain. In Albin MS (ed): Textbook of Neuroanesthesia with Neurosurgical and Neuroscience Perspectives, p 578. New York, McGraw-Hill Co., 1997
11. Greenfield JC, Rembert JC, Tindall GT: Transient changes in cerebral vascular resistance during the Valsalva maneuver in man. Stroke 15:76, 1984
12. Joshi S, Ornstein E, Young WL: Cerebral and spinal cord blood flow. In Cottrell JE, Smith DC (eds): Anesthesia and Neurosurgery, 4th ed., p 19. St Louis, Mosby Inc., 2001
13. Strandgaard S, Olesen J, Skinhoj E *et al*: Autoregulation of brain circulation in severe arterial hypertension. Br Med J 1:507, 1973
14. Artru AA: Cerebrospinal fluid. In Cottrell JE, Smith DS (eds): Anesthesia and Neurosurgery, 4th ed., p 83. St. Louis, Mosby Inc., 2001
15. Artru AA: Cerebrospinal fluid dynamics. In Cucchiara RF, Michenfelder JD (eds): Clinical Neuroanesthesia, p 41. New York, Churchill Livingstone, 1990
16. Miller JD, Garibi J, Pickard JD: The effects of induced changes of cerebrospinal fluid volume during continuous monitoring of ventricular pressure. Arch Neurol 28:265, 1973
17. Siesjo BK: Cerebral circulation and metabolism. J Neurosurg 60:883, 1984
18. Meldrum B: Epileptic seizures. In Siegel G, Agranoff RW, Albers BW *et al* (eds): Basic Neurochemistry, p 885. New York, Raven Press, 1994
19. Gopinath SP, Robertson CS: Management of severe head injury. In Cottrell JE, Smith DS (eds): Anesthesia and Neurosurgery, p 661. St. Louis, CV Mosby, 1994
20. Lipton P: Ischemic cell death in brain neurons. Physiological Rev 79:1431, 1999
21. Minghetti L, Levi G: Microglia as effector cells in brain damage and repair: Focus on prostanoids and nitric oxide. Prog Neurobiol 54:99, 1998
22. Friedlander RM: Apoptosis and caspases in neurodegenerative diseases. N Engl J Med 348:1365, 2003
23. Lodish H, Berk A, Matsudaira P *et al*: Cell interactions in development. In Molecular Cell Biology, 5th ed, p 924. New York, W. H. Freeman & Co, 2004
24. Sakabe T, Nakakimura K: Effects of anesthetic agents and other drugs on cerebral blood flow, metabolism and intracranial pressure. In Cottrell JE, Smith DS (eds): Anesthesia and Neurosurgery, p 129. St. Louis, Mosby, 2001
25. Ornstein E, Young WL, Fleischer LH *et al*: Desflurane and isoflurane have similar effects on cerebral blood flow in patients with intracranial mass lesions. Anesthesiology 79:498, 1993
26. Scheller MS, Tateishi A, Drummond JC *et al*: The effects of sevoflurane on cerebral blood flow, cerebral metabolic rate for oxygen, intracranial pressure, and the electroencephalogram are similar to those of isoflurane in the rabbit. Anesthesiology 68:548, 1988
27. DeDeyne C, Joly LM, Ravussin P: Newer inhalation anaesthetics and neuroanaesthesia: What is the place for sevoflurane or desflurane. Ann Fr Anesth Reanim 23:367, 2004
28. Holmstrom A, Akeson J: Cerebral blood flow at 0.5 and 1.0 minimal alveolar concentrations of desflurane or sevoflurane compared with isoflurane in normoventilated pigs. J Neurosurg Anesthesiol 15:90, 2003
29. Bedforth NM, Girling KJ, Skinner HJ *et al*: Effects of desflurane on cerebral autoregulation. Br J Anaesth 87:193, 2001
30. Holmstrom A, Akeson J. Desflurane increases intracranial pressure more and sevoflurane less than isoflurane in pigs subjected to intracranial hypertension. J Neurosurg Anesthesiol 16:136, 2004
31. Petersen KD, Landsfeldt U, Cold GE *et al*: Intracranial pressure and cerebral hemodynamic in patients with cerebral tumors: a randomized prospective study of patients subjected to craniotomy in propofol-fentanyl, isoflurane-fentanyl or sevoflurane-fentanyl anesthesia. Anesthesiology 98:329, 2003
32. Oshima T, Karasawa F, Okazaki Y *et al*: Effects of sevoflurane on cerebral blood flow and cerebral metabolic rate of oxygen in human beings: a comparison with isoflurane. Eur J Anaesthesiol 20:543, 2003
33. Michenfelder JD, Cucchiara RF: Canine cerebral oxygen consumption during enflurane anesthesia and its modification during induced seizures. Anesthesiology 40:575, 1974
34. Muzzi DA, Losasso TJ, Dietz NM *et al*: The effect of desflurane and isoflurane on cerebrospinal fluid pressure in humans with supratentorial mass lesions. Anesthesiology 76:720, 1992
35. Ebert TJ, Perez F, Uhrich TD *et al*: Desflurane-mediated sympathetic activation occurs in humans despite preventing hypotension and baroreceptor unloading. Anesthesiology 88:1227, 1998
36. Jaaskelainen SK, Kaisti K, Suni L *et al*: Sevoflurane is epileptogenic in healthy subjects at surgical levels of anesthesia. Neurology 61:1073, 2003
37. Werner C, Kochs E, Hoffman WE *et al*: The effects of sevoflurane on neurological outcome from incomplete ischemia in rats. J Neurosurg Anesth 3:237, 1991
38. Pellegrino DA, Miletich DJ, Hoffman WE *et al*: Nitrous oxide markedly increases cerebral cortical metabolic rate and blood flow in the goat. Anesthesiology 60:405, 1984
39. Baughman VL: N_2O: Of questionable value. J Neurosurg Anesth 7: 1995.
40. Michenfelder JD: The interdependency of cerebral function and metabolic effects following massive doses of thiopental in the dog. Anesthesiology 41:231, 1974
41. Rockoff MA, Goudsouzian NG: Seizures induced by methohexital. Anesthesiology 54:333, 1981
42. Fragen KJ, Shanks CA, Molteni A *et al*: Effects of etomidate on hormonal responses to surgical stress. Anesthesiology 61:652, 1984
43. Kaisti KK, Langsjo JW, Aalto S *et al*: Effects of sevoflurane, propofol and adjunct nitrous oxide on regional cerebral blood flow, oxygen consumption and blood volume in humans. Anesthesiology 99:603, 2003
44. Pinaud M, Lelausque J-N, Chetanneau A *et al*: Effects of propofol on cerebral hemodynamics and metabolism in patients with brain trauma. Anesthesiology 73:404, 1990
45. Kawano Y, Kawaguchi M, Inoue S *et al*: Jugular bulb oxygen saturation under propofol or sevoflurane/nitrous oxide anesthesia during deliberate mild hypothermia in neurosurgical patients. J Neurosurg Anesthesiol 16:6, 2004
46. Blouin RT, Conard PF, Gross JB: Time course of ventilatory depression following induction doses of propofol and thiopental. Anesthesiology 75:940, 1991

47. Fleischer JE, Milde JH, Moyer TP *et al*: Cerebral effects of high-dose midazolam and subsequent reversal with RO-1788 in dogs. Anesthesiology 68:234, 1988
48. Young WL, Prohovnik I, Correll JW *et al*: A comparison of the cerebral hemodynamic effects of sufentanil and isoflurane in humans undergoing carotid endarterectomy. Anesthesiology 71:863, 1989
49. Hanel F, Werner C, von Knobelsdorff G *et al*: The effects of fentanyl and sufentanil on cerebral hemodynamics. J Neurosurg Anesthesiol 9:223, 1997
50. Marx W, Shah N, Long C *et al*: Sufentanil, alfentanil, and fentanyl: Impact on cerebrospinal fluid pressure in patients with brain tumors. J Neurosurg Anesth 1:3, 1989
51. Lutz LJ, Milde JH, Milde LN: Cerebral effects of alfentanil in dogs with reduced intracranial compliance. J Neurosurg Anesth 1:169, 1989
52. Jung R, Free K, Shah N *et al*: Cerebrospinal fluid pressure in anesthetized patients with brain tumors: Impact of fentanyl vs alfentanil. J Neurosurg Anesth 1:136, 1989
53. Ostapkovich ND, Baker KZ, Fogarty-Mack P *et al*: Cerebral blood flow and CO_2 reactivity is similar during remifentanil/N_2O and fentanyl/N_2O anesthesia. Anesthesiology 89:358, 1998
54. Viviand X, Garnier F: Opioid anesthetics (sufentanil and remifentanil) in neuroanesthesia. Ann Fr Anesth Reanim 23:383, 2004
55. Kadoi Y, Saito S, Kunimoto F *et al*: Comparative effects of propofol versus fentanyl on cerebral oxygenation state during normothermic cardiopulmonary bypass and postoperative cognitive dysfunction. Ann Thorac Surg 75:840, 2003
56. Maze M, Scarfini C, Cavaliere F: New agents for sedation in the intensive care unit. Crit Care Clin 7:88, 2001
57. Prielipp RC, Wall MH, Tobin JR *et al*: Dexmedetomidine-induced sedation in volunteers decreases regional and global cerebral blood flow. Anesth Analg 95:1052, 2002
58. Davis DW, Mans AM, Biebuyck JF *et al*: The influence of ketamine on regional brain glucose use. Anesthesiology 69:199, 1988
59. Takeshita H, Okuda Y, Sari A: The effects of ketamine on cerebral circulation and metabolism in man. Anesthesiology 36:69, 1972
60. Barbe MF, Tytell M, Gower DJ *et al*: Hyperthermia protects against light damage in the rat retina. Science 241:1817, 1988
61. Chopp M, Chen H, Ho KL *et al*: Transient hyperthermia protects against subsequent forebrain ischemic cell damage in the rat. Neurology 39:1396, 1989
62. For additional references, see Cottrell JE: Brain protection for neurosurgery. In Annual Refresher Course Lectures, Am Soc Anesthesiologists, 2004.
63. Stenzel-Poore MP, Stevens SL, Ziong Z *et al*: Effect of ischaemic preconditioning on genomic response to cerebral ischaemia: Similarity to neuroprotective strategies in hibernation and hypoxia-tolerant states. Lancet 362(9389):1007, 2003
64. Ehrenreich H, Hasselblatt M, Dembowski C *et al*: Erythropoietin therapy for acute stroke is both safe and beneficial. Molecular Medicine 8(8):495, 2002
65. Sharp FR, Liu J, Bernabeu R: Neurogenesis following brain ischemia. Brain Res Interactive. Developmental Brain Research 134:23, 2002
66. Zhang R, Zhang Z, Wang L *et al*: Activated neural stem cells contribute to stroke-induced neurogenesis and neuroblast migration toward the infarct boundary in adult rats. J Cereb Blood Flow Metab 24(4):441, 2004
67. Kempermann G, Wiskott l, Gage FH: Functional significance of adult neurogenesis. Curr Opin Neurobiol 14(2):186, 2004
68. Carmichael ST, Tatsukawa K, Katsman D *et al*: Evolution of diaschisis in a focal stroke model. Stroke 35:758–763, 2003
69. Berntman L, Welsh FA, Harp JR: Cerebral protective effect of low-grade hypothermia. Anesthesiology 55:495, 1981
70. Hartung J, Cottrell JE: Mild hypothermia and cerebral metabolism. J Neurosurg Anesth 6:1, 1994
71. Hartung J, Cottrell JE: In reply to: Effects of hypothermia on cerebral metabolic rate for oxygen. J Neurosurg Anesth 6:222, 1994
72. Todd M, Hindman B, Clark W et al: Intraoperative Hypothermia for Intracranial aneurysm surgery (IHAST): Initial Results. Presented at the 29th International Stroke Conference, San Diego, CA, February 7, 2004
73. Cottrell JE, Hartung J: Cool it on cooling—At least during aneurysm surgery. J Neurosurg Anesthesiol 16(2):113, 2004
74. Clifton GL, Miller ER, Choi SC *et al*: Lack of effect of induction of hypothermia after acute brain injury. N Eng J Med 344(8):556, 2001
75. Polderman K, Peerdeman S, Girbies AR: Hypophosphatemia and hypomagnesemia induced by cooling in patients with severe head injury. J Neurosurg 94:697, 2001
76. Bernard SA, Gray TW, Buist MD *et al*: Treatment of comatose survivors of out-of-hospital cardiac arrest with induced hypothermia. N Engl J Med 326(8):557, 2002
77. The Hypothermia After Cardiac Arrest Study Group: Mild therapeutic hypothermia to improve the neurologic outcome after cardiac arrest. N Engl J Med 346(8):549, 2002
78. Amorim P, Cottrell JE, Kass IS: Effect of small changes in temperature on CA1 pyramidal cells from rat hippocampal slices during hypoxia: implications about the mechanism of hypothermic protection against neuronal damage. Brain Res 844(1–2):143, 1999
79. Wang J, Chambers G, Cottrell JE *et al*: Differential fall in ATP accounts for effects of temperature on hypoxic damage in rat hippocampal slices. J Neurophysiology 83(6):3462, 2000
80. Knoll T, Wimmer MLJ, Gumpinger F *et al*: The low normothermia concept: maintaining a body temperature between 36.0 and 37.0 C in acute stroke unit patients. J Neurosurg Anesth 14(4):304, 2002
81. Bayona NA, Gelb AW, Jiang Z *et al*: Propofol neuroprotection in cerebral ischemia and its effects on low-molecular-weight antioxidants and skilled motor tasks. Anesthesiology 100(5):1151, 2004
82. Elsersy H, Sheng H, Lynch JR *et al*: Effects of isoflurane versus fentanyl-nitrous oxide anesthesia on long-term outcome from severe forebrain ischemia in the rat. Anesthesiology 100(5):1160, 2004
83. Hindman JB, Todd MM: Editorial views: Improving neurologic outcome after cardiac surgery. Anesthesiology 90:1243, 1990
84. Nakashima K, Todd MM, Warner DS: The relation between cerebral metabolic rate and ischemic depolarization. A comparison of the effects of hypothermia, pentobarbital, and isoflurane. Anesthesiology 82:1199, 1995
85. Verhaegen M, Laizzo PA, Todd MM: A comparison of the effects of hypothermia, pentobarbital, and isoflurane on cerebral energy stores at the time of ischemic depolarization. Anesthesiology 82:1209, 1995
86. Goodman JC, Valadka AB, Gopinath SP *et al*: Lactate and excitatory amino acids measured by microdialysis are decreased by pentobarbital coma in head-injured patients. J Neurotrauma 13:549, 1996
87. Zhu H, Cottrell JE, Kass IS: The effect of thiopental and propofol on NMDA- and AMPA-mediated glutamate excitotoxicity. Anesthesiology 87(4):944, 1997
88. Lei B, Popp S, Capuano-Waters C *et al*: Effects of low-dose lidocaine on cytochrome C release and caspase-3 activation after transient focal cerebral ischemia in rats. ASA 2002 Meeting Abstract A-800.
89. Fried E, Amorim P, Chambers G *et al*: The importance of sodium for anoxic transmission damage in rat hippocampal slices: mechanisms of protection by lidocaine. J Physiol (Lond) 489:557, 1995
90. Raley-Susman KM, Kass IS, Cottrell JE *et al*: Sodium influx blockade and hypoxic damage to CA1 pyramidal neurons in rat hippocampal slices. J Neurophysiology 86(6):2715, 2001
91. Lei B, Cottrell JE, Kass IS. Neuroprotective effect of low-dose lidocaine in a rat model of transient focal cerebral ischemia. Anesthesiology 96(2):445, 2001
92. Lei B, Popp S, Capuano-Waters C *et al*: Effects of delayed administration of low-dose lidocaine on transient focal cerebral ischemia in rats. ASA 97:1534, 2002
93. Mitchell SJ, Pellett O, Gorman DF1: Cerebral protection by lidocaine during cardiac operations. Ann Thor Surg 67:1117, 1999
94. Wang D, Wu X, Li J *et al*: The effect of lidocaine on early postoperative cognitive dysfunction after coronary artery bypass surgery. Anesthes Analg 95:1134, 2002
95. Mathew J, Grocott H, Phillips-Bute B *et al*: Lidocaine does not prevent cognitive dysfunction after cardiac surgery. Presented at the 26th Annual Meeting of the Society of Cardiovascular Anesthesiologists, Honolulu, April 24, 2004
96. Kass IS, Cottrell JE, Chambers G: Magnesium and cobalt, not nimodipine, protect against anoxic damage in the rat hippocampal slice. Anesthesiology 69:710, 1988
97. Saver JL, Kidwell C, Eckstein M *et al*: Prehospital neuroprotective therapy for acute stroke: Results of the field administration of stroke therapy-magnesium (FAST-MAG) Pilot Trial. Stroke 2004 (March 11) epub ahead of print DOI: 10.1161/01.STR.0000124458.98123.52
98. IMAGES Study Investigators: Magnesium for acute stroke: Randomized controlled trial. Lancet 363:439, 2004
99. Arrowsmith JE *et al*: Neuroprotection of the brain during cardiopulmonary bypass. Stroke 29:2357, 1998
100. Cruz J, Minoja G, Okuchi K *et al*: Successful use of the new high-dose mannitol treatment in patients with Glasgow Coma Scale scores of 3 and bilateral abnormal pupillary widening: a randomized trial. J Neurosurg 100:376, 2004
101. Marshall LF: High-dose mannitol. J Neurosurg 100:367, 2004
102. Barker FG, Ogilvy CS: Efficacy of prophylactic nimodipine for delayed ischemic deficit after subarachnoid hemorrhage: A meta-analysis. J Neurosurg 84:405, 1996
103. Ahmed N, Nasman P, Wahlgren NG: Effect of intravenous nimodipine on blood pressure and outcome after acute stroke. Stroke 31:1250, 2000
104. Horn J, de Haan RJ, Vermeulen M *et al*: Very early nimodipine use in stroke (VENUS): A randomized, double-blind, placebo-controlled trial. Stroke 32:461, 2001
105. Horn J, de Haan RJ, Vermeulen M *et al*: Nimodipine in animal model experiments of focal cerebral ischemia: A system review. Stroke 32:2433, 2001
106. Amadeu ME, Abramowicz AE, Chambers G *et al*: Etomidate does not alter recovery after anoxia of evoked population spikes recorded from the CA1 region of rat hippocampal slices. Anesthesiology 88:1274, 1998
107. Hoffman WE, Charbel FT, Edelman G *et al*: Comparison of the effect of etomidate and desflurane on brain tissue gases and pH during prolonged middle cerebral artery occlusion. Anesthesiology 88:1188, 1998
108. Courville CB: The pathogenesis of necrosis of the cerebral grey matter following nitrous oxide anesthesia. Ann Surg 107:371, 1938
109. Jevtovic-Todorovic V, Todorovic SM, Mennerick S *et al*: Nitrous oxide (laughing gas) is an NMDA antagonist, neuroprotectant and neurotoxin. Nature Med 4:460, 1998

110. Maze M, Fuijinaga M. Editorial: Recent advance in understanding the actions and toxicity of nitrous oxide. Anesthesia 55:311, 2000
111. Jevtovic-Todorovic V, Wozniak DF, Benshoff ND: A comparative evaluation of the neurotoxic properties of ketamine and nitrous oxide. Brain Res 859(1–2):264, 2001
112. Arnfred I, Secher O: Anoxia and barbiturates: Tolerance to anoxia in mice influenced by barbiturates. Arch Int Pharmacodyn 139:67, 1962
113. Wilhjelm BJ, Arnfred I: Protective action of some anaesthetics against anoxia. Acta Pharmacol 22:93, 1965
114. Hartung J, Cottrell JE: Nitrous oxide reduces thiopental-induced prolongation of survival in hypoxic and anoxic mice. Anesth Analg 66:47, 1987
115. Baughman VL, Hoffman WE, Thomas C *et al*: The interaction of nitrous oxide and isoflurane with incomplete cerebral ischemia in the rat. Anesthesiology 70(5):767, 1989
116. Jevtovic-Todorovic V, Benshoff N, Olney JW: Ketamine potentiates cerebrocortical damage induced by the common anaesthetic agent nitrous oxide in adult rats. Brit J Pharmacol 130(7):1692, 2000
117. Jevtovic-Todorovic V, Hartman RE, Izumi Y *et al*: Early exposure to common anesthetic agents causes widespread neurodegeneration in the developing rat brain and persistent learning deficits. J Neuroscience 23(3):876, 2003
118. Amorim P, Chambers G, Cottrell J *et al*: Nitrous oxide impairs electrophysiologic recovery after severe hypoxia in rat hippocampal slices. Anesthesiology 87:642, 1997
119. Hadzic A, Glab K, Sauborn KC *et al*: Severe neurologic deficit after nitrous oxide anesthesia. Anesthesiology 83:863, 1995
120. Enlund M: Is nitrous oxide a real gentleman? ACTA Anaesthesiologica Scandinavica 944:922, 2001
121. Kassell NF, Haley EC Jr., Apperson-Hansen C *et al*: Randomized, double-blind vehicle controlled trial of tirilazad mesylate in patients with aneurysmal subarachnoid hemorrhage: A cooperative study. J Neurosurg 84:221, 1996
122. Haley EC, Kassell NF, Apperson-Hansen *et al*: A randomized double-blind, vehicle-controlled trial of tirilazad mesylate in patients with aneurysmal subarachnoid hemorrhage: a cooperative study in North America. J Neurosurg 86:467, 1997
123. Lanzino G, Kassell NF, Dorsch NW *et al*: Double-blind randomized, vehicle-controlled study of high-dose tirilazad mesylate in women with aneurysmal subarachnoid hemorrhage. Part II. A comparative study in North America. J Neurosug 90:1018, 1999
124. Hartung J, Cottrell JE: Letters to the editor: Tirilazad and subarachnoid hemorrage. J Neurosurg 92:508, 2000
125. Bath PM, Iddenden R, Bath FJ *et al*: The Tirilazad International Steering Committee. Tirilazad for acute ischaemic stroke. Cochrane Database Syst Rev (4):CD002087, 2001
126. Rampil IJ: A primer for EEG signal processing in anesthesia. Anesthesiology 89:980, 1998
127. White PF, Ma H, Tang J *et al*: Does the use of electroencephalographic bispectral index or auditory evoked potential index monitoring facilitate recovery after desflurane anesthesia in the ambulatory setting? Anesthesiology 100:811, 2004
128. Vakkuri A, Yli-Hankala A, Talja P *et al*: Time-frequency balanced spectral entropy as a measure of anesthetic drug effect in central nervous system during sevoflurane, propofol, and thiopental anesthesia. Acta Anaesthesiol Scand 48:145, 2004
129. Nishiyama T, Matsukawa T, Hanaoka K: A comparison of the clinical usefulness of three different electroencephalogram monitors. Bispectral index, processed electroencephalogram, and alaris auditory evoked potentials. Anesth Analg 98:341, 2004
130. Myles PS, Leslie K, McNeil J *et al*: Bispectral index monitoring to prevent awareness during anesthesia: the B-Aware randomised controlled trial. Lancet 363:1757, 2004
131. Stockard JJ, Bickford RG: The neurophysiology of anesthesia. In Gordon E (ed): A Basis and Practice of Neuroanesthesia, 2nd ed, p 3. Amsterdam, Elsevier, 1981.
132. Banoub M, Tetzlaff JE, Schubert A: Pharmacology and physiologic influences affecting sensory evoked potentials. Anesthesiology 99:716, 2003
133. Peterson DO, Drummond JC, Todd MM: Effects of halothane, enflurane, isoflurane and nitrous oxide on somatosensory evoked potentials in humans. Anesthesiology 65:35, 1986
134. Lotto ML, Banoub M, Schubert A: Effects of anesthetic agents and physiologic changes on intraoperative motor evoked potentials. J Neurosurg Anesthesiol 16:32, 2004
135. Lundberg N: Continuous recording and control of ventricular fluid pressure in neurosurgical practice. Acta Psychiatr Neurol Scand 36(suppl 149):1, 1960
136. Patteson SK, Chesney JT: Anesthetic management for magnetic resonance imaging: Problems and solutions. Anesth Analg 74:121, 1992
137. Shellock FG, Crues JV: MR procedures: Biologic effects, safety, and patient care. Radiology 232:635, 2004
138. Hashimoto T, Gupta DK, Young WL: Interventional neuroradiology-anesthetic considerations. Anesthesiology Clin N Am 20:347, 2002
139. Castagnini HE, van Eijs F, Salevsky FC *et al*: Sevoflurane for interventional neuroradiology procedures is associated with more rapid early recovery than propofol. Can J Anesth 51:486, 2004
140. Qureshi AI, Suarez JI: Use of hypertonic saline solutions in treatment of cerebral edema and intracranial hypertension. Crit Care Med 28:3301, 2000
141. Vialet R, Albanese J, Thomachot L *et al*: Isovolume hypertonic solutes (sodium chloride or mannitol) in the treatment of refractory posttraumatic intracranial hypertension: 2 ml/kg 7% saline is more effective than 2 ml/kg 20% mannitol. Crit Care Med 31:1683, 2003
142. Obrist WD, Langfitt TW, Jaggi JL *et al*: Cerebral blood flow and metabolism in comatose patients with acute head injury. Relationship to intracranial hypertension. J Neurosurg 61(2):241, 1984
143. Coles JP, Minhas PS, Fryer TD *et al:* Effect of hyperventilation on cerebral blood flow in traumatic head injury: Clinical relevance and monitoring correlates. Crit Care Med 30:1950, 2002
144. For additional references, see Bendo AA, Kass IS, Hartung J *et al*: Anesthesia for neurosurgery. In Barash PG, Cullen BF, Stoelting RK (eds): Clinical Anesthesia, 4th ed, p 743. Lippincott Williams & Wilkins, Philadelphia, 2001
145. Lanier WL, Iaizzo PA, Milde JH. Cerebral function and muscle afferent activity following IV succinylcholine in dogs anesthetized with halothane: The effects of pretreatment with defasciculating doses of pancuronium. Anesthesiology 71:87, 1989
146. Kaye A, Kucera IJ, Heavner J *et al*: The comparative effects of desflurane and isoflurane on lumbar cerebrospinal fluid pressure in patients undergoing craniotomy for supratentorial tumors. Anesth Analg 98:1127, 2004
147. Larsen B, Seitz A, Larsen R: Recovery of cognitive function after remifentanil-propofol anesthesia: A comparison with desflurane and sevoflurane anesthesia. Anesth Analg 90:168, 2000
148. Cenic A, Craen RA, Lee T-Y *et al*: Cerebral blood volume and blood flow responses to hyperventilation in brain tumors during isoflurane or propofol anesthesia. Anesth Analg 94:661, 2002
149. Jansen GFA, van Praagh BH, Kadaria MB *et al*: Jugular bulb oxygen saturation during propofol and isoflurane/nitrous oxide anesthesia in patients undergoing brain tumor surgery. Anesth Analg 89:358, 1999
150. Kawano Y, Kawaguchi M, Horiuchi T *et al*: Jugular bulb oxygen saturation under propofol or sevoflurane/nitrous oxide anesthesia during deliberate mild hypothermia in neurosurgical patients. J Neurosurg Anesthesiol 16:6, 2004
151. Bruder N, Ravassin P: Recovery from anesthesia and postoperative extubation of neurosurgical patients: A review. J Neurosurg Anesthesiol 11:282, 1999
152. Basali A, Mascha EJ, Kalfas I *et al*: Relationship between perioperative hypertension and intracranial hemorrhage after craniotomy. Anesthesiology 93:48, 2000
153. Manninen PH, Tan TK: Postoperative nausea and vomiting after craniotomy for tumor surgery: A comparison between awake craniotomy and general anesthesia. J Clin Anesth 14:279, 2002
154. Bendo AA: Supratentorial tumors: Anesthetized, awake and computer-assisted management. In Schwartz AJ, et al (eds): ASA Refresher Courses in Anesthesiology, vol. 33, Lippincott Williams & Wilkins, Philadelphia, 2005
155. Mack PF, Perrine K, Kobylarz E *et al*: Dexmedetomidine and neurocognitive testing in awake craniotomy. J Neurosurg Anesth 16:20, 2004
156. Sarang A, Dinsmore J: Anesthesia for awake craniotomy—Evolution of a technique that facilitates awake neurological testing. Br J Anaesth 90:161, 2003
157. Porter JM, Pidgeon C, Cunningham AJ: The sitting position in neurosurgery: A critical appraisal. Br J Anaesth 82:117, 1999
158. Black S, Ockert DB, Oliver WC *et al*: Outcome following posterior fossa craniectomy in patients in the sitting or horizontal positions. Anesthesiology 69:49, 1988
159. Kwapisz MM, Deinsberger W, Müller M *et al*: Transesophageal echocardiography as a guide for patient positioning before neurosurgical procedures in semi-sitting position. J Neurosurg Anesthesiol 16:277, 2004
160. Ciric I, Ragin A, Baumgartner C *et al*: Complications of transsphenoidal surgery: Results of a national survey, review of the literature, and personal experience. Neurosurgery 40:225, 1997
161. Schievink WI: Intracranial aneurysms. N Engl J Med 336(1):28, 1997
162. Wardlaw JM, White PM: The detection and management of unruptured intracranial aneurysms. Brain 123:205, 2000
163. The International Study of Unruptured Intracranial Aneurysms Investigators. Unruptured intracranial aneurysms—Risk of rupture and risks of surgical intervention. N Engl J Med 339:1725, 1998
164. Bederson JB, Awad IA, Wiebers DO *et al*: Recommendations for the management of patients with unruptured intracranial aneurysms, from the Stroke Council of the AHA. Circulation 102:2300, 2000
165. The International Study of Unruptured Intracranial Aneurysms Investigators. Unruptured intracranial aneurysms: Natural history, clinical outcome, and risks of surgical and endovascular treatment. Lancet 362:103, 2003
166. Kassell NF, Torner JC: Aneurysmal rebleeding: A preliminary report from the Cooperative Aneurysm Study. J Neurosurg 13:479, 1983
167. Kassell NF, Torner JC, Haley EC *et al*: The International Cooperative Study on the Timing of Aneurysm Surgery. Part I: Overall management results. J Neurosurg 73:18, 1990
168. Kassell NF, Torner JC, Jane JA *et al*: The International Cooperative Study on the Timing of Aneurysm Surgery. Part II: Surgical results. J Neurosurg 73:37, 1990

169. Haley EC Jr, Kassell NF, Torner JC: The International Cooperative Study on the Timing of Aneurysm Surgery. The North American Experience. Stroke 23:205, 1992
170. Sen J, Belli A, Alban H *et al*: Triple-H therapy in the management of aneurysmal subarachnoid hemorrhage. Lancet Neurol 2(10):614, 2003
171. Treggiari MM, Walder B, Suter PM *et al*: Systematic review of the prevention of delayed ischemic neurologic deficits with hypertension, hypervolemia, and hemodilution therapy following subarachnoid hemorrhage. J Neurosurg 98(5):978, 2003
172. Feng L, Fitzsimmons B-F, Young WL *et al*: Intraarterially administered verapamil as adjunct therapy for cerebral vasospasm: Safety and 2-year experience. AJNR 23:1284, 2002
173. Rajshekhar V, Harbaugh RE: Results of routine ventriculostomy with external ventricular drainage for acute hydrocephalus following subarachnoid hemorrhage. Acta Neurochir (Wien) 115:8, 1992
174. Molyneux A: International Subarachnoid Aneurysm Trial (ISAT) of neurosurgical clipping versus endovascular coiling in 2143 patients with ruptured intracranial aneurysms: A randomized trial. Lancet 360(9342):1267, 2002
175. Nichols DA, Brown RD Jr, Meyer FB: Coils or clips in subarachnoid haemorrhage? Lancet 360(9342):1262, 2002
176. Todd MM, Hindman BJ, Clark WR *et al*: Mild inoperative hypothermia during surgery for intracranial aneursym. N Engl J Med 352(2):135, 2005
177. Dodson BA: Interventional neuroradiology and the anesthetic management of patients with arteriovenous malformations. In Cottrell JE, David DS (eds): Anesthesia and Neurosurgery, 4th ed, p 399. St. Louis, Mosby, Inc., 2001
178. Taylor CL, Dutton K, Rappard G *et al*: Complications of preoperative embolization of cerebral arteriovenous malformations. J Neurosurg 100:810, 2004
179. Young WL, Kader A, Ornstein E *et al*: Cerebral hyperemia after arteriovenous malformation resection is related to "breakthrough" complications but not to feeding artery pressure. Neurosurgery 38:1085, 1996
180. Miller JD: Assessing patients with head injury. Br J Surg 77:241, 1990
181. Chesnut RM, Marshall LF, Klauber MR *et al*: The role of secondary brain injury in determining outcome from severe head injury. J Trauma 34:216, 1993
182. Hastings RH, Marks JD: Airway management for trauma patients with potential cervical spine injuries. Anesth Analg 73:471, 1991
183. Crosby ET, Lui A: The adult cervical spine: Implications for airway management. Can J Anaesth 37:77, 1990
184. Hoffman JR, Mower WR, Wolfson AB *et al*: Validity of a set of clinical criteria to rule out injury to the cervical spine in patients with blunt trauma. N Engl J Med 343(2):94, 2000
185. Lennarson PJ, Smith D, Todd MM *et al*: Segmental cervical spinal motion during orotracheal intubation of the intact and injured spine with and without external stabilization. J Neurosurg (Spine 2) 92:201, 2000
186. Zornow MH, Todd MM, Moore SS: The acute cerebral effects of changes in plasma osmolality and oncotic pressure. Anesthesiology 67:936, 1987
187. Kaieda R, Todd MM, Cook LN *et al*: Acute effects of changing plasma osmolality and colloid oncotic pressure on the formation of brain edema after cryogenic injury. Neurosurgery 24:671, 1989
188. Kaieda R, Todd MM, Warner DS: Prolonged reduction in colloid oncotic pressure does not increase brain edema following cryogenic injury in rabbits. Anesthesiology 72:554, 1989
189. Drummond JC, Patel PM, Cole DJ *et al*: The effect of the reduction of colloid oncotic pressure, with and without reduction of osmolality, on post-traumatic cerebral edema. Anesthesiology 88:993, 1998
190. Prough DS, Whitley JM, Taylor CL *et al*: Regional cerebral blood flow following resuscitation from hemorrhagic shock with hypertonic saline. Anesthesiology 75:319, 1991
191. The Brain Trauma Foundation Update Notice: Guidelines for the management of severe traumatic brain injury: Cerebral perfusion pressure. 2002. Available from http://www2.braintrauma.org/guidelines/
192. Guidelines for the Management of Severe Head Injury: Brain Trauma Foundation, American Association of Neurologic Surgery, Joint Section on Neurotrauma and Critical Care. J Neurotrauma 13:641, 1996
193. Bullock RM, Chesnut RM, Clifton GL *et al*: Part 1: Guidelines for the management of severe traumatic brain injury. J Neurotrauma 17:451, 2000
194. Martin NA, Patwardhan RV, Alexander MJ *et al*: Characterization of cerebral hemodynamic phases following severe head trauma: Hypoperfusion, hyperemia, and vasospasm. J Neurosurgery 87:9, 1997
195. Matjasko MJ: Multisystem sequelae of severe head injury. In Cottrell JE, Smith DS (eds): Anesthesia and Neurosurgery, 4th ed, p 693. St. Louis, Mosby, Inc., 2001

CHAPTER 28 ■ RESPIRATORY FUNCTION IN ANESTHESIA

M. CHRISTINE STOCK

KEY POINTS

1. In a person with normal lungs, both breathing and coughing can be performed exclusively by the diaphragm.
2. In the adult, the tip of an orotracheal tube moves an average of 3.8 cm with flexion and extension of the neck, but can travel as much as 6.4 cm. In infants and children, displacement of even 1 cm can move the tube above the vocal cords or below the carina.
3. The following anatomy should be considered when contemplating the use of a double-lumen tube. The adult right main-stem bronchus is ~2.5 cm long before it branches into lobar bronchi. In 10% of adults, the right upper lobe bronchus departs from the right main-stem bronchus less than 2.5 cm above the carina. In 2 to 3% of adults, the right upper lobe bronchus opens into the trachea, above the carina.
4. When lung compliance is small, larger changes in pleural pressure are needed to create the same Vt. Patients with low lung compliance breathe with smaller Vt and more rapidly, making spontaneous respiratory rate the most sensitive clinical index of lung compliance.
5. Carotid and aortic bodies are stimulated by PaO_2 values less than 60 to 65 mm Hg. Thus, patients who depend on hypoxic ventilatory drive do not have PaO_2 values >65 mm Hg. The peripheral receptors' response will not reliably increase ventilatory rate or minute ventilation to herald the onset of hypoxemia during general anesthesia or recovery.
6. There are three etiologies of hyperventilation: arterial hypoxemia, metabolic acidemia, and central etiologies (e.g., intracranial hypertension, hepatic cirrhosis, anxiety, pharmacologic agents).
7. Increases in dead space ventilation primarily affect CO_2 elimination (with minimal influence on arterial oxygenation), and physiologic shunt increase primarily affects arterial oxygenation (with minimal influence on CO_2 elimination).
8. During spontaneous ventilation, the ratio of alveolar ventilation to dead space ventilation is 2:1. The alveolar-to-dead space ventilation ratio during positive-pressure ventilation is 1:1. Thus, minute ventilation during mechanical ventilatory support must be greater than that during spontaneous ventilation to achieve the same $PaCO_2$.
9. $PaCO_2 \geq PETCO_2$ unless the patient inspires or receives exogenous CO_2. The difference between $PaCO_2$ and $PETCO_2$ is due to dead space ventilation. The most common reason for an acute increase in dead space ventilation is decreased cardiac output.
10. The best evaluation of the efficiency with which the lungs oxygenate the arterial blood is the calculation of shunt fraction. It is the only index of oxygenation that takes into account the contribution of mixed venous blood to arterial oxygenation.
11. When functional residual capacity (FRC) is reduced, lung compliance falls and results in tachypnea, and venous admixture increases, creating arterial hypoxemia.

12 There is no compelling evidence that defines rules or parameters for ordering preoperative pulmonary function tests. Rather, they should be obtained to ascertain the presence of the reversible pulmonary dysfunction (bronchospasm) or to define the severity of advanced pulmonary disease.

13 Smoking patients should be advised to *stop* smoking at least 2 months prior to an elective operation to decrease the risk of postoperative pulmonary complications (PPCs).

14 The operative site is one of the most important determinants of the risk of PPC. The highest risk for PPC is associated with nonlaparoscopic upper abdominal operations, followed by lower abdominal and intrathoracic operations.

15 The single most important aspect of postoperative pulmonary care and prevention of PPC is getting the patient out of bed, preferably walking.

Anesthesiologists directly manipulate pulmonary function. Thus, a sound and thorough working knowledge of applied pulmonary physiology is essential to the safe conduct of anesthesia. This chapter discusses pulmonary anatomy, the control of ventilation, oxygen and carbon dioxide transport, ventilation–perfusion relationships, lung volumes and pulmonary function testing, abnormal physiology and anesthesia, the effect of smoking on pulmonary function, and assessing risk for PPCs.

FUNCTIONAL ANATOMY OF THE LUNGS

This section emphasizes functional lung anatomy, with structure described as it applies to the mechanical and physiologic function of the lungs.

Thorax

The thoracic cage is shaped like a truncated cone, with small superior and large inferior openings and diaphragms attached at the base. The sternal angle is located in the horizontal plane that passes through the vertebral column at the T4 or T5 level. This plane separates the superior from the inferior mediastinum. The predominant ventilatory changes in thoracic diameter occur in the anteroposterior direction in the upper thoracic region and in the lateral or transverse direction in the lower portion of the thorax.

Muscles of Ventilation

The ventilatory muscles are endurance muscles. Poor nutrition, chronic obstructive pulmonary disease (COPD) with gas trapping, and increased airway resistance predispose to the development of ventilatory failure due to ventilatory muscle fatigue. The ventilatory muscles include the diaphragm, intercostal muscles, abdominal muscles, cervical strap muscles, sternocleidomastoid muscles, and the large back and intervertebral muscles of the shoulder girdle. The primary ventilatory muscle is the diaphragm, with minor contributions from the intercostal muscles. Normally, at rest, inspiration requires work and expiration is passive. As ventilatory effort increases, abdominal muscles assist with rib depression and increase intra-abdominal pressure to facilitate forced exhalation causing the "stitch" athletes experience when they actively exhale. With a further increase in effort, the cervical strap muscles help elevate the sternum and upper portions of the chest. Finally, the large back and paravertebral muscles of the shoulder girdle become
1 important during maximum ventilatory effort. In a person with normal lungs, both breathing and coughing can be performed exclusively by the diaphragm.

Ventilatory muscles must create sufficient force to lift the ribs to create subatmospheric pressure in the intrapleural space. Breathing is an endurance phenomenon, thus involving fatigue-resistant fibers, characterized by a slow-twitch response to electrical stimulation. They comprise approximately 50% of the diaphragmatic fibers and, because of their high oxidative capacity, function mostly as endurance units.[1] Fast-twitch muscle fibers, which are susceptible to fatigue, have rapid responses to electrical stimulation, impart strength, and allow the muscle to produce greater force over a short period of time. Thus, the diaphragm is composed of fast-twitch fibers that are useful during brief periods of maximal ventilatory effort (coughing, sneezing) and slow-twitch fibers provide endurance (breathing without rest).[2] The muscles of the abdominal wall, the most powerful muscles of expiration, are important for expulsive efforts such as coughing.[3]

To perform work, a muscle must be firmly anchored at both its origin and insertion. The diaphragm is unique because its insertion is mobile—an untethered central tendon that originates from fibers directly attached to the vertebral bodies and the costal portions of the lower ribs and sternum. Diaphragmatic contraction results in descent of the diaphragmatic dome and expansion of the thoracic base. These changes result in decreased intrathoracic and intrapleural pressure, with a corresponding increase in intra-abdominal pressure.

The cervical strap muscles are active even during breathing at rest. They are the most important inspiratory accessory muscles, and become the primary inspiratory muscles when diaphragmatic function is impaired, as in patients with cervical spinal cord transection.

Lung Structures

With an intact respiratory system, the expandable lung tissue completely fills the pleural cavity. The visceral and parietal pleurae are constantly in contact with each other, creating a potential intrapleural space in which pressure decreases when the diaphragm descends and the rib cage expands. At passive end inspiration, the resultant subatmospheric intrapleural pressure is a reflection of the opposing and equal forces between the tendency of the lung to collapse and the chest wall musculature to remain expanded. These equal and opposing forces at end inspiration result in the functional residual capacity (FRC), the volume of gas in the lungs at passive end expiration. The intrapleural space normally has a slightly subambient pressure (−2 to −3 mm Hg) at FRC. With inspiration, the intrapleural pressure becomes more negative as the chest wall expands. Major divisions of the right and left lung are listed in Table 28-1. Working knowledge of the bronchopulmonary segments is important for localizing lung pathology, interpreting lung radiographs, identifying lung regions during bronchoscopy, and operating on the lung. Each bronchopulmonary segment is separated from its adjacent segments by well-defined connective tissue planes. Therefore, pulmonary pathology initially tends to remain segmental.

The lung parenchyma can be subdivided into three airway categories based on functional lung anatomy (Table 28-2). The conductive airways provide basic gas transport but no gas exchange. The next group, which has smaller diameters, is transitional airways. Transitional airways are conduits for gas movement, and additionally perform limited gas diffusion and

TABLE 28-1

MAJOR DIVISIONS OF THE LUNG

■ LUNG SIDE/LOBE	■ BRONCHOPULMONARY SEGMENT
■ RIGHT	
Upper	Apical
	Anterior
	Posterior
Middle	Medial
	Lateral
Lower	Superior
	Medial basal
	Lateral basal
	Anterior basal
	Posterior basal
■ LEFT	
Upper	Apical posterior
	Anterior
Lingula	Superior
	Inferior
Lower	Superior
	Posterior basal
	Anteromedial basal
	Lateral basal

exchange. Finally, the smallest respiratory airways' primary function is gas exchange.

Conventionally, large airways with diameters of >2 mm create 90% of total airway resistance. The number of alveoli increases progressively with age, starting at approximately 24 million at birth and reaching the final adult count of 300 million by the age of 8 to 9 years. The alveoli are associated with about 250 million precapillaries and 280 billion capillary segments, resulting in a surface area of ~70 m² for gas exchange.

Conductive Airways

In the adult, the trachea is a fibromuscular tube ~10 to 12 cm long with an outside diameter of ~20 mm. Structural support is provided by 20 U-shaped hyaline cartilages, with the open part of the U facing posteriorly. The cricoid membrane tethers the trachea to the cricoid cartilage at the level of the sixth cervical vertebral body. The trachea enters the superior mediastinum and bifurcates at the sternal angle (the lower border of the fourth thoracic vertebral body). Normally, half of the trachea is intrathoracic and half is extrathoracic. Both ends of the trachea are attached to mobile structures. Thus, the adult carina can move superiorly as much as 5 cm from its normal
2 resting position. Airway "motion" becomes important in the intubated patient. In the adult, the tip of an orotracheal tube moves an average of 3.8 cm with flexion and extension of the neck but can travel as far as 6.4 cm.[4] In infants and children, tracheal tube movement with respect to the trachea is even more critical: displacement of even 1 cm can move the tube above the cords or below the carina.

The next airway generation is composed of the right and left main-stem bronchi. The diameter of the right bronchus is generally greater than that of the left. In the adult, the right bronchus leaves the trachea at ~25° from the vertical tracheal axis, whereas the angle of the left bronchus is ~45°. Thus, inadvertent endobronchial intubation or aspiration of foreign material is more likely to occur in the right lung than the left. Furthermore, the right upper lobe bronchus dives almost directly posterior at ~90° from the right main bronchus. Foreign bodies and fluid aspirated by a supine subject usually fall into the right upper lobe. In children younger than 3 years of age, the angles created by the right and left main-stem bronchi are approximately equal, with takeoff angles of about 55°.

3 The adult right main bronchus is ~2.5 cm long before it initially branches into lobar bronchi. However, in 10% of adults, the right upper lobe bronchus departs from the right main-stem bronchus less than 2.5 cm from the carina. Furthermore, in ~2 to 3% of adults, the right upper lobe bronchus opens into the trachea, above the carina. Patients with these anomalies require special consideration when placing double-lumen tracheal tubes, especially if one contemplates inserting a right-sided endobronchial tube. After the right upper and middle lobe bronchi divide from the right main bronchus, the main channel becomes the right lower lobe bronchus.

The left main bronchus is ~5 cm long before its initial branching point to the left upper lobe and the lingual. Then, it continues on as the left lower lobe bronchus.

The bronchioles, typically 1 mm in diameter, are devoid of cartilaginous support and have the highest proportion of smooth muscle in the wall. Of the three to four bronchiolar generations, the final generation is the terminal bronchiole, which is the last airway component that does not participate in gas exchange.

Transitional Airways

The respiratory bronchiole, which follows the terminal bronchiole, is the first site in the tracheobronchial tree where gas exchange occurs. In adults, two or three generations of respiratory bronchioles lead to alveolar ducts, of which there are four to five generations, each with multiple openings into alveolar sacs. The final divisions of alveolar ducts terminate in alveolar sacs that open into alveolar clusters.

Respiratory Airways and the Alveolar–Capillary Membrane

The pulmonary capillary beds are the densest capillary networks in the body. This extensive vascular branching system starts with pulmonary arterioles in the region of the respiratory bronchioles. Each alveolus is closely associated with ~1,000 short capillary segments.

The alveolar–capillary interface is complicated but well designed to facilitate gas exchange. Viewed with electron microscopy, the alveolar wall consists of a thin capillary epithelial cell, a basement membrane, a pulmonary capillary endothelial cell, and a surfactant lining layer. The flattened, squamous type I alveolar cells cover ~80% of the alveolar surface. Type I cells contain flattened nuclei and extremely thin cytoplasmic extensions that provide the surface for gas exchange. Type I cells are

TABLE 28-2

FUNCTIONAL AIRWAY DIVISIONS

■ TYPE	■ FUNCTION	■ STRUCTURE
Conductive	Bulk gas movement	Trachea to terminal bronchioles
Transitional	Bulk gas movement Limited gas exchange	Respiratory bronchioles Alveolar ducts
Respiratory	Gas exchange	Alveoli Alveolar sacs

highly differentiated and metabolically limited, which makes them highly susceptible to injury. When type I cells are damaged severely (during acute lung injury or adult respiratory distress syndrome), type II cells replicate and modify to form new type I cells.[5]

Type II alveolar cells are interspersed among type I cells, primarily at alveolar–septal junctions. These polygonal cells have vast metabolic and enzymatic activity, and manufacture surfactant. The enzymatic activity required to produce surfactant is only 50% of the total enzymatic activity present in type II alveolar cells.[6] The remaining enzymatic activity modulates local electrolyte balance, as well as endothelial and lymphatic cell functions. Both type I and type II alveolar cells have tight intracellular junctions, thus providing a relatively impermeable barrier to fluids.

Type III alveolar cells, alveolar macrophages, are an important element of lung defense. Their migratory and phagocytic activities result in the ingestion of foreign materials within alveolar spaces.[7] Although functional pulmonary macrophages reduce the incidence of lung infection,[8] they are also an integral part of the lung inflammatory response. Therefore, whether their presence is good (to reduce the change of infection) or bad (because they contribute to the inflammatory response) is highly controversial.[9]

Finally, numerous finger-like projections of the capillary endothelial cells greatly increase their surface area. They also provide intimate contact between the capillary endothelial cell and the entire circulating blood volume. Thus, the alveolar-capillary membrane has two primary functions: transport of respiratory gases (oxygen and carbon dioxide), and the production of a wide variety of local and humoral substances.

Pulmonary Vascular Systems

Two major circulatory systems supply blood to the lungs: the pulmonary and bronchial vascular networks. The pulmonary vascular system delivers mixed-venous blood from the right ventricle to the pulmonary capillary bed via the pulmonary arteries. After gas exchange occurs in the pulmonary capillary bed, oxygen-rich and carbon dioxide-poor blood is returned to the left atrium via the pulmonary veins. The pulmonary veins run independently along the intralobar connective tissue planes. The pulmonary capillary system adequately provides for the metabolic and oxygen needs of the alveolar parenchyma. However, the bronchial arterial system must provide oxygen to the conductive airways and pulmonary vessels. Anatomic connections between the bronchial and pulmonary venous circulations create an absolute shunt of ~2 to 5% of the total cardiac output, and represents "normal" shunt.

LUNG MECHANICS

Lung movement is entirely passive and responds to forces external to the lungs. During spontaneous ventilation, the external forces are produced by ventilatory muscles. The lungs' response is governed by the impedance of the chest wall and by the airways. This impedance, or hindrance, falls mainly into two categories: (1) elastic recoil of the lung and gas–liquid interface, and (2) resistance to gas flow.

Elastic Work

The lungs' natural tendency is to collapse; thus, expiration at rest is normally passive because gas flows out of the lungs when they elastically recoil. The thoracic cage exerts an outward-directed force, and the lungs exert an inward-directed force. Together these forces result in a subatmospheric intrapleural pressure. Because the outward force of the thoracic cage exceeds the inward force of the lung, the overall tendency of the lung is to remain inflated when it resides within the thoracic cage. At FRC, the outward and inward forces on the lung are equal. Thus, at passive end-exhalation, the respiratory muscles are relaxed and the lung returns to its resting volume within the relaxed thorax: FRC. Gravitational forces create a more subatmospheric pressure in nondependent areas of the lung than in dependent areas. In the upright adult, the difference in intrapleural pressure from the top to the bottom of the lung is ~7 cm H_2O.

Surface tension at an air–fluid interface produces forces that tend to further reduce the area of interface. The gas pressure within a bubble is always higher than the surrounding gas pressure because of the bubble's surface tension. Thus, the bubble remains inflated. The alveoli resemble bubbles in this respect, although alveolar gas communicates with the atmosphere via the airways, unlike a bubble. The Laplace equation describes this phenomenon: $P = 2T/R$, where P is the pressure within the bubble (dyn $\cdot$ cm^{-2}), T is the surface tension of the liquid (dyn $\cdot$ cm^{-1}), and R is the radius of the bubble (cm).

During inspiration, the surface tension of the liquid in the lung increases to 40 mN/m, a value close to that of plasma. During expiration, this surface tension falls to 19 mN/m, a value lower than that of most other fluids. The alveoli experience hysteresis, that is, different pressure–volume relationships during inspiration and expiration. In contrast to a bubble, the pressure within an alveolus decreases as the radius of curvature decreases. Thus, gas tends to flow from larger to smaller alveoli, thereby maintaining stability and preventing lung collapse.

The alveolar transmural pressure gradient, or transpulmonary pressure, is the difference between intrapleural and alveolar pressure and is directly proportional to lung volume. Intrapleural pressure can be safely measured with a percutaneously inserted catheter;[10] however, clinicians rarely perform this technique. Esophageal pressure can be used as a reflection of intrapleural pressure, but the esophageal balloon must reside in the midesophagus to avoid inaccurate measurement.[11] Commercially available esophageal pressure monitors increase the ease and accuracy of measuring esophageal pressure as a reflection of intrapleural pressure.[12] These monitors are useful for estimating the elastic work performed by the patient during spontaneous ventilation, mechanical ventilation, or a combination of spontaneous and mechanical ventilation. By estimating intrapleural pressure on a real-time basis, it is possible to quantitate the patient's work of breathing as one intervenes. For example, low levels of inspiratory pressure support can compensate for the work of breathing imposed by the endotracheal tube.[13]

Physiologic work of breathing includes elastic work (inspiratory work required to overcome the elastic recoil of the pulmonary system) and resistive work (work to overcome resistance to gas flow in the airway). For a patient in whom breathing apparatus is employed, the concept of total work of breathing encompasses physiologic work plus equipment-imposed ventilatory work: the work performed by the patient to overcome the resistance imposed by the breathing apparatus. Examples of imposed work include the resistance imposed by tracheal tubes and demand valves.

If the lungs are slowly inflated and deflated, the pressure–volume curve during inflation differs from that obtained during deflation. The two curves form a hysteresis loop that becomes progressively broader as the tidal volume is increased (Fig. 28-1). A greater pressure than anticipated is required during inflation, and recoil pressure is less than expected during deflation. Thus, the lung accepts deformation poorly and, once deformed, assumes its original shape slowly. This elastic hysteresis is important for the maintenance of normal lung compliance

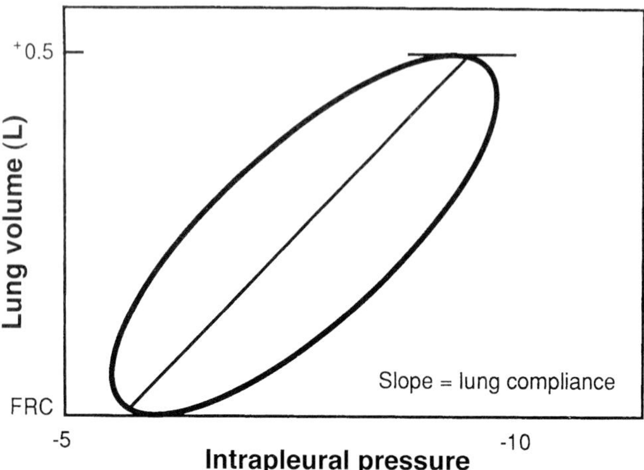

FIGURE 28-1. Dynamic pressure–volume loop of resting tidal volume. Quiet, normal breathing is characterized by hysteresis of the pressure–volume loop. The lung is more resistant to deformation than expected and returns to its original configuration less easily than expected. The slope of the line connecting the zenith and nadir lung volumes is lung compliance, ~500 mL/3 cm H_2O = 167 mL/cm H_2O.

but is not clinically significant. Thus, in the following discussion, it is ignored.

The sum of the pressure–volume relationships of the thorax and lung results in a sigmoidal curve (Fig. 28-2). The vertical line drawn at end expiration coincides with FRC. Normally, humans breathe on the steepest part of the sigmoidal curve, where compliance is highest. The compliance of the curve is represented by the slope of the curve ($\Delta V/\Delta P$). In restrictive diseases, the curve shifts to the right, the slope is depressed, or both. These changes result in smaller FRCs and lower lung compliance. When lung compliance is small, larger changes in

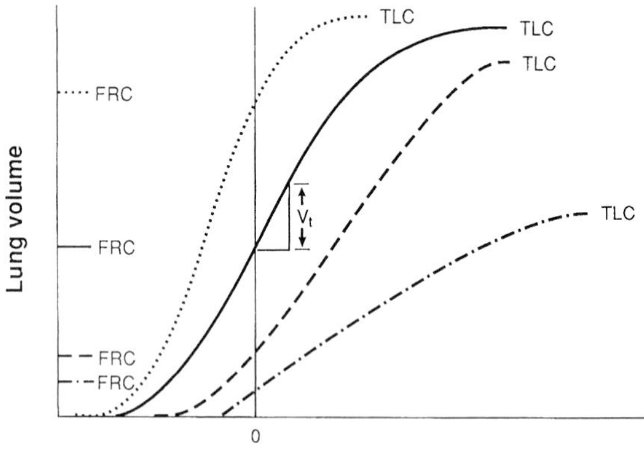

FIGURE 28-2. Pulmonary pressure–volume relationships at different values of total lung capacity (TLC), ignoring hysteresis. The *solid line* depicts the normal pulmonary pressure–volume relationships. Humans normally breathe on the linear, steep part of this sigmoidal curve, where the slope, which is equal to compliance, is greatest. The *vertical line* at zero defines functional residual capacity (FRC), regardless of the position of the curve on the graph. Mild restrictive lung disease, indicated by the *dashed line*, shifts the curve to the right with little change in slope. However, with restrictive disease, the patient breathes on a lower FRC, at a point on the curve where the slope is less. Severe restrictive pulmonary disease profoundly depresses the FRC and diminishes the slope of the entire curve (*dashed-dotted line*). Obstructive disease (*dotted line*) elevates both FRC and compliance.

intrapleural pressure are needed to create the same tidal volume; that is, the thorax has to suck harder to get the same volume of gas into the lungs. The body, being a smart organism, prefers to move less gas with each breath rather than sucking
4 harder to achieve the same tidal volume. Thus, patients with low lung compliance typically breathe with smaller tidal volumes at more rapid rates, making spontaneous ventilatory rate one of the most sensitive indices of lung compliance.

Continuous positive airway pressure (CPAP) will shift the vertical line to the right, thus allowing the patient to breathe on a steeper and more favorable portion of the volume–pressure curve, resulting in a slower ventilatory rate with a larger tidal volume.

At the other end of the spectrum, patients with diseases that increase lung compliance experience larger than normal FRC (gas trapping), and their pressure–volume curves shift to the left and steepen. These patients expend less elastic work to inspire, but elastic recoil is reduced significantly. Chronic obstructive lung disease and acute asthma are the most common examples of diseases with high lung compliance. If lung compliance and FRC are sufficiently high that elastic recoil is minimal, the patient must use ventilatory muscles to actively expire. The difficulty these patients experience in emptying the lungs is compounded by the increased airway resistance.

Both compliance and inspiratory elastic work can be measured for a single breath by measuring airway (Paw), intrapleural (Ppl) pressures, and tidal volume. If esophageal pressure is measured carefully, the esophageal pressure values can be substituted for Ppl values. Lung compliance, C_L, the slope of the volume–pressure curve, is given by the equation

$$C_L = \frac{\Delta V}{\Delta P_L} + \frac{Vt}{P_{L_i} - P_{L_e}} = \frac{Vt}{(Paw_i - Ppl_i) - (Paw_e - Ppl_e)} \quad (28\text{-}1)$$

where P_L is transpulmonary pressure, PL_i and PL_e are transpulmonary pressure at end-inspiratory and end-expiratory, Vt is tidal volume, Paw_e and Paw_i are expiratory and inspiratory airway pressures, and Ppl_e and Ppl_i are expiratory and inspiratory intrapleural pressures.

Elastic work (W_{el}) is performed during inspiration only because expiration is passive during normal breathing. The area within the triangle in Figure 28-2 describes the work required to inspire. The equation that yields elastic work (and the area of the triangle) is

$$\begin{aligned} W_{el} &= \tfrac{1}{2}(Vt)(PL_i - PL_e) \\ &= \tfrac{1}{2}(Vt)[(Paw_i - Ppl_i) - (Paw_e - Pple)] \end{aligned} \quad (28\text{-}2)$$

Resistance to Gas Flow

Both laminar and turbulent flows exist within the respiratory tract, usually in mixed patterns. The physics of each, however, is significantly different and worth consideration.

Laminar Flow

Below critical flows, gas proceeds through a straight tube as a series of concentric cylinders that slide over one another. Fully developed flow has a parabolic profile with a velocity of zero at the cylinder wall and a maximum velocity at the center of the advancing "cone." Peripheral cylinders tend to be stationary, and the central cylinder moves fastest. This type of streamlined flow is usually inaudible. The advancing conical front means that some fresh gas reaches the end of the tube before the tube has been completely filled with fresh gas. A clinical implication of laminar flow in the airways is that significant alveolar ventilation can occur even when the tidal volume (Vt) is less than anatomic dead space. This phenomenon, noted by Rohrer in 1915,[14] is important in high-frequency ventilation.

Laminar gas flows in a straight, unbranched tube encounter meets resistance that can be calculated by the following equation:

$$R = \frac{8 \times \text{length} \times \text{viscosity}}{\pi \times (\text{radius})^4} = \frac{P_B - P_A}{\text{flow}} \quad (28\text{-}3)$$

where P_B and P_A are barometric and alveolar pressures. The inverse relationship between resistance and the fourth power of the radius explains the critical importance of narrowed air passages. Viscosity is the only physical gas property that is relevant under conditions of laminar flow. Helium has a low density, but its viscosity is close to that of air. Therefore, helium will not improve gas flow if the flow is laminar. Usually, flow is turbulent when there is critical airway narrowing or abnormally high airway resistance, making low-density helium useful therapy (see next section).

Turbulent Flow

High flow rates, particularly through branched or irregularly shaped tubes, disrupt the orderly flow of laminar gas. Turbulent flow is usually audible and is almost invariably present when high resistance to gas flow is problematic. Turbulent flow usually presents with a square front so fresh gas will not reach the end of the tube until the amount of gas entering the tube is almost equal to the volume of the tube. Thus, turbulent flow effectively purges the contents of a tube. Four conditions that will change laminar flow to turbulent flow are high gas flows, sharp angles within the tube, branching in the tube, and a change in the tube's diameter.

Resistance during laminar flow is inversely proportional to gas flow rate. Conversely, during turbulent flow, resistance increases in proportion to the flow rate. A detailed description of these phenomena is beyond the scope of this chapter, but the reader is referred to descriptions by Nunn.[15]

Increased Airway Resistance

Bronchiolar smooth muscle hyperreactivity (true bronchospasm), mucosal edema, mucous plugging, epithelial desquamation, tumors, and foreign bodies all increase airway resistance. The normal response to increased inspiratory resistance is increased inspiratory muscle effort, with little change in FRC.[16] Accessory muscles act according to the degree of resistance. The conscious subject can detect small increases in inspiratory resistance.[17]

Emphysematous patients retain remarkable ability to preserve an adequate alveolar ventilation, even with gross airway obstruction. In patients with preoperative FEV_1 values <1 L, Pa_{CO_2} is normal in most patients. Furthermore, asthmatic patients compensate well for increased airway resistance and also keep the mean Pa_{CO_2} in the lower end of normal range.[18] Thus, an increased Pa_{CO_2} in the setting of increased airway resistance deserves serious attention and may signal that the patient's compensatory mechanisms are nearly exhausted.

Mild expiratory resistance does not result in activation of the expiratory muscles in conscious or anesthetized subjects. The initial work to overcome expiratory resistance is performed by augmenting inspiratory force until a sufficiently high lung volume is achieved so elastic recoil overcomes expiratory resistance.[19] The immediate effects of excessive expiratory resistance are to use accessory muscles to force gas from the lungs. This response is useful during acute increases in expiratory resistance. However, patients who chronically use accessory muscles to expire are at risk for ventilatory muscle fatigue if they experience an acute worsening of ventilatory work, most commonly precipitated by pneumonia or heart failure.

Physiologic Changes in Respiratory Function Associated With Aging[20]

Physiologic aging of the lung is associated with dilation of the alveoli, enlargement of the airspaces, decrease in exchange surface area, and loss of supporting tissue. Changes in the aging lung and chest wall result in decreased lung recoil, and increased residual volume and FRC. Compliance of the chest wall diminishes, thereby increasing the work of breathing compared with younger subjects. Respiratory muscle strength decreases with aging and is strongly correlated with nutritional status and cardiac index. Expiratory flow rates decrease with a flow–volume curve suggestive of small airway resistance. Despite these changes, the respiratory system is able to maintain adequate gas exchange at rest and during exertion throughout life, with only modest decrements in Pa_{O_2} and no change in Pa_{CO_2}. The respiratory centers lose sensitivity to hypoxemia and hypercapnia; thus, the elderly exhibit a blunted ventilatory response when challenged by heart failure, airway obstruction, or pneumonia.

CONTROL OF VENTILATION

Mechanisms that control ventilation are extremely complex, requiring integration with many parts of the central and peripheral nervous systems (Fig. 28-3). LeGallois, who localized the respiratory centers in the brainstem in 1812, demonstrated that breathing does not depend on an intact cerebrum. Rather, breathing depends on a small region of the medulla near the origin of the vagus nerves.[21] Countless studies in the past two centuries have greatly increased our knowledge and understanding of the anatomic components of ventilatory control. However, experimental work performed in animals is difficult to apply to humans because of interspecies variation.

Generation of Ventilatory Pattern

Refer to Table 28-3 for definitions of terms used in this section. A *respiratory center* is a specific area in the brain that integrates any neural traffic resulting in spontaneous ventilation. Within the pontine and medullary reticular formations, there are several discrete respiratory centers that function as the control system (see Fig. 28-3).

Initial descriptions of brainstem respiratory functions are based on classic ablation and electrical stimulation studies. Another method for localizing respiratory centers entails recording action potentials from different areas of the brainstem with microelectrodes. This method is based on the assumption that local brain activity that occurs in phase with respiratory activity is evidence that the area under study has "respiratory neurons."[22] These techniques are imperfect for precisely localizing discrete respiratory centers.

Medullary Centers

The medulla oblongata contains the most basic ventilatory control centers in the brain. Specific medullary areas are active primarily during inspiration or during expiration, with many neural inspiratory or expiratory interconnections. The inspiratory centers that reside in the dorsal respiratory group (DRG) are located in the dorsal medullary reticular formation. The DRG is the source of elementary ventilatory rhythmicity[23,24] and serves as the "pacemaker" for the respiratory system.[25] Whereas resting lung volume occurs at end expiration, the electrical activity of the ventilatory centers is at rest at end inspiration. The rhythmic activity of the DRG persists even when all incoming

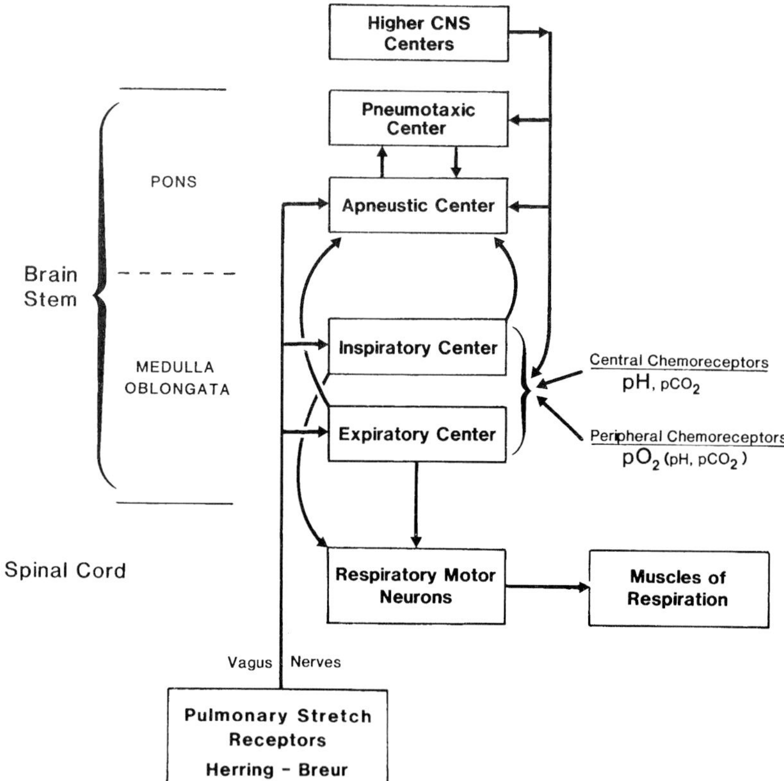

FIGURE 28-3. Classic central nervous system (CNS) respiratory centers. Diagram illustrates major respiratory centers, neurofeedback circuits, primary neurohumoral sensory inputs, and mechanical outputs.

peripheral and interconnecting nerves are sectioned or blocked completely. Isolating the DRG in this manner results in ataxic, gasping ventilation with frequent maximum inspiratory efforts: apneustic breathing.

The ventral respiratory group (VRG), which is located in the ventral medullary reticular formation, serves as the expiratory coordinating center. The inspiratory and expiratory neurons function by a system of reciprocal innervation, or negative feedback.[22] When the DRG creates an impulse to inspire, inspiration occurs and the DRG impulse is quenched by a reciprocating VRG impulse. This VRG transmission prohibits further use of the inspiratory muscles, thus allowing passive expiration to occur.

TABLE 28-3

DEFINITION OF RESPIRATORY PATTERN TERMINOLOGY

WORD	DEFINITION
Eupnea	"Good breathing": continuous inspiratory and expiratory movement without interruption
Apnea	"No breathing": cessation of ventilatory effort at passive end-expiration (lung volume = FRC)
Apneusis	Cessation of ventilatory effort with lungs filled at TLC
Apneustic ventilation	Apneusis with periodic expiratory spasms
Biot	Ventilatory gasps interposed between periods of ventilation apnea; *also* "agonal ventilation"

FRC, fucntional residual capacity; TLC, total lung capacity.

Pontine Centers

The pontine centers process information that originates in the medulla. The apneustic center is located in the middle or lower pons. With activation, this center sends impulses to inspiratory DRG neurons and is designed to sustain inspiration. Electrical stimulation results in inspiratory spasm.[26] The middle and lower pons contain specific areas for phase-spanning neurons.[27] These neurons assist with the transition between inspiration and expiration, and do not exert direct control over ventilatory muscles.

The pneumotaxic respiratory center is in the rostral pons. A simple transection through the brainstem that isolates this portion of the pons from the upper brainstem reduces ventilatory rate and increases tidal volume. If both vagus nerves are additionally transected, apneusis results.[28] Thus, the primary function of the pneumotaxic center is to limit the depth of inspiration. When maximally activated, the pneumotaxic center secondarily increases ventilatory frequency. The pneumotaxic center performs no pacemaking function and has no intrinsic rhythmicity.

Higher Respiratory Centers

Many higher brain structures clearly affect ventilatory control processes. In the midbrain, stimulation of the reticular activating system increases the rate and amplitude of ventilation.[29] The cerebral cortex also affects breathing pattern, although precise neural pathways are not known. Occasionally, the ventilatory control process becomes subservient to other regulatory centers. For example, the respiratory system plays an important role in the control of body temperature because it supplies a large surface area for heat exchange. This is especially important in animals in which panting is a primary means of dissipating heat. Then, ventilatory pattern is influenced by neural input from descending pathways from the anterior and posterior hypothalamus to the pneumotaxic center of the upper pons.

Vasomotor control and certain respiratory responses are closely linked. Stimulation of the carotid sinus not only decreases vasomotor tone, but also inhibits ventilation. Alternatively, stimulation of the carotid body chemoreceptors (see Chemical Control of Ventilation section) results in an increase in both ventilatory activity and vasomotor tone.

Reflex Control of Ventilation

Reflexes that directly influence ventilatory pattern usually do so to prevent airway obstruction. *Deglutition*, or swallowing, involves the glossopharyngeal and vagus nerves. Stimulation of the anterior and posterior pharyngeal pillars of the posterior pharynx induces swallowing. During swallowing, inspiration ceases momentarily, is usually followed by a single large breath, and briefly increases ventilation.

Vomiting significantly modifies normal ventilatory activity.[30] Swallowing, salivation, gastrointestinal reflexes, rhythmic spasmodic ventilatory movements, and significant diaphragmatic and abdominal muscular activity must be coordinated over a very brief interval. Because of the obvious risk of aspirating gastric contents, it is advantageous to inhibit inspiration during vomiting. Input into the respiratory centers occurs from both cranial and spinal cord nerves.

Coughing results from stimulation of the tracheal subepithelium, especially along the posterior tracheal wall and carina.[31] Coughing also requires coordination of both airway and ventilatory muscle activity. An effective cough requires deep inspiration and then forced exhalation against a momentarily closed glottis to increase intrathoracic pressure, thus allowing an expulsive expiratory maneuver.

Proprioception in the pulmonary system, the qualitative knowledge of the gas volume within the lungs, probably arises from smooth muscle spindle receptors. These proprioceptors, which are located within the smooth muscle of all airways, are sensitive to pressure changes. Airway stretch reflexes can be demonstrated during distention of isolated airways so airway pressure, rather than volume distention, appears to be the primary stimulation.[32] Clinical conditions in which pulmonary airway stretch receptors are stimulated include pulmonary edema and atelectasis.

Golgi tendon organs (tendon spindles), which occur in series arrangements within ventilatory muscles, facilitate proprioception. The intercostal muscles are rich in tendon spindles, whereas the diaphragm has a limited number. Thus, the pulmonary stretch reflex primarily involves the intercostal muscles but not the diaphragm. When the lungs are full and the chest wall is stretched, these receptors send signals to the brainstem that inhibit further inspiration.

In 1868, Hering and Breuer reported that lightly anesthetized, spontaneously breathing animals would cease or decrease ventilatory effort during sustained lung distention.[33] This response was blocked by bilateral vagotomy. The *Hering–Breuer reflex* is prominent in lower-order mammals and is sufficiently active in lower mammals that even 5 cm H_2O CPAP will induce apnea. In humans, however, the reflex is only weakly present, as evidenced by the fact that humans will continue to breathe spontaneously with CPAP in excess of 40 cm H_2O.

Chemical Control of Ventilation

Peripheral Chemoreceptors

In a simplistic view of chemical ventilatory control, the peripheral chemoreceptors primarily respond to lack of oxygen, and the central nervous system (CNS) receptors primarily respond to changes in PCO_2, pH, and acid-base disturbances.

The peripheral chemoreceptors are composed of the carotid and aortic bodies. The carotid bodies, located at the bifurcation of the common carotid artery, have predominantly ventilatory effects. The aortic bodies, which are scattered about the aortic arch and its branches, have predominantly circulatory effects. The neural output from the carotid body reaches the central respiratory centers via the afferent glossopharyngeal nerves. Output from the aortic bodies travels to the medullary centers
5 via the vagus nerve. Both carotid and aortic bodies are stimulated by decreased PaO_2, but not by decreased SaO_2 or CaO_2. When PaO_2 falls to less than 100 mm Hg, neural activity from these receptors begins to increase. However, it is not until the PaO_2 reaches 60 to 65 mm Hg that neural activity increases sufficiently to substantially augment minute ventilation. Thus, patients who depend on hypoxic ventilatory drive have PaO_2 values in the mid-60s. Once these patients' PaO_2 values exceed 60 to 65 mm Hg, ventilatory drive diminishes and PaO_2 falls until ventilation is again stimulated by arterial hypoxemia. When we withdraw mechanical ventilation from the patient who depends on hypoxic ventilatory drive, the PaO_2 must fall to less than 65 mm Hg so the patient will regain hypoxic ventilatory drive.

The carotid bodies are also sensitive to decreased pH_a, but this response is minor. Similarly, changes in $PaCO_2$ do not stimulate these receptors sufficiently to alter minute ventilation. Increases in blood temperature, hypoperfusion of the carotid bodies themselves, and some chemicals will stimulate these receptors. Sympathetic ganglion stimulation by nicotine or acetylcholine will stimulate the carotid and aortic bodies; this effect is blocked by hexamethonium. Blockade of the cytochrome electron transport system by cyanide will prevent oxidative metabolism and thus stimulate these receptors.

Ventilatory effects resulting from stimulation of these receptors cause increased ventilatory rate and tidal volume. Hemodynamic changes resulting from stimulation of these receptors include bradycardia, hypertension, increases in bronchiolar tone, and increases in adrenal secretion. The carotid body chemical receptors have been termed *ultimum moriens* ("last to die"). Although the peripheral receptors' response to hypoxemia was formerly believed to be resistant to the influences of anesthesia, potent inhaled anesthetics appear to depress hypoxic ventilatory response by depressing carotid body response to hypoxemia.[34] The peripheral receptors' response is not sufficiently robust to reliably increase ventilatory rate or minute ventilation to herald the onset of arterial hypoxemia during general anesthesia or recovery from anesthesia. Furthermore, flumazenil, in a 1-mg intravenous dose, only partially reversed the diazepam-induced depression of hypoxic ventilatory drive.[35] Mora's data further suggest that humans may develop tolerance to respiratory depressant effects of diazepam.

Central Chemoreceptors

Approximately 80% of the ventilatory response to inhaled carbon dioxide originates in the central medullary centers. Acid-base regulation involving carbon dioxide, H^+, and bicarbonate is related primarily to chemosensitive receptors located in the medulla close to or in contact with the cerebrospinal fluid (CSF). The chemosensitive areas of the brainstem are in the infralateral aspects of the medulla near the origin of cranial nerves IX and X. The area just beneath the surface of the ventral medulla is exquisitely sensitive to the extracellular fluid H^+ concentration.[36] Although the central response is the major factor in the regulation of breathing by carbon dioxide, carbon dioxide has little direct stimulating effect on these chemosensitive areas. These receptors are primarily sensitive to changes in H^+ concentration. Carbon dioxide has a potent but indirect effect by reacting with water to form carbonic acid, which dissociates into hydrogen and bicarbonate ions.[37]

Increased $Paco_2$ is a more potent ventilatory stimulus than increased arterial H^+ concentration from a metabolic source. Carbon dioxide, but not H^+, passes readily through the blood-brain and blood-CSF barriers. Local buffering systems immediately neutralize H^+ in arterial blood and body fluids. In contrast, the CSF has minimal buffering capacity. Thus, once carbon dioxide crosses into the CSF, H^+ are created and trapped in the CSF, resulting in a CSF H^+ concentration considerably greater than that found in the blood. Because carbon dioxide crosses the blood-brain barrier readily, the Pco_2 values in the CSF, cerebral tissue, and jugular venous blood rise quickly and to the same degree as the $Paco_2$, although the central values are ~10 mm Hg higher than those measured in arterial blood.

The ventilatory response to changes in $Paco_2$ (increased Vt, increased respiratory rate) is rapid and peaks within 1 to 2 minutes after the change in $Paco_2$. With the same level of carbon dioxide stimulation, the resultant increase in ventilation declines over a period of several hours, probably as a result of bicarbonate ions that are actively transported from the blood into the CSF through the arachnoid villi.[38] Central medullary chemoreceptors also respond to temperature change. Cold CSF (with normal pH) or local anesthetic applied to the medullary surface will depress ventilation.

Ventilatory Response to Altitude

Ventilatory response and adaptation to high altitude are good examples of the integration of peripheral and central chemoreceptor control of ventilation. The following mechanism of acclimatization was proposed by Severinghaus and coworkers in 1963 and has since been confirmed.[39]

Following ascent from sea level to 4,000 m, acute exposure to high altitude and low Pio_2 results in arterial hypoxemia. This decrease in Pao_2 activates the peripheral hypoxemic ventilatory drive by stimulating the carotid and aortic bodies, and causes increased minute ventilation. As minute ventilation increases, $Paco_2$ and CSF Pco_2 decrease, causing concomitant increases in pH_a and CSF pH. The alkaline shift of the CSF decreases ventilatory drive via medullary chemoreceptors, partially offsetting hypoxemic drive. A temporary equilibrium is attained within minutes, with $Paco_2$ only 2 to 5 mm Hg less than normal and Pao_2 approximately 45 mm Hg. This initially profound hypoxemia probably causes the acute respiratory distress and other associated symptoms (headache, diarrhea) associated with rapid ascent. However, the CNS is able to restore CSF pH to normal (7.326) by pumping bicarbonate ions out of the CSF over 2 to 3 days. In 2 to 3 days, CSF bicarbonate concentration decreases approximately 5 mEq/L and restores CSF pH to within 0.01 pH unit of values at sea level. Then, centrally mediated ventilatory drive returns to normal, and hypoxic drive and stimulation of peripheral receptors can proceed unopposed. Thus, after 3 days' exposure to 4,000 m altitude, ventilatory adaptation would result in a new equilibrium, with $Paco_2$ approximately 30 mm Hg and Pao_2 approximately 55 mm Hg. Following descent to sea level, the low CSF bicarbonate concentration persists for several days, and the climber "overbreathes" until CSF bicarbonate and pH values return to normal.

Breath-Holding

Most adults with normal lungs and gas exchange can hold their breath for ~1 minute when breathing room air without previously hyperventilating. After 1 minute of breath-holding under these circumstances, Pao_2 decreases to ~65 to 70 mm Hg and $Paco_2$ increases by ~12 mm Hg. In the absence of supplemental oxygen and hyperventilation, the "breakpoint" at which normal people are compelled to breathe is remarkably constant at a $Paco_2$ of 50 mm Hg.[40,41] However, if the individual breathes 100% oxygen prior to breath-holding, he or she should be able to hold his or her breath for 2 to 3 minutes, or until $Paco_2$ rises to 60 mm Hg. Hyperventilation sufficient to reduce $Paco_2$ to 20 mm Hg can lengthen the period of breath-holding to 3 to 4 minutes.[42] Hyperventilation with 100% oxygen prior to breath-holding should extend the apneic period to 6 to 10 minutes. The $Paco_2$ rate of rise in awake, preoxygenated adults with normal lungs who hold their breath without previous hyperventilation is 7 mm Hg/min in the first 10 seconds, 2 mm Hg/min in the next 10 seconds, and 6 mm Hg/min thereafter.[41]

The duration of voluntary breath-holding is directly proportional to lung volume at onset, and is probably related both to oxygen stores in the alveoli and to the rate at which $Paco_2$ rises. With smaller lung volumes, the same amount of carbon dioxide is emptied into a smaller volume during the apneic period, thus increasing the carbon dioxide concentration more rapidly than occurs with larger lung volumes. Of note, apneic patients during general anesthesia actually "breath-hold" at FRC rather than at vital capacity, which would tend to accelerate the rate of rise of carbon dioxide. Despite this difference in lung volume, the rate of rise of $Paco_2$ in apneic anesthetized patients is 12 mm Hg during the first minute and 3.5 mm Hg/min thereafter, significantly lower than in the awake state.[42,43] During anesthesia, metabolic rate and carbon dioxide production are significantly less than during ambulatory wakefulness, which probably accounts for the different rates of rise in carbon dioxide levels.

Hyperventilation with room air prior to prolonged breath-holding during exercise is inadvisable. During underwater swimming after poolside hyperventilation, the urge to breathe is first stimulated by a rising $Paco_2$. Swimmers who hyperventilate with room air prior to swimming long distances underwater frequently lose consciousness from arterial hypoxemia before the $Paco_2$ is sufficiently increased to stimulate the "need" to breathe.

Hyperventilation rarely is followed by an apneic period in awake humans, despite a markedly depressed $Paco_2$. However, minute ventilation may decrease significantly. Aggressive intermittent positive-pressure breathing treatments for patients with COPD can depress minute ventilation sufficiently to create arterial hypoxemia if they breathe room air after cessation of therapy.[44] In contrast, even mild hyperventilation during general anesthesia will produce prolonged apneic periods.[45]

Quantitative Aspects of Chemical Control of Breathing

The ventilatory responses to oxygen and carbon dioxide can be assessed quantitatively. Unfortunately, the quantitative indices of hypoxemic sensitivity are not clinically useful because the normal range is wide and confounded by many environmental factors. The reader is referred to a classical discussion of the quantitative indices of hypoxemic sensitivity.[46]

Ventilatory responses to $Paco_2$ changes are measured in several ways, provided that carbon dioxide production remains constant. When subjects voluntarily increase minute ventilation to a prescribed level, the $Paco_2$ decreases hyperbolically. The plot of minute ventilation (independent variable) and $Paco_2$ (dependent variable) is the metabolic hyperbola

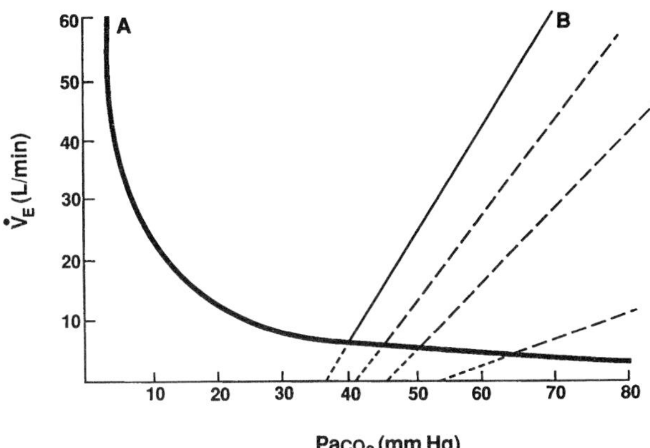

FIGURE 28-4. Carbon dioxide–ventilatory response curve. The metabolic hyperbola, curve A, is generated by varying $\dot{V}_E$ and measuring changes in carbon dioxide concentration. The hyperbolic configuration makes it cumbersome for clinical use. The carbon dioxide–ventilatory response curve, B is linear between approximately 20 and 80 mm Hg. It is generated by varying $PaCO_2$ (usually by controlling inspired carbon dioxide concentration) and measuring the resultant $\dot{V}_E$. This is the most commonly used test of ventilatory response. The slope defines "sensitivity"; the setpoint, or resting $PaCO_2$, occurs at the intersection of the metabolic hyperbola and the carbon dioxide–ventilatory response curve; and the apneic threshold can be obtained by extrapolating the carbon dioxide–ventilatory response curve to the x-intercept. In the absence of surgical stimulation, increasing doses of potent inhaled anesthesia or opioids will shift the curve to the right and eventually depress the slope (*dashed lines*). Painful stimulation will reverse these changes to varying and unpredictable degrees.

(Fig. 28-4). The metabolic hyperbola is cumbersome to evaluate and difficult to use clinically.

The curve more commonly used is the $PaCO_2$ ventilatory response curve (see Fig. 28-4). It describes the effect of changing $PaCO_2$ on the resultant minute ventilation. Usually, subjects inspire carbon dioxide to raise $PaCO_2$, and the effect on minute ventilation is measured. Creating these curves and observing how they change in various circumstances allows quantitative study of factors that affect the chemical carbon dioxide control of ventilation. The carbon dioxide response curve approaches linearity in the range most often encountered in life: at $PaCO_2$ values between 20 and 80 mm Hg. Once the $PaCO_2$ exceeds 80 mm Hg, the curve becomes parabolic, with its peak ventilatory response at a $PaCO_2$ between 100 and 120 mm Hg. Increasing the $PaCO_2$ to higher than 100 mm Hg allows carbon dioxide to act as a ventilatory and CNS depressant, the origin of the term "carbon dioxide narcosis," with 1 minimum alveolar concentration (MAC) being approximately 200 mm Hg.

The slope of the carbon dioxide response curve is considered to represent carbon dioxide sensitivity. Normal carbon dioxide sensitivity ranges from 0.5 to 0.7 L/min/mm Hg CO_2. When $PaCO_2$ reaches 100 mm Hg, carbon dioxide sensitivity is at its peak and normally reaches as high as 2.0 L/min/mm Hg CO_2. The *setpoint*, the point of intersection of the carbon dioxide response curve and the metabolic hyperbola, defines normal resting $PaCO_2$. Extrapolation of the carbon dioxide response curve to the x-intercept (where minute ventilation is 0) defines the apneic threshold. In awake, normal adults, the apneic threshold normally occurs at a $PaCO_2$ of ~32 mm Hg, although adults usually continue to breathe when they achieve the apneic threshold because the sensation of apnea is disturbing to awake adults. The slope of the curve is a measure of the response of the entire ventilatory mechanism to carbon dioxide stimulation.

Once PaO_2 exceeds 100 mm Hg, it no longer influences the carbon dioxide response curve. When the PaO_2 is between 65 and 100 mm Hg, its effect on the carbon dioxide response curve is small. However, when PaO_2 falls to less than 65 mm Hg, the carbon dioxide response curve shifts to the left and its slope increases, probably as a result of increased ventilatory drive stimulated by the peripheral chemoreceptors. Thus, during measurements of carbon dioxide ventilatory response, the subject should breathe supplemental oxygen.

The carbon dioxide response curve can be generated rapidly by increasing the fraction of inspired carbon dioxide ($FICO_2$) by requiring the subject to rebreathe exhaled gas. The results obtained with this technique are less pure because the $FICO_2$ is not controlled.

Three clinical states result in a left shift and/or a steepened slope of the carbon dioxide response curve. These same three situations are the only causes of true hyperventilation, that is, an increase in minute ventilation such that the decreased $PaCO_2$ creates respiratory alkalemia (either primary or com-
6 pensatory). The three causes of hyperventilation (enhanced carbon dioxide response) are arterial hypoxemia, metabolic acidemia, and central etiologies. Examples of central etiologies that cause hyperventilation include drug administration, intracranial hypertension, hepatic cirrhosis, and nonspecific arousal states such as anxiety and fear. Aminophylline, salicylates, and norepinephrine stimulate ventilation independent of peripheral chemoreceptors. Opioid antagonists, given in the absence of opioids to presumably normal people, do not stimulate ventilation. However, when given after opiate administration, they do reverse the effects of opioids on the carbon dioxide response curve.

Ventilatory depressants displace the carbon dioxide response curve to the right or decrease its slope or both. Changes in physiology that depress ventilation include metabolic alkalemia, denervation of peripheral chemoreceptors, normal sleep, and drugs. During normal sleep, the carbon dioxide response curve is displaced to the right, with the degree of displacement depending on the depth of sleep. Usually, $PaCO_2$ increases up to 10 mm Hg during deep sleep. Hypoxemic responses are not impaired by sleep, which is convenient for continued survival at high altitude.

Opioids displace the carbon dioxide response curve to the right with little change in slope at sedative doses. With higher, "anesthetic" doses, the curve shifts farther to the right and its slope is depressed, simulating the effect of potent inhalation agents on the carbon dioxide response curve (see Fig. 28-4). In the absence of other ventilatory depressant drugs, opioids induce pathognomonic changes in ventilatory patterns: a decreased ventilatory rate with an increased tidal volume. Not until opioids nearly induce apnea is tidal volume decreased. Large narcotic doses usually result in apnea before consciousness is lost. Like sex, breathing requires both ability and desire.

Barbiturates in sedative or light hypnotic doses have little effect on the carbon dioxide response curve. In doses adequate to allow skin incision, barbiturates shift the carbon dioxide response curve to the right. The ventilatory pattern resulting from barbiturate administration is characterized by decreased tidal volume and increased ventilatory rate. Potent inhaled anesthetics displace the carbon dioxide response curve to the right and decrease the slope, the degree depending on the anesthetic dose and the level of surgical stimulation. As the inhaled anesthetic dose increases, the carbon dioxide response curve eventually becomes horizontal (slope = 0), resulting in essentially no ventilatory response to $PaCO_2$ changes.

Potent inhaled anesthetics and opioids displace the setpoint to the right, implying that the resting, steady-state $PaCO_2$ is higher and minute ventilation lower. Furthermore, when the carbon dioxide response curve shifts to the right, the apneic threshold also increases (see Fig. 28-4). Surgical stimulation reverses the ventilatory response changes induced by inhaled anesthetics and opioids, but the degree of reversal is not predictable.

OXYGEN AND CARBON DIOXIDE TRANSPORT

This chapter discusses only external respiration, in which oxygen moves from the ambient environment into the pulmonary capillaries, and carbon dioxide leaves the pulmonary capillaries to enter the atmosphere. The movement of gas across the alveolar–capillary membrane depends on the integrity of the pulmonary and cardiac systems. Unless it is otherwise stated, the reader should assume the ventilation and perfusion of alveolar–capillary units are normal. Abnormal distribution of ventilation or perfusion of the lungs is discussed later (see Ventilation–Perfusion Relationships section).

Bulk Flow of Gas (Convection)

Convection, in which all gas molecules move in the same direction, is the primary mechanism responsible for gas flow in large and most small airways, down to the bronchi and bronchiolar airways of the fourteenth or fifteenth generation. Because the cross-sectional area of the airways progressively increases as gas moves toward the lung periphery, the average velocity of gas particles decreases as they travel toward the alveoli. As a result, the greatest part of airway resistance occurs in the larger airways, where gas molecules travel more quickly. During normal quiet ventilation, gas flow within convective airways is mainly laminar, thus reducing resistance to gas flow (see Resistance to Gas Flow section).

Gas Diffusion

Diffusion within a gas-filled space is random molecular motion that results in complete mixing of all gases. In the lung, diffusion gradually becomes the predominant mode of gas transport, beginning with the terminal bronchioles (sixteenth airway generation). Once gas reaches the small alveolar ducts, alveolar sacs, and alveoli, both diffusion and regional $\dot{V}/\dot{Q}$ relationships influence gas transport. Historically, clinicians assumed defects in gas diffusion were responsible for arterial hypoxemia. However, the most frequent cause of arterial hypoxemia is physiologic shunt (see Ventilation–Perfusion Relationships section).[47]

The other usage of "diffusion" refers to the passive movement of molecules across a membrane that is governed primarily by concentration gradient. In this sense, carbon dioxide is 20 times more diffusible across human membranes than is oxygen; therefore, carbon dioxide crosses membranes easily. As a result, hypercarbia is never the result of defective diffusion; rather, it is the result of inadequate alveolar ventilation with respect to carbon dioxide production.

True diffusion defects that create arterial hypoxemia are rare. The most common reason for a measured decrease in diffusing capacity (see Pulmonary Function Testing section) is mismatched ventilation and perfusion, which functionally results in a decreased surface area available for diffusion.

Distribution of Ventilation and Perfusion

The efficiency with which oxygen and carbon dioxide exchange at the alveolar–capillary level highly depends on the matching of capillary perfusion and alveolar ventilation. At this level, the marriage between the lung and the circulatory system must be well matched and intimate.

Distribution of Blood Flow

Blood flow within the lung is mainly gravity dependent. Because the alveolar–capillary beds are not composed of rigid vessels, the pressure of the surrounding tissues can influence the resistance to flow through the individual capillaries. Thus, blood flow depends on the relationship between pulmonary artery pressure (Ppa), alveolar pressure (PA), and pulmonary venous pressure (Ppv) (Fig. 28-5). West created a lung model that divides the lung into three zones.[47,48] Zone 1 conditions occur in the most gravity-independent part of the lung above the level where pulmonary artery pressure is equal to alveolar pressure. Because alveolar pressure is approximately equal to atmospheric pressure, pulmonary artery pressure in zone 1 is subatmospheric but necessarily greater than pulmonary venous pressure (PA > Ppa > Ppv). Alveolar pressure that is transmitted to the pulmonary capillaries promotes their collapse, with a consequent theoretical blood flow of zero to this lung region. Thus, zone 1 receives ventilation in the absence of perfusion and creates alveolar dead space ventilation. Normally, zone 1 areas exist only to a limited extent. However, in conditions of decreased pulmonary artery pressure, such as hypovolemic shock, zone 1 enlarges.

Zone 3 occurs in the most gravity-dependent areas of the lung where Ppa > Ppv > PA and blood flow is primarily governed by the pulmonary arterial to venous pressure difference. Because gravity also increases pulmonary venous pressure, the pulmonary capillaries become distended. Thus, perfusion in

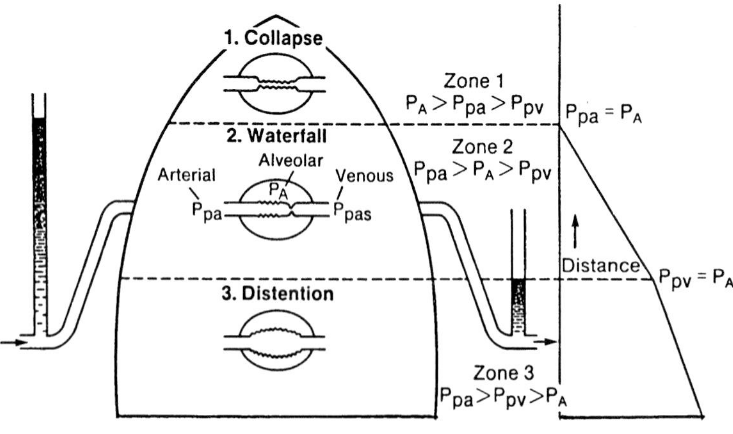

FIGURE 28-5. Distribution of blood flow in the isolated lung. In zone 1, alveolar pressure (P_A) exceeds pulmonary artery pressure (P_{pa}), and no flow occurs because the vessels are collapsed. In zone 2, arterial pressure exceeds alveolar pressure, but alveolar pressure exceeds pulmonary venous pressure (P_{pv}). Flow in zone 2 is determined by the arterial–alveolar pressure difference ($P_{pa} - P_A$), which steadily increases down the zone. In zone 3, pulmonary venous pressure exceeds alveolar pressure, and flow is determined by the arterial–venous pressure difference ($P_{pa} - P_{pv}$), which is constant down this pulmonary zone. However, the pressure across the vessel walls increases down the zone so their caliber increases, as does flow. (From West JB, Dollery CT, Naimark A: Distribution of blood flow in isolated lung: Relation to vascular and alveolar pressures. J Appl Physiol 19:713, 1964.)

zone 3 is lush, resulting in capillary perfusion in excess of ventilation, or physiologic shunt.

Finally, zone 2 occurs from the lower limit of zone 1 to the upper limit of zone 3, where Ppa > PA > Ppv. The pressure difference between pulmonary artery and alveolar pressure determines blood flow in zone 2. Pulmonary venous pressure has little influence. Well-matched ventilation and perfusion occur in zone 2, which contains the majority of alveoli.

Distribution of Ventilation

Alveolar pressure is the same throughout the lung; therefore, the more negative intrapleural pressure at the apex (or the least gravity-dependent area) results in larger, more distended apical alveoli than in other areas of the lung. The transpulmonary pressure (Paw – Ppl), or distending pressure of the lung, is greater at the top and lower at the bottom, where intrapleural pressure is less negative. Despite the smaller alveolar size, more ventilation is delivered to dependent pulmonary areas. The decrease in intrapleural pressure at the base of the lungs during inspiration is greater than at the apex because of diaphragmatic proximity. Thus, more gas is sucked into dependent areas of the lung.

Ventilation–Perfusion Relationships

As discussed previously, the majority of blood flow is distributed to the gravity-dependent part of the lung. During a spontaneous breath, the largest portion of the tidal volume also reaches the gravity-dependent part of the lung. Thus, the nondependent area of the lung receives a lower proportion of both ventilation and perfusion, and dependent lung receives greater proportions of ventilation and perfusion. Nevertheless, ventilation and perfusion are not matched perfectly, and various $\dot{V}A/\dot{Q}$ ratios result throughout the lung. The ideal $\dot{V}A/\dot{Q}$ ratio of 1 is believed to occur at approximately the level of the third rib. Above this level, ventilation occurs slightly in excess of perfusion, whereas below the third rib the $\dot{V}A/\dot{Q}$ ratio becomes less than 1 (Fig. 28-6).

In a simplified model, gas exchange units can be divided into normal ($\dot{V}A/\dot{Q} = 1{:}1$), dead space ($\dot{V}A/\dot{Q} = 1{:}0$), shunt ($\dot{V}A/\dot{Q} = 0{:}1$), or a silent unit ($\dot{V}A/\dot{Q} = 0{:}0$) (Fig. 28-7). Although this model is helpful in understanding $\dot{V}A/\dot{Q}$ relationships and their influences on gas exchange, $\dot{V}A/\dot{Q}$ really occurs as a continuum. In the lungs of a healthy, upright, spontaneously breathing individual, the majority of alveolar-capillary units are normal gas exchange units. The $\dot{V}A/\dot{Q}$ ratio varies between absolute shunt (in which $\dot{V}A/\dot{Q} = 0$) to absolute dead space (in which $\dot{V}A/\dot{Q} = \infty$). Rather than absolute shunt, most units with low $\dot{V}A/\dot{Q}$ mismatch receive a small amount of ventilation relative to blood flow. Similarly, most dead space units are not absolute, but rather are characterized by low blood flow relative to ventilation.

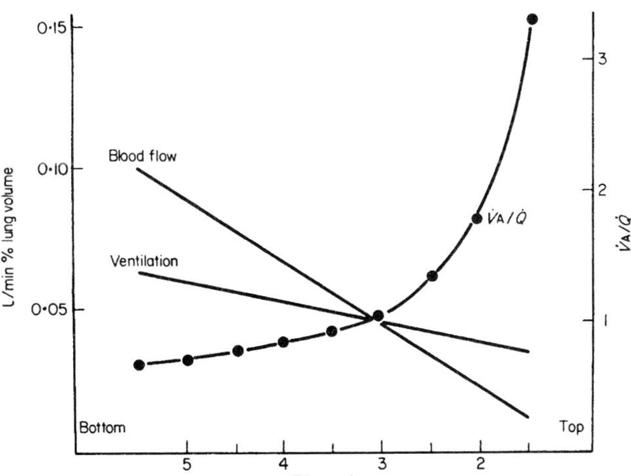

FIGURE 28-6. Distribution of ventilation, blood flow, and ventilation–perfusion ratio in the normal, upright lung. Straight lines have been drawn through the ventilation and blood flow data. Because blood flow falls more rapidly than ventilation with distance up the lung, ventilation–perfusion ratio rises, slowly at first, then rapidly. (From West JB: Ventilation/Blood Flow and Gas Exchange, 4th ed. Oxford, England, Blackwell Scientific, 1985.)

Hypoxic pulmonary vasoconstriction, stimulated by alveolar hypoxia, severely decreases blood flow. Thus, poorly ventilated alveoli also receive minuscule blood flow. Furthermore, decreased regional pulmonary blood flow results in bronchiolar constriction and diminishes the degree of dead space ventilation.[49,50] When either phenomena occurs, the shunt or dead space units effectively become silent units in which little ventilation or perfusion occurs.

Many pulmonary diseases result in both physiologic shunt and dead space abnormalities. However, most disease processes can be characterized as producing either primarily shunt or dead space in their early stages. Increases in dead space ventilation primarily affect carbon dioxide elimination and have 7 little influence on arterial oxygenation until dead space ventilation exceeds 80 to 90% of minute ventilation ($\dot{V}E$). Similarly, physiologic shunt primarily affects arterial oxygenation with little effect on carbon dioxide elimination until the physiologic shunt fraction exceeds 75 to 80% of the cardiac output. Defective to absent gas exchange can be the net effect of either abnormality in the extreme.

Physiologic Dead Space

Each inspired breath is composed of gas that contributes to alveolar ventilation (V_A) and gas that becomes dead space ventilation (VD). Thus, tidal volume (Vt) = VA + VD. In the normal, spontaneously breathing person, the ratio of alveolar-to-dead space ventilation for each breath is 2:1. Conveniently, the rule of "1, 2, 3" applies to normal, spontaneously breathing persons. For each breath, 1 mL/lb (lean body weight) becomes VD, 2 mL $\cdot$ lb^{-1} becomes VA, and 3 mL $\cdot$ lb^{-1} constitutes the Vt.

Physiologic dead space consists of anatomic and alveolar dead space. Anatomic dead space ventilation, approximately 2 mL/kg ideal body weight, accounts for the majority of physiologic dead space. It arises from ventilation of structures that do not exchange respiratory gases: the oronasopharynx to the terminal and respiratory bronchioles. Clinical conditions that modify anatomic dead space include tracheal intubation, tracheostomy, and large lengths of ventilator tubing between the tracheal tube and the ventilator Y-piece.

Alveolar dead space ventilation arises from ventilation of alveoli where there is little or no perfusion. Because disease changes anatomic dead space little, physiologic dead space is primarily influenced by changes in alveolar dead space. Rapid changes in physiologic dead space ventilation most often arise from changes in pulmonary blood flow, resulting in decreased perfusion to ventilated alveoli. The most common etiology of acutely increased physiologic dead space is an abrupt decrease in cardiac output. Another pathologic condition that interferes with pulmonary blood flow, and thereby creates dead space, is pulmonary embolism, whether due to thrombus or to fat, air, or amniotic fluid. Although there may be obstruction to blood flow with some types of pulmonary emboli, the greatest decrease in pulmonary blood flow is due to vasoconstriction

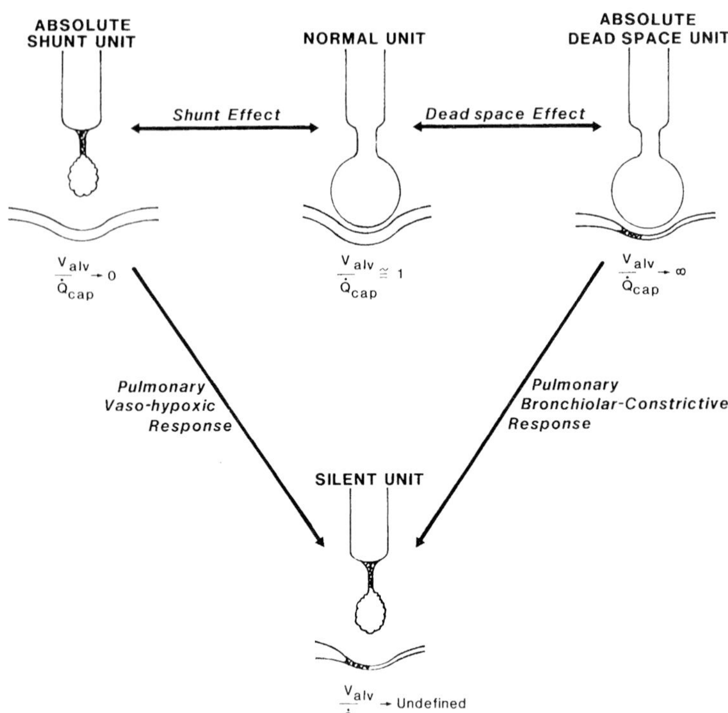

FIGURE 28-7. Continuum of ventilation–perfusion relationships. Gas exchange is maximally effective in normal lung units and only partially effective in shunt and dead space effect units. It is totally absent in silent units, absolute shunt, and dead space units.

induced by locally released vasoactive substances such as leukotrienes.

Chronic pulmonary diseases create dead space ventilation by irreversibly changing the relationship between alveolar ventilation and blood flow; this alteration is especially prominent in patients with COPD. Furthermore, acute diseases such as adult respiratory distress syndrome can cause an increase in dead space ventilation owing to intense pulmonary vasoconstriction. Finally, therapeutic or supportive manipulations such as positive-pressure ventilation or positive airway pressure therapy can increase alveolar dead space because depressed venous return to the right heart will decrease cardiac output. Intravenous fluid administration will usually overcome this problem.

Assessment of Physiologic Dead Space

Because the lung receives nearly 100% of the cardiac output, assessment of physiologic dead space ventilation in the acute setting yields valuable information about pulmonary blood flow and, ultimately, about cardiac output. If pulmonary blood flow decreases, the most likely cause is a decreased cardiac output. Thus, it is clinically useful to be able to readily assess the degree of physiologic dead space ventilation.

There are two easy and several difficult ways to assess dead space ventilation. A comparison of minute ventilation and $Paco_2$ allows a gross qualitative assessment of physiologic dead space ventilation. The $Paco_2$ is determined only by alveolar ventilation and $\dot{V}co_2$. If $\dot{V}co_2$ remains constant, $Paco_2$ also will remain constant as long as minute ventilation supplies the same degree of alveolar ventilation. If the spontaneously breathing individual must increase minute ventilation to maintain the same $Paco_2$, he or she has experienced an increase in dead space ventilation because less of the minute ventilation is contributing to alveolar ventilation. Alternatively, a mechanically ventilated patient with a fixed minute ventilation and no increase in $\dot{V}co_2$ also experiences an increased dead space ventilation if the $Paco_2$ rises. Hence, when $Paco_2$ in a mechanically ventilated patient increases, it is necessary to determine if the cause is increased dead space ventilation or an increased $\dot{V}co_2$.

The mechanically ventilated patient with normal lungs has a dead space to alveolar ventilation ratio (V_D/V_A) of 1:1 rather than 1:2, as during spontaneous ventilation. If mechanical Vt
8 is 1,000 mL, 500 mL contributes to $\dot{V}_A$, and 500 mL contributes to V_D. At rest, the required $\dot{V}_A$ with normal $\dot{V}co_2$ is approximately 60 mL/kg/min. A 70-kg man would then require a $\dot{V}_A$ of 4,200 mL/min. During spontaneous breathing, the required $\dot{V}_E$ would be 6,300 mL/min, but during mechanical ventilation $\dot{V}_E$ would have to be 8,400 mL/min. Using this calculation, if a 70-kg resting patient requires $\dot{V}_E$ much in excess of 8,400 mL/min, either $\dot{V}_D$ or $\dot{V}co_2$ is increased. A rule of thumb for mechanically ventilated patients is that doubling baseline minute ventilation decreases $Paco_2$ from 40 to 30 mm Hg, and quadrupling minute ventilation decreases $Paco_2$ from 40 to 20 mm Hg.

9 The $Paco_2$ will be greater than or equal to end-tidal $Paco_2$ ($P_{ET}co_2$) unless the patient inspires or receives exogenous carbon dioxide (e.g., from peritoneal insufflation). The difference between $P_{ET}co_2$ and $Paco_2$ is due to dead space ventilation. Measurement of this difference—which is simple, readily obtainable, and fairly inexpensive—yields reliable information relative to the degree of dead space ventilation. Clinical situations that change pulmonary blood flow sufficiently to increase dead space ventilation can be detected by comparing $P_{ET}co_2$ with temperature-corrected $Paco_2$. Yamanaka and Sue[51] found that the $P_{ET}co_2$ in ventilated patients varied linearly with the dead space to tidal volume ratio (V_D/Vt) and that $P_{ET}co_2$ correlated poorly with $Paco_2$. Thus, in the critically ill, mechanically ventilated patient, and in anesthetized patients, monitoring $P_{ET}co_2$ gives far more information about ventilatory efficiency or dead space ventilation than it does about the absolute value of $Paco_2$.

Anesthesiologists commonly measure $P_{ET}co_2$ to detect venous air embolism during anesthesia. A lowered cardiac output alone, in the absence of venous air embolism, may sufficiently decrease pulmonary perfusion so dead space ventilation increases and $PETCO_2$ falls. Thus, a depressed $PETCO_2$ is a sensitive but nonspecific monitor. Air in the pulmonary arteries mechanically interferes with blood flow and also causes pulmonary arterial constriction, further decreasing pulmonary blood flow. A decreased $PETCO_2$ suggests that a physiologically significant air embolism has occurred. The same physiologic considerations apply to detecting pulmonary thromboembolism.

Some clinicians use the divergence of $PETCO_2$ from $PaCO_2$ as a reflection of pulmonary blood flow for other applications. During intentional pharmacologic or surgical manipulation of pulmonary blood flow, the difference between $PaCO_2$ and $PETCO_2$ serves as a useful physiologic monitor of the effectiveness of these interventions. Furthermore, regarding $PETCO_2$ as a reflection of pulmonary perfusion is a useful tool for studying and monitoring the effectiveness of resuscitation efforts and may provide a marker for survival after resuscitation.[52]

The most quantitative technique used to measure physiologic dead space uses a modification of the Bohr equation:

$$\frac{V_D}{V_t} = \frac{PaCO_2 - P\bar{E}CO_2}{PaCO_2} \quad (28\text{-}4)$$

where $P\bar{E}CO_2$ is the PCO_2 from the mixture of all expired gases over the period of time during which measurements are made. This calculation estimates the fraction of each breath that does not contribute to gas exchange. In spontaneously breathing patients, normal V_D/V_t is between 0.2 and 0.4, or ~0.33. In patients receiving positive-pressure ventilation, V_D/V_t becomes ~0.5. The major limitation of performing this calculation is the difficulty in collecting exhaled gas for $P\bar{E}CO_2$ measurement. Exhaled gases, collected in cumbersome 8–l bags, can easily be contaminated with inspired air or supplemental oxygen. The measurement will also be inaccurate if the patient does not maintain a steady ventilatory pattern. Therefore, extreme care must be taken to ensure all measurements are performed accurately. In practice, this measurement is rarely performed.

Physiologic Shunt

Whereas physiologic dead space ventilation applies to areas of the lung that are ventilated but poorly perfused, physiologic shunt occurs in lung that is perfused but poorly ventilated. The physiologic shunt ($\dot{Q}_{SP}$) is that portion of the total cardiac output ($\dot{Q}_T$) that returns to the left heart and systemic circulation without receiving oxygen in the lung. When pulmonary blood is not exposed to alveoli or when those alveoli are devoid of ventilation, the result is *absolute shunt,* in which $\dot{V}_A/\dot{Q} = 0$. *Shunt effect,* or *venous admixture,* is the more common clinical phenomenon and occurs in areas where alveolar ventilation is deficient compared with the degree of perfusion: $0 < \dot{V}_A/\dot{Q} < 1$.

Because blood passing through areas of absolute shunt receives no oxygen, arterial hypoxemia resulting from absolute shunt is minimally reversed with supplemental oxygen. Alternatively, supplemental oxygen supplied to patients with arterial hypoxemia due to venous admixture will increase the PaO_2. Although ventilation to these alveoli is deficient, they do carry a small amount of oxygen to the capillary bed.

A small percentage of venous blood normally bypasses the right ventricle and empties directly into the left atrium. This anatomic, absolute shunt arises from the venous return from the pleural, bronchiolar, and thebesian veins. This venous drainage accounts for 2 to 5% of total cardiac output and explains the small shunt that normally occurs. Anatomic shunts of greatest magnitude are usually associated with congenital heart disease that causes right-to-left shunt. Intrapulmonary anatomic shunts can also cause anatomic shunt. For example, the arterial hypoxemia associated with advanced hepatic failure (hepatopulmonary syndrome) is due, in part, to arteriovenous malformations.[53,54] Diseases that may cause absolute shunt include acute lobar atelectasis, extensive acute lung injury, advanced pulmonary edema, and consolidated pneumonia. Disease entities that tend to produce venous admixture include mild pulmonary edema, postoperative atelectasis, and COPD.

Assessment of Arterial Oxygenation and Physiologic Shunt

The simplest assessment of oxygenation is qualitative comparison of the patient's FIO_2 and PaO_2. The highest possible PaO_2 for any given FIO_2 (and $PaCO_2$) can be calculated from the alveolar gas equation:

$$P_{AO_2} = F_{IO_2}(P_b - P_{H_2O}) - \frac{P_{ACO_2}}{R} \quad (28\text{-}5)$$

where PAO_2 and $PACO_2$ are alveolar PO_2 and PCO_2, PH_2O is water vapor pressure at 100% saturation and 37°C, P_b is barometric pressure, and R is respiratory quotient. Assuming one makes the calculation for a well-perfused alveolus, the alveolar and arterial PCO_2 are equal. Therefore, $PaCO_2$ can be substituted for $PACO_2$. Respiratory quotient (R) is the ratio of O_2 consumed ($\dot{V}O_2$) to CO_2 produced ($\dot{V}CO_2$):

$$\frac{\dot{V}CO_2}{\dot{V}O_2} = \frac{200\ \text{mL/min}}{250\ \text{mL/min}} = 0.8 \quad (28\text{-}6)$$

Oxygen tension–based indices do not reflect mixed venous contribution to arterial oxygenation and can be misleading.[55] Even if venous admixture is small, mixed venous blood with very low oxygen content will magnify the effect of a small shunt. Oxygen tension–based indices, for example, PaO_2/FIO_2, alveolar to arterial PO_2 difference (DA-aO_2), and ratio PaO_2/PAO_2, do not take into account the influence of $C\bar{v}O_2$ on arterial oxygenation. Therefore, in critically ill patients who are hypoxemic, the insertion of a pulmonary artery catheter to assess shunt and to measure cardiac output may be essential to understanding the influence of cardiac function on arterial oxygenation.

DA-aO_2 is a useful quantitative assessment of arterial oxygenation mainly when arterial hemoglobin is well saturated when normal DA-aO_2 is <5 mm Hg. When PaO_2 is less than 150 mm Hg (and certainly when it is less than 100 mm Hg), the relationship between oxygen content and oxygen tension is nonlinear, thus making DA-aO_2 more difficult to interpret.

The assessment of arterial oxygenation requires, at least, knowledge of FIO_2 and either PaO_2 or SaO_2. Oxygen tension–based indices of oxygenation are useful, but they do not take into account the contribution of mixed venous blood to arterial oxygenation. Mixed venous blood can become extremely desaturated in the critically ill patient owing to inadequate cardiac
10 output, anemia, arterial hypoxemia, or increased $\dot{V}O_2$. The best knowledge of the efficiency with which the lungs oxygenate the arterial blood can be obtained only by calculating shunt fraction or ventilation–perfusion ratio (VQI).

Physiologic Shunt Calculation

The clinical reference standard for the calculation of physiologic shunt fraction is derived from a two-compartment pulmonary blood flow model where one compartment performs ideal gas exchange and contains perfectly married alveolar–capillary units. The other compartment is the shunt compartment and contains pulmonary capillaries that enjoy no exposure to ventilated alveoli. Using the Fick relationship, the following equation can be derived:

$$\frac{\dot{Q}_{SP}}{\dot{Q}_T} = \frac{Cc'O_2 - CaO_2}{Cc'O_2 - C\bar{v}O_2} \tag{28-7}$$

where $\dot{Q}_{SP}/\dot{Q}_T$ is the shunt fraction ($\dot{Q}_{SP}$ is blood flow through the physiologic shunt compartment, $\dot{Q}_T$ is total cardiac output), and $Cc'O_2$ and $C\bar{v}O_2$ are end-capillary and mixed-venous oxygen contents, respectively. Normal intrapulmonary shunt is approximately 5%. Because this equation is based on an artificial two-compartment model, the absolute value is physically meaningless. A calculated $\dot{Q}_{SP}/\dot{Q}_T$ of 25% means that if the lung existed in two compartments, 25% of the cardiac output would travel through the shunt compartment. Because the lung does not exist in two compartments, this equation only grossly estimates pulmonary oxygen exchange defects. Nevertheless, it remains our best tool for clinically evaluating the efficiency with which the lungs oxygenate arterial blood. Observing shunt fraction change with therapeutic intervention or with the progress of disease is more valuable than knowing the absolute value per se.

Because hemoglobin concentration is uniform throughout the vascular system, the oxygen contents in the shunt equation are determined primarily by oxyhemoglobin saturation. Thus, the shunt equation can be approximated by substituting saturation values for each term; the new value, called *ventilation–perfusion ratio* (VQI),[55] is determined as follows:

$$VQI = \frac{Sc'O_2 - SaO_2}{Sc'O_2 - S\bar{v}O_2} \cong \frac{1 - SaO_2}{1 - S\bar{v}O_2} \tag{28-8}$$

If the patient is neither breathing a hypoxic gas mixture nor has a methemoglobin or carboxyhemoglobin value in excess of 5 to 6%, $Sc'O_2$ must equal 1 because the model requires a perfect alveolar–capillary interface. This substitution results in the final expression in the previous equation. The absolute values of VQI are meaningless, although "normal" should be 0 to 4%. Like $\dot{Q}_{SP}/\dot{Q}_T$, the importance of these values lies in their trend as disease and treatment progress.

SaO_2 and $S\bar{v}O_2$ can be estimated continuously with pulse oximetry and by using a pulmonary artery catheter with oximetry capability. By interfacing the outputs of these two devices with a computer, VQI can be calculated continuously. The greatest advantage of calculating $\dot{Q}_{SP}/\dot{Q}_T$ or VQI to assess arterial oxygenation is that these values include the contribution of mixed venous blood.

PULMONARY FUNCTION TESTING

Anesthesiologists frequently care for patients with significant pulmonary dysfunction. It is important for the anesthesiologist to be able to interpret tests of pulmonary function intelligently and to know which tests will help define dysfunction if the patient's history and physical are suggestive of disease. This section discusses lung volumes, tests of pulmonary mechanics, and diffusing capacity.

Lung Volumes and Capacities

Known, reproducible pulmonary gas volumes and capacities provide a reliable basis for comparison between normal and abnormal measurements.[56] Because normal measurements vary with size, height is most frequently used to define "normal." Lung capacities are composed of two or more lung volumes.

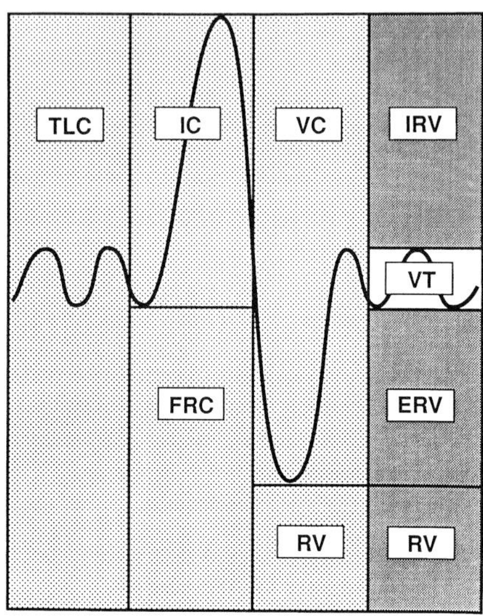

FIGURE 28-8. Lung volumes and capacities. The darkest bar on the far right depicts the four basic lung volumes that sum to create TLC. Other lung capacities are composed of two or more lung volumes. The overlying spirographic tracing orients the reader to the relationship between the lung volumes and capacities and the spirogram. ERV, expiratory reserve volume; FRC, functional residual capacity; IC, inspiratory capacity; IRV, inspiratory reserve volume; RV, residual volume; TLC, total lung capacity; VC, vital capacity; VT, tidal volume.

Lung volumes and capacities are schematically illustrated in Figure 28-8.

Tidal volume is the volume of gas that moves in and out of the lungs during quiet breathing and is ~6 to 8 mL/kg. Tidal volume falls with decreased lung compliance or when the patient has reduced ventilatory muscle strength.

Vital capacity is usually ~60 mL/kg but may vary as much as 20% from normal in healthy individuals. Vital capacity correlates well with the capability for deep breathing and effective coughing. It usually is decreased by restrictive pulmonary disease such as pulmonary edema or atelectasis. Vital capacity may also be reduced by the mechanically induced restriction that occurs with problems such as pleural effusion, pneumothorax, pregnancy, large ascites, or ventilatory muscle weakness.

The *inspiratory capacity* is the largest volume of gas that can be inspired from the resting expiratory level and is frequently decreased in the presence of significant extrathoracic airway obstruction. This measurement is one of the few simple tests that can detect extrathoracic airway obstruction. Most routine pulmonary function tests measure only exhaled flows and volumes, which may be relatively unaffected by extrathoracic obstruction until it is severe. Changes in the absolute volume of inspiratory capacity usually parallel changes in vital capacity. *Expiratory reserve volume* is not of great diagnostic value.

Functional residual capacity (FRC) is the volume of gas remaining in the lungs at passive end expiration. *Residual volume* is that gas remaining within the lungs at the end of forced maximal expiration. The FRC serves two primary physiologic functions. It determines the point on the pulmonary volume-pressure curve for resting ventilation (see Fig. 28-2). The tangent defined by the midportion pulmonary volume–pressure curve at FRC defines lung compliance. Thus, FRC determines the elastic pressure–volume relationships within the lung. Furthermore, FRC is the resting expiratory volume of the lung. As
11 such, it greatly influences ventilation–perfusion relationships within the lung. When FRC is reduced, venous admixture (low

$\dot{V}A/\dot{Q}$) increases and results in arterial hypoxemia (see Oxygen and Carbon Dioxide Transport and Lung Mechanics sections).

Further, the FRC may be used to quantify the degree of pulmonary restriction. Disease processes that reduce FRC and lung compliance include acute lung injury, pulmonary edema, pulmonary fibrotic processes, and atelectasis. Mechanical factors also reduce FRC, for example, pregnancy, obesity, pleural effusion, and posture. The FRC decreases 10% when a healthy subject lies down. Ventilatory muscle weakness or paralysis will also decrease FRC. In contrast, patients with COPD have excessively compliant lungs that recoil less forcibly. Their lungs retain an abnormally large volume at the end of passive expiration, a phenomenon called *gas trapping*.

FRC Measurement

The FRC and residual volume must be measured indirectly because residual volume cannot be removed from the lung. The multiple-breath nitrogen washout test is performed by having the subject breathe 100% oxygen for several minutes so alveolar nitrogen is gradually "washed out." With each breath, the volume of gas and the concentration of nitrogen in the exhaled gas are measured. A rapid nitrogen analyzer coupled to a spirometer or pneumotachometer provides a breath-by-breath analysis of nitrogen washout. Electronic signals proportional to nitrogen concentrations and exhaled volumes (or flow, if a pneumotachometer is used) are integrated to derive the exhaled volume of nitrogen for each breath. Then, the values for all breaths are summed to provide a total volume of nitrogen washed out of the lungs. The test proceeds until the alveolar nitrogen concentration is reduced to less than 7%, usually requiring 7 to 10 minutes. FRC is calculated using the equation:

$$FRC = N_2\ \text{volume} \times \frac{[N_2]_f}{[N_2]_i} \quad (28\text{-}9)$$

where $[N_2]_i$ and $[N_2]_f$ are the fractional concentrations of alveolar nitrogen at the beginning and end of the test, respectively.

Pulmonary Function Tests

Forced Vital Capacity

The forced vital capacity (FVC) is the volume of gas that can be expired as forcefully and rapidly as possible after maximal inspiration. Normally, FVC is equal to vital capacity. Because forced expiration significantly increases intrapleural pressures but changes airway pressure little, bronchiolar collapse, obstructive lesions, and gas trapping are exaggerated. Thus, FVC may be reduced in chronic obstructive diseases even when the vital capacity appears near normal. FVC is nearly always decreased by restrictive diseases. FVC values <15 mL/kg are associated with an increased incidence of PPCs, probably because these patients cough ineffectively.[57] FVC reduced to this level represents a profound defect, most commonly seen in quadriplegics or severe neuromuscular disease. Finally, FVC is largely dependent on patient effort and cooperation.

Forced Expiratory Volume

FEV_T is the forced expiratory volume of gas over a given time interval during the FVC maneuver. The interval, described by the subscript T, is the time elapsed in seconds from the onset of expiration. Because FEV_T records a volume of gas expired over time, it is actually a measure of flow. By measuring expiratory flow at specific intervals, the severity of airway obstruction can be ascertained. Decreased FEV_T values are common in both obstructive and restrictive disease patterns. The most important application of FEV_T is its comparison with the patient's FVC. Normal subjects can expire at least three-fourths of FVC within the first second of the forced expiratory maneuver. The FEV_1, the most frequently employed value, is normally greater than or equal to 75% of the FVC, or $FEV_1/FVC \geq 0.75$.

Normally, an individual can expire 50 to 60% of FVC in 0.5 second, 75 to 85% in 1 second, 94% in 2 seconds, and 97% in 3 seconds. Cooperative patients with obstructive disease will exhibit a reduced FEV_1/FVC in most cases. However, patients with restrictive disease usually have normal FEV_1/FVC ratios. The validity of the evaluation of the FEV_1/FVC is highly dependent on patient cooperation and effort. It is possible to deliberately produce an artificially low FEV_1/FVC.

Forced Expiratory Flow

$FEF_{25-75\%}$ is the average forced expiratory flow during the middle half of the FEV maneuver. This test is also called maximum midexpiratory flow rate. The length of time required for a subject to expire the middle half of the FVC is divided into 50% of the FVC. The spirogram in Figure 28-9 marks the place from 25 to 75% of FVC, constituting the middle 50% of FVC. The straight line connecting the 25% and 75% volumes has a slope approximately equal to average flow. A normal value for a healthy 70-kg man is approximately 4.7 L/sec (or 280 mL/min). Normally, both the absolute value and the percentage of predicted value for the individual being studied are recorded. A normal value is 100 ± 25% of predicted. Decreased flow rates indicate medium-size airway obstruction. This value is typically normal in restrictive diseases. This test is fairly sensitive in the early stages of obstructive airway disease. Decreased $FEV_{25-75\%}$ frequently will be observed before other obstructive manifestations occur. Although somewhat effort dependent, the test is much more reliable and reproducible than FEV_1/FVC.

Maximum Voluntary Ventilation

Maximum voluntary ventilation (MVV) is the largest volume of gas that can be breathed in 1 minute by voluntary effort. The MVV is measured by having the subject breathe as deeply and as rapidly as possible for 10, 12, or 15 seconds. The results are extrapolated to 1 minute. The subject is instructed to set his or her own ventilatory rate and move more than tidal volume but less than vital capacity in each breath.

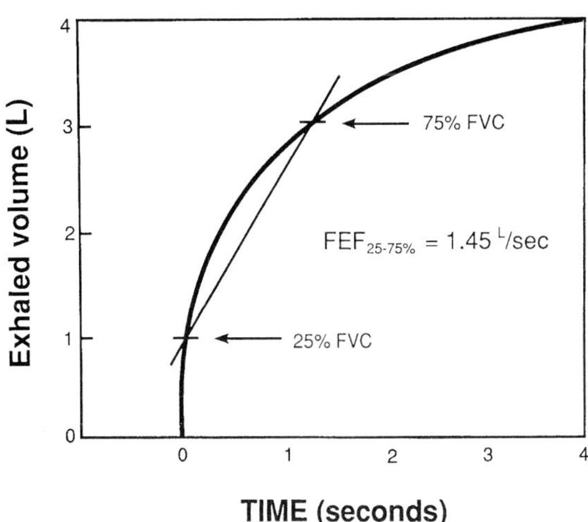

FIGURE 28-9. $FEF_{25-75\%}$. The spirogram depicts a 4 L FVC on which the points representing 25% and 75% FVC are marked. The slope of the line connecting these points is the $FEF_{25-75\%}$.

MVV measures the endurance of the ventilatory muscles and indirectly reflects lung–thorax compliance and airway resistance. MVV is the best ventilatory endurance test that can be performed in the laboratory. Values that vary by as much as 30% from predicted values may be normal so only large reductions in MVV are significant. Healthy, young adults average ~170 L/min. Values are lower in women and decrease with age in both sexes. Because this maneuver exaggerates air trapping and exerts the ventilatory muscles, MVV is decreased greatly in patients with moderate to severe obstructive disease. MVV is usually normal in patients with restrictive disease.

Flow–Volume Loops

The flow–volume loop graphically demonstrates the flow generated during a forced expiratory maneuver followed by a forced inspiratory maneuver, plotted against the volume of gas expired (Fig. 28-10). The subject forcefully exhales completely, then immediately and forcefully inhales to vital capacity. The expired and inspired volumes are plotted on the abscissa and flow is plotted on the ordinate. Although various numbers can be generated from the flow–volume loop, the configuration of the loop itself is probably the most informative part of the test.

Flow–volume loops were formerly useful in the diagnosis of large airway and extrathoracic airway obstruction prior to the availability of precise imaging techniques. Imaging techniques such as MRI give more precise and useful information in the diagnosis of upper airway and extrathoracic obstruction and superceded the use of flow–volume loops for diagnosis of these conditions. Therefore, it is rare that flow–volume loops are useful for preoperative pulmonary evaluation in the modern era of imaging.

Carbon Monoxide Diffusing Capacity

Because P_{O_2} in the pulmonary capillary blood varies with time as it moves through the pulmonary capillary bed, oxygen cannot be used to assess diffusing capacity. A gas mixture containing carbon monoxide is the traditional diagnostic gas used to measure diffusing capacity. Its partial pressure in the blood is nearly zero, and its affinity for hemoglobin is 200 times that of oxygen.[58] Carbon monoxide diffusing capacity (DLCO) collectively measures all the factors that affect the diffusion of gas across the alveolar–capillary membrane. The DLCO is recorded in mL CO/min/mm Hg at STPD.

In persons with normal hemoglobin concentrations and normal $\dot{V}_A/\dot{Q}$ matching, the main factor limiting diffusion is the alveolar–capillary membrane. Small amounts of carbon dioxide and inspired gas can produce measurable changes in the concentration of inspired gas compared with expired gas. There are several methods for determining DLCO, but all methods measure diffusing capacity according to the equation

$$D_{LCO} = \frac{\text{mL CO transferred/min}}{\text{mean } P_{ACO_2} - \text{mean capillary } P_{CO_2}} \qquad (28\text{-}10)$$

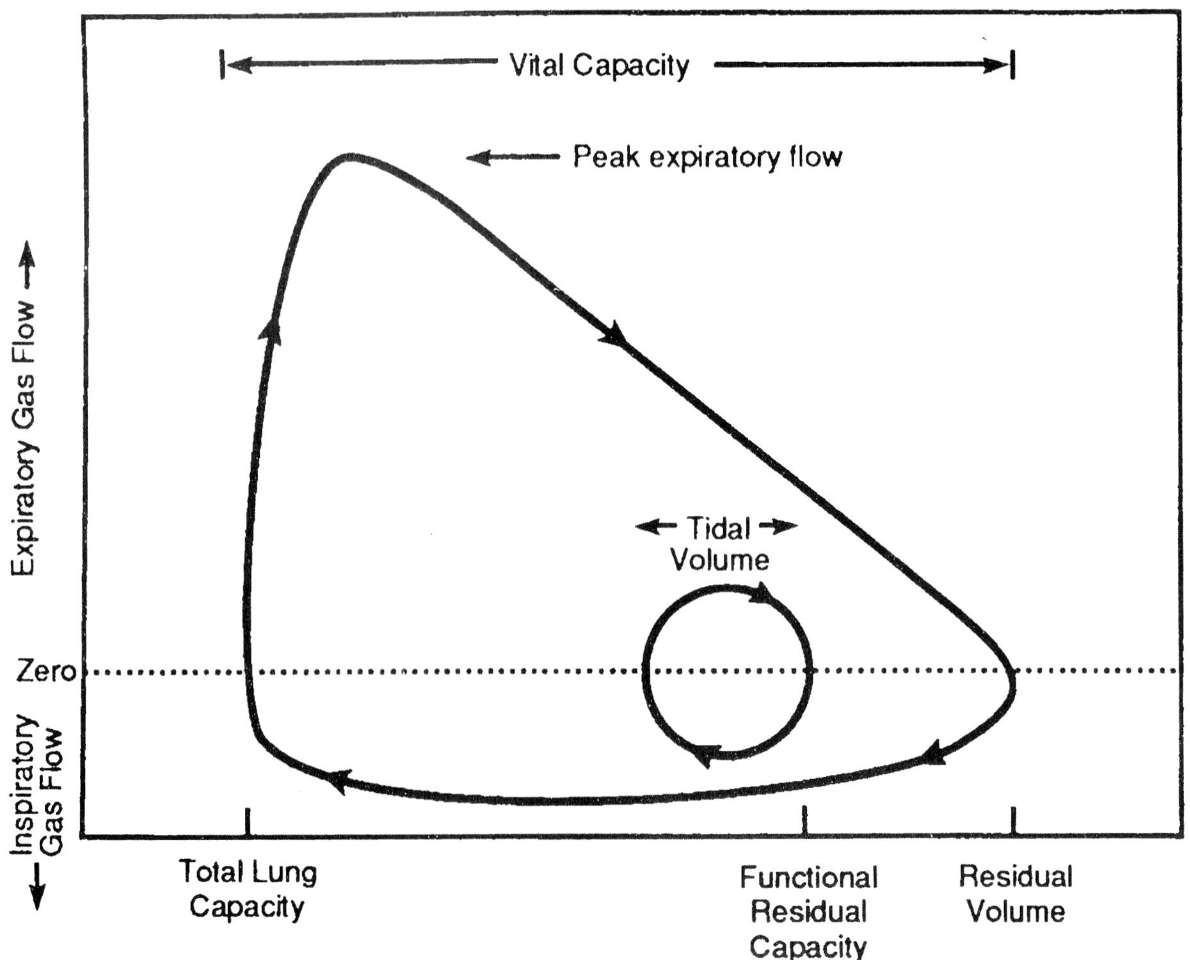

FIGURE 28-10. Flow–volume loop. The figure depicts a normally configured adult flow–volume loop. The slope of the loop after the subject reaches peak expiratory flow is nearly linear.

TABLE 28-4

PULMONARY FUNCTION TESTS IN RESTRICTIVE AND OBSTRUCTIVE LUNG DISEASE

■ VALUE	■ RESTRICTIVE DISEASE	■ OBSTRUCTIVE DISEASE
Definition	Proportional decreases in all lung volumes	Small airway obstruction to expiratory flow
FVC	↓↓↓	Normal or slightly ↑
FEV_1	↓↓↓	Normal or slightly ↓
FEV_1/FVC	Normal	↓↓↓
$FEF_{25-75\%}$	Normal	↓↓↓
FRC	↓↓↓	Normal or ↑ if gas trapping
TLC	↓↓↓	Normal or ↑ if gas trapping

FEV, forced expiratory volume; FRC, functional residual capacity; FVC, forced vital capacity; TLC, total lung capacity; ↓↓↓, ↑↑↑ = large decrease or increase, respectively; ↓, ↑ = small/moderate decrease or increase, respectively.

The average value for resting subjects when the single-breath method is used is 25 mL CO/min/mm Hg. DLCO values can increase to two or three times normal during exercise.

The DLO_2 may be estimated from the DLCO by multiplying DLCO by 1.23, although the DLCO is usually the reported value. DLCO can be divided by the lung volume at which the measurement was made to obtain an expression of diffusing capacity per unit lung volume.

Some of the other factors that can influence DLCO are as follows:

1. Hemoglobin concentration: decreased hemoglobin concentration decreases the DLCO
2. Alveolar PCO_2: an increased $PACO_2$ raises DLCO
3. Body position: the supine position increases DLCO
4. Pulmonary capillary blood volume

Diffusing capacity is decreased in alveolar fibrosis associated with sarcoidosis, asbestosis, berylliosis, oxygen toxicity, and pulmonary edema. These states are frequently categorized as diffusion defects, but low DLCO is probably more closely related to loss of lung volume or capillary bed perfusion. DLCO is decreased in obstructive disease because of the decreased alveolar surface area, loss of capillary bed, the increased distance from the terminal bronchiole to the alveolar–capillary membrane, and $\dot{V}A/\dot{Q}$ mismatching. Space-occupying lesions and lung resection also decrease diffusing capacity. In short, the decrease in measured DLCO is actually caused by abnormal $\dot{V}A/\dot{Q}$ matching in most cases. Few disease states truly inhibit oxygen diffusion across the alveolar–capillary membrane.

Pulmonary Function Tests Summary

Although we have a host of pulmonary function tests from which to choose, spirometry is the most useful, cost-effective, and commonly used test.[59] Screening spirometry yields VC, FVC, and FEV_1. From these values, two basic types of pulmonary dysfunction can be identified and quantitated: obstructive defects and restrictive defects. The primary criterion for airflow obstruction is decreased FEV_1/FCV ratio. Other measurements, such as $FEF_{25-75\%}$, can be used to support the diagnosis of an obstructive defect or to assist in making decisions (e.g., whether to institute bronchodilation). A restrictive defect is a proportional decrease in all lung volumes; thus, VC, FVC, and FEV_1 all are reduced, but FEV_1/FVC remains normal. When there is a question about whether a decreased VC is due to restriction, TLC should be measured. Reduced TLC defines a restrictive defect but is not necessary unless VC on screening spirometry is reduced. The American Thoracic Society published an experts' consensus concerning interpretation of lung function tests.[60] Table 28-4 summarizes the distinction between pulmonary function results obtained from those with restrictive and obstructive defects. Refer to the "Pulmonary Function Postoperatively" section for a discussion on the use of pulmonary testing.

Preoperative Pulmonary Assessment

Markedly impaired pulmonary function is likely in patients who have the following:

1. Any chronic disease that involves the lung
2. Smoking history, persistent cough, and/or wheezing
3. Chest wall and spinal deformities
4. Morbid obesity
5. Requirement for single-lung anesthesia or lung resection
6. Severe neuromuscular disease

Preoperative pulmonary evaluation must include history and physical examination, and may include chest radiograph, arterial blood gas analysis, and screening spirometry, depending on the patient's history. A history of sputum production, wheezing or dyspnea, exercise intolerance, or limited daily activities may yield more practical information than does formal testing. Arterial blood analysis, which should be sampled while the patient breathes room air, adds information regarding gas exchange and acid-base balance. Arterial blood gas sampling is primarily useful if the patient's history suggests that he or she may be chronically hypoxemic or may "retain" CO_2 (ie, a patient with a chronic, compensated arterial academia).

Preoperative assessment of pulmonary function may alert the anesthesiologist to the special needs of a patient with respiratory disease and may allow improvement of pulmonary function before an elective operation. The goals one might hope to achieve through preoperative pulmonary function would be to predict the likelihood of pulmonary complications, obtain quantitative baseline information concerning pulmonary function, and identify patients who may benefit from therapy to improve pulmonary function preoperatively. For patients who will have lung resections, pulmonary function testing does provide some predictive benefit.[61] For all other patients, however, overwhelming evidence suggests that preoperative pulmonary function testing does not predict or assign risk for PPCs.[62,63]

In 2002, the American Society of Anesthesiologists' Taskforce on Preanesthetic Evaluation published a practice
12 advisory[64] wherein they recommended that "there is insufficient evidence to identify explicit decision parameters or rules for ordering preoperative tests on the basis of specific clinical characteristics." Review of the literature[65] also reveals that specific measurements of lung function do not predict PPCs.

TABLE 28-5

RESPIRATORY FORMULAS

	■ NORMAL VALUES (70 kg)
Alveolar oxygen tension	110 mm Hg
$PAO_2 = (PB - 47)\ FIO_2 - (PACO_2/R)$	($FIO_2 = 0.21$)
Alveolar-arterial oxygen gradient	<10 mm Hg
$A\text{-}aO_2 = PAO_2 - PaO_2$	($FIO_2 = 0.21$)
Arterial-to-alveolar oxygen ratio, a/A ratio	>0.75
Arterial oxygen content	20 mL/100 mL blood
$CaO_2 = (SaO_2)(Hb \times 1.34) + PaO_2\ (0.0031)$	
Mixed venous oxygen content	15 mL/100 mL blood
$C\bar{v}O_2 = (S\bar{v}O_2)(Hb \times 1.34) + P\bar{v}O_2\ (0.0031)$	
Arterial-venous oxygen content difference	4–6 mL/100 mL blood
$Ca\text{-}\bar{v}O_2 = CaO_2 - C\bar{v}O_2$	
Intrapulmonary shunt	<5%
$\dot{Q}sp/\dot{Q}T = (Cc'O_2 - CaO_2)/(Cc'O_2 - C\bar{v}O_2)$	
where $Cc'O_2 = (Hb \times 1.34) + (PAO_2 \times 0.0031)$	
Physiologic dead space	0.33
$VD/VT = (PaCO_2 - P\bar{E}CO_2)/PaCO_2$	
Oxygen consumption	250 mL/min
$\dot{V}O_2 = CO\ (CaO_2 - C\bar{v}O_2)$	
Oxygen transport	1,000 mL/min
$O_2T = CO\ (CaO_2)$	
Respiratory quotient	0.8
$\dfrac{\dot{V}CO_2}{\dot{V}O_2}$	

CaO_2, arterial oxygen content; $C\bar{v}O_2$, mixed venous oxygen content; $Cc'O_2$, end-pulmonary capillary oxygen content; CO, cardiac output; FIO_2, fraction inspired oxygen; Hb, hemoglobin concentration; O_2T, oxygen transport; PB, barometric pressure; $\dot{Q}sp/\dot{Q}T$, intrapulmonary shunt; $PACO_2$, alveolar carbon dioxide tension; $PaCO_2$, arterial carbon dioxide tension; PAO_2, alveolar oxygen tension; PaO_2, arterial oxygen tension; $P\bar{E}CO_2$, mixed expired carbon dioxide tension; $P\bar{v}O_2$, mixed venous oxygen tension; SaO_2, arterial oxygen saturation; $S\bar{v}O_2$, mixed venous oxygen saturation; VD, dead space gas volume; VT, tidal volume; $\dot{V}O_2$, oxygen consumption (mL/min); $\dot{V}CO_2$, carbon dioxide production (mL/min); R, respiratory quotient.

Rather, the clinician obtains more information from the patient's history. In a series of 272 adults undergoing nonthoracic surgery, McAlister et al.[66] found that the following historical factors independently increased the risk of PPC: age >65 years, smoking >40 pack-years, COPD, asthma, productive cough, and exercise intolerance of less than one flight of stairs.

The need to obtain baseline pulmonary function data should be reserved for those patients with severely impaired preoperative pulmonary function, such as quadriplegics or myasthenics, so assessment for weaning from mechanical ventilation and/or tracheal extubation might be based on the patient's baseline pulmonary function. Ideally, tests should be chosen to quantify specific pulmonary problems.

Arterial blood gases (ABG) are not indicated unless the patient's history suggests arterial hypoxemia or severe enough COPD that one suspects CO_2 retention. Then, the ABG should be used in essentially the same manner as one might use preoperative PFTs: to look for reversible disease, or to define the severity of the disease at its baseline. Defining baseline PaO_2 and $PaCO_2$ is particularly important if one anticipates postoperatively ventilating a patient who has severe COPD. Table 28-5 summarizes the respiratory physiology formulas discussed in this chapter.

ANESTHESIA AND OBSTRUCTIVE PULMONARY DISEASE

Patients with marked obstructive pulmonary disease are at increased risk for both intraoperative and PPCs. For example, patients with reduced FEV_1/FVC or reduced midexpiratory flow not only suffer airway obstruction, but also usually exhibit increased airway reactivity. Because of the hazard of provoking reflex bronchoconstriction during laryngoscopy and tracheal intubation, patients with COPD or asthma should receive aggressive bronchodilator therapy preoperatively. High alveolar concentrations of potent inhalational anesthetics will blunt airway reflexes and reflex bronchoconstriction but require a fairly robust cardiovascular system. Adjunctive intravenous administration of opioids and lidocaine prior to airway instrumentation will decrease airway reactivity. Furthermore, a single dose of corticosteroids may help prevent postoperative increases in airway resistance.

Spontaneous ventilation during general anesthesia in patients with severe obstructive disease is more likely to result in hypercarbia than in patients with normal pulmonary function.[67] Preoperative FEV_1 reduction correlates with the $PaCO_2$ increase during anesthesia. Slower rates of mechanical ventilation (8–10 breaths $\cdot$ min^{-1}) should be used to allow time for exhalation. Low ventilatory rates necessitate larger tidal volume if one desires a normal $PaCO_2$, but larger V_t and resultant higher peak airway pressure may predispose the patient to pulmonary barotrauma. Tidal volume and inspiratory flows should be adjusted to keep peak airway pressure less than 40 cm H_2O,[68,69] if possible. Higher inspiratory flows produce a shorter inspiratory time and, usually, a high peak airway pressure. Thus, a balance that avoids high peak airway pressure and excessively large V_t that allows the longest possible expiratory time should be sought.

Ideally, depending on the procedure and the duration of anesthesia, one would extubate the patient's trachea at the end of the operation. The irritating tracheal tube increases both airway resistance and reflex bronchoconstriction, limits the ability of the patient to clear secretions effectively, and increases the risk of iatrogenic infection. For some patients with obstructive disease (eg, the young asthmatic), many advocate tracheal extubation during deep anesthesia at the conclusion of the operation.

ANESTHESIA AND RESTRICTIVE PULMONARY DISEASE

Restrictive disease is characterized by proportional decreases in all lung volumes. The decreased FRC produces low lung compliance and also results in arterial hypoxemia because of low $\dot{V}_A/\dot{Q}$ mismatching. These patients typically breathe rapidly and shallowly.

Positive-pressure ventilation of patients with restrictive disease is fraught with high peak airway pressures because more pressure is required to expand stiff lungs. Lower mechanical tidal volumes at more rapid rates reduce the risk of barotrauma but augment ventilation-induced cardiovascular depression and increase the chances of developing atelectasis. Larger tidal volumes should be avoided, because of the increased risk of both barotrauma[70] and volutrauma.[71] Various lung protective strategies have been developed to ventilate patients with profound restrictive lung disease (see Chapter 56).

Because the FRC is small, a lower oxygen store is available during apneic periods. Even preoxygenation with an F_{IO_2} of 1.0 can result in arterial hypoxemia seconds after the cessation of breathing or disconnection from a ventilator circuit. Patients with severe restrictive diseases tolerate apnea poorly. Because arterial hypoxemia develops so rapidly, transportation of these patients within the hospital should be performed with a pulse oximeter.

Even healthy individuals develop mild restrictive defects during anesthesia. FRC decreases 10 to 15% when healthy, spontaneously breathing individuals lie supine. Controlled ventilation further reduces FRC only slightly. General anesthesia consistently decreases FRC by a further 5 to 10%,[72] which usually results in decreased lung compliance.[73] The FRC reaches its nadir within the first 10 minutes of anesthesia[72,74,75] and is independent of whether ventilation is spontaneous or controlled. The diminished FRC persists in the postoperative period but may be restored postoperatively by the use of positive end-expiratory pressure or CPAP.[72,76,77] However, once positive airway pressure is removed, FRC plummets to previously diminished levels, which reach a postoperative nadir 12 hours after operation.[78]

EFFECTS OF CIGARETTE SMOKING ON PULMONARY FUNCTION

Smoking affects pulmonary function in many ways. The irritant smoke decreases ciliary motility and increases sputum production. Thus, these patients have a high volume of sputum and decreased ability to clear it effectively. As smoking habits persist, airway reactivity and the development of obstructive disease become problematic. Studies of the pathogenesis of COPD suggest that smoking results in an excess of pulmonary proteolytic enzymes, which directly cause damage to the lung parenchyma.[79] Exposure to smoke increases synthesis and release of elastolytic enzymes from alveolar macrophages—cells instrumental in the genesis of COPD due to smoking. Further damage to the lung tissue is probably caused by reactive metabolites of oxygen, such as hydroxyl radicals and hydrogen peroxide, which are usually used by the macrophages to kill microorganisms. The immunoregulatory function of the macrophages is also changed by cigarette smoking, with changes occurring in the presentation of antigens and interaction with T lymphocytes.[80] Other direct effects on lung tissue caused by smoking include increased epithelial permeability[81] and changed pulmonary surfactant.[82] The airway irritation or small airway reactivity evoked by inhaling cigarette smoke is the result of activation of sensory endings located in the central airways, which is primarily caused by nicotine.[83]

Early in the disease, mild $\dot{V}_A/\dot{Q}$ mismatch, bronchitic disease, and airway hyperreactivity are primary problems. Later, these problems are accompanied by the hallmarks of COPD: gas trapping, flattened diaphragmatic configuration (which decreases the efficiency with which the diaphragm functions), and barrel chest deformity. Lung compliance increases significantly so limited elastic recoil prevents complete passive emptying. As a result, many patients exhale forcibly to reduce gas trapping.

With gas trapping, ventilation and perfusion become increasingly mismatched. Large areas of dead space ventilation and venous admixture occur. Carbon dioxide elimination is inefficient because of dead space ventilation. The typical minute ventilation for patients with advanced obstructive lung disease can be one and one-half to two times normal. In addition, venous admixture produces arterial hypoxemia that is exquisitely sensitive to low concentrations of supplemental oxygen. Gas exchange is further impaired by the increased carboxyhemoglobin concentration that results from inspiring smoke. Normal carboxyhemoglobin concentration in nonsmokers is approximately 1%; in smokers, however, it can be as high as 8 to 10%. Cessation of smoking, even for 12 to 24 hours preoperatively, can decrease CO concentration to near normal.

Smoking is one of the main and most prevalent risk factors associated with postoperative morbidity.[84] COPD patients who smoke have a twofold to sixfold[85] risk of developing postoperative pneumonia compared with nonsmokers. Further, smokers' relative risk of PPC is doubled, even if they do not have evidence of clinical pulmonary disease or abnormal pulmonary function.[86] The incidence of PPC in smokers can be reduced by abstinence from smoking, although there is no consensus on the minimal or optimal duration of preoperative smoking abstinence.[87–89] Warner et al.[84] studied 200 patients undergoing coronary artery bypass grafting and found that patients who continued to smoke or stopped less than 8 weeks before the operation had a complication rate nearly four times that of patients who had quit smoking more than 8 weeks preoperatively. These data further demonstrated that those who quit smoking less than 8 weeks preoperatively had a higher rate of complication than those who continued to smoke. Normalization of mucociliary function requires 2 to 3 weeks of abstinence from smoking, during which time sputum increases. Several months of smoking abstinence is required to return sputum clearance to normal.[90] In a study of brupopion-assisted smoking cessation, Hurt and coworkers demonstrated decreased risk of postoperative complications even after 4 weeks of abstinence from smoking.[91]

Smokers who decrease, but do not stop, cigarette consumption without the aid of nicotine replacement therapy, continue to acquire equal amounts of nicotine from fewer cigarettes by changing their technique of smoking to maximize nicotine intake.[92] Levels of serum nicotine and cotinine and urinary mutagenesis levels remain unchanged. Thus, *reduction* in the number of cigarettes smoked will likely have little effect on the
13 risk of developing PPCs.[85] Smoking patients should be advised to *stop* smoking 2 months prior to elective operations to maximize the effect of smoking cessation,[84] or for at least 4 weeks

to benefit from improved mucociliary function and some reduction in PPC rate. If patients cannot stop smoking for 4 to 8 weeks preop, it is controversial whether they should be advised to stop smoking 24 hours preoperatively. A 24-hour smoking abstinence would allow carboxyhemoglobin levels to fall to normal but may increase the risk of PPC.

PULMONARY FUNCTION POSTOPERATIVELY

Risk of Postoperative Pulmonary Complications

Postoperative Pulmonary Function

The changes in pulmonary function that occur postoperatively are primarily restrictive, with proportional decreases in all lung volumes and no change in airway resistance. The decrease in FRC, however, is the yardstick by which the severity of the restrictive defect is gauged. This defect is generated by abdominal contents that impinge on and prevent normal movement of the diaphragm, and by an abnormal respiratory pattern devoid of sighs and characterized by shallow, rapid respirations. The normal resting respiratory rate for adults is 12 breaths per minute, whereas the postoperative patient in the ward usually breathes approximately 20 breaths per minute. Furthermore, most (but not all) factors that tend to make the restrictive defect worse are also those associated with a higher risk of PPCs.

14 The operative site is one of the single most important determinants of the degree of pulmonary restriction and the risk of PPCs. Nonlaparoscopic upper abdominal operations cause the most profound restrictive defect, precipitating a 40 to 50% decrease in FRC compared with preoperative levels, when conventional postoperative analgesia is employed. Lower abdominal and thoracic operations cause the next most severe change in pulmonary function, with decreases in FRC to 30% of preoperative levels. Most other operative sites—intracranial, peripheral vascular, otolaryngologic—have approximately the same effect on FRC, with reductions to 15 to 20% of preoperative levels.

Postoperative Pulmonary Complications

Two problems confound interpretation of the literature examining PPCs. First, there is no clear definition of what constitutes a PPC. For example, some clinical studies include only pneumonia, whereas others add atelectasis and/or ventilatory failure. Thus, to interpret data concerning rates of PPCs, it is important to discern what complications are specifically being addressed. Second, the criteria by which the diagnosis of postoperative pneumonia or atelectasis is made vary from study to study. For this discussion, PPCs include atelectasis and pneumonia only. Reasonable, well-accepted diagnostic criteria for these diagnoses include change in the color and quantity of sputum, oral temperature exceeding 38.5°C, and a new infiltrate on chest radiograph.

The operative site is an important risk factor for the development of PPCs. Nonlaparoscopic upper abdominal operations increase risk for PPC at least twofold,[88] with rates of occurrence varying from 20 to 70%.[93] Lower abdominal and intrathoracic operations are associated with slightly less risk, but still higher risk than extremity, intracranial, and head/neck operations.

Patients with COPD are at risk for PPC. These patients' risks can be minimized by ensuring they do not have an active pulmonary infection and any increased resistance associated with reactive airways disease is minimized by the use of therapeutic bronchodilation. Interestingly, those with asthma are not at increased risk for atelectasis or pneumonia. However, exacerbation of asthma in the postoperative period can be problematic. Careful attention must be given to ensuring the continuation of bronchodilating regimens and steroid administration through the perioperative period.

There are several strategies by which it is possible to reduce risk of PPC: the use of lung-expanding therapies postoperatively, choice of analgesia,[94] and cessation of smoking. After upper abdominal operations, which are associated with the highest incidence of PPCs, FRC recovers over 3 to 7 days. With the use of intermittent CPAP by mask, FRC will recover within 72 hours.[95] Patients correctly use incentive spirometers only 10% of the time unless therapy is supervised.[96] Stir-up regimens are as effective as incentive spirometry at preventing PPCs,[95] and they are less expensive than supervised incentive spirometry; thus, they are preferred over incentive spirometry therapy.

After median sternotomy for cardiac operations, FRC does not return to normal for several weeks, regardless of postoperative pulmonary therapy.[97] The persistently low FRC in this population is probably due to mechanical factors such as a widened mediastinum, intrapleural fluid, and altered chest wall compliance. The single most important aspect of postoperative
15 pulmonary care is getting the patient out of bed, preferably walking.

The choice of anesthetic technique for intraoperative anesthesia does not change the risk for PPC independent of the operative site or duration of the operation. Operations exceeding 3 hours are associated with a higher rate of PPC. Choice of postoperative analgesia strongly influences the risk of PPC.[88] The use of postoperative epidural analgesia, particularly for abdominal and thoracic operations, markedly decreases the risk of PPC and appears to decrease length of stay in the hospital.

Although obesity is associated with marked restrictive defects, some studies demonstrate that obesity does not independently increase the risk of PPC, whereas others do demonstrate increased independent risk for PPCs in the obese population.[98] Similarly, there are data both to support[98] and refute advanced age as an independent risk factor for PPCs.

Several authors have attempted to assess the influence of overall health on PPC risk. The use of indices that weight and score various aspects of physiology and health shows that patients who are in a poor state of health preoperatively tend to be at higher risk of PPC.[89]

Patients with obstructive airway disease and decreased expiratory flows may benefit from preoperative bronchodilator therapy and formal pulmonary toilet.[99] High-risk patients with COPD who receive bronchodilation, chest physical therapy, deep breathing, forced oral fluids (>3 L/day), and preoperative instruction in postoperative respiratory techniques, as well as those who stop smoking for more than 2 months preoperatively, experience a PPC rate approximately equal to that observed in normal patients.[100] Interestingly, although a regimen of this nature significantly reduces the incidence of PPCs,[101] airway obstruction and arterial hypoxemia are not measurably reversed during the 48 to 72 hours of preoperative therapy.[102] It is possible that the reduced complication rate results from the additional attention that these patients receive rather than from the specific regimen employed.

References

1. Lieberman DA, Falkner JA, Craig AB Jr *et al*: Performance and histochemical composition of guinea pig and human diaphragm. J Appl Physiol 34:233, 1973

2. Roussos C, Macklin PT: Diaphragmatic fatigue in man. J Appl Physiol 43:189, 1977
3. Campbell EJM, Green JH: The behavior of the abdominal muscles and intra-abdominal pressure during quiet breathing and increased pulmonary ventilation: A study in man. J Physiol (Lond) 127:423, 1955
4. Conrardy PA, Goodman CR, Lainge F *et al:* Alteration of endotracheal tube position: Flexion and extension of the neck. Crit Care Med 4:8, 1976
5. Bachoven M, Weibel ER: Basic pattern of tissue repair in human lungs following unspecific injury. Chest 65:145, 1974
6. Fishman AP: Non-respiratory function of lung. Chest 72:84, 1977
7. Hocking WG, Golden DW: The pulmonary-alveolar macrophage. N Engl J Med 301:580, 1979
8. Whitehead TC, Zhang H, Mullen B, Slutsky AS: Effect of mechanical ventilation on cytokine response to intratracheal hypopolysaccharide. Anesthesiology 101(1):1, 2004
9. Dreyfuss D, Rouby J-J: Mechanical ventilation-induced lung release of cytokines: A key for the future or Pandora's box? Anesthesiology 101:1, 2004
10. Downs JB: A technique for direct measurement of intrapleural pressure. Crit Care Med 4:207, 1976
11. Baydur A, Behrakis P, Zin WA: A simple method for assessing the validity of the esophageal balloon technique. Am Rev Respir Dis 126:788, 1982
12. Blanch MJ, Kirby RR, Gabrielli A *et al*: Partially and totally unloading the respiratory muscles based on real time measurements of work of breathing. Chest 106:1835, 1994
13. Brochard L, Rua F, Lorino H: Inspiratory pressure support compensates for the additional work of breathing caused by the endotracheal tube. Anesthesiology 75:739, 1991
14. Rohrer F: Der Strömungswiderstand in den menschlichen Atemwegen. Pflugers Arch 162:225, 1915
15. Nunn JF: Resistance to gas flow and airway closure. In: Applied Respiratory Physiology, p 50. Boston, Butterworths, 1987
16. Fink BR, Ngai SH, Holiday DA: Effect of air flow resistance on ventilation and respiratory muscle activity. JAMA 168:2245, 1958
17. Campbell EJM, Freedman S, Smith PS, Taylor ME: The ability of man to detect added elastic loads to breathing. Clin Sci 20:223, 1961
18. Palmer KNV, Diament ML: Effect of aerosol isoprenaline on blood-gas tensions in severe bronchial asthma. Lancet 2:1232, 1967
19. Campbell EJM: The effects of increased resistance to expiration on the respiratory behavior of the abdominal muscles and intraabdominal pressure. J Physiol 136:556, 1957
20. Janssens JP, Pache JC, Nicod LP: Physiologic changes in respiratory function associated with aging. Eur Respir J 13:107, 1999
21. LeGallois CJJ: Expériences sur le Principe de la Vie, p 325. Paris, D'Hautel, 1812
22. Salmoiraghi GC, Burns BD: Localization and patterns of discharge of respiratory neurons in the brainstem of a cat. J Neurophysiol 23:2, 1960
23. Cohen MI: Neurogenesis of respiratory rhythm in the mammal. Physiol Rev 59:1105, 1979
24. Guz A: Regulation of respiration in man. Ann Respir Physiol 37:303, 1975
25. Pitts RF, Magoun HW, Ranson SW: The origin of respiratory rhythmicity. Am J Physiol 127:654, 1939
26. Lumsden TL: Observations on the respiratory centers in the cat. J Physiol (Lond) 57:153, 1923
27. Cohen MI, Wang SC: Respiratory neuronal activity in the pons of the cat. J Neurophysiol 22:33, 1959
28. Stella G: On the mechanism of production and the physiologic significance of "apneusis." J Physiol (Lond) 93:10, 1938
29. Kabat H: Electrical stimulation of points in the forebrain and mid-brain: The resultant alterations in respiration. J Comp Neurol 64:187, 1936
30. Wang SC, Borison HL: The vomiting center: A critical experimental analysis. Arch Neurol Psychiatry 63:928, 1950
31. Gaylor JB: The intrinsic nervous mechanisms of the human lung. Brain 57:143, 1934
32. Davis HL, Fowler WS, Lambert EH: Effect of volume and rate of inflation and deflation on transpulmonary pressure and response of pulmonary stretch receptors. Am J Physiol 187:558, 1956
33. Hering E, Breuer J: Die Sebsteuerung der Atmung durch den Nervus vagus. Stizber Akad Wiss Wien 57:672, 1868
34. Ide T, Sakurai Y, Aono M, Nishino T: Contribution of peripheral chemoreception to the depression of the hypoxic ventilatory response during halothane anesthesia in cats. Anesthesiology 90:1084, 1998
35. Mora CT, Torjman M, White PF: Effects of diazepam and flumazenil on sedation and hypoxic ventilatory response. Anesth Analg 68(4):473, 1989
36. Leusen I: Regulation of cerebrospinal fluid composition with reference to breathing. Physiol Rev 52:1, 1972
37. Cohen MI: Discharge patterns of brainstem respiratory neurons in relation to carbon dioxide tension. J Neurophysiol 31:142, 1968
38. Heinemann HO, Golaring RM: Bicarbonate and the regulation of ventilation. Am J Med 57:361, 1974
39. Severinghaus JW, Mitchell RA, Richardson BW *et al*: Respiratory control at high altitude suggesting active transport regulation of CSF pH. J Appl Physiol 18:1155, 1166, 1963
40. Ferris EB, Engel GL, Stevens CD, Webb J: Voluntary breath holding. J Clin Invest 25:734, 1946
41. Stock MC, Downs JB, McDonald JS *et al:* The carbon dioxide rate of rise in awake apneic man. J Clin Anesth 1:96, 1988
42. Eger EI, Severinghaus JW: The rate of rise of $Paco_2$ in the apneic anesthetized patient. Anesthesiology 22:419, 1961
43. Stock MC, Schisler JQ, McSweeney TD: The $Paco_2$ rate of rise in anesthetized patients with airway obstruction. J Clin Anesth 1:328, 1989
44. Wright FG, Foley MF, Downs JB *et al:* Hypoxemia and hypocarbia following intermittent positive-pressure breathing. Anesth Analg 55:555, 1976
45. Fink BR: The stimulant effect of wakefulness on respiration: Clinical aspects. Br J Anaesth 33:97, 1961
46. Berger AJ, Mitchell RA, Severinghaus JW: Regulation of respiration: III. N Engl J Med 297:194, 1977
47. West JB, Dollery CT, Naimark A: Distribution of blood flow in isolated lung: Relation to vascular and alveolar pressures. J Appl Physiol 19:713, 1964
48. West JB, Dollery CT: Distribution of blood flow and the pressure-flow relations of the whole lung. J Appl Physiol 20:175, 1965
49. Benumof JL, Pirla AF, Johanson I *et al:* Interaction of Pvo_2 with Pao_2 on hypoxic pulmonary vasoconstriction. J Appl Physiol 51:871, 1981
50. Swenson EW, Finley TN, Guzman SV: Unilateral hypoventilation in man during temporary occlusion of one pulmonary artery. J Clin Invest 40:828, 1961
51. Yamanaka MK, Sue DY: Comparison of arterial-end-tidal Pco_2 difference and deadspace/tidal volume ratio in respiratory failure. Chest 92:832, 1987
52. Tyburski JG, Collinge JD, Wilson RF, Carlin AM, Albaran RG, Steffes CP: End-tidal CO_2-derived values during emergency trauma surgery correlated with outcome: A prospective study. J Trauma 53(4):738, 2002
53. Mazzeo AT, Lucanto T, Santamaria LB: Hepatopulmonary syndrome: A concern for the anesthetist? Preoperative evaluation of hypoxemic patients with liver disease. Acta Anaesthesiol Scand 48(2):178, 2004
54. Gaines DI, Faloon MB: Hepatopulmonary syndrome. Liver Int 24(5):397, 2004.
55. Räsänen J, Downs JB, Malec DJ, Oates K: Oxygen tensions and oxyhemoglobin saturations in the assessment of pulmonary gas exchange. Crit Care Med 15:1058, 1987
56. Christi RV: Lung volume and its subdivisions. J Clin Invest 11:1099, 1932
57. Tisi GM: Preoperative evaluation of pulmonary function. Am Rev Respir Dis 119:293, 1979
58. Apthorp GH, Marshall R: Pulmonary diffusing capacity: A comparison of breath-holding and steady-state methods using carbon monoxide. J Clin Invest 40:1775, 1961
59. Crapo RO: Pulmonary function testing. N Engl J Med 331:25, 1994
60. American Thoracic Society: Lung function testing: Selection of reference values and interpretive strategies. Am Rev Respir Dis 144:1202, 1991
61. Kearney DJ, Lee TH, Reilly JJ *et al:* Assessment of operative risk in patients undergoing lung resection: Importance of predicted pulmonary function. Chest 105:753, 1994
62. Ferguson MK: Preoperative assessment of pulmonary risk. Chest 115:58S, 1999
63. Lawrence VA, Dhanda R, Hilsenbeck SG, Page CP: Risk of pulmonary complications after elective abdominal surgery. Chest 110:744, 1996
64. Task Force on Preanesthetic Evaluation. Practice advisory for preanesthetic evaluation: A report by the American Society of Anesthesiologists. Anesthesiology 96:485, 2002
65. Zollinger A, Hofer C, Pasch T: Preoperative pulmonary evaluation: Fact and myth. Curr Opin Anaesth 14:59, 2002
66. McAlister FA, Khan NA, Strauss SE, Papaioakim M, Fisher BW, Majumdar SR, *et al*: Accuracy of the preoperative assessment in predicting pulmonary risk after non-thoracic surgery. Am J Respir Crit Care Med 167:7412003
67. Pietak W, Weenig CS, Hickey RF *et al:* Anesthetic effects on ventilation in patients with chronic obstructive pulmonary disease. Anesthesiology 42:160, 1975
68. Connors AF, McAferee D, Gray BA: Effect of inspiratory flow rate on gas exchange during mechanical ventilation. Am Rev Respir Dis 124:537, 1981
69. Tuxen DV, Lane S: The effects of ventilatory pattern on hyperinflation, airway pressures, and circulation in mechanical ventilation of patients with severe airflow obstruction. Am Rev Respir Dis 136:872, 1987
70. Petersen GW, Baier H: Incidence of pulmonary barotrauma in a medical ICU. Crit Care Med 11:67, 1983
71. Brower RG, Rubenfeld GD: Lung-protective ventilation strategies in acute lung injury. Crit Care Med 31(4 suppl):S312, 2003
72. Brisner B, Hedenstierna G, Lundquist H *et al:* Pulmonary densities during anesthesia with muscular relaxation: A proposal of atelectasis. Anesthesiology 62:422, 1985
73. Don HF, Robson JG: The mechanics of the respiratory system during anesthesia. Anesthesiology 26:168, 1965
74. Don HF, Wahba M, Cuadrado L *et al:* The effects of anesthesia and 100 percent oxygen on the functional residual capacity of the lungs. Anesthesiology 32:251, 1970
75. Westbrook PR, Stubbs SE, Sessler AD *et al:* Effects of anesthesia and muscle paralysis on respiratory mechanics in normal man. J Appl Physiol 34:81, 1973
76. Wyche MQ, Teichner RL, Kallost T *et al:* Effects of continuous positive-pressure breathing on functional residual capacity and arterial oxygenation during intra-abdominal operation. Anesthesiology 38:68, 1973
77. Rose DM, Downs JB, Heenen TJ: Temporal responses of functional residual

capacity and oxygen tension to changes in positive end-expiratory pressure. Crit Care Med 9:79, 1981

78. Craig DB: Postoperative recovery of pulmonary function. Anesth Analg 60:46, 1981
79. Diamond L, Lai YL: Augmentation of elastase-induced emphysema by cigarette smoke: Effects of reducing tar and nicotine content. J Toxicol Environ Health 20:287, 1987
80. Deshazo RD, Banks DE, Diem JE, *et al.* Broncho-alveolar lavage cell–lymphocyte interactions in normal nonsmokers and smokers. Am Rev Respir Dis 127:545, 1983
81. Hogg JC: The effect of smoking on airway permeability. Chest 83:1, 1983
82. Clements JA: Smoking and pulmonary surfactant. N Engl J Med 286:261, 1972
83. Lee L-Y, Gerhardstein DC, Wang AL, Burki NK: Nicotine is responsible for airway irritation evoked by cigarette smoke inhalation in men. J Appl Physiol 75:1955, 1993
84. Warner MA, Divertie MB, Tinker JH: Preoperative cessation of smoking and pulmonary complications in coronary artery bypass patients. Anesthesiology 60:380, 1984
85. Bluman LG, Mosca L, Newman N, Simon DG: Preoperative smoking habits and postoperative pulmonary complications. Chest 113:883, 1998
86. Chalon J, Tayyab MA, Ramanathan S: Cytology of respiratory complications after operation. Chest 67:32, 1975
87. Lillington GA, Sachs DPL: Preoperative smoking reduction: All or nothing at all? Chest 113:856, 1998
88. Celli BR: Perioperative care of patients undergoing upper abdominal surgery. Clin Chest Med 14:227, 1993
89. Warner MA, Offord KP, Warner ME *et al:* Role of postoperative cessation of smoking and other factors in postoperative pulmonary complications: A blinded prospective study of coronary artery bypass patients. Mayo Clin Proc 64:609, 1989
90. Beckers S, Camu F. The anesthetic risk of tobacco smoking. Acta Anaesthesiol Belg 42:45, 1991
91. Hurt RD, Sachs DPL, Gover ED *et al:* A comparison of sustained-release bupropion and placebo of smoking cessation. N Engl J Med 337:1195, 1997
92. Benowitz NL, Jacob P, Kozlowski LT *et al:* Influence of smoking fewer cigarettes on exposure to tar, nicotine and carbon monoxide. N Engl J Med 3115:1310, 1986
93. Hall JC, Tarala RA, Hall JL *et al:* A multivariate analysis of the risk of pulmonary complications after laparotomy. Chest 99:923, 1991
94. Gust R, Pecher S, Gust A *et al:* Effect of patient-controlled analgesia on pulmonary complications after coronary artery bypass grafting. Crit Care Med 27:2218, 1999
95. Stock MC, Downs JB, Gauer PK *et al:* Prevention of postoperative pulmonary complications with CPAP, incentive spirometry and conservative therapy. Chest 87:151, 1985
96. Lyager S, Wernberg M, Rajani N *et al:* Can postoperative pulmonary complications be improved by treatment with BartlettEdwards incentive spirometer after upper abdominal surgery? Acta Anaesthesiol Scand 23:312, 1979
97. Stock MC, Downs JB, Cooper RB *et al:* Comparison of continuous positive airway pressure, incentive spirometry, and conservative therapy after cardiac operations. Crit Care Med 12:969, 1984
98. Brooks-Brunn JA: Predictors of postoperative pulmonary complications following abdominal surgery. Chest 111:564, 1997
99. Chumillas S, Pace JL, Delgado F *et al:* Prevention of postoperative pulmonary complications through respiratory rehabilitation: A controlled clinical trial. Arch Phys Med Rehab 79:5, 1998
100. Brooks-Brunn JA: Validation of a predictive model for postoperative pulmonary complications. Heart Lung 27:151, 1998
101. Gracey DR, Divertie MB, Didier EP: Preoperative pulmonary preparation of patients with chronic obstructive pulmonary disease: A prospective study. Chest 76:123, 1979
102. Petty TL, Brink GA, Miller NW, Corsello PR: Objective functional improvement in chronic airway obstruction. Chest 57:216, 1970

CHAPTER 29 ■ ANESTHESIA FOR THORACIC SURGERY

EDMOND COHEN, STEVEN M. NEUSTEIN, AND JAMES B. EISENKRAFT

KEY POINTS

1. It is important to determine prior to the onset of anesthesia and surgery whether the patient will be able to tolerate the planned lung resection.
2. Preoperative assessment of vital capacity (VC) is critical because at least three times the tidal volume (VT) is necessary for an effective cough.
3. Smoking increases airway irritability, decreases mucociliary transport, and increases secretions. It also decreases forced vital capacity (FVC) and forced expiratory flow $(FEF)_{25-75\%}$, thereby increasing the incidence of postoperative pulmonary complications.
4. A lobectomy or pneumonectomy is a relative indication for lung separation using a double-lumen tube (DLT).
5. The most important advance in checking the proper position of a DLT is the introduction of the pediatric flexible fiberoptic bronchoscope.
6. During one-lung ventilation (OLV), the dependent lung should be ventilated using a VT that results in a plateau airway pressure <25 cm H_2O at a rate adjusted to maintain Pa_{CO_2} at 35 ± 3 mm Hg.
7. The choice of anesthetic technique for OLV must take into consideration the effects on oxygenation and therefore on hypoxic pulmonary vasoconstriction (HPV).
8. The need for OLV is much greater with video-assisted thoracoscopic surgery (VATS) than with open thoracotomy because it is not possible to retract the lung during VATS as it is during an open thoracotomy.
9. The potential advantages offered by high-frequency positive-pressure ventilation (HFPPV) during thoracic anesthesia are that lower VT and inspiratory pressures result in a quiet lung field for the surgeon, with minimal movements of airway, lung tissue, and mediastinum.
10. Myasthenia gravis, a disorder of the neuromuscular junction, is a chronic disorder characterized by weakness and fatigability of voluntary muscles with improvement following rest.
11. The key disadvantage of inadequate pain relief is postoperative atelectasis, limited inspiratory thoracic cage expansion, and great discomfort on the part of the patient.

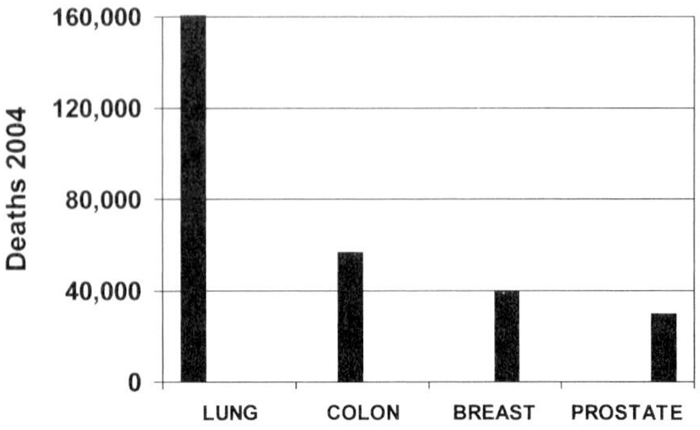

FIGURE 29-1. Lung cancer is the leading cause of cancer-related mortality. (Based on data from Jemal A, Tiwari RC, Murray T *et al*: Cancer statistics. CA Cancer J Clin 54:8, 2004.)

The number of noncardiac thoracic surgical operations has dramatically increased in more recent years and is expected to increase further in the future.[1] This is because lung cancer is currently the most common cause of cancer mortality in the United States and throughout the world. The American Cancer Society estimates that lung cancer will be responsible for approximately 160,440 deaths in the United States during 2004 (28% of all cancer deaths), in comparison with 127,210 deaths from the combined mortality due to colorectal, breast, and prostate cancer[2,3] (Fig. 29-1). Approximately 173,770 new cases of lung cancer will be diagnosed in 2004, accounting for 13% of all new cancer cases. In 2004, an estimated 91,000 males in the United States will die from lung cancer. Worldwide, almost 600,000 deaths were due to lung cancer in 1995, and it is projected that this number will continue to increase. Although lung cancer has long been the leading cause of cancer death in men, it surpassed breast cancer as the leading cause of cancer death in women only relatively recently. Although overall cancer incidence rates are declining, lung cancer incidence rates among women continues to increase. However, it is now far ahead of breast cancer, more than 50% of women in the United States will die from lung cancer than from breast cancer in 2004 (68,510 versus 40,110). Since the mid-1970s, it represents an increase of 400% among women.

The increase in noncardiac thoracic surgery has been associated with, and sometimes has been made possible by, advances in anesthesia care. Indeed, thoracic anesthesia is developing into a subspecialty in its own right, with several texts dedicated exclusively to this subject.[4,5] The physiologic, pharmacologic, and clinical considerations for the patient undergoing pulmonary surgery are reviewed, followed by sections on anesthesia for diagnostic and therapeutic procedures, high-frequency ventilation, and special situations, including bronchopleural fistula and tracheal reconstruction. A discussion of myasthenia gravis is included because of the relationship between the thymus gland and myasthenia, and because thymectomy is one of the most commonly performed surgical procedures in these patients. The chapter concludes with a review of the postoperative management of the patient who has undergone noncardiac thoracic surgery.

PREOPERATIVE EVALUATION

In addition to the routine assessment for any type of major surgery, the preoperative evaluation of the patient for thoracic surgery should focus on the extent and severity of pulmonary
1 disease and cardiovascular involvement. Prior to the onset of anesthesia and surgery, it is important to determine whether the patient will be able to tolerate the planned lung resection. To find out postoperatively that the patient cannot tolerate the resection would be catastrophic.

History

Dyspnea. Dyspnea occurs when the requirement for ventilation is greater than the patient's ability to respond appropriately. Dyspnea is quantitated as to the degree of physical activity required to produce it, the level of activity possible (e.g., ability to walk on level ground or climb stairs), and management of daily activities. Severe exertional dyspnea usually implies a significantly diminished ventilatory reserve and a forced expiratory volume in 1 second (FEV_1) of less than 1,500 mL, with possible need for postoperative ventilatory support.

Cough. Recurrent productive cough for 3 months of the year for 2 consecutive years is necessary to make the diagnosis of chronic bronchitis. Cough indirectly increases airway irritability. If the cough is productive, the volume, consistency, and color of the sputum should be assessed. Sputum should be cultured to rule out infection and to establish whether there is a need for preoperative antibiotic therapy. Blood-stained sputum or episodes of gross hemoptysis should alert the anesthesiologist to the possibility of a tumor invading the respiratory tract (e.g., the main-stem bronchus), which might interfere with endobronchial intubation.

Cigarette Smoking. Cigarette smoking increases the risk of chronic lung disease and malignancy, as well as the incidence of postoperative pulmonary complications. The number of pack-years (packs smoked per day multiplied by the number of years) is directly related to measurable changes in respiratory gas flow and closing capacity, making these patients prone to postoperative atelectasis and arterial hypoxemia.

Exercise Tolerance. Patients who can walk up three or more flights of stairs are at reduced risk, and those unable to climb two flights are generally at increased risk.[6] The best evaluation is actually the history of the patient's quality of life.[7] An otherwise healthy patient, with good exercise tolerance, generally does not require additional screening tests.

Risk Factors for Acute Lung Injury. In some cases, thoracic surgery may lead to acute lung injury postoperatively. Perioperative risk factors that have been identified include preoperative alcohol abuse and patients undergoing pneumonectomy. Intraoperative risk factors include high ventilatory pressures and excessive amounts of fluid administration.[8]

Physical Examination

The physical examination of the patient should address the following aspects.

Respiratory Pattern

The presence of cyanosis and clubbing, the breathing pattern, and the type of breath sounds should be noted.

Cyanosis. The presence of peripheral cyanosis (in the fingers, toes, or ears) should be distinguished from causes of poor circulation (acrocyanosis). The presence of central cyanosis (in the buccal mucosa) is usually secondary to arterial hypoxemia. If cyanosis is present, the arterial hemoglobin saturation with oxygen is 80% or less ($Pa{O_2} < 50$ to 52 mm Hg), which indicates a limited margin of respiratory reserve.

Clubbing. Clubbing is often seen in patients with chronic lung disease, malignancies, or congenital heart disease associated with right-to-left shunt.

Respiratory Rate and Pattern. A patient's inability to complete a normal sentence without pausing for breath is an indication of severe dyspnea. Inspiratory paradox, the abdomen moving in while the chest moves out, suggests diaphragmatic fatigue and respiratory dysfunction. The patient should be assessed for paroxysmal retraction (Hoover's sign), limited diaphragmatic movement because of hyperinflation, and asymmetry of chest movement secondary to phrenic nerve involvement, hemothorax, pleural effusion, and pneumothorax. The pattern and rate of breathing have important roles in distinguishing between obstructive and restrictive lung disease. For constant minute ventilation, the work done against airflow resistance decreases when breathing is slow and deep. Work done against elastic resistance decreases when breathing is rapid and shallow (e.g., as in pulmonary infarct or pulmonary fibrosis).

Breath Sounds. Wet sounds (crackles) are usually caused by excessive fluid in the airways and indicate sputum retention or edema. Dry sounds (wheezes) are produced by high-velocity gas flow through bronchi and are a sign of airway obstruction. Distant sounds are an indication of emphysema and possibly bullae. The trachea should be in the midline. Displacement of the trachea may be secondary to a number of causes, including mediastinal mass, and should alert the anesthesiologist to a potentially difficult intubation of the trachea or airway obstruction on induction of anesthesia.

Evaluation of the Cardiovascular System

One of the most important factors in the evaluation of a patient scheduled for thoracic surgery is the presence of an increase in pulmonary vascular resistance secondary to a fixed reduction in the cross-sectional area of the pulmonary vascular bed. The pulmonary circulation is a low-pressure, high-compliance system capable of handling an increase in blood flow by recruitment of normally underperfused vessels. This acts as a compensatory mechanism that normally prevents an increase in pulmonary arterial pressure. In chronic obstructive pulmonary disease (COPD), there is distention of the pulmonary capillary bed with decreased ability to tolerate an increase in blood flow (decreased compliance). Such patients demonstrate an increase in pulmonary vascular resistance when cardiac output increases because of a decreased ability to compensate for an increase in pulmonary blood flow. This results in pulmonary hypertension, signs of which include a narrowly split second heart sound, increased intensity of the pulmonary component of the second heart sound, and right ventricular and atrial hypertrophy.

An increase in pulmonary vascular resistance is of significance in the management of the patient during anesthesia because several factors, such as acidosis, sepsis, hypoxia, and application of positive end-expiratory pressure (PEEP), all further increase the pulmonary vascular resistance and increase the likelihood of right ventricular failure.

In patients with ischemic or valvular heart disease, the function of the left side of the heart should also be carefully evaluated (see Chapter 31).

Electrocardiogram

A patient with COPD may present with electrocardiographic features of right atrial and ventricular hypertrophy and strain. These include a low-voltage QRS complex due to lung hyperinflation and poor R-wave progression across the precordial leads. An enlarged P wave ("P pulmonale") in standard lead II is diagnostic of right atrial hypertrophy. The electrocardiographic changes of right ventricular hypertrophy are an R/S ratio of greater than 1.0 in lead V_1 (i.e., R-wave voltage exceeds S-wave voltage).

Chest Radiography

Hyperinflation and increased vascular markings are usually present with COPD. Prominent lung markings often occur in bronchitis, whereas they are decreased in emphysema, particularly at the bases, where actual bullae may be present in severe cases. Hyperinflation, with an increased anteroposterior chest diameter, may be present, together with an enlarged retrosternal air space of greater than 2 cm in diameter seen in a lateral chest radiograph.

The location of the lung lesion should be assessed by posteroanterior and lateral projections on chest radiography. In addition to tracheal or carinal shift, a mediastinal mass may indicate difficulty with ventilation, a difficult and bloody dissection, difficulty in placing a double-lumen tube (DLT) (because of deviation of the main-stem bronchus), or a collapsed lobe owing to bronchial obstruction with possible sepsis. Review of a computed tomography (CT) study is also useful, and often provides more information about tumor size and location than the chest radiograph.

Arterial Blood Gas Analysis

A common finding in arterial blood gas analysis of patients with COPD is hypoventilation and CO_2 retention. The "blue bloaters" (chronic bronchitics) are cyanotic, hypercarbic, hypoxemic, and usually overweight. They are in a state of chronic respiratory failure and have a decreased ventilatory response to CO_2. In these patients, the high $Paco_2$ increases cerebrospinal fluid bicarbonate concentration, the medullary chemoreceptors become reset to a higher level of CO_2, and sensitivity to CO_2 is decreased. Such patients hypoventilate when given high oxygen concentrations to breathe because of a decreased hypoxic drive.

The "pink puffers" (patients with emphysema) are typically thin, dyspneic, and pink, with essentially normal arterial blood gas values. They present with an increase in minute ventilation to maintain their normal $Paco_2$, which explains the increase in work of breathing and dyspnea. The preoperative Pao_2 correlates with the intraoperative Pao_2 during one-lung ventilation (OLV), but the intraoperative Pao_2 during two-lung ventilation correlates more closely.[9]

Pulmonary Function Testing and Evaluation for Lung Resectability

There are three goals in performing pulmonary function tests in a patient scheduled for lung resection. The first is to identify the patient at risk of increased postoperative morbidity and mortality. In thoracic surgery for lung cancer, the specific question is: How much lung tissue may be safely removed without making the patient a pulmonary cripple?" This should be weighed against the 1-year mean survival rate of the patient with surgically untreated lung carcinoma. The second goal is to identify the patient who will need short-term or long-term postoperative ventilatory support. The third goal is to evaluate the beneficial effect and reversibility of airway obstruction with the use of bronchodilators.

Effects of Anesthesia and Surgery on Lung Volumes

Anesthesia and postoperative medications can cause changes in lung volumes and ventilatory pattern. Total lung capacity (TLC) decreases after abdominal surgery but not after surgery on an extremity. Vital capacity is decreased by 25 to 50% within 1 to 2 days after surgery and generally returns to normal after 1 to 2 weeks. Residual volume (RV) increases by 13%, whereas expiratory reserve volume decreases by 25% after lower abdominal surgery and 60% after upper abdominal and thoracic surgery. Tidal volume (VT) decreases by 20% within 24 hours after surgery and gradually returns to normal after 2 weeks. Pulmonary compliance decreases by 33% with similar reductions in functional residual capacity (FRC) secondary to small airway closure. Most of the patients who undergo lung resection are smokers with a certain degree of COPD and are prone to postoperative complications in direct relation to the amount of lung to be resected (lobectomy or pneumonectomy) and to the severity of the preoperative lung disease.

Spirometry

Forced vital capacity (FVC), forced expired volume in one second (FEV_1), and peak expiratory flow can be measured at the patient's bedside using a spirometer. The measurement can be
2 recorded as a volume–time trace or as a flow–volume loop. A vital capacity of at least three times the VT is necessary for an effective cough. A vital capacity of <50% of predicted or <2 L is an indication of increased risk.[10] An abnormal preoperative vital capacity can be identified in 30 to 40% of postoperative deaths. A patient with an abnormal vital capacity has a 33% likelihood of complications and a 10% risk of postoperative mortality.

FEV_1 is a more direct indication of airway obstruction. In the past, an FEV_1 of less than 800 mL in a 70-kg male had been considered an absolute contraindication to lung resection. However, with the advent of thoracoscopic surgery and improved postoperative pain management, patients with smaller lung volumes are now successfully undergoing surgery. It is preferable to indicate the percentage of predicted, rather than just using the absolute value. The percentage of predicted takes into account the age and size of the patient, and the same number may have a different implication in another patient. Mortality in patients with an FEV_1 >2 L is 10%, and in patients whose FEV_1 is <1 L is between 20% and 45%.[11]

The ratio FEV_1/FVC is useful in differentiating between restrictive and obstructive pulmonary disease. It is normal in restrictive disease because both FEV_1 and FVC decrease, whereas in obstructive disease the ratio is usually low because the FEV_1 is markedly decreased. Maximum voluntary ventilation (MVV) is a nonspecific test, and is an indicator of both restriction and obstruction. Although MVV has not been systematically evaluated as a predictor of morbidity, it is generally accepted that an MVV <50% of predicted value is an indication of high risk. A ratio of RV to TLC (RV/TLC) of >50% is generally indicative of a high-risk patient for pulmonary resection. Mittman[12] found that an RV/TLC ratio of >40% was associated with a 30% mortality rate, compared with a 7% mortality when RV/TLC was <40% (normal range 20 to 25%). By multiplying the preoperative FEV_1 by the percentage of lung tissue expected to remain following resection, a predicted postop (PPO) FEV_1 can be calculated. Patients with a PPO FEV_1 value >40% are at reduced risk, and those with PPO FEV_1 <30% are at increased risk.[13] Those patients who fall into the latter category are more likely to need postoperative ventilation.

Flow–Volume Loops

The flow–volume loop displays essentially the same information as a spirometer but is more convenient for measurement of specific flow rates (Fig. 29-2). The shape and peak airflow rates during expiration at high lung volumes are effort dependent, but indicate the patency of the larger airways. Effort-independent expiration occurs at low lung volumes and usually reflects small airways resistance, best measured by forced expiratory flow (FEF) during the middle half of the FVC ($FEF_{25-75\%}$).

In general, patients with obstructive airways disease (Fig. 29-3), such as asthma, bronchitis, and emphysema, have

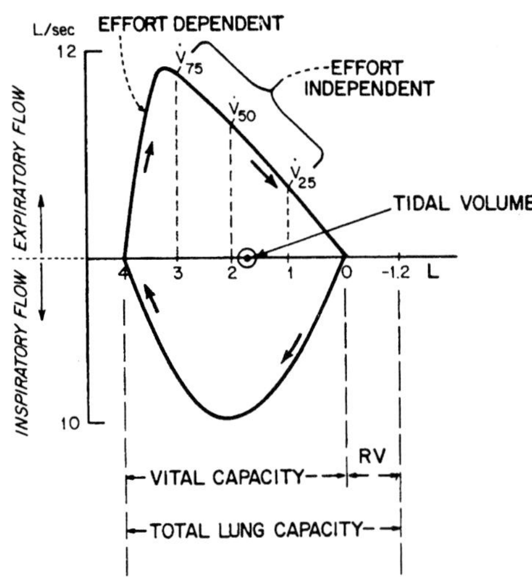

FIGURE 29-2. Flow–volume loop in a normal subject. $\dot{V}_{75}$, $\dot{V}_{50}$, and $\dot{V}_{25}$ represent flow at 75%, 50%, and 25% of vital capacity, respectively. RV, residual volume. (Reproduced with permission from Goudsouzian N, Karamanian A: Physiology for the Anesthesiologist, 2nd ed. Norwalk, CT, Appleton-Century-Crofts, 1984.)

grossly decreased FEV_1/FVC ratios because of increased airways resistance and a decrease in FEV_1. Peak expiratory flow rate and MVV are usually decreased, whereas total lung capacity increases secondary to increases in RV. In these patients, the effort-independent portion of the flow–volume curve is markedly depressed inward, with reduction of the flow rate at 25 to 75% of FVC.

In patients with restrictive disease (see Fig. 29-3), such as pulmonary fibrosis and scoliosis, there is a decrease in FVC with a relatively normal FEV_1. Because the airways resistance is normal, FEV_1/FVC is also normal. TLC is markedly decreased, whereas MVV and $FEF_{25-75\%}$ are usually normal. The flow–volume curves of these patients are normal in shape, but the lung volumes and peak flow rates are decreased.

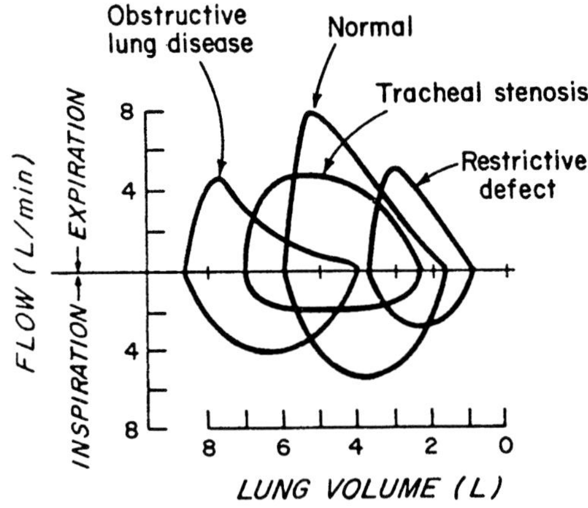

FIGURE 29-3. Flow–volume loops relative to lung volumes (1) in a normal subject, (2) in a patient with chronic obstructive pulmonary disease (COPD), (3) in a patient with fixed obstruction (tracheal stenosis), and (4) in a patient with pulmonary fibrosis (restrictive defect). Note the concave expiratory form in the patient with COPD and the flat inspiratory curve in the patient with a fixed obstruction. (Reprinted with permission from Goudsouzian N, Karamanian A: Physiology for the Anesthesiologist, 2nd ed. Norwalk, CT, Appleton-Century-Crofts, 1984.)

Significance of Bronchodilator Therapy. Pulmonary function tests are usually performed before and after bronchodilator therapy to assess the reversibility of the airways obstruction. This is useful in the assessment of the degree of airways obstruction and the patient's effort ability. After treatment with bronchodilators, increases in peak expiratory flow compared with a baseline indicate reversibility of airways obstruction (often seen in asthmatic patients). A 15% improvement in pulmonary function tests may be considered a positive response to bronchodilator therapy and indicates that this therapy should be initiated before surgery. The overall prognosis of COPD is better related to the level of spirometric function after bronchodilator therapy than to a baseline function.

Split-Lung Function Tests

Regional lung function studies serve to predict the function of the lung tissue that would remain after lung resection. A whole (two)-lung test may fail to estimate whether the amount of postresection lung tissue will allow the patient to function at a reasonable level of activity without disabling dyspnea or cor pulmonale.

Regional Perfusion Test. This involves the intravenous injection of insoluble radioactive xenon (^{133}Xe). The peak radioactivity of each lung is proportional to the degree of perfusion of each lung.

Regional Ventilation Test. Using an inhaled, insoluble radioactive gas, the peak radioactivity over each lung is proportional to the degree of ventilation. Combining radiospirometry with whole-lung testing (FEV_1, FVC, maximal breathing capacity) has resulted in a fair degree of correlation between predicted volumes and pulmonary function tests measured after pneumonectomy.

Regional Bronchial Balloon-Occlusion Test. This test simulates the postresection condition preoperatively by using balloon occlusion of the bronchus to the segment of the lung to be resected. Spirometry and arterial blood gas analysis are then performed with the remaining functional lung.

Computed Tomography and Positron Emission Tomography Scans. Patients normally undergo CT scanning. The CT scan provides anatomic sections through the chest. It can delineate the size of the tumor. It can also reveal if there is airway or cardiovascular compression,

Positron emission tomography (PET) scans use a glucose analog that is labeled with a radionuclide positron emitter. This scan can detect tumor based on the metabolic activity. Because malignant tumors are growing at such a fast rate compared with healthy tissue, the tumor cells will use up more of the sugar that has the radionuclide attached to it. There is greater uptake by malignant mediastinal lymph nodes than benign nodes. PET may be more accurate than CT for mediastinal staging.[14] Currently, PET scans can be used to further evaluate lesions that are seen on a CT scan. The PET scan can also be used to follow the results of lung cancer treatments.[15]

The CT and PET scans can be done at the same time to produce a PET-CT scan. A mass that is seen on the CT scan is more likely to be malignant if it also demonstrates enhanced glucose uptake on the PET scan.

Pulmonary Artery Balloon-Occlusion Test

The postoperative stress on the right ventricle and remaining pulmonary vascular bed can be simulated by occluding the pulmonary artery of the lung to be resected using a specially designed balloon-tipped pulmonary artery (PA) catheter that has a pressure-sensing port just proximal to the balloon. This test may be performed with or without exercise. If, on balloon occlusion of the pulmonary artery of the lung to be resected, the mean pulmonary artery pressure increases to >40 mm Hg, $Pa{O_2}$ is <60 mm Hg, or $Pa{CO_2}$ is >45 mm Hg, it is unlikely that the patient will be able to tolerate pneumonectomy without experiencing postoperative respiratory failure or cor pulmonale. Due to the usefulness of the noninvasive split-lung function tests, the bronchial and pulmonary artery balloon occlusion tests are rarely performed for clinical evaluation.

Diffusing Capacity for Carbon Monoxide

The ability of the lung to perform gas exchange is reflected by the diffusing capacity for carbon monoxide (DLCO). It is impaired in such disorders as interstitial lung disease, which affects the alveolar-capillary site. A predicted postoperative DLCO <40% is associated with increased risk. Predicted postoperative diffusing capacity percent is the strongest single predictor of risk of complications and mortality after lung resection. There is little interrelationship of predicted postoperative diffusing capacity percent and predicted postoperative FEV_1, indicating that these values should be assessed independently when estimating operative risk.[16]

Maximal Oxygen Consumption. The maximal oxygen consumption (VO_2 max) is a predictor of postoperative complications. Patients with a VO_2 max >15 to 20 mL/kg per minute are at reduced risk.[17] A VO_2 max <10 mL/kg per minute indicates very high risk for lung resection.[18] A simpler test that can be performed is exercise oximetry—a decrease of 4% during exercise is associated with increased risk.[19] A 6-minute walk test less than 2,000 feet has been correlated both with a VO_2 max < 15 mL/kg per minute, and with a decrease in oximetry reading during exercise.

The preoperative evaluation of the patient for lung resection is summarized in Fig. 29-4.

PREOPERATIVE PREPARATION

The wide spectrum of physiologic changes that occurs during thoracic surgery puts patients at great risk of developing postoperative complications. Morbidity and mortality increase when these changes are superimposed on an acutely or chronically compromised patient. Several conditions, including infection, dehydration, electrolyte imbalance, wheezing, obesity, cigarette smoking, cor pulmonale, and malnutrition, show particular correlations with postoperative complications. Proper, vigorous preoperative preparation can improve the patient's ability to face the surgery with a decreased risk of morbidity and mortality. It is important that conditions predisposing to postoperative complications be rigorously treated before surgery.

Smoking

Approximately 33% of adult patients presenting for surgery are smokers, and there is extensive evidence that they are at increased risk for development of postoperative respiratory
3 tory complications.[20] Smoking increases airway irritability, decreases mucociliary transport, decreases FVC and $FEF_{25-75\%}$, and increases secretions, thereby increasing the incidence of postoperative pulmonary complications. In contrast, cessation of smoking for a period of longer than 4 to 6 weeks before surgery is associated with a decreased incidence of postoperative complications.[21] Furthermore, cessation of smoking for 48 hours before surgery has been shown to decrease the percentage of carboxyhemoglobin, to shift the oxyhemoglobin dissociation curve to the right, and to increase oxygen availability. It should be emphasized, however, that most of the beneficial effects of cessation of smoking, such as improvement in ciliary function, improvement in closing volume, increase in

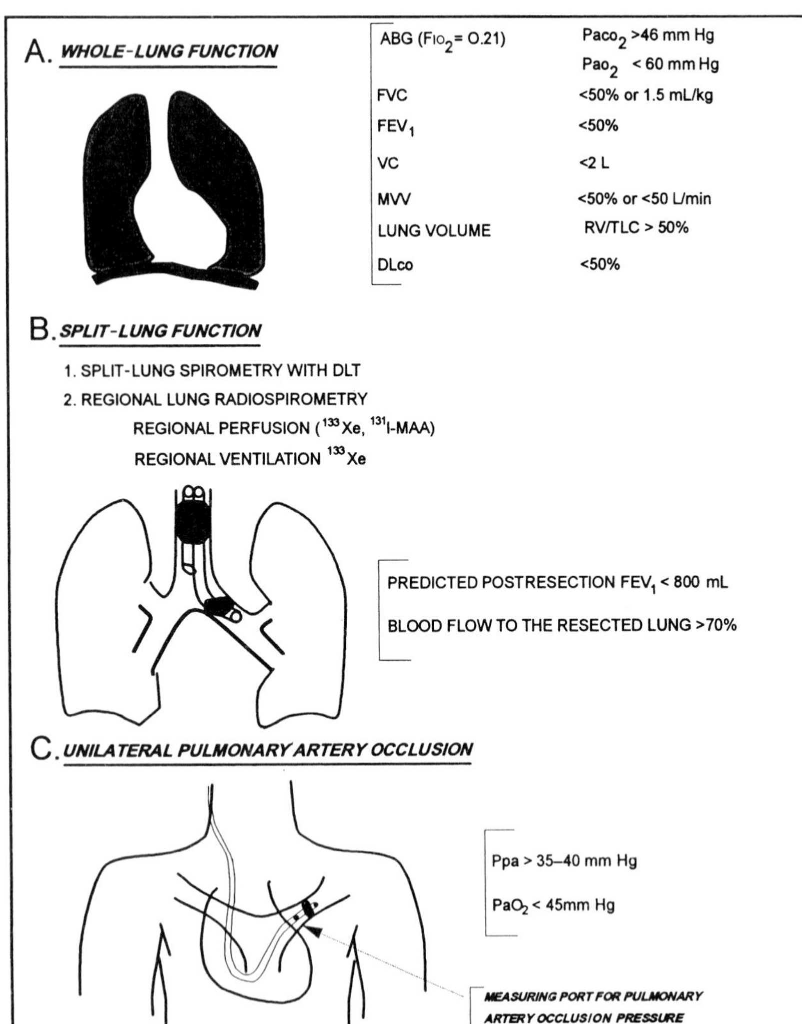

FIGURE 29-4. The order of tests to determine the cardiopulmonary status of the patient and the extent of lung resection that would be tolerated. **A.** The whole-lung function test is a basic screening test. **B.** The split-lung function tests are regional tests to determine the involvement of the diseased lung to be removed. **C.** Tests that mimic the postoperative cardiopulmonary function are the decisive tests to determine if the patient will be able to tolerate the planned resection. (Adapted with permission from Neustein SM, Cohen E: Preoperative evaluation of thoracic surgical patients. In Cohen E [ed]: The Practice of Thoracic Anesthesia, p 187. Philadelphia, JB Lippincott, 1995.)

$FEF_{25-75\%}$, and reduction in sputum production, usually occur 2 to 3 months after smoking has ceased.

Infection

Acute or chronic infection should be vigorously treated before surgery. Broad-spectrum antibiotics are commonly used. Treatment of the acutely ill patient depends on the results of the Gram's stain of the sputum and blood cultures. In one prospective study, the incidence of mortality was lower in the group treated with prophylactic antibiotics compared with the untreated group (9% versus 17%), and a lower incidence of postoperative pulmonary infection was also found.[22] Although not all surgeons routinely administer antibiotics prophylactically to their patients, any infection present before surgery should be vigorously treated.

Hydration and Removal of Bronchial Secretions

Correction of hypovolemia and electrolyte imbalance should be accomplished before surgery because adequate hydration decreases the viscosity of bronchial secretions and facilitates their removal from the bronchial tree. Humidification of inspired gas is extremely useful. The use of mucolytic drugs, such as acetylcysteine (Mucomyst), or oral expectorants (potassium iodide) can be beneficial to patients with viscous secretions. Commonly used methods for removing secretions from the bronchial tree include postural drainage, vigorous coughing, chest percussion, deep breathing, and the use of an incentive spirometer. These modalities often require patient cooperation and frequent verbal encouragement to maximize the benefit.

Wheezing and Bronchodilation

The presence of acute wheezing represents a medical emergency, and elective surgery should be postponed until effective treatment has been instituted. Chronic wheezing is often seen in patients with COPD and is attributable to the presence of gas flow obstruction secondary to smooth muscle contraction, accumulation of secretions, and mucosal edema. Smooth muscle contraction may occur in small airways only (detectable by changes in $FEF_{25-75\%}$) or may be widespread, with a large reduction of FEV_1 and FVC. The efficacy of bronchodilators in reversing the bronchospastic component is extremely important. A trial of bronchodilators and measurement of their effects on pulmonary function should be performed in any patient who shows evidence of air flow obstruction. Several classes of bronchodilators are available.

Sympathomimetic Drugs. Sympathomimetic drugs increase the formation of 3′5′-cyclic adenosine monophosphate (cAMP). The balance between cAMP, which produces bronchodilation, and cyclic guanosine monophosphate, which produces bronchoconstriction, determines the state of contraction of the bronchial smooth muscle. Increasing cAMP production therefore causes relaxation of the bronchial tree. Sympathomimetic drugs, such as epinephrine, isoproterenol, isoetharine, and ephedrine, all have mixed β_1 and β_2 sympathetic agonist effects. The β_1 (cardiac effects) of these drugs are often undesirable in patients with COPD. Selective β_2 sympathomimetic drugs, such as albuterol, terbutaline, and metaproterenol, given as inhaled aerosols, are the preferred drugs for the treatment of bronchospasm, particularly in patients with cardiac disease.

Phosphodiesterase Inhibitors. Phosphodiesterase inhibitors inhibit the breakdown of cAMP by cytoplasmic phosphodiesterase. The methylxanthines, such as aminophylline, increase the level of cAMP, resulting in bronchodilation. In addition, aminophylline improves diaphragmatic contractility and increases the patient's resistance to fatigue. Therapeutic blood levels of aminophylline are 5 to 20 μg/mL and can be achieved by infusing a loading dose of 5 to 7 mg/kg over 20 minutes, followed by a continuous intravenous infusion of 0.5 to 0.7 mg/kg/hr. Aminophylline may cause ventricular arrhythmias, and this side effect should be borne in mind when treating patients who have myocardial ischemia. Because newer medications have fewer side effects, aminophylline is now rarely used.

Steroids. Although not true bronchodilators, steroids are traditionally considered to decrease mucosal edema and may prevent the release of bronchoconstricting substances. They are of questionable benefit in acute bronchospasm. Steroids may be administered orally, parenterally, or in aerosol form, such as beclomethasone by inhaler.

Cromolyn Sodium. Cromolyn sodium stabilizes mast cells and inhibits degranulation and histamine release. It is useful in the prevention of bronchospastic attacks but is of little value in the treatment of the acute situation.

Parasympatholytic Drugs. Parasympatholytics include atropine and ipratropium. In the past, atropine has been avoided in patients with COPD and bronchitis because of concern regarding increases in the viscosity of mucus produced by this agent. However, atropine blocks the formation of cyclic guanosine monophosphate and therefore has a bronchodilator effect. Marini et al.[23] found that inhaled atropine alone improved FEV_1 in 85% of patients with COPD. When atropine was given in combination with terbutaline, the FEV_1 improved in 93% of patients, whereas terbutaline alone improved FEV_1 in only 56% of patients. Antimuscarinic drugs such as atropine therefore potentiate the bronchodilator effect of the sympathomimetic agents.

In conclusion, the preoperative preparation of the patient for thoracic surgery should focus on those conditions that are treatable before surgery so the patient is in optimal condition at the time of surgery.

INTRAOPERATIVE MONITORING

All patients undergoing anesthesia for thoracic surgical procedures require use of standard American Society of Anesthesiologists or ASA monitors. These include an electrocardiogram (lead II and, if possible, V_5), chest or esophageal stethoscopes for heart and breath sound auscultation, and a temperature probe. A chest stethoscope may be placed over the dependent hemithorax to assess dependent lung ventilation. Pulse oximetry, which is a standard of care, is especially valuable during thoracic surgery because hypoxemia may occur during OLV.

Arrhythmias occur commonly both during and after thoracic surgery, making the usual need for continuous electrocardiographic monitoring even more important. Intraoperative supraventricular tachyarrhythmias may be caused by cardiac manipulation. Arrhythmias that occur during OLV may be a sign of inadequate oxygenation or ventilation. Postoperative arrhythmias may be related to sympathetic nervous system stimulation from pain or to a decreased pulmonary vascular bed following lung resection. Patients who present for lung resection often have COPD owing to cigarette smoking, have right-sided heart strain, and are prone to multifocal atrial tachyarrhythmias.

The axis of electrocardiogram lead II parallels that of the P wave, making this lead useful for arrhythmia detection. The simultaneous monitoring of lead V_5 also allows for monitoring of anterolateral wall myocardial ischemia. The use of multiple leads increases the sensitivity for ischemia detection.[24] The following invasive monitors are also indicated and have led to marked improvements in patient care.

Direct Arterial Catheterization

Peripheral arterial catheterization has become an essential tool for the anesthesiologist in the management of patients undergoing major thoracic surgical procedures. It allows for continuous beat-to-beat measurement of blood pressure and frequent sampling for the determination of arterial blood gases. Continuous blood pressure readings are critical during thoracic surgery because surgical manipulations or intravascular volume shifts can cause sudden major changes in the blood pressure. Immediate recognition of these changes allows time for proper identification of the etiology and the institution of appropriate treatment.

Serial arterial blood gas determinations are performed as needed in the management of patients undergoing one-lung anesthesia or during cases in which a part of the lung may be "packed away" for a period. Arterial hypoxemia may occur because of shunting through the collapsed lung and inadequate hypoxic pulmonary vasoconstriction (HPV). Significant changes in acid-base status and hyperventilation or hypoventilation can also be identified.

A radial artery catheter can be placed in either extremity during thoracic surgery. For a mediastinoscopic examination, one approach is to place the catheter in the right arm and to use it to monitor for possible compression of the innominate artery by the mediastinoscope.[25] This can help avoid central nervous system complications that might result from inadequate cerebral blood flow via the right carotid artery (see Mediastinoscopy section). The other approach would be to place the arterial catheter in the left radial artery, allowing for continuous blood pressure measurements, uninterrupted by innominate artery compression. If this is done, a pulse oximeter probe should be placed on the right upper extremity to monitor for innominate artery compression. During thoracotomy, the radial artery catheter is often placed in the dependent arm to aid in stabilizing the catheter. However, an "axillary roll" must be placed under the patient's dependent hemithorax to protect the axilla and avoid compression of the axillary artery and brachial plexus in the dependent ("down") arm. Placement of the arterial catheter in the dependent arm can be used to monitor for possible axillary artery compression, which may occur if the patient is not properly positioned. In rare cases, the arterial catheter can be placed in the brachial, femoral, or dorsalis pedis artery if the ulnar collateral circulation is believed to be inadequate.

Central Venous Pressure Monitoring

The continuous venous pressure (CVP) reflects the patient's blood volume, venous tone, and right ventricular performance; however, it is also affected by central venous obstructions and alterations of intrathoracic pressure (e.g., PEEP). Serial measurements are more useful than an individual number, and the response of the CVP to a volume infusion is a useful test of right ventricular function. The CVP reflects right-sided heart function, not left ventricular performance. Catheters for measuring CVP may be placed for thoracotomies, and in particular, patients undergoing pneumonectomy. Uses of CVP catheters or large-bore introducers include (1) insertion of a transvenous pacemaker where necessary, (2) infusion of vasoactive drugs, and (3) insertion of a PA catheter, which may subsequently be required during surgery or in the postoperative period.

The CVP catheter can be placed centrally from either the external or the internal jugular vein, from the subclavian veins, or from one of the arm veins. The success rate is highest using the right internal jugular vein, and a pacemaker or PA catheter can be inserted most easily from this vein. The major disadvantage of using the external jugular vein during thoracotomy is that the catheter often kinks when the patient is turned to the lateral decubitus position. The subclavian technique leads to a high incidence of pneumothorax, which can be disastrous if it occurs in the dependent lung during OLV.

Pulmonary Artery Catheterization

The PA catheter is most reliably inserted through the right internal jugular vein using a modified Seldinger technique. Insertion of the PA catheter through either the external jugular vein or the subclavian vein often leads to obstruction of the catheter when the patient is placed in the lateral decubitus position. Pulmonary artery rupture is the most serious complication associated with the use of the PA catheter. Risk factors for this complication include hypothermia, pulmonary hypertension, anticoagulation, and being elderly or female. Pulmonary artery perforation most commonly manifests as hemoptysis. Misinterpretation of data from a PA catheter is a real risk in a patient with cardiac and pulmonary disease undergoing thoracic surgery with OLV. These errors can be produced by altered ventilatory modes, the location of the PA catheter tip, ventricular compliance changes, or ventricular interdependence.[26] A major limitation of the PA catheter is the assumption that the pulmonary capillary wedge pressure (PCWP) provides a good approximation of left ventricular end-diastolic volume. The use PCWP directly to assess preload assumes a linear relationship between ventricular end-diastolic volume and ventricular end-diastolic pressure. However, alterations in ventricular compliance affect this pressure–volume relationship during surgery. Decreases in ventricular compliance can occur with myocardial ischemia, shock, right ventricular overload, or pericardial effusion. Numerous investigators have demonstrated a poor correlation between PCWP and left ventricular end-diastolic volume in acutely ill patients.[27] This correlation is further worsened by the application of PEEP. Therefore, whenever PCWP is used to estimate left ventricular preload, the number must be interpreted in light of the clinical situation. The interdependence of the right and left ventricles must also be remembered when interpreting PCWP. Ventricular interdependence can cause misdiagnosis when the interventricular septum encroaches on the left ventricular cavity, leading to increased values of PCWP. A PCWP associated with a decreased cardiac output can be interpreted as left ventricular failure, when, in fact, left ventricular end-diastolic volume may not be increased but decreased because of compression of the left ventricle by a distended right ventricle. This situation can occur with acute respiratory failure and high levels of PEEP. Techniques such as echocardiography, which directly measure ventricular dimensions, are necessary to resolve this complex situation.

Because most of the pulmonary blood flow is to the right lower lobe, the tip of a flow-directed PA catheter is usually located in the right lower lobe. During a left thoracotomy with OLV, the catheter tip would then be in the dependent lung and should provide accurate hemodynamic measurements. However, during a right thoracotomy with OLV, the catheter tip should be in the nondependent lung. Cohen et al.[28] reported that during right thoracotomies with the tip of the PA catheter in a West zone 1 or zone 2 region of the right lung, hemodynamic measurements may be inaccurate. These authors found that values for cardiac output measurements were lower during right thoracotomies than left thoracotomies, and the derived parameters of stroke volume index and oxygen delivery were also inappropriately low. Therefore, hemodynamic data derived from a PA catheter whose tip is located in the nondependent collapsed lung must be carefully evaluated.

A PA catheter capable of monitoring $S\bar{v}O_2$ is also available. Four mechanisms can account for a decreased $S\bar{v}O_2$: (1) decreased SaO_2, (2) decreased cardiac output, (3) increased oxygen consumption, and (4) decreased hemoglobin concentration. $S\bar{v}O_2$ represents a measure of global tissue oxygen extraction and consumption and is, in general, directly related to cardiac output *via* the Fick formula. The monitoring of $S\bar{v}O_2$ has been evaluated in patients undergoing one-lung anesthesia.[29] Changes in $S\bar{v}O_2$ were mainly dependent on changes in SaO_2.

Transesophageal Echocardiography

Transesophageal echocardiography (TEE) is a useful intraoperative monitor for ventricular function, valvular function, and wall motion changes that might reflect ischemia. Its use in thoracic surgical patients has been limited, but it is widely used in patients undergoing lung transplant. In one study, central lung tumors were seen with TEE in nine of nine patients, peripheral lung tumors in one of three patients, and an anterior mediastinal mass in one of one patients.[30] In this study, TEE revealed pulmonary artery compression in five patients and pulmonary artery infiltration in two patients. In another study investigating echocardiographic recognition of mediastinal tumors, TEE revealed that the tumors were often adjacent to the heart and identified those patients in whom there was compression of the innominate vein or pulmonary artery, or infiltration of the heart.[31]

Intraoperative TEE has also revealed tumor invasion of the heart, indicating that a resection by thoracotomy without cardiopulmonary bypass was not feasible.[32] In one case report, TEE monitoring during an attempted resection of a tumor invading the left atrium showed embolization of the tumor.[33] Fragments of the tumor were seen to pass through the aortic valve. This patient subsequently died of disseminated metastases. In an exploratory thoracotomy for hemothorax, intraoperative TEE revealed the presence of a subacute aortic dissection, which was believed to be the etiology of the hemothorax.[34]

Monitoring of Oxygenation and Ventilation

Oxygenation

During the administration of all thoracic surgical anesthetics, the concentration of inspired oxygen in the breathing system must be measured using an oxygen analyzer with a low oxygen concentration limit alarm. Such analyzers vary in sophistication from fuel cells, polarographic and paramagnetic analyzers, to mass and Raman spectrometers that can monitor all the gases used during anesthesia. Adequacy of blood oxygenation must also be ensured, and adequate illumination and exposure of the patient are necessary to assess the color of shed blood or the presence of cyanosis of the lips, nail beds, or mucous membranes. Most patients undergoing thoracic surgical or diagnostic procedures have an arterial catheter in place for continuous monitoring of blood pressure and sampling of arterial blood for blood gas determinations. In such cases, baseline arterial blood gas values should be obtained when breathing room air ($FIO_2 = 0.21$) before starting the procedure and repeated regularly and/or whenever indicated during surgery. Arterial blood is usually analyzed for oxygen tension (PaO_2), and a value for saturation is calculated from the oxyhemoglobin dissociation curve, correcting for temperature, pH, and $PaCO_2$.

The oxygen *content* of arterial blood can be measured by analyzing arterial blood in a laboratory cooximeter or calculated (see Chapter 28). Pulse oximetry is a standard of care for noninvasive assessment of blood oxygenation. The pulse oximeter reading (SpO_2) is fairly accurate in predicting hemoglobin saturation with oxygen over the range of 70 to 100%. The importance of pulse oximetry has also been demonstrated during OLV, when rapid assessment of oxygenation is extremely important, and when arterial blood gas analysis may involve some delay.[35] Pulse oximetry does not, however, eliminate the need for arterial blood gas analysis during thoracic surgery. A low SpO_2 reading provides the clinician with an indication for sampling and laboratory analysis of arterial blood, but an erroneously high SpO_2 reading may also occur.[36]

Ventilation

All patients must be continually monitored to ensure adequacy of ventilation. Monitoring includes qualitative signs such as chest excursion (visual observation of the lungs when the chest is open) and auscultation of breath sounds. In addition, during OLV, a stethoscope can be placed on the chest wall under the ventilated dependent lung. During controlled ventilation, circuit low-pressure and high-pressure alarms with an audible signal must be used. The respiratory rate, VT, minute volume, and inflation pressures should be observed.

Adequacy of ventilation should be confirmed by monitoring arterial blood gases and $PaCO_2$, in particular. This may be estimated continuously and noninvasively by using a capnograph. The end-tidal CO_2 concentration represents alveolar CO_2 ($PACO_2$), which approximates $PaCO_2$. There is normally a small arterial-to-alveolar CO_2 difference (4 to 6 mm Hg), depending on alveolar dead space. The capnogram waveform is also helpful in diagnosing airway obstruction, incomplete relaxation, and even malposition of the DLT. In the latter application, a capnograph is coupled with each port of the DLT (one or two capnographs may be used), and the correct position of the DLT is identified by simultaneous and synchronous CO_2 readings on each of the two analyzers. The waveforms from each lung are examined for shape, height, and rhythm, depending on the correct position of the tube and on the ventilation/perfusion ($\dot{V}/\dot{Q}$) ratio for each lung.[37] During two-lung ventilation, a decrease in end-tidal CO_2 in the gas from one lumen of the DLT suggests that the tube may be malpositioned. During OLV, systemic hypoxemia is usually a greater problem than hypercarbia.[38] This is because CO_2 is approximately 20 times more diffusible than oxygen and $PaCO_2$ is more dependent on ventilation, compared with PaO_2, which is more dependent on perfusion.

More recently, devices have been introduced clinically that use one small noninvasive digital sensor clipped to the earlobe to provide continuous monitoring of $PaCO_2$, SpO_2, and pulse rate. Optoelectronic components, micro-pH electrode, temperature sensors, and a mixed-signal microcontroller reside on a digital sensor print. The measurement principles used are the Severinghaus-type PCO_2 electrode and a two-wavelength reflectance pulse oximeter.

Physiology of One-Lung Ventilation

Physiology of the Lateral Decubitus Position. Ventilation and blood flow in the upright position are discussed in Chapter 28. These variables will now be considered as they pertain to the lateral decubitus position under six circumstances that are encountered during thoracic surgery.

Lateral position, awake, breathing spontaneously, chest closed. In the lateral decubitus position, the distribution of blood flow and ventilation is similar to that in the upright position, but turned by 90 degrees (Fig. 29-5). Blood flow and ventilation to the dependent lung are significantly greater than to the nondependent lung. Good V/Q matching at the level of the dependent lung results in adequate oxygenation in the awake patient who is breathing spontaneously. There are two important concepts in this situation. First, because perfusion is gravity dependent, the vertical hydrostatic pressure gradient is smaller in the lateral than in the upright position; therefore, zone 1 is usually less extended. Second, in regard to ventilation, the dependent hemidiaphragm is pushed higher into the chest by the abdominal contents compared with the nondependent lung hemidiaphragm. During spontaneous ventilation, the conserved ability of the dependent diaphragm to contract results in an adequate distribution of VT to the dependent lung. Because most of the perfusion is to the dependent lung, the V/Q matching in this position is maintained similar to that in the upright position.

Lateral position, awake, breathing spontaneously, chest open. Controlled positive-pressure ventilation is the most common way to provide adequate ventilation and ensure gas exchange in an open chest situation. Frequently, thoracoscopy is performed using intercostal blocks with the patient breathing spontaneously to allow proper lung examination. The thoracoscope provides an adequate seal of the open chest to prevent a

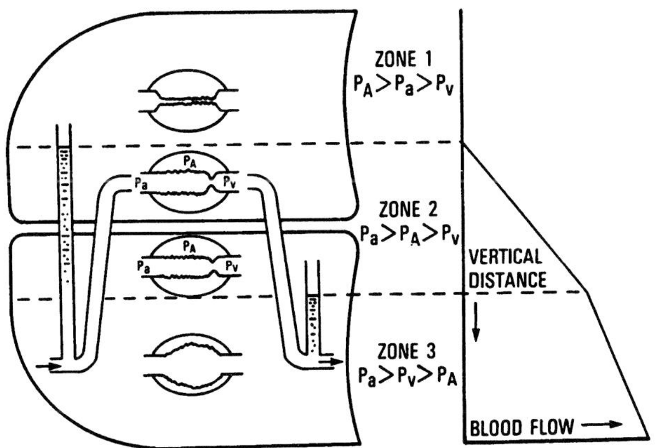

FIGURE 29-5. Schematic representation of the effects of gravity on the distribution of pulmonary blood flow in the lateral decubitus position. Vertical gradients in the lateral decubitus position are similar to those in the upright position and cause the creation of West zones 1, 2, and 3. Consequently, pulmonary blood flow increases with lung dependency, and is largest in the dependent lung and least in the nondependent lung. P_a, pulmonary artery pressure; P_A, alveolar pressure; P_v, pulmonary venous pressure. (From Benumof JL: Physiology of the open-chest and one lung ventilation. In: Thoracic Anesthesia, p 288. New York, Churchill Livingstone, 1983.)

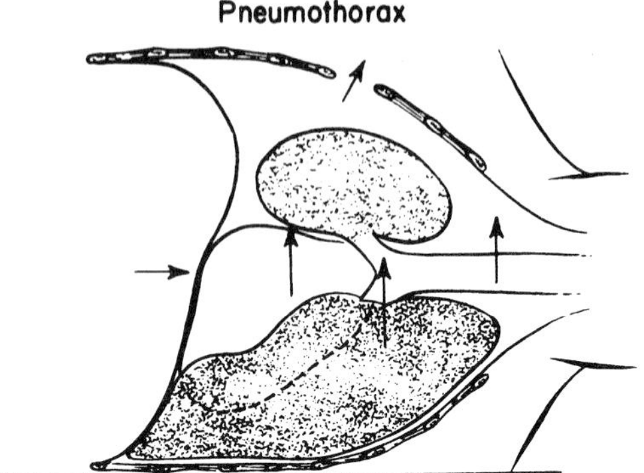

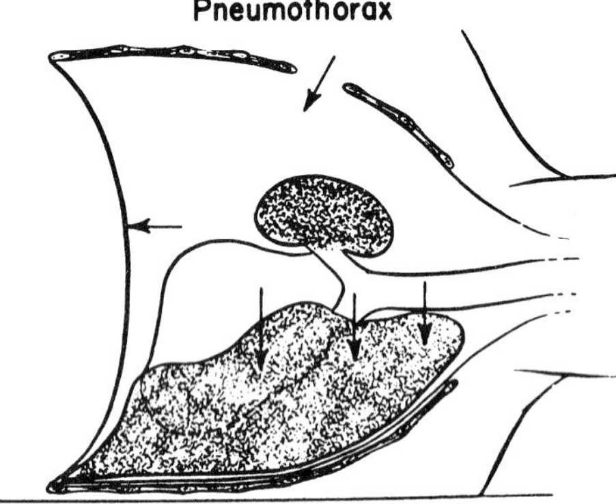

FIGURE 29-6. Schematic representation of mediastinal shift in the spontaneously breathing, open-chested patient in the lateral decubitus position. During inspiration, negative pressure in the intact hemithorax causes the mediastinum to move downward. During expiration, relative positive pressure in the intact hemithorax causes the mediastinum to move upward. (From Tarhan S, Moffitt EA: Principles of thoracic anesthesia. Surg Clin North Am 53:813, 1973.)

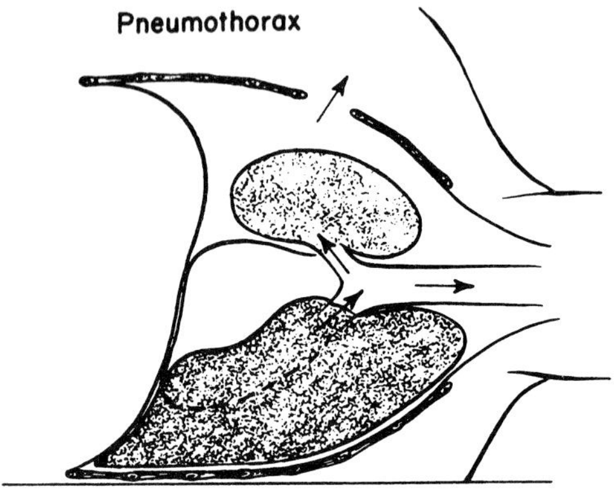

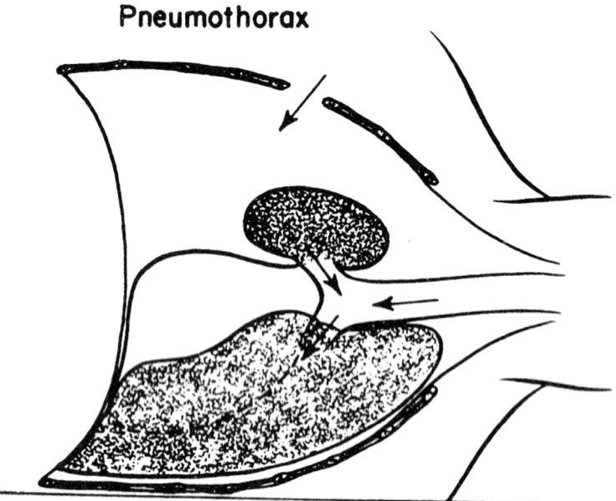

FIGURE 29-7. Schematic representation of paradoxical respiration in the spontaneously breathing, open-chested patient in the lateral decubitus position. During inspiration, movement of gas from the exposed lung into the intact lung and movement of air from the environment into the open hemithorax cause collapse of the exposed lung. During expiration, the reverse occurs, and the exposed lung expands. (From Tarhan S, Moffitt EA: Principles of thoracic anesthesia. Surg Clin North Am 53:813, 1973.)

"free" open-chest situation. Two complications can arise from the patient breathing spontaneously with an open chest. The first is mediastinal shift, usually occurring during inspiration (Fig. 29-6). The negative pressure in the intact hemithorax, compared with the less negative pressure of the open hemithorax, can cause the mediastinum to move vertically downward and push into the dependent hemithorax. The mediastinal shift can create circulatory and reflex changes that may result in a clinical picture similar to that of shock and respiratory distress. Sometimes, depending on the severity of the distress, the patient needs to be tracheally intubated immediately, with initiation of positive-pressure ventilation, and the anesthesiologist must be prepared to intubate in this position without disturbing the surgical field. The second phenomenon is paradoxical breathing (Fig. 29-7). During inspiration, the relatively negative pressure in the intact hemithorax compared with atmospheric pressure in the open hemithorax can cause movement of air from the nondependent lung into the dependent lung. The opposite occurs during expiration. This gas movement reversal from one lung to the other represents wasted ventilation and can compromise the adequacy of gas exchange. Paradoxical breathing is increased by a large thoracotomy or by an increase in airways resistance in the dependent lung. Positive-pressure ventilation or adequate sealing of the open chest eliminates paradoxical breathing.

Lateral position, anesthetized, breathing spontaneously, chest closed. The induction of general anesthesia does not cause significant change in the distribution of blood flow, but it has an important impact on the distribution of ventilation. Most of the V_T enters the nondependent lung, and this results in a significant $\dot{V}/\dot{Q}$ mismatch. Induction of general anesthesia causes a reduction in the volumes of both lungs secondary to a reduction in FRC. Any reduction in volume in the dependent lung is of a greater magnitude than that in the nondependent lung for several reasons. First, the cephalad displacement of the dependent diaphragm by the abdominal contents is more pronounced and is increased by paralysis. Second, the mediastinal structures pressing on the dependent lung or poor positioning of the dependent side on the operating table prevents the lung from expanding properly. The aforementioned factors will move lungs to a lower volume on the S-shaped volume-pressure curve (Fig. 29-8). The nondependent lung moves to a steeper position on the compliance curve and receives most of the V_T, whereas the dependent lung is on the flat (noncompliant) part of the curve.

Lateral position, anesthetized, breathing spontaneously, chest open. Opening the chest has little impact on the distribution of perfusion. However, the upper lung is now no longer restricted by the chest wall and is free to expand, resulting in

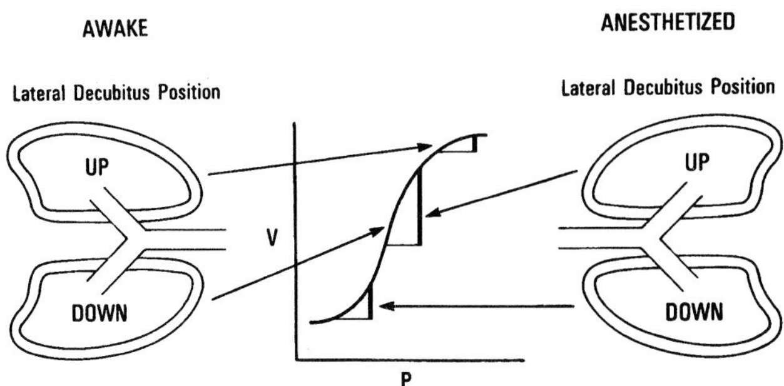

FIGURE 29-8. The left-hand side of the schematic shows the distribution of ventilation in the awake patient (closed chest) in the lateral decubitus position, and the right-hand side shows the distribution of ventilation in the anesthetized patient (closed chest) in the lateral ducubitus position. The induction of anesthesia has caused a loss in lung volume in both lungs, with the nondependent (up) lung moving from a flat, noncompliant portion to a steep, compliant portion of the pressure–volume curve, and the dependent (down) lung moving from a steep, compliant part to a flat, noncompliant part of the pressure–volume curve. Thus, the anesthetized patient in the lateral decubitus position has most tidal ventilation in the nondependent lung (where there is the least perfusion) and less tidal ventilation in the dependent lung (where there is the most perfusion). V, volume; P, pressure. (From Benumof JL: Anesthesia for Thoracic Surgery, p 112. Philadelphia, WB Saunders, 1987.)

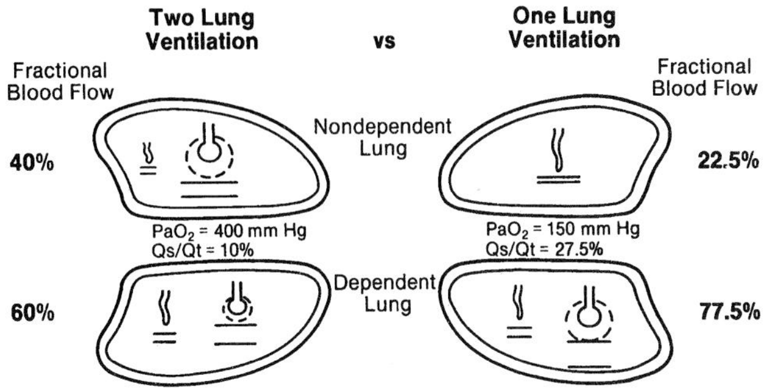

FIGURE 29-10. Schematic representation of two-lung ventilation versus one-lung ventilation (OLV). Typical values for fractional blood flow to the nondependent and dependent lungs, as well as PaO_2 and $\dot{Q}s/\dot{R}t$ for the two conditions, are shown. The $\dot{Q}s/\dot{R}t$ during two-lung ventilation is assumed to be distributed equally between the two lungs (5% to each lung). The essential difference between two-lung ventilation and OLV is that, during OLV, the nonventilated lung has some blood flow and therefore an obligatory shunt, which is not present during two-lung ventilation. The 35% of total flow perfusing the nondependent lung, which was not shunt flow, was assumed to be able to reduce its blood flow by 50% by hypoxic pulmonary vasoconstriction. The increase in $\dot{Q}s/\dot{R}t$ from two-lung to OLV is assumed to be due solely to the increase in blood flow through the nonventilated, nondependent lung during OLV. (From Benumof JL: Anesthesia for Thoracic Surgery, p 112. Philadelphia, WB Saunders, 1987.)

a further increase in $\dot{V}/\dot{Q}$ mismatch as the nondependent lung is preferentially ventilated, owing to a now increased compliance.

Lateral position, anesthetized, paralyzed, chest open. During paralysis and positive-pressure ventilation, diaphragmatic displacement is maximal over the nondependent lung, where there is the least amount of resistance to diaphragmatic movement caused by the abdominal contents (Fig. 29-9). This further compromises the ventilation to the dependent lung and increases the V/Q mismatch.

One-lung ventilation, anesthetized, paralyzed, chest open. During two-lung ventilation in the lateral position, the mean blood flow to the nondependent lung is assumed to be 40% of cardiac output, whereas 60% of cardiac output goes to the dependent lung (Fig. 29-10). Normally, venous admixture (shunt) in the lateral position is 10% of cardiac output and is equally divided as 5% in each lung. Therefore, the average percentage of cardiac output participating in gas exchange is 35% in the nondependent lung and 55% in the dependent lung.

OLV creates an obligatory right-to-left transpulmonary shunt through the nonventilated, nondependent lung because the V/Q ratio of that lung is zero. In theory, an additional 35% should be added to the total shunt during OLV. However, assuming active HPV, blood flow to the nondependent hypoxic lung will be decreased by 50% and therefore is (35/2) = 17.5%. To this, 5% must be added, which is the obligatory shunt through the nondependent lung. The shunt through the nondependent lung is therefore 22.5% (see Fig. 29-10). Together with the 5% shunt in the dependent lung, total shunt during OLV is 22.5% + 5% = 27.5%. This results in a PaO_2 of approximately 150 mm Hg (FIO_2 = 1.0).[39]

Because 72.5% of the perfusion is directed to the dependent lung during OLV, the matching of ventilation in this lung

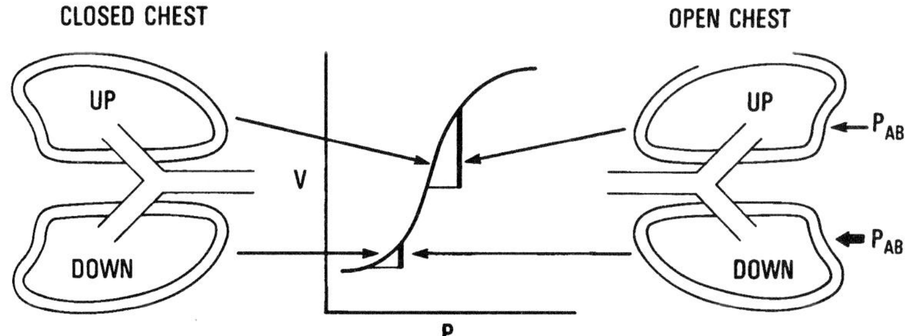

FIGURE 29-9. This schematic of a patient in the lateral decubitus position compares the closed-chested anesthetized condition with the open-chested anesthetized and paralyzed condition. Opening the chest increases nondependent lung compliance and reinforces or maintains the larger part of the tidal ventilation going to the nondependent lung. Paralysis also reinforces or maintains the larger part of tidal ventilation going to the nondependent lung because the pressure of the abdominal contents (P_{AB}) pressing against the upper diaphragm is minimal, and it is therefore easier for positive-pressure ventilation to displace this less resisting dome of the diaphragm. V, volume; P, pressure. (From Benumof JL: Anesthesia for Thoracic Surgery, p 112. Philadelphia, WB Saunders, 1987.)

is important for adequate gas exchange. The dependent lung is no longer on the steep (compliant) portion of the volume-pressure curve because of reduced lung volume and FRC. There are several reasons for this reduction in FRC, including general anesthesia, paralysis, pressure from abdominal contents, compression by the weight of mediastinal structures, and suboptimal positioning on the operating table. Other considerations that impair optimal ventilation to the dependent lung include absorption atelectasis, accumulation of secretions, and the formation of a fluid transudate in the dependent lung. All these create a low V/Q ratio and a large $P(A\text{-}a)O_2$ gradient.

ONE-LUNG VENTILATION

Absolute Indications for One-Lung Ventilation

Separation of the lungs to prevent spillage of pus or blood from an infected or bleeding source is an absolute indication for OLV (Table 29-1). Life-threatening complications, such as massive atelectasis, sepsis, and pneumonia, can result from bilateral contamination. Bronchopleural and bronchocutaneous fistulae both represent low-resistance pathways for the V_T delivered by positive-pressure ventilation, and both prevent adequate alveolar ventilation. Giant cysts or unilateral bullae may rupture under positive-pressure ventilation. This can be avoided by selective lung ventilation. During bronchopulmonary lavage, an effective separation of the lungs is mandatory to avoid accidental spillage of fluid from the lavaged lung to the nondependent ventilated lung. Video-assisted thoracoscopic surgery (VATS) requires lung separation and is becoming the most common indication for OLV. Finally, minimally invasive cardiac procedures require the lung to be collapsed.

TABLE 29-1

INDICATIONS FOR ONE-LUNG VENTILATION

■ ABSOLUTE

1. Isolation of each lung to prevent contamination of a healthy lung
   a. Infection (abscess, infected cyst)
   b. Massive hemorrhage
2. Control of distribution of ventilation to only one lung
   a. Bronchopleural fistula
   b. Bronchopleural cutaneous fistula
   c. Unilateral cyst or bullae
   d. Major bronchial disruption or trauma
3. Unilateral lung lavage
4. Video-assisted thoracoscopic surgery

■ RELATIVE

1. Surgical exposure—high priority
   a. Thoracic aortic aneurysm
   b. Pneumonectomy
   c. Upper lobectomy
2. Surgical exposure—low priority
   a. Esophageal surgery
   b. Middle and lower lobectomy
   c. Thoracoscopy under general anesthesia

Modified from Benumof JL: Physiology of the open-chest and one lung ventilation. In Kaplan JA (ed): Thoracic Anesthesia, p 299. New York, Churchill Livingstone, 1983.

Relative Indications for One-Lung Ventilation

4 In clinical practice, a DLT is commonly used for a lobectomy or pneumonectomy; these represent relative indications for lung separation. Upper lobectomy, pneumonectomy, and thoracic aortic aneurysm repair are relatively high-priority indications. These procedures are technically difficult, and optimal surgical exposure and a quiet operative field are highly desirable. Lower or middle lobectomy and esophageal resection are of lower priority. Nevertheless, many surgeons are accustomed to operating with the lung collapsed, which minimizes lung trauma from retractors and manipulation, improves visualization of lung anatomy, and facilitates identification and separation of anatomic structures and lung fissures. Thoracoscopy, if not performed with an intercostal block in the spontaneously breathing patient, is greatly facilitated by collapse of the lung under examination.

Methods of Lung Separation

Bronchial Blockers

Bronchial Blocker. Lung separation can be achieved with a reusable bronchial blocker. Magill described an endobronchial blocker that is placed using a bronchoscope and directed to the nonventilated lung. Inflation of the cuff at the distal end of the blocker serves to block ventilation to that lung. The lumen of the blocker permits suctioning of the airway distal to the catheter tip. Depending on the clinical circumstance, oxygen can be insufflated through the catheter lumen. A conventional endotracheal tube is then placed in the trachea. This technique can be useful in achieving selective ventilation in children younger than 12 years of age. However, because the blocker balloon requires a high distending pressure, it easily slips out of the bronchus into the trachea, obstructing ventilation and losing the seal between the two lungs. This displacement can be secondary to changes in position or to surgical manipulation. The loss of lung separation can be a life-threatening situation if it was performed to prevent spillage of pus, blood, or fluid from bronchopulmonary lavage. For this reason, bronchial blockers are rarely used in current practice.

Arterial Embolectomy (Fogarty) Catheter. Selective airway occlusion can be achieved by the use of a Fogarty catheter designed for embolectomy procedures (Fig. 29-11). Placement of the embolectomy catheter is best performed under direct vision with the aid of a fiberoptic bronchoscope. A conventional endotracheal tube is then placed alongside the catheter after withdrawing the bronchoscope. Alternatively, the bronchial blocker may be inserted through the lumen of a standard tracheal tube if the rubber diaphragm in a swivel connector is first perforated for passage of the blocker. The swivel connector is then placed between the tracheal tube and the Y-piece of the breathing circuit. A fiberscope can be inserted through the lumen of the tracheal tube to facilitate positioning of the blocker under direct vision.

Univent Tube. The Univent (Fuji Systems Corp., Tokyo, Japan) is a single-lumen endotracheal tube with a movable endobronchial blocker (Fig. 29-12). In the Univent tube, the bronchial blocker is housed in a small channel bored in the wall of the tube. After intubation of the trachea, the movable blocker is manipulated into the desired main-stem bronchus with the aid of a fiberoptic bronchoscope.[40] Disadvantages of the Univent tube are that correct positioning of the blocker may be difficult to achieve or maintain. The Univent tube may be ideal for cases in which a tube change (e.g., from single to double lumen) may be difficult (e.g., mediastinoscopy followed by thoracotomy), or in cases of bilateral lung transplantation. The Univent tube has the advantage common to all bronchial

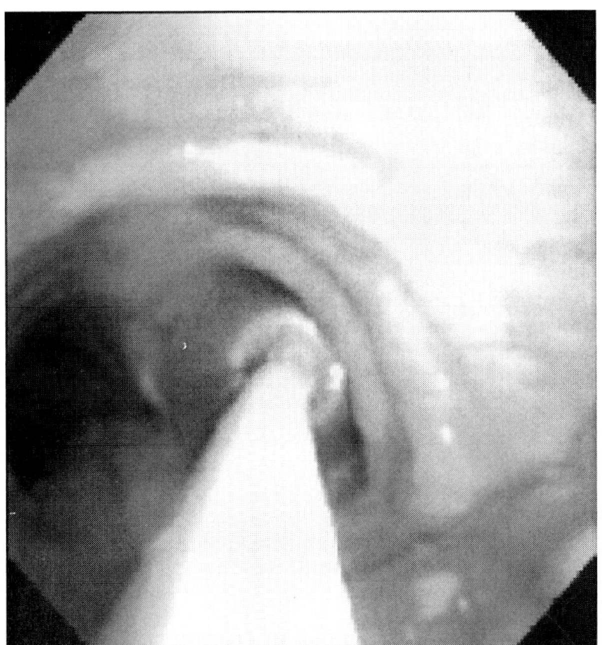

FIGURE 29-11. Use of a Fogarty catheter to block the right main-stem bronchus.

blockers: it is a single-lumen tube, and there is no need to change the tube at the end of the procedure if postoperative ventilatory support is required. This is particularly important in cases of difficult intubation, prolonged surgery with airway edema, such as thoracic aortic aneurysm surgery or extensive neurosurgical procedures on the spine with massive fluid replacement, and altered anatomy of the airway. It is also possible to suction through the blocker lumen or to apply continuous positive airway pressure (CPAP) to improve oxygenation in cases of hypoxemia.

The disadvantages of the Univent tubes are that the external diameter is relatively large, the blocker can dislocate during surgical manipulation, and satisfactory bronchial seal and lung separation are sometimes difficult to achieve. The bronchial blocker is somewhat stiff and sometimes will not easily be directed into the main bronchus. This is particularly true for the left side. The bulky external diameter can also make it difficult to pass the tube between the vocal cords.

The first-generation Univent tube's bronchial blocker was difficult to direct into the selected main bronchus. The blocker would spin (torque) on its long axis, which made it difficult to control. The second generation, the Torque Control Blocker (TCB) Univent, was more recently introduced. It consists of a silicon endotracheal tube that has a high friction coefficient. The TCB provides better control, which facilitates direction of the blocker into the target main-stem bronchus.

Double-Lumen Endobronchial Tubes

Double-lumen endobronchial tubes are currently the most widely used means of achieving lung separation and OLV. There are several different types of DLT, but all are essentially similar in design in that two catheters are bonded together. One lumen is long enough to reach a main-stem bronchus, and the second lumen ends with an opening in the distal trachea. Lung separation is achieved by inflation of two cuffs: a proximal tracheal cuff, and a distal bronchial cuff located in the main-stem bronchus (see Positioning Double-Lumen Tubes section). The endobronchial cuff of a right-sided tube is slotted or otherwise designed to allow ventilation of the right upper lobe because the right main-stem bronchus is too short to accommodate both the right lumen tip and a right bronchial cuff.

Robertshaw Tube. The Carlens tube (which had a carinal hook) was the first clinically available DLT and was used by pulmonologists for split function spirometry testing (Fig. 29-13A). Subsequently, the Robertshaw design DLT (which lacked a carinal hook) was developed to facilitate thoracic surgery (Fig. 29-13B). This DLT is available in left-sided and right-sided forms. The absence of a carinal hook facilitates insertion. This tube design has the advantages of having D-shaped, large-diameter lumens that allow easy passage of a suction catheter, offer low resistance to gas flow, and have a fixed curvature to facilitate proper positioning and reduce the possibility of kinking. The original red rubber Robertshaw tubes were available in three sizes: small, medium, and large. Red rubber tubes are rarely used now and have been replaced by clear, polyvinyl chloride (PVC) disposable Robertshaw-design DLTs. These are available in both right-sided and left-sided versions and in 35F,

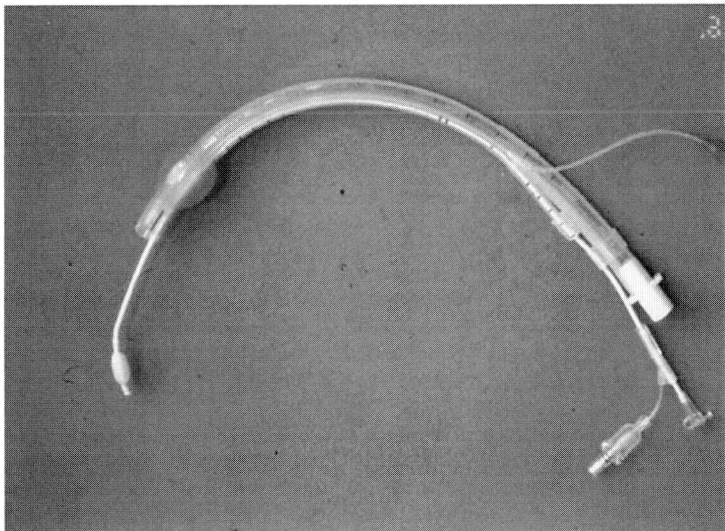

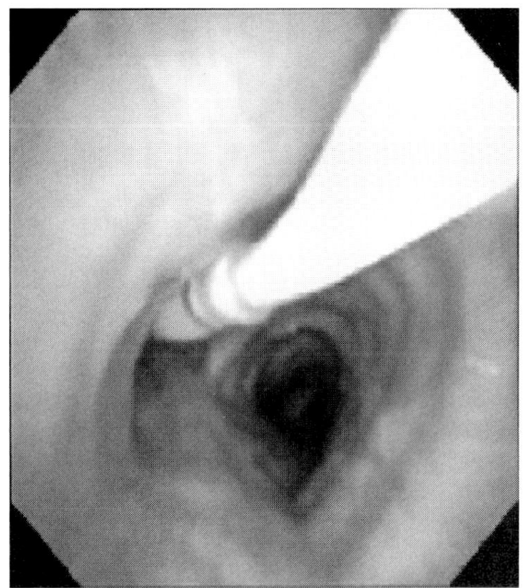

FIGURE 29-12. **A.** The Univent tube also allows lung separation using a single-lumen endotracheal tube. **B.** The Univent bronchial blocker positioned in left main-stem bronchus.

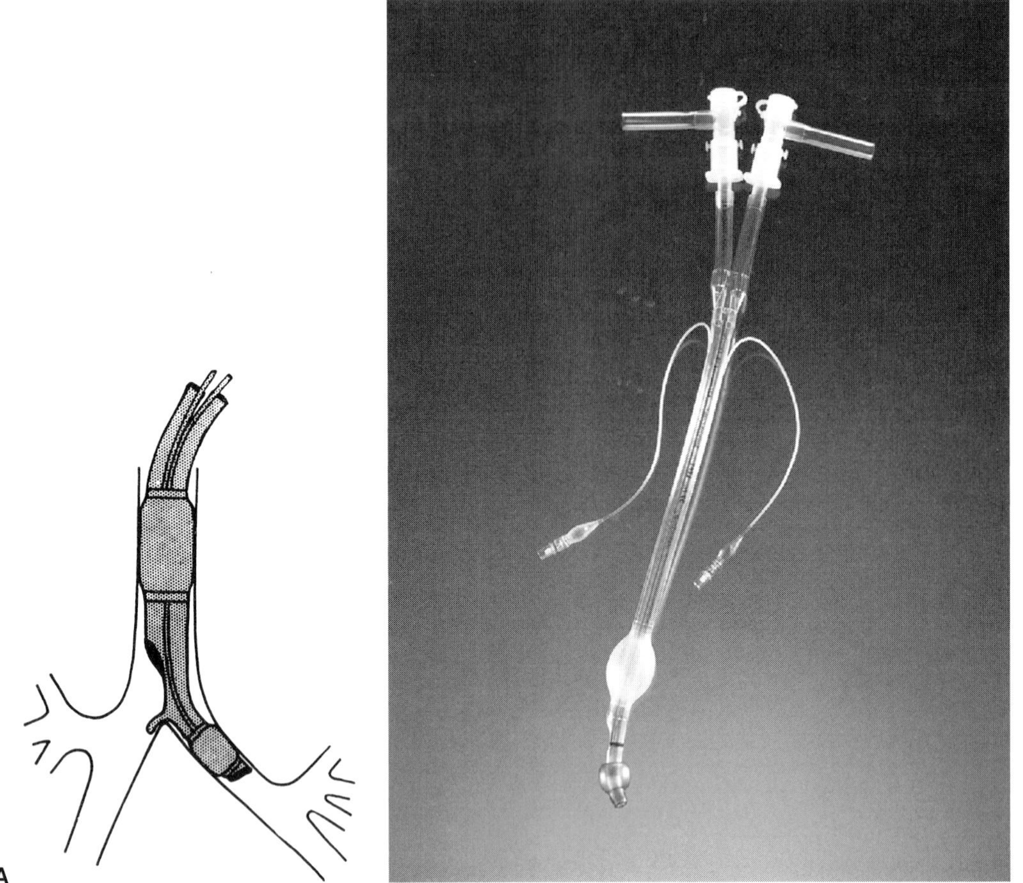

FIGURE 29-13. A. Left main-stem endobronchial intubation using a Carlens tube. Note carinal "hook" used for correct positioning. B. A left-sided Robertshaw type double-lumen tube constructed from PVC. (A: From Hillard EK, Thompson PW: Instruments used in thoracic anaesthesia. In Mushin WW [ed]: Thoracic Anaesthesia, p 315. Oxford, Blackwell Scientific, 1963. B: Courtesy of Nellcor Puritan Bennett, Inc., Pleasanton, California.)

37F, 39F, and 41F. A 28F is available for use in pediatric cases. The advantages of the disposable tubes include relative ease of insertion and proper positioning, easy recognition of the blue color of the endobronchial cuff when fiberoptic bronchoscopy is used, confirmation of position on a chest radiograph using the radiopaque lines in the wall of the tube, and continuous observation of tidal gas exchange and respiratory moisture through the clear plastic. The right-sided endobronchial tube is designed to minimize occlusion of the opening of the right upper lobe bronchus. The right endobronchial cuff is doughnut-shaped and allows the right upper lobe ventilation slot to ride over the opening of the right upper lobe bronchus. The tube is also suitable for use in long-term ventilation in the intensive care unit because it has a high-volume, low-pressure cuff. These disposable PVC tubes are generally considered the tubes of choice for achieving lung separation and OLV.[41]

Positioning Double-Lumen Tubes. This section concentrates on the insertion of Robertshaw-design DLTs (both disposable and nondisposable) because they are the most widely used. Before insertion, the DLT should be prepared and checked. The tracheal cuff (high-volume, low-pressure) can accommodate up to 20 mL of air, and the bronchial cuff should be checked using a 3-mL syringe. The tube should be coated liberally with water-soluble lubricant, and the stylet should be withdrawn, lubricated, and gently placed back into the bronchial lumen without disturbing the tube's preformed curvature. The Macintosh 3 blade is preferred for intubation of the trachea because it provides the largest area through which to pass the tube. The insertion of the tube is performed with the distal concave curvature facing anteriorly. After the tip of the tube is past the vocal cords, the stylet is removed and the tube is rotated through 90 degrees. A left-sided tube is rotated 90 degrees to the left, and a right-sided tube is rotated to the right. Advancement of the tube ceases when moderate resistance to further passage is encountered, indicating that the tube tip has been firmly seated in the main-stem bronchus. It is important to remove the stylet before rotating and advancing the tube to avoid tracheal or bronchial laceration. Rotation and advancement of the tube should be performed gently and under continuous direct laryngoscopy to prevent hypopharyngeal structures from interfering with proper positioning. Once the tube is believed to be in the proper position, a sequence of steps should be performed to check its location.

First, the tracheal cuff should be inflated, and equal ventilation of both lungs established. If breath sounds are not equal, the tube is probably too far down, and the tracheal lumen opening is in a main-stem bronchus or is lying at the carina. Withdrawal of the tube by 2 to 3 cm usually restores equal breath sounds. The second step is to clamp the right side (in the case of the left-sided tube) and remove the right cap from the connector. Then, the bronchial cuff is slowly inflated to prevent an air leak from the bronchial lumen around the bronchial cuff into the tracheal lumen. This ensures excessive pressure is not applied to the bronchus and helps avoid laceration. Inflation of the bronchial cuff rarely requires more than 2 mL of air. The third step is to remove the clamp and check that both lungs are ventilated with both cuffs inflated. This ensures the bronchial cuff is not obstructing the contralateral hemithorax, either totally or partially. The final step is to clamp each side selectively and watch for absence of movement and breath sounds on the ipsilateral (clamped) side; the ventilated side should have clear breath sounds, chest movement that feels compliant, respiratory gas moisture with each tidal ventilation, and no gas leak. If peak airway pressure during two-lung ventilation is 20 cm H_2O, it should not exceed 40 cm H_2O for the same VT during OLV.

Other methods that have been used for ensuring the correct placement of a DLT include fluoroscopy, chest radiography, selective capnography, and use of an underwater seal. Determination of the presence of gas leaks when positive pressure is applied to one lumen of a DLT is easily done in the operating room. If the bronchial cuff is not inflated and positive pressure is applied to the bronchial lumen of the DLT, gas leaks past the bronchial cuff and returns through the tracheal lumen. If the tracheal lumen is connected to an underwater seal system, gas will be seen to bubble up through the water. The bronchial cuff can then be gradually inflated until no gas bubbles are seen and the desired cuff seal pressure can be attained. This test is of extreme importance when absolute lung separation is needed, such as during bronchopulmonary lavage.

5 The most important advance in checking for proper position of a DLT is the introduction of the pediatric flexible fiberoptic bronchoscope (Fig. 29-14). Smith et al.[42] showed that when the disposable DLT was believed to be in correct position by auscultation and physical examination, subsequent fiberoptic bronchoscopy showed that 48% of tubes were, in fact, malpositioned. Such malpositions, however, are usually of no clinical significance.[43] When using a left-sided DLT, the bronchoscope is usually first introduced through the tracheal lumen. The carina is visualized, but no bronchial cuff herniation should be seen. The upper surface of the blue endobronchial cuff should be just below the tracheal carina. The bronchial cuff of the disposable DLT is easily visualized because of its blue color. The bronchoscope should then be passed through the bronchial lumen, and the left upper lobe bronchial orifice should be identified. When a right-sided DLT is used, the carina should be visualized through the tracheal lumen but, more important, the orifice of the right upper lobe bronchus should be identified when the bronchoscope is passed through the right upper lobe ventilating slot of the DLT. Pediatric fiberoptic bronchoscopes are available in several sizes: 5.6, 4.9, and 3.6 mm in external diameter. The 4.9-mm diameter bronchoscope can be passed through DLTs of 37F and larger. The 3.6-mm diameter bronchoscope is easily passed through all sizes of DLT. In general, it is recommended that the largest size that can pass through the lumen of a DLT be used because it provides better visualization and facilitates identification of the bronchial anatomy.

Problems of Malposition of the Double-Lumen Tube. The use of a DLT is associated with a number of potential problems, the most important of which is malposition. There are several

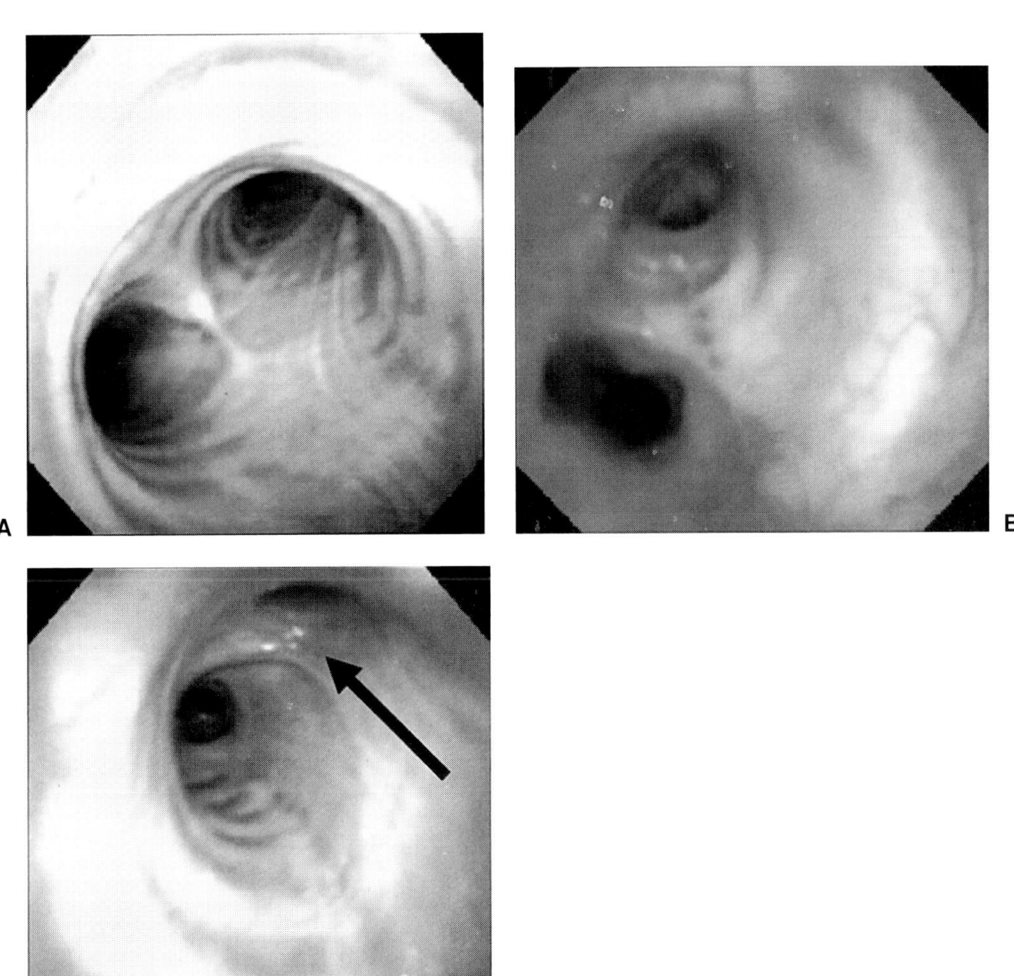

FIGURE 29-14. Fiberoptic bronchoscopic view of the main carina (A), the "left bronchial carina" (B), and the right bronchus (C). Note right upper lobe orifice *(arrow)*.

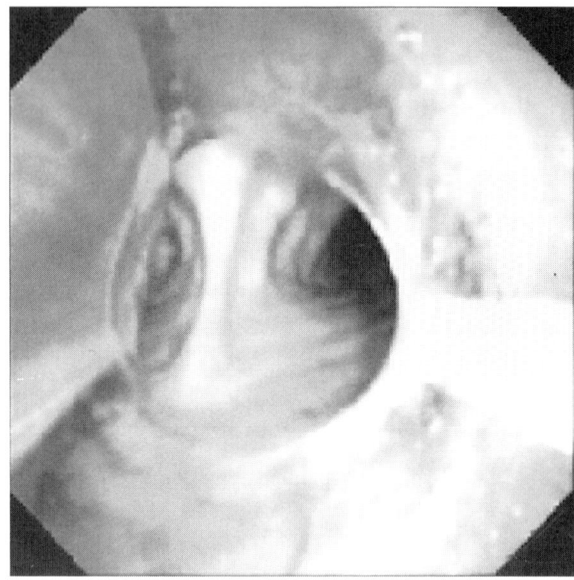

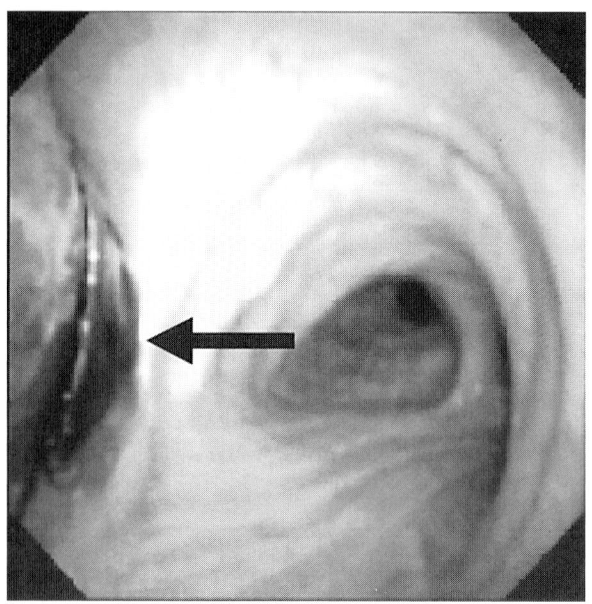

FIGURE 29-15. Malposition of the left bronchial limb of the double-lumen tube (DLT). A. The limb is too far into the left bronchus because the cuff if not evident. B. DLT withdrawn and balloon is now in view, indicating appropriate position of the DLT.

possibilities for tube malposition. The DLT may be accidentally directed to the side opposite the desired main-stem bronchus. In this case, the lung opposite the side of the connector clamp will collapse. Inadequate separation, increased airway pressures, and instability of the DLT usually occur. In addition, because of the morphology of the DLT curvatures, tracheal or bronchial lacerations may result. If a left-sided DLT is inserted into the right main-stem bronchus, it obstructs ventilation to the right upper lobe. It is therefore essential to recognize and correct such a malposition as soon as possible.

Second, the DLT may be passed too far down into either the right or the left main-stem bronchus (Fig. 29-15). In this case, breath sounds are very diminished or not audible over the contralateral side. This situation is corrected when the tube is withdrawn and until the opening of the tracheal lumen is above the carina.

Third, the DLT may not be inserted far enough, leaving the bronchial lumen opening above the carina. In this position, good breath sounds are heard bilaterally when ventilating through the bronchial lumen, but no breath sounds are audible when ventilating through the tracheal lumen because the inflated bronchial cuff obstructs gas flow arising from the tracheal lumen. The cuff should be deflated and the DLT rotated and advanced into the desired main-stem bronchus.

Fourth, a right-sided DLT may occlude the right upper lobe orifice. The mean distance from the carina to the right upper lobe orifice is 2.3 ± 0.7 cm in men and 2.1 ± 0.7 cm in women.[44] With right-sided DLTs, the ventilatory slot in the side of the bronchial catheter must overlie the right upper lobe orifice to permit ventilation of this lobe. The margin of safety, however, is extremely small, and varies from 1 to 8 mm.[44] It is, therefore, difficult to ensure proper ventilation to the right upper lobe and avoid dislocation of the DLT during surgical manipulation. When right endobronchial intubation is required, a disposable right-sided DLT is perhaps the best choice because of the slanted doughnut shape of the bronchial cuff, which allows the ventilation slot to ride off the right upper lobe ventilation orifice and increases the margin of safety.

Fifth, the left upper lobe orifice may be obstructed by a left-sided DLT. Traditionally, it was believed the take-off of the left upper lobe bronchus was at a safe distance from the carina and that it would not be obstructed by a left-sided DLT. However, the mean distance between the left upper lobe orifice and the carina is 5.4 ± 0.7 cm in men and 5.0 ± 0.7 cm in women.[44] The average distance between the openings of the right and left lumens on the left-sided disposable tubes is 6.9 cm.[44] Therefore, an obstruction of the left upper lobe bronchus is possible while the tracheal lumen is still above the carina. There is also a 20% variation in the location of the blue endobronchial cuff on the disposable tubes because this cuff is attached to the tube at the end of the manufacturing process.

Finally, bronchial cuff herniation may occur and obstruct the bronchial lumen if excessive volumes are used to inflate the cuff. The bronchial cuff has also been known to herniate over the tracheal carina, and in the case of a left-sided DLT, to obstruct ventilation to the right main-stem bronchus.

Another rare complication with DLTs is tracheal rupture. Overinflation of the bronchial cuff, inappropriate positioning, and trauma owing to intraoperative dislocation that resulted in bronchial rupture have been described in association with the Robertshaw tube and the disposable DLT.[45] Therefore, the pressure in the bronchial cuff should be assessed and decreased if the cuff is found to be overinflated. If absolute separation of the lungs is not needed, the bronchial cuff should be deflated and then reinflated slowly to avoid excessive pressure on the bronchial walls. The bronchial cuff should also be deflated during any repositioning of the patient unless lung separation is absolutely required during this time.

Lung Separation in the Patient With a Tracheostomy

Occasionally, a patient with a permanent tracheotomy is scheduled for surgery on the lung that requires isolation. Examples of such patients include those who have undergone resection of a tumor in the floor of the mouth or on the base of the tongue, followed by extensive reconstructive surgery with creation of a permanent tracheal stoma. Routine follow-up may

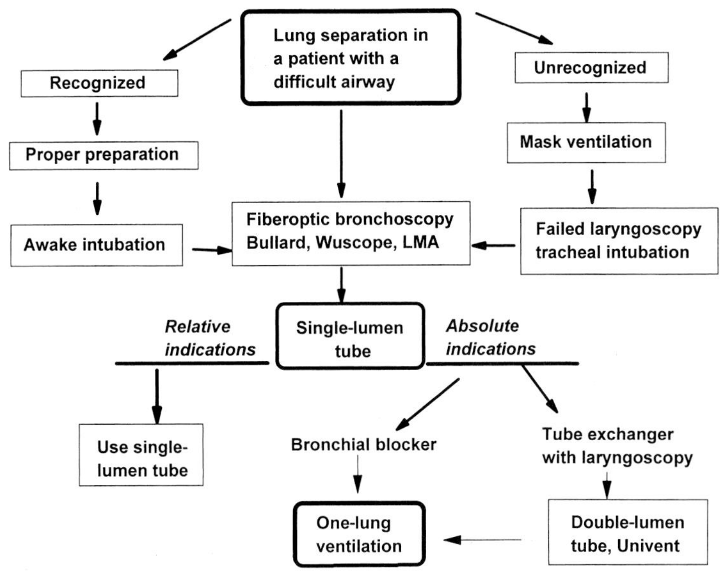

FIGURE 29-16. Lung separation in a patient with a difficult airway. (Adapted from Cohed E, Benumot JL. Lung separation in the patient with a difficult airway. Curr Opin Anesthesiol 12:1, 29–35, 1999.)

reveal a lung lesion that requires a diagnostic procedure. Conventional double-lumen endobronchial tubes are designed to be inserted through the mouth, not through a tracheal stoma. The standard DLTs are usually too stiff to negotiate the curve required for insertion through a tracheal stoma and are difficult to position.[46]

A separately inserted bronchial blocker, either within or alongside a single-lumen tube that has been placed through the tracheostomy, may permit adequate lung separation.[47] Compared with an orotracheal or nasotracheal single-lumen tube, passing a Fogarty catheter (to function as a bronchial blocker) through a tracheostomy into a main-stem bronchus may be easier because of the shorter distances involved.

Saito et al.[48] described a spiral, wire-reinforced, double-lumen endobronchial tube made of silicone (Koken Medical, Tokyo, Japan) that is designed for placement through a tracheostomy. The middle section of the tube consists of two thin-walled silicone catheters with an internal diameter of 5 mm, glued together and reinforced with a stainless steel spiral wire and covered with a silicone coating with two pilot balloons. The distal section, which contains the bronchial lumen and the bronchial cuff, is made of wire-reinforced silicone to avoid excessive flexibility. The dimensions are based on the Mallinckrodt DLT. The bronchial cuff is located 1.2 cm from the tip, and the distance between the tip orifice and the tracheal orifice is 4.9 cm. In a clinical trial in patients with permanent tracheal stomas, the tubes functioned well in achieving lung separation, with no sign of kinking or movement, and permitted easy passage of a suction catheter.

Lung Separation in the Patient With a Difficult Airway

An airway may be recognized initially as difficult when conventional laryngoscopy reveals a grade III or IV view. When separation of the lungs is required and the patient has a clearly recognized difficult airway, then awake intubation using a flexible fiberoptic bronchoscope can be planned to place a double-lumen, Univent, or single-lumen tube. The single-lumen tube may then be exchanged for a double-lumen or Univent tube using a tube exchanger plus laryngoscopy, or a Fogarty embolectomy catheter may be passed through the lumen of the single-lumen tube to act as an independent bronchial blocker. Furthermore, depending on the expected extent and the duration of the surgical procedure and the degree of fluid shift, an airway not initially classified as difficult may become difficult secondary to facial edema, secretions, and laryngeal trauma from the initial intubation.[49,50]

A logical approach to lung separation is shown in Fig. 29-16. When lung separation is mandated and the patient has a recognized difficult airway, awake intubation using flexible fiberoptic bronchoscopy can be attempted using a DLT, Univent, or single-lumen tube. The same approach may be used for the patient with an unrecognized difficult airway and a failure to intubate with conventional laryngoscopy. When using a DLT over a fiberoptic bronchoscope, the anesthesiologist should keep in mind that it is a bulky tube with a large external diameter, and because of the length of the DLT, only a limited part of the fiberoptic bronchoscope is available for manipulation. In addition, the mismatch between the flexibility of the fiberoptic bronchoscope and the rigidity of the DLT makes it harder to advance over the fiberoptic bronchoscope. The Univent tube has the same bulky external diameter and is also often difficult to pass between the vocal cords, particularly in a patient who is awake.

Single-Lumen Tube Can Be Successfully Placed. If a failure to provide lung separation could result in a life-threatening situation, there are two possibilities to provide OLV when a single-lumen tube is already in place. First, depending on the indication for lung isolation, a tube exchanger can be used to switch to a DLT or a Univent tube. The second possibility is to direct a bronchial blocker through the single-lumen tube into the selected main-stem bronchus. These two methods, however, offer limited protection or an inadequate seal in cases such a lung lavage, pulmonary abscess, or hemoptysis, where a DLT would be the tube of choice.

Use of a tube exchanger. Several tube exchangers are commercially available (Cook Critical Care, Bloomington, IN; Sheridan Catheter Corporation, Argyle, NY). On these tube exchangers, the depth is marked in centimeters, and they are available in a wide range of external diameters and easily adapted for either oxygen insufflation or jet ventilation. The size of the tube exchanger and the size of the tube to be inserted should be tested before use in a patient. The 11F tube changer will pass through a 35 to 41F DLT, whereas the 14F tube exchanger does not pass through a 35F. To prevent lung laceration, the tube exchanger should never be inserted against resistance. Finally, when passing any tube over an airway guide, a laryngoscope

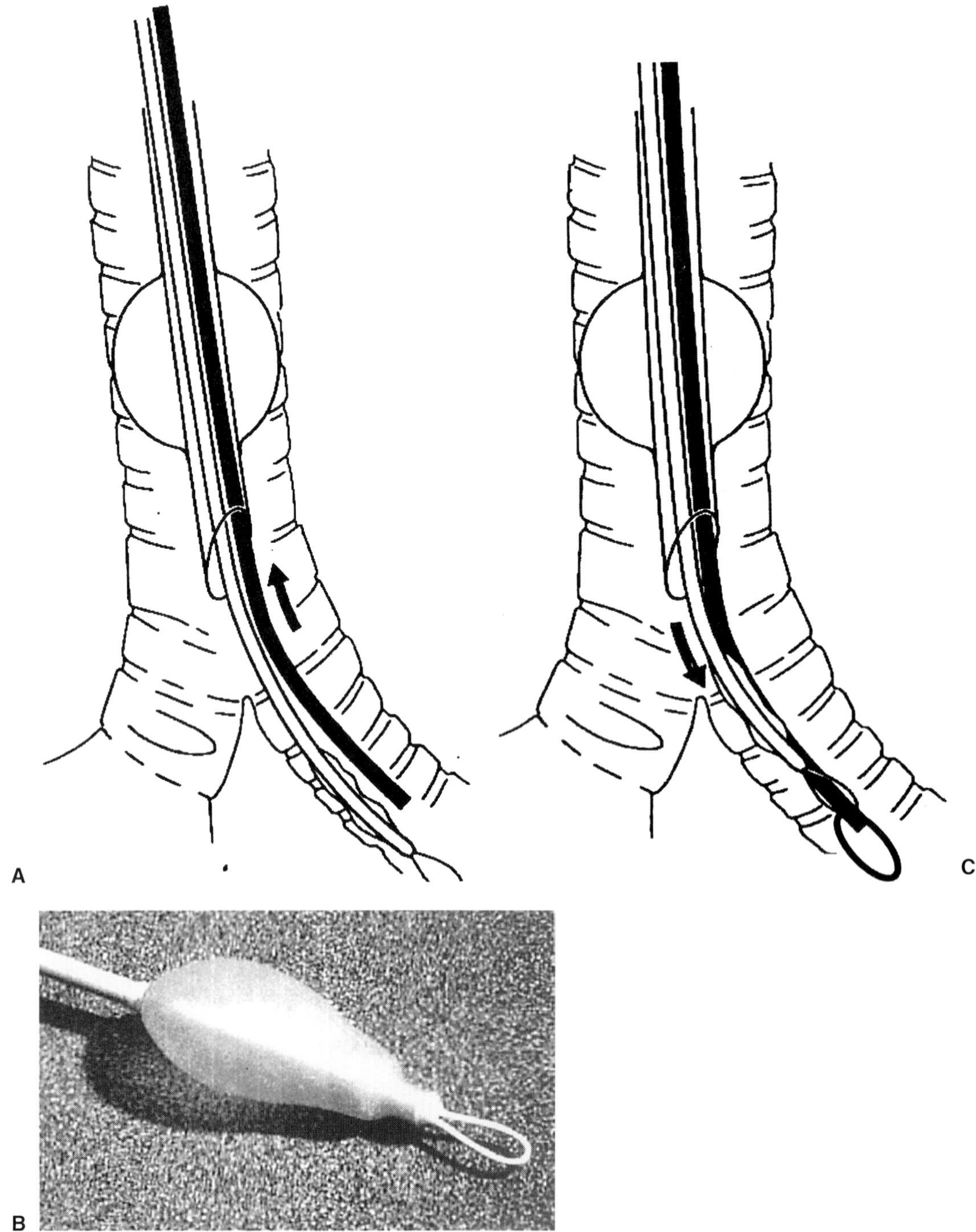

FIGURE 29-17. The Arndt endobronchial blocker is a wire-guided blocker that allows a direct placement with the use of a fiberoptic bronchoscope. The fiberoptic bronchoscope is inserted through the wire loop at the tip of the blocker, which is then slid over the bronchoscope into the selected bronchus. **A.** The fiberoptic bronchoscope is passed through the wire loop and guided into the left main bronchus. **B.** The wire loop at the tip of the blocker with the high-volume, low-pressure cuff. **C.** The bronchoscope is retracted leaving the blocker in place.

should be used to facilitate passage of the tube over the airway guide past supraglottic tissues.

Use of modern bronchial blockers. The use of a bronchial blocker is discussed earlier in this chapter. An independently passed bronchial blocker may be used with a single-lumen tube to obtain lung isolation, thereby avoiding the use of a double-lumen or Univent tube in a patient with a difficult airway. The most commonly used independent bronchial blocker was a number 7.0 Fogarty embolectomy catheter, which has an occlusion balloon that can range in volume from 5.0 to 8.0 mL (see Fig. 29-11). The balloon should be inflated to a volume sufficient to occlude the lumen of the main-stem bronchus and to hold the catheter in place. The fiberoptic bronchoscope is passed through a bronchoscopy elbow, down a single-lumen tube to visualize the carina, and past the Fogarty balloon-tipped catheter into the appropriate main-stem bronchus. The

Fogarty catheter is supplied with a wire stylet in place, which can be curved at the distal end to facilitate passage through the bronchoscopy elbow and down the single-lumen tube. The catheter balloon is then inflated under direct vision using the bronchoscope, with enough volume to occlude the main bronchus. The balloon of the Fogarty catheter is a high-pressure, low-volume design and can exert significant pressure on the mucosa of the bronchial wall.

Drawbacks to the use of the Fogarty catheter as a bronchial blocker include difficulty in directing the blocker into the desired bronchus, even with help of a fiberscope, and the inability to effectively suction the airway distal to the blocker. Also, during the surgical manipulation, the blocker may slip into the trachea, resulting in life-threatening acute airway obstruction.

The Arndt endobronchial blocker. In an attempt to overcome the potential problems described previously, a snare-guided bronchial blocker has been introduced (Cook Critical Care, Bloomington, IN) (Fig. 29-17). A fiberscope is passed through the loop of the bronchial blocker and then guided into the desired bronchus. The blocker is then slid distally over the fiberscope and into the selected bronchus. Bronchoscopic visualization confirms blocker placement and bronchial occlusion. The string (snare) is then removed through the blocker and the 1.8-mm diameter lumen may then be used as a suction port or for insufflation of oxygen. Disadvantages of the Arndt blocker are its high cost and the inability to reinsert the snare (string) once it has been pulled out, making it impossible to redirect the blocker should this become necessary. Finally, the external diameter is somewhat larger, which requires it to be passed through a single-lumen tube of at least 7.5 to 8.0 mm in internal diameter. In a more recent study, the effectiveness of these devices to provide lung isolation during elective thoracic procedures was evaluated. A left-sided double-lumen tube (Mallinckrodt Medical, Tyco.) was compared with the Fogarty catheter and the wired-snare Arndt blocker. The study found that the Arndt blocker took longer to position and, because of the limited size of the suction lumen, lung deflation took longer even with application of suction. It is important that time needed to position and to collapse the lung should be evaluated. Although the additional 5 minutes to deflate the lung may be statistically significant, it is of little clinical significance. Once the lung was collapsed, the management was similar in all three groups.[51]

The Cohen Flexitip endobronchial blocker is designed for use as an independent bronchial blocker inserted through a single-lumen endotracheal tube with the aid of a small diameter (4.0-mm) fiberoptic bronchoscope (Fig. 29-18). The blocker has a rotating wheel that deflects the soft tip by more than 90 degrees and easily directs it into the desired bronchus. The blocker cuff is a high-volume, low-pressure balloon inflated via 0.4-mm lumen inside the wall of the blocker. It has a pear shape that provides adequate seal of the bronchus. Generally, it takes between 6 and 8 mL of air to seal the bronchus with the cuff. The cuff is a distinctive blue color that is easily recognizable by fiberoptic bronchoscopy. It is best to inflate the cuff under "direct vision" via the fiberoptic bronchoscope. The blocker size is 9F. It has a central main lumen (1.6 mm) that allows limited suctioning of secretions and insufflation of oxygen to the collapsed lung in case of hypoxemia.

Conclusion of the Surgical Procedure

Depending on the extent and the duration of the surgical procedure and the degree of fluid shift, an airway, initially not classified as difficult, may become difficult secondary to facial edema, secretions, and laryngeal trauma from the original intubation. In these cases, when planning to provide lung separation, the postoperative period should be considered and the appropriate tube placed. Many procedures that are not considered to represent absolute indications for lung separation are lengthy and complex. Complex lung resection, with or without chest wall resection, thoracoabdominal esophagogastrectomy, thoracic aortic aneurysm resection with or without total circulatory arrest, or an extensive vertebral tumor resection, may result in facial edema, secretion, and hemoptysis, requiring postoperative ventilatory support. Other indications for postoperative ventilatory support are marginal respiratory reserve, unexpected blood loss or fluid shift, hypothermia, and inadequate reversal of residual neuromuscular blockade.

If a Univent tube was used to provide OLV, the blocker may be fully retracted and the Univent tube can be used as a single-lumen tube. If an independent bronchial blocker was used, then the blocker is removed, leaving the single-lumen tube in place. The problem arises when a DLT was inserted for lung separation. In a patient with a difficult airway and subsequent facial edema, the DLT may be left in place after surgery.

If the decision to leave the DLT in place is made, it is important to keep in mind that the intensive care unit staff is usually less experienced in managing such a tube, which may easily become dislocated. In addition, it is more difficult to suction through the lumens, and a longer, narrower suction catheter is needed to reach the tip of the endobronchial lumen. Another possibility is to withdraw the DLT to place the 19- to 20-cm mark at the teeth so the endobronchial lumen is above the carina and both lungs can be ventilated via the bronchial lumen. Tracheal extubation from the DLT should be considered after diuresis and steroid therapy to allow reduction of the facial and airway edema.

If it is necessary to change the DLT to a single-lumen tube, a tube exchanger must be used to maintain access to the airway, as previously discussed. Tube exchange may be performed under direct vision using a Bullard or Wu laryngoscope. With these laryngoscopes, the tube exchanger or a stylet can be placed under direct vision through the vocal cords alongside the existing tube to permit passage of a single-lumen tube (Fig. 29-19).

In summary, the clinician should be able to master different methods of lung separation and make himself or herself familiar with the devices available to provide OLV. In addition, one should always plan in advance for the postoperative period when choosing the method of lung separation. Finally, in these cases, a close dialog with the surgical team is of vital importance.

MANAGEMENT OF ONE-LUNG VENTILATION

This section discusses the management of OLV in a paralyzed patient in the lateral decubitus position with an open chest. Inspired oxygen fraction (F_{IO_2}), VT and respiratory rate, dependent lung, PEEP, and nondependent lung CPAP are reviewed, and an approach to the management of OLV is presented.

Inspired Oxygen Fraction

An F_{IO_2} of 1.0 is usually used during OLV. This high oxygen concentration serves to protect against hypoxemia during the procedure. In many studies, an F_{IO_2} of 1.0 has been used and resulted in a shunt of 25 to 30% and mean Pa_{O_2} values between 150 and 210 mm Hg during OLV.[52] In addition to a higher margin of safety, high F_{IO_2} values cause vasodilatation of the vessels in the dependent lung, which increases the capability of this lung to accept blood flow redistribution due to

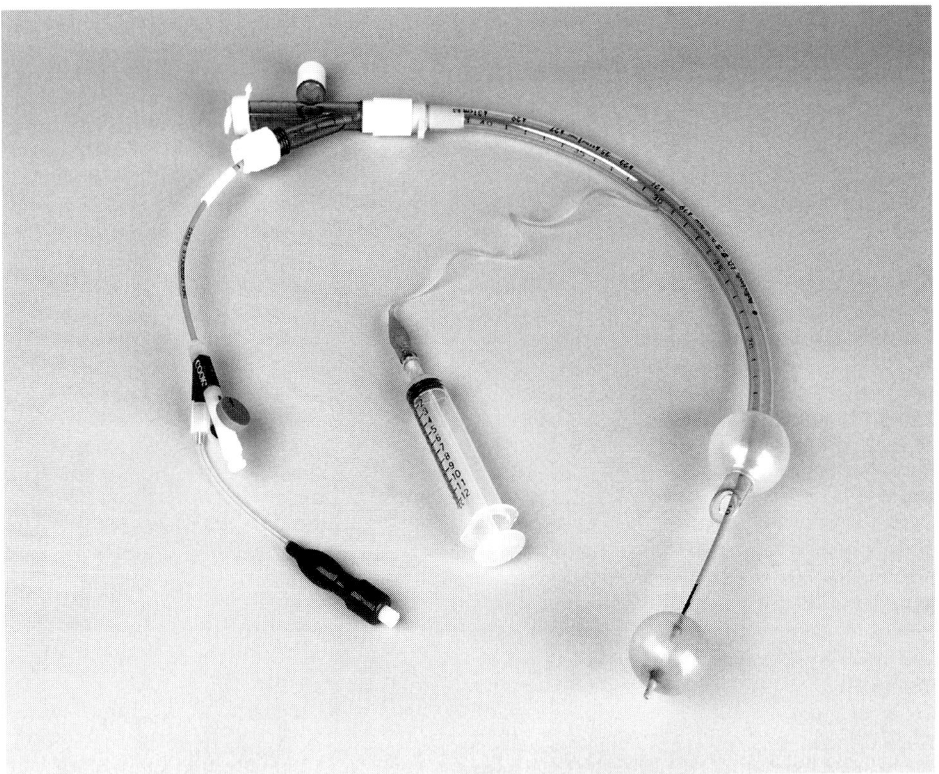

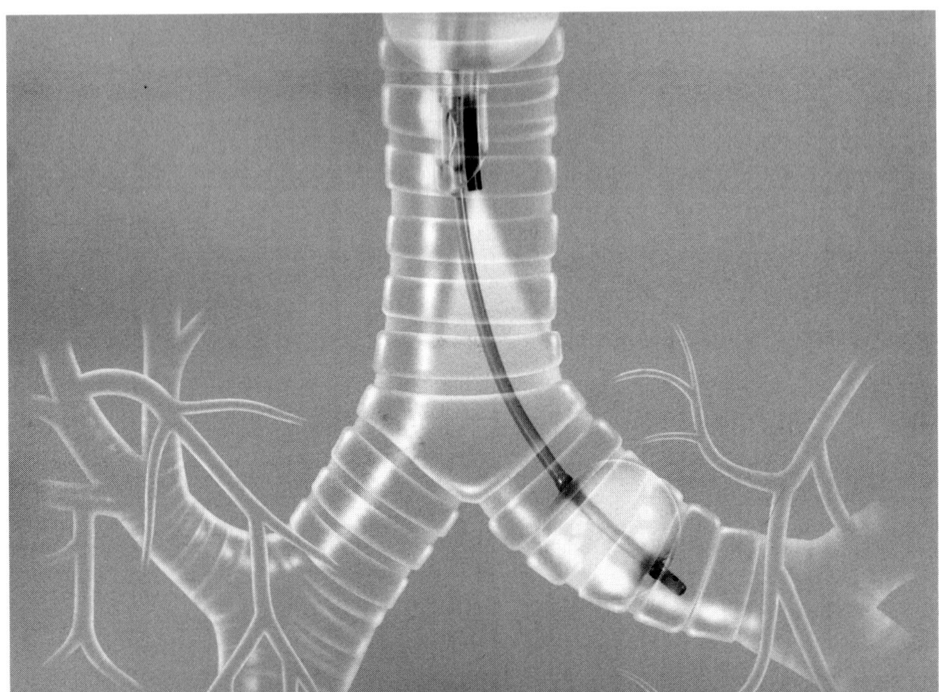

FIGURE 29-18. Cohen Flexitip endobronchial blocker (**A**) allows flexion of the bronchial blocker tip and passage into the appropriate bronchial lumen (**B**). (Courtesy of Cook, Bloomington, Indiana.)

nondependent lung HPV. A high FIO_2 may, however, cause absorption atelectasis and potentially further increase the degree of shunt because of the collapsed alveoli. The risk can be reduced by using a lower FIO_2, by the application of positive-pressure ventilation, or by the use of a high V_T and PEEP. Theoretically, a high FIO_2 can also cause lung injury owing to oxygen toxicity, although this complication is unlikely to occur in the time frame of a surgical operation. Lower FIO_2 values (0.25 to 0.50) have also been used, with resulting mean PaO_2 values between 62 and 87 mm Hg.[53,54]

The use of an FIO_2 less than 1.0 during OLV offers the benefits of reducing the risk of absorption atelectasis and may permit use of lower concentrations of potent inhaled anesthetics, which in higher concentrations might be more depressant

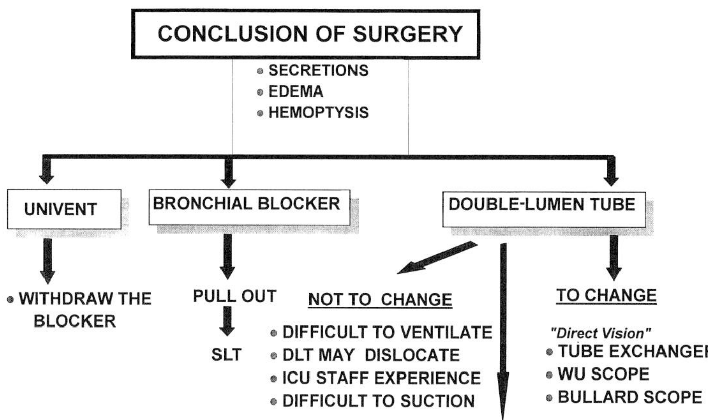

FIGURE 29-19. Conclusion of the surgical procedure. See text for discussion. DLT, double-lumen tube; SLT, single-lumen tube.

to the myocardium, particularly in high-risk patients. An FIO_2 <1.0 may also be indicated in patients with bleomycin toxicity. The combination of N_2O/O_2 with pulse oximetry monitoring may represent an optimal solution in such cases. However, the risk-benefit ratio for each patient should always be carefully considered.

Tidal Volume and Respiratory Rate

6 It was recommended that during OLV, the dependent lung be ventilated with a VT of 10 to 12 mL/kg. Tidal volumes ranging between 8 and 15 mL/kg produced no significant effect on transpulmonary shunt or PaO_2.[55] A VT <8 mL/kg can result in a decrease in FRC and enhanced formation of atelectasis in the dependent lung. A VT >15 mL/kg can increase the pulmonary vascular resistance of the dependent lung (similar to the application of PEEP) and divert blood flow into the nondependent lung. The value of 10 to 12 mL/kg is a middle range between 8 and 15 mL/kg and appears to have the smallest effect on PaO_2 and shunt fraction. In a more recent study, Tugrul et al.[56] compared pressure-controlled ventilation with volume-controlled ventilation. They suggested that pressure control may be preferred for management of OLV because the lower peak airway pressure was associated with perfusion of the dependent lung and less transpulmonary shunt. More recently, there is a trend for clinicians to decrease the VT as necessary to avoid increases in airway pressure, thereby making acute lung injury less likely to occur.

The respiratory rate should be adjusted to maintain a $PaCO_2$ of 35 ± 3 mm Hg. Elimination of CO_2 is usually not a problem during OLV if the DLT is positioned correctly. The shunt during OLV has little influence on $PaCO_2$ values because the arteriovenous PCO_2 difference is normally only 6 mm Hg. Furthermore, CO_2 is 20 times more diffusible than O_2 and will be eliminated faster. It is also important not to hyperventilate the patient's lungs because hypocapnia increases vascular resistance in the dependent lung, inhibits nondependent lung HPV, increases shunt, and decreases PaO_2. Hypocarbia is believed to inhibit HPV secondary to a vasodilator effect. Because hypocarbia can only be achieved by hyperventilating the dependent lung, it raises the mean intra-alveolar pressure and therefore increases the vascular resistance in that lung. Finally, OLV decreases the deadspace-to-tidal volume (VD/VT) ratio and enhances CO_2 elimination.[57]

Positive End-Expiratory Pressure to the Dependent Lung

The beneficial effect of selective PEEP 10 cm H_2O ($PEEP_{10}$) to the dependent lung is caused by an increased lung volume at end expiration (FRC), which improves the V/Q relationship in the dependent lung. The increase in FRC prevents airway and alveolar closure at end expiration. Therefore, it is not surprising that attempts have been made to improve oxygenation OLV by the application of PEEP to the dependent lung. However, the results were somewhat disappointing. Most of the studies showed either no change in PaO_2, a decrease, or a slight increase in PaO_2,[52,57] probably owing to the PEEP inducing an increase in lung volume that caused compression of the small interalveolar vessels and increased pulmonary vascular resistance. If this increase in resistance is limited to the dependent lung, blood flow can be diverted only to the nondependent (nonventilated) lung, increasing shunt fraction and further decreasing PaO_2.

The studies of PEEP cited previously used an FIO_2 of 1.0 with a mean PaO_2 OLV of between 150 and 200 mm Hg, at which further improvement in PaO_2 is clinically unnecessary. The possibility that the application of PEEP can improve PaO_2 in a diseased dependent lung (low lung volume and low V/Q ratio) with a low PaO_2 (<80 mm Hg) during OLV has been addressed by Cohen et al.[58] They found that application of $PEEP_{10}$ during OLV in patients with a low PaO_2 may increase FRC to normal values, resulting in a lower pulmonary vascular resistance and in an improved V/Q ratio and PaO_2. Presumably, patients with a higher PaO_2 had a dependent lung with an adequate FRC, and the application of PEEP had the negative effect of redistributing blood flow away from the dependent ventilated lung (Fig. 29-20).

Continuous Positive Airway Pressure to the Nondependent Lung

7 The single most effective maneuver to increase PaO_2 during OLV is the application of CPAP to the nondependent lung. This has been clearly demonstrated in several studies.[52,54,59] A lower level of CPAP (5 to 10 cm H_2O) maintains the patency of the nondependent lung alveoli, allowing some oxygen uptake to occur in the distended alveoli. CPAP should be applied after delivering an inspiratory VT to the nondependent lung to keep it slightly expanded. CPAP, applied by insufflation of oxygen

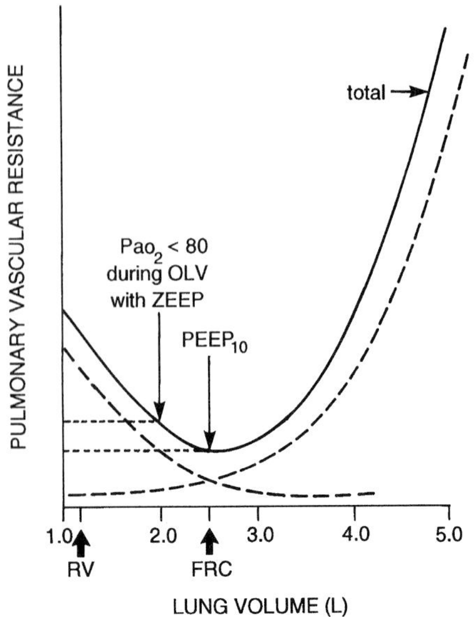

FIGURE 29-20. Effect of 10 cm H_2O PEEP on FRC. It is postulated that, in patients having Pao_2 <80 mm Hg with ZEEP, FRC is low. $PEEP_{10}$ increases FRC and thereby increases Pao_2. $PEEP_{10}$, positive end-expiratory pressure [10 cm H_2O]; OLV, one-lung ventilation; FRC, functional residual capacity; RV, residual volume; ZEEP, zero end-expiratory pressure.

under positive pressure, keeps this lung "quiet" and prevents it from collapsing completely. Insufflation of oxygen without maintaining a positive pressure failed to improve Pao_2,[52] although some improvement in Pao_2 occurred after 45 minutes of OLV (from 140 ± 107 to 206 ± 76 mm Hg) with oxygen insufflation only.[60] Intermittent reinflation of the collapsed (nondependent) lung with oxygen also resulted in a significant improvement in Pao_2.[61] The beneficial effects of CPAP 10 cm H_2O ($CPAP_{10}$) are not attributable solely to the effect of positive pressure in diverting blood flow away from the collapsed lung because (in dogs) the hyperinflation of nitrogen into the nondependent lung under 10 cm H_2O failed to improve Pao_2.

The application of high-level CPAP (15 cm H_2O) is not beneficial. At this pressure, the lung becomes overdistended, which interferes with surgical exposure. Also, this level of CPAP might have hemodynamic consequences, whereas $CPAP_{10}$ has been shown to have no significant hemodynamic effects.[54]

CPAP can be applied to the nondependent lung using a number of simple systems, all of which have essentially the same features: an oxygen source, tubing to connect the oxygen source to the nonventilated lung, a pressure relief valve, and a pressure gauge.[5] The catheter to the nondependent lung is usually insufflated with 5 L/min of oxygen using a modified Ayres T-piece (pediatric) circuit, and the valve on the expiratory limb is adjusted to the desired pressure as read on the attached gauge. Instead of a pressure gauge or manometer inserted into the circuit, a weighted pop-off valve, such as a ball or spring-loaded PEEP valve, can be used.

High-frequency ventilation with oxygen to the nondependent lung and conventional ventilation to the dependent lung has also been used to improve Pao_2 during OLV (see High-Frequency Ventilation section).

Clinical Approach to Management of One-Lung Ventilation

Once the patient is in the lateral position, the position of the DLT should be rechecked. Two-lung ventilation should be maintained for as long as possible, and when OLV needs to be instituted, it is generally recommended that an Fio_2 of 1.0 be used. The lung should be ventilated using a VT that results in a plateau airway pressure <25 cm H_2O at a rate adjusted to maintain $Paco_2$ at 35 ± 3 mm Hg. This is usually monitored with the use of a capnometer or other multigas analyzer.

After initiation of OLV, depending on the lung pathology and the intensity of hypoxic pulmonary vasoconstriction, Pao_2 can continue to decrease for up to 45 minutes.[57] Frequent monitoring of arterial blood gases and use of a pulse oximeter continue throughout the operative period. It is also essential to work closely with the surgeon. If there are any questions concerning the position of the DLT, and if fiberoptic bronchoscopy is not available, the surgeon can palpate the tube and help manipulate it into the correct position with direct digital guidance.

If hypoxemia occurs during OLV, the position of the DLT should be rechecked using a fiberoptic bronchoscope. If the dependent lung is not severely diseased, a satisfactory Pao_2 on two-lung ventilation should not decrease to dangerously hypoxic levels on OLV. If a left thoracotomy is being performed using a right-sided DLT, ventilation to the right upper lobe should be ensured. After the tube position has been confirmed as correct, $CPAP_{10}$ should be applied to the nondependent lung after a VT that expands the lung. In most cases, the Pao_2 increases to a safe level. During thoracoscopy, application of CPAP is usually not possible because it impedes the surgeon. This is especially so during VATS procedures. In this case, PEEP to the ventilated lung may be tried.

In the very rare case in which the Pao_2 remains low despite these maneuvers, intermittent two-lung ventilation can be reinstituted with the surgeon's cooperation. Also, depending on the stage of surgical dissection, if a pneumonectomy is being performed, ligation of the pulmonary artery eliminates the shunt.

During OLV, the peak airway pressure, the actual VT delivered (measured by a spirometer), the shape of the capnogram, and, if available, the pressure–volume loop, should be checked continuously. A sudden increase in peak airway pressure may be secondary to tube dislocation because of surgical manipulation, resulting in impaired ventilation. In addition, the ability to auscultate by a stethoscope over the dependent lung is extremely important.

If any questions arise about the stability of the patient, or if the patient becomes hypotensive, dusky, or tachycardic, two-lung ventilation should be resumed until the problem has been resolved. Because of pericardial manipulation (during left thoracotomy in particular) and pulling on the great vessels, cardiac arrhythmias and hypotension are not uncommon. Cardiotonic drugs should be prepared and kept available for use during any thoracic surgical procedure. Most thoracic surgical procedures represent only relative indications for OLV, and the benefits of OLV should always be weighed against the risks to the patient.

CHOICE OF ANESTHESIA FOR THORACIC SURGERY

The choice of anesthesia technique for a thoracic surgical procedure must take into account the patient's cardiovascular and respiratory status and the particular effects of anesthetic drugs on these and other organ systems. Thoracic surgical patients are more likely than others to have increased airway reactivity and a propensity to develop bronchoconstriction. This is because many of these patients are cigarette smokers and have chronic bronchitis or COPD. In addition, surgical manipulation of the airways and bronchial tree by instruments, a DLT, or the surgeon makes bronchoconstriction more likely to occur. The potent inhaled anesthetic agents have all been shown to decrease airway reactivity and bronchoconstriction provoked by hypocapnia or inhaled or irritant aerosols. Their mechanism of action is probably a direct one on the airway musculature itself, and potent inhaled anesthetic agents are therefore the drugs of choice in patients with reactive airways. For an inhalation induction, halothane or sevoflurane might be preferable because they are the least pungent of the three drugs, although once the patient is asleep isoflurane may be the preferred drug because it raises the cardiac arrhythmia threshold and provides greater cardiovascular stability than halothane. Fentanyl does not appear to influence bronchomotor tone, but morphine may increase tone by a central vagotonic effect and by releasing histamine.

In most patients, anesthesia is safely induced with thiopental or propofol. In patients with reactive airways, ketamine may be the drug of choice for induction because it has a bronchodilator effect and has been successfully used in the treatment of asthma. Thiopental has been associated with bronchospasm in asthmatic patients, although the reactivity in such cases may be related to inadequate levels of anesthesia before instrumentation of the airway. Shimizu et al.[62] compared the effects of isoflurane and sevoflurane on PaO_2 during OLV in 20 patients undergoing thoracotomy and found no significant difference between the groups in PaO_2, concluding that both agents can be used safely. In an in vitro study, Loer et al.[63] showed that desflurane inhibits HPV, with an ED_{50} of 1.6 minimum alveolar concentration (MAC). Thus, overall, the potent inhaled anesthetics are the drugs of choice during thoracic surgery.

Propofol infused in doses of 6 to 12 mg/kg/hr does not abolish HPV during OLV in humans.[64] Propofol infusion in combination with remifentanil is probably the technique of choice for producing a stable OLV with no effect on HPV. Propofol is widely used during OLV and has been investigated in terms of its effect on oxygenation. Kellow et al.[65] compared the effects of propofol and isoflurane anesthesia on right ventricular function and shunt fraction during thoracic surgery, and found that isoflurane, but not propofol, was associated with an increase in shunt fraction due to HPV inhibition. However, propofol was associated with a reduction in cardiac index and right ventricular ejection fraction.

The neuromuscular blocking drugs of choice for thoracic procedures are those that lack a histamine-releasing or vagotonic effect and that have some sympathomimetic effect. In this respect, pancuronium, vecuronium, rocuronium, and cisatracurium probably represent the drugs of choice. Succinylcholine is useful to provide rapid profound relaxation for intubation of the trachea and is not associated with an increase in airways reactivity.

Intravenous lidocaine (1.0 to 1.5 mg/kg) can be used before manipulations of the airway to prevent reflex bronchospasm. It has also been given by infusion to depress airway reactivity in patients who have poor cardiovascular function and cannot tolerate normal doses of the potent inhaled agents. Intravenous lidocaine has also been used to treat bronchospasm occurring during anesthesia. Lidocaine nebulized and administered via the airways has a similar salutary effect on bronchial tone.

Atropine may be used to block the antimuscarinic effects of acetylcholine and thereby protect against cholinergically induced bronchoconstriction. It may be administered intravenously or in nebulized form (see Bronchoscopy section).

HYPOXIC PULMONARY VASOCONSTRICTION

General anesthesia may impair pulmonary gas exchange, and arterial hypoxemia may occur as a result. In patients undergoing halothane–oxygen anesthesia with spontaneous two-lung ventilation, Nunn[66] found a calculated shunt of 14% of pulmonary blood flow as compared with a calculated shunt of 1% in normal, conscious, supine patients measured using the same techniques. He suggested that the large shunt observed was probably due to perfusion of totally unventilated parts of the lung. Marshall et al.[67] confirmed this and concluded that postoperative hypoxemia may also be a result of the residual effects of the anesthetic on venous admixture. With this background, many investigators have studied the regulation of the pulmonary circulation through a homeostatic mechanism called HPV, which normally diverts blood away from hypoxic regions of the lung and thereby optimizes the gas exchange function of the lung.

Hypoxic pulmonary vasoconstriction was first described by Von Euler and Liljestrand in 1946.[68] They were studying changes in the pulmonary circulation of the cat in response to changes in inspired gas mixtures and found that 10.5% inspired O_2 (in N_2) mixtures caused an increase in pulmonary artery pressure. Breathing 100% O_2 caused a decrease in pulmonary artery pressure. They concluded that the increased pressure during hypoxia was caused by a direct effect on the pulmonary vessels. Whereas they delivered hypoxic gas mixtures to both lungs, others have studied the effects of the size of the hypoxic segment and the size of the hypoxic stimulus on perfusion pressure and on flow diversion. Pulmonary perfusion pressure (in dogs) increased with the size of the hypoxic segment from zero (smallest hypoxic segment) to approximately 2.2 times baseline for the hypoxic whole lung. Flow diversion, as a percentage of flow to the test segment under normoxic conditions, decreased with increasing size of the hypoxic test segment from a maximum of 75% for very small segments to zero when the whole lung was made hypoxic. Flow diversion increased linearly as PaO_2 was decreased over the range of 128 to 28 mm Hg. In both flow diversion and changes in perfusion pressure, the response to HPV was predictable, continuous, and maximal at a predicted PaO_2 of 30 mm Hg (4% oxygen). Thus, HPV causes an increase in both perfusion (pulmonary artery) pressure and flow diversion.[69]

7 The choice of anesthetic technique for OLV must take into consideration the effects on oxygenation and therefore on HPV. Normally, collapse of the nonventilated, nondependent lung results in activation of reflex HPV in this lung. This causes local increases in pulmonary vascular resistance and diversion of blood flow to other, better oxygenated parts of the pulmonary vascular bed (i.e., the dependent oxygenated and ventilated lung). The stimulus to HPV appears to be a function of both PaO_2 and $P\bar{v}O_2$ in isolated rat lungs ventilated with hypoxic mixtures, but in the atelectatic lung the stimulus is the $P\bar{v}O_2$.[70] A decrease in cardiac output may potentiate HPV by lowering $S\bar{v}O_2$. The response is believed to be accounted for by each smooth muscle cell in the pulmonary arterial wall responding to the oxygen tension in its vicinity. Because HPV causes flow diversion, PaO_2 should be higher than if there were no HPV. The relationship between PaO_2 and the size of the hypoxic segment (Fig. 29-21) shows that, when not much of the lung is hypoxic, HPV has little effect on PaO_2 because shunt is small in this situation. When most of the lung is hypoxic, there is no significant normoxic region to which the hypoxic region can divert flow, and then it does not matter, in terms of PaO_2, whether the hypoxic region has active HPV. When the amount of lung made hypoxic is 30 to 70%, such as occurs during OLV, there may be a large difference between the PaO_2 to be expected with normal HPV compared with that expected in its absence. HPV can raise PaO_2 from potentially dangerous levels to higher and safer ones. Conversely, inhibition of HPV may cause or contribute to hypoxemia during anesthesia.

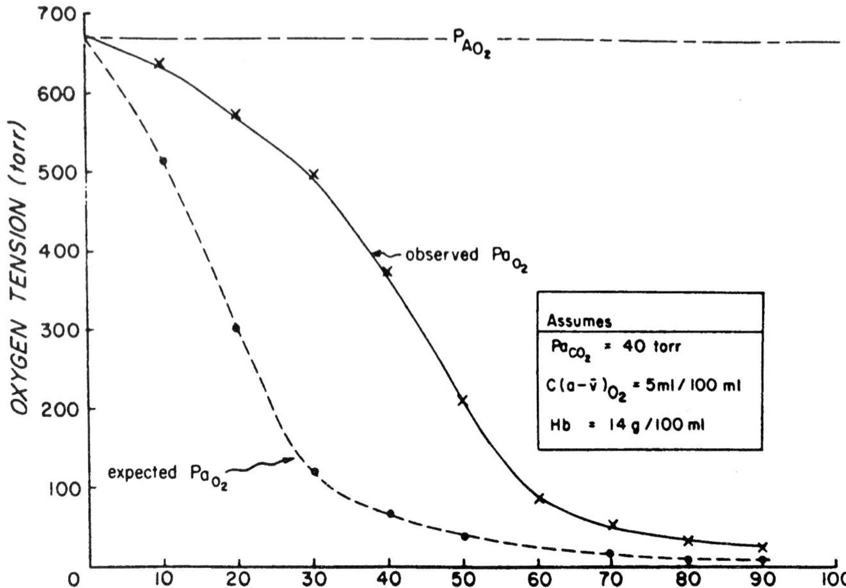

FIGURE 29-21. Role of hypoxic pulmonary vasoconstriction (HPV) in preserving PaO_2 (in dogs). Assumptions are shown in insert. Lung is ventilated with $FIO_2 = 1.0$, while increasing portions of lung are subjected to hypoxia or atelectasis. In the absence HPV, the expected PaO_2 would follow the broken line, whereas in the presence of an active HPV response, observed PaO_2 is maintained close to the solid line. PAO_2, alveolar PO_2; PaO_2, arterial PO_2. (Adapted from Marshall BE, Marshall C, Benumof JL *et al*: Hypoxic pulmonary vasoconstriction in dogs: Effects of lung segment size and alveolar oxygen tension. J Appl Physiol 51:1543, 1981.)

Effects of Anesthetics on Hypoxic Pulmonary Vasoconstriction

The inhalation anesthetics and many of the intravenous drugs used in anesthesia have been studied for their effects on HPV. The results have not always been consistent. Benumof[71] classified the preparations used to study these effects as in vitro, in vivo nonintact, in vivo intact, and human studies. Based on the results of these three types of preparation, it is generally believed that inhaled agents inhibit HPV, whereas intravenous drugs do not have this effect.[72]

Human studies are perhaps the most significant because of their applicability to the clinical situation. Bjertnaes[73] used perfusion scans (scintigraphy) to assess the effect of anesthetics on human HPV. In his patients, lung separation was achieved using a DLT. One lung could then be ventilated with 100% O_2 and the other with 100% nitrogen. HPV was assessed in the presence and absence of ether, halothane, and intravenous drugs (thiopental and fentanyl). Based on his scintigraphic findings, Bjertnaes concluded that the inhaled agents, in clinically useful concentrations, inhibited HPV in humans.

Jolin Carlsson et al.[74] used separate lung ventilation and a triple-gas washout technique to study HPV in eight patients. They demonstrated the presence of HPV in response to 8% O_2 in 92% nitrogen in the test lung but found no further change with the addition of 1.0% or 1.5% end-tidal isoflurane, and blood gas readings remained essentially unaltered. Attempts to use higher concentrations caused unacceptable hypotension. These authors concluded that isoflurane might be indicated for anesthesia in the presence of lung disease or during OLV because arterial oxygenation might be better preserved than would be the case with an anesthetic that more effectively inhibited HPV. Thus, although it is possible that higher concentrations of isoflurane might have caused a clear change in the differential blood flow distribution, at clinically used concentrations the effect of HPV in their subjects was all but unmeasurable.

Weinreich et al.[75] used a ketamine infusion and found a lower incidence of hypoxemia (defined as PaO_2 <70 mm Hg) than other studies reporting the use of halothane for OLV. Rees and Gaines[76] compared a ketamine–oxygen technique with an enflurane (1 to 3% inspired)–oxygen technique for OLV and found no differences between the groups in PaO_2 or shunt. These findings suggested that ketamine afforded no advantage over enflurane during OLV.

Rogers and Benumof[77] compared the effects of inhaled (isoflurane and halothane) with intravenous (methohexital and ketamine) anesthesia during OLV and concluded that the inhaled anesthetics at approximately 1 MAC do not significantly affect HPV in humans, as evidenced by a lack of significant differences in PaO_2 between use of the two techniques. The conclusions of this study have been questioned because the period of clinical exposure to the potent inhaled agents was very short. Thus, clinically relevant tissue concentrations of anesthetic may not have been achieved.

In a subsequent study, Benumof et al.[78] investigated the changes in PaO_2 and shunt that occurred after conversion from 1 MAC halothane or isoflurane anesthesia to intravenous anesthesia (fentanyl, diazepam, and sodium thiopental) during OLV for thoracic surgery in 12 patients. In this study, they found that during one-lung atelectasis, 1 MAC halothane anesthesia slightly but significantly increased shunt and decreased PaO_2 (compared with intravenous anesthesia), whereas 1 MAC isoflurane anesthesia very slightly but nonsignificantly increased shunt and decreased PaO_2 (compared with intravenous anesthesia). Fundamental differences between the two studies[77,78] were in the duration of the periods of OLV with the potent inhaled agent and in the MAC multiples of the drugs used. In the earlier study,[78] end-tidal concentrations of halothane and isoflurane were kept constant for approximately 20 minutes at 1.45 and 1.15 MAC, respectively. In the later study,[78] patients were maintained on one-lung anesthesia with the potent inhaled agent (1 MAC) for 40 minutes before final measurements under these conditions were taken. The authors also concluded that halothane and isoflurane had only a small inhibitory effect on the one-lung HPV response.[78] A randomized crossover study during OLV with an FIO_2 of 1.0 found that 1 MAC isoflurane anesthesia was associated with greater PaO_2 values than was 1 MAC enflurane.[79] Shimizu et al.[62] compared the effects of isoflurane and sevoflurane on PaO_2 during OLV in 20 patients undergoing thoracotomy and found no significant difference between the groups in PaO_2, concluding that both agents can be used safely. In an in vitro study, Loer et al.[63] showed that desflurane inhibits HPV, with an ED_{50} of 1.6 MAC.

Beck et al.[80] studied 40 patients requiring OLV randomized to receive propofol (4–6 mg/kg per hour) or sevoflurane

(1 MAC) for anesthesia maintenance. During OLV shunt fraction increased in both groups, but there was no significant difference between groups. It was concluded that inhibition of HPV by sevoflurane may only account for small increases in shunt fractions and that much of the overall shunt fraction during OLV has other causes.

Overall, the potent inhaled anesthetics are the drugs of choice during thoracic surgery. The technique chosen should, however, always be dictated by the needs of the particular patient, so in the presence of cardiovascular instability or poor oxygenation when depression of HPV is a possibility, a balanced technique may be chosen. Propofol in doses of 6 to 12 mg/kg per hour does not appear to abolish HPV during OLV in humans.[64]

Other Determinants of Hypoxic Pulmonary Vasoconstriction

Aside from potent inhaled agents, other drugs and maneuvers used during anesthesia may also have an inhibitory effect on regional or whole-lung HPV. Factors associated with an increase in pulmonary artery pressure antagonize the effect of increased resistance caused by HPV and result in increased flow to the hypoxic region. Such indirect inhibitors of HPV include mitral stenosis, volume overload, thromboembolism, hypothermia, vasoconstrictor drugs, and a large hypoxic lung segment. Direct inhibitors of HPV include infection; vasodilator drugs, such as nitroglycerin and nitroprusside; hypocarbia; and metabolic alkalemia. All these potential inhibitors should be considered when evaluating a patient for hypoxemia during thoracic surgery.

Potentiators of Hypoxic Pulmonary Vasoconstriction

Whereas in the past most research effort has been directed to studying inhibition of HPV, more recent research has investigated substances that may potentiate it. Almitrine, a respiratory stimulant drug, has been found to improve PaO_2 in patients with COPD and to have this effect in the absence of ventilatory stimulation. Indirect evidence suggested that it may potentiate HPV in intact dogs, although a subsequent and more extensive study in dogs concluded that almitrine caused nonspecific pulmonary vasoconstriction that was greater in the 100% oxygen-ventilated lung than in the hypoxic lung regions, thus causing a reduction of the HPV response.[81]

It has been suggested that prostaglandins may play a role in HPV inhibition, and therefore, prostaglandin inhibitors have been investigated as potentiators of HPV. Ibuprofen, a cyclooxygenase inhibitor, has been found to potentiate HPV in hypoxic isolated rat lung preparations and to reverse the inhibition of HPV caused by halothane. In an animal model, lidocaine has also been found to have salutary effects in terms of reversing depression of HPV. The value, if any, of such potentiators in humans undergoing one-lung anesthesia has not yet been reported.

Nitric Oxide and One-Lung Ventilation

Nitric oxide is an endothelial-derived relaxing factor that appears to be an important mediator for smooth muscle relaxation.[82] HPV is inhibited by inhaled nitric oxide. Inhibition of nitric oxide synthase improved, but did not completely restore, HPV in dogs suffering from sepsis.[83] Frostell et al.[84] showed that inhalation of nitric oxide selectively induced vasodilation and reversed HPV in healthy humans without causing systemic vasodilatation. It was theorized that intravenous administration of almitrine (to increase HPV) causing vasoconstriction throughout the lung, together with inhalation of nitric oxide to inhibit HPV locally and cause increased flow in the ventilated regions, would improve V/Q matching and PaO_2 in patients with V/Q mismatching or during OLV.[85]

Moutafis et al.[86] studied the effects of inhaled nitric oxide in combination with almitrine infusion during OLV in 40 patients undergoing thoracoscopic procedures. They found that inhaled nitric oxide alone did not affect PaO_2 during OLV, but the additional infusion of almitrine 16 mg/kg/min caused a marked increase in PaO_2. These authors suggested that this nonventilatory technique should be of value during special thoracic procedures, such as thoracoscopy, where there is a need to manipulate the pulmonary circulation to improve PaO_2 but measures such as PEEP and CPAP cannot be used. Moutafis et al.[87] also reported the use of almitrine infusion/nitric oxide inhalation to improve PaO_2 during OLV for bronchopulmonary lavage.

Although the use of almitrine appears to be attractive, this drug is not without side effects.[88] Also, the manufacturer has not made it available outside France. Possible alternatives to almitrine might be phenylephrine[89] and prostaglandin $F_{2\alpha}$.[90]

ANESTHESIA FOR DIAGNOSTIC PROCEDURES

Bronchoscopy

Early bronchoscopes were of the rigid type, but in 1966, the Machida and Olympus Companies introduced the first practical bronchofiberscopes. Since then, they have been improved dramatically and have simplified many otherwise complicated bronchoscopies. The indications for bronchoscopy are shown in Table 29-2 and the instruments of choice in Table 29-3. Operator preferences and experience may play a major role in the choice of instrument.

TABLE 29-2

INDICATIONS FOR BRONCHOSCOPY

■ DIAGNOSTIC	■ THERAPEUTIC
Cough	Foreign bodies
Hemoptysis	Accumulated secretions
Wheeze	Atelectasis
Atelectasis	Aspiration
Unresolved pneumonia	Lung abscess
Diffuse lung disease	Reposition endotracheal tubes
Preoperative evaluation	Placement of endobronchial tubes
Rule out metastases	Laser surgery of the airway
Abnormal chest radiograph	
Assess local disease recurrence	
Recurrent laryngeal nerve palsy	
Diaphragm paralysis	
Acute inhalation injury	
Exclude tracheoesophageal fistula	
During mechanical ventilation	
Selective bronchography	

Adapted from Landa JF: Indications for bronchoscopy. Chest 73(suppl): 686, 1978, with permission of author and publisher.

TABLE 29-3

INSTRUMENTS OF CHOICE FOR BRONCHOSCOPY

RIGID
Foreign bodies
Massive hemoptysis
Vascular tumors
Small children
Endobronchial resections
FIBEROPTIC/FLEXIBLE
Mechanical problems of neck
Upper lobe and peripheral lesions
Limited hemoptysis
During mechanical ventilation
Pneumonia, for selective cultures
Positioning of double-lumen tubes
Difficult intubation
Checking position of endotracheal tube
Bronchial blockade
COMBINATION
Positive cytologic findings with negative chest radiographic results

Adapted from Landa JF: Indication for bronchoscopy. Chest 73(suppl): 686, 1978, with permission of author and publisher.

Before bronchoscopy is performed, the patient must be evaluated for chronic lung disease, respiratory obstruction, bronchospasm, coughing, hemoptysis, and infectivity of secretions. Medications should be reviewed, and the need for a more major procedure should always be anticipated. Thus, bronchoscopy may lead to thoracotomy or sternotomy. The planned technique for bronchoscopy should be discussed with the surgeon before the operation, and all equipment and connectors should be checked for compatibility. Monitoring during bronchoscopy should include an electrocardiogram, a blood pressure cuff, a precordial stethoscope, and a pulse oximeter. If thoracotomy is planned, an arterial cannula should also be placed, as well as other monitors (e.g., PA or CVP catheters) that may be indicated by the patient's condition. Many anesthetic techniques are useful for bronchoscopy.

Local Anesthesia

The patient should first be pretreated with a drying agent. The local anesthetics most commonly used are lidocaine and tetracaine. In all cases, the total dose of anesthetic must be considered and the potential for toxicity recognized. A nebulizer can be used to spray the oropharynx and base of the tongue, or the patient may gargle with viscous (2%) lidocaine. The tongue is then held forward, and pledgets soaked in local anesthetic are held in each piriform fossa using Krause forceps to achieve block of the internal branch of the superior laryngeal nerve. Tracheal anesthesia is achieved by a transtracheal injection of local anesthetic, or by spraying the vocal cords and trachea under direct vision using a laryngoscope or through the suction channel of the bronchofiberscope. Alternatively, a superior laryngeal nerve block can be performed by an external approach, and a glossopharyngeal block can be used to depress the gag reflex. These blocks cause depression of airway reflexes, so that patients must be kept on nothing by mouth for several hours after the examination. If fiberoptic bronchoscopy is to be performed transnasally, the nasal mucosa should be pretreated topically with 4% cocaine, or viscous lidocaine may be administered through the nares. Local anesthesia for bronchoscopy has the advantages of a patient who is awake, cooperative, and breathing spontaneously. Sedatives may be added to make the patient more comfortable. Disadvantages of local anesthesia include poor tolerance of any bleeding by the patient and the occasional lack of patient cooperation.

General Anesthesia

General anesthesia for bronchoscopy is often combined with topical laryngeal anesthesia so less general anesthesia is needed. A balanced technique uses N_2O/O_2, incremental doses of an intravenous drug such as thiopental, an opioid, and a neuromuscular blocking drug. A potent inhaled anesthetic technique is also satisfactory. The use of N_2O and potent inhaled agents may create an operating room atmosphere contamination problem for the waste anesthesia gases, but limited scavenging may be possible by placing a suction catheter in the patient's oropharynx. Unless there is some contraindication, ventilation of the lungs is usually controlled. In any patient undergoing a thoracic diagnostic procedure for a suspected malignancy, the possibility of the myasthenic syndrome with sensitivity to nondepolarizing muscle relaxants must always be considered. The doses of neuromuscular blocking drugs should be titrated to effect using a neuromuscular monitoring system.

Rigid Bronchoscopy

A modern rigid ventilating bronchoscope is essentially a hollow tube with a blunted, beveled tip. Various sizes and designs are available; however, in all of them, a side arm is provided for connection to an anesthesia source. A number of techniques have been described for maintaining ventilation and oxygenation during rigid bronchoscopic examination.

Apneic Oxygenation. After preoxygenation and induction of general anesthesia, skeletal muscle paralysis and cessation of intermittent positive-pressure breathing, the $Paco_2$ increases. During the first minute the increase is ~6 mm Hg. Subsequently, the average rate of increase is 3 mm Hg/min. Oxygen is insufflated at 10 to 15 L/min through a small catheter placed above the carina. If the patient has been adequately denitrogenated, this technique can provide adequate oxygenation for more than 30 minutes.[91] The apneic period should not be allowed to extend beyond 5 minutes, however, because the technique is limited by buildup of CO_2, respiratory acidosis, and cardiac dysrhythmias.

Apnea and Intermittent Ventilation. Oxygen and anesthesia gases are delivered to the bronchoscope via the anesthesia circuit. Ventilation is possible only when the eyepiece is in place, which limits the period for instrumentation by the surgeon. Intermittent ventilation of the lungs is achieved by squeezing the reservoir bag. In this way, assuming a good bronchoscope fit in the airway, compliance is constantly monitored, the risk of barotrauma is reduced, and VT may be estimated. The disadvantage of this technique is that there may be a leak around the bronchoscope, which could lead to hypoventilation and hypercarbia. Packing of the oropharynx can reduce the leak, and improve ventilation in the case of such a gas leak.

Sanders Injection System. Sanders applied the Venturi principle to provide ventilation of the lungs by attaching a jet ventilator to the bronchoscope.[92] Oxygen from a high-pressure source (50 psig) is delivered, using a controllable pressure-reducing valve and toggle switch, to a 2.5 to 3.5-cm 18- or 16-gauge needle inside and parallel to the long axis of the bronchoscope. When the toggle switch is depressed, the jet of oxygen entering the bronchoscope entrains room air, and the air–oxygen mixture resulting at the distal tip of the bronchoscope emerges at a pressure to provide adequate ventilation and oxygenation. The intraluminal tracheal pressure depends on the driving pressure from the reducing valve; the size of the needle jet; and the length, internal diameter, and design of the bronchoscope. Increasing the size of the needle jet increases the total gas flow for any given driving pressure. For each combination of gas driving pressure, jet orifice, and bronchoscope diameter, only one inflation pressure can be attained, regardless of the volume or compliance of the lung. As long as the proximal end of the bronchoscope is open, the system is strictly pressure limited, and the pressure does not increase because of obstruction at the distal end. Pressure varies inversely with the cross-sectional area of the bronchoscope so insertion of a suction catheter or biopsy forceps into the lumen causes the intratracheal pressure to increase. Provided there is not a tight fit between the bronchoscope and the airway, the risk of barotrauma is low. If the fit is tight, driving pressure should be decreased.

The advantages of the Sanders system are that because continuous ventilation is possible (because the presence of an eyepiece is not necessary for ventilation of the lungs), the duration of the bronchoscopy procedure is minimized, but the efficiency also permits extended bronchoscopy. A disadvantage is that entrainment of air by the oxygen jet results in a variable FIO_2 at the distal end of the bronchoscope, ventilation of the lungs may be inadequate if compliance is poor, and adequacy of ventilation may be difficult to assess. A comparison between the intermittent ventilation and Sanders techniques found that PaO_2 was satisfactory with either method but was higher in the intermittent ventilation group.[93] $PaCO_2$ was lower and arterial pH higher in the Sanders group, indicating superiority of this method, particularly for long procedures.

The basic Sanders technique has been modified to increase FIO_2 and to deliver N_2O and potent inhaled anesthetics. The 16-gauge oxygen jet has been replaced with a longer jet (Carden side arm) that allows ventilation with 100% oxygen and the development of much higher pressures at the tracheal end of the bronchoscope, while using a driving pressure of 50 psig. The Sanders injector system may also be used with a ventilating bronchoscope, the side arm of which is connected to a supply of anesthesia gases so the injection jet entrains the anesthesia gases.[94]

Mechanical Ventilator. Ventilation of the lungs may be achieved by connecting a mechanical ventilator to an anesthesia circuit that is connected to the bronchoscope side arm.

High-Frequency Positive-Pressure Ventilation. HFPPV has been used in conjunction with rigid bronchoscopy and has been compared with the Sanders injector in patients with tracheobronchial stenosis. With HFPPV of up to 150 breaths/min, blood gases were identical with both techniques. At a frequency of 500 breaths/min, oxygenation deteriorated and CO_2 was not removed effectively. HFPPV has the advantage that the tracheobronchial wall remains perfectly immobilized during ventilation.[95]

Other Techniques. Cuirass ventilation, external chest compression, and a ventilating catheter or endotracheal tube placed alongside the bronchoscope have also been used to provide ventilation during bronchoscopy.

Fiberoptic Bronchoscopy

The recent generations of fiberscopes, with their improved optics and smaller diameters, have revolutionized bronchoscopy. Examination of the fifth order of bronchial branching is now possible, and the diagnostic potential of this instrument is thereby enhanced. The flexibility has also been applied in preoperative assessment of the airway, management of difficult tracheal intubations, endotracheal tube positioning and change, bronchial toilet, correct positioning of DLTs, bronchial blockade, and evaluation of the larynx and trachea.

Nasal fiberoptic bronchoscopy under topical anesthesia is well tolerated by most awake patients. A suction catheter in the mouth is useful to remove oral secretions. Oral insertion is also possible in both awake and asleep patients and should be performed via a specially designed airway, which guides the fiberscope over the back of the tongue and prevents potential damage to it by the patient's teeth.

Physiologic Changes Associated With Fiberoptic Bronchoscopy. In all patients, insertion of the fiberoptic bronchoscope is associated with hypoxemia. The average decline in PaO_2 is 20 mm Hg and lasts for 1 to 4 hours after the procedure. By 24 hours, the blood gas tensions are usually back to normal. It is therefore recommended that if the initial PaO_2 is 70 mm Hg ($FIO_2 = 0.21$), bronchoscopy should be performed only with the administration of supplemental oxygen. This can be provided using mouth-held nasal prongs, a special face mask with a diaphragm through which the fiberscope can be passed, or an endotracheal tube with a T-piece diaphragm adapter.

During and after fiberoptic bronchoscopy, patients experience increased airway obstruction. Thus, in 35 patients, insertion of the bronchoscope was associated with an increase in FRC (17 to 30%) and decreases in PaO_2, vital capacity, FEV_1, and forced inspiratory flow.[96] All returned to baseline by 24 hours. These changes are believed to be secondary to direct mechanical activation of irritative reflexes in the airway and, possibly, to mucosal edema. They may be avoided if atropine, either intramuscular or aerosolized into the airway, is administered before the procedure. Isoproterenol has a similar salutary effect on lung function but is associated with an increased incidence of cardiac arrhythmias. Overall, atropine is recommended as premedication for fiberoptic bronchoscopy. Concern that atropine may have an overall undesirable effect by increasing viscosity of secretions in patients with COPD is unsubstantiated.

The standard adult fiberoptic bronchoscope has an external diameter of 5.7 mm and a 2-mm diameter suction channel. If suction at 1 atm is applied to the fiberscope, air is removed at a rate of 14 L/min. If the fiberscope is in the airway, this causes decreases in FIO_2, PAO_2, and FRC, leading to decreased PaO_2. Suctioning should therefore be kept brief. The adult fiberscope can be passed through endotracheal tubes of 7 mm or greater internal diameter. Clearly, passage through an endotracheal tube decreases the cross-sectional area available for ventilating the patient, so if fiberoscopy is planned, an endotracheal tube of the largest possible diameter should be used.

Insertion of the bronchoscope also causes a significant PEEP effect that may result in barotrauma in ventilated patients. If PEEP is already being used, it should be discontinued before passage of the fiberscope. A postendoscopy chest radiograph is advisable to exclude the presence of mediastinal emphysema or pneumothorax. In patients whose tracheas are intubated with endotracheal tubes of less than 8 mm internal diameter, use of pediatric fiberscopes, which have smaller diameters, would be more appropriate.

The suction channel of the adult fiberoptic bronchoscope has been used to oxygenate and ventilate the lungs of patients. By attaching a jet ventilation system (similar to that used to drive the Sanders injector for rigid bronchoscopy) to the suction connection at the head of a fiberoptic bronchoscope, successful ventilation of the lungs of patients undergoing gynecologic procedures was achieved.[97] A driving pressure of 50 psig of oxygen was used with a ventilatory rate of 18 to 20 breaths/min. This technique permitted adequate ventilation of patients with normally compliant lungs and chest walls. Ventilation of the lungs should be performed only with the tip of the instrument in the trachea because a more peripheral location may produce barotrauma.

Neodymium-yttrium-aluminum garnet (Nd-YAG) lasers are used for the resection of obstructing and endobronchial lesions. This procedure is performed under general anesthesia. The lasers may be introduced into the bronchial tree through a fiberoptic bundle passed via the suction port of the fiberoptic bronchoscope. During laser resection, FIO_2 should be kept to a minimum and titrated against oxygen saturation (as continuously monitored by pulse oximeter) to make endotracheal fire less likely (see Chapter 8). Laser therapy of bronchial tumors is also possible using a rigid bronchoscope. HFPPV through a rigid bronchoscope provides satisfactory operating conditions for laser resection of tracheal tumors and has the advantage of producing airway immobility.

Complications of Bronchoscopy

Complications of rigid bronchoscopy include mechanical trauma to the teeth, hemorrhage, bronchospasm, loss of a sponge, bronchial or tracheal perforation, subglottic edema, and barotrauma. The incidence of complications is much lower with fiberoptic bronchoscopy. Nevertheless, complications may arise owing to overdose with topical anesthetic, insertion trauma, local trauma, hemorrhage, upper airway obstruction related to passage of the instrument through an area of tracheal stenosis, hypoxemia, and bronchospasm. In most cases, it is best to intubate the trachea with an endotracheal tube after bronchoscopy under general anesthesia. This permits avoidance or treatment of some of these problems, particularly the increased airway irritability. Intubation also facilitates effective suctioning of the trachea and bronchi, and allows the patient to recover more gradually from general anesthesia.

DIAGNOSTIC PROCEDURES FOR MEDIASTINAL MASS

Patients with an anterior mediastinal mass present a special problem for the anesthesiologist. Although such masses may cause obvious superior vena cava obstruction, they may also cause obstruction of major airways and cardiac compression, which are less obvious and may become apparent only on induction of anesthesia. Many cases of anesthetic related airway compression from anterior mediastinal mass have been reported. In one case, total occlusion of the trachea starting 2 to 3 cm above the carina and extending to both main-stem bronchi was observed, and a bronchoscope was passed through the obstruction.[98] In the second case of this report, extrinsic compression of the left main-stem bronchus occurred on inspiration during recovery from anesthesia. In the third case, flow–volume studies were performed with the patient in the upright and supine positions, with marked reductions in FEV_1 and peak expiratory flow in the latter position. These findings suggested potential obstruction with onset of anesthesia; radiation therapy to the mediastinum was commenced, after which the flow–volume studies showed improved function. The planned surgical procedure was then performed under local anesthesia. In a more recent series of 105 patients with mediastinal masses, the incidence of intraoperative cardiorespiratory complications was 38%, and the incidence of postoperative respiratory complications was 11%.[99] No cases of airway collapse were reported during anesthesia. In this series, patients were at increased risk of complications if there were preoperative cardiorespiratory signs and symptoms, obstructive and restrictive dysfunction on PFTs, and greater than 50% tracheal compression on CT scan.[99] In another series of patients with mediastinal mass, four patients had abnormal spirometry, but underwent general anesthesia without sequealae.[100] In severe cases of airway compression, femoral vessels may be cannulated prior to induction to institute cardiopulmonary bypass.[101]

The mass may be sensitive to radiation therapy, which could shrink the tumor and make an induction of general anesthesia less hazardous. However, a serious potential disadvantage of preoperative radiation therapy is that it may affect tissue histologic appearance, thereby preventing an accurate diagnosis. Furthermore, if the patient is a child, it may be difficult to obtain tissue samples under local anesthesia. In a series of 44 patients ages 18 years of age or younger with anterior mediastinal masses who underwent general anesthesia before radiation or chemotherapy, no fatalities occurred. However, seven patients did have airway compromise.[102] This report concluded that general anesthesia may be safely induced before radiation therapy and that the benefits of obtaining an accurate tissue diagnosis outweighed the risks. Others have disagreed with these conclusions, stating that anesthesia is not safe when the reported rate of life-threatening complications is 16 to 20%. In another report in a series of children, it was found to be safe to induce general anesthesia if the CT scan revealed that the tracheal cross-sectional area and peak expiratory flow rates were at least 50% of predicted.[103]

Airway obstruction caused by an anterior mediastinal mass has been attributed to changes in lung and chest wall mechanics associated with changes in position or to onset of paralysis in muscles that previously maintained airway patency. Preoperative evaluation of a patient with an anterior mediastinal mass to avoid life-threatening total airway obstruction is shown in Fig. 29-22.[98] It is important to determine in the history if the patient has dyspnea in the supine position and to examine the CT scan to determine the extent of the tumor and its effect on surrounding structures. If such obstruction occurs, it may be relieved by passage of a rigid bronchoscope or anode tube past the obstruction, by direct laryngoscopy,[104] or by changing the position of the patient.

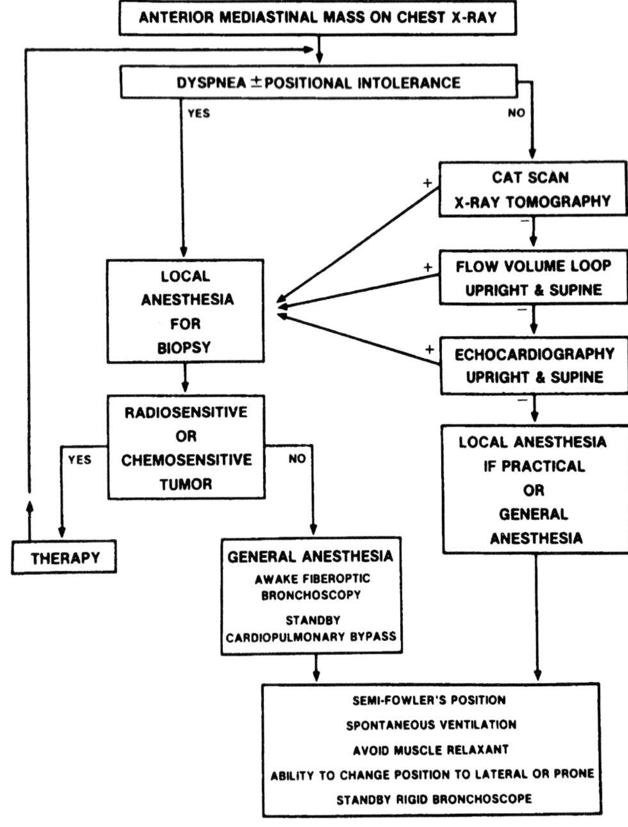

FIGURE 29-22. Flow chart describing the preoperative evaluation of the patient with an anterior mediastinal mass. +, indicates positive finding; –, indicates negative workup. (Reprinted from Neuman GC, Weingarten AE, Abramowitz RM *et al:* Anesthetic management of the patient with an anterior mediastinal mass. Anesthesiology 60:144, 1984.)

In a situation in which the biopsy procedure cannot be performed under local anesthesia and there is concern that muscle paralysis may result in airway compression, fiberoptic intubation of the awake patient followed by general anesthesia with spontaneous ventilation has been described for thoracotomy. Thus, during spontaneous inspiration, the normal transpulmonary pressure gradient distends the airways and helps maintain their patency, even in the presence of extrinsic compression.

Mediastinoscopy

Mediastinoscopy was introduced as a means of assessing spread of bronchial carcinoma. The lymphatics of the lung drain first to the subcarinal and paratracheal areas, and then to the sides of the trachea, the supraclavicular areas, and the thoracic duct. Examination of these nodes has provided a tissue diagnosis and greater selectivity of patients for thoracotomy. It is most useful in right-lung tumors because left-lung cancers tend to spread to subaortic nodes that are more accessible by an anterior mediastinoscopy in the second or third interspace (Chamberlain procedure). The transcervical approach to the thymus is an adaptation of mediastinoscopy.

The anesthetic considerations for mediastinoscopy follow naturally from an understanding of the anatomy of this procedure and its potential complications. For cervical mediastinoscopy, the patient is placed in a reverse Trendelenburg (i.e., head-up) position, and the mediastinoscope is inserted into the superior mediastinum through a transverse incision just above the suprasternal notch. The instrument is advanced along the anterior aspect of the trachea and passes behind the innominate vessels and the aortic arch (Fig. 29-23). The left recurrent nerve is vulnerable as it loops around the aortic arch, and any of these structures may be traumatized. Because of scarring, previous mediastinoscopy may be considered a contraindication to a repeat examination. Relative contraindications include superior vena cava obstruction, tracheal deviation, and aneurysm of the thoracic aorta.

Preoperative evaluation should include a search for airway obstruction or distortion. Review of a CT scan is very helpful in this regard. Evidence of impaired cerebral circulation, history of stroke, or signs of the Eaton-Lambert syndrome resulting from oat cell carcinoma should be sought. Blood must be available for the procedure because hemorrhage is a real risk and may be life threatening.

Most surgeons and anesthesiologists prefer general anesthesia using an endotracheal tube and continuous ventilation because this offers a more controlled situation and greater flexibility in terms of surgical manipulation. The anesthetic technique should include a muscle relaxant to prevent the patient from coughing because this may produce venous engorgement in the chest or trauma by the mediastinoscope to surrounding structures.

The incidence of morbidity with mediastinoscopy has been reported as 1.5 to 3.0%, and that of mortality, 0.09%. The most common complication is hemorrhage (0.73%) because of the proximity of major vessels and the vascularity of certain tumors. Tamponade may be the only recourse, and thoracotomy or median sternotomy may be required to achieve hemostasis. Needle aspiration of any structure is essential before any biopsy is taken. If severe bleeding occurs, induced arterial hypotension may be helpful in reducing the size of the tear in a vessel. If bleeding is venous, fluids given via an upper limb vein may enter the mediastinum, in which case a large-bore catheter should be placed in a lower limb vein. A venous laceration may also result in air embolism, particularly if the patient is breathing spontaneously. Some recommend the use of a precordial Doppler probe if the risk of air embolism is likely.

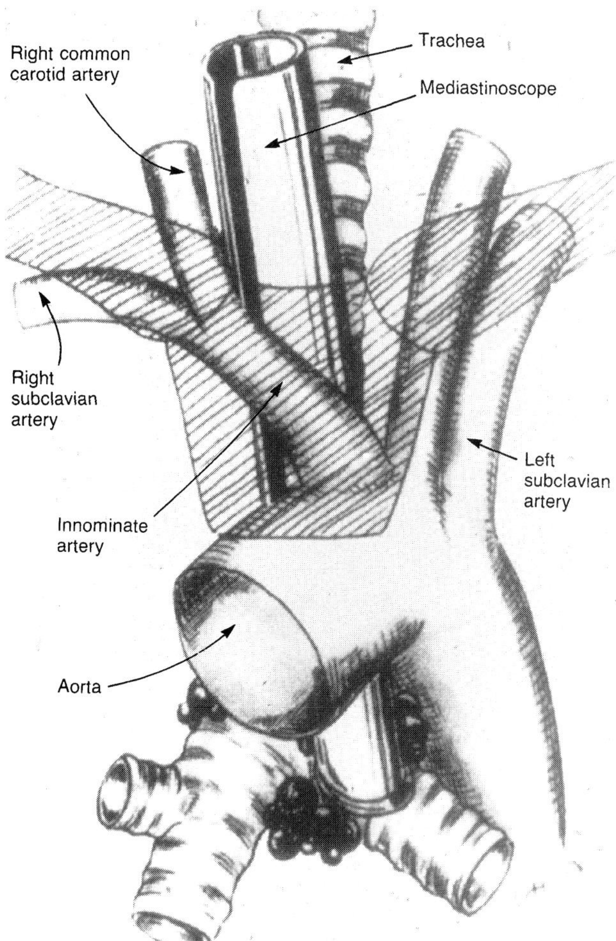

FIGURE 29-23. Anatomic relationships during mediastinoscopy. Note the position of the mediastinoscope behind the right innominate artery and aortic arch and anterior to the trachea. (From Carlens E: Mediastinoscopy: A method for inspection and tissue biopsy in the superior mediastinum. Dis Chest 36:343, 1959.)

Pneumothorax is the second most common complication (0.66%). It is usually right sided, often recognized at the time of the occurrence, and is treated according to size. A symptomatic pneumothorax should be treated by chest tube decompression.

Recurrent laryngeal nerve injury occurred in 0.34% of cases and was permanent in 50% of these cases. The nerve may be damaged by the mediastinoscope or be involved in tumor. Such injury is not a problem unless both nerves are damaged, in which case upper airway obstruction may result. Autonomic reflexes may be initiated by manipulation of the trachea or the aorta, the latter having pressor receptors located in the arch. Vagally mediated reflexes may be blocked by atropine.

"Factitious" cardiac arrest has been reported when the right radial pulse was monitored using a plethysmograph, and the tracing suddenly disappeared in the presence of a normal electrocardiogram. A normal pulse returned after the mediastinoscope was removed, and the cause of the apparent arrest was pressure on the innominate artery by the instrument. Decreases in right arm as compared with left arm blood pressure have been reported in cases undergoing mediastinoscopy. Duration was 15 to 360 seconds. This is of particular significance if there is a history of impaired cerebral circulation or transient ischemic attacks, or if a carotid bruit is present, because transient left hemiparesis may occur after mediastinoscopy. It is therefore recommended that blood pressure be monitored in the left arm and that the right radial pulse be monitored continuously during mediastinoscopy. A decrease in the right radial pulse amplitude is an indication for repositioning the mediastinoscope, especially in a patient with a history of cerebrovascular disease.

Other reported complications include acute tracheal collapse, tension pneumomediastinum, mediastinitis, hemothorax, and chylothorax. A chest radiograph taken in the immediate postoperative period is a useful precaution in all patients after mediastinoscopy.

Thoracoscopy

Thoracoscopy (medical thoracoscopy) involves the insertion of an endoscope into the thoracic cavity and pleural space. It is used for the diagnosis of pleural disease, effusions, and infectious disease (especially in immunosuppressed patients and those with acquired immunodeficiency syndrome) and for staging procedures, chemical pleurodesis, and lung biopsy. It is usually performed by the pulmonary physician in the clinic, under local anesthesia. It is also used in therapeutic procedures such as CO_2 laser treatment of spontaneous pneumothorax or bullous emphysema[105] and Nd-YAG laser vaporization of malignant pleural tumors. A small incision is made in the lateral chest wall, and with the insertion of the instrument, fluid and biopsy specimens are easily obtained.

This procedure may be performed using local, regional, or general anesthesia, the choice depending on the expected duration of the procedure and the physical status of the patient. The most common methods are local anesthetic infiltration or intercostal nerve blocks two spaces above and below the usual sixth intercostal space. Intercostal blocks also anesthetize the parietal pleura. Pneumothorax is a potential complication of an intercostal block, but it would not have clinical sequelae during a thoracoscopy because it is created as part of the surgical procedure. The collapse of the lung provides the surgeon with a working space, and a chest tube is placed at the conclusion of the surgery. The addition of a stellate ganglion block helps suppress the cough reflex that is sometimes provoked during manipulation of the hilum of the lung.

When air enters the pleural cavity under inspection, a partial pneumothorax occurs, permitting good surgical visualization. Changes in $Pa{O_2}$, $Pa{CO_2}$, and cardiac rhythm are usually minimal when the procedure is performed using local or regional anesthesia. (The physiology of this situation was discussed in the Lateral Position, Awake, Breathing Spontaneously, Chest Open section.)

With local anesthesia, the spontaneous pneumothorax is usually well tolerated because the skin and chest wall form a seal around the thoracoscope and limit the degree of lung collapse. Occasionally, however, the procedure is poorly tolerated, and general anesthesia must be induced. The insertion of a DLT with the patient in the lateral position may be difficult, in which case the patient may be temporarily placed in the supine position for the intubation.

If general anesthesia is required, either a single-lumen tube or a DLT may be used. Because positive-pressure ventilation interferes with endoscopic visualization, a DLT is preferable. In addition, if pleurodesis is being performed, general anesthesia through a DLT allows for complete reexpansion of the lung and avoids the pain associated with instillation of talc for recurrent pneumothorax.

Video-Assisted Thoracoscopic Surgery

Video-assisted thoracoscopic surgery (VATS) (see Chapter 38) entails making small incisions in the chest wall, which allows the introduction of a video camera and surgical instruments into the thoracic cavity.[106] Generally, it is performed by a thoracic surgeon in the operating room under general anesthesia. Although the first thoracoscopy was performed by Jacobeus in 1910, using what was at that time a cystoscope, in more recent years the surgical techniques, instruments, and video technology have been improved to permit a wide variety of procedures to be performed using VATS. These now include diagnostic procedures for evaluation of pleural disease and effusions, staging of lung cancer, and the identification of parenchymal disease, including nodules, mediastinal tumors, and pericardial disease. They also include therapeutic procedures such as operations for pleural disease, including pleurodesis, decortication and drainage of empyema, resection of lung tissue or bullae, pericardial window or stripping, and esophageal surgery. Even lung lobectomies can now be performed by VATS.

Anesthesia Considerations

As with a traditional thoracotomy, the patient needs to be in the lateral decubitus position, and lung collapse is needed for adequate surgical exposure. This generally mandates the use of a lung separation technique. VATS is most commonly per-
8 formed under general anesthesia with OLV. The need for OLV is much greater with VATS than with open thoracotomy because it is not possible to retract the lung during VATS as it is during an open thoracotomy. The operated lung should be deflated as soon as possible after tracheal intubation and positioning because it may take over 30 minutes for complete lung collapse to occur. Also, the surgeon enters the thoracic cavity much sooner during VATS than with open thoracotomy. Suction applied to the airway can help facilitate a more rapid deflation of the lung. In some cases, carbon dioxide is insufflated into the pleural cavity to facilitate visualization. Insufflation pressures should be maintained as low as possible and the CO_2 inflow rate kept less than 2 L/min. Higher pressures can cause mediastinal shift, hemodynamic compromise, increases in airway pressure, and increases in end-tidal CO_2. Hemodynamic compromise presents a picture similar to that due to tension pneumothorax. Significant hemodynamic changes can be produced when pressures of as little as 5 mm Hg are used to insufflate CO_2 into the chest cavity.[107]

CPAP is commonly used for the treatment of hypoxemia during OLV for thoracotomy and is usually very effective. However, during VATS, CPAP interferes with the surgical exposure and is therefore best avoided. It would be preferable to use PEEP to the nonoperated (dependent lung). In addition, a lower $Pa{O_2}$ may have to be tolerated during VATS compared with a thoracotomy.

Postoperative Concerns

There is less pain after VATS than open thoracotomy, and an epidural catheter is usually placed before surgery only if there is a likelihood that a thoracotomy may need to be performed. After a positive biopsy during VATS, an open thoracotomy may be required to perform a lobectomy or pneumonectomy. The patient's respiratory function is better preserved after VATS, and their recovery is faster. However, postoperative arrhythmias, which commonly occur after thoracotomy, have also been reported after VATS.[108] Other complications that may occur include bleeding, pulmonary edema, and pneumonia.

ANESTHESIA FOR SPECIAL SITUATIONS

Management of patients with bronchopleural fistula (BPF), empyema, cysts, and bullae, as well as those requiring tracheal reconstruction, is considered here. Many of these cases are appropriately managed using high-frequency ventilatory techniques; therefore, these techniques are described first.

High-Frequency Ventilation

With conventional positive-pressure ventilation, V_T and rates usually exceed or approach those in the normal, spontaneously breathing patient. Gas transport to the alveoli occurs by convection in the larger airways, and then by convection and molecular diffusion in the more distal airways and alveoli. High-frequency ventilation differs from conventional positive-pressure ventilation in that smaller V_T and more rapid rates are used. Gas transport may depend more on molecular diffusion, high-velocity flow, and coaxial gas flow in the airways, with gas in the center moving distally and that in the periphery moving proximally.

There are three different types of high-frequency ventilation. HFPPV uses small V_T at rates of 60 to 120 breaths/min (1 to 2 Hz). The ventilator used (e.g., Bronchovent) has a negligible internal compliance so the V_T generated, which usually approximates the dead space volume, equals the volume set on the ventilator and represents all fresh gas. The high instantaneous gas flows generated facilitate gas exchange and movement in the conducting airways.

HFPPV may be delivered by an open or a closed system. An example of the former is the percutaneous placement of a transtracheal catheter or placement of a catheter through the nose or mouth with its distal end above the carina. Inflow is intraluminal and outflow is extraluminal. This technique has been used during bronchoscopy, tracheal resection, and reconstructive surgery. When open systems are used, the gas outflow pathway is not established mechanically and depends on natural airway patency. It is therefore subject to compromise. Also, aspiration is a potential complication with open systems.

The closed system is superior because it integrates both airway patency and outflow protection. A closed system is represented by a catheter placed in a short segment of an endotracheal tube for delivery of the HFPPV, whereas the remainder of the tube lumen represents the exit pathway for gas. A quadruple-lumen endotracheal tube (Hi-Lo Jet Tracheal Tube, Mallinckrodt, Inc., Argyle, NY) has been designed specifically for delivery of HFPPV. One lumen is for the HFPPV delivery, one for gas outflow, one for cuff inflation, and one for measuring airway pressures at the distal end of the tube. The use of a closed system also permits application of PEEP, a situation not possible with an open arrangement.

High-frequency jet ventilation (HFJV) uses a pulse of a small jet of fresh gas introduced from a high-pressure source (50 psig) into the airway through a small catheter or additional lumen in an endotracheal tube. Rates used are usually 100 to 400 breaths/minute. The fresh gas jet entrains gas from an injection cannula side-port reservoir. This system is somewhat analogous to the Sanders injector system described in the Bronchoscopy section, and FiO_2 is similarly variable. The jet and entrained gas flows cause forward motion of the mass of gas in the airways. HFJV can be used with an open system or with a closed arrangement, as described earlier. In the latter, PEEP may be added to enhance oxygenation. Also, with use of high fresh gas flows from an anesthesia circuit, inhaled anesthetics may be delivered as an entrained gas mixture.

High-frequency oscillation ventilation uses a mechanism that oscillates gas at rates of 400 to 2,400 breaths/minute. It has not been described in association with thoracic surgical procedures. In this system, V_T is small (50 to 80 mL), and gas exchange occurs through enhanced molecular diffusion and coaxial airway flow.

9 The potential advantages offered by HFPPV during thoracic anesthesia are that lower V_T and inspiratory pressures result in a quiet lung field for the surgeon, with minimal movements of airway, lung tissue, and mediastinum. Thus, HFPPV has been used to ventilate both the nondependent and the dependent lung during thoracic surgical procedures, with adequate arterial blood gas measurements obtained throughout. At high frequencies (>6 Hz), however, CO_2 retention may become a problem.

High-frequency jet ventilation has been used to ventilate the nondependent lung to improve PaO_2 during one-lung anesthesia, whereas the dependent lung was ventilated with conventional intermittent positive-pressure ventilation. PaO_2 increased compared with that obtained during simple collapse of the nondependent lung. A study comparing HFJV with CPAP to the nondependent lung during conventional intermittent positive-pressure ventilation to the dependent lung found that both improved PaO_2 significantly during closed and open stages of the surgery. When the chest was open, HFJV maintained satisfactory cardiac output, whereas CPAP usually decreased cardiac output; however, there were no significant differences in $PaCO_2$ between HFJV and CPAP. Because similar increases in PaO_2 may be obtained using selective CPAP to the nondependent lung and much simpler equipment than that necessary to deliver high-frequency ventilation, the use of CPAP would seem preferable to high-frequency ventilation to increase PaO_2 during most one-lung anesthesia situations.

The lower pressures and V_Ts associated with high-frequency ventilation result in a small leak through BPFs, and HFJV is now generally considered the conservative treatment of choice in this condition. Another advantage of high-frequency ventilation is that the rapid rate small V_T can be delivered through small tubes or catheters so if an airway has to be divided, the passage of a small tube across the surgical field permits ventilation of the distal airway and lung tissue. This use has been applied during sleeve resection of the lung, tracheal reconstruction, and surgery for tracheal stenosis. In all three situations, the surgeon is able to work easily around the small catheter used to provide the high-frequency ventilation.

Bronchopleural Fistula and Empyema

A bronchopleural fistula (BPF) is an abnormal communication between the bronchial tree and the pleural cavity. Occasionally, there is an additional communication to the surface of the chest, a cutaneous BPF. BPF occurs most commonly after pulmonary resection for carcinoma. Other causes include traumatic rupture of a bronchus or bulla (sometimes caused by barotrauma or PEEP), penetrating chest wound, or spontaneous drainage into the bronchial tree of an empyema cavity or lung cyst. The incidence of BPF is higher after pneumonectomy than following other types of lung resection. The problems associated with BPF and empyema are that positive-pressure ventilation may result in contamination of healthy lung, loss of air, decreased alveolar ventilation leading to CO_2 retention, and the development of a tension pneumothorax.

If an empyema is present, it should be drained under local anesthesia before any surgery to close the BPF. Drainage is performed with the patient sitting up and leaning toward the affected side. Empyemas are often loculated, and complete drainage is not always possible. A drain to an underwater seal system is left in the cavity before administration of anesthesia for surgery of the BPF, and after drainage of an empyema, a chest radiograph should be obtained to determine the efficacy of the procedure.

The priorities in the anesthetic management of BPF are the isolation of the affected side in terms of contamination and ventilation. The ideal approach is intubation of the trachea while the patient is awake using a DLT with the patient breathing spontaneously. Supplemental oxygen should be administered, and the patient should be constantly reassured. Neuroleptanalgesia is satisfactory in providing a suitably cooperative patient, and the airway is then pretreated with topical anesthesia. The endobronchial tube selected should be such that the bronchial lumen is on the side opposite the BPF. Selection of the largest possible tube provides a close fit in the trachea, which helps stabilize the tube. Once the tube is adequately positioned in the trachea, there may be a considerable outpouring of pus from the tracheal lumen if an empyema is present; therefore, this lumen should be immediately suctioned using a large-bore suction catheter. The healthy and possibly the affected lung may then be ventilated; adequacy of oxygenation and ventilation is assessed by pulse oximetry and arterial blood gas analysis.

An alternative technique is to insert the DLT under general anesthesia, with the patient breathing spontaneously to avoid a tension pneumothorax. With either technique, the chest drainage tube must be left unclamped to avoid any bouts of coughing and to prevent the buildup of a tension pneumothorax in the event that a predisposing valvular mechanism exists. In patients who do not have an empyema, use of a single-lumen tube has been described and may be satisfactory if the BPF and air leak are small. A rapid-sequence induction with ketamine or thiopental followed by a relaxant has also been described, but is associated with considerable risk of contamination and tension pneumothorax.

BPF may also be treated conservatively using various ventilatory techniques. Thus, the bronchus of the normal lung may be intubated and ventilated, allowing the BPF to rest and heal. This approach may result in an intolerable shunt, however, and PEEP may be necessary to maintain PaO_2. Differential lung ventilation using a DLT has also been described, the healthy lung being ventilated with normal V_T, while the affected lung is exposed to a smaller V_T or to CPAP with oxygen at pressures just below the critical opening pressure of the fistula. The critical opening pressure of the BPF can be assessed by determining the lowest level of CPAP that must be applied to the bronchus on the affected side to produce continuous bubbling through the underwater seal chest drain.

For a large BPF, HFJV may be the nonsurgical treatment of choice. The use of small V_Ts results in minimal gas loss through the fistula, which may heal more quickly. In addition, hemodynamic effects are usually minimal and spontaneous efforts at ventilation are usually abolished, thereby decreasing the work of breathing and eliminating the need for relaxants or excessive sedation.

Lung Cysts and Bullae

Air-filled cysts of the lung are usually bronchogenic, postinfective, infantile, or emphysematous. They may be associated with COPD or be an isolated finding. A bulla is a thin-walled space filled with air that results from the destruction of alveolar tissue. The walls are, therefore, composed of visceral pleura, connective tissue septa, or compressed lung tissue. In general, bullae represent an area of end-stage emphysematous destruction of the lung.

Patients may be considered for surgical bullectomy when dyspnea is incapacitating, when the bullae are expanding, when there are repeated pneumothoraces owing to rupture of bullae, or if the bullae compress a large area of normal lung. Most of these patients have severe COPD and CO_2 retention, and little functional respiratory reserve. The first consideration in management is maintenance of a high FIO_2. If the bulla or cyst communicates with the bronchial tree, positive-pressure ventilation may cause it to expand or even to rupture if it is compliant, producing a situation analogous to tension pneumothorax. If the bulla is very compliant, most of the applied V_T may be wasted in this additional dead space. Nitrous oxide should be avoided because it causes expansion of any air spaces in the body, including bullae. Once the chest is open, even more of the V_T may enter the compliant bulla, which is no longer limited by chest wall integrity, and an increase in ventilation is needed until the bulla is controlled.

The anesthetic management of these patients is challenging, particularly if the disease is bilateral. Ideally, a DLT is inserted with the patient awake or under general anesthesia but breathing spontaneously. The avoidance of positive-pressure ventilation (when possible) helps decrease the likelihood of the potential problems described previously, although oxygenation may be precarious with spontaneous ventilation. Once the endotracheal tube is in place, each lung may be controlled separately, and adequate ventilation can be applied to the healthy lung if bilateral disease is not present. Gentle positive-pressure ventilation with rapid, small V_T and pressures not to exceed 10 cm H_2O may be used during the induction and maintenance of anesthesia, especially if the bullae have been shown to have no or only poor bronchial communication by preoperative ventilation scanning. While the surgery is being performed, as each bulla is resected, the operated lung can be separately ventilated to check for air leaks and the presence of additional bullae.

If positive-pressure ventilation is to be applied before the chest is opened, the possibility of a tension pneumothorax must be kept in mind, and treatment should be readily available. The diagnosis of pneumothorax may be made by a unilateral decrease in breath sounds (this may be difficult to distinguish in a patient with bullous disease), increase in ventilatory pressure, progressive tracheal deviation, wheezing, or cardiovascular changes. Treatment of a pneumothorax involves the rapid placement of a chest tube. An added risk of chest tube placement is the creation of a cutaneous BPF, which causes problems for ventilation. Alternatively, general anesthesia is induced only after the surgeon has prepared the operative field and draped the patient. In the event of sudden deterioration in the patient's condition during induction, the surgeon may perform an immediate median sternotomy. In any event, the time from induction of anesthesia to sternotomy must be kept to a minimum. Thoracoscopic laser ablation of bullae has also been described.[108]

To avoid these problems in a patient with known bullae, HFJV has been used in a patient with a large bulla undergoing coronary artery bypass graft and in another patient undergoing bilateral bullectomy. If bilateral bullectomy is to be performed, a median sternotomy is usually used. Benumof[109] described the use of sequential OLV using a DLT in the management of a patient needing bilateral bullectomy. The side with the largest bulla and least lung function, as assessed before surgery by ventilation and perfusion scans, should be operated on first. In this way, the lung with the better function should support gas exchange first. If hypoxemia develops during this one-lung situation, application of CPAP to the nonventilated lung during the deflation phase of a tidal breath should increase PaO_2.

Unlike most cases of pulmonary resection, patients after bullectomy are left with a greater amount of functional lung tissue than was previously available to them, and the mechanics of respiration are improved. At the end of the procedure, the DLT is replaced by a single-lumen tube, and the patients generally require several days to be weaned from the ventilator. During this time, the positive airway pressure used should be minimized to avoid causing a pneumothorax owing to rupture of suture or staple lines or of residual bullae.

Lung Volume Reduction Surgery

Emphysematous changes are common in the general population, occasionally resulting in pneumothoraces. A significant number of these patients require surgical intervention. Many surgical procedures have been performed to alleviate the dyspnea in severely emphysematous patients, some with beneficial effect and others without any proven beneficial outcome. More recently, laser and videoscopic technology have been used to ablate small bullae.[105,110,111] Lung volume reduction surgery (LVRS) should not be confused with excision of giant bullae. In these (bullae) cases, the presumed mechanism of improvement in lung function, exercise tolerance, and oxygenation is secondary to reexpansion of more normal, underlying compressed lung.[111]

In 1959, Brantigan et al.[112] reported on the surgical management of diffuse emphysema:

> In patients with distended lungs caused by severe COPD, the normal outward circumferential pull on the bronchioles had been lost, causing their collapse during expiration. Reducing overall lung volume, by means of multiple wedge excisions or plications, would restore the elastic pull on the small airways and reduce expiratory airway obstruction. . . . Thus, in these patients with severe dyspnea, a distended chest, and a flattened diaphragm, surgical excision of a functionless but nonbullous area by multiple wedge resections, can relieve the dyspnea. Thus, lung volume reduction results in the use of "bilateral multiple wedge excisions of bullous and nonbullous areas of the lung in patients with diffuse emphysema to improve pulmonary mechanics."

The Brantigan procedure did not receive wide acceptance. In the absence of an automated stapler, surgery was performed with a hand-sutured line of resection, which resulted in a high incidence of persistent air leak and an 18 to 20% mortality rate. The procedure was resurrected by Cooper et al.[113] after their experience with lung transplantation in patients with severe emphysema. The critical issue was to determine the optimal size of donor lungs for emphysematous recipients. The TLC of the recipient is much larger than that of the donor lung. If the lung does not fill the recipient chest, complications such as prolonged air leak and pleural effusion will persist. Their conclusion was that the ability of the chronically distended chest to configure to a smaller volume gave credence to the notion that downsizing the lungs in an emphysematous patient might improve respiratory mechanics by alleviating the overdistention. This is the basis of a resurgence of interest in the Brantigan proposal as to the surgical options for diffuse bullous emphysema (e.g., lung volume reduction).

Outcome of Lung Volume Reduction Surgery

LVRS rapidly gained popularity.[114–117] Evidence of a short-term beneficial effect was observed. By decreasing the FRC and returning the diaphragm to a more normally curved and lengthened configuration, improvement in the mechanical function of the diaphragm and intercostal muscles was noted.[118] These benefits may be evidenced by an increased contribution of the abdominal compartment to tidal volume and diminished paradoxical motion of the chest wall and abdomen during inspiration in postoperative patients.[119] In addition, recovery of ventricular function (cardiopulmonary interdependence) was seen.[120] A decreased central respiratory drive and ventilatory response to CO_2 was also noted.[121] Inspiratory lung resistance correlated significantly (and inversely) with the improvement in FEV_1 after surgery.[122] This suggests that patients with a greater loss of elastic recoil, but with intact airway structure, may derive the most benefit from the procedure.

Finally, the RV/TLC ratio was the only preoperative predictor of the increase in forced vital capacity following LVRS, and an increase in FEV_1 was largely attributable to the increase in FVC.[123–130]

The National Emphysema Treatment Trial

Due to the large number of potential procedures that could be performed in the Medicare patient population, in the absence of sufficient evidence of beneficial outcome, the National Institutes of Health (NIH) and the Health Care Financing Administration (HCFA) concluded in 1995 that "although initial results were promising, LVRS was often being performed with sufficient evaluation and a randomized study should be undertaken to evaluate the procedure critically." (Note: The HCFA has been renamed The Centers for Medicare & Medicaid Services.) The National Emphysema Treatment Trial (NETT) was established as a randomized multicenter prospective clinical trial of medical versus surgical treatment of patients with severe bilateral emphysema. In addition, comparison of the surgical approaches, sternal split versus bilateral video-assisted thoracoscopy, would be evaluated.[117,131] Twenty-five hundred ($n = 2{,}500$) patients were to be enrolled in the trial, with survival as the primary outcome. The other parameters to be evaluated included the maximum exercise capacity, pulmonary function, and oxygen requirement for distance walking 6 minutes; quality of life; and costs. The study was designed to determine which patients would benefit from the procedure and what is the best surgical approach (median sternotomy or bilateral video-assisted thoracoscopy); to establish the cost-effectiveness; and finally, to assess the utility as an alternative, or more likely as a bridge, to lung transplantation.

In 2001, the NETT Research Group published a preliminary report ($n = 1{,}033$ patients) entitled "Patients at High Risk of Death After Lung Volume–Reduction Surgery."[131] This report recommended not performing surgery on the highest-risk patients with emphysema. The investigators concluded that the operation harmed some patients and did not benefit those who survived. In an accompanying editorial, Dr. Jeffrey Drazen, the Editor-in-Chief of the *New England Journal of Medicine*, agreed: "At this time, it does not make sense to use lung-volume–reduction surgery in patients whose emphysema is so severe that they meet these exclusion criteria."[132]

However, a subsequent report from the NETT that described the results of all 1,228 randomized patients divided the subjects into four groups, depending on the extent of the emphysema and their exercise capacity.[133] The first group with upper lobe emphysema and a low exercise capacity had a significant reduction in mortality with surgery. The other two groups, those with upper lobe emphysema and high exercise capacity and those with non–upper lobe emphysema and low exercise capacity, had similar mortality with surgery or medical therapy. Only the fourth group with non–upper lobe emphysema and high exercise capacity had a higher mortality with surgery (Fig. 29-24). The place of LVRS in the management of emphysema remains controversial and should be applied selectively.

Patient Selection

The patient selection criteria are summarized in Table 29-4. Indications for a good outcome include age younger than 75 years, $FEV_1 > 0.5$ L (FEV_1 of 15 to 20% of predicted is less useful as a predictor of postoperative respiratory support), $PaO_2 > 55$ mm Hg, and $PaCO_2$ 40 to 45 mm Hg (>50 mm Hg is of concern).

Lung Volume Measurement. Body plethysmography (BP) versus inert gas (IG) technique provides some information on the degree of trapped gas in the emphysematous lung (trapped gas index = IG/BP).

Ventilation–Perfusion Scan. The ideal candidate presents with 30 to 40% reduction in perfusion to the upper lobes. In the case of α_1-antitrypsin deficiency, decreased perfusion is also evident in the lower lobes. The least favorable candidates by

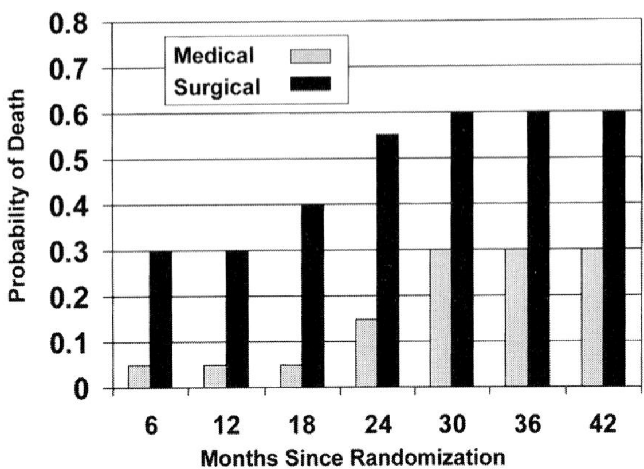

FIGURE 29-24. Mortality rates in the medical versus surgical treatment for the NETT trial. (Based on data from Fishman A, Martinez F, Naunheim K *et al*: A randomized trial comparing lung-volume-reduction surgery with medical therapy for severe emphysema. N Engl J Med 348:2059, 2003.)

scanning are those with a patchy, mottled pattern, uniformly affecting the lung.[134]

Anesthetic Management

Bronchodilator therapy is continued until the morning of surgery. Morphine and atropine premedication is administered to facilitate insertion of bronchoscopes and tracheal intubation. In addition to steroids, bronchodilators are commonly used intraoperatively. A thoracic epidural catheter is best placed before induction of anesthesia in the sitting position at T3–T4 level.[135,136] During induction of anesthesia, increases in intrathoracic pressure after neuromuscular blockade should be avoided. These patients are intravascularly depleted and have large wasted muscle mass. They commonly present with polycythemia, which may give a false impression of adequate hydration. Therefore, hydration, stable hemodynamic induction with an agent such as etomidate, and gentle ventilation may attenuate the increase in intrathoracic pressure and the degree of hypotension. Patients who have undergone surgery for emphysematous conditions are best managed with spontaneous ventilation as soon as possible after the procedure. Therefore, short-acting neuromuscular blocking agents (rocuronuim, cisatracurium, vecuronium) are indicated. Pain relief must be optimal as soon as possible because it enables early tracheal extubation and early mobilization, which is crucial to the recovery of these patients. OLV is an absolute requirement, whether the procedure is performed by sternal split or bilateral thoracoscopy.[137] This author (EC) prefers using a double-lumen tracheal tube over endobronchial blockers for complete and reliable isolation and rapid lung deflation. However, whichever tube is used in these patients with a marginal respiratory reserve, perfect isolation and confirmation with fiberoptic bronchoscopy are mandatory.

In the post anesthesia care unit (PACU), it is important to recognize the early signs of tension pneumothorax and dynamic hyperinflation as possible complications. Adequate analgesia, chest physiotherapy, incentive spirometry, and early ambulation are all important for a successful outcome.

TABLE 29-4

LUNG VOLUME REDUCTION SURGERY

■ PATIENT SELECTION
Progressive emphysema
Severe, symptomatic dyspnea
Radiographic evidence of diffuse emphysema
Identifiable distention and hyperinflated lung tissue
FEV_1 <40%, RV >150%, TLC >120% predicted
No previous chest surgery
Smoking cessation
Acceptable cardiac function
■ CONTRAININDICATIONS
Age >75 years
Uniformly destroyed lungs
FEV_1 <15% of predicted
$Paco_2$ >55 mm Hg
O_2 >6 L/min
Pulmonary hypertension
Severe kyphoscoliosis
Predominance of chronic bronchitis, asthma
Active infection
Inability to complete preoperative rehabilitation program

FEV_1, forced expiratory volume in 1 second; RV, residual volume; TLC, total lung capacity.

Anesthesia for Resection of the Trachea

Tracheal resection and reconstruction are technically difficult for the surgeon and challenging for the anesthesiologist. Indications for this type of procedure include congenital lesions (agenesis, stenosis), neoplasia (primary or secondary), injuries (direct or indirect), infections, and postintubation injuries (caused by an endotracheal tube or tracheotomy). For the surgical team, the major problems are maintenance of ventilation to the lungs while the airway is being operated on and postoperative integrity of the anastomoses. In this respect, the presence of lung disease sufficiently severe to require postoperative ventilatory support is a relative contraindication to tracheal resection or reconstruction.

Monitoring of these patients should include placement of an arterial cannula in the left radial artery to permit continuous measurement of blood pressure during periods of innominate artery compression. Steroids should be administered to help reduce any tracheal edema, and a high FIO_2 should be used throughout the procedure to ensure an adequate oxygen reserve at all times in the FRC so temporary interruptions of ventilation are less likely to produce hypoxemia.

Numerous methods have been reported to provide oxygenation and ventilation of the lungs during these procedures. A small-bore anode tube may be placed through and distal to an upper tracheal lesion so resection may occur around the tube. This technique is useful only in mild stenoses. Alternatively, an endotracheal tube may be passed through the glottis to above the stenosis, and a sterile endotracheal or bronchial tube may later be inserted into the trachea opened distal to the site of stenosis, with the sterile anesthesia tubing being led across the surgical field. After resection of the lesion, the sterile and distally placed endotracheal tube is withdrawn, and the upper tube (originally passed through the glottis) is advanced across the anastomosis. With low tracheal or bronchial lesions, resection and reconstruction may be performed around an endobronchial or DLT. During these procedures, the patient is kept in a head-down position to minimize aspiration of blood and debris into the alveoli, and ventilation must be carefully monitored throughout.

Clearly, the presence of a large-bore tube in the airway may make these resections technically difficult, and the use of high-frequency ventilation techniques may improve surgical access.

Thus, a small-diameter catheter or catheters may be placed across or through the stenotic lesion or transected airway(s) and ventilation to the distal airways and lungs maintained using HFPPV or HFJV. Potential disadvantages of these high-frequency ventilation techniques are that, by necessity, the system is "open" (see High-Frequency Ventilation section), and egress of gas during exhalation may be compromised if the stenosis is tight. Also, the catheter may become occluded by blood and become displaced, and distal aspiration of debris or blood may occur. With complex resections, two anesthesia teams with two machines and anesthesia circuits or sets of ventilating equipment may be necessary to ensure adequate ventilation of the two distal airway segments, although during carinal resections, HFPPV to the left lung alone usually provides adequate oxygenation and ventilation.

After tracheal resection or reconstructive surgery, patients should be kept with their neck and head flexed to reduce tension on the anastomotic suture lines. In some cases, this is maintained by using sutures between the chin and the anterior chest wall. Extubation of the trachea is performed as early as possible to minimize tracheal trauma due to the endotracheal tube and cuff.

Bronchopulmonary Lavage

This procedure involves irrigation of the lung and bronchial tree, and is used as a treatment for alveolar proteinosis, radioactive dust inhalation, cystic fibrosis, bronchiectasis, and asthmatic bronchitis. Lung lavage is performed under general anesthesia using a DLT so one lung may be ventilated while the other is being treated with lavage fluid.[138]

The preoperative assessment of these patients should include ventilation–perfusion scans so lavage can be performed first on the more severely affected lung (i.e., the one with the least ventilation). If involvement is equal, the left lung is generally lavaged first because gas exchange should be better through the larger, right lung. Patients are premedicated and supplied with supplemental oxygen en route to the operating room.

Anesthesia is induced with an intravenous drug and maintained with an inhaled agent in oxygen to maintain the highest possible FIO_2. Muscle relaxation facilitates placement of the DLT, and the cuff seal should be checked to maintain perfect separation at a pressure of 50 cm H_2O to prevent leakage of lavage fluid around the cuff. A fiberoptic bronchoscope is useful to check the position of the bronchial cuff of the DLT. Monitoring should include an arterial catheter, and a stethoscope should be placed over the ventilated lung to check for rales, the presence of which may indicate leakage of lavage fluid into this lung.

The patient is maintained on an FIO_2 of 1.0 throughout the procedure. Before lavage, this serves to denitrogenate the lungs so only oxygen and carbon dioxide remain. Instillation of fluid then allows these gases to be absorbed, resulting in greater access by the fluid to the alveolar spaces than if the more insoluble nitrogen bubbles remained.

Once the trachea is intubated, the patient is turned so the side to be lavaged is lowermost, and the DLT position and seal are checked once again. With the patient in a head-up position, warmed heparinized isotonic saline is infused by gravity from a reservoir 30 cm above the midaxillary line into the catheter to the dependent lung, while the nondependent lung is ventilated. When fluid ceases to flow in (usually after 700 to 1,000 mL in an adult), the patient is placed in a head-down position and fluid is allowed to drain out. The lavage is continued until the effluent is clear (as opposed to the milky fluid that drains initially when lavage is being performed for alveolar proteinosis), at which point the lung is suctioned and ventilation is reestablished with large VT (and pressures) because compliance is decreased owing to loss of surfactant. With each lavage, inflow and outflow volumes are monitored so the patient is not "drowned" in fluid, and there is no excessive absorption or leakage to the ventilated side. At least 90% of the saline volume should be recovered with each lavage. Two-lung ventilation is reestablished and, as compliance improves, an air–oxygen mixture (addition of nitrogen) may be introduced to help maintain alveolar patency. After a further period of ventilation, in most patients, the trachea can be extubated in the operating room. In the posttreatment period, patients are encouraged to cough and engage in breathing exercises to fully reexpand the treated lung. From 3 days to 1 week after lavage of the first lung, the patient may return to the operating room for lavage of the other lung.

Problems sometimes encountered with this procedure include spillage of lavage fluid from the treated to the ventilated lung. This must be managed by stopping the lavage and ensuring functional separation of the lungs before continuing. DLT positioning is critical. Spillage may cause profound decreases in oxygenation, which may necessitate terminating the procedure and maintaining two-lung ventilation with oxygen and PEEP.

During periods when lavage fluid is being instilled into the dependent lung, oxygenation usually improves because the increased intra-alveolar pressure caused by the fluid produces diversion of the pulmonary blood flow to the nondependent, ventilated lung. Conversely, when the fluid is drained out of the dependent lung, hypoxemia may occur.[138] In some cases in which severe hypoxemia was anticipated during right lung lavage, the risk has been reduced by passing a balloon-tipped catheter into the right main pulmonary artery (checked by radiography) and inflating the balloon during periods of right lung drainage. In this way, blood flow to the dependent, right, nonventilated lung is minimized during periods of drainage. This technique is not without risk (e.g., pulmonary artery rupture) and is reserved for those patients considered to be at greatest risk for hypoxemia during lavage. Almitrine by infusion and nitric oxide by inhalation have also been reported to improve oxygenation during bronchopulmonary lavage.[88]

If the patient has recently had a diagnostic open lung biopsy, a BPF may be present. If this is a possibility, a chest tube should be inserted on the side of the BPF, and this side should be lavaged first. The chest drain is removed several days later.

Limitations in the sizes of available DLTs preclude their use for lavage in patients weighing less than 40 kg. In such cases, cardiopulmonary bypass may be required to provide oxygenation during lavage.

Myasthenia Gravis

The thoracic anesthesiologist will most likely have to manage patients with myasthenia gravis (MG) for thymectomy, which is now considered the treatment of choice in most cases of MG.
10 MG is a disorder of the neuromuscular junction, the function of which is altered routinely in the modern practice of anesthesia. The worldwide prevalence of the disease is 1 per 20,000 to 30,000 of the population; it is more common in women than men in a 6:4 ratio. People of any age may be affected, but peaks of incidence occur in the third decade for women and the fifth decade for men. MG is a chronic disorder characterized by weakness and fatigability of voluntary muscles with improvement following rest.[139] Onset is usually slow and insidious, any skeletal muscle or group of muscles may be affected, and the condition is associated with relapses and remissions. The most common onset is ocular; if the disease remains localized to the eyes for 2 years, the likelihood of progression to generalized MG is low. In some cases, the disease is generalized and may involve the bulbar musculature, causing problems with breathing and swallowing. Peripheral muscle involvement may cause

TABLE 29-5

CLINICAL CLASSIFICATION OF MYASTHENIA GRAVIS

I	Ocular myasthenia—Involvement of ocular muscles only. Mild with ptosis and diplopia. Electrophysiologic testing of other musculature is negative for MG.
IA	Ocular myasthenia with peripheral muscles showing no clinical symptoms but showing a positive electromyogram for MG.
II	Generalized myasthenia
IIA	Mild—Slow onset, usually ocular, spreading to skeletal and bulbur muscles. No respiratory involvement. Good response to drug therapy. Low mortality rate.
IIB	Moderate—As IIA but progressing to more severe involvement of skeletal and bulbar muscles. Dysarthria, dysphagia, difficulty chewing. No respiratory involvement. Patient's activities limited. Fair response to drug therapy.
III	Acute fulminating myasthenia—Rapid onset of severe bulbar and skeletal weakness with involvement of muscles of respiration. Progression usually within 6 months. Poor response to therapy. Patient's actvities limited. Low mortality rate.
IV	Late severe myasthenia—Severe MG developing at least 2 years after onset of group I or group II symptoms. Progression of disease may be gradual or rapid. Poor response to therapy and poor prognosis.

MG, myasthenia gravis.
Adapted from Osserman KE, Genkins G: Studies in myasthenia gravis—A review of a 20-year experience in over 1200 patients. Mt Sinai J Med 38:497, 1971.

TABLE 29-6

ANTICHOLINESTERASE DRUGS USED TO TREAT MYASTHENIA GRAVIS

	DOSE (mg)			
DRUG	ORAL	IV	IM	EFFICACY
Pyridostigmine (Mestinon)	60	2.0	2.0–4.0	1
Neostigmine (Prostigmine)	15	0.5	0.7–1.0	1

iv, intravenous; im, intramuscular.

weakness, clumsiness, and difficulty in holding up the head or in walking. The most commonly used clinical classification of MG is shown in Table 29-5.

In MG, there is a decrease in the number of postsynaptic acetylcholine receptors at the end plates of affected muscles. This causes a decrease in the margin of safety of neuromuscular transmission. MG is an autoimmune disorder, and most of the affected patients have circulating antibodies to the acetylcholine receptors. These antibodies may cause complement-mediated lysis of the postsynaptic membrane or direct blockade of the receptors, or may modulate the receptor turnover such that the degradation rate exceeds the resynthesis rate. Studies of the end plate area show loss of synaptic folds and a widening of the synaptic cleft.

The diagnosis of MG is suspected from the history and confirmed by pharmacologic, electrophysiologic, or immunologic testing. Patients cannot sustain or repeat muscular contraction. The electrical counterpart of this is a decrement in the muscle action potentials evoked by repetitive stimulation of a motor nerve. Mechanical and electrical (electromyography) decrements improve with 2 to 10 mg of intravenous edrophonium (Tensilon test). MG patients characteristically are sensitive to *d*-tubocurarine. When the routine electromyographic results are equivocal, a regional curare test may be performed using a tourniquet to isolate the limb and limit the action of the drug. In the regional curare test, electromyograms are performed before and after the administration of 0.2 mg of curare. In equivocal cases, a positive result of a test for antiacetylcholine receptor antibodies is considered diagnostic.

Medical Therapy

Anticholinesterases are used to prolong the action of acetylcholine at the postsynaptic membrane and may also exert their own agonist effect at the acetylcholine receptors. They are the most commonly used therapy in MG (Table 29-6). Myasthenic patients learn to regulate their medication and titrate dose against optimum effect. Overdosage causes the muscarinic effects of acetylcholine and may cause a cholinergic crisis. Underdosage causes weakness or a myasthenic crisis. In a patient with weakness, distinction between the two types of crisis may be made by performing a Tensilon test or by examining pupillary size, which will be large (mydriatic) in a myasthenic crisis but small (miotic) in a cholinergic crisis. Muscarinic side effects are treatable with atropine.

The immunologic basis of MG has led to the use of immunosuppressive drugs such as steroids, azathioprine, cyclophosphamide, and, most recently, cyclosporine. Steroids often produce initial deterioration before an improvement. The usual regimen is prednisone 1 mg/kg on alternate days. The other drugs mentioned represent third and fourth lines of treatment.

Plasma exchange or plasmapheresis may produce dramatic but transient improvements in muscle strength with decreases in antiacetylcholine receptor antibody titers. Usually reserved for severe MG, plasma exchange has been shown to improve respiratory function in both operated and nonoperated patients with MG. Plasmapheresis causes a decrease in plasma cholinesterase levels that may prolong the effect of drugs such as succinylcholine that are normally broken down by this enzyme system.

Abnormalities are found in 75% of thymus glands removed from patients with MG (85% show hyperplasia, 15% thymoma). After thymectomy, approximately 75% of patients either go into remission or show some improvement. Thymectomy is now considered the treatment of choice in most patients with MG, except for those in Osserman class I (see Table 29-5).

Management of General Anesthesia

When possible, patients with MG should be admitted for elective surgery while in remission.[140] On admission, the patient's physical and emotional states should be optimized. Other diseases occasionally associated with MG should be excluded (Table 29-7). The patient's current drug therapy should be reviewed and possible drug interactions considered. Because patients are less active while in the hospital, their anticholinesterase dosage may need to be decreased. If the patient has a history of respiratory disease or bulbar involvement, preoperative evaluation should include respiratory function studies. Breathing exercises and instruction in the use of incentive spirometers may be indicated. Patients should be told of the possible need for postoperative intubation of the trachea and ventilation of the lungs. Ideally, patients with MG should be scheduled to be the first case of the day in the operating room. Patients receiving steroid therapy should receive perioperative coverage.

Because the trachea is to be intubated and the lungs ventilated for the planned procedure in the patient with MG, anticholinesterase therapy should be withheld on the morning of

TABLE 29-7

DISORDERS ASSOCIATED WITH MYASTHENIA GRAVIS

Thymoma	Multiple sclerosis
Thyroid disease	Ulcerative colitis
Hyperthyroidism	Leukemia
Hypothyroidism	Lymphoma
Thyroiditis	Convulsive disorders
Idiopathic thrombocytopenic purpura	Extrathymic neoplasia
Rheumatoid arthritis	Sjögren's syndrome
Systemic lupus erythematosus	Scleroderma
Anemias	
Pernicious	
Hemolytic	

surgery so the patient is weak on arrival at the operating room. This avoids interactions with other drugs used in the operating room. Anticholinesterase therapy may be continued if the patient is physically or psychologically dependent on it. Premedication is satisfactorily achieved with a benzodiazepine or barbiturate. Opioids are usually avoided because of the risk of producing respiratory depression.

Monitoring should be dictated by the patient's state and planned surgical procedure, but should include an assessment of neuromuscular transmission (by means of a mechanomyogram/twitch monitor, an integrated electromyographic monitor, or an accelograph monitor) if agents affecting neuromuscular transmission are to be used.

Induction of anesthesia is readily achieved with a short-acting barbiturate or propofol. In elective cases, intubation of the trachea, maintenance, and relaxation are readily achieved using potent inhaled anesthetics. Anesthesia may be deepened using a potent inhaled agent and the trachea intubated under its effect. Myasthenic patients are more sensitive than normal patients to the neuromuscular depressant effects of the potent inhaled agents. In patients with MG, isoflurane at 1.9 MAC end-tidal concentration induced a neuromuscular block of 30 to 50%, whereas halothane at 1.8 MAC induced a block of 10 to 20%. Both agents produced fade in the train-of-four ratio of 41% and 28%, respectively.[141] Because these inhaled agents are easily administered and withdrawn, they are the most commonly used anesthetic drugs for patients with MG. At the end of the procedure, the drug is discontinued and recovery of neuromuscular function begins.

Nondepolarizing Relaxants. In some cases, patients with MG cannot tolerate the cardiovascular depressant effects of the potent inhaled anesthetics, in which case neuromuscular blocking drugs may be used, titrating dose against monitored effect. Patients with MG are sensitive to the nondepolarizing relaxants. A usual defasciculating dose in a normal patient may represent an ED_{90} in a patient with MG.[140] All nondepolarizing relaxants have been successfully and uneventfully used with careful monitoring in patients with MG. They should be titrated in 1/10 to 1/20 of the usual dose. Atracurium is probably the preferred agent because of its short elimination half-life (20 minutes), small volume of distribution, lack of cumulative effect, and high clearance. The Hofmann elimination pathway results in atracurium having very reproducible pharmacodynamics and kinetics, and most patients do not require reversal if monitored carefully. The ED_{90} of atracurium in patients with MG is approximately one-fifth of that in normal patients.[142] Relaxation is readily maintained thereafter using an atracurium infusion, and recovery time is not prolonged with this drug. Cisatracurium is also an appropriate choice.[143] Sensitivity to nondepolarizing relaxants is increased during the coadministration of a potent inhaled anesthetic.[144]

Although other short-duration or intermediate-duration nondepolarizing agents may be used, they do have cumulative effects, which may represent a potential disadvantage. Long-acting relaxants are probably best avoided in patients with MG. Myasthenic patients show increased sensitivity to mivacurium. Because mivacurium is metabolized by cholinesterase, anticholinesterase drugs prolong the recovery from this relaxant.[145] If necessary, the other nondepolarizers may be reversed by increments of anticholinesterase drugs, while neuromuscular transmission is carefully monitored to obtain maximum antagonism yet avoid a cholinergic crisis. All anticholinesterases have been safely used. Edrophonium may be the drug of choice because its onset of action is rapid and higher doses have a prolonged duration of action. Because of the risk of cholinergic crisis with anticholinesterase agents, the rapid, predictable, spontaneous recovery from atracurium (or cisatracurium) may represent an additional advantage in that reversal may not be necessary.[140]

The sensitivity of patients with MG to nondepolarizing relaxants is very variable, depending on the individual patient, the severity of MG, and the treatment. Mann et al.[146] showed that MG patients who have a T4/T1 ratio <0.9 in the preanesthetic period show increased sensitivity to atracurium. They suggest that neuromuscular monitoring using TOF stimulation should begin in the preinduction period following administration of adequate analgesia (fentanyl 2 μg/kg). Itoh et al.[147] found that patients with ocular MG were less sensitive to vecuronium than were those with generalized MG. They also found that in patients with clinical MG, sensitivity to vecuronium was unrelated to presence or absence of antibodies to the acetylcholine receptor. Seronegative patients were as sensitive to vecuronium as seropositive patients.[148] There are conflicting reports as to the sensitivity of patients with MG in remission. All such patients should be considered sensitive to nondepolarizers until proven otherwise.

Succinylcholine. Myasthenic patients are resistant to the neuromuscular blocking effects of succinylcholine. The ED_{95} is 2.6 times normal in these patients.[149] Clinically, however, the use of succinylcholine has been without incident, with the usual clinical doses producing adequate relaxation for endotracheal intubation and a normal recovery time, despite the occasionally reported early onset of phase II block. Doses of 0.2 to 1.0 mg/kg have been used in a number of patients with MG, and most did not show fasciculation before becoming paralyzed. Fade in response to train-of-four stimulation was observed in some patients during recovery, but recovery was not delayed. Prior administration of an anticholinesterase may complicate the response to succinylcholine by delaying its metabolism.

When a rapid-sequence intubation of the trachea is required, rapid onset of muscle relaxation may be achieved with succinylcholine or with moderate doses of a nondepolarizer in the latter case, with an associated prolongation of effect. A succinylcholine (1.5 mg/kg)–vecuronium (0.01 mg/kg) sequence has been safely used in three patients with MG for thymectomy. The authors suggested that this technique may be particularly advantageous when rapid-sequence induction of anesthesia is indicated.[150]

Nonrelaxant Techniques. Because of concerns over the use of muscle relaxants in MG patients, there are many reports of successful use of nonrelaxant techniques. Della Rocca et al.[151] studied 68 consecutive MG patients undergoing transsternal thymectomy randomized to receive propofol/O_2/N_2O/fentanyl or sevoflurane/N_2O/O_2/fentanyl. All were tracheally extubated in the operating room, and none required intubation for postoperative respiratory depression. Madi-Jebara et al.[152] described the use of sevoflurane as the sole anesthetic combined with intrathecal sufentanil-morphine for analgesia in an adult patient who underwent transsternal thymectomy. Abe et al.[153] described propofol anesthesia combined with thoracic epidural anesthesia for thymectomy in 11 patients with MG. Chevalley et al.[154] reported use of propofol combined with epidural bupivacaine and sufentanil in 12 MG patients undergoing similar procedures. They commented that the shift away from use of muscle relaxants provided optimal operating condition and improved patient comfort. Lorimar and Hall[155] used a total intravenous anesthetic (TIVA) technique with propofol and remifentanil for transsternal thymectomy in an MG patient. Baraka et al.[156] described a 19-year-old myasthenic patient with a thymoma who received remifentanil and sevoflurane anesthesia for a 2-hour thymectomy. Although the trachea was extubated 10 minutes after discontinuation of remifentanil, the patient was unresponsive to verbal stimuli and remained somnolent for 12 hours. Because the patient had been receiving pyridostigmine for the months prior to surgery, they suggest that the delayed arousal may have been due to possible inhibition by pyridostigmine of the nonspecific esterases that normally hydrolyze remifentanil. Ingersoll-Weng et al.[157] reported use of a dexmedetomidine infusion/isoflurane technique for transsternal thymectomy in a 52-year-old female. The patient was stable at the start of surgery but became asystolic on sternal retraction and received open cardiac massage. Resuscitation was successful, the dexmedetomidine infusion was discontinued, and surgery was completed uneventfully. Several factors may have contributed to the asystolic arrest, including a centrally mediated increase in parasympathetic activity resulting from dexmedetomidine in a patient who was also being treated with pyridostigmine, which also increases vagal tone. Thus, pyridostigmine may have interacted with dexmedetomidine in an additive or synergistic manner.

Other Drug Interactions. Medications with neuromuscular blocking properties should be used with caution in patients with MG, particularly if relaxants are being used concurrently. Such drugs include antiarrhythmics (quinidine, procainamide, calcium channel blockers), diuretics (by causing hypokalemia), nitrogen mustards, quinine, and aminoglycoside antibiotics. Dantrolene has been used safely in a patient with MG.

Recovery From Anesthesia. Recovery from anesthesia must be carefully monitored in these patients. Extubation of the trachea should be performed when the patients are responsive and able to generate negative inspiratory pressures of greater than −20 cm H_2O. After extubation of the trachea, patients are carefully observed in the recovery area or the intensive care unit. As soon as possible, patients should resume their usual pyridostigmine regimen. Cases of mild respiratory depression may be treatable with parenteral anticholinesterase; more severe cases may require reintubation of the trachea and mechanical ventilation of the lungs. In the immediate postoperative period, postthymectomy patients often show a marked improvement in their condition and a decreased need for anticholinesterase therapy.

Postoperative Respiratory Failure

Myasthenic patients are at increased risk for development of postoperative respiratory failure. There have been several attempts to predict before surgery which patients with MG will require prolonged postoperative ventilation of the lungs.[158] For patients who underwent transsternal thymectomy, positive predictors were a duration of MG >6 years; history of chronic respiratory disease, other than that directly caused by MG; pyridostigmine dosage >750 mg/day; and a preoperative vital capacity <2.9 L. This predictive system was not found useful when applied in patients with MG undergoing transsternal thymectomy at other centers, and of no value in patients with MG undergoing other types of surgical procedure.[158] In a study of 52 MG patients following thymectomy, Mori et al.[159] concluded that those patients who received >250 mg of pyridostigmine were at greater risk for respiratory failure requiring reintubation. Each patient should therefore be treated on his or her own merits.

A study of patients undergoing transsternal thymectomy suggested that the need for postoperative mechanical ventilation correlated best with preoperative maximum static expiratory pressure. It was concluded that expiratory weakness, by reducing cough efficacy and ability to clear secretions, was the main predictive determinant. Adequate clearance of secretions is essential in these patients and may occasionally necessitate bronchoscopy.

In general, the postoperative morbidity in terms of respiratory failure is lower after transcervical rather than transsternal thymectomy.[158] Techniques described that may be useful in reducing postoperative ventilatory failure include preoperative plasma exchange and high-dose perioperative steroid therapy. If the anticipated duration of the surgical procedure is 1 to 2 hours, preoperative oral anticholinesterase therapy may be of value because the peak effect of the drug coincides with the conclusion of the surgical procedure and attempts at tracheal extubation.

Postoperative Care

In the immediate postoperative period, pain relief for patients with MG is usually provided by opioid analgesics, such as meperidine, but in reduced doses. The analgesic effect of morphine and other opioid analgesics has been reported to be increased by anticholinesterases, which has led to the recommendation that the dose of opioid analgesics be reduced by one-third in patients receiving anticholinesterase therapy. Combined regional and general anesthesia techniques have also been used to provide good surgical conditions and improved postoperative analgesia in patients with MG undergoing thymectomy. Combined epidural–general anesthesia has been reported to provide excellent intraoperative and postoperative conditions for both surgeon and patient.[160,161]

Myasthenic Syndrome (Eaton-Lambert Syndrome)

The myasthenic syndrome is a very rare disorder of neuromuscular transmission that is sometimes associated with small cell carcinoma of the lung. Complaints of weakness may be mistaken for MG, but in Eaton-Lambert syndrome, symptoms do not respond to administration of anticholinesterases or steroids, and activity improves strength. The defect in this condition is believed to be prejunctional, associated with diminished release of acetylcholine from nerve terminals, and improved by agents such as 4-aminopyridine, guanidine, and germine that increase repetitive firing. Affected patients are particularly sensitive to the effects of all muscle relaxants, which should be used with great caution or avoided entirely.[162] The possibility of Eaton-Lambert syndrome should be considered in all patients with known malignant disease and those patients undergoing diagnostic procedures for suspected carcinoma of the lung. Anesthesia considerations in these patients are essentially the same as in those with MG.[163]

POSTOPERATIVE MANAGEMENT AND COMPLICATIONS

Postoperative Pain Control

After extubation of the trachea, respiratory therapy and pain management become critical components of postoperative care. Adequate postoperative pain control is necessary to

ensure a good respiratory effort.[144,164] Administration of intravenous opioids has been the standard form of pain management for years. These drugs may improve pulmonary function slightly or allow respiratory therapy maneuvers; however, meperidine (50 mg) has been shown to be relatively ineffective at allowing patients to increase their ability to cough. Advantages of intravenous opioids are the ease of administration, relatively low toxicity, and the lack of a need for close medical
11 supervision. The key disadvantage is the inadequate pain relief leading to postoperative atelectasis and great discomfort on the part of the patient. The administration of sufficient opioid to treat pain adequately is likely to cause sedation and respiratory depression.

Patient-controlled analgesia (PCA) has been reported to decrease the amount of postoperative pain, drug use, sedation, and pulmonary complications.[165] PCA also eliminates the delays associated with personnel-administered medications and in general is very well accepted by patients. Subcutaneous PCA with hydromorphone has been reported to be as effective as intravenous PCA. Complications related to the use of PCA are presented elsewhere in this volume (see Chapter 55).

Many clinicians have suggested the use of intercostal nerve blocks before, during, or after thoracic surgery to decrease pain and improve postoperative respiratory function. Studies have documented a decrease in requirements for postoperative opioids, improved respiratory function, and some decrease in time of hospital stay. The intercostal blocks can be performed externally before or after surgery using a standard technique. However, the easiest method during thoracic surgery is to have the surgeon perform the blocks under direct vision from inside the thorax while the chest is open. Bupivacaine 0.5%, in doses of 2 to 3 mL, can be placed in the five intercostal spaces around the incision and in intercostal spaces where chest tubes will be placed. This provides 6 to 24 hours of moderate pain relief, but patients still complain of diaphragmatic and shoulder discomfort caused by the chest tubes. Larger volumes of local anesthetic (e.g., 5 to 10 mL) should not be used in the intercostal space because of the high absorption rate and attendant systemic toxicity that can be produced, as well as the possibility of pushing the drug centrally and producing a paravertebral sympathetic or epidural block with central sympatholysis and severe hypotension. The intraoperative placement of catheters in intercostal grooves allows for a continuous postoperative intercostal nerve block. The technique reduces pain and improves pulmonary function. Although bupivacaine has been used in most reports, use of lidocaine has also been described.

A prolonged intercostal nerve block may be obtained by cryoanalgesia, a technique of freezing the nerve under direct vision at the time of thoracotomy. A cryoprobe is applied directly to the nerve to disrupt the axon but not the support structures. In this way, conduction is interrupted until the nerve regenerates over the next 1 to 6 months, by which time full structure and function are usually restored. Hypoesthesia in the scar and adjacent skin is a common late finding. During the postoperative period, the patients are numb in the segments thus treated. Ideally, any drains or chest tubes should be located within the area made analgesic with the cryoprobe to minimize immediate postoperative discomfort. Cryoanalgesia provides excellent analgesia when supplemented with other pain treatments. Because cryoanalgesia is of prolonged duration, it is not used routinely after thoracotomy but rather in cases in which prolonged analgesia would be necessary, such as after surgery for chest trauma.

Another approach to postoperative pain control after thoracic surgery is the use of epidural or subarachnoid opioids. Epidural morphine produces profound analgesia lasting from 16 to 24 hours after thoracotomy and does not cause a sympathetic block or sensory or motor loss. These are significant advantages over other methods of administering opioids or local anesthetics. The opioids have been successfully used by both the thoracic and lumbar epidural routes. Morphine, in a dose of 5 to 7 mg diluted in 15 to 20 mL of fluid, has been used in the lumbar epidural technique. This technique has led to a 30% increase in postoperative expiratory flow rates without significant side effects, even in patients with chronic lung disease.

Epidural morphine has been shown to decrease pain and improve respiratory function in postthoracotomy patients.[164] The successful use of lumbar epidural sufentanil or fentanyl diluted to 20 mL has also been reported.[165] There have been reports of severe respiratory depression with epidural fentanyl and several reports with sufentanil. The addition of epinephrine, 5 mg/mL, to sufentanil administered in the thoracic epidural space decreases the plasma concentration of sufentanil and increases the duration of block. Lumbar epidural hydromorphone (1.25 to 1.5 mg) has been reported to provide excellent analgesia, with fewer side effects than epidural morphine. Severe respiratory depression was reported in one patient who received hydromorphone via a thoracic epidural catheter. A prophylactic low-dose infusion of naloxone, or nalbuphine, an agonist–antagonist drug, can reduce the incidence of respiratory depression.

Subarachnoid (intrathecal) morphine, in a dose of 10 to 12 μg/kg, has been successfully used after thoracic surgery.[166] With this technique, the drug acts directly on the spinal cord, and analgesia can be produced with a smaller dose than by the epidural or intravenous routes. When morphine is given intrathecally before the induction of anesthesia, a decrease in the dose of anesthetic drugs required may occur. All patients who have received subarachnoid or epidural opioids must be closely observed for potential side effects, including delayed respiratory depression, urine retention, pruritus, nausea, and vomiting. These effects appear to be dose related and may be reversed with naloxone.

Noxious stimuli, including surgical incision, may lead to changes in the central nervous system that exacerbate postoperative pain. The administration of analgesic agents before surgery is termed preemptive analgesia and may prevent these neuroplastic changes, thereby decreasing postoperative pain. The administration of lumbar epidural fentanyl before thoracotomy incision reduced postoperative pain scores and use of PCA morphine by a small but significant amount, compared with administration of lumbar epidural fentanyl after skin incision.[167]

Intrapleural analgesia is another technique for postoperative pain treatment. Although the mechanism has not been fully elucidated, the injection of local anesthetic between the pleural layers is believed to block multiple intercostal nerves or the pain fibers traveling with the thoracic sympathetic chain. The surgeon can place the catheter under direct vision while the chest is open. Catheter malposition has been documented after percutaneous placement, especially if the patient is not breathing spontaneously. The chest tubes should not be suctioned for approximately 15 minutes after injection of local anesthetic to avoid loss of the anesthetic into the drainage. The efficacy of interpleural blockade for postthoracotomy pain relief has been reported to be both poor and good.[164]

Complications Following Thoracic Surgery

Atelectasis

Patients who require thoracotomy often have preexisting pulmonary disease that, when combined with the operative procedure, is likely to result in significant pulmonary dysfunction and possibly pneumonia. Atelectasis, the most significant cause of postoperative morbidity, has been reported to occur in up to 100% of patients undergoing thoracotomy for pulmonary resection. It occurs more commonly in the basal lobes than in the middle or upper lung regions. It may be secondary to reduction of normal respiratory effort due to splinting from pain, obesity, intrathoracic blood and fluid accumulation, and decreased compliance, all of which lead to rapid, shallow, constant V_T. Such a respiratory pattern produces small airway closure and obstruction with inspissated secretions, resulting ultimately in alveolar air resorption and terminal airway collapse. A poor cough and limited clearance of secretions add to the problem. Other sources of atelectasis include mucous plugging, which can obstruct a lobe or even an entire lung, and incomplete reexpansion of the remaining lung tissue after one-lung anesthesia. The diagnosis of atelectasis can be made by clinical findings, chest radiography, or arterial blood gas analysis. This problem is best resolved by increasing resting lung volume or FRC. The latter can be increased by an increase in transpulmonary pressure (difference between airway pressure and interpleural pressure) or in lung compliance.

The tracheas of many patients can be extubated shortly after thoracic surgical procedures using standard extubation criteria. These patients should be observed in the operating room for at least 5 minutes following extubation, and many will require a high F_{IO_2} by facemask. Some patients with COPD undergoing extensive thoracic surgical procedures require postoperative ventilation to avoid atelectasis and other pulmonary complications. Mechanical ventilation increases airway pressure and, to a lesser extent, interpleural pressure; therefore, transpulmonary pressure increases.

In addition to the use of incentive spirometry and bronchodilators, coughing and clearance of secretions, and mobilizing the patient, adequate analgesia is essential to the prevention and treatment of atelectasis. Atelectasis caused by collapse of lung tissue distal to a mucous plug can be treated by positioning the patient in the lateral decubitus position with the fully expanded lung in the dependent position. This improves V/Q matching and facilitates clearance of mucus from the nondependent obstructed lung. However, the patient should not be placed with the operative side in the dependent position after a pneumonectomy because of the risk of cardiac herniation.

The other major complications after thoracic surgery can be grouped into cardiovascular, pulmonary, and related problems.

Cardiovascular Complications

Cardiovascular complications are often the most difficult to manage in patients with associated respiratory insufficiency. The low cardiac output syndrome and postoperative cardiac arrhythmias are the most common and life threatening of these problems. In the postoperative period, advanced hemodynamic monitoring is used to make the differential diagnosis of left or right ventricular failure and the low output syndrome. A key monitor is the PA catheter, which facilitates assessment of hemodynamics. Other diagnostic modalities, such as echocardiography, may be required to rule out the presence of pericardial effusions or tamponade after opening the pericardium during certain types of thoracic surgical procedure. The low cardiac output syndrome must be differentiated from hypovolemia resulting from intrathoracic hemorrhage, tamponade, pulmonary emboli, or the effects of mechanical ventilation with PEEP. Postoperative fluid administration can lead to pulmonary edema resulting from the resection of lung tissue and the concomitant reduction of the pulmonary vascular bed. A postoperative pulmonary embolism can originate from the remaining pulmonary artery stump or tumor tissue. Therapeutic interventions for postoperative myocardial dysfunction include inotropic drugs, vasodilators, and combinations of these drugs, as needed, to improve ventricular function. The goal is to shift the Starling function curve up and to the left by reducing preload of either the left or right side of the heart and increasing cardiac output. Vasodilators are very effective at decreasing right ventricular afterload and improving right ventricular function because this side of the heart is especially afterload dependent. Combinations of inotropes and vasodilators, such as isoproterenol and nitroglycerin, or combined drugs, such as amrinone, can be especially useful in the treatment of right-sided heart failure.

Postoperative cardiac arrhythmias are common after thoracic surgery. Patients following pulmonary resection have postoperative supraventricular tachycardias with a frequency and severity proportional to both their age and the magnitude of the surgical procedure. Many factors contribute to these arrhythmias, including underlying cardiac disease, degree of surgical trauma, intraoperative cardiac manipulation, stimulation of the sympathetic nervous system by pain, a reduced pulmonary vascular bed, effects of anesthetics and cardioactive drugs, and metabolic abnormalities.

In a series of 300 thoracotomies for lung resection, atrial fibrillation occurred in 20% of patients with malignant disease but in only 3% with benign disease.[168] A similar incidence of arrhythmias is observed after pneumonectomies. Multifocal atrial tachycardia often occurs in patients with COPD and concomitant right-sided cardiac dysfunction. The right side of the heart may be further strained by the reduction in the size of the pulmonary vasculature from the lung resection, especially after right pneumonectomy. The prophylactic use of digitalis in thoracic surgical patients is controversial, particularly in patients with signs of congestive heart failure. Arguments against its use include the potential toxic effects of the drug and the difficulty in assessing adequacy of digitalization in the absence of heart failure. A prospective, placebo-controlled, randomized study demonstrated no advantage to prophylactic digitalization of patients undergoing thoracic surgery.[169] Part of the argument for its use is the drug's efficacy in reducing the incidence of potentially fatal complications in older patients. In some studies, it has been reported to reduce the incidence of perioperative arrhythmias. If digitalis therapy is to be instituted, normokalemia should be ensured to reduce the likelihood of digitalis toxicity.

Supraventricular tachycardias can also be treated with either beta-blocking or calcium channel-blocking drugs after ruling out underlying reversible physiologic abnormalities, such as hypoxia. Verapamil has been the standard treatment for these problems until the introduction of the ultrashort-acting beta-blocker, esmolol. Esmolol has been shown to be equally effective in controlling the ventricular rate in patients with postoperative atrial fibrillation or flutter and in increasing the conversion rate to regular sinus rhythm from 8 to 34%. Owing to its short duration of action (beta elimination half-life of 9 minutes) and β_1-cardioselectivity, it is the drug of choice in the postoperative period to control these arrhythmias. Esmolol, in an intravenous loading dose of 500 μg/kg given over 1 minute followed by an infusion of 50 to 200 μg/kg/min, has been shown to be effective in the control of supraventricular tachycardias.

Bleeding and Respiratory Complications

Hemorrhage and pneumothorax are always major concerns after intrathoracic surgery. Because of these problems, interpleural thoracostomy tubes with an underwater seal system are routinely used after thoracic surgery. Slippage of a suture on any major vessel or airway in the chest can lead to the slow or rapid development of hypovolemic shock or a tension pneumothorax. Drainage of more than 200 mL/hr of blood is an indication for surgical reexploration for hemorrhage. Management of the pleural drainage system is fraught with confusion. The chest bottles must be kept below the level of the chest, and the tubes should not be clamped during patient transport. These tubes can be lifesaving, but errors in technique can lead to serious complications. The creation of a pneumothorax in the nonoperative chest by central venous catheter placement is very hazardous because this lung is essential both intraoperatively during one-lung anesthesia and postoperatively after contralateral lung resection. Dehiscence of the bronchial stump may lead to the formation of a BPF, which carries a mortality rate of 20%. Surgical treatment may be needed, in which case ventilation of the patient's lungs may be difficult because of loss of VT through the fistula. A double-lumen endobronchial tube positioned in the contralateral main-stem bronchus or the use of HFJV may be required for safe management. HFJV allows ventilation with lowered peak airway pressures. However, there have been reports in which ventilation by HFJV was difficult. If a double-lumen endobronchial tube is placed, the lung with the fistula can be ventilated independently with either CPAP or HFJV.

Neurologic Complications

Central and peripheral neurologic injuries can occur during intrathoracic procedures. Such injuries often result in serious and disabling loss of function and are very distressing to the patient. Peripheral nerves can be injured, either in the chest or in other parts of the body, by pressure or stretching. It has been recognized for years that most of these postoperative neuropathies are caused by malpositioning of the patient on the operating table, with subsequent stretching or compression of the nerves. The nerve injury may be apparent immediately after surgery or may not become obvious until several days later. These patients often complain of a variety of unpleasant sensations, including paresthesias, cold, pain, or anesthesia in the area supplied by the affected nerves. The brachial plexus is especially vulnerable to trauma during thoracic surgery, owing to its long superficial course in the axilla between two points of fixation, the vertebrae above and the axillary fascia below. Stretching is the chief cause of damage to the brachial plexus, with compression playing only a secondary role. Branches of the brachial plexus may also be injured lower in the arm by compression against objects such as an ether screen or other parts of the operating table. Intrathoracic nerves can be directly injured during a surgical procedure by being transected, crushed, stretched, or cauterized. The intercostal nerves are the ones most frequently injured during intrathoracic surgical procedures. The recurrent laryngeal nerve can become involved in lymph node tissue and injured at the time of a node biopsy, especially when the biopsy is performed through a mediastinoscope. This nerve can also be injured during tracheostomy or radical pulmonary dissections. The phrenic nerve is frequently injured during pericardiectomy, radical pulmonary hilar dissections, division of the diaphragm during esophageal surgery, or dissection of mediastinal tumors.

Prevention is the treatment of choice for these intraoperative nerve injuries. Analgesics may be necessary to control postoperative pain in the distribution of the nerve injury and to aid in maintaining joint mobility during the healing phase. Subsequent surgical procedures may be necessary to move a swollen ulnar nerve at the elbow or to stent a partially paralyzed vocal cord.

References

1. Rutkow IM: Thoracic and cardiovascular operations in the United States, 1979 to 1984. J Thorac Cardiovasc Surg 92:181, 1986
2. Travis WD, Lubin J, Ries L, Devesa S: United States lung cancer incidence trends. Cancer 77:2464, 1996
3. Jemal A, Tiwari RC, Murray T *et al*: Cancer statistics. CA Cancer J Clin 54:8, 2004
4. Cohen E (ed): The Practice of Thoracic Anesthesia. Philadelphia, JB Lippincott, 1995
5. Benumof JL: Anesthesia for Thoracic Surgery, 2nd ed. Philadelphia, WB Saunders, 1995
6. Slinger, PD: Preoperative assessment for pulmonary resection. J Cardiothorac Vasc Anesth 4:202, 2000
7. Reilly JJ: Evidence-based preoperative evaluation of candidates for thoracotomy. Chest 116:474s, 1999
8. Licker M, Perrot M, Spiliopulos A: Risk factors for acute lung injury after thoracic surgery for lung cancer. Anesth Analg 97:1558, 2003
9. Slinger PD, Susssa S, Triolet W: Predicting arterial oxygenation during one-lung anaesthesia. Can J Anaesth 39:1030, 1992
10. Gass GD, Olsen GN: Clinical significance of pulmonary function tests. Preoperative pulmonary function testing to predict postoperative morbidity and mortality. Chest 89:127, 1986
11. Lockwood P: Lung function test results and the risk of post-thoracotomy complications. Respiration 30:529, 1973
12. Mittman C: Assessment of operative risk in thoracic surgery. Am Rev Respir Dis 84:197, 1961
13. Nakahara K, Ohno K, Hashimoto J *et al*: Prediction of postoperative respiratory failure in patients undergoing lung resection for cancer. Ann Thorac Surg 46:549, 1988
14. Vansteenkiste J, Fischer BM, Dooms C *et al*: Positron-emission tomography in prognostic and therapeutic assessment of lung cancer: Systematic review. Lancet Oncol 5:531, 2004
15. Gould MK, Kuschner WG, Rydzak CE, Maclean CC, Demas AN, Shigemitsu H, Chan JK, Owens DK: Test performance of positron emission tomography and computer tomography for mediastinal staging in patients with non-small-cell lung cancer: A meta-analysis. Ann Intern Med 139:879, 2003
16. Ferguson MK, Reeder LB, Mick R: Optimizing selection of patients for major lung resection. J Thorac Cardiovasc Surg 109:275, 1995
17. Walsh GL, Morice RC, Putnam JB: Resection of lung cancer is justified in high-risk patients selected by oxygen consumption. Ann Thorac Surg 58:704, 1994
18. Bollinger CT, Wyser C, Roser H *et al*: Lung scanning and exercise testing for the prediction of postoperative performance in lung resection candidates at increased risk for complications. Chest 108:341, 1995
19. Ninan M, Sommers KE, Landranau RJ *et al*: Standardized exercise oximetry predicts post pneumonectomy outcome. Ann Thorac Surg 64:328, 1997
20. Jones RM, Rosen M, Seymour L: Smoking and anaesthesia (editorial). Anaesthesia 42:1, 1987
21. Pearce AC, Jones RM: Smoking and anesthesia: Preoperative abstinence and preoperative morbidity. Anesthesiology 61:576, 1984
22. Cooper DKL: The incidence of postoperative infection and the role of antibiotic prophylaxis in pulmonary surgery: A review of 221 consecutive patients undergoing thoracotomy. Br J Dis Chest 75:154, 1981
23. Marini JJ, Lakshmimara Y, Kradyan WA: Atropine and terbutaline aerosols in chronic bronchitis. Chest 80:285, 1981
24. Landesberg G, Mosseri M, Wolf Y *et al*: The probability of detecting perioperative myocardial ischemia in vascular surgery by continuous 12-lead ECG. Anesthesiology 96:264, 2002
25. Petty C: Right radial artery pressure during mediastinoscopy. Anesth Analg 58:428, 1979
26. Iberti TJ, Fischer EP, Leibowitz AB *et al*: A multicenter study of physician's knowledge of the pulmonary artery catheter. JAMA 264:2928, 1990
27. Raper R, Sibbald WJ: Misled by the wedge. Chest 89:427, 1986
28. Cohen E, Eisenkraft JB, Thys D *et al*: Hemodynamics and oxygenation during OLA: Right vs. left. Anesthesiology 63(3A):A566, 1985
29. Thys DM, Cohen E, Eisenkraft JB: Mixed venous oxygen saturation during thoracic anesthesia. Anesthesiology 69:1005, 1988
30. Pothoft G, Curtius JM, Wassermann K *et al*: Transesophageal echography in staging of bronchial cancers. Pneumologie 446:111, 1992
31. Manguso L, Pitrolo F, Bond F *et al*: Echocardiographic recognition of mediastinal masses. Chest 93:144, 1988
32. Neustein SM, Cohen E, Reich DL, Kirschner PA: Transesophageal echocardiography and the intraoperative diagnosis of left atrial invasion by carcinoid tumor. Can J Anaesth 40:664, 1993
33. Suriani RJ, Konstadt SN, Camunas J, Goldman M: Transesophageal echocardiographic detection of left atrial involvement in a lung tumor. J Cardiothorac Vasc Anesth 7:73, 1993
34. Neustein SM, Narang J: Spontaneous hemothorax due to subacute aortic dissection. J Cardiothorac Vasc Anesth 7:79, 1993
35. Brodsky JB, Shulman MS, Swan M *et al*: Pulse oximetry during one-lung ventilation. Anesthesiology 63:212, 1985
36. van Norman G, Cheney FW: Falsely elevated oximeter reading dangerous on one lung. Anesthesia Patient Safety Foundation Newsletter 4:23, 1989
37. Shafieha MA, Sit J, Kartha R *et al*: End-tidal CO_2 analyzers in proper positioning of double-lumen tubes. Anesthesiology 64:844, 1986
38. Yam PCI, Innes PA, Jackson M *et al*: Variation in the arterial to end-tidal P_{CO_2} difference during one-lung thoracic anaesthesia. Br J Anaesth 72:21, 1994
39. Benumof JL: Isoflurane anesthesia and arterial oxygenation during one-lung ventilation. Anesthesiology 64:419, 1986
40. MacGillivay RG: Evaluation of a new tracheal tube with a movable bronchus blocker. Anaesthesiology 43:687, 1988
41. Hurford WE, Alfille PH: A quality improvement study of the placement and complications of double-lumen endobronchial tubes. J Cardiothorac Vasc Anesth 7:517, 1993
42. Smith G, Hirsch N, Ehrenwerth J: Sight and sound: Can double-lumen endotracheal tubes be placed accurately without fiberoptic bronchoscopy? Br J Anaesth 58:1317, 1987

43. Cohen E, Neustein SM, Goldofsky S, Camunas J: Incidence of malposition of PVC and red rubber left-sided double lumen tubes and clinical sequelae. J Cardiothorac Vasc Anesth 9:122, 1995
44. Benumof JL, Partridge BL, Salvatierra C *et al*: Margin of safety in positioning modern double-lumen endotracheal tubes. Anesthesiology 67:729, 1987
45. Wagner DL, Gammage GW, Wong ML: Tracheal rupture following the insertion of a disposable double-lumen endotracheal tube. Anesthesiology 63:698, 1985
46. Andros TG, Lennon PF: One-lung ventilation in a patient with a tracheostomy and severe tracheobronchial disease. Anesthesiology 79:1127, 1993
47. Bellver J, Garcia-Aguado A, Andres JD *et al*: Selective bronchial intubation with the Univent system in patients with a tracheostomy. Anesthesiology 79:1453, 1993
48. Saito T, Naruke T, Carney E *et al*: New double-lumen intrabronchial tube (Naruke tube) for tracheostomized patients. Anesthesiology 89:1038, 1998
49. Cohen E, Benumof JL: Lung separation in the patient with a difficult airway. Curr Opin Anesthesiol 12:29, 1999
50. Benumof JL: Difficult tubes and difficult airways. J Cardiothorac Vasc Anesth 12:131, 1998
51. Campos JH, Kernstine KH: A comparison of a left-sided Broncho-Cath with the torque control blocker Univent and the wire-guided blocker. Anesth Analg 96:283, 2003
52. Capan LM, Turndorf H, Patel K *et al*: Optimization of arterial oxygenation during one-lung anesthesia. Anesth Analg 59:847, 1980
53. Lunding M, Fernandes A: Arterial oxygen tensions and acid-base status during thoracic anaesthesia. Acta Anaesthesiol Scand 11:43, 1967
54. Cohen E, Eisenkraft JB, Thys DM *et al*: Oxygenation and hemodynamic changes during one-lung ventilation. J Cardiothorac Vasc Anesth 2:34, 1988
55. Katz JA, Larlane RG, Fairly HB *et al*: Pulmonary oxygen exchange during endobronchial anesthesia: Effect of tidal volume and PEEP. Anesthesiology 56:164, 1982
56. Tugrul M, Camici E, Karadeniz H *et al*: Comparison of volume control with pressure control ventilation during one-lung anaesthesia. Br J Anaesth 79:306, 1997
57. Tarhan S, Lundborg RO: Effects of increased expiratory pressure on blood gas tensions and pulmonary shunting during thoracotomy with use of the Carlens catheter. Can Anaesth Soc J 17:4, 1970
58. Cohen E, Thys DM, Eisenkraft JB *et al*: PEEP during one-lung anesthesia improves oxygenation in patients with low Pa_{O_2}. Anesth Analg 64:200, 1985
59. Hogue CW: Effectiveness of low levels of nonventilated lung continuous positive airway pressure in improving arterial oxygenation during one-lung ventilation. Anesth Analg 79:364, 1994
60. Rees DI, Wansbrough SR: One-lung anesthesia and arterial oxygen tension during continuous insufflation of oxygen to the nonventilated lung. Anesth Analg 61:501, 1982
61. Malmkvist G: Maintenance of oxygenation during one-lung ventilation. Effect of intermittent reinflation of the collapsed lung with oxygen. Anesth Analg 68:763, 1989
62. Shimizu T, Abe K, Kinovchik, Yoshiya I: Arterial oxygenation during one-lung ventilation. Can J Anaesth 44:1162, 1997
63. Loer SA, Scheeren TWL, Tarnow J: Desflurane inhibits HPV in isolated rabbit lungs. Anesthesiology 83:552, 1995
64. Van Keer L, Van Aken H, Vandermeersch E, Vermaut G: Propofol does not inhibit HPV in humans. J Clin Anesth 1:284, 1989
65. Kellow NH, Scott AD, White SA, Feneck RO: Comparison of the effects of propofol and isoflurane anaesthesia on right ventricular function and shunt fraction during thoracic surgery. Br J Anesth 75:578, 1995
66. Nunn JF: Factors influencing the arterial oxygen tension during halothane anesthesia with spontaneous respiration. Br J Anaesth 36:327, 1964
67. Marshall BE, Cohen PJ, Klingenmaier CH *et al*: Pulmonary venous admixture before, during and after halothane: Oxygen anesthesia in man. J Appl Physiol 27:653, 1967
68. Von Euler US, Liljestrand G: Observations on the pulmonary arterial blood pressure in the cat. Acta Physiol Scand 12:301, 1946
69. Marshall BE, Marshall C, Benumof JL *et al*: Hypoxic pulmonary vasoconstriction in dogs: Effects of lung segment size and alveolar oxygen tensions. J Appl Physiol 51:1543, 1981
70. Domino KB, Wetstein L, Glasser SA *et al*: Influence of mixed venous oxygen tension (Pv_{O_2}) on blood flow to atelectatic lung. Anesthesiology 59:428, 1983
71. Benumof JL: One-lung ventilation and hypoxic pulmonary vasoconstriction: Implications for anesthetic management. Anesth Analg 64:821, 1985
72. Eisenkraft JB: Effects of anesthetics on the pulmonary circulation. Br J Anaesth 65:63, 1990
73. Bjertnaes LJ: Hypoxia-induced pulmonary vasoconstriction in man: Inhibition due to diethyl ether and halothane anaesthesia. Acta Anaesthesiol Scand 22:578, 1978
74. Jolin Carlsson A, Bindslev L, Hedenstierna G: Hypoxia-induced pulmonary vasoconstriction in the human lung: The effect of isoflurane anesthesia. Anesthesiology 66:312, 1987
75. Weinreich AI, Silvay G, Lumb PD: Continuous ketamine infusion for one-lung ventilation. Can Anaesth Soc J 27:485, 1980
76. Rees DI, Gaines GY: One-lung anesthesia: A comparison of pulmonary gas exchange during anesthesia with ketamine or enflurane. Anesth Analg 63:521, 1984
77. Rogers SM, Benumof JL: Halothane and isoflurane do not decrease Pa_{O_2} during one-lung ventilation in intravenously anesthetized patients. Anesth Analg 64:946, 1985
78. Benumof JL, Augustine SD, Gibbons JA: Halothane and isoflurane only slightly impair arterial oxygenation during one-lung ventilation in patients undergoing thoracotomy. Anesthesiology 67:910, 1987
79. Slinger P, Scott WAC: Arterial oxygenation during one-lung ventilation: A comparison of enflurane and isoflurane. Anesthesiology 82:940, 1995
80. Beck DH, Doepfmer UR, Sinemus C *et al*: Effects of sevoflurane and propofol on pulmonary shunt fraction during one-lung ventilation for thoracic surgery. Br J Anaesth 86:38, 2001
81. Chen L, Miller FL, Malmkvist G *et al*: High-dose almitrine bimesylate inhibits hypoxic pulmonary vasoconstriction in closed-chest dogs. Anesthesiology 67:534, 1987
82. Furchgott RF, Vanhoutte PM: Endothelium derived relaxing and contracting factors. FASEB J 3:2007, 1989
83. Fischer SR, Deyo DJ, Bone HG *et al*: Nitric oxide synthase inhibition restores HPV in sepsis. Am J Respir Crit Care Med 156:833, 1997
84. Frostell CG, Blomqvist H, Hedenstierna G *et al*: Inhaled nitric oxide selectively reverses human HPV without causing systemic vasodilation. Anesthesiology 78:427, 1993
85. Troncy E, Francoeur M, Blaise G: Inhaled nitric oxide: Clinical applications, indications and toxicology. Can J Anaesth 44:973, 1997
86. Moutafis M, Liu N, Dalibon N *et al*: The effects of inhaled nitric oxide and its combination with intravenous almitrine on Pa_{O_2} during one-lung ventilation in patients undergoing thoracoscopic procedures. Anesth Analg 85:1130, 1997
87. Moutafis M, Dalibon N, Colchen A, Fischler M: Improving oxygenation during bronchopulmonary lavage using nitric oxide inhalation and almitrine infusion. Anesth Analg 89:302, 1999
88. B'chir A, Mebassa A, Losserm MR *et al*: Intravenous almitrine bimesylate reversibly inhibits lactic acidosis and hepatic dysfunction in patients with lung injury. Anesthesiology 89:823, 1998
89. Doering EB, Hanson CW, Reily D *et al*: Improvement in oxygenation by phenylephrine and nitric oxide in patients with adult respiratory distress syndrome. Anesthesiology 87:18, 1997
90. Scherer R, Vigfusson G, Lawin P: Pulmonary blood flow reduction by prostaglandin $F_{2\alpha}$ and pulmonary artery balloon manipulation during one-lung ventilation in dogs. Acta Anaesth Scand 30:2, 1986
91. Frumin MJ, Epstein R, Cohen G: Apneic oxygenation in man. Anesthesiology 20:789, 1959
92. Sanders RD: Two ventilating attachments for bronchoscopes. Del Med J 39:170, 1967
93. Giesecke AH, Gerbershagen H, Dortman C *et al*: Comparison of the ventilating and injection bronchoscopes. Anesthesiology 38:298, 1973
94. Carden E: Recent improvements in anesthetic techniques for use during bronchoscopy. Otol Rhinol Laryngol 83:777, 1974
95. Vourc'h G, Fishler M, Michon F *et al*: Manual jet ventilation vs. high-frequency jet ventilation during laser resection of tracheo-bronchial stenosis. Br J Anaesth 55:973, 1983
96. Matsushima Y, Jones RL, King EG *et al*: Alterations in pulmonary mechanics and gas exchange during routine fiberoptic bronchoscopy. Chest 86:184, 1984
97. Satyanarayana T, Capan L, Ramanathan S *et al*: Bronchofiberscopic jet ventilation. Anesth Analg 59:350, 1980
98. Neuman G, Weingarten AE, Abramowitz RM *et al*: The anesthetic management of the patient with an anterior mediastinal mass. Anesthesiology 60:144, 1984
99. Bechard P, Letourneau L, Lacasse Y. Perioperative cardiorespiratory complications in adults with mediastinal mass: Incidence and risk factors. Anesthesiology 100:826, 2004
100. Oley LTC, Hnatiuk MC, Corcoran MC *et al*: Spirometry in surgery for anterior mediastinal masses. Chest 120:1152, 2001
101. Tempe DK, Arya R, Dubey S *et al*: Mediastinal mass resection: Femorofemoral cardiopulmonary bypass before induction of anesthesia in the management of airway obstruction. J Cardiothorac Vasc Anesth 15:233, 2001
102. Ferrari LR, Bedford RF: General anesthesia prior to treatment of anterior mediastinal masses in pediatric cancer patients. Anesthesiology 72:991, 1990
103. Shamberger RC: Preanesthetic evaluation of children with anterior mediastinal masses. Semin Pediatr Surg 8:61, 1999
104. DeSoto H: Direct laryngoscopy as an aid to relieve airway obstruction in a patient with a mediastinal mass. Anesthesiology 67:116, 1987
105. Barker SJ, Clarke C, Trivedi N *et al*: Anesthesia for thoracoscopic laser ablation of bullous emphysema. Anesthesiology 78:44, 1993
106. Brodsky JB, Cohen E: Video-assisted thoracoscopic surgery. Curr Opin Anaesthesiol 13:41, 2000
107. Plummer S, Hartley M, Vaughan RS: Anaesthesia for telescopic procedures in the thorax. Br J Anaesth 80:223, 1998
108. Neustein SM, Kahn P, Krellenstein DJ *et al*: Incidence of arrhythmias and

predisposing factors after thoracic surgery: Thoracotomy versus video-assisted thoracoscopy. J Cardiothorac Vasc Anesth 12:659, 1998
109. Benumof JL: Sequential one-lung ventilation for bilateral bullectomy. Anesthesiology 67:268, 1987
110. Argenziano M, Moazami N, Thomashow B *et al*: Extended indications for lung volume reduction surgery in advanced emphysema. Ann Thorac Surg 62:1588, 1996
111. Cohen E, Kirshner PA, Benumof JL: Case conference: Anesthesia for bullectomy. J Cardiothorac Anesth 4:119, 1990
112. Brantigan OC, Mueller E, Kress MB: A surgical approach to pulmonary emphysema. Am Rev Respir Dis 80:194, 1959
113. Cooper JD, Trulock EP, Triantafillou AN *et al*: Bilateral pneumonectomy (volume reduction) for chronic obstructive pulmonary disease. J Thorac Cardiovac Surg 109:106, 1995
114. Geddes D, Davies M, Koyama H *et al*: Effect of lung-volume-reduction surgery in patients with severe emphysema. N Engl J Med 343:239, 2000
115. Davies L, Calverley PMA: Lung volume reduction surgery in chronic obstructive pulmonary disease. Thorax 51(suppl 2):S29, 1996
116. Deslauriers J: History of surgery for emphysema. Semin Thorac Cardiovasc Surg 8:43, 1996
117. National Emphysema Treatment Trial Research Group: Rationale and design of the National Emphysema Treatment Trial: A prospective randomized trial of lung volume reduction surgery. The National Emphysema Treatment Trial Research Group. Chest 116:1750, 1999
118. Lando Y, Boiselle PM, Shade D *et al*: Effect of lung volume reduction surgery on diaphragm length in severe chronic obstructive pulmonary disease. Am J Respir Crit Care Med 159(3):796, 1999
119. Bloch KE, Li Y, Zhang J *et al*: Effect of surgical lung volume reduction on breathing patterns in severe pulmonary emphysema. Am J Respir Crit Care Med 156(2 Pt 1):553, 1997
120. Jorgensen K, Houltz E, Westfelt U, Nilsson F, Schersten H, Ricksten SE: Effects of lung volume reduction surgery on left ventricular diastolic filling and dimensions in patients with severe emphysema. Chest 124:1863, 2003
121. Celli BR, Montes de Oca M, Mendez R, Stetz J: Lung reduction surgery in severe COPD decreases central drive and ventilatory response to CO_2. Chest 112:902, 1997
122. Ingenito EP, Loring SH, Moy ML, Mentzer SJ, Swanson SJ, Reilly JJ: Interpreting improvement in expiratory flows after lung volume reduction surgery in terms of flow limitation theory. Am J Respir Crit Care Med 163:1074, 2001
123. McKenna RJ Jr, Brenner M, Fischel RJ *et al*: Patient selection criteria for lung volume reduction surgery. J Thorac Cardiovasc Surg 114:957, 1997
124. Slone RM, Pilgram TK, Gierada DS *et al*: Lung volume reduction surgery: Comparison of preoperative radiologic features and clinical outcome. Radiology 204:685, 1997
125. Hunsaker A, Ingenito E, Topal U, Pugatch R, Reilly J: Preoperative screening for lung volume reduction surgery: Usefulness of combining thin-section CT with physiologic assessment. Am J Roentgenol 170:309, 1998
126. Ingenito EP, Evans RB, Loring SH *et al*: Relation between preoperative inspiratory lung resistance and the outcome of lung-volume-reduction surgery for emphysema. N Engl J Med 338:1181, 1998
127. Wesley JR, Macleod WM, Mullard KS: Evaluation and surgery of bullous emphysema. J Thorac Cardiovasc Surg 63:945, 1972
128. Flaherty KR, Kazerooni EA, Curtis JL *et al*: Short-term and long-term outcomes after bilateral lung volume reduction surgery: Prediction by quantitative CT. Chest 119:1337, 2001
129. Fessler HE, Scharf SM, Permutt S: Improvement in spirometry following lung volume reduction surgery: Application of a physiologic model. Am J Respir Crit Care Med 165:34, 2002
130. Cederlund K, Tylen U, Jorfeldt L, Aspelin P: Classification of emphysema in candidates for lung volume reduction surgery: A new objective and surgically oriented model for describing CT severity and heterogeneity. Chest 122:590, 2002
131. National Emphysema Treatment Trial Research Group: Patients at high risk of death after lung-volume-reduction surgery. N Engl J Med 345:1075, 2001
132. Drazen JN: Surgery for emphysema—not for everyone. N Engl J Med 345:1126, 2001
133. Fishman A, Martinez F, Naunheim K *et al*: A randomized trial comparing lung-volume-reduction surgery with medical therapy for severe emphysema. N Engl J Med 348:2059, 2003
134. Gaissert HA, Trulock EP, Cooper JD *et al*: Comparison of early functional results after volume reduction or lung transplantation for chronic obstructive pulmonary disease. J Thorac Cardiovasc Surg 111:296, 1996
135. Triantafillou AN: Anesthetic management for bilateral volume reduction surgery. Semin Thorac Cardiovasc Surg 8:94, 1996
136. Hurford WE, Dutton RP, Alfille PH *et al*: Comparison of thoracic and lumbar epidural infusions of bupivacaine and fentanyl for post-thoracotomy analgesia. J Cardiothorac Vasc Anesth 5:521, 1993
137. Wakabayashi A: Thoracoscopic technique for management of giant bullous disease. Ann Thorac Surg 56:708, 1993
138. Cohen E, Eisenkraft JB: Bronchopulmonary lavage: Effects on oxygenation and hemodynamics. J Cardiothorac Anesth 4:119, 1990
139. Drachman DB: Myasthenia gravis: Review article. N Engl J Med 330:1797, 1994
140. Eisenkraft JB, Neustein SM: Anesthesia for esophageal and mediastinal surgery. In Kaplan JA (ed): Thoracic Anesthesia, 3rd ed, p 269.New York, Churchill-Livingstone, 2003.
141. Nilsson E, Muller K: Neuromuscular effects of isoflurane in patients with myasthenia gravis. Acta Anaesthesiol Scand 34:126, 1990
142. Smith CE, Donati F, Bevan DR: Cumulative dose-response curves for atracurium in patients with myasthenia gravis. Can J Anaesth 36:402, 1989
143. Baraka A, Siddik S, Kawkabani N: Cisatracurium in a myasthenic patient undergoing thymectomy. Can J Anaesth 46:779, 1999
144. Baraka AS, Taha SK, Kawkabani NI: Neuromuscular interaction of sevoflurane—cisatracurium in a myasthenic patient. Can J Anaesth 47:562, 2000
145. Seigne RD, Scott RPF: Mivacurium chloride and myasthenia gravis. Br J Anaesth 72:468, 1994
146. Mann R, Blobner M, Jelen-Esselborn *et al*: Preanesthetic train-of-four fade predicts the atracurium requirement of myasthenia gravis patients. Anesthesiology 93:346, 2000
147. Itoh H, Shibata K, Nitta S: Difference in sensitivity to vecuronium between patients with ocular and generalized myasthenia gravis. Br J Anaesth 87:885, 2001
148. Itoh H, Shibata K, Nitta S: Sensitivity to vecuronium in seropositive and seronegative patients with myasthenia gravis. Anesth Analg 96:1842, 2003
149. Eisenkraft JB, Book WJ, Papatestas AE, Hubbard M: Resistance to succinylcholine in myasthenia gravis: A dose-response study. Anesthesiology 69:760, 1988
150. Baraka A, Tabboush Z: Neuromuscular response to succinylcholine-vecuronium sequence in three myasthenic patients undergoing thymectomy. Anesth Analg 72:827, 1991
151. Della Rocca G, Coccia C, Diana L *et al*: Propofol or sevoflurane anesthesia without muscle relaxants allow the early extubation of myasthenic patients. Can J Anesth 50:547, 2003
152. Madi-Jebara, Yazigi A, Hayek M *et al*: Sevoflurane anesthesia and intrathecal sufentanil-morphine for thymectomy in myasthenia gravis. J Clin Anesthesia 14:558, 2002
153. Abe S, Takeuchi C, Kaneko T *et al*: Propofol anesthesia combined with thoracic epidural anesthesia for thymectomy for myasthenia gravis—a report of eleven cases. Masui 50:1217, 2001
154. Chevalley C, Spiliopoulos A, dePerrot M *et al*: Perioperative medical management and outcome following thymectomy for myasthenia gravis. Can J Anesth 48:446, 2001
155. Lorimer M, Hall R: Remifentanil and propofol total intravenous anaesthesia for thymectomy in myasthenia gravis. Anaesth Intens Care 26:210, 1998
156. Baraka AS, Haroun-Bizri ST, Georges FJ: Delayed postoperative arousal following remifentanil-based anesthesia in a myasthenic patient undergoing thymectomy. Anesthesiology 100:460, 2004
157. Ingersoll-Weing E, Manecke GR, Thistlethwaite PA: Dexmedetomidine and cardiac arrest. Anesthesiology 100:758, 2004
158. Eisenkraft JB, Papatestas AE, Kahn CH *et al*: Predicting the need for postoperative mechanical ventilation in myasthenia gravis. Anesthesiology 65:79, 1986
159. Mori T, Yoshioka M, Watanabe K *et al*: Changes in respiratory condition after thymectomy for patients with myasthenia gravis. Ann Thorac Cardiovasc Surg 9:93, 2003
160. Burgess FW, Wilcosky B: Thoracic epidural anesthesia for transsternal thymectomy in myasthenia gravis. Anesth Analg 69:529, 1989
161. Gorback MS: Analgesic management after thymectomy. Anesthesiol Rep 2:262, 1990
162. Itoh H, Shibata K, Nitta S: Neuromuscular monitoring in myasthenic syndrome. Anesthesia 56:562, 2001
163. Telford RJ, Hollway TE: The myasthenic syndrome: Anesthesia in a patient treated with 3,4 diaminopyridine. Br J Anaesth 64:363, 1990
164. Kavanagh BP, Katz J, Sandler AN: Pain control after thoracic surgery: A review of current techniques. Anesthesiology 81:737, 1994
165. Whiting WG, Sandler AN, Lau LC *et al*: Analgesic and respiratory effects of epidural sufentanil in post-thoracotomy patients. Anesthesiology 69:36, 1988
166. Cohen E, Neustein SM: Intrathecal morphine during thoracotomy. J Thorac Cardiovasc Anesth 7:154, 1993
167. Katz J, Kavanagh BP, Sandler AN *et al*: Preemptive analgesia. Anesthesiology 77:439, 1992
168. Beck-Nielsen J, Sorensen HR, Alstrup P: Atrial fibrillation following thoracotomy for non-cardiac cases, in particular, cancer of the lung. Acta Med Scand 193:425, 1973
169. Ritchie J, Bowe P, Gibbons JRP: Prophylactic digitalization for thoracotomy: A reassessment. Ann Thorac Surg 50:86, 1990

CHAPTER 30 ■ CARDIOVASCULAR ANATOMY AND PHYSIOLOGY

CAROL L. LAKE

KEY POINTS

1. The two coronary arteries originate from the sinuses of Valsalva in the cusps of the aortic valve. The left coronary artery branches into the anterior descending and circumflex branches, whereas the right coronary artery branches to the sinus and atrioventricular (AV) nodes.
2. Cardiac innervation includes sympathetic fibers from the stellate ganglion and caudal cervical sympathetic trunks, as well as parasympathetic fibers from the recurrent laryngeal and thoracic vagus. Vagal innervation affects the atrial musculature, sinoatrial (SA) and AV nodes, and ventricular myocardium, whereas sympathetic fibers are in all portions of the atria, ventricles, and conduction system.
3. The venous pressure waveform (seen in the right atrium [RA], left atrium [LA], and pulmonary wedge pressure tracings) includes the a wave of atrial contraction, the *V* wave representing the gradual increase in atrial blood volume as blood returns from the periphery, and the *Y* wave resulting from opening of the AV valve combined with ventricular relaxation.
4. Extracellular ions cross the cell membranes of myocardial cells through specialized membrane proteins called the ion channels, which are named for the ion most rapidly transferred and characterized by conductance, selectivity, gating, and density. Density is the number of channels per square micrometer. Gating is the property of the channel that allows it to be activated or inactivated in response to voltage changes or binding of an agonist.
5. Coronary perfusion is 4% of the cardiac output or about 250 mL/minute. Coronary circulation consists of large, low-resistance epicardial vessels and higher resistance intramyocardial arteries and arterioles. Coronary perfusion mainly occurs during diastole.
6. Myocardial oxygen consumption is 8 to 10 mL/100 g per minute; therefore, coronary venous blood is only 30% saturated, and its po_2 is 18 to 20 mm Hg. Coronary perfusion is autoregulated to maintain a constant flow over a range of perfusion pressure between 50 and 120 mm Hg at any myocardial oxygen demand. Above and below these limits, coronary flow varies with perfusion pressure.
7. Cardiac output, the volume of blood pumped by the heart each minute, is the product of heart rate and stroke volume. It is determined by preload, afterload, heart rate, contractility, and ventricular compliance.
8. Cardiac output is distributed to the systemic circulation as follows: brain 12%, heart 4%, liver 24%, kidneys 20%, muscle 23%, skin 6%, and intestines 8%. The veins accommodate 64% of the blood, and 15% is in the heart and pulmonary circulation at any time.
9. Arterial pressure is the lateral pressure exerted by contained blood on the walls of the vessels. Mean arterial pressure is the product of cardiac output and systemic vascular resistance. As blood moves peripherally in circulation, pulse pressure and systolic pressure increase, while mean pressure remains constant.
10. Peripheral vascular tone is controlled by central and autonomic nervous function, cardiac output, peripheral vascular resistance, hormonal mechanisms (catecholamines, renin-angiotensin system, atrial natriuretic peptide, antidiuretic hormone), and nitric oxide.

Perioperative management of patients during either cardiac or noncardiac surgery requires an extensive knowledge of cardiovascular anatomy and physiology. In addition, knowledge of genomics and proteomics will be essential as these fields revolutionize their approaches to diagnosis, risk assessment, and therapies for cardiovascular disease.[1] Whereas genomics is the sequencing, modification, and functioning of the DNA and messenger RNA (mRNA) of the genome, proteomics is the sequence, modification, and function of the proteins of a biological system (see Chapter 7).

ANATOMY

Heart

Transesophageal echocardiography[2] (Fig. 30-1) visualizes the functional anatomy of the four cardiac chambers, four valves, and great vessels.

Right Atrium

Systemic veins drain into the right atrium (RA) via the superior vena cava (SVC), inferior vena cava (IVC), and coronary sinus. The ostium of the IVC is guarded by the eustachian valve, whereas the ostium of the coronary sinus is guarded by the Thebesian valve. The right and left atria are separated by the interatrial septum with its central fossa ovalis, the remnant of the fetal foramen ovale.

Blood leaving the RA passes through the anterior, posterior, and medial leaflets of the tricuspid valve. The anterior leaflet, the largest, is attached to the crista supraventricularis (the structure dividing the inflow [sinus] and outflow [infundibular] portions of the right ventricle [RV]) and controlled by the anterior papillary muscle (APM). The APM originates from a prominent intraventricular muscle, the moderator band, and the anterolateral ventricular wall. Connecting the papillary muscles to the valve leaflets are strong, fibrous structures known as the chordae tendineae.

Right Ventricle

The RV is a pocket wrapped around one-third of the left ventricle (LV), and its muscle fibers are continuous with those of the LV. The inflow portion contains prominent muscle bands (moderator, septal, and parietal) and muscle bundles known as trabeculae carneae. The crista supraventricularis also joins the interventricular septum and LV to the right ventricular free wall.

Pulmonary Artery and Peripheral Pulmonary Circulation

The pulmonic valve separates the right ventricular infundibulum (right ventricular outflow tract) from the main pulmonary artery (PA). It is a trileaflet valve (right, left, and anterior cusps) normally about 4 cm^2 in area. As it originates from the superior portion of the RV, the PA passes under the aorta before it bifurcates into the right and left pulmonary arteries. The remnant of the fetal ductus arteriosus, the ligamentum arteriosum, connects the upper aspect of the bifurcation to the inferior aortic surface.

Most pulmonary arteries run adjacent to the airways. Pulmonary arteries branch into arterioles and thence into capillaries, which spread over the alveolar surfaces between two alveolar endothelial layers. Larger pulmonary arteries (>1 mm internal diameter) are elastic, but the smooth muscle layer is reduced distal to the respiratory bronchioles. The pulmonary arteries and veins of the lower lobes are normally larger and more prominent than those of the upper lobes. The pulmonary circulation is innervated by the sympathetic system, and α_2 and probably α_1 receptors are present.[3]

The size of the peripheral pulmonary vessels indicates pulmonary blood volume and flow. With left-to-right cardiac shunts, the main PA and hilar vessels are prominent. With pulmonary hypertension, however, dilation of the main PA and abrupt tapering of the peripheral pulmonary vessels are noted.

Left Atrium

The left atrium (LA) is slightly larger than the right, and receives one or two pulmonary veins on its left and two or three on its right side. It has three major functions: (1) reservoir for pulmonary venous blood, (2) conduit to empty its contents into the LV, and (3) active contractile chamber.[4] Leaving the LA, blood traverses the mitral valve consisting of two major anteromedial and posterolateral leaflets, papillary muscles, and chordae tendineae. The normal adult mitral valve is about 6 to 8 cm^2 in area. The blood supply to the mitral chordae and papillary muscles is often quite tenuous.[5]

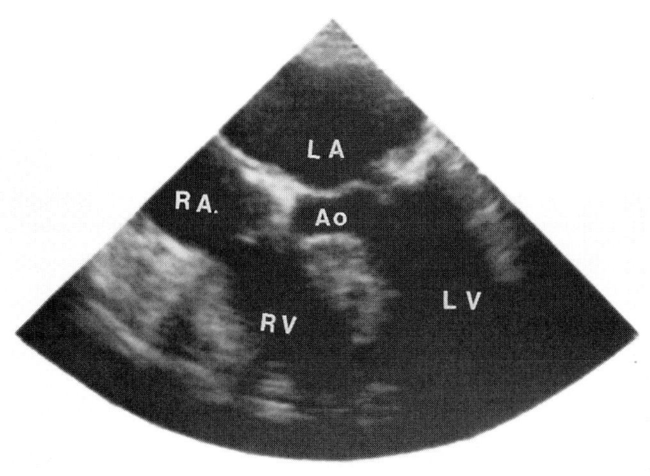

FIGURE 30-1. The functional anatomy of all four cardiac chambers, atrioventricular valves, aortic outflow track, and interatrial and interventricular septa are easily visualized using either transthoracic or transesophageal echocardiography. LA, left atrium; RA, right atrium; Ao, aorta; RV, right ventricle; LV, left ventricle.

Left Ventricle

Normally, the LV is thicker (8 to 15 mm) and more densely trabeculated than the right. Its internal dimension is also greater, about 4.5 cm compared with 3.5 cm for the RV.[6] The interventricular septum has a membranous superior portion near the aortic valve and a muscular inferior portion. Both ventricles consist of an inner layer, the endocardium covered with endothelium, the myocardium or muscle layer, and the outer layer, the epicardium.

Aorta and Its Branches

1 The aortic valve is adjacent to the mitral valve, separated only by the fibrous tissue framework that comprises the annuli of both valves. Three cusps, the right and left (coronary) and posterior (noncoronary) cusps, form the valve. A normal aortic valve is about 3 to 4 cm^2 in area. The aorta at the level of the valve dilates to form the Sinuses of Valsalva in which the coronary ostia are located.

The ascending aorta just beyond the aortic valve has no branches. Major branches of the aorta, the innominate, left carotid, and left subclavian arteries, arise from the aortic arch. The innominate artery subdivides into the right subclavian and right carotid arteries.

Coronary Circulation

1 Two coronary arteries, right and left, originate from the sinuses of Valsalva in the aortic valve to supply blood to the myocardium. The left coronary artery usually has a short common or left main coronary artery before bifurcation into anterior descending and circumflex branches. The anterior descending artery courses downward over the anterior left ventricular wall and supplies the interventricular groove through its diagonal and septal perforator branches. Occlusive disease in the anterior descending distribution produces ischemic electrocardiographic changes in leads V_3 to V_5. The circumflex branch follows the AV groove, giving off the obtuse marginal branch and supplying all the posterior LV and part of the right ventricular wall.[7] Electrocardiogram (ECG) changes resulting from circumflex coronary artery disease are seen in leads I and aV_L (Fig. 30-2 and Table 30-1).

TABLE 30-1

CORONARY ARTERY DISTRIBUTION

■ LEFT CORONARY ARTERY
Anterior descending branch
Right bundle branch
Left bundle branch
Anterior and posterior papillary muscles (mitral)
Anterolateral left ventricle
■ CIRCUMFLEX BRANCH
Lateral left ventricle
■ RIGHT CORONARY ARTERY
SA and AV nodes
Right atrium and ventricle
Posterior interventricular septum
Posterior fascicle of left bundle branch
Interatrial septum

AV, atrioventricular; SA, sinoatrial.

The sinus node and AV nodal arteries originate from the right coronary artery. The right atrial myocardium is also supplied by the sinus node artery. The right coronary artery terminates on the diaphragmatic surface of the heart as the posterior descending artery[8] (see Fig. 30-2). The blood supply to the AV node and common bundle of His is the AV branch of the right coronary artery (in 90% of hearts) and the septal perforating branches of the left anterior descending coronary artery (in 10% of hearts).[9] Branches to the interatrial septum and posterior interventricular septum also arise from the AV nodal artery. The right bundle branch and the left anterior fascicle are supplied by branches of the left anterior descending artery but can be supplied by the AV nodal artery. Both the left anterior and posterior descending coronary arteries supply the posterior fascicle.[9] Significant right coronary artery occlusion causes ischemic changes in ECG leads II, III, and aV_F, as well as conduction abnormalities.

Coronary Dominance. Descriptions of the coronary circulation often refer to the dominance of one or the other coronary artery. Dominance is determined by which artery crosses the

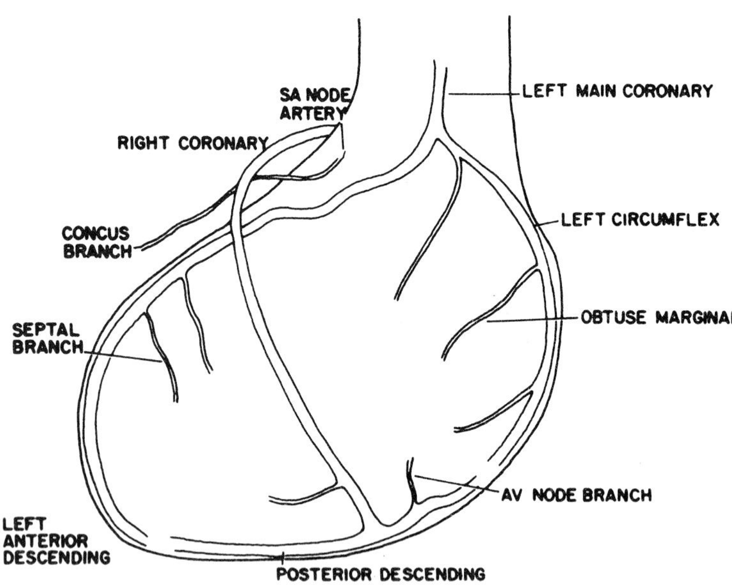

FIGURE 30-2. In this lateral view, the normal left coronary artery divides into the anterior descending and circumflex coronary arteries. The right coronary artery usually gives off the arteries to the sinoatrial (SA) and atrioventricular (AV) nodes before terminating on the inferior surface of the heart as the posterior descending artery.

crux or junction between atria and ventricles to supply the posterior descending coronary branch. In about 50% of humans, the right coronary artery is dominant; in 20%, the left; and in 30%, a balanced pattern exists. Areas of the myocardium affected by stenosis or occlusion of individual coronary arteries are listed in Table 30-1. Collateral vessels may develop between the major coronary arteries in response to myocardial ischemia.

Peripheral Venous Circulation

Major veins follow a course similar to that of the arteries. From the head, the internal and external jugular veins join the subclavian veins of either side. The course of the external jugular vein is often tortuous and variable, and it has two sets of valves, one at the entrance to the subclavian vein and the other about 4 cm superior to the clavicle. From the arms, the basilic (medial aspect) and cephalic veins join as the brachial vein. This vein becomes the axillary vein in the axilla and thence the subclavian. Normally, subclavian veins from both sides unite to form the SVC.

Cardiac veins, the great and middle cardiac veins and the posterior left ventricular vein, drain into the coronary sinus. Near the orifice of the great cardiac vein, the oblique vein of Marshall (vein of the LA) enters the coronary sinus. Anterior cardiac veins and the small cardiac vein may enter the RA independently of the coronary sinus. Thebesian veins, which traverse the myocardium, drain into various cardiac chambers. Thebesian venous flow, coupled with bronchial and pleural venous flows, contributes the normal 1 to 3% arteriovenous shunt.

Cardiac Conduction System

The system for electrical activation of the heart, the conduction system, consists of the SA node, the AV node, the bundle of His, right and left bundle branches, and the Purkinje system. Nodal cells of both spider and spindle pacemaker cell types are found in the center of the SA node, whereas atrial cells are found near the periphery.[10] The SA node is in the right atrial wall at the junction of the RA with the SVC. The SA and AV nodes are connected via the internodal conduction system, which consists of three tracts: the anterior (Bachmann's bundle), middle, and posterior internodal systems.[11] Conduction also spreads rapidly through the atrial musculature to the LA via Bachmann's bundle. In human hearts, the AV node is located in the floor of the RA, near the ostium of the coronary sinus.[7] The AV node consists of four areas, the A-N transitional zone containing cells smaller than normal atrial cells, the compact node, the posterior nodal extension, and a lower nodal cell bundle.[12] The fibers forming the common bundle of His pass along the superior edge of the membranous interventricular septum to the apex of the muscular portion of the septum. Here the bundle divides into right and left bundle branches, which extend subendocardially along the surfaces of both ventricles. The right bundle branch emerges in the right ventricular endocardium near the moderator band at the base of the anterior papillary muscle. It usually extends for some distance without dividing, but one branch passes through the moderator band and the other passes over the right ventricular endocardial surface. Subdivision of the left bundle into anterior and posterior fascicles occurs shortly after its origin. There is also a small collection of short medial fascicles that originate from the left bundle just after the anterior fascicle and activate the septal myocardium. The posterior fascicle terminates in the posterior papillary muscle.

Peripherally, the fascicles of both right and left bundle branches subdivide to form the Purkinje network. The left bundle branch fascicles make their initial functional contact with the endocardium of the interventricular septum below the aortic valve. Right bundle branch fascicles contact ventricular subendocardium near the base of the anterior papillary muscle.

Cardiac and Vascular Nerves

Sympathetic System

Nerves to the heart and blood vessels originate from sympathetic neurons of the thoracolumbar region and parasympa-
2 thetic nerves originate from the cervical region. Sympathetic fibers come from the stellate ganglion and the caudal cervical sympathetic trunks. From these trunks arise the right dorsal medial and dorsal lateral cardiac nerves, which frequently unite to form one large nerve that follows the course of the left main coronary artery. It further separates into branches along the anterior descending and circumflex coronary arteries.

Parasympathetic System

Parasympathetic preganglionic neurons arise in the medulla oblongata in the dorsal vagal nucleus and the nucleus ambiguous. These fibers enter the thorax as branches from the recurrent laryngeal and thoracic vagus nerve. The dorsal and ventral cardiopulmonary plexuses between the aortic arch and the tracheal bifurcation receive both sympathetic and parasympathetic branches. From the plexuses emerge three large cardiac nerves, the right and left coronary cardiac nerves and the left lateral cardiac nerve. Parasympathetic nerves are particularly abundant near the coronary sinus and SVC. Ganglia occur within the heart, usually close to the structures innervated by the short postganglionic neurons. Postganglionic transmission occurs from stimulation of nicotinic cholinergic receptors at the postganglionic junction by acetylcholine. Release of acetylcholine at the neuroeffector junction activates muscarinic receptors in the heart.

Cerebral Vasomotor Center

Afferent nerves from the heart ascend via the tenth cranial nerve (vagus) and spinal cord to the nucleus tractus solitarius and the dorsal vagal nucleus and nucleus ambiguous to form the parasympathetic motor efferent system of the medullary vasomotor center. Sympathetic activation of heart and vasculature originates in the rostral ventrolateral (RVL) medulla, ventromedial rostral medulla, and parvocellular region of the paraventricular nucleus. The RVL neurons receive multiple inputs from other medullary nuclei and modulate sympathetic output.[13] Although the vasomotor center independently regulates arterial pressure, blood flow distribution, and cardiac contractility, higher centers such as the cerebral cortex, hypothalamus, and pons also influence cardiovascular responses (Fig. 30-3).

Cardiac Receptors. Vagal receptors located in various cardiac chambers are sensitive to changes in heart rate or chamber pressure. Vagal innervation affects the atrial musculature, the SA and AV nodes, and the ventricular myocardium.[14] The greatest concentrations of parasympathetic nerves are in the SA node, with lesser numbers in the AV node, RA, LA, and ventricles. Parasympathetic α_1 but not α_2 receptors have been identified. Stimulation of cardiac parasympathetic nerves causes negative chronotropic and dromotropic effects.[15]

Sympathetic fibers extend to all portions of the atria, ventricles, and conduction system. α_1, α_2, β_1, and β_2 subtypes of adrenergic receptors are present. Human RA contains about 74% β_1 and 26% β_2 receptors.[16] The proportions of β receptors differ in the ventricle, with 86% β_1 and 14% β_2.

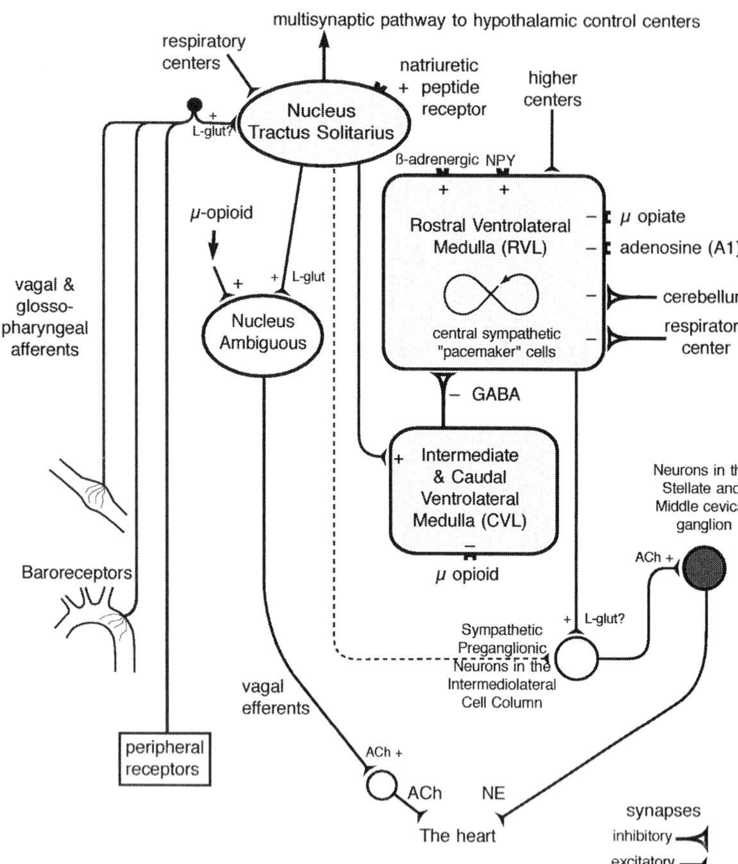

FIGURE 30-3. The central nervous system exerts considerable control over the heart and circulation via the rostral ventrolateral medulla (RVL), nucleus tractus solitarius, and intermediate and caudal ventrolaterial medulla. The RVL contains neurons that provide regular output to sympathetic preganglionic neurons like a pacemaker. The baroreceptor pathway, effects of GABAergic input, and opioid effects on RVL are also depicted. (Reprinted with permission from Lynch C, Lake CL: Cardiovascular anatomy and physiology. In Youngberg J, Lake C, Roizen M *et al* (eds): Cardiac, Vascular and Thoracic Anesthesia, p 136. Philadelphia, Churchill Livingstone, 2000.)

Neural Supply of the Peripheral Vasculature

Innervation of the peripheral circulation, with the exception of the cerebral and coronary vasculature, originates from the thoracolumbar sympathetic fibers. Vasodilation results from reduced sympathetic tone or activation of vasodilatory receptors. Stimulation of α-adrenergic fibers causes constriction in the arterial vascular beds of the skin, skeletal muscle, splanchnic organs, kidneys, and systemic veins. Stimulation of β_2 receptors dilates systemic veins and arteries of the muscle, splanchnic, and renal circulations.

Pericardium

The normal pericardium consists of thick fibrous and serous visceral layers. It has certain anatomic functions, among which are the isolation of the heart from other mediastinal structures, maintenance of the heart in optimal functional shape and position, minimization of cardiac dilatation, and prevention of adhesions.[17] The pericardium also contains vagal nerve branches.

CARDIOVASCULAR DIAGNOSTIC PROCEDURES

Abnormalities of both the anatomy and physiology of the cardiovascular system are diagnosed by invasive catheterization when noninvasive procedures such as echocardiography (cross reference section on echocardiography) or magnetic resonance angiography insufficiently define the defects.

Cardiac Magnetic Resonance Imaging

Cardiac magnetic resonance imaging (CMRI) is rapidly becoming the most comprehensive technique for evaluation and quantification of global and regional wall motion, wall thickening (contractility), ejection fraction, myocardial mass, ejection fraction, and blood flow (magnitude, direction, and shunt).[18] It is complementary to echocardiography for diagnosis of congenital cardiac defects.[19] The combination of CMRI and pharmacologic stress with dobutamine or adenosine stress assesses contractile reserve. Thus, its use may replace resting/stress echocardiography, thallium scintigraphy, and positron emission tomography for evaluation of myocardial viability (stunning, hibernating, or scarring).[20] However, it cannot substitute for coronary angiography in the evaluation of small branch arteries.

Catheterization

In all age groups, cardiac catheterization is usually performed via the femoral vessels. Occasionally, the brachial vessels are used in adults if the femoral vessels cannot be entered or catheters cannot be manipulated through the abdominal aorta.[21] The passage of catheters through either the venous or the arterial system is guided by fluoroscopy. Pressure measurements are made in each cardiac chamber or great vessel, their pressure waveforms recorded, and vascular or ventricular angiography performed. Normal pressure values and oxygen saturations are presented in Table 30-2. Oxygen saturation is greater in the IVC than in the SVC, owing to the contribution of blood from the renal veins. Normal pressure waveforms are

TABLE 30-2

NORMAL CATHETERIZATION DATA

■ SITE	■ PRESSURE (mm Hg)	■ OXYGEN SATURATION (%)
Inferior vena cava	0–8	80 ± 5
Superior vena cava	0–8	70 ± 5
Right atrium	0–8	75 ± 5
Right ventricle	15–30/0–8	75 ± 5
Pulmonary artery	15–30/4–12	75 ± 5
Pulmonary wedge	5–12 (mean)	75 ± 5
Left atrium	12 (mean)	95 ± 1
Left ventricle	100–140/4–12	95 ± 1
Aorta	100–140/60–90	95 ± 1

seen in Figure 30-4. Measurements commonly made or calculated during cardiac catheterization are detailed in Tables 30-3 and 30-4. These include cardiac output, measurement of valve areas,[22] and calculation of shunt flows.

Angiography

Cineangiography with iodinated dyes is performed to quantitate ventricular contractility, to evaluate shunting between cardiac chambers, to demonstrate valvular regurgitation, or to delineate vascular outlines (e.g., pulmonary venous return, aortic dissection, pulmonary embolism). Angiography assesses the amount of valvular regurgitation by grading the amount of contrast agent reentering the chamber preceding the valve. For instance, in the case of aortic regurgitation, 1+ regurgitation is a small amount of contrast material entering the LV during diastole but clearing with each systole. The LV is faintly opacified during diastole and fails to clear with systole with 2+ regurgitation. In 3+ aortic regurgitation, the LV is progressively opacified during diastole and eventually completely opacified, whereas in 4+ aortic regurgitation, the LV is completely opacified on the first diastole and remains opacified for several beats. A similar grading system is used during echocardiography.

Coronary Arteriography

Selective coronary angiography using either the retrograde brachial technique of Sones or the percutaneous femoral approach of Amplatz or Judkins selectively evaluates each coronary artery for the presence and extent of coronary occlusive disease, aneurysm formation, or congenital anomalies (see Fig. 30-2). Coronary arteriography occasionally causes ventricular ectopy, the Bezold-Jarisch reflex, ventricular asystole, or fibrillation. More common are T-wave changes, bradycardia, and mild hypotension. Even in normal coronary arteries, injection of the right coronary artery produces T-wave inversion in lead II and injection of the left artery produces T-wave peaking in lead II.[23] These changes revert to normal when the catheter is removed from the coronary ostia or the blood pressure is increased by having the patient cough.

Determination of Shunts

A shunt exists when arterial and venous blood mix at either an intracardiac or an extracardiac location, usually as a result of a congenital cardiac malformation. The site of a shunt can be determined by measurement of oxygen saturations in various cardiac chambers. A 10% step-up in oxygen saturation at the atrial level indicates left-to-right shunting into the RA. A 5% step-up at the ventricular or aorticopulmonary level indicates shunting at that site.

PHYSIOLOGY

Cardiac Cycle

The cardiac cycle begins with the filling of the right and left atria while the tricuspid and mitral valves are closed (see
3 Fig. 30-4).[24,25] The V wave on the venous pressure waveform represents the gradual increase in atrial blood volume as blood returns from the periphery. Once the aortic valve has closed but ventricular pressure still exceeds atrial pressure, the ventricle undergoes isovolumetric relaxation. About 0.02 to 0.04 seconds after closure of the aortic valve, atrial and ventricular pressures equalize, and a small gradient develops across the AV valves as ventricular pressure decreases further. The AV valve cusps bulge into the ventricle and separate slightly. After crossover of the atrial and ventricular pressure waves, the AV valves open completely. The V wave of the atrial pressure waveform crests when the atria are filled, and the tricuspid and mitral valves open to initiate ventricular filling. The Y wave results from opening of the AV valves combined with ventricular relaxation. Effective atrial systole at resting heart rates contributes about 5 to 20% of the stroke volume. Acute atrial fibrillation increases atrial pressures, reduces atrial compliance, increases atrial oxygen consumption, and eliminates the contribution of the atria to ventricular filling.[26]

During initial ventricular filling, ventricular volume increases rapidly, the rapid filling phase, during which time the ventricular pressure continues to decrease because ventricular expansion exceeds filling. Peak ventricular filling in early diastole occurs at 500 to 700 mL/sec as ventricular relaxation actually produces a negative intracavitary pressure (diastolic suction). The elastic recoil of the heart and great vessels during diastole contributes to the accelerated filling phase of the ventricle, particularly during tachycardia.

A period of reduced ventricular filling follows the rapid filling phase. The third heart sound, S_3, occurs at the point of transition from rapid ventricular filling to reduced filling. The nadir of the ventricular pressure curve at the end of the rapid filling phase probably marks the end of ventricular relaxation and the beginning of elastic distention of the ventricle. The upswing in the ventricular pressure abolishes forward movement of blood and can force the AV valves into a semiclosed position unless venous return is great. The previous ventricular contraction provides much of the energy for the subsequent diastolic expansion through the energy expenditure of the gross movement and deformation of the heart during systole.[27] Atrial systole, the A wave on the venous pressure waveform, which coincides with the P wave on the ECG, concludes ventricular filling.

Right atrial pressure, a guide to right atrial and right ventricular function, is indirectly assessed by observation of the level of jugular venous pressure, the end-expiratory peak pulsation of the internal jugular vein above the sternal angle with the subject in a 30° reverse Trendelenburg position. Normally, the level is <4 cm. A sustained increase in the level of >1 cm during abdominal compression (hepatojugular reflux) indicates abnormal right ventricular function. Only when biventricular function is normal can the central venous pressure be used as a guide to left ventricular function.

There are three phases of activity in the LA: (1) the reservoir phase of inflow during ventricular diastole, (2) a conduit phase of passive emptying during ventricular end diastole, and (3) contraction and active emptying during ventricular end

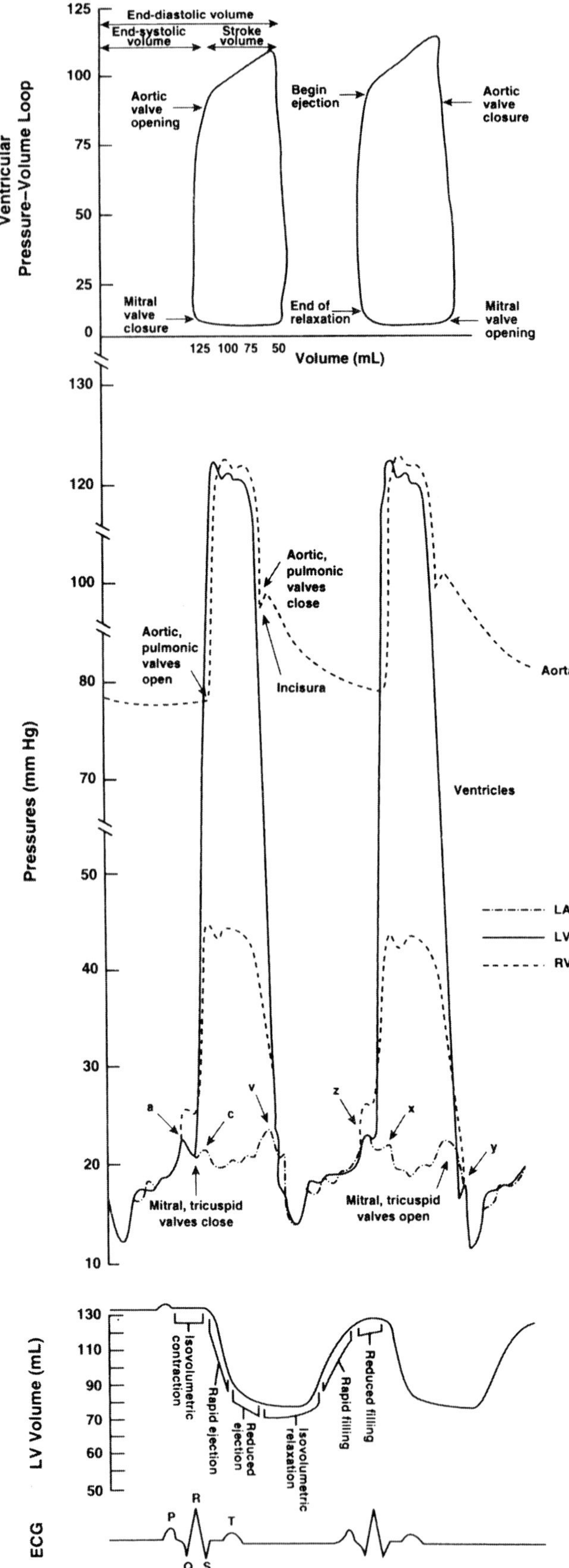

FIGURE 30-4. The events of the cardiac cycle from filling of the atria to ventricular emptying are demonstrated using waveforms from the aorta, pulmonary artery, right and left ventricles, and central veins. The relationship between the electrocardiogram and the phases of the cardiac cycle shows that ventricular systole occurs immediately following the QRS complex. The changes in ventricular pressure–volume waveform coincide with ventricular ejection and filling. ECG, electrocardiogram; LV, left ventricle.

TABLE 30-3

MEASUREMENTS DURING CARDIAC CATHERIZATION

FICK PRINCIPLE CARDIAC OUTPUT

$$\text{Cardiac Output (Q) (L/min)} = \frac{\dot{V}o_2}{Cao_2 - Cvo_2} \times 100$$

$\dot{V}o_2$ = oxygen consumption
Cao_2 = arterial oxygen content
Cvo_2 = venous oxygen content
Oxygen Content = $\alpha po_2 + 1.34\,\text{Hb} \times \%\text{Hb saturation}$
($\alpha = .0031$)

INDICATOR—DILUTION CARDIAC OUTPUT

$$\frac{60 \times \text{indicator dose (mg)}}{\text{average concentration} \times \text{time (sec)}}$$

Example: thermodilution (Stewart-Hamilton equation)

$$Q = \frac{V_1(T_B - T_1)K_1K_2}{\int_0^\infty T_B(t)\,dt}$$

V_1 = injectate volume
T_B = blood temperature
T_1 = injectate temperature
K_1 = density factor and is a function of the specific heat and specific gravity of injectate and specific heat and specific gravity of blood
K_2 = computation constant for deadspace of catheter, heat change in transit, injection rate
$\int T_B(t)\,dt$ = change in blood temperature as a function of time

SHUNT FLOWS

Qp = Qs = 1 No shunt
Bidirectional shunt

$$Qpe = \frac{\dot{V}o_2}{CPVo_2 - CMVo_2}$$

$CPVo_2$ = pulmonary venous oxygen content
$CMVo_2$ = mixed venous oxygen content
Qp − Qpe = L → R shunt
Qs − Qpe = R → L shunt
Qpe = effective pulmonary flow
Qp = pulmonary flow
Qs = systemic flow

VALVE AREAS

Aortic

$$\text{Valve area} = \frac{\text{Aortic Valve Flow (AVF)}}{1 \times 44.5\sqrt{AVG_{(systolic)}}}$$

$AVF = CO/SEP_{minute}$

$$SEP = \frac{\text{Systolic ejection period}}{\text{beat}} \times HR$$

Mitral

$$\text{Valve area} = \frac{\text{Mitral Valve Flow}}{0.7 \times 44.5\sqrt{MVG_{(diastolic)}}}$$

$MVF = CO/DFP_{minute}$

$$DFP = \frac{\text{Diastolic filling period}}{\text{beat}} \times HR$$

diastole.[28] Each left atrial function is affected by atrial relaxation, stiffness, and contractility.[28]

In hearts with poorly functioning ventricles, atrial contraction is important and a fourth heart sound, S_4, which occurs 0.04 seconds after the P wave, results from vibrations of left ventricular muscle and mitral valve. The S_4 is most likely to occur with vigorous atrial contraction. The adequacy of ventricular filling is determined by the distensibility (compliance) of the ventricles, the filling time, and the effective filling pressure. The effective filling pressure is the transmural ventricular pressure. Tachycardia also decreases the time available for ventricular filling, decreasing filling time from 400 to 500 milliseconds at a heart rate of 60 beats per minute to 10 milliseconds or less at 160 beats per minute. Mitral stenosis, ischemic heart

TABLE 30-4

HEMODYNAMIC VARIABLES: CALCULATIONS AND NORMAL VALUES

VARIABLE	CALCULATION	NORMAL VALUES
Cardiac index (CI)	CO/BSA	2.5–4.0 L/min/m^2
Stroke volume (SV)	CO/HR	60–90 mL/beat
Stroke index (SI)	SV/BSA	40–60 mL/beat/m^2
Mean arterial pressure (MAP)	Diastolic pressure + one-third pulse pressure	80–120 mm Hg
Systemic vascular resistance (SVR)	MAP – CVP/CO × 79.9	1200–1500 dyn/cm/s^5
Pulmonary vascular resistance (PVR)	PAP – PWP/CO × 79.9	100–300 dyn/cm/s^5
Right ventricular stroke work index (RVSWI)	0.0136 (PAP – CVP) SI	5–9 g/m/beat/m^2
Left ventricular stroke work index (LVSWI)	0.0136 (MAP – PWP) SI	45–60 g/m/beat/m^2

BSA, body surface area; CO, cardiac output; CVP, mean central venous pressure; MAP, mean arterial blood pressure; PAP, mean pulmonary artery pressure; PWP, pulmonary wedge pressure.

disease, and hypertrophic cardiomyopathy slow ventricular filling and alter ventricular distensibility. The intraventricular pressure just prior to the beginning of ventricular contraction is end-diastolic pressure (Table 30-2). However, normal end-diastolic pressures do not imply normal ventricular function. Increased end-diastolic pressures occur with hypervolemia or changes in ventricular compliance as well as decreased contractility.

The period just before the sudden increase in ventricular pressure is presystole, which includes atrial systole and the time just before isovolumetric ventricular contraction. The Z point on the venous pressure waveform is the period when atrial and ventricular pressures are essentially equal immediately preceding ventricular systole. The isovolumetric phase of ventricular contraction is marked by the C wave on the venous waveform. Isovolumetric contraction is the period between closure of the AV valves and opening of the semilunar (aortic, pulmonic) valves. Intraventricular pressure increases, but there is no change in intraventricular volume. After this point, the AV valves close, atrial diastole begins, the ventricles begin to contract, and ventricular pressure soon exceeds atrial pressure. Ventricular systole occurs immediately after the QRS complex on the ECG, about 0.12 to 0.20 seconds after atrial contraction. AV valve closure is facilitated by the increased ventricular pressure and the cessation of atrial systole. Closure of the AV valves is noted clinically by the normally split first heart sound, S_1.

Once the ventricular pressure exceeds the aortic pressure, the aortic and pulmonic valves open (at the summit of the C wave of the venous pressure waveform). The majority of ventricular ejections occur during the rapid ejection phase. The pressure in the aorta is slightly lower, whereas ventricular pressure increases rapidly. The atrial pressure decreases, resulting in the X descent because blood goes into the aorta and PA. Initially the output into the aorta exceeds the runoff into the peripheral circulation. Peak aortic pressure occurs slightly after peak aortic blood flow. As aortic runoff and ventricular output equilibrate, the period of reduced ventricular ejection occurs. Forward flow continues until the end of ventricular diastole, protodiastole, when a brief period of retrograde flow initiates aortic and pulmonic valve closure. On pressure waveforms, semilunar valve closure is marked by a notch or incisura. The second heart sound, S_2, results from rapid deceleration of blood causing vibration of the outflow tracks and great vessels and closure of the semilunar valves.

Cardiac Electrophysiology

Cellular Electrophysiology

Cardiac pacemaker cells have an intracellular ionic composition that differs from that found in the extracellular fluid. The most important ions are calcium, sodium, and potassium. An active transport system in the cell membrane, the sodium–potassium pump, maintains normal concentration gradients for sodium and potassium by pumping sodium ions out of the
4 cell and potassium ions into the cell. Extracellular ions cross the cell membrane through specialized membrane proteins, the ion channels, which are characterized by their conductance, selectivity, gating, and density. Because a more detailed discussion of the cardiac channels is beyond the scope of this chapter, the reader is referred to reviews on specific channels.[29–31] Conductance is the rate (ions/msec) at which ions pass through the channel. In a given channel, each ion has a particular conductance. Channels are named for the ion most rapidly transferred because some ions, but not others, are transported. Some channels rectify or pass current in one direction across the membrane more easily than the other. Density is described as the number of channels per square micrometer. However, density may be variable over the cellular sarcolemma.

Channels have three states: resting, open (activated), and inactivated. Gating is the property of the channel that allows it to be activated or inactivated in response to voltage changes or binding of an agonist. If gating kinetics are rapid, the channel activates or opens quickly. If the change in channel conformation is slow, channel activation is delayed as with delayed rectifier potassium channels. Examples of cardiac channels, which directly or indirectly control cardiac function, are given in Table 30-5. After an ion channel is activated, it may stay open until closed by another stimulus such as repolarization or inactivated (closed) in response to a continued stimulus.

The central portion of the SA node contains spider cells that have a faster intrinsic phase 4 depolarization rate, a less negative maximum diastolic potential (~−50 mV), and a longer action potential duration than other portions of the node or atrial, AV nodal, or His-Purkinje cells. The longer action potential duration and shorter interval between spontaneous action potentials preserves SA dominance and limits invasion by ectopic impulses.

β Receptors, consisting of the receptor, the G protein (guanosine triphosphate binding protein) system,[26] and adenylate cyclase are also located in the cell membrane. Receptors recognize and bind agonists, activating the G protein Gs, which, in turn, activates adenylate cyclase to stimulate hydrolysis of adenosine triphosphate (ATP) to cyclic adenosine monophosphate (cAMP). cAMP opens the calcium channel, permitting calcium influx. The entire complex forms a transmembrane signaling system (Fig. 30-5). β-Adrenergic receptor stimulation augments subsarcolemmal calcium release via the ryanodine receptors during diastolic depolarization and during the action potential upstroke.

The SA node is normally the dominant pacemaker because, in it, automaticity is most highly developed and impulses are initiated at the fastest rate. Activation of the sodium-calcium exchanger during diastolic depolarization, as well as cyclic variation in subsarcolemmal calcium release via the ryanodine receptor, act together with the cardiac ion channels to ensure the sinus node is the dominant pacemaker. Cardiac pacemaker regulation is critically dependent on the calcium release via ryanodine receptors.[32] In SA nodal cells, when the internal membrane potential reaches −50 mV, the depolarization rate increases to 1 to 2 V/sec, causing a slowly depolarizing action potential. Automaticity decreases in order from SA node, AV node, His bundle, proximal Purkinje fibers, and distal Purkinje fibers. The rate of phase 4 depolarization is faster in the SA node than in the AV node and faster in the AV node than in the terminal Purkinje fibers, causing less highly developed pacemakers to be depolarized by the propagated wave from above before they spontaneously depolarize. Interactions between sympathetic and parasympathetic innervations also affect the intrinsic depolarization rate.

The compound action potential in cells results from the integrated activity of different ionic transmembrane currents at different times in the cardiac cycle (see Fig. 30-5). Ionic transfer is facilitated by the energy released from the hydrolysis of ATP. The cardiac potassium current has four subunits: ether-a-go-go, mink-related channel subunit 1, long QT interval-related subunit, and beta subunit of I_{Ks} (minK). Pacemaker cells in the unexcited state are maintained at a resting potential of −80 mV by the selective inward rectifier current I_{K1}. These channels with inward rectification pass inward current more easily than outward and thus limit outward current flow. Thus, the resting membrane potential is around the equilibrium potential for potassium. As the slow spontaneous depolarization of phase 4 proceeds, there is an increase in the permeability of the membrane, which permits positively charged sodium ions

TABLE 30-5

CARDIAC ION CHANNELS

■ CHANNEL SUBUNITS	■ ION CURRENT	■ FUNCTION
Sodium (Nav 1.5)	I_{Na}	Conduction atrium, ventricle, Purkinje
HCN (hyperpolarization-activated, cyclic nucleotide binding)	If (pacemaking)	Diastolic depolarization
Kir 2.1	IK_1	Terminal repolarization, resting potential
Kir 3.1/3.4	IK_{ACH}	Mediation of acetylcholine effects
Ca_v3.1/3.3	$I_{Ca.t}$	Role uncertain
Ca_v1.2 I_{CaL}	α subunit	
Ether-a-go-go related (ERG)	I_{Kr}(α subunit)	Phase 3 repolarization
Kv4.2/4.3	I_{to}(α subunit)	Early phase 1 repolarization
minK	I_{ks}(β subunit)	Necessary to form I_{ka} with KvLQT1
MIRP1 (minK-related channel subunit)	Modulates I_{kr}, I_f, I_{to}	Function unclear
KvLQT1	I_{ka}(α subunit)	Phase 3 repolarization
KChIP2	I_{to} (β subunit)	Necessary to form I_{to}
Kv1.5/3.1	I_{kur}	Phase 1–2 repolarization

Data from Schram G, Pourrier M, Melnyk P, Nattel S: Differential distribution of cardiac ion expression as a basis for regional specialization in electrical function. Circ Res 90:939, 2002.

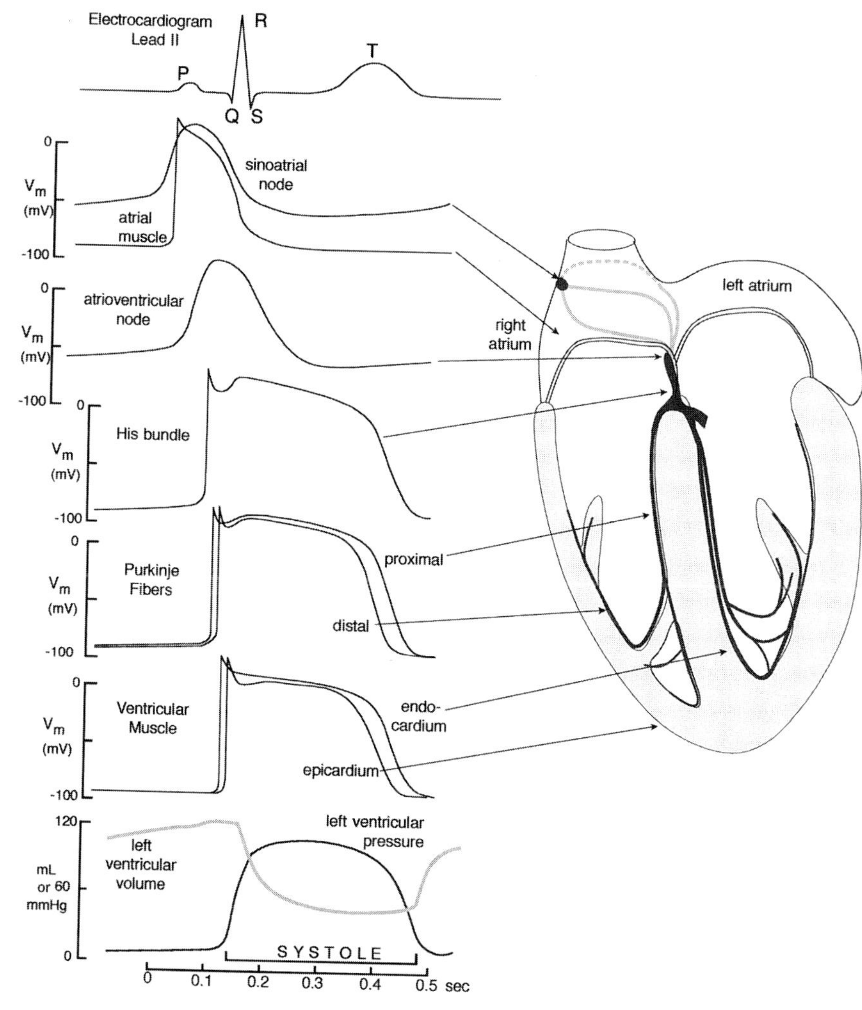

FIGURE 30-5. The action potential of an automatic cell such as the sinoatrial node differs from that of the ventricular muscle cell in that the cell slowly depolarizes spontaneously during phase 4. The inward current I_f is responsible for diastolic depolarization. The action potential in a Purkinje cell has the most rapid rate of depolarization, 400 to 800 V/sec. When the cell is stimulated, an action potential occurs due to a rapid influx of sodium ions (inward current) into the cell (phase 0). Phase 1 includes a notch caused by the "early outward current," I_{to}, which is a transient K efflux, probably activated by an intracellular calcium increase. Phase 2 is the plateau of the action potential resulting principally from calcium entry (inward currents I_{CaL} and I_{CaT}) through the slow channel of the cell membrane. During phase 3, repolarization of the cell occurs (outward current I_{K1}), while during phase 4, the sodium entering during phase 0 is actively pumped out of the cell. In a ventricular muscle cell, unlike the automatic cells, there is no spontaneous phase 4 depolarization. (Reprinted with permission from Lynch C, Lake CL: Cardiovascular anatomy and physiology. In Youngberg J, Lake C, Roizen M *et al* (eds): Cardiac, Vascular, and Thoracic Anesthesia, p 87. Philadelphia, Churchill Livingstone, 2000.)

to move across the cell membrane into the cell, resulting in depolarization at a threshold potential of ∼−65 to 70 mV. This sodium influx (fast sodium current, I_{Na}) reverses the transmembrane potential from −80 mV to +20 to 30 mV and initiates the rapid depolarization (phase 0) of the action potential in a cardiac pacemaker cell (see Fig. 30-5). Phase 0 lasts only 1 to 2 milliseconds. The sodium channels open and sodium ions enter the cell, causing the cell membrane potential to move toward the sodium equilibrium potential of +50 mV. During phase 0, there is also a decrease in permeability to potassium. At about −30 mV, inward calcium transfer (I_{CaL}) begins through the L-type (long-lasting, high-threshold) channels that require greater than −40 mV to activate for opening. The spread of depolarization throughout the atrial and ventricular muscle results in the P wave and the QRS complex of the ECG, respectively. After excitation, the cell membrane undergoes an initial period of rapid repolarization (phase 1), followed by a variable period when the membrane potential is close to 0, the plateau of the action potential. Early repolarization results from inactivation of the sodium current and activation of the potassium current I_{TO}. The principal subunits of I_{TO} are Kv1.4, Kv4.2, and Kv4.3. The plateau is caused by low potassium conductance with inward rectification of I_{K1} causing a small outward current. The outward current is balanced by inward current through the L-type calcium channel I_{Ca-L}, inward flux of chloride ions through the ATP-dependent cystic fibrosis transmembrane regulator channel, and slowly inactivating sodium channels.

Four K^+ currents participate in repolarization, including I_{TO_1}, the transient outward current during the initial phase of repolarization; I_{TO2}, the slow inactivating current; and delayed rectifier K currents I_{Kr} and I_{Ks} during final repolarization.[33] Rapid repolarization during phase 3 results from inactivation of L-type calcium current and increasing outward current through the delayed rectifier potassium channels. The duration of the action potential is rate dependent, owing to enhanced calcium entry. During phase 4, the resting membrane potential is generated by active exchange of intracellular sodium for potassium through the sodium-potassium adenosine triphosphatase or sodium pump. The resting potassium conductance that maintains the resting potential is G_{K1}, the inward (anomalous) rectifier. In the latter part of phase 4, the resting membrane potential is stable in ventricular muscle cells until the cell is excited again. In automatic cells such as the SA and AV nodes, slow, spontaneous depolarization occurs during phase 4 as a result of the hyperpolarization-activated inward current I_f and I_{K2}. The hyperpolarization-activated cation channel is more abundant in the SA node than in Purkinje cells or ventricular myocardium.

During depolarization, the cell membrane is absolutely refractory to other stimuli because almost all the sodium channels inactivate. The end of the absolute refractory period is signaled by the earliest transient depolarization that can be elicited because sufficient numbers of sodium channels that can be activated are present. The absolute refractory period ends at the beginning of the T wave of the ECG. Once repolarization reaches the threshold potential, the cell is relatively refractory, although an unusually strong stimulus can produce depolarization. This period is marked by the T wave of the ECG. The earliest propagated action potential defines the end of the effective or functional refractory period.

Action Potential Alterations

Changes in the action potential itself or factors that affect the action potential alter the rate of firing of an automatic cell. The rate of an automatic cell depends on the slope of phase 4 depolarization, the resting membrane potential [RMP], and the threshold potential.[34] The RMP is the maximum diastolic potential achieved at the end of repolarization. The variable expression of the previously described ion channels in different parts of the heart produces the characteristic electrophysiology of the pacemakers, conduction tissue, atria, and ventricles. Factors affecting the action potential are listed in Table 30-6.[34–37] In addition to effects on the action potential, alterations in potassium current affect membrane electrical stability. Low extracellular K^+ reduces conductance through the inward rectifier channel (G_{K1}). Thus, there is greater cellular excitability and tendency for ectopy. With increased extracellular K, more potassium current escapes from the cell and the membrane is relatively stable.

TABLE 30-6

ACTION POTENTIAL ALTERATIONS[30–32]

■ EFFECTS ON PHASE 4
Hypothermia ↓ slope
Hypothermia ↑ rate
Hypoxia ↑ slope
Ischemia ↑ slope
Hyperkalemia ↓ rate
Hypokalemia ↑ rate
Hyponatremia ↓ slope
Hypercarbia ↑ slope
Increased pH ↑ slope
■ EFFECTS ON ACTION POTENTIAL DURATION
Hypercalcemia ↓
Hypocalcemia ↑
■ EFFECTS ON DIASTOLIC DEPOLARIZATION
Hypoxia ↓ max diastolic potential
Hyperkalemia ↓ max diastolic potential
Hypercarbia ↓ max diastolic potential (Purkinje only)
Hypercarbia ↓ diastolic depolarization
Increased pH ↓ diastolic depolarization

Clinical Electrophysiology

The first wave of the normal ECG is the P wave, which is produced by atrial depolarization resulting from an action potential in the SA node. It is usually upright, except in lead aV_R, and 0.11 seconds in duration. Sinus node rate exhibits a circadian rhythm, decreasing nocturnally. Sinus node recovery time is also prolonged at night.[38]

An electrical impulse travels from the SA node to the AV node in 0.04 seconds via atrial tissue, specialized atrial conducting tissue, or the anterior, middle, and posterior tracts of the RA. Transmission is further delayed in the AV node because its conduction velocity is about 0.2 m/sec. The effective refractory period of the AV node demonstrates circadian rhythm and is increasingly prolonged at night. The P-R interval (normally 0.2 milliseconds or less), which occupies the time between atrial and ventricular depolarization, is nearly isoelectric, because atrial repolarization is not recordable. Significant interactions between the parasympathetic and sympathetic nervous systems control the conduction through the AV node with predominantly sympathetic activity.[39]

Ventricular depolarization begins ∼0.12 to 0.20 seconds in adults and 0.15 to 0.18 seconds in children after depolarization of the SA node to produce the QRS complex.[40] The entire QRS complex should be <0.10 seconds. The first negative wave of the QRS complex is the Q wave, which should be ≤0.04 seconds in duration and less than one-fourth of the subsequent R wave in amplitude. The first positive wave in the QRS is the R wave, and the second negative wave is the S wave. The right and left branches of the bundle of His connecting with the Purkinje fibers conduct the depolarizing impulse rapidly over the endocardial surface of the heart. Normally, in sinus rhythm the earliest area of ventricular activation is the trabecular area on the anterior right ventricular surface about 18 to 25 milliseconds after the surface QRS complex. Activation then spreads toward the apex and base of the heart, with the latest activation at the cardiac base. Electrical activation also spreads from endocardium to epicardium.

On the ECG, the time from the end of ventricular depolarization to the beginning of repolarization, the ST segment, is isoelectric. More than 1 mm of elevation in the standard leads or 2 mm of elevation in the precordial leads is abnormal in this segment. No more than 0.5 mm of depression should be seen in any lead. The J point, the junction between the QRS complex and the ST segment, is depressed or elevated with the ST segment. Ventricular repolarization results in the T wave. T waves are normally upright in leads I, II, and V_3 to V_6, inverted in lead aV_R, and variable in leads II, aV_L, aV_F, V_1, and V_2. The T wave should not exceed 5 mm in height in the standard leads or 10 mm in the precordial leads. The QT interval, varying inversely with heart rate, should be slightly less than one-half of the RR interval.[41] The U wave, a small upright deflection after the T wave, is usually nondetectable.

Physiology of the Cardiac Nerves

Neural Regulation

Neural regulation of the heart is complex. The dominance of either the sympathetic or the parasympathetic system varies with age and physical condition, but the inhibitory parasympathetic system usually predominates.[42,43] Parasympathetic stimulation, particularly of the right vagus nerve, decreases heart rate by slowing the SA node. Lower pacemakers such as the AV node or His bundle may take over, causing "nodal rhythm." Vagal stimulation tends to suppress ventricular automaticity, which may facilitate termination of ventricular dysrhythmias. Intense vagal stimulation depresses both atrial and ventricular contractility by stimulation of cardiac muscarinic receptors that alter the myocyte cAMP level, by inhibition of norepinephrine release from nearby sympathetic nerve terminals by acetylcholine, and by inhibition of adrenergic receptor activation. One of the G proteins, Gi, which inhibits adenylcyclase, lowering the levels of cAMP, is coupled with the muscarinic receptor to control potassium channels and decrease heart rate.

Stimulation of the stellate ganglion or other sympathetic cardiac fibers increases heart rate, contractility, and ejection fraction. The right stellate ganglion has a greater effect on heart rate, whereas the left has more effect on contractility. Abnormalities of sympathetic cardiac nerve tone occur in long QT interval syndromes.[44]

The role of the cardiac α receptors is unclear, but their action is modulated by G protein signal transduction (Fig. 30-6). β_1 Receptors of the heart have positive chronotropic, inotropic, and lusitropic effects on the heart by stimulation of adenylcyclase. Action potentials may be restored by β_1 stimulation owing to increased numbers of calcium channels that can be activated in sufficient density to permit regenerative ionic flux along a fiber. Activation of cardiac β_2 receptors also increases rate and contractility, particularly in end-stage heart failure. The effects of norepinephrine on contractility are mediated by increased calcium entry through more active calcium

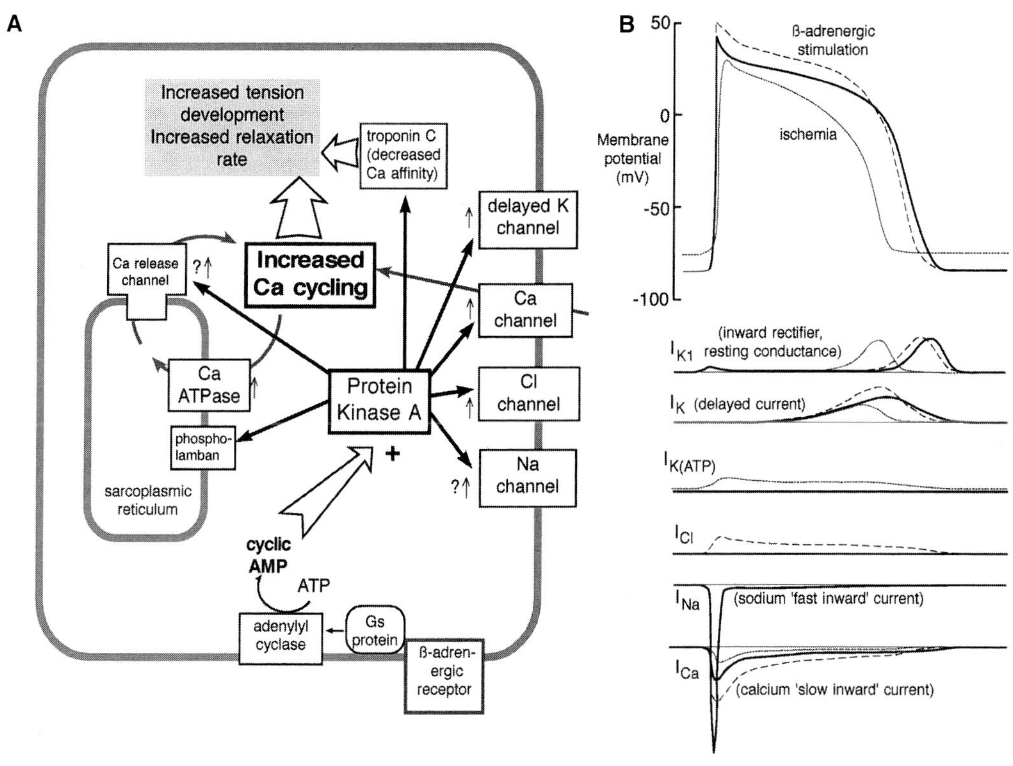

FIGURE 30-6. Effects of adrenergic stimulation on the heart. β-Adrenergically stimulated protein phosphorylation occurs owing to activation of protein kinase A and increased cyclic adenosine monophosphate production. Increased cycling of Ca^{2+} and phosphorylation of multiple ion channels (Ca, Cl, Na, and delayed K) occurs. AMP, adenosine monophosphate; ATP, adenosine triphosphate; ATPase, adenosine triphosphatase. (Reprinted with permission from Lynch C, Lake CL: Cardiovascular anatomy and physiology. In Youngberg J, Lake C, Roizen M *et al* (eds): Cardiac, Vascular, and Thoracic Anesthesia, p 100. Philadelphia, Churchill Livingstone, 2000.)

channels and increased sarcoplasmic reticular uptake of calcium. Increased sarcoplasmic uptake of calcium has a lusitropic effect, while making the increased calcium (in the sarcoplasmic reticulum [SR]) available for subsequent contractions (see Fig. 30-10).

Atrial Receptors

Parasympathetic receptors type A, type B, and receptors innervated by group C fibers reflexly alter intravascular volume or heart rate. The primary locations of type A and B receptors are the cavoatrial junction, pulmonary venous–atrial junction, atrial appendage, and atrial body.[45] Type A receptors may actually respond to heart rate rather than atrial pressure.[45] Type B receptors are stretch receptors whose discharge is closely related to atrial volume and varies with the rate of atrial pressure increase.

Ventricular Receptors

Stimulation of ventricular receptors causes either cardiovascular excitation or depression. Types of ventricular receptors include the pressure-sensitive coronary baroreceptors, mechanoreceptors (innervated by nonmyelinated vagal afferent fibers), and sympathetic mechanosensitive or chemosensitive receptors.[45]

The Bainbridge reflex, described later in this chapter, is mediated by the parasympathetic receptors. Myocardial ischemia increases discharge of both vagal and sympathetic receptors. The sympathetic afferent fibers may transmit the pain sensation associated with coronary occlusion. Postcardiotomy hypertension results from a cardiogenic reflex transmitted through the sympathetic afferent fibers of the stellate ganglion.[45] Finally, opiate receptors of the K type, found in vagus, cardiac, and sympathetic ganglia, may mediate dysrhythmias, particularly during ischemia and reperfusion.[46,47]

Both cardiac contraction and conduction are modulated through the β-adrenergic receptors and guanine nucleotide binding proteins or G proteins. G protein molecules consist of seven transmembrane α-helical segments, which create a central cleft to which various ligands can bind. When binding occurs, the receptor undergoes a conformational change. An example of the G protein signaling system in the heart is the binding of catecholamines to the β-adrenergic receptor, which in turn, activates the stimulatory G protein and adenyl cyclase, increasing intracellular cAMP, cardiac contractility, and heart rate (see Fig. 30-6). However, a detailed discussion of the G proteins is beyond the scope of this chapter and may be found in other sources.[48]

Coronary Circulatory Physiology

5 About 4% of the cardiac output, or 250 mL/min, perfuses the coronary arteries of a 70-kg person. Physiologically, the coronary circulation consists of large, low-resistance epicardial vessels and higher-resistance intramyocardial arteries and arterioles. Myocardial flow, pressure, and oxygen consumption are integrally related. Coronary blood flow is locally regulated by metabolic, mechanical, anatomic, and possibly myogenic factors.[49] Numerous methods to measure human myocardial blood flow have been described.[50] Coronary flow is determined by the duration of diastole and the difference between diastolic aortic pressure and left ventricular end-diastolic pressure. During systole, about 15 to 25% of the coronary flow distends and is stored in the extramural coronary arteries. Only a small amount actually perfuses the myocardium. During diastole, this stored blood perfuses the myocardium[51] (Fig. 30-7). The majority of left coronary artery flow occurs in diastole because intramyocardial pressure is lowest at that time.[52] Right

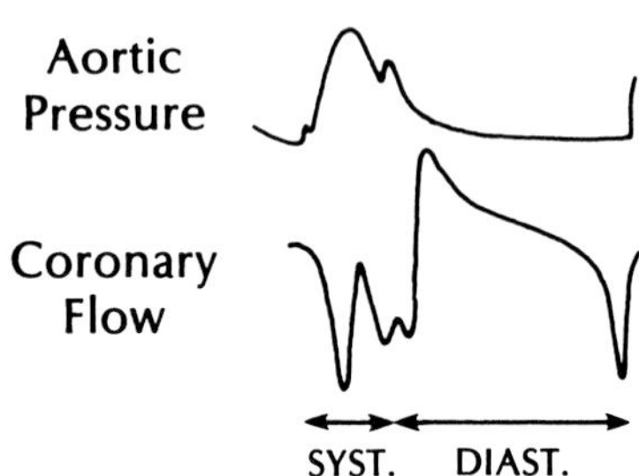

FIGURE 30-7. This diagrammatic relationship between aortic pressure and coronary flow demonstrates that little coronary flow occurs during systole, while the majority occurs during diastole. This relationship is particularly true to the left coronary artery that supplies the left ventricle. The right ventricle, being thinner and developing less pressure, produces less impediment to systolic coronary flow.

coronary artery flow occurs in both systole and diastole because intramyocardial pressure is lower in the thinner RV. Intramyocardial pressure affects coronary flow to a small extent because of the varying stiffness of ventricular muscle over the cardiac cycle.[52] Coronary flow also decreases from epicardium to endocardium as a consequence of extravascular pressure.

The zero flow pressure, normally about 12 to 50 mm Hg, is a minimum coronary pressure required to initiate flow. The source of this pressure is the collapsed intramyocardial coronary microvessels when tissue pressures exceed intraluminal pressures and intracavitary back pressure. At least half of coronary vascular resistance results from vessels larger than 100 μm in diameter, whereas 10% results from coronary veins.[53] Coronary flow ceases completely at 20 mm Hg, the critical closure or critical flow pressure.[54]

6 Myocardial oxygen consumption is high; therefore, coronary venous blood is only 30% saturated and its PO_2 of 18 to 20 mm Hg is the lowest anywhere in the body. Because oxygen extraction cannot be increased further, coronary flow must increase if the heart requires additional oxygen.

Coronary Autoregulation

Coronary perfusion is autoregulated to maintain a constant flow over a range of perfusion pressures (usually between 50 and 120 mm Hg) at any given myocardial oxygen demand.[55] Above and below these limits, coronary flow varies with perfusion pressure. The term *autoregulation* refers strictly to pressure-dependent changes in coronary resistance unrelated to changes in myocardial metabolism.[55] The principal site of coronary autoregulation is the coronary arteriole, a <150-μm–diameter vessel, although small coronary arteries (>150 μm) can be recruited to increase flow during hypoperfusion.[56] Nevertheless, the coronary arterioles are not fully dilated even during hypoperfusion states.[57]

However, changes in myocardial oxygen demand alter autoregulation. The involved metabolite, therefore, is oxygen (specifically, myocardial oxygen tension, PO_2) acting through mediators such as adenosine.[51] Adenosine-induced vasodilation is inversely related to arterial diameter, with the greatest dilation occurring in smaller vessels.[56] Hyperoxia decreases, and a low PO_2 of 49 mm Hg increases coronary blood flow and myocardial oxygen consumption independently of changes in oxygen content or delivery.[58] The threshold oxygen tension for autoregulation is 32 mm Hg.[59] Coronary autoregulation is also closely coupled with coronary venous PO_2, particularly at PO_2 <25 mm Hg.[51,59] Decreased heart rate attenuates autoregulation, whereas pharmacologic coronary constriction augments it.[59]

The autoregulatory mechanism extends into different myocardial layers.[51] Autoregulation is greater in the subepicardium than in the subendocardium, possibly because of the transmural gradient to which the subendocardial vessels are exposed.[59] Autoregulation in the right coronary artery may be less than in the left coronary artery. Pressure and flow-dependent changes in myocardial oxygen consumption in the RV explain this difference.[59]

Immediately after occlusion of a coronary artery, reperfusion flow increases beyond preocclusion levels, a process termed *reactive hyperemia*. In a related process, *reactive dilation,* large coronary arteries dilate after relief of occlusion; however, unlike in reactive hyperemia, the onset is delayed to 60 seconds and sustained for 150 seconds after relief of occlusion.[60]

The most important regulators of coronary vascular tone are metabolic and involve multiple pathways. Modulation of basal tone and normal autoregulation is mediated by glybenclamide-sensitive K_{ATP} channels, which are enhanced by adenosine receptor activation.[61,62] Other mediators and pathways such as oxygen, potassium, pH, carbon dioxide, endothelium-derived relaxing factor, prostaglandins, prostacyclin, histamine, and ATP may also be involved in regulating coronary tone.[49] Prostaglandin E_1 dilates the coronary arteries, probably acting through adenosine as a mediator. Prostaglandin E_2, however, is a coronary vasoconstrictor.[63] Acetylcholine increases coronary flow. Acting through the H_1 receptor, histamine contracts epicardial coronary arteries, provoking spasm, but the H_2 receptor mediates vasodilation.[64] Histamine also promotes production of prostaglandin in the heart.[64] Although norepinephrine (or sympathetic cardiac nerve stimulation) causes coronary constriction through its α effects, the associated increase in myocardial contractility increases coronary flow. Similarly, vagal stimulation may directly produce coronary vasodilation, but the associated decrease in heart rate and contractility causes secondary coronary vasoconstriction.

Coronary Flow Reserve

Coronary flow increases during maximal dilation of the coronary arteries. The difference between resting and maximal coronary flow is the coronary flow reserve. Coronary flow is heterogeneous throughout the myocardium, although there is correlation between regional flows in neighboring myocardial areas.[65] Although coronary vasodilation occurs in response to ischemia or other endogenous stimuli, maximal flow, which is normally unavailable to the heart, may be achieved with pharmacologic agents. Exhaustion of autoregulatory vasodilator reserve does not necessarily mean that exhaustion of pharmacologic vasodilator reserve has occurred. Coronary flow reserve can be decreased by decreased maximal flow and increased regulated coronary flow.[66] Maximal coronary flow is decreased by tachycardia, increased blood viscosity, increased myocardial contractility, and myocardial hypertrophy.[51]

As epicardial coronary artery stenosis occurs, so does arteriolar vasodilation to maintain flow at normal levels. Once the vasodilator reserve is exhausted (usually at stenoses of >90%), however, an increase in the stenosis of the coronary artery will decrease flow. Administration of a vasodilator to a vascular bed served by a normal and a stenotic coronary artery connected by collaterals will dilate the normal arterioles but produce little change in the arterioles served by the stenotic artery because they are maximally dilated. The increased flow to the normal arterioles is termed "coronary steal."

Endocardial/Epicardial Flow Ratio

The distribution of coronary flow is as important as total flow. The ratio of flow in the endocardium to that in the epicardium, the endo/epi ratio, is used to assess flow distribution. Subepicardial flow is usually adequate; thus, if the endo/epi ratio remains constant, adequate subendocardial blood flow is inferred.[65] However, with maximal coronary vasodilation, the endo/epi ratio varies with the coronary perfusion pressure.[51] The ratio is minimally affected by changes in afterload but reduced by increased left ventricular preload. The latter results either from a disproportionate increase in subendocardial diastolic tissue pressure or an increase in coronary sinus pressure.[51] However, increased right ventricular preload decreases right ventricular blood flow without altering its intramyocardial distribution.[67]

Transient subendocardial ischemia accompanies the onset of severe exercise. Although anemia increases coronary blood flow by autoregulation, severe anemia decreases the endo/epi ratio, indicating subendocardial ischemia.[51] Hypoxia, in contrast, increases both coronary blood flow and the endo/epi ratio.

Neural Influences

Coronary arteries are also responsive to neural stimuli.[68] Parasympathetic and sympathetic nerves extend to the precapillary coronary vessels. Parasympathetic stimulation directly activates coronary muscarinic receptors, inducing dilation.

Sympathetic stimulation causes coronary dilatation as a result of the metabolic factors produced by increased $M\dot{V}O_2$ and direct β receptor stimulation. α_2 Adrenoceptors or muscarinic receptors are present in the sympathetic nerve endings of coronary arteries. Activation of α-adrenergic receptors by norepinephrine and acetylcholine (via the vagus nerve) reduces sympathetic neurotransmitter output, which would reduce the dilation of these vessels causing coronary vasoconstriction. α_2 Agonists also mediate release of endothelial-derived relaxing factor in coronary arteries. β_1-Adrenergic receptors predominate over α_1 receptors in canine circumflex coronary artery.[69] Termination of the sympathetic cardiac effects results from extensive neuronal uptake of norepinephrine.[70] Only small amounts of the norepinephrine released by the heart enter the systemic circulation.[70]

Coronary artery spasm may result from unopposed α_1-adrenoceptor stimulation in the presence of β-adrenergic blockade or when a pure α agonist is given. Acute coronary occlusion attenuates the baroreflex responses of heart rate and systemic vascular resistance.[57]

Cardiac Output

7 Cardiac output is the volume of blood pumped by the heart each minute. It is the product of the heart rate and the volume of each beat (stroke volume) but is determined by preload, afterload, heart rate, contractility, and ventricular compliance. Cardiac output measurements are usually corrected for the size of the patient by dividing the output by the body surface area to give the cardiac index. A normal cardiac index is 2.5 to 3.5 L/min/m^2 and may be determined by the Fick principle or indicator-dilution methods (Fig. 30-8 and see Table 30-4). Cardiac output increases with increased heart rate, preload, or contractility and decreased afterload.

Determinants

Preload. Preload is defined as the end-diastolic stress on the ventricle (end-diastolic fiber length or end-diastolic volume). The determinants of preload are blood volume, venous tone, ventricular compliance, ventricular afterload, and myocardial contractility. The distribution of the blood volume between intrathoracic and extrathoracic compartments also affects preload. Extrathoracic blood volume increases with

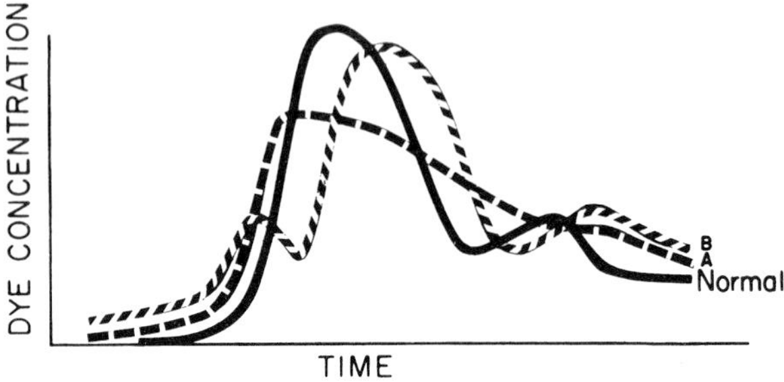

FIGURE 30-8. A normal dye dilution cardiac output curve has an uninterrupted build-up slope, a steep disappearance slope with a short disappearance time, and a prominent recirculation peak. In right-to-left shunts (*A*), there is a deformity on the build-up slope by the abnormal early appearance of the dye in the arterial circulation. Left-to-right (*B*) shunting causes a decreased peak dye concentration, absence of the recirculation peak, and prolongation of the disappearance time. (Reprinted with permission from Lake CL: Cardiovascular Anesthesia, p 70. New York, Springer-Verlag, 1985.)

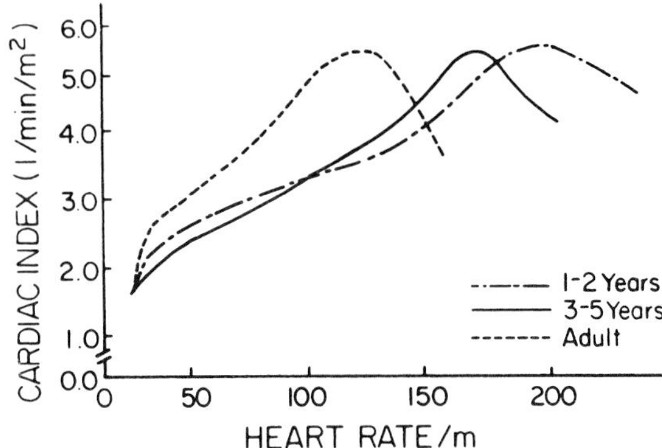

FIGURE 30-9. The effect of heart rate on cardiac output varies with age. In children, an increase in heart rate increases cardiac output because the immature heart is relatively noncompliant and does not increase its stroke volume in response to increased demands. In the adult, however, an increase in heart rate over 120 beats per minute does not increase cardiac index. (Reprinted with permission from Wetsel RC: Critical Care State of the Art. p 9. Fullerton, Society of Critical Care Medicine, 1981.)

standing, whereas the negative intrathoracic pressure during inspiration increases intrathoracic blood volume.

Stroke volume is determined by the volume of blood in the heart at the beginning of systole (end-diastolic volume [EDV]) and the amount of blood remaining in the ventricle at closure of the aortic valve at the end of systole (end-systolic volume [ESV]). The degree of stretch of the left ventricular fibers, influenced by the amount of blood in the ventricle, determines the amount of work the ventricle can do.[71] An increase in preload increases EDV and wall tension.

EDV is not synonymous with end-diastolic pressure, nor are the two linearly related. The ejection fraction, normally 0.6 to 0.7, is the ratio of the stroke volume to the EDV:

$$\text{Ejection fraction} = \text{EDV} - \text{ESV/EDV}$$

Severe impairment of ventricular function is present when the ejection fraction is <0.4.

Afterload. Afterload is the wall stress or tension faced by the myocardium during ventricular ejection. It is the force opposing ventricular fiber shortening during ejection. Left ventricular afterload depends on the shape, size, radius, and wall thickness of the ventricle, the principal factors being the radius (related to preload and chamber volume) and aortic impedance (controlled by arterial compliance and systemic vascular resistance). Other factors involved in afterload include arterial wall stiffness (aortic), blood viscosity, and the mass of blood in the aorta. Usually, the ejection phase stress is implied in discussions of afterload, although there are wall stresses during the isovolumetric contraction phase.

Clinically, systemic vascular resistance is frequently used as an estimate of afterload (Table 30-4). However, systemic vascular resistance reflects only peripheral arteriolar tone rather than left ventricular systolic wall tension. A true measure of left ventricular afterload, such as left ventricular end-systolic wall stress, which incorporates left ventricular chamber pressure, ventricular dimensions, wall thickness, and peripheral loading conditions, should be used to accurately assess afterload.[72] However, these measurements require direct intraventricular pressure determination and echocardiographic evaluation of wall thickness and ventricular dimensions. Compared with left ventricular end-systolic wall stress, systemic vascular resistance underestimates afterload when afterload is increased or decreased or contractility is improved.[72]

When afterload is reduced, the ventricle shortens more quickly and completely.[73] An increase in afterload decreases the extent and velocity of shortening and increases active tension and the time to peak tension in cardiac muscle. Wall tension, ventricular radius, and EDV are also increased to maintain stroke volume. In the poorly contractile heart, acute increases in afterload severely reduce stroke volume. Hypertrophy occurs in ventricles facing a chronic increase in afterload so wall stress and shortening characteristics return toward normal.

Heart Rate. Heart rate is primarily determined by the automaticity of the sinus node. However, its intrinsic rate depends on neural and humoral influences. An increase in heart rate increases cardiac output, even if the stroke volume remains constant, by increasing the extent and velocity of shortening and dP/dt.[74] The increase of dP/dt with heart rate is even more pronounced if end-diastolic dimensions are maintained by volume infusion.[74] At heart rates between 120 and 160 beats/min, cardiac output increases but not as much as at more optimal heart rates (Fig. 30-9). An increase in heart rate shortens the filling time between beats, reducing EDV. Because most cardiac filling occurs during the first half-second of the rapid filling phase, cardiac output decreases at heart rates >160 beats/min because of inadequate filling time.

Cardiac output is also increased during the heartbeat after a ventricular extrasystole. This extrasystolic potentiation results from increased ejection fraction, decreased left ventricular EDV, and enhanced diastolic filling. The mechanism is probably increased availability of calcium to the contractile mechanism.[75]

Contractility. Contractility is the inotropic state independent of changes in preload, afterload, or heart rate.

Cardiac Systole. Myocardial contraction begins when the action potential, acting through the T-tubule system of the SR, results in calcium release into the sarcoplasm. A cAMP-dependent protein kinase in the heart stimulates calcium transport by the vesicles of the SR (Fig. 30-10). Intracellular cAMP protein kinase is activated and transfers the terminal phosphate of ATP to troponin I, phospholamban, or other intracellular proteins. Troponin has three components: troponin I, the inhibitory factor inhibiting the magnesium-stimulated adenosine triphosphatase of actomyosin; troponin C, which is the calcium-sensitive factor; and troponin T, the tropomyosin-binding subunit.

The actin and myosin filaments forming the myofibrils of the cardiac myocyte are functionally divided into sarcomeres. The sarcomere is further divided into three major subdomains, the electron-lucent I band composed primarily of actin; the

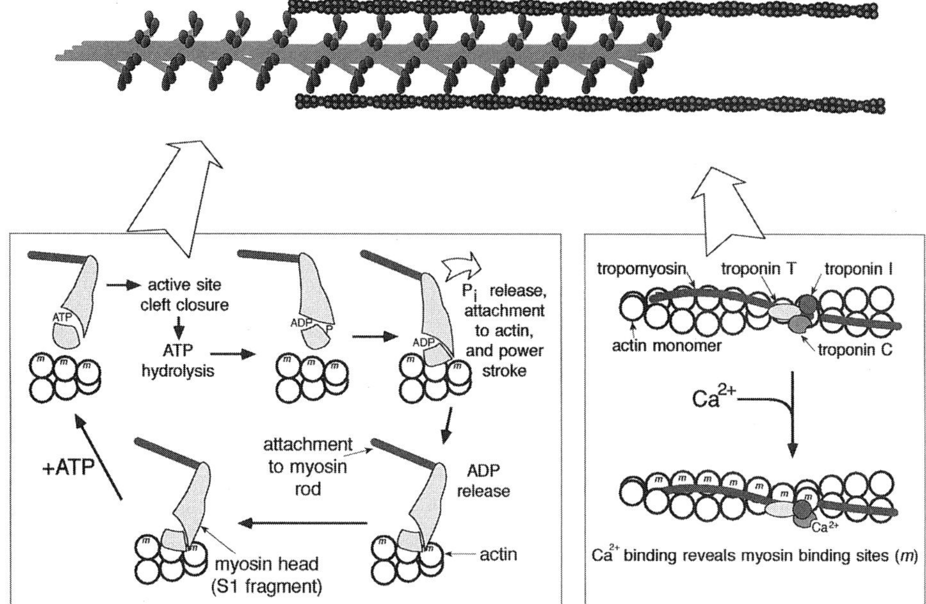

FIGURE 30-10. **Left.** A schematic diagram of the actin filament with its individual monomers and active myosin binding sites (*m*). The myosin head (S1 fragment) is dissociated from actin by binding with adenosine triphopshate (ATP). Subsequent ATP hydrolysis and release of inorganic phosphate (P_i) "cocks" the head group into a tension-generating conformation. Attachment of the myosin head to actin allows the head to apply tension to the myosin rod and to the actin filament. **Right.** Calcium binding to troponin C causes troponin I, the inhibitory subunit, to decrease its affinity for actin. Via tropomyosin, seven *m* sites on actin monomers are revealed. ADP, adenosine diphosphate. (Adapted from Rayment I, Holden HM, Whitaker M *et al*: Structure of the actin–myosin complex and implications for muscle contraction. Science 261:58, 1993, with permission of C. Lynch III.)

Z line, where actin filaments from adjacent sarcomeres meet and SR is juxtaposed to the T-tubule system (junctional SR); and the electron-dense A band composed of myosin thick filaments (further subdivided by the M band into two symmetric bundles). Junctional SR is characterized by a larger lumen containing calsequestrin, a protein that provides extra "releasable" calcium and has low calcium-binding affinity. Calcium entering the myocyte through the L-type calcium channels primarily activates release of SR calcium, a process called calcium-induced calcium release. A portion of the entering calcium binds to calcium release channels to activate their opening, permitting rapid efflux of stored calcium from the SR lumen into the myoplasm to bind to troponin C.

Phospholamban, a membrane-bound protein that modulates the activity of calcium-stimulated magnesium adenosine triphosphatase, permits increased calcium uptake and calcium release by the SR in its phosphorylated state.[76] Adenosine triphosphatase from the calcium pump, which couples hydrolysis of one molecule of ATP with the active transport of two calcium ions, is the channel through which the activator calcium is released to initiate systole. The increased free calcium is bound to troponin C, releasing the inhibition of actin-myosin interaction by the troponin–tropomyosin complex. Contraction of actin and myosin occurs (see Fig. 30-10). The strength of contraction depends on the length of the sarcomere and the amount of activator calcium because cardiac contractility is controlled by the degree of activation of the myocytes. Likewise, relaxation depends on the rate of calcium delivery to troponin, the quantity of available calcium, and the rate of calcium removal from troponin.[77]

Diastole. Myocardial relaxation occurs as a result of reuptake of or binding of calcium ion by the SR, a lusitropic or relaxing effect of cAMP.[78] Relaxation is a load-dependent process. In the relaxing heart, load is the premature lengthening of cardiac muscle. Myocardial relaxation depends on internal restoring forces such as cardiac fibers, hemodynamic loading such as the impedance of the arterial system, and external restoring forces resulting from deformation of the wall of the intact heart.[79]

Alterations in Contractility. Cardiac output is increased by increasing load, either volume or pressure (heterometric autoregulation); by the Anrep effect (homeometric autoregulation); the treppe phenomenon; or by a change in the inotropic state independent of the previous mechanisms.

The Anrep effect improves ventricular performance several beats after the initial stretching of the myocardial fibers, owing to abruptly increased aortic or left ventricular pressure. It results from increased contractility with more rapid activation of the contractile process, increased developed force, and increased velocity of shortening. Homeometric autoregulation is operative for only a few minutes as the initially increased ventricular EDV and circumference decrease with recovery of stroke work.[79]

Rate-dependent variations in contractility, collectively known as force-frequency relationships (FFRs), include the treppe phenomenon, positive staircase effect, or Bowditch's phenomenon. An increase in heart rate increases the developed tension, whereas a decreased stimulation frequency reduces tension development. FFRs result from a variation in myofibril calcium sensitivity and an alteration in activator calcium. The ratio of systolic pressure to echocardiographic measurement of ESV plotted against various heart rates during exercise permits clinical evaluation of myocardial contractility.[80]

A long pause between beats also increases the force of contraction; this is known as the Woodworth phenomenon or reverse (negative) staircase effect.[81] Increasing contractility increases the ejection fraction if ESV decreases while EDV remains the same. Contractility is decreased by hypoxia, cardiomyopathy, myocardial ischemia, or infarction.

Compliance. Compliance is the nonlinear change in ventricular EDV/change in end-diastolic pressure. The rapidity of diastolic filling is a major determinant of cardiac output, which is reduced by decreased compliance. Although ventricular contractility may be normal, reduced relaxation from coronary artery disease, hypertrophic cardiomyopathy, cardiac tamponade, and hypertensive heart disease impairs diastolic filling, which, in turn, limits cardiac output.

Myocardial Mechanics

The mechanical function of the heart is evaluated by *ejection phase indices* (Starling stroke volume versus end-diastolic pressure curves, stroke work versus end-diastolic pressure, force-velocity curves, ejection fraction, velocity of circumferential fiber shortening), *preload recruitable stroke work, isovolumic phase indices* (rate of left ventricular pressure development at 40 mm Hg pressure, [dP/dtP_{40}]; maximum dP/dt; maximal velocity of contractile element shortening, V_{max}; point of maximum $dP/dt/P$ or Vpm), and *end-systolic indices* (pressure–volume or pressure–length relationship at end systole). Many of these measurements are complicated and affected by preload or afterload as noted in Table 30-7. A measurement of the coupling between ventricular performance and the peripheral arterial circulation is obtained by measurement of ventricular time-varying elastance.[82]

Starling (Ventricular Function) Curve

If the cardiac muscle is stretched, it develops greater contractile tension because of changes in myofibril calcium sensitivity and alterations in the amount of activator calcium. This observation is the basis of Starling's law: "The law of the heart is therefore the same as that of skeletal muscle, namely, that the mechanical energy set free on passage from the resting to the contracted state depends . . . on the length of the muscle fibers."[83] Atrial and ventricular muscle obeys Starling's law. Increased preload or initial fiber length increases resting tension, velocity of tension development, and peak tension. An increase in venous return stretches the muscle fibers to increase contractility and improve cardiac output. However, this process occurs only at subnormal filling pressures. In the upright position, ventricular filling pressures decrease to ~4 mm Hg, and the normal heart operates on the ascending limb of the ventricular function curve. Peak ventricular output occurs at filling pressures of ~10 mm Hg in normal humans.[84] Whether the heart can fall onto a descending limb of the length–stroke volume curve like skeletal muscle is unclear.[84] On the descending limb, the heart decompensates and further increases in EDV decrease stroke volume, but disengagement of actin and myosin does not occur. In all probability, the heart moves to a different curve.

Ventricular function curves are influenced by afterload, although they incorporate the effects of preload alterations (Fig. 30-11). Starling curves are used clinically when weaning patients from cardiopulmonary bypass, to assess the effects of anesthetic agents on the heart, and to guide fluid and pharmacologic therapy in the perioperative period. The increased stretch and end-diastolic length produced by atrial (atrial kick) or early contracting ventricular fibers (idioventricular kick) increase ventricular stroke volume. Both of these effects are manifestations of Starling's law.

Pressure–Volume Loops

Another index of contractility that is less affected by preload, afterload, or other conditions is the pressure–volume loop, an end-systolic index (Fig. 30-12). At end systole, ejection ceases, and the aortic valve closes with the ventricle at minimum dimension and volume.

In such loops, the height and width of the loop are determined by the ventricular systolic pressure and stroke volume. The area subtended by the systolic portion of the curve provides a measure of stroke work during ejection, whereas the area of the diastolic limb is a measure of diastolic work performed during ventricular filling and distention. The volume

TABLE 30-7

MEASURES OF MYOCARDIAL CONTRACTILITY

INDICES	USEFULNESS
EJECTION PHASE INDICES	
Stroke volume versus EDP	Useful for acute contractility if ventricular function curve obtained Afterload sensitive
Stroke work versus EDP	Not useful for basal contractility
Ejection fraction (EF)	Useful for basal contractility when EDV is known Afterload dependent
Maximum acceleration of aortic blood flow	Afterload dependent
Mean velocity of circumferential fiber shortening (V_{cf})	Afterload dependent More sensitive for basal contractility than EF
Mean normalized systolic ejection rate	Afterload dependent Less useful than mean V_{cf}
Maximum chamber elastance	Useful for acute contractility changes Nonlinear behavior complicates interpretation
ISOVOLUMIC PHASE INDICES	
$dP/dt/P_{40}$ mm Hg pressure	Useful in acute contractility changes Not useful for basal contractility
Maximum dP/dt	Dependent on timing of aortic valve opening
V_{pm}	Useful in acute contractility changes Most reliable measure for acute contractility changes Dependent on preload/afterload if increased
V_{max}	Not as useful as $dP/dt/P_{40}$ Decreases with increased preload or afterload Useful for basal contractility

P, intraventricular pressure; V_{pm}, velocity of shortening of contractile elements.
Prepared by C. Lynch with data from Strobeck JE, Sonnenblick EH: Pathophysiology of heart failure: Deficiency in cardiac contraction. In Cohn JN (ed): Drug Treatment in Heart Failure, p 13. Secaucus, NJ, Advanced Therapeutics Communications International, 1988.

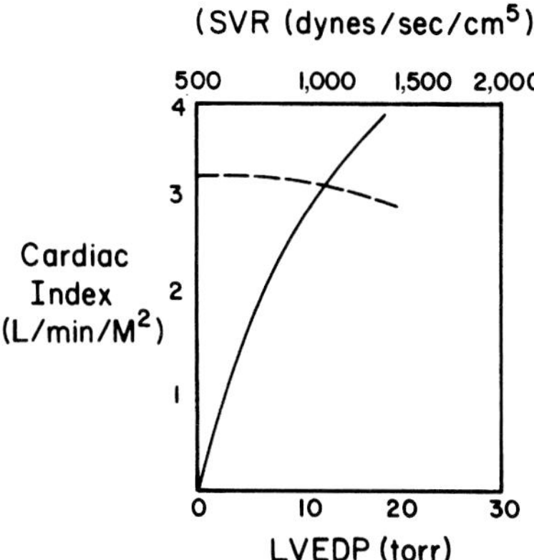

FIGURE 30-11. The ventricular function (Starling) curve of the normal left ventricle (*solid line*) is affected much more by changes in preload (left ventricular end-diastolic pressure) than it is by an increase in afterload (*dotted line*). The failing heart moves to a curve downward and to the right of the normal heart. Venodilator therapy decreases preload without increasing cardiac index (the heart moves to the left on the curve), while reduction of afterload increases cardiac index without a change in preload. Combined preload and afterload reduction decrease filling pressure and increase cardiac index. SVR, systemic vascular resistance; LVEDP, left ventricular end diastolic pressure.

between the systolic and diastolic portions of the loop is the stroke volume. Cardiac work, the product of pressure and volume, is the area of the pressure–volume loop, which is linearly related to myocardial oxygen consumption under various hemodynamic conditions.[85] In a given ventricle, all the end-systolic points are positioned on the same line, which represents the elastance of that ventricle (the change in end-systolic pressure/change in ESV, although elastance is actually the linear relationship between length and force). Contractility is directly proportional to elastance, with the slope of this relationship becoming steeper with increased contractility and flatter with decreased contractility. The slope of the end-systolic pressure–volume relation is linear and correlates well with the ejection fraction.[86]

Pressure–volume loops also reveal information about ventricular compliance. Compliance actually changes during each contraction. The normal relationship between diastolic pressure and volume is curvilinear. There is a relatively gentle slope at low end-diastolic pressures (e.g., little change in pressure for large changes in volume). At end-diastolic pressures at the upper limits of normal (≥12 mm Hg), the curve becomes steeper, and pressure is almost exponentially related to EDV. Ventricular compliance decreases under such conditions. The ventricular end-systolic pressure–volume relationship may be dependent on the type of loading intervention but can be used to assess left ventricular performance under various conditions[87] (see Figs. 30-12 and 30-13). However, one limitation of pressure–volume loops is that pressure may

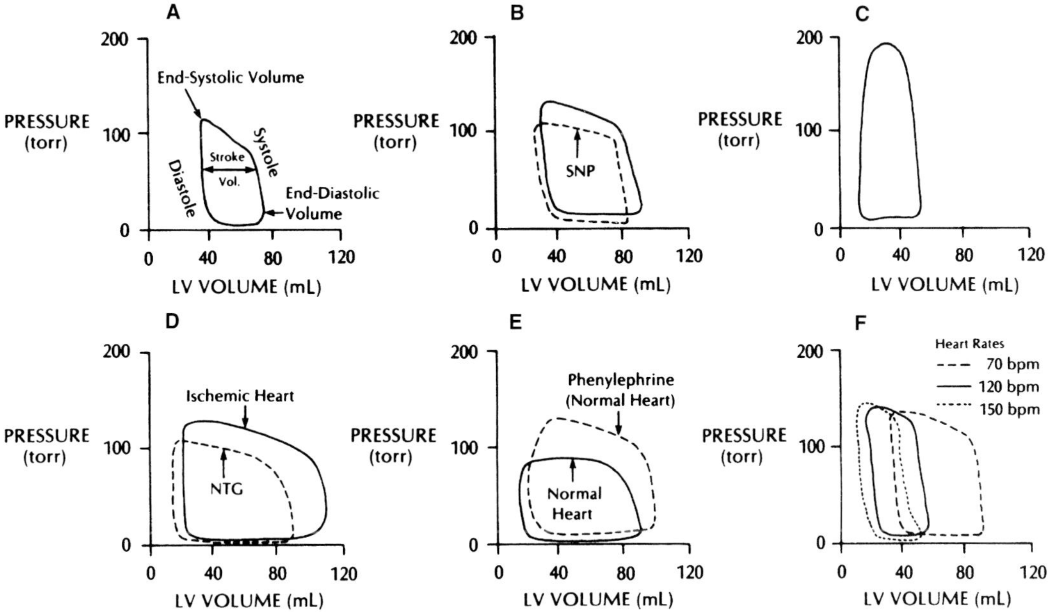

FIGURE 30-12. Ventricular pressure–volume loops. **A.** The relationship of ventricular pressure and volume over the entire cardiac cycle. The loop begins on the bottom left with opening of the mitral valve and filling of the ventricle to end-diastolic volume. When multiple pressure–volume loops are created, the slope of the individual end-systolic pressure–volume relations indicates myocardial contractility. An extension of the bottom portion of the loop (without ventricular systole) would give a diastolic pressure–volume relation for the ventricle. Isovolumetric contraction begins at the lower right portion of the curve with closure of the mitral valve. The aortic valve opens at the upper right portion of the loop and ventricular ejection begins. At the upper left of the loop, the aortic valve closes (end-systolic volume) and isovolumetric relaxation returns the loop to the starting point. Stroke volume is the difference between the volume at the end of diastole and the end of systole. The area of the loop is stroke work. **B.** The effects of afterload reduction with sodium nitroprusside (SNP) on the pressure–volume loop. **C.** The changes in the pressure–volume loop in a patient with aortic stenosis with a high peak systolic pressure and steep diastolic slope representing reduced ventricular compliance. **D.** An ischemic heart has its pressure–volume shifted upward and to the right. **E.** The effects of increasing the afterload of a normal heart with phenylephrine. **F.** In a normal heart, an increase in heart rate markedly reduces left ventricular volume. LV, left ventricle; NTG, nitroglycerin. See also Figure 30-13.

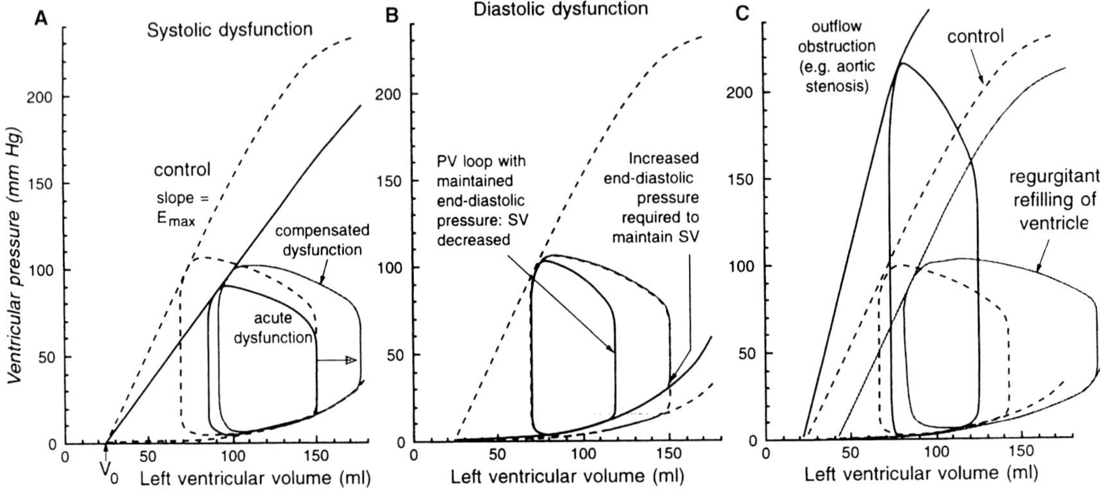

FIGURE 30-13. A. The ventricular pressure–volume relationship in systolic dysfunction demonstrates depressed E_{max} and decreased stroke volume (SV). With compensation, the SV is restored by an increased end-diastolic volume. B. With diastolic dysfunction, SV is decreased unless end-diastolic pressure increases to maintain it. C. As in Figure 30-12C, ventricular outflow obstruction usually enhances systolic function because of ventricular hypertrophy, but associated diastolic dysfunction decreases SV while increasing total ventricular work. With regurgitant ventricular filling, a compensatory increase in stroke volume occurs. (Reprinted with permission from Lynch C, Lake CL: Cardiovascular anatomy and physiology. In Youngberg J, Lake C, Roizen M *et al* (eds): Cardiac, Vascular, and Thoracic Anesthesia, p 119. Philadelphia, Churchill Livingstone, 2000.)

inaccurately reflect end-systolic afterload. The ratio of pressure to volume at end systole can also be used as an index of contractile function. However, this assumes that at higher pressures there are larger volumes at a given inotropic state.

Although pressure–volume loops are most often used to consider ventricular function, they can also be used to analyze atrial function (stroke volume [EDV-ESV] and emptying fraction [stroke volume/EDV], particularly of the LA)[4] (Fig. 30-14). However, these measures are dependent on LA loading conditions. The LA pressure–volume loop consists of two horizontal loops in a figure-of-eight pattern, including an active or A loop and the passive V loop. The A loop begins at atrial end diastole (the pressure immediately before atrial contraction), with the active component proceeding in a counterclockwise direction during atrial systole until blood is ejected through the mitral valve into the LV (active LA stroke work). The passive V loop proceeds in a clockwise direction over time. The total reservoir volume of the LA can be determined from the maximum and minimum volumes of the A and V loops.

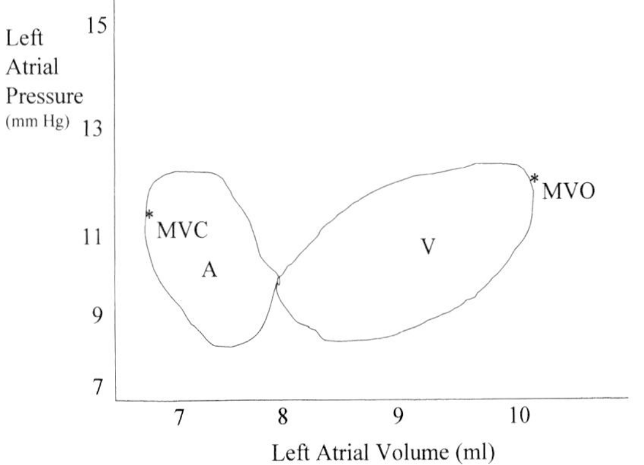

FIGURE 30-14. An atrial pressure–volume loop has the appearance of a figure eight. *A* represents active atrial contraction and proceeds in a counterclockwise direction. *V* represents left atrial reservoir function and proceeds in a clockwise direction over time. Mitral valve opening (MVO) and closure (MVC) are depicted. (Adapted from Pagel PS, Kehl F, Gare M *et al*: Mechanical functions of the left atrium. Anesthesiology 98:975, 2003.)

Pressure–Length Loops

Measurement of a pressure–length loop is a reproducible and sensitive method to evaluate total or regional systolic and diastolic myocardial function. However, it requires direct measurement of changes in myocardial length and intraventricular pressure. Ventricular segment length is plotted on the *x*-axis and ventricular pressure on the *y*-axis (Fig. 30-15). Normal loops are rectangular and include four segments: isovolumic contraction (*right*), ejection (*top*), isovolumic relaxation (*left*), and filling (*bottom*). The area of the loop represents ventricular stroke work.[88] Pressure–length loops are altered by changes in preload, afterload, inotropic state, and ischemia. Ischemia increases postsystolic shortening and systolic lengthening, as depicted in Figure 30-15 (*inset*).[89]

Force–Velocity Curve

Myocardial contractility can also increase when the myocardial fibers increase their developed force or velocity of shortening without a change in fiber length. Force–velocity curves evaluate contractility (velocity of shortening) at constant fiber length in a passively stretched muscle (preloaded), which is stimulated to contract against either no load or an afterload. Force–velocity curves are much more sensitive indicators of contractility than Starling curves and are based on the Hill model of isolated muscle.

As afterload is increased, the initial rate of shortening follows a hyperbolic relationship (Fig. 30-16). The force or tension developed during contraction is measured by dP/dt_{max}, the maximum rate of rise of intraventricular pressure during the isometric phase of ventricular contraction. The point of the curve where no shortening occurs, although the muscle develops maximal force, is termed P_0. Extrapolation of

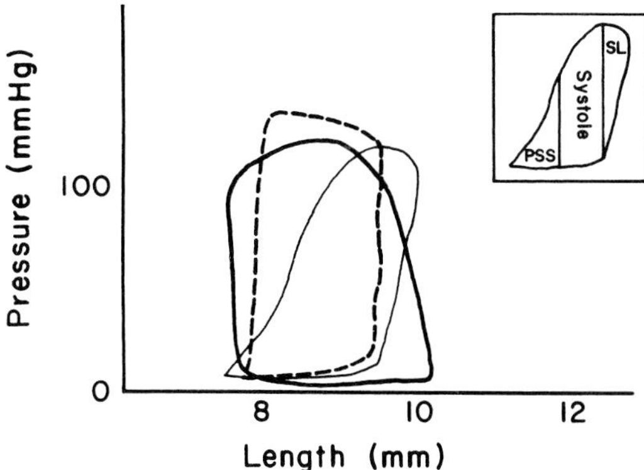

FIGURE 30-15. The normal pressure–length loop (*thick black line*) is a rectangle whose area indicates total ventricular work. Ischemia (*thin solid line*) causes the loop to lean toward the right because of increased systolic lengthening and postsystolic shortening (*inset*). Increased afterload (*dotted line*) causes the loop to become taller at a similar preload. Post systolic shortening (PSS); systolic lengthening (SL). (Reprinted with permission from Lake CL (ed): Clinical Monitoring for Anesthesia and Critical Care, p 181. Philadelphia, WB Saunders, 1994.)

the curve back to zero load where the maximal velocity of shortening occurs is termed V_{max}. Both preload and afterload affect dP/dt_{max}. As preload increases, the maximum isometric tension that the muscle develops increases, but the maximal velocity of shortening is unchanged. An increase in myocardial contractility increases both the developed tension and the maximum velocity of shortening, shifting the force–velocity curve upward and to the right.

Preload Recruitable Stroke Work

Stroke work is linearly related to left ventricular EDV. A plot of EDV against stroke work demonstrates that stroke work increases with increased preload and decreases with unloading.

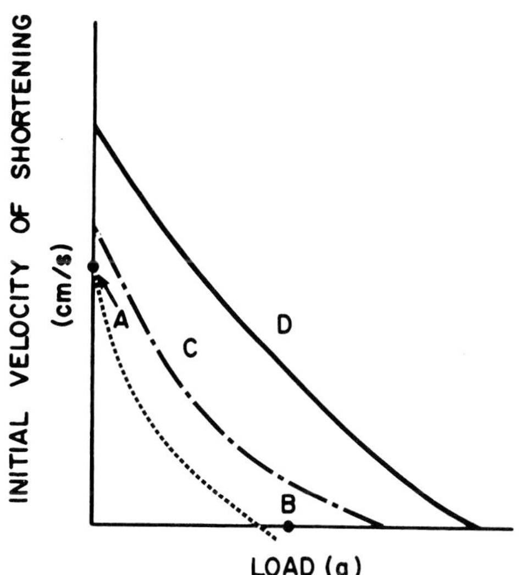

FIGURE 30-16. A force velocity curve of cardiac muscle shows the point of maximal shortening with no load or V_{max} (point A). Point B is P_0 where no shortening occurs, although tension development is maximal. Curve C is a force–velocity curve with increased preload. Curve D demonstrates increased myocardial contractility. On any curve, load (afterload) increases from left to right. (Reprinted with permission from Lake CL: Cardiovascular Anesthesia, p 10. New York, Springer-Verlag, 1985.)

Thus, the preload recruitable stroke work is determined by plotting stroke work from successive pressure–volume loops during alterations in preload.

Cardiac Work

Because of the difficulties in obtaining the data for pressure–volume loops or force–velocity curves under clinical conditions, cardiac work is often measured as a substitute. Cardiac work describes pump function in terms of the load carried and the distance moved. Calculation of cardiac work standardized to body surface area (left and right ventricular stroke work indexes) is shown in Table 30-4. Using cardiac work instead of cardiac output or stroke volume to describe pump function has several advantages: (1) calculation includes heart rate, preload, and afterload—the major variables affecting cardiac function; (2) stroke work index defines the area of the pressure–volume loop; and (3) stroke work index measures both systolic and diastolic performance.[90]

Ventricular End-Systolic Elastance

Direct measurements of end-systolic elastance are complicated and impractical clinically. However, Hayashi and coworkers developed a method to estimate this parameter using only ventricular and aortic pressures. The derived equation $k = (E_{es}/E_a)^{0.51}$, where k is the slope of the two straight lines (one for the isovolumic phase and the second for the ejection phase). E_{es} is ventricular elastance, and E_a is arterial elastance. However, the complexity of the measurements, the substitition of end-ejection pressure for end-systolic pressure, and the determination of the method in animals may not permit application in patients.

Right Ventricular Function

The functional significance of the RV in normal circulatory homeostasis is minimal. Although the right ventricular spiral muscles contract during systole, direct left ventricular assistance to right ventricular contraction has been demonstrated.[91] Compared with the LV, intraventricular pressure develops more gradually in the RV and declines more slowly during diastole. Right ventricular pumping capability depends on (1) pressure against which it ejects, (2) filling volume, and (3) right ventricular contractility.[92] The RV obeys Starling's law except that its curve is upward and to the left of the left ventricular curve. At higher end-diastolic pressures, the RV response is flatter than that of the LV. Increases in filling volume increase right ventricular stroke volume up to the limit imposed by the restraint of the pericardium (normally, ~20% acute increase in cardiac volume).[93] The contractility of the RV depends on sympathetic tone, myocardial structural integrity, and chemical content of the coronary perfusate.[92] Normal right ventricular systolic pressures are only 30 to 40 mm Hg because the recruitable vasculature of the pulmonary circulation allows between 5 and 20 L of blood to flow within it. Peak ejection occurs later than in the LV, and the ejection fraction is only 0.4. This difference in function results because the right ventricular free wall is flattened by the pull of the interventricular septum toward the LV during systole, giving a bellows-like action for expulsion of blood.[93] Because of this mechanism, right ventricular function is less likely to be impaired during right coronary arterial occlusion.[93]

During systole, right ventricular stroke volume is more sensitive to afterload than left ventricular stroke volume. Factors that oppose blood flow from the RV (afterload) include the resistance of the pulmonary vascular bed, pulmonary arterial impedance, the mass of the pulmonary blood, blood viscosity, and pulse wave reflection altering PA pressure. In diastole, the RV is twice as distensible (more compliant) as the LV.[92]

Under conditions of pressure overload, such as increased pulmonary vascular resistance or left ventricular failure, the RV hypertrophies to generate systemic pressures. Although acute right ventricular failure is compatible with life, the symptoms caused by increased venous pressure suggest that right ventricular function is important for maintenance of normal venous pressures.[93]

Ventricular Interdependence

Because the ventricles are anatomically associated, alterations of volume and pressure in one ventricle affect these parameters in the other.[94] During normal respiration with negative intrathoracic pressure, increased venous return increases right ventricular EDV during inspiration, pulmonary vascular capacitance increases, left ventricular diastolic volume decreases, and left ventricular stroke volume increases, but left ventricular transmural pressure is unchanged. Important factors in ventricular interdependence are septal position and deformability, pulmonary venous capacitance, right ventricular distensibility, the transseptal pressure gradient, and the presence of the pericardium.

In vitro experimental animal models confirm that when left ventricular pressure increases, diastolic compliance and systolic ventricular function decrease in the RV and vice versa. The mechanisms are the Frank-Starling effect caused by decreased ventricular diastolic volume and decreased systolic ventricular function.[95] The etiology of the depressed systolic function is unclear.[95] Computer models confirm that hypertrophy from right ventricular pressure overload, which increases septal thickness and decreases septal compliance, decreases transfer of pressure and volume between the ventricles, limiting ventricular interdependence.

Myocardial Metabolism

Knowledge of myocardial metabolism is essential to the preservation of the heart during conditions of stress, cardiac arrest, or elective asystole during cardiac surgery. Metabolism includes both substrate utilization and oxygen consumption.

Sources of Energy

The energy supply of the heart is derived primarily from lactate and fatty acids delivered by the coronary blood. Free or nonesterified fatty acids (palmitic and oleic acids) are the preferred fuel. Myocardial uptake of fatty acids is almost linear, with the plasma concentration above the threshold of 345 μmol/L.[96] Fatty acid uptake by the heart from either fatty acid–albumin complexes or lipoprotein triglyceride occurs by passive diffusion or carrier-mediated transport. During fasting, free fatty acids are always used as fuel. The heart has a limited ability to synthesize fatty acids from acetyl coenzyme A, except for the formation of structural lipids. The oxidation of fatty acids and ketone bodies inhibits uptake of glucose, pyruvate oxidation, and glycolysis while facilitating glycogen synthesis.[96] Oxidation of nonesterified fatty acids accounts for 90% of myocardial oxygen consumption.

Fuel selection by the heart probably depends on regulatory enzymes controlled by factors other than substrate availability and product removal. Myocardial lactate utilization is regulated by the arterial lactate concentrations and pyruvate oxidation in the Krebs tricarboxylic acid cycle. Glucose, pyruvate, acetate, and triglycerides can also be used by the heart as energy sources. Utilization of glucose by the myocardium depends on the arterial glucose and insulin concentrations. Glucose is normally used postprandially. However, glucose use by the myocardium as the primary energy source occurs only with high glucose levels, insulin secretion, or hypoxia. Glucose is the only substrate used by the heart anaerobically. As long as the entry of acetyl coenzyme A into the Krebs cycle is not inhibited, the heart will use as much pyruvate as it is given. Substrates such as fructose, glycogen, or proteins are used for energy only during special circumstances, such as starvation, diabetic ketoacidosis, or anoxia.

Myocardial Oxygen Consumption

The heart has one of the highest metabolic rates of any organ. At rest it uses 8 to 10 mL of oxygen per 100 g of myocardium per minute. The subendocardium requires about 20% more oxygen than the epicardium. Myocardial oxygen consumption ($M\dot{V}O_2$) is determined by heart rate, wall tension, and myocardial contractility. The relative importance of each factor is difficult to evaluate because they are interrelated through wall tension.[97] Less important factors include the oxygen costs of shortening of muscle fibers, electrical activation, and catecholamines, as well as the basal oxygen requirements and the level of arterial oxygenation. Tension development constitutes about 50% of $M\dot{V}O_2$ (Table 30-8).

Myocardial wall tension is related to the tension–time index, left ventricular end-diastolic pressure, and ventricular size. Wall tension can be divided into its components: the rate of force development, the magnitude of force development, the interval during which force is generated and maintained for each contraction, and the frequency with which force is developed per unit time.[97] Wall tension is measured according to Laplace's law:

$$T = Pr/2h$$

where radius (r) is cardiac radius, T is cardiac tension, P is interventricular pressure, and h is ventricular muscle thickness. Increases in ventricular chamber pressure or volume increase both the magnitude of force development and the force maintained during ejection.

Myocardial Supply–Demand Ratio

A balance must always exist between oxygen consumption (demand) and myocardial oxygen supply if ischemia is to be avoided. Factors important to this relationship are shown in Table 30-8. Myocardial oxygen supply depends on the diameter of the coronary arteries, left ventricular end-diastolic pressure, aortic diastolic pressure, and arterial oxygen content. In the normal heart, the coronary perfusion pressure is the difference between the aortic diastolic pressure and the left ventricular

TABLE 30-8

FACTORS INVOLVED IN MYOCARDIAL OXYGEN SUPPLY AND DEMAND

■ MYOCARDIAL OXYGEN CONSUMPTION (DEMAND)
Heart rate
Contractile state
Myocardial wall tension
Arterial oxygen content
Basal oxygen requirements
Oxygen cost of muscle fiber shortening
Oxygen cost of electrical activation
■ MYOCARDIAL OXYGEN SUPPLY
Aortic diastolic pressure
Left ventricular end-diastolic pressure
Coronary artery diameter
Arterial oxygen content

end-diastolic pressure. Myocardial blood flow is determined by the blood pressure at the coronary ostia, arteriolar tone, intramyocardial pressure or extravascular resistance, coronary occlusive disease, heart rate, coronary collateral development, and blood viscosity.

Myocardial blood flow is reduced by a low aortic diastolic pressure and increased pulmonary wedge pressure (both of which increase subendocardial tissue pressure), and tachycardia, which shortens diastole, reducing the duration of blood flow. Increasing preload or intracavitary pressure increases wall tension and oxygen demand, while decreasing subendocardial perfusion.

Myocardial oxygen supply is also affected by the level of arterial oxygenation. Oxygen content resulting from Pa_{O_2}; hemoglobin; 2,3-diphosphoglycerate; and pH, P_{CO_2}, or temperature effects on the oxyhemoglobin dissociation curve can be an important factor in patients with obstructive lung disease or severe anemia. Normal oxygen extraction by the heart is 60 to 70% and changes little with increased cardiac work because coronary vascular resistance decreases. However, if the coronary vascular resistance response is limited, oxygen extraction can be increased to more than 90%.[97] An increase in oxygen extraction and coronary vasodilation constitutes the metabolic reserve of the heart in the case of increased demand.

Heart rate and diastolic ventricular volume are the two factors most likely to produce ischemia if either or both are increased. Increased myocardial contractility or afterload, by increasing arterial pressure and myocardial oxygen supply, offsets their tendency to increase myocardial oxygen consumption.

Distribution of Cardiac Output

8 The cardiac output is distributed to the systemic circulation as follows: brain 12%, heart 4%, liver 24%, kidneys 20%, muscle 23%, skin 6%, and intestines 8%. About 15% of the blood volume remains in the heart and pulmonary circulation, with the remainder in the systemic circulation. Of the blood in the systemic circulation, about 64% is in the veins. The total tissue blood flow in a given vascular bed is a function of the effective perfusion pressure and vascular resistance. Effective perfusion pressure is the difference between arterial and venous pressure across the vascular bed. Autoregulation maintains a constant blood flow in the face of changes in perfusion pressure in the cerebral, renal, coronary, hepatic arterial, intestinal, and muscle circulations. Reflexes that alter circulatory distribution are in Table 30-9.[98–106] The carotid sinus, a dilated portion of the common carotid artery just before its bifurcation, contains two types of receptors that sense pressure in the carotid sinus, providing the most important aspect of reflex circulatory control. The cardiovascular reflexes may interact to regulate blood pressure. An example is when there is decreased activity and firing of fibers in the afferent limb of the von Bezold-Jarisch reflex, causing release of vasomotor inhibition, increased medulary outflow, and increased blood pressure, but the baroreceptor reflex attenuates the increased blood pressure response so no effective change in blood pressure occurs.[104]

Peripheral Circulatory Physiology

The peripheral circulation consists of resistance and capacitance vessels. The majority of the resistance is in the arterial circulation, which consists of the Windkessel vessels, the precapillary resistance vessels, and the capillary exchange vessels. The Windkessel vessels are distensible elastic arteries such as the aorta and large muscular arteries that damp the pulsatile output of the ventricle. The arterioles, the precapillary resistance vessels, are muscular vessels that provide more than 60% of the peripheral resistance. At the most distal portion of the terminal, arterioles are precapillary sphincters that regulate the flow of blood into specific capillary beds. The capillary exchange vessels contribute about one-fourth of the total peripheral resistance, although most capillaries consist of a single endothelial cell layer without any surrounding smooth muscle. The systemic veins are the capacitance system.

Arterial Pulses and Blood Pressure

Arterial Pulse

The arterial pulse is a wave of vascular distention resulting from the impact of the stroke volume of each beat being ejected into a closed system. The wave of distention begins at the base of the aorta and passes over the entire arterial system with each heartbeat. The pulse is not caused by the passage of the blood itself. The pulse waveform is the result of the combined effects of the forward-propagating pressure wave and its reflectance back toward the heart from various parts of the vasculature. Wave reflection may occur in high-resistance arterioles, branching points, or sites of changes in arterial distensibility, but the major source is the arteriole. The velocity of the pulse wave depends on the elasticity of the vessel. The pulse wave velocity is most rapid in the least distensible arteries. In the aortic arch, the pulse wave travels 3 to 5 m/sec, and the aortic pulse waveform precedes the brachial waveform by about 0.05 seconds. In large distensible arteries such as the subclavian, the pulse wave travels 7 to 10 m/sec, whereas in the small nondistensible peripheral arteries it travels about 15 to 30 m/sec. Such differences become important when timing the counterpulsation of an intraaortic balloon.

The arterial pressure waveform changes as it moves peripherally (Fig. 30-17). In central aortic waveforms, the closure of the aortic valve is indicated by a notch or incisura on the descending limb. In contrast, peripheral pulse waveforms have greater amplitude, more pronounced diastolic wave, and lower mean pressure, and the foot of the wave is delayed.[107] The dicrotic notch, corresponding to the incisura, is more prominent. Systolic pressure is higher, whereas mean and diastolic pressures are slightly lower in the periphery. Such changes are best explained by a tubular model of the vascular system. In such a system, the contour of the pressure wave depends on the velocity of the pressure wave, the duration of the pulse, and the length of the tube.[107]

Pulse contour also changes with hemodynamic conditions. In children, wave reflection facilitates cardiac performance by a relative decrease in arterial pressure during systole and a relative increase during diastole. As aging occurs, wave reflection occurs earlier in the cardiac cycle, increasing systolic pressure and decreasing diastolic pressure. In shock, the pulse wave velocity is reduced by hypotension, increased heart rate reduces the duration of cardiac systole, and peripheral vasoconstriction increases the peripheral reflection coefficient. Pulse waveforms vary in atrial fibrillation; beats with short systolic durations demonstrating diastolic waves and those with long durations having accentuated systolic peaks. Patients with hypertrophic cardiomyopathy have double systolic pulse waveforms because the initial systolic wave of ventricular ejection occurs during the first half of systole and the reflected wave returns during the same systole.[107]

Blood Pressure

9 Arterial pressure is the lateral pressure exerted by the contained blood on the walls of the vessels. Mean arterial pressure is the

TABLE 30-9

CARDIOVASCULAR REFLEXES[98–106]

CAROTID SINUS (PRESSORECEPTOR, BARORECEPTOR)	
Anatomy:	Carotid-afferent nerve of Hering (glossopharyngeal) Aortic-vagus Cardiovascular centers in medulla
Stimulus:	Increased blood pressure
Response:	Inhibition of sympathetic and increase in parasympathetic activity, causing decreased cardiac contractility, heart rate, and vasoconstrictor tone
Other:	Gain determined by pulse pressure Reduces arterial pressure fluctuation to one-third of expected threshold 60 torr, limits 175–300 torr
VALSALVA MANEUVER	
Anatomy:	Same as pressoreceptor reflex
Stimulus:	Forced expiration against closed glottis
Response:	Increased venous pressure in head, upper extremities, with decreased right heart venous return causing decreased blood pressure and cardiac output, and reflex increase in heart rate; the tachycardia coupled with coupling of the E and A waves on the mitral transvelocity curve indicates normal left ventricular filling pressures[132]
Other:	Glottic opening increases venous return to right heart, resulting in forceful right and then left ventricular contraction, followed by transient bradycardia
MÜLLER MANEUVER	
Anatomy:	Decreased pleural pressure increasing left ventricular volume through afterload reduction
Stimulus:	Inspiratory effort against a closed airway
Response:	Right ventricular end-diastolic volume and left ventricular end-diastolic pressure increase, while left ventricular end-diastolic volume is unchanged or decreased, and ejection fraction is unchanged
Other:	Net effect on left ventricular function depends on ventricular interdependence, heart rate, and contractility (position of the heart on diastolic pressure–volume curve) Müller maneuver may cause ventricular akinesis due to increased wall stress, increasing myocardial oxygen demand, or increased left ventricular transmural pressure, decreasing motion in nonfunctional ventricular myocardium
von BEZOLD–JARISCH[103,104]	
Anatomy:	Ventricular chemoreceptors and mechanoreceptors with afferent pathway in unmyelinated vagal C fibers
Stimulus:	Noxious stimuli to either ventricle associated with myocardial ischemia, profound hypovolemia, coronary reperfusion, aortic stenosis, neuraxial anesthesia associated with sympathetic blockade and "empty" ventricle, or even vasovagal syncope
Response:	Hypotension, bradycardia, parasympathetically induced coronary vasodilation, and inhibition of sympathetic outflow from vasomotor centers
Other:	Reperfusion of previously ischemic tissue elicits reflex
CARDIOGENIC HYPERTENSIVE CHEMOREFLEX[105]	
Anatomy:	Chemoreceptors located between the aorta and pulmonary artery and supplied by the left coronary artery Afferent reflex pathway is intrathoracic vagal branches and the efferent path is via phrenic, vagal, and sympathetic routes
Stimulus:	Serotonin
Response:	Arterial pressure increases markedly in 4–6 sec owing to increased inotropy and peripheral vasoconstriction
Other:	Reflex may be responsible for hypertension during angina, myocardial infarction, and after coronary bypass grafting and is abolished by vagotomy, atropine, or local anesthesia of the intertruncal space
CUSHING'S REFLEX	
Anatomy:	Increased cerebrospinal fluid (CSF) pressure compresses cerebral arteries
Stimulus:	Cerebral ischemia secondary to increased CSF pressure
Response:	An increase in arterial pressure sufficient to reperfuse the brain Intense sympathetic activity causes severe peripheral vasoconstricion as a result of this reflex
BAINBRIDGE ATRIAL REFLEX[106]	
Anatomy:	Primarily mediated through vagal myelinated afferent fibers; activation of sympathetic afferent fibers may also occur[39] Increased right atrial pressure directly stretches the SA node and enhances its automaticity, increasing the heart rate
Stimulus:	Increased vagal tone and distention of the right atrium or central veins
Response:	Depends upon the preexisting heart rate With preexisting tachycardia, there is no effect Volume loading at a slow heart rate causes progressive tachycardia Global atrial distention in response to high pressures causes bradycardia, hypotension, and decreased systemic vascular resistance
Other:	Experimental distention of the cavoatrial junctions or other small portions of the atria increases heart rate, but clinical conditions such as heart failure usually do not produce such locally increased atrial pressure[106]

(continued)

TABLE 30-9

CONTINUED

■ CHEMORECEPTOR	
Anatomy:	Carotid and aortic bodies chemoreceptors whose nerve fibers pass through the nerve of Hering and the vagus nerve to the medullary vasomotor centers
Stimulus:	Decreasing oxygen tension or increased hydrogen ion concentrations
Response:	Increased pulmonary ventilation and blood pressure with decreased heart rate (carotid body chemoreceptors) Stimulation of the aortic bodies causes tachycardia
Other:	Normally, the peripheral chemoreceptors are minimally active
■ OCULOCARDIAC	
Anatomy:	Afferent fibers run with the short or long ciliary nerves to the ciliary ganglion, and then with the ophthalmic division of the trigeminal nerve to the gasserian ganglion
Stimulus:	Traction on the extraocular muscles (more especially the medial rather than the lateral rectus) or pressure on the globe
Response:	Bradycardia and hypotension as a consequence of this reflex
Other:	Demonstrated in 30–90% of patients undergoing ophthalmic surgery and attenuated by IV atropine
■ CELIAC (VAGOVAGAL)	
Anatomy:	Vagal stimulation via mesenteric traction, rectal distention, traction on gallbladder, respiratory tract receptors
Response:	Bradycardia, apnea, hypotension with narrowed pulse pressure
Other:	Traction on the mesentery or gallbladder, stimulation of vagal nerve fibers in the respiratory tract, or rectal distention stimulates afferent vagal nerve endings to cause bradycardia, apnea, and hypotension (vagovagal reflex) Manipulation around the celiac plexus decreases systolic pressure, narrows pulse pressure, and slightly decreases heart rate

SA, sinoatrial.

product of the cardiac output and the systemic vascular resistance. If a normal arterial waveform is present, mean pressure is about one-third the difference between the systolic and diastolic pressures. However, mean pressure remains constant, whereas pulse pressure and systolic pressure increase as blood moves peripherally in the circulation.

Arterial pressure varies with the respiratory cycle. It normally decreases 6 mm Hg or less during inspiration because pulmonary venous capacitance increases during inspiration to a greater extent than the increase in right-sided heart venous return and output, thus causing a decrease in left ventricular stroke output and pressure. These changes are exaggerated in pericardial tamponade, causing pulsus paradoxus. Clinically, auscultation of the blood pressure is performed until the first heart sound is heard intermittently. Further deflation of the cuff to the pressure where all beats are heard yields the difference known as the paradoxical pulse.

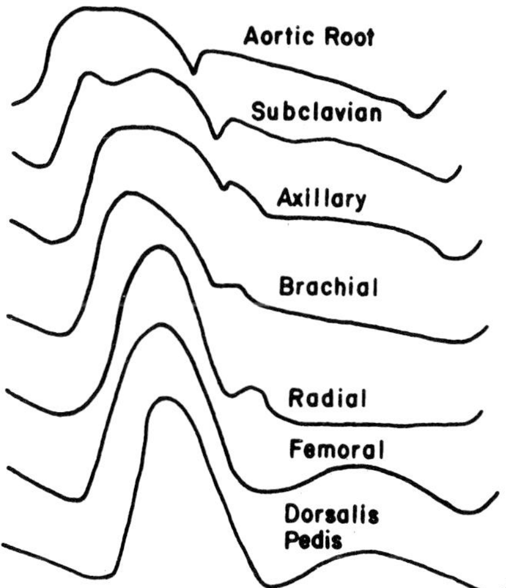

FIGURE 30-17. The change in the pulse waveform as it moves from the aortic root to the dorsalis pedis artery is dramatic. These changes result from both forward wave propagation and wave reflection at branch points in the circulation. The waveform has a greater amplitude, higher systolic pressure, lower diastolic pressure, and reduced mean pressure in the peripheral circulation. (Reprinted with permission from Shah N, Bedford RF: Invasive and noninvasive blood pressure monitoring. In Lake CL, Hines R, Blitt CD (eds): Clinical Monitoring: Practical Applications for Anesthesia and Critical Care, p 182. Philadelphia, WB Saunders, 2001.)

Factors Controlling Peripheral Vascular Tone

10 Factors controlling blood pressure include central and autonomic nervous function, cardiac output, peripheral vascular resistance, and hormonal mechanisms, including antidiuretic hormone, catecholamines, the renin-angiotensin system, and atrial natriuretic peptide.[108] Three medullary centers—the nucleus tractus solitarius, the caudal ventrolateral medulla, and the rostal ventrolateral medulla—are important in blood pressure control. Arteriolar tone is regulated by intrinsic and extrinsic mechanisms. The intrinsic mechanism is the inherent myotonic activity of vascular smooth muscle cells and vascular endothelial cells. Extrinsic factors include neural (sympathetic) and humoral factors. Sympathetic neural activity provides rapid alteration of tone in response to a need for greater blood flow. During normal conditions, sympathetic tone maintains blood vessels in a partially constricted state, vasomotor tone. Figure 30-18 details the intracellular mechanisms for peripheral vasodilation and vasoconstriction. Nitric oxide (NO) and prostacyclin production and endothelin release from endothelial cells produce vasodilation and vasoconstriction, respectively, in large arteries. The natriuretic peptides and NO are two major pathways for synthesis of cyclic guanosine monophosphate (cGMP). The effectors of cGMP are the cGMP-regulated phosphodiesterases and cGMP-dependent protein kinase (cGK or PKG) in vascular smooth muscle cells and platelets. Relaxation of vascular smooth muscle occurs through the Rho pathway of vascular smooth muscle by phosphorylation of Rho A to inhibit Rho kinase and, in turn,

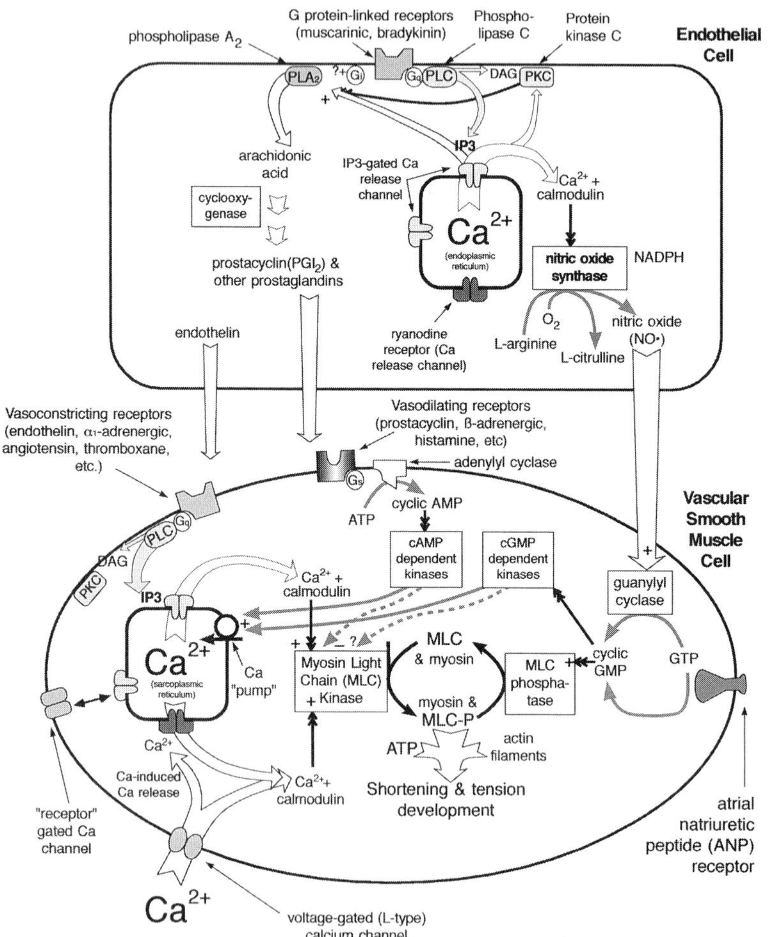

FIGURE 30-18. Vascular smooth muscle and endothelial function. Both endothelial cells and vascular smooth muscle cells have intracellular stores of calcium that can be released by the production of inositol triphosphate (IP_3). In both types of cells, agonist binding to specific receptors results in activation of phospholipase C (PLC) via guanine protein Gq (α). In the vascular smooth muscle cell, PLC activation results in IP_3 formation and release of intracellular calcium. Calcium binds to calmodulin, activating myosin light chain kinase (MLC), which then phosphorylates, causing myosin to interact with actin, producing shortening or tension generation. In contrast, in the endothelial cell, calcium binds to calmodulin to activate nitric oxide synthase, producing nitric oxide (NO). NO can diffuse to the vascular smooth muscle and modulate its behavior via activation of guanylate cyclase. Phospholipase A can be activated by G protein–linked pathways or by phosphokinase C and calcium, resulting in production of arachidonic acid. Arachidonic acid generates prostacyclin via the cyclooxygenase system, allowing relaxation of vascular smooth muscle. ATP, adenosine triphosphate; AMP, adenosine monophosphate; cAMP, cyclic adenosine monophosphate; cGMP, cyclic guanosine monophosphate; GMP, guanosine monophosphate; GTP, guanosine triphosphate. (Reprinted with permission from Lynch C, Lake CL: Cardiovascular anatomy and physiology. In: Youngberg J, Lake C, Roizen M *et al* (eds): Cardiac, Vascular, and Thoracic Anesthesia, p 126. Philadelphia, Churchill Livingstone, 2000.)

activate myosin light-chain phosphate to dephorylate myosin light chain.[109]

Endothelin

There are four active endothelin isoforms (1–4) of which endothelin-1 (ET-1) exerts a major effect on blood pressure through its actions on vascular smooth muscle.[110] It is formed by cleavage of preproendothelin-1 to big ET-1 and by ET-converting enzymes to ET-1. ET-1 acts by binding to two specific receptor subtypes: endothelin-A and endothelin-B in vascular smooth muscle and in atrial and ventricular smooth muscle layers. Endothelin-A is the major subtype producing vasoconstriction. Although endothelin-B also produces vasoconstriction through actions on vascular smooth muscle cells, it produces vasodilation via the release of NO and prostacyclin in endothelial cells. In addition to vasoconstriction, ET-1 stimulates production of vascular endothelial growth factor and potentiates the effects of platelet-derived growth factor and transforming growth factor-β. ET-1 is particularly abundant in pulmonary vasculature, where its production is stimulated by hypoxia.[111]

Nitric Oxide (NO)

NO, the endothelium-derived relaxing factor (EDRF), is a short-lived substance that activates soluble guanylate cyclase to increase intracellular cyclic guanosine 3′,5′-monophosphate, causing relaxation of vascular smooth muscle. It is formed from L-arginine by the enzyme nitric oxide synthase (NOS) in various mammalian tissues, particularly vascular endothelium. All three NOS isoforms—endothelial (e or NOSIII), inducible (i or NOSII), neuronal (n)—are expressed in cardiac myocytes. The calcium-sensitive enzymes nNOS and eNOS, as well as NO are activated when intracellular calcium increases as a result of extracellular calcium entry or intracellular calcium release. Basal release of NO occurs in all except cerebral and coronary vessels. Atherosclerosis impairs endothelium-dependent relaxation. Decreased production of NO may also contribute to both systemic and pulmonary hypertension. Hypoxia impairs endothelium-dependent vasodilation owing to inhibition of NO production and decreased half-life.[112] It also inhibits platelet adhesion and aggregation.

NO also has significant cardiac effects through both vascular-dependent and vascular-independent pathways.[113] The vascular-dependent effects include regulation of coronary tone, thrombogenicity, and angiogenesis, whereas the independent effects are fine regulation of excitation-contraction coupling, mitochondrial respiration, and modulation of autonomic signaling. The multiple effects of NO in myocardial cells are shown in Figure 30-19. In addition to the vascular effects, NO has a positive inotropic effect at low concentrations and a negative inotropic effect at higher concentrations.[113] Although the chronotropic effects are dependent on the experimental model, it appears that NO promotes negative chronotropic effects through nNOS-mediated effects in the cardiac ganglia and eNOS effects in the myocytes.[113] Activation of eNOS causes increased resistance to ventricular arrhythmias in dogs, and mice deficient in eNOS have lower thresholds to arrhythmogenic drugs.[114,115]

Natriuretic Peptides

Atrial natriuretic peptide (ANP) is a peptide stored in the perinuclear granules of human atrial myocytes and to a lesser extent

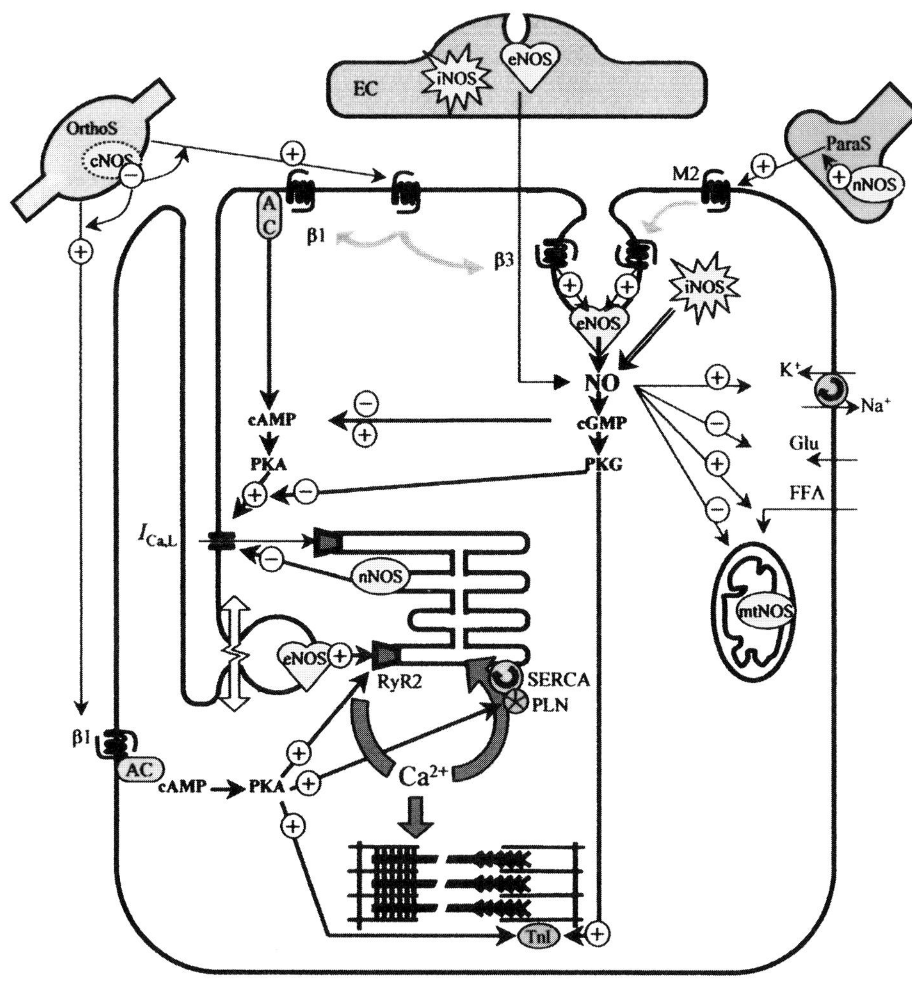

FIGURE 30-19. Effects of endogenous nitric oxide (NO) on myocardial cells. The intracellular effectors of endogenous NO are expressed in sympathetic (orthoS), parasympathetic (paraS), or the myocardial cells themselves. On the left side is the classic stimulatory effect on excitation-contraction coupling acting through β-adrenergic signaling. β-Adrenoceptor activation activates adenylcyclase and subseqently protein kinase A (PKA)-dependent phosphorylation of voltage-operated calcium channels (L-type calcium current I_{CaL}), ryanodine receptors (RyR2), and phospholamban (PLN) to de-repress the sarcoplasmic and endoplasmic reticulum Ca^{++}-ATPase (SERCA) to produce positive inotropic effects and phosphorylation of troponin I (TnI) to produce positive lusitropic effects. The right side of the figure shows modulating effects of NO on the β-adrenergic pathway, including phosphodiesterase regulation of cAMP levels through phosphodiesterase II (PDEII)-induced decreases and phosphokinase G (PKG)-mediated downregulation of L-type calcium current (all cyclic guanosine monophosphate [cGMP]-mediated effects). (Reprinted with permission from Massion PB, Feron O, Dessy C *et al*: Nitric oxide and cardiac function. *Circ Res* 93:388, 2003.)

in the ventricle.[116] Brain or B-type natriuretic peptide (BNP) is also produced primarily in atrium, whereas natriuretic peptide C is localized in the central nervous system. Natriuretic peptide receptors A, B, and C are receptor guanylyl cyclases, consisting of intracellular and extracellular domains. ANP is released in response to increased vascular volume (atrial distention), epinephrine, vasopressin, morphine, and increased atrial pressure. Normal circulating plasma levels are 25 to 100 μg/mL.[117]

The primary effects of ANP are direct peripheral vasodilation, suppression of antidiuretic hormone (ADH) release when the ADH is elevated by hemorrhage or dehydration, inhibition of aldosterone release, and direct renal effects such as increased glomerular filtration, natriuresis, and diuresis. Factors such as renal perfusion pressure and renal sympathetic nerve activity in conjunction with physiologic plasma concentrations of ANF produce natriuresis.[118] Kaliuresis does not occur. Atrial natriuretic factor affects not only blood pressure (by decreasing cardiac output and vascular resistance), but also water and electrolyte balance and blood volume. It has no direct inotropic or chronotropic properties.

Renin–Angiotensin System

Renin is a proteolytic enzyme produced in the granular juxtaglomerular cells of the kidney. Its release is governed by the macula densa, an intrarenal stretch-type receptor, circulating potassium, angiotensin II, epinephine, and concentrations of ADH, and by the renal sympathetic nerves. Renin secretion is also inversely related to renal perfusion.[119] The half-life of renin is 4 to 15 minutes, during which it initiates the formation of angiotensin I from angiotensinogen, which is synthesized in the liver. Angiotensin I is biologically inactive until it is cleaved by angiotensin-converting enzyme in lung and other tissues to angiotensin II. Angiotensin II and angiotensin III, formed by hydrolysis of angiotensin II, stimulate the secretion of aldosterone and inhibit renin release through a negative-feedback loop. The half-life of angiotensin II is about 30 seconds.

Sympathetic Nervous System

Norepinephrine is the important agonist at the α_1 receptor, mediating smooth muscle vasoconstriction in arteries and veins independently of neural supply. Epinephrine is more potent as a β_2 receptor agonist than is norepinephrine. β_2 Receptors, located in both presynaptic and postsynaptic regions, dilate arteries by stimulation of adenylcyclase.

Specific Peripheral Circulations

Pulmonary Circulation

The pulmonary circulation is a low-pressure, high-flow system that has five principal functions: (1) metabolic transport of humoral substances and drugs;[120] (2) transport of blood through the lungs; (3) reservoir for the LV; (4) filtration of venous drainage; and (5) transport of gas, fluid, and solutes across the walls of exchanging vessels. Normally, all circulating blood passes through the pulmonary circulation at least once each minute, but only 500 mL is present at a given time. Pulmonary pressures and resistances are only 80 to 90% of those in the systemic circulation. However, the pulmonary vessels are very reactive to hypoxia, sympathetic activation, and endogenous constrictors.

Metabolic Transport

The pulmonary vascular endothelium is important for removal, biosynthesis, and release of various vasoactive hormones, including biogenic amines, prostaglandins, leukotrienes, and peptides. Norepinephrine is removed by the lung by a carrier-mediated, temperature-sensitive and drug-sensitive transport process. Epinephrine, histamine, vasopressin, and dopamine, however, are unaltered by transpulmonary passage.[120] Almost complete removal of 5-hydroxytryptamine, ATP, and monophosphate occurs in the lungs. Acetylcholine and bradykinin are inactivated by the lungs. Prostaglandins of the E and F series are also removed either by a carrier-mediated, energy-requiring process or by rapid degradation by 15-hydroxyprostaglandin dehydrogenase. Prostacyclin is not inactivated in the lung. Many drugs such as propranolol, lidocaine, bupivacaine, captopril, and fentanyl are removed extensively during transpulmonary passage.

Intravascular Transport

The passage of blood and its distribution to various segments of the lung depend on pulmonary blood flow, pulmonary vascular resistance or impedance, left atrial pressure, transmural distending pressure, and distensibility of the pulmonary vessel walls. Blood flow to the lung apex is less than that to the base because of regional differences in pulmonary venous, alveolar, and arterial pressures. However, the pulmonary circulation accommodates a large increase in flow with little change in pressure by a substantial decrease in resistance. Pulmonary resistance is about one-fifth systemic and pulmonary impedance is about one-half systemic; pulse wave reflections are stronger in the pulmonary beds—although the reflecting sites are similar, the vascular bed is smaller. Abundant vascular smooth muscle is present in pulmonary vessels, distributed evenly between arteries and veins. Muscular arterioles are absent in the lung.

Capillary endothelium, endothelial basement membrane, interstitial space, epithelial basement membrane, and alveolar epithelium form the alveolocapillary membrane, which separates the blood and gas phases in the lung. The pulmonary veins perform primarily a reservoir function, preventing pulmonary edema in the event of reduced left ventricular compliance.[121]

Measurements of Pulmonary Tone

Measurements of pulmonary tone are essential to therapeutic investigations. However, the available measurement methods are either difficult or have significant limitations. Normal values for pulmonary vascular resistance are given in Table 30-4.

PA pressures are clinically measured using flow-directed catheters. Wedging of the tip of these catheters in a small branch of the PA measures the pulmonary wedge pressure or occluded pressure (PAoP) (Table 30-2). As the pressure of the column of blood from the tip of the catheter (beyond the point of balloon occlusion) equilibrates with left atrial pressure, PAoP is achieved. Normally, left atrial pressure is similar to left ventricular end-diastolic pressure in the absence of mitral valvular stenosis. Other reasons for a PAoP that is greater than left ventricular end-diastolic pressure include increased airway pressures or the presence of an intra-atrial mass. Normally, the PAoP is 1 to 4 mm Hg lower than pulmonary end-diastolic pressure. However, with tachycardia or increased pulmonary resistance, the pulmonary wedge pressure may be the same or slightly higher than pulmonary end-diastolic pressure.

PA pressure is not linearly related to either flow or left atrial pressure. An increase in pulmonary flow or left atrial pressure is unaccompanied by a proportional increase in pulmonary arterial pressure. Therefore, calculated pulmonary vascular resistance decreases when either pulmonary flow or left atrial pressure increases. The nonlinearity results from distention or recruitment of vessels when flow or pressure increases. However, in zone 3 of the lung (where left atrial pressure is greater than airway pressure), PA pressure is the most important factor determining pulmonary blood flow.[122] Therefore, regardless of the effect on the pulmonary vascular tone, agents or manipulations that change pulmonary flow or left atrial pressure will change calculated pulmonary vascular resistance. Only if a particular intervention does not change pulmonary flow or left atrial pressure, or if the changes in pulmonary resistance can be explained only by active changes in pulmonary tone (e.g., a decrease in PA pressure accompanied by an increase in pulmonary blood flow), is pulmonary vascular resistance unchanged. Even in these circumstances, however, reflex effects caused by the drug or maneuver cannot be eliminated.[123]

Another major factor affecting indirect measurements is airway pressure because the degree of lung inflation and the ventilatory pressure directly influence pulmonary pressure–flow relationships. Either increases or decreases in lung volume beyond normal functional residual capacity increase pulmonary resistance because of compression of small intra-alveolar vessels.

Effects of Drugs and Maneuvers on Pulmonary Tone

Baseline pulmonary tone, stimulation of pulmonary chemoreceptors, autonomic influences, bronchospasm, and other physiologic or nonphysiologic conditions actively or passively affect the pulmonary vasculature or modify its response to drugs. These factors are summarized in Table 30-10.

Alveoli in a poorly ventilated area of lung that contains hypoxic gas cause the precapillary arterial vessels supplying that area to constrict to divert blood away from the area. This process is termed hypoxic pulmonary vasoconstriction. Pulmonary hypertension does not occur because the hypoxia is localized. If hypoxia is generalized, pulmonary hypertension ensues.[124] Metabolic acidosis slightly enhances hypoxic pulmonary vasoconstriction, whereas respiratory acidosis has no effect.[125] Metabolic and respiratory alkalosis decrease it.[125] Drugs such as nitroprusside, nitroglycerin, and inhalation anesthetics decrease hypoxic pulmonary vasoconstriction, resulting in worsening of venous admixture and arterial PO_2.[126] However, increased PA pressure from whatever mechanism inhibits hypoxic pulmonary vasoconstriction.

Renal Circulation

Renal blood flow is well in excess of the amount needed for renal perfusion. It is autoregulated so glomerular filtration remains relatively constant despite changes in arterial pressure between 70 and 180 mm Hg. The autoregulatory mechanisms operate sluggishly so oscillations in pressure of even several seconds' duration are not compensated by constant flow.[127] Mechanisms proposed to explain renal autoregulation include (1) tubuloglomerular feedback (vasoactive hormonal release from the juxtaglomerular apparatus in response to the quantity or quality of filtrate reaching the macula densa), and (2) myogenic response of renal vascular smooth muscle (changes in afferent/efferent arteriole tone). The myogenic response causes renal resistance vessels to constrict when perfusion pressure increases. The tubuloglomerular feedback mechanism provides fine-tuning via sensing of the distal tubule sodium chloride by the macula densa. Preglomerular or postglomerular resistance is then altered by vasoactive substances

TABLE 30-10

ALTERATIONS IN PULMONARY VASCULAR RESISTANCE

FACTORS	CHANGES
ACTIVE CHANGES	
Sympathetic stimulation	Increased or unchanged
Parasympathetic stimulation	Unchanged
Catecholamines	Increased
Angiotensin	Increased
Acetylcholine	Decreased
Histamine	Increased/decreased
Bradykinin	Decreased
Serotonin	Increased
Prostaglandin E_1	Decreased
Prostaglandin F	Increased
Hypoxia	Increased
Hypercarbia	Increased or unchanged
Acidemia	Increased
PASSIVE CHANGES	
Pulmonary hypertension	Decreased
Left atrial hypertension	Decreased
Increased pulmonary interstitial pressure	Increased
Increased blood viscosity	Increased
Increased pulmonary blood volume	Decreased

Data from Murray JP: The Normal Lung, p 128. Philadelphia, WB Saunders, 1976; Perloff WH: Physiology of the heart and circulation. In Swedlow DB, Raphaely RC (eds): Cardiovascular Problems in Pediatric Critical Care, p 1. New York, Churchill Livingstone, 1986; Stalcup A *et al*: Inhibition of angiotensin-converting enzyme activity in cultured endothelial cells by hypoxia. J Clin Invest 63:966, 1979; Hyman AL *et al*: Autonomic regulation of the pulmonary circulation. J Cardiovasc Pharmacol 7(suppl 3)S80, 1985.

such as adenosine, NO, ATP, or renin. In particular, the renal medulla may have impaired autoregulatory capacity because it receives only a small fraction of total renal blood flow and its oxygen tension is low. Glomerular capillary pressure, about two-thirds of systemic pressure, is increased by dilation of the afferent arteriole or constriction of the efferent arteriole. Other factors affecting glomerular filtration include the total surface area available for filtration and the permeability of the glomerular membrane.

The main purpose of the excessive renal flow is to provide energy for active renal tubular reabsorption of sodium. Renal oxygen consumption is high, and the arteriovenous oxygen content difference is low. Of the blood delivered to the glomeruli, about 20% is filtered to form an ultrafiltrate of plasma. The main driving force is the glomerular hydrostatic pressure, which is essentially the systemic arterial pressure modified by the renal vasculature. The ultrafiltrate collects in Bowman's space before passing into the renal tubular system.

Physiology of the Venous System

Systemic veins have a conduit and a reservoir function. Because the smallest postcapillary venules lack muscular layers, and venules and small veins have only small amounts of muscle, the postcapillary resistance is usually small. However, postcapillary resistance is important because the ratio of precapillary to postcapillary resistance determines the capillary filtration pressure. The major capacitance vessels include medium and large veins, as well as the venae cavae. About 60% of the systemic blood volume is in small veins and venules whose diameters range from 20 μm to 2 mm.[128]

The term *vascular capacitance* is used for the vascular pressure–volume relationship at a given level of venous tone. Venous tone is normally at 70% of maximum in the erect human. Venodilation to accommodate as much as 70 to 75% of the systemic blood volume buffers sudden increases in arterial blood pressure by allowing sequestration of blood in systemic veins. The compliance of the venous system is regulated by venomotor tone, which is controlled by cerebral autonomic impulses. Sympathetically mediated venoconstriction adds about 1 L of blood to the circulation, but passive constriction from a reduction in venous pressure contributes about two-thirds of the total volume mobilized. Individual organs contribute about 30 to 50% of their blood volume by sympathetically mediated venoconstriction.

Venous return (VR), the rate of flow of blood from the periphery to the heart, is a major determinant of cardiac preload. In a steady state, cardiac output is equal to VR. It is determined by the pressure gradient from the peripheral vascular beds (P_{MS} or mean systemic pressure) to the right side of the heart (P_{RA}) and the resistance to venous return (R_V).[129] This gradient is described by $P_{MS} - P_{RA}$ resulting in the formula

$$VR = (P_{MS} - P_{RA})/R_V$$

The upstream driving pressure from the peripheral tissue to the RA is the mean circulatory filling pressure or mean systemic pressure. The term *mean systemic pressure* should not be confused with *mean arterial pressure*. The mean circulatory filling pressure, which is an equalization of pressures between the venous and arterial beds when flow is 0, is usually about 10 mm Hg, similar to the mean systemic filling pressure. It is increased by catecholamines or increased sympathetic activity.[128] An increase in right atrial pressure decreases the pressure gradient and venous return. The resistance to venous return is primarily determined by large veins, such as the venae cavae and peripheral large and medium-size veins that are responsive to autonomic influences or vasoactive mediators. Factors that increase VR include redistribution of blood from vascular beds with low volume and high flows to those with high volume and low flow, polycythemia or conditions increasing blood viscosity, and venous constriction.[129] Cutaneous venous tone is determined by thermoregulatory mechanisms rather than systemic pressure regulatory mechanisms.

Loss of venous tone, as in autonomic neuropathy or during anesthesia, limits the normal compensatory increases in venous tone to changes in posture, positive airway pressure, or decreased blood volume. If these factors are excessive, ventricular preload is adversely affected. Venoconstriction induced by hypovolemia, anxiety, or exercise augments intrathoracic blood volume and preload.

Physiology of the Pericardium

The pericardium has limited but important physiologic functions in the maintenance of biventricular systolic and diastolic function.[130] As dilatation of the LV occurs, intrapericardial pressure limits right ventricular filling and reduces forward flow to the lungs, possibly preventing pulmonary edema. Shifts of the left ventricular diastolic pressure–volume relationship are equal to changes in pericardial pressure and volume. During cardiac tamponade, increased intrapericardial fluid causes hypotension, decreased cardiac output, myocardial ischemia, and tachycardia. However, a vagally mediated depressive reflex is also operative, contributing further to the decreased cardiac output resulting from the presence of pericardial fluid.[131] Increased intrapericardial pressure results in an underfilled ventricle, which operates on the ascending limb of Starling's curve.

References

1. Loscalzo J: Proteomics in cardiovascular biology and medicine. Circulation 108:380, 2003
2. Stumper O, Fraser AG, Anderson RH *et al*: Transesophageal echocardiography in the longitudinal axis: Correlation between anatomy and images and its clinical implications. Br Heart J 64:282, 1990
3. Blaise G, Langleben D, Hubert B: Pulmonary arterial hypertension. Anesthesiology 99:1415, 2003
4. Pagel PS, Kehl F, Gare M *et al*: Mechanical functions of the left atrium. Anesthesiology 98:975, 2003
5. Lam JHS, Ranganathan N, Wiggle ED, Silver MD: Morphology of the human mitral valve. I. Chordae tendineae. Circulation 41:449, 1970
6. Byrd BF, Schiller NB, Botvinick EH, Higgins CB: Normal cardiac dimensions by magnetic resonance imaging. Am J Cardiol 55:1440, 1985
7. James TN: Blood supply of the human interventricular septum. Circulation 17:391, 1958
8. Nerantzis CE, Toutouzas P, Avgoustakis D: The importance of the sinus node artery in the blood supply of the atrial myocardium. Acta Cardiol 38:35, 1983
9. James TN: Morphology of the human atrioventricular node, with remarks pertinent to its electrophysiology. Am Heart J 62:756, 1961
10. Schram G, Pourrier M, Melnyk P, Nattel S: Differential distribution of cardiac ion channel expression as a basis for regional specialization in electrical function. Circ Res 90:939, 2002
11. Bachmann G: The inter-auricular time interval. Am J Physiol 41:309, 1916
12. Medkour D, Becker AE, Khalife K, Billette J: Anatomic and functional characteristics of a slow posterior AV nodal pathway: Role in dual-pathway physiology and reentry. Circulation 98:164, 1998
13. Brown DL, Guyenet FG: Electrophysiological study of cardiovascular neurons in the rostral ventrolateral medulla in rats. Circ Res 56:359, 1985
14. DeGeest H, Levy MN, Zieske H, Lipman RI: Depression of ventricular contractility by stimulation of the vagus nerves. Circ Res 17:222, 1965
15. Schauerte P, Mischke K, Plisiene J *et al*: Catheter stimulation of cardiac parasympathetic nerves in humans. Circulation 104:2430, 2001
16. Stiles GL, Taylor S, Lefkowitz RJ: Human cardiac beta adrenergic receptors: Subtypes heterogeneity delineated by direct radiological binding. Life Sci 33:467, 1983
17. Spodick DH: The normal and diseased pericardium: Current concepts of pericardial physiology, diagnosis and treatment. J Am Coll Cardiol 1:240, 1983
18. Poon M, Fuster V, Fayad Z: Cardiac magnetic resonance imaging: A "one-stop-shop" evaluation of myocardial dysfunction. Curr Opin Cardiol 17:663, 2002
19. Pohost GM, Hung L, Doyle M: Clinical use of cardiovascular magnetic resonance. Circulation 108:647, 2003
20. Khandheria BK: Noninvasive imaging. J Am Coll Cardiol 44(suppl A):25A, 2004
21. Kennedy JW: Registry Committee of the Society for Cardiac Angiography: Complications associated with cardiac catheterization and angiography. Cathet Cardiovasc Diagn 8:5, 1982
22. Cannon SR, Richards Kl, Crawford M: Hydraulic estimation of stenotic orifice area: A correction of the Gorlin formula. Circulation 71:1170, 1985
23. Conti CR: Coronary angiography. Circulation 55:227, 1977
24. Pagel PS, Grossman W, Haering JM, Warltier DC: Left ventricular diastolic function in the normal and diseased heart. Anesthesiology 79:836, 1993
25. Pagel PS, Grossman W, Haering JM, Warltier DC: Left ventricular diastolic function in the normal and diseased heart. Anesthesiology 79:1104, 1993
26. White CW, Holida MD, Marcus ML: Effects of acute atrial fibrillation on the vasodilator reserve of the canine atrium. Cardiovasc Res 20:683, 1986
27. Robinson TF, Factor SM, Sonnenblick EH: The heart as a suction pump. Sci Am 254:84, 1986
28. Barbier P, Solomon SB, Schiller NB, Glantz SA: Left atrial relaxation and left ventricular systolic function determine left atrial reservoir function. Circulation 100:427, 1999
29. Perez-Reyes E, Schneider T: Molecular biology of calcium channels. Kidney Int 48:1111, 1995
30. Po S, Roberds S, Snyders DJ, Tamkun MM, Bennett PB: Heteromultimeric assembly of human potassium channels. Molecular basis of a transient outward current? Circ Res 72:1326, 1993
31. Krapivinsky G, Gordon EA, Wickman K, Velimirovic B, Krapivinskly L, Clapham DE: The G-protein-gated atrial K+ channel IKA Ch is a heteromultimer of two inwardly rectifying K(+)-channel proteins. Nature 374:135, 1995
32. Lakatta EG, Maltsev VA, Bogdanov KY *et al*: Cyclic variation of intracellular calcium. A critical factor for cardiac pacemaker cell dominance. Circ Res 92:e45, 2003
33. Carmeliet E: Mechanisms and control of repolarization. Eur Heart J 14(suppl H):3, 1993
34. Wendt DJ, Martin JB: Autonomic neural regulation of intact Purkinje system of dogs. Am J Physiol 258:H1420, 1990
35. Coraboeuf E, Weidman S: Temperature effects on the electrical activity of Purkinje fibers. Helv Physiol Pharmacol Acta 12:32, 1954
36. Kohlhardt M, Mnich Z, Maier G: Alteration of the excitation process of the sinoatrial pacemaker cell in the presence of anoxia and metabolic inhibitors. J Mol Cell Cardiol 9:477, 1977
37. Fisch C, Knoebel SB, Feigenbaum H, Greenspan K: Potassium and the monophasic action potential, electrocardiogram, conduction, and arrhythmias. Prog Cardiovasc Dis 8:387, 1966
38. Cinca J, Morja A, Figueras J *et al*: Circadian variations in the electrical properties of the human heart assessed by sequential bedside electrophysiologic testing. Am Heart J 112:315, 1986
39. Urthaler F, Neely BH, Hageman GR, Smith LR: Differential sympathetic-parasympathetic interactions in sinus node and AV junction. Am J Physiol 250:H43, 1986
40. Hoffman BF, Moore EN, Stuckey JH *et al*: Functional properties of the atrioventricular conduction system. Circ Res 13:308, 1963
41. Kovacs SJ: The duration of the QT interval as a function of heart rate: A derivation based on physical principles and comparison to measured values. Am Heart J 110:876, 1985
42. De Marneffe M, Jacobs P, Haardt R, Englert M: Variation of normal sinus node function in relation to age: Role of autonomic influence. Eur Heart J 7:662, 1986
43. Evans JM, Randall DC, Funk JN, Knapp CF: Influence of cardiac innervation on intrinsic heart rate in dogs. Am J Physiol 258:H1132, 1990
44. Medak R, Benumof JL: Perioperative management of prolonged Q-T interval syndrome. Br J Anaesth 55:361, 1983
45. Longhurst JC: Cardiac receptors: Their function in health and disease. Prog Cardiovasc Dis 27:201, 1984
46. Wong TM, Lee AY-S, Tai KK: Effects of drugs interacting with opioid receptors during normal perfusion or ischemia and reperfusion in the isolated rat heart. An attempt to identify cardiac opioid receptor subtypes involved in arrhythmogenesis. J Mol Cell Cardiol 22:1167, 1997
47. Lee AY-S: Endogenous opioid pepetides and cardiac arrhythmias. Int J Cardiol 27:145, 1990
48. Lynch C, Jaeger JM: The G protein cell signaling system. In Lake CL, Barash PG, Sperry RJ (eds): Advances in Anesthesia, vol 11, p 65. Chicago, Mosby–Year Book, 1994
49. Feigl EO, Neat GW, Huang AH: Interrelations between coronary artery pressure, myocardial metabolism and coronary blood flow. J Mol Cell Cardiol 22:375, 1990
50. White CF, Wilson RF, Marcus ML: Methods of measuring myocardial blood flow in humans. Prog Cardiovasc Dis 31:79, 1988
51. Hoffman JIE: Determinants and prediction of transmural myocardial perfusion. Circulation 58:381, 1978
52. Westerhof N: Physiological hypotheses—intramyocardial pressure. A new concept, suggestions for measurement. Basic Res Cardiol 85:105, 1990
53. Marcus ML, Chilian WM, Kanatsuka H *et al*: Understanding the coronary circulation through studies at the microvascular level. Circulation 82:1, 1990
54. Rubio P, Berne RM: Regulation of coronary blood flow. Progr Cardiovasc Dis 43:105, 1975
55. Dole WP: Autoregulation of the coronary circulation. Prog Cardiovasc Dis 29:293, 1987
56. Chilian WM, Layne SM: Coronary microvascular responses to reductions in perfusion pressure. Circ Res 66:1227, 1990
57. Trimarco B, Ricciardelli B, Cuocolo A *et al*: Effects of coronary occlusion on arterial baroreflex control of heart rate and vascular resistance. Am J Physiol 252:H749, 1987
58. Baron JF, Vicaut E, Hou X, Duvelleroy M: Independent role of arterial O_2 tension in local control of coronary blood flow. Am J Physiol 258:H1388, 1990
59. Dole WP, Nuno DW: Myocardial oxygen tension determines the degree and pressure range of coronary autoregulation. Circ Res 59:202, 1986
60. Vatner SF: Regulation of coronary resistance vessels and large coronary arteries. Am J Cardiol 56:16E, 1985
61. Samaha FF, Heineman W, Ince C *et al*: ATP-sensitive potassium channel is essential to maintain basal coronary vascular tone in vivo. Am J Physiol 31:C1220, 1992
62. Narishige T, Egashira K, Akatsuka Y *et al*: Glibenclamide, a putative ATP-sensitive K+ channel blocker, inhibits coronary autoregulation in anesthetized dogs. Circ Res 73:771, 1993
63. Karmazyn M, Dhalla NS: Physiological and pathophysiological aspects of cardiac prostaglandins. Can J Physiol Pharmacol 61:1207, 1983
64. Marone G, Triggiani M, Cirillo R *et al*: Chemical mediators and the human heart. Prog Biochem Pharmacol 20:38, 1985
65. Austin RE, Aldea GS, Coggins DL *et al*: Profound spatial heterogeneity of coronary reserve. Circ Res 67:319, 1990
66. Hoffman JIE: Transmural myocardial perfusion. Progr Cardiovasc Dis 29:429, 1987
67. Dyke CM, Brunsting LA, Salter DR *et al*: Preload dependence of right ventricular blood flow. I. The normal right ventricle. Ann Thorac Surg 43:478, 1987
68. Vatner SF: Alpha adrenergic regulation of the coronary circulation in the conscious dog. Am J Cardiol 52:15A, 1983
69. Shepherd JT, Vanhoutte PM: Mechanisms responsible for contrary vasospasm. J Am Coll Cardiol 8:50A, 1986
70. Goldstein DS, Brush JE, Eisenhofer G *et al*: In vivo measurement of neuronal uptake of norepinephrine in the human heart. Circulation 78:41, 1988

71. Little RC, Little WC: Cardiac preload, afterload, and heart failure. Arch Intern Med 142:819, 1982
72. Lang RM, Borow KM, Neumann A, Janzen D: Systemic vascular resistance: An unreliable index of left ventricular afterload. Circulation 74:1114, 1986
73. Prewitt RM, Wood LDH: Effect of altered resistive load on left ventricular systolic mechanics in dogs. Anesthesiology 56:195, 1982
74. Shaeffer S, Taylor AL, Lee HR *et al*: Effect of increasing heart rate on left ventricular performance in patients with normal cardiac function. Am J Cardiol 61:617, 1988
75. Wisenbaugh T, Nissen S, DeMaria A: Mechanics of postextrasystolic potentiation in normal subjects and patients with valvular heart disease. Circulation 74:10, 1986
76. Hathaway DR, March KL, Lash JA *et al*: Vascular smooth muscle. A review of the molecular basis of contractility. Circulation 83:382, 1991
77. Braunwald E, Sonnenblick EH, Ross J: Contraction of the normal heart. In Braunwald E (ed): Textbook of Cardiovascular Medicine, 2nd ed, p 409, Philadelphia, WB Saunders, 1983
78. Katz AM: Cyclic adenosine monophosphate effects on the myocardium: A man who blows hot and cold with one breath. J Am Coll Cardiol 2:143, 1983
79. Brutsaert DL, Rademakers FE, Sys SU *et al*: Analysis of relaxation in the evaluation of ventricular function of the heart. Prog Cardiovasc Dis 28:143, 1985
80. Bombardini T, Joao-Correia J, Cicerone C *et al*: Force-frequency relationship in the echocardiography laboratory: A noninvasive assessment of Bowditch treppe. J Am Soc Echocardiogr 16:646, 2003
81. Woodworth RS: Maximal contraction, "staircase" contraction, refractory period, and compensatory pause of the heart. Am J Physiol 8:213, 1902
82. Hayashi K, Shigemi K, Shishido T *et al*: Single-beat estimation of ventricular end-systolic elastance—effective arterial elastance as an index of ventricular mechanoenergetic performance. Anesthesiology 92:1769, 2000
83. Starling EH: The Lineacre lecture on the law of the heart. In Chapman CB, Mitchell JH (eds): Starling on the Heart, p 119. London, Pall Mall, 1965
84. Parker JO, Case RB: Normal left ventricular function. Circulation 60:4, 1979
85. Chung N, Wu X, Bailey KR, Ritman EL: LV pressure–volume area and oxygen consumption. Evaluation by intact dog by fast CT. Am J Physiol 258:H1208, 1990
86. Jacob R, Kissling G: Ventricular pressure–volume relations as the primary basis for evaluation of cardiac mechanics. Return to Frank's diagram. Basic Res Cardiol 84:227, 1989
87. Van der Linden LP, Van der Wilde ET, Bruschke AVG, Baan J: Comparison between force-velocity and end-systolic pressure volume characterization of intrinsic LV function. Am J Physiol 259:H1419, 1990
88. Foex P, Francis CM, Cutfield GR, Leone B: The pressure-length loop. Br J Anaesth 60:65S, 1988
89. Safwat A, Leone BJ, Norris RM, Foex P: Pressure-length loop area: Its components analyzed during graded myocardial ischemia. J Am Coll Cardiol 17:790, 1991
90. Barash PG, Kopriva CJ: Cardiac monitoring. In Thomas SJ, Kramer JL (eds): Manual of Cardiac Anesthesia, 2nd ed, p 23. New York, Churchill Livingstone, 1993
91. Damino RJ, Cox JL, Lowe JE, Santamore WP: Left ventricular pressure effects on right ventricular pressure and volume outflow. Cathet Cardiovasc Diagn 19:269, 1990
92. Weber KT, Janicki JS, Shroff SG *et al*: The right ventricle: Physiologic and pathophysiologic considerations. Crit Care Med 11:323, 1983
93. Barnard D, Alpert JS: Right ventricular function in health and disease. Curr Probl Cardiol 12:423, 1987
94. Santamore WP, Shaffer T, Papa L: Theoretical model of ventricular interdependence: Pericardial effects. Am J Physiol 259:H181, 1990
95. Maruyama Y, Nunokawa T, Kiowa T *et al*: Mechanical interdependence between the ventricles. Basic Res Cardiol 78:544, 1993
96. Berne RM (ed): Handbook of Physiology. The Cardiovascular System, p 873, Baltimore, Williams & Wilkins, 1979
97. Weber KT, Janicki JS: The metabolic demand and oxygen supply of the heart: Physiologic and clinical considerations. Am J Cardiol 44:722, 1979
98. Shoukas AA: Overall systems analysis of the carotid sinus baroreceptor reflex control of the circulation. Anesthesiology 79:1402, 1993
99. Hering HE: Der karotisdruckversuch. Munch Med Wochenschr 70:1287, 1923
100. Schmidt RM, Kumada M, Sagewa K: Cardiovascular responses to various pulsatile pressures in the carotid sinus. Am J Physiol 223:1, 1972
101. Von Bezold A, Hirt L: Uber die physiologischen wirkungen des essigsauren veratrins. Physiol Lab Wuerzburg Untersuchungen 1:75, 1867
102. Mark AL: The Bezold Jarisch reflex revisited: Clinical implications of inhibitory reflexes originating in the heart. J Am Coll Cardiol 1:90, 1983
103. Jarisch A, Richter H: Die afferenten bahnen des veratrins effektes in den herznerven. Arch Exp Pathol Pharmacol 193:355, 1939
104. Campagna JA, Carter C: Clinical relevance of the Bezold-Jarisch reflex. Anesthesiology 98:1250, 2003
105. James TN: A cardiogenic hypertensive chemoreflex. Anesth Analg 69:633, 1989
106. Ledsome JR, Linden RJ: A reflex increase in heart rate from distention of the pulmonary vein-atrial junction. J Physiol 170:456, 1964
107. O'Rourke MF, Yaginuma T: Wave reflections and the arterial pulse. Arch Intern Med 144:366, 1984
108. Burnstock G: Integration of factors controlling vascular tone. Anesthesiology 79:1368, 1993
109. Munzel T, Feil R, Mulsch A *et al*: Physiology and pathophysiology of vascular signaling controlled by cyclic guanosine-3′,5′-cyclic monophosphate-dependent protein kinase. Circulation 108:2172, 2003
110. McEniery CM, Qasem A, Schmitt M *et al*: Endothelin-1 regulates arterial pulse wave velocity in vivo. J Am Coll Cardiol 42:1975, 2003
111. Rich S, McLaughlin VV: Endothelin receptor blockers in cardiovascular disease. Circulation 108:2184, 2003
112. Johns RA: Endothelium-derived relaxing factor: Basic review and clinical implications. J Cardiothorac Vasc Anesth 5:69, 1991
113. Massion PB, Feron O, Dessy C, Balligand J-L: Nitric oxide and cardiac function. Circ Res 93:388, 2003
114. Fei L, Baron AD, Henry DP, Zipes DP: Intrapericardial delivery of L-arginine reduces the increased severity of ventricular arrhythmias during sympathetic stimulation in dogs with acute coronary occlusion: Nitric oxide modulates sympathetic effects on ventricular electrophysiological properties. Circulation 96:4044, 1997
115. Kubota I, Han X, Opel DJ, *et al*: Increased susceptibility to development of triggered activity in myocytes from mice with targeted disruption of endothelial nitric oxide synthase. J Mol Cell Cardiol 32:1239, 2000
116. Ferrari R, Agnoletti G: Atrial natriuretic peptide: Its mechanism of release from the atrium. Int J Cardiol 25:S3, 1989
117. de Bold AJ: Atrial natriuretic factor: A hormone produced by the heart. Science 230:767, 1985
118. Blaine EH: Atrial natriuretic factor plays a significant role in body fluid homeostasis. Hypertension 15:2, 1990
119. Reid IA: The renin-angiotensin system and body function. Arch Intern Med 145:1475, 1985
120. Said SI: Metabolic functions of the pulmonary circulation. Circ Res 50:325, 1982
121. Goto M, Arakawa M, Suzuki T *et al*: A quantitative analysis of reservoir function of the human pulmonary "venous" system for the left ventricle. Jpn Circ J 50:222, 1986
122. Thorvaldson J, Ilebekk A, Loraand S, Kiil F: Determinants of pulmonary blood volume. Effects of acute changes in pulmonary vascular pressure and flow. Acta Physiol Scand 121:45, 1984
123. Rich S, Martinez J, Lam W *et al*: Reassessment of the effects of vasodilator drugs in primary pulmonary hypertension. Guidelines for determining a pulmonary vasodilator response. Am Heart J 105:119, 1983
124. Rudolph AM, Yuan S: Response of the pulmonary vasculature to hypoxia and H+ ion concentration changes. J Clin Invest 45:399, 1966
125. Brimioulle S, Lejeune P, Vachiery J-L *et al*: Effects of acidosis and alkalosis on hypoxic pulmonary vasoconstriction in dogs. Am J Physiol 258:347, 1990
126. Marshall BE, Marshall C: Anesthesia and the pulmonary circulation. In Covino BG, Fozzard HA, Strichartz G (eds): Effects of Anesthesia, p 121, Bethesda, MD, American Physiological Society, 1985
127. Persson PB: Renal blood flow autoregulation in blood pressure control. Curr Opin Nephrol Hypertens 11:67, 2002
128. Rothe CF: Physiology of venous return. Arch Intern Med 146:977, 1986
129. Jacobsohn E, Chorn R, O'Connor M: The role of the vasculature in regulating venous return and cardiac output: Historical and graphical approach. Can J Anaesth 44:849, 1997
130. Lake CL: Anesthesia and pericardial disease. Anesth Analg 62:431, 1983
131. Friedman HS, Lajam F, Gomes JA *et al*: Demonstration of a depressor reflex in acute cardiac tamponade. J Thorac Cardiovasc Surg 73:278, 1977
132. Maniu CV, Nishimura RA, Tajik AJ: Tachycardia during the Valsalva maneuver: A sign of normal diastolic filling pressures. J Am Soc Echocardiogr 17:634, 2004

CHAPTER 31 ■ ANESTHESIA FOR CARDIAC SURGERY

NIKOLAOS SKUBAS, ADAM D. LICHTMAN, AARTI SHARMA, AND STEPHEN J. THOMAS

KEY POINTS

1. Decreasing O_2 demand is as important as modifying O_2 supply.
2. Intraoperative ischemia is usually silent and is not always accompanied by hemodynamic changes.
3. A slow, small in size, and well-perfused heart are the goals.
4. The pulmonary artery catheter does not always reliably detect ischemia.
5. Echocardiography is more sensitive than electrocardiogram (ECG) in detecting ischemia: a myocardial segment is healthy if it moves inward and thickens.
6. Echocardiographic ejection fraction does not always represent contractility.
7. Impaired relaxation mandates volume augmentation and relatively slow, sinus rhythm, while a dilated ventricle requires unloading and inotropes.
8. There is no "ideal" anesthetic.
9. In aortic stenosis, a preload-dependent, hypertrophic ventricle requires adequate diastolic time and perfusion pressure.
10. In chronic aortic insufficiency, a dilated ventricle requires increased preload and decreased afterload.
11. In mitral stenosis, the left ventricle (LV) is "lazy" and "under used," and requires a slow heart rate to fill.
12. In mitral regurgitation, a preload-dependent and dilated LV benefits from afterload reduction and fast heart rate.
13. Maintenance of perfusion pressure should not take precedence over ventilation (never forget your ABCs).
14. Fast-track anesthetic techniques depend on higher concentration of inspired volatile agents, use of vasoactive medications (beta-blockers) and smaller doses of benzodiazepines and opioids.
15. The combination of systolic systemic and diastolic pulmonary pressures characterize the performance of the LV, and the combination of systolic pulmonary and central venous pressures the performance of the right ventricle (RV).

Anesthetizing patients for open heart surgery is exciting, intellectually challenging, and emotionally rewarding. Competent and skillful clinical management requires a thorough understanding of normal and altered cardiac physiology; an intimate knowledge of the pharmacology of anesthetic, vasoactive, and cardioactive drugs; and a familiarity with the physiologic derangements associated with cardiopulmonary bypass and the surgical procedures themselves. This chapter presents a brief overview of the subject to familiarize the reader with the critical physiologic and technical considerations when caring for cardiac surgical patients. The initial discussions concerning coronary artery and valvular heart disease lay the physiologic and some of the pharmacologic groundwork on which anesthetic planning and therapeutic decisions are based. First, we describe the balance of myocardial oxygen supply and demand, with particular reference to the patient with coronary artery disease. Next, we focus on those variables that regulate myocardial performance, specifically myocardial contractility, heart rate, and loading conditions (both preload and afterload). Then, we discuss the mechanics of cardiopulmonary bypass. Following this, we describe anesthetic considerations relevant to all adults undergoing cardiac surgery either with or without cardiopulmonary bypass (CPB), including preoperative evaluation, choice of monitoring techniques, selection of anesthetic drugs, and the actual conduct of the anesthetic before, during, and after bypass. The chapter concludes with some special topics, as well as a brief introduction to the child with congenital heart disease. Some of the issues discussed are controversial because the field is continuously evolving. We have tried, whenever possible, to suggest what is the consensus about these topics, but, inevitably, our own preferences will be apparent. For the sake of brevity, numerous tables are included that summarize data and provide readily accessible guidelines for the various phases of the operative procedure. Many monographs are available for those who desire more detailed analysis of any aspect of cardiac anesthesia.[1,2]

CORONARY ARTERY DISEASE

Prevention or treatment of ischemia during coronary artery bypass graft (CABG) surgery reduces the incidence of perioperative myocardial infarction. Hemodynamic management is tailored to avoid factors known to increase myocardial oxygen demand ($\dot{M}VO_2$), particularly during the vulnerable pre-CPB period. Optimizing oxygen delivery to the myocardium is equally important for the successful management of these patients because it is well recognized that most ischemic events occur with minimal or no change in $\dot{M}VO_2$.[3,4] The determinants of myocardial oxygen supply and demand are shown in Figure 31-1 and are also discussed in Chapter 30.

Myocardial Oxygen Demand

The principal determinants of $\dot{M}VO_2$ are wall tension and contractility.[5] Laplace's law states that wall tension is directly proportional to intracavitary pressure and ventricular radius, and inversely proportional to wall thickness. Therefore, myocardial oxygen demand can be reduced by interventions that (1) prevent or promptly treat ventricular distention, and (2) decrease myocardial oxygen consumption.

Myocardial Oxygen Supply

Increases in myocardial oxygen requirements can be met only by raising coronary blood flow. Blood oxygen content is important, as is oxygen extraction by the myocardium, but these are infrequent reasons for intraoperative ischemia because oxygenation and blood volume are usually well maintained during anesthesia. Blood in the coronary sinus is 50% saturated (PO_2 ~27 mm Hg), and although extraction can be increased somewhat under conditions of stress, it is inadequate to meet the continuously increasing demand. Therefore, the principal mechanism for matching oxygen supply to alterations in $\dot{M}VO_2$ is exquisite regulation and control of coronary blood
1 flow.

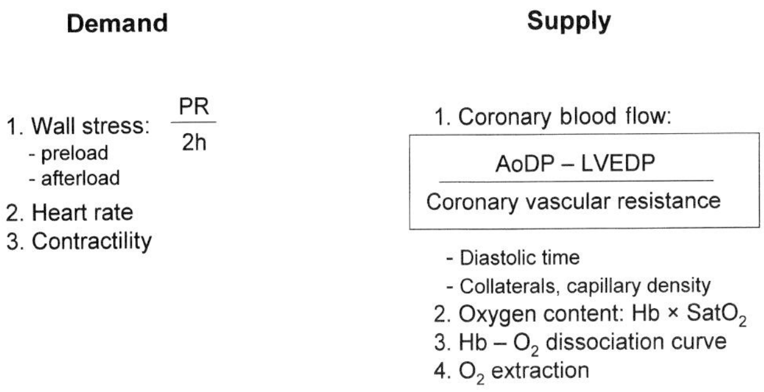

Demand

1. Wall stress: $\frac{PR}{2h}$
   - preload
   - afterload
2. Heart rate
3. Contractility

Supply

1. Coronary blood flow: $\frac{\text{AoDP} - \text{LVEDP}}{\text{Coronary vascular resistance}}$
   - Diastolic time
   - Collaterals, capillary density
2. Oxygen content: Hb × $SatO_2$
3. Hb – O_2 dissociation curve
4. O_2 extraction

FIGURE 31-1. Myocardial oxygen balance. P, intracavitary pressure; R, ventricular radius; h, wall thickness; AoDP, diastolic arterial pressure; LVEDP, left ventricular end-diastolic pressure; Hb, hemoglobin; $SatO_2$, arterial oxygen saturation.

Coronary Blood Flow

The critical factors that modify coronary blood flow are the perfusion pressure and vascular tone of the coronary circulation, the time available for perfusion (determined namely by heart rate), the severity of intraluminal obstructions, and the presence of (any) collateral circulation. The area most vulnerable to ischemia is the subendocardium of the left ventricle (LV), where the metabolic requirements are increased because of greater systolic shortening.[6]

Perfusion of the left ventricular subendocardium takes place almost entirely during diastole, whereas the right ventricular subendocardium is perfused mostly during systole, provided there is no pulmonary hypertension. This temporal disparity is explained by the different intraventricular pressures developing during systole.

The left ventricular coronary perfusion pressure is often defined as the difference between aortic diastolic pressure (AoDP) and left ventricular end-diastolic pressure (LVEDP). This is an oversimplification because there is no single AoDP. Rather, it is likely that there is a range of pressures that drive blood to the subendocardium. In the presence of intraluminal obstruction or increased vascular tone, this pressure gradient is reduced (Fig. 31-2). It is convenient and useful to consider ventricular filling pressure (the pulmonary artery occlusion pressure as the closest surrogate) as the end pressure. Therefore, a low ventricular filling pressure is ideal both in terms of improving perfusion (higher pressure gradient) and of reducing $\dot{M}VO_2$ (decreased ventricular volume and wall tension). The consequences of systemic pressure are more difficult to predict because the cost of increasing perfusion pressure (~afterload) is an increase in $\dot{M}VO_2$. However, it has been shown experimentally that at any given heart rate, ischemia is induced more likely by hypotension than hypertension.

Alterations in the tone of the small intramyocardial arterioles regulate diastolic vascular resistance, allowing the matching of oxygen supply with metabolic demand over a wide range of perfusion pressures. The difference between autoregulated,

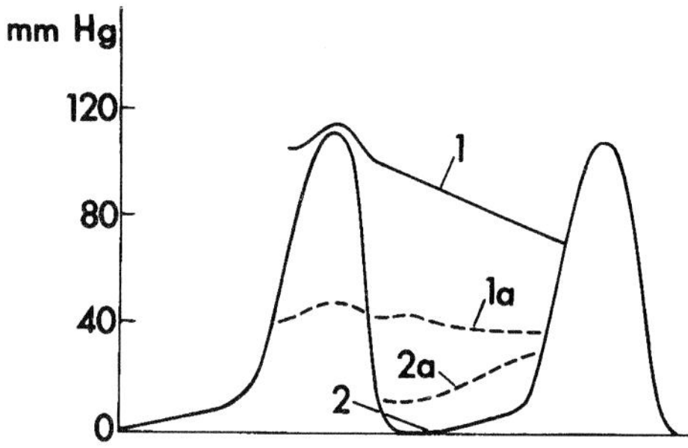

FIGURE 31-2. The pressure relationships between the aorta (*1*) and the left ventricle (*2*) determine coronary perfusion pressure. In coronary artery disease, myocardial perfusion may be compromised by decreased pressure distal to a significant stenosis (*1a*) (not quantifiable clinically) and/or by an increase in left ventricular end-diastolic pressure (*2a*). (Reprinted with permission from Gorlin R: Coronary Artery Disease, p 75. Philadelphia, WB Saunders, 1976.)

baseline flow and blood flow available under conditions of maximal vasodilation is termed coronary vascular reserve, and is normally three to five times higher than basal flow. As epicardial stenosis becomes more pronounced, progressive vasodilation of these resistance vessels allows preservation of basal flow, but at the cost of reduced reserve. Whenever demand increases above available reserve, signs, symptoms, and metabolic evidence of ischemia develop.

Prinzmetal et al.[7] first described angina and myocardial infarction in patients with angiographically normal coronary vessels. Subsequently, Maseri et al. and others have repeatedly emphasized the frequency with which reductions in oxygen supply cause ischemia so small adjustments in coronary vascular tone at the site of existing obstructions can cause substantial reductions in luminal cross-sectional area.[8] Alterations in vessel diameter at the stenotic area are possible because at least two-thirds of plaques or atheromas are not concentric. It is now apparent that anesthesia is not protective against "supply" ischemia, which occurs frequently during surgery (Fig. 31-3).[4] The etiology of this is unclear, but it may be caused by circulating catecholamines, local effects of blood components such as

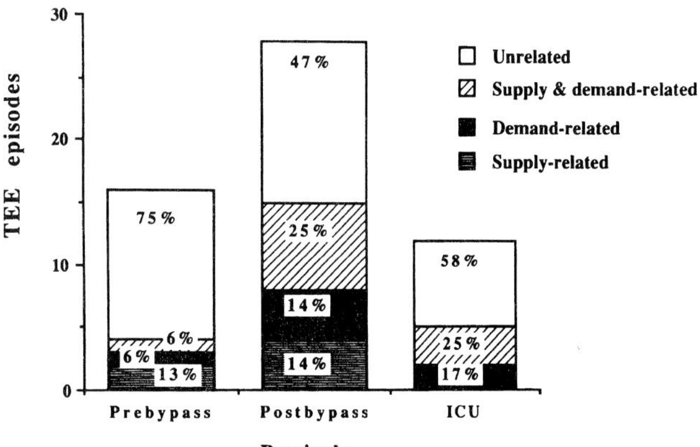

FIGURE 31-3. Association of transesophageal echocardiographic (TEE) wall motion changes with hemodynamic indices of supply and demand from continuous monitoring of 50 patients undergoing coronary artery bypass surgery. (Reproduced with permission from Leung JM, O'Kelly BV, Mangano DT *et al:* Relationship of regional wall motion abnormalities to hemodynamic indices of myocardial oxygen supply and demand in patients undergoing CABG surgery. Anesthesiology 73:802, 1990.)

platelets at areas of unstable atherosclerotic plaques, or other as yet undetermined factors. It is not uncommon for an anesthetized patient to show signs of ischemia without any change in heart rate, blood pressure, or ventricular filling pressures. In fact, most ischemic episodes are not accompanied by hemodynamic changes.[4] Drugs such as nitroglycerin or calcium entry blockers may be used to prevent and/or treat such episodes of coronary spasm,[9] although prophylactic use of these agents is
2 usually ineffective.

Hypotension, vasospasm, and acute thrombosis decrease coronary perfusion pressure, reduce coronary blood flow, and limit oxygen delivery to the myocardium. Unstable angina pectoris and/or acute coronary thrombosis are the results of plaque rupture with ensuing platelet activation and thrombus formation. The presence of the potentially hyperreactive normal vessel wall adjacent to the thrombus may result in vasospasm and total occlusion of the vessel lumen in the presence of a previously nonocclusive eccentric plaque or thrombus. This type of acute thrombosis is believed to be the cause of acute myocardial infarction and sudden death (generally ischemia-induced cardiac dysrhythmias).

Hemodynamic Goals

Although the precise relationship between intraoperative ischemia and postoperative myocardial infarction remains controversial, there is consensus that one of the primary goals of any successful anesthetic is prevention of myocardial ischemia.[10] Failing that, prompt identification and treatment of new ischemic episodes is essential. As is evident from the previous discussion and from the summary in Table 31-1, anesthetic decisions are designed to reduce and control those factors that increase myocardial oxygen demand (heart rate, contractility, and wall tension). At the same time, every attempt is made to optimize coronary blood flow, notably, maintaining coronary perfusion pressure and increasing diastolic time. The buzz words for patients with coronary artery disease are "slow, small, and well perfused." Combinations of anesthetics, sedatives, muscle relaxants, and vasoactive drugs are selected to provide this hemodynamic milieu. Techniques to effectively prevent or treat alterations in coronary vascular tone—antiplatelet drugs, specific bradycardic agents, and so on—are still evolving and await further clinical trial before definitive
3 recommendations can be made.[10]

TABLE 31-1

CORONARY ARTERY DISEASE—HEMODYNAMIC GOALS

P	Keep the heart small: ↓wall tension (diameter) and LVEDP; ↑perfusion pressure gradient
A	Maintain: hypertension better than hypotension
C	Depression (if LV function is within normal)
R	Slow
Rhythm	Sinus
MVO_2	Monitor for and treat "supply"-related disturbances; control of myocardial O_2 demand is not enough
CPB	Elevated filling pressures are usually not needed after CABG

A, afterload; C, contractility; CABG, coronary artery bypass graft; CPB, cardiopulmonary bypass; LVEDP, left ventricular end-diastolic pressure; MVO_2, myocardial oxygen consumption; P, preload; R, rate; ↑, increase; ↓, decrease.

Monitoring for Ischemia

Electrocardiogram

The ideal monitoring technique is not yet available. Analysis of the ST segment in multiple leads (most commonly leads II and V_4 or V_5) is currently the standard. Patients likely to develop right ventricular ischemia[19] or those with disease of the right coronary artery might benefit from monitoring of leads V_{4R} or V_{5R}. Computerized ST segment trending and interactive monitors that alarm when the ST segment deviates from the programmed algorithm aid in the detection of intraoperative events overlooked by even the most astute observer.

Heart Rate and Blood Pressure

Multiple attempts have been made to determine ischemic thresholds using commonly measured hemodynamic variables. Among the earliest of these was the rate–pressure product (RPP = heart rate × peak systolic arterial pressure). The RPP was considered an easily determined index of $M\dot{V}O_2$. Although RPP may correlate with oxygen demand, especially during exercise, it is not a sensitive or specific indicator of intraoperative ischemia; identical RPPs can be produced from multiple combinations of heart rate and blood pressure. Favorable conditions for oxygen balance are more likely those of lower heart rate and higher blood pressure than tachycardia and hypotension.

Neither the pressure–rate *ratio* (P/RR), nor the mean arterial pressure (MAP)/heart rate ratio are any more predictive or reliable than the RPP.

Pulmonary Artery Catheter

Sudden elevations in pulmonary artery or capillary wedge pressure indicating systolic and/or diastolic left ventricular dysfunction, large a waves reflecting decreased ventricular compliance, and v waves signaling the development of ischemia-induced papillary muscle dysfunction and/or mitral regurgitation are purported signs of ischemia that may be detected with a pulmonary artery catheter (PAC). Several studies contradict this long-held dogma and demonstrate that the PAC is of little value as a monitor of myocardial ischemia. Leung et al.[11] found that only 10% of all regional wall motion abnormalities were associated with an acute rise in pulmonary capillary wedge pressure in 40 patients undergoing elective CABG surgery. Haggmark et al.[12] found that neither an increase in the pulmonary capillary wedge pressure nor the occurrence of an abnormal pulmonary capillary wedge pressure waveform was a sensitive indicator for myocardial ischemia in 53 patients with coronary artery disease undergoing vascular surgery. A prospective study of 1,094 patients by Tuman et al.[13] showed that even high-risk cardiac surgical patients may be safely managed without routine use of a PAC, and if the need for it developed intraoperatively, delayed placement of a PAC did not influence outcome. Fontes et al. assessed the limitations of PAC in the management of critically ill patients in the ICU. Compared with transesophageal echocardiography, PAC predicted normal left ventricular function well, but performed poorly in judging preload and ventricular dysfunction.[14] A more recent study showed no benefit from PACs in high-risk surgical patients.[15] Nevertheless, the PAC is still frequently used in cardiac surgical patients to measure cardiac output and as a guide, albeit not ideal, to
4 volume status.

Intraoperative Transesophageal Echocardiography

Since its introduction in the 1980s, transesophageal echocardiography (TEE) has become an invaluable diagnostic and monitoring tool during cardiac surgery. TEE permits assessment of ventricular volume, global and regional function, estimation and quantitation of valvular pathology, measurement of valve gradients and calculation of filling pressures, visualization of the thoracic aorta, and detection of intracardiac air.

Basics. Multiple image planes are necessary to reconstruct the three-dimensional (3D) structure of the heart. The American Society of Echocardiography (ASE)/Society of Cardiovascular Anesthesiologists task force for intraoperative echocardiography has published guidelines for performing a comprehensive intraoperative echocardiographic examination.[16] These recommendations describe a series of 20 standard tomographic views of the heart and great vessels that should be included in a comphrehensive intraoperative echocardiographic examination. With experience, a thorough examination can be performed in less than 10 minutes.

Evaluation of Ventricular Function. Although various techniques are available to quantify ventricular function, qualitative assessment currently predominates in the clinical arena. The transgastric midpapillary short-axis view of the LV (Fig. 31-4) is the standard initial view for evaluation of size and function. The presence of the papillary muscles ensures the same view is consistently obtained on repeated examinations. Using two-dimensional (2D) echocardiography, global left ventricular function is usually evaluated by calculating the ejection fraction.

Ischemia. The ventricular distribution of the coronary arteries and their branches are depicted in Figure 31-5. All major branches of the coronary arteries supply segments of the ventricle viewed in the transgastric midpapillary short-axis level, enhancing the utility of this view as a monitor for ischemia. The grading of the wall motion is shown in Figure 31-6 and Table 31-2.

The TEE diagnosis of segmental wall motion abnormalities (SWMAs) is based on visual assessment of wall motion *and* wall thickness. The use of cine loops (side-by-side comparison of the ventricle over time) of the transgastric midpapillary short-axis view of LV improves the ability to recognize new wall motion abnormalities. In one study, however, the short-axis

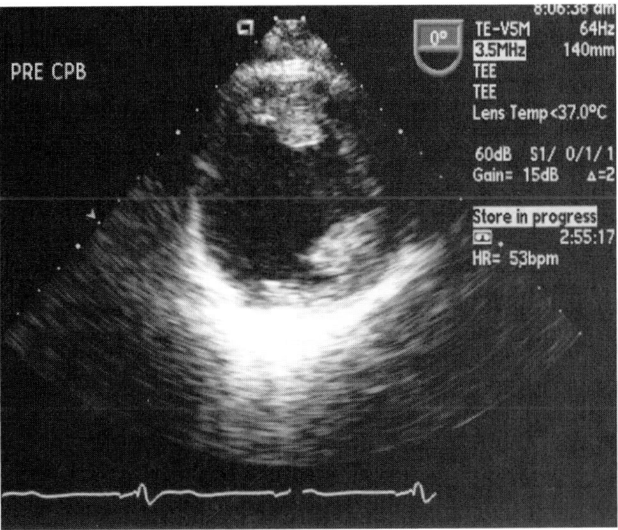

FIGURE 31-4. Transgastric short-axis view of the left ventricle at the midpapillary level. The body of the anterolateral papillary muscle is seen at 5 o'clock, and that of the posteromedial at 12 o'clock. In this case, the imaging depth is set at 14 cm, rather than the typical 12 cm so that the entire left ventricle is visualized.

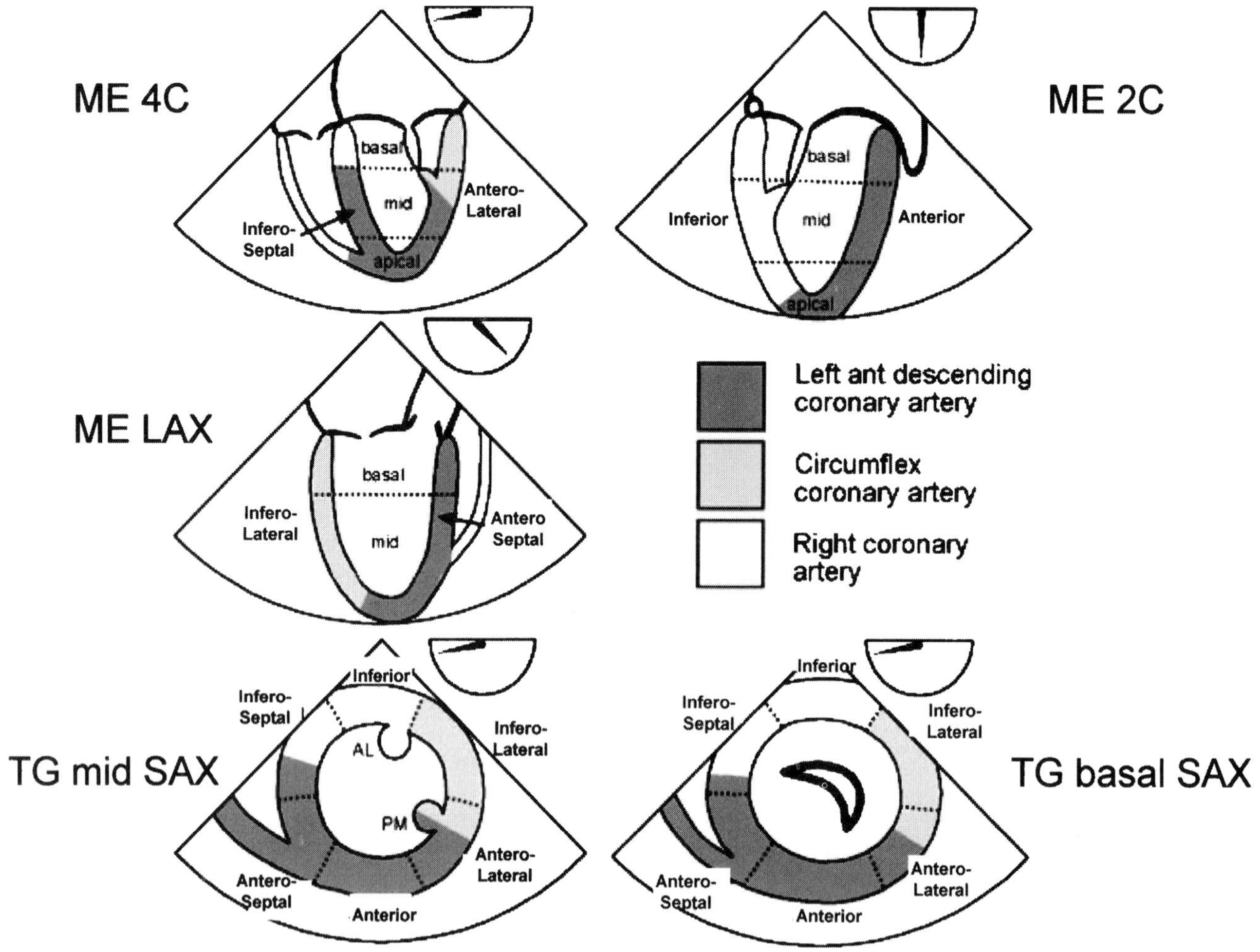

FIGURE 31-5. The distribution of the three major coronary arteries in relation to two-dimensional TEE images. The left ventricle (LV) is divided vertically into three levels: basal, mid, and apical. The basal and mid levels are each divided circumferentially into six segments, the apical level into four (for a total of 16 segments). For the LV midesophageal (ME) views, the transducer is positioned posterior to the LA at the level of the mitral valve, and the imaging depth is adjusted to include the entire LV. By rotating the multiplane transducer to different angles, the following views are obtained: ME 4C (four chamber) at 10° to 20° (until the aortic valve is not in view), ME 2C at 80° to 100° (until the right atrium and ventricle disappear), and ME long axis (LAX) view at 120° to 160° (until the LV outflow tract and the proximal aorta come into view). The transgastric (TG) views of the LV are obtained by advancing the probe into the stomach: At an angle of 0° the short axis (SAX) view appears, and the probe is withdrawn or advanced as needed to reach the basal or midpapillary (mid) level. (Modified with permission from Sidebotham D, Legget AMM: Practical Perioperative Transesophageal Echocardiography. Edinburgh, Scotland, Butterworth Heinemann, 2003.)

midpapillary view detected only 17% of all SWMAs, emphasizing the importance of evaluating the ventricle in multiple planes with careful standardization of location and edge definition.[17] Training will increase the operator's ability to attain the required images and to recognize new SWMA in real time.

Although ventricular wall motion is clearly very sensitive to coronary blood flow, the definition of ischemia is difficult. There is little agreement on a "gold standard" for the diagnosis of ischemia. Most studies have compared SWMA with changes in ST segments recorded on ECG. The concordance between SWMA and ECG evidence of ischemia is variable, ranging from 30% to 100%.[18,19] This discrepancy may exist for a number of reasons, for example, because SWMAs are more sensitive to compromised coronary blood flow than is ECG. Thus, SWMAs on TEE can appear when the compromise in coronary flow is still insufficient to produce ECG changes. If the compromise in coronary flow is enough to produce ECG evidence of ischemia,
5 TEE SWMAs will precede these ECG changes.

Not all SWMAs are indicative of ischemia. Nonischemic myocardium adjacent to ischemic or infarcted myocardium may be interpreted as SWMAs, a phenomenon known as "tethering." SWMAs also occur with pacing, bundle branch blocks, and myocarditis, as well as tachycardia and hypovolemia. Differentiating stunned myocardium (postischemic ventricular dysfunction despite adequate blood flow that shows gradual improvement) from ischemia is important because treatment differs. Stunned myocardium requires supportive measures such as inotropic infusions until function returns, whereas inadequate revascularization with ongoing ischemia requires an assessment of graft patency and consideration of further revascularization. In the future, echocardiographic contrast agents that delineate coronary perfusion territories may refine this evaluation. Newer ultrasound techniques, such as

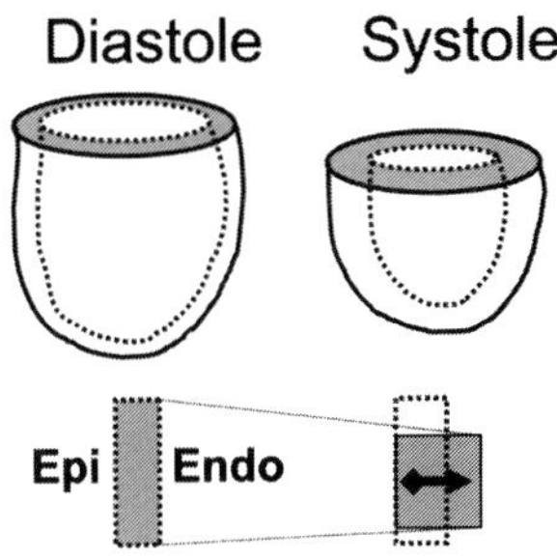

1 = normal (>30% thickening)

2 = hypokinetic (10 to 30% thickening)

3 = akinetic (<10% thickening)

4 = dyskinetic (moves paradoxically during systole)

FIGURE 31-6. Definitions for changes in regional wall motion. During systole, the base of the left ventricle descends toward the apex and the myocardium thickens while the endocardium moves toward the center of the left ventricular cavity. The systolic segmental wall motion is evaluated for both inward excursion and thickening. The grading scale has been used extensively in the intraoperative echocardiograpic literature. All 16 segments are examined by obtaining five cross-sectional views of the LV.

the deformation (strain), deformation rate (strain rate), and timing of systolic and diastolic events, if applicable in the operating room, will offer more objective insight into regional myocardial function.[20]

Quantification of Ventricular Function. A range of 2D echocardiographic methods are employed to define ventricular systolic function (Table 31-3). The LV is often enlarged/dilated with chronic systolic dysfunction and in regurgitant valvular lesions with chronic volume overload. A disproportional increase in wall thickness (concentric hypertrophy) suggests the chronic pressure overload of aortic stenosis or systemic hypertension. Marked septal hypertrophy and abnormal anterior systolic motion of the anterior mitral leaflet are signs indicative of hypertrophic cardiomyopathy. The discovery of thrombus or outpouching of the free wall of the LV implies the presence of ischemic heart disease.

Most experienced anesthesiologists rely on a visual estimate of the LV global function using the transgastric short-axis view at the midpapillary level. Although subjective, it is the preferred method in the often demanding cardiac operating room environment.

The fractional area of change (FAC) infers the systolic decrease in ventricular volume measured along the short axis, and is a reliable and quick index of systolic function.[21] Nevertheless, FAC still demonstrates intraobserver variability of 10% and an interobserver variability of 6 to 23%.[22] Because the FAC method assesses global left ventricular function based on a single short-axis view, it is inherently inaccurate in the setting of ventricular assymetry. In addition, FAC does not take into account the apical contraction nor does it represent systole along the long axis of the ventricle. Such variability, coupled with the time required to manually trace the endocardial border, limits the clinical utility of the FAC method. 6

A single measurement of the LV short-axis diameter from the TG SAX view at midpapillary level is sufficient for calculation of EF (Quinones method), provided the wall motion is either normal or diffusely abnormal (i.e., there are no distinct SWMAs). When the formula was tested against angiography, the authors found excellent correlation.[23]

More sophisticated and complex approaches to determine left ventricular systolic function calculate ventricular volumes. The end-diastolic volume and end-systolic volume are then used to calculate the EF. The methods recommended by the ASE[16] are the method of discs and the area-length method (Fig. 31-7). Alternatively, the stroke volume can be measured by a combination of 2D and pulsed-Doppler measurements.

The Tei index incorporates systolic (isovolumic contraction and ejection) and diastolic (isovolumic relaxation) time intervals, measured by Doppler, to derive a number representing global LV function, both systolic and diastolic. The index is independent of heart rate or blood pressure and can be easily obtained with two simple measurements from the conventional Doppler echocardiogram. The index correlates well with both peak positive and negative dP/dt and reflects the overall cardiac function better because patients more commonly have features of both systolic and diastolic dysfunction.[24]

The rate of rise of LV intraventricular pressure (dP/dt) during systole can be used as a less load dependent index of systolic function.[25] Normal values are >1,200 mm Hg/second and severely depressed systolic function is present if <800 mm Hg/second.

Tissue Doppler imaging is a new techique to quantify tissue contraction and relaxation. For example, the average peak systolic velocity from six sites of the base of the LV at the mitral annulus correlates well with LV ejection fraction, and a cutoff value of mean systolic mitral annular velocity of ≥7.5 cm/second has a sensitivity of 79% and a specificity of 88% in predicting preserved global systolic function.[26]

Currently, there is no echocardiographic measurement of global ventricular function that is both quick and accurate. Therefore, qualitative assessment remains the most frequently used modality. An experienced observer can reasonably estimate ejection fraction if there is good endocardial definition and the ventricular areas of interest are well visualized. One should bear in mind that the echocardiographically derived ejection fraction is not always proportional to cardiac output: hypovolemia reduces cardiac output in the presence of unchanged ejection fraction (normal inotropic state), whereas stroke volume may be normal in the presence of depressed ejection fraction (dilated ventricle with poor systolic function). This emphasizes that EF is dependent not only on contractility, but also on preload and afterload.

Right Ventricle. The right ventricle (RV) is a complex anatomic structure draped over the anteromedial portion of the LV. There are no accepted 3D representations of the RV. In the transgastric short-axis midpapillary view, the RV appears crescent shaped, with the septum forming the medial wall. In the midesophageal four-chamber view, the tricuspid vavle plane is anchored slightly lower than the mitral annulus, and the right ventricular apex reaches to about two-thirds the length of the the interventricular septum. The right ventricular border is irregular due to trabeculation. Contraction of the RV is also complex. It involves a shortening of the long axis and an

TABLE 31-2

GRADES OF SEGMENTAL SYSTOLIC MOTION

CLASS OF MOTION	SYSTOLIC WALL THICKENING	RADIAL (INWARD) SHORTENING
1. Normal	Marked	>30%
2. Hypokinetic	Minimal to moderate	10 to 30%
3. Akinetic	None	None or <10%
4. Dyskinetic	Thinning	Outward motion

TABLE 31-3

EVALUATION OF LEFT VENTRICULAR SYSTOLIC FUNCTION

	TEE VIEW	COMMENT
A. Initial estimation		
Size of ventricle—2D		
Dilated if —ESd >4.5 cm —EDd >7 cm	TG SAX	Seek coexisting valvular or ventricular structural abnormalities
B. Global function		
"Eyeball"—2D		
Visual evaluation of LV global function	TG SAX (usually)	Quick, easy, and widely used. Accuracy affected by echocardiographer's experience
Fractional area change—2D FAC = [(EDA − ESA) / EDA] × 100)		
% change of LV area	TG mid SAX	Quick, widely used, and accurate, provided there are no regional abnormalities
Ejection fraction (Quinones method)—M-Mode EF = $(EDd^2 - ESd^2) / EDd^2$		
% change of LV internal diameters between ESd and EDd	TG mid SAX	Easy and accurate calculation, provided that there are no regional motion abnormalities in base or apex
Ejection fraction—2D EF = [(EDV − ESV) / EDV] × 100		
Volume calculation using — Area-length method: volume = $8A^2/3\pi L$ (A, area; L, length) — Method of discs (modified Simpson's)	ME 2C and 4C	Planimetry (tracing) of endocardial border, calculation performed by software. Very accurate but tedious and time-consuming
Stroke volume (2D and Doppler) SV = CSA × VTI		
Cross-sectional area (CSA = D^2 × 0.785) from diameter (D), and VTI at LV outflow tract	DTG	Easy to perform but prone to errors if D or VTI wrongly measured/traced
Tei index—Doppler = [(ICT + IRT) / ET]		
Global myocardial performance index based on ICT, IRT, and ET	Combination of any ME and DTG	Quick, inversely related to heart function, not "real" time measurement
dP/dt—Doppler		
Maximum rate of LV pressure change over time (calculated from change of MR velocity from 1 to 3 m/sec during ICT)	Any ME	Afterload independent, requires mitral regurgitation signal
C. Regional function		
Regional wall motion abnormalities—2D		
Visual evaluation of wall thickening	ME and TG	Widely used and reliable but dependent on echocardiographer's experience. Drop-out of echo signal in regions parallel to ultrasound propagation introduces inaccuracy. Cannot differentiate actively contracting from passively drawn (scar) segments. The epicardium is not always visible for evaluation of thickening
Tissue velocities—tissue Doppler		
Longitudinal myocardial shortening velocity reflects subendocardial contraction and is a more sensitive marker of impaired contractile function than reduced wall motion	ME at periphery of MA	Requires newer echocardiographic machines (cannot distinguish between actively contracting or passively following tissue). Velocities decrease toward apex
Strain—tissue Doppler		
Deformation of a myocardial segment	Any view	Allows objective comparison between different segments, difficult to implement in real time in OR environment, requires newer echocardiographic machines

2D, two-dimensional; DTG, deep transgastric; EDd, end-diastolic diameter; ESd, end-systolic diameter; ET, ejection time; ICT, isovolumic contraction time; IRT, isovolumic relaxation time; LV, left ventricle; MA, mitral valve annulus; ME, midesophageal; MR, mitral regurgitation; SAX, short axis; TEE, transesophageal echocardiography; TG, transgastric; VTI, velocity time integral.

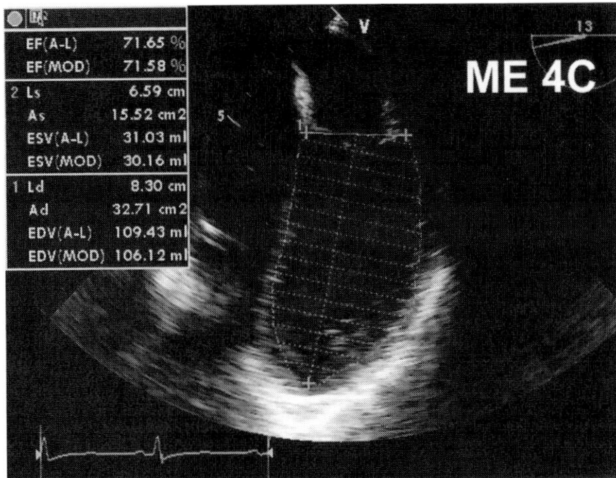

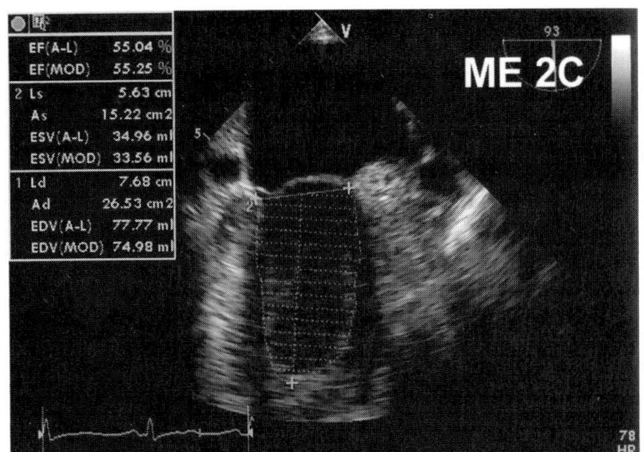

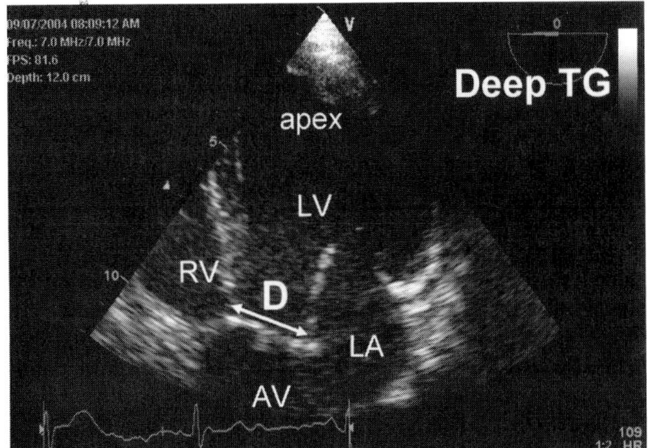

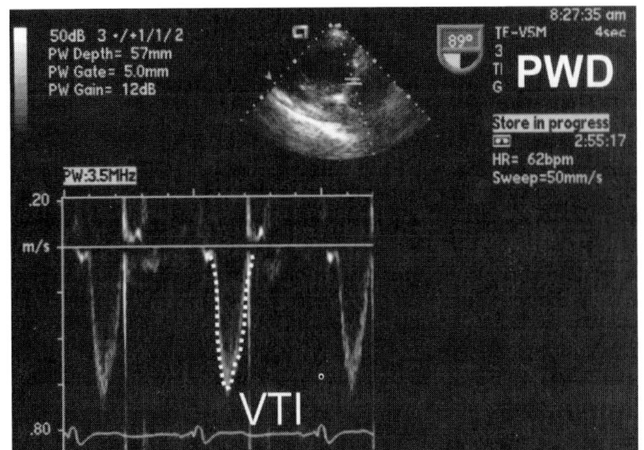

FIGURE 31-7. Evaluation of ventricular systolic function. **A, B.** Calculation of *ventricular* volume. The ME 4C and ME 2C of the left ventricle (LV) are obtained, and the endocardial border is traced in end-systole and end-diastole, from one side of the mitral annulus to the opposite. The *method of discs* (MOD) or modified Simpson's method assumes that the LV cavity contains twenty discs, centered along the long axis of the ventricle. The discs have the same thickness, but different diameter. The volume of each disc is calculated from its cross-sectional area and thickness. The *area-length* (A-L) method calculates the ventricular volume from the same traced area (A) and the length (L) of the LV long axis. Using either method, the stroke volume (SV) is calculated as the difference between end-diastolic volume (EDV) and end-systolic volume (ESV), and ejection fraction (EF) is calculated as SV/EDV. **C, D.** Calculation of *stroke* volume. The diameter (D) of the LV outflow tract is measured just proximal to the aortic valve using the deep transgastric (deep TG) view of the LV (**C**). The cross-sectional area is then calculated as $\pi (D/2)^2$ or $D^2 \times 0.785$. The velocity of the blood passing through this area is displayed with pulsed wave Doppler (PWD) (**D**), its envelope is traced and the velocity time integral (VTI) obtained. SV is calculated as $D^2 \times 0.785 \times VTI$. Other cylindrical sites (ascending aorta, main pulmonary artery) can be also used. It is important to measure D accurately as any error is subsequently squared. The SV calculation assumes the blood flow at this location is laminar and parallel to the ultrasound beam (any deviation in the angle between the ultrasound beam and the blood flow will underestimate the VTI). RV, right ventricle; LV, left ventricle; AV, aortic valve; LA, left atrium.

inward movement of the free wall, which is primarily responsible for the ejection of blood. Collectively, these properties make it difficult to accurately evaluate RV function.[27]

The diagnosis of right ventricular infarct requires a change in right ventricular function from normal to akinesis or dyskinesis.[28] If the right ventricular apex extends as deep as the left ventricular apex, the RV is moderately dilated, and if it extends beyond the LV apex, the dilation is severe. Abnormalities of shape and motion of the interventricular septum (normally curved toward the RV) signify volume (diastolic flattening) and pressure (systolic bulging toward the LV) overload. A leftward bulging of the interatrial septum, the presence of tricuspid regurgitation, or pulmonary hypertension are surrogate findings in pressure or volume overload of the RV. Quantitative measurements of the RV with linear parameters have not been found to accurately reflect right ventricular function. Automated border detection has been applied to normovolemic RVs to generate pressure–area loops to evaluate right ventricular contractility.[29] It is not clear if this method is accurate with hypervolemic ventricles.[30] The myocardial systolic velocity (measured at the lateral border of the tricuspid annulus with tissue Doppler) significantly correlates with the right ventricular ejection fraction (assessed by ventriculography), and a value of <11.5 cm/second predicts right ventricular dysfunction (EF $<45\%$) with good sensitivity and specificity.[31]

If the RV appears dilated, this should trigger an evaluation for a culprit lesion such as an atrial septal defect, tricuspid, or pulmonic regurgitation. Long-standing right ventricular pressure overload can result in right ventricular dilation; however, hypertrophy is more common. Right ventricular hypertrophy is diagnosed with a diastolic right ventricular free wall thickness greater than 0.5 cm.

Diastolic Function and Filling Pressures. Although not well recognized, diastolic heart failure is common as an isolated disease in the elderly, increases the burden of heart failure among patients with systolic dysfunction, and is associated with increased morbidity and mortality.[32] The gold standards for evaluation of diastolic heart function (i.e., the rate of relaxation and pressure–volume loops are not feasible for daily perioperative practice). Doppler echocardiography has emerged as the principal tool for assessment of LV diastolic function.

Pulsed-wave Doppler examination of transmitral flow demonstrates an early (E) and a late (A) diastolic velocity, corresponding to early, rapid diastolic filling and atrial contraction, respectively. Faster relaxation results in an increased pressure gradient and greater filling in early diastole. The E/A ratio is usually about 2, decreasing with normal aging to 0.75 to 1.5 around the sixth decade of life. In disease states, relaxation is impaired reducing early LV filling. Simultaneously, there is a compensatory increase in filling with atrial contraction (E/A < 1) (Fig. 31-8). These patients depend on a relatively slow sinus rhythm and adequate preload to maintain a normal cardiac output. When the chamber compliance is decreased (stiff myocardium, increased pericardial restraint, increased volume), the associated increased left artial (LA) pressure results in proportionally greater filling in early diastole, resulting in a normal E/A pattern (pseudonormal pattern). The Valsalva maneuver is simple to perform in a mechanically ventilated patient and helps in unmasking the underlying abnormal LV relaxation. In cases of pseudonormal pattern, the decreased cardiac filling during Valsalva maneuver lowers the LA pressure resulting in an E/A ratio <1.[33] With disease progression, there is severe decrease in LV compliance, which leads to a further increase in LA pressure and results in a very high E/A ratio (restrictive pattern). These patients become more sensitive to alterations in filling volume, with relatively small increases in volume reflected by marked increases in filling pressures.

Pulmonary venous flow Doppler echocardiography provides additional information for the evaluation of diastolic function. The flow from the pulmonary veins to the LA occurs both during ventricular systole (LA relaxation, as well as downward motion of the mitral annulus and base of the heart produce a systolic [S] velocity) and diastole ([D] velocity). There is also a retrograde (rA) velocity back into the pulmonary veins during atrial contraction. When LA pressure is normal, LA filling occurs primarily in systole (S/D > 1), whereas with increasing LA pressure, LA filling occurs during diastole (S/D < 1). Comparison of the atrial contraction events (A and rA waves) provide additional information: rA > 35 cm/second, rA duration > 30 milliseconds or rA duration > A duration predict an LA pressure >15 mm Hg, usually found in moderate
7 and severe diastolic dysfunction.[34]

Aorta. Neurologic dysfunction in cardiac surgical patients continues to be a devastating complication.[35] Stroke, defined as a fixed neurologic deficit lasting longer than 24 hours, occurs with an incidence of 2 to 5% in patients undergoing CABG with CPB, whereas more subtle neurologic dysfunction is detected in 30 to 60% of these patients.[35,36] Risk factors that have been identified include a history of neurologic disease, older age, and presence of aortic atherosclerosis.[37] Detecting aortic atherosclerotic disease allows surgical modifications that may decrease a patient's morbidity and mortality. Prior to echocardiography, detection of aortic atherosclerotic disease relied on surgical palpation or radiographic evidence of its presence. Although successful for detection of severe aortic calcification, these techniques do not reliably predict aortic atheromas.[38] TEE can accurately detect the presence of both aortic

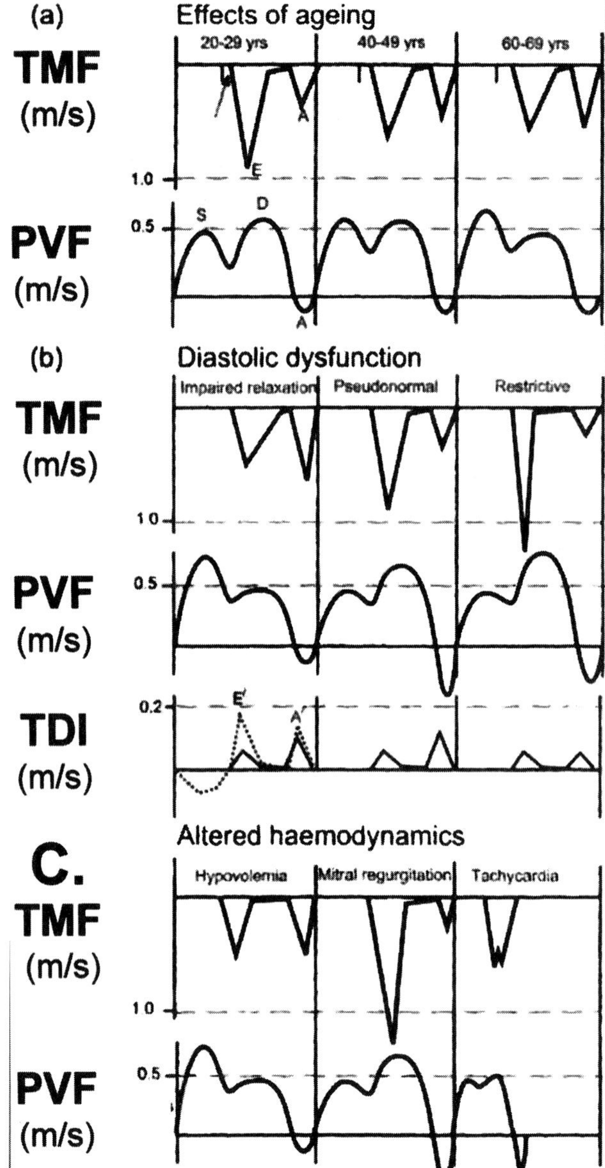

FIGURE 31-8. Echocardiographic evaluation of diastolic function. **a.** With increasing age the myocardium becomes progressively thicker and less compliant, and left venticular (LV) filling depends more on atrial contribution. This is reflected in transmitral flow (TMF): early diastolic filling velocity (E) decreases, and the ratio between early and late (A, atrial) velocities decreases. These changes are also reflected in the pulmonary venous flow (PVF) velocities: the ratio between systolic and diastolic (S/D) velocities increases with aging. **b.** With impaired relaxation, early LV filling is reduced, and the E/A ratio is <1. As LV compliance progressively worsens, left atrial pressure increases. There is proportionally greater filling in early diastole and less with atrial contraction (E/A > 1 in pseudonormal, and E/A > 2 in restrictive diastolic dysfunction). PVF: the S/D ratio remains <1. Although the classic Doppler velocities (TMF and PVF) do not always distinguish between healthy and disease states (compare velocities in the age group 20 to 29 years with the pseudonormal pattern of diastolic dysfunction), tissue Doppler imaging (TDI) velocities remain persistently reduced once diastolic dysfunction occurs. **c.** The Doppler velocities are affected not only by the intrinsic diastolic function of the LV, but also by various other factors. Hypovolemia reduces the initial gradient between the LA and LV (E reduced, S/D > 1), a full LA (e.g., in moderate or severe mitral regurgitation) will create a pattern similar to one found in restrictive diastolic dysfunction (E/A > 2, S/D < 1), whereas tachycardia reduces the diastolic time interval and causes fusion of E and A velocities. (Reproduced with permission from Sidebotham D, Legget AMM: Practical Perioperative Transesophageal Echocardiography. Edinburgh, Scotland, Butterworth Heinemann, 2003.)

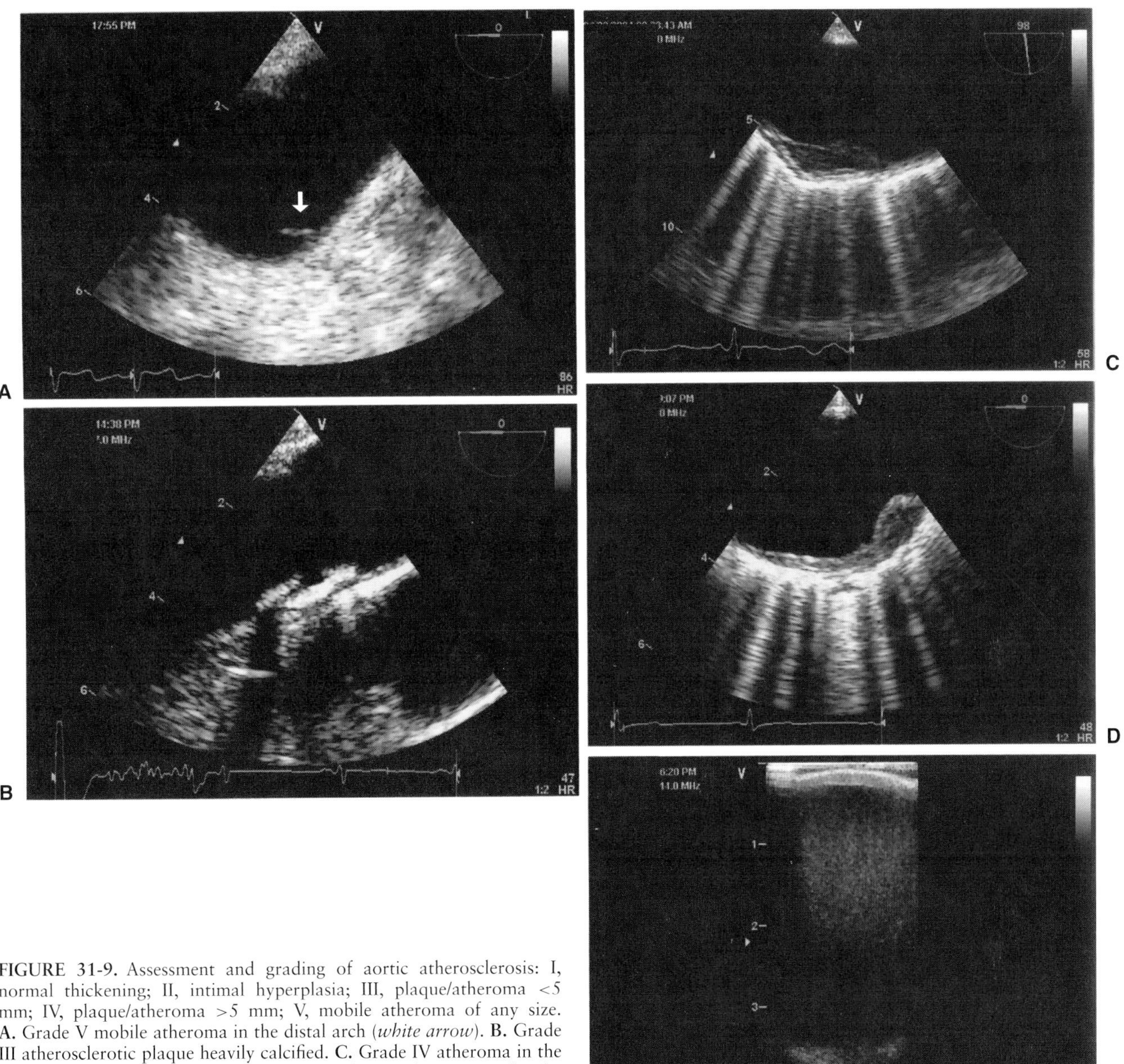

FIGURE 31-9. Assessment and grading of aortic atherosclerosis: I, normal thickening; II, intimal hyperplasia; III, plaque/atheroma <5 mm; IV, plaque/atheroma >5 mm; V, mobile atheroma of any size. **A.** Grade V mobile atheroma in the distal arch (*white arrow*). **B.** Grade III atherosclerotic plaque heavily calcified. **C.** Grade IV atheroma in the descending aorta (short-axis view). **D.** Grade IV atheroma in the descending aorta (long-axis view). **E.** Grade I (epiaortic scan) of ascending aorta.

calcification and atherosclerosis.[39] Because TEE is easy to perform, reproducible, quantifiable, and carries minimum risk, it has become the diagnostic method of choice for detecting aortic atheromas. The severity of aortic atherosclerotic disease is graded according to the scale depicted in Figure 31-9.

TEE completely and accurately images the descending thoracic aorta. However, owing to the interposition of the trachea and/or the right mainstem bronchus between the esophagus and the ascending aorta, the distal ascending aorta and proximal aortic arch are almost invisible. Complete and accurate examination of this segment of the aorta requires direct examination with an epiaortic probe. The presence of a grade III, IV, or V descending thoracic aorta is associated with an increased incidence of postoperative morbidity (stroke) and mortality.[37,40] In a series of 189 patients who underwent a CABG with CPB and intraoperative TEE examination of the descending aorta, no strokes were noted in individuals with grades I and II aortas, whereas stroke rates of 5.5% (2/36), 10.5% (2/19), and 45% (5/11) were documented for descending aortas grades 3, 4, and 5[37] (Fig. 31-10). In a subsequent study, an epiaortic examination of the ascending aorta was performed in all patients with a grade 4 or 5 descending thoracic aorta. If a grade V ascending thoracic aorta was documented, there was a 71% (5/7) incidence of stroke. It has been shown that if a complete TEE examination of the thoracic aorta is negative for atheromatosis, it is highly unlikely that there is significant atherosclerotic disease in the ascending aorta and proximal aortic arch. If the TEE examination reveals significant atheromatosis (>3 mm) in the descending aorta, there is a 34% chance of significant disease in the ascending aorta, and epiaortic scanning is applicable.[41] Thus, TEE is a very sensitive, but only mildly specific, method of determining the extent of atherosclerosis in the thoracic aorta.

Despite the shortcomings of TEE in imaging the thoracic aorta for atherosclerosis, it remains a primary tool for rapid and accurate evaluation of patients with suspected thoracic aortic pathology, especially aortic dissections. TEE has consistently demonstrated a 95 to 100% sensitivity and specificity

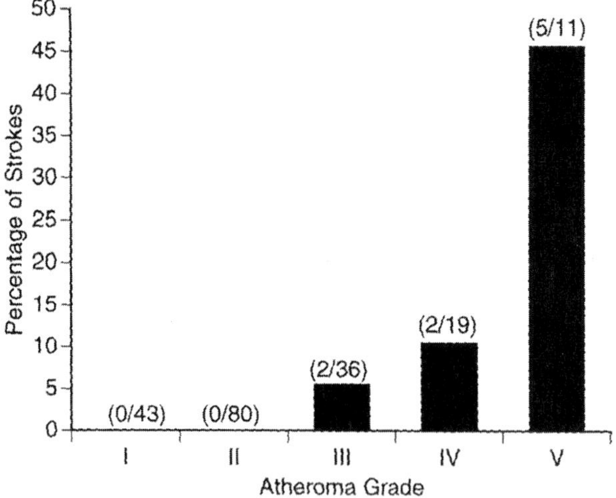

FIGURE 31-10. Risk of perioperative stroke versus descending thoracic aortic grade. Numbers in parentheses represent the number of patients who suffered a stroke out of the total number of patients with that descending aortic grade. (Reproduced with permission from Hartman GS, Yao FS, Bruefach M *et al:* Severity of aortic artheromatous disease diagnosed by transesophageal echocardiography predicts stroke and other outcomes associated with coronary artery surgery: A prospective study. Anesth Analg 83:701, 1996.)

in diagnosing an acute aortic dissection[42] (Fig. 31-11). It is important to recognize that artifacts may appear as an aortic dissection. These artifacts can be classified as linear artifacts or mirror-image artifacts. Linear artifacts may mimic intimal flaps. They frequently occur in the ascending aorta when the aortic diameter is greater than the left atrial diameter. Mirror-image artifacts are more common in the transverse and descending aorta and appear as a double-barrel aorta. These are produced by the aortic-lung tissue interface. Numerous methods can be used to decrease the risk of interpreting an artifact as a dissection. Performing a complete 2D assessment of the aorta in multiple image planes will eliminate the majority of artifacts. Applying color flow Doppler to the aorta may also distinguish a dissection from an artifact. Dissections will disrupt the blood flow pattern to produce a mosaic color flow image, a pattern not seen with artifacts. Finally, M-mode echocardiography can be used to demonstrate independent movement of the true aortic flap, a property not consistent with an artifact. Epiaortic evaluation of the ascending aorta should be performed if an acute dissection is suspected secondary to surgical cannulation of the aorta.

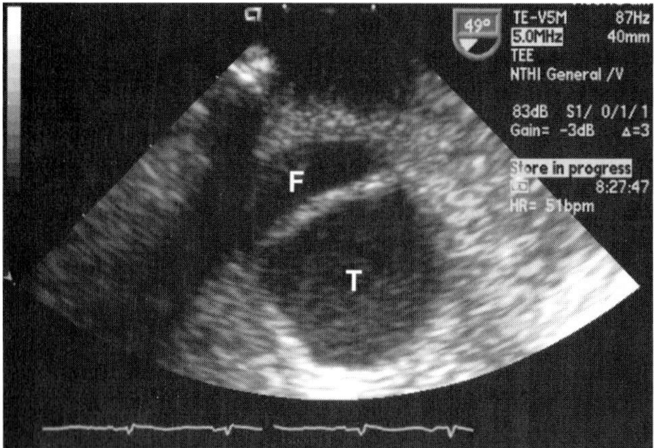

FIGURE 31-11. Aortic dissection. Two-dimensional short-axis view of the descending aorta demonstrates the presence of an intimal flap separating the true lumen (T) from the false lumen (F).

Selection of Anesthetic

8 There is no one "ideal" anesthetic for patients with coronary artery disease. The choice of anesthetic should depend primarily on the extent of preexisting myocardial dysfunction and the pharmacologic properties of the drugs themselves. The fit patient who has angina only on heavy exertion and good ventricular function profits from having $M\dot{V}O_2$ decreased with a volatile-based technique. Conversely, the patient with severe congestive heart failure and a scarred myocardium might be better served by a less depressant technique. These examples illustrate the point that myocardial depression is harmful only in the patient whose heart cannot be further depressed without fear of precipitating overt heart failure. Most patients with mild or even moderate dysfunction may benefit from some degree of myocardial depression, decreasing oxygen demand, and alleviating or at least decreasing episodes of ischemia.

Early extubation is popular for both on as well as off-pump cardiac procedures. There are multiple approaches to achieve early extubation in the cardiac surgical patient. The choice of anesthetic should be based on known hemodynamic, pharmacologic, and pharmacokinetic effects of each drug as they apply to the particular patient, the experience of the anesthesiologist, and the relative cost-benefit of each agent. Volatile anesthetics with low-dose narcotics and total intravenous anesthesia with short-acting drugs (e.g., midazolam, alfentanil, remifentanil, propofol) have been used to effect early extubation. Another interesting approach is the combination of the opiates, sufentanil and morphine, instilled intrathecally before induction.

Opioids

The primary advantages of opioids are lack of myocardial depression, maintenance of a stable hemodynamic state, and reduction of heart rate (except for meperidine). Problems include (1) hypertension and tachycardia during surgical stimulation (sternotomy and aortic manipulation), especially in patients with good ventricular function; (2) predictable hypotension when combined with benzodiazepines; (3) lack of titratability when used in high doses; and (4) a low incidence of intraoperative recall. An opioid-based technique may be of value in the patient with severe myocardial dysfunction, whereas in a patient with normal ventricle, it may be inadequate and need to be combined with other anesthetics or vasoactive drugs. The planned time of extubation is now one of the major factors determining the selection and dosage of opioid.

Inhalation Anesthetics

The desirable features of volatile anesthetics include dose dependency, easy reversibility, titratable myocardial depression, amnesia, and suppression of sympathetic responses to surgical stress and cardiopulmonary bypass. Disadvantages include myocardial depression, systemic hypotension (whether induced by decreased contractility or vasodilation), and lack of postoperative analgesia. Combinations of opioids and volatile anesthetics retain their advantages with minimal untoward effects. It is likely that any volatile anesthetic agent could be used in a balanced technique.

Isoflurane is a coronary vasodilator, as are the other volatile anesthetics (although to a lesser degree). This dose-related effect is clinically insignificant in doses less than 1 minimum alveolar concentration (MAC). Clinical studies using isoflurane to clinical rather than pharmacologic endpoints have not shown increased episodes of ischemia or a worsened outcome.

Desflurane and sevoflurane have the fastest recovery of all volatile anesthetics. Desflurane has a rapid uptake and distribution, allowing it to be useful in cases where hemodynamic swings are dramatic. It has a cardiac profile similar to that of isoflurane. Of concern is the fact that a sudden increase in inspired concentration can lead to a marked increase in heart rate, mean arterial pressure, and plasma epinephrine levels, making it riskier for use in patients with coronary artery disease. In patients undergoing noncardiac surgery, desflurane does increase pulmonary artery pressure, wedge pressure, and pulmonary vascular resistance compared with isoflurane.[43] Studying sympathetic nervous system activity, Helman et al. found an increase in sympathetic activity and myocardial ischemia in patients anesthetized with desflurane as the sole anesthetic agent for coronary artery bypass surgery compared with patients anesthetized with sufentanil.[44] In contrast, the hemodynamic profile of sevoflurane also resembles that of isoflurane.[45] Compared with isoflurane, in a technique combining fentanyl with the inhalational anesthetic, sevoflurane had an acceptable cardiovascular profile prior to cardiopulmonary bypass and had similar outcome data to isoflurane.[46]

Intravenous Sedative Hypnotics

An alternative adjuvant anesthetic to a low-dose opioid technique is a titratable intravenous infusion of a short-acting sedative, such as midazolam, propofol, or dexmedatomidine. These can be continued postoperatively in the intensive care unit (ICU), and afford a predictable and fairly rapid awakening after discontinuation.

Treatment of Ischemia

The use of anesthetics or vasoactive drugs that enable the heart to return to the slower-rate, smaller-size, and well-perfused state is frequently essential during anesthesia. The principal vasoactive drugs are nitrates, β-blockers, peripheral vasoconstrictors, and calcium-entry blockers. Clinical scenarios for their use are given in Table 31-4. These drugs are discussed extensively in Chapter 12 and are reviewed only briefly here. Volatile anesthetics can also be used to control blood pressure and reduce contractility.

Nitrates

Nitroglycerin is the drug of choice for the acute treatment of coronary vasospasm. It is a systemic venodilator (reduces venous return and decreases wall tension and $M\dot{V}O_2$) and a coronary arterial dilator (effective in both stenosed coronaries and in collateral beds). The evidence for the prophylactic use of nitroglycerin is unconvincing for prevention of either intraoperative ischemic episodes or postoperative cardiac complications. At higher doses, it dilates arterial beds and may cause systemic hypotension. The recommended trynitroglycerol (nitroclycerin) (TNG) dose is 0.5 to 3 mcg/kg per minute and is reduced in the presence of hepatic and/or renal disease. TNG may cause methemoglobinemia, especially in patients with methemoglobin reductase deficiency. TNG is administered via special intravenous tubing that does not adsorb the drug.

Sodium Nitroprusside

Sodium nitroprusside (SNP), which is comparable to other nitrovasodilators, decreases peripheral vascular resistance by metabolic or spontaneous reduction to nitric oxide. Similar to TNG, SNP improves ventricular compliance in the ischemic myocardium. The recommended SNP dose is 0.5 to 3 mcg/kg per minute, and is reduced in the presence of hepatic and/or renal disease. Adverse effects include cyanide and thiocyanate toxicity, rebound hypertension, intracranial hypertension, blood coagulation abnormalities, increased pulmonary shunting, and hypothyroidism. Cyanide is produced when SNP is metabolized; 1 mg of SNP contains 0.44 mg of cyanide. Toxic blood levels (>100 mg/dL) occur when >1 mg/kg SNP is administered within 2 hours or when >0.5 mg/kg/hr is administered within 24 hours. The presenting signs of cyanide toxicity include the triad of elevated mixed venous O_2 (P_{VO_2}), requirements for increasing SNP dose (tachyphylaxis), and metabolic acidosis.[47] In addition, the patient may appear flushed. Greater risk of cyanide toxicity exists in patients who are nutritionally deficient in cobalamine (vitamin B_{12} compounds) or in dietary substances containing sulfur. Measurement of blood cyanide and pH will enable detection of abnormalities in high-risk patients for whom larger than recommended amounts of SNP have been used (8 to 10 mcg/kg per minute). Treatment should consist of discontinuing infusion, administering 100% O_2, and administering amyl nitrate (inhaler) or intravenous sodium nitrite and intravenous thiosulfate, except in those patients with abnormal renal function, for whom hydroxocobalamin is recommended. A cyanide antidote kit is commercially available (Eli Lilly Co.). Circulating levels of thiocyanate increase when renal function is compromised, and central nervous system abnormalities result when thiocyanate levels reach 5 to 10 mg/dL. Lowering the SNP dose requirement can be achieved with captopril, trimethaphan,

TABLE 31-4

TREATMENT OF INTRAOPERATIVE ISCHEMIA

■ DEMAND: INCREASED	■ CLINICAL MANIFESTATION	■ SUPPLY: DECREASED
Rx usual suspects, β-blocker	↑ HR ↓	Atropine, pacing
↑ Anesthetic depth	↑ BP ↓	↓ Anesthetic depth, vasoconstrictor
NTG	↑ PCWP ↓	NTG, inotrope
	No changes	NTG, calcium channel blockers, ?heparin

↑, increase; ↓, decrease; BP, blood pressure; HR, heart rate; NTG, nitroglycerin; PCWP, pulmonary capillary wedge pressure.

diltiazem, nicardipine, metoprolol, and esmolol, thereby reducing the consequent buildup of cyanide. SNP can also cause inhibition of platelet aggregation; however, more recent evidence indicates that this complication is reversible and transitory.[48] Once dissolved, SNP deteriorates in the presence of light. The container, therefore, should be wrapped in aluminum foil. An unstable SNP ion in aqueous solution reacts with various substances within 3 to 4 hours, forming colored salts. Other drugs should not be infused in the same solution as SNP.

Vasoconstrictors

Vasoconstrictors are useful adjuncts in the prevention and treatment of ischemia because they increase systemic blood pressure. Administration of an α-adrenergic agent such as phenylephrine improves coronary perfusion pressure, albeit at the expense of increasing afterload and $M\dot{V}O_2$. In addition, concomitant venoconstriction increases venous return and left ventricular preload. Nitroglycerin is sometimes added to counteract any increase in preload. In most situations, the increase in coronary perfusion pressure more than offsets any increase in wall tension. Peripheral vasoconstriction is indicated during episodes of systemic hypotension, especially those caused by reduced surgical stimulation or drug-induced vasodilation (e.g., when nitroglycerin results in unacceptably low arterial pressure).

Beta Blockers

β-Adrenergic blockade improves myocardial oxygen balance by preventing or treating tachycardia and by decreasing contractility. Myocardial depression can result in increased ventricular end-systolic volume and wall tension. Clinically, this is not usually a problem. Indications for β-blockers include treatment of sinus tachycardia not resulting from the usual causes (e.g., light anesthesia, hypovolemia), slowing the ventricular response to supraventricular dysrhythmias, decreasing heart rate and contractility in hyperdynamic states, and control of ventricular dysrhythmias. The use of atenolol has been shown to improve long-term survival in patients with heart disease undergoing noncardiac surgery.[49,50] Intravenous preparations include propranolol, metoprolol, labetalol, and esmolol. Propranolol is a nonselective β-blocker with an elimination half-life of 4 to 6 hours. Metoprolol is similar to propranolol but has the purported advantage of β_1 selectivity. Labetalol combines β-blocking properties with those of α-blockade and is useful in treating hyperdynamic and hypertensive situations. Esmolol is a short-acting β_1-blocker that is cardioselective, with a half-life of only 9.5 minutes. It is particularly useful in treating transient increases in heart rate owing to episodic sympathetic stimulation.

Calcium Channel Blockers

Calcium channel blockers are useful in slowing the ventricular response in atrial fibrillation and flutter, as coronary vasodilators, and in the treatment of postoperative hypertension. In vitro, all calcium entry blockers depress contractility, reduce coronary and systemic vascular tone, decrease sinoatrial node firing rate, and impede atrioventricular conduction. Unlike the β-blockers, which are similar both in structure and pharmacodynamic effect, the calcium entry blockers vary remarkably in their predominant pharmacologic action. The negative inotropic effect is greatest with verapamil and less with nifedipine, diltiazem, and isradipine (in decreasing order). Verapamil is useful in the treatment of supraventricular tachycardia and slowing the ventricular response in atrial fibrillation and/or flutter; however, its myocardial depressant effects may limit its usefulness in some patients. In patients with reduced myocardial function, intravenous diltiazem is effective in the treatment of atrial fibrillation and flutter by slowing atrioventricular conduction with minimal myocardial depression. It is also useful in decreasing sinus rate. Nifedipine and diltiazem are coronary vasodilators used as antianginal agents and in the prevention of coronary vasospasm.

Nifedipine, isradipine, amlodipine, and nicardipine are prominent peripheral vasodilators. Owing to their systemic vasodilatory effects, intravenous isradipine and nicardipine have been shown to be effective in the treatment of postoperative hypertension in cardiac surgical patients, with minimal side effects.[51,52] Magnesium has use in the treatment of myocardial ischemia. It has coronary artery vasodilating properties, reduces the size of myocardial infarction in the setting of acute ischemia, and decreases mortality associated with infarction.[53] In addition, it is an antiarrhythmic and minimizes myocardial reperfusion injury.

VALVULAR HEART DISEASE

Alterations in loading conditions are the initial physiologic burdens imposed by valvular heart lesions, both stenotic and regurgitant. For example, the LV is pressure overloaded in aortic stenosis and volume overloaded in aortic insufficiency and mitral regurgitation. In mitral stenosis, however, the LV is both volume-underloaded and pressure-underloaded, whereas the RV faces progressively increasing left atrial and pulmonary artery pressure. Compensatory mechanisms consist of chamber enlargement, myocardial hypertrophy, and variations in vascular tone and level of sympathetic activity. These mechanisms in turn induce secondary alterations, including altered ventricular compliance, development of myocardial ischemia, chronic cardiac dysrhythmias, and progressive myocardial dysfunction.[54] Myocardial contractility is often transiently depressed but may progress to irreversible impairment even in the absence of clinical symptoms. Conversely, the patient with aortic stenosis may complain of dyspnea, not because of impaired systolic function, but because of reduced ventricular compliance, increased left ventricular end-diastolic pressure, and increased pulmonary pressure.

The patient presenting for valve repair or replacement often has pulmonary hypertension, severe ventricular dysfunction, and chronic rhythm disorders. Anesthetic management is predicated on understanding the altered loading conditions, preserving the compensatory mechanisms, maintaining circulatory homeostasis, and anticipating problems that may arise during and after valve surgery. In this section, we briefly describe the pathophysiology, the desirable hemodynamic profile, and other pertinent anesthetic considerations for each valvular lesion.

TEE has become the standard of care in the perioperative management of patients undergoing valve surgery.[55] TEE can further refine the preoperative diagnosis, identify valvular pathology and the mechanism of disease, and quantify the degree of stenosis and/or regurgitation. Studies have shown a change in the perioperative plan regarding valve surgery in as many as 19% of cases as a result of the prebypass echocardiographic exam.[54,55] Prompt evaluation of the surgical results by TEE also affects the operative course: depending on the surgical intervention, 5 to 18% of the time TEE reveals findings that result in an immediate return to CPB.[56] However, the detailed assessment of valvular function pre-CPB and post-CPB is complex. 2D echocardiography and color flow Doppler can provide a gross evaluation of valve function, but complete assessment requires Doppler evaluation of blood flow velocities. Comprehensive reviews of these topics can be found in standard textbooks of echocardiography. Ultimately, the decision to intervene is clinical and must take into account the patient's individual situation. Both valve replacement and repair result in a level of valve pathology that may or may not be in the best interest of the patient.

Aortic Stenosis

In a normal adult, the aortic valve (AV) is composed of three semilunar cusps attached to the wall of the aorta. The normal AV diameter is 1.9 to 2.3 cm with an aortic valve area (AVA) of 2 to 4 cm^2. The outpouchings of the aortic wall immediately above the valve cusps are called the sinuses of Valsalva. These are symmetric with a diameter 0.2 to 0.3 cm greater than the AV annular diameter. The cusps and the corresponding sinuses are named according to their relation to the coronary ostia: left, right, and noncoronary. On the ventricular side of the aortic valve is the cylindrical outflow tract. Its borders are the inferior surface of the anterior leaflet of the mitral valve, the interventricular septum, and the left ventricular free wall. The normal diameter of the left ventricular outflow tract (LVOT) is 2.2 cm $\pm$ 0.2 cm.

Etiologies of aortic stenosis include (1) bicuspid AV, a congenital lesion, where the mechanical shear stress leads to injury and stenosis of the valve orifice; (2) degeneration of normal, tricuspid AV from autoimmune phenomena (rheumatic fever), leading to calcification and fusion along the commissures; (3) cardiovascular risk factors (hypercholesterolemia, male gender, smoking), which initiate a "response to injury" similar to that seen in atherosclerosis, where the cusps become calcified, thickened, and deformed, with a decreased ability to separate; and (4) conditions associated with chronically elevated stroke volume and altered calcium metabolism (Paget's disease, hyperparathyroidism, renal failure associated with arteriovenous fistula). Rheumatic disease causes mixed aortic stenosis and AV regurgitation, and coexists with mitral valve disease.[57]

Pathophysiology

The progressive narrowing of the AV orifice results in chronic obstruction to left ventricular ejection. Intraventricular systolic pressure increases to preserve forward flow. "Concentric" ventricular hypertrophy, in which the wall gradually thickens but the chamber size remains unchanged, is the compensatory response normalizing the concomitant increase in wall tension. Contractility is preserved and ejection fraction is maintained at a normal range until late in the disease process (Fig. 31-12). Signs and symptoms of aortic stenosis occur when the AV orifice is reduced to 0.8 cm^2.[58]

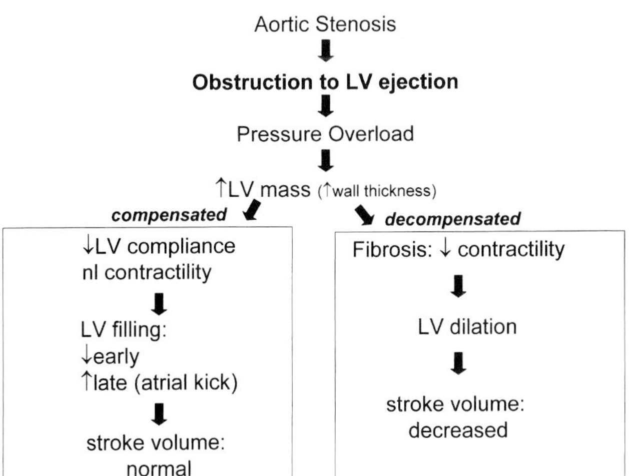

FIGURE 31-12. The physiologic consequences of aortic stenosis. LV, left ventricle.

The cost of this concentric hypertrophy is decreased diastolic compliance and a precarious balance between myocardial oxygen supply and $M\dot{V}O_2$. Hypertrophy-induced impairment of diastolic relaxation ("stiff" ventricle) impedes early left ventricular filling and atrial contraction is often critical for maintaining adequate ventricular filling and stroke volume. The "atrial kick" may account for up to 30 to 40% of left ventricular end-diastolic volume. The ventricular filling pressure, as reflected by pulmonary capillary wedge pressure, may vary widely with only small changes in ventricular volume.

The enlarged muscle mass has increased basal myocardial oxygen requirements, while demand per beat rises because of the elevated intraventricular systolic pressure. Simultaneously, with a capillary density often inadequate for the hypertrophic muscle, supply may be further compromised, when perfusion pressure is reduced (as when the aortic diastolic pressure is decreased and/or the ventricular filling pressure is increased), and total vasodilator reserve may be impaired. This situation is compounded in the presence of coronary obstruction. Often, patients with aortic stenosis will present in heart failure.

Anesthetic Considerations

9 The ideal hemodynamic environment for the patient with aortic stenosis is summarized in Table 31-5. Maintenance of adequate ventricular volume and sinus rhythm is crucial. Hypotension must be prevented and treated promptly if it develops. Anticipation of likely hemodynamic changes is essential (e.g., expected decreases in blood pressure following spinal anesthesia). Coronary perfusion pressure must be maintained to prevent the catastrophic cycle of hypotension-induced ischemia, subsequent ventricular dysfunction, and worsening hypotension. Bradycardia is a common clinical etiology for hypotension in the patient with aortic stenosis. Slowing the heart rate and increasing diastolic time will not increase stroke volume in the thick, concentrically hypertrophied LV. Therefore, bradycardia will induce a fall in total cardiac output and systemic arterial pressure. This is especially pertinent in the elderly patient, in whom sinus node disease and reduced sympathetic responses may predispose to significant bradycardia. Tachycardia must be avoided because it reduces the duration of diastolic coronary perfusion.

Ischemia may be difficult to detect because the characteristic electrocardiographic changes are often obscured by signs of LV hypertrophy and strain. Elevated LV filling pressures, although not necessarily reflecting increased volume, often require

TABLE 31-5

AORTIC STENOSIS—HEMODYNAMIC GOALS

P	Full
A	Maintain coronary perfusion gradient
C	Usually not a problem, may require inotropic support if persistent hypotension
R	Avoid bradycardia (↓CO) and tachycardia (ischemia)
Rhythm	Sinus: may need cardioversion or β-blockers
$M\dot{V}O_2$	Avoid tachycardia and hypotension (ischemia is an ever-present risk)
CPB	Contractility augmentation may be required transiently secondary to myocardial stunning; blood pressure may need to be controlled later

A, afterload; C, contractility; CPB, cardiopulmonary bypass; $M\dot{V}O_2$, myocardial oxygen consumption; P, preload; R, rate.

treatment to optimize coronary perfusion pressure.[59] Nitroglycerin is useful in this regard, but it must be remembered that minimal reductions in ventricular volume are required; therefore, very low doses of nitroglycerin should be used and titrated to effect. As an alternative, an arterial dilator, such as nicardipine or sodium nitroprusside[60] will lower afterload without affecting ventricular volume.

Transesophageal Echocardiography in Aortic Stenosis

The short-axis view of the aortic valve during systole can provide both a diagnosis and the mechanism of aortic stenosis. All three cusps of the aortic valve should be identified during systolic excursion. In degenerative calcification, the systolic orifice becomes smaller as the leaflet cusps become calcified, thickened, and deformed, resulting in a decreased ability to separate. In contrast, rheumatic valve calcification is along the commissures resulting in fusion and a progressive decrease in the valve orifice area. Although the rheumatic process usually involves the mitral valve, it can simultaneously or in isolation affect the aortic valve. A bicuspid aortic valve occurs in 2% of the population and predisposes the individual to aortic stenosis, as well as aortic regurgitation and endocarditis. Frequently, bicuspid valves have a raphe in the large cusp, which may be mistaken as a commissure during diastole. Trileaflet valves, if heavily calcified and fibrotic, may be indistinguishable from biscuspid valves.

The systolic AVA can be accurately estimated by planimetery. In the midesophageal aortic valve long-axis view, a systolic leaflet separation >1.3 cm reliably excludes severe aortic stenosis. Associated 2D findings with aortic stenosis may include concentric hypertrophy of the LV, left ventricular diastolic dysfunction, and a poststenotic aortic root dilatation that can become severe enough to require surgical correction.

Doppler interrogation across the stenotic aortic valve permits determination of the pressure gradient and AVA. Color flow Doppler across a stenotic aortic valve will show a mosaic of aliased turbulent flow. In about 90% of the patients, the deep transgastric long-axis view allows excellent alignment of the ultrasound beam with aortic blood flow angle (<30). If this view cannot be obtained, rotation to an angle between 60° to 120° from the transgastric midpapillary short-axis view may align the ultrasound beam with the aortic blood flow. Using the modified Bernoulli equation ($4V^2$ = pressure gradient), the peak and mean aortic valve gradients can be determined from the peak and mean blood flow velocities across the stenotic valve. It is important to note that the cardiac catheterization data frequently report the left ventricular peak to aortic peak pressure gradient. These pressures occur at different times in the cardiac cycle, and the gradient is consistently less than the peak instantaneous gradient measured by Doppler. However, the mean gradients measured by echocardiography and catheterization should be the same. The pressure gradient depends on the flow through the orifice. The severity of the stenosis may be underestimated if the cardiac output is reduced; conversely, it is overestimated if flow is increased from aortic regurgitation or inotropic support. If one of these scenarios is suspected, the AVA should be calculated using the continuity equation (Fig. 31-13).[61] The continuity equation assumes the flow across any two orifices should be the same. In this case, LVOT flow equals aortic valve flow. Doppler-derived flow measurements are the product of the velocity time integral

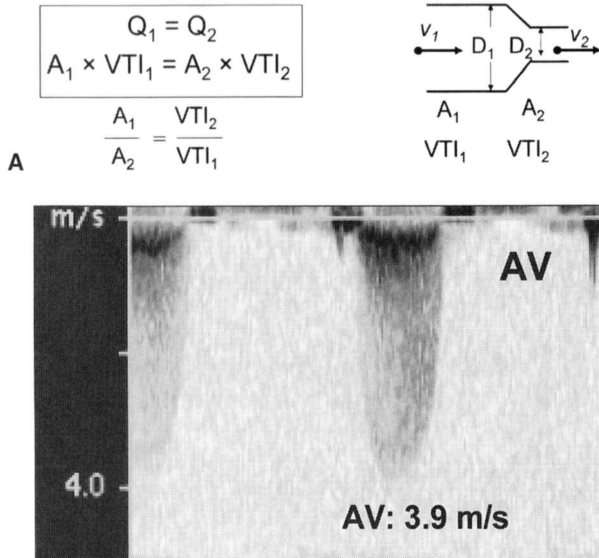

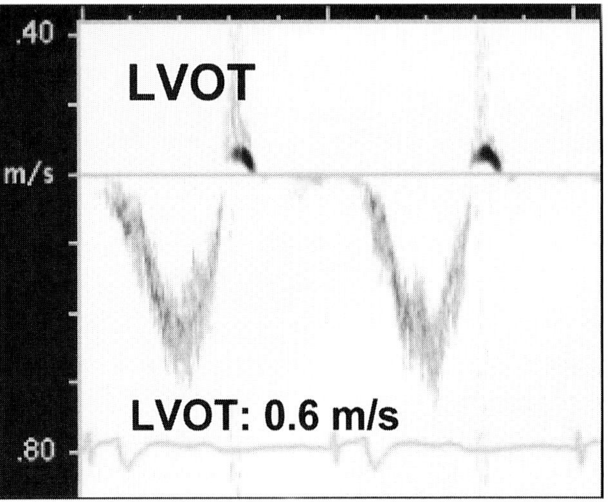

FIGURE 31-13. Transesophageal echocardiography (TEE) in aortic stenosis. **A.** The continuity equation calculates the orifice of a stenotic aortic valve, using the concept of conservation of flow. The volume across any orifice is the product of the orifice area (A) and the integral of its velocity (VTI). Therefore, flow Q_1 across an orifice with diameter D_1 and surface A_1 has a velocity v_1 and VTI_1 and is equal to flow Q_2 across an orifice with diameter D_2, surface A_2, and velocity v_2 and VTI_2. By rearranging the continuity equation, $A_2 = (A_1 \times VTI_1)$, VTI_2. **B, C.** If A_1 is the orifice of the left ventricular outflow tract (LVOT) and A_2 is the orifice of the aortic valve (AV), then area of AV = (LVOT × VTI_{LVOT}), VTI_{AV}. Because the flow duration across the LVOT and the AV is the same, VTI can be replaced by AVA = LVOT × (V_{LVOT}, V_{AV}). The AVA is inversely related to the VTI (or v) ratio of the LVOT and the AV. In the above TEE pictures, the LVOT velocity is 0.6 m/s (**B**), the AV velocity is 3.9 m/s (**C**), and the LVOT diameter was measured 2.12 cm. The continuity equation calculated an AVA of 0.54 cm^2. In general, if the ratio $Vmax_{AV}/Vmax_{LVOT}$ is >4, then the AVA is probably <1 cm^2 (assuming an LVOT diameter of ~2 cm).

TABLE 31-6

ECHOCARDIOGRAPHIC FINDINGS IN AORTIC STENOSIS

■ 2D		
• Valve anatomy and structure • Planimetry of orifice	Systolic orifice is star shaped (tricuspid) or elliptical/circular (bicuspid) Absence of calcification makes significant AS unlikely	
• Cusp excursion (use M-mode)	<8 mm: suggestive of AS >13 mm: unlikely AS	
• LV, LVOT, and aorta	Concentric LV hypertrophy, poststenotic dilation of ascending aorta in AS	
■ DOPPLER		
• Color flow	Turbulence (mosaic flow) in ascending aorta is suggestive of poststenotic flow	
• Continuous wave		
◦ V_{max} of AV	2.5 to 3.5 m/sec (mild AS)	>4.5 m/sec (severe AS)
◦ PG = 4 × v^2 max	25 to 50 mm Hg (mild AS)	>80 mm Hg (severe AS)

2D, two-dimensional; AS, aortic stenosis; LV, left ventricle; LVOT, left ventricular outflow tract; PG, pressure gradient; v, velocity.

(VTI) and the area of the orifice. The VTI of the LVOT is measured with pulsed Doppler, whereas the LVOT diameter is measured with 2D echocardiography. Continuous-wave Doppler can measure the peak velocity through the stenotic lesion. The AVA is then calculated from the continuity equation:

$$VTI_{AV} \times Area_{AV} = VTI_{LVOT} \times Area_{LVOT}$$
$$Area_{AV} = VTI_{LVOT} \times Area_{LVOT}/VTI_{AV}$$

The severity of aortic stenosis can be estimated by employing these echocardiographic modalities and the grading criteria outlined in Table 31-6.

Hypertrophic Cardiomyopathy

Hypertrophic cardiomyopathy (or idiopathic hypertrophic subaortic stenosis or asymmetric septal hypertrophy) is a genetically determined disease characterized by histologically abnormal myocytes and myocardial hypertrophy developing a priori, in the absence of a pressure or volume overload. The hypertrophic LV is not dilated.[62]

Pathophysiology

The physiologic consequences of hypertrophic cardiomyopathy (similar to those detailed for aortic stenosis) are depicted in Figure 31-14. Some degree of subvalvular obstruction is present in 20 to 30% of patients. During systole, the left ventricular outflow tract is narrowed by apposition of the hypertrophic interventricular septum to the anterior leaflet of the mitral valve. Blood is ejected rapidly through this area, creating a Venturi effect, and the anterior mitral valve leaflet is pulled even closer to the septum (systolic anterior motion [SAM]). The timing and duration of septal–leaflet contact determine the severity and clinical significance of the obstruction: early, prolonged

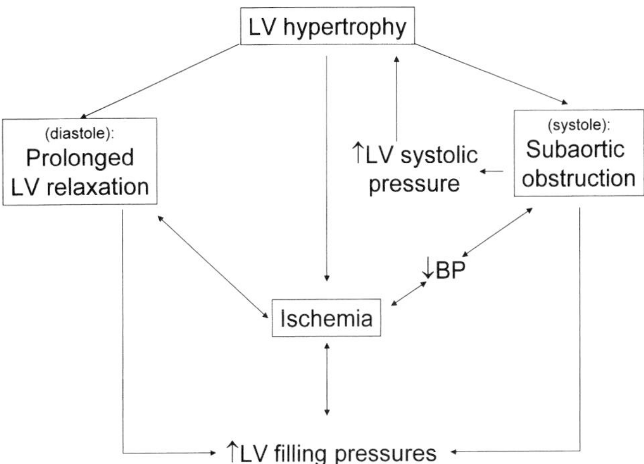

FIGURE 31-14. The physiologic interrelationships of primary left ventricular hypertrophy in hypertrophic cardiomyopathy. LV, left ventricle; BP, blood pressure.

contact can generate pressure gradients of 100 mm Hg. If the apposition occurs later, it is of little importance, even if a pressure gradient still exists, because most of the stroke volume has already been ejected. This type of obstruction is dynamic, and is accentuated by any intervention that reduces ventricular size. Therefore, increases in contractility and heart rate or decreases in either preload or afterload are harmful because they facilitate septal–leaflet contact. Another hypothesis proposed for systolic anterior motion of the mitral valve is an abnormally displaced mitral apparatus. The systolic anterior motion of the anterior mitral valve leaflet results in a posteriorly directed mitral regurgitation jet.

The ventricles are hypertrophic, even in the absence of a pressure gradient. In addition, there is evidence of alterations in the small intramyocardial vessels. As expected, myocardial oxygen balance is tenuous, and the development of ischemia is an ever-present possibility.

Anesthetic Considerations

Treatment options for HCM include alcohol ablation of the interventricular septum, dual-chamber cardiac pacing, and septal myectomy. Anesthetic management for patients undergoing septal myectomy focuses on maintenance of ventricular filling and reduction in the factors predisposing to outflow tract obstruction or ischemia (Table 31-7). Myocardial depression is desirable, and volatile anesthetics are useful, although their

TABLE 31-7

HYPERTROPHIC CARDIOMYOPATHY—HEMODYNAMIC GOALS

P	Full, one of first treatments for hypotension
A	Increased: treat aggressively if hypotension
C	Prefer depression
R	Normal range
Rhythm	Sinus rhythm crucial. Atrial pacing modalities (PA cath, transesophageal) may be helpful
$M\dot{V}O_2$	Not a problem
CPB	Start with volume and vasoconstrictors: avoid inotropes. Check carefully for residual gradient and SAM

A, afterload; C, contractility; CPB, cardiopulmonary bypass; $M\dot{V}O_2$, myocardial oxygen consumption; P, preload; PA, pulmonary artery; R, rate; SAM, systolic anterior motion of the mitral valve.

tendency to cause junctional rhythm is of some concern. Because of the dependence of preload on atrial contraction, these patients will benefit from atrial pacing if junctional rhythm occurs. Methods to achieve this include transesophageal pacing or use of a pulmonary artery catheter with pacing capability. This permits the administration of volatile anesthetics without fear of compromising sinoatrial conduction. In addition, control of atrial rate and rhythm is beneficial during the prebypass period.

Although infrequent, hypertrophic cardiomyopathy occasionally coexists with valvular aortic stenosis and may explain unanticipated difficulties in separating from bypass following seemingly uncomplicated aortic valve replacement. If this is suspected, measurement of the gradient between the LV and the outflow tract will resolve this dilemma. In addition, dynamic left ventricular outflow obstruction is occasionally observed following mitral valve repair. In this case, anterior septal motion of the mitral valve can be observed echocardiographically. Pharmacologic management of hypotension is with volume replacement and vasoconstrictors rather than inotropes and vasodilators.

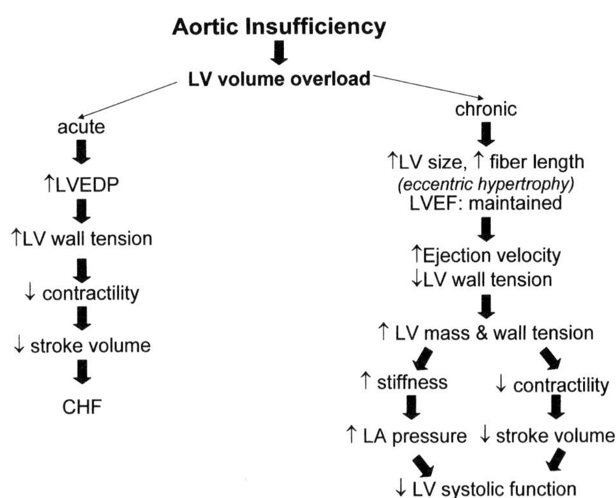

FIGURE 31-15. The physiologic consequences of aortic insufficiency. CHF, congestive heart failure; LA, left atrium; LV, left ventricle; LVEDP, left ventricular end-diastolic pressure; LVEF, left ventricular ejection fraction.

Aortic Insufficiency

Aortic valve insufficiency is the result of annular dilatation or abnormal leaflet motion.[63] Annular dilatation can occur with aneurysms or dissections of the ascending aorta. Because the aortic cusp area is 40% greater than the cross-sectional area of a normal aortic root, small increases in the diameter of the aortic annulus can be accommodated before the valve becomes incompetent. Abnormal leaflet motion and coaptation can be noted with calcific degeneration, rheumatic disease, bicuspid aortic valves, and endocarditis.

Pathophysiology

The fundamental physiologic derangement is chronic volume overload (Fig. 31-15). Chamber size increases gradually, sometimes to massive proportions, increasing wall stress and inducing mural hypertrophy. The chamber enlargement is of a greater magnitude than the increase in ventricular wall thickness and is termed *eccentric hypertrophy.* Despite the enormous increases in end-diastolic volume, end-diastolic pressures are usually within the normal range, evidence of a significant increase in chamber compliance. As a result, and in contrast to aortic stenosis, considerable alterations in left ventricular volume can occur with only minimal changes in left ventricular filling pressure. Although the ventricle may pump three to four times the normal cardiac output, $\dot{M}VO_2$ does not increase extraordinarily because the oxygen cost for muscle shortening is low. The diastolic runoff and the moderate vasodilation reduce the ventricular afterload. This will allow patients to be relatively symptom-free even when contractility is reduced so it is difficult to evaluate the myocardial contractile state from clinical signs and symptoms. This is important in terms of planning the anesthetic, but perhaps even more so with respect to the timing of aortic valve replacement. Ideally, the valve should be replaced just prior to the onset of irreversible myocardial damage. Therefore, continued follow-up of these patients emphasizes repeated noninvasive measurements of contractility, usually after some form of afterload stress, either pharmacologic-induced or exerciseinduced.

In acute aortic insufficiency the previously normal-size and normally compliant LV is presented with a large regurgitant volume. As a result left ventricular end-diastolic pressure rises rapidly (along the steep portion of the diastolic pressure–volume relation). Severe congestive heart failure is the cardinal clinical sign (Table 31-8). Myocardial contractility becomes impaired as left ventricular end-diastolic pressure increases. Compensatory mechanisms include tachycardia and peripheral vasoconstriction, but occasionally hypotension and low cardiac output ensue. In acutely ill patients, emergency aortic valve replacement is required, whereas in less severe circumstances mild systemic vasodilation and inotropic support can return hemodynamics toward normal.

Anesthetic Considerations

10 Full, mildly vasodilated, and modestly tachycardic describe the optimal cardiovascular state for patients with aortic insufficiency (Table 31-9). Vasodilation promotes forward flow, although additional intravascular volume may be necessary to maintain preload. The ideal heart rate is somewhat controversial. It is likely that changes in heart rate alone will not alter forward or regurgitant flow; each will be proportionately reduced. Tachycardia reduces the diastolic run-off from the aorta to the LV and results in a reduction of the ventricular volume and wall tension, and increase in the diastolic blood pressure and coronary perfusion gradient, offsetting any increase in oxygen demand secondary to an increased heart rate.

TABLE 31-8

ACUTE VERSUS CHRONIC AORTIC INSUFFICIENCY

	CHRONIC	ACUTE
Left ventricular size	↑	—
Left ventricular compliance	↑	—
Left ventricular end-diastolic pressure	—	↑
Effective cardiac output	Normal	↓
Systemic vascular resistance	—	↑
Pulmonary edema	No	Yes
Pulse pressure	↑	↑/—
Heart rate	—	↑

↑, increase; ↓, decrease; —, no change.

TABLE 31-9

AORTIC INSUFFICIENCY—HEMODYNAMIC GOALS

P	Normal to slightly ↑
A	Reduction beneficial with anesthetics or vasodilators; increases augment regurgitant flow
C	Usually adequate
R	Modest tachycardia reduces ventricular volume, raises aortic diastolic pressure
Rhythm	Usually sinus; not a problem
$M\dot{V}o_2$	Not usually a problem
CPB	Observe for ventricular distention (↓ HR, ↑ VFP) when going onto CPB

P, preload; A, afterload; C, contractility; R, rate; $M\dot{V}o_2$, myocardial oxygen balance; CPB, postcardiopulmonary bypass; HR, heart rate; VFP, ventricular filling pressure.

Bradycardia should be avoided as it results in ventricular distention and elevations in left atrial pressure and pulmonary congestion.

Ventricular distention may occur with the onset of CPB if the heart rate slows or if there is unexpected ventricular fibrillation. Monitoring of the heart size, rate, rhythm, and ventricular filling pressure are especially important in these patients. If distention occurs, the insertion of a left ventricular vent or the immediate application of an aortic cross-clamp should relieve the problem. The presence of moderate to severe aortic insufficiency (AI) affects the surgeon's approach to CPB. An incompetent aortic valve may prevent the delivery of cardioplegia to the coronary system to produce diastolic arrest of the heart. After application of the aortic cross-clamp, the cardioplegia is normally injected into the aortic root, delivering this solution to the coronary system, producing a diastolic arrest of the heart. If moderate to severe AI is present, the cardioplegia will fill and distend the LV, increasing the ischemic insult incurred during CPB. As a result, in the presence of AI the surgeon may elect to arrest the heart by injecting cardioplegia directly into the coronary ostia or the coronary sinus.

Transesophageal Echocardiography in Aortic Insufficiency

Echocardiographic examination will demonstrate the structural findings associated with aortic regurgitation mentioned previously and the effects of volume overload on the LV. Doppler will identify the aortic regurgitant jet, localize its site, and help grade its severity (Table 31-10 and Fig. 31-16).

Accurate evaluation of aortic insufficiency is essential in determining the feasibility of performing an AV repair. Successful AV repairs are often performed during repair of aortic dissections and have been reported with aneurysms and bicuspid aortic valves.

Mitral Stenosis

Stenosis of the mitral valve (MV) is usually of rheumatic origin, and clinical symptoms develop within 3 to 5 years following initial infection. Debilitating symptoms such as fatigue and dyspnea on exertion do not begin for another decade or two.

TABLE 31-10

ECHOCARDIOGRAPHIC FINDINGS IN AORTIC INSUFFICIENCY

2D	
• Valve anatomy and structural deformities	Perforations, vegetations in endocarditis
• Leaflet motion, coaptation	Usually abnormal, flail leaflet, wide coaptation defect
• LV size	Normal (acute AI), significantly enlarged (severe AI)
DOPPLER	
• Color flow	
○ Regurgitant flow	
○ Ratio AI jet width/LVOT diameter	<25% in mild (1+), ≥ 65% in severe (4+)
• Continuous wave	Diastolic jet deceleration (PHT): >500 msec in mild, <200 msec in severe
• Pulsed wave	Thoracic aorta flow: brief, early reversal (mild AI), prominent holodiastolic (severe AI)

2D, two-dimensional; AI, aortic insufficiency; LV, left ventricle; LVOT, left ventricular diameter; PHT, pressure half time.

Pathophysiology

The spectrum of physiologic disruption in patients with mitral stenosis is presented in Figure 31-17. Distal to the obstructed MV and unlike any other valvular lesion, the LV is not subjected to either pressure or volume overload. It is small, relatively underloaded, with preserved systolic function. However, one-third of patients may demonstrate contractile abnormalities on angiography, presumably as a result of rheumatic carditis or involvement of the subvalvular apparatus. Proximally, the narrowed MV orifice results in increased left atrial pressure (LAP) and volume.

The relationship between LAP and the size of the MV orifice area (MVA) is expressed in the formula derived by Gorlin and Gorlin:

$$\text{Valve area} = \text{flow}/K \cdot \sqrt{(\text{pressure gradient})}$$

where flow (i.e., flow during time that MV is open) is cardiac output/diastolic filling time; pressure gradient is LAP minus left ventricular diastolic pressure (LVDP); and K is the hydraulic pressure constant. This calculation assumes no regurgitant flow. If we consider a constant MVA, rearrange terms, and eliminate the constant, we have a more useful expression of the clinical variables determining atrial and ventricular pressures:

$$\text{LAP} - \text{LVDP} = [(\text{cardiac output})/(\text{diastolic time})]^2$$

Therefore, whenever cardiac output increases or the diastolic filling period decreases, the gradient across the MV is altered by the square of the original changes. This explains why tachycardia or increases in forward flow, seen classically with pregnancy, thyrotoxicosis, or infection, can precipitate pulmonary edema. As LAP increases, left ventricular filling pressure may actually decrease. Thus, the development of atrial fibrillation causes hemodynamic embarrassment, not so much because of the loss of atrial kick but because of the rapid rate that ensues.

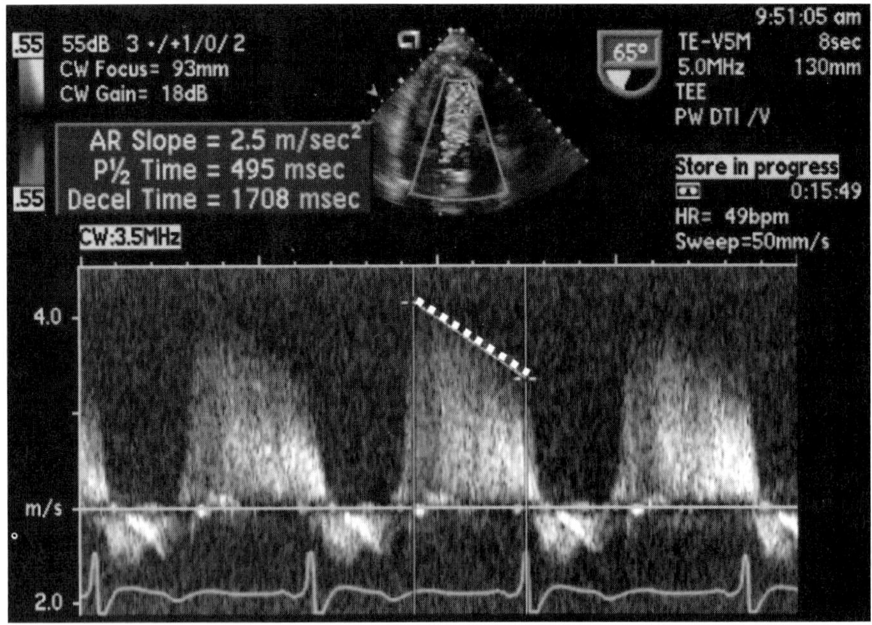

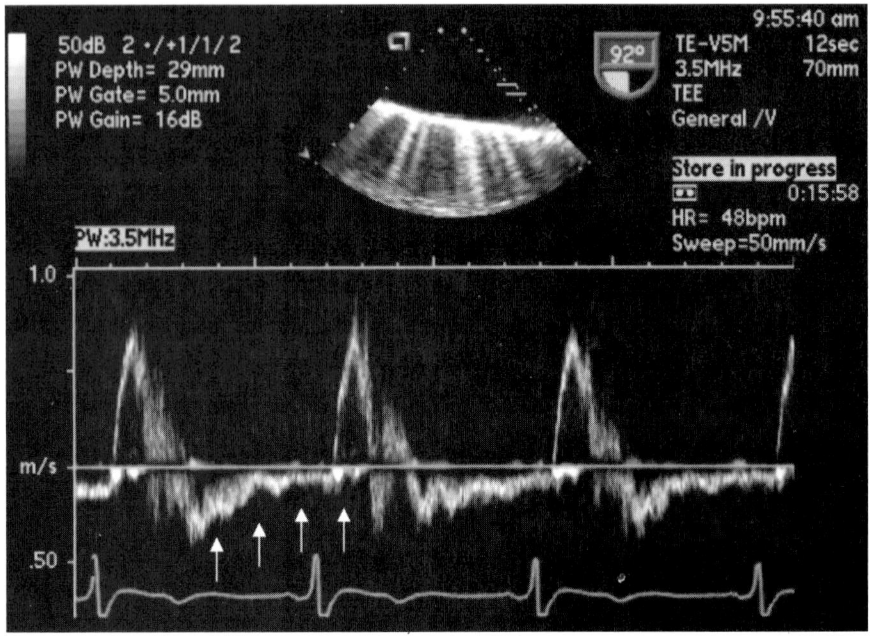

FIGURE 31-16. Transesophageal echocardiography (TEE) in aortic insufficiency. **A.** Continuous wave Doppler across the jet of aortic insufficiency (AI) typically demonstrates a pandiastolic flow signal (the systolic portion is forward flow across the aortic valve). The peak velocity in early diastole corresponds to the peak aortic to left ventricular diastolic pressure gradient as defined by the modified Bernoulli equation ($P = 4v^2$). The slope or decay of this pressure gradient reflects the severity of AI. When AI is severe, the equilibration of pressure between the aorta and the left ventricle is rapid and the PHT (the time it takes for the pressure gradient to decrease by 50%) shorter. With less severe AI, the equilibration of pressures between the aorta and the left ventricle is slower, resulting in a relatively flat slope and a prolonged PHT. **B.** Aortic diastolic flow reversal. Flow reversal is best recorded with pulsed wave Doppler in the lower descending aorta. As AI increases in severity, the duration and the velocity of the flow reversal (*arrows*) increase.

In mitral stenosis, the paradoxical situation exists of a patient in pulmonary edema with a relatively empty LV. Therefore, the treatment is not inotropic or vasodilator therapy, but rather attempts to reduce the heart rate or diagnose and treat the cause responsible for the increased flow. The pulmonary capillary wedge pressure can be used as an index of left ventricular filling, even during episodes of tachycardia or increased flow, keeping in mind that it is higher than the true left ventricular end-diastolic pressure, at least by the amount of the pressure gradient.

Upstream from the LA, the persistently elevated LAP is reflected through the pulmonary circulation, leading to right ventricular pressure overload with compensatory right ventricular hypertrophy and elevated strain. The progression and severity of pulmonary hypertension are variable and reflect further narrowing of the valve orifice and irreversible reactive changes in the pulmonary vasculature. Right ventricular dysfunction may develop in response to this increase in afterload. Tricuspid annular dilatation and insufficiency may result from this hemodynamic nightmare.

Chronically elevated LAP causes perivascular edema in the lung, increased vascular pressure in the dependent portions of the lung, redistribution of blood to the upper lung fields, and an increased work of breathing.

Anesthetic Considerations

11 Preemption is the cornerstone of prebypass anesthetic management (Table 31-11). Avoiding tachycardia precludes episodes of left atrial and pulmonary hypertension with potential right ventricular dysfunction, as well as inadequate left ventricular filling with concomitant systemic hypotension. Preoperative maintenance of digitalis and beta-blocking drugs, selection of anesthetics with no propensity to increase heart

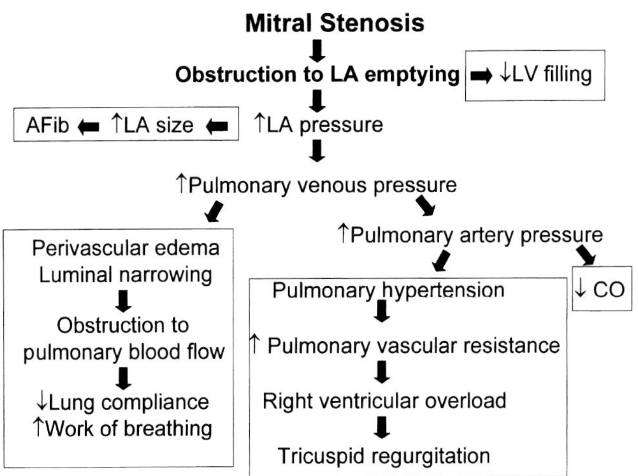

FIGURE 31-17. The cardiovascular and pulmonary effects of mitral stenosis. CO, cardiac output; LA, left atrium; LV, left ventricle.

rate, and attainment of anesthetic levels deep enough to suppress autonomic responses are methods to achieve these goals. Episodes of pulmonary hypertension and potential right-sided heart failure stemming from pulmonary vasoconstriction must also be prevented. It is wise to avoid hypoxia, hypercarbia, and acidosis because they increase pulmonary vascular resistance.

Treatment of hypotension in patients with mitral stenosis can present a challenging dilemma. Although these patients normally take diuretics, hypovolemia is not usually the cause; hence, the response to volume administration is often disappointing. Use of a vasoconstrictor to offset mild peripheral vasodilation is acceptable, bearing in mind the effect of pulmonary vasoconstriction on right ventricular function. It is often prudent to select a drug with some inotropic effect such as ephedrine or epinephrine instead of relying on a pure vasoconstrictor, such as phenylephrine. In separating from CPB, much is made of right ventricular failure (discussed subsequently); more commonly, however, it is the LV that is dysfunctional. This may be because of intraoperative injury or sudden increase in flow to and distention of the chronically underloaded LV. After bypass, prominent V waves may be present in the left atrial pressure curve. This almost always reflects increased left atrial filling from the right side rather than mitral regurgitation because cardiac output is increased after bypass when compared with preinduction values.

TABLE 31-11

MITRAL STENOSIS—HEMODYNAMIC GOALS

P	Maintain, avoid hypovolemia
A	Prevent pulmonary vasoconstriction (hypoxia, hypercarbia) Inotropes may be required for systemic hypotension
C	Usually okay. RV dysfunction may be a problem with long-standing pulmonary hypertension
R	Low end of normal. Avoid tachycardia
Rhythm	Keep ventricular response controlled in atrial fibrillation
$M\dot{V}O_2$	Not a problem
CPB	LV seeing higher preloads—filling pressures may be elevated. Heart not immediately "better"

A, afterload; C, contractility; CPB, cardiopulmonary bypass; LV, left ventricle; $M\dot{V}O_2$, myocardial oxygen consumption; P, preload; R, rate; RV, right ventricle.

Transesophageal Echocardiography in Mitral Stenosis

The normal MV consists of a semilunar-shaped anterior leaflet, comprising two-thirds of the total MV surface area and neighboring the noncoronary aortic cusp and a crescent-shaped posterior leaflet. The leaflets are composed of thin, flexible, fibrous tissue, thicker in the base and tips and thinner in their centrum, and are connected to each other at the anterolateral and posteromedial commissures (the closure "lines" of the two mitral leaflets). The mitral annulus is D-shaped, and the posterior leaflet is continous with the atrial and the ventricular myocardium, making this leaflet more pone to being displaced when either chamber enlarges. During diastole, the leaflets open and "drop" inside the LV, forming a funnel-shaped orifice, 4 to 6 cm^2 in diameter. In systole, the LV systolic pressure and the contraction of the two papillary muscles cause the two leaflets to coapt along their free edges. Strong, fibrous cords (chordae tendinae) connected to the anterolateral and posteromedial papillary muscles, create a tensor mechanism and prevent the prolapse of the closed leaflets into the LA during systole.

The grading of the severity of mitral stenosis is outlined in Table 31-12. The echocardiographic signs of mitral stenosis are seen in Figure 31-18.

Mitral Regurgitation

Mitral regurgitation (MR) results from several mechanisms permitting blood to flow from the LV to the LA during systole. Mechanical etiologies of MR include annular dilatation (chronic ischemic heart disease), leaflet prolapse, restricted leaflet motion (rheumatic heart disease), and leaflet perforation (endocarditis). Acute MR occurs with papillary muscle dysfunction or chordal rupture following myocardial infarction and may require emergency surgical repair[64] (Table 31-13).

Pathophysiology

Chronic volume overload similar to that described with AI is the cardinal feature of MR[65] (Fig. 31-19). The LA acts as a low-pressure vent during left ventricular ejection: there is no isovolumetric contraction period because blood is immediately ejected retrograde with the onset of ventricular systole. Total left ventricular stroke volume consists of the forward flow via the aorta and the retrograde flow into the LA. Atrial and ventricular chamber enlargement, ventricular wall hypertrophy, and increased blood volume are the compensatory responses. Ventricular compliance increases; thus, the large end-diastolic volume does not cause striking increases in left ventricular end-diastolic pressure. Despite progressive myocardial damage (decreased contractility), patients may have minimal symptoms because of reduced afterload. The increase in oxygen cost (required for additional muscle shortening) is small because there is little pressure development. Ejection fraction, a parameter heavily afterload dependent, can be misleading in patients with MR: normal or minimally reduced ejection fractions can be present even with severe impairment of contractile function. The regurgitant blood volume is related to the size of the regurgitant orifice, the time available for retrograde flow, and the pressure gradient across the valve. Regurgitant orifice size, in turn, depends on ventricular size. Therefore, both increases in heart rate and preload reduction decrease the amount of regurgitant flow by diminishing ventricular volume. Arteriolar

TABLE 31-12

ECHOCARDIOGRAPHIC FINDINGS IN MITRAL STENOSIS

MODALITY	MILD MS (MVA > 1.5 cm^2)	SEVERE MS (MVA < 1 cm^2)
2D		
• Valve anatomy and structural deformities	Thickened, calcified, diastolic doming	
• Leaflet motion, coaptation		
• Left atrium	In severe MS (MVA <1 cm^2): dilated with spontaneous echo contrast and/or thrombus in left atrial appendage	
• Right ventricle	In severe MS: signs of failure (dilatation, tricuspid regurgitation, pulmonary hypertension)	
DOPPLER		
• Continuous wave		
○ Diastolic deceleration (PHT)	Fast: <150 msec (mild MS), slow: >220 msec (severe MS)	
○ Mean transmitral pressure gradient	Low: <6 mm Hg (mild MS), high: >12 mm Hg (severe MS)	

2D, two-dimensional; MS, mitral stenosis; MVA, mitral valve area; PHT, pressure half time.

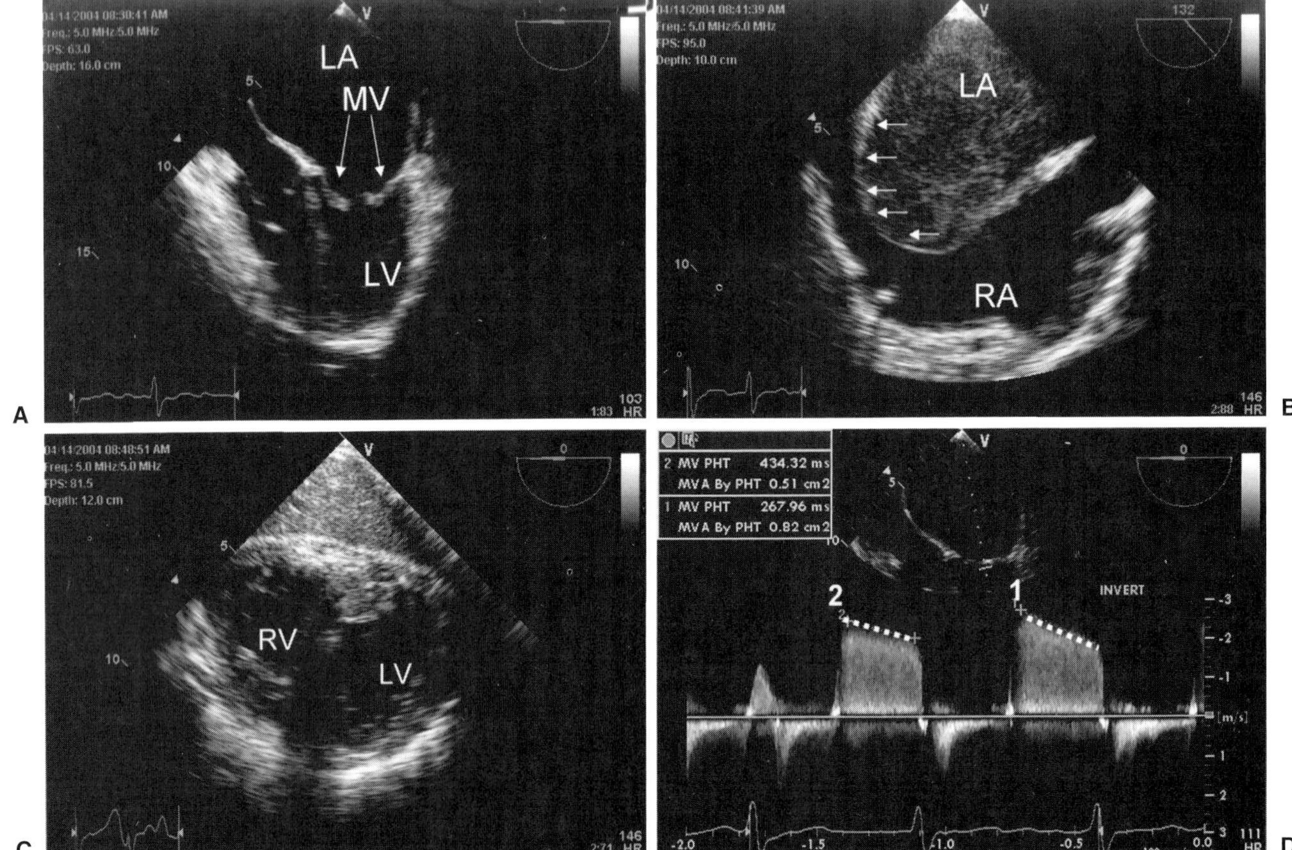

FIGURE 31-18. Echocardiographic signs of mitral stenosis. **A–C.** Two-dimensional echocardiography. **A.** Midesophageal four-chamber view. The mitral valve (MV) leaflets (*arrows*) appear thickened and barely separate in diastole. Left atrium (LA) size is increased. **B.** Midesophageal bicaval view. LA pressure is much higher than the right atrium (RA) pressure: interatrial septum (*arrows*) bulges towards the RA. There is sluggish blood flow that presents as vague, diffuse echo contrast ("smoke"). **C.** Transgastric short-axis view. The left ventricle (LV) is underfilled, small in size and the right ventricle (RV) demonstrates hypertrophy (pressure overload). **D.** Continuous wave Doppler echocardiography across the MV. The mitral valve area (MVA) is calculated using the pressure half-time method (PHT). Notice the dependence of the method on the duration of the diastolic period: beat 2 (which is shorter than beat 1 in this patient with atrial fibrillation and variable R-R interval) has a longer PHT and a smaller calculated MVA than beat 1.

TABLE 31-13

ETIOLOGIES OF MITRAL REGURGITATION

	■ ETIOLOGY	■ CHARACTERISTICS	■ LOCATION
Primary (structural)	MV prolapse	Myxomatous degeneration	Leaflet
	Redundant tissue	Ruptured chordae	Leaflet
	Rheumatic	Thickened, calcified, restricted leaflets	Leaflet
		Commissural fusion	Leaflet
	Congenital	Cleft MV, double orifice MV	Leaflet
	Miscellaneous	Fenfluramine	Leaflet
	Endocarditis	Perforated leaflets, vegetations	Leaflet
	Papillary muscle rupture	Post myocardial infarction	Tensor apparatus
Functional	Annular dilatation	Dilated cardiomyopathy	Annulus
	LV wall regional ischemia	Ischemic heart disease	Tensor apparatus

LV, left ventricle; MV, mitral valve.

dilators are effective by reducing the ventriculoatrial pressure gradient.

Repairing or replacing the valve increases left ventricular afterload and that often unmasks the dysfunction of the myocardium. However, the decrease in left ventricular systolic function is mostly due to decreased preload after the correction of MR and does not necessarily indicate true impairement of left ventricular systolic performance. Administration of inotropes and/or vasodilators, as well as judicious increase in preload, may be necessary to successfully separate from bypass.

When MR is of acute onset, the hemodynamic picture is different. Volume overload of the LA and ventricle occurs in the absence of compensatory ventricular enlargement. Ventricular filling pressures increase dramatically, as do pulmonary pressures. Cardiac output decreases, and pulmonary edema develops. If this occurs in the setting of acute myocardial infarction, cardiac performance may be inadequate despite pharmacologic support. Intra-aortic balloon assistance and emergency surgery may be lifesaving.

Anesthetic Considerations

12 Selection of anesthetics that promote vasodilation and tachycardia is ideal in the patient with MR (Table 31-14). Active pharmacologic intervention is usually unnecessary because most patients are not teetering on the brink of myocardial failure. However, in some patients, especially those with acute MR, aggressive pharmacologic management may be required. In the absence of acute deterioration, difficulties in management are usually limited to the postbypass period. Paradoxically, after the administration of vasodilators and inotropes, a patient occasionally deteriorates even further. This is seen after valve repair, not replacement. In these patients, the pathophysiologic and clinical picture is that of hypertrophic cardiomyopathy, and systolic anterior motion of the anterior mitral leaflet is demonstrable by echocardiography. The risk of systolic anterior motion after repair is increased when the anteroposterior length of the anterior leaflet is longer than the transverse diameter, when there is excessive leaflet tissue, a nondilated LV cavity or/and a narrow angle between the mtitral and aortic annuli. If this scenario is suspected, a trial of volume expansion and vasoconstrictors is indicated.

Transesophageal Echocardiography in Mitral Regurgitation

The presence and severity of MR are major determinants of outcome in cardiac surgical patients. The etiology of the regurgitation and the accurate localization of the site of MR are two important factors in deciding if the mitral valve should be repaired or replaced. In the suitable patient population, a repair has become the treatment of choice. It avoids the morbidity associated with valvular prostheses and long-term anticoagulation, late valve-related events are lower, and there

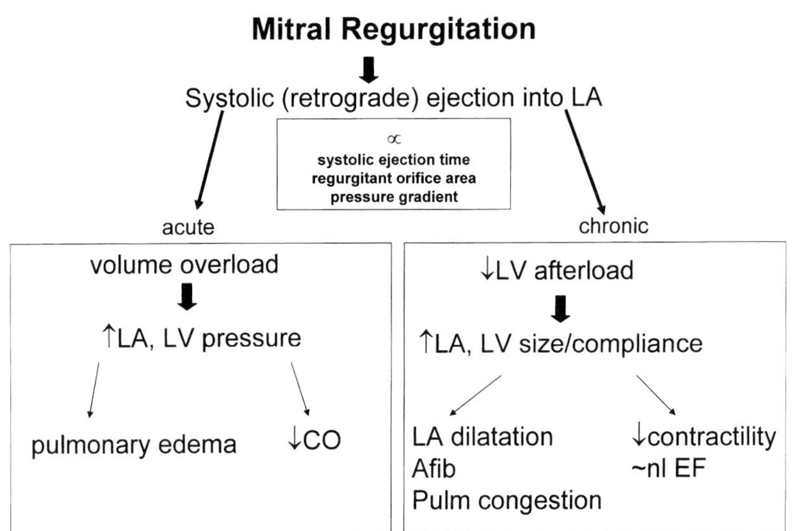

FIGURE 31-19. The physiologic consequences of mitral regurgitation.

TABLE 31-14

MITRAL REGURGITATION—HEMODYNAMIC GOALS

P	Usually slightly increased; however, preload reduction may reduce regurgitant flow
A	Decrease with anesthetics, vasodilators
C	May be depressed, titrate myocardial depressants carefully
R	Slightly increased
Rhythm	If atrial fibrillation present, control ventricular response
$M\dot{V}O_2$	Compromised if MR coexists with ischemic heart disease
CPB	Newly competent valve increases afterload, often necessitating inotropic support

A, afterload; C, contractility; CPB, cardiopulmonary bypass; MR, mitral regurgitation; $M\dot{V}O_2$, myocardial oxygen consumption; P, preload; R, rate.

is better long-term survival. Pathology localized to the posterior leaflet or to a focal portion of the anterior leaflet is most amenable to repair. Conversely, mitral repair is more difficult when there is heavy calcification of the annulus or extensive disease of the anterior leaflet of the MV. This has resulted in the desire for increasingly sophisticated TEE evaluation of mitral regurgitation.

Because of close proximity of the ultrasound probe to the MV, higher resolution, and multiplane capabilities, TEE is particularly well suited to identify the underlying mechanism of MR. Successful valve repair depends on accurate description of the location and identification of the mechanism of regurgitation. Therefore, precise and reliable functional information about the valve is necessary. A systematic TEE examination of the MV using standard, universally accepted, cross-sectional views is necessary.

The approach to evaluation of MR severity should integrate multiple parameters rather than depend on a single measurement (Table 31-15). It is also important to distinguish between the amount of MR and its hemodynamic consequences: a modest regurgitant volume that develops acutely into a small, noncompliant LA may cause severe pulmonary congestion and systemic hypotension. Conversely, some patients with chronic, severe MR remain asymptomatic due to compensatory mechanisms and a dilated, compliant LA. Maximum regurgitant flow rate, regurgitant orifice area, and proximal jet width provide the best results compared with contrast angiography, and they are superior to Doppler color flow jet area and pulmonary venous flow ratio, and should be systematically used whenever image quality is sufficient[66] (Fig. 31-20).

CARDIOPULMONARY BYPASS

On May 6, 1953, Dr. John Gibbon, Jr., used CPB with an oxygenator to successfully close an atrial septal defect in an 18-year-old girl. This first successful use of CPB brought about the dawn of modern cardiac surgery. Since that day in 1953, technology has evolved but the fundamental components of the CPB machine remain unchanged.

Circuits

CPB systems require large-bore cannulae that drain systemic venous blood into a reservoir (Fig. 31-21). This is accomplished by placing a large two-stage cannula in the right atrium that drains blood from both the atrium and the inferior vena cava. This single cannula allows most venous blood to be drained into the CPB machine reservoir; however, some systemic venous return is able to enter the heart. In open cardiac chamber procedures such as valve surgery or when a bloodless field is required, separate cannulae are placed into the superior and

TABLE 31-15

ECHOCARDIOGRAPHIC FINDINGS IN MITRAL REGURGITATION

■ MODALITY	■ MILD MR	■ SEVERE MR
■ 2D		
• Valve and leaflet anatomy	Flail leaflet and ruptured papillary muscle (severe MR)	
• Left atrium	Enlarged (in severe but not acute MR)	
• Left ventricle	Enlarged in chronic, significant MR Regional wall motion abnormalities, dysfunctional papillary muscle	
■ DOPPLER		
Color flow		
• Jet area (% LA area)	<4 cm^2 ($<20\%$): mild MR, >10 cm^2 ($>40\%$): severe MR	
• Vena contracta	<0.3 cm (mild MR), ≥ 0.7 cm (severe MR)	
• EROA by PISA	<0.2 cm^2(mild MR), >0.4 cm^2(severe MR)	
Pulsed wave		
• Mitral inflow	Prominent atrial (A) wave	Dominant early (E) wave >1.2 m/sec
• Pulmonary venous flow	Systolic dominance (mild MR)	Systolic flow reversal (severe MR)
Continuous wave		
• Jet density	Incomplete, faint jet (mild MR)	Dense jet (severe MR)

2D, two-dimensional; EROA, effective regurgitant orifice area; LA, left atrium; MR, mitral regurgitation; PISA, proximal isovelocity surface area.

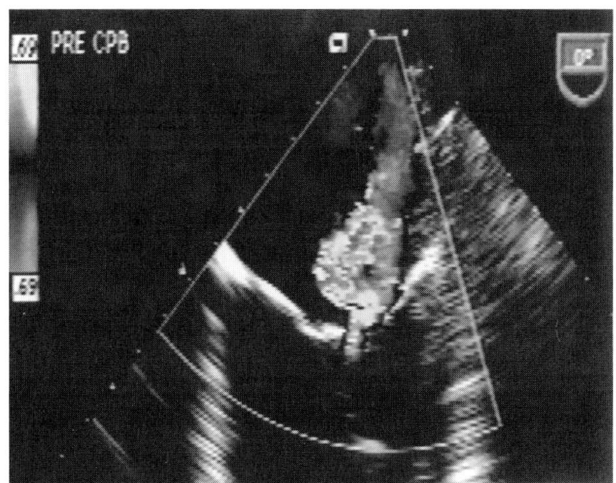

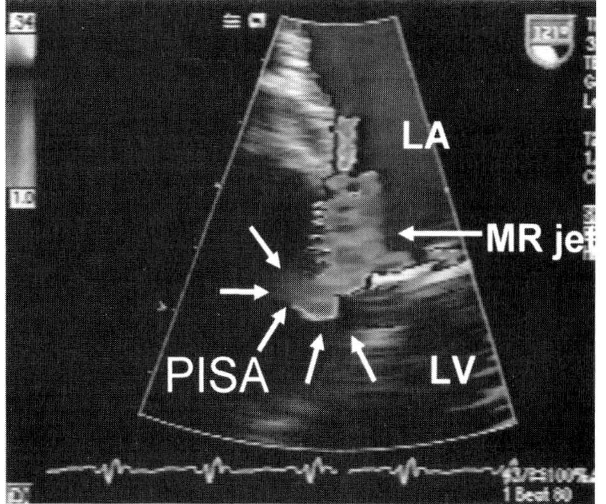

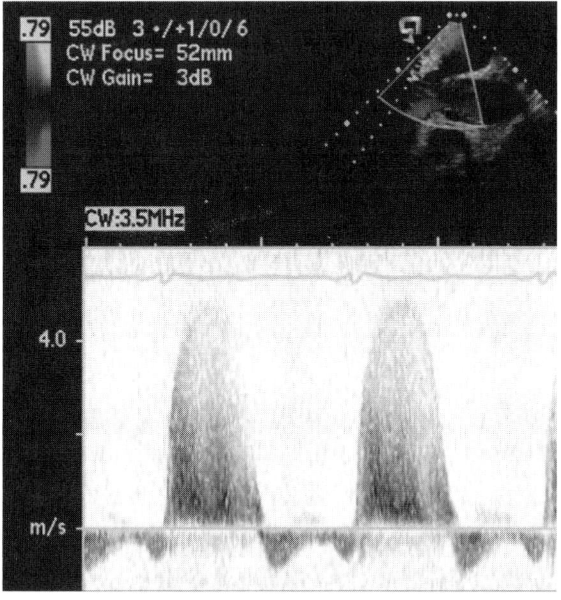

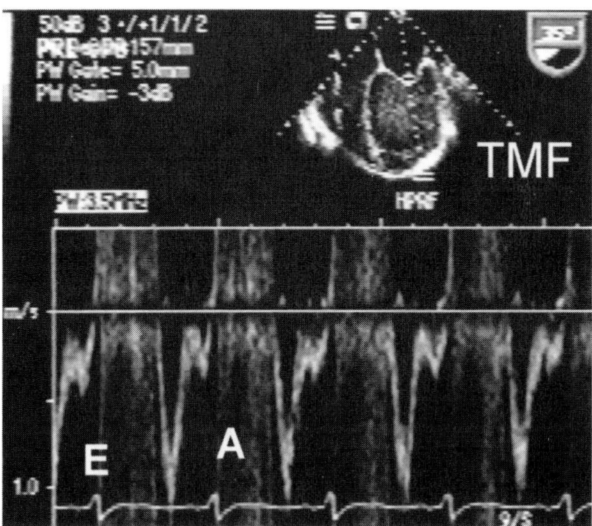

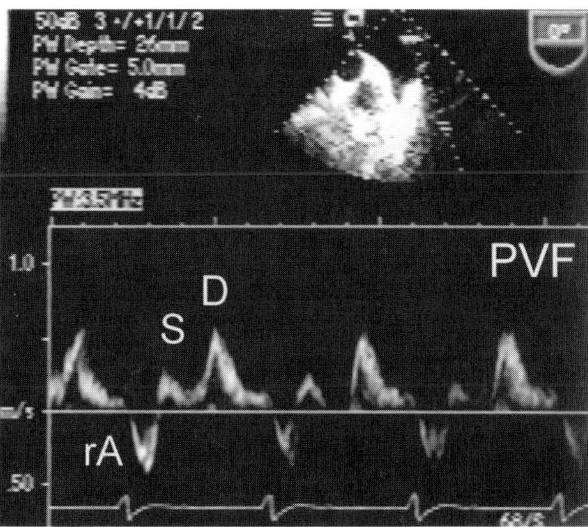

FIGURE 31-20. Echocardiographic evaluation of mitral regurgitation severity. **A.** Jet area: the visual examination of the mitral regurgitation (MR) jet by color Doppler flow is the most widely used method, but also the least accurate. More accurate measurements include width of the vena contracta and effective regurgitant orifice area (EROA) calculated from PISA. The vena contracta is the width of the neck (or narrowest portion) of the MR jet. It is often dynamic and may change during systole. **B.** Proximal isovelocity surface area (PISA): the PISA method is based on the principle of flow = velocity × area. As flow approaches an orifice, it forms concentric shells of decreasing surface area and increasing velocity. Doppler color flow mapping can depict such shells. The flow through any such hemispheric shell (*arrows*) equals its surface area π the velocity that defines the shell ($2\pi^2 \times$ [velocity]). The EROA is equal to PISA flow ÷ MR jet peak velocity. **C.** The maximal velocity and intensity of the MR jet are depicted with continuous wave Doppler. An early peaking, dense, triangular in shape MR jet characterizes severe MR. **D, E.** The hemodynamic effects of MR on the left ventricle (LV) filling are shown using pulsed wave Doppler recordings of the transmitral flow (TMF) and pulmonary venous flow (PVF). The increased gradient between the left atrium (LA) and the LV in early diastole gives rise to accelerated blood flow, whereas the atrial contraction fails to generate adequate velocity as it contracts against a full LV (E:A > 1). Therefore, retrograde flow into the pulmonary vein during atrial contraction (rA) is accentuated. During systole, the more severe the MR, the more the LA fills retrograde from the LV, reducing pulmonary systolic (S) venous flow. During diastole, as the LA empties into the LV, blood enters from the pulmonary veins (S < D). Sampling through all pulmonary veins is recommended because the MR jet may selectively affect one or more pulmonary vein(s), depending on the orientation of the regurgitant jet. Elevation of LA pressure of any etiology (e.g., atrial fibrillation) also results in blunting of the systolic forward pulmonary vein flow.

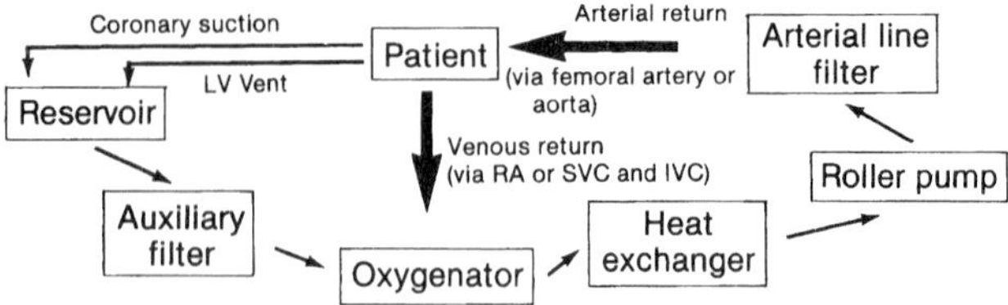

FIGURE 31-21. The basic circuit for cardiopulmonary bypass. IVC, inferior vena cava; LV, left ventricle; RA, right atrium; SVC, superior vena cava. (Reprinted with permission from Thomson IR: Technical aspects of cardiopulmonary bypass. In Thomas SJ (ed): Manual of Cardiac Anesthesia, 2nd ed, p 480. New York, Churchill Livingstone, 1993.)

inferior vena cava directly. Caval snares can effectively prevent systemic venous blood from entering the heart.

During CPB, the rate of venous drainage depends on several factors. These include proper placement of the cannulas, intravascular volume, and the hydrostatic pressure gradient (height of the right atrium above the venous reservoir). CPB machines are low to the floor to create a greater potential difference in driving pressure between the right atrium and the venous reservoir. In the event of poor venous drainage, this differential may be augmented by raising the height of the operating table. From this reservoir, the blood enters a heat exchanger/oxygenator where the blood is warmed/cooled and oxygenated, and carbon dioxide is removed. The now oxygenated blood is returned to the arterial circulation via another large cannulae, and the cycle continues for the duration of CPB. Arterial cannulas may be placed in the ascending aorta, femoral, or axillary arteries. Surgeon preference, patient anatomy, and surgical procedure will dictate the location of the arterial cannula.

In addition to systemic venous blood, additional sources of blood may be returned back to the CPB machine. Coronary suction scavenges waste blood from the surgical field. Vents are used to decompress the LV and aspirate air from the heart during de-airing procedures. Ventricular venting is particularly important in patients with aortic insufficiency, large coronary sinus or bronchial blood flow, or when heart positioning restricts drainage. Venting prevents the development of myocardial ischemia secondary to ventricular distention. Common vent sites include the left superior pulmonary vein across the MV into the LV, the LV apex, or cardioplegia cannula in the aortic root. In the event of acute ventricular distention, the surgeon may make a stab wound in the LV apex to decompress a rapidly dilating heart.

In addition to the basic components, modern CPB systems have extra optional components. These include bubble and debris filters on the arterial side of the circuit, inline blood gas monitoring, separate circuits to deliver cardioplegia, and volatile agent vaporizers. In addition, monitors may be placed in key locations in the circuit to detect problems such as low blood levels in the oxygenator (to prevent pumping of air to the arterial side of the circuit) and systemic line pressure (to detect possible arterial cannula obstruction/aortic dissection).

Oxygenators

Oxygenators serve two main purposes: (1) to oxygenate deoxygenated venous blood and (2) to remove carbon dioxide. Older bubble oxygenators are very efficient and work on the principle of direct gas–blood contact. Oxygen is relatively insoluble compared with carbon dioxide and requires either a high partial pressure or a large surface area to ensure diffusion. This surface interaction is the source of its efficiency. By altering the size of the bubbles, the total surface area of the interface may be altered (i.e., smaller bubbles, larger interface). This large surface area aids in the transfer of gases. Factors that effect diffusion of gases include the differential partial pressures of each gas at the liquid-bubble interface and gas solubility.

Bubble oxygenators are divided into two sections. The first is a mixing chamber where fresh gas flows through a perforated plate or screen that forms the gas bubbles. The second is a reservoir/heat exchanger. After gas exchange occurs in the mixing chamber, the oxygenated blood is directed into the reservoir, allowed to settle, and then passed through a defoaming matrix. This causes the gas bubbles to destabilize and break down prior to the blood return to the patient.

Bubble oxygenators are not without problems. With long CPB times, there is time-dependent destruction of formed blood elements due to the very nature of the bubble–blood interface. This interface is responsible for hemolysis, platelet destruction, protein denaturation, microemboli, and activation of the complement cascade via the alternate pathway. With bypass times less than 90 minutes, this is seldom observed.

Membrane oxygenators eliminate the blood–gas interface. Membrane oxygenators use microporous membranes that allow a transient blood–gas interface. After a brief time, protein deposition over the membrane prevents a continued blood–gas interface, but allows continued gas diffusion. These micropores act as channels in the membrane, allowing the diffusion of both oxygen and carbon dioxide. Membrane oxygenators use bundles of hollow microporous polypropylene fibers contained in a plastic housing.[67] In this housing, blood flows around the fibers, while fresh gas is passed through the microporous fibers. This allows fresh gas to diffuse through the micropores into the passing blood. With this arrangement, oxygen tension is controlled by FIO_2 and carbon dioxide elimination by total gas flow.

Pumps

In extracorporeal circulation, a pump is required to circulate blood through the circuit tubing and back to the patient. Roller and centrifugal pumps are the most commonly seen types in clinical practice. Roller pumps are the earliest type of pump and were the first used in extracorporeal circulation. In the roller pump, a length of tubing (polyvinyl chloride, silicone rubber, latex rubber) is placed in the periphery of a 210° rigid curved housing. In the center of this housing are two metal arms set 180° apart with rollers at each end. This permits constant flow over a range of arterial inflow resistance. When the arm rotates, the tubing is alternately compressed and released against the housing so one side of the arm is compressing while the other is releasing the tubing. Alternately compressing and releasing the tubing generates forward flow without the possibility of retrograde flow. It is important to note that the tubing must not be totally compressed because unacceptable destruction of blood elements will result. The advantages of roller pumps are their simplicity and ease of use. Disadvantages include destruction of blood elements, spallation (development of plastic microemboli due to tubing compression), and complications from inflow and outflow occlusion of the pump. If pump inflow is occluded, negative pressure will develop in the roller head, causing cavitation or the development of microscopic bubbles. If pump outflow becomes occluded, excessive pressure may develop proximal to the occlusion, causing the tubing connections to separate or causing the tubing to burst. Roller pumps are seldom used as the primary pump in CPB. They are most frequently used for delivering cardioplegia and vent/cardiotomy suction. In the event of power failure in the operating room, a hand crank may be used to operate the pump to develop adequate pump flow and systemic blood pressure.

Increasingly, centrifugal pumps are replacing roller head pumps. These pumps use a magnetically controlled impeller housed within a rigid plastic cone. This impeller is either composed of vanes or stacked smooth plastic cones that rotate to provide flow. By magnetically coupling the impeller to an electric motor located in the CPB machine, the speed of the electric motor (rpm) equals rotational speed of the drive head. By rotating rapidly, a pressure drop across the impeller occurs, causing blood to be sucked into the housing and then be ejected. One major difference between roller head and centrifugal pumps is that flow from centrifugal pumps will vary with changes in pump preload and afterload. It is for this reason that a flow meter must be placed on the downstream side of the bypass circuit. Advantages of centrifugal pumps include less blood trauma, lower line pressures, less cavitation, lower risk of massive air emboli, and elimination of tubing wear and spallation.

Despite the reliability of both roller and centrifugal pumps to provide systemic pressure on CPB, neither is able to deliver physiologically significant pulsatile blood flow. Pulsatile flow is the native pattern of blood flow in the human body, and the lack of this type of flow has been cited as a cause of renal dysfunction, production of ischemic metabolic byproducts, and higher need for inotropic and mechanical support. Studies show that the use of pulsatile flow on bypass confers increased survival in high-risk patients and decreases the inflammatory response seen with bypass.[68,69] Despite years of speculation, controversy still exists as to whether pulsatile flow is in fact better than standard flow. Until these controversies are resolved, nonpulsatile flow will remain the most common type seen in cardiac surgery.

Heat Exchanger

Systemic hypothermia is used in cardiac surgery as a method of myocardial and neurologic protection. Hypothermia's beneficial effects include reduction in metabolic rate and oxygen consumption, preservation of high-energy phosphate substrates, and reduction in excitatory neurotransmitter release. For each degree centigrade reduction in temperature, there is a reduction of 8% in metabolic rate. At 28°C, there is approximately a 50% reduction in metabolic rate. Both passive and active cooling can achieve moderate systemic hypothermia. Using passive cooling, patients' core temperatures are allowed to equalize with ambient temperature. This may be either a slow or a rapid process, depending on variables such as body surface area exposed and ambient temperature. More commonly, patients undergoing cardiac surgery are actively cooled and then rewarmed at the conclusion of the surgical repair. This is accomplished by using a heat exchanger. A heat exchanger is a device where either heated or cooled nonsterile water is circulated around a conducting material with good thermal properties, such as aluminum or stainless steel, in contact with the patient's blood. This method allows uniform warming and cooling without hot or cold spots and delivers consistent thermal regulation over a spectrum of temperatures. Separate heat exchangers are used in CPB circuits for the delivery of cardioplegia. Often, to increase the efficiency of heat exchangers, a countercurrent system is employed.

Prime

The most common prime used in adult cardiac surgery is a balanced salt solution. This solution attempts to mimic the composition of blood plasma. Using crystalloid solutions such as lactated Ringer's allows the pump prime to achieve similar osmolarity and electrolyte composition as blood plasma. In addition to using lactated Ringer's, many institutions add albumin to decrease postoperative edema, mannitol to promote diuresis, additional electrolytes (calcium to prevent hypocalcemia due to citrate in transfused blood), corticosteroids (antiinflammatory), and extra heparin (ensure a safety level of anticoagulation). Many institutions use a standard volume prime for all adult patients, whereas others use a minimum volume based on body weight or body surface area. Priming volumes may also vary due to circuit configurations and individual specifications, but the average prime volume is 1,500 to 2,500 mL. Of note, there is active research into the area of oxygen-carrying compounds that may be added to pump prime. These substances include perflurocarbons and hemoglobin-based compounds that may extend the ability of patients to tolerate anemia on CPB that would otherwise require blood transfusion.

In infants, children, small adults, and patients with preoperative anemia, blood may be added to the pump prime prior to going on CPB. This is done to prevent excessive dilutional anemia and resulting drop in oxygen-carrying capacity. The exact hematocrit that can be tolerated on CPB has been debated, but hematocrits of as low as 17% have been reported to be well tolerated by patients undergoing cardiac operations. However, the trend currently seems to favor higher levels to avoid renal and neurologic consequences.[70–72] If hypothermia is used on CPB, then some degree of anemia is desirable.[73] Decreases in hematocrit help offset changes in blood viscosity due to hypothermia and may improve systemic flow.

Anticoagulation

To prevent patient death and thrombosis of the CPB circuit, systemic anticoagulation is required prior to insertion of cannulas and initiation of CPB. Contact between patient blood and components of the CPB circuit initiate activation of the coagulation cascade. To avoid this effect, heparin is used as the anticoagulant of choice. Heparin is a polyionic mucopolysaccharide extracted from either bovine lung or porcine intestinal mucosa. Anticoagulant activity varies between commercial preparations and between the bovine and porcine versions. Heparin is provided in units with 1 U, according to the U.S. Pharmacopoeia, maintaining fluidity of 1 mL of citrated sheep plasma for 1 hour after recalcification. Following intravenous injection, the peak onset of heparin is less than 5 minutes, with a half-life of approximately 90 minutes in normothermic patients. In hypothermic patients, there is a progressive increase in the half-life proportional to the degree of hypothermia. Heparin's anticoagulant effect is derived from its ability to potentiate the activity of antithrombin III (AT III), a plasma glycoprotein that contains a lysine residue. Heparin binding at this site alters the structural configuration of AT III, increasing its thrombin inhibitory potency greater than 1,000-fold. By inhibiting thrombin, AT III prevents the formation of fibrin clot via both the intrinsic and extrinsic pathways, in addition to inhibiting factors IX, Xa, XIa, XIIa, kalikrein, and plasmin. In addition, heparin also binds to factor II, which, independent of AT III, inhibits thrombin. In patients receiving heparin preoperatively and those with congenital deficiencies of AT III, higher than expected, doses of heparin may be required to adequately achieve anticoagulation. In the event of inadequate anticoagulation due to relative or absolute deficiency of AT III, exogenous AT III can be administered by transfusing fresh frozen plasma or by administering a commercial preparation of human AT III concentrate (Thrombate III).

The dosing and measurement of heparin has changed over many years. In the past, heparin was dosed empirically using doses between 200 and 400 U/kg; redosing was time based. One common question that occurs frequently is why is the partial thromboplastin (PTT) not used clinically in cardiac surgery to measure heparin level. Modern PTT assays are so sensitive that heparin levels far lower than those required for safe initiation of CPB cause the sample blood to become almost unclottable within the time frame of the test. Currently, the two methods for determining adequate heparinization are the measuring activated clotting time (ACT) or blood heparin concentration. The ACT consists of adding blood to tubes containing either diatomaceous earth (celite) or kaolin, warming and rotating the tube, and recording the time until clot formation. Generally, ACTs greater than 480 seconds are considered acceptable for the initiation of CPB. The exception to this is when the serine protease inhibitor aprotinin is used. If celite-containing tubes are used, ACTs of 700 seconds are required due to the effect of aprotinin on the test. Aprotinin delays activation of the intrinsic pathway via factor XIIa, in addition to inhibiting kallikrein. This will prolong the celite ACT artifactually. Many early case reports of thrombosis with "adequate" ACTs were written prior to this understanding of how aprotinin interacts with the celite ACT test. Adding kaolin activates the intrinsic pathway and binds to aprotinin, reducing its anticoagulant effect in vitro and producing a more accurate ACT.

An alternative method to the ACT test uses heparin/protamine titration. In this method, a known dose of protamine is added to a heparinized sample of blood and followed until the optimum dose of protamine that produces a clot in the shortest amount of time is determined. By knowing the neutralization ratio of heparin and protamine (usually 1 mg to 100 U of heparin), the heparin concentration in the sample can be determined. The advantages cited with this method include the fact that conditions such as hypothermia, hemodilution, and even surgical incision alter ACTs. However, because heparin levels do not always correlate with anticoagulant effect, many centers prefer to use qualitative tests of heparin function such as the ACT. Using the ACT method is also easier and less expensive.

Allergies to heparin are rare; more commonly, patients may present with a history of heparin-induced thrombocytopenia (HIT). HIT contains two subtypes; the first is generally mild in which there is a transient decrease in platelet count. The second type is a more severe autoimmune-mediated decrease in the platelet count due to the formation of antigenic heparin compounds that activate platelets in the face of endothelial injury. This endothelial injury predisposes to the formation of platelet clots and microvascular thrombosis. In patients with HIT that require systemic anticoagulation, alternatives to heparin are required. These include defibrinogenating agents (ancrod obtained from pit viper venom), hirudin, bivalirudin, and factor inhibitors. Hirudin, which is isolated from the salivary gland of the medicinal leech (Hirudo medicinalis) and bivalirudin (Hirulog), are direct inhibitors of thrombin. This action is independent of AT III. The use of these agents is uncommon, and the reader is advised to consult one of the several reviews on this subject.[74]

Blood Conservation in Cardiac Surgery

Due to declining donation and restrictions on those that may donate, blood and its component products are a finite resource that are increasingly difficult to replace. In addition, the costs associated with the processing of blood are high and affect the economics of health care. In concert with the decrease in the supply of blood products, patients are increasingly demanding "bloodless" surgeries to lessen the risks of blood transfusion (infection, incompatibility reactions, transfusion error). Due to the nature of cardiac surgery, there is often a high risk of transfusion. Bleeding that may be significant can be encountered during reoperation from the use of anticoagulants and platelet function inhibitors preoperatively, and ill-defined surgical bleeding. The inherent risk of platelet dysfunction and derangements in coagulation due to extracorporeal circulation cannot be minimized. In the past, blood conservation included the use of intraoperative autologous blood donation, as well as the scavenging of shed blood and reinfusion. New techniques have emerged to reduce the need for homologous blood. These include the use of antifibrinolytics (ε-aminocaproic acid, tranexemic acid, aprotinin, desmopressin [DDAVP]), ultrafiltration, blood fractionization, and the use of improved topical hemostaic agents.

Intraoperative autologous hemodilution is a well-described method of removing whole blood from a patient prior to systemic heparinization and coagulopathy from CPB. Using blood collection bags containing anticoagulant whole blood is removed, and crystalloid or colloid fluids are administered, making up for the circulating volume removed. Following CPB, the blood is transfused returning red blood cells, active platelets, and coagulation factors. Contraindications for the use of intraoperative autologous blood donation include preoperative anemia, unstable angina/high-grade left main coronary artery disease, and aortic stenosis.

Intraoperative blood salvage is another method of blood conservation that is used in cardiac surgery. This method is as simple as blood suctioned from the surgical field being anticoagulated, filtered, and reinfused, or as complicated as cell washing machines. The first method is simple and easy to perform with a minimum of equipment needed. Unfortunately, shed blood may worsen the coagulopathy associated with CPB because factors that cause coagulopathy are not removed in the filtering process. Cell washing is the more frequently seen method of cell salvage seen in the operating room. Cell washing is composed of four steps: harvesting of the patient's blood, processing of the shed blood and removal of the serum, storage of the red blood cells, and reinfusion of the high hematocrit red blood cells. Final hematocrits of reinfused red cells may reach 70%. Contraindications to the use of intraoperative cell salvage include infection, malignancy, and use of topical hemostatic agents.

Antifibrinolytic agents such as aprotinin and ε-aminocaproic acid have become the standard in most cardiac centers. These protease inhibitors and lysine analogs bind to plasminogen and plasmin, blocking the ability of fibrinolytic enzymes to bind at lysine residues of fibrinogen. The administration of these antifibrinolytics decreases bleeding after bypass and reduces the risk of blood transfusion.[75] Aprotinin is a naturally occurring fibrinolytic that possesses properties that the synthetic lysine analogs do not. These include aprotinin's ability to inhibit kallikrein, preservation of platelet glycoprotein receptors (Gib, GIIb/IIIa), inhibition of the proinflammatory cytokine release seen on CPB, and the inhibition of plasmin and protein C. These actions have a remarkable effect on intraoperative bleeding, post-CPB coagulopathy, and transfusion requirements.[76] The use of aprotinin is not without risks. There is a small but significant risk of anaphylaxis on reexposure due to its animal-derived protein structure. It is significantly more costly to use compared with the lysine analogs and despite studies refuting the fact, there is concern that aprotinin many cause graft thrombosis and renal failure, especially following hypothermia and circulatory arrest.[77]

One of the unwanted effects of extracorporeal circulation is the hemodilution associated with the pump prime. One method that has been used with success to avoid excess hemodilution and reduce the need for blood transfusion is retrograde autologous priming (RAP). In RAP, the crystalloid prime contained within the arterial and venous lines is drained into a recirculation bag prior to the initiation of CPB and replaced by blood-drained retrograde via the arterial cannula. This reduces hemodilution and the drop in systemic vascular resistance associated with the initiation of CPB. When using this technique, care must be taken to avoid acute hypovolemic hypotension due to the patient exsanguination. Other reported benefits of RAP include reduced extravascular lung water and weight gain.[78,79]

Another technique used in conjunction with CPB to reduce postoperative bleeding and the need for transfusion is ultrafiltration. During ultrafiltration/hemoconcentration, plasma water is separated from low molecular weight solutes, intravascular cell components, and plasma proteins using a semipermeable membrane. Using a hydrostatic pressure difference created by external suction plasma, water is removed by the gradient created across the ultrafiltration membrane. Most ultrafiltration devices are composed of a rigid plastic housing containing bundles of semipermeable hollow fibers, which is placed inline with the CPB circuit. The exact timing of the ultrafiltration process depends on the technique employed. Conventional ultrafiltration is initiated during rewarming and is based on the volume within the CPB circuit and exogenous fluid given. Modified ultrafiltration used commonly in pediatric cardiac surgery consists of ultrafiltration after separation from CPB when blood is pumped retrograde from the aortic cannula through the hemofilter/hemoconcentrator and returned to the right atrium. Advantages of hemoconcentration include a reduction in free water, preservation of hemostasis, and decrease in levels of circulating inflammatory mediators. By employing hemoconcentration, levels of formed blood elements including erythrocytes, platelets, and coagulation factors are augmented. This translates into a net increase in hemoglobin and hematocrit, and a decrease in postoperative bleeding and need for transfusion.[80]

Similar to hemoconcentration is blood fractionation. In this process, blood elements are removed and made into a concentrate that is removed from the patient prebypass. These concentrates are then retuned to the patient following CPB, thereby avoiding dilutional coagulopathy and activation of these blood elements while on CPB.

Much work is also being done in the field of blood substitutes. These hemoglobin-based compounds are made from blood in which the hemoglobin is chemically extracted for its oxygen-carrying capacity. The goal being a shelf-stable product devoid of the infectious complications of transfusion. Although not possessing all the qualities of banked blood, these compounds show great promise and are being actively studied.[81]

Myocardial Protection

The most common method of myocardial protection used today is that of intermittent hyperkalemic cold cardioplegia and moderate systemic hypothermia. The fundamental concept of cold cardioplegia is that a cold solution (10 to 15°C) of either blood or crystalloid with a supranormal concentration of potassium is injected into the coronary arteries or veins to induce diastolic electrical arrest. Cardioplegia may be delivered by using a separate roller head circuit from the CPB machine, a pneumatic infusion device, or a handheld gravity system. Cardioplegia is injected anterograde, retrograde, or as a combination of the two. Anterograde cardioplegia solution is injected via the aortic root into the native coronaries. The cardioplegia follows the normal anatomic flow of blood. In coronary artery bypass surgery, individual grafts may be used to deliver cardioplegia once distal anastamoses have been completed. In patients with significant aortic insufficiency, the anterograde technique is not effective due to the incompetent AV allowing cardioplegia to flow into the LV bypassing the coronary ostia. In this case, following aortic cross-clamp, an aortotomy is made and handheld cannulae are placed in the individual coronary ostia under direct vision and cardioplegia is delivered. In addition, in patients with severe coronary disease due to diffuse multiple or high-grade ostial lesions, anterograde cardioplegia may provide inadequate myocardial protection. In this case, retrograde cardioplegia may be employed. Retrograde cardioplegia is injected via a ballon-tipped catheter placed in the coronary sinus, bypassing the obstructed coronaries and achieving greater myocardial protection. Often, both anterograde and retrograde are used in combination to maximize the effects of cardioplegia.

Depending on the time required for surgical repair, multiple injections of cardioplegia may be necessary. This washes out metabolic by-products, adds new high-energy and oxygen-carrying substrates, and continues hypothermic diastolic arrest.

In addition to anterograde and retrograde cardioplegia, many other techniques have been used for myocardial protection. These include single-injection hyperkalemia with aortic cross-clamp, intermittent cross-clamp with periods of reperfusion, and hypothermic ventricular fibrillation. Many different solutions of cardioplegia exist. Some use osmotically active agents—albumin, energy substrates such as glucose-containing and phosphate-containing compounds citrate to chelate calcium, and nitroglycerin or nitroprusside—to facilitate uniform perfusion of the solution.

For the anesthesiologist monitoring a patient on CPB, the sentinel events of cardioplegic electrical arrest and resumption of electrical activity must be keenly followed. Events that must be watched for, are left ventricular distention and lack of rapid electrical arrest. These events may be evidence of poor myocardial protection and the possibility of difficulty in separation from CPB. Transesopegeal echocardiography is particularly helpful in diagnosing ventricular distention and its relief by venting or manual decompression.

PREOPERATIVE EVALUATION

The preoperative visit appropriately concentrates on the cardiovascular system but should also focus on the assessment of pulmonary, renal, hepatic, neurologic, endocrine, and hematologic functions. Equally invaluable is discussing with the patient the anticipated events on the day of surgery, including transport to the operating room, preoperative routines (O_2 mask, vascular cannulation, anesthetic induction), and by finally, the awakening process in the recovery room or ICU. The importance of communicating to the anesthesiologist any symptoms such as chest pain, shortness of breath, or the need for nitroglycerin during transport or the preinduction period should be emphasized to the patient. The depth and detail of the explanation should be custom tailored to each patient.

Data from history, physical examination, and laboratory investigations are used to define the cardiovascular anatomy and functional state. Pertinent findings suggestive of left and/or right ventricular dysfunction are described in Table 31-16. Increases in the severity or frequency of anginal attacks or the presence of ischemia-induced ventricular dysfunction suggest that large areas of myocardium are at risk. A history of arrhythmias should be obtained, including the type, severity, associated symptoms, prior intervention, and successful treatment. Integration of this information leads to appropriate selection of monitoring devices and anesthetic techniques.

Conditions commonly associated with heart disease, such as hypertension, diabetes mellitus, and cigarette smoking, must also be evaluated. The latter is extremely important and may be useful in differentiating whether episodes of intraoperative pulmonary hypertension are caused primarily by pulmonary

TABLE 31-16

PREOPERATIVE FINDINGS SUGGESTIVE OF VENTRICULAR DYSFUNCTION

History
- CAD: previous MI, chest pain/pressure
- CHF (intermittent or chronic): fatigue, DOE, orthopnea, PND, ankle swelling

Physical examination
- Vital signs: hypotension, tachycardia (severe CHF)
- Engorged neck veins, apical impulse displaced laterally, S_3, S_4, rales, pitting edema, pulsatile liver, ascites

Electrocardiogram
- Ischemia/infarct, rhythm, conduction abnormalities

Chest radiograph
- Cardiomegaly, pulmonary vascular congestion/pulmonary edema, pleural effusion, Kerley B lines

Cardiovascular testing
- Catheterization data: LVEDP > 18 mm Hg, EF < 0.4, CI < 2.0 L/min/m^2

CAD, coronary artery disease; CHF, congestive heart failure; CI, cardiac index; DOE, dyspnea on exertion; EF, ejection fraction; LVEDP, left ventricular end-diastolic pressure; MI, myocardial infarction; PND, paroxysmal nocturnal dyspnea.

or cardiac factors. Higher systemic arterial pressures may be desirable throughout surgery in patients with a history or other evidence of carotid artery disease. Evidence for renal dysfunction must be sought because the most common cause of postoperative renal failure is preexisting renal insufficiency. If renal reserve is reduced, intraoperative measures such as diuretics or dopamine may be used, although no data showing an improved outcome are available.

Current Drug Therapy

Almost without exception, cardiovascular drugs, including cardiac antiarrhythmics (e.g., amiodarone), β-blockers or calcium channel blockers, and nitrates are continued until the time of surgery. Interactions between these drugs and anesthetics are more often beneficial than harmful in maintaining hemodynamic control during periods of surgical stress.

Concern about intraoperative hypotension and increased requirement for vasopressor support in patients receiving β-blockers or calcium channel blockers or angiotensin-converting enzyme inhibitors is unwarranted. Digoxin is prescribed less frequently to suppress cardiac dysrhythmias, control the ventricular response to atrial fibrillation, and improve contractility in patients with congestive heart failure. Continuation until the time of surgery seems advisable for those patients in whom it is being used for rate or rhythm control. Signs or symptoms of digoxin excess, including ventricular ectopy, atrial tachydysrhythmias, and variable degrees of atrioventricular block should be sought. The latter is typically manifested by slowing and regularization of the ventricular response to atrial fibrillation. This represents digoxin-induced atrioventricular blockade with a regular junctional escape rhythm. Noncardiac symptoms include gastrointestinal distress or visual disturbances. Toxicity is more common in patients concomitantly receiving drugs that increase digoxin levels (e.g., nifedipine, verapamil, amiodarone) or reduce potassium levels (e.g., diuretics). Most cardiac antidysrhythmics should also be continued to the time of surgery. Their pharmacology is well known (see Chapters 12 and 21), and they usually present little problem with anesthetic management.

Physical Examination

As mentioned previously, the physical examination seeks to elicit signs of cardiac decompensation such as an S_3 gallop, rales, jugular venous distention, or pulsatile liver. Routes for vascular access should be assessed, and the status of peripheral arteries should be evaluated. As always, the airway should be carefully evaluated with respect to ease of mask ventilation and intubation of the trachea. Other pertinent points are described in Table 31-17.

Premedication

Even the most thorough preoperative psychological preparation is often inadequate to assuage the anxieties and apprehensions of a patient facing cardiac surgery. Premedication will assist in providing a calm, anxiety-free but arousable and hemodynamically stable patient who is prepared for surgery. Selection of drug and dosage is predicated on the patient's age, cardiovascular state, level of anxiety, and location. If the patient is coming from home, often there is inadequate time for adequate premedication. Heavy premedication is ideal for the

TABLE 31-17

PREOPERATIVE PHYSICAL EXAMINATION

Vital Signs
- Current values and range

Height, weight
- For calculations of drug dosages, pump flow, cardiac index

Airway
- Evaluate, identify difficulties for ventilation, intubation

Neck
- Landmarks for jugular vein cannulation
- Vein engorgement (CHF)
- Bruits (carotid artery disease)

Heart
- Murmurs: characteristic of valve lesions, S_3 (elevated LVEDP), S_4 (decreased compliance), click (MVP prolapse)
- Lateral PMI displacement (cardiomegaly)
- Precordial heave, lift (hypertrophy, wall motion abnormality)

Lungs
- Rales (CHF)
- Rhonchi, wheezes (COPD, asthma)

Vasculature
- Peripheral pulses
- Sites for venous and arterial access

Abdomen
- Pulsatile liver (CHF, tricuspid regurgitation)

Extremities
- Peripheral edema (CHF)

Nervous System
- Motor or sensory deficits

CHF, congestive heart failure; COPD, chronic obstructive pulmonary disease; LVEDP, left ventricular end-diastolic pressure; MVP, mitral valve prolapse; PMI, point of maximum impulse.

fit person scheduled for CABG. Inadequate sedation may predispose to hypertension, tachycardia, or coronary vasospasm, all potential causes of myocardial ischemia. However, the frail, 50-kg cachetic patient with severe valvular dysfunction fares better with light premedication to avoid possible respiratory depression or loss of endogenous catecholamine support. Additional sedation can always be given in the operating room under direct observation by the anesthesiologist.

Premedication for cardiac surgery often combines the sedative and analgesic properties of an opioid (morphine, 0.1 to 0.2 mg/kg) with the sedative and amnestic properties of scopolamine (0.006 mg/kg) or a benzodiazepine (diazepam 0.05 to 0.1 mg/kg, midazolam 0.03 to 0.05 mg/kg, or lorazepam 0.04 mg/kg). The possibility of oversedation, hypercarbia, or hypoxia following premedication is always of concern.

Premedication may have a previously unappreciated but profound effect on intraoperative hemodynamics. Thomson et al.[82] administered a standard high-dose fentanyl anesthetic to patients premedicated with either morphine and scopolamine or lorazepam. In general, the patients receiving lorazepam were hemodynamically less responsive in that they had less hypertension, more hypotension, and a greater requirement for vasoactive drugs. Clonidine has also been used as a premedication with similar intraoperative effects. The difficulty with premedication currently is that the patients arrive in the hospital on the same day of surgery.

Monitoring

We emphasize only those aspects of monitoring particularly relevant to cardiac surgery because the subject is discussed extensively in Chapter 24.

Pulse Oximeter

The need for multiple vascular cannulations and applications of numerous monitoring devices often prolongs the preinduction period. The pulse oximeter should be positioned prior to catheter insertion to detect clinically unsuspected episodes of hypoxemia, especially if additional intravenous sedation has been administered. Attention must be focused on the whole patient, even during the hunt for successful vascular access.

Electrocardiogram

Regional ischemia may be localized by appropriate lead monitoring: lead II (and/or leads III, AVF: right coronary artery distribution) for the inferior, leads V_4, V_5 (left anterior descending [LAD] artery) for the anterior, and leads I and AVL (circumflex artery) for the lateral wall of the LV. If the standard leads prove inadequate for detection and analysis of cardiac dysrhythmia, esophageal or epicardial leads may be used. Occasionally, intraoperative myocardial injury causes substantial reductions in QRS voltage. Monitoring an ECG via a surgically placed ventricular pacing wire provides adequate voltage to facilitate dysrhythmia analysis or to trigger an intra-aortic balloon pump, if necessary. A strip-chart recorder documents and facilitates detailed analysis of both ST segment alterations and complex dysrhythmias.

Temperature

Central temperature can be measured with esophageal, tympanic, urinary bladder catheter probes or with a thermistor from a pulmonary artery catheter. Obviously, this last method is not reliable during the period of aortic cross-clamping when there is no flow through the heart. Rectal and toe probes record peripheral temperatures, which lag behind central measurements during both cooling and rewarming periods.

Arterial Blood Pressure

Systemic arterial pressure is always monitored invasively. The radial or femoral artery is usually cannulated, although the brachial and axillary arteries may also be used. The exact site is often a matter of personal or institutional preference. Criteria include convenience, selection of the fullest or most bounding pulse, and avoidance of the dominant hand. In addition, during dissection of the internal mammary artery, the ipsilateral radial or brachial artery pulse may be transiently occluded; therefore, an artery opposite a planned internal mammary artery is selected. Occasionally, the site of surgery dictates appropriate placement; for example, the right radial artery should be used for procedures involving the descending thoracic aorta because the left subclavian artery may be included in the proximal aortic clamp. Following cardiopulmonary bypass, radial artery pressure is often misleading and may be as much as 30 mm Hg lower than central aortic pressure.[83] The mechanism is believed to be peripheral vasodilation during rewarming. Whenever such a discrepancy is suspected, aortic pressure can be estimated by palpation by the surgeon, or if direct measurement is needed, a needle may be placed directly into the aorta. The gradient between aortic and radial pressure usually disappears within 45 minutes of separation from bypass.

Central Venous Pressure/Pulmonary Artery Catheter

Access to the central circulation is mandatory for infusion of cardioactive drugs. In addition, right atrial or central venous pressure accurately reflects right ventricular filling pressure and is of critical importance whenever right ventricular dysfunction is suspected. In patients with normal LV function, transduced right atrial pressure is often assumed to be a reliable guide of left-sided filling. This relationship is less predictable in the presence of severe left ventricular dyssynergy, pulmonary hypertension, or reduced left ventricular compliance. In these instances, insertion of a pulmonary artery catheter for measurement of pulmonary capillary wedge pressure provides a somewhat better index of left ventricular filling, although TEE data are far more valid. In addition, determination of cardiac output and calculation of derived hemodynamic indices offer additional information to guide hemodynamic and anesthetic management.

Indications for pulmonary artery catheterization vary greatly among institutions. In some these catheters are used routinely, whereas in others they are limited to patients with specific disease states such as severe left ventricular dysfunction or pronounced pulmonary hypertension. Additional indications include combined procedures (valvular plus coronary) or those that require prolonged intraoperative time (cardiac reoperations or use of one or both internal mammary arteries). Insertion of a pacing pulmonary artery catheter can be helpful whenever exact control of rate and rhythm is desirable, for example, in patients with hypertrophic cardiomyopathy or those with significant bradycardia secondary to β blockade.

When pulmonary artery catheters are used, disagreement still exists as to whether they should be placed before or after the induction of anesthesia. In some patients, early insertion of the catheter and determination of baseline hemodynamic values can beneficially influence anesthetic selection and guide the induction sequence. However, the anxious and uncomfortable hypertensive patient is better served by a smooth anesthetic induction followed by catheter placement.

It must be remembered that the catheter often migrates toward the periphery of the lung with cardiac manipulation before and during CPB. Therefore, it seems prudent to pull the catheter back a few centimeters prior to the initiation of bypass to prevent permanent wedging or possible pulmonary artery rupture. Despite the controversy concerning the routine use of these catheters, there is no disagreement that the capability to measure both cardiac output and ventricular filling pressures must be available in any institution performing cardiac surgery. Whether this is done with a pulmonary artery catheter, direct cannulation of the LA and dye dilution techniques, or TEE is immaterial. The critically ill patient requires these measurements to determine the effectiveness of vasoactive drugs, adjust dosage, and evaluate the need for further pharmacologic or mechanical intervention.

Echocardiography

2D TEE is the newest, most complex, and most expensive diagnostic device. Detection of ischemia by online evaluation of new regional wall motion abnormalities and its utility in assessing valvular lesions (before and after repair) and the ascending aorta have been mentioned. Other applications specific to cardiac surgical patients are also useful. It is well known that, following CPB, ventricular filling pressure, irrespective of site of measurement (left ventricular end-diastolic pressure, LA, pulmonary capillary wedge pressure), is a poor and often misleading indicator of ventricular volume status.[84,85] Direct estimation of left ventricular volume with 2D TEE more appropriately directs fluid infusion and selection of vasoactive drugs in patients who are difficult to wean from bypass. In addition, residual valve lesions, intracardiac air, or new areas of ischemia are readily identified. Global dysfunction suggesting residual cross-clamp effect, inadequate cardioplegia, or reperfusion injury can be detected.

Central Nervous System Function and Complications

Monitoring of the brain during extracorporeal bypass is difficult, with a lack of standardized equipment or criteria. Neurologic complications after cardiac surgery can be devastating to patients and their families, significantly affecting their quality of life, while exponentially increasing the economic cost of recovery after cardiac surgery. Thus, many investigators have more recently focused on methods to determine the etiology and improve the detection, prevention, and treatment of postoperative neurologic complications in patients undergoing cardiac surgery.

The incidence of stroke after CABG surgery is approximately 3% (1 to 5%). There is a much higher incidence (60 to 70%) of subtle cognitive deficits that can be elicited by detailed neuropsychometric testing. It is known that the neuropsychiatric deficits do improve over the initial 2 to 6 months after cardiac surgery; however, a significant percentage of patients (13 to 39%) have residual impairment. The etiology of perioperative neurologic complications is believed to be predominantly secondary to emboli (air, atheroma, other particulate matter) than to hypoperfusion in susceptible patients (e.g., preexisting cerebrovascular disease). Most overt strokes after cardiac surgery are focal and likely due to macroemboli, whereas the cognitive changes are subtle and probably result from microemboli. Risk factors for neurologic complications include advanced age (>70 years), preexisting cerebrovascular disease (e.g., carotid artery stenosis >80%), history of prior stroke, peripheral vascular disease, ascending aortic atheroma, and diabetes. Operative factors include the duration of CPB, intracardiac procedure (e.g., valve replacement), excessive warming during and following CPB, and perhaps perfusion pressure on CPB.[86–89] Intraoperative hyperglycemia, which could theoretically result in worsened neurologic damage, has not been associated with poorer neurologic outcome.[90]

Historically, intracardiac (e.g., valvular) procedures are associated with a greater risk of neurologic complications (presumably secondary to greater risk of air emboli) than closed cardiac (i.e., CABG) procedures. As discussed earlier, TEE has given both anesthesiologists and surgeons an appreciation for the adequacy of the de-airing process after intracardiac procedures. From studies using transcranial Doppler to detect cerebral emboli, it is now known that the time points of maximal risk for embolization are at aortic cannulation, onset of CPB, weaning from CPB, and decannulation.[91]

The role of TEE in evaluating the ascending and descending aorta is described previously. There are several management options undergoing investigation for patients with severely diseased aortas, especially those with mobile atheromas who are at increased risk of stroke. These include hypothermic fibrillatory arrest with left ventricular vent and no cross-clamp, single cross-clamp (i.e., distal and proximal grafts performed during same cross-clamp), relocation of proximal grafts to area of nondiseased aorta, no proximal grafts (internal mammary arteries only) either on CPB or using off-pump coronary artery bypass, hypothermic ischemic arrest with resection, and graft replacement of diseased aorta.

Cerebral protection is rather limited. Hypothermia is excellent in that it decreases cerebral metabolic rate and prolongs ischemic tolerance; however, profound hypothermia is not practical for routine cardiac surgery. Unfortunately, during routine CPB the patient is normothermic when the highest risk of embolization exists, (unclamping, during rewarming, and with initial ventricular ejection). Sodium thiopental has been shown to be cerebroprotective in intracardiac procedures,[92] but not in CABG surgery.[93] This difference may be a result of the "reversible" neurologic impairment secondary to gas emboli, which is more likely during intracardiac procedures than CABG surgery.

Selection of Anesthetic Drugs

The task confronting the anesthesiologist is to render the patient undergoing cardiac surgery analgesic, amnesic, and unconscious, while suppressing the endocrine and autonomic responses to intraoperative stress. Equally important is preservation of compensatory cardiovascular mechanisms and prevention of perioperative episodes of myocardial ischemia. Although these goals are not unique to the cardiac surgical patient, they are sometimes a bit more difficult to accomplish because of the severity of ischemic and/or valvular disease. Notwithstanding institutional and personal bias with respect to choice of anesthetic, there are no data that document superiority of any anesthetic for either coronary or valvular surgery. The large outcome studies of Tuman et al. and Slogoff and Keats indicate that the choice of anesthetic has no effect on outcome in CABG patients.[93a,93b] As was previously emphasized, the most critical factor governing anesthetic selection is the degree of ventricular dysfunction. Anticipated difficulties during the tracheal intubation sequence, the expected length of surgery, and the anticipated time until extubation of the trachea also influence choice of anesthetic. It is desirable to be able to alter anesthetic depth to accommodate the varying intensity of surgical stress. During intubation of the trachea, incision, sternotomy, pericardiotomy, and manipulation of the aorta, there is intense stimulation and sympathetic response. The period of prepping and draping following intubation of the trachea requires minimal levels of anesthetic, as does the period of hypothermic bypass.

There is no one best technique. Familiarity with all anesthetics and their physiologic and pharmacologic effects in the patient with severe cardiac disease allows great flexibility in anesthetic selection. In addition, it provides numerous options applicable to the cardiac patient undergoing noncardiac surgery.

Potent Inhalation Anesthetics

These drugs are useful both as primary anesthetic drugs and as adjuvants to treat or prevent "breakthrough" hypertension associated with high-dose opioid techniques. The balance of myocardial oxygen supply and $M\dot{V}O_2$ is usually altered favorably by reduction in contractility and afterload. Deleterious declines in perfusion must be prevented or treated, and the possibilities of increases in wall tension must be considered. These agents have been used successfully in all types of valve surgery without untoward effects, although they are sometimes associated with more hemodynamic variability than is seen with opioids. Use of these drugs involves no more hemodynamic intervention than upfront loading with opioids, and the ability to rapidly increase and decrease concentrations permits easy adjustment to variable levels of surgical stimulation. Volatile anesthetics can be administered during bypass through a vaporizer mounted on the pump; they are also appropriate in the postbypass period, assuming cardiac function is adequate. Volatile anesthetics seem to be more important now, in combination with short-acting opiates or hypnotics, because the volume of off-bypass procedures is increasing and the urge to fast-track continues.

Opioids

The opioids lack negative inotropic effects in the doses used clinically and have thus found widespread use as the primary agents for cardiac surgery. This era began in 1969, when high doses of morphine were used to anesthetize patients for aortic valve replacement.[94] However, hypotension, histamine release, increased fluid requirements and, often, inadequate anesthesia resulted in a decline in the use of morphine in favor of the more potent fentanyl derivatives. Aside from bradycardia, fentanyl and its analogs are relatively devoid of cardiovascular effects and have proved to be effective anesthetics. As a primary anesthetic agent, fentanyl (50 to 100 μg/kg) or sufentanil (10 to 20 μg/kg) and oxygen provide hemodynamic stability, although they do not consistently prevent a hypertensive response to periods of increased surgical stimulation. In patients with good ventricular function, although high doses of opioids produce unconsciousness and characteristic electrocardiographic slowing, patient recall of intraoperative events remains a potential problem. Adjuvant agents are frequently used to supplement the opioids—benzodiazepines to provide amnesia and volatile anesthetics or vasodilators to control hypertension. Superiority of any one opioid has not been demonstrated for either coronary or valvular surgery. The use of high-dose opioids prolongs the time until emergence and extubation when compared with techniques primarily based on volatile anesthetics and is no longer in fashion. Alfentanil, with an elimination half-life shorter than that of fentanyl or sufentanil, is suitable for infusion techniques and may provide optimal conditions for early extubation of the trachea. Remifentanil, an ultrashort-acting opioid, is 30 times more potent than alfentanil and undergoes hydrolysis by nonspecific esterases in minutes. Its predictable and rapid elimination is unaffected by hepatic or renal disease, making it an optimal drug for infusion techniques.

Combinations of the fentanyl-type drugs and benzodiazepines, whether given concomitantly or as premedication, result in hypotension secondary to a fall in systemic vascular resistance.[95] Any opioid in high doses can produce excessive bradycardia. Vecuronium or cisatracurium may magnify this problem, whereas pancuronium is often useful in preventing it. Abdominal and chest wall rigidity commonly occur with rapid injection of high doses of opioids and can be severe enough to render ventilation impossible. A low dose (priming) of nondepolarizing muscle relaxant should be given prior to opioid administration.

Nitrous Oxide

In many centers, nitrous oxide is not used during cardiac surgery. Increases in pulmonary vascular resistance associated with nitrous oxide have been demonstrated, with the greatest response in patients with preexisting pulmonary hypertension. Nitrous oxide is also a mild myocardial depressant and elicits a compensatory sympathetically mediated increase in systemic vascular resistance. These minimal changes may not be well tolerated in patients with minimal cardiovascular reserve.

It is well known that nitrous oxide increases the size of any air-filled cavity. The possibility of expansion of air introduced into the circulation either before or during bypass should preclude its use immediately before, during, or after bypass.

Induction Drugs

The benzodiazepines, barbiturates, propofol, and etomidate can be used as supplements to either inhalation or opioid anesthetics and, more important, are excellent as sole induction drugs in patients with cardiac disease. Obviously, dosage requirements must be altered to fit the clinical situation.

Neuromuscular Blocking Drugs

Muscle relaxants are part of an anesthetic plan for cardiac surgery. Although they are not essential to surgical exposure of the heart, muscle paralysis facilitates intubation of the trachea, prevents shivering, and attenuates skeletal muscle contraction during defibrillation. In addition, muscle relaxants are necessary to prevent or treat opioid-induced truncal rigidity. The chief criteria for selection are the hemodynamic and pharmacokinetic properties associated with each relaxant, the patient's myocardial function, the presence of coexisting disease, current pharmacologic regimen, and anesthetic technique.

Intraoperative Management

In this section, we describe the anesthetic management of a patient undergoing a cardiac surgical procedure from the time of arrival in the operating room until care is transferred to ICU personnel. Because the physiologic and pharmacologic rationales for anesthetic selection are previously discussed, this is rather a sequential description of what occurs and what is required during surgery. Anticipation of needs specific to each stage of the procedure and ready availability of necessary equipment and drugs prevents untoward hemodynamic aberrations and last-minute scrambling.

Preparation

The operating room must be readied prior to arrival of the patient. The anesthesia machine is checked, and all supplies necessary for airway management (or any additional equipment if a difficult tracheal intubation is anticipated) should be available. Drugs—anesthetic, emergency, and infusions—should be prepared and ready for use. Heparin must be drawn up prior to induction of anesthesia in the unlikely event of the need to "crash" onto bypass. All monitoring equipment should be switched on, be working, and be calibrated. Typed and crossmatched blood should be available in the operating suite. Table 31-18 provides a checklist to aid in proper preoperative preparation of the operating room.

TABLE 31-18

ANESTHETIC PREPARATION FOR CARDIAC SURGERY

Anesthesia machine
- Routine check

Airway
- Nasal cannula for O_2
- Ventilation/intubation equipment
- Suction
- Difficult airway anticipated?: special equipment
- Inspired gas humidifier

Circulatory access
- Catheters for peripheral and central IV and arterial access
- IV fluids and infusion tubing and pumps
- Fluid warmer

Monitors
- Standard ASA: ECG leads, blood pressure cuff, pulse oximeter, neuromuscular blockade monitor
- Temperature: various probes (nasal, tympanic, bladder, rectal)
- Transducers (arterial, pulmonary, and central venous pressure): calibrated and zeroed
- Cardiac output computer: proper constant inserted
- Anticoagulation (ACT)
- Recorder

Medications
- General anesthetic: hypnotic/induction, amnestic/benzodiazepine-volatile, opioid, muscle relaxant
- Heparin (predrawn)
- Cardioactive
  —In syringes: nitroglycerin, $CaCl_2$, phenylephrine/ephedrine, epinephrine
  —Infusions: nitroglycerin, inotrope
- Antibiotics

Miscellaneous
- Pacemaker with battery
- Compatible blood in operating room

ASA, American Society of Anesthesiologists; ACT, activated clotting time; ECG, electrocardiogram.

Preinduction Period

A conversation prior to entering the operating room serves to evaluate the patient's general status and level of anxiety, and to assess the effectiveness of premedication (if ordered). The patient is reminded to report if chest pain, shortness of breath, or other symptoms occur. Supplemental oxygen via nasal cannula should be administered once the patient has been transferred to the operating table; electrocardiographic leads, noninvasive blood pressure, and peripheral oxygen saturation cuff are placed; and a set of initial vital signs is recorded. Angina should be promptly treated with oxygen, sublingual or intravenous nitroglycerin, additional sedation, or if related to anxiety-induced hypertension or tachycardia, with prompt induction of general anesthesia.

One or two large-bore intravenous cannulas are inserted after site infiltration with local anesthetic (additional routes for infusion are desirable in patients undergoing repeat cardiac surgery). In some centers, anesthesia is then induced, and following intubation of the trachea, arterial and central venous cannulas are inserted. In other centers, however, these cannulae are inserted prior to the anesthetic. Preinduction or postinduction insertion of central venous or pulmonary artery catheters has been discussed previously. Once they are inserted, however, initial values for all pressures and cardiac output should be recorded, and baseline determinations of arterial blood gases, hematocrit, and activated coagulation time should be obtained.

Throughout the preinduction period, while the intravenous and pressure monitoring catheters are inserted, the anesthesiologist must never divert his or her attention from the patient. Placing a functioning pulse oximeter with the volume loud enough to be easily heard should precede line placement. Continuous monitoring of the vital signs, careful observation of the patient, and periodic verbal contact facilitate detection of hemodynamic or electrocardiographic abnormalities, increased anxiety, or excessive response to intravenous sedation.

Induction and Intubation

The exact choice and sequence of drugs are a subtle—sometimes not so subtle—combination of art and science. The choice of specific agents (e.g., sedative, opioid, volatile drug, muscle relaxant), dose, and speed of administration depend primarily on the patient's cardiovascular reserve and desired cardiovascular profile. A smooth transition from consciousness to blissful sleep is desired without untoward airway difficulties (e.g., coughing, laryngospasm, truncal rigidity) or hemodynamic responses (e.g., hypotension from relative overdose, loss of sympathetic tone, or myocardial depression; or hypertension caused by airway insertion; or jaw thrust). A "slow cardiac induction" sometimes causes, rather than alleviates, these potential problems. However, an awake tracheal intubation, after proper sedation, may be appropriate in a bull-necked, obese patient if ventilation and intubation appear to be difficult. The necessity for individual approach to each patient
13 cannot be overemphasized.

Deep planes of anesthesia, brief duration of laryngoscopy, and innumerable pharmacologic regimens have been proposed for eliminating the hypertension and tachycardia associated with intubation of the trachea. None is uniformly successful, and all drug interventions carry some degree of risk, small though they may be. In addition, in some patients, especially those with a slow heart rate prior to induction of anesthesia, the reflex response to intubation of the trachea is primarily vagal, and severe bradycardia and rarely sinus arrest can occur. Furthermore, more recent evidence suggests that intubation of the trachea is a strong stimulus for coronary vasoconstriction irrespective of the anesthetic because left ventricular blood flow is dramatically altered in the absence of hemodynamic changes. Therefore, the response to tracheal intubation may be variable, although usually short lived. Nevertheless, identification of persistently abnormal hemodynamics or ischemia should be sought and treated.

After verification of successful intubation of the trachea, the endotracheal tube is secured, and the eyes and all pressure points are protected. The importance of frequent checks of all monitors during these busy minutes cannot be overemphasized.

Preincision Period

The period of time from tracheal intubation until skin incision is one of minimal stimulation as the surgical team attends to insertion of a bladder catheter, temperature probe, positioning, prepping, and draping. As a result, hypotension often develops, regardless of the anesthetic used. It may be necessary to reduce the anesthetic depth or alternatively support the systemic pressure with a vasoconstrictor. The potential risks of vasoconstriction in patients with poor left or right ventricular performance must be kept in mind. Deeper planes of anesthesia are obviously necessary immediately prior to incision and sternotomy.

Incision to Bypass

As previously emphasized, the prebypass period is characterized by periods of intense surgical stimulation that may cause hypertension and tachycardia, or induce ischemia. Anticipating these events and deepening the anesthetic may be effective, but a vasodilator or other adjuvant is often required. Hypotension can occur during the less stressful moments before bypass, but it is more commonly associated with cardiac manipulation in preparation for, and during, atrial cannulation. This may interfere with venous return or produce episodic ectopic beats or sustained supraventricular dysrhythmias. Atrial fibrillation is not uncommon. Depending on the blood pressure and heart rate response, appropriate treatment may range from nothing to vasoconstrictors, cardioversion, or rapid cannulation and institution of bypass. Maintaining adequate intravascular volume may attenuate the extent of blood pressure decrease. This is a critical period, and continual observation of the surgical field is essential.

Prebypass, ST segment analysis and frequent TEE observation (if used) is important in identifying and localizing new ischemia. If it occurs, it should be treated appropriately and the surgeon notified. During all cardiac procedures (perhaps more so than with any other type of surgery), hemodynamic change must be immediately correlated with events in the surgical field. The hemodynamic consequences of sometimes necessary manipulations (retracting, lifting, and, in general, "mugging" the heart) are unpredictable. This occurs more often during reoperations, when dissection may be difficult, tedious, and time consuming, and when retraction of the heart is necessary. Also, following CPB when grafts and suture lines are inspected and, if necessary, repaired. Bleeding, sometimes unexpectedly profuse, may compound the problem. In rare cases in which a cardiac chamber is entered and bleeding is uncontrollable, heparin is administered, the femoral vessels are cannulated, and cardiopulmonary bypass is begun using coronary suction from the field as the major means of venous return. Communication between the anesthesiologist and the surgeon is necessary to keep both apprised of the situation and to ensure the heart gets a periodic "rest."

Cardiopulmonary Bypass

After heparin administration, the cannulas are inserted, and adequate levels of anticoagulation are checked to ensure the patient is ready for the institution of CPB (Table 31-19). Attention is focused on adequacy of venous drainage, unobstructed arterial return, sufficient gas exchange, and provision of necessary anesthetics and muscle relaxants. The anesthetic requirements are decreased if systemic hypothermia is used.

There is complete agreement that once full CPB is established, it is no longer necessary to ventilate the lungs. However, there is no such consensus about what exactly to do with the lungs during the period of bypass. Some anesthesiologists completely disconnect the patient from the anesthesia machine; others maintain the lungs slightly inflated with low levels of positive end-expiratory pressure using 100% oxygen or various mixtures of room air. No specific method is associated with superior postoperative pulmonary function.

During the initial minutes of bypass, systemic pressure initially drops to 30 to 40 mm Hg as pulsatile flow ceases and the hemodilution effect of the dilute prime becomes apparent. Once adequate mixing is obtained, blood pressure increases to levels determined primarily by flow rate, and secondary by total vascular resistance (Table 31-20). There is no consensus as to what constitutes the ideal blood pressure or flow rate for adequate vital organ perfusion, especially of the brain, during bypass. Commonly, flow rates are maintained at approximately 50 to 60 mL/kg/min, with systemic blood pressures in the 50 to 60 mm Hg range. Some surgeons believe that a higher perfusion pressure affords better myocardial protection for the cold fibrillating heart, rather than cardioplegia. Others opt for a mean pressure equal to patient's age!

TABLE 31-19

CHECKLIST BEFORE INITIATING CARDIOPULMONARY BYPASS

Laboratory values
- Heparinization: adequate (ACT or other method)
- Hematocrit

Anesthetic
- Maintenance: amnestics, opioids, muscle relaxants are supplemented

Monitors
- Arterial pressure: initial hypotension and then return
- CVP: indicates adequate venous drainage
- PCWP:
  —Elevated?: LV distention (inadequate drainage, AI)
  —Pull back PAC 1 to 2 cm

Patient/field
- Cannulas in place:
  —No kinks or clamps or air locks
  —Arterial cannula is free of bubbles
- Face:
  —Suffusion?: inadequate SVC drainage
  —Unilateral blanching?: innominate artery cannulation
- Heart:
  —Signs of distention (AI, ischemia)

Support
- Usually not required

ACT, activated clotting time; AI, aortic insufficiency; CVP, central venous pressure; LV, left ventricle; PAC, pulmonary artery catheter; PCWP, pulmonary capillary wedge pressure; SVC, superior vena cava.

Monitoring and Management During Bypass

The common etiologies of blood pressure changes during CPB are listed in Table 31-20. Of primary importance is continuous observation of the surgical field and cannulas to ensure nothing mechanical is awry. Attention can then be directed to other causes of hypotension or hypertension and their appropriate treatment. Additional areas that require periodic monitoring and occasional intervention during bypass are also described in Table 31-20. Maintenance of adequate depths of anesthesia is obviously important during bypass, although clinical signs are few. Use of bispectral monitoring may aid in determing the approximate anesthetic depth. Anesthetic requirements are decreased during the period of hypothermia but return toward normal when the patient is rewarmed.

Arterial pH and mixed venous oxygen saturation, often measured online, are used to assess the adequacy of perfusion. Urine output is also monitored, but so many variables (e.g., arterial and venous pressure, flow rate, temperature, diuretic history) influence this that it is difficult to draw meaningful conclusions from this measurement. In addition, postoperative renal failure develops from either aggravation of preexisting renal dysfunction or persistent low cardiac output following bypass. Although many institutions administer diuretics routinely, they are just as assiduously avoided elsewhere.

Rewarming

When surgical repair is nearly complete, gradual rewarming of the patient begins. A gradient of approximately 10°C is

TABLE 31-20

CHECKLIST DURING CARDIOPULMONARY BYPASS

Laboratory Values
- Heparinization: adequate (ACT or other method)
- ABGs (uncorrected): is there acidosis?
- Hematocrit, Na^+, K^+, ionized Ca^{++}, glucose

Anesthetic
- Discontinue ventilation

Monitors
- Arterial hypotension:
  - —Inadequate venous return
    - Venous cannula: malposition, clamp, kink, air lock
    - Bleeding, hypovolemia, IVC obstruction, table too low
  - —Pump: poor occlusion, low flow
  - —Arterial cannula: misdirected, kinked, partially clamped, aortic dissection
  - —Decreased vascular tone: anesthetics, hemodilution, idiopathic
  - —Transducer/monitor malfunction: radial artery cannula malpositioned, dampened waveform
- Arterial hypertension:
  - —Pump: high flow
  - —Arterial cannula: misdirected
  - —Vasoconstriction: light anesthetic plane, response to hypothermia
  - —Transducer/monitor malfunction: radial artery cannula malpositioned/kinked
- Venous pressure:
  - —Transducer higher than atrial level?
  - —True obstruction to chamber drainage? (CVP: right, PCWP/LA: left heart)
- EEG
- Adequate body perfusion:
  - —Flow and pressure?
  - —Acidosis
  - —Mixed venous blood oxygen saturation
- Temperature
- Urine output

Patient/field
- Conduct of the operation
- Heart: distention, fibrillation
- Cyanosis, venous engorgement, skin temperature
- Movement
- Signs of light anesthesia/hypercapnia: breathing/diaphragmatic movement

Support
- Assist adequacy of pump flow:
  - —Anesthetics/vasodilators for hypertension
  - —Constrictors for hypotension

ACT, activated clotting time; CVP, central venous pressure; EEG, electroencephalogram; IVC, inferior vena cava; LA, left atrium; PCWP, pulmonary capillary wedge pressure.

maintained between the patient and the perfusate to prevent formation of gas bubbles. Patient awareness becomes a possibility as the potentiation of anesthetic effects due to hypothermia dissipates. If adequate doses of anesthetics have not been given, administration during rewarming should be considered to prevent recall of intraoperative events. Use of volatile anesthetics is helpful if a smooth postbypass course is anticipated and early weaning from mechanical ventilation and extubation are planned. On completion of the surgical repair, various maneuvers are performed to remove any residual air in the ventricles. The anesthesiologist is called on to vigorously inflate the lungs to remove air from the pulmonary veins and aid in filling the cardiac chambers. TEE is particularly useful in assessing the effectiveness of the de-airing process. The heart is defibrillated (if needed) and allowed to beat to replace some of the oxygen debt. The field is tidied up, and preparations are made to separate from CPB.

Discontinuation of Cardiopulmonary Bypass

Prior to discontinuing CPB, the patient should be normothermic, the surgical field must be dry, the appropriate laboratory values must be checked, the pulmonary compliance must be evaluated, and ventilation of the lungs begun (Table 31-21). If necessary, heart rate and rhythm are regulated either pharmacologically or electrically (appropriate pacing, defibrillation, cardioversion). The venous cannula(s) are then occluded incrementally and sufficient pump volume is transfused into the patient, while the bypass flow is slowly decreased (Fig. 31-22). During this time, the cardiac function is constantly evaluated from hemodynamic data and direct inspection of the heart, and the need for vasoactive or cardioactive drugs is assessed. The potential disparity, previously alluded to, between radial artery and aortic pressures must be kept in mind. Contractility, rhythm, and ventricular filling can all be estimated by careful observation of the beating heart. For example, a low blood pressure and a vigorously contracting, relatively empty ventricle suggest that volume and perhaps a vasoconstrictor are all that is needed to wean the patient from bypass, whereas adequate blood pressure in the presence of a sluggish and overdistended heart may be treated with a vasodilator and/or a small dose of an inotrope. See Figure 31-23 for a general approach
14 to termination of cardiopulmonary bypass.

TABLE 31-21

CHECKLIST BEFORE SEPARATION FROM CARDIOPULMONARY BYPASS

Laboratory values
- Hematocrit, ABGs
- K^+: ?elevated (cardioplegia)
- Ionized Ca^{2+}

Anesthetic/machine
- Lung compliance: evaluate (hand ventilation)
- Lungs are ventilated (manual or mechanical)
- Vaporizers: off
- Alarms: on

Monitors
- Normothermia (37°C nasopharyngeal, 35.5°C bladder, 35°C rectal)
- ECG: rate, rhythm, ST
- Transducers recalibrated and zeroed
- Arterial and filling pressures
- Recorder (if available)

Patient/field
- *Look at the heart!*
- De-aired: check lead II, TEE
- Eyeball contractility, size, rhythm
- LV vent clamped/removed, caval snares released
- Bleeding: no major sites (grafts, suture lines, LV vent site)
- Vascular resistance: CPB flow $\propto$ MAP $\div$ resistance

Support
- As needed

ABG, arterial blood gas; CPB, cardiopulmonary bypass; ECG, electrocardiogram; LV, left ventricle; MAP, mean arterial pressure; TEE, transesophageal echocardiography.

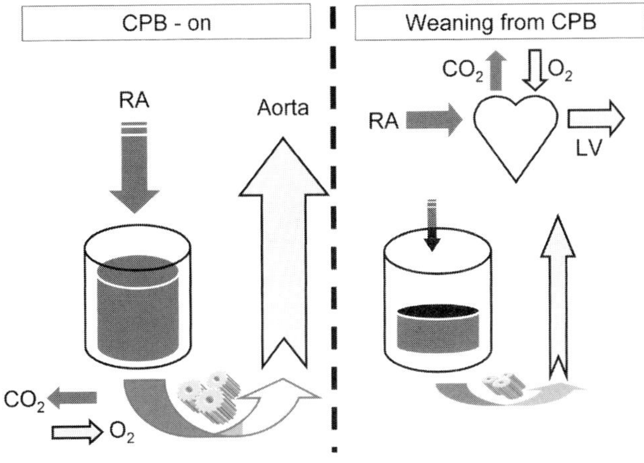
CPB - on
Weaning from CPB
RA
Aorta
CO_2
O_2
RA
LV
CO_2
O_2

FIGURE 31-22. Weaning from cardiopulmonary bypass (CPB). While on CPB, the venous return to the heart is diverted from the right atrium (RA) to the CPB reservoir. The drainage is passive (by gravity). From the venous reservoir, the blood is "ventilated," CO_2 is removed and O_2 is added, and then returned to the patient, usually into the aorta but occasionally via the femoral or axillary arteries. During weaning from CPB, the venous return to the CPB is reduced by gradually occluding the venous cannula, directing more of its contents to the right heart and lungs. LV, left ventricle.

Inadequate cardiac performance must prompt a search for possible etiologies (Table 31-22); structural defects require more than mere regulation of inotropes or vasodilators. If the clinical picture is suggestive of coronary air emboli with diffuse ST segment elevation and a hypocontractile heart, continuous support on CPB with a high perfusion pressure and an empty ventricle is indicated.

Our approach to patients with inadequate cardiac output is summarized in Table 31-23. The heart rate is adjusted as much as possible. Following that, ventricular filling is optimized by transfusing blood from the pump. It is important not to overdistend the heart by transfusing to an arbitrary level of filling pressure because this may result in further myocardial dysfunction. Looking at the heart to monitor the response to small incremental volume infusions is important. The ratio of systemic to pulmonary artery pressure is also helpful: both pressures should increase in the same direction (as in Fig. 31-24A). Change in opposite directions (e.g., pulmonary pressure increases and systemic pressure decreases) (see Fig. 31-24C) is suggestive of left ventricular failure.

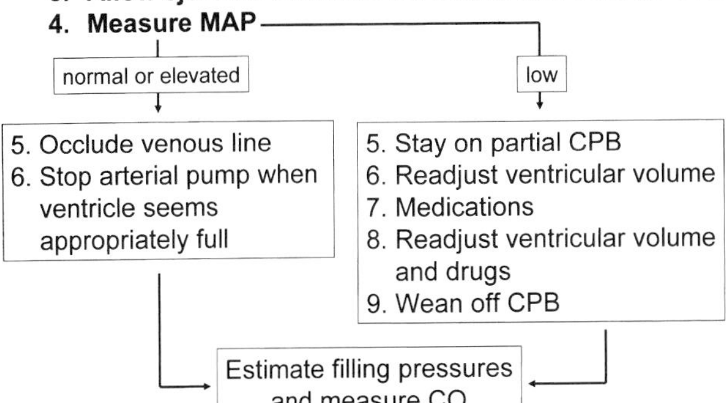
1. Rate & rhythm: adjust, pace if needed
2. Fill the heart: partially occlude the venous line
3. Allow ejection: decrease the arterial flow from the CPB
4. Measure MAP
normal or elevated
low
5. Occlude venous line
6. Stop arterial pump when ventricle seems appropriately full
5. Stay on partial CPB
6. Readjust ventricular volume
7. Medications
8. Readjust ventricular volume and drugs
9. Wean off CPB
Estimate filling pressures and measure CO

FIGURE 31-23. General approach to termination of cardiopulmonary bypass (CPB). CO, cardiac output; MAP, mean arterial pressure.

TABLE 31-22

ETIOLOGY OF RIGHT OR LEFT VENTRICULAR DYSFUNCTION AFTER CARDIOPULMONARY BYPASS

Ischemia
- Inadequate myocardial protection
- Intraoperative infarction
- Reperfusion injury
- Coronary spasm
- Coronary embolism (air, thrombus, calcium)
- Technical difficulties (kinked or clotted grafts)

Uncorrected structural defects
- Nongraftable vessels, diffuse coronary artery disease
- Residual or new valve pathology
- Hypertrophic cardiomyopathy
- Shunts
- Preexisting cardiac dysfunction

CPB-related factors
- Excessive cardioplegia
- Unrecognized cardiac distention

CPB, cardiopulmonary bypass.

If pharmacologic support is required, an integration of cardiac physiology (see Chapter 31) and pharmacology (see Chapter 12) will lead to the rational selection of an appropriate drug or drugs. Numerous algorithms are available to guide decision making; one is described in (Fig. 31-25). This algorithm uses systemic arterial and pulmonary artery pressures, and cardiac output. If TEE is available, myocardial contractility and valvular function can be more readily assessed. A search for new wall motion changes, paravalvular leaks, or new mitral insufficiency is appropriate. After integrating available data, a diagnosis is made and appropriate treatment is begun. Continual reassessment of the situation is necessary to document the efficacy of treatment or to suggest new diagnoses and therapeutic approaches. If cardiac output is low and systemic pressure is adequate (see Fig. 31-24A, B), an arteriolar dilator may improve forward flow by decreasing afterload. If systemic pressure is too low (see Fig. 31-24C, D), thus prohibiting the use of vasodilators, an inotrope should be selected instead. Each inotropic drug has a distinct profile with respect to its effects on rate, contractility, systemic and pulmonary vascular resistance, and cardiac dysrhythmogenic potential. By first defining the hemodynamic problem and then deciding what needs treatment and in what order, the most suitable drug for the situation should be selected, rather than always selecting the standard

TABLE 31-23

STEPS FOR IMPROVING SYSTEMIC FLOW

1	Heart rate (A-, V-, A/V-pacing) and rhythm
2	Preload: optimize (beware of altered compliance postbypass)
3–4	Afterload reduction if blood pressure is high and/or contractility augmentation (inotrope if low CO)
5	Preload: recheck and adjust
6	Combine therapies
7	IABP
8	VAD

A, atrial; IABP, intraaortic balloon pump; V, ventricular; VAD, ventricular assist device.

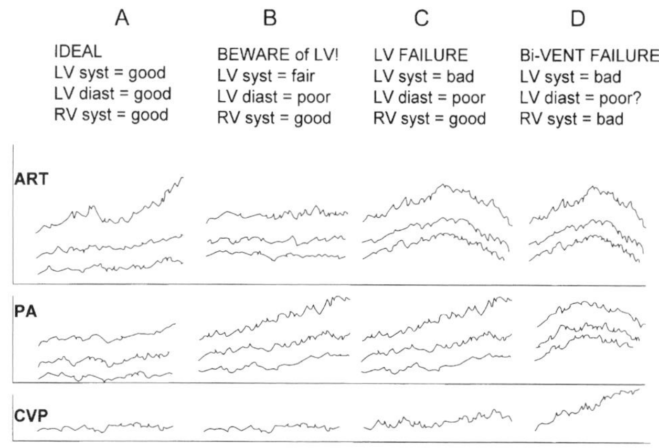

FIGURE 31-24. Hemodynamic abnormalities at termination of cardiopulmonary bypass. ART, arterial pressure; bi-vent, biventricular; CVP, central venous pressure; diast, diastolic function; LV, left ventricle; PA, pulmonary artery pressure; RV, right ventricle; syst, systolic function.

"institutional inotrope." If these initial therapies are insufficient to promote adequate forward flow, various combinations of drugs may be tested. If systemic perfusion is still inadequate, mechanical circulatory support is required.

A therapeutic approach to right ventricular failure (see Fig. 31-24D) is outlined in Table 31-24. When pulmonary arterial pressure is normal or decreased, the etiology is usually severe right ventricular ischemia secondary to intraoperative events or air. The initial response is to return to full bypass, improve perfusion, and await recovery and improvement of contractility. If this does not occur, inotropic and vasodilator therapy is established. In patients who have right ventricular failure secondary to high pulmonary vascular resistance, the mainstay of therapy is reduction of pulmonary vascular resistance with vasodilators, such as prostaglandin E_1 (PGE_1) or nitric oxide, and inotropic support. The phosphodiesterase III inhibitors, amrinone and milrinone, are particularly useful because they significantly decrease pulmonary vascular resistance and increase contractility. Overdistention of the ventricle must be assiduously avoided. Combination therapy with differential infusions refers to infusion of inotropes with vasoconstrictive properties into the left side of the circulation to maintain systemic perfusion, while avoiding an increase of the pulmonary circulation resistance. Persistent right ventricular failure

mm Hg

150
120
90
60
30
0

	A	B	C	D
Systemic	140/70	140/70	90/70	90/70
Pulmonary	30/15	60/30	60/30	30/15

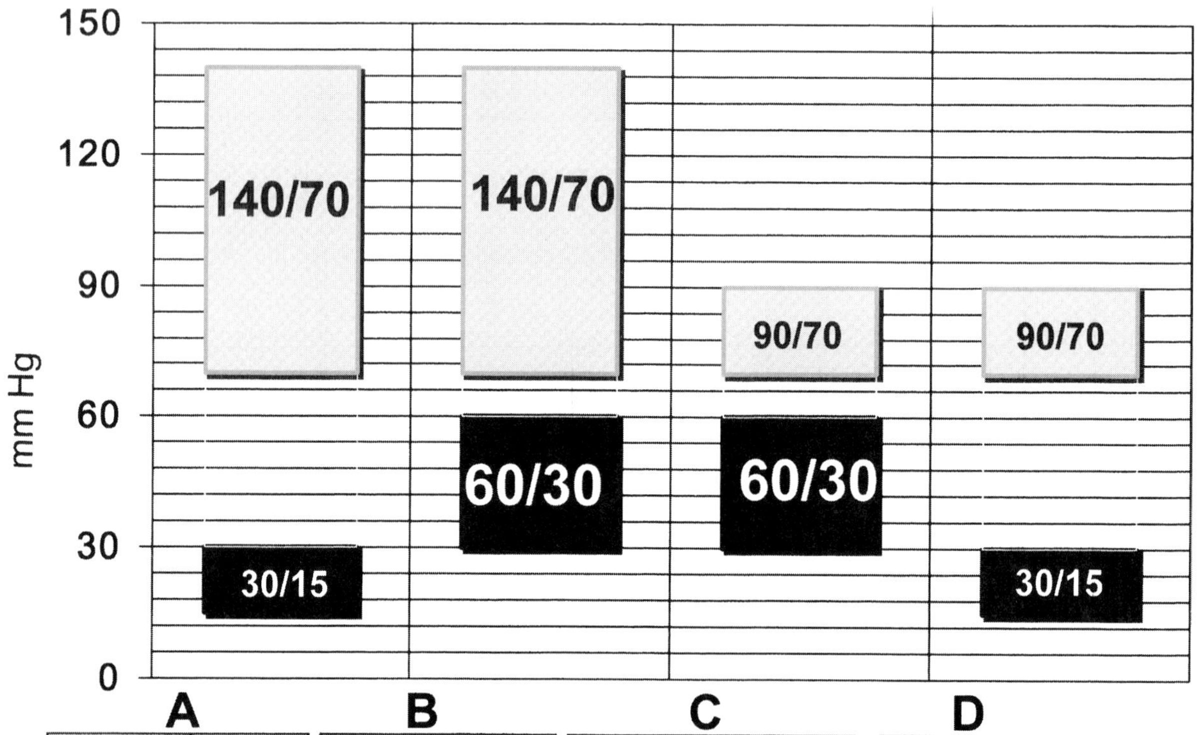

A

CO ↑	CO ↓
hyperdynamic	↑↑SVR ?↓ volume
wait ↑ depth	dilate ±volume

B

CO ↑	CO ↓
too full	↑vasc tone ?contractility
wait dilate	dilate ±inotrope

C

CO ↑	CO ↓
↓SVR too full	↓↓ contractility ALARM
wait ↑vasc tone	adjust preload inotrope (?IABP, LVAD) ↑tone

D

CO ↑	CO ↓
↓↓SVR	↓volume ↓contractility ↑ CVP: RV failure?
↑ tone	↑ preload, Inotrope NO, PGI_2 (unload RV) (?IABP, LVAD) ↑perfusion pressure

FIGURE 31-25. Algorithm for the diagnosis and treatment of hemodynamic abnormalities at termination of cardiopulmonary bypass. CO, cardiac output; CVP, central venous pressure; IABP, intra-aortic balloon pump; LVAD, left ventricular assist device; NO, nitric oxide; PGI_2, prostacyclin; RV, right ventricle; SVR, systemic vascular resistance.

TABLE 31-24

RIGHT VENTRICULAR FAILURE

	■ PAP			
	■ INCREASED		■ NORMAL OR DECREASED	
CVP	Increased	Decreased	Increased	Decreased
Diagnosis	RV and LV failure	LV failure	RV failure	
Management	PGE_1, inhaled NO, PDE-III Inotropes Differential infusions RVAD		Support on CPB High perfusion pressure Volume (if CVP low) ? CABG	

CABG, coronary artery bypass graft; CVP, central venous pressure; LV, left ventricle; NO, nitric oxide; PAP, pulmonary artery pressure; PDE-III, phosphodiesterase-III inhibitor; PGE_1, prostaglandin E_1; RV, right ventricle; RVAD, right ventricular assist device.

precluding separation from CPB may require the insertion of a right ventricular assist device.

Intra-aortic Balloon Pump

The simplest and most readily available mechanical support device is the intra-aortic balloon pump. It consists of a 25-cm long sausage-shaped balloon composed of nonthrombogenic polyurethane mounted on a 90-cm vascular catheter. It is usually inserted into the femoral artery, either percutaneously or after surgical exposure, and advanced so the distal tip is below the left subclavian artery (to prevent emboli to the head vessels) and the proximal above the renal arteries. Occasionally, when peripheral vascular disease prohibits passage of the balloon via the femoral artery, it is inserted via the ascending aorta. The intra-aortic balloon pump is the only method that decreases myocardial oxygen demand and increases oxygen supply to the myocardium.

The intra-aortic balloon pump does not pump blood. Rather, it uses the principle of synchronized counterpulsation to assist a beating, ejecting heart: blood volume is moved in a direction "counter" to normal flow. The balloon is inflated during diastole and deflated during systole. The balloon inflation elevates aortic diastolic blood pressure (diastolic augmentation), thus increasing the coronary perfusion gradient proximally, and enhances forward flow distally. During the subsequent systole, the LV will eject facing a lower systemic diastolic pressure (afterload reduction, reduced $M\dot{V}O_2$) (Fig. 31-26). Proper timing of balloon deflation is necessary to reduce end-diastolic pressure as much as possible to maximally off-load the ventricle. The indications and contraindications for intra-aortic balloon pump placement are listed in Table 31-25. Myocardial function often improves with the use of the intra-aortic balloon pump, and systemic perfusion and vital organ function are preserved.[96] It is crucial to control heart rate and suppress atrial and ventricular dysrhythmias to ensure proper balloon timing. As cardiac function returns, the assist ratio is gradually weaned from every beat to every other beat and so on and, assuming no further cardiac deterioration, it is removed.

Complications associated with the intra-aortic balloon pump are primarily related to ischemia distal to the site of balloon insertion. Direct trauma to the vessel, arterial obstruction, and thrombosis are most common, although aortic perforation and balloon rupture occur rarely. Platelet destruction and thrombocytopenia may also occur.

Ventricular Assist Device

Infrequently (1%), the heart is unable to meet systemic metabolic demands despite maximal pharmacologic therapy and insertion of the intra-aortic balloon pump. Under these circumstances, devices that actually pump blood and bypass either the LV or RV are required. These devices are effective when the injury that produced myocardial dysfunction took place intraoperatively and, more important, if it is reversible. Markedly impaired cardiac function after bypass is not necessarily synonymous with cell death but, rather, may represent temporary "stunning" of the myocardium. Survival ranges from 20 to 30%, often with minimal or no decline in cardiac function.

A second group of patients who have shown benefit from assist devices are those with chronic heart failure. These devices allow for hemodynamic support as a temporizing measure prior to heart transplantation. In the failing heart, it is important to make decisions promptly, and move swiftly to an assist device after the various therapeutic options are exhausted. Very often, mechanical support for one ventricle unmasks previously unrecognized failure in the other, necessitating additional pharmacologic or mechanical intervention.

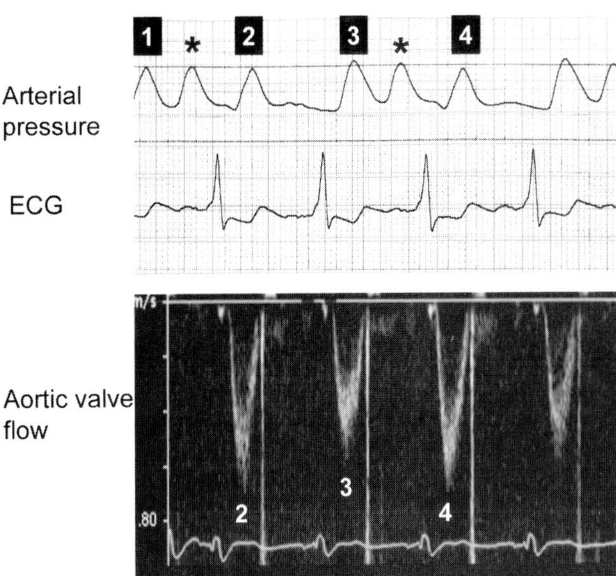

FIGURE 31-26. The physiologic effects of intra-aortic balloon pump (IABP) counterpulsation. The IABP is inflated during diastole (*asterisk*), every other beat (rate 1:2). The arterial systolic pressure is decreased after IABP augmentation (compare beats 2 and 4 to beats 1 and 3). The diastolic arterial pressure is augmented during IABP inflation (*asterisk*). The flow through the aortic valve (~stroke volume) as demonstrated when pulsed wave Doppler echocardiogram (ECG) shows the increased forward flow after augmentation (beats 2 and 4).

TABLE 31-25

INTRA-AORTIC BALLOON PUMP INDICATIONS AND CONTRAINDICATIONS

Indications

Complications of myocardial ischemia
- Hemodynamic: cardiogenic shock
- Mechanical: mitral regurgitation, ventricular septal defect
- Intractable dysrhythmias
- Extension of infarct: postinfarction angina

Acute cardiac instability
- Angina: unstable, preinfarction
- Cath lab mishap: failed PTCA
- Bridge to transplantation
- Cardiac contusion
- ?Septic shock

Open heart surgery
- Separation from cardiopulmonary bypass
- Ventricular failure: right or left
- Increasing inotropic requirement
- Progressive hemodynamic deterioration
- Refractory ischemia

Contraindications
- Severe aortic insufficiency
- Inability to insert
- Irreversible cardiac disease (patient is not a transplant candidate)
- Irreversible brain damage

PTCA, percutaneous transluminal coronary angioplasty.

Postcardiopulmonary Bypass

The procedure is not over when the patient is safely "off pump." Continued vigilance is mandatory during decannulation, protamine administration, "drying up," and chest closure. Anesthetics are administered when clinically indicated. Atrial or junctional dysrhythmias may be caused by removal of the atrial cannulas, but often disappear once they are out. Heparin is reversed with protamine following removal of the atrial cannulas; the arterial return cannula remains in place for continued transfusion of pump contents. When this is completed and bleeding is controlled, the arterial cannula is removed, and after bleeding is considered to be under control, the chest is closed. During decannulation, the possibility exists for unexpected bleeding from the atrial or aortic suture lines, and this sometimes requires rapid transfusion. Continued vigilance for new ischemia (manifested by ST segment changes, ectopy, atrial arrhythmia, regional wall motion abnormalities by TEE) is important because it may indicate a correctable problem with the grafts. Valve patients should have the adequacy of the repair or replacement (i.e., perivalvular leak, residual stenosis) assessed by TEE.

Reversal of Anticoagulation

Protamine, a polycationic protein derived from salmon sperm, is used to neutralize heparin. The initial and total doses administered vary widely. Some use a fixed ratio of protamine to heparin, others use 2 to 4 mg/kg, and still others look to automated protamine titrations to suggest the initial dose. Regardless of the method selected, further requirements are assessed by repeated measures of the activated coagulation time or other clotting assay(s), as well as by the appearance of the surgical field.

Protamine administration is associated with a broad spectrum of hemodynamic effects.[97,98] Idiosyncratic responses include type I anaphylactic reactions and both immediate and delayed anaphylactoid responses. True anaphylaxis, mercifully rare, is characterized by increased airway pressure, decreased systemic vascular resistance with systemic hypotension, and skin flushing.[99] Increased incidence of reactions has been reported in patients sensitized to protamine from previous cardiac catheterization, hemodialysis, cardiac surgery, or exposure to neutral protamine Hagedorn insulin. Perhaps the most devastating complication associated with protamine is sudden and profound pulmonary hypertension accompanied by an elevated central venous pressure, a flaccid distended RV, and systemic hypotension. This complication, which may occur in approximately 1% of patients, is mediated by release of thromboxane and C5a anaphylatoxin.[100,101] The reaction is extremely short lived, and although reinstitution of bypass is required on rare occasions, it is usually not necessary. Whether protamine is administered via the right atrium, LA, or aorta or peripherally probably makes no difference. However, slow administration into a peripheral venous site is advisable. Monitoring of the effectiveness of anticoagulation and its reversal is the subject of a more recent review.[102]

Postbypass Bleeding

Persistent oozing following heparin reversal is not uncommon. The usual causes include inadequate surgical hemostasis or reduced platelet count or function, and neither is identified by a prolonged activated coagulation time. Insufficient doses of protamine, dilution of coagulation factors, and, very rarely, "heparin rebound" belong in the differential diagnosis.

After adequate hemostasis is obtained, the chest is closed. This is occasionally associated with transient decreases in blood pressure, which usually respond to volume infusion. If hypotension persists, the chest should be reopened to rule out cardiac tamponade, a kinked graft, or other serious problems.

As the surgeon completes skin closure, the anesthesiologist prepares for an orderly, unhurried transfer of the patient from the operating room to the recovery room or ICU. Medicated infusions must be regulated, as clinically indicated, with portable infusion pumps. Additional syringes with emergency cardiac medications and necessary equipment for airway management should be carried, and blood pressure(s) and ECG are constantly monitored.

MINIMALLY INVASIVE CARDIAC SURGERY

Despite advantages in cardiac surgery and perfusion technology, the deleterious effects of CPB are well documented. These include stroke and neurocognitive defects, renal failure, pulmonary insufficiency, coagulopathy, and activation of a systemic inflammatory response. The desire to avoid these complications, as well as complications associated with sternotomy, were factors leading to development of techniques not requiring CPB. In addition to the medical concerns, patients and insurance providers are demanding shorter hospital stays, faster recuperation, and less painful and invasive surgery. As the population ages, older patients with multiple comorbid medical conditions have become increasingly common. Avoidance of aortic manipulation and cross-clamping, especially in the el-
15 derly, is associated with lower stroke rates.[103]

New procedures include minimally invasive direct coronary artery bypass (MIDCAB) followed by the off-pump coronary artery bypass (OPCAB), robotic surgery, and, in the not too distant future, percutaneous valve repair/replacement performed in the cath lab. Initially, MIDCAB was described as an alternative to angioplasty for single-vessel LAD coronary artery disease because internal mammary artery grafts have higher patency rates than angioplasty. To access the LAD and provide adequate exposure for graft anastamosis, MIDCABs were initially performed via a left thoracotomy using one-lung ventilation. MIDACB success allowed the development of other forms of minimally invasive surgery. These include the use of parasternal and inframammary incisions, minithoracotomies, and partial sternotomy. Despite effectively decreasing complications seen from sternotomy (large scar, infection, brachial plexus palsy, and 4- to 8-week recovery period), these alternate incisions provide limited exposure and increasing surgical difficulty. As a result, use of these incisions is more limited and may be supplanted in time by robotic exposure. Another type of minimally invasive cardiac surgery uses port access technology.[104] A small sternotomy is made and catheters are placed percutaneously in the femoral artery and internal jugular vein to facilitate CPB. These catheters include an endovascular aortic balloon that acts as cross-clamp, a pulmonary artery catheter to act as vent, and a coronary sinus catheter placed for retrograde cardioplegia administration. In most cases, the anesthesiologist is required to place these. This technique is used in only a few centers and is not commonly seen. Readers are directed to more recent review articles on this subject.[104]

Following success with minimally invasive surgery, the time was right for the development of off-bypass cardiac surgery, where exposure is via a sternotomy but CPB is not used. The first experiences with off-pump surgery were "simple" left internal mammary artery (LIMA) to LAD grafts supplemented with angioplasty. Off pump then developed into multivessel complete coronary revascularizations. During this period, the lack of specialized cardiac stabilization devices required the use of pharmacologic manipulation of heart rate and myocardial contractility. Heart rates between 40 and 50 beats per minute were considered ideal. This facilitated surgery by allowing the surgeon to operate on a relatively slow and stable target, while not causing undue hypotension. Agents such as short-acting β-blockers, calcium channel blockers, adenosine, and anticholinesterases were used to achieve optimal surgical conditions. With the development of improved retractors and stabilization devices, the need for bradycardia has for the most part disappeared. Other advances include the use of intracoronary shunts, blowers to improve visualization, and sutureless anastomotic devices.

Changes in surgical technique also forced changes in anesthetic technique. High-dose narcotics were abandoned in favor of shorter-acting agents that facilitate early extubation. In addition, the lull period seen on CPB was replaced by the need to constantly monitor hemodynamics and intervene rapidly in the face of changing hemodynamics. Monitoring for OPCAB is well described. Use of an arterial line is mandatory because changes in hemodynamics occur rapidly and may be catastrophic during cardiac manipulation. Central access is also necessary for the infusion of drugs and volume. The use of a pulmonary artery catheter is not mandatory but does provide information about cardiac output and other indices. One major problem associated with OPCAB is that exposure of the diseased coronaries and subsequent graft placement often requires positioning of the heart that is associated with hypotension and ischemia. Unfortunately, standard monitors used in cardiac surgery may not be useful in detecting this ischemia. In OPCAB, positioning and retraction of the heart often results in a low amplitude ECG with axis deviation. These changes may cause ST-T-wave changes to be obscured or falsely minimized. Due to the heart being obscured by lap pads in the pericardial well or being lifted out of the chest, TEE may be unreliable in detecting regional wall motion changes signifying ischemia. Changes in pulmonary artery pressure may signify acute MR due to positioning. However, displacement of the heart may cause falsely elevated central venous and pulmonary pressures despite hypovolemia. Direct observation of the heart and communication with the surgeon are critical in avoiding hemodynamic swings.

The coronary artery to be anastamosed must be isolated proximally and distally. This is performed using either an occluder clip or a snare. Following occlusion, there is usually a period of myocardial ischemia distal to the occlusion. The location of the coronary lesion will determine severity of ischemia. Preexisting high-grade lesions will predispose to collateral formation, which may ameliorate potential ischemia. Right coronary lesions may predispose to bradycardia, atrial arrhythmias, and heart block. The availability of cardiac pacing and rapid cardioversion are essential. Left-sided lesions may cause malignant ventricular arrhythmias and hemodynamic collapse. Sudden hemodymaic collapse may be rescued using inotropes, vasoconstrictors, and volume but may necessitate placement of an intra-aortic balloon pump or conversion to full CPB. The sequence of graft placement must be understood in light of each patient's unique situation. As a rule, the most critical lesion is bypassed last and the least critical performed first. This allows for the greatest amount of blood to be redirected to the myocardium prior to the largest ischemic insult.

Several techniques may be used to avoid rapid hemodynamic changes: optimizing preload prior to positioning, judicious use of inotropes and α-agonists, and changing table position to include the Trendelenburg position. The Trendelenburg position redistribution of intravascular volume facilitates to the heart. Noromthermia contributes to early extubation and the prevention of coagulopathy. Aggressive pain control improves patient satisfaction and contributes to early extubation. Techniques for pain control in OPCAB and minimally invasive surgery include systemic opioids and nonsteroidal agents such as ketorolac (in patients without renal insufficiency), local infiltration of the surgical incision, and regional anesthesia. Regional techniques including thoracic epidurals, and neuraxial narcotic are used with great success, although anticoagulation is a concern in patients with neuraxial regional anesthetics.[105]

Anticoagulant protocols are controversial. Both heparin and protamine doses vary between centers. Some do not routinely reverse heparin or give half doses of protamine due to the suspicion that OPCAB may cause hypercoagulability.[106]

Despite great interest in OPCAB as a way to decrease the complications associated with CPB, many remain skeptical of the benefits. Several studies have shown the superiority of OPCAB in regard to improved neurologic outcome, whereas others have not.[107] Many have argued that the advantages of CABG on CPB include a still bloodless field allowing for a better anastamosis and long-term graft patency.[108] Other studies have refuted this to prove equal long-term graft patency rates and decreased length of hospital stays.[109,110] These proponents of OPCAB tend to be very familiar with the technique and perform off-pump surgery frequently. This frequency seems to make them technically facile in the peculiarities unique to off-pump surgery. As such, this may account for varying results from center to center. Currently, there is no consensus as to the superiority of standard CABG versus OPCAB. Approximately 20% of centers that perform CABG do so off bypass with the majority of centers performing it infrequently or not at all.

Relatively new to the area of minimally invasive cardiac surgery is that of endoscopic and robotic cardiac surgery. In these techniques, trocars are placed in the chest in anatomic locations to allow the use of long-handled surgical instruments or manipulators. Supporters of its routine use cite decreased pain, faster healing, and greater patient satisfaction. For the most part, the anesthetic considerations for endoscopic and robotic surgery are similar to standard minimally invasive off-pump surgery.[111] These include one-lung ventilation, positioning issues, and normothermia. One major difference is that, just as in port access surgery, TEE is crucial in the placement of percutaneous cannulas.

Due to the high cost of the equipment and training required, few centers perform robotic surgery. However, just as endoscopic and video-assisted surgery has become ubiquitous in general surgery, it may have a larger role in cardiac surgery in the future.

POSTOPERATIVE CONSIDERATIONS

Bring Backs

Postoperative reexploration is needed in 4 to 10% of cases. The indications are persistent bleeding, excessive blood loss, cardiac tamponade, and, infrequently, unexplained poor cardiac performance (rule out tamponade). Surgery is usually required within the first 24 hours but also later in cases of delayed tamponade. The possibility of cardiac tamponade must always be included in the differential diagnosis of the postoperative "dwindles" because the classic symptoms and signs are often absent.

Tamponade

Cardiac tamponade exists when venous return is impaired because of elevated intrapericardial pressure. Normally, the pressure surrounding the heart is within 1 to 3 mm Hg of atmospheric, and the intracavitary pressures can be monitored using atmospheric pressure as the zero reference point. In tamponade, the intracardiac pressures are deceptively elevated and do not reflect the actual volume state. Because the surrounding (intrapericardial) pressure is increased, the distending pressure (transmural pressure = intracavitary pressure − extracavitary pressure) is actually decreased. Cardiac chamber collapse is a critical feature of cardiac tamponade, and the chambers with the lowest intracardiac pressure (atria and RV in diastole) are most likely to be compressed. The stroke volume is limited, and cardiac output depends on heart rate. Compensatory mechanisms include peripheral vasoconstriction to preserve venous return and systemic blood pressure, as well as tachycardia. Myocardial ischemia may occur because of the tachycardia and reduced coronary perfusion pressure.

Clinically, patients present with dyspnea, orthopnea, tachycardia, paradoxical pulse, and hypotension, but the intubated, sedated, mechanically ventilated patient in the postanesthesia care unit following cardiac surgery may have varied clinical and hemodynamic presentations. Owing to its often atypical presentation in the cardiac surgical patient, the diagnosis of tamponade should be considered whenever hemodynamic deterioration or signs of low output failure occur in these patients. In postoperative cardiac patients, the pericardium is no longer intact, and loculated areas of clot may compress only one chamber, causing isolated increases in filling pressure (i.e., mimicking right and/or left ventricular dysfunction). Urine output is usually diminished. Serial chest films typically show progressive mediastinal widening. The diagnosis of tamponade may be confirmed by transthoracic echocardiography (TTE) or TEE. Despite the usually present diastolic collapse of the right atrium, RV and/or LV diastolic collapse are the most sensitive and specific signs of cardiac tamponade.[112] In addition, there is excessive respiratory variation of the Doppler flow velocities across the tricuspid and mitral valves. Because of the existing extracardiac compression, respiration increases the ventricular interdependence and affects the diastolic filling of the two ventricles differently. During mechanical inspiration, the increased intrathoracic pressure will impede the RV and augment the LV filling, respectively. The pulsed-wave Doppler echocardiographic examination of the diastolic tricuspid flow will show marked decrease in the velocity of the early (E) wave as the already compromised filling gradient between the extrathoracic veins and the intrathoracic RV is further reduced. During the same time, the early diastolic mitral flow will increase as the increased intrathoracic pressure is transmitted to the intrathoracic pulmonary veins, increasing the filling gradient of the LV. The opposite effects take place during mechanical exhalation, when the effects of positive ventilation dissipate. The TTE approach may have important limitations: a retrosternal collection may be very difficult to be visualized in a postoperative patient, and subcostal views are rarely feasible early in the postoperative period because of the presence of chest tubes, pacemaker wires, and/or local tenderness in the subxyphoid area. Therefore, TEE is a better diagnostic tool in the immediate postoperative period.

The cure for cardiac tamponade is surgical; anesthetics can only further depress cardiac function. Therefore, drugs are selected that will preserve the compensatory mechanisms sustaining forward flow. Drugs with vasodilator (either venous or arteriolar) or myocardial depressant properties should be avoided in patients with serious hemodynamic compromise; dosages of induction agents should be appropriately reduced. Ketamine, because of its sympathomimetic effects, may be helpful in preserving heart rate and blood pressure response. It is not, however, a panacea and can induce hypotension in patients under maximal sympathetic stress. If on reopening the chest there is minimal fluid or if the patient shows little improvement, a thorough search for other causes of inadequate cardiac performance, such as clotted or kinked grafts, myocardial ischemia, or valve malfunction, is indicated.

Postoperative Pain Management

Early awakening and extubation have brought the problem of postoperative pain management in cardiac surgery into focus. The standard practice has been intravenous opioids given as needed followed by conversion to oral pain medications. However, the quest is on to find an ideal postoperative pain management technique to complement the goal of early extubation and maximize patient satisfaction. Several studies have shown the benefits of intrathecal administration of opioids. The addition of nonsteroidal anti-inflammatory agents may play an increasing role. In cardiac patients with severe pain associated with sternal fractures due to the sternal retraction device during internal mammary harvest, epidural analgesia has been shown to be safe and effective, and results in improved postoperative pulmonary function.

ANESTHESIA FOR CHILDREN WITH CONGENITAL HEART DISEASE

Because "anatomy dictates physiology," the anesthetic management of children with congenital heart disease requires knowledge of anatomic defects, planned surgical procedures, and comprehensive understanding of the altered physiology. The overall incidence of congenital heart diseases varies between 4 and 12 per 1,000 live births.

The best way to understand the impact of a congenital defect and how anesthetic agents will interact with this defect is

TABLE 31-26

PHYSIOLOGIC EFFECTS OF CONGENITAL CARDIAC LESIONS

Volume Overload of Ventricle or Atrium Resulting in Increased Pulmonary Blood Flow
Atrial septal defect (high flow, low pressure)
Ventricular septal defect (high flow, high pressure)
Patent ductus arteriosus (high flow, high pressure)
Endocardial cushion defect (high flow, high pressure)

Cyanosis Resulting From Obstruction to Pulmonary Blood Flow
Tetralogy of Fallot
Tricuspid atresia
Pulmonary atresia

Pressure Overload to Ventricle
Aortic stenosis
Coarctation of the aorta
Pulmonary stenosis

Cyanosis Due to Common Mixing Chamber
Total anomalous venous return
Truncus arteriosus
Double outlet right ventricle
Single ventricle

Cyanosis Due to Separation of Systemic and Pulmonary Circulation
Transposition of the great vessels

to envision the path blood must follow to maintain flow to the pulmonary arteries and aorta. Congenital cardiac lesions can be cyanotic or acyanotic. Cyanotic lesions can be due a common mixing chamber, obstruction to pulmonary blood flow, or due to separation of the systemic and pulmonary circulation. Shunting of blood causes volume overload on the ventricle; and obstruction of blood flow causes pressure overload. Table 31-26 classifies various types of lesions by their physiologic impact. However, it must be remembered that there is often more than one defect present.

Preoperative Evaluation

History

Symptoms. Infants who have heart failure present with feeding difficulties and symptoms of respiratory distress, often take frequent small feeds, and rapidly become exhausted. Poor weight gain is often a consequence of this. In warmer climates infants may perspire profusely, particularly with feeds. Parents may notice that their baby is breathing rapidly and suffers from recurrent chest infections. Cyanosis may not be recognized until quite severe. The cyanosis may be continuous and unchanging or intermittent and progressive. Cyanotic episodes that are occurring more frequently and with less stimulation suggest the potential for rapid cardiorespiratory decompensation. In older children, heart failure manifests as breathlessness and exercise intolerance. This can be assessed by comparison with peers or by formal exercise testing. Orthopnea and nocturnal dyspnea indicate severe failure. Overt syncope or presyncope, light headedness, vertigo, and blurred vision may be the symptoms of an arrhythmia or, much less commonly, of significant outflow obstruction or myocardial dysfunction. The presence of an upper respiratory tract infection in a child may be associated with an increased incidence of postoperative respiratory complications and an extended stay in the ICU.[113]

Medications. It is important to obtain a detailed history of medications the patient is currently receiving and be aware of their potential interactions with anesthetic agents.

Previous Surgical Procedures. It is vital to understand the patient's original and "corrected" anatomy, as well as his or her response to previous surgery and anesthesia.

Physical Examination

The physical examination of a child should seek signs and symptoms of cardiac dysfunction and failure. Failure to thrive due to pulmonary hypertension, poor peripheral oxygenation, or metabolite delivery is a common finding. Obstructive lesions without congestive failure, such as coarctation, aortic stenosis, or pulmonary stenosis, are associated with normal growth. Patients with cyanotic lesions such as tetralogy of Fallot may exhibit generalized growth retardation; for those who have lesions associated with congestive heart failure, such as left-to-right shunts, weight is more often affected than height. Complete cessation of growth, even weight loss, is seen in patients with severe congestive heart failure.[114] The physical examination should seek to discover other signs of congestive heart failure, such as irritability, diaphoresis, rales, jugular venous distention, and hepatomegaly.

The possibility of associated congenital anomalies must be considered. The overall incidence of extracardiac anomalies among children with congenital heart disease may be as high as 20%.[115]

Assessment of extremities should include evaluation of cyanosis, clubbing, edema, pulse volume, and blood pressure. In children with Blalock-Taussig shunts, the pulse may be absent or reduced on the side of the shunt. It is important to measure blood pressure in the arms and in the legs in all patients in whom congenital heart disease is suspected; thus, coarctation of aorta will not be missed.

Auscultation of the heart in these patients can reveal different types of murmurs, depending on the lesions as shown in Table 31-27.

All children undergoing cardiac surgery should have a complete examination of their airway. Presence of macroglossia, hypoplastic mandible, narrow palate, enlarged tonsils, and

TABLE 31-27

CLASSIFICATION OF CARDIAC MURMURS

Systolic
- Stenotic semilunar valves
- Regurgitant atrioventricular valves
- Atrial septal defect
- Ventricular septal defect
- Coarctation of the aorta
- Still's murmur

Diastolic
- Regurgitant semilunar valves
- Stenotic atrioventricular valves
- Mitral flow rumble
- Tricuspid flow rumble

Continuous
- Patent ductus arteriosus
- Arteriovenous fistula
- Excessive bronchial collaterals
- Aortopulmonary window
- Venous hum
- Surgical shunt
- Severe peripheral pulmonic stenosis

laryngotracheal anomalies may compromise the anesthesiologist's ability to maintain a patent airway. This attention is particularly important in small children and in patients with compromised hemodynamic status because their small functional residual capacity, in combination with higher oxygen consumption, provides a mechanism for rapid desaturation and the potential for cardiovascular collapse.

Laboratory Evaluation

Hemoglobin. The presence of anemia in these patients may require priming of the extracorporeal circuit with red blood cells. Children with cyanotic lesions are polycythemic. Polycythemia results as a consequence of bone marrow stimulation (via release of erythropoietin from the kidneys) from arterial desaturation. This increase in red cell mass can lead to hyperviscosity. The increase in blood's viscosity predisposes to peripheral sludging and reduced oxygen delivery. The sludging is augmented by the presence of dehydration from preoperative fasting and by hypothermia from low ambient operating room temperatures. Children brought into the operating room with increased levels of hemoglobin are at risk for the development of a sudden hyperviscosity crisis that can lead to progressive acidosis, cardiovascular decompensation, and end-organ thrombosis. In patients with hematocrit of more than 70%, consideration should be given to preoperative electrophoresis if symptomatic hyperviscosity is present. Cyanotic children with low hematocrit may exhibit hypoxic spells more readily than if the oxygen-carrying capacity were normal.

Coagulation Profile. All children with congenital heart disease undergoing open heart surgical procedures are at risk for perioperative hemostatic derangements. Polycythemia can induce a low-grade disseminated intravascular coagulation with activation of fibrinolysis, degranulation of platelets, and consumption of coagulation factors.[116]

Newborns often have inadequate liver-dependent coagulation factors due to immaturity of hepatic function. A platelet count, prothrombin time, and partial thromboplastin time should be evaluated in every child.

Other Laboratory Evaluations. Children on diuretic therapy are at risk for hypokalemia, particularly if they are digitalized. Infants, particularly those in congestive heart failure, are also at risk for both hypoglycemia and hypocalcemia. Many children who have undergone major cardiac procedures earlier in their lives may have been exposed to blood or blood products. These children are at increased risk of having abnormal serum antibodies to various blood antigens. Hence, samples of the child's blood should be sent to the blood bank for possible cross matching, which will allow proper identification of any abnormal antibodies.

Preoperative arterial blood gases obtained in patients with cardiorespiratory compromise indicate the amount of respiratory reserve present. Arterial PO_2 values of 30 to 40 mm Hg and peripheral O_2 saturations of less than 70% indicate a severe reduction of cardiovascular reserve to the point where progressive metabolic acidosis may be expected.

Chest Radiograph

The chest radiograph of a child with congenital heart disease should be evaluated for cardiac position, size, shape, abnormal vessels, right aortic arch, scimitar syndrome (hypoplasia/aplasia of one or more lobes of right lung and hypoplasia of right pulmonary artery), aberrant pulmonary vessels, abnormal position of bronchi, vascular rings, or associated pulmonary abnormalities (e.g., pneumonia, atelectasis, or emphysema).

Electrocardiogram

ECG should be reviewed for rate and rhythm abnormalities.

Echocardiography and Cardiac Catheterization

Echocardiography delineates most of the cardiac anatomy and permits noninvasive measurement of ventricular size and function, of cardiac output, and of the severity of valve dysfunction. Cardiac catheterization is reserved for patients with poor echocardiographic windows and when there is intervening bone or air-filled lung (e.g., scoliosis or abnormalities of the peripheral pulmonary arteries). The physiologic and anatomic data from echocardiography and cardiac catheterization provides invaluable insight into the formulation of the anesthetic plan.

Premedication

The primary purpose of the premedication is to calm the child without hemodynamic compromise. This will facilitate the separation of the child from the parents, as well as ease the fear and anxiety associated with the perioperative period. The choice of premedicant drug should be based on the child's physiology. The primary danger of premedication is oversedation, which leads to the loss of protective airway reflexes. Medications used for premedication include midazolam, fentanyl, ketamine, and atropine.

Small infants, particularly those scheduled later in the day, should not be kept without fluids while awaiting surgery.

Monitoring

Monitors typically used during the open heart procedures include ECG, peripheral and central temperatures, noninvasive and invasive blood pressure monitoring, central venous pressure monitoring (which can include right atrial and left atrial pressure lines placed by the surgeon intraoperatively), arterial oxygen saturation, and end-expiratory capnography. Intraoperative TEE has become an invaluable diagnostic and monitoring tool.

Induction

Inhalational agents hold a prominent place as induction agents for pediatric cardiac anesthesia and may also be continued for maintenance. Nitrous oxide can be used in conjunction with one of the potent inhalational agents. It does not increase pulmonary artery pressures except in those with preexisting pulmonary hypertension. The use of nitrous oxide in children with intracardiac shunts is primarily limited to the induction period because of the risk of enlarging bubbles of air. In addition, nitrous oxide has direct cardiac depressant effects that are more pronounced in infants and children than in adults.[117]

Ketamine has enjoyed some popularity as an induction agent in children with cyanotic lesions. Its popularity stems from its hemodynamic effects, combined with the facts that it can be given intramuscularly and spontaneous respiration can be maintained while intravenous and arterial cannulae are placed. In children studied postoperatively, ketamine was shown to have no significant effects on pulmonary vascular resistance as long as ventilation is preserved.[118] Ketamine is the agent of choice for induction of anesthesia in patients with cardiac tamponade. Ketamine usually produces a tachycardia and rise in blood pressure. Oxygenation is usually not impaired.

Maintenance

The choice of anesthetic agents following induction is governed by ventricular function, the use of CPB, and the anticipation of continued mechanical ventilation or tracheal extubation at the end of the case.

Intravenous Agents

Opioids are used routinely to eliminate the stress response in the prebypass phase of pediatric cardiac surgery. Stress responses to surgery (as measured by plasma concentration of epinephrine, norepinephrine, insulin, glucagons, and glucocorticoids) were blocked with high doses of fentanyl compared with surgery without fentanyl.[119] Large-dose synthetic opioid anesthesia with fentanyl 50 to 100 μg/kg is commonly used for neonates and infants undergoing congenital cardiac surgery, particularly if the patients have limited hemodynamic reserve, are at risk of pulmonary hypertension, or are expected to have a prolonged postoperative recovery. Sufentanil is similarly effective.[120] Remifentanil is a unique opioid allowing a rapidly titrable effect. In infants and children younger than 5 years of age, infusions of 1.0 μg/kg/min and greater can suppress glucose increase and tachycardia, and reduce plasma cortisol levels associated with the prebypass phase of cardiac surgery, whereas 0.25 μg/kg/min infusion does not. Remifentanil should be used with caution in neonates with complex congenital heart disease because it can be associated with severe bradycardia.[120] No specific relationship between opioid dose and stress response has been established. A balanced anesthetic technique containing fentanyl 25 to 50 μg/kg is sufficient to blunt hemodynamic and stress response to the prebypass phase of surgery. Higher doses of fentanyl 100 to 150 μg/kg offer little advantage over 50 μg/kg and can necessitate intervention to prevent hypotension.[121]

Inhalational Agents

Halothane depresses the cardiac output and blood pressure in a dose-dependent manner.[122] Halothane must be used cautiously in children with severe left ventricular failure or severe cyanosis because the myocardial depression from the drug may further compromise the already poorly contractile ventricle. Dose-dependent beta-blocking action of halothane may actually be beneficial in certain circumstances such as idiopathic hypertrophic subaortic stenosis or infundibular pulmonic stenosis.

Isoflurane causes a decrease in blood pressure that appears to be similar in magnitude to that caused by halothane when administered at equipotent doses. However, with isoflurane, myocardial function appears to be better preserved than with halothane.[123] Sevoflurane use may be associated with a decrease in blood pressure. The incidence of hypotension (defined as >30% decrease from baseline) at 1 MAC is highest in neonates and infants younger than 1 year of age. With incision, blood pressure tends to return toward baseline in all groups except neonates. Sevoflurane use is associated with a lower incidence of arrhythmias than is halothane. The ability to use sevoflurane for an inhalation induction, together with its lack of significant myocardial depression, makes it a good choice for induction when an inhalation agent is used.

Neuromuscular Blocking Drugs

Succinylcholine has often been used to facilitate tracheal intubation. Because infants have an increased extracellular fluid space compared with adults and succinylcholine is distributed throughout this fluid space, a dose of 2 mg/kg is required to provide muscle relaxation for intubation in infants. The drug's major side effects are bradycardia and, very infrequently, asystole. These events are more common with repeated doses. Because of the potential for bradycardia and the ability to use other agents, succinylcholine should have little place in pediatric cardiac anesthesia.

A nondepolarizing relaxant can be used both to facilitate tracheal intubation and to provide muscle relaxation during the operative procedure. The choice among nondepolarizing relaxants is based on their hemodynamic effects and duration of action. When an increased heart rate would be beneficial, as in the case of a small infant, pancuronium is the preferred agent. The popularity of the intermediate-acting agents such as cis-atracurium and vecuronium has spilled over into cardiac anesthesia. They are more suitable for procedures where patients are expected to be extubated within a short postoperative period. Neuromuscular blocking agents should be titrated to effect. This is especially important in the case of a reoperation, in which the phrenic nerve may be encased in scar tissue. If excessive relaxants have been given and the diaphragm does not respond to electrical stimulation of the phrenic nerve, it is possible to transect the phrenic nerve with the electrocautery. In the small infant, loss of diaphragmatic activity can cause respiratory failure.

Cardiopulmonary Bypass

The many advances in the CPB, together with improved surgical and anesthetic techniques, have significantly improved the survival of children with congenital heart disease. Hemostatic derangement due to CPB is of particular significance in pediatric cardiac surgery and may result in a more pronounced bleeding tendency than that seen in adult patients. Specific influences include a greater degree of hemodilution, the use of deep hypothermic circulatory arrest, the influence of cyanosis on hemostasis and coagulation, and the immature coagulation system of the neonate. These factors can exacerbate activation of the hemostatic and inflammatory cascades and the impaired platelet function that result from a period of extracorporeal circulation. The protease inhibitor aprotinin has shown its capacity to block fibrinolysis in low doses and to attenuate contact activation in higher doses. Despite the proven efficacy of aprotinin to reduce bleeding and the need for blood and blood product transfusions in adult cardiac surgery, the results in pediatric cardiac surgery are conflicting.[124] Aprotinin has the ability to provoke an antibody response in the recipient, and children who are having repeat procedures are at risk for anaphylaxis, if aprotinin was used in previous operations.[125]

During the course of CPB, vasodilating agents may be employed to promote uniform cooling and rewarming. The adequacy of flow during CPB can be assessed by the difference between esophageal and rectal temperatures. If deep hypothermia is planned (temperature <20°C), a tympanic temperature probe may also be placed.

Separation from CPB will require pharmacologic inotropic and/or chronotropic support in some patients. Pacing should be employed in the presence of a heart rate that is slow for age. In lesions where the presence of increased pulmonary vascular resistance is known or suspected, the patient may benefit from addition of nitric oxide. Nitric oxide, a low molecular weight, lipophilic molecule with a rapid onset of action and a very short intravascular half-life, increases intracellular cyclic guanosine monophosphate, causing pulmonary vasodilation. The response among patients with pulmonary hypertension to inhaled NO (iNO) is variable. A favorable response is defined as a reduction in pulmonary arterial pressure and improvement in systemic arterial saturation (by virtue of increased pulmonary blood flow). Left ventricular filling and cardiac output may also increase, and may be evidenced as an increase in urine output or a decrease in arterial base deficit. The presence of a dose-response relationship for iNO has been observed between the concentrations 2 and 80 ppm. Patients with higher pulmonary artery pressure or pulmonary vascular resistance have the most consistent and pronounced vasodilatory response. Nitric oxide is rapidly inactivated in the bloodstream by either binding to iron-rich oxyhemoglobin to form methemoglobin and nitrate or binding with oxygen to form nitrite. Methemoglobin is reduced by methemoglobin reductase to its oxygen-carrying form, and nitrites and nitrates are excreted in the urine. Clinical use of iNO should include various precautionary measures. Because of the risk of nitrite production, the concentration of iNO should be titrated to the smallest concentration that achieves the desired clinical response. Concentrations of nitrites and methemoglobin levels should be monitored.[126]

Drugs useful in the postbypass period are listed in Table 31-28.

Tracheal Extubation and Postoperative Ventilation

Children with simple lesions who have undergone surgery (atrial septal defect, ventricular septal defect without failure repaired across the tricuspid valve) that does not involve ventricular incisions can often be extubated at the conclusion of surgery, or shortly thereafter in the ICU.[127,128] Those with risk factors for ventilatory failure must fulfill traditional extubation criteria. Risks factors include complex surgery, circulatory arrest, pulmonary hypertension, and preexisting pulmonary disease.

Criteria for tracheal extubation following complex repairs are as follows: (1) ability to maintain oxygenation during spontaneous ventilation; (2) coordination of thoracic and abdominal components of respiration; (3) chest radiograph without significant atelectasis, effusions, or infiltrates; (4) short period of time without caloric input, or supplementation with enteral or intravenous feeding for patients requiring ventilation for a long period; and (5) stable inotropic support.

TABLE 31-28

MEDICATIONS GIVEN BY CONTINUOUS INFUSION

DRUGS	USUAL INITIAL DOSE (μg/kg/min)	USUAL DOSE RANGE (μg/kg/min)
Amrinone[a]	2–5	2–20
Dobutamine	2–5	2–20
Dopamine	2–5	2–20
Epinephrine	0.01	0.01–0.1
Isoproterenol[b]	0.05–1	0.1–1
Lidocaine	20	20–50
Milrinone	50 μg/kg over 3 min	0.3–0.7
Nitroglycerin	0.5	0.5–5
Nitroprusside	0.5	0.5–5
Norepinephrine	0.1	0.1–1
Phentolamine	0.1–1	0.5–5
Phenylephrine	1	1–3
Prostaglandin E_1	0.05–0.1	0.05–0.2
Trimethaphan	5	5–10
Vasopressin	(1 μg–4 U)	0.0004

[a]Requires initial bolus of 750 μg/kgover 3 min before start of infusion.
[b]For chronotropic effect following cardiac transplantation, doses of 0.005 to 0.010 μg/kg/min are used.

A thoracotomy incision in a young infant, for ligation of a patent ductus arteriosus or placement of a Blalock shunt, has been shown to decrease functional residual capacity in this population, and postoperative respiratory support is indicated. In some cases, nasal continuous positive airway pressure can be employed instead of mechanical ventilation.

The effects of mechanical ventilation on cardiac performance can be judged by changes in arterial oxygenation and right atrial (central venous) or mixed venous oxygenation.

In patients with Fontan physiology with passive pulmonary circulatory arrangement, decreasing pulmonary vascular resistance is of paramount importance, and very much depends on adequate ventilation, usually through mechanical ventilation. The potentially detrimental effects of endotracheal intubation and positive-pressure ventilation offset this. Positive-pressure ventilation is known to have a deleterious effect on pulmonary blood flow in patients with Fontan physiology. Resumption of pain-free spontaneous respiration does enhance hemodynamic performance in these patients.[129]

References

1. Kaplan J (ed): Cardiac Anesthesia, 4th ed. Philadelphia, WB Saunders, 1999
2. Thomas SJ (ed): Manual of Cardiac Anesthesia, 3rd ed. New York, Churchill Livingstone, 2005 (in press)
3. Mangano DT, Hollenberg M, Fegert G *et al*: Perioperative myocardial ischemia in patients undergoing noncardiac surgery: I. Incidence and severity during the 4 day perioperative period. J Am Coll Cardiol 17:843, 1991
4. Leung JM, O'Kelly BF, Mangano DT *et al*: Relationship of regional wall motion abnormalities to hemodynamic indices of myocardial oxygen supply and demand in patients undergoing CABG surgery. Anesthesiology 73:802, 1990
5. Weber KT, Janicki JS: The metabolic demand and oxygen supply of the heart: Physiologic and clinical considerations. Am J Cardiol 44:22, 1979
6. Hoffman J: Transmural myocardial perfusion. Prog Cardiovasc Dis 29:429, 1987
7. Prinzmetal M, Kennamer R, Merliss R: Angina pectoris: A variant form of angina pectoris. Am J Med 27:375, 1959
8. Maseri A, Chierchia S: Coronary artery spasm, definition, diagnosis and consequences. Prog Cardiovasc Dis 25:169, 1982
9. Seitelberger R, Hannes W, Gleichauf M *et al*: Effects of diltiazem on perioperative ischemia, arrhythmias, and myocardial function in patients undergoing elective coronary bypass grafting. J Thorac Cardiovasc Surg 107:811, 1994
10. Warltier DC, Pagel PS, Versten JR: Approaches to prevention of perioperative myocardial ischemia. Anesthesiology 92:253, 2000
11. Leung JM, O'Kelly B, Browner WS *et al*: Prognostic importance of postbypass regional wall-motion abnormalities in patients undergoing coronary artery bypass graft surgery. Anesthesiology 71:16, 1989
12. Haggmark S, Hohner P, Ostman M *et al*: Comparison of hemodynamic, electrocardiographic, mechanical, and metabolic indicators of intraoperative myocardial ischemia in vascular surgical patients with coronary artery disease. Anesthesiology 70:19, 1989
13. Tuman KJ, McCarthy RJ, Spiess BD *et al*: Effect of pulmonary artery catheterization on outcome in patients undergoing coronary artery surgery. Anesthesiology 70:199, 1989
14. Fontes ML *et al*: Assessment of ventricular function in critically ill patients: Limitations of pulmonary artery catheterization. J Cardiothorac Vasc Anesth 13:521, 1999
15. Sandham JD, Hull RD, Brant RF *et al.* A randomized, controlled trial of the use of pulmonary-artery catheters in high-risk surgical patients. N Engl J Med 348:5, 2003
16. Shanewise JS, Cheung AT *et al*: ASE/SCA guidelines for performing a comprehensive intraoperative multiplane transesophageal echocardiographic examination: Recommendations of the American Society of Echocardiography council for intraoperative echocardiography and the Society of Cardiovascular Anesthesiologists task force for certification in perioperative transesophageal echocardiography. Anesth Analg 89:870, 1999
17. Shah PM, Kyo S, Matsumura M *et al*: Utility of biplane transesophageal echocardiography in left ventricular wall motion analysis. J Cardiothorac Vasc Anesth 5:316, 1991
18. Wohlgelernter D, Jaffe C, Cabin HS *et al*: Silent ischemia during coronary occlusion produced by balloon inflation: Relation to regional myocardial dysfunction. J Am Coll Cardiol 10:491, 1987
19. Hauser AM, Gangadharan V, Ramos RG *et al*: Sequence of mechanical, electrocardiographic and clinical effects of repeated coronary artery occlusion in human beings: Echocardiographic observations during coronary angioplasty. J Am Coll Cardiol 5:193, 1985

20. Hattle L, Sutherland GR. Regional myocardial function—a new approach. Eur Heart J 21:1337, 2000
21. Urbanowicz JH, Shaaban MJ, Cohen NH *et al*: Comparison of transesophageal echocardiographic and scintigraphic estimates of left ventricular end-diastolic volume index and ejection fraction in patients following coronary artery bypass grafting. Anesthesiology 72:607, 1990
22. Liu N, Darmon PL, Saada M *et al*: Comparison between radionuclide ejection fraction and fractional area changes derived from transesophageal echocardiography using automated border detection. Anesthesiology 85:468, 1996
23. Quinones MA, Waggoner AD, Reduto LA *et al*: A new, simplified and accurate method for determining ejection fraction with two-dimensional echocardiography. Circulation 64:744, 1981
24. Tei C, Nishimura RA, Seward JB, Tajik AJ. Noninvasive Doppler-derived myocardial performance index: correlation with simultaneous measurements of cardiac catheterization measurements. J Am Soc Echocardiogr 10:169, 1997
25. Loutfi H, Nishimura RA. Quantitative evaluation of left ventricular systolic function by Doppler echocardiographic techniques. Echocardiography 11:305, 1994
26. Pellerin D, Sharma R, Elliott P, Veyrat C. Tissue Doppler, strain, and strain rate echocardiography for the assessment of left and right systolic ventricular function. Heart 89(suppl III):iii9, 2003
27. Aebischer N, Meuli R, Jeanrenaud X *et al*: An echocardiographic and magnetic resonance imaging comparative study of right ventricular volume determination. Int J Card Imaging 14:271, 1998
28. D'Arcy B, Nanda NC: Two-dimensional echocardiographic features of right ventricular infarction. Circulation 65:167, 1982
29. Ochiai Y, Morita S, Tanoue Y *et al*: Use of transesophageal echocardiography for postoperative evaluation of right ventricular function. Ann Thorac Surg 67:146, 1999
30. Rafferty T: Invited commentary regarding use of transesophageal echocardiography for postoperative evaluation of right ventricular function. Ann Thorac Surg 67:153, 1999
31. Meluzin J, Špinarová L, Bakala J *et al*. Pulsed Doppler tissue imaging of the velocity of tricuspic annular systolic motion. A new, rapid, and noninvasive method of evaluation right ventricular systolic function. Eur Heart J 22:340, 2001
32. Redfield MM, Jacobsen SJ, Burnett JC Jr, Mahoney DW, Bailey KR, Rodeheffer RJ. Burden of systolic and diastolic ventricular dysfunction in the community. JAMA 289:194, 2003
33. Ommen SR, Nishimura RA, Appleton CP, Miller FA, Oh JK, Redfield MM, *et al*. Clinical utility of Doppler echocardiography and tissue Doppler imaging in the estimation of left ventricular filling pressures: A comparative simultaneous Doppler-catheterization study. Circulation 102:1788, 2000
34. Rossvoll O, Hatle LK. Pulmonary venous flow velocities recorded by transthoracic Doppler ultrasound: Relation to left ventricular diastolic pressures. J Am Coll Cardiol 21:1687, 1993
35. Roach GW *et al*: Adverse central nervous system outcomes following coronary artery bypass graft surgery in a multicenter study: Incidence, predictors and resource utilization. 335:1857, 1996
36. CASS Principal Investigators: Myocardial infarction and mortality in the coronary artery surgery study (CASS) randomized trial. N Engl J Med 310:750, 1984.
37. Hartman GS, Yao FS, Bruefach M *et al*: Severity of aortic artheromatous disease diagnosed by transesophageal echocardiography predicts stroke and other outcomes associated with coronary artery surgery: A prospective study. Anesth Analg 83:701, 1996
38. Royse C, Toyse A, Blake D, Grigg L: Screening the thoracic aorta for atheroma: A comparison of manual palpation, transesophageal and epiaortic ultrasonography. Ann Thorac Cardiovasc Surg 4:347, 1998
39. Konstadt SN, Reich DL, Quintana C, Levy M: The ascending aorta: How much does transesophageal echocardiography see? Anesth Analg 78:240, 1994
40. Paul D, Hartman GS, Barbut MD *et al*: Neurologic risk associated with severe aortic atheromatosis is based on the distribution of disease within the three regions of the thoracic aorta. Anesthesiology 87:A127, 1997
41. Konstadt SN, Reich DL, Kahn R, Viggiani RF: Transesophageal echocardiography can be used to screen for ascending aortic atherosclerosis. Anesth Analg 81:225, 1995
42. Nienaber CA, Spielmann RP, VonKodolitsch Y *et al*: Diagnosis of thoracic aortic dissection: Magnetic resonance imaging versus transesophageal echocardiography. Circulation 85:434, 1992
43. Pagel S *et al*: Desflurane and isoflurane produce similar alterations in systemic and pulmonary hemodynamics and arterial oygenation in patients undergoing one-lung ventilation during thoracotomy. Anesth Analg 87:800, 1998
44. Helman JD *et al*: The risk of myocardial ischemia in patients receiving desflurane versus sufentanil anesthesia for coronary artery bypass graft surgery. Anesthesiology 77(1):47, 1992
45. Graf BM *et al*: The comparative effects of equimolar sevoflurane and isoflurane in isolated hearts. Anesth Analg 81:1026, 1995
46. Searle N *et al*: Comparison of sevoflurane/fentanyl and isoflurane/fentanyl during elective coronary artery bypass surgery. Can J Anaeth 43(9):890, 1996
47. Zerbe NF, Wagner BKJ: Use of vitamin B_{12} in the treatment and prevention of nitroprusside-induced cyanide toxicity. Crit Care Med 21:465, 1993
48. Harris SN, Rinder CS, Rinder HM, *et al*. Nitroprusside inhibition of platelet function is transient and reversible by catecholamine priming. Anesthesiology 83:1145, 1995
49. Mangano DT, Layug EL, Wallace A, Tateo I: Effect of atenolol on mortality and cardiovascular morbidity after noncardiac surgery. Multicenter study of perioperative ischemia research group [see comments]. N Engl J Med 335:1713, 1996
50. Warltier DC: β-Adrenergic-blocking drugs: Incredibly useful, incredibly underutilized [editorial comment]. Anesthesiology 88:2, 1998
51. Brister NW, Barnette RE, Schartel SA *et al*: Isradipine for treatment of acute hypertension after myocardial revascularization. Crit Care Med 19:334, 1991
52. Kaplan J: Clinical considerations for the use of intravenous nicardipine in the treatment of postoperative hypertension. Am Heart J 119:443, 1990
53. Garcia LA *et al*: Magnesium reduces free radicals in an in vivo coronary occlusion-reperfusion model. J Am Coll Cardiol 32:536, 1998
54. Ross J: Afterload mismatch in aortic and mitral valve disease: Implications for surgical therapy. J Am Coll Cardiol 5:811, 1985
55. Grimm RA, Stewart WJ: The role of intraoperative echocardiography in valve surgery. Cardiol Clin 16:477, 1998
56. Ungerleider RM, Greeley WJ, Sheikh KH *et al*: Routine use of intraoperative epicardial echocardiography and Doppler color flow imaging to guide and evaluate repair of congenital heart lesions. A prospective study. J Thorac Cardiovasc Surg 100:297, 1990
57. Rajamannan NM, Gersh B, Bonow RO. Calcific aortic stenosis: From bench to the bedside—emerging clinical and cellular concepts. Heart 89:801, 2003
58. Carabello BA: Clinical practice. Aortic stenosis. N Engl J Med 346(9):677, 2002
59. Zile MR, Gaasch WH. Heart failure in aortic stenosis-improving diagnosis and treatment. N Engl J Med 348:1735, 2003
60. Khot UN, Novato GM, Popović ZB, Mills RM *et al*. Nitroprusside in critically ill patients with left ventricular dysfunction and aortic stenosis. N Engl J Med 348:1756, 2003
61. Smith MD, Dawson PL, Elion JL *et al*: Systematic correlation of continuous-wave Doppler and hemodynamic measurements in patients with aortic stenosis. Am Heart J 111:245, 1986
62. Ommen SR, Nishimura RA. Hypertrophic caridomyopathy. Curr Probl Cardiol 29(5):239, 2004
63. Carabello BA. Progress in mitral and aortic regurgitation. Prog Cardiovasc Dis 43(6):457, 2001
64. Irvine T, Li XK, Sahn DJ, Kenny A. Assessment of mitral regurgitation. Heart 88(suppl IV):iv11, 2002
65. Carabello BA. The pathophysiology of mitral regurgitation. J Heart Valve Dis 9(5):600, 2000
66. Flachskamph FA, Frieske R, Engelhard B *et al*. Comparison of transesophageal Doppler methods with angiography for evaluation of the severity of mitral regurgitation. J Am Soc Echocardiogr 11:882, 1998
67. Turri F, Della Volpe A, Leirner AA: Clinical comparison of blood oxygenators: A retrospective study. Artif Organs 19:263, 1995
68. Driessen JJ, Dhaese H, Fransen G *et al*: Pulsatile compared with non pulsatile perfusion using a centrifugal pump for cardiopulmonary bypass during coronary artery bypass grafting. Effects on systemic haemodynamics, oxygenation, and inflammatory response parameters. Perfusion 10:3, 1995
69. Song Z, Wang C, Stammers AH: Clinical comparison of pulsatile and nonpulsatile perfusion during cardiopulmonary bypass. J Extra Corpor Technol 29:170, 1997
70. Fang WC, Helm RE, Krieger KH *et al*: Impact of minimum hematocrit during cardiopulmonary bypass on mortality in patients undergoing coronary artery surgery. Circulation 96(9 suppl):II-194, 1997
71. Swaminathan M, Phillips-Bute BG, Conlon PJ, Smith PK, Newman MF, Stafford-Smith M: The association of lowest hematocrit during cardiopulmonary bypass with acute renal injury after coronary artery bypass surgery. Ann Thorac Surg 76(3):784, 2003
72. Habib RH, Zacharias A, Schwann TA, Riordan CJ, Durham SJ, Shah A: Adverse effects of low hematocrit during cardiopulmonary bypass in the adult: Should current practice be changed? J Thorac Cariovasc Surg 125(6):1438, 2003
73. Jonas RA, Wypij D, Roth SJ *et al:* The influence of hemodilution on outcome after hypothermic cardiopulmonary bypass: Results of a randomized trial in infants. J Thorac Cardiovasc Surg 126(6):1765, 2003
74. Greinacher A: The use of direct thrombin inhibitors in cardiovascular surgery in patients with heparin-induced thrombocytopenia. Semin Thromb Hemost 30:315, 2004
75. Hardy JF, Belisle S, Dupont C *et al*: Prophylactic tranexamic acid and epsilon-aminocaproic acid for primary myocardial revascularization. Circulation 108(suppl 1):II15, 2003
76. Sedrakyan A, Treasure T, Elefteriades JA: Effects of aprotinin on clinical outcomes in coronary artery bypass surgery: A systematic review and meta-analysis randomized clinical trials. J Thoracic Cardiovascular Surg 128:442, 2004
77. Mora Mangano CT, Neville MJ, Hsu PH *et al*: Aprotinin, blood loss, and renal dysfunction in deep hypothermic circulatory arrest. Circulation 104(12 suppl 1):I276, 2001

78. Eising GP, Pfauder M, Niemeyer M *et al*: Retrograde autologous priming: is it useful in elective on-pump coronary artery bypass surgery? Ann Thorac Surg 75(1):23, 2003
79. Rosengart TK, Debois W, O'Hara M *et al*: Retrograde autologous priming for cardiopulmonary bypass: A safe and effective means for decreasing hemodilution and transfusion requirements. J Thorac Cardiovasc Surg 115:426, 1998.
80. Fujita M, Ishihara M, Kusama Y *et al*: Effect of modified ultrafiltration on inflammatory mediators, coagulation factors, and other proteins in blood after an extracorporeal circuit. Artif Organs 28(3):310, 2004
81. Lamy ML, Daily EK, Brichant JF: Randomized trial of diaspirin cross-linked hemoglobin solution as an alternative to blood transfusion after cardiac surgery. The DCLHb Cardiac Surgery Trial Collaborative Group. Anesthesiology 92(3):646, 2000
82. Thomson IR, Bergstrom RG, Rosenbloom M *et al*: Premedication and high-dose fentanyl anesthesia for myocardial revascularization: A comparison of lorazepam versus morphine–scopolamine. Anesthesiology 68:194, 1988
83. Bazaral MG, Welch M, Golding LAR *et al*: Comparison of brachial and radial artery pressure monitoring in patients undergoing coronary artery bypass surgery. Anesthesiology 73:38, 1990
84. Douglas PS, Edmunds LH, Sutton MS *et al*: Unreliability of hemodynamic indexes of left ventricular size during cardiac surgery. Ann Thorac Surg 44:31, 1987
85. Hansen RM, Viquerat CE, Matthy MA *et al*: Poor correlation between pulmonary arterial wedge pressure and left ventricular end-diastolic volume after coronary artery bypass graft surgery. Anesthesiology 64:764, 1986
86. Gold JP, Charlson ME, Williams-Russo P *et al:* Improvement of outcomes after coronary artery bypass a randomized trial comparing intraoperative high versus low mean arterial pressure. J Thorac Cardiovasc Surg 110:1302, 1995
87. Mack MJ, Magee MJ, Dewey TM *et al:* Neurocognitive function after coronary-artery bypass surgery. N Engl J Med 345:543, 2001
88. Newman MF, Kirchner JL, Phillips-Bute B *et al:* The Neurological Outcome Research Group and the Cardiothoracic Anesthesiology Research Endeavors Investigators. Longitudinal assessment of neurocognitive fuction after coronary-artery bypass surgery. N Engl J Med 344:395, 2001
89. Grocott HP, Mackensen GB, Grigore AM, Mathew J *et al:* Postoperative hyperthermia is associated with cognitive dysfunction after coronary artery bypass graft surgery. Stroke 33:537, 2002
90. Metz S, Keats AS: Benefits of a glucose-containing priming solution for cardiopulmonary bypass. Anesth Analg 72:428, 1991
91. van der Linden J, Casimir-Ahn H: When do cerebral emboli appear during open heart operations? A transcranial Doppler study. Ann Thorac Surg 51:237, 1991
92. Nussmeier NA, Arlund C, Slogoff S: Neuropsychiatric complications after cardiopulmonary bypass: Cerebral protection by a barbiturate. Anesthesiology 64:165, 1986
93. Zaidan JR, Klochany A, Martin WN *et al*: Effect of thiopental on neurologic outcome of coronary artery bypass grafting. Anesthesiology 74:406, 1991
93a. Tuman KJ, McCarthy RJ, Spiess BD *et al*: Does choice of anesthetic agent significantly affect outcome after coronary artery surgery? Anesthesiology 70(2):189, 1989
93b. Slogoff S, Keats AS, Dear WS *et al*: Steal-prone coronary anatomy and myocardial ischemia associated with four primary anesthetic agents in humans. Anesth Analg 72(1):22, 1991
94. Lowenstein E, Hallowell P, Levine FH *et al*: Cardiovascular response to large doses of intravenous morphine in man. N Engl J Med 281:1389, 1969
95. Tomicheck RC, Rosow CE, Philbin DM *et al*: Diazepam–fentanyl interaction: Hemodynamic and hormonal effects in coronary artery surgery. Anesth Analg 62:881, 1983
96. Buckley MJ, Craver JM, Gold HK *et al*: Intra-aortic balloon pump assist for cardiogenic shock after cardiopulmonary bypass. Circulation 48(suppl 3):90, 1973
97. Horrow J: Protamine: A review of its toxicity (review). Anesth Analg 64:348, 1997
98. Jobes DR: Safety issues in heparin and protamine administration for extracorporeal circulation. J Cardiothorac Vasc Anesth 12(2)(suppl 1):17, 1998
99. Moorthy SS, Pond W, Rowland RG: Severe circulation shock following protamine (and anaphylactic reaction). Anesth Analg 59:77, 1980
100. Morel DR, Zapol WM, Thomas SJ *et al*: C5a and thromboxane generation associated with pulmonary vaso- and broncho-constriction during protamine reversal of heparin. Anesthesiology 66:597, 1987
101. Morel DR, Costabella PMM, Pittet JF: Adverse cardiopulmonary effects and increased plasma thromboxane concentrations following the neutralization of heparin with protamine in awake sheep are infusion rate-dependent. Anesthesiology 73:415, 1990
102. Despotis GJ, Gravlee G *et al*: Anticoagulation monitoring during cardiac surgery: A review of current and emerging techniques. Anesthesiology 91:1122, 1999
103. Trehan N, Mishra M, Sharma OP: Further reduction in stroke after off-pump coronary artery bypass grafting: a 10-year experience. Ann Thorac Surg 72(3):S1026:2001
104. Yozu R, Shin H, Maehara T: Minimally invasive cardiac surgery by the port-access method. Artif Organs 26(5):430, 2002
105. Fillinger MP, Yeager MP, Dodds *et al*: Epidural anesthesia and analgesia: Effects on recovery from cardiac surgery. J Cardiothorac Vasc Anesth 16(1):15, 2002
106. Kurlansky PA: Is there a hypercoagulable state after off-pump coronary artery bypass surgery? What do we know and what can we do? J Thorac Cardiovasc Surg 126(1):7, 2003
107. Lev-Ran O, Ben-Gal Y, Matsa M *et al*: 'No touch' techniques for porcelain ascending aorta: comparison between cardiopulmonary bypass with femoral artery cannulation and off-pump myocardial revascularization. J Card Surg 17(5):370, 2002
108. Kim KB, Lim C, Lee C *et al*: Off-pump coronary artery bypass may decrease the patency of saphenous vein grafts. Ann Thorac Surg 72(3):S1033, 2001
109. Puskas JD, Williams WH, Mahoney EM *et al*: Off-pump vs conventional coronary artery bypass grafting: Early and 1-year graft patency, cost, and quality-of-life outcomes: A randomized trial. JAMA 291(15):1841, 2004
110. Matsuura K, Kobayashi J, Tagusari O *et al*: Rationale for off-pump coronary revascularization to small branches—Angiographic study of 1,283 anastomoses in 408 patients. Ann Thorac Surg 77(5):1530, 2004
111. D'Attellis N, Loulmet D, Carpentier A *et al*: Robotic-assisted cardiac surgery: Anesthetic and postoperative considerations. J Cardiothorac Vasc Anesth 16(4):397, 2002
112. Chuttani K, Pandian N, Mohanty P *et al:* Left ventricular diastolic collapse: An echocardiographic sign of regional cardiac tamponade. Circulation 83:1999, 1991
113. Malviya S, Voepel-Lewis T, Siewert M, Pandit UA, Riegger LQ, Tait AR. Risk factors for adverse postoperative outcomes in children presenting for cardiac surgery with upper respiratory tract infections. Anesthesiology 98(3):628, 2003
114. Bauer LM, Robinson SJ. Growth history of children with congenital heart defects. Am J Dis Child 117:564, 1969
115. Greenwood RD, Rosenthal LA, Parisi L *et al*: Extracardiac abnormalities in infants with congenital heart disease. Pediatrics 55:485, 1975
116. Colon-Otero G, Gilchrist G, Holcomb G, Ilstrup DM, Bowie EJ: Preoperative evaluation of hemostasis in patients with congenital heart disease. Mayo Clin Proc 62:379, 1987
117. Goldberg A, Sohn Y, Phear W. Direct myocardial effects of nitrous oxide. Anesthesiology 37:373, 1972
118. Hickey PR, Hansen DD, Cramolini GM *et al*: Pulmonary and systemic hemodynamic responses to ketamine in infants with normal and elevated pulmonary vascular resistance. Anesthesiology 62:287, 1985
119. Gruber EM, Laussen PC, Casta A *et al*: Stress response in infants undergoing cardiac surgery: A randomized study of fentanyl bolus, fentanyl infusion, and fentanyl-midazolam infusion. Anesth Analg 92:882, 2001
120. Weale NK, Rogers CA, Cooper R, Nolan J, Wolf AR. Effect of remifentanil infusion rate on stress response to the prebypass phase of paediatric cardiac surgery. Br J Anaesth 92(2):187, 2004
121. Duncan HP, Cloote A, Weir PM *et al:* Reducing stress responses in the pre-bypass phase of open heart surgery in infants and young children: A comparison of different fentanyl doses. Br J Anaesth 84(5):556, 2000
122. Barash P, Glanz S, Katz J *et al*: Ventricular function in children during halothane anesthesia. Anesthesiology 49:79, 1978
123. Wolf W, Neal M, Peterson M. The hemodynamic and cardiovascular effects of isoflurane and halothane anesthesia in children. Anesthesiology 64:328, 1986
124. Mössinger H, Dietrich W. Activation of hemostasis during cardiopulmonary bypass and pediatric aprotinin dosage. Ann Thorac Surg 65:S45, 1998
125. Scheule AM, Beierlein W, Wendel HP *et al*: Fibrin sealant, aprotinin, and immune response in children undergoing operations for congenital heart disease. J Thorac Cardiovasc Surg 115:883, 1998
126. Hermon MM, Burda G, Golej J *et al:* Methemoglobin formation in children with congenital heart disease treated with inhaled nitric oxide after cardiac surgery. Intens Care Med. 29(3):447, 2003
127. Davis S, Worley S, Mee R, Harrison MA. Factors associated with early extubation after cardiac surgery in young children. Pediatr Crit Care Med 5(1):63, 2004
128. Kloth RL, Baum VC. Very early extubation in children after cardiac surgery. Crit Care Med 30(4):787, 2002
129. Lofland GK. The enhancement of hemodynamic performance in Fontan circulation using pain free spontaneous ventilation. Eur J Cardiothorac Surg 20:114, 2001

CHAPTER 32 ■ ANESTHESIA FOR VASCULAR SURGERY

JOHN E. ELLIS, MICHAEL F. ROIZEN, SRINIVAS MANTHA, MARGARET L. SCHWARZE, DAVID A. LUBARSKY, AND CHARBEL A. KENAAN

KEY POINTS

1. The heart is the major focus of the anesthesiologist's attention because myocardial dysfunction remains the single most important cause of morbidity following vascular surgery.
2. Excellent medical therapy, including use of antihypertensives such as beta-blockers and angiotensin-converting enzyme (ACE) inhibitors, statin drugs, aspirin, and control of hyperglycemia with hypoglycemics and/or insulin, may reduce perioperative morbidity and mortality in vascular surgery.
3. The multicenter Coronary Artery Revascularization Prophylaxis (CARP) trial randomized patients with coronary disease (except left main disease or ejection fraction <20%) before elective vascular surgery to either coronary revascularization or medical therapy. With state-of-the-art aggressive medical therapy (>80% of patients on beta-blockers, >70% on aspirin, and >50% on statins in both groups), they could find no benefit to coronary revascularization
4. Of the various risk-reducing strategies, evidence suggests that perioperative beta-blockade provides benefit in preventing cardiac morbidity and mortality.
5. Hypotension and hypoperfusion may not be the precipitating or sole cause of stroke after carotid endarterectomy (CEA); embolic events may be just as or even more important, and often occur postoperatively.
6. Phenylephrine doubles the incidence of wall motion abnormalities observed by echocardiography compared with the incidence in patients whose blood pressure is maintained simply by light anesthesia and endogenous vasoconstrictors.
7. The definitive preventive measures for spinal cord ischemia are short cross-clamping time, fast surgery, maintenance of normal cardiac function, and higher perfusion pressures. Other methods such as cerebrospinal fluid (CSF) drainage, distal perfusion, and hypothermia may be beneficial in high aortic clamping.
8. As opposed to elective aortic reconstruction, in which preserving myocardial function is the primary goal, in emergency resection of the aorta the crucial factor for patient survival is first rapid control of blood loss and reversal of hypotension, and then preservation of myocardial function.
9. Regional anesthesia may offer several advantages, including avoidance of hyperdynamic responses to tracheal intubation and extubation, reduced incidences of postoperative respiratory and infectious complications, and reduced postoperative hypercoagulability and graft thrombosis.

GOALS OF ANESTHESIA

The goals of anesthesia for vascular surgery are similar to those for any procedure: to minimize patient morbidity and maximize surgical benefit. In the current environment, we must also achieve these goals in the most cost-effective manner. The increasing age of the population in Western societies and our desire to restore functional status to the elderly will likely increase the number of vascular procedures performed in the United States. The morbidity from these procedures has decreased rapidly, from a 6-day mortality of >25% for major aortic reconstruction in the mid-1960s to as low as 3% mortality today. We believe that advances in preoperative preparation and anesthetic management are responsible for much of these improvements. The anesthesiologist may have a greater influence in reducing the morbidity and costs of vascular surgery than in any other surgical procedure.

This chapter begins with a discussion of the pathophysiology of atherosclerotic vascular disease and the general medical problems common in patients with peripheral vascular dis-
1 ease, particularly coronary artery disease (CAD). We believe the heart should be the major focus of the anesthesiologist's attention insofar as myocardial dysfunction remains the single most important cause of morbidity following vascular surgery. More recent studies have identified and emphasized the stressful nature of the postoperative period, whereas other workers have refined preoperative risk stratification and risk-reducing strategies. However, preservation of other organ systems (particularly renal and central nervous) is also crucial. Outcome after vascular surgery is determined essentially by patient factors, surgical factors, and institution-specific factors. The National Veterans Affairs Surgical Risk Study found that low serum albumin values and high American Society of Anesthesiologists (ASA) physical classification were among the best predictors of morbidity and mortality after vascular surgery (Table 32-1). Thus, this chapter reviews current controversies in the selection of anesthetic techniques, monitoring modalities, and organ protection strategies. The specific surgical goals, anatomy, and complications for cerebrovascular, thoracic aortic, visceral, abdominal aortic, and lower-extremity revascularization are placed in the context of optimal anesthetic management. New surgical techniques such as angioplasty and endovascular repair with the placement of stent grafts promise to further reduce morbidity and mortality.[1] The anesthetic implications of these new techniques are discussed. The different scenarios that lead to emergency surgery for these conditions and their appropriate management are also discussed.

TABLE 32-1

THE 10 MOST IMPORTANT PREOPERATIVE PREDICTORS OF POSTOPERATIVE 30-DAY MORTALITY AFTER VASCULAR SURGERY IN VETERAN'S AFFAIRS MEDICAL CENTERS

■ PREDICTOR	■ ODDS RATIO
Ventilator dependent	2.71
ASA class	1.89
Emergency operation	2.40
DNR status	2.96
BUN >40 mg/dL	1.47
Albumin	0.61
Age	1.03
Creatinine >1.2 mg/dL	1.48
Esophageal varices	4.30
Operative complexity score	1.32

BUN, blood urea nitrogen; DNR, do not resuscitate.
All variables are statistically significant ($P < .05$) and were selected after stepwise multivariable analysis.
Modified from Khuri SF, Daley J, Henderson W *et al:* Risk adjustment of the postoperative mortality rate for the comparative assessment of the quality of surgical care: Results of the National Veterans Affairs surgical risk study. J Am Coll Surg 185(4):315, 1997.

VASCULAR DISEASE: EPIDEMIOLOGIC, MEDICAL, AND SURGICAL ASPECTS

Pathophysiology of Atherosclerosis

Atherosclerosis is a generalized inflammatory disorder of the arterial tree with associated endothelial dysfunction.[3] As a major regulator of vascular homeostasis, the endothelium exerts numerous vasoprotective effects such as vasodilation, suppression of smooth muscle cell growth, and inhibition of inflammatory responses. Many of these are mediated by nitric oxide, the most potent endogenous vasodilator. Inflammatory and degenerative processes characterized by the formation of intimal plaques composed of oxidized lipid accumulation, inflammatory cells, smooth muscle cells, connective tissue fibers, and calcium deposits play an important role in the pathogenesis of atherosclerosis. Putative etiologies are endothelial damage caused by hemodynamic shear stress, inflammation from chronic infections, hypercoagulability resulting in thrombosis, and the destructive effects of oxidized low-density lipoproteins (LDLs). Disruption of the fibrous cap over a lipid deposit can lead to plaque rupture and ulceration. Vasoactive influences can result in spasm and acute thrombosis.

In atherosclerosis, the normal homeostatic functions of endothelium are altered, promoting an inflammatory response. In fact, chronic inflammation has been implicated at every stage of atherosclerosis, from initiation to progression and eventually, plaque rupture. Adhesion molecules expressed by inflamed endothelium recruit leukocytes, including monocytes which then penetrate into the intima, predisposing the vessel wall to lipid accretion and vasculitis. Markers of inflammation (e.g., acute-phase reactants such as high-sensitivity C-reactive protein [hs-CRP]) may be useful in predicting an increased risk of coronary heart disease. Predisposing risk factors for atherosclerosis include many aspects of the metabolic syndrome: abdominal obesity, atherogenic dyslipidemia, raised blood pressure, insulin resistance, proinflammatory state, and prothrombotic state.[4] Major risk factors also include cigarette smoking, elevated low-density lipoprotein cholesterol (LDL-C), low high-density lipoprotein (HDL), family history of premature coronary heart disease, and aging; emerging risk factors include elevated triglycerides, and small LDL particles. More recent recommendations for more aggressive treatment of hypertension reflect studies that suggest that this will delay the progression atherosclerotic disease; beginning at 115/75 mm Hg, cardiovascular disease risk doubles for each increment of 20/10 mm Hg throughout the blood pressure range.[5]

Morbidity associated with atherosclerosis arises from plaque enlargement and lumen obstruction (e.g., lower-extremity arterial occlusion with limb ischemia) or plaque ulceration, embolization, and thrombus formation (e.g., transient ischemic attacks in patients with carotid disease). Alternatively, atrophy of the media due to atherosclerotic disease may weaken the arterial wall, producing aneurysmal dilatation. The clinical expression of atherosclerosis tends to be focal, with clinical symptoms caused by localized interference with circulation occurring in several critical sites. Major arterial sites that are particularly prone to the development of advanced atherosclerotic lesions include the coronary arteries, carotid bifurcation, infrarenal abdominal aorta, and iliofemoral vessels.

Natural History of Patients with Peripheral Vascular Disease

Atherosclerotic vascular disease (AVD) is one of the most important and common causes of death and disability in the United States and throughout the world. More than 25 million persons in the United States have at least one clinical manifestation of atherosclerosis. Throughout the last half of the twentieth century, coronary artery atherosclerosis has been a major focus for basic and clinical investigation. As a result, considerable strides have been made in the development of programs to prevent and treat the clinical manifestations of CAD. Yet atherosclerosis is a systemic disease with important sequelae in many other regional circulations, including those supplying the brain, kidneys, mesentery, and limbs. Elderly patients with symptomatic or even asymptomatic peripheral vascular disease have greatly increased mortality rates, particularly from cardiovascular causes (6- to 15-fold increases).

The prevalence of >25% carotid stenosis in patients older than 65 years of age was 43% in men and 34% in women in one of the Framingham studies. Patients with cerebral atherosclerosis are at increased risk for ischemic stroke. Stroke is the third leading cause of death and principal cause of long-term disability in the United States today, with 600,000 new or recurrent strokes occurring annually. Presence of carotid artery disease also identifies patients at risk for fatal and nonfatal myocardial infarction (MI). Stroke risk is most strongly associated with previous stroke history and greater degree of illness. The risk of stroke is relatively uncommon (0.4% to 0.6% of patients) after noncarotid peripheral vascular surgery, but when it does occur it is associated with longer length of stay and higher mortality.[6] Patients with renal artery atherosclerosis are at risk for severe and refractory hypertension and renal failure. The principal clinical syndromes associated with aortic atherosclerosis are abdominal aortic aneurysms (AAAs), aortic dissection, peripheral atheroembolism, penetrating aortic ulcer, and intramural hematoma. Patients with atherosclerosis affecting the limb (i.e., peripheral arterial disease [PAD]) can develop disabling symptoms of claudication or critical limb ischemia and its associated threat to limb viability. The prevalence of claudication is 2% among older adults, but 10 times as many elderly patients have asymptomatic lower-extremity atherosclerosis, which can be detected by comparing blood pressure in the legs with blood pressure in the arms (ankle-brachial index). Moreover, once disease is apparent in one vascular territory, there is increased risk for adverse events in other territories. For example, patients with PAD have a fourfold greater risk of MI and a twofold to threefold greater risk of stroke than patients without PAD.

AAAs occur in up to 5% of men older than 65 years of age; most of them are small and require only infrequent follow-up. Data suggest that the risk of rupture is very low for AAAs 4.0 cm in diameter or less but rises exponentially for AAAs greater than 5 cm. AAAs between 4 and 5 cm in diameter should be followed every 6 to 12 months to determine whether they are increasing in size.

Medical Therapy for Atherosclerosis

The goals of medical therapy for atherosclerotic peripheral vascular disease are to improve functional status, prevent stroke, prevent limb loss, and reduce potential atherosclerotic progression
2 and cardiovascular morbidity. Excellent medical therapy, including use of antihypertensives such as beta-blockers and angiotensin-converting enzyme (ACE) inhibitors, statin drugs, aspirin, and control of hyperglycemia with hypoglycemics and/or insulin, may reduce perioperative morbidity and mortality in vascular surgery. Prevention, including meticulous foot care in diabetic patients, is important to avoid infections and tissue loss. Lifestyle changes such as weight loss and exercise can forestall claudication. The use of statin drugs may reduce progression or even cause regression of atherosclerotic plaques, improve endothelial function, and reduce cardiovascular events in high-risk patients.[7] In the presence of oxidative stress, LDL particles can become oxidized to form a lipoprotein species that are particularly atherogenic and proinflammatory, and cause endothelial dysfunction as they readily accumulate within the arterial wall. Statins reduce the production of reactive oxygen species and increase the resistance of LDL to oxidation. The beneficial effects of statins on clinical events also involve other nonlipid mechanisms that modify endothelial function, inflammatory responses, plaque stability on the vascular wall, and thrombus formation. Patients with acute coronary events or undergoing major noncardiac surgery who received statins in the hospital were less likely to experience complications or die.[8] Statin use is also associated with improved graft patency, limb salvage, and decreased amputation rate in patients undergoing infrainguinal bypass for AVD.[9] The use of antioxidant vitamins such as C and E may also improve endothelial function, and folate supplementation may be of benefit for patients with hyperhomocysteinemia. Exercise programs improve vascular endothelial function and may delay the need for vascular surgery in those with claudication. ACE inhibitors have numerous beneficial effects in patients with AVD, including plaque stabilization, by increasing collagen synthesis in a thin, friable fibrous cap. Such action may explain beneficial effects of ACE inhibitors with regard to acute vascular events (e.g., stroke) that are independent of antihypertensive effect. ACE inhibitor use is also associated with decreased long-term mortality in patients undergoing infrainguinal bypass for AVD.[9] Cessation of smoking may be the most effective "medical" therapy. Cessation rates are approximately 25% after major surgery. Despite the low success rates, the benefits of smoking cessation are so great that such programs may be cost effective.[10] Our recommendations for management of concomitant medical therapy in the perioperative period are listed in Table 32-2.

Antiplatelet therapy is a mainstay of medical therapy for peripheral vascular disease. Chronic therapy with aspirin or other anti-inflammatory drugs may retard the progression of atherosclerosis and prevent morbid cardiovascular events. Therefore, many patients presenting for vascular surgery will be taking aspirin, clopidogrel, ticlopidine, or COX-2 inhibitors. The benefits of aspirin in reducing heart attack and ischemic stroke after vascular surgery may outweigh the risks of gastrointestinal bleeding and hemorrhagic stroke. COX-2 inhibitors are useful in providing perioperative analgesia, and although they may reduce inflammation, their negative properties in vasculopathic patients include inhibition of prostacyclin production, increased blood pressure, and thrombotic potential. The use in COX-2 inhibitors of patients with AVD is controversial at present, with studies suggesting increased cardiovascular events leading to drug recall and black box warnings.[2] Clopidogrel irreversibly inhibits ADP-induced platelet aggregation, and reduces formation of both arterial and venous thrombi. Oral platelet glycoprotein IIb/IIIa inhibitors may also be used acutely during percutaneous coronary intervention and as adjunctive treatment of acute coronary syndromes. In general, we recommend that patients continue to take aspirin until the day of surgery for carotid and lower-extremity surgery, and individualize the choice for larger operations. In urgent

TABLE 32-2

CONCOMITANT MEDICAL THERAPY, SIDE EFFECTS OF POTENTIAL CONCERN PERIOPERATIVELY, AND THE AUTHORS' CURRENT RECOMMENDATIONS

MEDICATION OR DRUG CLASS	SIDE EFFECT OF POTENTIAL CONCERN IN THE PERIOPERATIVE PERIOD	RECOMMENDATION FOR PERIOPERATIVE USE
Aspirin	Platelet inhibition may increase bleeding; decreased GFR	Continue until day of surgery, especially for carotid and peripheral cases; monitor fluid and urine status
Clopidogrel	Platelet inhibition may increase bleeding Very rare thrombotic thrombocytopenic purpura	Hold for 7 d before surgery except for CEA and severe CAD. Consider additional cross-match of blood. Avoid neuraxial anesthesia if not held at least 7 d
HMG CoA reductase inhibitors (statins)	Liver function test abnormalities Rhabdomyolysis	Assess liver function tests and continue through morning of surgery Check CPK if myalgias
Beta-blockers	Bronchospasm Hypotension Bradycardia, heart block	Continue through perioperative period
ACE inhibitors	Induction hypotension, cough	Continue through perioperative period; consider one-half dose on day of surgery
Diuretics	Hypovolemia, electrolyte abnormalities	Continue through morning of surgery; monitor fluid and urine status
Calcium channel blockers	Perioperative hypotension, especially with amlodipine	Continue through perioperative period; consider withholding amlodipine on the morning of surgery
Oral hypoglycemics	Hypoglycemia preoperatively and intraoperatively Lactic acidosis with metformin	When feasible switch over to insulin preoperatively. Monitor glucose status perioperatively

ACE, angiotension-converting enzyme; CAD, coronary artery disease; CEA, carotid endarterectomy; CPK, creatine phosphokinase; GFR, glomerular filtration rate; HMG, 3-hydroxy-3-methylglutaryl–coenzyme A reductase.

situations when patients develop acute ischemia, systemic anticoagulation may be instituted. The agents used may range from heparin, Coumadin, or thrombolytics. Therefore, when patients present to us for urgent surgery to reverse acute ischemia, we specifically ask them and their surgeons about recent or planned anticoagulation. If the answer is "yes," we almost always forego regional anesthesia. The implications of new antiplatelet agents on the use of regional anesthesia are unclear. However, the use of low-molecular-weight heparins (LMWHs) may be dangerous when combined with regional anesthesia, as discussed in this section.

A primary concern with the use of anticoagulation and antiplatelet therapy is the risk of spinal hematoma after spinal–epidural anesthesia. Therapeutic anticoagulation with intravenous heparin is routine during vascular surgery and may also be continued into the postoperative period. Concomitant use of other anticoagulants (antiplatelet medications, LMWH, and oral anticoagulants) is common. Guidelines have been proposed to improve safety in such situations. Spinal and epidural anesthesia may be safely performed in a patient undergoing subsequent therapeutic heparinization, provided that heparinization occurs at a minimum of 60 minutes after the needle placement. However, the authors of the most often quoted study (with ~3,100 patients) in support of such practice postponed surgery for 1 day for patients who had a "bloody tap" during attempted epidural catheterization.[11] The surgery was then subsequently performed under general anesthesia. In addition, some have suggested that heparin effect be monitored and maintained within acceptable levels (activated clotting time or activated partial thromboplastin time one and one-half to two times baseline), and indwelling catheters be removed at a time when heparin activity is low or completely reversed. More recently, concern has been growing about the use of LMWHs and the occurrence of spinal and epidural hematoma. In these cases, even when emergency decompressive laminectomy is performed to evacuate the hematoma, permanent neurologic deficit may occur (especially if diagnosis or surgical treatment is delayed). Factors suspected of predisposing patients to epidural hematoma include a dose of enoxaparin that exceeds the recommended dose (30 mg every 12 hours), use of indwelling epidural catheters, administration of concomitant medications known to increase bleeding, presence of vertebral column abnormalities, older age, and female gender. Because plasma half-life and bioavailability are higher for LMWHs as compared with conventional unfractionated heparin, the guidelines for spinal and epidural anesthesia are different. A single-dose spinal anesthetic may be the safest neuraxial technique in patients receiving preoperative LMWHs. Needle placement should occur at least 10 to 12 hours after the last dose of LMWH. Subsequent dosing of the anticoagulant should be delayed for at least 2 hours after the needle placement. Presence of blood during needle placement may warrant an additional delay in initiation of postoperative therapy. If a continuous technique is selected, the epidural catheter should be left indwelling overnight and removed the following day, with the first dose of LMWH administered 2 hours after catheter removal.[12] It is important to remember that not only the needle puncture, but also neuraxial catheter removal poses a potential risk for development of spinal–epidural hematoma in an anticoagulated patient.

We refer the reader to the guidelines produced by the Consensus Conference on Neuraxial Anesthesia and Anticoagulation convened by the American Society of Regional Anesthesia and Pain Medicine (Table 32-3).[12] In summary, for any given scenario, concomitant use of other anticoagulants, including antiplatelet medications and dextran, increase the risk of spinal hematoma. It must be remembered that identification of risk factors and establishment of guidelines will not completely eliminate the complication of spinal hematoma. The type of analgesic solution should be tailored to minimize the degree of sensory and motor blockade. Vigilance in monitoring is critical to allow early evaluation of neurologic dysfunction

TABLE 32-3

NEURAXIAL ANESTHESIA IN THE PATIENT RECEIVING THROMBOPROPHYLAXIS

	ANTIPLATELET MEDICATIONS	UNFRACTIONATED HEPARIN		LMWH	WARFARIN	THROMBOLYTICS	HERBAL THERAPY
		SUBCUTANEOUS	INTRAVENOUS				
German Society of Anesthesiology and Intensive Care Medicine	No contraindication	Needle placement 4 hr after heparin; heparin 1 hr after needle placement or catheter removal	Needle placement and/or catheter removal 4 hr after discontinuing heparin; heparinize 1 hr after neuraxial technique, delay surgery 12 hr if traumatic	Neuraxial technique 10–12 hr after LMWH; next dose 4 hr after needle or catheter placement	Discontinue in advance, remove catheter prior to initiation of warfarin	Not discussed	Not discussed
Spanish Consensus Forum	Discontinue in advance	Not discussed	Neuraxial technique 4 hr after heparin dose; heparinize 30 min after needle placement; delay heparinization 6 hr if traumatic	Needle placement 12+ hr after LMWH; first postoperative dose 4–12 hr; catheters removed 10–12 hr after LMWH and 4 hr prior to next dose; postpone LMWH 24 hr if traumatic	INR < 1.5 for performance of neuraxial techniques; no INR guidelines for catheter removal	Not discussed	Not discussed
American Society of Regional Anesthesia and Pain Medicine	No contraindication; with NSAIDs; discontinue ticlopidine 14 d, clopidogrel 7 d, GP IIb/IIIa inhibitors 8–48 hr in advance	No contraindication, consider delaying heparin until after block if technical difficulty anticipated	Heparinize 1 hr after neuraxial technique, remove catheter 2–4 hr after last heparin dose; no mandatory delay if traumatic	Twice daily dosing: LMWH 24 hr after surgery, regardless of technique; remove neuraxial catheter 2 hr before first LMWH dose. Single daily dosing: according to European statements	Document normal INR after discontinuation (prior to neuraxial technique); remove catheter when INR $\leq$ 1.5 (initiation of therapy)	No data on safety interval for performance of neuraxial technique or catheter removal; follow fibrinogen level	No evidence for mandatory discontinuation prior to neuraxial technique; be aware of potential drug interactions

NSAIDs, nonsteroidal anti-inflammatory drugs; GP IIb/IIIa, platelet glycoprotein receptor IIb/IIIa inhibitors; INR, international normalized ratio; LMWH, low-molecular-weight heparin.
Data from the German Society of Anesthesiology and Intensive Care Medicine Consensus guidelines, the Spanish Consensus Forum. Horlocker TT, Wedel DJ, Benzon H *et al*: Regional anesthesia in the anticoagulated patient: defining the risks (the second ASRA consensus conference on neuraxial anesthesia and anticoagulation). Reg Anesth Pain Med 28:172, 2003.

and prompt intervention. The guidelines focus not only on the prevention of spinal hematoma, but also optimization of neurologic outcome. Finally, it must be noted that the guidelines represent general recommendations, but in a given case, direct communication with the surgeon and specific risk–benefit decision about the management are warranted.

In patients who have previously undergone procedures during which heparin was administered, heparin antibodies may be present. When undiagnosed patients with heparin antibodies receive heparin, platelet counts may drop several days following surgery. In the most severe cases, thrombosis may occur due to platelet activation. Heparin-induced thrombosis (HIT) is one of the most common immune-mediated adverse drug reactions. HIT is caused by IgG antibodies that recognize complexes of heparin and platelet factor 4, leading to platelet activation via platelet Fc gamma IIa receptors. Two types of assays for HIT, washed platelet activation assays and commercial platelet factor 4/polyanion enzyme immunoassays, are sensitive for detecting clinically relevant HIT antibodies; thus, a negative test generally rules out HIT. However, weak antibodies can also be detected.[13] If HIT is suspected, heparin therapy should be stopped, including heparin in the "flush" of invasive monitors. Procoagulant, platelet-derived microparticles, and possibly the activation of endothelium cause thrombin generation in vivo. The central role of thrombin generation in this syndrome provides a rationale for the use of anticoagulants that inhibit thrombin (lepirudin and argatroban). Fondaparinux produces its antithrombotic effect through factor Xa inhibition. These drugs may be given to provide anticoagulation during surgery instead of heparin; however, their half-lives are longer than those of heparin, and their metabolism depends on renal (lepirudin) or hepatic (argatroban) function, which requires dose adjustment in the setting of end-organ dysfunction. Their interactions with regional anesthesia are unclear; we advise clinicians to limit regional anesthesia in their presence and to follow future Consensus Statements.

Chronic Medical Problems and Risk Prediction in Peripheral Vascular Disease Patients

Many disorders are associated with vascular disease; however, diabetes, smoking and its sequelae, chronic pulmonary disease, hypertension, renal insufficiency, and ischemic heart disease are the most common. Understanding the end-organ effects of these diseases can guide appropriate perioperative therapy. It would be suboptimal to administer anesthesia to patients with uncontrolled medical conditions such as severe hypertension, a recent MI, uncontrolled diabetes and hyperglycemia, or untreated pulmonary infections. However, an expanding aneurysm, crescendo transient ischemic attacks, or threatened limb loss can force one's hand. In such situations, attempts to rapidly control chronically deranged blood pressure (which could precipitate cerebral ischemia) or electrolytes (which could, for example, result in accidental administration of a bolus of potassium) may be more hazardous than leaving the condition untreated or trying to control the abnormality slowly.

Whereas chronic medical conditions increase the likelihood of postoperative morbidity and mortality, postoperative complications have even greater predictive value for adverse outcomes. Other causes of morbidity following vascular surgery include bleeding, pulmonary infections, graft infections, renal insufficiency and failure, hepatic failure, cerebrovascular accidents, and spinal cord ischemia resulting in paraplegia. The incidence of these other causes of morbidity has declined substantially in the past 20 years; in particular, death from renal failure after abdominal aortic reconstruction has declined from 25 to <1% at present. Much of the decline in renal failure has been the result of better perioperative fluid management. Although multisystem organ failure may account for an increasing proportion of deaths after vascular surgery, we believe that maintaining adequate cardiac function and perfusion of vital organs remains a vital aspect of reducing perioperative mortality. The factors that limit patient prognosis after vascular surgery remain primarily related to the heart. We therefore more closely examine the effects of known or suspected CAD on patient management before, during, and after vascular surgery.

Coronary Artery Disease in Patients with Peripheral Vascular Disease

Hertzer et al.[14] performed coronary angiography in 1,000 consecutive patients presenting for vascular surgery and identified severe correctable CAD in 25% of the entire series. The incidence of significant CAD (stenosis >70%) detected by angiography was 78% in those with clinical indications of CAD and 37% in patients without any clinical indications. However, subsequent analysis demonstrated that clinical risk factors still predicted the severity of CAD (Fig. 32-1). The absence of severe coronary stenoses can be predicted with a positive predictive value of 96% for patients without diabetes, prior angina, previous MI, or congestive heart failure (CHF).

Short-term postoperative morbidity and mortality after vascular surgery is higher than after other types of noncardiac surgery. Cardiac-related death, MI, cardiogenic pulmonary edema, unstable angina, and dysrhythmias may occur after vascular surgery. Complications after carotid endarterectomy (CEA) are generally less frequent, regardless of the presence or absence of known CAD. However, even after carotid surgery, cardiac causes produce 50 to 100% of the mortality encountered. Patients undergoing lower-extremity revascularization often have more severe medical conditions as a group than patients undergoing abdominal aortic surgery, resulting in equal aggregate risks for cardiac complications in one series.[15]

Long-term morbidity and mortality following vascular surgery are also greatly influenced by the presence of CAD. The presence of uncorrected CAD appears to double 5-year

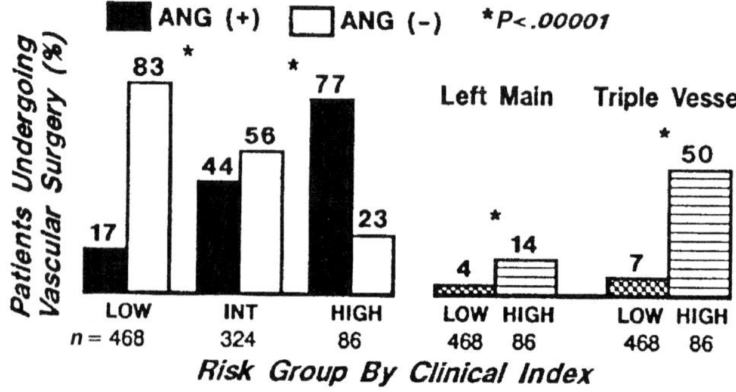

FIGURE 32-1. Clinical risk factors predict severe (left main or triple vessel) coronary artery disease. A preoperative clinical index (diabetes mellitus, prior myocardial infarction, angina, age older than 70 years, congestive heart failure) was used to stratify patients. ANG (+), angiogram positive for coronary artery disease; ANG (−), angiogram negative for coronary artery disease; INT, intermediate. (Based on data from Paul SD, Eagle KA, Kuntz KM *et al*: Concordance of preoperative clinical risk with angiographic severity of coronary artery disease in patients undergoing vascular surgery. Circulation 94(7):1561, 1966; secondary analysis of data from Hertzer NR, Beven EG, Young JR *et al*: Coronary artery disease in peripheral vascular patients: A classification of 1000 coronary angiograms and results of surgical management. Ann Surg 199:223, 1984.)

mortality after vascular surgery. Coronary artery bypass graft (CABG) is associated with improved survival in peripheral vascular disease patients who have triple-vessel but not single-vessel or double-vessel CAD.[16] Previous percutaneous transluminal coronary angioplasty (PTCA) and stenting may or may not protect against perioperative cardiac events after vascular surgery. However, in the first 6 weeks after coronary stent placement, noncardiac surgery carries considerable risks. Because clopidogrel (Plavix) is usually prescribed to reduce stent thrombosis, clinicians are left with difficult choices: continue the clopidogrel and risk increased surgical bleeding, or stop it with an increased risk of acute perioperative coronary stent thrombosis and MI. Whenever possible, noncardiac surgery should be delayed until 6 weeks after coronary stent placement, by which time stents are generally endothelialized, and a course of antiplatelet therapy to prevent stent thrombosis has been completed.[17] Drug-eluting stents may simplify these problems in the future.

The prevalence of asymptomatic CAD and the substantial short-term and long-term cardiac morbidity and mortality in patients undergoing vascular surgery have led investigators and clinicians to propose and undertake extensive preoperative workups to detect underlying CAD. Controversy persists as to whether preoperative identification of patients most likely to have perioperative cardiovascular events related to myocardial ischemia benefits patients. Preoperative evaluation of the electrocardiogram (ECG) is more often abnormal than not in elderly patients and does not appear to be independently associated with adverse events, when ASA and heart failure status are considered.[18] Despite this, we continue to obtain an ECG before surgery to have a baseline with which to compare any ECGs obtained after surgery in the event of adverse outcomes. Invasive coronary interventions may benefit patients with vascular disease but are generally more risky than in other groups of patients. Many believe that preparatory coronary revascularization may be "survival tests" that are accompanied by increased short-term morbidity; others believe that these procedures lead to better long-term survival. In contrast, patients who have survived recent coronary revascularization (CABG <5 years, PTCA <2 years) have fewer cardiac complications after vascular surgery.

The timing and character of perioperative MI reported in the literature seems to have shifted from classical reports with a predominance of Q-wave MI peaking between postoperative days 2 and 3 with high mortality to more modern series with non–Q-wave MI occurring earlier (operative day/day 1 postsurgery) with lower mortality. In addition, MI occurring in the perioperative period is associated with sustained elevation of heart rate, absence of chest pain, and prolonged premonitory episodes of ST segment depression before overt MI.[19] The pathophysiology of perioperative MI differs somewhat from that of MI occurring in the usual nonoperative setting. In the latter, rupture of a coronary atherosclerotic plaque leads to platelet aggregation and thrombus formation. In contrast, plaque rupture occurs only in about one-half of perioperative infarctions. The remainder is due to a prolonged imbalance between myocardial oxygen demand and supply in the setting of CAD. Myocardial oxygen supply may be diminished by anemia or hypotension, whereas oxygen demand may be increased by tachycardia and hypertension resulting from postoperative pain, withdrawal of anesthesia, or shifts in intravascular volume. Even small changes in cardiac troponin-I (cTn-I) or cardiac troponin-T (cTn-T) after surgery are associated with a worse perioperative and 6-month outcome, with a dose-response relationship.[20] This led to a shift in the current diagnostic definitions of MI with greater emphasis on elevation of cardiac troponins (either cTn-I or cTn-T).

Three essential purposes are served by preoperative cardiac risk stratification. The first would be to forego surgery or perform a more conservative surgical procedure in those at high risk. The second goal would be to determine which patients should undergo myocardial revascularization. This goal requires that we identify patients with left main CAD, as well as those with triple-vessel CAD and poor left ventricular function, because these patients are most likely to benefit from coronary revascularization in the long run. Finally, because most perioperative myocardial ischemia and MI occur early in the postoperative period, a third rationale for preoperative segregation of high-risk patients is to target those who might benefit from aggressive therapy in the first 24 to 72 hours after surgery. Risk-reducing interventions may include invasive monitoring in an intensive care unit (ICU), forced-air warming, stress-reducing anesthetic techniques, and/or perioperative beta-blockade. These attempts to reduce morbidity vary widely in cost, and their effectiveness is controversial. The choice of risk-reducing strategies depends on the surgical procedures, the discretion of the anesthesiologists and surgeons, and institutional protocols (clinical pathways).

The patient's history and bedside examination before vascular surgery serve not only to predict coronary anatomy, but also to provide important prognostic information. Studies have consistently identified CHF, previous MI, advanced age, severely limited exercise tolerance, chronic renal insufficiency, and diabetes as risk factors for the development of perioperative cardiac morbidity. The presence of three or more of these risk factors makes an individual patient "high risk." Patients who need emergency or urgent surgery are also at greatly increased risk for cardiac complications.

Previous work has suggested that risk of reinfarction depends primarily on the amount of time passed since infarction, with reduced reinfarction rate after 6 months. In the modern era, however, acute thrombolysis or angioplasty during MI reduces infarct size, as do ACE inhibitors and control of hyperglycemia. Therefore, given appropriate acute care of an MI, and subsequent risk stratification and quantification of ischemic burden with noninvasive testing (as described later in this seciton), we may identify patients who are at relatively low risk despite a recent infarction. In addition, studies using aggressive hemodynamic monitoring and intensive postoperative care suggest that the rate of reinfarction after a recent infarction is currently much lower in some centers. Thus, the long waiting period of 6 months after an MI before surgery may no longer apply to most patients. However, if coronary stenting has been performed, a 6-week wait would seem prudent if feasible.[17]

Exercise tolerance is also a useful prognostic indicator, although claudication, orthopedic problems, and frailty may limit a patient's capabilities. Patients with limited exercise capacity (<4 metabolic equivalents levels [METS]; 4 METS is represented by being able to do light household work such as dusting and washing clothes) have greatly increased perioperative risk. We believe that if patients can walk briskly for two blocks with neither angina nor dyspnea, and have no other indicators of CAD, they are very unlikely to have left main disease, triple-vessel disease, or severe left ventricular dysfunction. Such patients can probably undergo surgery without specialized noninvasive testing because they are unlikely to be at risk for adverse perioperative outcomes. However, because claudication and arthritis can limit the evaluation of functional capacity and CAD by conventional exercise testing, other noninvasive tests have become popular for cardiac risk stratification in the past two decades.

Routine coronary angiography is impractical to use routinely before vascular surgery because of the costs and risks involved. The use of screening tests has remained controversial, with some studies showing great prognostic value (Table 32-4) and others showing that these tests do not perform better than the basic clinical evaluation. In 2002, the American Heart

TABLE 32-4

SUMMARY OF CLINICAL CHARACTERISTICS AND SENSITIVITY AND SPECIFICITY OF THE STUDIES INCLUDED IN THE META-ANALYSIS

TYPE OF TEST	NO. OF STUDIES	NO. OF PATIENTS	MEAN AGE (YEARS)	PROPORTION OF MEN (%)	HISTORY OF CAD (%)	PROPORTION OF DM (%)	SENSITIVITY (%; 95% CI)	SPECIFICITY (%; 95% CI)
Radionuclide ventriculography	8	532	67.0	83	45	25	50 (32 to 69)	91 (87 to 96)
Ambulatory electrocardiography	8	893	68.0	72	55	32	52 (21 to 84)	70 (57 to 83)
Exercise electrocardiography	7	685	64.5	72	36	28	74 (60 to 88)	69 (60 to 78)
Dipyridamole stress echocardiography	4	850	66.8	78	28	33	74 (53 to 94)	86 (80 to 93)
Myocardial perfusion scintigraphy	23	3,119	65.5	78	40	30	83 (77 to 89)	49 (41 to 57)
Dobutamine stress echocardiography	8	1,877	67.3	76	37	16	85 (74 to 97)	70 (62 to 79)

Tests are sorted according to ascending sensitivities.
CAD, coronary artery disease; CI, confidence interval; DM, diabetes mellitus.
From Kertai MD, Boersma E, Bax JJ, et al. A meta-analysis comparing the prognostic accuracy of six diagnostic tests for predicting perioperative cardiac risk in patients undergoing major vascular surgery. Heart. 2003 Nov;89(11):1327–34.

Association and American College of Cardiology (AHA/ACC) published revised guidelines for perioperative cardiovascular evaluation before noncardiac surgery.[21] The algorithm incorporates clinical history, exercise tolerance, and surgical procedure in the decision to perform further evaluation. Application of Bayes' theorem also suggests that as the prior probability of a disease in a population increases, the predictive value of a positive test increases and predictive value of a negative test decreases. The guidelines classified the clinical predictors of increased perioperative cardiovascular risk (MI, CHF, and death) as "major," "intermediate," and "minor." The major risk factors include acute MI (<7 days), recent MI (7 to 30 days), unstable angina, decompensated CHF, and significant arrhythmias. Major risk factors, when present, mandate intensive management, which may result in delay or cancellation of surgery unless it is emergent. "Intermediate risk factors" include current or prior angina pectoris, prior MI, CHF, advanced age (70 years or older), severely limited exercise tolerance, chronic renal insufficiency (serum creatinine >2.0 mg%), cerebrovascular accident, and diabetes (preoperative insulin therapy) as risk factors for the development of perioperative cardiac morbidity.[22] Generally, patients presenting for vascular surgery can be categorized by these clinical criteria as follows: at least 1 risk factor, "low risk"; 2 risk factors, "intermediate risk"; 3 or more risk factors, "high risk." The guidelines placed aortic and peripheral vascular surgery in the "high-risk" surgery category with an estimated cardiac risk (MI or cardiac-related death) exceeding 5%. CEA is regarded as the "intermediate-risk" category, with an estimated cardiac risk ranging from 1 to 5%. By applying the principles of Bayes' theorem, traditional recommendations made more than a decade ago proposed the use of noninvasive cardiac testing in patients with intermediate clinical risk category, "no testing" in low clinical risk category, and coronary angiography in high clinical risk category and in those tested positive by noninvasive test. However, the current recommendations seem to have shifted the paradigm toward perioperative drug therapy aimed at reducing the cardiac risk either with no noninvasive cardiac testing or only very highly selective noninvasive testing.[23] Studies where the AHA/ACC guidelines were used to guide preoperative testing have conflicted as to whether using the guidelines can improve outcome. Figure 32-2 summarizes our recommendations for vascular surgery patients.

Dipyridamole-thallium scintigraphy is based on the principle of coronary steal. Dipyridamole is an antiplatelet drug and a coronary artery vasodilator. At rest, coronary arteries supplying the normal myocardium have a great vasodilatory reserve and are able to increase blood flow up to 10 times the normal to meet any extra demand. In the areas of critical stenosis, however, the coronary arteries are vasodilated in nonstressed state and have diminished reserve. Therefore, dipyridamole can vasodilate normal coronary arteries but cannot vasodilate those in areas with stenosis. When thallium radioisotope is injected, stenotic areas of myocardium will have lower concentration of the isotope (cold spot) after dipyridamole administration. When the effect of dipyridamole wears off, the isotope redistributes to ischemic zones. These areas with redistribution are considered ischemic but viable zones, whereas those with persistent defects with no redistribution are indicative of infarction. Both redistribution (reversible) and persistent (fixed) defects may be abnormal test results. Reversible defects are more important in risk stratification.

CHF is a strong predictor of morbid postoperative events. Determination of systolic left ventricular function may therefore provide prognostic information. In the past, some clinicians would place a pulmonary artery catheter preoperatively to measure hemodynamics and perform risk stratification. This approach is rarely used today because catheter placement requires preoperative admission to an ICU, and most patients are now admitted on the day of surgery. In addition, preoperative transthoracic echocardiography can provide noninvasive preoperative evaluation of cardiac function. Pulmonary artery catheterization may still occasionally prove useful for preoperative optimization of unstable patients who require relatively urgent surgery; however, more recently, its use and safety have been increasingly questioned.

Radionuclide ventriculography can be used to define systolic and diastolic function. Our meta-analysis showed that patients who have an ejection fraction <35% by radionuclide ventriculography are 3.7 times more likely to have a postoperative cardiac event.[24] However, radionuclide ventriculography has generally been supplanted by echocardiography, which can define myocardial structure and function, and can also be combined with exercise or pharmacologic stress.

Dobutamine (5 to 30 μg/kg/min, with or without atropine) stress echocardiography (DSE) can produce changes in regional wall motion in patients with underlying CAD. In our meta-analysis, we found that a positive dobutamine stress test increased the risk of a postoperative cardiac event by 6.2-fold. Semiquantitative interpretation (high-risk, intermediate-risk, or low-risk results) of both dipyridamole-thallium scintigraphy and DSE may allow us to refer only high-risk patients for cardiac catheterization. By convention, marked changes in prior disease probability can be assumed in likelihood ratio (LR) for positive test exceeding 10.0 and LR for negative test falling below 0.1. Abnormality in five or more segments during DSE is considered as "strongly-positive" test result for risk stratification with a likelihood ratio of 13.09. Redistribution in >50% of the left ventricle during DTS has an LR of 11. Therefore, although severely positive patients might benefit from coronary angiography and revascularization, less severe cases of CAD identified by weakly positive (low-risk) results on these tests may benefit from current state-of-the-art perioperative care and risk reduction. However, these less severe cases will still require careful follow-up after surgery to look for progression of CAD. These results have been largely corroborated by another more recent meta-analysis, which suggests that DSE may be the best preoperative test.[25]

Endothelial dysfunction as evaluated preoperatively by noninvasive ultrasound assessment of brachial artery flow-mediated dilation is useful in predicting the short-term and long-term adverse cardiovascular outcomes following vascular surgery.[26] Decreased endothelium-dependent flow-mediated dilation reflects endothelial dysfunction in patients with AVD. Coronary calcium detected by CT is a hallmark of CAD and has been shown to predict MI following vascular surgery.[27]

One limitation of specialized testing, including coronary angiography, is the fact that MI and cardiac-related mortality are not necessarily due to severely narrowed coronary arteries. More recent evidence suggests that the rupture of previously nonocclusive lipid-laden, macrophage-rich coronary plaques can cause spasm and initiate unstable angina, acute MI, and sudden death. Therefore, testing that attempts to induce ischemia will miss some patients who have nonobstructive plaques that can rupture and cause transmural infarction; this appears to be the mechanism of a significant minority of perioperative MI.

Preoperative Coronary Revascularization

Myocardial revascularization may have long-term benefits in patients with triple-vessel coronary disease or poor left ventricular function. The range of options for preparatory coronary revascularization continues to expand. These include traditional surgical revascularization (CABG) with or without cardiopulmonary bypass (CPB), transmyocardial laser therapy, and PTCA with or without coronary stent placement. However, mortality rates associated with these techniques are

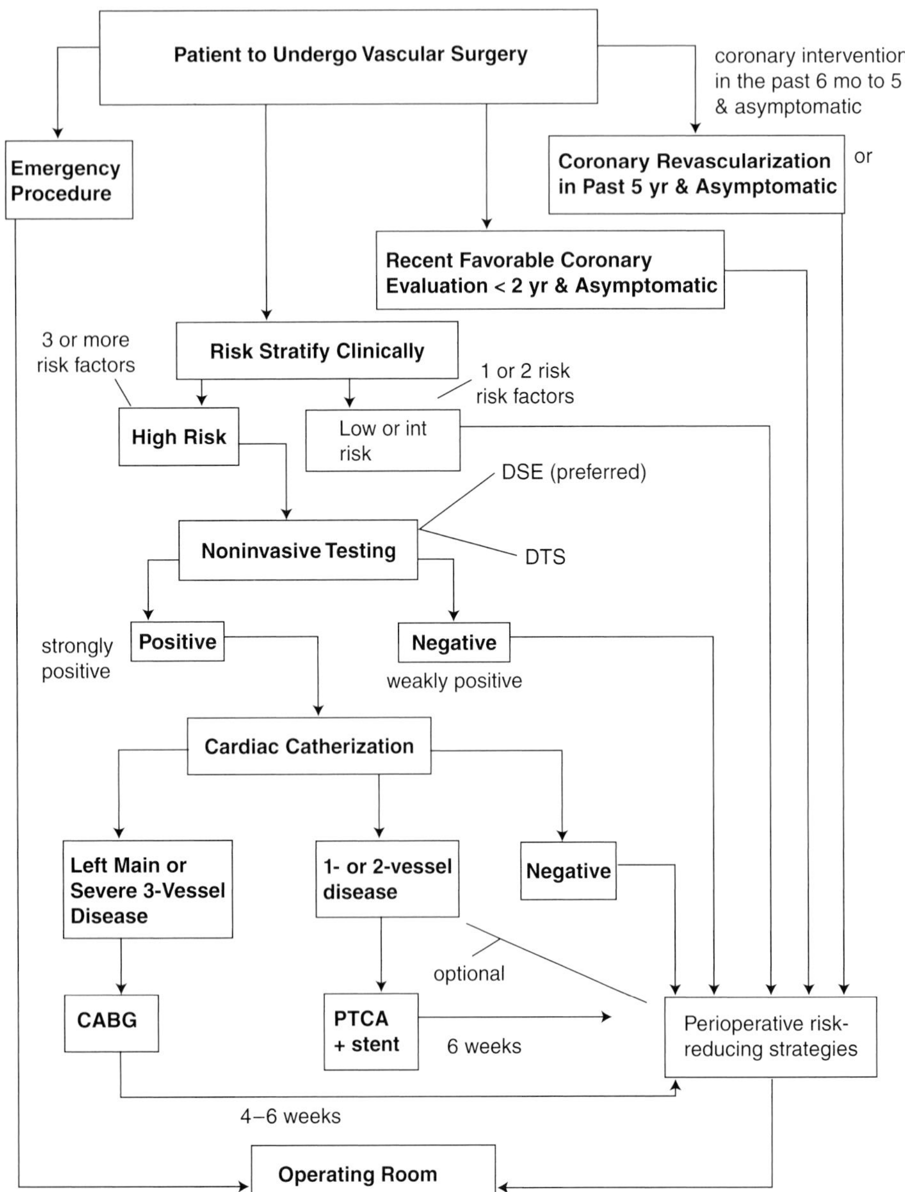

FIGURE 32-2. Our recommended algorithm for preoperative assessment. This may change as future randomized trials compare aggressive medical therapy with coronary revascularization. CABG, coronary artery bypass graft; DSE, dobutamine stress echocardiography; DTS, dipyridamole thallium scan; PTCA, percutaneous transluminal coronary angioplasty.

consistently higher in patients with peripheral vascular disease compared with those without.

Initial observational studies of PTCA performed before major noncardiac surgery suggest that patients who survive successful PTCA do well. Anticoagulation and antiplatelet therapy may be continued after these procedures and may preclude the use of regional anesthesia. Stent thrombosis and increased surgical bleeding from clopidogrel are concerns in the patient with a recent coronary stent.

Whether preoperative coronary revascularization actually protects against the perioperative cardiac events is controversial. The benefits likely diminish as time goes on; CABG more than 5 years or PTCA more than 2 years before vascular surgery may actually be associated with a high risk of complications because CAD is a recurrent disease.[28] Even if one considers coronary revascularization to be protective, an obligate delay in performing the planned vascular surgical procedure must be considered. Once the patient has recovered from successful coronary revascularization (1 week after angioplasty and 6 to 8 weeks after coronary stenting or CABG, typically), peripheral vascular surgery is usually then performed. In some cases, CABG can be combined with vascular surgery, most commonly with CEA. However, patients with both symptomatic coronary and carotid disease are at high risk of both cardiac and neurologic complications following surgery, whether combined or
3 staged; their management remains controversial.[29] The multicenter CARP trial randomized patients with coronary disease (except left main disease or ejection fraction <20%) before elective vascular surgery to either coronary revascularization or medical therapy. With state-of-the-art aggressive medical therapy (>80% of patients on beta-blockers, >70% on aspirin, and >50% on statins in both groups), they could find no benefit to coronary revascularization.[30] This trial may contribute further to the trend of aggressive prophylactic treatment rather than routine stress testing of vascular surgery patients.

Perioperative Cardiac Monitoring

The goals of perioperative cardiac monitoring are to detect myocardial ischemia and to identify abnormalities of preload, afterload, and ventricular function. Such monitoring may prevent MI and allow better perfusion and preservation of other organs such as the liver, kidney, gut, and spinal cord.

Detection of Perioperative Myocardial Ischemia

ECG monitoring remains the mainstay of perioperative detection of myocardial ischemia. ECG evidence of ST segment depression is a more common indicator of myocardial ischemia in vascular surgery patients than is ST segment elevation. ST segment depression occurs in 20 to 50% of patients undergoing vascular surgery. Landesberg et al. documented that a multilead system is required to detect ischemia (V3, V4, V5 for maximal detection). Further, leads V3 to V4 have a higher incidence and a greater degree of maximal myocardial ischemia than does lead V5.[31] Because clinicians often fail to detect intraoperative ischemic ECG changes when viewing oscilloscopes, automated ST segment monitors promise to increase the detection of such ECG changes. We have documented that the sensitivity of ST segment monitors for transesophageal echocardiography (TEE)-diagnosed myocardial ischemia is 40% and for ECG-diagnosed ischemia, 75%.[32] Although these monitors are not always accurate, we believe they are useful as alarms for busy clinicians.

Perioperative Holter monitoring has shown that the intraoperative period may be the least stressful for patients with CAD. Patients undergoing vascular surgery are most likely to manifest myocardial ischemia in the immediate postoperative period, with its associated pain, adrenergic stress, hypothermia, hypercoagulability, anemia, shivering, and sleep deprivation. Several studies have shown that postoperative myocardial ischemia begins earlier than previously believed, usually on the day of vascular surgery or the next day. At present, our clinical practice is to obtain a 12-lead ECG in the first 24 hours following surgery in high-risk patients, and then perhaps daily for the next 2 to 3 days. We believe such a strategy will detect most ischemia that is severe and protracted enough to represent a prodrome to infarction. Unfortunately, many vascular surgery patients will have baseline ECG abnormalities (left bundle branch block, paced rhythm, digoxin effect, left ventricular hypertrophy with strain) that preclude the detection of myocardial ischemia.

Other monitoring devices for detecting myocardial ischemia have been proposed. Pulmonary capillary wedge pressure (PCWP) monitoring in patients undergoing vascular surgery has low sensitivity and specificity in detecting ischemia; most elevations in PCWP appear to be associated with tachycardia and hypertension, which suggests inadequate anesthesia. Our own group found that 90% of patients developed wall motion abnormalities on TEE when the aorta was cross-clamped above the celiac artery. However, the PCWP remained normal in >80% of these episodes.[33] We therefore do not routinely use PCWP as a monitor for myocardial ischemia, but we believe the pulmonary artery catheter provides useful information about a patient's intravascular volume status, myocardial performance, and organ perfusion.

TEE has also been proposed as a monitor for intraoperative myocardial ischemia. In animal studies and in models of coronary angioplasty during balloon inflation, mechanical dysfunction precedes surface ECG changes when myocardial ischemia is produced. Supporting these observations, Smith et al.[34] found that regional wall motion abnormalities were more sensitive than ST segment change on the ECG in detecting intraoperative ischemia in patients with CAD undergoing major vascular and coronary surgery. However, others have concluded that ischemia monitoring with TEE during noncardiac surgery appeared to have little incremental clinical value over preoperative clinical data and Holter monitoring in predicting perioperative ischemic outcomes.

Traditionally, creatine kinase myocardial band isoenzyme determination has been used to document myocardial damage after vascular surgery. Limitations of this method include false-positive results owing to skeletal muscle damage during surgery. The cardiac troponins appear to offer increased sensitivity, primarily because of their prolonged diagnostic window, and may offer enhanced specificity in patients with surgical skeletal muscle damage. Troponin leak after vascular surgery dramatically increases perioperative and 6-month MI and death risk, with a dose-response relationship; in this study, 12% of patients had postoperative cTnI > 1.5 ng/mL, which was associated with a 6-fold increased risk of 6-month mortality and a 27-fold increased risk of MI.[20]

Management of Perioperative Myocardial Ischemia and Infarction in Vascular Patients

In the modern era, rates of MI in patients undergoing major vascular surgery can be reduced to <10%, but the rates are significantly lower for patients undergoing elective vascular repair. Perioperative myocardial ischemias (PMIs) are much more likely to occur in patients undergoing urgent or emergent surgery, who are presumably sicker and do not have the luxury of undergoing extensive preoperative evaluation and preparation. MIs in the modern era are more likely to occur in the first 24 hours following surgery. Badner et al. found that 5.6% of patients with known CAD undergoing major surgery had a PMI, of which 17% were fatal. Only 3 of 18 patients had chest pain, whereas 10 of 18 patients (56%) had other clinical findings. The PMIs occurred on the day of operation in nearly one-half the cases.[19] Patients who have PMIs after vascular surgery have a mortality of approximately 20% in a series at the Cleveland Clinic; Sprung et al. stated,

> The in-hospital cardiac mortality rate is high for patients who undergo vascular surgery and experience clinically significant PMI. Stress of surgery (increased intraoperative bleeding and aortic, peripheral vascular, and emergency surgery), poor preoperative cardiac functional status (CHF, lower ejection fraction, diagnosis of CAD), and preoperative history of coronary artery bypass grafting (protective) are the factors that determine perioperative cardiac morbidity and mortality rates.[35]

Stable coronary ischemic syndromes presumably occur with increased oxygen demand by the myocardium in a setting of fixed coronary plaques. Unstable syndromes are believed to be the result of active lesions caused by plaque rupture with local thrombus and vasoreactivity that produce intermittent critical decreases in coronary oxygen supply. The period following vascular surgery is characterized by adrenergic stress (Fig. 32-3).[36] The postoperative adrenergic response can predispose to myocardial ischemia in numerous ways, including tachycardia and decreased diastolic time, coronary vasoconstriction, and platelet aggregation. Factors increasing the likelihood of postoperative myocardial ischemia that the anesthesiologist can control include tachycardia, hypertension, hypotension, anemia, hypothermia, shivering, endotracheal suctioning, and less than optimal analgesia. Other factors, such as postoperative hypercoagulability, rapid eye movement (REM) sleep rebound, and mild postoperative hypoxemia are more speculative culprits.

Postoperative myocardial ischemia confers increased risk to vascular surgical patients. Landesberg et al. found that patients experienced twice as much ischemia after vascular surgery than before or during.[37] Ischemia that lasted longer than 2 hours was associated with a 32-fold increase in the risk of postoperative morbid cardiac events. In this study, postoperative MI was usually preceded by long periods of severe ST segment depression. Aggressive efforts at prevention or treatment of ischemia

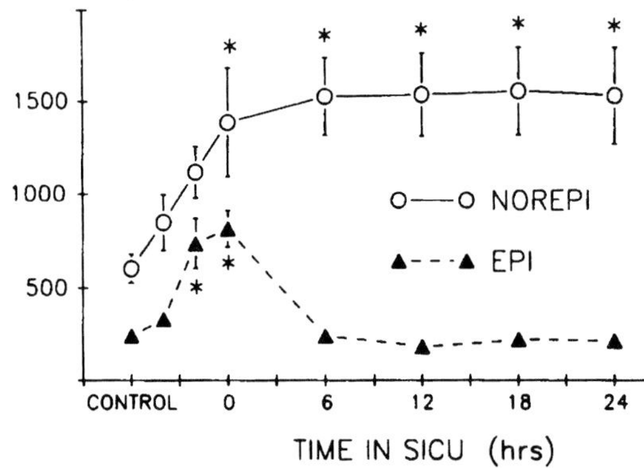

FIGURE 32-3. Aortic reconstructive surgery is associated with markedly elevated adrenergic tone. Epinephrine levels (pg/mL) rise with emergence from anesthesia but begin to fall by 6 hr after surgery. Norepinephrine levels (pg/mL) remain elevated for at least 1 day following surgery. SICU, Surgical ICU; NOREPI, norepinephrine; EPI, epinephrine. (Reprinted with permission from Breslow MJ: The role of stress hormones in perioperative myocardial ischemia. Int Anesthesiol Clin 30:81, 1992.)

during these periods may improve patient outcome. We refer patients with documented severe postoperative myocardial ischemia (lasting longer than 2 hours; 2 mm ST segment depression) to a cardiologist because most adverse cardiac outcomes in a 2-year follow-up program were preceded by in-hospital postoperative ischemia.

Various strategies have been proposed to reduce cardiac morbidity during and after vascular surgery, including the prophylactic use of antianginal drugs and special anesthetic techniques. It is crucial that patients continue to receive their chronic antianginal and antihypertensive medications before and after surgery.

4 Of the various risk-reducing strategies (Table 32-5), growing evidence suggests that perioperative beta-blockade provides benefit in preventing cardiac morbidity and mortality.[38,39] Benefits of the therapy are best observed when oral preoperative therapy is extended to intraoperative and postoperative periods by intravenous therapy to titrate the heart rate $\leq$65 beats/minute. Typically, oral therapy has been initiated 7 to 30 days before surgery with either 50 to 100 mg atenolol daily or 5 to 10 mg of bisoprolol,[40] whereas intraoperative and postoperative periods are best managed by intravenous administration of 5 to 10 mg atenolol or metoprolol twice daily. Alternatively, esmolol 500 μg/kg may be given intravenously over 1 minute followed by infusion of 50 to 300 μg/kg per minute to achieve the target heart rate. In patients already taking beta-blockers, they are continued to the day of surgery followed by intravenous therapy to achieve the target heart rate as described previously. Although older literature warns against use with any degree of reactive airway disease, insulin-dependent diabetes, and even peripheral vascular disease, newer data suggest that careful titration of β1-selective agents is well tolerated in many of these patients. However, severe asthma or a strong reversible component with chronic obstructive airway disease remains a major contraindication, as do cardiac conduction disease in the absence of a pacemaker and previous documented drug

TABLE 32-5

PHARMACOLOGIC PROPHYLAXIS AGAINST ACUTE VASCULAR EVENTS IN PATIENTS UNDERGOING VASCULAR SURGERY

INTERVENTION	REGIMEN AND REMARKS	RECOMMENDATION[a]
Perioperative beta-blockade	Preoperative oral beta-1-selective beta-blocker (bisoprolol, metoprolol, or atenolol) initiated at least 30 d before surgery and IV therapy during intraoperative and postoperative period (metoprolol, atenolol, or esmolol).	Class I
Alpha-2-agonists	Pretreatment with oral clonidine 300 μg at least 90 min before surgery and therapy continued for 72 hr (oral or transdermal, 0.2 mg/d). IV clonidine 300 μg daily can also be administered for 72 hr.	Class IIa
Statin therapy	Typical dose of atorvastatin is 20 mg once daily initiated at least 45 d prior to surgery. Continued use after surgery for at least 2 wk. Statin use is also associated with improved graft patency, limb salvage, and decreased amputation rate in patients undergoing infrainguinal bypass for atherosclerotic vascular disease.	Class I
ACE inhibitors	Potential benefits include decreased stroke rate (e.g., ramipril), limitation of ventricular remodeling that follows acute ST elevation MI, decreased long-term mortality following infrainguinal bypass surgery, etc. Ability to stabilize the atherosclerotic plaque by upregulating type III collagen of the fibrous cap of the unstable plaque may explain some of these benefits.	Class IIb
Calcium channel blockers	Reduced perioperative adverse cardiac events; including supraventricular tachycardia in patients undergoing various types of noncardiac surgery (primarily diltiazem). Evidence limited in patients undergoing vascular surgery.	Class IIb
Nitroglycerin	Not indicated for myocardial ischemia prophylaxis or initial treatment. May be used to treat arterial hypertension or elevated cardiac filling pressures or suspected coronary vasospasm	Class III

ACE, angiotension converting enzyme; MI, myocardial infarction.

[a]Class I recommendation refers to conditions for which there is evidence or general agreement that a given procedure or treatment is useful or effective, class III refers to conditions for which there is evidence and/or general agreement that the procedure/treatment is not useful/effective or in some cases may be harmful. Class II recommendations fall in between and indicate conditions for which there is conflicting evidence or a divergence of opinion about the usefulness/efficacy of a procedure/treatment. Class IIa indicates that the weight of evidence/opinion is in favor of usefulness/efficacy. Class IIb indicates that the usefulness/efficacy is less well established by evidence/opinion. In simple terms, class I recommendations are the "dos," class III recommendations are "don'ts," and class II recommendations are the "maybes." Refer to Figure 32-2 for the algorithm. Calcium channel blockers and ACE inhibitors, although not recommended as independent agents for the purpose, should be continued if a patient is receiving them. Refer to Table 32-1 for suggestions for precautions on their perioperative use.

sensitivities. It must be noted that hypovolemia can be poorly tolerated in the presence of beta-blockade and also that racial difference in response to beta-blockade can exist (Blacks may respond less favorably).[39]

Alpha-2-adrenergic blockers (clonidine or mivazerol) have been in use aimed at controlling the perioperative cardiac morbidity and mortality for more than a decade. In our study, we used a regimen of a transdermal clonidine system (0.2 mg/day) the night prior to surgery, which was left in place for 72 hours, and 0.3 mg oral clonidine administered 60 to 90 minutes before surgery. Clondine not only reduced intraoperative myocardial ischemia, but also reduced catecholamine (adrenaline and noradrenaline) levels as measured on the first postoperative day.[41] More recently, a meta-analysis demonstrated beneficial effects of perioperative alpha-blockers with regard to cardiac morbidity and death in patients undergoing vascular surgery (evidence level B).[42] In addition, a randomized trial suggested that perioperative clonidine administration during high-risk noncardiac surgery reduces mortality[43] in a fashion similar to atenolol.

Interest has more recently focused on the use of statins aimed at controlling adverse cardiac events perioperatively and on those occurring during long-term follow-up for vascular surgery patients. A randomized trial demonstrated beneficial effects of statin use (atorvastatin 20 mg daily started 30 days before surgery and continued for roughly 2 weeks after surgery) with regard to primary end points (cardiac-related death, nonfatal MI, unstable angina, stroke) at 6-month follow-up.[44]

ACE inhibitors also have several beneficial actions with regard to acute vascular events independent of their antihypertensive action in patients with atherosclerotic vascular disease. Currently, there are no studies to provide evidence for their independent ability to reduce perioperative cardiac problems for their therapy aimed at risk reduction. However, if a patient is already taking ACE inhibitors, he or she is best to continue, taking care to limit the morning dose of the drug.

A more recent meta-analysis suggested beneficial effects of calcium channel blockers in reducing perioperative adverse cardiac events (cardiac-related death, MI, ischemia, or supraventricular tachycardia) in patients undergoing different types of noncardiac surgery. The majority of these effects were attributable to diltiazem. Limited evidence was available from this meta-analysis for patients undergoing vascular surgery. Large randomized trials are required to establish their benefits in vascular surgery patients. Currently, we do not recommend their use as independent drug therapeutic modality for the perioperative cardiac risk reduction. Similarly, prophylactic intravenous nitroglycerin 0.9 μg/kg/min failed to reduce the incidence of PMI in patients with known or suspected CAD undergoing noncardiac surgery.[45] In this study, the preponderance of myocardial ischemia occurred during emergence from anesthesia, which is associated with acute increases in heart rate.

High-dose narcotic anesthetics reduce the stress response and may improve overall outcome after major surgery. Postoperative infusion of sufentanil 1 μg/kg/hr can reduce the severity of myocardial ischemia (ST segment changes) following CABG, although clinical outcome was not improved. High-dose narcotics may mandate overnight ventilation, which may not be cost effective. Another approach using intensive analgesia involves the use of epidural analgesia. Epidural local anesthetics may reduce perioperative myocardial ischemia because preload and afterload are reduced, the postoperative adrenergic and coagulation responses are reduced, and, with thoracic administration, the coronary arteries are dilated. Despite these effects on intermediate variables, improvement in cardiac outcomes has generally not been demonstrated in well-designed trials, suggesting that anesthetic technique does not affect cardiac outcome after abdominal aortic surgery, especially if heart rate is well controlled in the ICU.[46] Concerns about respiratory depression, neuraxial/epidural hematomas, and the expense and reimbursement for surveillance have limited the use of peridural narcotics in greater numbers of patients. Although epidural anesthesia may improve outcome in other organ systems, especially the lungs, its ability to reduce MI remains speculative. Last, a meta-analysis suggests that thoracic epidurals may reduce PMI.[47]

Given the prominent role of coronary thrombosis in causing acute coronary syndromes and the hypercoagulable state after vascular surgery, future development in the treatment of postoperative myocardial ischemia may include drugs with antiplatelet or anticoagulant effects, such as aspirin and newer platelet inhibitors, warfarin, or heparin. Increased postoperative hemorrhage, however, makes the use of anticoagulant therapy problematic in surgical patients. At present, we do not know how to balance these risks and benefits, or which patients might benefit most from such therapy.

Anemia (hematocrit <28%) may increase the incidence of postoperative myocardial ischemia and cardiac events in high-risk patients undergoing noncardiac surgery.[48] Therefore, we are more likely to transfuse high-risk patients, or those who demonstrate myocardial ischemia with packed red blood cells, to augment the hematocrit to 30%. We continue this practice, although some work in ICU patients (with a relatively low percentage of patients with CAD) suggests that lower transfusion thresholds may be beneficial.[49] Hypothermia is also associated with increased adrenergic tone and postoperative myocardial ischemia and events in vascular surgery patients.[50] We therefore aggressively warm patients and conserve heat during and after such surgery. Suctioning, extubation, and weaning from mechanical ventilation may also produce myocardial ischemia. Therefore, we attempt to extubate patients in the operating room with the same attention to the control of hemodynamics as during induction. If patients require postoperative ventilation, we provide adequate sedation, analgesia, and occasionally even paralysis (which can prevent shivering and its attendant increases in oxygen consumption). We treat tachycardia aggressively, most often with β-adrenergic blocking agents, while we attempt to correct other potential causes such as fever, pain, anemia, and hypovolemia.

Occasionally, in patients with evolving MI, we have resorted to using an intra-aortic balloon pump (IABP) to improve coronary blood flow while decreasing workload. Definitive studies of its effectiveness are lacking, and IABP placement can be difficult and risky in patients with peripheral vascular disease. We have also referred some patients to interventional cardiologists immediately after surgery for emergent cardiac catheterization, selective thrombolysis, and PTCA for unstable angina or evolving postoperative MI.

Other Medical Problems in Vascular Surgery Patients

Hypertension occurs in the majority of vascular surgery patients and may produce end-organ damage to the heart and kidneys. One benefit of the modern system of same-day admission is that it allows us to interview many patients in a preanesthesia clinic a week or so before surgery. At that time, if hypertension is poorly controlled, we consult with the patient's internist or cardiologist and adjust or begin the antihypertensive regimen. Most often, this is accomplished with oral doses of atenolol or metoprolol 25 to 200 mg daily, which we may start in our clinic. Additional risk-reducing therapy prescribed more commonly by internists or cardiologists may include ACE inhibitors and statin drugs. Lowering blood pressure gradually in this way before surgery allows for restoration of normal intravascular volume and results in a more stable perioperative course. In the past few decades, many clinicians have chosen to postpone surgery in patients with elevated blood pressure before surgery, regardless of whether they receive chronic treatment for hypertension. A more recent meta-analysis of 30 observational trials of cardiovascular outcomes after surgery in hypertensive patients suggests a statistically but "not clinically significant" increase in events.[51]

Diabetic patients have a greatly increased risk for peripheral vascular disease. Aggressive chronic treatment to maintain euglycemia promotes wound healing and forestalls retinopathy and the development of proteinuria, but its effects on the progression of large vessel peripheral vascular disease and CAD are unknown. Coronary disease is ubiquitous in diabetic patients requiring vascular surgery. Diabetic patients generally have higher risks of MI and wound infection compared with nondiabetics undergoing abdominal aortic aneurysm. The dramatic increase in the risk of postoperative death (7%) in diabetic patients with autonomic neuropathy suggests that simple tests to identify such patients might be part of the preoperative workup.[52] Patients with diabetes and severe CAD may live longer if they undergo CABG rather than PTCA. We are especially fastidious about glucose management during carotid and thoracic aortic procedures, where hyperglycemia may exacerbate neurologic injury. In addition, more recent randomized trials and large observational trials have suggested mortality reduction in surgical ICU patients and improved outcomes in cardiovascular surgery when insulin infusions are used to provide "tight" glucose control.[53] Possible mechanisms of these beneficial effects include reduced immunosupression, maintenance of ischemic preconditioning, improved cholesterol and fat metabolism, reduced inflammatory mediators, reduced free radical production, reduced nitric oxide scavenging and less hypercoagulability. More recent studies suggest that best results may be obtained by keeping glucose <110 mg/dL. Although in the past our practice was to give one-half the morning dose of insulin and treat with "sliding scale" insulin to keep glucose 150 to 200, we are now more likely to employ insulin infusions, usually at 1 to 2 U/hour, especially in those patients who will be in an ICU after surgery. We attempt to maintain a glucose <150 mg/dL. Frequent monitoring of glucose levels is required in patients receiving insulin infusions.

Patients with peripheral vascular disease may have hypercoagulable states. Hypercoagulable states are more common in younger patients presenting for vascular surgery and in those with vascular thrombosis in unusual locations. Hypercoagulable responses to surgery may also predispose patients to vascular graft occlusion after surgery. Postoperative abnormalities include elevated fibrinogen levels, antithrombin III deficiency, impaired fibrinolysis, protein C deficiency, and protein S deficiency. HIT can occur paradoxically on an immunologic basis (IgG) after several days of exposure to heparin.[13] Treatment includes cessation of all heparin, full anticoagulation with argatroban, and 3 weeks of Coumadin to prevent arterial thrombosis. Coumadin alone is not recommended as it depletes protein C and may increase thrombosis.

Patients with peripheral vascular disease have frequently abused tobacco. Preoperative spirometry may help identify patients likely to have postoperative pulmonary complications. In vascular surgery patients, the incidence of postoperative pulmonary complications (pneumonia, ventilator dependence >48 hours, or the adult respiratory distress syndrome) may be significant. Patients with forced expiratory volume in 1 second (FEV_1) <2.0 L/sec have a much higher incidence of pulmonary complications. Not surprisingly, respiratory failure was much more common in patients undergoing repair of aortic aneurysm than surgery for lower-extremity occlusive disease or for carotid procedures. Chronic obstructive pulmonary disease (COPD) is more common in patients with aortic aneurysms than in patients presenting for other vascular surgery.[54]

Renal insufficiency or failure exists in many patients who present for arterial reconstruction. Patients with preexisting renal insufficiency have an increased risk of postoperative renal failure, as well as cardiac complications and death. Postoperative renal failure markedly increases the chance of death. If patients receive chronic dialysis treatments, we prefer that they receive dialysis on the day before or the same day as surgery. Some patients will actually be hypovolemic as a result, which can contribute to hypotension upon induction of general or regional anesthesia. Many dialysis patients receive recombinant erythropoietin, which normally increases the hematocrit to ~30%. Left ventricular hypertrophy and mitral annular calcification are more common in dialysis patients and may predispose to pulmonary edema in the perioperative period; ECG and echocardiography may help the clinician to make these diagnoses. In addition, we usually seek laboratory and electrocardiographic evidence of hyperkalemia, and avoid succinylcholine when possible if we suspect hyperkalemia. We are careful when positioning patients to avoid putting pressure on the arm used for hemodialysis; we also do not measure blood pressure in that arm. Vascular access may be difficult in patients who have had multiple arteriovenous fistulae placed for hemodialysis. Central venous access may be more difficult in those who have had multiple central venous dialysis catheters. We also anticipate a more difficult abdominal dissection in some patients who have received peritoneal dialysis.

CAROTID ENDARTERECTOMY

Anesthetic management of CEA involves attempts to optimize cerebral perfusion in patients with a high prevalence of CAD. During the period of interruption of flow to allow vascular repair, cerebral ischemia may occur. Approaches to this problem include preoperative testing to predict cerebral ischemic potential, routine shunting of every patient, neurologic monitoring of the awake patient, and specialized intraoperative testing. These specialized tests detect electrical integrity (electroencephalogram [EEG], somatosensory-evoked potential [SSEP], auditory-evoked potentials), flow velocities (transcranial Doppler), and perfusion (jugular vein oxygenation, stump pressure, and cerebral oximetry). Specialized testing or evaluation of the awake patient is undertaken in the hopes of limiting shunting to only those patients believed likely to benefit.

In addition to traditional CEA, carotid angioplasty and stenting (CAS) is increasingly used. The challenge for angioplasty is to limit stroke from distal embolization of plaque. It has been shown with transcranial Doppler that embolic events are far more common with angioplasty as compared with CEA[55] but may not be associated with increased rates of cognitive dysfunction.[56] "Umbrella" devices that allow capture of embolic particles may improve the results of angioplasty. The ischemic time for angioplasty and stenting, however, is much shorter than for CEA, which may have benefits. Large randomized trials have more recently been reported, with initial promising results for stenting compared with traditional CEA.

Carotid atherosclerosis is the leading cause of extracranial vascular cerebral events. Carotid disease is bilateral in about one-half of all cases. Atherosclerotic plaque usually develops at the lateral aspect of the carotid artery bifurcation (where shear stress is lowest), and commonly extends into the internal and external carotid arteries. The disease is primarily a problem of embolization and rarely occlusion or insufficiency. Plaque rupture or embolization can lead to transient ischemic attack (TIA)/cerebrovascular accident (CVA). Risk factors for carotid disease include advanced age, hypertension, and tobacco abuse. Elevated serum lipid levels and a history of diabetes mellitus are less powerful predictors. Patients with left main CAD and other peripheral vascular disease are also more likely to have carotid disease.

Carotid disease may manifest itself only as an asymptomatic bruit, or as amaurosis fugax (transient attacks of monocular blindness) when the ophthalmic artery is embolized. Other patients may experience episodes of paresthesias, clumsiness of the extremities, or speech problems, which resolve spontaneously after a short period of time. These are the classic TIAs. The differentiation between a TIA and a reversible ischemic neurologic deficit (RIND) is one of degree and is somewhat arbitrary. A TIA resolves within 24 hours, whereas a RIND will last longer than 24 hours before complete resolution.

An isolated, cervical bruit in asymptomatic patients also seems to be associated with a higher risk of stroke, but the correlation between the location of the bruits and the type of subsequent stroke is poor. A bruit per se does not define the presence of a critical carotid lesion, nor are critical carotid lesions always associated with bruits. Therefore, a bruit may prompt further testing. The most common noninvasive test is the duplex scan, which combines B-mode anatomic imaging and pulse Doppler spectral analysis of blood flow velocity. The presence of high velocities and turbulent flow is used to predict the extent of carotid stenosis. The accuracy of duplex scanning reaches 95% in experienced hands when compared with angiography. Angiography provides measurements of the size and morphology of the atheromatous plaque and can also document aortic arch or intracranial disease, which may occur in conjunction with carotid disease and can cause strokes that are not prevented by CEA. Because of the risks of contrast angiography, most surgeons will now operate based on duplex findings and reserve angiography for special situations such as a string sign (pseudoocclusion of the extracranial internal carotid artery, a "diagnostic trap," often angiographically misdiagnosed as complete occlusion), or suspected proximal disease. Also, many surgeons use magnetic resonance angiography as the sole modality to detect disease.

There are pharmacologic and surgical treatments for carotid artery disease. Combined administration of aspirin and dipyridamole, when compared with placebo, reduces the incidence of TIAs more so than either drug alone.[57] More potent platelet inhibitors such a clopidogrel may offer further protection. Therefore, it is essential that patients presenting for CEA continue to receive aspirin and/or clopidogrel in the perioperative period. Discontinuation of these medications may promote perioperative thrombosis and stroke or other morbid cardiovascular events. In contrast, CEA, in conjunction with aspirin therapy, has proven superior to medical therapy alone in a large trial of symptomatic patients with a stenosis >70% in the North American trial (NASCET).[58] In this trial, major or fatal ipsilateral stroke was significantly reduced from 13.1% in the medical group to 2.5% in the surgical group. Estimates of the cumulative risk of any ipsilateral stroke at 2 years were 26% in the medical patients and 9% in the surgical patients. For asymptomatic patients with a stenosis of >60%, the Asymptomatic Carotid Atherosclerosis (ACAS) study also detected a substantial outcome benefit. However, the overall risk of stroke was lower in both medical and surgical groups than for symptomatic patients in NACSET. In ACAS, ipsilateral stroke and any perioperative stroke or death was estimated to be 11.0% for patients treated medically and 5.1% for surgical patients after 5 years.[59] Patients with ulcerated soft plaques seem to have a higher risk of stroke that approaches 7 to 8% per year. The serious nature of cerebrovascular disease is underscored by the fact that about one-third of all acute strokes are fatal and another third result in significant residual functional deficit. Of course, CEA is justifiable only if the operative morbidity and mortality are lower than the natural risk for ischemic events in the untreated patient. Also, repair of asymptomatic disease may not be beneficial in patients who do not have a reasonable chance of living 5 years. The number of asymptomatic patients who need to undergo CEA to prevent one stroke is approximately 20 to 40, leading some investigators to question its cost effectiveness in this setting. The guidelines published for CEA by the AHA were last revised in 1998.[60]

More recently, the SAPPHIRE trial of high-risk patients randomized to angioplasty plus stenting or traditional surgery reported noninferiority of stenting with a suggestion of important outcome benefits.[61] These benefits included a trend toward a lower cumulative incidence of a major cardiovascular event at 1 year—a composite of death, stroke, or MI within 30 days after the intervention or death or ipsilateral stroke between 31 days and 1 year. The primary end point occurred in 12.2% of patients randomly assigned to undergo carotid artery stenting and in 20.1% of patients randomly assigned to undergo endarterectomy ($P = .004$ for noninferiority, and $P = .053$ for superiority of stenting). It is important to point out that these results were obtained with the use of "umbrella" devices to retrieve atheromatous debris. Previous series of angioplasty and stenting performed without such protection were associated with high rates of asymptomatic (detected by transcranial Doppler and/or postprocedure surveillance magnetic resonance imaging [MRI]) and symptomatic distal embolization.[55] Patients will generally receive clopidogrel and aspirin before stenting, plus periprocedural heparin to maintain the activated clotting time (ACT) at twice normal. Others have added glycoprotein IIb–IIIa receptor inhibitors to their antithrombotic "cocktails." To prevent bradycardia and hypotension during balloon inflation and stent deployment, prophylactic atropine is often administered as a routine, although some centers choose to treat only after a patient evidences bradycardia.[62]

Factors that consistently predict neurologic and cardiac morbidity and mortality after CEA include age ≥75 years, experience of the surgeon, preoperative neurologic symptoms or previous stroke, history of angina, diastolic blood pressure >110 mm Hg, CEA performed in preparation for CABG, internal carotid artery thrombus, stenosis near the carotid siphon, or contralateral carotid occlusion. Patients undergoing CEA for lesions of the left carotid artery may suffer stroke more often, possibly due to technical difficulties, because most surgeons are right handed.

Preoperative Evaluation and Preparation

Although the most common cause of TIAs is occlusive carotid disease, other neurologic disease such as intracerebral tumor or cerebrovascular malformation may produce similar symptoms. Cardiac diseases also may produce neurologic symptoms, including atrial fibrillation, valvular heart disease, dilated cardiomyopathy, or an MI with akinetic ventricular segments leading to intracardiac thrombus formation and cerebral embolization. CAD is common in patients presenting for CEA. We are less likely to request special studies (DSE or dipyridamole-thallium scintigraphy) or cardiac catheterization before CEA than for other major vascular procedures. Our rationale is that CEA can prevent stroke, is less stressful, and does not result in death as frequently as other vascular operations. Indeed, it has been proposed that preoperative risk can be based not only on the presence of CAD, but also on the basis of exercise tolerance and extent of the surgical procedure.[21]

In the NASCET trial, the 30-day results were as follows: death, 1.1%; disabling stroke, 1.8%; nondisabling stroke, 3.7%; and cardiac death, 0.3%. These values are clearly lower than those reported for CABG, even in patients free of significant carotid disease. Therefore, it is difficult to recommend a CABG procedure to a patient with symptomatic carotid disease and stable coronary disease because the combined mortality and stroke rate after CABG may be higher than that of an expertly performed CEA. Cerebrovascular disease is associated with increased mortality after CABG. In contrast, patients who have had previous CABG may have lower mortality following CEA.

We therefore usually undertake CEA in patients for whom the operation offers benefits, even if they have stable CAD. Our classification of stable CAD is based on a thorough history, physical examination, and review of basic laboratory tests, not specialized testing. We do not delay urgent surgery that might prevent a stroke for extensive cardiac evaluation in the patient with stable cardiac disease. However, the long-term risks of adverse cardiac events after CEA are related to progression of CAD. Identification and coronary revascularization or aggressive medical therapy of patients with triple-vessel or left main CAD and those with very low ejection fractions may prolong their lives.

The approach to patients with both severe CAD and carotid occlusive disease is controversial. The risk of stroke in patients with symptomatic carotid disease undergoing CABG surgery has been reported to range from 8.7 to 17%. Options include either a concurrent (performed under one anesthetic) operation or two separate, staged procedures. A medical record review of 10,561 CEA procedures randomly selected from Medicare patients undergoing CEA in 10 states found worse outcomes in 226 CEAs performed in combination with CABG in the same operative event.[29] The combined stroke and death rate was 17.7%; 80% of the nonfatal strokes were disabling. Proximal aortic arch atherosclerosis and symptomatic carotid stenosis were associated with stroke ($P < .05$). Female gender, emergent operation, redo CABG, blood pressure on pump, total pump time, presence of left main disease, and number of diseased coronaries were associated with mortality ($P < .05$). The strokes appeared to be associated with the operative event, but diagnosis was delayed and postevent carotid patency was not documented. Operative strategies used in concurrent operations vary among surgeons. Some surgeons will begin with a simultaneous CEA and a saphenous vein harvest. After these procedures have been completed, coronary artery bypass is initiated. This technique avoids the potential threats posed to the brain by hypotension at the initiation of CPB or during cardiac manipulation during off-pump CABG. This strategy presumes hypoperfusion is the dominant mechanism of stroke after CABG. However, studies suggest that embolic events may predominate. Emboli may occur when the ascending aorta is cannulated or occluded with a cross-clamp and protruding aortic arch atheromas are dislodged; mobile atheromas are seen using TEE in 15% of patients with severe carotid artery disease. Therefore, other surgeons will perform a simultaneous correction of both the coronary and carotid arteries during the aortic cross-clamp period. They seek to protect the brain with systemic hypothermia of 20 to 25°C. With this strategy, several investigators have reported extremely low rates of perioperative strokes. Although these reports are encouraging, rigorous scientific proof for a preferred operative strategy in patients with severe coronary and carotid disease is not yet available.

Monitoring and Preserving Neurologic Integrity

The two main goals of intraoperative management are to protect the brain and to protect the heart, yet these two goals often conflict. For example, increasing arterial blood pressure to augment cerebral blood flow can increase afterload or myocardial contractility, thereby increasing the oxygen demand of the heart. Also, although hypothermia might provide effective cerebral protection, it also poses a significant challenge to myocardial well-being if patients wake up shivering. General approaches to myocardial protection have been summarized previously. Our approaches to neurologic and myocardial protection during CEA involve compromises that must be made if both organs are to be protected.

Routine aspects of anesthetic care that may affect cerebral outcome if hemispheric ischemia occurs during CEA include blood pressure augmentation, manipulation of $Paco_2$, glucose management, and choice of intraoperative fluid administration. Whether further interventions to reduce cerebral metabolism and cerebral oxygen requirements are neuroprotective is controversial. More recent research suggests that the outcome of cerebral ischemia may be improved by antagonizing or modifying processes that normally occur after reperfusion rather than during ischemia. Shunts may be used if cerebral hypoperfusion is suspected. Percutaneous approaches using carotid stenting are no panacea; neurologic events also occur during and after these procedures.

The rationale behind maintaining a stable, high-normal blood pressure throughout the procedure is based on the assumption that blood vessels in ischemic or hypoperfused areas of brain have lost normal autoregulation. Flow in such areas is believed to be mainly pressure dependent. Under these circumstances, prolonged, severe hypotension may jeopardize the brain. Consequently, we maintain blood pressure in the
5 patient's high-normal range. Nonetheless, hypotension and hypoperfusion may not be the precipitating or sole cause of stroke after CEA; embolic events may be just as or even more important, and often occur postoperatively (Fig. 32-4).[63] In addition, blood pressure augmentation with sympathomimetic drugs is not without risk to the heart. Indiscriminate use of phenylephrine to raise blood pressure during deep general anesthesia with a volatile anesthetic increases the incidence of intraoperative segmental wall abnormalities detected by TEE compared with light anesthesia without the use of phenylephrine. However, the judicious use of phenylephrine to raise blood pressure only in specific instances of EEG-detected reversible cerebral ischemia seems to be without detriment to the heart. Although phenylephrine lowers ejection fraction measured with TEE and causes cardiac dilatation in patients with CAD, norepinephrine maintains cardiac function while raising blood pressure. Phenylephrine and norepinephrine both raise cerebral blood flow velocities to a similar extent, and the increase is proportional to increases in systemic blood pressure. Despite this, we almost never use norepinephrine during CEA due to

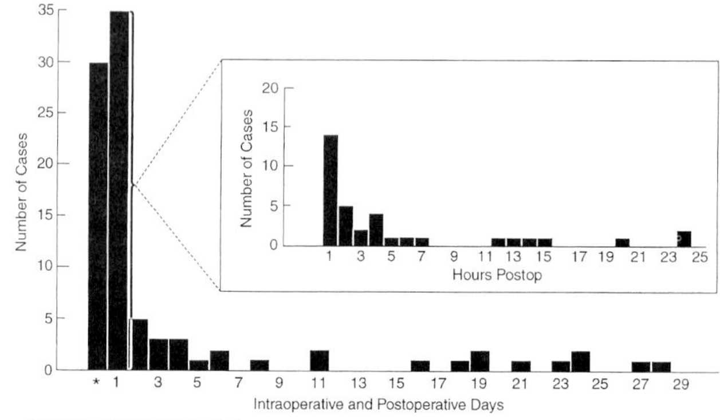

FIGURE 32-4. Data from the North American Symptomatic Carotid Trial (NASCET). Of the perioperative strokes, 35% (30/85) occurred intraoperatively, whereas 65% (55/85) occurred after the patient left the operating room (delayed events). The figure illustrates the time of onset of the 92 surgical outcome events.

its potent effects and the possibility of raising blood pressure more than desired. Whatever the choice of vasopressor, we believe one benefit of EEG or other neurophysiologic monitoring is that it allows the anesthesiologist to use less vasopressor and to maintain a lower blood pressure during the period of temporary carotid occlusion than would be otherwise feasible. Thus, as long as the patient is without new neurologic deficits or the EEG or other neurophysiologic monitor is unchanged, the anesthesiologist may decrease the afterload in the patient who is at risk for myocardial ischemic events. Based on these studies, limited vasopressor use during hypotensive episodes associated with a change in neurophysiologic monitoring appears defensible, allowing the clinician to treat only those patients who might benefit most and sparing others from its risks.

Hypercapnia dilates cerebral blood vessels and thus increases cerebral blood flow. However, hypercapnia during CEA may be detrimental if it dilates vessels in normal areas of the brain while vessels in ischemic brain areas that are already maximally dilated cannot respond. The net effect, then, is a "steal" phenomenon (i.e., a diversion of blood flow from hypoperfused brain regions to normally perfused brain regions). Most authorities recommend the maintenance of normocarbia or moderate hypocarbia at best.

Moderate hyperglycemia may worsen ischemic brain injury. Increased cerebral lactic acidosis resulting from the anaerobic glycolysis of increased brain glucose stores is postulated to be directly or indirectly responsible for the adverse effect. Because of the neuroendocrine response to surgery, with its resultant breakdown of glycogen, and the relatively high incidence of diabetes in this patient population, blood sugar levels will often already be mildly elevated during CEA. The administration of dextrose-containing intravenous fluid may exacerbate hyperglycemia. A similar effect may result from lactated solutions because lactate is metabolized to dextrose. Although there is no proof that the focal neurologic injury that may follow CEA is actually augmented by hyperglycemia, we nonetheless prefer normal saline for intraoperative fluid substitution. Isovolemic hemodilution with dextran or hetastarch is of theoretical interest in cerebral ischemia because blood viscosity is reduced and attendant microcirculatory disturbances ameliorated.

Almost all commonly used anesthetic agents reduce cerebral metabolism, thereby decreasing the brain's requirements for oxygen. It has been assumed that under anesthesia the brain's tolerance of temporary ischemia is enhanced. However, the notion that reduced cerebral metabolism is associated with cerebral protection has been challenged. Nonetheless, we believe that as long as this method of pharmacologic brain protection is not clearly refuted, there is no good justification to deny its potential benefits to a patient. The following section reviews the putative benefits of inhalational and intravenous anesthetic agents, as well as hypothermia in reducing cerebral metabolism.

Compared with older inhalational anesthetics, isoflurane may have more potential protective effect against cerebral ischemia, whereas compared with enflurane and halothane, isoflurane decreased the frequency of EEG-detected cerebral ischemic changes during CEA.[64] Nonetheless, clinical neurologic outcome was not different among the anesthetic groups. However, isoflurane's protective effects are maximal only at ~2 minimal alveolar concentrations (MAC). At this MAC level, systemic hypotension will occur in many patients; therefore, maximal protection may not be clinically achievable. Desflurane and sevoflurane also reduce cerebral oxygen requirements at MAC values comparable to those with isoflurane, resulting in faster emergence and recovery than isoflurane.[65]

Barbiturates may offer a degree of brain protection during periods of regional ischemia. Thiopental decreases cerebral metabolic oxygen requirements to about 50% of baseline. These maximally achievable reductions in oxygen requirements correspond to a silent (i.e., isoelectric) EEG. Beyond this point, additional doses of barbiturates are neither necessary nor helpful. In cases of massive global ischemia where basal cellular metabolism has already deteriorated, even high doses of barbiturates will not improve neurologic outcome. Therefore, some clinicians use thiopental not only for induction of anesthesia, but also for continuous infusion and/or as a 4 to 6 mg/kg bolus just before carotid occlusion. The cardiac depressant effects of the barbiturates may require inotropic support. Unfortunately, no rigorous proof is available that the use of barbiturates in the described manner can improve neurologic outcome after CEA. Excellent results have been obtained for CEA using high doses of barbiturates during carotid occlusion, without neurophysiologic monitoring or shunt placement; on average, tracheal extubation was delayed until 2 hours after surgery was completed.

Both etomidate and propofol decrease brain electrical activity and thus decrease cellular oxygen requirements. Etomidate preserves cardiovascular stability and may be beneficial in a patient population whose cardiac reserves are often limited. Propofol also allows rapid awakening of the patient and neurologic assessment at the end of surgery. Propofol may also be associated with a lower incidence of myocardial ischemia than is a volatile-based anesthetic but does not appear to affect overall clinical outcome.[66] Although the available evidence for the protective effects of etomidate or propofol during CEA is inconclusive, a small series in patients undergoing temporary ischemia for intracranial aneurysm clipping suggests that etomidate, propofol, or barbiturate use prolongs tolerable ischemia and reduces brain infarction.[67] Some animal studies have supported, and others refuted, the utility of α_2-agonists in reducing cereberal infarction in animal models.

Hypothermia can depress neuronal activity sufficiently to decrease cellular oxygen requirements below the minimum levels normally required for continued cell viability. In theory, hypothermia represents the most effective method of cerebral protection. Even a mild decrease in temperature of about 2 to 3°C at the time of arterial hypoxemia may reduce ischemic damage to the brain. The first reported CEA was performed with the patient's head covered by ice packs. Unfortunately, this method is cumbersome, unpredictable, and rarely used. We allow patients to cool passively in the operating room and avoid warming the operating suite, intravenous fluids, or inspired gases until the carotid repair has been completed. Afterward, forced-air warming may counteract the adrenergic response and increased incidence of myocardial ischemia associated with hypothermia in vascular surgery patients. We do not currently have clinical evidence to support the hypothesis that hypothermia protects the brain sufficiently to justify the myocardial risks imposed by hypothermia and shivering.

Effective pharmacologic brain protection is still theoretical. The outcome of cerebral ischemia may be improved by preventing activation of the neuron's excitatory amino acid receptor after reperfusion. However, to date no conclusive data exist for use of this method in humans. Ischemia also leads to neuronal calcium overload, which in turn sets off a series of harmful biochemical intracellular events. Given early after the onset of stroke symptoms, nimodipine, a calcium channel blocker, may confer some benefit to patients. Nitric oxide synthesis and free-radical scavengers may also have important therapeutic roles. Volatile anesthetics may provide preconditioning and neuronal protection by inducing nitric oxide synthase.[68] Some centers still use intravenous steroids to protect the brain from the effects of hypoxia, as well as for prevention and treatment of hyperperfusion syndrome.

Temporary occlusion ("cross-clamping") of the carotid artery acutely disrupts blood flow, even if flow to the ipsilateral hemisphere of the brain was already markedly diminished by severe stenosis. Continued blood supply to the brain will depend entirely on adequate collateral blood flow through the circle of Willis if no shunt is used. If carotid stenosis has worsened gradually before CEA is performed, collaterals from the circle of Willis may have had time to develop, and the cerebral circulation may not be compromised by carotid occlusion during surgery. However, if collateral flow is compromised because of occlusive disease of the contralateral carotid artery and/or the vertebral arteries, the chances are greater that marked hypoperfusion of the brain will occur during carotid clamping. Indeed, patients with bilateral carotid disease have a higher risk of perioperative stroke after CEA than patients with unilateral disease only.

There are practice variations among surgeons in the use of shunts in carotid surgery. Some surgeons never use shunts, others use them routinely, and still others use them only selectively. Surgeons who never use shunts usually rely on expedient surgery to avoid neurologic problems and do not report worse overall outcome statistics than those who do. The routine use of shunts is not risk free. Placement of a shunt is associated with an embolism-related stroke rate of at least 0.7% from the dislodgment and embolization of atheroma. The technical problems of shunting include air embolism, kinking of the shunt, shunt occlusion against the side of the vessel wall, and injury or disruption of the distal internal carotid artery. Patients with shunts may still develop EEG abnormalities; in these situations, we alert surgeons that shunt adjustments may be necessary. The shunt may impair surgical access to the artery, thereby increasing cross-clamp time. Most important, the use of a shunt is beneficial only if the cause of neurologic dysfunction is inadequate blood flow. However, the majority of studies suggest that as many as 65 to 95% of all neurologic deficits during CEA may be caused by thromboembolic events (see Fig. 32-4), which may occur when the carotid artery is dissected, at which point insertion of a shunt will not prevent a deficit. Not surprisingly, there is no rigorous proof that the routine insertion of a shunt reduces the incidence of postoperative neurologic deficits. In the NASCET trial, shunting (used in 41% of patients) was not associated with a change in risk of stroke.

Surgeons who use shunts selectively will need a monitoring device of cerebral perfusion to help them decide when to place the shunt. To this end, various cerebral perfusion monitors are used. Monitoring approaches include assessment of the awake patient, transcranial Doppler, SSEP, EEG, cerebral oximetry, and direct xenon cerebral blood flow measurement. In each case, the goal is to avoid routine shunting, which can cause air embolism and thromboembolism. Different techniques individually or in combination may be used by different centers.

Processed EEG monitoring is often used. However, as in all the previous techniques, its sensitivity in detecting perioperative stroke is limited by the fact that most strokes occur following surgery and are likely related to thromboembolic phenomena.[69] Rapid changes in anesthetic depth may also complicate interpretation.[70] This is particularly relevant in centers where barbiturates or propofol infusions are used to induce EEG suppression in hopes of reducing $CMRO_2$. In the North American trial, 93% of patients underwent CEA with general anesthesia; 51% of patients had intraoperative cerebral monitoring (31% EEG, 14% stump pressure, 7% evoked potentials, and 3% transcranial Doppler). However, the use of monitoring was not associated with reduced risk of stroke.[63] In summary, none of the previous procedures or neurophysiologic monitors has been shown to improve outcome. Because embolism, not hypoperfusion, is probably the most common cause of perioperative stroke, the real value of cerebral monitoring may lie in the avoidance of interventions such as the placement of shunts (which can cause stroke) and blood pressure augmentation (with its detrimental effects on the heart).

The interpretation of the information gained from the scalp-recorded EEG has been simplified by the use of computerized data reduction methods. The EEG reflects the spontaneous electrical activity of cortical (surface) neurons. Increasing levels of ischemia lead to a decrease in recorded electrical activity. EEG deterioration begins usually below a cerebral blood flow rate of about 15 mL/min/100g brain tissue, but cellular metabolic failure does not seem to occur until blood flow falls below 10 to 12 mL/min/100g brain tissue.[71] Under conditions of focal cortical ischemia, the frequency of the recorded EEG waves over the affected area of the brain will slow significantly (i.e., >50%). In addition, the amplitude of the waves may decrease (attenuate) to a comparable extent. The appearance of a disorganized background rhythm may also be a sign of ischemia. Finally, as ischemia becomes severe, the EEG will become isoelectric. Ischemic EEG changes occur in 28% of all monitored patients during CEA.[72] When they occur, they define a patient subgroup with a significantly increased risk of perioperative stroke. The most common manifestations of EEG ischemia during CEA are ipsilateral attenuation, ipsilateral slowing with attenuation, and ipsilateral slowing without attenuation.

In practice, the EEG can be obtained using a 16-channel strip-chart recording or a processed EEG monitor with 2 or 4 channels. A 16-channel strip-chart EEG generally requires a technician to set up the monitor, and to monitor and interpret the large amount of (unprocessed) data generated. In contrast, a 2-channel or 4-channel processed EEG monitor provides less data but can be monitored more easily. Figure 32-5 shows a processed EEG reflecting acute cerebral ischemia following left carotid artery occlusion; the placement of a shunt in this case promptly reversed the ischemic changes.

However, EEG monitoring has several limitations. For one, deep brain structures are not monitored by EEG. Also, in patients with preexisting or fluctuating neurologic deficits the EEG may be false negative; that is, these patients can develop perioperative strokes despite the absence of major intraoperative EEG changes. In these patients, there may be cell populations that are electrically silent or immediately adjacent to regions of infarction, and therefore, not monitored by the EEG. The still viable regions may progress to irreversible deterioration in the course of the operative procedure. Furthermore, the EEG may not be an ischemia-specific monitor because decreases in temperature and blood pressure, as well as increases in the depth of anesthesia, produce EEG changes that mimic

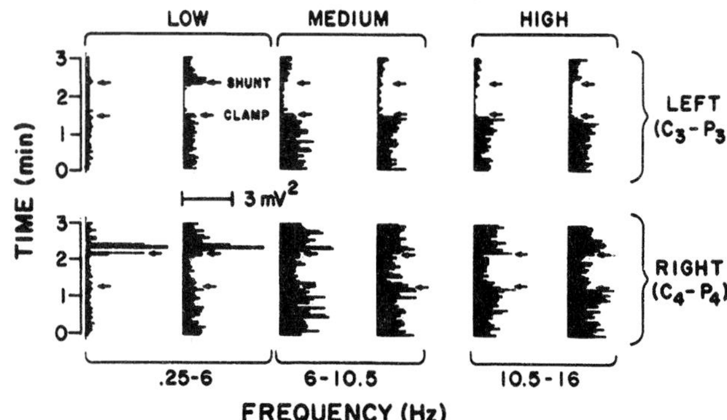

FIGURE 32-5. Acute cerebral ischemia following left carotid artery occlusion detected with processed electroencephalogram. The placement of a shunt in this case promptly reversed the ischemic changes. (Courtesy of Dr. Bruce L. Gewertz.)

ischemic changes. However, EEG changes secondary to anesthetics or hypothermia are more likely to be bilateral, whereas hemispheric ischemia is more likely to affect the electrical activity of only one side of the brain. Thus, we are compulsive in informing the encephalographer about adjustments to the anesthetic regimen.

Most importantly, the value of relatively costly EEG monitoring has not been rigorously established. Even if the advanced warning of an EEG can prevent some strokes, it would presumably do so only in the minority of patients who suffer strokes from intraoperative hypoperfusion (see Fig. 32-4).

Transcranial Doppler (TCD) measures middle cerebral artery blood flow velocities. TCD can also detect and quantify embolic signals, which almost always arise during dissection and/or angioplasty. A large series of 1,058 patients found the following TCD predictors of stroke after CEA: emboli during wound closure, >90% decrease of middle cerebral artery peak systolic velocity at cross-clamping, and >100% increase of the pulsatility index of the Doppler signal at clamp release. Emboli during dissection did not quite reach significance. The area under the ROC curve for stroke prediction was 0.69.[73] In a small case series, TCD predicted neurologic events despite a normal EEG.[74] However, compared with the awake patient as a gold standard, TCD may have a low positive predictive value for neurologic deficit accompanying carotid occlusion.[75] Other workers suggested that TCD is particularly useful in postoperative surveillance because most strokes occur after and not during CEA. TCD may also predict patients at risk of cerebral hyperperfusion syndrome following CEA/CAS.[76]

SSEP monitoring may be particularly useful in patients with cerebral ischemia in whom EEG interpretation is more difficult.[77] SSEP monitoring is based on the detection of cortical potentials after electrical stimuli are presented to a peripheral nerve. Detecting the potentials requires computer-assisted mathematic analysis and considerable expertise. In contrast to the EEG, which interrogates only cortical function, SSEP monitoring also evaluates deep brain structures. Any damage to these neural structures results in characteristic changes in the SSEP, usually in a decrease in amplitude and/or an increase in latency. If neural damage is severe, the cortical-evoked potential is completely abolished. Severe damage occurs at about one-third of normal cerebral blood flow (i.e., at 15 mL/min/100g brain tissue).

Whereas some studies have been optimistic about the value of SSEP monitoring in the detection of cerebral ischemia, other investigators have concluded that SSEP is neither sensitive nor specific for the detection of ischemic injury during CEA. Virtually all commonly used anesthetics lead to SSEP changes that mimic changes produced by cerebral hypoxia. Therefore, a constant light plane of anesthesia needs to be maintained if increased latencies and decreased amplitudes of evoked potentials are to be ascribed to inadequate cerebral perfusion. False-negative results may also occur. Based on the available data, we conclude that this monitoring system cannot yet be considered essential for a safe CEA.

Cerebral oximetry has had mixed results. One study of 100 patients suggests that "a 20% decrease in rSO_2 (regional frontal lobe saturation) reading from the preclamp baseline, as a predictor of neurologic compromise, resulted in a sensitivity of 80% and specificity of 82.2%. The false-positive rate using this cutoff point was 66.7%, and the false-negative rate was 2.6%, providing a positive predictive value of 33.3% and a negative predictive value of 97.4%." Monitoring rSO_2 with INVOS-3100 to detect cerebral ischemia during CEA has a high negative predictive value, but the positive predictive value is low.[78] With SSEP considered a "gold standard," the predictive value of cerebral oximetry was low, and "substantial interindividual variability of rSO_2 and derived change of rSO_2 did not allow the definition of a threshold value indicating need of shunt placement."[79] Others added that "relying on RSO_2 alone would increase the number of unnecessary shunts because of the low specificity. Accepting higher decreases in RSO_2 does not appear reasonable because it bears the risk of a low sensitivity."[80]

Anesthetic and Monitoring Choices for Elective Surgery

General discussions of cardiac function and myocardial ischemia monitoring can be found earlier in this chapter. Our practice with patients undergoing CEA, summarized in this section, is somewhat different. Our intraoperative monitors include the usual monitors employed during all major, general, or regional anesthetics: temperature probe, blood pressure cuff, pulse oximeter, and an end-tidal carbon dioxide tension monitor. We routinely place an intra-arterial catheter for blood pressure monitoring so beat-to-beat changes in pressure are detected and treated promptly. However, in some patients, particularly elderly females, cannulation of the radial artery may be difficult. Before surgery, we also measure the blood pressures noninvasively in both arms because generalized peripheral vascular disease in this patient population can produce striking differences between the two upper extremities.

We routinely monitor leads II and V_5 of the ECG for ST-T segment changes because of the high incidence of perioperative myocardial ischemia after carotid reperfusion. In high-risk patients, we may rarely use TEE as an additional monitor, especially in those with acute stroke where source of embolus may be an issue. Rarely is it necessary to use a central venous or pulmonary artery catheter, even if TEE is not available. We seek to avoid central venous or pulmonary artery catheterization because of the risk of an accidental carotid artery puncture during cannulation of the internal jugular vein. We restrict the use of central venous access to the rare patient with uncompensated CHF undergoing urgent CEA, and then may insert it from the contralateral brachial or subclavian vein. Finally, in our experience, intravenous access for volume administration is generally sufficient with one well-secured and well-running, medium-bore, intravenous catheter because major blood loss or fluid shifts during CEA are rare.

For most patients, the assurance provided by the preoperative interview obviates the need for sedative drugs to prevent anxiety-induced myocardial ischemia. If sedatives are deemed indispensable, the smallest effective dose of midazolam is chosen for premedication to facilitate early perioperative neurologic assessment. Equally important, we obtain blood pressure and heart rate determinations from the preoperative clinic, other hospital or clinic visits, and at the time of admission, thus determining the range of a patient's acceptable values. We seek to maintain hemodynamics within this range intraoperatively. Chronic antianginal, antihypertensive, and aspirin medications are generally continued on the day of surgery. Patients who come to the hospital the same day as surgery must be reminded to take their medications at home. This is especially true for antiplatelet therapy. When patients forget to take their medications, we give them readily available oral or parenteral substitutes.

Our experience is that many patients present after an overnight fast slightly hypovolemic. They often present hypertensive despite having taken their morning antihypertensive and antianginal medications. These patients appear to be the most prone to hypotension after the induction of general anesthesia. For procedures performed under general anesthesia, we typically use propofol for induction, although thiopental or etomidate may be used. If thiopental is used, esmolol is particularly valuable to blunt hypertensive and tachycardic responses to intubation. However, when a patient has a diastolic blood pressure >100 mm Hg in the operating room or is not well hydrated (often, both conditions exist simultaneously), induction of general anesthesia may result in hypotension. The clinician can anticipate this possibility and induce general anesthesia slowly, being prepared to use pharmacologic blood pressure augmentation if blood pressure decreases excessively. Despite this, in the operating room, we generally avoid administering more than 10 mL/kg of crystalloid in a typical 2-hour operation because fluid overload may contribute to postoperative hypertension. Diastolic filling abnormalities are common in elderly surgical patients,[81] and limiting fluid administration may also lessen symptoms of congestion following surgery.

Because the respiratory depression and sedation caused by opioids may persist into the postoperative period and may confound the results of early neurologic assessment, we generally restrict the use of opioids whenever possible (e.g., fentanyl ≤3 mg/kg) or use remifentanil. The combined use of a cervical plexus block and/or surgeon-administered local anesthetic helps considerably in almost eliminating opiate requirements.

We provide patients with a "light" general anesthetic that permits EEG monitoring and results in blood pressures in the high range of normal. We may spray the trachea with 100 mg lidocaine to minimize stimulation by the endotracheal tube during surgery. Others have described the use of the laryngeal mask airway (LMA) during CEA, which may reduce hypertensive and tachycardic episodes. Anesthesia is maintained with 50% nitrous oxide in oxygen and light levels of a volatile anesthetic because of its salutary effects on the incidence of cerebral ischemia.[65] The newer volatile agents, desflurane and sevoflurane, may be used to facilitate rapid awakening and assessment of neurologic status.

We do not routinely use continuous infusions of vasopressors (e.g., phenylephrine) to augment blood pressure, but rather reduce the inhaled concentrations of volatile anesthetics and thereby rely on a patient's endogenous pressure-sustaining responses. Vasopressors are used to treat hypotension or EEG changes. Because sudden onset of bradycardia and hypotension may be caused by activation of baroreceptor reflexes with surgical irritation of the carotid sinus, some surgeons may infiltrate the carotid bifurcation with 1% lidocaine to attenuate this response. However, this practice may result in more postoperative hypertension. The vagal response may also occur during CAS, and atropine should be readily available. We typically use a medium-duration relaxant to provide muscle relaxation, although the choice of muscle relaxant depends on the heart rate we want to obtain. One of us administers no muscle relaxant except as necessary for intubation. Another usually gives an additional dose of muscle relaxant immediately before carotid occlusion when the concentration of volatile anesthetic is decreased to allow the blood pressure to rise. One limitation of this technique is that it lessens the potential neuroprotective effects of volatile anesthesia because the cerebral metabolic depression it produces is dose dependent. Our patients are almost always extubated at the end of the surgical procedure before or after we confirm neurologic integrity. In patients who were easy to intubate, we may perform a deep extubation in an attempt to limit the explosive hypertension that may accompany extubation. If this is done, we wait until neurologic integrity is verified before we leave the operating room. New neurologic deficits may lead to noninvasive imaging, contrast angiography, and/or surgical re-exploration. Our overall institutional results are good (mortality, 1%; stroke and MI, both 0.76%). Others achieved similar results using a nitrous oxide/opioid technique or a continuous infusion of thiopental. Intravenous techniques (propofol/remifentanil) may offer more hemodyanamic stability[82] than volatile anesthetic techniques. However, volatile anesthetic techniques allow easy titration of anesthetic depth and rapid awakening. In addition, animal and human studies suggest that volatile anesthetics may limit brain[83] and myocardial infarct[84] size at clinical doses. There is no proof that any one general anesthetic technique provides a superior outcome.

Regional anesthesia is used by many centers for CEA. The necessary sensory blockade of the C2 to C4 dermatomes can be achieved by superficial or deep cervical block or by subcutaneous infiltration of the surgical field. Superficial and deep plexus blocks appear to be equivalent in providing good surgical conditions and patient satisfaction; deep plexus blocks are more effective when a paresthesia is obtained.[85] Proponents of regional anesthetic techniques claim the following advantages: greater stability of blood pressure during surgery, inexpensive and easy cerebral monitoring, avoidance of tracheal intubation in patients with chronic obstructive lung disease, and avoidance of negative inotropic anesthetic agents in patients with limited cardiac reserves. The use of regional techniques appears to be associated with fewer episodes of EEG ischemia compared with general anesthesia.[86] In addition, overall hospital costs associated with the use of regional anesthesia may be lower. A systematic analysis has suggested lower stroke rates with regional anesthesia for CEA[87]; most published series are either not randomized and/or have too little power to detect outcome differences.

Disadvantages of regional anesthesia are that potential pharmacologic brain protection with anesthetics cannot be provided and that, in the case of panic, sudden loss of consciousness, or onset of seizures, control of the airway may be difficult. Although emergent intubation is uncommon, it may be difficult under these circumstances and complicate surgical management. Regional anesthesia requires that the patient remain highly cooperative throughout the operation, and sedation can be provided only to a limited extent during carotid occlusion. The NASCET study found no difference in event rate between regional and general anesthesia, although only 7% of the 1,415 patients received a regional anesthetic. Based on the currently available evidence, the choice of anesthetic technique should take into account the preference of the surgeon and the experience and expertise of the anesthesiologist.

Initially, the internal carotid artery is isolated where the plaque or ulcerative lesion has been identified radiographically (usually starting near the bifurcation). Heparin is typically given in a dose of 50 to 100 U/kg. The surgeon isolates the diseased carotid segment with clamps or ties placed on the proximal and distal internal carotid artery and on the external carotid artery. After a period of test occlusion during which the adequacy of cerebral blood flow may be assessed with the modalities previously described, an incision is made into the artery. A shunt may be inserted at this time. The surgeon then endarterectomizes the ulcerated or plaque-containing area. Occasionally, a long or tortuous region is shortened by resection and reanastomosis, or if the remaining portion of the intima is too thin, a vein (often from the leg) or a Dacron patch is used. The use of a patch has been shown to improve long-term patency rates, particularly in women. Because suturing of the patch requires more time than suturing of the native vessel, an internal shunt is used more often during these procedures. Time is of the essence to help prevent neurologic deficits. If the shunt has been placed, it is then removed just prior to completing the repair. Shunt placement and removal usually takes between 1 and 4 minutes, and the total occlusion time rarely exceeds 40 minutes.

CAS may be performed by vascular surgeons, cardiologists, and/or radiologists. In some cases, this will involve sedation and monitoring provided by anesthesiologists; in other cases, no anesthesiologist will be involved. Adequate heparinization is crucial, with most protocols seeking to maintain ACT > 300 seconds. Both open CEA and CAS may cause blood pressure to fall immediately after reperfusion and into the postoperative period, due to alterations in baroreceptor function.[88] Postoperative hypertension is common following CEA and may predispose to wound hematoma. Our experience has been that more aggressive antiplatelet therapy, especially with clopidogrel increasingly continued up until the time of surgery, is associated with greater bleeding in the Postanesthesia Care Unit (PACU). Wound hematoma may compromise the airway[89]; it is associated more with edema of the larynx than extrinsic compression and represents an emergency airway challenge.[90]

Postoperative Management

Common problems arising after CEA include the onset of new neurologic dysfunction, hemodynamic instability during emergence from general anesthesia, and respiratory insufficiency. Patients who have undergone general anesthesia may be awakened while still on the operating table to permit early neurologic evaluation. We may choose to extubate the trachea while the patient is breathing spontaneously but still anesthetized ("deep extubation"). We may do this in a patient who was easy to intubate, in an attempt to prevent emergence hypertension. However, even in these cases, we do not leave the operating room until the patient is awake enough to undergo neurologic assessment. A new neurologic deficit may demand immediate reexploration, or at least arteriography. A few surgeons routinely perform arteriography after restoring blood flow, but most believe that the complications of routine arteriography (emboli, allergic reactions, vasospasm, bleeding from the puncture hole, and stroke) are greater than its benefits (the detection of inadequate repairs, suture lines, or flow). With another method, duplex ultrasonography, the resutured vessel may be imaged at the end of surgery. The neurologic examination should also seek to identify cranial nerve (hypoglossal and facial) injuries arising from surgical manipulation.

Hyperperfusion syndrome is believed to result from blood flow to the brain that is greatly in excess of its metabolic needs following CEA. It may not occur until several days after surgery, when patients present with severe ipsilateral headache and can progress to develop signs of increased cerebral excitability or frank seizures. Transcranial Doppler may have a role in predicting which patients will develop this syndrome. Steroids may be used in the treatment of hyperperfusion syndrome.

Blood pressure abnormalities are common after CEA; hypertension is more common than hypotension. Severe hypertension seems to occur more often in patients with poorly controlled preoperative hypertension. Both acute tachycardia and hypertension may precipitate acute myocardial ischemia and failure, and hypertension may lead to cerebral edema and/or hemorrhage. Post-CEA hypertension is significantly associated with adverse events (stroke or death, with a statistical trend toward reduced cardiac complications), whereas postoperative hypotension and bradycardia do not appear to correlate with primary or secondary outcomes. We therefore routinely treat hypertension to reduce the work of the heart and in hopes of decreasing neck hematoma. Thus, having excluded and/or treated other causes of hypertension such as bladder distention, pain, hypoxemia, and hypercarbia, we lower systolic pressures of >140 mm Hg and diastolic pressures of >90 mm Hg to within the range of a patient's perioperative values. We write "as required" orders in the PACU, most often for labetalol in 5-mg increments; because labetalol is not beta-1-selective, we use other drugs in patients with reactive airways disease. Hyperdynamic responses accompanying emergence and extubation may be attenuated by prophylactic administration of intravenous lidocaine, esmolol, labetalol, or nitroglycerin. We prefer to use drugs with short half-lives that can be titrated to avoid undue hypotension. We believe that by supplementing with a regional anesthetic and/or tracheal lidocaine spray, these responses are suppressed. The incidence of myocardial ischemia is higher in the first few hours after CEA, even in patients who have been "awake" during CEA with a deep cervical block and prophylactic nitroglycerin infusions. Patients who undergo carotid artery stenting also manifest intraprocedural and postprocedural hemodynamic abnormalities similar to surgical patients. Bradycardia occurs frequently when right carotid lesions are angioplastied. The causes of postoperative hypertension are unclear. Our clinical experience suggests less postoperative hypertension when regional blocks are used, either alone or combined with a general anesthetic. Overzealous administration of intravenous fluid or surgical or chemical denervation of the baroreceptors of the carotid sinus nerve may also be responsible. Postoperative hypertension may be associated with an increased incidence of neurologic deficits. Usually, the hypertensive episode has its peak 2 to 3 hours after surgery, but in individual cases it may persist for 24 hours.

Postoperative hypotension and bradycardia after CEA are less frequent than hypertension. Surgical removal of the atheroma reexposes the baroreceptors of the carotid sinus nerve to higher levels of transmural pressure and causes brainstem-mediated vagal bradycardia and hypotension. Chemical denervation of the carotid baroreceptors with a local anesthetic by the surgeon results in fewer hypotensive patients but increases the incidence of postoperative hypertension. Over time, the baroreceptors seem to adjust and the hypotensive phase resolves within 12 to 24 hours. For patients who are hypotensive, some argue against any treatment as long as the ECG is unchanged and the patient's neurologic status is stable. Other clinicians, however, typically administer intravenous fluids and/or vasopressors such as ephedrine, dopamine, or phenylephrine to restore blood pressure to the low range of normal. Because significant hypertension and hypotension can be due to or caused by myocardial ischemia or infarction, we may obtain a 12-lead ECG in the recovery room in hemodynamically unstable patients.

Postoperative respiratory insufficiency may be caused by recurrent laryngeal nerve or hypoglossal nerve injury, a massive hematoma, or deficient carotid body function. Wound hematomas develop in up to 2% of patients after CEA. Whereas small hematomas caused by venous oozing usually can be treated by reversing residual heparin with protamine or by applying gentle digital compression for a few minutes, an expanding hematoma must be carefully and immediately evaluated because tracheal compression and loss of the airway may ensue rapidly. In some cases, evacuation of the hematoma may not relieve the airway obstruction if lymphatic obstruction has produced massive pharyngolaryngeal edema.[89,90] Indeed, four patients (0.3%) in the NASCET trial died directly due to neck hematomas. Risk factors for neck hematoma may also include failure to reverse heparin and the presence of an endotracheal tube beyond the end of surgery. Hematomas are more common and delayed if a patch angioplasty has been performed. Therefore, some clinicians routinely reverse heparin with protamine in patients who have had a patch angioplasty. Some studies, however, have suggested protamine may contribute to postoperative stroke. However, in the NASCET trial, heparin reversal using protamine (used in 40% of patients) was not associated with a change in risk of stroke.[63]

Surgical manipulation may also damage the nerve supply to the carotid body. Although unilateral loss of carotid body function is unlikely to be significant, a bilateral loss may prevent the patient from increasing ventilation in response to a decrease in PaO_2. Therefore, supplemental oxygen should be routinely used in the recovery area. Similarly, drugs that depress respiratory drive should be avoided as much as possible in postoperative pain management. It is our experience that administration of acetaminophen constitutes effective pain relief in most patients when skin infiltration or plexus block with local anesthetic was performed in the operating room.

In experienced centers, CEA causes only minor postoperative physiologic derangements in most patients. As a consequence, routine postoperative intensive care is unusual in our practice and has been questioned. In one study, postoperative intensive care surveillance was necessary only for patients with four or more of the following risk factors: stroke, CHF, chronic kidney failure, hypertension, arrhythmia, and MI. Equally important, all patients requiring interventions or with adverse outcomes could be identified by the eighth postoperative hour.[91] We believe routine admission of all patients to the ICU is probably not necessary and that intensive care surveillance can be limited to high-risk patients. Certain complications of CEA, such as hyperperfusion syndrome or bleeding after a patch angioplasty, may not occur until several days after CEA.

Management of Emergent Carotid Surgery

The patient who awakens with a major new neurologic deficit or who develops a suspected stroke in the immediate postoperative period represents a surgical emergency. Although postoperative neurologic deficits may be due to inadequate collateral flow, carotid thrombosis may cause postoperative stroke; prompt surgical reexploration can produce significant neurologic improvement. If a new neurologic deficit occurs in the postanesthesia recovery unit, most surgeons believe immediate reexploration is indicated, and logic would dictate utilization of pharmacologic methods of "cerebral protection;" however, this "logic" is controversial. Alternatively, if the deficit is deemed only focal and minor, it is most commonly due to microembolization. Consequently, noninvasive assessment of internal carotid flow and anticoagulation after exclusion of a hemorrhagic brain lesion usually constitute indicated treatment.

A patient undergoing emergency CEA may have a full stomach and thus may require protection against aspiration of gastric contents. The main goal is to minimize the hemodynamic stress of a rapid-sequence induction while maintaining adequate perfusion pressure across the stenotic lesion. General anesthesia is maintained with any of a variety of techniques aimed at attenuating hemodynamic fluctuations, achieving normocarbia (or a carbon dioxide level slightly below normal, as in elective operations), and maintaining adequate carotid artery perfusion pressure. An anesthetic technique similar to one for elective situations is used.

For patients undergoing neck exploration for a wound hematoma following CEA, oxygen is given at high concentration by face mask. In the event of acute airway obstruction, a high concentration of oxygen in the functional residual volume of the lung may provide additional protection against hypoxemia until the airway is secured by intubation or even by tracheostomy, or until the hematoma is evacuated surgically. A tracheostomy or cricothyroidotomy tray should be immediately available, as well as other devices for management of the difficult airway. It may be difficult to visualize the trachea because of edema or because of deviation caused by pressure of the hematoma.

If the hematoma does not obstruct the airway and the patient is not having difficulty breathing spontaneously, induction may be accomplished as in an elective procedure. If the airway appears compromised, topical anesthesia of the tongue, posterior pharynx, and epiglottis is provided. The larynx may then be visualized traditionally or with fiberoptic laryngoscopy. Esmolol is particularly useful to control hyperdynamic cardiovascular responses during awake intubation. If no difficulty with tracheal intubation is anticipated, induction is performed as described previously. However, if any difficulty is expected, the wound is opened and drained externally, and tracheal intubation is performed before general anesthesia is induced.

AORTIC RECONSTRUCTION

In vascular surgery, understanding the pathophysiology of the disease and anticipating the surgical approach and techniques allow the anesthesiologist to serve the patient most effectively. The surgical goal in these operations is to create an enduring restoration of the normal circulation while minimizing the duration of ischemia to viscera, especially to the renal circulation. This goal is difficult to achieve: each possible surgical approach compromises some aspects while optimizing others. Surgery may be undertaken to correct aneurysmal or occlusive disease; sometimes the two coexist.

Aneurysmal Disease

Aneurysms pose an ever-present threat to life because of their unpredictable tendency to rupture or embolize. Mortality from rupture may be as high as 85%, and even patients who receive emergent surgery have mortality rates one-half that. Therefore, early recognition and aggressive surgical management are warranted, even in the absence of symptoms.

Epidemiology and Pathophysiology of Abdominal Aortic Aneurysm

There are approximately 200,000 new AAAs diagnosed annually with approximately 45,000 undergoing surgical repair per year in the United States. A population-based study in Norway in 1994 to 1995 used ultrasound to measure renal and infrarenal aortic diameters; an aneurysm was present in 263 (8.9%) of men and 74 (2.2%) of women ($P < .001$). Risk factors for aneurysm included advanced age, smoking >40 years, hypertension, low serum HDL cholesterol, high level of plasma fibrinogen, and low blood platelet count. This study indicates that risk factors for atherosclerosis are also associated with increased risk for AAA.[92] Thoracoabdominal aneurysms also occur in patients with hypertension or other risk factors for atherosclerotic disease.

AAA represents a dilatation of the abdominal aorta generally below the level of the renal arteries. The risk of rupture of the AAA is directly related to the luminal diameter of the aortic aneurysm. The aneurysm can develop an inner lining of mural thrombus, thereby decreasing the effective luminal diameter, but the size of the mural thrombus has not been shown to significantly decrease the risk of rupture. The risk of aortic rupture is only related to the absolute diameter of the aortic aneurysm sac. The risk of rupture increases once the aneurysm is greater than 4.5 to 5 cm in diameter. The size of the aneurysm is the most important predictor of subsequent rupture and mortality. A prospective study followed 300 consecutive patients (mean age 70 years; 70% men) who presented with AAA (average size, 4.1 cm) and were initially managed nonoperatively. The diameter of the aneurysm increased by a median of 0.3 cm per year. The 6-year cumulative incidence of rupture was 1% among patients with aneurysms <4.0 cm and 2% for aneurysms 4.0 to 4.9 cm in diameter. By comparison, the 6-year cumulative incidence of rupture was 20% among patients with aneurysms >5.0 cm in diameter.[93] Larger aneurysms expand even more rapidly. Patients with AAAs that do not undergo operation have an 80% 5-year mortality, predominantly owing to rupture. Generally, it has been recommended that in good-risk patients with aneurysms greater than 4.5 to 5 cm they should be considered for surgical repair.

Although traditional thinking has been that the lowered rate of mortality after elective AAA resection might justify elective repair of aneurysms as small as 4 cm, more recent evidence questions this practice. Although screening allows identification of larger numbers of patients with asymptomatic aneurysms, it also provides a mechanism for "watchful waiting." A randomized trial of 1,136 patients randomized to immediate repair versus surveillance with CT scanning and ultrasonography found similar survival in the two groups. In the immediate repair group, standard open repair was performed. In the surveillance group, patients were followed without repair until the aneurysm reached at least 5.5 cm in diameter or enlarged by at least 0.7 cm in 6 months or at least 1.0 cm in 1 year, or until symptoms developed that were attributed to the aneurysm. When one of these criteria was met, open repair was to be carried out. The actual results showed that 80% of the "immediate" group had surgery within 6 weeks, while approximately 75% of patients in the "watchful waiting" group eventually had repair performed, but in this group it was delayed by an average of approximately 4 years after randomization. Although 11 patients in the surveillance group had rupture of AAAs (0.6% per year), resulting in seven deaths, the rate of hospitalization related to abdominal aortic aneurysm was actually 39% lower in the surveillance group.[94] This was true even though operative mortality was less than 3%. Therefore, these results may even be applicable to endovascular repair: watchful waiting may be preferable to repair in patients with AAAs of 4.0 to 5.4 cm in diameter.

The argument for aggressive surgical treatment is based on the fact that traditional surgery for ruptured AAA is still associated with mortality approaching 50%, roughly an order of magnitude greater than elective AAA surgery. Risk factors for mortality in patients with rupture include advanced age, APACHE (Acute Physiology and Chronic Health Evaluation) II score, initial hematocrit, and preoperative cardiac arrest. Unfortunately, in most patients with rupture, the diagnosis of AAA was unknown beforehand. These data reinforce the importance of screening of the high-risk population to permit elective repair.

Pathophysiology of Aortic Occlusion and Reperfusion

Aortic cross-clamping and unclamping is associated with complex cardiovascular, renal, humoral, and hemostatic changes. The intensity of these changes varies proportionally with the level of aortic clamping.

Cardiovascular Changes

The classic investigations of Gelman form the basis of our understanding of the pathophysiology of hemodynamic changes during aortic cross-clamping and unclamping.[95] Aortic cross-clamping increases mean arterial pressure and systemic vascular resistance up to 50%. This is attributed to a sudden increase in impedance to aortic flow (afterload); activation of renin; and release of cathecolamines, prostaglandins, and other active vasoconstrictors. Cardiac output initially decreases in the face of high systemic vascular resistance, and that decrease may be reinforced by the decrease in oxygen consumption below the aortic cross-clamp (Figs. 32-6 to 32-8 and Table 32-6). Some of the initial changes in hemodynamics associated with cross-clamping can be offset by boluses of a vasodilator

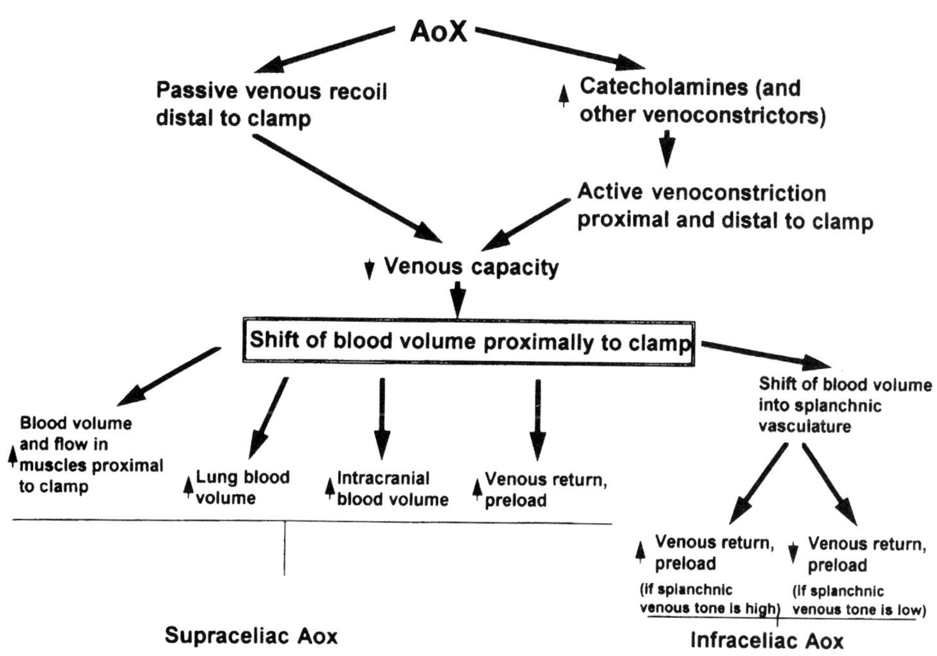

FIGURE 32-6. Blood volume redistribution during aortic cross-clamping. This schedule depicts the reason for the decrease in venous capacity, which results in blood volume redistribution from the vasculature distal to aortic occlusion to the vasculature proximal to aortic occlusion. If the aorta is occluded above the splanchnic system, the blood volume travels to the heart, increasing preload and blood volume in all organs and tissues proximal to the clamp. However, if the aorta is occluded below the splanchnic system, blood volume may shift into the splanchnic system or into the vasculature of other tissues proximal to the clamp. The distribution of this blood volume between the splanchnic and nonsplanchnic vasculature determines changes in preload. AoX, aortic cross-clamping; ↑ and ↓, increase and decrease, respectively. (Reprinted with permission from Gelman S: The pathophysiology of aortic cross-clamping and unclamping. Anesthesiology 82:1026, 1995.)

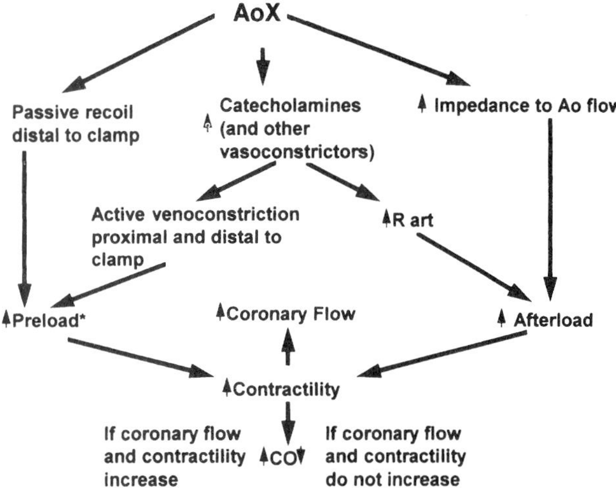

FIGURE 32-7. Systemic hemodynamic response to aortic cross-clamping. Preload does not necessarily increase. If during infrarenal aortic cross-clamping blood volume shifts into the splanchnic vasculature, preload does not increase (see Fig. 32-6). AoX, aortic cross-clamping; Ao, aortic; R art, arterial resistance; CO, cardiac output; ↑ and ↓, increase and decrease, respectively; *, different patterns are possible (see Fig. 32-6). (Reprinted with permission from Gelman S: The pathophysiology of aortic cross-clamping and unclamping. Anesthesiology 82:1026, 1995.)

administered immediately prior to placement of the clamp (e.g., 0.3 to 0.7 mcg/kg of nitroprusside or milrinone 5 mcg/kg over 10 minutes). In this case, mechanical and pharmacologic actions cancel each other out while the body is allowed to adapt.

Preload changes are more variable than blood pressure changes. Higher central venous pressure (CVP) and pulmonary artery occlusion pressures do not accompany the decrease in cardiac index in the healthy heart. However, in those with

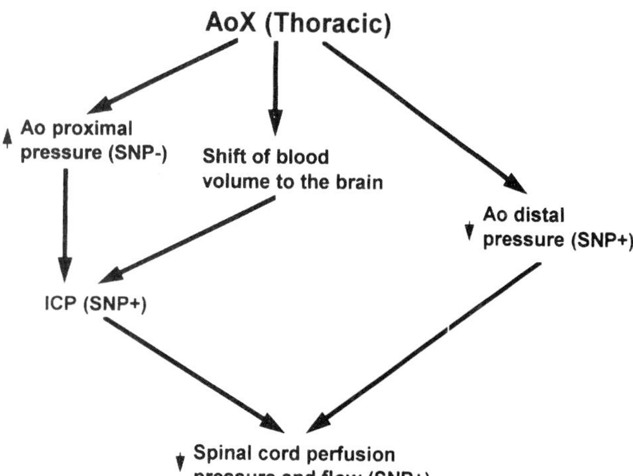

FIGURE 32-8. Spinal cord blood flow and perfusion pressure during thoracic aortic occlusion, with or without sodium nitroprusside (SNP) infusion. The changes (*arrows*) represent the response to aortic cross-clamping per se. SNP+, SNP aggravates the effect of cross-clamping; SNP–, SNP counteracts the effect of cross-clamping; AoX, aortic cross-clamping; Ao, aortic; ICP, intercranial pressure; ↑ and ↓, increase and decrease, respectively. (Reprinted with permission from Gelman S: The pathophysiology of aortic cross-clamping and unclamping. Anesthesiology 82:1026, 1995.)

CAD, myocardial dysfunction may be associated with cross-clamping and may lead to an increase in filling pressures as documented by TEE studies.[96]

The level of clamping affects hemodynamic response. Infrarenal aortic cross-clamping is well attenuated compared with suprarenal clamping, and during occlusive disease repair, aortic clamping usually has limited systemic hemodynamic effect. With lower clamping, blood volume from the infrasplanchnic vasculature may shift to the compliant splanchnic vasculature limiting preload changes, and vasodilation above the level of the clamp offsets the mechanical impedance to aortic flow. Clamping an occluded artery obviously is expected to have minimal effect. Existing collateral circulation remains intact during clamping and is responsible for maintaining lower body perfusion despite aortic cross-clamping. For higher clamps, nitrate therapy will not necessarily prevent wall motion abnormalities, and care should be exercised when using any vasodilator so perfusion pressure below the aortic cross-clamp remains at a level that will not potentiate visceral/spinal cord ischemia. It may be acceptable to allow a systolic blood pressure as high as 180 to 200 mm Hg as long as there is no other contraindication (e.g., intracerebral hemorrhage) and the surgeon has acceptable operating conditions. Even relative hypotension (<20% below resting pressure) probably should be avoided unless other means (shunts) are used to perfuse the lower part of the body.

Unclamping of the aorta can result in severe arterial hypotension unless aggressive therapy is undertaken prior to unclamping (Fig. 32-9). Various therapies are employed by anesthesiologists and surgeons, with no evidence one is superior to another. Most anesthesiologists employ some degree of fluid loading with or without vasoconstrictors such as neosynephrine (often 100 to 200 mcg) or drugs such as calcium chloride (300 to 500 mg) that can offset the negative inotropic/dromotropic effects of an acute potassium and acid load (and possibly other mediators) on the heart immediately following reperfusion. Much preferable to pharmacologic manipulation is gradual unclamping, which allows the body to adapt without much pharmacologic support. Whenever possible, unclamping should be gradual, either through actual staged release of the clamp, compression and gradual release of the femoral arteries by the surgical assistant, or restoring flow to one leg at a time in aortobifemoral grafts.

Renal Hemodynamics and Renal Protection

Renal protection is still a controversial topic, with no therapies proven to yield superior outcome. The level of aortic clamping is probably the most important of all the factors, as it markedly impacts renal blood flow. The incidence of acute renal failure is approximately 5% postinfrarenal clamping but approaches 13% postsuprarenal clamping. A major postoperative complication such as renal failure necessitating dialysis is probably the strongest predictor of mortality. Postoperative mortality is fourfold to fivefold higher in those who develop acute renal failure when compared with those who do not. It is imperative to understand routine regulation of renal perfusion (see Chapter 35), as well as the effect of aortic clamping on renal perfusion. With suprarenal occlusion, renal blood flow decreases by 80%. Blood flow is not only reduced with aortic cross-clamping, but also redistributed, favoring the cortical and juxtamedullary layers over the hypoxia-prone renal medulla.[97] Even with an infrarenal aortic clamping, renal blood flow is 45% lower during cross-clamping. Renal vascular resistance increases by almost 70%. Interestingly, these renal hemodynamic changes do not immediately revert after the release of cross-clamping and persisted for at least 30 minutes beyond the systemic cardiovascular return to baseline.

TABLE 32-6

EFFECT OF LEVEL OF AORTIC OCCLUSION ON CHANGES IN CARDIOVASCULAR VARIABLES

■ CARDIOVASCULAR VARIABLE	■ % CHANGE IN VARIABLE, BY LEVEL OF AORTIC OCCLUSION		
	■ SUPRACELIAC	■ SUPRARENAL–INFRACELIAC	■ INFRARENAL
Mean arterial blood pressure	54	5[a]	2[a]
Pulmonary capillary wedge pressure	38	10[a]	0[a]
End-diastolic area	28	2[a]	9[a]
End-systolic area	69	10[a]	11[a]
Ejection fraction	−38	−10[a]	−3[a]
Abnormal motion of wall, % of patients	92	33	0
New myocardial infarctions, % of patients	8	0	0

[a]Statistically different ($P < .05$) from group undergoing supraceliac aortic occlusion.
Adapted with permission from Roizen MF, Ellis JE, Foss JF *et al:* Intraoperative management of the patient requiring supraceliac aortic occlusion. In Veith FJ, Hobson RW, Williams RA, Wilson SE (eds): Vascular Surgery, 2nd ed, p 256. New York, McGraw-Hill, 1994.

Many different methods of renal protection have been advocated, most of them centering on improving renal blood flow or glomerular flow. These include dopamine (dopaminergic receptor dose 2 to 3 mcg/kg per minute), fenoldopam,[98] ACE inhibitors, prostaglandins, thoracic epidurals for renal arterial sympatholysis,[99] vasodilators, isovolemic hemodilution (for increased blood flow in the face of increased vascular resistance), furosemide, and mannitol. Mannitol increases diuresis (although physiologically unimportant, it often satisfies the surgeon's need to hear that there is some urine output) and functions as a hydroxyl free radical scavenger. Outcomes have not been shown to improve with its use. Dopamine has been shown to lack specific renal hemodynamic effects and does not appear to improve postoperative renal dysfunction. Fenoldopam is gaining more interest due to its specific DA-1 activity. Animal studies are promising, and human studies have shown better intermediate variables (e.g., creatinine clearance) but have not shown a reduction in need for dialysis.[98] One of the most important factors for preventing postoperative renal failure remains good hydration (as the most important factor for maintaining renal blood flow) during clamping and postclamp release.

Previous work from our group has shown that intraoperative urinary output is not predictive of postoperative renal function. In 137 patients undergoing aortic reconstruction (38 at the supraceliac level), we found no significant correlation between intraoperative mean urinary output, or lowest hourly urinary output, and changes from preoperative to postoperative levels of creatinine or blood urea nitrogen (Fig. 32-10).[100] Thus, urinary output, which is believed to be an index of perfusion and is therefore monitored routinely during surgery, was not predictive of postoperative renal function in normovolemic patients. When patients who underwent aortic occlusion at the suprarenal level were compared with those who underwent occlusion at the infrarenal level, there was no difference in postoperative renal function. Rather, preoperative renal dysfunction was the most powerful predictor of postoperative renal dysfunction. If prolonged renal ischemia is anticipated, selective

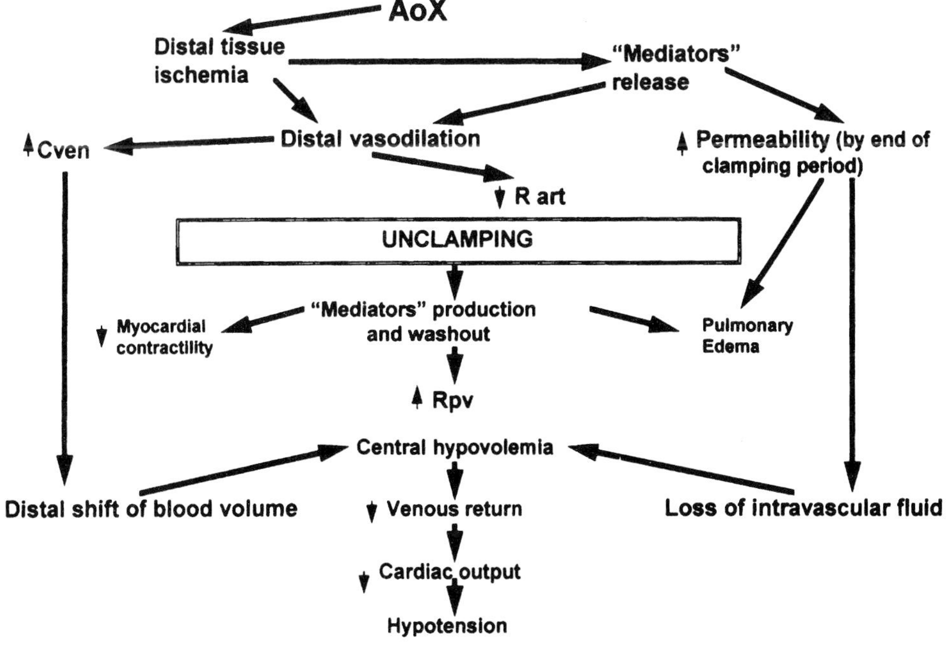

FIGURE 32-9. Systemic hemodynamic response to aortic unclamping. Preload does not necessarily increase. AoX, aortic cross-clamping; Cven, venous capacitance; R art, arterial resistance; Rpv, pulmonary vascular resistance; ↑ and ↓, increase and decrease, respectively. (Reprinted with permission from Gelman S: The pathophysiology of aortic cross-clamping and unclamping. Anesthesiology 82:1026, 1995.)

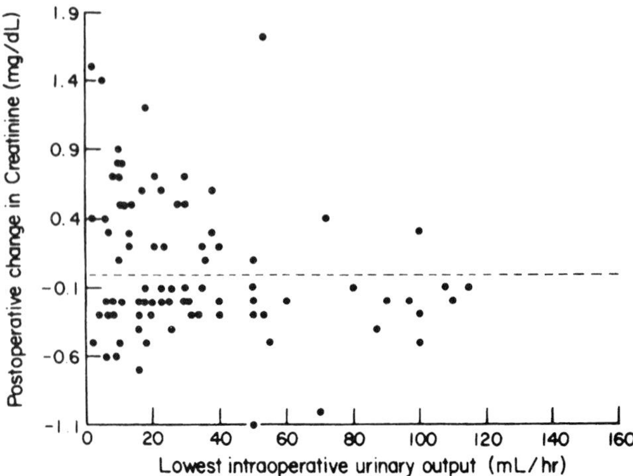

FIGURE 32-10. Lowest hourly intraoperative urinary output and maximal adverse change in renal function as assayed by change in creatinine from preoperatively to 7 days postoperatively. There was no correlation between lowest intraoperative urinary output and change in renal function postoperatively. (Modified with permission from Alpert RA, Roizen MF, Hamilton WK *et al*: Intraoperative urinary output does not predict postoperative renal function in patients undergoing abdominal aortic revascularization. Surgery 95:707, 1984.)

profound hypothermia and the direct intra-arterial infusion of mannitol into the kidneys may decrease the incidence of postoperative renal impairment.

Humoral and Coagulation Profiles

Although the most evident factor contributing to hypotension is volume redistribution to the lower body after aortic cross-clamp release, many humoral mediators are released from the underperfused areas and contribute to the hemodynamic changes. Among the many factors described are renin, angiotensin, epinephrine, norepinephrine, PGI_2, endothelin, PGF-1, thromboxane A2 and B2, lactate, potassium, oxygen-free radicals, platelets activator, cytokines, activated complement (C3 and C4), and neutrophil sequestration. Administration of bicarbonate does not prevent immediate postunclamping hypotension and, in our anecdotal experience, can exacerbate it, probably due to the initial increase in intracellular myocardial acidity. Mannitol administration before and after unclamping may be beneficial because of its function as a hydroxyl free radical scavenger. Nonsteroidal anti-inflammatory drugs may counteract the effect of prostaglandins; however, their use remains controversial due to their potential detrimental antiplatelet and renal perfusion effects. The use of COX-2 inhibitors augments postoperative pain control and avoids any platelet effect, but still may have some renal perfusion effects that have not been studied in this context. Regardless, we have used preoperative COX-2 inhibitors as part of a multimodal approach to postoperative pain control if a thoracic epidural is not employed, although more recent controversy suggests that COX-2 drugs may be contraindicated in patients with cardiovascular disease.

A high incidence (5 to 14%) of pulmonary complications is a fact in thoracoabdominal aneurysm repair. Sequestration of microaggregates and neutrophils contribute to postoperative pulmonary dysfunction. Aortic reperfusion may result in pulmonary vasoconstiction due to liberation of thromboxane A2 and other vasoactive substances. Increased permeability and pulmonary edema are not uncommon. As noted previously, mannitol may attenuate these responses.

Thirty minutes after aortic cross-clamping, t-PA and t-PA Ag levels in the peripheral vascular bed are increased. This reflects the increase in adrenergic state. TEG studies have documented an increase in clotting factor activity during cross-clamping and decreased speed of solid clot formation after unclamping. These changes, along with a low fibrinogen level, are consistent with clotting factor consumption rather than fibrinolysis.

Visceral and Mesenteric Ischemia

As with postoperative renal failure, bowel ischemia is associated with a higher postoperative mortality rate, approaching 25%. Factors contributing to the pathogenesis of visceral ischemia include preexisting medical conditions, renal dysfunction, stage of aortic disease and level of aortic cross-clamping, perioperative hypotension, and last but not least the duration of cross-clamping.

Besides the acute ischemic injury to the organ, hypoxic insult to the intestines during aortic occlusion leads to gut permeability and bacterial translocation as evidenced by activation of polymorphonuclear leukocytes. This may predict respiratory and renal failure. Peak plasma level of tumor necrosis factor and interleukin-6 are significantly higher in hypotensive patients and in those who die. With endovascular repair, intestinal ischemic events seem less profound. High doses of methylprednisolone at induction of anesthesia may be beneficial in reducing the inflammatory response, including C-reactive protein and T-cell activation levels. Anesthetic techniques appear to minimally influence inflammatory cytokine stress responses, which correlate most with increasing operative times. Further research is needed to determine if anti-inflammatory therapy can reduce morbidity and mortality after aortic reconstructive surgery.

CNS and Spinal Cord Ischemia and Protection

Few studies address the effect of abdominal aortic cross-clamping and unclamping on cerebral circulation. Middle cerebral artery blood velocity decreases during aortic occlusion. Unclamping is followed by a transient dilation of cerebral pial arterioles, followed by a sustained vasoconstriction. These changes are due to the hemodynamic changes, CO_2 accumulation and washout, decreased pH, and release of thromboxane A2, which is a powerful vasoconstrictor on cerebral vessels.

Spinal cord ischemia occurs in 1 to 11% of operations involving a distal aortic repair. The spinal cord is supplied by two posterior arteries; together, both supply 25% of spinal cord blood flow. The anterior spinal artery (Fig. 32-11), which supplies 75% of spinal cord blood flow, is the primary supplier to the anterolateral cord. The anterior spinal artery is fed by a series of radicular arteries arising from the aorta, and collateralization is poor. The blood supply to the thoracolumbar cord is derived from the radicular artery of Adamkiewicz. In 75% of cases, it joins the anterior spinal artery between T8 and T12, and in 10% it joins between L1 and L2. Much of the blood flow in the anterior spinal artery depends on the artery of Adamkiewicz. Because the flow in the spinal arteries depends on collateralization and is often bidirectional, the blood supply to the spinal cord can be shunted to the rest of the body when perfusion pressures are low. Such a situation may arise when a single high aortic occlusion clamp is applied.

6 The definitive preventive measures to spinal cord ischemia are short cross-clamping time, fast surgery, maintenance of normal cardiac function, and higher perfusion pressures. Other methods such as cerebrospinal fluid (CSF) drainage, distal perfusion, and hypothermia may be beneficial in high aortic clamping.

Surgical Procedures for Aortic Reconstruction

Perioperative (i.e., 30-day) mortality in elective aortic surgeries ranges between 0% and 12%, with a much higher probability

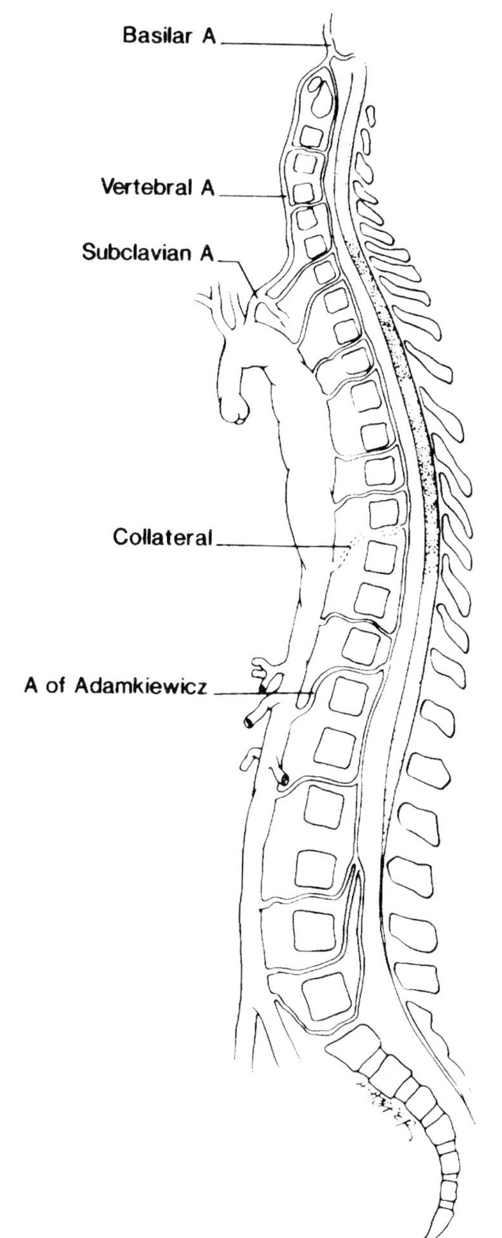

FIGURE 32-11. The artery of Adamkiewicz usually arises at the T11–T12 level and provides the blood supply to the lower spinal cord. Its variable location and the uncertainty of additional collateral blood supply explain, in part, the unpredictability of paraplegia following descending aortic surgery. (Reprinted with permission from Piccone W, DeLaria GA, Najafi H: Descending thoracic aneurysms. In Bergan JJ, Yao JST (eds): Aortic Surgery, p 249. Philadelphia, WB Saunders, 1989.)

of death in emergent surgery especially in those situations where preoperative hypotension (systolic blood pressure (SBP) < 90 mm Hg) exists. Hypotension increases the risk by 3-fold, whereas preexisting heart disease including coronary artery disease (CAD) and congestive heart failure (CHF) increase the risk of mortality by 2.5- to 5-fold. Other identifiable risks for increased mortality are gender, with slight increase in female, serum creatinine above 2 mg/dL, and age older than 80 years. The size of an aneurysm does not appear to influence operative mortality by itself. Expeditious surgery with better graft materials, minimal clamp time, and blood conservation, along with better understanding of the pathophysiology of the disease, have made aortic surgery safer.

Arterial reconstruction surgery was developed based on normal anatomy. Although this is usually the easiest and best option, situations do occur that require circuitous revascularization procedures, such as axillofemoral or femoral-femoral bypass. These situations include graft infection, repeat surgery, and a hostile abdomen, such as one encounters with postradiation states, adhesions, sepsis, and malignancy. It should be emphasized that overall these procedures have lower long-term patency rates than anatomically correct procedures.

Approach

Abdominal aortic reconstruction can be performed through a transperitoneal or retroperitoneal exposure. In the first case, a thoracoabdominal midline incision is performed and the aorta is accessed through the peritoneum. This generous exposure is usually favored for complex aortic reconstruction or replacement. In the retroperitoneal approach, incision is made over the lateral border of the left rectus muscle, 2 cm below the umbilicus to the twelfth rib. This will allow the access to the aorta from the crux of the diaphragm to its bifurcation. The debate continues between advocates of transperitoneal versus the retroperitoneal approach. In more recent randomized studies, the retroperitoneal technique allowed a surgical exposure as good as the transperitoneal approach and was associated with less fluid shift, faster return of bowel function, lower pulmonary complications, shorter ICU stay, and lower overall hospital cost with an average savings of $4,000 to $5,000.[101] The retroperitoneal approach is considered by many to be more appropriate in cases of truncal obesity, serious COPD, hostile abdomen (e.g., previous surgeries), and juxtarenal aneurysm. However, the flank approach is not a panacea, as frequent chronic wound pain, incisional hernias, and abdominal bulges have been reported. Intraoperative blood loss during open AAA repair varies between 500 to several thousand milliliters of blood, depending on the size and complexity of the AAA. The postoperative course many times requires admission to the ICU for several days and hospital admission for 5 to 7 days. The postoperative recovery period after the open repair can be several months.

Clamp Level

Infrarenal aortic clamping carries the lowest risk for patients; supraceliac clamping carries the highest. Anesthesiologists should be aware that 10 to 20% of "infrarenal" aortic disease will actually involve the suprarenal portion of the aorta, necessitating suprarenal clamping. Ruptured aneurysms often must be controlled initially by supraceliac clamping. In these cases, great care must be taken so atheromatous material is not dislodged in the renal arteries during surgical manipulation and clamping.

Thoracic Aneurysm Repair

These operations are among the most challenging for anesthesiologists. Coincident CAD and COPD are common. Lung separation is required to facilitate surgical access to the aneurysm and to avoid an iatrogenic pulmonary contusion in the left lung. Lung separation may be provided with either double-lumen tubes or bronchial blockers. Bronchial blockers may be advantageous because they facilitate postoperative ventilation without the need to change a double-lumen tube at the end of surgery. Because of edema of the head and neck frequently occur after high cross-clamping (even with distal perfusion), reintubation may be difficult at the end of the procedure, and we have seen patients require emergent tracheostomy when an endotracheal tube could not be passed. Generous exposure of the thoracic and abdominal aorta and its major branches can be obtained with a left thoracoabdominal incision and retroperitoneal dissection. The thoracoabdominal approach is favored for complex thoracoabdominal aortic replacement in the presence of stenotic or aneurysmal disease. The visceral branches are often excised from the parent aorta with a button of aortic wall. If the patient also has mesenteric occlusive disease, endarterectomy of these branch vessels is performed before they are attached as "buttons" to the graft at appropriate positions. If only mesenteric revascularization is to be performed and aortic replacement is not used, endarterectomy of any or all the major branches of the aorta may be performed with this exposure.

Aortomesenteric Revascularization

Chronic mesenteric ischemia occurs due to atherosclerosis or dissection. Surgical revascularization is indicated only in symptomatic disease. This will occur when two of the main mesenteric vessels become occluded. Elective surgery for asymptomatic occlusive disease is not justified because of the high risk of perioperative mortality, which can range from 7 to 18%. Cardiac events, hemorrhage, and bowel infarction are the most dreaded complications. In symptomatic cases, elective surgical reconstruction with or without concomitant aortic replacement remains the best choice because percutaneous transluminal angioplasty and stenting are associated with a significant incidence of recurrence and should be reserved to specific cases. Partial cross-clamping of the aorta is preferred if possible and may mitigate hemodynamic changes.

Acute mesenteric ischemia differs in its genesis. It is usually the result of an acute embolic event or trauma. The presence or absence of intestinal infarction plays a major role in the patient's overall prognosis in this setting. Endarterectomy of the mesenteric arteries may be performed through a transaortic access for isolated disease, or before the attachment of the vessels to the aortic graft at appropriate positions. If single-vessel endarterectomy is performed, it may be carried out for either the celiac axis or the superior mesenteric artery.

Aortorenal Revascularization

Renal artery revascularization can be performed by several surgical techniques. These techniques include endarterectomy, reimplantation, bypass, and ex vivo renal artery reconstruction. Extra-anatomical renal artery bypass may be the perfect choice in sick, debilitated patients who do not tolerate aortic clamping. Percutaneous approaches have largely replaced surgery for isolated renal artery revascularization.

Infrarenal Operations

Reconstruction of the infrarenal aorta is performed by exposing the relevant portion of the aorta and the iliac arteries. Heparin is commonly administered in a central line to reduce the risk of thromboembolic events before aortic clamping. Although it is generally recognized that distal ischemic complications are due to dislodgment of atheromatous material off the diseased aorta and that the systemic use of heparin in the absence of distal occlusive disease is unnecessary, many centers still religiously employ heparin before aortic clamping. Aortic repair is carried out by interposition of a graft with an end-to-end anastomosis. Collagen impregnated polyester fibers (Dacron) grafts make the majority of implanted grafts. Dacron grafts appear to be associated with rare episodes of anaphylactic reactions, which may be related to the stabilizers used in their manufacture. Polytetrafluoroethylene (PTFE) grafts are less porous and are gaining more widespread use. Aortobiiliac, aortobifemoral, and aortoiliac/femoral grafts are used in most

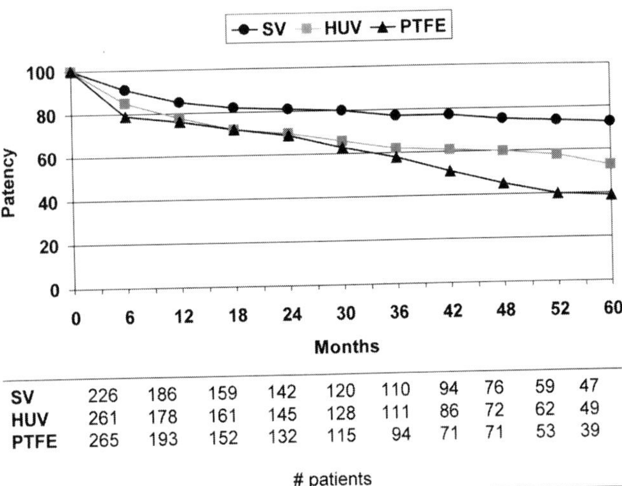

SV	226	186	159	142	120	110	94	76	59	47
HUV	261	178	161	145	128	111	86	72	62	49
PTFE	265	193	152	132	115	94	71	71	53	39

patients

FIGURE 32-12. Superiority of saphenous vein bypass grafts for femorial-popliteal, above-knee bypass. Life table analysis for the patency of saphenous vein (SV), human umbilical vein (HUV), and polytetrafluoroethylene (PTFE). *N* represents the number of bypass grafts being observed for patency at that time. (Modified with permission from Johnson WC, Lee KK: A comparative evaluation of polytetrafluoroethylene, umbilical vein, and saphenous vein bypass grafts for femoral-popliteal above-knee revascularization: A prospective randomized Department of Veterans Affairs cooperative study. J Vasc Surg 32:268, 2000.)

cases. Straight grafting constitutes approximately 30% of cases (see Fig. 32-12).

Thoracic Aortic Surgery

Traditional surgery for thoracic aortic aneurysm continues to be associated with higher morbidity and mortality than infrarenal AAAs. The analysis of large databases suggests that population-based perioperative mortality is higher than that reported in series from selected institutions.[102] Mortality may approach 20%; risk factors include diabetes mellitus, cerebrovascular disease, and renal insufficiency. Median hospital charges ($64,000) are also high. Therefore, endovascular thoracoabdominal aortic aneurysm repair (endoTAAR) has been advocated as an alternative to open surgery with its stresses and frequent complications. Complications may be lower with endovascular approaches, with blood loss averaging only 450 cc and ICU stay 1 day in uncomplicated cases. Although paraplegia still may occur after endoTAAR, its incidence seems reduced compared with open abdominal aortic aneurysm repair (AAAR).[103] One approach to attempt to lessen paraplegia after endoTAAR has been to place a temporary stent under SSEP monitoring; if SSEP is unchanged, then the thinking goes, a permanent stent may be placed. However, motor evoked potential (MEP) monitoring would seem more appropriate for monitoring function of the anterior spinal column.[104] Drainage of CSF may be performed in attempt to rescue patients with paraplegia, as has been reported after open thoracoabdominal aortic aneurysm (TAAA) repair. Successful treatment of paraplegia with induced hypertension and CSF drainage following endoTAAR has been reported by several authors. The use of a single continuous subarachnoid catheter, first for local anesthetic injection to facilitate femoral or iliac arterial access in the groins, and later for prophylactic removal of CSF has been described during endoTAAR.[105] Aspiration of CSF does not result in loss of the sensory or motor blockade if performed 15 to 20 minutes after local anesthetic instillation. Paraplegia has also been reported after endovascular repair of AAA (endoAAAR);

atheroembolization to the spinal cord appears to have been the underlying cause.

Endovascular Surgery of Aortic Aneurysms

There has been an explosion in the use of endovascular therapy of aortic and peripheral vascular disease. Approximately one-half of patients with AAA appear to be candidates for endoAAAR. Experienced centers have not noted a decrease in open AAA repair accompanying the growth of endoAAAR programs. This growth in endovascular repair has been occasioned by hopes of lower morbidity and mortality, shorter hospital stays and convalescence, and screening programs. In addition, manufacturers have driven the growth of endovascular procedures. Despite the shorter length of stay (LOS) after endoAAAR, the costs of the implant and radiologic procedures for follow-up actually may result in higher costs than open surgery; however, anesthesia costs are lower for endovascular repair. Vascular surgeons, cardiac surgeons, interventional radiologists, and/or cardiologists (with turf battles not uncommon) may perform procedures. When they are performed outside the main operating room (ours are performed by vascular surgeons in a specialized suite built in the ambulatory suite), appropriate equipment must be provided. This may include a blood refrigerator, the ability to obtain arterial blood gases and other labs, fluid warmers, forced-air warming, and so on. When faced with new technologies, clinicians caring for patients undergoing such procedures must exercise good judgment. That means being prepared for the rare disaster, especially during the "learning curves" of new practioners. It is also our experience that as technology is used for expanded indications and outside specialized centers and hospitals, complication rates may be higher.

In 1991, Juan Parodi, reported a small series of high-risk patients who underwent minimally invasive endoluminal repair of their aortic aneurysm through catheter delivery of grafts from remote cutdowns in the femoral arteries.[106] His initial report triggered significant interest within the vascular surgical community on the minimally invasive repair of AAAs. Initially, homemade devices were used to bridge the area of the aortic aneurysm with an expandable stent and Dacron-coated grafts. Commercially produced grafts initially started clinical trials in the United States in 1994. These grafts had hooks that were embedded with balloons into the aorta and iliac vessels, mimicking the effect of conventional surgical suturing. The body of the graft was unsupported, again consistent with the conventional open aortic aneurysm repair. Other graft designs quickly became available which involve the use of supported grafts with first expandable stainless steel stents and then the Nitinol stent that implemented the use the radial force of the stent to hold the stent graft in place. Generally, a neck below the renal arteries of approximately 15 mm is required for adequate fixation of the stent graft to the infrarenal aorta. The distal attachment of these grafts would either be to the distal abdominal aorta if an adequate neck was noted above the aortic bifurcation or, in most cases, into the common iliac vessels distal to the aneurysmal dilatation.

The technique for implantation of the endovascular aortic grafts generally requires bilateral common femoral artery or iliac artery cut down in the supine position. Arterial sheaths between 16F and 27F are then advanced into the iliac arteries and up into the AAA sac. This can be performed using local anesthetic, regional with epidural or general endotracheal anesthetic, as discussed later in this section. If the patient has small common femoral or external iliac arteries, the introducer sheath may be too large to safely advance to the abdominal aorta. In these cases, a retroperitoneal cutdown to the distal common iliac artery or the proximal external iliac artery can be performed to access a more suitable caliber vessel for graft implantation. This can be done with a small retroperitoneal incision, dissection down to the iliac vessels, and the suturing of a synthetic conduit onto the common iliac artery or the junction of the common and external iliac artery. The graft is then introduced through this conduit and deployed either into the common iliac artery or, in some cases, actually into the conduit itself. The conduit can then either be ligated or implanted into the femoral artery as an ileal femoral bypass graft. In isolated cases with extension of the aneurysm to the bifurcation of the common iliac into the external and internal iliac artery, embolization of the internal iliac artery or reimplantation of the internal iliac artery into the external iliac artery by a retroperitoneal cutdown have been employed, as well as placement of the iliac stent graft into the external iliac artery.

Preimplantation calibrated angiography is required to identify the renal vessels, the potential for an accessory renal artery, the length from the renal arteries to the aortic bifurcation, and the distance from the aortic bifurcation to the bifurcation of the common iliac artery to the external and internal iliac artery. Dye loads may be considerable (100 to 250 cc); especially in diabetic patients, we may pretreat with N-acetyl cysteine, fluid loading (with bicarbonate added),[107] and/or mannitol in an attempt to reduce postoperative renal insufficiency. These measurements coupled with the diameter measurements allow the selection of the appropriate size endovascular stent graft. The device is then positioned just below the renal artery orifices and then fully deployed. Each type of stent graft has a unique method of deployment and specialized training is required for each device.

Major complications in endovascular stent grafting have included aneurysm rupture during the time of graft implantation, renal insufficiency secondary to contrast use, and the late complications include migration of the graft with changes in configuration of the aortic aneurysm sac, endoleak, or late AAA rupture.

Endoleak is defined as a persistent perfusion of the aneurysm sac through an attachment site leakage points (type 1 endoleak) or through lumbar or mesenteric artery branches (type 2 endoleak). A tear in the fabric of the aortic stent graft or a modular disconnect between the pieces of the endovascular aortic stent graft is classified as a type 3 endoleak. The significance of aortic endoleak is still uncertain. It has been shown that type 1 endoleaks have a high potential for aortic expansion or even rupture, and should be repaired with an additional stent, covered stent, or conversion to an open AAA repair. The significance of type 2 endoleak is uncertain. The general consensus is that in the presence of a type 2 endoleak the patient should be followed with serial CT scans and only intervened on if there are signs of progression or enlargement of the aortic aneurysm sac. Endoleaks may require subsequent repair in a significant percentage (up to 10%) of patients.

The potential for the need for retroperitoneal cutdown to the iliac arteries, or worst-case scenario, injury to the iliac vessels or the aortic aneurysm, necessitates that these procedures be performed in a setting that is suitable for urgent transfer to the operating facility or preferably within the operating room itself. This way, if either open aortic conversion or iliac repair is required, this can be accomplished with greatest efficiency and safety. One of the major U.S. Food and Drug Administration-approved device has shown that there is approximately a 0.8% risk of rupture in the perioperative or long-term postoperative period after aortic stent graft placement. Many of these cases are actually due to lack of follow-up and failure to intervene on changes of the aortic morphology that could have prevented AAA rupture.

Follow-up is critical in the patients undergoing endovascular aortic stent grafting. Generally, patients are followed with plain radiograph and serial CT scans at 1, 3, 6, 12, 18, and

24 months, and then yearly thereafter. This differs from the standard open aneurysm repair in which the patient may receive an ultrasound or no follow-up except for physical examination. The follow-up CT scan after endovascular aortic stent grafts is to detect signs of endoleak, aneurysmal sac enlargement, or graft migration. Graft migration can occur due to a technical problem with the stent graft itself or due to changes in the configuration of the aortic aneurysm as it decreases in size from lack of perfusion and then kinking or migration of the graft. Many late complications of aortic stent grafting can be repaired through endovascular techniques of embolization or addition of additional cuffs without necessitating open surgical conversion.

There are still many questions regarding the long-term patency and durability of endovascular aortic stent grafts,[108] but the preliminary data appear good. Changes in the design and configuration of aortic stent graft have shown significant improvement in the patency and ability to implant these devices into the abdominal aorta. As the grafts continue to progress into their third and fourth generation, the authors are optimistic that this will continue to improve and become a safe and effective way of managing AAAs. A more recent randomized trial has confirmed what several large registries have shown: reduced combined mortality and severe complications, and reduced hospital length of stay with endovascular repair compared with traditional repair.[109]

Goals of Anesthesia for Endovascular Aneurysm Repair

As in open AAAR, the primary goal of perioperative management is to preserve organ function. This is particularly important, because endoAAAR patients may be sicker and have more end-organ disease than candidates for open repair. Even when performed under MAC, preparation for endoAAAR must anticipate significant blood loss and fluid requirements. In a series of 47 patients (from one of the most experienced centers in the United States), the average blood loss was 623 mL (range, 100 to 2,500 mL), and fluid requirements averaged 2,491 mL.[110] Therefore, the choice of a local or regional anesthetic may still require placement of invasive monitors in patients.

At the time of deployment, mild hypotension and lack of patient movement are important goals. In early series, induction of VF or atrioventricular block with adenosine was used to induce brief asystole. These are more feasible under general anesthesia (GA) compared with regional anesthesia (RA). However, more recently, mild hypotension is used, which can be induced with infusions of vasodilators such as nitroglycerin. In the patient receiving RA or monitored anesthesia MAC, brief induction of GA with a bolus of propofol and mask ventilation may accomplish these goals.

Managing Intraoperative Complications During Endovascular Thoracoabdominal Aortic Aneurysm Repair

EndoAAAR, although likely representing a significance advance, is not benign. Rupture may rarely occur during endoAAAR. In a case report, intraoperative monitored rupture, despite rapid inflation of a proximal balloon to effectively "cross-clamp" the aorta, was associated with hemorrhagic shock typical of ruptures occurring outside the hospital. In this patient, endotracheal intubation was performed after rupture because a regional anesthetic technique was originally chosen.[111] However, we are more likely to provide GA for patients with complicated anatomy (especially iliac arteries), where conversion might be more likely.

Misdeployment may result in immediate onset of visceral ischemia. Alternatively, atheroembolization may occur with resultant ischemic complications. Blood loss may be considerable in patients with severely diseased and tortuous femoral or iliac arteries. Injury to these arteries may require repair. A proactive approach in such a patient with severe iliac disease was described in a case report. In this report, an open iliac artery reconstruction (under RA) was initially performed, followed by stent deployment via the reconstructed artery. Other workers suggested arterial access via the brachial or carotid arteries.

Mortality in patients with ruptured AAA remains high after traditional surgery. More recently, reports suggest significantly better results with a novel, multifaceted approach, which includes endovascular repair with a proprietary device, balloon inflation above the site of rupture to mimic "cross-clamping," hypotensive hemostasis, limited fluid resuscitation, and monitored anesthesia care. Using this approach, 23 of 25 patients with ruptured aortoiliac aneurysms survived. Median hospital stay was 6 days, and the preoperative symptoms resolved in all patients. This approach tends to contradict traditional notions of the importance of aggressive volume resuscitation and normalization of blood pressure. However, this approach has been adapted from one shown successful in surgical patients suffering penetrating trauma.[112] The endovascular approach to patients with ruptured AAAs may be limited because of the need for time-consuming measurement (angiography) and the expense of keeping multiple-size grafts in inventory. Future studies will define the role of endovascular therapy in emergent and rupture situations.

Complications of Anesthetics

Various anesthetic techniques have been used for endoAAAR, including general, epidural, combined epidural/spinal, spinal, and continuous spinal. Because most endoAAAR are associated with less hemodynamic stress, endocrine stress, cytokine release, decline in respiratory function, and prolonged convalescence compared with open repair, regional anesthesia might have less incremental benefit in endoAAAR. Of course, controversy persists even for open AAAR as to whether RA improves outcome.[113]

EndoAAAR is often advocated for patients with chonic obstructive pulmonary disease (COPD). Respiratory function and outcome is better after endoAAAR under GA compared with openAAA repair under GA. Although RA may or may not offer pulmonary benefits for patients undergoing open repair, it is not so clearly the case in endoAAAR. This may be because the hemodynamic[114] and endocrine metabolic response[115] to endoAAAR is far less than for open repair. Therefore, the potential amount of stress reduction produced by using RA for endoAAAR is likely to be much less than for openAAAR.

Local/sedation techniques have been be used successfully for endoAAAR and endoTAAR. It has been suggested that the use of epidural anesthesia, as opposed to local/sedation, may prolong stay and costs after ambulatory endovascular repair, perhaps because of greater administration of intravenous fluids in the epidural group.[116] However, interpretation of this and other retrospective studies may be confounded by the likely selection of epidural techniques for more extensive, complicated procedures and those earlier in the "learning curve." Similarly, the validity of retrospective studies of outcome after endoAAAR under GA versus RA techniques may be limited.

In traditional femoral-distal surgery, failure rates as high as 10% for spinal and 15% for epidural anesthesia have been reported.[117] Failure was defined as the need to convert to general aesthesia. In our experience, most conversions from regional to general have occurred either during long procedures when patients became restless or because of complications of the procedure (i.e., hemorrhage), which required aggressive management.

Anticoagulation management can complicate regional anesthesia in endoAAAR patients. One disadvantage of using epidural or continuous spinal catheter techniques is the need to wait until heparin effect has dissipated before removing the catheter. In most patients, postoperative pain is not a significant issue after successful endoAAAR, particularly if the groin incisions have been infiltrated with local anesthetic. Therefore, maintaining an epidural or subarachnoid catheter after surgery is not generally necessary to provide analgesia, unless more extensive adjuvant procedures such as iliac artery repair have been performed. Obviously, the normal cautions that apply to regional anesthesia in patients receiving preoperative anticoagulation therapy apply to those undergoing endoAAAR.

Endovascular repair likely represents an advance in care but not a panacea. Clinicians caring for these patients must be prepared for complications. Regional and local anesthesia with sedation may be a key part of the management of these patients if the caveats discussed previously are kept in mind.

Protecting the Spinal Cord and Visceral Organs

Thoracic aortic occlusion reduces distal blood flow tremendously. Various strategies have been used to protect the spinal cord from ischemia, including maintenance of proximal hypertension during cross-clamping, local, or systemic hypothermia, CSF drainage, and various drugs (including magnesium, steroids, papaverine, naloxone, and barbiturates) to protect the brain and spinal cord during resection of abdominal or thoracoabdominal aneurysms, or coarctation repairs. Spinal cord sensory-evoked, motor-evoked potentials and CSF lactate concentrations may prove useful in predicting patients at risk for spinal cord ischemia and in gauging spinal cord protection, but there is limited experience in the use of the techniques. Spinal cord metabolism can be reduced by moderate hypothermia and high-dose barbiturates. Local hypothermia achieved by infusion of cold saline into the epidural space, when combined with CSF drainage, has been reported to significantly reduce paraplegia rate. Alternatively, femoral-femoral bypass and deep hypothermic cardiac arrest may be used in patients at high risk of paraplegia. Reperfusion injury may be addressed by the use of mannitol, steroids, calcium channel blockers, and avoidance of hyperglycemia. The multitude of proposed pharmacologic and surgical maneuvers to reduce spinal cord ischemia and neurologic deficits after thoracic aortic occlusion highlights the serious nature of this complication and the lack of consensus on its prevention. Table 32-7 summarizes some of these approaches. We still believe short cross-clamp times are the common element of successful regimens.

Some surgeons place a Gott shunt, a heparinized tube that can decompress the heart and also provide distal perfusion. The Gott shunt can be placed proximally into the ascending aorta (the most common site), aortic arch, descending aorta, or left ventricle and inserted distally into the descending aorta (most commonly), femoral artery, or abdominal aorta. Even with a Gott shunt or partial bypass, there is an obligatory time of visceral ischemia when the visceral blood supply arises from a point between the proximal and distal clamps. Placement of a shunt may result in atheroembolism, which can produce rather than prevent ischemic injury and death. Other surgeons may place a temporary ex vivo right axillofemoral bypass graft before positioning for thoracotomy. After the thoracic aortic surgery is completed, the axillofemoral graft is removed. The placement of a shunt or distal perfusion attenuates the hemodynamic response to aortic unclamping, reduces acidosis, and could conceivably ameliorate the hormonal and metabolic changes that accompany aortic occlusion.

TABLE 32-7

METHODS OF SPINAL CORD PROTECTION DURING DESCENDING THORACIC AORTIC SURGERY[170]

- Limitation of cross-clamp duration
- Distal circulatory support
- Reattachment of critical intercostal arteries
- CSF drainage
- Hypothermia
  - Moderate systemic (32–34°C)
  - Epidural cooling
  - Circulatory arrest
- Maintenance of proximal blood pressure
  - Pharmacotherapy
    - Systemic:
      - Corticosteroids, barbiturates, naloxone, calcium channel antagonists, O_2 free radical scavengers, NMDA antagonists, mannitol, magnesium, vasodilators (adenosine papaverine, prostacyclin), perfluorocarbons, colchicine
    - Intrathecal:
      - Papaverine, magnesium, tetracaine, perfluorocarbons
- Avoidance of postoperative hypotension
- Sequential aortic clamping
- Enhanced monitoring for spinal cord ischemia
  - Somatosensory-evoked potentials
  - Motor-evoked potentials
  - Hydrogen-saturated saline
  - Avoidance of hyperglycemia

CSF, cerebrospinal fluid; NMDA, N-methyl-D-aspartate.

Other groups have chosen to use partial bypass, either from the left atrium or ascending aorta to the iliac or femoral artery to provide distal perfusion and decompress the heart. A heat exchanger may be used to induce hypothermia, which may be neuroprotective. Segmental sequential surgical repair may minimize the duration of ischemia to any given vascular bed. Intercostal artery reattachment in hopes of preserving blood flow to the anterior spinal cord may also be beneficial. After reperfusion, the heat exchanger can be used to warm the patient. Other potential advantages of left atrial–left femoral artery shunt with centrifugal pump support are better operative field exposure, afterload reduction, maintenance of stable distal aortic perfusion, and reduced (but not eliminated) head and neck edema.

A markedly reduced incidence of neurologic deficits has been reported when distal aortic perfusion is combined with drainage of CSF.[118] CSF drainage is used in the hope of improving the pressure gradient, allowing spinal cord blood flow as aortic occlusion lowers distal arterial pressures and increases the CVP. The new endovascular techniques represent an alternative therapy when anatomy permits; lower paraplegia rates have been reported compared with open surgery.[103]

Monitoring and Anesthetic Choices for Aortic Reconstruction

We routinely place arterial catheters in patients undergoing aortic reconstruction. In patients undergoing thoracic aortic clamping with distal perfusion, we may also measure distal arterial pressure and CSF pressure. We may place a pulmonary artery catheter (PAC) in patients undergoing suprarenal aortic cross-clamp, but rarely in patients when the clamp will be infrarenal. However, we may place PACs in patients with a history of CHF or poor left ventricular function on preoperative or intraoperative echocardiography, diabetes with end-organ damage, cor pulmonale, or renal insufficiency. We recognize, however, that more recent large randomized trials and observational studies have not been able to demonstrate any improvements in outcome with pulmonary artery catheters.[119] Therefore, although we occasionally use them in major vascular surgery in patients with associated end-organ dysfunction, we do not believe that pulmonary artery catheterization is required for vascular surgery.

For patients undergoing thoracic or thoracoabdominal aortic resection, we may place a large double-lumen introducer in an internal jugular or subclavian vein. This large catheter provides two very large-bore routes for volume resuscitation and allows passage of a PAC if desired. For a patient undergoing an infrarenal procedure, we are generally satisfied with a simple 9F introducer in the right internal jugular vein (with a triple-lumen central venous catheter or a PAC) and a large-bore peripheral intravenous catheter.

If we elect to drain CSF, we place specialized silastic lumbar drainage catheters into the intrathecal space at L3–L4 or L4–L5. These catheters have a one-way pressure valve that allow drainage only when the CSF pressure exceeds 5 to 10 mm Hg. Some clinicians have placed them the night before surgery in case a "bloody tap" results so clotting may be assured. We generally wait until after the likelihood of paraplegia has declined and until after coagulopathy (which is common after thoracoabdominal repair) has resolved to remove CSF drains, usually on the second or third postoperative day.

Virtually all anesthetic techniques and drugs have been used for aortic reconstructive surgery. We believe our ability to maintain hemodynamic equilibrium and attend to detail is more crucial to outcome than is the choice of drugs.

Halogenated agents produce vasodilation that has advantages and disadvantages. It provides an additional means of controlling afterload and preload but can lead to an increased need for intravascular volume. Volatile drugs also permit careful, deliberate induction, manipulation of hemodynamic variables, and adjustment of dose. They can also be used to treat stress-induced increases in left ventricular filling pressures.[120] They provide a moderate degree of muscle relaxation, decreasing the need for muscle relaxants and increasing the ease of reversing paralysis. Volatile anesthetics also facilitate tracheal extubation at the end of surgery. Thus, the stressful stimuli and hypertension associated with continued intubation of the trachea after surgery are avoided. Also, this approach permits early assessment of neurologic function and the presence of angina (although the vast majority of episodes of postoperative myocardial ischemia are "silent"). Perhaps the most important reason to routinely include volatile agents into general anesthetics is the increasing awareness that volatile anesthetics improve preconditioning mechanisms and reduce the size of MI should it occur.[121] These effects have been documented in animal models and on-pump CABG models, although we await specific information in vascular surgery patients.

All commonly used opioids produce similar cardiovascular effects unless they are administered rapidly in large doses. Induction of anesthesia with opioids, which can be accomplished quickly, decreases the cardiac index by a small amount. In sufficient doses, opioids produce analgesia and hypnosis, with only slight decreases in cardiac contractility and blood pressure. Higher doses predictably decrease peripheral vascular resistance, especially when administered after benzodiazepines. With continual infusion of opioids or other drugs, anesthesia can be maintained throughout the surgical procedure. Surgical stimulation after opioid induction significantly increases the heart rate, arterial blood pressure, and systemic vascular resistance. Nitroglycerin, nitroprusside, or a volatile anesthetic (our usual choice) can be added to the opioid for manipulation of the circulation during cross-clamping and unclamping.

Nitrous oxide can be used with opioids or with the inhalational drugs. However, it increases afterload and myocardial work, while depressing myocardial inotropic performance and output. In one study of patients undergoing abdominal aortic surgery, nitrous oxide increased the need for nitroglycerin to treat elevated PCWP and myocardial ischemia, although clinical outcome was not affected. Nitrous oxide may decrease renal and splanchnic blood flows, and may have long-lasting toxic effects by causing nutritional, neurologic, and immunologic deficits. Nitrous oxide acutely increases homocyteine concentrations, and this can be associated with increased perioperative myocardial ischemia in vascular surgery; pretreatment with B vitamins can mitigate this response.[122] Nitrous oxide can also contribute to bowel distention.

Our work suggests that large doses (15 to 20 mcg/kg) of the synthetic narcotic sufentanil improve patient outcome after aortic reconstruction. High-dose sufentanil anesthesia alone was associated with less major (cardiac and renal) morbidity than isoflurane anesthesia (Table 32-8). Sufentanil may have a protective effect because of its superior blockade of the

TABLE 32-8

MORBIDITY AFTER AORTIC RECONSTRUCTION WITH ONE OF TWO DIFFERENT ANESTHETIC AGENTS

MORBIDITY	ISOFLURANE-BASED ANESTHETIC ($n = 50$)	SUFENTANIL-BASED ANESTHETIC ($n = 46$)
Renal insufficiency	16	4*
Congestive heart failure	13	4*
Ventilation >24 hr	9	4
Pneumonia	2	1
Renal failure	3	1
Stroke	2	0
Myocardial ischemia	0	1
Death	2	1
Important or severe complications	20	9*
Important or severe complications and failure	17	7*

*$P < .05$ by Fisher exact test.

Modified with permission from Benefiel DJ, Roizen MF, Lampe GH *et al:* Morbidity after aortic surgery with sufentanil versus isoflurane anesthesia. Anesthesiology 65:A516, 1986.

adrenergic stress response. Further study is needed to determine whether all opioids are protective. A disadvantage of the opioids is that most linger into the postoperative period. However, in more than 50% of the patients who received a high-dose, opioid-nitrous oxide anesthetic technique (sufentanil 15 to 20 μg/kg) for suprarenal aortic reconstruction, tracheal extubation was accomplished in the operating room. High-dose opioid anesthetics also produce excellent postoperative analgesia. Our current practice relies on smaller doses of sufentanil (2 to 5 mcg/kg), combined with 0.5 to 1.0 MAC volatile agent if an epidural is not used.

Combined general epidural and general spinal anesthetics have been used successfully for aortic reconstruction. A detailed description of the advantages and disadvantages of regional anesthetics can be found below in lower-extremity revascularization. For patients requiring thoracotomy, the analgesia provided by thoracic epidural infusion of narcotics and/or local anesthetics may be particularly helpful in improving spirometric function. Thoracic epidural local anesthetics can also dilate coronary arteries and help prevent stress-induced elevations in PCWP. Some clinicians are reluctant to use epidural anesthesia for supraceliac aortic reconstruction because of concerns about concurrent heparinization and the associated incidence of paraplegia. In such patients, the use of peridural narcotics without local anesthetics can preserve sensory and motor function and can allow early assessment of neurologic integrity. Because urinary catheters are typically left in place for at least 36 hours after aortic reconstruction surgery, urinary retention is not a major issue. We often use intrathecal or epidural narcotics after supraceliac aortic occlusion. Animal studies have shown that intrathecal naloxone improves neurologic function after thoracic aortic occlusion, but results in humans have been inconclusive. Another disadvantage of epidural local anesthetics is that although patients must receive increased amounts of intravenous fluids, they are still likely to become hypotensive after reperfusion.[123] Therefore, we are prepared for the possibility of fluid overload toward the end of the procedure. Alternatively, infusions of dopamine or dobutamine may be used to maintain systemic vascular resistance and contractility in the presence of the sympathectomy induced by the use of local anesthetics for regional block.

We believe prophylaxis of stress and pain by any mechanism (epidural anesthetics, opiate infusion, or α_2-agonists) may result in lower morbidity in those least able to tolerate the myocardial and cardiovascular demands of stress.

Management of Elective Aortic Surgery

We believe prehydration reduces variations in blood pressure on induction of anesthesia. After the patient's preoperative condition has been optimized, the range of hemodynamic variables for that patient is determined. The anesthetic management is then planned to keep the patient within 20% of this range, as long as the PCWP does not exceed 15 mm Hg, the heart rate does not exceed 80 to 90 beats/min, and signs of organ ischemia are absent. In the preoperative holding area or in the operating room, the monitors and catheters that are needed for induction of anesthesia are placed, usually a radial artery catheter in the nondominant hand, a manual blood pressure cuff, pulse oximeter, ECG (leads II and V_5), ST segment trend monitor, precordial stethoscope, a 16-gauge intravenous line, and, occasionally, a central venous or pulmonary artery catheter. We generally induce anesthesia with small incremental doses of propofol and judicious amounts of opiates, lidocaine, or esmolol to blunt responses to intubation; we are aware that the combination of propofol and beta-blockers or ACE inhibitors can cause hypotension in elderly or hypovolemic patients. The remainder of the pre–cross-clamping phase is devoted to meticulous attention to the details of maintaining temperature homeostasis (unless hypothermia is desired for its potential spinal cord protection): maintaining volume homeostasis as judged by heart rate, blood pressure, pulmonary capillary pressure, or CVP; maintaining left ventricular end-diastolic volume as assessed by echocardiography; ensuring absence of organ ischemia; monitoring (but usually not treating) urine output; and keeping systemic and pulmonary blood pressures and heart rate in the patient's usual range. Every increase in blood pressure or heart rate is either anticipated or treated as soon as it occurs with 25 to 50 μg of sufentanil.

For the half-hour immediately before cross-clamping and aortic occlusion, the patient is kept slightly hypovolemic by examining the ventricular volume by means of echocardiography or by keeping PCWP at 5 to 15 mm Hg. At the time of occlusion we are prepared to give a vasodilating drug through an intravenous catheter placed specifically for that purpose to avoid hypotension from an accidental bolus of vasodilator. Alternatively, we may increase the concentration of volatile anesthetic, or inject local anesthetics into the epidural catheter. Both of these approaches require careful attention to avoid hypotension. A novel approach to reduce blood pressure in the face of aortic occlusion has been described using placement of 15 cm positive end-expiratory pressure immediately before cross-clamp, with removal just before unclamping.[124] This approach facilitates volume loading and reduces hypotension after unclamping. Our approach is different when we are concerned about spinal cord perfusion in patients whose aorta will be occluded at the thoracic level without distal perfusion. In these instances, we will accept some proximal hypertension while the aorta is occluded in the hope of obtaining higher distal perfusion pressures and preventing distal ischemia. This choice may come at the expense of myocardial well-being. In fact, 92% of the patients we studied had ischemia, as evidenced by abnormal motion and thickening of the left ventricle (see Table 32-6). More distal levels of temporary occlusion are less stressful hemodynamically.

Administration of exogenous vasoconstrictors is avoided, if
7 possible. Phenylephrine doubles the incidence of wall motion abnormalities observed by echocardiography compared with the incidence in patients whose blood pressure is maintained simply by light anesthesia and endogenous vasoconstrictors.[34] Rather than relying on vasoconstrictors, we ensure adequate volume at the time of cross-clamp removal by replacing blood lost during occlusion with crystalloid or colloid, warmed cell-saver blood, or banked blood to keep the hematocrit slightly above 30% because it will decrease to 30% in the postocclusion period. We believe that this is the minimal acceptable value for patients in this risk group.[48] Guided by filling pressures or echocardiographic estimates of volume, we are careful not to dilate the left ventricle to an abnormal size.

We routinely use autotransfusion devices and prefer to have a technician to operate them. We continue to do this even though autotransfusion devices may not reduce transfusion of allogenic blood but only delay it.[125] After the sixth unit of blood has been given and if more blood loss is anticipated, or after 8 units of blood have been administered, 10 units of platelets are requested for the patient (and occasionally 2 units of fresh frozen plasma). Because a large part of the vascular tree is excluded from circulation during temporary aortic occlusion, blood loss can be considerable during supraceliac cross-clamping without the onset of hypotension or tachycardia. Evisceration of bowel, often necessary for optimal exposure of the thoracoabdominal aorta, further depletes intravascular volume. Blood loss into the pleural or retroperitoneal cavity may not be readily detected.

Immediately before and during removal of the cross-clamp, we stop infusing vasodilators. We allow blood pressure, PCWP, and filling volumes to go as high as possible without the occurrence of myocardial ischemia. The surgeon then opens the aorta gradually to ensure that severe hypotension does not develop and that there is not too much bleeding from the suture line. Pathophysiologic events on removal of the aortic cross-clamp are associated with inadequate preload. We therefore infuse crystalloid, colloid, or blood just before reperfusion. Guided by filling pressures or echocardiographic estimates of volume, or both, we are careful not to dilate the left ventricle.

Volume replacement and maintenance are mainstays of therapy before, during, and immediately after removal of the aortic cross-clamp. At this point in the procedure, pulmonary artery pressures or CVP may increase because reperfusion of ischemic tissues is associated with the release of lactic acid and other unknown mediators that can cause pulmonary vasoconstriction. Mannitol prophylaxis may prevent part of this response, and we frequently give mannitol 0.5 to 1.0 g/kg immediately before release of the clamp.

During closure, we again ensure adequate organ perfusion, as well as hemodynamic and temperature homeostasis, and we reverse the effects of muscle relaxants. Reversal is easier when patients are warm. Hypothermia after aortic reconstruction is associated with other complications, including coagulopathy, low cardiac output states, and significantly higher incidences of organ dysfunction and death. We routinely use forced-air warming on the upper portion of the body in these patients, although their lateral position and extensive exposure during thoracic procedures make maintaining normothermia difficult.

During emergence from anesthesia, we use infusions of nitroglycerin and esmolol or another β-adrenergic blocking agent to prevent hemodynamic variations outside the patient's normal range. If ventilation is adequate and fluid replacements have been modest and we do not suspect airway edema, the trachea is extubated; otherwise, controlled ventilation is maintained until spontaneous ventilation is judged adequate. If we elect to use a predominantly inhalational anesthetic technique, we often place a thoracic epidural catheter and administer epidural local anesthetics and opioids for postoperative analgesia. When the sufentanil-based technique described previously is used, rarely is much additional pain therapy needed for 24 hours. We continue to provide prophylactic beta-blockade into the postoperative period, as tolerated. In unstable patients, esmolol may be infused; in more stable patients, we will often prescribe metoprolol 5 to 10 mg intravenously q6h, as long as heart rate >55 beats/minute and blood pressure >110 mm Hg.

Anesthesia for Emergency Aortic Surgery

The most common cause of emergency aortic reconstruction is a leaking or ruptured aortic aneurysm. Ruptured aneurysms can be atherosclerotic, mycotic, syphilitic, or inflammatory, or may occur in patients with the marfanoid syndrome. Ruptured aneurysms carry associated mortality roughly 10 times greater than elective repair. Therefore, efforts should be made to increase the number of elective operations performed for aortic aneurysms before they rupture, as urgent/emergent surgery is associated with increased mortality even in the absence of frank rupture.

Symptoms of ruptured AAAs include pain, faintness or frank collapse, and vomiting. Pain in the back, abdomen, or both is almost always present. Therefore, many surgeons believe pain in combination with a known AAA or pulsatile abdominal mass indicates dissection or rupture and the immediate need for surgical exploration until proved otherwise. Ruptures most commonly occur into the retroperitoneum. This site permits tamponade of the hemorrhage; however, retroperitoneal hemorrhage and subsequent hematoma can displace the left renal vein, inferior vena cava, and intestine, possibly leading to damage to these structures during the surgical approach. Venous hemorrhage is often much more difficult to control than arterial hemorrhage.

Approximately 25% of aneurysms rupture into the peritoneal cavity, a site associated with a great degree of exsanguination. Other sites of rupture include adjacent structures after formation of fistulae with the inferior vena cava, iliac veins, or renal veins. Aortoenteric fistulae can occur. The mortality from these fistulae is high, often exceeding 50%. The importance of controlling bleeding gives credence to the inescapable sense of urgency that accompanies such events.

Management of hemodynamically unstable patients is challenging. Shock frequently accompanies rupture. However, the absence of hypotension does not rule out the possibility of rupture, and shock may occur suddenly. Rapid diagnosis with immediate laparotomy and control of the proximal aorta are of the highest priority. If systolic blood pressure is <90 mm Hg, some clinicians advocate the administration of oxygen by face mask, with tracheal intubation performed only after proximal control of the aorta has been achieved. We prefer an awake intubation, with very slow induction of anesthesia after the airway is secured. However, in uncooperative patients we may perform a rapid-sequence tracheal intubation after small doses of etomidate (0.1 mg/kg) and a steroid. Almost simultaneously, laparotomy is begun so the surgeon can clamp the aorta.

We attempt to replace volume to normalize systemic blood pressure. However, when rupture is suspected, rapid control of the proximal portion of the aorta is probably more important than optimizing the patient's preoperative condition. Alternatively, a balloon may be passed from the femoral artery under fluoroscopic control to occlude the aorta above the site of rupture. The patient is resuscitated quickly (before induction of anesthesia, if possible) with crystalloid, colloid, packed red blood cells, and even type-specific non–cross-matched blood if necessary, administered via large-bore peripheral or central venous catheters by roller pumps or pressured bags. If type-specific blood is not available, O-negative washed red blood cells may be given. We emphasize the importance of large-bore peripheral catheters placed in the most easily accessible vein, often 14-gauge catheters in each antecubital fossa. We recommend the use, when possible, of fluid warmers that deliver rapid volumes of normothermic fluids.

Once the aorta is controlled with a cross-clamp, and blood pressure and perfusion are restored, additional venous access and a radial, brachial, or axillary arterial line are secured. Attention may then be turned to placing a CVP or pulmonary artery catheter once blood pressure is adequate. Even more quickly, an echocardiographic probe can be inserted for rapid assessment of left ventricular volume and contractility. At this point, volume administration is guided by means of PCWP or by TEE. High-normal filling pressures are desirable for attenuation of hypotension after removal of the aortic clamp. Some patients with hemorrhagic shock will require infusions of dopamine, epinephrine, or norepinephrine to sustain an adequate blood pressure even after restoration of normal blood volume. Vasopressin may be particularly effective in restoring blood pressure when hemorrhagic shock is resistant to catecholamines. These patients are often profoundly acidotic; if we administer sodium bicarbonate, we increase ventilation to help eliminate the extra carbon dioxide produced. We do not hesitate to paralyze and administer propofol, midazolam, and/or opioids to these patients if they are hemodynamically stable because they usually require postoperative mechanical ventilation of the lungs and sedation to minimize cardiovascular stress. Acute respiratory distress syndrome develops frequently in patients who survive surgery for a ruptured aneurysm.

Due to hypothermia from massive fluid resuscitation and the aortic occlusion above the hepatic artery, replacement blood may not pass through the liver in amounts adequate to allow for metabolism of citrate. Therefore, if hypotension due to poor myocardial contractility (which may be easily assessed with TEE) or coagulopathy develops, administration of calcium may be therapeutic. It has been suggested that the aggressive fluid resuscitation of trauma patients in the emergency room before transport to the operating room may result in increased mortality, perhaps by causing hypothermia or dilutional coagulopathy, or by raising blood pressure and increasing bleeding. At present, however, we cannot recommend allowing patients to remain hypotensive but believe attention should be paid to maintaining temperature, adequate hematocrit, and coagulation, in addition to simply normalizing intravascular volume.

We routinely use autotransfusion in patients with actual or suspected rupture of an aortic aneurysm, even though some have questioned its effectiveness in reducing transfusion requirements.[125]

The complications that occur during aortic occlusion can usually be linked to the heart, central nervous system, or kidneys. Organ dysfunction can be minimized by maintaining intraoperative values for hemodynamic variables within the normal preoperative range, ensuring cardiac dilation does not occur at any point, and minimizing episodes of tachycardia. Attention to the details of preoperative drug therapy, preoperative hydration, and temperature homeostasis may also promote an improved outcome. Further, vigilance must continue into the postoperative period if morbidity and mortality are
8 to be minimized. As opposed to elective aortic reconstruction, in which preserving myocardial function is the primary goal, in emergency resection the crucial factor for patient survival is first rapid control of blood loss and reversal of hypotension, and then preservation of myocardial function.

LOWER-EXTREMITY REVASCULARIZATION

The number of patients undergoing lower-extremity revascularization has increased as surgeons attempt to improve functional status in elderly patients. Many patients undergo revision or repeat operations. They often have complex medical histories and diseases of multiple organ systems that present additional challenges beyond those of routine anesthetic management. Despite this fact, patients are now frequently admitted to the hospital on the day of surgery. For others, surgery is emergent or urgent. In all these situations, the primary goal of anesthetic management is to prevent the development of perioperative complications. These patients are at particularly high risk for perioperative cardiac complications, including myocardial ischemia and infarction, low cardiac output (forward failure), and pulmonary edema (backward failure). Krupski et al.[15] showed that the incidence of cardiac morbidity after infrainguinal procedures may exceed that associated with abdominal aortic procedures because patients scheduled for distal procedures often have more preoperative cardiac risk factors than patients scheduled for aortic procedures. Yet, patients undergoing lower-extremity revascularization may receive less attentive care than patients undergoing "major" procedures.

Increasingly, endovascular repair may involve angioplasty and or stenting of smaller vessels, including femoral arteries. However, restenosis after stenting may necessitate repeated percutaneous or surgical revascularization procedures. Increasingly, these procedures may be performed by cardiologists, and they may be performed without an anesthesiologist present. The use of drug-eluting stents that deliver drugs such as paclitaxel to the site of vascular injury may reduce the incidence of neointimal hyperplasia and restenosis. Their use in the coronary circulation reduces restenosis and may or may not reduce morbid events.[126]

In addition to maintaining adequate cardiac function, another goal of our anesthetic and perioperative care is to ensure adequate perfusion and to prevent hypercoagulable responses to surgery to maintain graft patency in the immediate postoperative period. Pulmonary, renal, neurologic, and hepatic dysfunction may occur following vascular surgery; proper intraoperative and postoperative management may also help prevent these adverse outcomes. Anesthetic techniques that reduce the stress response may improve outcome. We believe ideal anesthetic management of these patients may decrease morbidity and mortality, as well as hasten recovery and hospital discharge.

Because some patients may undergo multiple procedures, anesthesiologists may become cynical about the effectiveness of lower-extremity revascularization; however, long-term patency and limb salvage rates are good, demanding that anesthesiologists do all they can to optimize outcome in these procedures. The typical cost of a limb salvage procedure approaches $20,000, which may be less than the cost of amputation when rehabilitation and the loss of independence are considered.

There are three clinical indications for elective surgery for chronic peripheral occlusive disease: (1) claudication, (2) ischemic rest pain or ulceration, and (3) gangrene. Patients with claudication have symptoms on walking that are relieved by rest. Such patients are not at significant risk for imminent limb loss. Patients with rest pain, ulceration, or gangrene are at variable risk for imminent limb loss and may have severe progressive ischemia. Thus, reconstruction for such patients is semi-urgent or urgent. When a patient presents with a gangrenous (black) or pregangrenous (blue) toe, several causes other than progression of chronic arteriosclerotic occlusive disease must be considered. Emboli may originate from the heart, a proximal aneurysm, or any proximal atherosclerotic lesion. Intra-arterially administered lytic agents, particularly urokinase, may have been administered, precluding regional anesthesia. Local infection is particularly common in diabetic patients.

Vascular reconstruction procedures are generally categorized as either inflow or outflow procedures. Inflow reconstruction involves bypass of the obstruction in the aortoiliac segment, whereas outflow procedures are those performed distal to the inguinal ligament for bypass of femoral-popliteal or distal obstructions. The most common inflow reconstruction procedure for obstructions in the aortoiliac segment is aortofemoral bypass. The usual vascular reconstruction below the inguinal ligament is a bypass graft that originates in the common femoral artery and extends to the popliteal or tibial artery. Such a bypass may be performed with a reversed saphenous vein, the saphenous vein in situ, or a prosthetic graft.

The complexity of femoral-popliteal and femorotibial bypass varies widely. The site for distal anastomosis and the quality of the outflow vessels are assessed by preoperative contrast or magnetic resonance angiography. Prosthetic bypasses can be performed more quickly and require less dissection than the saphenous vein bypass because it is not necessary to make multiple incisions for vein harvest. Prosthetic bypasses, however, have significantly lower patency rates than saphenous vein bypasses when they extend below the knee. The best short-term and long-term results are achieved with the saphenous vein, but this technique requires longer operative time and greater technical expertise than are needed for prosthetic grafts. The duration and complexity of the operation are usually determined by the quality of the saphenous vein, as well as the quality and size of the distal outflow vessels. In the past, the choice of a vascular prosthesis for a femoral-popliteal, above-knee, arterial bypass graft reflected the surgeon's preference. However, a Veterans Affairs randomized trial of different bypass graft materials for patients with femoral-popliteal, above-knee bypass grafts found that after 5 years, above-knee saphenous vein bypass grafts had a significantly better patency rate (73%) than cryopreserved human umbilical vein bypass grafts (53%), which had a significantly better patency rate than PTFE bypass grafts (39%).[127] Limb salvage was worse with prosthetic conduits, whereas bypass graft thromboses and amputations within the first 30 days were highest in the umbilical vein group. Therefore, although the anesthesiologist may rightly perceive that saphenous vein harvest and preparation prolong the surgery and anesthetic, this is done for the patient's benefit.

In a reversed saphenous vein bypass, the vein is dissected, all branches are ligated and divided, and the vein is excised. The direction of the saphenous vein is reversed to permit blood flow in the direction of the valves, and the vein is tunneled from the femoral artery to the distal vessel. The use of the vein in situ offers significant advantages over the reversed-vein bypass; because the vein is not removed from its bed, it is subjected to little trauma; twisting or kinking is unlikely. These advantages have improved patency rates. The use of intraluminal angioscopy is reported to result in better vein preparation, smaller incisions, improved patency, and shorter hospital stay. The quality of the repair is determined from the pulse quality, Doppler ultrasound studies, or completion angiography.

The surgeons' concerns for patients with peripheral vascular insufficiency include not only those problems involving the cardiovascular system, but also specific problems related to the operative repair. Tunneling of the graft between the incisions may be more stimulating than other parts of the procedure and may cause hypertension under general anesthesia. The patient is usually given heparin during the procedure. In most cases, the heparin effect is not antagonized because bleeding problems are rare and graft reocclusion is a concern. Graft patency is evaluated carefully in the recovery room. Most surgeons believe the patient's feet should be kept warm and that the patient should be well hydrated so peripheral vasoconstriction, which may limit outflow from the new graft, is prevented. If graft thrombosis develops early in the postoperative period, the patient is promptly returned to the operating room for graft thrombectomy, as well as for evaluation and correction of the cause of the thrombosis. It can be anticipated that, during graft thrombectomy, significant blood loss will occur with flushing of the graft.

Anesthetic Management of Elective Lower-Extremity Revascularization

There is perhaps no other disease entity about which the anesthesiologist can be misled so easily than vascular disease of the lower extremity. One is apt to hear, "Oh, it's just a local procedure," or "Just put a spinal in and let's get on with it; you don't have to read the chart." However, the morbidity and mortality following distal operations approach those following infra-aortic reconstruction and are mainly of cardiac origin.[15] Thus, although we often use epidural or spinal anesthetics and opioids for pain relief, we pay close attention to body temperature, oxygen delivery, and hemodynamic homeostasis during peripheral vascular procedures and during aortic procedures that involve much greater hemodynamic fluctuations. The devices and the concerns previously described apply, with special attention to the postoperative period. It is during the postoperative period that most cardiac problems arise, and pain relief and correction of hemodynamic and fluid disequilibria are most likely to be needed. Care must be taken not to allow overhydration to occur intraoperatively in support of blood pressure, and then to cause CHF as the epidural sympathectomy wears off. Dye loads given for "completion angiography" also contribute to fluid shifts; thus, monitoring of cardiac preload is important for a successful outcome.

We often monitor hemodynamic variables invasively in patients undergoing lower-extremity revascularization. We place a radial arterial line in many patients, because the associated morbidity is low. An arterial line provides real-time information on blood pressure that can guide pharmacologic therapy for the rapid hemodynamic fluctuations that accompany induction of, and emergence from, anesthesia. Arterial cannulation also facilitates blood drawing in the crucial first 24 hours after surgery, especially in diabetics. If percutaneous radial artery catheterization is impossible, we rely instead on noninvasive blood pressure measurement.

We may place CVP catheters for various reasons. Blood loss may be insidious and unrecognized during prolonged, revision, infrapopliteal, or in situ procedures. Rapid blood loss or hemodynamic changes are not usually encountered with distal reconstruction, but the procedures tend to be lengthy, making intraoperative urinary drainage advisable. Our experience is that blood loss may be underestimated, and we may measure the CVP and obtain a hematocrit every 2 hours in patients undergoing below-knee procedures. Because the major morbidity and mortality with this procedure are related to the cardiovascular system, with rates above 8% and 2%, respectively, the noninvasive nature and the absence of hemodynamic alterations should not lull the anesthesiologist into a casual attitude.

Cardiac preload is reduced by epidural and spinal anesthesia due to the venodilation caused by their sympatholytic properties. Later, as the spinal or epidural anesthetic recedes, the patient's blood volume is distributed back to the central circulation. This "autotransfusion" can lead to elevated filling pressures, which may precipitate CHF if not recognized and treated appropriately. In our experience, CVP monitoring is helpful in diagnosing and treating postoperative hypovolemia. The early diagnosis and treatment of even subtle hypovolemia may be important in preventing postoperative renal dysfunction and early graft thrombosis. In some patients, the placement of a triple-lumen catheter allows for concurrent volume loading, multiple drug infusions, and CVP monitoring. Central venous catheters are also useful in the patient who will have vein harvested from the upper extremities. The risks associated with central catheter placement can be minimized by attention to strict aseptic technique during placement by an experienced or closely supervised practitioner. The risks associated with an indwelling catheter can be minimized by inserting a single-lumen or double-lumen catheter where feasible and removing the catheter as soon as it is no longer needed.

We do not believe the information obtained from a PAC justifies the additional risks (including heart block, dysrhythmia, pulmonary artery rupture, and pulmonary infarction) associated with routine use of this monitor in this patient population. Berlauk et al.[128] found that patients who were monitored during lower-extremity revascularization with PACs had a lower incidence of early graft occlusion than did patients with CVP monitoring. This study has been criticized because patients in the PAC group received nitroglycerin and volume loading (which have been previously shown to reduce morbidity from vascular surgery), whereas those in the CVP group did not. Also, the investigators and practitioners were not blinded to the randomization groups, so the potential for introduction of bias during diagnosis and treatment was very high. We believe the prophylactic use of nitrates and volume loading in this study may have contributed more to the observed improved outcome than did the use of PACs. Therefore, we rarely use PACs. We may use PACs in patients with severe left ventricular dysfunction, renal failure, diabetes mellitus with autonomic neuropathy, and severe cor pulmonale and pulmonary hypertension. Further discussions about invasive monitoring can be found earlier in the chapter.

The choice of anesthetic for lower-extremity revascularization is individualized for each patient. Table 32-9 summarizes

TABLE 32-9

REGIONAL ANESTHESIA VERSUS GENERAL ANESTHESIA

ANESTHETIC TECHNIQUE	ADVANTAGES	DISADVANTAGES
Regional	Effective blockade of stress response Patient as monitor (dyspnea, angina) Improved graft blood flow Possible prevention of postoperative hypercoagulability Postoperative analgesia Possible prevention or improvement of chronic pain syndromes (RSD) Possible improved cardiopulmonary morbidity	Time-consuming May be technically difficult May be inadequate for the surgery Patient discomfort during long cases Sympathectomy requires volume loading Respiratory depression (from sedation or high level of blockade) Rare neurologic sequelae Precludes thrombolytic therapy
General	Controlled airway Hemodynamics easily controlled Reliable Patient comfort ensured for long cases	Hyperdynamic state after surgery Large fluctuations in cathecholamine levels Postoperative hypercoagulability not inhibited Greater perturbation of respiratory mechanics

From Tzeng GF: Hemostatic interventions and regional anesthesia for vascular surgery. Prob Anesth 11:207, 1999.

the advantages and disadvantages of regional versus general anesthesia for this procedure.[129] The patient may have a preference for one technique over another based on previous experiences. Technical factors may contribute to the decision: obesity, previous laminectomy, or severe kyphoscoliosis may make it difficult to establish neuraxial blockade. Septicemia, local infection, anticoagulation, and certain neurologic diseases provide varying degrees of relative and absolute contraindications to regional anesthetic techniques. Regional anesthesia may be poorly tolerated by patients who are orthopneic, uncomfortable lying still for many hours, or demented and uncooperative. Indeed, failed regional anesthesia (11% of spinals and 16% of epidurals) is associated with 9% mortality, compared with 2% for successful regional or general anesthesia for femoral bypass.[117] Sedation allows patients to better tolerate a regional anesthetic for a long procedure, but we administer sedation judiciously because these patients are often frail or at risk for pulmonary aspiration. The combination of a high level of regional blockade and sedation may rarely produce cardiovascular collapse. The patient with rest pain who has received narcotic premedication may become very sedated or even apneic when the pain is suddenly relieved by a regional anesthetic. The argument that regional anesthesia allows the patient to be a monitor for myocardial ischemia by being able to complain of angina may be specious because the vast majority of episodes of perioperative myocardial ischemia are painless. 9 Regional anesthesia may offer several advantages, however, including avoidance of hyperdynamic responses to tracheal intubation and extubation, reduced incidences of postoperative respiratory and infectious complications, and reduced postoperative hypercoagulability and graft thrombosis[130] (see Table 32-9). Other studies refute any effects of regional anesthesia on thrombotic outcomes and suggest only higher costs for postoperative surveillance. In some cases, the combination of regional and general anesthesia may provide patients with the benefits of each technique. To reduce the incidence of pruritus and respiratory depression from epidural narcotic analgesia, some anesthesiologists routinely infuse naloxone or place partial opiate agonists into the epidural space.

The operative procedure may also dictate the choice of anesthetic. Prolonged in situ and/or repeat procedures may not be amenable to a single-shot spinal technique; catheter spinal or continuous epidural techniques may be useful in these situations. The use of microcatheters for continuous spinal anesthesia was abandoned after reports of cauda equina syndrome, but the use of continuous spinal anesthesia through a larger catheter (e.g., those intended for use in the epidural space) does not appear to be a problem because it permits better dispersal and dilution of local anesthetic in the CSF. The incidence of postdural puncture headache is low in elderly patients. At times, we have combined spinal and epidural anesthesia for lengthy procedures. If the procedure takes longer than the 4 to 6 hours of surgical anesthesia provided by long-acting local anesthetics (often supplemented with 0.1 to 0.15 mg of preservative-free morphine), then the epidural catheter can be used to supplement surgical anesthesia and provide postoperative analgesia. Alternatively, an LMA may be placed for the duration of the procedure.

The formation of an epidural hematoma or abscess is a dreaded complication of any neuroaxial anesthetic technique. We try to ensure every health care provider who participates in the care of patients who have had epidural or spinal anesthesia is vigilant for the signs of an epidural hematoma and is aware of the need for its emergent operative evacuation. Severe back pain or pressure is the earliest symptom of epidural hematoma formation. The pain often develops a radicular component, and the patient may develop focal neurologic findings that correlate with injury to the spinal cord or nerve root. Both CT and MRI are acceptable imaging modalities for the diagnosis of a lumbar epidural hematoma. Time is of the essence, for if the spinal cord compression persists for longer than 6 to 12 hours, catastrophic paralysis may result. One must realize that if the patient is recovering from a general or a regional anesthetic, the spinal cord may have been compressed long before the patient started to complain. If a hematoma is diagnosed by CT, MRI, or myelography, the patient must have an emergent laminectomy and decompression if the risk of paralysis is to be minimized.[129]

Coagulopathy therefore represents a relative contraindication to regional anesthesia. The degree of coagulopathy at which it becomes unsafe to perform regional anesthesia is unknown, is highly controversial, and must be part of the risk–benefit calculation in each patient. Table 33-12 summarizes some suggestions for management of regional anesthetics and anticoagulation therapy; they have been reviewed earlier in the chapter.[12]

General anesthesia for lower-extremity revascularization has the advantage of obviating patient discomfort and lack of cooperation (see Table 32-9). It allows for adequate oxygenation and ventilation, and facilitates hemodynamic manipulation. Its use is virtually mandated in patients who are to have vein harvested from an arm (unless spinal and brachial plexus blocks are performed coincidentally). General anesthesia has been associated with a higher incidence of postoperative respiratory complications in some studies. However, although reduction in cardiac complications is often a stated reason for avoiding general anesthesia, more recent series have been unable to show such an effect in patients undergoing lower-extremity revascularization. Regional anesthetics may or may not reduce postoperative thrombotic complications. We do not believe the evidence favoring regional anesthesia is so overwhelming that we would withhold a general anesthetic from most patients to whom we have offered a regional anesthetic. Peripheral nerve blocks ("3-in-1," femoral sciatic block) may also be useful during and after lower-extremity revascularization.[131]

Specific types of general anesthetic may be preferred for patients undergoing vascular surgery. High-dose narcotic anesthetics may be associated with less renal insufficiency and CHF after aortic reconstruction than are volatile anesthetics.[132] This effect may be attributed to the superior ability of narcotics to blunt the adrenergic response to surgery. Despite these findings, we usually provide general anesthesia with doses of narcotics, which, although generous, still permit extubation in the operating room. Patients who receive general anesthesia can have a carefully controlled emergence and extubation, whether in the operating room or later in the ICU. We prefer to perform tracheal extubation at the end of surgery in the operating room, with the same intense monitoring of hemodynamics used during induction of anesthesia. We believe it is important to appreciate the complex physiology of the anesthetic emergence. This period is punctuated by large increases in catecholamine levels (see Fig. 32-3) and a high incidence of myocardial ischemia.[130] Emergence is a period of careful titration: opiates are infused to control pain and blunt sympathetic discharge, while still allowing the patient to ventilate effectively. Therefore, while still intubated and breathing spontaneously, patients receive incremental doses of narcotics titrated to adequate respiration (respiratory rate 8 to 16 min^{-1}; end-tidal P_{CO_2} <50 mm Hg). However, the anesthesiologist does not have the luxury of administering large amounts of opiates to blunt this response during the anesthetic emergence if he or she wants to extubate the patient in the operating room. Therefore, additional intravenous drugs are often required to control hemodynamics during emergence. Our usual practice is to titrate intravenous labetalol, metoprolol, dexmedetomidine infusion, or esmolol for extubation to keep heart rate below 80 beats · min^{-1} in the vast majority of patients who can tolerate β-adrenergic receptor blockade.

Anesthesia for Emergency Surgery for Peripheral Vascular Insufficiency

Emergency surgery for peripheral vascular insufficiency is required when acute arterial occlusion results in severe ischemia and threatens the viability of a limb. Immediate operation and restoration of blood flow are needed if limb loss is to be avoided. Depending on the etiology of the occlusion, the patient may or may not be at very high risk. Although this problem may appear to be localized to an extremity, the occluding material may originate in the heart or in major arteries. Therefore, peripheral vascular occlusion may be the result of a more serious cardiovascular problem. In fact, some patients with acute peripheral vascular occlusion are the sickest patients we have ever anesthetized.

With acute arterial occlusion, the involved extremity suddenly becomes cold and pulseless. Patients usually complain of coldness, pain, numbness, and paresthesias, and they may lose motion and sensation. Abnormal sensation in the toes, feet, and legs in response to light touch and pinprick, as well as abnormal proprioception and loss of motor function in the feet and toes, are hallmarks of acute ischemia and nonviability. If the ischemia is not reversed in a matter of hours, irreversible loss of viability is likely to result.

Acute arterial occlusion may develop in patients with preexisting peripheral occlusive or aneurysmal disease caused by thrombosis of a stenotic or ulcerated atherosclerotic artery. Acute arterial occlusion can also occur in patients with normal peripheral arteries that contain emboli. Such embolism is usually of cardiac origin in patients with cardiac dysrhythmias, recent MIs, or ventricular aneurysms.

The cause is important in planning operative treatment. If the cause is an arterial embolus, Fogarty embolectomy through a groin incision with or without angioscopy under local anesthesia may suffice. However, if the cause is thrombosis of severely diseased atherosclerotic arteries, bypass reconstruction will be required. Although preoperative angiography may be of help in the differential diagnosis, often the cause is not uncovered until the vessel is opened. Thus, the anesthesiologist must be prepared for either a simple procedure or a complex, extended procedure. An incision in the groin is usually made for exposure of the femoral artery. Attempts to pass Fogarty catheters proximally and distally are made in the effort to establish flow and extract the thrombus. If flow is not restored in this manner, more complex reconstructive procedures such as aortofemoral, axillofemoral, or femoral-popliteal bypass may be required. Femoral venous drainage (into the autotransfusion suction if available) on restoration of flow to the femoral artery can aid in management by washing the initial venous effluent from an acutely ischemic extremity. Drainage may entail significant blood loss, but subsequent washing in a cell salvage device before reinfusion may prevent hyperkalemia. Significant fluid losses can also be anticipated when the artery is flushed during thrombectomy and fluid is sequestered in edematous revascularized tissue. Serum potassium levels can change quickly because cell death and release of intracellular potassium into the circulation can be anticipated. Myoglobin may also be released into the circulation, and the development of a compartment syndrome is a possibility. Skill and intensive care as meticulous as that given patients with visceral ischemia may also benefit patients with peripheral vascular insufficiency. Free radical scavengers such as mannitol and N-acetyl cysteine may be given to mitigate reperfusion responses; sodium bicarbonate may or may not be given at the time of reperfusion.

Anticoagulants are commonly administered to patients suspected of having peripheral vascular occlusion. If a patient has received anticoagulants, the appropriateness of using a major conduction block (subarachnoid or epidural block with or without catheter placement) is controversial. We believe regional anesthesia should be avoided when patients have received thrombolytic therapy.[12]

CONCLUSION

Patients undergoing vascular reconstruction are generally persons who are elderly. Vascular disease is a generalized process; thus, patients having surgery for a specific vascular disorder are likely to have atherosclerotic disease elsewhere in the vascular system. Most of the patients have CAD. The skills of the anesthesiologist can therefore greatly influence outcome in vascular surgery. The considerations for preoperative patient evaluation are the same as for patients with cardiac disease undergoing other noncardiac procedures. Many have a history of smoking and COPD; renal insufficiency, and lipid abnormalities are frequently present. The major morbidity in each operation relates to myocardial well-being; therefore, the heart should be the major focus of the anesthesiologist's attention.

Attempts to segregate patients who have significant CAD by use of preoperative testing are controversial. The benefits of coronary revascularization are likely to persist long after vascular surgery in patients with triple-vessel CAD.

In cerebrovascular surgery, the goals in anesthesia management (i.e., ensuring adequate myocardial and brain perfusion and a rapidly arousable patient) may be facilitated with the use of neurophysiologic monitoring as a guide to afterload reduction. In aortic reconstruction, ensuring intact myocardial function is probably the best way of making certain that spinal cord, visceral, and renal perfusion will be adequate.

In the case of peripheral occlusive disease, the absence of hemodynamic changes should not lull the anesthesiologist into loss of vigilance with regard to myocardial well-being. In addition, vigilance in ensuring routine prehydration and use of a warming device are probably more important to outcome than is occasional brilliance. We prefer the diligent, compulsive practitioner to the occasionally brilliant one. Nowhere is such diligence needed more than in the postoperative period, when most morbidity related to the heart occurs. Perhaps it is most important to remember that the best patient results are achieved when intraoperative vigilance is extended to the preoperative and postoperative periods as well. Technologic changes in endovascular surgery will reduce the stress of revascularization, but the patient population presenting for repair may evidence even greater comorbidity as selection criteria for surgical candidates become more permissive.

References

1. Khuri SF, Daley J, Henderson W *et al*: Risk adjustment of the postoperative mortality rate for the comparative assessment of the quality of surgical care: Results of the National Veterans Affairs surgical risk study. J Am Coll Surg 185(4):315, 1997
2. Fitzgerald GA: Coxibs and cardiovascular disease. N Engl J Med 351(17): 1709, 2004
3. Faxon DP, Creager MA, Smith SC Jr *et al*: Atherosclerotic vascular disease conference: Executive summary: Atherosclerotic vascular disease conference proceeding for healthcare professionals from a special writing group of the American Heart Association. Circulation 109:2595, 2004
4. Grundy SM, Brewer HB Jr, Cleeman JI *et al*: Definition of metabolic syndrome: Report of the National Heart, Lung, and Blood Institute/American Heart Association conference on scientific issues related to definition. Circulation 109:433, 2004
5. Chobanian AV, Bakris GL, Black HR *et al*: Seventh report of the Joint National Committee on Prevention, Detection, Evaluation, and Treatment of High Blood Pressure. Hypertension 42:1206, 2003
6. Axelrod DA, Stanley JC, Upchurch GR Jr *et al*: Risk for stroke after elective noncarotid vascular surgery. J Vasc Surg 39(1):67, 2004
7. Spencer FA, Allegrone J, Goldberg RJ *et al*: Association of statin therapy with outcomes of acute coronary syndromes: The GRACE study. Ann Intern Med 140:857, 2004
8. Lindenauer PK, Pekow P, Wang K, Gutierrez B, Benjamin EM: Lipid-lowering therapy and in-hospital mortality following major noncardiac surgery. JAMA 291(17):2092, 2004
9. Henke PK, Blackburn S, Proctor MC *et al*: Patients undergoing infrainguinal bypass to treat atherosclerotic vascular disease are underprescribed cardioprotective medications: Effect on graft patency, limb salvage, and mortality. J Vasc Surg 39:357, 2004
10. Parrott S, Godfrey C: Economics of smoking cessation. BMJ 328(7445): 947, 2004
11. Rao TLK, El-Etr AA: Anticoagulation following placement of epidural and subarachnoid catheters: An evaluation of neurologic sequelae. Anesthesiology 55:618, 1981
12. Horlocker TT, Wedel DJ, Benzon H *et al*: Regional anesthesia in the anticoagulated patient: Defining the risks (the second ASRA Consensus Conference on Neuraxial Anesthesia and Anticoagulation). Reg Anesth Pain Med 28:172, 2003
13. Warkentin TE: Heparin-induced thrombocytopenia: Diagnosis and management. Circulation. 110(18):e454, 2004
14. Hertzer NR, Beven EG, Young JR *et al*: Coronary artery disease in peripheral vascular patients: A classification of 1000 coronary angiograms and results of surgical management. Ann Surg 199:223, 1984
15. Krupski WC, Layug EL, Reilly LM *et al*: Comparison of cardiac morbidity rates between aortic and infrainguinal operations: Two-year follow-up. Study of perioperative ischemia research. J Vasc Surg 18:609, 1993
16. Rihal CS, Eagle KA, Mickel MC *et al*: Surgical therapy for coronary artery disease among patients with combined coronary artery and peripheral vascular disease. Circulation 91:46, 1995
17. Kaluza GL, Joseph J, Lee JR, Raizner ME, Raizner AE: Catastrophic outcomes of noncardiac surgery soon after coronary stenting. J Am Coll Cardiol 35(5):1288, 2000
18. Liu LL, Dzankic S, Leung JM: Preoperative electrocardiogram abnormalities do not predict postoperative cardiac complications in geriatric surgical patients. J Am Geriatr Soc 50(7):1186, 2002
19. Badner NH, Knill RL, Brown JE *et al*: Myocardial infarction after noncardiac surgery. Anesthesiology 88:572, 1998
20. Kim LJ, Martinez EA, Faraday N, Dorman T, Fleisher LA, Perler BA, Williams GM, Chan D, Pronovost PJ: Cardiac troponin I predicts short-term mortality in vascular surgery patients. Circulation 106(18):2366, 2002
21. Eagle KA, Berger PB, Calkins H *et al*: ACC/AHA guideline update for perioperative cardiovascular evaluation for noncardiac surgery—executive summary. A report of the American College of Cardiology/American Heart Association Task Force on Practice Guidelines (Committee to Update the 1996 Guidelines on Perioperative Cardiovascular Evaluation for Noncardiac Surgery). Anesth Analg 94(5):1052, 2002
22. Lee TH, Marcantonio ER, Mangione CM *et al*: Derivation and prospective validation of a simple index for prediction of cardiac risk of major noncardiac surgery. Circulation 100:1043, 1999
23. Grayburn PA, Hillis LD: Cardiac events in patients undergoing noncardiac surgery: Shifting the paradigm from noninvasive risk stratification to therapy. Ann Intern Med 138(6):506, 2003
24. Mantha S, Roizen MF, Barnard J *et al*: Relative effectiveness of four preoperative tests for predicting adverse cardiac outcome after vascular surgery: A meta-analysis. Anesth Analg 79:422, 1994
25. Kertai MD, Boersma E, Bax JJ *et al*: A meta-analysis comparing the prognostic accuracy of six diagnostic tests for predicting perioperative cardiac risk in patients undergoing major vascular surgery. Heart 89(11):1327, 2003
26. Gokce N, Keaney JF Jr, Hunter LM *et al*: Predictive value of noninvasively determined endothelial dysfunction for long-term cardiovascular events in patients with peripheral vascular disease. J Am Coll Cardiol 41:1769, 2003
27. Mahla E, Vicenzi MN, Schrottner B *et al*: Coronary artery plaque burden and perioperative cardiac risk. Anesthesiology 95(5):1133, 2001
28. Back MR, Stordahl N, Cuthbertson D *et al*: Limitations in the cardiac risk reduction provided by coronary revascularization prior to elective vascular surgery. J Vasc Surg 36:526, 2002
29. Brown KR, Kresowik TF, Chin MH, Kresowik RA, Grund SL, Hendel ME: Multistate population-based outcomes of combined CEA and coronary artery bypass. J Vasc Surg 37(1):32, 2003
30. McFalls EO, Ward HB, Moritz TE *et al*: Coronary-artery revascularization before elective major vascular surgery. N Engl J Med 351:2795, 2004
31. Landesberg G, Mosseri M, Wolf Y *et al*: The probability of detecting perioperative myocardial ischemia in vascular surgery by continuous 12-lead ECG. Anesthesiology 96:264, 2002
32. Ellis JE, Shah MN, Briller JE *et al*: A comparison of methods for the detection of myocardial ischemia during noncardiac surgery: Automated ST-segment analysis systems, electrocardiography, and transesophageal echocardiography. Anesth Analg 75:764, 1992
33. Roizen MF, Beaupre PN, Alpert RA *et al*: Monitoring with two-dimensional transesophageal echocardiography: Comparison of myocardial function in patients undergoing supraceliac, suprarenal-infraceliac, or infrarenal aortic occlusion. J Vasc Surg 1:300, 1984
34. Smith JS, Cahalan MK, Benefiel DJ *et al*: Intraoperative detection of myocardial ischemia in high-risk patients: Electrocardiography versus two-dimensional transesophageal echocardiography. Circulation 872:1015, 1985
35. Sprung J, Abdelmalak B, Gottlieb A *et al*: Analysis of risk factors for myocardial infarction and cardiac mortality after major vascular surgery. Anesthesiology 93(1):129, 2000
36. Breslow MJ: The role of stress hormones in perioperative myocardial ischemia. Int Anesthesiol Clin 30:81, 1992
37. Landesberg G, Luria MH, Cotev S: Importance of long-duration postoperative ST-segment depression in cardiac morbidity after vascular surgery. Lancet 341:715, 1993
38. Auerbach AD, Goldman L: Beta-blockers and reduction of cardiac events in noncardiac surgery: Scientific review. JAMA 287:1435, 2002
39. London MJ, Zaugg M, Schaub MC *et al*: Perioperative beta-adrenergic receptor blockade: Physiologic foundations and clinical controversies. Anesthesiology 100:170, 2004
40. Poldermans D, Boersma E, Bax JJ *et al*: The effect of bisoprolol on perioperative mortality and myocardial infarction in high-risk patients undergoing vascular surgery. Dutch echocardiographic cardiac risk evaluation applying stress echocardiography study group. N Engl J Med 341(24):1789, 1999
41. Ellis JE, Drijvers G, Pedlow S *et al*: Premedication with oral and transdermal clonidine provides safe and efficacious postoperative sympatholysis. Anesth Analg 79:1133, 1994
42. Wijeysundera DN, Naik JS, Beattie WS: Alpha-2 adrenergic agonists to prevent perioperative cardiovascular complications: A meta-analysis. Am J Med 114:742, 2003

43. Wallace AW, Galindez D, Salahieh A *et al*: Effect of clonidine on cardiovascular morbidity and mortality after noncardiac surgery. Anesthesiology 101(2):284, 2004
44. Durazzo AE, Machado FS, Ikeoka DT *et al*: Reduction in cardiovascular events after vascular surgery with atorvastatin: A randomized trial. J Vasc Surg 39:967, 2004
45. Dodds TM, Stone JG, Coromilas J *et al*: Prophylactic nitroglycerin infusion during noncardiac surgery does not reduce perioperative ischemia. Anesth Analg 76:705, 1993
46. Norris EJ, Beattie C, Perler BA *et al*: Double-masked randomized trial comparing alternate combinations of intraoperative anesthesia and postoperative analgesia in abdominal aortic surgery. Anesthesiology 95(5):1054, 2001
47. Beattie WS, Badner NH, Choi P: Epidural analgesia reduces postoperative myocardial infarction: A meta-analysis. Anesth Analg 93(4):853, 2001
48. Nelson AH, Fleisher LA, Rosenbaum SH: Relationship between postoperative anemia and cardiac morbidity in high-risk vascular patients in the intensive care unit. Crit Care Med 21:860, 1993
49. Hebert PC, Wells G, Blajchman MA *et al*: A multicenter, randomized, controlled clinical trial of transfusion requirements in critical care. Transfusion requirements in critical care investigators, Canadian Critical Care Trials Group. N Engl J Med 340(6):409, 1999
50. Frank SM, Fleisher LA, Breslow MJ *et al*: Perioperative maintenance of normothermia reduces the incidence of morbid cardiac events. A randomized clinical trial. JAMA 277(14):1127, 1997
51. Howell SJ, Sear JW, Foex P: Hypertension, hypertensive heart disease and perioperative cardiac risk. Br J Anaesth 92(4):570, 2004
52. Charlson ME, MacKenzie CR, Gold JP: Preoperative autonomic function abnormalities in patients with diabetes mellitus and patients with hypertension. J Am Coll Surg 179:1, 1994
53. van den Berghe G, Wouters P, Weekers F *et al*: Intensive insulin therapy in the critically ill patients. N Engl J Med 345:1359, 2001
54. Sakamaki F, Oya H, Nagaya N, Kyotani S, Satoh T, Nakanishi N: Higher prevalence of obstructive airway disease in patients with thoracic or abdominal aortic aneurysm. J Vasc Surg 36(1):35, 2002
55. Jordan WD Jr, Voellinger DC, Doblar DD, Plyushcheva NP, Fisher WS, McDowell HA: Microemboli detected by transcranial Doppler monitoring in patients during carotid angioplasty versus carotid endarterectomy. Cardiovasc Surg 7(1):33, 1999
56. Crawley F, Stygall J, Lunn S, Harrison M, Brown MM, Newman S: Comparison of microembolism detected by transcranial Doppler and neuropsychological sequelae of carotid surgery and percutaneous transluminal angioplasty. Stroke 31(6):1329, 2000
57. Diener HC, Cunha L, Forbes C, Sivenius J, Smets P, Lowenthal A: European stroke prevention study: 2. Dipyridamole and acetylsalicylic acid in the secondary prevention of stroke. J Neurol Sci 143:1, 1996
58. North American Symptomatic Carotid Endarterectomy Trial Collaborators: Beneficial effect of carotid endarterectomy in symptomatic patients with high grade stenosis. N Engl J Med 325:445, 1991
59. Executive Committee for the Asymptomatic Carotid Atherosclerosis Study: Endarterectomy for asymptomatic carotid artery stenosis. JAMA 273:1421, 1995
60. Biller J, Feinberg WM, Castaldo JE *et al*: Guidelines for carotid endarterectomy: A statement for healthcare professionals from a Special Writing Group of the Stroke Council, American Heart Association. Circulation 97(5):501, 1998
61. Yadav JS, Wholey MH, Kuntz RE *et al*: Stenting and angioplasty with protection in patients at high risk for endarterectomy investigators. Protected carotid-artery stenting versus endarterectomy in high-risk patients. N Engl J Med 351(15):1493, 2004
62. Theiss W, Hermanek P, Mathias K *et al*: German Societies of Angiology and Radiology. Pro-CAS: A prospective registry of carotid angioplasty and stenting. Stroke 35(9):2134, 2004
63. Ferguson GG, Eliasziw M, Barr HW *et al*: The North American symptomatic carotid endarterectomy trial: Surgical results in 1415 patients. Stroke 30(9):1751, 1999
64. Michenfelder JD, Sundt TM, Fode N *et al*: Isoflurane when compared to enflurane and halothane decreases the frequency of cerebral ischemia during carotid endarterectomy. Anesthesiology 67:336, 1987
65. Umbrain V, Keeris J, D'Haese J *et al*: Isoflurane, desflurane and sevoflurane for carotid endarterectomy. Anaesthesia 55:1052, 2000
66. Jellish WS, Sheikh T, Baker WH, Louie EK, Slogoff S: Hemodynamic stability, myocardial ischemia, and perioperative outcome after carotid surgery with remifentanil/propofol or isoflurane/fentanyl anesthesia. J Neurosurg Anesthesiol 15(3):176, 2003
67. Lavine SD, Masri LS, Levy ML, Giannotta SL: Temporary occlusion of the middle cerebral artery in intracranial aneurysm surgery: Time limitation and advantage of brain protection. J Neurosurg 87(6):817, 1997
68. Kapinya KJ, Lowl D, Futterer C *et al*: Tolerance against ischemic neuronal injury can be induced by volatile anesthetics and is inducible NO synthase dependent. Stroke 33(7):1889, 2002
69. de Borst GJ, Moll FL, van de Pavoordt HD *et al*: Stroke from carotid endarterectomy: When and how to reduce perioperative stroke rate? Eur J Vasc Endovasc Surg 21(6):484, 2001
70. Heyer EJ, Adams DC, Moses C, Quest DO, Connolly ES: Erroneous conclusion from processed electroencephalogram with changing anesthetic depth. Anesthesiology 92(2):603, 2000
71. Sundt TM Jr, Sharbrough FW, Piepgras DG *et al*: Correlation of cerebral blood flow and electroencephalographic changes during carotid endarterectomy: With results of surgery and hemodynamics of cerebral ischemia. Mayo Clin Proc 56:533, 1981
72. Kearse LA Jr, Lopez-Bresnahan M, McPeck K, Zaslavsky A: Preoperative cerebrovascular symptoms and electroencephalographic abnormalities do not predict cerebral ischemia during carotid endarterectomy. Stroke 26(7):1210, 1995
73. Ackerstaff RG, Moons KG, van de Vlasakker CJ *et al*: Association of intraoperative transcranial doppler monitoring variables with stroke from carotid endarterectomy. Stroke 31(8):1817, 2000
74. Costin M, Rampersad A, Solomon RA, Connolly ES, Heyer EJ: Cerebral injury predicted by transcranial Doppler ultrasonography but not electroencephalography during carotid endarterectomy. J Neurosurg Anesthesiol 14(4):287, 2002
75. McCarthy RJ, McCabe AE, Walker R, Horrocks M: The value of transcranial Doppler in predicting cerebral ischaemia during carotid endarterectomy. Eur J Vasc Endovasc Surg 21(5):408, 2001
76. Dalman JE, Beenakkers IC, Moll FL, Leusink JA, Ackerstaff RG: Transcranial Doppler monitoring during carotid endarterectomy helps to identify patients at risk of postoperative hyperperfusion. Eur J Vasc Endovasc Surg 18(3):222, 1999
77. Manninen PH, Tan TK, Sarjeant RM: Somatosensory evoked potential monitoring during carotid endarterectomy in patients with a stroke. Anesth Analg 93(1):39, 2001
78. Samra SK, Dy EA, Welch K, Dorje P, Zelenock GB, Stanley JC: Evaluation of a cerebral oximeter as a monitor of cerebral ischemia during carotid endarterectomy. Anesthesiology 93(4):964, 2000
79. Beese U, Langer H, Lang W, Dinkel M: Comparison of near-infrared spectroscopy and somatosensory evoked potentials for the detection of cerebral ischemia during carotid endarterectomy. Stroke 29(10):2032, 1998
80. Grubhofer G, Plochl W, Skolka M, Czerny M, Ehrlich M, Lassnigg A: Comparing Doppler ultrasonography and cerebral oximetry as indicators for shunting in carotid endarterectomy. Anesth Analg 91(6):1339, 2000
81. Phillip B, Pastor D, Bellows W, Leung JM: The prevalence of preoperative diastolic filling abnormalities in geriatric surgical patients. Anesth Analg 97(5):1214, 2003
82. De Castro V, Godet G, Mencia G, Raux M, Coriat P: Target-controlled infusion for remifentanil in vascular patients improves hemodynamics and decreases remifentanil requirement. Anesth Analg 96(1):33, 2003
83. Homi HM, Mixco JM, Sheng H, Grocott HP, Pearlstein RD, Warner DS: Severe hypotension is not essential for isoflurane neuroprotection against forebrain ischemia in mice. Anesthesiology 99(5):1145, 2003
84. Julier K, da Silva R, Garcia C *et al*: Preconditioning by sevoflurane decreases biochemical markers for myocardial and renal dysfunction in coronary artery bypass graft surgery: A double-blinded, placebo-controlled, multicenter study. Anesthesiology 98(6):1315, 2003
85. Stoneham MD, Doyle AR, Knighton JD *et al*: Prospective, randomized comparison of deep or superficial cervical plexus block for carotid endarterectomy surgery. Anesthesiology 89(4):907, 1998
86. Illig KA, Sternbach Y, Zhang R *et al*: EEG changes during awake carotid endarterectomy. Ann Vasc Surg 16(1):6, 2002
87. Zvara DA: Pro: Regional anesthesia is the best technique for carotid endarterectomy. J Cardiothorac Vasc Anesth 12(1):111, 1998
88. McKevitt FM, Sivaguru A, Venables GS *et al*: Effect of treatment of carotid artery stenosis on blood pressure: A comparison of hemodynamic disturbances after carotid endarterectomy and endovascular treatment. Stroke 34(11):2576, 2003
89. Carmichael FJ, McGuire GP, Wong DT, Crofts S, Sharma S, Montanera W: Computed tomographic analysis of airway dimensions after carotid endarterectomy. Anesth Analg 83(1):12, 1996
90. Munro FJ, Makin AP, Reid J: Airway problems after carotid endarterectomy. Br J Anaesth 76(1):156, 1996
91. Lipsett PA, Tierney S, Gordon TA *et al*: Carotid endarterectomy: Is intensive care unit care necessary? J Vasc Surg 20:403, 1994
92. Singh K, Bonaa KH, Jacobsen BK, Bjork L, Solberg S: Prevalence of and risk factors for abdominal aortic aneurysms in a population-based study: The Tromso study. Am J Epidemiol 154(3):236, 2001
93. Guirguis EM, Barber GG: The natural history of abdominal aortic aneurysms. Am J Surg 162:481, 1991
94. Lederle FA, Wilson SE, Johnson GR *et al*: Immediate repair compared with surveillance of small abdominal aortic aneurysms. N Engl J Med 346:1437, 2002
95. Gelman S: The pathophysiology of aortic cross-clamping and unclamping. Anesthesiology 82:1026, 1995.
96. Roizen MF, Ellis JE, Foss JF *et al*: Intraoperative management of the patient requiring suproceliac aortic occlusion. InVeith FJ, Hobson RW, William RA, Wilson SE (eds): Vascular Surgery, 2nd ed, p 256. New York, McGraw-Hill, 1994.
97. Wahlberg E, DiMuzio PJ, Stoney RJ *et al*: Aortic clamping during elective operations for infrarenal disease: The influence of clamping time on renal function. J Vasc Surg 36(1):13, 2002

98. Miller Q, Peyton BD, Cohn EJ *et al*: The effects of intraoperative fenoldopam on renal blood flow and tubular function following suprarenal aortic cross-clamping. Ann Vasc Surg 17:656, 2003
99. Reiz S, Nath S, Ponten E *et al*: Effects of thoracic epidural block and the beta-1-adrenoreceptor agonist prenalterol on the cardiovascular response to infrarenal aortic cross-clamping in man. Acta Anaesthesiol Scand 23:395, 1979
100. Alpert RA, Roizen MF, Hamilton WK *et al*: Intraoperative urinary output does not predict postoperative renal function in patients undergoing abdominal aortic revascularization. Surgery 95:707, 1984
101. Ballard JL, Yonemoto H, Killeen JD: Cost-effective aortic exposure: A retroperitoneal experience. Ann Vasc Surg 14(1):1, 2000
102. Derrow AE, Seeger JM, Dame DA *et al*: The outcome in the United States after thoracoabdominal aortic aneurysm repair, renal artery bypass, and mesenteric revascularization. J Vasc Surg 34(1):54, 2001
103. Glade GJ, Vahl AC, Wisselink W, Linsen MA, Balm R: Mid-term survival and costs of treatment of patients with descending thoracic aortic aneurysms: Endovascular vs. open repair: A case-control study. Eur J Vasc Endovasc Surg 29(1):28, 2005
104. Meylaerts SA, Jacobs MJ, van Iterson V, De Haan P, Kalkman CJ: Comparison of transcranial motor evoked potentials and somatosensory evoked potentials during thoracoabdominal aortic aneurysm repair. Ann Surg 230(6):742, 1999
105. Kim SS, Leibowitz AB: Endovascular thoracic aortic aneurysm repair using a single catheter for spinal anesthesia and cerebrospinal fluid drainage. J Cardiothorac Vasc Anesth 15(1):88, 2001
106. Parodi JC, Palmaz JC, Barone HD: Transfemoral intraluminal graft implantation for abdominal aortic aneurysms. Ann Vasc Surg 5(6):491, 1991
107. Merten GJ, Burgess WP, Gray LV *et al*: Prevention of contrast-induced nephropathy with sodium bicarbonate: A randomized controlled trial. JAMA 291(19):2328, 2004
108. Ohki T, Veith FJ, Shaw P *et al*: Increasing incidence of midterm and long-term complications after endovascular graft repair of abdominal aortic aneurysms: A note of caution based on a 9-year experience. Ann Surg 234(3):323, 2001
109. Prinssen M, Verhoeven EL, Buth J *et al*: Dutch Randomized Endovascular Aneurysm Management (DREAM) Trial Group. A randomized trial comparing conventional and endovascular repair of abdominal aortic aneurysms. N Engl J Med 351(16):1607, 2004
110. Henretta JP *et al*: Feasibility of endovascular repair of abdominal aortic aneurysms with local anesthesia with intravenous sedation. J Vasc Surg 29(5):793, 1999
111. Moskowitz DM *et al*: Intraoperative rupture of an abdominal aortic aneurysm during an endovascular stent-graft procedure. Can J Anaesth 46(9):887, 1999
112. Siegel JH, Veech RL, Lessard MR *et al*: Immediate versus delayed fluid resuscitation in patients with trauma. N Engl J Med 332:681, 1995
113. Baron JF, Bertrand M, Barre E *et al*: Combined epidural and general anesthesia versus general anesthesia for abdominal aortic surgery. Anesthesiology 75(4):611, 1991
114. Kahn RA *et al*: Endovascular aortic repair is associated with greater hemodynamic stability compared with open aortic reconstruction. J Cardiothorac Vasc Anesth 13(1):42, 1999
115. Salartash K *et al*: Comparison of open transabdominal AAA repair with endovascular AAA repair in reduction of postoperative stress response. Ann Vasc Surg 15(1):53, 2001
116. Shindelman LE *et al*: Ambulatory endovascular surgery: Cost advantage and factors influencing its safe performance. J Endovasc Surg 6(2):160, 1999
117. Bode RH Jr, Lewis KP, Zarich SW *et al*: Cardiac outcome after peripheral vascular surgery. Comparison of general and regional anesthesia. Anesthesiology 84(1):3, 1996
118. Cheung AT, Pochettino A, Guvakov DV, Weiss SJ, Shanmugan S, Bavaria JE: Safety of lumbar drains in thoracic aortic operations performed with extracorporeal circulation. Ann Thorac Surg 76(4):1190, 2003
119. Sandham JD, Hull RD, Brant RF *et al*: Canadian Critical Care Clinical Trials Group. A randomized, controlled trial of the use of pulmonary-artery catheters in high-risk surgical patients. N Engl J Med 348(1):5, 2003
120. Eyraud D, Benmalek F, Teugels K, Bertrand M, Mouren S, Coriat P: Does desflurane alter left ventricular function when used to control surgical stimulation during aortic surgery? Acta Anaesthesiol Scand 43(7):737, 1999
121. Tanaka K, Ludwig LM, Kersten JR, Pagel PS, Warltier DC: Mechanisms of cardioprotection by volatile anesthetics. Anesthesiology 100(3):707, 2004
122. Badner NH, Freeman D, Spence JD: Preoperative oral B vitamins prevent nitrous oxide-induced postoperative plasma homocysteine increases. Anesth Analg 93(6):1507, 2001
123. Lunn JK, Dannemiller FJ, Stanley TH: Cardiovascular responses to clamping of the aorta during epidural and general anesthesia. Anesth Analg 58:372, 1979
124. Johnston WE, Conroy BP, Miller GS, Lin CY, Deyo DJ: Hemodynamic benefit of positive end-expiratory pressure during acute descending aortic occlusion. Anesthesiology 97(4):875, 2002
125. Clagett GP, Valentine RJ, Jackson MR *et al*: A randomized trial of intraoperative autotransfusion during aortic surgery. J Vasc Surg 29(1):22, 1999
126. Moses JW, Leon MB, Popma JJ *et al*: Sirolimus-eluting stents versus standard stents in patients with stenosis in a native coronary artery. N Engl J Med 349:1315.2003
127. Johnson WC, Lee KK: A comparative evaluation of polytetrafluoroethylene, umbilical vein, and saphenous vein bypass grafts for femoro-popliteal above-knee revascularization: A prospective randomized Department of Veterans Affairs cooperative study. J Vasc Surg 32:268, 2000
128. Berlauk JF, Abrams JH, Gilmour IJ *et al*: Preoperative optimization of cardiovascular hemodynamics improves outcome in peripheral vascular surgery: A prospective, randomized clinical trial. Ann Surg 214:289, 1991
129. Tzeng GF: Hemostatic interventions and regional anesthesia for vascular surgery. Prob Anesth 11:207, 1999
130. Breslow MJ, Parker SD, Frank SM *et al*: Determinants of catecholamine and cortisol responses to lower extremity revascularization: The PIRAT study group. Anesthesiology 79:1202, 1993
131. Griffith JP, Whiteley S, Gough MJ: Prospective randomized study of a new method of providing postoperative pain relief following femoropopliteal bypass. Br J Surg 83(12):1735, 1996
132. Benefiel DJ, Roizen MF, Lampe GH *et al*: Morbidity after aortic surgery with sufentanil versus isoflurane anesthesia. Anesthesiology 65:A516, 1986

CHAPTER 33 ■ ANESTHESIA AND THE EYE

KATHRYN E. McGOLDRICK AND and STEVEN I. GAYER

KEY POINTS

1. Although apprehension is predictable in potentially blind patients awaiting surgery, this problem is often exacerbated in the elderly whose coping mechanisms may be diminished by depression or dementia.
2. Inhalation anesthetics cause dose-related reductions in IOP. The exact mechanisms are unknown, but postulated etiologies include depression of a control center in the diencephalon, reduction of aqueous humor production, enhancement of aqueous outflow, or relaxation of the extraocular muscles.
3. The oculocardiac reflex is triggered by pressure on the globe and by traction on the extraocular muscles, as well as on the conjunctiva or on the orbital structures. This reflex, the afferent limb of which is trigeminal and the efferent limb vagal, may also be elicited by performance of a retrobulbar block, by ocular trauma, and by direct pressure on tissue remaining in the orbital apex after enucleation.
4. Ophthalmic drugs may significantly alter the patient's reaction to anesthesia. Similarily, anesthetic drugs and maneuvers may dramatically influence intraocular dynamics.
5. Several anesthetic options are available for many types of ocular procedures, including general anesthesia, retrobulbar block, peribulbar anesthesia, sub-Tenon's (episcleral) block, topical analgesia, and intracameral injection.
6. The complications of ophthalmic anesthesia can be both vision and life threatening.
7. With intraocular procedures, profound akinesia and meticulous control of intraocular pressure (IOP) are requisite. However, with extraocular surgery, the significance of IOP fades, whereas concern about elicitation of the oculocardiac reflex assumes prominence.

Anesthesia for ophthalmic surgery presents many unique challenges (Table 33-1). In addition to possessing technical expertise, the anesthesiologist must have detailed knowledge of ocular anatomy, physiology, and pharmacology. It is essential to appreciate that ophthalmic drugs may significantly alter the reaction to anesthesia and that, concomitantly, anesthetic drugs and maneuvers may dramatically influence intraocular dynamics. Patients undergoing ophthalmic surgery may represent extremes of age and coexisting medical diseases (e.g., diabetes mellitus, coronary artery disease, essential hypertension, chronic lung disease), but they are likely to be in the elderly age group. Indeed, the elderly constitute the most rapidly growing subset of the U.S. population, with the 2002 Census reporting 4.2 million Americans age 85 years or older, an increase of 30% since 1990. Moreover, the elderly are a uniquely vulnerable group with reduced functional reserve and a myriad of age-related diseases. The economic implication of these age-related diseases is staggering. For example, age-related

TABLE 33-1

REQUIREMENTS OF OPHTHALMIC SURGERY

Safety
Akinesia
Profound analgesia
Minimal bleeding
Avoidance or obtundation of oculocardiac reflex
Control of intraocular pressure
Awareness of drug interactions
Smooth emergence

macular degeneration is the leading cause of blindness in individuals older than 65 years of age in the United States, affecting more than 1.75 million people. Because of the rapid aging of our population, this number will increase to almost 3 million by 2020.[1] More recent prevalence studies suggest that the number of persons with Alzheimer's disease in the United States is 4.5 million. Given that the percentage of individuals with Alzheimer's disease increases by a factor of two with approximately every 5 years of age, 1% of 60 year olds and about 30% of 85 year olds have the disease. Without advances in therapy, the number of symptomatic cases in the United States is predicted to increase to 13.2 million by 2050.[2] Current annual expenditures on care for patients with Alzheimer's disease exceed $84 billion,[3] a statistic that underscores the urgency of seeking more effective therapeutic and prophylactic interventions. 1 Moreover, although apprehension is predictable in blind or potentially blind patients awaiting surgery, this problem is often exacerbated in the elderly whose coping mechanisms may be diminished by depression or dementia.

It is mandatory to be knowledgeable about the numerous surgical procedures unique to the specialty of ophthalmology. Whereas the list of ocular surgical interventions is lengthy, these procedures may, in general, be classified as extraocular or intraocular. This distinction is critical because anesthetic considerations are different for these two major surgical categories. For example, with intraocular procedures, profound akinesia (relaxation of recti muscles) and meticulous control of intraocular pressure (IOP) are requisite. However, with extraocular surgery, the significance of IOP fades, whereas concern about elicitation of the oculocardiac reflex assumes prominence.

OCULAR ANATOMY

The anesthesiologist should be knowledgeable about ocular anatomy to enhance his or her understanding of surgical procedures and to aid the surgeon in the performance of regional blocks when needed[4] (Fig. 33-1). Salient subdivisions of ocular anatomy include the orbit, the eye itself, the extraocular muscles, the eyelids, and the lacrimal system.

The orbit is a bony box, or pyramidal cavity, housing the eyeball and its associated structures in the skull. The walls of the orbit are composed of the following bones: frontal, zygomatic, greater wing of the sphenoid, maxilla, palatine, lacrimal, and ethmoid. A familiarity with the surface relationships of the orbital rim is mandatory for the skilled performance of regional blocks.

The optic foramen, located at the orbital apex, transmits the optic nerve and the ophthalmic artery, as well as the sympathetic nerves from the carotid plexus. The superior orbital fissure transmits the superior and inferior branches of the oculomotor nerve; the lacrimal, frontal, and nasociliary branches of the trigeminal nerve; and the trochlear and abducens nerves and

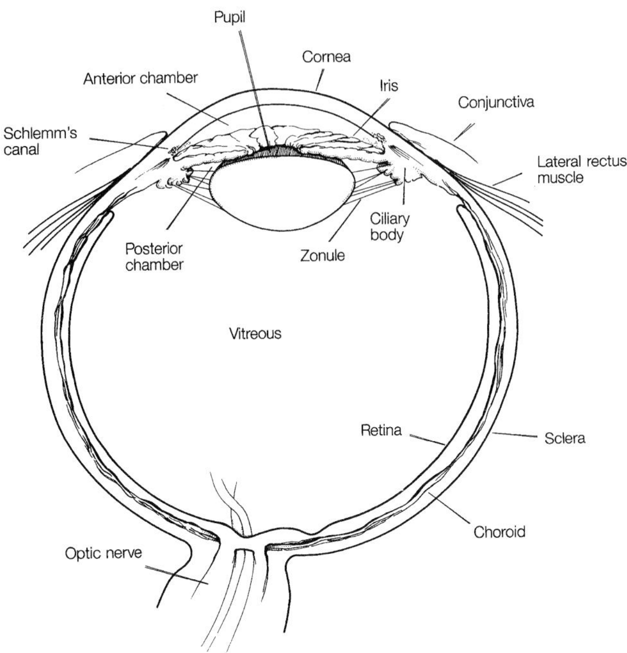

FIGURE 33-1. Diagram of ocular anatomy.

the superior and inferior ophthalmic veins. The inferior orbital or sphenomaxillary fissure contains the infraorbital and zygomatic nerves and communication between the inferior ophthalmic vein and the pterygoid plexus. The infraorbital foramen, located about 4 mm below the orbital rim in the maxilla, transmits the infraorbital nerve, artery, and vein. The lacrimal fossa contains the lacrimal gland in the superior temporal orbit. The supraorbital notch, located at the junction of the medial one-third and temporal two-thirds of the superior orbital rim, transmits the supraorbital nerve, artery, and vein. The supraorbital notch, the infraorbital foramen, and the lacrimal fossa are clinically palpable and function as major landmarks for administration of regional anesthesia.

The eye itself is actually one large sphere with part of a smaller sphere incorporated in the anterior surface, constituting a structure with two different radii of curvature. The coat of the eye is composed of three layers: sclera, uveal tract, and retina. The fibrous outer layer, or sclera, is protective, providing sufficient rigidity to maintain the shape of the eye. The anterior portion of the sclera, the cornea, is transparent, permitting light to pass into the internal ocular structures. The double-spherical shape of the eye exists because the corneal arc of curvature is steeper than the scleral arc of curvature. The focusing of rays of light to form a retinal image commences at the cornea.

The uveal tract, or middle layer of the globe, is vascular and in direct apposition to the sclera. A potential space, known as the suprachoroidal space, separates the sclera from the uveal tract. This potential space, however, may become filled with blood during an expulsive or suprachoroidal hemorrhage, often associated with surgical disaster. The iris, ciliary body, and choroid compose the uveal tract. The iris includes the pupil, which, by contractions of three sets of muscles, controls the amount of light entering the eye. The iris dilator is sympathetically innervated; the iris sphincter and the ciliary muscle have parasympathetic innervation. Posterior to the iris lays the ciliary body, which produces aqueous humor (see Formation and Drainage of Aqueous Humor section). The ciliary muscles, situated in the ciliary body, adjust the shape of the lens to accommodate focusing at various distances. Large vessels and a network of small vessels and capillaries known as the choriocapillaris constitute the choroid, which supplies nutrition to the outer part of the retina.

The retina is a neurosensory membrane composed of 10 layers that convert light impulses into neural impulses. These neural impulses are then carried through the optic nerve to the brain. Located in the center of the globe is the vitreous cavity, filled with a gelatinous substance known as vitreous humor. This material is adherent to the most anterior 3 mm of the retina, as well as to large blood vessels and the optic nerve. The vitreous humor may pull on the retina, causing retinal tears and retinal detachment.

The crystalline lens, located posterior to the pupil, refracts rays of light passing through the cornea and pupil to focus images on the retina. The ciliary muscle, whose contractile state causes tautness or relaxation of the lens zonules, regulates the thickness of the lens.

In addition, six extraocular muscles move the eye within the orbit to various positions. The bilobed lacrimal gland provides most of the tear film, which serves to maintain a moist anterior surface on the globe. The lacrimal drainage system—composed of the puncta, canaliculi, lacrimal sac, and lacrimal duct—drains into the nose below the inferior turbinate. Blockage of this system occurs frequently, necessitating procedures ranging from lacrimal duct probing to dacryocystorhinostomy, which involves anastomosis of the lacrimal sac to the nasal mucosa.

Covering the surface of the globe and lining the eyelids is a mucous membrane called the *conjunctiva*. Because drugs are absorbed across the membrane, it is a popular site for administration of ophthalmic drugs.

The eyelids consist of four layers: (1) the conjunctiva, (2) the cartilaginous tarsal plate, (3) a muscle layer composed mainly of the orbicularis and the levator palpebrae, and (4) the skin. The eyelids protect the eye from foreign objects; through blinking, the tear film produced by the lacrimal gland is spread across the surface of the eye, keeping the cornea moist.

Blood supply to the eye and orbit is by means of branches of both the internal and external carotid arteries. Venous drainage of the orbit is accomplished through the multiple anastomoses of the superior and inferior ophthalmic veins. Venous drainage of the eye is achieved mainly through the central retinal vein. All these veins empty directly into the cavernous sinus.

The sensory and motor innervations of the eye and its adnexa are very complex, with multiple cranial nerves supplying branches to various ocular structures. A branch of the oculomotor nerve supplies a motor root to the ciliary ganglion, which in turn supplies the sphincter of the pupil and the ciliary muscle. The trochlear nerve supplies the superior oblique muscle. The abducens nerve supplies the lateral rectus muscle. The trigeminal nerve constitutes the most complex ocular and adnexal innervation. In addition, the zygomatic branch of the facial nerve eventually divides into an upper branch, supplying the frontalis and the upper lid orbicularis, whereas the lower branch supplies the orbicularis of the lower lid.

OCULAR PHYSIOLOGY

Despite its relatively diminutive size, the eye is a complex organ, concerned with many intricate physiologic processes. The formation and drainage of aqueous humor and their influence on IOP in both normal and glaucomatous eyes are among the most important functions, especially from the anesthesiologist's perspective. An appreciation of the effects of various anesthetic manipulations on IOP requires an understanding of the fundamental principles of ocular physiology.

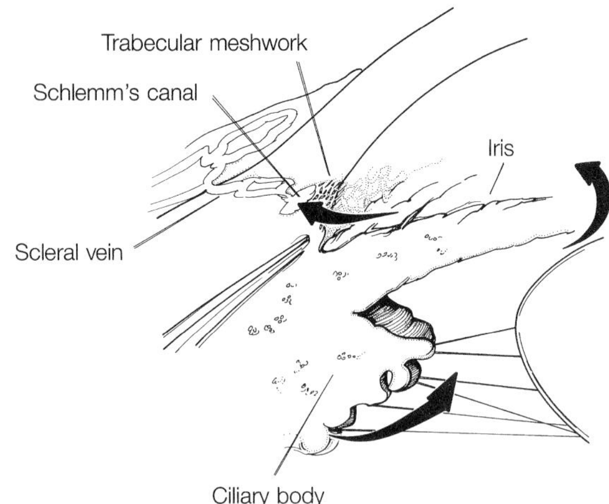

FIGURE 33-2. Ocular anatomy concerned with control of intraocular pressure.

Formation and Drainage of Aqueous Humor

Two-thirds of the aqueous humor is formed in the posterior chamber by the ciliary body in an active secretory process involving both the carbonic anhydrase and the cytochrome oxidase systems (Fig. 33-2). The remaining third is formed by passive filtration of aqueous humor from the vessels on the anterior surface of the iris.

At the ciliary epithelium, sodium is actively transported into the aqueous humor in the posterior chamber. Bicarbonate and chloride ions passively follow the sodium ions. This active mechanism results in the osmotic pressure of the aqueous being many times greater than that of plasma. It is this disparity in osmotic pressure that leads to an average rate of aqueous humor production of 2 μL/min.

Aqueous humor flows from the posterior chamber through the pupillary aperture and into the anterior chamber, where it mixes with the aqueous formed by the iris. During its journey into the anterior chamber, the aqueous humor bathes the avascular lens and, once in the anterior chamber, it also bathes the corneal endothelium. Then, the aqueous humor flows into the peripheral segment of the anterior chamber and exits the eye through the trabecular network, Schlemm's canal, and episcleral venous system. A network of connecting venous channels eventually leads to the superior vena cava and the right atrium. Thus, obstruction of venous return at any point from the eye to the right side of the heart impedes aqueous drainage, elevating IOP accordingly.

Maintenance of Intraocular Pressure

IOP normally varies between 10 and 21.7 mm Hg and is considered abnormal above 22 mm Hg. This level varies 1 to 2 mm Hg with each cardiac contraction. Also, a diurnal variation of 2 to 5 mm Hg is observed, with a higher value noted on awakening. This higher awakening pressure has been ascribed to vascular congestion, pressure on the globe from closed lids, and mydriasis—all of which occur during sleep. If IOP is too high, it may produce opacities by interfering with normal corneal metabolism.

During anesthesia, a rise in IOP can produce permanent visual loss. If the IOP is already elevated, a further increase can trigger acute glaucoma. If penetration of the globe occurs when the IOP is excessively high, rupture of a blood vessel with subsequent hemorrhage may transpire. IOP becomes atmospheric once the eye cavity has been entered, and any sudden rise in pressure may lead to prolapse of the iris and lens, and loss of vitreous. Thus, proper control of IOP is critical.

Three main factors influence IOP: (1) external pressure on the eye by the contraction of the orbicularis oculi muscle and the tone of the extraocular muscles, venous congestion of orbital veins (as may occur with vomiting and coughing), and conditions such as orbital tumor; (2) scleral rigidity; and (3) changes in intraocular contents that are semisolid (lens, vitreous, or intraocular tumor) or fluid (blood and aqueous humor). Although these factors are significant in affecting IOP, the major control of intraocular tension is exerted by the fluid content, especially the aqueous humor.

Sclerosis of the sclera, not uncommonly seen in the elderly, may be associated with decreased scleral compliance and increased IOP. Other degenerative changes of the eye linked with aging can also influence IOP, the most significant being a hardening and enlargement of the crystalline lens. When these degenerative changes occur, they may lead to anterior displacement of the lens–iris diaphragm. A resultant shallowness of the anterior chamber angle may then occur, reducing access of the trabecular meshwork to aqueous. This process is usually gradual, but, if rapid lens engorgement occurs, angle-closure glaucoma may transpire.

Changes in the nature of the vitreous that affect the amount of unbound water also influence IOP. Myopia, trauma, and aging produce liquefaction of vitreous gel and a subsequent increase in unbound water, which may lower IOP by facilitating fluid removal. However, under different circumstances, the opposite may occur, that is, the hydration of more normal vitreous may be associated with elevation of IOP. Hence, it is often prudent to produce a slightly dehydrated state in the surgical patient with glaucoma.

Intraocular blood volume, determined primarily by vessel dilation or contraction in the spongy layers of the choroid, contributes significantly to IOP. Although changes in arterial or venous pressure may secondarily affect IOP, excursions in arterial pressure have much less importance than do venous fluctuations. In chronic arterial hypertension, ocular pressure returns to normal levels after a period of adaptation brought about by compression of vessels in the choroid as a result of increased IOP. Thus, a feedback mechanism reduces the total volume of blood, keeping IOP relatively constant in patients with systemic hypertension.

However, if venous return from the eye is disturbed at any point from Schlemm's canal to the right atrium, IOP increases substantially. This is caused both by increased intraocular blood volume and distention of orbital vessels, as well as by interference with aqueous drainage. Straining, vomiting, or coughing greatly increase venous pressure and raise IOP as much as 40 mm Hg or greater. The deleterious implications of these activities cannot be overemphasized. Laryngoscopy and tracheal intubation may also elevate IOP, even without any visible reaction to intubation, but especially when the patient coughs. Topical anesthetization of the larynx may attenuate the hypertensive response to laryngoscopy but does not reliably prevent associated increases in IOP.[5] Ordinarily the pressure elevation from such increases in blood volume or venous pressure dissipates rapidly. However, if the coughing or straining occurs during ocular surgery when the eye is open, as in penetrating keratoplasty, the result may be a disastrous expulsive hemorrhage, at worst, or a disconcerting loss of vitreous, at best.

Despite the significant role of venous pressure, scleral rigidity, and vitreous composition, maintenance of IOP is determined primarily by the rate of aqueous formation and the rate of aqueous outflow. The most important influence on formation of aqueous humor is the difference in osmotic pressure between aqueous and plasma. This fact is illustrated by the equation:

$$\text{IOP} = K[(\text{OPaq} - \text{OPpl}) + \text{CP}] \qquad (33\text{-}1)$$

where K is coefficient of outflow, OPaq is osmotic pressure of aqueous humor, OPpl is osmotic pressure of plasma, and CP is capillary pressure. Hypertonic solutions such as mannitol are used to lower IOP because a small change in the solute concentration of plasma can markedly influence the formation of aqueous humor and hence IOP.

Fluctuations in aqueous outflow may also produce a dramatic alteration in IOP. The most significant factor controlling aqueous humor outflow is the diameter of Fontana's spaces, as illustrated by the equation:

$$A = \frac{r^4(\text{Piop} - \text{Pv})}{8\eta L} \qquad (33\text{-}2)$$

where A is volume of aqueous outflow per unit of time, r is radius of Fontana's spaces, Piop is IOP, Pv is venous pressure, η is viscosity, and L is length of Fontana's spaces. When the pupil dilates, Fontana's spaces narrow, resistance to outflow is increased, and IOP rises. Because mydriasis is undesirable in both closed-angle and open-angle glaucoma, miotics such as pilocarpine are applied conjunctivally in patients with glaucoma.

Glaucoma

Glaucoma is a condition characterized by elevated IOP, resulting in impairment of capillary blood flow to the optic nerve with eventual loss of optic nerve tissue and function. Two different anatomic types of glaucoma exist: open-angle or chronic simple glaucoma, and closed-angle or acute glaucoma. (Other variations of these processes occur but are not especially germane to anesthetic management.)

With open-angle glaucoma, the elevated IOP exists with an anatomically open anterior chamber angle. It is believed that sclerosis of trabecular tissue results in impaired aqueous filtration and drainage. Treatment consists of medication to produce miosis and trabecular stretching. Commonly used eyedrops are epinephrine, timolol, dipivefrin, and betaxolol. Closed-angle glaucoma is characterized by the peripheral iris moving into direct contact with the posterior corneal surface, mechanically obstructing aqueous outflow. People who have a narrow angle between the iris and posterior cornea are predisposed to this condition. In these patients, mydriasis can produce such increased thickening of the peripheral iris that corneal touch occurs and the angle is closed. Another mechanism producing acute, closed-angle glaucoma is swelling of the crystalline lens. In this case, pupillary block occurs, with the edematous lens blocking the flow of aqueous from the posterior to the anterior chamber. This situation can also develop if the lens is traumatically dislocated anteriorly, thus physically blocking the anterior chamber.

It was previously believed by some clinicians that patients with glaucoma should not be given atropine. However, this claim is untenable. Atropine in the dose range used clinically has no effect on IOP in either open-angle or closed-angle glaucoma. When 0.4 mg of atropine is given parenterally to a 70-kg person, approximately 0.0001 mg is absorbed by the eye.[6] Garde et al.[7] reported, however, that scopolamine has a greater mydriatic effect than atropine and recommended not using scopolamine in patients with known or suspected closed-angle glaucoma.

Equation 33-2, describing the volume of aqueous outflow per unit of time, clearly demonstrates that outflow is exquisitely sensitive to fluctuations in venous pressure. Because a rise in venous pressure produces an increased volume of ocular blood and decreased aqueous outflow, it is obvious that considerable elevation of IOP occurs with any maneuver that increases venous pressure. Hence, in addition to preoperative instillation of miotics, other anesthetic goals for the patient with glaucoma include perioperative avoidance of venous congestion and overhydration. Furthermore, hypotensive episodes are to be avoided because these patients are allegedly vulnerable to retinal vascular thrombosis.

Primary congenital glaucoma is classified according to age of onset, with the infantile type presenting any time after birth until 3 years of age. The juvenile type presents between the ages of 37 months and 30 years. Moreover, childhood glaucoma may also occur in conjunction with various eye diseases or developmental anomalies such as aniridia, mesodermal dysgenesis syndrome, and retinopathy of prematurity.

Successful management of infantile glaucoma is crucially dependent on early diagnosis. Presenting symptoms include epiphora, photophobia, blepharospasm, and irritability. Ocular enlargement, termed *buphthalmos,* or "ox eye," and corneal haziness secondary to edema are common. Buphthalmos is rare, however, if glaucoma develops after 3 years of age because by then the eye is much less elastic.

Because infantile glaucoma is frequently associated with obstructed aqueous outflow, management of it often requires surgical creation, by goniotomy or trabeculotomy, of a route for aqueous humor to flow into Schlemm's canal. However, advanced disease may be unresponsive to even multiple goniotomies, and the more radical trabeculectomy or some other variety of filtering procedure may be necessary.

The juvenile form of glaucoma, in which the cornea and eye size are normal, is commonly associated with a family history of open-angle glaucoma and is treated similarly to primary open-angle glaucoma.

In cases of pediatric secondary glaucoma, goniotomy and filtering may be unsuccessful, whereas cyclocryotherapy may affect a reduction in IOP, pain, and corneal edema. The ciliary body is destroyed with a cryoprobe cooled to −70°C, thus dramatically decreasing aqueous formation.

It is essential to appreciate that the high IOP frequently encountered in infantile glaucoma can be reduced by more than 15 mm Hg when surgical anesthesia is achieved. One study, however, demonstrated minimal effect of halothane on IOP when the concentration ranged narrowly between 0.5% and 1.0%.[8] Some clinicians maintain that ketamine is a useful drug to use for examination under anesthesia when infantile glaucoma is part of the differential diagnosis because ketamine does not appear to reduce IOP, giving a spuriously low reading. Moreover, even normal infants sporadically have pressures in the mid-20s. Hence, diagnosis is not based exclusively on the numerical pressure recorded under anesthesia. Other factors such as corneal edema and increased corneal diameter, tears in Descemet's membrane, and cupping of the optic nerve are considered in making the diagnosis. If these aberrations are noted, surgical intervention may be mandatory, even in the setting of a reputedly normal IOP.

EFFECTS OF ANESTHESIA AND ADJUVANT DRUGS ON INTRAOCULAR PRESSURE

Central Nervous System Depressants

Inhalation anesthetics purportedly cause dose-related decreases in IOP. The exact mechanisms are unknown, but postulated etiologies include depression of a central nervous system (CNS) control center in the diencephalon, reduction of aqueous hu-
2 mor production, enhancement of aqueous outflow, or relaxation of the extraocular muscles.[6] Moreover, virtually all CNS depressants, including barbiturates, neuroleptics, opioids, tranquilizers,[6] and hypnotics, such as etomidate and propofol, lower IOP in both normal and glaucomatous eyes. Etomidate, despite its proclivity to produce pain on intravenous injection and skeletal muscle movement, is associated with a significant reduction in IOP.[9] However, etomidate-induced myoclonus may be hazardous in the setting of a ruptured globe.

Controversy, however, surrounds the issue of ketamine's effect on IOP. Administered intravenously or intramuscularly, ketamine initially was believed to increase IOP significantly, as measured by indentation tonometry.[10] Corssen and Hoy[11] also reported a slight but statistically significant increase in IOP that appeared unrelated to changes in blood pressure or depth of anesthesia. However, nystagmus made proper positioning of the tonometer difficult and may have resulted in less-than-accurate measurements.

Conflicting results arose from a study in which 2 mg/kg of ketamine given intravenously to adults failed to have a significant effect on IOP.[12] Furthermore, a pediatric study reported no increase in IOP after an intramuscular ketamine dose of 8 mg/kg. Indeed, values obtained were similar to those reported with halothane and isoflurane.[13,14]

Some of the confusion may arise from differences in premedication practices and from the use of different instruments to measure IOP. More recent studies have used applanation tonometry rather than indentation tonometry. However, even if future studies should confirm that ketamine has minimal or no effect on IOP, ketamine's proclivity to cause nystagmus and blepharospasm makes it a less-than-optimal agent for many types of ophthalmic surgery.

Ventilation and Temperature

Hyperventilation decreases IOP, whereas asphyxia, administration of carbon dioxide, and hypoventilation have been shown to elevate IOP.[15]

Hypothermia lowers IOP. On initial consideration, hypothermia might be expected to raise IOP because of the associated increase in viscosity of aqueous humor. However, hypothermia is linked with decreased formation of aqueous humor and with vasoconstriction; hence, the net result is a reduction in IOP.

Adjuvant Drugs

Ganglionic Blockers, Hypertonic Solutions, and Acetazolamide

Ganglionic blockers such as tetraethylammonium and pentamethonium cause a dramatic decrease in IOP. Trimethaphan also significantly lowers IOP in normal subjects, despite mydriasis.

Intravenous administration of hypertonic solutions such as dextran, urea, mannitol, and sorbitol elevates plasma osmotic pressure, thereby decreasing aqueous humor formation and reducing IOP. As effective as urea is in reducing IOP, intravenous mannitol has the advantage of fewer side effects. Mannitol's onset, peak (30 to 45 minutes), and duration of action (5 to 6 hours) are similar to those of urea. Moreover, both drugs may produce acute intravascular volume overload. Sudden expansion of plasma volume secondary to efflux of intracellular water into the vascular compartment places a heavy workload on the kidneys and heart, often resulting in hypertension and dilution of plasma sodium. Furthermore, mannitol-associated diuresis, if protracted, may trigger hypotension in volume-depleted patients.

Intravenous administration of acetazolamide inactivates carbonic anhydrase and interferes with the sodium pump. The resultant decrease in aqueous humor formation lowers IOP. However, the action of acetazolamide is not limited to the eye, and systemic effects include loss of sodium, potassium, and water secondary to the drug's renal tubular effects. Such electrolyte imbalances may then be linked to cardiac dysrhythmias during general anesthesia.

An advantage of acetazolamide is its relative ease of administration. Whereas large volumes of hypertonic solutions must be infused to reduce IOP, acetazolamide is easily given as a typical adult dose of 500 mg dissolved in 10 mL of sterile water. Acetazolamide may also be given orally, and topical carbonic anhydrase inhibitors are commercially available.

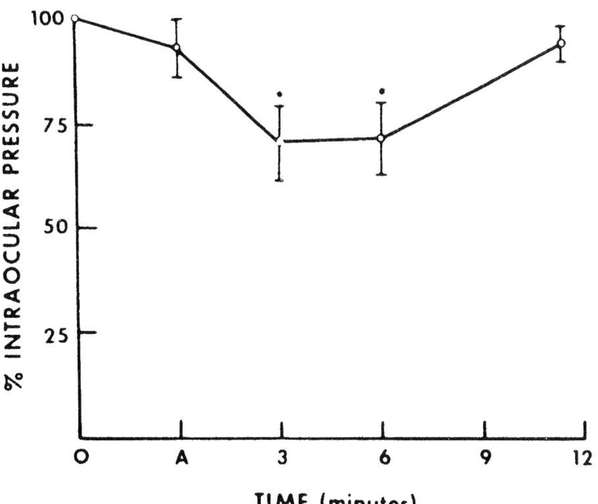

FIGURE 33-3. Mean intraocular pressure after administration of thiopental, 3 to 4 mg/kg, and pancuronium, 0.08 mg/kg at 0. A, loss of lid reflex; $^*P < .05$. (Reprinted with permission from Litwiller RW, DeFazio CA, Rushia EF: Pancuronium and intraocular pressure. Anesthesiology 42:750, 1975.)

Neuromuscular Blocking Drugs

Neuromuscular blocking drugs have both direct and indirect actions on IOP. Hence, a paralyzing dose of *d*-tubocurarine directly lowers IOP by relaxing the extraocular muscles. The same is true of equipotent doses of the other nondepolarizing drugs, including pancuronium[16] (Fig. 33-3). However, if paralysis of the respiratory muscles is accompanied by alveolar hypoventilation, the latter secondary effect may supervene to increase IOP.

In contrast to nondepolarizing drugs, the depolarizing drug succinylcholine elevates IOP. Lincoff et al.[17] reported extrusion of vitreous after succinylcholine administration to a patient with a surgically open eye. An average peak IOP increase of about 8 mm Hg is produced within 1 to 4 minutes of an intravenous dose. Within 7 minutes, return to baseline usually transpires.[18] The ocular hypertensive effect of succinylcholine has been attributed to several mechanisms, including tonic contraction of extraocular muscles,[6] choroidal vascular dilation, and relaxation of orbital smooth muscle. One study speculates that the succinylcholine-induced increase in IOP is multifactorial but primarily the result of the cycloplegic action of succinylcholine, producing a deepening of the anterior chamber and increased outflow resistance.[19] Because they studied eyes with the extraocular muscles detached and still observed an elevation in IOP, these investigators proposed that changes in extraocular muscle tone do not contribute significantly to the increase in IOP observed after succinylcholine administration.

A variety of methods have been advocated to prevent succinylcholine-induced elevations in IOP. However, although some attenuation of the increase results, none of these techniques consistently and completely block the ocular hypertensive response. Prior administration of such drugs as acetazolamide, propranolol, and nondepolarizing neuromuscular blocking drugs has been suggested. The efficacy of pretreatment with nondepolarizing drugs is controversial.

In 1968, using indentation tonometry, Miller et al.[20] reported that pretreatment with small amounts of gallamine or *d*-tubocurarine prevented succinylcholine-associated increases in IOP. However, in 1978, using the more sensitive applanation tonometer, Meyers et al.[21] were unable to consistently circumvent the ocular hypertensive response after similar pretreatment therapy (Table 33-2). In addition, Verma[22] claimed that a "self-taming" dose of succinylcholine was protective, but in a controlled study using applanation tonometry, Meyers et al.[23] challenged this claim. Although intravenous pretreatment with lidocaine, 1 to 2 mg/kg, may blunt the hemodynamic response to laryngoscopy,[5,24] such therapy does not reliably prevent the ocular hypertensive response associated with succinylcholine and intubation.[25] However, Grover and associates[26] claimed that pretreatment with lidocaine, 1.5 mg/kg intravenously, 1 minute before induction with thiopental and succinylcholine offered protection from IOP increases

TABLE 33-2

EFFECTS OF SUCCINYLCHOLINE ON INTRAOCULAR PRESSURE: DOUBLE-BLIND *d*-TUBOCURARINE OR GALLAMINE PRETREATMENT

Pretreatment[a]	MEAN AGE (yr)	INTRAOCULAR PRESSURE (mm Hg, MEAN ± SE)		
		BASELINE	3 MIN AFTER PRETREATMENT	1 MIN AFTER SUCCINYLCHOLINE[b]
d-Tubocurarine	13.4	13.0 ± 1.0	12.3 ± 1.2	24.0 ± 1.3
Gallamine	8.7	10.9 ± 1.1	10.6 ± 1.0	23.4 ± 2.3

[a] *d*-Tubocurarine, 0.09 mg · kg^{-1}, or gallamine, 0.3 mg/kg.
[b] 1 to 1.5 mg/kg IV.
Reprinted with permission from Meyers EF, Krupin T, Johnson M *et al*: Failure of nondepolarizing neuromuscular blockers to inhibit succinylcholine-induced increased intraocular pressure: A controlled study. Anesthesiology 48:149, 1978.

due to succinylcholine and may therefore be of value in rapid-sequence induction for open eye injuries.

Certainly, no one would disagree that succinylcholine—if unaccompanied by pretreatment with a nondepolarizing neuromuscular blocking drug—is contraindicated in patients with penetrating ocular wounds and should not be given for the first time after the eye has been opened. Nonetheless, it is no longer valid to recommend that succinylcholine be used only with extreme reluctance in ocular surgery. Clearly, any succinylcholine-induced increment in IOP is usually dissipated before surgery is started. Of concern, however, is Jampolsky's[27] warning that succinylcholine be avoided in patients undergoing repeat strabismus surgery because the forced duction test (FDT) does not return to baseline for approximately 30 minutes after administration of the drug. More recent and quantitatively sophisticated studies by France et al.[28] supported this caveat, although the latter investigators suggest waiting only 20 minutes after administration of succinylcholine before performing the FDT.

OCULOCARDIAC REFLEX

Bernard Aschner and Giuseppe Dagnini first described the oculocardiac reflex in 1908. This reflex is triggered by pressure on
3 the globe and by traction on the extraocular muscles, as well as on the conjunctiva or the orbital structures. Moreover, the reflex may also be elicited by performance of a retrobulbar block,[29] by ocular trauma, and by direct pressure on tissue remaining in the orbital apex after enucleation. The afferent limb is trigeminal, and the efferent limb is vagal. Although the most common manifestation of the oculocardiac reflex is sinus bradycardia, a wide spectrum of cardiac dysrhythmias may occur, including junctional rhythm, ectopic atrial rhythm, atrioventricular blockade, ventricular bigeminy, multifocal premature ventricular contractions, wandering pacemaker, idioventricular rhythm, asystole, and ventricular tachycardia.[30] This reflex may appear during either local or general anesthesia; however, hypercarbia and hypoxemia are believed to augment the incidence and severity of the problem, as may inappropriate anesthetic depth.

Reports on the alleged incidence of the oculocardiac reflex are remarkable in their striking variability. Berler's study[29] reported an incidence of 50%, but other sources quote rates ranging from 16 to 82%. Commonly, those articles disclosing a higher incidence included children in the study population, and children tend to have more vagal tone.

A variety of maneuvers to abolish or obtund the oculocardiac reflex have been promulgated. None of these methods has been consistently effective, safe, and reliable. Inclusion of intramuscular anticholinergic drugs such as atropine or glycopyrrolate in the usual premedication regimen for oculocardiac reflex prophylaxis is ineffective.[31]

Atropine given intravenously within 30 minutes of surgery is believed to reduce incidence of the reflex. However, reports differ concerning dosage and timing. Moreover, some anesthesiologists claim that prior intravenous administration of atropine may yield more serious and refractory cardiac dysrhythmias than the reflex itself. Clearly, atropine may be considered a potential myocardial irritant. A variety of cardiac dysrhythmias[32] and several conduction abnormalities,[33] including ventricular fibrillation, ventricular tachycardia, and left bundle-branch block, have been attributed to intravenous atropine.

Although administration of retrobulbar anesthesia may provide some cardiac antidysrhythmic value by blocking the afferent limb of the reflex arc, such a regional technique is not devoid of potential complications, which include, but are not limited to, optic nerve damage, retrobulbar hemorrhage, and stimulation of the oculocardiac reflex arc by the retrobulbar block itself.

It is generally believed that, in adults, the aforementioned prophylactic measures, fraught with inherent hazards, are usually not indicated. If a cardiac dysrhythmia appears, initially the surgeon should be asked to cease operative manipulation. Next, the patient's anesthetic depth and ventilatory status are evaluated. Commonly, heart rate and rhythm return to baseline within 20 seconds after institution of these measures. Moreover, Moonie et al.[34] noted that, with repeated manipulation, bradycardia is less likely to recur, probably secondary to fatigue of the reflex arc at the level of the cardioinhibitory center. However, if the initial cardiac dysrhythmia is especially serious or if the reflex tenaciously recurs, atropine should be administered intravenously, but only after the surgeon stops ocular manipulation.

During pediatric strabismus surgery, however, some anesthesiologists administer intravenous atropine, 0.02 mg/kg, before commencing surgery.[35] Alternatively, glycopyrrolate, 0.01 mg/kg administered intravenously, may be associated with less tachycardia than atropine in this setting.

ANESTHETIC RAMIFICATIONS OF OPHTHALMIC DRUGS

There is considerable potential for drug interactions during
4 administration of anesthesia for ocular surgery. Topical ophthalmic drugs may produce undesirable systemic effects or may have deleterious anesthetic implications. Systemic absorption of topical ophthalmic drugs may occur from either the conjunctiva or the nasal mucosa after drainage through the nasolacrimal duct. In addition, from spillover, some percutaneous absorption through the immature epidermis of the premature infant may transpire.[36] Occluding the nasolacrimal duct by pressing on the inner canthus of the eye for a few minutes after each instillation greatly decreases systemic absorption. Some of the potentially worrisome topical ocular drugs include acetylcholine, anticholinesterases, cocaine, cyclopentolate, epinephrine, phenylephrine, and timolol. In addition, intraocular sulfur hexafluoride and other intraocular gases have important anesthetic ramifications. Furthermore, certain ophthalmic drugs given systemically may produce untoward sequelae germane to anesthetic management. Drugs in this category include glycerol, mannitol, and acetazolamide.

Acetylcholine

Acetylcholine is sometimes used intraocularly after lens extraction to produce miosis. The local use of this drug may occasionally result in such systemic effects as bradycardia, increased salivation, and bronchial secretions, as well as bronchospasm. The side effects, including hypotension and bradycardia, that may develop in patients given acetylcholine after cataract extraction may be rapidly reversed with intravenous atropine. Furthermore, vagotonic anesthetic agents such as halothane can accentuate the effects of acetylcholine.

Anticholinesterase Agents

Echothiophate is a long-acting anticholinesterase miotic that lowers IOP by decreasing resistance to the outflow of aqueous humor. Useful in the treatment of glaucoma, echothiophate is absorbed into the systemic circulation after instillation in the conjunctival sac. Any of the long-acting anticholinesterases may prolong the action of succinylcholine because, after 1 month or more of therapy, plasma pseudocholinesterase activity may be less than 5% of normal. It is said, moreover, that normal enzyme activity does not return until 4 to 6 weeks after discontinuation of the drug.[37] Hence, the anesthesiologist should anticipate prolonged apnea if these patients are given a usual dose of succinylcholine. In addition, a delay in metabolism of ester local anesthetics should be expected.

Cocaine

Cocaine, introduced to ophthalmology in 1884 by Koller, has limited topical ocular use because it can cause corneal pits and erosion. However, as the only local anesthetic that inherently produces vasoconstriction and shrinkage of mucous membranes, cocaine is commonly used in nasal packs during dacryocystorhinostomy. The drug is so well absorbed from mucosal surfaces that plasma concentrations comparable to those after direct intravenous injection are achieved. Because cocaine interferes with catecholamine uptake, it has a sympathetic nervous system potentiating effect.

Historically, epinephrine had often been mixed with cocaine in hopes of augmenting the degree of vasoconstriction produced. This practice is both superfluous and deleterious because cocaine is a potent vasoconstrictor in its own right, and the combination of epinephrine with cocaine may trigger dangerous cardiac dysrhythmias. It has been shown that cocaine used alone, without topical epinephrine, to shrink the nasal mucosa in conjunction with halothane or enflurane does not sensitize the heart to endogenous epinephrine during halothane or enflurane anesthesia. However, animal studies have shown that after pretreatment with exogenous epinephrine, cocaine facilitates the development of epinephrine-induced cardiac dysrhythmias during halothane anesthesia.[38]

The usual maximal dose of cocaine used in clinical practice is 200 mg for a 70-kg adult, or 3 mg/kg. However, 1.5 mg/kg is preferable because this lower dose has been shown not to exert any clinically significant sympathomimetic effect in combination with halothane.[39] Although 1 g is considered to be the usual lethal dose for an adult, considerable variation occurs. Furthermore, systemic reactions may appear with as little as 20 mg.

Meyers[40] described two cases of cocaine toxicity during dacryocystorhinostomy, underscoring that cocaine is contraindicated in hypertensive patients or in patients receiving drugs such as tricyclic antidepressants or monoamine oxidase inhibitors. In addition, sympathomimetics such as epinephrine or phenylephrine should not be given with cocaine.

Obviously, before administering cocaine or another potent vasoconstrictor for dacryocystorhinostomy, the physician should carefully search out possible contraindications. To avoid toxic levels, doses of dilute solutions should be meticulously calculated and carefully administered. If serious cardiovascular effects occur, labetalol should be used to counteract them.[41] In the past, propranolol was widely used to control cocaine-induced hypertension,[42] but a lethal hypertensive exacerbation has been ascribed to unopposed α-adrenergic stimulation.[43] Labetalol offers the advantage of combined α-blockade and β-blockade.

Cyclopentolate

Despite the popularity of cyclopentolate as a mydriatic, it is not without side effects, which include CNS toxicity. Manifestations include dysarthria, disorientation, and frank psychotic reactions. Purportedly, CNS dysfunction is more likely to follow use of the 2% solution as opposed to the 1% solution. Furthermore, cases of convulsions in children after ocular instillation of cyclopentolate have been reported. Hence, for pediatric use, 0.5 to 1.0% solutions are recommended. At higher concentrations, cyclopentolate also causes cycloplegia.

Epinephrine

Although topical epinephrine has proved useful in some patients with open-angle glaucoma, the 2% solution has been associated with such systemic effects as nervousness, hypertension, angina pectoris, tachycardia, and other dysrhythmias.[44]

Some anesthesiologists have maintained that it is unwise to use topical or intraocular epinephrine in patients being anesthetized with a halogenated hydrocarbon. However, the iris, with its rich supply of adrenergic receptors, is able to capture with extreme rapidity the epinephrine given into the eye. Apparently, there is not much systemic absorption from the globe.

Phenylephrine

Pupillary dilation and capillary decongestion are reliably produced by topical phenylephrine. Although systemic effects secondary to topical application of prudent doses are rare,[45] severe hypertension, headache, tachycardia, and tremulousness have been reported.

In patients with coronary artery disease, severe myocardial ischemia, cardiac dysrhythmias, and even myocardial infarction may develop after topical 10% eyedrops. Those with cerebral aneurysms may be susceptible to cerebral hemorrhage after phenylephrine in this concentration. In general, a safe systemic level follows absorption from either the conjunctiva or the nasal mucosa after drainage by the tear ducts. However, phenylephrine should not be given in the eye after surgery has begun and venous channels are patent.

Children are especially vulnerable to overdose and may respond in a dramatic and adverse fashion to phenylephrine drops. Hence, the use of only 2.5%, rather than 10%, phenylephrine is recommended in infants and the elderly, and the frequency of application should be strictly limited in these patient populations.

Timolol and Betaxolol

Timolol, a nonselective β-adrenergic blocking drug, historically has been a popular antiglaucoma drug. Because significant conjunctival absorption may occur, timolol should be administered with caution to patients with known obstructive airway disease, congestive heart failure, or greater than first-degree heart block. Life-threatening asthmatic crises have been reported after the administration of timolol drops to some patients with chronic, stable asthma.[46] The development of severe sinus bradycardia in a patient with cardiac conduction defects (left anterior hemiblock, first-degree atrioventricular block, and incomplete right bundle branch block) has been reported after timolol.[47] Moreover, timolol has been implicated in the exacerbation of myasthenia gravis[48] and in the production of postoperative apnea in neonates and young infants.[49]

In contrast to timolol, a newer antiglaucoma drug, betaxolol, a β_1-blocker, is said to be more oculospecific and have minimal systemic effects. However, patients receiving an oral beta-blocker and betaxolol should be observed for potential additive effect on known systemic effects of β-blockade. Caution should be exercised in patients receiving catecholamine-depleting drugs. Although betaxolol has produced only minimal effects in patients with obstructive airways disease, caution should be exercised in the treatment of patients with excessive restriction of pulmonary function. Moreover, betaxolol is contraindicated in patients with sinus bradycardia, congestive

TABLE 33-3

DIFFERENTIAL SOLUBILITIES OF GASES

	BLOOD: GAS PARTITION COEFFICIENTS
Sulfur hexafluoride	0.004
Nitrogen	0.015
Nitrous oxide	0.468

heart failure, greater than first-degree heart block, cardiogenic shock, and overt myocardial failure.

Intraocular Sulfur Hexafluoride

For a patient with a retinal detachment, intraocular sulfur hexafluoride or other gases such as certain perfluorocarbons may be injected into the vitreous to facilitate reattachment mechanically. These recommendations do not apply to open-eye procedures, during which volume and pressure changes are readily compensated for by fluid and gas leak.

Stinson and Donlon[50] suggested terminating nitrous oxide 15 minutes before gas injection to prevent significant changes in the size of the intravitreous gas bubble. The patient is then given virtually 100% oxygen, or a combination of oxygen and air (admixed with a small percentage of volatile agent), for the balance of the operation without adversely affecting intravitreous gas dynamics. Furthermore, if a patient requires reoperation and general anesthesia after intravitreous gas injection, nitrous oxide should be avoided for 5 days subsequent to air injection and for 10 days after sulfur hexafluoride injection[51] (Table 33-3).

Perfluoropropane and octafluorocyclobutane may also be used in vitreoretinal surgery to support the retina. Like sulfur hexafluoride, these gases are relatively insoluble and require discontinuance of nitrous oxide at least 15 minutes before injection. If the patient requires reoperation, it must be remembered that perfluoropropane lingers in the eye for longer than 30 days.[52] A Medic-Alert bracelet might be helpful in these circumstances.

Systemic Ophthalmic Drugs

In addition to topical and intraocular therapies, various ophthalmic drugs given systemically may result in complications of concern to the anesthesiologist. These systemic drugs include glycerol, mannitol, and acetazolamide. For example, oral glycerol may be associated with nausea, vomiting, and risk of aspiration. Hyperglycemia or glycosuria, disorientation, and seizure activity may also occur after oral glycerol.

The recommended intravenous dose of mannitol is 1.5-2 g/kg given over a 30- to 60-minute interval. However, serious systemic problems may result from rapid infusion of large doses of mannitol. These complications include renal failure, congestive heart failure, pulmonary congestion, electrolyte imbalance, hypotension or hypertension, myocardial ischemia, and, rarely, allergic reactions. Clearly, the patient's renal and cardiovascular status must be thoroughly evaluated before mannitol therapy.

Acetazolamide, a carbonic anhydrase inhibitor with renal tubular effects, should be considered contraindicated in patients with marked hepatic or renal dysfunction or in those with low sodium levels or abnormal potassium values. As is well known, severe electrolyte imbalances can trigger serious cardiac dysrhythmias during general anesthesia. Furthermore, people with chronic lung disease may be vulnerable to the development of severe acidosis with long-term acetazolamide therapy. Topically active carbonic anhydrase inhibitors have been developed, are now commercially available, and appear to be relatively free of clinically important systemic effects.

PREOPERATIVE EVALUATION

Establishing Rapport and Assessing Medical Condition

Preoperative preparation and evaluation of the patient begin with the establishment of rapport and communication among the anesthesiologist, the surgeon, and the patient. Most patients realize that surgery and anesthesia entail inherent risks, and they appreciate a candid explanation of potential complications, balanced with information concerning probability or frequency of permanent adverse sequelae. Such an approach also fulfills the medicolegal responsibilities of the physician to obtain informed consent.

A thorough history of the patient and physical examination are the foundation of safe patient care. A complete list of medications that the patient is currently taking, both systemic and topical, must be obtained so potential drug interactions can be anticipated and essential medication will be administered during the hospital stay. Naturally, a history of any allergies to medicines, foods, or tape should be documented. Clearly, knowledge of any personal or family history of adverse reactions to anesthesia is mandatory. The requisite laboratory data vary, depending on the medical history and physical status of the patient, as well as the nature of the surgical procedure. Indeed, the American Society of Anesthesiologists (ASA) task force on preoperative evaluation concluded that routine preoperative tests are commonly not useful in assessing and managing patients' perioperative experience. In a more recent multicenter study of cataract patients, for example, Schein[53] demonstrated that "routine" testing does not improve patient safety or outcome. Some physicians and laypersons misinterpreted the results and conclusions of this investigation, believing that patients having cataract surgery need no preoperative evaluation. It is vital to note that all patients in this trial received regular medical care and were evaluated by a physician preoperatively. Patients whose medical status indicated a need for preoperative lab tests were excluded from the study. Clearly, testing should be based on the results of the history and physical examination. Because "routine" testing for the more than 1.5 million cataract operations in the United States is estimated to cost $150 million annually, the favorable economic impact of this "targeted" approach is obvious.

Many elderly adult candidates for ophthalmic surgery are on antiplatelet or anticoagulant therapy because of a history of coronary or vascular pathology. Such patients are at higher risk for perioperative hemorrhagic events, including retrobulbar hemorrhage, circumorbital hematoma, intravitreous bleeding, and hyphema. Traditionally, antiplatelet and anticoagulant medications were withheld for an appropriate length of time before eye surgery. However, this strategy may increase the risk of such adverse events as myocardial ischemia or infarction, cerebrovascular accident, and deep venous thrombosis. Several studies exploring this controversial issue suggest that cataract surgery can be safely performed under regional anesthesia without discontinuing anticoagulants,[54,55] especially if the prothrombin time is approximately 1.5 times control.[56] A more recent multicenter study of almost 20,000 cataract patients older than 50 years of age attempted to establish the risks and benfits of continuing aspirin or Coumadin therapy.[57] Despite the large population studied, the rate of complications was so low that absolute differences in risk were minimal. Patients who continued therapy did not have more ocular hemorrhage; those who discontinued treatment did not have a greater incidence of medical events. Nonetheless, it is critical to appreciate that these investigations focused specifically on cataract operations. Retinal surgery may be another matter.

Patients presenting for ocular surgery are often at the extremes of age—ranging from premature babies with retinopathy of prematurity to nonagenarians. Hence, special age-related considerations such as altered pharmacokinetics and pharmacodynamics apply. In addition, elderly patients frequently have multiple comorbitities that include thyroid dysfunction, cardiopulmonary, and renal diseases. Hypertension is encountered in the majority of geriatric patients. Those with poorly controlled blood pressure should not receive dilating eye drops, such as phenylephrine, without consulting an anesthesiologist. Systemic absorption of high concentrations (e.g., >2.5% phenylephrine) or improperly instilled mydriatics can precipitate a hypertensive crisis with potentially devastating consequences.

The anesthesiologist must be aware of the anesthetic implications of congenital and metabolic diseases with ocular manifestations. Diabetics often present with ocular complications, and the anesthesiologist must be knowledgeable about the systemic disturbances of physiology that affect these patients. Indeed, the list of congenital and metabolic diseases associated with ocular pathologic effects that have significant anesthetic implications is lengthy. A partial summary includes syndromes such as Crouzon's, Apert's, Goldenhar's (oculoauriculovertebral dysplasia), Sturge-Weber, Marfan's, Lowe's (oculocerebrorenal syndrome), Down (trisomy 21), Wagner-Stickler, and Riley-Day (familial dysautonomia). Other diseases in this category are homocystinuria, malignant hyperthermia, myotonia dystrophica, and sickle cell disease.[58]

Anesthesia Options

The requirements of ophthalmic surgery include safety, akinesia, profound analgesia, minimal bleeding, avoidance or obtundation of the oculocardiac reflex, prevention of intraocular hypertension, awareness of drug interactions, and a smooth emergence devoid of vomiting, coughing, or retching (see Table 33-1). Moreover, the exigencies of ophthalmic anesthesia mandate that the anesthesiologist be positioned remote from the patient's airway, sometimes creating certain logistic problems.

A number of anesthetic options exist, including general anesthesia, retrobulbar block, peribulbar anesthesia, sub-Tenon's (episcleral) block, topical anesthesia, and intracameral injection. General anesthesia is administered for the vast ma-
5 jority of children. Some adolescent and most adult patients can be cared for with regional or topical anesthesia and monitored anesthesia care (MAC), with or without sedation. The choice of anesthesia technique should be individualized based on the patient's needs and preferences, the nature and duration of the procedure, and the preferences and skills of the anesthesiologist and the surgeon.

Traditionally, the most commonly selected regional anesthetic technique for cataract surgery had been the retrobulbar block. Since the mid-1990s, peribulbar injection has surpassed retrobulbar block in popularity because of a relatively superior safety profile. Recently, however, topical analgesia has become more commonly used for cataract surgery in the United States (59% versus 41% for block techniques),[59] and sub-Tenon's blocks have surged in popularity in the United Kingdom and New Zealand.[60] Anesthesia for adult patients undergoing retina surgery is still accomplished primarily with peribulbar or retrobulbar block,[61] although some surgeons prefer general anesthesia for certain patients. More recently, anesthesiologists have had increasing interest in administering ocular anesthesia, and workshops in ophthalmic regional anesthesia are often conducted at major regional and national meetings. Many ophthalmologists and administrators encourage anesthesiologists to administer the blocks to facilitate operating room efficiency.

When a regional anesthetic of the orbit is administered, either by the anesthesiologist or the ophthalmologist, it is the responsibility of the anesthesiologist to monitor the patient's vital signs, electrocardiogram (ECG), and oxygen saturation. Sedation may be administered before performance of the block and/or initiation of surgery. The anesthesiologist must be vigilant for the oculocardiac reflex, signs of brainstem anesthesia, and the need for airway support or other interventions.

Anesthesia Techniques

More than 40 years ago, it was common for ophthalmic procedures to involve large ocular incisions. General endotracheal anesthesia, with deep and sustained neuromuscular paralysis and placement of sandbags to surround the patient's head, were typical strategies to ensure perioperative immobility. In more recent years, general anesthesia typically has been reserved for children and adults who are unabe to communicate, cooperate, or remain suitably stationary. Although endotracheal anesthesia is necessary for patients at risk of aspiration, the laryngeal mask airway (LMA) has been increasingly accepted as a means to secure the airway in patients with no risk factors for aspiration who are having eye surgery with general anesthesia.[62] The LMA is not only safe and effective in this setting, but it also offers the advantage of less increase in IOP on insertion and removal than is encountered with an endotracheal tube.[63] Similarly, less bucking and coughing on emergence and during the recovery phase has been noted.[64] Vigilance must be maintained, however, to detect initial misplacement or intraoperative displacement of the LMA. In addition, intraoperative laryngospasm in infants and neonates is not uncommon with an LMA.

Retrobulbar and Peribulbar Blocks. Needle-based ophthalmic regional anesthesia was first described by Knapp in 1884.[65] Then, in the early twentieth century, Atkinson introduced the retrobulbar block.[66] Retrobulbar block is a practical means to achieve analgesia and profound akinesia of the globe. The peribulbar block is a more recently introduced needle-based technique that varies from the retrobulbar block in terms of the depth and angulation of needle placement within the orbit. Traditionally, the four rectus muscles, along with connective tissue septae, were believed to create a defined compartment known as the orbital cone. This so-called cone extends from the rectus muscle origins around the optic foramen at the apex of the orbit to the attachment of the muscles to the globe anteriorly. Retrobulbar blocks are accomplished by directing a needle toward the orbital apex with sufficient depth and angulation such that the cone is penetrated (Figs. 33-4 and 33-5). Local anesthetic is then instilled in the cone, behind the eye. Cadaveric dissections, however, have shown the fallacy of the classic concept of the cone. There is no complete intermuscular septum encircling the rectus muscles, linking them together to form an impermeable compartment behind the globe akin to the brachial plexus sheath in the axilla.[67] Ripart and colleagues[68] clearly demonstrated that extraconal injections of dye into cadaveric specimens diffused into the intraconal space, and solutions placed within the cone distributed to the extraconal space. Thus, the peribulbar block is executed by directing

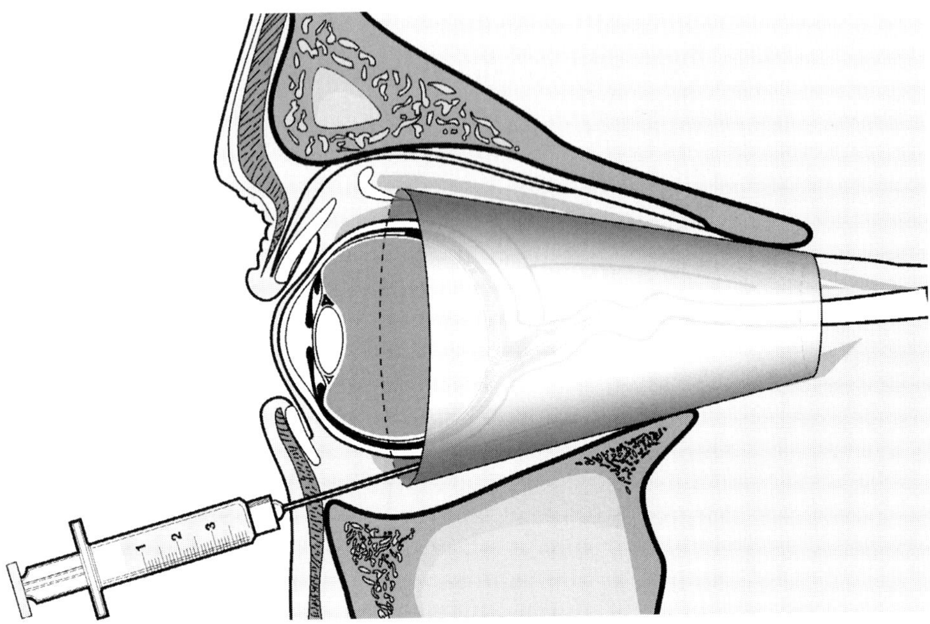

FIGURE 33-4. Retrobulbar (intraconal) block and schematic representation of the intraorbital muscle cone.

a needle to less depth and with minimal angulation, parallel to the globe, toward the greater wing of the sphenoid bone (Figs. 33-6 and 33-7). Local anesthetic instilled in this extraconal space will eventually penetrate toward the optic nerve and other structures, establishing conduction anesthesia. The peribulbar block is theoretically safer because the needle tip is kept at a greater distance from vital intraorbital structures and brain.

A retrobulbar or so-called intraconal block positions local anesthetics deep within the orbit proximate to the nerves and muscle origins. Thus, it requires low volume, has rapid onset, and yields intense depth of anesthesia. The peribulbar, or extraconal block, placed further from the optic and other orbital nerves, requires larger volumes of local anesthetic and has longer latency of onset. The needle entry point for both blocks is at the same inferotemporal location. The junction of the lateral third and medial two-thirds of the inferior orbital rim in line with the lateral limbal margin has been the conventional access point. However, locating the needle entry point more laterally may serve to decrease the likelihood of injecting local anesthetics into the delicate inferior rectus muscle. This is important because intramuscular injection of anesthetics has been postulated as a potential cause of postoperative strabismus.[69] Medial approaches at the caruncle have also been popularized more recently.[70] Supplementation of anesthesia with an injection above the globe may not be prudent because the preponderance of vessels lie in the superior orbit. In addition, the belly of the superior oblique muscle and the trochlear muscle can be encountered superonasally. Katsev and colleagues[71] demonstrated that the tips of commonly used 1.5–in. (38-mm) needles can reach critical structures in the densely packed apex of the orbit in almost 20% of retrobulbar blocks. Consequently, 1.25-in. (31-mm) needles are appropriate. Controversy exists over the advantages of sharp versus dull needles. Dull needles may require more force to penetrate the globe. However, sharp needles are less painful to insert and may cause less damage in the face of inadvertent globe puncture.[72] In the past, patients were asked to gaze superonasally while a block was conducted. Unsold and colleagues[73] found, however, that this maneuver caused the optic nerve to stretch directly in the path of the incoming needle during retrobulbar injection, exposing it to risk of needle trauma. Patients should be instructed to maintain gaze in the neutral position, leaving the optic nerve lax within the orbit in the course of needle insertion.[74]

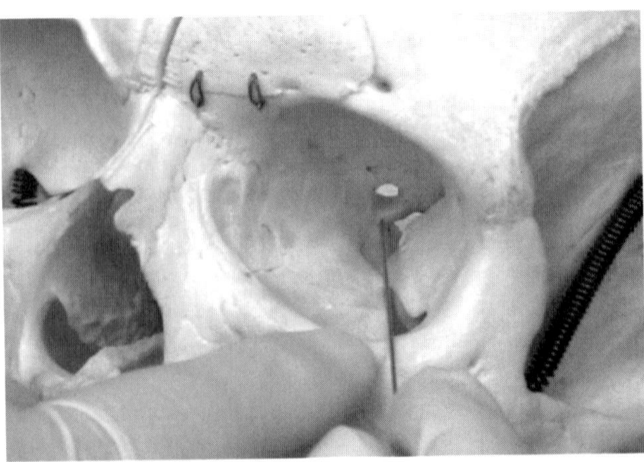

FIGURE 33-5. Needle placement for retrobulbar block.

Akinesia of the eyelids is obtained by blocking the branches of the facial nerve supplying the orbicularis muscle. Lid akinesia is often a direct consequence of the larger volume of local anesthetic used for peribulbar blocks. Retrobulbar blocks, in contrast, often leave the orbicularis oculi fully functional. Thus, a facial nerve block is performed in conjunction with retrobulbar block to prevent squeezing of the eyelid that could result in extrusion of intraocular contents during corneal transplantation, for example. Since first used for ophthalmic surgery by Van Lint in 1914, numerous methods of facial nerve blockade have been described. These techniques block the facial nerve after its exit point from the skull in the stylomastoid foramen. Moving distally to proximally to the foramen, the techniques include the Van Lint, Atkinson, O'Brien, and Nadbath-Rehman methods. Although each has advantages and disadvantages, the Nadbath-Rehman approach can potentially produce the most serious systemic consequences. With this approach, a 27-gauge, 12-mm needle is inserted between the mastoid process and the posterior border of the mandibular ramus. Due to the proximity of the jugular foramen (10 mm medial to the stylomastoid foramen) to the injection site, ipsilateral paralysis of cranial

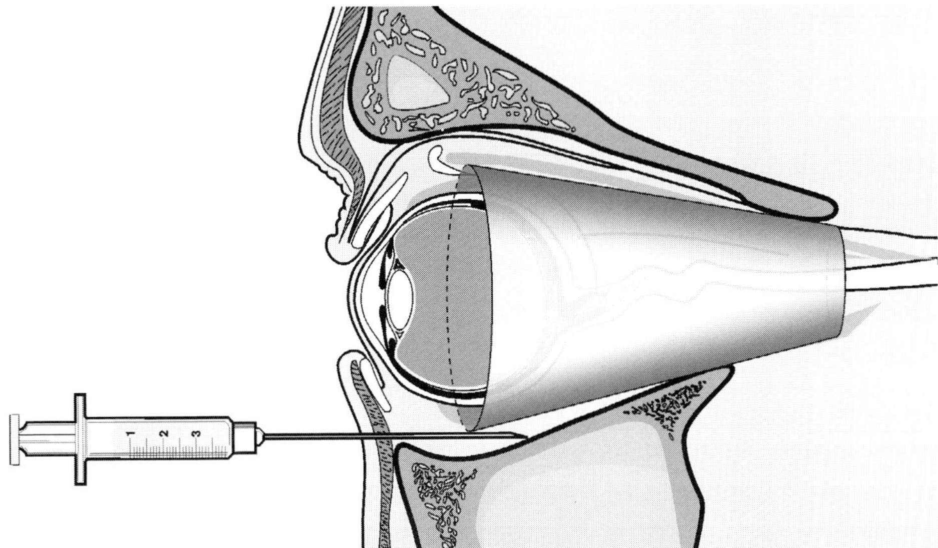

FIGURE 33-6. Peribulbar (extraconal) block and schematic representation of the intraorbital muscle cone.

nerves IX, X, and XI can occur, producing hoarseness, dysphagia, pooling of secretions, agitation, respiratory distress, or
6 laryngospasm. Moreover, because the Nadbath-Rehman block produces complete hemifacial akinesia that interferes with oral intake, this approach is not recommended for outpatients.

Complications associated with needle-based ophthalmic anesthetics may be local or systemic, and may result in blindness or even death (Table 33-4). Bleeding may be superficial or deep, arterial or venous. Superficial hemorrhage may produce an unsightly circumorbital hematoma. Retrobulbar hemorrhage, when arterially based, may produce precipitous bleeding and a palpable, dramatic increase in IOP, as well as globe proptosis and entrapment of the upper lid. With the globe's vascular supply in jeopardy, the patient's long-term ultimate visual acuity may be quickly compromised. Consultation with an ophthalmologist should be immediately sought, and fundoscopic examination, tonometric measurement of IOP, ultrasound to assess presence/location of blood, and even a lateral canthotomy may be warranted. Continuous ECG monitoring is indicated because the oculocardiac reflex may appear as blood extravasates from the muscle cone. The decision to proceed with surgery in the presence of a mild or moderate hemorrhage is dependent on numerous factors, including the degree of bleeding, the nature of the planned ophthalmologic surgery, and the patient's condition.

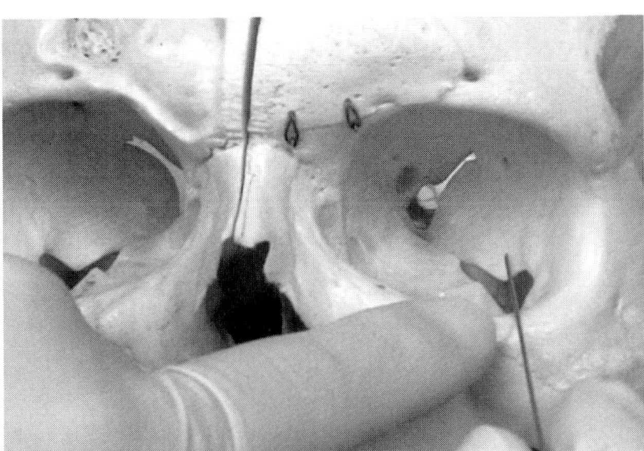

FIGURE 33-7. Needle placement for peribulbar block.

Penetration of the sclera is a distinct possibility with needle-based anesthesia techniques. Mechanical trauma, with potential retinal detachment, and chemical injury by local anesthetics to delicate retina tissue can occur. Blindness or very poor vision may be the result. Globe puncture is defined as a single entry into the eye, whereas perforation is caused by two full-thickness wounds—an entry and a subsequent exit. The globe's posterior pole is the most commonly penetrated area. Risk factors for posterior pole needle injury include presence of an elongated globe, recessed orb, and/or atypical-shaped eye. The AP distance of an eye may be long because of myopia or presence of globe-enveloping intraorbital hardware such as a scleral buckle. Some patients have an abnormal outpouching of the eye termed staphyloma. Most staphyloma are located at the posterior of the globe, surrounding the juncture of the eye with the optic nerve. By definition, a retrobulbar anesthetic is conducted by purposefully angling the needle steeply and deeply within the orbit behind the globe. If the globe is longer than one assumes, then it is at greater risk of penetration or puncture by the retrobulbar needle. In one more recent study, ultrasound detection determined that often the tip of the needle, placed in retrobulbar fashion, is much closer to the posterior pole of the globe than presupposed by physicians.[75] Peribulbar anesthesia entails shallower placement of the needle without directing the

TABLE 33-4

COMPLICATIONS OF NEEDLE-BASED OPHTHALMIC ANESTHESIA

- Stimulation of oculocardiac reflex arc
- Superficial hemorrhage → circumorbital hematoma
- Retrobulbar hemorrhage ± retinal perfusion compromise → loss of vision
- Globe penetration ± intraocular injection → retinal detachment, loss of vision
- Trauma to optic nerve or orbital cranial nerves → loss of vision
- Optic nerve sheath injection → orbital epidural anesthesia
- Extraocular muscle injury, leading to postoperative strabismus, diplopia
- Intra-arterial injection, producing immediate convulsions
- Central retinal artery occlusion
- Inadvertent brainstem anesthesia → contralateral amaurosis, neurocardiopulmonary compromise

needle inward toward the orbital apex; thus, it is associated with a lower incidence of globe-needle injury. Be aware, however, that it is still possible to engage the needle with sclera laterally.

The risk of penetrating the sclera with a needle is also inversely proportional to the anesthesiologist's education and experience. This is affirmed by several reports of globe injuries rendered by inadequately educated or trained personnel in the early 1990s.[76] In a survey of 284 directors of anesthesiology and ophthalmology programs, no formal training or education in ophthalmic regional anesthesia techniques was provided to anesthesia residents in the vast majority of academic programs.[77] This survey concluded that anesthesiologists who perform needle-based ophthalmic blocks should have knowledge of orbital anatomy and the ocular risk factors that were noted previously. Thus, appropriate preanesthesia history-taking includes direct interrogation concerning myopia or previous scleral buckle surgery, as both imply increased globe length. Physical exam of surface anatomy should note the position of the globe within the orbit and whether enophthalmos is present. A recessed eye is at greater risk of needle-tip misadventure. The most important laboratory exam is the preoperative ultrasound. For patients undergoing cataract surgery, an ultrasound is *always* performed to calculate the appropriate intraocular lens to insert intraoperatively. This ultrasound reveals the length and shape of the eye. An axial length greater than 26 mm confers greater risk of perforation. In the event that the ultrasound report is not found in the patient's chart, the anesthesiologist should inquire about the results before embarking on a needle-based block.

Brainstem anesthesia and inadvertent intravascular injection of local anesthetics are two additional potentially devastating consequences of needle-based ocular anesthesia. In the course of accidental intravascular arterial injection, local anesthetics flow from the needle via a branch of the ophthalmic artery in retrograde fashion to the internal carotid artery and then to the circle of Willis. Rapid redistribution of local anesthetic to the brain results in immediate onset of convulsions, and cardiopulmonary instability may also occur. Although the incidence of brainstem anesthesia is rare, it is even less common with peribulbar versus retrobulbar blocks. Brainstem anesthesia is a consequence of the direct spread of local anesthetic agents to the brain along the meningeal sheath surrounding the optic nerve. In contradistinction to intra-arterial injection, symptoms are not always immediate. There is a continuum of sequelae dependent on the concentration and volume of drug that gains access centrally, as well as the specific areas where the anesthetics spread (Fig. 33-8). One case report described the insidious onset of unconsciousness and apnea over 7 minutes, without concomitant seizures or cardiovascular collapse.[78] Nicoll et al.[79] reported 16 cases of apparently central spread of anesthetics in a series of 6,000 retrobulbar blocks. Eight patients developed respiratory arrest. Other protean CNS signs may include violent shivering; contralateral amaurosis; eventual loss of consciousness; apnea; and hemiplegia, paraplegia, quadriplegia, or hyperreflexia. Blockade of cranial nerves VIII to XII results in deafness, vertigo, vagolysis, dysphagia, aphasia, and loss of neck muscle power. It is axiomatic that personnel skilled in airway maintenance and ventilatory and circulatory support should be immediately available whenever retrobulbar or other needle-based anesthetic blocks are administered.

Cannula-Based Techniques. Cannula-based ophthalmic regional anesthesia was first described by Swan in 1956.[80] The sub-Tenon's block was rediscovered and popularized in the 1990s as another practical means to achieve analgesia and akinesia of the globe, while offering potential advantages in certain circumstances over needle-based blocks. Magnetic resonance imaging (MRI) studies have shown that local anesthetics, instilled beneath Tenon's capsule, spread into the posterior orbit.[81] The block is accomplished by inserting a blunt cannula through a small incision in the conjunctiva and Tenon's capsule, also known as the episcleral membrane, with subsequent infusion of local anesthetics (Fig. 33-9). Onset of analgesia is rapid. The ultimate extent of globe akinesia is proportional to the volume of local anesthetic injected. One large prospective study by Guise[82] of 6,000 such blocks found this technique to be highly effective. Advantages, particularly for very myopic patients who have elongated axial lengths, include decreased risk of posterior pole perforation because needles are not placed into the posterior orbit.

After application of topical anesthetic, the episcleral space can be accessed from all quadrants with blunt-tipped scissors; however, the incision is most commonly made in the inferonasal

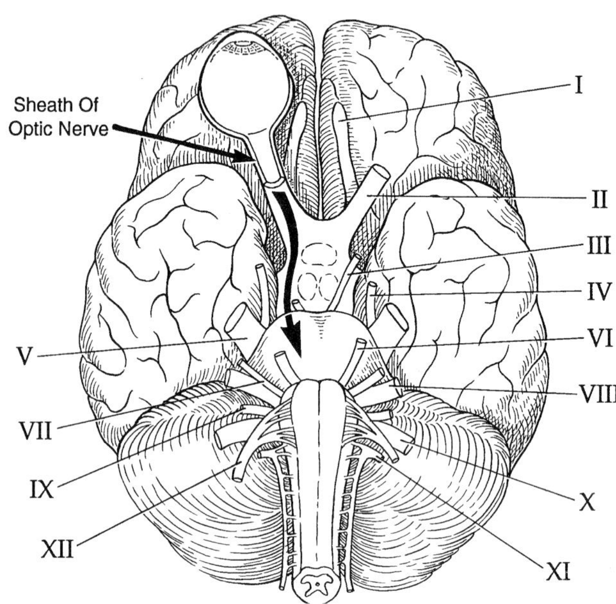

FIGURE 33-8. Base of the brain and the path that local anesthetic agents might follow if inadvertently injected into the subarachnoid space. This route includes the cranial nerves, pons, and midbrain. (Reprinted with permission from Javitt JC, Addiego R, Friedberg HL *et al*: Brain stem anesthesia after retrobulbar block. Ophthalmology 94:718, 1987.)

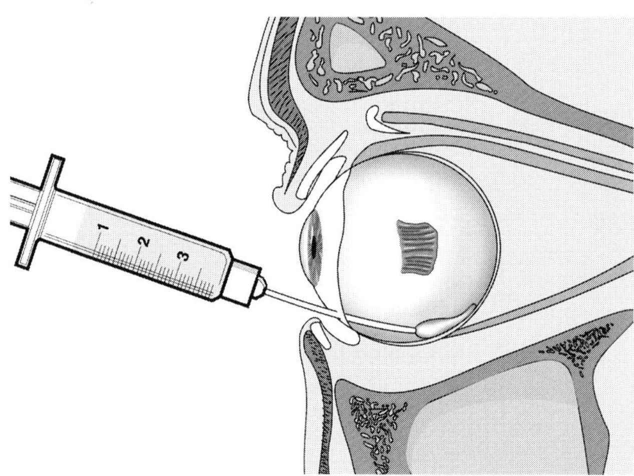

FIGURE 33-9. Sub-Tenon's (episcleral) block with blunt cannula.

quadrant. The cannula is guided through the opening with the aid of a toothless forceps. It is common for local anesthetics to leak retrograde out of the incision site. Conjunctival bleeding (especially if diathermy is not used), chemosis, and ballooning up of the conjunctiva and Tenon's capsule are common. Fortunately, these are cosmetic issues that rarely affect outcome. Guise[82] estimated the incidence of minor hemorrhage to be less than 10% and had to abandon only one case because of a large subconjunctival hemorrhage that was not sight threatening. Thus, the sub-Tenon's block may be a prudent ocular anesthesia technique for the anticoagulated patient at risk for retrobulbar hemorrhage.

Major complications of sub-Tenon's ocular anesthesia include globe perforation,[83] major orbital hemorrhage, rectus muscle trauma, postoperative strabismus, orbital cellulitis, and brainstem anesthesia.[84] A greater proportion of complications seem to be associated with longer (18 to 25 mm), more rigid, metallic cannulae. Shorter (12 mm), more flexible, plastic cannulae may be preferable. However, they are associated with a higher incidence of conjunctival hemorrhage and chemosis. Variations of sub-Tenon's blocks include a more recently introduced ultrashort cannula (6 mm) and needle-based episcleral block techniques.[85]

Topical Analgesia. Ophthalmologists have also been returning to a technique that was popularized during the early 1900s—the use of topical anesthetic agents, particularly when the surgical incision is being made through clear cornea. Indeed, surface analgesia was the technique of choice for cataract surgery until the evolution of effective needle-based methods of regional anesthesia and improved safety of general anesthesia in the 1930s. Multiple advances in cataract surgery that have enabled faster operations, with greater control and less trauma, have allowed ophthalmologists to reexamine the use of topical anesthesia for this procedure. Phacoemulsification, with its small incisions, is clearly the procedure of choice in using topical anesthesia; however, planned extracapsular procedures can also be performed under topical anesthesia, thereby circumventing potential complications of peribulbar or retrobulbar block. Certainly, fully anticoagulated patients are excellent candidates for topical analgesia, as are monocular patients who are spared the trauma of prolonged local anesthetic-induced postoperative amaurosis. Potential disadvantages of topical anesthesia include eye movement during surgery, patient anxiety, and, rarely, allergic reactions. Patient selection is critical and should be restricted to individuals who are alert and able to follow instructions, and who can control their eye movements. Patients who are demented or photophobic, or who cannot communicate, are inappropriate candidates, as are those with an inflamed eye. Similarly, patients with small pupils who may require significant iris manipulation or those who need large scleral incisions may be contraindicated for topical anesthesia.

Topical analgesia can be achieved with local anesthetic drops or gels. Anesthetic gels produce greater levels of drug in the anterior chamber than equal doses of drops and may afford superior surface analgesia.[86] Intracameral injection of 0.1 to 0.2 mL of 1% preservative-free lidocaine into the anterior chamber supplements the analgesia effects but may be deleterious to cornal endothelium.[87] Concerns about increased potential for postoperative endophthalmitis with gel-based topical analgesia exist because gels might theoretically form a barrier to bactericidal agents. Therefore, if administered, gels should be applied after antiseptic solutions, taking care to apply anesthetic drops before the use of caustic bactericidal preps.

Choice of Local Anesthetics, Block Adjuvants, and Adjuncts. Anesthetics for ocular surgery are selected based on onset and duration needed. Fast-onset, brief duration local anesthetics are optimal for procedures such as cataract surgery or pterygium excision. Longer-acting agents are indicated for lengthier operations such as vitreoretinal surgery. A tradition of mixing different local anesthetics to produce a block with shorter latency of onset, yet longer duration of effect, has been a paradigm of ophthalmic anesthesia. Vasoconstrictors may improve the quality of the block by delaying washout of drug from the orbit. There is concern, however, that epinephrine, the most common vasoconstrictor additive, may compromise retinal perfusion.[88]

Sodium bicarbonate, morphine sulfate, clonidine, and even vecuronium have been used as local anesthetic adjuvants in ophthalmic surgery. Without question, however, hyaluronidase has been the most popular ancillary agent used to modify ocular local anesthetic actions since it was introduced by Atkinson in 1949. It acts by hydrolyzing hyaluronic acid, a natural substance that binds cells together, keeping them cohesive. Thus, hyaluronidase increases tissue permeability, serves to promote dispersion of local anesthetics through tissues within the orbit, reduces the increase in orbital pressure associated with the volume of injected anesthetics, and enhances the quality of orbital blockade. Furthermore, hyaluronidase may reduce the risk of local anesthetic-induced extraocular muscle injury because clustered increases of postoperative diplopia were reported after national shortages of the drug in 1998 and 2000.[89] However, this is a controversial claim because it is possible, if not likely, that many who were administering orbital blocks may have modified their technique in response to the shortage, placing needles deeper, using more injections, or depositing larger volumes of local anesthetics.

Intravenous osmotic agents, such as mannitol and glycerin, as well as carbonic anhydrase inhibitors can be given to reduce vitreous volume and decrease IOP after it is artificially increased by local anesthetics. Digital pressure to soften the globe was described almost 50 years ago.[90] Mechanical means developed shortly thereafter and a number of devices are available. Essentially, they are all variations on a ball, balloon, or bag theme. The Super Pinky ball, the Honan IOP Reducer, and the Buys Mercury Reducer (soon to be eliminated because of pollutant concerns expressed by the U.S. Environmental Protection Agency) are examples. Immediately after administration of regional orbital anesthesia, the compression device may be positioned on the eye for 5 to 20 minutes. Reduction of IOP to below baseline levels is not uncommon. However, excessive pressure on the globe by these devices may impede blood flow, causing ischemic optic neuropathy or central retinal artery occlusion, possibly leading to blindness.[91] The Honan device addresses this potentially catastrophic complication with a pneumatic bellows that maintains even compression of the globe coupled to a manometric gauge that indicates a numeric value of applied pressure. A safety valve limits the amount of inflation of the bellows. With the increasing popularity of smaller incisions, lower-profile prosthetic lenses, and topical analgesia for cataract surgery, there is less need for IOP-reducing devices.

General Principles of Monitored Anesthesia Care. Many advocate the intravenous administration of an appropriate agent immediately before performance of ocular regional anesthesia to provide comfort and amnesia. What should be avoided at all costs, however, is the combination of local anesthesia with heavy sedation in the form of high doses of opioids, benzodiazepines, and hypnotics. This polypharmacology is highly unsatisfactory because of the pharmacologic vagaries in the geriatric population and the attendant risks of respiratory depression, airway obstruction, hypotension, CNS aberrations, and prolonged recovery time. This undesirable technique has all the disadvantages of a general anesthetic in the absence of a tracheal tube or LMA without the advantage of controllability that general anesthesia offers. After the block has been performed, the patient should be relaxed but awake to avoid head movement associated with snoring or sudden abrupt movement on awakening. Clearly, patients under conscious sedation must be capable of responding rationally to commands and must be able to maintain airway patency. Undersedation should likewise be avoided because tachycardia and hypertension may have deleterious effects, especially in patients with coronary artery disease. Moreover, patients with orthopedic deformities or arthritis must be meticulously positioned and given comfortable padding on the operating table. Adequate ventilation about the face is essential for all patients to avoid carbon dioxide accumulation, and each must be comfortably warm. (The hazards of shivering in patients with cardiac disease and, for that matter, in any patient having delicate eye surgery are well known.) Continuous ECG monitoring is vital, lest performance of the retrobulbar block, pressure on the orbit, or tugging on the extraocular muscles stimulates the oculocardiac reflex arc and produces dangerous cardiac dysrhythmias. Likewise, pulse oximetry is essential.

Studies have confirmed that most cataract operations performed in the United States are conducted with the patient under some form of local anesthesia (either retrobulbar, peribulbar, or parabulbar injection, or topical analgesia), with monitoring equipment used in 97% of cases and an anesthesiologist present in 78% of cases.[92] Indeed, many anesthesiologists have long wondered whether CMS will decide not to reimburse for monitored anesthesia care for "routine" cataract cases.

An important study by Rosenfeld and colleagues[93] is the first to assess the need for monitored anesthesia care in cataract surgery. These investigators prospectively studied the incidence and the nature of interventions required by anesthesia personnel in 1,006 consecutive cataract operations (both phacoemulsification and extracapsular techniques were included) performed under peribulbar block. They also analyzed the risk factors for intervention, including patient demographic data, medical history, and preoperative laboratory tests, for reliability in predicting those patients at greatest risk for intervention. They found that 37% of patients required some type of intervention and that, in general, the majority of those interventions could not have been predicted before surgery. The interventions ranged from minor forms, such as verbal reassurance and hand holding, to administering such intravenous medications as supplemental sedation or antihypertensive, pressor, or antiarrhythmic agents, or to providing respiratory assistance. Although hypertension, lung disease, renal disease, and a diagnosis of cancer were related to interventions, these four conditions combined accounted for only a small portion of the needed interventions. Moreover, although many of the interventions were relatively minor, several were more serious, and 30% of the interventions were considered (by the involved anesthesia personnel) to be critical to the success of the operation. The investigators concluded that monitored anesthesia care by qualified anesthesia personnel is reasonable and justified and contributes to the quality of patient care when cataract surgery is performed with local anesthesia. Although there were few, if any, injection-related problems, one wonders if the conclusion regarding need for anesthesia involvement would be different if the majority of cases had received topical analgesia. Given that analgesia is less profound with a topical approach, it seems likely that anesthesia care is equally appropriate to provide comfort, support, and indicated drugs for these patients. For both ethical and technical reasons, the ophthalmologist's attention must not be distracted from the microsurgical field.

ANESTHETIC MANAGEMENT IN SPECIFIC SITUATIONS

General Concepts and Objectives

Most patients undergoing eye surgery are either younger than 10 years of age or older than 55 years of age. In children, operations on the ocular adnexa, including lid surgery, repair of lacrimal apparatus, and adjustment of extraocular muscles, are common. However, surgery on the anterior segment, such as cataract removal, glaucoma procedures, and trauma repair, is definitely not limited to the adult population. Nor are posterior segment operations such as scleral buckling and vitrectomy the exclusive domain of geriatrics.

Most ocular procedures demand profound analgesia but minimal skeletal muscle relaxation. The airway must be protected from obstruction, and the anesthesiologist must distance himself or herself—along with anesthetic apparatus—from the surgical field. Depending on whether the patient is a child or an adult and various other factors previously discussed, a decision is reached regarding selection of local or general anesthesia. Additional preparation must include, of course, identification of underlying diseases, such as asthma, diabetes mellitus, or nephropathy. The patient should also be prepared emotionally for the recovery period, when he or she may awaken with one or both eyes closed by bandages. This is important not only to spare him or her fear and anxiety but to prevent much of the thrashing about that fright might produce, to the detriment of the eye.

Preoperative sedation is chosen carefully and is usually administered intravenously immediately before surgery because the vast majority of ophthalmic procedures are performed on an ambulatory basis. Except for strabismus correction, retinal detachment surgery, and cryosurgery, ophthalmic procedures are usually associated with little pain. Thus, the routine use of opioid premedication, replete with emetic potential, is ill advised. Rather, premedication should be prescribed with a view toward amnesia, sedation, and antiemesis.

Analgesia and akinesis are then secured through either local or general anesthesia, with careful attention paid to proper control of IOP and to the possible appearance of the oculocardiac reflex. The anesthesiologist strives to provide a smooth intraoperative course and to prevent coughing, retching, and vomiting, lest harmful increases in IOP transpire that could hinder successful surgery. If general anesthesia is elected, extubation of the trachea should be accomplished before there is a tendency to cough. The administration of intravenous lidocaine, 1.5 to 2 mg/kg, before extubation of the trachea is helpful in attenuating coughing. Likewise, prophylactic intravenous droperidol—the "black box" warning issued by the U.S. Food and Drug Administration (FDA) not withstanding—is valuable in reducing the incidence and severity of nausea and vomiting. If droperidol is ineffective as a prophylactic agent, then the more expensive ondansetron or dolasetron may be administered as a "rescue" antiemetic. If the patient is deemed to be at extremely high risk for postoperative nausea and vomiting, prophylactic multimodal antiemetic therapy may be selected in conjunction with total intravenous anesthesia with propofol.

"Open-Eye, Full-Stomach" Encounters

The anesthesiologist involved in caring for a patient with a penetrating eye injury and a full stomach confronts special challenges. He or she must weigh the risk of aspiration against the risk of blindness in the injured eye that could result from elevated IOP and extrusion of ocular contents.

As in all cases of trauma, attention should be given to the exclusion of other injuries, such as skull and orbital fractures, intracranial trauma associated with subdural hematoma formation, and the possibility of thoracic or abdominal bleeding.

Although regional anesthesia is often a valuable alternative for the management of trauma patients who have recently eaten, this option had traditionally been considered contraindicated in patients with penetrating eye injuries because of the potential to extrude intraocular contents via pressure generated by local anesthetics. Nonetheless, some anecdotal case reports of successful use of ophthalmic blocks in this setting have been published. Recognizing that there are several distinct permutations of eye injuries, Gayer and colleagues developed techniques to safely block patients with *select* open-globe injuries.[94] In a 4-year period, 220 disrupted eyes were repaired via regional anesthesia at Bascom Palmer Eye Institute. A significant number of injuries were caused by intraocular foreign bodies and dehiscence of cataract or corneal transplant incisions. Blocked eyes tended to have more anterior, smaller wounds than those repaired via general anesthesia. There was no outcome difference—that is, change of visual acuity from initial evaluation until final examination—between the eyes repaired via regional versus general anesthesia. Moreover, combined topical anesthesia and sedation for *selected* patients with open-globe injuries has also been reported.[95]

Nonetheless, it is not always possible to determine the extent of disruption preoperatively, and general anesthesia is typically considered prudent in this setting. Preoperative prophylaxis against aspiration may involve administering H_2 receptor antagonists to elevate gastric fluid pH and to reduce gastric acid production. Metoclopramide may be given to induce peristalsis and enhance gastric emptying.

Frequently, a barbiturate, nondepolarizing neuromuscular blocking drug technique is described as the method of choice for the emergency repair of an open eye injury; the nondepolarizing drug pancuronium in a dose of 0.15 mg/kg has been shown to lower IOP. However, this method has its disadvantages, including risk of aspiration and death during the relatively lengthy period—ranging from 75 to 150 seconds—that the airway is unprotected. Performance of the Sellick maneuver during this interval affords some protection. Furthermore, a premature attempt at intubation of the trachea produces coughing, straining, and a dramatic rise in IOP, emphasizing the need to confirm the onset of drug effect with a peripheral nerve stimulator while appreciating, nonetheless, that muscle groups vary in their response to muscle relaxants. Moreover, the cardiovascular side effects of tachycardia and hypertension may prove worrisome in patients with coronary artery disease. Also, the long duration of action of intubating doses of pancuronium may mandate postoperative mechanical ventilation of the lungs. Intermediate-acting nondepolarizing drugs such as vecuronium have briefer durations of action, and less dramatic, if any, circulatory effects, but nevertheless have an onset of action similar to that of pancuronium.

Several studies have explored the use of extremely large doses of nondepolarizing muscle relaxants to accelerate the onset of adequate relaxation for endotracheal intubation. Using vecuronium doses of 0.2 and 0.4 mg/kg, Casson and Jones[96] found mean onset times of 95 and 87 seconds, respectively. Ginsberg et al.[97] found comparable albeit slightly longer onset times.

Succinylcholine offers the distinct advantages of swift onset, superb intubating conditions, and brief duration of action. If administered after careful pretreatment with a nondepolarizing drug and an induction dose of thiopental (4 to 6 mg/kg), succinylcholine produces only small increases in IOP.[98] Although the advisability of this technique has been debated vociferously, there are no published reports of loss of intraocular contents from a pretreatment barbiturate–succinylcholine sequence when used in this setting.[99] Moreover, in 1993, McGoldrick[100] pointed out that Lincoff's 1957 watershed article states: "Various communications have been received from ophthalmologists who have used succinylcholine in surgery. This includes several reports of cases in which succinylcholine was given *to forestall impending vitreous prolapse* only to have a prompt expulsion of vitreous occur" (our italics).[17] Under such desperate circumstances, it is extremely difficult to attribute the expulsion of vitreous directly to succinylcholine.[100]

What about the so-called priming principle?[101] This concept involves using approximately one-tenth of an intubating dose of nondepolarizing drug, followed 4 minutes later by an intubating dose. Then, after waiting an additional 90 seconds, intubation of the trachea may be performed. However, studies in this area demonstrate wide variability and disconcerting scatter of data. Future investigations should use a randomized, double-blind design because studies of intubating conditions are notoriously difficult to interpret. Moreover, priming is not devoid of risk; a case of pulmonary aspiration after a priming dose of vecuronium has been reported.[102]

Rocuronium, with its purportedly rapid onset, may prove to be a useful drug in these circumstances provided adequate doses (1.2 mg/kg intravenously) are administered. However, additional data are needed before rocuronium can be enthusiastically recommended in this challenging situation. Moreover, rocuronium has an intermediate duration of action that could be disadvantageous, compared with succinylcholine, in a patient with an unrecognized difficult airway. It was hoped that rapacuronium (Org 9487), with its swift onset, would emerge as a viable alternative to succinylcholine. However, rapacuronium is no longer available in the United States because of its role in triggering intractable bronchospasm in some patients. A new ultrashort-acting nondepolarizing alternative (GW280430A) to succinylcholine is currently undergoing clinical investigation in human volunteers.

Perhaps the wisest approach to the management of open-eye, full-stomach situations is summarized by Baumgarten and Reynolds,[103] who wrote in 1985:

> It may be possible to devise a combination of intravenous anesthetics and nondepolarizing relaxants that totally prevents coughing after rapid intubation. Until this combination is devised and confirmed in a large, controlled double-blind series, clinicians should not apply the priming principle to the open eye-full stomach patient. Use of a blockade monitor to predict intubating conditions may be unreliable, since muscle groups vary in their response to nondepolarizing relaxants. At this time, succinylcholine with precurarization probably remains the most tenable compromise in the open eye-full stomach challenge.

Strabismus Surgery

Approximately 3% of the population has malalignment of the visual axes, which may be accompanied by diplopia, amblyopia, and loss of stereopsis (Table 33-5). Indeed, strabismus surgery is the most common pediatric ocular operation performed in the United States, and it entails a variety of techniques to weaken an extraocular muscle by moving its insertion on the globe (recession) or to strengthen an extraocular muscle by eliminating a short strip of the tendon or muscle (resection).

Infantile strabismus occurs within the first 6 months of life and is often observed in the neonatal period. Although most patients with strabismus are healthy, normal children, the incidence of strabismus is increased in those with CNS dysfunction such as cerebral palsy and meningomyelocele with hydrocephalus. Moreover, strabismus may be acquired secondary to oculomotor nerve trauma or sensory abnormalities such as cataracts or refractive aberrations.

In addition to the well-known propensity of strabismus surgery to trigger the oculocardiac reflex (previously discussed), there is also an increased incidence of malignant hyperthermia in patients with conditions such as strabismus or ptosis. This observation is consistent with the impression that people susceptible to malignant hyperthermia often have localized areas of skeletal muscle weakness or other musculoskeletal abnormalities. Other aspects of strabismus surgery of interest

TABLE 33-5

CONCERNS WITH VARIOUS OCULAR PROCEDURES

PROCEDURE	CONCERNS
Strabismus repair	Forced duction testing Oculocardiac reflex Oculogastric reflex Malignant hyperthermia
Intraocular surgery	Proper control of IOP Akinesia Drug interactions Associated systemic disease
Retinal detachment surgery	Oculocardiac reflex Proper control of IOP Nitrous oxide interaction with air, sulfur hexafluoride, or perfluorocarbons

IOP, intraocular pressure.

to anesthesiologists include succinylcholine-induced interference with the FDT and an increased incidence of postoperative nausea and vomiting.

In formulating a surgical treatment plan for incomitant strabismus, ophthalmologists often find the FDT to be exquisitely helpful in differentiating between a paretic muscle and a restrictive force preventing ocular motion. To perform the FDT, the surgeon grasps the sclera of the anesthetized eye with a forceps near the corneal limbus and moves the eye into each field of gaze, concomitantly assessing tissue and elastic properties. This simple test provides valuable clues to the presence and site of mechanical restrictions of the extraocular muscles and is most valuable in patients who have previously undergone strabismus surgery, in those who may have paralysis of one of the extraocular muscles, and in those who have sustained orbital trauma.

France et al.[28] quantitated the magnitude and duration of change of the FDT after succinylcholine administration. They demonstrated that quantitation of the force necessary to rotate the globe remained significantly elevated over control for 15 minutes, even though the rise in IOP and the skeletal muscle paralysis lasted less than 5 minutes. Because succinylcholine interferes with FDT, its use is contraindicated less than 20 minutes before testing. Hence, France et al. suggested performing the FDT on the anesthetized patient either while mask inhalation anesthesia is being administered, before intubation of the trachea; after intubation, facilitated by nondepolarizing neuromuscular blocking drugs; or after intubation under moderately deep inhalation anesthesia, unaided by succinylcholine.

Eye movement under general anesthesia is well documented, and in nonaligned eyes this tendency is augmented such that divergent squints diverge more and convergent squints converge less. A more recent report discloses that surgeons at a regional eye teaching hospital in the United Kingdom who specialize in strabismus surgery are increasingly requesting that, if the FDT is being used, nondepolarizing neuromuscular blockade be incorporated into the anesthetic management so muscle tone is minimal or absent during testing.[104]

Once intubation of the trachea has been accomplished, anesthesia is commonly maintained with halothane; desflurane; sevoflurane; or isoflurane, nitrous oxide, and oxygen. The patient is carefully monitored with a precordial stethoscope, ECG, blood pressure device, pulse oximeter, end-tidal carbon dioxide measurement, and temperature probe. If bradycardia occurs, the surgeon is asked to discontinue ocular manipulation, and the patient's ventilatory status and anesthetic depth are quickly assessed. If additional intravenous atropine is indicated, it is not given while the oculocardiac reflex is active in case even more dangerous cardiac dysrhythmias are triggered.

The laryngeal mask airway is gaining popularity for strabismus surgery in the United States, provided the patient is not at risk for aspiration. The laryngeal mask can be inserted without the use of muscle relaxants, causes less hemodynamic perturbation, and is associated with less straining and coughing on removal.

Vomiting after eye muscle surgery is common, giving credibility to the existence of the oculogastric reflex. The administration of droperidol, 0.075 mg/kg at induction of anesthesia before manipulation of the eye, has been shown to reduce the incidence of vomiting after strabismus surgery to a clinically acceptable level of approximately 10% without prolonging recovery time.[105] Moreover, a lower dose of droperidol, 0.02 mg/kg intravenously, administered immediately after anesthetic induction in patients with strabismus may decrease both the incidence and severity of nausea and vomiting.[106]

Prophylactic intravenous administration of ondansetron also appears to be efficacious. More studies are needed to document the efficacy of some of the other serotonin receptor antagonists, such as dolasetron, granisetron, tropisetron, and ramosetron in this setting. Combination therapy consisting of one or two antiemetics, each with a different mechanism of action, plus a glucocorticoid such as dexamethasone is also gaining popularity.[107] Moreover, a total intravenous technique with proprofol has also been associated with a low incidence of emesis after strabismus surgery.[108] In addition, avoiding narcotics may be helpful. One study demonstrates that the nonopioid analgesic ketorolac, in a dose of 0.75 mg/kg intravenously, provides analgesia comparable with that of morphine in pediatric patients with strabismus, but with a much lower incidence of nausea and vomiting in the first 24 hours.[109]

Intraocular Surgery

Advances in both anesthesia and in technology now permit a level of controlled intraocular manipulation not possible one-quarter century ago (see Table 33-5).

Proper control of IOP is crucial for such intraocular procedures as glaucoma drainage surgery, open sky vitrectomy, penetrating keratoplasty (corneal transplantation), and traditional intracapsular cataract extraction. Before scleral incision (when
7 IOP becomes equal to atmospheric pressure), a low-normal IOP is essential because abrupt decompression of a hypertensive eye could result in iris or lens prolapse, vitreous loss, or expulsive choroidal hemorrhage. Available data have not demonstrated a major difference in the rate of complications such as vitreous loss and iris prolapse between local anesthesia and general anesthesia.

Many anesthetic techniques may be safely used for elective intraocular surgery. If general anesthesia is selected, virtually any of the inhalation drugs may be given after intravenous induction of anesthesia with a barbiturate or propofol, neuromuscular blocking drug, and topical laryngeal lidocaine. Because complete akinesia is essential for delicate intraocular surgery, nondepolarizing drugs are administered, followed by neuromuscular function monitoring to ensure a 90 to 95% twitch suppression level during surgery. Because proper control of IOP is critical, controlled ventilation of the lungs is used, along with end-tidal carbon dioxide monitoring to ensure avoidance of hypercarbia.

Maximal pupillary dilation is important for many types of intraocular surgery and can be induced by continuous infusion of epinephrine 1:200,000 in a balanced salt solution, delivered through a small-gauge needle placed in the anterior chamber. Almost simultaneous with its administration, the drug is removed by aspirating it from the anterior chamber. The iris usually dilates immediately on contact with the epinephrine infusion, and drug uptake is presumably limited by the associated intense vasoconstriction of the iris and ciliary body. However, epinephrine may also be potentially absorbed by drainage through Schlemm's canal into the venous system or by spillover of the infusion into the conjunctival vessels or drainage to the nasal mucosa.

At the completion of surgery, any residual neuromuscular blockade is reversed. On resumption of spontaneous ventilation, the patient's trachea is extubated (often in the lateral position) with the patient still deeply anesthetized and after intravenous administration of lidocaine to prevent coughing. Atropine and neostigmine may be safely used to reverse neuromuscular blockade, even in patients with glaucoma because this combination of drugs, in conventional doses, has minimal effects on pupil size and IOP.

Retinal Detachment Surgery

Surgery to repair retinal detachments involves procedures affecting intraocular volume, frequently using a synthetic silicone band or sponge to produce a localized or encircling scleral indentation (see Table 33-5). Furthermore, internal tamponade of the retinal break may be accomplished by injecting an expandable gas such as sulfur hexafluoride into the vitreous. Because of blood gas partition coefficient differences, the administration of nitrous oxide may enhance the internal tamponade effect of sulfur hexafluoride intraoperatively, only to be followed by a dramatic drop in IOP and volume on discontinuation of nitrous oxide. The injected sulfur hexafluoride bubble, in the presence of concomitant administration of nitrous oxide, can cause a rapid and dramatic rise in IOP, reaching a peak within 20 minutes[50,51] (see Intraocular Sulfur Hexafluoride section). Because the resultant rise in IOP may compromise retinal circulation, Stinson and Donlon[50] recommended cessation of nitrous oxide administration 15 minutes before gas injection to prevent significant changes in the volume of the intravitreous gas bubble. Furthermore, Wolf et al.[51] stated that if a patient requires anesthesia after intravitreous gas injection, nitrous oxide should be omitted for 5 days after an air injection and for 10 days after sulfur hexafluoride injection. Perfluoropropane, moreover, remains in the eye longer than 30 days.

Alternatively, silicone oil, a vitreous substitute, may be injected to achieve internal tamponade of a retinal break.

Retinal detachment operations are basically extraocular but may briefly become intraocular if the surgeon elects to perforate and drain subretinal fluid. Furthermore, rotation of the globe with traction on the extraocular muscles may elicit the oculocardiac reflex so the anesthesiologist must be vigilant about potential cardiac dysrhythmias. In addition, because it is desirable to have a soft eye while the sclera is being buckled, intravenous administration of acetazolamide or mannitol is common during retinal surgery to lower IOP.

These patients are usually managed in the same manner as those having intraocular surgery, except that maintenance of intraoperative skeletal muscle paralysis is not as critical as during intraocular surgery. Hence, inhalational anesthetics need not be accompanied during surgery by nondepolarizing neuromuscular blocking drugs.

POSTOPERATIVE OCULAR COMPLICATIONS

The incidence of eye injuries associated with nonocular surgery is low. In a study by Roth and colleagues[110] of 60,965 patients undergoing nonocular surgery from 1988 to 1992, the incidence of eye injury was 0.056% (34 patients). Twenty-one of these 34 patients sustained corneal abrasion, although other injuries included conjunctivitis, blurry vision, red eye, chemical injury, direct ocular trauma, and blindness. Independent risk factors for greater relative risk of ocular injury were protracted surgical procedures, lateral intraoperative positioning, head or neck surgery, general anesthesia, and (for some unknown reason) surgery on a Monday. A specific mechanism of injury could be identified in only 21% of cases. In the ASA Closed Claims Study published in 1992 (which analyzed only cases involving litigation), eye injuries represented merely 3% of all claims, but the serious nature of some of the injuries were reflected in large financial awards.[111] Similar to the findings of Roth et al., in the Closed Claims Study the specific mechanism of injury could be ascertained in only a minority of cases. A more recent Closed Claims Study published in 2004 examining injuries associated with regional anesthesia reported that the proportion of regional anesthesia claims linked to eye blocks increased from 2% in the 1980s to 7% in the 1990s.[112] These injuries were typically permanent and related to the block technique. More than half of the claims resulted in blindness. Almost all these claims involved retrobulbar or peribulbar block performed by anesthesiologists. Topical anesthesia for cataract removal is becoming more common and may result in a reduced prevalence of these complications.

Although infrequent and often transient, eye injuries can result occasionally in blindness or more limited, but nonetheless permanent, visual impairment. Postoperative complications after nonocular surgery include corneal abrasion and minor visual disturbances, chemical injuries, thermal or photic injury, and serious visual disturbances, including blindness. Serious injury may result from such diverse conditions as acute corneal epithelial edema, glycine toxicity and other visual disturbances associated with transurethral resection of the prostate, retinal ischemia, ischemic optic neuropathy, cortical blindness, and acute glaucoma. It appears that certain types of surgery, including complex spinal surgery in the prone position; operations involving extracorporeal circulation; and neck, nasal, or sinus surgery may increase the risk of serious postoperative visual complications.

Corneal Abrasion

Although the most common ocular complication of general anesthesia is corneal abrasion,[113] the incidence varies widely, depending on the perioperative circumstances. In a prospective study, Cucchiara et al.[114] found a 0.17% incidence of corneal abrasion in 4,652 neurosurgical patients whose eyes were protected, whereas Batra and Bali[113] one decade earlier reported a 44% incidence of corneal abrasion when eyes were left unprotected and partly open. A variety of mechanisms can result in corneal abrasion, including damage caused by the anesthetic mask, surgical drapes, and spillage of solutions. During intubation of the trachea, moreover, the end of plastic watch bands or hospital ID cards clipped to the laryngoscopist's vest pocket can injure the cornea. Ocular injury may also occur due to loss of pain sensation, obtundation of protective corneal reflexes, and decreased tear production during anesthesia. Therefore, it may be prudent to tape the eyelids closed immediately after induction, and during mask ventilation and laryngoscopy. In addition to taping the eyelids closed, applying protective goggles, and instilling petroleum-based ointments into the conjunctival sac may provide protection. Disadvantages of ointments include occasional allergic reactions; flammability, which may make their use undesirable during surgery around the face and contraindicated during laser surgery; and blurred vision in the early postoperative period. The blurring and foreign-body sensation associated with ointments may actually increase the incidence of postoperative corneal abrasions if they trigger excessive rubbing of the eyes while the patient is still emerging from anesthesia. Moreover, halothane absorption into paraffin-based ointments can damage the cornea, and even water-based (methylcellulose) ointments may be irritating and cause scleral erythema. It would seem prudent, therefore, to close the eyelids with tape during general anesthesia for procedures away from the head and neck. For certain procedures on the face, ocular occluders or tarsorrhaphy may be indicated. Special attention should also be devoted to frequent checking of the eyes during procedures on a prone patient.

Patients with corneal abrasion usually complain of a foreign-body sensation, pain, tearing, and photophobia. The pain is typically exacerbated by blinking and ocular movement. It is wise to have an ophthalmologic consultation immediately. Treatment typically consists of the prophylactic application of antibiotic ointment and patching the injured eye shut. Although permanent sequelae are possible, healing usually occurs within 24 hours.

Chemical Injury

Spillage of solutions during skin preparation may result in chemical damage to the eye. The FDA reported serious corneal damage from eye contact with Hibiclens, a 4% chlorhexidine gluconate solution formulated with a detergent. Again, with meticulous attention to detail, this misadventure is preventable. Treatment consists of liberal bathing of the eye with balanced salt solution to remove the offending agent. After surgery, it may be desirable to have an ophthalmologist examine the eye to document any residual injury or lack thereof.

Photic Injury

Direct or reflected light beams may permanently damage the eye. The potential for serious injury to the cornea or retina from certain laser beams requires that the patient's eyes be protected with moist gauze pads and metal shields, and that operating room personnel wear protective glasses. These goggles must be appropriately tinted for the specific wavelength they are intended to block. Clear goggles may be worn when working with the carbon dioxide laser, whereas for work with the argon, Nd-YAG, or Nd-YAG-KTP laser, the goggles must be tinted orange, green, and orange-red, respectively.

Mild Visual Symptoms

After anesthesia, transient, mild visual disturbances such as photophobia or diplopia are common. Blurred vision in the early postoperative period may reflect residual effects of petroleum-based ophthalmic ointments or ocular effects of anticholinergic drugs administered in the perioperative period (see Corneal Abrasion section).

In contrast, the complaint of postoperative visual loss is rare and is cause for alarm. Several of the following conditions may be associated with visual loss after anesthesia and surgery, and should be included in the differential diagnosis: hemorrhagic retinopathy, retinal ischemia, retinal artery occlusion, ischemic optic neuropathy, cortical blindness, and acute glaucoma.

Hemorrhagic Retinopathy

Retinal hemorrhages that occur in otherwise healthy people secondary to hemodynamic changes associated with turbulent emergence from anesthesia or protracted vomiting are termed Valsalva retinopathy. Fortunately, these venous hemorrhages are usually self-limiting and resolve completely in a few days to a few months.

Because no visual changes occur unless the macula is involved, most cases are asymptomatic. However, if bleeding into the optic nerve occurs, resulting in optic atrophy, or if the hemorrhage is massive, permanent visual impairment may ensue. In some instances of massive hemorrhage, vitrectomy may offer some improvement.

Retinal venous hemorrhage has also been described after injections of local anesthetics, steroids, or saline into the lumbar epidural space, and these cases have been summarized by Purdy and Ajimal.[115] The patients all received large injections ($\geq$40 mL) into the epidural space, and they subsequently developed blurry vision or headaches. On funduscopic examination, retinal hemorrhage was consistently observed. Eight of the nine patients described had complete recovery. It is believed that the hemorrhage is produced by rapid epidural injection, which causes a sudden increase in intracranial pressure. This increase in cerebrospinal fluid pressure causes an increase of retinal venous pressure, which may cause retinal hemorrhages. It is possible that obesity, hypertension, coagulopathies, preexisting elevated cerebrospinal fluid pressure (as seen in pseudotumor cerebri), and such retinal vascular diseases as diabetic retinopathy may be risk factors. Caution is recommended when injecting drugs or fluid into the epidural space; a slow injection rate and using the minimal volume necessary to accomplish the desired objective are strongly recommended.

Retinal Ischemia

Retinal bleeding may also originate from the arterial circulation. This bleeding may be associated with extraocular trauma. Funduscopic examination shows cotton-wool exudates, and this condition is known as Purtscher's retinopathy. Purtscher's retinopathy should be ruled out when a trauma patient complains of postanesthetic visual loss. This condition is associated with a poor prognosis, and most patients sustain permanent visual impairment.

Retinal ischemia or infarction may also result from direct ocular trauma secondary to external pressure exerted by an ill-fitting anesthetic mask, especially in a hypotensive setting, and from embolism during cardiac surgery, or from the intraocular injection of a large volume of sulfur hexafluoride in the presence of high concentrations of nitrous oxide. It may also result from increased ocular venous pressure associated with impaired venous drainage or elevated IOP.

The importance of carefully positioning patients and scrupulously monitoring external pressure on the eye cannot be overemphasized, especially when the patient is in the prone or jackknife positions. When the head is dependently positioned, venous pressure may be elevated. If external pressure is applied to the globe from improper head support, perfusion pressure to the eye is likely to be reduced. An episode of systemic hypotension in this setting could further decrease perfusion pressure and thereby decrease intraocular blood flow, resulting in possible retinal ischemia.

It is imperative that for procedures in the prone position, a padded or foam headrest be used. The patient's eyes must be in the opening of this headrest and they must be checked at frequent intervals for pressure. If the patient's head is too large to fit properly into the headrest, then a pin head-holder should be used. During some spine procedures, a steep head-down position may be used to decrease venous bleeding and enhance surgical exposure. This position, in combination with deliberate hypotension and infusion of large quantities of crystalloid, may increase the risk of compromising the ocular circulation.

It seems prudent to avoid combining these three risk factors to any significant degree.

Central retinal arterial occlusion and branch retinal arterial occlusion are important, and frequently preventable, causes of postoperative visual loss. Cases have occurred following spinal, nasal, sinus, or neck surgery, as well as after coronary artery bypass graft (CABG) surgery. In addition to external pressure on the eye, causes can include emboli from carotid plaques or other sources, as well as vasospasm or thrombosis after radical neck surgery complicated by hemorrhage and hypotension, and after intranasal injection of α-adrenergic agonists. Several cases have followed intra-arterial injections of corticosteroids or local anesthetics in branches of the external carotid artery, with possible retrograde embolization to the ocular blood supply.[116] Mabry[117] suggested that, to produce retrograde flow into the branches of the ophthalmic artery, the needle must be positioned intra-arterially, and the perfusion pressure must be overcome during the injection. Therefore, when injecting in the nasal and sinus areas, topical vasoconstrictors should be applied to decrease the size of the vascular bed, and a small (25-gauge) needle on a low-volume syringe should be used to minimize injection pressure. Moreover, because some cases have followed injections of corticosteroids combined with other drugs, it is believed that this practice may predispose to formation of drug crystals and should therefore be discouraged.

In cases of central retinal arterial occlusion, funduscopic examination discloses a pale, edematous retina and a cherry-red spot. Platelet-fibrin, cholesterol, calcific, or crystalloid emboli may be found in narrowed retinal arterioles. Computed tomography (CT) and MRI studies are negative.

Prevention is much more successful than treatment. It may be possible to apply ocular massage (contraindicated if glaucoma is a possibility) to dislodge an embolus to more peripheral sites, and intravenous acetazolamide and 5% carbon dioxide inhalation have been used to increase retinal blood flow. The prognosis, however, is typically poor, and approximately 50% of patients with central retinal arterial occlusion eventually have optic atrophy.

Ischemic Optic Neuropathy

Ischemic optic neuropathy (ION) in the nonsurgical setting is the most common cause of *sudden* visual loss in patients older than 50 years of age, and it may be either arteritic or nonarteritic. Our discussion is limited to postoperative ION and contrasts the similarities and differences between anterior ischemic optic neuropathy (AION) and posterior ischemic optic neuropathy (PION). Due to a perceived increase in the incidence of postoperative visual loss since the mid-1990s, the Committee on Professional Liability of the ASA established the Postoperative Visual Loss Database on July 1, 1999, to better identify associated risk factors so these tragic complications might be prevented in the future.[118] Because the incidence of postoperative vision loss after spine surgery in the prone position may be as high as 1%, it would seem prudent to discuss this potential complication preoperatively with the patient during the informed consent process.

Anterior Ischemic Optic Neuropathy

Although the multifactorial pathophysiology of AION has not been completely established, it is believed to involve temporary hypoperfusion or nonperfusion of the vessels supplying the anterior portion of the optic nerve, although intra-axonal edema and disturbed autoregulation to the optic nerve head may also play a role.[116] Coexisting systemic disease, especially involving the cardiovascular system and (to a lesser extent) the endocrine system, is common in patients in whom AION develops. Male gender also strongly predominates. Other risk factors for postoperative AION include CABG and other thoracovascular operations, as well as spinal surgery. Although massive bleeding, anemia, and hypotension are commonly described intraoperative risk factors, a retrospective survey of surgeons who perform spinal fusion surgery disclosed that hypotension and anemia were equally prevalent in patients in whom ION developed and in those in whom it did not.[119] Other possible risk factors are increased IOP or orbital venous pressure. Although emboli may also play a role, AION is not usually caused by emboli because emboli preferentially lodge in the central retinal artery rather than in the short posterior ciliary arteries that supply the anterior optic nerve.

Increased IOP caused by extrinsic compression of the eye decreases retinal blood flow that can produce both retinal and optic nerve injury. Moreover, increased IOP can result from large infusions of crystalloid when the head is steeply dependent, as during many spinal operations.[120] Increased orbital venous pressure results in a decreased perfusion pressure gradient to the optic nerve head. Interestingly, one patient who had ION despite perioperative normotension had marked facial edema after surgery of protracted duration.[120] Similarly, a study in cardiac surgery patients revealed that increases in IOP correlated with the degree of hemodilution and the use of crystalloid priming solution.[121] Patients with AION were more likely to have significant weight gain within 24 hours of open heart surgery, again suggesting the role of elevated ocular venous pressure in impeding blood flow to the optic nerve.

According to Roth and Gillesberg,[116] a complex interaction of factors such as ocular venous pressure, hemodilution, hypotension, release of endogenous vasoconstrictors, and individual risk factors such as atherosclerosis and aberrant optic nerve circulation may be implicated in the development of AION. Therefore, specific recommendations for preventative strategies are elusive. Clearly, however, external pressure on the eyes must be meticulously avoided. It also seems prudent to minimize time in the prone position when the head is notably dependent. In patients with preexisting cardiovascular disease, significant hypertension, or glaucoma, it seems advisable to maintain systemic blood pressure as close to baseline as possible.[116] Recommendations about specific hematocrit levels are difficult to make at this time and should be individualized based on a constellation of circumstances, but it seems prudent to have a different "transfusion threshold" in high-risk patients.

Patients with AION typically have painless visual loss that may not be noted until the first postoperative day (or possibly later), an afferent pupillary defect, altitudinal field defects, and optic disc edema or pallor. MRI or CT initially show enlargement of the optic nerve. However, optic atrophy is detected by MRI later.

The prognosis for AION varies but is often grim. Although there is no recognized treatment for AION, Williams et al.[122] reviewed the various therapies that may be instituted. These include intravenous acetazolamide, furosemide, mannitol, and steroids. Maintaining the head-up position could be helpful if increased ocular venous pressure is operative. Surgical optic nerve sheath fenestration or decompression is not only ineffective, but may actually be harmful.[123]

Posterior Ischemic Optic Neuropathy

The posterior optic nerve has a less luxuriant blood supply than the anterior optic nerve. In contrast to AION, relatively few cases have been reported after CABG, and PION appears to be less related to coexisting cardiovascular disease. As with AION, male patients outnumber female patients four to one. Many cases have been associated with surgery involving the neck, nose, sinuses, or spine. In approximately one-third of cases reported, facial edema has been noted.[116] Approximately 11% of cases were associated with cardiopulmonary bypass procedures.

PION is produced by reduced oxygen delivery to the retrolaminar part of the optic nerve. Most likely, compression of the pial vessels (supplied by small collaterals from the ophthalmic artery) or embolic phenomena produce ischemia. However, severe systemic hypotension, anemia, or venous stasis may also be contributory.[116]

A hypoxic insult in this region results in a slower development of ischemic damage so a symptom-free period often precedes the loss of vision. In some patients, the onset of symptoms may be delayed several days. Typical findings include an afferent pupillary defect or nonreactive pupil. Disc edema is not a feature of PION because of its retroorbital position. CT scan in the early postoperative period may reveal enlargement of the intraorbital portion of the optic nerve. Bilateral blindness is more common with PION than AION, possibly indicating involvement of the optic chiasm. Concomitant disease of the eye or ocular blood supply may be related to PION.[116] Some cases may show partial improvement spontaneously, but often no improvement is noted. Steroids may be considered for treatment. Preventative strategies are as outlined for AION.

Cortical Blindness

Brain injury rostral to the optic nerve may cause cortical blindness. The impairment is produced by damage to the visual path beyond the lateral geniculate nucleus or the visual cortex in the occipital lobe. Similar to AION, cortical blindness is a significant concern in patients undergoing CABG, and systemic disease is often present. Emboli and sustained, profound hypotension are common causes. Other events implicated in the pathophysiology include cardiac arrest, hypoxemia, intracranial hypertension, exsanguinating hemorrhage, vascular occlusion, thrombosis, and vasospasm.

Differential diagnostic features include a normal optic disc on fundoscopy and normal pupillary responses. There is, however, loss of optokinetic nystagmus with normal eye motility. CT and MRI are helpful in delineating the extent of brain infarction associated with cortical blindness. Occipital lesions are frequently bilateral and CT findings typically indicate posterior cerebral artery thrombosis, basilar artery occlusion, posterior cerebral artery branch occlusion, or watershed infarction. Lesions after CABG often include the parietooccipital area.

Whereas most cases of ION do not improve significantly or completely, visual recovery from cortical blindness in previously healthy patients may be considerable but prolonged. Preventive strategies include maintenance of adequate systemic perfusion pressure and, in cardiac surgery, minimizing manipulation of the aorta, meticulous removal of air and particulate matter during valvular procedures, and use of an arterial line filter in selected patients during bypass.

Visual Symptoms After Transurethral Resection of the Prostate

Visual disturbances associated with transurethral resection of the prostate (TURP) are transient and often the result of the TURP syndrome, wherein excessive absorption of irrigating fluid can produce cardiac failure, hyponatremia, serious dysrhythmias, seizures, and coma. Visual disturbances can extend the gamut from subtle changes, such as seeing halos or a bluish hue, to complete absence of light perception.

Liberal bladder irrigation is required during TURP to remove clots and other detritus to enhance visibility for the surgeon. Factors postulated to influence the volume of irrigant absorbed include the extent of opening of the prostatic venous sinuses, the hydrostatic pressure of the irrigation fluid, the venous pressure at the irrigant–blood interface, and, arguably, the duration of the resection.

Glycine 1.5%, although slightly hypoosmolar, does not cause clinically significant hemolysis and is one of the most commonly used irrigating solutions. Glycine toxicity is probably the most important mechanism resulting in TURP-associated visual dysfunction, although the disturbance may be multifactorial. An inhibitory neurotransmitter in the CNS, glycine freely crosses the blood–brain barrier and depresses the spontaneous and evoked activity of retinal neurons. In addition, glycine is metabolized to serine and ammonia, both of which have been linked to CNS disturbances after TURP. Serine is known to have inhibitory effects on the retina similar to those produced by glycine.

Hyponatremia can occur independently of glycine toxicity and produce hypoosmolality-induced CNS dysfunction. The degree of brain dysfunction is determined by the rapidity and the severity of the reduction in sodium concentration. Symptoms include hallucinations, psychosis, focal neurologic signs, seizures, and coma. It has been suggested that TURP-associated hypoosmolality produces occipital cortical edema, but this has not been definitively established.

Preventive strategy should focus on taking all possible measures to avoid excessive absorption of irrigating solution. Moreover, a high index of suspicion is necessary because significant amounts of irrigant may be absorbed even if the surgeon does not see any open venous sinuses. Thus, it is difficult, if not impossible, to estimate the degree of fluid absorption without confirmatory laboratory data.

Acute Glaucoma

Although topical application of such mydriatic drugs as atropine and scopolamine is contraindicated in patients with known, chronic glaucoma, the systemic use of anticholinergics in usual premedicating doses is safe for glaucomatous eyes. The use of an atropine–neostigmine combination for reversal of neuromuscular blockade is also safe in patients with glaucoma. Topical ophthalmic medications that are being administered to control glaucoma should be continued through the perioperative period.

Acute angle-closure glaucoma typically occurs spontaneously but has been reported, albeit rarely, after both spinal and general anesthesia. Acute angle-closure glaucoma caused by pupillary block is a serious, multifactorial disease. Risk factors include genetic predisposition, shallow anterior chamber depth, increased lens thickness, small corneal diameter, female gender, and advanced age. One study[124] explored possible precipitating events in at-risk patients and found no evidence that the type of anesthetic agent, the duration of surgery, the volume of parenteral fluids, or the intraoperative blood pressure were related to the development of acute angle-closure glaucoma.

Despite its seriousness, acute angle-closure glaucoma may be difficult to recognize. However, physicians should be knowledgeable about this potential complication because diagnostic delay may detrimentally affect visual outcome and cause permanent optic nerve damage. Fazio et al.[125] recommended that the preoperative evaluation include a thorough ocular history and a penlight examination to detect a shallow anterior chamber. Those patients considered at risk should then undergo a preoperative ophthalmic evaluation and perioperative miotic therapy. After surgery, these patients should be scrupulously watched for red eye or a fixed dilated pupil, as well as for complaints of pain and blurred vision. Acute glaucoma is a true emergency, and ophthalmologic consultation should be secured immediately to acutely decrease IOP with systemic and topical therapy. The intense periorbital pain typically described by these patients is an important aid in differential diagnosis.

Postcataract Ptosis

Ptosis after cataract surgery is not uncommon, and multiple factors have been implicated in its etiology.[126,127] These include the presence of a preexisting ptosis, injection of anesthetic solution into the upper lid when performing facial nerve block, retrobulbar injection, injection of peribulbar anesthesia through the upper eyelid at the 12 o'clock position, ocular compression or massage, the eyelid speculum, placement of a superior rectus bridle suture with traction on the superior rectus–levator complex, creation of a large conjunctival flap, prolonged or tight patching in the postoperative period, and postoperative eyelid edema. Feibel and colleagues[126] believed that the development of postcataract ptosis is multifactorial and that no single aspect of cataract surgery is the sole contributor. More recently, Taylor et al. used MRI immediately after diagnosis of diplopia in four patients who received peribulbar block.[127] They found peribulbar edema consistent with direct local anesthetic-induced myotoxicity after presumed inadvertent intramuscular injection. Although local anesthetics are clearly myotoxic, the local anesthetic injection cannot be isolated as the primary factor because postsurgical ptosis is also seen in patients undergoing surgery with general anesthesia.

References

1. Eye Diseases Prevalence Research Group: Prevalence of age-related macular degeneration in the United States. Arch Ophthalmol 122:564, 2004
2. Hebert LE, Scherr PA, Bienias JL *et al*: Alzheimer disease in the US population: Prevalence estimates using the 2000 Census. Arch Neurol 60:119, 2003
3. Wimo A, Winblad B: Health economical aspects of Alzheimer disease and its treatment. Psychogeriatrics 1:189, 2001
4. Bruce RA: Ocular anatomy. In Bruce RA, McGoldrick KE, Oppenheimer P (eds): Anesthesia for Ophthalmology, p 3. Birmingham, AL, Aesculapius, 1982
5. Stoelting RK: Circulatory changes during direct laryngoscopy and tracheal intubation: Influence of duration of laryngoscopy with or without prior lidocaine. Anesthesiology 47:381, 1977
6. Duncalf D, Foldes FF: Effect of anesthetic drugs and muscle relaxants on intraocular pressure. In Smith RB (ed): Anesthesia in Ophthalmology, p 21. Boston, Little, Brown, 1973
7. Garde JF, Aston R, Endler GC *et al*: Racial mydriatic response to belladonna preparations. Anesth Analg 57:572, 1978
8. Watcha MF, Chu FC, Stevens JL *et al*: Effects of halothane on intraocular pressure in anesthetized children. Anesth Analg 71:181, 1990
9. Thompson MF, Brock-Utne JG, Bean P *et al*: Anaesthesia and intraocular pressure: A comparison of total intravenous anaesthesia using etomidate with conventional inhalational anaesthesia. Anaesthesia 37:758, 1982
10. Yoshikawa K, Murai Y: Effect of ketamine on intraocular pressure in children. Anesth Analg 50:199, 1971
11. Corssen G, Hoy JE: A new parenteral anesthetic—CI581: Its effect on intraocular pressure. J Pediatr Ophthalmol 4:20, 1967
12. Peuler M, Glass DD, Arens JF: Ketamine and intraocular pressure. Anesthesiology 43:575, 1975
13. Ausinsch B, Rayburn RL, Munson ES *et al*: Ketamine and intraocular pressure in children. Anesth Analg 55:773, 1976
14. Ausinsch B, Graves SA, Munson ES *et al*: Intraocular pressure in children during isoflurane and halothane anesthesia. Anesthesiology 42:167, 1975
15. Duncalf D, Weitzner SW: Ventilation and hypercapnia on intraocular pressure in children. Anesth Analg 43:232, 1963
16. Litwiller RW, Difazio CA, Rushia EL: Pancuronium and intraocular pressure. Anesthesiology 42:750, 1975
17. Lincoff HA, Ellis CH, DeVoe AG *et al*: Effect of succinylcholine on intraocular pressure. Am J Ophthalmol 40:501, 1955
18. Pandey K, Badolas RP, Kumar S: Time course of intraocular hypertension produced by suxamethonium. Br J Anaesth 44:191, 1972
19. Kelly RE, Dinner M, Turner LS *et al*: Succinylcholine increases intraocular pressure in the human eye with the extraocular muscles detached. Anesthesiology 79:948, 1993
20. Miller RD, Way WL, Hickey RF: Inhibition of succinylcholine-induced increased intraocular pressure by nondepolarizing muscle relaxants. Anesthesiology 29:123, 1968
21. Meyers EF, Krupin T, Johnson M *et al*: Failure of nondepolarizing neuromuscular blockers to inhibit succinylcholine-induced increased intraocular pressure: A controlled study. Anesthesiology 48:149, 1978
22. Verma RS: "Self-taming" of succinylcholine-induced fasciculations and intraocular pressure. Anesthesiology 50:245, 1979
23. Meyers EF, Singer P, Otto A: A controlled study of the effect of succinylcholine self-taming on IOP. Anesthesiology 53:72, 1980
24. Stoelting RK: Blood pressure and heart rate changes during short duration laryngoscopy for tracheal intubation: Influences of viscous or intravenous lidocaine. Anesth Analg 57:197, 1978
25. Smith RB, Babinski M, Leano N: Effect of lidocaine on succinylcholine-induced rise in IOP. Can Anaesth Soc J 26:482, 1979
26. Grover VK, Lata K, Sharma S *et al*: Efficacy of lignocaine in the suppression of the intraocular pressure response to suxamethonium and tracheal intubation. Anaesthesia 44:22, 1989
27. Jampolsky A: Strabismus: Surgical overcorrections. Highlights Ophthalmol 8:78, 1965
28. France NK, France TD, Woodburn JD *et al*: Succinylcholine alteration of the forced duction test. Ophthalmology 87:1282, 1980
29. Berler DK: Oculocardiac reflex. Am J Ophthalmol 12(56):954, 1963
30. Alexander JP: Reflex disturbances of cardiac rhythm during ophthalmic surgery. Br J Ophthalmol 59:518, 1975
31. Mirakur RK, Clarke RSJ, Dundee JW *et al*: Anticholinergic drugs in anaesthesia: A survey of their present position. Anaesthesia 33:133, 1978
32. Massumi RA, Mason DT, Amsterdam EA *et al*: Ventricular fibrillation and tachycardia after intravenous atropine for treatment of bradycardias. N Engl J Med 287:336, 1972
33. McGoldrick KE: Transient left bundle branch block during local anesthesia. Anesthesiol Rev 8(6):36, 1981
34. Moonie GT, Rees DI, Elton D: Oculocardiac reflex during strabismus surgery. Can Anaesth Soc J 11:621, 1964
35. Steward DJ: Anticholinergic premedication for infants and children. Can Anaesth Soc J 30:325, 1983
36. Nachman RL, Esterly NB: Increased skin permeability in preterm infants. J Pediatr 79:628, 1971
37. Ellis EP, Esterdahl M: Echothiophate iodide therapy in children: Effect upon blood cholinesterase levels. Arch Ophthalmol 77:598, 1967
38. Koehntop DE, Liao J, Van Bergen FH: Effects of pharmacologic alterations of adrenergic mechanisms by cocaine, tropolone, aminophylline, and ketamine on epinephrine-induced arrhythmias during halothane–N_2O anesthesia. Anesthesiology 46:83, 1977
39. Barash PG, Kopriva CJ, Langou R *et al*: Is cocaine a sympathetic stimulant during general anesthesia? JAMA 243:1437, 1980
40. Meyers EF: Cocaine toxicity during dacryocystorhinostomy. Arch Ophthalmol 98:842, 1980
41. Gay GR, Loper KA: Control of cocaine-induced hypertension with labetalol (letter). Anesth Analg 67:92, 1988
42. Rappolt RT, Gay GR, Inaba DS: Propranolol: A specific antagonist to cocaine. Clin Toxicol 10:265, 1977
43. Ramoska E, Sacchetti AD: Propranolol-induced hypertension in treatment of cocaine intoxication. Ann Emerg Med 14:1112, 1985
44. Lansche RK: Systemic effects of topical epinephrine and phenylephrine. Am J Ophthalmol 49:95, 1966
45. Brown MM, Brown GC, Spaeth GL: Lack of side effects from topically administered 10% phenylephrine eye drops: A controlled study. Arch Ophthalmol 98:487, 1980
46. Jones FL, Eckberg NL: Exacerbation of asthma by timolol. N Engl J Med 301:170, 1979
47. Kim JW, Smith PH: Timolol-induced bradycardia. Anesth Analg 59:301, 1980
48. Shavitz SA: Timolol and myasthenia gravis. JAMA 242:1612, 1979
49. Bailey PL: Timolol and postoperative apnea in neonates and young infants. Anesthesiology 61:622, 1984
50. Stinson TW, Donlon JV: Interaction of SF6 and air with nitrous oxide. Anesthesiology 51:S16, 1979
51. Wolf GL, Capriano C, Hartung J: Effects of nitrous oxide on gas bubble volume in the anterior chamber. Arch Ophthalmol 103:418, 1985
52. Chang S, Lincoff HA, Coleman DJ *et al*: Perfluorocarbon gases in vitreous surgery. Ophthalmology 92:651, 1985
53. Schein OD, Katz J, Bass EB *et al*: The value of routine preoperative medical testing before cataract surgery. N Engl J Med 342:168, 2000
54. Hall DL, Steen WH, Drummond JW *et al*: Anticoagulants and cataract surgery. Ophthalmic Surg 19:221, 1988
55. Robinson GA, Nylander A: Warfarin and cataract extraction. Br J Ophthalmol 73:702, 1989
56. Feitl ME, Krupin T: Retrobulbar anesthesia. Ophthalmol Clin North Am 3:83, 1990
57. Katz J, Feldman MA, Bass EB *et al*: Risks and benefits of anticoagulant and antiplatelet medication use before cataract surgery. Ophthalmology 110:1784, 2003

58. McGoldrick KE: Ocular pathology and systemic diseases: Anesthetic implications. In McGoldrick KE (ed): Anesthesia for Ophthalmic and Otolaryngologic Surgery, p 210. Philadelphia, WB Saunders, 1992
59. Leaming DV: Practice styles and preferences of ASCRS members: 2002 survey. J Cataract Refract Surg 29:1421, 2003
60. Guise PA: Sub-Tenon anesthesia: A prospective study of 6000 blocks. Anesthesiology 98:964, 2003
61. Gayer S, Flynn HW Jr: Sub-Tenon's injection for local anesthesia in posterior segment surgery (discussion). Ophthalmology 107:46, 2000
62. Wainwright AC: Positive pressure ventilation and the laryngeal mask airway in ophthalmic anaesthesia. Br J Anaesth 75:249, 1995
63. Lamb K, James MFM, Janicki PK: The laryngeal mask airway for intraocular surgery: Effects on intraocular pressure and stress responses. Br J Anaesth 69:143, 1992
64. Thomson KD: The effect of the laryngeal mask airway on coughing after eye surgery under general anesthesia. Ophthalmic Surg 23:630, 1992
65. Knapp H: On cocaine and its use in ophthalmic and general surgery. Arch Ophthalmol 13:402, 1884
66. Atkinson WS: Retrobulbar injection of anesthetic within the muscular cone. Arch Ophthalmol 16:494, 1936
67. Korneef L: The architecture of the musculofibrous apparatus in the human orbit. Acta Morphol Neerl Scand 15:35, 1977
68. Ripart J, Lefrant J, de la Coussaye J *et al*: Peribulbar versus retrobulbar anesthesia for ophthalmic surgery. Anesthesiology 94:56, 2001
69. Capó H, Roth E, Johnson T *et al*: Vertical strabismus after cataract surgery. Ophthalmology 103:918, 1996
70. Ripart J, Lefrant J, Lalourcey L *et al*: Medial canthus (caruncle) single injection periocular anesthesia. Anesth Analg 83:1234, 1996
71. Katsev DA, Drews RC, Rose BT: An anatomic study of retrobulbar needle path length. Ophthalmology 96:1221, 1989
72. Waller SG, Taboada J, O'Connor P: Retrobulbar anesthesia risk: Do sharp needles really perforate the eye more easily than blunt needles? Ophthalmology 100:506, 1993
73. Unsold R, Stanley JA, DeGroot J: The CT topography of retrobulbar anesthesia. Graefes Arch Clin Exp Ophthalmol 217:125, 1981
74. Liu C, Youl B, Moseley I: Magnetic resonance imaging of the optic nerve in extremes of gaze. Implications for the positioning of the globe for retrobulbar anesthesia. Br J Ophthalmol 76:728, 1992
75. Birch A, Evans M, Redembo E: The ultrasonic localiazation of retrobulbar needles during retrobulbar block. Ophthalmology 102:824, 1995
76. Grizzard WS, Kirk NM, Pavan PR *et al*: Perforating ocular injuries caused by anesthesia personnel. Ophthalmology 98:1011, 1991
77. Miller-Meeks MJ, Bergstrom T, Karp KO: Prevalent attitudes regarding residency training in ocular anesthesia. Ophthalmology 101:1353, 1994
78. Nicoll JMV, Acharya PA, Ahlen K *et al*: Central nervous system complications after 6000 retrobulbar blocks. Anesth Analg 66:1298, 1987
79. Chang J-L, Gonzalez-Abola E, Larson CE: Brain stem anesthesia following retrobulbar block. Anesthesiology 61:789, 1984
80. Swan KC: New drugs and techniques for ocular anesthesia. Trans Am Acad Ophthalmol Otolaryngol 60:368, 1956
81. Niemi-Murola L, Krootila K, Kivisaari R *et al*: Localization of local anesthetic solution by magnetic resonance imaging. Ophthalmology 111:342, 2004
82. Guise PA: Sub-Tenon anesthesia: A prospective study of 6,000 blocks. Anesthesiology 98:964, 2003
83. Frieman BJ, Friedberg MA: Globe perforation associated with subtenon's anesthesia. J Ophthalmol 131:520, 2001
84. Ruschen H, Bremner FD, Carr C: Complications after sub-Tenon's eye block. Anesth Analg 96:273, 2003
85. Ripart J, Metge L, Prat-Pradal D *et al*: Medial canthus single-injection episcleral (sub-Tenon) anesthesia: Computed tomography imaging. Anesth Analg 87:42, 1998
86. Bardocci A, Lofoco G, Perdicaro *et al*: Lidocaine 2% gel versus lidocaine 4% unpreserved drops for topical anesthesia in cataract surgery: A randomized controlled trial. Ophthalmology 110:144, 2003
87. Eggeling P, Pleyer U, Hartman C *et al*: Corneal endothelial toxicity of different lidocaine concentrations. J Cataract Refract Surg 26:1403, 2000
88. Netland PA, Harris A: Color Doppler ultrasound measurements after topical and retrobulbar epinephrine in primate eyes. Invest Ophthalmol Vis Sci 38:2655, 1997
89. Brown SM, Coats DK, Collins MLZ *et al*: Second cluster of strabismus cases after periocular anesthesia without hyaluronidase. J Cataract Refract Surg 27:1876, 2001
90. Kirsch RE: Further studies on the use of digital pressure in cataract surgery. Optimal length of time for application of digital pressure. Arch Ophthalmol 58:641, 1957
91. Jay WM, Aziz MZ, Green K: Effect of intraocular pressure reducer on ocular and optic nerve blood flow in phakic rabbit eyes. Acta Ophthalmologica 64:52, 1986
92. Norregaard JC, Schein OD, Bellan L *et al*: International variation in anesthesia care during cataract surgery: Results from the International Cataract Surgery Outcomes Study. Arch Ophthalmol 115:1304, 1997
93. Rosenfeld SI, Litinsky SM, Snyder DA *et al*: Effectiveness of monitored anesthesia care in cataract surgery. Ophthalmology 106:1256, 1999
94. Scott IU, McCabe CM, Flynn HW Jr, Gayer S *et al*: Local anesthesia with intravenous sedation for surgical repair of selected open globe injuries. Am J Ophthalmol 134:707, 2002
95. Boscia F, La Tegola MG, Columbo G *et al*: Combined topical anesthesia and sedation for open-globe injuries in selected patients. Ophthalmology 110:1555, 2003
96. Casson WR, Jones RM: Vecuronium induced neuromuscular blockade. Anaesthesia 41:354, 1986
97. Ginsberg B, Glass PS, Quill T *et al*: Onset and duration of neuromuscular blockade following high-dose vecuronium administration. Anesthesiology 71:201, 1989
98. Konchiergeri HN, Lee YE, Venugopal K: Effect of pancuronium on intraocular pressure changes induced by succinylcholine. Can Anaesth Soc J 26:479, 1979
99. Libonati MM, Leahy JJ, Ellison N: The use of succinylcholine in open eye surgery. Anesthesiology 62:637, 1985
100. McGoldrick KE: The open globe: Is an alternative to succinylcholine necessary? (editorial). J Clin Anesth 5:1, 1993
101. Foldes FF: Rapid tracheal intubation with nondepolarizing neuromuscular blocking drugs: The priming principle. Br J Anaesth 56:663, 1984
102. Musich J, Walts LF: Pulmonary aspiration after a priming dose of vecuronium. Anesthesiology 64:517, 1986
103. Baumgarten RK, Reynolds WJ: Priming principle and the open eye-full stomach. Anesthesiology 63:561, 1985
104. Dell R, Williams B: Anesthesia for strabismus surgery: A regional review. Br J Anaesth 82:761, 1999
105. Lerman MD, Eustis S, Smith DR: Effect of droperidol pretreatment on postanesthetic vomiting in children undergoing strabismus surgery. Anesthesiology 65:322, 1986
106. Brown RE, James DG, Weaver RG *et al*: Low-dose droperidol versus standard-dose droperidol for prevention of postoperative vomiting after pediatric strabismus surgery. J Clin Anesth 3:306, 1991
107. Gan TJ, Meyer T, Apfel CC *et al*: Consensus guidelines for managing postoperative nausea and vomiting. Anesth Analg 97:62, 2003
108. Watcha MF, Simeon RM, White PF *et al*: Effect of propofol on the incidence of postoperative vomiting after strabismus surgery in pediatric outpatients. Anesthesiology 75:204, 1991
109. Munro HM, Riegger LQ, Reynolds PI *et al*: Comparison of the analgesic and emetic properties of ketorolac and morphine for paediatric outpatient strabismus surgery. Br J Anaesth 72:624, 1994
110. Roth S, Thisted RA, Erickson JP *et al*: Eye injuries after nonocular surgery: A study of 60,965 anesthetics from 1985–1992. Anesthesiology 85:1020, 1996
111. Gild WA, Posner KL, Caplan RA *et al*: Eye injuries associated with anesthesia. Anesthesiology 76:204, 1992
112. Lee LA, Posner KL, Domino KB *et al*: Injuries associated with regional anesthesia in the 1980s and 1990s: A Closed Claims analysis. Anesthesiology 101:143, 2004
113. Batra YK, Bali M: Corneal abrasions during general anesthesia. Anesth Analg 56:363, 1977
114. Cucchiara R, Black S: Corneal abrasion during anesthesia and surgery. Anesthesiology 69:978, 1988
115. Purdy EP, Ajimal GS: Vision loss after lumbar epidural steroid injection. Anesth Analg 86:119, 1998
116. Roth S, Gillesberg I: Injuries to the visual system and other sense organs. In Benumof JL, Saidman LJ (eds): Anesthesia and Perioperative Complications, 2nd ed, p 377. St. Louis, Mosby, 1999
117. Mabry RL: Visual loss after intranasal corticosteroid injection. Arch Otolaryngol 107:484, 1981
118. Lee LA: Postoperative visual loss data gathered and analyzed. ASA Newsletter 64:25, 2000
119. Myers MA, Hamilton SR, Bogosian AJ *et al*: Visual loss as a complication of spinal surgery. Spine 22:1325, 1997
120. Dilger JA, Tetzlaff JE, Bell GR *et al*: Ischemic optic neuropathy after spinal fusion. Can J Anaesth 45:63, 1998
121. Shapira OM, Kimmel WA, Lindsey PS *et* al: Anterior ischemic optic neuropathy after open heart operations. Ann Thorac Surg 61:660, 1996
122. Williams EL, Hart WM, Tempelhoff R: Postoperative ischemic optic neuropathy. Anesth Analg 80:1018, 1995
123. The Ischemic Optic Neuropathy Decompression Trial Research Group: Optic nerve decompression surgery is not effective and may be harmful. JAMA 273:625, 1995
124. Drance SM: Angle-closure glaucoma among Canadian Eskimos. Can J Ophthalmol 8:252, 1973
125. Fazio DT, Bateman JB, Christensen RE: Acute angle-closure glaucoma associated with surgical anesthesia. Arch Ophthalmol 103:360, 1985
126. Feibel RM, Custer PL, Gordon MO: Postcataract ptosis: A randomized, double-masked comparison of peribulbar and retrobulbar anesthesia. Ophthalmology 100:660, 1993
127. Taylor G, Devys JM, Heran F, Plaud B. Early exploration of diplopia with magnetic resonance imaging after peribulbar anaesthesia. Br J Anaesth 92:899, 2004

CHAPTER 34 ■ ANESTHESIA FOR OTOLARYNGOLOGIC SURGERY

LYNNE R. FERRARI AND ALEXANDER W. GOTTA

KEY POINTS

1. The restricted spaces in the airway require an understanding and cooperative relationship between surgeon and anesthesiologist, and the use of specially adapted equipment suitable to these cramped areas.
2. Despite only mild to moderate tonsillar enlargement on physical examination, children with obstructive sleep apnea have upper airway obstruction while awake and apnea during sleep. The clinician should not underestimate the severity of the problem based on tonsillar size alone.
3. Posttonsillar hemorrhage may result in unappreciated large volumes of swallowed blood originating from the tonsillar fossa. These patients must be considered to have a full stomach, and anesthetic precautions addressing this situation must be taken.
4. The middle ear and sinuses are air-filled, nondistensible cavities. During procedures in which the eardrum is replaced or perforation is patched, N_2O should be discontinued or, if this is not possible, limited to a maximum of 50% during the application of the tympanic membrane graft to avoid pressure-related displacement.
5. In a LeFort III fracture, the fracture line may pass through the cribriform plate of the ethmoid bone, creating a fistula between the nasopharynx and the subarachnoid space within the skull. Clinical and radiographic studies are mandated to determine the integrity of the cribriform plate.
6. Upper airway tumors may be friable and lead to significant hemorrhage during intubation. Prior radiation therapy may lead to fibrosis and ankylosis in the temporomandibular joint, rendering orotracheal intubation difficult.
7. Prior to extubation after temporomandibular arthroscopy, the oral cavity and neck must be examined carefully to rule out the presence of extracapsular extravasation of irrigation fluid. Extravasation can lead to airway closure.
8. After extensive facial trauma or resection of tumors of the upper airway, it is prudent to keep the patient intubated until edema has subsided. Extraoral facial edema should lead the physician to suspect intraoral edema and possible airway compromise.

1 The anesthetic management of a patient undergoing surgery of the head, neck, ear, nose, and throat challenges the anesthesiologist to devise an anesthetic plan that will accommodate the needs of the surgeon, anesthesiologist, and patient. Among the problems that must be solved are the following:

1. Diagnosing alterations in a patient's airway created by infection, tumor, trauma, or congenital defect
2. Establishing and maintaining the airway in a patient whose anatomy has been distorted
3. Creating a shared operative field that enables the anesthesiologist to ventilate the patient's lungs and monitor the patient safely, and allows the surgeon to perform his or her tasks
4. Selecting appropriate anesthetic drugs compatible with the surgical procedure
5. Defining the appropriate moment for extubating the trachea of the postoperative patient

EVALUATING THE AIRWAY

In the healthy human, air flows through the upper respiratory passages; into the trachea, bronchi, and bronchioles; and into alveoli. This occurs seemingly without either thought or effort, and the actual work of respiration in the unobstructed airway is minimal. However, airway obstruction due to tumor, infection,

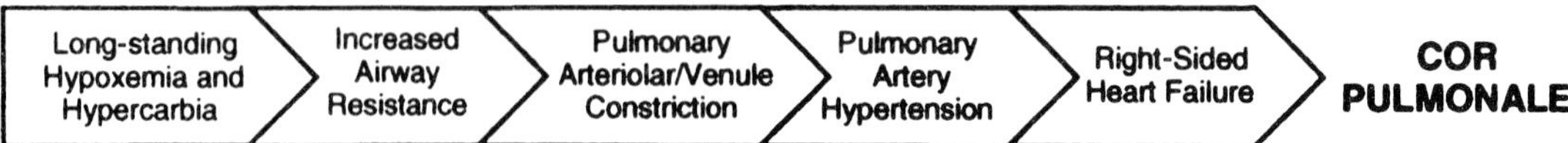

FIGURE 34-1. Events leading to cor pulmonale.

or trauma may significantly alter the clinical presentation and make gas exchange a laborious, energy-consuming process. This may leave the patient exhausted, incapable of maintaining adequate gas exchange, and finally succumbing to respiratory failure. Clinically, evident upper airway obstruction is a late sign, significant obstruction and anatomic distortion may be present in a patient with minimal evidence of disease. It is a most unwelcome experience for the anesthesiologist to discover a large, unexpected, obstructed upper airway at the time of attempted tracheal intubation.

In the presence of tumor, other mass lesions, or infection in the airway, it may be useful to obtain radiologic evaluation of the airway with plain films of the tracheal and laryngeal air columns or computed tomography (CT) and magnetic resonance imaging studies of the airway. Significant anatomic distortion is usually evident and may help the anesthesiologist determine the most appropriate technique for securing the airway.

ANESTHESIA FOR PEDIATRIC EAR, NOSE, AND THROAT SURGERY

Particularly challenging to the anesthesiologist is the safe management of the pediatric patient undergoing surgery of the ear, nose, and throat (ENT). The restricted spaces in the airway of the child require an understanding and cooperative relationship between surgeon and anesthesiologist, and the use of specially adapted equipment suitable to these cramped areas.

Tonsillectomy and Adenoidectomy

Untreated adenoidal hyperplasia may lead to nasopharyngeal obstruction, causing failure to thrive, speech disorders, obligate mouth breathing, sleep disturbances, orofacial abnormalities with a narrowing of the upper airway, and dental abnormalities. Surgical removal of the adenoids is usually accompanied by tonsillectomy; however, purulent adenitis, despite adequate medical therapy, and recurrent otitis media with effusion secondary to adenoidal hyperplasia are improved with adenoidectomy alone.

Tonsillectomy is one of the more commonly performed pediatric surgical procedures today.[1] Chronic or recurrent acute tonsillitis, peritonsillar abscess, tonsillar hyperplasia, and obstructive sleep apnea syndrome are the major indications for surgery.[2–4] In addition, patients with cardiac valvular disease are at risk for endocarditis from recurrent streptococcal bacteremia secondary to infected tonsils. Tonsillar hyperplasia may lead to chronic airway obstruction resulting in sleep apnea, CO_2 retention, cor pulmonale, failure to thrive, swallowing disorders, and speech abnormalities. These risks are eliminated with removal of the tonsils.

Obstruction of the oropharyngeal airway by hypertrophied tonsils leading to apnea during sleep is an important clinical syndrome referred to as *obstructive sleep apnea syndrome*. Despite only mild to moderate tonsillar enlargement on physical examination, these patients have upper airway obstruction while awake and apnea during sleep. The goals of treatment are to relieve airway obstruction and increase the cross-sectional area of the pharynx, which is successful in two-thirds of cases.[5] Some patients require the use of nasal constant positive airway pressure during sleep, whereas others may require a tracheostomy to bypass the chronic upper airway obstruction that is present. The two most frequent levels of obstruction during sleep are at the soft palate and the base of the tongue.[6] Most children will have tremendous improvement in their symptoms after tonsillectomy.

In children with long-standing hypoxemia and hypercarbia, increased airway resistance can lead to cor pulmonale (Fig. 34-1). Patients have electrocardiographic evidence of right ventricular hypertrophy, with one-third of them having chest radiographs consistent with cardiomegaly. Each apneic episode causes progressively increasing pulmonary artery pressure with
2 significant systemic and pulmonary artery hypertension leading to ventricular dysfunction and cardiac dysrhythmias.[7] Often, these patients have dysfunction in the medulla or hypothalamic areas of the central nervous system causing persistently elevated CO_2, despite relief of airway obstruction. This group of patients has a hyperreactive pulmonary vascular bed, and the increased pulmonary vascular resistance and myocardial depression in response to hypoxia, hypercarbia, and acidosis are far greater than what is expected for that degree of physiologic alteration in the normal population. Cardiac enlargement is frequently reversible with digitalization and surgical removal of the tonsils and adenoids.

Preoperative Evaluation

A thorough history is the basis for the preoperative evaluation. Because patients requiring tonsillectomy and adenoidectomy have frequent infections, the parent should be questioned for current use of antibiotics, antihistamines, or other medicines. A history of sleep apnea should be sought. The physical examination should begin with observation of the patient. The presence of audible respirations, mouth breathing, nasal quality of the speech, and chest retractions should be noted. Mouth breathing may be the result of chronic nasopharyngeal obstruction. An elongated face, retrognathic mandible, and a high-arched palate may be present.[8] The oropharynx should be inspected for evaluation of tonsillar size to determine the ease of mask ventilation and tracheal intubation (Fig. 34-2). The presence of wheezing or rales on auscultation of the chest may be a result of lower respiratory manifestation of pharyngitis or tonsillitis. The presence of inspiratory stridor or prolonged expiration may indicate partial airway obstruction from hypertrophied tonsils or adenoids.

Measurement of hematocrit and coagulation parameters is suggested. Many nonprescription cold medications and antihistamines contain aspirin, which may affect platelet function, and this should be taken into consideration. Chest radiographs and electrocardiograms (ECGs) are not required unless specific history of abnormalities in these areas is elicited, such as recent pneumonia, bronchitis, upper respiratory infection (URI), or history consistent with cor pulmonale. In those children with a history of cardiac abnormalities, an echocardiogram may be indicated.

Anesthetic Management

The goals of the anesthesia for tonsillectomy and adenoidectomy are to render the child unconscious in the most atraumatic manner possible, provide the surgeon with optimal operating conditions, establish intravenous access to provide a route for

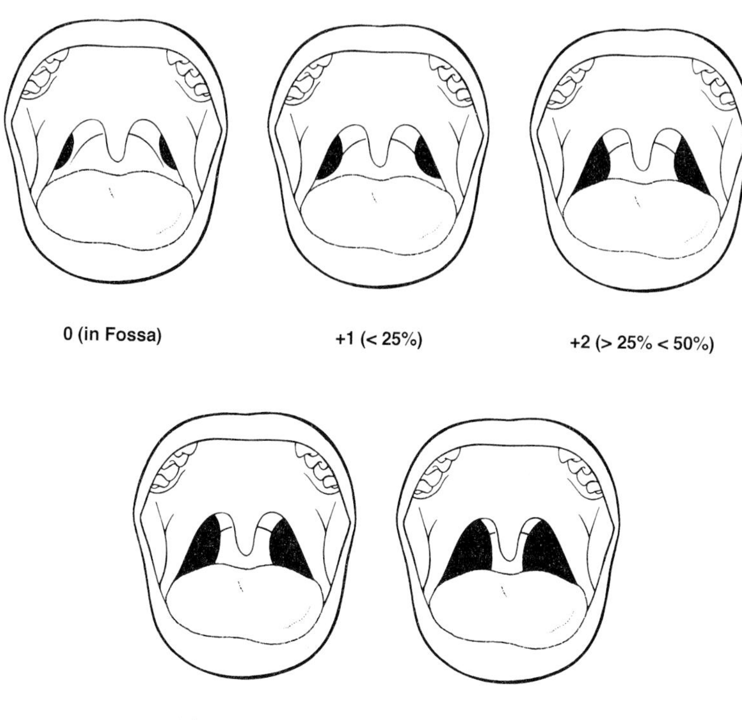

FIGURE 34-2. Classification of tonsil size, including percentage of oropharyngeal area occupied by hypertrophied tonsils.

volume expansion and medications should they be necessary, and to provide rapid emergence so the patient is awake and able to protect the recently instrumented airway. Premedication may be used as determined by the anesthesiologist during the preanesthetic visit. Sedative premedication should be avoided in children with obstructive sleep apnea, intermittent obstruction, or very large tonsils. An antisialagogue is often included to minimize secretions in the operative field.

Anesthesia is usually induced with a volatile drug, oxygen, and nitrous oxide (N_2O) by mask. Parental presence in the operating room (OR) during mask induction is often helpful in the anxious unpremedicated child. Tracheal intubation is best accomplished under deep inhalation anesthesia or aided by a short-acting nondepolarizing muscle relaxant. The possibility exists for blood in the pharynx to enter the trachea during the surgical procedure. For this reason, the supraglottic area may be packed with petroleum gauze, or a cuffed endotracheal tube may be used provided an appropriate leak around the endotracheal tube is obtained. Monitoring consists of precordial stethoscope, ECG, automated blood pressure, pulse oximetry, and end-tidal CO_2.

Emergence from anesthesia should be rapid, and the child should be alert before transfer to the recovery area. The child should be awake and able to clear blood or secretions in the oropharynx as efficiently as possible before removal of the endotracheal tube. Maintenance of airway and pharyngeal reflexes is of utmost importance in the prevention of aspiration, laryngospasm, and airway obstruction. There is no difference in the incidence of airway complications on emergence between patients who are extubated awake or deep.[9]

The use of the laryngeal mask airway (LMA) for adenotonsillectomy was described in 1990; however, it was not until the widespread availability of a streamlined flexible model that it was widely used.[10,11] The wide, rigid tube of the original model did not fit under the mouth gag and was easily compressed or dislodged during full mouth opening. The newer, flexible model has a soft, reinforced shaft that easily fits under the mouth gag without becoming dislodged or compressed. Adequate surgical access can be achieved, and the lower airway is protected from exposure to blood during the procedure.[12,13]

Insertion is possible after either the intravenous administration of 3.5 mg/kg propofol or when sufficient depth of anesthesia is achieved using a volatile agent administered by mask. The same depth of anesthesia should be obtained during insertion of the LMA as would be required for performing laryngoscopy and endotracheal intubation. Positive-pressure ventilation should be avoided when the LMA is used during tonsillectomy, although gentle assisted ventilation is both safe and effective if peak inspiratory pressure is kept below 20 cm H_2O.[14]

Tonsillar enlargement can make LMA insertion difficult, so care in placement is essential.[15] Maneuvers to overcome this difficulty include increased head extension, lateral insertion of the mask, anterior displacement of the tongue, pressure on the tip of the LMA using the index finger as it negotiates the pharyngeal curve, or use of the laryngoscope if all else fails. Dislodgment of the device does not occur during extreme head extension, assuming good position and ventilation were obtained before changes in head position.[16]

Advantages of the LMA over traditional endotracheal intubation are a decrease in the incidence of postoperative stridor and laryngospasm and an increase in immediate postoperative oxygen saturation. If the child is breathing spontaneously at a regular rate and depth, the LMA may be removed before emergence from anesthesia. The oropharynx should be gently suctioned with a soft, flexible catheter, the LMA deflated and removed, an oral airway inserted, and the respirations assisted with 100% oxygen delivered by mask. It is often distressing for young children to awaken with the LMA still in place, and although the device is an appropriate substitute for oral airway in the adult population, the same is not so in children. If the practitioner wants to remove the LMA when the child has emerged from anesthesia, it should be deflated and removed as soon as possible after the return to consciousness.

Complications

The incidence of emesis after tonsillectomy ranges from 30 to 65%.[17] Whether this is due to irritant blood in the stomach or interference with the gag reflex by inflammation and edema at the surgical site remains unclear. Central nervous system stimulation from the gastrointestinal tract, as may be seen with gastric distention from the introduction of swallowed or insufflated air, may trigger the emetic center. Decompressing the stomach with an orogastric tube may be helpful in preventing this response. Treatment with ondansetron 0.10 to 0.15 mg/kg either with or without dexamethasone has been shown to be very effective in reducing posttonsillectomy nausea and vomiting.[18] Postoperative administration of meperidine increases the probability of emesis, and other analgesic agents should be administered. Dehydration secondary to poor oral intake as a result of nausea, vomiting, or pain can occur after tonsillectomy in 1% of cases. Vigorous intravenous hydration during surgery can offset the physiologic effects of later decreases in fluid intake.

The most serious complication of tonsillectomy is postoperative hemorrhage, which occurs at a frequency of 0.1 to 8.1%.
3 Approximately 75% of postoperative tonsillar hemorrhage occurs within 6 hours of surgery. Most of the remaining 25% occurs within the first 24 hours of surgery, although bleeding may be noted until the sixth postoperative day.[19] Sixty-seven percent of postoperative bleeding originates from the tonsillar fossa, 27% in the nasopharynx, and 7% in both. Initial attempts to control bleeding may be made using pharyngeal packs and cautery. If this fails, patients must return to the OR for exploration and surgical hemostasis.

Unappreciated large volumes of blood originating from the tonsillar bed may be swallowed. These patients must be considered to have a full stomach, and anesthetic precautions addressing this situation must be taken. A rapid sequence induction accompanied by cricoid pressure and a styletted endotracheal tube is often recommended. Because the amount of blood swallowed can be considerable, blood pressure must be checked in both the erect and supine positions to look for orthostatic changes resulting from decreases in vascular volume. Intravenous access and hydration must be established before the induction of anesthesia. A variety of laryngoscope blades and endotracheal tubes, as well as functioning suction apparatus, should be prepared in duplicate because blood in the airway may impair visualization of the vocal cords and cause plugging of the endotracheal tube.

Pain after adenoidectomy is usually minimal but is severe after tonsillectomy. This contributes to poor fluid intake and overall discomfort of patients. An increase in postoperative pain medication requirements has been noted in patients having laser or electrocautery as part of the operative tonsillectomy compared with those who have had sharp surgical dissection and ligation of blood vessels to achieve hemostasis.[20] Intraoperative administration of corticosteroids may decrease edema formation and subsequent patient discomfort. Although infiltration of the peritonsillar space with local anesthetic and epinephrine has been shown to be effective in reducing intraoperative blood loss, it does not decrease postoperative pain.[21]

Peritonsillar abscess, or quinsy tonsil, is a condition that may require immediate surgical intervention to relieve potential or existing airway obstruction. An acutely infected tonsil may undergo abscess formation, producing a large mass in the lateral pharynx that can interfere with swallowing and breathing (Figs. 34-3 to 34-5). Fever, pain, and trismus are frequent symptoms. Treatment consists of surgical drainage of the abscess, either with or without tonsillectomy, and intravenous antibiotic therapy. Although the airway seems compromised, the peritonsillar abscess is usually in a fixed location in the lateral pharynx and does not interfere with ventilation of the patient by mask after induction of general anesthesia. Visualization of the vocal cords should not be impaired because the pathologic process is supraglottic and well above the laryngeal inlet. Laryngoscopy must be carefully performed, avoiding manipulation of the larynx and surrounding structures. Intubation should be gentle because the tonsillar area is tense and friable and inadvertent rupture of the abscess can occur, leading to spillage of purulent material into the trachea.

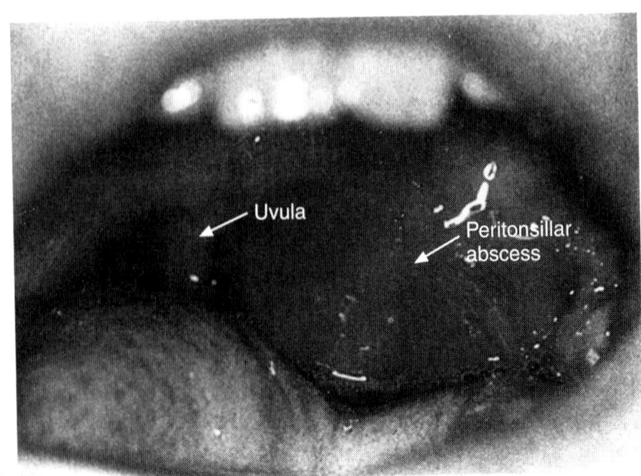

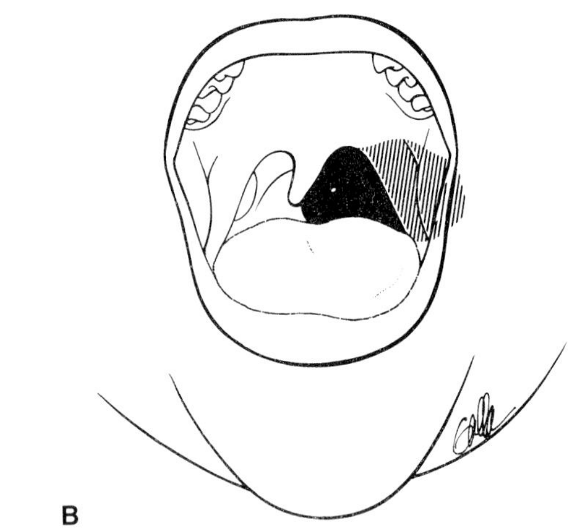

FIGURE 34-3. A. Patient with a peritonsillar abscess on the left side. B. Note the displacement of the uvula. (Courtesy of Michael Cunningham, MD, Boston, MA.)

Acute postoperative pulmonary edema is an infrequent but potentially life-threatening complication encountered when airway obstruction is suddenly relieved. One proposed mechanism is that during inspiration before adenotonsillectomy, the negative intrapleural pressure that is generated causes an increase in venous return, enhancing pulmonary blood volume. In the healthy child without airway obstruction, pleural pressure ranges from −2.5 cm to −10.0 cm H_2O during inspiration. Intrapleural pressure generated in the child with airway obstruction can be as much as −30 cm H_2O, which when transmitted to the interstitial peribronchial and perivascular spaces causes disruption of the capillary walls of the pulmonary microvasculature. Concurrent with a negative transpulmonary gradient is an increase in venous return to the right side of the heart, thus increasing preload, which in the setting of "leaky capillaries" facilitates transudation of fluid into the alveolar space. To counterbalance this, positive intrapleural and alveolar pressure is generated during exhalation, which decreases pulmonary venous return and blood volume. This is similar to an expiratory "grunt" mechanism in which the transpleural pressures generated are similar to those present during a Valsalva maneuver.

The rapid relief of airway obstruction results in decreased airway pressure, an increase in venous return, an increase in pulmonary hydrostatic pressure, hyperemia, and finally

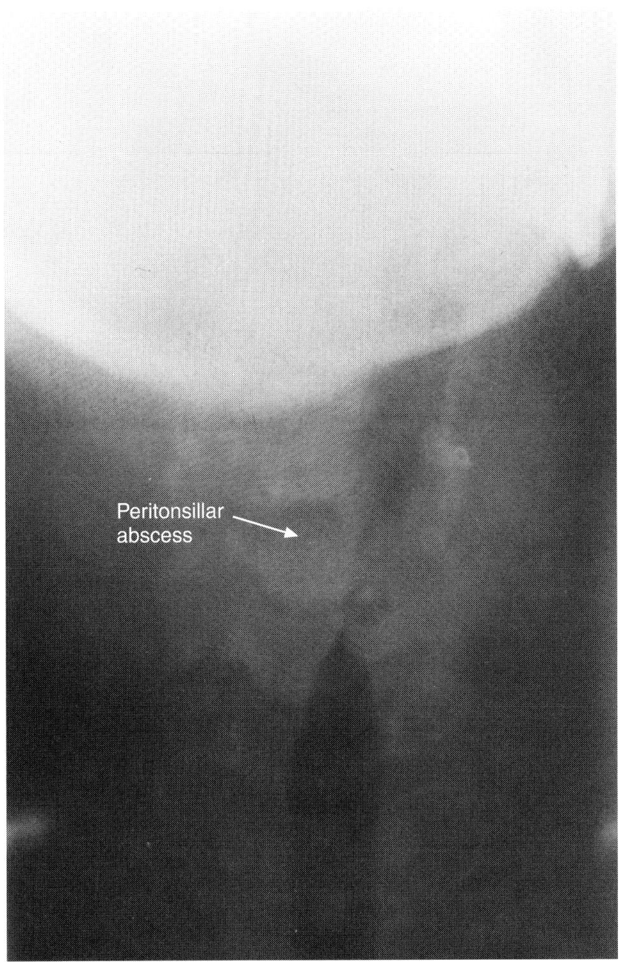

FIGURE 34-4. Neck radiograph of a patient with a peritonsillar abscess.

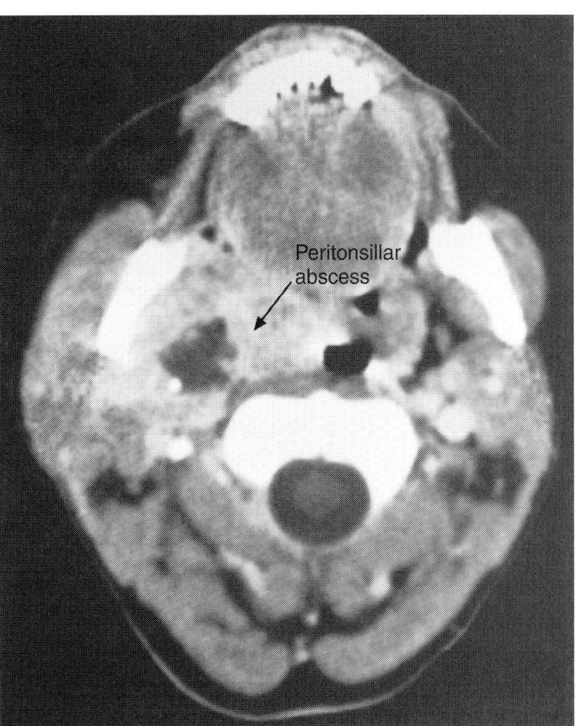

FIGURE 34-5. Computed tomography scan of a patient with a peritonsillar abscess.

pulmonary edema. The all-important counterbalance of the expiratory "grunt" in limiting pulmonary venous return is lost when the obstruction is relieved. Contributing factors are the increased volume load on both ventricles, as well as the inability of the pulmonary lymphatic system to remove acutely large amounts of fluid. The anesthesiologist may attempt to prevent this situation during induction of anesthesia by applying moderate amounts of continuous positive pressure to the airway, thus allowing time for circulatory adaptation to take place. This physiologic sequence is similar to that seen in patients with severe acute airway obstruction secondary to epiglottitis or laryngospasm.

Negative-pressure pulmonary edema is signaled by the appearance of frothy pink fluid in the endotracheal tube of an intubated patient or the presence of a decreased oxygen saturation, wheezing, dyspnea, and increased respiratory rate in the immediate postoperative period in a previously extubated patient. Mild cases may present with minimal symptoms. The differential diagnosis of negative-pressure pulmonary edema includes aspiration of gastric contents, adult respiratory distress syndrome, congestive heart failure, volume overload, and anaphylaxis. A chest radiograph illustrating diffuse, usually bilateral interstitial pulmonary infiltrates combined with an appropriate clinical history will confirm the diagnosis.[22]

Treatment is usually supportive, with maintenance of a patent airway, oxygen administration, and diuretic therapy in some cases. Endotracheal intubation and mechanical ventilation with positive end-expiratory pressure may be necessary in severe cases. Resolution is usually rapid and may occur within hours of surgery. Most cases resolve without treatment within 24 hours. There is currently no reliable method for predicting which children will experience this clinical syndrome after their airway obstruction has been resolved.[23]

Adenoidectomy patients may be safely discharged on the same day after recovering from anesthesia. Tonsillectomy has been a procedure that warranted postoperative admission of the patient to the hospital for observation, administration of analgesics, and hydration. Many centers are discharging tonsillectomy patients on the day of surgery without adverse outcomes, and this trend will likely continue.[19,20,24,25] It is recommended that patients be observed for early hemorrhage for a minimum of 6 hours and be free from significant nausea, vomiting, and pain prior to discharge. Ability to take fluid by mouth is not a requirement for discharge home. However, intravenous hydration must be adequate to prevent dehydration. Excessive somnolence and severe vomiting are indications for hospital admission. There is a set of patients in whom early discharge is not advised, and those patients should be admitted to the hospital after tonsillectomy. The characteristics of such patients are listed in Table 34-1.[26]

Ear Surgery

The ear and its associated structures are target organs for many pathologic conditions. General anesthesia for surgery of the ear has its own set of unique considerations that must be addressed.

Myringotomy and Tube Insertion

Chronic serous otitis in children can lead to hearing loss, and drainage of accumulated fluid in the middle ear is effective treatment for this condition. Myringotomy, which creates an

TABLE 34-1

TONSILLECTOMY AND ADENOIDECTOMY INPATIENT GUIDELINES: RECOMMENDATION OF THE AMERICAN ACADEMY OF OTOLARYNGOLOGY–HEAD AND NECK SURGERY PEDIATRIC OTOLARYNGOLOGY COMMITTEE

Admit patients to the hospital after adenotonsillectomy if they meet any of the following criteria:

- Age ≤3 yr
- Abnormal coagulation values with or without an identified bleeding disorder in the patient or family
- Evidence of obstructive sleep disorder or apnea due to tonsillar or adenoidal hypertrophy
- Systemic disorders that put the patient at increased preoperative cardiopulmonary, metabolic, or general medical risk
- Child with craniofacial or other airway abnormalities, including, but not limited to, syndromic disorders such as Treacher Collins syndrome, Crouzon's syndrome, Goldenhar syndrome, Pierre Robin anomalad, C.H.A.R.G.E. association, achondroplasia, and, most prominently, Down syndrome, as well as isolated airway abnormalities such as choanal atresia and laryngotracheal stenosis
- When the procedure is being done for acute peritonsillar abscess
- When extended travel time, weather conditions, and home social conditions are not consistent with close observation, cooperation, and ability to return to the hospital quickly at the discretion of the attending physician

opening in the tympanic membrane for fluid drainage, may be performed alone. During healing, the drainage path may become occluded. Therefore, tube placement is usually included. The insertion of a small plastic tube in the tympanic membrane serves as a vent for the ostium and allows for continued drainage of the middle ear until the tubes are naturally extruded in 6 months to 1 year or surgically removed at an appropriate time (Fig. 34-6).

Myringotomy and tube insertion is a relatively short procedure, and anesthesia may be effectively accomplished with a potent inhalation drug, oxygen, and N_2O administered by mask. Premedication is not recommended because most sedative drugs used for premedication will far outlast the duration of the surgical procedure. Patients with chronic otitis frequently have accompanying recurrent URIs. It is often the eradication of middle ear fluid that resolves the concomitant URI. Because tracheal intubation is not required for routine patients, the criteria for cancellation of surgery and anesthesia may be different for this procedure. No significant difference in perioperative morbidity between asymptomatic patients and those fulfilling URI criteria has been demonstrated.[27,28] It is recommended that patients with URI symptoms receive supplemental postoperative oxygen.[29]

Middle Ear and Mastoid

Tympanoplasty and mastoidectomy are two of the most common procedures performed on the middle ear and accessory structures. To gain access to the surgical site, the head is positioned on a head rest, which may be lower than the operative table, and extreme degrees of lateral rotation may be required. Extreme tension on the heads of the sternocleidomastoid muscles must be avoided. The laxity of the ligaments of the cervical spine and the immaturity of odontoid process in children make them especially prone to C1–C2 subluxation.

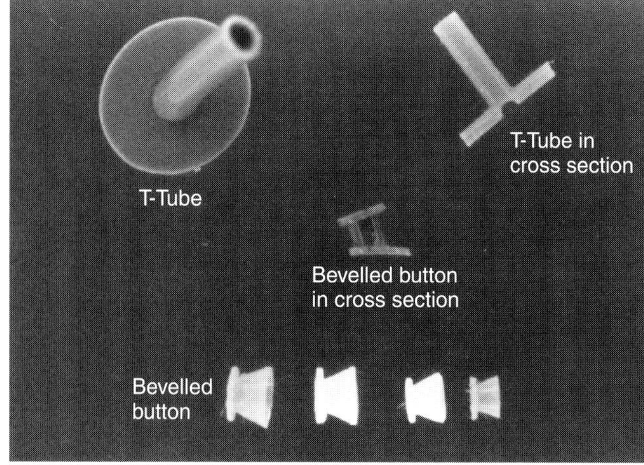

FIGURE 34-6. Two types of myringotomy tubes, both are 2.5 mm in internal diameter. Both the ventilating T-tube and the beveled-button ventilating tube (large and small) are shown in full and cross-sectional views. (Courtesy of Michael Cunningham, MD, Boston, MA.)

Ear surgery often involves surgical identification and preservation of the facial nerve, which requires isolation of the nerve by the surgeon and verification of its function by means of electrical stimulation (Fig. 34-7). This is accomplished by brainstem auditory-evoked potential and electrocochleogram monitoring, which requires that muscle relaxation be avoided and a volatile drug is the primary anesthetic.[30] If an opioid-relaxant technique is chosen, however, at least 30% of the muscle response, as determined by a twitch monitor, should be preserved. This suggests that it is not mandatory to avoid skeletal muscle relaxants in the anesthetic management of patients undergoing surgical procedures when monitoring of facial nerve function is necessary.

Bleeding must be kept to a minimum during surgery of the small structures of the middle ear. Relative hypotension, keeping the mean arterial pressure 25% below baseline, is effective. Concentrated epinephrine solution, often 1:1,000, can be injected in the area of the tympanic vessels to produce

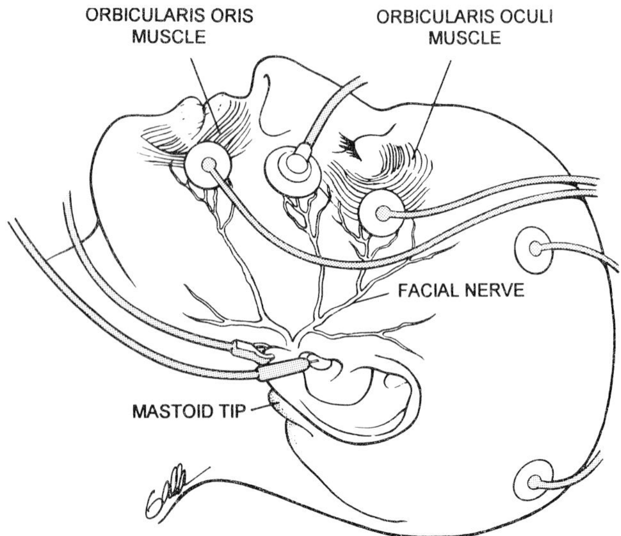

FIGURE 34-7. Illustration of facial nerve and monitoring electrodes. (Courtesy of Steve Ronner, PhD, Boston, MA.)

vasoconstriction. Close attention should be paid to the volume of injected epinephrine to avoid dysrhythmias and wide swings in blood pressure.

The middle ear and sinuses are air-filled, nondistensible cavities. An increase in the volume of gas in these structures results in an increase in pressure. N_2O diffuses along a concentration gradient into the air-filled middle ear spaces more rapidly than
4 nitrogen moves out. Passive venting occurs at 20 to 30 cm H_2O pressure, and it has been shown that use of N_2O results in pressures that exceed the ability of the eustachian tube to vent the middle ear within 5 minutes, leading to pressure buildup.[31] During procedures in which the eardrum is replaced or perforation is patched, N_2O should be discontinued or, if this is not possible, limited to a maximum of 50% during the application of the tympanic membrane graft to avoid pressure-related displacement.

After N_2O is discontinued, it is quickly reabsorbed, creating a void in the middle ear with resulting negative pressure. This negative pressure may result in serous otitis, disarticulation of the ossicles in the middle ear (especially the stapes) and hearing impairment, which may last up to 6 weeks after surgery. The use of N_2O is related to a high incidence of postoperative nausea and vomiting, which is a direct result of negative middle ear pressure during recovery. The vestibular system is stimulated by traction placed on the round window by the negative pressure that is created. Although all patients have the potential for nausea and vomiting after surgery, children younger than 8 years of age seem to be most affected. If the use of N_2O cannot be avoided, vigorous use of antiemetics is warranted.

Airway Surgery

Stridor

Noisy breathing due to obstructed airflow is known as *stridor*. Inspiratory stridor results from upper airway obstruction; expiratory stridor results from lower airway obstruction; and biphasic stridor is present with midtracheal lesions. The evaluation of a patient with stridor begins with a thorough history. The age of onset suggests a cause because laryngotracheomalacia and vocal cord paralysis are usually present at or shortly after birth, whereas cysts or mass lesions develop later in life (Table 34-2). Information indicating positions that make the stridor better or worse should be obtained, and placing a patient in a position that allows gravity to aid in reducing obstruction can be of benefit during anesthetic induction.

Physical examination reveals the general condition of a patient and the degree of the airway compromise. Laboratory examination may include assessment of hemoglobin, a chest radiograph, and barium swallow, which can aid in identifying lesions that may be compressing the trachea. CT scan and tomograms may be indicated in isolated instances but are not routinely ordered. Specific note of the signs and symptoms listed in Table 34-3 should be made.

TABLE 34-3

CLINICAL EVALUATION OF PATIENTS WITH STRIDOR

Respiratory rate
Heart rate
Wheezing
Cyanosis
Chest retractions
Nasal flaring
Level of consciousness

Laryngomalacia is the most common cause of stridor in infants. It is most often due to a long epiglottis that prolapses posteriorly and prominent arytenoid cartilages with redundant aryepiglottic folds that obstruct the glottic opening during inspiration.[32] The definitive diagnosis is obtained by direct laryngoscopy and rigid or flexible bronchoscopy. Preliminary examination is usually carried out in the surgeon's office. A small, flexible fiberoptic bronchoscope is inserted through the nares into the oropharynx, and the movement of the vocal cords is observed. Alternatively, it may be accomplished in the OR before anesthetic induction in an awake patient or in a lightly anesthetized patient during spontaneous respiration. Patients must be spontaneously breathing so the vocal cords move freely. After deepening anesthesia, a rigid bronchoscope is inserted through the vocal cords and the subglottic area is inspected; the lower trachea and bronchi are evaluated with a rigid or flexible fiberoptic bronchoscope.

Bronchoscopy

Small infants may be brought into the OR unpremedicated. Older children and adults may experience respiratory depression and worsening of airway obstruction if heavy premedication is administered, so light sedation is suggested. The airway must be protected from aspiration of gastric contents during prolonged airway manipulation; therefore, premedication with the full regimen of acid aspiration prophylaxis may be indicated.

The goals of anesthesia are analgesia, an unconscious patient, and a "quiet" surgical field.[33] Coughing, bucking, or straining during instrumentation with the rigid bronchoscope may cause difficulty for the surgeon and result in damage to the patient's airway. At the conclusion of the procedure,

TABLE 34-2

CAUSES OF STRIDOR

SUPRAGLOTTIC AIRWAY	LARYNX	SUBGLOTTIC AIRWAY
Laryngomalacia	Laryngocele	Tracheomalacia
Vocal cord paralysis	Infection (tonsillitis, peritonsillar abscess)	Vascular ring
Subglottic stenosis	Foreign body	Foreign body
Hemangiomas	Choanal atresia	Infection (croup, epiglottitis)
Cysts	Cyst	
	Mass	
	Large tonsils	
	Large adenoids	
	Craniofacial abnormalities	

TABLE 34-4

COMPARISON OF EXTERNAL DIAMETER OF STANDARD ENDOTRACHEAL TUBES VERSUS RIGID BRONCHOSCOPE

ENDOTRACHEAL TUBE		RIGID BRONCHOSCOPE
INTERNAL DIAMETER (mm)	EXTERNAL DIAMETER (mm)	EXTERNAL DIAMETER (mm)
2.5	3.5	4.2
3.0	4.3	5.0
3.5	4.9	5.7
4.0	5.5	6.7
5.0	6.8	7.8
6.0	8.2	8.2

Adapted with permission from Mallinckrodt Medical, Inc., St. Louis, MO.

patients should be returned to consciousness quickly, with airway reflexes intact. For most patients, a pulse oximeter, blood pressure cuff, ECG, and precordial stethoscope are applied before induction of anesthesia. Inhalation induction by mask is accompanied by oxygen and a volatile agent administered in increasing concentrations in children and intravenous drugs in adults. Patients should be placed in the position that produces the least adverse effect on airway symptoms (often the sitting position). An intravenously administered antisialagogue may help decrease secretions that can obscure the view through the bronchoscope.

The size of a bronchoscope refers to the internal diameter. Because the external diameter may be significantly greater than in an endotracheal tube of similar size (Table 34-4), care must be taken to select a bronchoscope of proper external diameter to avoid damage to the laryngeal structures.

A rigid bronchoscope can be used for ventilation of the lungs during examination of the airway. It is inserted through the vocal cords, and ventilation is accomplished through a side port, which can be attached to the anesthesia circuit. During ventilation with the viewing telescope in place, high resistance may be encountered as a result of partial occlusion of the lumen. High fresh gas flow rates, large tidal volumes, and high inspired volatile anesthetic concentrations are often necessary to compensate for leaks around the ventilating bronchoscope and the high resistance encountered when the viewing telescope is in place. Manual ventilation at higher-than-normal rates is most effective in achieving adequate ventilation. Adequate time for exhalation must be provided for passive recoil of the chest.

An alternative method of ventilation is the jet ventilation technique, which involves intermittent bursts of oxygen delivered under pressure through a 16-gauge catheter attached to a rigid bronchoscope.[34] Intermittent flow is accomplished by depressing the lever of an on–off valve. The use of jet ventilation techniques is associated with the additional risks of pneumothorax or pneumomediastinum due to rupture of alveolar blebs or a bronchus.[35]

Because ventilation may be intermittent and at times suboptimal, it is recommended that oxygen be used as the carrier gas during bronchoscopic examination. Intravenous drugs that cause excessive respiratory depression should be avoided. It is wise to ask the surgeon if movement of the vocal cords will be observed at the conclusion of the procedure or if tracheal or bronchial dynamics will be evaluated during the procedure so the anesthetic may be planned accordingly (i.e., spontaneous respirations preserved during light levels of anesthesia versus no respiratory efforts and the use of short-acting muscle relaxants).

Maintenance of anesthesia is usually accomplished with a volatile anesthetic. Intravenous anesthetics combined with muscle relaxation best maintain a constant level of anesthesia because the delivery of volatile anesthetics through the bronchoscope may be interrupted, and anesthetic depth can vary. At the conclusion of rigid bronchoscopy, an endotracheal tube is usually placed in the trachea to control the airway during recovery of anesthesia. This tube is particularly important if muscle relaxants have been used because passive regurgitation of gastric contents may be more likely to occur in paralyzed patients. An additional advantage of placing an endotracheal tube is that if the surgeon should want to examine the distal airways, a small, flexible fiberoptic bronchoscope can be passed through the endotracheal tube.

Pediatric Airway Emergencies

Upper airway emergencies may be life threatening and demand immediate treatment. Rapid respiratory failure can occur in patients with croup, epiglottitis, or foreign body aspiration, and few clinical situations are more challenging to the anesthesiologist.

Epiglottitis

Acute epiglottitis is one of the most feared infectious diseases in children and adults, and is the result of *Haemophilus influenzae* type B. It can progress with extreme rapidity from sore throat to airway obstruction to respiratory failure and ultimately to death if proper diagnosis and intervention are not rapidly implemented. Patients are usually between 2 and 7 years of age, although epiglottitis has been reported in younger children and adults. Vaccination against *H. influenzae* type B polysaccharide is now recommended before 2 years of age to provide immunity before the greatest period of vulnerability in pediatric patients.

Characteristic signs and symptoms of acute epiglottitis include sudden onset of fever; dysphagia; drooling; thick, muffled voice; and preference for the sitting position with the head extended and leaning forward. Retractions, labored breathing, and cyanosis may be observed in cases where respiratory obstruction is present. However, in the early stages, the patient may be pale and toxic without respiratory distress. *Supraglottitis* may be a more appropriate designation because it is the tissues of the supraglottic structures—from the vallecula to the arytenoids—that are involved in the infectious process. At no time (in the emergency room or radiography suite) should direct visualization of the epiglottis be attempted in the unanesthetized patient. The differential resulting from negative pressure inside and atmospheric pressure outside the extrathoracic airway results in slight narrowing during normal inspiration. The pressure differential on inspiration is exaggerated in the patient with airway obstruction. This dynamic collapse of the airway may become life threatening in the struggling, agitated patient, and every attempt should be made to keep him or her calm. Blood drawing, intravenous catheter insertion, and excessive manipulation of the patient, as well as sedation, should be avoided before securing the airway to avoid the possibility of total obstruction.

If the clinical situation allows, oxygen should be administered by mask, and lateral radiographs of the soft tissues in the neck may be obtained. Thickening of the aryepiglottic folds and swelling of the epiglottis may be noted. Radiologic examination should only be carried out if skilled personnel and adequate equipment accompany the patient at all times. The patient with severe airway compromise should proceed from the emergency department directly to the operating suite, accompanied by both the anesthesiologist and surgeon. Parental presence in this situation may calm an anxious and frightened child.

In all cases of epiglottitis, an artificial airway is established by means of tracheal intubation. In some centers where personnel experienced in the management of the compromised airway are not available, tracheostomy is a less favored alternative. In the OR, the child is kept in the sitting position while monitors are placed. A pulse oximeter and precordial stethoscope are essential. If it is believed to be helpful, one parent may accompany the child and remain in the OR during the induction of general anesthesia. The OR must be prepared with equipment and personnel for laryngoscopy, rigid bronchoscopy, and tracheostomy. Anesthetic induction is accomplished by inhalation of oxygen and increasing concentrations of halothane or sevoflurane. After loss of consciousness occurs, intravenous access should be secured and the child lowered into the supine position. Laryngoscopy followed by oral tracheal intubation is then accomplished without the use of muscle relaxants. The endotracheal tube chosen should be at least one size (0.5 mm) smaller than would normally be chosen, and a stylette is often useful. Once the surgeon has examined the larynx, noting the appearance of the epiglottis, aryepiglottic folds, and surrounding tissues, the endotracheal tube may be changed to a nasotracheal tube and secured. Tissue and blood cultures are taken, and antibiotic therapy is initiated. The child is then transferred to the intensive care unit for continued observation and radiographic confirmation of tube placement. Sedation is appropriate at this time. Tracheal extubation is usually attempted 48 to 72 hours later in the OR, when a significant leak around the nasotracheal tube is present and visual inspection of the larynx by flexible fiberoptic bronchoscopy confirms reduction in swelling of the epiglottis and surrounding tissues.

Laryngotracheobronchitis

Laryngotracheobronchitis (LTB), or croup, occurs in children from 6 months to 6 years of age, but is primarily seen in children younger than 3 years of age. It is usually viral in etiology, and its onset is more insidious than that of epiglottitis. The child presents with low-grade fever, inspiratory stridor, and a "barking" cough. Radiologic examination confirms the diagnosis, and subglottic narrowing of the airway column secondary to circumferential soft-tissue edema produces the "steeple" sign characteristic of LTB. Approximately 6% of patients with LTB require admission to the hospital. Treatment includes cool, humidified mist and oxygen therapy, usually administered in a tent for mild to moderate cases. More severe cases of LTB are accompanied by tachypnea, tachycardia, and cyanosis. Racemic epinephrine administered by nebulizer is beneficial. The use of steroids has been surrounded by a great deal of controversy, but current opinion is that a short course of steroids may be beneficial. In rare circumstances, thick secretions are present in the airway, and the child requires intubation to allow pulmonary toilet and suctioning to be carried out. Management in the intensive care unit and extubation are carried out in the same fashion as for epiglottitis.

Foreign Body Aspiration

A major cause of morbidity and mortality in children and adults is aspiration of a foreign body. Any history of coughing, choking, or cyanosis while eating (peanuts, popcorn, jelly beans, hot dogs) should suggest the possibility of foreign body aspiration. Any patient who presents to the emergency room with refractory wheezing should be suspected of this diagnosis. Physical findings include decreased breath sounds, tachypnea, stridor, wheezing, and fever. These signs indicate an obstructive–inflammatory process in the airway. Some foreign bodies are identifiable on radiologic examination; however, 90% are radiolucent, and air trapping, infiltrate, and atelectasis are all that are noted. The most common site of foreign body aspiration is the main-stem bronchus, the right being more frequent than the left. Food particles comprise the majority of aspirated items; however, beads, pins, and small toys are not unusual. Each type of aspirated item has potential complications associated with it. Vegetable items expand with moisture encountered in the respiratory tract and can fragment into multiple pieces, thus creating a situation where the original foreign body is in one bronchus and, with coughing, a fragment is dislodged and transported to the other bronchus. Oil-containing objects, such as peanuts, cause a chemical inflammation and sharp objects cause bleeding in addition to the obstruction.

All aspirated foreign bodies in the airway should be removed in the OR and considered to be emergency situations. No sedation should be administered to patients before removal of the foreign body. If the patient has recently eaten, full stomach precautions must be taken and anesthesia should be induced intravenously (topical EMLA cream may be applied to the skin before intravenous catheter insertion in small children) by rapid sequence, and gentle cricoid pressure maintained during intubation of the trachea. If the child has not recently eaten, anesthesia may be induced by inhalation of sevoflurane in oxygen by mask. Inhalation induction can be prolonged secondary to obstruction of the airway, and N_2O should be avoided to reduce air trapping distal to the obstruction. After evacuation of the stomach by orogastric tube, the airway may be given over to the surgeon, who replaces the endotracheal tube with a rigid bronchoscope and removes the aspirated object.

Spontaneous ventilation should be preserved until the location and nature of the foreign body have been determined. Ventilation via the bronchoscope requires careful attention. Hypoxia and hypercarbia may occur because of inadequate ventilation caused by an excessively large leak around the bronchoscope or, more commonly, inability to provide adequate gas exchange through a narrow-lumen bronchoscope fitted with an internal telescope. These conditions are remedied by frequent removal of the telescope and withdrawal of the bronchoscope to the midtrachea, allowing effective ventilation. Bronchospasm may occur during examination of the respiratory tract and should be treated with increasing depths of anesthesia, nebulized albuterol, or intravenous bronchodilators. Although rare, pneumothorax should be suspected if acute deterioration occurs during the procedure.

Once the foreign body has been removed, examination of the entire tracheobronchial tree is carried out to detect any additional objects or fragments. Often, vigorous irrigation and suctioning distal to the obstruction are required to remove secretions and prevent the possibility of postobstructive pneumonia. Steroids are administered if inflammation of the airway mucosa is observed. Close postoperative observation of the patient is required so that early intervention may be instituted in the event of respiratory compromise secondary to airway edema or infection.

ANESTHESIA FOR PEDIATRIC AND ADULT SURGERY

Certain surgical procedures are commonly performed in both adults and children, including nasal surgery and laser surgery of the airway. Surgery for maxillofacial trauma and upper airway tumors or infection, as well as temporomandibular joint (TMJ) arthroscopy, are conducted more commonly in adults.

Laser Surgery of the Airway

One of the greatest advances in airway surgery has been the use of the laser (*l*ight *a*mplification by *s*timulated *e*mission of *r*adiation). For use in the airway, the laser provides precision in targeting lesions, minimal bleeding and edema, preservation of surrounding structures, and rapid healing. The laser consists of a tube with reflective mirrors at either end and an amplifying medium between them to generate electron activity, resulting in the production of light.[36] The CO_2 laser is the most widely used in medical practice, having particular application in the treatment of laryngeal or vocal cord papillomas, laryngeal webs, resection of redundant subglottic tissue, and coagulation of hemangiomas. The laser is an especially useful modality for the surgeon because the invisible beam of light affords an unobstructed view of the lesion during resection. The energy emitted by a CO_2 laser is absorbed by water contained in blood and tissues. Human tissue is approximately 80% water, and laser energy absorbed by tissue water rapidly increases the temperature, denaturing protein and vaporizing the target tissue. The thermal energy of the laser beam cauterizes capillaries as it vaporizes tissues; thus, bleeding and postoperative edema are minimized.

The properties that give the laser a high degree of specificity also supply the route by which a misdirected laser beam may cause injury to a patient or to unprotected OR personnel.[37] The eyes are especially vulnerable, and all OR personnel should wear laser-specific eye goggles with side protectors to prevent injury. Due to the limited penetration (0.01 mm) of the CO_2 laser, it may cause injury only to the cornea. Other lasers such as the neodymium–yttrium-aluminum-garnet (Nd-YAG) have deeper penetration, and may cause retinal injury and scarring. The eyes of a patient undergoing laser treatment must be protected by taping them shut, followed by the application of wet gauze pads and a metal shield. Any stray laser beam is absorbed by the wet gauze, preventing penetration of the eyes. Laser radiation increases the temperature of absorbent material, and flammable objects such as surgical drapes must be kept away from the path of the laser beam. To avoid cutaneous burns from deflected beams, wet towels should be applied to exposed skin of the face and neck when the laser is being used in the airway. Laser smoke plumes may cause damage to the lungs, with interstitial pneumonia has been reported with long-term exposure. In addition, it has been postulated that during laser application cancer cells and virus particles, including human immunodeficiency virus, are vaporized, and the resultant smoke plume, if inhaled, may be a vehicle for spread. The use of specially designed surgical masks for filtering laser smoke is recommended.

Most anesthetic techniques are suitable for laser surgery provided that patients are immobile and the laser beam can be directed at a target that is entirely still and in full view. Both N_2O and oxygen support combustion. The primary gas for anesthetic maintenance should consist of blended air and oxygen or helium and oxygen. A pulse oximeter should be used at all times.

Anesthesia during laser surgery may be administered with or without an endotracheal tube. The choice of endotracheal tube used during laser surgery can affect the safety of the technique. All standard polyvinyl chloride (PVC) endotracheal tubes are flammable, and can ignite and vaporize when in contact with the laser beam. Red rubber endotracheal tubes wrapped with reflective metallic tape do not vaporize, but instead deflect the laser beam. The unwrapped cuff below the vocal cords is still vulnerable to laser injury. Cuffed endotracheal tubes should be inflated with sterile saline to which methylene blue has been added so a cuff rupture from a misdirected laser spark is readily detected by the blue dye and extinguished by the saline.[38] Endotracheal tubes have been manufactured specifically for use during laser surgery. Some have a double cuff to ensure protection of the airway in the event of a cuff rupture, whereas others have a special matte finish that is effective in deflecting the laser beam throughout the entire length. Nonreflective flexible metal endotracheal tubes are also specifically manufactured for use during laser surgery. The outer diameter of each size of metal laser tube is considerably greater than the PVC counterpart, especially in the small sizes used for pediatric anesthesia (Figs. 34-8 and 34-9, Table 34-5).

An apneic technique is preferred by some surgeons, especially when working on the airway of small infants and children. The advantage of this technique is an unobstructal

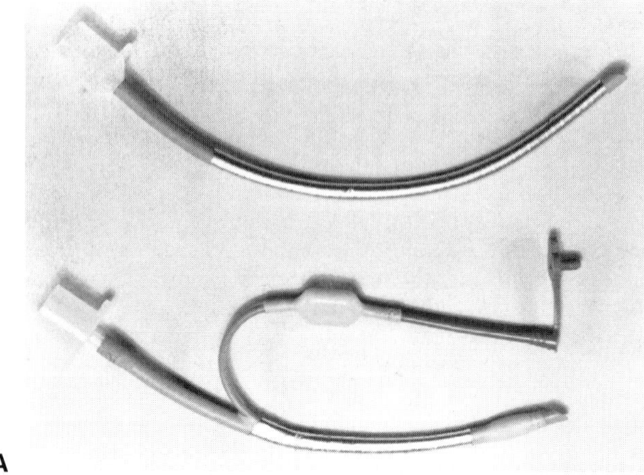

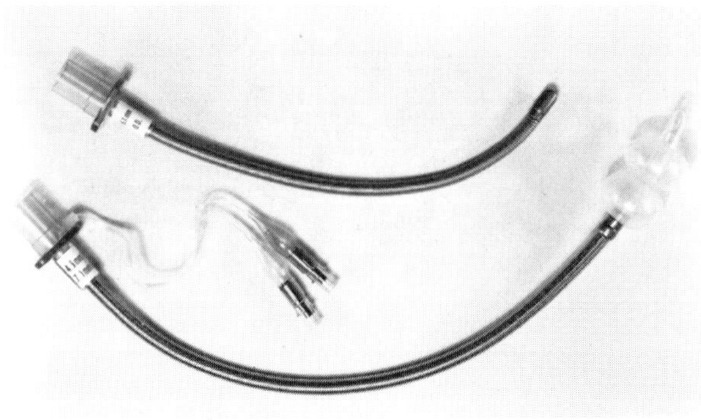

FIGURE 34-8. **A.** Cuffed and uncuffed rubber endotracheal tubes wrapped with reflective metallic tape. **B.** Cuffed and uncuffed flexible metal endotracheal tubes for use during laser surgery of the airway. (Reprinted with permission from Ferrari LR: Anesthesia for otorhinolaryngology procedures. In Cote C, Ryan J, Todres D, Goudsouzian N [eds]: A Practice of Anesthesia for Infants and Children, 2nd ed, Chapter 18, Philadelphia, WB Saunders, 1993.)

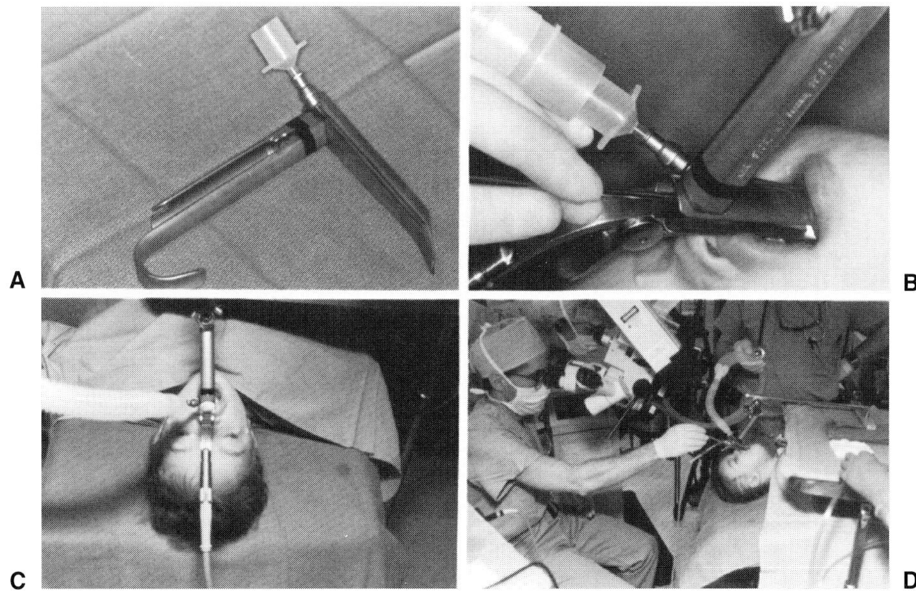

FIGURE 34-9. A. The surgical laryngoscope fitted with an endotracheal tube connector. B. The surgical laryngoscope positioned in the patient's pharynx and connected to the anesthesia circuit. C. Surgical view of the anesthetized, spontaneously breathing patient. D. Laser-aided resection of vocal cord lesion.

surgical field to the absence of an endotracheal tube, which may obscure the surgical field. In this circumstance, a child is anesthetized and rendered immobile by use of a muscle relaxant or deep inhalation of a volatile anesthetic. The patient's trachea is not intubated, and the airway is given over to the surgeon, who uses the laser for brief periods. Between laser applications, the patient's lungs are ventilated by mask. Because apnea is a component of this technique, it is prudent to ventilate the lungs with oxygen. Although this technique has been widely used with safety, there is a greater potential for debris and resected material to enter the trachea.

The use of a jet ventilator is a modification of the apneic technique that does not require tracheal intubation but does provide for oxygenation during laser surgery uses a jet ventilator. The operating laryngoscope is fitted with a catheter through which oxygen is delivered under pressure through a variable reducing value (see Fig. 34-9). Additional room air is entrained, and the patient's lungs are ventilated with this combination of gases. This technique produces a quiet surgical field because large chest excursions of the diaphragm are eliminated and ventilation is uninterrupted. In morbidly obese patients and those with severe small airway disease, effective ventilation is not accomplished with this technique, and an alternate technique should be used.

The final technique that may be used without the aid of an endotracheal tube is spontaneous ventilation with the "oxiscope." In this technique, a surgical laryngoscope fitted with an oxygen insufflation port is inserted into the larynx. The volatile anesthetic gas is mixed with oxygen and administered through the side port. Anesthesia is maintained without muscle relaxant in the spontaneously breathing patient in this manner. Propofol may be infused to decrease the concentration of inhaled volatile anesthetic, and the vocal cords may be sprayed with 4% lidocaine to decrease reactivity. This technique is advantageous in that longer periods of uninterrupted laser application may be provided. Disadvantages include the absence of complete control of the airway, limited protection from laryngospasm, limited protection from debris entering the airway, presence of vocal cords motion and difficult scavenging.

TABLE 34-5

COMPARISON OF STANDARD PLASTIC VERSUS METAL ENDOTRACHEAL TUBES

■ INTERNAL DIAMETER (mm)	■ EXTERNAL DIAMETER (mm)	
	■ PLASTIC	■ METAL
3.0 (uncuffed)	4.3	5.2
3.5 (uncuffed)	4.9	5.7
4.0 (uncuffed)	5.5	6.1
4.5 (cuffed)	6.2	7.0
5.0 (cuffed)	6.8	7.5
5.5 (cuffed)	7.5	7.9
6.0 (cuffed)	8.2	8.5

Nasal Surgery

Nasal surgery may be successfully accomplished under either general anesthesia or conscious sedation. Whichever method is selected, profound vasoconstriction is required. Cocaine packs, local anesthetics, and epinephrine infiltration are often used simultaneously. All three of these agents can cause cardiac irritability, and both epinephrine and cocaine are known to produce varying degrees of hypertension. The simultaneous use of these medications causes cumulative and often dangerous side effects. Young, healthy patients may be able to tolerate these effects. The older patient, or one who has known cardiovascular compromise, may benefit from slow, sequential administration of these medications guided by heart rate, cardiac rhythm, and blood pressure. The potent inhalation anesthetics do have varying degrees of dysrhythmogenic potential and should be used with caution in the face of pharmacologically induced alterations in cardiac rhythm.

A moderate degree of controlled hypotension combined with head elevation decreases bleeding in the surgical site, but some blood may passively enter the stomach. The placement of an oropharyngeal pack or suctioning of the stomach at the conclusion of surgery may attenuate postoperative retching and vomiting.

Maxillofacial Trauma

Traumatic disruption of the bony, cartilaginous, and soft-tissue components of the face and upper airway challenge the anesthesiologist to recognize the nature and extent of the injury and consequent anatomic alteration, create a plan for securing the airway safely, implement the plan without doing further damage, maintain the airway during the administration of an anesthetic, and determine when and how to extubate the patient's trachea. Also necessary is the creation of a comfortable environment for both surgeon and anesthesiologist in a limited work space.

Anatomy

It is conventional to divide the facial skeleton into thirds. The lower third consists of the mandible, with its subdivisions of midline symphysis, body, angle, ramus, condyle, and coronoid process. The middle third contains the zygomatic arch of the temporal bone, blending into the zygomaticomaxillary complex, the maxillae, nasal bones, and orbits. The superior third consists of the frontal bone. Actually, there are two skeletons, facial and cranial, each one in contiguity with the other. Great forces are generated within the facial skeleton during the normal physiologic process of mastication. To prevent injury of one skeleton against the other, there is a series of bony buttresses built into the relationship between the two skeletons. Horizontal posterior displacement of the facial skeleton is limited by the zygomatic process of the temporal bone, oblique posterior displacement by the pterygoid process of the sphenoid bone, and vertical posterior displacement by the greater wing of the sphenoid bone. Upward displacement is held in check by the zygomatic process of the frontal bone, the nasal part of the frontal bone, and the roof of the mandibular fossa.

In addition to the buttresses, there are two arches lending stability to the craniofacial skeleton. An arch extends from the mandibular condyle to the coronoid process, and another arch is created by the zygomatic arch of the temporal bone extending into the zygomaticomaxillary complex.

This combination of bony buttresses and arches creates a normal vector of force dispersion and distribution. Thus, a blow to the mandible may be of sufficient magnitude to fracture the mandible at the point of impact or elsewhere, but does not extend the fracture line into the base of the skull. However, a blow to the midface, especially from in front and above, does not follow a normal vector of force dispersion and redistribution and tends to create an abnormal shearing force, which may tear the facial skeleton from the cranial skeleton and extend the fracture into the base of the skull. In any patient with severe midfacial trauma, a fracture of the base of the skull must be considered.

The mandible is a tubular bone and, as such, derives its strength from the cortices and is least vulnerable to fracture where the cortex is thickest (i.e., at the anteroinferior margin).[39] Moving posteriorly, the cortex thins and a greater incidence of fractures is found at the angle of the mandible, the ramus, and the condyle.[40–42] Another common point of fracture is in the body of the mandible at the level of the first or second molar. These are laboratory observations, but clinical experience indicates that this distribution occurs after high-velocity, high-impact trauma, such as in an automobile accident. After personal trauma, such as inflicted by a fist, a blunt weapon, or a fall, there is a greater tendency for a fracture of the symphysis, parasymphysis, and body to occur. This may not only result from lesser versus greater energy impact and redistribution, but also from the person's tendency to turn the head away from an impending blow and thus take the force of impact on the side of the face and the body of the mandible rather than on the symphysis.[43]

The mandible has a unique, horseshoe shape that causes forces to gather at points of vulnerability, often distant from the point of impact.[41] If this phenomenon is unrecognized, it can create serious problems in diagnosis. It may be known, for example, that the patient was struck on the symphysis, but it must also be recognized that he or she may have a fracture of the condyle, perhaps with involvement of the TMJ and limitation of jaw mobility.

LeFort Classification of Fractures

In 1901, Rene LeFort of Lille, France, published the results of a series of rather bizarre experiments.[44] He attempted to determine if there is a reliable means of detecting facial fractures by examining facial soft-tissue injuries and by using the nature and extent of these injuries as indicators of bony disruption. This relationship does not exist. Extensive soft-tissue injury does not necessarily indicate bony trauma, and conversely, serious fractures may exist with relatively little soft-tissue disruption. In the course of his studies, LeFort determined the common lines of midface fracture, which are thus eponymous and called LeFort I, LeFort II, and LeFort III fractures.

The LeFort I fracture is a horizontal fracture of the maxilla, passing above the floor of the nose but involving the lower third of the septum, mobilizing the palate, maxillary alveolar process, and the lower third of the pterygoid plates and parts of the palatine bones. The fracture segment may be displaced posteriorly or laterally or rotated about a vertical axis.

The LeFort II fracture is pyramidal, beginning at the junction of the thick upper part of the nasal bone, with the thinner portion forming the upper margin of the anterior nasal aperture. The fracture crosses the medial wall of the orbit, including the lacrimal bone beneath the zygomaticomaxillary suture; crosses the lateral wall of the antrum; and passes posteriorly through the pterygoid plates. The fracture segment may be displaced posteriorly or rotated about an axis.

In a LeFort III fracture, the line of fracture parallels the base of the skull, separating the midfacial skeleton from the base of the cranium. The line of fracture passes through the base of
5 the nose and the ethmoid bone in its depth, and through the orbital plates. The cribriform plate of the ethmoid may or may not be fractured. The fracture line crosses the lesser wing of the sphenoid, then downward to the pterygomaxillary fissure and sphenopalatine fossa. From the base of the inferior orbital fissure, the fracture extends laterally and upward to the frontozygomatic suture and downward and backward to the root of the pterygoid plates. A LeFort III fracture results from massive force applied to the midface. The zygomata are displaced and rotational force applied to the zygomatic arches. The arches are usually fractured as a result.

With this fracture, the midface is mobilized and often distracted posteriorly. The normal convexity of the face may be replaced by a concavity, giving rise to the characteristic "dish face deformity" of a LeFort III fracture. Even if this facial concavity is not clinically evident, the presence of a LeFort III fracture should be suspected if the incisive edges of the maxillary and mandibular teeth are apposed, instead of the normal position in which the maxillary incisors shingle over the mandibular incisors. This apposition serves as a subtle clue to minimal posterior displacement of the midface.

Tumors

Neoplastic growths can occur anywhere within the upper air-
6 way and may achieve significant size with little evidence of airway obstruction. These tumors are often friable and bleed readily. Attempted tracheal intubation can induce significant hemorrhage and edema and cause severe compromise of the airway. Prior radiation therapy may cause extensive fibrosis, increased intraoperative bleeding, and ankylosis of the TMJ, making tracheal intubation under direct vision difficult or impossible. Consultation with a surgeon as to the nature and

extent of the tumor, and its potential to bleed, together with review of appropriate radiographs and prior therapy, are important in determining techniques for airway management. Tumors of the head and neck are usually associated with abuse of both cigarettes and alcohol, with consequent abnormalities of both pulmonary and hepatic function.

Upper Airway Infection

Infectious processes in the upper airway may be of sufficient size to mimic neoplasms and present the same problems of airway distortion, compression, and compromise. The same precautions must be taken in dealing with airway abscesses as with tumors. An added problem is the ability of an abscess to leak spontaneously, dribbling pus into the lungs, contaminating and infecting them, and producing scattered areas of pneumonitis; or to rupture during tracheal intubation, flooding the lungs with purulent material.

Ludwig's Angina

Ludwig's angina is an overwhelming generalized septic cellulitis of the submandibular region.[45,46] It generally occurs after dental extraction, especially of the second or third mandibular molars, whose roots lie below the attachment of the mylohyoid muscle. The infection is bilateral and involves three fascial spaces: submandibular, submental, and sublingual. Ludwig's angina is characterized by brawny induration of the upper neck, usually without obvious fluctuation, and the patient has a typical open-mouthed appearance. Involvement of the sublingual space pushes the tongue upward and backward, and it usually protrudes from the open mouth. Soft-tissue swelling in the suprahyoid region, coupled with upward and posterior displacement of the tongue, as well as the frequent presence of laryngeal edema, can close the airway and asphyxiate the patient.

Early signs and symptoms include chills, fever, drooling of saliva, inability to open the mouth, and difficulty in speaking. The cause is often hemolytic streptococci, but may be a mixture of aerobic and anaerobic organisms, including gas-forming bacteria.[47] Although fluctuation is rarely appreciated, abscesses may be present but their presence hidden by the thick, indurated tissue of the neck. The infectious process may spread into the thorax, causing empyema, pericarditis, pericardial effusion, and pulmonary infiltrates. Patients with Ludwig's angina often require incision and drainage of whatever purulent material is present, coupled with airway decompression. Airway management may be extremely difficult. Although inhalation anesthesia and intubation have been advocated,[48] preliminary tracheostomy using local anesthesia in the awake patient is the safest course. The patient with Ludwig's angina is commonly septic, extremely ill, and often poorly hydrated.

Temporomandibular Joint Arthroscopy

Open surgery of the human TMJ was first described in 1887, in a discussion of operative repair of displaced interarticular cartilage of the joint.[49] Although open surgery of the joint is still sometimes considered necessary, the development of small-gauge arthroscopes and lasers has made arthroscopic surgery of the TMJ an increasingly popular technique, frequently performed on an ambulatory basis.[50] Common indications for arthroscopic correction of TMJ lesions include the following[50]: (1) internal joint derangement with closed lock, (2) internal joint derangement with painful clicking, (3) osteoarthritis, (4) hypermobility, (5) fibrous ankylosis, and (6) arthralgia. Other less common indicators include chondromalacia and synovitis.

TMJ disease is usually caused by spasm of the muscles of mastication secondary to chronic tensing of these muscles as an involuntary mental tension–relieving mechanism. The patient population is unique in that 86% of patients with chronic TMJ dysfunction have significant psychopathology, with major depression in 74% and somatoform disorder in 50%.[51] A total of 40% of the patients are preoccupied with facial pain, yet have no physical findings accounting for the pain. Many of these patients habitually use mood-altering or tension-abating drugs such as benzodiazepines, phenothiazines, or lithium.

Nasotracheal intubation is usually preferred, allowing the surgeon the option of intraoral manipulation during surgery. Complications of TMJ arthroscopy are rare but include partial or total hearing loss, infection, hemorrhage requiring open arthrotomy, and temporary or permanent deficits of the fifth and eighth cranial nerves and temporary seventh nerve paresis.[51,52]

Of particular importance to the anesthesiologist is partial or even complete closure of the airway due to extracapsu-
7 lar extravasation of the fluid used to irrigate the joint during arthroscopy.[53] Significant amounts of fluid can leak into the soft tissues of the neck and compromise the airway. After TMJ arthroscopy, the patient's trachea should not be extubated until the oral cavity, especially on the affected side, and neck have been examined carefully and no evidence of unusual swelling that might indicate extravasated fluid is found.

Patient Evaluation

The patient who has sustained facial trauma or whose airway is clearly distorted by tumor or infection may present with an obvious pathologic process that can distract the physician from completing a total evaluation of the patient. In the patient with facial trauma, other injuries may not be as apparent but may represent a greater threat to the patient's well-being. In patients with maxillofacial injury due to low-velocity, low-impact blows (as from a fist), 4% had major (life-threatening) other injuries, and 10% had minor (non–life-threatening) injuries. With high-velocity, high-impact (motor vehicle) accidents, 32% had major and 31% minor other injuries.[54] Of great importance, cervical spine fractures occurred in 1.2% of high-velocity injuries. Other studies have reported a 5.5% incidence of cervical spine injury in patients with facial skeletal trauma.[55] Any level of the cervical spine may be involved, but injuries at C2 (31%) and C6–C7 (50%) predominate. Cranial fractures and intracranial injury are also not uncommon.

SECURING THE AIRWAY

In most instances of anesthesia for head and neck surgery, tracheal intubation is effected without significant problems. Grave difficulties can arise in patients with tumor or infection or other facial trauma. If any of these processes has so altered the airway that attempted tracheal intubation risks airway compromise and an inability to ventilate the lungs, then awake tracheal intubation or preliminary tracheostomy is mandated. History, physical examination, appropriate radiographs, and surgical consultation are the foundation of airway evaluation and choice of intubating technique. The technique of an "awake look" before a decision to anesthetize and paralyze a patient is particularly hazardous and misleading. Muscle tone and labored respiration in the awake patient help identify the rima glottis or some seemingly familiar anatomic structure but disappear once anesthesia and paralysis have been induced, and it may be impossible to identify the entrance to the airway and intubate the trachea.

For the anesthesiologist to be able to intubate the trachea of a patient under direct vision, the patient must be able, at a minimum, to open the mouth and extend the tongue beyond the incisors. After maxillofacial trauma, there may be serious limitation in mobility owing to one or more factors, including pain, trismus, edema, and mechanical dysfunction of the TMJ. Pain yields to an anesthetic and muscle relaxant, presenting no problem.

Trismus is spasm of the masseter muscles, binding the jaw closed, secondary to trauma or infection. Trismus, too, succumbs to an anesthetic and muscle relaxant, but with an important caveat. If the trismus has been present for 2 weeks or if the jaw has been closed for some other reason for 2 weeks, the masseters acquire a degree of fibrosis that limits their response to an anesthetic and relaxant. A jaw closed for 2 weeks for whatever cause merits consideration for awake tracheal intubation. Edema varies in severity and consequences from mild to extreme and may occasionally cause serious limitation in jaw mobility.

Mechanical dysfunction in the jaw arises from several causes. A fracture of the condyle in its articulation in the TMJ may create a situation in which the jaw is locked closed and is unresponsive to an anesthetic and muscle relaxant. A fracture of the zygomatic arch of the temporal bone will always causes some decrease in jaw mobility. This bone is well protected, enveloped in the tough temporal fascia. Nonetheless, a severe blow to the side of the head may fracture the bone, pushing bony segments down onto the coronoid process of the mandible. There is a biphasic motion in the mandible, rotation about an axis passing through the condyles, and anterior-posterior motion (translation). This anterior motion is limited by the bony impingement on the coronoid process, and TMJ function is thus restricted by the limitation in translation. Usually, the decrease in function is not severe enough to make tracheal intubation impossible, but it may be, making the decision as to whether to anesthetize and paralyze the patient or perform awake tracheal intubation difficult. The anesthesiologist in doubt is cautioned to err on the side of conservatism.

Patients with TMJ dysfunction undergoing arthroscopic surgery may present with either closed or open lock and be unsuitable for intubation of the trachea after induction of anesthesia. Patients with large cervical abscesses may require awake intubation or tracheostomy. If the abscess has caused anatomic distortion or respiratory difficulty, awake intubation or tracheostomy is usually mandatory. Early tracheostomy in Ludwig's angina is preferred, and no patient should ever be observed to the point of airway compromise.[56] In any instance in which awake intubation is elected in the infected patient, provision must be available for immediate tracheostomy.

Awake Intubation

Passing an endotracheal tube through the mouth or nose and into the larynx and trachea of an awake patient is a formidable procedure that the patient resists fiercely, stimulated by the protestations of highly sensitive airway reflexes. To overcome these reflexes, the airway must be anesthetized using a combination of topical local anesthetic and superior laryngeal nerve block.

The *superior laryngeal nerve* is a branch of the vagus arising from the nodose ganglion and coursing with the main trunk of the vagus until it reaches the level of the larynx, where it springs forward and terminates in two branches, internal and external. The external branch of the superior laryngeal nerve penetrates and innervates the cricothyroid muscle, a tensor of the vocal cords. The internal branch penetrates the thyrohyoid membrane, ramifies, and provides sensory innervation from the base of the tongue to the vocal cords.[57] Once it has penetrated the thyrohyoid membrane, it lies in a closed space, bounded medially by the laryngeal mucosa, laterally by the thyrohyoid membrane, superiorly by the inferior border of the hyoid bone, and inferiorly by the superior surface of the thyroid cartilage. The anatomic landmarks for superior laryngeal nerve block are as follows:

1. The hyoid bone, a freely movable bone in the upper part of the neck, articulating with no other bone
2. The thyroid cartilage, the largest component of the larynx, usually easily identified
3. The thyrohyoid membrane binding the two together

With the patient lying supine, a 22-gauge needle attached to a syringe containing 2 mL of 2% lidocaine is aimed directly at the hyoid, traveling parallel to the operating table. When the needle strikes the hyoid, the operator can appreciate the characteristic gritty feeling of a needle on bone, similar to striking the rib while doing an intercostal block. The needle is then walked caudad until it just slips off the bone, penetrating the thyrohyoid membrane. After negative aspiration, lidocaine may be injected and the block repeated on the other side.[58]

Contraindications to a superior laryngeal nerve block are relative, not absolute, and include the following:

1. A full stomach, because of the possibility of vomiting and aspiration into an airway whose protective reflexes have been partially obtunded
2. Tumor at the site of block
3. Infection at the site of block

Tumor and infection are considered to be relative contraindications because of the possibility of dissemination of either tumor or infection secondary to the manipulation associated with the block. Risks must be weighed against benefit, and very often benefit wins. Protection against aspiration can be increased by the presence of knowledgeable help, an operating table that can swing quickly into the Trendelenburg position, and efficient suction apparatus.

Local anesthetic may be instilled into the nose for nasotracheal intubation and into the mouth and oropharynx for either nasal or oral intubation. A vasoconstrictor, such as 0.5% phenylephrine hydrochloride or 0.05% oxymetazoline, should also be instilled in the nose to shrink the nasal mucosa, decrease the risk of trauma, and create a larger passage for tracheal intubation. Topical anesthetic may be applied to the trachea below the level of the vocal cords by introducing a 22-gauge needle attached to a syringe containing 4 mL of 2% lidocaine and injecting the drug rapidly into the trachea at the end of the maximal expiration. The injection of the drug excites a vigorous cough reflex, spraying the local anesthetic along the tracheal side walls and inferior surface of the vocal cords. As a supplement to direct tracheal instillation of local anesthetic and bilateral superior laryngeal nerve block, local anesthetic (e.g., 2% lidocaine) may be nebulized in a handheld nebulizer and inhaled by the patient. This is a tedious process, demanding long, slow breaths and inhalation of the nebulized anesthetic over the course of at least 20 minutes. The endotracheal tube may then be passed into the anesthetized airway using a guided, fiberoptic technique or blindly. Complications of superior laryngeal nerve block include intravascular injection of local anesthetic. The carotid sheath lies just posterior to the site of block and, if the needle is angled posteriorly, the sheath may be entered and the anesthetic injected directly into the carotid artery or internal jugular vein.

The role of the LMA in head and neck surgery awaits clarification. The LMA may be useful in temporarily securing a compromised airway. In any situation, however, where the airway is jeopardized by blood or pus, or the anatomy distorted by trauma, the airway must be secured with a cuffed endotracheal or tracheostomy tube. The intubating LMA may facilitate awake intubation.[59] The flexible LMA is unsafe in head and neck surgery in the presence of foreign material such as blood, bone fragments, or pus.[60]

A modification of the LMA is the LMA-ProSeal, which has a double cuff and a double-lumen design that separates the airway and the alimentary tract, thus providing a safe escape channel for regurgitated fluids. Incorporated in its design is an independent drain tube that opens at the upper esophageal sphincter, permitting drainage of gastric fluids and allowing blind insertion of an orogastric tube. However, only a properly placed endotracheal tube offers complete airway protection.

The LMA-Fastrach is a modification of the intubating LMA, designed specifically for the anatomically difficult airway, especially the patient who cannot open his or her mouth fully. When used with the LMA-Fastrach, endotracheal tube intubation can be effected without moving the patient. This tube is a straight, silicone, wire-reinforced, cuffed tube, not exceeding 8 mm internal diameter, and capable of being passed entirely through an LMA-Fastrach. The use of this device may make possible an otherwise very difficult intubation.

LeFort III Fractures

A LeFort III fracture may involve the cribriform plate of the ethmoid bone, thus violating the separation of nasopharynx and base of the skull and allowing entrance into the intracranial subarachnoid space. Nasotracheal intubation risks the introduction of foreign material from the nasopharynx into the subarachnoid space and the consequent development of meningitis. More important, it risks the introduction of the endotracheal tube into the substance of the brain, with direct mechanical damage. Even positive-pressure bag and mask ventilation is contraindicated because the increase in volume and pressure within the nasopharynx can force foreign material[61] or air into the skull.[62]

The problems of securing the airway in a patient with a LeFort III fracture are ordinarily obviated by doing a preliminary tracheostomy using local anesthetic in an awake patient. This has the added advantage of separating surgeon and anesthesiologist and allowing each an adequate working space. Nasotracheal intubation can be performed in a patient with a LeFort III fracture provided three criteria are met: (1) absence of clinical signs of basal skull fracture, (2) absence of radiographic evidence of basal skull fracture, and (3) a compelling reason for doing so. Occasionally (rarely), these three criteria are fulfilled.

Anesthetic Management of the Traumatized Upper Airway

After tracheal intubation has been achieved or tracheostomy performed, general or intravenous anesthetics may be used. The use of ketamine as a sole anesthetic in an attempt to obviate the necessity of performing a difficult tracheal intubation is perilous and should be avoided. Ketamine is a potent respiratory depressant[63] in bolus doses, increases intracranial pressure[64] (ICP), and causes focal alterations in the cerebral metabolic rate.[65] Because there is a significant incidence of intracranial trauma associated with maxillofacial trauma, the brain must be protected and alterations in ICP avoided. Opioids have little effect on ICP and are useful in anesthetic management. However, the dose may be difficult to determine because of the high incidence of drug abuse associated with trauma. Inhalation anesthetics are safe and effective, and ICP can be moderated by altering the Pa_{CO_2}. The halogenated ethers are particularly useful, but the halogenated alkane halothane should be avoided because of the high incidence of cardiac arrhythmias associated with its use.[66]

Extubation

When tracheostomy has been incorporated into the anesthetic-surgical plan, it is maintained at the termination of the procedure, and the only decision facing the anesthesiologist is whether to allow spontaneous respiration or to create suitable conditions for continued mechanical ventilation by maintaining the patient anesthetized and paralyzed. This decision is contingent on such factors as the nature and duration of surgery, the patient's prior physical condition, and concurrent respiratory disease, a frequent concomitant of head and neck tumors.

After trauma, infection, or extensive oral resection for tumor, the endotracheal tube must not be removed until there is clearly subsidence of any edema that might compromise the unprotected airway. Particular attention must be given to
8 the submandibular area, where extensive edema pushes the tongue upward and posteriorly and risks the airway. An edematous tongue protruding past the incisors is an ominous warning of dangerous edema. If substantial edema is present, a waiting period of 24 to 36 hours is usually indicated. Serious infection may require a longer period of time to resolve. An oral endotracheal tube may be removed over a tube changer. When removing a nasotracheal tube, a useful technique is to place a fiberoptic bronchoscope through the tube and into the airway and to remove the tube over the bronchoscope so it can be replaced immediately if necessary.

References

1. Brodsky L: Modern assessment of tonsils and adenoids. Pediatr Clin North Am 36:1551, 1989
2. Berkowitz RG, Zalzal GH: Tonsillectomy in children under 3 years of age. Arch Otolaryngol Head Neck Surg 116:685, 1990
3. Ferrari LR: Anesthesia for pediatric ENT procedures. Danamiller Memorial Education Foundation. Prog Anesthesiol 15:15, 2001
4. Strauss SG, Lynn AM, Bratton SL *et al*: Ventilatory response to CO_2 in children with obstructive sleep apnea from adenotonsillar hypertrophy. Anesth Analg 89:328, 1999
5. Clinical practice guideline: Diagnosis and management of childhood obstructive sleep apnea syndrome. Pediatrics 109:704, 2002
6. Chaban R, Cole P, Hoffstein V: Site of upper airway obstruction in patients with idiopathic obstructive sleep apnea. Laryngoscope 98:641, 1988
7. Blum RH, McGowan FX Jr: Chronic upper airway obstruction and cardiac dysfunction: Anatomy, pathophysiology and anesthetic implications. Paediatr Anaesth 14:75, 2004
8. Smith RM, Gonzalez C: The relationship between nasal obstruction and craniofacial growth. Pediatr Clin North Am 36:1423, 1989
9. Patel RI, Hannallah RS, Norden J *et al*: Emergence airway complications in children: A comparison of tracheal extubation in awake and deeply anesthetized patients. Anesth Analg 73:266, 1991
10. Alexander CA: A modified Intavent laryngeal mask for ENT and dental anaesthesia. Anaesthesia 45:892, 1990
11. Haynes SR, Morton NS: The laryngeal mask airway: A review of its use in paediatric anaesthesia. Paediatr Anaesth 3:65, 1993
12. Nair I, Bailey PM: Review of uses of the laryngeal mask in ENT anaesthesia. Anaesthesia 50:898, 1995
13. Williams PJ, Bailey PM: Comparison of the reinforced laryngeal mask airway and tracheal intubation for adenotonsillectomy. Br J Anaesth 70:30, 1993
14. Hatcher IS, Stack CG: Postal survey of the anaesthetic techniques used for paediatric tonsillectomy surgery. Paediatr Anaesth 9:311, 1999
15. Mason DG, Bingham RM: The laryngeal mask airway in children. Anaesthesia 45:760, 1990
16. Goudsouzian NG, Cleveland R: Stability of the laryngeal mask airway during marked extension of the neck. Paediatr Anaesth 3:117, 1993
17. Ferrari LR, Donlon JV: Metoclopramide reduces the incidence of vomiting after tonsillectomy in children. Anesth Analg 75:351, 1992

18. Sukhani R, Pappas AL, Lurie J *et al*: Ondansetron and dolasetron provide equivalent postoperative vomiting control after ambulatory tonsillectomy in dexamethasone-pretreated children. Anesth Analg 95:1230, 2002
19. Crysdale WS, Russel D: Complications of tonsillectomy and adenoidectomy in 9409 children observed overnight. CMAJ 135:1139, 1986
20. Linden BE, Gross CW, Long TE *et al*: Morbidity in pediatric tonsillectomy. Laryngoscope 100:120, 1990
21. Broadman LM, Patel RI, Feldman BA *et al*: The effects of peritonsillar infiltration on the reduction of intraoperative blood loss and post-tonsillectomy pain in children. Laryngoscope 99:578, 1989
22. Galvis AG, Stool SE, Bluestone CD: Pulmonary edema following relief of acute upper airway obstruction. Ann Otol Rhinol Laryngol 89:124, 1980
23. Allen SJ: New concepts in the management of pulmonary edema. ASA Refresher Courses 22:11, 1994
24. Colclasure JB, Graham SS: Complications of outpatient tonsillectomy and adenoidectomy: A review of 3,340 cases. Ear Nose Throat J 69:155, 1990
25. Guida RA, Mattucci KF: Tonsillectomy and adenoidectomy: An inpatient or outpatient procedure? Laryngoscope 100:491, 1990
26. Brown OE, Cunningham MJ: Tonsillectomy and adenoidectomy inpatient guidelines. Am Acad Otololaryngol Head Neck Surg Bull 15:13, 1996
27. Tait AR, Knight PR: The effects of general anesthesia on upper respiratory tract infections in children. Anesthesiology 67:930, 1987
28. Tait AR, Malviya S, Voepel-Lewis T *et al*: Risk factors for perioperative adverse respiratory events in children with upper respiratory tract infections. Anesthesiology 95:299, 2001
29. DeSoto H, Patel RI, Soliman IE *et al*: Changes in oxygen saturation following general anesthesia in children with upper respiratory infection signs and symptoms undergoing otolaryngological procedures. Anesthesiology 68:276, 1988
30. Levine RA, Ronner SF, Ojemann RG: Auditory evoked potential and other neurophysiologic monitoring techniques during tumor surgery in the cerebellopontine angle. In Levine RA, Ronner SF, Ojemann RG (eds): Intraoperative Monitoring Techniques in Neurosurgery, p 175. New York, McGraw-Hill, 1994
31. Casey WF, Drake-Lee AB: Nitrous oxide and middle ear pressure. A study of induction methods in children. Anaesthesia 37:896, 1982
32. Zalzal GH: Stridor and airway compromise. Pediatr Clin North Am 36:1389, 1989
33. Woods AM: Pediatric bronchoscopy, bronchography and laryngoscopy. In Woods AM (ed): Anesthetic Management of Difficult and Routine Pediatric Patients, p 189. New York, Churchill Livingstone, 1986
34. Sanders RD: Two ventilating attachments for bronchoscopes. Del Med J 39:170, 1967
35. Steward DJ: Percutaneous transtracheal ventilation for laser endoscopic procedures in infants and small children. Can J Anaesth 34:429, 1987
36. Hermens JM, Bennett MJ, Hirshman CA: Anesthesia for laser surgery. Anesth Analg 62:218, 1983
37. McLesky CH: Anesthetic management of patients undergoing endoscopic laser surgery. In McLesky CH (ed): IARS Review Course Lectures, p 135. Cleveland, International Anesthesia Research Society (IARS), 1988
38. Sosis MB, Dillon FX: Saline-filled cuffs help prevent laser-induced polyvinylchloride endotracheal tube fires. Anesth Analg 72:187, 1991
39. Haskell R: Applied surgical anatomy. In Haskell R (ed): Maxillo Facial Injuries, p 3. Edinburgh, Churchill Livingstone, 1985
40. Huelke DF, Patrick LM: Mechanics in the production of mandibular fractures: Strain-gauge measurements of impacts to the chin. J Dent Res 43:437, 1964
41. Halazonetis JA: The 'weak' regions of the mandible. Br J Oral Surg 6:37, 1968
42. Nahum AM: The biomechanics of facial bone fracture. Laryngoscope 85:140, 1975
43. Olson RA, Fonseca RJ, Zeitler DL *et al*: Fractures of the mandible: A review of 580 cases. J Oral Maxillofac Surg 40:23, 1982
44. LeFort R: Etude experimentale sur les fractures de la machoire superieure. Rev Chir 23:208, 1901
45. Burke J: Angina Ludovici A translation, together with a biography of Wilhelm Frederick von Ludwig. Bull Hist Med 7:1115, 1939
46. Ballenger JJ: Diseases of the Nose, Throat, Ear, Head and Neck, 14, p 240. Philadelphia, Lea & Febiger, 1991
47. Moreland LW, Corey J, McKenzie R: Ludwig's angina. Report of a case and review of the literature. Arch Intern Med 148:461, 1988
48. Loughnan TE, Allen DE: Ludwig's angina. The anaesthetic management of nine cases. Anaesthesia 40:295, 1985
49. Annandale T: On displacement of the inter-articular cartilage of the lower jaw, and its treatment by operation. Lancet 1:411, 1887
50. McCain JP, Sanders B, Koslin MG *et al*: Temporomandibular joint arthroscopy: A 6-year multicenter retrospective study of 4,831 joints. J Oral Maxillofac Surg 50:926, 1992
51. Kinney RK, Gatchel RJ, Ellis E *et al*: Major psychological disorders in chronic TMD patients: Implications for successful management. J Am Dent Assoc 123:49, 1992
52. Sanders B: Arthroscopic surgery of the temporomandibular joint: Treatment of internal derangement with persistent closed lock. Oral Surg Oral Med Oral Pathol 62:361, 1986
53. Hendler BH, Levin LM: Postobstructive pulmonary edema as a sequela of temporomandibular joint arthroscopy: A case report. J Oral Maxillofac Surg 51:315, 1993
54. Luce EA, Tubb TD, Moore AM: Review of 1,000 major facial fractures and associated injuries. Plast Reconstr Surg 63:26, 1979
55. Davidson JS, Birdsell DC: Cervical spine injury in patients with facial skeletal trauma. J Trauma 29:1276, 1989
56. Har-El G, Aroesty JH, Shaha A *et al*: Changing trends in deep neck abscess. A retrospective study of 110 patients. Oral Surg Oral Med Oral Pathol 77:446, 1994
57. Durham CF, Harrison TS: The surgical anatomy of the superior laryngeal nerve. Surg Gynecol Obstet 118:38, 1964
58. Gotta AW, Sullivan CA: Superior laryngeal nerve block: An aid to intubating the patient with fractured mandible. J Trauma 24:83, 1984
59. Ferson DZ, Brimacombe J, Brain AI *et al*: The intubating laryngeal mask airway. Int Anesthesiol Clin 36:183, 1998
60. Bailey P, Brimacombe JR, Keller C: The flexible LMA: Literature considerations and practical guide. Int Anesthesiol Clin 36:111, 1998
61. Kitahata LM, Collins WF: Meningitis as a complication of anesthesia in a patient with a basal skull fracture. Anesthesiology 32:282, 1970
62. Dacosta A, Billard JL, Gery P *et al*: Posttraumatic intracerebral pneumatocele after ventilation with a mask: Case report. J Trauma 36:255, 1994
63. Zsigmond EK, Matsuki A, Kothary SP *et al*: Arterial hypoxemia caused by intravenous ketamine. Anesth Analg 55:311, 1976
64. Gardner AE, Olson BE, Lichtiger M: Cerebrospinal-fluid pressure during dissociative anesthesia with ketamine. Anesthesiology 35:226, 1971
65. Takeshita H, Okuda Y, Sari A: The effects of ketamine on cerebral circulation and metabolism in man. Anesthesiology 36:69, 1972
66. Gotta AW, Sullivan CA, Pelkofski J *et al*: Aberrant conduction as a precursor to cardiac arrhythmias during anesthesia for oral surgery. J Oral Surg 34:421, 1976

CHAPTER 35 ■ THE RENAL SYSTEM AND ANESTHESIA FOR UROLOGIC SURGERY

JEROME F. O'HARA Jr., JACEK B. CYWINSKI, AND TERRI G. MONK

KEY POINTS

1. Renal filtration and reabsorption are susceptible to alterations by surgical illness and anesthesia. Autoregulation of renal blood flow (RBF) is effective over a wide range of mean arterial pressure (50 to 150 mm Hg). Autoregulation of urine flow does not occur, but a linear relationship between mean arterial pressure above 50 mm Hg and urine output is observed.
2. Renal medullary blood flow is low (receives 2% of total RBF) but essential to the kidneys' ability to concentrate urine. During periods of reduced RBF, the metabolically active medullary thick ascending limb (mTAL) may be especially vulnerable to ischemic injury.
3. Patient response to surgical stress uses intrinsic mechanisms for sodium and water conservation. Renal cortical vasoconstriction, shift in RBF to salt-and-water-conserving juxtamedullary nephrons, decrease in glomerular filtration rate (GFR), retention of salt and water result.
4. The patient's stress response may induce a decrease in RBF and GFR, causing afferent arteriolar constriction. If an extreme situation is not reversed, ischemic damage to the kidney may result in acute renal failure (ARF).
5. Anesthetic-induced reductions in RBF have been described for many agents, but are usually clinically insignificant and reversible. Likewise, anesthetic agents have not been shown to interfere with renal neurohumoral responses to physiologic stress.
6. Overall, there are no conclusive comparative studies demonstrating superior renal protection or improved renal outcome with general versus regional anesthesia.
7. Isolated ARF carries a mortality of up to 10% in surgical patients, with acute tubular necrosis (ATN) being the etiology for ARF in most of these patients.
8. Surgical patients with nondialysis chronic renal failure (CRF) are at higher risk to develop end-stage renal disease (ESRD). The single most reliable predictor of postoperative renal dysfunction is preoperative renal dysfunction.
9. Maintaining adequate intravascular volume and hemodynamic stability with aggressive management of kidney hypoperfusion is a basic tenet of anesthetic care to prevent ARF.
10. Irrigation fluid absorption during the transurethral resection of the prostate (TURP) procedure is directly related to the number and size of venous sinuses opened, duration of the resection, hydrostatic pressure of the irrigating fluid, and venous pressure at the irrigant–blood interface. Studies comparing general with spinal anesthesia reveal no difference in mortality and morbidity.

The kidney plays a central role in implementing and controlling a variety of homeostatic functions, including excreting metabolic waste products in the form of urine, while keeping extracellular fluid volume and composition constant. Renal dysfunction can occur perioperatively as a direct result of surgical or medical disease, prolonged reduction in renal oxygen delivery, nephrotoxin insult, or, frequently, a combination of the three. The first part of this chapter reviews renal physiology and pathophysiologic states as they relate to anesthetic practice, and then addresses strategies for recognizing and managing patients at risk for renal failure. The second part describes current urological procedures and their attendant anesthetic management issues.

RENAL ANATOMY AND PHYSIOLOGY

Anatomy and Innervation of the Genitourinary System

The kidneys and ureters are located in the retroperitoneal space, with their center at the L2 vertebral body. Renal pain sensation is conveyed back to spinal cord segments T10–L1 by sympathetic fibers. Sympathetic innervation is supplied by preganglionic fibers from T8–L1. The vagus nerve provides parasympathetic innervation to the kidney, and the S2–S4 spinal segments supply the ureters (Fig. 35-1).

The bladder is located in the retropubic space and receives its innervation from sympathetic nerves originating from T11–L2, which conduct pain, touch, and temperature sensations, whereas bladder stretch sensation is transmitted via parasympathetic fibers from segments S2–S4. Parasympathetics also provide the bladder with most of its motor innervation (Fig. 35-2).

The prostate, penile urethra, and penis also receive sympathetic and parasympathetic fibers from the T11–L2 and S2–S4 segments, respectively. The pudendal nerve provides pain sensation to the penis via the dorsal nerve of the penis. Sensory innervation of the scrotum is via cutaneous nerves, which project to lumbosacral segments, whereas testicular sensation is conducted to lower thoracic and upper lumbar segments (see Fig. 35-2).

Anatomy of the Nephron

The *nephron* is the microscopic functional unit of the kidney and is elegantly designed to carry out its excretory and regulatory roles (Fig. 35-3). The *glomerulus* is a capillary network that serves as the basic filtering unit of the nephron and is situated in the outer cortex of the kidney. Blood to be filtered enters the glomerular tuft through the afferent arteriole and eventually exits the glomerulus through the efferent arteriole. The initial segment of the renal tubular system, called *Bowman's capsule,* envelops the glomerulus. The glomerular filtrate passes from Bowman's capsule into the proximal tubule and then into the descending loop of Henle, which dips deep into the medullary portion of the kidney. The ascending limb of the loop ascends back to the cortex. In the cortex, the distal tubule comes into contact with the afferent and efferent arterioles to form the juxtaglomerular apparatus. The distal tubule then proceeds through the cortex to join with other tubules to form cortical collecting ducts. These collecting ducts again plunge into the medulla, coalesce, and eventually empty urine into the renal pelvis, which is drained by the ureters. Blood supply to the entire tubular system comes from the glomerular efferent arteriole, which branches into an extensive capillary network. Some of these peritubular capillaries, the *vasa recta,* descend deep into the medulla to parallel the loops of Henle. The vasa recta then return in a cortical direction with the loops, join other peritubular capillaries, and empty into the cortical veins.

Renal Physiology

The kidney fulfills its dual roles of waste excretion and body fluid management by filtering large amounts of fluid and solutes from the blood, reabsorbing needed components of this filtrate, and secreting waste products into the tubular fluid.[1] Filtration and reabsorption are susceptible to alterations by surgical illness and anesthesia and are the focus of this discussion.

Glomerular Filtration

Urine production begins with filtration of water and solutes from blood flowing through the afferent arteriole. The glomerular membrane serves as the filter, whereas Bowman's capsule acts as the initial receptacle for the filtrate. The kidneys receive ~20% of the systemic cardiac output and are able to filter 10% of this volume to produce 180 L/day of glomerular filtrate. More than 99% of the filtered fluid is reabsorbed and returned to the circulation, resulting in 1 to 2 L of urine output per day in healthy adults.

The *glomerular filtration rate* (GFR) is a measure of glomerular function expressed as milliliters of filtrate produced per minute. GFR can be thought of as the product of the tendency of the glomerular membrane to allow filtration to occur

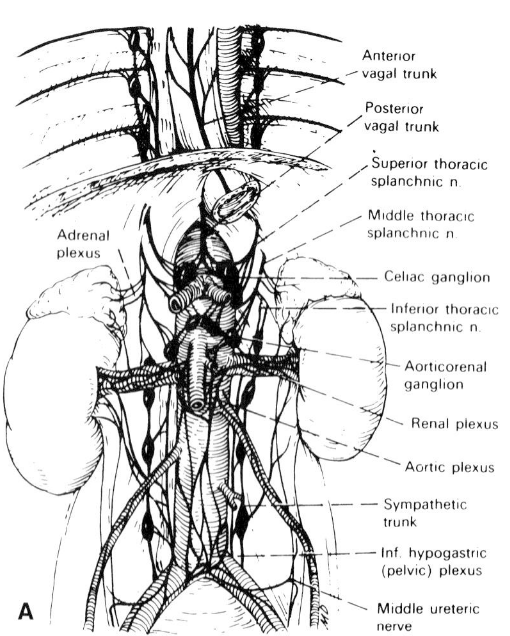

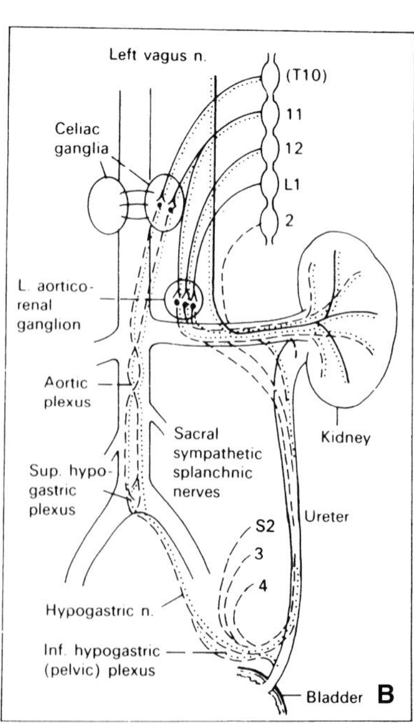

FIGURE 35-1. **A.** Anatomy and innervation of the kidney and ureters. **B.** Schematic illustration of the autonomic and sensory nerve pathways supplying the kidney and ureters. (Reprinted with permission from Ansell JS, Gee WF: Diseases of the kidney and ureter. In Bonica JJ [ed]: The Management of Pain, p 1233. Philadelphia, Lea & Febiger, 1990.)

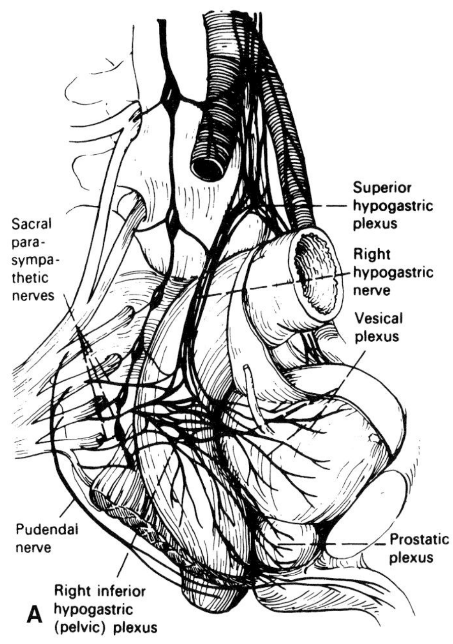

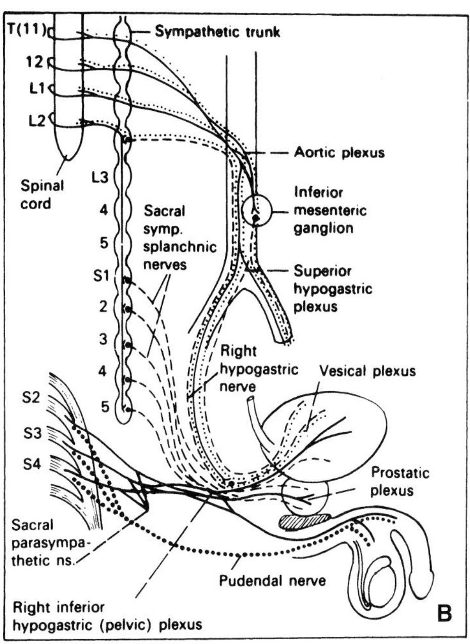

FIGURE 35-2. A. Anatomy and innervation of the urinary bladder and prostate. B. Schematic illustration of the innervation of the bladder, penis, and scrotum. Solid lines, preganglionic fibers; dashed lines, postganglionic fibers; dotted lines, sensory fibers. (Reprinted with permission from Gee WF, Ansell JS: Pelvic and peritoneal pain of urologic origin. In Bonica JJ [ed]: The Management of Pain, p 1369. Philadelphia, Lea & Febiger, 1990.)

(i.e., glomerular permeability and surface area) and the pressure inside the glomerular capillary that forces fluid through the filter.

The *ultrafiltration constant* (Kf) is directly related to glomerular capillary permeability and glomerular surface area. Glomerular capillary permeability is relatively constant, but the glomerular surface area can be reduced by intense sympathetic or angiotensin II stimulation, which in turn decreases GFR.

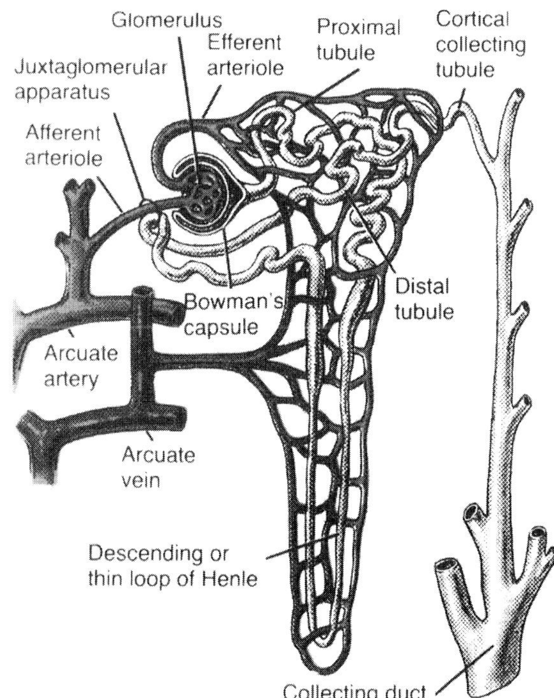

FIGURE 35-3. Anatomy of the nephron. (Reprinted with permission from Guyton AC: Formation of urine by the kidney: Renal blood flow, glomerular filtration, and their control. In Guyton AC [ed]: Textbook of Medical Physiology, 8th ed, p 287. Philadelphia, WB Saunders, 1991.)

Changes in glomerular filtration pressure exercise the greatest influence on GFR in the normal and pathologic states. The two major determinants of filtration pressure are glomerular capillary pressure (P_{GC}) and glomerular oncotic pressure (π_{GC}). P_{GC} is directly related to renal artery pressure, but is heavily influenced by arteriolar tone at points upstream (afferent) and downstream (efferent) from the glomerulus. An increase in afferent arteriolar tone, as occurs with intense sympathetic or angiotensin II stimulation, causes filtration pressure and GFR to fall. Milder degrees of sympathetic or angiotensin activity cause a selective increase in efferent arteriolar tone, which tends to increase filtration pressure and GFR. The π_{GC} is directly dependent on plasma oncotic pressure. Afferent arteriolar dilatation enhances GFR by increasing glomerular flow, which in turn elevates glomerular capillary pressure. Efferent arteriolar constriction intense enough to slow glomerular blood flow produces opposing effects on the GFR.

Autoregulation of Renal Blood Flow and Glomerular Filtration Rate

From the preceding discussion, it is apparent that renal blood flow (RBF) and perfusion pressure determine GFR, in large part. To maintain relatively constant rates of RBF and glomerular filtration over a wide range of physiologic demands, the kidney must exercise some control over its own performance. Renal autoregulation of blood flow and filtration is accomplished by local feedback signals that modulate glomerular arteriolar tone.

1 Autoregulation of RBF is effective over a wide range of arterial pressure (Fig. 35-4). Two separate mechanisms for regulating blood flow to the glomerulus have been proposed, and both involve modulation of afferent arteriolar tone. A myogenic reflex has been postulated in which an increase in arterial pressure causes the afferent arteriolar wall to stretch and then through the reflex to constrict, whereas a decrease in arterial pressure causes arteriolar dilatation. The other proposed mechanism of RBF autoregulation is a phenomenon called *tubuloglomerular feedback,* which is also responsible for autoregulation of GFR.

Tubuloglomerular feedback control of RBF and GFR works by using the composition of distal tubular fluid to influence glomerular function through the *juxtaglomerular apparatus.* When RBF falls, the concomitant decrease in GFR results in

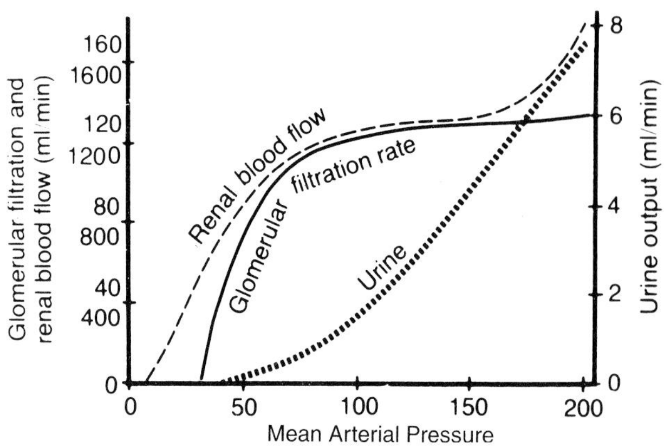

FIGURE 35-4. Autoregulation of glomerular filtration rate and renal blood flow over a wide range of arterial pressures. Note that urine output is not subject to autoregulation. (Reprinted with permission from Guyton AC: Formation of urine by the kidney: Renal blood flow, glomerular filtration, and their control. In Guyton AC [ed]: Textbook of Medical Physiology, 8th ed, p 293. Philadelphia, WB Saunders, 1991.)

less chloride ion delivery to the juxtaglomerular apparatus, which then signals the afferent arteriole to dilate. Glomerular flow and pressure then increase, and GFR returns to previous levels. Chloride ion also acts as the feedback signal for control of efferent arteriolar tone. When GFR falls, declining chloride ion delivery to the juxtaglomerular apparatus triggers release of *renin,* which causes formation of *angiotensin II.* In response to angiotensin, efferent arteriolar constriction increases glomerular pressure, which increases glomerular filtration. Simultaneous afferent arteriolar dilatation and efferent arteriolar constriction allow glomerular flow and filtration to increase.

Note from Fig. 35-4 that autoregulation of urine flow does not occur and that there is a linear relationship between mean arterial pressure above 50 mm Hg and urine output.

Tubular Reabsorption of Sodium and Water

The renal tubular system is responsible for selectively reabsorbing the vast quantities of fluid and solutes filtered by the glomeruli. Waste materials are thereby separated from essential solutes and excreted in the minimum volume of water possible.

The active, energy-dependent reabsorption of sodium begins almost immediately as filtrate enters the proximal tubule. Here, an adenosine triphosphatase pump drives the sodium into tubular cells while chloride ions passively follow. Glucose, amino acid, and other organic compound reabsorption is strongly coupled to sodium in the proximal tubule. Normally, the proximal tubule reabsorbs ~65% of the filtered sodium, but no active sodium transport occurs in the loop of Henle until the medullary thick ascending limb (mTAL) is reached. Cells of the mTAL are metabolically active in their role of reabsorbing sodium and chloride, and have a high oxygen consumption compared with the thin portions of the descending and ascending limbs. Sodium pumps in the distal tubule and collecting duct are unique in that they are under control of the adrenal hormone aldosterone.

Reabsorption of water is a passive, osmotically driven process tied to sodium and other solute reabsorption. Water reabsorption also depends on peritubular capillary pressure; high capillary pressure opposes water reabsorption in the proximal tubule and tends to increase urine output. The proximal tubule reabsorbs ~65% of filtered water in an isosmotic fashion with sodium and chloride. The descending limb of the loop of Henle allows water to follow osmotic gradients into the renal interstitium. However, the thin ascending limb and mTAL are relatively impermeable to water and play a key role in producing concentrated urine. Only approximately 15% of filtered water is reabsorbed by the loop of Henle, and the remaining 20% of the filtrate volume flows into the distal tubule. There, and in the collecting duct, water reabsorption is controlled entirely by antidiuretic hormone (ADH) secreted by the pituitary gland.

Conservation of water and excretion of excess solute by the kidneys would become untenable without the ability to produce concentrated urine. This is accomplished by establishing a hyperosmotic medullary interstitium and regulating water permeability of the distal tubule and collecting duct with ADH.

The medullary interstitium would eventually lose its hyperosmolarity by washout of solutes were it not for the unique role of the vasa recta. The vasa recta prevents medullary solute washout by providing for a countercurrent exchange of ions, which continually "recycles" solutes between its descending
2 and ascending arms. Medullary blood flow is low (it receives 2% of total RBF) but essential to renal concentrating ability. During periods of reduced RBF, the metabolically active mTAL may be especially vulnerable to ischemic injury.[2]

All that is now necessary to produce concentrated urine is to alter the water permeability of the distal tubule and collecting duct in response to bodily needs. ADH increases the water permeability of these structures and allows for passive diffusion of water (under considerable osmotic pressure) back into the circulation. The posterior pituitary releases ADH in response to an increase in either extracellular sodium concentration or extracellular osmolality. In addition, ADH release can be triggered by a perceived reduction in intravascular fluid volume. The arterial baroreceptors are activated when hypovolemia leads to a decrease in blood pressure, whereas atrial receptors are stimulated by a decline in atrial filling pressure. Both of these circulatory reflex systems stimulate release of ADH from the pituitary and cause retention of water by the kidney in an effort to return the intravascular volume toward normal. ADH also causes renal cortical vasoconstriction when it is released in large amounts, such as during the physiologic stress response to trauma, surgery, or other critical illness. This induces a shift of RBF to the hypoxia-prone renal medulla.

Neurohumoral regulation of sodium reabsorption by the kidney is another important component of the physiologic response to stress. The hormonal messengers involved in sodium management also have potent vasoactive effects on both the renal and systemic vasculature.

Renin-Angiotensin-Aldosterone System. Renin-angiotensin activity plays an important role in regulating RBF and GFR. Renin release by the renal afferent arteriole may be triggered by hypotension, increased tubular fluid chloride ion concentration, or sympathetic stimulation. Renin enhances angiotensin II production, which induces renal efferent arteriolar vasoconstriction. Angiotensin II also promotes ADH release from the posterior pituitary, sodium reabsorption by the proximal tubule, and aldosterone release by the adrenal medulla. Aldosterone, in turn, stimulates the distal tubule and collecting duct to actively reabsorb sodium (and water), resulting in intravascular volume expansion. Sympathetic nervous system stimulation may also directly cause release of aldosterone. Thus, response of the body to surgical stress uses existing mechanisms for sodium and water conservation. This results in renal cortical vasoconstriction, a shift in RBF to salt-and-water–conserving juxtamedullary nephrons, a decrease in GFR, and salt and water retention. Clinically, this tendency toward oliguria and edema formation may persist for several days into the postoperative period because of ongoing stress (pain, sepsis, hypovolemia).

Renal Vasodilator Mechanisms. Opposing the salt and water retention and vasoconstriction observed in stress states and mediated by the sympathetic nervous system, ADH, and the renin-angiotensin-aldosterone system are the actions of *atrial natriuretic peptide* (ANP), *nitric oxide*, and the renal *prostaglandin* system. ANP is released by the cardiac atria in response to increased stretch under conditions of relative hypervolemia. Both salt and water excretion increase as ANP blocks reabsorption of sodium in the distal tubule and collecting duct. ANP also increases GFR, causes systemic vasodilatation, inhibits release of renin, opposes production and action of angiotensin II, and decreases aldosterone secretion.[3–5] Nitric oxide produced by the kidney opposes the renal vasoconstrictor effects of angiotensin II and the adrenergic nervous system, increases sodium and water excretion, and participates in the tubuloglomerular feedback system.[6]

Prostaglandins are produced by the kidney as part of a complex system that modulates RBF and opposes the actions of ADH, norepinephrine, and the renin-angiotensin-aldosterone system.[7] Stress states, renal ischemia, and hypotension stimulate the production of renal prostaglandins through the enzymes phospholipase A_2 and cyclooxygenase. Prostaglandins produced by cyclooxygenase activity cause dilatation of renal arterioles (antiangiotensin II), whereas their distal tubular effects result in an increase in sodium and water excretion (anti-ADH and aldosterone). The renal prostaglandin system is important in maintaining RBF and sodium and water excretion during times of high physiologic stress and poor renal perfusion.[7] This defensive role for the prostaglandins has been confirmed by experiments demonstrating that cyclooxygenase inhibition has damaging effects in the ischemic kidney, but not in the unstressed state.[8] Conversely, stimulation of prostaglandin synthesis or administration of exogenous prostaglandin E_2 protects the kidney from hypoxic injury.[9]

RENAL DYSFUNCTION AND ANESTHESIA

Altered renal function can be represented as a clinical continuum that ranges from normal compensatory changes during stress to frank renal failure. Clinically, there is considerable overlap between compensated and decompensated renal dysfunctional states.

The kidney under stress reacts in a predictable manner to help restore intravascular volume and maintain blood pres-
3 sure. The sympathetic nervous system reacts to trauma, shock, or pain by releasing norepinephrine, which acts much like angiotensin II on the renal arterioles. Norepinephrine also activates the renin-angiotensin-aldosterone system and causes ADH release. The net result of modest activity of the stress response system is characterized by a shift of blood flow from the renal cortex to the medulla, avid sodium and water reabsorption, and decreased urine output. A more intense stress response may induce a decrease in RBF and GFR by causing afferent arteriolar constriction. If this extreme situation is not reversed, ischemic damage to the kidney may result, and acute renal failure (ARF) may become clinically manifest. More often,
4 some other insult contributes to renal failure in the "stressed" patient with coexisting renal vasoconstriction.[10]

With the exception of methoxyflurane and possibly enflurane, anesthetic agents do not directly cause renal dysfunction or interfere with normal compensatory mechanisms activated by the stress response. Nephrotoxicity of methoxyflurane appears to be due to its metabolism, which results in release of fluoride ions believed to be responsible for the renal injury.[11] It has been suggested that renal, not hepatic, metabolism of methoxyflurane may be responsible for generating fluoride ions locally that contribute to nephrotoxicity.[12] Enflurane nephrotoxicity may occur,[13] but it seems to be of minor clinical importance, even in patients with preexisting renal dysfunction.[14] Controversy over sevoflurane-induced nephrotoxicity appears to be waning and is discussed in Chapter 15. Anesthetic-induced reductions in RBF have been described for many agents, but are clinically insignificant and
5 reversible.[15,16] Likewise, anesthetic agents have not been shown to interfere with renal neurohumoral responses to physiologic stress.

Although direct anesthetic effects on the kidney are usually not harmful, indirect effects may combine with hypovolemia, shock, nephrotoxin exposure, or other renal vasoconstrictive states to produce renal dysfunction. If the chosen anesthetic technique causes a protracted reduction in cardiac output or sustained hypotension that coincides with a period of intense renal vasoconstriction, renal dysfunction or failure could result. This is true for either general or regional anesthesia. There
6 are no comparative studies demonstrating superior renal protection or improved renal outcome with general versus regional anesthesia.

Acute Renal Failure

ARF is a sudden decrease in renal function resulting in inability of the kidneys to excrete nitrogenous and other wastes. This is manifested by accumulation of creatinine and urea in the blood (uremia) and is often accompanied by reduced urine production, although nonoliguric forms of postoperative ARF are common.[17] Isolated ARF carries a mortality of <10%.[18] In surgical patients, acute tubular necrosis (ATN) is the most common etiology of ARF. ARF frequently occurs in the setting
7 of critical surgical illness with multiple organ failure (MOF) (it is rarely an isolated event), mortality is alarmingly high (up to 90%), and the mortality rate may be higher for surgical patients than for medical patients with renal failure.[19]

A contributing factor to poor outcome is the fact that extracorporeal renal support appears to have had little success in altering the course of ARF in critically ill surgical patients.[20,21] Even studies that advocate use of extracorporeal technology report mortality of between 50% and 70%.[22–25]

Active renal failure can be classified as arising from *prerenal* factors causing renal hypoperfusion, numerous *intrinsic* renal etiologies, or *postrenal* causes (obstructive uropathy). There are many pathophysiologic similarities between the various causes of renal failure that ultimately lead to a common syndrome referred to as *organic ARF* (Fig. 35-5).

Prerenal Azotemia and Acute Tubular Necrosis

Prerenal azotemia is the increase in blood urea nitrogen (BUN) associated with renal hypoperfusion or ischemia that has not caused renal parenchymal damage. As such, it forms a continuum with ATN. The metabolically active cells of the mTAL of Henle are especially vulnerable to hypoxic damage because of their relatively high oxygen consumption-to-delivery ratio.[2] Necrosis of tubular cells releases debris into the tubules, causing flow obstruction, increased tubular pressure, and back leak of tubular fluid (see Fig. 35-5). Often, prerenal failure is precipitated in patients with preexisting renal vasoconstriction (e.g., volume depletion, heart failure, sepsis) by nephrotoxin exposure or reduction in cardiac output.[26]

Intrinsic Acute Renal Failure

The term "intrinsic" not only implies a primary renal etiology of ARF, but also includes ischemia, toxins, and renal parenchymal diseases. ATN remains the most common ischemic lesion and represents an extension of prerenal azotemia, whereas cortical necrosis may follow a massive renovascular insult such as prolonged suprarenal aortic clamping or renal artery

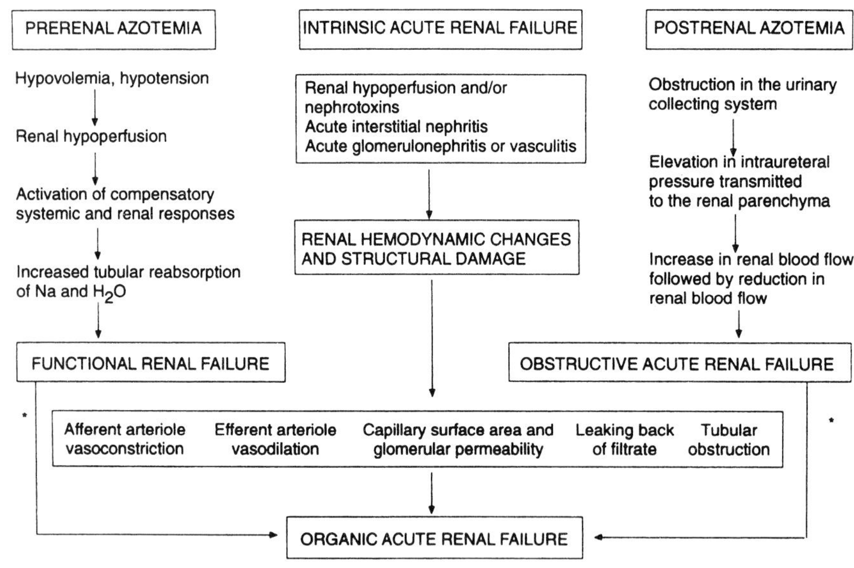

FIGURE 35-5. Mechanisms of acute renal failure. *, Depending on severity and duration of injury. (Reprinted with permission from Pelanda MV, Fabris A, Ronco C: Etiology and pathophysiology of acute renal failure. In Pinsky MR, Dhainaut JFA [eds]: Pathophysiologic Foundations of Critical Care, p 575. Baltimore, Williams & Wilkins, 1993.)

embolism. Nephrotoxins often act in concert with hypoperfusion or underlying renal vasoconstrictive states to damage renal tubules or microvasculature. Several common nephrotoxins, some of which are difficult to avoid in a hospitalized patient population, are listed in Table 35-1. Renal parenchymal diseases may affect either the glomerulus or interstitium, and are frequently immune mediated or part of a more systemic disorder that targets the kidney.

Postrenal Azotemia: Obstructive Uropathy

Downstream obstruction of the urinary collecting system is the least common pathway to organic ARF, accounting for <5% of cases.[26] The obstructing lesion may occur at any level of the collecting system, from the renal pelvis to the distal urethra. Intraluminal pressure then rises and is eventually transmitted back to the glomerulus, thereby reducing its filtration pressure.

TABLE 35-1

NEPHROTOXINS COMMONLY FOUND IN THE HOSPITAL SETTING

EXOGENOUS	ENDOGENOUS
Antibiotics	Calcium (hypercalcemia)
Aminoglycosides, cephalosporins, amphotericin B, sulfonamide, tetracyclines, vancomycin	Uric acid (hyperuricemia and hyperuricosuria)
Anesthetic agents	Myoglobin (rhabdomyolysis)
Methoxyflurane, enflurane	Hemoglobin (hemolysis)
Nonsteroidal anti-inflammatory drugs	Bilirubin (obstructive jaundice)
Aspirin, ibuprofen, naproxen, indomethacin, ketorolac	Oxalate crystals
Chemotherapeutic–immunosuppressive agents	Paraproteins
Cisplatinum, cyclosporin A, methotrexate, mitomycin, nitrosoureas, tacrolimus	
Contrast media	

Intraoperative Oliguria: Prerenal Azotemia or Acute Tubular Necrosis

Several real-time RBF monitors are being developed for intraoperative and critical care use (see Perioperative Assessment of Renal Function section). However, urine flow rate has traditionally been used as a measure of renal "well-being," a job for which it is ill suited.[27] Nevertheless, oliguria (urine flow rate of <0.5 mL/kg/hr) may be a useful sign of renal hypoperfusion when other objective signs of reduced systemic blood flow are present and the overall clinical scenario is appropriate. The presumption should be that intraoperative oliguria is a normal response to the stress of surgery and ongoing blood and fluid losses. If a fluid bolus improves the urine flow rate, or the heart rate and blood pressure indicate hypovolemia, further fluid administration is indicated. Isolated hypovolemia can usually be corrected relatively quickly as long as ongoing loss of blood and intravascular fluid are also replaced. If oliguria persists and signs of heart failure or volume overload appear, the patient's hemodynamic profile can be further assessed with a pulmonary artery catheter or transesophageal echocardiography to optimize cardiac output and systemic oxygen delivery and to improve renal perfusion.

When sepsis is responsible for poor urine output, hypotension is a common finding and is usually secondary to systemic vasodilation, hypovolemia, and depressed myocardial contractility. Hypovolemia should be corrected with vigorous fluid resuscitation, while combinations of inotropic–vasopressor agents, such as dopamine, norepinephrine, phenylephrine, or dobutamine, are given to increase cardiac output, systemic vascular resistance, and renal perfusion pressure.[28–30]

Chronic Renal Failure

Patients with nondialysis chronic renal failure (CRF) are at increased risk of developing *end-stage renal disease* (ESRD). ESRD is the term used to describe a clinical syndrome characterized by multiple organ dysfunction that would prove fatal without dialysis. These patients have GFRs <25% of normal. Lesser degrees of renal dysfunction are categorized as renal insufficiency (25 to 40% of normal GFR) or decreased renal reserve (60 to 75% of normal GFR). Patients with decreased renal reserve are asymptomatic and frequently do not have

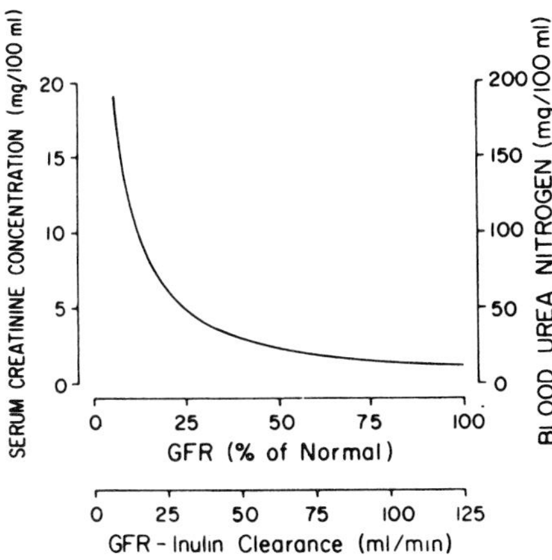

FIGURE 35-6. Relationship of serum creatinine concentration and blood urea nitrogen levels to glomerular filtration rate (GFR). (Reprinted with permission from Valtin H: Renal Dysfunction: Mechanisms Involved in Fluid and Solute Imbalance, p 206, Boston, Little, Brown, 1979.)

abnormally elevated blood levels of creatinine or urea (Fig. 35-6). Renal insufficiency results in clearly abnormal creatinine and BUN values, but nocturia (due to decreased concentrating ability) may be the only symptom.

The *uremic syndrome* represents the most extreme form of CRF, which occurs as the surviving nephron population and GFR decrease below 10% of normal. It results in inability of the kidney to perform its two major duties: regulating the volume and composition of extracellular fluid and excreting waste products. The loss of homeostasis, accumulation of cellular toxins, and inability of the kidney to maintain water balance causes multiple organ system dysfunction in the uremic syndrome[31] (Table 35-2). Water balance in ESRD becomes difficult to manage because the number of functioning nephrons is too small either to concentrate or to fully dilute the urine. This results in the inability to conserve water and to excrete excess water. Patients with uremic syndrome usually require frequent or continuous dialysis.

Life-threatening hyperkalemia may occur in CRF because of slower-than-normal potassium clearance. Situations predisposing patients with renal failure to hyperkalemia are presented in Table 35-3. Derangements in calcium, magnesium, and phosphorus metabolism are also commonly seen in CRF (see Table 35-2).

Metabolic acidosis occurs in two forms in ESRD: a hyperchloremic, normal–anion-gap acidosis and a high-gap acidosis due to inability to excrete titratable acids. Both render patients susceptible to an endogenous acid load as may occur in shock states, hypovolemia, or an increase in catabolism.

Cardiovascular complications of the uremic syndrome are primarily due to volume overload, high renin–angiotensin activity, autonomic nervous system hyperactivity, acidosis, and electrolyte disturbances. Hypertension due to extracellular fluid volume expansion, autonomic factors, and hyperreninemia is an almost universal finding in ESRD. Together with volume overload, acidemia, anemia, and high-flow arteriovenous fistulae created for dialysis access, hypertension contributes to development of myocardial dysfunction and heart failure. Pericarditis may occur secondary to uremia or dialysis, with pericardial tamponade developing in 20% of the latter group.[32] Pulmonary problems associated with CRF are limited to changes in lung water and control of ventilation. Pulmonary edema and restrictive pulmonary dysfunction are commonly seen in patients with renal failure and are responsive to dialysis. Hypervolemia, heart failure, reduced serum oncotic pressure, and increased pulmonary capillary permeability are factors in the development of pulmonary edema. Chronic metabolic acidosis may be responsible, in part, for the hyperventilation seen in patients with ESRD, but increased lung water and poor pulmonary compliance also stimulate ventilation.

The anemia of CRF is due to reduced levels of erythropoietin, red cell damage, ongoing gastrointestinal blood loss, and iron or vitamin deficiencies. Recombinant human erythropoietin has improved the management of anemia in ESRD.[33] Platelet dysfunction may aggravate blood loss, but it is responsive to dialysis, cryoprecipitate, and desmopressin acetate (or DDAVP). Acquired defects in both cellular and humoral immunity probably account for the high prevalence of serious infections (60%) and high mortality due to sepsis in CRF (30%).

Issues related to the gastrointestinal, neuromuscular, and endocrine-metabolism organ systems are listed in Table 35-2.

TABLE 35-2

THE UREMIC SYNDROME

■ WATER HOMEOSTASIS
Extracellular fluid expansion
■ ELECTROLYTE AND ACID-BASE
Hyponatremia Hyperkalemia Hypercalcemia or hypocalcemia Hyperphosphatemia Hypermagnesemia Metabolic acidosis
■ CARDIOVASCULAR
Heart failure Hypertension Pericarditis Myocardial dysfunction Dysrhythmias
■ RESPIRATORY
Pulmonary edema Central hyperventilation
■ HEMATOLOGIC
Anemia Platelet hemostatic defect
■ IMMUNOLOGIC
Cell-mediated and humoral immunity defects
■ GASTROINTESTINAL
Delayed gastric emptying, anorexia, nausea, vomiting, hiccups, upper gastrointestinal tract inflammation/hemorrhage
■ NEUROMUSCULAR
Encephalopathy, seizures, tremors, myoclonus Sensory and motor polyneuropathy Autonomic dysfunction, decreased baroreceptor responsiveness, dialysis-associated hypotension
■ ENDOCRINE-METABOLISM
Renal osteodystrophy ↓ Glucose intolerance Hypertriglyceridemia, ↑ atherosclerosis

TABLE 35-3

FACTORS CONTRIBUTING TO HYPERKALEMIA IN CHRONIC RENAL FAILURE

■ POTASSIUM INTAKE
Increased dietary intake
Exogenous IV supplementation
Potassium salts of drugs
Sodium substitutes
Blood transfusion
Gastrointestinal hemorrhage
■ POTASSIUM RELEASE FROM INTRACELLULAR STORES
Increased catabolism, sepsis
Metabolic acidosis
β-Adrenergic blocking agents
Digitalis intoxication (Na-K-ATPase inhibition)
Insulin deficiency
Succinylcholine
■ POTASSIUM EXCRETION
Acute decrease in GFR
Constipation
Potassium-sparing diuretics
Angiotensin-converting enzyme inhibitors (decreased aldosterone secretion)
Heparin (decreased aldosterone effect)

Na-K-ATPase, Na-K-adenosine triphosphatase; GFR, glomerular filtration rate; IV, intravenous.

Anesthetic Agents in Renal Failure

Significant renal impairment may affect the disposition, metabolism, and excretion of commonly used anesthetic agents. Inhalational anesthetics are, of course, an exception to the rule that drugs with central nervous system activity (which generally are lipid soluble) must be converted to more hydrophilic compounds by the liver before being excreted by the kidney. Water-soluble metabolites of agents that are not inhaled may accumulate in renal failure and contribute to prolongation of clinical effects if they possess even a small percentage of the pharmacologic activity of the parent drug. Drugs that are eliminated unchanged by the kidneys (e.g., certain nondepolarizing muscle relaxants, the cholinesterase inhibitors, many antibiotics, digoxin) may have a prolonged elimination half-life when given to patients with renal failure. Many drugs used in the practice of anesthesia are highly protein bound and may demonstrate exaggerated clinical effects when protein binding is reduced by uremia. Renal failure may also increase the volume of distribution of certain agents, thereby prolonging their elimination half-life. There is a paucity of data concerning the effects of renal failure on anesthetic drug metabolism,[34,35] and suspected pharmacodynamic changes in patients with renal failure have proved difficult to document for most drugs.[36]

Induction Agents and Sedatives

Thiopental serves as an example of how reduced protein binding in CRF may affect clinical use of an anesthetic agent. Burch and Stanski[37] showed that the free fraction of a thiopental induction dose is nearly doubled in patients with renal failure. This accounts for the exaggerated clinical effects of thiopental in these patients and explains the need for a decreased induction dose in uremic patients compared with normal patients.

Ketamine is less extensively protein bound than thiopental, and renal failure appears to have minimal influence on its free fraction. Redistribution and hepatic metabolism are largely responsible for termination of the anesthetic effects, with <3% of the drug excreted unchanged in the urine. Norketamine, the major metabolite, has one-third the pharmacologic activity of the parent drug and is further metabolized before it is excreted by the kidney.[38] Poor renal function is not known to alter the pharmacokinetics or clinical profile of ketamine.[39]

Etomidate, although only 75% protein bound in normal patients, has a larger free fraction in ESRD.[40] The decrease in protein binding does not seem to alter the clinical effects of an etomidate anesthetic induction in patients with renal failure.

Propofol undergoes extensive, rapid hepatic biotransformation to inactive metabolites that are renally excreted. Its pharmacokinetics appear to be unchanged in patients with renal failure,[41,42] and there are no reports of prolongation of its effects in ESRD.

The benzodiazepines, as a group, are extensively protein bound. CRF increases the free fraction of benzodiazepines in plasma, which may potentiate their clinical effect. Certain benzodiazepine metabolites are pharmacologically active and have the potential to accumulate with repeated administration of the parent drug to anephric patients. For example, 60 to 80% of midazolam is excreted as its (active) α-hydroxy metabolite,[43] which accumulates during long-term infusions in patients with renal failure.[44] ARF appears to slow the plasma clearance of midazolam,[44] whereas repeated diazepam or lorazepam administration in CRF may carry a risk of active metabolite-induced sedation.[35] Alprazolam is one of the few drugs related to anesthesia practice that has undergone pharmacodynamic studies in patients with CRF. Schmith et al.[45] found that when decreased protein binding and increased free fraction of alprazolam are taken into account, patients with CRF are actually more sensitive to its sedative effects than normal persons.

Dexmedetomidine is a relatively new sedative agent primarily metabolized in the liver. Volunteers with renal impairment receiving dexmedetomidine experienced a longer-lasting sedative effect than subjects with normal kidney function. The most likely explanation is that less protein binding of dexmedetomidine occurs in subjects with renal dysfunction.[46]

Opioids

Single-dose studies of morphine pharmacokinetics in renal failure demonstrate no alteration in its disposition. However, chronic administration results in accumulation of its 6-glucuronide metabolite, which has potent analgesic and sedative effects.[47] There is also a decrease in protein binding of morphine in ESRD, which mandates a reduction in its initial dose. Meperidine is remarkable for its neurotoxic, renally excreted metabolite (normeperidine) and is not recommended for use in patients with poor renal function. Hydromorphone is metabolized to hydromorphone-3-glucuronide, which is excreted by the kidneys. This active metabolite accumulates in patients with renal failure and may cause cognitive dysfunction and myoclonus.[48] Oxycodone elimination was found to be prolonged in a single-dose study of patients with CRF.[49] Repeated dosing of oxycodone should result in prolonged opioid effects. Codeine also has the potential for causing prolonged narcosis in patients with renal failure and cannot be recommended for long-term use.[47]

Fentanyl appears to be an excellent opioid for use in ESRD because of its lack of active metabolites, unchanged free fraction, and short redistribution phase.[35] Small to moderate doses, titrated to effect, are well tolerated by uremic patients. However, a dose of 25 μg/kg given to patients undergoing renal transplantation resulted in prolonged opioid effect that correlated with preoperative BUN.[50] Alfentanil has been shown to

TABLE 35-4

NONDEPOLARIZING MUSCLE RELAXANTS IN RENAL FAILURE[54,56,57,63,65,69,70,236–238]

DRUG	% RENAL EXCRETION	HALF-LIFE (hr) NORMAL/ESRD	RENALLY EXCRETED ACTIVE METABOLITE	USE IN ESRD
d-Tubocurarine	60	1.4–2.2	–	Avoid
Metocurine	45–60	6/11.4	–	Avoid
Pancuronium	30	2.3/4–8	+	Avoid
Gallamine	>85	2.5/6–20	–	Avoid
Pipecuronium	37	1.8–2.3/4.4	+	Avoid
Doxacurium	30	1.7/3.7	–	Avoid
Vecuronium	30	0.9/1.4	+	Normal single, smaller repeat doses; avoid prolonged CI
Rocuronium	30	1.2–1.6/1.6–1.7	–	Normal single, repeat doses, increased variability
Atracurium/ *cis*-atracurium	<5	0.3/0.4	–	Normal single, repeat, CI doses
Mivacurium	<7	2 min/2 min	–	Duration 1.5 × normal, lower CI dose
Rapacuronium	<12	0.5/0.5	++	Normal single dose, much smaller repeat dose, avoid CI

CI, continuous infusion; ESRD, end-stage renal disease.

have reduced protein binding but no change in its elimination half-life or clearance in ESRD, and is extensively metabolized to inactive compounds.[51] Therefore, caution should be exercised in administering a loading dose, but the total dose and infusion dose should be similar to those for patients with normal renal function. The free fraction of sufentanil is unchanged in ESRD; however, its pharmacokinetics are variable, and it has been reported to cause prolonged narcosis.[52]

Remifentanil is rapidly metabolized by blood and tissue esterases to a weakly active (about 4,600 times less potent as μ-opioid agonist), renally excreted metabolite, and remifentanil acid. Renal failure has no effect on clearance of remifentanil, but elimination of the principal metabolite, remifentanil acid, is markedly reduced. However, the clinical implications of this metabolite are limited.[53]

Muscle Relaxants

Muscle relaxants are the most likely group of drugs used in anesthetic practice to produce prolonged effects in ESRD because of their reliance on renal excretion (Table 35-4). (See also Chapter 16.) Only succinylcholine, atracurium, *cis*-atracurium, and mivacurium appear to have minimal renal excretion of the unchanged parent compound. Most nondepolarizing muscle relaxants must be either hepatically excreted or metabolized to inactive forms to terminate their activity in the absence of renal function. Some muscle relaxants have renally excreted, active metabolites that may contribute to their prolonged duration of action in patients with ESRD. Although the following discussion focuses on the pharmacology of individual muscle relaxants, coexisting acidosis and electrolyte disturbances, as well as drug therapy (e.g., aminoglycosides, diuretics, immunosuppressants, magnesium-containing antacids), may alter the pharmacodynamics of muscle relaxants in patients with renal failure.[54]

Succinylcholine has a long history of use in CRF that has been somewhat confused by conflicting reports of plasma cholinesterase activity in renal failure.[55,56] Its use can be justified as part of a rapid-sequence intubation technique because its duration of action in ESRD is not significantly prolonged. Use of a continuous infusion of succinylcholine, however, is more problematic because the major metabolite, succinylmonocholine, is weakly active and excreted by the kidney. Concern about the increase in serum potassium levels after succinylcholine administration (0.5 mEq/L in normal subjects) implies that the serum potassium should be normalized to the extent possible in patients with renal failure, but clinical experience has shown that the acute small increase in potassium following administration of succinylcholine is well tolerated in patients with persistently elevated potassium levels. Use of the long-acting muscle relaxants, doxacurium and pipecuronium, might also be questioned in patients with known renal insufficiency. In a single-dose study of doxacurium, Cook et al.[57] demonstrated an increased elimination half-life, reduced plasma clearance, and prolonged duration of effect in patients with renal failure. These data support the observations of Cashman et al.[58] that renal failure nearly doubles the clinical duration of doxacurium. Similar findings have been reported for the pharmacokinetics of pipecuronium.

Intermediate-acting muscle relaxants (atracurium, *cis*-atracurium, vecuronium, and rocuronium) have a distinct advantage in ESRD because of their shorter duration. The risk of a clinically significant, prolonged block is reduced. Atracurium and its derivative, *cis*-atracurium, undergo enzymatic ester hydrolysis and spontaneous nonenzymatic (Hoffman) degradation with minimal renal excretion of the parent compound. Their elimination half-life, clearance, and duration of action are not affected by renal failure,[59] nor have they been reported to cause prolonged clinical effects in ESRD. These characteristics strongly recommend the use of atracurium and *cis*-atracurium in patients with renal disease. One potential concern is that an atracurium metabolite, laudanosine, causes seizures in experimental animals and may accumulate with repeated dosing or continuous infusion.[60] This, however, has not been realized in intensive care patients with renal failure receiving prolonged infusions of atracurium.[61] Consistent with its greater potency and lower dosing requirements, *cis*-atracurium metabolism results in lower laudanosine blood levels than does atracurium in ESRD patients.[62]

The pharmacokinetics of vecuronium were initially reported as unchanged in renal failure, but it was later demonstrated that its duration of action was prolonged as a result of reduced plasma clearance and increased elimination half-life.[63] In addition, the active metabolite, 3-desmethylvecuronium, was shown to accumulate in anephric patients receiving a continuous vecuronium infusion who subsequently had prolonged neuromuscular blockade.[64] An intubating dose would be expected to last ~50% longer in patients with ESRD.[63]

Rocuronium, a rapid-onset muscle relaxant, has a pharmacokinetic profile in normal subjects similar to that of vecuronium.[65] Single-dose pharmacokinetic studies in patients with renal failure have reported conflicting results. Szenhradszky et al.[66] reported that renal failure increased the volume of distribution and elimination half-life of rocuronium, but had no effect on its clearance. Cooper et al.[67] found that clearance was reduced and duration of block widely variable in patients with renal failure, although mean duration of clinical relaxation and spontaneous recovery was not statistically different from that in control subjects. Wide variation in the duration of neuromuscular block has been reported by others, who also found that repeated maintenance doses of rocuronium were well tolerated in patients with ESRD.[68]

The short-acting muscle relaxant mivacurium is enzymatically eliminated by plasma pseudocholinesterase at a somewhat slower rate than succinylcholine. Low pseudocholinesterase activity correlates with slower recovery from a bolus dose of mivacurium in anephric patients.[56,69,70] The maintenance infusion dose has been reported to be both lower[69] and similar[70] to that in normal control subjects.

The pharmacokinetics of clinically available anticholinesterases are affected by renal failure.[71] They have a prolonged duration of action in ESRD because of their heavy reliance on renal excretion. The anticholinergic agents atropine and glycopyrrolate, used in conjunction with the anticholinesterases, are similarly excreted by the kidney.[72] Therefore, no dosage alteration of the anticholinesterases is required when antagonizing neuromuscular blockade in patients with reduced renal function.

PRESERVATION OF RENAL FUNCTION

Preventing renal failure in surgical patients is preferable to treating established ARF, given the poor outcome of these patients. To prevent ARF, the clinician must first identify those patients who are particularly at risk for perioperative renal damage and then focus on preserving renal function in that group. Certain patient-based indicators, nephrotoxin exposures, and surgical procedures are known risk factors for postoperative ARF (Table 35-5). Identifying these factors prior to surgery allows the anesthesiologist an opportunity to devise an anesthetic plan emphasizing renal preservation.

TABLE 35-5

RISK FACTORS FOR POSTOPERATIVE RENAL FAILURE

PATIENT-BASED INDICATORS
Preoperative renal dysfunction
Perioperative cardiac dysfunction
Sepsis
Hepatic failure, obstructive jaundice, ascites
Hypovolemia
Advanced age
NEPHROTOXIN EXPOSURE (SEE TABLE 35-1)
HIGH-RISK SURGICAL PROCEDURES
Cardiopulmonary bypass
Aortic clamping
Trauma/burn (emergency)
Hepatic transplantation
Renal transplantation
Partial nephrectomy

Patient-Based Risk Factors for Acute Renal Failure

Large, prospective studies of preoperative patient-based risk factors for ARF are lacking. Most often, retrospective reviews of ARF in surgical patients have revealed conflicting data that may be pertinent to a select patient population, but cannot be generalized to a larger group of patients. Novis et al.[73] published a review of the available prospective and retrospective studies examining patient-based risk factors for postoperative renal failure. Their report serves as the basis for the following discussion on preoperative risk factors, which can be easily identified with history, physical examination, and appropriate laboratory screening tests.

The single most reliable predictor of postoperative renal dysfunction is preoperative renal dysfunction.[73] Elevated BUN or creatinine levels, a history of renal dysfunction, or other ev-
8 idence of preexisting renal problems successfully predict postoperative ARF. It is likely that preexisting renal disease predisposes patients to further renal insult, but it may also make further loss of function easier to recognize.[73] The presumption, of course, is that it is essential to preserve what renal function the patient has. The alternative (frank renal failure) is potentially catastrophic. Identifying patients with preexisting renal dysfunction requires appropriate screening of BUN and creatinine in those who have other renal risk factors (history of renal problems, cardiac disease, or sepsis) or who are facing high-risk surgical procedures.

Preoperative cardiac dysfunction is another important predictor of postoperative ARF.[73] Shusterman et al.[74] identified heart failure as a risk factor in a mixed, surgical–medical population. Specifically, evidence of left ventricular dysfunction or elevated pulmonary capillary wedge pressure has predictive value in identifying patients at risk for ARF. This is intuitively obvious when one considers that poor cardiac output reduces RBF and increases the potential for renal vasoconstriction and ischemic injury. If left ventricular dysfunction is confirmed, medical management should be optimized before surgery whenever possible. Perioperative invasive monitoring can be helpful in managing fluid administration, oliguria, respiratory dysfunction, or further deterioration in cardiac performance.

Volume depletion has been reported to be a risk factor for ARP in both medical and surgical patients.[74] As with heart failure and sepsis, hypovolemia may induce renal vasoconstriction and render the kidney vulnerable to nephrotoxin exposure or further reduction in oxygen delivery. Patients with diabetes mellitus (and microangiopathy) are particularly prone to developing ARF when they become volume depleted.[74]

Cholestatic jaundice has long been suspected to be a risk factor for postoperative ARF.[75] Patients with severe cirrhosis and ascites or hepatic failure are clearly predisposed to renal dysfunction as a result of portal vein sepsis. In up to 75% of patients with hepatic failure, associated renal dysfunction/failure (hepatorenal syndrome) develops.[76]

Twenty-five percent of patients presenting for liver transplantation have some degree of renal dysfunction; posttransplantation, this percentage rises to almost 70%.[77] Preoperative serum creatinine levels can predict short-term survival of liver transplant recipients.[78]

Numerous investigators cite advanced age as a risk factor for postoperative ARF.[73] Patients who are elderly are frequently found to have reduced GFR, RBF, and renal reserve, making them less able to withstand a renal insult.[79] They also have a high incidence of cardiovascular disease and flow-limiting renal arterial atherosclerosis, which may account for their apparent increased risk of ARF. One study has convincingly demonstrated that advanced age increases the risk of ARF due to aminoglycoside toxicity.[74] However, age as an isolated risk factor has not been shown to predict postoperative ARF.[73]

Other risk factors for postoperative ARF were reviewed by Novis et al.,[73] but could not be conclusively shown to be significant. These included aortic aneurysm, acute bacterial endocarditis, decreased serum albumin, malignancy, emergency surgery, and previous cardiac surgery.

Perioperative Assessment of Renal Function

Although an accurate preoperative assessment of renal function is important in identifying high-risk patients, it would be advantageous to be able to differentiate prerenal azotemia from early ATN and predict impending ARF. Kellen et al.[27] examined the ability of commonly used renal function measures to predict and diagnose early ARF in critically ill patients. The findings of their meta-analysis of the specificity, sensitivity, and positive predictive value of renal function tests are summarized in Table 35-6.

Kellen et al. found that urine flow rate, specific gravity, and osmolality are poor indicators of renal dysfunction because they are influenced by many nonrenal variables. Serum creatinine and BUN are good screening tools for preoperative renal dysfunction, but they are late warning signs of reduced GFR. A sizable loss of GFR may occur before serum creatinine and BUN levels become abnormal (see Fig. 35-6). Unfortunately, creatinine and BUN are influenced by nonrenal variables such as catabolic rate and muscle mass, making isolated serum determinations unreliable in a rapidly changing scenario of critical illness. This is also true for tests based on creatinine and urea levels, such as urine-to-plasma ratios of these compounds. Urine sodium excretion should increase when tubular injury results in a loss of reabsorptive ability, but in the acute setting, isolated urine sodium (urine Na^+) values are more accurate reflectors of the composition of resuscitative fluids than tubular function. Fractional excretion of sodium (percentage of filtered sodium excreted) can reliably distinguish prerenal azotemia from established ATN, but it is unable to serve as an early indicator or predictor of ARF. Free water clearance (CH_2O) measures the diluting–concentrating ability of the kidney and should reflect tubular integrity. As a predictor of impending ARF, however, CH_2O cannot be used by itself and should be combined with a creatinine clearance (Ccr) determination.[80] It would appear that Ccr, as a sole indicator of imminent ARF, is the best test available to the clinician.[27]

Ccr is a direct reflection of GFR and may be either measured or calculated. Measured determination requires that urine and plasma creatinine (cr) levels be obtained and that the urine volume for 24 hours be collected and measured, such that

$$\text{Ccr} = \frac{\text{Urine cr} \times \text{Urine volume}}{\text{Plasma cr}}$$

Traditionally, the need for a 24-hour urine collection has limited the usefulness of Ccr in the acute situation. However, a 2-hour Ccr correlates reasonably well with the standard 24-hour collection in critically ill surgical patients [81] and nonoliguric intensive care patients.[82] A major advantage of the abbreviated Ccr determination is that it facilitates sequential monitoring of renal function during periods of rapidly changing patient status. Therapeutic interventions directed at improving renal function may be quickly assessed in this way.

Measured Ccr remains the most reliable predictor of renal dysfunction in critically ill surgical patients, regardless of the urine collection duration. The ideal renal function monitor would provide real-time data using noninvasive, easily transportable, and interpretable technology. Real-time monitoring of renal function is under development using ultrasonography[83] and nuclear medicine[84] technology.

Nephrotoxins and Perioperative Acute Renal Failure

Nephrotoxin exposure is a common occurrence in hospitalized patients and frequently plays a role in etiology of ARF in this population. Nephrotoxins may take the form of drugs, nontherapeutic chemicals, heavy metals, poisons, and endogenous compounds; a partial list is found in Table 35-1. The nephrotoxins most likely to contribute to renal dysfunction/failure in the perioperative period are certain antimicrobial and chemotherapeutic–immunosuppressive agents, radiocontrast media, nonsteroidal anti-inflammatory drugs (NSAIDs), and the endogenous heme pigments myoglobin and hemoglobin. These diverse groups of renal toxins share a common pathophysiologic characteristic: they disturb either renal oxygen delivery or oxygen utilization and thereby promote renal ischemia.

Antimicrobial and chemotherapeutic–immunosuppressive agents are effective for their designed purpose because they are cellular toxins. When these drugs are filtered, reabsorbed, secreted, and eventually excreted by the kidney, toxic concentrations in renal cells can be realized.[85] The aminoglycoside antibiotics (neomycin, gentamicin, tobramycin, amikacin) and amphotericin B are particularly difficult to avoid because they are effective antimicrobials, with few available alternatives.[86]

TABLE 35-6

CLINICAL USEFULNESS OF RENAL FUNCTION TESTS

RENAL FUNCTION TEST	DISTINGUISH ATN VERSUS PRA	PREDICT EARLY ATN	COMMENTS
Urine flow rate	Poor	Poor	
Urine-specific gravity	Poor	Poor	Many nonrenal factors
Urine osmolality	Poor	Poor	Many nonrenal factors
Serum creatinine, BUN	Poor	Late findings	Rapid preoperative screen
Urine/plasma creatinine, BUN	Poor	Poor	
Urine Na^+	Poor	Poor	
Fractional excretion Na^+	Good in late ATN	Poor	
Free water clearance	—	Good with Ccr	Less sensitive than Ccr
Ccr	Good	Good	24-hr collection

ATN, acute tubular necrosis; BUN, blood urea nitrogen; Ccr, creatinine clearance; PRA, prerenal azotemia.

They are filtered into the proximal tubule and, when reabsorbed into intracellular lysosomes, inhibit mitochondrial phosphorylation and deplete tubular cells' ATP stores. Their effect can be additive to other nephrotoxic factors, causing impairment of kidney function. Hypovolemia, fever, renal vasoconstriction, and concomitant therapy with other nephrotoxic agents should be avoided. Electrolyte disorders such as hypercalcemia, hypomagnesemia, hypokalemia, and metabolic acidosis can further enhance toxic effect on the kidney.

Cyclosporin A and tacrolimus are similarly indispensable agents, but in combination with other nephrotoxins and clinical factors, they cause both acute and chronic renal injury in transplant recipients.[87]

Radiocontrast media pose a threat to the renal function of patients with diabetic nephropathy, preexisting renal vasoconstriction (heart failure, hypovolemia), or renal insufficiency.[88] Radiocontrast dye effects on renal function develop 24 to 48 hours after exposure and peak at 3 to 5 days. Measures that can prevent ARF or lessen the severity of renal damage include prehydration, smaller contrast doses, and withholding of other nephrotoxins, such as NSAIDs. Elective surgery should be postponed until the effects of dye resolve. There is some evidence that pretreatment with N-acetylcysteine can prevent radiocontrast nephropathy in patients with renal insufficiency.[89]

NSAIDs produce reversible inhibition of prostaglandin synthesis and are well-known nephrotoxins.[90] Except in cases of massive overdose, NSAIDs produce renal dysfunction only in patients with coexisting renal hypoperfusion or vasoconstriction. Advanced age, hypovolemia, end-stage hepatic disease, heart failure, sepsis, renal insufficiency, and major surgery are risk factors for development of NSAID-induced ARF.[86] Of particular interest to anesthesiologists is *ketorolac*, a parenterally administered NSAID. Ketorolac may predispose critically ill and elderly patients to ischemic ARF and acute, life-threatening hyperkalemia when given perioperatively.[86]

Myoglobin and hemoglobin are both capable of causing ARF in the context of critical surgical illness. Myoglobin seems to be a more potent nephrotoxin than hemoglobin because it is more readily filtered at the glomerulus and can be reabsorbed by the renal tubules, where it inhibits nitric oxide and induces medullary vasoconstriction and ischemia.[2,91] Hypovolemia and acidemia potentiate the toxicity of both pigments. Reduced intravascular volume causes a decrease in RBF and GFR, which results in a smaller volume of tubular fluid with a relatively higher concentration of pigment. Myoglobin and hemoglobin dissociate more easily to ferrihemate (a potent nephrotoxin) in acidic tubular fluid. There is also evidence suggesting that pigment precipitation inside the tubular lumen is enhanced under acidotic conditions and that tubular obstruction plays a role in the pathogenesis of ARF.[91,92]

Myoglobinuric renal failure occurs in the clinical setting of massive rhabdomyolysis that may follow from a number of insults. The most common causes of massive rhabdomyolysis in surgical patients are major crush, thermal, or electrical injuries, acute muscle ischemia due to arterial occlusion or compartment syndrome, malignant hyperpyrexia, extreme lithotomy position, and hyperlordotic position.[92–95] Potassium, phosphorus, and creatinine are released in large quantities from the necrotic muscle. The clinical picture of myoglobinuric ARF is one of oligoanuria, rapidly rising creatinine, and life-threatening hyperkalemia. Unfortunately, the diagnosis of rhabdomyolysis is not straightforward, and a high index of suspicion is necessary to identify patients at risk for ARF. A creatine phosphokinase level of >15,000 U/L is predictive of hyperkalemic ARF and a high risk of death.[96]

Hemoglobinuric ARF usually results from massive hemolysis in association with renal hypoperfusion, as seen during exposure to extracorporeal circulation or cardiopulmonary bypass (CPB). Major transfusion reactions that occur in hypovolemic, acidemic, septic, or hemodynamically unstable patients may lead to renal injury, but rarely does isolated hemoglobinemia cause renal failure.[92]

Preventive treatment of pigmenturia-induced ARF is directed at increasing RBF and tubular (urine) flow while correcting any existing acidosis. These goals are accomplished by expanding the intravascular fluid volume with crystalloid infusion, stimulating an osmotic diuresis with mannitol, and increasing urine pH with alkali therapy.[97] Adequate systemic resuscitation from shock cannot be overemphasized as a prerequisite for preventing ARF, especially in massive crush injuries and electrical burns. Forced mannitol–alkali diuresis is indicated as the second step in preventive treatment of myoglobinuric renal failure, with urine flow rates of up to 300 mL/hr and urine pH of 6.5 advocated for patients with massive crush injuries.[97]

The nephrotoxicity of volatile agents remains debatable. Inhalation anesthetics such as enflurane, isoflurane, and sevoflurane can generate free fluoride ions during their metabolism, which (when levels are >150 μg/L) may cause polyuric ARF by interfering with tubular concentrating ability. However, peak fluoride levels during administration of these agents seldom reach toxic levels, and there are few reports describing only enflurane-induced nephrotoxicity.[98] The potential of sevoflurane-induced nephrotoxicity has been related to production of compound A during prolonged, low gas flow, sevoflurane anesthesia.[99] There are not enough data to support sevoflurane-induced renal injury in the human population, even during low gas flow anesthesia. However, maintaining fresh gas flow of at least 2 L/min to inhibit compound A formation during sevoflurane anesthesia is recommended.[100]

High-Risk Surgical Procedures

Several common surgical procedures can place renal function at risk. These include surgery of the heart and aorta, trauma surgery, and hepatic transplantation. Renal transplantation poses other special problems for renal preservation and is discussed in more detail in Chapter 53.

Emergency surgery has been reported as a possible risk factor for ARF, with trauma surgery figuring as a prominent subgroup of emergency procedures.[73] ATN is the preeminent renal lesion associated with trauma, and it may be produced by a number of ischemic mechanisms. Most often, hypovolemic shock, pigmenturia, MOF, or exogenous nephrotoxins are responsible for sequential or simultaneous insults to the kidney.[101] ARF that develops in the trauma patient may be characterized by either an early, oliguric picture related to inadequate volume resuscitation, or a later, often nonoliguric syndrome associated with MOF, nephrotoxin exposure, or sepsis.[102] The outcomes of these two posttraumatic ARF scenarios are dramatically different. The early form is associated with up to 90% mortality, whereas only 20 to 30% of patients die with nonoliguric ARF.[103] Not surprisingly, trauma victims with preexisting renal insufficiency experience higher mortality than previously healthy patients.[104]

Preventing ARF in patients presenting for emergency
9 surgery begins with proper management of intravascular volume depletion and shock. Restoring euvolemia and maintaining cardiac output, systemic oxygen delivery, and RBF obviate renal vasoconstriction. Urine flow, once established, is maintained at ≥0.5 mL/kg/hr. Invasive hemodynamic monitoring may be required to guide intraoperative management of ongoing cardiovascular instability due to surgical manipulation, blood loss, fluid shifts, and anesthetic effects. Intraoperative transesophageal echocardiography provides excellent assessment of left and right ventricular function, as well as therapeutic guidance of fluid resuscitation.

Nephrotoxin exposure should be kept to a minimum in the unstable trauma victim. Radiocontrast media, NSAIDs, and myoglobin pose the greatest threat in this patient group. There is no place for either furosemide or mannitol therapy in the early, resuscitative phase of trauma management, except in the case of head injury with elevated intracranial pressure or when massive rhabdomyolysis is suspected. After surgery, 1- or 2-hour Ccr determinations can help identify patients with impending ARF.[80]

Vascular surgery requiring aortic clamping has deleterious effects on renal function regardless of the level of clamp placement. Suprarenal clamping results in an attenuated ATN-like lesion.[105] Infrarenal clamping causes a smaller, short-lived reduction in GFR and is associated with a lower risk of ARF, whereas surgery involving the thoracic aorta has a 25% incidence of renal failure.[106] Two major predictors of ARF following aortic surgery appear to be preexisting renal dysfunction and perioperative hemodynamic instability.[107] Olsen et al.[21] reported that in a large series of patients undergoing abdominal aortic aneurysm repair, overall incidence of ARF was 12%. Patients who had emergency surgery for ruptured aneurysm had a very high incidence of hemodynamic instability, and ARF developed in 26%; in contrast, elective aortic surgery was associated with good hemodynamic control and a 4% incidence of renal failure. Atheromatous renal artery emboli and prolonged aortic clamp time may contribute to ischemic renal injury.

Efforts to improve renal outcome in aortic surgery should begin in the preoperative period by identification of patients with renal dysfunction. Ideally, these high-risk patients should not receive radiocontrast media or other nephrotoxins in the immediate preoperative period.

An endovascular approach to major aortic surgery has gained popularity. The etiology of renal dysfunction after endovascular and open repair of aortic aneurysm is multifactorial (renal ischemia, atheroembolism, hemodynamic instability). Although hemodynamic changes during endovascular procedures on the aorta may be less dramatic than those accompanying open repair, prevalence of renal complications is similar.[108] During endovascular procedures, patients are exposed to a substantial amount of radiocontrast dye, which can exacerbate postoperative renal dysfunction, especially in those with preexisting renal insufficiency. The long-term incidence of renal insufficiency/failure (followed up to 24 months postoperatively) is similar after endovascular and open repair of aortic aneurysm.[108,109] It is important that before endovascular procedures, patients are adequately hydrated and the total dose of radiocontrast dye is limited.

Most efforts to preserve renal function in aortic surgery have centered on diuretic and renal vasodilator therapy. Unfortunately, is little to support the use of either mannitol or low-dose dopamine to prevent the renal injury associated with aortic surgery. Indeed, a clinical study of infrarenal aortic clamping found that combined mannitol and low-dose dopamine treatment was no more effective in preventing renal dysfunction than volume expansion with saline.[110] Although other investigators have demonstrated an increase in urine flow rate with low-dose dopamine in sick postoperative patients,[111] evidence that this can preserve renal function during aortic surgery is lacking. Nifedipine prevented a postoperative decrease in GFR in a small, placebo-controlled study of aortic surgery patients.[112] Larger outcome trials are needed to confirm this preliminary finding. Insulin-like growth factor-1 has been shown to speed healing in experimental ischemic ARF,[113] and to improve renal function in patients with ESRD[114] and in those undergoing aortic or renal artery surgery.[115] A synthetic form of ANP may be useful in managing established oliguric ARF,[116] but it has not been used prophylactically in high-risk surgical patients. Fenoldopam, a selective dopamine-1 receptor agonist, shows great promise as a renal protective agent and should be the subject of future perioperative studies.[117]

Cardiac operations requiring CPB can be expected to result in renal dysfunction or failure in up to 7% of patients.[118–122] Preoperative renal dysfunction is a major risk factor for postoperative ARF in this population,[118,121–123] yet patients with preoperative CRF appear to tolerate surgery and CPB well.[119] Renal hypoperfusion is considered the primary pathogenic mechanism involved in precipitating ARF. Preoperative left ventricular dysfunction[121,122,124]and duration of CPB[118,121,122] are associated with post–CPB renal failure.

Early experience with non-CPB ("off pump") coronary artery bypass grafting (CABG) suggests that it offers better renal preservation than the traditional, "on-pump" technique.[125] However, despite the fact that pulsatile CPB suppresses plasma renin activity, postoperative renal function in patients with normal kidneys undergoing pulsatile or nonpulsatile CPB was equivalent.[126]

There are reports that patients on hemodialysis recover more quickly after off-pump than on-pump CABG.[127] Higgins et al.[128] found that preoperative renal function is an important predictor of postoperative renal morbidity and mortality in patients undergoing cardiac surgery. In particular, a preoperative serum creatinine level above 1.9 mg/dL was associated with a high prevalence of postoperative renal complications.[128]

When CPB is used, mannitol can protect against hemoglobin-induced ARF, promote urine flow, and reduce renal cell swelling.[129] Dopamine has been used as a renal vasodilator in cardiac surgery with mixed success. Costa et al.[130] administered low-dose dopamine during CPB to patients with preoperative renal dysfunction and were able to induce a saluresis without affecting GFR or protecting the kidney from ischemic injury. Dopexamine has been shown to improve Ccr and systemic oxygen delivery in cardiac surgery patients,[131] but studies examining the renal protective effects of fenoldopam, ANP, and insulin-like growth factor-1 in this population are not yet available.

As previously discussed, patients with hepatic failure or cholestatic jaundice are particularly susceptible to renal dysfunction. When conjugated bilirubin exceeds 8 mg/dL, endotoxins from the gastrointestinal tract are absorbed into the portal circulation, causing intense renal vasoconstriction. Intravenous mannitol and/or oral administration of bile salts in the preoperative period seem to limit renal dysfunction in patients with cholestatic jaundice. This probably accounts for the high incidence of ARF after liver transplantation and biliary surgery.[75,132–134] Renal dysfunction/failure may occur in up to two-thirds of liver transplant recipients.[77] Many transplantation candidates have overt hepatorenal syndrome, asymptomatic renal dysfunction, or underlying renal vasoconstriction. When such patients are exposed to intraoperative hemodynamic instability, massive transfusion, and nephrotoxins, ARF frequently follows.[133,134] Both preoperative and postoperative renal dysfunction contribute to early and long-term mortality.[78,133,135,136] Maintenance of adequate intravascular volume and aggressive management of hypoperfusion are basic tenets of anesthetic care of the liver transplant recipient, but investigators have also sought a role for low-dose dopamine. Low-dose dopamine has been shown to be no better than preoperative hydration in preserving renal function in patients with obstructive jaundice.[137]

Perioperative sepsis is a common cause of renal dysfunction. The mechanism of kidney damage in sepsis is multifactorial and includes hypotension, vasomotor nephropathy, and effects of endotoxins. During sepsis, renal autoregulation is impaired. Decrease in RBF, GFR, sodium excretion, and urine flow is related to hypotension-induced activation of the neurohormonal cascade, including renin-angiotensin system, vasopressin, and thromboxane.[138]

ANESTHESIA FOR ENDOUROLOGIC PROCEDURES

Medical care continues to evolve toward nonoperative or minimally invasive surgical procedures. Incisional surgery in urology is being replaced by endoscopic procedures in which endoscopes are passed along natural pathways (e.g., urethra, ureter) or through small incisions.[139] Economic considerations, patient convenience, and advances in instrumentation have all supported the trend toward endoscopy in urologic surgery (Table 35-7).

Cystourethroscopy and Ureteral Procedures

Cystourethroscopy is commonly used to examine and treat lower urinary tract disease. It provides direct visualization of the anterior and posterior urethra, bladder neck, and bladder. In the past, cystourethroscopy was performed with rigid endoscopes. General or regional anesthesia was required for patient comfort. In 1973, the flexible endoscope was introduced, which can be gently passed over anatomic angles with less patient discomfort.[140] For brief cystoscopic procedures, 5 to 10 mL of lubricant anesthetic jelly (2% lidocaine hydrochloride jelly) can be instilled into the urethra preoperatively.[141] This local anesthetic technique provides adequate anesthesia for many patients undergoing simple cystoscopy. For longer or more extensive procedures, conscious sedation techniques using a wide variety of sedative–hypnotic, anxiolytic, and analgesic drugs have been shown to combine excellent patient comfort and operating conditions with rapid patient recovery.[142,143] If general anesthesia is required for cystoscopy or urethral procedures, laryngeal mask airways are an alternative to the traditional facemask.

Numerous therapeutic procedures may also be performed using endoscopic techniques. Strictures of the bladder neck or urethra are treated with internal optical urethrotomy, which uses a "cold knife" to excise the scar. Ureteroscopy is an extension of cystoscopic techniques, providing access to the upper urinary tract and kidney for diagnostic endoscopy and biopsy, removal of ureteral and renal calculi, passage of a ureteral stent, dilatation and incision of strictures, fulguration of tumors, and laser treatments.[139] Ureteroscopy usually requires dilatation of the ureteral orifice and intramural ureter, often necessitating regional or general anesthesia.

Transurethral Resection of the Prostate

Benign prostatic hyperplasia (BPH) is the most common benign tumor in men and refers to regional nodular growth that occurs in the prostate gland as men age.[144] The prostate is a pear-shaped gland that surrounds the urethra at the base of the bladder (Fig. 35-7). Because of its anatomic position, hypertrophy of the prostate gland can compress the proximal urethra, resulting in urinary retention. BPH is responsible for the majority of urinary symptoms in men older than the age of 50 and results in need for prostatectomy in approximately one-third of all men who live to age 80.[145]

TABLE 35-7

COMMON ENDOUROLOGIC PROCEDURES

Cystourethroscopy
Internal optical urethrotomy
Ureteroscopy
Placement of ureteral stent
Distal stone manipulation/laser lithotripsy
Transurethral resection of the prostate
Transurethral incision of the prostate
Balloon dilation of the prostate
Transurethral resection of bladder tumors
Percutaneous nephrostomy, nephroscopy, and nephrolithotomy

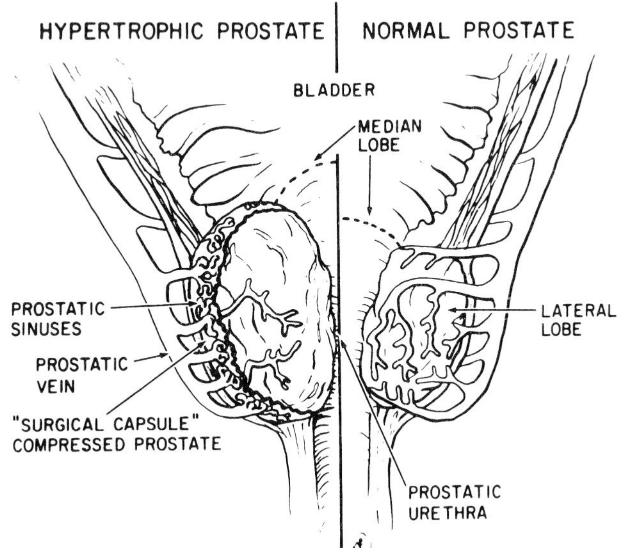

FIGURE 35-7. Anatomy of the normal and hypertrophic prostate gland. (Reprinted from Stoelting RK, Barash PG, Gallagher TJ: Advances in Anesthesia, p. 379, Chicago, Year Book Medical Publishers, 1986.)

Transurethral resection of the prostate (TURP) is the primary treatment for symptomatic BPH. This procedure commences with an initial cystoscopy to rule out concomitant disease and evaluate the size of the prostate gland.[146] The resectoscope, a specialized instrument with an electrode capable of both coagulating and cutting tissue, is then introduced through a modified cystoscope into the bladder, and the tissue protruding into the prostatic urethra is resected. Continuous irrigation of the bladder and prostatic urethra is required to maintain visibility, distend the operative site, and remove dissected tissue and blood.[147]

The prostate gland contains a rich plexus of veins that can be opened during surgical resection (see Fig. 35-7). If the pressure of the irrigating fluid during TURP procedures exceeds venous pressure, intravascular absorption of the fluid may occur via these open venous sinuses. The need for large volumes of irrigating fluid during the procedure and the potential for absorption of this fluid into the intravascular space may result in unique perioperative complications.

Irrigating Solutions for Transurethral Resection of the Prostate

The ideal irrigating fluid for use during TURP would be isotonic and nonhemolytic if absorbed. In addition, it would be nonelectrolytic to disperse the electrical current, transparent to allow clear visibility for the surgeon, nonmetabolized, nontoxic, rapidly excreted, and inexpensive.[148] A variety of irrigating solutions are available for transurethral procedures (Table 35-8), but most are hypoosmolar (normal serum osmolality is 280 to 300 mOsm/L) and acidic (pH of 4.5 to 6.5).[149]

Distilled water was the irrigating solution used by urologists in the past because it was nonconductive and interfered least

TABLE 35-8

PROPERTIES OF COMMONLY USED IRRIGATING SOLUTIONS FOR TRANSURETHRAL RESECTION PROCEDURES

■ SOLUTION	■ OSMOLALITY (mOsm/L)	■ ADVANTAGES	■ DISADVANTAGES
Distilled water	0	Improved visibility	Hemolysis Hemoglobinemia Hemoglobinuria Hyponatremia
Glycine (1.5%)	200	Less likelihood of transurethral resection syndrome	Transient postoperative visual syndrome Hyperammonemia Hyperoxaluria
Sorbitol (3.3%)	165	Same as glycine	Hyperglycemia, possible lactic acidosis Osmotic diuresis
Mannitol (5%)	275	Isosmolar solution Not metabolized	Osmotic diuresis Possibility of acute intravascular volume expansion

Adapted with permission from Krongrad A, Droller MJ: Complications of transurethral resection of the prostate. In Marshall FF (ed): Urologic Complications: Medical and Surgical, Adult and Pediatric, 2nd ed, p 305. St. Louis, Mosby–Year Book, 1990.

with surgical visibility. However, because of its low tonicity, water absorbed into the circulation can cause massive intravascular hemolysis, hemoglobinemia, and renal failure, and result in dilutional hyponatremia.[150] Distilled water can be used for transurethral procedures that do not open venous sinuses, such as cystoscopy and transurethral resection of bladder tumor, but it is no longer used in TURP procedures.

Solutes such as sorbitol, mannitol, glycine, urea, and glucose have been added to water to make its osmolality closer to that of plasma[148] (see Table 35-8). It is essential that the anesthesiologist be aware of the type of irrigating solution being used during an endoscopic procedure, because absorption of this fluid can be associated with numerous perioperative complications. Electrolyte solutions such as Ringer's lactate or normal saline should not cause electrolyte imbalance if absorbed into the circulation, but they cannot be used in conjunction with an electrocautery device because they are ionized and able to conduct electrical currents. Sorbitol is metabolized to fructose, and use of this solution can produce hyperglycemia. Glycine is a nonessential amino acid that is normally present in the circulation. It is metabolized in the liver by oxidative deamination into ammonia and glyoxylic acid.[151] Depressed mental status and coma secondary to hyperammonemia have been reported following TURP procedures in which glycine was used as the irrigating solution.[151,152] Blood ammonia levels as high as 834 μM/L (normal 11 to 35 μM/L) have been documented, although the central nervous system depression was transient in these patients and they recovered within 24 to 48 hours.[152] Other investigators have observed development of hyperoxaluria in association with glycine irrigation.[153]

Visual disturbances, including blurred vision and transient blindness, have been reported following TURP procedures with glycine-containing irrigation fluid.[154] Loss of vision after transurethral procedures was traditionally believed to be secondary to cerebral edema from the hypervolemia and hyponatremia that developed as irrigating fluid was absorbed. However, when a centrally acting mechanism, such as cerebral edema, is the cause of visual impairment, patients have normal pupillary light reflexes. A review of patients with blindness after TURP revealed that some had sluggish or nonreactive pupils, suggesting an anterior pathway disturbance rather than cerebral edema.[154] Glycine acts as an inhibitory neurotransmitter in the brain, spinal cord, and retina. Elevated serum glycine levels could exert an inhibitory action on the retina and result in transient blindness consistent with the clinical picture seen in these patients.[154] It would appear that the visual disturbance after TURP may have more than one etiology.

Transurethral Resection Syndrome

Transurethral resection (TUR) syndrome (water intoxication syndrome) is a general term used to describe a wide range of neurologic and cardiopulmonary symptoms that occur when irrigating fluid is absorbed during TUR procedures, especially TURP. Its principal components are respiratory distress secondary to volume expansion from rapid intravascular absorption of the irrigating fluid, dilution of electrolytes and proteins by the electrolyte-free irrigating fluid, and symptoms related to the type of irrigating solution used.[148,155,156]

The average amount of irrigating fluid absorbed during TURP is ~20 mL/min of resection time.[150,157] The volume of fluid absorbed during the procedure can be estimated with the following formula[155]:

$$\text{Volume absorbed} = \frac{\text{preoperative serum Na}^+}{\text{postoperative serum Na}^+ \times \text{ECF}} - \text{ECF}$$

where ECF is extracellular fluid volume.

The amount of irrigation fluid absorbed during the pro-
10 cedure is directly related to the number and size of venous sinuses opened, duration of resection, hydrostatic pressure of the irrigating fluid, and venous pressure at the irrigant–blood interface.[147] To prevent excessive fluid absorption, it is recommended that resection time be limited to <1 hour and that the bag of irrigating fluid be suspended no more than 30 cm above the operating table at the beginning of the resection and 15 cm in the final stages of resection.[147,157] Investigations have demonstrated that ethanol-labeled irrigating fluid can be used to accurately assess the degree of fluid absorption during TUR procedures by measuring the ethanol content of the patient's exhaled breath.[158] Clinical manifestations of TUR syndrome range from mild (restlessness, nausea, shortness of breath, dizziness) to severe (seizures, coma, hypertension, bradycardia, cardiovascular collapse). In the awake patient with a regional block, a classic triad of symptoms has been described that consists of an increase in both systolic and diastolic pressures associated with an increase in pulse pressure, bradycardia, and mental status changes.[148,149] During general anesthesia, many of the more subtle signs of TUR syndrome are obscured, making early diagnosis more difficult. The initial hypertension and bradycardia are the result of acute volume overload, which may

TABLE 35-9

SIGNS AND SYMPTOMS ASSOCIATED WITH ACUTE CHANGES IN SERUM Na^+ LEVELS

SERUM Na^+	CENTRAL NERVOUS SYSTEM CHANGES	ELECTROCARDIOGRAM CHANGES
120 mEq/L	Confusion Restlessness	Possible widening of QRS complex
115 mEq/L	Somnolence Nausea	Widened QRS complex Elevated ST segment
110 mEq/L	Seizures Coma	Ventricular tachycardia or fibrillation

Adapted with permission from Jensen V: The TURP syndrome. Can J Anaesth 38:90, 1991.

lead to left heart failure, pulmonary edema, and cardiovascular collapse.[159] With the continued absorption of electrolyte-free irrigation fluid, dilutional hyponatremia and cerebral edema develop. The acute decrease in serum sodium concentration is responsible for many of the signs and symptoms of TUR syndrome[148] (Table 35-9).

Symptoms related to absorption of a specific irrigating solution during the procedure may further complicate TUR syndrome. For example, if excessive amounts of glycine are absorbed, the patient may become encephalopathic secondary to high blood ammonia concentrations. Likewise, absorption of large volumes of sorbitol may produce hyperglycemia and coma, especially in diabetic patients.

Prompt intervention is necessary when neurologic or cardiovascular complications of TUR procedures are recognized (Table 35-10). Oxygenation, ventilation, and circulatory support must be ensured, and other potentially treatable conditions such as diabetic coma, hypercarbia, or drug interactions should be considered.[148] The surgeon should be informed of a change in the patient's status so the procedure can be terminated as quickly as possible. Treatment with hypertonic saline has been associated with development of demyelinating central nervous system lesions due to rapid increases in plasma osmolality and should be reserved for patients with severe, life-threatening symptoms.[160] Three percent sodium chloride solution should be infused at a rate no greater than 100 mL/hr and discontinued as soon as the serum sodium is >120 mEq/L. Once this goal is reached, treatment can continue with fluid restriction and diuretic therapy. The rate at which serum sodium is increased should not exceed 12 mEq/L in a 24-hour period.[160]

TABLE 35-10

TREATMENT OF THE TRANSURETHRAL RESECTION SYNDROME

Ensure oxygenation and circulatory support.
Notify surgeon and terminate procedure as soon as possible.
Consider insertion of invasive monitors if cardiovascular instability occurs.
Send blood to laboratory for electrolytes, creatinine, glucose, and arterial blood gases.
Obtain 12-lead electrocardiogram.
Treat mild symptoms (with serum Na^+ concentration >120 mEq/L) with fluid restriction and loop diuretic (furosemide).
Treat severe symptoms (if serum Na^+ <120 mEq/L) with 3% sodium chloride IV at a rate <100 mL/hr.
Discontinue 3% sodium chloride when serum Na^+ >120 mEq/L.

Other Complications of Transurethral Resection of the Prostate

Bleeding comes from either open venous sinuses or unrecognized arterial bleeding sites and typically ranges from 2 to 4 mL/min during the resection.[147] Blood loss is difficult to assess because of mixing with the irrigating fluid. Therefore, serial hemoglobin or hematocrit levels and the patient's vital signs should be evaluated to determine the need for transfusion.[149] The incidence of intraoperative blood transfusion is reported to be ~2.5%.

Abnormal bleeding after TURP occurs in <1% of resections[147] and may be caused by release of thromboplastin, which is found in high concentrations in prostate cancer cells.[149] This thrombogenic stimulus can produce disseminated intravascular coagulation. Treatment of this condition is supportive and may include transfusion of coagulation factors and platelets.[161] Another cause of postoperative bleeding after TURP is release of tissue plasminogen activators from the prostate. These factors activate the coagulation system and convert plasminogen to plasmin, which in turn causes fibrinolysis.

Perforation of the prostatic capsule occurs in ~1 to 2% of patients undergoing TURP, usually resulting in extraperitoneal extravasation of fluid.[149,162] This complication occurs more commonly during transurethral resection of the bladder, and management of this problem is discussed in that section of this chapter.

Fever in the perioperative period suggests bacteremia secondary to spread of bacteria through open prostatic venous sinuses. Hypothermia can occur if large volumes of room-temperature irrigating fluids are not warmed to body temperature. Body temperature decreases ~1°C/hr of surgery, and shivering occurs in 16% of patients who receive room-temperature irrigation fluids; hypothermia does not develop if the irrigation solution is warmed to body temperature (95 to 100°F).[163]

Anesthetic Techniques for Transurethral Resection of the Prostate

Regional anesthesia has long been considered the anesthetic technique of choice for TURP and is used in >70% of these procedures in the United States.[164] It allows the patient to remain awake, which should facilitate early diagnosis of TUR syndrome or extravasation of irrigation fluid. Some studies have demonstrated decreased blood loss when TURP procedures are performed using regional anesthesia, whereas others have found no difference in blood loss between regional and general anesthesia.[165,166]

Bowman et al.[167] found that only 15% of patients receiving spinal anesthesia for TURP required any pain medication other than acetaminophen, whereas the need for analgesics was increased approximately fourfold after general anesthesia.

A prospective study comparing the effect of general versus spinal anesthesia on cognitive function after TURP found a significant decrease in mental status in both groups at 6 hours after surgery, but no differences in mental function at any time in the first 30 days after surgery.[168] Perioperative morbidity and mortality among patients older than 90 years of age who underwent TURP did not depend on the type of anesthesia used.[169] A study of the occurrence of perioperative myocardial ischemia in patients undergoing transurethral surgery, assessed by Holter monitoring, determined that both the incidence and duration of myocardial ischemia increased following TUR surgery, but there was no difference between general or spinal anesthesia.[170] A second study confirmed these findings and concluded that presence of short-duration silent myocardial ischemia did not correlate with adverse outcome in elderly patients undergoing TURP procedures.[171] Thus, it appears that TURP can be performed safely with either type of anesthesia, and the choice of anesthetic technique should be tailored to the individual patient.

If spinal or epidural anesthesia is used for the procedure, a T10 dermatome anesthetic level is needed to block the pain from bladder distention by the irrigating fluid. Spinal anesthesia is usually preferred over lumbar epidural anesthesia because sacral segments are sometimes inadequately blocked with lumbar epidural techniques. Local anesthesia has also been used for TURP procedures in patients with small to moderate size prostate glands, with limited success.[172]

Morbidity and Mortality After Transurethral Resection of the Prostate

An American Urological Association (AUA) cooperative study evaluated postoperative complications in 3,885 patients after TURP[162]; average patient age was 69 years, and most patients (>75%) had coexisting medical problems that involved many of the major organ systems. The prevalence of complications in the intraoperative period was 6.9%. These included bleeding requiring transfusion (2.5%), TUR syndrome (2%), cardiac dysrhythmias (1%), and extravasation of irrigating fluid (0.9%). No intraoperative deaths occurred. Immediate postoperative problems following TURP occurred in 18% of patients, with the most common being failure to void. Other common postoperative problems were bleeding, clot retention, and infection. Patients at an increased risk for perioperative morbidity after TURP were those with large prostate glands (>45 g), resection times exceeding 90 min, acute urinary retention, or age >80 years.

Despite the high incidence of coexisting medical problems in patients undergoing TURP, 30-day mortality has declined over the years. In 1962, it was 2.5%, whereas the AUA cooperative study evaluating these procedures during 1978 to 1987 reported a much lower mortality of 0.2%, even though patient age and amount of prostate tissue resected had not changed from earlier surveys.[162] An evaluation of 181,161 TURP Medicare beneficiaries between 1991 and 1997 revealed a 30-day mortality of 0.39% for those ages 65 to 69 years. Age-specific mortality for those older than age 70 years was compared with 1984 to 1990 mortality and was also found to be lower (Table 35-11).[173]

TABLE 35-11

THIRTY-DAY MORTALITY RATE FOLLOWING TRANSURETHRAL RESECTION OF THE PROSTATE

PT. AGE	BPH COHORTS (95% CI)	
	1991–1997	1984–1990
65–69	0.39 (0.32–0.46)	0.39 (0.34–0.44)
70–74	0.52 (0.45–0.59)	0.67 (0.61–1.74)
75–79	0.90 (0.81–100)	1.10 (1.01–1.19)
80–84	1.34 (1.19–1.48)	1.92 (1.76–2.07)
85+	2.52 (2.26–2.78)	3.54 (3.26–3.82)

BPH, benign prostatic hyperplasia; CI, confidence interval.

The Future of Transurethral Resection of the Prostate

TURP began to decline in 1987 for all age groups older than 65 years, likely because of less invasive medical and surgical treatments, changes in reimbursement, and greater involvement of patients in the decision-making process.[173] Less invasive surgical treatments include balloon dilatation, prostate stents, transurethral incision of the prostate, and laser prostatectomy. These procedures can usually be done on an outpatient basis, decrease the risk of TUR syndrome, and may be preferred for elderly patients with significant comorbidity risk factors.[174]

Transurethral Resection of Bladder Tumors

Bladder cancer is the second most common urologic malignancy, with nearly 50,000 new cases diagnosed in the United States each year.[175,176] Superficial transitional cell carcinoma accounts for ~90% of bladder cancers. In diagnosing and treating this cancer, most patients undergo endoscopic transurethral resection.[175,176] This procedure can be performed with either regional or general anesthesia. If a regional anesthetic is employed, an anesthetic level to T10 is required to block the pain associated with bladder distention. If the bladder tumor lies near the obturator nerve, the electrocautery may cause the thigh muscles to contract violently, resulting in inadvertent bladder perforation, regardless of whether general or regional anesthesia is used.[177] General anesthesia with addition of a muscle relaxant is the preferred technique when this is anticipated or occurs intraoperatively.

Complications During Transurethral Resection of the Bladder

Perforation of the bladder has been reported during transurethral surgery.[178] This can result in intraperitoneal or extraperitoneal extravasation of the fluid used to irrigate the bladder. Clinical diagnosis of bladder perforation is simplified if the procedure is performed under regional anesthesia. The conscious patient describes sudden, severe abdominal pain, often associated with referred pain from the diaphragm to the shoulder.[150,178] Associated symptoms include pallor, sweating, abdominal rigidity, nausea, and vomiting. If extravasation is suspected, the operation should be terminated as quickly as possible. Small perforations with minimal intraperitoneal leakage rarely cause hemodynamic changes and can usually be managed with catheter drainage and diuretics. The consequences of a large intraperitoneal accumulation of irrigating fluid (especially sterile water) can be life threatening. Open laparotomy for drainage and bladder perforation repair is recommended in these cases.[150,178,179]

Extracorporeal Shock Wave Lithotripsy

In the United States, the annual incidence of urolithiasis is 16.4 per 10,000 persons, and it is estimated that 12% of the population will experience calculus disease in their lifetime.[180] This disease is three times more common in men than women, with a peak age incidence in the third to fourth decade of life.[181] Several therapeutic modalities exist for surgical treatment of urinary calculi. The final treatment decision is based on the size of the stone being treated (<4.0 mm usually pass spontaneously), location in the urinary tract, and composition.[181]

Introduction of extracorporeal shock wave lithotripsy (SWL) in 1980 dramatically changed the management of urolithiasis. Before development of this modality, open surgical removal was the most common technique for treating urethral and renal calculi.[182] Now, only 5% of all urinary calculi require open surgical procedures. SWL has the advantages of being a minimally invasive technique that is performed on an outpatient basis and is associated with minimal perioperative morbidity and a significant reduction in treatment costs.[183]

Technical Aspects of Shock Wave Lithotripsy

Lithotripters have four main components: an energy source, focusing device, coupling medium, and multiplane stone localization system. The original, first-generation lithotripter was the Dornier HM-3, which required the patient to be placed in a hydraulically supported gantry chair and immersed in a water bath (Fig. 35-8). Its energy source is a spark plug generator that creates an explosive impact and transmits high pressures (shock waves) to the water when discharged. An ellipsoidal reflector aims the shock waves at a focal point. Two fluoroscopes are oriented so their beam paths intersect at the focal point above the ellipsoidal reflector, and the patient's position in the tub is adjusted so the calculus is centered in these beam paths.[184] The water bath transmits the shock wave to the patient. It serves as the coupling medium, allowing the shock wave to pass into the body without dissipation because the acoustic impedance of body tissue is close to that of water.[183]

Initial SWL treatments were associated with ventricular ectopic beats and even ventricular tachycardia.[185] It was postulated that these dysrhythmias were caused by stimulation of the myocardium when shock waves were delivered during the repolarization phase of the heart. To avoid this problem, shock waves can be synchronized and triggered off the electrocardiogram to occur 20 milliseconds after the R wave during the refractory period of the heart.[185] The average treatment on the Dornier HM-3 lithotripter uses 1,500 to 2,000 shocks.[183]

Physiologic Effects of Immersion Lithotripsy

Placing a patient into the water bath during lithotripsy produces a number of physiologic alterations in the cardiopulmonary system, with immersion causing peripheral venous compression that results in increased central blood volume (Table 35-12). Central venous pressure (CVP) and pulmonary capillary wedge pressure increases are linearly related to depth of immersion, with immersion to the clavicles increasing CVP by 10 to 14 cm H_2O.[186] Despite the increase in venous return during immersion, some patients experience hypotension as a result of vasodilatation from the warm water.[187]Placing a patient in water to the level of the clavicles increases the work of breathing and can result in respirations becoming shallow and rapid because of extrinsic pressure on the upper abdomen and thorax, which causes a decrease in vital capacity and functional reserve capacity.[188] Continuous monitoring of hemodynamics, respiratory gas exchange, and oxygenation should be used in all patients undergoing SWL, but are of paramount importance in patients with cardiopulmonary disease. In these patients, immersion should be achieved in a gradual fashion, or the procedure can be performed with minimal immersion so only the shock wave entry site is covered with water. Alternatively, a nonimmersion (second-generation or third-generation) lithotripter may be used.

Problems involving temperature regulation may occur during immersion SWL, especially in elderly patients with impaired thermoregulatory systems. Water in the lithotripter tub should be maintained in the temperature range of 35.8 to 37.5°C, and temperature monitoring should be used in every patient.[189]

Modifications of the original Dornier HM-3 have produced second-generation and third-generation lithotripters with several advantages[182] (see Fig. 35-8). Newer devices generate shock waves within a "shock tube" coupled to the body surface with a water cushion. This eliminates the water bath and all problems associated with patient immersion in water. They also have decreased power, causing less pain; however, most patients still require IV sedation or a "light" general anesthetic during treatment. One disadvantage of the newer lithotripters is that by decreasing power, efficiency of stone fragmentation is reduced, and thus the prevalence of retreatment is higher.[182]

Patient Selection and Complications of Shock Wave Lithotripsy

Absolute and relative contraindications to SWL are listed in Table 35-13. It was initially believed that presence of a cardiac pacemaker was a contraindication secondary to electrical interference from the shock wave energy's ability to inhibit, reprogram, or damage the pacemaker.[183] However, a review of 142 SWL treatments in pacemaker-dependent patients found a low (<1%) incidence of major pacemaker complications, with only one pacemaker deprogrammed during the treatment period.[190] Based on these findings, patients with pacemakers are considered acceptable candidates for lithotripsy provided that certain precautions are taken, including (1) preoperative determination of the type of pacemaker and its functional status; (2) availability of a magnet or programming device in the operating room, along with a person skilled in its use; (3) availability of an alternative pacing device; and (4) positioning of the patient so the pacemaker is not in the shock wave path. SWL can be performed safely in patients with an automatic implantable cardioverter-defibrillator with appropriate precautions and deactivation of the unit during lithotripsy.[191]

Renal parenchymal damage is believed to be responsible for the hematuria that occurs in nearly all patients, whereas subcapsular hematoma is seen in only 0.5% of patients after lithotripsy.[182] These problems usually resolve spontaneously, and bleeding that requires transfusion is rare.[192] Transient renal failure after SWL has been reported; however, there is no evidence that lithotripsy is associated with permanent renal dysfunction.

After treatment, many patients complain of flank pain, which may be severe for several days.[192,193] Petechia and soft-tissue swelling can be seen at the entry site of the shock wave, especially in thin patients treated with first-generation lithotripters. Up to 10% of patients have significant urinary tract colic, occasionally requiring hospitalization and opioid analgesics. Broken stone fragments can also collect in the ureter and form a column of stone, which is commonly referred to as *steinstrasse* or "stone street." If *steinstrasse* results in total ureteral obstruction, rising creatinine levels, or severe pain, the patient may require an endoscopic procedure with ureteral stent placement to relieve the obstruction.[192]

SWL may be problematic in children or patients of small stature (height <48 in.) because of position in the immersion lithotripter chair and a higher risk of pulmonary contusion by shock waves.[194] Lungs of small patients can be shielded by foam padding during the treatment to help prevent this complication.

Other potential complications following lithotripsy include damage to adjacent organs by the shock waves.[182] Several cases of pancreatitis and transient gastrointestinal injury have been reported. Approximately 1% of patients have septic

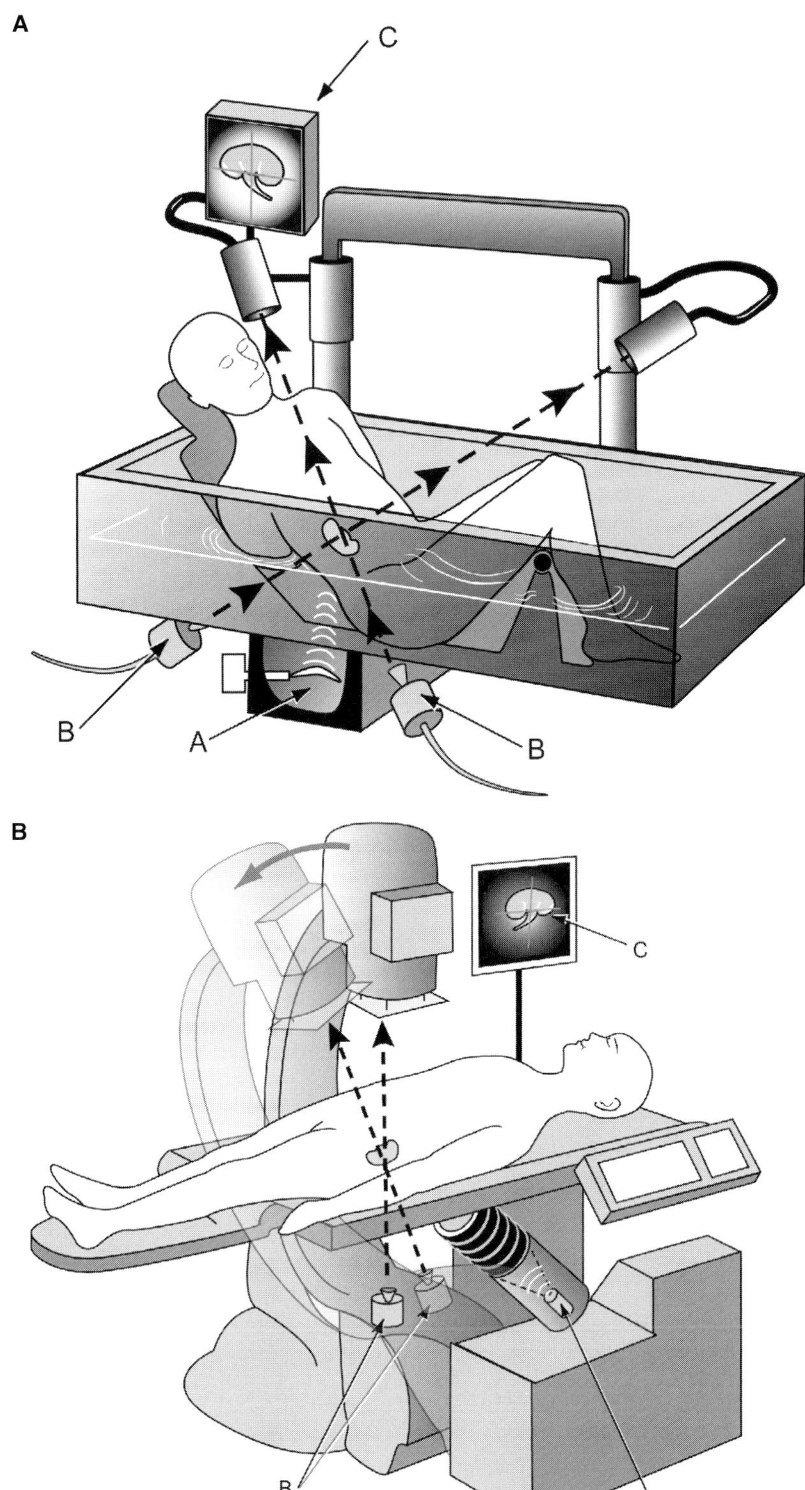

FIGURE 35-8. Schematics of patient positioned in (A) first-generation water bath immersion and (B) second-generation non-water bath lithotripter. A, energy source; B, multiplane fluoroscopy; C, focusing device. (Reprinted The Cleveland Clinic Foundation Copyright © 2004.)

complications after SWL. Brachial plexus injuries have also occurred from improper positioning of patients in the lithotripter chair. Despite the wide array of potential complications, mortality after SWL was only 0.02% in a review of more than 62,000 patients.[182] It appears that with proper patient selection and cautious intraoperative management, most patients can safely undergo lithotripsy procedures.

Radiation and auditory exposure of anesthesiology personnel during SWL appears to be safe with proper precautions. These include avoiding direct patient contact during fluoroscopy.[195,196]

Anesthetic Techniques for Shock Wave Lithotripsy

Shock wave impact and propagation through the skin and viscera are responsible for the pain experienced during SWL.[197]

TABLE 35-12

CARDIOPULMONARY CHANGES ON IMMERSION DURING LITHOTRIPSY

SYSTEM	VARIABLE	DIRECTION OF CHANGE
Cardiovascular	Central blood volume	Increased
	Central venous pressure	Increased
	Pulmonary artery pressure	Increased
Respiratory	Pulmonary blood flow	Increased
	Vital capacity	Decreased
	Functional residual	Decreased
	Tidal volume	Decreased
	Respiratory rate	Increased

Modified from Atlee JL. Complications in Anesthesia, © 1998 Elsevier Inc. and Miller RD: Anesthesia, © 1994 Elsevier Inc.

The initial approach to anesthesia for lithotripsy on the Dornier HM-3 used either a regional or general technique. General anesthesia offers the advantages of controlling patient ventilation and movement, rapid induction of anesthesia, and quicker recovery from anesthesia compared with epidural anesthesia.[198] However, patients have to be positioned in the lithotripter chair while unconscious, increasing the risk of peripheral nerve injuries. With regional anesthesia, the patient is awake and cooperative during transport, simplifying patient positioning. Regional anesthetic techniques for this procedure require a sensory level of T6. Neurologic damage has been reported after SWL when air was introduced into the epidural space during epidural anesthesia.[199]

Conscious sedation techniques have been developed for use during lithotripsy.[193,200] Monk et al.[193] examined the use of propofol and fentanyl or midazolam and alfentanil for intravenous sedation during treatments on the Dornier HM-3. Both sedative–analgesic combinations provided good treatment conditions and were associated with a high degree of patient satisfaction. When this intravenous sedation technique was compared with epidural anesthesia for the same procedures, anesthesia and recovery times were significantly shortened and hospital costs decreased with use of IV sedation.[193] Local anesthetic infiltration of the flank alone or in combination with intercostal blocks and topical application of local anesthetic cream have also been used during lithotripsy on the Dornier HM-3 to decrease intravenous analgesic requirements.[197,201] Although both local anesthetic techniques produced cutaneous analgesia, intravenous analgesics were still required for intraoperative patient comfort.

TABLE 35-13

CONTRAINDICATIONS TO EXTRACORPEAL SHOCK WAVE LITHOTRIPSY

Absolute contraindications	Obstruction distal to the renal calculi
	Bleeding disorder or anticoagulation
	Pregnancy
Relative contraindications	Large calcified aortic or renal artery aneurysms
	Untreated urinary tract infection
	Pacemaker or AICD implant
	Morbid obesity

AICD, automatic implantable cardioverter-defibrillator.

SWL has revolutionized the standard of treatment of nephrolithiasis. Currently, general or regional anesthesia is used with first-generation lithotripters, and conscious sedation or "light" general anesthesia is used with the second-generation or third-generation devices.

Percutaneous Renal Procedures

Percutaneous nephrostomy (PCN) is commonly performed to diagnose and treat a wide variety of urologic problems, including relief of renal obstruction, stone removal, biopsy of tumors, and ureteral stent placement.[139] During a PCN procedure, a needle-guidewire-catheter sequence technique is used to enter the renal collecting system under fluoroscopic guidance to establish access and drainage of the kidney. This procedure is performed with the patient prone, and local anesthesia with intravneous sedation is used for analgesia.[139] PCN involves passing an endoscope through the nephrostomy tract. Percutaneous nephrolithotomy, a procedure to remove renal calculi too large to be treated with lithotripsy, is one of the most common urologic endosurgical procedures, requiring dilatation of a nephrostomy tract and usually general or regional anesthesia.

Although percutaneous surgical techniques are considerably less invasive than open surgical procedures, a variety of complications can occur.[202] During insertion of the nephrostomy tube, trauma to the spleen, liver, or kidney can result in acute blood loss necessitating an emergency open surgical procedure. Colon injury has been reported if a retrorenal colon overlies the lower pole of the kidney.[139] Pleural injury may occur during nephrostomy tube placement when access is created above the twelfth rib or the kidney lies in a more cephalad position than normal. Nephrostomy tract dilatation causes bleeding in most patients, with hemoglobin declining an average of 1.2 g/dL. If excessive intraoperative bleeding occurs, it is wise to stop the procedure and insert a large-caliber nephrostomy tube or high-pressure balloon nephrostomy catheter to tamponade the bleeding.[202] In a study of 50 patients undergoing PCN for stone removal, prevalence of complications was 12%, with pleural effusion and hydropneumothorax being the most common problems encountered.[203]

During nephroscopy procedures, continuous irrigation of fluid through the endoscope is necessary to prevent blood and debris from obscuring the surgeon's vision. If a significant discrepancy exists between the amount of irrigating fluid infused and output from the patient, then clinical evaluation of the patient for extravasation of irrigation fluid into the retroperitoneal, intraperitoneal, intravascular, or pleural spaces is warranted. Intravenous absorption of irrigation fluid during percutaneous renal procedures can create a situation similar to that seen with TUR syndrome, in which electrolyte abnormalities and fluid overload can occur. Because electrocautery is rarely used during percutaneous renal procedures, the preferred irrigating solution is 0.9% sodium chloride.[204] If an electrocautery device is needed, irrigation fluid is temporarily changed to a nonelectrolyte solution.

LASER SURGERY IN UROLOGY

Laser therapy has been shown to be effective in treating a multitude of urologic problems, including condyloma acuminatum of the external genitalia and urethra; ureteral stricture or bladder neck contracture; interstitial cystitis; BPH; ureteral calculi, and superficial carcinoma of the penis, bladder, ureter, and renal pelvis.[205] Major advantages of laser surgery over traditional surgical approaches include minimal blood loss, decreased postoperative pain, and tissue denaturation, a process that reduces risk of tumor implantation.

Because lasers are an integral part of urologic surgery, understanding the indications and limitations of each type of laser is essential.[206] The *carbon dioxide (CO_2) laser* produces intense heat with vaporization, but has minimal tissue penetration and is unable to penetrate water. Thus, its use is limited to treating cutaneous lesions of the external genitalia. The *argon laser* is poorly absorbed by water, but is selectively absorbed by hemoglobin and melanin, making it useful for procedures in the bladder requiring coagulation of bleeding sites. The *pulsed dye laser* generates a pulsed output and is useful for destroying ureteral calculi. One of the most versatile and widely used lasers in urologic surgery is the *Nd-YAG laser.*[205] This device produces deep tissue penetration via protein denaturation with minimal vaporization. It can be used in water or urine without loss of effectiveness and delivered with a fiber-optic laser delivery system for endourologic surgery. Excellent results have been reported after treatment of lesions of the penis, urethra, bladder, ureters, and kidneys. The *KTP-532 laser* is a frequency-doubled Nd-YAG laser that does not penetrate tissue as deeply as the Nd-YAG but has a better cutting effect.[206] It is extremely effective in treating urethral strictures and bladder neck contractures.

Safety issues assume paramount importance during laser surgery. Damage to the eye is the potential injury that requires the greatest attention because both direct and reflected laser beams can cause eye injury.[207] Protective goggles with appropriate filtering lenses are available for each type of laser, and laser equipment should not be activated until all operating room personnel and the patient are wearing glasses. Although less critical than eye damage, inadvertent thermal injury to the skin may also occur during laser treatments. Thermal injuries are avoidable if the laser is placed in the "standby" mode when not in operation and is activated only by the surgeon performing the procedure. During CO_2 laser therapy for condyloma acuminatum, the plume (smoke) from the vaporization of tissue contains active human papilloma virus particles.[208] To avoid inhalation of infectious agents, all operating room personnel involved in CO_2 laser procedures for genital lesions should wear protective laser masks that prevent small particles from being inhaled. In addition, the laser plume should be removed from the operating room with a smoke evacuation system.

UROLOGIC LAPAROSCOPY

Urologic laparoscopy techniques are minimally invasive and have rapidly gained acceptance because they are associated with decreased postoperative pain, shorter hospital stays, lower hospital costs, and more rapid convalescence than open surgical procedures.[139] Laparoscopic procedures performed in urology include diagnostic procedures for evaluating undescended testis, orchiopexy, varicocelectomy, bladder suspension, pelvic lymphadenectomy, nephrectomy, partial nephrectomy, nephroureterectomy, adrenalectomy, prostatectomy, and cystectomy.

Unique cardiopulmonary changes may occur during laparoscopic surgery (see Chapter 38). Physiologic alterations during laparoscopy are often related to the surgical technique itself, in particular, the creation of the pneumoperitoneum and absorption of insufflating gas.[209] A wide variety of intraoperative complications are also possible during laparoscopy (Table 35-14). Occurrence of complications for large laparoscopy series is reported to range from 0.6 to 2.4%, with approximately one-third being cardiopulmonary in nature.[210]

Laparoscopic urologic procedures differ from conventional laparoscopy in several respects. Many structures in the genitourinary system are extraperitoneal (i.e., pelvic lymph nodes, bladder, ureters, adrenal glands, kidneys), and urologists often prefer extraperitoneal insufflation during laparoscopic surgery on these organs. Several studies have reported that CO_2 absorption is greater with extraperitoneal (76%) compared with intraperitoneal (15 to 25%) insufflation.[211]

Some laparoscopic procedures in urology, namely, cystectomy and nephrectomy, tend to be lengthy. Prolonged insufflation times during these procedures increase the amount of CO_2 absorbed and also necessitate use of general anesthesia to guarantee patient comfort. Increased absorption of CO_2 during extraperitoneal laparoscopic techniques mandates that the anesthesiologist carefully monitor and adjust ventilation to maintain normocarbia. Oliguria has been associated with prolonged duration of pneumoperitoneum during laparoscopic nephrectomy surgery.[212] A possible mechanism for intraoperative oliguria during laparoscopic surgery is an increase in stress hormone levels, such as ADH.[213] Intraoperative oliguria is often treated with fluid administration; thus, it is important that the anesthesiologist be aware that oliguria during prolonged laparoscopic procedures may not reflect intravascular volume depletion.

TABLE 35-14

POTENTIAL INTRAOPERATIVE COMPLICATIONS DURING LAPAROSCOPIC SURGERY

■ PULMONARY
Pneumothorax
Pneumomediastinum
Hypoxemia
Hypercapnia
Aspiration
■ CARDIOVASCULAR
Dysrhythmias
Hypotension
Hypertension
Venous gas embolus
Venous thrombosis
■ MISCELLANEOUS
Vascular injury
Visceral perforation
Oliguria
Hypothermia
Peripheral nerve injury

RADICAL CANCER SURGERY

Most major, open surgical procedures in urology are performed to treat cancer of the prostate, bladder, or kidney. These procedures are often lengthy and require intraoperative patient positions associated with significant impact on cardiorespiratory function. Radical urologic surgery also carries a potential for hemorrhage and large intraoperative blood and fluid requirements. In addition, patients undergoing these procedures are often elderly with preexisting medical conditions.

Radical Prostatectomy

Prostate cancer is the most commonly diagnosed cancer in men, as well as the second most common cause of prostate-related mortality in American men.[214] Localized prostate cancer (stage A or B) is treated with radical prostatectomy, radioactive implants, or radiation therapy. In the United States, men with clinically localized prostate cancer whose life expectancy is 10 years or longer tend to undergo radical prostatectomy, whereas patients older than 70 years of age or with a life expectancy of less than 10 years usually opt for radiation therapy or observation. The outcome of the two approaches is similar.[215]

Radical prostatectomy can be performed by a perineal, retropubic, or laparoscopic surgical approach. The anesthetic technique for radical prostatectomy is influenced by whether an open or laparoscopic surgical approach is planned. The surgical procedure involves en bloc removal of the entire prostate gland, seminal vesicles, ejaculatory ducts, and a portion of the bladder neck, while attempting to preserve nerves controlling sexual function. After en bloc removal of these structures, the remaining bladder neck is anastomosed to the membranous urethra over an indwelling urethral catheter. Limited pelvic lymphadenectomy is usually performed during the procedure to aid in cancer staging.[216]

Proponents of radical perineal prostatectomy claim it is associated with less intraoperative blood loss, better exposure for the vesicourethral anastomosis, and a shorter convalescent time than with retropubic prostatectomy.[217] During a radical perineal prostatectomy, the patient is positioned in the exaggerated lithotomy position, slight flexion of the trunk, and a Trendelenburg tilt. This extreme lithotomy position compresses abdominal contents on the diaphragm and may cause respiratory embarrassment. Rhabdomyolysis with secondary ARF has also been reported after perineal prostatectomy in the exaggerated lithotomy position.[93–95] These reports suggest muscle damage is probably secondary to ischemia of the muscles in the elevated legs or the lumbar and pelvic muscles that were compressed by the exaggerated position. Lower-extremity nerve injury due to intraoperative leg positioning is another potential complication of the lithotomy position. In the exaggerated lithotomy, most anesthesiologists prefer either general or a combined epidural–general anesthetic for the procedure.[164]

Radical retropubic prostatectomy is performed through a midline lower abdominal incision, with the patient in a slight hyperextended supine position to distance the symphysis pubis from the umbilicus. General or regional (epidural or spinal) anesthesia with sedation may be used for this procedure. If regional anesthesia is used, a sensory block of T6–T8 is adequate.[164] Advocates of general anesthesia believe it provides greater intraoperative patient comfort, improved airway control, faster onset, and a more controllable duration of action. Other anesthesiologists suggest that regional anesthesia is preferable for radical retropubic prostatectomy. Epidural anesthesia and analgesia has been described to favorably affect operative blood loss, postoperative pain control, and patient activity level after surgery.[218–220] A review of the current literature reveals no difference in patient mortality between regional and general anesthesia for radical prostatectomy.[220,221]

Preoperative administration of erythropoietin, preoperative autologous blood donation, acute normovolemic hemodilution, and intraoperative cell salvage are recommended perioperative techniques to avoid allogenic blood transfusion in radical retropubic prostatectomy. Autologous blood donation (3 U) versus preoperative erythropoietin and acute normovolemic hemodilution versus acute normovolemic hemodilution alone have been compared to determine which blood conservation strategy for radical retropubic prostatectomy was most efficient.[222] The authors concluded that all three blood conservation strategies resulted in similar allogenic blood exposure, but acute normovolemic hemodilution was the least costly technique. The need for allogenic blood transfusion in patients who participate in autologous blood donation is reported to be 0 to 14% and is similar to that in patients who do not donate blood (2.4 to 11%).[223]

Another technique to prevent allogenic blood transfusion for radical retropubic prostatectomy is intraoperative cell salvage. Gray et al.[224] evaluated the safety of this technique compared with preoperative autologous blood donation. They concluded that intraoperative cell salvage using leucocyte reduction filters in radical retropubic prostatectomy resulted in higher preoperative hematocrit levels with a low occurrence (3% versus 14%) of allogenic blood transfusion. Intraoperative cell salvage did not appear to be associated with increased risk of any early biochemical cancer progression. The safety of intraoperative cell salvage in malignant fields has not been clearly established, but there is some evidence that it is safe.[225,226]

General anesthesia is the technique of choice for laparoscopic prostatectomy. Endotracheal intubation with muscle relaxation provides a secure airway with controlled ventilation during pneumoperitoneum to facilitate the surgical procedure. Pulmonary implications of laparoscopy include management of decreased compliance and increased $Paco_2$ produced from CO_2 absorption during pneumoperitoneum. It may be advisable to insert an intra-arterial catheter to facilitate arterial blood gas measurement and to monitor arterial pressure during the procedure. Major cardiovascular complications during CO_2 pneumoperitoneum include dysrhythmia and CO_2 embolism.[227]

Laparoscopic prostatectomy may take longer to perform than conventional open surgery, but less blood loss, shorter hospital stay, and quicker return of normal patient function is expected. Uncontrollable hemorrhage can occur, however, so at least one large-bore intravenous catheter should be inserted.

The head-down (Trendelenburg) position is used in perineal, retropubic, and laparoscopic prostatectomy surgery. This position produces physiologic changes in the cardiopulmonary and cerebrovascular systems in proportion to the degree of head-down tilt[228] (see Chapter 23). Head-down positioning during open prostatectomy procedures places the operative site in the pelvis above the heart, creating a gravitational gradient between the prostatic fossa and the heart. If the prostatic venous network is opened while the patient is in this position, then venous air embolism may occur.[229,230] The most common intraoperative problem during radical prostatectomy is hemorrhage.[216] Massive blood loss may occur if one of the branches of the hypogastric vein is inadvertently torn during pelvic lymphadenectomy or transection of the dorsal venous complex. With the potential for rapid blood loss, invasive monitoring or echocardiography may be needed to further assess cardiac filling pressures and overall hemodynamic status in patients with severe preexisting cardiopulmonary disease.

Length of hospital stay for radical retropubic prostatectomy is currently expected to be 2 to 3 days with an open procedure and 1 to 2 days with the laparoscopic approach. Choice of anesthesia for future radical prostatectomy surgeries may depend on whether a specific surgical approach (open versus laparoscopic) is determined to deliver superior patient outcome.

Radical Cystectomy

The standard of care for treating muscle-invasive bladder cancer is a radical cystectomy.[231] In men, this surgery involves en bloc removal of the bladder, prostate, seminal vesicles, and proximal urethra. In women, it is necessary to remove the bladder, urethra, and anterior vaginal wall, as well as to perform a total hysterectomy and bilateral salpingo-oophorectomy. At completion of the procedure, a urinary diversion is performed, most commonly as an ileal or colon conduit.

Significant intraoperative hemorrhage can occur, suggesting the need for large-bore intravneous access and invasive monitoring (arterial line and CVP) for intraoperative management. This intraperitoneal procedure is similar to a major bowel procedure, resulting in increased fluid requirements. The urinary diversion also prolongs the procedure, and most anesthesiologists find that the additional length and extent of surgery mandate a general or combined general–epidural anesthetic.[164] Patients with bladder cancer may have been treated with chemotherapy before their procedure. The most commonly used chemotherapeutic agents are methotrexate, vinblastine, cisplatinum, and doxorubicin. The anesthesiologist should be aware of prior use of any chemotherapeutic agent so any possible drug toxicity can be elucidated. In particular, doxorubicin has cardiotoxic effects, methotrexate may cause hepatic toxicity, and both cisplatinum and methotrexate are associated with neurotoxicity and renal injury.

Radical Nephrectomy

Renal cell carcinoma accounts for ~3% of all adult malignancies.[232] Surgery is the only effective treatment, with radical or partial nephrectomy the treatment of choice. Radical nephrectomy involves en bloc removal of the kidney and surrounding fascia, the ipsilateral adrenal gland, and the upper ureter. The tumor extends into the vena cava in ~5% of patients, and aggressive surgical therapy is warranted if there is no evidence of metastasis. On occasion, CPB and circulatory arrest have been used to treat extensive caval tumor invasion.

The kidney can be approached through a lumbar, transabdominal, or thoracoabdominal incision.[164] If a lumbar approach is used, the patient is placed in the flexed lateral decubitus position with the operative side up and the mechanical kidney support elevated beneath the twelfth rib. General anesthesia or combined epidural–general anesthesia is used for patients placed in the "kidney position" because the position is extremely uncomfortable. It may also predispose patients to nerve damage or cardiopulmonary alterations (see Chapter 23). During radical nephrectomy procedures, the anesthesiologist needs to be prepared for acute blood loss because of the proximity of the kidney to large blood vessels. The patient also needs to be adequately hydrated to optimize blood flow to the remaining kidney and to prevent hypotension from inferior vena caval compression during positioning. Pneumothorax can occur during surgery if the chest is inadvertently entered. A chest radiograph should be obtained in the postanesthesia care unit if a pneumothorax is suspected. Venous air embolisms are also possible during nephrectomy procedures if the positioning places the operative site above the heart.

Radical Surgery for Testicular Cancer

Although testicular cancer accounts for only 1% of all cancers in men, it is the most common malignancy in men between 15 and 34 years of age.[233] All intratesticular masses are considered cancerous until proven otherwise, and radical orchiectomy is performed for both definitive diagnosis and as the initial step of most treatment regimens. Either regional or general anesthesia can be used for this procedure.

Subsequent treatment depends on the stage and histology of the testicular tumor. Potential treatment options include observation, radiation to the inguinal and retroperitoneal areas, chemotherapy, or retroperitoneal lymph node dissection. Because chemotherapy regimens change frequently, the National Cancer Institute's CancerNet website (http://cancernet.nci.nih.gov) carries current treatment protocols for each type and stage of testicular cancer.

Prior to surgery, the anesthesiologist should identify the chemotherapeutic agents used and be aware of the side effects of these drugs. One commonly used chemotherapeutic agent, bleomycin, is an antitumor antibiotic used against germ cell tumors of the testis. Its use is associated with pulmonary toxicity, and there are numerous reports of postoperative respiratory failure after retroperitoneal lymph node dissection in patients treated with it.[234,235] The onset of respiratory failure usually occurs 3 to 10 days after surgery. Risk factors for postoperative respiratory distress include preoperative evidence of pulmonary injury, recent exposure to bleomycin (within 1 to 2 months), a total dose of bleomycin >450 mg, or a Ccr of <35 mL/min.[235] Although intraoperative exposure to hyperoxia (inspired oxygen concentrations >30%) has been linked to postoperative pulmonary toxicity, this relationship is controversial.[234,235] A retrospective study found that intravenous fluid management, including blood transfusion, was the most significant factor affecting postoperative pulmonary morbidity and clinical outcome.[234] The authors recommend that intravenous fluid administration consist primarily of colloid and be limited to the minimum volume necessary to maintain hemodynamic stability and adequate renal output.

References

1. Guyton AC: Formation of urine by the kidney: Renal blood flow, glomerular filtration, and their control. In Guyton AC (ed): Texbook of Medical Physiology, 8th ed, p 286. Philadelphia, WB Saunders, 1991
2. Brezis M, Rosen S: Hypoxia of the renal medulla—Its implications for disease. N Engl J Med 332:647, 1995
3. Awazu M, Ichikawa I: Biological significance of atrial natriuretic peptide in the kidney. Nephron 63:1, 1993
4. Espiner EA: Physiology of natriuretic peptides. J Intern Med 235:527, 1994
5. McIntyre RW, Schwinn DA: Atrial natriuretic peptide. J Cardiothorac Anesth 3:91, 1989
6. Gabbai FB, Blantz RC: Role of nitric oxide in renal hemodynamics. Semin Nephrol 19:242, 1999
7. Mene P, Dunn MJ: Vascular, glomerular and tubular effects of angiotensin II, kinins and prostaglandins. In Seldin DW, Giebisch G (eds): The Kidney: Physiology and Pathophysiology, 2nd ed, p 1205. New York, Raven Press, 1992
8. Satoh S, Zimmerman BG: Influence of the renin-angiotensin system on the effect of prostaglandin synthesis inhibitors in the renal vasculature. Circ Res 36:89, 1975
9. Silva P, Rosen S, Spokes K *et al*: Influence of endogenous prostaglandins on mTAL injury. J Am Soc Nephrol 1:808, 1990
10. Badr KF, Ichikawa I: Prerenal failure: A deleterious shift from renal compensation to decompensation. N Engl J Med 319:623, 1988
11. Crandell WB, Pappas SG, Macdonald A: Nephrotoxicity associated with methoxyflurane anesthesia. Anesthesiology 27:591, 1966
12. Kharasch ED, Hankins DC, Thummel KE: Human kidney methoxyflurane and sevoflurane metabolism. Intrarenal fluoride production as a possible mechanism of methoxyflurane nephrotoxicity. Anesthesiology 82:689, 1995
13. Mazze RI, Calverley RK, Smith NT: Inorganic fluoride nephrotoxicity: Prolonged enflurane and halothane anesthesia in volunteers. Anesthesiology 46:265, 1977
14. Mazze RI, Sievenpiper TS, Stevenson J: Renal effects of enflurane and halothane in patients with abnormal renal function. Anesthesiology 60:161, 1984
15. Priano LL: The effects of anesthetic agents on renal function. In Barash PG (ed): ASA Refresher Courses in Anesthesiology, p 240. Philadelphia, JB Lippincott, 1985
16. Halperin BD, Feeley TW: The effect of anesthesia and surgery on renal function. Int Anesthesiol Clin 22:157, 1984
17. Anderson RJ, Linas SL, Berns AS *et al*: Nonoliguric acute renal failure. N Engl J Med 19(296):1134, 1977
18. Cameron JS: Acute renal failure in the intensive care unit today. Intensive Care Med 12:64, 1986
19. Firmat J, Zucchini A, Martin R *et al*: A study of 500 cases of acute renal failure (1978–1991). Ren Fail 16:91, 1994
20. Baudouin SV, Wiggins J, Keogh BF *et al*: Continuous veno-venous haemofiltration following cardio-pulmonary bypass. Indications and outcome in 35 patients. Intensive Care Med 19:290, 1993
21. Olsen PS, Schroeder T, Perko M *et al*: Renal failure after operation for abdominal aortic aneurysm. Ann Vasc Surg 4:580, 1990
22. Storck M, Hartl WH, Zimmerer E *et al*: Comparison of pump-driven and spontaneous continuous haemofiltration in postoperative acute renal failure. Lancet 337:452, 1991
23. Gordon AC, Pryn S, Collin J *et al*: Outcome in patients who require renal

support after surgery for ruptured abdominal aortic aneurysm. Br J Surg 81:836, 1994
24. Tominaga GT, Ingegno MD, Scannell G *et al*: Continuous arteriovenous hemodiafiltration in postoperative and traumatic renal failure. Am J Surg 166:612, 1993
25. Bellomo R, Farmer M, Boyce N: A prospective study of continuous venovenous hemodiafiltration in critically ill patients with acute renal failure. J Intensive Care Med 10:187, 1995
26. Pellanda MV, Fabris A, Ronco C: Etiology and pathophysiology of acute renal failure. In Pinsky MR, Dhainaut JFA (eds): Pathophysiologic Foundations of Critical Care, p 571. Baltimore, Williams & Wilkins, 1993
27. Kellen M, Aronson S, Roizen MF *et al*: Predictive and diagnostic tests of renal failure: A review. Anesth Analg 78:134, 1994
28. Desjars P, Pinaud M, Bugnon D *et al*: Norepinephrine therapy has no deleterious renal effects in human septic shock. Crit Care Med 17:426, 1989
29. Martin C, Papazian L, Perrin G *et al*: Norepinephrine or dopamine for the treatment of hyperdynamic septic shock? Chest 103:1826, 1993
30. Vincent JL, Preiser JC: Inotropic agents. New Horiz 1:137, 1993
31. Martinez-Maldonado M, Benabe JE, Cordova HR: Chronic clinical intrinsic renal failure. In Seldin DW, Giebisch G (eds): The Kidney: Physiology and Pathophysiology, 2nd ed. New York, Raven Press, 3227–3288, 1992
32. Kuruvila KC, Schrier RW: Chronic renal failure. Int Anesthesiol Clin 22:101, 1984
33. Eschbach JW: The anemia of chronic renal failure: Pathophysiology and the effects of recombinant erythropoietin. Kidney Int 35:134, 1989
34. Touchette MA, Slaughter RL: The effect of renal failure on hepatic drug clearance. DICP 25:1214, 1991
35. Sear JW: Kidney transplants: Induction and analgesic agents. Int Anesthesiol Clin 33:45, 1995
36. St. Peter WL, Halstenson CE: Pharmacologic approach in patients with renal failure. In Chernow B (ed): The Pharmacologic Approach to the Critically Ill Patient, 3rd ed, p 41. Baltimore, Williams & Wilkins, 1994
37. Burch PG, Stanski DR: Decreased protein binding and thiopental kinetics. Clin Pharmacol Ther 32:212, 1982
38. Trevor AJ: Biotransformation of ketamine. In Domino EF (ed): Status of Ketamine in Anesthesiology, p 93. Ann Arbor, MI, NPP Books, 1990
39. Reich DL, Silvay G: Ketamine: An update on the first twenty-five years of clinical experience. Can J Anaesth 36:186, 1989
40. Carlos R, Calvo R, Erill S: Plasma protein binding of etomidate in patients with renal failure or hepatic cirrhosis. Clin Pharmacokinet 4:144, 1979
41. Morcos WE, Payne JP: The induction of anaesthesia with propofol ('Diprivan') compared in normal and renal failure patients. Postgrad Med J 61(suppl 3):62, 1985
42. Kirvela M, Olkkola KT, Rosenberg PH *et al*: Pharmacokinetics of propofol and haemodynamic changes during induction of anaesthesia in uraemic patients. Br J Anaesth 68:178, 1992
43. Vinik HR, Reves JG, Greenblatt DJ *et al*: The pharmacokinetics of midazolam in chronic renal failure patients. Anesthesiology 59:390, 1983
44. Driessen JJ, Vree TB, Guelen PJ: The effects of acute changes in renal function on the pharmacokinetics of midazolam during long-term infusion in ICU patients. Acta Anaesthesiol Belg 42:149, 1991
45. Schmith VD, Piraino B, Smith RB *et al*: Alprazolam in end-stage renal disease. II. Pharmacodynamics. Clin Pharmacol Ther 51:533, 1992
46. De Wolf AM, Fragen RJ, Avram MJ *et al*: The pharmacokinetics of dexmedetomidine in volunteers with severe renal impairment. Anesth Analg 93:1205, 2001
47. Chan GL, Matzke GR: Effects of renal insufficiency on the pharmacokinetics and pharmacodynamics of opioid analgesics. Drug Intell Clin Pharm 21:773, 1987
48. Babul N, Darke AC, Hagen N: Hydromorphone metabolite accumulation in renal failure. J Pain Symptom Manage 10:184, 1995
49. Kirvela M, Lindgren L, Seppala T *et al*: The pharmacokinetics of oxycodone in uremic patients undergoing renal transplantation. J Clin Anesth 8:13, 1996
50. Koehntop DE, Rodman JH: Fentanyl pharmacokinetics in patients undergoing renal transplantation. Pharmacotherapy 17:746, 1997
51. Davis PJ, Stiller RL, Cook DR *et al*: Effects of cholestatic hepatic disease and chronic renal failure on alfentanil pharmacokinetics in children. Anesth Analg 68:579, 1989
52. Wiggum DC, Cork RC, Weldon ST *et al*: Postoperative respiratory depression and elevated sufentanil levels in a patient with chronic renal failure. Anesthesiology 63:708, 1985
53. Breen D, Wilmer A, Bodenham A *et al*: Offset of pharmacodynamic effects and safety of remifentanil in intensive care unit patients with various degrees of renal impairment. Crit Care 8:R21, 2004
54. Smith CE, Hunter JM: Anesthesia for renal transplantation: Relaxants and volatiles. Int Anesthesiol Clin 33:69, 1995
55. Ryan DW: Preoperative serum cholinesterase concentration in chronic renal failure. Clinical experience of suxamethonium in 81 patients undergoing renal transplant. Br J Anaesth 49:945, 1977
56. Cook DR, Freeman JA, Lai AA *et al*: Pharmacokinetics of mivacurium in normal patients and in those with hepatic or renal failure. Br J Anaesth 69:580, 1992
57. Cook DR, Freeman JA, Lai AA *et al*: Pharmacokinetics and pharmacodynamics of doxacurium in normal patients and in those with hepatic or renal failure. Anesth Analg 72:145, 1991
58. Cashman JN, Luke JJ, Jones RM: Neuromuscular block with doxacurium (BW A938U) in patients with normal or absent renal function. Br J Anaesth 64:186, 1990
59. Boyd AH, Eastwood NB, Parker CJ *et al*: Pharmacodynamics of the 1R cis-1'R cis isomer of atracurium (51W89) in health and chronic renal failure. Br J Anaesth 74:400, 1995
60. Fahey MR, Rupp SM, Canfell C *et al*: Effect of renal failure on laudanosine excretion in man. Br J Anaesth 57:1049, 1985
61. Yate PM, Flynn PJ, Arnold RW *et al*: Clinical experience and plasma laudanosine concentrations during the infusion of atracurium in the intensive therapy unit. Br J Anaesth 59:211, 1987
62. Eastwood NB, Boyd AH, Parker CJ *et al*: Pharmacokinetics of 1R-cis 1'R-cis atracurium besylate (51W89) and plasma laudanosine concentrations in health and chronic renal failure. Br J Anaesth 75:431, 1995
63. Lynam DP, Cronnelly R, Castagnoli KP *et al*: The pharmacodynamics and pharmacokinetics of vecuronium in patients anesthetized with isoflurane with normal renal function or with renal failure. Anesthesiology 69:227, 1988
64. Segredo V, Caldwell JE, Matthay MA *et al*: Persistent paralysis in critically ill patients after long-term administration of vecuronium. N Engl J Med 20(327):524, 1992
65. Wierda JM, Kleef UW, Lambalk LM *et al*: The pharmacodynamics and pharmacokinetics of Org 9426, a new non-depolarizing neuromuscular blocking agent, in patients anaesthetized with nitrous oxide, halothane and fentanyl. Can J Anaesth 38:430, 1991
66. Szenohradszky J, Fisher DM, Segredo V *et al*: Pharmacokinetics of rocuronium bromide (ORG 9426) in patients with normal renal function or patients undergoing cadaver renal transplantation. Anesthesiology 77:899, 1992
67. Cooper RA, Maddineni VR, Mirakhur RK *et al*: Time course of neuromuscular effects and pharmacokinetics of rocuronium bromide (Org 9426) during isoflurane anaesthesia in patients with and without renal failure. Br J Anaesth 71:222, 1993
68. Khuenl-Brady KS, Pomaroli A, Puhringer F *et al*: The use of rocuronium (ORG 9426) in patients with chronic renal failure. Anaesthesia 48:873, 1993
69. Phillips BJ, Hunter JM: Use of mivacurium chloride by constant infusion in the anephric patient. Br J Anaesth 68:492, 1992
70. Blobner M, Jelen-Esselborn S, Schneider G *et al*: Effect of renal function on neuromuscular block induced by continuous infusion of mivacurium. Br J Anaesth 74:452, 1995
71. Morris RB, Cronnelly R, Miller RD *et al*: Pharmacokinetics of edrophonium in anephric and renal transplant patients. Br J Anaesth 53:1311, 1981
72. Ali-Melkkila T, Kanto J, Iisalo E: Pharmacokinetics and related pharmacodynamics of anticholinergic drugs. Acta Anaesthesiol Scand 37:633, 1993
73. Novis BK, Roizen MF, Aronson S *et al*: Association of preoperative risk factors with postoperative acute renal failure. Anesth Analg 78:143, 1994
74. Shusterman N, Strom BL, Murray TG *et al*: Risk factors and outcome of hospital-acquired acute renal failure. Clinical epidemiologic study. Am J Med 83:65, 1987
75. Blamey SL, Fearon KC, Gilmour WH *et al*: Prediction of risk in biliary surgery. Br J Surg 70:535, 1983
76. Ring-Larsen H: Associated renal failure. In Williams R (ed): Liver Failure, p 72. New York, Churchill Livingstone, 1986
77. Rimola A, Gavaler JS, Schade RR *et al*: Effects of renal impairment on liver transplantation. Gastroenterology 93:148, 1987
78. Cuervas-Mons V, Millan I, Gavaler JS *et al*: Prognostic value of preoperatively obtained clinical and laboratory data in predicting survival following orthotopic liver transplantation. Hepatology 6:922, 1986
79. Lindeman RD: Overview: Renal physiology and pathophysiology of aging. Am J Kidney Dis 16:275, 1990
80. Shin B, Mackenzie CF, Helrich M: Creatinine clearance of early detection of posttraumatic renal dysfunction. Anesthesiology 64:605, 1986
81. Wilson RF, Soullier G, Antonenko D: Creatinine clearance in critically ill surgical patients. Arch Surg 114:461, 1979
82. Sladen RN, Endo E, Harrison T: Two-hour versus 22-hour creatinine clearance in critically ill patients. Anesthesiology 67:1013, 1987
83. Taylor GA, Barnewolt CE, Adler BH *et al*: Renal cortical ischemia in rabbits revealed by contrast-enhanced power Doppler sonography. AJR Am J Roentgenol 170:417, 1998
84. Bauman LA, Watson NE Jr, Scuderi PE *et al*: Transcutaneous renal function monitor: Precision during unsteady hemodynamics. J Clin Monit Comput 14:275, 1998
85. Walker RS, Duggin GG: Cellular mechanisms of drug nephrotoxitcity. In Seldin DW, Giebisch G (eds): The Kidney: Physiology and Pathophysiology, 2nd ed, p 3571. New York, Raven Press, 1992
86. Hock R, Anderson RJ: Prevention of drug-induced nephrotoxicity in the intensive care unit. J Crit Care 10:33, 1995
87. Wilkinson AH, Cohen DJ: Renal failure in the recipients of nonrenal solid organ transplants. J Am Soc Nephrol 10:1136, 1999
88. Barrett BJ: Contrast nephrotoxicity. J Am Soc Nephrol 5:125, 1994
89. Alonso A, Lau J, Jaber BL *et al*: Prevention of radiocontrast nephropathy with N-acetylcysteine in patients with chronic kidney disease: A meta-analysis of randomized, controlled trials. Am J Kidney Dis 43:1, 2004
90. Garella S, Matarese RA: Renal effects of prostaglandins and clinical

adverse effects of nonsteroidal anti-inflammatory agents. Medicine (Baltimore) 63:165, 1984
91. Abassi ZA, Hoffman A, Better OS: Acute renal failure complicating muscle crush injury. Semin Nephrol 18:558, 1998
92. Dubrow A, Flamenbaum W: Acute renal failure associated with myoglobinuria and hemoglobinuria. In Brenner BM, Lazarus JM (eds): Acute Renal Failure, 2nd ed, p 279. New York, Churchill Livingstone, 1988
93. Ali H, Nieto JG, Rhamy RK *et al*: Acute renal failure due to rhabdomyolysis associated with the extreme lithotomy position. Am J Kidney Dis 22:865, 1993
94. Gabrielli A, Caruso L: Postoperative acute renal failure secondary to rhabdomyolysis from exaggerated lithotomy position. J Clin Anesth 11:257, 1999
95. Guzzi LM, Mills LM, Greenman P: Rhabdomyolysis, acute renal failure, and the exaggerated lithotomy position. Anesth Analg 77:635, 1993
96. Veenstra J, Smit WM, Krediet RT *et al*: Relationship between elevated creatine phosphokinase and the clinical spectrum of rhabdomyolysis. Nephrol Dial Transplant 9:637, 1994
97. Better OS, Stein JH: Early management of shock and prophylaxis of acute renal failure in traumatic rhabdomyolysis. N Engl J Med 322:825, 1990
98. Eichhorn JH, Hedley-Whyte J, Steinman TI *et al*: Renal failure following enflurane anesthesia. Anesthesiology 45:557, 1976
99. Eger EI, Gong D, Koblin DD *et al*: Dose-related biochemical markers of renal injury after sevoflurane versus desflurane anesthesia in volunteers. Anesth Analg 85:1154, 1997
100. Conzen PF, Kharasch ED, Czerner SF *et al*: Low-flow sevoflurane compared with low-flow isoflurane anesthesia in patients with stable renal insufficiency. Anesthesiology 97:578, 2002
101. Sirinek KR, Hura CE: Renal failure. In Moore EE, Mattox KL, Feliciano DV (eds): Trauma, 2nd ed. Norwalk, CT, Appleton & Lange, 927–940, 1991
102. Baxter CR: Acute renal insufficiency complicating trauma and surgery. In Shires GT (ed): Principles of Trauma, 3rd ed, p 502. New York, McGraw-Hill, 1985
103. Stene JK: Renal failure in the trauma patient. Crit Care Clin 6:111, 1990
104. Cachecho R, Millham FH, Wedel SK: Management of the trauma patient with pre-existing renal disease. Crit Care Clin 10:523, 1994
105. Myers BD, Miller DC, Mehigan JT *et al*: Nature of the renal injury following total renal ischemia in man. J Clin Invest 73:329, 1984
106. Godet G, Fleron MH, Vicaut E *et al*: Risk factors for acute postoperative renal failure in thoracic or thoracoabdominal aortic surgery: A prospective study. Anesth Analg 85:1227, 1997
107. Svensson LG, Coselli JS, Safi HJ *et al*: Appraisal of adjuncts to prevent acute renal failure after surgery on the thoracic or thoracoabdominal aorta. J Vasc Surg 10:230, 1989
108. Greenberg RK, Chuter TA, Lawrence-Brown M *et al*: Analysis of renal function after aneurysm repair with a device using suprarenal fixation (Zenith AAA Endovascular Graft) in contrast to open surgical repair. J Vasc Surg 39:1219, 2004
109. Greenberg RK, Chuter TA, Sternbergh WC III *et al*: Zenith AAA endovascular graft: Intermediate-term results of the US multicenter trial. J Vasc Surg 39:1209, 2004
110. Paul MD, Mazer CD, Byrick RJ *et al*: Influence of mannitol and dopamine on renal function during elective infrarenal aortic clamping in man. Am J Nephrol 6:427, 1986
111. Flancbaum L, Choban PS, Dasta JF: Quantitative effects of low-dose dopamine on urine output in oliguric surgical intensive care unit patients. Crit Care Med 22:61, 1994
112. Antonucci F, Calo L, Rizzolo M *et al*: Nifedipine can preserve renal function in patients undergoing aortic surgery with infrarenal crossclamping. Nephron 74:668, 1996
113. Ding H, Kopple JD, Cohen A *et al*: Recombinant human insulin-like growth factor-I accelerates recovery and reduces catabolism in rats with ischemic acute renal failure. J Clin Invest 91:2281, 1993
114. Vijayan A, Franklin SC, Behrend T *et al*: Insulin-like growth factor I improves renal function in patients with end-stage chronic renal failure. Am J Physiol 276:R929, 1999
115. Franklin SC, Moulton M, Sicard GA *et al*: Insulin-like growth factor I preserves renal function postoperatively. Am J Physiol 272:F257, 1997
116. Allgren RL, Marbury TC, Rahman SN *et al*: Anaritide in acute tubular necrosis. Auriculin Anaritide Acute Renal Failure Study Group. N Engl J Med 20(336):828, 1997
117. Singer I, Epstein M: Potential of dopamine A-1 agonists in the management of acute renal failure. Am J Kidney Dis 31:743, 1998
118. Abel RM, Buckley MJ, Austen WG *et al*: Etiology, incidence, and prognosis of renal failure following cardiac operations. Results of a prospective analysis of 500 consecutive patients. J Thorac Cardiovasc Surg 71:323, 1976
119. Anderson LG, Ekroth R, Bratteby LE *et al*: Acute renal failure after coronary surgery—A study of incidence and risk factors in 2009 consecutive patients. Thorac Cardiovasc Surg 41:237, 1993
120. Zanardo G, Michielon P, Paccagnella A *et al*: Acute renal failure in the patient undergoing cardiac operation. Prevalence, mortality rate, and main risk factors. J Thorac Cardiovasc Surg 107:1489, 1994
121. Mangano CM, Diamondstone LS, Ramsay JG *et al*: Renal dysfunction after myocardial revascularization: Risk factors, adverse outcomes, and hospital resource utilization. The Multicenter Study of Perioperative Ischemia Research Group. Ann Intern Med 128:194, 1998
122. Conlon PJ, Stafford-Smith M, White WD *et al*: Acute renal failure following cardiac surgery. Nephrol Dial Transplant 14:1158, 1999
123. Anderson RJ, O'Brien M, MaWhinney S *et al*: Renal failure predisposes patients to adverse outcome after coronary artery bypass surgery. VA Cooperative Study #5. Kidney Int 55(3):1057, 1999
124. Hilberman M, Myers BD, Carrie BJ *et al*: Acute renal failure following cardiac surgery. J Thorac Cardiovasc Surg 77:880, 1979
125. Ascione R, Lloyd CT, Underwood MJ *et al*: On-pump versus off-pump coronary revascularization: Evaluation of renal function. Ann Thorac Surg 68:493, 1999
126. Badner NH, Murkin JM, Lok P: Differences in pH management and pulsatile/nonpulsatile perfusion during cardiopulmonary bypass do not influence renal function. Anesth Analg 75:696, 1992
127. Tashiro T, Nakamura K, Morishige N *et al*: Off-pump coronary artery bypass grafting in patients with end-stage renal disease on hemodialysis. J Card Surg 17:377, 2002
128. Higgins TL, Estafanous FG, Loop FD *et al*: Stratification of morbidity and mortality outcome by preoperative risk factors in coronary artery bypass patients. A clinical severity score. JAMA 267:2344, 1992
129. Hilberman M: The kidneys: Function, failure and protection in the perioperative period. In Ream A, Fogdall R (eds): Acute Cardiovascular Management Anesthesia and Intensive Care, p 806. Philadelphia, JB Lippincott, 1982
130. Costa P, Ottino GM, Matani A *et al*: Low-dose dopamine during cardiopulmonary bypass in patients with renal dysfunction. J Cardiothorac Anesth 4:469, 1990
131. Berendes E, Mollhoff T, Van Aken H *et al*: Effects of dopexamine on creatinine clearance, systemic inflammation, and splanchnic oxygenation in patients undergoing coronary artery bypass grafting. Anesth Analg 84:950, 1997
132. Dawson JL: The incidence of postoperative renal failure in obstructive jaundice. Br J Surg 52:663, 1965
133. Pascual E, Gomez-Arnau J, Pensado A *et al*: Incidence and risk factors of early acute renal failure in liver transplant patients. Transplant Proc 25:1837, 1993
134. Haller M, Schonfelder R, Briegel J *et al*: Renal function in the postoperative period after orthotopic liver transplantation. Transplant Proc 24:2704, 1992
135. Brown RJ, Lombardero M, Lake J: Outcome of patients with renal insufficiency undergoing liver or liver-kidney transplantation. Transplantation 27:1788, 1996
136. Fraley DS, Burr R, Bernardini J *et al*: Impact of acute renal failure on mortality in end-stage liver disease with or without transplantation. Kidney Int 54:518, 1998
137. Parks RW, Diamond T, McCrory DC *et al*: Prospective study of postoperative renal function in obstructive jaundice and the effect of perioperative dopamine. Br J Surg 81:437, 1994
138. Schrier RW, Wang W: Acute renal failure and sepsis. N Engl J Med 351:159, 2004
139. Clayman RV, Kavoussi LR: Endosurgical techniques for the diagnosis and treatment of noncalculus disease of the ureter and kidney. In Walsh P, Retik A, Stamey T *et al* (eds): Campbell's Urology, 6th ed, p 2231. Philadelphia, WB Saunders, 1992
140. Kennedy TJ, Preminger GM: Flexible cystoscopy. Urol Clin North Am 15:525, 1988
141. Clayman RV: Diagnostic and therapeutic applications of outpatient cystourethroscopy. In Kaye KW (ed): Outpatient Urologic Surgery, p. 111. Philadelphia, Lea & Febiger, 1985
142. Monk TG: Clinical applications of monitored anaesthesia care. Minim Invasive Ther 3(suppl 2):17, 1994
143. Schow DA, Jackson TL, Samson JM *et al*: Use of intravenous alfentanil-midazolam anesthesia for sedation during brief endourologic procedures. J Endourol 8:33, 1994
144. Walsh P: Benign prostatic hyperplasia. In Walsh P, Retik A, Stamey T *et al* (eds): Campbell's Urology, 6th ed, p 1009. Philadelphia, WB Saunders, 1992
145. Riehmann M, Bruskewitz R: Evaluation of benign prostatic hyperplasia. In Brahnson RR (ed): Management of Urologic Disorders, p 12. London, Wolfe, 1994
146. Freiha F, Deem S, Pearl RG: Urology: Transurethral resection of the prostate (TURP). In Jaffe RA, Samuels SI (eds): Anesthesiologist's Manual of Surgical Procedures, p 553. New York, Raven Press, 1994
147. Hatch PD: Surgical and anaesthetic considerations in transurethral resection of the prostate. Anaesth Intensive Care 15:203, 1987
148. Jensen V: The TURP syndrome. Can J Anaesth 38:90, 1991
149. Krongrad A, Droller MJ: Complications of transurethral resection of the prostate. In Marshall FF (ed): Urologic Complications: Medical and Surgical, Adult and Pediatric, 2nd ed, p 305. St. Louis, Mosby–Year Book, 1990
150. Marx GF, Orkin LR: Complications associated with transurethral surgery. Anesthesiology 23:802, 1962
151. Roesch RP, Stoelting RK, Lingeman JE *et al*: Ammonia toxicity resulting from glycine absorption during a transurethral resection of the prostate. Anesthesiology 58:577, 1983

152. Hoekstra PT, Kahnoski R, McCamish MA *et al*: Transurethral prostatic resection syndrome—A new perspective: Encephalopathy with associated hyperammonemia. J Urol 130:704, 1983
153. Fitzpatrick JM, Kasidas GP, Rose GA: Hyperoxaluria following glycine irrigation for transurethral prostatectomy. Br J Urol 53:250, 1981
154. Barletta JP, Fanous MM, Hamed LM: Temporary blindness in the TUR syndrome. J Neuroophthalmol 14:6, 1994
155. Agin C: Anesthesia for transurethral prostate surgery. In Lebowitz P (ed): Anesthesia for Urological Surgery, p 25. Boston, Little, Brown, 1993
156. Gravenstein D: Transurethral resection of the prostate (TURP) syndrome: A review of the pathophysiology and management. Anesth Analg 84:438, 1997
157. Rippa A: Transurethral resection of the prostate: Aids and accessories. In Smith AD (ed): Smith's Textbook of Endourology, p 1190. St. Louis, Quality Medical, 1996
158. Hahn RG, Larsson H, Ribbe T: Continuous monitoring of irrigating fluid absorption during transurethral surgery. Anaesthesia 50:327, 1995
159. Hahn RG: The transurethral resection syndrome. Acta Anaesthesiol Scand 35:557, 1991
160. Black RM: Disorders of plasma sodium and plasma potassium. In Rippe JM, Irwin RS, Alpert J *et al* (eds): Intensive Care Medicine, 2nd ed, p 794. Boston, Little, Brown, 1991
161. Ansell JE: Acquired bleeding disorders. In Rippe JM, Irwin RS, Alpert J *et al* (eds): Intensive Care Medicine, 2nd ed, p 1013. Boston, Little, Brown, 1991
162. Mebust WK, Holtgrewe HL, Cockett AT *et al*: Transurethral prostatectomy: Immediate and postoperative complications. A cooperative study of 13 participating institutions evaluating 3,885 patients. J Urol 141:243, 1989
163. Allen T: Body temperature changes during prostatic resection as related to the temperature of the irrigating solution. J Urol 110:443, 1973
164. Raj PP, Gesund P, Phero J: Rationale and choice for surgical procedures. In Raj PP (ed): Clinical Practice of Regional Anesthesia, p 197. New York, Churchill Livingstone, 1991
165. Mackenzie AR: Influence of anaesthesia on blood loss in trasurethral prostatectomy. Scot Med J 35:1, 1990
166. McGowan SW, Smith GF: Anaesthesia for transurethral prostatectomy. A comparison of spinal intradural analgesia with two methods of general anaesthesia. Anaesthesia 35:847, 1980
167. Bowman GW, Hoerth JW, McGlothlen JS *et al*: Anesthesia for transurethral resection of the prostate: Spinal or general? AANA J 49:63, 1981
168. Chung FF, Chung A, Meier RH *et al*: Comparison of perioperative mental function after general anaesthesia and spinal anaesthesia with intravenous sedation. Can J Anaesth 36:382, 1989
169. Hosking MP, Lobdell CM, Warner MA *et al*: Anaesthesia for patients over 90 years of age. Outcomes after regional and general anaesthetic techniques for two common surgical procedures. Anaesthesia 44:142, 1989
170. Edwards ND, Callaghan LC, White T *et al*: Perioperative myocardial ischaemia in patients undergoing transurethral surgery: A pilot study comparing general with spinal anaesthesia. Br J Anaesth 74:368, 1995
171. Windsor A, French GW, Sear JW *et al*: Silent myocardial ischaemia in patients undergoing transurethral prostatectomy. A study to evaluate risk scoring and anaesthetic technique with outcome. Anaesthesia 51:728, 1996
172. Sinha B, Haikel G, Lange PH *et al*: Transurethral resection of the prostate with local anesthesia in 100 patients. J Urol 135:719, 1986
173. Wasson JH, Bubolz TA, Lu-Yao GL *et al*: Transurethral resection of the prostate among Medicare beneficiaries: 1984 to 1997. For the Patient Outcomes Research Team for Prostatic Diseases. J Urol 164:1212, 2000
174. Watson G: Lasers. In Smith AD (ed): Smith's Textbook of Endourology, p 78. St. Louis, Quality Medical, 1996
175. Catalona WJ: Urothelial tumors of the urinary tract. In Walsh P, Retik A, Stamey T *et al* (eds): Campbell's Urology, 6th ed, p 1094. Philadelphia, WB Saunders, 1992
176. Paola AS, Lamm DL: Bladder: Superficial transitional cell carcinoma. In Resnick M, Kursh E (eds): Current Therapy in Genitourinary Surgery, 2nd ed, p 68. St. Louis, Mosby–Year Book, 1992
177. Prentiss RJ, Harvey GW, Bethard WF *et al*: Massive adductor muscle contraction in transurethral surgery: Cause and prevention; Development of electrical circuity. J Urol 93:263, 1965
178. Smith RB: Complications of transurethral surgery. In Smith RB, Ehrlich RM (eds): Complications of Urologic Surgery, 2nd ed, p 355. Philadelphia, WB Saunders, 1990
179. Dorotta I, Basali A, Ritchey M *et al*: Transurethral resection syndrome after bladder perforation. Anesth Analg 97:1536, 2003
180. Van Arsdalen KN, Levy JB: Urolithiasis. In Hanno PM, Wein AJ (eds): Clinical Manual of Urology, 2nd ed, p 229. New York, McGraw-Hill, 1994
181. Drach GW: Urinary lithiasis: Etiology, diagnosis and medical management. In Walsh P, Retik A, Stamey T *et al* (eds): Campbell's Urology, 6th ed, p 2085. Philadelphia, WB Saunders, 1992
182. McCullough DL: Extracorporeal shock wave lithotripsy. In Walsh P, Retik A, Stamey T *et al* (eds): Campbell's Urology, 6th ed, p 2157. Philadelphia, WB Saunders, 1992
183. Eide TR: Anesthetic considerations for extracorporeal shock wave lithotripsy. In Lebowitz P (ed): Anesthesia for Urological Surgery, p 47. Boston, Little, Brown, 1993
184. Hunter PT: II: The physics and geometry pertinent to ESWL. In Riehle RA Jr, Newman RC (eds): Principles of Extracorporeal Shock Wave Lithotripsy, p 13. New York, Churchill Livingstone, 1987
185. Carlson CA, Gravenstein JS, Gravenstein N: Ventricular tachycardia during ESWL: Etiology treatment and prevention. In Gravenstein JS, Peter K (eds): Extracorporeal Shock-Wave Lithotripsy for Renal Stone Disease, p 119. Boston, Butterworths, 1986
186. Weber W, Madler C, Keil B: Cardiovascular effects of ESWL. In Gravenstein JS, Peter K (eds): Extracorporeal Shock-Wave Lithotripsy for Renal Stone Disease, p 101. Boston, Butterworths, 1986
187. Abbott MA, Samuel JR, Webb DR: Anaesthesia for extracorporeal shock wave lithotripsy. Anaesthesia 40:1065, 1985
188. Bromage PR, Bonsu AK, el Faqih SR *et al*: Influence of Dornier HM3 system on respiration during extracorporeal shock-wave lithotripsy. Anesth Analg 68:363, 1989
189. Malhotra V: Hyperthermia and hypothermia as complications of extracorporeal shock wave lithotripsy. Anesthesiology 67:448, 1987
190. Drach GW, Weber C, Donovan JM: Treatment of pacemaker patients with extracorporeal shock wave lithotripsy: Experience from 2 continents. J Urol 143:895, 1990
191. Chung MK, Streem SB, Ching E *et al*: Effects of extracorporeal shock wave lithotripsy on tiered therapy implantable cardioverter defibrillators. Pacing Clin Electrophysiol 22:738, 1999
192. Segura JW: Complications of shock wave lithotripsy. In Marshall FF (ed): Urologic Complications: Medical and Surgical, Adult and Pediatric, 2nd ed, p 215. St. Louis, Mosby–Year Book, 1990
193. Monk TG, Boure B, White PF *et al*: Comparison of intravenous sedative-analgesic techniques for outpatient immersion lithotripsy. Anesth Analg 72:616, 1991
194. Fuchs GJ, David RD, Fuchs AM *et al*: Complications of extracorporeal shock wave lithotripsy (ESWL). In Smith RB, Ehrlich RM (eds): Complications of Urologic Surgery, p 181. Philadelphia, WB Saunders, 1990
195. Bush WH, Jones D, Gibbons RP: Radiation dose to patient and personnel during extracorporeal shock wave lithotripsy. J Urol 138:716, 1987
196. Newman RC, Riehle RA: Principles of Treatment. In Riehle RA (ed): Principles of Extracorporeal Shock Wave Lithotripsy, p 79. New York, Churchill Livingstone, 1987
197. Monk TG, Ding Y, White PF *et al*: Effect of topical eutectic mixture of local anesthetics on pain response and analgesic requirement during lithotripsy procedures. Anesth Analg 79:506, 1994
198. Richardson MG, Dooley JW: The effects of general versus epidural anesthesia for outpatient extracorporeal shock wave lithotripsy. Anesth Analg 86:1214, 1998
199. Saberski LR, Kondamuri S, Osinubi OY: Identification of the epidural space: Is loss of resistance to air a safe technique? A review of the complications related to the use of air. Reg Anesth 22:3, 1997
200. Monk TG, Rater JM, White PF: Comparison of alfentanil and ketamine infusions in combination with midazolam for outpatient lithotripsy. Anesthesiology 74:1023–1028, 1991
201. Malhotra V, Long CW, Meister MJ: Intercostal blocks with local infiltration anesthesia for extracorporeal shock wave lithotripsy. Anesth Analg 66:85, 1987
202. Segura JW: Complications of endourology. In Marshall FF (ed): Urologic Complications: Medical and Surgical Adult, 2nd ed, pp 200. St. Louis, Mosby–Year Book, 1990
203. Picus D, Weyman PJ, Clayman RV *et al*: Intercostal-space nephrostomy for percutaneous stone removal. AJR Am J Roentgenol 147:393, 1986
204. Schultz RE, Hanno PM, Wein AJ *et al:* Percutaneous ultrasonic lithotripsy: Choice of irrigant. J Urol 130:858, 1983
205. Smith JA Jr: Urologic laser surgery. In Walsh P, Retik A, Stamey T et al. (eds): Campbell's Urology, 6th ed, p 2923. Philadelphia, WB Saunders, 1992
206. Malloy TR, Wein AJ: Complications of lasers in urology. In Marshall FF (ed): Urologic Complications: Medical and Surgical, Adult and Pediatric, 2nd ed, p 411. St. Louis, Mosby–Year Book, 1990
207. Smith JA Jr: Complications of laser surgery. In Smith RB, Ehrlich RM (eds): Complications of Urologic Surgery, p 629. Philadelphia, WB Saunders, 1990
208. Gloster HM Jr, Roenigk RK: Risk of acquiring human papillomavirus from the plume produced by the carbon dioxide laser in the treatment of warts. J Am Acad Dermatol 32(3):436, 1995
209. Monk TG, Weldon BC: Anesthetic considerations for laparoscopic urology. In Das S, Crawford ED (eds): Urologic Laparoscopy, p 45. Philadelphia, WB Saunders, 1994
210. Wolf JS Jr, Monk TG: Anesthetic considerations. In Smith AD (ed): Smith's Textbook of Endourology, p 731. St. Louis, Quality Medical Publishing, 1996
211. Mullett CE, Viale JP, Sagnard PE *et al*: Pulmonary CO^2 elimination during surgical procedures using intra- or extraperitoneal CO^2 insufflation. Anesth Analg 76:622, 1993
212. Kerbl K, Clayman RV, McDougall EM *et al*: Laparoscopic nephrectomy: The Washington University experience. Br J Urol 73:231, 1994
213. Ortega AE, Peters JH, Incarbone R *et al*: A prospective randomized comparison of the metabolic and stress hormonal responses of laparoscopic and open cholecystectomy. J Am Coll Surg 183:249, 1996

214. Brawer MK: How to use prostate-specific antigen in the early detection or screening for prostatic carcinoma. CA Cancer J Clin 45:148, 1995
215. Potosky AL, Davis WW, Hoffman RM *et al*: Five-year outcomes after prostatectomy or radiotherapy for prostate cancer: The prostate cancer outcomes study. J Natl Cancer Inst 96(18):1358, 2004
216. Walsh P: Radical retropubic prostatectomy. In Walsh P, Retik A, Stamey T *et al* (eds): Campbell's Urology, 6th ed, p 2865. Philadelphia, WB Saunders, 1992
217. Frazier HA, Robertson JE, Paulson DF: Radical prostatectomy: The pros and cons of the perineal versus retropubic approach. J Urol 147:888, 1992
218. Frank E, Sood OP, Torjman M *et al*: Postoperative epidural analgesia following radical retropubic prostatectomy: Outcome assessment. J Surg Oncol 67:117, 1998
219. Gottschalk A, Smith DS, Jobes DR *et al*: Preemptive epidural analgesia and recovery from radical prostatectomy: A randomized controlled trial. JAMA 279:1076, 1998
220. Shir Y, Frank SM, Brendler CB *et al*: Postoperative morbidity is similar in patients anesthetized with epidural and general anesthesia for radical prostatectomy. Urology 44:232, 1994
221. Monk TG: Cancer of the prostate and radical prostatectomy. In Malhotra V (ed): Renal Anesthesia for Renal and Genito-urologic Surgery, p 177. New York, McGraw-Hill, 1996
222. Monk TG, Goodnough LT, Brecher ME *et al*: A prospective randomized comparison of three blood conservation strategies for radical prostatectomy. Anesthesiology 91:24, 1999
223. O'Hara JF Jr, Whalley D: Anesthetic considerations for contemporary radical prostatectomy. In Klein EA (ed): Management of Prostate Cancer, 2nd ed, p 297. Totowa, NJ, Humana Press, 2004
224. Gray CL, Amling CL, Polston GR *et al*: Intraoperative cell salvage in radical retropubic prostatectomy. Urology 58:740, 2001
225. Thomas MJ: Infected and malignant fields are an absolute contraindication to intraoperative cell salvage: Fact or fiction? Transfus Med 9:269, 1999
226. Davis M, Sofer M, Gomez-Marin O *et al*: The use of cell salvage during radical retropubic prostatectomy: Does it influence cancer recurrence? Br J Urol Int 91:474, 2003
227. Morison DH, Riggs JR: Cardiovascular collapse in laparoscopy. Can Med Assoc J 111:433, 1974
228. Martin JT: The Trendelenburg position. In Martin JT (ed): Positioning in Anesthesia and Surgery, 2nd ed, p 127. Philadelphia, WB Saunders, 1987
229. Albin MS, Ritter RR, Reinhart R *et al*: Venous air embolism during radical retropubic prostatectomy. Anesth Analg 74:151, 1992
230. Razvi HA, Chin JL, Bhandari R: Fatal air embolism during radical retropubic prostatectomy. J Urol 151:433, 1994
231. Freiha F: Open bladder surgery. In Walsh P, Retik A, Stamey T *et al* (eds): Campbell's Urology, 6th ed, p 2750. Philadelphia, WB Saunders, 1992
232. Dekernion JB, Belldegrun A: Renal tumors. In Walsh P, Retik A, Stamey T *et al* (eds): Campbell's Urology, 6th ed, p 1053. Philadelphia, WB Saunders, 1992
233. Kinkade S: Testicular cancer. Am Fam Physician 59:2539, 1999
234. Donat SM, Levy DA: Bleomycin associated pulmonary toxicity: Is perioperative oxygen restriction necessary? J Urol 160:1347, 1998
235. Mathes DD: Bleomycin and hyperoxia exposure in the operating room. Anesth Analg 81:624, 1995
236. Wierda JM, Szenohradszky J, De Wit AP *et al*: The pharmacokinetics, urinary and biliary excretion of pipecuronium bromide. Eur J Anaesthesiol 8:451, 1991
237. Schiere S, Proost JH, Schuringa M *et al*: Pharmacokinetics and pharmacokinetic–dynamic relationship between rapacuronium (Org 9487) and its 3-desacetyl metabolite (Org 9488). Anesth Analg 88:640, 1999
238. Szenohradszky J, Caldwell JE, Wright PM *et al*: Influence of renal failure on the pharmacokinetics and neuromuscular effects of a single dose of rapacuronium bromide. Anesthesiology 90:24, 1999

CHAPTER 36 ■ ANESTHESIA AND OBESITY

BABATUNDE O. OGUNNAIKE AND CHARLES W. WHITTEN

KEY POINTS

1. Many morbidly obese patients have clinically significant obstructive sleep apnea (OSA), which in the long term can result in the obesity hypoventilation syndrome (OHS). OSA predisposes to airway difficulties during anesthesia.
2. Angina or exertional dyspnea may rarely present because morbidly obese patients often have limited mobility and may appear asymptomatic even when they have significant cardiovascular disease.
3. Nonalcoholic fatty liver disease and elevated liver function tests (mostly elevated ALT) are seen in a significant number of obese patients. Despite these histologic and enzymatic changes, no clear correlation exists between abnormalities of routine liver function tests and the capacity of the liver to metabolize drugs.
4. Rhabdomyolysis is sometimes seen in morbidly obese patients undergoing prolonged operative procedures. Unexplained elevations in serum creatinine and creatine phosphokinase (CPK) levels or complaints of buttock, hip, or shoulder pain in the postoperative period may indicate that rhabdomyolysis has occurred.
5. Patients scheduled for repeat bariatric surgery may have long-term vitamin and nutritional abnormalities, which can lead to acute postgastric reduction surgery (APGARS) neuropathy, a polynutritional multisystem disorder characterized by protracted postoperative vomiting, hyporeflexia, and muscular weakness.
6. Morbid obesity is a major independent risk factor for deep venous thrombosis (DVT) and sudden death from acute postoperative pulmonary embolism. Subcutaneous heparin reduces the risk of DVT; however, low molecular weight heparins are currently popular for thromboembolism prophylaxis because of their bioavailability when injected subcutaneously.
7. Neck circumference has been identified as the single best predictor of problematic intubation in morbidly obese patients. A larger neck circumference is associated with the male sex, a higher Mallampati score, grade 3 views at laryngoscopy, and obstructive sleep apnea.
8. Forearm blood pressure is a fairly good predictor of upper arm blood pressure in most patients, but in obese patients, forearm measurements with a standard cuff may overestimate both systolic and diastolic blood pressures.
9. The head-elevated laryngoscopy position (HELP) elevates the obese patient's head, upper body, and shoulders above the chest to the extent that an imaginary horizontal line connects the sternal notch with the external auditory meatus to better improve laryngoscopy and intubation.

OBESITY

Obesity is a condition of excessive body fat with adverse health implications, including increased risk for hypertension, coronary artery disease, hyperlipidemia, diabetes mellitus, gall bladder disease, degenerative joint disease, obstructive sleep apnea (OSA), and psychological and socioeconomic impairment. *Obesity* defines an abnormally high percentage of body weight as fat while *overweight* means an increased body weight above a standard related to height.

Varying pathophysiologic consequences are associated with the anatomic distribution of body fat. In *android* (central) obesity, adipose tissue is located predominantly in the upper body (truncal distribution) and is associated with increased oxygen consumption and increased incidence of cardiovascular disease. In *gynecoid* (peripheral) obesity, adipose tissue is located predominantly in the hips, buttocks, and thighs. This fat is less metabolically active so it is less closely associated with cardiovascular disease. Intra-abdominal fat is particularly associated with cardiovascular risk and left ventricular dysfunction.

Ideal body weight (IBW) is the weight associated with the lowest mortality rate for a given height and gender and can be estimated using Broca's index:

IBW (kg) = height (cm) − *x;* where *x* is 100 for adult males and 105 for adult females. In clinical practice, *body mass (Quetelet's) index* (BMI) is used to estimate the degree of obesity

$$\text{BMI} = \frac{\text{body weight (kg)}}{\text{height}^2\ \text{(m)}}$$

Obesity and *morbid obesity* are BMI >30 and 40 kg/m^2, respectively, while BMI >55 kg/m^2 denotes *super morbid obesity*. BMI differentiates obese from nonobese adults and it reliably measures body fat because it adjusts for height while strongly correlating with body weight; however, it cannot distinguish between overweight and overfat as heavily muscled people can be easily classified as overweight using BMI. Other factors such as age and fat distribution should therefore be taken into consideration, among other health risk predictors that utilize the concept of BMI. Weight loss reduces the risk associated with obesity and men are at a higher risk than women for a given level of obesity. Immediate preoperative weight loss has not been shown to reduce overall perioperative morbidity and mortality.

Body circumference indices such as waist circumference, waist-to-height ratio, and waist-to-hip ratio can identify patterns of obesity (e.g., android obesity) and correlate strongly with mortality and the risk for developing obesity-related diseases. Waist circumference strongly correlates with abdominal fat and is an independent risk predictor of disease. A waist circumference exceeding 102 cm (40 in) in men and 89 cm (35 in) in women indicates increased risk in overweight and obese individuals. A waist-to-hip ratio (WHR) >0.9 in women and >1.0 in men is associated with a higher risk of morbidity and mortality than a more peripheral distribution of body fat (WHR <0.75 in women and <0.85 in men). Alcohol encourages central (android) fat.

Pathophysiology of Obesity

Respiratory System

Fat accumulation on the thorax and abdomen decreases chest wall and lung compliance. Decreased lung compliance is partially explained by increased pulmonary blood volume because of an overall increase in blood volume as more volume is required to perfuse the additional body fat. Polycythemia from chronic hypoxemia contributes to increased total blood volume. Increased elastic resistance and decreased compliance of the chest wall further reduces total respiratory compliance while supine, leading to shallow and rapid breathing, increased work of breathing, and limited maximum ventilatory capacity. Respiratory muscle efficiency is below normal in obese individuals. Decreased pulmonary compliance leads to decreased functional residual capacity (FRC), vital capacity (VC), and total lung capacity (TLC). Reduction in FRC is primarily a result of reduced expiratory reserve volume (ERV) but the relationship between FRC and closing capacity (CC), the volume at which small airways begin to close, is adversely affected (Fig. 36-1). Residual volume and CC are unchanged. Reduced FRC can result in lung volumes below CC in the course of normal tidal ventilation, leading to small airway closure, ventilation-perfusion mismatch, right-to-left shunting, and arterial hypoxemia. Anesthesia worsens this situation such that up to a 50% reduction in FRC occurs in the obese anesthetized patient compared with 20% in the nonobese. Forced expiratory volume in one second (FEV_1) and forced vital capacity (FVC) are usually within normal limits.

Obesity increases oxygen consumption and carbon dioxide production because of the metabolic activity of excess fat and the increased workload on supportive tissues. The body attempts to meet these metabolic demands by increasing both cardiac output and alveolar ventilation. Basal metabolic activity is usually within normal limits in relation to body surface area and normocapnia is usually maintained by an increase in minute ventilation. This requires increased oxygen

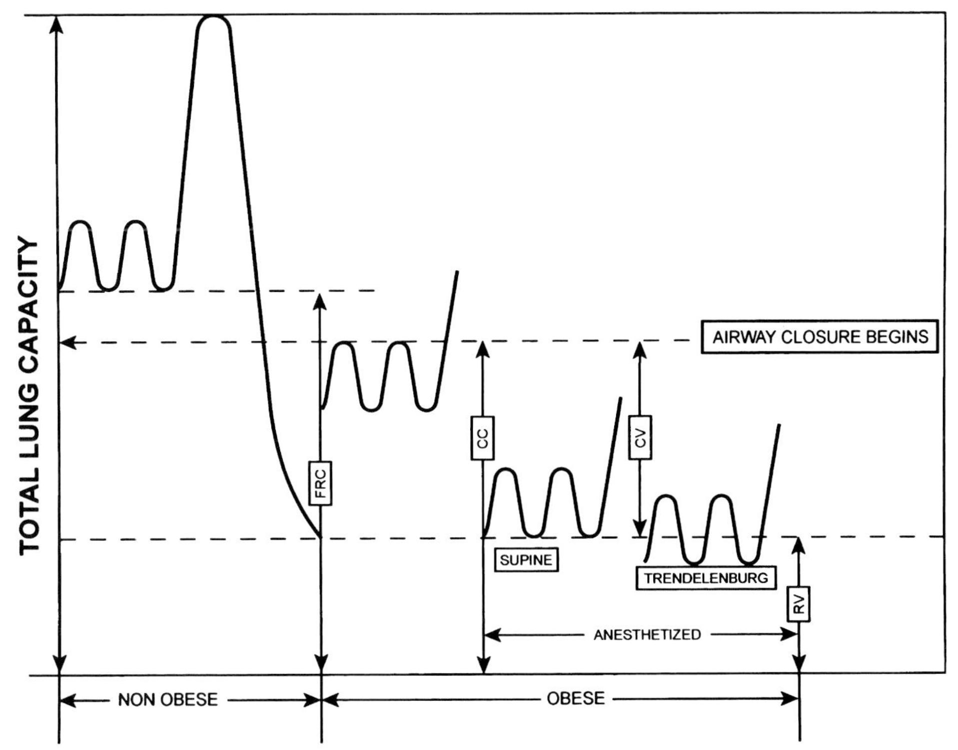

FIGURE 36-1. Effects of obesity, positioning, and anesthesia on lung volumes. FRC, functional residual capacity; CC, closing capacity; CV, closing volume; RV, residual volume.

consumption because most obese patients retain their normal response to hypoxemia and hypercapnia. Arterial oxygen tension in morbidly obese patients and breathing room air is lower than that predicted for similarly aged nonobese subjects in both sitting and supine positions. Chronic hypoxemia may lead to pulmonary hypertension and cor pulmonale.

Obstructive Sleep Apnea. Up to 5% of obese patients have
1 clinically significant *obstructive sleep apnea*. OSA is characterized by frequent episodes of apnea or hypopnea during sleep, snoring, and daytime symptoms, which include sleepiness, impaired concentration, memory problems, and morning headaches. Apnea is defined as 10 seconds or more of total cessation of airflow despite continuous respiratory effort against a closed glottis. A 50% reduction in airflow or a reduction sufficient enough to cause a 4% decrease in arterial oxygen saturation defines hypopnea. Resultant physiologic abnormalities include hypoxemia, hypercapnia, pulmonary and systemic vasoconstriction, and secondary polycythemia (from recurrent hypoxemia), which is associated with an increased risk of ischemic heart disease and cerebrovascular disease.[1] Right ventricular failure can occur from hypoxic pulmonary vasoconstriction. Respiratory acidosis is initially limited to sleep with a return to normal homeostasis during the awake state.

Long-term OSA can lead to the *obesity hypoventilation (Pickwickian) syndrome* (OHS), which is seen in 5 to 10% of morbidly obese patients. Prolonged OSA results in altered control of breathing, with central apneic events as the main feature. This leads to increasing reliance on hypoxic drive for ventilation. The main ventilatory impairment of OHS is alveolar hypoventilation independent of intrinsic lung disease in a patient with obesity, daytime hypersomnolence, hypercapnia, hypoxemia, and polycythemia. Right ventricular failure eventually ensues. These patients also have an increased sensitivity to respiratory depressant effects of general anesthetics.

Cardiovascular System

Total blood volume is increased in the obese, but on a volume-to-weight basis, it is less than in nonobese individuals (50 mL/kg compared with 70 mL/kg). Most of this extra volume is distributed to the fat organ. Renal and splanchnic blood flows are increased. Cardiac output increases with increasing weight by as much as 20 to 30 mL/kg of excess body fat because of ventricular dilatation and increases in stroke volume. The resulting increased left ventricular wall stress leads to hypertrophy, reduced compliance, and impairment of left ventricular filling (diastolic dysfunction) with elevated left ventricular and diastolic pressure and pulmonary edema, but when left ventricular wall thickening fails to keep pace with dilatation, systolic dysfunction ("obesity cardiomyopathy") results with eventual biventricular failure (Fig. 36-2). Obesity accelerates atherosclerosis. Symptoms such as angina or exertional dyspnea occur
2 only occasionally because morbidly obese patients often have very limited mobility and may appear asymptomatic even when they have significant cardiovascular disease.

Blood flow to fat is 2 to 3 mL/100 g of tissue. An excess of fat requires an increase in cardiac output, to parallel an increase in oxygen consumption, leading to a systemic arteriovenous oxygen difference that remains normal or slightly above normal. Intraoperative ventricular failure may occur from rapid

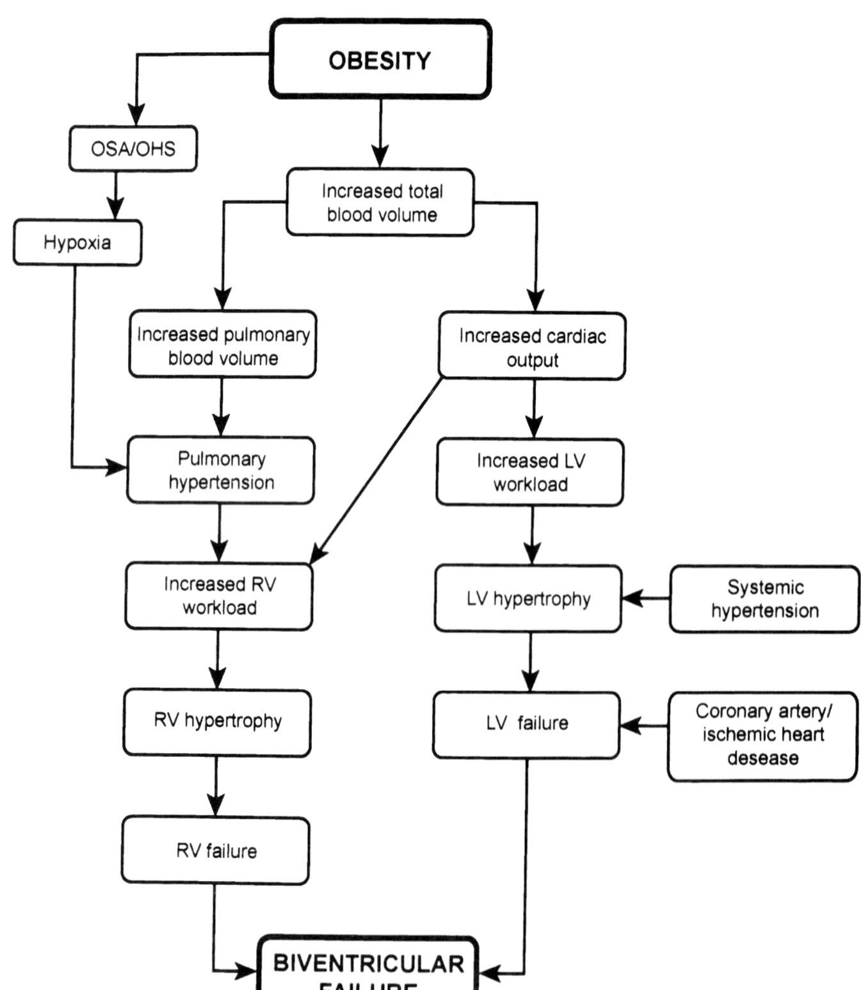

FIGURE 36-2. Interrelationship of cardiovascular and pulmonary sequelae of obesity. LV, left ventricular; RV, right ventricular; OSA, obstructive sleep apnea; OHS, obesity hypoventilation syndrome.

intravenous fluid administration (indicating left ventricular diastolic dysfunction), negative inotropy of anesthetic agents, or pulmonary hypertension precipitated by hypoxia or hypercapnia. Dysrhythmias can also be caused by hypoxia, hypercapnia, electrolyte imbalance, coronary artery disease, increased circulating catecholamines, OSA, myocardial hypertrophy, and fatty infiltration of the conduction system.

Cardiac output rises faster in response to exercise in the morbidly obese and is often associated with a rise in left ventricular end-diastolic pressure and pulmonary capillary wedge pressure. Similar changes occur during the perioperative period, which should prompt a low threshold for performing detailed cardiac investigations. Many obese patients have mild to moderate hypertension, with a 3- to 4-mm Hg increase in systolic and a 2-mm Hg increase in diastolic arterial pressure for every 10 kg of weight gained. Normotensive obese patients have reduced systemic vascular resistance (SVR), which rises with the onset of hypertension. Their expanded blood volume causes an increased cardiac output with a lower calculated SVR for the same level of arterial blood pressure.

Gastrointestinal System

Gastric volume and acidity are increased, hepatic function altered, and drug metabolism adversely affected by obesity. Most fasted morbidly obese patients presenting for elective surgery have gastric volumes in excess of 25 mL and gastric fluid pH less than 2.5 (the generally accepted volume and pH indicative of high risk for pneumonitis should regurgitation and aspiration occur). Delayed gastric emptying occurs because of increased abdominal mass that causes antral distension, gastrin release, and a decrease in pH with parietal cell secretion. An increased incidence of hiatal hernia and gastroesophageal reflux also increase aspiration risk.

Gastric emptying has been said to be actually faster in the obese, especially with high energy content intake such as fat emulsions, but because of their larger gastric volume (up to 75% larger), the residual volume is larger. Both the faster gastric emptying and the larger gastric volume can be partially reversed by weight loss.[2] Nonpremedicated, nondiabetic fasting obese surgical patients who are free from significant gastroesophageal pathology are significantly less likely to have high volume, low pH gastric contents than are lean patients at the time of general anesthetic induction after routine preoperative fasting.[3] They should follow the same fasting guidelines as nonobese patients and be allowed to drink clear liquids until up to 2 hours before elective surgery. Up to 300 mL of clear liquid 2 hours before elective surgery in the fasting obese patient does not adversely affect the pH and volume of gastric contents at induction of anesthesia.[4]

3 Peculiar morphologic and biochemical abnormalities of the liver that are associated with obesity include fatty infiltration (high prevalence of nonalcoholic fatty liver disease), inflammation, focal necrosis, and cirrhosis. Fatty infiltration reflects the duration rather than the degree of obesity. Histological and liver function test abnormalities are relatively common in the obese, but clearance is usually not reduced. Abnormal liver function tests are seen in up to one-third of obese patients who have no evidence of concomitant liver disease, of which increased alanine aminotransferase (ALT) is most frequently seen. Weight loss results in sustained improvement in liver enzymes in direct proportion to the extent of weight reduction.[5] Despite these histologic and enzymatic changes, no clear correlation exists between routine liver function tests and the capacity of the liver to metabolize drugs.[6] Morbidly obese patients who have undergone intestinal bypass surgery have a particularly high prevalence of hepatic dysfunction and cholelithiasis, which is also common in the general obese population and of which abnormal cholesterol metabolism is partially to blame.

Renal and Endocrine Systems

Impaired glucose tolerance in the morbidly obese is reflected by a high prevalence of type II diabetes mellitus as a result of resistance of peripheral fatty tissues to insulin. Greater than 10% of obese patients have an abnormal glucose tolerance test, which predisposes them to wound infection and an increased risk of myocardial infarction during periods of myocardial ischemia.[7] Exogenous insulin may be required perioperatively even in obese patients with type II diabetes mellitus to oppose the catabolic response to surgery. Abnormal serum lipid profiles explain the high prevalence of ischemic heart disease.

Obesity is associated with glomerular hyperfiltration as evidenced by increased renal plasma flow (RPF) and increased glomerular filtration rate (GFR). Excessive weight gain increases renal tubular resorption and impairs natriuresis through activation of the sympathetic and renin–angiotensin system as well as physical compression of the kidney. With prolonged obesity, there may be a loss of nephron function, with further impairment of natriuresis and further increases in arterial pressure. Obesity-related glomerular hyperfiltration decreases after weight loss, which decreases the incidence of overt glomerulopathy.[8,9]

Airway

Anatomic changes of obesity that affect the airway include limitation of movement of the atlantoaxial joint and cervical spine by upper thoracic and low cervical fat pads; excessive tissue folds in the mouth and pharynx; short thick neck; suprasternal, presternal, and posterior cervical fat; and a very thick submental fat pad. All these factors contribute to potential difficult airway management. The history obtained from the patient and examination of previous records may help predict airway difficulties. OSA predisposes to airway difficulties during anesthesia. Obese patients with OSA have excess pharyngeal tissue deposited in their lateral pharyngeal walls, which may not be noticed during routine airway examination. Even with the presence of these anatomic and pathologic changes, the magnitude of BMI does not seem to have much influence on the difficulty of laryngoscopy. Such difficulty correlates better with increased age, male sex, temperomandibular joint (TMJ) pathology, Mallampati classes 3 and 4, history of OSA, and abnormal upper teeth.[10]

PHARMACOLOGY

The volume of the central compartment in which drugs are first distributed remains unchanged in obese patients, but absolute body water content and lean body and adipose tissue mass are increased, affecting lipophilic and polar drug distribution. The volume of distribution (V_D) in obese patients is affected by reduced total body water, increased total body fat, increased lean body mass (LBM), altered protein binding, increased blood volume, increased cardiac output, increased blood concentrations of free fatty acids, triglycerides, cholesterol, and alpha-1-acid glycoprotein, lipophilicity of the drug, and organomegaly.[11] Increased distribution of a drug prolongs its elimination half-life even when clearance is unchanged or increased. Hyperlipidemia and an increased concentration of alpha-1-acid glycoprotein may affect protein binding, leading to a reduction in free drug concentration. Plasma albumin and total plasma protein concentration and binding are not significantly changed by obesity, but when compared to normal weight individuals, a relative increase in plasma protein binding may be evident. Splanchnic blood flow, blood volume, cardiac size, cardiac output, organ adipose tissue, and LBM are all increased in obese patients. In contrast to the expected decrease in bioavailability of orally administered medication because of increased splanchnic blood flow in obese people, there is no significant difference in absorption and bioavailability when comparing obese and normal weight subjects. Drugs that undergo phase I metabolism (oxidation, reduction, hydrolysis) are generally unaffected by changes induced by obesity while phase II reactions (glucuronidation, sulfation) are enhanced. Acetylation, a phase II reaction, is, however, unaltered.[11]

Histologic abnormalities of the liver are common in the obese, with concomitant deranged liver function tests, but drug clearance is not usually affected. Renal clearance of drugs is increased in obesity because of increased renal blood flow and glomerular filtration rate.[8,9] Increase in GFR is an important contributing factor to proteinuria, a commonly cited renal abnormality in obese patients.[9] As a result of both increased GFR and increased tubular secretion, drugs such as cimetidine and aminoglycoside antibiotics that depend on renal excretion may require increased dosing. Highly lipophilic substances such as barbiturates and benzodiazepines show significant increases in V_D for obese individuals.[11] These drugs have a more selective distribution to fat stores and therefore a longer elimination half-life but with comparable clearance values to normal people. Less lipophilic compounds have little or no change in V_D with obesity. Exceptions to this rule include the highly lipophilic drugs digoxin, procainamide, and remifentanil.[12–14] Drugs with weak or moderate lipophilicity can be dosed on the basis of IBW or LBM. About 20 to 40% of an obese patient's increase in total body weight can be attributed to an increase in LBM. Adding 20% to the estimated IBW dose of hydrophilic medications is sufficient to include the extra lean mass. Nondepolarizing muscle relaxants can be dosed in this manner.

Specific Intravenous Agents (Table 36-1)

1. **Thiopental:** Prolonged somnolence with thiopental is expected because it is highly lipophilic and has a larger V_D in the obese patient. However, increased blood volume, cardiac output, and muscle mass necessitates an increase in the initial induction dose.
2. **Propofol:** There is no difference in initial V_D between obese and nonobese patients with propofol. Increased

TABLE 36-1

DETERMINANTS OF DOSING FOR INTRAVENOUS DRUGS IN THE OBESE PATIENT

DRUG	DOSING	COMMENTS
Propofol	Induction: IBW Maintenance: TBW	Systemic clearance and V_D at steady state correlates well with TBW. High affinity for excess fat and other well-perfused organs. High hepatic extraction and conjugation relates to TBW.
Thiopental	TBW	Increased V_D. Increased blood volume, cardiac output, and muscle mass. Increased absolute dose. Prolonged duration of action.
Midazolam	TBW	Central V_D increases in line with body weight. Increased absolute dose. Prolonged sedation because higher loading doses needed to achieve adequate serum concentrations.
Succinylcholine	TBW	Plasma cholinesterase activity increases in proportion to body weight. Increased absolute dose.
Vecuronium	IBW	Recovery may be delayed if given according to TBW because of increased volume of distribution and impaired hepatic clearance.
Rocuronium	IBW	Faster onset and longer duration of action. Pharmacokinetics and pharmacodynamics not altered in obese subjects.
Atracurium Cisatracurium	TBW	Absolute clearance, V_D, and elimination half-life do not change. Unchanged dose per unit body weight without prolongation of recovery because of organ independent elimination.
Fentanyl Sufentanil	TBW Induction: TBW Maintenance: IBW	Increased V_D and elimination half-time which correlates positively with the degree of obesity. Distributes as extensively in excess body mass as in lean tissues. Dose should account for total body mass. Fentanyl dosing based on a derived pharmacokinetic mass correlates better with clearance.
Remifentanil	IBW	Systemic clearance and V_D corrected per kg of TBW—significantly smaller in the obese. Pharmacokinetics are similar in obese and nonobese patients. Age and lean body mass should be considered for dosing.

IBW, ideal body weight; TBW, total body weight; V_D, volume of distribution.
Adapted from Ogunnaike BO, Jones SB, Jones DB *et al*: Anesthetic considerations for bariatric surgery. Anesth Analg 95:1793, 2002.

V_D at steady state and increased clearance offsets any increase in elimination half-life without evidence of accumulation. Total clearance and V_D at steady state correlate to body weight during maintenance infusion. The dose should be increased based on lean body weight. Propofol has high affinity for excess fat and other well-perfused organs. High hepatic extraction and conjugation relates to total body weight.[15]

3. **Benzodiazepines:** Benzodiazepines persist long after discontinuation because they are highly lipophilic drugs with a larger V_D in obese patients. Midazolam, although considered short acting, has the potential for prolonged sedation in obese patients because larger initial doses are required to achieve adequate serum concentrations.
4. **Neuromuscular Blocking Agents:** Pseudocholinesterase activity increases linearly with increasing weight and larger extracellular fluid compartment; therefore, the dose of succinylcholine should be increased somewhat. Nondepolarizing muscle relaxants should be administered according to lean body weight to prevent delayed recovery because of increased V_D and impaired hepatic clearance. The pharmacokinetics and pharmacodynamics of rocuronium are not altered by obesity in female subjects; however, in the general obese population, the onset time is shorter and duration slightly prolonged.[16,17] The V_D, absolute clearance, and elimination half-life of atracurium are unchanged and dosing can be based on actual body weight without prolongation of recovery because of organ function–independent breakdown.[18] Cisatracurium duration may be prolonged in light of more recent references.
5. **Opioids:** Application of nonweight-scaled pharmacokinetic models for fentanyl derived from normal-weight patients overestimates the plasma concentration of fentanyl as body weight increases from normal to morbid obesity. Fentanyl dosing based on a derived pharmacokinetic mass (derived pharmacokinetic body weight for dosing) is clinically more useful than that based on total body weight because of the strong linear correlation between this pharmacokinetic mass and total body clearance.[20] Sufentanil is highly lipid soluble; therefore, it has an increased V_D and a prolonged elimination half-life that correlates positively with the degree of obesity. It distributes extensively in excess body fat as in lean tissues; therefore, dosing should account for total body mass. Pharmacokinetic parameters derived from nonobese subjects accurately predict plasma sufentanil concentrations in morbidly obese subjects, but at the morbidly obese range, overestimation of plasma sufentanil concentration rises with increasing BMI.[21] Remifentanil pharmacokinetics are more closely related to lean body mass than to total body weight; therefore, dosing should be based on ideal body weight.[12]

Increased blood volume in the obese patient decreases the plasma concentrations of rapidly injected intravenous drugs. Fat, however, has poor blood flow, and doses calculated on actual body weight could lead to excessive plasma concentrations. Calculating initial doses based on lean body weight with subsequent doses determined by pharmacologic response to the initial dose is a reasonable approach.[22] Repeated injections may accumulate in fat, leading to a prolonged response because of subsequent release from this large depot.

MEDICAL THERAPY FOR OBESITY

Medications used to treat obesity are formulated to reduce energy intake, increase energy utilization, or decrease absorption of nutrients. Indications for drug treatment include a BMI $\geq$30 kg/m^2 or a BMI between 27 and 29.9 kg/m^2 in conjunction with an obesity-related medical complication. The combination of phentermine and fenfluramine (Phen-Fen) was popular for the treatment of obesity until it became evident that it was associated with valvular heart disease and pulmonary hypertension.

Sibutramine and orlistat are newer antiobesity medications approved for long-term use. Sibutramine inhibits the reuptake of norepinephrine to increase satiety after the onset of eating rather than reduce appetite. It does not promote the release of serotonin unlike fenfluramine and dexfenfluramine, which primarily increase the release of serotonin in brain synapses and also inhibit reuptake to cause anorexia. These differences in mechanisms of action may explain why thus far there have been no reports of sibutramine causing cardiac valvular lesions. Because sibutramine does not deplete neural synapses of catecholamines, dangerous hypotension unresponsive to indirectly acting vasopressors, as seen with fenfluramine and dexfenfluramine, does not generally occur.[23] The most frequent adverse effects of sibutramine include dry mouth, insomnia, anorexia, and constipation. Sibutramine also results in transient dose-related increases in systolic and diastolic blood pressure by an average of 2 to 4 mmHg and a slight increase in heart rate of 3 to 5 bpm.[24]

Orlistat blocks the absorption and digestion of dietary fat by binding lipases in the gastrointestinal (GI) tract. Cardiovascular risk factors associated with obesity, including blood pressure, waist circumference, fasting blood glucose levels, and lipid profile, all improve with orlistat treatment.[25] Low density lipoprotein (LDL) and total cholesterol levels also decrease. Gastrointestinal complaints of oily spotting, liquid stools, fecal urgency, flatulence, and abdominal cramping are most common and are induced by fat malabsorption. Chronic dosing of orlistat results in an increase in warfarin's anticoagulant effect because of decreased absorption of vitamin K.[26] This leads to an abnormal prothrombin time (PT) with a normal partial thromboplastin time (PTT), because of deficiency of clotting factors II, VII, IX, and X. The resulting coagulopathy should be corrected 6 to 24 hours before elective surgery with a vitamin K analogue such as phytonadione and fresh frozen plasma for emergency surgery or active bleeding.

BARIATRIC SURGERY

Bariatric surgery encompasses a variety of surgical procedures used to treat morbid obesity. They are classified as malabsorptive, restrictive, or combined. *Malabsorptive procedures* (jejuno-ileal bypass and biliopancreatic diversion) are rarely used today. *Restrictive procedures* include the vertical banded gastroplasty (VBG) and the adjustable gastric banding (AGB). Roux-en-Y gastric bypass (RYGB) combines gastric restriction with a minimal degree of malabsorption. VBG, AGB, and RYGB can all be performed laparoscopically, albeit with difficulty in patients weighing >180 kg, because of technical considerations.

Gastric restriction (gastroplasty) creates a small upper pouch (15 to 30 mL) in the stomach, which restricts food intake and communicates with the remainder of the stomach through a narrow channel, or stoma. RYGB, the most commonly performed bariatric procedure in the United States, involves anastomizing the proximal gastric pouch to a segment of the proximal jejunum, bypassing most of the stomach and the entire duodenum (Fig. 36-3). It is the most effective bariatric procedure to produce safe short- and long-term weight loss in severely obese patients. With RYGB, patients lose an average of 50 to 60% excess body weight and show a BMI decrease of approximately 10 kg/m^2 during the first 12 to 24 postoperative months. Type II diabetes resolves in the majority of patients.[27] Adjustable gastric banding is a restrictive gastric operation usually done by a minimally invasive laparoscopic approach.

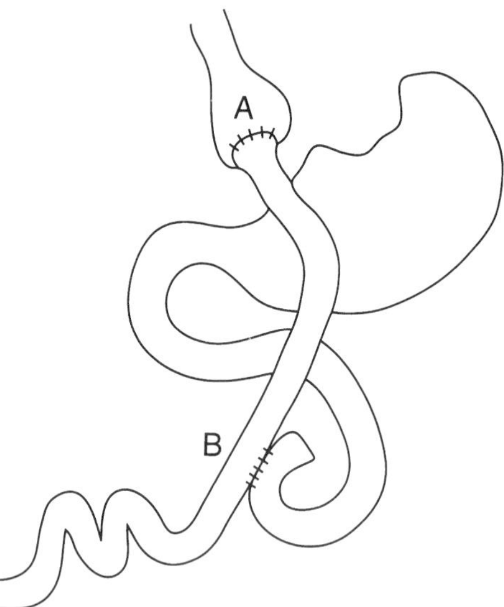

FIGURE 36-3. Roux-en-Y gastric bypass. **A.** A 15- to 30-mL gastric pouch with connected jejunal limb. **B.** Site of jejuno-jejunostomy. (Reprinted with permission from Ogunnaike BO, Jones SB, Jones DB *et al*: Anesthetic considerations for bariatric surgery. Anesth Analg 95;1794, 2002.)

An adjustable inflatable band is placed around the proximal stomach to limit stomach capacity (Fig. 36-4). The band can be made tighter or less so by adding or removing saline with adjustments made to meet patients' individual weight loss needs.

Laparoscopic bariatric surgery is minimally invasive with less postoperative pain, lower morbidity, and faster recovery. It is performed through five or six small abdominal incisions while pneumoperitonem is used to create a working space and gravity displacement for the abdominal viscera. Operative trauma is reduced when compared to open procedures, because the need for mechanical retraction of the abdominal wall is eliminated and because the surgical incision is smaller. Patients appreciate laparoscopic bariatric surgery because it reduces postoperative pain and the duration of convalescence.[28] Accumulation of "third-space" fluid, which correlates with the extent of surgical trauma, is significantly lower after laparoscopic RYGB than after open RYGB.[28] Laparoscopic gastric bypass patients also have a reduced incidence of wound infection and an early return to daily activities.

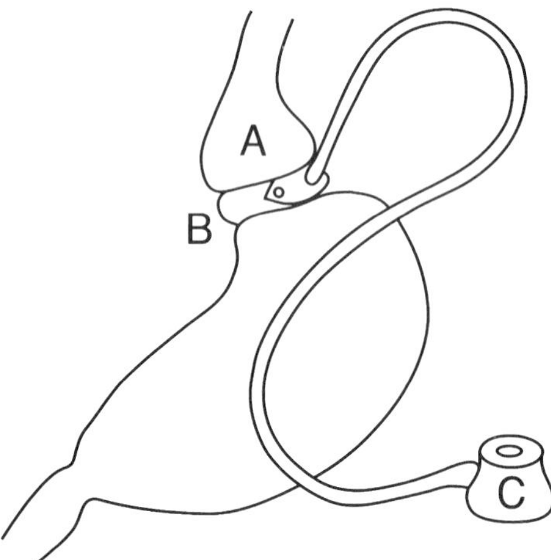

FIGURE 36-4. Adjustable gastric banding. **A.** Proximal pouch. **B.** Adjustable band. **C.** Needle access port through which saline is injected or removed to vary the size of the adjustable band. (Reprinted with permission from Ogunnaike BO, Jones SB, Jones DB *et al*: Anesthetic considerations for bariatric surgery. Anesth Analg 95;1795, 2002.)

Profound muscle relaxation is important during laparoscopic bariatric procedures to facilitate ventilation and to maintain an adequate working space for visualization and safe manipulation of laparoscopic instruments. It also facilitates extraction of excised tissues. Collapse of the pneumoperitoneum and tightening of the patient's musculature around port sites are early indications of inadequate muscle relaxation.[29]

Laparoscopic bariatric surgery requires maneuvering the operating table into various surgically favorable positions. These maneuvers could contribute to a very large patient slipping off the operating table, with disastrous consequences. The use of a malleable "bean-bag," in addition to belts and straps, may help to keep the patient secured. Anesthesia personnel may be asked to facilitate the proper placement of an intragastric balloon to help the surgeon size the gastric pouch and also facilitate performance of leak tests with saline or methylene blue through a nasogastric (NG) tube. Care should be taken to ensure a tight seal of the endotracheal tube cuff, otherwise aspiration of saline or methylene blue can occur. All endogastric tubes should be completely removed (not just merely pulled back into the esophagus) before gastric division to avoid unplanned stapling and transection of these devices (Fig. 36-5). After the gastric pouch is created, blind insertion of an NG tube should be avoided by viewing the laparoscope monitor and carefully watching to avoid disruption of the anastomosis.[29] Cephalad displacement of the diaphragm and carina from a pneumoperitoneum during laparoscopy can cause a firmly secured endotracheal tube to displace into a main-stem bronchus.[30]

Rhabdomyolysis is more common in morbidly obese pa-
4 tients undergoing laparoscopic procedures when compared to the open procedure. Long duration of surgery is one of the risk factors. Unexplained elevations in serum creatinine and

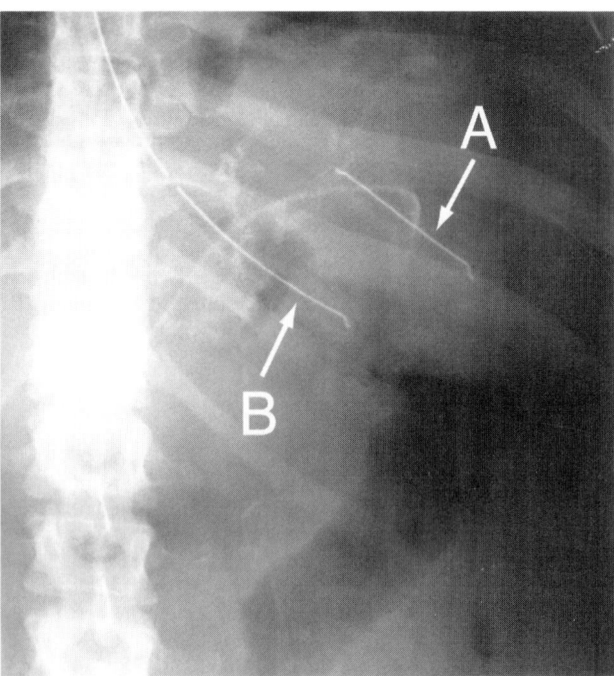

FIGURE 36-5. Radiograph of postoperative gastrograffin swallow. **A.** Transected end of nasogastric (NG) tube left in the gastric remnant. **B.** New properly placed NG tube replacing the transected one. (Reprinted with permission from Ogunnaike BO, Jones SB, Jones DB *et al*: Anesthetic considerations for bariatric surgery. Anesth Analg 95;1801, 2002.)

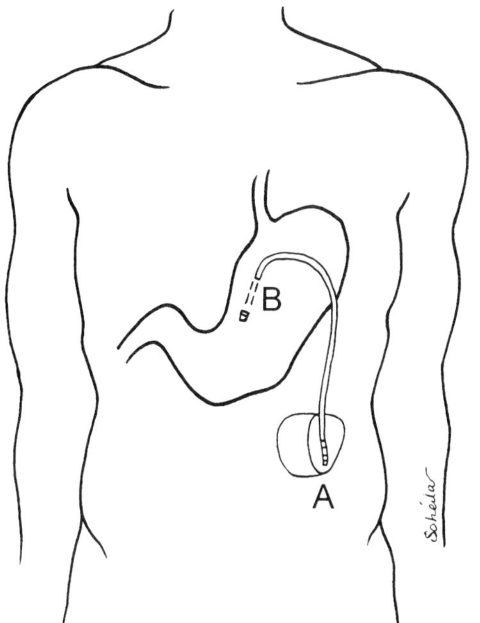

FIGURE 36-6. Illustration of the implantable gastric stimulator (IGS). A pulse generator (**A**) implanted subcutaneously sends impulses to a lead with two electrodes (**B**) implanted in the lesser curvature of the stomach.

creatine phosphokinase (CPK) levels or complaints of buttock, hip, or shoulder pain in the postoperative period should raise suspicion of rhabdomyolysis and should be investigated. Serum CPK measured pre- and postoperatively aids in early diagnosis and treatment, which helps reduce further complications such as myoglobinuric acute renal failure that can be as high as 30% with serum CPK >5,000 IU/L.[31]

Gastric electrical stimulation by means of an implantable gastric stimulator (IGS) is a newer weight-loss procedure being performed laparoscopically. Electrical impulses stimulate smooth muscles of the stomach to stop peristalsis so that the patient feels full.[32] A lead with two electrodes implanted in the lesser curvature of the stomach is connected to an electrical pulse generator implanted subcutaneously on the abdominal wall (Fig. 36-6). Implications of this procedure for the anesthesiologist include possible lead dislodgement from violent stomach contractions during postoperative nausea and vomiting. The stimulating pulses emitted by the IGS can be picked up on the electrocardiogram (ECG), which may lead to false readings. The IGS can also be adversely affected by defibrillation, electrocautery, lithotripsy, magnetic resonance imaging, and therapeutic radiation.

PREOPERATIVE CONSIDERATIONS

Preoperative Evaluation

Attention should focus on issues peculiar to the obese patient including evaluation of the cardiorespiratory systems and the airway. Previous anesthetic experiences as detailed by the patient and previous anesthetic records are useful sources of information.

Obese patients should be evaluated for systemic hypertension, pulmonary hypertension, signs of right and/or left ventricular failure, and ischemic heart disease. Signs of cardiac failure such as elevated jugular venous pressure (JVP), added heart sounds, pulmonary crackles, hepatomegaly, and peripheral edema may all be difficult to detect because of masking by excess adiposity. Pulmonary hypertension is fairly common in this patient population because of the chronicity of their pulmonary impairment. The most common features of pulmonary hypertension are exertional dyspnea, fatigue, and syncope (which reflect an inability to increase cardiac output during activity). Tricuspid regurgitation on echocardiography is the most useful confirmatory test of pulmonary hypertension but should be combined with clinical evaluation.[33] An ECG may demonstrate signs of right ventricular hypertrophy such as tall precordial R waves, right axis deviation, and right ventricular strain. The higher the pulmonary artery pressure the more sensitive the ECG. Chest radiographs may show evidence of underlying lung disease and prominent pulmonary arteries.

Patients scheduled for repeat bariatric surgery may have long-term metabolic and nutritional abnormalities that should
5 be investigated during the preoperative visit. Common deficiencies include vitamin B_{12}, iron, calcium, and folate. Vitamin and nutritional deficiencies can lead to a collective form of postoperative polyneuropathy, known as acute postgastric reduction surgery (APGARS) neuropathy, a polynutritional multisystem disorder characterized by protracted postoperative vomiting, hyporeflexia, and muscular weakness.[34] Differential diagnoses of this disorder include thiamine deficiency (Wernicke's encephalopathy, beriberi), vitamin B_{12} deficiency, and Guillain-Barré syndrome. APGARS neuropathy should cause anesthesiologists to pay close attention to dosing and monitoring neuromuscular blocking agents. Electrolyte and coagulation indices should be checked before surgery, particularly in poorly compliant or acutely ill patients because chronic vitamin K deficiency can lead to coagulation abnormalities. Administration of a vitamin K analog or fresh frozen plasma may be needed.

Evidence of OSA and OHS should be sought preoperatively because they are frequently associated with difficult laryngoscopy. OSA patients on a continuous positive airway pressure (CPAP) device at home should be instructed to bring it with them to the hospital as it may be needed postoperatively. The possibility of invasive monitoring, prolonged intubation, and postoperative mechanical ventilation should be discussed with the patient. Arterial blood gas measurement will help evaluate ventilation, as well as the need for perioperative oxygen administration and postoperative ventilation. Routine pulmonary function tests (PFTs) and liver function tests (LFTs) are not cost-effective in asymptomatic obese patients. Blood glucose abnormalities should be corrected if present.

Concurrent, Preoperative, and Prophylactic Medications

Patients' usual medications should be continued until the time of surgery with the possible exception of insulin and oral hypoglycemics. Antibiotic prophylaxis is important because of an increased incidence of wound infections in the obese.[35] Anxiolysis and prophylaxis against both aspiration pneumonitis and deep vein thrombosis (DVT) should be addressed at premedication. Oral benzodiazepines are reliable for anxiolysis and sedation. Intravenous midazolam can also be titrated in small doses for anxiolysis during the immediate preoperative period. Pharmacologic intervention with H_2-receptor antagonists, nonparticulate antacids, or proton pump inhibitors will reduce gastric volume, acidity, or both, thereby reducing the risk and severity of aspiration pneumonitis.

Morbid obesity is a major independent risk factor for sud-
6 den death from acute postoperative pulmonary embolism (PE). Subcutaneous heparin 5,000 IU administered before surgery and repeated every 8 to 12 hours until the patient is fully

mobile reduces the risk of DVT. Four important risk factors, namely venous stasis disease, BMI ≥60, truncal obesity, and obesity hypoventilation syndrome (OHS)/sleep apnea syndrome (SAS), are significant in the development of postoperative venous thromboembolism, and if present, preoperative prophylactic placement of an IVC filter should be considered.[36] Many bariatric surgeons prefer low-dose unfractionated heparin as their method of thromboprophylaxis.[37] Use of a protocol for heparin dosing in gastric bypass patients, as opposed to a fixed dose, is preferred. Dosing based on height and weight initially, and then adjusted based on peak antifactor Xa activity, results in better thromboprophylaxis and few side effects.[38] Low molecular weight heparins (LMWH) have gained popularity for thromboembolism prophylaxis during bariatric surgery because of their bioavailability when injected subcutaneously. Enoxaparin, 40 mg, injected subcutaneously every 12 hours rather than the often recommended 30 mg every 12 hours decreases the incidence of postoperative DVT without an increase in bleeding complications.[39] It has also been suggested that enoxaparin dosing in the obese be varied with age and lean body mass.[40]

AIRWAY

7 Neck circumference has been identified as the single biggest predictor of problematic intubation in morbidly obese patients.[41] The probability of a problematic intubation is approximately 5% with a 40-cm neck circumference compared with a 35% probability at 60-cm neck circumference. A larger neck circumference is associated with the male sex, a higher Mallampati score, grade 3 views at laryngoscopy, and OSA.

INTRAOPERATIVE CONSIDERATIONS

Positioning

Specially designed tables or two regular operating tables may be required for safe anesthesia and surgery in obese patients. Regular operating tables have a maximum weight limit of approximately 205 kg, but operating tables capable of holding up to 455 kg, with a little extra width to accommodate the extra girth, are available. Electrically operated or motorized tables facilitate maneuvering into various surgically favorable positions. Strapping obese patients to the operating table in combination with a malleable bean bag helps keep them from falling off the operating table. Particular care should be paid to protecting pressure areas because pressure sores and neural injuries are common in this group. Brachial plexus and lower extremity nerve injuries are frequent. A documented association between ulnar neuropathy and increasing BMI quoted as much as one-third incidence of ulnar neuropathy in patients with a BMI ≥38 kg/m^2 compared with only 1% in the control group.[42]

Supine positioning causes ventilatory impairment and inferior vena cava and aortic compression in obese patients. FRC and oxygenation are decreased further with supine positioning. Trendelenburg positioning, often required during bariatric procedures, further worsens FRC and should be avoided if possible. Simply changing the obese patient from a sitting to supine position can cause a significant increase in oxygen consumption, cardiac output, and pulmonary artery pressure. The head-up reverse Trendelenburg position provides the longest safe apnea period (SAP) during induction of anesthesia.[43] The extra time gained may help preclude hypoxemia if intubation is delayed. Both intraoperative positive end-expiratory pressure (PEEP) and reverse Trendelenburg positions significantly decrease alveolar–arterial oxygen tension difference and increase total respiratory compliance to a similar degree in the obese, but reverse Trendelenburg position results in lower airway pressures. Both, however, decrease cardiac output significantly, which partially counteracts the beneficial effects on oxygenation.[44] Prone positioning, when required in the obese patient, should be correctly performed with freedom of abdominal movement to prevent detrimental effects on lung compliance, ventilation, and arterial oxygenation. Prone positioning increases intra-abdominal pressure, worsening IVC and aortic compression and further decreasing FRC. Lateral decubitus positioning allows for better diaphragmatic excursion and should be favored over prone positioning whenever the surgical procedure permits.

Monitoring

Invasive arterial pressure monitoring may be indicated for the super morbidly obese patient, for those patients with cardiopulmonary disease, and for those patients where the noninvasive blood pressure cuff may not fit properly. Blood pressure measurements can be falsely elevated if a cuff is too small. Cuffs with bladders that encircle a minimum of 75% of the upper arm circumference or, preferably, the entire arm, should be used. Forearm measurements with a standard cuff overestimate
8 both systolic and diastolic blood pressures in obese patients.[45]
Central venous and pulmonary artery catheters can be used in patients with significant cardiopulmonary disease or in patients undergoing extensive surgery where significant fluid shifts are anticipated. Central venous catheterization may also be required for intravenous access, which can be problematic in this patient population, although insertion of peripheral lines is almost always successful.[46]

Induction, Intubation, and Maintenance

Adequate preoxygenation is vital in obese patients because of rapid desaturation after loss of consciousness because of increased oxygen consumption and decreased FRC. Application of positive pressure ventilation during preoxygenation decreases atelectasis formation and improves oxygenation in morbidly obese patients.[47] Four vital capacity breaths with 100% oxygen within 30 seconds have been suggested as superior to the usually recommended 3 minutes of 100% preoxygenation in obese patients.[48] Larger doses of induction agents may be required by obese patients because blood volume, muscle mass, and cardiac output increase linearly with the degree of obesity. An increased dose of succinylcholine is necessary because of an increase in activity of pseudocholinesterase. Any of the intravenous induction agents can be used after taking into consideration problems peculiar to individual patients.

If a difficult intubation is anticipated, awake intubation utilizing topical or regional anesthesia is a prudent approach. During awake intubation, sedative–hypnotic medications should be reduced to a minimum. If endotracheal intubation under general anesthesia is selected, hypoxia and aspiration of gastric contents should be prevented at all costs. An experienced colleague who is immediately available or, better still, in the room during induction and airway management can help with mask ventilation or attempts at intubation. A surgeon capable of accessing the airway surgically should be readily available. Towels or folded blankets under the shoulders and head can compensate for the exaggerated flexed position of posterior cervical fat (Fig. 36-7). The object of this maneuver, known as "stacking," is to position the patient so that the tip of the chin is at a higher level than the chest to facilitate laryngoscopy and

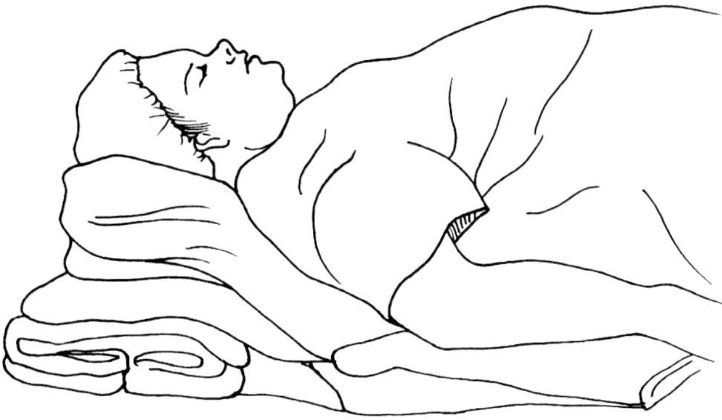

FIGURE 36-7. "Stacking" using towels and blankets.

9 intubation. The head-elevated laryngoscopy position (HELP) is a step beyond stacking. It significantly elevates the obese patient's head, upper body, and shoulders above the chest to the extent that an imaginary horizontal line connects the sternal notch with the external auditory meatus to better improve laryngoscopy and intubation.[49] To facilitate proper HELP placement, the preformed Troop Head Elevation Pillow® (C&R Enterprises, Frisco, TX) in combination with a standard intubation pillow can be used in place of folded towels or blankets (Fig. 36-8A and 36-8B). The advantage of the preformed pillow is that it can be prepositioned, inserted, and removed much faster with less effort than that required to build and dismantle a ramp made from blankets and towels.[50]

Continuous infusion of a short-acting intravenous agent, such as propofol, or any of the inhalational agents or a combination may be used to maintain anesthesia. Desflurane, sevoflurane, and isoflurane are minimally metabolized and are therefore useful agents in the obese patient, with desflurane possibly providing better hemodynamic stability.[51] Sevoflurane provides rapid recovery, good hemodynamic control, infrequent incidence of nausea and vomiting, and prompt regaining of psychological and physical functioning when compared to isoflurane.[52] Metabolism of volatile anesthetics is greater in obese than in normal-weight patients, which is reflected by a greater increase in serum inorganic fluoride, including with sevoflurane, whose biotransformation has not been shown to result in significant differences in plasma fluoride levels nor differences in pre- and postoperative liver function and renal function tests between obese and nonobese patients.[53] A potentially hepatotoxic reductive pathway metabolizes halothane in obese patients, resulting in an increased incidence of "halothane hepatitis." Fortunately, halothane is rarely needed in modern-day practice. Evidence does not support the suggestion that significant delayed recovery and awakening from volatile

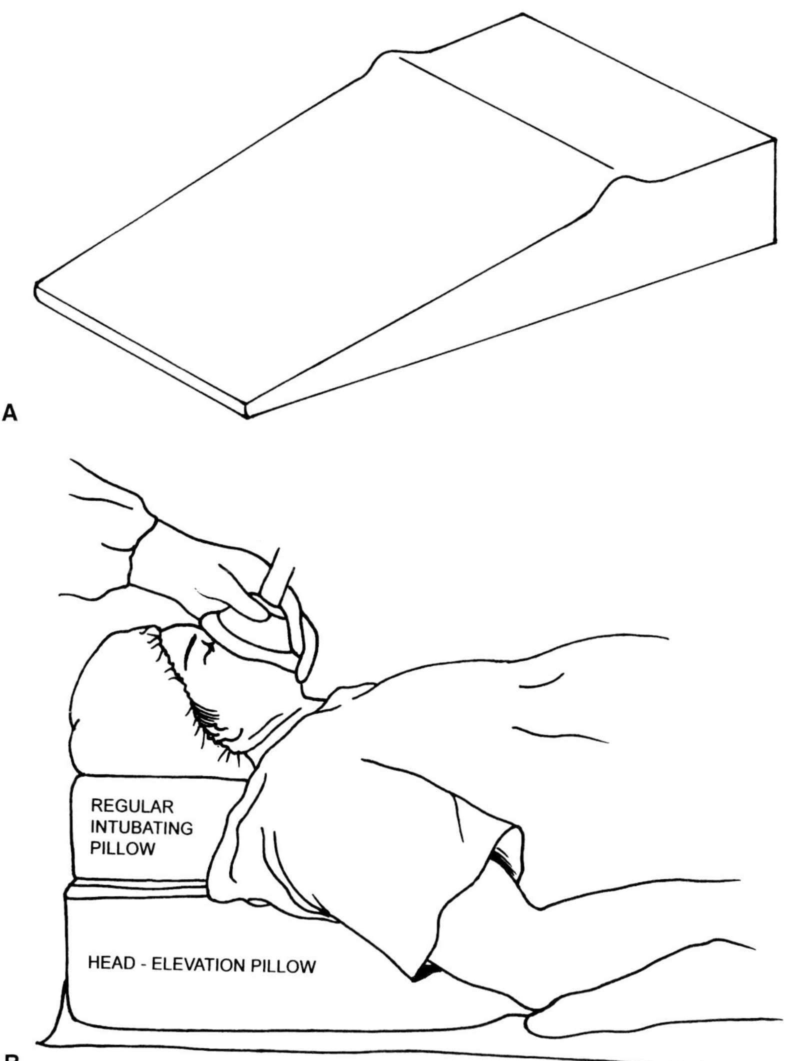

FIGURE 36-8. **A.** The preformed head elevation pillow. **B.** Proper head-elevated laryngoscopy position (HELP) placement with the head elevation pillow combined with a standard intubating pillow as described in the text.

anesthetic agents occurs in obese patients when compared to the nonobese. Rapid elimination and analgesic properties make nitrous oxide an attractive choice for anesthesia in obese patients, but high oxygen demand in this patient population limits its use.

Short-acting opioids at the lowest possible dose, combined with a low solubility inhalation anesthetic, facilitate a more rapid emergence without increasing opioid-related side effects.[54] Cisatracurium possesses an organ-independent elimination profile and is a favorable nondepolarizing muscle relaxant for use during maintenance of anesthesia. Vecuronium and rocuronium are also useful choices. Dexmedetomidine, an alpha-2 agonist with sedative and analgesic properties, provides hemodynamic stability without myocardial depression. It has no clinically significant adverse effects on respiration, which makes it an attractive agent for use as an anesthetic adjunct in obese patients.[55] Furthermore, it reduces the postoperative opioid analgesic requirements and their subsequent detrimental respiratory depressant effects.[56]

Ventilatory tidal volumes greater than 13 mL/kg offer no added advantages during ventilation of anesthetized morbidly obese patients. Increasing tidal volumes further only increases the peak inspiratory airway pressure, end-expiratory (plateau) airway pressure, and lung compliance without significantly improving arterial oxygen tension.[57] Arterial oxygenation during laparoscopy in morbidly obese patients is affected mainly by body weight and not body position, pneumoperitoneum, or mode of ventilation, and oxygenation is not significantly improved by increasing either the respiratory rate or tidal volume.[58] Positive end-expiratory pressure is the only ventilatory parameter that has consistently been shown to improve respiratory function in obese subjects.[59] PEEP may, however, decrease venous return and cardiac output.

Excess adipose tissue may mask peripheral perfusion, making fluid balance difficult to assess. Blood loss is usually greater in the obese than in the nonobese for the same type of surgery, because technical difficulties of accessing the surgical site necessitate larger incisions and more extensive dissection. Early infusion of colloids and blood products may be necessary because obese patients are less able to compensate for small volumes lost, but rapid infusion of excessive amounts should be avoided because preexisting congestive cardiac failure is common in the obese.

Regional Anesthesia

A regional technique is a useful alternative to general anesthesia in the morbidly obese patient as it may help avoid potential intubation difficulties. It can, however, be technically difficult because of inability to identify usual bony landmarks. A peripheral nerve stimulator with an insulated needle may be of use. Central neuraxial block is easier in the lumbar region because the midline in this area has a thinner layer of fat than other areas of the spinal column. Longer needles and the sitting position are other useful tools that facilitate induction of central neuraxial anesthesia. Ultrasound[60] and fluoroscopy[61] can be used to guide the needle or continuous infusion catheter into the epidural space. Low current electrical epidural stimulation through an epidural catheter, to achieve trunk or limb movement, can also be used for confirmation of epidural catheter placement.[62] Epidural vascular engorgement and fatty infiltration reduce the volume of the space, making dose requirements of local anesthetics for epidural anesthesia 20 to 25% less in obese patients. Subarachnoid blocks are not technically as difficult as epidural blocks but the height of a subarachnoid block in obese patients can be unpredictable because it may spread considerably upward within a short time, causing cardiovascular and respiratory embarrassment. A continuous catheter subarachnoid block therefore seems an attractive choice that allows careful titration of the local anesthetic to desired effect and level.[63]

Combined epidural and balanced general anesthesia allows for better titration of anesthetic drugs, use of larger oxygen concentration, and optimal muscle relaxation. It also allows for continuation of postoperative analgesia through the same catheter used to provide surgical anesthesia, thereby facilitating early postoperative mobilization.

POSTOPERATIVE CONSIDERATIONS

Emergence

Prompt extubation reduces the likelihood that the morbidly obese patient, who may have underlying cardiopulmonary disease, will become ventilator dependent. The patient should be preferably extubated in the semirecumbent position, which has less adverse effect on respiration. Supplemental oxygen should be administrated after extubation. Lifting devices such as the HoverMatt® (Patient Handling Technologies, Allentown, PA) and the Patient Transfer Device (PTD®; Alimed, Dedham, MA) are useful for transporting morbidly obese patients onto or off the operating table. The PTD can be combined with the Walter Henderson Maneuver (Fig. 36-9) to safely and gently transfer obese patients onto their postoperative beds.[64]

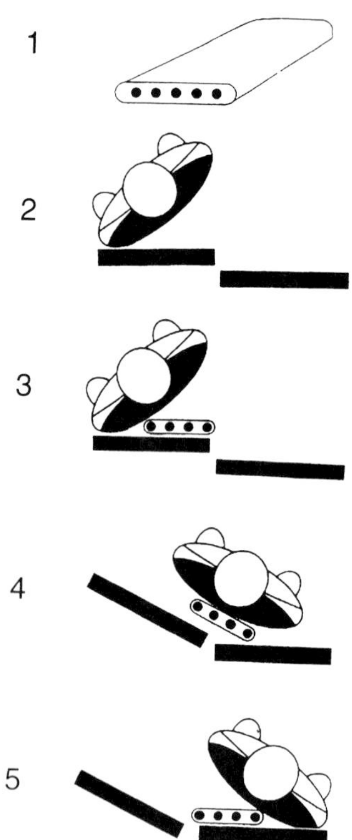

FIGURE 36-9. Illustration of the Walter Henderson maneuver. 1 = Patient Transfer Device—PTD® (a.k.a. patient roller); 2 = patient tilted to slip roller under; 3 = roller slipped under patient; 4 = table tilted to roll patient downhill onto bed; 5 = patient rolled onto bed. (Reprinted with permission from Ogunnaike BO, Whitten CW: In response to Rosenblatt MA, Reich DL, Roth R *et al* [Letter]. Anesth Analg 98;1809, 2004.)

There is an increased incidence of atelectasis in morbidly obese patients after general anesthesia, which persists into the postoperative period.[65] Consequently, initiation of continuous positive airway pressure (CPAP) or bi-level positive airway pressure (Bi-PAP) has been advocated to combat airway obstruction. Postoperative CPAP does not increase the incidence of major anastomotic leakage after gastric bypass surgery despite a theoretical risk.[66] The obese patient may avoid taking deep breaths because of pain after abdominal surgery. Adequate analgesia and a properly fitted elastic binder for abdominal support may encourage them to cooperate with early ambulation and deep breathing exercises with the aid of incentive spirometry. Pulse oximetry and arterial blood gases should be monitored appropriately.

Postoperative Analgesia

Perioperative use of regional anesthesia and analgesia reduces the incidence of postoperative respiratory complications. Epidural analgesia with local anesthetics, opioids, or both is an effective form of analgesia. Intrathecal opioid is also a viable option. Potential advantages of epidural analgesia in obese patients include prevention of DVT, improved analgesia, and earlier recovery of intestinal motility. Lesser oxygen consumption and decreased left ventricular stroke work are other benefits. PCA morphine is equivalent to low thoracic/high lumbar continuous infusions of bupivacaine/fentanyl epidural analgesia in morbidly obese patients undergoing gastric bypass surgery with regards to the quality of pain control at rest, the frequency of nausea and pruritius, the time to ambulation, time to return of GI function, and the length of hospital stay.[67] Multimodal analgesia (incisional local anesthetic infiltration plus PCA) was found to produce lower pain scores when compared to epidural anesthesia and analgesia and postoperative PCA for gastric bypass surgery. In addition, infiltration analgesia as part of a multimodal regimen offers a simple, safe, and inexpensive alternative to epidural analgesia alone.[68] A combination of intraoperative nonopioid analgesics and anesthetic adjuvants (ketorolac, clonidine, ketamine, lidocaine, magnesium sulfate, and methylprednisolone) that produce analgesia by mechanisms different from opioids decreases sedation during recovery from anesthesia and reduces postoperative morphine requirements when compared to intraoperative fentanyl anesthesia in morbidly obese patients.[69] Delayed respiratory depression is one of the known complications of central neuraxial opioids. When this is coupled with a potentially difficult airway in the obese patient, closer monitoring in a step-down or intensive care unit is a wise choice until this complication is no longer a threat.

RESUSCITATION

The possible need for cardiopulmonary resuscitation should be entertained during anesthesia for the morbidly obese. Of concern are the equipment and technical aspects of resuscitation. Chest compressions may not be effective and mechanical compression devices may be required. The maximum 400 joules of energy on regular defibrillators is sufficient for the morbidly obese,[70] because their chest wall is usually not much thicker, but the higher transthoracic impedance from the fat may obligate several attempts. The laryngeal mask airway (LMA)® and the esophageal tracheal Combitube® are temporary supraglottic airway devices that are useful during resuscitation of the obese. Tracheostomy and percutaneous cricothyrotomy are time-consuming and technically difficult options in such emergency situations. Fiberoptic or retrograde wire intubation may be quicker alternatives in the absence of, or inadequate ventilation with, supraglottic devices.

References

1. Adams JP, Murphy PG: Obesity in anaesthesia and intensive care. Br J Anaesth 85:91, 2000
2. Tosetti C, Corinaldesi R, Stranghellini V *et al*: Gastric emptying of solids in morbid obesity. Int J Obes Relat Metab Disord 20:200, 1996
3. Harter RL, Kelly WB, Kramer MG *et al*: A comparison of the volume and pH of gastric contents of obese and lean surgical patients. Anesth Analg 86:147, 1998
4. Maltby JR, Pytka S, Watson NC *et al*: Drinking 300 ml of clear fluid two hours before surgery has no effect on gastric fluid volume and pH in fasting and non-fasting obese patients. Can J Anesth 51:111, 2004
5. Hickman IJ, Jonsson JR, Prins JB *et al*: Modest weight loss and physical activity in overweight patients with chronic liver disease results in sustained improvements in alanine aminotransferase, fasting insulin, and quality of life. Gut 53:413, 2004
6. Cheymol G: Effects of obesity on pharmacokinetics: implications for drug therapy. Clin Pharmacokinet 39:215, 2000
7. Raucoles-Aime M, Brimaud D: Diabetes mellitus: Implications for the anesthesiologist. Curr Opin Anaesth 9:247, 1996
8. Chagnac A, Weinstein T, Herman M *et al*: The effects of weight loss on renal function in patients with severe obesity. J Am Soc Nephrol 14:1480, 2003
9. Hall JE: The kidney, hypertension, and obesity. Hypertension 41:625, 2003
10. Ezri T, Medalion B, Weisenberg M *et al*: Increased body mass per se is not a predictor of difficult laryngoscopy. Can J Anesth 50:179, 2003
11. Blouin RA, Warren GW: Pharmacokinetic considerations in obesity. J Pharm Sci 88:1, 1999
12. Egan TD, Huizinga B, Gupta SK *et al*: Remifentanil pharmacokinetics in obese versus lean patients. Anesthesiology 89:562, 1998
13. Abernethy DR, Greenblatt DJ, Smith TW: Digoxin disposition in obesity: Clinical pharmacokinetic investigation. Am Heart J 102:740, 1981
14. Christoff PB, Conti DR, Naylor C *et al*: Procainamide disposition in obesity. Drug Intell Clin Pharm 17:516, 1983
15. Servin F, Farinotti R, Haberer JP *et al*: Propofol infusion for maintenance of anesthesia in morbidly obese patients receiving nitrous oxide. A clinical pharmacokinetic study. Anesthesiology 78:657, 1993
16. Leykin Y, Pellis T, Lucca M, *et al*. The pharmacodynamic effects of rocuronium when dosed according to real body weight or ideal body weight in morbidly obese patients. Anesth Analg 99:1086, 2004
17. Puhringer FK, Keller C, Kleinsasser A *et al*: Pharmacokinetics of rocuronium bormide in obese female patients. Eur J Anaesthesiol 16:507, 1999
18. Varin F, Ducharme J, Theoret Y *et al*: Influence of extreme obesity on the body disposition and neuromuscular blocking effect of atracurium. Clin Pharmacol Ther 48:18, 1990
19. Leykin Y, Pellis T, Lucca M, *et al*. The effects of cisatracurium on morbidly obese women. Anesth Analg 99:1090, 2004
20. Shibutani K, Inchiosa MA, Sawada K *et al*: Accuracy of pharmacokinetic models for prediction plasma fentalyl concentrations in lean and obese surgical patients. Derivation of dosing weight ("pharmacokinetic mass"). Anesthesiology 101:603, 2004
21. Slepchenko G, Simon N, Goubaux B *et al*: Performance of target-controlled sufentanil infusion on obese patients. Anesthesiology 98:65, 2003
22. Bouillon T, Shafer SL: Does size matter? Anesthesiology 89:557, 1998
23. Rich JM, Njo L, Roberts KW *et al*: Unusual hypotension and bradycardia in a patient receiving fenfluramine, phentermine, and fluoxetine. Anesthesiology 88:529, 1997
24. Weigle DS: Pharmacological therapy of obesity: past, present, and future. J Clin Endocrinol Metab 88:2462, 2003
25. Krempf M, Louvet JP, Allanic H *et al*: Weight reduction and long-term maintenance after 18 months treatment with orlistat for obesity. Int J Obes Relat Metal Disord 27:591, 2003
26. MacWalter RS, Fraser HW, Armstrong KM: Orlistat enhances warfarin effect. Ann Pharmacother 37:510, 2003
27. Rubino F, Gagner M, Gentileschi P *et al*: The early effect of the Roux-en-Y gastric bypass on hormones involved in body weight regulation and glucose metabolism. Ann Surg 240:236, 2004
28. Nguyen NT: Open vs. laparoscopic procedures in bariatric surgery. J Gastrointest Surg 8:393, 2004
29. Ogunnaike BO, Jones SB, Jones DB *et al*: Anesthetic considerations for bariatric surgery. Anesth Analg 95:1793, 2002
30. Ezri T, Hazin V, Warters D *et al*: The endotracheal tube moves more often in obese patients undergoing laparoscopy compared with open abdominal surgery. Anesth Analg 96:278, 2003
31. Mognol P, Vignes S, Chosidow D *et al*: Rhabdomyolysis after laparoscopic bariatric surgery. Obes Surg 14:19, 2004
32. Cigaina V: Gastric pacing as therapy for morbid obesity: preliminary results. Obes Surg 12:S12, 2002
33. Elliot C, Kiely DG: Pulmonary hypertension: Diagnosis and treatment. Clin Med 4:211, 2004

34. Chang C, Adams-Huet B, Provost DA: Acute post-gastric reduction surgery (APGARS) neuropathy. Obes Surg 14:182, 2004
35. Kabon B, Nagele A, Reddy D *et al*: Obesity decreases perioperative tissue oxygenation. Anesthesiology 100:274, 2004
36. Sapala JA, Wood MH, Schuhknecht MP *et al*: Fatal pulmonary embolism after bariatric operations for morbid obesity: A 24-year retrospective analysis. Obes Surg 13:819, 2003
37. Wu EC, Barba CA: Current practices in the prophylaxis of venous thromboembolism in bariatric surgery. Obes Surg 10:7, 2000
38. Shepherd MF, Rosborough TK, Schwartz ML: Heparin thromboprophylaxis in gastric bypass. Obes Surg 13:249, 2003
39. Scholten DJ, Hoedema RM, Scholten SE: A comparison of two different prophylactic dose regimens of low molecular weight heparin in bariatric surgery. Obes Surg 12:19, 2002
40. Green B, Duffull SB: Development of a dosing strategy for enoxaparin in obese patients. Br J Clin Pharmacol 56:96, 2003
41. Brodsky JB, Lemmons HJM, Brock-Utne JG *et al*: Morbid obesity and tracheal intubation. Anesth Analg 94:732, 2002
42. Warner MA, Warner ME, Martin JT: Ulnar neuropathy: Incidence, outcome and risk factors in sedated or anesthetized patients. Anesthesiology 81:1332, 1994
43. Boyce JR, Ness T, Castroman P: A preliminary study of the optimal positioning for the morbidly obese patient. Obes Surg 13:4, 2003
44. Perilli V, Sollazzi L, Modesti C *et al*: Comparison of positive end-expiratory pressure with reverse Trendelenburg position in morbidly obese patients. Obes Surg 13:605, 2003
45. Pierin AM, Alavarce DC, Gusmao JL *et al*: Blood pressure measurement in obese patients: Comparison between upper arm and forearm measurements. Blood Press Monit 9:101, 2004
46. Juvin P, Blarel A, Bruno F *et al*: Is peripheral line placement more difficult in obese than in lean patients? Anesth Analg 96:1218, 2003
47. Coussa M, Proietti S, Schnyder P *et al*: Prevention of atelectasis formation during the induction of general anesthesia in morbidly obese patients. Anesth Analg 98:1491, 2004
48. Goldberg ME, Norris MC, Larijani GE *et al*: Preoxygenation in the morbidly obese: A comparison of two techniques. Anesth Analg 68:520, 1989
49. Levitan RM, Mechem CC, Ochroch EA *et al*: Head-elevated laryngoscopy position: Improving laryngeal exposure during laryngoscopy by increasing head elevation. Ann Emerg Med 41:322, 2003
50. Rich JM: Use of an elevation pillow to produce the head-elevated laryngoscopy position for airway management in morbidly obese and large-framed patients. Anesth Analg 98:264, 2004
51. De Baerdemaeker LE, Struys MM, Jacobs S *et al*: Optimization of desflurane administration in morbidly obese patients: A comparison with sevoflurane. Br J Anaesth 91:638, 2003
52. Torri G, Casati A, Albertin A *et al*: Randomized comparison of isoflurane and sevoflurane for laparoscopic banding in morbidly obese patients. J Clin Anesth 13:565, 2001
53. Frink EJ, Malan TP, Brown EA *et al*: Plasma inorganic fluoride levels with sevoflurane anesthesia in morbidly obese and nonobese patients. Anesth Analg 76:1333, 1993
54. Song D, Whitten CW, White PF: Remifentanil infusion facilitates early recovery for obese outpatients undergoing laparoscopic cholecystectomy. Anesth Analg 90:1111, 2000
55. Ramsay MA, Jones CC, Cancemi MR *et al*: Hemodynamic and respiratory changes related to the use of dexmedetomidine in bariatric surgical patients. Anesthesiology 96:A165, 2002
56. Hofer RE, Sprung J, Sarr MG *et al*. Anesthesia for a patient with morbid obesity using dexmedetomidine without narcotics. Can J Anesth 52:176, 2005
57. Bardoczky GI, Yernault JC, Houben JJ *et al*: Large tidal volume ventilation does not improve oxygenation in morbidly obese patients during anesthesia. Anesth Analg 81:385, 1995
58. Sprung J, Whalley DG, Falcone T *et al*: The effects of tidal volume and respiratory rate on oxygenation and respiratory mechanics during laparoscopy in morbidly obese patients. Anesth Analg 97:268, 2003
59. Pelosi P, Ravagnan I, Giurati G *et al*: Positive end-expiratory pressure improves respiratory function in obese but not in normal subjects during anesthesia and paralysis. Anesthesiology 91:1221, 1999
60. Grau T, Leipold RW, Fatehi S *et al*: Real time ultrasonic observation of combined spinal-epidural anaesthesia. Eur J Anaesthesiol 21:25, 2004
61. Johnson TW, Morgan R, Smalley P: Radiographic guided epidural placement. Anaesthesia 58:485, 2003
62. Tsui BC, Gupta S, Finucane B: Confirmation of epidural catheter placement using nerve stimulation. Can J Anesth 45:640, 1998
63. Michaloudis D, Fraidakis O, Petrou A *et al*: Continuous spinal anesthesia/analgesia for perioperative management of morbidly obese patients undergoing laparotomy for gastroplastic surgery. Obes Surg 10:220, 2000
64. Ogunnaike BO, Whitten CW: Bariatric surgery and the prevention of postoperative respiratory complications (In reply). Anesth Analg 98:1809, 2004
65. Eichenberger A, Proietti S, Wicky S *et al*: Morbid obesity and postoperative pulmonary atelectasis: An underestimated problem. Anesth Analg 95:1788, 2002
66. Huerta S, DeShields S, Shpiner R *et al*: Safety and efficacy of postoperative continuous positive airway pressure to prevent pulmonary complications after Roux-en-y gastric bypass. J Gastrointest Surg 6:354, 2002
67. Charghi R, Backman S, Christou N *et al*: Patient controlled IV analgesia is an acceptable pain management strategy in morbidly obese patients undergoing gastric bypass surgery. A retrospective comparison with epidural analgesia. Can J Anesth 50:672, 2003
68. Schumann R, Shikora S, Weiss JM *et al*: A comparison of multimodal perioperative analgesia to epidural pain management after gastric bypass surgery. Anesth Analg 96:469, 2003
69. Feld JM, Laurito CE, Beckerman M *et al*: Non-opioid analgesia improves pain relief and decreases sedation after gastric bypass surgery. Can J Anesth 50:336, 2003
70. DeSilva RA, Lown B: Energy requirement for defibrillation of a markedly overweight patient. Circulation 57:827, 1978

CHAPTER 37 ■ ANESTHESIA AND GASTROINTESTINAL DISORDERS

BABATUNDE O. OGUNNAIKE AND CHARLES W. WHITTEN

KEY POINTS

1. The difference between the lower esophageal sphincter (LES) pressure and gastric pressure is "barrier pressure," which is more important than the LES tone in the production of gastroesophageal reflux.
2. Epidural analgesia that includes local anesthetics has been most effective in minimizing postoperative ileus. Other beneficial adjuncts include minimally invasive surgery, early enteral nutrition, and early mobilization.
3. Carcinoid crises can be precipitated by physical or chemical stimulation, stress, tumor necrosis from hepatic artery ligation or embolization, chemotherapy, and succinylcholine-induced fasciculations, which can potentially trigger mediator release. Octreotide effectively treats intraoperative carcinoid crises.

GASTROINTESTINAL DISORDERS

Esophagus

The adult esophagus extends from the cricophargyngeal sphincter at the level of the C6 vertebra to the gastroesophageal (GE) junction. An inner circular layer surrounded by an outer longitudinal layer makes up the musculature. The upper one-third of the inner circular muscle is striated while the lower two-thirds are smooth.

The cricopharyngeus muscle, one of the two inferior muscles of the pharynx, together with the circular fibers of the upper esophagus, acts as the functional *upper esophageal sphincter* (UES) at the pharyngoesophageal junction. The UES extends from one side of the cricoid arch to the other and is continuous with the circular muscular coat of the esophagus. This sphincter is in a state of tonic contraction with a resting pressure of 15 to 60 cm H_2O, preventing air from entering the esophagus under normal circumstances. The UES also helps prevent aspiration by sealing off the upper esophagus from the hypopharynx in conscious healthy patients. UES function is impaired during both normal sleep and anesthesia. Most anesthetic agents, except ketamine, will reduce UES tone and increase the likelihood of regurgitation of material from the esophagus into the hypopharynx. Impaired swallowing and reduction in tone of the UES from partial neuromuscular blockade increase the risk of aspiration.[1] Video manometry studies have shown a significant delay in relaxation of the UES following contraction of the inferior constrictor muscle during partial neuromuscular blockade, suggesting that conscious patients in the recovery room may still be at risk of aspiration even with clinically adequate neuromuscular transmission.[2] Subhypnotic concentrations of intravenous (IV) and inhalational anesthetics increase the incidence of pharyngeal dysfunction.[3] Both intrinsic and extrinsic nerves supply the esophagus. The intrinsic nerve supply includes the myenteric plexus of Auerbach (which lies between the outer longitudinal and middle circular layers of muscle) and the submucosal plexus of Meissner (which lies between the circular layer and the mucosa). The extrinsic nerve supply is derived from parasympathetic fibers from the vagi with sympathetic fibers from the superior and inferior cervical and fourth and fifth thoracic sympathetic ganglia.

The border between the stomach and esophagus is formed by the *lower esophageal sphincter* (LES). It is a band of circular muscle fibers surrounding the lower end of the esophagus and has a resting tone of 10 to 15 cm H_2O with an approximate length of 3 cm. The left margin of the lower esophagus makes an acute angle with the gastric fundus and contraction of the right crus of the diaphragm forms a sling around the abdominal esophagus. The LES, the major barrier to gastroesophageal reflux, is histologically similar to the rest of the esophagus but functionally different. The LES appears as an area of increased pressure on gastroesophageal manometry. During swallowing, the LES is relaxed whereas there is peristalsis in the remainder of the esophagus. The major physiological derangement in gastroesophageal reflux is a reduction in LES pressure. The sphincteric pressure is affected by both the intrinsic nerve plexus and by gastrin released by the mucosa of the gastric antrum in response to the presence of acid. Gastrin increases the sphincter pressure, as well as α-adrenergic agents, acetylcholine, serotonin, histamine, and pancreatic polypeptide. Dopamine, secretin, glucagons, and β-adrenergic agents decrease the LES sphincter pressure among other factors (Table 37-1).

The difference between the LES pressure and gastric pres-
1 sure is "barrier pressure" and is more important than the LES tone in the production of gastroesophageal reflux. Adequately high intragastric pressure can overcome the LES and lead to reflux. This is unlikely in healthy individuals whose LES pressure usually rises in response to increased intragastric pressure. Low to normal barrier pressures are characteristic of patients with gastroesophageal reflux with no distinct cut-off point. Vagal denervation does not seem to affect the active function or resting tone of the LES but reduced tone can be clinically seen with obesity, hiatal hernia, and pregnancy. Anesthetic agents that may reduce the barrier pressure, thereby reducing LES pressure, include thiopental, propofol, opioids, anticholinergics, and inhaled anesthetics, while antiemetics, cholinergics, antacids, and succinylcholine increase LES pressure. Nondepolarizing muscle relaxants and H_2-receptor antagonists have no effect on LES pressure. Cricoid pressure in both conscious and unconscious patients decreases LES tone as a result of a significant reduction in esophageal barrier pressure while gastric pressure remains normal.[4] The evidence that succinylcholine increases LES tone, while cricoid pressure decreases LES tone, makes the necessity for application of cricoid pressure during a rapid sequence induction questionable.

Stomach

Digestion begins in the stomach by mixing of ingested food with gastric secretions. It is very distensible with the capacity to store large amounts of material (up to 1.5 L of fluid) without a significant increase in intragastric pressure. Electrical activity that originates at a "pacemaker" located near the midpoint of the greater curvature of the stomach initiates mechanical activity that spreads toward the pylorus. Pyloric relaxation, in response to the waves of gastric activity, expels gastric contents into the duodenum in small amounts.

Obesity, bedridden states, pregnancy, shock, trauma, and pain are examples of pathologic states associated with high gastric content volume. Bowel handling during laparotomy increases gastric emptying time for up to 24 hours. Gastric secretion is predominantly hydrochloric acid with a pH of between 1.0 and 3.5, high potassium content, and a rate of production of about 50 to 100 mL per hour. A gastric volume of 0.4 mL/kg and gastric pH of <2.5 increase the risk and severity of aspiration pneumonitis; however, the volume of fluid aspirated does not necessarily relate to the volume in the stomach. Adequately starved patients have been anesthetized with greater than 0.5 mL/kg gastric volumes without evidence of aspiration. There is a dose-response relationship in the severity of aspiration pneumonitis for both gastric volume and acidity that directly reaches the lung. Human breast milk predisposes to an increased severity of aspiration pneumonitis when compared to other types of milk. Soy-based formula causes a less severe form of acute lung injury than human milk or dairy formula.[5]

Protective Airway Reflexes

The main protective airway reflexes include (1) Apnea with laryngospasm, which causes closure of both the false and true vocal cords. Prolonged laryngospasm maintains the true cords in spasm while the false cords relax. (2) Coughing, which is a brief period of inspiration followed by a forceful expiratory effort. Expiration is accompanied by wider opening of the false cords than inspiration. (3) Expiration reflex, which induces a closure of the false cords preceded by sudden opening of the glottis. It is a forceful expiration without prior preceding inspiration. (4) Spasmodic panting is a reflex involving the glottis

TABLE 37-1

FACTORS AFFECTING LOWER ESOPHAGEAL SPHINCTER TONE

DECREASE TONE	INCREASE TONE	NO CHANGE IN TONE
• Inhaled anesthetics	• Anticholinesterases—neostigmine, edrophonium	• H_2-receptor antagonists—cimetidine, ranitidine
• Opioids	• Cholinergics	• Nondepolarizing muscle relaxants—atracurium, vecuronium
• Anticholinergics—atropine, glycopyrrolate	• Acetylcholine	• Propranolol
• Thiopental	• Succinylcholine	
• Propofol	• α adrenergic stimulants	
• β-agonists	• Antacids	
• Ganglion blockers	• Metoclopramide	
• Tricyclic antidepressants	• Gastrin	
• Secretin	• Serotonin	
• Glucagon	• Histamine	
• Cricoid pressure	• Pancreatic polypeptide	
• Obesity	• Metoprolol	
• Hiatal hernia		
• Pregnancy		

opening and closing rapidly and involves shallow breathing at approximately 60 breaths per minute for less than 10 seconds. These reflexes, except for laryngospasm, can be blunted by opioids such as fentanyl. Premedicated and anesthetized patients, and the elderly, have reduced airway reflexes, putting them at an increased risk for perioperative aspiration pneumonitis.[6]

REDUCING PERIOPERATIVE ASPIRATION RISK

This involves the control of gastric contents (volume and acidity) and prevention of pulmonary aspiration (e.g., cricoid pressure and cuffed endotracheal intubation). Controlling gastric volume and acidity helps minimize the effects of aspiration if it occurs (Table 37-2).

Control of Gastric Contents

Control of gastric contents involves (1) minimizing intake, (2) increasing gastric emptying with prokinetics, and (3) reducing gastric volume and acidity with a nasogastric tube, antacids, H_2-receptor antagonists, and proton pump inhibitors (PPIs). Clear liquids can be administered to children and adults up to 2 and 3 hours respectively prior to anesthesia without increased risk for regurgitation and aspiration.[7] Gastric emptying is slower for milk than for clear liquids. Human breast milk is cleared more rapidly than other milk products.[8] Altered physiological states (e.g., pregnancy and diabetes mellitus) and GI pathology (e.g., bowel obstruction and peritonitis) adversely affect the rate of gastric emptying, thereby increasing aspiration risk. The extent of delayed gastric emptying with diabetes mellitus correlates well with the presence of autonomic neuropathy, but not with age, duration of disease, preprandial HbA_{1C}, or peripheral neuropathy. The time difference in the delay between diabetic and healthy patients ranges from 30 minutes to 2 hours.[9] The American Society of Anesthesiologists (ASA) recommends a fasting period of 4 hours for breast milk, 6 hours for both nonhuman milk and infant formula, and also 6 hours for a light solid meal.[7]

TABLE 37-2

METHODS TO REDUCE THE RISK OF REGURGITATION AND PULMONARY ASPIRATION

1. Minimize intake
   - Adequate preoperative fasting
   - Clear liquids only if necessary
2. Increase gastric emptying
   - Prokinetics (e.g., metoclopramide)
3. Reduce gastric volume and acidity
   - Nasogastric tube
   - Nonparticulate antacid (e.g., sodium citrate)
   - H_2-receptor antagonists (e.g., famotidine)
   - Proton pump inhibitors (e.g., lansoprazole)
4. Airway management and protection
   - Cricoid pressure
   - Cuffed endotracheal intubation
   - Esophageal-tracheal combitube®
   - Proseal LMA®

LMA, laryngeal mask airway.

Reduction of gastric acidity can be achieved with the aid of H_2-receptor antagonists and PPIs, which also reduce gastric volume. Famotidine effectively reduces gastric volume and increases gastric pH better than ranitidine given a few hours before surgery.[10] The PPIs rabeprazole, lansoprazole, and omeprazole are most effective when given in two successive doses, in the evening before and on the morning of anesthesia.[11,12] When given in a single dose, rabeprazole and lansoprazole should be administered on the morning of anesthesia as they are not sufficiently effective when given the previous night, but single-dose omeprazole can be given on the previous night because it is not as effective when given on the morning of anesthesia.[11–13] Sodium citrate, best administered within 1 hour preoperatively in a dose of 15 to 30 mL, increases gastric pH to greater than 2.5, and when combined with metoclopramide (10-mg IV), it reduces gastric contents to less than 25 mL. A nasogastric (NG) tube can be used to reduce gastric volume prior to induction of anesthesia, especially in an emergency situation, but also in elective patients with a high risk of regurgitation and aspiration. Presence of an NG tube does not guarantee an empty stomach and may impair the function of the LES and UES, but it does not diminish the effectiveness of cricoid pressure.[14] The NG tube also provides a direct connection to the outside for passive drainage of gastric contents and is best left in place and open to freely drain during induction of anesthesia.

Prevention of Pulmonary Aspiration

Cricoid pressure may be used to occlude the upper end of the esophagus to prevent passive regurgitation of gastric contents and decrease the risk of pulmonary aspiration during rapid sequence induction intubation technique. The technique has not been subjected to outcome analysis as to its effectiveness in patients. Also, application of cricoid pressure reduces LES tone and may cause the esophagus to be displaced to the side rather than to be compressed.[15] Application of cricoid pressure was first described by Sellick in 1961. He wrote that, "the maneuver consists in temporary occlusion of the upper end of the esophagus by backward pressure of the cricoid cartilage against the bodies of the cervical vertebrae."[16] It was described as compression generated with downward pressure exerted by the forefinger while the thumb and middle finger prevent lateral displacement of the cricoid ring (Fig. 37-1). Compression in the backward and upward direction has since been found to improve laryngoscopy. The force applied to the cricoid cartilage should be sufficient to prevent aspiration but not so great as to cause airway obstruction or allow the possibility of esophageal rupture if vomiting occurs. The recommended force is estimated to range between 20 and 44 newtons (N); however, cricoid deformation occurs at 44 N with associated cricoid occlusion, vocal cord closure, and difficult ventilation. A force of 1 N will give a mass of 1 kilogram an acceleration of 1 meter per second per second (i.e., $1\ N = 1\ kg\ ms^{-2}$). Cricoid occlusion may also occur at 20 N and 30 N but to a lesser degree.[17] Cricoid deformation, vocal cord closure, and associated difficult ventilation may be caused by improperly applied cricoid pressure. Awake patients experience pain, coughing, and retching with pressures greater than 20 N, so this amount of force should be applied only after loss of consciousness. A reasonable approach is to apply 10 N force to the cricoid in the awake state and increase to 30 N after loss of consciousness.[14] Cricoid pressure by itself, before laryngoscopy and intubation, increases the incidence of hypertension and tachycardia during induction of anesthesia.[18] The upward and backward direction of application of cricoid pressure has been associated with improved laryngoscopy but with a reduction in manual

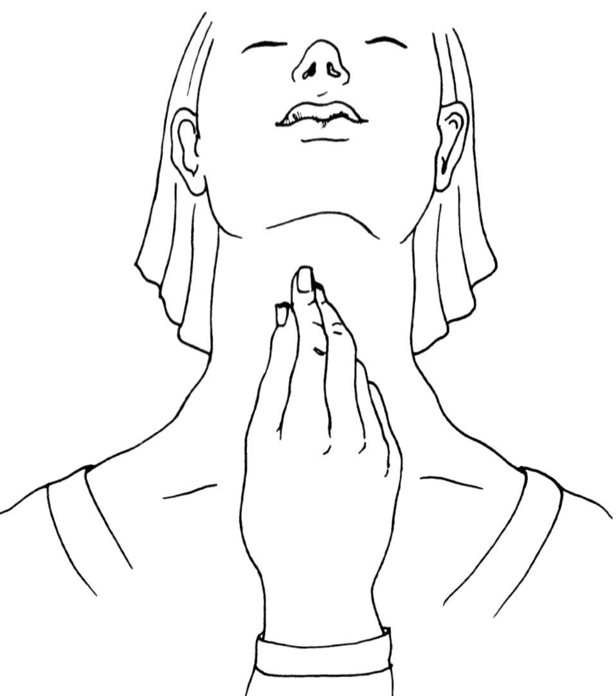

FIGURE 37-1. Cricoid pressure (Sellick's maneuver). Pressure is exerted by the forefinger while the thumb and middle finger prevent lateral displacement of the cricoid ring.

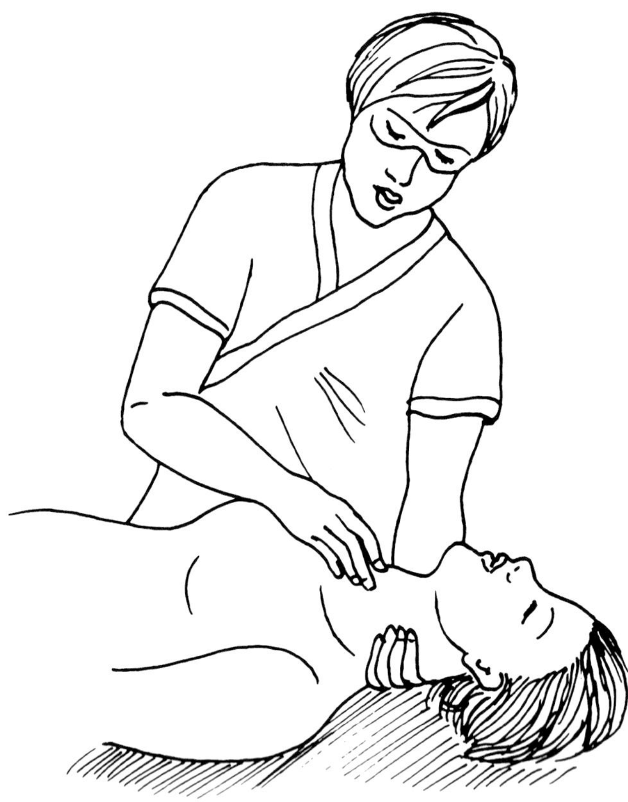

FIGURE 37-2. Bimanual cricoid pressure. Counterpressure with a hand beneath the cervical vertebrae supporting the neck and minimizing distortions of the head position.

ventilatory tidal volumes, suggesting that the upward direction should be omitted if ventilation becomes necessary and continue application of pressure in the backward direction only.[19] Cricotracheal injury, active vomiting, and unstable cervical spine are some contraindications to cricoid pressure. Uncommon complications include esophageal rupture and cricoid ring fracture. In cases of failure to intubate, cricoid pressure may impede ventilation and should be released.[20]

Bimanual cricoid pressure (Fig. 37-2), described as counterpressure with a hand beneath the cervical vertebrae to support the neck, minimizes the distortions of the position of the head and the alignment of the trachea, which can complicate cricoid pressure performed with one hand. A hyperextended vertebral column forms an arch based on the scapulae fixed below and a mobile rotating occiput above. The cricoid forms the apex of this arch, which if disrupted, complicates the maintenance of an unobstructed airway and good glottic view at laryngoscopy. Significant cricoid pressure with the neck extended tends to collapse the arch by downward apical pressure, making the occipital base of the arch rotate and causing the head to flex on the neck, reducing the glottic view with the tongue blocking the pharynx. The use of two hands balances pressure, facilitates the "sniffing" position, and aids laryngoscopy and intubation. Caution should be exercised with this technique in patients with suspected cervical spine trauma or fracture, cervical spine arthritis, immobile neck, and laryngotracheal pathology. No difference in laryngoscopic view has been found in some patients with bimanual cricoid pressure when compared to the single-handed technique.[21]

Airway Protection

Cuffed endotracheal intubation tube is the mainstay of prevention of regurgitated material from reaching the trachea and lungs. The high-volume low-pressure cuffs in current widespread use may not completely prevent regurgitated material from reaching the airway. Leakage from the subglottis via the longitudinal folds of the cuff into the trachea can be prevented by cuff lubrication.[22] Of the other airway devices used, the laryngeal mask airway (LMA) reduces barrier pressure at the LES with an increased incidence of reflux in comparison with the cuffed endotracheal tube.[23] The use of the LMA with unusual positions, such as the lithotomy position, increases the incidence of GE reflux.[24] Other studies have found no evidence of regurgitation in LMA-anesthetized patients during either mechanical or spontaneous ventilation.[25,26] Some LMA devices have an esophageal vent for passage of a nasogastric tube and through which regurgitated material can pass to the outside. An incorporated dorsal cuff also allows for provision of a better seal around periglottic tissues. These improvements may help to better isolate the airway from the GI tract.

THE INTESTINES

The small intestine (SI) is the site of most of the absorption of fluids and nutrients from the GI tract. Parasympathetic stimulation and antagonism increases and decreases the activity of the SI respectively. Suppression of sympathetic activity increases SI activity while stimulation results in a decrease. Bowel denervation results in minimal change in intestinal activity, lending credence to the possibility that humoral secretions (e.g., somatostatin and pancreatic polypeptides) play a major role in intestinal activity. Hypokalemia, peritonitis, and laparotomy all suppress intestinal activity for up to 48 hours. In addition, laparotomy decreases SI absorptive ability.

Absorption is the predominant function of the colon. A pacemaker in the transverse colon controls colonic motility. The vagus nerve supplies neural control to the colon down to the splenic flexure after which the sacral parasympathetic outflow takes over. Sympathetic supply is from T_{6-10}, which decreases colonic motility when stimulated in contrast to parasympathetic stimulation, which increases motility. Neostigmine increases colonic activity while morphine and other opioids decrease both activity and tone.

Splanchnic Blood Flow

Splanchnic blood flow is influenced predominantly by the autonomic nervous system. Alpha-adrenergic stimulation leads to vasoconstriction and ß-2 adrenergic stimulation causes vasodilation. Stimulation of dopaminergic receptors produces vasoconstriction, which predominates over the mild vasodilation produced by ß-2 adrenergic stimulation. Parasympathetic stimulation increases metabolism, which increases blood flow. Autoregulation normally maintains blood flow to the small intestine. With prolonged sympathetic stimulation, there is an initial decrease in blood flow, which is not sustained because of an "escape" phenomenon in the mesenteric circulation whereby the blood flow gradually increases toward normal after a few minutes. Severe stress induces the release of vasoconstrictors including vasopressin, angiotensin II, and catecholamines, which all reduce visceral blood flow. Reduced blood flow results in sympathetic stimulation, which preferentially diverts blood to the muscularis while reducing mucosal perfusion.

It is difficult to maintain adequacy of blood flow after colonic resection, especially in the sigmoid region. This is not usually a problem with small intestinal or stomach surgery. Hypoxia, inadequate oxygen carrying capacity from anemia or impairment of blood supply, may lead to further reductions in oxygen supply, causing ischemia at the anastomotic suture line and consequent anastomotic damage. Splanchnic vascular resistance increases with severe hemorrhage, which helps divert blood flow to other vital organs. Hypocapnia significantly reduces splanchnic blood flow while hypercapnia does the opposite; therefore, hyperventilation to produce hypocapnia is better avoided during colonic surgery and in the perioperative period. Neostigmine reduces mesenteric blood flow because of induced exaggerated contraction. Atropine partially offsets the blood flow reduction. Morphine decreases splanchnic vascular resistance thereby increasing splanchnic blood flow, an effect that can be reversed by naloxone. Thoracic epidural block reduces mean colonic serosal red cell flux and inferior meseneteric artery flow in proportion to a reduction in the mean arterial blood pressure, a situation that does not improve with fluid resuscitation but responds to vasopressor therapy.[27]

Postoperative Anastomotic Leakage

Anastomotic leakage after colon surgery can be related to patient factors (anemia, comorbidity), surgical factors (bowel preparation, operative expertise), and anesthesia- and pain management–related factors (morphine, epidural analgesia, neostigmine).[28] Anesthesia-related factors increase the incidence of anastomotic dehiscense by increasing intestinal motility and intraluminar pressure. In addition, epidural analgesia may reduce blood supply to the anastomotic site. No statistically significant difference in the incidence of anastomotic leakage has been observed in comparing epidural local anesthetics or opioids to intravenous opioids.[29] Neostigmine is an anticholinesterase that increases parasympathetic activity, which increases bowel peristalsis. Vagotomy reduces this effect. Postoperative use of neostigmine after bowel anastomosis has generated controversy as a result of the suggestion that it increases the incidence of anastomotic disruption because of its prokinetic effect. Neostigmine increases the frequency and magnitude of colonic pressure waves, an effect that can be magnified by bowel disease. Anticholinergics like atropine and glycopyrrolate reduce these effects. Prokinetics like metoclopramide have been associated with colonic anastomotic dehiscence during the early postoperative period,[30] however, clinical observations and animal studies have largely discounted the suggestions that neostigmine has a deleterious effect on bowel anastomosis.[31]

Postoperative Ileus

Multiple mechanisms contribute to ileus after intestinal surgery. Abdominal pain activates a spinal reflex that inhibits GI motility, which is further inhibited by the stress of surgery that induces sympathetic hyperactivity. Other contributing factors include excessive handling of bowel, parenteral opioids, electrolyte imbalance, immobility, lack of enteral feeding, and intestinal wall swelling from excessive fluid administration.[32] Thoracic epidural blockade of sympathetic outflow increases GI parasympathetic activity with subsequent increased motility. Low thoracic and lumbar epidural blockade are not as beneficial for minimizing postoperative ileus as is upper thoracic epidural blockade. The colon, beyond the splenic flexure, and the rectum receive their parasympathetic supply from sacral nerve roots and are therefore more susceptible to ileus when lumbar epidural blockade is initiated. Opioids depress
2 GI motility through μ-opioid receptors within the bowels, an effect that can be reversed by naloxone. Epidural analgesia that includes local anesthetics has been most effective in minimizing postoperative ileus. Minimally invasive surgery (including laparoscopy) reduces inflammatory responses, thereby reducing ileus; as does early enteral nutrition and early mobilization.[33]

Mesenteric Traction Syndrome

The mesenteric traction syndrome consists of sudden tachycardia, hypotension, and cutaneous hyperemia occurring during mesenteric traction. In addition, PaO_2 decreases.[34] Clinical features suggest the syndrome results from a release of vasoactive amines (mainly prostacyclin [PGI_2]) from the mesenteric vascular bed because the hemodynamic changes coincide with an increase in plasma concentrations of 6-keto-prostaglandin F_1 (a stable metabolite of prostacyclin) and thromboxane B_2 (a stable metabolite of thromboxane). In addition, even traction of the small intestine can cause histamine release from the mesenteric mast cells. Nonsteroidal anti-inflammatory drugs and aspirin, which inhibit cyclooxygenase, significantly ameliorate these clinical features, further suggesting a prostacyclin-mediated etiology. Intravenous ketorolac has been successfully used to treat persistent hypotension and flushing associated with mesenteric traction syndrome.[35] Prophylactic administration of H_1 and H_2 antihistamines also reduce the incidence of dysrhythmias because of the mesenteric traction syndrome. In addition, they reduce the need for stabilizing interventions.[34] Significant decreases in mean arterial pressure related to central and/or autonomic nervous reflexes occur during operations on upper abdominal viscera.[36] These hypotensive responses to visceral traction appear to be transmitted along afferent fibers contained within the splanchnic nerves. However, deafferentation of the splanchinc nerves, as occurs with epidural anesthesia, does not influence prostacyclin release, hypotension, or hypoxemia during mesenteric traction, lending further credence that prostacyclin is involved in the etiology of the syndrome.

Nitrous Oxide and the Bowel

Because nitrous oxide is 30 times more soluble than nitrogen in blood, nitrous oxide diffuses into gas-containing body cavities from the bloodstream faster than the nitrogen in those cavities can diffuse out into circulation. This can contribute to excessive distension of gas-containing bowels, possible bowel ischemia,[37] and increased difficulty with surgical exposure. Factors that determine the extent of distension include the amount of gas within the bowel, the duration of nitrous oxide administration, and the concentration of nitrous oxide used. There is a linear increase in bowel cavity size with time during administration of nitrous oxide such that after about 4 hours a 100 to 200% increase in gaseous bowel volume is observed with nitrous oxide anesthesia.[38] Use of 80% nitrous oxide can potentially result in a fivefold increase in bowel gas, whereas use of a 50% concentration can result in no more than a doubling of bowel gas. Nitrous oxide is best avoided in situations when the bowels are distended. On the other hand, use of low concentrations of nitrous oxide during elective abdominal operations where no significant amount of gas is present in the bowels is reasonable.[39,40]

CARCINOID TUMORS

Carcinoid tumor was so named for its resemblance to carcinoma. It was earlier recognized as a slow-growing benign small intestinal tumor capable of metastasis, but with a good prognosis. The GI tract is the usual site of origin of carcinoid tumors, which are derived from enterochromaffin cells but can be found in any tissue derived from the endoderm. Intestinal carcinoid (appendix and ileum) is the usual source of metastasis.[41] Carcinoid tumors are usually asymptomatic, although nonspecific symptoms such as abdominal pain, diarrhea, intermittent intestinal obstruction, and GI bleeding are occasionally seen. Nonmetastatic carcinoid tumors secrete hormones that are usually transported to the liver through the portal vein where they are subsequently inactivated. Although symptoms are sometimes caused by mechanical effects of the tumors, most symptoms are produced by the effects of hormones and substances secreted into the GI tract or into the systemic circulation. Carcinoid tumors, especially those arising in the midgut, secrete a variety of hormones, mediators, and biogenic amines including large quantities of serotonin that produce increased platelet serotonin levels and increased urinary levels of 5-hydroxy-indole-acetic-acid (5-HIAA), a metabolite of serotonin. Other secreted substances include histamine, substance P, catecholamines (including dopamine), bradykinin, tachykinin, motilin, corticotrophin, prostaglandins, kallikrein, and neurotensin. Bradykinin produces cutaneous flushing, bronchospasm and hypotension while serotonin causes hypertension or hypotension. Histamine also produces flushing.

Carcinoid Syndrome

Metastatic carcinoid tumor releases vasoactive peptides into the systemic circulation, which leads to signs and symptoms collectively known as the *carcinoid syndrome*. It generally indicates the presence of pulmonary or hepatic metastasis, although access to the systemic circulation can occur without hepatic metastasis. Carcinoid syndrome occurs when massive amounts of circulating hormones produced by the tumor reach the systemic circulation. It occurs in approximately 20% of patients with carcinoid tumors.[41] The overall clinical manifestations of carcinoid syndrome include cutaneous flushing of the head, neck, and upper thorax (most common); bronchoconstriction; hypotension; diarrhea; and carcinoid heart disease. Hypertension can also occur. Serotonin increases the chronotropic and inotropic activity of the heart, and when coupled with vasoconstriction, will lead to hypertension. The diagnosis of carcinoid syndrome can be confirmed by urinary excretion of 5-HIAA, and serial values of this metabolite can be used to monitor tumor progression. A 24-hour urine sample with >30 mg of 5-HIAA suggests carcinoid syndrome. There is, however, no correlation between the blood level of serotonin and the severity of symptoms. Serotonin increases the tone and motility of the jejunum causing diarrhea, which is the major feature of increased serotonin level.

Carcinoid Heart Disease

Carcinoid heart disease is seen in up to 60% of patients with carcinoid syndrome. Cardiac involvement combines with flushing and diarrhea to make up the classic "carcinoid triad." Cardiac involvement is usually right-sided, affecting tricuspid and pulmonary valves. Left-sided cardiac involvement is rare. Tricuspid regurgitation is the predominant finding, although tricuspid stenosis and pulmonary valve regurgitation or stenosis can also occur. The pathology is described as tricuspid and/or pulmonary valve fibrosis with retraction and fixation of the leaflets leading to regurgitation.[42] Intramyocardial metastases and cardiac dysrhythmias are also seen. Over 50% of carcinoid deaths are a result of cardiac failure. The predominance of right-sided cardiac lesions suggests that the substances secreted from liver metastasis into the hepatic vein never reach the left side of the heart because of pulmonary metabolism. Carcinoid plaques damage valvular integrity and are caused by fibroblast proliferation and valvulitis because of the actions of serotonin and tachykinin on platelets and endothelium. The now banned appetite-suppressant drugs fenfluramine and dexfenfluramine interfere with serotonin metabolism to produce cardiac valve lesions similar to carcinoid valvular lesions.[43] Patients with carcinoid heart disease have higher levels of serum serotonin and urinary 5-HIAA, but it is debatable whether serotonin is responsible for the cardiac lesions. Also, treatment that reduces 5-HIAA excretion does not lead to regression of cardiac lesions.

Perioperative Management of the Carcinoid Patient

Complete surgical excision is the most effective treatment for carcinoid tumors. Chemotherapy results are marginal at best. Biotherapy with interferon and octreotide may reduce tumor bulk and attenuate the release of vasoactive amines. Management should focus on blocking histamine and serotonin receptors and avoidance of drugs that facilitate mediator release from tumor cells. Mediator release can be triggered by opioids and muscle relaxants that release histamine, including succinylcholine, mivacurium, atracurium, and d-tubocurarine. Epinephrine, norepinephrine, histamine, dopamine, and isoproterenol have also been known to provoke carcinoid crises. Perioperative management should include acquisition of the knowledge and severity of the specific features of the syndrome in each specific patient. Therapy should be directed at preventing the release of mediator substances from the tumor or antagonizing their effects. There is a positive correlation between the presence of carcinoid heart disease or high urinary output of 5-HIAA and postoperative complications.[44] Patients with carcinoid may have diarrhea and high gastric output.[45] Therefore, fluid resuscitation may be required, and serum electrolytes and glucose should be measured at regular intervals.

Many carcinoid tumor specimens contain somatostatin receptors. Somatostatin is a GI regulatory peptide that reduces the production and release of gastropancreatic hormones. It reduces the amount of serotonin released from carcinoid tumors, which subsequently reduces the levels of urinary 5-HIAA. Somatostatin has a very short half-life of about 3 minutes and must therefore be given as infusion. Octreotide is a synthetic somatostatin analogue with approximately 50 times the half-life of somatostatin and is useful in treatment of symptoms and perioperative management of carcinoid syndrome. It has a half-life of approximately 2.5 hours. Subcutaneous octreotide at a dose of 50 to 500 mcg every 8 hours can be titrated to effect for relief of symptoms or prevention of hypotension. Alternatively, 10 to 100 mcg IV can be administered slowly 1 hour preoperatively. Preoperative preparation should also include 100 mg octreotide subcutaneously three times daily in the preceding 2 weeks and, if necessary, should be weaned slowly over 1 week postoperatively. Preoperative anxiolytics should be administered to prevent stress-triggered release of serotonin, and patients receiving octreotide preoperatively should continue with their normal dose on the morning of surgery. A combination of H_1- and H_2-blocking drugs can be used to block the effects of histamine. Histamine release is most likely to occur with gastric carcinoids; therefore, antihistamines may not be needed for carcinoid tumors originating in other areas.[41] H_2-blockers, diphenhydramine, and steroids inhibit the action of bradykinin.

Carcinoid crises can be precipitated by physical or chemical stimulation, stress, or tumor necrosis from hepatic artery
3 ligation or embolization or chemotherapy. Succinylcholine-induced fasciculations can potentially trigger mediator release. Octreotide effectively treats intraoperative carcinoid crises. An octreotide infusion at a rate of 50 to 100 mcg/hr can be administered during surgery and if more is required, intravenous boluses of 25 to 100 mcg can be administered to the desired effect. Aprotinin, a kallikrein inhibitor, may be employed for hypotension if there is a refractory response to octreotide.[46]

Availability of newer titratable and short-acting anesthetic agents precludes the use of potentially histamine-releasing and longer acting anesthetic agents. Any of the currently available induction agents and muscle relaxants including propofol, etomidate, vecuronium, cisatracurium, and rocuronium can be used successfully. Caution should be exercised with drugs such as thiopental and succinylcholine that can release histamine. The short-acting synthetic opioids sufentanil, alfentanil, fentanyl, and remifentanil are all acceptable for use.[47] All current inhalation agents can be used successfully; however, desflurane may be the better choice in patients with liver metastasis because of its low rate of metabolism. Increased levels of serotonin have been associated with delayed awakening from general anesthesia. Administration of octreotide prior to manipulation of the tumor will attenuate adverse hemodynamic responses. Use of epidural analgesia in patients that have been adequately treated with octreotide is a safe technique provided the local anesthetic is administered in a graded manner with careful hemodynamic monitoring and a diluted concentration of local anesthetic is used.[47] The sympathetic blockade produced by epidural or spinal anesthesia may worsen hypotension, which can be minimized by dosing the epidural catheter with opioids or dilute local anesthetic solutions. Intraoperative hypotension from sympathetic blockade should be treated with volume expansion and intravenous infusion of octreotide rather than with sympathomimetics like ephedrine, which can trigger release of vasoactive substances from carcinoid tumors. Octreotide infusion can also be used for intraoperative hypertension in combination with increasing doses of volatile anesthetic. Ondansetron, a serotonin antagonist, is a useful and logical antiemetic choice.

Invasive arterial blood pressure monitoring may be necessary during the intraoperative management of patients with carcinoid syndrome because of rapid changes in hemodynamic variables. Other useful monitors may include central venous or pulmonary artery catheters and transesophageal echocardiography (TEE). Intense hemodynamic monitoring and octreotide administration should continue into the postoperative period as secretion of vasoactive substances can still occur from residual tumor or metastasis. Emotional and physical stress that can trigger vasoactive substance release can be minimized by effective postoperative analgesia.

References

1. Ng A, Smith G: Gastroesophageal reflux and aspiration of gastric contents in anesthetic practice. Anesth Analg 93:494, 2001
2. Sundman E, Witt H, Olsson R *et al*: The incidence and mechanisms of pharyngeal and upper esophageal dysfunction in partially paralyzed humans: pharyngeal videoradiography and simultaneous manometry after atracurium. Anesthesiology 92:977, 2000
3. Sundman E, Witt H, Sandin R *et al*: Pharyngeal function and airway protection during sybhypnotic concentrations of propofol, isoflurane and sevoflurane: volunteers examined by pharyngeal videoradiography and simultaneous manometry. Anesthesiology 95:1125, 2001
4. Garrard A, Campbell AE, Turley A *et al*: The effect of mechanically induced cricoid force on lower esophageal sphincter pressure in anaesthetized patients. Anaesthesia 59:435, 2004
5. Chin C, Lerman J, Endo J: Acute lung injury after tracheal instillation of acidified soy-based or Enfalac formula or human breast milk in rabbits. Can J Anaesth 46:282, 1999
6. Caranza R, Nandwani N, Tring JP *et al*: Upper airway reflex sensitivity following general anesthesia for day-case surgery. Anaesthesia 55:367, 2000
7. American Society of Anesthesiologists Task Force on Preoperative Fasting. Practice guidelines for preoperative fasting and the use of pharmacologic agents to reduce the risk of pulmonary aspiration: Application to healthy patients undergoing elective procedures. Anesthesiology 79:482, 1999
8. Van Den Driessche M, Peeters K, Marien P *et al*: Gastric emptying in formula-fed and breast-fed infants measured with 13C-octanoic acid breath test. J Pediatr Gastroenterol Nutr 29:46, 1999
9. Merio R, Festa A, Bergmann H *et al*: Slow gastric emptying in Type I diabetes: Relation to autonomic and peripheral neuropathy, blood glucose, and glycemic control. Diabetes Care 20:419, 1997
10. Kulkarni PN, Batra YK, Wig J: Effects of different combinations of H2 receptor antagonist with gastrokinetic drugs on gastric fluid pH and volume in children—a comparative study. Int J Pharmacol Ther 35:561, 1997
11. Nishina K, Mikawa K, Takao Y *et al*: A comparison of rabeprazole, lansoprazole and ranitidine for improving preoperative gastric fluid property in adults undergoing elective surgery. Anesth Analg 90:717, 2000
12. Nishina K, Mikawa K, Maekawa N *et al*: A comparison of lansoprazole, omeprazole and ranitidine for reducing preoperative gastric secretion in adult patients undergoing elective surgery. Anesth Analg 82:832, 1996
13. Escolano F, Castano J, Lopez R *et al*: Effects of omeprazole, ranitidine, Famotidine and placebo on gastric secretion in patients undergoing elective surgery. Br J Anaesth 69:404, 1992
14. Vanner RG, Asai T: Safe use of cricoid pressure. Anaesthesia 54:1, 1999
15. Smith KJ, Dobranowski J, Yip G, Dauphin A, Choi PT: Cricoid pressure displaces the esophagus: An observational study using magnetic resonance imaging. Anesthesiology 99:60, 2003
16. Sellick BA: Cricoid pressure to control regurgitation of stomach contents during induction of anaesthesia. Lancet 2:404, 1961
17. MacG Palmer JH, Ball DR: The effect of cricoid pressure on the cricoid cartilage and vocal cords: An endoscope study in anaesthetized patients. Anaesthesia 55:263, 2000
18. Saghaei M, Masoodifar M: The pressor response and airway effects of cricoid pressure during induction of general anesthesia. Anesth Analg 93:787, 2001
19. Hartsilver EL, Vanner RG: Airway obstruction with cricoid pressure. Anaesthesia 55:208, 2000
20. Harry RM, Nolan JP: The use of cricoid pressure with the intubating laryngeal mask. Anaesthesia 54:656, 1999
21. Vanner RG, Clarke P, Moore WJ *et al*: The effect of cricoid pressure and neck support on the view at laryngoscopy. Anaesthesia 52:896, 1997
22. Young PJ, Basson C, Hamilton D *et al*: Prevention of tracheal aspiration using the pressure-limited tracheal tube cuff. Anaesthesia 54:559, 1999
23. Valentine J, Stakes AF, Bellamy MC: Reflux during positive pressure ventilation through the laryngeal mask. Br J Anaesth 73:543, 1994
24. McCrory CR, McShane AJ: Gastroesophageal reflux during spontaneous respiration with the laryngeal mask airway. Can J Anaesth 46:268, 1999

25. Bapat PP, Verghese C: Laryngeal mask airway and the incidence of regurgitation during gynecological laprascopies. Anesth Analg 85:139, 1997
26. Joshi GP, Morrison SG, Okonkwo NA *et al*: Continuous hypopharyngeal pH measurements in spontaneous breathing anesthetized outpatients: laryngeal mask airway versus tracheal intubation. Anesth Analg 82:254, 1996
27. Gould TH, Grace K, Thorne G *et al*: Effect of thoracic epidural anaesthesia on colonic blood flow. Br J Anaesth 89:446, 2002
28. Ng A, Smith G: Anesthesia and the gastrointestinal tract. J Anesth 16:51, 2002
29. Holte K, Kehlet H: Epidural analgesia and risk of anastomotic leakage. Reg Anesth Pain Med 26:111, 2001
30. Garcia-Olmo D, Paya J, Lucas FJ *et al*: Effects of the pharmacological manipulation of postoperative intestinal motility on colonic anastomosis. An experimental study in a rat model. Int J Colorectal Dis 12:73, 1997
31. Garcia-Olmo DC, Garcia-Rivas M, Garcia-Olmo D: Does neostigmine have deleterious effect on the resistance of colonic anastomoses? Eur J Anaesthesiol 15:38, 1998
32. Fotiadis RJ, Badvie S, Weston MD *et al*: Epidural analgesia in gastrointestinal surgery. Br J Surg 91:828, 2004
33. Baig MK, Wexner SD: Postoperative ileus: a review. Dis Colon Rectum 47:516, 2004
34. Duda D, Lorenz W, Celik I: Histamine release in mesenteric traction syndrome during abdominal aortic aneurysm surgery: prophylaxis with H1 and H2 antihistamines. Inflamm Res 51:495, 2002
35. Latson JW, Reinhart DJ, Allison PM *et al*: Ketorolac tromethamine may be efficacious in treating hypotension from mesenteric traction. J Cardiothorac Vasc Anesth 6:456, 1992
36. Brinkmann A, Seeling W, Wolf CF *et al*: The effect of thoracic epidural anesthesia on the pathophysiology of the eventration syndrome. Anaesthesist 43:235, 1994
37. Reinelt H, Marx T, Schirmer U *et al*: Diffusion of xenon and nitrous oxide into bowel during mechanical ileus. Anesthesiology 96:512, 2002
38. Akca O, Lenhardt R, Fleischmann E *et al*: Nitrous oxide increases the incidence of bowel distension in patients undergoing elective colon resection. Acta Anaesthesiol Scand 48:894, 2004
39. Krogh B, Jorn Jensen P, Henneberg SW *et al*: Nitrous oxide does not influence operating conditions or postoperative course in colonic surgery. Br J Anaesth 72:55, 1994
40. Taylor E, Feinstein R, White PF *et al*: Anesthesia for laparoscopic cholecystectomy. Is nitrous oxide contraindicated? Anesthesiology 76:541, 1992
41. Dierdorf SF: Carcinoid tumor and carcinoid syndrome. Curr Opin Anaesthesiol 16:343, 2003
42. Simula DV, Edwards WD, Tazolaar HD *et al*: Surgical pathology of carcinoid heart disease: a study of 139 values from 75 patients spanning 20 years. Mayo Clin Proc 77:139, 2002
43. Khan MA, Herzog CA, St Peter JV *et al*: The prevalence of cardiac valvular insufficiency assessed by transthoracic echocardiography in obese patients treated with appetite suppressant drugs. N Engl J Med 339:713, 1998
44. Kinney MA, Warner ME, Nagorney DM *et al*: Perianesthetic risks and outcomes of abdominal surgery for metastatic carcinoid tumors. Br J Anaesth 87:447, 2001
45. Pandharipande PP, Reichard PS, Vallee MF: High gastric output as a perioperative sign of carcinoid syndrome. Anesthesiology 96:755, 2002
46. Cortinez FLI: Refractory hypotension during carcinoid resection surgery. Anaesthesia 55:505, 2000
47. Farling PA, Durairaju AK: Remifentanil and anaesthesia for carcinoid syndrome. Br J Anaesth 92:893, 2004

CHAPTER 38 ■ ANESTHESIA FOR MINIMALLY INVASIVE PROCEDURES

ANTHONY J. CUNNINGHAM AND CATHAL NOLAN

KEY POINTS

1. Minimal-access surgical procedures produce significantly less trauma than conventional open procedures, with the potential advantages of reduced postoperative pain, shorter hospital stays, more rapid return to normal activities, and significant cost savings.
2. Laparoscopic cholecystectomy is increasingly being performed in older patients with coexisting cardiopulmonary disease. Careful perioperative monitoring of ASA III and IV patients is advised during peritoneal insufflation.
3. Minimal-access surgical techniques are now routine for cholecystectomy, Nissen fundoplication for refractory gastroesophageal reflux disease, splenectomy, and adrenalectomy.
4. The physiological consequences of laparoscopy relate to the combined effects of intraperitoneal insufflation of carbon dioxide (CO_2) to create a pneumoperitoneum, alteration of patient position, and the effects of systemic absorption of carbon dioxide.
5. The principal physiologic responses are an increase in systemic vascular resistance (SVR), mean arterial blood pressure (MAP), and myocardial filling pressures, accompanied by an initial fall in cardiac index (CI), with little change in heart rate.
6. Pneumoperitoneum, changes in patient position, reductions in cardiac output, and systemic carbon dioxide absorption influence splanchnic, renal, and cerebral blood flow during minimal-access procedures.
7. The direct mechanical effects of pneumoperitoneum in reducing splanchnic circulation may be counterbalanced by the direct splanchnic vasodilating effects of carbon dioxide.
8. Although laparoscopic cholecystectomy is considered a minimally invasive procedure, it is associated with intra-abdominal, incisional, and shoulder pain after surgery.
9. A multimodal analgesic regimen combining opioids, nonsteroidal anti-inflammatory drugs (NSAIDs), and local anesthetic infiltration may be most effective, allowing reduction of opioid dose and minimizing side effects.
10. The selective 5HT3 receptor antagonist ondansetron may provide effective prophylaxis against postoperative emesis following laparoscopic procedures.
11. Intraoperative complications may arise because of the physiologic changes associated with patient positioning and pneumoperitoneum creation. Traumatic injuries during blind trocar insertion, extraperitoneal insufflation, pneumothorax, and gas embolism are additional risks.
12. Caution is urged, however, against overenthusiastic ambulatory laparoscopic cholecystectomy, as early discharge may lead to occasional delays in diagnosis and management of postoperative complications.

MINIMAL ACCESS INTRA-ABDOMINAL GYNECOLOGIC PROCEDURES

Over the past decade, there has been an enormous expansion in the use of minimally invasive surgical procedures that aim to minimize the trauma of the interventional process but still
1 achieve a satisfactory therapeutic result.[1] Minimal-access surgical procedures produce significantly less trauma than conventional open procedures, with the potential advantages of reduced postoperative pain, shorter hospital stays, more rapid return to normal activities, and significant cost savings.[2]

Laparoscopic cholecystectomy was first described in 1987 by Phillipe Mouret; the first series was reported by Perissat et al[3] and the technique was introduced into the United States in 1988 by Reddick and Olsen.[4] Laparoscopic cholecystectomy rapidly emerged as an alternative to traditional open cholecystectomy. It is now a routinely performed procedure and has replaced conventional open cholecystectomy as the procedure of choice for symptomatic cholelithiasis.[5,6] The evolution of laparoscopic cholecystectomy has represented a departure from traditional surgical development. Few prospective randomized controlled trials comparing laparoscopic and open procedures have been performed. Public expectation and perception of the superiority of minimally invasive techniques led to poorly controlled and audited introduction of laparoscopic surgical procedures. However, a significant body of experience and literature has emerged in the 1990s confirming the safety and efficacy of laparoscopic cholecystectomy. Several studies demonstrated that the introduction of laparoscopic cholecystectomy was associated with significant growth in cholecystectomy rates, possibly because of patient demand and lower surgical threshold. However, in 43 tertiary-care university-affiliated Veteran Administration Medical Centers participating in the National Veterans Affairs Surgical Risk Study 1991–1993, the number of cholecystectomies remained stable and the proportion of patients with acute cholecystitis, emergent cholecystectomies, and technically difficult procedures did not change significantly.[7]

2 Increasingly laparoscopic cholecystectomy is being performed in older patients with coexisting cardiopulmonary disease, in pregnancy, in morbid obesity, and in pediatric patients. Laparoscopy produces significant physiological changes associated with peritoneal insufflation and alteration in patient position, which can have a major impact on cardiopulmonary function, particularly in American Society of Anesthesiologists (ASA) class III or IV patients. Specific intraoperative complications as a result of traumatic injuries and gas embolism may also occur and present significant challenges in anesthetic management. The duration of some procedures, the risk of vascular or visceral injury, and difficulty in evaluating blood loss add to the anesthetic challenge.

Increasing surgical experience and improvements in instrumentation, including developments in optics, laser, and electrosurgical technology, has resulted in an expansion of both the range of surgical procedures performed by the laparoscopic approach[8–11] and the patient population to whom such
3 procedures are offered. Laparoscopic techniques have been applied not only in gastrointestinal (gastric, colonic, splenic, hepatic) but also in gynecologic (hysterectomy) and urologic (nephrectomy) surgery. Public expectation and technology developments have fueled these changes. The physiologic effects of intraperitoneal carbon dioxide insufflation combined with variations in patient positioning can have a major impact on cardiorespiratory function, particularly in elderly patients with comorbidities. Intraoperative complications may include traumatic injuries associated with blind trocar insertion, gas embolism, pneumothorax, and surgical emphysema associated with extraperitoneal insufflation. Appropriate monitoring and a high index of suspicion can result in early diagnosis of and treatment of complications.

SURGICAL TECHNIQUE

Laparoscopic operative techniques involve intraperitoneal insufflation of carbon dioxide. Techniques for pneumoperitoneum creation include insufflation after insertion of the Veress needle infra-umbilicus or open laparoscopy involving dissection through the linea alba and opening of the peritoneum under direct vision.[12] The Veress needle consists of a blunt-tipped, spring-loaded inner stylet and sharp outer needle that penetrates the tissue layers of the abdominal wall. The abdominal wall may be elevated by hand or by clamps placed on the margins of the umbilicus. The Veress needle is inserted at an angle of 45 to 90 degrees depending on operator preference, patient habitus, and previous lower abdominal surgery. The aortic bifurcation lies directly beneath the umbilicus, especially if the Trendelenburg position has already been established. Most practitioners insert the needle and trocar directed toward the pelvis with the patient still horizontal, with or without elevating the anterior abdominal wall. Once inserted, a number of tests are used to test for correct needle placement within the peritoneal cavity, including hanging drop of saline or "hiss test" of gas being sucked into peritoneum upon elevation of anterior abdominal wall.

Hasson, in 1971, described a technique for open insertion of the trocar, thereby guaranteeing pneumoperitoneum and avoiding dangers of blind trocar insertion.[13] Perone confirmed the efficacy of this technique in 585 patients, 173 of whom (29.5%) had undergone previous abdominal surgery. No technical failure or major complications (major vascular injury, bowel or urinary tract trauma) were reported.[14] Modern laparoscopic insufflators automatically terminate gas flow when a preset intra-abdominal pressure (IAP) of 10- to 15 mm Hg is reached. An access port is then inserted in place of the needle to maintain insufflation during surgery. A video laparoscope, inserted through the port, allows visualization of the operative field. Additional access ports are inserted through a number of small skin incisions, which allow the introduction of surgical dissection instruments.

Patient position during minimal-access procedures varies. Patients are usually placed in the Trendelenburg position for laparoscopic gynecologic procedures while laparoscopic cholecystectomy usually involves change to a steep reverse Trendelenburg (rT), with left lateral tilt to facilitate retraction of the gallbladder fundus and to minimize the diaphragmatic dysfunction associated with the induced pneumoperitoneum. The cystic duct and artery are identified and ligated. The diseased gallbladder is dissected from the hepatic bed and removed through the periumbilical cannula. Despite concerns about technical difficulties because of tissue edema and inflammation, acute cholecystitis is no longer considered a contraindication to laparoscopic cholecystectomy.[15] The conversion rate to an open procedure is, however, high, particularly in older patients with a history of biliary disease and acute gangrenous gallbladder.[16]

Physiological Effects of Laparoscopy

4 The physiological consequences of laparoscopy relate to the combined effects of intraperitoneal insufflation of carbon dioxide (CO_2) to create a pneumoperitoneum, alteration of patient position, and the effects of systemic absorption of carbon

TABLE 38-1

HEMODYNAMIC EFFECTS OF LAPAROSCOPY

■ PATIENT FACTORS
Preexisting cardiorespiratory status Intravascular volume
■ INTRA-ABDOMINAL PRESSURE
■ PATIENT POSITION
■ SYSTEMIC CO_2 ABSORPTION
■ NEUROHUMORAL RESPONSES

dioxide. In addition, reflex increase in vagal tone and arrhythmias can develop.

Cardiovascular Effects

The hemodynamic response to peritoneal insufflation has been well described and depends on the interaction of factors including the IAP achieved[17], patient positioning[18], neurohumoral response[19], and patient factors including cardiorespiratory status[20] and intravascular volume[21] (Table 38-1).

5 The principal physiologic responses are an increase in systemic vascular resistance (SVR), mean arterial blood pressure (MAP), and myocardial filling pressures, accompanied by an initial fall in cardiac index (CI), with little change in heart rate[22–24] (Table 38-2).

A characteristic phasic hemodynamic response is described with initial reduction in cardiac index after CO_2 insufflation and subsequent recovery.[23] Using flow-directed pulmonary artery catheters in healthy patients during laparoscopic cholecystectomy, Joris and colleagues[24] observed a significant (35 to 40%) reduction in CI with induction of anesthesia and rT positioning, which was further decreased to 50% of baseline following peritoneal insufflation. Gradual restoration of CI and reduction of SVR occurred. A similar phasic hemodynamic response to pneumoperitoneum was observed by Branche and colleagues[25] using echocardiographic assessment. Left ventricular fractional area of shortening decreased significantly immediately after insufflation and returned to preinsufflation value after 30 minutes of pneumoperitoneum.

TABLE 38-2

SUMMARY OF HEMODYNAMIC CHANGES

■ CARDIAC OUTPUT
Variable-decreased–depending on CO_2 insufflation/patient position/measurement technique
■ CARDIAC FILLING
Venous return—reduced—pooling in extremities **Left ventricular end-diastolic volume**—reduced **Intrathoracic pressure**—increased **Right atrial and pulmonary artery occlusion pressures**—increased during insufflation
■ HEART RATE
Unchanged/minimal increase
■ ARTERIAL PRESSURE
Increased mechanical/neurohumoral (catecholamines, renin-angiotensin/vasopressin)
■ SYSTEMIC AND PULMONARY VASCULAR RESISTANCE
Increased mechanical/neurohumoral (catecholamines, renin-angiotensin/vasopressin)

Mechanical Effects of Pneumoperitoneum

6 Increased IAP associated with pneumoperitoneum may compress venous capacitance vessels causing an initial increase, followed by a sustained decrease in preload.[25] Compression of the arterial vasculature increases afterload and may result in a marked increase in calculated SVR.[23] Cardiac index may be significantly reduced and the magnitude of this effect is proportional to the intra-abdominal pressure achieved. In healthy subjects undergoing laparoscopic cholecystectomy, Dexter et al[27] using transesophageal Doppler found that cardiac output was depressed to a maximum of 28% at an insufflation pressure of 15 mm Hg but was maintained at an insufflation pressure of 7 mm Hg. In an animal model, Ishizaki et al[18] report the threshold IAP that had minimal effects on hemodynamic function was $\leq$12 mm Hg and recommend this pressure limit to avoid cardiovascular compromise during CO_2 insufflation.

Neurohumoral Response

Potential mediators of the increased SVR observed during pneumoperitoneum include vasopressin and catecholamines. Hypercapnia and pneumoperitoneum are likely to cause stimulation of the sympathetic nervous system and catecholamine release.[27,28] A number of investigators have reported activation of the renin–angiotensin system with vasopressin production.[25–27] Joris and colleagues[24] observed a marked increase in plasma vasopressin immediately after peritoneal insufflation in healthy patients and the profile of vasopressin release paralleled the time course of changes in SVR. A fourfold increase in plasma renin and aldosterone concentrations correlating with increases in MAP was reported by O'Leary and colleagues[28]. The time course of vasopressin release paralleling observed changes in CI and SVR suggest a possible cause-and-effect relationship.

CO_2 Absorption

Significant hypercapnia and acidosis may occur during laparoscopy as a result of CO_2 absorption.[29] Hypercapnia may cause a decrease in myocardial contractility and lower arrhythmia threshold.
7 The anticipated direct vascular effect of hypercapnia, producing arteriolar dilation and decreased SVR, is modulated by mechanical and neurohumoral responses including catecholamine release.

Effect of Patient Position

Intraperitoneal insufflation of CO_2 for laparoscopic cholecystectomy is performed with the patient in a horizontal or 15- to 20-degree Trendelenburg position. The patient's position is then changed to a steep rT position with left lateral tilt to facilitate retraction of the gallbladder fundus and to minimize diaphragmatic dysfunction (Fig. 38-1).[11] Patient

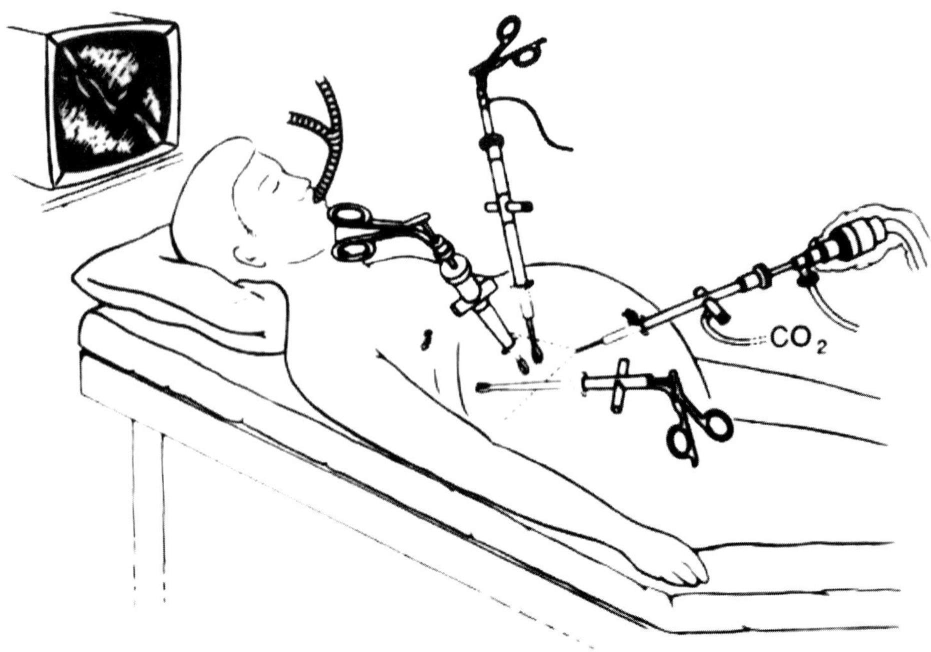

FIGURE 38-1. Patient positioning for laparoscopic colocystectomy.

position may have significant effects on the hemodynamic consequences of pneumoperitoneum. In a series of 13 patients undergoing laparoscopic cholecystectomy, Cunningham and colleagues[19] using TOE monitoring reported a significant reduction in left ventricular end-diastolic area on assumption of rT position, indicating reduced venous return. Left ventricular ejection fraction was maintained throughout in these otherwise healthy patients. However, such changes in left ventricular loading conditions might have adverse consequences in patients with cardiovascular disease. The pattern of changes in cardiac output and arterial pressures in those with mild to severe cardiac disease are similar to otherwise healthy patients.[32] However, quantitatively these changes appear to be more marked.[29]

Increased IAP and the head-up position results in reduced femoral vein blood flow, lower limb venous stasis, predisposing to thromboembolism.[29]

RESPIRATORY EFFECTS

Mechanical

Changes in pulmonary function during abdominal insufflation include reduction in lung volumes, decrease in pulmonary compliance, and increase in peak airway pressure.[30–32] Reduction in functional residual capacity (FRC) and lung compliance associated with supine positioning and induction of anesthesia is further aggravated by CO_2 insufflation and cephalad shift of the diaphragm during head-down tilt[30,33] Hypoxemia because of reduction in FRC is uncommon in healthy patients during laparoscopy.[34] However, reduction in FRC may result in significant hypoxemia because of ventilation-perfusion mismatch and intrapulmonary shunting in obese patients or in patients with preexisting pulmonary disease.[35]

Gas Exchange Effects—CO_2 Absorption

Surgical exposure and access is facilitated during laparoscopic surgery by peritoneal gas insufflation. CO_2 is the insufflation gas of choice for laparoscopic surgery. Unlike nitrous oxide (N_2O), it does not support combustion and therefore can be used safely with diathermy. Compared to helium, the high blood solubility of CO_2 and its capability for pulmonary excretion reduces the risk of adverse outcome in the event of gas embolism.[36] CO_2 insufflation into the peritoneal cavity increases arterial carbon dioxide tension[30] ($PaCO_2$), which is managed by increasing minute ventilation.

The absorption of gas from the peritoneal cavity depends on its diffusibility, the absorption area, and vascularity of insufflation site. Carbon dioxide absorption is greater during extraperitoneal (pelvic) insufflation than during intraperitoneal insufflation. Mullet and colleagues[37] examined end-tidal CO_2 ($ETCO_2$) and pulmonary CO_2 elimination during CO_2 insufflation for laparoscopic cholecystectomy and pelviscopy. CO_2 absorption reached a plateau within 10 minutes after initiation of intraperitoneal insufflation, but continued to increase slowly throughout extraperitoneal insufflation. During uneventful pneumoperitoneum creation, $PaCO_2$ progressively rises to reach a plateau 15 to 30 minutes after insufflation. Any significant subsequent increase in $PaCO_2$ should prompt a search for a cause, either independent of or related to CO_2 insufflation, such as CO_2-subcutaneous emphysema.

The resulting rise in $PaCO_2$ is unpredictable, particularly in patients with severe pulmonary disease. Wittgen and colleagues[38] observed significant decreases in pH and decreases in $PaCO_2$ in ASA III patients during pneumoperitoneum, and these patients had significantly higher minute ventilation requirements and peak airway pressures. Furthermore, $ETCO_2$ levels may not correlate with arterial concentrations in this patient population. The $PETCO_2$ gradient remained stable during laparoscopy in ASA III patients[38], while other investigators have found $PETCO_2$ gradient to be variable in patients with cardiopulmonary disease.[37] Therefore, $ETCO_2$ may not be a reliable index of $PaCO_2$ during CO_2 insufflation in this patient population.

Splanchnic, Renal, and Cerebral Blood Flow

Pneumoperitoneum, changes in patient position, reductions in cardiac output, and systemic carbon dioxide absorption

TABLE 38-3

REGIONAL HEMODYNAMICS

■ SPLANCHNIC
Unchanged—mechanical pneumoperitoneum compression balanced by hypercarbic vasodilatation
■ RENAL
Glomerular filtration—reduced
Renal plasma flow—reduced
Urine output—reduced during pneumoperitoneum/recovery following deflation
■ CEREBRAL
Cerebral blood flow velocity—increased
Intracranial pressure—increased

influence splanchnic, renal, and cerebral blood flow during minimal-access procedures (Table 38-3).

The clinical consequences of these changes depend largely on the patient's preexisting status. The direct mechanical effects of pneumoperitoneum in reducing splanchnic circulation may be counterbalanced by the direct splanchnic vasodilating effects of carbon dioxide. Notwithstanding occasional reports of mesenteric ischemia following laparoscopy,[39] the effects of pneumoperitoneum on the splanchnic circulation are not clinically significant. The mechanical compressive effects of pneumoperitoneum may account for the more than 50% reduction in glomerular filtration, renal plasma flow, and urine output during laparoscopic cholecystectomy.[40] Urine output increases significantly following pneumoperitoneum deflation. Cerebral blood flow velocity and intracranial pressure both increase during CO_2 pneumoperitoneum, with implications for patients with intracranial mass lesions undergoing minimal access surgery.[41]

ANESTHETIC TECHNIQUE

Anesthetic technique for intra-abdominal general surgical and gynecologic procedures has been mostly limited to general anesthesia. Diagnostic laparoscopic procedures have been performed under spinal anesthesia,[42,43] and successful performance of laparoscopic cholecystectomy under continuous epidural anesthesia has been reported in patients with chronic respiratory disease[44] including cystic fibrosis.[45] However, the high level of sympathetic denervation required, the frequent need for change of patient position, and the mandatory pneumoperitoneum may be associated with adverse ventilatory and circulatory responses complicating perioperative management.

Airway Management

Endotracheal intubation and controlled mechanical ventilation comprise the accepted anesthetic technique to reduce the increase in $PaCO_2$ and avoid ventilatory compromise because of pneumoperitoneum and initial Trendelenburg position.[46] The laryngeal mask airway (LMA) has been used widely during pelvic laparoscopy. Continuous esophageal pH[47,48] and clinical monitoring[49,50] failed to detect gastroesophageal reflux in patients undergoing gynecologic laparoscopy using LMA. However, this evidence cannot be extrapolated to upper abdominal laparoscopy, and high intra-abdominal pressures during laparoscopic cholecystectomy may increase the risk of passive regurgitation of gastric contents. Cuffed endotracheal tube placement minimizes the risk of acid aspiration should reflux occur.

Choice of neuromuscular blocking drug depends on anticipated duration of surgery and the individual drug side effect profile. Reversal of residual neuromuscular blockade with neostigmine has been reported to increase the incidence of postoperative nausea and vomiting (PONV) following laparoscopy compared with spontaneous recovery,[50] and some practitioners avoid its use. However, other investigators have found no effect on the incidence of PONV associated with the use of neostigmine,[51] and specifically, in patients undergoing outpatient gynecological laparoscopy, use of neostigmine and glycopyrrolate did not increase the incidence or severity of PONV.[52] Even minor degrees of residual neuromuscular blockade can produce distressing symptoms and must be avoided. Therefore any benefit from omitting neostigmine must be balanced against the risk of inadequate reversal of neuromuscular blockade.

Monitoring

Standard intraoperative monitoring is recommended for all patients undergoing minimal-access procedures. Invasive hemodynamic monitoring may be appropriate in ASA III or IV patients to monitor the cardiovascular response to pneumoperitoneum and position changes and to institute therapy.[45] $ETCO_2$ is most commonly used as a noninvasive indicator of $PaCO_2$ in assessing the adequacy of ventilation during laparoscopic procedures. Wahba and colleagues[54] found that increasing minute ventilation by 12 to 16% maintained $PaCO_2$ close to preinsufflation levels, and that $ETCO_2$ provided a reasonable approximation of $PaCO_2$ in healthy patients undergoing laparoscopic cholecystectomy. McKinstry et al[55] similarly observed equal and proportional increases in $ETCO_2$ and $PaCO_2$ following CO_2 insufflation in healthy patients. In contrast, patients with preexisting cardiopulmonary disease sustained significant increases in $PaCO_2$ during CO_2 insufflation that were not reflected by comparable increases in $ETCO_2$.[37] Online compliance and pressure-volume loop monitoring may be helpful in diagnosing complications resulting in increase airway pressure, such as bronchospasm, endobronchial intubation, and pneumothorax.

Preoperative pulmonary function tests showing low forced expiratory and vital capacity volumes and high ASA status may predict those patients at risk for development of hypercapnia and acidosis during laparoscopic cholecystectomy.[40] For such patients it would seem prudent to monitor $PaCO_2$ at times during the procedure to avoid adverse outcome. Persistent refractory hypercapnia or acidosis may require deflation of the pneumoperitoneum, lowering of the insufflation pressure, or conversion to an open procedure.

Nitrous Oxide

The use of N_2O during laparoscopic procedures has been controversial as a result of concerns regarding its ability to diffuse into bowel lumen causing distension and to increase postoperative nausea. As N_2O is more soluble than nitrogen (N_2), a closed air-containing space may accumulate N_2O more rapidly than it can eliminate N_2. Eger and Saidman[56] noted an increase of more than 200% in intestinal luminal size after 4 hours of N_2O breathing. The safety and efficacy of N_2O, specifically during laparoscopic cholecystectomy, were investigated by Taylor et al.[65] Surgical conditions during procedures lasting 70 to 80 minutes were identical regardless of whether N_2O was used. In particular, bowel distension did not increase over time in those patients who received N_2O and surgeons were unable to distinguish between patients who had received N_2O compared to air. In a laboratory experimental study, N_2O was shown to diffuse into a CO_2 pneumoperitoneum and the N_2O fraction exceeded 29%, a level that can support combustion, within two hours.[66] The clinical risk associated with prolonged laparoscopy remains unclear. However, in practice, leakage of intraperitoneal gas and replacement with fresh CO_2 is likely to reduce risk.

Although N_2O can contribute to PONV, Muir and colleagues,[67] in a large randomized, blind study, found no association between the use of N_2O and the subsequent development of PONV. Omission of N_2O failed to reduce the occurrence of PONV after laparoscopic cholecystectomy[65] or pelvic laparoscopy.[68] As conclusive evidence is lacking demonstrating a significant effect of N_2O on the incidence of postoperative emesis after laparoscopic cholecystectomy, any benefit from its elimination must be balanced against the potential increased risk of awareness.

Analgesia

Opioids remain an important component of a balanced general anesthetic technique for minimal-access procedures. Concern has been raised regarding narcotic-induced spasm of the sphincter of Oddi,[69] leading to misinterpretation of intraoperative cholangiographic findings during laparoscopic cholecystectomy. Many opioids, including fentanyl, have been implicated and there are conflicting reports regarding the relative effect of individual opioids.[70,71] Opioid-induced spasm of the sphincter of Oddi may be antagonized by several drugs including glucagon[71] and naloxone.[72]

8 Although laparoscopic cholecystectomy is considered a minimally invasive procedure, it is associated with intra-
9 abdominal, incisional, and shoulder pain after surgery. A multimodal analgesic regimen combining opioids, nonsteroidal anti-inflammatory drugs (NSAIDs), and local anesthetic infiltration may be the most effective approach, allowing reduction of opioid dose, thereby minimizing side effects. The intraperitoneal route of administration of local anesthetics is simple, does not involve central neuraxial block, and may be particularly suited to ambulatory anesthesia.[73] Of 13 clinical trials in a systematic review of intraperitoneal administration of bupivacaine 50 to 200 mg in volumes of 10 to 100 mL, significant reduction in overall pain occurred in seven trials but not in the other six.[74] Joris and colleagues[76] found that visceral pain accounted for most of the discomfort after laparoscopic cholecystectomy and was not attenuated by intraperitoneal administration of 80 mL of 0.125% bupivicaine.

10 PONV is a common and distressing symptom following laparoscopy. Reduction of opioid dose with multimodal analgesia regimes may reduce the incidence of PONV. The selective 5HT3 receptor antagonist ondansetron was reported to provide effective prophylaxis against postoperative emesis following laparoscopic procedures.[76] Other investigators found no difference in antiemetic efficacy between ondansetron and cyclizine in patients undergoing ambulatory laparoscopy.[77] The timing of ondansetron administration was found to be significant, with administration at the end of surgery producing a significantly greater antiemetic effect compared to preinduction dosing.[78]

SPECIFIC INTRAOPERATIVE COMPLICATIONS

11 Intraoperative complications during minimal-access procedures as a consequence of creation and maintenance of carbon dioxide pneumoperitoneum are included in Table 38-4.

Major vascular injuries may occur during surgical instrumentation, particularly during insertion of the Veress needle or trocars. The incidence of vascular injury during upper abdominal laparoscopy is reported to be approximately 0.03% to 0.06%[79] and has decreased with increasing surgical experience. Hemorrhage may occur because of insertion of the Veress needle or trocar into major intra-abdominal vessels[80] or because of injury to abdominal wall vasculature.[81] Disruption or avulsion of the cystic or hepatic artery may cause major bleeding during laparoscopic cholecystectomy. Concealed bleeding, particularly into the retroperitoneal space, may result in delayed diagnosis of vascular injury, which may be indicated initially by unexplained hypotension. The anesthesiologist may therefore play a crucial role in early diagnosis of this potentially fatal complication of laparoscopic procedures.[82] Uncontrollable hemorrhage requires immediate conversion to an open procedure to control bleeding and repair the vascular injury. Other reported intra-abdominal injuries associated with trocar insertion include gastrointestinal tract perforations, hepatic and splenic tears, and mesenteric lacerations.[83] Unrecognized gastrointestinal (GI) injuries may be associated with significant morbidity and mortality. Risk factors for GI injuries include gastric distension and adhesions because of previous abdominal surgery. Placement of the Veress needle using a minilaparotomy approach[84] should be considered in patients at increased risk.

TABLE 38-4

INTRAOPERATIVE COMPLICATIONS

■ VASCULAR INJURIES
Veress needle/trocar insertion—aorta, inferior vena cava, iliac vessels, retroperitoneal hematoma
■ GASTROINTESTINAL
Veress needle/trocar insertion—small and large bowel, liver and spleen, mesenteric
■ CARDIAC ARRHYTHMIAS
Hypercarbia
Reflex increased vagal tone—peritoneal stretch
■ SUBCUTANEOUS EMPHYSEMA
Intentional extraperitoneal insufflation—inguinal hernia repair/pelvic lymphadenectomy
Unintentional-accidental extraperitoneal CO_2 insufflation
■ PNEUMOTHORAX/PNEUMOMEDIASTINUM/PNEUMOPERICARDIUM
Embryonic defects
Diaphragm defects—aortic/esophageal hiatus
Pleural tears
Emphysematous bullae rupture
CARBON DIOXIDE EMBOLISM
Direct needle placement in vessel—induction of pneumoperitoneum
Gas insufflation into abdominal organ—hysteroscopy

Cardiac Arrhythmias

Arrhythmias during laparoscopic procedures may be multifocal and include hypercapnia as a result of intraperitoneal CO_2 insufflation and increased vagal tone following peritoneal stretching, especially associated with light levels of anesthesia. Bradycardia, cardiac arrhythmias, and asystole have all been reported.[84]

Inadvertent Extraperitoneal Insufflation

Access to the peritoneal cavity is achieved during laparoscopy by blind insertion of the Veress needle through a small subumbilical incision. Extraperitoneal insufflation of CO_2 may occur if the needle tip lies in the subcutaneous, preperitoneal, or retroperitoneal tissue during insufflation. The reported incidence of this complication varies from 0.4 to 2%.[85] As there is a continuum of fascial planes, extensive subcutaneous emphysema can develop involving the abdomen, chest, neck, and groin. Subcutaneous emphysema is indicated by the development of crepitus over the abdominal wall. Increased CO_2 absorption may cause a sudden rise in $ETCO_2$ and significant hypercapnia and respiratory acidosis has been reported in association with subcutaneous emphysema because of extraperitoneal insufflation.[86–87] In most cases, no specific intervention is required and the subcutaneous emphysema resolves soon after the abdomen is deflated. Careful surgical technique during Veress needle insertion and verification of intraperitoneal location prior to insufflation[88] will reduce the incidence of these complications.

Pneumothorax, Pneumomediastinum, and Pneumopericardium

Pneumothorax has been reported during both intraperitoneal and extraperitoneal laparoscopic procedures,[34,90] and although rare, is a potentially life-threatening complication. During laparoscopic cholecystectomy, pneumothorax has occurred during Veress needle or trocar insertion, CO_2 insufflation, or gallbladder dissection.[91]

The suggested mechanisms include tracking of insufflated CO_2 around the aortic and esophageal hiatuses of the diaphragm into the mediastinum with subsequent rupture into the pleural space. Passage of gas through anatomic defects in the diaphragm occurring at the outer crus or through a congenital defect at the pleuroperitoneal hiatus (patent pleuroperitoneal canal) is also a likely mechanism.[92] Tension pneumothorax has been described during laparoscopic cholecystectomy[93,94] and has been attributed to such a congenital diaphragmatic defect. Alternatively, rupture of a lung bulla or bleb could produce a tension pneumothorax independent of the pneumoperitoneum.

Clinical signs are variable. Pneumothorax may be undetected intraoperatively, or may present as unexplained increased airway pressure, hypoxemia–hypercapnia, surgical emphysema, or, if tension pneumothorax occurs, severe cardiovascular compromise with profound hypotension. Maintaining a high index of suspicion will facilitate early diagnosis and treatment, which can be life saving. If pneumothorax is suspected, a chest radiograph should be obtained to confirm the diagnosis. In the event of hemodynamic instability or clinical evidence of tension pneumothorax, immediate abdominal deflation and chest tube decompression are indicated prior to chest radiograph. Further management depends on hemodynamic status. If the patient remains stable, the abdomen may be insufflated and the procedure continued. Small pneumothoraces detected at the end of surgery and not associated with hemodynamic compromise may be treated conservatively. CO_2 in the pleural cavity is rapidly resorbed following deflation of the abdomen obviating the need for chest tube placement.

Pneumomediastinum and pneumopericardium have also been reported during laparoscopic procedures. Hasel[95] reports three cases of extravasation of CO_2 during laparoscopic cholecystectomy resulting in subcutaneous emphysema, associated with pneumomediastinum, pneumothorax, and ocular emphysema, all of which resolved spontaneously over 24 hours. High IAPs during insufflation may have contributed to these complications. Management depends on the degree of hemodynamic compromise that results. Deflation of the pneumoperitoneum and close observation is adequate in many patients.[91]

Gas Embolism

Serious adverse intraoperative events attributed to gas embolism during laparoscopic procedures are widely reported.[96,97] Venous CO_2 embolism in these cases was associated with profound hypotension, cyanosis, and asystole after creation of the pneumoperitoneum. The proposed mechanisms of gas embolism include inadvertent intravenous placement of the Veress needle, passage of CO_2 into abdominal wall and peritoneal vessels during insufflation, or into open vessels on the liver surface during gallbladder dissection. Signs and severity of effects of CO_2 embolism are variable and may include hypotension with cardiovascular collapse, hypoxemia, detection of a "mill-wheel" murmur, and an associated decrease in $ETCO_2$ because of reduction in pulmonary blood flow. Paradoxical embolism through a probe-patent foramen ovale or an atrial septal defect[98] may result in cerebral CO_2 embolism.

The incidence of gas embolism during laparoscopy is unclear. Using transesophageal echocardiography, Derouin and colleagues[99] reported CO_2 embolism occurring in 69% of patients during laparoscopic cholecystectomy but without significant cardiopulmonary effects. In contrast Wadhwa and colleagues, using precordial Doppler, did not observe any gas embolism in 100 patients undergoing gynecologic laparoscopic procedures.[101]

Appropriate monitoring and maintenance of a high index of suspicion can result in early detection and prevention of serious adverse sequelae from CO_2 embolism.

POSTOPERATIVE CONSIDERATIONS

It has been suggested that laparoscopic surgery reduces postoperative pulmonary complications by avoiding the restrictive pattern of respiration that usually follows upper abdominal surgery. Although there have been few prospective randomized trials comparing laparoscopic and open cholecystectomy, many early studies[82,101] report a lower incidence of pulmonary complications with the laparoscopic approach. Diaphragmatic dysfunction occurs following laparoscopic cholecystectomy and may last for up to 24 hours postoperatively.[102,103] Visceral afferents originating in the gallbladder area or somatic afferents arising from the abdominal wall that exert an inhibitory action on phrenic discharge may cause this diaphragmatic dysfunction.[91] However, although spirometric measures of lung function are decreased following both procedures, compared with patients undergoing open cholecystectomy, the laparoscopic approach was associated with 30 to 38% less impairment of postoperative pulmonary function including FRC, forced expiratory volume in 1 second (FEV_1), and vital capacity.[93] In addition, global respiratory muscle strength is greater 24 and 48 hours after laparoscopic compared with open cholecystectomy as determined by mouth pressure measurements during maximal inspiratory and expiratory efforts.[94]

Increased IAP during pneumoperitoneum has been reported to cause venous stasis that can increase the potential for deep vein thrombosis and pulmonary embolism (PE). The reported incidence of fatal PE following laparoscopic cholecystectomy (0.016%) is lower than after open surgery (0.8%).[95] Measures to reduce venous stasis such as graduated elastic compression stockings are indicated in the perioperative period. Minimal tissue trauma with laparoscopic techniques, facilitating early postoperative ambulation, also reduces risk.

Bile duct injuries are more common after laparoscopic compared with open cholecystectomy[96] and tend to be more extensive and located higher in the duct system. Pain and jaundice associated with bile collections are typical presenting features in the postoperative period. MacFadyen et al[96] analyzed a total of 114,005 laparoscopic cholecystectomies performed in the United States from 1989 to 1995. Major bile duct injuries occurred in 561 patients (0.5%). The common bile duct/common hepatic duct were most frequently injured (61.8%), and the majority of injuries required a surgical drainage procedure with either biliary-enteric anastomosis (41.8%) or T-tube placement (27.5%).

AMBULATORY LAPAROSCOPIC CHOLECYSTECTOMY

The minimally invasive nature of laparoscopic surgery facilitating earlier mobilization, and feeding, and reduced hospital stay has extended the range of procedures that can be performed on a day-case basis to include laparoscopic cholecystectomy. Some centers report successful same-day discharge for laparoscopic cholecystectomy in 68 to 94% of patients.[109–111] Concerns have been raised regarding the safety of outpatient laparoscopic cholecystectomy. In a series of 506 patients undergoing this procedure, 7.5% experienced postoperative complications, 61% of which had not become evident by 24 hours.[112] In an Australian report of 725 laparoscopic procedures, there was a 1.37% incidence of intensive care unit (ICU) admission.[113] Surgical complications were associated with delayed diagnosis and 12 longer ICU admissions. Therefore, caution is urged against overenthusiastic ambulatory laparoscopic cholecystectomy based on the logical if unproven assumption that early discharge will lead to occasional delays in diagnosis and management of postoperative complications.

VIDEO-ASSISTED THORACIC SURGERY (VATS)

Video-assisted thoracic surgery (VATS) presents new challenges for the surgeon and anesthesiologist. Potential advantages include less postoperative pain, improved postoperative pulmonary function, shorter hospitalization, and earlier return to work.[115] Applications of VATS include lobectomy, pneumonectomy, esophagectomy, and pericardial resection (Table 38-5). More innovative applications include implantation of the implantable cardioverter–defibrillator, excision of mediastinal masses, transthoracic endoscopic sympathectomy for the treatment of upper limb hyperhydrosis, and painful causalgias and splanchnicectomy (celiac plexus block) for intractable pain from pancreatic cancer and pancreatitis. VATS has been reported in the management of multiple diseases of the thoracic spine, including disc herniation, disc space abscesses, and spinal deformities.[116]

TABLE 38-5

VIDEO-ASSISTED THORACIC SURGERY

LUNGS
Pneumonectomy
Lobectomy
Wedge, subsegmental, segmental resection
Resection of pulmonary metasteses
Excision of blebs and bullae
HEART
Pericardiocentesis
Pericardiectomy
Insertion of implantable cardioverter–defibrillator
ESOPHAGUS
Esophagectomy
Repair of esophageal perforation
Fundoplication
MEDIASTINUM
Excision of tumors/cysts
SYMPATHETIC NERVOUS SYSTEM
Transthoracic endoscopic sympathectomy
VAGUS
Truncal vagotomy
THORACIC SPINE
Disc herniation
Deformity correction
Abscess drainage

Anesthetic techniques for thoracoscopy were reviewed by Horswell.[117] Most VATS are performed under general anesthesia with one-lung ventilation (OLV) provided through a double-lumen endobronchial tube placed in the left main stem bronchus and verified bronchoscopically (Fig. 38-2). Anesthesia is maintained by a combination of intravenous (IV) and inhaled agents. A radial artery cannula is usually placed for continuous blood pressure measurement and blood gas analysis.

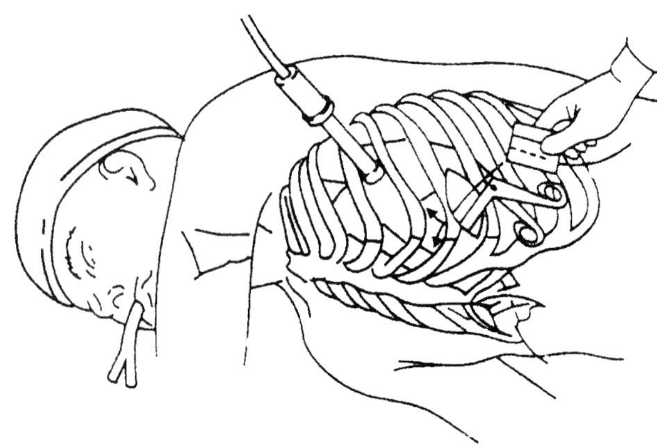

FIGURE 38-2. Patient positioning for thoracoscopic surgery.

Continuous pulse oximetry and end-tidal carbon dioxide tension ($PETCO_2$) are measured. Postoperative pain is managed by patient-controlled opioid analgesia, NSAIDs, or regional techniques. VATS-assisted placement of paravertebral catheters during thoracoscopic procedures has been reported in the management of postoperative pain.

SUMMARY

Laparoscopic cholecystectomy has proven to be a major advance in the treatment of patients with symptomatic gallbladder disease. The minimal-access nature of the surgical insult results in less pain and less postoperative ileus, facilitating faster recovery, shorter hospital stay, and more rapid return to normal activities.

General anesthesia and controlled ventilation comprise the accepted anesthetic technique to control arterial carbon dioxide tension. There is no conclusive evidence demonstrating a significant effect of N_2O on surgical conditions during laparoscopic cholecystectomy or on the incidence of postoperative emesis. Opioids remain an important component of a balanced anesthetic technique for laparoscopic cholecystectomy. A multimodal analgesic regimen combining opioids, NSAIDs, and local anesthetic infiltration may be the most effective approach, allowing a reduction of opioid dose, thereby minimizing side effects. Postoperative nausea and vomiting is common and requires appropriate prophylaxis and treatment.

The physiologic changes associated with patient positioning and pneumoperitoneum creation may cause significant cardiorespiratory compromise, particularly in ASA III and IV patients, and careful monitoring during CO_2 insufflation is recommended. Intraoperative complications may also arise because of traumatic injuries sustained during blind trocar insertion, CO_2 embolism, extraperitoneal insufflation and surgical emphysema, pneumothorax, and pneumomediastinum. Increasingly laparoscopic cholecystectomy is being performed in pregnancy, morbid obesity, and in older patients with coexisting cardiopulmonary disease presenting significant challenges in anesthetic management. Appropriate monitoring and maintenance of a high index of suspicion can result in early diagnosis of complications and prevent serious adverse sequelae.

Increasing surgical experience and improvements in instrumentation, including developments in optics, laser, and electrosurgical technology, has resulted in an expansion of both the range of surgical procedures performed by the laparoscopic approach to include gastrointestinal (gastric, colonic, splenic, hepatic), gynecologic (hysterectomy), and urologic (nephrectomy) procedures.

References

1. Darzi A, Mackay S: Recent advances in minimal access surgery. Br Med J 324:31, 2002
2. Soper NJ, Barteau JA, Clayman RV *et al*: Comparison of early postoperative results for laparoscopic versus standard open cholecystectomy. Surg Gynecol Obstet 174:114, 1992
3. Perissat J, Collet DR, Belliard R: Gallstones: Laparoscopic treatment, intracorporeal lithotripsy followed by cholecystostomy or cholecystectomy—A personal technique. Endoscopy 21:373, 1989
4. Reddick EJ, Olsen DO: Laparoscopy laser cholecystectomy, a comparison with mini-lap cholecystectomy. Surg Laparosc Endosc 3:131, 1989
5. NIH Consensus Conference: Gallstones and laparoscopic cholecystectomy. JAMA 269:1018, 1993
6. The E.A.E.S. Consensus Development Conferences on laparoscopic cholecystectomy, appendectomy and hernia repair. Consensus statements—September 1994. Surg Endosc 9:550, 1995
7. Chen AY, Daley J, Pappas TN, Henderson WG, Khuri SF: Growing use of laparoscopic cholecystectomy in the National Veterans Affairs Surgical Risk Study: Effects on volume, patient selection and selected outcomes. Ann Surg 227:12, 1998
8. Liem MSL, van der Graaf Y, van Steensel CJ *et al*: Comparison of conventional anterior surgery and laparoscopic surgery for inguinal hernia repair. N Engl J Med 336:1541, 1997
9. Smith CD, Weber CJ, Amerson JR: Laparoscopic adrenalectomy. New gold standard. World J Surg 23:389, 1999
10. Conacher ID, Soomro NA, Rix D: Anaesthesia for laparoscopic urological surgery. Br J Anaesth 93:859, 2004
11. Hunter JG, Trus Tl, Branum GD *et al*: A physiologic approach to laparoscopic fundoplication for gastroesophageal reflux disease. Ann Surg 223:673, 1996
12. Rosen DM, Lam AM, Chapman M, Carlton M, Cario GM: Methods of creating pneumoperitoneum: A review of techniques and complications. Obstet Gynecol Surv 53:167, 1998
13. Hasson HM: A modified instrument and method for laparoscopy. Am J Obstet Gynecol 110:886, 1971
14. Perone N: Laparoscopy using a simplified open technique. A review of 585 cases. J Reprod Med 37:921, 1992
15. Holohan TV: Laparoscopic cholecystectomy. Lancet 338:801, 1991
16. Lujan JA, Parilla P, Robles R *et al*: Laparoscopic cholecystectomy vs open cholecystectomy in the treatment of acute cholecystitis: A prospective study. Arch Surg 133:173, 1998
17. Eldar S, Sabo E, Nash E *et al*: Laparoscopic cholecystectomy for acute cholecystitis. Prospective trial. World J Surg 21:540, 1997
18. Ishizaki Y, Bandai Y, Shimomura K *et al*: Safe intraabdominal pressure of pneumoperitoneum during laparoscopic surgery. Surgery 114:549, 1993
19. Cunningham AJ, Turner J, Rosenbaum S *et al*: Transoesophageal assessment of haemodynamic function during laparoscopic cholecystectomy. Br J Anaesth 70:621, 1993
20. Rasmussen JP, Dauchot PJ, De Palma RG: Cardiac function and hypercarbia. Arch Surg 113:1196, 1978
21. Safran D, Sgambati S, Orlando R III. Laparoscopy in high-risk cardiac patients. Surg Gynecol Obstet 176:548, 1993
22. Ho HS, Saunders CJ, Corso FA *et al*: The effects of CO_2 pneumoperitoneum on haemodynamics in haemorrhaged animals. Surgery 114:381, 1993
23. Wahba RW, Beique F, Kleiman SJ: Cardiopulmonary function and laparoscopic cholecystectomy. Can J Anaeth 42:51, 1995
24. Joris Jl, Noirot DP, Legrand MJ *et al*: Hemodynamic changes during laparoscopic cholecystectomy. Anesth Analg 76:1067, 1993
25. Branche PE, Duperret SL, Sagnard PE *et al*: Left ventricular loading modifications induced by pneumoperitoneum: A time course echocardiographic study. Anesth Analg 86:482, 1998
26. Goodale RL, Beebe DS, McNevin MP *et al*: Hemodynamic, respiratory and metabolic effects of laparoscopic cholecystectomy. Am J Surg 166:533, 1993
27. Dexter SP, Vucevic M, Gibson J *et al*: Hemodynamic consequences of high- and low-pressure capnoperitoneum during laparoscopic cholecystectomy. Surg Endosc 13:376, 1999
28. Aoki T, Tanii M, Takahashi K *et al*: Cardiovascular changes and catecholamine levels during laparoscopic surgery. Anesth Analg 78:88, 1994
29. Hein HA, Joshi GP, Ramsey MA: Hemodynamic changes during laparoscopic cholecystectomy in patients with severe cardiac disease. J Clin Anesth 9:261, 1997
30. Safran D, Sgambati S, Orlando R: Laparoscopy in high-risk cardiac patients. Surg Gynecol Obstet 176:548, 1993
31. Joris JL, Chiche JD, Canivet JL *et al*: Hemodynamic changes during laparoscopy and their endocrine correlates: Effects of clonidine. J Am Coll Cardiol 32:1389, 1998
32. Walder AD, Aitkenhead AR: Role of vasopressin in the haemodynamic response to laparoscopic cholecystectomy. Br J Anaesth 78:264, 1997
33. O'Leary E, Hubbard K, Tormey W *et al*: cholecystectomy: Haemodynamic and neuroendocrine responses after pneumoperitoneum and changes in position. Br J Anaesth 76:640, 1996
34. Jorgensen JO, Lalak NJ, North L: Venous stasis during laparoscopic cholecystectomy. Surg Laparosc Endosc 2:128, 1994
35. Holzman M, Sharp K, Richards W: Hypercarbia during carbon dioxide gas insufflation for therapeutic laparoscopy: A note of caution. Surg Laparosc Endosc 2:11, 1992
36. Makinen MT, Yli-Hankala A: Respiratory compliance during laparoscopic hiatal and inguinal hernias repair. Can J Anaesth 45:865, 1998
37. Bardoczky GI, Engelman E, Levarlet M *et al*: Ventilatory effects of pneumoperitoneum monitored with continuous spirometry. Anaesthesia 48:309, 1993
38. Fahy BG, Barnas GM, Nagle SE *et al*: Changes in lung and chest wall properties with abdominal insufflation of carbon dioxide are immediately reversible. Anesth Analg 82:501, 1996
39. Schiller WR: The Trendelenburg position. Surgical aspects. In Martin JT (ed): Positioning in Anesthesia and Surgery, 2nd ed., pp 117–126. Philadelphia, WB Saunders, 1987
40. Puri GD, Singh H: Ventilatory effects of laparoscopy under general anaesthesia. Br J Anaesth 68:211, 1992
41. Wolf JS Jr, Carrier S, Stoller S: Gas embolism: Helium is more lethal than carbon dioxide. J Laparoendoscopic Surg 4:173, 1994

42. Mullett CE, Viale JP, Sagnard PE *et al*: Pulmonary CO_2 elimination during surgical procedures using intra- or extraperitoneal CO_2 insufflation. Anesth Analg 76:622, 1993
43. Wittgen CM, Andrus CH, Fitzgerald SD *et al*: Analysis of the hemodynamic and ventilatory effects of laparoscopic cholecystectomy. Arch Surg 126:997, 1991
44. Dwerryhouse SJ, Melsome DS, Burton PA: Acute intestinal ischaemia after laparoscopic cholecystectomy. Br J Surg 82:1413, 1993
45. Iwase K, Takenaka H, Ishizaka T: Serial changes in renal function during laparoscopic cholecystectomy. Eur Surg Res 25:203, 1993
46. Rosenthal RJ, Hiatt JR, Phillips EH: Intracranial pressure. Effects of pneumoperitoneum in a large-animal model. Surg Endosc 11:376, 1997
47. Dhoste K, Lacoste L, Karayan J *et al*: Haemodynamic and ventilatory changes during laparoscopic cholecystectomy in elderly ASA III patients. Can J Anaesth 43:783, 1996
48. Feig BW, Berger BH, Dougherty TB *et al*: Pharmacological intervention can re-establish baseline hemodynamic parameters during laparoscopy. Surgery 116:733, 1994
49. Wittgen CM, Naunhein KS, Andrus CH *et al*: Preoperative pulmonary evaluation for laparoscopic cholecystectomy. Arch Surg 128:880, 1993
50. Solylo MA, Vaghadia H, Henderson C *et al*: Walk-in/walk-out spinal anesthesia for laparoscopy: Return of spinal cord function. Can J Anaesth 46:39, 1999
51. Viskari D, Berrill A, Vaghadia H: Walk-in/walk-out spinal anesthesia for out-patient laparoscopy: Evaluation of three hypobaric solutions. Can J Anaesth 44:A26, 1997
52. Pursnani KG, Bazza Y, Calleja M *et al*: Laparoscopic cholecystectomy under epidural anaesthesia in patients with chronic respiratory disease. Surg Endosc 12:1082, 1998
53. Edelman DS: Laparoscopic cholecystectomy under continuous epidural anesthesia in patients with cystic fibrosis. Am J Dis Child 145:723, 1991
54. Cunningham AJ: Anesthetic implications of laparoscopic surgery. Yale J Biol and Med 71(6):551, 1999
55. Bapat PP, Verghese C: Laryngeal mask airway and the incidence of regurgitation during gynaecological laparoscopies. Anesth Analg 85:139, 1997
56. Ho BY, Skinner HJ, Mahajan RP: Gastro-oesophageal reflux during day case gynaecological laparoscopy under positive pressure ventilation. Laryngeal mask vs tracheal intubation. Anaesthesia 53:921, 1998
57. Malins AF, Cooper GM: Laparoscopy and the laryngeal mask airway [letter]. Br J Anaesth 73:121, 1994
58. Verghese C, Brimacombe JR: Survey of laryngeal mask airway usage in 11,910 patients. Safety and efficacy of conventional and nonconventional usage. Anesth Analg 82:129, 1996
59. Ding Y, Fredman B, White PF: Use of mivacurium during laparoscopic surgery: Effect of reversal drugs on postoperative recovery. Anesth Analg 78:450, 1994
60. Hovorka J, Korttila K, Nelskyla K *et al*: Reversal of neuromuscular blockade with neostigmine has no effect on the incidence or severity of postoperative nausea and vomiting. Anesth Analg 85:1359, 1997
61. Nelskyla K, Yli-Hankala A, Soikkeli A *et al*: Neostigmine with glycopyrrollate does not increase the incidence or severity of postoperative nausea and vomiting in outpatients undergoing gynaecological laparoscopy. Br J Anaesth 81:757, 1998
62. Wahba RW, Mamazza J: Ventilatory requirements during laparoscopic cholecystectomy. Can J Anaesth 40:206, 1993
63. McKinstry LJ, Perverseff RA, Yip RW: Arterial and end-tidal carbon dioxide in patients undergoing laparoscopic cholecystectomy. Anesthesiology 77:A108, 1992
64. Eger EI II, Saidman LJ: Hazards of nitrous oxide anaesthesia in bowel obstruction and pneumothorax. Anesthesiology 26:61, 1965
65. Taylor E, Feinstein R, White PF: Anesthesia for laparoscopic cholecystectomy: Is nitrous oxide contraindicated? Anesthesiology 76:541, 1992
66. Diemunsch PA, Torp KD, Van Dorsselaer T *et al*: Nitrous oxide fraction in the carbon dioxide pneumoperitoneum during laparoscopy under general inhaled anaesthesia in pigs. Anesth Analg 90:951, 2000
67. Muir JJ, Warner Ma, Offord KP *et al*: Role of nitrous oxide and other factors in postoperative nausea and vomiting: A randomised and blinded prospective study. Anesthesiology 66:513, 1987
68. Sukhani R, Lurie J, Jabamoni R: Propofol for ambulatory gynaecological laparoscopy: Does omission of nitrous oxide alter postoperative sequelae and recovery? Anesth Analg 78:831, 1994
69. Chessick KC, Black S, Hoye SJ: Spasm and operative cholangiography. Arch Surg 110:53, 1975
70. Radnay PA, Brodman E, Mankikar D *et al*: The effect of equi-analgesic doses of fentanyl, morphine, meperidine, and pentazocine on common bile duct pressure. Anaesthetist 29:26, 1980
71. Jones RM, Detmer M, Hill AB *et al*: Incidence of choledochoduodenal sphincter spasm during fentanyl supplemented anesthesia. Anesth Analg 60:638, 1981
72. McCammon RL, Viegas OJ, Stoelting RK *et al*: Naloxone reversal of choledochoduodenal sphincter spasm associated with narcotic administration. Anesthesiology 48:437, 1978
73. Michaloliakou C, Chung F, Sharma S: Peroperative multimodal analgesia facilitates recovery after ambulatory laparoscopic cholecystectomy. Anesth Analg 82: 44, 1996
74. Moiniche S, Jorgensen H, Wetterslev J, Berg J: Local anesthetic infiltration for postoperative pain relief after laparoscopy: A qualitative and quantitative systematic review of intraperitoneal, port-site infiltration and mesosalpinx block. Anesth Analg 90:899, 2000
75. Ng A: Intraperitoneal administration of analgesia: Is this practice of any utility? Br J Anaesth 89:535, 2002
76. Joris J, Thiry E, Paris P *et al*: Pain after laparoscopic cholecystectomy: Characteristics and effect of intraperitoneal bupivicaine. Anesth Analg 81:379, 1995
77. Raphael JH, Norton AC: Antiemetic efficacy of prophylactic ondansetron in laparoscopic surgery. Randomized double-blind comparison with metoclopramide. Br J Anaesth 71:845, 1993
78. Cholwill JM, Wright W, Hobbs GJ *et al*: Comparison of ondansetron and cyclizine for prevention of nausea and vomiting after day-case gynaecological laparoscopy. Br J Anaesth 83:611, 1999
79. Tang J, Wang B, White PF *et al*: The effect of timing of ondansetron administration on its efficacy, cost-effectiveness and cost-benefit as a prophylactic antiemetic in the ambulatory setting. Anesth Analg 86:274, 1998
80. Hashizume M, Sugimachi K: Study group of endoscopic surgery in Kyushu Japan: Needle and trocar injury during laparoscopic surgery in Japan. Surg Endosc 11:1198, 1997
81. Katz M, Beck P, Tancer ML: Major vessel injury during laparoscopy: Anatomy of two cases. Am J Obstet Gynecol 135:544, 1979
82. Hurd WW, Pearl ML, DeLancey JO *et al*: Laparoscopic injury of abdominal wall blood vessels: A report of three cases. Obstet Gynecol 82:673, 1993
83. Noga J, Fredman B, Olsfanger D *et al*: Role of the anesthesiologist in early diagnosis of life-threatening complications during laparoscopic surgery. Surg Laparosc Endosc 7:63, 1997
84. Ponsky JL: Complications of laparoscopic cholecystectomy. Am J Surg 161:393, 1991
85. Hasson H: A modified instrument and method for laparoscopy. Am J Obstet Gynecol 70:886, 1971
86. Kabukoba JJ, Skillern LH: Coping with extraperitoneal insufflation during laparoscopy. A new technique. Obstet Gynecol 80:144, 1992
87. Kent III RB: Subcutaneous emphysema and hypercarbia following laparoscopic cholecystectomy. Arch Surg 126:1154, 1991
88. Leonard IE, Cunningham AJ: Anaesthetic considerations for laparoscopic cholecystectomy. Clin Anaesthesiol 16:1, 2002
89. Pearce DJ: Respiratory acidosis and subcutaneous emphysema during laparoscopic cholecystectomy. Can J Anaesth 41:314, 1994
90. Deziel DJ: Avoiding laparoscopic complications. Int Surg 79:361, 1994
91. Gabbott DA, Dunckley AB, Roberts FL: Carbon dioxide Pneumothorax occurring during laparoscopic cholecystectomy. Anaesthesia 47:587, 1992
92. Joshi GP: Complications of laparoscopy. Anesth Clin N Am 19(1):89, 2001
93. Calverley RK, Jenkins LC: The anaesthetic management of pelvic laparoscopy. Can Anaesth Soc J 20:679, 1973
94. Dawson R, Ferguson CJ: Life-threatening tension pneumothorax during laparoscopic cholecystectomy. Surg Laparosc Endosc 7:271, 1997
95. Whiston RJ, Eggers KA, Morris RW *et al*: Tension pneumothorax during laparoscopic cholecystectomy. Br J Surg 78:1325, 1991
96. Hasel R, Arora SK, Hickey DR: Intraoperative complications of laparoscopic cholecystectomy. Can J Anaesth 40:459, 1993
97. Root B, Levy MN, Pollack S *et al*: Gas embolism death after laparoscopy delayed by "trapping" in the portal circulation. Anesth Analg 57:232, 1978
98. de Plater RM, Jones IS: Non-fatal carbon dioxide embolism during laparoscopy. Anaesth Intens Care 17:359, 1989
99. Schindler E, Muller M, Kelm C: Cerebral carbon dioxide embolism during laparoscopic cholecystectomy. Anesth Analg 81:643, 1995
100. Derouin M, Couture P, Boudreault D *et al*: Detection of gas embolism by transoesophageal echocardiography during laparoscopic cholecystectomy. Anesth Analg 82:119, 1996
101. Wadhwa RK, McKenzie R, Wadhwa SR *et al*: Gas embolism during laparoscopy. Anesthesiology 48:74, 1978
102. Frazee RC, Roberts JW, Okeson GC *et al*: Open versus closed cholecystectomy: A comparison of postoperative pulmonary function. Ann Surg 213:651, 1991
103. Erice F, Fox GF, Salib YM *et al*: Diaphragmatic function before and after laparoscopic cholecystectomy. Anesthesiology 79:966, 1993
104. Sharma RR, Axelsson H, Oberg A *et al*: Diaphragmatic activity after laparoscopic cholecystectomy. Anesthesiology 91:406, 1999
105. Schauer PR, Luna J, Ghiatas AA *et al*: Pulmonary function after laparoscopic cholecystectomy. Surgery 114:389, 1993
106. Rovina N, Bouros D, Tzanakis N *et al*: Effects of laparoscopic cholecystectomy on global respiratory muscle strength. Am J Respir Crit Care Med 153:458, 1996
107. Scott TR, Zucker KA, Bailey RW: Laparoscopic cholecystectomy: A review of 12,397 patients. Surg Laparosc Endosc 2:191, 1992
108. Collins R, Scrimgeour A, Yusuf S *et al*: Reduction in fatal pulmonary embolism and venous thrombosis by perioperative administration of subcutaneous heparin. N Engl J Med 318:1162, 1988

109. MacFayden Jr BV, Vecchio R, Ricardo AE *et al*: Bile duct injury after laparoscopic cholecystectomy. The United States experience. Surg Endosc 12(4):315, 1998
110. Singleton RJ, Rudkin GE, Osborne GA *et al*: Laparoscopic cholecystectomy as a day surgery procedure. Anaesth Intens Care 24:231, 1996
111. Taylor E, Gaw F, Kennedy C: Outpatient laparoscopic cholecystectomy feasibility. J Laparoendosc Surg 6:73, 1996
112. Voitk AJ: Outpatient cholecystectomy. J Laparoendosc Surg 6:79, 1996
113. Saunders CJ, Leary BF, Wolfe BM: Is outpatient laparoscopic cholecystectomy wise? Surg Endosc 9:1263, 1995
114. Hayes C, Ambazidis S, Gani JS: Intensive care unit admissions following laparoscopic surgery: What lessons can be learned? Aust NZ J Surg 66:206, 1996
115. Allen MS: Video-assisted thoracic surgical procedures: The Mayo experience. Mayo Clin Proc 71:351, 1996
116. Cunningham AJ, Dowd N: Anesthesia for minimally invasive procedures in clinical anesthesia. Barash PG, Cullen BF, Stoelting RK (eds): Clinical Anesthesia, 4th ed, pp 1051–1065. Philadelphia, Lippincott Williams & Wilkins, 2001
117. Horswell JL. Anesthetic technique for thoracoscopy. Ann Thoracic Surg 56:624, 1993

CHAPTER 39 ■ ANESTHESIA AND THE LIVER

BRIAN S. KAUFMAN AND J. DAVID ROCCAFORTE

KEY POINTS

1. The hepatic buffer response, in which the hepatic artery blood flow changes reciprocally with changing portal venous flow, is the mechanism by which total oxygen delivery to the liver is maintained. This response is limited in its ability to compensate during conditions of hypoperfusion, inflammation, or shock.
2. Hepatitis associated with volatile anesthetics is rare overall and is most commonly associated with halothane. The disorder appears to be immune mediated and is best avoided by eliminating halothane from clinical use.

3 Because of the liver's central role in the inflammatory response, the metabolic demands greatly increase whenever acute-phase proteins are being produced. These demands occur when hepatic oxygen delivery is likely to be compromised, placing the liver in a highly vulnerable situation.

4 The risk of developing perioperative hepatic dysfunction varies with the preexisting hepatic reserve status; presence of comorbid conditions; and the type, duration, and location of surgery. Commonly employed general and regional anesthetic techniques impart minimal additional stress to the liver.

5 Currently, there is no commonly available hepatic replacement therapy for acute liver failure. The most effective support for the liver, maintaining adequate perfusion and oxygenation, as well as avoiding secondary toxic insults, must occur before it fails.

The liver occupies the center of a diverse spectrum of vital physiologic functions and plays an essential role in maintaining perioperative homeostasis. Patients with advanced liver disease are at high risk of excessive morbidity and mortality following surgery due to failure of one or more of these essential functions. For example, the normal liver moderates the hypotensive response to acute blood loss and hypovolemia through its reservoir function, and helps minimize blood loss through synthesis of coagulation factors and degradation of fibrinolytic substances. Failure of these functions contributes to intraoperative and postoperative hypoperfusion, tissue ischemia, and activation of the systemic inflammatory response, setting the stage for the postoperative development of multisystem organ failure. The liver is the primary regulatory site for metabolism. After oral intake, all nutrients are brought to the liver for processing, followed by controlled distribution to extrahepatic tissues. The liver also helps sustain energy supplies during fasting, is the site of synthesis of almost all the body's proteins, plays a central role in the individual's defense against infection, and modulates inflammatory processes. Predictable termination of the pharmacologic effects of many anesthetic agents depends on the liver for metabolic biotransformation into inactive products that can be eliminated.

The liver is a remarkably resilient organ, with unparalleled regenerative capacity and substantial physiologic reserves. Normal function may be present in humans when as much as 80% of the organ has been resected. Insidious hepatic diseases such as chronic hepatitis C can progress silently and destroy the majority of the liver before symptoms develop. Identifying patients with marked limitation of hepatic reserve, but without overt hepatic failure is important, but often difficult. A careful preoperative history and physical examination will help identify patients in whom laboratory evaluation of liver function is appropriate. These patients are often at increased risk for perioperative morbidity and mortality, including development of overt liver dysfunction postoperatively, particularly after major procedures.

As therapy for chronic hepatic diseases improves and the number of patients with chronic hepatitis C continues to rapidly increase, it can be expected that the number of patients with moderate-to-severe liver disease presenting for surgery will rise. These patients may be at extremely high risk for perioperative complications, and it is essential that the anesthesiologist understands the interactions between liver disease, surgical procedures, and anesthetic interventions so an appropriate therapeutic plan can be developed and implemented to optimize patient outcome.

HEPATIC ANATOMY

The liver is the largest gland in the human body with a median weight of 1.8 kg in men and 1.4 kg in women.[1] The liver is covered by peritoneum (Glisson's capsule), except for the gallbladder bed, the inferior vena cava (IVC), the bare area, and the porta hepatis. At the porta hepatis, the connective tissue of the capsule is continuous with the fibrous sheath, which invests the portal vessels and ducts. The capsular peritoneum reflects onto the diaphragm and continues as the parietal peritoneum. The reflections form various ligaments (coronary, triangular, and falciform), which firmly attach the liver to the anterior abdominal wall and diaphragm.

Lobes Versus Segments of the Liver

The customary division of the liver into the right, left, caudate, and quadrate lobes is derived from the topographic anatomy, with the falciform ligament separating the right and left lobes (Fig. 39-1). This anatomic description does not correspond to the branches of the liver's vascular supply and therefore is of limited clinical and physiologic significance. The liver can be divided on a different plane into right and left hemilivers, which have their own blood supplies and duct drainage. The liver can be further divided into a total of eight functionally independent segments, each with its own vascular inflow and outflow, and biliary drainage (Fig. 39-2). The segmental division of the liver was devised by Couinaud, based on the divisions of the portal vein, and more recently modified by Strasberg, based on the more consistent divisions of the hepatic artery and biliary ducts.[2] This anatomic arrangement facilitates limited segmental resection of the liver with relatively bloodless surgical dissection along the planes between segments, and thereby prevents major disruption of hepatobiliary function. With current imaging techniques, radiologists can construct precise, three-dimensional models of a patient's liver, defining the segmental location of lesions and their relation to the vasculature. Such information can help the surgeon decide on the most appropriate operative approach, while enhancing the resectability of a variety of lesions and improving outcome for patients undergoing operations for neoplasm or trauma.[3]

Vascular Supply of the Liver

The liver receives about 25% of the cardiac output, and therefore, has an average blood flow between 100 and 130 mL/minute per 100 g. There are two major sources of blood to the liver: the hepatic artery and the portal vein. The common hepatic artery arises from the celiac trunk and sends off the cystic artery before entering the liver (Fig. 39-3). The portal vein is formed by the confluence of the splenic and superior mesenteric veins, and receives blood from the entire digestive tract, spleen, pancreas, and gallbladder. The hepatic artery delivers about 25% of the total hepatic blood flow but nearly 50% of the hepatic oxygen delivery. The portal vein provides the remaining 75% of total hepatic blood flow and 50% of hepatic oxygen delivery. Because portal venous blood has already perfused the preportal organs (stomach, intestines, spleen, and pancreas) (see Fig. 39-3), it is partially deoxygenated and enriched with nutrients and other substances absorbed from the gastrointestinal tract.

The portal vein has numerous tributaries, which are usually of little importance (see Fig. 39-1). When patients develop portal hypertension, however, these normally rudimentary connections form large portosystemic shunts, permitting portal

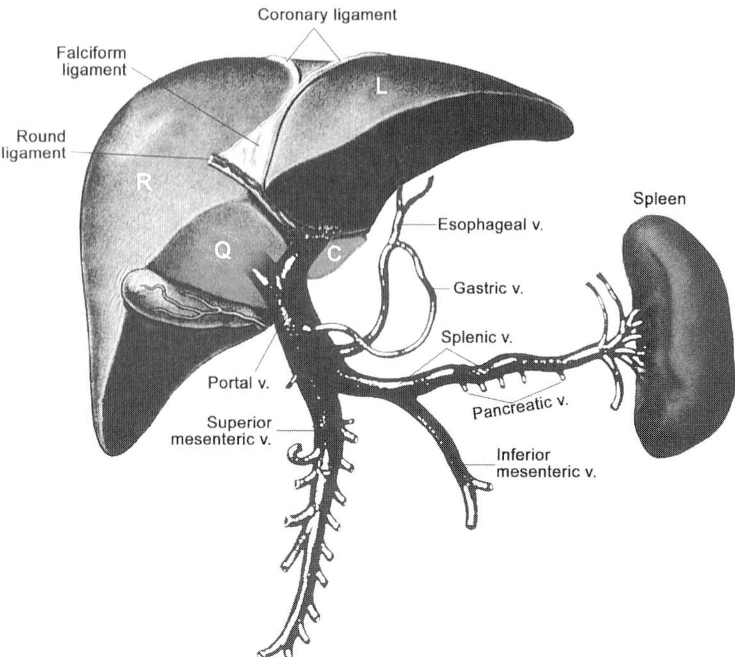

FIGURE 39-1. Schematic representation depicting the lobar classification of the liver and the extrahepatic portal venous circulation.

venous blood to return to the systemic circulation without traversing the liver. These shunts produce many of the pathologic findings and severe complications of portal hypertension (e.g., esophageal varices).

Intrahepatic Circulation

The portal vein and hepatic artery enter the liver at the porta hepatis, where the larger bile ducts join and accompany them. Both vessels bifurcate into left and right branches, which arborize in parallel while diminishing in caliber as they penetrate the hepatic parenchyma to end as terminal hepatic arterioles and portal venules (Fig. 39-4). Most terminal vessels drain directly into the hepatic sinusoids, delivering substrates to, and removing products from, adjacent parenchymal cells. Before this, some arteriolar blood flows through the peribiliary capillary plexus, which plays a major role in bile secretion and absorption (see Fig. 39-4). Hepatic arterial pressure is similar to aortic pressure, while the mean portal vein pressure is approximately 6 to 10 mm Hg. These two afferent vascular systems merge in the sinusoids where the pressure is normally 2 to 4 mm Hg above that of the IVC. The hepatic sinusoids connect the terminal portal vessels with the hepatic venules. The continuity of the sinusoidal wall is interrupted by fenestrations, which facilitate transfer of solutes to the space of Disse for uptake by hepatocytes. Flow through the sinusoids is influenced by several factors, the most important of which may be local control by shrinking or swelling of endothelial and Kupffer cells.

Blood drains from the hepatic sinusoids into the central vein and then flows through sublobular veins that join to form one of the three major hepatic veins (right, middle, and left) (Fig. 39-5). A short extrahepatic segment joins each major hepatic vein to the IVC. The caudate lobe drains directly into the IVC through small posterior caudate veins. If thrombosis of the major hepatic veins occurs (Budd-Chiari syndrome), the caudate veins become the key to drainage of hepatic blood into the IVC.

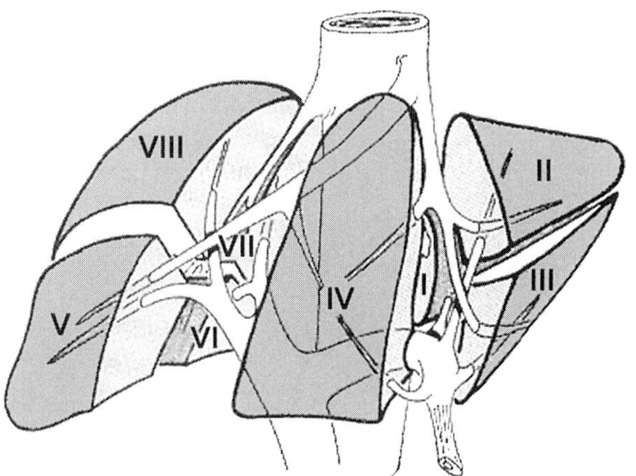

FIGURE 39-2. Segmental division of the liver according to Couinaud's nomenclature. (Reprinted with permission from Parks RW, Chrysos E, Diamond T: Management of liver trauma. Br J Surg 86:1121, 1999.)

Hepatic Microanatomy: Classic Liver Lobule Versus Acinar Lobule

The functional units of the liver have defied delineation. The organization of the hepatic parenchyma has been conceptualized in two contrasting models: Kierman's classic lobule and Rappaport's acinus.[4] Each model can successfully explain some of the pathologic and physiologic processes in the liver, but neither explains them all.

The classic liver lobule is hexagonal on cross section, with six vertically aligned portal canals at the corners and a hepatic venule (central vein) in its center (see Fig. 39-5). Each canal contains connective tissue, lymphatics, nerves, and a portal triad (terminal branches of portal vein, hepatic artery, and bile duct). A lobule consists of an array of anastomosing cords of hepatocytes, separated by vascular channels (lacunae) that radiate from the six portal areas and converge on the hepatic venule at the center of the hexagon. The lacunae contain the capillaries (sinusoids), which are lined by endothelium and scattered Kupffer cells, which protrude into the sinusoidal lumen.

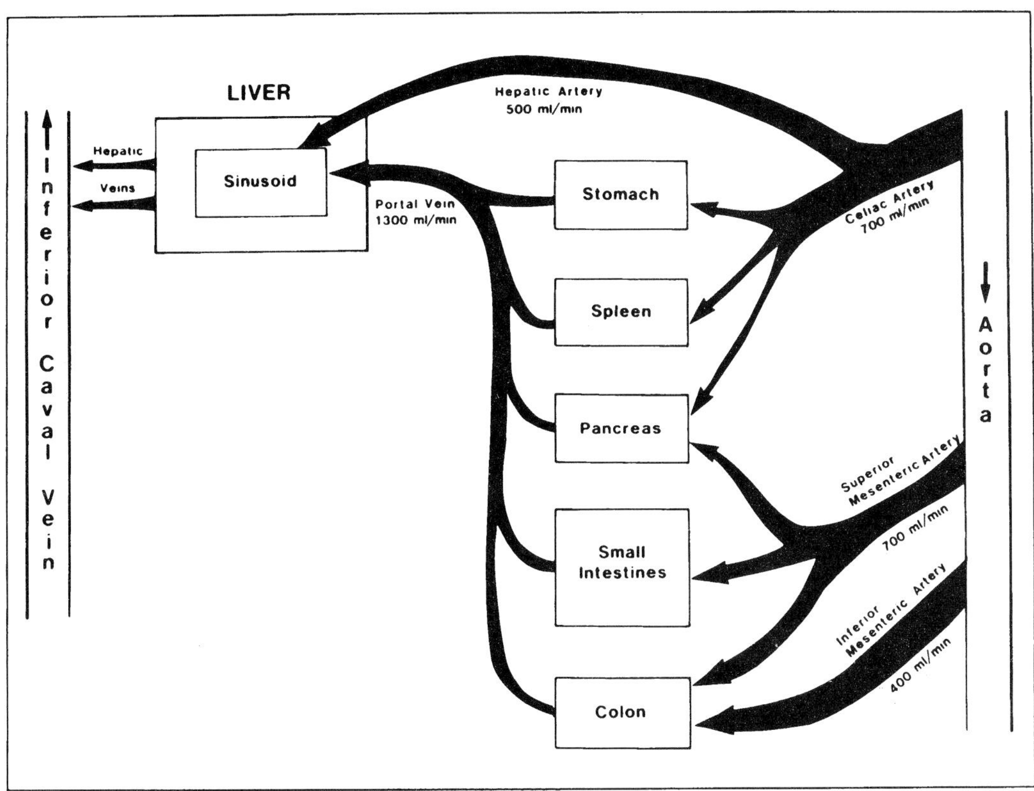

FIGURE 39-3. Schematic representation of splanchnic circulation. (Reprinted with permission from Gelman S: Effects of anesthetics on splanchnic circulation. In Altura BM, Halevy S [eds]: Cardiovascular Action of Anesthetics and Drugs Used in Anesthesia, p 127. Basel, Karger, 1986.)

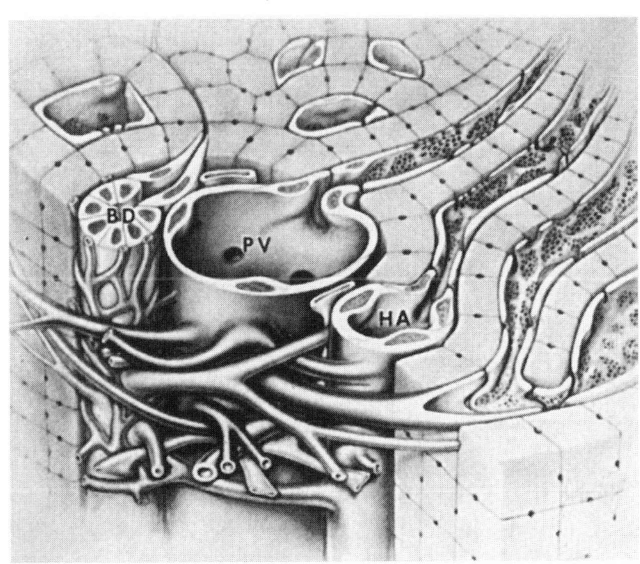

FIGURE 39-4. Relationship of branches of the portal vein (PV), hepatic artery (HA), and bile duct (BD). Notice the peribiliary capillary plexus that envelops the bile ducts. These three structures constitute a portal triad, which is a transverse section of a portal canal. (Reprinted with permission from Jones AL: Anatomy of the normal liver. In Zakim D, Boyer T [eds]: Hepatology: A Textbook of Liver Disease, 3rd ed, p 3. Philadelphia, WB Saunders, 1996.)

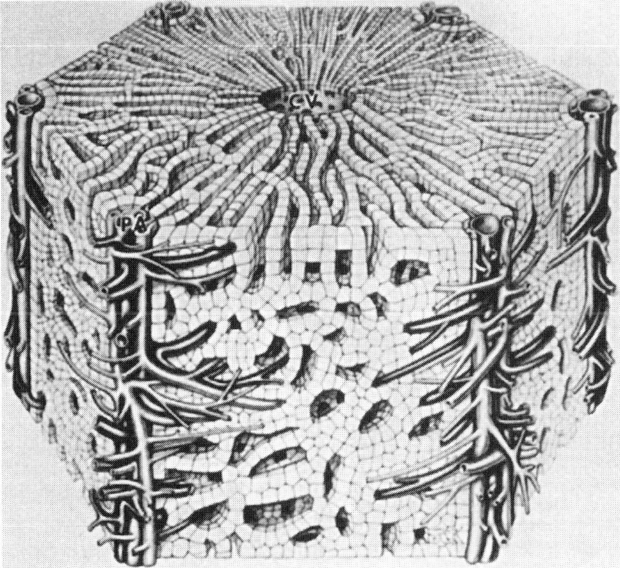

FIGURE 39-5. Schematic view of liver lobule: The central vein (CV) lies in the center of the figure surrounded by anastomosing cords of block-like hepatocytes. About the periphery of this schema are six portal areas (PAs) consisting of branches of the portal vein, the hepatic artery, and the bile duct. (Reprinted with permission from Jones AL: Anatomy of the normal liver. In Zakim D, Boyer T [eds]: Hepatology: A Textbook of Liver Disease, 3rd ed, p 3. Philadelphia, WB Saunders, 1996.)

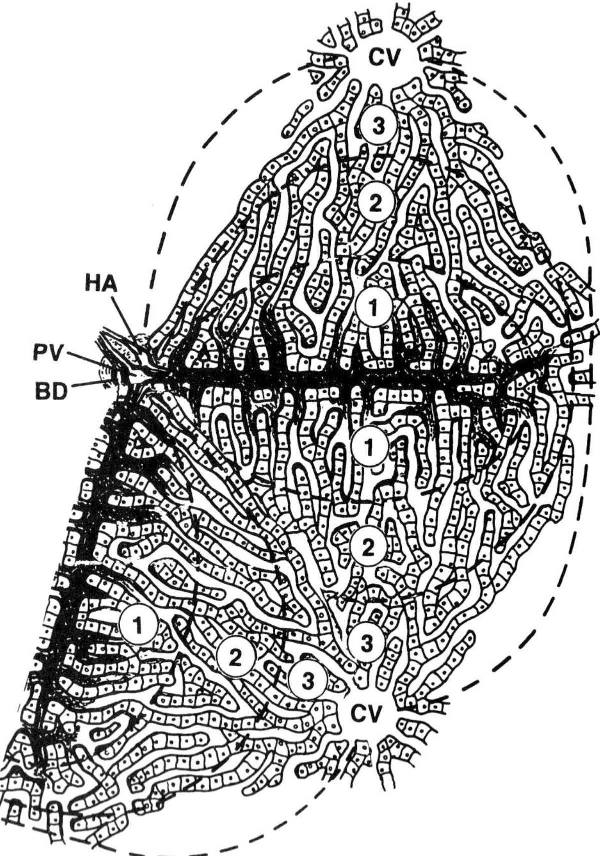

FIGURE 39-6. Blood supply of the simple liver acinus. The oxygen tension and the nutrient level of the blood in sinusoids decrease from zone 1 through zone 3. Note that the lower left side of the figure also depicts zones 1, 2, and 3 in a portion of an adjacent acinar unit. BD, bile duct; HA, hepatic artery; PV, portal vein; CV, central vein. (Reprinted with permission from Jones AL: Anatomy of the normal liver. In Zakim D, Boyer T [eds]: Hepatology: A Textbook of Liver Disease, 3rd ed, p 3. Philadelphia, WB Saunders, 1996.)

A lacunar labyrinth penetrates the entire lobule, except for the first row of hepatocytes in contact with the portal tract (the limiting plate), where a near continuous wall of hepatocytes separates the interior of the lobule from the portal canal.

Human livers do not have well-defined interlobular connective tissue, making it difficult to visualize the classic lobule. The quest to identify the boundaries of the classic lobule led to the discovery of circumferential terminal hepatic arterioles, portal venules, and bile ductules. Reasoning that these encircling vessels supply segments of contiguous classic lobules that lie between two terminal hepatic venules, Rappaport developed the acinus lobule (acinus) concept.[4] The simple liver acinus is a small parenchymal mass, irregular in size and shape, and arranged around a central axis consisting of a terminal hepatic arteriole, portal venule, bile ductule, lymph vessels, and nerves (Fig. 39-6). Blood enters the center of the acinus and flows centrifugally to the hepatic venules. In contrast to the direction of blood flow, bile flows in the opposite direction from perivenular hepatocytes to the portal tract bile ducts.

The simple liver acinus lies between two (or more) terminal hepatic venules. The terminal hepatic venule is therefore at the center of a classic liver lobule, but at the periphery of several simple liver acini. The dividing line between adjacent acini would be the watershed of biliary drainage (i.e., distinct acini empty their biliary secretions into distinct axial bile ducts). The conceptual advantage of the acinus concept is that the blood supply and biliary drainage of a portion of parenchyma reside in the same portal tract, whereas multiple portal vein branches and arteries supply each classic lobule.

The physiologic functions of the liver are performed at the liver cell plate, where interaction between the blood and hepatocytes occurs. The liver cell plates are formed by cords of hepatocytes extending as one-cell-thick plates, 12 to 25 hepatocytes in length, between two vascular structures, the portal tract and the terminal hepatic venule. The liver cell plate receives unidirectional perfusion from the portal tract to the hepatic venule via the hepatic sinusoids. This structural organization allows an orderly interaction between blood and hepatocytes. There is a zonal relationship between the cells that constitute the lobule or acinus and their blood supply (see Fig. 39-6). Periportal hepatocytes located close to the terminal vascular branches of the portal vein and hepatic artery are the first to be supplied with oxygen and nutrients (zone 1). The perivenular (centrilobular) area, which is most distant from these terminal vascular branches, has the least resistance to metabolic and anoxic damage (zone 3). The intermediate area is termed zone 2. The oxygen content and nutritive value of the blood progressively decreases as blood flows from zone 1 to zone 3.

The sequential perfusion of hepatocytes in the liver cell plate allows a progressive qualitative and quantitative modification of the composition of sinusoidal blood as it traverses the liver. There are ultrastructural differences between hepatocytes located in zones 1 and 3, and these hepatocytes attain different functional capabilities. Hepatocytes in zone 1 contain numerous large mitochondria and have the highest concentrations of Krebs cycle enzymes. These cells are adapted for high oxidative activities such as gluconeogenesis, beta-oxidation of fatty acids, amino acid catabolism, ureagenesis, cholesterol synthesis, and bile acid secretion. Zone 3 hepatocytes are relatively anaerobic. Smooth endoplasmic reticulum is more abundant in these cells. Zone 3 is a primary site for glycolysis and lipogenesis. It is also the site for general detoxification and biotransformation of drugs, chemicals, and toxins. The anaerobic milieu of zone 3, however, is also its Achilles heel because these cells are exquisitely susceptible to injury from systemic hypoperfusion and hypoxemia. Sharply defined zone 3 necrosis is also characteristic of injury resulting from accumulation of toxic products of biotransformation as seen in toxicity from acetaminophen and halothane.

Innervation of the Liver

The liver is predominantly innervated by two plexuses that enter at the hilum and supply both sympathetic and parasympathetic nerve fibers. The anterior plexus surrounds the hepatic artery and is composed of postganglionic sympathetic fibers from the celiac ganglia and parasympathetic fibers from the anterior vagus nerve. The posterior plexus surrounds the portal vein and bile duct, and is formed from branches of the right celiac ganglia and posterior vagus. Sympathetic nerve fibers predominate and form a rich perivascular plexus around large hilar blood vessels, and follow these vessels to each lobule to reach the sinusoids and hepatocytes. Stimulation of the sympathetic fibers alters hemodynamics and metabolism of the liver. Hepatic vascular resistance increases and blood volume decreases, whereas glycogenolysis and gluconeogenesis increase, producing an increase in the blood glucose concentration. Parasympathetic stimulation increases glucose uptake and glycogen synthesis.

Hepatic Lymphatic System

The site of hepatic lymph formation is uncertain, but the most accepted hypothesis is that lymph is formed by filtration of plasma through the sinusoids into the perisinusoidal space of

Disse. This lymph travels through the periportal space of Mall (between the limiting plate and portal connective tissue), permeates the connective tissue, and drains into the lymphatic vessels of the portal canal. About 80% of hepatic lymph then travels through a rich plexus of lymphatic channels that surround the hepatic arteries, portal vein, and bile ducts until converging to form 12 to 15 lymph vessels that exit the porta hepatis and ultimately drain into the thoracic duct. The remaining 20% of hepatic lymph either leaves the liver through lymphatic vessels that accompany the hepatic veins to the IVC, or drain via lymphatic trunks within the coronary, triangular, and falciform ligaments that pierce the diaphragm and anastomose with esophageal and retrosternal lymph nodes. Portal hypertension and increased hepatic venous pressure can markedly increase hepatic lymph flow and lead to transudation through the hepatic capsule into the peritoneal cavity, producing ascites.

REGULATION OF HEPATIC BLOOD FLOW

Blood flow and oxygen supply to the liver are regulated to fulfill two separate demands. The first is to supply the liver itself with necessary energy substrates and oxygen for its own maintenance needs. The second is from the rest of the body, for which the liver provides vital services. Although the liver as a whole receives 25% of the cardiac output, regional blood flow within the organ is such that certain areas are highly prone to ischemia. The hepatic circulation is regulated by both intrinsic (regional microvascular) and extrinsic (neural and hormonal) mechanisms.[5]

Intrinsic Circulatory Regulation

The liver lacks the ability to directly regulate portal venous flow; therefore, regional microvascular regulatory mechanisms must operate almost exclusively by modulating hepatic arteriolar tone. The primary mechanism by which this occurs is called the hepatic arterial buffer response, whereby hepatic arterial flow varies reciprocally with changes in portal venous flow. This response is limited, however, to a 50% reduction of portal venous flow and a corresponding twofold increase
1 in hepatic artery flow. Fortunately, because the hepatic artery carries higher oxygen content, this is an effective mechanism for protecting the liver from ischemic insults.

The hepatic buffer response appears to be mediated via adenosine. Presumably, this potent arteriolar dilator is synthesized at a constant rate and continuously secreted in the vicinity of the terminal hepatic arterioles and portal venules.[5] As flow through the portal vein decreases, less of the perivascular adenosine is "washed out," leading to its accumulation around hepatic arterioles. The result is increased arteriolar dilatation and an increase in hepatic arterial flow. Conversely, an increase in portal vein flow decreases the periarteriolar adenosine, leading to a corresponding decrease in hepatic artery flow.

The hepatic arterial system undergoes flow autoregulation when the liver is very active metabolically (postprandial), but not during the fasted state. The metabolic state modifies the composition of portal venous and systemic blood, thereby influencing hepatic blood flow. Decreases in pH and O_2 content, or increases in $P\text{CO}_2$ of the portal blood promote increases of hepatic arterial flow.[6] Postprandial hypersomolarity can increase both hepatic arterial and portal venous blood flow, but this effect would not be relevant in fasted patients. Thus, hepatic flow autoregulation is not likely to be an important mechanism during most anesthetics, given that they are performed in fasted patients.

Extrinsic Circulatory Regulation

Extrinsic factors regulate blood flow through the portal vein indirectly by modulating the tone of arterioles in the preportal splanchnic organs. Portal venous pressure (normally 7 to 10 mm Hg), therefore, reflects both splanchnic arteriolar tone and intrahepatic resistance to flow. Portal venules (presinusoidal sphincters) affect the distribution of blood flow to the sinusoids; however, the hepatic venules (postsinusoidal sphincters) control venous resistance in the liver. Extrinsic mechanisms modulate this postsinusoidal tone, with the sympathetic nervous system as the primary physiologic regulator. Stimulation of α_1-adrenergic receptors increases vascular tone, leading to constriction and a reduction in both blood flow and blood volume in the sinusoids.

Hepatic arteriolar tone is the main determinant of resistance in the hepatic arterial tree. Blood flow through the liver decreases with stimulation of certain arteriolar receptors (α_1-adrenergic and type 1 dopaminergic) and increases with activation of others (β_2-adrenergic).

Humoral Regulators

Myriad humoral substances alter liver blood flow, including gastrin, glucagon, secretin, bile salts, angiotensin II, vasopressin, and catecholamines. In addition, during inflammatory or septic states, cytokines, interleukins, and other inflammatory mediators have been implicated in the alteration of normal splanchnic and hepatic blood flow. Of the systemic hormones, epinephrine is most likely to attain concentrations producing vasoactive effects. Both α-adrenergic and β-adrenergic receptors exist in the hepatic arterial bed, whereas the portal vasculature has only α receptors. An injection of epinephrine directly into the hepatic artery causes vasoconstriction (α_1-adrenergic effect), followed by vasodilitation (β_2-adrenergic effect). When injected into the portal vein, epinephrine produces only vasoconstriction. During activation of the sympathetic nervous system, the hepatic circulatory effects of epinephrine and norepinephrine far exceed those of dopamine, which probably has little if any importance as a physiologic modulator of the hepatic circulation. Glucagon induces a graded, long-lasting dilation of hepatic arterioles; it also antagonizes arterial constrictor responses to a wide range of physiologic stimuli, including stress-induced sympathoadrenal outflow. Angiotensin II markedly constricts both hepatic arterial and portal beds, and significantly reduces mesenteric outflow; the result is a substantial decrease in total hepatic blood flow. Vasopressin also intensely constricts splanchnic vessels, markedly reducing flow into the portal vein. This action accounts for the efficacy of high-dose vasopressin (0.2 to 0.4 U/minute intravenously) to alleviate portal hypertension and decrease bleeding from esophageal varices. The splanchnic and hepatic effects of low-dose (0.02 to 0.04 U/minute intravenously) vasopressin for endogenous vasopressin deficiency replacement therapy in sepsis remain controversial. Animal studies document splanchnic vasoconstriction and increases in lactate; however, human studies, although supporting positive renal effects, have documented inconsistent benefits on splanchnic perfusion and hepatic function.[7,8]

MAJOR PHYSIOLOGIC FUNCTIONS OF THE LIVER

Blood Reservoir

The liver is a vital reservoir of blood in humans. It contains nearly 25 to 30 mL of blood per 100 g of tissue, which represents 10 to 15% of the total blood volume. The autonomic innervation of the liver, coupled with neurohumoral input from the systemic circulation, allows for rapid, precise control of the reservoir volume. Intense sympathetic nervous system stimulation (e.g., pain, hypoxia, hypercarbia) abruptly decreases hepatic blood flow and blood volume; 80% of the hepatic blood volume (approximately 400 to 500 mL) can be expelled within a matter of seconds.

Anesthetics that suppress sympathetic nervous system outflow impair this reservoir function and predispose the patient to circulatory decompensation when significant decreases of intravascular volume occur without immediate replacement. Severe liver disease exacerbates the hypotensive effects of hypovolemia by impairing vasoconstrictor responses to catecholamines. A total failure of vasoconstriction not only incapacitates the splanchnic reservoir, but also prevents the redirection of blood flow from skeletal muscle beds and splanchnic tissues to the heart and brain.

Regulator of Blood Coagulation

The liver helps maintain normal blood clotting in numerous ways. It is responsible for the synthesis of factors involved in coagulation, anticoagulation, and fibrinolysis. All procoagulation factors derive from the liver, with the exception of the endothelial product, Von Willebrand factor (VIIIvWF). Although factor VIII clotting factor is produced mostly by hepatocytes, it is also produced in endothelial cells, and adequate functional levels of this factor are often present in patients with liver disease. Precursor proteins for vitamin K-dependent coagulation are synthesized in the liver. Vitamin K catalyzes the activation of these factors (II, VII, IX, and X). Vitamin K_1 absorption depends on bile secretion into the gastrointestinal tract and transformation to active vitamin K_2 by the action of gut bacteria. Vitamin K deficiency results in the production of nonfunctional factors II, VII, IX, and X. The liver also modulates platelet production through the synthesis of thrombopoietin.

The liver synthesizes anticoagulant factors such as antithrombin III, proteins C and S, and fibrinolytic factors. The liver is also responsible for clearance of activated coagulation factors, fibrinolysins, and tissue plasminogen activators. Appropriate clearance of these activated factors is essential for prevention or control of fibrinolytic states.

Endocrine Organ

The liver has important endocrine functions. It synthesizes and secretes essential hormones, including insulin-like growth factor-1 (IGF-1), angiotensinogen, and thrombopoietin. IGF-1, formerly called somatomedin, mediates the peripheral actions of hormones produced by other endocrine glands. Angiotensinogen is a precursor of angiotensin II, playing a major role in the regulation of fluid and electrolyte balance. Thrombopoietin stimulates bone marrow precursor cells to differentiate into platelet-generating megakaryocytes.

The liver is also a principal site of hormone biotransformation and catabolism. Thyroxine (T_4) is actively taken up by the liver, where it is converted to tri-iodothyronine (T_3). In addition, the liver synthesizes thyroid-binding globulin. Thus, the liver can influence the distribution of thyroid hormones between intracellular and extracellular compartments. Corticosteroids, aldosterone, estrogen, androgens, insulin, and antidiuretic hormone are all inactivated by the liver. The interaction of altered hormone levels and diminished hepatic synthesis of hormone-binding globulins with altered metabolism and receptor regulation leads to significant endocrine abnormalities in patients with liver disease.

Erythrocyte Breakdown and Bilirubin Excretion

Bilirubin is an end product of heme degradation. About 300 mg is formed daily, with approximately 75% of bilirubin precursors derived from breakdown of the heme moiety of hemoglobin from senescent erythrocytes by the reticuloendothelial system, and the remainder from breakdown of nonerythrocytic hemoproteins, including cytochrome P450. After reticuloendothelial cells phagocytize senescent erythrocytes and separate the protein portion of hemoglobin from the heme moiety, the heme is oxidized by the microsomal heme oxygenase system to biliverdin. Biliverdin is then rapidly converted to unconjugated bilirubin, which is then released into the bloodstream, where it avidly binds to albumin while being transported to the liver. The albumin–bilirubin complex passes through fenestrations in the sinusoidal-lining cells to enter into the space of Disse where direct contact with the hepatocyte plasma membrane occurs. Binding proteins on the plasma membrane dissociate the unconjugated bilirubin from albumin before uptake into the hepatocyte where the bilirubin binds to cytoplasmic protein and is transported to the endoplasmic reticulum. The bilirubin is then conjugated with carbohydrate moieties, especially glucuronic acid. This reaction is catalyzed by the enzyme uridine diphosphate-glucuronyl transferase; this water-soluble conjugated bilirubin is actively excreted into bile canaliculi, and only a small portion enters the plasma. Conjugated bilirubin passes unchanged through the biliary tree and proximal small intestine. In the terminal ileum and large intestine, bacteria convert most of the conjugated bilirubin to urobilinogen. The intestinal mucosa reabsorbs some urobilinogen, which reaches the liver by mesenteric blood. The liver efficiently extracts the urobilinogen and returns it to the intestine (enterohepatic circulation). Eighty percent of urobilinogens are excreted in the stool. Ten percent is excreted in the urine, and the rest is reabsorbed.

The liver also scavenges free hemoglobin from blood, helping conserve body iron. It synthesizes haptoglobin, which forms complexes with dimers of free intravascular hemoglobin. Receptors on hepatocytes remove these complexes from plasma and thereby prevent the loss of hemoglobin dimers in the urine.

Metabolic Functions of the Liver

Receiving blood from the intestine through the portal vein, the liver is ideally positioned to play a major role in the regulation of carbohydrate, protein, and lipid metabolism. The liver is also the major site for catabolism of various hormones involved in regulating metabolism, including insulin, glucagon, glucocorticoids, thyroxin, and growth hormone.

Carbohydrate Metabolism

The liver plays an important role in maintaining euglycemia. The normal liver receives the dietary carbohydrate intake through the portal circulation. Following a carbohydrate-containing meal, hyperglycemia is prevented by insulin-mediated hepatic extraction of glucose from the portal blood. Excess glucose in the liver is converted to glycogen. The liver can maximally store approximately 75 g of glycogen, which, when broken down, can provide up to 24 hours of available glucose. During fasting, hypoglycemia is initially prevented by glucagon-mediated glycogenolysis: glycogen stores are rapidly mobilized and converted to glucose, which is released into the circulation.

Once glycogen stores are depleted, the continued production of glucose requires muscle catabolism to provide the liver with amino acids. Through the process of gluconeogenesis, certain amino acids (e.g., alanine) undergo oxidative deamination and are converted to glucose. More limited amounts of glucose may be formed by conversion from lactate and glycerol. In patients with chronic liver disease, hyperglycemia occurs commonly because portosystemic shunting allows direct entry of glucose-rich portal venous blood into the systemic circulation. Hypoglycemia is a late manifestation of advanced liver disease, and when present, a variety of mechanisms may be involved, including impaired glycogen storage, glycogenolysis, and gluconeogenesis. Hypoglycemia may also be seen in patients with large hepatocellular carcinomas secondary to increased glucose uptake by the tumor.

Lipid Metabolism

The liver is the major site of synthesis of fatty acids from excess sugar, protein, and lipid. Fatty acids in the liver are esterified to form triglycerides, cholesterol esters, and phospholipids, and are incorporated into lipoproteins for transport to storage sites in adipocytes. Fatty acids are vital for cellular function because they represent a major energy source for heart and skeletal muscle. Cholesterol is an essential constituent of biological membranes and an important precursor of steroid hormones, vitamins, and bile acids. The body pool of cholesterol in the adult is kept fairly constant by balancing absorption and endogenous synthesis with metabolism and excretion. The liver plays a central role in cholesterol and lipoprotein metabolism. It regulates uptake and excretion of cholesterol and synthesizes the various enzymes and apoproteins needed for cholesterol transport. Biliary secretion of cholesterol and its degradation product, bile acid, represents the major mechanism for elimination of cholesterol from the body.

In the fasted state, fatty acid beta-oxidation to acetylcoenzyme A (acetyl-CoA) in the liver is markedly stimulated by increased glucagon secretion. Acetyl-CoA is further oxidized to carbon dioxide and water or converted to ketone bodies, which are important fuels for extrahepatic organs (e.g., brain, muscle, kidney). Liver dysfunction may result in significant disturbances of cholesterol and lipoprotein metabolism.

Amino Acid Metabolism

The liver is the major site of protein and amino acid metabolism. After ingestion of protein, proteolytic enzymes in the digestive tract efficiently hydrolyze ingested proteins, yielding free amino acids that are absorbed by the gut and transported to the liver via the portal vein. Several distinct sinusoidal membrane transport systems then convey the amino acids into the hepatocyte. When necessary, the liver is able to synthesize the nonessential amino acids and use them to synthesize a large number of biologically essential proteins.

Protein catabolism occurs primarily in the liver. Proteins enter the hepatocyte through endocytosis and are then degraded into their component amino acids in the lysosomes. These may then form substrates for glucose production through gluconeogenesis, enter lipid metabolic pathways, or be further catabolized via transamination and deamination to form keto-acids, ammonia (NH_3), and glutamine. The urea cycle converts ammonia and most other nitrogenous excretory products into urea, which is excreted by the kidney. Patients with significant liver dysfunction may not have the capacity to eliminate nitrogen equivalents adequately through the urea cycle. Consequently, the serum ammonia level rises and hepatic encephalopathy may develop. Because urea is synthesized in the liver, a normal or low blood urea nitrogen concentration in patients with advanced liver disease provides no assurance that glomerular filtration rate (GFR) is normal.

Synthesis of Important Proteins

The liver produces a vast assortment of proteins with important extrahepatic functions. Hepatocytes synthesize albumin; acute-phase proteins; all the coagulation factors and their inhibitors, except for factor VIII; ceruloplasmin; and most of the alpha-globulins and beta-globulins. Albumin accounts for nearly 10% of the protein synthesized by the liver. It constitutes about 60% of total plasma protein and is the primary determinant of the colloid oncotic pressure. Approximately 40% of the total exchangeable albumin pool is located intravascularly, and its serum half-life is about 20 days. This long half-life is one reason why the serum albumin level is not a reliable indicator of the liver's residual synthetic capacity in acute hepatic disease. The serum albumin level is affected by disturbances in synthesis, catabolism, and distribution. The normal liver synthesizes albumin at a rate of approximately 200 g/kg per day. Synthesis may be affected by several factors, including liver disease, dietary availability of amino acids, hormonal balance, plasma oncotic pressure, and heavy alcohol intake. Albumin serves as an important transport vehicle for metabolites (e.g., unconjugated bilirubin, heme, fatty acids), hormones (e.g., thyroxine, cortisol), and metals. Albumin also binds to a variety of pharmacologic agents; therefore, hypoalbuminemia has important consequences for the pharmacokinetics and pharmacodynamics of commonly administered drugs.

Immunologic Function

The liver is the largest organ in the reticuloendothelial system. Sinusoidal and perisinusoidal cells of the liver defend the body against microbial invaders and modulate inflammatory and immune responses to foreign materials. Pit cells, sparsely located in the perisinusoidal spaces, possess natural killer and neuroendocrine activities. Kupffer cells may constitute up to 10% of the total hepatic mass. These tissue macrophages police sinusoidal blood flow, filtering out toxins, bacteria, and debris that gain access from the gastrointestinal tract. They are aggressively involved in immune surveillance, participating in phagocytosis, cytolysis, and antigen presentation to T cells, and also may be involved in regulation of T-cell proliferation. Kupffer cells produce a variety of inflammatory mediators and cytokines that initiate and modulate both local and systemic effects of hepatic injury. Impairment of Kupffer cell function may be an important harbinger of sepsis or multiorgan system failure, particularly in the setting of severe gastrointestinal pathology or splanchnic ischemia.

Pharmacokinetics

Drug metabolism is primarily a hepatic event. The liver influences the plasma concentration and systemic availability of most orally and parenterally administered drugs. Through its synthesis of drug-binding proteins, the liver affects the partitioning of drugs into the various compartments of the body (apparent volume of distribution, V_d). Plasma proteins, especially albumin and α_1-acid glycoprotein, act as sinks to decrease free drug concentrations. Consequently, changes in the concentration of plasma proteins often modify dose–response relationships of drugs.

Hepatic clearance is the sum of all processes by which the liver eliminates a drug from the body. Hepatic biotransformation refers to the metabolism of drugs by hepatocytes with the goal of changing them into inactive water-soluble substances that can be excreted into the bile or urine for elimination from the body. A series of reactions that have been classified as phase

1 and phase 2 participate in these processes. Most drugs contain lipophilic functional groups to facilitate penetration of membrane barriers, thereby expediting gastrointestinal absorption. These same lipophilic groups inhibit excretion, owing to a high degree of protein binding and renal tubular reabsorption. By converting lipophilic substances to metabolites that can be excreted, hepatic enzymes detoxify drugs and terminate their pharmacologic activity. In general, phase 1 reactions (oxidation, reduction, *N*–dealkylation) modify structural features of drugs to render them more polar than the original compound. Most phase I reactions involve the participation of a group of cytochrome P450 isozymes, which are localized in the hepatic microsomes. In phase 2 reactions, catalyzed by transferase enzymes, the water solubility of the product is enhanced beyond that achieved by phase 1 reactions alone. The chemical groups generated by phase 1 reactions serve as receptors for conjugation with polar substances such as sulfate, glucuronic acid, and glutathione. The products of phase 2 reactions are usually less toxic and less biologically active than those of the parent compound. Phase 1 reactions are much more susceptible to inhibition by advanced age or hepatic diseases than are phase 2 reactions.

The ability of the liver to metabolize a drug is referred to as its intrinsic metabolic clearance.[9] Intrinsic clearance, which reflects the fraction of the delivered drug load that is metabolized or extracted during a single pass through the liver, provides the basis for classifying drugs as high-, intermediate-, or low-clearance compounds. High-clearance drugs (e.g., lidocaine, diphenhydramine, or metoprolol) are so efficiently metabolized that their hepatic clearance approaches the rates at which they traverse the liver (i.e., total hepatic blood flow) (Fig. 39-7). Therefore, hepatic blood flow determines the liver's ability to eliminate high-clearance drugs. Low-clearance drugs (e.g., diazepam), however, are metabolized at rates that are usually far below their flow rates through the liver; therefore, their hepatic clearances are relatively independent of hepatic blood flow (see Fig. 39-7). Factors that increase the free fraction of drugs (e.g., hypoalbuminemia) are much more consequential for low-extraction than high-extraction drugs. The clearance of low-extraction drugs increases almost linearly as the free fraction increases (Fig. 39-8). Patients with significant liver disease may have marked alterations of pharmacokinetics and pharmacodynamics. Portosystemic shunts allow orally administered drugs to bypass the liver, thereby reducing first-pass clearance. This and the reduction in total hepatic blood flow seen in patients with liver disease prolong the terminal half-life and increases the systemic effects of high-extraction drugs. The dosage of these agents should be reduced by as much as 50%. Hypoalbuminemia causes an increase in the free plasma drug concentration, not only increasing drug effects, but also facilitating elimination of compounds with low hepatic extraction ratios. The volume of distribution of some drugs will be increased in patients with hypoalbuminemia and ascites.

The complex and poorly quantifiable effects of hepatic dysfunction on drug disposition may render pharmacokinetic, and even pharmacodynamic, predictions precarious. The rational selection of medications for patients with severe liver dysfunction mandates a careful risk–benefit analysis that integrates both pharmacodynamic and pharmacokinetic concerns. At times, cirrhotic patients with coexisting diseases will be better served by use of a hepatically cleared agent (superior efficacy, fewer untoward effects) than by one whose clearance is primarily extrahepatic. In such cases, careful titration of medication is imperative to achieve the desired pharmacologic responses with minimal adverse effects.

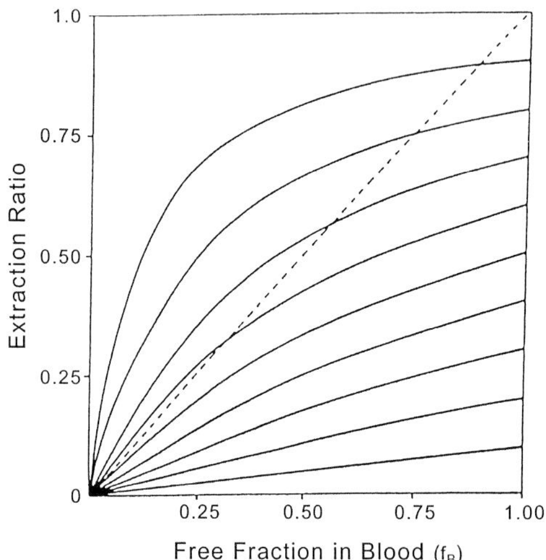

FIGURE 39-8. Relationship between hepatic extraction and fraction of unbound drug in blood: increasing free fraction (more unbound drug) usually produces increased extraction. This phenomenon is of greater importance for low-extraction drugs (with almost a direct linear change in extraction ratio with increasing free fraction) than for high-extraction drugs because the latter are almost completely cleared, regardless of extent of binding (nonrestrictive binding). The hepatic clearance (CL) reflects the changes in extraction ratio (E) if blood flow (Q) is constant ($CL = Q \cdot E$). (Reprinted with permission from Wilkinson GR, Shand DG: A physiological approach to hepatic drug clearance. Clin Pharmacol Ther 18:377, 1975.)

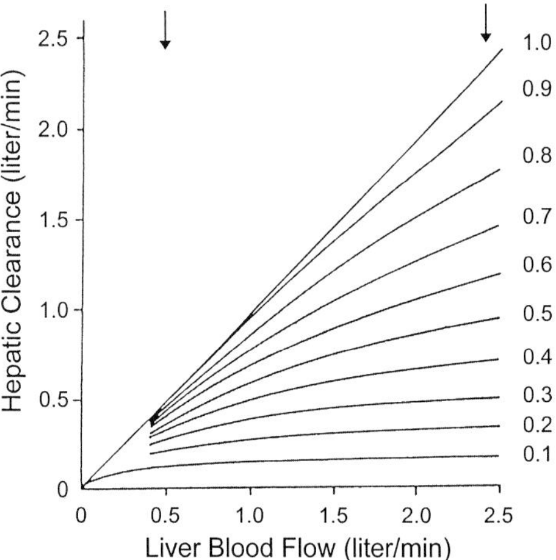

FIGURE 39-7. Relationship between hepatic clearance (*ordinate, on left*) and liver blood flow (*abscissa*) as determined by the extraction ratios (ERs) of the drug (*ordinate, on right*). Hepatic clearances of compounds with low extraction ratios are nearly independent of liver blood flow, whereas the clearances of compounds with high extraction ratios vary almost directly with changes in hepatic blood flow. The *arrows* indicate the normal physiologic range of liver blood flow. (Reprinted with permission from Wilkinson GR, Shand DG: A physiological approach to hepatic drug clearance. Clin Pharmacol Ther 18:377, 1975.)

ASSESSMENT OF HEPATIC FUNCTION

Laboratory Evaluation of Hepatic Function

A broad array of biochemical tests is available to assess the multiple functions of the liver and evaluate patients with suspected or established liver disease (Table 39-1).[10] Although

TABLE 39-1

BLOOD TESTS AND THE DIFFERENTIAL DIAGNOSIS OF HEPATIC DYSFUNCTION

	■ BILIRUBIN OVERLOAD (HEMOLYSIS)	■ PARENCHYMAL DYSFUNCTION	■ CHOLESTASIS
Aminotransferases	Normal	Increased (may be normal or decreased in advanced stages)	Normal (may be increased in advanced stages)
Alkaline phosphatase	Normal	Normal	Increased
Bilirubin	Unconjugated	Conjugated	Conjugated
Serum proteins	Normal	Decreased	Normal (may be decreased in advanced stages)
Prothrombin time	Normal	Decreased (may be normal in early stages)	Normal (may be prolonged in advanced stages)
Blood urea nitrogen	Normal	Normal (may be decreased in advanced stages)	Normal
Sulfobromophthalein/indocyanine green	Normal	Retention	Normal or retention

From Gelman S: Anesthesia and the liver. In Barash P, Cullen B, Stoelting, R (eds): Clinical Anesthesia, 3rd ed, p 1011. Philadelphia, Lippincott-Raven, 1997.

collectively called "liver function tests" (LFTs), many (e.g., aspartate aminotransferase [AST] and alanine aminotransferase [ALT]) do not assess a function of the liver but rather are indicative of liver cell injury or dysfunction. LFTs are used to screen for the presence of liver disease, suggest a general category of disease as the etiology, assess prognosis, and monitor the effectiveness of therapy. Many of the routine tests are not specific for liver disease; however, when combined in a battery of tests, the sensitivity and specificity for liver disease is high.

LFTs can be classified into several broad categories. These include tests that reflect (1) hepatocellular damage; (2) obstructed bile flow; (3) hepatic synthetic function; (4) hepatic uptake, conjugation, and excretion; and (5) other aspects of liver function.

Indices of Hepatocellular Damage

Increased serum activities of AST (formerly, serum glutamic oxalacetic transaminase or SGOT) and ALT (formerly, serum glutamic pyruvic transaminase or SGPT) are detected when there is hepatocellular injury and necrosis. Serum levels of AST and ALT are elevated in almost all types of hepatic disease. ALT is localized primarily to the liver, whereas AST is present in a wide variety of tissues, including liver, heart, skeletal muscle, kidney, and brain. An isolated elevation of the AST level is typically seen in cardiac or muscle disease. Mild elevations of ALT and AST (less than 3-fold) are seen in fatty liver, nonalcoholic steatohepatitis, drug toxicity, and chronic viral hepatitis. Larger increases (3- to 22-fold) are seen in patients with acute hepatitis or exacerbation of chronic hepatitis (alcoholic hepatitis). The highest concentrations are seen in drug-induced or toxin-induced hepatocellular necrosis (including anesthetics), severe viral hepatitis, and ischemic hepatitis complicating circulatory shock.

AST and ALT levels do not correlate with prognosis. A declining level may reflect either recovery from injury or a poor prognosis because of a paucity of surviving hepatocytes. The serum AST/ALT ratio may be helpful diagnostically. A ratio of >2 is characteristically found in alcoholic liver disease, while in viral hepatitis the ratio is typically <1.

Lactate dehydrogenase (LDH) is usually included in liver biochemistry panels. Markedly increased serum levels may be seen in hepatocellular necrosis, shock liver, or hemolysis associated with liver disease. However, LDH has poor diagnostic specificity for liver disease and even measurement of LDH isoenzymes has limited clinical usefulness.

Glutathione S-transferase (GST) is found in multiple organs, but plasma elevation of isoenzyme B is a sensitive indicator of liver damage. GST is rapidly released into the circulation following hepatic injury, and because of its short plasma half-life (90 minutes), monitoring of plasma GST concentrations permits rapid identification of continuing or resolving cellular damage. GST is most abundant in centrolobular (zone 3) hepatocytes, which are most susceptible to injuries from circulatory disturbances and toxic products of drug metabolism.[11] Following such injuries, GST elevations may be disproportionately greater than increases of serum transaminases, which are more highly localized to the periportal (zone 1) hepatocytes.

Indices of Obstructed Bile Flow

Alkaline phosphatase (AP) is a family of isoenzymes found in multiple organs, including the liver, bone, kidney, intestines, placenta, and leukocytes. In healthy individuals, most circulating AP originates from the liver or bone. In the liver, AP is concentrated in the microvilli of the bile canaliculi and the sinusoidal surface of hepatocytes. Elevations of serum AP disproportionate to changes of AST and ALT occur with intrahepatic or extrahepatic obstruction to bile flow. It is a highly sensitive test for assessing the integrity of the biliary system. Elevated serum levels of AP may also result from infiltrative liver diseases such as metastatic cancer. Mildly elevated levels of serum AP are nonspecific and may be seen in cirrhosis, hepatitis, or congestive heart failure. The liver is the source of an elevated AP in the majority of cases, but in up to one-third, no evidence of liver disease is found. During pregnancy, AP can nearly double from placental release of the enzyme.

5′-Nucleotidase (5′NT) is an alkaline phosphatase that degrades specific nucleotides. Although it is present in most human tissues, elevated serum levels are believed to be solely of hepatobiliary origin and may reflect the detergent action of bile salts on plasma membranes, which is needed for release of the enzyme into the circulation. 5′NT is markedly increased with intrahepatic or extrahepatic biliary obstruction, with more modest increases seen with other hepatocellular

TABLE 39-2

CAUSES OF HYPERBILIRUBINEMIA

■ UNCONJUGATED (INDIRECT)

Excessive bilirubin production (hemolysis)
Immaturity of enzyme systems
  Physiologic jaundice of newborn
  Jaundice of prematurity
Inherited defects
  Gilbert's syndrome
  Crigler-Najjar syndrome
Drug effects

■ CONJUGATED (DIRECT)

Hepatocellular disease (hepatitis, cirrhosis, drugs)
Intrahepatic cholestasis (drugs, pregnancy)
Benign postoperative jaundice, sepsis
Congenital conjugated hyperbilirubinemia
  Dubin-Johnson syndrome
  Rotor's syndrome
Obstructive jaundice
  Extrahepatic (calculus, stricture, neoplasm)
  Intrahepatic (sclerosing cholangitis, neoplasm, primary biliary cirrhosis)

From Friedman L, Martin P, Munoz S: Liver function tests and the objective evaluation of the patient with liver disease. In Zakim D, Boyer T (eds): Hepatology: A Textbook of Liver Disease, 3rd ed, p 791. Philadelphia, WB Saunders, 1996, with permission.

disorders. Serum levels correlate closely with AP levels, and because serum 5′NT is so specific for liver diseases, it is used to determine if an elevated serum AP level is of hepatic origin.

Gamma glutamyl transferase (GGT) is a membrane-bound enzyme widely distributed in a variety of tissues, including the liver. It is found in high concentrations in epithelial cells lining biliary ductules. Serum GGT is the most sensitive laboratory indicator of biliary tract disease. However, because it is ubiquitous, an elevated GGT has limited usefulness due to its poor specificity and has largely been replaced by 5′NT measurements to determine if an elevated AP is of hepatic origin.

Bilirubin is an endogenous organic anion derived primarily from the degradation of hemoglobin released from aging red blood cells. Measurement of serum bilirubin levels is central to the evaluation of hepatobiliary disorders. Serum levels of bilirubin are determined by the van den Bergh reaction, which separates bilirubin into two fractions: a water-soluble direct-reacting form representing conjugated bilirubin and a lipid-soluble indirect-reacting form representing unconjugated bilirubin.

Serum bilirubin levels are measured to confirm the severity of jaundice and to determine the extent of its conjugation. Hyperbilirubinemia has a wide variety of causes (Table 39-2) and is classified as either predominantly unconjugated or predominantly conjugated. Serum concentrations of unconjugated bilirubin between 1 and 4 mg/dL usually indicate a disorder of bilirubin metabolism, such as excessive production (hemolysis), impaired transport into hepatocytes, or defective conjugation by hepatocytes. Even in cases of severe hemolysis, the total serum bilirubin is rarely above 5 mg/dL in the presence of normal liver function. Serum bilirubin levels above 5 mg/dL, or lower levels in association with other LFT abnormalities, usually signify the presence of liver disease. Conjugated hyperbilirubinemia results from impaired intrahepatic excretion of bilirubin or extrahepatic obstruction. With complete biliary tract obstruction, the maximal serum bilirubin level will rarely exceed 35 mg/dL due to renal excretion of conjugated bilirubin. Therefore, total bilirubin levels above 35 mg/dL usually signify severe parenchymal liver disease in association with hemolysis or renal failure.

Indices of Hepatic Synthetic Function

The liver synthesizes and releases a variety of proteins, including albumin and the coagulation factors. Measurement of serum albumin level and assays of coagulation function are the most widely used methods for assessing hepatic synthetic function. Proper interpretation of these tests requires an understanding of the patient's clinical status. Many factors influence the serum albumin level independent of hepatic synthesis. Protein-losing enteropathy, burns, nephrotic syndrome, increased vascular permeability, nutritional deficiency, increased catabolism, and fluid retention can all depress serum albumin levels. A decreasing serum albumin concentration indicates worsening hepatic function in patients with chronic liver disease if none of these other factors is present. Because the half-life in serum is as long as 20 days, the serum albumin level is not a reliable indicator of hepatic protein synthesis in acute liver disease.

In contrast, the prothrombin time (PT) and international normalized ratio (INR) are sensitive indicators of severe hepatic dysfunction (whether patients have acute or chronic liver disease) because of the short half-life of factor VII. However, because most of the coagulation factors are present in quantities that far exceed requirements for normal coagulation, mild-to-moderate hepatic disease may not be detected by measurement of the PT. In acute or chronic hepatocellular disease, the PT may be a useful prognostic indicator. A progressively increasing PT is usually ominous in patients with acute hepatocellular disease, suggesting an increased likelihood of acute hepatic failure. Prolongation of the PT also suggests a poor long-term prognosis in chronic liver disease.

PT depends on normal hepatic synthesis of clotting factors and sufficient uptake of vitamin K. Absorption of vitamin K from the gastrointestinal tract requires adequate biliary secretion of bile salts. In patients with obstructive jaundice, a prolonged PT may be a manifestation of vitamin K deficiency rather than of impaired hepatic synthetic function. Prolongation of the PT is not specific for liver disease. It may result from congenital coagulation factor deficiencies, disseminated intravascular coagulopathy, vitamin K deficiency, or the use of drugs that antagonize the prothrombin complex, such as Coumadin.

Indices of Hepatic Blood Flow and Metabolic Capacity

Elimination of the dye indocyanine green (ICG) from the blood provides an estimate of hepatic perfusion and hepatocellular function because it is highly extracted (70 to 95% by the liver following an intravenous injection). Acute changes in hepatic circulation and function can be detected by this test and the ICG method has been a standard technique for comparing effects of various anesthetics on hepatic blood flow.

Hepatic function can also be assessed with substances that are metabolized selectively by the liver. Lidocaine is metabolized by oxidative N-demethylation to monoethylglycinexylidide (MEGX). Its concentration 15 to 30 minutes after intravenous injection of a single dose of lidocaine can be used as a quantitative measure of liver function. The MEGX test may have prognostic value in patients with end-stage liver disease; in one study of well-compensated cirrhotic patients, this test was able to identify patients at increased risk for developing postoperative complications following hepatic resection for carcinoma.[12]

Additional metabolic tests for assessing hepatic function include antipyrine clearance from plasma, aminopyrine breath test, caffeine breath test, galactose elimination capacity, and the maximum rate of urea synthesis. These tests have not gained wide acceptance in the United States, and their precise role in clinical practice remains uncertain.

Miscellaneous Tests

Several other laboratory tests are available for the diagnosis of liver disease but provide no specific information about hepatic function. These include specific serologic tests for hepatitis viruses, autoantibody measurements useful for the diagnosis of primary biliary cirrhosis and the classification of autoimmune hepatitis; specific protein measurements (ceruloplasmin, ferritin, α1-antitrypsin, and α-fetoprotein) useful for the diagnosis of Wilson's disease; hemochromatosis; α1-antitrypsin deficiency and hepatocellular carcinoma, respectively; and serum ammonia often followed in patients with, or at risk for, developing hepatic encephalopathy.

Hepatobiliary Imaging

Selection of the most appropriate hepatobiliary imaging technique in a patient depends on the clinical presentation (history, physical examination, and LFT results), an understanding of the uses and limitations of each technique, and whether the test is for diagnosis alone or for therapeutic intervention as well.

Plain radiography has a limited role in the evaluation of hepatobiliary disease. Abdominal radiographs can be useful for calcified or gas-containing lesions that may be overlooked or misinterpreted by ultrasonography. These lesions include calcified gallstones, chronic calcific pancreatitis, gas-containing liver abscesses, portal venous gas, and emphysematous cholecystitis.

Ultrasonography is the most commonly used hepatobiliary imaging technique. It has the advantages of low cost, portability, and avoidance of the use of ionizing radiation. Ultrasonography is the primary screening test for hepatic disease, gallstones, and biliary tract disease that may be suspected because of symptoms, abnormal LFT, hepatomegaly, jaundice, or suspicion of a mass lesion. It is the best method for detecting gallstones and confirming the presence of extrahepatic biliary obstruction. It also may be useful for determining the thickness of the gallbladder wall, detecting the presence of ascites, demonstrating portal or hepatic vein thrombosis, evaluating the patency of portosystemic shunts in patients with recurrent variceal bleeding after shunt surgery, and directing thin-needle biopsy of hepatic mass lesions. Its major limitations are its dependence on the operator's skill and its inability to penetrate bone or air (including bowel gas), which may prevent complete examination of the abdominal organs.

A variety of radioisotopes can be used to study the anatomy and function of the liver and biliary system. Radioisotope scanning of the liver seldom provides a precise diagnosis, and these tests have largely been supplanted by ultrasonography and computed tomography (CT) scanning. However, radioisotope scanning of the biliary tract remains an important investigative tool in patients with suspected acute cholecystitis. Radioisotopes that are cleared rapidly by hepatocytes and excreted into bile permit rapid visualization of the biliary tract. Visualization of the gallbladder rules out obstruction of the cystic duct, while visualization of the biliary tree and common bile duct without the gallbladder confirms obstruction of the cystic duct and presence of cholecystitis.

CT is a complementary examination to ultrasonography and provides information on liver texture, gallbladder disease, bile duct dilatation, and mass lesions of the liver and pancreas. It provides better and more complete anatomic definition than ultrasonography and is less operator dependent. Lesions can be biopsied under CT guidance. The disadvantages of CT scanning are radiation exposure and cost.

The role of magnetic resonance imaging (MRI) for the evaluation of hepatobiliary disease is continually evolving. The algorithm for noninvasive biliary imaging has been markedly altered by the development of magnetic resonance cholangiopancreatography, which has dramatically reduced the need for direct cholangiography for visualization of the bile and pancreatic ducts, and for delineating the most proximal extent of biliary tract obstruction when planning for operative resection or drainage.

Percutaneous transhepatic cholangiography (THC) involves the direct percutaneous injection, through a 22-gauge needle, of contrast into bile ducts in the liver under fluoroscopic guidance. THC may be used to determine the level and cause of biliary obstruction, confirm the presence of cholestasis without obstruction, and evaluate whether a proximal cholangiocarcinoma is surgically resectable. THC can be used for balloon dilation of biliary strictures via a catheter inserted through the tract, for placement of an internal stent to relieve obstruction, or for placement of an external drain.

Endoscopic retrograde cholangiopancreatography (ERCP) uses endoscopy to visualize the ampulla of Vater and guide insertion of a guidewire and catheter through the ampulla to permit selective injection of contrast material into the pancreatic and common bile ducts, which are then imaged radiographically. ERCP has the advantage over THC of not requiring dilation of the biliary tree to achieve a very high procedural success rate. ERCP is the imaging technique of choice in patients with choledocholithiasis because a sphincterotomy and stone extraction can often be performed. Stones can also be removed with this technique in patients with acute cholangitis and severe gallstone pancreatitis. ERCP also permits biopsies, brushings, balloon dilation, and stent insertion to relieve biliary obstruction caused by tumors.

Liver Biopsy

Liver biopsy continues to have a central role in the evaluation of patients with suspected liver disease because it provides the only means of determining the precise nature of hepatic damage (necrosis, inflammation, steatosis, or fibrosis). Liver biopsy plays a key role in the evaluation of otherwise unexplained abnormalities of liver enzymes in patients with or without hepatomegaly. It is used in patients with chronic hepatitis to determine the nature and extent of hepatic injury and degree of inflammation, which for patients with chronic hepatitis C, will be used to determine if antiviral therapy should be initiated. Liver biopsy is also an important tool for determining the etiology of abnormal LFT in the post liver transplant patient (see chapter 53). The presence of coagulopathy (e.g., PT that is 3 seconds greater than control, platelet count $<$60,000 cells/μL), however, contraindicates percutaneous liver biopsy, although transjugular liver biopsy can be performed safely in these patients.

HEPATIC AND HEPATOBILIARY DISEASES

Classification of Liver Diseases

For the purposes of the following discussion, liver diseases are divided into two large heterogeneous groups: parenchymal diseases (e.g., viral hepatitis, steatohepatitis, cirrhosis) and cholestatic diseases (e.g., intrahepatic and extrahepatic biliary obstruction). Some diseases are characterized by features of both parenchymal dysfunction and cholestasis.

Prevalence of Hepatobiliary Disease

More than 100 distinct hepatic diseases have been described. Currently, nearly 10% of the American population (25 million) has some form of hepatobiliary disease. Hepatitis B or C afflicts more than 5 million Americans. About 50% of those with hepatitis C may develop cirrhosis, which currently accounts for between 13,000 to 15,000 deaths each year. Alcoholic liver disease remains a problem, becoming severe in 10 to 15% of those who consume large amounts of alcohol over a prolonged period.

PARENCHYMAL DISEASES

Viral Hepatitis

Acute hepatitis usually results from a viral infection, although it may also be caused by drugs and toxins. Viral hepatitides are important causes of perioperative hepatic dysfunction. The diagnosis of viral hepatitis depends on the appearance of clinical signs and symptoms, laboratory findings, serologic assays, and, on occasion, liver biopsy. During the incubation period, patients are often asymptomatic and may undergo surgical procedures. When increased ALT and AST and/or jaundice develop postoperatively, it is essential that a comprehensive serologic evaluation be performed to document the viral origin for the liver damage.

Classic acute hepatitis is caused by one of five viruses: hepatitis A (HAV), hepatitis B (HBV), hepatitis C (HCV), hepatitis D (HDV, delta), and hepatitis E (HEV). In the United States, approximately 50% of reported cases of acute viral hepatitis are caused by HBV, 30% by HAV, and 20% by HCV. Chronic hepatitis can occur following HBV, HCV, and HDV infections. All five types of viral hepatitis have similar clinical and laboratory features. Patients may remain asymptomatic, develop influenza-like symptoms, became jaundiced, or develop acute hepatic failure.

HAV infection (infectious hepatitis) is a highly contagious enterovirus transmitted by the intake of fecal-contaminated food. It is not transmitted by blood transfusion. Viremia is present for several days prior to the onset of clinical symptoms. Virus is shed in stool for 14 to 21 days before the onset of jaundice. Patients are usually not infectious after 21 days. There are no chronic carriers, and chronic liver disease does not occur. Fulminant hepatic failure is rare (0.14 to 2%) in the absence of preexisting liver disease. Patients with HBV who acquire a HAV infection typically have an uncomplicated clinical course. In contrast, 41% of patients with chronic hepatitis C who acquire a HAV superinfection progress to fulminant hepatitis with a 35% fatality rate.[13]

HBV is primarily transmitted through percutaneous inoculation of infected serum or blood products. HBV is present in the serum and body secretions of most patients early in the course of acute hepatitis B. The surface coat of the virus is composed of a polypeptide that acts as the major hepatitis B surface antigen (HBsAg). Development of serum antibodies to HbsAg (anti-HbsAg) confirms immunity. Individuals who have detectable HbsAg for more than 6 months have a chronic HBV infection.

HCV (formerly, non-A, non-B hepatitis), which was discovered in 1989, was the major cause of transfusion-related hepatitis until the 1990s. It is also transmitted by percutaneous inoculation of infected serum or blood products, occupational exposure to blood or blood products, and intravenous drug abuse. Hepatitis C is the most common bloodborne infection in the United States; it accounts for 40% of chronic liver disease. Fortunately, serologic tests for HCV now exist. Because of their use in screening donated blood, HCV has almost been eliminated as a cause of posttransfusion hepatitis. HDV is an RNA strand that coinfects with and requires the helper function of HBV for its replication and expression. HDV may be acquired simultaneously with HBV or may be a superinfection of a patient with prior HBV infection. HBV and HDV coinfection substantially increases the likelihood of fulminant hepatitis and death.

HEV is an enterically transmitted virus that has epidemiologic features resembling HAV. HEV infections occur primarily in Asia, Africa, and Central America.

Other important but infrequent causes of viral hepatitis include cytomegalovirus, Epstein-Barr virus, and herpes simplex. These viruses typically produce benign, anicteric disease and often escape detection preoperatively. However, in rare circumstances, particularly in immunocompromised patients, they can disseminate, causing acute hepatitis, fulminant hepatic failure, and death.[14]

Acute viral hepatitis occurs after an incubation period that varies with the specific virus involved. The mean incubation period for HAV is 4 weeks, for HBV 12 weeks, and for HCV 7 weeks. Clinical disease is often heralded by the development of constitutional symptoms such as anorexia, nausea, vomiting, and low-grade fever. Dark urine and clay-colored stools usually precede the onset of jaundice. At this point, the liver may be enlarged and tender. Recovery usually takes weeks to months. Many patients with acute viral hepatitis never become clinically jaundiced. AST and ALT levels begin to rise during the prodromal phase and usually reach a peak between 400 to 4,000 IU when the patient is clinically jaundiced. Serologic tests are the mainstay for the diagnosis of viral hepatitis. The diagnosis of hepatitis A is based on the detection of serum immunoglobulin M (IgM) antibody to the HAV capsid or HAV RNA in stool during acute illness; recovery is associated with immunoglobulin G anti-HAV antibody, which confers long-lasting immunity to recurrent HAV infection. The diagnosis of HBV infection is usually made by identifying HbsAg in serum. HbsAg may be present in serum as early as 7 days after HBV infection. Infrequently, levels of HbsAg are too low to be detected during acute HBV infection, and in such cases, the diagnosis can be established by the identification of IgM antibody to the HBV core antigen (IgM anti-Hbc). Hepatitis Be antigen (HbeAg) follows the pattern of HbsAg, and recovery is heralded by the disappearance of this antigen, while persistence of HbeAg identifies patients whose blood remains infective. Development of antibody to HbsAg (anti-Hbs) is seen in recovered patients.

The serologic diagnosis of hepatitis C can be made by demonstrating the presence in serum of anti-HCV or the presence of HCV RNA. HBD infection can be identified by demonstrating the presence of anti-HDV antibody.

Nonviral Hepatitis

Toxin and Drug-Induced Hepatitis

Acute hepatitis may follow the ingestion, inhalation, or parenteral administration of pharmacologic and chemical agents. Drugs and chemicals that are directly toxic to the liver (carbon tetrachloride, acetaminophen, α-amanitin from the toxic mushroom, *Amanita phalloides*) predictably produce dose-dependent liver injury. Each of these direct hepatotoxins produces a pattern of histologic injury that is reasonably characteristic and reproducible. Clinical manifestations of liver injury usually occur within 1 to 2 days of exposure. Acetaminophen not only causes fulminant hepatic failure following ingestion of extremely large doses (suicide attempts), but can also produce chronic liver injury with analgesic doses in susceptible individuals (malnutrition, chronic alcoholism).[15]

Other drugs (nonsteroidal anti-inflammatory agents, volatile anesthetics, antibiotics, antihypertensives, anticonvulsants) infrequently cause liver injury. These idiosyncratic drug reactions are unpredictable, and the response is not dose dependent. Hepatitis may develop during or shortly after exposure to the drug, but more commonly, clinical signs of liver dysfunction occur 2 to 6 weeks after initiation. Treatment of toxin-induced and drug-induced hepatitis is largely supportive. Failure to discontinue the offending drug promptly may result in progressive hepatitis and death. Hemodialysis may be useful following ingestion of *Amamita phalloides,* whereas *N*-acetylcysteine is used to treat patients with potentially hepatotoxic ingestions of acetaminophen. Liver transplantation may be lifesaving in patients with fulminant hepatitis, resulting from toxin or drug ingestion.

Toxic Acute Hepatitis and Volatile Anesthetics

Halothane was introduced in the United States in 1958; concerns linking this agent to acute hepatitis were raised shortly thereafter. To determine the incidence of massive hepatic necrosis after halothane anesthesia, the Committee on Anesthesia of the National Academy of Sciences launched one of the largest epidemiologic studies ever completed: the National Halothane Study.[16] From 1959 to 1962, 856,000 anesthetics were retrospectively reviewed. The incidence of fulminant hepatic necrosis terminating in death associated with halothane was found to be 1 per 35,000 anesthetics. The incidence of nonfatal hepatitis, however, may be as low as 1 in 3,000.[17] The association prompted a dramatic decrease in the use of halothane, especially in adult patients. Other volatile anesthetic agents have been reported to cause hepatitis, but at a much lower rate (Table 39-3).

The classic presentation of volatile anesthetic-associated hepatitis includes fever, anorexia, nausea, chills, myalgias, and rash, followed by the appearance of jaundice 3 to 6 days later. The syndrome characteristically develops after minor uneventful procedures of brief duration (<30 minutes). Overt jaundice indicates severe disease and portends a mortality rate as high as 40%. Other predictors of poor prognosis include a short latency between the anesthetic and the onset of symptoms, certain demographic factors (age >40, obesity), and severe hepatic dysfunction.[18]

The single most important risk factor for halothane hepatitis is prior exposure to halothane. Previous exposure has also been reported as a factor in isoflurane-associated hepatitis.[19] Of the patients who develop jaundice after halothane, 71 to 95% have had at least one prior exposure to this agent.[20] Severe reactions occur nearly 10 times more often in patients who have had multiple exposures to halothane than in those having their first halothane anesthetic.[21]

Demographic factors also provide important information about the risk of developing halothane hepatitis. Obese women appear to be more likely than their nonobese counterparts to contract halothane hepatitis. The disease may also have a genetic basis.[22] Some ethnic groups, such as Mexican Americans, seem to be at greater risk, and chromosomal differences have been noted between patients who recovered from halothane hepatitis and halothane-treated patients who never had the disease.[23,24] For reasons that are not yet clear, age is also a significant risk factor. Approximately 50% of the cases of halothane-associated fulminant hepatic failure occur in patients older than 50, whereas children are highly resistant to the development of halothane hepatitis.[21,25,26] The rare cases documented in children have involved multiple exposures to halothane.[27] Notably, neither preexisting liver disease nor concomitant administration of medication has been identified as a risk factor for halothane hepatitis.

Although the incidence of hepatitis appears to correlate with the degree of metabolism of the various agents, the paucity of cases reported with anesthetics other than halothane has cast doubt that any of these anesthetics was actually involved in the hepatic complications (see Table 39-3).

The observation that halothane hepatitis is associated with repeated exposure has led investigators to postulate an immune reaction. Of the halothane taken up during anesthesia, 20 to 46% is metabolized, compared with 2.5 to 8.5% for enflurane, 2 to 5% for sevoflurane, 0.2 to 2% for isoflurane, and 0.02% for desflurane.[28–30] Each anesthetic, with the exception of sevoflurane, is oxidized via cytochrome P450 2E1 to yield highly reactive intermediates that bind covalently (acylation) to a variety of hepatocellular macromolecules (Fig. 39-9). Halothane anesthesia induces both neoantigens (arising via the reaction of TF-acetyl chloride with hepatic proteins) and autoantigens (lacking TF-acetyl adducts).[31–35] Presumably, the TF-acetyl moiety acts as a hapten and enhances the immune recognition of the carrier protein. In susceptible people, these altered hepatic proteins may trigger an immunologic response that causes massive hepatic necrosis.[36]

Halothane hepatitis is idiosyncratic, affecting only a tiny fraction of those anesthetized with this agent. Neither the incidence nor the severity of the reaction correlates with the dose

TABLE 39-3

RELATIONSHIP BETWEEN METABOLISM OF VOLATILE HALOGENATED AGENTS AND ANESTHETIC-INDUCED HEPATITIS

AGENT	YEAR INTRODUCED IN UNITED STATES	NO. OF CASES OF HEPATITIS	PERCENTAGE OF ANESTHETIC METABOLIZED	FLUOROACETYL METABOLITES
Halothane	1958	>500	20–46	Yes
Enflurane	1972	~50	2.5–8.5	Yes
Isoflurane	1981	6	0.2–2	Yes
Desflurane	1993	1	0.02	Yes
Sevoflurane	1995	3	2–5	No

From Mushlin PS, Gelman S: Liver dysfunction after anesthesia. In Benumof JL, Saidman LJ (eds): Anesthesia and Perioperative Complications, 2nd ed, p 440. St Louis, Mosby, 1999, with permission.

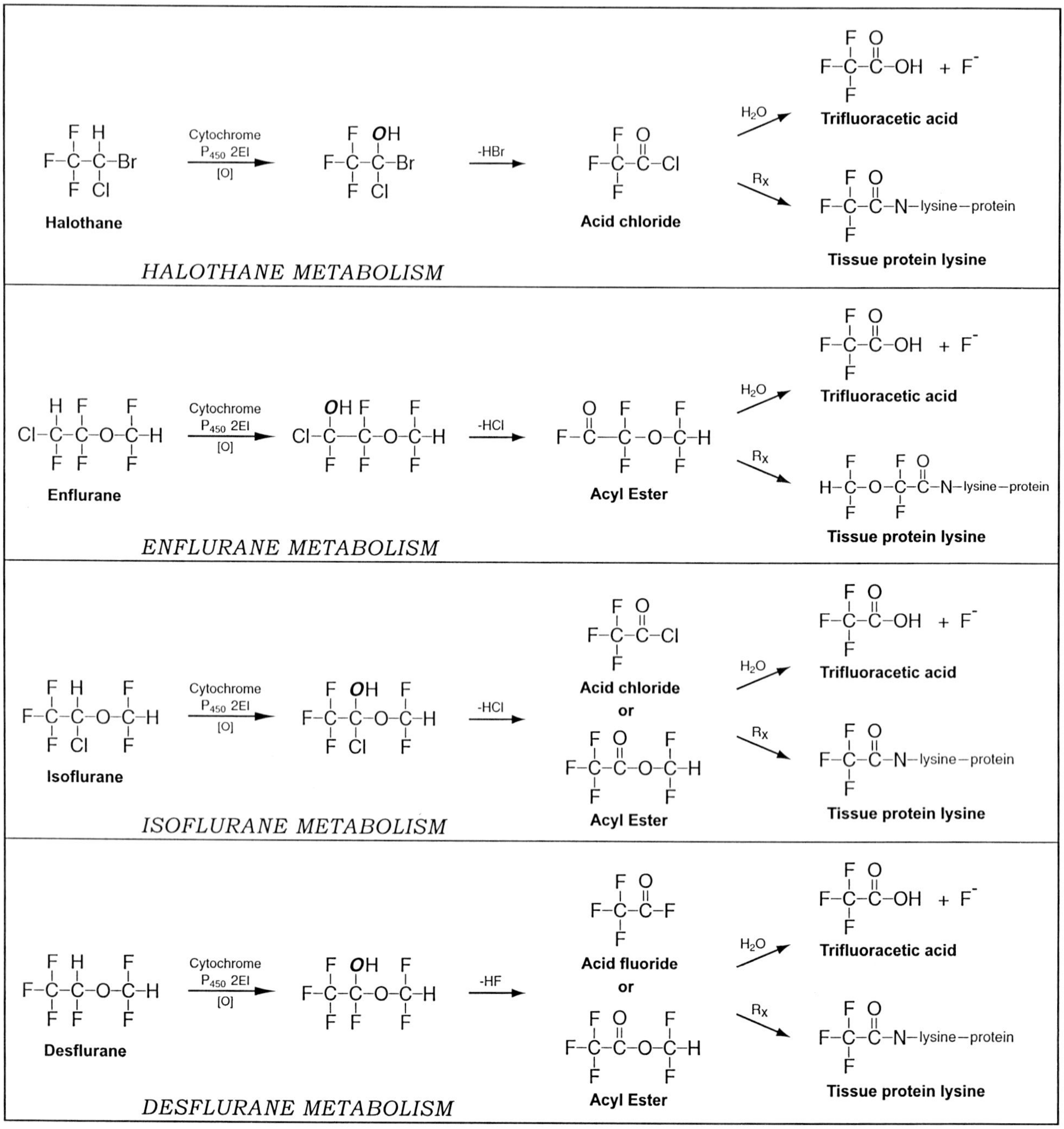

FIGURE 39-9. Proposed pathways of cytochrome P450 2E1-catalyzed metabolism of halothane, enflurane, isoflurane, and desflurane that are involved in the production of highly reactive intermediates that acylate hepatic proteins. The acylated moieties of the liver proteins appear to function as haptens to elicit an immune response. Sevoflurane metabolism is not included in this figure (see Fig. 39-10) because there is no evidence that it produces an acylating intermediate. (Modified with permission from Mushlin PS, Gelman S: Liver dysfunction after anesthesia. In Benumof JL, Saidman LJ [eds]: Anesthesia and Perioperative Complications, 2nd ed, p 442. St Louis, Mosby, 1999; modified from Frink EJ Jr: The hepatic effects of sevoflurane. Anesth Analg 81[suppl 6]:S46, 1995; Kenna JG, Jones RM: The organ toxicity of inhaled anesthetics. Anesth Analg 81[suppl 6]:S51, 1995.)

of halothane administered. The disease has a latency of days, unlike the hepatic injury produced by severe hypoxia or a potent cytotoxin, which typically appears within hours of the insult. Moreover, it is usually accompanied by laboratory findings that are characteristic of an immunologically mediated disorder, such as peripheral eosinophilia, circulating immune complexes, organ nonspecific autoantibodies, and antibodies that bind to antigens isolated from halothane-treated animals (rabbits).[37,38] Approximately 70% of patients have antibodies that recognize neoantigens (TF-acetyl-modified epitopes), and 90% have antibodies that recognize autoantigens (non–TF-acetyl–modified epitopes). Therefore, preoperative testing for halothane antibodies might identify patients at risk for developing hepatitis, whereas postoperative testing could help determine if halothane was the likely cause of unexplained postoperative hepatitis. Currently, however, no tests exist that are totally sensitive or specific for detecting the disease. The ELISA test for antibodies has been reported to be approximately 75% sensitive and 88% specific.[33] Obviously, the easiest way to avoid the risk of halothane-induced hepatitis is to avoid the use of halothane completely, especially in adults. Fortunately, alternative agents are readily available; thus, there has been decreased interest in developing preoperative tests.

2 Other volatile agents besides halothane also have immunogenic potential. Enflurane metabolism produces acyl adducts (difluoromethoxydifluoroacetyl halide) that are similar, but not identical, to those derived from halothane (TF-acetyl halide). Nonetheless, antibodies isolated from patients with halothane hepatitis can bind to hepatic proteins that contain enflurane-induced adducts (neoantigens).[39]

Isoflurane metabolism also yields highly reactive intermediates (TF-acetyl chloride; acyl ester) that bind covalently to hepatic proteins (see Fig. 39-9). The likelihood that isoflurane causes hepatitis via production of these intermediates appears to be extremely low, however, as just 0.2% of the isoflurane taken up into the body is actually metabolized. Only trace amounts of isoflurane-derived adducts are bound to hepatic proteins following isoflurane anesthesia.

Desflurane, which is similarly biotransformed to trifluoroacyl metabolites, appears even less likely than isoflurane to cause immune injury because only 0.02 to 0.2% of this agent is metabolized (1/1,000th that of halothane). Desflurane metabolites are usually undetectable in plasma, except after prolonged administration. Furthermore, although antibodies from patients with halothane hepatitis clearly react with proteins isolated from halothane-treated or enflurane-treated rats, they do not appear to react with hepatic proteins from desflurane-treated or isoflurane-treated rats.[36]

Sevoflurane is metabolized more extensively than is isoflurane or desflurane, slightly less than enflurane, and much less than halothane.[40] The metabolism of sevoflurane (primarily via cytochrome P450 2E1) is rapid (1.5 to 2 times faster than enflurane), and produces detectable plasma concentrations of fluoride and hexafluoroisopropanol (HFIP) within minutes of initiating the anesthetic. The liver conjugates most of the HFIP with glucuronic acid, which is then excreted by the kidney (Fig. 39-10). An important distinction between sevoflurane and the other volatile agents is that sevoflurane produces neither highly reactive metabolites nor fluoroacetylated liver proteins.[29] There is no evidence that any sevoflurane metabolites cause severe hepatic injury.

At present, the preponderance of evidence supports the immune theory (via TF-acetyl-hapten) of halothane-induced hepatitis. Nonetheless, it is conceivable that the antigen–antibody responses that accompany anesthesia-induced hepatitis are the result of the hepatic injury, rather than the cause. Most (if not all) patients anesthetized with halothane form the same or similar TF-acetylated liver proteins, but few develop halothane hepatitis. In fact, pediatric anesthesiologists, like halothane hepatitis patients, have been shown to have higher serum autoantibody levels of P450 2E1 than general anesthesiologists and controls, possibly because of their increased occupational exposure to anesthetics. The female pediatric anesthesiologists in this study had higher levels of P450 2E1 autoantibodies than all other anesthesiologists.[41] Despite one female anesthesiologist demonstrating evidence of hepatic injury in the aforementioned study, there are no reports of fulminant halothane hepatitis attributable to occupational exposure. Explanations for these observations, which proponents of the hapten theory must reconcile, include the following: only a few of the TF-acetyl proteins are actually immunogenic, the triggering of an immune response requires a critical threshold of TF-acetylated proteins (antigenic threshold), and only a small fraction of patients are genetically susceptible to these antigens.

Volatile Agents and Hepatic Blood Flow and Oxygen Delivery

Insofar as all halogenated anesthetic agents depress cardiac output and most surgical procedures stimulate a stress response with resultant catecholamine-induced vasoconstriction, it is predictable that hepatic blood flow and oxygen delivery will decrease during general anesthesia with volatile agents. The degree to which hepatic metabolic demands are also depressed with the various agents determines the relative impact on the hepatic supply–demand relationship, and consequently, the potential of each agent for causing hepatic ischemia.

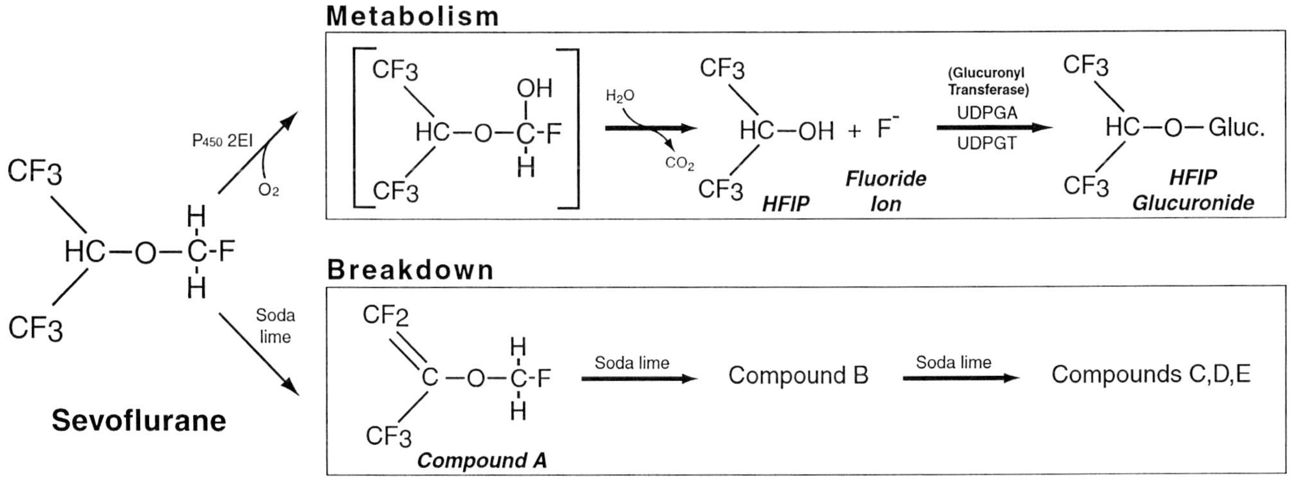

FIGURE 39-10. Cytochrome P450 2E1-catalyzed biotransformation of sevoflurane produces inorganic fluoride and hexafluoroisopropanol (HFIP). The liver rapidly metabolizes HFIP to HFIP-glucuronide. Sevoflurane also undergoes breakdown in soda lime, yielding compound A, which is nephrotoxic but does not appear to be hepatotoxic. (Modified with permission from Mushlin PS, Gelman S: Liver dysfunction after anesthesia. In Benumof JL, Saidman LJ [eds]: Anesthesia and Perioperative Complications, 2nd ed, p 442. St Louis, Mosby, 1999; modified from Frink EJ Jr: The hepatic effects of sevoflurane. Anesth Analg 81[suppl 6]:S46, 1995.)

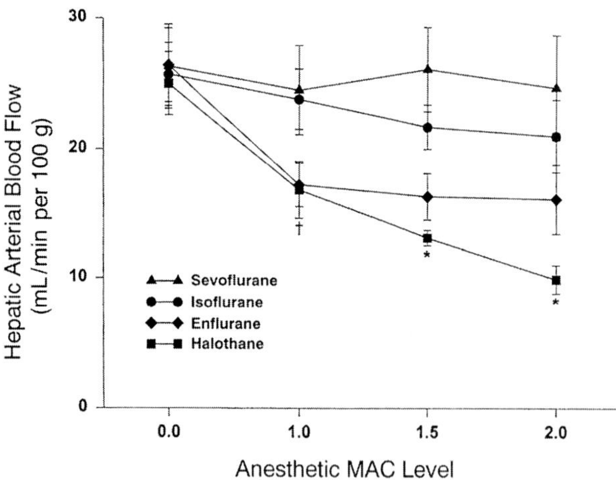

FIGURE 39-11. Dose-dependent effects of inhaled anesthetics on hepatic arterial flow in chronically instrumented dogs in the absence of a surgical stress. Sevoflurane and isoflurane preserve hepatic arterial flow even at the higher minimum alveolar concentration (MAC) levels. *Differs from sevoflurane and isoflurane at same MAC values ($p < .05$). †Differs from sevoflurane at same MAC value ($p < .05$). (Reprinted with permission from Frink EJ Jr: The hepatic effects of sevoflurane. Anesth Analg 8[suppl 6]:S46, 1995.)

Other perioperative conditions also contribute to hepatic blood flow, oxygen delivery, and metabolic requirements: hemoglobin concentration, oxygen saturation, systemic inflammation, volume status, and temperature. Additional insults such as direct hepatic trauma and hepatotoxic drug exposure, as well as occult preexisting hepatic insufficiency, can obscure the independent effects of the volatile agent.

Both animal and human studies indicate that halothane is more likely than other inhaled anesthetics to produce liver injury, probably because it causes the most cardiovascular and respiratory depression, as well as the greatest reduction in hepatic arterial flow (Fig. 39-11). Consequently, halothane is the most likely of the clinically used vapors to produce, or exacerbate, hepatic hypoxia when blood flow to the liver is critically limited and the adequacy of the oxygen supply-to-demand balance is in question.

Excluding halothane, enflurane decreases hepatic blood flow and splanchnic perfusion more than any other halogenated vapor in clinical use. It induces dose-dependant decreases in portal venous blood flow and either reduces or leaves unchanged hepatic arterial blood flow.[42,43] Splanchnic perfusion decreases in parallel with decreased mean arterial pressure and cardiac output. Enflurane also increases splanchnic oxygen extraction, and lowers both hepatic venous and mixed venous oxygen saturation.

Desflurane decreases hepatic blood flow in both experimental and clinical settings. Administration of 1 minimum alveolar concentration (MAC) desflurane to patients prior to skin incision reportedly decreases hepatic blood flow by 30% (measured by ICG), similar to the reduction associated with 1 MAC of halothane or isoflurane.[44] Desflurane can markedly reduce oxygen delivery to the liver and small intestine without producing comparable reductions of hepatic oxygen uptake or hepatic and mesenteric metabolism. Therefore, desflurane anesthesia may decrease the oxygen reserve capacity of both the liver and the small intestine.

Isoflurane is much less likely than halothane or enflurane to cause or contribute to hepatic injury. It undergoes minimal biodegradation, and preserves hepatic blood flow[45] and oxygen delivery even during open laparotomy.[46]

Sevoflurane anesthesia usually preserves blood flow and oxygen delivery to the liver, even in the presence of positive-pressure ventilation.[47] Patients having elective operations under sevoflurane anesthesia (1 or 2 MAC) experience significant reductions in mean arterial blood pressure, but maintain the hepatic blood flow at preanesthetic levels. Animal data suggest that the hepatic arterial buffer response remains intact.[48] Sevoflurane appears to be the most effective of the inhaled anesthetics for maintaining both blood flow and oxygen delivery to the liver. Thus, it is less likely than either halothane or enflurane to induce liver injury and is no more toxic than desflurane or isoflurane. Its metabolic products are less reactive, and therefore probably less injurious, than those resulting from halothane, enflurane, isoflurane, or even desflurane.[49] Sevoflurane better preserves hepatic blood flow and oxygen delivery than halothane, enflurane, or desflurane; its effects on hepatic perfusion and metabolic function are similar to those of isoflurane.

Other than sevoflurane, desflurane is the least likely of the halogenated vapors to cause severe hepatic injury, based on the immune theory of anesthesia-induced hepatitis. Nonetheless, desflurane produces a greater reduction of hepatic blood flow and oxygen delivery than either isoflurane or sevoflurane. Hence, it may be more likely than the latter agents to cause liver injury in the setting of marginal hepatic oxygenation.

Other Anesthetics and Hepatic Function

Nitrous Oxide

Nitrous oxide produces a mild increase in sympathetic nervous system tone. Consequently, one would expect mild vasoconstriction of the splanchnic vasculature, leading to a decrease in portal blood flow, and mild vasoconstriction of the hepatic arterial system. In addition, N_2O is a known inhibitor of the enzyme methionine synthase, which could potentially produce toxic hepatic effects. Even brief exposures to N_2O at concentrations used clinically are sufficient to produce time-related decreases in methionine synthase activity in the livers of animals and humans, and prolonged exposure will induce a functional vitamin B_{12} deficiency.[50] Whether the resultant abnormalities in folate and methionine metabolism actually injure the liver is unclear. In a survey of more than 60,000 dentists and chairside assistants, Cohen and coworkers found a higher prevalence of liver disease in professionals who were chronically exposed to nitrous oxide: 1.7-fold higher in dentists, and 1.6-fold higher in their assistants.[51] Other studies suggest that N_2O-containing anesthetics do not cause liver injury in the absence of impaired hepatic oxygenation. In one study, no hepatocellular injury resulted from up to 4 hours of anesthesia with 67% N_2O (in oxygen) and infusions of methohexital.[52] In another, no hepatic dysfunction developed when patients with mild alcoholic hepatitis received N_2O-opioid or N_2O-enflurane anesthetics for peripheral or superficial operations.[53] There is no convincing evidence that nitrous oxide per se causes hepatotoxicity in the absence of a precarious oxygen supply–demand ratio in the liver.[54]

Nonopioid Sedative-Hypnotic Agents

Because it is a sympathomimetic agent, ketamine may produce a moderate increase in serum concentrations of some liver enzymes.[55] Patients anesthetized with ketamine infusion plus oxygen show a dose-dependent increase in biochemical markers of hepatic injury.[56] Despite these findings, it remains unclear whether ketamine causes liver dysfunction by exerting direct hepatotoxic effects, by altering hepatic metabolism, or by increasing serum catecholamines, which would be expected to decrease hepatic blood flow and oxygen delivery.

Other intravenous agents, such as propofol, etomidate, and midazolam, have not been shown to alter hepatic function significantly in patients undergoing minor operative procedures. Although very large doses of thiopental (>750 mg) may cause hepatic dysfunction, usual induction doses have little effect on the liver.[57]

Opioids

Opioids have little effect on hepatic function, provided they do not impair hepatic blood flow and oxygen supply. All opioids increase tone of the common bile duct and the sphincter of Oddi, as well as the frequency of phasic contractions, leading to increases in biliary tract pressure and biliary spasm. The effect on the sphincter of Oddi does not favor one opioid over another and is not considered an absolute contraindication to narcotic analgesia, even in cases of pancreatitis.[58]

NONPHARMACOLOGIC CAUSES OF PERIOPERATIVE LIVER DYSFUNCTION

Inflammation and Sepsis

The liver occupies a central position in the inflammatory response, especially when the inflammation is secondary to intra-abdominal sepsis. Because of its location downstream from the splanchnic circulation, bacteria, endotoxin, and proinflammatory cytokines (IL-1, IL-6, and TNF-α) are carried directly to the liver. These interact with sinusoidal Kupffer cells and stimulate hepatocytes to decrease production of certain proteins (mainly albumin), called negative acute-phase reactants, and increase production of others (mainly C-reactive protein and serum amyloid A), called acute-phase reactants. In addition, especially following blunt trauma and burns, complement and coagulation factor production also increase in the liver. Some, such as C-reactive protein and serum amyloid A, up to 30,000-fold, greatly increase the liver's metabolic demands (Fig. 39-12). With inflammation, the resulting changes in systemic vascular resistance; regional blood flow distribution; tissue oxygen extraction; coagulation status; glucose, fat, and protein metabolism; and catecholamine sensitivity can be far reaching and profound.[59] In sepsis, hepatic arterial flow changes in a biphasic manner: an initial transient decrease followed by a marked and sustained increase in flow. The increase in hepatic artery flow occurs independent of changes in portal venous flow, suggesting a dysregulation of the physiologic hepatic arterial buffer response.[60] In sepsis, and inflammation in general, hypovolemia and splanchnic hypoperfusion are com-
3 mon, predictably decreasing oxygen delivery to the liver.

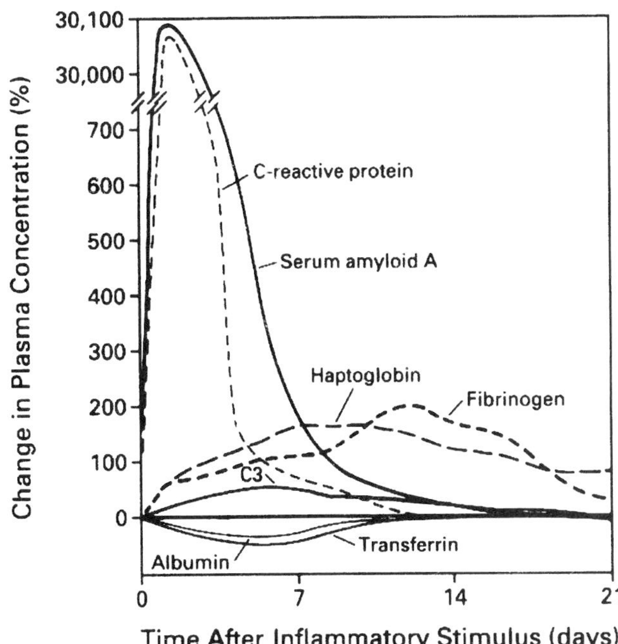

FIGURE 39-12. Characteristic patterns of change in plasma concentrations of some acute-phase proteins after a moderate inflammatory stimulus. (Reprinted with permission from Giltin JD, Colten HR. Molecular biology of the acute phase plasma proteins. In: Pick E, Landy M [eds]: Lymphokines. Vol. 14., pp. 123–153. San Diego, CA, Academic Press, 1987.)

Hypoxia and Ischemia

The liver is exquisitely sensitive to hypoxia. In one study, patients with chronic lung disease whose blood oxygen content fell below 9 mL/dL all developed liver injury without developing overt myocardial or cerebral damage.[61] The detrimental effects of oxygen deprivation on perioperative hepatic function can occur independent of anesthetic techniques.[62] In addition, if moderate hypotension occurs, a hepatitis-like illness (ischemic hepatitis) may follow. Patients develop jaundice, systemic symptoms, and large increases of serum transaminases, which may persist for 3 to 11 days. Liver biopsy shows centrilobular necrosis with little or no inflammatory response.[63]

Patients with ischemic hepatitis typically have a history of inadequate systemic perfusion, along with marked increases of serum aminotransferases. The increases are usually of greater magnitude than those associated with viral hepatitis. Prolonged shock or sepsis can cause extreme liver injury; a hepatic lobe or the entire liver may become infarcted, even in the absence of portal venous or hepatic arterial occlusion.[64] The mechanism of ischemic hepatitis is unknown, but it may involve free radical production because hepatocytes contain very high concentrations of xanthine oxidase. Ischemia and reperfusion increase xanthine oxidase activity; this enzyme catalyzes the oxidation of purines to uric acid and the associated reduction of O_2 to superoxide anion, which initiates toxic free radical reactions.

Cardiac Disease

Severe congestive heart failure may be associated with liver dysfunction.[65] The most common cause is ischemic hepatitis from decreased hepatic blood flow secondary to low cardiac output. Cardiac cirrhosis (fibrosis) may result from prolonged recurrent congestive heart failure. Acute liver failure is more likely to occur in patients with preexisting cirrhosis, severe chronic heart failure, or sustained hepatic ischemia, although passive hepatic congestion and fulminant hepatocellular necrosis has been reported from acute, severe elevations of central venous pressures.[67]

Surgical Stress

The surgical stress response includes stimulation of the sympathetic nervous system, activation of the renin-angiotensin-aldosterone system, and the nonosmotic release of vasopressin;

each of these responses may compromise the splanchnic circulation. These effects may persist for many hours or even days after surgery. Laboratory studies indicate that laparotomy, in particular, induces marked mesenteric vasoconstriction and decreases gastrointestinal and hepatic blood flow; acute hypophysectomy and administration of an angiotensin II antagonist can abolish these changes.[67] In addition to the surgical stress response, laparotomy independently decreases blood flow through the intestine and the liver, probably as a result of traction and manipulation of the viscera.[68]

Although reducing the surgical stress response and minimizing tissue injury and inflammation, laparoscopic procedures are not entirely benign with respect to the liver. The increased intra-abdominal pressures induced with insufflation appear to significantly decrease splanchnic perfusion and hepatic blood flow.[69]

Procedures performed under cardiopulmonary bypass, with low-flow states and nonpulsatile perfusion, can aggravate preexisting hepatic dysfunction. Administration of catecholamines to improve cardiac performance, either before or after bypass, may decrease hepatic oxygen delivery. Hypothermia during cardiopulmonary bypass probably limits the hepatic injury caused by the abnormal hemodynamics. Hypotension and hemorrhage decrease portal blood flow, but the hepatic arterial buffer response and pressure-flow autoregulation tend to preserve hepatic arterial flow and oxygen delivery. Perfusion at 28°C increases portal flow and slightly decreases hepatic arterial flow. A pump flow rate of 2.4 L/minute per m^2 maintains total blood flow to the liver better than does a rate of 1.2 L/minute per m^2. Only at low rates does pulsatile flow appear to be more advantageous than nonpulsatile perfusion in terms of hepatic blood flow.[70]

CHRONIC HEPATITIS

Chronic hepatitis refers to a group of liver disorders of varying etiologies and severity in which hepatic inflammation and necrosis continue for at least 6 months. Chronic hepatitis was previously classified based on liver biopsy as chronic persistent or chronic active hepatitis. When this early classification was devised, chronic persistent hepatitis was considered to have a good prognosis, whereas chronic active hepatitis was considered a progressive disorder with a poor outcome. However, the prognostic value of these histologic distinctions has been found to be limited; thus, this classification has been supplanted by one based on cause, grade, and stage. Clinical and serologic features allow the establishment of an etiology for chronic hepatitis caused by HBV, HBV plus HDV, HCV, autoimmune hepatitis, drug-associated chronic hepatitis, and a category of cryptogenic chronic hepatitis. Histologic features on liver biopsy are necessary for grading and staging chronic hepatitis. The grade is determined by an assessment of the degree of necrosis and inflammation, and the stage reflects the level of progression of the disease, which is determined by an assessment of the degree of fibrosis.

Patients with chronic HBV infection who are asymptomatic and have normal serum transaminases are called HbsAg carriers. Those with chronic HBV infection who have clinical, laboratory, or pathologic evidence of chronic hepatic disease are diagnosed as chronic hepatitis B. An estimated 0.2 to 0.5% of the American population are chronic carriers of HbsAg. These HBV carriers are at risk for developing cirrhosis and hepatocellular carcinoma. The goal of treatment of chronic hepatitis B is to eradicate HBV infection, and thereby prevent the development of cirrhosis and hepatocellular carcinoma. Current therapy of chronic hepatitis B has limited long-term efficacy and does not yet achieve these goals. However, available therapies can suppress HBV replication and lead to laboratory and histologic improvement.[71,72] The decision to initiate treatment depends on balancing the patient's age, severity of disease, likelihood of response, and potential adverse effects and complications. Treatment is not recommended for inactive HbsAg carriers. To date, three drugs have been approved for treatment of chronic hepatitis B: injectable interferon α, and two oral agents, lamivudine and adefovir.[73]

Chronic HCV infection follows acute HCV infection in 85% of patients; an estimated 1.8% of the United States population are carriers of HCV. Although the progression of chronic hepatitis C infection to cirrhosis is characteristically slow, end-stage liver disease due to HCV-associated cirrhosis is the most common indication for liver transplantation. At least six distinct genotypes of HCV have been identified by nucleotide sequencing, and differences exist among these genotypes in responsiveness to antiviral therapy. Chronic HCV infection is usually treated with the combination of ribavirin and interferon.[74]

Autoimmune hepatitis is a chronic disease characterized by a wide spectrum of clinical symptoms, seroimmunologic manifestations, and continued hepatocellular necrosis and inflammation, which often progresses to cirrhosis. Extrahepatic features of autoimmunity, seroimmunologic abnormalities, and association with other autoimmune disorders all support an autoimmune pathogenesis. The clinical and laboratory features of autoimmune hepatitis are often similar to those described for chronic hepatitis. Patients with autoimmune hepatitis, however, usually have hypergammaglobulinemia, rheumatoid factor, and other circulating autoantibodies. Immunosuppressive therapy using corticosteroids with or without azathioprine is the mainstay of treatment and leads to symptomatic, clinical, biochemical, and histologic improvement, along with increased survival.

Fatty Liver Disease

Nonalcoholic fatty liver disease (NAFLD) is the most common cause of chronic liver disease in the United States.[75] NAFLD is defined as fat accumulation in the liver exceeding 5% by weight.[76] It has been estimated that up to 24% of American adults have NAFLD. It usually becomes manifest in the fifth and sixth decades of life and is more common in women.[77] The two major risk factors for NAFLD are type II diabetes and obesity. In a consecutive autopsy series, 70% of obese patients had fatty liver. Among type II diabetics, it is estimated that 75% have some form of fatty liver.

NAFLD includes a spectrum of hepatic pathology that ranges from fatty liver (steatosis) at its most clinically indolent extreme to the intermediate stage of nonalcoholic steatohepatitis (NASH), characterized by steatosis with lobular inflammation and perisinusoidal fibrosis, to its most severe form, cirrhosis. NAFLD is now believed to be responsible for most cases of what was once classified as cryptogenic cirrhosis, a form that accounts for half of the annual liver-related deaths.

Most patients with NAFLD are asymptomatic, and the presence of an abnormality is often detected by abnormal LFT or hepatomegaly on a routine physician's office visit. The most common LFT abnormality is a 2- to 5-fold elevation of the AST and ALT. The AST/ALT ratio is reported to be <1 in 65 to 90% of patients with NAFLD, which distinguishes it from alcohol-related liver injury.

The pathophysiology of NAFLD is unknown, but present data suggest a multihit hypothesis in which common initial insults promote hepatic steatosis (e.g., obesity, subclinical insulin resistance), and the increased hepatic fat appears to stress the hepatocyte and render it more vulnerable to subsequent insults. This eventually produces some degree of hepatocyte necrosis, which promotes the accumulation of inflammatory cells within the liver (NASH). In some patients, a fibrotic response predominates, leading to cirrhosis.

The natural history of NAFLD varies according to its histologic type. Patients with steatosis alone usually have a benign clinical course. Significant adverse clinical sequelae, however, occur in patients with NASH and cryptogenic cirrhosis.

There are no proven treatments for NAFLD. Exercise and diet are recommended. Several studies have reported beneficial effects of bariatric surgery when NAFLD is secondary to obesity. When the disease is advanced, the patient is often a poor candidate for liver transplantation due to comorbid conditions such as obesity and the complications of diabetes.

Alcoholic Liver Disease

Alcoholic liver disease is defined by the development of three types of liver damage following chronic heavy alcohol consumption: (1) steatosis (fatty liver), (2) alcoholic hepatitis, and (3) cirrhosis.[78] The clinical features and laboratory values frequently do not distinguish among these because compensatory mechanisms can mask extensive liver disease. A liver biopsy is often necessary to arrive at a definitive diagnosis.

Alcoholic steatosis occurs commonly after ingestion of moderate to large amounts of alcohol for even a short period of time. When severe, patients may be symptomatic, with malaise, nausea, anorexia, weakness, abdominal discomfort, and tender hepatomegaly. Mild transaminase and AP elevations may be present. Alcoholic steatosis is usually a benign disorder, and the liver abnormalities will usually resolve with abstinence from alcohol. In contrast, alcoholic hepatitis is a precursor of cirrhosis. Although symptoms may overlap with those of alcoholic steatosis, patients with alcoholic hepatitis may be febrile and jaundiced. There may be up to a 10-fold elevation of the aminotransferases with the AST level characteristically higher than the ALT. Hypoalbuminemia, prolongation of the PT, and marked elevations of the AP may be present. Treatment of alcoholic hepatitis consists of abstinence from alcohol, bed rest, and intake of a normal or high protein diet if hepatic encephalopathy is not present. Corticosteroids are often used to treat patients with severe alcoholic hepatitis, although their use for this indication remains controversial. It should be noted that alcohol abusers have a 2- to 3-fold increase in perioperative morbidity (Fig. 39-13).[79]

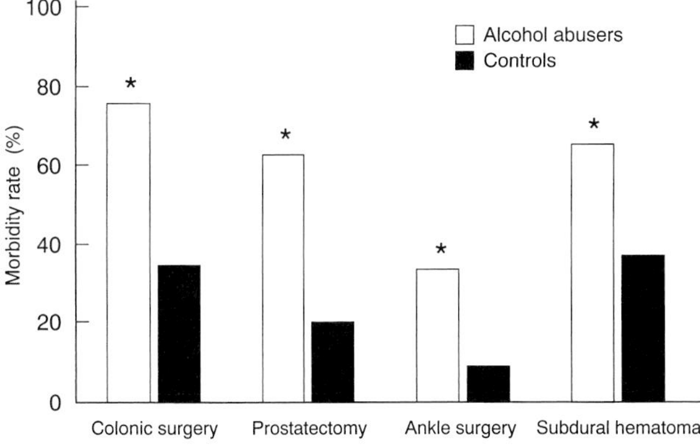

FIGURE 39-13. Prospective studies of postoperative morbidity in alcohol abusers and control subjects. $^*p < 0.05$ vs. control subjects. (Reprinted with permission from Tonnesen H, Kehlet H: Preoperative alcoholism and postoperative morbidity. Br J Surg 86:869, 1999.)

CIRRHOSIS: A PARADIGM FOR END-STAGE PARENCHYMAL LIVER DISEASE

This section discusses the pathophysiology of parenchymal liver disease, typified by hepatic cirrhosis, as it relates to anesthesia. Cirrhosis affects more than 3 million Americans and is the twelfth leading cause of death. The most frequent etiologies of cirrhosis in the United States are chronic hepatitis C infection and alcoholism. The most common symptoms are anorexia, weakness, nausea, vomiting, and abdominal pain. Signs include hepatosplenomegaly, ascites, jaundice, spider nevi, and metabolic encephalopathy. Advanced parenchymal hepatic disease alters the function of nearly every organ and body system.

Cardiovascular Abnormalities

Characteristically, patients with cirrhosis and portal hypertension have a hyperdynamic circulation with a high cardiac output, low peripheral vascular resistance, low to normal arterial blood pressure, normal to increased stroke volume, normal filling pressures, and a mildly elevated heart rate (Table 39-4).[80] The total blood volume is usually increased, but with an altered distribution in which the central "effective" blood volume is decreased, while the splanchnic bed is hypervolemic. Extensive arteriovenous collateralization occurs in many organs and tissues, leading to increased oxygen tension and saturation of the peripheral and mixed venous blood, and a decrease in the arteriovenous oxygen content difference. The mechanism by which these collaterals develop is complex and not completely understood, but may be related to increased plasma levels of glucagon and vasoactive intestinal polypeptide, which can induce peripheral vasodilation, decrease vascular resistance, and increase arteriovenous shunting. Glucagon also reduces the vascular responsiveness to infused catecholamines and other vasopressors in experimental animals.[81] Nitric oxide may also be an important mediator of the hyperdynamic changes that occur in cirrhosis and portal hypertension. Data from normal subjects and patients with cirrhosis reveal a positive correlation between exhaled concentrations of nitric oxide and cardiac index (Fig. 39-14).[82] Some causes of liver disease are also associated with cardiomyopathy (alcoholic liver disease, hemochromatosis); these patients may develop signs and symptoms of congestive heart failure, including decreased peripheral blood flow.

TABLE 39-4

CARDIOVASCULAR FUNCTION IN HEPATIC CIRRHOSIS

Decreased vascular resistance (peripheral vasodilation, increased arteriovenous shunting)
Increased cardiac output
Maintained arterial blood pressure, filling pressures, and heart rate (deterioration is late)
Blood volume maintained or increased, but redistributed (splanchnic hypervolemia, central hypovolemia)
Possible cardiomyopathy
Increased O_2 content in mixed venous blood; decreased difference in the O_2 contents of arterial and venous blood
Diminished responsiveness to catecholamines
Increased blood flow in splanchnic (extrahepatic), pulmonary, muscular, and cutaneous tissues
Decreased total hepatic blood flow
  Maintained hepatic arterial blood flow
  Decreased portal venous blood flow
Maintained or decreased renal blood flow

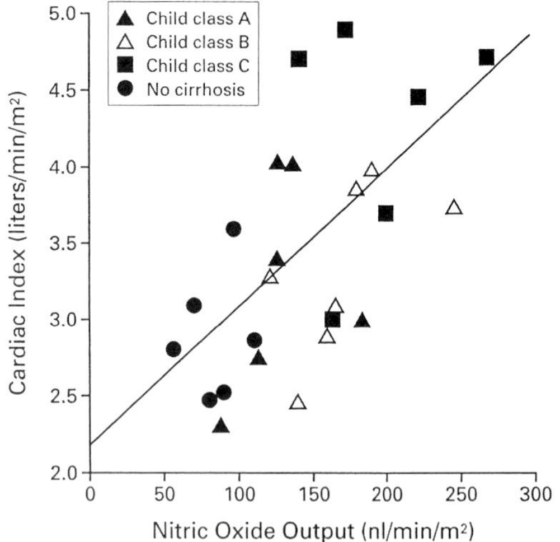

FIGURE 39-14. Relationship between nitric oxide in exhaled air and the cardiac index in 25 patients who had either normal hepatic function or cirrhosis with varying degrees hepatic dysfunction. (Severity of liver dysfunction increases progressively from Child class A to class C.) A positive correlation exists between nitric oxide output (expressed in nanoliters per minute per square meter of body surface area) and cardiac index (expressed in liters per minute per square meter). $r = 0.62$ and $p < 0.001$. (Reprinted with permission from Matsumoto A, Ogura K, Hirata Y *et al:* Increased nitric oxide production in the exhaled air of patients with decompensated cirrhosis. Ann Intern Med 123:110, 1995.)

Hepatic Circulatory Dysfunction

Portal hypertension can complicate the course of many chronic liver diseases but is a hallmark of end-stage cirrhosis. Portal hypertension is a pathologic increase in portal venous pressure, resulting in the formation of portosystemic collaterals, which develop by dilatation and hypertrophy of preexisting vascular channels. It plays an important role in the pathogenesis of ascites and hepatic encephalopathy, leads to the development of esophageal varices, and contributes to the enhanced susceptibility to bacterial infections and altered drug metabolism found in these patients.

In patients with cirrhosis, portal hypertension may result from increased vascular resistance to portal blood flow, which is believed to be the initial factor responsible for an increase in portal pressure. In cirrhotics, this increased resistance occurs mainly in the hepatic sinusoids. Subsequently, increased portal venous inflow occurs as a result of marked splanchnic arteriolar vasodilation. Several humeral vasodilators have been suspected of contributing to splanchnic hyperemia, including glucagon, prostacyclin, endotoxin, and nitric oxide.[83] Eventually, the majority of the blood entering the portal system flows through the collateral circulation, and under these circumstances, the resistance of these vessels markedly influences portal pressure. As portal blood flow to the liver decreases substantially, hepatic arterial flow remains the same or increases. Thus, although the total circulation of the liver decreases, the hepatic oxygen supply is preserved. This decrease in total hepatic blood flow has pharmacokinetic implications that have been previously discussed.

Variceal Hemorrhage

Gastroesophageal variceal hemorrhage is probably the most dreaded complication of portal hypertension. Varices are portosystemic collaterals formed after preexisting vascular channels have been dilated by portal hypertension. They permit the passage of splanchnic venous blood from the high-pressure portal venous system to the low-pressure azygos and hemiazygous veins. Gastroesophageal varices are present in 40 to 60% of cirrhotics, and 25 to 35% of these will bleed. Up to 30% of initial bleeding episodes are fatal, and as many as 70% of survivors of an initial hemorrhage will have a recurrence.[84]

Variceal ruptures typically present as acute severe upper gastrointestinal hemorrhage. Prompt aggressive fluid resuscitation, blood transfusion, and correction of hemostatic abnormalities are essential, and are usually implemented in an intensive care unit. Endotracheal intubation for airway protection is frequently necessary. Empiric pharmacologic therapy (e.g., with octreotide) is indicated in situations in which variceal bleeding is likely. Subsequent esophagogastroduodenoscopy will define the site of bleeding and permit endoscopic therapy if appropriate.

Treatment of patients with gastroesophageal varices includes prevention of the initial bleeding episode (primary prophylaxis), control of active hemorrhage, and prevention of recurrent bleeding after a first episode (secondary prophylaxis).[85]

The goal of pharmacologic treatment is to reduce portal and intravariceal pressures. The nonselective beta-blockers, propranolol and nadolol, are effective agents for primary prophylaxis as they produce sustained decreases in portal venous pressure and decrease the risk of bleeding by 40 to 50%. Isosorbide mononitrate added to a beta-blocker may not only produce a further decrease in portal pressure, but also cause increased side effects. Endoscopic band ligation is an acceptable option for primary prophylaxis in patients at high risk for variceal bleeding who cannot tolerate medical therapy.

Patients with acute gastrointestinal bleeding of probable variceal origin are initially treated with intravenous somatostatin or its synthetic analogue octreotide. These drugs stop variceal hemorrhage in up to 80% of patients by reducing portal pressure. The variceal origin of the bleeding is then confirmed endoscopically, and the varices are subsequently treated either by band ligation or sclerotherapy. Current endoscopic therapies are capable of stopping bleeding in approximately 90% of patients.

If variceal bleeding persists or recurs despite endoscopic and pharmacologic therapy, balloon tamponade with a Sengstaken-Blakemore or Minnesota tube may be attempted. These modified nasogastric tubes are infrequently used, but when applied properly, achieve hemostasis in most cases. Because rebleeding frequently occurs after balloon decompression, it should be used as a rescue technique and a bridge to more definitive treatment.

Transjugular intrahepatic portal systemic shunt (TIPS) was introduced in the 1990s, and its use has nearly eliminated the need for emergency shunt surgery. TIPS has become the preferred therapy for most bleeding patients who are not controlled by other nonoperative therapies. TIPS effectively decompresses the portal venous circulation with low short-term mortality, but late TIPS failure rates are high.[86]

A surgical portocaval shunt is considered in cases of continued hemorrhage or recurrent bleeding that cannot be controlled by endoscopic and pharmacologic means, and when TIPS is not available or technically feasible. When performed emergently, mortality approaches 40% but is substantially less when the procedure can be performed electively. Liver transplantation is often offered to patients with Childs B and C cirrhosis soon after or even before they bleed from varices. Secondary prophylaxis with nonselective beta-blockers, plus isosorbide mononitrate and band ligation of varices, reduces the incidence of rebleeding.

Pulmonary Dysfunction

A variety of disorders may produce hypoxemia in patients with advanced cirrhosis, including intrinsic cardiopulmonary

TABLE 39-5

HYPOXEMIA IN PATIENTS WITH CIRRHOSIS

Intrapulmonary shunting caused by intrapulmonary vascular dilatations (precapillary or arteriovenous)
Ventilation-perfusion mismatch caused by impaired hypoxic pulmonary vasoconstriction, pleural effusions, ascites, and diaphragm dysfunction
Decreases in pulmonary diffusion capacity secondary to increased extracellular fluid, interstitial pneumonitis, and/or pulmonary hypertension

disorders such as congestive heart failure, interstitial lung disease, obstructive airway disease, pleural effusions, and pulmonary vascular disease (Table 39-5). Fluid retention may cause interstitial edema, airway edema, and large volume ascites, all of which may contribute to the development of hypoxemia through ventilation-perfusion mismatch and intrapulmonary shunting from compression of the basal regions of the lung.

In the absence of primary lung disease, the major causes of arterial hypoxemia in patients with advanced cirrhosis may be intrapulmonary vascular dilatations (IPVDs). The clinical triad of chronic liver disease, increased alveolar-arterial oxygen gradient, and evidence of IPVDs is defined as the hepatopulmonary syndrome (HPS). IPVD encompasses two types of vascular abnormalities: (1) vascular dilatation at the precapillary level close to the alveoli, and (2) vascular dilatation resulting in larger arteriovenous communications that may or may not be in proximity to gas exchange units.[87] Supplemental oxygen significantly increases the Pa_{O_2} when precapillary IPVD is contributing to hypoxemia, but has minimal effects when larger arteriovenous communications are the primary etiology of hypoxemia. The pathogenesis of IPVD in HPS is incompletely understood, but enhanced pulmonary production of nitric oxide likely plays a role.

IPVD is most commonly detected using contrast-enhanced echocardiography. In normal patients, injection of microbubbles results in transient echogenicity in the right heart with no contrast in the left heart. Patients with dilated precapillary pulmonary vessels show delayed opacification in the left atrium approximately three to six contractions after visualization of the right ventricle.[87]

As many as 40% of patients with cirrhosis have detectable IPVD, and up to 15% have hypoxemia and functional limitation.[88] Survival of patients with HPS is reduced compared with cirrhotic patients of similar Child-Pugh class without HPS. Severe hypoxemia from HPS increases intraoperative and postoperative risks in liver transplantation. IPVD often resolves completely after liver transplantation.

Hepatic hydrothorax occurs in 4 to 10% of cirrhotic patients. These patients characteristically have pleural effusions in the absence of cardiopulmonary disease, secondary to transfer of ascitic fluid from the peritoneal cavity into the pleural space through diaphragmatic defects.[89] The initial treatment of hepatic hydrothorax consists of sodium restriction, diuretics, and thoracentesis; TIPS may be required in refractory cases. Because most of these patients have end-stage liver disease, liver transplantation becomes the preferred treatment if the previous options fail.[89]

Portopulmonary hypertension refers to the development of pulmonary artery hypertension in patients with portal hypertension. It is usually defined as a mean pulmonary artery pressure >25 mm Hg with a normal pulmonary capillary wedge pressure and an elevated pulmonary vascular resistance (>120 dyne/second per cm^{-5}). Portopulmonary hypertension affects between 4 to 6% of patients referred for liver transplantation. Patients with mean pulmonary artery pressures >35 mm Hg are considered to be high-risk transplant candidates.[90]

Ascites, Renal Dysfunction, and the Hepatorenal Syndrome

Ascites and Edema

Ascites is the most common of the major complications of cirrhosis. Nearly 50% of cirrhotic patients develop ascites within 10 years of being diagnosed.[91] Because 50% of cirrhotic patients with ascites die within 3 years, the development of ascites is a clear indication for evaluation for liver transplantation.

The pathogenesis of ascites in cirrhosis is complex and not completely understood. Sodium and water retention plays a key role. Three theories have evolved over time to explain the enhanced sodium and water avidity in patients with cirrhosis. Initially, the "underfilling" theory was proposed. The primary abnormality with this theory is cirrhosis-related hepatic venous block and portal hypertension leading to formation of ascites. This transudation of fluid decreases the effective intravascular volume. The neurohumoral response to "ineffective" plasma volume triggers the kidney to retain sodium and water. Thus, the underfilling hypothesis explains renal sodium retention as a secondary rather than a primary phenomenon (Fig. 39-15).

Subsequent studies determined that total blood volumes were increased in cirrhotic patients with ascites, and this finding led to the proposal of the "overflow" hypothesis to explain the development of ascites in cirrhotics.[92] The primary abnormality with this proposal is sodium and water retention induced by a hepatorenal reflex promoted by portal hypertension. The resulting hypervolemia and increased portal pressure produces "overflow" ascites. Thus, this hypothesis contends that renal sodium retention and plasma volume expansion, rather than

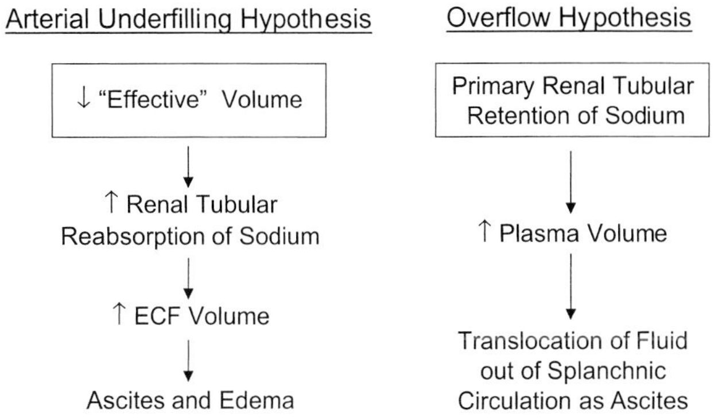

FIGURE 39-15. The presumed sequences of events that result in ascites formation according to the arterial underfilling hypothesis and the overflow hypothesis. The proposed primary disorders are shown in the boxes. According to the underfilling hypothesis, cirrhosis induces abnormal Starling forces in the portal venous circulation that cause an unfavorable distribution of the circulating blood volume (decreased effective blood volume). The diminished "effective" volume constitutes an afferent signal to the renal tubules to augment salt and water reabsorption. The attempt to replenish the diminished effective volume results in an expansion of the total blood volume to values far in excess of normal, with resultant ascites and edema formation. The overflow hypothesis holds that the primary disorder is retention of excessive sodium by the kidneys. In the setting of abnormal Starling forces in the portal venous bed, the expanded plasma volume is sequestered preferentially in the peritoneal sac. ECF, extracellular fluid. (Reprinted with permission from Epstein M: Renal functional abnormalities in cirrhosis: Pathophysiology and management. In Zakim D, Boyer TD [eds]: Hepatology: A Textbook of Liver Disease, p 448. Philadelphia, WB Saunders, 1982.)

plasma volume reduction, are responsible for ascites formation (see Fig. 39-15).

The "peripheral arterial vasodilation hypothesis" was proposed by Schrier and associates in 1988.[93] This theory contends that the primary event leading to sodium and water retention in cirrhosis is splanchnic arterial vasodilation secondary to portal hypertension induced production of vasodilatory mediators such as nitric oxide. At this phase of the disease, ascites has not yet developed, and a hyperdynamic circulation helps maintain systemic perfusion. With disease progression, this compensatory mechanism becomes insufficient to maintain circulatory homeostasis. Enlargement of the intravascular compartment decreases the effective arterial blood volume. Arterial blood pressure decreases, leading to baroreceptor activation, which stimulates three vasoconstrictor systems: the sympathetic nervous system, the renin-angiotensin-aldosterone system, and the nonosmotic release of vasopressin. Renal sodium and water retention increases and contributes to the development of ascites.

The most important initial treatment for patients with ascites resulting from cirrhosis is reduction of sodium intake and diuretic therapy. Fluid intake should be restricted to approximately 1,000 mL per day if the patient also has dilutional hyponatremia.[94] If the patient has significant anasarca, there is no limit to the amount of edema that can be safely mobilized. However, once the edema has resolved, 0.5 kg is probably a reasonable daily maximum weight loss, as ascitic fluid is much more slowly mobilized than edema. The diuretics of choice are either spironolactone or amiloride. Furosemide should be used with caution because of the risk of excessive diuresis, which may lead to potentially serious complications including renal failure of prerenal origin, precipitation of hepatorenal syndrome, hyponatremia, hypokalemia, and encephalopathy.

Refractory ascites occurs in 5 to 10% of ascitic patients and is defined as a lack of response to high dose of diuretics (spironolactone, 400 mg/day plus furosemide 160 mg/day).[95] The main clinical features include marked abdominal distension, frequent recurrence of ascites after paracentesis, an increased risk of developing hepatorenal syndrome, and a poor prognosis. Repeated large-volume paracentesis with use of plasma volume expanders is the most widely accepted therapy for refractory ascites.[96] Removal of large amounts of ascitic fluid without the administration of plasma volume expanders is associated with paracentesis-induced circulatory dysfunction (PICD), characterized by reduction of effective arterial blood volume due to shift of intravascular fluid to the peritoneal cavity, with progressive reaccumulation of ascites and marked activation of the renin-angiotensin-aldosterone system.[97]

The hemodynamic status of patients with tense ascites who undergo rapid total paracentesis without fluid resuscitation typically improves for the first 3 hours following the procedure, as a result of release of compression of the IVC and right atrium. Cardiac output increases, whereas pulmonary artery wedge pressure is unchanged and right atrial pressure decreases.[97] Other studies have demonstrated that along with the early increase in cardiac output, there is a decrease in plasma renin and aldosterone levels, a decrease in serum creatinine and BUN, and reduced portal pressures.[98] However, these beneficial effects are transient.

After 3 hours, the hemodynamic status is determined by the development of a relative hypovolemia caused by progressive reaccumulation of ascites. Twenty-four hours after total paracentesis, there is a significant decrease in cardiac output and cardiac filling pressures, accompanied by increased plasma renin and aldosterone concentrations. This effect is prevented by intravenous albumin infusion.[99] Although the use of albumin in this setting remains controversial because of its high cost and the lack of documented improvement in survival, albumin has a greater protective effect on the circulatory system than other expanders. More recent studies suggest that 50% of the plasma expander should be infused immediately after paracentesis, and the other half, 6 hours later.[100] The prevalence of PICD also depends on the amount of ascitic fluid removed because it is an uncommon complication following a low-volume paracentesis. It can be anticipated that similar hemodynamic changes may occur following emergent laparotomy in patients with tense ascites.

Placement of a peritoneal-venous shunt (Le Veen or Denver) was the first treatment specifically designed for patients with refractory ascites. Le Veen introduced the first prosthesis in 1974. It consists of a perforated intra-abdominal tube connected via a one-way valve to a second tube that traverses the subcutaneous tissue to the jugular vein. This creates a continuous passage of ascites into the systemic circulation. Poor long-term patency and excessive complications have led to the near abandonment of this procedure. A TIPS procedure is effective for preventing recurrence of ascites in patients with refractory ascites. TIPS decreases the activity of sodium-retaining mechanisms and improves the renal response to diuretics. This procedure is better than repeated large-volume paracentesis for the long-term control of ascites, but it has several disadvantages, including a high rate of shunt stenosis, which can lead to recurrence of ascites; a high incidence of severe hepatic encephalopathy; a high cost; and lack of availability in some centers. Survival is not improved by TIPS compared with repeated large-volume paracentesis. Thus, TIPS is not considered the first-line treatment for refractory ascites. Liver transplantation may also be a consideration in these patients.

Spontaneous Bacterial Peritonitis

Spontaneous bacterial peritonitis (SBP) is characterized by the spontaneous infection of ascitic fluid in the absence of an intra-abdominal source of infection. Its prevalence among patients with ascites ranges between 10 and 30%. SBP is diagnosed when there are ≥250 polymorphonuclear (PMN) cells/mm^3 of ascitic fluid. Bacterascites is diagnosed when there are positive ascitic fluid cultures and the neutrophil count is <250 cells/mm^3. SBP develops secondary to translocation of bacteria from the intestinal lumen to regional lymph nodes with subsequent bacteremia and infection of the ascitic fluid. Aerobic Gram-negative bacteria are most commonly isolated, but Gram-positive isolates are being recovered with increasing frequency. Ascitic fluid should be obtained by paracentesis and should be directly inoculated into blood culture bottles at the bedside rather than be cultured by conventional methods. Prospective clinical trials have demonstrated that cultures will be positive in approximately 80% of instances with the former approach versus 50% with the latter in patients with ≥250 PMN cells/mm^3 of ascitic fluid.

Because ascitic fluid PMN count can be assessed much more rapidly than cultures and accurately determines who can benefit from empiric antibiotic coverage, patients with a PMN count ≥250 cells/mm^3 in a clinical setting that is compatible with ascitic fluid infection should receive empiric antibiotic therapy. Delaying antibiotic therapy until positive ascitic fluid cultures are present likely increases the risk of the patient developing severe sepsis. Patients with ascitic PMN counts <250 cells mm^3 with clinical signs or symptoms of infection should also be treated with empiric antibiotics until ascitic culture results are available. Cefotaxime, a third-generation cephalosporin, appears to be the antibiotic of choice for suspected SBP because it covers 95% of the responsible flora, including the three most common isolates, which are *Escherichia coli*, *Klebsiella pneumonia*, and the pneumococcus.

In a retrospective analysis of 252 episodes of SBP, renal insufficiency developed in 33%.[101] The renal dysfunction was transient in 25%, stable in 33%, and progressive in 42%. The overall mortality for an episode of SBP was 24%, but was 54% versus 9% in those with and without the development of renal insufficiency. The development of renal impairment is therefore an important clinical event in the course of SBP. Sepsis-induced decrease in the effective arterial blood volume with subsequent baroreceptor-mediated stimulation of the renin-angiotensin and sympathetic nervous systems, and vasopressin release contribute toward the development renal dysfunction. Direct stimulation of renal vasoconstrictors by endotoxin may also play a role. Sort and associates demonstrated in a randomized, controlled clinical trial of 126 patients with SBP that interventions directed at maintaining effective arterial blood volume (1.5 g/kg albumin within 6 hours of diagnosis of SBP followed by 1 g/kg on day 3) were associated with a significant decrease in development of HRS, and in both the in-hospital and 30-day mortality rates.[102] Data do not exist regarding the efficacy of lower doses of albumin or other plasma volume expanders in preventing HRS.

Long-term antibiotic prophylaxis with a quinolone is recommended following resolution of SBP because there is an estimated 70% probability of recurrence within the first year, and antibiotic prophylaxis has a beneficial effect on patient survival. Short-term quinolone prophylaxis is also recommended for patients with low-protein ascites and gastrointestinal bleeding because bleeding increases bacterial translocation and SBP.

Pathogenesis of Renal Dysfunction

The three main renal functional abnormalities in cirrhosis are reduction in sodium excretion, reduction in free water excretion, and a decrease in renal perfusion and glomerular filtration.[94]

The arterial vasodilation characteristic of cirrhosis, with its associated decrease in effective plasma volume, leads to baroreceptor-mediated activation of the sympathetic nervous system. This causes the kidney to release renin, which results in an increased production of angiotensin II and aldosterone. Both aldosterone and increased sympathetic nervous system outflow enhance tubular sodium resorption. In addition, through their vasoconstrictive actions, norepinephrine and angiotensin II cause a redistribution of renal blood flow, which further decreases sodium elimination.

Water homeostasis is disturbed in up to 75% of patients with advanced cirrhosis and ascites (decompensated cirrhosis). In these patients, water retention, increased total body water, and dilutional hyponatremia develop when fluid intake exceeds the impaired renal capacity to excrete free water. Reduced glomerular filtration secondary to impaired perfusion, elevated vasopressin levels caused by nonosmotic hypersecretion and decreased metabolic clearance, and impaired renal production of prostaglandin E2 also contribute to the impairment of free water excretion.

The major consequence of reduced sodium excretion is the development of edema and ascites. When free water clearance becomes significantly reduced, dilutional hyponatremia develops. The main consequence of decreased renal perfusion and GFR is development of the hepatorenal syndrome.

Hepatorenal Syndrome

HRS is a functional prerenal failure that occurs in up to 10% of patients with advanced cirrhosis and ascites, and less commonly in patients with acute liver failure. HRS is characterized by intense vasoconstriction of the renal circulation, low glomerular filtration, preserved renal tubular function, and normal renal histology.

HRS may be diagnosed after other causes of renal failure are ruled out. The International Ascites Club has suggested five major criteria to confirm the diagnosis of HRS: (1) chronic or acute liver disease with advanced hepatic failure and portal hypertension; (2) a low GFR as assessed by serum creatinine >1.5 mg/dL or creatinine clearance below 40 mL/min; (3) absence of shock, ongoing bacterial infection, fluid losses, or treatment with nephrotoxic drugs; (4) no sustained improvement in renal function after oral diuretic withdrawal and plasma volume expansion; and (5) less than 500 mg/day proteinuria with no ultrasonographic evidence of parenchymal renal disease or urinary obstruction.[103]

HRS has been classified clinically into two types based on its intensity and presentation. Type 1 HRS is characterized by progressive oliguria and a rapid rise in the serum creatinine concentration. Type 1 HRS develops in 5% of cirrhotics hospitalized for acute upper gastrointestinal bleeding, 30% of those admitted for SBP, 10% of patients with ascites treated with total paracentesis, and 25% of patients with severe acute alcoholic hepatitis.[104] SBP commonly precipitates the development of type 1 HRS. The prognosis of type 1 HRS is poor, with a median survival of less than 1 month without therapeutic intervention. Type 2 HRS is usually seen in patients with refractory ascites, and is characterized by a moderate and more stable impairment of renal function.

Pathophysiologically, intense renal vasoconstriction is the final consequence of extreme vasodilation of the splanchnic arterial circulation that reduces the effective arterial blood volume (that sensed by the central arterial circulation). The resulting abnormal distribution of arterial volume is associated with reduced flow to all extrasplanchnic areas, including the kidneys. Splanchnic arterial vasodilation is related to an increased level of both endothelial (prostacyclin and nitric oxide) and nonendothelial vasodilators (e.g., glucagon). Increased activity of both the renin-angiotensin and sympathetic nervous systems mediate the renal vasoconstriction, as well as other intrarenal vasoconstrictor factors such as endothelin, adenosine, and leukotrienes.[105]

Until more recently, the development of type 1 HRS was considered to be an irreversible clinical condition, which in the absence of an emergent liver transplant, was associated with rapid progression to death. Because HRS develops as a consequence of splanchnic arterial vasodilation, drugs that produce splanchnic vasoconstriction have been proposed for treatment of this condition. Several different vasoconstrictors (vasopressin analogs, catecholamines), usually combined with albumin infusion, have been evaluated in small nonrandomized clinical trials. Vasoconstrictor therapy results in an increased arterial blood pressure, near-normalization of the activity of the major endogenous vasoconstrictor systems, and marked increases in renal plasma flow, GFR, and urine volume in approximately two-thirds of patients. These studies have demonstrated that a prolonged improvement in circulatory function, with 1 to 2 weeks of administration of intravenous albumin and vasoconstrictors, is required to reverse HRS, with a lag between the normalization of systemic circulation and the improvement in renal perfusion and GFR. Recurrence of HRS in responding patients after withdrawal of therapy is uncommon.[106,107]

Octreotide, an inhibitor of the release of gastrointestinal vasodilator peptides such as glucagon and vasoactive intestinal peptide, when combined with midodrine and intravenous albumin, has been shown to have beneficial effects on renal function in a clinical study of five patients with type 1 HRS.[107]

Patients showing an improvement in renal function after vasoconstrictor therapy survive significantly longer than patients who do not respond. Treatment with vasoconstrictors may thus increase the likelihood that patients with HRS will survive long enough to undergo liver transplantation. Transplant survival may be significantly reduced in cirrhotic patients with preoperative renal failure. Reversal of HRS with vasoconstrictor therapy is, therefore, an important tool in patients waiting for a liver transplant.

TABLE 39-6

DIFFERENTIAL DIAGNOSIS OF ACUTE AZOTEMIA IN PATIENTS WITH LIVER DISEASE: IMPORTANT DIFFERENTIAL URINARY FINDINGS

	PRERENAL AZOTEMIA	HEPATORENAL SYNDROME	ACUTE RENAL FAILURE (ACUTE TUBULAR NECROSIS)
Urinary sodium concentration	<10 mEq/L	<10 mEq/L	>30 mEq/L
Urine-to-plasma creatinine ratio	>30:1	>30:1	<20:1
Urinary osmolality	Exceeds plasma osmolality by at least 100 mOsm	Exceeds plasma osmolality by at least 100 mOsm	Equal to plasma osmolality
Urinary sediment	Normal	Unremarkable	Casts, cellular debris

From Epstein M: Renal functional abnormalities in cirrhosis: Pathophysiology and management. In Zakim D, Boyer TD (eds): Hepatology: A Textbook of Liver Disease, p 460. Philadelphia, WB Saunders, 1982, with permission.

Acute Renal Failure and Acute Tubular Necrosis

Cirrhotic patients are also at risk for developing acute renal failure from acute tubular necrosis (ATN), especially following infection or hypotensive episodes. ATN occurs more frequently after surgical procedures to relieve obstructive jaundice than it does following similar operations on nonjaundiced patients. The impaired vasoconstrictor response to hypovolemia seen in patients with hepatic parenchymal disease and obstructive jaundice limits the normal redistribution of splanchnic blood to the central circulation that occurs with hemorrhage. Therefore, even moderate hemorrhage may produce severe hypotension and cause ATN. In addition, conjugated bilirubin appears to be toxic to renal tubules and may contribute to the development of ATN in jaundiced patients.

The differential diagnosis of acute azotemia in patients with liver disease is outlined in Table 39-6. Of note is the remarkable similarity of the urinary characteristics of prerenal azotemia and HRS. Prompt detection and treatment of hypovolemia may rapidly improve renal function in prerenal azotemia, but this response does not if HRS is present.

Hematologic and Coagulation Disorders

The liver is the site of synthesis of all clotting factors with the exception of von Willebrand factor (vWF), an endothelial product. Anticoagulant (antithrombin III, proteins C and S), and fibrinolytic factors are also products of the liver. Acute or chronic liver disease results in a variable level of impairment of hemostasis from multiple causes: decreased production of coagulation and inhibitor factors, synthesis of dysfunctional clotting factors, quantitative and qualitative platelet defects, vitamin K deficiency, decreased clearance of activated factors, hyperfibrinolysis, and disseminated intravascular coagulation.

Vitamin K is an essential cofactor for the production in the liver of factors II, VII, IX, and X, and also proteins C and S. The precursors of vitamin K-dependent coagulation factors are also synthesized in the liver. Vitamin K is needed for conversion of these factors to active forms by gamma carboxylation of glutamic acid residues in the amino-terminal region of the precursors. The carboxylated residues permit the binding of calcium ions that are essential for their functional activity.

Vitamin K is a fat-soluble vitamin requiring bile salts for absorption from the intestines. Thus, deficiency of the vitamin K-dependent factors results when there is impaired bile secretion from either intrahepatic or extrahepatic cholestasis.

Thrombocytopenia occurs in approximately 30 to 64% of patients with advanced chronic liver disease; however, the platelet count is rarely less than 30,000 cells/μL, and spontaneous bleeding is uncommon. The primary cause of thrombocytopenia in cirrhosis is portal hypertension-induced splenomegaly because up to 90% of circulating platelets may be sequestered in the enlarged spleen. Decreased hepatic synthesis and serum levels of the cytokine thrombopoietin are also believed to have a causative role in cirrhotics with thrombocytopenia. Increased destruction of platelets by immune mechanism; coexistent, low-grade, disseminated intravascular coagulation; sepsis; and direct suppression of bone marrow thrombopoiesis by ethanol, folate deficiency, and other drugs may all contribute to the development of thrombocytopenia in patients with chronic liver disease.

Dysfibrinogenemia is the most common qualitative abnormality of clotting factors in patients with liver disease. The abnormal functioning of fibrinogen is caused by an increased degree of sialylation of the molecule. This produces abnormal polymerization of fibrin monomers and leads to a disproportionate prolonged thrombin time, despite mild prolongation of the PT and partial thromboplastin (PTT) and normal amount of fibrinogen.

Hyperfibrinolysis is a common finding in patients with advanced liver disease and results from decreased hepatic clearance of plasminogen activator. This complication may be documented by the finding of decreased whole blood euglobulin clot lysis time, with elevated levels of D-dimer, fibrin, and fibrinogen degradation products.

Diagnosing disseminated intravascular coagulation in cirrhotic patients is difficult. The diagnosis is suggested when there is a known triggering event associated with progressive worsening of coagulation test results and platelet counts, as well as a disproportionate reduction of factor V with a concomitant decreased level of a previously normal factor VIII.

Disorders of coagulation rapidly develop in patients with severe acute liver failure because of the brief half-life of some of the clotting factors. Factors II, V, VII, IX and X are all reduced in acute liver failure. As a consequence, the PT and INR become markedly elevated, serving as prognostic indicators and predictors of the need for transplantation. Reduced concentrations of the vitamin K-dependent factors are due predominantly to a combination of decreased hepatic synthesis and increased consumption of coagulation factors, rather than to vitamin K deficiency.

Thrombocytopenia is also a frequent finding in patients with acute liver failure with platelet counts below 100,000 cells/μL, developing in approximately 66% of patients at some point in their clinical course.

Quantitative and qualitative abnormalities of fibrinogen are also seen, and there is often evidence of excessive thrombin activity, increased fibrinogen turnover, and fibrinolysis, but the relative contributions of disseminated intravascular coagulopathy and impaired hepatic synthesis/clearance to the development of hemostatic abnormalities in acute liver failure remains unclear.

Spontaneous bleeding occurs infrequently in patients with advanced liver disease, and prophylactic treatment is not generally required. Bleeding, however, accounts for 60% of all deaths in cirrhotics having abdominal surgery; therefore, correction of coagulation abnormalities is appropriate prior to major surgical procedures and invasive diagnostic studies. A PT prolonged by >3 seconds or a platelet count of <50,000 cells/μL are considered contraindications to elective surgery.[108]

Perioperative management includes blood component therapy guided by laboratory studies. Fresh frozen plasma contains all the clotting factors, and administration of 10 to 20 mL/kg will usually correct the PT to nearly normal levels, but the effect lasts for no more than 12 to 24 hours. Vitamin K may improve the PT in patients with cholestatic disease. In these instances, 10 mg subcutaneous vitamin K should be given for 3 consecutive days. Platelets should be infused prophylactically prior to elective surgery when the platelet count is less than 60,000 cells/μL.[109]

Endocrine Disorders

The presence of advanced cirrhosis invariably leads to abnormal regulation and function of multiple endocrine systems. The prevalence and severity of endocrine dysfunction are increased in diseases such as hemochromatosis, in which both the liver and endocrine organs are damaged by a common pathophysiologic process. Cirrhotic patients often have abnormal glucose utilization. The mechanism of this phenomenon is rather complex and includes increased fatty acid concentration in the plasma, which antagonizes the effects of insulin on glucose uptake by skeletal muscles. In addition, plasma levels of growth hormone and glucagon are often increased, and undoubtedly contribute to the glucose intolerance and other derangements of intermediary metabolism that occur in patients with hepatic dysfunction. Patients with cirrhosis are also prone to hypoglycemia. This may reflect glycogen depletion secondary to malnutrition or alcohol-induced glycogenolysis and interference with gluconeogenesis. Severe cirrhosis may also impair hepatic conversion of lactate to glucose.

Abnormal metabolism of sex hormones causes gonadal dysfunction in both men and women. Men undergo feminization, often developing gynecomastia along with a decrease in the size of their testes and prostate gland. The frequency of impotence increases, and sperm counts typically decrease. Women with liver dysfunction commonly exhibit oligomenorrhea or amenorrhea.

Hepatic Encephalopathy

Hepatic encephalopathy (HE) is a complex reversible metabolic encephalopathy presenting as a wide spectrum of neuropsychiatric abnormalities in patients with hepatocellular failure and/or increased portal-systemic shunting. The clinical manifestations are highly variable and range from minimal changes in personality or altered sleep patterns without overt signs of HE (minimal HE), to confusion, lethargy, somnolence, and coma. Thirty to 60% of cirrhotics have at least minimal HE. Several well-recognized factors can precipitate HE in patients with cirrhosis who were previously stable (Table 39-7). A large dietary protein load, gastrointestinal hemorrhage, constipation, hypokalemia, diuretics, and azotemia produce an increased blood ammonia level. Surgery, associated with anesthesia and dehydration, can precipitate an episode of HE because of decreased hepatic perfusion. Sepsis can precipitate HE through increased ammonia production due to protein catabolism, impaired hepatic perfusion, and the effects of cytokines on the central nervous system. Psychoactive drugs can also precipitate HE. The diagnosis has to be made on the basis of clinical findings. Several other conditions that may present in a similar fashion must be excluded, including chronic subdural hematoma, Wernicke's encephalopathy, and electrolyte disturbances.

TABLE 39-7

FACTORS THAT MAY PRECIPITATE HEPATIC ENCEPHALOPATHY

PRECIPITATING FACTOR	POSSIBLE MECHANISMS
Excessive dietary protein Constipation Gastrointestinal bleeding Infection Azotemia	Increased ammonia production
Diarrhea and vomiting Diuretic therapy Paracentesis	Dehydration with electrolyte and acid-base imbalance, increased ammonia generation, and decreased hepatic perfusion, increasing blood ammonia level
Hypoxia Hypotension Anemia Hypoglycemia	Adverse effect on liver and brain function
Sedatives/hypnotics	Action at the $GABA_A$/benzodiazepine receptor complex
Creation of portal-systemic shunt	Reduced hepatic metabolism

It is commonly believed that HE is caused by substances that under normal circumstances are efficiently metabolized by the liver, rather than by insufficient synthesis of substrates essential for normal neurologic function. This notion is consistent with the development of HE in patients following portosystemic bypass who do not have significant intrinsic liver disease. More than 20 different compounds have increased blood concentrations when liver function is impaired. Of these, ammonia has been considered the most important factor in the genesis of HE. Ammonia is produced in the intestine by catabolism of proteins, amino acids, and biogenic amines. Forty percent is derived from intestinal bacterial metabolism of nitrogenous substances, and most of the remainder from digestion of dietary protein. The concentration of ammonia in portal venous blood is high, and a high degree of extraction occurs in the liver where the ammonia is converted to urea and glutamine. This detoxification is impaired in cirrhotics as a result of impaired conversion by the liver and marked portal-systemic shunting. Increased ammonia levels in blood result in increased diffusion of ammonia into the brain. Variation in the transfer of ammonia across the blood-brain barrier may explain the poor relationship between the blood ammonia level and the degree of hepatic encephalopathy. Ammonia has many deleterious effects on brain function. Although this ion seems to play a central role, the clinical features of HE differ from those of pure ammonia intoxication, and therefore, other mechanisms must be involved.

The clinical and neurophysiologic manifestations of HE seem to reflect a global depression of central nervous system function caused by an increase in inhibitory neurotransmission. The observation of an improvement in mental status after the administration of flumazenil, a benzodiazepine receptor antagonist, in some patients with advanced HE who have not taken benzodiazepines supports a role for an increased GABAergic tone. One possible mechanism is an increased availability of agonist ligands of the GABA receptor complex. These are called natural benzodiazepines and bind to the benzodiazepine site of the GABA receptor. Natural benzodiazepines accumulate in the brains of patients with HE, and it has been suggested that they may induce a decrease in consciousness.

Other putative mechanisms include the effects of a group of potentially neurotoxic compounds of colonic origin (mercaptans, short-chain fatty acids, manganese), impairment of cerebral energy metabolism, gliopathy secondary to astrocyte swelling, and disruption of the blood-brain barrier. Patients with liver failure have an increase in plasma levels of aromatic amino acids and a decrease in branched-chain amino acids. It has been proposed that this imbalance enhances the entry of aromatic amino acids into the brain and that these are channeled into the synthesis of abnormal biogenic amines, which are released along with, or instead of, normal neurotransmitters. These *false neurotransmitters* (octopamine, phenylethanolamine) are relatively inactive. However, this hypothesis has not been supported by in vivo or postmortem studies. Administration of intravenous branched-chain amino acids does not produce beneficial effects in acute HE.

The main principles of treatment of HE have not been evaluated by randomized clinical trials but rather have been accepted on the basis of clinical observation.[110,111] Most episodes of HE in patients with cirrhosis are initiated by an identifiable precipitating factor. Because effective methods exist to control most of these, a key component of the treatment of HE is to identify and treat the precipitating cause. Often, the elimination of these factors leads to an improvement without need for any additional therapy. If no precipitating factor can be identified or if rapid improvement does not occur with treatment, therapy should be initiated to reduce the production and absorption of ammonia. Dietary protein intake should be restricted, to an extent dependent on the severity of HE. However, severe restriction of dietary protein is no longer recommended because of the adverse effects of severe malnutrition on liver function and short-term prognosis.[112]

Lactulose (*B*-galactosidofructose) is a nonabsorbable disaccharide that is not broken down by intestinal enzymes following oral administration, but is metabolized by enteric bacteria in the cecum to lactate and acetate. This produces a reduction of ammonia absorption from the large intestine (because it is converted to ammonium) and net movement of NH_3 from the blood into the bowel. In addition, lactulose enhances the growth of non–urease-producing bacteria, thereby reducing the bacterial production of ammonia, and it also has cathartic activity.

Neomycin is an alternative to lactulose for patients who do not tolerate the disaccharide or have unsatisfactory results. It reduces the intestinal production of ammonia by reducing the population of urease-producing bacteria and may also have nonbacterial effects. Prolonged use should be avoided because of possible toxicity from the small amount of drug that is absorbed. Neomycin is as effective as lactulose.

Zinc deficiency is common in cirrhotics due to increased urinary excretion and malnutrition. Two of the five enzymes responsible for the metabolism of ammonia to urea are zinc dependent; thus, it has been suggested that zinc deficiency contributes to the development of HE. Whether zinc supplementation in this population is beneficial has not been established. Flumazenil, a selective antagonist of the central benzodiazepine receptor, produces a transient improvement in the mental status of some patients with HE, but has no sustained benefits. The dopamine agonists, bromocriptine and levodopa, were introduced to restore the decreased activity of central neurotransmitters caused by false neurotransmitters. Although the false neurotransmitter hypothesis is now questioned, these drugs may help chronic HE patients with extrapyramidal manifestations, which are believed to develop as a result of manganese accumulation in the basal ganglia.

It appears clear that encephalopathic changes are associated with clinically important alterations in pharmacodynamics and pharmacokinetics of various medications. For example, cerebral uptake of benzodiazepines increases substantially, which may reflect an increase in the density or affinity of benzodiazepine receptors or a leaky blood-brain barrier. Drugs administered to patients with advanced hepatic disease require careful titration against effect.

Orthotopic liver transplantation cures HE. Medical management for HE is mainly used for patients who do not yet meet the criteria for liver transplantation, who are waiting for a transplant, or who are not transplant candidates. Without transplantation, overt HE in the patient with chronic liver disease has a poor prognosis, with a survival rate of 42% at 1 year and 23% at 3 years.

Uncommon Causes of Cirrhosis

Wilson's Disease

Wilson's disease (hepatolenticular degeneration) is a hereditary disease characterized by decreased hepatocellular excretion of copper into the bile and decreased binding of copper to apoceruloplasmin, resulting in hepatic copper accumulation, hepatic injury, and decreased ceruloplasmin levels in the blood. Eventually, copper is released into the bloodstream and is deposited in various organs, especially the brain, cornea, and kidneys. Untreated, it is a lethal disease with progressive lenticular degeneration, accompanied by chronic liver disease leading to cirrhosis.[113] Wilson's disease has an autosomal recessive pattern of inheritance. Homozygotes have a defect of the hepatic enzyme required for transmembrane transport of copper into the bile. Wilson's disease occurs worldwide with an average prevalence of approximately 30 affected individuals per million population. It can present clinically as liver disease, as a progressive neurologic disorder, or as a psychiatric illness.

The clinical presentation of liver dysfunction in patients with Wilson's disease can range from asymptomatic, with only biochemical evidence of damage, to fulminant liver failure requiring urgent liver transplantation for survival. Histologically, steatosis and focal hepatocellular necrosis occur early, with progression to fibrosis and cirrhosis, which is present in most untreated patients by the second decade of life. Neurologic dysfunction typically becomes evident later than liver disease. Tremors, gait disturbances, and slurring of speech are common manifestations, simulating Parkinson's disease. Kayser-Fleischer rings are a pathognomonic sign but are present in only 50 to 62% of patients with Wilson's disease at the time of diagnosis.[113] They represent copper deposition in Decemet's membrane of the cornea and usually require a slit-lamp examination for their identification.

A combination of clinical findings and biochemical testing is necessary to establish the diagnosis of Wilson's disease. Recognition of Kayser-Fleischer rings, increased liver copper concentrations on percutaneous biopsy samples, reduced concentration of ceruloplasmin in the blood, and increased urinary copper excretion can point to the correct diagnosis prior to development of neurologic symptoms. A hepatic copper content of $\geq$250 μg/g dry weight is the best biochemical evidence for Wilson's disease. The combination of a blood ceruloplasmin level <200 mg/L associated with the presence of Kayser-Fleischer rings is also diagnostic.

Lifelong pharmacologic treatment is given to symptomatic patients or to those with active disease. The oral chelating drugs D-penicillamine or trientine bind copper and thereby promote urinary excretion. Liver transplantation corrects the underlying hepatic defect, but is reserved for patients with decompensated liver disease unresponsive to medical therapy and for patients presenting with fulminant hepatic failure.

Hereditary Hemochromatosis

Hemochromatosis is a hereditary disease characterized by excessive iron absorption from the duodenum and subsequent tissue deposition producing organ damage, which is frequently irreversible. Hemochromatosis may be the most common autosomal-recessive genetic disease in Caucasians. It is estimated that 1 in 10 to 20 Caucasians carry the disease gene, and 1 in 400 are homozygotes who are at risk of clinical disease. It is currently impossible to predict whether and to what extent the mutation will be expressed and, in a small percentage of homozygotes, laboratory evidence of altered iron metabolism never develops.[114]

Hemochromatosis occurs when intestinal absorption of dietary iron exceeds bodily needs. The primary site for regulating iron absorption is in duodenal mucosa cells. Duodenal iron absorption is normally minimized when body iron stores are increased. In hemochromatosis, this step is inappropriately controlled, and although iron overload is present, enterocytes continue to transfer unneeded iron into the bloodstream. A gradual and progressive expansion of the plasma iron compartment occurs that produces an increased transferrin-saturation value (the earliest detectable biochemical abnormality in hemochromatosis).

Symptomatic organ involvement usually does not begin until the fourth or fifth decade of life, and reflects injury induced by parenchymal iron deposition. The nonspecific initial symptoms often found in these patients, such as unexplained weakness, lethargy, and arthralgias, makes consideration of hemochromatosis unlikely. Subsequently, liver disease often predominates and may range from transaminitis to end-stage cirrhosis with signs of portal hypertension. Hepatomegaly is the most common physical finding on presentation, found in 80% of patients, followed by increased skin pigmentation in 75%.[115] Once the patient has developed cirrhosis, the chances of developing hepatocellular carcinoma are increased 200-fold.

In addition to hepatic infiltration, iron deposition frequently affects: (1) islet cells of the pancreas producing diabetes mellitus; (2) the pituitary gland, producing hypogonadotrophic hypogonadism, impotence, and hypothyroidism; (3) the myocardium, frequently with dysrhythmias, while up to one-third of untreated patients die of cardiac failure; and (4) the skin, with a characteristic bronze discoloration.

Thanks to increasingly early diagnosis, the classic triad of cirrhosis, diabetes mellitus, and bronze skin is now rare in adult-onset hemochromatosis. The best diagnostic test is the serum transferrin saturation level, which is normally less than 50%. In the absence of significant liver disease, which would lead to decreased hepatic transferrin synthesis, a transferrin saturation level consistently greater than 62% is associated with a greater than 90% chance of hemochromatosis. Suggestive laboratory results should be followed by a liver biopsy; the presence of substantial stainable iron in parenchymal liver cells is characteristic of hemochromatosis.

Once the diagnosis is confirmed by liver biopsy, the patient should be treated by repeated phlebotomy to remove excess iron from tissues and the blood. If initiated early in the course of the disease, organ damage can be prevented and survival improved. Established organ damage cannot be reversed, but progression can be slowed.

Primary Biliary Cirrhosis

Primary biliary cirrhosis (PBC) accounts for up to 2% of worldwide deaths from cirrhosis. It is a chronic progressive cholestatic liver disease of unknown etiology that most commonly affects middle-age women. Genetic factors play a role in the development of PBC, but it is not inherited in a simple dominant or recessive pattern. PBC is characterized by portal inflammation, destruction of the small intrahepatic bile ducts, and progressive scarring. It commonly presents as unexplained hepatomegaly or an elevated alkaline phosphatase level in an asymptomatic patient. Fatigue and pruritus are often the initial symptoms. Jaundice is a late manifestation of the disease. The antimitochondrial antibody test is positive in 95% of patients and is relatively specific for the disease. There is a strong association between PBC and other autoimmune diseases. The diagnosis should be confirmed by percutaneous liver biopsy, which also provides staging and prognostic data. The median survival of symptomatic patients is approximately 7 years. There is no generally accepted effective medical treatment, although cholestyramine may alleviate pruritus. Liver transplantation is the only treatment that improves survival.[116]

α-1-Antitripsin Deficiency

Patients with homozygous deficiency of serum α-1-antitrypsin (α-1-AT) develop a slowly progressive liver disease that most commonly progresses to asymptomatic cirrhosis, which may be complicated by the development of hepatocellular carcinoma. Adult patients with this disorder often have emphysema. The molecular basis for the disease is related to a single nucleic acid substitution. The diagnosis is suggested by the presence of hepatomegaly, mild LFT abnormalities, and the absence of α-1-AT on serum protein electrophoresis. The diagnosis is confirmed by direct measurement of serum α-1-AT and/or demonstration of characteristic periodic acid-Schiff-positive, diastase-resistant globules adjacent to portal tracts on liver biopsy.

Budd-Chiari Syndrome

Budd-Chiari syndrome is a heterogeneous group of disorders characterized by outflow obstruction of blood, from the liver to the right heart. The pathologic processes responsible for the syndrome can be categorized into three groups: those that affect the hepatic venules, those obstructing the major hepatic veins, and those preventing the flow of blood from the hepatic veins into the right atrium.[117]

Hepatic veno-occlusive disease refers to obstruction of hepatic venous outflow at the level of the central or sublobular veins. Cytotoxic agents used in preparation of patients for bone marrow transplantation are the most common causes of the disease in the United States. Obstruction of the major hepatic veins is most commonly related to an underlying hypercoagulable state, including myeloproliferative disorders or malignancies that involve the hepatic veins either directly or by extension of tumor thrombus. Obstruction of the IVC proximal to the right atrium is commonly the result of either a membranous intracaval web or caval thickening.

Obstruction of venous outflow results in increased hepatic sinusoidal pressure and portal hypertension. Hepatic venous stasis and congestion causes hypoxic damage to adjacent hepatic parenchymal cells and cells lining the sinusoids. Hepatocyte necrosis develops in centrilobular regions followed by fibrosis, nodular regeneration, and ultimately, cirrhosis.

The clinical presentation is highly variable, and depends on the extent and rapidity of hepatic vein occlusion and on the development of a collateral circulation to decompress the sinusoids. Symptoms include right upper quadrant tenderness secondary to hepatomegaly and abdominal distension due to ascites. Laboratory evaluation usually reveals modest alteration in liver function tests and low serum albumin. Rarely, fulminant liver failure occurs if there is rapid and complete occlusion of the hepatic veins and secondary thrombosis of the portal vein as the result of hepatic outflow obstruction.

A variety of noninvasive tests can be used to support the diagnosis of Budd-Chiari syndrome. Doppler ultrasonography of the liver is the most cost-effective radiographic tool for initial evaluation when the syndrome is suspected. It will reveal absent or diminished hepatic venous blood flow, thrombosis of the IVC, and liver and spleen enlargement. CT and MRI scanning are more expensive alternatives. Once the diagnosis is suggested by its clinical features and noninvasive radiographic evaluation, venography with cannulation of the hepatic veins is usually performed. The diagnosis is confirmed by a "spiderweb." If appropriate, a number of interventional procedures can then be performed, including thrombolytic therapy and balloon angioplasty.[117]

Untreated, Budd-Chiari syndrome will result in death within months to years. Therapy includes medical management and relief of hepatic venous outflow obstruction to prevent further hepatic injury or liver transplantation in selected patients, especially those with fulminant liver failure.

Medical therapy is limited primarily to anticoagulation and thrombolysis. The latter is considered in patients with acute onset of the syndrome, especially if angiography reveals fresh thrombus in the hepatic veins and IVC. The thrombolytic agent is infused directly into the thrombosed vein for approximately 24 hours. Percutaneous transluminal angioplasty of localized segments of narrowed hepatic veins or inferior vena caval webs may result in dramatic improvement, although the risk of restenosis is high. This may be prevented with intravascular metal stent placement.

The mainstay of therapy involves surgical intervention. By relieving sinusoidal hypertension, portosystemic shunting may reverse hepatic necrosis and prevent the development of cirrhosis. The most commonly used technique is a side-to-side portocaval shunt. Liver transplantation is usually reserved for those patients with decompensated cirrhosis, fulminant hepatic failure, or failure of a portosystemic shunt.[117]

HEPATOCELLULAR CARCINOMA

Primary hepatocellular carcinoma (HCC) is one of the most common tumors in the world and the third most frequent cause of death from cancer. It occurs in the United States with an incidence of 2.4 individuals per 100,000 population. HCC usually arises in a cirrhotic liver. Cirrhosis secondary to chronic viral hepatitis accounts for the large majority of HCC worldwide but only 30 to 40% of reported cases in America. Thus, there are many individuals in whom no obvious cause can be identified. Inherited metabolic diseases, including hemochromatosis, α-1-antitrypsin deficiency, and Wilson's disease, are well known to be risk factors for the development of HCC. Another implicated factor is alcohol. Alcoholic cirrhosis may clearly result in HCC, but it is uncertain whether alcohol is directly carcinogenic or whether associated hepatocellular injury and regeneration, iron accumulation, or coexistent hepatitis C infection is responsible.

HCC may escape early clinical detection because it occurs in patients with underlying cirrhosis, and the clinical findings may suggest progression of the underlying disease. The most common presenting complaint is abdominal pain, and the most frequent finding on physical examination is an abdominal mass. Serum alpha fetoprotein (AFP) values are greater than 500 μg/L in about 70 to 80% of patients with HCC. Unfortunately, AFP has a low specificity and levels may be elevated in pregnancy, germ cell tumors, and acute or chronic hepatitis. Hepatic ultrasound has greater sensitivity and specificity than AFP levels when used for HCC screening. Three imaging procedures are in common use for diagnosing HCC, ultrasonography, helical CT, and MRI. The sensitivity and specificity of radiologic studies for detection of HCC is unknown.

Chemoembolization is widely used for treatment of HCC. No studies have shown a long-term survival advantage in treated versus untreated patients. Surgical resection offers a chance for cure; however, few patients have a resectable tumor at the time of presentation. Patients with two or fewer lesions, each smaller than 5 cm, which are encapsulated and have no evidence of macroscopic vascular invasion are the best candidates for hepatic resection. Operative mortality in cirrhotics is approximately 10%.[118] Liver transplantation may be considered as a therapeutic option for patients who have a single lesion $\leq$5 cm or three or fewer lesions $\leq$3 cm. Survival after transplantation in these groups is similar to that of patients transplanted for nonmalignant disease.

PREGNANCY-RELATED DISORDERS

Well-known disorders of pregnancy that can cause fulminant hepatic failure during the third trimester or in the immediate postpartum period include acute fatty liver of pregnancy (AFLP) and the HELLP syndrome (Hemolysis, Elevated Liver enzymes, Low Platelets). In addition, parturients are unusually susceptible to morbidity and mortality from hepatitis E infection and herpes simplex hepatitis.

Acute Fatty Liver of Pregnancy

AFLP occurs in the late stages of pregnancy. Although severe cases are rare (frequency of 1/6,659 deliveries in a 1999 report), it is now recognized to exist in a broad clinical spectrum ranging from mild to severe hepatic disease. The pathogenesis is unclear, but an association between inherited defects in beta-oxidation of fatty acids and AFLP is now well established. Some affected patients have an inherited long-chain 3-hydroxyacyl-CoA dehydrogenase deficiency, which causes a defect in intramitochondrial beta-oxidation of fatty acids. Other patients with AFLP have a defect in beta-oxidation caused by deficiency of carnitine palmitoyltransferase I.

Affected women usually present in the third trimester with symptoms related to hepatic failure. Initial symptoms are variable, and include nausea, vomiting, abdominal pain, and encephalopathy. Modest elevations of serum transaminases (<750 U/L) are usual. Jaundice is common as is laboratory evidence of renal dysfunction and leukocytosis. Prolongation of the prothrombin time and other laboratory findings of disseminated intravascular coagulation are often present and help distinguish AFLP from HELLP syndrome. Severely affected patients have complications typical of any form of fulminant hepatic failure, including hepatic coma and renal failure. Some patients are asymptomatic, with the diagnosis made during evaluation of abnormal liver function tests. Imaging techniques have not been consistently useful for confirming the diagnosis of AFLP. Although a liver biopsy can be diagnostic, it is often contraindicated because of coagulopathy. Therefore, the diagnosis of AFLP is clinical. When a biopsy is available, the characteristic histologic finding is microvesicular fatty infiltration most prominent in the central zone, with sparing of the periportal hepatocytes.

When AFLP is diagnosed, delivery of the fetus is expedited, usually by induction of labor or, occasionally, cesarean section, because AFLP improves in response to termination of pregnancy. After delivery, maximal supportive care is required as the liver recovers. Most affected women recover completely, although severe cases may require prolonged intensive care. On rare occasions, liver transplantation has been necessary. Recurrence of AFLP with future pregnancy is uncommon.

Preeclampsia and HELLP Syndrome

HELLP syndrome was defined by Weinstein in 1982. It is now recognized to be a common and potentially ominous complication of preeclampsia, affecting 10% of women with this disorder, and 20% of women with severe preeclampsia. The presence of HELLP syndrome is associated with an increased risk of maternal (1%) and perinatal (up to 20.4%) death.[119] The diagnosis of HELLP syndrome is made clinically by the presence of signs of preeclampsia and laboratory evidence of hemolysis (elevated serum LDH level, schistocytes and burr cells on peripheral smear), elevated serum transaminases due to ischemic hepatocellular necrosis (up to several thousand IU), and thrombocytopenia (<100,000 cells/μL). Hyperbilirubinemia occurs in approximately 40% of cases of HELLP, and may be caused by hemolysis and liver dysfunction. The presence of full-blown coagulopathy is rare and should raise concern for the presence of hepatic failure caused by AFLP. It should be noted that there is considerable disagreement in the medical literature about the diagnostic criteria for the HELLP syndrome.[119]

Liver biopsy is rarely warranted, but when performed, the specimens usually demonstrate periportal hemorrhage and fibrin deposition with periportal hepatic necrosis. Both macrovesicular and microvesicular fat are present, but steatosis is usually modest and is unlike the pericentral microvesicular fat seen in AFLP. The liver involvement in HELLP syndrome is most frequently misdiagnosed as viral hepatitis, although thrombocytopenia is an uncommon finding in the latter disease. AFLP also should be considered, but is usually associated with more severe liver failure and not necessarily with thrombocytopenia. All affected patients should be considered to have severe preeclampsia. Once the diagnosis is made, management is primarily supportive. There is a consensus of opinion that prompt delivery is indicated if the syndrome develops beyond 34 weeks' gestation or earlier if life-threatening morbidity develops in the mother. When HELLP syndrome develops prior to 34 weeks' gestation, management is controversial with the choice of either providing supportive care with close monitoring of mother and fetus until the fetus is mature, or administration of corticosteroids to accelerate fetal lung maturity followed by delivery after 24 hours.[119]

In most affected patients, all abnormalities associated with preeclampsia and HELLP syndrome resolve after delivery, leaving no hepatic sequelae. Rarely, the condition worsens progressively after delivery with further diminution of the platelet count and development of sepsis with multisystem organ failure.

Hepatic Rupture, Hematoma, and Infarct

These conditions occur in preeclampsia and may be the extreme end of the spectrum of HELLP syndrome. Patients with spontaneous rupture of the liver present close to term with abdominal pain and distension, as well as cardiovascular collapse. The rupture results from extravasation of blood, presumably from one or several microscopic areas of periportal hemorrhage with subsequent separation of Glisson's capsule from the liver surface and eventual capsule rupture. The diagnosis depends on a high index of suspicion and identification of hemoperitoneum on abdominal ultrasonography, CT scan, or MRI. If the rupture goes undiagnosed, death results for both mother and fetus. Aggressive management is essential, with vigorous hemodynamic support, rapid delivery of the fetus, and surgical repair of the liver. Some patients may have a contained subcapsular hematoma without frank rupture into the peritoneum. These patients may be managed expectantly with serial hepatic CT scans.

Hepatic infarction typically occurs in the third trimester and presents with right upper quadrant pain, fever, leukocytosis, and marked elevations of serum transaminases. The infarcts can be seen on abdominal CT scan. Management is supportive.

CHOLESTATIC DISEASE

Cardiovascular Dysfunction

The presence of bile salts in circulating blood (cholemia) can impair myocardial contractility.[120] Cholemia also blunts the response to norepinephrine, angiotensin II, and isoproterenol, probably by interfering with their binding to membrane receptors.[121] Less severe hemodynamic perturbations occur in patients with biliary obstruction than in those with cirrhosis. However, the pattern of the pathophysiologic change is remarkably similar: increases in peripheral vasodilatation, cardiac output, and portal venous pressure, and a decrease in portal venous blood flow.

Coagulation Disorders

Cholestatic disease predisposes the patient toward development of coagulopathy primarily related to vitamin K deficiency. During even brief episodes of biliary obstruction, coagulopathy can result from a deficiency of coagulation factors whose activation depends on the presence of vitamin K. Absorption of vitamin K depends on the excretion of bile into the gastrointestinal tract. Long-lasting biliary obstruction can cause liver injury, with subsequent deterioration in the hepatic synthesis of proteins, including coagulation factors. Usually, the coagulation disorders are moderate, and parenteral vitamin K corrects the problem. If this treatment is not fully effective, one should suspect that the disease is not purely cholestatic and that hepatic parenchymal injury exists. If such patients need urgent surgery, the coagulopathy will require immediate treatment with fresh frozen plasma. The failure of parenteral vitamin K to correct a prolonged prothrombin time typically indicates the presence of severe hepatic parenchymal dysfunction and portends a poor prognosis.

PERIOPERATIVE MANAGEMENT

PREOPERATIVE

Hepatic Evaluation and Preparation

As with any preoperative evaluation, the history, physical exam, and laboratory tests are the initial modalities employed. While obtaining the history, inquiry should be made about risk factors and the presence of symptoms attributable to chronic liver disease. The history should include questions about prior episodes of jaundice and their relationship to surgical procedures and the anesthetic techniques used, blood product transfusions, use of alcohol and other recreational drugs, current medications (including herbal preparations), family history of jaundice or liver disease, travel history, and an occupational history (exposure to hepatotoxins). In the review of systems, the patient should be asked about easy bruising, anorexia, weight loss or gain, fatigue, nausea, vomiting, pain with fatty meals, pruritus, abdominal distension, and episodes of gastrointestinal bleeding.

The usage of prescription, over-the-counter medications, and herbal preparations is ubiquitous. Polypharmacy is unfortunately the rule, rather than the exception, especially in elderly and debilitated patients who undergo major operations. Thus, the capacity of pharmacologic agents to injure the liver is an important perioperative concern. Some 500 to 1,000 therapeutic agents have been implicated in causing a broad spectrum of liver diseases.[122] These diseases may be classified in accordance with whether the drug produces primarily direct cell toxicity (necrosis), cholestasis, or steatosis. Most forms of drug-induced liver disease are benign and of little consequence (e.g., estrogen-induced cholestasis), producing only transient alterations of LFT. Severe drug toxicities, which are typically dose related (acetaminophen), or idiosyncratic (halothane), are responsible for 15 to 30% of cases of fulminant hepatic failure and 20 to 50% of cases of chronic nonviral hepatitis. Moreover, when drug reactions produce hepatocellular necrosis, the estimated case fatality approaches 50%.

Drugs known to produce hepatocellular injury and centrilobular necrosis include acetaminophen, isoniazid, and methyldopa. Other cytotoxic drugs include oxyphenisatin, rifampin, papaverine, phenytoin, indomethacin, monoamine oxidase inhibitors, and amitriptyline. The use of dantrolene for treatment of muscle spastic disorders has been associated with the development of hepatic failure in patients receiving the drug for more than 60 days. Cholestatic reactions often result from drugs such as chlorpromazine, phenylbutazone, and androgenic and anabolic steroids. In at least one case, erythromycin (ethylsuccinate form) has caused hepatic failure that had initially been attributed to halothane administration.

A drug's potential to cause hepatotoxicity is influenced by various pharmacologic (other drugs) or pathophysiologic (hepatitis) factors. For example, the combination of trimethoprim and sulfamethoxazole is nearly five times more frequently associated with hepatotoxicity than sulfamethoxazole alone. By inducing hepatic microsomal drug-metabolizing systems, some drugs can markedly increase the injurious potential of others by altering their metabolism to favor the production of toxic metabolites. For example, phenobarbital increases the hepatotoxicity of various drugs, including chemotherapeutic agents (methotrexate) and antibiotics (tetracycline).[123]

Ethanol is obviously an important hepatotoxin. Although elective surgery is not contraindicated in patients with alcoholic steatosis, the mortality from acute alcoholic hepatitis, even without surgery, is significant. Animal studies indicate that alcohol ingestion increases the likelihood that centrilobular necrosis will develop after halothane anesthesia, which may relate to the ability of ethanol to increase hepatic hypoxia. Therefore, if alcoholic hepatitis is suspected, further examination of liver function is warranted before performing an elective operation.

The physical examination of the patient with chronic liver disease is particularly valuable because the patient may appear ill before there is laboratory evidence of hepatic dysfunction. The examination should focus on signs such as scleral icterus, jaundice, ascites, splenomegaly, palmar erythema, gynecomastia, asterixis, testicular atrophy, spider angiomata, petechiae, and ecchymosis. The liver may be enlarged with a tender soft and smooth edge if the patient has hepatitis, or firm and nodular with cirrhosis or malignancy. Patients with chronic hepatitis often have extrahepatic manifestations, including arthritis, skin rashes, and thyroiditis.

Acute liver failure has a distinct clinical presentation. Typically, nonspecific symptoms such as nausea and malaise are followed by the rapid onset of jaundice and subsequently altered mental status, which may progress to coma with clinical and radiologic evidence of cerebral edema.

If no suspicion of liver dysfunction arises from a thorough history and physical exam, then laboratory tests for liver function do not need to be routinely sent because of the low prevalence of disease. Routine testing may yield false-positive results, engendering patient anxiety and prompting the performance of expensive, unnecessary, and potentially dangerous invasive tests. If, however, hepatic dysfunction is known or suspected, then the degree of dysfunction should be quantified by applying either the Child-Pugh or Model of End-stage Liver Disease (MELD) scoring system. A dilemma arises when a patient without any risk factors or stigmata of liver disease is found to have one more abnormal LFT abnormalities on a recent blood test (e.g., routine yearly employment health assessment). The prudent action may be to delay surgery and repeat the tests later. This conservative approach helps ensure a patient is not in the early stages of a disease process (e.g., hepatitis) that may abruptly worsen and may minimize the medical-legal risk for the anesthesiologist. Acute hepatitis (viral, alcoholic, ischemic, or drug related) is associated with increased perioperative risk and mortality. For nonemergent procedures, supportive care allowing an improvement in their overall condition will diminish their perioperative risk. Therefore, in the presence of acute hepatic disease, elective surgery should be postponed (Fig. 39-16).

Perioperative Risk Associated With Acute and Chronic Liver Disease

Because of our limited ability to support a failing liver, the perioperative risks associated with acute and chronic liver disease present significant challenges.[124] The increased surgical morbidity and mortality associated with varying degrees of liver insufficiency have been described in detail for over four decades.[125–130] What remains less clear, however, is whether perioperative outcomes can be improved with proactive interventions.

Regardless of the etiology, an increased magnitude of liver dysfunction is associated with a higher probability of morbidity and mortality.[131] Thus, it is important to quantify and grade preoperative liver dysfunction. Most risk assessment studies about liver disease address expected life span in reference to the prioritization of candidates for liver transplant. In 1999, a new classification system called MELD was designed to predict the outcome of decompressive therapy for portal hypertension.[132] MELD integrates weighted values of three parameters: serum bilirubin, INR, and serum creatinine:

$$\text{MELD score} = 0.957 \times \log_e(\text{creatinine mg/dL}) + 0.378 \times \log_e(\text{bilirubin mg/dL}) + 1.120 \times \log_e(\text{INR}) + 0.643$$

The model was developed from prospective data. MELD has since been adopted by the United Network of Organ Sharing in the United States to prioritize patients for liver transplantation.

Child and Turcotte first described their classification system in 1964.[125] They selected five parameters—serum albumin, serum bilirubin, ascites, encephalopathy, and nutritional status—each graded at one of three levels of severity, and combined to generate an assignment to one of three classes (A to C). Mortality was assessed following portosystemic shunt operations. In 1972, Pugh modified the Child-Turcotte system, replacing the subjective assessment of nutritional status with the more objective PT (Table 39-8).[133]

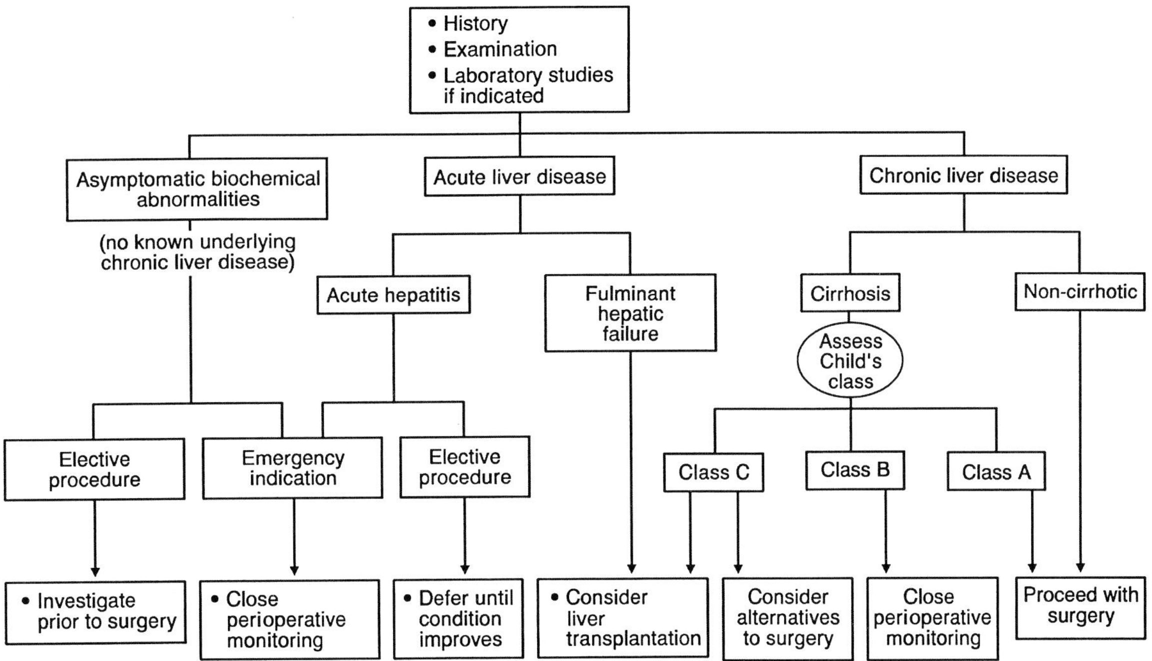

FIGURE 39-16. Preoperative approach to patient with known or suspected liver disease. (Modified with permission from Patel T: Surgery in the patient with liver disease. Mayo Clin Proc 74:593, 1999.)

It is important to note that surgical mortality from hepatic shunt and transplant procedures is less than that from other major surgery.[134,135] In 1997, Rice et al. reported a retrospective analysis of 40 consecutive patients over a 5-year period undergoing general anesthesia for surgery, including 28 abdominal procedures, 2 coronary artery bypass grafts, 5 orthopaedic procedures, and 5 miscellaneous procedures.[129] By multiple logistic regression analysis, an INR greater than 1.6 and encephalopathy were associated with a greater than 10- and 35-fold increased mortality risk, respectively. However, Child classification and Pugh score failed to predict 30-day mortality. Also in 1997, Mansour and associates studied mortality of patients with liver disease undergoing abdominal surgery.[130] Their retrospective analysis from a single institution reported operative 30-day mortality on 92 cirrhotic patients during a 12-year period. Types of surgery were divided into four categories: cholecystectomy, hernia repair, gastrointestinal, and miscellaneous procedures. Twenty-six percent of operations were performed as emergencies. Child class A was associated with 10% mortality, class B with 30%, and class C with 82%. Gastrointestinal procedures and emergent operations were associated with the highest mortality. For comparison, the 3-month mortality in patients hospitalized for liver complications but not undergoing surgery was 4% for Child class A, 14% for class B, and 51% for class C.

MELD score has shown comparable prediction of short-term, nonoperative mortality in advanced cirrhosis when compared with the Child classification. Except for liver transplantation and shunt procedures, MELD is not commonly used to predict perioperative morbidity and mortality.[136]

TABLE 39-8

MODIFIED CHILD-PUGH SCORE

	POINTS[a]		
PRESENTATION	1	2	3
Albumin (g/dL)	>3.5	2.8–3.5	<2.8
Prothrombin time			
Seconds prolonged	<4	4–6	>6
International normalized ratio	<1.7	1.7–2.3	>2.3
Bilirubin (mg/dL)[b]	<2	2–3	>3
Ascites	Absent	Slight–moderate	Tense
Encephalopathy	None	Grade I–II	Grade III–IV

[a]Class A = 5–6 points; B = 7–9 points; C = 10–15 points.
[b]Cholestatic diseases (e.g., primary biliary cirrhosis) produce bilirubin elevations that are disproportionate to the hepatic dysfunction. Thus, the following adjustments should be made: assign 1 point for a bilirubin level of 4 mg/dL; points for bilirubin concentrations between 4 and 10 mg/dL; and 3 points for bilirubin >10 mg/dL.
From Kamath PS: Clinical approach to the patient with abnormal liver test results. Mayo Clin Proc 71:1089, 1996, with permission.

The scoring of liver disease is only one component of evaluating perioperative risks. Other considerations are the patient's age; coexisting diseases; and the type, location, and duration of the surgery. Accurate assessment and communication of perioperative risks is an essential condition of informed consent.

4 Scant data exist to support lengthy preoperative admissions for "optimization," especially for patients with mild hepatic dysfunction having minor operative procedures. Patients with severe or long-standing hepatic dysfunction, however, may benefit from aggressive inpatient correction of certain abnormalities. Liver-related conditions that may benefit from preoperative correction or optimization include ethanol dependency, coagulopathy, malnutrition, anemia, SBP, and hepatic encephalopathy.[137] Esophageal varices can be treated as previously discussed. Preoperative coagulopathy warrants particular attention. Ideally, coagulation abnormalities should be corrected preoperatively, and this should help minimize intraoperative blood loss and thereby decrease the risk of major complications, including development of postoperative HRS. Significant coagulation abnormalities must be corrected prior to performing a spinal or epidural anesthetic. Increased PT or INR in patients with either cholestasis or obstructive jaundice may respond to a few days of vitamin K therapy, but if unsuccessful or if the urgency of surgery does not allow adequate time for a response, administration of fresh frozen plasma is indicated. Platelet transfusion should be considered for patients with evidence of platelet dysfunction or thrombocytopenia ($<$100,000 cells/μL).

Minor operations do not cause postoperative liver dysfunction in healthy patients. Even patients with marginal hepatic function usually tolerate peripheral procedures without hepatic complications, including those who receive halothane anesthesia.[138] A randomized study in patients with mild alcoholic hepatitis compared spinal versus general anesthesia (enflurane plus N_2O plus opioid) and found no anesthesia-related differences in values of LFTs following peripheral or superficial surgery.[139]

Major operations (especially laparotomy) are often associated with hepatic dysfunction or injury. The magnitude of the abnormality depends more on the type of operation than on a particular anesthetic technique.[140] Nonetheless, hepatic dysfunction subsequent to major surgery is rarely of concern in healthy patients. In contrast, patients with advanced hepatic disease (marginal hepatic function) who undergo major operations, such as laparotomy, have extremely high postoperative morbidity and mortality.[141] These patients are probably unable to tolerate the surgical stress, which contributes to decreased hepatic oxygen supply.

Medications needed to control the myriad complications of severe liver disease should be continued throughout the perioperative period. Preoperative sedatives, when indicated, should be used in lower doses because of the marked derangements in pharmacokinetics and pharmacodynamics associated with advanced liver disease. These patients may have a full stomach, even if they have not taken food or fluid for several hours, because of hiatal hernia, massive ascites, and decreased gastric and intestinal motility. Therefore, premedication may include an H_2-receptor blocker, metoclopramide, as well as sodium citrate.

Anticipated Pharmacokinetic and Pharmacodynamic Alterations

Drugs administered to patients with advanced hepatic disease require careful titration against effect. It appears clear that encephalopathic changes are associated with clinically important alterations in the pharmacodynamics and pharmacokinetics of various medications. For example, cerebral uptake of benzodiazepines increases substantially, which may reflect an increase in the density or affinity of benzodiazepine receptors or a leaky blood-brain barrier. Data concerning the pharmacokinetics of midazolam in patients with advanced liver disease are conflicting. One study demonstrated a significant decrease in clearance and elimination half-life, whereas another study demonstrated only slightly impaired disposition in cirrhotic patients.[142,143] The pharmacokinetics of single doses of sufentanil and propofol were found to be similar in cirrhotic patients and those with normal hepatic function, although some differences in elimination time were observed.[144,145] Such findings imply that administering infusions or multiple doses of certain intravenous drugs can result in prolonged pharmacologic effects because of impaired hepatic elimination in patients with advanced hepatic disease. The differences in the results of these studies are probably a consequence of certain differences in the binding proteins, as well as in the accumulation of endogenous binding inhibitors such as bilirubin. These findings might explain a smaller degree of midazolam protein binding in cirrhotic individuals, with a subsequent increase in the free fraction of the drug and enhancement of the pharmacologic effect in cirrhotic patients.

For thiopental, total plasma clearance and total apparent volume of distribution at the steady state are unchanged in cirrhotic patients. Therefore, the elimination half-life is not prolonged.[146] Thiopental has a low extraction ratio, so its clearance is independent of hepatic blood flow. Nonetheless, decreases in plasma protein binding, which are often unpredictable, may cause excessive pharmacologic responses to standard doses of the various agents used to induce anesthesia.

The plasma clearance of fentanyl is significantly lower in cirrhotic patients than in control subjects. The total apparent volume of distribution does not change, but the elimination half-life increases owing to decreased plasma clearance. With alfentanil, the free fraction also increases, and this agent exerts prolonged and pronounced effects in cirrhotic patients with advanced liver disease.[147]

The data regarding morphine pharmacokinetics in cirrhotic patients are contradictory. For example, Patwardhan and associates reported that the pharmacokinetics of morphine in cirrhotic patients and healthy people are similar. They suggested that the "reported intolerance to the central effects of morphine cannot be explained by impaired drug elimination and increased availability of morphine to cerebral receptors."[148] Other investigators, however, reported that the clearances of free morphine and its metabolites are decreased and their half-lives prolonged in cirrhotic patients compared with healthy control subjects.[149]

Although hepatic disease often produces substantial pharmacokinetic changes, it can also lead to important pharmacodynamic alterations. Patients with cirrhosis, particularly those with hepatic encephalopathy, are much more sensitive to sedatives (e.g., opioids, benzodiazepines) than are healthy people. For example, at equal plasma concentrations of diazepam, more pronounced encephalographic alterations occur in those with severe hepatic disease than in healthy people.[150] By contrast, pharmacologic responses to some medications decrease in patients with cirrhosis and portal hypertension as a result of the pathophysiologic changes associated with the disease. Increases in plasma concentrations of certain vasodilatory substances antagonize responses to catecholamines and other vasoconstrictors. Patients, as well as animals with portal hypertension, have elevations of plasma glucagon, which substantially reduces the responses of a variety of blood vessels to catecholamines.[81,83] Thus, while patients with advanced liver disease often require reduced doses of central nervous system depressants, they require increased doses of catecholamine or addition of a nonadrenergic vasoconstrictor (vasopressin) when such therapy is needed to support blood pressure.

INTRAOPERATIVE

Monitoring and Vascular Access

In addition to using the routine array of monitors required by the American Society of Anesthesiologists (ASA), the need for invasive monitoring and degree of vascular access will be dictated by the severity of the liver disease and type of surgery. For severely ill patients or major operative procedures, cannulation of an artery is important for direct and continuous blood pressure monitoring, as well as for periodic determinations of blood gases, electrolytes, hematocrit, and other laboratory data as needed during surgery. Because patients with advanced liver disease may present with multiple complex hemodynamic abnormalities, a central venous catheter, or even a pulmonary artery catheter may be of utility for confirming diagnoses of hypovolemia, abdominal compartment syndrome, distributive shock, or congestive heart failure, as well as for following responses to therapeutic intervention and for monitoring trends as the case progresses. In addition, because coagulopathies can accompany even mild hepatic insufficiency, the surgical bleeding encountered may be far in excess of that anticipated based on normal circumstances. Large-bore vascular access is encouraged for all but the most minor of procedures. Intraoperative monitoring of coagulation status presents formidable challenges; baseline values may be abnormal despite lack of bleeding. Intraoperative PT, PTT, and platelet count usually take too long for results to be of much utility during a large blood-loss operation. Assessing the activated clotting time and thromboelastography may be helpful, although clinical assessment remains the standard for intraoperative diagnosis of coagulopathy.[151]

Selection of Anesthetic Technique

For most cases, the presence of liver disease will not alter the choice of anesthetic technique based on other common considerations. Regional anesthesia is generally the preferred technique in patients without coagulation abnormalities who are undergoing peripheral surgery. However, it would be difficult to justify using regional anesthesia or analgesia for patients with overt coagulopathies or for those having major or lengthy operations. Local anesthesia with sedation is usually the least invasive for relatively minor procedures, such as sclerotherapy. Adequate sedation is essential to minimize sympathetic stimulation and resultant decreases in hepatic blood flow and oxygen delivery. A short-acting benzodiazepine, such as midazolam combined with remifentanil, or a low dose of fentanyl, will usually provide sedation, anxiolysis, and analgesia. As mentioned, patients with advanced hepatic disease have extensive pharmacodynamic and pharmacokinetic abnormalities, so each medication should be titrated carefully to achieve the desired effect.

Induction of General Anesthesia

Rapid-sequence induction (or awake intubation of the trachea) is indicated in patients perceived to be at risk for aspiration pneumonitis (full stomach). All widely used intravenous induction agents have been administered to patients with advanced hepatic disease. For patients who do not require rapid-sequence induction, careful titration of the anesthetic will minimize hemodynamic lability while achieving the desired anesthetic effect. Succinylcholine is a reasonable choice to facilitate endotracheal intubation, after screening for the usual contraindications (e.g., prolonged immobility or critical illness, hyperkalemia). Although severe liver dysfunction can markedly decrease cholinesterase activity and may prolong the effect of succinylcholine somewhat, this rarely causes a clinical problem. When using nondepolarizing neuromuscular blocking agents to induce anesthesia, consider that the initial dose to achieve total relaxation may be higher than in healthy patients. This increased dose requirement results primarily from pharmacokinetic alterations and pertains to relaxants such as rocuronium, atracurium, and pancuronium, but not to vecuronium.

Maintenance of Anesthesia

Intraoperative liver injury can develop from oxygen deprivation, the stress response, drug toxicity, blood transfusion, and infection. An impairment of hepatic oxygen supply can occur at any step in the process of delivering oxygen to the liver. Hypoxic hypoxia may result from inadequate FIO_2, right-to-left-shunting, or $\dot{V}/\dot{Q}$ mismatch. Anemic hypoxia may develop when the oxygen-carrying capacity of the blood (hematocrit) is inadequate. Circulatory hypoxia may result from systemic (hypovolemia, arterial hypotension, reduction in cardiac output) or regional (decrease in hepatic blood flow and oxygen supply) hemodynamic disorders. Delivery of blood and oxygen to the liver may decrease owing to systemic circulatory disturbances, surgical manipulation of the liver or adjacent structures, or from endogenous vasoconstrictors (e.g., renin-angiotensin, catecholamines, antidiuretic hormone). Anesthetics, exogenous vasoconstrictors, and other medications that impair electron transport or cellular metabolism could also induce histotoxic hypoxia.

In addition to ensuring adequate blood flow and oxygen supply, one must always consider the oxygen supply–demand relations in the liver. Experimental data indicate that severe surgical stress during fentanyl (moderate dose) anesthesia can produce a somewhat higher hepatic oxygen supply and uptake than an identical stress during isoflurane anesthesia; this results in similar values of hepatic oxygen supply–uptake ratio with the two anesthetics.[152] Taking this into consideration, the guiding principle is to maintain adequate pulmonary and cardiovascular function, including cardiac output, blood volume, and perfusion pressures. One should strive to prevent arterial hypotension by adequate blood and volume replacement, and by avoidance of relative overdoses of anesthetics or other blood pressure-lowering drugs. Vasodilation, a reduced perfusion pressure, and a decrease in blood velocity will inevitably increase oxygen extraction in all tissues, including those in the preportal area. A decrease in blood velocity and increased oxygen extraction will cause a decrease in venous oxygen content—in this case, decreased oxygen content in the portal venous blood. A reduction in portal blood oxygen content or flow usually leads to a compensatory increase in hepatic arterial flow. Thus, hepatic injury after moderate systemic arterial hypotension is a relatively rare event. However, in the presence of severe liver dysfunction, the ability of autoregulatory mechanisms to increase hepatic arterial blood flow may be diminished or abolished. Therefore, with severe hepatic disease, the hepatic arterial blood flow may not increase appropriately when portal blood flow or oxygen content decreases. This might lead to hepatic oxygen deprivation. Thus, the lesson is clear: take all precautions to avoid arterial hypotension and low cardiac output states.

A particular challenge exists when the operative procedure is on the splanchnic tissues or on the liver itself. In these cases, one objective is to minimize potential for hemorrhage by decreasing the portal blood pressures. Judicious limitation of fluids during the operative resection to maintain a low CVP (<5 mm Hg) has been associated with significantly decreased blood loss, while maintaining renal function in a retrospective analysis of hepatic resection cases.[153]

When performing general anesthesia, it seems prudent to avoid halothane, and possibly enflurane, because they cause the most prominent decreases in hepatic blood and oxygen supply, and are associated with the highest incidences of postoperative hepatic dysfunction. Isoflurane and probably sevoflurane appear to be the anesthetics of choice for inhalational anesthesia. Nitrous oxide does not appear to be associated with major hepatic complications in patients with advanced liver disease, despite its abilities to produce sympathomimetic effects and to limit the maximum oxygen content of arterial blood.

Consideration for the clinical use of halothane should take into account the following issues and concerns:

1. In children, halothane hepatitis is extremely uncommon, even after repeated exposures to halothane.
2. In adults, the disease rarely occurs after a single exposure to halothane; repeated anesthetics, however, especially in obese, middle-age women, over a brief period (<6 weeks) seem to substantially increase the risk of the disease.
3. No totally reliable tests exist for detecting halothane hepatitis or susceptibility to the disease.
4. Halothane can markedly decrease hepatic blood flow and oxygen supply, and often causes mild, transient liver injury.
5. Halothane anesthetics have potential legal liability implications, which may plague anesthesiologists whenever unexplained hepatic dysfunction develops in the postoperative period.

Why use halothane? The main advantages of halothane over other agents appear to be its low cost and its utility as an inhalational induction agent. However, when potential legal costs are factored into the equation, the cost–benefit analysis might actually favor the elimination of halothane from anesthesia practice.[(18)] Sevoflurane has emerged as the alternative inhalation induction agent of choice.

Opioids are reasonable to include in the anesthetics of patients with hepatic disease. Despite certain pharmacokinetic concerns (decreased clearance and prolonged half-life), fentanyl is probably the opioid of choice. Interestingly, fentanyl neither decreases the hepatic oxygen or blood supply nor prevents an increase in hepatic oxygen requirements when used in moderate doses. Therefore, the oxygen supply–demand relation in the liver is no better with a fentanyl-based anesthetic than during anesthesia with isoflurane.[152] It seems that anesthetic management using inhaled agents (especially isoflurane or sevoflurane) alone or in combination with nitrous oxide, and small doses of fentanyl would be the method of choice, provided that adequate hemodynamic parameters are maintained. Many other agents also have favorable risk–benefit profiles for patients with advanced hepatic disease.

Because substantial alterations in pharmacokinetics occur in patients with advanced hepatic disease, dose requirements for a variety of medications can be unpredictable. For example, the hepatic clearance of lidocaine may be increased by more than 300% and benzodiazepines by more than 100%. Drugs that bind to proteins usually have a decreased volume of distribution, so a lower initial dose would be required. The volume of distribution of other agents, such as muscle relaxants, may increase substantially for various reasons, including an increase in γ-globulin concentration or the presence of edema. These factors appear to account for the so-called "resistance" to such agents and explain why the initial dose requirements of these medications are increased in cirrhotic patients. However, subsequent dose requirements may be decreased, and drug effects prolonged, owing to decreases in hepatic blood flow and impaired hepatic clearance, and possible concurrent renal dysfunction. Advanced hepatic disease does not appear to significantly affect the pharmacokinetics of vecuronium, although some dose-dependent pharmacokinetic alterations may occur. These alterations may be the result of a limited hepatic uptake capacity, which is usually exceeded at doses greater than 0.15 mg/kg. At lower doses, hepatic dysfunction does not affect the pharmacokinetics or duration of action of vecuronium.[154]

Severe hepatic dysfunction per se does not contraindicate the use of any specific muscle relaxant. Atracurium (and cisatracurium) have a theoretical advantage because their elimination occurs mainly by Hofmann decomposition, making their clearance relatively independent of renal or hepatic function. Despite elimination and clearance profiles, which match those in healthy patients, the volumes of distribution of these agents are larger in cirrhosis and, accordingly, the distribution half-life is shorter in patients with hepatorenal dysfunction compared with normal individuals. The only situation that appears to prolong the elimination half-life of atracurium is marked metabolic acidosis, which may decrease the rate of Hofmann decomposition.[155]

The pharmacokinetics of many muscle relaxants in conditions of cholestasis and obstructive jaundice may be altered: prolonged duration of action has been demonstrated.[156] However, especially when postoperative ventilation is planned, any nondepolarizing agent can be used successfully. Titration of any relaxant must be made according to transcutaneous nerve stimulation monitoring. Although pharmacokinetic studies in patients with hepatic cirrhosis provide interesting data that are helpful in understanding the pathogenic aspects of chronic liver disease, the results do not necessarily have significant value for predicting the safety of a drug. The degree of hepatic dysfunction affects the degree of pharmacokinetic disorder, and both are dynamic processes that may vary during the course of a procedure; therefore, the best way to avoid complications when administering medications is to titrate to effect.

Fluids and Blood Products

Standard indications for intravascular resuscitation and transfusion of blood products apply to the patient with hepatic insufficiency. No prospective data exist, demonstrating superiority of either a crystalloid-based or colloid-based resuscitation strategy. Because of this lack of conclusive data, the choice of fluid continues to engender spirited opinion and debate. Clearly, colloids represent a higher cost, and some may contribute to coagulopathy, especially at higher doses; however, despite these limitations and lack of documented benefit, they remain the resuscitation fluid of choice for some practitioners.[157] Normovolemic hemodilution has been described as a blood conservation technique for hepatic resections with some success, but is not routinely used for nonhepatic cases in patients with liver insufficiency.[158]

Monitoring of central filling pressures may assist in administering proper fluid therapy and maintaining renal perfusion. The contents of infused solutions should be initially selected and then adjusted based on periodic determinations of serum electrolyte concentrations.

Vasopressors

Patients with hepatic disease, either parenchymal or cholestatic, have peripheral vasodilatation, systemic shunting, and a reduced sensitivity to vasopressor drugs. The exact reason for the decreased pressor sensitivity is unclear. However, data from in vitro and in vivo experiments indicate that bile acids contribute to the vasodilatation and hypotension that often occur in patients with biliary obstruction.[120] Conceivably, a decreased responsiveness to vasoactive substances (including catecholamines) is responsible for the interesting and clinically important observation that patients with biliary obstruction are often intolerant of even small blood losses. A moderate loss (10%) of blood volume in animals with experimentally induced biliary obstruction causes severe (~50%) arterial hypotension. Intact animals respond to such blood loss with an approximately 15% decrease in blood volumes in both the pulmonary and splanchnic vascular beds. Animals with biliary obstruction have only a 7% decrease of their pulmonary blood volume and no change in splanchnic blood volume.[121] If we can extrapolate these results to humans, patients with biliary obstruction would have an impaired hemodynamic response to blood loss. An impairment of the ability to translocate blood from pulmonary and splanchnic blood reservoirs to the systemic circulation would render patients highly susceptible to arterial hypotension from bleeding. Furthermore, the results would indicate the urgency of expeditiously replacing perioperative volume losses in this patient population. The anesthesiologist should be aware that biliary decompression can be accompanied by severe cardiovascular collapse.[159]

POSTOPERATIVE

Liver Dysfunction and Management

Postoperative liver dysfunction is common but rarely severe (Table 39-9). Although it is usually asymptomatic, it may progress to overt liver failure on rare occasions. Mild, transient increases in serum concentrations of hepatic enzymes are often detectable within hours of surgery, but do not usually persist for more than 2 days. Such subclinical hepatocellular injury occurs in as many as 20% of patients who receive enflurane anesthesia, and in nearly 50% of those receiving halothane. Jaundice rarely occurs in healthy patients following minor operations, but appears in up to 20% of patients after major surgical procedures.[160] Jaundice is typically the earliest sign of serious hepatic or hepatobiliary dysfunction, and therefore, requires prompt medical attention. Marked increases of serum aminotransferase activities are an ominous finding, reflecting extensive hepatocellular necrosis.

TABLE 39-9

CAUSES OF POSTOPERATIVE LIVER DYSFUNCTION

Hepatocellular	Drugs
	Anesthetics
	Ischemia
	Shock, hypotension, iatrogenic injury
	Viral hepatitis
Cholestasis	Benign postoperative cholestasis
	Sepsis
	Bile duct injury
	Drugs
	Antibiotics, antiemetics
	Choledocholithiasis or pancreatitis
	Cholecystitis
	Gilbert syndrome

Some cases of severe postoperative liver dysfunction are apparent hours after surgery (e.g., with hypoxic injury), whereas other cases are delayed in onset for days to weeks (e.g., with anesthesia-induced hepatitis). With severe postoperative liver dysfunction, residual liver function may fall below a critical threshold, leading to the development of hepatic encephalopathy. If encephalopathy occurs within 2 weeks of the onset of jaundice or within 8 weeks of the initial manifestation of hepatic disease, the disorder is defined as fulminant hepatic failure. Fulminant hepatic failure has a variety of causes.[161] The mortality rate from fulminant hepatic failure correlates with the severity of encephalopathy. The shorter the interval between the appearance of jaundice and presentation of encephalopathy, the worse the prognosis.

Successful treatment of patients with fulminant hepatic failure requires the clinician to make prompt and accurate predictions about the outcome of the disease. Proper recognition of reversible disease obviates unnecessary orthotopic liver transplantation (OLT). Irreversible cases of fulminant hepatic failure require immediate identification. Otherwise, the severe complications of fulminant hepatic failure that develop may render patients unacceptable candidates for OLT. Several bioartificial liver (BAL) devices are in various stages of development to provide "liver replacement therapy."[162] Most use porcine or human hepatocytes as a bridge to transplantation or regeneration. Other artificial liver devices are based on albumin dialysis and are undoubtedly effective in removing protein-bound toxins, and uncontrolled evidence shows 5 some survival benefit. Although initial animal studies demonstrated survival benefit of BAL devices, to date, no prospective randomized trial has shown improved survival using these devices.[163]

Hemolysis and Transfusion

Reabsorption of large surgical or traumatic hematomas and transfusions of red blood cells are major causes of postoperative jaundice in the absence of overt hepatocellular dysfunction. At least 10% of transfused erythrocytes hemolyze within the initial 24 hours following a blood transfusion (the bilirubin load is about 250 mg per unit transfused). A normal liver readily clears the bilirubin that results from mild hemolysis. With severe hemolysis, the excessive bilirubin leads to unconjugated hyperbilirubinemia, which persists until the liver conjugates and excretes the excess bilirubin. Excessive bilirubin loads can also result from severe hemolytic disorders, including hemoglobinopathies (e.g., sickle cell disease) or derangements of erythrocyte metabolism (e.g., glucose-6-phosphate dehydrogenase [G6PD] deficiency). These problems may be seen in the perioperative period as a result of hypovolemia, hypoxia, hypothermia or stress, exacerbations of sickle cell disease, or G6PD deficiency. Other causes of significant hemolysis include transfusion reactions and prosthetic cardiac valves.

CAUSES OF POSTOPERATIVE LIVER DYSFUNCTION UNRELATED TO PERIOPERATIVE FACTORS

Asymptomatic and Preexisting Hepatic Injury

Although postoperative liver dysfunction can clearly result from anesthetic or surgical interventions, it is often unrelated to perioperative factors. For example, it can arise from preexisting liver disease that has escaped preoperative detection. According to a study by Schemel, the prevalence of acute, asymptomatic liver disease in a healthy-appearing surgical population may approach 0.25%.[164] During a 1-year period, Schemel and coworkers performed multiple laboratory screening tests in 7,620 patients (ASA Physical Status I) scheduled for elective surgical procedures. Eleven of these patients (approximately 1 per 700) were found to have abnormal increases of AST, ALT, and LDH, and the proposed surgeries were cancelled. All 11 proved to have overt hepatic disorders (infectious mononucleosis, viral hepatitis, cirrhosis, or alcoholic hepatitis), and three later became clinically jaundiced (overall incidence of jaundice of 1:2,540). If any of these three patients actually received a halogenated anesthetic, with the subsequent development of overt hepatic disease between the 6th and 14th postoperative days, their diseases may well have been diagnosed erroneously as anesthesia-induced hepatitis. None of the 7,609 patients who underwent anesthesia and surgery exhibited laboratory evidence of preexisting hepatic disease, and none developed unexplained postsurgical jaundice. Another clinical study has documented a prevalence of unsuspected preoperative hepatic dysfunction similar to that reported by Schemel.[(165)] Thus, it appears that approximately 1 of every 2,500 healthy patients who undergo surgery and anesthesia may have clinically significant postoperative liver dysfunction that is totally unrelated to surgery or anesthesia, and that a preexisting disease is more likely than an anesthetic agent to cause severe postoperative liver dysfunction.

Congenital Disorders

Gilbert's syndrome (familial unconjugated hyperbilirubinemia) is the most common cause of jaundice in the United States. It is a benign metabolic disorder characterized by a decrease in the activity of the hepatic enzyme bilirubin glucuronyltransferase, which is required for hepatocyte uptake of unconjugated bilirubin. Affected individuals may have modest increases in their unconjugated bilirubin level preoperatively, but become jaundiced postoperatively secondary to exacerbation of the condition by commonly occurring postoperative factors such as stress, fasting, fever, and infection. The diagnosis is suggested by the combination of clinical (jaundice without dark urine) and laboratory (unconjugated hyperbilirubinemia) abnormalities.

Crigler-Najjar syndrome (congenital nonhemolytic jaundice) is a much less common congenital disorder that exhibits either an absence (type 1) or marked decrease (type 2) of bilirubin glucuronyltransferase producing unconjugated hyperbilirubinemia. Surgical and anesthesia-related problems are apparently minimal in patients with either Gilbert's or Crigler-Najjar syndrome.

Conjugated bilirubin is excreted into the bile by a rate-limited, energy-requiring mechanism. Dubin-Johnson and Rotor's syndromes are congenital disorders that exhibit a defect in the biliary excretory mechanism, resulting in an increased conjugated bilirubin level. Surgery can exacerbate these abnormalities.

CONCLUSION: PREVENTION AND TREATMENT OF POSTOPERATIVE LIVER DYSFUNCTION

Identifying patients at high risk for developing liver dysfunction or for having an exacerbation of preexisting liver disease is of utmost importance for minimizing the morbidity and mortality in such patients. Thus, a careful preoperative evaluation is required to detect preexisting liver disease and to identify important risk factors for anesthesia-induced hepatic injury. Perioperative physicians who are armed with an understanding of the interactions among liver disease, surgical procedures, the physiologic stress response, and anesthetic interventions can formulate and orchestrate therapeutic plans to optimize patient outcome.

When liver abnormalities are recognized preoperatively, it is prudent to defer elective procedures until the course of the disease can be determined. For operations that cannot be deferred, clinically significant pathophysiologic changes associated with the liver disease (e.g., coagulopathy, fluid and electrolyte abnormalities) should be corrected as soon as practical.

Which anesthetic technique best preserves the function of the liver? The choice of anesthesia is usually an insignificant issue for peripheral or minor surgery (operations that do not affect splanchnic blood flow), even in patients with severe liver disease. Regional anesthetic techniques, when appropriate (e.g., absence of coagulopathy), are often preferred because they minimize the cardiovascular and pulmonary perturbations associated with anesthesia. In addition, at least for certain types of procedures such as laparoscopic cholecystectomy, the addition of epidural anesthesia to a general anesthetic technique may decrease the circulating levels of endogenous catecholamines by mitigating the surgical stress response.[166] This effect seems to persist into the postoperative period, when epidural pain management is maintained.[167] The selection of pharmacologic anesthetic agents may also have important implications, especially in patients undergoing major operations. A rational approach to general anesthesia would include the use of agents that preserve cardiac output and do not adversely affect the oxygen supply–demand relationships of the liver (e.g., isoflurane, sevoflurane, fentanyl, remifentanil). Throughout the perioperative period, medications must be carefully titrated to achieve the desired pharmacologic effects while minimizing untoward effects; this can be challenging because pharmacokinetics and pharmacodynamics of many drugs are often unpredictable in patients with hepatobiliary dysfunction.

A primary goal during the maintenance of anesthesia is to ensure the adequacy of splanchnic, hepatic, and renal perfusion, especially in patients with severe liver disease who undergo major abdominal operations. Although well tolerated in the absence of liver disease, hepatic hypoperfusion in patients recovering from infectious hepatitis or chronic alcoholics can have devastating consequences. These patients may be highly susceptible to hepatic ischemia because of critically compromised liver blood flow, impaired pressure-flow autoregulation, and a dysfunctional hepatic arterial buffer response. In such cases, invasive monitoring of the circulation may be indicated so acute hypoperfusion can be rapidly detected and expeditiously treated.

Although anesthesia-induced hepatitis rarely occurs, we must remain aware of the association between this disorder and the use of halogenated vapors. As halothane usage for inhalation inductions and general anesthesia maintenance is increasingly supplanted by sevoflurane, the incidence of this complication decreases with each passing year.[168] In the final analysis, completely avoiding the use of halothane is perhaps the single most effective way to decrease the incidence of anesthesia-induced hepatitis.

When postoperative hepatic injury occurs, the mainstay of therapy is supportive. A thorough search is required to identify any reversible cause of the injury. The hepatotoxic potentials of all medications merit consideration. Discontinue any medication that is suspect. Investigate all potential sources of sepsis because the presence of sepsis mandates rapid, aggressive therapy. Consider extrahepatic biliary obstruction in the differential diagnosis because this may require prompt surgical intervention. In some cases, identifying the pathogen or documenting the type of hepatic injury requires a percutaneous liver biopsy. Judicious use of biochemical tests and imaging studies, which can help delineate hepatocellular from cholestatic dysfunction, usually shortens the list of diagnostic possibilities and provides useful prognostic information.

Unfortunately, fulminant hepatic failure is often survived only with orthotopic liver transplantation. Given that organ donors are far fewer than those in need, many must endure our currently inadequate means of supporting this essential organ when it fails. Caring for patients whose liver is failing can be a frustrating endeavor. Perhaps the future holds promise for a supportive intervention as dialysis has provided for renal failure. In the mean time, our efforts at mitigating the tragedy of liver failure will continue to be best directed at prevention.

ACKNOWLEDGMENT

The authors are indebted to Dr. Simon Gelman for his permission to use text, figures, and tables from this chapter in previous editions of *Clinical Anesthesia*.

References

1. Jones AL: Anatomy of the normal liver. In Zakim D, Boyer T (eds): Hepatology: A Textbook of Liver Disease, 3rd ed, p 3. Philadelphia, WB Saunders, 1996
2. Strasberg SM: Terminology of liver anatomy and liver resections: Coming to grips with hepatic Babel. J Am Coll Surg 184:413, 1997
3. Parks RW, Chrysos E, Diamond T: Management of liver trauma. Br J Surg 86:1121, 1999
4. Rappaport AM, Wanless IR: Physioanatomic considerations. In Schiff L, Schiff ER (eds): Diseases of the Liver, 7th ed. Philadelphia, JB Lippincott, 1993
5. Lautt WW: The 1995 Ciba-Geigy award lecture: Intrinsic regulation of hepatic blood flow. Can J Physiol Pharmacol 74:233, 1996
6. Gelman S, Ernst EA: Role of pH, PCO_2, and O_2 content of portal blood in hepatic circulatory autoregulation. Am J Physiol 233:E255, 1977
7. Martikainen TJ, Tenhunen JJ, Uusaro A, Ruokonen E: The effects of vasopressin on systemic and splanchnic hemodynamics and metabolism in endotoxin shock. Anesth Analg 97:1756, 2003
8. Asfar P, De Backer D, Meier-Hellmann A, Radermacher P, Sakka SG: Clinical review: Influence of vasoactive and other therapies on intestinal and hepatic circulations in patients with septic shock. Crit Care 8:170, 2004
9. Adedoyin A, Branch RA: Pharmacokinetics. In Zakim D, Boyer T (eds): Hepatology: A Textbook of Liver Disease, 3rd ed, p 307. Philadelphia, WB Saunders, 1996
10. Friedman LS, Martin P, Munoz SJ: Laboratory evaluation of the patient with liver disease. In Zakim D, Boyer T (eds): Hepatology: A Textbook of Liver Disease, 3rd ed, p 791. Philadelphia, WB Saunders, 1996
11. Redick JA, Jakoby WB, Baron J: Immunohistochemical localization of glutathione S-transferases in livers of untreated rats. J Biol Chem 257:15200, 1982
12. Ercolani G, Grazi GL, Calliva R *et al*: The lidocaine (MEGX) test as an index of hepatic function: Its usefulness in liver surgery. Surgery 127:464, 2000
13. Vento S, Garofano T, Renzini C *et al*: Fulminant hepatitis associated with hepatitis A virus superinfection in patients with chronic hepatitis C. N Engl J Med 338:286, 1998
14. Kaufman B, Gandhi SA, Louie E *et al*: Herpes simplex viral hepatitis: Case report and review. Clin Infect Dis 24:334, 1997
15. Eriksson LS, Broome U, Kalin M, Lindholm M: Hepatotoxicity due to repeated intake of low doses of paracetamol. J Intern Med 231:567, 1992
16. Anonymous: Summary of the National Halothane Study: Possible association between halothane anesthesia and postoperative hepatic necrosis. JAMA 197:775, 1966
17. Kenna JG, Jones RM: The organ toxicity of inhaled anesthetics. Anesth Analg 81(suppl 6):S51, 1995
18. Mushlin PS, Gelmen S: Liver dysfunction after anesthesia. In Benumof JL, Saidman LJ (eds): Anesthesia and Perioperative Complications, 2nd ed, p 441. St Louis, Mosby, 1999
19. Turner GB, O'Rourke D, Scott GO, Beringer TR: Fatal hepatotoxicity after re-exposure to isoflurane: A case report and review of the literature. Eur J Gastroenterol Hepatol 12:955, 2000
20. Inman WH, Mushin WW: Jaundice after repeated exposure to halothane: An analysis of reports to the Committee on Safety of Medicines. BMJ 1:5, 1974
21. Neuberger J, Williams R: Halothane anaesthesia and liver damage. BMJ 289:1136, 1984
22. Hoft R, Bunker JP, Goodman HI, Gregory PB: Halothane hepatitis in three pairs of closely related women. N Engl J Med 304:1023, 1981
23. Brown BJ, Gandolfi A: Adverse effects of volatile anaesthetics. Br J Anaesth 59:14, 1987
24. Otsuka S, Yamamoto S, Kasuya H *et al*: HLA antigens in patients with unexplained hepatitis following halothane anesthesia. Acta Anaesthesiol Scand 29:497, 1985
25. Warner LO, Beach TP, Garvin JP, Warner EJ: Halothane and children: The first quarter century. Anesth Analg 63:838, 1984
26. Hassall E, Israel DM, Gunasekaran T, Steward D: Halothane hepatitis in children (see comments). J Pediatr Gastroenterol Nutr 11:553, 1990
27. Kenna J, Neuberger J, Mieli-Vergeni G *et al*: Halothane hepatitis in children. BMJ 294:1209, 1987
28. Carpenter RL, Eger EI, Johnson BH *et al*: The extent of metabolism of inhaled anesthetics in humans. Anesthesiology 65:201, 1986
29. Kharasch ED: Biotransformation of sevoflurane. Anesth Analg 81:S27, 1995
30. Sutton TS, Koblin DD, Gruenke LD *et al*: Fluoride metabolites after prolonged exposure of volunteer and patients to desflurane. Anesth Analg 73:180, 1991
31. Callis AH, Brooks SD, Roth TP *et al*: Characterization of a halothane-induced humoral immune response in rabbits. Clin Exp Immunol 67:343, 1987
32. Hals J, Dodgson MS, Skulberg A, Kenna JG: Halothane-associated liver damage and renal failure in a young child. Acta Anaesthesiol Scand 30:651, 1986
33. Martin JL, Kenna JG, Pohl LR: Antibody assays for the detection of patients sensitized to halothane. Anesth Analg 70:154, 1990
34. Neuberger J, Gimson AES, Davis M, Williams R: Specific serologic markers in the diagnosis of fulminant hepatic failure associated with halothane anesthesia. Br J Anaesth 55:15, 1983
35. Kenna JG, Neuberger J, Williams R: Specific antibodies to halothane-induced liver antigens in halothane-associated hepatitis. Br J Anaesth 59:1286, 1987
36. Njoku D, Laster MJ, Gong DH *et al*: Biotransformation of halothane, enflurane, isoflurane, and desflurane to trifluoroacetylated liver proteins: Association between protein acylation and hepatic injury. Anesth Analg 84:173, 1997
37. Fujiwara M, Watanabe A, Sato Y *et al*: Clinical significance of eosinophilia in the diagnosis of halothane-induced liver injury. Acta Med Okayama 38:35, 1984
38. Hubbard AK, Roth TP, Gandolfi AJ *et al*: Halothane hepatitis patients generate an antibody response toward a covalently bound metabolite of halothane. Anesthesiology 68:791, 1988
39. Christ DD, Kenna JG, Kammerer W *et al*: Enflurane metabolism produces covalently bound liver adducts recognized by antibodies from patients with halothane hepatitis. Anesthesiology 69:833, 1988
40. Shiraishi Y, Ikeda K: Uptake and biotransformation of sevoflurane in humans: A comparative study of sevoflurane with halothane, enflurane, and isoflurane (see comments). J Clin Anesth 2:381, 1990
41. Njoku DB, Greenberg RS, Bourdi M *et al*: Autoantibodies associated with volatile anesthetic hepatitis found in the sera of a large cohort of pediatric anesthesiologists. Anesth Analg 94:243, 2002
42. Frink EJ Jr, Morgan SE, Coetzee A *et al*: The effects of sevoflurane, halothane, enflurane, and isoflurane on hepatic blood flow and oxygenation in chronically instrumented greyhound dogs. Anesthesiology 76:85, 1992
43. Bernard JM, Doursout MF, Wouters P *et al*: Effects of enflurane and isoflurane on hepatic and renal circulation in chronically instrumented dogs. Anesthesiology 74:298, 1991
44. Schindler E, Muller M, Zickmann B *et al*: Blood supply to the liver after 1 MAC desflurane in comparison with isoflurane and halothane (in German). Anasthesiol Intensivmed Notfallmed Schmerzther 31:344, 1996
45. Kanaya N, Nakayama M, Fujita S, Namiki A: Comparison of the effects of sevoflurane, isoflurane and halothane on indocyanine green clearance. Br J Anaesth 74:164, 1995
46. Gelman S, Dillard E, Bradley EL Jr: Hepatic circulation during surgical stress and anesthesia with halothane, isoflurane, or fentanyl. Anesth Analg 66:936, 1987
47. Conzen PF, Vollmar B, Habazettl H *et al*: Systemic and regional hemodynamics of isoflurane and sevoflurane in rats. Anesth Analg 74:79, 1992
48. Bernard JM, Doursout MF, Wouters P *et al*: Effects of sevoflurane and isoflurane on hepatic circulation in the chronically instrumented dog. Anesthesiology 77:541, 1992
49. Frink EJ Jr: The hepatic effects of sevoflurane. Anesth Analg 81(suppl 6):S46, 1995
50. Nunn JF: Clinical aspects of the interaction between nitrous oxide and vitamin B12. Br J Anaesth 59(1):3, 1987
51. Cohen EN, Gift HC, Brown BW *et al*: Occupational disease in dentistry and chronic exposure to trace anesthetic gases. J Am Dent Assoc 101:21, 1980
52. Prys-Roberts C, Sear JW, Low JM *et al*: Hemodynamic and hepatic effects of methohexital infusion during nitrous oxide anesthesia in humans. Anesth Analg 62:317, 1983
53. Zinn SE, Fairley HB, Glenn JD: Liver function in patients with mild

alcoholic hepatitis, after enflurane, nitrous oxide-narcotic, and spinal anesthesia. Anesth Analg 64:487, 1985
54. Brodsky JB: Toxicity of nitrous oxide. In Eger EI (ed): Nitrous Oxide/N_2O, p 265. New York, Elsevier, 1985
55. Gelman S: General anesthesia and hepatic circulation. Can J Physiol Pharmacol 65:1762, 1987
56. Dundee JW, Fee JP, Moore J *et al*: Changes in serum enzyme levels following ketamine infusions. Anaesthesia 35:12, 1980
57. Clarke RS, Kirwin MJ, Dundee JW *et al*: Clinical studies of induction agents: XIII. Liver function after propanidad and thiopentone anaesthesia. Br J Anaesth 37:415, 1965
58. Thompson DR: Narcotic analgesic effects on the sphincter of Oddi: A review of the data and therapeutic implications in treating pancreatitis. Am J Gastroenterol 96:1266, 2001
59. Tenhunen JJ, Uusaro A, Karja V *et al*: Apparent heterogeneity of regional blood flow and metabolic changes within splanchnic tissues during experimental endotoxin shock. Anesth Analg 97:555, 2003
60. Schiffer ER, Mentha G, Schwieger IM, Morel DR: Sequential changes in the splanchnic circulation during continuous endotoxin infusion in sedated sheep: Evidence for a selective increase of hepatic artery blood flow and loss of the hepatic arterial buffer response. Acta Physiol Scand 147:251, 1993
61. Refsum H: Arterial hypoxaemia, serum activity of GO-T, GP-T and LDH, and central lobular liver cell necrosis in pulmonary insufficiency. Clin Sci 25:369, 1963
62. Sims J, Morris L, Orth O *et al*: The influence of oxygen and carbon dioxide levels during anesthesia upon postsurgical hepatic damage. J Lab Clin Med 38:388, 1951
63. Gibson PR, Dudley FJ: Ischemic hepatitis: Clinical features, diagnosis and prognosis. Aust N Z J Med 14:822, 1984
64. Bynum TE, Boitnott JK, Maddrey WC: Ischemic hepatitis. Dig Dis Sci 24:129, 1979
65. Giallourakis CC, Rosenberg PM, Friedman LS: The liver in heart failure. Clin Liver Dis 6:947, 2002
66. Szawarski P, Sensky PR, Doshi M, Hudson I: Fulminant liver failure: An indicator of silent myocardial rupture. Postgrad Med J 80:553, 2004
67. McNeill JR, Pang CC: Effect of pentobarbital anesthesia and surgery on the control of arterial pressure and mesenteric resistance in cats: Role of vasopressin and angiotensin. Can J Physiol Pharmacol 60:363, 1982
68. Gelman SI: Disturbances in hepatic blood flow during anesthesia and surgery. Arch Surg 111:881, 1976
69. Kotake Y, Takeda J, Matsumoto M *et al*: Subclinical hepatic dysfunction in laparoscopic cholecystectomy and laparoscopic colectomy. Br J Anaesth 87:774, 2001
70. Mathie RT: Hepatic blood flow during cardiopulmonary bypass. Crit Care Med 21:S72, 1993
71. Liaw YF, Sung JJY, Chow WC *et al*: Lamivudine for patients with chronic hepatitis B and advanced liver disease. N Engl J Med 351:1521, 2004
72. Lok ASF, McMahon BJ: AASLD practice guideline: Chronic hepatitis B: Update of recommendations. Hepatology 39:857, 2004
73. Ganem D, Prince AM: Hepatitis B virus infection-natural history and clinical consequences. N Engl J Med 350:1118, 2004
74. Branch AD, Seeff LB: Hepatitis C: State of the art at the millennium. Semin Liver Dis 20:127, 2000
75. Solga SF, Diehl AM: Non-alcoholic fatty liver disease: Lumen–liver interactions and possible role for probiotics. J Hepatol 38:681, 2003
76. Neuschwander-Tetri BA, Caldwell SH: Nonalcoholic steatohepatitis: Summary of an AASLD single topic conference. Hepatology 37:1202, 2003
77. Falck-Ytter Y, Younossi ZM, Marchesini G, McCullough AJ: Clinical features and natural history of nonalcoholic steatosis syndromes. Semin Liver Dis 21:17, 2001
78. Stewart SF, Day CP: The management of alcoholic liver disease. J Hepatol 38:S2, 2003
79. Tonnesen H, Kehlet H: Preoperative alcoholism and postoperative morbidity. Br J Surg 86:869, 1999
80. Murray JF, Dawson AM, Sherlock S: Circulatory changes in chronic liver disease. Am J Med 24:358, 1958
81. Bomzon A, Blendis L: Vascular reactivity in experimental portal hypertension. Am J Physiol 252:G158, 1987
82. Matsumoto A, Ogura K, Hirata Y *et al*: Increased nitric oxide production in the exhaled air of patients with decompensated cirrhosis. Ann Intern Med 123:110, 1995
83. Benoit JN, Granger DN: Splanchnic hemodynamics in chronic portal hypertension. Semin Liver Dis 6:287, 1986
84. Sharara AI, Rockey DC: Gastroesophageal variceal hemorrhage. N Engl J Med 345:669, 2001
85. Bosch J, Abraldes JG, Groszmann R: Current management of portal hypertension. J Hepatol 38:S54, 2003
86. Shiffman ML, Jeffers L, Hoofnagle JH, Tralka TS: The role of transjugular intrahepatic portosystemic shunt for treatment of portal hypertension and its complications: A conference sponsored by the National Digestive Diseases Advisory Board. Hepatology 22:1591, 1995
87. Krowka MJ, Cortese DA: Hepatopulmonary syndrome: An evolving perspective in the era of liver transplantation. Hepatology 11:138, 1990
88. Lange PA, Stoller JK: The hepatopulmonary syndrome. Ann Intern Med 122:521, 1995
89. Lazaridis KN, Frank JW, Krowka MJ, Kamath PS: Hepatic hydrothorax: Pathogenesis, diagnosis, and management. Am J Med 107:262, 1999
90. Krowka M, Plevak D, Findlay J *et al*: Pulmonary hemodynamics and perioperative cardiopulmonary-related mortality in patients with portopulmonary hypertension undergoing liver transplantation. Liver Transpl 6:443, 2000
91. Jalen R, Hayes PC: Hepatic encephalopathy and ascites (see comments). Lancet 350:1309, 1997
92. Lieberman FL, Denison EK, Reynolds TB: The relationship of plasma volume portal hypertension, ascites, and renal sodium and retention in cirrhosis: The "overflow" theory of ascites formation. Ann N Y Acad Sci 170:202, 1970
93. Schrier RW, Arroyo V, Bernardi M *et al*: Peripheral arterial vasodilation hypothesis: A proposal for the initiation of renal sodium and water retention in cirrhosis. Hepatology 8:1151, 1988
94. Gines P, Berl T, Bernardi M *et al*: Hyponatremia in cirrhosis: From pathogenesis to treatment. Hepatology 28:851, 1998
95. Runyon BA: AASLD practice guidelines: Management of adult patients with ascites caused by cirrhosis. Hepatology 27:264, 1998
96. Moore KP, Wong F, Gines P *et al*: The management of ascites in cirrhosis: Report on the consensus conference of the International Ascites Club. Hepatology 38:258, 2003
97. Panos MZ, Moore K, Vlavianos P *et al*: Single total paracentesis for tense ascites: Sequential hemodynamic changes and right atrial size. Hepatology 11:662, 1990
98. Luca A, Garcia-Pagan JC, Bosch J *et al*: Beneficial effects of intravenous albumin infusion on the hemodynamics and humoral changes after total paracentesis. Hepatology 22:753, 1995
99. Sola-Vera J, Minana J, Ricart E *et al*: Randomized trial comparing albumin and saline in the prevention of paracentesis-induced circulatory dysfunction in cirrhotic patients with ascites. Hepatology 37:1147, 2003
100. Gines A, Fernandez-Esparrach G, Monescillo A *et al*: Randomized trial comparing albumin, dextran 70, and polygeline in cirrhotic patients with ascites treated by paracentesis. Gastroenterology 111:1002, 1996
101. Follo A, Llovet JM, Navasa M *et al*: Renal impairment after spontaneous bacterial peritonitis in cirrhosis: Incidence, clinical course, predictive factors and prognosis. Hepatology 20:1495, 1994
102. Sort P, Navasa M, Arroyo V *et al*: Effect of intravenous albumin on renal impairment and mortality in patients with cirrhosis and spontaneous bacterial peritonitis. N Engl J Med 341:403, 1999
103. Arroyo V, Gines P, Gerbes AL *et al*: Definition and diagnostic criteria of refractory ascites and hepatorenal syndrome in cirrhosis. Hepatology 23:164, 1996
104. Moreau R, Lebrec D: Acute renal failure in patients with cirrhosis: Perspectives in the age of MELD. Hepatology 37:233, 2003
105. Arroyo V, Colmenero J: Ascites and hepatorenal syndrome in cirrhosis: Pathophysiological basis of therapy and current management. J Hepatol 38:S69, 2003
106. Duvoux C, Zanditenas D, Hezode C *et al*: Effects of noradrenalin and albumin in patients with type I hepatorenal syndrome: A pilot study. Hepatology 36:374, 2002
107. Angeli P, Volpin R, Gerunda G *et al*: Reversal of type I hepatorenal syndrome with the administration of midodrine and octreotide. Hepatology 29:1690, 1999
108. Friedman LS: The risk of surgery in patients with liver disease. Hepatology 29:1617, 1999
109. Amitrano L, Guardascione MA, Brancaccio V, Balzano A: Coagulation disorders in liver disease. Semin Liver Dis 22:83, 2002
110. Ferenci P, Herneth A, Steindl P: Newer approaches to therapy of hepatic encephalopathy. Semin Liver Dis 16:329, 1996
111. Riordan SM, Williams R: Treatment of hepatic encephalopathy. N Engl J Med 337:473, 1997
112. Plauth M, Merli M, Weimann A *et al*: ESPEN guidelines for nutrition in liver disease and transplantation. Clin Nutr 16:43, 1997
113. Roberts EA, Schilsky ML: A practice guideline on Wilson disease. Hepatology 37:1475, 2003
114. Pietrangelo A: Hereditary hemochromatosis—A new look at an old disease. N Engl J Med 350:2383, 2004
115. Rouault TA: Hereditary hemochromatosis. JAMA 269:3152, 1993
116. Kaplan MM: Primary biliary cirrhosis. N Engl J Med 335:1570, 1996
117. Menon KVN, Shah V, Kamath PS: The Budd-Chiari syndrome. N Engl J Med 350:578, 2004
118. Di Bisceglie AM, Carithers RL, Gores GJ: Hepatocellular carcinoma. Hepatology 28:1161, 1998
119. Sibai BM: Diagnosis, controversies, and management of the syndrome of hemolysis, elevated liver enzymes, and low platelet count. Obstet Gynecol 103:981, 2004
120. Better OS: Renal and cardiovascular dysfunction in liver disease (clinical conference). Kidney Int 29:598, 1986
121. Bomzon A, Monies-Chass I, Kamenetz L, Blendis L: Anesthesia and pressor responsiveness in chronic bile-duct-ligated dogs. Hepatology 11:551, 1990
122. Bass N, Ockner R: Drug-induced liver disease. In Zakim D, Boyer T (eds): Hepatology: A Textbook of Liver Disease, 3rd ed, p 962. Philadelphia, WB Saunders, 1996
123. GilmanA: In Gilman A *et al* (eds): The Pharmacological Basis of Therapeutics, 7th ed. New York, Macmillan, 1985

124. Ziser A, Plevak DJ, Wiesner RH *et al*: Morbidity and mortality in cirrhotic patients undergoing anesthesia and surgery. Anesthesiology 90:42, 1999
125. Child CG, Turcotte JG: Surgery and portal hypertension. In Child CG (eds): The Liver and Portal Hypertension, Vol I, Major Problems in Clinical Surgery, p 50. Philadelphia, WB Saunders, 1964
126. Aranha GV, Sontag SJ, Greenlee HB: Cholecystectomy in cirrhotic patients: A formidable operation. Am J Surg 143:55, 1982
127. Doberneck RC, Sterling WA, Allison DC: Morbidity and mortality after operation in nonbleeding cirrhotic patients. Am J Surg 146:306, 1983
128. Garrison RN, Cryer HM, Howard DA, Polk HC: Clarification of risk factors for abdominal operations in patients with hepatic cirrhosis. Ann Surg 199:648, 1984
129. Rice HE, O'Keefe GE, Helton WS, Johanson K: Morbid prognostic features in patients with chronic liver failure undergoing nonhepatic surgery. Arch Surg 132:880, 1997
130. Mansour A, Watson W, Shayani V, Pickleman J: Abdominal operations in patients with cirrhosis: Still a major surgical challenge. Surgery 122:730, 1997
131. Knaus WA, Draper EA, Wagner DP, Zimmerman JE: APACHE II: A severity of disease classification system. Crit Care Med 13:818, 1985
132. Freeman RB Jr, Wiesner RH, Harper A *et al:* UNOS/OPTN Liver Disease Severity Score, UNOS/OPTN Liver and Intestine, and UNOS/OPTN Pediatric Transplantation Committees. The new liver allocation system: Moving toward evidence-based transplantation policy. Liver Transpl 8:851, 2002
133. Pugh RNH, Murray-Lyon IM, Dawson JL *et al*: Transection of the oesophagus for bleeding oesophageal varices. Br J Surg 60:646, 1973
134. Iwatsuki S, Starzl TE, Todo S *et al*: Liver transplantation in the treatment of bleeding esophageal varices. Surgery 104:697, 1988
135. Orloff MJ, Orloff MS, Rambotti M, Girard B: Is portal-systemic shunt worthwhile in Child's class C cirrhosis? Long-term results of emergency shunt in 94 patients with bleeding varices. Ann Surg 216:256, 1992
136. Kamath PS, Wiesner RH, Malinchoc M *et al*: A model to predict survival in patients with end-stage liver disease. Hepatology 33:464, 2001
137. Wiklund RA: Preoperative preparation of patients with advanced liver disease. Crit Care Med 32:S106, 2004
138. Clarke RS, Doggart JR, Lavery T: Changes in liver function after different types of surgery. Br J Anaesth 48:119, 1976
139. Zinn SE, Fairley HB, Glenn JD: Liver function in patients with mild alcoholic hepatitis, after enflurane, nitrous oxide-narcotic, and spinal anesthesia. Anesth Analg 64:487, 1985
140. Viegas O, Stoelting RK: LDH5 changes after cholecystectomy or hysterectomy in patients receiving halothane, enflurane, or fentanyl. Anesthesiology 51:556, 1979
141. Ziser A, Plevak DJ, Wiesner RH *et al*: Morbidity and mortality in cirrhotic patients undergoing anesthesia and surgery. Anesthesiology 90:42, 1999
142. MacGilchrist AJ, Birnie GG, Cook A *et al*: Pharmacokinetics and pharmacodynamics of intravenous midazolam in patients with severe alcoholic cirrhosis. Gut 27:190, 1986
143. Trouvin JH, Farinotti R, Haberer JP *et al*: Pharmacokinetics of midazolam in anesthetized cirrhotic patients. Br J Anaesth 60:762, 1988
144. Chauvin M, Ferrier C, Haberer JP *et al*: Sufentanil pharmacokinetics in patients with cirrhosis. Anesth Analg 68:1, 1989
145. Servin F, Desmonts JM, Haberer JP *et al*: Pharmacokinetics and protein binding of propofol in patients with cirrhosis. Anesthesiology 69:887, 1988
146. Pandele G, Chaux F, Salvadori C *et al*: Thiopental pharmacokinetics in patients with cirrhosis. Anesthesiology 59:123, 1983
147. Ferrier C, Marty J, Bouffard Y *et al*: Alfentanil pharmacokinetics in patients with cirrhosis. Anesthesiology 62:480, 1985
148. Patwardhan RV, Johnson RF, Hoyumpa A Jr *et al*: Normal metabolism of morphine in cirrhotics. Gastroenterology 81:1006, 1981
149. Mazoit JX, Sandouk P, Zetlaoui P, Scherrmann JHM: Pharmacokintics of unchanged morphine in normal and cirrhotic subjects. Anesth Analg 66:293, 1987
150. Branch R, Morgan M, James J *et al*: Intravenous administration of diazepam in patients with chronic liver disease. Gut 17:975, 1976
151. Clayton DG, Miro AM, Kramer DJ *et al*: Quantification of thromboelastographic changes after blood component transfusion in patients with liver disease in the intensive care unit. Anesth Analg 81:272, 1995
152. Gelman S, Dillard E, Bradley ER Jr: Hepatic circulation during surgical stress and anesthesia with halothane, isoflurane, or fentanyl. Anesth Analg 66:936, 1987
153. Melendez JA, Arsian V, Fischer ME *et al*: Perioperative outcomes of major hepatic resection under low central venous pressure anesthesia: Blood loss, blood transfusion, and the risk of postoperative renal dysfunction. J Am Coll Surg 187:620, 1998
154. Arden J, Cannon J, Lynam D *et al*: Vecuronium pharmacokinetics and pharmacodynamics in hepatocellular disease. Anesth Analg 66:S3, 1987
155. Ward S, Neill E: Pharmacokinetics of atracurium in acute hepatic failure (with acute renal failure). Surv Anesth 28:364, 1984
156. Westra P, Houwertjes C, DeLange A *et al*: Effect of experimental cholestasis on neuromuscular blocking drugs in cats. Br J Anaesth 52:747, 1980
157. Redai I, Emond J, Brentjens T: Anesthetic considerations during liver surgery. Surg Clin North Am 84:401, 2004
158. Matot I, Scheinin O, Jurim O, Eid A: Effectiveness of acute normovolemic hemodilution to minimize allogeneic blood transfusion during major liver resections. Anesthesiology 97:794, 2002
159. Tamakuma S, Wada N, Ishiyama M *et al*: Relationship between hepatic hemodynamics and biliary pressure in dogs: Its significance in clinical shock following biliary decompression. Jap J Surg 5:255, 1975
160. Evans C, Evans M, Pollack AV: The incidence and causes of postoperative jaundice: A prospective study. Br J Anaesth 46:520, 1974
161. Lee WM: Acute liver failure in the United States. Semin Liver Dis 23:217, 2003
162. Van de Kerkhove MP, Hoekstra R, Chamuleau RA, Van Gulik TM: Clinical application of bioartificial liver support systems. Ann Surg 240:216, 2004
163. Sens S, Williams R: New liver support devices in acute liver failure: A critical evaluation. Semin Liver Dis 23:283, 2003
164. Schemel WH: Unexpected hepatic dysfunction found by multiple laboratory screening. Anesth Analg 55:810, 1976
165. Wataneeyawech M, Kelly K: Hepatic disease: Unsuspected before surgery. N Y State J Med 75:1278, 1975
166. Aono H, Takeda A, Tarver SD, Goto H: Stress responses in three different anesthetic techniques for carbon dioxide laparoscopic cholecystectomy. J Clin Anesth 10:546, 1998
167. Adams HA, Saatweber P, Schmitz CS, Hecker H: Postoperative pain management in orthopaedic patients: No differences in pain score, but improved stress control by epidural anaesthesia. Eur J Anaesthesiol 19:658, 2002
168. Tarpey J, Lawler PG: Volatile agent use: Perception and practice. A survey of agent use over a 3-year period. Anesthesia 44:596, 1989

CHAPTER 40 ■ ANESTHESIA FOR ORTHOPAEDIC SURGERY

TERESE T. HORLOCKER AND DENISE J. WEDEL

KEY POINTS

1. Orthopaedic surgery is well suited to neuraxial and peripheral regional anesthetic techniques. Improved surgical outcomes have increased their popularity.
2. The frequency of neurologic injuries following scoliosis correction is approximately 1%, with half of these resulting in partial or complete paraplegia. Neurophysiologic monitoring and the wake-up test are often used to monitor spinal cord integrity.
3. Orthopaedic procedures are frequently associated with significant blood loss. The anesthesia care provider must be knowledgeable of blood salvage techniques, induced hypotension, and normovolemic hemodilution to decrease blood loss and transfusion requirements.
4. Visual changes, including blindness, may occur following major spine surgery.
5. Continuous brachial plexus infusions may be used during hospitalization or at home with disposable pumps.
6. Proper positioning for orthopaedic procedures is paramount to providing optimal surgical conditions, as well as avoiding potential stretch and compression injuries.
7. Neuraxial and peripheral continuous blockade improve surgical outcome, including increased joint range of motion and decreased hospital stay, following total knee replacement.
8. Orthopaedic patients are at high risk for thromboembolic complications, with the highest risk reported among hip fracture patients.
9. Regional anesthetic techniques reduce the risk of thromboembolism. However, they do not currently replace the need for pharmacologic prophylaxis.

Surgical procedures involving bone, muscle, and related soft tissues require similar monitoring and anesthetic techniques, regardless of the patient's age. For example, many orthopaedic surgical procedures lend themselves to the use of regional anesthesia. Regional anesthetic techniques allow intraoperative surgical anesthesia and postoperative pain relief, and create a further subspecialty within orthopaedic anesthesia. Another seemingly trivial but vitally important part of orthopaedic anesthesia is patient positioning. Unusual patient positioning is a common feature in orthopaedic cases. Experience and specific knowledge are required to produce optimal surgical conditions and avoid potential injuries. Orthopaedic procedures are frequently associated with major blood loss. The orthopaedic anesthesiologist must be experienced in techniques that decrease these risks, must be able to use intraoperative hypotension and blood salvage techniques, and must be able to manage transfusion-related complications. The orthopaedic surgical patient is also at risk for deep venous thrombosis and pulmonary embolus. Knowledge of the current pharmacologic and mechanical methods of thromboprophylaxis is required to prevent the occurrence of these thromboembolic complications. Likewise, potential interactions between anticoagulants and anesthetic drugs or regional anesthetic techniques must be thoroughly understood to reduce the risk of perioperative bleeding.

Knowledge of specific orthopaedic surgical techniques, including duration, extent, predicted blood loss, and associated complications, is invaluable for providing the best possible patient care. Orthopaedic surgical patients usually require early mobilization and rehabilitation, both of which can be expedited by appropriate selection of anesthetic techniques and management of postoperative analgesia. In this chapter, we discuss the various aspects of orthopaedic anesthesia, emphasizing the anesthetic techniques and patient management issues unique to this practice.

PREOPERATIVE ASSESSMENT

The anesthesiologist's preoperative assessment is crucial to the formulation and execution of the anesthetic plan. The patient must be evaluated for preexisting medical problems, previous anesthetic complications, potential airway difficulties, and considerations relating to intraoperative positioning. This evaluation, coupled with an appreciation of the surgeon's needs, is used to formulate the anesthetic plan.

Patients with *coronary artery disease* pose unique problems to the anesthesiologist. Overall, patients undergoing orthopaedic procedures are considered at intermediate risk for cardiac complications perioperatively. However, it is often difficult to assess exercise tolerance or a recent progression of cardiac symptoms because of the limitations in mobility induced by the underlying orthopaedic condition. As a result, pharmacologic functional cardiovascular testing may be warranted based on clinical history. Perioperative cardiac morbidity may be decreased by the initiation of beta-blockade.[1]

Many patients undergoing orthopaedic surgery have *rheumatoid arthritis*. Systemic manifestations of this disease include pulmonary, cardiac, and musculoskeletal involvement. Particularly significant to the anesthesiologist is involvement of the cervical spine, temporomandibular joint, and larynx. Rheumatoid involvement of the cervical spine may result in limited neck range of motion, which interferes with airway management. Atlantoaxial instability, with subluxation of the odontoid process, can lead to spinal cord injury during neck extension. Patients with rheumatoid arthritis are often on chronic steroid therapy and may require perioperative steroid replacement.

Preoperative evaluation should include a focused *physical examination*. Patients should be assessed for limitation in mouth opening or neck extension, adequacy of thyromental distance (measured from the lower border of the mandible to the thyroid notch), and state of dentition. The heart and lungs should be auscultated. In addition, the site of proposed injection for regional anesthesia should be assessed for evidence of infection and anatomic abnormalities or limitations. At this time, the patient should also be evaluated for any potential positioning difficulties related to arthritic involvement of other joints or body habitus.

CHOICE OF ANESTHETIC TECHNIQUE

1 Many orthopaedic surgical procedures, because of their localized peripheral site, lend themselves to regional anesthetic techniques. Neural structures may be blocked at the peripheral nerve, plexus, or neuraxial level. Regional anesthetics offer several advantages over general anesthetics among these patients, including improved postoperative analgesia, decreased incidence of nausea and vomiting, less respiratory and cardiac depression, improved perfusion via sympathetic block, reduced blood loss, and decreased risk of thromboembolism. It is important to explain these benefits and encourage regional anesthesia where appropriate. The regional technique and local anesthetic solution used depend on a variety of factors, including duration of surgery, length of desired postoperative analgesia, and indication for postoperative sympathectomy. Likewise, any patient who has an absolute contraindication to regional anesthesia (patient refusal, infection at the site of needle placement, systemic anticoagulation) is a candidate for general anesthesia. The risks and benefits of regional and general anesthesia are discussed in the following sections.

SURGERY TO THE SPINE

Spinal Cord Injuries

Spinal injury occurs at a rate of 11,000 cases per year. Approximately one-half of these are at the cervical level. The examination of a person with a suspected spinal cord injury begins with a prompt neurologic examination and a rapid assessment for possible injury to other systems. Cervical injuries are frequently associated with head injury, thoracic fractures with pulmonary and cardiovascular injury, and lumbar fractures with abdominal and long bone injuries. The patient should be examined immediately for signs of respiratory insufficiency, airway obstruction, rib fractures, and chest wall or facial trauma.

Serial neurologic examination is necessary to assess function of the spinal cord above the level of the fracture. The fifth cervical segment is perhaps the most important in providing clinical evidence of cervical spinal injury. This segment controls motor function of the deltoid, biceps, brachialis, and brachioradialis muscles. If these muscles are flaccid, the fifth cervical nerve is involved, and there will be partial diaphragmatic paralysis. A complete lesion at the fourth cervical segment is not compatible with survival unless artificial respiration is initiated. Spinal shock occurs acutely and results in complete cessation of spinal cord functions below the level of the lesion. This results in flaccid paralysis, loss of visceral and somatic sensation, and paralytic ileus. Vasopressor reflexes are also lost. Spinal shock may persist from a few days to 3 months.

Surgical treatment of spinal cord injuries is based on the presence or absence of neurologic function and the radiographic evaluation of vertebral displacement and instability. Patients with unstable spines who are not quadriplegic or paraplegic may become so during transport or positioning for surgery.

Tracheal Intubation

Airway management is critical in patients with cervical spinal cord injury. The most common cause of death with acute cervical spinal cord injury is respiratory failure. All patients with severe trauma or head injuries should be assumed to have an unstable cervical fracture until proven otherwise radiographically. During transport, the patient should be moved on a spine board with the neck immobilized to prevent further injury. Awake fiberoptic-assisted intubation may be necessary, with general anesthesia induced only after voluntary upper- and lower-extremity movement is confirmed. Blind nasotracheal intubation may be used if there is no evidence of facial or basal skull fractures. In a truly emergent situation, oral intubation with direct laryngoscopy is the usual approach. The trachea should be intubated with minimum flexion or extension of the neck.

Respiratory Considerations

Ventilatory impairment increases with the higher level of spinal injury. A high cervical lesion that includes the diaphragmatic segments (C4–C5) results in respiratory failure, and death occurs unless artificial pulmonary ventilation is used. Lesions between C5 and T7 cause significant alterations in respiratory function, owing to the loss of abdominal and intercostal support. The indrawing of flaccid thoracic muscles during inspiration produces paradoxical respirations, resulting in a vital capacity reduction of 60%. Inability to cough and effectively clear secretions results in atelectasis and infection.

Cardiovascular Considerations

During spinal shock, there is loss of sympathetic vascular tone below the injury. If the cardioaccelerator fibers (T1–T4) are damaged, bradycardia results. Therefore, hemorrhagic shock may not produce a compensatory tachycardia in these patients; the rate may remain at 40 to 60 beats/min. Monitoring of central venous or pulmonary artery pressures may be necessary as an aid to fluid management in a patient with a high cervical lesion. Autonomic instability should be treated with vasoconstrictors, vasodilators, and positive chronotropic drugs as needed.

Succinylcholine-Induced Hyperkalemia

Hyperkalemia may develop after administration of succinylcholine to a patient with spinal cord injury. The amount of potassium released depends on the extent of the patient's motor deficit. It is usually safe to administer succinylcholine for the first 48 hours. After that time, there is a proliferation of acetylcholine receptors in muscle, and they become supersensitive to depolarizing muscle relaxants.[2] The increases in serum potassium are maximal between 4 weeks and 5 months after spinal injury. Serum potassium levels may increase from normal to as high as 14 mEq/L, causing ventricular fibrillation or cardiac arrest. Therefore, succinylcholine should be avoided in all spinal cord-injured patients after 48 hours. There are no contraindications to the nondepolarizing agents.

Temperature Control

Disruption of the sympathetic pathways carrying temperature sensation, and subsequent loss of vasoconstriction below the level of injury, causes spinal cord-injured patients to be poikilothermic. Maintenance of normal temperature can be achieved by applying exogenous heat to the skin, increasing ambient air temperature, warming intravenous fluids, and humidifying gases.

Maintaining Spinal Cord Integrity

All patients with spinal cord trauma should be considered to have compromised spinal cords, and an important component of anesthetic management is the preservation of spinal cord blood flow. Blood pressure and intravascular volume should be maintained within normal levels to ensure adequate spinal cord perfusion pressure. Sustained hypotension may worsen neurologic deficits. Hyperventilation should be avoided because hypocarbia decreases spinal cord blood flow.

Autonomic Hyperreflexia

After recovery from spinal shock, 85% of patients exhibit autonomic hyperreflexia when there has been complete cord transection above T5. The syndrome, which can also occur with injuries at lower levels, is characterized by severe paroxysmal hypertension with bradycardia (baroreceptor reflex), dysrhythmias, and cutaneous vasoconstriction below, and vasodilation above, the level of the injury. The episode is typically precipitated by distention of the bladder or rectum, but can be induced by any noxious stimulus. Many patients with spinal injuries and autonomic hyperreflexia will report characteristic headaches with bladder distention. The lack of supraspinal inhibition allows the sympathetic outflow below the lesion to react to the stimulus unopposed. If autonomic hyperreflexia occurs, it should be treated by removal of the stimulus, deepening anesthesia, and administration of direct-acting vasodilators. Untreated, the hypertensive crisis may progress to seizures, intracranial hemorrhage, or myocardial infarction.

Scoliosis

Scoliosis is a deformity of the spine resulting in lateral curvature and rotation of the vertebrae, as well as deformity of the rib cage (Fig. 40-1). The incidence of scoliosis predominantly reflects the incidence of idiopathic scoliosis, which

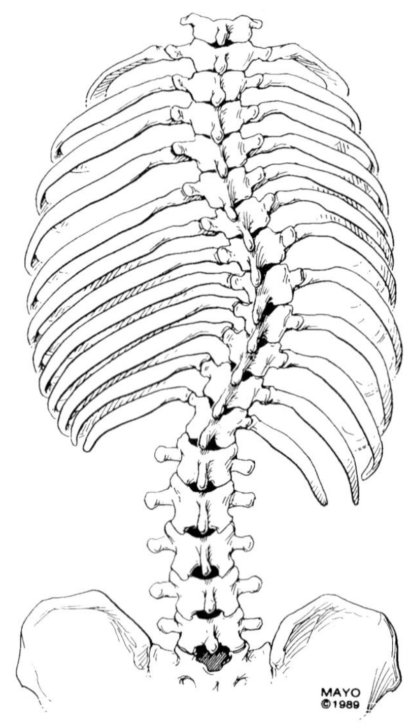

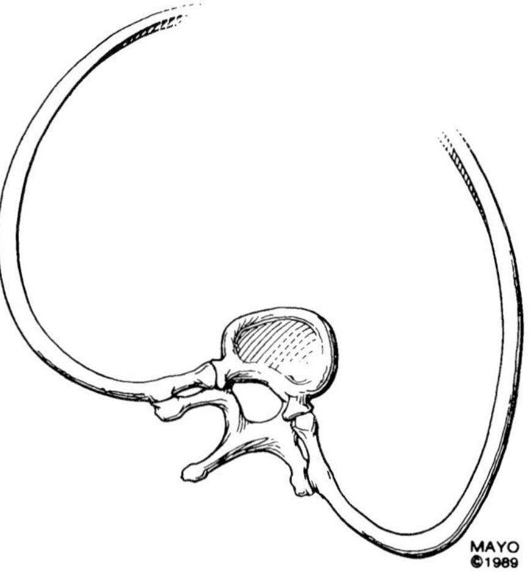

FIGURE 40-1. Deformity of the vertebrae and rib cage in scoliosis. Primary curvature occurs most frequently in the thoracic and lumbar regions. The vertebral bodies are wedge shaped, and the posterior angles of the ribs are shallow on the side of concavity. On the convex side, the rib angles are more acute. (Reprinted with permission from Horlocker TT, Cucchiara RF, Ebersold MJ: Vertebral column and spinal cord surgery. In Cucchiara RF, Michenfelder JD [eds]: Clinical Neuroanesthesia, p 325. New York, Churchill Livingstone, 1990.)

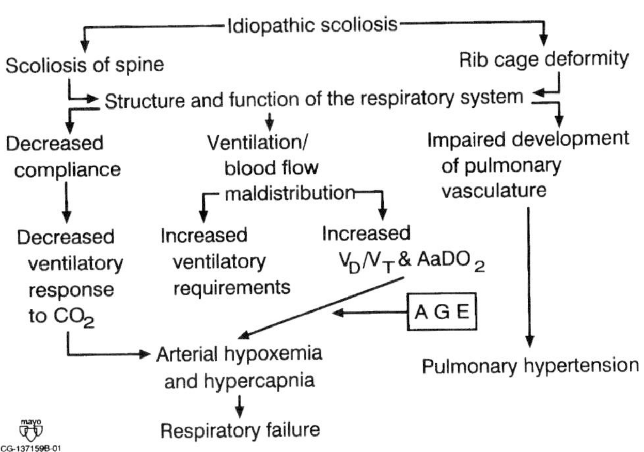

FIGURE 40-2. The factors in idiopathic scoliosis that contribute to respiratory function abnormalities and failure. (Reprinted with permission from Kafer ER: Respiratory and cardiovascular functions in scoliosis. Bull Eur Physiopathol Respir 13:299, 1977.)

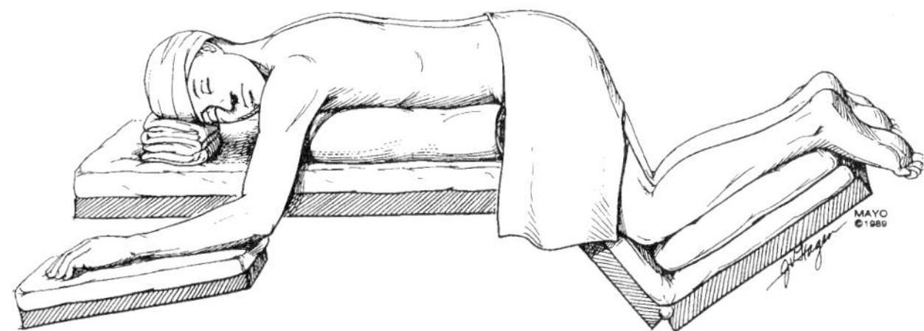

FIGURE 40-3. Prone position. The head is turned with the dependent ear and eye protected from pressure. Chest rolls are in place, the arms are brought forward without hyperextension, and the knees are flexed. (Reprinted with permission from Horlocker TT, Cucchiara RF, Ebersold MJ: Vertebral column and spinal cord surgery. In Cucchiara RF, Michenfelder JD [eds]: Clinical Neuroanesthesia, p 325. New York, Churchill Livingstone, 1990.)

represents 75 to 90% of cases. The remaining 10 to 25% of cases are associated with neuromuscular diseases and congenital abnormalities, including congenital heart disease, trauma, and mesenchymal disorders. A diagnosis of scoliosis in a patient should therefore include a family history and physical examination, with particular attention to the respiratory, cardiac, and neuromuscular systems. The severity of scoliosis is defined by the angle of scoliosis, or *Cobb angle*. Surgical correction is performed for Cobb angles greater than 50 degrees, with the intent of halting progression of respiratory and cardiac dysfunction.

Pulmonary Considerations

Scoliosis has profound effects on the respiratory and cardiovascular systems (Fig. 40-2). In patients with untreated scoliosis, respiratory failure and death usually occur by 45 years of age. Vital capacity appears to be a reliable prognostic indicator of perioperative respiratory reserve. Postoperative ventilation will most likely be required for patients with a vital capacity less than 40% of predicted. Although the long-term effect of scoliosis repair is to halt the decline in respiratory function, pulmonary function acutely deteriorates for 7 to 10 days after surgery.

The primary abnormality in gas exchange is ventilation–perfusion maldistribution, which contributes to hypoxemia. However, hypercapnia develops with increasing age as compensatory mechanisms fail. Prolonged hypoxia, hypercapnia, and pulmonary vascular constriction may result in irreversible pulmonary vascular changes and pulmonary hypertension. In general, the prognosis of scoliosis associated with neuromuscular disease is worse than that of idiopathic scoliosis. These patients frequently need postoperative ventilatory support.

Cardiovascular Considerations

Cardiovascular function is also affected in patients with scoliosis. At autopsy, these patients exhibit right ventricular hypertrophy and hypertensive pulmonary vascular changes. Prolonged alveolar hypoxia due to hypoventilation and ventilation–perfusion mismatch eventually causes irreversible vasoconstriction and pulmonary hypertension. Scoliosis is also associated with congenital heart conditions, including mitral valve prolapse, coarctation, and cyanotic heart disease, suggesting a common embryonic insult or collagen defect.

Surgical Approach and Positioning

The prone position is used for the posterior approach to the spine. Pressure points should be carefully padded. An orthopaedic frame, such as the Jackson table or Wilson frame, can be used to free the chest and abdomen. In correct prone positioning for thoracolumbar spine surgery, the head is turned, the neck is slightly flexed, and the arms are anteriorly flexed and abducted to reduce tension on the brachial plexus (Fig. 40-3). If only one arm is abducted, the head should be laterally rotated toward the ipsilateral arm to prevent stretch injury to the brachial plexus. Because rotation of the neck in patients with cervical spondylosis may alter carotid or vertebral circulation and compromise the spinal cord, patients should be evaluated for neck pain or neurologic symptoms with neck rotation before surgery. The chest and iliac crest are supported by chest rolls or other supports to leave the abdomen free. Breasts should be positioned medially to avoid traumatic injury. The dependent ear and eye should be checked frequently during surgery to avoid injury and ischemia. Necrosis of the dependent ear cartilage may occur if the pinna is doubled back on itself. Eyes should be taped closed to avoid corneal abrasion, which occurs in the dependent eye with a frequency of 0.17%.

The anterior approach to the spine is achieved with the patient in the lateral position, usually with the convexity of the curve uppermost. Removal of one or more ribs may be necessary for adequate surgical exposure. Likewise, placement of a double-lumen endotracheal tube, with collapse of the lung on the operative side may be required for surgery above T8. Thus, the thoracolumbar approach for anterior spinal fusion may be associated with more postoperative respiratory insufficiency than posterior fusion due to lung and diaphragmatic manipulation.

Combined anterior and posterior spinal procedures yield higher union rates and greater correction in patients undergoing scoliosis correction. It remains unclear whether these two major procedures should be performed on the same day or whether the posterior fusion should be delayed to allow the patient to recover from the anterior (first) procedure. Furthermore, the actual timing of the second procedure remains controversial. Although the degree of correction and the arthrodesis rates are similar for one-stage or two-stage procedures, the morbidity and number of complications, such as increased blood loss and transfusion requirements, decreased nutritional parameters, and longer hospital stays, may be increased for staged procedures.[3] However, these results are not consistent.[4] Because the risk of significant complications is present with either same-day or staged anterior–posterior fusion, prospective studies are needed to clarify this issue.

Anesthetic Management

The primary aim of preoperative evaluation of patients with scoliosis is to detect the presence and extent of cardiac or pulmonary compromise. Respiratory reserve is assessed by exercise tolerance, vital capacity, and arterial blood gases. Cardiac studies are performed as indicated to optimize preoperative cardiovascular status. A brief neurologic examination will document preexisting neurologic deficits. Finally, cervical mobility and upper airway anatomy are assessed to discover any potential airway or positioning difficulties. Patients should also be encouraged to participate in preoperative autologous blood donation. Usually four or more units of blood can be collected in the month before surgery.

Anesthetic considerations for surgical correction of scoliosis by *spinal fusion and instrumentation* include management of a patient in the prone position, hypothermia secondary to a long procedure with an extensive exposed area, and replacement of blood and fluid losses, which may be extensive.[5] More recently, attention has been focused on the maintenance of spinal cord integrity, the prevention and treatment of venous air embolism (VAE), and reduction of blood loss through hypotensive anesthetic techniques.

Monitoring

Adequate monitoring and venous access are essential in management of patients undergoing spinal fusion and instrumentation. The radial artery is cannulated for direct blood pressure measurement and assessment of blood gases. A central venous catheter is helpful in evaluating blood and fluid management, and can be used to aspirate air if VAE occurs. Patients with evidence of pulmonary hypertension, or severe coexistent cardiovascular or pulmonary disease, may require a pulmonary artery catheter. Neurophysiologic monitoring, such as the use of somatosensory-evoked potentials (SSEPs), motor-evoked potentials (MEPs), or electromyography, assists in prompt diagnosis of neurologic changes and early intervention in situations of potential neurologic ischemia. The wake-up test may also be used to confirm neurologic dysfunction in the presence of changes in MEP or SSEP waveforms.

Degenerative Vertebral Column Disease

Spinal stenosis, spondylosis, and spondylolisthesis are all forms of degenerative vertebral column disease. It is not unusual for more than one of these degenerative changes in the spine to occur concomitantly, leading to a more rapid progression of neurologic symptoms and the need for surgical intervention.

Surgical Approach and Positioning

Cervical laminectomy is performed in the prone, lateral, or sitting position, whereas thoracolumbar laminectomy is usually performed prone. Considerations for positioning a prone patient have been previously discussed. Patients undergoing cervical laminectomy should be assessed before surgery for cervical range of motion and the presence of neurologic symptoms during flexion, extension, or rotation. Fiberoptic-assisted intubation may be necessary in patients with severely limited cervical movement. With the anterior approach, the surgical incision approximates the anterior border of the sternocleidomastoid muscle, and is therefore near critical anatomic structures. Lateral retraction of the carotid artery may endanger blood flow to the brain, particularly in the elderly patient.[6] Retraction of the esophagus and trachea medially may cause pharyngeal laceration, laryngeal edema, and recurrent laryngeal nerve paralysis. Cerebrospinal fluid leaks and trauma to the vertebral artery have also been reported.

The use of the sitting position for cervical laminectomy has become increasingly popular. Blood flows away from the site of operation, producing a clear operative field and better surgical exposure. In this position, the patient sits with head, arms, and chest supported. The patient must be carefully positioned and dependent areas padded to prevent compression injuries to nerves and skin. Extreme cervical flexion may obstruct the airway. Hypotension can be minimized by gradual attainment of the sitting position. A disadvantage of the sitting position is the increased occurrence of VAE. Although the incidence of VAE in sitting posterior fossa cases is 40%, the incidence is only 5 to 25% in sitting cervical spine procedures.[7] This decreased incidence may alter the need for a central venous pressure catheter.

Anesthetic Management

Either general or neuraxial anesthesia may be safely administered for relatively uncomplicated lower thoracic and lumbar spine surgery. However, general anesthesia is preferred for essentially all thoracic and cervical procedures because of the high spinal level that would be required with a regional technique. The advantages of regional anesthesia include a reduction in blood loss and improved operating conditions by contraction of epidural vasculature. Both spinal and epidural techniques have been described. Epidural catheters may be placed under direct vision by the surgeon to provide intraoperative anesthesia and postoperative analgesia. Likewise, the accessibility of the dural sac facilitates intrathecal reinjection by the surgeon for extended procedures. Despite these considerations, most spine surgery is performed under general anesthesia. General anesthesia ensures airway access, is associated with greater patient acceptance, and can be used for prolonged operations. Succinylcholine should be avoided if there are progressive neurologic deficits because of the possible hyperkalemic response.

Spinal Cord Monitoring

2 Paraplegia is one of the most feared complications of spinal surgery. The incidence of neurologic injuries associated with scoliosis correction is 1.2%, with partial or complete paraplegia occurring in one-half of cases. When patients awaken paraplegic, neurologic recovery is unlikely, although immediate removal of instrumentation improves the prognosis. It is therefore essential that any intraoperative compromise of spinal cord function be detected as early as possible and reversed immediately. The two methods developed to accomplish this are the wake-up test and neurophysiologic monitoring.

The *wake-up test*, first described by Vauzelle et al,[8] consists of the intraoperative awakening of patients after completion of spinal instrumentation. Surgical anesthesia is typically provided with a balanced technique of nitrous oxide, a volatile drug, and opioids, although use of opioids and a short-acting volatile anesthetic (e.g., sevoflurane) alone is also possible. The opioids are important to provide analgesia while the patient is awake and to permit the patient to tolerate the endotracheal tube. During the 30 to 45 minutes before intraoperative wake-up, the volatile anesthetic and muscle relaxants are discontinued and the patient is allowed to gradually awaken. The patient is addressed by name and asked to move both hands, and after a positive response, both feet. Patients usually respond within 5 minutes. If there is satisfactory movement of the hands, but not the feet, the distraction on the rod is released one notch, and the wake-up test repeated. Although recall of the event occurs in only 0 to 20% of patients and is rarely viewed as unpleasant,[9] it is important to describe what will transpire to the patient before surgery so anxiety will be minimized if the patient is fully aware. It is extremely rare for a patient who was neurologically intact when awakened during surgery to have a neurologic deficit on completion of the procedure. However, certain hazards of the wake-up test do exist and include recall, pain, air embolism, dislocation of spinal instrumentation, and accidental tracheal extubation or removal of intravenous and arterial lines.

An adjunct or alternative to the wake-up test is neurophysiologic monitoring. Neurophysiologic monitoring, including SSEPs, MEPs, and electromyography, is also discussed in Chapter 24. Somatosensory stimulation follows the dorsal column pathways of proprioception and vibration: pathways supplied by the posterior spinal artery. The motor pathway, which is supplied by the anterior spinal artery, is not monitored. MEPs, in contrast, monitor motor pathways but are technically more difficult to use. Muscle relaxants cannot be used in patients having MEP monitoring. It is of critical importance to note that postoperative paraplegia has occurred in at least one patient with preserved intraoperative SSEPs.[10]

Acute alterations in SSEP amplitude or latency signify spinal cord compromise and may be the result of direct trauma, ischemia, compression, or hematoma. If changes occur, it is recommended that surgery be discontinued, blood pressure returned to normal or 20% above normal, and volatile agents decreased or discontinued. Arterial blood gases may be drawn to rule out a metabolic derangement. If the waveform does not return to normal, the surgeon should release distraction on the cord. A wake-up test is often performed at this time definitely to exclude neurologic deficits. In addition to neural injury, SSEPs are altered by volatile anesthetics, hypercarbia, hypoxia, hypotension, and hypothermia.[11,12]

Blood Loss

3 Most of the blood loss in spinal instrumentation and fusion occurs with decortication and is proportional to the number of vertebral levels decorticated.[13] Blood loss and transfusion requirements may be reduced through proper positioning and the use of intraoperative blood salvage, induced hypotension, intraoperative hemodilution, and the administration of aprotinin, although reported results are inconsistent.[14–16] However, induced hypotension is not without risk, and has been reported to cause cord ischemia and neurologic deficit, including blindness.[18–20] The various agents used to induce hypotension in scoliosis surgery include trimethaphan, nitroglycerin, sodium nitroprusside, volatile anesthetics, calcium channel blockers, and α-antagonists and β-antagonists.[21] The volatile agents provide anesthesia and hypotension. However, all volatile anesthetics produce a dose-dependent deterioration of evoked potential waveforms. Therefore, a combination of intravenous hypotensive agents and volatile anesthetics is frequently used.

Finally, patients undergoing major spine surgery may acquire a perioperative coagulopathy from dilution of coagulation factors and/or platelets or fibrinolysis. The mechanisms of the coagulopathy and the role of coagulation testing during these procedures are poorly defined. However, it appears that a significant deviation from normal values of either the prothrombin time, or the activated partial thromboplastin time, are predictive of bleeding and may be used to guide transfusion therapy.[22]

Another rare etiology of bleeding during spine surgery is trauma to the aorta, vena cava, or iliac vessels. Unexplained hypotension or signs of hypovolemia without obvious blood loss should alert the anesthesiologist to this possibility.

Visual Loss After Spine Surgery

4 Unilateral and bilateral blindness have been reported in case reports and small series after spinal surgery.[18–20] The diagnoses included optic neuropathy, retinal artery occlusion, and cerebral ischemia. Most cases were associated with complex instrumented fusions.[19] Although no definitive risk factors have been identified, many cases were associated with significant (prolonged) intraoperative hypotension, anemia, large intraoperative blood loss, and prolonged surgery.[20] However, these conditions are present during many major spine procedures, without visual sequelae. Therefore, actual risk factors remain unidentified at this time (see Chapter 5).

Venous Air Embolus

VAE is a catastrophic event that may occur during spine surgery. The large amount of exposed bone and the elevated location of the surgical incision relative to the heart predispose to VAE. The use of capnography, mass spectrometry, and precordial Doppler are noninvasive, yet effective, in detecting VAE. VAE can occur in all positions associated with laminectomies because the wound is above the cardiac level. Incidences of VAE (defined by aspiration of air through a central venous catheter) in patients undergoing neurosurgical procedures in the sitting, supine, prone, and lateral positions are 25, 18, 10, and 8%, respectively.[7] The actual incidence of VAE in scoliosis surgery is unknown; however, six cases have been reported in the literature, four of which were fatal.[23–26] The presenting sign in all cases was unexplained hypotension and an increase in the end-tidal nitrogen concentration. The anesthesiologist, therefore, should be aware of the possibilities of VAE because prompt diagnosis and treatment increase patient survival. If VAE is suspected, the wound should be irrigated with saline, nitrous oxide discontinued, and vasopressors administered. Massive embolism may necessitate turning the patient supine and initiating cardiopulmonary resuscitation.

Postoperative Care

Most patients undergoing posterior spinal fusion can be extubated immediately after the operation if the procedure was relatively uneventful and preoperative vital capacity values were acceptable. Residual opioid or muscle relaxant may lead to hypoventilation or apnea, especially in patients with an associated neuromuscular disease. Some patients who have experienced considerable blood loss and who have received large amounts of intravenous fluids, particularly if they were prone, may have severe facial edema that renders immediate tracheal extubation unwise. Aggressive postoperative pulmonary care, including incentive spirometry, is necessary to avoid atelectasis and pneumonia. Continued hemorrhage in the postoperative period is another concern. Careful monitoring of systemic and central venous pressures, urine output, and wound drainage is essential. Neurologic status must also be monitored closely for deterioration.

Postoperative analgesia is typically provided by systemic opioids. However, wound instillation with local anesthetic or injection of intrathecal morphine is associated with improved pain scores and decreased side effects in the early postoperative period.[27,28]

Epidural and Spinal Anesthesia After Major Spine Surgery

Previous spinal surgery has been considered to represent a relative contraindication to the use of regional anesthesia. The presence of postoperative spinal stenosis or other degenerative changes in the spine or preexisting neurologic symptoms may preclude the use of regional anesthesia in these patients. Likewise, many of these patients experience chronic back pain and are reluctant to undergo epidural or spinal anesthesia, fearing exacerbation of their preexisting back complaints. Finally, postoperative anatomic changes make needle or catheter placement more difficult and complicated after major spinal surgery; needle insertion can be accomplished only at nonfused segments.

Spread of epidural local anesthetic following spinal surgery may be affected by adhesions, producing an incomplete or "patchy" block. Obliteration of the epidural space may increase the incidence of dural puncture and make subsequent epidural blood patch placement impossible. Several retrospective studies have demonstrated that epidural anesthesia may be successfully performed in patients with previous spinal surgery; however, successful catheter placement was possible on the first attempt in only 50% of patients, even with an experienced anesthesiologist. In addition, although adequate epidural anesthesia was eventually produced in 40 to 95% of patients, there appeared to be a higher incidence of traumatic needle placement, inadvertent dural puncture, and unsuccessful epidural needle or catheter placement, especially if spinal fusion extended to L5–S1.[29–31]

Spinal anesthesia may produce a more reliable block and cause less trauma than epidural anesthesia. Although needle placement may be more difficult or traumatic in these patients, the spread of local anesthetic in the subarachnoid space and quality of block would not be affected. A spinal anesthetic may be more desirable after spinal surgery because the technique does not depend on a subjective loss of resistance, but instead has a definite end point—the presence of cerebrospinal fluid.

SURGERY TO THE UPPER EXTREMITIES

Orthopaedic surgical procedures to the upper extremity are well suited to regional anesthetic techniques. In addition to intraoperative anesthesia, brachial plexus and peripheral nerve blocks may be used in the treatment and prevention of reflex sympathetic dystrophy. Continuous catheter techniques provide postoperative analgesia and allow early limb mobilization. Conversely, although the benefits of regional anesthesia in this patient population are well established, orthopaedic surgical procedures often involve peripheral nerves with preexisting deficits, such as ulnar nerve transposition and carpal tunnel release. In addition, the operative site may be adjacent to neural structures, as with total shoulder arthroplasty or fractures of the proximal humerus. The decision to perform regional anesthesia in a patient with preexisting neurologic deficits or who is at risk for perioperative neuropraxia should be made on an individual basis after discussion with the patient and surgeon. Meticulous regional anesthetic technique with appropriate use of local anesthetic solutions and vasoconstrictors, careful patient positioning, and serial postoperative neurologic examinations may reduce the incidence of neurologic dysfunction.

Local anesthetic selection is based on the duration and degree of sensory or motor block required. Although prolonged blockade of the lower extremities interfere with ambulation and therefore delay outpatient discharge, persistent upper-extremity block is not a contraindication to hospital dismissal. However, the patient should be informed of the anticipated duration of analgesia during the postoperative visit and instructed to protect the blocked extremity until block resolution.

Surgery to the Shoulder and Upper Arm

Reconstructive shoulder surgery, including total shoulder arthroplasty and rotator cuff repair, presents unique management and positioning considerations to the anesthesiologist. For example, 4% of patients undergoing total shoulder arthroplasty have a documented postoperative neurologic deficit, including 3% of patients with injury to the brachial plexus. The level of injury is at the level of the nerve trunks, which is the level at which an interscalene block is performed, making it impossible to determine the etiology of the nerve injury (surgical versus anesthetic). Most of these nerve injuries represent a neurapraxia; 90% resolve in 3 to 4 months.[32] In addition, nerve injury often occurs in association with upper-extremity trauma. Radial nerve palsy is identified in up to 18% of patients with humeral shaft fractures, whereas injury to the axillary nerve and brachial plexus is associated with proximal humerus fractures. However, the significant incidence of neurologic deficits demonstrates the importance of clinical examination before regional anesthetic techniques in these patients.

Surgical Approach and Positioning

Surgical procedures to the upper arm and shoulder are typically performed with the patient in the "beach chair" position. The patient is flexed at the hips and knees and placed in a 10- to 20-degree reverse Trendelenburg position to promote venous return. The patient is shifted laterally to the edge of the operating table to allow unrestricted surgical access to the upper extremity. The patient's head, neck, and hips must be secured to prevent additional lateral movement. The head and neck must remain firmly supported by the operating table and secured in a neutral position; excessive rotation or flexion of the head away from the operative side results in stretch injury to the brachial plexus. Care also must be taken to avoid pressure on the eyes and ears. All airway connections should be tightened and possibly reinforced with tape because after surgical draping, access to the patient's face and airway is limited. Hypotension and bradycardia, which occur in up to 20% of cases, can be minimized by gradual assumption of the beach chair position, hydration, and administration of atropine or beta-blockade.

A tourniquet cannot be used during proximal upper-extremity surgical procedures, and significant blood loss may occur. Therefore, arterial cannulation may be helpful for direct blood pressure measurement and monitoring of intraoperative hemoglobin concentrations during total shoulder arthroplasty and reduction of humeral fractures. In theory, VAE may occur during surgical procedures to the shoulder because the operative site is higher than the heart. However, this complication has not been reported in the literature. Patients with a documented right-to-left shunt may be monitored with a precordial Doppler to allow prompt diagnosis and treatment of VAE.

Anesthetic Management

Surgery to the shoulder and humerus may be performed under regional or general anesthesia.[33] With careful positioning and appropriate sedation, interscalene or supraclavicular blockade alone can provide excellent surgical anesthesia. However, general anesthesia or a combination of regional and general anesthesia is often chosen because of limited access to the patient's airway during these surgical procedures. Interscalene brachial plexus block may be performed before surgical incision or after postoperative upper-extremity neurologic function has been determined. Although preoperative interscalene block reduces the intraoperative requirement of volatile anesthetic and opioids, and in theory provides preemptive analgesia, postoperative evaluation of neurologic function will not be possible until block resolution.

Interscalene block should be performed with caution in patients with a preexisting brachial plexopathy because of the risk of perioperative exacerbation of neurologic deficits. The ipsilateral diaphragmatic paresis and 25% loss of pulmonary function produced by interscalene block also contraindicates this block in patients with severe pulmonary disease.[34] The reduction in pulmonary function is present for the duration of the interscalene block.

Surgery to the Elbow

Surgical procedures to the distal humerus, elbow, and forearm are commonly performed under regional anesthetic techniques. Infraclavicular and supraclavicular approaches to the brachial plexus are the most reliable and provide consistent anesthesia to the four major nerves of the brachial plexus: median, ulnar, radial, and musculocutaneous. However, the small but definite risk of pneumothorax associated with supraclavicular and infraclavicular blocks usually makes this approach unsuitable for outpatient procedures. Typically, the pneumothorax occurs 6 to 12 hours after hospital discharge; therefore, a postoperative chest radiograph is not helpful. Although chest tube placement is advised for pneumothorax greater than 20% of lung volume, the lung may also be reexpanded with a small Teflon catheter under fluoroscopic guidance, eliminating the need for hospital admission. The axillary approach to the brachial plexus eliminates the risk of pneumothorax and reliably provides adequate anesthesia for surgery near the elbow.[35]

Surgery to the Wrist and Hand

Surgery to the distal forearm, wrist, and hand may be performed under general or regional anesthesia. Brachial plexus block provides comprehensive and consistent regional anesthesia for the distal upper extremity.[36] Although the brachial plexus may be successfully blocked at several sites, the interscalene approach is seldom used for wrist and hand procedures because incomplete anesthesia of the ulnar nerve is noted in 15 to 30% of patients. In addition, although the supraclavicular approach results in blockade of all four major nerves, the risk of pneumothorax reduces its suitability for outpatient procedures. Therefore, the axillary approach is most commonly used for surgical procedures to the forearm, wrist, and hand.

Minor hand procedures such as carpal tunnel release, reduction of phalanx fractures, and superficial wound debridements may require only local infiltration or peripheral blockade at the midhumeral, elbow, or wrist level. Inflation of an upper arm tourniquet in these patients causes significant discomfort in 45 to 60 minutes and limits the duration of the surgical procedure. Intravenous regional anesthesia (Bier block) using a double tourniquet permits more extensive surgery and longer tourniquet times than distal peripheral block, but does not provide postoperative analgesia.

Continuous Brachial Plexus Anesthesia

5 Brachial plexus catheters may be inserted using interscalene, infraclavicular, and axillary approaches. However, the axillary approach is most common. A 20-gauge catheter is advanced 5 to 10 cm through a medium-gauge needle after elicitation of a paresthesia (or motor response if the nerve stimulator technique is used), and 45 to 50 mL of local anesthetic is injected. Although *analgesia* is produced in all nerve distributions, the block may not provide satisfactory surgical *anesthesia,* even with administration of more potent local anesthetic solutions. Therefore, for surgical procedures, the continuous brachial plexus block is often supplemented with a general anesthetic. After surgery, the catheters may be left indwelling for 4 to 7 days without adverse effects. A continuous infusion of local anesthetic solution, such as bupivacaine 0.125%, prevents vasospasm and increases circulation after limb replantation or vascular repair. More concentrated solutions result in complete sensory block and allow early joint mobilization after painful surgical procedures to the elbow. Ambulatory (at-home) applications provide superior analgesia with fewer side effects than conventional systemic analgesic therapy.[37]

SURGERY TO THE LOWER EXTREMITIES

Although orthopaedic procedures to the lower extremity may be performed under both general and regional anesthesia, the ability to provide superior postoperative analgesia, rapid postoperative rehabilitation, and reduced cost of medical care may result from thoughtfully implemented regional anesthetic and analgesic techniques.

Multiple studies demonstrate significantly reduced intraoperative blood loss during total hip arthroplasty (THA) completed under central neuraxial blockade compared with general anesthesia.[38] The reasons for this reduction are unproved but may be influenced by the decrease in mean arterial pressure, blood flow redistribution to larger-caliber vessels, and locally reduced venous pressure. Decreased postoperative blood loss can be demonstrated when the epidural local anesthetic is continued for analgesia. Likewise, postoperative pulmonary thromboembolism (PTE) from deep venous thrombosis (DVT) is an important cause of morbidity and mortality in orthopaedic surgical patients. Historical investigations reported a decreased incidence of DVT and PTE in patients whose surgery was conducted under regional anesthesia.[39,40] However, these patients did not receive anticoagulants. The potential benefit of regional anesthesia in reducing thromboembolic complications is discussed later in this chapter.

Surgery to the Hip

More than 200,000 total hip replacements are performed annually in North America. Patients undergoing surgical procedures to the hip for arthritic conditions typically are elderly and often have preexisting medical conditions that may affect perioperative outcome. In addition, because hospital costs appear to be directly related to the length of hospital stay, anesthetic techniques associated with improved recovery and reduced complications may decrease the total hospital costs among these patients.

Surgical Approach and Positioning

The lateral decubitus position is frequently used to facilitate
6 surgical exposure for THA, whereas the fracture table is often used for repair of femur fractures. In transferring the patient from the supine to lateral decubitus position, care must be taken to maintain the head and shoulders in a neutral position. The patient is supported while the position is secured with hip rests or other mechanical devices. The dependent arm is abducted and placed on a padded arm rest; a rolled towel or wrapped intravenous fluid bag is placed in the axilla to avoid

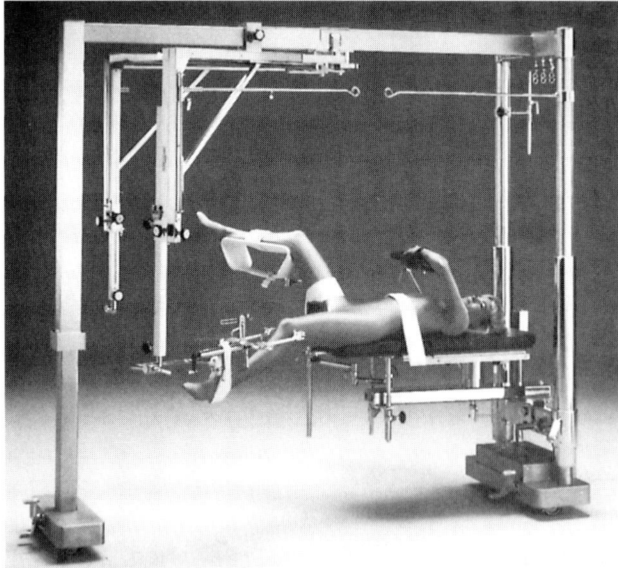

FIGURE 40-4. The fracture table. The patient must be moved carefully with continuous traction on the fractured limb. The ipsilateral arm is positioned on an arm board or sling without stretching the brachial plexus. (Courtesy of Midmark Corporation, Versailles, OH.)

compression of the brachial plexus and vascular structures. The upper arm is placed on a padded over-arm board.

Positioning on the fracture table (Fig. 40-4) also requires adequate personnel to move the patient, with one person assigned to apply traction to the fractured limb. The fracture table affords two advantages: maintenance of traction on the fractured extremity, allowing manipulation for closed reduction and fixation; and access to the fracture site for radiography in several planes. The patient must be carefully monitored for hemodynamic changes during positioning, whether under regional or general anesthesia. Care must be taken to pad the perineal post before positioning the patient's pelvis. Usually, the arm ipsilateral to the fractured hip is placed on an arm board or in a sling to keep it from obstructing the fluoroscopic view.

Anesthetic Technique

Regional anesthetic techniques are well suited to procedures involving the hip. Central neuraxial blockade, including spinal and epidural blockade, is commonly used. Regional anesthesia may be instituted with the patient sitting or in the lateral decubitus position. Both hypobaric and isobaric spinal anesthetic solutions are effective. Adequate intravenous hydration before placing the spinal block protects against a precipitous drop in blood pressure that can occur secondary to sympathetic blockade and peripheral vasodilation. Epidural blockade also provides excellent surgical anesthesia. Placement of a catheter allows prolonged anesthesia as well as postoperative analgesia. More recently, both single-dose and continuous lumbar plexus techniques have been performed to provide postoperative analgesia in patients undergoing major hip surgery. Psoas compartment block was associated with decreased postoperative pain and facilitated hospital discharge in a series of 660 patients.[41] The lumbar plexus block also contributes to the intraoperative anesthetic, allowing decreased dosing of volatile agents, opioids, and/or spinal anesthetic solutions.

Blood Loss

Regional anesthetic techniques reduce blood loss in patients undergoing hip surgery. Deliberate hypotension can also be used with general anesthesia as a means of reducing surgical blood loss and has been recommended when the benefits can be expected to outweigh the risks.[42] Diltiazem, nitroprusside with and without captopril, beta-blockers, and nitroglycerin have also been used to induce hypotension.

Total Knee Arthroplasty

More than 300,000 total knee arthroplasties are performed annually in North America. Patients undergoing total knee arthroplasty (TKA) experience significant postoperative pain. Failure to provide adequate analgesia impedes aggressive physical therapy and rehabilitation, which is critical to maintaining joint range of motion and potentially delays hospital dismissal. Thus, the anesthesiologist must devise a plan for not only intraoperative anesthesia, but also postoperative analgesia.

Surgical anesthesia for operative procedures on the knee in which a tourniquet will be used requires blockade of all four nerves (femoral, lateral femoral cutaneous, obturator, and sciatic nerves) innervating the leg. Although it is possible to perform major knee surgery under peripheral nerve blocks, more often a femoral three-in-one or lumbar plexus (psoas) block is combined with a spinal or general anesthetic. This is less difficult technically, reduces the amount of local anesthetic (and associated systemic toxicity), and provides postoperative analgesia for 12 to 24 hours. Continuous lumbar plexus and sciatic techniques allow for prolonged postoperative analgesia.

Regional anesthetic techniques that can be used for surgical procedures about the knee include neuraxial and peripheral leg blocks. Spinal anesthesia can be accomplished with hyperbaric or isobaric solutions, although the latter are favored by most orthopaedic anesthesiologists. Injection of hyperbaric solutions often results in a higher level of sensory and motor blockade than needed for the surgical procedure, with subsequent earlier offset of anesthesia. Epidural blockade offers the advantage of a continuous catheter technique that can be continued into the postoperative period. These procedures are often associated with significant postoperative pain, particularly when continuous-motion machines are applied to the affected joint.

7 Although numerous methods of providing postoperative analgesia after total knee arthroplasty have been reported, the optimal technique based on efficacy, number/type of side effects, surgical outcome, and resource utilization is unknown. Several studies have suggested that aggressive postoperative regional analgesic techniques maintained for 48 to 72 hours result in a shorter rehabilitation period and increased joint mobility compared with conventional systemic opioids.[43,44]

Positioning

The supine position optimizes surgical exposure during knee arthroscopy or arthroplasty, lower-extremity amputations, and procedures to the tibia and fibula. Care must be taken to cushion the extremities and bony prominences.

Knee Arthroscopy and Anterior Cruciate Ligament Repair

Outpatient knee surgery may be performed under a variety of regional anesthetic techniques. Traditionally, neuraxial or general anesthesia is used. Because diagnostic knee arthroscopy is a relatively minor procedure that may be performed under local anesthesia with sedation, the performance of a single-dose or continuous lower-extremity block is probably not warranted in the majority of patients. The optimal anesthetic technique would allow rapid operating suite turnover and patient

TABLE 40-1

ANESTHETIC TECHNIQUES FOR COMMON FOOT AND ANKLE OPERATIONS

	ANESTHETIC TECHNIQUES FOR COMMON FOOT AND ANKLE OPERATIONS		
	SURGICAL PROCEDURE	REGIONAL TECHNIQUE	COMMENTS
Forefoot[a]	Hallux valgus	Metatarsal, ankle, popliteal blockade	Sural nerve block not necessary for surgery
	Amputations	Ankle, popliteal blockade	Popliteal blockade is the technique of choice in the presence of infection or swelling
Midfoot[a]	Transmetatarsal amputations	Popliteal, ankle blockade	
Hindfoot[a]	Ankle arthroscopy	Spinal, epidural or general anesthesia	Operation typically requires good muscle relaxation for manipulation; thigh tourniquet
	Achilles tendon repair	Spinal, epidural, or popliteal blockade	Spinal or epidural anesthesia whenever thigh tourniquet is required
	Triple arthrodesis	Spinal or epidural	Neuraxial technique preferred for bone graft harvesting; popliteal blockade for postoperative analgesia

[a]Femoral or saphenous block required if the incision extends to the medial aspect of the foot or ankle.
From Hadzic A, Vloka JD: Anesthesia for ankle and foot surgery. Tech Reg Anesth Pain Manage 3:113, 1999.

recovery, excellent operating conditions, and minimal side effects. Unfortunately, each approach is associated with advantages and disadvantages. For example, concerns over transient neurologic symptoms propelled a search for an alternative to intrathecal lidocaine; to date, its reliable sensory and motor block (of limited duration) have not been duplicated. Bupivacaine has a low incidence of transient neurologic symptoms. However, the time to hospital discharge following administration of low-dose bupivacaine (5 to 7.5 mg) with fentanyl (10 μg) may be as long as 3 hours. Epidural 2-chloroprocaine may be an alternative to spinal lidocaine, but experience remains limited. Finally, general anesthesia is associated with nausea and vomiting, side effects prevalent in the patient population undergoing knee arthroscopy. Meta-analyses have failed to demonstrate a clinically significant difference in patient outcome with respect to anesthetic technique.[45]

ACL repair is also performed as an outpatient procedure. However, the surgery is more extensive than knee arthroscopy and postoperative pain may be significant. The anesthetic considerations are similar to those of diagnostic knee arthroscopy with the addition of providing substantial analgesia. Although few data exist on the use of lower-extremity blocks for patients undergoing ACL repair, one study suggests that lumbar plexus block (combined with a spinal or sciatic block) dramatically reduces postoperative opioids requirements and opioid-related side effects.[46] Patients may be discharged home with an indwelling femoral catheter to provide sustained pain relief for 48 hours.[47] Thus, for outpatient procedures, the complexity/duration of the surgical procedure will determine the usefulness of peripheral blocks compared with neuraxial or general anesthesia.

Surgery to the Ankle and Foot

Innervation of the foot is provided by the femoral nerve (via the saphenous nerve) and by the sciatic nerve (via the posterior tibial, sural, and deep and superficial peroneal nerves). Therefore, central neuraxial blockade and peripheral nerve blocks at the upper leg, knee, or ankle are appropriate regional anesthetic techniques for foot surgery. The selection of the regional technique is based on the surgical site, use of a calf or thigh tourniquet, degree of weight bearing/ambulation, and the need for postoperative analgesia. For example, inflation of a thigh tourniquet for longer than 15 to 20 minutes necessitates a general or neuraxial anesthetic, regardless of surgical site. Common surgical procedures and considerations regarding the choice of regional technique are discussed in Table 40-1.[48]

The distal surgical site and the ability to block the pain pathways at multiple sites give regional anesthesia an advantage over general anesthesia for surgery to the ankle and foot. Peripheral blockade avoids the cardiovascular and respiratory side effects, as well as the urinary retention associated with neuraxial and general anesthesia. Often, patients undergoing lower-extremity peripheral techniques may be discharged directly from the operating room to the outpatient nursing station, reducing recovery time and charges. The use of long-acting local anesthetics and the addition of epinephrine or clonidine allow prolongation of postoperative analgesia. However, additional onset time is required with bupivacaine and ropivacaine. Mepivacaine and lidocaine may be more appropriate in the ambulatory setting, where fast-onset and reliable surgical anesthesia is essential. The main disadvantage of peripheral blocks is the technical expertise required for consistent success; neuraxial techniques are a suitable alternative.

Postoperative Analgesia

Systemic Analgesics

Systemic opioids remain a popular postoperative regimen for major orthopaedic surgery because they are relatively simple to administer, safe, and cost-effective. Delivery of opioids using patient-controlled analgesia (PCA) devices results in improved analgesia, decreased total opioid consumption, and increased patient and nurse satisfaction. However, the pain after total joint replacement, particularly total knee arthroplasty, is severe. Adequate analgesia achieved with systemic opioids is frequently associated with side effects, including sedation, nausea, and pruritus. Anti-inflammatory medications and acetaminophen are valuable adjuvants to systemic opioids. The addition of nonopioid analgesics reduces opioid use, improves analgesia, and decreases opioid-related side effects.

Neuraxial and Peripheral Blockade

Studies have demonstrated that epidural analgesia or peripheral nerve blocks provide better pain relief and faster postoperative rehabilitation than intravenous PCA with morphine after total joint replacement. For example, after total knee arthroplasty, patients receiving epidural analgesia or continuous femoral three-in-one block reported lower pain scores, better knee flexion, faster ambulation, and shorter hospital stays compared with patients who received intravenous PCA morphine.[43,44] These landmark studies demonstrate the long-term effects of an aggressive postoperative analgesic technique following orthopaedic surgery—continuous femoral and epidural analgesia hastened rehabilitation and improved joint mobility. An additional relevant result of these investigations is the finding that continuous femoral block provided a quality of analgesia and surgical outcomes similar to that of continuous epidural analgesia, but was associated with fewer side effects. These studies support the movement toward continuous peripheral technique as the optimal analgesic method following total knee arthroplasty.

Intra-Articular Injection

Intra-articular injections of local anesthetics, opioids, or combinations have become routine for perioperative pain management after arthroscopic knee surgery. A number of reports enthusiastically recommend the use of this technique; however, the results remain conflicting.[49,50] Comparison of reports is difficult because of variability in underlying anesthetic techniques, different dosages and concentrations of local anesthetic, and lack of control groups. The safety of injecting large volumes of intra-articular bupivacaine has been ascertained,[51] and side effects are rare after intra-articular doses of morphine. Because these techniques are simple and low risk and seem to afford pain relief under some conditions, they will likely be continued.

MICROVASCULAR SURGERY

Microvascular surgery includes both replantation, the reattachment of a completely severed body part, and revascularization, the reestablishment of blood flow through a severed body part. Most replantation surgery involves the upper extremity. Anesthetic management in microvascular surgery includes maintenance of blood flow through microvascular anastomoses, positioning considerations associated with a long surgical procedure during which the patient must lie completely still, and replacement of blood and fluid losses, which may be extensive.

Maintenance of blood flow through microvascular anastomoses is paramount to limb or graft viability. Blood flow may be improved by increasing the perfusion pressure, preventing hypothermia, and using vasodilators and sympathetic blockade. Microvascular perfusion pressure depends on both adequate intravascular volume and oncotic pressure. Blood loss during microvascular surgery is typically continual and insidious. Unrecognized bleeding and migration of intravascular fluid into the third space reduce microvascular perfusion pressure, and must be corrected. However, overzealous use of crystalloid results in generalized edema, including the replanted body part, whereas excessive transfusion of blood products increases blood viscosity and therefore decreases flow. Evidence suggests that use of phenylephrine to support blood pressure does not jeopardize blood flow to the tissue being replanted.[52] Rheologically, the oxygen-carrying capacity of blood is optimized with a hematocrit of 30%. Arterial cannulation allows frequent assessment of hemoglobin levels and acid-base status, as well as direct blood pressure measurement.

Body temperature is also a determinant of blood flow. Hypothermia not only results in peripheral vasoconstriction, but causes sympathetic activation, shivering, increased oxygen demand, a leftward shift of the oxygen–hemoglobin dissociation curve, and altered coagulation. Therefore, hypothermia must be prevented in microvascular surgical patients. The operating room temperature should be increased to 21°C, intravenous solutions should be warmed,[53] and the patient covered with a forced-air warming blanket.

The use of vasodilators has also been studied in the treatment of perioperative vasospasm. Local anesthetics and papaverine, applied topically, may be used to provide relaxation of vascular smooth muscle in the intraoperative setting.[54] All the volatile anesthetics are potent vasodilators and can increase tissue blood flow 200 to 300%, even at typical expired anesthetic concentrations. Direct-acting vasodilating agents, such as sodium nitroprusside, trimethaphan, and hydralazine, produce vasodilation but do not prevent vasospasm due to direct surgical stimulation. Nitroprusside has been shown to reduce perfusion in a microvascular free flap.[52] In addition, the volatile anesthetics and intravenous agents may also result in hypotension and decreased microvascular perfusion pressure. Regional anesthetic techniques provide sympathectomy and vasodilation to the proximal (innervated) segment of an extremity, but have no effect on vasospasm in the replanted (denervated) tissue. Antithrombotics (heparin), fibrinolytics (streptokinase, urokinase, low molecular weight dextran), and smooth muscle relaxants (papaverine, local anesthetics) are also used to preserve blood flow in microvascular anastomoses.

Microvascular surgery may be performed under regional or general anesthesia. Regional anesthesia has several advantages over general anesthesia. The sympathectomy associated with local anesthetic blockade results in vasodilation and increased blood flow. A single-injection regional anesthetic technique may be of insufficient duration for many microvascular procedures. However, placement of an indwelling catheter (intrathecal, epidural, or axillary) provides extended intraoperative anesthesia and continuous postoperative analgesia. General anesthesia ensures airway access and reduces the possibility of patient movement during critical surgical events. A combination of general and continuous regional anesthesia allows prolonged intraoperative anesthesia and postoperative analgesia, reduces the amount of inhalational agent, and increases the patient's acceptance of lengthy surgical procedures. However, regardless of anesthetic technique, conditions that stimulate vasospasm or vasoconstriction, such as pain, hypotension, and hypovolemia, must be avoided. Whether administration of a vasopressor with vasoconstrictive qualities or addition of epinephrine to local anesthetic solutions may decrease anastomotic blood flow is controversial.[52]

PEDIATRIC ORTHOPAEDIC SURGERY

Pediatric patients present with a variety of orthopaedic conditions, including congenital deformities, traumatic injuries, infections, and malignancies. Anesthetic management of the pediatric orthopaedic patient involves not only the usual pediatric patient considerations, such as airway management, fluid replacement, and maintenance of body temperature, but also the unique concerns associated with orthopaedic surgery. Coexisting neuromuscular conditions, such as arthrogryposis or myelomeningocele, may predispose pediatric orthopaedic patients to latex allergy and malignant hyperthermia. In addition, patient positioning and the use of regional techniques for intraoperative anesthesia and postoperative analgesia must be considered.

Regional techniques are readily adaptable to the pediatric orthopaedic patient. Often, regional anesthetic procedures are technically easier to perform on children because the relative lack of subcutaneous tissue facilitates identification of bony and vascular landmarks as well as spread of local anesthetic solutions. The advantages of regional anesthesia in children are similar to those in adults and include earlier ambulation and hospital discharge, decreased incidence of nausea and vomiting, and prolonged postoperative analgesia. However, pediatric patients often are not considered candidates for regional techniques. The preoperative visit is essential in building a patient–parent–physician relationship and establishing an anesthetic plan. The use of preoperative and preblock sedation (oral and intranasal midazolam, intramuscular ketamine, and rectal methohexital) decreases anxiety and increases acceptance of regional anesthesia in the pediatric patient.

Orthopaedic procedures may be performed with children anesthetized with regional, general, or a combination of anesthetic techniques. The patient's age, operative site and positioning, and surgical duration are important factors in selection of an anesthetic. Children older than 7 years of age may tolerate a primary regional anesthetic technique, whereas younger children may benefit from a general or combination regional/general anesthesia. Neural blockade may be initiated after induction of general anesthesia and before surgical incision, to provide possible preemptive analgesia, or, on completion of the surgical procedure, to extend the duration of postoperative analgesia.

Surgical procedures to the lower extremity may be safely and successfully performed under caudal, epidural, and spinal anesthesia.[55] However, the anatomic differences between the pediatric and adult spine and spinal cord must be appreciated.[56] In addition, femoral, lateral femoral cutaneous, and sciatic nerve blocks allow prolonged anesthesia and analgesia to the blocked extremity, but often require additional intraoperative supplementation with intravenous or inhalational agents.[57]

Upper-extremity procedures may be performed with any of the anesthetic techniques previously described for adults. The superficial location of the brachial plexus, decreased neural diameter, and rapid diffusion of local anesthetics contribute to the high success rate, which approaches 100%, even with a variety of techniques.[58] Blockade of the brachial plexus is usually accomplished with perivascular, sheath, or nerve stimulator techniques in children younger than 7 years of age because elicitation of paresthesias is regarded as uncomfortable (and therefore unacceptable) by the younger pediatric patients. Intravenous regional (Bier) block is particularly useful in the pediatric population for limited procedures such as closed reduction of forearm fractures. The use of local anesthetic eutectic creams minimizes patient discomfort during intravenous catheter placement.

OTHER CONSIDERATIONS

Anesthesia for Nonsurgical Orthopaedic Procedures

Many orthopaedic procedures requiring anesthesia are carried out in areas other than the operating room. These include cast and dressing changes in pediatric patients, pin removal, hip and shoulder relocation, closed reduction of fractures, and joint manipulations. Although some of the minor procedures require only light sedation, those procedures involving bone and joint manipulation usually require a full anesthetic intervention. It is critically important that patients undergoing these procedures be managed with the same careful attention afforded those scheduled for a standard operating room. Regional anesthesia, usually with a short-acting local anesthetic, can be a good choice for these procedures, especially when the patient wants to leave the hospital on the same day with minimal residual anesthetic effects.

Regional Anesthesia in the Outpatient Setting

Hospital discharge criteria generally include successful oral intake, ambulation, and voiding by the patient. Thus, patients who have undergone a neuraxial technique will not be discharged until complete block resolution (although the requirement to void is somewhat controversial). Return of full neurologic function may be less important immediately after peripheral nerve blocks. Persisting peripheral or plexus blockade provides excellent pain relief and increased blood flow to the surgical site, both of which may be desirable side effects. However, the risk of accidental nerve trauma in an anesthetized extremity is theoretically higher outside the hospital environment. The patient should be informed of the risks and instructed in appropriate care of the extremity. Patients who are unable or unwilling to comply with recommended medical care may not be good candidates for regional anesthesia techniques and/or should be fully recovered before discharge.

In all cases, a follow-up telephone call on the first postoperative day should include questions concerning residual areas of neural blockade or altered neural function, such as paresthesias. Any patient concerns regarding the anesthetic or surgery should also be discussed. Patients with indwelling plexus or peripheral catheters should be queried regarding the presence of residual block, signs of local anesthetic toxicity, and catheter migration.[37,47] Following spinal anesthesia or accidental dural puncture during epidural anesthesia, the patient should be informed of the risk of postspinal headache and given a contact person in the anesthesia department to call if problems arise.

Tourniquets

Tourniquets are often used to minimize blood loss and provide a bloodless operating field. The cuff should be applied over limited padding or none at all. Appropriate selection of tourniquet cuff size and inflation pressure is paramount in reducing the risk of neuromuscular injury related to tourniquet ischemia. The cuff should be large enough to comfortably circle the limb to ensure circumferentially uniform pressure. The point of overlap should be placed 180 degrees from the neurovascular bundle because there is some area of decreased compression at the overlap point. The width of the inflated cuff should be more than half the limb diameter. Before tourniquet inflation, the limb should be elevated for approximately 1 minute and tightly wrapped with an elastic bandage distally to proximally.

Opinions differ as to the pressure required in tourniquets to prevent bleeding. In general, a cuff pressure 100 mm Hg above a patient's measured systolic pressure is adequate for the thigh, and 50 mm Hg above systolic pressure is adequate for the arm, with the understanding that if hypertensive episodes occur, the cuff pressure should be increased. Bleeding from the surgical site after cuff inflation may rarely be due to inadequate occlusion of the major arterial inflow, which is corrected by cuff reapplication and use of the proper degree of inflation. Bleeding during tourniquet inflation is more commonly due to intramedullary blood flow in the long bones, particularly in the skeletally immature, and to small arterial vessels between the two bones of distal extremities. Overinflation of the tourniquet does *not* resolve these problems. Likewise, the duration of safe tourniquet inflation is unknown. Recommendations range from 30 minutes to 4 hours. Five minutes of intermittent perfusion between 1- and 2-hour inflations, followed by repeated exsanguination through elevation and compression, may allow more extended use.[59]

Damage to underlying vessels, nerves, and skeletal muscles has been reported following tourniquet inflation.[60] Injury is a function of both inflation pressure and duration of inflation.[61,62] Direct pressure from the cuff is more damaging than the ischemia distally.[61,63] Arterial spasm, venous thrombosis, and nerve injury are all demonstrable after several hours. Clinical examination, electromyography, and effluent blood analysis all show completely reversible changes for inflations of 1 to 2 hours, which is the basis for the recommendation of this period as the safe duration for tourniquet use; longer inflation times are associated with prolonged or irreversible changes in neurologic and/or muscular function.[64]

Transient systemic metabolic acidosis and increased arterial carbon dioxide levels have been demonstrated after tourniquet deflation, and do not cause deleterious effects in healthy patients.[65,66] Measurable changes include a 10 to 15% increase in heart rate, a 5 to 10% increase in serum potassium, and a rise of 1 to 8 mm Hg in carbon dioxide tension in blood. Prolonged inflation or the simultaneous release of two tourniquets may produce clinically significant acidosis, particularly in patients with an underlying acidosis due to other causes. Tourniquet release has also been associated with cerebral embolic phenomena.[67]

When a pneumatic tourniquet is used with regional anesthetic techniques, some patients complain of dull, aching pain or become restless, even though seemingly adequate analgesia exists for the operation itself. Patient discomfort usually appears approximately 45 minutes after the tourniquet is inflated and becomes more intense with time. No satisfactory explanation for its genesis has been found. Current explanations involve pain transmission through both A delta and C fibers, and its modulation in the dorsal horn synapses. The C (slow pain) fibers recover faster as the block wanes. Analogous phenomena may be observed at the same time point during general anesthesia. Evidence of lightening anesthesia (increase in blood pressure and pulse rate) may appear even though the same concentrations of anesthetic are being delivered.[68,69] The definitive treatment for tourniquet pain is release of the tourniquet. Relief of pain is prompt and complete. During surgery, however, opioids and hypnotics are usually effective.

Fat Embolus Syndrome

Fat embolus syndrome (FES) is associated with multiple traumatic injuries and surgery involving long bone fractures.[70] Risk factors include male gender, age (20 to 30 years), hypovolemic shock, intramedullary instrumentation, rheumatoid arthritis, THA using the technique of cementing femoral stems designed for press-fit application, and bilateral total knee surgery. The incidence of FES in isolated long bone fractures is 3 to 4%, and the mortality rate associated with this condition is significant, ranging from 10 to 20%.

Clinical and laboratory signs of FES have been classified by Gurd[71] as major or minor (Table 40-2), with a diagnosis requiring at least one major and four minor criteria, as well as the exclusion of other posttraumatic causes of hypoxemia. Major signs of the syndrome include the presence of axillary or subconjunctival petechiae, significant hypoxemia, central nervous system depression in excess of that expected due to the level of hypoxemia, and pulmonary edema. Classified as minor signs are tachycardia, hyperthermia, retinal fat emboli on funduscopic examination, urinary fat globules, an unexplained decrease in hematocrit or platelets, an increased erythrocyte sedimentation rate, and fat globules in the sputum. Symptoms usually occur 12 to 40 hours after the injury and can range from mild dyspnea to frank coma. Decreased arterial oxygen tension is the most consistent abnormal laboratory value. Fulminant episodes can occur within hours of the traumatic injury, causing severe hypoxemia, respiratory failure, and severe neurologic impairment. Disseminated intravascular coagulation can also occur in conjunction with FES. Not all trauma patients who have demonstrated evidence of fat emboli fit the criteria for diagnosis of FES. Two theories are hypothesized to explain the mechanism of this syndrome: the mechanical theory and the biochemical theory. The mechanical theory proposes that long bone trauma results in release of fat droplets that enter the vascular system through torn veins. These droplets are transported to the pulmonary vascular bed where they act as microemboli. The biochemical theory can be divided into two mechanisms: toxic and obstructive. The toxic mechanism proposes that free fatty acids released at the time of trauma directly affect pneumocytes in the lung and cause adult respiratory distress syndrome. This effect would be enhanced by the trauma-induced release of catecholamines, which would result in further mobilization of free fatty acids. The obstructive theory hypothesizes that an unspecified chemical event at the site of the fracture releases mediators that affect lipid solubility, resulting in coalescence of lipids and consequent embolization. Some or all these theories may play a role in development of FES. Other predisposing or aggravating factors such as shock, hypovolemia, sepsis, or disseminated intravascular coagulation may be required to trigger the conversion of fat emboli to FES.

TABLE 40-2

CRITERIA FOR DIAGNOSIS OF FAT EMBOLUS SYNDROME

MAJOR
Axillary/subconjunctival petechiae
Hypoxemia (Pa_{O_2} < 60 mm Hg; FI_{O_2} < 0.4)
Central nervous system depression (disproportionate to hypoxemia)
Pulmonary edema
MINOR
Tachycardia (>110 beats/min)
Hyperthermia
Retinal fat emboli
Urinary fat globules
Decreased platelets/hematocrit (unexplained)
Increased erythrocyte sedimentation rate
Fat globules in sputum

Diagnosis of fat embolus syndrome requires at least one sign from the major and four signs from the minor criteria categories.
From Gurd AR: Fat embolism: An aid to diagnosis. J Bone Joint Surg Br 52:732, 1970, with permission.

Appropriate treatment of FES requires early recognition of the syndrome, reversal of possible aggravating factors such as hypovolemia, early surgical stabilization of fracture sites, and aggressive respiratory support. Corticosteroid therapy is controversial but may be beneficial. Other pharmacologic interventions, including heparin and dextran, have not been shown to be effective in treating FES.

Methyl Methacrylate

Methyl methacrylate is an acrylic bone cement used during arthroplastic procedures. Insertion of this cement is associated with sudden onset of hypotension in some patients. This

TABLE 40-3

8 VENOUS THROMBOEMBOLISM PREVALENCE AFTER MAJOR ORTHOPAEDIC SURGERY

	DEEP VENOUS THROMBOSIS[a]		PULMONARY EMBOLISM	
PROCEDURE	TOTAL (%)	PROXIMAL (%)	TOTAL (%)	FATAL (%)
Total hip replacement	42–57%	18–36%	0.9–28%	0.14–2.0%
Total knee replacement	41–85%	5–22%	1.5–10%	0.1–1.7%
Hip fracture surgery	46–60%	23–30%	3–11%	2.5–7.5%

[a]Total or proximal deep venous thrombosis prevalence based on the use of mandatory venography in prospective randomized clinical trials in which patients received either prophylaxis or a placebo.
From Geerts WH, Pineo GF, Heit JA *et al*: Prevention of venous thromboembolism: The seventh ACCP conference on antithrombotic and thrombolytic therapy. Chest 126(3 suppl):338S, 2004, with permission.

hypotension has been attributed to absorption of the volatile monomer of methyl methacrylate, embolization of air and bone marrow during femoral reaming, lysis of blood cells and marrow induced by the exothermic reaction, and conversion of methyl methacrylate to methacrylate acid. Adequate hydration and maximizing inspired oxygen concentration minimize the hypotension and hypoxemia that can accompany cementing of the prosthesis. Because air can be entrained during this procedure, nitrous oxide should be discontinued several minutes before this point.

Deep Venous Thrombosis and Pulmonary Embolus

Orthopaedic surgical procedures are associated with a variety of complications due to embolic phenomena. Reported emboli occurring during and after surgery include fat, cement, air, and thrombus. These may be caused by multiple factors such as positioning, fracture of long bones, injection of cement under pressure, and predisposing medical conditions. VAE can occur in orthopaedic surgical patients undergoing spinal surgery in the prone position and shoulder surgery in the sitting position, and is discussed earlier in this chapter.

Venous thromboembolism is a major cause of death after surgery or trauma to the lower extremities. Without prophylaxis, venous thrombosis develops in 40 to 80% of orthopaedic patients, and 1 to 28% show clinical or laboratory evidence of pulmonary embolism. Fatal pulmonary embolism occurs in 0.1 to 8% of patients[72] (Table 40-3). The incidence of fatal pulmonary embolism is highest in patients who have undergone surgery for hip fracture. Although fatal pulmonary embolism may be the most common preventable cause of hospital death, many physicians fail to use prophylaxis appropriately because of concern about bleeding complications from anticoagulation. Effective thromboprophylaxis requires knowledge of clinical risk factors in individual patients, such as advanced age, prolonged immobility or bed rest, prior history of thromboembolism, cancer, preexisting hypercoagulable state, and major surgery. In many patients, multiple risk factors may be present, and the risks are cumulative. After identification of the risk of thromboembolism, an assessment may be made regarding the risks and benefits of physical or pharmacologic techniques used to prevent thromboembolic complications.

Antithrombotic Prophylaxis

Patients undergoing major orthopaedic surgery are at high risk for thromboembolism. Thromboprophylaxis is based on identification of risk factors. Guidelines for antithrombotic therapy, including selection of pharmacologic agent, degree of anticoagulation desired, and duration of therapy continue to evolve.[72] Recommendations from the Seventh American College of Chest Physicians in 2004 are based on prospective randomized studies that assess the efficacy of therapy, using contrast venography or fibrinogen leg scanning to diagnose asymptomatic thrombi (Table 40–4).

Multiple thromboprophylaxis regimens for patients undergoing total joint replacement and hip fracture surgery have

TABLE 40-4

ANTITHROMBOTIC REGIMENS TO PREVENT THROMBOEMBOLISM IN ORTHOPAEDIC SURGICAL PATIENTS

HIP AND KNEE ARTHROPLASTY AND HIP FRACTURE SURGERY

- LMWH[a] started 12 hr before surgery or 12 to 24 hr after surgery, or 4 to 6 hr after surgery at half the usual dose and then increasing to the usual high-risk dose the following day
- Fondaparinux (2.5 mg started 6 to 8 hr after surgery)
- Adjusted-dose warfarin started preoperatively or the evening after surgery (INR target, 2.5; INR range, 2.0 to 3.0)
- Intermittent pneumatic compression is an alternative option to anticoagulant prophylaxis in patients undergoing total knee (but not hip) replacement

SPINAL CORD INJURY

- LMWH once primary hemostasis is evident
- Intermittent pneumatic compression is an alternative option when anticoagulation is contraindicated early after the injury
- During the rehabilitation phase, conversion to adjusted-dose warfarin (INR target, 2.5; INR range, 2.0 to 3.0)

ELECTIVE SPINE SURGERY

- Routine use of thromboprophylaxis, apart from early and persistent mobilization, not recommended

KNEE ARTHROSCOPY

- Routine use of thromboprophylaxis, apart from early and persistent mobilization, not recommended

INR, international normalized ratio; LMWH, low molecular weight heparin.
[a]Use with caution in patients receiving neuraxial anesthesia/analgesia. Enoxaparin and dalteparin are LMWH approved by the U.S. Food and Drug Administration.
From Geerts WH, Pineo GF, Heit JA *et al*: Prevention of venous thromboembolism: The seventh ACCP conference on antithrombotic and thrombolytic therapy. Chest 126(3 suppl):338S, 2004, with permission.

been studied. Although aspirin, subcutaneous unfractionated heparin, and the presence of a neuraxial block are more efficacious than placebo, the risk of thromboembolism remains significant, and a higher level of anticoagulation is required. In addition, although adjusted-dose administration of unfractionated heparin (to attain an activated partial thromboplastin time in the upper normal range) is effective, most orthopaedic surgeons consider adjusted-dose heparin prophylaxis impractical. Rather, administration of low molecular weight heparin (LMWH), warfarin, or fondaparinux is recommended. Similar recommendations are made for patients with acute spinal cord injury. Conversely, other orthopaedic patients are considered low risk, and no pharmacologic prophylaxis is warranted.

Neuraxial Anesthesia and Analgesia in the Patient Receiving Antithrombotic Therapy

Several studies show a decrease in the incidence of both DVT
9 and PTE in patients undergoing hip surgery under epidural[38–40] and spinal[73–75] anesthesia. Similar findings have been reported for knee surgery performed under epidural anesthesia.[76,77] Proposed mechanisms for this effect include (1) rheologic changes resulting in hyperkinetic lower-extremity blood flow, reducing venous stasis and preventing thrombus formation; (2) beneficial circulatory effects from epinephrine added to the local anesthetic solutions; (3) altered coagulation and fibrinolytic responses to surgery under central neural blockade, resulting in a decreased tendency for blood to clot and better fibrinolytic function[78]; (4) the absence of positive-pressure ventilation and its concomitant effects on circulation; and (5) direct local anesthetic effects such as decreased platelet aggregation. It is important to note that most of the studies examining the value of epidural and spinal anesthesia in preventing DVT and PTE involved patients who were not receiving currently recommended pharmacologic prophylaxis.

Despite the advantages of neuraxial techniques, patients receiving perioperative anticoagulants and antiplatelet medications are often not considered candidates for spinal or epidural anesthesia/analgesia because of the risk of neurologic compromise from expanding spinal hematoma. The actual incidence of neurologic dysfunction resulting from hemorrhagic complications associated with neuraxial blockade is unknown; however, the incidence cited in the literature is estimated to be less than 1 in 150,000 epidural and less than 1 in 220,000 spinal anesthetics.[79] The frequency of spinal hematoma is increased in patients who receive perioperative anticoagulation.[80] The more recent introduction of more efficacious anticoagulants and antiplatelet agents has further increased the complexity of patient management. Anesthesiologists must balance the risk of thromboembolic and hemorrhagic complications.

Spinal hematoma was considered a rare complication of neuraxial blockade until the introduction of LMWH as a thromboprophylactic agent in the 1990s. The calculated incidence (approximately 1 in 3,000 epidural anesthetics), along with the catastrophic nature of spinal bleeding (only 30% of patients had good neurologic recovery)[81] warranted an alternate approach to analgesic management following total hip and knee replacement. Although psoas compartment and femoral catheters are suitable (if not superior) alternatives to neuraxial infusions, there are no investigations that examine the frequency and severity of hemorrhagic complications following plexus or peripheral blockade in anticoagulated patients. All cases of major bleeding (significant decreases in hemoglobin and/or blood pressure) associated with nonneuraxial techniques occurred after psoas compartment or lumbar sympathetic blockade and have involved heparin, LMWH, warfarin, and thienopyridine derivatives. These cases suggest that significant blood loss, rather than neural deficits, may be the most serious complication of nonneuraxial regional techniques in the anticoagulated patient. Additional information is needed to make definitive recommendations. The current information focuses on neuraxial blocks and anticoagulants (Table 40-5).[82] Conservatively, these neuraxial guidelines may be applied to plexus and peripheral techniques. However, this may be more restrictive than necessary.

In summary, thromboembolism is a serious complication of total joint replacement. The development of new antithrombotic drugs, mechanical devices, and postoperative rehabilitation regimens is paramount in improving patient outcome. Neuraxial and peripheral techniques, which allow for early ambulation and earlier hospital discharge may prove to be an integral component of patient care. However, at this time, they do not replace the need for pharmacologic thromboprophylaxis.

TABLE 40-5

NEUERAXIAL ANESTHESIA AND ANALGESIA IN THE ORTHOPAEDIC PATIENT RECEIVING ANTITHROMBOTIC THERAPY

■ LMWH
Needle placement should occur 10–12 hr after a dose. Indwelling neuraxial catheters are allowed with once (but not twice daily) dosing of LMWH. In general, it is optimal to place/remove indwelling catheters in the morning and administer LMWH in the evening to allow normalization of hemostasis to occur prior to catheter manipulation.
■ WARFARIN
Adequate levels of all vitamin K-dependent factors should be present during catheter placement and removal. Patients chronically on warfarin should have normal INR prior to performance of regional technique. Monitor prothrombin time and INR daily. Remove catheter when INR <1.5.
■ FONDAPARINUX
Neuraxial techniques are not advised in patients who are anticipated to receive fondarinux perioperatively.
■ NONSTEROIDAL ANTI-INFLAMMATORY DRUGS
No significant risk of regional anesthesia-related bleeding is associated with aspirin-type drugs. However, for patients receiving warfarin or LMWH, the combined anticoagulant and antiplatelet effects may increase the risk of perioperative bleeding. In addition, other medications affecting platelet function such as the thienopyridine derivatives and glycoprotein IIb/IIIa platelet receptor inhibitors should be avoided.

INR, international normalized ratio; LMWH, low molecular weight heparin.
Adapted from Horlocker TT, Wedel DJ, Benzon H *et al*: Regional anesthesia in the anticoagulated patient: Defining the risks (the second ASRA consensus conference on neuraxial anesthesia and anticoagulation). Reg Anesth Pain Med 28:172, 2003.

References

1. Eagle KA, Brundage BH, Chaitman BR *et al*: Guidelines for perioperative cardiovascular evaluation for noncardiac surgery. Report of the American College of Cardiology/American Heart Association Task Force on Practice Guidelines. Committee on Perioperative Cardiovascular Evaluation for Noncardiac Surgery. Circulation 93: 1278, 1996
2. Martyn JA, White DA, Gronert GA *et al*: Up-and-down regulation of skeletal muscle acetylcholine receptors: Effects on neuromuscular blockers. Anesthesiology 76: 822, 1992
3. Ferguson RL, Hansen MM, Nicholas DA, Allen BL: Same-day versus

staged anterior-posterior spinal surgery in a neuromuscular scoliosis population: The evaluation of medical complications. J Pediatr Orthop 16: 293, 1996
4. McDonnell MF, Glassman SD, Dimar JR *et al:* Perioperative complications of anterior procedures on the spine. J Bone Joint Surg Am 78: 839, 1996
5. Winkler M, Marker E, Hetz H: The peri-operative management of major orthopaedic procedures. Anaesthesia 53(suppl 2): 37, 1998
6. Sloan TB, Ronai AK, Koht A: Reversible loss of somatosensory evoked potentials during anterior cervical spinal fusion. Anesth Analg 65: 96, 1986
7. Albin MS, Chang JL, Babinski M *et al:* Intracardiac catheters in neurosurgical anesthesia. Anesthesiology 50: 67, 1979
8. Vauzelle C, Stagnara P, Jouvinroux P: Functional monitoring of spinal cord activity during spinal surgery. Clin Orthop 93: 173, 1973
9. Pathak KS, Brown RH, Nash CL, Cascorbi HF: Continuous opioid infusion for scoliosis fusion surgery. Anesth Analg 62: 841, 1983
10. Ginsburg HH, Shetter AG, Raudzens PA: Postoperative paraplegia with preserved intraoperative somatosensory evoked potentials. J Neurosurg 63: 296, 1985
11. Burke D, Hicks RG: Surgical monitoring of motor pathways. J Clin Neurophysiol 15: 194, 1998
12. Pathak KS, Ammadio M, Kalamchi A *et al:* Effects of halothane, enflurane, and isoflurane on somatosensory evoked potentials during nitrous oxide anesthesia. Anesthesiology 66: 753, 1987
13. Nuttall GA, Horlocker TT, Santrach PJ *et al*: Predictors of blood transfusions in spinal instrumentation and fusion surgery. Spine 25: 596, 2000
14. Copley LA, Richards BS, Safavi FZ, Newton PO: Hemodilution as a method to reduce transfusion requirements in adolescent spine fusion surgery (see discussion). Spine 24: 219, 1999
15. Murray DJ, Forbes RB, Titone MB, Weinstein SL: Transfusion management in pediatric and adolescent scoliosis surgery: Efficacy of autologous blood. Spine 22: 2735, 1997
16. Brodsky JW, Dickson JH, Erwin WD, Rossi CD: Hypotensive anesthesia for scoliosis surgery in Jehovah's Witnesses. Spine 16: 304, 1991
17. Lentschener C, Cottin P, Bouaziz H *et al*: Reduction of blood loss and transfusion requirement by aprotinin in posterior lumbar spine fusion. Anesth Analg 89: 590, 1999
18. Dilger JA, Tetzlaff JE, Bell GR *et al*: Ischaemic optic neuropathy after spinal fusion. Can J Anaesth 45: 63, 1998
19. Myers MA, Hamilton SR, Bogosian AJ *et al*: Visual loss as a complication of spine surgery. A review of 37 cases. Spine 22: 1325, 1997
20. Warner ME, Warner MA, Garrity JA *et al*: The frequency of perioperative vision loss. Anesth Analg 93: 1417, 2001
21. Patel NJ, Patel BS, Paskin S, Laufer S: Induced moderate hypotensive anesthesia for spinal fusion and Harrington-rod instrumentation. J Bone Joint Surg Am 67: 1384, 1985
22. Horlocker TT, Nuttall GA, Dekutoski MB, Bryant SC: The accuracy of coagulation tests during spinal fusion and instrumentation. Anesth Analg 93: 33, 2001
23. Lang SA, Duncan PG, Dupius PR: Fatal air embolism in an adolescent with Duchenne muscular dystrophy during Harrington instrumentation. Anesth Analg 69: 132, 1989
24. Frankel AS, Holzman RS: Air embolism during posterior spinal fusion. Can J Anaesth 35: 511, 1988
25. McCarthy RE, Lonstein JE, Mertz JD, Kuslich SD: Air embolism in spinal surgery. J Spinal Disord 3: 1, 1990
26. Horlocker TT, Wedel DJ, Cucchiara RF: Venous air embolism during spinal instrumentation and fusion in the prone position (letter). Anesth Analg 75: 152, 1992
27. Bianconi M, Ferraro L, Ricci R *et al*: The pharmacokinetics and efficacy of ropivacaine continuous wound instillation after spine fusion surgery. Anesth Analg 98: 166, 2004
28. France JC, Jorgenson SS, Lowe TG, Dwyer AP: The use of intrathecal morphine for analgesia after posterolateral lumbar fusion: A prospective, double-blind, randomized study. Spine 22: 2272, 1997
29. Daley MD, Morningstar BA, Rolbin SH *et al:* Epidural anesthesia for obstetrics after spinal surgery. Reg Anesth 15: 280, 1990
30. Crosby ET, Halpern SH: Obstetric epidural anaesthesia in patients with Harrington instrumentation. Can J Anaesth 36: 693, 1989
31. Hubbert CH: Epidural anesthesia in patients with spinal fusion. Anesth Analg 64: 843, 1985
32. Lynch NM, Cofield RH, Silbert PL, Hermann RC: Neurologic complications after total shoulder arthroplasty. J Shoulder Elbow Surg 5: 53, 1996
33. Conn RA, Cofield RH, Byer DE, Linstromberg JW: Interscalene block anesthesia for shoulder surgery. Clin Orthop 216: 94, 1987
34. Urmey WF, Talts KH, Sharrock NE: One hundred percent incidence of hemidiaphragmatic paresis associated with interscalene brachial plexus anesthesia as diagnosed by ultrasonography. Anesth Analg 72: 498, 1991
35. Schroeder LE, Horlocker TT, Schroeder DR: The efficacy of axillary block for surgical procedures about the elbow. Anesth Analg 83: 747, 1996
36. Davis WJ, Lennon RL, Wedel DJ: Brachial plexus anesthesia for outpatient surgical procedures on an upper extremity. Mayo Clin Proc 66: 470, 1991
37. Ilfeld BM, Morey TE, Wright TW *et al*: Interscalene perineural ropivacaine infusion: A comparison of two dosing regimens for postoperative analgesia. Reg Anesth Pain Med 29: 9, 2004
38. Sculco TP: Global blood management in orthopaedic surgery. Clin Orthop 357: 43, 1998
39. Modig J, Borg T, Karlstrom G *et al*: Thromboembolism after total hip replacement: Role of epidural and general anesthesia. Anesth Analg 62: 174, 1983
40. Modig J, Borg T, Bagge L, Saldeen T: Role of extradural and of general anaesthesia in fibrinolysis and coagulation after total hip replacement. Br J Anaesth 55: 625, 1983
41. Pagnano MW, Trousdale RJ, Hanssen A *et al*: A comprehensive regional anesthesia protocol markedly improves patient care and facilitates early discharge after total knee and total hip arthroplasty. Abstract 043. Annual meeting of the American Academy of Orthopaedic Surgeons, February 23–27, 2005. http://www.aaos.org/wordhtml/anmt2005/sciexh/se043.htm.
42. Rosberg B, Fredin H, Gustafson C: Anesthetic techniques and surgical blood loss in total hip arthroplasty. Acta Anaesthesiol Scand 26: 189, 1982
43. Singelyn FJ, Deyaert M, Joris D *et al*: Effects of intravenous patient-controlled analgesia with morphine, continuous epidural analgesia, and continuous three-in-one block on postoperative pain and knee rehabilitation after unilateral total knee arthroplasty. Anesth Analg 87: 88, 1998
44. Capdevila X, Barthelet Y, Biboulet P *et al*: Effects of perioperative analgesic technique on the surgical outcome and duration of rehabilitation after major knee surgery. Anesthesiology 91: 8, 1999
45. Horlocker TT, Hebl JR: Anesthesia for outpatient knee arthroscopy: Is there an optimal technique? Reg Anesth Pain Med 28: 58, 2003
46. Matheny JM, Hanks GA, Rung GW *et al*: A comparison of patient-controlled analgesia and continuous lumbar plexus block after anterior cruciate ligament reconstruction. Arthroscopy 9: 87, 1993
47. Klein SM, Greengrass RA, Gleason DH *et al*: Major ambulatory surgery with continuous regional anesthesia and a disposable infusion pump. Anesthesiology 91: 563, 1999
48. Hadzic A, Vloka JD: Anesthesia for ankle and foot surgery. Tech Reg Anesth Pain Manage 3: 113, 1999
49. Stein C, Comisel K, Haimeri E *et al*: Analgesic effect of intraarticular morphine after arthroscopic knee surgery. N Engl J Med 325: 1123, 1991
50. Hughes DG: Intra-articular bupivacaine for pain relief in arthroscopic surgery. Anaesthesia 40: 84, 1985
51. Reuben SS, Sklar J: Pain management in patients who undergo outpatient arthroscopic surgery of the knee. J Bone Joint Surg 82: 1754, 2000
52. Banic A, Krejci V, Erni D *et al*: Effects of sodium nitroprusside and phenylephrine on blood flow in free musculocutaneous flaps during general anesthesia. Anesthesiology 90: 147, 1999
53. Bird TM, Strunin L: Anaesthetic considerations for microsurgical repair of limbs. Can Anaesth Soc J 31: 51, 1984
54. Geter RK, Winters RRW, Puckett CL: Resolution of experimental microvascular spasm and improvement in anastomotic patency by direct topical agent application. Plast Reconstr Surg 66: 690, 1980
55. Yaster M, Maxwell LG: Pediatric regional anesthesia. Anesthesiology 70: 324, 1989
56. Dalens B: Regional anesthesia in children. Anesth Analg 68: 654, 1989
57. Wedel DJ: Femoral and lateral femoral cutaneous nerve block for muscle biopsies in children. Reg Anesth 14: 63, 1989
58. Wedel DJ, Krohn JS, Hall J: Brachial plexus anesthesia in pediatric patients. Mayo Clin Proc 66: 583, 1991
59. Sapega A, Heppenstall RB, Chance B *et al*: Optimizing tourniquet application and release times in extremity surgery. J Bone Joint Surg Am 67: 303, 1985
60. Hamilton WK, Sokoll MD: Tourniquet paralysis. JAMA 199: 37, 1967
61. Patterson S, Klenerman L: The effect of pneumatic tourniquets on ultrastructure of skeletal muscle. J Bone Joint Surg Br 61: 178, 1979
62. Hurst LN, Weinglein O, Brown WF, Campbell GJ: The pneumatic tourniquet: A biomechanical and electrophysiologic study. Plast Reconstr Surg 67: 648, 1981
63. Miller SH, Price G, Buck D *et al:* Effects of tourniquet ischemia and postischemic edema on muscle metabolism. J Hand Surg 4: 547, 1979
64. Heppenstall RB, Balderston R, Goodwin C: Pathophysiologic effects distal to a tourniquet in the dog. J Trauma 19: 234, 1979
65. Kadoi Y, Ide M, Saito S *et al*: Hyperventilation after tourniquet deflation prevents an increase in cerebral blood flow velocity. Can J Anaesth 46: 259, 1999
66. Bourke DL, Silberberg MS, Ortega R, Willock MM: Respiratory responses associated with release of intraoperative tourniquets. Anesth Analg 69: 541, 1989
67. Della Valle CJ, Jazrawi LM, Di Cesare PE, Steiger DJ: Paradoxical cerebral embolism complicating a major orthopaedic operation: A report of two cases. J Bone Joint Surg Am 81: 108, 1999
68. Valli H, Rosenberg PH: Effects of three anaesthetic methods on haemodynamic responses connected with the use of thigh tourniquets in orthopaedic patients. Acta Anaesthesiol Scand 29: 142, 1985
69. Hagenouw RPM, Bridenbaugh PO, van Egmond J, Stuebing R: Tourniquet pain: A volunteer study. Anesth Analg 65: 1175, 1986
70. Parisi DM, Koval K, Egol K: Fat embolism syndrome. Am J Orthop 31(9): 507, 2002
71. Gurd AR: Fat embolism: An aid to diagnosis. J Bone Joint Surg Br 52: 732, 1970
72. Geerts WH, Pineo GF, Heit JA *et al*: Prevention of venous thromboembolism: The seventh ACCP conference on antithrombotic and thrombolytic therapy. Chest 126(3 suppl): 338S, 2004

73. Thorburn J, Louden JR, Vallance R: Spinal and general anaesthesia in total hip replacement: Frequency of deep vein thrombosis. Br J Anaesth 52: 1117, 1980
74. Donadoni R, Baele G, Devulder J, Rolly G: Coagulation and fibrinolytic parameters in patients undergoing total hip replacement: Influence of the anaesthesia technique. Acta Anaesthesiol Scand 33: 588, 1989
75. Davis FM, Laurenson VG, Gillespie WJ *et al*: Deep vein thrombosis after total hip replacement: A comparison between spinal and general anaesthesia. J Bone Joint Surg 71: 181, 1989
76. Sharrock NE, Haas SB, Hargett MJ *et al*: Effects of epidural anesthesia on the incidence of deep-vein thrombosis after total knee arthroplasty. J Bone Joint Surg 73: 502, 1991
77. Nielsen PT, Jorgensen LN, Albrecht-Beste E *et al*: Lower thrombosis risk with epidural blockade in knee arthroplasty. Acta Orthop Scand 61: 29, 1990
78. Simpson PJ, Radford SG, Forster SJ *et al*: The fibrinolytic effects of anaesthesia. Anaesthesia 37: 3, 1982
79. Tryba M: Epidural regional anesthesia and low molecular heparin: Pro (in German). Anasthesiol Intensivmed Notfallmed Schmerzther 28: 179, 1993
80. Vandermeulen EP, Van Aken H, Vermylen J: Anticoagulants and spinal-epidural anesthesia. Anesth Analg 79: 1165, 1994
81. Horlocker TT, Wedel DJ: Neuraxial block and low molecular weight heparin: Balancing perioperative analgesia and thromboprophylaxis. Reg Anesth Pain Med 23: 164, 1998
82. Horlocker TT, Wedel DJ, Benzon H *et al*: Regional anesthesia in the anticoagulated patient: Defining the risks (the second ASRA consensus conference on neuraxial anesthesia and anticoagulation). Reg Anesth Pain Med 28: 172, 2003

CHAPTER 41 ■ ANESTHESIA AND THE ENDOCRINE SYSTEM

JEFFREY J. SCHWARTZ AND STANLEY H. ROSENBAUM

KEY POINTS

1. Asymptomatic or mild hypothyroidism does not appear to significantly increase anesthetic risk and is not a contraindication to surgery. Moderate to severe hypothyroidism should be corrected before surgery to prevent multisystem complications.
2. The major risk of anesthesia in the poorly controlled thyrotoxic patient is thyroid storm, which must be aggressively treated with beta-blockers, iodide, and antithyroid drugs.
3. Patients who have received corticosteroids for more than 1 week in the past year may have adrenal suppression and should receive supplemental steroids in the perioperative period.
4. Preoperative preparation of the pheochromocytoma patient with alpha-blockers decreases intraoperative hemodynamic instability.
5. Tumor manipulation is associated with severe hypertension that should be treated aggressively with nitroprusside, phentolamine, or other rapidly acting vasodilators.
6. The major perioperative risks to the diabetic patient come from coexisting disease, especially coronary artery disease. Coexisting disease must be aggressively sought and optimized.
7. Maintenance of blood glucose levels near euglycemia appears to reduce cardiac, wound, neurologic, and septic complications.
8. Patients with acromegaly may be difficult intubations that cannot be anticipated by physical examination.

THYROID GLAND

The thyroid gland secretes thyroid hormones, thyroxine (T_4), and 3,5,3′-1-tri-iodothyronine (T_3), which are the major regulators of cellular metabolic activity. Thyroid hormones exert a variety of actions by regulating the synthesis and activity of various proteins. They are necessary for proper cardiac, pulmonary, and neurologic function during both health and illness.

Thyroid Metabolism and Function

The production of thyroid hormone is initiated by the active uptake and concentration of iodide in the thyroid gland (Fig. 41-1). Dietary iodine is reduced to iodide in the gastrointestinal (GI) tract. Circulating iodide is taken up by the thyroid gland, where it is then bound to tyrosine residues to form various iodotyrosines. After organification, monoiodotyrosine or diiodotyrosine is coupled enzymatically by thyroid peroxidase

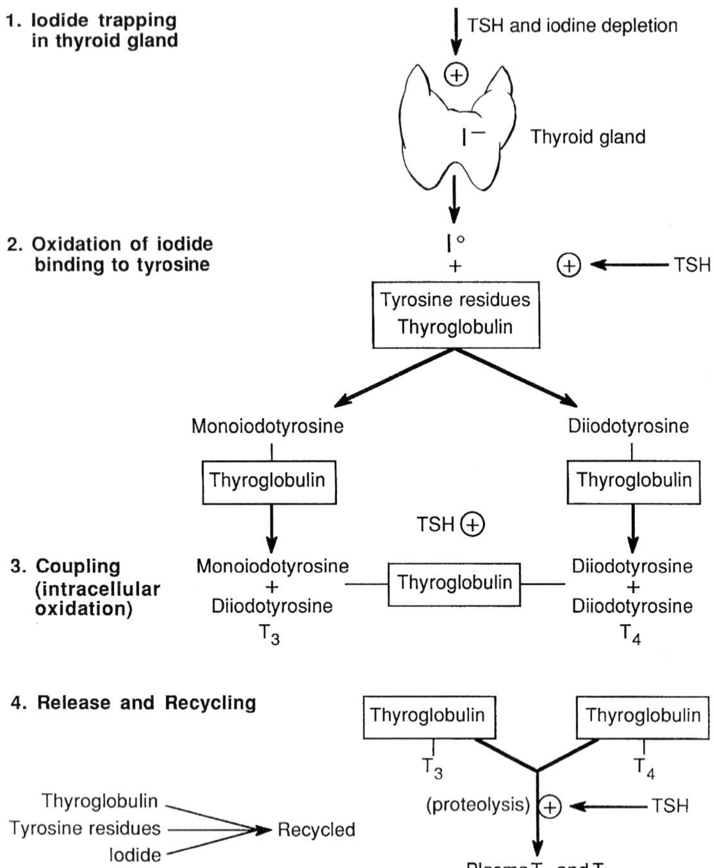

FIGURE 41-1. Thyroid hormone biosynthesis consists of four stages: (1) organification, (2) binding, (3) coupling, and (4) release. TSH, thyroid-stimulating hormone; T_3, triiodothyronine; T_4, thyroxine.

to form either T_3 or T_4. These hormones are attached to the thyroglobulin protein and stored as colloid in the gland. The release of T_3 and T_4 from the gland is accomplished through proteolysis from the thyroglobulin and diffusion into the circulation. Thyrotropin (thyroid-stimulating hormone or TSH) is produced in the anterior pituitary gland, and its secretion is regulated by thyrotropin-releasing hormone, produced in the hypothalamus. TSH is responsible for maintaining the uptake of iodide and proteolytic release of thyroid hormone. Excess iodine inhibits the synthesis and secretion of thyroid hormone. Circulating thyroid hormone inhibits thyroid-releasing hormone and TSH secretion in a negative feedback loop. The thyroid gland is solely responsible for the daily secretion of T_4 (80 to 100 μg/day). The half-life of T_4 in the circulation is 6 to 7 days.

Approximately 80% of T_3 is produced by the extrathyroidal deiodination of T_4 and 20% by direct thyroid secretion. The half-life of T_3 is 24 to 30 hours. Most of the effects of thyroid hormones are mediated by the more potent and less protein-bound T_3. The degree to which these hormones are protein bound in the circulation is the major factor influencing their activity and degradation. T_4 is metabolized by monodeiodination to either T_3 or reverse T_3 (rT_3). T_3 is biologically active, whereas rT_3 is inactive. The major fraction of circulating hormone is bound to thyroid-binding globulin (TBG), with a smaller fraction bound to albumin and thyroid-binding prealbumin. Less than 0.1% is present as free, unbound hormone. Changes in serum-binding protein concentrations have a major effect on total T_3 and T_4 serum concentrations. The plasma normally contains 5 to 12 μg/dL of T_4 and 80 to 220 ng/dL of T_3. Many drugs can affect thyroid function, including amiodarone and dopamine.[1]

Although the thyroid hormone is important to many aspects of growth and function, the anesthesiologist is most often concerned with the cardiovascular manifestations of thyroid disease. Thyroid hormones affect tissue responses to sympathetic stimuli and increase the intrinsic contractile state of cardiac muscle. β-Adrenergic receptors are increased in number, and cardiac α-adrenergic receptors are decreased by thyroid hormone.

Tests of Thyroid Function

Serum Thyroxine

The serum T_4 assay is the standard screening test for evaluation of thyroid gland function (Table 41-1). The total T_4 is elevated in approximately 90% of patients with hyperthyroidism, and it is low in 85% of those who are hypothyroid. The concentration of T_4 is measured by radioimmunoassay (RIA). The serum T_4 concentration is influenced by thyroid hormone protein-binding capacity. An increase or decrease in TBG levels or in protein binding may therefore alter the total T_4 but not the concentration of the free T_4. Because of the effect of TBG on circulating total T_4, T_4 levels should never be used alone to evaluate thyroid disease. Elevations in the TBG concentration are the most common cause of hyperthyroxinemia in euthyroid patients. Increases in TBG due to acute liver disease, pregnancy, or drugs (oral contraceptives, exogenous estrogens, clofibrate, opioids) may be responsible. Because a total T_4 can be misleadingly high in euthyroidism or normal in hypothyroidism, some measure of free thyroid hormone activity (free T_4) must also be used.

TABLE 41-1

TESTS OF THYROID GLAND FUNCTION

	T_4	T_3	THBR	TSH
Hyperthyroidism	Elevated	Elevated	Elevated	Normal or low
Primary hypothyroidism	Low	Low or normal	Low	Elevated
Secondary hypothyroidism	Low	Low	Low	Low
Sick euthyroidism (decreased peripheral conversion of T_4 to T_3)	Normal	Low	Normal	Normal
Pregnancy	Elevated	Normal	Low	Normal

T_4, total serum thyroxine; T_3, serum triiodothyronine; THBR, thyroid hormone-binding rate; TSH, thyroid-stimulating hormone.

Serum Triiodothyronine

The serum T_3 is also measured by RIA. Serum T_3 levels are often determined to detect disease in patients with clinical evidence of hyperthyroidism in the absence of elevations of T_4. T_3 may be the only thyroid hormone produced in excess. T_3 concentrations may be depressed by factors that impair the peripheral conversion of T_4 to T_3 (sick euthyroid syndrome). In 50% of hypothyroid patients, the serum T_3 concentration is low; in the remaining 50%, it is normal.

Tests for Assessing Thyroid Hormone Binding

It is necessary to find some measure of thyroid-binding proteins, mostly TBG, to interpret correctly total thyroxine levels. The "T uptake" test measures the ability of the patient's serum to bind exogenously introduced T_4 and reflects the amount of TBG and the extent of T_4 saturation on TBG. The T uptake is inversely related to the degree of unsaturation of TBG. The T uptake can be used to calculate the T_4-binding capacity, which is directly related to the degree of unsaturation of TBG. The T uptake or T_4-binding capacity can be used to calculate the estimated free T_4 or free T_4 index, which reflects the free T_4 concentration in the blood independent of binding proteins.

Thyroid-Stimulating Hormone

The RIA for this hormone has proved most useful in detecting patients who are hypothyroid. It is often higher than 20 μIU/mL in primary hypothyroidism (normal, 8 μIU/mL). Current assays are sensitive enough to diagnose hyperthyroidism by depressed levels of TSH. A condition characterized by elevated TSH and normal T_4 may represent subclinical hypothyroidism. A low TSH level in a clinically hypothyroid patient indicates disease at the pituitary or hypothalamic level. The goal of thyroid replacement therapy is to normalize TSH levels.[2] Starvation, fever, stress, corticosteroids, and T_3 or T_4 can all depress TSH levels.

Radioactive Iodine Uptake

The thyroid gland has the ability to concentrate large amounts of inorganic iodide. The oral administration of radioactive iodine (^{131}I) can be used to indicate thyroid gland activity. Thyroid uptake is elevated in hyperthyroidism unless the hyperthyroidism is caused by thyroiditis, in which case the uptake is low or absent. Because of overlap in values, it is difficult to distinguish euthyroid from hypothyroid people. Radioactive iodide uptake may be increased by a variety of factors, including dietary iodine deficiency, renal failure, and congestive heart failure. Because uptake is under TSH control, elevated free T_4 levels and corticosteroids decrease radioactive iodide uptake. Functioning ("hot") thyroid tissue is rarely malignant. Nonfunctioning ("cold") tissue may be malignant or benign.

Hyperthyroidism

Hyperthyroidism results from the exposure of tissues to excessive amounts of thyroid hormone (Table 41-2). The most common etiology is the multinodular diffuse goiter of Graves' disease. This typically occurs between the ages of 20 and 40 years, and is predominant in women. Most of these patients demonstrate a syndrome characterized by diffuse glandular enlargement, ophthalmopathy, dermopathy, and clubbing of the fingers. A thyroid-stimulating autoantibody may be present. Thyroid adenoma is the second most common cause. Another cause of increased thyroid hormone synthesis is thyroiditis. Subacute thyroiditis frequently follows a respiratory illness and is characterized by a viral-like illness with a firm, painful gland. This type of thyroiditis is frequently treated with

TABLE 41-2

CAUSES OF HYPERTHYROIDISM

INTRINSIC THYROID DISEASE
Hyperfunctioning thyroid adenoma
Toxic multinodular goiter
ABNORMAL TSH STIMULATOR
Graves' disease
Trophoblastic tumor
DISORDERS OF HORMONE STORAGE OR RELEASE
Thyroiditis
EXCESS PRODUCTION OF TSH
Pituitary thyrotropin (rare)
EXTRATHYROIDAL SOURCE OF HORMONE
Struma ovarii
Functioning follicular carcinoma
EXOGENOUS THYROID
Iatrogenic
Iodine induced

TSH, thyroid-stimulating hormone.

anti-inflammatory agents alone. Rarely, subacute thyroiditis may occur in a patient with a normal-size, painless gland. Hashimoto's thyroiditis is a chronic autoimmune disease that usually produces hypothyroidism but may occasionally produce hyperthyroidism. Hyperthyroidism may also be associated with pregnancy, ^{131}I therapy, thyroid carcinoma, trophoblastic tumors, or TSH-secreting pituitary adenomas. Iatrogenic hyperthyroidism may follow thyroid hormone replacement or may occur after iodide exposure (angiographic contrast media) in patients with chronically low iodide intake (Jod-Basedow phenomenon). The antiarrhythmic agent amiodarone is iodine rich and is another cause of iodine-induced thyrotoxicosis.[3]

The major manifestations of hyperthyroidism are weight loss; diarrhea; skeletal muscle weakness and stiffness; warm, moist skin; heat intolerance; and nervousness. Cardiovascular manifestations include increased left ventricular contractility and ejection fraction, tachycardia, elevated systolic blood pressure, and decreased diastolic blood pressure. Hypercalcemia, thrombocytopenia, and a mild anemia may be present. Elderly patients may present with heart failure, atrial fibrillation, or other cardiac dysrhythmias. They may also present with apathetic hyperthyroidism characterized by depression and withdrawal, without the usual systemic signs or symptoms.

Treatment and Anesthetic Considerations

The most important goal in managing the hyperthyroid patient is to make the patient euthyroid before any surgery, if possible. The drugs propylthiouracil and methimazole are thiourea derivatives that inhibit organification of iodide and the synthesis of thyroid hormone.[4] Propylthiouracil also decreases the peripheral conversion of T_4 to T_3. Normal thyroid glands usually contain a store of hormone that is large enough to maintain a euthyroid state for several months, even if synthesis is abolished. Therefore, hyperthyroid patients are unlikely to be regulated to a euthyroid state with antithyroid drugs alone in less than 6 to 8 weeks. Toxic reactions from these drugs are uncommon, but include skin rash, nausea, fever, agranulocytosis, hepatitis, and arthralgias.

Inorganic iodide inhibits iodide organification and thyroid hormone release—the Wolff-Chaikoff effect. Iodide is also effective in reducing the size of the hyperplastic gland and has a role in the preparation of the patient for emergency thyroid surgery. Antithyroid drugs should be started before iodide treatment because of the possibility of worsening the thyrotoxicosis.

β-Adrenergic antagonists are effective in attenuating the manifestations of excessive sympathetic activity and should be used in all hyperthyroid patients unless contraindicated. β-Adrenergic blockade alone does not inhibit hormone synthesis, but propranolol does impair the peripheral conversion of T_4 to T_3 over 1 to 2 weeks. Propranolol given over 12 to 24 hours decreases tachycardia, heat intolerance, anxiety, and tremor. Any beta-blocker may be used, and long-acting agents may be more convenient. The combination of propranolol (in doses titrated to effect) plus potassium iodide (two to five drops every 8 hours) is frequently used before surgery to ameliorate cardiovascular symptoms and reduce circulating concentrations of T_4 and T_3. Preoperative preparation usually requires 7 to 14 days. Heart failure secondary to poorly controlled paroxysmal atrial fibrillation may improve with slowing of the ventricular rate, but abnormalities of left ventricular function secondary to hyperthyroidism may not be corrected with the use of β-antagonists. If a hyperthyroid patient with clinically apparent disease requires emergency surgery, β-adrenergic blockade should be administered to achieve a heart rate less than 90 beats/min. Beta-blockers do not prevent thyroid storm. Glucocorticoids such as dexamethasone (8 to 12 mg/day) are used in the management of severe thyrotoxicosis because they reduce thyroid hormone secretion and the peripheral conversion of T_4 to T_3.

Iopanoic acid, a radiographic contrast agent that decreases peripheral conversion of T_4 and releases iodine that inhibits synthesis, is useful for emergency preparation.

Radioactive iodine therapy is an effective treatment for some patients with thyrotoxicosis.[5] It should not, however, be administered to patients who are pregnant because it crosses the placenta and may destroy the fetal thyroid. A side effect of RIA therapy is hypothyroidism; 10 to 60% of cases occur in the first year of therapy, and an additional 2% occur per year thereafter.

A variety of anesthetic techniques and drugs have been used for hyperthyroid patients undergoing surgery. All antithyroid medications are continued through the morning of surgery. The goal of intraoperative management in the hyperthyroid patient is to achieve a depth of anesthesia that prevents an exaggerated sympathetic response to surgical stimulation, while avoiding the administration of medication that stimulates the sympathetic nervous system. Pancuronium should be avoided. It is best to avoid using ketamine, even when a patient is clinically euthyroid. Hypotension that occurs during surgery is best treated with direct-acting vasopressors rather than a medication that provokes the release of catecholamines. The incidence of myasthenia gravis is increased in hyperthyroid patients; thus, the initial dose of muscle relaxant should be reduced, and a twitch monitor should be used to titrate subsequent doses. Regional anesthesia is an excellent alternative when appropriate; however, epinephrine-containing solutions should be avoided.

Thyroid storm is a life-threatening exacerbation of hyperthyroidism that most commonly develops in the undiagnosed or untreated hyperthyroid patient because of the stress of
1 surgery or nonthyroid illness.[6] Operating on an acutely hyperthyroid gland may provoke thyroid storm, although this is probably not due to mechanical release of hormone.[7] Its manifestations include hyperthermia, tachycardia, dysrhythmias, myocardial ischemia, congestive heart failure, agitation, and confusion. It must be distinguished from, or considered with, pheochromocytoma, malignant hyperthermia, and light anesthesia. Although free T_4 levels are often markedly elevated, no laboratory test is diagnostic. Treatment involves large doses of propylthiouracil and supportive measures to control fever and restore intravascular volume. Hemodynamic monitoring (pulmonary artery catheter, arterial catheter) is especially useful in guiding the treatment of patients with significant left ventricular dysfunction (Table 41-3). Again, it is essential to remove or treat the precipitating event.

TABLE 41-3

MANAGEMENT OF THYROID STORM

- Administer IV fluids.
- Administer sodium iodide, 250 mg PO or IV q6h.
- Administer propylthiouracil, 200–400 mg PO or via NGT q6h.
- Administer hydrocortisone, 50–100 mg IV q6h.
- Administer propranolol, 10–40 mg PO q4–6h, or esmolol infusion to treat hyperadrenergic signs.
- Cooling blankets and acetaminophen and meperidine (25–50 mg) IV q4–6h may be used to prevent shivering.
- Use digoxin for heart failure especially in the presence of atrial fibrillation with rapid ventricular response.

IV, intravenous(ly); PO, oral(ly); NGT, nasogastric tube.

Anesthesia for Thyroid Surgery

Subtotal thyroidectomy as an alternative to prolonged medical therapy is used less frequently now than in the past. Indications include failed medical therapy, underlying cancer, and symptomatic goiter. It is usually performed under general endotracheal anesthesia, although the use of the laryngeal mask airway is increasing.[8] Use of a laryngeal mask airway allows real-time visualization of vocal cord function because the patient is allowed to breathe spontaneously. Limited thyroidectomy may also be performed under bilateral superficial cervical plexus block. The anesthesiologist must be prepared to manage an unexpected difficult intubation because the incidence of difficult intubation during goiter surgery is 5 to 8%.[9] Thyroid cancer increases the risk, but the size of the goiter is not predictive. Airway obstruction is a potential problem in the patient with a large substernal goiter, although rarely a problem with goiters exclusively in the neck. Evidence of significant airway obstruction or tracheal deviation or narrowing may warrant inhalation induction or awake fiberoptic intubation. The complications after subtotal thyroidectomy include recurrent laryngeal nerve damage, tracheal compression secondary to hematoma or tracheomalacia, and hypoparathyroidism. Hypoparathyroidism secondary to the inadvertent surgical removal of parathyroid glands is most frequently seen after total thyroidectomy. The symptoms of hypocalcemia develop within the first 24 to 96 hours after surgery.[10] Laryngeal stridor progressing to laryngospasm may be one of the first indications of hypocalcemic tetany. The intravenous administration of calcium chloride or calcium gluconate is warranted in this situation. Magnesium levels should also be monitored and corrected if low. Bilateral recurrent laryngeal nerve injury is an extremely rare injury and necessitates reintubation. Unilateral nerve injury is more common and is often transient.[11] Unilateral damage to the recurrent laryngeal nerve is characterized by hoarseness and a paralyzed vocal cord, whereas bilateral injury causes aphonia. It is wise to evaluate vocal cord function before and after surgery by laryngoscopy or by asking the patient to phonate by saying the letter "e". Routine postoperative visualization of the vocal cords is not warranted. Postoperative extubation of the trachea should be performed under optimal conditions. Intraoperative laryngeal nerve injury or collapse of the tracheal rings from previous weakening may mandate emergency reintubation.

Hypothyroidism

Hypothyroidism is a relatively common disease (0.5 to 0.8% of the adult population) that results from inadequate circulating levels of T_4 or T_3, or both.[12] The development of hypothyroidism is often slow and progressive, making the clinical diagnosis difficult, especially in the more subtle cases. Hypofunctioning of the thyroid gland has many causes (Table 41-4). Primary failure of the thyroid gland refers to decreased production of thyroid hormone, despite adequate TSH production, and accounts for 95% of all cases of thyroid dysfunction. The remainder is caused by either hypothalamic or pituitary disease (secondary hypothyroidism) and is associated with other pituitary deficiencies.

A lack of thyroid hormone produces a variety of signs and symptoms. These early findings are often nonspecific and difficult to recognize. A history of RIA therapy, external neck irradiation, or the presence of a goiter is helpful in diagnosis. There is a generalized reduction in metabolic activity, resulting in lethargy, slow mental functioning, cold intolerance, and slow movements. The cardiovascular manifestations of hypothyroidism reflect the importance of thyroid hormone for myocardial contractility and catecholamine function. These patients exhibit bradycardia, decreased cardiac output, and increased peripheral resistance.[13] The accumulation of a cholesterol-rich pericardial fluid produces low voltage on the electrocardiogram (ECG). Heart failure only rarely occurs in the absence of coexisting heart disease. Angina pectoris itself is unusual in hypothyroidism but can appear when thyroid hormone treatment is initiated. Ventilatory responsiveness to hypoxia and hypercapnia is depressed in hypothyroid patients. This depression is potentiated by sedatives, opioids, and general anesthesia. Postoperative ventilatory failure requiring prolonged ventilation is rarely seen in hypothyroid patients in the absence of coexisting lung disease, obesity, or myxedema coma. Other abnormalities found in hypothyroidism include anemia, coagulopathy, hypothermia, sleep apnea, and impaired renal free water clearance with hyponatremia. Decreased gastrointestinal motility can compound the effect of postoperative ileus. In long-standing or severe disease, the stress response may be blunted and adrenal depression may occur.

TABLE 41-4

CAUSES OF HYPOTHYROIDISM

■ PRIMARY HYPOTHYROIDISM
Autoimmune
Irradiation to the neck
Previous ^{131}I therapy
Surgical removal
Thyroiditis (Hashimoto's disease)
Severe iodine depletion
Medications (iodines, propylthiouracil, methimazole)
Hereditary defects in biosynthesis
Congenital defects in gland development
■ SECONDARY OR TERTIARY HYPOTHYROIDISM
Pituitary
Hypothalamic

Reproduced with permission from Petersdorf RG (ed): Harrison's Principles of Internal Medicine, 10th ed. New York, McGraw-Hill, 1983.

Treatment and Anesthetic Considerations

Treatment of symptomatic hypothyroidism is with hormone replacement therapy.[14] Controversy remains regarding the preoperative anesthetic management of the hypothyroid patient. Although it seems logical, given the multisystem effects of thyroid hormone, to recommend that all hypothyroid surgical candidates be restored to a euthyroid state before surgery, such a recommendation is, in general, based on individual case reports. There have been few controlled studies to support the position that most hypothyroid patients are unusually sensitive to anesthetic drugs, have prolonged recovery times, or have a higher incidence of cardiovascular instability or collapse.

No increase in serious complications in patients with mild or moderate hypothyroidism undergoing general anesthesia has been noted.[15] One study[16] noted a higher incidence of intraoperative hypotension and postoperative GI and neuropsychiatric complications in mild and moderately hypothyroid patients undergoing noncardiac surgery, but still noted there were no compelling clinical reasons to postpone surgery in these patients. Surgery in severely hypothyroid patients should be postponed when possible until these patients are at least partially
2 treated.

The management of hypothyroid patients with symptomatic coronary artery disease has been a subject of particular controversy.[17] The need for thyroid hormone replacement therapy must be weighed against the risk of precipitating

TABLE 41-5

MANAGEMENT OF MYXEDEMA

Tracheal intubation and controlled ventilation as needed
Levothyroxine, 200–300 μg IV over 5–10 min initially, and 100 μg IV q24h
Hydrocortisone, 100 mg IV, then 25 mg IV q6h
Fluid and electrolyte therapy as indicated by serum electrolytes
Cover to conserve body heat; no warming blankets

IV, intravenous(ly).

myocardial ischemia. Several studies and a literature review found no differences in the frequency of intraoperative or postoperative complications when mild or moderately hypothyroid patients underwent cardiac surgery. In symptomatic patients or unstable patients with cardiac ischemia, thyroid replacement should probably be delayed until after coronary revascularization.

There appears to be little reason to postpone elective surgery in patients who have mild or moderate hypothyroidism. Thyroid replacement therapy is, however, indicated for patients with severe hypothyroidism or myxedema coma and for pregnant patients who are hypothyroid. Untreated hypothyroidism in pregnant patients is associated with an increased incidence of spontaneous abortion and mental and physical abnormalities in the offspring.

A number of anesthetic medications have been used without difficulty in hypothyroid patients. Although ketamine has been proposed as the ideal induction agent, thiopental has also been used in the hypothyroid patient. The maintenance of anesthesia may be safely achieved with either intravenous or inhaled anesthetics. There appears to be little if any decrease in the minimum alveolar concentration for volatile agents. Regional anesthesia is a good choice in the hypothyroid patient, provided the intravascular volume is well maintained. Monitoring is directed toward the early recognition of hypotension, congestive heart failure, and hypothermia. Scrupulous attention should be paid to maintaining normal body temperature.

Myxedema coma represents a severe form of hypothyroidism characterized by stupor or coma, hypoventilation, hypothermia, hypotension, and hyponatremia. This is a medical emergency with a high mortality rate (25 to 50%), and as such, requires aggressive therapy (Table 41-5). Only lifesaving surgery should proceed in the face of myxedema coma. Intravenous thyroid replacement is initiated as soon as the clinical diagnosis is made. An intravenous loading dose of T_4 (sodium levothyroxine, 200 to 300 μg) is given initially and followed by a maintenance dose of T_4, 50 to 200 mg/day intravenously.[18] Alternatively, T_3 may be used because it has a more rapid onset. Improvements in heart rate, blood pressure, and body temperature may occur within 24 hours. However, replacement therapy with either form of thyroid hormone may precipitate myocardial ischemia. There is also an increased likelihood of acute primary adrenal insufficiency in these patients, and they should receive stress doses of hydrocortisone. Steroid replacement continues until normal adrenal function can be confirmed.

PARATHYROID GLANDS

Calcium Physiology

The normal adult body contains approximately 1 to 2 kg of calcium (Ca^{2+}), of which 99% is in the skeleton.[19] Plasma calcium is present in three forms: (1) a protein-bound fraction (50%); (2) an ionized fraction (45%); and (3) a diffusible but nonionized fraction (5%) that is complexed with phosphate, bicarbonate, and citrate. This division is interesting because it is the ionized fraction that is physiologically active and homeostatically regulated. The normal total serum calcium concentration is 8.8 to 10.4 mg/dL. Albumin binds approximately 90% of the protein-bound fraction of calcium, and total serum Ca^{2+} consequently depends on albumin levels. In general, an increase or decrease in albumin of 1 g/dL is associated with a parallel change in total serum Ca^{2+} of 0.8 mg/dL. The serum ionized Ca^{2+} concentration is affected by temperature and blood pH through alterations in Ca^{2+} protein binding to albumin. Acidosis decreases protein binding (increases ionized Ca^{2+}), and alkalosis increases protein binding (decreases ionized Ca^{2+}). The concentration of free Ca^{2+} ion is of critical importance in regulating skeletal muscle contraction, coagulation, neurotransmitter release, endocrine secretion, and a variety of other cellular functions. As a consequence, the maintenance of serum Ca^{2+} concentration is subject to exquisite hormonal control by parathyroid hormone (PTH) and vitamin D (Fig. 41-2).

Parathyroid hormone acts to maintain the extracellular fluid Ca^{2+} concentration through direct effects on bone resorption and renal Ca^{2+} resorption at the distal tubule, and indirectly through its effects on the synthesis of 1,25-dihydroxyvitamin D. The renal effects of PTH include phosphaturia and bicarbonaturia, in addition to enhanced Ca^{2+} and magnesium resorption. Most evidence suggests that rapid changes in blood Ca^{2+} levels are due primarily to hormonal effects on bone and, to a lesser extent, to renal Ca^{2+} clearance, whereas maintenance of Ca^{2+} balance depends more on the indirect effects of the hormone on intestinal calcium absorption.

Parathyroid hormone secretion is primarily regulated by the serum ionized Ca^{2+} concentration. This negative feedback mechanism is exquisitely sensitive in maintaining calcium levels in a normal range. Release of PTH is also influenced by phosphate, magnesium, and catecholamine levels. Acute hypomagnesemia directly stimulates PTH release, whereas chronic magnesium depletion appears to inhibit proper functioning of the parathyroid gland. The plasma phosphate concentration has an indirect influence on PTH secretion by causing reciprocal changes in the serum ionized Ca^{2+} concentration.

Vitamin D is absorbed from the GI tract and can be produced enzymatically by ultraviolet irradiation of the skin. Vitamin D (cholecalciferol) is made from cholesterol metabolites and is inactive. Calciferol is hydroxylated in the liver to 25-hydroxycholecalciferol (25-OHD) and in the kidney is further hydroxylated to 1,25-dihydroxycholecalciferol [1,25 $(OH)_2D$] or 24,25-dihydroxycholecalciferol [24,25$(OH)_2D$]. 25-OHD is the major circulating form of vitamin D. The synthesis of this hormone is not regulated by a hormone or by Ca^{2+} or phosphate levels. 1,25$(OH)_2D$ and 24,25$(OH)_2D$ are the major active metabolites of vitamin D, and their production is reciprocally regulated at the kidney. Hypocalcemia and hypophosphatemia cause an increased production of 1,25$(OH)_2D$ and a decreased production of 24,25$(OH)_2D$. 1,25$(OH)_2D$ stimulates bone, kidney, and intestinal absorption of calcium and phosphate. Vitamin D deficiency can lead to decreased intestinal absorption of Ca^{2+} and secondary hyperparathyroidism.

Hyperparathyroidism

Primary hyperparathyroidism is most commonly due to a benign parathyroid adenoma (90% of cases) or hyperplasia (9%) and very rarely to a parathyroid carcinoma. Primary hyperparathyroidism may also exist as part of a multiple endocrine neoplastic (MEN) syndrome. Hyperplasia usually involves all four glands. Although most patients with primary hyperparathyroidism are hypercalcemic, most are asymptomatic

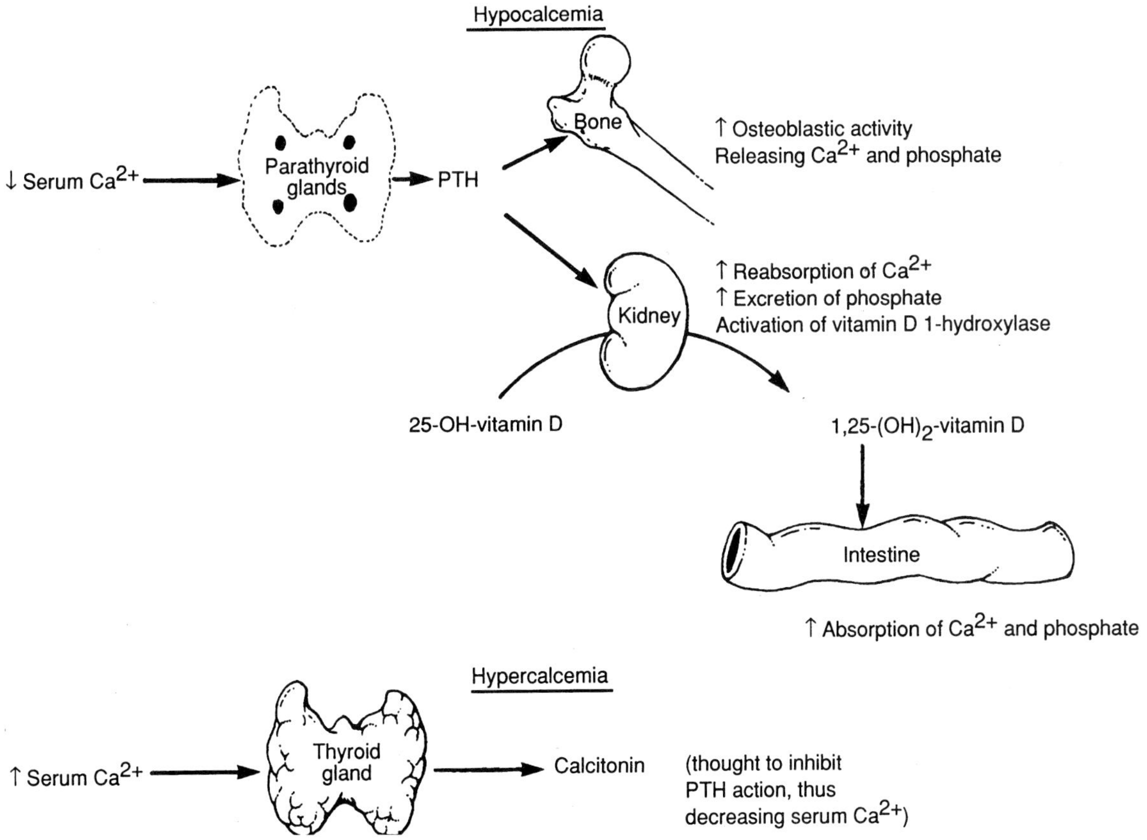

FIGURE 41-2. Parathyroid hormone (PTH) and vitamin D metabolism and action. (From McClatchey KD: Clinical Laboratory Medicine, 2nd ed. Philadelphia, Lippincott Williams & Wilkins, 2002.)

at the time of diagnosis. When symptoms occur, they usually result from the hypercalcemia that accompanies the disease. Primary hyperparathyroidism occurring during pregnancy is associated with a high maternal and fetal morbidity rate (50%). The placenta allows the fetus to concentrate calcium, promoting fetal hypercalcemia and leading to hypoparathyroidism in the newborn. Pregnant women with primary hyperparathyroidism should be treated with surgery.

Hypercalcemia is responsible for a broad spectrum of signs and symptoms. Nephrolithiasis is the most common manifestation, occurring in 60 to 70% of patients. Polyuria and polydipsia are also common complaints. An increase in bone turnover may lead to generalized demineralization and subperiosteal bone resorption; however, only a small group of patients (10 to 15%) have clinically significant bone disease. Patients may experience generalized skeletal muscle weakness and fatigability, epigastric discomfort, peptic ulceration, and constipation. Psychiatric manifestations include depression, memory loss, confusion, or psychosis. Between 20 and 50% of patients are hypertensive, but this usually resolves with successful treatment of the disease. Cardiac function is enhanced in the early stages of hypercalcemia. Calcium flux into the cells is reflected in the plateau phase of the action potential (phase 2). As extracellular calcium increases, the inward flux is more rapid, and phase 2 is shortened. The corresponding ECG change is a shorter QT interval. Cardiac contractility may increase until a level between 15 and 20 mg/dL is reached. At this point, there is a prolongation of the PR segment and QRS complex that can result in heart block or bundle-branch block. Bradycardia also occurs.

An elevated serum Ca^{2+} concentration is a valuable diagnostic indicator of primary hyperparathyroidism. The serum phosphate concentration is nonspecific, with many patients having normal or near-normal levels. The reported incidence of hyperchloremic acidosis varies widely in primary hyperparathyroidism, but most patients usually have a serum chloride concentration in excess of 102 mEq/L. Rarely does a patient with hypercalcemia secondary to ectopic PTH production (malignancy) present with hyperchloremic acidosis. The definitive diagnosis of primary hyperparathyroidism is made by RIA demonstration of an elevation in PTH levels in the presence of hypercalcemia. An elevated nephrogenous cyclic adenosine monophosphate is noted in more than 90% of patients with primary hyperparathyroidism.

Hypercalcemia may also result from the ectopic production of PTH or PTH-like substances from lung, genitourinary, breast, GI, and lymphoproliferative malignancies. Tumors may also produce hypercalcemia through direct bone resorption or the production of osteoclast-activating factor. In the absence of a clinically obvious neoplasm, there may be difficulty in differentiating between PTH-producing malignancies and primary hyperparathyroidism. PTH fragments from malignant tissue differ from native PTH and aid in distinguishing between ectopic PTH production and primary hyperparathyroidism.

Secondary hyperparathyroidism represents an increase in parathyroid function as a result of conditions that produce hypocalcemia or hyperphosphatemia. Chronic renal disease is a common cause of hyperphosphatemia (due to decreased phosphate excretion) and decreased vitamin D metabolism. The hypocalcemia that results leads to an increased production of PTH. GI disorders accompanied by malabsorption may also lead to a secondary increase in parathyroid activity. Tertiary hyperparathyroidism refers to the development of hypercalcemia in a patient who has had prolonged secondary hyperparathyroidism that has caused adenomatous changes in the parathyroid gland and unregulated PTH.

Treatment and Anesthetic Considerations

Surgery is the treatment of choice for the patient with symptomatic disease. Considerable controversy, however, surrounds the choice of treatment in the asymptomatic patient. It is not clear that mild primary hyperparathyroidism decreases longevity. Surgery is often chosen over medical therapy because it offers definitive treatment and is generally safe.

Preoperative preparation focuses on the correction of intravascular volume and electrolyte irregularities. It is particularly important to evaluate the patient with chronic hypercalcemia for abnormalities of the renal, cardiac, or central nervous systems. Emergency treatment of hypercalcemia is undertaken before surgery, when the serum Ca^{2+} concentration exceeds 15 mg/dL (7.5 mEq/L). Lowering of the serum Ca^{2+} concentration is initially accomplished by expanding the intravascular volume and establishing a sodium diuresis. This is achieved with the intravenous administration of normal saline and furosemide. Rehydration alone is capable of lowering the serum Ca^{2+} level by $\geq$2 mg/dL. Hydration dilutes the serum Ca^{2+}, and a sodium diuresis promotes Ca^{2+} excretion through an inhibition of sodium and Ca^{2+} resorption in the proximal tubule. Hypokalemia and hypomagnesemia may result. Another element in the treatment of hypercalcemia is the correction of hypophosphatemia. Hypophosphatemia increases GI absorption of Ca^{2+}, stimulates the breakdown of bone, and impairs the uptake of Ca^{2+} by bone. Low serum phosphate levels impair cardiac contractility and may contribute to congestive heart failure. Hypophosphatemia also causes skeletal muscle weakness, hemolysis, and platelet dysfunction.

Other medications that have a role in lowering the serum Ca^{2+} include bisphosphonates, mithramycin, calcitonin, and glucocorticoids. Bisphosphonates are pyrophosphate analogs that inhibit osteoclast action. They are the drugs of choice for severe hypercalcemia. Toxic effects include fever and hypophosphatemia. Mithramycin, a cytotoxic agent, inhibits PTH-induced osteoclast activity and can lower the serum Ca^{2+} levels by $\geq$2 mg/dL in 24 to 48 hours. Toxic effects include azotemia, hepatotoxicity, and thrombocytopenia. Calcitonin is useful in transiently lowering the serum Ca^{2+} level 2 to 4 mg/dL through direct inhibition of osteoclastic bone resorption. The advantages of calcitonin are that side effects are mild (urticaria, nausea) and the onset of activity is rapid. Calcitonin resistance usually develops within 24 to 48 hours. Glucocorticoids are effective in lowering the serum Ca^{2+} concentration in several conditions (sarcoidosis, some malignancies, hyperthyroidism, vitamin D intoxication) through their actions on osteoclast bone resorption, GI absorption of calcium, and the urinary excretion of calcium. Glucocorticoids are usually of no benefit in the treatment of primary hypercalcemia. Finally, hemodialysis or peritoneal dialysis can be used to lower the serum Ca^{2+} level when alternative regimens are ineffective or contraindicated.

There is no evidence that a specific anesthetic drug or technique has advantages over another. A thorough knowledge of the clinical manifestations attributable to hypercalcemia is of the greatest value in choosing an anesthetic technique. Special monitoring is usually not required. Because of the unpredictable response to neuromuscular blocking drugs in the hypercalcemic patient, a conservative approach to muscle paralysis makes sense. There is an increased requirement for vecuronium, and probably all nondepolarizing muscle relaxants, during onset of neuromuscular blockade.[20] Careful positioning of the osteopenic patient is necessary to avoid pathologic bone fractures.

Anesthesia for Parathyroid Surgery

General anesthesia is most commonly used, but cervical plexus block and local anesthesia with hypnosis have been used successfully.[21] Postoperative complications include recurrent laryngeal nerve injury, bleeding, and transient or complete hypoparathyroidism. Unilateral recurrent laryngeal nerve injury is characterized by hoarseness and usually requires no intervention. Bilateral recurrent laryngeal nerve injury is a rare complication, producing aphonia and requiring immediate tracheal intubation. After successful parathyroidectomy, a decrease in the serum Ca^{2+} level should be observed within 24 hours. Patients with significant preoperative bone disease may have hypocalcemia after removal of the PTH-secreting glands. This "hungry bone" syndrome comes as a result of the rapid remineralization of bone.[22] Thus, serum Ca^{2+}, magnesium, and phosphorus levels should be closely monitored until stable. The serum Ca^{2+} nadir usually occurs within 3 to 7 days.

Hypoparathyroidism

An underproduction of PTH or resistance of the end-organ tissues to PTH results in hypocalcemia (<8 mg/dL). The normal physiologic response to hypocalcemia is an increase in PTH secretion and $1,25(OH)_2D$ synthesis with an increase in Ca^{2+} mobilization from bone, GI absorption, and renal tubule reclamation. The most common cause of acquired PTH deficiency is inadvertent removal of the parathyroid glands during thyroid or parathyroid surgery. Other causes of acquired hypoparathyroidism include ^{131}I therapy for thyroid disease, neck trauma, granulomatous disease, or an infiltrating process (malignancy or amyloidosis). Severe hypomagnesemia (<0.8 mEq/L) from any cause can produce hypocalcemia by suppressing PTH secretion and interfering with PTH action. Renal insufficiency leads to phosphorus retention and impaired $1,25(OH)_2D$ synthesis, and this results in hypocalcemia. These patients are commonly treated with vitamin D, which increases intestinal calcium absorption and suppresses secondary increases in PTH secretion. Hypocalcemia due to pancreatitis and burns results from the suppression of PTH and from the sequestration of calcium.

Clinical Features and Treatment

The clinical features of hypoparathyroidism are a manifestation of hypocalcemia. Neuronal irritability and skeletal muscle spasms, tetany, or seizures reflect a reduced threshold of excitation. Latent tetany may be demonstrated by eliciting Chvostek's or Trousseau's sign. Chvostek's sign is a contracture of the facial muscle produced by tapping the facial nerve as it passes through the parotid gland. Trousseau's sign is contraction of the fingers and wrist after application of a blood pressure cuff inflated above the systolic blood pressure for approximately 3 minutes. Other common complaints of hypocalcemia include fatigue, depression, paresthesias, and skeletal muscle cramps. The acute onset of hypocalcemia after thyroid or parathyroid surgery may manifest as stridor and apnea. Cardiovascular manifestations of hypocalcemia include congestive heart failure, hypotension, and a relative insensitivity to the effects of β-adrenergic agonists. Delayed ventricular repolarization results in a prolonged QT interval on the ECG. Although prolongation of the QT interval may be a reliable sign of hypocalcemia in an individual patient, the ECG is relatively insensitive for the detection of hypocalcemia.

The treatment of hypoparathyroidism consists of electrolyte replacement. The objective is to have the patient's clinical symptoms under control before anesthesia and surgery. Hypocalcemia caused by magnesium depletion is treated by correcting the magnesium deficit. Serum phosphate excess is corrected by the removal of phosphate from the diet and the oral administration of phosphate-binding resins (aluminum hydroxide). The urinary excretion of phosphate can be increased with a saline volume infusion. Ca^{2+} deficiencies are corrected with Ca^{2+} supplements or vitamin D analogs. Patients with severe symptomatic hypocalcemia are treated with intravenous calcium gluconate (10 to 20 mL of 10% solution) given over several minutes and followed by a continuous infusion (1 to 2 mg/kg/hr) of elemental Ca^{2+}. The correction of serum Ca^{2+} levels should be monitored by measuring serum Ca^{2+} concentrations and following clinical symptoms. When oral or intravenous calcium is inadequate to maintain a normal serum ionized calcium level, vitamin D is added to the regimen.

ADRENAL CORTEX

The adrenal cortex functions to synthesize and secrete three types of hormones. Endogenous and dietary cholesterol is used in the adrenal biosynthesis of glucocorticoids (cortisol), mineralocorticoids (aldosterone and 11-deoxycorticosterone), and androgens (dehydroepiandrosterone). Cortisol and aldosterone are the two essential hormones, whereas adrenal androgens are of relatively minor physiologic significance in adults. The major biologic effects of adrenal cortical hyperfunction or hypofunction occur as a result of cortisol or aldosterone excess or deficiency. Abnormal function of the adrenal cortex may render a patient unable to respond appropriately during a period of surgical stress or critical illness.

Glucocorticoid Physiology

Cortisol (hydrocortisone) is the most potent endogenous glucocorticoid and is produced by the inner portions of the adrenal cortex. Cortisone is a glucocorticoid produced in small amounts. Cortisol is produced under the control of adrenocorticotropic hormone (ACTH; corticotropin), a polypeptide synthesized and released by the anterior pituitary gland. Glucocorticoids exert their biological effects by diffusing into the cytoplasm of target cells and combining with specific high-affinity receptor proteins.

The daily production of endogenous cortisol is approximately 20 mg. The maximal output is 150 to 300 mg/dL. Most of the circulating hormone is bound to the α-globulin transcortin (cortisol-binding globulin). It is the relatively small amount of free hormone that exerts the biological effects. Endogenous glucocorticoids are inactivated primarily by the liver and are excreted in the urine as 17-hydroxycorticosteroids. Cortisol is also filtered at the glomerulus and may be excreted unchanged in the urine. Although the rate of cortisol secretion is decreased by approximately 30% in the elderly patient, plasma cortisol levels remain in a normal range because of a corresponding decrease in hepatic and renal clearance.

Cortisol secretion is directly controlled by ACTH, which in turn is regulated by the corticotropin-releasing factor (CRF) from the hypothalamus. ACTH is synthesized in the pituitary gland from a precursor molecule that also produces β-lipotropin and β-endorphin. The secretion of ACTH and CRF is governed chiefly by glucocorticoids, the sleep–wake cycle, and stress. Cortisol is the most potent regulator of ACTH secretion, acting by a negative feedback mechanism to maintain cortisol levels in a physiologic range. ACTH release follows a diurnal pattern, with maximal activity occurring soon after awakening. This diurnal pattern of activity occurs in normal subjects and in those with adrenal insufficiency. Psychological or physical stress (trauma, surgery, intense exercise) also promotes ACTH release, regardless of the level of circulating cortisol or the time of day.

Cortisol has multiple effects on intermediate carbohydrate, protein, and fatty acid metabolism, as well as maintenance and regulation of immune and circulatory function. Glucocorticoids enhance gluconeogenesis, elevate blood glucose, and promote hepatic glycogen synthesis. The catabolic effect of glucocorticoids is partially blocked by insulin. The net effect on protein metabolism is enhanced degradation of muscle tissue and negative nitrogen balance. In supraphysiologic amounts, glucocorticoids suppress growth hormone secretion and impair somatic growth. The anti-inflammatory actions of cortisol relate to its effect in stabilizing lysosomes and promoting capillary integrity. Cortisol also antagonizes leukocyte migration inhibition factor, thus reducing white cell adherence to vascular endothelium and diminishing leukocyte response to local inflammation. Phagocytic activity does not decrease, although the killing potential of macrophages and monocytes is diminished. Other diverse actions include the facilitation of free water clearance, maintenance of blood pressure, a weak mineralocorticoid effect, promotion of appetite, stimulation of hematopoiesis, and induction of liver enzymes.

Mineralocorticoid Physiology

Aldosterone is the most potent mineralocorticoid produced by the adrenal gland. This hormone binds to receptors in sweat glands, the alimentary tract, and the distal convoluted tubule of the kidney. Aldosterone is a major regulator of extracellular volume and potassium homeostasis through the resorption of sodium and the secretion of potassium by these tissues. The major regulators of aldosterone release are the renin–angiotensin system and serum potassium (Fig. 41-3). The juxtaglomerular apparatus that surrounds the renal afferent arterioles produces renin in response to decreased perfusion pressures and sympathetic stimulation. Renin splits the hepatic precursor angiotensinogen to form the decapeptide, angiotensin I, which is then altered enzymatically by converting enzyme (primarily in the lung) to form the octapeptide angiotensin II. Angiotensin II is the most potent vasopressor produced in the body. It directly stimulates the adrenal cortex to produce aldosterone. The renin–angiotensin system is the body's most important protector of volume status. Other stimuli that increase the production of aldosterone include hyperkalemia and, to a limited degree, hyponatremia, prostaglandin E, and ACTH.

Glucocorticoid Excess (Cushing's Syndrome)

Cushing's syndrome, caused either by the overproduction of cortisol by the adrenal cortex or exogenous glucocorticoid therapy, results in a syndrome characterized by truncal obesity, hypertension, hyperglycemia, increased intravascular fluid volume, hypokalemia, fatigability, abdominal striae, osteoporosis, and muscle weakness. Most cases of Cushing's syndrome that occur spontaneously are due to bilateral adrenal hyperplasia secondary to ACTH produced by an anterior pituitary microadenoma or nonendocrine tumor (e.g., of the lung, kidney, or pancreas). The primary overproduction of cortisol and other adrenal steroids is caused by an adrenal neoplasm in approximately 20 to 25% of patients with Cushing's syndrome. These tumors are usually unilateral, and approximately half are malignant. When Cushing's syndrome occurs in patients older than 60 years of age, the most likely cause is an adrenal carcinoma or ectopic ACTH produced from a nonendocrine tumor. Finally, an increasingly common cause of Cushing's syndrome is the prolonged administration of exogenous glucocorticoids to treat a variety of illnesses.

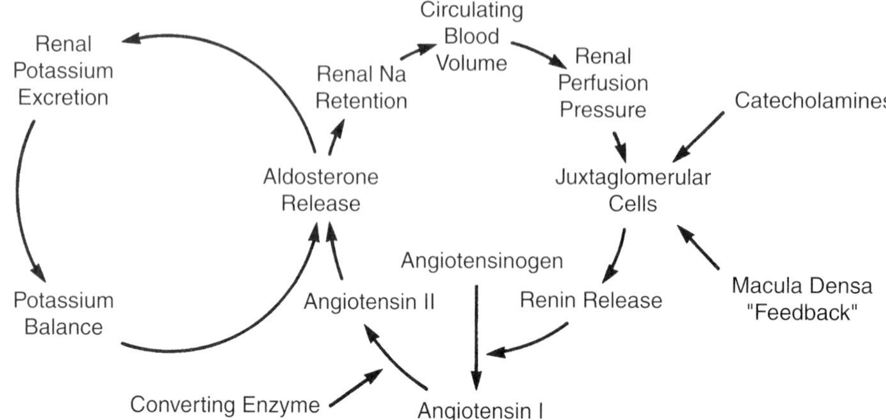

FIGURE 41-3. The interrelationship of the volume and potassium feedback loops on aldosterone secretion. (Reprinted with permission from Petersdorf RG [ed]: Harrison's Principles of Internal Medicine, 10th ed. New York, McGraw-Hill, 1983.)

The signs and symptoms of Cushing's syndrome follow from the known actions of glucocorticoids. Truncal obesity and thin extremities reflect increased muscle wasting and a redistribution of fat in facial, cervical, and truncal areas. Impaired calcium absorption and a decrease in bone formation may result in osteopenia. Sixty percent of patients have hyperglycemia, but overt diabetes mellitus occurs in less than 20%. Hypertension and fluid retention are seen in most patients. Profound emotional changes ranging from emotional lability to frank psychosis may be present. An increased susceptibility to infection reflects the immunosuppressive effects of corticosteroids. Hypokalemic alkalosis without distinctive physical findings is common when adrenal hyperplasia is caused by ectopic ACTH production from a nonendocrine tumor.

The laboratory diagnosis of hyperadrenocorticism is based on a variable elevation in plasma and urinary cortisol levels, urinary 17-hydroxycorticosteroids, and plasma ACTH. Once the diagnosis is established, simultaneous measurement of plasma ACTH and cortisol levels can determine whether the Cushing's syndrome is due to primary pituitary or adrenal disease.[23] Alternatively, a dexamethasone suppression test can be used. Patients with pituitary adenomas frequently show depression in cortisol and 17-hydroxycorticosteroid levels when a high dose of dexamethasone is administered because the tumor retains some negative feedback control, while adrenal tumors do not.

Anesthetic Management

General considerations for the preoperative preparation of the patient include treating hypertension and diabetes and normalizing intravascular fluid volume and electrolyte concentrations. Diuresis with the aldosterone antagonist spironolactone helps mobilize fluid and normalize the potassium concentration. Careful positioning of the osteopenic patient is important to avoid fractures. Intraoperative monitoring is planned after evaluation of the patient's cardiac reserve and consideration of the site and extent of the proposed surgery. When either unilateral or bilateral adrenalectomy is planned, glucocorticoid replacement therapy is initiated at a dose equal to full replacement of adrenal output during periods of extreme stress (see Steroid Replacement During the Perioperative Period section). The total dosage is reduced by approximately 50% per day until a daily maintenance dose of steroids is achieved (20 to 30 mg/day). Hydrocortisone given in doses of this magnitude exerts significant mineralocorticoid activity, and additional exogenous mineralocorticoid is usually not necessary during the perioperative period. After bilateral adrenalectomy, most patients require 0.05 to 0.1 mg/day of fludrocortisone (9-α-fluorohydrocortisone) starting around day 5 to provide mineralocorticoid activity. Slightly higher doses may be needed if prednisone is used for glucocorticoid maintenance because it has little intrinsic mineralocorticoid activity. The fludrocortisone dose is reduced if congestive heart failure, hypokalemia, or hypertension develops. For the patient with a solitary adrenal adenoma, unilateral adrenalectomy may be followed by normalization of function in the contralateral gland over time. Treatment plans should therefore be individualized, and adjustments in dosage may be necessary. The production of glucocorticoids or ACTH by a neoplasm may not be eliminated if the tumor is unresectable. These patients often need continuous medical therapy with steroid inhibitors such as metyrapone to control their symptoms.

There are no specific recommendations regarding the use of a particular anesthetic technique or medication in patients with hyperadrenocorticism. When significant skeletal muscle weakness is present, a conservative approach to the use of muscle relaxants is warranted. Etomidate has been used for temporizing medical treatment of severe Cushing's disease because of its inhibition of steroid synthesis.

Mineralocorticoid Excess

Hypersecretion of the major adrenal mineralocorticoid aldosterone increases the renal tubular exchange of sodium for potassium and hydrogen ions. This leads to hypertension, hypokalemic alkalosis, skeletal muscle weakness, and fatigue. Possibly as many as 1% of unselected hypertensive patients have primary hyperaldosteronism. The increase in renal sodium reabsorption and extracellular volume expansion is in part responsible for the high incidence of diastolic hypertension in these patients. Patients with primary hyperaldosteronism (Conn's syndrome) characteristically do not have edema. Secondary aldosteronism results from an elevation in renin production. The diagnosis of primary or secondary hyperaldosteronism should be entertained in the nonedematous hypertensive patient with persistent hypokalemia who is not receiving potassium-wasting diuretics. Hyposecretion of renin that fails to increase appropriately during volume depletion or salt restriction is an important finding in primary aldosteronism. The measurement of plasma renin levels is useful in distinguishing primary from secondary hyperaldosteronism. It is of limited value in differentiating patients with primary aldosteronism from those with other causes of hypertension because renin activity is also suppressed in approximately 25% of patients with essential hypertension.

Anesthetic Considerations

Preoperative preparation for the patient with primary aldosteronism is directed toward restoring the intravascular volume and the electrolyte concentrations to normal. Hypertension and hypokalemia may be controlled by restricting sodium intake and administration of the aldosterone antagonist spironolactone. This diuretic works slowly to produce an increase in potassium levels, with dosages in the range of 25 to 100 mg every 8 hours. Total body potassium deficits are difficult to estimate and may be in excess of 300 mEq. Whenever possible, potassium should be replaced slowly to allow equilibration between intracellular and extracellular potassium stores. The usual complications of chronic hypertension need to be assessed.

Adrenal Insufficiency (Addison's Disease)

The undersecretion of adrenal steroid hormones may develop as the result of a primary inability of the adrenal gland to elaborate sufficient quantities of hormone or as the result of a deficiency in the production of ACTH.

Clinically, primary adrenal insufficiency is usually not apparent until at least 90% of the adrenal cortex has been destroyed. The predominant cause of primary adrenal insufficiency used to be tuberculosis; however, today, the most frequent cause of Addison's disease is idiopathic adrenal insufficiency secondary to autoimmune destruction of the gland. Autoimmune destruction of the adrenal cortex causes both a glucocorticoid and a mineralocorticoid deficiency. A variety of other conditions presumed to have an autoimmune pathogenesis may also occur concomitantly with idiopathic Addison's disease. Hashimoto's thyroiditis in association with autoimmune adrenal insufficiency is termed *Schmidt's syndrome*. Other possible causes of adrenal gland destruction include certain bacterial, fungal, and advanced HIV infections; metastatic cancer; sepsis; and hemorrhage. Secondary adrenal insufficiency occurs when the anterior pituitary fails to secrete sufficient quantities of ACTH. Pituitary failure may result from tumor, infection, surgical ablation, or radiation therapy.

Patients receiving chronic corticosteroid therapy will not generally have frank adrenal insufficiency, but may have hypothalamic-pituitary-adrenal (HPA) suppression and may develop acute adrenal insufficiency during the stress of the perioperative period. Adrenal insufficiency is a common finding in critically ill surgical patients with hypotension requiring vasopressors.[24]

Clinical Presentation

The cardinal symptoms of idiopathic Addison's disease include chronic fatigue, muscle weakness, anorexia, weight loss, nausea, vomiting, and diarrhea. Hypotension is almost always encountered in the disease process. Female patients may exhibit decreased axillary and pubic hair growth due to the loss of adrenal androgen secretion. An acute crisis can present as abdominal pain, severe vomiting and diarrhea, hypotension, decreased consciousness, and shock. Diffuse hyperpigmentation occurs in most patients with primary adrenal insufficiency and is secondary to the compensatory increase in ACTH and β-lipotropin. These hormones stimulate an increase in melanocyte production. Mineralocorticoid deficiency is characteristically present in primary adrenal disease; as a result, there is a reduction in urine sodium conservation. Hyperkalemia may be a cause of life-threatening cardiac dysrhythmias. Adrenal insufficiency secondary to pituitary disease is not associated with cutaneous hyperpigmentation or mineralocorticoid deficiency. Salt and water balance is usually maintained unless severe fluid and electrolyte losses overwhelm the subnormal aldosterone secretory capacity. Organic lesions of pituitary origin require a diligent search for coexisting hormone deficiencies. Acute adrenal insufficiency from inadequate replacement of steroids on chronic steroid therapy is rare and can present as refractory, distributive shock. In critically ill patients, adrenal insufficiency may not present with classic symptoms. The clinical picture may resemble that of sepsis without a source of infection.[25] A high degree of suspicion must be maintained if the patient has cardiovascular instability without a defined cause.[26,27]

Diagnosis

The patient's pituitary-adrenal responsiveness should be determined when the diagnosis of primary or secondary adrenal insufficiency is first suspected. Biochemical evidence of impaired adrenal or pituitary secretory reserve unequivocally confirms the diagnosis. Patients who are clinically stable may undergo testing before treatment is initiated. Those believed to have acute adrenal insufficiency should receive immediate therapy.

Plasma cortisol levels are measured before and 30 and 60 minutes after the intravenous administration of 250 μg of synthetic ACTH. In patients with adequate adrenal reserve, plasma cortisol rises at least 7 mg/dL (or to a total of 18 mg/dL) 60 minutes after the injection of the synthetic ACTH.[28] Patients with adrenal insufficiency usually demonstrate little or no adrenal response.

Treatment and Anesthetic Considerations

Normal adults secrete about 20 mg of cortisol (hydrocortisone) and 0.1 mg of aldosterone per day. Glucocorticoid therapy is usually given twice daily in sufficient dosage to meet physiologic requirements. A typical regimen may consist of prednisone, 5 mg in the morning and 2.5 mg in the evening, or hydrocortisone, 20 mg in the morning and 10 mg in the evening. The daily glucocorticoid dosage is typically 50% higher than basal adrenal output to cover the patient for mild stress. Replacement dosages are adjusted in response to the patient's clinical symptoms or the occurrence of intercurrent illnesses. Mineralocorticoid replacement is also administered on a daily basis; most patients require 0.05 to 0.1 mg/day of fludrocortisone. The mineralocorticoid dose may be reduced if severe hypokalemia, hypertension, or congestive heart failure develops, or it may be increased if postural hypotension is demonstrated.

Secondary adrenal insufficiency often occurs in the presence of multiple hormone deficiencies. A decrease in ACTH production results in the decreased secretion of cortisol and adrenal androgens, but aldosterone control by more dominant mechanisms remains intact. A liberal salt diet is encouraged. Glucocorticoid substitution follows the same guidelines previously outlined for primary adrenal insufficiency.

Immediate therapy of acute adrenal insufficiency is mandatory, regardless of the etiology and consists of electrolyte resuscitation and steroid replacement (Table 41-6). Initial therapy begins with the rapid intravenous administration of an isotonic

TABLE 41-6

MANAGEMENT OF ACUTE ADRENAL INSUFFICIENCY

- Hydrocortisone 100 mg IV bolus followed by hydrocortisone 100 mg q6h for 24 hr
- Fluid and electrolyte replacement as indicated by vital signs, serum electrolytes, and serum glucose

IV, intravenous(ly).

crystalloid solution (D_5NS). One hundred milligrams of hydrocortisone is administered as an intravenous bolus over several minutes. Steroid replacement is continued during the first 24 hours with 100 mg intravenous hydrocortisone given every 6 hours. If the patient is stable, the steroid dose is reduced starting on the second day. After adequate fluid resuscitation, if the patient continues to be hemodynamically unstable, inotropic support may be necessary. Invasive monitoring is extremely valuable as a guide to both diagnosis and therapy.

Steroid Replacement During the Perioperative Period

Perioperatively, patients with adrenal insufficiency and those with HPA suppression from chronic steroid use require additional corticosteroids to mimic the increased output of the normal adrenal gland during stress. The normal adrenal gland can secrete up to 200 mg of cortisol per day or more during the perioperative period. During periods of extreme stress, the adrenal gland may be exogenously stimulated to secrete between 200 and 500 mg/day of cortisol.[29] The pituitary-adrenal axis is usually considered to be intact if a plasma cortisol level of greater than 22 mcg/dL is measured during acute stress. The degree of adrenal responsiveness has been correlated with the duration of surgery and the extent of surgical trauma. The mean maximal plasma cortisol level measured during major surgery (colectomy, hip osteotomy) was 47 mcg/dL. Minor surgical procedures (herniorrhaphy) resulted in mean maximal plasma cortisol levels of 28 mcg/dL. Adrenal activity may also be affected by the anesthetic technique used. Regional anesthesia is effective in postponing the elevation in cortisol levels during surgery of the lower abdomen and extremities.[30] Deep general anesthesia may also suppress the elevation of stress hormones such as ACTH and cortisol during the surgical procedure.

Although symptoms indicative of clinically significant adrenal insufficiency have been reported during the perioperative period, these clinical findings have rarely been documented in direct association with glucocorticoid deficiency.[31] There is evidence in adrenally suppressed primates that subphysiologic steroid replacement causes perioperative hemodynamic instability and increased mortality.

Identifying which patients require steroid supplementation
3 can be difficult. Provocative testing with ACTH stimulation is too costly to justify compared with the risk of brief steroid supplementation. HPA suppression can occur after five daily doses of prednisone 20 mg or more. Recovery of HPA function occurs gradually and can take up to 9 to 12 months. HPA suppression can occur with topical, regional, and inhaled steroids. Alternate-day therapy decreases the risk of HPA suppression.[32]

The clinical problem is how much steroid to give. There is no proven optimal regimen for perioperative steroid replacement (Table 41-7). A "low-dose" cortisol replacement program using an intravenous infusion of 25 mg of cortisol before the induction of anesthesia, followed by a continuous infusion of cortisol (100 mg) in the next 24 hours has been advocated[33] (Fig. 41-4). This low-dose cortisol replacement program was used in patients with proven adrenal insufficiency and resulted in plasma cortisol levels as high as those seen in healthy control subjects subjected to a similar operative stress. One study with a limited number of patients found no problems with cardiovascular instability if patients received their usual dose of steroids.[34] Although the low-dose approach appears logical, many clinicians are unwilling to adopt this regimen until further trials have been undertaken in patients receiving physiologic steroid replacement. A popular regimen calls for the administration of 200 to 300 mg of hydrocortisone per 70 kg body weight in divided doses on the day of surgery. The lower dose is adjusted upward for longer and more extensive surgical procedures. Patients who are using steroids at the time of surgery receive their usual dose on the morning of surgery and are supplemented at a level that is at least equivalent to the usual daily replacement. Glucocorticoid coverage is rapidly tapered to the patient's normal maintenance dosage during the postoperative period. Although no conclusive evidence supports an increased incidence of infection or abnormal wound healing when supraphysiologic doses of supplemental steroids are used acutely, the goal of therapy is to use the minimal drug dosage necessary to adequately protect the patient.

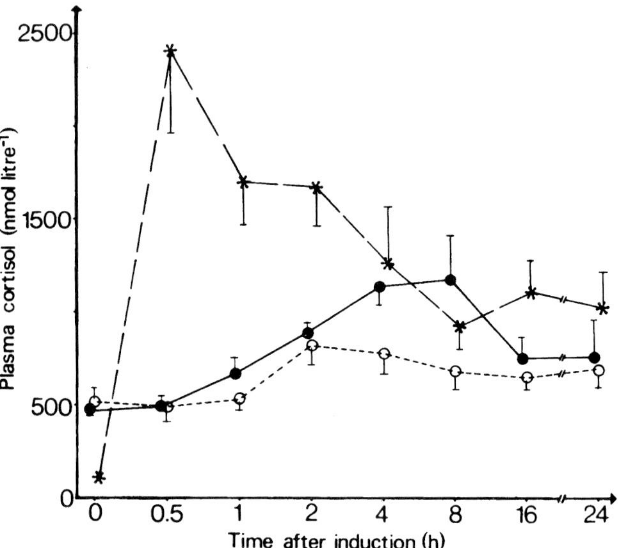

FIGURE 41-4. Plasma cortisol concentrations (mean ± SEM) were measured in three groups of patients undergoing elective surgery. Group I control patients, $n = 8$ (*closed circles*), had never received corticosteroids. Group II patients, $n = 8$ (*open circles*), received preoperative corticosteroids with a normal response to preoperative adrenocorticotropic hormone (ACTH; corticotropin) stimulation testing. These patients and control patients received no corticosteroid substitution during the perioperative period. Group III, $n = 6$ (*asterisks*), consisted of patients receiving long-term corticosteroid therapy with an abnormal response to ACTH stimulation testing during the perioperative period. These patients (group III) received intravenous (IV) cortisol, 25 mg, after the induction of anesthesia plus a continuous IV infusion of cortisol, 100 mg, during the next 24 hours. Plasma cortisol levels in group III were significantly lower than in the other two groups before the induction of anesthesia. After IV administration of cortisol to group III patients, plasma concentrations were significantly higher than in groups I and II for the next 2 hours ($p < .01$). Thereafter, the mean plasma concentrations were similar for all groups. There were no clinical signs of circulatory insufficiency in any group. (Reprinted with permission from Symreng T, Karlberg BE, Kagedol B, Schildt B: Physiological cortisol substitution of long-term steroid-treated patients undergoing major surgery. Br J Anaesth 53:949, 1981.)

TABLE 41-7

MANAGEMENT OPTIONS FOR STEROID REPLACEMENT IN THE PERIOPERATIVE PERIOD

Hydrocortisone 25 mg IV at time of induction followed by hydrocortisone infusion 100 mg over 24 hr
Hydrocortisone 100 mg IV before, during, and after surgery

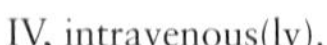
IV, intravenous(ly).

TABLE 41-8

GLUCOCORTICOID PREPARATIONS

GENERIC NAME	ANTI-INFLAMMATORY	MINERALOCORTICOID	APPROXIMATE EQUIVALENT DOSE (mg)
SHORT ACTING			
Hydrocortisone	1.0	1.0	20.0
Cortisone	0.8	0.8	25.0
Prednisone	4.0	0.25	5.0
Prednisolone	4.0	0.25	5.0
Methylprednisolone	5.0	—	4.0
INTERMEDIATE ACTING			
Triamcinolone	5.0	—	4.0
LONG ACTING			
Dexamethasone	30.0	—	0.75

Relative milligram comparisons with cortisol. The glucocorticoid and mineralocorticoid properties of cortisol are set as 1.0.

Exogenous Glucocorticoid Therapy

The therapeutic use of supraphysiologic doses of glucocorticoids has expanded, and the anesthesiologist should be familiar with the various preparations (Table 41-8). Dexamethasone, methylprednisolone, and prednisone have less mineralocorticoid effect than cortisone or hydrocortisone. Prednisone and methylprednisolone are precursors that must be metabolized by the liver before anti-inflammatory activity can occur and should be used cautiously in the presence of liver disease.

Mineralocorticoid Insufficiency

Isolated mineralocorticoid insufficiency has been reported as a congenital biosynthetic defect, after unilateral adrenalectomy for removal of an aldosterone-secreting adenoma, during protracted heparin therapy, and in patients with a deficiency in renin production. This syndrome is commonly seen in patients with mild renal failure and long-standing diabetes mellitus. A feature common to all patients with hypoaldosteronism is a failure to increase aldosterone production in response to salt restriction or volume contraction.

Most patients present with hypotension, hyperkalemia that may be life threatening, and a metabolic acidosis that is out of proportion to the degree of coexisting renal impairment. Patients with low renin secretion, hypoaldosteronism, and renal dysfunction respond to ACTH stimulation. Nonsteroidal anti-inflammatory drugs, which inhibit prostaglandin synthesis, may further inhibit renin release and exacerbate the condition. Patients with isolated hypoaldosteronism are given fludrocortisone orally in a dose of 0.05 to 0.1 mg/day. Patients with low renin secretion usually require higher doses to correct the electrolyte abnormalities. Caution should be observed in patients with hypertension or congestive heart failure. An alternative approach in these patients is the administration of furosemide alone or in combination with mineralocorticoid.

ADRENAL MEDULLA

The adrenal medulla is derived embryologically from neuroectodermal cells. As a specialized part of the sympathetic nervous system, the adrenal medulla synthesizes and secretes the catecholamines epinephrine (80%) and norepinephrine (20%). Preganglionic fibers of the sympathetic nervous system bypass the paravertebral ganglia and pass directly from the spinal cord to the adrenal medulla. The adrenal medulla is analogous to a postganglionic neuron, although the catecholamines secreted by the medulla function as hormones, not as neurotransmitters.

The synthesis of norepinephrine begins with hydroxylation of tyrosine to dopa (Fig. 41-5). This rate-limiting step in catecholamine biosynthesis is regulated so synthesis is coupled to release. In the adrenal medulla and in those rare central neurons using epinephrine as a neurotransmitter, most of the norepinephrine is converted to epinephrine by the enzyme phenylethanolamine-*N*-methyltransferase. It is likely that the capacity of the adrenal medulla to synthesize epinephrine

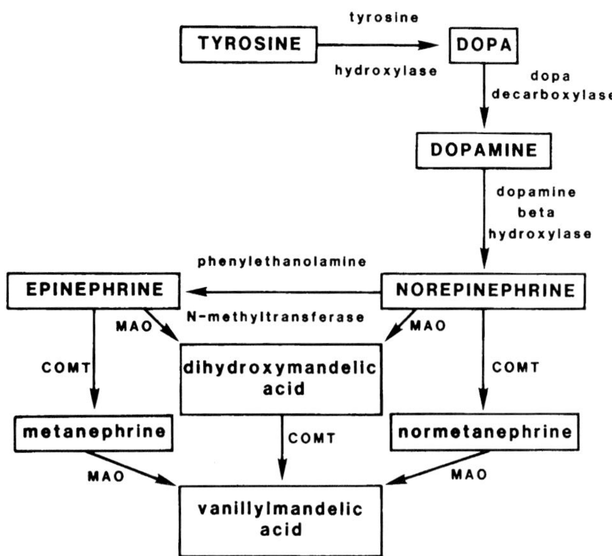

FIGURE 41-5. The synthesis and metabolism of endogenous catecholamines. COMT, catechol-O-methyltransferase; MAO, monoamine oxidase. (Reprinted with permission from Stoelting RK, Dierdorf SF [eds]: Anesthesia and Co-existing Disease. New York, Churchill-Livingstone, 1983.)

is influenced by the flow of glucocorticoid-rich blood from the adrenal cortex through the intra-adrenal portal system because it is known that high concentrations of glucocorticoid are able to induce the enzyme phenylethanolamine-*N*-methyltransferase.

In the adrenal medulla, catecholamines are stored in chromaffin granules complexed with adenosine triphosphate and Ca^{2+}. The normal adrenal releases epinephrine and norepinephrine by exocytosis in response to stimulation by preganglionic sympathetic neurons. The circulatory half-life (10 to 30 seconds) of these catechols is considerably longer than the brief receptor activity of norepinephrine released as a neurotransmitter from postganglionic sympathetic nerve endings. Biotransformation of circulating norepinephrine and epinephrine is accomplished chiefly by the enzyme catechol-O-methyltransferase, located in the liver and kidney. Monoamine oxidase is of less importance in the metabolism of circulating catechols. Metanephrine and vanillylmandelic acid (VMA) are the major end products of catecholamine metabolism. These metabolites and a small amount of unchanged catecholamine (1%) appear in the urine.

The outflow of postganglionic sympathetic neurotransmitters and circulating catecholamine from the adrenal medulla is coordinated by higher cortical centers connected to the brainstem. The intrinsic activity of the brainstem sympathetic areas is modulated by higher cortical functions, emotional reactions (anger, fear), and various physiologic stimuli, including changes in the physical and chemical properties of the extracellular fluid (hypoglycemia, hypotension). The adrenal medulla and sympathetic nervous system are often stimulated together in a generalized fashion, although many physiologic conditions exist in which they act independently.

Pheochromocytoma

The only important disease process associated with the adrenal medulla is pheochromocytoma. These tumors produce, store, and secrete catecholamines. Most pheochromocytomas secrete both epinephrine and norepinephrine, with the percentage of secreted norepinephrine being greater than that secreted by the normal gland. Although pheochromocytomas occur in less than 0.2% of hypertensive patients, it is important to aggressively evaluate the patient with clinically suspect symptoms because surgical extirpation is curative in more than 90% of patients and complications are often lethal in undiagnosed cases.[35] Postmortem series have reported high perioperative mortality rates in undiagnosed patients undergoing relatively minor surgical procedures. Most deaths are from cardiovascular causes. Perioperative morbidity is related to tumor size and the degree of catecholamine secretion.[36]

Most (85 to 90%) pheochromocytomas are solitary tumors localized to a single adrenal gland, usually the right. Approximately 10% of adults and 25% of children have bilateral tumors. The tumor may originate in extra-adrenal sites (10%), anywhere along the paravertebral sympathetic chain; however, 95% are located in the abdomen, and a small percentage is located in the thorax, urinary bladder, or neck. Malignant spread of these highly vascular tumors occurs in approximately 10% of cases.

In approximately 5% of cases, this tumor is inherited as a familial autosomal dominant trait. It may be part of the polyglandular syndrome referred to as MEN type IIA or IIB. Type IIA includes medullary carcinoma of the thyroid, parathyroid hyperplasia, and pheochromocytoma; Type IIB consists of medullary carcinoma of the thyroid, pheochromocytoma, and neuromas of the oral mucosa. Pheochromocytomas may also arise in association with von Recklinghausen's neurofibromatosis or von Hippel-Lindau disease (retinal and cerebellar angiomatosis). The pheochromocytoma of the familial syndromes is rarely extra-adrenal or malignant. Bilateral tumors occur in approximately 75% of cases. When these patients present with a single adrenal pheochromocytoma, the chances of subsequent development of a second adrenal pheochromocytoma are sufficiently high that bilateral adrenalectomy should be considered. Every member of a MEN family should be considered at risk for pheochromocytoma.

Clinical Presentation

Pheochromocytoma may occur at any age, but it is most common in young to midadult life. The clinical manifestations are mainly due to the pharmacologic effects of the catecholamines released from the tumor. These tumors are not innervated, and catecholamine release is independent of neurogenic control. Most patients have sustained hypertension, although occasionally it is paroxysmal.[37] When true paroxysms occur, the blood pressure may rise to alarmingly high levels, placing the patient at risk for cerebrovascular hemorrhage, heart failure, dysrhythmias, or myocardial infarction. Headache, palpitations, tremor, profuse sweating, and either pallor or flushing may accompany an attack. Pheochromocytoma can masquerade as malignant hyperthermia. Physical examination of the patient with pheochromocytoma may be unrevealing during the period between attacks unless the patient presents with symptoms and signs of sequelae related to long-standing hypertension. A catecholamine-induced cardiomyopathy may manifest as myocarditis accompanied by heart failure and cardiac dysrhythmias. Paroxysms are commonly not associated with clearly defined events but may be precipitated by displacement of the abdominal contents or, in the case of a bladder tumor, by micturition.

Diagnosis

Biochemical determination of free catecholamine concentration and catecholamine metabolites in the urine is the most common screening test used to establish the diagnosis of pheochromocytoma.[38] Urinary VMA and unconjugated norepinephrine and epinephrine levels are measured in a 24-hour urine collection and are expressed as a function of the creatinine clearance. Excess production of catecholamines is diagnostic for pheochromocytoma. Free catecholamines represent less than 1% of the originally released hormone, and urinary levels are not always elevated to a significant degree. Hence, differentiation from normal subjects may be difficult. A change in the ratio of unconjugated epinephrine to norepinephrine may be the only biochemical finding. Certain drugs interfere with urinary assays, and some patients with paroxysmal hypertension have normal values between attacks.

Although routine laboratory data are unlikely to provide specific diagnostic insight, the ECG, chest radiograph, and complete blood cell count can provide valuable information to the clinician who entertains the diagnosis. Left ventricular hypertrophy and nonspecific T-wave changes are two of the more common ECG findings. Evidence of acute myocardial infarction or tachyarrhythmia has also been reported. The chest radiograph may reveal cardiomegaly, and the blood count often shows an elevated hematocrit consistent with a reduced intravascular volume and hemoconcentration. Standardized imaging methods such as computed tomography and magnetic resonance imaging (MRI) are used in the noninvasive localization of these tumors.[39] Improvements in imaging may obviate the need for abdominal exploration or venous sampling to localize the tumor in selected patients.[40] Ultrasound and MRI are especially useful in pregnant patients. ^{131}I-Metaiodobenzylguanidine (^{131}I-MIBG) scintigraphy is also effective in localizing recurrent or

TABLE 41-9

DRUGS USED IN THE MANAGEMENT OF PHEOCHROMOCYTOMA

DRUG	ACTION	PREOPERATIVE BLOOD PRESSURE CONTROL	PRESSOR CRISIS	COMMENT
Phentolamine	Nonselective α-antagonist	—	1–5 mg IV; 0.5–1 mg/min IV	Short duration of action ~5 min
Phenoxybenzamine	Nonselective α-antagonist	20 mg/d PO up to 160 mg/d in divided doses	—	Long half-life; may accumulate
Doxazosin (terazosin dosing similar)	Selective α_1-antagonist	1 mg/d PO up to 8 mg/d PO	—	First-dose phenomena; may cause syncope
Propranolol	Nonselective β-antagonist	40 mg/d PO up to 480 mg/d in divided doses to control tachycardia	1–2 mg IV bolus	Should never be given without first creating α-blockade
Atenolol	Selective β_1-antagonist	50–100 mg/d PO	—	Long-acting drug eliminated; unchanged by kidney
Esmolol	Selective β_1-antagonist	—	250–500 mcg/kg/min IV loading followed by maintenance infusion 25–250 mcg/kg/min	Short acting; elimination half-life ~9 min
Labetalol	α-antagonist and β-antagonist	200 mg/d PO in divided doses up to 800 mg/d	10 mg IV bolus	A much weaker alpha-blocker than beta-blocker; may cause hypertensive response
Nitroprusside	Direct vasodilator	—	0.5–1.5 mcg/kg/min initially, increased to maximum of 8 mcg/kg/min; titrate to effect	Powerful vasodilator; short acting
Magnesium sulfate	Direct vasodilator and membrane stabilizer	—	2–4 g IV bolus followed by 1–2 g/hr and additional 1–2 g boluses as needed	May potentiate neuromuscular blockade
Nicardipine	Calcium channel antagonist		1–2 mcg/kg/min increased to 7.5 mcg/kg/min; titrate to effect	
α-Methyltyrosine	Inhibitor of biosynthesis of catecholamine	1–4 g/d PO in divided doses	~	Suitable for patients not amenable to surgery; may be nephrotoxic

IV, intravenous(ly); PO, oral(ly).

extra-adrenal masses. Arteriography must be performed with extreme care in these patients because a hypertensive crisis can be precipitated.

Anesthetic Considerations

Preoperative Preparation. The reduction in perioperative mortality rates from a high of 45% to between 0% and 3% with the excision of pheochromocytoma is followed the 4 introduction of α-antagonists for preoperative therapy. Perioperative blood pressure fluctuations, myocardial infarction, congestive heart failure, cardiac dysrhythmias, and cerebral hemorrhage all appear to be reduced in frequency when the patient has been treated before surgery with alpha-blockers and the intravascular fluid compartment has been reexpanded. Extended treatment with α-antagonists is also effective in treating the clinical manifestations of catecholamine myocarditis. However, alpha-blocker therapy has never been studied in a controlled way, and there are some groups that question its necessity in light of the availability of potent titratable vasodilators for intraoperative use.[41] A list of drugs frequently used in the management of pheochromocytoma is given in Table 41-9.

α-Adrenergic blockade is initiated once the diagnosis of pheochromocytoma is established. Phenoxybenzamine, a long-acting (24 to 48 hours), noncompetitive presynaptic (α_2) and postsynaptic (α_1) blocker, has traditionally been used at doses of 10 mg every 8 hours. Increments are added until the blood pressure is controlled and paroxysms disappear. Most patients need between 80 and 200 mg/day. The absorption after oral administration is variable, and side effects are common. Certain cardiovascular reflexes, such as the baroreceptor reflex, are blunted, and postural hypotension is common. Selective competitive α-1-blockers, such as doxazosin, terazosin, and prazosin, have also been used effectively. Because postural hypotension can be pronounced with the commencement of therapy, the initial 1-mg dose is given at bedtime. Postural changes are also seen with maintenance therapy. A comparison of patients with pheochromocytoma receiving phenoxybenzamine and prazosin has shown both drugs to be equally effective in controlling the blood pressure. Although the optimal period of preoperative treatment has not been established, most clinicians recommend beginning α-blockade therapy at least 10 to 14 days before the proposed surgery; however, periods as short as 3 to 5 days have been used.[42] During this time, the contracted intravascular volume and hematocrit return toward normal, and the blood pressure is stabilized. Despite the real possibility of hypotension after vascular isolation of the tumor, most clinicians continue alpha-blockers up until the morning of surgery.

β-Adrenergic blockade is occasionally added after α-blockade has been established. This addition is considered in patients with persistent tachycardia or cardiac dysrhythmias that may be caused by nonselective α-blockade or epinephrine-secreting tumors. Beta-blockers should not be given until adequate α-blockade is ensured to avoid the possibility of unopposed α-mediated vasoconstriction. There is no clear preoperative advantage of one β antagonist over another, although the short half-life of esmolol may allow better control of heart rate and arrhythmias in the perioperative setting. Labetalol, a β-adrenergic antagonist with α-blocking activity, is effective as a second-line medication, but can increase blood pressure when this drug is used alone.

α-Methyl tyrosine is an agent that inhibits the enzyme tyrosine hydroxylase, the rate-limiting step in catecholamine biosynthesis. This medication is currently reserved for patients with metastatic disease, or for situations in which surgery is contraindicated and long-term medical therapy is required. When α-methyl tyrosine is used in combination with α-adrenergic-blocking agents, there is a significant reduction in catecholamine biosynthesis.

Unrecognized pheochromocytoma during pregnancy may be life threatening to the mother and fetus. Although the safety of adrenergic-blocking agents during pregnancy has not been established, these agents probably improve fetal survival in pregnant patients with pheochromocytoma. The trend is to perform surgery during the first trimester or at the time of cesarean delivery. There is no reason to terminate an early pregnancy, but the patient should be aware of the risk of spontaneous abortion resulting from abdominal surgery to remove the tumor.[43]

Perioperative Anesthetic Management. Symptomatic patients continue to receive medical therapy until tachycardia, cardiac dysrhythmias, and paroxysmal elevations in blood pressure are well controlled. If it is not possible to initiate α-blocking therapy before surgery, or if the patient has received less than 48 hours of intensive treatment, it may be necessary to infuse nitroprusside during the induction of anesthesia. A low-dose infusion is often initiated in anticipation of the marked blood pressure elevations that can occur with laryngoscopy and surgical stimulation.

Improvements in imaging now allow most patients with solitary tumors without evidence of metastases or local invasion to undergo a laparoscopic retroperitoneal approach. If the surgeon needs to assess for bilateral disease or the dissection is too difficult, then the procedure can be converted to an open one. During laparoscopic surgery, creation of the pneumoperitoneum may cause release of catecholamines and large changes in hemodynamics that can be controlled with a vasodilator.[44]

Although there is no clear advantage to one anesthetic technique over another, drugs that are known to liberate histamine are avoided. Because of the potential for ventricular irritability, halothane is not administered. A potent sedative-hypnotic, in combination with an opioid analgesic, is used for induction. It is extremely important to achieve an adequate depth of anesthesia before proceeding with laryngoscopy to minimize the sympathetic nervous system response to this maneuver. Maintenance is provided with an opioid analgesic and a potent inhalation agent. Manipulation of the tumor may produce marked elevations in blood pressure. Acute hypertensive crises are treated with intravenous infusions of nitroprusside
5 or phentolamine. Phentolamine is a short-acting α-adrenergic antagonist that may be given as an intravenous bolus (2 to 5 mg) or by continuous infusion. Tachydysrhythmia is controlled with intravenous boluses of propranolol (1-mg increments) or by a continuous infusion of the ultrashort-acting selective β_1-adrenergic antagonist esmolol. The disadvantage of long-acting beta-blockers may be persistence of bradycardia and hypotension after the tumor is removed. Even esmolol may be problematic because there are cases of cardiac arrest after clamping of the venous drainage in patients on large doses of esmolol. Almost every vasodilator has been tried and recommended as an adjuvant to control hypertension. Magnesium sulfate given as an infusion with intermittent boluses has successfully controlled blood pressure.[45] Nicardipine, nitroglycerin, diltiazem, fenoldopam, and prostaglandin E_1 have all been used anecdotally. The reduction in blood pressure that may occur after ligation of the tumor's venous supply can be dangerously abrupt and should be anticipated through close communication with the surgical team. Restitution of any intravascular fluid deficit is the initial therapy in this situation. After replenishment of the intravascular volume, if the patient remains hypotensive, phenylephrine is administered. After surgery, catecholamine levels return to normal over several days. Approximately 75% of patients become normotensive within 10 days.

DIABETES MELLITUS

Diabetes mellitus (DM) is the most commonly occurring endocrine disease found in surgical patients.[46] Twenty-five to 50% of diabetics will require surgery. It has a broad spectrum of severity, and its manifestations can be altered in reaction to the patient's metabolic stress. Although the most serious complications of DM are related to its character as a chronic disease, it can cause difficulties in the short-term management of acute illness. Occasionally, DM remains clinically inapparent until exacerbated by the stress of trauma or surgery.

The principles of the treatment of DM will be easier to understand if we review the physiology of glucose metabolism and the stress response, and then consider some of the specific pathologic entities that comprise the clinical picture of DM.

Classification

DM is primarily a disease of glucose metabolism; however, it has numerous manifestations and interactions with a large range of hormonal and endocrinologic functions. Despite a variety of etiologic factors, its hallmark is a deficiency, either absolute or relative, in the amount of insulin effect to the tissues.

DM is often divided into two broad types. Type I, formerly called insulin-dependent diabetes mellitus, is distinguished from type II, formerly called non–insulin-dependent diabetes mellitus. The patient with type I DM typically experiences the onset of disease early in life.[47] Consequently, this form is also referred to as juvenile-onset diabetes. In general, the patient with type I DM is not obese, had an abrupt onset of the disease, and has very low levels of circulating insulin.

Disease in these patients cannot be controlled with diet or oral hypoglycemic agents; rather, it mandates treatment with insulin. Patients in this group are often difficult to maintain in good glucose balance, are more likely to become ketotic, and are likely to sustain the end-organ complications of diabetes if they live long enough.

Patients with type II DM, also called adult-onset diabetes, typically experience a gradual onset of the disease later in life. They are often obese and have some resistance to the effects of insulin. They may have normal or even elevated levels of insulin. In milder forms, this version of diabetes can often be treated with diet or oral hypoglycemic agents. Because these patients are relatively resistant to ketosis, their disease may be clinically inapparent until exacerbated by the stress of surgery or intercurrent illness.

This classification of DM is only a generalization. The milder, type II form occasionally occurs in young people, and many older adults acquire a severe and brittle form of type I. Secondary DM can be a result of a disease that damages the pancreas and thus impairs insulin secretion. Pancreatic surgery, chronic pancreatitis, cystic fibrosis, and hemochromatosis can damage the pancreas and impair insulin secretion sufficiently to produce clinical DM. DM can result from one of the endocrine diseases that produces a hormone that opposes the action of insulin. Hence, a patient with a glucagonoma, pheochromocytoma, or acromegaly may be diabetic. An increased effect of glucocorticoids, either from Cushing's disease or steroid therapy, may also oppose the effect of insulin enough to elicit clinical diabetes and would certainly complicate the management of preexisting diabetes. Gestational diabetes is a common medical problem of pregnancy and may presage future type II DM.

Physiology

Insulin has multiple and complex interactions with lipid, protein, and glucose metabolism. For our purposes, it is easiest to regard the effects of insulin on glucose metabolism as primary and to view its effects on other metabolic functions only as they relate to glucose.

Insulin is a small protein produced by the β cells of the islets of Langerhans in the pancreas. Normal production in the adult human is approximately 40 to 50 U/day. Insulin acts through receptor sites on cells. The half-life of insulin in the circulation is only a few minutes. However, it may clinically appear to have a longer duration of action, owing to delays in binding and release from the cellular receptors. These facts lead us to the important principle that once a high level of insulin saturates all the binding sites, insulin will not have a more potent effect, just a more long-lasting effect. This is crucial to understanding insulin therapy, which is discussed in the following paragraphs.

Insulin is metabolized in the liver and kidney. In patients with hepatic dysfunction, the loss of gluconeogenesis and a prolongation of insulin effect increase the risk of hypoglycemia. Renal disease may prolong the action of insulin, is another risk factor for hypoglycemia, and is an important consideration in managing the use of exogenous insulin in diabetic patients.

Insulin release is related to a number of events. First is the direct effect of glucose and amino acids to stimulate insulin release. The mechanism involves interaction with hormones from the GI tract released during enteral feeding. The autonomic nervous system, also through vagal stimulation, increases insulin release, as does β-adrenergic stimulation and α-adrenergic blockade.

The most fundamental action of insulin is to stimulate increased cellular uptake of glucose. This is particularly important in skeletal muscle cells, where muscle activity also increases glucose uptake and is an important variable in the management of the physically active diabetic patient. The brain and liver are exceptions where insulin does not affect glucose transport. Hence, the diabetic patient has hyperglycemia because of inadequate cellular uptake of glucose. Along with glucose, potassium enters the cells under the influence of insulin, so the diabetic patient is also likely to have an imbalance of potassium concentrations across cell membranes.

Other important metabolic functions of insulin include the stimulation of glycogen formation, as well as the suppression of gluconeogenesis and lipolysis. The patient with insulin deficiency has low glycogen stores and active gluconeogenesis. This implies that in the diabetic patient, due to an absence of glycogen, protein must be broken down to make glucose. Insulin also increases the uptake of amino acids into muscle cells. Hence, an insulin deficiency leads to catabolism and negative nitrogen balance.

Fat metabolism is also abnormal in the diabetic state, with acceleration of lipid catabolism and increased formation of ketone bodies. A deficiency of insulin leads to increased fatty acid liberation from adipose tissue. These fatty acids have multiple metabolic effects, including interference with carbohydrate phosphorylation in muscle, which leads to further hyperglycemia. Low concentrations of insulin, which may be inadequate to prevent hyperglycemia, are often sufficient to block lipolysis. This effect explains the common clinical situation in which a patient is hyperglycemic without being ketotic.

Glucagon is a polypeptide released from the α cells of the pancreas, and acts both to stimulate the release of insulin and oppose some of the effects of insulin. Hence, it has both a direct and an indirect ability to increase circulating glucose levels. In some patients, after total pancreatic resection, glucose balance is not as poor as might be expected because of the concomitant absence of glucagon. Glucagon release is stimulated by hypoglycemia, as well as by epinephrine and cortisol, and is suppressed by glucose ingestion.

The metabolic effects of stress are intricately involved with the same pathways as those involved in DM. During stress, elevations in the circulating levels of cortisol, glucagon, catecholamines, and growth hormone all act to cause hyperglycemia. In addition, glucagon and α-adrenergic stimulation exert a suppressive effect on insulin release. Mild hyperglycemia may occur in the stressed patient who does not have DM. In the diabetic patient, stress makes the diabetes more difficult to control. In a patient with minimal or subclinical DM before the stressful episode, the glucose balance may become difficult to manage during the stress-related event.

Treatment

Patients with type I DM require insulin to survive. Further, the risk of microvascular complications can be decreased if tight glycemic control maintains near-normal levels of blood glucose. Patients may be on a range of doses of both short-acting and intermediate-acting insulin, with doses given one to six times per day, depending on the desire for tight control.

Patients with type II DM may initially be treated with diet control and exercise. If this fails to control glucose levels or the diabetes worsens, therapy with an oral agent is indicated.[48] Sulfonylureas enhance β-cell insulin secretion. Metformin is a biguanide that enhances the sensitivity of both hepatic and peripheral tissues to insulin.[49] Rosiglitazone (Avandia) and pioglitazone (Actos) are thiazolidinediones that also increase insulin sensitivity. α-Glucosidase inhibitors decrease postprandial glucose absorption. If oral agents cannot maintain acceptable glucose levels, insulin is used.

Anesthetic Management

Successful management of the diabetic patient depends as much, if not more, on the proper management of the chronic
6 complications of the disease as on acute glycemic management.

Preoperative

A thorough preoperative search must be done for end-organ complications of DM. In addition to a thorough history and physical, a recent ECG, blood urea nitrogen, potassium, creatinine, glucose, and urinalysis are essential.

Atherosclerosis develops earlier and is more widespread in diabetic patients compared with nondiabetics. Manifestations include coronary artery disease, peripheral vascular disease, cerebrovascular disease, and renovascular disease. The incidence of postoperative myocardial infarction is increased in diabetic patients, and the complication rate is higher. Coronary artery disease can manifest at a young age or atypically in type I diabetics. Silent myocardial ischemia and infarction occur more commonly in diabetic patients, perhaps because of sensory neuropathy of the visceral afferents to the heart. DM may be associated with a cardiomyopathy in the face of angiographically normal coronary arteries, possibly with diffuse disease in arteries too small to be visualized. The American College of Cardiology (ACC)/American Heart Association guidelines recognize DM as an intermediate risk factor when evaluating patients for noncardiac surgery.

In up to 40% of juvenile patients with DM presenting for renal transplantation, laryngoscopy can be difficult.[50] This may be due to diabetic stiff joint syndrome, a frequent complication of type I DM, leading to decreased mobility of the atlanto-occipital joint. The "prayer sign," an inability to approximate the palmar surfaces of the interphalangeal joints, is associated with stiff joint syndrome and may predict difficult laryngoscopy.

Diabetic nephropathy eventually occurs in up to 40 to 50% of patients with DM. Albuminuria usually precedes a steady decline in renal function.

Diabetic patients with autonomic neuropathy are at increased risk for intraoperative hypotension, requiring vasopressor support, and perioperative cardiorespiratory arrest.[51–53] There may be an exaggerated pressor response to tracheal intubation.[54] Autonomic function may be tested by measuring the beat-to-beat variation in heart rate during breathing, heart rate response to a Valsalva maneuver, and orthostatic changes in diastolic blood pressure and heart rate. Autonomic neuropathy predisposes to intraoperative hypothermia.[55]

Diabetic patients may have delayed gastric emptying as a result of diabetic autonomic neuropathy, and therefore, they may be at increased risk of aspiration. Autonomic function tests can predict the presence of solid food particles in gastric contents but not increased gastric volume or acidity.[56] Metoclopramide may be useful in emptying the stomach of solid food.

It is axiomatic that the patient should attain the best possible preoperative metabolic control. If the patient's glucose level has been unstable, especially with episodes of hypoglycemia, adjustment of insulin therapy is required. Traditionally, oral hypoglycemics have been held before surgery because of fear of hypoglycemia in the fasted patient. With today's shorter-acting agents, this may be unnecessary because the risk is much reduced. Metformin should be discontinued preoperatively because it has been associated with severe lactic acidosis during episodes of hypotension, poor perfusion, or hypoxia. Unless the patient has a surgical emergency, patients with diabetic ketoacidosis or hyperosmolar coma should receive intensive medical management before coming to the operating room (see Emergencies section).

Intraoperative

The details of the anesthetic plan depend intimately on the end-organ complications. Invasive monitoring may be indicated for the patient with heart disease, awake intubation may be necessary if a difficult intubation is predicted, fluid management and drug choices may depend on renal function, and aspiration must be considered if there is gastroparesis.

Blood glucose levels should be measured before and after surgery. The need for additional measurements is determined by the duration and magnitude of surgery, as well as the brittleness of the diabetes. Hourly measurements are reasonable in high-risk patients.

On the basis of a preoperative osmotic diuresis, the diabetic patient may reach the operating room with clinically significant dehydration. In addition to the usual principles of perioperative fluid management, it is important to note the amount of glucose administered intravenously to avoid a massive overdose of glucose. The standard glucose dosage for an adult patient is 5 to 10 g/hr (100 to 200 mL of 5% dextrose solution hourly). It is best to monitor and record the dextrose administered separately from the fluids given. It would be wrong to give large amounts of dextrose (contained in the intravenous solutions) just because that patient needed vigorous fluid replacement. If this happens, the patient is likely to be extremely hyperglycemic in the postanesthesia care unit. It is difficult to determine the proper dose of insulin to correct this iatrogenic hyperglycemia, so prolonged observation and therapy may be required.

Monitoring of the patient who arrives in the operating room with significant metabolic impairment, such as diabetic ketoacidosis, is similar to management in the medical intensive care unit, including hourly determinations of blood glucose, arterial pH, electrolytes, and fluid balance. Frequent reassessments with medical consultation as necessary guide the use of fluids; electrolytes, especially potassium; insulin; phosphate; and glucose.

Another area of patient monitoring that is extremely important in the diabetic patient is positioning on the operating table. Injuries to the limbs or nerves are more likely in the patient who arrives in the operating room already compromised by diabetic peripheral vascular disease or neuropathy. The peripheral nerves may already be partly ischemic and therefore particularly vulnerable to pressure or stretch injuries.[57]

Glycemic Goals

Traditionally, intraoperative glucose management has been a laissez-faire approach, where mild hyperglycemia would not be treated unless blood glucose was greater than 200 to 250 mg/dL or even higher. It was widely believed that short-term, mild hyperglycemia was not detrimental and the risk from inadvertent hypoglycemia too great. Over the past few years, there has been increasing evidence that even mild hyperglycemia is associated with increased perioperative morbidity, and tight control to achieve euglycemia can reduce complica-
7 tions in many groups of medical and surgical patients.

One study looked at 1,548 critically ill surgical patients, many of whom had cardiac surgery, and found that patients who had conventional therapy as opposed to intensive insulin therapy (goal 80 to 110 mg/dL) had increased risk of sepsis, renal failure, neuropathy, and mortality.[58] One study of 3,500 diabetic patients undergoing coronary artery bypass graft (CABG) surgery found decreased mortality and infections in patients who received continuous insulin infusions.[59] Similarly, a study of 141 diabetic patients undergoing CABG surgery found improved survival, decreased episodes of recurrent ischemia, and fewer recurrent wound infections in those who received a glucose-insulin-potassium infusion to maintain blood glucose less than 200 mg/dL.[60] This study was notable because tight control began during the intraoperative period and continued for 12 hours afterward. Hyperglycemia exacerbates neuronal ischemic damage. Patients undergoing surgical procedures associated with cerebral ischemia such as intracranial surgery, carotid endarterectomy, and cardiopulmonary bypass may benefit from euglycemia.[61] On the strength of these and other studies,[62,63] there is a growing trend toward recommending tight control of glucose in critically ill and perioperative patients. The American College of Endocrinology has published a position paper stating that the goal for maintaining blood glucose should be less than 110 mg/dL.[64]

There are limitations in applying these data to the intraoperative period. Most of the studies looked at glucose control over days to weeks. The specific importance of the few hours of the intraoperative period is not addressed, although it is reasonable to assume good intraoperative metabolic control will help achieve good postoperative metabolic control. Further, these studies included heterogeneous populations undergoing a variety of procedures. The majority of studies are in cardiac surgical patients. Some studies had diabetics and nondiabetics. It may be possible to stratify the risk and select patients for intensive therapy. As the desired glycemic end point gets lower, the incidence of hypoglycemia will increase. Although no complications have been reported from hypoglycemia during intensive therapy, outside the rigid protocols and monitoring of a study there may be serious neurologic complications.

The mechanisms by which intensive insulin therapy reduces complications are likely multifactorial. Hyperglycemia impairs neutrophil, fibroblast, and endothelial function. Insulin decreases inflammation and reduces fatty acids, which can have detrimental effects on myocardial metabolism.

Therefore, it seems reasonable to keep perioperative glucose levels lower than in the past, certainly below 200 mg/dL, and probably close to 110 mg/dL. Further studies may identify which patients will benefit from resource-intensive, tight control and provide empirical or consensus guidelines for managing intraoperative glucose.

Management Regimens

There is no consensus about the optimal way to manage perioperative metabolic changes in diabetic patients; many options are available. Factors to consider in selecting a plan include the type of DM, how aggressively euglycemia will be sought, whether the patient takes insulin, whether the surgery is minor and in an ambulatory unit, whether the surgery is elective or an emergency, and the ability of hospital resources to safely administer a complex plan. The goal of any regimen should be to minimize metabolic derangements and, most obviously, to avoid hypoglycemia.

Type I Diabetes

Type I diabetics require insulin or they will rapidly develop ketoacidosis and its complications. This can be given by administering one-half to two-thirds of the patient's usual intermediate-acting insulin subcutaneously on the morning of surgery. In addition to this basal insulin, a regular insulin sliding scale (RISS) can be added and titrated to blood glucose measurement.[65] Alternatively, an insulin infusion of 0.5 to 2 U/hr (100 U regular insulin in 1,000 mL normal saline at 5 to 20 mL/hr) can meet basal metabolic needs and be adjusted to maintain blood glucose at the desired level.[66] With either method, a slow glucose infusion (D5W at 75 to 125 mL/hr) will prevent hypoglycemia while the patient is fasting. Some authorities recommend a combination glucose-insulin or glucose-insulin-potassium infusions.

Type II Diabetes

The hospitalized type II diabetic may find glucose control improved because of stricter dietary control. Fasting patients will not have postprandial hyperglycemia. Sulfonylureas should be held while the patient is NPO (nothing per mouth) to decrease the risk of hypoglycemia and because they interfere with the cardioprotective effect of ischemic preconditioning. Metformin should probably also be held, especially if there is a risk of decreased renal function perioperatively because of a risk of lactic acidosis. Thiazolidinediones can be continued because they do not predispose to hypoglycemia. α-Glucosidase inhibitors should be held because they only work when taken with meals. For type II patients on oral agents alone, RISS can be added to titrate blood glucose levels.

Patients on chronic insulin can be treated similarly to the type I patient by giving one-half the usual NPH dose the morning of surgery, supplemented by a RISS, or an insulin infusion titrated to blood glucose. The use of a RISS as the sole method of control is to be discouraged because it can predispose to wide glucose variations.[67]

At Yale-New Haven Hospital, the Department of Medicine has implemented an effective insulin infusion protocol designed to achieve strict glycemic control in medical intensive care unit patients.[68] It emphasizes the need to consider the current blood glucose value, as well as the rate of change of blood glucose level when adjusting the infusion.

Postoperatively, as the patient resumes oral intake, therapy can be transitioned to the patient's chronic regimen. Type II diabetics who have had gastric bypass can have rapid resolution of their glucose intolerance, and will often need their oral agents and insulin reduced or even discontinued in the postoperative period. This effect appears to be due to changes in the enteric hormones such as glucose-dependent insulinotropic polypeptide and glucagon-like peptide-1, rather than weight loss.[69]

Emergencies

Patients may present with metabolic instability, or it may develop perioperatively. Stress, trauma, and infection may all lead to increased insulin requirements and insulin resistance.

Hyperosmolar Nonketotic Coma

An occasional elderly patient with minimal or mild DM may present with remarkably high blood glucose levels (>600 mg/dL) and profound dehydration. Such patients usually have enough endogenous insulin activity to prevent ketosis; even with blood sugar concentrations of 1,000 mg/dL, they are not in ketoacidosis. Presumably, it is the combination of an impaired thirst response and mild renal insufficiency that allows the hyperglycemia to develop. The marked hyperosmolarity may lead to coma and seizures, with the increased plasma viscosity producing a tendency to intravascular thrombosis. It is characteristic of this syndrome that the metabolic disturbance responds quickly to rehydration and small doses of insulin. One to 2 L of normal saline, or equivalent, should be infused over 1 to 2 hours if there are no cardiovascular contraindications. Insulin, by bolus or infusion, should be administered. With rapid correction of the hyperosmolarity, cerebral edema is a risk, and recovery of mental acuity may be delayed after the blood glucose level and circulating volume have been normalized.

Diabetic Ketoacidosis

If the diabetic patient has insufficient insulin effect to block the mobilization and metabolism of free fatty acids, the metabolic byproducts acetoacetate and β-hydroxybutyrate accumulate.[70]

TABLE 41-10

MANAGEMENT OF DIABETIC KETOACIDOSIS

- Regular insulin 10 U IV bolus followed by an insulin infusion nominally at (blood glucose/150) U/hr
- Isotonic IV fluids as guided by vital signs and urine output; anticipate 4–10 L deficit
- When urine output is >0.5 mL/kg/hr, give potassium chloride 10–40 mEq/hr (with continuous ECG monitoring when the rate is greater than 10 mEq/hr)
- When serum glucose decreased to 250 mg/dL, add dextrose 5% at 100 mL/hr
- Consider sodium bicarbonate to correct pH < 6.9

ECG, electrocardiogram; IV, intravenous(ly).

These ketone bodies are organic acids and cause a metabolic acidosis with an increased unmeasured anion gap. Clinically, the patient often presents because of intercurrent illness, trauma, or the untoward cessation of insulin therapy. Although hyperglycemia is almost always present, the degree of hyperglycemia does not correlate with the severity of the acidosis. Blood sugar levels are often in the 300 to 500 mg/dL range. The patient is always dehydrated because of the combination of the hyperglycemia-induced osmotic diuresis and the nausea and vomiting typical of this syndrome. Because leukocytosis, abdominal pain, GI ileus, and mildly elevated amylase levels are all common in ketoacidosis, an occasional patient is misdiagnosed as having an intra-abdominal surgical problem.

Treatment of diabetic ketoacidosis includes insulin administration and fluid and electrolyte replacement (Table 41-10). An intravenous bolus of 10 to 20 U of insulin achieves rapid maximal effect. Further insulin can be administered by intravenous infusion or intermittent bolus every 30 to 60 minutes. When blood glucose levels decrease below 250 mg/dL, glucose should be added to the intravenous fluid while insulin therapy continues. Fluid requirements can be marked; 1 to 2 L of normal saline, or equivalent, should be given over 1 to 2 hours. Further deficits can be replaced more gradually. Potassium replacement is a key concern in patients with diabetic ketoacidosis. Because of the diuresis, the total body potassium stores are reduced. However, acidosis by itself causes a shift of potassium ions out of the cell. Thus, the serum potassium concentration may be normal or even slightly elevated while the patient is acidotic. As soon as the metabolic acidosis is corrected, the potassium ions shift back into the cells. Consequently, the serum potassium concentration can decline acutely. Therefore, early and vigorous potassium replacement is required in these patients, with the exception of those patients in renal failure. Hypophosphatemia also occurs with the correction of the acidosis and, if severe, may cause impairment of ventilation, resulting from skeletal muscle weakness in the vulnerable patient. Instead of diabetic ketoacidosis, the diabetic patient with a metabolic acidosis may have lactic acidosis, which results from poor tissue perfusion or sepsis. It is diagnosed by the presence of an increased serum lactate concentration without an elevated ketone concentration.

Diabetic ketoacidosis must also be distinguished from the syndrome of alcoholic ketoacidosis. This typically occurs in the poorly nourished alcoholic patient after acute intoxication. Except for the presence of chemical ketoacidosis, alcoholic ketoacidosis is not clinically related in any way to DM. The alcoholic patient may be hypoglycemic or mildly hyperglycemic. The predominant ketone in this syndrome is β-hydroxybutyrate, which tends to react less sensitively in the standard laboratory nitroprusside reaction measurement of ketones. Hence, the diagnosis may be obscured. Administration of dextrose and parenteral fluids is the specific treatment for alcoholic ketoacidosis; insulin is not indicated (except in the rare circumstance in which the patient also has clear-cut DM).

Hypoglycemia

Hypoglycemia is the clinical occurrence most feared in the management of diabetic patients. The precise level at which symptomatic hypoglycemia occurs is variable. The normal, fasted patient may have blood sugar levels lower than 50 mg/dL without symptoms. However, the diabetic patient who has a chronically elevated blood sugar level may be symptomatic at levels significantly above this glucose concentration. Hypoglycemia is almost impossible to diagnose clinically in the unconscious patient.

In the awake patient, hypoglycemia often produces central nervous system changes ranging from light-headedness to coma with seizures. Often, the patient recognizes the symptoms and can tell that the blood sugar is low before any overt clinical signs develop. With hypoglycemia, there is a reflex catecholamine release that produces overt sympathetic hyperactivity causing tachycardia, lacrimation, diaphoresis, and hypertension. In the anesthetized patient, these signs of sympathetic hyperactivity can easily be misinterpreted as inadequate or "light" anesthesia. In the anesthetized, sedated, or seriously ill patient, the mental changes of hypoglycemia are also unrecognizable. Furthermore, in patients being treated with β-adrenergic blocking agents or in patients with advanced diabetic autonomic neuropathy, the sympathetic hyperactivity of hypoglycemia may be obscured. Thus, the clinical diagnosis of hypoglycemia in the surgical patient may be difficult to make, and only a high degree of suspicion and frequent blood glucose checks can prevent this complication.

Hypoglycemia is more likely to occur in the diabetic surgical patient if insulin or sulfonylureas are given without supplemental glucose. With renal insufficiency, the action of insulin and oral hypoglycemic agents is prolonged.

PITUITARY GLAND

The pituitary gland is located below the base of the brain in a bony structure called the sella turcica. The pituitary gland and the hypothalamus together form a central unit that regulates the release of various hormones. The pituitary gland is divided into two components. The anterior pituitary (adenohypophysis) secretes prolactin, growth hormone, gonadotropins (luteinizing hormone and follicle-stimulating hormone), TSH, and ACTH. The posterior pituitary (neurohypophysis) secretes the hormones vasopressin and oxytocin. Hormone release from the anterior and posterior pituitary is regulated by the hypothalamus. Regulatory peptides or preformed hormones from the hypothalamus are transported to the pituitary gland through vascular or tissue connections.

Anterior Pituitary

Hyposecretion of anterior pituitary hormones is usually due to compression of the gland by tumor. This may begin as an isolated deficiency, but it usually develops into multiglandular dysfunction. Male impotence or secondary amenorrhea in the woman is an early manifestation of panhypopituitarism. Panhypopituitarism after postpartum hemorrhagic shock (Sheehan's syndrome) is due to necrosis of the anterior pituitary gland. Radiation therapy delivered to the sella turcica or nearby structures and surgical hypophysectomy are other causes of panhypopituitarism. Panhypopituitarism is treated with specific hormone replacement therapy, which should be continued in the perioperative period. Stress doses of corticosteroids are necessary for patients receiving steroid replacement due to inadequate ACTH.

The hypersecretion of various anterior pituitary hormones is usually caused by an adenoma. Excess prolactin secretion with galactorrhea is a common hormonal abnormality associated with pituitary adenoma. Cushing's disease may occur secondary to excess ACTH production, and gigantism or acromegaly may occur as a consequence of excess growth hormone production in the child or adult, respectively. Excessive secretion of TSH is rare.

Acromegaly in the adult patient may pose several problems for the anesthesiologist.[71] Excess hypertrophy occurs in skeletal, connective, and soft tissues.[72] The tongue and epiglottis are enlarged, making the patient susceptible to upper airway obstruction. The incidence of difficult intubation is 20 to 30%, and it is difficult to predict which patients will be
8 difficult.[73] Hoarseness may reflect thickening of the vocal cords or paralysis of a recurrent laryngeal nerve due to stretching. Dyspnea or stridor is associated with subglottic narrowing. Peripheral nerve or artery entrapment, hypertension, and DM are other common findings. The anesthetic management of these patients is complicated by distortion of the facial anatomy and upper airway. Induction of general anesthesia may put the patient at increased risk if mask fit or vocal cord visualization is impaired. When the preoperative history suggests upper airway or vocal cord involvement, it is prudent to consider intubation of the trachea while the patient is awake.

Posterior Pituitary

The posterior pituitary, or neurohypophysis, is composed of terminal nerve endings that extend from the ventral hypothalamus. Vasopressin (antidiuretic hormone or ADH) and oxytocin are the two principal hormones secreted by the posterior pituitary. Both hormones are synthesized in the supraoptic and paraventricular nuclei of the hypothalamus. They are bound to inactive carrier proteins, neurophysins, and transported by axons to membrane-bound storage vesicles located in the posterior pituitary. ADH is a nonapeptide that circulates as a free peptide after its release. The primary functions of ADH are the maintenance of extracellular fluid volume and regulation of plasma osmolality. Oxytocin elicits contraction of the uterus and promotes milk secretion and ejection by the mammary glands.

Vasopressin

ADH promotes resorption of solute-free water by increasing cell membrane permeability to water alone. The target sites for ADH are the collecting tubules of the kidneys. A decrease in free water clearance causes a decrease in serum osmolality and a corresponding increase in circulating blood volume. Under normal conditions, the primary stimulus for the release of ADH is an increase in serum osmolality.

Osmoreceptors located in the hypothalamus are sensitive to changes in the normal serum osmolality of as little as 1% (normal osmolality is approximately 285 mOsm/L). Stretch receptors in the left atrium and perhaps pulmonary veins, which are sensitive to moderate reductions in the blood volume, are also capable of stimulating ADH secretion. The need to restore plasma volume may at times override osmotic inhibition of ADH release. Various physiologic and pharmacologic stimuli also influence the secretion of ADH. Positive-pressure ventilation of the lungs, stress, anxiety, hyperthermia, β-adrenergic stimulation, and any histamine-releasing stimulus can promote the release of ADH.

ADH also has other actions. It can increase blood pressure by constricting vascular smooth muscle. This activity is most significant in the splanchnic, renal, and coronary vascular beds, and provides the rationale for administering exogenous vasopressin in the management of hemorrhage due to esophageal varices. Caution must be taken when this drug is used in patients with coronary artery disease. ADH (even in small doses) can precipitate myocardial ischemia through vasoconstriction of the coronary arteries. It is unclear whether selective arterial infusion is safer than systemic administration with regard to cardiac and vascular side effects. ADH is also often used in vasodilatory shock as an adjuvant to other pressor agents.

ADH also promotes hemostasis through an increase in the level of circulating von Willebrand factor and factor VIII. Desmopressin (DDAVP), an analog of ADH administered to patients after cardiopulmonary bypass in a dose of 0.3 μg/kg, significantly decreased blood loss and reduced transfusion requirements compared with a group of patients who did not receive the drug. DDAVP is also frequently used to reverse the coagulopathy of renal failure.

Diabetes Insipidus

This disorder results from inadequate secretion of ADH or resistance on the part of the renal tubules to ADH (nephrogenic diabetes insipidus). Failure to secrete adequate amounts of ADH results in polydipsia, hypernatremia, and a high output of poorly concentrated urine. Hypovolemia and hypernatremia may become so severe as to be life threatening. This disorder usually occurs after destruction of the pituitary gland by intracranial trauma, infiltrating lesions, or surgery. Patients in whom diabetes insipidus develops secondary to severe head trauma or subarachnoid hemorrhage often have impending brain death.[74] The treatment of diabetes insipidus depends on the extent of the hormonal deficiency. During surgery, the patient with complete diabetes insipidus receives an intravenous infusion of aqueous ADH (100–200 mU/hr), combined with administration of an isotonic crystalloid solution. The serum sodium and plasma osmolality are measured on a regular basis, and therapeutic changes are made accordingly. ADH may also be given intramuscularly (as vasopressin tannate in oil). DDAVP administered intranasally has prolonged antidiuretic activity (12 to 24 hours) and is associated with a low incidence of pressor effects. As a consequence of the large outpouring of ADH in response to surgical stress, patients with a residually functioning gland usually do not need parenteral ADH during the perioperative period unless the plasma osmolality rises above 290 mOsm/L. Nonhormonal agents that have efficacy in the treatment of incomplete diabetes insipidus include the oral hypoglycemic chlorpropamide (200 to 500 mg/day). This drug stimulates the release of ADH and sensitizes the renal tubules to the hormone. Hypoglycemia is a serious side effect that limits the usefulness of the drug. Clofibrate, a hypolipidemic agent, is also capable of stimulating ADH release and has been used in the outpatient setting. None of these medications is effective in the patient with nephrogenic diabetes insipidus. Paradoxically, the thiazide diuretics exert an antidiuretic action in patients with this disorder.

Inappropriate Secretion of Antidiuretic Hormone

The inappropriate and excessive secretion of ADH may occur in association with a number of diverse pathologic processes, including head injuries, intracranial tumors, pulmonary infections, small cell carcinoma of the lung, and hypothyroidism. The clinical manifestations occur as a result of a dilutional hyponatremia, decreased serum osmolality, and a reduced urine output with a high osmolality. Weight gain, skeletal muscle weakness, and mental confusion or convulsions are presenting symptoms. Peripheral edema and hypertension are rare. The diagnosis of the syndrome of inappropriate ADH (SIADH) secretion is one of exclusion, and other causes of hyponatremia must first be ruled out. The prognosis is related to the underlying cause of the syndrome.

The treatment of patients with mild or moderate water intoxication is restriction of fluid intake to 800 mL/day. Patients with severe water intoxication associated with hyponatremia and mental confusion may require more aggressive therapy, with the intravenous administration of a hypertonic saline solution. This may be administered in conjunction with furosemide. Caution must be observed in patients with poor left ventricular function. Isotonic saline is substituted for hypertonic solutions once the serum sodium is brought into a safe range. Too-rapid correction of hyponatremia may induce central pontine myelinolysis and cause permanent brain damage. Serum sodium should not be raised by more than 12 mEq/L in 24 hours. Other drugs that may be used in the patient with SIADH are demeclocycline and lithium. Demeclocycline interferes with the ability of the renal tubules to concentrate urine and is frequently used in outpatients. Lithium usually is not used because of the high incidence of toxicity.

ENDOCRINE RESPONSE TO SURGICAL STRESS

Anesthesia, surgery, and trauma elicit a generalized endocrine metabolic response characterized by an increase in the plasma levels of cortisol, ADH, renin, catecholamines, and endorphins, and by metabolic changes such as hyperglycemia and a negative nitrogen balance.[75,76] Various neural and humoral factors (e.g., pain, anxiety, acidosis, local tissue factors, hypoxia) play a role in activating this stress response.

The induction of anesthesia increases the levels of circulating catecholamines and is a form of metabolic stress. Regional anesthesia may block part of the metabolic stress response during surgery, probably by blockade of the neural communications from the surgical area. It is theorized that the persistently high levels of circulating catecholamines in trauma and critical illness lead to stress hyperglycemia through a direct inhibition of insulin release. Bypass of the gut hormonal actions in patients receiving intravenous glucose feedings, especially if given in large amounts, contributes to the impairment of insulin release during illness and can create a particularly difficult management problem for diabetic patients.

Endorphins are a group of endogenous peptides with opioid activity that have been isolated from the central nervous system. It is well documented that β-endorphin is released from the anterior pituitary, where it is contained as part of β-lipoprotein, a 91-chain amino acid, which is a cleavage product of the precursor peptide for ACTH. Large increases in the central nervous system and plasma concentrations of endorphins in response to emotional or surgical stimuli suggest that these substances play a role in the body's response to stress. These substances modulate painful stimuli by binding to opiate receptors located throughout the brain and spinal cord.

Numerous experiments have focused on the stress response and its relationship to the depth of anesthesia. Regional anesthesia and general anesthesia appear to blunt the release of various stress hormones during the period of surgical stimulation in a dose-dependent fashion. Historically, anesthesiologists have relied on the indirect measurement of hemodynamic variables such as blood pressure and heart rate to evaluate the level of autonomic activity in response to anesthesia and surgery. It is assumed that the physiologic manifestations of stress are potentially harmful, especially in patients with limited functional reserve. As such, our anesthetic techniques and pain management strategies are designed to limit this neurohormonal response, in the hope of providing the patient with some benefit. Further investigations are needed to assess the impact of these efforts on perioperative morbidity and mortality.

References

1. Surks MI, Sievert R: Drugs and thyroid function. N Engl J Med 333:1688, 1995
2. Mandel SJ, Brent GA, Larsen PR: Levothyroxine therapy in patients with thyroid disease. Ann Intern Med 119:492, 1993
3. Mulligan DC, McHenry CR, Kinney W, Esselstyn CB Jr: Amiodarone-induced thyrotoxicosis: Clinical presentation and expanded indications for thyroidectomy. Surgery 114:1114, 1993
4. Langley RW, Burch HB: Perioperative management of the thyrotoxic patient. Endocrinol Metab Clin of North America 32:519, 2003
5. Franklyn JA: The management of hyperthyroidism. N Engl J Med 330:1731, 1994
6. Smallridge RC: Metabolic and anatomic thyroid emergencies: A review. Crit Care Med 20:276, 1992
7. Hermann M, Richter B, Roka R, Freissmuth M: Thyroid surgery in untreated severe hyperthyroidism: Perioperative kinetics of free thyroid hormones in the glandular venous effluent and peripheral blood. Surgery 115:240, 1994
8. Farling PA: Thyroid disease. Br J Anaesth 85:15, 2000
9. Bouaggad A, Nejmi SE, Bouderka MA, Abbassi O: Prediction of difficult tracheal intubation in thyroid surgery. Anesth Analg 99:603, 2004
10. Szubin L, Kacker A, Kakani R *et al*: The management of post-thyroidectomy hypocalcemia. Ear Nose Throat J 75:612, 1996
11. Wagner HE, Seiler C: Recurrent laryngeal nerve palsy after thyroid gland surgery. Br J Surg 81:226, 1994
12. Lindsay RS, Toft AD: Hypothyroidism. Lancet 349:413, 1997
13. Stathatos N, Wartofsky L: Perioperative management of patients with hypothyroidism. Endocrinol Metab Clin of North America 32:503, 2003
14. Toft AD: Thyroxine therapy. N Engl J Med 331:174, 1994
15. Bennett-Guerrero E, Kramer DC, Schwinn DA: Effect of chronic and acute thyroid hormone reduction on perioperative outcome. Anesth Analg 85:30, 1997
16. Ladenson PW, Levin AA, Ridgway EC, Daniels GH: Complications of surgery in hypothyroid patients. Am J Med 77:261, 1984
17. Whitten CW, Latson TW, Klein KW *et al*: Anesthetic management of a hypothyroid cardiac surgical patient. J Cardiothorac Vasc Anesth 5:156, 1991
18. Weinberg AD, Ehrenwerth J: Anesthetic considerations and perioperative management of patients with hypothyroidism. Adv Anesth 4:185, 1987
19. Mihai R, Farndon JR: Parathyroid disease and calcium metabolism. Br J Anaesth 85:29, 2000
20. Roland EJ, Wierda JM, Eurin BG, Roupie E: Pharmacodynamic behaviour of vecuronium in primary hyperparathyroidism. Can J Anaesth 41:694, 1994
21. Meuriaaw M, Hamoir E, Defechereux T *et al*: Bilateral neck exploration under hypnosedation. Ann Surg 229:401, 1999
22. Al-Zahrani A, Levine MA: Primary hyperparathyroidism. Lancet 349:1233, 1997
23. Vaughan ED Jr: Diseases of the adrenal gland. Med Clin North Am 88:443, 2004
24. Rivers EP, Gaspari M, Abi Saad G *et al*: Adrenal insufficiency in high-risk surgical ICU patients. Chest 119:889, 2001
25. Lamberts SWJ, Bruining HA, DeJong FH: Corticosteroid therapy in severe illness. N Engl J Med 337:1285, 1997
26. Bennett N, Gabrielli A: Hypotension and adrenal insufficiency. J Clin Anesth 11:425, 1999
27. Sutherland FWH, Naik SK: Acute adrenal insufficiency after coronary artery bypass grafting. Ann Thorac Surg 62:1516, 1996
28. Oelkers W: Adrenal insufficiency. N Engl J Med 335:1206, 1996
29. Chin R: Adrenal crisis. Crit Care Clin 7:23, 1991
30. Engquist A, Brandt MR, Fernandes A, Kehlet H: The blocking effect of epidural analgesia on the adrenocortical and hyperglycemic responses to surgery. Acta Anaesthesiol Scand 21:330, 1977
31. Salem M, Tainsh RE Jr, Bromberg J *et al*: Perioperative glucocorticoid coverage: A reassessment 41 years after emergence of a problem. Ann Surg 219:416, 1994
32. Axelrod L: Perioperative management of patients treated with glucocorticoids. Endocrinol Metab Clin of North America 32:367, 2003
33. Symreng T, Karlberg BE, Kagedal B, Schildt B: Physiological cortisol substitution of long-term steroid-treated patients undergoing major surgery. Br J Anaesth 53:949, 1981
34. Glowniak JV, Loriaux DL: A double-blind study of perioperative steroid requirements in secondary adrenal insufficiency. Surgery 121:123, 1997
35. Prys-Roberts C: Phaeochromocytoma: Recent progress in its management. Br J Anaesth 85:44, 2000
36. Kinney MAO, Warner ME, vanHeerden JA *et al*: Perianesthetic risks and

outcomes of pheochromocytoma and paraganglioma resection. Anesth Analg 91:1118, 2000
37. Kinney MAO, Narr BJ, Warner MA: Perioperative management of pheochromocytoma. J Cardiothorac Vasc Anesth 16:359, 2002
38. Giffird RW Jr, Manger WM, Bravo EL: Pheochromocytoma. Endocrinol Metab Clin North Am 23:387, 1994
39. Witteles RM, Kaplan EL, Roizen MF: Sensitivity of diagnostic and localization tests for pheochromocytoma in clinical practice. Arch Int Med 160:2521, 2000
40. Geoghegan JG, Emberton M, Bloom R, Lynn JA: Changing trends in the management of phaeochromocytoma. Br J Surg 85:117, 1998
41. Ulchaker JC, Goldfarb DA, Bravo EL, Novick AC: Successful outcomes in pheochromocytoma surgery in the modern era. J Urol 161:764, 1999
42. Russell WJ, Metecalfe IR, Tonkin AL, Frewin DB: The preoperative management of phaeochromocytoma. Anaesth Intensive Care 26:196, 1998
43. Hamilton A, Sirrs S, Schmidt N, Onrot J: Anaesthesia for phaeochromocytoma in pregnancy. Can J Anaesth 44:654, 1997
44. Joris JL, Hamoir EE, Hartstein GM *et al*: Hemodynamic changes and catecholamine release during laparoscopic adrenalectomy for pheochromocytoma. Anesth Analg 88:16, 1999
45. James MF, Cronje L: Pheochromocytoma crisis: The use of magnesium sulfate. Anesth Analg 99:680, 2004
46. Gusberg RJ, Moley J: Diabetes and abdominal surgery. Yale J Biol Med 56:285, 1983
47. Atkinson MA, Maclaren NK: The pathogenesis of insulin-dependent diabetes mellitus. N Engl J Med 331:1428, 1994
48. DeFronzo RA: Pharmacologic therapy for type 2 diabetes mellitus. Ann Intern Med 131:281, 1999
49. Bailey CJ, Turner RC: Metformin. N Engl J Med 334:574, 1996
50. Hogan K, Rusy D, Springman SR: Difficult laryngoscopy and diabetes mellitus. Anesth Analg 67:1162, 1988
51. Charlson ME, MacKenzie CR, Gold JP: Preoperative autonomic function abnormalities in patients with diabetes mellitus and patients with hypertension. J Am Coll Surg 179:1, 1994
52. Latson TW, Ashmore TH, Reinhart DJ *et al*: Autonomic reflex dysfunction in patients presenting for elective surgery is associated with hypotension after anesthesia induction. Anesthesiology 80:326, 1994
53. Page MM, Watkins PJ: Cardiorespiratory arrest and diabetic autonomic neuropathy. Lancet 1:14, 1978
54. Vohra A, Kumar S, Charlton AJ *et al*: Effect of diabetes mellitus on the cardiovascular responses to induction of anesthesia and tracheal intubation. Br J Anaesth 71:258, 1993
55. Kitamura A, Hoshino T, Kon Tadashi T *et al*: Patients with diabetic neuropathy are at risk of a greater intraoperative reduction in core temperature. Anesthesiology 92:1311, 2000
56. Ishihara H, Singh H, Giesecke AH: Relationship between diabetic autonomic neuropathy and gastric contents. Anesth Analg 78:943, 1994
57. Harati Y: Diabetic peripheral neuropathies. Ann Intern Med 107:546, 1987
58. Van den Berghe G, Wouters P, Weekers F *et al*: Intensive insulin therapy in critically ill patients. N Engl J Med 345:1359, 2001
59. Furnary AP, Gao G, Grunkemeier GL *et al*: Continuous insulin infusion reduces mortality in patients with diabetes undergoing coronary artery bypass grafting. J Thorac Cardiovasc Surg 125:1007, 2003
60. Lazar HL, Chipkin SR, Fitzgerald CA *et al*: Tight glycemic control in diabetic coronary artery bypass graft patients improves perioperative outcomes and decreases recurrent ischemic events. Circulation 109:1497, 2004
61. Sieber FE: The neurologic implications of diabetic hyperglycemia during surgical procedures at increased risk for brain ischemia. J Clin Anesth 9:334, 1997
62. Malmberg K, Norhammar A, Wedel H, Ryden L: Glycometabolic state at admission: Important risk marker of mortality in conventionally treated patients with diabetes mellitus and acute myocardial infarction: Long-term results from the diabetes and insulin-glucose infusion in acute myocardial infarction (DIGAMI) study. Circulation 99:2626, 1999
63. Carvalho G, Moore A, Qizilbash B *et al*: Maintenance of normoglycemia during cardiac surgery. Anesth Analg 99:319, 2004
64. Garber AJ, Moghissi ES, Bransome ED Jr *et al*: American College of Endocrinology Task Force on Inpatient Diabetes Metabolic Control. Endocr Prac 10:77, 2004
65. Coursin DB, Connery LE, Ketzler JT: Perioperative diabetic and hyperglycemic management issues. Crit Care Med 32:S116, 2004
66. Inzucchi SE: Glycemic management of diabetes in the perioperative setting. Int Anesth Clin 40:77, 2002
67. Metchick LN, Petit WA Jr, Inzucchi SE: Inpatient management of diabetes mellitus. Am J Med 113:317, 2002
68. Goldberg PA, Siegel MD, Sherwin RS *et al*: Implementation of a safe and effective insulin infusion protocol in a medical intensive care unit. Diabetes Care 27:461, 2004
69. Cummings DE, Overduin J, Foster-Schubert KE: Gastric bypass for obesity: Mechanisms of weight loss and diabetes resolution. J Clin Endocrinol Metabol 89:2608, 2004
70. Foster DW, McGarry JD: The metabolic derangements and treatment of diabetic ketoacidosis. N Engl J Med 309:159, 1983
71. Melmed S: Acromegaly. N Engl J Med 322:966, 1990
72. Kitahata LM: Airway difficulties associated with anaesthesia in acromegaly. Br J Anaesth 43:1187, 1971
73. Schmitt H, Buchfelder M, Radespiel-Troger M *et al*: Difficult intubation in acromegalic patients: Incidence and predictability. Anesthesiology 93:110, 2000
74. Wong MF, Chin NM, Lew TW: Diabetes insipidus in neurosurgical patients. Ann Acad Med Singapore 27:340, 1998
75. Weissman C: The metabolic response to stress: An overview and update. Anesthesiology 73:308, 1990
76. Woolf PD: Hormonal responses to trauma. Crit Care Med 20:216, 1992

CHAPTER 42 ■ OBSTETRIC ANESTHESIA

ALAN C. SANTOS, FERNE R. BRAVEMAN, AND MIECZYSLAW FINSTER

KEY POINTS

1. As oxygen consumption increases during pregnancy, the maternal cardiovascular system adapts to meet the metabolic demands of a growing fetus.
2. Airway edema may be particularly severe in women with preeclampsia, in patients placed in the Trendelenburg position for prolonged periods, or with concurrent use of tocolytic agents.
3. A rapid-sequence induction of anesthesia, application of cricoid pressure, and intubation with a cuffed endotracheal tube are required for all pregnant women receiving general anesthesia after the first trimester.
4. The driving force for placental drug transfer is the concentration gradient of free drug between the maternal and fetal blood.
5. For cesarean section, the choice of anesthesia depends on the urgency of the procedure, in addition to the condition of the mother and fetus.
6. The case fatality rate (maternal mortality) with general anesthesia is 16.7 times greater than that with regional anesthesia.
7. By virtue of age and gender, as well as reduced epidural pressure after delivery, pregnant women are at a higher risk for developing postdural puncture headache (PDPH).
8. Pregnancy and parturition are considered "high risk" when accompanied by conditions unfavorable to the well-being of the mother, fetus, or both.
9. Preeclampsia is classified as severe if it is associated with severe hypertension, proteinuria, or end-organ damage.
10. Antepartum hemorrhage occurs most commonly in association with placenta previa.
11. Heart disease during pregnancy is a leading nonobstetric cause of maternal mortality.
12. Substance abuse with cocaine has the greatest implications for anesthetic management because it causes a heightened sympathetic state.
13. Fetal asphyxia develops as a result of interference with maternal or fetal perfusion of the placenta.
14. There is an increased incidence of adverse obstetric outcome, particularly after nonobstetric operations during the first trimester.

PHYSIOLOGIC CHANGES OF PREGNANCY

During pregnancy, there are major alterations in nearly every maternal organ system. These changes are initiated by hormones secreted by the corpus luteum and placenta. The mechanical effects of the enlarging uterus and compression of surrounding structures play an increasing role in the second and third trimesters. This altered physiologic state has relevant implications for the anesthesiologist caring for the pregnant patient. The most relevant changes, involving hematologic, cardiovascular, ventilatory, metabolic, and gastrointestinal functions, are considered in Table 42-1.

Hematologic Alterations

Increased mineralocorticoid activity during pregnancy produces sodium retention and increased body water content.[1] Thus, plasma volume and total blood volume begin to increase in early gestation, resulting in a final increase of 40 to 50% and 25 to 40%, respectively, at term. The relatively smaller increase in red blood cell volume (20%) accounts for a reduction in hemoglobin (to 11 to 12 g/dL) and hematocrit (to 35%).[1] The leukocyte count ranges from 8,000 to 10,000 per mm^3 throughout pregnancy, whereas the platelet count remains unchanged. Plasma fibrinogen concentrations increase during normal pregnancy by approximately 50%, whereas clotting factor activity is variable.[2] Serum cholinesterase activity declines to a level of 20% below normal by term and reaches a nadir in the puerperium. However, it is doubtful that moderate succinylcholine doses lead to prolonged apnea in otherwise normal circumstances.[3] Total plasma protein concentration declines to less than 6 g/dL at term, whereas the total amount in the circulation increases.[4] The albumin–globulin ratio declines because of the relatively greater reduction in albumin concentration. A decrease in serum protein concentration may be clinically significant in that the free fractions of protein-bound drugs can be expected to increase.

TABLE 42-1

SUMMARY OF PHYSIOLOGIC CHANGES OF PREGNANCY AT TERM

■ VARIABLE	■ CHANGE	■ AMOUNT
Total blood volume	Increase	25–40%
Plasma volume	Increase	40–50%
Fibrinogen	Increase	50%
Serum cholinesterase activity	Decrease	20–30%
Cardiac output	Increase	30–50%
Minute ventilation	Increase	50%
Alveolar ventilation	Increase	70%
Functional residual capacity	Decrease	20%
Oxygen consumption	Increase	20%
Arterial carbon dioxide tension	Decrease	10 mm Hg
Arterial oxygen tension	Increase	10 mm Hg
Minimum alveolar concentration	Decrease	32–40%

Cardiovascular Changes

1 As oxygen consumption increases during pregnancy, the maternal cardiovascular system adapts to meet the metabolic demands of a growing fetus. Decreased vascular resistance due to estrogens, progesterone, and prostacyclin may be the initiating factor.[5] Lowered resistance is found in the uterine, renal, and other vascular beds; at term, there is an increase in heart rate (15 to 25%), and cardiac output (up to 50%) above that of the nonpregnant state. Arterial blood pressure decreases slightly because the decrease in peripheral resistance exceeds the increase in cardiac output. Additional increases in cardiac output occur during labor (when cardiac output may reach 12 to 14 L/min) and also in the immediate postpartum period due to added blood volume from the contracted uterus.

From the second trimester, aortocaval compression by the enlarged uterus becomes progressively more important, reaching its maximum at 36 to 38 weeks, after which it may decrease as the fetal head descends into the pelvis.[6] Studies of cardiac output, measured with the patient in the supine position during the last weeks of pregnancy, have indicated a decrease to nonpregnant levels; however, this decrease was not observed when patients were in the lateral decubitus position.[6] Supine hypotensive syndrome, which occurs in 10% of pregnant women because of venous occlusion, results in maternal tachycardia, arterial hypotension, faintness, and pallor. Compression of the lower aorta in this position may further decrease uteroplacental perfusion and result in fetal asphyxia. Therefore, uterine displacement or lateral pelvic tilt should be applied routinely during the second and third trimesters of pregnancy.

Changes in the electrocardiogram may also occur. Left axis deviation results from the upward displacement of the heart by the gravid uterus, and there is also a tendency toward premature atrial contractions, sinus tachycardia, and paroxysmal supraventricular tachycardia.

Ventilatory Changes

Increased extracellular fluid and vascular engorgement may not only lead to edema of the extremities, but may also compromise the upper airway. Many pregnant women complain of difficulty with nasal breathing, and the friable nature of the mucous membranes during pregnancy can cause severe bleeding, especially on insertion of nasopharyngeal airways or naso-
2 gastric and endotracheal tubes. Airway edema may be particularly severe in women with preeclampsia, in patients placed in the Trendelenburg position for prolonged periods, or with concurrent use of tocolytic agents. It may also be difficult to perform laryngoscopy in obese, short-necked parturients with enlarged breasts. Use of a short-handled laryngoscope has proved helpful.

The level of the diaphragm rises as the uterus increases in size, and is accompanied by an increase in the anteroposterior and transverse diameters of the thoracic cage. From the fifth month, the expiratory reserve volume, residual volume, and functional residual capacity (FRC) decrease, the latter to 20% less than in the nonpregnant state. Concomitantly, there is an increase in inspiratory reserve volume so total lung capacity remains unchanged. In most pregnant women, a decreased FRC does not cause problems, but those with preexisting alterations in closing volume as a result of smoking, obesity, or scoliosis may experience early airway closure with advancing pregnancy, leading to hypoxemia. The Trendelenburg and supine positions also exacerbate the abnormal relationship between closing volume and FRC. The residual volume and FRC return to normal shortly after delivery.

Progesterone-induced relaxation of bronchiolar smooth muscle decreases airway resistance, whereas lung compliance remains unchanged. Minute ventilation increases from the beginning of pregnancy to a maximum of 50% above normal at term.[7] This is accomplished by a 40% increase in tidal volume and a 15% increase in respiratory rate. Dead space does not change significantly, and thus alveolar ventilation is increased by 70% at term. After delivery, as blood progesterone levels decline, ventilation returns to normal within 1 to 3 weeks.[8]

Metabolism

Basal oxygen consumption increases during early pregnancy, with an overall increase of 20% by term.[7] However, increased alveolar ventilation leads to a reduction in the partial pressure of carbon dioxide in arterial blood ($Paco_2$) to 32 mm Hg and an increase in the partial pressure of oxygen in arterial blood (Pao_2) to 106 mm Hg. The plasma buffer base decreases from 47 to 42 mEq/L, and therefore, the pH remains practically unchanged. The maternal uptake and elimination of inhalational anesthetics is enhanced because of the increased alveolar ventilation and decreased FRC.[8] However, the decreased FRC and increased metabolic rate predispose the mother to development of hypoxemia during periods of apnea/hypoventilation, such as may occur during airway obstruction or prolonged attempts at tracheal intubation.[9]

Human placental lactogen and cortisol increase the tendency toward hyperglycemia and ketosis, which may exacerbate preexisting diabetes mellitus. The patient's ability to handle a glucose load is decreased, and the transplacental passage of glucose may stimulate fetal secretion of insulin, leading in turn to neonatal hypoglycemia in the immediate postpartum period.[10]

Gastrointestinal Changes

Enhanced progesterone production may cause slower absorption of food. Gastric secretions are more acidic and lower esophageal sphincter (LES) tone is decreased. Controversy exists as to when a pregnant woman becomes at risk for aspiration. A delay in gastric emptying can be demonstrated by the end of the first trimester,[11] whereas other studies suggest that gastric emptying is not delayed in pregnancy.[12] Earlier studies showing delayed emptying in the first trimester may have been a result of the patients' pain, anxiety, or opioid administration.[11]

The risk of regurgitation on induction of general anesthesia depends, in part, on the gradient between the LES and intragastric pressures. In most patients, the gradient increases after succinylcholine administration because the increase in LES pressure exceeds the increase in intragastric pressure. However, in parturients with "heartburn," the LES tone is greatly reduced.[13] The efficacy of prophylactic nonparticulate antacids is diminished by inadequate mixing with gastric contents, improper timing of administration, and the tendency for antacids to increase gastric volume. Administration of histamine (H_2) receptor antagonists, such as cimetidine and ranitidine, requires careful timing. A good case can be made for the administration of intravenous metoclopramide before elective cesarean section. This dopamine antagonist hastens gastric emptying and increases resting LES tone in both nonpregnant and pregnant women.[14] However, conflicting reports have appeared on its efficacy and on the frequency of side effects such as extrapyramidal reactions and transient neurologic dysfunction.[15] Although no routine prophylactic regimen can be recommended with certainty, it is the authors' preference to administer at least a nonparticulate antacid before cesarean section and to use
3 regional anesthesia whenever possible. A rapid-sequence induction of anesthesia, application of cricoid pressure, and intubation with a cuffed endotracheal tube are required for all pregnant women receiving general anesthesia from the twelfth week of gestation.[12] These recommendations also pertain to women in the immediate postpartum period because there is uncertainty as to when gastric volume returns to normal.

Altered Drug Responses

The minimum alveolar concentration (MAC) for inhalational agents is decreased by 8 to 12 weeks' gestation and may be related to an increase in progesterone levels.[16] In addition, lower doses of local anesthetic are needed per dermatomal segment of epidural or spinal block. This has been attributed to an increased spread of local anesthetic in the epidural and subarachnoid spaces, which occurs as a result of epidural venous engorgement. An increased neural sensitivity to local anesthetics has also been suggested, which may be mediated by progesterone.[17]

PLACENTAL TRANSFER AND FETAL EXPOSURE TO ANESTHETIC DRUGS

Most drugs, including anesthetic agents, readily cross the placenta. Several factors influence the placental transfer of drugs, including physicochemical characteristics of the drug itself, maternal drug concentrations in the plasma, properties of the placenta, and hemodynamic events within the fetomaternal unit.

Drugs cross biologic membranes by simple diffusion, the rate of which is determined by the Fick principle, which states that:

$$Q/t = KA\,(C_m - C_f)/D$$

where Q/t is rate of diffusion, K is diffusion constant, A is surface area available for exchange, C_m is concentration of free drug in maternal blood, C_f is concentration of free drug in fetal blood, and D is thickness of diffusion barrier.

The diffusion constant (K) of the drug depends on physicochemical characteristics such as molecular size, lipid solubility, and degree of ionization. Compounds with a molecular weight of less than 500 daltons are unimpeded in crossing the placenta, whereas those with molecular weights of 500 to 1,000 daltons are more restricted. Most drugs commonly used by the anesthesiologist have molecular weights that permit easy transfer.

If blood flow to the fetal side of the placenta can be measured, as in some animal models, calculating the placental clearance may be a more appropriate way of expressing drug transfer to the fetus.

Drugs that are highly lipid soluble cross biological membranes more readily, and the degree of ionization is important because the nonionized moiety of a drug is more lipophilic than the ionized one. Local anesthetics and opioids are weak bases, with a relatively low degree of ionization and considerable lipid solubility. In contrast, muscle relaxants are less lipophilic and more ionized, and their rate of placental transfer is therefore more limited. The relative concentrations of drug existing in the nonionized and ionized forms can be predicted from the Henderson-Hasselbalch equation:

$$\text{pH} = \text{pKa} + \log(\text{base})/(\text{cation})$$

The ratio of base to cation becomes particularly important with local anesthetics because the nonionized form penetrates tissue barriers, whereas the ionized form is pharmacologically

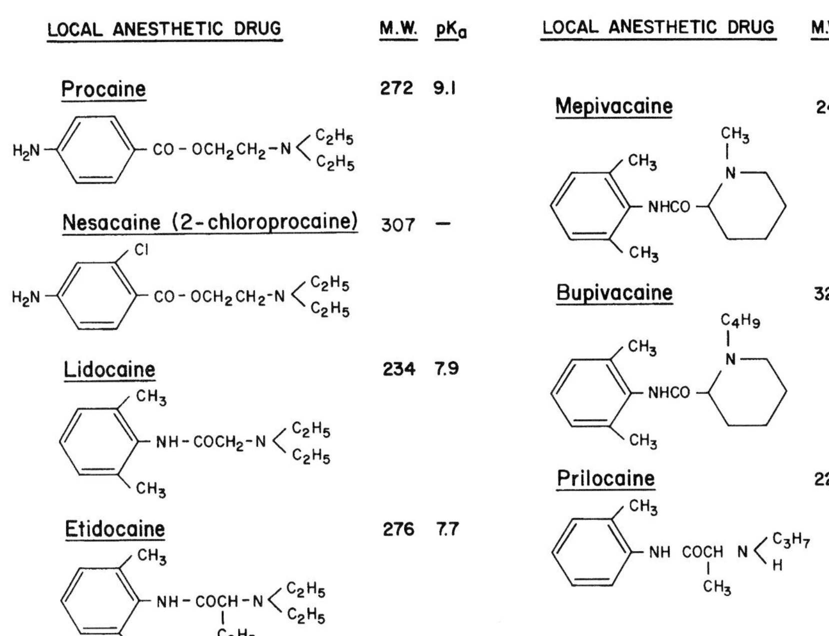

LOCAL ANESTHETIC DRUG M.W. pKa
Procaine 272 9.1
Nesacaine (2-chloroprocaine) 307 –
Lidocaine 234 7.9
Etidocaine 276 7.7
LOCAL ANESTHETIC DRUG M.W. pKa
Mepivacaine 246 7.7
Bupivacaine 325 8.1
Prilocaine 220 7.9

FIGURE 42-1. Chemical structures, pKa, and molecular weights (MWs) of commonly used local anesthetics. (Reprinted with permission from Finster M, Pedersen H: Placental transfer and fetal uptake of local anesthetics. Clin Obstet Gynecol 18:556, 1975.)

active in blocking nerve conduction. The pKa is the pH at which the concentrations of free base and cation are equal. For the amide local anesthetics, the pKa values (7.7 to 8.1) are sufficiently close to physiologic pH that changes in maternal or fetal biochemical status may significantly alter the proportion of ionized and nonionized drug present (Fig. 42-1). At equilibrium, the concentrations of nonionized drug in the fetal and maternal plasma are equal. In the case of the acidotic fetus, a greater tendency for drug to exist in the ionized form, which cannot diffuse back across the placenta into the maternal plasma, causes a larger total amount of drug to accumulate in the fetal plasma and tissues. This is the mechanism for the phenomenon termed *ion trapping*.[18]

The effects of maternal plasma protein binding on the rate and amount of drug transferred to the fetus are not so well understood. Animal studies have shown that the transfer rate is slower for drugs that are extensively bound to maternal plasma proteins, such as bupivacaine.[19] In sheep, the low fetomaternal ratio of bupivacaine plasma concentrations has been attributed to the difference between fetal and maternal plasma protein binding, rather than to extensive fetal tissue uptake.[20] However, if enough time is allowed for fetomaternal equilibrium to be approached, substantial accumulation of highly protein-bound drugs, such as bupivacaine, can occur in the fetus.[21]

4 As already stated, the driving force for placental drug transfer is the concentration gradient of free drug between the maternal and fetal blood. On the maternal side, the following factors interact: the dose administered, the mode and site of administration, and, in the case of local anesthetics, the use of vasoconstrictors. The rates of distribution, metabolism, and excretion of the drug, which may vary at different stages of pregnancy, are equally important. In general, higher doses result in higher maternal blood concentrations. The absorption rate varies with the site of drug injection. Compared with other forms of administration, an intravenous bolus results in the highest blood concentrations. It was believed that intrathecal administration of local anesthetics resulted in negligible plasma concentrations because of the small doses used and the relatively poor vascularity of this area. However, spinal anesthesia may also result in significant maternal and umbilical venous plasma concentrations of drug.

Increased maternal blood concentrations after repeated administration of a drug greatly depend on the dose and frequency of reinjection, in addition to the kinetic characteristics of the drug. The elimination half-life of amide local anesthetic agents is relatively long so repeated injection may lead to accumulation in the maternal plasma[22] (Fig. 42-2). In contrast, 2-chloroprocaine, an ester local anesthetic, undergoes rapid enzymatic hydrolysis in the presence of pseudocholinesterase. After epidural injection, the mean half-life in the mother was shown to be approximately 3 minutes; after reinjection, 2-chloroprocaine could be detected in the maternal plasma for only 5 to 10 minutes, and no accumulation of this drug was evident[23] (Fig. 42-3).

Pregnancy is associated with physiologic changes that may influence maternal pharmacokinetics and the action of anesthetic drugs. These changes may be progressive during the course of gestation and are often difficult to predict. Alterations in ventilation and lung volumes have a significant effect on the rate of uptake and excretion of inhalation agents. Of most concern to the anesthesiologist is a 20% reduction in FRC.[7] As a result, the equilibration time between the alveolar and inspired concentrations of inhalation agents is shortened.

Placenta

Maturation of the placenta can affect the rate of drug transfer to the fetus, as the thickness of the trophoblastic epithelium decreases from 25 to 2 mm at term. Uptake and biotransformation of anesthetic drugs by the placenta would decrease the amount transferred to the fetus. However, placental drug uptake is limited, and there is no evidence to suggest that this organ metabolizes any of the agents commonly used in obstetric anesthesia.

Hemodynamic Factors

Any factor decreasing placental blood flow, such as aortocaval compression, hypotension, or hemorrhage, can decrease drug delivery to the fetus. During labor, uterine contractions intermittently reduce perfusion of the placenta. If a uterine

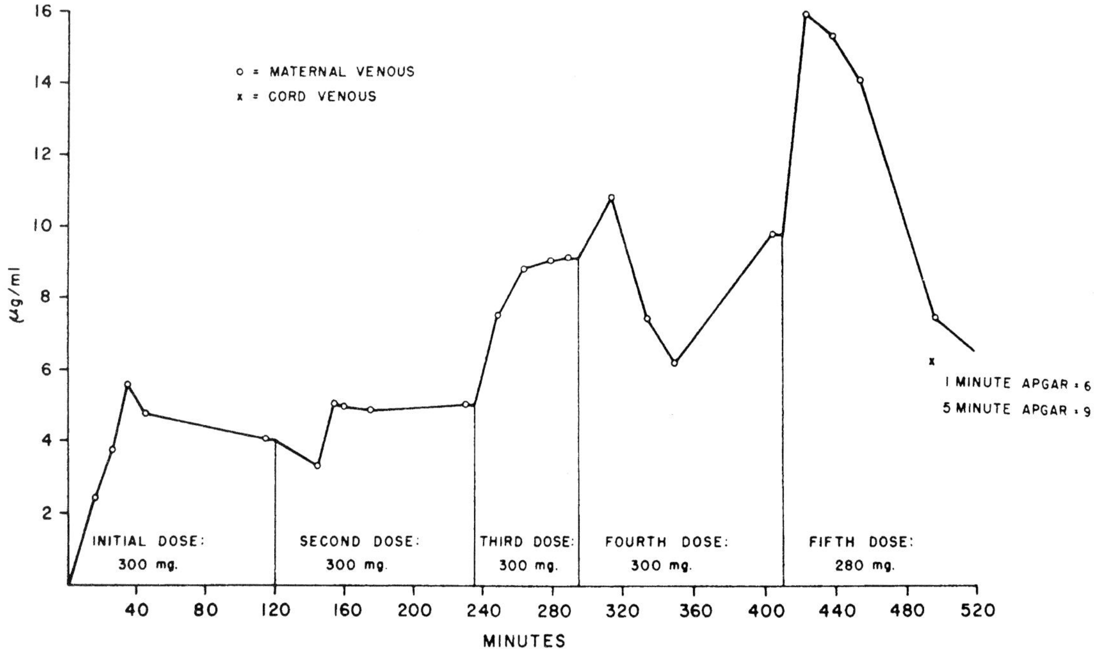

FIGURE 42-2. Increased levels of mepivacaine with each reinforcing dose in a patient receiving continuous caudal anesthesia during parturition. (Reprinted with permission from Moore DC, Bridenbaugh LD, Bagdi PA *et al*: Accumulation of mepivacaine hydrochloride during caudal block. Anesthesiology 29:585, 1968.)

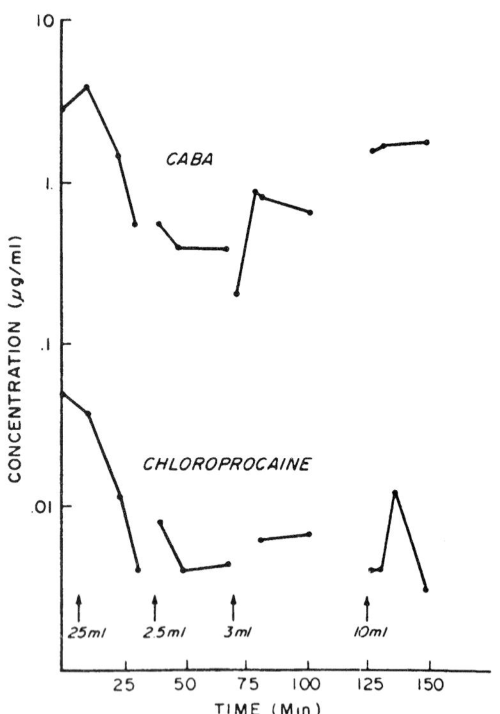

FIGURE 42-3. Plasma concentrations of chloroprocaine and chloroaminobenzoic acid (CABA) in a typical patient after epidural anesthesia (multiple injections) for vaginal delivery. (Reprinted with permission from Kuhnert BR, Kuhnert PM, Prochaska AL *et al*: Plasma levels of 2-chloroprocaine in obstetric patients and their neonates after epidural anesthesia. Anesthesiology 53:21, 1980.)

contraction coincides with a rapid decline in plasma drug concentration after an intravenous bolus injection, by the time perfusion has returned to normal, the concentration gradient across the placenta has been greatly reduced. When women were given an intravenous injection of diazepam, administered at the onset of contraction in one group and during uterine diastole in the other, less drug was found in infants born to mothers in the former group.[24]

Several characteristics of the fetal circulation delay equilibration between the umbilical arterial and venous blood, and thus delay the depressant effects of anesthetic drugs (Fig. 42-4). The liver is the first fetal organ perfused by umbilical vein blood, which carries drug to the fetus. Substantial uptake by this organ has been demonstrated for a variety of drugs, including thiopental, lidocaine, and halothane. During its transit to the arterial side of the fetal circulation, the drug is progressively diluted as blood in the umbilical vein becomes admixed with fetal venous blood from the gastrointestinal tract, the lower extremities, the head and upper extremities, and, finally, the lungs. Because of this unique pattern of fetal circulation, continuous administration of anesthetic concentrations of nitrous oxide during elective cesarean sections caused newborn depression only if the induction-to-delivery interval exceeded 5 to 10 minutes. Rapid transfer of inhalational agents, including halothane, enflurane, and isoflurane, result in detectable umbilical arterial and venous concentrations after 1 minute.[25] Because of the rapid decline in maternal plasma drug concentrations, administration of thiopental or thiamylal as a single bolus injection not exceeding 4 mg/kg was followed by fetal arterial concentrations of barbiturate below a level that would result in neonatal depression[26] (Fig. 42-5).

Fetal regional blood flow changes can also affect the amount of drug taken up by individual organs. For example, during asphyxia and acidosis, a greater proportion of the fetal cardiac output perfuses the fetal brain, heart, and placenta. Infusion of lidocaine resulted in increased drug uptake in the heart, brain, and liver of asphyxiated baboon fetuses compared with nonasphyxiated control fetuses.[27]

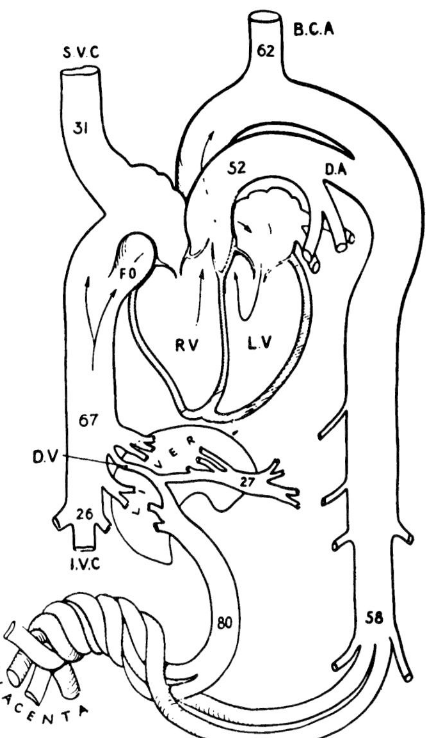

FIGURE 42-4. Diagram of the circulation in the mature fetal lamb. The numerals indicate the mean oxygen saturation (%) in the great vessels of six lambs: right ventricle (RV), left ventricle (LV), superior vena cava (SVC), inferior vena cava (IVC), brachiocephalic artery (BCA), foramen ovale (FO), ductus arteriosus (DA), ductus venosus (DV). (Reprinted with permission from Born GVR, Dawes GS, Mott JC *et al*: Changes in the heart and lungs at birth. Cold Spring Harbor Symp Quant Biol 19:103, 1954.)

Fetus and Newborn

Any drug that reaches the fetus undergoes metabolism and excretion. In this respect, the fetus has an advantage over the newborn in that it can excrete the drug back to the mother once the concentration gradient of the free drug across the placenta has been reversed. With the use of local anesthetics, this may occur even though the total plasma drug concentration in the mother may exceed that in the fetus because there is lower protein binding in fetal plasma.[20] There is only one drug, 2-chloroprocaine, that is metabolized in the fetal blood so rapidly that even in acidosis, substantial accumulation in the fetus is avoided.[23]

In both the term and the preterm newborn, the liver contains enzymes essential for the biotransformation of amide local anesthetics. A study comparing the pharmacokinetics of lidocaine among adult ewes and lambs (fetal and neonatal) showed that the metabolic clearance in the newborn was similar to, and renal clearance greater than, that in the adult.[28] Nonetheless, the elimination half-life was prolonged in the newborn. This was attributed to a greater volume of distribution and tissue uptake of the drug so at any given time the neonate's liver and kidneys were exposed to a smaller fraction of lidocaine accumulated in the body. Similar results were reported in another study involving lidocaine administration to human infants in a neonatal intensive care unit.[29] Prolonged elimination half-lives in the newborn compared with the adult have been noted for other amide local anesthetics.

The question remains whether the fetus and newborn are more sensitive than adults to the depressant and toxic effects of drugs. Laboratory investigations have shown that the newborn is, in fact, more sensitive to the depressant effects of opioids. The relative central nervous and cardiorespiratory toxicity of several local anesthetics has been studied in adult ewes and lambs (fetal and neonatal).[30] The doses required to produce toxicity in the fetus and newborn were greater than those required in the adult. In the fetus, this difference was attributed to placental clearance of drug into the mother and better maintenance of blood gas tensions during convulsions, whereas in the newborn, a larger volume of distribution is probably responsible for the higher doses needed to induce toxic effects.

Bupivacaine has been implicated as a possible cause of neonatal jaundice because its high affinity for fetal erythrocyte membranes may lead to a decrease in filterability and deformability, rendering them more prone to hemolysis. However, a more recent study has failed to show increased bilirubin production in newborns whose mothers received bupivacaine for epidural anesthesia during labor and delivery.[31] Finally, neurobehavioral studies have revealed subtle changes in newborn neurologic and adaptive function. In the case of most anesthetic agents, these changes are minor and transient, lasting for only 24 to 48 hours.

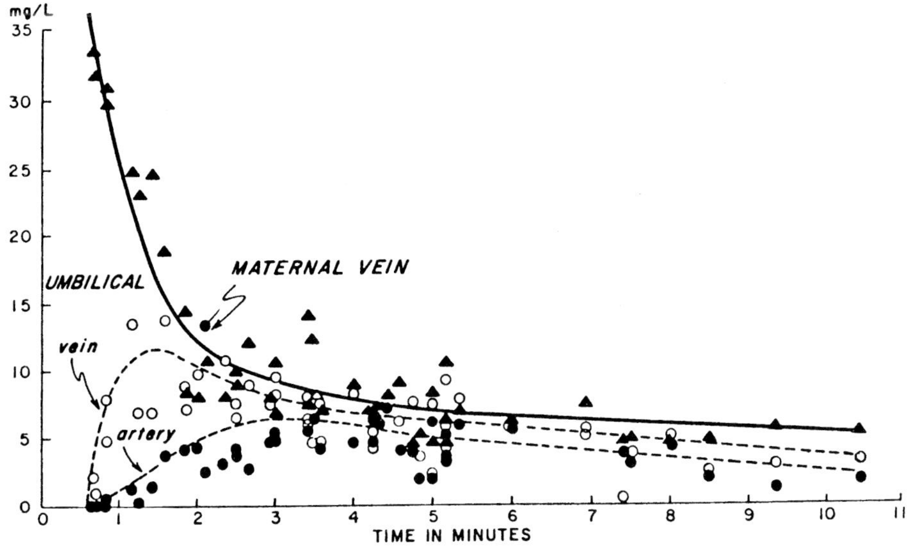

FIGURE 42-5. Cesarean section. Thiamylal concentrations in maternal vein (▲—▲), umbilical vein (○—○), and umbilical artery (●—●). Curves drawn by inspection. (Reprinted with permission from Kosaka Y, Takahashi T, Mark LS: Intravenous thiobarbiturate anesthesia for cesarean section. Anesthesiology 31:489, 1969.)

ANESTHESIA FOR LABOR AND VAGINAL DELIVERY

Most women experience moderate to severe pain during parturition. In the first stage of labor, pain is caused by uterine contractions, associated with dilation of the cervix and stretching of the lower uterine segment. Pain impulses are carried in visceral afferent type C fibers accompanying the sympathetic nerves. In early labor, only the lower thoracic dermatomes (T11–T12) are affected, but with progressing cervical dilation in the transition phase, adjacent dermatomes may be involved and pain referred from T10 to L1. In the second stage, additional pain impulses due to distention of the vaginal vault and perineum are carried by the pudendal nerves, composed of lower sacral fibers (S2–S4).

Well-conducted obstetric analgesia, in addition to relieving pain and anxiety, may benefit the mother. Pain may result in maternal hypertension and reduced uterine blood flow. During the first and second stages of labor, epidural analgesia blunts the increases in maternal cardiac output, heart rate, and blood pressure that occur with painful uterine contractions and "bearing-down" efforts.[32] In reducing maternal secretion of catecholamines, epidural analgesia may convert a previously dysfunctional labor pattern to normal. Maternal analgesia may also benefit the fetus by eliminating maternal hyperventilation, which often leads to a reduced fetal arterial oxygen tension because of a leftward shift of the maternal oxygen-hemoglobin dissociation curve.

The most frequently chosen methods for relieving the pain of parturition are psychoprophylaxis, systemic medication, and regional analgesia. Inhalational analgesia, conventional spinal analgesia, and paracervical blockade are less commonly used. General anesthesia is rarely necessary, but may be indicated for uterine relaxation in some complicated deliveries.

Psychoprophylaxis

The philosophy of prepared childbirth maintains that lack of knowledge, misinformation, fear, and anxiety can heighten a patient's response to pain and consequently increase the need for analgesics. The most popular method of prepared childbirth is that introduced by Lamaze. It provides an educational program on the physiology of parturition and attempts to diminish cortical pain perception by encouraging responses such as specific patterns of breathing and focused attention on a fixed object.[33] However, labors do vary in length and intensity; thus, it is realistic to encourage the mother in the Lamaze method, while recognizing individual variations in pain tolerance and need for pain relief. Of course, medication should not be withheld if required. Neonatal outcome appears to be similar for women who deliver infants solely with the Lamaze technique and for women who receive appropriate supplementary analgesia.

Systemic Medication

The advantages of systemic analgesics include ease of administration and patient acceptability. However, the drug, dose, time, and method of administration must be chosen carefully to avoid maternal or neonatal depression. Drugs used for systemic analgesia are opioids, tranquilizers, and occasionally ketamine.

Opioids

Meperidine is the most commonly used systemic analgesic and is reasonably effective in ameliorating pain during the first stage of labor. It can be administered by intravenous injection (effective analgesia in 5 to 10 minutes) or intramuscularly (peak effect in 40 to 50 minutes). The major side effects are a high incidence of nausea and vomiting, dose-related depression of ventilation, orthostatic hypotension, and the potential for neonatal depression. Meperidine may cause transient alterations of the fetal heart rate (FHR), such as decreased beat-to-beat variability and tachycardia. Among other factors, the risk of neonatal depression is related to the interval from the last drug injection to delivery. The placental transfer of an active metabolite, normeperidine, which has a long elimination half-life in the neonate (62 hours), has also been implicated in contributing to neonatal depression and subtle neonatal neurobehavioral dysfunction.

Experience with the newer synthetic opioids such as fentanyl, alfentanil, and remifentanil has been limited. Although they are potent, their use during labor is restricted by their short duration of action. For example, a single intravenous injection of fentanyl, up to 1 μg/kg, results in prompt pain relief without severe neonatal depression.[34] These drugs offer an advantage when analgesia of rapid onset but short duration is necessary (e.g., with forceps application). For more prolonged analgesia, fentanyl or remifentanil can be administered with patient-controlled delivery devices. Patient-controlled analgesia administration of opioid does carry with it the potential for drug accumulation and the risk of neonatal depression.[35] Opioid agonists–antagonists, such as butorphanol and nalbuphine, have also been used for obstetric analgesia. These drugs have the proposed benefits of a lower incidence of nausea, vomiting, and dysphoria, as well as a "ceiling effect" on depression of ventilation. Butorphanol 1 to 2 mg or nalbuphine 10 mg by intravenous or intramuscular injection are probably most popular. Unlike meperidine, these are biotransformed into inactive metabolites and have a ceiling effect on depression of ventilation. A potential disadvantage is a high incidence of maternal sedation.

Naloxone, a pure opioid antagonist, should not be administered to the mother shortly before delivery to prevent neonatal ventilatory depression because it reverses maternal analgesia at a time when it is most needed and, in some instances, has caused maternal pulmonary edema and even cardiac arrest. If necessary, the drug should be given directly to the newborn intramuscularly (0.1 mg/kg).

Ketamine

Ketamine is a potent analgesic. However, it may also induce unacceptable amnesia that may interfere with the mother's recollection of the birth. Nonetheless, ketamine is a useful adjuvant to incomplete regional analgesia during vaginal delivery or for obstetric manipulations. In low doses (0.2 to 0.4 mg/kg), ketamine provides adequate analgesia without causing neonatal depression. In higher doses, ketamine may induce general anesthesia. Thus, constant communication is required with the patient to ensure she is awake and able to protect her airway.

Regional Analgesia

Regional techniques provide excellent analgesia with minimal depressant effects on mother and fetus. The regional techniques most commonly used in obstetric anesthesia include central neuraxial blocks (spinal, epidural, and combined spinal/epidural or CSE), paracervical and pudendal blocks, and, less frequently, lumbar sympathetic blocks (LSBs). Hypotension resulting from sympathectomy is the most frequent complication that occurs with central neuraxial blockade. Therefore, maternal blood pressure should be monitored at regular intervals, typically every 2 to 5 minutes for approximately 15 to 20 minutes after the initiation of the block and at routine intervals thereafter. The use of regional analgesia may be contraindicated in the presence of severe coagulopathy, acute hypovolemia, or infection at the site of needle insertion. Chorioamnionitis itself, without frank sepsis, is not a contraindication to central neuraxial blockade in obstetrics.

Epidural Analgesia

Epidural analgesia may be used for pain relief during labor and vaginal delivery, and converted to anesthesia for cesarean delivery, if required. Effective analgesia during the first stage of labor may be achieved by blocking the T10–L1 dermatomes with low concentrations of local anesthetic and/or with the use of opioids, which have their effect at the opioid receptors in the dorsal horn of the spinal cord. For the second stage of labor and delivery, because of pain due to vaginal distention and perineal pressure, the block should be extended to include the S2–S4 segments.

Because of ethical considerations and methodological difficulties, it is difficult to design clinical studies to examine the effects of epidural analgesia on the progress of labor and mode of delivery. The first stage of labor may be slightly prolonged by epidural analgesia. However, this is not of clinical significance, provided aortocaval compression is avoided.[36–40] There has been concern that early initiation of epidural analgesia during the latent phase of labor (2 to 4 cm cervical dilation) in nulliparous women may result in a higher incidence of dystocia and cesarean delivery.[38–41] However, this has largely been dispelled by several large, randomized, prospective studies. Chestnut et al.[36,37] demonstrated that there was no significant difference in the incidence of cesarean delivery between nulliparous women having epidural analgesia initiated during the latent phase (<4 cm dilation) compared with control group whose analgesia was initiated during the active phase. Similarly, other investigators have demonstrated that epidural analgesia was not associated with an increased incidence of cesarean delivery compared with patient-controlled intravenous analgesia in nulliparous women.[39,40] However, a prolongation of the second stage of labor has been reported in nulliparous women, possibly owing to a decrease in expulsive forces or malposition of the vertex.[36–41] Thus, with use of epidural analgesia, the American College of Obstetricians and Gynecologists have redefined an abnormally prolonged second stage of labor as greater than 3 hours in nulliparous and 2 hours in multiparous women. Prolongation of the second stage may be minimized by the use of an ultradilute local anesthetic solution in combination with opioid. Long-acting amides such as bupivacaine, ropivacaine, or levobupivacaine are most frequently used because they produce excellent sensory analgesia while sparing motor function, particularly at the low concentrations used for epidural analgesia during labor. Analgesia for the first stage of labor may be achieved with 5 to 10 mL of bupivacaine, ropivacaine, or levobupivacaine (0.125 to 0.25%), followed by a continuous infusion (8 to 12 mL/hr) of 0.0625% bupivacaine or levobupivacaine, or 0.1% ropivacaine. Addition of fentanyl 1 to 2 μg/mL or sufentanil 0.3 to 0.5 μg/mL is often required and will allow for more dilute local anesthetic solutions to be administered. During the delivery, the sacral dermatomes may be blocked with 10 mL of 0.5% bupivacaine, 1% lidocaine, or, if a rapid effect is required, 2% chloroprocaine, in the semirecumbent position. Many parturients have adequate analgesia, particularly if epidural analgesia has been in place for a long interval, and thus do not require an additional dose of local anesthetic at the time of delivery.

There is controversy regarding the need for a test dose when using an ultradilute solution of local anesthetic.[42] Because catheter aspiration is not always diagnostic, some authors believe a test dose should be administered to improve detection of an intrathecally or intravascularly placed catheter (see Lumbar Epidural Anesthesia section under Cesarean Section).

Patient-controlled epidural analgesia (PCEA) is a safe and effective alternative to conventional bolus or infusion techniques. Maternal satisfaction is excellent and demands on anesthesia manpower reduced.

Spinal Analgesia

A single subarachnoid injection for labor analgesia has the advantages of a fast and reliable onset of neural blockade, but repeated intrathecal injections may be required for a long labor, thus increasing the risk of postdural puncture headache (PDPH). Spinal analgesia with fentanyl 10 μg or sufentanil 2 to 5 μg, alone or in combination with 1 mL isobaric bupivacaine 0.25%, may be appropriate in the multiparous patient whose anticipated course of labor does not warrant a catheter technique (duration 1.5 hours). Although infrequent, a potential disadvantage of a single-shot spinal is that the duration of labor, even in a rapidly progressing multiparous woman, may be longer than anticipated. Furthermore, if the woman requires an urgent cesarean delivery, a new anesthetic will need to be initiated. However, spinal anesthesia (a "saddle block") is a safe and effective alternative to general anesthesia for instrumental delivery.

Combined Spinal/Epidural Analgesia

CSE is an ideal analgesic technique for use during labor. CSE combines the rapid, reliable onset of profound analgesia resulting from spinal injection with the flexibility and longer duration associated with a continuous epidural technique. After identification of the epidural space using a conventional (or specialized) needle, a longer (127-mm), pencil-point spinal needle is advanced into the subarachnoid space through the epidural needle. After intrathecal injection, the spinal needle is removed, and an epidural catheter is inserted. Intrathecal injection of fentanyl 10 to 20 μg or sufentanil 2.5 to 5 μg, alone or more commonly in combination with 1 mL of isobaric bupivacaine 0.25%, produces profound analgesia lasting for 90 to 120 minutes with minimal motor block. Although opioid alone may suffice for the early latent phase, addition of bupivacaine is usually necessary for satisfactory analgesia during advanced labor. An epidural infusion of bupivacaine 0.03 to 0.0625% with added opioid may be started within 10 to 20 minutes of spinal injection. Alternatively, the epidural component may be activated when necessary. Women with hemodynamic stability and preserved motor function who do not require continuous fetal monitoring may ambulate with assistance. Before ambulation, women should be observed for 30 minutes after intrathecal or epidural drug administration to assess maternal and fetal well-being.

The most common side effects of intrathecal opioids are pruritus, nausea, vomiting, and urinary retention. Rostral spread resulting in delayed respiratory depression is rare with fentanyl and sufentanil, and usually occurs within 30 minutes of injection. Transient nonreassuring FHR patterns may occur because of uterine hyperstimulation, presumably as a result of a rapid decrease in maternal catecholamines, or because of hypotension after sympatholysis. Fetal bradycardia may occur in the absence of uterine hyperstimulation or hypotension and is unrelated to uteroplacental insufficiency. The incidence of fetal heart rate abnormalities may be greater in multiparous women with rapidly progressing, painful labors.[43] However, the incidence of emergency cesarean delivery is no greater after CSE than after conventional epidural analgesia.[44]

PDPH is always a risk after intrathecal injection. However, it has been demonstrated that the incidence of cephalalgia is no greater with CSE than with standard epidural analgesia.[45] Unintentional intrathecal catheter placement through the dural puncture site is also extremely rare after use of a 26-gauge spinal needle for CSE.[45] The potential exists for epidurally administered drug to leak into the subarachnoid space after dural puncture, particularly if large volumes of drug are rapidly injected. Indeed, epidural drug requirements are approximately 30% less with CSE than with standard lumbar epidural techniques.[46]

Mothers in early labor may particularly benefit from CSE. In early labor, spinal opioid may provide sufficient analgesia without the need for local anesthetic and almost always allows the woman to ambulate because there is no motor block—although ambulation has little effect, positive or negative, on the course of labor.[47] Because the epidural component of a CSE is not initially tested, a CSE should be used with caution in those women who may require an urgent cesarean section and are most at increased risk, such as a morbidly obese parturient with a poor airway.

Paracervical Block

Although paracervical block effectively relieves pain during the first stage of labor, the technique has fallen out of favor because it was associated with a high incidence of fetal asphyxia and poor neonatal outcome, particularly with the use of bupivacaine. This may be related to uterine artery constriction or increased uterine tone. The technique is basically simple and involves a submucosal injection of local anesthetic at the vaginal fornix, near the neural fibers innervating the uterus.

Paravertebral Lumbar Sympathetic Block

Paravertebral LSB is a reasonable alternative when contraindications exist to central neuraxial techniques. LSB interrupts the painful transmission of cervical and uterine impulses during the first stage of labor.[48] Although there is less risk of fetal bradycardia with LSB compared with paracervical blockade, technical difficulties associated with the performance of the block and risks of intravascular injection have decreased its use in standard practice.

Pudendal Nerve Block

The pudendal nerves, derived from the lower sacral nerve roots (S2–S4), supply the vaginal vault, perineum, rectum, and parts of the bladder. The nerves are easily anesthetized transvaginally where they loop around the ischial spines. Ten milliliters of local anesthetic deposited behind each sacrospinous ligament can provide adequate anesthesia for outlet forceps delivery and episiotomy repair.

Inhalation Analgesia

Inhalation analgesia is easily administered and, although it does not relieve pain completely, it may make uterine contractions more tolerable. During delivery, a combination of inhalation analgesia with a pudendal block or infiltration of the perineum with a local anesthetic may be satisfactory. A particular advantage of inhalation analgesia is that the desired level of analgesia can be easily and rapidly titrated. However, a major disadvantage of inhalational analgesia is the need for a waste gas scavenging system. Nitrous oxide, 50% by volume, is the most commonly used inhalation agent for analgesia during labor. However, the analgesia provided by intermittently self-administered 50% nitrous oxide alone has been shown to be equivalent to that of a placebo.[49]

General Anesthesia

General anesthesia is rarely used for vaginal delivery, and precautions against gastric aspiration must always be observed (see General Anesthesia section under Cesarean Section). It may be required when time constraints prevent induction of regional anesthesia. Potent inhalation drugs (1.5 to 2.0 MAC for short periods) can provide uterine relaxation for obstetric maneuvers such as second twin delivery, breech presentation, or postpartum manual removal of a retained placenta. After obstetric manipulation is completed, an intravenous infusion of oxytocin 10 to 20 U should be commenced to promote uterine contraction. In current practice, intravenous nitroglycerin (50 to 500 μg) has replaced the need for general anesthesia for uterine relaxation.

ANESTHESIA FOR CESAREAN SECTION

The most common indications for cesarean section include failure to progress, nonreassuring fetal status, cephalopelvic disproportion, malpresentation, prematurity, prior cesarean de-
5 livery, and prior uterine surgery involving the corpus.[50] The choice of anesthesia depends on the urgency of the procedure, in addition to the condition of the mother and fetus. After a comprehensive discussion of the risks and benefits of all anesthesia options, the mother's wishes should be considered.

Regional Anesthesia

A 1992 survey of obstetric anesthesia practices in the United States revealed that most patients undergoing cesarean section do so under spinal or epidural anesthesia.[51] Regional techniques have several advantages: they lessen the risk of gastric aspiration, avoid the use of depressant anesthetic drugs, and allow the mother to remain awake during delivery.[52] It has also been suggested that operative blood loss is less with regional than general anesthesia. In elective cesarean sections, the duration of antepartum anesthesia does not affect neonatal outcome provided there is no protracted aortocaval compression or hypotension. The risk of hypotension is greater than during vaginal delivery because the block must extend to at least the T4 dermatome. Proper positioning and prehydration with up to 20 mL/kg of a crystalloid solution is recommended.[53] If hypotension occurs despite these measures, left uterine displacement should be increased, the rate of intravenous infusion augmented, and intravenous ephedrine 10 to 15 mg administered incrementally, or phenylephrine 20 to 50 μg, may be used.

Spinal Anesthesia

Subarachnoid block is probably the most commonly administered regional anesthetic for cesarean delivery because of its speed of onset and reliability. It has become an alternative to general anesthesia for emergency cesarean section.[54] Hyperbaric 0.75% bupivacaine, 1.6 to 1.8 mL, is perhaps the most commonly used local anesthetic lasting approximately 120 to 180 minutes. Using 0.75% hyperbaric bupivacaine, Norris[55] showed that it is not necessary to adjust the dose of drug based on the patient's height. Hemodynamic monitoring during cesarean section should be similar to that used for other surgical procedures. Before delivery, oxygen should be routinely administered to optimize fetal oxygenation.

Despite an adequate dermatomal level for surgery, women may experience varying degrees of visceral discomfort, particularly during exteriorization of the uterus and traction on abdominal viscera. Improved perioperative analgesia can be provided with the addition of fentanyl 6.25 μg or 0.1 mg of preservative-free morphine to the local anesthetic solution. Fentanyl is short acting and provides little additional postoperative analgesia. However, morphine 0.1 mg, in addition to intraoperative anesthesia, will also provide anesthesia into the postoperative period. Nausea and vomiting may be alleviated by the administration of metoclopramide. Maternal sedation should be avoided if possible.

Lumbar Epidural Anesthesia

In contrast to spinal anesthesia, epidural anesthesia is associated with a slower onset of action and a larger drug requirement to establish an adequate sensory block. The advantages are a reduced risk of PDPH and the ability to titrate the local anesthetic through the epidural catheter. To avoid inadvertent intrathecal or intravascular injection, correct placement of the epidural catheter is essential. This is especially a concern when administering the large doses of local anesthetic required for cesarean delivery.

Aspiration of the epidural catheter for blood or cerebrospinal fluid is not reliable for detection of catheter misplacement. Thus, administration of a test dose has become popular. A small dose of local anesthetic, lidocaine 45 mg or bupivacaine 5 mg, produces a readily identifiable sensory and motor block if injected intrathecally. Addition of epinephrine (15 μg) with careful hemodynamic monitoring may signal intravascular injection if followed by a transient increase in heart rate and blood pressure. However, the use of an epinephrine test dose is controversial because false-positive results do occur in the presence of uterine contractions. In addition, epinephrine may reduce uteroplacental perfusion. Electrocardiography and application of a peak-to-peak heart rate criterion may improve detection.[56] Rapid injection of 1 mL of air with simultaneous precordial Doppler monitoring appears to be a reliable indicator of intravascular catheter placement.[57] A negative test, although reassuring, does not eliminate the need for fractional administration of local anesthetic.

The most commonly used agents are 2-chloroprocaine 3% and lidocaine 2% with epinephrine 1:200,000. Adequate anesthesia is usually achieved with 15 to 25 mL of the solution, given in divided doses. Alternatively, 0.5% bupivacaine, ropivacaine or levobupivacaine may be used if a prolonged block is desired. The patient should be monitored as with spinal anesthesia. Because of its extremely high rate of metabolism in maternal and fetal plasma, 2-chloroprocaine provides a rapid-onset, reliable block with minimal risk of systemic toxicity. It is the local anesthetic of choice in the presence of fetal acidosis and when a preexisting epidural block is to be rapidly extended for an urgent cesarean section. There has been controversy as to whether chloroprocaine antagonizes the effects of spinally administered opioids or whether the chloroprocaine block recedes so rapidly before the full onset of neuraxial morphine analgesia. Transient neurologic deficits after massive inadvertent intrathecal administration of the drug have occurred with the formulation containing a relatively high concentration of sodium bisulfite, at a low pH.[58] The most recent formulation of 2-chloroprocaine contains no additives and is packaged in an amber vial to prevent oxidation. Bupivacaine 0.5% provides profound anesthesia for cesarean section of slower onset but longer duration of action. Considerable attention has been focused on the drug since it was reported that unintentional intravascular injection could result not only in convulsions, but also in almost simultaneous cardiac arrest, with patients often refractory to resuscitation.[59] The greater cardiotoxicity of bupivacaine (and etidocaine) compared with other amide local anesthetics has been well established.[60] Lidocaine has an onset and duration intermediate to those of 2-chloroprocaine and bupivacaine. The need to include epinephrine in the local anesthetic solution to ensure adequate lumbosacral anesthesia may be of concern in women with maternal hypertension and uteroplacental insufficiency.

Prolonged postoperative pain relief can be provided by epidural administration of an opioid, such as preservative free morphine 0.3 to 0.5 mg. PCEA is another option. Delayed respiratory depression is rare, but it may occur with the use of morphine; thus, the patient must be monitored carefully in the postoperative period.

General Anesthesia

General anesthesia may be necessary when contraindications exist to regional anesthesia or when time precludes central neuraxial blockade. General anesthesia with a potent halogenated agent may also be useful in situations where uterine relaxation will facilitate delivery, as with some types of breech presentation, transverse lie, or in women with multiple gestation who may not tolerate regional blocks owing to dyspnea and supine hypotension syndrome. General anesthesia should be used cautiously in women with asthma, upper respiratory tract infection, obesity, or a history of difficult tracheal intubation. Preoperative airway evaluation is particularly important in pregnant women because inability to intubate the trachea and provide effective ventilation is the leading cause of maternal death related to anesthesia.[51] Airway assessment should include removal of all oral jewelry in anticipation of the need for general anesthesia.[52] If airway difficulties are anticipated, a regional anesthetic technique should be considered or an awake tracheal intubation performed. Premedication is usually not necessary, except for oral administration of 15 to 30 mL of a nonparticulate antacid within 30 minutes of induction of anesthesia and an H_2 receptor antagonist administered intravenously. The patient should be positioned with a wedge in place to prevent aortocaval compression. Routine monitoring should be the same as with regional anesthetic techniques and should comply with national standards.

To minimize the risk of hypoxemia during induction, denitrogenation for 3 to 5 minutes with a tight-fitting mask is essential. In an emergency, four deep breaths with 100% oxygen suffice. A "defasciculating" dose of a nondepolarizing muscle relaxant is not necessary. Rapid-sequence induction is performed with thiopental (4 mg/kg), propofol (2 mg/kg), ketamine (up to 1 mg/kg), or a combination of thiopental (2 to 3 mg/kg) and ketamine (0.5 mg/kg), followed by succinylcholine (1 to 1.5 mg/kg) to facilitate intubation. Succinylcholine is the preferred muscle relaxant. However, when its use is contraindicated, rocuronium (0.6 mg/kg) is an acceptable alternative. Cricoid pressure is applied by a trained assistant until the airway is properly secured with a cuffed endotracheal tube. If there is difficulty in securing the airway, cricoid pressure should be maintained throughout, and the mother ventilated with 100% oxygen before a subsequent attempt at tracheal intubation is made. It is safer to allow the mother to awaken and to reassess the method of induction than to persist with traumatic efforts at tracheal intubation, which may result in loss of the airway because of edema and bleeding (Fig. 42-6). Once placement of the endotracheal tube is confirmed, with capnography and auscultation, the obstetrician may proceed

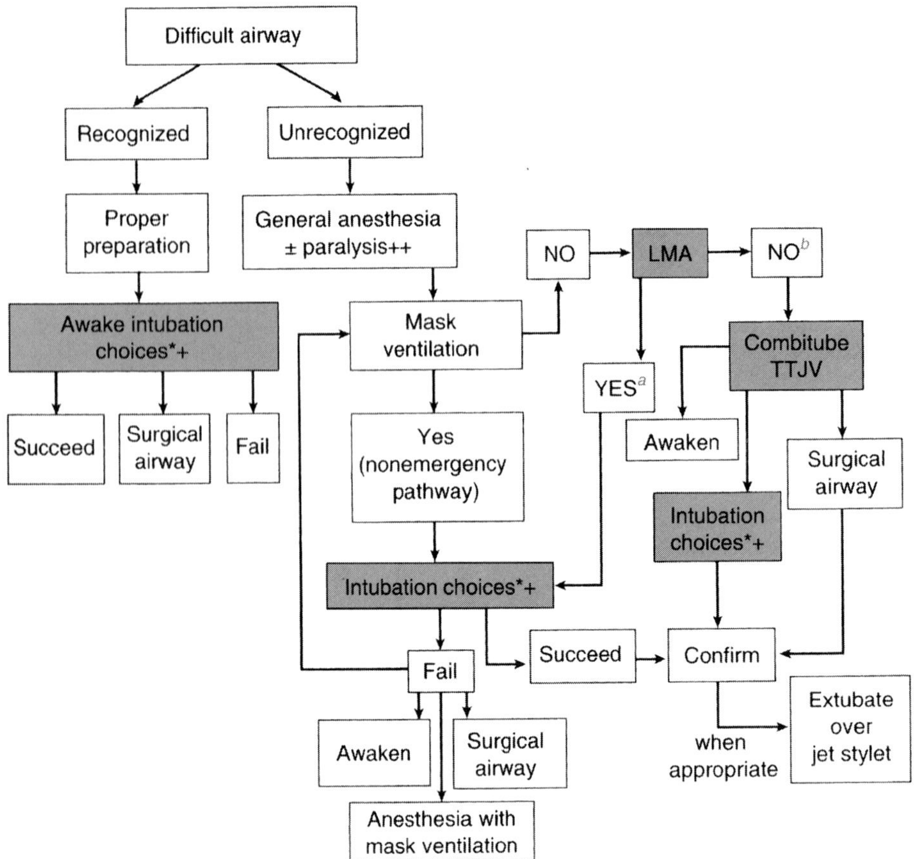

FIGURE 42-6. Management of the difficult airway in pregnancy with special reference to the presence or absence of fetal distress. When mask ventilation is not possible, the clinician is referred to the American Society of Anesthesiologists algorithm for the emergency airway management found in Chapter 22. LMA, laryngeal mask airway; TTJV, transtracheal jet ventilation [a], Ventilation through LMA adequate; [b], ventilation through LMA inadequate. (Adapted with permission from Kuczkowski KM, Reisner LS, Benumof JL, Cooper SD: The difficult airway: Risk, prophylaxis, and management, p 607. In Chestnut DH [ed]: Obstetric Anesthesia: Principles and Practice, 3rd ed. St Louis, Elsevier-Mosby, 2004.)

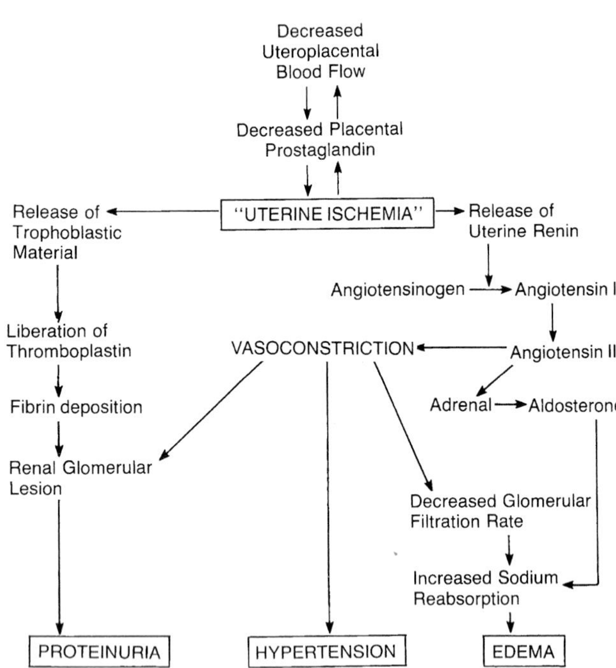

FIGURE 42-7. Proposed scheme of pathophysiologic changes in toxemia of pregnancy. (Reprinted with permission from Speroff L: Toxemia of pregnancy: Mechanism and therapeutic management. Am J Cardiol 32:582, 1973.)

with incision. If difficulty is encountered in securing the airway, it should be managed according to the American Society of Anesthesiologists algorithm for difficult airway (Fig. 42-6). It is crucial to maintain ventilation/oxygenation by mask ventilation and cricoid pressure, if necessary, by other means such as the laryngeal mask airway.[61,62] In the predelivery interval, anesthesia is maintained with a 50:50 mixture of nitrous oxide in oxygen and 0.5 MAC of a potent agent. Severe maternal hyperventilation should be avoided because it may reduce uterine blood flow. A few minutes before delivery is anticipated, the concentration of the potent agent may be increased temporarily to 2 MAC, if uterine relaxation is desired to facilitate delivery, or nitroglycerin may be used.

The newborn's condition after cesarean section with general anesthesia is comparable with that seen with regional techniques.[63] The uterine incision-to-delivery interval seems to be more important to neonatal outcome than the induction of anesthesia-to-delivery interval. Lower Apgar scores at 1 minute and acidosis were reported in cases in which the uterine incision-to-delivery time interval exceeded 180 seconds, whereas anesthesia for up to 30 minutes before delivery appears to have no adverse effects on the infant.[64] In contrast, with use of nitrous oxide 70 to 75% in oxygen, neonatal depression has been reported to occur within approximately 10 minutes of anesthesia. Increasing the FIO_2 to 50% has the additional benefit of increasing the fetal PaO_2.[57]

After delivery of the infant, 20 U of oxytocin should be added to the infusion and anesthesia is deepened with an opioid and benzodiazepine, as necessary. At the end of the procedure, the mother's trachea is extubated once she is awake and extubation criteria have been met. The usual blood loss at a cesarean section is 750 to 1,000 mL, and transfusion is rarely necessary.

ANESTHETIC COMPLICATIONS

Maternal Mortality

6 A study of anesthesia-related deaths in the United States between 1979 and 1990 revealed that the case fatality rate with general anesthesia was 16.7 times greater than that with regional anesthesia. Most anesthesia-related deaths were a result of cardiac arrest due to hypoxemia when difficulties securing the airway were encountered.[65,66] Pregnancy-induced anatomic and physiologic changes, such as reduced FRC, increased oxygen consumption, and oropharyngeal edema, may expose the patient to serious risks of desaturation during periods of apnea and hypoventilation (see Physiologic Changes of Pregnancy).

Pulmonary Aspiration

The risk of inhalation of gastric contents is increased in pregnant women, as discussed previously, particularly if difficulty is encountered establishing the airway. Measures to decrease the risks of aspiration include comprehensive airway evaluation, prophylactic administration of nonparticulate antacids, and preferred use of regional anesthesia. Occasionally, general anesthesia may be unavoidable in obstetric anesthesia practice, and therefore, awake intubation may be indicated in women in whom airway difficulties are anticipated.

Hypotension

Regional anesthesia may be associated with hypotension. The risk of hypotension is lower in women who are in labor compared with nonlaboring women.[67] Maternal prehydration up to 20 mL/kg of lactated Ringer's solution before initiation of regional anesthesia and avoidance of aortocaval compression after induction may decrease the incidence of hypotension.[53] It has been demonstrated that for effective prevention of hypotension, the blood volume increase from preloading must be sufficient to result in a significant increase in cardiac output.[68] This was possible only with the administration of hetastarch, 0.5 to 1 L.[68] Nonetheless, controversy exists regarding the efficacy of volume loading in the prevention of hypotension.[69] If hypotension does occur despite prehydration, therapeutic measures include increased displacement of the uterus, rapid infusion of intravenous fluids, titration of intravenous ephedrine (5 to 10 mg) or phenylephrine (20 to 50 μg), oxygen administration, and placement of the patient in the Trendelenburg position. Continued vigilance and active management of hypotension can prevent serious sequelae in both mother or neonate.[67]

Total Spinal Anesthesia

High or total spinal anesthesia is a rare complication of intrathecal injection that occurs after excessive cephalad spread of local anesthetic in the subarachnoid space. Unintentional intrathecal administration of epidural medication as a result of dural puncture or catheter migration may also result in this complication. Left uterine displacement, placement in the Trendelenburg position, and continued fluid and vasopressor administration may be necessary to achieve hemodynamic stability. Rapid control of the airway is essential, and endotracheal intubation may be necessary to ensure oxygenation without aspiration.

Local Anesthetic-Induced Seizures

Unintended intravascular injection or drug accumulation after repeated epidural injection can result in high serum levels of local anesthetic. Rapid absorption of local anesthetic from highly vascular sites of injection may also occur after paracervical and pudendal blocks.

Resuscitation equipment should always be available when any major nerve block is undertaken. Intravenous access, airway equipment, emergency drugs, and suction equipment should be immediately accessible. To avoid systemic toxicity of local anesthetic agents, strict adherence to recommended dosages, methods to detect misplaced needles and catheters, and fractional administration of the induction dose are essential.

Despite these precautions, life-threatening convulsions and, more rarely, cardiovascular collapse may occur. Seizure activity should be treated with intravenous thiopental 50 to 100 mg or diazepam 5 to 10 mg; larger doses may enhance local anesthetic-induced myocardial depression. The maternal airway should be secured and oxygenation maintained. If cardiovascular collapse does occur, cesarean delivery may be required to relieve aortocaval compression and to ensure the efficiency of cardiac massage.[70]

Postdural Puncture Headache

7 By virtue of age and gender, pregnant women are at a higher risk for developing PDPH. In addition, after delivery, the reduced epidural pressure increases the risk of cerebrospinal fluid leakage through the dural opening.

The frequency of PDPH is related to the diameter of the dural puncture, ranging from in excess of 70% after use of 16-gauge needles to less than 1% with the smaller 25- or 26-gauge spinal needles. The incidence of cephalalgia is reduced with the use of atraumatic pencil-point needles (Whitacre or Sprotte), which are believed to separate the dural fibers, rather than the diamond-shaped (Quincke) cutting needles. Conservative treatment is indicated in the presence of mild to moderate discomfort, and includes bed rest, hydration, and simple analgesics. Caffeine (500 mg intravenously or 300 mg orally) or theophylline have also been used in treatment of PDPH. Severe headache that does not respond to conservative measures is best treated with autologous blood patch. Using aseptic technique, 10 to 15 mL of the patient's blood is injected into the epidural space close to the site of dural puncture. This procedure may be repeated as necessary and is associated with excellent success rates. If an epidural catheter is in place after delivery, there is sufficient evidence to support the efficacy of injecting 15 to 20 mL of autologous blood may be injected through the catheter before removal.[71]

Nerve Injury

Neurologic sequelae of central neuraxial blockade, although rare, have been reported. Pressure exerted by a needle or catheter on spinal nerve roots produces immediate pain and requires repositioning. Infections such as epidural abscess or meningitis are rare and may be a manifestation of systemic sepsis. Epidural hematoma can also occur, usually in association with coagulation defects. Nerve root irritation may have a protracted recovery, lasting weeks or months. Peripheral nerve injury as a result of instrumentation, lithotomy position, or compression by the fetal head may occur even in the absence of neuraxial technique.[72]

MANAGEMENT OF HIGH-RISK PARTURIENTS

8 Pregnancy and parturition are considered "high risk" when accompanied by conditions unfavorable to the well-being of the mother, the fetus, or both. Maternal problems may be related to pregnancy, such as preeclampsia–eclampsia and other hypertensive disorders of pregnancy, or antepartum hemorrhage resulting from placenta previa or abruptio placentae. Diabetes mellitus; cardiac, chronic renal, neurologic, or sickle cell disease; and asthma, obesity, and drug abuse are not related to pregnancy but are often affected by it. Prematurity (gestation of less than 37 weeks), postmaturity (42 weeks or longer), intrauterine growth retardation, and multiple gestation are fetal conditions associated with risk. During labor and delivery, fetal malpresentation (breech, transverse lie), placental abruption, compression of the umbilical cord (prolapse, nuchal cord), precipitous labor, or intrauterine infection (prolonged rupture of membranes) may increase the risk to the mother or the fetus.

In general, the anesthetic management of the high-risk parturient is based on the same maternal and fetal considerations as the management of healthy mothers and fetuses. These include maintenance of maternal cardiovascular function and oxygenation, maintenance and possibly improvement of uteroplacental blood flow, and creation of optimal conditions for a painless, atraumatic delivery of an infant without significant drug effects. However, there is less room for error because many of these functions may be compromised before the induction of anesthesia. For example, significant acidosis is prone to develop in fetuses of diabetic mothers when delivered by cesarean section with spinal anesthesia complicated by even brief maternal hypotension.[10] Because the high-risk parturient may have received a variety of drugs, anesthesiologists must be familiar with potential interactions between these drugs and the anesthetic drugs they plan to administer.

Preeclampsia–Eclampsia

Hypertensive disorders, which occur in approximately 7% of all late pregnancies, are among the major causes of maternal mortality. Preeclampsia is diagnosed on the basis of development of hypertension with proteinuria. The added appearance of convulsions makes for the diagnosis of eclampsia. Preeclampsia–eclampsia is a disease unique to human pregnancy, occurring predominantly in young nulliparas. Symptoms usually appear after the twentieth week of gestation, occasionally earlier than that if in association with a hydatidiform mole. The condition requires the presence of a trophoblast but not a fetus.

The origin of preeclampsia–eclampsia is unknown. Many of the symptoms associated with preeclampsia, including placental ischemia, systemic vasoconstriction, and increased platelet aggregation, may result from an imbalance between the placental production of prostacyclin and thromboxane (Figs. 42-7 and 42-8). During normal pregnancy the placenta produces equivalent quantities of these prostaglandins, whereas in preeclamptic pregnancy, there is seven times more thromboxane than prostacyclin.[73] Endothelial cell injury is central to the development of preeclampsia. This injury occurs as a result of reduced placental perfusion leading to a production and release of substances (possibly lipid peroxidases), and causing endothelial cell injury. Abnormal endothelial cell function contributes to an increase in peripheral resistance and other abnormalities noted in preeclampsia through a release of fibronectin, endothelin, and other substances.

Placental ischemia related to preeclampsia results in a release of uterine renin and an increase in angiotensin activity

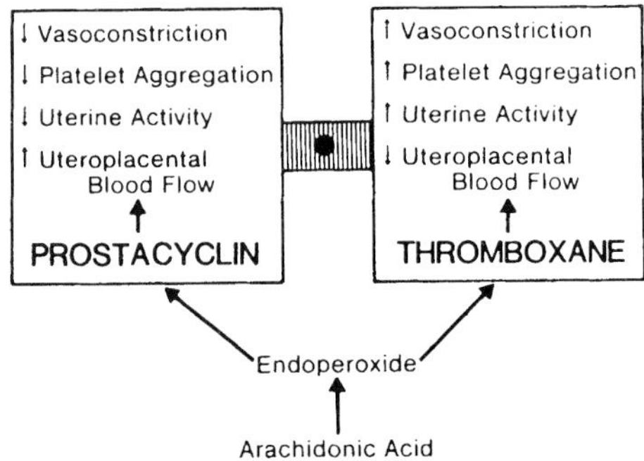

PREECLAMPSIA

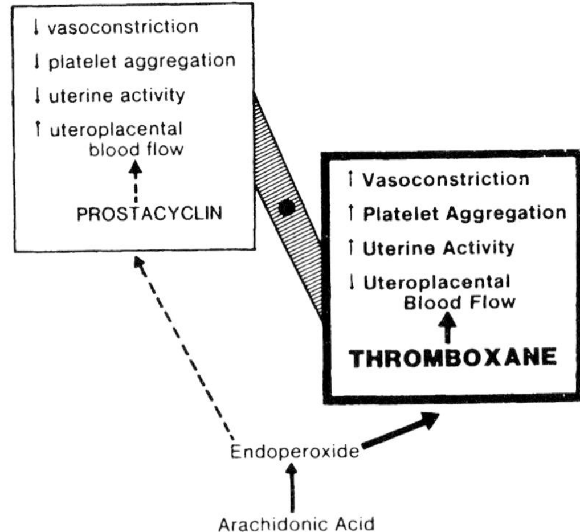

FIGURE 42-8. Comparison of the balance in the biological actions of prostacyclin and thromboxane in normal pregnancy with the imbalance of increased thromboxane and decreased prostacyclin in preeclamptic pregnancy. (Reprinted with permission from Walsh SW: Preeclampsia: An imbalance in placental prostacyclin and thromboxane production. Am J Obstet Gynecol 152:335, 1985.)

(see Fig. 42-7). This would lead to a widespread arteriolar vasoconstriction, causing hypertension, tissue hypoxia, and endothelial damage. Adherence of platelets at sites of endothelial damage would result in coagulopathies, occasionally in disseminated intravascular coagulation. Enhanced angiotensin-mediated aldosterone secretion would lead to an increased sodium reabsorption and edema. Proteinuria, another symptom of preeclampsia, may also be attributed to placental ischemia, which would lead to local tissue degeneration and a release of thromboplastin with subsequent deposition of fibrin in constricted glomerular vessels, as well as increased permeability to albumin and other plasma proteins. Furthermore, there is believed to be a decreased production of prostaglandin E, a potent vasodilator secreted in the trophoblast, which normally would balance the hypertensive effects of the renin–angiotensin system. The HELLP syndrome is a particular form of severe preeclampsia characterized by *h*emolysis, *e*levated *l*iver enzymes, and *l*ow *p*latelet count (thrombocytopenia). In contrast to preeclampsia, elevations in blood pressure and proteinuria may be mild.

9 Preeclampsia is classified as severe if it is associated with any of the following:

1. Severe hypertension
   a. Systolic blood pressure of 160 mm Hg
   b. Diastolic blood pressure of 110 mm Hg
2. Severe proteinuria of 5 g/24 hr

3. Evidence of severe end-organ damage
   a. Refractory oliguria (400 mL/24 hr)
   b. Cerebral or visual disturbances
   c. Pulmonary edema or cyanosis
   d. Epigastric pain
   e. Intrauterine growth retardation

In severe preeclampsia–eclampsia, all major organ systems are affected because of widespread vasospasm. Global cerebral blood flow is not diminished, but focal hypoperfusion may occur. Indeed, postmortem examination has revealed hemorrhagic necrosis in the proximity of thrombosed precapillaries, suggesting intense vasoconstriction. Cerebral edema and small foci of degeneration have been attributed to hypoxia. Petechial hemorrhages are common after the onset of convulsions. Symptoms related to these changes include headache, vertigo, cortical blindness, hyperreflexia, and convulsions. The extent of blood pressure elevation correlates poorly with the incidence of seizures, which are commonly generalized. Cerebral hemorrhage and edema are the leading causes of death in preeclampsia–eclampsia, together accounting for approximately 50% of deaths.

In the eyes, intense arteriolar constriction may result in blurred vision, even temporary blindness. Heart failure may occur in severe cases as a result of peripheral vasoconstriction and increased blood viscosity secondary to hemoconcentration. Changes described in autopsy specimens include left ventricular hypertrophy, subendocardial hemorrhages, cloudy swelling, and fatty and hyaline degeneration.

Decreased blood supply to the liver may lead to periportal necrosis of variable extent and severity. Subcapsular hemorrhages account for the epigastric pain encountered in severe cases. Rarely, there is rupture of the overstretched liver capsule and massive hemorrhage into the abdominal cavity. Hepatic function tests show elevated plasma levels of aspartate aminotransferase, lactate dehydrogenase, and alkaline phosphatase, whereas bilirubin is unaltered.

In the kidneys, there is swelling of glomerular endothelial cells and deposition of fibrin, leading to a constriction of the capillary lumina. Renal blood flow and glomerular filtration rate decrease, resulting in reduced uric acid clearance and, in severe cases, reduced clearance of urea and creatinine. As already stated, oliguria and proteinuria are among the characteristic symptoms of severe preeclampsia. The severity of renal involvement is reflected in the degree of proteinuria, which may reach nephrotic levels of 10 to 15 g/24 hr.

A mild degree of pulmonary ventilation–perfusion imbalance has been reported in severe cases. It is not believed to be clinically important because the arterial oxygen tension was within normal limits. In contrast, airway edema, which may also occur in severe preeclampsia, is of great concern because it may lead to respiratory embarrassment and difficulty in tracheal intubation. Pulmonary edema is commonly found at autopsy. It may result from heart failure, circulatory overload, or aspiration of gastric contents during convulsions.

In the placenta, a reduction in intervillous blood flow may result from vasoconstriction or the development of occlusive lesions in decidual arteries, despite the elevated maternal blood pressure. Histologic examination of the placenta often reveals nodular ischemia and varying stages of infarction. Necrosis of the supporting tissues may lead to a rupture of fetal cotyledonary vessels and hemorrhage. If the hemorrhage is extensive, it may extend retroplacentally, initiating the process of abruption. Reduced placental blood flow leads to chronic fetal hypoxia and malnutrition. The risks of intrauterine growth retardation, premature birth, and perinatal death are substantially higher than in normal pregnancies and correlate with the severity of preeclampsia.

Although preeclampsia is accompanied by exaggerated retention of water and sodium, a shift of fluid and proteins from the intravascular into the extravascular compartment may result in hypovolemia, hypoproteinemia, and hemoconcentration. This phenomenon may be further aggravated by proteinuria. The risk of uteroplacental hypoperfusion and poor fetal outcome correlates with the degree of maternal plasma and protein depletion. The mean plasma volume in women with preeclampsia was found to be 9% less than normal, and in those with severe disease it was as much as 30 to 40% below normal.[66] The inverse relationship between the intravascular volume and the severity of hypertension was confirmed with measurements of central venous pressure (CVP; Fig. 42-9). Patients with a diastolic pressure of 110 mm Hg may have a CVP as low as –4 cm H_2O and may require careful hydration to increase the CVP. A significant reduction in maternal plasma volume may precede the clinical appearance of preeclampsia in previously normotensive patients.

Hemodynamic changes in preeclampsia may vary with the progression of the disease, whether patients are in labor or have received therapy. Earlier studies, using pulmonary artery flow-directed catheters, suggested patients with severe preeclampsia were in a hyperdynamic state. However, these investigations were performed when patients were in labor or in the postpartum period, after treatment had been instituted. More

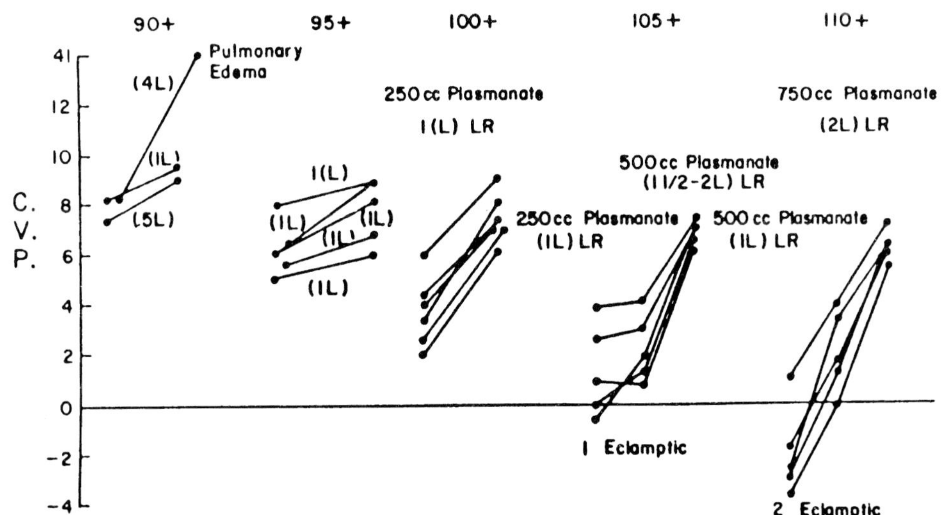

FIGURE 42-9. Initial central venous pressure (CVP) measurements (three or more recordings of maternal diastolic pressure) and intravenous volume replacement required to attain the range of 6 to 8 cm H_2O in five groups of women with preeclampsia classified according to the severity of the disease (by diastolic BP). LR, lactated Ringer's solution. (Reprinted with permission from Joyce TH III, Debnath KS, Baker EA: Preeclampsia: Relationship of CVP and epidural analgesia. Anesthesiology 51:S297, 1979.)

TABLE 42-2

HEMODYNAMIC VARIABLES (MEAN AND RANGE) IN PREECLAMPTIC PATIENTS AND CONTROL SUBJECTS

VARIABLE	PREECLAMPTIC PATIENTS ($n = 10$) INITIAL	AFTER VOLUME EXPANSION	p^a	AFTER VASODILATION	p^b	CONTROL SUBJECTS ($n = 4$)
Diastolic blood pressure (mm Hg)	106 (100–120)	102 (90–120)	NS	85 (75–100)	<.01	77 (70–90)
Mean arterial pressure (mm Hg)	121 (113–136)	116 (103–136)	<.02	102 (97–116)	<.01	95 (93–106)
Heart rate (beats/min)	100 (90–130)	81 (60–110)	<.02	82 (70–100)	NS	84 (70–90)
Pulmonary capillary wedge pressure (mm Hg)	3.3 (1–5)	8 (7–10)	<.01	8 (7–9)	NS	9 (6–12)
Systemic vascular resistance (dyne/sec/cm^5)	1,943 (1,480–2,580)	1,284 (1,073–1,600)	<.01	947 (782–1,028)	<.01	886 (805–1,021)
Cardiac index (L/min/m^2)	2.75 (1.97–3.33)	3.77 (3.26–4.05)	<.01	4.40 (3.94–5.00)	<.01	4.53 (3.96–4.97)

NS, not significant. Wilcoxon signed-rank test (two-tailed).
[a]As compared with initial values.
[b]As compared with values after volume expansion.
Reproduced with permission from Groenendijk R, Trimbos MJ, Wallenberg HCS: Hemodynamic measurements in pre-eclampsia: Preliminary observations. Am J Obstet Gynecol 150:232, 1984.

recently, hemodynamic data were obtained in 10 preeclamptic and 4 healthy pregnant women near term who were not in labor[75] (Table 42-2). In the preeclamptic women, measurements were made before treatment, after volume expansion, and after vasodilation was achieved with a continuous intravenous infusion of dihydralazine. Initial measurements revealed a low pulmonary capillary wedge pressure, a low cardiac index, a high systemic vascular resistance, and an increased heart rate, indicating the existence of a low-output state in untreated preeclamptic women. Volume expansion resulted in a significant increase in pulmonary capillary wedge pressure and cardiac index, whereas the systemic vascular resistance and maternal heart rate decreased. The mean arterial pressure was significantly reduced, mainly because of a decrease in systolic pressure. Subsequent infusion of dihydralazine did not alter the capillary wedge pressure but led to an additional increase in cardiac index and a decrease in systemic vascular resistance. These data indicate that careful volume expansion may improve maternal tissue perfusion in severe preeclampsia.

Simultaneous determinations of CVP and pulmonary capillary wedge pressure were obtained in another group of 18 patients with severe preeclampsia.[76] In approximately half of the cases, there was a linear relation between the two modalities, but even in these women it was difficult to predict the pulmonary capillary wedge pressure from the CVP because of wide interindividual variations.

Adherence of platelets at sites of endothelial damage may result in consumption coagulopathy. Thrombocytopenia is the most frequent finding. It is usually mild, with the platelet count in the range of 100,000 to 150,000 per mm^3. The use of high dose steroids (>24 mg of beta or dexamethasone in 24 hours) to accelerate fetal lung maturity has been shown in a retrospective study to prevent a further decrease in platelet count or even increase platelet count in women with HELLP[77] (Fig. 42-10). Elevated levels of fibrin degradation products are found less frequently, and plasma fibrinogen concentrations remain normal unless there is a placental abruption. Prolongation of prothrombin and partial thromboplastin times indicates consumption of procoagulant. Bleeding time is no longer considered a reliable test of clotting.

General Management

Because the origin of preeclampsia–eclampsia is not known, management is symptomatic, until such time as the obstetrician determines that delivery is appropriate for the fetus. The definitive treatment of preeclampsia–eclampsia remains delivery of the fetus and placenta. The goals are to prevent or control convulsions, improve organ perfusion, normalize blood pressure, and correct clotting abnormalities. Mild cases may be managed expectantly with bed rest, antihypertensive medication, and fetal surveillance until the pregnancy is closer to term. Delivery is indicated in refractory cases, if there is nonreassuring fetal status or if the pregnancy is already close to term. In severe cases, aggressive management should continue for at least 24 to 48 hours after delivery.

The mainstay of anticonvulsant therapy in the United States is magnesium sulfate. Although its efficacy in preventing seizures has been well substantiated, its mechanism of action remains controversial. The patient usually receives an intravenous loading dose of 4 g in a 20% solution, administered

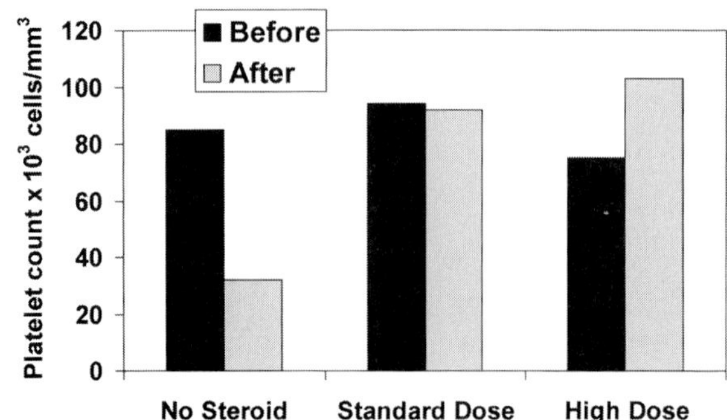

FIGURE 42-10. Mean platelet count in women with HELLP syndrome without steroids, and before and after standard steroid (<24 mg/day) and high steroid (>24 mg/day) therapy. (Adapted from O'Brien JM, Milligan DA, Barton JR. Impact of high dose corticosteroid therapy for patients with HELLP [hemolysis, elevated liver function tests, and low platelets] syndrome. Am J Obstet Gynecol 183:921, 2000.)

over 5 minutes. Therapeutic blood levels are maintained by continuous infusion of 1 to 2 g/hr. In addition to its anticonvulsant properties, by causing mild peripheral arterial vasodilation, magnesium sulfate may affect the maternal hemodynamic state. Magnesium ions cross the placenta readily, and may lead to fetal and neonatal hypermagnesemia. There is poor correlation between magnesium concentrations in the umbilical cord blood and the incidence of low Apgar scores and depression of ventilation at birth, which are more likely due to fetal asphyxia and prematurity.

Magnesium potentiates the duration and intensity of action of depolarizing and nondepolarizing muscle relaxants by decreasing the amount of acetylcholine liberated from the motor nerve terminals, diminishing the sensitivity of the endplate to acetylcholine, and depressing the excitability of the skeletal muscle membrane. Magnesium may also increase the severity of hypotension under regional anesthesia and make it more difficult to treat. Judicious hydration with a balanced salt solution may be required to replace intravascular volume. In all cases, careful monitoring of arterial pressure and urine output should be started as soon as possible. In severe cases, invasive central pressure monitoring may be required.[76] A pulmonary artery catheter is preferred in patients with pulmonary edema, refractory hypertension, or oliguria.[76] Monitoring should also be carried out in the postpartum period, preferably in the recovery room or intensive care setting.

Antihypertensive therapy in preeclampsia is used to lessen the risk of cerebral hemorrhage in the mother while maintaining, even improving, tissue perfusion. Plasma volume expansion combined with vasodilation fulfills these goals.[75] Hydralazine is the most commonly used vasodilator in preeclampsia because it increases uteroplacental and renal blood flows. It can be administered orally, intramuscularly, or intravenously. Nitroprusside, a potent vasodilator of resistance and capacitance vessels, with an immediate but evanescent action, is useful in preventing dangerous elevations in systemic and pulmonary artery blood pressure during laryngoscopy and intubation, and is ideal for treatment of hypertensive emergencies. Nitroprusside infusion can be decreased gradually in the interim as a longer-acting agent, such as hydralazine, begins to take effect. Infusion rates of nitroprusside less than 5 to 10 mg/kg/min, depending on the length of administration, can be maintained without undue risk of cyanide toxicity to the mother and fetus. Other agents used to control maternal blood pressure in preeclampsia include nitroglycerin and labetalol, a nonselective beta-blocker with some α_1-blocking effects.

Consumption coagulopathy may require corrective measures such as infusion of fresh whole blood, platelet concentrates, fresh frozen plasma, and cryoprecipitate. The administration of conduction anesthesia is contraindicated in patients with severe coagulopathy because of the increased risk of an epidural hematoma, leading to permanent neurologic damage.

Anesthetic Management

Epidural anesthesia (or CSE) for labor and delivery should no longer be considered contraindicated, provided there is no severe clotting abnormality or plasma volume deficit.[78] In volume-repleted patients positioned with left uterine displacement, regional anesthesia does not cause an unacceptable reduction in blood pressure and leads to a significant improvement in placental perfusion.[79] With the use of radioactive xenon, it was shown that the intervillous blood flow increased by approximately 75% after the induction of epidural analgesia (10 mL of bupivacaine 0.25%).[80] The total maternal body clearance of amide local anesthetics may be prolonged in preeclampsia, and repeated administration of these drugs can lead to higher blood concentrations than in normotensive patients.[81]

For cesarean section, the sensory level of regional anesthesia must extend to T3–T4, making adequate fluid therapy and left uterine displacement even more vital. In two more recent studies, the incidence of hypotension, perioperative fluid and ephedrine administration, and neonatal conditions were found to be similar in preeclamptic women who received either epidural or spinal anesthesia for cesarean delivery.[82,83]

General anesthesia in preeclamptic patients has its particular hazards. Rapid-sequence induction of anesthesia and intubation of the trachea necessary to avoid aspiration are occasionally difficult because a swollen tongue, epiglottis, or pharynx distorts the anatomy. In patients with impaired coagulation, laryngoscopy and intubation of the trachea may provoke profuse bleeding. Marked systemic and pulmonary hypertension occurring at intubation and extubation enhance the risk of cerebral hemorrhage and pulmonary edema (Fig. 42-11). However, these hemodynamic changes can be minimized with appropriate antihypertensive therapy, such as administration of labetalol or nitroprusside infusion. The use of ketamine and ergot alkaloids should be avoided. As already mentioned, magnesium sulfate may prolong the effects of all muscle relaxants through its actions on the myoneural junction. Therefore, relaxants should be administered with caution (using a nerve stimulator) to avoid overdosage. General anesthesia may be necessary in acute emergencies, such as abruptio placentae, and in patients who do not meet the criteria for regional anesthesia.

Antepartum Hemorrhage

10 Antepartum hemorrhage occurs most commonly in association with placenta previa (abnormal implantation on the lower uterine segment and partial to total occlusion of the internal cervical os) or abruptio placentae. Placenta previa occurs in 0.1 to 1.0% of all pregnancies, resulting in up to a 0.9% incidence of maternal and a 17 to 26% incidence of perinatal mortality. Placenta previa may be associated with abnormal fetal presentation, such as transverse lie or breech. It should be suspected whenever a patient presents with painless, bright red vaginal bleeding, usually after the seventh month of pregnancy. The diagnosis is confirmed by ultrasonography. If the bleeding is not profuse and the fetus is immature, obstetric management is conservative to prolong pregnancy. In severe cases, or if the fetus is mature at the onset of symptoms, prompt delivery is indicated, usually by cesarean section. An emergency hysterectomy may be required because of severe hemorrhage, even after delivery of the placenta, because of uterine atony. The risk of severe hemorrhage after attempted removal of a placenta previa is greatly increased in patients who have undergone prior uterine surgery, including cesarean section. This is due to a higher incidence of placenta accreta, which results from the penetration of myometrium by placental villi. After one previous cesarean delivery, placenta accreta was reported to occur in 20 to 25% of patients with placenta previa, and after four or more prior cesarean sections, the incidence is greater than 67%.[84]

Abruptio placentae occurs in 0.2 to 2.4% of pregnant women, usually in the final 10 weeks of gestation and usually in association with hypertensive diseases. Complications include Couvelaire uterus (when extravasated blood dissects between the myometrial fibers), renal failure, disseminated intravascular coagulation, and anterior pituitary necrosis (Sheehan's syndrome). The maternal mortality rate is high (1.8 to 11.0%), and the perinatal mortality rate is even higher, in excess of 50%. The diagnosis of abruptio placentae is based on the presence of uterine tenderness and hypertonus, as well

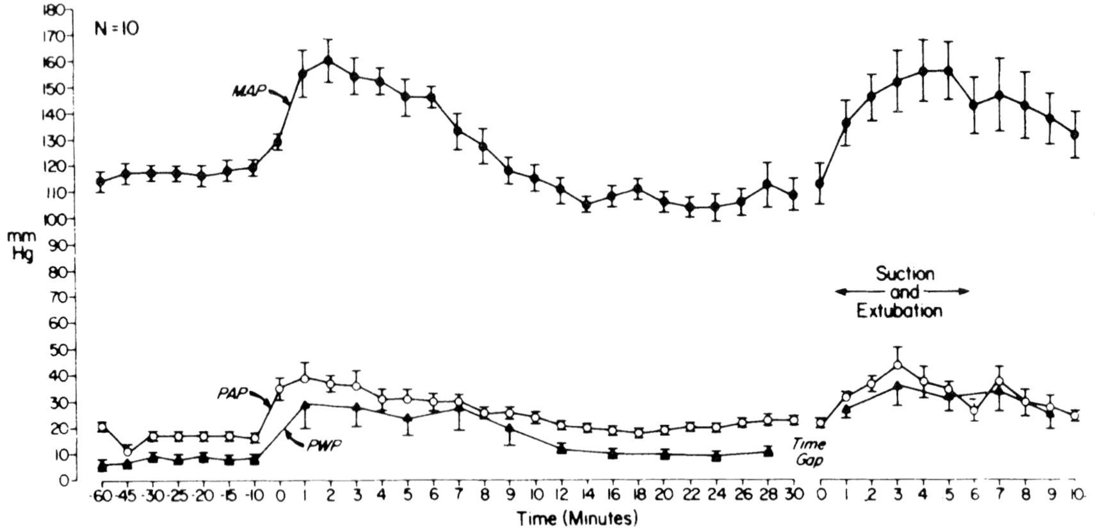

FIGURE 42-11. Mean and SE of mean arterial pressure (MAP), mean pulmonary artery pressure (PAP), and pulmonary wedge pressure (PWP) in patients with severe preeclampsia receiving thiopental and nitrous oxide (40%) with 0.5% halothane anesthesia for cesarean section. (Reprinted with permission from Hodgkinson R, Husain FJ, Hayashi RH: Systemic and pulmonary blood pressure during cesarean section in parturients with gestational hypertension. Can Anaesth Soc J 27:389, 1980.)

as vaginal bleeding of dark, clotted blood. Bleeding may be concealed if the placental margins have remained attached to the uterine wall. If the blood loss is severe (>2 L), there may be changes in the maternal blood pressure and pulse rate indicative of hypovolemia. Fetal movements may increase during acute hypoxia or decrease if hypoxia is gradual. Fetal bradycardia and death may ensue. Management of milder cases of abruption includes artificial rupture of amniotic membranes and oxytocin augmentation of labor, if required. In the presence of nonreassuring fetal status, an emergency cesarean section may be performed.

The anesthesiologist is involved in both maternal resuscitation and provision of anesthesia. This may include establishment of invasive monitoring (an arterial and a central venous catheter are usually adequate) and blood volume replacement, preferably through 14- or 16-gauge cannulae. If clotting abnormalities are present, fresh frozen plasma, cryoprecipitate, and platelet concentrates may be required. The anesthesiologist also performs the traditional role of providing appropriate anesthesia for a cesarean section or a cesarean hysterectomy. The choice of anesthetic technique depends on the anticipated duration of surgery, maternal condition and volume status, the potential for coagulopathy and urgency of the procedure. General anesthesia is indicated in the presence of uncontrolled hemorrhage and/or severe coagulation abnormalities.[85] However, continuous epidural anesthesia has been successfully used for hysterectomy in planned, controlled situations.[85]

Heart Disease

11 Heart disease during pregnancy occurs in 0.4 to 4.1% of patients and is a leading nonobstetric cause of maternal mortality, with a mortality rate ranging from 0.4% among patients in class I or II of the New York Heart Association's functional classification to 6.8% among those in classes III and IV. The following lesions pose the greatest risk for the mother: pulmonary hypertension, particularly with Eisenmenger's syndrome; mitral stenosis with atrial fibrillation; tetralogy of Fallot; Marfan's syndrome; and coarctation of the aorta. Cardiac decompensation and death occur most commonly at the time of maximum hemodynamic stress, that is, in the third trimester of pregnancy, during labor and delivery, and particularly during the immediate postpartum period. During labor, cardiac output increases above antepartum levels. Between contractions, this increase is approximately 15% in the early first stage, approximately 30% during the late first stage, approximately 45% during the second stage, and after delivery 30 to 50%. With each uterine contraction, approximately 200 mL of blood is squeezed out of the uterus into the central circulation. Consequently, stroke volume, cardiac output, and left ventricular work increase, and each contraction consistently increases cardiac output by 10 to 25% above that of uterine diastole. The greatest change occurs immediately after delivery of the placenta, when cardiac output increases to an average of 80% above prepartum values, and in some patients, it may increase by as much as 150%. These changes in cardiac output can be reduced by administration of regional anesthesia. In patients managed with continuous caudal anesthesia, cardiac output increased only 24% above prepartum control values during the second stage and 59% immediately postpartum.[30] A multidisciplinary approach is best when managing patients with complicated cardiac disease. All members of the team should be aware of the management plan for when the patient arrives in labor or requires a cesarean section. For the anesthesiologist, it is particularly important to know how the hemodynamic consequences of different anesthetic techniques could adversely affect mothers with specific cardiac lesions.

PRETERM DELIVERY

Preterm labor and delivery present a significant challenge to the anesthesiologist because the mother and the infant may be at risk. The definition of prematurity was altered to distinguish between the preterm infant, born before the thirty-seventh week of gestation is completed, and the small-for-gestational-age infant, who may be born at term but whose weight is more than 2 standard deviations below the mean. Although preterm deliveries occur in 8 to 10% of all births, they account for approximately 80% of early neonatal deaths. In general, the mortality and morbidity rates are higher among preterm infants than among small-for-gestational-age infants of comparable weight. Severe problems, including respiratory distress syndrome, intracranial hemorrhage, hypoglycemia, hypocalcemia, and hyperbilirubinemia, are prone to develop in preterm infants. Fortunately, with improved neonatal intensive care, severe, lasting impairment, such as cerebral palsy, mental retardation, or chronic lung disease, has become infrequent among the survivors.

Obstetricians frequently try to inhibit preterm labor to enhance fetal lung maturity. Delaying delivery by even 24 to 48 hours may be beneficial if glucocorticoids are administered to the mother. Various agents have been used to suppress uterine activity (tocolysis), including ethanol, magnesium sulfate, prostaglandin inhibitors, β-sympathomimetics, and calcium channel blockers. β-Adrenergic drugs, such as ritodrine and terbutaline, are the most commonly used tocolytics. These agents are initially administered by an intravenous infusion at the rate of 0.05 to 0.1 mg/min for ritodrine and 0.01 mg/min for terbutaline. Their predominant effect is β_2 receptor stimulation, resulting in myometrial inhibition, vasodilation, and bronchodilation. Numerous maternal complications may occur: hypotension, hypokalemia, hyperglycemia, myocardial ischemia, pulmonary edema, and death.[86] Complications also may occur because of interactions with anesthetic drugs and techniques. With the use of regional anesthesia, peripheral vasodilation caused by β-adrenergic stimulation increases the risk of hypotension. Acute prehydration must be managed carefully to avoid pulmonary edema. General anesthesia may be associated with increased risks of hemodynamic instability in the presence of preexisting tachycardia, hypotension, and hypokalemia. Caution should be exercised with use of halothane (cardiac dysrhythmias), atropine, and pancuronium (tachycardia). In nonemergent situations, delay of anesthesia by at least 3 hours from the cessation of tocolysis allows β-mimetic effects to dissipate. Potassium supplementation is usually not necessary because the intracellular potassium concentration is normal, despite a reduction in serum concentrations.

It has become axiomatic that the premature infant is more vulnerable than the term newborn to the effects of drugs used in obstetric analgesia and anesthesia. However, there have been few systematic studies to determine the maternal and fetal pharmacokinetics and dynamics of drugs throughout gestation. There are several postulated causes of enhanced drug sensitivity in the preterm newborn: less protein available for drug binding; higher levels of bilirubin, which may compete with the drug for protein binding; greater drug access to the central nervous system (CNS) because of a poorly developed blood-brain barrier; greater total body water and lower fat content; and a decreased ability to metabolize and excrete drugs. However, these deficiencies of the preterm infant should not be as serious as we have been led to believe. Although the serum albumin and α_1-acid glycoprotein concentrations are lower in the preterm fetus, this would primarily affect drugs that are highly bound to these proteins. However, most drugs used in anesthesia exhibit only low to moderate degrees of binding in the fetal serum: approximately 50% for etidocaine and bupivacaine, 25% for lidocaine, 52% for meperidine, and 75% for thiopental.

The placenta efficiently eliminates fetal bilirubin. Thus, the hyperbilirubinemia of prematurity normally occurs in the postpartum period. With the exception of diazepam, bilirubin does not compete with anesthetic drugs because most are bound to other serum proteins (e.g., meperidine and local anesthetics to α_1-acid glycoproteins). It seems likely that the human blood-brain barrier develops substantially in early gestation. Thus, factors such as tissue affinity changes may account for differences between immature and mature brain uptake of highly lipid-soluble drugs.

Greater total body water in the preterm fetus results in a greater volume of distribution for drugs. Thus, to achieve equal blood concentrations, the immature fetus must receive a greater amount of drug transplacentally than the mature fetus. A study of age-related toxicity of lidocaine in sheep showed that the greater the volume of distribution, the greater the dose required to achieve toxic blood concentrations of the drug.[30] Decreased ability to metabolize or excrete drugs, associated with prematurity, is certainly not a universal phenomenon. In a study comparing the pharmacokinetics of lidocaine in preterm newborns and adults, plasma clearance was similar in both groups.[29] Neonates excreted much more unchanged lidocaine than did adults. Similarly, although meperidine metabolism is more limited in the neonate than in the adult, urinary excretion of the unchanged drug is greater in the neonate.

Another factor is gestational changes in maternal serum albumin and α_1-acid glycoprotein concentrations, which tend to decrease. Serial determinations of protein binding of diazepam, phenytoin, and valproic acid in maternal serum, performed in early (8 to 16 weeks), middle (17 to 32 weeks), and late pregnancy, showed a progressive increase in the unbound fraction of these drugs.[87] This increases drug availability for placental transfer. Placental permeability itself increases as pregnancy progresses because of the increased area and decreased thickness of tissue barriers.

In a largely ignored, prospective study of more than 1,000 premature labors, during which mothers received meperidine alone or with scopolamine, medication had no effect on the perinatal death rate, the incidence of respiratory distress syndrome, Apgar scores, the need for resuscitation, and the incidence of severe neurologic defects within 1 year.[88]

Therefore, it appears that in selection of the anesthetic drugs and techniques for delivery of a preterm infant, concerns regarding drug effects on the newborn are far less important than prevention of asphyxia and trauma to the fetus. For labor and vaginal delivery, well-conducted epidural anesthesia is advantageous in providing good perineal relaxation. The anesthesiologist should ascertain that the fetus is neither hypoxic nor acidotic before induction of epidural blockade. Asphyxia results in a redistribution of fetal cardiac output, which increases oxygen delivery to vital organs such as the brain, heart, and adrenals. These changes in the preterm fetus may be better preserved with bupivacaine or chloroprocaine than with lidocaine.[89,90] Preterm infants with breech presentation are usually delivered by cesarean section. General anesthesia with uterine relaxation, provided by a halogenated drug, facilitates delivery of the aftercoming head. If regional anesthesia is used, nitroglycerin should be available for uterine relaxation.

HIV AND AIDS

HIV infection is tragically not an uncommon occurrence in women of reproductive age. Fortunately, the use of combination antiretroviral therapy has improved the long-term outlook for women with HIV. Unfortunately, some of these women will become pregnant. There is no evidence that pregnancy itself accelerates the progression of the disease. However, there is compelling interest to prevent vertical transmission of HIV from mother to fetus. Neonatal detection is difficult because maternal antibody can persist in the neonate for up to 18 months. The factors associated with increased vertical transmission are a high viral load (or AIDS), rupture of amniotic membranes, coexisting sexually transmitted disease, chorioamnionitis, and obstetric interventions, such as with amniocentesis or cervical cerclage. The greatest success in reducing vertical transmission has been with combination antiretroviral therapy to reduce the maternal viral load and elective cesarean delivery prior to rupture of membranes/labor. Intravenous antiretroviral therapy usually administered prior to delivery.

The choice of anesthetic technique should be based on maternal condition, obstetric considerations, and patient desires. There has been concern that regional anesthesia may spread HIV infection to the CNS or accelerate the course of the disease. However, spread of HIV to the CNS occurs rapidly after initial infection, and there is no evidence linking the use of regional anesthesia (epidural or spinal) to progression of the disease.[91,92] A PDPH should be managed conservatively with caffeine, theophylline, or sumatriptan. If these modalities fail, an epidural blood patch (EBP) may be considered. There has been concern that an EBP, particularly if the viral load is high, may accelerate neurologic symptoms of the disease. In a more recent case series of six patients with HIV infection and PDPH requiring EBP, there was no evidence of acceleration of HIV symptoms.[93]

SUBSTANCE ABUSE

Substance abuse with amphetamines, ecstasy, opioid, marijuana, or cocaine is also not uncommon among women of re-
12 productive age. Of these, cocaine has the greatest implications for anesthetic management because it causes a heightened sympathetic state. Women abusing cocaine generally display euphoria, tachycardia, and hypertension. More serious manifestations may include seizure and coma, myocardial infarction, pulmonary edema, or subarachnoid hemorrhage. Sudden death may occur due to a lethal ventricular arrhythmia. For the fetus as well, maternal cocaine use is harmful. For instance, cocaine use in the first trimester may cause congenital anomalies. Later in pregnancy, cocaine use may be associated with premature labor, intrauterine growth retardation, and nonreassuring fetal status due to uteroplacental insufficiency or placental abruption. Therapy is supportive primarily aimed at controlling CV and CNS consequences of cocaine use. Pure β-antagonist drugs should be avoided because of the potential for worsening hypertension due to unopposed pure α-receptor stimulation by cocaine. The choice of anesthetic depends on maternal and fetal condition, the planned procedure (vaginal delivery or cesarean section), and urgency. General anesthesia may be associated with uncontrolled hypertension/tachycardia and life-threatening arrhythmias in women using cocaine.[94] Regional anesthesia is not without its hazards. Cocaine is a local anesthetic, and systemic toxicity may be additive when using amide local anesthetics for epidural anesthesia. Chronic cocaine use may also be associated with thrombocytopenia. The incidence and severity of hypotension related to regional anesthesia may be greater in cocaine using parturients compared with controls, and hypotension may be more difficult to treat.[94]

FETAL AND MATERNAL MONITORING

The development of biophysical and biochemical monitoring of the fetus during labor and delivery has had a tremendous impact on obstetric practice since the early 1970s. Monitoring procedures are now performed routinely, and it is important that the anesthesiologist understand the basic principles of the technology, as well as the interpretation of results, because they relate to both mother and fetus.

During the same period, there has been an explosion in monitoring technology in the fields of anesthesiology and intensive care. The mother with serious medical problems requiring intensive care or the one whose infant is delivered in an operating room under an anesthesiologist's care is subject to the same standards of monitoring as any other surgical patient. It is generally agreed that the use of intensive peripartum monitoring is appropriate in a high-risk pregnancy. In contrast, patients with routine labor are frequently observed in the same way that patients were many generations ago (i.e., with intermittent blood pressure readings). With the growing sophistication of electronic devices, and specifically the science of telemetry, we can look forward to better surveillance of both mother and fetus without the loss of maternal freedom and activity that monitoring currently entails.

Biophysical Monitoring

A fetal monitor is a two-channel recorder of FHR and uterine activity. In the direct system, the fetal ECG is obtained from an electrode attached to the presenting part. Intrauterine pressure is measured continuously with a transducer connected to a saline-filled catheter that is inserted transcervically. Direct monitoring is quantitative but requires rupture of the membranes and a cervical dilation of at least 1.5 cm. In addition, the presenting part must dip into the true pelvis. Indirect fetal monitoring uses data obtained from transducers secured to the mother's abdomen with adjustable straps. Ultrasound cardiography is the most commonly used indirect method of obtaining FHR signals. Uterine activity is monitored with a tocodynamometer triggered by the changing shape of the uterus during the contraction. Indirect monitoring is mostly qualitative. Its advantage is that it can be applied without rupture of membranes, even before the onset of labor.

The following variables are considered when fetal well-being is determined: baseline heart rate, beat-to-beat variability, periodic patterns, and uterine activity. The baseline FHR is measured between contractions and ranges between 120 and 160 beats/min in the normal fetus. An acceleration of FHR in response to fetal stimulation, such as during vaginal examination or fetal capillary blood sampling, is a reassuring sign that the fetus is not acidotic. Persistently elevated rates may be associated with chronic fetal distress, maternal fever, or administration of drugs such as ephedrine and atropine. Abnormally low rates may be encountered in fetuses with congenital heart block or as a late occurrence during the course of fetal hypoxia and acidosis.

The baseline FHR variability, which is normally present, reflects the beat-to-beat adjustments of the parasympathetic and sympathetic nervous systems to a variety of internal and external stimuli. Fetal CNS depression by asphyxia may decrease baseline variability. Therefore, a smooth FHR tracing may be an ominous finding. However, drugs can also decrease FHR variability by depressing mechanisms in the CNS that integrate cardiac control (tranquilizers, opioids, barbiturates, anesthetics) or by blocking the transmission of control impulses to the cardiac pacemaker (atropine). In contrast, ephedrine administration may increase beat-to-beat variability.

Periodic FHR patterns consist of decelerations or accelerations of relatively brief duration in association with uterine contractions (Fig. 42-12). There are three major forms of FHR deceleration: early, late, and variable. Early decelerations are U shaped, with the heart rate usually not decreasing to less than 100 beats/min. The fetal heart begins to slow with the onset of the contraction, the low point coincides with the peak of the contraction, and the rate usually returns to the baseline as the uterus relaxes. This type of deceleration has been attributed to fetal head compression, leading to increased vagal tone. It is not ameliorated by increasing fetal oxygenation but is blocked by atropine administration. Early decelerations are transient and well tolerated by the fetus because there is no systemic hypoxemia or acidosis.

Late decelerations are also U shaped. However, they begin 20 to 30 seconds or more after the onset of uterine contraction,

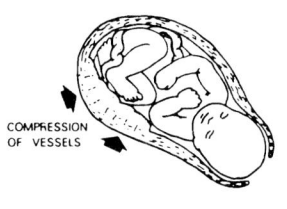

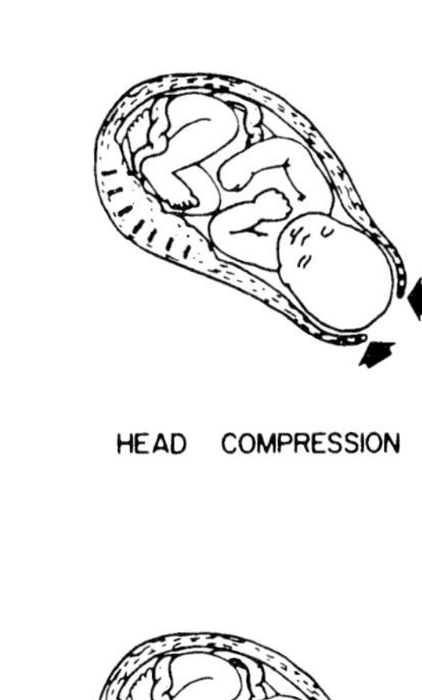

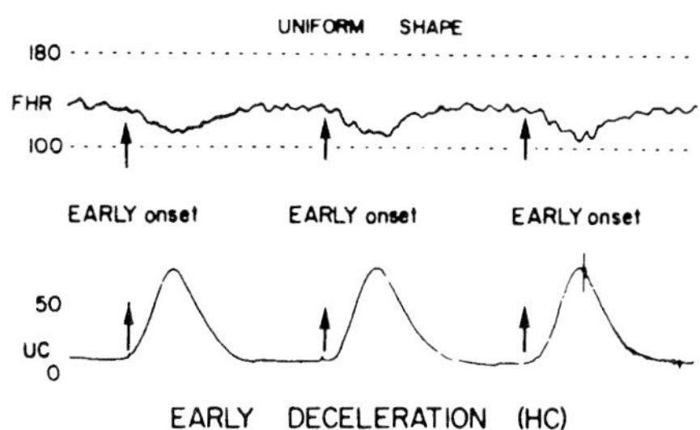

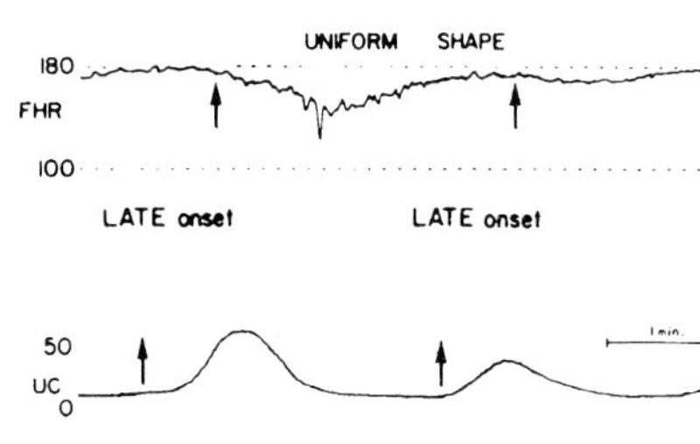

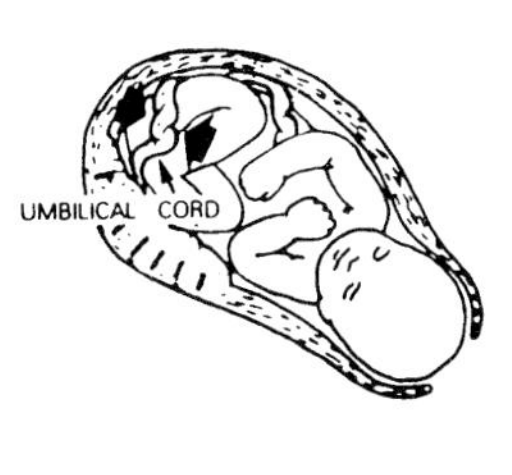

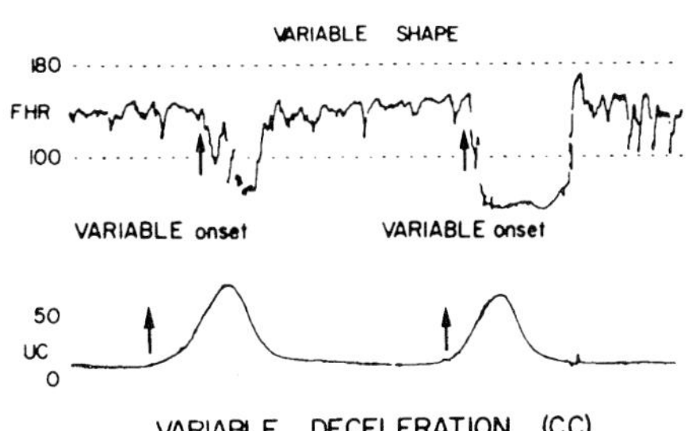

FIGURE 42-12. Classification and mechanism of fetal heart rate patterns. (Reprinted with permission from Hon EH: An Introduction to Fetal Heart Rate Monitoring, p 29. New Haven, CT, Harty Press, 1969.)

and the low point of the deceleration occurs well after the peak of the contraction. Myocardial ischemia resulting from uteroplacental insufficiency is believed to cause late decelerations. Late deceleration can be corrected by improving fetal oxygenation, which may be accomplished with oxygen administration to the mother, correction of maternal hypotension, or aortocaval compression, or by taking measures that reduce uterine activity. If late decelerations are repetitive, continuous, and progressive in severity, there is a significant correlation with fetal acidosis, and delivery may be required.

Variable decelerations, which result from umbilical cord compression, are the most common periodic patterns observed in the intrapartum period. They are variable in shape and onset, with the rate usually decreasing to less than 100 beats/min and >15 beats/min below baseline. Although the initial FHR changes are of reflex origin, if the cord compressions are frequent or prolonged, fetal asphyxia may result in direct myocardial depression.

A prolonged deceleration is defined as a FHR decrease lasting longer than 2 minutes but less than 10 minutes. All decelerations should be quantified based on deviation from baseline and duration.[95]

Cervical dilation and descent of the presenting part during the first stage of labor result primarily from uterine contractions. During the active phase, contractions should occur every 2 to 3 minutes, with peak intrauterine pressures of 50 to 80 mm Hg and resting pressures of 5 to 20 mm Hg. Uterine activity may be abnormally elevated in association with abruptio placentae or the injudicious use of oxytocics. Tetanic uterine contractions have been reported after the use of methoxamine, a pure α-adrenergic agonist. In the first and second trimesters of pregnancy, increased uterine tone may occur with ketamine in doses greater than 1.1 mg/kg. At term, ketamine does not appear to have this effect.

Poor uterine contractility may result from overdistention (polyhydramnios, multiple pregnancy) or aortocaval compression. During early labor, administration of opioids, sedatives, or regional anesthesia may delay the onset of the active phase by diminishing uterine activity. However, regional anesthesia instituted during the active phase has no untoward effects on uterine activity as long as hypotension and the supine position are avoided. The addition of epinephrine to a local anesthetic solution may have a dose-related inhibitory effect on uterine activity.

Fetal Pulse Oximetry

Fetal pulse oximetry (FPO) is a newer technique to evaluate intrapartum fetal oxygenation. Currently, it remains an adjunct to electronic FHR monitoring. The fetal pulse oximeter is currently being used when the electronic FHR monitor shows a nonreassuring FHR tracing or if the tracing is unreliable (i.e., fetal arrhythmia). Fetal O_2 saturation between 30% and 70% is considered normal. Saturation readings consistently <30% for a prolonged period of time (i.e., 10 to 15 min) are suggestive of fetal acidemia. Fetal blood scalp sampling and/or prompt obstetric intervention may be indicated.

As of September 2001, the American College of Obstetrics and Gynecology failed to endorse the routine use of the FPO in clinical practice related to concerns over increased health costs without clear-cut improvement in obstetric outcome. Others suggest that simultaneous monitoring with a combination of fetal ECG and FPO is easily feasible, and reliable in indicating signs of intermittent hypoxia.[96]

Biochemical Monitoring

Before labor, the normal fetus is neither hypoxic nor acidotic. During labor, many events, including repeated uterine contractions, cord compression, aortocaval compression, and maternal hypotension from any cause, may decrease uteroplacental blood flow sufficiently to produce fetal hypoxia and acidosis. Acidosis associated with short-term placental hypoperfusion primarily results from carbon dioxide accumulation (respiratory acidosis). With prolonged asphyxia, hypercarbia is accompanied by metabolic acidosis resulting from anaerobic metabolism. Thus, fetal acid-base indices, such as PCO_2 and base deficit, usually reflect the degree and duration of asphyxia.

Assessment of fetal acid-base status became possible in the early 1960s, with the development of a fetal capillary blood sampling technique. Blood is usually obtained from the scalp, but it may also be sampled from the breech. It is collected into a heparinized glass capillary tube, and pH, PCO_2, PO_2, and base deficit are determined immediately with an appropriate electrode system adapted to the small sample size.

This technique has been validated in animal and clinical studies. It has been shown that fetal blood values obtained from the scalp of fetal monkeys are closely correlated with those in simultaneously obtained samples from the carotid artery and jugular vein.[97] A fetal capillary blood pH of 7.25 is the lowest limit of normal. A pH below 7.20 indicates fetal acidosis, and values between 7.20 and 7.24 are considered preacidotic. The last predelivery fetal pH correlated with the Apgar score at 1 or 2 minutes after birth.[98,99] Ninety-two percent of infants scored 7 or better when the pH was above 7.25. With the pH below 7.16, 80% of infants scored 6 or less.[88] In general, when the pH is normal immediately before delivery, it can be assumed the infant will be in good condition. However, there is a small incidence of false-positive and false-negative results. In one study, normal pH was associated with low Apgar scores (false-positive results) in approximately 10% of cases[99] (Fig. 42-13). In approximately 8% of cases (false-negative results), a vigorous infant was born despite a low capillary scalp pH. The major factors contributing to false-positive outcomes are administration of sedative drugs or anesthetics, infection, airway obstruction, and congenital anomalies. False-negative outcomes are usually associated with maternal acidosis, which may occur after prolonged labor, excessive muscular activity, or inadequate fluid and caloric intakes. Obtaining a maternal sample (arterial or free-flowing venous blood) for the evaluation of the acid-base status helps identify this group. If fetal acidosis is of maternal origin, the mother's blood shows a large base deficit value, and the difference between the fetal and maternal base deficit values is small. In contrast, fetal acidosis resulting from prolonged asphyxia is reflected in a large fetal, but normal maternal, base deficit value; consequently, the difference in base deficit values is large. Fetal acidosis of maternal origin can be treated by correcting the maternal acid-base imbalance.

NEWBORN RESUSCITATION IN THE DELIVERY ROOM

Of the approximately 3.5 million infants born in the United States each year, 6% require resuscitation in the delivery room.

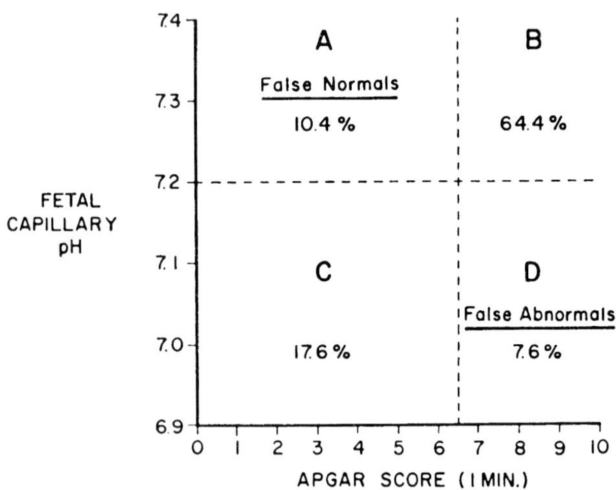

FIGURE 42-13. Fetal pH as an index of infant's condition at birth in 355 patients during labor. *Segment A:* depressed infants with normal pH; *segment B:* vigorous infants with normal pH; *segment C:* depressed infants with low pH; *segment D:* vigorous infants with low pH. (Reprinted with permission from Bowe ET, Beard RW, Finster M *et al:* Reliability of fetal blood sampling. Am J Obstet Gynecol 107:279, 1970.)

Among those weighing 1,500 g or less, the incidence is approximately 80%. The following factors may contribute to depression of the newborn: drugs used in labor or during delivery, including anesthetic agents; trauma of precipitate labor and operative obstetrics; and birth asphyxia (i.e., hypoxia and hypercapnia with acidosis).

Fetal Asphyxia

13 Fetal asphyxia, the best-studied cause of neonatal depression, usually develops as a result of interference with maternal or fetal perfusion of the placenta. As stated previously, the normal fetus is neither hypoxic nor acidotic before labor. Experimental data have revealed that transplacental gradients for pH and PCO_2 are approximately 0.05 pH units and 5 mm Hg, respectively. Although oxygen tension is low, oxygen saturation is relatively high (80 to 85%) by virtue of the shift to the left of the fetal oxyhemoglobin dissociation curve.

During labor, uterine contractions decrease the blood flow through the intervillous space of the placenta or may stop it completely. On the fetal side, cord compression occurs during the final stages of approximately one-third of vaginal deliveries. Thus, mild degrees of hypoxia and acidosis occur even during normal labor and delivery, and play an important role in initiation of ventilation. On average, healthy, vigorous infants (at birth) have an oxygen saturation of 21%, a pH of 7.24, and a PCO_2 of 56 mm Hg.

Severe fetal asphyxia occasionally develops as a result of fetal and maternal complications, such as a tight nuchal cord, prolapsed cord, premature separation of the placenta, uterine hyperactivity, or maternal hypotension. During asphyxia, changes in blood gases and hydrogen ion concentration are rapid. The decrease in pH results from accumulation of carbon dioxide and end products of anaerobic glycolysis. After oxygen stores are exhausted, the ability of fetal brain and myocardium to derive energy from anaerobic metabolism is essential for survival. However, anaerobic glycolysis is pH dependent, and its rate is greatly diminished when the pH decreases below 7.0. Other untoward effects of severe hypoxia and acidosis include depression of the myocardium resulting from a decrease in its

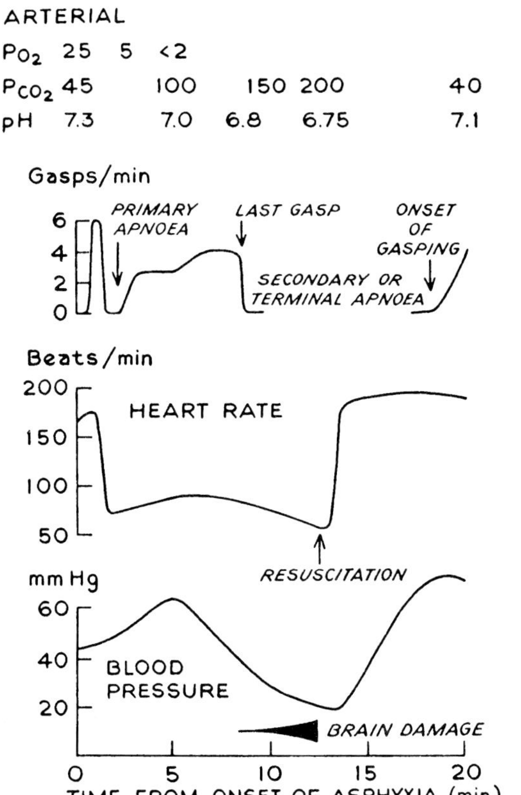

FIGURE 42-14. Schematic diagram of changes in rhesus monkeys during asphyxia and with resuscitation by positive-pressure ventilation. Brain damage was assessed by histologic examination some weeks or months later. (Reprinted with permission from Dawes GS: Foetal and Neonatal Physiology: A Comparative Study of the Changes at Birth, p 149. Chicago, Year Book Medical, 1968.)

responsiveness to catecholamines; a shift to the right of the fetal oxyhemoglobin dissociation curve, resulting in reduced oxygen-carrying capacity; and an increase in pulmonary vascular resistance, which plays an important role during circulatory readjustment after birth.

Ventilatory and cardiovascular responses to controlled experimental asphyxia have been investigated extensively in newborn monkeys (Fig. 42-14). During the initial phase of asphyxia, the unanesthetized animal exhibits respiratory efforts that increase in depth and frequency for up to 3 minutes. This period, called primary hyperpnea, is followed by primary apnea, which lasts for approximately 1 minute. Rhythmic gasping then begins and is maintained at a fairly constant rate of approximately 6 gasps/min for 4 to 5 minutes. Thereafter, the gasps become weaker and slower. Their cessation at approximately 8.5 minutes after the onset of asphyxia marks the beginning of secondary apnea. Administration of opioids and systemic anesthetic agents to the mother can abolish the period of primary hyperpnea and prolong primary apnea.

There is a linear relationship between the duration of asphyxia and the onset of gasping and rhythmic spontaneous breathing. In the newborn monkey, for each minute of asphyxia beyond the last gasp, 2 additional minutes of artificial ventilation is required before gasping begins again and 4 minutes before rhythmic breathing is established.[100] This indicates that the longer artificial ventilation of the lungs is delayed during secondary apnea, the longer it will take to resuscitate the infant. Furthermore, in the newborn monkey, prolongation of asphyxia for 4 minutes beyond the last gasp is accompanied by extensive damage to brainstem nuclei, whereas animals resuscitated before the last gasp show little or no brain damage. Thus, a relatively short delay in resuscitation can have serious sequelae.

Neonatal Adaptations at Birth

During this period, and through the early hours and days of life, many morphologic and functional changes take place, with the cardiovascular and ventilatory systems undergoing the most dramatic alterations. In the normal newborn, two events occur almost simultaneously, and within seconds of delivery: the end of umbilical circulation through the placenta and expansion of the lungs. These events change the fetal circulation toward the adult type. Survival of the neonate depends primarily on prompt expansion of the lungs and establishment of effective ventilation.

The onset of ventilation and expansion of the lungs dilates the pulmonary vascular bed, resulting in decreased resistance and a significant increase in pulmonary blood flow. Pulmonary vascular resistance decreases as oxygen tension increases and carbon dioxide levels decrease. As soon as pulmonary perfusion increases, the foramen ovale, which is a communication between the inferior vena cava and the left atrium, undergoes functional closure because of pressure changes across the valve of the foramen (see Fig. 42-4). Cessation of the umbilical circulation reduces pressure in the inferior vena cava and right atrium, whereas the increase in pulmonary blood flow increases venous return and pressure in the left atrium. The ductus arteriosus does not constrict abruptly or completely after birth; functional closure may take hours, even days. Thus, shunting may still occur in the neonatal period, its direction depending on relative resistances in the pulmonary and systemic vascular beds. The smooth muscle of the ductus arteriosus constricts in response to increased oxygen tension in the newborn's blood. Catecholamines, which exist in increased concentrations in the newborn, particularly during the first 3 hours of life, also constrict the ductus arteriosus. In contrast, prostaglandins PGI_2 and PGE_2, produced by the wall of the ductus arteriosus, relax the ductal smooth muscle. Administration of prostaglandin synthesis inhibitors to fetal animals promotes constriction of the ductus arteriosus.

Cardiac output and its distribution also increase; left ventricular output increases ~150 to 400 mL/kg/min, whereas right ventricular output increases less significantly. Cardiac output changes closely parallel the increase in oxygen consumption. The redistribution of cardiac output also leads to increases in myocardial, renal, and gastrointestinal blood flow, and decreases in cerebral, adrenal, and carotid flow.

During fetal life, respiratory gas exchange takes place through the placenta. Delivery of the infant's trunk relieves the thoracic compression that occurs as the infant passes through the birth canal, and the thorax and the lungs expand. Most infants initiate respiratory efforts a few seconds after birth. After the first inspiration, a cry usually results as the infant exhales against a partially closed glottis, thus increasing intrathoracic pressure significantly. Negative pressures in excess of 40 cm H_2O bring about the initial entry of air into fluid-filled alveoli. In the mature, normal neonate, the lungs expand almost completely after the first few breaths, and the pressure–volume changes achieved with each respiration resemble those of the adult. After lung expansion, the FRC approximates 70 mL in the term newborn and changes little over the first 6 days of life. The tidal volume varies between 10 and 30 mL, the breathing frequency ranges from 30 to 60 breaths/min, and minute ventilation exceeds 500 mL. After delivery and prompt lung expansion, reoxygenation is rapid, but it takes 2 or 3 hours to achieve a relatively normal acid-base balance, primarily by pulmonary excretion of carbon dioxide. By 24 hours, the healthy

TABLE 42-3

RESUSCITATION EQUIPMENT IN THE DELIVERY ROOM

Radiant warmer
Suction with manometer and suction trap
Suction catheters
Wall oxygen with flow meter
Resuscitation bag (≤750 mL)
Infant facemasks
Infant oropharyngeal airways
Endotracheal tubes, 2.5, 3.0, 3.5, and 4.0 mm
Endotracheal tube stylets
Laryngoscope(s) and blade(s)
Sterile umbilical artery catheterization tray
Needles, syringes, three-way stopcocks
Medications and solutions
1:10,000 Epinephrine
Naloxone hydrochloride
Sodium bicarbonate
Volume expanders

neonate has reached the same acid-base state as that of the mother before labor.

Resuscitation

The delivery room must be prepared for adequate and prompt treatment of severe neonatal depression at birth. All members of the delivery room team should be trained in resuscitation methods because both mother and infant may encounter difficulty simultaneously. Every piece of apparatus necessary for emergency resuscitation should be checked carefully before delivery (Table 42-3). An overview of resuscitation in the delivery room is provided in >Fig. 42-15.

Initial Treatment and Evaluation of All Infants

Immediately after delivery, the infant should be held head down while the cord is clamped and cut. The infant should then be placed supine under a radiant heat source, with the head kept low with a slight lateral tilt, and the skin should be dried promptly. A nurse or assistant should listen to the heartbeat immediately, indicating the rate by finger movement. If help is not available, the rate can be detected from pulsation of the umbilical cord. At the same time, the resuscitator should aspirate the mouth, pharynx, and nose with a catheter. This suction should be brief, not exceeding 30 seconds. Slapping the infant's soles lightly or rubbing its back frequently aids in initiating a deep breath or cry. The initial appraisal of the newborn should start from the moment of birth, with particular attention paid to the first few breaths and the evenness and ease of respiration. Most infants are vigorous and cough or cry within seconds of delivery. Their heart rate is above 100 beats/min. The administration of free-flowing oxygen rapidly improves their oxygenation and decreases pulmonary vascular resistance. Mildly to moderately depressed infants constitute the largest group requiring some form of resuscitation at birth. These infants are pale or cyanotic, have not established sustained respiration even at 1 minute after delivery, and may be nearly flaccid. However, their heart rate is usually above 100 beats/min. The severely depressed infant is flaccid, unresponsive, and pale, and may often have a heart rate below 100 beats/min. The scoring system introduced by Apgar is a useful method of clinically evaluating the infant, particularly at 1 and 5 minutes after delivery (Table 42-4).

Treatment of Moderately Depressed Infants

If initial resuscitative methods, including rubbing the back or slapping the feet once or twice, have produced no response, that is, the infant is apneic or its heart rate remains below 100 beats/min, positive-pressure ventilation by bag and mask should be instituted at a rate of 40 breaths/min. The initial breath may require pressures of 30 to 40 cm H_2O. Subsequently, the inflation pressures should be reduced to 15 to 20 cm H_2O in an infant with normal lungs. A small plastic oropharyngeal airway may be needed to maintain patency of the upper airway. If after 15 to 30 seconds of ventilation the heart rate is below 60 beats/min, or maintained between 60 and 80 beats/min, chest compressions should be initiated.[101]

Treatment of Severely Depressed Infants

Ventilation should be established without delay. The glottis should be inspected immediately with the laryngoscope. If meconium or thick meconium-stained mucus has been aspirated into the trachea, it should be suctioned out at once through an endotracheal tube before the lungs are inflated. It is usually possible to accomplish this within 1 to 2 minutes of delivery. Severely depressed infants may require 3 to 8 minutes of artificial ventilation before a spontaneous gasp is taken. The endotracheal tube can be removed as soon as quiet and sustained respiration is established.

Use of Cardiac Massage

If the blood pressure or heart rate is unduly low at the beginning of resuscitation, positive-pressure ventilation is unlikely to be successful unless cardiac massage is used. Chest compressions should be provided if heart rate is less than 60 beats/min, despite adequate ventilation for 30 seconds. The technique preferred by the authors consists of intermittent compression of the lower third of the sternum. The ratio of chest compression to ventilation should be approximately 3:1 or 100 compressions to 30 breaths per min. Cardiac massage and ventilation should be maintained until the heart rate exceeds 100 beats/min.

Rapid Correction of Acidosis

Sodium bicarbonate use is not recommended during brief cardiopulmonary resuscitation. The hyperosmolarity and CO_2 generated may be detrimental to cerebral and myocardial function. After ensuring adequate ventilation and perfusion, severe acidosis (pH $<$ 7.0 or a base deficit $>$ 15 mEq/mL) may need to be corrected. For that purpose, a 3.5F or 5F catheter should be inserted, under sterile conditions, into the umbilical vein and advanced until the tip of the catheter is just below the skin level. A solution of sodium bicarbonate, 0.5 mEq/mL (4.2%), is then infused over at least 2 minutes, up to a total dose of 2 mEq/mL (Fig. 42-16).

Other Drugs and Fluids

If it is believed that persistent depression has resulted from maternal opioid medication, naloxone should be given after adequate ventilation has been established (Table 42-5). The recommended dose of 0.1 mg/kg may be injected intravenously, intramuscularly, subcutaneously, or by endotracheal tube. The initial dose may be repeated as needed. Naloxone should be avoided in infants born to opioid-addicted mothers so as not to precipitate acute withdrawal. A severely asphyxiated newborn might require cardiotonic drugs during early resuscitation. Epinephrine should be used to treat asystole or persistent bradycardia despite 30 seconds of effective ventilation and external cardiac massage. A dose of 0.1 to 0.3 mL/kg of a

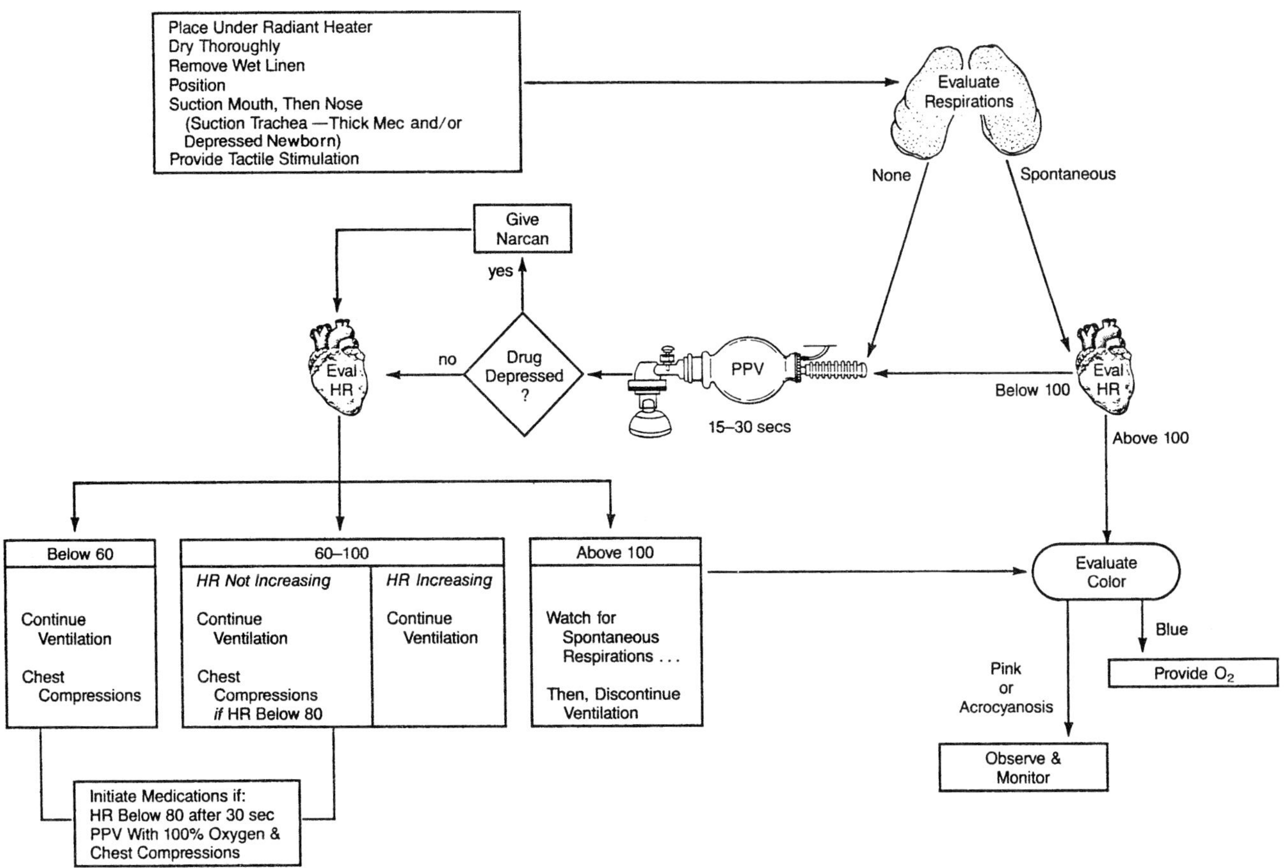

FIGURE 42-15. Overview of resuscitation in the delivery room. HR, heart rate; PPV, positive-pressure ventilation. (Adapted from Bloom RS, Copley C: Textbook of Neonatal Resuscitation. Elk Grove Village, IL, American Heart Association/American Academy of Pediatrics, 1990.)

1:10,000 solution should be injected intravenously or by endotracheal tube, and repeated every 5 minutes if necessary.

Hypovolemia frequently follows severe birth asphyxia because a greater than normal portion of fetal blood remains in the placenta. The infant appears pale and has low arterial pressure, tachycardia, and tachypnea. Acute blood volume expansion may be accomplished with the intravenous administration of the following solutions over 5 to 10 minutes: O negative blood, cross-matched with the mother's blood, 10 mL/kg; and normal saline or lactated Ringer's solution, 10 mL/kg. Albumin is no longer indicated because it is associated with increased mortality.

Diagnostic Procedures

After the neonate is successfully resuscitated and stabilized, several diagnostic procedures are indicated. To rule out choanal atresia, each nostril should be obstructed. Because newborns must breathe through their noses, occlusion of the nostril on the patent side causes respiratory obstruction. To rule out esophageal atresia, a suction catheter is inserted into the stomach. Gastric contents are aspirated; volume in excess of 12 mL after vaginal delivery and 20 mL after cesarean section may result from an abnormality of the upper gastrointestinal tract.

ANESTHESIA FOR NONOBSTETRIC SURGERY IN THE PREGNANT WOMAN

Approximately 1.6 to 2.2% of pregnant women undergo surgery for reasons unrelated to parturition.[102,103] Apart from trauma, the most common emergencies are abdominal, involving torsion or rupture of an ovarian cyst and acute appendicitis,

TABLE 42-4

APGAR SCORES

SIGN	0	1	2
Heart rate	Absent	<100 beats/min	>100 beats/min
Respiratory effort	Absent	Slow, irregular	Good, crying
Muscle tone	Limp	Some flexion of extremities	Active motion
Reflex irritability	No response	Grimace	Cough, sneeze, or cry
Color	Pale, blue	Body pink, extremities blue	Completely pink

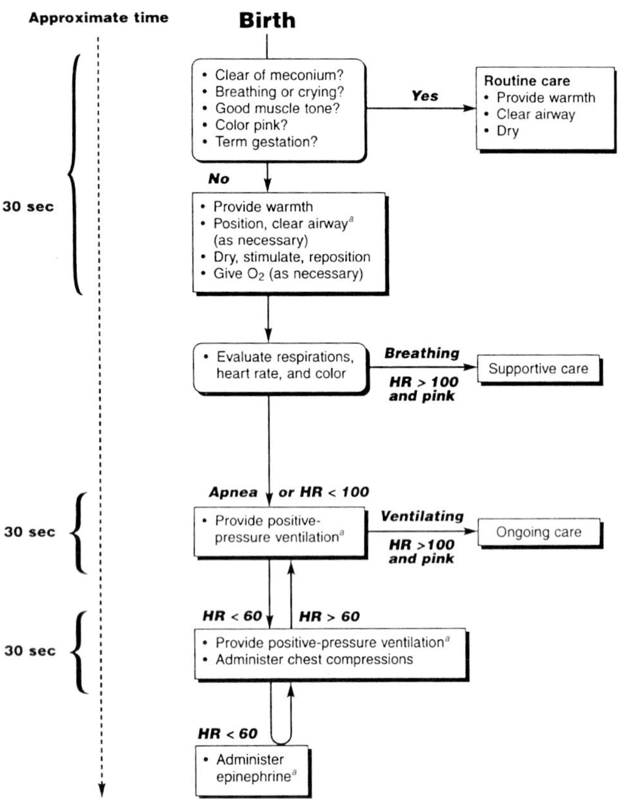

FIGURE 42-16. Algorithm for resuscitation of the newly born heart. [a]Endotracheal intubation may be considered at several steps. (From Neonatal Resuscitation. Guidelines 2000 for Cardiopulmonary resuscitation and emergency cardiovascular care: International consensus on science. Part II. Circulation 102:I-343, 2000.)

but breast tumors are not uncommon, as are serious conditions such as intracranial aneurysms, cardiac valvular disease, and pheochromocytoma. Surgery to correct an incompetent cervix with Shirodkar or McDonald sutures is more related to the pregnancy itself.

When the necessity for surgery arises, anesthetic considerations are related to the alterations in maternal physiologic condition with advancing pregnancy, the teratogenicity of anesthetic drugs, the indirect effects of anesthesia on uteroplacental blood flow, and the potential for abortion or premature delivery. The risks must be balanced to provide the most favorable outcome for mother and child.

Five major studies have attempted to relate surgery and anesthesia during human pregnancy to fetal outcome as determined by anomalies, premature labor, or intrauterine death.[102–106] Although they failed to correlate surgery and
14 anesthetic exposure with congenital anomalies, all of them demonstrated an increased incidence of fetal death, particularly after operations during the first trimester. No particular anesthetic agent or technique was implicated, and it seemed that the condition that necessitated surgery was the most relevant factor, with fetal mortality greatest after pelvic surgery or procedures performed for obstetric indications (i.e., cervical incompetence).

Two studies deserve mention. A review was taken of the entire population of the province of Manitoba, Canada, between the years 1971 and 1978.[105] State health insurance records were used to identify approximately 2,500 pregnant women who had undergone surgery during this period. Each patient was matched with a woman of similar age, living in the same area, with a pregnancy-related condition but no surgical intervention. As in earlier studies, there was no increase in the incidence of congenital anomalies in the offspring of mothers who had had surgery. However, there was an increased risk of spontaneous abortion in women who had received general anesthesia during the first or second trimesters, which was most evident after gynecologic operations. Few of the surgical group had had procedures to treat cervical incompetence, suggesting that factors other than the obstetric condition itself might be important. The results also might have been influenced by the fact that a small number of gynecologic procedures were performed with anesthesia other than general so the effect of the surgical site alone could not be distinguished. The authors emphasized a multiplicity of factors other than choice of anesthetic agent (e.g., diagnostic radiologic procedures, antibiotics, analgesics, infection, decreased uterine perfusion, stress) that might have been responsible for the increased risk of abortion.

TABLE 42-5

THERAPEUTIC GUIDELINES FOR NEONATAL RESUSCITATION

DRUG OR VOLUME EXPANDER	CONCENTRATION TO ADMINISTER	PREPARATION (BASED ON RECOMMENDED CONCENTRATION)	DOSAGE	ROUTE/RATE
Epinephrine	1:10,000	1 mL in a syringe Can dilute 1:1 with normal saline if given IT	0.1–0.3 mL/kg	IV or IT Give rapidly
Volume expanders	Whole blood 5% solution Normal saline Lactated Ringer's	40 mL to be given by syringe or IV drip	10 mL/kg	Give over 5–10 min
Sodium bicarbonate	0.5 mEq/mL (4.2% solution)	20 mL in a syringe or two 10-mL prefilled syringes	2 mEq/kg	IV Give slowly over at least 2 min (1 mEq/kg/min)
Naloxone hydrochloride	Narcan Neonatal 0.02 mg/mL	2 mL in a syringe	0.5 mL/kg	IV, IM, SC, or IT Give rapidly

IM, intramuscular(ly); IV, intravenous(ly); IT, intratracheal(ly); SC, subcutaneous(ly).
Adapted from Bloom RS, Cropley C, Drew CR: Textbook of Neonatal Resuscitation. Reproduced with permission of the American Heart Association, American Academy of Pediatrics, Dallas, 1987.

The largest study to date regarding reproductive outcome after surgery during pregnancy is a Swedish registry review covering the years 1973 to 1981.[106] During this period, there were a total of 720,000 births, 5,405 of them after anesthesia and surgery during pregnancy. The results of this study are reassuring in that there was no increased incidence of congenital anomalies or stillbirths among infants exposed in utero to maternal surgery and anesthesia. However, in this group there was an increased frequency of very low and low birth weights, and of deaths within 168 hours after delivery. The reasons for this are unclear and are not related to any specific type of operation. The authors postulated that the maternal illness itself may have been a major contributor to adverse neonatal outcome.

Direct Effects of Anesthetic Agents on Embryo and Fetus

The idea that surgical anesthesia, although deemed necessary for the patient, might have detrimental effects on the growth and development of the human fetus has led to a great deal of investigation, both in vitro and in experimental animals. These studies present difficulties in interpretation because the concentrations of anesthetic and the duration of exposure are frequently far in excess of what is clinically used and because most of the studies were performed in lower animals.

Animals exposed to toxic substances and anesthetics show a dose-related response, the first change being decreased fertility and increased fetal death. The teratogenic effects between species and also within the same species vary significantly. The developmental stage is crucial, with dramatic sensitivity to exposure at certain times and little or no effect at a later time. The period of organogenesis is most critical. In humans, it corresponds to the fifteenth to fifty-sixth days of gestation.

Many congenital malfunctions show a pattern of multifactorial inheritance. In this mode, maldevelopment may result from a combination of factors in one person, such as hereditary predisposition, sensitivity to a given drug, and exposure at a vulnerable time in development. There are numerous other factors contributing to the potential teratogenicity of anesthesia. The cytotoxicity of anesthetic agents is closely associated with biodegradation, which, in turn, is influenced by oxygenation and hepatic blood flow. Thus, the complications associated with anesthesia, such as maternal hypoxia, hypotension, administration of vasopressors, hypercarbia, hypocarbia, and electrolyte disturbances, may possibly be a greater cause for concern as regards teratogenesis than the use of the agents themselves. Hypoxia is certainly a well-documented teratogen in the incubating chick embryo.[107] The role of maternal carbohydrate metabolism on embryonic development is also important. For example, the effects of 48 hours of fasting and administration of insulin to pregnant rats have included a large number of skeletal deformities.[108]

Experimental evidence on exposure to specific drugs and agents is highlighted briefly, with the consideration that it is difficult to extrapolate laboratory data to the clinical situation in humans. Large numbers of patients must be exposed to a suspected teratogen before its safety can be ascertained. Complicating factors include the frequency of maternal exposure to a multiplicity of drugs; the difficulty in separating the effects of the underlying disease process and surgical treatment from those of the drug administered; differing degrees of risk with stage of gestation; and the variety, rather than the consistency, of anomalies that appear in association with one agent. Of the premedicants, anticholinergics have not been found to be teratogenic, whereas tranquilizers and sedatives such as phenothiazines and barbiturates produce anomalies in some species.[109] Several reports have described a specific relationship between diazepam and oral clefts, but another study has not confirmed this.[110,111] Intravenous agents such as thiopental, methohexital, and ketamine in doses normally used in the operating room have not been associated with birth defects. Only one study has shown musculoskeletal deformities involving the joints after infusion of a muscle relaxant (*d*-tubocurarine) in the chick embryo between the seventh and fifteenth day of incubation.[112] Local anesthetics have not been shown to be teratogenic in animals or humans. Halogenated inhalation drugs have produced conflicting results. Pregnant rats exposed to halothane 0.8% for 12 hours at various times during gestation have increased incidences of anomalous skeletal development and fetal death.[113] Other investigators have failed to show teratogenic effects of halothane in rats, rabbits, and mice exposed to subanesthetic concentrations for brief periods. Subanesthetic concentrations of enflurane do not appear to be teratogenic.[114] However, mice exposed to 1% enflurane for 4 hr/day on days 6 to 15 of gestation showed an increased incidence of cleft palates and minor skeletal and visceral abnormalities.[103] In a subsequent study by the same authors, teratogenic changes after exposure to 0.6% isoflurane in mice were similar to those found with enflurane, but the incidence of cleft palate was six times more frequent (12% vs. 1.9%).[115] Cleft palate readily develops in mice, and its occurrence as an isolated finding suggests that this might be a species-specific response. To clarify the results from earlier studies, rats were exposed to 0.75 MAC halothane, isoflurane, or enflurane; 0.55 MAC nitrous oxide; or a known teratogen, retinoic acid, for two 6-hour periods at three different stages of pregnancy.[116] No major morphologic abnormalities occurred in any of the anesthetic-exposed groups.

Nitrous oxide has been the most extensively investigated agent since the 1955 observation that leukopenia developed in patients with tetanus after they inhaled nitrous oxide for several days. Numerous studies have demonstrated significant effects on fetal growth, skeletal development, and death rate in both pregnant rats and incubating chicks exposed to concentrations of between 50% and 80%, for periods ranging from hours to days.[117] The question arises as to whether adverse effects at such high doses resulted from the anesthetic itself or from the accompanying physiologic derangements.

Although the mechanism of the teratogenic effect of nitrous oxide has not been determined, it may be related to the inhibitory effect of the agent on methionine synthetase activity and vitamin B_{12}. A dose-dependent decrease in both maternal and fetal methionine synthetase activity occurred in pregnant rats receiving 10% or 50% nitrous oxide for periods ranging from 60 to 240 minutes.[118] It is possible that failure of this enzyme to convert homocysteine to the essential amino acid methionine may lead to abnormalities of myelination of nerve fibers (Fig. 42-17). Furthermore, inhibition of methionine synthesis results in decreased thymidine production, which in turn can lead to decreased DNA synthesis and inhibition of cell division. Because there is evidence that nitrous oxide adversely affects methionine synthetase activity, it has been recommended that it not be administered to pregnant women in the first two trimesters. However, a more recent human study demonstrated no significant changes in plasma methionine concentrations after anesthesia with 60 to 70% nitrous oxide for up to 4 hours.[119] Two other reviews of exposure to this agent, this time for cervical cerclage procedures, showed no effects on fetal outcome.[120,121] Further, in the already mentioned Swedish birth registry study, nitrous oxide was administered to almost all 2,929 patients receiving general anesthesia without adverse fetal consequences.[106] In rats, the teratogenic effects of nitrous oxide could be prevented by the concomitant administration of isoflurane or halothane.[122] It is controversial whether pretreatment with folinic acid, the concentration of which is

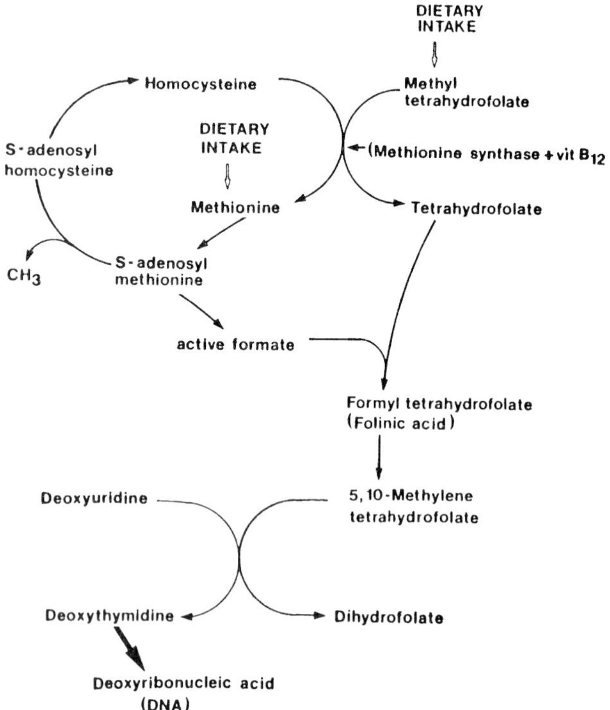

FIGURE 42-17. Abridged metabolic map showing the relationship between methionine and deoxythymidine syntheses. (Reprinted with permission from Nunn JF: Interaction of nitrous oxide and vitamin B_{12}. Trends Pharmacol Sci 5:225, 1984.)

reduced when methionine synthetase is inhibited, affords protection against the effects of nitrous oxide.[122] Because a single exposure to anesthetic agents seems unlikely to result in fetal abnormality, the selection of agent should be based on specific surgical requirements.

Indirect Effects of Agents and Techniques

The adequacy of the uteroplacental circulation, so vital to the well-being of the fetus, is easily affected by drugs and anesthetic procedures. As discussed previously, perfusion of the intervillous space of the placenta may be diminished consequently on maternal systemic hypotension, which in turn may result from the use of epidural or spinal anesthesia, from aortocaval compression with the patient in the supine position, or from hemorrhage. Similarly, increased uterine activity may result in reduced placental perfusion. Thus, the use of α-adrenergic drugs to correct maternal hypotension and anesthetics such as ketamine (in doses above 1 mg/kg) may produce increased uterine tone sufficient to endanger the fetus. Severe hyperventilation of the mother may also reduce uterine blood flow. Finally, it has been shown in experimental animals that epinephrine or norepinephrine infusion results in decreased uterine blood flow and deterioration of fetal condition. Maternal pain and apprehension may similarly affect the fetus.[123]

Practical Suggestions

It is generally agreed that only surgeries that cannot be delayed for months, including emergency surgery, should be performed during pregnancy, particularly in the first trimester. The possibility of pregnancy should be considered in all female surgical patients of reproductive age. Based on the maternal and fetal hazards already described, the following approach to anesthesia seems indicated:

1. The patient's apprehension should be allayed as much as possible by personal reassurance during the preanesthetic visit and by adequate sedation and premedication.
2. Pain should be relieved whenever present.
3. An antacid, 15 to 30 mL, should be administered within half an hour before induction of anesthesia. Ranitidine and metoclopramide may be useful.
4. Beginning in the second trimester, uterine displacement must be maintained at all times.
5. Hypotension related to spinal or epidural anesthesia should be prevented as much as possible by rapid intravenous infusion of crystalloid solution before induction. If the mother becomes hypotensive, ephedrine or phenylephrine should be promptly administered intravenously.
6. General anesthesia should be preceded by careful denitrogenation.
7. The risk of aspiration should be minimized by application of cricoid pressure and rapid tracheal intubation with a cuffed tube.
8. To reduce fetal hazard, particularly during the first trimester, it appears preferable to choose drugs with a long history of safety; these drugs include thiopental, morphine, meperidine, muscle relaxants, and low concentrations of nitrous oxide.
9. Avoid maternal hyperventilation and monitor end-expiratory $Pa{CO_2}$ or arterial blood gases.
10. FHR may be monitored continuously or intermittently throughout surgery and anesthesia, provided that placement of the transducer does not encroach on the surgical field[113] (this becomes technically feasible from the sixteenth week of pregnancy). The decision to monitor the fetus should be made in conjunction with the obstetrician based on the severity of maternal disease, the potential for fetal jeopardy and whether the fetus is viable or not. Uterine tone may also be monitored with an external tocodynamometer if the uterus reaches the umbilicus or above.
11. Monitoring of uterine activity should be continued after operation, and tocolytic agents may be required.
12. Special procedures such as hypothermia and induced hypotension might be necessary to facilitate surgery, despite the potential fetal hazard. It is reassuring to know that there was successful fetal outcome after both procedures for intracranial operations.[114] There are numerous reports of cardiopulmonary bypass being performed during pregnancy, with generally good maternal and fetal results.[115,116]

References

1. Lund CJ, Donovan JC: Blood volume during pregnancy. Am J Obstet Gynecol 98:393, 1967
2. Maternal adaptations to pregnancy. In Cunningham G, Grant NF, Leveno KJ *et al* (eds): Williams Obstetrics, p 167. New York, Appleton-Century-Crofts, 2001
3. Wildsmith JAW: Serum pseudocholinesterase, pregnancy and suxamethonium. Anaesthesia 27:90, 1972
4. Coryell MN, Beach EF, Robinson AR *et al*: Metabolism of women during the reproductive cycle: XVII. Changes in electrophoretic patterns of plasma proteins throughout the cycle and following delivery. J Clin Invest 29:1559, 1950
5. Goodman RP, Killom AP, Brash AR *et al*: Prostacyclin production during pregnancy: Comparison of production during normal pregnancy and pregnancy complicated by hypertension. Am J Obstet Gynecol 142:817, 1982

6. Kerr MG, Scott DB, Samuel E: Studies of the inferior vena cava in late pregnancy. BMJ 1:532, 1964
7. Prowse CM, Gaensler EA: Respiratory and acid-base changes during pregnancy. Anesthesiology 26:381, 1965
8. Moya F, Smith BE: Uptake, distribution and placental transport of drugs and anesthetics. Anesthesiology 26:465, 1965
9. Archer GW, Marx GF: Arterial oxygenation during apnoea in parturient women. Br J Anaesth 46:358, 1974
10. Datta S, Kitzmiller JL, Naulty JS *et al*: Acid-base status of diabetic mothers and their infants following spinal anesthesia for cesarean section. Anesth Analg 61:662, 1982
11. Chiloiro M, Darconza G, Piccioli E *et al*: Gastric emptying and orocecal transit time in pregnancy. J Gastroenterol 36:538, 2001
12. Simpson KH, Stakes AF, Miller M: Pregnancy delays paracetamol absorption and gastric emptying in patients undergoing surgery. Br J Anaesth 60:24, 1988
13. Brock-Utne JG, Dow TGB, Dimopoulos GE *et al*: Gastric and lower oesophageal sphincter (LOS) pressures in early pregnancy. Br J Anaesth 53:381, 1981
14. Wyner J, Cohen SE: Gastric volume in early pregnancy: Effect of metoclopramide. Anesthesiology 57:209, 1982
15. Cohen SE, Woods WA, Wyner J: Antiemetic efficacy of droperidol and metoclopramide. Anesthesiology 60:67, 1984
16. Gin T, Chan MTV: Decreased minimum alveolar concentration of isoflurane in pregnant humans. Anesthesiology 81:829, 1994
17. Datta S, Lambert DH, Gregus J *et al*: Differential sensitivities of mammalian nerve fibers during pregnancy. Anesth Analg 62:1070, 1983
18. Brown WU, Bell GC, Alper MH: Acidosis, local anesthetics and the newborn. Obstet Gynecol 48:27, 1976
19. Hamshaw-Thomas A, Rogerson N, Reynolds F: Transfer of bupivacaine, lignocaine and pethidine across the rabbit placenta: Influence of maternal protein binding and fetal flow. Placenta 5:61, 1984
20. Kennedy RL, Miller RP, Bell JU *et al*: Uptake and distribution of bupivacaine in fetal lambs. Anesthesiology 65:247, 1986
21. Kuhnert PM, Kuhnert BR, Stitts BS *et al*: The use of a selected ion monitoring technique to study the disposition of bupivacaine in mother, fetus and neonate following epidural anesthesia for cesarean section. Anesthesiology 55:611, 1981
22. Morishima HO, Daniel SS, Finster M *et al*: Transmission of mepivacaine hydrochloride (Carbocaine) across the human placenta. Anesthesiology 27:147, 1966
23. Kuhnert BR, Kuhnert PM, Prochaska AL *et al*: Plasma levels of 2-chloroprocaine in obstetric patients and their neonates after epidural anesthesia. Anesthesiology 53:21, 1980
24. Haram K, Bakke OM, Johannessen KH *et al*: Transplacental passage of diazepam during labor: Influence of uterine contractions. Clin Pharmacol Ther 24:590, 1978
25. Dwyer R, Fee JP, Moore J: Uptake of halothane & isoflurane by mother and baby during cesarean section. Br J Anesth 74:379, 1995
26. Kosaka Y, Takahashi T, Mark LC: Intravenous thiobarbiturate anesthesia for cesarean section. Anesthesiology 31:489, 1969
27. Morishima HO, Covino BG: Toxicity and distribution of lidocaine in nonasphyxiated and asphyxiated baboon fetuses. Anesthesiology 54:182, 1981
28. Morishima HO, Finster M, Pedersen H *et al*: Pharmacokinetics of lidocaine in fetal and neonatal lambs and adult sheep. Anesthesiology 50:431, 1979
29. Mihaly GW, Moore RG, Thomas J *et al*: The pharmacokinetics and metabolism of the anilide local anaesthetics in neonates. Eur J Clin Pharmacol 13:143, 1978
30. Morishima HO, Pedersen H, Finster M *et al*: Toxicity of lidocaine in adult, newborn and fetal sheep. Anesthesiology 55:57, 1981
31. Gale R, Ferguson JE II, Stevenson D: Effect of epidural analgesia with bupivacaine hydrochloride on neonatal bilirubin production. Obstet Gynecol 70:692, 1987
32. Ueland K, Hansen JM: Maternal cardiovascular dynamics: III. Labor and delivery under local and caudal analgesia. Am J Obstet Gynecol 103:8, 1969
33. Scott JR, Rose NB: Effect of psychoprophylaxis (Lamaze preparation) on labor and delivery in primiparas. N Engl J Med 294:1205, 1976
34. Eisele JH, Wright R, Rogge P: Newborn and maternal fentanyl levels at cesarean section. Anesth Analg 61:179, 1982
35. Morley-Forester PK, Weber J: ALS neonatal effects of patient controlled analgesia using fentanyl in labor. Int J Obstet Anesth 7:103, 1998
36. Chestnut DH, Vincent RD, McGrath JM *et al*: Does early administration of epidural analgesia affect obstetric outcome in nulliparous women who are receiving intravenous oxytocin? Anesthesiology 80:1193, 1994
37. Chestnut DH, McGrath JM, Vincent RD *et al*: Does early administration of epidural analgesia affect obstetric outcome in nulliparous women who are in spontaneous labor? Anesthesiology 80:1201, 1994
38. Thorp JA, Hu DH, Albin RM *et al*: The effect of intrapartum epidural analgesia on nulliparous labor: A randomized, controlled, prospective trial. Am J Obstet Gynecol 169:851, 1993
39. Sharma SK, Sidawi JE, Ramin SM *et al*: Cesarean delivery: A randomized trial of epidural versus patient controlled meperidine analgesia during labor. Anesthesiology 87:487, 1997
40. Halpern SH, Leighton BL, Ohlsson A *et al*: Effect of epidural vs parenteral opioid analgesia in the progress of labor: A metaanalysis. JAMA 280:2105, 1998
41. Halpern SH, Muir H, Breen TW *et al*: A multi-center randomized controlled trial comparing patient-controlled epidural with intravenous analgesia for pain relief in labor. Anesth Analg 99:1532, 2004
42. Norris MC, Ferrenbach D, Dalman H *et al*: Does epinephrine improve the diagnostic accuracy of aspiration during labor epidural analgesia? Anesth Analg 88:1073, 1999
43. Cohen SE, Cherry CM, Holbrook RH *et al*: Intrathecal sufentanil for labor-analgesia—Sensory changes, side-effects and fetal heart rate changes. Anesth Analg 77:1155, 1993
44. Nielson PE, Erickson R, Abouleish E *et al*: Fetal heart rate changes after intrathecal sufentanil or epidural bupivacaine for labor analgesia: Incidence and clinical significance. Anesth Analg 83:742, 1996
45. Norris MC, Grieco WM, Borkowski M *et al*: Complications of labor analgesia: Epidural versus combined spinal epidural techniques. Anesth Analg 79:529, 1995
46. Leighton BL, Arkoosh VA, Haffnagle S *et al*: The dermatomal spread of epidural bupivacaine with and without prior intrathecal sufentanil. Anesth Analg 83:526, 1996
47. Bloom SL, McIntire DD, Kelly MA *et al*: Lack of effect of walking on labor and delivery. N Engl J Med 339(2):76, 1998
48. Leighton BL, Halpern SH, Wilson DB: Lumbar sympathetic blocks speed early and second stage induced labor in nulliparous women. Anesthesiology 90:1039, 1999
49. Carstoniu J, Levytam S, Norman P *et al*: Nitrous oxide in early labor: Safety and analgesic efficacy assessed by a double-blind, placebo controlled study. Anesthesiology 80:30, 1994
50. Landon MB, Hauth JC, Leveno KJ *et al*: Maternal and perinatal outcomes associated with a trial of labor after prior cesarean delivery. N Engl J Med 351(25):2581, 2004
51. Hawkins JL, Gibbs CP, Orleans M *et al*: Obstetric anesthesia workforce survey: 1992 vs 1981. Anesthesiology 87:135, 1994
52. Kuczkowski KM, Benumof JL: Tongue piercing and obstetric anesthesia: Is there cause for concern? J Clin Anesth 14(16):447, 2002
53. Rout CC, Rocke DA, Levin J *et al*: A reevaluation of the role of crystalloid preload in the prevention of hypotension associated with spinal anesthesia for elective cesarean section. Anesthesiology 79:262, 1993
54. Marx GF, Luykx WM, Cohen S: Fetal-neonatal status following cesarean section for fetal distress. Br J Anaesth 56:1009, 1984
55. Norris MC: Height, weight and the spread of subarachnoid hyperbaric bupivacaine in the term parturient. Anesth Analg 67:555, 1988
56. Leighton BL, Norris MC, Sosis M *et al*: Limitations of epinephrine as a marker of intravascular injection in laboring women. Anesthesiology 66:688, 1987
57. Leighton BL, Norris MC, DeSimone CA *et al*: The air test as a clinically useful indicator of intravenously placed epidural catheters. Anesthesiology 73:610, 1990
58. Gissen AJ, Datta S, Lambert D: The chloroprocaine controversy: Is chloroprocaine neurotoxic? Reg Anesth 9:135, 1984
59. Albright GA: Cardiac arrest following regional anesthesia with etidocaine or bupivacaine. Anesthesiology 51:285, 1979
60. Tanz RD, Heskett T, Loehning RW *et al*: Comparative cardiotoxicity of bupivacaine and lidocaine in the isolated perfused mammalian heart. Anesth Analg 63:549, 1984
61. Crosby ET, Cooper RM, Douglas MJ *et al*: The unanticipated difficult airway with recommendations for management. Can J Anaesth 45:757, 1998
62. Awan R, Nolan JP, Cook TM: Use of proseal laryngeal mask airway for airway maintenance during emergency caesarean section after failed tracheal intubation. Br J Anaesth 92:144, 2004
63. Ong BV, Cohen MM, Palahniuk RJ: Anesthesia for cesarean section: Effects on neonates. Anesth Analg 68:270, 1989
64. Datta S, Ostheimer GW, Weiss JB *et al*: Neonatal effect of prolonged anesthetic induction for cesarean section. Obstet Gynecol 58:331, 1981
65. Marx GF, Mateo CV: Effects of different oxygen concentrations during general anaesthesia for elective caesarean section. Can Anaesth Soc J 18:587, 1971
66. Hawkins JL, Koonin LM, Palmer SK, Gibbs CP: Anesthesia related deaths during obstetric delivery in the US, 1979–1990. Anesthesiology 86:277, 1997
67. Emmett RS, Cyna AM, Andrew M, Simmons SW: Techniques for preventing hypotension during spinal anesthesia for cesarean delivery. Cochrane Database Syst Rev 3:CD002251, 2002
68. Ueyama H, He YL, Tanigami H *et al*: Effects of crystalloid and colloid preload or blood volume in the parturient undergoing spinal anesthesia for elective cesarean section. Anesthesiology 91:1571, 1999
69. Rout CC, Roche DA: Spinal hypotension associated with cesarean section: Will preload ever work? Anesthesiology 91:1565, 1999
70. Kasten GW, Martin ST: Resuscitation from bupivacaine-induced cardiovascular toxicity during partial inferior vena cava occlusion. Anesth Analg 65:341, 1986
71. Duffy PJ, Crosby ET: The epidural blood patch. Resolving the controversies. Can J Anaesth 46:878, 1999

72. Cheney FW: Injuries associated with regional anesthesia in the 1980's and 1990's. Anesthesiology 101:143, 2004
73. Wang Y, Walsh SW, Kay HH: Placental lipid peroxides and thromboxane are increased and prostacyclin is decreased in women with preeclampsia. Am J Obstet Gynecol 167:946, 1992
74. Chesley LC: Plasma and red cell volumes during pregnancy. Am J Obstet Gynecol 112:440, 1972
75. Bosio PM, McKenna PJ, Conroy R, O'Herlihy C: Maternal central hemodyanamics in hypertensive disorders of pregnancy. Obstet Gynecol 94:978, 1999
76. Cotton DB, Gonik B, Dorman K *et al*: Cardiovascular alterations in severe pregnancy-induced hypertension: Relationship of central venous pressure to pulmonary capillary wedge pressure. Am J Obstet Gynecol 151:762, 1985
77. O'Brien JM, Milligan DA, Barton JR: Impact of high dose corticosteroid therapy for patients with HELLP (hemolysis, elevated liver function tests, and low platelets) syndrome. Am J Obstet Gynecol 183:921, 2000
78. Hogg B, Hauth JC, Caritis SN *et al*: Safety of labor epidural anesthesia for women with severe hypertensive disease. Am J Obstet Gynecol 181:1099, 1999
79. Newsome LR, Bramwell RS, Curling PE: Severe preeclampsia: Hemodynamic effects of lumbar epidural anesthesia. Anesth Analg 65:31, 1986
80. Jouppila P, Jouppila R, Hollmen A *et al*: Lumbar epidural analgesia to improve intervillous blood flow during labor in severe preeclampsia. Obstet Gynecol 59:158, 1982
81. Ramanathan J, Botorff M, Jeter JN *et al*: The pharmacokinetics and maternal and neonatal effects of epidural lidocaine in preeclampsia. Anesth Analg 65:120, 1986
82. Wallace DH, Leveno KJ, Cunningham FG *et al*: Randomized comparison of general and regional anesthesia for cesarean delivery in pregnancies complicated by severe preeclampsia. Obstet Gynecol 86:193, 1995
83. Hood DD, Curry R: Spinal versus epidural anesthesia for cesarean section in severely preeclamptic patients: A retrospective survey. Anesthesiology 90:1276, 1999
84. Clark SL, Koonings PP, Phelan JP: Placenta previa/accreta and prior cesarean section. Obstet Gynecol 66:89, 1985
85. Chestnut DH, Dewan DM, Redick LF *et al*: Anesthetic management for obstetric hysterectomy: A multi-institutional study. Anesthesiology 70:607, 1989
86. Benedetti TJ: Maternal complications of parenteral beta-sympathomimetic therapy for premature labor. Am J Obstet Gynecol 145:1, 1983
87. Krauer B, Krauer F, Hytten F: Drug prescribing in pregnancy. In Current Reviews in Obstetrics and Gynaecology, Vol 7, p 44. Edinburgh, Churchill Livingstone, 1984
88. Kaltreider DF: Premature labor and meperidine analgesia. Am J Obstet Gynecol 99:989, 1967
89. Santos AC, Yun EM, Bobby PD *et al*: The effects of bupivacaine, L nitro-L-arginine-methyl-ester and phenylephrine on cardiovascular adaptations to asphyxia in the preterm fetal lamb. Anesth Analg 84:1299, 1997
90. Morishima HO, Pedersen H, Santos AC *et al*: Adverse effects of maternally administered lidocaine on the asphyxiated preterm fetal lamb. Anesthesiology 71:110, 1989
91. Hughes SC, Dailey PA, Landers D *et al*: Parturients infected with human immunodeficiency virus and regional anesthesia: Clinical and immunologic response. Anesthesiology 97:320, 2002
92. Avidan MS, Groves P, Blott M *et al*: Low complication rate associated with cesarean section under spinal anesthesia for HIV-1 infected women on anti-retroviral therapy. Anesthesiology 97:320, 2002
93. Tom DJ, Gulevich SJ, Shapiro HM *et al*: Epidural blood patch in the HIV positive patient: Review of clinical experience. Anesthesiology 76:943, 1992
94. Birnbach DJ, Stein DJ: The substance abusing parturient. Implications for analgesia and anesthetic management. Baillieres Clin Obstet Gynaecol 12:443, 1998
95. Parer JT. Efficacy and safety of intrapartum electronic fetal monitoring: An update. Obstet Gynecol 87:476, 1996
96. Luttkus AK, Stupin JH, Callsen TA, Dudenhausen JW: Feasibility of simultanoeus application of fetal electrocardiography and fetal pulse oximetry. Acta Obstet Gynecol Scand 82:443, 2003
97. Adamsons K, Beard RW, Cosmi EV *et al*: The validity of capillary blood in the assessment of the acid-base state of the fetus. In Adamsons K (ed): Diagnosis and Treatment of Fetal Disorders, p 175. New York, Springer-Verlag, 1968
98. Beard RW: Fetal blood sampling. Br J Hosp Med 3:523, 1970
99. Bowe ET, Beard RW, Finster M *et al*: Reliability of fetal blood sampling. Am J Obstet Gynecol 107:279, 1970
100. Adamsons K, Behrman R, Dawes GS *et al*: Resuscitation by positive pressure ventilation and tris-hydroxymethylaminomethane of rhesus monkeys asphyxiated at birth. J Pediatr 65:807, 1964
101. Neonatal resuscitation. Guidelines 2000 for cardiopulmonary resuscitation and emergency cardiovascular care: International consensus on science. Part II. Circulation 102(8):I-343, 2000
102. Shnider SM, Webster GM: Maternal and fetal hazards of surgery during pregnancy. Am J Obstet Gynecol 92:891, 1965
103. Brodsky JB, Cohen EN, Brown BW Jr *et al*: Surgery during pregnancy and fetal outcome. Am J Obstet Gynecol 138:1165, 1980
104. Smith BE: Fetal prognosis after anesthesia during gestation. Anesth Analg 42:521, 1963
105. Duncan PG, Pope WDB, Cohen MM *et al*: Fetal risk of anesthesia and surgery during pregnancy. Anesthesiology 64:790, 1986
106. Mazze RI, Källén B: Reproductive outcome after anesthesia and operation during pregnancy: A registry study of 5405 cases. Am J Obstet Gynecol 161:1178, 1989
107. Grabowski CT, Paar JA: The teratogenic effects of graded doses of hypoxia on the chick embryo. Am J Anat 103:313, 1958
108. Hannah RS, Moore KL: Effects of fasting and insulin on skeletal development in rats. Teratology 4:135, 1971
109. Hartz SC, Heinonen OP, Shapiro S *et al*: Antenatal exposure to meprobamate and chlordiazepoxide in relation to malformations, mental development and childhood mortality. N Engl J Med 292:726, 1975
110. Sáxen I, Sáxen L: Association between maternal intake of diazepam and oral clefts. Lancet 2:498, 1975
111. Safra MJ, Oakley GP: Association between cleft lip with or without cleft palate and prenatal exposure to diazepam. Lancet 2:478, 1975
112. Drachman DB, Coulombre AJ: Experimental clubfoot and arthrogryposis multiplex congenita. Lancet 2:523, 1962
113. Basford AB, Fink BR: The teratogenicity of halothane in the rat. Anesthesiology 29:1167, 1968
114. Wharton RS, Mazze RI, Wilson AI: Reproduction and fetal development in mice chronically exposed to enflurane. Anesthesiology 54:505, 1981
115. Mazze RI, Wilson AI, Rice SA *et al*: Effects of isoflurane on reproduction and fetal development in mice. Anesth Analg 63:249, 1984
116. Mazze RI, Fujinaga M, Rice SA *et al*: Reproductive and teratogenic effects of nitrous oxide, halothane, isoflurane and enflurane in Sprague-Dawley rats. Anesthesiology 64:339, 1986
117. Smith BE, Gaub MI, Moya F: Teratogenic effects of anesthetic agents: Nitrous oxide. Anesth Analg 44:726, 1965
118. Baden JM, Serra M, Mazze RI: Inhibition of fetal methionine synthase by nitrous oxide. Br J Anaesth 56:523, 1984
119. Nunn JF, Sharer NM, Battiglieri T *et al*: Effect of short-term administration of nitrous oxide on plasma concentration of methionine, tryptophan, phenylalanine, and S-adenosyl methionine in man. Br J Anaesth 58:1, 1986
120. Crawford JS, Lewis M: Nitrous oxide in early human pregnancy. Anaesthesia 41:900, 1986
121. Aldridge LM, Tunstall ME: Nitrous oxide and the fetus: A review and the results of a retrospective study of 175 cases of anaesthesia for insertion of Shirodkar suture. Br J Anaesth 58:1348, 1986
122. Fujinaga M, Baden JM, Yhap EO *et al*: Halothane and isoflurane prevent the teratogenic effects of nitrous oxide in rats, folinic acid does not. Anesthesiology 67:A456, 1987
123. Adamsons K, Mueller-Heubach E, Myers RE: Production of fetal asphyxia in the rhesus monkey by administration of catecholamines to the mother. Am J Obstet Gynecol 109:148, 1971
124. Katz JD, Hook R, Barash PG: Fetal heart rate monitoring in the pregnant patient under surgery. Am J Obstet Gynecol 125:267, 1976
125. Kofke WA, Wuest HP, McGinnis LA: Cesarean section following ruptured cerebral aneurysm and neuroresuscitation. Anesthesiology 60:242, 1984
126. Estafanous FG, Buckley S: Management of anesthesia for open heart surgery during pregnancy. Cleve Clin Q 43:121, 1976
127. Trimakas AP, Maxwell KD, Berkay S *et al*: Fetal monitoring during cardiac pulmonary bypass for removal of a left atrial myxoma during pregnancy. Johns Hopkins Med J 144:156, 1979

CHAPTER 43 ■ NEONATAL ANESTHESIA

FREDERIC A. BERRY AND BARBARA A. CASTRO

KEY POINTS

1. Understanding the physiologic changes that occur during the transition from fetal to neonatal life is crucial to the anesthetic management of the neonate. The circulatory, pulmonary, hepatic, and renal systems are all affected.
2. Persistent pulmonary hypertension (PPH) is a pathologic condition that can be primary but is often secondary to other conditions, including meconium aspiration, sepsis, congenital diaphragmatic hernia, or pneumonia. Understanding the pathophysiologic characteristics of PPH helps guide therapy.
3. Knowledge of the major anatomic differences between the infant and adult airway helps one understand why the infant's airway is often described as "anterior" and why airway management may be challenging. These differences include a relatively large tongue, a higher glottis with anterior slanting vocal folds, a larger occiput, and a narrowing at the cricoid ring.
4. Four important physiologic factors account for the rapid rate of desaturation observed in neonates. These include an increase in oxygen consumption, a high closing volume, a high ratio of minute ventilation to FRC, and a pliable rib cage.
5. Careful attention must be given to the choice of anesthetic agents and dosing of such agents in the neonatal population. Ongoing maturational changes in the renal and hepatobiliary systems, which occur during the first 30 days of life, will affect the metabolism and elimination of many anesthetic agents.
6. Although a host of anesthetic techniques are available, including regional, multiple factors are considered when choosing an anesthetic plan for the neonate. These include the surgical requirements, the need for postoperative ventilation, the cardiovascular stability of the neonate, and the anticipated method of postoperative pain control.
7. Special considerations must be addressed when planning an anesthetic for a neonate. Some of the most common and controversial issues include the risk of postoperative apnea and the use of caffeine in treatment and prophylaxis, the role of oxygen concentration in the development of retinopathy of prematurity, and the neurodevelopmental effects of anesthetic agents on the developing brain.
8. True surgical emergencies are uncommon in the neonatal period. Knowledge of conditions with comorbidities, such as tracheoesophageal fistula, omphalocele, and congenital diaphragmatic hernia, and a thorough preoperative evaluation and stabilization of such neonates cannot be overemphasized.

PHYSIOLOGY OF THE INFANT AND THE TRANSITION PERIOD

The first year of life is characterized by an almost miraculous growth in size and maturity. The body weight alone changes by a factor of three, and there is no other period in extrauterine life when changes occur so rapidly. Before birth, fetal growth and development depend on the genetic composition of the fetus, the mother's placental function, and potential exposure to chemicals or infectious agents that can affect mother, fetus, or both. The journey down the birth canal (or through the abdominal wall)—called the most dangerous trip in a person's life—ends the fetal period, and the newborn must adapt to extrauterine life. This change from fetal to extrauterine life is called the period of transition or adaptation.

The infant is considered a newborn in the first 24 hours of life. This chapter focuses on the neonatal period, which is defined as the first 30 days of extrauterine life and includes the newborn period. The most significant part of transition occurs in the first 24 to 72 hours after birth. All systems of the body change during transition, but the most important to the anesthesiologist are the circulatory, pulmonary, hepatic, and renal systems. The circulatory and pulmonary systems are so interdependent that they are discussed together.

Transition of the Cardiopulmonary System

Fetal Circulation

Fetal circulation is characterized by the presence of three main shunts (Fig. 43-1A). These shunts are the placenta, foramen ovale, and ductus arteriosus. The placenta oxygenates the blood, which then courses up the inferior vena cava into the right atrium. The right atrium is divided by a structure called the crista dividends so this relatively well-oxygenated blood is shunted from the right atrium through the foramen ovale into the left atrium, thereby bypassing the right ventricle and the pulmonary vascular bed. This blood, the best oxygenated in the fetus, progresses from the left atrium to the left ventricle and out the ascending aorta to provide oxygenation for the brain and upper extremities. Blood returns from the upper body to the right heart by the superior vena cava, where it is directed

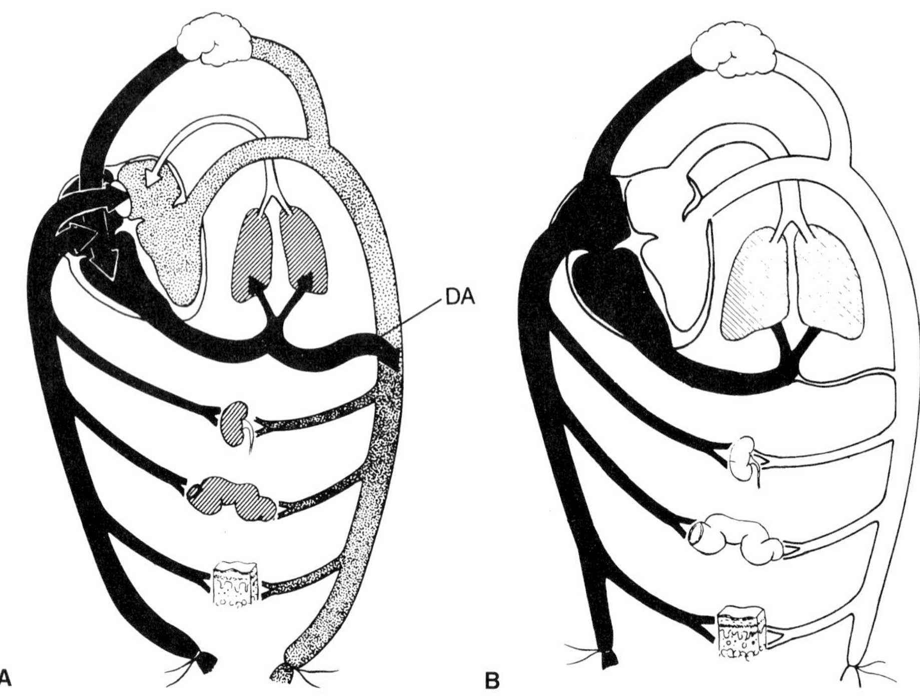

FIGURE 43-1. **A.** Schematic representation of the fetal circulation. Oxygenated blood leaves the placenta in the umbilical vein (*vessel without stippling*). Umbilical vein blood joins blood from the viscera (represented here by the kidney, gut, and skin) in the inferior vena cava. Approximately half of the inferior vena cava flow passes through the foramen ovale to the left atrium, where it mixes with a small amount of pulmonary venous blood, and this relatively well-oxygenated blood (*light stippling*) supplies the heart and brain by way of the ascending aorta. The other half of the inferior vena cava stream mixes with superior vena cava blood and enters the right ventricle (blood in the right atrium and ventricle has little oxygen, which is denoted by *heavy stippling*). Because the pulmonary arterioles are constricted, most of the blood in the main pulmonary artery flows through the ductus arteriosus (DA) so the descending aorta's blood has less oxygen (*heavy stippling*) than does blood in the ascending aorta (*light stippling*). **B.** Schematic representation of the circulation in the normal newborn. After expansion of the lungs and ligation of the umbilical cord, pulmonary blood flow and left atrial and systemic arterial pressures increase. When left atrial pressure exceeds right atrial pressure, the foramen ovale closes so all inferior and superior vena cava blood leaves the right atrium, enters the right ventricle, and is pumped through the pulmonary artery toward the lung. With the increase in systemic arterial pressure and decrease in pulmonary artery pressure, flow through the ductus arteriosus becomes left to right, and the ductus constricts and closes. The course of circulation is the same as in the adult. (Reprinted with permission from Phibbs R: Delivery room management of the newborn. In Avery GB [ed]: Neonatology, Pathophysiology and Management of the Newborn, p 184. Philadelphia, JB Lippincott, 1981.)

by the crista dividends into the right ventricle, from which it is then pumped out the pulmonary artery. The relatively low pressure in the left atrium and the high pressure in the right atrium result in the foramen ovale being open. The pulmonary vascular bed has a high vascular resistance because the alveoli are relatively closed and filled with fluid, and the blood vessels are compressed. In addition, decreased $Pa{O_2}$ and low pH increase pulmonary vascular resistance. The ductus arteriosus represents a low-resistance system because it is dilated secondary to a low $Pa{O_2}$. Therefore, the blood that leaves the right ventricle by the pulmonary artery is shunted preferentially (90%) through the ductus arteriosus and down the descending aorta, whereas only 10% of the output of the right ventricle flows through the pulmonary artery into the pulmonary vascular bed. The pulmonary vascular bed requires only enough blood flow to ensure growth and development of the lungs, including surfactant production.

1 Clamping of the umbilical cord and initiation of ventilation produce enormous circulatory changes in the newborn (Fig. 43-1B). The transition of the alveoli from a fluid-filled to an air-filled state results in a reduced compression of the pulmonary alveolar capillaries with a reduction in pulmonary vascular resistance over the first several hours of life. However, it takes 3 to 4 days for the pulmonary vascular resistance to decrease to normal levels. Nitric oxide is an integral part of the reduction in pulmonary vascular resistance; its clinical use is discussed later in the chapter. The initial moderate decrease in pulmonary vascular resistance is accompanied by constriction of the ductus arteriosus secondary to oxygenation. This results in an increase in pulmonary blood flow and an increase in left atrial pressure so the foramen ovale functionally closes. Closure of these two neonatal shunts (i.e., the ductus arteriosus and the foramen ovale) is initially only a functional closure. Both shunts usually close permanently in the first several months of life. However, an autopsy study of normal hearts has demonstrated a 30% incidence of patent foramen ovale during the first 30 years of life and a 20% incidence for people 30 years of age and older.[1]

Transition of the Pulmonary System

The pulmonary system transition occurs more quickly than the circulatory system. The primary event is the initiation of ventilation, which changes the alveoli from a fluid-filled to an air-filled state. During the first 5 to 10 minutes of extrauterine life, normal ventilatory volumes develop and normal tidal ventilation is established. The initial negative intrathoracic pressures that the newborn generates are often in the range of 40 to 60 cm H_2O. By 10 to 20 minutes of life, the newborn has achieved its near-normal functional residual capacity (FRC) and the blood gases are well stabilized. Table 43-1 lists the normal blood gases for the various periods of life. One study in preterm infants older than 26 weeks' gestational age demonstrated that a single dose of dexamethasone given within 2 hours of delivery resulted in lower ventilator settings and a higher mean blood pressure during the first week of life.[2] In addition, fewer infants in this group received indomethacin to treat a patent ductus arteriosus (PDA).

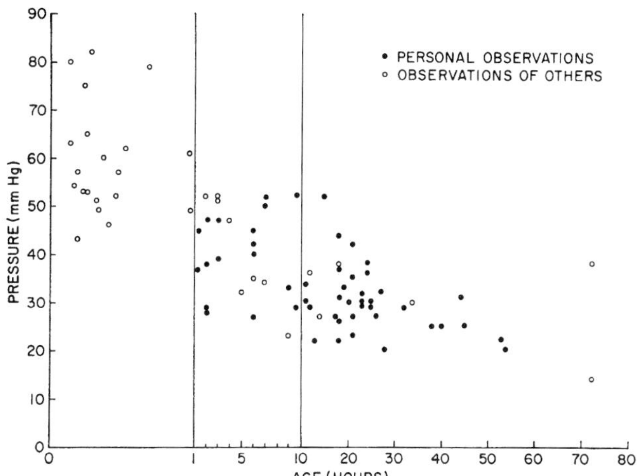

FIGURE 43-2. Correlation of mean pulmonary arterial pressure with age in 85 normal-term infants studied during the first 3 days of life. (Reprinted with permission from Emmanouilides GC, Moss AJ, Duffie ER, Adams FH: Pulmonary arterial pressure changes in human newborn infants from birth to 3 days of age. J Pediatr 65:327, 1964.)

Patent Ductus Arteriosus

A study by Reller et al.[3] demonstrated that a PDA on or beyond the fourth day of life is abnormal, regardless of gestational age. Prematurity, unless complicated by acute asphyxia or the respiratory distress syndrome, is not a risk factor for persistent PDA. In their study, 95% of premature infants, regardless of gestational age, had closure of the ductus by day 4. The incidence of a PDA in premature infants with respiratory distress syndrome without a history of birth asphyxia was 11%, a percentage that is somewhat less than is commonly assumed.

Persistent Pulmonary Hypertension

2 The pulmonary circulation is extremely sensitive to oxygen, pH, and nitric oxide. Figure 43-2 illustrates the correlation of the mean pulmonary artery pressure with age during the first 3 days of life. Hypoxia and acidosis, along with inflammatory mediators, may cause pulmonary artery pressure either to persist at a high level or, after initially decreasing, to increase to pathologic levels. The result is termed *persistent pulmonary hypertension* (PPH). The pathophysiologic characteristics of

TABLE 43-1

NORMAL BLOOD GAS VALUES IN THE NEONATE

SUBJECT	AGE	PO_2 (mm Hg)	PCO_2 (mm Hg)	pH
Fetus (term)	Before labor	25	40	7.37
Fetus (term)	End of labor	10–20	55	7.25
Newborn (term)	10 min	50	48	7.20
Newborn (term)	1 hr	70	35	7.35
Newborn (term)	1 wk	75	35	7.40
Newborn (preterm, 1,500 g)	1 wk	60	38	7.37

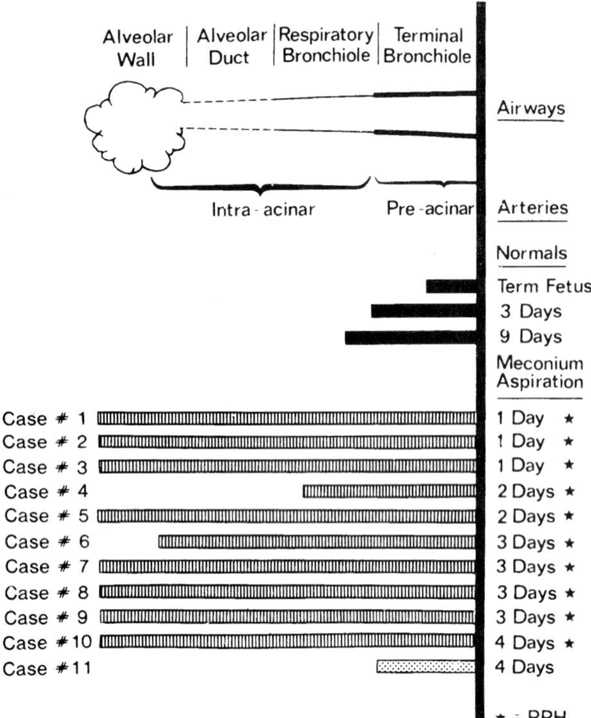

FIGURE 43-3. Diagram of muscle extension along pulmonary arterial branches (*shaded bars*). In the normal newborn, virtually no intra-acinar artery is muscular. In 9 of 10 infants with meconium aspiration and persistent pulmonary hypertension (PPH), muscle extended into the most peripheral arteries; the infant with meconium aspiration without PPH (case # 11) had normal intra-acinar arteries. (Reprinted with permission from Murphy JD, Vawter GF, Reid LM: Pulmonary vascular disease in fetal meconium aspiration. J Pediatr 104:758, 1984.)

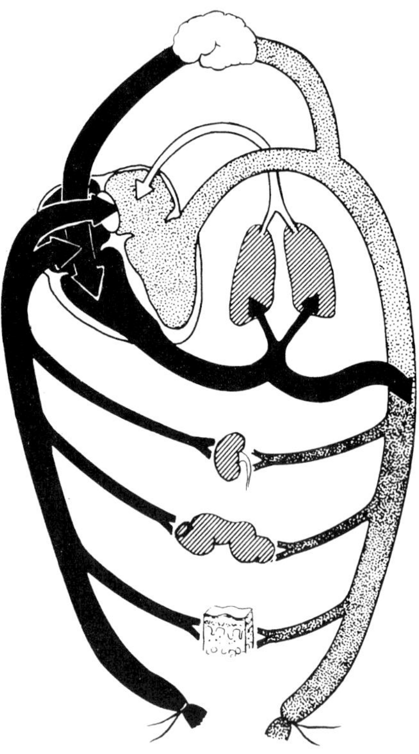

FIGURE 43-4. Schematic representation of the circulation in an asphyxiated newborn with incomplete expansion of the lungs. Pulmonary vascular resistance is high, pulmonary blood flow is low (note the small caliber of the pulmonary vein), and flow through the ductus arteriosus is high. With little pulmonary venous flow, left atrial pressure decreases below right atrial pressure, the foramen ovale opens, and vena cava blood flows through the foramen into the left atrium. This partially venous blood flows to the brain by the ascending aorta. The descending aorta blood that flows to the viscera has less oxygen than that of the ascending aorta (*heavy stippling*) because of the right-to-left flow through the ductus arteriosus. The circulation is the same in the fetus, except there is no oxygenated blood in the inferior vena cava from the umbilical vein. (Reprinted with permission from Phibbs R: Delivery room management of the newborn. In Avery GB [ed]: Neonatology, Pathophysiology and Management of the Newborn, p 184. Philadelphia, JB Lippincott, 1981.)

pulmonary hypertension comprise a spectrum, ranging from normal pulmonary vasculature to abnormal pulmonary vasculature that is characterized by extension of smooth muscle into the distal respiratory units (Fig. 43-3). Vasoconstriction of the muscle in the blood vessels of the pulmonary vascular bed results in pulmonary hypertension with a right-to-left shunt through the foramen ovale and/or the ductus arteriosus (Fig. 43-4).

Problems of PPH or hypoxemic respiratory failure involve not only preterm, but also term infants. PPH may be primary with no recognized etiology, or it may be secondary to meconium aspiration, sepsis, pneumonia, respiratory distress, and congenital diaphragmatic hernia (CDH). Currently, the basic treatment depends on the degree of respiratory failure and the response to therapy. The goals of therapy are to achieve a Pa_{O_2} between 50 and 70 mm Hg and a Pa_{CO_2} between 40 and 60 mm Hg. There have been major changes in therapy since the 1990s, with the introduction of surfactant, high-frequency ventilation, inhaled nitric oxide, and extracorporeal membrane oxygenation (ECMO). The technique and degree of intervention depend on the response to supportive care. Surfactant and various ventilatory techniques are used as the first-line treatment. These techniques include intermittent mandatory ventilation, assist control ventilation, and proportional assist ventilation.[4–6] Studies with proportional assist ventilation demonstrate that gas exchange can be maintained with smaller transpulmonary pressure changes, which may reduce the incidence of chronic lung disease in low-birth-weight infants.[6]

Meconium Aspiration

Interference with the normal maternal placental circulation in the third trimester may cause fetal hypoxia. Fetal hypoxia can result in an increase in the amount of muscle in the blood vessels of the distal respiratory units. Figure 43-3 illustrates the muscle increase found in blood vessels of a series of 11 infants who died of PPH.[7] Chronic fetal hypoxia leads to the passage of meconium in utero. The fetus breathes in utero so the meconium mixed with amniotic fluid enters the pulmonary system. Meconium aspiration can be a marker of chronic fetal hypoxia in the third trimester. This condition is different from the meconium aspiration that occurs during delivery. This meconium at birth is thick and tenacious, and mechanically obstructs the tracheobronchial system. Meconium aspiration syndrome leads to varying degrees of respiratory failure, which can be fatal in spite of all treatment modalities.

Until relatively recently, tracheal intubation and suctioning were recommended for all infants with frank meconium aspiration or meconium staining (approximately 10% of newborns). Now a more conservative approach should be used because routine intubation may cause unnecessary respiratory complications.[8–10] Routine oropharyngeal suctioning of meconium is recommended immediately at the time of delivery, but tracheal intubation and suctioning should be performed selectively, depending on the condition of the infant. Infants with a high Apgar score (i.e., 7-9) need no additional airway management. Infants with a low Apgar score or who are clinically obstructed with meconium should have the appropriate resuscitative measures taken.

Transition and Maturation of the Renal System

The fetal kidneys and the fetal lungs have certain similarities. During the fetal period, both have a relatively low blood flow compared with that during the newborn and neonatal periods because both organs need only enough blood flow for growth and development. The maternal placenta removes fetal waste material. The major function of the fetal kidneys is the production of urine; this contributes to the formation of amniotic fluid, which is important for the normal development of the fetal lung, and acts as a shock absorber for the fetus. The fetal kidney is characterized by a low renal blood flow (RBF) and glomerular filtration rate (GFR).[11] There are four major reasons for the low RBF and GFR: low systemic arterial pressure, high renal vascular resistance, low permeability of the glomerular capillaries, and the small size and number of glomeruli. The low systemic arterial pressure and high vascular resistance are the two characteristics that are similar to those found in the fetal lung. This results in a low RBF, which in turn results in a low GFR. Transition changes the first two factors: the systemic arterial pressure increases and the renal vascular resistance decreases. Again, this is similar to what occurs in the lung. The other two factors are changed through maturation. The limited ability of the newborn's kidney to concentrate or dilute urine results from the low GFR at birth. However, during the first 3 to 4 days, the circulatory changes increase RBF and GFR and improve the neonate's ability to concentrate and dilute the urine. The maturation continues, and by the time the normal full-term infant is 1 month of age, the kidneys are approximately 60% mature. This is sufficient renal function to handle almost any contingency.

The neonatal kidney does have certain limitations. The renin-angiotensin-aldosterone system is the primary compensatory system for the reabsorption of sodium and water to compensate for the loss of plasma, blood, gastrointestinal tract fluid, and third-space fluid. Aldosterone facilitates the reabsorption of sodium in the distal tubule. The immature tubular cells cannot completely reabsorb sodium under the stimulus of aldosterone so the neonate continues to excrete sodium in the urine, even in the presence of a severe sodium defect. For this reason, the neonate is considered an "obligate sodium loser." In the mature state, the distal tubule can reabsorb essentially all the sodium so the urine has less than 5 to 10 mEq of sodium per liter of urine. In the neonate, this number may be as high as 20 to 25 mEq of sodium per liter of urine.

Fluid and Electrolyte Therapy in the Neonate

The inability of the neonatal distal tubule to respond fully to aldosterone results in the obligatory sodium loss in the urine. Therefore, intravenous fluids in the neonate must contain sodium. Most operations on neonates involve loss of blood and extracellular fluid, which must be replaced with a fluid of similar electrolyte content (i.e., a balanced salt solution such as lactated Ringer's or Plasmalyte).

The other problems of the neonate are those of appropriate glucose administration. Infants of diabetic mothers and those small for gestational age have particular problems with hypoglycemia. These infants need to have their blood glucose values monitored. Neonates who are scheduled for surgery and have been receiving hyperalimentation fluids or supplementary glucose must continue to receive that fluid during surgery or must have their glucose levels monitored because of concerns of hypoglycemia. There is no consensus on the issue of what constitutes hypoglycemia.[12] This concern must be balanced against the potential augmentation of ischemic injury by the administration of glucose leading to hyperglycemia. Interestingly, in a more recent study in infants undergoing cardiac surgery, low glucose concentrations tended to relate to electroencephalographic seizures, and high glucose concentrations were not associated with worse neurodevelopmental outcomes. The authors concluded that avoiding hypoglycemia was preferable to restricting glucose in infants having cardiac surgery.[13]

Premature infants and neonates must receive full-strength balanced salt solution for the replacement of third-space and blood losses during the perioperative period.[14] There is a misconception that these infants cannot tolerate the salt load; therefore, they are often given hypotonic fluids. It is not unusual to see premature infants with postoperative sodium values of 125 to 130 mEq/L. Alone, these levels may not be a major problem, but when added to the residual effects of muscle relaxants and antibiotics in a sick infant, they may result in depression of neuromuscular function.

ANATOMIC AND MATURATIONAL FACTORS OF NEONATES AND THEIR CLINICAL SIGNIFICANCE

Anatomy of the Neonatal Airway

The anatomic and maturational factors unique to the neonatal airway have far-reaching clinical implications (Fig. 43-5). Neonates are obligate nose breathers; therefore, anything that obstructs the nares compromises the neonate's ability to

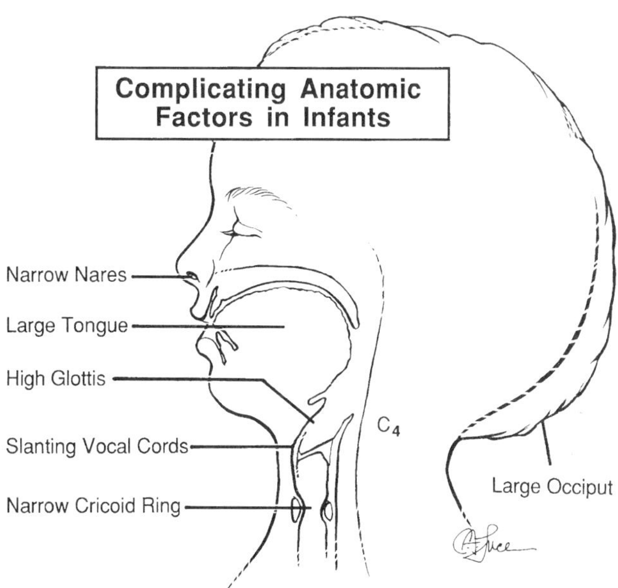

FIGURE 43-5. Complicating anatomic factors in infants. (Modified with permission from Smith RM: Anesthesia for Infants and Children, 4th ed, p 16. St Louis, Mosby, 1980.)

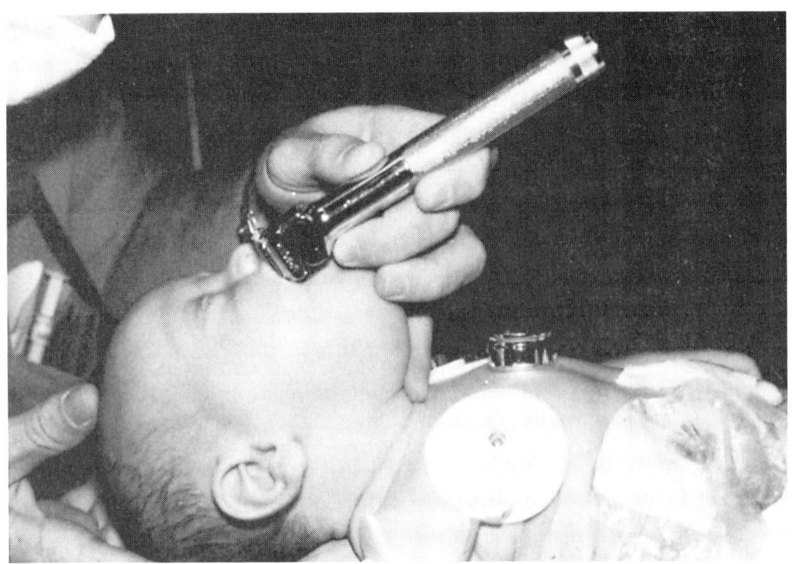

FIGURE 43-6. Cricoid pressure applied with little finger. (Reprinted with permission from Physiology and surgery of the infant. In Berry FA [ed]: Anesthetic Management of Difficult and Routine Pediatric Patients, Fredrick A. Berry Chapter 5 Physiology and Surgery of the Infant. p 129. New York, Churchill Livingstone, 1990.)

breathe. For this reason, choanal atresia is a life-threatening surgical problem for the neonate. The large tongue occupies relatively more space in the infant's airway and makes it diffi-
3 cult to conduct a laryngoscopic examination and intubate the infant's trachea. In the normal adult, the glottis is at the level of C5. In the full-term infant, the glottis is at the level of C4, and in the premature infant, it is at the level of C3. The combination of a large tongue and a relatively high glottis means that on laryngoscopic examination it is more difficult to establish a line of vision between the mouth and larynx; there is relatively more tissue in less distance. Therefore, the infant's larynx appears to be anterior. When combined with the anterior-slanting vocal cords, the result is a more difficult laryngoscopic examination and intubation. Application of cricoid pressure by the anesthesiologist or an assistant improves visualization of the neonate's larynx. If the anesthesiologist's hand is large enough, cricoid pressure can be applied with the little finger (Fig. 43-6).

A narrow cricoid ring is significant because it means that the narrowest portion of the neonate's airway is not the vocal cords but the cricoid ring. In the mature state, the airway from the vocal cords down the trachea is of equal dimensions (Fig. 43-7),

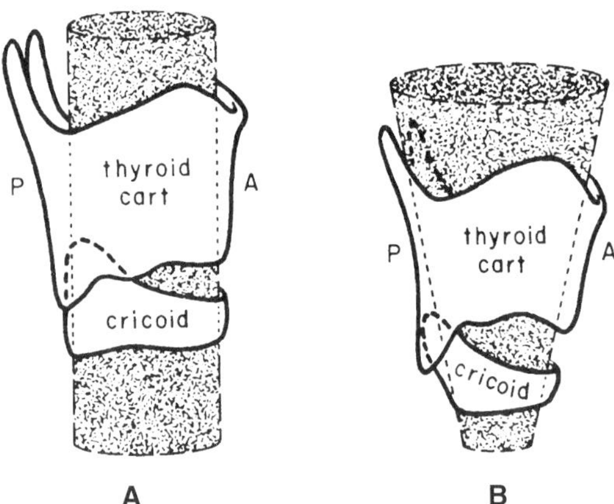

FIGURE 43-7. Configuration of the adult (A) versus the infant larynx (B). The adult larynx has a cylindrical shape. The infant larynx is funnel shaped because of the narrow, undeveloped cricoid cartilage. (Reprinted with permission from The pediatric airway. In Ryan JF, Charles J. Coté and I. David Todres [eds]: A Practice of Anesthesia for Infants and Children, 2nd ed, p 61. Orlando, FL, Grune & Stratton, 1992.)

and if the endotracheal tube passes comfortably through the vocal cords, it will not be tight within the cricoid cartilage. However, the neonate's laryngeal structures resemble a funnel; even though the endotracheal tube may pass through the vocal cords, which are at the midpoint of the funnel, the endotracheal tube may be tight within the cricoid ring. This tight fit may cause temporary or permanent damage to the cricoid cartilage, resulting in short-term or long-term airway difficulties.

Finally, the infant has a large occiput so the head flexes forward onto the chest when the infant is lying supine with its head in the midline (Fig. 43-8A). Extreme extension can also obstruct the airway, so a midposition of the head with slight extension is preferred for airway maintenance. This is accomplished by placing a small roll at the base of the neck and shoulders (Fig. 43-8B).

The Pulmonary System

Anatomically and physiologically, the neonate's pulmonary system differs in at least four respects from that of the adult: high oxygen consumption, high closing volumes, high ratio of minute ventilation to FRC, and pliable ribs. The oxy-
4 gen consumption of the infant is 7 to 9 mL/kg/min, whereas in the adult it is 3 mL/kg/min. Therefore, varying degrees of airway obstruction have more impact on oxygen delivery and reserve in the neonate and in the infant in the mature state.

The high closing volumes of the neonate's lungs are within the range of the normal tidal volume (Fig. 43-9). Closing volumes are the lung volumes at which alveoli close, resulting in the shunting of blood by a closed alveolus. If an infant experiences mild laryngospasm and a reduction in lung volume, the high closing volume contributes to shunting of blood and rapid desaturation. When a high oxygen consumption is combined with a high closing volume in the presence of laryngospasm, the rapidity with which desaturation occurs is breathtaking not only for the infant, but also for the anesthesiologist. When coughing and breath-holding occur with an endotracheal tube in place, the situation is not much different because there is an inability to ventilate the alveoli. Positive pressure ventilates the large airways, but there is no oxygen delivery to the closed alveoli. Therefore, even though an endotracheal tube may be in the appropriate anatomic location, severe desaturation can occur in infants who are lightly anesthetized and are coughing on the

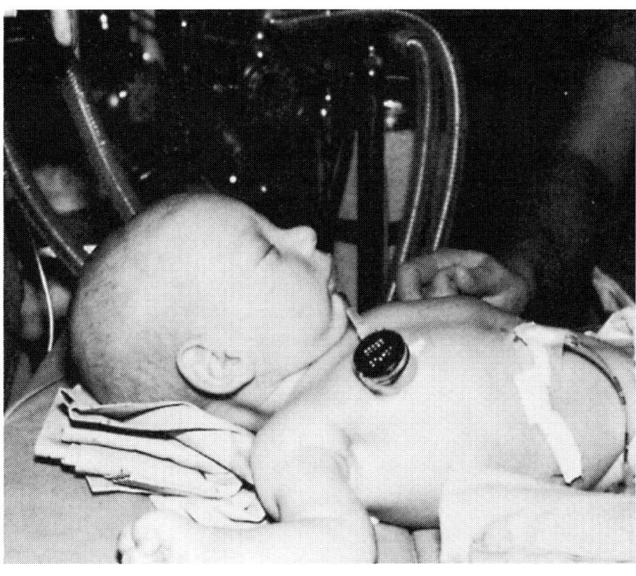
A

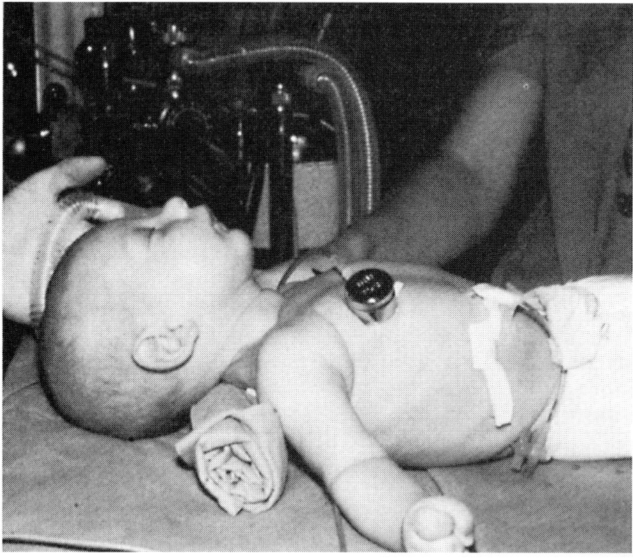
B

FIGURE 43-8. **A.** Pad placed under occiput in an attempt to achieve a "sniffing" position obstructs the infant's airway. **B.** Pad is placed under infant's neck to improve the airway patency and for laryngoscopic examination.

endotracheal tube. At times, because of inability to oxygenate the infant, it might be incorrectly believed that the endotracheal tube has come out of the trachea. The high intrathoracic pressure along with hypoxia, which increases pulmonary vascular resistance, may well cause right-to-left shunting either through the ductus arteriosus or through the foramen ovale. Management of the patient in this situation entails deepening the anesthesia or paralysis. This can be done with either small intravenous doses of succinylcholine, 0.5 mg/kg, or intravenous lidocaine, 1.5 mg/kg. Caution must be taken not to exceed this dose of lidocaine in the neonate.

The third unique pulmonary feature of the neonate is the high ratio of minute ventilation to FRC, which is similar to that of the term pregnant woman but occurs for different reasons. The pregnant woman has a reduction in FRC because of elevation of the diaphragm by the uterus. The neonate has increased alveolar ventilation because of the need to increase oxygen delivery secondary to the high oxygen consumption. Table 43-2 compares the normal respiratory values for newborns and adults.

The tidal ventilation for an infant is the same, in milliliters per kilogram, as for the adult; therefore, with oxygen consumption that is three times greater, the respiratory rate must be three times greater, which results in alveolar ventilation that is three times greater. Consequently, the ratio of minute ventilation to FRC is 5:1 in the neonate, whereas in adults it is 1.5:1. The clinical implication of the high ratio of minute ventilation to FRC is that there is a much more rapid induction of inhalational anesthesia, as well as more rapid awakening. The more rapid induction of anesthesia also results from a higher percentage of the neonate's body weight consisting of vessel-rich tissues.

The fourth anatomic difference of the neonate is a pliable rib cage. When increased minute ventilation is needed, which requires an increase in respiratory frequency or tidal volume, the pliable ribs of the neonate are a disadvantage. The neonate's diaphragm is the major ventilatory muscle. To increase oxygen

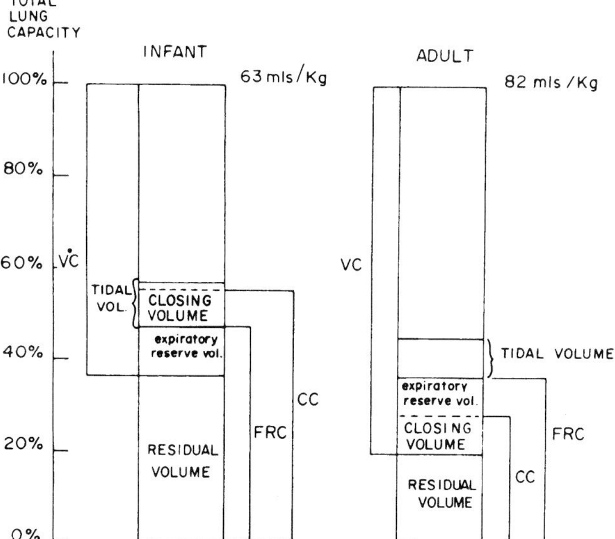

FIGURE 43-9. Static lung volumes of infants and adults. (Reprinted with permission from Smith CA, Nelson NM: Physiology of the Newborn Infant, 4th ed, p 207. Springfield, IL, Charles C Thomas, 1976.)

TABLE 43-2

COMPARISON OF NORMAL RESPIRATORY VALUES IN INFANTS AND ADULTS

PARAMETER	INFANT	ADULT
Respiratory frequency	30–50	12–16
Tidal volume (mL/kg)	7	7
Dead space (mL/kg)	2–2.5	2.2
Alveolar ventilation (mL/kg/min)	100–150	60
Functional residual capacity (mL/kg)	27–30	30
Oxygen consumption (mL/kg/min)	7–9	3

delivery by either an increase in frequency or excursion, the contraction of the diaphragm results in greater negative intrathoracic pressures. In older infants and children with a fixed rib cage, this results in an increase in air movement. However, with a pliable rib cage, the resulting increase in negative intrathoracic pressure results in retractions of ribs, as well as retraction in the subcostal and supraclavicular area. This results in less efficient ventilation and a high-energy price for the effort involved. This is one of the reasons why neonates are susceptible to fatigue with airway obstruction, pneumonia, and any other conditions that result in interference with pulmonary function.

There are two types of muscles: type 1, slow-twitch, high-oxidative muscles, which are necessary for sustained muscle activity; and type 2, fast-twitch, low-oxidative muscles, which have an immediate but short activity.[15] The development of type 1 muscles is necessary for sustained ventilatory activity. The premature infant has 10% type 1 and the newborn 25% type 1 muscles in the diaphragm, which is the primary muscle for ventilation. The infant's diaphragm achieves maturity of type 1 muscles at approximately 8 months of age. At that point, he or she has approximately 55% type 1 muscles. The intercostal muscles are the other ventilatory muscles. The premature infant has 20% type 1 intercostal muscles and the newborn, 46%. The age of maturity for these muscles is 2 months, when type 1 muscles comprise 65% of the total.

The Cardiovascular System

Heart and Sympathetic Nervous System

The ability of the neonate's immature cardiovascular system to respond to stress is limited by the relatively low contractile mass per gram of cardiac tissue, which results in a limited ability to increase myocardial contractility and a reduction in ventricular compliance.[16] The clinical implication of this limited compliance of the ventricle means that, although there may be some ability to increase stroke volume, it is extremely limited. Therefore, any increase in cardiac output must be accomplished by an increase in heart rate. For this reason, the infant is said to be rate dependent for its cardiac output. Thus, any slowing of the heart rate is reflected in a reduction in cardiac output. This is why bradycardia has such serious consequences for the infant. Hypoxia is a major cause of bradycardia in the neonate. Even in the absence of stress, the neonatal heart has limited ability to increase cardiac output compared with the mature heart (Fig. 43-10). The resting cardiac output of the immature heart is close to the maximal cardiac output, so there is a limited reserve. The mature heart can increase cardiac output by 300%, whereas the immature heart can only increase cardiac output by 30 to 40%.

In summary, the neonatal heart has some significant limitations. The resting cardiac output is much higher relative to body weight than in the adult because of the higher O_2 consumption per kg body weight. Stimulation of the myocardium produces a limited increase in contractility and cardiac output. The sympathetic nervous system, which usually provides the important chronotropic and inotropic support to the mature circulation during stress, is severely limited in the neonate because of immaturity.

Baroresponse

Neonates have immature baroreceptors. The baroreceptor is responsible for the reflex tachycardia that occurs in response to hypotension. Therefore, the immaturity of this reflex would limit the neonate's ability to compensate for hypotension. In addition, the baroresponse of the neonate is more depressed than that of the adult at the same level of anesthesia.

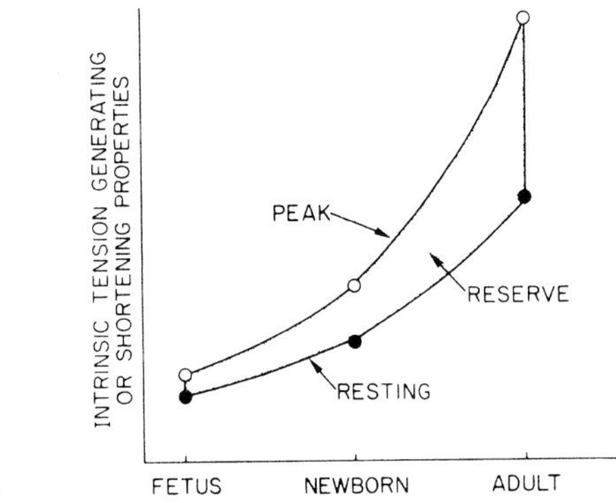

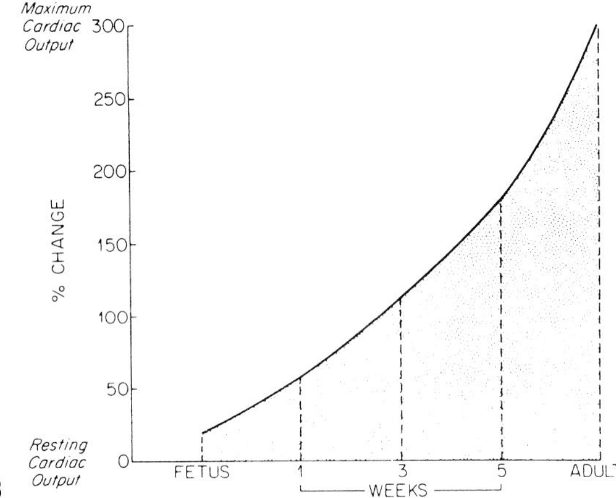

FIGURE 43-10. Schema of reduced cardiac reserve in fetal and newborn animal hearts compared with adult hearts. A. In the newborn infant, resting cardiac muscle performance is close to a peak of ventricular function because of limitations in diastolic, systolic, and heart rate reserve. B. Similarly, pump reserve early in life is limited by these factors and by much higher resting cardiac output relative to body weight, compared with that in adults. (Reprinted with permission from Friedman WF, George BL: Treatment of congestive heart failure by altering loading conditions of the heart. J Pediatr 106:700, 1985.)

ANESTHETIC DRUGS AND THE NEONATE

Anticholinergic Drugs

There is controversy about the need for routine premedication with anticholinergics. The neonate is at risk for developing bradycardia due to increased vagal activity. This may manifest during induction, with suctioning, during laryngoscopy, or after administration of succinylcholine. Because of these concerns, many anesthesiologists routinely administer anticholinergics either before or during surgery to infants younger than 6 months of age. We administer anticholinergics only for specific indications. One of the major indications for anticholinergics is to reduce secretions. The management of a difficult infant airway can be simplified by reducing secretions. The dose of atropine in the neonate is 0.02 mg/kg; for glycopyrrolate, it is 0.01 mg/kg. These drugs can be administered orally, rectally, intravenously, or intramuscularly.

Inhalational Agents

Nitrous oxide is usually considered a reasonably benign anesthetic drug from the standpoint of the cardiovascular system. However, in adult patients, when nitrous oxide is combined with opioids, the cardiac index and arterial pressure decrease because of myocardial depression. Nitrous oxide has mild depressant effects on systemic hemodynamics in sedated infants, similar to those reported in adults, but does not produce the elevations in pulmonary artery pressure and pulmonary vascular resistance that are seen in adults. Therefore, it appears that nitrous oxide is a reasonable drug in neonates if there is no concern for expanding gas pockets within the body (i.e., pneumocephalus, intestinal obstruction, pneumothorax) and no need for a high FIO_2 to maintain saturation.

All the volatile anesthetics affect the cardiovascular system. Halothane has little effect on peripheral vascular resistance; therefore, the decrease in blood pressure that accompanies the administration of halothane results from myocardial depression.[17] However, isoflurane, desflurane, and sevoflurane decrease systemic vascular resistance so the major effect on blood pressure is a decrease in peripheral vascular resistance.[18]

Neuromuscular Blocking Agents

Neuromuscular blocking agents (NMBAs) are frequently used during neonatal anesthesia to facilitate tracheal intubation, assist with controlled ventilation, relax abdominal musculature, and ensure immobility. Factors that influence the choice of agent include the time of onset, duration of action, cardiovascular effects, and mechanism of clearance/elimination.

Succinylcholine

Succinylcholine, the only depolarizing muscle relaxant available, has the most rapid onset time of all the NMBAs. The neonate and infant have a larger extracellular fluid volume leading to a larger volume of distribution and an increased dose requirement compared with children and adults.[19] The recommended intravenous dose of succinylcholine for neonates and infants is 3 mg/kg, compared with 2 mg/kg in children, with an onset time of 30 to 45 seconds and duration of 5 to 10 minutes. The recommended intramuscular dose of succinylcholine is 4 mg/kg, with an onset time of 3 to 4 minutes and duration of approximately 20 minutes. Caution should be exercised when administering a second dose of succinylcholine because this can lead to vagally mediated bradycardia or sinus arrest. Pretreatment with atropine is recommended.

The more recent succinylcholine controversy has called into question the use of succinylcholine in male children younger than 8 years of age.[20] The reports of hyperkalemia with cardiac arrest in such children with unrecognized muscular dystrophy has led some clinicians to take the position that succinylcholine should not be used routinely for this group of patients. The occurrence of this problem is somewhere in the range of 1 in 250,000 anesthetics, with a mortality rate of 50%. However, succinylcholine is still recommended in rapid-sequence situations, a potentially difficult airway, or if there are airway emergencies with a developing desaturation. In the emergency airway situation, the clinician should not wait to use succinylcholine until the patient becomes severely desaturated and bradycardic. When it is evident that a neonate is obstructed by laryngospasm or any other reason and no progress is made in ventilation, then either intramuscular or intravenous succinylcholine should be administered. The anesthesiologist must know how to recognize and treat hyperkalemia.[21] Hyperkalemia can be recognized by peaked T waves. However, the clinician may not see this particular electrocardiographic change because it occurs 2 to 3 minutes after drug administration, when the anesthesiologist is attending to the airway. The hyperkalemia interferes with conduction, leading to a bradycardia and, if severe enough, cardiac arrest. The drug of first choice is epinephrine 5 to 10 μmg/kg. One of the actions of epinephrine is to stimulate the sodium–potassium pump and cause the potassium to reenter the cell, thereby reducing the serum level. If there is no response at this dose level, it should be increased incrementally until there is a response. Magnesium has been described as a treatment for hyperkalemia because it also antagonizes the effects of hyperkalemia, as does calcium.[22] The use of sodium bicarbonate to treat any metabolic acidosis that may occur with arrest is also believed to be useful because alkalosis decreases hyperkalemia. At the same time, the patient should be hyperventilated to reduce the CO_2, thereby encouraging a respiratory alkalosis.

Nondepolarizing Agents

5 The neonate's neuromuscular junction is more sensitive to nondepolarizing muscle relaxants, and the neonate has a larger volume of distribution because of a large extracellular fluid volume. These two effects tend to balance each other so, roughly speaking, the dose of a nondepolarizing muscle relaxant for an infant is similar to that for a child on a milligram per kilogram basis. The ongoing organ maturation, which continues during the neonatal period, has a tremendous impact on the metabolism and clearance of the nondepolarizing agents. As a result, there is considerable variability and unpredictability in the duration of action of these agents in the neonatal period. Dosing should be titrated to effect and, when possible, guided by monitoring neuromuscular function with a nerve stimulator.

Rocuronium appears to be the drug of choice among the intermediate-acting, nondepolarizing muscle relaxants. The dose of rocuronium is 0.6 mg/kg. The length of action of rocuronium in the neonate is similar to that in the older infant or child following an equipotent dose.[23] However, if a larger dose of rocuronium, 1.0 to 1.2 mg/kg, is administered to avoid using succinylcholine during a rapid-sequence induction, then rocuronium will be a relatively long-acting muscle relaxant. Rocuronium is metabolized by the liver; however, unlike vecuronium there are no active metabolites. Rocuronium has mild vagolytic properties and may slightly increase heart rate.

Although vecuronium is considered an intermediate-acting muscle relaxant in children and adults, in infants younger than 1 year of age it is considered a long-acting muscle relaxant.[24] The duration of action of vecuronium is approximately twice that observed in children because of liver immaturity. Vecuronium undergoes primarily hepatic metabolism with production of active metabolites that are dependent on renal excretion. The recommended dose of vecuronium is 0.1 to 0.15 mg/kg with an onset time of 90 seconds and duration of action of 60 to 90 minutes in the neonate. Even with increased doses, vecuronium has no effect on the cardiovascular system.[25]

Pancuronium is a long-acting NMBA with a pharmacokinetic profile similar to vecuronium. The recommended dose of 0.1 to 0.15 mg/kg has an onset time of 120 seconds and duration of 60 to 75 minutes. Unlike vecuronium, however, pancuronium primarily undergoes renal excretion. Pancuronium has vagolytic and sympathomimetic actions that cause tachycardia and an increase in blood pressure.[26] If a neonate is moribund or in shock, or there is concern about the volume status, then pancuronium may well be the muscle relaxant of choice. However, in a relatively normal neonate with a normal blood pressure and normal blood volume, the use of pancuronium may result in hypertension, which has the potential to increase blood loss and increase the risk of hemorrhage in the extremely premature neonate.

Reversal Agents

Due to the unpredictable nature of the NMBAs in the neonatal population, as well as the inability to accurately assess neuromuscular function in many situations, it has become common practice to reverse all nondepolarizing NMDAs in neonates. The two commonly used reversal agents are edrophonium and neostigmine. Edrophonium in a dose of 1 mg/kg achieves a 90% reversal of a neuromuscular block in 2 minutes, whereas neostigmine in a dose of 0.07 mg/kg requires 10 minutes for a 90% reversal of neuromuscular block. This difference in time to peak effect allows the anesthesiologist to decide which agent is needed. A word of caution: when edrophonium is used to reverse neuromuscular blockade, the effect is so rapid that atropine should be administered before the edrophonium; some believe that atropine is superior to glycopyrrolate for this reversal. The dose of atropine is 0.01 to 0.02 mg/kg. Neostigmine is a suitable alternative for reversal of nondepolarizing muscle relaxants in neonates. The muscarinic effects of neostigmine can be blocked with atropine or glycopyrrolate (0.01 mg/kg), and the drugs can be given concurrently. The two advantages of edrophonium over neostigmine are a more rapid reversal and fewer muscarinic side effects.

Opioids

Opioids are mild vasodilators but have little direct effect on cardiac function. Cholinergic side effects of fentanyl may decrease the heart rate. If the neonate is hypovolemic, the administration of opioids may decrease blood pressure. However, if the infant is adequately volume resuscitated, the administration of opioids should have little effect on the blood pressure.[27,28]

A study of the dose-response relationship of fentanyl in neonates undergoing surgery demonstrated that, in doses of 10 to 12.5 μg/kg, fentanyl produced a stable hemodynamic state and reliable anesthesia as determined by the heart rate and blood pressure.[28] The doses were given in increments of 2.5 μg/kg. In all infants in the study, heart rate and systolic blood pressure decreased with the administration of fentanyl. One of the concerns with the administration of opioids in neonates is the altered pharmacokinetics and pharmacodynamics.[29,30] In one study, 25 to 50 μg/kg of fentanyl resulted in unpredictable respiratory effects and, in some neonates, postoperative respiratory depression. There was a prolonged metabolism of the fentanyl, particularly in those with increased intra-abdominal pressure. This was believed to be due to a reduction in liver blood flow and hence metabolism of fentanyl—evidence of altered pharmacokinetics. In addition, it also appeared that newborns were more sensitive at the same plasma level to the respiratory depressant effects of fentanyl—evidence of altered pharmacodynamics.

Traditionally, morphine has been avoided in neonates because of adverse side effects, including respiratory depression. On a pharmacokinetic basis, morphine has been shown to have a longer half-life and decreased plasma clearance in neonates compared with children and adults. Pharmacodynamically, the plasma concentration of morphine required to produce adequate analgesia is higher in neonates than infants and children. Studies have failed to detect morphine-6-glucuronide, a metabolite of morphine with potent analgesic properties, in neonates. This has been attributed to the immaturity of the neonate's liver.[31]

Intravenous Agents

Ketamine has unique cardiovascular effects.[32] Its action is centrally mediated through the sympathetic nervous system, and it can cause a release of norepinephrine. Ketamine in vitro has negative inotropic effects. However, on balance, ketamine can override the depressant effects on the myocardium and overall results in support of the cardiovascular system. Therefore, ketamine is a useful agent for the infant who has an unstable cardiovascular system or in whom there is some question about volume repletion. The intravenous induction dose of ketamine is 1 to 2 mg/kg in titrated doses, followed by 0.5 to 1 mg/kg every 15 to 30 minutes.

ANESTHETIC MANAGEMENT OF THE NEONATE

The anesthesiologist has a host of anesthetic techniques from
6 which to choose and can tailor the anesthetic to the requirements of the surgery and the condition of the neonate. The three major factors to consider in selecting an anesthetic technique are (1) whether it is anticipated that the neonate will be extubated at the end of surgery or shortly thereafter, (2) the need to control blood pressure, and (3) the need for postoperative pain relief. The drugs and techniques available to achieve these goals are many, and include inhalational anesthetics, regional techniques, muscle relaxants, opioids, and ketamine. If extubation is anticipated at the end of surgery or shortly thereafter, the anesthetic must be tailored so there are minimal residual effects from inhalational agents and muscle relaxants, thereby allowing the infant to be awake and in control of its airway reflexes, which promotes early extubation. The use of a regional anesthesia technique, such as a caudal technique, reduces the need for inhalational agents, opioids, and muscle relaxants. There are great advantages to using a combined general and regional technique when early extubation is anticipated. Yet, if the management plan is to leave the infant intubated and ventilated for a longer time, then the choice of anesthetic technique and muscle relaxant depends on other factors, such as the need to control blood pressure and the length of postoperative ventilation.

The neonate who is moribund or who has a severely compromised cardiovascular status needs resuscitation. The use of ketamine or opioids and a muscle relaxant can be advantageous when caring for the hemodynamically unstable infant. The normal full-term neonate has a systolic blood pressure between 60 and 70 mm Hg. For purposes of controlled hypotension, a blood pressure of 50 to 60 mm Hg is desired. As the neonate's status improves, anesthetic drugs may be titrated. Nitrous oxide can be added, providing oxygenation is closely monitored and expansion of any gas pocket in the body is considered. In the case of intestinal obstruction, the use of air along with appropriate concentrations of oxygen and a volatile drug is indicated.

Tracheal Intubation

One of the frequently asked questions about the anesthetic management of neonates is whether tracheal intubation is routinely needed or if the airway and ventilation can be managed with the laryngeal mask airway. The answer to this question depends on the skill of the anesthesiologist and the surgical procedure, but in most clinical situations, the neonate should be intubated because of various anatomic and physiologic considerations. If the anesthesiologist is skilled and the surgery is short, intubation may not be necessary and a laryngeal mask airway can be used. Another question is whether to control the ventilation of all neonates. If the overall condition of the neonate is healthy and the procedure is short, then spontaneous ventilation is certainly acceptable. However, if the neonate is debilitated, has had a relatively long-standing illness, has circulatory instability, and requires muscle relaxation for the surgery, then intraoperative controlled ventilation of the lungs is indicated.

Opinion on whether to perform an awake tracheal intubation in the neonate has changed in the last several years. There is concern that awake tracheal intubation causes hypertension and that the hypertension can rupture the fragile intracerebral vessels, particularly in premature infants. There are times when awake tracheal intubation would seem to be the technique of choice, such as in neonates who are critically ill and need resuscitation.

Topical anesthesia is used to reduce laryngospasm during intubation with volatile agents. Topical anesthesia of the larynx may be achieved with 4 to 5 mg/kg of 2% lidocaine sprayed on the larynx and vocal cords. Lidocaine 2% is preferred to higher concentrations in these small infants because it is easier to control the dose.

The question of extubation of the trachea is considerably easier to answer. The awake state is associated with control of the airway reflexes. Partially anesthetized infants are susceptible to laryngospasm and its associated apnea. Laryngospasm, apnea, and high oxygen consumption are a devastating combination. Therefore, the trachea should be extubated when the neonate is awake. An awake neonate opens his or her eyes, grasps the endotracheal tube, and cries. Crying cannot be heard because of the endotracheal tube but can be readily visualized. Any of these findings indicates that the infant is ready for extubation. If there is any doubt, however, the neonate should remain intubated until the clinician feels comfortable that the neonate can be extubated.

Impact of Surgical Requirements on Anesthetic Technique

Blood loss and muscle relaxation are two areas of concern for the surgeon and anesthesiologist. Parents and health care workers are also concerned about the transmission of AIDS and hepatitis through transfusions of blood and blood products. The use of blood and blood products should be minimized whenever possible. One way to minimize blood replacement is to minimize blood loss. This can be achieved through the control of blood pressure by the various anesthetics and muscle relaxants. Volatile anesthetics reduce blood pressure by 20 to 30%. Blood replacement is indicated if the neonate has demonstrated circulatory instability and considerable blood loss is anticipated. However, if the neonate is basically healthy, the anticipated blood loss is 25 to 30% of the blood volume, and the final hemoglobin is in the range of 8 to 9 g/dL, then blood transfusion probably can be avoided. The anesthesiologist can tailor the anesthetic to control the blood pressure and thereby reduce blood loss.

Uptake and Distribution of Anesthetics in Neonates

Various reasons for the faster uptake of anesthetics in infants have been proposed: (1) the ratio of alveolar ventilation to FRC is 5:1 in the infant and 1.5:1 in the adult; (2) in the neonate, more of the cardiac output goes to the vessel-rich group of organs, which includes the heart and brain; (3) the neonate has a greater cardiac output per kilogram of body mass; and (4) the infant has a lower blood gas partition coefficient for volatile anesthetics. One not well-recognized factor that may result in higher concentrations of volatile anesthetics being administered to infants has to do with the use of nonrebreathing systems such as the Bain or a Mapleson "D" circuit. When an adult circle system is used with infant tubes and bag, the clinician experienced with this equipment is used to reading the inspired, end-tidal, and dialed concentrations of the volatile anesthetic. In the circle system, the inspired concentration is a result of the combination of the end-tidal concentration that is rebreathed through the soda lime absorber and the dialed concentration. The inspired concentration is always lower than the dialed concentration, unless the flow rates are so high that a nonrebreathing system has been created. In the nonrebreathing system, the dialed concentration is the inspired concentration. Clinicians who use both systems are accustomed to these subtle differences. However, if the clinician switches back and forth between the circle system and a nonrebreathing circuit, but does so infrequently, there is a danger of not recognizing the possibility of excessive overpressure of volatile anesthetics with the nonrebreathing systems.

Anesthetic Dose Requirements of Neonates

Neonates and premature infants have lower anesthetic requirements than older infants and children.[33] The easiest way to remember the MAC values is that the MAC value in the mature state (i.e., late teenager or adult) is the same as for a full-term infant. By 6 months of age, the MAC value has increased by 50%. In the premature infant, the MAC value decreases by 20 to 30%.[33,34] The reasons for the lower MAC requirements are believed to be an immature nervous system, progesterone from the mother, and elevated blood levels of endorphins, coupled with an immature blood-brain barrier. The neonate has an immature central nervous system with attenuated responses to nociceptive cutaneous stimuli. These responses rapidly mature in the first several months of an infant's life, along with an increase in the MAC. Progesterone has been shown to reduce the MAC of the pregnant mother. The newborn infant has elevated progesterone levels, similar to those of the mother. Elevated levels of β-endorphin and β-lipotropin have been demonstrated in infants in the first few days of postnatal life. Endorphins do not cross the blood-brain barrier in adults; however, it is believed that the neonate's blood-brain barrier is more permeable and that endorphins might well pass into the central nervous system, thus elevating the pain threshold and reducing the MAC requirement.

Regional Anesthesia

There has been a tremendous increase in the use of regional anesthesia in children. In general, the regional techniques are combined with general anesthesia to permit early extubation and provide postoperative pain relief. Early extubation is possible because the use of regional anesthetic techniques eliminates the need for intraoperative narcotics in neonates, reduces or eliminates the need for muscle relaxants, and reduces the concentration of volatile agents needed for relaxation. Spinal anesthesia has been reported to be effective when used as the sole anesthetic technique in premature and high-risk infants, but this technique requires excellent cooperation between the anesthesiologist and an experienced surgeon. Even at a dose of 0.5 mg/kg, the effects of tetracaine last only approximately 90 minutes in the neonate. Total spinal anesthesia, produced either with a primary spinal technique or secondary to an attempted epidural puncture, presents as respiratory insufficiency rather than as hypotension because of the lack of sympathetic tone in infants.[35] The exact mechanism for the lack of cardiovascular change with spinal anesthesia in infants and young children is not clear. One study suggests that the sympatholysis is offset by a decrease in parasympathetic activity, resulting in the withdrawal of cardiac vagal activity. The overall effect is no change in heart rate and blood pressure.[36] The first indication of a high spinal is falling oxygen saturation rather than a falling blood pressure. Sedation can be added to regional anesthesia but may cause problems of apnea in ex-premature infants.

The techniques of caudal, spinal, brachial plexus, and other blocks should be considered in all neonates. Caudal epidural block is frequently used for abdominal and thoracic surgery in neonates. There are several different techniques described for performing a caudal. We prefer the 22-gauge, short-bevel needle; the caudal space is identified both by the loss of resistance and the ease of administering the anesthetic. Once the sacrococcygeal membrane is penetrated and there is a loss of resistance, gentle aspiration is applied to the needle to determine if there is blood or cerebrospinal fluid (CSF). Injection of the anesthetic is then attempted. If there is difficulty in injecting the solution, the tip of the needle is not in the caudal space and it needs to be repositioned. If the anesthetic can be injected easily, this confirms placement in the epidural space. The needle is not advanced up the caudal canal after proper placement in the caudal epidural space has been accomplished. In one study that uses Longwell catheters for the caudal epidural, the catheter is advanced up the caudal canal.[37] They report an intravenous injection incidence of approximately 6% with this technique. Epinephrine is added to local anesthetic solutions for the purposes of determining if there is an intravascular injection of the anesthetic. Evidence of an intravascular injection includes (1) peaked T waves (which may be of relatively short duration, e.g., 30 seconds), and (2) increase in heart rate. The other technique to minimize the potential difficulties of an intravascular injection is to fractionate the dose by dividing the dose into three aliquots and waiting approximately 20 to 30 seconds between each aliquot before continuing the injection.

Caudal anesthesia is particularly effective at reducing the concentrations of volatile anesthetics needed, as well as relaxants and opioids. In addition, a single-injection caudal anesthetic can provide analgesia for 6 to 8 hours. The two local anesthetics currently in use are 0.25% bupivacaine or 0.2% ropivacaine. Epinephrine is added to local anesthetics to assist in determining if there has been an intravenous injection. The amount of epinephrine added should result in a 1:200,000 dilution of epinephrine (5 μmg/mL). Although ropivacaine has not been approved for use in infants, it does have several theoretical advantages. Because it is used in a concentration of 0.2%, compared with 0.25% for bupivacaine, less drug is being administered per milliliter of injectate. In addition, ropivacaine has been reported to be less cardiodepressant than equipotent doses of bupivacaine. If a caudal catheter is placed, an infusion of ropivacaine can be administered and provide analgesia for several days. Current recommendations for infusions in neonates and young infants are for an initial loading dose of 0.2 to 0.25 mg/kg; after 1 to 2 hours, an infusion can be begun in a dose of 0.2 mg/kg/hr. For older infants, toddlers, and children, the dosage range is 0.4 to 0.5 mg/kg/hr. The addition of clonidine, 1.0 to 2.0 μg/kg, to local anesthetic for caudal block has prolonged the duration of analgesia in small children.[38] However, there has been some controversy as to whether the addition of clonidine has contributed to postoperative apnea in neonates and preterm infants.[39,40]

Another block that has become popular is a simple ring block of the penis for circumcision. Bupivacaine 0.25% is injected subcutaneously in a ring about the base of the penis. This way, there is no danger of causing a hematoma, which occasionally occurs with a penile block.

Postoperative Ventilation

The choice of an anesthetic drug should also be determined by the need for postoperative management of ventilation and by the drug's effects on the circulation. If the surgical procedure or the neonate's condition is such that postoperative ventilation is likely, the prolonged respiratory effects of opioids or any other drug are of little concern. However, if the surgical procedure is relatively short and by itself does not require postoperative ventilation, the clinician should carefully select drugs, as well as doses of anesthetic drugs and relaxants, that will not necessitate prolonged postoperative ventilation or intubation. Postoperative ventilation places the neonate at added risk because of the problems associated with mechanical ventilation, the trauma to the subglottic area, and the potential development of postoperative subglottic stenosis or edema. However, if there is any question about the neonate's ability to maintain protective airway reflexes or normal ventilation after anesthesia, the neonate should be returned to the recovery room or newborn intensive care unit with the trachea intubated, and either ventilated or treated with a small amount of positive end-expiratory pressure (PEEP) (2 to 4 cm H_2O).

Postoperative Pain Management

The concepts of postoperative pain management are well known to most anesthesiologists. The use of intraoperative epidural anesthesia followed by postoperative epidural local anesthetics or opioids has been popular in older children and adults, and these techniques are being applied to neonates. In addition, most neonatologists are experienced with the intravenous administration of opioids for patient comfort. Each technique has its own risks and benefits.

SPECIAL CONSIDERATIONS

Maternal Drug Use During Pregnancy

Maternal cocaine and marijuana use during pregnancy leads to a host of problems for the neonate. These drugs result in a reduced catecholamine reuptake, which may result in the accumulation of catecholamines. This has circulatory effects on the uterus, the umbilical blood vessels, and the fetal cardiovascular system. The three major problems affecting the infant are premature birth, intrauterine growth retardation, and cardiovascular abnormalities, including low cardiac output.[41,42] The cardiac output and stroke volume are reduced on the first day of life but return to normal by the second day. The clinical implication of this finding is that in infants of these mothers it may be advantageous to postpone any surgery until the second or third day of life. There is an increase in structural cardiovascular malformations and electrocardiographic abnormalities. The most frequent lesions are peripheral pulmonic stenosis, right ventricular conduction delay, right ventricular hypertrophy, and ST segment and T-wave changes.

Respiratory Distress Syndrome

Because of the enormous technical ability of the neonatologist and the resources of neonatal intensive care units (NICUs), many small infants survive who need surgery. One of the frequent problems of these infants is the occurrence of the respiratory distress syndrome secondary to a deficiency of surfactant. Respiratory distress syndrome is not an all-or-none disease; there are varying degrees of the disease and various treatments for it. Exogenous surfactant has been widely used in premature infants of low birth weight either to prevent or to treat respiratory distress syndrome.[43] As a result, fewer infants now die of this entity, and the incidence of bronchopulmonary dysplasia in survivors has fallen. However, the use of exogenous surfactant appears to have had little impact on other complications of prematurity such as PDA, necrotizing enterocolitis (NEC), or intraventricular hemorrhage.

Postoperative Apnea

7 A major concern with surgery in neonates is the development of apnea in the postoperative period. The infants at highest risk are those born prematurely, those with multiple congenital anomalies, those with a history of apnea and bradycardia, and those with chronic lung disease. The etiology of this apnea is multifactorial. Decreased ventilatory control and hyporesponsiveness to hypoxia and hypercarbia may be potentiated by anesthetic agents. Respiratory muscle fatigue may also play a role because neonates have a smaller percentage of type I fibers in their diaphragm and intercostal muscles. Hypothermia and anemia may also contribute to the development of postoperative apnea.[44–47] The treatment of postoperative apnea may be as simple as tactile stimulation with "blow by" oxygen. However, some infants require prolonged intubation and ventilatory support. Infants with life-threatening apnea and bradycardia before surgery may be on central nervous system stimulants. Caffeine and theophylline both act by increasing central respiratory drive and lowering the threshold of response to hypercarbia, as well as stimulating contractility in the diaphragm. Caffeine is favored because of its wider therapeutic margin and decreased propensity for toxicity. Administering caffeine prophylactically to infants at risk of postoperative apnea to ensure adequate serum levels may prevent the need for prolonged periods of postoperative ventilatory support. The recommended loading dose is 10 mg/kg caffeine base.[48–50]

Those infants at high risk for development of postoperative apnea may benefit from the use of a regional anesthetic as opposed to general anesthesia. Multiple studies have shown that spinal anesthesia without supplemental sedation decreases the incidence of postoperative apnea and bradycardia in high-risk infants. Once supplemental sedation is used, inhalation or ketamine, this advantage is lost.[51,52]

The question remains as to which infant should be admitted and monitored after outpatient surgery and for how long. The most conservative approach is to monitor all infants younger than 60 weeks postconceptual age for 24 hours after surgery.[44] Many reports show that the incidence of significant apnea and bradycardia is highest in the first 4 to 6 hours after surgery, but they have been reported up to 12 hours after surgery. In addition, the incidence of apnea directly correlates to postconceptual age. Therefore, the most widely accepted guideline is to monitor all infants younger than 50 weeks' postconceptual age for at least 12 hours after surgery, even infants who have had a spinal as their sole anesthetic.[45,46]

Retinopathy of Prematurity

Advances in neonatal medicine have led to the survival of extremely premature infants (i.e., infants weighing <1,000 g and infants <28 weeks' gestation). These infants are at high risk for development of retinopathy of prematurity (ROP).[53] ROP is a common cause of blindness in these extremely premature infants. Although the exact etiology is unknown, variations in arterial oxygenation (hypoxia or hyperoxia) and prolonged exposure to bright light are believed to play a significant role. Hyperoxic vasoconstriction of retinal vessels, induction of vascular endothelial growth factor, and damage to spindle cells by oxygen-free radicals are some of the currently supported hypotheses in the pathogenesis of ROP.[54] Advances in the treatment of ROP have followed the advances in neonatal care that led to the increased incidence of ROP. ROP is staged as follows:

Stage 1: Presence of a demarcation line between vascularized and avascularized retina
Stage 2: Presence of a demarcation line that has height, width, and volume (ridge)
Stage 3: Presence of a ridge with extraretinal fibrovascular proliferation
Stage 4: Partial retinal detachment
Stage 5: Total retinal detachment

The early stages are treated with cryotherapy or laser. These treatments may be performed with sedation in the NICU or under general anesthesia in the operating room. The later stages require retinal surgery (scleral buckle or vitrectomy) to be performed under general anesthesia.[55] In addition, the anesthesiologist may be called on to anesthetize an infant with ROP for an unrelated surgery, such as hernia repair, ventriculoperitoneal shunt, or central line placement.

The question the anesthesiologist faces is what inspired oxygen concentration is safe under general anesthesia. There are no studies that document some threshold PaO_2 above which ROP develops. In addition, there are no studies that document the length of time that the PaO_2 has to remain above some threshold number. A study by Flynn et al.[56] suggested that the longer time the premature infant had a documented TcO_2 (transcutaneous oxygen) above 80 mm Hg, the higher the incidence of ROP. The guidelines for the administration of oxygen in premature infants is a goal of 50 to 80 mm Hg.[57] An oxygen saturation of 90 to 95% represents a PaO_2 of somewhere between 60 and 80 mm Hg. Therefore, it seems reasonable to try to maintain an oxygen saturation of 95% with minimal inspired oxygen while these premature infants are under general anesthesia. If the infant is experiencing episodes of hypotension or problems with ventilation, then attempts to micromanage the oxygen saturation should be secondary to the management of the primary problems. However, if an infant is stable, it might be appropriate to dilute the inspired oxygen with room air, nitrogen, or nitrous oxide until the saturation is in the neighborhood of 95%.

Sudden Infant Death Syndrome

Sudden infant death syndrome (SIDS) is defined as the sudden death of an infant younger than 1 year of age that remains unexplained after complete autopsy, death scene investigation, and review of family history. SIDS is the most frequent cause of death in infants between the ages of 1 month and 1 year. Death from SIDS is relatively rare in the first month of life, with the peak occurring at the third to fourth months of life. Premature infants are known to be at increased risk. However, studies have failed to prove a relationship between apnea of prematurity and SIDS.[58] Data from the Collaborative Home Infant Monitoring Evaluation (CHIME) study suggest that preterm infants are at increased risk of having at least one extreme event until about 43 weeks' postconceptual age (PCA) compared with term infants. However, given the peak timing of SIDS deaths, these extreme events are not likely to be precursors to SIDS.[59] Epidemiologic studies suggest that the risk factors for SIDS include low birth weight, maternal smoking, maternal cocaine use, young maternal age, low socioeconomic status, and African American race.[60] There is currently no evidence that general anesthesia triggers SIDS.[61]

The relationship between infant sleep position and SIDS was evaluated in the early 1990s. It was noted that there was a 50% reduction of SIDS rates in those countries where there was a decline in prone positioning of infants. As a result, the American Academy of Pediatrics recommended that all well infants at term with no other problems be placed either on their side or on their back when sleeping.[62,63]

SIDS remains a mystery in many ways. Multiple theories have been proposed over the years, including the "infant apnea syndrome." Many current theories focus on abnormalities of cardiorespiratory control during sleep states. In addition, more recent evidence suggests an abnormality in the maturational process of brainstem nuclei, particularly the arcuate nucleus. As a result, it is believed that these infants lack the normal homeostatic mechanisms necessary to respond to exogenous stressors during sleep.[64] A separate theory focuses on abnormalities in autonomic control during obstructive sleep events in infants at risk.[65]

Neurodevelopmental Effects of Anesthetic Agents

Parents will frequently ask whether anesthesia will harm their infant. More recent studies suggesting that anesthetic agents may be harmful to the developing brain are inconclusive. These studies primarily performed in animals were done with prolonged exposure to high doses of agents; therefore, correlation to humans is difficult, and further investigation is warranted.[66]

SURGICAL PROCEDURES IN NEONATES

Surgical procedures in neonates are arbitrarily divided into two
8 periods: those performed in the first week and those performed in the first month. Except for gastroschisis, which should be attended to within 12 to 24 hours, there are really no acute emergency operations in the neonate. This means that a period of 2 to 3 days can be allowed for stabilization or transport to an appropriate pediatric center for treatment. There is more to neonatal emergency surgery than just the immediate anesthetic and surgical procedure. Many of these infants require the support services of specialized nursing units, pediatric radiologists, pediatric intensive care physicians, and so forth. Managed care considerations should never take precedence over the appropriate care of infants and children.

Surgical Procedures in the First Week of Life

The five most frequent major surgical procedures performed in the first week of life are for CDH, omphalocele and gastroschisis, tracheoesophageal fistula (TEF), intestinal obstruction, and meningomyelocele. Some of these conditions, such as CDH, omphalocele and gastroschisis, and meningomyelocele, are obvious at birth. It may take hours or days for a TEF or intestinal obstruction to become manifest.

Two confounding factors in neonatal surgery are prematurity and associated congenital anomalies. The presence of one congenital anomaly increases the likelihood of another congenital anomaly. In conditions such as TEF, the mortality rate from the associated congenital heart defect is far higher than that from the surgical correction of the TEF. Prematurity, particularly when associated with the respiratory distress syndrome, may adversely affect surgical outcome. The use of surfactant in the treatment of the respiratory distress syndrome has greatly increased the number of survivors and has decreased the complexity of the issues of the infant with a combination of TEF and the respiratory distress syndrome. A neonatologist should be consulted in the case of any neonate with a congenital defect who is considered for surgery. The most serious associated congenital lesion is that of the cardiovascular system. Approximately 25 to 30% of infants with CDH have a cardiac anomaly,[67] whereas approximately 15 to 25% of infants with TEF have an associated congenital cardiac anomaly.[68]

Congenital Diaphragmatic Hernia

CDH occurs with an incidence of approximately 1 in 4,000 live births. Traditionally, the mortality rate from CDH was in the range of 40 to 50%. The new strategy of permissive hypercapnia and delayed surgical repair has resulted in survival rates of >75% in some centers. However, the morbidity remains high in survivors. A brief discussion of the embryologic characteristics of CDH will help the clinician understand the potentially enormous postoperative problems that may be encountered. It will become evident that the defect is more than a hernia of the diaphragm.

Early in fetal development, the pleuroperitoneal cavity is a single compartment. The gut is herniated or extruded to the extraembryonic coelom during the ninth to tenth weeks of fetal life (Fig. 43-11). During this period, the diaphragm develops to separate the thoracic and abdominal cavities (Fig. 43-12). The development of the diaphragm is usually completed by the seventh fetal week. In the ninth to tenth weeks, the developing gut returns to the peritoneal cavity. If there is delay or incomplete closure of the diaphragm, or if the gut returns early and prevents normal closure of the diaphragm, a diaphragmatic hernia will develop, producing varying degrees of herniation of the intestinal contents into the chest. The left side of the diaphragm closes later than the right side, which results in the higher incidence of left-sided diaphragmatic hernias (foramen of Bochdalek). Approximately 90% of hernias detected in the first week of life are on the left side.

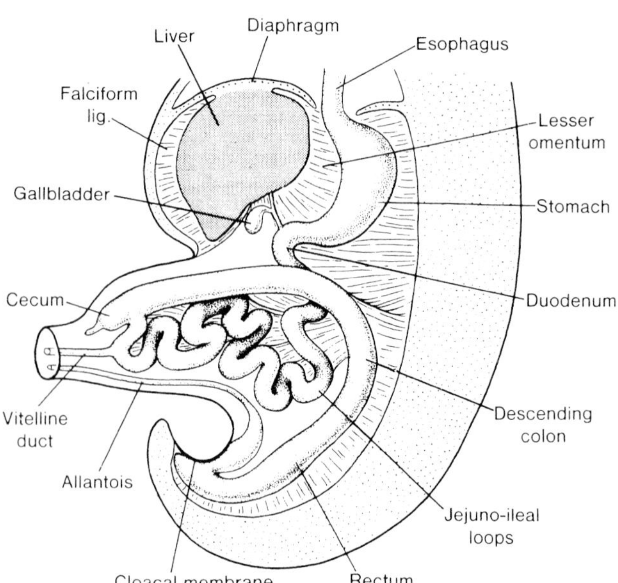

FIGURE 43-11. Umbilical herniation of the intestinal loops in an embryo of approximately 8 weeks' gestation (crown-rump length, 35 mm). Coiling of the small intestinal loops and formation of the cecum occur during the herniation. (Reprinted with permission from Langman J, Body cavities and serous membranes. In Sadler TW: Langman's Medical Embryology, 5th ed, p 150. Baltimore, Williams & Wilkins, 1985.)

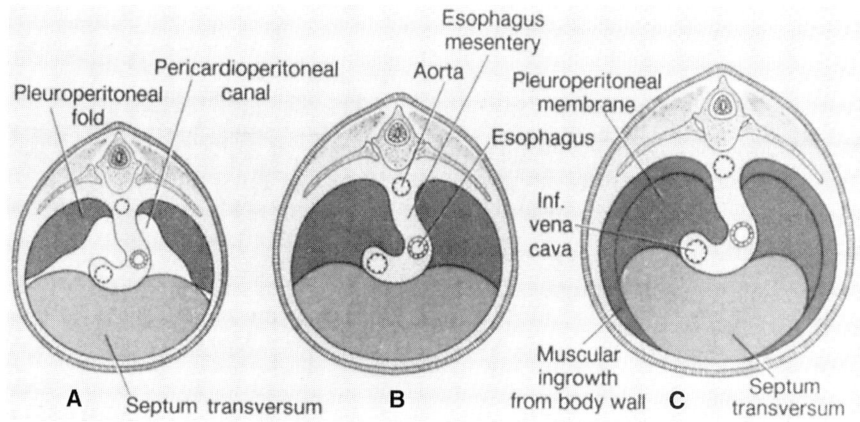

FIGURE 43-12. Schematic drawings illustrating the development of the diaphragm. A. The pleuroperitoneal folds appear at the beginning of the sixth week. B. The pleuroperitoneal folds have fused with the septum transversum and the mesentery of the esophagus in the seventh week, thus separating the thoracic cavity from the abdominal cavity. C. In a transverse section at the fourth month of development, an additional rim derived from the body wall forms the most peripheral part of the diaphragm. (Reprinted with permission from Langman J, Body cavities and serous membranes. In Sadler TW: Langman's Medical Embryology, 5th ed, p 147. Baltimore, Williams & Wilkins, 1985.)

The clinical presentation and the outcome from a diaphragmatic hernia are varied. At one end of the spectrum, the diaphragmatic hernia may develop early in fetal life so the abdominal contents compress the developing lung bud, resulting in an extremely small, hypoplastic lung. In severe cases, bilateral hypoplastic lungs may be found, with no chance for survival. At the other end of the spectrum, a moderately small diaphragmatic hernia may develop later in fetal life so the lung is normal but compressed by the abdominal viscera. In between is a large range of possibilities. At the mild end of the scale, the infant might have a relatively normal pulmonary vascular bed with varying degrees of PPH that may rapidly revert to normal. At the more serious end of the spectrum are severe pulmonary hypoplasia and abnormal pulmonary vasculature with a low chance for survival. As a result, there is an irreducible mortality rate associated with CDH; some infants will just not survive no matter what treatment is provided.

After closure of the pleuroperitoneal membrane, muscular development of the diaphragm occurs. Incomplete muscularization of the diaphragm results in the development of a hernia sac because of intra-abdominal pressure. The condition is known as eventration of the diaphragm, and the diaphragm may extend well up into the thoracic cavity. The other possibility is that the innervation of the diaphragm is incomplete and the muscle atonic. Eventration of the diaphragm is usually not symptomatic in the first week of life.

Antenatal Diagnosis

The diagnosis of CDH can be made prenatally by fetal ultrasonography or ultrafast fetal magnetic resonance imaging. Antenatal diagnosis has led to the identification of a "hidden mortality" in CDH, fetuses who did not survive gestation and neonates who died before diagnosis. One of the hopes of prenatal diagnosis is to identify predictors of poor postnatal outcome. Various factors have been proposed, including early gestation diagnosis, severe mediastinal shift, polyhydramnios, a small lung-to-thorax transverse area ratio, and the herniation of liver or stomach. New techniques in fetal surgery, such as temporary fetal tracheal occlusion, may prove beneficial to fetuses with CDH who are identified to be at risk for not surviving to term.[69,70] The other obvious advantage of prenatal diagnosis is that plans can be made for maternal or neonatal transport to a center with advanced neonatal critical care.

Clinical Presentation

Because the infant's status immediately at birth is determined primarily by the oxygenation by the placenta, the 1-minute Apgar score may well be normal. The occurrence of symptoms depends on the degree of herniation and interference with pulmonary function. At times, the degree of interference is so great that the neonate's clinical condition begins to deteriorate immediately, whereas in other situations it may be several hours before the infant's condition is fully appreciated. In the severely involved newborn, the initial clinical findings are usually classic and readily discerned. The infant has a scaphoid abdomen secondary to the absence of intra-abdominal contents, which have herniated into the chest (Fig. 43-13). Breath sounds on the affected side are reduced or absent. The diagnosis can be confirmed with a radiograph. Immediate supportive care entails tracheal intubation and control of the airway, along with decompression of the stomach. Excessive airway pressure carries a high risk for pneumothorax and worsening of a bad situation.

Preoperative Care

CDH was traditionally treated as a surgical emergency. The infants were taken immediately to surgery for decompression and repair. The thought was that removing the abdominal viscera from the thorax would allow for reexpansion of the atelectatic lung and improved oxygenation. However, as the pathophysiology of CDH was more clearly defined—pulmonary hypoplasia associated with a hyperreactive pulmonary vasculature—a strategy of preoperative stabilization with delayed surgical repair was adopted.

The stabilization of an infant with CDH may require multiple treatment modalities. The use of aggressive ventilation strategies to induce hyperventilation alkalosis has been

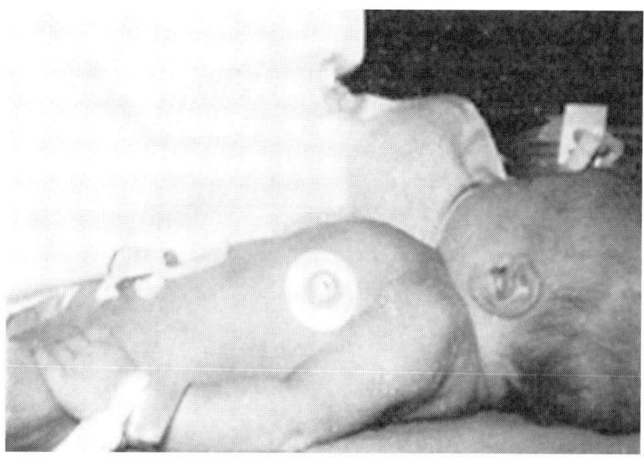

FIGURE 43-13. Infant with congenital diaphragmatic hernia. Note scaphoid abdomen.

abandoned secondary to the high incidence of iatrogenic lung injury. Conventional ventilation with permissive hypercapnia is now favored. The goal is to maintain preductal arterial saturation above 85% using peak inspiratory pressures below 25 cm H_2O and allowing the PCO_2 to rise to 45 to 55 mm Hg.[71,74] High-frequency oscillatory ventilation has been used in place of conventional ventilation in an attempt to reduce barotrauma, but has not been shown to improve survival.[72] The Neonatal Inhaled Nitric Oxide Study Group (NINOS) was unable to demonstrate a beneficial effect for inhaled nitric oxide in infants with CDH and hypoxic respiratory failure unresponsive to aggressive conventional therapy, although it may have some benefit post-ECMO.[73] Neonates born with CDH may also have a component of surfactant deficiency, and studies have shown improvement in oxygenation in those infants given surfactant prophylactically.[72]

The use of ECMO in infants with CDH was initiated in the mid-1980s. Since then, more than 2,000 infants with CDH have been placed on ECMO. Despite extensive literature on the subject, there remains an ongoing debate as to whether ECMO improves survival in neonates with CDH. The Congenital Diaphragmatic Hernia Study Group analyzed data from the multicenter CDH Registry and determined that ECMO improves the survival rate in CDH neonates with a predicted high risk of mortality ($\geq$80%) based on birth weight and 5-minute Apgar score.[75]

Perioperative Care

Because delayed surgical repair of CDH is now the norm, neonates with CDH frequently present to the operating room already intubated and on some form of ventilatory support. Despite a period of preoperative stabilization, some infants still have a component of reactive pulmonary hypertension. The goals of ventilatory management are to ensure adequate oxygenation and avoid barotrauma. Any sudden deterioration in oxygen saturation with or without associated hypotension should raise suspicion of pneumothorax. It is important to avoid hypothermia because this increases the oxygen requirement and could precipitate pulmonary hypertension. Blood loss and fluid shifts are usually not a problem, although maintenance of intravascular volume is essential to avoid acidosis, which could also precipitate pulmonary hypertension.

The anesthetic technique chosen depends on the size of the defect and the anticipated postoperative respiratory status. In those infants who will remain intubated after surgery, inhalational agents and narcotics may be used as tolerated. In those infants with a small defect who present to the operating room with little or no respiratory distress, it may be beneficial to avoid intraoperative narcotics and provide regional analgesia in anticipation of extubation. The use of nitrous oxide should be avoided, particularly in those situations in which abdominal closure could be difficult. Muscle relaxation is often needed to facilitate abdominal closure.

Some centers are performing repairs of CDH while the neonate is on ECMO. This may be performed in the operating room or in the NICU. The anesthetic technique usually consists of narcotics with muscle relaxation. Surgical repair while on ECMO can be associated with significant bleeding, making fluid management more challenging and increasing the mortality rate.

Postoperative Care

Most infants with CDH require intensive postoperative care. Recovery depends on the degree of pulmonary hypertension and pulmonary hypoplasia. It was previously believed that pulmonary hypoplasia was responsible for most deaths; however, it is now believed that potentially reversible pulmonary hypertension may be responsible for as much as 25% of reported deaths.[76]

There is evidence to suggest that cardiac development is impaired in infants with CDH. Relative left ventricular hypoplasia with an attenuated muscle mass and cavity size have been described. Many studies have confirmed that a calculated left ventricular mass less than 2 g/kg on pre-ECMO echocardiography was predictive of subsequent death.[77]

Omphalocele and Gastroschisis

Although omphalocele and gastroschisis sometimes appear similar and may be confused, they have entirely different origins and associated congenital anomalies.[78] During the fifth to tenth weeks of fetal life, the abdominal contents are extruded into the extraembryonic coelom, and the gut returns to the abdominal cavity at approximately the tenth week (see Fig. 43-11). Failure of part of or all the intestinal contents to return to the abdominal cavity results in an omphalocele that is covered with a membrane called the *amnion*. The amnion protects the abdominal contents from infection and the loss of extracellular fluid. The umbilical cord is found at approximately the apex of the sac (Fig. 43-14). Gastroschisis, in contrast, develops later in fetal life, after the intestinal contents have returned to the abdominal cavity. It results from interruption of the omphalomesenteric artery, which results in ischemia and atrophy of the various layers of the abdominal wall at the base of the umbilical cord. The gut then herniates through this tissue defect (Fig. 43-15). The degree of herniation may be slight, or major amounts of the abdominal viscera may be found outside the peritoneal cavity. The umbilical cord is found to one side of the intestinal contents. The intestines and viscera are not covered by any membrane and therefore are highly susceptible to infection and loss of extracellular fluid. There is a high incidence of associated congenital anomalies with omphalocele, but not with gastroschisis. The Beckwith-Wiedemann syndrome consists of mental retardation, hypoglycemia, congenital heart disease, a large tongue, and an omphalocele. Congenital heart lesions are found in approximately 20% of infants with omphalocele. Other associated congenital defects are found with gastroschisis and omphalocele; most involve the gastrointestinal

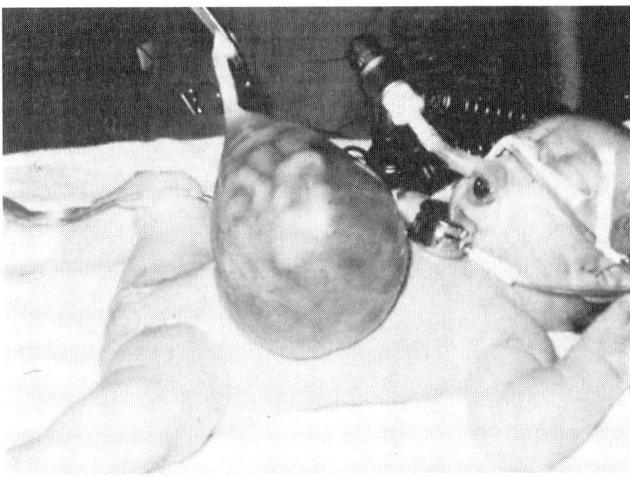

FIGURE 43-14. Omphalocele. (Reprinted with permission from Berry FA, Physiology and surgery of the infant. In Berry FA [ed]: Anesthetic Management of Difficult and Routine Pediatric Patients, p 152. New York, Churchill Livingstone, 1990.)

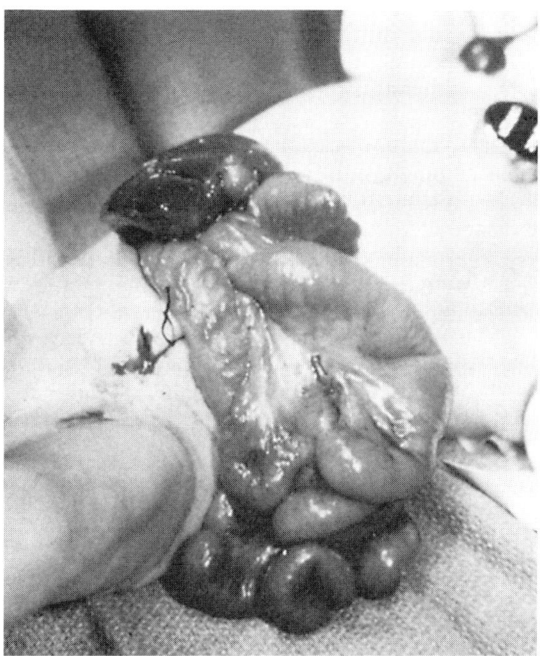

FIGURE 43-15. Gastroschisis.

tract and consist primarily of intestinal atresia or stenosis and malrotation.

Antenatal Diagnosis

Alpha-fetoprotein (AFP) is a normal protein present in fetal tissues during fetal development. Closure of the abdominal wall and the neural tube (see Meningomyelocele section) prevents release of large quantities of this protein into the amniotic fluid. High levels of AFP in the amniotic fluid can cross the placenta and be detected in maternal blood. Thus, abnormal levels of AFP in the mother raise concerns over the possibility of either an abdominal wall defect or a neural tube defect in the fetus, as do high levels of AFP in fluid obtained during amniocentesis. Ultrasonography is reliable in helping diagnose either condition.

Preoperative Care

There is controversy over the appropriate mode of delivery, vaginal or cesarean section, in parturients in whom the antenatal diagnosis has been made. Advocates of operative delivery maintain that it is necessary to prevent trauma to the exposed bowel and that it allows better coordination of the various medical specialties needed for immediate surgical management of the defect. Advocates of vaginal delivery point out that most infants with abdominal wall defects are born without injury to the bowel. The aspect of delivery room care unique to an infant with gastroschisis is the need to protect the exposed bowel and minimize fluid and temperature loss. This is best achieved by "bagging" the neonate by placing its lower body in a sterile, clear plastic bag. The bag is then filled with warm saline and a drawstring is used to tighten the bag against the infant's body.

Preoperative stabilization of the neonate with an abdominal wall defect includes management of respiratory insufficiency, establishment of adequate intravenous access, and an assessment for associated congenital anomalies. Respiratory failure at birth in infants with omphalocele is a significant predictor of mortality.[79] Lung hypoplasia and abnormal thoracic development may be significant in infants with large omphaloceles. A difficult airway can be anticipated in the patient with Beckwith-Wiedemann syndrome.

Surgery is not urgent in the neonate with an omphalocele, and can be delayed for several days until the infant is assessed and stabilized. In those infants with severe respiratory distress or congenital heart disease who are too unstable for surgery, nonsurgical treatment with topical antiseptics and delayed closure is an option.

Perioperative Care

The two major perioperative concerns are fluid loss and ventilation. The fluid volume management of the infant often entails administration of large amounts of full-strength, balanced salt solution. The adequacy of the peripheral circulation and urine output is an indicator of the adequacy of the volume resuscitation. Both conditions may present an intraoperative challenge to the anesthesiologist because with an omphalocele, after the amniotic membrane is removed, large volumes of fluid may transude or exude from the exposed abdominal viscera. The fluid that is lost is extracellular fluid, which should be replaced with full-strength, balanced salt solution. An arterial line is often used for blood pressure monitoring and frequent blood gas monitoring to assess acid-base status.

If the defect in the abdominal wall is small, a primary repair of the deficit can be accomplished. However, with a large defect, it may be difficult to return the abdominal viscera to the peritoneal cavity because the muscle and peritoneum are underdeveloped. Because of concern for the increase in the volume of gas in the intestine, nitrous oxide should not be used. Muscle relaxation is necessary to allow closure of the abdomen. With moderate-size abdominal wall defects, it may not be possible to close the peritoneum, but there may be sufficient skin to close the defect. With large defects, the peritoneal cavity may be too small to contain the viscera, and attempted closure can impair circulation to the bowel, kidneys, and lower extremities, as well as compromise respiration. A pulse oximeter probe on the foot can be helpful in monitoring circulation to the lower extremities during abdominal wall closure.

Attempts have been made to find objective criteria by which to determine whether the infant will tolerate primary closure of the defect, and to avoid or minimize the circulatory and ventilatory problems. One study that measured intragastric pressure in infants who underwent primary closure found that if the intragastric pressure was 20 mm Hg or more, the infant needed reoperation and placement of a Dacron silo (Fig. 43-16) within 24 hours of the primary closure.[80] If the intragastric pressure was less than 20 mm Hg, the defect was successfully closed primarily. Intragastric pressure is measured by placing a nasogastric tube in the stomach and using a column of saline to measure the pressure.

If primary closure is impossible, a silo is incorporated into the abdominal wall to contain and cover the abdominal viscera. The repair is then staged from this point onward. Every 2 or 3 days, the size of the silo is reduced, in much the same fashion that a tube of toothpaste is squeezed. The infant may feel some degree of discomfort as the peritoneum and skin are stretched. Small doses of ketamine, 0.5 to 1.0 mg/kg, are titrated as the silo is reduced. The infant is allowed to breathe spontaneously and without intubation. Oxygen saturation should be monitored with a pulse oximeter, and the infant's pulse and blood pressure are also monitored. These measurements help the surgeon and anesthesiologist determine the appropriate silo reduction that allows adequate ventilation and circulation. This is a situation that requires clinical judgment. After several stages of silo reduction, the final operation is complete closure of the abdominal wall defect under full anesthesia with complete muscle relaxation.

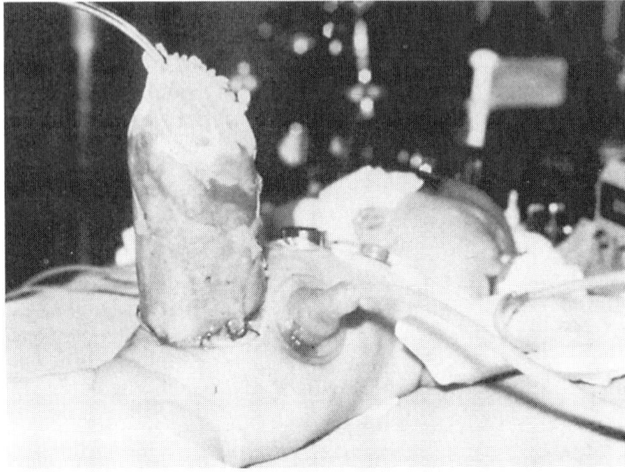

FIGURE 43-16. Dacron silo for extruded viscera. (Reprinted with permission from Berry FA, Physiology and surgery of the infant. In Berry FA [ed]: Anesthetic Management of Difficult and Routine Pediatric Patients, p 154. New York, Churchill Livingstone, 1990.)

Postoperative Care

The postoperative care of infants with omphalocele or gastroschisis is critical. Some need tracheal intubation and assisted ventilation of the lungs for as long as 3 to 7 days. Additional complications include postoperative hypertension and edema of the extremities. The increased abdominal pressure can reduce the circulation to the kidneys, which results in a release of renin. Renin activates the renin-angiotensin-aldosterone system, which is believed to cause the hypertension.

Tracheoesophageal Fistula

The treatment of esophageal atresia and TEF can be both challenging and satisfying for the anesthesiologist. Death in the perioperative period typically results from prematurity or from an associated congenital heart defect. TEF occurs in approximately 1 in 3,000 live births. Approximately 85% consist of a fistula from the distal trachea to the esophagus and a blind proximal esophageal pouch. In 10% of cases, there is a blind proximal esophageal pouch with no TEF (Fig. 43-17). The embryologic defect results from imperfect division of the foregut into the anteriorly positioned larynx and trachea and the posteriorly positioned esophagus; the division should occur between the fourth and fifth weeks of intrauterine life. Fifty percent of affected infants have associated congenital anomalies, of which approximately 15 to 25% involve the cardiovascular system.

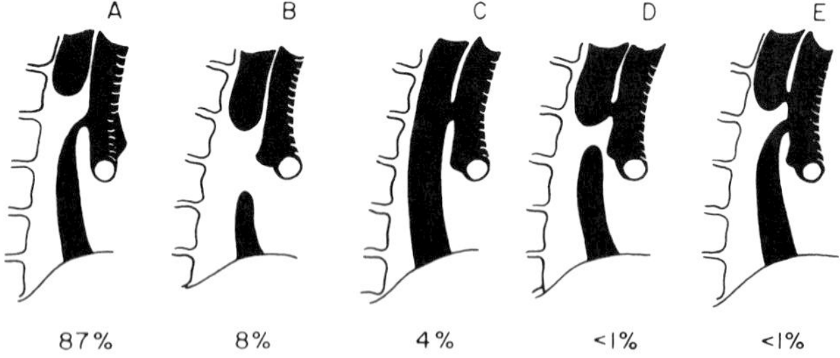

FIGURE 43-17. Diagrams of the five most commonly encountered forms of esophageal atresia and tracheoesophageal fistula, shown in order of frequency. (Reprinted with permission from Herbst JJ: Gastrointestinal tract. In Behrman RE, Kleigman RM, Nelson WE, Vaughan WC III [eds]: Nelson Textbook of Pediatrics, 14th ed, p 942. Philadelphia, WB Saunders, 1992.)

Clinical Presentation

Atresia of the esophagus leads to inability of the fetus to swallow amniotic fluid and the subsequent development of polyhydramnios. Ultrasound may well raise the possibility of a congenital anomaly. For that reason, if polyhydramnios is present, attempts should be made to pass a nasogastric tube shortly after delivery. Passing a nasogastric tube is not routine in the delivery room; therefore, the diagnosis may not become apparent until the infant is fed. Cyanosis and choking with oral feedings should raise suspicion.

There are two major complications of esophageal atresia with a distal tracheal fistula: aspiration pneumonia and dehydration. The presence of a distal TEF increases the likelihood of reflux of gastric juice up the esophagus and into the pulmonary system. Dehydration results from the fact that the proximal esophagus does not communicate with the stomach. Therefore, preoperative preparation of these infants is aimed at evaluation and treatment of the pulmonary system, as well as at ensuring adequate hydration and electrolyte balance. Rarely, the degree of reflux and pneumonia is so great that a gastrostomy must be performed to protect the pulmonary system, and a period of several days is needed to improve the general condition of the infant. However, if the infant is in good condition, primary repair can be performed at 24 to 48 hours. This consists of ligation of the fistula and a primary repair with approximation of the two ends of the esophagus.

Anesthetic Considerations

The presence of a gastrostomy reduces the potential for reflux of gastric juice during the surgical procedure. If a gastrostomy is present, the gastrostomy tube should be open to air and left at the head of the table under the anesthesiologist's observation to avoid kinking and obstruction.

There are two approaches to tracheal intubation after induction of anesthesia. One is to use an inhalation induction, followed by topical spray of lidocaine and intubation while the infant is breathing spontaneously. The other technique is to use an intravenous or inhalation induction and intubate the trachea after muscle paralysis. This technique may lead to distention of the fistula and stomach with excessive positive-pressure ventilation. When controlled ventilation of the lungs is used, attempts must be made to minimize the distention of the stomach and the potential for reflux. If a gastrostomy tube is in place, the point is moot. Alternatively, because the fistula is usually located just above the carina on the posterior wall of the membranous trachea, the endotracheal tube can be placed just distal to the TEF. To do this, the endotracheal tube is inserted until it enters one or the other main-stem bronchi. This is judged by unilateral expansion of the chest and unilateral breath sounds. The endotracheal tube is then slowly withdrawn until bilateral chest movement and breath sounds are confirmed.

The endotracheal tube might inadvertently enter the fistula, when the infant is turned or during surgical manipulation. This should be suspected if there is increased difficulty in ventilation of the lungs, as well as decreased oxygen saturation and end-tidal CO_2. Because these findings may also be present when the lung is packed away to perform the surgery and because there are other explanations for these findings, intubation of the fistula should always be included in the differential diagnosis. Any time ventilation is difficult and desaturation is occurring, the surgeon must stop the procedure while the situation is clarified. The surgeon will be able to palpate the tip of the tube in the fistula if this is the problem.

The localization and isolation of H-type fistulas can be difficult. In this situation, bronchoscopy is performed by the surgeon, the fistula is identified, and a guidewire is fed through the fistula tract into the esophagus. The infant is then intubated, with care taken not to dislodge the guidewire. Once intubated esophagoscopy is performed, the guidewire is visualized and brought out through the mouth. In this way, the surgeon can use fluoroscopy to determine the level of the fistula and decide whether a cervical or thoracic approach is necessary. During surgery, the anesthesiologist can apply traction to the wire loop to facilitate the localization of the fistula by the surgeon.[81]

Postoperative Care

Although there have been great advances in the treatment of TEF and esophageal atresia, postoperative care can be complicated by associated congenital heart disease, respiratory distress syndrome, and a need for continued postoperative ventilation. The compression of the lung for several hours, along with preexisting aspiration pneumonia in some of these infants, suggests the need in the more difficult cases for a short period of postoperative ventilation, or at least intubation with PEEP, as the most conservative technique for postoperative airway management. Some infants are in excellent condition at the time of surgery with no complicating factors, and therefore, should be considered for extubation immediately at the end of surgery or shortly thereafter. If extubation of the trachea is planned for the end of surgery, the anesthetic technique must be tailored accordingly. Caudal anesthesia as part of the technique is useful in these situations, reducing the concentration of maintenance volatile anesthetics, the amount of muscle relaxants, and the need for intraoperative narcotics.

A high percentage of infants with esophageal atresia have residual difficulties of the tracheobronchial tree and esophagus for many years. These include tracheomalacia, gastroesophageal reflux, esophageal stricture, and recurrent fistulas.

Intestinal Obstruction

Obstruction of the gastrointestinal system can be arbitrarily divided into obstruction of the upper gastrointestinal tract (i.e., duodenum) and obstruction of the lower gastrointestinal tract (i.e., terminal ileum, colon, imperforate anus). Obstruction of the upper gastrointestinal tract is usually evident within the first 24 hours of life, when the institution of feedings leads to vomiting, whereas obstruction of the lower gastrointestinal tract becomes evident somewhere between 2 and 7 days of age as the infant becomes progressively distended, little or no stool is passed, and there is vomiting.

Upper Gastrointestinal Tract Obstruction

If there has been persistent vomiting, this usually means that a deficit of fluids or electrolytes will develop in the infant. The stomach contains approximately 100 to 130 mEq/L of sodium and 5 to 10 mEq/L of potassium. The greatest deficit is for sodium. Another major concern in the infant with upper gastrointestinal tract obstruction is aspiration of gastric contents.

The anesthetic management of these patients is directed toward ensuring adequate relaxation for abdominal exploration, repair of the congenital defect, and closure of the abdomen. Nitrous oxide can be used in high intestinal obstruction because there is essentially no gas in the gastrointestinal tract. The next concern is whether the infant's trachea should be extubated at the end of surgery. If the infant is robust, extubation of the trachea at the end of surgery can be anticipated. The preferred technique is for general anesthesia combined with caudal epidural anesthesia. This allows light levels of volatile agent and minimal muscle relaxant use, resulting in an early extubation. Opioids are not administered until the postoperative period. However, if the infant is moderately debilitated or if the surgical incision is extensive, a period of postoperative intubation with PEEP may well be indicated, particularly if moderate doses of opioids have been used.

Lower Gastrointestinal Tract Obstruction

The problems associated with lower gastrointestinal tract obstruction usually develop within 1 to 7 days after birth. It may take this long for the lesion to become evident because it is low in the gastrointestinal tract. An imperforate anus should be recognizable shortly after birth. Some of these infants may have vomiting secondary to the obstruction, which poses a problem for fluid and electrolyte management. An enormous amount of fluid can be sequestered within the intestinal tract. This fluid is essentially extracellular fluid and has high sodium content. Therefore, these infants should be prepared carefully for surgery and have a serum sodium level of at least 130 mEq/L and a urine volume of 1 to 2 mL/kg/hr.

Nitrous oxide should not be used in any infant who has gaseous distention of the intestine, which is easily determined from the preoperative radiograph. Providing adequate muscle relaxation for surgery can be accomplished with various anesthetic techniques, such as volatile anesthesia, muscle relaxants, and caudal epidural block.

The criteria for tracheal extubation at the end of surgery are the same as those described for upper gastrointestinal tract obstruction. When in doubt, leave the tracheal tube in place with PEEP.

Meningomyelocele

Clinical Presentation

Myelomeningocele is the most common congenital primary neural tube defect, occurring in approximately 1 of every 1,000 live births. It results from failure of neural tube closure during the fourth week of gestation. Neural tube defects can be identified on prenatal ultrasound. Elevated maternal serum AFP detects 50 to 90% of open neural tube defects but has a false-positive rate of 5%. Amniotic fluid AFP is more reliable. Evidence also supports a relation between folic acid deficiency and the development of neural tube defects.

By definition, the lesion involves both the meninges and neural components, as compared with a meningocele, which does not contain neural elements. The infant is born with a cystic mass on the back comprising a neural placode, arachnoid, dura, nerve tissue and roots, and CSF. The lesion most commonly occurs in the lumbosacral or sacral region. The bony canal is also malformed, leading to multiple orthopaedic problems as the child matures. Urologic complications correlate with the level of the spinal lesion.

Most infants born with myelomeningocele have an associated anomaly of the brainstem known as the Arnold-Chiari II (Chiari II) malformation. The Chiari II malformation is characterized by caudal displacement of the cerebellar vermis through the foramen magnum, caudal displacement of the medulla oblongata and the cervical spine, kinking of the medulla, and obliteration of the cisterna magna. Hydrocephalus requiring shunting develops in approximately 90% of infants with myelomeningocele. In contrast, only 20% of patients have symptoms of brainstem dysfunction as a result of the Chiari II malformation, but the mortality rate among those symptomatic patients is high. Complications of brainstem dysfunction include stridor, apnea and bradycardia, aspiration pneumonia, sleep-disordered breathing patterns, vocal cord paralysis, lack of coordination, and spasticity. If the symptoms are not improved by shunting, posterior fossa decompression is necessary.[82–84]

The infant with a myelomeningocele is usually operated on within the first 72 hours of life. This reduces the risk for development of ventriculitis or progressive neurologic deficits. Most centers close the defect and place a shunt at the same time. However, some centers may delay placement of a shunt until the infant shows symptoms of hydrocephalus. There is some evidence that intrauterine repair of myelomeningocele may decrease the morbidity associated with the Chiari II malformation and brainstem dysfunction.[85]

Preoperative Care

The safest route of delivery of an infant with a myelomeningocele remains controversial. Some question whether labor and vaginal delivery can adversely affect neurologic outcome. However, there are studies suggesting no difference in neurologic deficits between infants delivered vaginally or by cesarean section.

The preoperative stabilization period focuses on the prevention of infection, maintenance of extracellular fluid volume, and assessment for other congenital anomalies. The exposed neural placode is susceptible to trauma, leakage, and infection. The infant is usually placed in the prone position, and the placode is covered with saline-soaked gauze to prevent desiccation. Because of the high risk of infection, antibiotic therapy is initiated in the preoperative period. Rupture of the cyst on the back can lead to ongoing CSF leakage. This fluid is replaced with full-strength balanced salt solution. The infant is also assessed for any potentially life-threatening congenital anomalies.

Perioperative Care

The high prevalence of clinical latex allergy and latex sensitization in children with myelomeningocele has drawn much attention. Studies show that the prevalence increases with increasing age. It is believed that an early, intense exposure to the allergen, as occurs with frequent surgery and bladder catheterization, contributes to this high prevalence. As a result, these infants are now labeled as latex sensitive and cared for in a latex-free environment.[86]

Positioning is critical in the infant with myelomeningocele. For induction of anesthesia, the infant may be placed supine with the defect resting in a "donut" to minimize trauma. Alternatively, the induction can be performed with the infant in the lateral position, although this makes intubation more challenging. The infant is turned prone for surgery. Rolls are positioned to ensure the abdomen and chest are free, avoiding pressure on the epidural venous plexus to minimize bleeding and allowing for adequate ventilation.

In most instances, the infant has an intravenous line placed before surgery and an intravenous induction is performed. Succinylcholine may be used to facilitate intubation without risking hyperkalemia.[87] Because increased intracranial pressure is rarely present before closure of the defect, inhalational induction is an alternative in the infant with difficult intravenous access. Identification of neural tissue may require nerve stimulation, and therefore, muscle relaxants are avoided. Narcotics are used with caution in these infants because of the abnormal response to hypoxia and hypercarbia, predisposing to apnea and bradycardia. The effects of general anesthesia in association with the abnormalities of respiratory control may warrant a prolonged period of respiratory support in some infants with myelomeningocele.

Regional anesthesia has been reported as a safe alternative to general anesthesia in the neonate with myelomeningocele. Viscomi et al.[88] successfully administered tetracaine spinals to 14 infants undergoing repair of myelomeningocele. In this small series, there was no evidence of anesthetic-induced neurologic damage. Two of the 14 infants had a postoperative respiratory event (1 transient apnea/bradycardia and 1 brief desaturation with bradycardia). Both of these infants had received intraoperative midazolam for sedation.

Postoperative Care

These infants must be monitored closely in the postoperative period. Respiratory complications, including stridor, apnea and bradycardia, cyanosis, and respiratory arrest, may develop after surgery in these infants with known brainstem abnormalities and potential disorders of central respiratory control. In addition, those infants who were not shunted during repair may show signs of hydrocephalus, including lethargy, vomiting, seizures, apnea and bradycardia, or cardiovascular instability. These infants need to return to the operating room for insertion of a shunt.

Hydrocephalus

Hydrocephalus may occur after closure of a meningomyelocele because of the Arnold-Chiari malformation. The cranial sutures in the neonate are open so intracranial pressure increases are blunted or minimized. However, infants with hydrocephalus eventually have an increase in head size and sometimes in intracranial pressure, resulting in lethargy, vomiting, and cardiorespiratory problems. The anesthetic approach and the technique for tracheal intubation depend on the infant's condition. The major concern is protection of the airway and control of intracranial pressure. Awake tracheal intubation, crying, struggling, and straining can increase intracranial pressure. A rapid-sequence induction of anesthesia to control the airway and intracranial pressure is preferred. Volatile drugs, nitrous oxide, and opioids are all reasonable choices for maintenance of anesthesia. Noninvasive intracranial pressure measurements in neurologically normal preterm neonates have shown a decrease in intracranial pressure with all drugs, including ketamine, fentanyl, and isoflurane. The failure of volatile anesthetics and ketamine to increase intracranial pressure as in adults is attributed to the compliance of the neonate's open-sutured cranium. After surgery, the trachea of these infants should remain intubated, and they should receive PEEP if they were experiencing periods of apnea or bradycardia before surgery because of the intracranial abnormalities. If not, the trachea can be extubated as soon as the protective reflexes have recovered.

Surgical Procedures in the First Month of Life

Surgical procedures in the first month also are considered emergent, or at least urgent, surgery. The six most frequent surgical procedures in the first month are exploratory laparotomy for NEC, inguinal hernia repair, correction of pyloric stenosis, PDA ligation, a shunt procedure for hydrocephalus, and placement of a central venous catheter.

Necrotizing Enterocolitis

Necrotizing enterocolitis is a disease that primarily affects premature infants who have survived the first days of life. One of the theories about NEC is that earlier, more rapid feeding places infants at greater risk for development of NEC. The incidence of NEC among very-low-birth-weight infants varies between 5 and 15%.[89,90]

The exact pathophysiology of NEC has yet to be determined.[91] The condition is characterized by a cascade of pathologic events, beginning with an immature intestine that has a decreased ability to absorb substrate, leading to stasis. Stasis encourages bacterial proliferation, which leads to local infection. The picture is complicated by further pooling of fluid. The ischemia and infection may lead to necrosis of the intestinal mucosa, followed by perforation. The perforation leads to gangrene, fluid loss, peritonitis, septicemia, and disseminated intravascular coagulation. The first signs that NEC may be developing are abdominal distention, irritability, and the development of metabolic acidosis. NEC is primarily a medical disease and is treated by cessation of oral intake, administration of antibiotics, fluid and electrolyte therapy, and recently the insertion of a peritoneal drain. In nonresponsive cases, the infant becomes more septic with severe peritonitis, and the only solution is to perform an exploratory laparotomy to remove the gangrenous bowel and create an ileostomy.

The preoperative problems are an acute abdomen with severe peritonitis, necrosis, and gangrene of the intestine; septicemia; metabolic acidosis; and hypovolemia. These neonates may also have a coagulopathy. Preparation of the patient is directed toward these problems. Often the septicemia, coupled with the distended abdomen and the overall clinical deterioration of the infant, also necessitates the use of intubation and ventilation in the NICU. The anesthetic requirements are continuation of resuscitation, provision of abdominal relaxation for the surgery, and careful titration of anesthetic drugs. These infants are often so critically ill that they tolerate minimal anesthesia. One choice is to start with small doses of ketamine, 0.5 to 1 μg/kg. This can be administered every 20 to 30 minutes. If the condition improves, fentanyl, 2 to 3 μg/kg, can be administered, up to a total dose of 10 to 12 μg/kg. If the infant's condition improves dramatically, small doses of volatile drug can also be added. The use of nitrous oxide should be avoided because of the gas pockets in the abdomen.

These infants are among the most challenging cases in pediatric anesthesia. Monitoring of intra-arterial pressure and arterial blood gases has usually been started in the NICU. The fluid loss can be enormous. They need full-strength, balanced salt solution for maintenance of blood pressure and urine output. If the hematocrit is below 30 to 35%, blood should be administered. These infants are returned to the NICU, and their postoperative care is coordinated carefully with the surgeon, neonatologist, or pediatrician.

Inguinal Hernia Repair in the Neonate

The development of a hernia in the premature infant or neonate is a different clinical problem from the development of a hernia in an infant older than 1 year of age.[92,93] In one study of 100 infants younger than 2 months of age who needed inguinal hernia repair, 30% were premature, 42% had a history of respiratory distress syndrome, 16% had been ventilated, and 19% had congenital heart disease.[92] Furthermore, 31% of the infants had incarcerated hernias, 9% had an intestinal obstruction, and 2% had gonadal infarction. These data preclude waiting until a premature infant or neonate is 6 months or 1 year of age before performing "elective" surgery. The potential for emergent or urgent intervention is so great that surgical repair should be accomplished within a reasonable amount of time after an inguinal hernia is discovered. The "reasonable" time depends on the infant's condition. If the infant is normal and has no other life-threatening medical problems, repair can be done within several days or weeks. If the infant has another problem, the waiting period should be sufficient to stabilize the infant's condition.

Anesthetic Techniques for Hernia Repair

Surgical procedures below the umbilicus can be performed with either general or regional anesthesia. The choice of whether to do general or regional depends on the preference of the surgeon and/or the anesthesiologist. Regional anesthesia can be used entirely for the surgery or as an adjunct to reduce general anesthetic requirements and provide postoperative analgesia. Other methods of providing intraoperative anesthesia and postoperative analgesia include the ilioinguinal-iliohypogastric nerve block or local infiltration. Ilioinguinal-iliohypogastric nerve block with 0.25% bupivacaine or 0.2% ropivacaine, with epinephrine, can be administered shortly after the induction of general anesthesia; it affords excellent postoperative analgesia without the need for opioids.

Pyloric Stenosis

Pyloric stenosis is a relatively frequent surgical disease of the neonate and infant. It can appear as early as the second week of life. The pathologic characteristics include hypertrophy of the pyloric smooth muscle with edema of the pyloric mucosa and submucosa. This process, which develops over a period of days to weeks, leads to progressive obstruction of the pyloric valve, causing persistent vomiting. The vomiting leads to varying losses of fluids and electrolytes. Pediatricians are now adept at the early diagnosis of pyloric stenosis with ultrasound, so it is rare to find an infant with severe fluid and electrolyte derangements. However, an infant is occasionally seen whose problem has developed slowly over a period of weeks, resulting in severe fluid and electrolyte derangements. The stomach contents contain sodium, potassium, chloride, hydrogen ions, and water. The classic electrolyte pattern in infants with severe vomiting is a hyponatremic, hypokalemic, and hypochloremic metabolic alkalosis with a compensatory respiratory acidosis. The anesthesiologist, pediatrician, and surgeon are all responsible for preparing these infants for surgery. Pyloric stenosis is a medical emergency and should not be converted into an anesthetic nightmare by premature surgical repair before adequate fluid and electrolyte homeostasis has been achieved. The infant should have normal skin turgor, and the correction of the electrolyte imbalance should produce a sodium level that is greater than 130 mEq/L, a potassium level that is at least 3 mEq/L, a chloride level that is greater than 85 mEq/L and increasing, and a urine output of at least 1 to 2 mL/kg/hr. These patients need a resuscitation fluid of full-strength, balanced salt solution and, after the infant begins to urinate, the addition of potassium.

Anesthetic Management

One of the concerns in the anesthetic management of patients with pyloric stenosis is the aspiration of gastric contents. A large orogastric tube is passed, and the stomach contents are aspirated.[94] This procedure greatly reduces the quantity of gastric fluid. Intubation of the trachea can be done while the patient is awake or after induction of anesthesia, which is preferred by most clinicians. The infant will most likely have an intravenous line in place for hydration. A rapid-sequence induction is performed using succinylcholine or rocuronium for muscle relaxation. Cricoid pressure is applied as soon as tolerated, and the infant's trachea is intubated. If an intravenous line is not present and cannot be placed with reasonable ease, then a careful inhalation induction can be done using sevoflurane. An intravenous line should be started as soon as possible;

however, if this is not accomplished, intubation can be facilitated by intramuscular succinylcholine or airway topicalization. Anesthesia can be maintained by almost any technique the clinician prefers. The point to remember is that surgeons need muscle relaxation twice: when they deliver the pylorus at the beginning of surgery and when they replace the pylorus into the abdomen at the end of surgery, shortly before closing the peritoneum. Administration of a caudal anesthetic (1.25 mL/kg of 0.25% ropivacaine with epinephrine) after the induction of general anesthesia with tracheal intubation provides intraoperative relaxation, reduces the anesthetic requirement, and provides postoperative analgesia without the need for narcotics. Controlled ventilation reduces or eliminates the need for muscle relaxants for this surgery. The infant's trachea should remain intubated until he or she is awake with eyes opened and is reaching for the endotracheal tube, or is crying. These infants do not appear to be at increased risk of postoperative apnea.[95]

Ligation of a Patent Ductus Arteriosus

As the number of small premature infants who survive has increased, so also has the number of infants who have PDA with heart failure and respiratory failure. Prostaglandins relax the smooth muscle of the ductus so it cannot constrict. Indomethacin, a prostaglandin synthetase inhibitor, is administered to encourage closure of the ductus. However, indomethacin is often unsuccessful in the small premature infant because of the lack of muscle within the ductus. Infants with a PDA and heart failure need maximal medical management with fluid restriction and diuretics. These infants are at special risk because of the reduced blood volume and precarious cardiopulmonary system. Fentanyl with pancuronium is a frequent choice for anesthesia. The clinician must be prepared to augment volume rapidly with 10 to 15 mL/kg of lactated Ringer's solution. If the lactated Ringer's solution accompanies the administration of 20 to 25 μg/kg of fentanyl and pancuronium, the pressure changes are minimal and the infant will be appropriately anesthetized. The tracheas of these infants usually remain intubated and the lungs ventilated in the postoperative period, so concern about the length of action of muscle relaxants and opioids is minimized.

A new technique for closing the PDA in low-birth-weight infants has been developed, called video-assisted ligation of the PDA.[96] Under general anesthesia, four small thoracotomy incisions are made that allow the insertion of an endoscope and various other instruments to ligate the PDA. The operation is accomplished without either spreading the ribs or cutting muscles, thereby offering a minimally traumatic and safe technique for the surgery. This operation has been accomplished both in the operating room and in the NICU; where the surgery is performed is more of a "turf" issue than a technical one.

Placement of a Central Venous Catheter

The use of a central venous catheter for monitoring serum electrolytes for hyperalimentation and for administering medications is increasing. It can be placed either as part of the surgical procedure or at some other time as a separate procedure. The three major concerns in central venous catheter placement are airway management, pneumothorax, and bleeding. The airway should be secured by an endotracheal tube in small infants because of the difficulty in sharing the head, neck, and upper chest with the surgeon and as an adjunct for treating complications such as pneumothorax and bleeding. The anesthetic technique depends on the infant's condition. A pneumothorax may occur with attempts at subclavian vein puncture. The first indication of trouble may be a decreasing oxygen saturation, hypotension, or difficulty with ventilation of the lungs. Because a fluoroscope is often used for central venous catheter placement, it can be used rapidly to diagnose a pneumothorax. If not, the chest should be rapidly aspirated for both diagnostic and therapeutic reasons. Bleeding is an unusual but serious complication of central venous catheter placement. It usually becomes manifest in the perioperative period as a hemothorax or as hypovolemia with a decreasing hematocrit or blood pressure. The question of whether an infant needs an intravenous catheter placed before proceeding with a central line has never been answered. The reason for the central line is usually that the infant has no veins and the clinician is left with a trade-off between prolonged attempts at starting an intravenous catheter versus proceeding without an intravenous line to obtain central venous line placement. The subclavian approach has a higher incidence of problems than an external or internal jugular approach. An intravenous catheter should be started when possible if it can be done within a reasonable time (i.e., 15 to 20 minutes). If not, then central catheter placement continues as described previously, without an intravenous catheter, after discussion and agreement with the surgeon.

References

1. Hagen PT, Scholz DG, Edwards WD: Incidence and size of patent foramen ovale during the first 10 decades of life: An autopsy study of 965 normal hearts. Mayo Clin Proc 59:17, 1984
2. Kopelman AE, Moise AA, Holbert D, Hegemier SE: A single very early dexamethasone dose improves respiratory and cardiovascular adaptation in preterm infants. J Pediatr 135:345, 1999
3. Reller MD, Rice MJ, McDonald RW: Review of studies evaluating ductal patency in the premature infant. J Pediatr 122:S59, 1993
4. Sahni R, Wung J-T, James LS: Controversies in management of persistent pulmonary hypertension of the newborn. Pediatrics 94:307, 1994
5. UK Collaborative ECMO Trial Group: UK collaborative randomised trial of neonatal extracorporeal membrane oxygenation. Lancet 348:75, 1996
6. Schulze A, Gerhardt T, Musante G *et al*: Proportional assist ventilation in low birth weight infants with acute respiratory disease: A comparison to assist/control and conventional mechanical ventilation. J Pediatr 135:339, 1999
7. Murphy JD, Vawter GF, Reid LM: Pulmonary vascular disease in fatal meconium aspiration. J Pediatr 104:758, 1984
8. Katz VL, Bowes WA: Meconium aspiration syndrome: Reflections on a murky subject. Am J Obstet Gynecol 166:171, 1992
9. Wiswell TE, Henley MA: Intratracheal suctioning, systemic infection, and the meconium aspiration syndrome. Pediatrics 89:203, 1992
10. Wiswell TE, Tuggle JM, Turner BS: Meconium aspiration syndrome: Have we made a difference? Pediatrics 85:715, 1990
11. Berry FA, Castro BA: Anesthesia for genitourinary anesthesia. In Gregory GA (ed): Pediatric Anesthesia, 4th ed. New York, Churchill Livingstone, 1999
12. Cornblath M, Schwartz R, Aynsley-Green A *et al*: Hypoglycemia in infancy: The need for a rational definition. Pediatrics 85:834, 1990
13. de Ferranti S, Gauvreua K, Hickey PR *et al*: Intraoperative hyperglycemia during infant cardiac surgery is not associated with adverse neurodevelopmental outcomes at 1, 4, and 8 years. Anesthesiology 100:1345, 2004
14. Berry FA: Practical aspects of fluid and electrolyte therapy. In Berry FA (ed): Anesthetic Management of Difficult and Routine Pediatric Patients, p 89. New York, Churchill Livingstone, 1990
15. Keens TG, Bryan AC, Levison H *et al*: Developmental pattern of muscle fiber types in human ventilatory muscles. J Appl Physiol 44:909, 1978
16. Friedman WF, George BL: Treatment of congestive heart failure by altering loading conditions of the heart. J Pediatr 106:697, 1985
17. Lerman J, Robinson S, Willis MM *et al*: Anesthetic requirements for halothane in young children 0–1 months and 1–6 months of age. Anesthesiology 59:421, 1983
18. Mannion D, Doherty P: Desflurane in paediatric anaesthesia. Paediatr Anaesth 4:301, 1994
19. Meakin G, McKiernan EP, Morris P, Baker RD: Dose-response curves for suxamethonium in neonates, infants and children. Br J Anaesth 62:655, 1989
20. Morell RC, Berman JM, Royster RI *et al*: Revised label regarding use of succinylcholine in children and adolescents (letter). Anesthesiology 80:242, 1994
21. Parker SF, Bailey A, Drake AF: Infant hyperkalemic arrest after succinylcholine. Anesth Analg 80:206, 1995

22. Kraft LF, Katholi RE, Woods WT, James TN: Attenuation by magnesium of the electrophysiologic effects of hyperkalemia on human and canine heart cells. Am J Cardiol 45:1189, 1980
23. Taivaineu T, Meretoja OA, Erkila O *et al*: Rocuronium in infants, children and adults during balanced anesthesia. Pediatr Anesth 6:271, 1996
24. Meretoja OA: Is vecuronium a long-acting neuromuscular blocking agent in neonates and infants? Br J Anaesth 62:184, 1989
25. Miller RD, Rupp SM, Fisher DM *et al*: Clinical pharmacology of vecuronium and atracurium. Anesthesiology 61:444, 1984
26. Cabal LA, Siassi B, Artal R *et al*: Cardiovascular and catecholamine changes after administration of pancuronium in distressed neonates. Pediatrics 75:284, 1985
27. Hickey PR, Hansen DD, Wessel DL *et al*: Pulmonary and systemic hemodynamic responses to fentanyl in infants. Anesth Analg 64:483, 1985
28. Yaster M: The dose response of fentanyl in neonatal anesthesia. Anesthesiology 66:433, 1987
29. Koehntop DE, Rodman JH, Brundage DM *et al*: Pharmacokinetics of fentanyl in neonates. Anesth Analg 65:227, 1986
30. Gauntlett IS, Fisher DM, Hertzka RE *et al*: Pharmacokinetics of fentanyl in neonatal humans and lambs: Effects of age. Anesthesiology 69:683, 1988
31. Chay P, Duffy BJ, Walker JS: Pharmacokinetic and pharmacodynamic relationship of morphine in neonates. Clin Pharmacol Ther 51:334, 1992
32. Friesen RH, Morrison JE Jr: The role of ketamine in the current practice of paediatric anaesthesia. Paediatr Anaesth 4:79, 1994
33. LeDez KM, Lerman J: The minimum alveolar concentration (MAC) of isoflurane in preterm neonates. Anesthesiology 67:301, 1987
34. Lerman J, Robinson S, Willis MM *et al*: Anesthetic requirements for halothane in young children 0–1 month and 1–6 months of age. Anesthesiology 59:421, 1983
35. Bailey A, Valley R, Bigler R: High spinal anesthesia in an infant. Anesthesiology 70:560, 1989
36. Oberlander TF, Berde CB, Lam KH *et al*: Infants tolerate spinal anesthesia with minimal overall autonomic changes: Analysis of heart rate variability in former premature infants undergoing hernia repair. Anesth Analg 80:20, 1995
37. Fisher QA, Shaffner DH, Yaster M: Detection of intravascular injection of regional anaesthetics in children. Can J Anaesth 44:592, 1997
38. Klinscha W, Chiari A, Michalek-Sauber A *et al*: The efficacy and safety of clonidine/bupivacaine combination in caudal blockade for pediatric hernia repair. Anesth Analg 86:54, 1998
39. Fellmann C, Gerber AC, Weiss M: Apnea in a former preterm infant after caudal bupivacaine with clonidine for inguinal herniorrhaphy. Pediatr Anaesth 12:637, 2002
40. Breschan C, Krumpholz R, Likar R *et al*: Can a dose of 2 μg/kg caudal clonidine cause respiratory depression in neonates? Pediatr Anaesth 9:81, 1999
41. Lipshultz SE, Frassica JJ, Orav EJ: Cardiovascular abnormalities in infants prenatally exposed to cocaine. J Pediatr 118:44, 1991
42. van de Bor M, Walther FJ, Ebrahimi M: Decreased cardiac output in infants of mothers who abused cocaine. Pediatrics 85:30, 1990
43. Willson DF: Surfactant in pediatric respiratory failure. Reviews, overviews, and updates. Respir Care 43:1070, 1998
44. Steward DJ: Preterm infants are more prone to complications following minor surgery than are term infants. Anesthesiology 56:304, 1982
45. Liu LMP, Coté CJ, Goudsouzian NG *et al*: Life-threatening apnea in infants recovering from anesthesia. Anesthesiology 59:506, 1983
46. Kurth CD, Spitzer AR, Broennle AM, Downes JJ: Postoperative apnea in preterm infants. Anesthesiology 66:483, 1987
47. Kurth CD, LeBard SE: Association of postoperative apnea, airway obstruction, and hypoxemia in former premature infants. Anesthesiology 75:22, 1991
48. Welborn LG, Hannallah RS, Fink R *et al*: High-dose caffeine suppresses postoperative apnea in former preterm infants. Anesthesiology 71:347, 1989
49. Lee TC, Charles B, Steer P *et al*: Population pharmacokinetics of intravenous caffeine in neonates with apnea of prematurity. Clin Pharmacol Ther 61:628, 1997
50. McNamara DG, Nixon GM, Anderson BJ: Methylxanthines for the treatment of apnea associated with bronchiolitis and anesthesia. Pediatr Anaesth 14:541, 2004
51. Welborn LG, Rice LJ, Hannallah RS *et al*: Postoperative apnea in former preterm infants: Prospective comparison of spinal and general anesthesia. Anesthesiology 72:838, 1990
52. Krane EJ, Haberkern CM, Jacobson LE: Postoperative apnea, bradycardia, and oxygen desaturation in formerly premature infants: Prospective comparison of spinal and general anesthesia. Anesth Analg 80:7, 1995
53. Hussain N, Clive J, Bhandari V: Current incidence of retinopathy of prematurity. Pediatrics 104:552, 1999
54. Spaeth JP, O'Hara IB, Kurth CD: Anesthesia for the micropremie. Semin Perinatol 22:390, 1998
55. Andrews AP, Hartnett ME, Hirose T: Surgical advances in retinopathy of prematurity. Int Ophthalmol Clin 39:275, 1999
56. Flynn JT, Bancalari E, Snyder ES *et al*: A cohort study of transcutaneous oxygen tension and the incidence and severity of retinopathy of prematurity. N Engl J Med 326:1050, 1992
57. Phelps DL: Retinopathy of prematurity. N Engl J Med 326:1078, 1992
58. Metzl K: Telephone advice: To charge or not to charge, that is the question. Pediatrics 102:969, 1998
59. Ramanathan R, Corwin MJ, Hunt CE *et al*: Cardiorespiratory events recorded on home monitors: Comparison of healthy infants with those at increased risk of SIDS. JAMA 285:2199, 2001
60. Gibson E, Cullen JA, Spinner S: Infant sleep position following new AAP guidelines. Pediatrics 96:69, 1995
61. Steward DJ: Is there a risk of general anesthesia triggering SIDS? Possibly not! Anesthesiology 63:326, 1985
62. Kattwinkel J, Brooks J, Myerberg D: Positioning and SIDS: AAP Task Force on Infant Positioning and SIDS. Pediatrics 89:1120, 1992
63. Willinger M, Hoffman HJ, Hartford RB: Infant sleep position and risk for sudden infant death syndrome: Report of meeting held January 13 and 14, 1994, National Institutes of Health, Bethesda, MD. Pediatrics 93:814, 1994
64. Gaultier C: Early disturbances in cardiorespiratory control. Pediatr Pulmonol 16:225, 1997
65. Franco P, Szliwowski H, Dramaix M, Kahn A: Decreased autonomic responses to obstructive sleep events in future victims of sudden infant death syndrome. Pediatr Res 46:33, 1999
66. Davidson A, Soriano S: Does anaesthesia harm the developing brain—Evidence or speculation? Pediatr Anesth 14:199, 2004
67. Greenwood RD, Rosenthal A, Nadas AS: Cardiac anomalies associated with congenital diaphragmatic hernia. Pediatrics 57:92, 1976
68. Greenwood RD, Rosenthal A: Cardiovascular malformations associated with tracheoesophageal fistula and esophageal atresia. Pediatrics 57:87, 1976
69. Kitano Y, Adzick NS: New developments in fetal lung surgery. Curr Opin Pediatr 11:193, 1999
70. Skarsgard ED, Meuli M, Vanderwall KJ *et al*: Fetal endoscopic tracheal occlusion ("Fetendo-PLUG") for congenital diaphragmatic hernia. J Pediatr Surg 31:1335, 1996
71. Bohn D: Congenital diaphragmatic hernia. Am J Respir Crit Care Med 166:911, 2002
72. Katz AL, Wiswell TE, Baumgart S: Contemporary controversies in the management of congenital diaphragmatic hernia. Clin Perinatol 25:219, 1998
73. The Neonatal Inhaled Nitric Oxide Study Group (NINOS): Inhaled nitric oxide and hypoxic respiratory failure in infants with congenital diaphragmatic hernia. Pediatrics 99:838, 1997
74. Frenckner B, Ehren H, Granholm T *et al*: Improved results in patients who have congenital diaphragmatic hernia using preoperative stabilization, extracorporeal membrane oxygenation, and delayed surgery. J Pediatr Surg 32:1185, 1997
75. The Congenital Diaphragmatic Hernia Study Group: Does extracorporeal membrane oxygenation improve survival in neonates with congenital diaphragmatic hernia? J Pediatr Surg 34:720, 1999
76. Iocono JA, Cilley RE, Mauger DT *et al*: Postnatal pulmonary hypertension after repair of congenital diaphragmatic hernia: Predicting risk and outcome. J Pediatr Surg 34:349, 1999
77. Schwartz SM, Vermillion RP, Hirschl RB: Evaluation of left ventricular mass in children with left-side congenital diaphragmatic hernia. J Pediatr 125:447, 1994
78. Grosfeld JL, Weber TR: Congenital abdominal wall defects: Gastroschisis and omphalocele. Curr Probl Surg 19:158, 1982
79. Tsakayannis DE, Zurakowski D, Lillehei CW: Respiratory insufficiency at birth: A predictor of mortality for infants with omphalocele. J Pediatr Surg 31:1088, 1996
80. Yaster M, Buck JR, Dudgeon DL *et al*: Hemodynamic effects of primary closure of omphalocele/gastroschisis in human newborns. Anesthesiology 69:84, 1988
81. Garcia NM, Thompson JW, Shaul DB: Definitive localization of isolated tracheoesophageal fistula using bronchoscopy and esophagoscopy for guide wire placement. J Pediatr Surg 33:1645, 1998
82. McLone DG: Care of the neonate with a myelomeningocele. Neurosurg Clin North Am 1:111, 1998
83. Dias MS, Li V: Pediatric neurosurgical disease. Pediatr Clin North Am 45:1539, 1998
84. Rowe MI, O'Neill JA, Grosfeld JL, Fonkalsrud EW, Coran AG: Neurosurgical disorders. In Rowe MI. Essentials of Pediatric Surgery, p 831. St Louis, Mosby, 1995
85. Tulipan N, Hernanz-Schulman M, Bruner JP: Reduced hindbrain herniation after intrauterine myelomeningocele repair: A report of four cases. Pediatr Neurosurg 29:274, 1998
86. Shah S, Cawley M, Gleeson R *et al*: Latex allergy and latex sensitization in children and adolescents with meningomyelocele. J Allergy Clin Immunol 101:741, 1998
87. Dierdorf SF, McNiece WL, Rao CC *et al*: Failure of succinylcholine to alter plasma potassium in children with myelomeningocele. Anesthesiology 64:272, 1986
88. Viscomi CM, Abajian JC, Wald SL *et al*: Spinal anesthesia for repair of meningomyelocele in neonates. Anesth Analg 81:492, 1995
89. Kliegman RM: Neonatal necrotizing enterocolitis: Bridging the basic science with the clinical disease. J Pediatr 117:833, 1990
90. Fujiwara T, Konishi M, Chida S: Surfactant replacement therapy with a single postventilatory dose of a reconstituted bovine surfactant in preterm neonates with respiratory distress syndrome: Final analysis of a multicenter,

double-blind, randomized trial and comparison with similar trials. Pediatrics 86:753, 1990
91. Kosloske AM: Pathogenesis and prevention of necrotizing enterocolitis: A hypothesis based on personal observation and a review of the literature. Pediatrics 74:1086, 1984
92. Rescorla FJ, Grosfeld JL: Inguinal hernia repair in the perinatal period and early infancy: Clinical considerations. J Pediatr Surg 19:832, 1984
93. Peevy KJ, Speed FA, Hoff CJ: Epidemiology of inguinal hernia in preterm neonates. Pediatrics 77:246, 1986
94. Cook-Sather SD, Tulloch HV, Liacouras CA, Schreiner MS: Gastric fluid volume in infants for pyloromyotomy. Can J Anaesth 44:278, 1997
95. Chipps BE, Moynihan R, Schieble T *et al*: Infants undergoing pyloromyotomy are not at risk for postoperative apnea. Pediatr Pulmonol 27:278, 1999
96. Burke RP, Jacobs JP, Cheng W *et al*: Video-assisted thoracoscopic surgery for patent ductus arteriosus in low birth weight neonates and infants. Pediatrics 104:227, 1999

CHAPTER 44 ■ PEDIATRIC ANESTHESIA

JOSEPH P. CRAVERO AND ZEEV N. KAIN

KEY POINTS

1. There are numerous specific anatomic, physiologic, and psychological issues that should be understood prior to anesthetizing pediatric patients.
2. A child with an upper respiratory infection (URI) or who is recovering from a URI is at increased risk to develop laryngospasm, bronchospasm, oxygen desaturation, and postoperative atelectasis and croup.
3. Children with obstructive sleep apnea (OSA) may obstruct with the use of preoperative sedative premedication during the induction process. Muscle relaxants should be used carefully.
4. Healthy children undergoing elective minor surgery require no laboratory evaluation.
5. The American Society of Anesthesiologists has issued practice guidelines regarding preoperative fasting. Solids are prohibited within 6 to 8 hours of surgery (generally after midnight), formula within 6 hours, breast milk within 4 hours of surgery, and clear liquids within 2 hours of surgery.
6. Oral midazolam is the most commonly used sedative premedicant.
7. Mask induction of general anesthesia remains the most common induction technique for pediatric anesthesia.
8. Succinylcholine is recommended in situations where ultra-rapid onset and short duration of action is of paramount importance (laryngospasm), when relaxation is required, or when intravenous access is not available and intramuscular administration is required.
9. Perioperative fluid and blood product management for pediatric patients must take into account fluid deficits, translocation of fluids and blood loss during surgery, and maintenance fluid requirements.
10. Appropriate airway management remains the single most important aspect of delivering safe pediatric anesthesia.
11. The most commonly used form of regional anesthesia in children is the *caudal block*. This technique can provide postoperative analgesia following a wide variety of lower abdominal and genitourinary surgical procedures.
12. Recovery of the young child in the postanesthesia care unit (PACU) includes management of hypothermia, nausea and vomiting, and postoperative pain.

1 The provision of safe anesthesia for the pediatric patient requires a clear understanding of the anatomic, psychological, physiologic, and pharmacologic differences between patients in different age epochs from newborn to adolescent. These distinctive features form the basis for the techniques and pharmacology outlined in this chapter. A partial listing of the most important differences is presented in Table 44-1. Consideration of these differences when providing anesthesia care to children is critical to achieving high-quality and efficient care. Given its brief nature, this chapter focuses on only the most salient issues relating to anesthesia delivery for pediatric patients. The reader should note that relevant topics such as neonatal anesthesia, pediatric pharmacology, and pediatric equipment are covered elsewhere in this textbook.

THE PREOPERATIVE EVALUATION

The preoperative evaluation and preparation of the child for surgery is an integral part of the perioperative process. The preoperative evaluation of the pediatric patient should consist of all pertinent maternal history, birth and neonatal history, review of systems, physical examination and evaluation of height, weight, and vital signs. Preoperative use of bronchodilators, steroids, and chemotherapeutic agents has significant implications for the anesthetic management. The use of herbal medication, as well as other alternative and complementary medicine modalities, also has to be assessed.[1] Special attention should be paid to the existence of congenital malformations in the child and family. Issues such as anesthetic risks, anesthetic plans, recovery, and postoperative analgesia and discharge must be discussed in detail. Indeed, a more recent study found that most parents were interested in receiving all information about the surgery *and*, as a result of the detailed discussion regarding anesthetic plans and risks, the parents were not overly anxious.[2]

It is important to appreciate that anesthesia and surgery cause an enormous amount of stress and hardship on both the child and parents. Anxiety in children undergoing surgery is characterized by subjective feelings of tension, apprehension, nervousness, and worry, and may be expressed in many forms.[3]

TABLE 44-1

ANATOMIC AND PHYSIOLOGIC DISTINCTIONS BETWEEN ADULTS AND PEDIATRIC PATIENTS

PHYSICAL OR PHYSIOLOGIC VARIABLE	CONTRAST BETWEEN CHILD AND ADULT	ANESTHETIC IMPLICATION
Head size	Much larger head size relative to body	Consider roll under shoulders or neck for optimal intubation positioning
Tongue size	Larger size relative to mouth	Makes airway appear slightly anterior; oral airways particularly helpful during mask ventilation
Airway shape	Narrowest diameter is below the glottis at cricoid level in children	Uncuffed tubes can make seal when appropriately sized in children younger than 8 years of age
Respiratory physiology	Oxygen consumption is two to three times greater in infants than adults. FRC ranges from 8–13 $cm^3 \approx 1/3$ as large as adults	Oxygen desaturation is extremely rapid following apnea
Cardiac physiology	Relatively fixed stroke volume in neonates and infants	Bradycardia must be treated aggressively in young age groups; consider atropine prior to airway management; heart rates less than 60 require circulatory support
Renal function	Limited GFR at birth; does not reach adult levels until late infancy; total body water and % extracellular fluid are increased in the infant	Prolonged duration of action for hydrophilic drugs, particularly those that are renally excreted
Hepatic function	P450 system not fully developed in neonates and infants; liver blood flow decreased in newborns	Prolonged excretion for drugs, depending on hepatic metabolism
Body surface area	Larger surface-to-body ratio in newborns/infants/toddlers	Heat loss more prominent problem for these age groups
Psychological development	0–6 mo—stress on family 8 mo–4 yr—separation anxiety 4–6 yr—misconceptions of surgical mutilation 6–13 yr—fear of not "waking up" ≥13 yr—fear of loss of control, body image issues	Changes the manner in which each patient and family should be approached; must address issues with personal and systemic strategies

FRC, functional residual capacity; GFR, glomerular filtration rate.

Some children verbalize their fears explicitly, whereas for others anxiety is expressed only behaviorally. Many children look scared, become agitated, breathe deeply, tremble, stop talking or playing, and may start to cry. These behaviors, which may prolong the induction of anesthesia, could give children some sense of control in the situation and thereby diminish a damaging sense of helplessness.[3] Coping with this preoperative stress requires consistent communication between the child, the parents, and all health care providers involved in the perioperative period. Because parental anxiety increases a child's anxiety,[4] preoperative preparation should include the entire family.[5] Both behavioral and pharmacological interventions can be used to address the issue of preoperative anxiety in children and their parents. Behavioral interventions include tours of the operating room, written and audiovisual materials, coloring books, and patient care representatives skilled in the preoperative preparation of children.[6] To date, most studies suggest that preoperative preparation programs reduce anxiety and enhance coping in children.[6] Some hospitals allow parents to be present for the induction of anesthesia in their child, but the efficacy of this intervention is uncertain and the availability of such programs is limited.[6–10] Also, other nonpharmacological interventions such as music and acupuncture have been shown to reduce the anxiety of parents and children in the perioperative settings.[11,12] Pharmacological interventions such as midazolam are effective treatment for preoperative anxiety and are discussed later in this chapter. The anesthesiologist should also be aware that more recent research has documented that a child's fear on the day of surgery might extend beyond the immediate operative period.[13] About 50% of all children undergoing routine outpatient surgery present at 2 weeks postoperatively with new-onset anxiety, nighttime crying, enuresis, separation anxiety, temper tantrums, and sleep or eating disturbances.[4] Most of these behaviors disappear within 3 to 4 weeks postoperatively. It is important for the primary health care provider to be aware of these behaviors and to assure the parents that these behavioral changes are self-limited. Children with postoperative behavioral changes that persist beyond 3 to 4 weeks after surgery should be referred to a trained mental health provider.

Coexisting Health Conditions

Upper Respiratory Infection

2 Multiple investigations have found that a child with an upper respiratory infection (URI) or who is recovering from a URI is at increased risk to develop laryngospasm, bronchospasm, oxygen desaturation, and postoperative atelectasis and croup.[14,15] Although these complications usually do not cause significant morbidity in otherwise healthy children, they may be significant in children with underlying conditions such as asthma and sickle cell disease. More recent studies indicated that children with asthma, infants and young children with bronchopulmonary dysplasia, children younger than 1 year of age, children with sickle cell disease, children who live in a household

that includes smoking parents, and children who are to undergo bronchoscopy are at a higher risk of developing perioperative morbidity if suffering from a URI.[14] Patients in these categories should be carefully assessed, and strong consideration should be given to postponing elective surgery. It is unclear how long surgery should be delayed following a URI, however, because bronchial hyperreactivity may exist for up to 7 weeks after a URI.[16] The final decision would take into account the risk–benefit ratio of the surgical procedure. Finally, mask anesthetic, but not laryngeal mask airway, was clearly shown to be associated with a significantly lower rate of perioperative complications as compared with endotracheal tube and thus should be used whenever possible with these children.

Obstructive Sleep Apnea

Severe adenotonsillar hypertrophy with obstructive sleep apnea (OSA) is a frequent indication for children to undergo tonsil-
3 lectomy and adenoidectomy. Postoperatively, patients with severe OSA may exhibit worsening of their obstructive symptoms secondary to tissue edema, altered response to carbon dioxide, and residual anesthetic and analgesic agents.[17] Although most children who undergo tonsillectomy and adenoidectomy can be discharged home following 4 hours of postanesthesia care unit (PACU) observation, children with severe OSA may require postoperative observation in the hospital. Such issues have to be discussed a priori with the family and the surgeon.

Asthma

It is well established that children with asthma should be under optimal medical care prior to undergoing general anesthesia and surgery.[18] In fact, the more active the disease, as indicated by recent asthma symptoms, drug usage, and recent treatment in an emergency department, the greater probability of perioperative complications.[19] All oral and inhaled medications, such as corticosteroids and beta agonists, should be continued up to and including the day of surgery. More recent data have indicated that administration of inhaled short-acting beta agonists prior to induction of anesthesia eliminates the increase in airway pressure that is typically associated with intubation in asthmatic patients.[20]

The Former Preterm Infant

There are multiple concerns related to the perioperative period of preterm infants. Three frequent problems are the impact bronchopulmonary dysplasia might have on the patient's perioperative course, the presence of anemia, and the possibility of postoperative apnea. Bronchodilators and inhaled corticosteroids, which many of these patients require, affect treatment, and should be continued up to and including the day of surgery. The parents should be questioned about the need for oxygen therapy at home, and recent hematocrit data should be available. In fact, many institutions require preoperative hematocrit for all infants younger than 2 months of age. Data also indicate that former preterm infants are more likely to develop postoperative apnea following general anesthesia.[21,22] Reports indicate that risk of postoperative apnea is inversely related to postconceptional age, and that infants with a history of apnea and bradycardia, respiratory distress, and mechanical ventilation may be at increased risk.[23] Although which infants should be admitted to the hospital following anesthesia is controversial, the age generally is believed to be younger than 52 to 60 weeks' postconceptual age.[23] Arrangements for overnight hospital monitoring should be made for any child considered to be at significant risk for postoperative apnea.

Laboratory Evaluation

4 It is currently the standard of care that healthy children undergoing elective minor surgery require no laboratory evaluation, and thus can be spared the anxiety and pain of blood drawing.[24] Indeed, blood chemistry analyses are usually performed only for indications, such as measurement of ionized potassium in children on digoxin or diuretics. The arbitrary hemoglobin value of 10 g/dL has been cited for infants older than 3 months, with higher values for the younger infants, depending on gestational age and general health status. Children whose hemoglobin values are less than this arbitrary standard should have the cause of their anemia investigated and corrected. Outside this subgroup, there is little evidence that testing for hematocrit levels is helpful in the management of routine pediatric outpatients. Patients with sickle cell anemia or other hemoglobinopathies require special preoperative preparation. Routine chest radiographs and urinary analysis are also unnecessary. Coagulation screening has been among the most debated of all laboratory tests. Although an undiagnosed coagulopathy could result in serious surgical morbidity, commonly used screening tests, such as bleeding time and prothrombin time, do *not* reliably predict abnormal perioperative bleeding.[25] Laboratory testing should only be considered in children in whom either the history or medical condition suggests a possible hemostatic defect, in patients undergoing surgical procedures that might induce hemostatic disturbances (e.g., cardiopulmonary bypass), when the coagulation system is particularly needed for adequate hemostasis, and in patients for whom even minimal postoperative bleeding could be critical.

Although teratogenicity of anesthetic agents has not been firmly established, a determination of whether a female patient is pregnant should be ascertained before the administration of anesthesia. This may be a difficult task because parents might decline a request for a pregnancy test, and a reliable menstrual and sexual history may be difficult to obtain from an adolescent when a relationship of confidentiality with medical personnel has not been previously established. Because there are no clear national guidelines, whether pregnancy screening of all female patients of childbearing age before the administration of anesthesia is routine or selective is a matter of policy at individual facilities.

Preoperative Fasting Period

The risk of aspiration pneumonia in children is well recognized, and more recent reports found an incidence of about 1 in 10,000 for this clinical phenomenon.[26] These reports also indicate that the outcome of children who developed aspiration pneumonia is excellent, unless these children had some major underlying problem such as abdominal or thoracic trauma.[26]
5 As the importance of this issue is recognized, the American Society of Anesthesiologists issued practice guidelines regarding preoperative fasting. Solids are prohibited within 6 to 8 hours of surgery (generally after midnight), formula within 6 hours, breast milk within 4 hours of surgery, and clear liquids within 2 hours of surgery.[27] Indeed, liquids such as apple or grape juice, flat cola, and sugar water may be encouraged up to 2 hours prior to the induction of anesthesia because their consumption has been shown to decrease the gastric residual volume. It is important to note that some institutions have chosen to make the fasting period for clear liquids for 2 to 4 hours because this longer fasting time allows for flexibility in patient

TABLE 44-2

PREMEDICATION

MEDICATION	ROUTE	DOSE mg/kg	TIME TO ONSET (min)	ELIMINATION HALF-LIFE $T_{1/2}$ (hr)
Midazolam	Oral	0.25–1.0	10	2
	Intranasal	0.2–0.3	<10	2–3
	Rectal	0.3–1.0	10	2–3
Ketamine	Oral	3.0–6.0	10	2–3
	Intranasal	3.0–5.0	<10	3
	Rectal	5.0–6.0	20–30	3
Clonidine	Oral	0.002–0.004	45	8–12

scheduling. This issue of fasting time is important because the younger the child, the smaller the glycogen stores, and the more likely the occurrence of hypoglycemia with prolonged intervals of fasting. For this reason, fasting time should be reduced based on the previous recommendation. Regardless of the length of preoperative fasting, there still exists a defined population of children who are at an increased risk for regurgitation and aspiration of stomach contents. This group of children includes children with delayed gastric emptying times, and abdominal pathology associated with ileus, vomiting, or electrolyte disorders.

Preoperative Sedatives

Sedation before surgery is an effective method for decreasing anxiety that is widely used for young children (Table 44-2).[7,28] The primary goals of premedication in children are to facilitate a smooth and anxiety-free separation from the parents and induction of anesthesia. Other effects that may be achieved by pharmacological preparation of the patient include amnesia, anxiolysis, prevention of physiologic stress, and analgesia. In addition, children who are sedated before coming to the operating room may have fewer stress-related behavioral changes in the immediate postoperative time compared with groups of patients who receive no sedation (Fig. 44-1).

Oral

6 Midazolam is the most commonly used sedative premedicant used in the United States.[29] It has rapid onset and predictable effect, without causing cardiorespiratory depression. In a dose of 0.5 to 0.75 mg/kg, midazolam peaks approximately 30 minutes after administration, and its effect lasts approximately 30 minutes.[28] Midazolam has short duration that generally does not delay emergence from general anesthesia or discharge from the PACU. Although serious side effects after oral midazolam are uncommon, strict adult supervision is necessary in children who receive this drug. Midazolam has been shown to be superior to parental presence in decreasing perioperative stress for patients and families.[30] Midazolam can be reversed with flumazenil, which antagonizes benzodiazepines competitively. The initial recommended dose in children is 0.05 mg/kg given intravenously in a titrated fashion of up to 1.0 mg total.[31]

Oral ketamine has also been used as a sedation medication in doses of 5 to 6 mg/kg for children 1 to 6 years of age.[28] Maximal sedation occurred within 20 minutes. Investigators also evaluated a combination of ketamine and midazolam as an oral sedative premedication mixture. Funk et al reported that the combination of midazolam and ketamine administrated orally had a 90% success rate of satisfactory anxiolysis compared with less than 75% with either drug alone.[32] Nausea and vomiting rates were slightly increased in children who received oral ketamine.

Oral transmucosal fentanyl represents the first commercial attempt to deliver medication to children by the transmucosal oral route and was shown to sedate children prior to induction of anesthesia.[28] Its sedative effect is often, however, heralded by facial pruritus, higher incidence of postoperative nausea and vomiting, and arterial oxygen desaturation.[33] Thus, this drug is not currently used routinely in the perioperative settings.

Finally, clonidine is an α_2 agonist that, when given in combination with atropine, produces satisfactory preoperative sedation, easy separation from parents, and mask acceptance within 30 minutes.[33] Orally administrated clonidine in a dose of 4 μg/kg has been demonstrated to reliably cause sedation, decrease anesthetic requirements, and decrease requirement for postoperative analgesics. It also attenuates the hemodynamic response to tracheal intubation. With the recommended dose, perioperative hypotension is not observed.[28]

Nasal

A major disadvantage of intranasally administered sedative medications is that *most* children cry upon administration because it transiently irritates the nasal passages. Rapid absorption and avoidance of first-pass hepatic metabolism of medications are advantages of this route of administration. When required, midazolam can be administered intranasally in a dose of 0.2 mg/kg. The use of sufentanil and other sedatives intranasally has been abandoned because of untoward side effects.

Rectal

Rectal administration of midazolam in doses of 0.5 to 1.0 mg/kg effectively reduces the anxiety of children prior to induction.[28] Care must be taken, however, that the medication is not expelled immediately on placement. Both methohexital and thiopental have also been used in rectal formulations in a dose of 25 mg/kg. Onset of sedation requires approximately 10 minutes. Respiratory depression and oxygen desaturation may occur because of variable absorption of the medication in the rectum.

Intramuscular

Parenteral administration of sedation may be the only alternative in a child who refuses to cooperate with other modalities. Intramuscular midazolam in a dose of 0.3 mg/kg provides anxiolysis in 5 to 10 minutes. Ketamine in an intramuscular dose

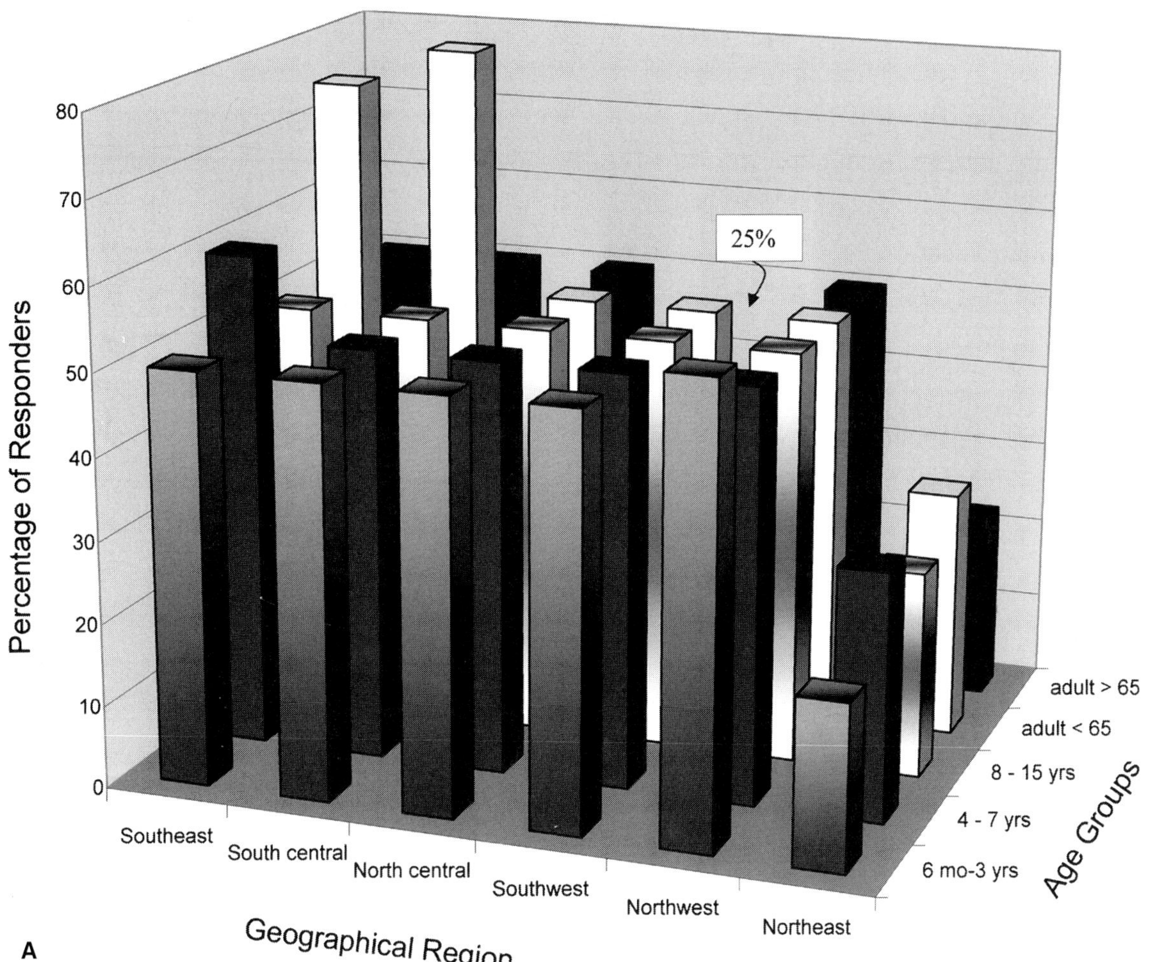

FIGURE 44-1. **A.** Frequency of sedative premedication practice in the United States as of 2002. **B.** Frequency of sedative premedication practice in the United States as of 1996. Data reported are medians (range, 0–100%). (From Kain ZN, Caldwell-Andrews AA, Krivutza DM *et al*: Trends in the practice of parental presence during induction of anesthesia and the use of preoperative sedative premedication in the United States, 1995–2002: Results of a follow-up national survey. Anesth Analg 98[5]:1252, 2004.)

of 3 to 4 mg/kg provides a quiet and breathing, yet minimally responsive, patient in approximately 5 minutes.

ANESTHETIC AGENTS

Potent Inhalation Agents

Mask Induction Pharmacology

7 Mask induction of general anesthesia remains the most common induction technique for pediatric anesthesia the United States. Although inhalation induction of anesthesia is safe, the incidence of bradycardia, hypotension, and cardiac arrest during this form of induction is higher in infants younger than 1 year of age than in older children and adults.[34] This difference in outcome is due to the extremely rapid uptake of inhalation agents in infants compared with adults as a result of the much greater ratio of alveolar ventilation to functional residual capacity and the altered distribution of cardiac output. In addition, high inspired concentrations (overpressure) are often used early in induction, yielding high tissue concentrations of anesthetic that can lead to severe cardiac depression and junctional rhythms.[35] In light of these facts, mask induction of anesthesia in this age group should be accompanied by monitoring of blood pressure, electrocardiogram (ECG), oxygenation, and ventilation.

Minimal Alveolar Concentration

The minimum alveolar concentration (MAC) of anesthetic required in pediatric patients differs with age. There is actually a small increase in MAC between birth and 2 to 3 months of age, which represents the age of highest MAC requirement. After that time, MAC slowly decreases with age. For sevoflurane, the change in MAC is marked—with a value of approximately 2.5% for young infants compared with 2% for adolescents and adults.[36]

Intracardiac Shunts

Children with unrepaired or partially repaired congenital heart malformations may safely undergo inhaled induction of anesthesia. Although intracardiac shunts can, in theory, alter the uptake of anesthetic agents and affect the speed of induction, this is rarely clinically evident. A right-to-left shunt slows the

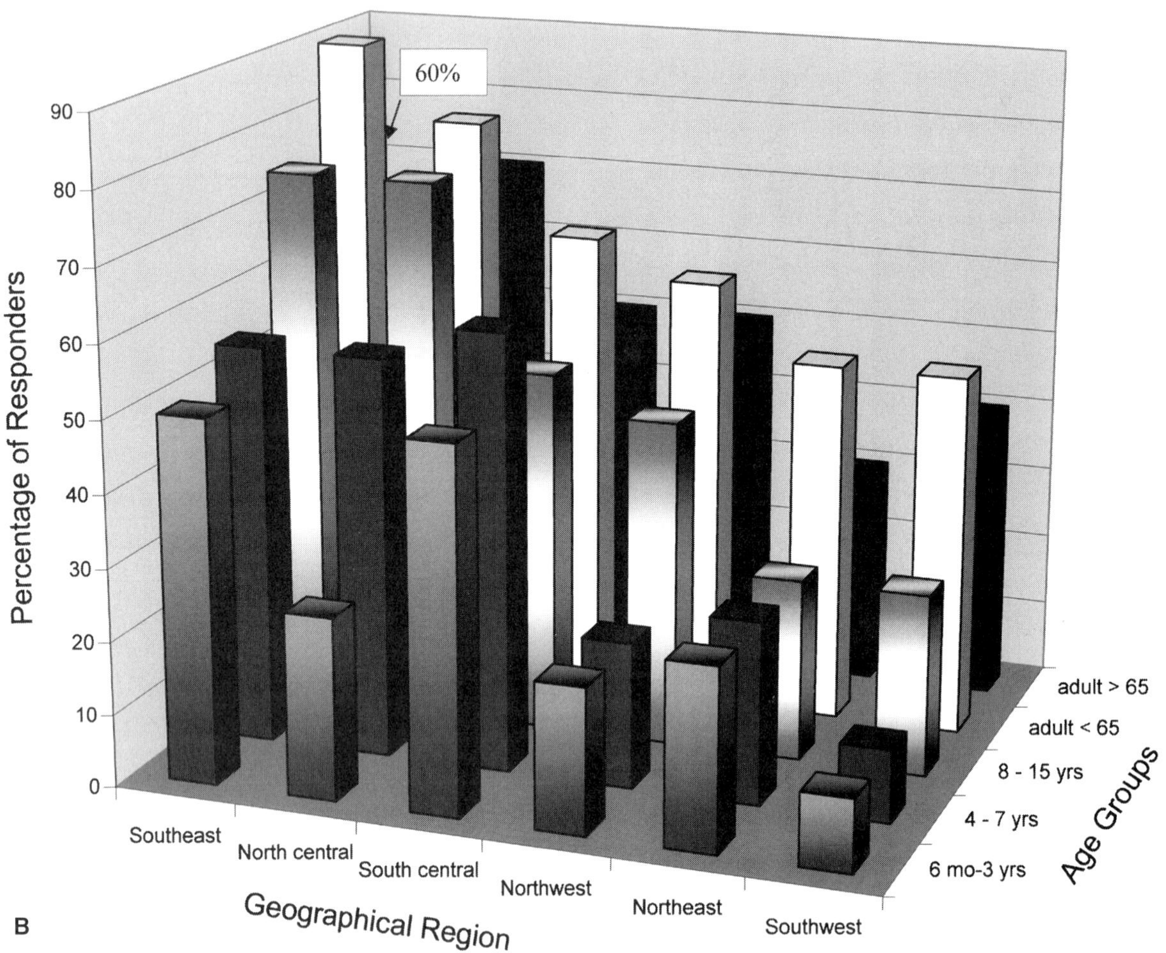

FIGURE 44-1. (*continued*)

inhaled induction of anesthesia because anesthetic concentration in the arterial blood increases more slowly. A left-to-right shunt should have the opposite effect; volatile agent induction is more rapid because the rate of anesthetic transfer from the lungs to the arterial blood is increased. In practice, decreased delivery of anesthetic to the target tissues largely negates the increased uptake with this type of shunt.

Inhaled Agents for Induction of Anesthesia

The only two potent anesthetic agents currently in use that are compatible with inhaled induction are sevoflurane and halothane.[37] Both of these agents have acceptable odor and can be used for smooth inhaled induction in children. Sevoflurane dominates this market in the United States where its advantages—including rapid onset and relatively *less frequent* junctional bradycardia associated with its use—are perceived as worth its added cost over halothane.[38] Some of these (clinically noted) differences may, in fact, be due to vaporizer design owing to the fact that it is possible to deliver a much higher MAC multiple of halothane versus sevoflurane.[39] Halothane has been shown to have a greater depressive effect on the myocardial contractility than sevoflurane during standard inhaled induction techniques.[40,41]

Inhaled Agents—General Points on Maintenance and Recovery in Pediatric Patients

The safety and efficacy of sevoflurane for maintenance of anesthesia in children has been established in hundreds of studies. Intubation and laryngeal mask airway (LMA) insertion under deep sevoflurane anesthesia has also been reported.[42–45] The rapid and extensive pulmonary elimination of sevoflurane minimizes the amount of anesthetic available for metabolism. In vivo studies suggest that only about 5% of the sevoflurane dose is metabolized by the hepatic cytochrome P4502E1 isoenzyme to hexafluoroisopropanol (HFIP) with the release of inorganic fluoride and carbon dioxide. Fluoride is primarily excreted in the urine, and no evidence of toxic levels or renal injury has been found in children after exposure to sevoflurane.[46]

Sevoflurane undergoes ex vivo degradation reaction in the clinical setting through direct contact with CO_2 absorbents (i.e., soda lime or Baralyme) in the anesthesia circuit. This reaction produces pentafluoroisopropenyl fluoromethyl ether (PIFE), also known as compound A, and trace amounts of pentafluoromethoxy isopropyl fluoromethyl ether (PMFE or compound B). Mean maximum concentrations in pediatric patients with soda lime are about half those found in adults. Although the level of compound A at which toxicity occurs is not known, sevoflurane use with fresh gas flows of 1 L/minute appears to be safe in children. Finally, although emergence from anesthesia is more rapid with sevoflurane than with more soluble agents such as halothane or isoflurane, there is a growing literature supporting the fact that agitation behaviors in children on emergence are more common with this agent. The exact reason for this disturbance is not known, but there is evidence that it may occur with or without pain as a factor.[47–49] The use of various medications to decrease the problem of emergence agitation after sevoflurane (including midazolam, ketorolac, fentanyl, propofol, and dexmedetomidine) have been reported.[50–54] Careful attention to pain control and supportive environments are indicated.

Halothane has a long history of safety and efficacy as an inhaled agent for pediatric anesthesia. Although there has been some concern regarding sensitization of the myocardium to catecholamines, there is little problem in the absence of hypercarbia or light anesthesia.[55] Up to 10 μg/kg of epinephrine may be used with minimal risk of cardiac dysrhythmia in the absence of hypercarbia.

Halothane can cause myocardial depression. This effect is exaggerated in young children and in those who are hypovolemic. Addition of muscle relaxants to a lighter halothane anesthetic (in conjunction with regional anesthetic techniques or opioids) can ameliorate this effect.

Isoflurane also has a long track record as a safe and efficacious agent for maintenance of anesthesia in infants and children. Like halothane, it decreases blood pressure in pediatric patients. Although myocardial depression in children is less than that caused by halothane, isoflurane reduces peripheral vascular resistance, whereas halothane does not. (In neonates, equal myocardial depression has been demonstrated with both drugs.[56] The major disadvantage of isoflurane is its pungent odor and high incidence of laryngospasm when this agent is used for inhaled induction of anesthesia. It should not be used for inhaled induction of anesthesia.

Desflurane is also a safe and effective agent for anesthesia[57] in infants and children. Unfortunately (like isoflurane), an unacceptable incidence of coughing, increased secretions, and laryngospasm preclude its use as a mask induction agent.[58] Although desflurane appears to be associated with faster initial awakening when used as a maintenance anesthetic agent in pediatric patients, studies have shown no difference between halothane and desflurane in time to discharge after ambulatory surgery. As is the case with sevoflurane, emergence agitation has been reported with desflurane use in children.[47]

Intravenous Agents

Sedative Hypnotics

Sedative hypnotic agents may be employed after inhaled induction of anesthesia (e.g., to deepen anesthesia for airway management), or they may be used as primary induction and maintenance agents in children who have an intravenous catheter in place. Intravenous line placement may be made easier for the awake patient through the use of topical anesthetics such as the eutectic mixture of local anesthetics, topical liposomal lidocaine cream, or lidocaine iontophoresis.[59,60] As with inhaled agents mentioned previously, the doses of intravenous agents used in infants and toddlers will often need to be increased by 25 to 40% to obtain the same level of sedation/anesthesia in children as compared with adults.

Propofol, thiopental, methohexital, etomidate, midazolam, and ketamine have all been used to produce effective intravenous induction of anesthesia or sedation in infants and children. Methohexital, midazolam, and ketamine have also been used through the rectal administration, whereas midazolam (in particular) and ketamine have been shown to have useful oral and intramuscular applications. In this chapter, we discuss only the two agents; the other drugs are reviewed in detail in other chapters of this text and elsewhere.

Propofol is the most widely reported agent for induction and maintenance of anesthesia or sedation in children. Its use is limited to the operating room environment and brief sedation outside the operating room as prolonged use in the intensive care environment (although not well understood) is believed to be linked to acidosis, heart failure, and several fatalities.[61,62] Propofol induction doses range from 3 to 4 mg/kg for children younger than 2 years of age to approximately 2.5 to 3 mg/kg for older children, whereas maintenance of anesthesia requires 200 to 300 mcg/kg per minute.[63] Onset is rapid, but may be accompanied by some random movement and cough. Bag-mask ventilation is generally easily performed. Pain on injection of propofol is marked. This problem may be minimized by infusing the largest vein possible and running carrier fluid as rapidly as possible. Other techniques for minimizing pain include small doses of lidocaine preceding or mixed with the propofol bolus, fentanyl premedication, ketamine premedication, and nitrous oxide inhalation at the time of propofol infusion.[64] Propofol will cause mild to moderate decreases in blood pressure when used at recommended doses.[65]

The emergence profile of propofol in children shows clear advantages over other intravenous agents and inhaled anesthetics. Emergence from deep sedation/anesthesia is clearly faster than that from most other sedative agents and most inhaled agents, especially after prolonged administration. In addition, although time to awakening may not be faster than sevoflurane or desflurane, the emergence from propofol is associated with less nausea and vomiting, and is accompanied by less emergence agitation so readiness for discharge is at least as rapid.[66]

Although it was first described 40 years ago, ketamine has been increasingly reported for use in anesthesia, procedural sedation, and sedation in the intensive care environment for children. It is the only agent that offers both hypnosis *and* analgesia. Other unique aspects include the fact that ketamine preserves airway reflexes, maintains respiratory drive, increases endogenous catecholamine release, and results in bronchodilation and pulmonary vasodilation. Induction doses of 1 mg/kg intravenously yields effective analgesia and sedation with rapid onset. Intramuscular doses of 3 to 4 mg/kg result in a similar state with significant analgesia appropriate for minor procedures such as intravenous catheter starts or fracture manipulation.[67] Simultaneous administration of an anticholinergic will minimize oral secretions. Emergence can be marked by diplopia, occasional disturbing dreams, and nausea/vomiting, although these are less common in children than in adults.[68] The use of concomitant midazolam 0.025 to 0.50 mg/kg to decrease some of these side effects has a mixed record of success and should not be considered reliable.

Opioids

Opioids are important elements of balanced anesthesia and sedation in children. Their use for surgical anesthesia will decrease MAC of inhaled agents, smooth hemodynamics during airway management or stimulating procedures, and provide postoperative analgesia. Usual recommended doses include fentanyl 0.5 to 1.0 mcg/kg, morphine 0.10 mg/kg, sufentanil 0.1 mcg/kg, and alfentanil 50 to 100 μg/kg. Remifentanil has also been shown to be an effective part of anesthesia and sedation protocols for a variety of procedures at 0.25 to 1.0 μg/kg per minute.[69,70] It should be noted that due to its short half-life, remifentanil does not offer effective postoperative analgesia when used in this manner.

Chest wall rigidity is not uncommon when administering bolus opioids, especially to drug-naïve neonates and infants. This effect can severely impair respiration, and providers must be prepared to provide muscle relaxation and general airway support when delivering these medications in this

TABLE 44-3

ONSET, DURATION, CARDIOVASCULAR EFFECTS, COST, AND SPECIAL CONSIDERATIONS OF NONDEPOLARIZING NEUROMUSCULAR-BLOCKING AGENTS IN CHILDREN

	RECOMMENDED DOSE (μg/kg)	ONSET	DURATION	CARDIOVASCULAR EFFECTS	COST	SPECIAL CONSIDERATIONS
Atracurium	500	Intermediate	Intermediate	Rare hypotension	Intermediate	Mild erythema common
Cisatracurium	80–200	Slow–intermediate	Intermediate–long	Absent	Inexpensive–intermediate	
Mivacurium	250–400	Intermediate	Short	Rare hypotension	Intermediate	Mild erythema common
Pancuronium	100	Intermediate	Intermediate–long	Tachycardia, occasional hypertension	Inexpensive	Effect prolonged in renal failure
Rocuronium	500–1,200	Rapid	Intermediate	Slight increase in heart rate	Intermediate	Deltoid injection facilitates tracheal intubation
Vecuronium	100–400	Intermediate (rapid with large doses)	Intermediate (long with doses >150 μg/kg)	Absent	Intermediate	

Doses are the authors' preference and, in some instances, exceed those recommended in the package insert. For onset and duration, specific values are omitted because of the difficulty in comparing studies and the influence of anesthetic technique.
From Fisher DM: Neuromuscular blocking agents in paediatric anaesthesia. Br J Anaesth 83:58, 1999.

manner. Opioids are also well known to depress central respiratory effort. Newborns and infants younger than 6 months are particularly susceptible to this effect due the immature blood-brain barrier and increased levels of free drug. These facts highlight the need to carefully monitor pediatric patients given opioids; however, they do not argue for withholding pain medications. In fact, after 6 months of age, there is evidence that infants and children are no more susceptible to central depression due to opioids than adults given equivalent doses.[71] It should be noted that opiate delivery via patient-controlled analgesia is well studied and effective in most developmentally normal patients 5 years of age or older.[72] Other modalities such as nurse-controlled analgesia and parent-controlled analgesia are also employed in some centers.[73]

Muscle Relaxants

Succinylcholine has been used as part of pediatric anesthesia and airway management for more than 60 years. When given in a dose of 1.5 to 2.0 mg/kg, it produces excellent intubating conditions (reliably) in 60 seconds. Recovery occurs in 6 to 7 minutes. Succinylcholine can also be given intramuscularly at 4 mg/kg in emergencies when intravenous access is not available. Its use is absolutely contraindicated in a variety of patients, particularly in those with muscular dystrophy, recent burn injury, spinal cord transection, and/or immobilization, as well as any child with a family history of malignant hyperthermia because of the risk of rhabdomyolysis, hyperkalemia, masseter spasm, and malignant hyperthermia. In addition, the drug is currently listed as relatively contraindicated for use in all children by the U.S. Food and Drug Administration (FDA). This is due to the infrequent but well-reported cases where succinylcholine has been inappropriately administered to children with risk factors (usually) that are not clinically appar-
8 ent or unappreciated. The requirement for succinylcholine has also been decreased by the availability of fast-acting nondepolarizing agents such as rocuronium. For these reasons, succinylcholine can only be recommended in situations where ultrarapid onset and short duration of action is of paramount importance (laryngospasm), or when relaxation is required or intravenous access is not available and intramuscular administration is required.

All nondepolarizing muscle relaxants used in adults are effective for pediatric patients. Because they have a larger percentage of total body water and larger extracellular fluid volume, neonates and young infants have a larger volume of distribution for these hydrophilic drugs than older children and adults. In contrast, these patients are slightly more sensitive to these drugs. The result is a pharmacokinetic and pharmacodynamic profile where the recommended doses of these agents are identical for children and adults, but the duration of action tends to be slightly longer (Table 44-3). In selecting a particular drug for a clinical scenario, one must consider the possible side effects of each medication, its route of metabolism, and the possible duration of action. For instance, pancuronium has a vagolytic effect that may be desirable in many neonates; however, it is renally excreted and therefore may have a markedly extended duration of action in this patient group where glomerular filtration rate is relatively decreased. Rocuronium has the fastest onset of action in this class (60 to 90 seconds for a 1 mg/kg dose) and is generally the choice for rapid-sequence intubation.

The need for reversal of muscle blockade should be carefully considered in each patient. The risks associated with inadequate ventilation in small children are great, especially in cases where the work of breathing may be increased, as is the case with intercurrent illness and chest/abdominal procedures. Muscle twitch should be monitored and reversal agents (i.e., neostigmine 0.05 mg/kg with 0.015 mg/kg of atropine or 0.01 mg/kg glycopyrrolate) administered if residual weakness is detected. Clinical signs of adequate strength for ventilation in this age group include the ability to flex the hips.

Antiemetics

Postoperative nausea and vomiting are among the most common causes of prolonged recovery stays and unanticipated hospitalization in children. Unfortunately, this is a complex clinical problem to manage, with many factors influencing its frequency. Postoperative nausea and vomiting (PONV) is particularly prominent after certain surgeries, such as orchidopexy, strabismus surgery, and tonsillectomy. In addition, certain age groups such as adolescent females are much more prone to postoperative nausea and vomiting than when compared with young infants. There is no one therapy that is universally

TABLE 44-4

MAINTENANCE FLUID REQUIREMENTS FOR PEDIATRIC PATIENTS

WEIGHT (kg)	HOURLY FLUID	24-hr FLUID
<10	4 mL/kg	100 mL/kg
11–20	40 mL + 2 mL/kg > 10 kg	1,000 mL + 50 mL/kg > 10 kg
>20	60 mL + 1 mL/kg > 20 kg	1,500 mL + 20 mL/kg > 20 kg

accepted as safe and effective. In fact, all antiemetic therapies for children are only shown to have efficacy in high-risk groups and surgeries; their use in lower-risk situations is suspect. The type of anesthetic employed for a particular surgery will also influence the incidence of PONV. For instance, when propofol is used in place of inhaled agents as the primary anesthetic, there is evidence that PONV is less common, particularly for high-risk surgeries such as tonsillectomy.[74] Opiate-based anesthetics are, conversely, more often associated with PONV.

All the antiemetics used in adults, including phenothiazines, antihistamines, anticholinergics, benzamides, butyrophenones, and 5-HT(3) antagonists, have been used in children and (to one extent or the other) have been shown to have some effectiveness. The 5-HT(3) antagonists are generally considered equivalent as a group; however, ondansetron has been most thoroughly studied in children, and at 0.05 to 0.15 mg/kg, has been found to be effective in tonsillectomy and strabismus models.[75] Its effectiveness as a "rescue" medication is not proven. Dexamethasone 0.15 to 1.0 mg/kg appears to be effective in limiting PONV after oral pharyngeal surgery (tonsillectomy), but there is much less data on its use in other types of procedures.[76]

Complete reviews of antiemetic use in children are available;[77,78] however, droperidol deserves special mention. Its use and effectiveness in children as an antiemetic is well documented.[79] However, in 2003, the FDA issued a report warning of prolonged QT syndrome and possible torsades de pointes with its use, suggesting prolonged monitoring (6 hours) for patients given this drug. A black box warning has been placed on this medication to this effect. The frequency of this problem in children is unknown but is believed to be extremely low; nevertheless, use of the drug has decreased significantly in light of this warning.

Unfortunately, the issue of antiemetic efficacy and cost effectiveness remains largely unanswered in spite of the hundreds of studies that exist concerning their use in children. The use of at least one of the drugs mentioned previously with known antiemetic action is indicated for surgeries associated with a high incidence of nausea and vomiting, especially in high-risk age groups. In addition, the practice of *requiring* patients to eat and/or drink prior to discharge will only increase PONV rates and does not appear to improve outcomes. Likewise, the use of pain control modalities in lieu of opioids (acetaminophen or nonsteroidal anti-inflammatory drugs [NSAIDs], and regional anesthesia) will likely decrease the overall risk of PONV.

FLUID AND BLOOD PRODUCT MANAGEMENT

9 Perioperative fluid and blood product management for pediatric patients must take into account fluid deficits, translocation of fluids and blood loss during surgery, and maintenance fluid requirements. A patient's fluid deficit prior to starting a case can be simply calculated by multiplying his or her calculated maintenance requirement by the number of hours since the last PO fluid intake. The calculation for maintenance fluids depends directly on metabolic demand; each calorie of energy expended requires 1 mL of H_2O for metabolism. Relating this energy requirement to patient weight results in an hourly fluid requirement that may be estimated as in Table 44-4.

Immediate intravascular volume expansion may be accomplished with a 10 cc/kg bolus of isotonic fluid. The balance of the calculated fluid deficit can be provided over 1 or 2 hours and is often provided in the form of isotonic fluid or a 5% dextrose solution in 0.9% normal saline. There is conflicting data concerning the need for glucose-containing solutions in this setting. In our current era with liberalized recommendations for intake of clear fluids (generally up to 2 hours prior to surgery), there is little evidence of hypoglycemia in children due to fasting prior to surgery. Indeed, most children who are given non–glucose-containing fluids during surgery actually experience a rise in blood glucose due to sympathetic activation. Hyperglycemia has been documented in children given 5% dextrose solutions to replace deficits or fluid losses intraoperatively. This is particularly problematic for patients with intracranial injury where hyperglycemia may result in worsening outcomes. In addition, hyperosmolar diuresis caused by significant hyperglycemia may also confuse diuretic and fluid therapy. In contrast, life-threatening *hypo*glycemia would be undetectable on clinical grounds under anesthesia.

To optimize fluid administration and glucose delivery, a balanced salt solution containing 2.5% glucose may be used (although not commercially available). Another approach would be to provide 5% dextrose in 0.45% normal saline (D_5 0.45 NS) for maintenance, piggybacked into a balanced salt solution for the deficit and third-space fluid. The exact composition of fluids used is less important than being aware of the issue of glucose control.[80] Intraoperative monitoring of blood glucose is appropriate for newborns, former premature infants, and any high-risk pediatric patients.

Surgical manipulation is associated with the isotonic transfer of fluids from the extracellular fluid compartment to the nonfunctional interstitial compartment. Estimated third-space loss during intra-abdominal surgery varies from 6 to 15 mL/kg per hour, whereas in intrathoracic surgery it is less (4 to 7 mL/kg per hour), and during intracranial or cutaneous surgery, it is negligible (1 to 2 mL/kg per hour). These third-space losses should be estimated and replaced on an hourly basis. These losses are derived from extracellular fluid; therefore, it is important to replace them with a balanced salt solution to avoid hyponatremia that would result from using hypotonic replacement. Lactated Ringer's solution is frequently used as normal saline contains an excessive chloride and acid load for infants.

Indications for blood or blood component therapy in pediatric patients are not always clear cut. Decisions must be based on considerations of the patient's blood volume, preoperative hematocrit, general medical condition, ability to provide oxygen to tissues, the nature of the surgical procedure, and the risks versus benefits of transfusion. All blood loss should be measured as accurately as possible and accounted for with some form of volume replacement to maintain intravascular volume and perfusion. If an isotonic solution is chosen to replace some element of blood loss it should be given in a ratio of 3 mL of solution for each milliliter of blood lost.

Many major procedures in children will be accompanied by significant blood loss and require transfusion of red blood cells and other blood products. In these cases, calculation of acceptable blood loss is vital to any replacement plan. The concept of the maximum allowable blood loss (MABL) takes into account the patient's total blood volume, starting hematocrit, and estimated "target" hematocrit—that which represents the lowest acceptable hematocrit for this patient considering age and comorbid conditions. In general, blood volume is estimated at 100 mL/kg for the preterm infant, 90 mL/kg for the term infant, 80 mg/kg for the child 3 to 12 months of age, and 70 mg/kg for the patient older than 1 year of age. These estimates of blood volume can be used in calculating the individual patient's blood volume by multiplying the child's weight by the estimated blood volume (EBV) per kilogram:

$$\text{MABL} = \frac{\text{EBV} \times (\text{starting hematocrit} - \text{target hematocrit})}{\text{starting hematocrit}}$$

As the MABL is approached, the patient's hematocrit should be checked to confirm estimated blood losses and volumes.

Packed red blood cells have a hematocrit between 55 and 70%. On average, 1 mL/kg of packed red blood cells increases the hematocrit by 1.5%. Units of blood can be subdivided into pediatric packs of 50 to 100 mL; thus, the remainder of a single unit is not wasted. Administration of other products such as cryoprecipitate or fresh frozen plasma should be based on laboratory evidence of coagulopathy and aimed at replacement of identifiable deficiencies of factors relating to hemostasis. Rapid administration of citrated blood products (particularly fresh frozen plasma) can result in hypocalcemia and hypothermia. Although under most circumstances, mobilization of calcium and hepatic metabolism of citrate are sufficiently rapid to prevent precipitous decreases in ionized calcium, infants have smaller stores of calcium.

As always, the end point of fluid and blood therapy is adequate blood pressure, tissue perfusion, and urine volume (0.5 to 1 mL/kg per hour). Careful attention to these goals through the examination of clinical (e.g., capillary refill time, urine output) and laboratory (e.g., blood gases) examination are more important than adherence to any one particular clinical protocol.

AIRWAY MANAGEMENT

10 Appropriate airway management remains the single most important aspect of delivering safe pediatric anesthesia. At any age, operative cases can be performed with facemask, LMA, or endotracheal tube placement. The choice of airway will depend on the age of the child, the time since last PO intake, coexisting illness, and the procedure to be performed. Each case must be considered on its own merits, but trends and guidelines have been established:

1. As a general rule, endotracheal tubes are preferred for premature infants and most neonates due to the slightly greater difficulty of providing effective facemask ventilation under appropriate levels of anesthesia and the risk of filling the stomach with air while providing mask ventilation.
2. Cases where recent oral intake or pathology (e.g., pyloric stenosis or intestinal obstruction) raise the probability that the stomach contains food or acid (and therefore risk aspiration injury) and are best managed with a rapid-sequence induction and intubation, regardless of age.
3. LMAs come in a range of full sizes and half sizes, and can be employed in infants, toddlers, and older children for almost any procedure that does not involve opening the abdomen or thoracic cavity. Although their use is standard for lower-extremity, inguinal, cutaneous, or eye procedures, comfort with this airway for oral procedures such as tonsillectomy/adenoidectomy varies from center to center. Use of the LMA in neonates and premature infants is less common, and depends on provider experience and preference. Aspiration and laryngospasm with the airway in place are not common but are possible, and plans to quickly manage these events must always be in place.[81] The LMA has become a critical part of the difficult airway algorithm for pediatric patients. This device can be used to ventilate patients where conventional mask ventilation is difficult, as well as to provide a conduit for fiberoptic–assisted intubation.
4. Because the narrowest portion of the pediatric airway is at the level of the cricoid cartilage (and is therefore round), uncuffed tubes can be used and will create a functional seal when appropriately sized.[82] Several formulas have been used for tube selection in children older than 1 year of age, the most common being (16 + age)/4 or variations thereof. One may also estimate the size by comparing the size of the fifth digit or of a nostril. Once the tube is in place, it should be checked to determine at what pressure air can escape around the tube. Air should leak out at no higher than 20 to 25 cm H_2O to minimize risk of postextubation croup. Cuffed tubes can also be safely used in children by selecting a tube 0.5 mm smaller in internal diameter than the uncuffed choice.[82] Care should be taken to check the pressure in the cuff to assure it does not exceed 20 cm H_2O.
5. Intubation in children can be safely accomplished after inhaled induction with or without the use of muscle relaxant. Intubating conditions after 3 minutes of 8% sevoflurane or a dose of propofol and opiate[43,83] may produce acceptable views of the larynx. In fact, a recent survey of pediatric anesthesiologists revealed the majority do not use muscle relaxants for elective surgery.[84] The use of muscle relaxants should be based on the specific issues related to the child and the procedure to be performed.

PEDIATRIC BREATHING CIRCUITS

Much has been written about the advantages and disadvantages of various anesthesia circuits for use in pediatric patients (see Chapter 21). Pediatric circuit design has been directed to the physiology of the neonate and ways of reducing the work of breathing while preventing rebreathing. Nonrebreathing circuits minimize the work of breathing because they have no valves to be opened by the patient's respiratory effort. In addition, because the total volume of the circuit is less, the partial pressure of inhaled agent increases faster. Compression and compliance volumes are also decreased compared with a standard breathing circuit.

A number of combinations of the simple T-piece tubing, reservoir bag, and sites of fresh gas entry and overflow are possible. Mapleson classified the various combinations into five types. The Jackson Rees modification is functionally identical to the Mapleson D, as are coaxial systems. Carbon dioxide is removed most effectively in the D configuration when controlled ventilation is used, whereas spontaneous ventilation is most effective in the A system.

Circle breathing systems can also be used effectively in infants and children. Newer anesthesia machines use valves with much less resistance than older models. In addition, most neonates and small infants (for whom resistance would be the biggest problem) are ventilated mechanically during surgery, making work of breathing a nonissue. Dead space in these systems is no more than that of the Mapleson circuits.

MONITORING

Monitoring decisions for pediatric patients are similar in many respects to those in adults. The pediatric patient should be monitored continuously with precordial or esophageal stethoscope. This simple device allows the anesthesiologist to detect changes in the rate, quality, and intensity of the heart sounds. Pulse oximetry, capnography, blood pressure (measured, *appropriately* sized cuffs), temperature, and ECG should also be monitored routinely in children as in adults. More invasive or sophisticated monitoring should be used in appropriate circumstances. One should note that patient pathophysiology may contribute to an increased gradient between end-tidal and arterial CO_2 measurements, usually by increasing shunt (V/Q mismatch) and increasing dead space (V_D/V_T). That is, in children with cyanotic congenital heart disease, $ETCO_2$ underestimates $AaCO_2$ as venous blood passes directly into the arterial circulation *without* going through the lungs.[57] Low tidal volumes, rapid respiratory rates, and changing intrapulmonary shunts make $ETCO_2$ accuracy also inaccurate for infants and premature neonates with respiratory distress syndrome. It is important to note that transesophageal echocardiography has become an important tool for intraoperative assessment of cardiac function, flow defects, cardiac morphology, and adequacy of repair during and after surgical procedures for congenital heart disease. Although placement of the probe in the anesthetized infant is usually the responsibility of the anesthesiologist, interpretation of the echocardiogram occurs in collaboration between surgeons, cardiologists and anesthesiologists. Finally, the use of pulmonary artery catheters (Swan-Ganz) is quite limited in the pediatric population because of size issues and because of the fact that left-sided and right-sided pressures are similar.

PAIN MANAGEMENT AND REGIONAL ANESTHESIA

It is important for the health care provider to note that children experience pain, just like adults, regardless of their age. More recent studies indicate that neonates have considerable maturation of pain transmission by 26 weeks' gestation and respond to injury with specific behavior and with autonomic, hormonal, and metabolic signs of stress and distress.[85] In fact, more recent data indicate that extreme pain experienced during the neonatal period may have lifelong lasting adverse effects.[85,86] Pain in children can be assessed by self-reporting, observational, and physiological assessment tools.[85,87] Although self-reporting pain is considered the gold standard, this assessment methodology cannot be used in infants, younger children, and children who suffer from developmental delay.[86] In these children, the clinicians often need to rely on parental report.[87] Children older than 4 to 6 years of age can usually self-report pain using a face scale. Younger children are usually assessed using a behavioral or physiologic-behavioral scale.[87]

The most common oral analgesic used in children continues to be acetaminophen (Table 44-5). This medication has been shown to be safe and efficacious in neonates and older children. Doses of 10 to 15 mg/kg orally every 4 hours.[88] The plasma concentrations effective for fever control and analgesia are 10 to 20 μg/mL.[89] Rectal administration is associated with delayed and erratic absorption; single doses of 35 to 45 mg/kg generally produce therapeutic plasma concentrations.[85] Subsequent rectal doses, however, should not exceed 20 mg/kg, and the interval between doses should be extended to at least 6 to 8 hours. The rectal route of administration can be particularly effective for children with no intravenous access, such as pressure-equalizing ear tube placement.

TABLE 44-5

MANAGEMENT OF POSTOPERATIVE PAIN

	DOSE			MAXIMAL DAILY DOSE	
DRUG	PATIENTS <60 kg (mg/kg)	PATIENTS ≥60 kg (mg)	INTERVAL (hr)	PATIENTS <60 kg (mg/kg)	PATIENTS ≥60 kg (mg)
Acetaminophen	10–15	650–1,000	4	100[a]	4,000
Ibuprofen	6–10	400–600[b]	6	40[b,c]	2,400[b]
Naproxen	5–6[b]	250–375[b]	12	24[b,c]	1,000[b]
Aspirin[d]	10–15[b,d]	650–1,000[b]	4	80[b–d]	3,600[b]

[a]The maximal daily doses of acetaminophen for infants and neonates are a subject of current controversy. Provisional recommendations are that daily dosing should not exceed 75 mg/kg per day for infants, 60 mg/kg per day for term neonates and preterm neonates of more than 32 weeks of postconceptional age, and 40 mg/kg per day for preterm neonates 28 to 32 weeks of postconceptional age. Fever, dehydration, hepatic disease, and lack of oral intake may all increase the risk of hepatotoxicity.
[b]Higher doses may be used in selected cases for treatment of rheumatologic conditions in children.
[c]Dosage guidelines for neonates and infants have not been established.
[d]Aspirin carries a risk of provoking Reye's syndrome in infants and children. If other analgesics are available, aspirin should be restricted to indications for which an antiplatelet or antiinflammatory effect is required, rather than being used as a routine analgesic or antipyretic in neonates, infants, or children. Dosage guidelines for aspirin in neonates have not been established.
From Berde CB, Sethna NF: Analgesics for the treatment of pain in children. N Engl J Med 347:1094, 2002.

Ketorolac has been shown to be an effective and safe analgesic for pediatric patients.[85,90] It may be administered intramuscularly (0.75 mg/kg) or intravenously with a loading dose of 1 mg/kg followed by a maintenance dose of 0.5 mg/kg every 6 hours. Ketorolac has the disadvantage of prolonging bleeding time because of its effect on platelet aggregation. As with other NSAIDs, ketorolac should be avoided in patients with preexisting nephropathy or bleeding diathesis. Ibuprofen is the most popular NSAID given orally to children. It comes in several palatable preparations. When given in the recommended oral dose of 10 mg/kg, it has similar analgesic effects as acetaminophen or ketorolac. Gastrointestinal side effects are uncommon.

The safety and efficacy of patient-controlled analgesia for children as young as 6 years has been shown.[91] Although routinely used in Children's Hospitals, this technique is to be used *only* by highly trained medical personnel who are knowledgeable in pediatric pain management. For infants and children younger than 6 years of age, nurse-controlled analgesia is now widely used as a pain management modality. Finally, it should be noted that although parent-controlled analgesia is now accepted in palliative care, its use for postoperative pain is controversial because of the potential for overdosing.

Regional Anesthesia

Chapters 25 and 26 discuss regional anesthesia and analgesia in detail. Most regional anesthetic techniques can be useful for children undergoing anesthesia and surgery.[92] Because of obvious developmental and cognitive issues, regional techniques are rarely used as a sole anesthetic and most often used as adjuncts to general anesthesia and to provide postoperative analgesia.[92] Regional anesthetic techniques may also be used as the sole anesthetic in premature infants at risk for postoperative apnea undergoing abdominal or lower-extremity procedures (spinal/epidural). Simple techniques such as ilioinguinal-iliohypogastric nerve block, ring block of the penis, or caudal block can be useful for common pediatric surgical procedures.[92] Direct local infiltration of surgical wounds can also be helpful. The types of blocks that can be used safely in children are limited only by the skill of the anesthesiologist.

Because of the unique anatomic and physiologic considerations, strict attention must be paid to the dose of local anesthetic, dose of epinephrine, and technique of administration. More sophisticated techniques such as continuous caudal or epidural analgesia using combinations of opioids and local anesthetics are useful for inpatients after thoracic, abdominal, or lower-extremity procedures. These regional techniques are usually used in combination with general anesthesia (catheters are placed after the child is induced), and the regional block is maintained for postoperative pain control. Close postoperative monitoring of the child must take place when these continuous infusions are used.[93]

The most commonly used form of regional anesthesia in
11 children is the *caudal block*. This technique can provide postoperative analgesia following a wide variety of lower abdominal and genitourinary surgical procedures. Usually, bupivacaine 0.175% solution in a dose of 1 mg/kg is used, and if larger volumes are needed, the use of 0.125% is recommended. Postoperative analgesia typically lasts 4 to 6 hours and is not associated with a motor paralysis. This route can be used for either a single-dose injection or for catheter advancement for continuous infusion.[94]

Spinal anesthesia may be used for procedures involving surgical dermatomes below T_6. It is important to note that the dural sac migrates cephalad during the first year of life and in a neonate it is at S_3, whereas over the age of 1 year it is at the S_1 level.[92] The sitting position may be especially helpful in neonates to maintain midline needle position and free flow of spinal fluid. It may be easier for the novice assistant to hold the infant more securely in the lateral decubitus position. As mentioned previously, spinal anesthetic is a particularly good option for premature infants who undergo surgery because the incidence of postoperative apnea has been shown to be reduced in these infants with the use of this technique.[94]

Epidural anesthesia can be used to provide postoperative analgesia for thoracic, lumbar, and sacral dermatomes. In young children, the epidural space can be reached easily by the caudal approach with less risk of dural puncture than with thoracic or lumbar approaches. This approach is ideal for analgesia/anesthesia of lumbar and sacral nerve roots. Higher dermatomes can be reached by either using a lumbar approach or increasing drug volume, or threading a catheter several centimeters into the epidural space.[92]

POSTANESTHESIA CARE

12 Recovery of the young child in the PACU can be hindered by a variety of challenges. Hypothermia is a common perioperative problem, particularly in infants and young children. The inability to regulate body temperature under general anesthesia, cold large operating rooms, and continued heat loss are major reasons for hypothermia. Although minor hypothermia (34 to 36°) has not been found to influence the recovery period,[95] it is best to restore normothermia prior to discharge from the PACU. More significant hypothermia can result in increased oxygen consumption, cardiovascular manifestations of hypothermia,[96] prolonged metabolism and excretion of anesthetic drugs, and delayed wound healing.

Nausea and vomiting occur frequently after eye or ear surgery but can occur after any surgical procedure or anesthetic. More recent studies quote an overall incidence of 20 to 30%,[6] whereas others have found that the problem is even more widespread (39 to 73%).[97] The physiologic mechanisms for postoperative nausea include central causes (opiates), gastrointestinal malfunction (ileus or gastric distention), the surgical procedure itself (eye and ear, most commonly), and postoperative pain.[98] Control of nausea and vomiting no longer remains purely within the domain of the PACU, but begins in the selection of agents/techniques used for anesthesia.[99] For example, induction and maintenance of anesthesia with propofol-air-oxygen is associated with only a 23% incidence of nausea and vomiting, as compared with a 50% incidence using halothane-N_2O-droperidol for strabismus surgery.[100] Pretreatment with ondansetron 0.15 mg/kg, droperidol 0.075 mg/kg, or metoclopramide 0.15 mg/kg has been successful in reducing nausea and vomiting for patients at higher risk, such as those undergoing tonsillectomy or strabismus repair. Ondansetron, a selective serotonin antagonist, is particularly effective in reducing postoperative nausea and vomiting when used prophylactically. Although more expensive than other antiemetics, its significant efficacy makes it cost effective when used for procedures with a high incidence of nausea and vomiting.

Special attention should be paid to the treatment of pain in the PACU. Although pain self-report is considered the best assessment modality in older children, physiologic responses such as tachycardia, hypertension, nausea, vomiting, and agitation may be important indicators of analgesic needs in the preverbal child. Intravenous opiates such as fentanyl or morphine are used most commonly to treat moderate to severe pain in the PACU. Carefully titrated intravenous narcotics present few untoward effects.

Finally, many children are terrified in the recovery room. They awaken in a strange place with unfamiliar people and may be disoriented from residual effects of the anesthesia. Some children may experience nightmares, develop enuresis, or have behavioral problems after a surgical procedure.[101] Measures taken to calm and comfort the child may reduce the incidence of these sequelae and aid in the overall recovery. Many institutions have found that allowing parents to soothe the child during recovery is beneficial.

References

1. Lin Y, Bioteau A, Ferrari L *et al*: The use of herbs and complementary and alternative medicine in pediatric preoperative patients. J Clin Anesth 16:4, 2004
2. Kain Z, Wang SM, Caramico LA *et al*: Parental desire for perioperative information and informed consent: A two-phase study. Anesth Analg 84:299, 1997
3. Kain Z, Mayes L: Anxiety in children during the perioperative period. In Borestein M, Genevro J (ed): Child Development and Behavioral Pediatrics, p 85. Mahwah, NJ, Erlbaum, 1996
4. Kain ZN, Mayes LC, O'Connor TZ, Cicchetti DV: Preoperative anxiety in children. Predictors and outcomes. Arch Pediatr Adolesc Med 150:1238, 1996
5. Kain Z, Caramico L, Mayes L *et al*: Preoperative preparation programs in children: A comparative study. Anesth Analg 87:1249, 1998
6. Kain ZN, Caldwell-Andrews A, Wang SM: Psychological preparation of the parent and pediatric surgical patient. Anesthesiol Clin North Am 20:29, 2002
7. Kain Z: Parental presence and premedication revisited. Curr Opinion Anesth 14:331, 2001
8. Kain ZN, Mayes LC, Caramico LA *et al*: Parental presence during induction of anesthesia. A randomized controlled trial. Anesthesiology 84:1060, 1996
9. Kain Z, Mayes L, Wang S *et al*: Parental presence during induction of anesthesia vs. sedative premedication: Which intervention is more effective? Anesthesiology 89:1147, 1998
10. Kain Z, Mayes L, Wang S *et al*: Parental presence and a sedative premedicant for children undergoing surgery: A hierarchical study. Anesthesiology 92:939, 2000
11. Kain ZN, Wang SM, Mayes LC *et al*: Sensory stimuli and anxiety in children undergoing surgery: A randomized, controlled trial. Anesth Analg 92:897, 2001
12. Wang SM, Kain ZN: Auricular acupuncture: A potential treatment for anxiety. Anesth Analg 92:548, 2001
13. Kain Z: Postoperative maladaptive behavioral changes in children: Incidence, risk factors and interventions. Acta Anaesth Scand 51:217, 2000
14. Tait AR, Malviya S, Voepel-Lewis T *et al*: Risk factors for perioperative adverse respiratory events in children with upper respiratory tract infections. Anesthesiology 95:299, 2001
15. Cohen M, Cameron C: Should you cancel the operation when a child has an upper respiratory tract infection? Anesth Analg 72:282, 1991
16. Collier A, Pimmel R, V.H *et al*: Spirometric changes in normal children with upper respiratory infections. Am Rev Respir Dis 117:47, 1978
17. Helfar M, Wilson D: Obstructive sleep apnea, control of ventilation, and anesthesia in children. Pediatr Clin North Am 41:131, 1994
18. Szefler S: Current concepts in asthma treatment in children. Curr Opin Pediatr 16:299, 2004
19. Warner D, Warner M, Barnes R *et al*: Perioperative respiratory complications in patients with asthma. Anesthesiology 85:460, 1996
20. Scalfaro P, Sly P, Sims C, Habre W: Salbutamol prevents the increase of respiratory resistance caused by tracheal intubation during sevoflurane anesthesia in asthmatic children. Anesth Analg 93:898, 2001
21. Kurth C, Spitzer A, Broennle A *et al*: Postoperative apnea in preterm infants. Anesthesiology 66:483, 1987
22. Welborn L, Ramirez N, Oh T *et al*: Postanesthetic apnea and periodic breathing in infants. Anesthesiology 65:658, 1986
23. Cote C, Zaslavsky A, Downes J *et al*: Postoperative apnea in former preterm infants after inguinal herniorrhaphy. A combined analysis. Anesthesiology 82:809, 1995
24. Maxwell L, Yaster M: Perioperative management issues in pediatric patients. Anesthesiol Clin North Am 18:601, 2000
25. Gabriel P, Mazoit X, Ecoffey C: Relationship between clinical history, coagulation tests, and perioperative bleeding during tonsillectomies in pediatrics. J Clin Anesth 12:288, 2000
26. Warner M, Warner M, Warner D *et al*: Perioperative pulmonary aspiration in infants and children. Anesthesiology 90:66, 1999
27. Practice guidelines for preoperative fasting and the use of pharmacologic agents to reduce the risk of pulmonary aspiration: Application to healthy patients undergoing elective procedures: A report by the American Society of Anesthesiologist Task Force on Preoperative Fasting. Anesthesiology 90:896, 1999
28. McCann ME, Kain ZN: The management of preoperative anxiety in children: An update. Anesth Analg 93:98, 2001
29. Kain ZN, Caldwell-Andrews AA, Krivutza DM *et al*: Trends in the practice of parental presence during induction of anesthesia and the use of preoperative sedative premedication in the United States, 1995–2002: Results of a follow-up national survey. Anesth Analg 98:1252, 2004
30. Kain ZN, Mayes LC, Wang SM *et al*: Parental presence during induction of anesthesia versus sedative premedication: Which intervention is more effective? Anesthesiology 89:1147, 1998
31. Shannon M, Albers G, Burkhart K *et al*: Safety and efficacy of flumazenil in the reversal of benzodiazepine-induced conscious sedation. J Pediatr 131:582, 1997
32. Funk W, Jakob W, Reidl T, Taeger K: Oral preanaesthetic medication for children: Double-blind randomized study of a combination of midazolam and ketamine vs midazolam or ketamine alone. Br J Anaesth 84:335, 2000
33. Nishina K, Mikawa K, Shiga M, Obara H: Clonidine in paediatric anaesthesia. Paediatr Anaesth 9:187, 1999
34. Keenan RL, Shapiro JH, Dawson K: Frequency of anesthetic cardiac arrests in infants: Effect of pediatric anesthesiologists. J Clin Anesth 3:433, 1991
35. Lerman J: Pharmacology of inhalational anaesthetics in infants and children. Paediatr Anaesth 2:191, 1992
36. Katoh T, Ikeda K: Minimum alveolar concentration of sevoflurane in children. Br J Anaesth 68:139, 1992
37. Black A, Sury MR, Hemington L *et al*: A comparison of the induction characteristics of sevoflurane and halothane in children. Anaesthesia 51:539, 1996
38. Goa KL, Noble S, Spencer CM: Sevoflurane in paediatric anaesthesia: A review. Paediatr Drugs 1:127, 1999
39. Lerman J: Inhalational anesthetics. Paediatr Anaesth 14:380, 2004
40. Holzman RS, van der Velde ME, Kaus SJ *et al*: Sevoflurane depresses myocardial contractility less than halothane during induction of anesthesia in children. Anesthesiology 85:1260, 1996
41. Wodey E, Pladys P, Copin C *et al*: Comparative hemodynamic depression of sevoflurane versus halothane in infants: An echocardiographic study. Anesthesiology 87:795, 1997
42. Wappler F, Frings DP, Scholz J *et al*: Inhalational induction of anaesthesia with 8% sevoflurane in children: Conditions for endotracheal intubation and side-effects. Eur J Anaesthesiol 20:548, 2003
43. Simon L, Boucebci KJ, Orliaguet G *et al*: A survey of practice of tracheal intubation without muscle relaxant in paediatric patients. Paediatr Anaesth 12:36, 2002
44. Politis GD, Frankland MJ, James RL *et al*: Factors associated with successful tracheal intubation of children with sevoflurane and no muscle relaxant. Anesth Analg 95:615, 2002
45. Erb T, Christen P, Kern C, Frei FJ: Similar haemodynamic, respiratory and metabolic changes with the use of sevoflurane or halothane in children breathing spontaneously via a laryngeal mask airway. Acta Anaesthesiol Scand 45:639, 2001
46. Levine MF, Sarner J, Lerman J, Davis P *et al*: Plasma inorganic fluoride concentrations after sevoflurane anesthesia in children. Anesthesiology 84:348, 1996
47. Cohen IT, Finkel JC, Hannallah RS *et al*: The effect of fentanyl on the emergence characteristics after desflurane or sevoflurane anesthesia in children. Anesth Analg 94:1178, 1998
48. Cohen IT, Finkel JC, Hannallah RS *et al*: Rapid emergence does not explain agitation following sevoflurane anaesthesia in infants and children: A comparison with propofol. Paediatr Anaesth 13:63, 2003
49. Cravero J, Surgenor S, Whalen K: Emergence agitation in paediatric patients after sevoflurane anaesthesia and no surgery: A comparison with halothane. Paediatr Anaesth 10:419, 2000
50. Cravero JP, Beach M, Thyr B, Whalen K: The effect of small dose fentanyl on the emergence characteristics of pediatric patients after sevoflurane anesthesia without surgery. Anesth Analg 97:364, 2003
51. Davis PJ, Greenberg JA, Gendelman M, Fertal K: Recovery characteristics of sevoflurane and halothane in preschool-aged children undergoing bilateral myringotomy and pressure equalization tube insertion. Anesth Analg 88:34, 1999
52. Galinkin JL, Fazi LM, Cuy RM *et al*: Use of intranasal fentanyl in children undergoing myringotomy and tube placement during halothane and sevoflurane anesthesia. Anesthesiology 93:1378, 2000
53. Ibacache ME, Munoz HR, Brandes V, Morales AL: Single-dose dexmedetomidine reduces agitation after sevoflurane anesthesia in children. Anesth Analg 98:60, 2004
54. Ko YP, Huang CJ, Hung YC *et al*: Premedication with low-dose oral midazolam reduces the incidence and severity of emergence agitation in pediatric patients following sevoflurane anesthesia. Acta Anaesthesiol Scand 39:169, 2001
55. Rolf N, Cote CJ: Persistent cardiac arrhythmias in pediatric patients: Effects of age, expired carbon dioxide values depth of anesthesia, and airway management. Anesth Analg 73:720, 1991
56. Friesen RH, Henry DB: Cardiovascular changes in preterm neonates receiving isoflurane, halothane, fentanyl, and ketamine. Anesthesiology 64:238, 1986
57. Lovell A: Anaesthetic implications of grown-up congenital heart disease. Br J Anesth 93:129, 2004
58. Welborn LG HR, McGill WA *et al*: Induction and recovery characteristics of desflurane and halothane anaesthesia in paediatric outpatients. Paediatr Anaesth 4:359, 1994

59. Eichenfield LF, Funk A, Fallon-Friedlander S, Cunnigham BB: A clinical study to evaluate the efficacy of ELA-Max (4% liposomal lidocaine) as compared with eutectic mixture of local anesthetics cream for pain reduction of venipuncture in children. Pediatrics 109:1093, 2002
60. Kleiber C, Sorenson M, Whiteside K *et al*: Topical anesthetics for intravenous insertion in children: A randomized equivalency study. Pediatrics 110:758, 2002
61. Wolf A, Weir P, Segar P *et al*: Impaired fatty acid oxidation in propofol infusion syndrome. Lancet 357:606, 2001
62. Vasile B, Rasulo F, Candiani A, Latronico N: The pathophysiology of propofol infusion syndrome: A simple name for a complex syndrome. Intens Care Med 29:1417, 2003
63. McFarlan CS, Anderson BJ, Short TG: The use of propofol infusions in paediatric anaesthesia: A practical guide. Paediatr Anaesth 9:209, 1999
64. Cox RG: Are children just little adults when it comes to propofol injection pain? Can J Anaesth 49:1016, 2002
65. Guard BC, Sikich N, Lerman J, Levine M: Maintenance and recovery characteristics after sevoflurane or propofol during ambulatory surgery in children with epidural blockade. Can J Anaesth 45:1072, 1998
66. Picard V, Dumont L, Pellegrini M: Quality of recovery in children: Sevoflurane versus propofol. Acta Anaesthesiol Scand 44:307, 2000
67. Bergman SA: Ketamine: Review of its pharmacology and its use in pediatric anesthesia. Anesth Prog 46:10, 1999
68. Kennedy RM, Porter FL, Miller JP, Jaffe DM: Comparison of fentanyl/midazolam with ketamine/midazolam for pediatric orthopedic emergencies. Pediatrics 102:956, 1998
69. Roulleau P, Gall O, Desjeux L *et al*: Remifentanil infusion for cleft palate surgery in young infants. Paediatr Anaesth 13:701, 2003
70. Ganidagli S, Cengiz M, Baysal Z: Remifentanil vs alfentanil in the total intravenous anaesthesia for paediatric abdominal surgery. Paediatr Anaesth 13:695, 2003
71. Bhatt-Mehta V, Rosen DA: Management of acute pain in children. Clin Pharm 10:667, 1991
72. Lehr VT, BeVier P: Patient-controlled analgesia for the pediatric patient. Orthop Nurs 22:305, 2003
73. Monitto CL, Greenberg RS, Kost-Byerly S *et al*: The safety and efficacy of parent-/nurse-controlled analgesia in patients less than six years of age. Anesth Analg 91:573, 2000
74. Ved SA, Walden TL, Montana J *et al*: Vomiting and recovery after outpatient tonsillectomy and adenoidectomy in children. Comparison of four anesthetic techniques using nitrous oxide with halothane or propofol. Anesthesiology 85:4, 1996
75. Culy CR, Bhana N, Plosker GL: Ondansetron: A review of its use as an antiemetic in children. Paediatr Drugs 3:441, 2001
76. Steward DL, Welge JA, Myer CM: Steroids for improving recovery following tonsillectomy in children. Cochrane Database Syst Rev 1:CD003997, 2003
77. Rose JB, Watcha MF: Postoperative nausea and vomiting in paediatric patients. Br J Anaesth 83:104, 1999
78. Baines D: Postoperative nausea and vomiting in children. Paediatr Anaesth 6:7, 1996
79. Henzi I, Sonderegger J, Tramer MR: Efficacy, dose-response, and adverse effects of droperidol for prevention of postoperative nausea and vomiting. Can J Anaesth 47:537, 2000
80. Berleur M, Dahan A, Murat I, Hazebroucq G: Perioperative infusions in paediatric patients: Rationale for using Ringer-lactate solution with low dextrose concentration. J Clin Pharm Ther 28:31, 2003
81. Tait AR, Pandit UA, Voepel-Lewis T *et al*: Use of the laryngeal mask airway in children with upper respiratory tract infections: A comparison with endotracheal intubation. Anesth Analg 86:706, 1998
82. Khine HH, Corddry DH, Kettrick RG *et al*: Comparison of cuffed and uncuffed endotracheal tubes in young children during general anesthesia. Anesthesiology 86:627, 1997
83. Blair JM, Hill DA, Bali IM, Fee JP: Tracheal intubating conditions after induction with sevoflurane 8% in children. A comparison with two intravenous techniques. Anaesthesia 55:774, 2000
84. Politis GD, Tobin JR, Morell RC *et al*: Tracheal intubation of healthy pediatric patients without muscle relaxant: A survey of technique utilization and perceptions of safety. Anesth Analg 88:737, 1999
85. Berde C, Sethna N: Analgesics for the treatment of pain in children. N Engl J Med 347:1094, 2002
86. Howard R: Current status of pain management in children. JAMA 290:2464, 2003
87. Franck L, Greenberg C, Stevens B: Pain assessment in infants and children. Pediatr Clin North Am 47:487, 2000
88. Anderson B, Holford N, Woollard G *et al*: Perioperative pharmacodynamics of acetaminophen analgesia in children. Anesthesiology 90:411, 1999
89. Schachtel B, Thoden W: A placebo-controlled model for assaying systemic analgesics in children. Clin Pharmacol Ther 53:593, 1993
90. Rusy L, Houck C, Sullivan L *et al*: A double-blind evaluation of ketorolac tromethamine versus acetaminophen in pediatric tonsillectomy: Analgesia and bleeding. Anesth Analg 80:226, 1995
91. Berde C, Lehn B, Yee J *et al*: Patient-controlled analgesia in children and adolescents: A randomized, prospective comparison with intramuscular administration of morphine for postoperative analgesia. J Pediatr 118:460, 1991
92. Suresh S, Wheeler M: Practical pediatric regional anesthesia. Anesthesiol Clin North Am 20:83, 2002
93. Giaufre E, Dalens B, Gombert A: Epidemiology and morbidity of regional anesthesia in children: A 1-year prospective survey of the French-Language Society of Pediatric Anesthesiologists. Anesth Analg 83:904, 1996
94. Gunter J, Watcha M, Forestner J *et al*: Caudal epidural anesthesia in conscious premature and high-risk infants. J Pediatr Surg 26:9, 1991
95. Bissonnette B, Sessler D: Mild hypothermia does not impair postanesthetic recovery in infants and children. Anesth Analg 76:168, 1993
96. Frank S, Higgins M, Breslow M *et al*: The catecholamine, cortisol, and hemodynamic responses to mild perioperative hypothermia. A randomized clinical trial. Anesthesiology 82:83, 1995
97. Cohen M, Duncan P, DeBoer D *et al*: The postoperative interview: Assessing risk factors for nausea and vomiting. Anesth Analg 78:7, 1994
98. Eberhart L, Morin A, Guber D *et al*: Applicability of risk scores for postoperative nausea and vomiting in adults to paediatric patients. Br J Anaesth 93:386, 2004
99. Olutoye O, Watcha M: Management of postoperative vomiting in pediatric patients. Int Anesthesiol Clin 41:99, 2003
100. Watcha M, Bras P, Cieslak G, Pennant J: The dose-response relationship of ondansetron in preventing postoperative emesis in pediatric patients undergoing ambulatory surgery. Anesthesiology 82:47, 1995
101. Kain ZN, Mayes LC, O'Connor TZ, Cicchetti DV: Preoperative anxiety in children. Predictors and outcomes. Arch Pediatr Adolesc Med 150:1238, 1996

CHAPTER 45 ■ ANESTHESIA FOR THE GERIATRIC PATIENT

STANLEY MURAVCHICK

KEY POINTS

1. Aging is a physiologic process associated with decreased functional reserve and an increase in the variability of clinical signs and symptoms.
2. At a cellular level, normal aging may be largely due to declining mitochondrial bioenergetics and the deleterious effects of oxidative stress.
3. Physiologic reserve provides a margin of safety that allows elderly surgical patients to meet the increased demands imposed by illness, surgical trauma, infection, and wound healing.
4. Decreased tissue elasticity, reduced lean tissue mass, neuronal attrition, and a loss of autonomic homeostasis explain much of the measurable physical decline associated with normal aging.
5. Aging is associated with a decline in anesthetic requirements and an increase in the duration of clinical effect for drugs that require organ-based elimination.
6. Adverse drug effects and other forms of perioperative morbidity are more common in older surgical patients than in younger adults.
7. In older adults, a higher likelihood of perioperative mortality and major adverse outcome are largely the result of age-related disease and site of surgery rather than of chronological age itself.

Advances in nutrition, public health, education, and social services have produced major changes in human longevity in industrialized societies, and elderly patients now account for more than one-half of all hospital care days in the United States. In addition, almost one-third of all surgical patients are 65 years of age or older, and an even larger fraction is anticipated in the next two decades. Therefore, unless intentionally limited to pediatrics or obstetric patients, every anesthesiologist in contemporary practice must acquire expertise in geriatric medicine. The following sections define the current concepts of aging that are relevant to anesthetic practice. They discuss the distinction between aging and age-related disease, present strategies useful for perioperative assessment of the elderly patient, and summarize practical aspects of anesthetic management and the perioperative care of geriatric surgical patients.

CONCEPTS OF AGING AND GERIATRICS

As they age, adults exhibit an increasingly varied array of physical responses to concurrent disease states. These, in turn, reflect life-long exposure to environmental and socioeconomic conditions, and to the accumulated stigmata of prior traumatic
1 injuries and medical therapies. Prolonged longevity also enables complete expression of intrinsic genetic qualities as subtle physiologic manifestations. Therefore, extreme variability of signs, symptoms, and physical presentation among older patients is an essential characteristic of geriatric medicine. Currently, however, there is no consensus as to when the "geriatric" era begins in human subjects or whether any single physiologic marker can identify an "elderly" patient. Therefore, establishing a rigid and finite chronological definition of the term "geriatric" has little medical value other than for administrative, actuarial, or epidemiologic applications. For clarity and consistency, however, the terms "elderly" and "geriatric" are used synonymously in this chapter to describe human subjects who are 65 years of age or older. The term "aged" will be used to describe individuals older than 80 years.

"Life span" is a species-specific biological parameter that quantifies maximum attainable individual age under optimal conditions. Human life span has remained nearly constant at about 120 years for the past 20 centuries, but this is only a brief epoch on the evolutionary scale and human life span may actually be increasing slightly.[1] In contrast, the term "life expectancy" describes typical longevity under prevailing conditions, and this has changed dramatically during short periods in history. More recent advances in medical science and health care have increased the relative "agedness" of voting populations in democratic societies to the point that the economics of health care for the elderly have, for the first time, assumed roles of major social and political importance.

Most studies of human aging are cross-sectional studies that measure physiologic parameters simultaneously in young and elderly subjects. Although straightforward in design and execution, even a comprehensive cross-sectional approach may not identify patients with subtle manifestations of disease. In addition, cross-sectional experimental design cannot be controlled for cohort-specific factors such as nutritional and environmental history, and the "young" and "old" patient groups being compared often differ not only in age, but also in their overall ethnic, anatomic, and biochemical characteristics for genetic background, or for prior exposure to infectious agents. Many changes now known to be due to age-related disease have, in the past, been attributed erroneously to aging. Therefore, data from cross-sectional studies rarely permit unambiguous conclusions regarding the effect of age itself on a measured parameter.

Longitudinal studies of aging, in contrast, require the investigator to obtain repeated measurements in each individual subject over several decades. Each subject therefore generates his or her own "young adult" control value for comparison with subsequent measurements. If any of the subjects in a longitudinal study eventually manifest signs of age-related disease, their data points can be excluded from the study, thereby leaving behind a smaller but more homogeneous group of healthy elderly subjects. Although difficult and expensive to organize and maintain, long-term longitudinal studies have produced substantial amounts of extremely valuable data related to human aging.

The mechanisms that control the aging process remain unknown. The impressive consistency of observed life span does not necessarily imply that there is a "biological clock" for each
2 species. Instead, age-related decline in organ and tissue function may simply be the inevitable accumulation of nonspecific degenerative phenomena. Declining mitochondrial bioenergetics may be the underlying mechanism for age-related deterioration of cellular and organ function.[2] Throughout adulthood, increasing levels of oxygen-derived free radicals or "reactive oxygen species" create oxidative stress within the mitochondria, and disrupt the structural and enzymatic machinery of oxidative phosphorylation. As the ability to scavenge these byproducts of aerobic metabolism declines, it creates a "vicious cycle of aging" within the mitochondria (Fig. 45-1).

Viewed from this perspective, the unique life span demonstrated by each species could be explained as the net result of interaction between the genetically determined biochemical and physiologic attributes of each species, as well as the randomly destructive environmental factors that produce disorder in biological systems. Two recent observations support this concept. First, the cellular resistance to oxidative stress has been shown to be intrinsically involved in both aging and longevity,[3] and second, mitochondrial DNA mutation has produced phenotypic aging in laboratory animals.[4]

AGING AND ORGAN FUNCTION

Contemporary definitions of aging remain conceptual rather than quantitative. The implied consequence of aging in all species is an increasing probability of death as a function of time. Aging manifests itself in mammalian species as degenerative changes in both the structure and the functional capacity of organs and tissues. At one time, global age-related physiologic degeneration was depicted as a linear decline of maximal function beginning in young adulthood and continuing inexorably downward thereafter. However, a more contemporary analysis describes nonlinear change in maximal organ function that first becomes apparent following the years that represent the peak of somatic maturation, in the fourth decade of human life (Fig. 45-2). Additional decrements of function during the middle adult years appear to be relatively subtle, but subsequently become progressively more dramatic during the traditional years of geriatric senescence, the seventh decade of life and beyond. Elderly patients who maintain greater than average functional
3 capacities are considered "physiologically young." When organ function declines at an earlier age than usual, or at a more rapid rate, elderly patients appear to be "physiologically old."

Nevertheless, the competence of integrated organ system function varies greatly from one elderly patient to the next, even in the absence of disease, and is significantly altered by activity level, social habits, diet, and genetic background. In all healthy geriatric patients, however, maximum organ system function is greater than basal demand at all ages. The difference between maximal organ system capacity and basal function represents organ system functional reserve (Fig. 45-3). Organ system functional reserve is the "safety margin" available to meet, for example, the additional demands for cardiac output, carbon dioxide excretion, or protein synthesis imposed on the patient by trauma or disease, or by surgery and convalescence.

Increased susceptibility of elderly patients to stress-induced and disease-induced organ system dysfunction is a defining characteristic of physiologic aging. Consequently, preoperative

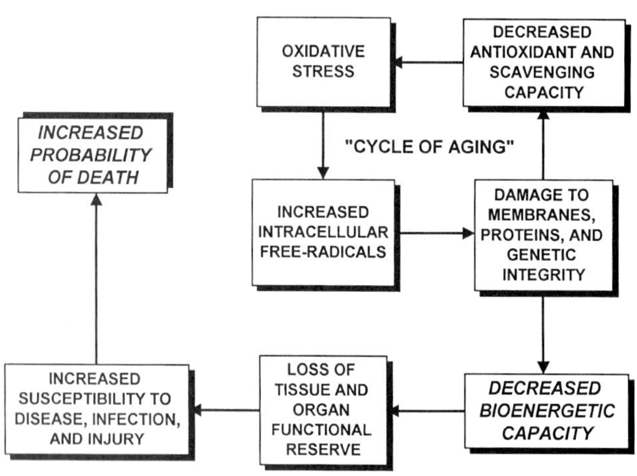

FIGURE 45-1. At a cellular level, there may be a self-sustaining "cycle of aging" within mitochondria in which oxidative stress damages the metabolic machinery needed to provide adequate bioenergetic capacity for full organ system functional reserve.

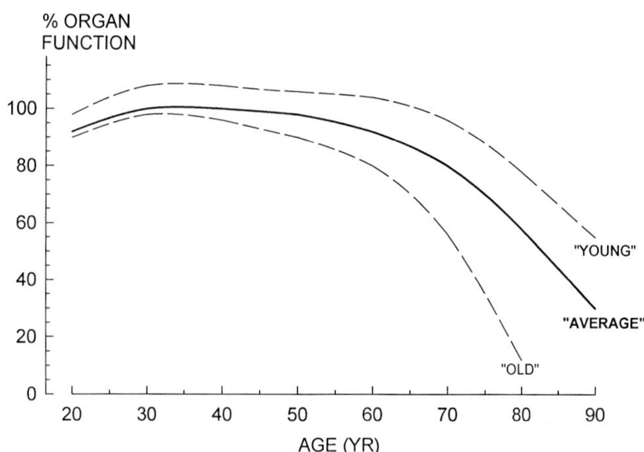

FIGURE 45-2. Differences in the rate at which maximal organ system functions decline with increasing age, and, to a lesser extent, differences in initial functional levels explain the inevitable variability seen in geriatric patients commonly described as physiologically "younger" or "older" than average.

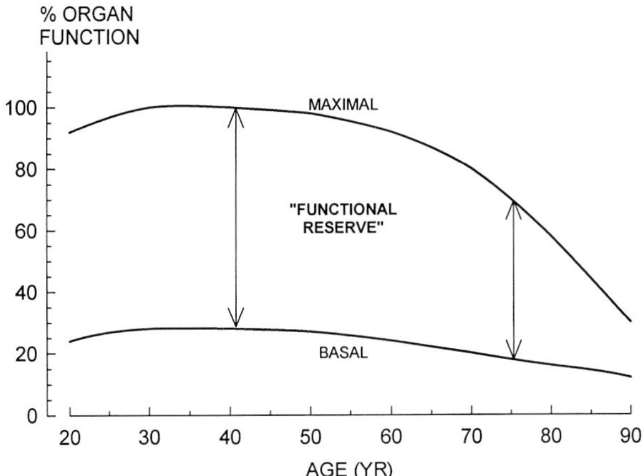

FIGURE 45-3. For any organ system, "functional reserve" represents the difference between basal (minimal) and maximal organ system function. The age-related decline in functional reserve may not be clinically apparent until demands made on the organ system are increased by stress, disease, polypharmacy, or surgical intervention.

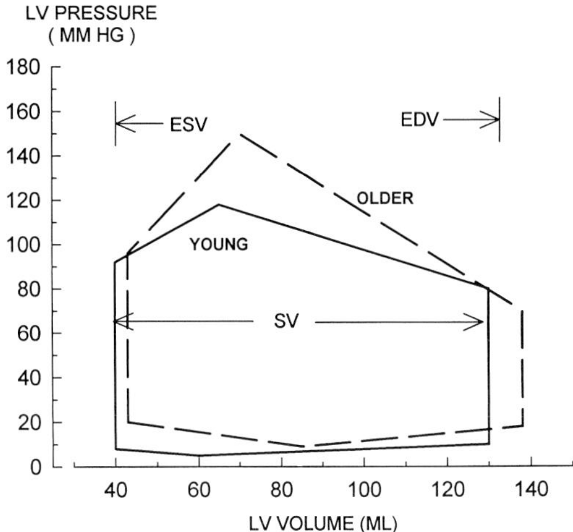

FIGURE 45-4. Left ventricular (LV) cardiac pressure–volume loops for fit subjects who are young (*solid line*) and elderly (*broken line*). Subjects who are elderly have a slightly higher end-diastolic ventricular volume (EDV) and larger end-diastolic stroke volume (ESV), as well as slightly elevated intracavitary pressures throughout the cardiac cycle due to increased myocardial stiffness and delayed active relaxation during diastole. SV, stroke volume.

testing in the elderly patient is most effective when it provides the anesthesiologist with a quantifiable assessment of organ system reserve. Testing should be clinically directed according to symptoms and complaints referable to age-related disease or functional decline, suggesting erosion of physiologic homeostasis. Cardiopulmonary functional reserve can be assessed clinically using various exercise or aerobic stress tests, but currently there are no comparable techniques for assessment of hepatic, immune, or nervous system functional reserve.

CARDIOPULMONARY FUNCTION

The aging heart increases output to meet imposed metabolic demands as needed within the limits of its maximal capacity. Consequently, the modest decrease in resting cardiac index observed in most healthy elderly subjects should not be considered as evidence of degenerative cardiovascular change. Rather, it represents an appropriate integrated response to the reduced requirements for perfusion and metabolism that occur with age-related atrophy of skeletal muscle and the loss of tissue mass in major organs with high intrinsic metabolic rates. From the perspective of integrated cardiovascular function, skeletal muscle energy expenditure and maximal breathing capacity, aging simply produces a progressively smaller "aerobic machine."

Under conditions of submaximal demand, myocardial contractility appears to remain uncompromised by increasing age at least until the eighth decade.[5] The heart, unlike other major organs, does not atrophy with age. Short-term demands for increased cardiac output are met at first by modest increases in heart rate, and then by increasing left ventricular end-diastolic volumes and pressures, changes that produce progressively larger stroke volumes. Because aging reduces the inotropic and chronotropic responses to adrenergic stimulation and beta-agonists, maximal heart rate is age limited, and unlike young adults, older adults exhibit little enhancement of ejection fraction under these conditions.

The aging left ventricle is also thicker and less elastic than its younger counterpart, exhibiting symmetric hypertrophy and an increase in collagen cross-linking in the myocardial cytoskeleton to which the myocytes are attached.[6] Cross-linking may reflect the buildup of advanced glycation end products produced by the chemical transformation of sugar moieties normally found in tissues.[7] Whatever the precise mechanism, the stiffer ventricle and atrium do not undergo complete relaxation until relatively late in diastole, and passive ventricular filling, which occurs during the early phase of diastole, is significantly reduced (Fig. 45-4). The progressive change in tissue quality imposes a form of diastolic dysfunction that makes the elderly depend more on the synchronous atrial contraction of sinus rhythm for complete ventricular filling.[8] Therefore, small decreases in venous return, such as those produced by positive-pressure ventilation, surgical hemorrhage, or venodilator drugs, may significantly compromise stroke volume when even minor cardiac dysrhythmias are present.

Systolic hypertension with increased arterial pulse pressure is common in the geriatric population. It is a major cardiovascular risk factor[9] caused by a gradual increase in large artery stiffness due to fibrotic replacement of elastic tissues during the adult years. This reduces the ability of the aorta and large arteries to store hydraulic energy, and increases vascular impedance to ejection of stroke volume. The end result of these changes is a progressive and sustained rise in left ventricular wall tension and myocardial workload that produces symmetric ventricular hypertrophy. Because vascular impedance is a frequency-dependent form of hydraulic resistance, increased impedance to the ejection of stroke volume occurs in older adults, even when systemic vascular resistance is unchanged.[10] Increased vascular stiffness and loss of arterial cross-sectional area also increase the reflection of arterial pressure waves that produces the familiar "ringing" characteristics of radial artery waveform tracings in geriatric patients.

Age-related loss of tissue elasticity occurs in the lung and the cardiovascular system. There is an increase in fibrous connective tissue within the lung parenchyma, as well as degeneration and cross-linking of lung elastin. Therefore, all elderly individuals
4 eventually demonstrate some degree of emphysema-like increases in lung compliance. However, calcification and stiffening of the costochondral joints of the thorax reduce chest wall compliance, so net pulmonary compliance is essentially unchanged.[11] Nevertheless, loss of lung elastic recoil is the primary anatomic mechanism by which aging exerts deleterious effects on pulmonary gas exchange. Breakdown of alveolar septae also reduces total alveolar surface area, increasing both anatomic and alveolar dead space. These changes are nonuniform and severely disrupt the normal matching of ventilation

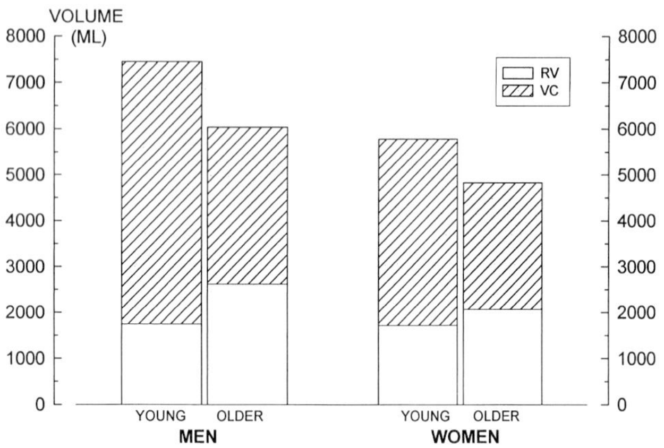

FIGURE 45-5. Total lung capacity, the sum of vital capacity (VC) and residual volume (RV), falls slowly in older adults of either gender. VC, however, the exchangeable gas volume, is markedly compromised by increases in thoracic rigidity and loss of ventilatory muscle power. RV increases because intrinsic lung elastic recoil is progressively reduced.

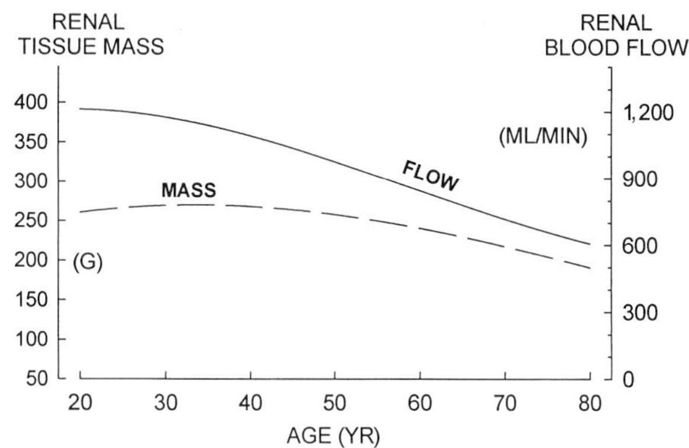

FIGURE 45-6. Renal blood flow (*solid line*) declines more rapidly than does renal tissue mass (*broken line*) with increasing age. Glomerular filtration rate (not shown) falls somewhat more slowly than plasma flow because filtration fraction actually increases in some individuals who are elderly.

and perfusion within the lungs, increasing both shunting and physiologic dead space. Small airway patency, normally maintained by elastic recoil, may also be compromised and closing capacity typically becomes greater than the volume of the lung at rest.[12]

Vital capacity is significantly and progressively compromised[13] because residual lung volume increases at the expense of inspiratory and expiratory reserve volumes (Fig. 45-5). Although the strength and endurance of the ventilatory apparatus remain adequate to meet moderate demands,[14] skeletal calcification and increased airway resistance increase work of breathing in subjects who are elderly and predispose them to acute postoperative ventilatory failure.[15] Moment-to-moment neural control of ventilation and the responses to changes in pH and respiratory gases appear to be essentially unchanged. Overall, pulmonary function in older adults during general anesthesia is best described as progressive ventilation–perfusion mismatch due to the deterioration of alveolar architecture and to anesthetic-induced depression of active hypoxic pulmonary vasoconstriction. The cardiovascular and ventilatory response to imposed hypoxia or hypercarbia is also delayed in onset and is smaller in geriatric patients.[16]

Opioid-induced rigidity of the chest wall occurs more frequently in older adults than in younger adults. The threshold stimulus magnitude needed for vocal cord closure is markedly elevated, increasing the risk of pulmonary injury due to aspiration of gastric contents in older patients, especially if level of consciousness is depressed. Consequently, geriatric surgical patients are clearly at increased risk of unrecognized respiratory failure in the typical postoperative setting of residual anesthetic depression and the use of opioids for pain management.

PHARMACOKINETICS, HEPATORENAL, AND IMMUNE FUNCTION

Hepatic enzyme activities are comparable to those of young adults, but liver tissue mass declines about 40% by the age of 80 years, and hepatic blood flow is proportionally reduced.[17] Loss of perfused hepatic tissue mass largely explains the reduced rates of plasma clearance and prolonged clinical effects of narcotics and many other xenobiotics in geriatric subjects.[18] In general, age-related differences in the binding of drugs to plasma proteins do not affect pharmacokinetics significantly in a clinical context. However, hepatic metabolism and drug biotransformation may be altered unpredictably in this patient subpopulation because of sustained exposure to the intense polypharmacy of age-related chronic disease. In addition, the hepatic synthetic reserve needed for wound healing or response to sepsis may be inadequate, especially if associated with arterial hypotension, low cardiac output, hypothermia, or any form of direct hepatic injury.

Almost one-third of renal tissue mass is lost by the eighth decade, and renal blood flow decreases by about 10% per decade beginning in early adulthood (Fig. 45-6). Atrophy is especially marked in the renal cortex, although the extent of parenchymal loss is often masked by diffuse interstitial fibrosis and a reciprocal increase in intrarenal fat. More than one-third of the glomeruli and tubular structures disappear in the elderly, and in some of the remaining glomeruli, sclerosis impairs effective filtration by producing tubular diverticuli and dysfunctional continuity between afferent and efferent glomerular arterioles.[19] The renal cortex suffers the greatest reduction in vascularity, with relative sparing of the medulla. Shifting perfusion from cortex to medulla produces a slight compensatory increase in filtration fraction in subjects who are elderly.[20] Serum creatinine concentration remains normal because loss of skeletal muscle mass imposes a progressively smaller creatinine load, and glomerular filtration rate is sufficient to avoid uremia and maintain normal plasma osmolarity and electrolyte concentrations.[21] Geriatric surgical patients do not appear to require a unique fluid replacement protocol, but their renal functional reserve is rarely adequate to withstand gross disruptions of water and electrolyte balance. Water retention through antidiuretic hormone secretion is less efficient than in young adults, and excretion of free water is delayed. Diminished thirst, poor diet, and the use of diuretic agents to decrease age-related hypertension also predispose debilitated, elderly surgical patients with chronic disease to intravascular and intracellular dehydration.

Aging appears to have little effect on macrophage and other phagocytic activity, but even fit subjects who are elderly exhibit evidence of decreased immune responsiveness.[22] There is shrinkage of thymic mass and progressive alteration of thymus cellular composition. Older adults have decreased B-cell and T-cell lymphocyte activity, as well as depressed serum titers of immunoglobulin E, depressed skin response to allergens, and impaired delayed hypersensitivity. Older adults are particularly predisposed to streptococcal pneumonia, meningitis, and septicemia. Sepsis is second only to respiratory failure as a cause of morbidity and mortality in trauma patients who are elderly.[23]

METABOLISM AND BODY COMPOSITION

Particularly in men, aging produces a progressive and generalized loss of skeletal muscle mass and atrophy of other metabolically active tissues in brain, liver, and kidney. Reciprocal increases in the lipid fraction of total body mass during the middle adult years are typical but extremely variable in magnitude. In general, changes in body composition reduce basal metabolic requirements by 10 to 15% compared with young adults. Reduction in body heat production and impairment of thermoregulatory vasoconstriction[24] place surgical patients who are elderly at increased risk for inadvertent intraoperative hypothermia. In fact, intraoperative core temperature decreases at a rate twice as great as that observed in young adults under comparable conditions,[25] and the time needed for spontaneous postoperative rewarming increases in direct proportion to patient age.[26] Because muscle and liver provide storage for carbohydrates, aging is also associated with impairment of the ability to handle a glucose challenge, even though the timing and the magnitude of insulin release appear to remain normal. Age-related glucose intolerance therefore may also reflect progressive impairment of insulin function or antagonism of its effect on target tissues.[27] Fluid replacement with glucose-containing solutions in patients who are elderly should be limited to environments that permit frequent measurement of blood sugar levels.

After the young adult years, men gain adipose tissue and lose skeletal muscle mass, changes that eventually result in the loss of 10 to 15% of their total body water (Fig. 45-7). In men who are aged, continuing loss of muscle and central organ atrophy eventually produces a significant decline in total body weight, often to levels less than those of young adulthood. In women, however, muscle and bone loss due to osteoporosis are largely offset by increasing body fat; therefore, total body weight usually returns toward, but rarely falls below, young adult values. Virtually all age-related changes in body water in men and women are limited to the intracellular compartments. Plasma volume, red cell mass, and extracellular fluid volumes are usually well maintained in nonhypertensive elderly individuals who maintain their habits of daily physical activity.

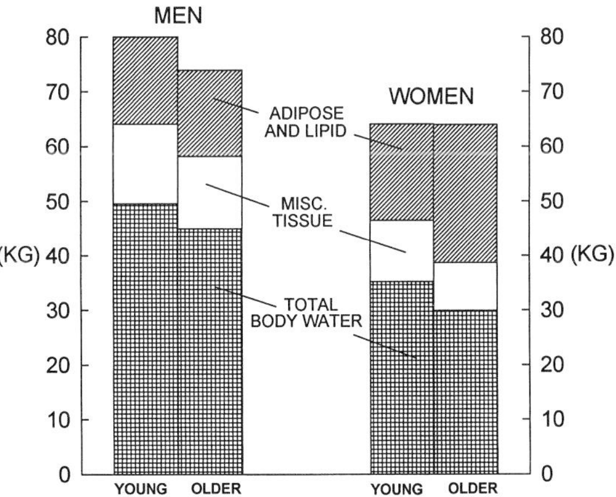

FIGURE 45-7. Age-related changes in body composition are gender specific. In women, total body mass remains constant because increases in body fat (*upper shaded segment*) offset bone loss (*middle segment*) and intracellular dehydration (*lower shaded segment*). In men, body mass declines despite maintenance of body lipid and skeletal tissue elements because accelerating loss of skeletal muscle and other components of lean tissue mass produces marked contraction of intracellular water (*lower shaded segment*).

Decreases in circulating blood volume are typical only in the bed-ridden and deconditioned elderly or those with essential hypertension.[28]

CENTRAL NERVOUS SYSTEM

Aging reduces brain size. Average adult brain mass is about 20% less by the age of 80 years than respective values measured postmortem in young adults.[29] The fraction of intracranial volume occupied by brain tissue falls from 92 to 82% over the same time period, with the most rapid reduction in gray matter tissue mass and the greatest rate of compensatory increase in cerebrospinal fluid occurring after the sixth decade. Aging, in effect, produces a form of low-pressure hydrocephalus. Most of the tissue loss reflects attrition of neurons because there is little decline in the number of glial cells that normally constitute almost half of total brain mass. Neuron loss is highly selective according to type and region, the rate of loss varies greatly at different ages, and some degree of neuronal regeneration may occur at any age.[30] In general, the most metabolically active, highly specialized neuronal subpopulations, particularly those that synthesize neurotransmitters, appear to suffer the most severe degree of attrition. The residual neutropil also develops a markedly simplified pattern of synaptic interconnection.[31]

These and other age-related changes within the brain and spinal cord are well described anatomically but their functional significance remains unclear. In the healthy elderly individual, decreased cerebral blood flow is a consequence, not a cause, of brain tissue atrophy, and it falls in proportion to reduced brain tissue mass. The mechanisms that couple regional cortical and subcortical perfusion to local variation of metabolic demands are maintained and the blood-brain barrier is functionally intact. Aging does not impair autoregulation of cerebrovascular resistance to changes in arterial blood pressure, and the cerebral vasoconstrictor response to hyperventilation remains intact in the healthy geriatric patient.[32]

As in other organ systems, it may be difficult to distinguish between aging and age-related nervous system disease. Many forms of "senile" dysfunction may eventually be established as age-related disease, and conversely, it has become increasingly clear that most neurodegenerative disorders and normal aging neurons share declining mitochondrial bioenergetics and rising levels of oxidative stress as common characteristics.[33] Nevertheless, most studies suggest that "crystallized intelligence," such as language skills and personality, do not decline with increasing age. General knowledge, comprehension, and long-term memory are well maintained even in individuals who are aged if they remain physically fit and mentally active. It remains unclear whether "fluid intelligence" and other cognitive functions that require immediate processing or rapid retrieval suffer intrinsic deterioration or whether they are compromised by age-related limitation of attention span. In general, however, anatomic and functional redundancy within the central nervous system appears to compensate adequately for attrition of cellular elements, reduction of neurotransmitter concentrations, and simplification of neuronal interconnections within the neuropil that occur in the aging brain.

PERIPHERAL NERVOUS SYSTEM

The threshold intensities of stimuli needed to initiate all forms of perception, including vision, hearing, touch, joint position sense, smell, peripheral pain, and temperature increase during senescence. This process of progressive age-related deafferentation is due, at least in part, to degenerative changes within specialized sense organs such as the pain-generating

Meissner's corpuscles in skin. However, there are also age-related changes at central sites of pain processing such as the thalamus and throughout peripheral pathways for conduction of pain impulses. In addition, attrition of the individual nerve fibers within afferent conduction pathways in both the peripheral nervous system and spinal cord reduce the velocity and amplitude of evoked sensory potentials. Peripheral motor nerve conduction velocity decreases steadily throughout adulthood, and impairment of efferent corticospinal transmission increases the latency between intention and onset of motor activity.

Isometric muscle strength appears to be well maintained, but failing proximodistal protoplasmic transport in aging motor neurons reduces the myotrophic support normally provided to skeletal muscle. Mitochondrial volume within skeletal muscle cells is reduced, and neurogenic skeletal muscle atrophy[34] causes the dynamic strength and steadiness of skeletal muscle in the extremities to decline 20 to 50% by the age of 80 years. Reduced neurotrophic support also produces disseminated neurogenic atrophy at the neuromuscular junction.[35] The postjunctional muscle membrane thickens, and atypical "extrajunctional" cholinoceptors appear on the skeletal muscle surface.[36] The increase in the total number of cholinoceptors at each end plate and in the surrounding areas of the muscle cell surface may mask the age-related decline in the number and the density of motor neuron and end-plate units.

AUTONOMIC NERVOUS SYSTEM

As in other parts of the peripheral nervous system, neurons in sympathoadrenal pathways are subject to significant cellular attrition. In addition, adrenal tissues atrophy and cortisol secretion declines at least 15% by the age of 80. Nevertheless, plasma concentrations of norepinephrine are two- to fourfold higher in subjects who are elderly than in younger adults during sleep, at rest, and even in response to exercise-induced physical stress.[37] High plasma levels of catecholamines are rarely apparent clinically in patients who are elderly, however, because aging markedly and progressively depresses beta-adrenergic end-organ responsiveness.[38] The response to beta agonists such as isoproterenol are markedly reduced. In effect, aging produces "endogenous beta-blockade." There appears to be little change in alpha adrenoceptor or muscarinic cholinoceptor activity in older adults and no intrinsic changes in the basic contractile properties of peripheral vascular smooth muscle.[39]

Nevertheless, the integrated autonomic reflex responses that maintain cardiovascular and metabolic homeostasis are progressively impaired in individuals who are elderly.[40] This may explain the increased incidence and severity of arterial hypotension seen in older patients following anesthetic induction. Baroreflex responsiveness, the vasoconstrictor response to cold stress, and beat-to-beat heart rate responses following postural change in subjects who are elderly become progressively less rapid in onset, smaller in magnitude, and less effective in stabilizing blood pressure under a variety of circumstances.[41] The autonomic nervous system in the elderly patient is effectively "underdamped," and is characterized by wider variation from homeostatic set points and delayed restabilization during hemodynamic stress.[42]

ANALGESIC AND ANESTHETIC REQUIREMENTS

The net effect of the age-related structural and functional changes within the nervous system described previously on pain-related neurologic function remains controversial. The study of amplification, modulation, and selectivity of afferent input within the spinal cord, thalamus, and other locations within the aging nervous system does not yet permit broad generalizations regarding aging and perception of pain.[43] Perceived intensity of pain perioperatively is extremely unpredictable and appears to depend far more on anxiety, personality, and the prospect of long-term debility than on age itself.[44] Nevertheless, parenteral morphine requirements are clearly inversely related to patient age and essentially independent of body weight.[45] Similarly, when a fixed dose and volume of local anesthetic is used, higher levels of sensory blockade occur in patients who are elderly than in young patients undergoing spinal anesthesia.[46] Segmental dose requirements for epidural analgesia are similarly reduced,[47] and more cephalad levels of neural blockade carry a greater risk of hypotension in the elderly.[48] Overall, however, the differences are small and considered to be clinically insignificant by some investigators.[49]

The effect of nervous system aging on requirements for general anesthesia is less controversial. Between young adulthood and the geriatric era, relative minimum alveolar concentration
5 (MAC) values for the newer inhalational agents decline by as much as 30%,[50,51] the same decrement seen with older anesthetics (Fig. 45-8). The mechanisms producing age-related increases in sensitivity to anesthetic agents remain unknown, but the consistency of this phenomenon for anesthetic agents with markedly different chemical characteristics suggests that it reflects a fundamental neurophysiologic process. Declining neuronal bioenergetics due to mitochondrial genetic mutation or to age-related oxidative stress have both been recently shown to reduce anesthetic requirement.[52,53]

The data for the effect of aging on the pharmacodynamics, or dose requirements, for opioids, barbiturates, and benzodiazepines are less consistent than that for inhalational anesthetics. There is considerable controversy as to whether the clinically apparent age-related increase in the potency of these drugs is truly a pharmacodynamic (drug sensitivity) phenomenon or whether it simply reflects age-related changes in "alpha" or early-phase redistribution pharmacokinetics (molecular drug disposition). Plasma drug concentrations immediately after intravenous injection are often higher in subjects who are elderly than in young adults.[54] This may reflect delayed intercompartmental transfer of drug rather than a decreased initial volume of distribution.[55] In any case, the concentrations of short-acting intravenous agents in plasma change so rapidly, and in such a complex manner, that the traditional two-compartment

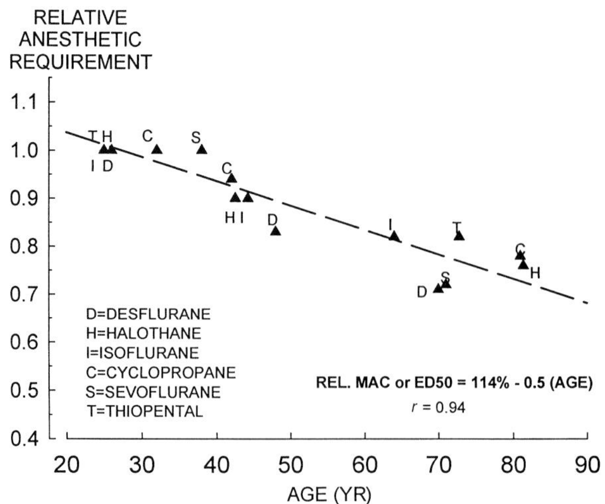

FIGURE 45-8. The age-related decline in relative anesthetic requirement (minimum alveolar concentration [MAC] or ED50) in unsedated human subjects is a consistent characteristic reported for a wide variety of inhaled and injected anesthetic agents.

pharmacokinetic model may be of little value for studying the early or "alpha-phase" behavior of these drugs and their subsequent redistribution in subjects who are elderly.[56]

Interpretation of data from clinical studies of intravenous agents is further complicated by difficulty in defining the anesthetic end point in a process that, in contrast to the conditions under which MAC is determined, does not represent pharmacokinetic equilibrium. Therefore, both onset and duration of clinical effects can be influenced by pharmacodynamic or pharmacokinetic processes. Clinical experience suggests that there are significant age-related reductions in the dose requirements for thiopental,[57] as well as virtually all other agents that depress consciousness. Most studies also suggest that aging increases brain sensitivity to narcotics,[58,59] with insignificant pharmacodynamic effects for barbiturates or etomidate.[60] Overall, there is a complex interaction between subtle changes in pharmacodynamics and altered "alpha-phase" redistribution pharmacokinetics due to age-related hemodynamic factors that must be characterized for each drug to predict the implications of aging for clinical drug action and drug dosage.[61]

Despite the inevitable loss of skeletal muscle mass in subjects who are elderly, the median effective doses (ED50) and steady-state plasma concentrations required for half-maximal neuromuscular-blocking effect (EC50) remain virtually unchanged or may actually increase slightly in the patient who is elderly.[62] Although the elderly have reduced skeletal muscle mass, disseminated neurogenic atrophy at the neuromuscular junction allows proliferation of extrajunctional cholinoceptors, and thereby may require increased local concentrations of neuromuscular-blocking drugs to produce competitive blockade. Maximal relaxant effect is clearly delayed in onset relative to that produced in young adults.[63,64] Duration of neuromuscular blockade is also markedly prolonged for relaxants with hepatic or renal elimination because plasma clearance declines with increasing age.[65,66] However, antagonism of the effects of blocking drugs and recovery of neuromuscular transmission should be unchanged. As in younger adults, the intensity of neuromuscular blockade at time of or "reversal" by neostigmine or edrophonium, not patient age, determines the speed and the completeness of recovery of neuromuscular transmission.

PERIOPERATIVE MANAGEMENT AND OUTCOME

There probably are no healthy patients who are "too old" for anesthesia, even ambulatory surgical procedures.[67] Age-related disease, and not aging itself, largely determines the morbidity and mortality that characterizes an elderly surgical population,[68–70] although advanced age itself may have additional negative prognostic significance if associated with severe multiple organ system dysfunction. Following orthopaedic surgery, the speed and extent to which a patient who is elderly
6 recovers full function has also been shown to depend on functional level prior to surgery.[71] Morbidity and mortality rates, therefore, are higher in elderly surgical patients largely because this surgical patient subpopulation has a greater incidence and severity of concurrent disease, and greater exposure to invasive medical interventions, than do younger adults. Polypharmacy also produces an age-related increase in adverse drug reactions that complicate perioperative management (Fig. 45-9).

The probability of a serious pulmonary or hemodynamic complication after surgery is determined both by the site of operation and by the patient's physical status (Fig. 45-10). Many members of the geriatric surgical population summarily
7 "cleared" for major surgery by medical consultants on empirical clinical grounds may later be found to have mild to severe cardiopulmonary functional deficits.[72] Adverse outcomes in geriatric surgical patients show a relative predominance of disorders of cardiac rate or rhythm,[73] myocardial ischemia, or general hemodynamic instability. Pulmonary complications, infections and sepsis, and renal failure also contribute significantly to morbidity.[74] In-hospital postoperative complications have also been identified as having negative prognostic implications with regard to long-term survival.[75] Consequently, adequate time for diagnosis, treatment, and preparation of the anesthetic plan is essential if the rate and severity of complications are to be reduced.[76]

Elderly patients at low risk may be able to proceed without further testing or preparation, and intermediate-risk patients are now believed to benefit substantially from perioperative beta-blockade.[77] For the elderly surgical patient at high cardiac risk, coronary angiography prior to elective major surgery may be indicated.[78] Newer inhalational agents such as sevoflurane and desflurane appear to be the agents of choice to

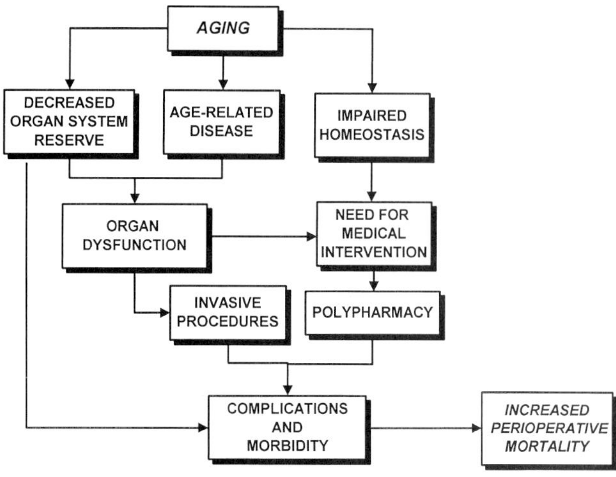

FIGURE 45-9. Increased rates of perioperative morbidity and mortality in surgical patients who are elderly can be attributed primarily to interactions between age-related decreases in organ system reserve, a high prevalence of disease in the elderly, and the inherent risk associated with therapy and surgical intervention.

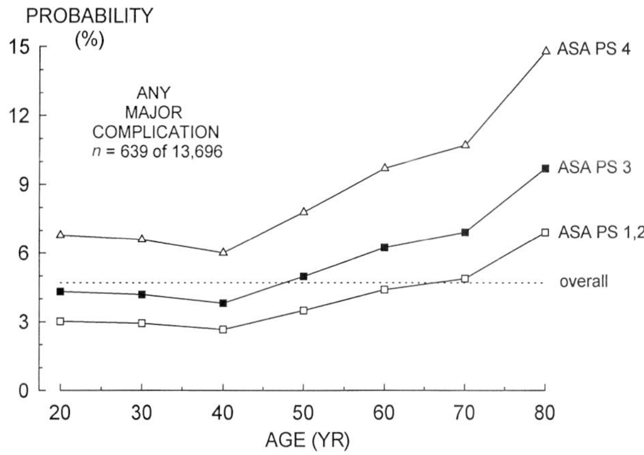

FIGURE 45-10. The probability of adverse postoperative outcome increases gradually with age across middle adulthood. Analyzed prospectively from a large series of randomized patients, preexisting cardiovascular or pulmonary disease and physical status (*solid lines*) were found to be the primary determinants of perioperative morbidity, although the widening of the separation between physical status lines shown here suggests that age itself may further amplify the negative prognostic value of impaired physical status in surgical patients who are well into the geriatric era.[68]

preserve left ventricular function after cardiopulmonary bypass in high-risk, elderly coronary surgery patients.[79] Nevertheless, although many clinical studies have shown that some perioperative complications are associated more frequently with one form of anesthesia than another,[80,81] it may not be possible to determine whether there is a single "best" anesthetic for patients who are elderly.[82]

No single anesthetic technique or agent appears to have universal advantage for the elderly surgical patient with regard to survival. Neither regional anesthesia nor general anesthesia has clearly demonstrable superiority of outcome in patients who are elderly, although one or the other may be preferred for use in specific procedures[83] or certain patients for other medical reasons.[84] In fact, the intraoperative period of anesthetic management is often only a small component of a prolonged, difficult, and complex hospital course. Nevertheless, more recent preliminary studies suggest that there may be value in careful titration of the depth of surgical anesthesia in older adults to the minimum value needed to avoid awareness. In older surgical patients, deeper maintenance anesthetic levels are associated with higher 1-year postoperative death rates.[85] Male gender and subnormal body mass index may be additional cofactors that, along with prolonged deep levels of anesthesia, increase long-term mortality in the geriatric surgical patient population.[86]

Prompt and complete postoperative recovery of mental function is particularly important in patients who are elderly if mentation is already compromised by age-related disease or drug therapy. The use of newer intravenous agents such as remifentanil[87,88] and cisatracurium[89] minimize dependence on organ system functional reserve for drug elimination.[90] Newer inhalation agents such as sevoflurane and especially desflurane[91] also provide more rapid recovery of consciousness in the adult who is aged than was possible with isoflurane.[92] There is less nausea and vomiting in older adults[93] after general anesthesia but a greater likelihood of prolonged postoperative confusion.[94] Full recovery of psychomotor function is somewhat delayed in older patients, even after typically brief outpatient anesthesia with propofol.[95] Local anesthesia or regional techniques, if they can be comfortably performed without heavy intravenous sedation, may significantly improve postoperative mental function immediately after surgery, although there is no clinical evidence of long-term benefits to this approach.[96] In addition, nerve palsies, residual paresthesias, and other neurapraxias associated with regional anesthesia occur more often than in young adults.[97–99]

Even when anesthetic management of the older patient is appropriate and surgical convalescence uncomplicated, full return of cognitive function to preoperative levels after a prolonged general anesthetic may require up to 2 weeks.[100] Perioperative environmental factors such as chronic medication and drug interaction,[101] disorientation due to sensory deprivation, or the disruption of normal routine needed to maintain "implicit" memory[102] have been identified as factors that predispose older surgical patients to "delirium."[103] However, the neurophysiologic or pharmacologic explanation for persistent disruption of nervous system function remains unknown. Psychometrically defined postoperative cognitive dysfunction can be demonstrated 3 months after apparently uncomplicated surgery in 10 to 15% of patients 60 years of age or older who have had major procedures and a hospital stay of 4 or more days.[104] This suggests that, at least in older adults with reduced central nervous system functional reserve, either the process of general anesthesia itself or the drugs used to produce it may produce residual neurologic dysfunction or perhaps even injury.[105] Impairment of learning long after the pharmacologic effects of anesthetic agents are dissipated has been clearly demonstrated in older laboratory animals given uncomplicated conventional general anesthesia.[106,107]

The physical management of patients who are elderly in the operating room and afterward also requires specific precautions. Aged skin and bones are fragile, joints are stiff, and their range of motion is limited, especially if compromised by age-related arthritic processes. The elderly surgical patient therefore requires gentle and expert routine care if traumatic injuries from improper positioning, bandaging, or enforced bed rest are to be avoided. Avoiding hypothermia is important; however, active heating devices in contact with poorly perfused skin or connective tissue pressure points can quickly produce ischemic lesions requiring surgical treatment. In all patients who are elderly, postoperative bleeding diatheses or hypercoagulable states and bacterial infection are more frequent than in younger adults. Because of diastolic dysfunction and increased ventricular stiffness, rates of intravenous fluid administration that would be modest for young adults may produce dangerous increases in atrial and pulmonary artery pressures in geriatric patients, precipitating congestive heart failure or pulmonary edema.

Whatever anesthetic approach is selected, surgical tissue injury produces extensive neuroendocrine and sympathoadrenal stress. Suppression of excessive sympathetic activity promotes prompt rewarming, wound healing, and a reduced period of increased cardiovascular and pulmonary demands. Careful attention to need for analgesia may eliminate the long periods of emotional stress due to persistent surgical pain sometimes imposed on geriatric patients because of exaggerated fears of opioid side effects. To some extent, "ageism" may influence caregivers to withhold diagnostic or therapeutic measures that would be offered routinely to a younger adult.[108] Untreated pain and related emotional stress itself may also significantly impair immune responsiveness in older adults and increase the risk of perioperative infection.[109] Therefore, an anesthetic plan that includes postoperative epidural sympathectomy and analgesia, or a parenteral sympathetic modulator such as dexmedetomidine,[110] may be of special value in the elderly surgical patient.

Overall, however, patients who are elderly and aged do not require a "special" kind of anesthetic. A well-conducted anesthetic of any type is a safe and appropriate anesthetic plan if attention to dosage and careful assessment of anesthetic depth are used.[111] Good perioperative care of the geriatric patient simply requires the highest standards of diagnosis and control of preexisting disease, as well as clinical vigilance and meticulous delivery of anesthetic and postoperative care.

References

1. Schneider EL, Reed JD Jr: Life extension. N Engl J Med 312:1159, 1985
2. Ozawa T: Genetic and functional changes in mitochondria associated with aging. Physiol Rev 77:425, 1997
3. Kapahi P, Boulton ME, Kirkwood TB: Positive correlation between mammalian life span and cellular resistance to stress. Free Radical Biol Med 26:495, 1999
4. Trifunovic A, Wredenberg A, Falkenberg M *et al*: Premature ageing in mice expressing defective mitochondrial DNA polymerase. Nature 429:417, 2004
5. Aronow WS, Stein PD, Sabbah HN, Koenigsberg M: Resting left ventricular ejection fraction in elderly patients without evidence of heart disease. Am J Cardiol 63:368, 1989
6. Folkow B, Svanborg A: Physiology of cardiovascular aging. Physiol Rev 73:725, 1993
7. Irich P, Cerami A: Protein glycation, diabetes, and aging. Recent Prog Horm Res 56:1, 2001
8. Pagel PS, Grossman W, Haering JM, Warltier DC: Left ventricular diastolic function in the normal and diseased heart. Perspectives for the anesthesiologist. Anesthesiology 79:836, 1104, 1993
9. Laurent S, Boutouyrie P, Benetos A: Pathophysiology of hypertension in the elderly. Am J Geriatr Cardiol 11:34, 2002
10. Nichols WW, O'Rourke MF, Avolio AP *et al*: Ventricular/vascular interaction in patients with mild systemic hypertension and normal peripheral resistance. Circulation 74:455, 1986

11. Dauchot PJ, Graber RG: The aging respiratory system. Prob Anesth 9:498, 1997
12. Allen SJ: Respiratory considerations in the elderly surgical patient. Clin Anaesthesiol 4:899, 1986
13. Wahba WM: Influence of aging on lung function—Clinical significance of changes from age twenty. Anesth Analg 62:764, 1983
14. Tolep K, Kelsen SG: Effect of aging on respiratory skeletal muscles. Clin Chest Med 14:363, 1993
15. Rose DK, Cohen MM, Wigglesworth DF, DeBoer DP: Critical respiratory events in the postanesthesia care unit. Anesthesiology 81:410, 1994
16. Peterson DD, Pack AI, Silage DA, Fishman AP: Effects of aging on ventilatory and occlusion pressure responses to hypoxia and hypercapnia. Am Rev Respir Dis 124:387, 1981
17. Zoli M, Iervese T, Abbati S *et al*: Portal blood velocity and flow in aging man. Gerontology 35:61, 1989
18. Swift CG, Homeida M, Halliwell M, Roberts CJ: Antipyrine disposition and liver size in the elderly. Eur J Clin Pharmacol 14:149, 1978
19. Lindeman RD: Renal physiology and pathophysiology of aging. Contrib Nephrol 105:1, 1993
20. Hollenberg NK, Adams DF, Solomon HS *et al*: Senescence and the renal vasculature in normal man. Circ Res 34:309, 1974
21. Lubran MM: Renal function in the elderly. Ann Clin Lab Sci 25:122, 1995
22. Miller RA: The aging immune system: Primer and prospectus. Science 273:70, 1996
23. Tornetta P III, Mostafavi H, Riina J *et al*: Morbidity and mortality in elderly trauma patients. J Trauma-Injury Infect Crit Care 46:702, 1999
24. Kurz A, Plattner O, Sessler DI *et al*: The threshold for thermoregulatory vasoconstriction during nitrous oxide/isoflurane anesthesia is lower in elderly than in young patients. Anesthesiology 79:465, 1993
25. Frank SM, Beattie C, Christopherson R *et al*: Epidural versus general anesthesia: Ambient operating room temperature, and patient age as predictors of inadvertent hypothermia. Anesthesiology 77:252, 1992
26. Carli F, Gabrielczyk M, Clark MM, Aber VR: An investigation of factors affecting postoperative rewarming of adult patients. Anaesthesia 41:363, 1986
27. Davidson MB: The effect of aging on carbohydrate metabolism: A review of the English literature and a practical approach to the diagnosis of diabetes in the elderly. Metabolism 28:688, 1979
28. Fulop T Jr, Worum I, Csongor J *et al*: Body composition in elderly people. Gerontology 31:6, 1985
29. Terry RD, DeTeresa R, Hansen LA: Neocortical cell counts in normal human aging. Ann Neurol 21:530, 1987
30. Schjeide OA: Relation of development and aging: Pre- and postnatal differentiation of the brain as related to aging. Adv Behav Biol 16:37, 1975
31. Feldman ML: Aging changes in the morphology of cortical dendrites. In Terry RD, Gershon S (eds): Neurobiology of Aging, p 11. New York, Raven Press, 1976
32. Meyer JS, Terayama Y, Takashima S: Cerebral circulation in the elderly. Cerebrovasc Brain Metab Rev 5:122, 1993
33. Calabrese V, Scapagnini G, Giuffrida Stella AM *et al*: Mitochondrial involvement in brain function and dysfunction: Relevance to aging, neurodegenerative disorders and longevity. Neurochem Res 26:739, 2001
34. Swash M, Fox KP: The effect of age on human skeletal muscle: Studies of the morphology and innervation of muscle spindles. J Neurol Sci 16:417, 1972
35. Gutmann E, Hanzlikova V, Jaboubek B: Changes in the neuromuscular system during old age. Exp Gerontol 3:141, 1968
36. Martyn JAJ, White DA, Gronert GA *et al*: Up-and-down regulation of skeletal muscle acetylcholine receptors: Effects on neuromuscular blockers. Anesthesiology 76:822, 1992
37. Ziegler MG, Lake CR, Kopin IJ: Plasma noradrenaline increases with age. Nature 261:333, 1976
38. Vestal RE, Wood AJJ, Shand DG: Reduced adrenoceptor sensitivity in the elderly. Clin Pharmacol Ther 26:181, 1979
39. Seals DR, Taylor JA, Ng AV, Esler MD: Exercise and aging: Autonomic control of the circulation. Med Sci Sports Exerc 26(5):568, 1994
40. Rooke GA, Robinson BJ: Cardiovascular and autonomic nervous system aging. Probl Anesth 9:482, 1997
41. Pfeifer MA, Weinberg CR, Cook D *et al*: Differential changes of autonomic nervous system function with age in man. Am J Med 75:249, 1983
42. Shannon RP, Maher KA, Santinga JT *et al*: Comparison of differences in the hemodynamic response to passive postural stress in healthy subjects greater than 70 years and less than 30 years of age. Am J Cardiol 67:1110, 1991
43. Melding PS: Is there such a thing as geriatric pain? (editorial). Pain 46:119, 1991
44. Hapidou EG, DeCatanzaro D: Responsiveness to laboratory pain in women as a function of age and childbirth pain experience. Pain 48:177, 1992
45. Bellville JW, Forrest WH, Miller E, Brown BW: Influence of age on pain relief from analgesics: A study of postoperative patients. JAMA 217:1835, 1971
46. Cameron AE, Arnold RW, Ghoris MW, Jamieson V: Spinal analgesia using bupivacaine 0.5% plain: Variation in the extent of block with patient age. Anaesthesia 36:318, 1981
47. Sharrock NE: Epidural dose responses in patients 20 to 80 years old. Anesthesiology 49:425, 1978
48. Simon MJ, Veering BT, Stienstra R *et al*: The effects of age on neural blockade and hemodynamic changes after epidural anesthesia with ropivacaine. Anesth Analg 94:1325, 2002
49. Curatolo M, Orlando A, Zbinden AM *et al*: A multifactorial analysis of the spread of epidural analgesia. Acta Anaesth Scand 38:646, 1994
50. Gold MI, Abello D, Herrington C: Minimum alveolar concentration of desflurane in patients older than 65 years. Anesthesiology 79:710, 1993
51. Nakajima R, Nakajima Y, Ikeda K: Minimum alveolar concentration of sevoflurane in elderly patients. Br J Anaesth 70:273, 1993
52. Hartman PS, Ishii N, Kayser EB *et al*: Mitochondrial mutations differentially affect aging, mutability and anesthetic sensitivity in *Caenorhabditis elegans*. Mech Ageing Devel 122:1187, 2001
53. Morgan PG, Hoppel CL, Sedensky MM: Mitochondrial defects and anesthetic sensitivity. Anesthesiology 96:1268, 2002
54. Singleton MA, Rosen JI, Fisher DM: Pharmacokinetics of fentanyl in the elderly. Br J Anaesth 60:619, 1988
55. Avram MJ, Krejcie TC, Henthorn TK: The relationship of age to the pharmacokinetics of early drug distribution: The concurrent disposition of thiopental and indocyanine green. Anesthesiology 72:403, 1990
56. Hull CJ: How far can we go with compartmental models? (editorial). Anesthesiology 72:399, 1990
57. Muravchick S: Effect of age and premedication on thiopental sleep dose. Anesthesiology 61:333, 1984
58. Scott JC, Stanski DR: Decreased fentanyl and alfentanil dose requirements with increasing age. A simultaneous pharmacokinetic and pharmacodynamic evaluation. J Pharmacol Exp Ther 240:159, 1987
59. Minto CF, Schnider TW, Egan TD *et al*: Influence of age and gender on the pharmacokinetics and pharmacodynamics of remifentanil. Anesthesiology 86:10, 1997
60. Arden JR, Holley FO, Stanski DR: Increased sensitivity to etomidate in the elderly: Initial distribution versus altered brain response. Anesthesiology 65:19, 1986
61. Bjorkman S, Wada DR, Stanski DR: Application of physiologic models to predict the influence of changes in body composition and blood flows on the pharmacokinetics of fentanyl and alfentanil in patients. Anesthesiology 88:657, 1998
62. Shanks CA: Pharmacokinetics of the nondepolarizing neuromuscular relaxants applied to calculation of bolus and infusion dosage regimens. Anesthesiology 64:72, 1986
63. Koscielniak-Nielsen ZJ, Bevan JC, Popovic V *et al*: Onset of maximum neuromuscular blockade following succinylcholine or vecuronium in four age groups. Anesthesiology 79:229, 1993
64. Sarooshian SS, Stafford MA, Eastwood NB *et al*: Pharmacokinetics and pharmacodynamics of cisatracurium in young and elderly adult patients. Anesthesiology 84:1083, 1996
65. Lien CA, Matteo RS, Ornstein E *et al*: Distribution, elimination, and action of vecuronium in the elderly. Anesth Analg 73:39, 1991
66. Matteo RS, Ornstein E, Schwartz AE *et al*: Pharmacokinetics and pharmacodynamics of rocuronium (Org 9426) in elderly surgical patients. Anesth Analg 77:1193, 1993
67. Kortilla K: Aging, medical disease, and outcome of ambulatory surgery. Curr Opin Anaesthesiol 6:546, 1993
68. Forrest JB, Rehder K, Cahalan MK, Goldsmith CH: Multicenter study of general anesthesia III: Predictors of severe perioperative adverse outcomes. Anesthesiology 76:3, 1992
69. Arvidsson S, Ouchterlony J, Nilsson S, et al: The Gothenburg study of perioperative risk I; preoperative findings, postoperative complications. Acta Anaesth Scand 38:679, 1994
70. Pedersen T: Complications and death following anaesthesia: A prospective study with special reference to the influence of patient-, anaesthesia-, and surgery-related risk factors. Danish Med Bull 41:319, 1994
71. Eisler J, Cornwall R, Strauss E *et al*: Outcomes of elderly patients with nondisplaced femoral neck fractures. Clin Orthopaed Rel Res 399:52, 2002
72. Beliveau MM, Multach M: Perioperative care for the elderly patient. Med Clin North Am 87:273, 2003
73. Amar D, Zhang H, Yeung DH *et al*: Older age is the strongest predictor of postoperative atrial fibrillation. Anesthesiology 96:352, 2002
74. Smetana GW: Preoperative pulmonary assessment of the older adult. Clin Geriatr Med 19:35, 2003
75. Manku K, Bacchetti P, Leung JM: Prognostic significance of postoperative in-hospital complications in elderly patients. I. Long-term survival. Anesth Analg 96:583, 2003
76. Kennedy RH, al Mufti RA, Brewster SF *et al*: The acute surgical admission: Is mortality predictable in the elderly? Ann Roy Coll Surg Engl 76:342, 1994
77. Romero L, de Virgilio C: Preoperative cardiac risk assessment: An updated approach. Arch Surg 136:1370, 2001
78. Eagle KA, Berger PB, Calkins H *et al*: ACC/AHA guideline update for perioperative cardiovascular evaluation for noncardiac surgery—Executive summary. A report of the American College of Cardiology/American Heart Association Task Force on Practice Guidelines (committee to update the 1996 guidelines on perioperative cardiovascular evaluation for noncardiac surgery). Anesth Analg 94:1052, 2002
79. De Hert SG, Cromheecke S, ten Broecke PW *et al*: Effects of propofol, desflurane, and sevoflurane on recovery of myocardial function after coronary surgery in elderly high-risk patients. Anesthesiology 99:314, 2003

80. Davis FM, Woolner DF, Frampton C *et al*: Prospective, multi-centre trial of mortality following general or spinal anaesthesia for hip fracture surgery in the elderly. Br J Anaesth 59:1080, 1987
81. Sutcliffe AJ, Parker M: Mortality after spinal and general anaesthesia for surgical fixation of hip fractures. Anaesthesia 49:237, 1994
82. Go AS, Browner WS: Cardiac outcomes after regional or general anesthesia: Do we have the answer? (editorial). Anesthesiology 84:1, 1996
83. Fredman B, Sheffer O, Zohar E *et al*: Fast-track eligibility of geriatric patients undergoing short urologic surgery procedures. Anesth Analg 94:560, 2002
84. Christopherson R, Beattie C, Frank SM *et al*: Perioperative morbidity in patients randomized to epidural or general anesthesia for lower extremity vascular surgery. Anesthesiology 79:422, 1993
85. Weldon BC, Mahla ME, van der Aa MT *et al*: Advancing age and deeper intraoperative anesthetic levels are associated with higher first year death rates. Anesthesiology 96:A1097, 2002
86. Lennmarken C, Lindholm M-L, Greenwald S *et al*: Confirmation that low intraoperative BIS^{TM} levels predict increased risk of post-operative mortality. Anesthesiology 99:A303, 2003
87. Westmoreland CL, Hoke JF, Sebel PS *et al*: Pharmacokinetics of remifentanil (GI87084B) and its major metabolite (GI90291) in patients undergoing elective inpatient surgery. Anesthesiology 79:893, 1993
88. Minto CF, Schnider TW, Egan TD *et al*: Influence of age and gender on the pharmacokinetics and pharmacodynamics of remifentanil. Anesthesiology 86:10, 1997
89. Wright PMC, Ornstein E: Pharmacokinetics, pharmacodynamics and safety of cisatracurium in elderly patients. Curr Opin Anaesth 9(Suppl 1):S30, 1996
90. Cope TM, Hunter JM: Selecting neuromuscular-blocking drugs for elderly patients. Drugs Aging 20:125, 2003
91. Heavner JE, Kaye AD, Lin BK *et al*: Recovery of elderly patients from two or more hours of desflurane or sevoflurane anaesthesia. Br J Anaesth 91:502, 2003
92. Nathanson MH, Fredman B, Smith I *et al*: Sevoflurane versus desflurane for outpatient anesthesia: A comparison of maintenance and recovery profiles. Anesth Analg 81:1186, 1995
93. Sinclair DR, Chung F, Mezel G: Can postoperative nausea and vomiting be predicted? Anesthesiology 91:109, 1999
94. Tzabar Y, Asbury AJ, Millar K: Cognitive failures after general anaesthesia for day-case surgery. Br J Anaesth 76:194, 1996
95. Shinozaki M, Usui Y, Yamaguchi S *et al*: Recovery of psychomotor function after propofol sedation is prolonged in the elderly. Can J Anaesth 49:927, 2002
96. Chung FF, Chung A, Meier RH *et al*: Comparison of perioperative mental function after general anaesthesia and spinal anaesthesia with intravenous sedation. Can J Anaesth 36:382, 1989
97. Warner MA, Martin JT, Schroeder DR *et al*: Lower-extremity motor neuropathy associated with surgery performed on patients in a lithotomy position. Anesthesiology 81:6, 1994
98. Hampl KF, Heinzmann-Wiedmer S, Luginbuehl I, et al: Transient neurologic symptoms after spinal anesthesia. Anesthesiology 88:629, 1998
99. Martinez-Bourio R, Arzuaza M, Quintana JM *et al*: Incidence of transient neurologic symptoms after hyperbaric subarachnoid anesthesia with 5% lidocaine and 5% prilocaine. Anesthesiology 88:624, 1998
100. Muravchick S: Immediate and long-term nervous system effects of anesthesia in elderly patients. Clin Anaesthesiol 4:1035, 1986
101. Jolles J, Verhey FR, Riedel WJ, Houx PJ: Cognitive impairment in elderly people: Predisposing factors and implications for experimental drug studies. Drugs Aging 7:459, 1995
102. Inouye SK, Bogardus ST, Charpentier PA *et al*: A multicomponent intervention to prevent delirium in hospitalized older patients. N Engl J Med 340:669, 1999
103. O'Keefe ST, Ni Conchubhair A: Postoperative delirium in the elderly. Br J Anaesth 73:673, 1994
104. Moller JT and the ISOPCD Investigators: Long-term postoperative cognitive dysfunction in the elderly: ISPOCD1 study. Lancet 351:857, 1998
105. Johnson T, Monk T, Rasmussen LS *et al*: Postoperative cognitive dysfunction in middle-aged patients. Anesthesiology 96:1351, 2002
106. Culley DJ, Baxter M, Yukhananov R, Crosby G: The memory effects of general anesthesia persist for weeks in young and aged rats. Anesth Analg 96:1004, 2003
107. Culley DJ, Baxter MG, Yukhananov R, Crosby G: Long-term impairment of acquisition of a spatial memory task following isoflurane-nitrous oxide anesthesia in rats. Anesthesiology 100:309, 2004
108. Giugliano RP, Camargo CA Jr, Lloyd-Jones DM *et al*: Elderly patients receive less aggressive medical and invasive management of unstable angina: Potential impact of practice guidelines. Arch Intern Med 158:1113, 1998
109. Esterling BA, Kiecolt-Glaser JK, Glaser R: Psychosocial modulation of cytokine-induced natural killer cell activity in older adults. Psychosom Med 58:264, 1996
110. Talke P, Richardson CA, Scheinin M, Fisher DM: Postoperative pharmacokinetics and sympatholytic effects of dexmedetomidine. Anesth Analg 85:1136, 1997
111. Wong J, Song D, Blanshard H *et al*: Titration of isoflurane using BIS index improves early recovery of elderly patients undergoing orthopedic surgeries. Can J Anaesth 49:13, 2002

CHAPTER 46 ■ ANESTHESIA FOR AMBULATORY SURGERY

J. LANCE LICHTOR

KEY POINTS

1. All individuals, whether young or old, deserve a careful preoperative history and physical examination.
2. Patients of American Society of Anesthesiologists (ASA) physical status III or IV patients are appropriate candidates for ambulatory surgery, providing their systemic diseases are medically stable.
3. Particularly when midazolam is combined with fentanyl, adult patients can remain sleepy for up to 8 hours.
4. Most surgeons that direct their patient's choice of anesthetic choose regional anesthesia, yet delay in establishing a block and unpredictable success detract from their enthusiasm. Unnecessary delays can be obviated by performing the block preoperatively in a preoperative holding area.
5. For those patients who do receive spinal anesthesia, it is incumbent on the anesthesiologist and the facility to have follow-up with telephone calls to ensure no disabling symptoms of headache have developed.
6. When the bispectral index (BIS) or other guide of anesthetic depth is used, the difference between drugs and wake-up times may not be as great.
7. Nausea, with or without vomiting, is probably the most important factor contributing to a delay in discharge of patients and an increase in unanticipated admissions of both children and adults after ambulatory surgery.
8. Inhalation agents are associated with an increased risk of postoperative nausea and vomiting (PONV), particularly in the early stages of recovery.
9. Combination therapy is probably the most effective way to control PONV.
10. BIS or another guide of anesthetic depth can decrease the incidence of awareness.

The first ether anesthetic was given for ambulatory surgery. James M. Venable, a school teacher, had a small cystic tumor removed from the back of his neck by Dr. Crawford W. Long on the evening of March 30, 1842, after school was dismissed. The patient described the procedure in this way: "I commenced inhaling the ether before the operation was commenced and continued it until the operation was over. I did not feel the slightest pain from the operation and could not believe the tumor was removed until it was shown to me."[1] The modern concept of an independent surgical center for outpatients was popularized in the early 1970s by Wallace Reed. Since then, ambulatory surgery has been so well accepted that the majority of patients currently return home within 24 hours of an operative procedure. Because of this fact, anesthesiologists have had to refine the method of performing anesthesia so the anesthetic is not responsible for hindering a patient from returning to normal activities.

Cost savings partially prompted the original ambulatory centers. In the late 1960s, in Arizona, an uninsured barber's two children needed myringotomies, which in those days meant 2 days of hospitalization before the procedure.[2] The surgeons, astounded by how many haircuts they would receive instead of payment, began the cost-reducing measure of ambulatory surgery. Patient selection today is based on the desire to reduce cost while maintaining quality of care, so morbidity from the procedure or preexisting disease is no greater than if the patient were hospitalized. The length and complexity of operations performed in an ambulatory setting have increased, especially with the arrival of many new procedures. In the past, only patients with American Society of Anesthesiologists (ASA) physical status class I or II were candidates for ambulatory surgery. Today, patients classified as ASA physical status III or IV and whose systemic disease is medically stable are considered for procedures as outpatients. Preoperative screening, preferably in a clinic or by telephone, is essential both for reduction of patient anxiety and to ensure medical management is appropriate. Specific laboratory tests that should be performed before these operations are discussed elsewhere (see Chapter 18). In this chapter, we review the patients and procedures suitable for ambulatory surgery, as well as how to manage anesthesia for outpatients.

PLACE, PROCEDURES, AND PATIENT SELECTION

Ambulatory surgery occurs in a variety of settings. Some centers are within a hospital or in a freestanding satellite facility that is either part or independent of a hospital. Physicians' offices may also serve for procedures. The independent facilities are often for-profit and not located in rural or inner-city areas. Although freestanding, independent facilities continue to grow, although some consumers prefer care in units affiliated with hospitals.

Procedures appropriate for ambulatory surgery are those associated with postoperative care that is easily managed at home and with low rates of postoperative complications that require intensive physician or nursing management. The definition of a low rate of postoperative complication depends on the relative aggressiveness of the facility, surgeon, patient, and payer. For example, procedures that postoperatively result in intense pain may be treated with continuous regional techniques that are continued at home, whereas in other settings these procedures are limited to inpatients.

Lists of ambulatory procedures quickly become outdated simply because they exclude certain procedures that in a short time may become routine in ambulatory settings. In 1986, a patient would have been hospitalized for cholecystectomy but not for cataract extraction. When laparoscopic cholecystectomy was first introduced, a much higher percentage of patients required open cholecystectomy afterward, hence inpatient admission. Now, this procedure is commonly performed as an outpatient procedure, particularly when patients are generally healthy, live nearby, and when an uneventful operative procedure is anticipated. Procedure costs can be significantly reduced when a hospital stay is avoided.

Length of surgery is not a criterion for ambulatory procedures because there is little relationship between length of anesthesia and recovery. Patients undergoing longer procedures, though, should have their operations earlier in the day. The need for transfusion is also not a contraindication for ambulatory procedures. Some patients undergoing liposuction as outpatients, for example, are given autologous blood. Some surgeons, however, are uneasy about performing transfusion-requiring operations in an ambulatory setting because blood loss is a factor in unexpected hospital admission after surgery.[3]

Preterm infants (gestation age 37 weeks) who are younger than 50 weeks' postconceptual age should not be discharged from an ambulatory surgery center for at least 23 hours after a procedure because they are at risk of developing apnea even without a history of apnea. Although some have found that spinal anesthesia without the use of other drugs intraoperatively or postoperatively is not associated with apnea; one study of 62 premature and former-premature infants who underwent surgery using spinal anesthesia, postoperative apnea was seen in 5 of 55 premature infants.[4] In a pooled study of 255 former preterm infants who underwent general anesthesia, taken from eight previously published studies from four institutions, it was seen that apnea was strongly and inversely related to gestational and postconceptual age, apnea at home, and anemia (Fig. 46-1).[5] Yet, apnea varied dramatically in different institutions: it was highest in those institutions that used continuous recording devices, compared with those that used impedance pneumography and nursing observation. Nonetheless, apnea may not be apparent up to 12 hours after anesthesia. Anemia (hematocrit <30%) was also predictive of apnea, yet the number of patients with anemia was small and they tended to be younger.

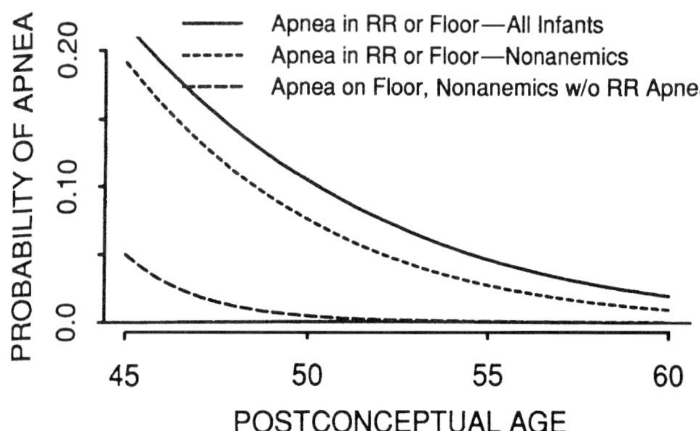

FIGURE 46-1. The risk for apnea after surgery is a function of gestational age, hematocrit, and the presence of apnea in the postanesthesia care unit (PACU). The predicted probability for apnea by weeks postconception is shown for all infants (*solid line*), nonanemic infants (*irregular line*), and infants who were not anemic and did not have apnea in the PACU (*broken line*).[5] (Reprinted with permission from Coté CJ, Zaslavsky A, Downes JJ *et al*: Postoperative apnea in former preterm infants after inguinal herniorrhaphy. A combined analysis. Anesthesiology 82:809, 1995.)

Some techniques have been tried to eliminate postoperative apnea in infants to allow them to go home on the same day of a procedure. When caffeine 10 mg/kg was administered immediately after induction of anesthesia, no preterm infants younger than or at 44 conceptual weeks of age developed postoperative apnea.[6]

At the other extreme of life, advanced age alone is not a reason to disallow surgery in an ambulatory setting. Age, however, does affect the pharmacokinetics of drugs. Even short-acting drugs such as midazolam and propofol have decreased clearance in older individuals. In addition, age may be a factor that affects the likelihood of unanticipated admission. In a study of 169 patients (of 3,152 patients), age was a factor that influenced unanticipated admission.[7] In a study of outcome after 6,000 procedures, some for patients older than 90 years, longer recovery time was not correlated with older age.[8] In a study of more than 6,000 patients undergoing ambulatory surgery, age was not a predictor of return; however, patients younger than 40 years of age who returned after ambulatory procedures were more likely to be treated in the emergency room, whereas patients older than 65 years were more likely to be hospitalized.[9] When age, gender, duration, and type of surgery were adjusted, hypertension, obesity, smoking, asthma, and gastroesophageal reflux were medical conditions that were associated with perioperative adverse events related to ambulatory anesthesia.[10] Admission, by itself, is not necessarily bad if it results in a better quality of care or uncovers the need for more extensive surgery. With proper patient selection for ambulatory procedures, which are usually elective, the incidence of readmission should be very low. Most medical problems that older individuals may experience after ambulatory procedures are not caused by age, but by specific organ dysfunction. For that rea-
1 son, all individuals, whether young or old, deserve a careful preoperative history and physical examination.

Whatever their age, ambulatory surgery is no longer restricted to patients of ASA physical status I or II. Patients of ASA physical status III or IV are appropriate candidates,
2 providing their systemic diseases are medically stable. In a review of ASA III patients who were compared with ASA I or II patients undergoing outpatient surgery, no significant increase in unplanned admissions, unplanned contact with health

professionals, and postoperative complications was found.[11] Certainly, not all life-threatening diseases have been studied as to how appropriate such patients with these diseases might be if they were to undergo ambulatory surgery. Yet, of those patients with such diseases who have been studied, the disease label itself does not seem to preclude an ambulatory surgical procedure. For example, in a review of 258 morbidly obese patients who underwent outpatient surgery, compared with patients who were not morbidly obese, there was not a greater incidence of unplanned admissions, minor complications, or unplanned contact with health care professionals.[12] Patients with diagnosed obstructive sleep apnea who underwent nonotorhinolaryngolic procedures were not found to have a greater risk for unanticipated hospital admission or for other adverse perioperative events.[13] Certainly, though, preexisting medical illness is a factor in both intraoperative difficulties and postoperative complications that require unexpected patient admission.[10] Patients who undergo ambulatory surgery should have someone to take them home and stay with them afterward to provide care. Before the procedure, the patient should receive information about the procedure itself, where it will be performed, laboratory studies that will be ordered, and dietary restrictions. The patient must understand that he or she will be going home on the day of surgery. The patient, or some responsible person, must ensure all instructions are carried out. Once at home, the patient must be able to tolerate the pain from the procedure, assuming adequate pain therapy is provided. The majority of patients are satisfied with early discharge, although a few prefer a longer stay in the hospital. Patients for certain procedures such as laparoscopic cholecystectomy or transurethral resection of the prostate should live close to the ambulatory facility because postoperative complications may require their prompt return. "Reasonable" distance and time for the patient to get care if problems arise are not easily defined. This issue must be addressed by each facility and by each patient, and depends on the type of surgery to be performed.

PREOPERATIVE EVALUATION AND REDUCTION OF PATIENT ANXIETY

Each outpatient facility should develop its own method of preoperative screening to be conducted before the day of surgery. The patient may visit the facility, or staff members may telephone to obtain necessary information about the patient, including a complete medical history of the patient and family, the medications the patient is taking, and the problems the patient or the patient's family may have had with previous anesthetics. In a study of the usefulness of a preoperative screening telephone call, patients were less likely to cancel surgery if they had been screened beforehand.[14] The screening may uncover the need for transportation to the facility or the need for child care. The process also provides the staff with an opportunity to remind patients of arrival time, suitable attire, and dietary restrictions (e.g., nothing to eat or drink after midnight, no jewelry or makeup). Staff members can determine whether a responsible person is available to escort the patient to and from the facility and care for the patient at home after surgery. The screening is the ideal time for the anesthesiologist to talk with the patient, but if that is not possible, the anesthesiologist may review the screening record to determine whether additional evaluation by other consultants is necessary and if laboratory tests must be obtained.

Automated history-taking may also prove beneficial during the screening of a patient. Computerized questionnaires or checklists with plastic overlays automate the taking of patient histories, flag problem areas, and suggest laboratory tests to be ordered. Such devices can also be used in a surgeon's office, both to guide the surgeon in the selection of laboratory tests and to serve as a medical summary for the anesthesiologist. Such devices are particularly useful to control the cost of preoperative testing. They enable test ordering based on information obtained from a patient's responses to health questions, thus eliminating requests for tests that are not warranted by history or physical examination.

Another important reason for preoperative screening is to help alleviate a patient's anxiety. Preoperative reassurance from nonanesthesia staff and the use of booklets also reduce preoperative anxiety. However, use of booklets is less effective than a preoperative visit by the anesthesiologist. Audiovisual instructions also reduce preoperative anxiety.

For children, information modeling and coping-based programs have been shown to reduce anxiety and enhance coping, particularly during the preoperative period. A child's anxiety seems to be maximally reduced if the effort to reduce it is made before surgery. However, behavior during induction, in the postanesthesia care unit (PACU), or postoperatively does not seem to be affected by this effort.

Upper Respiratory Tract Infection

A patient might be seen several days before surgery without any contraindication to the upcoming procedure. However, on the day of surgery, the patient may have an upper respiratory infection (URI). One study of 1,078 children 1 month to 18 years of age examined risk factors for adverse respiratory events in children with URIs.[15] The authors could find no difference in laryngospasm or bronchospasm if the children had active URIs, a URI within 4 weeks, or no symptoms. But children with active or recent URIs had more episodes of breath holding, incidences of desaturation <90%, and more respiratory events compared with children without symptoms (Fig. 46-2). Independent risk factors for adverse respiratory events in children with URIs included use of an endotracheal tube (versus use of a laryngeal mask airway [LMA] or facemask), a history of prematurity, a history of reactive airway disease, a history of paternal smoking, surgery involving the airway, presence of copious secretions, and nasal congestion. Generally, if a patient with a URI has a normal appetite, does not have a fever or an elevated respiratory rate, and does not appear toxic, it is probably safe to proceed with the planned procedure.

Restriction of Food and Liquids Before Ambulatory Surgery

To decrease the risk of aspiration of gastric contents, patients are routinely asked not to eat or drink anything (non per os [NPO] or "nothing by mouth") for at least 6 to 8 hours before surgery. However, prolonged fasting can be detrimental to a patient. One study actually showed that infants who fasted longer had greater drops in intraoperative blood pressure (Fig. 46-3).[16] No trial has shown that a shortened fluid fast increases the risk of aspiration. Gastric volumes are actually less when patients are allowed to drink some fluids before surgery. Admittedly, though, the majority of studies have not been specifically performed in individuals who are at an increased risk for aspiration. An excellent review of this topic has been published.[17]

The ASA has published practice guidelines for preoperative fasting.[18] The guidelines allow a patient to have a light meal up to 6 hours before an elective procedure. In one survey of anesthesiologists' practice in an outpatient setting based on the practice guidelines, only 35% of those surveyed said that

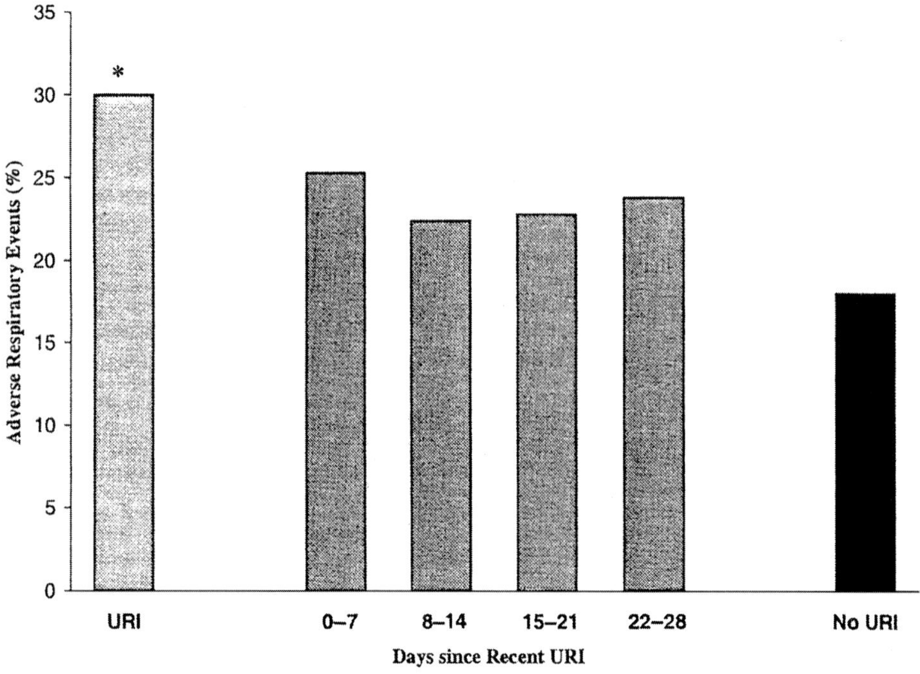

FIGURE 46-2. Adverse respiratory events are similar between children with an upper respiratory infection (URI) and a recent URI, and this similarity persists for at least 4 weeks after the URI.[15] *$P < .05$ vs. no URI. (Reprinted with permission from Tait AR, Malviya S, Voepel-Lewis T *et al*: Risk factors for perioperative adverse respiratory events in children with upper respiratory tract infections. Anesthesiology 95:299, 2001.)

their institution had a policy that would allow a light breakfast 6 hours before elective surgery, although 65% said they would proceed without delay.[19] The guidelines support a fasting period for clear liquids of 2 hours for all patients. Coffee is not transparent but is free of particulate matter and is accepted as a clear liquid. Coffee drinkers should follow fasting guidelines but should be encouraged to drink coffee prior to their procedure because physical signs of withdrawal (e.g., headache) can easily occur.[20] Some surgeons are not aware of these guidelines, so some patients are still fasting for longer periods of time. There is some evidence that shorter periods of preoperative fasting are accompanied by less postoperative nausea and vomiting (PONV). Yet, it is unclear whether rehydration during surgery is equivalent to a shorter fast before surgery in relation to PONV.

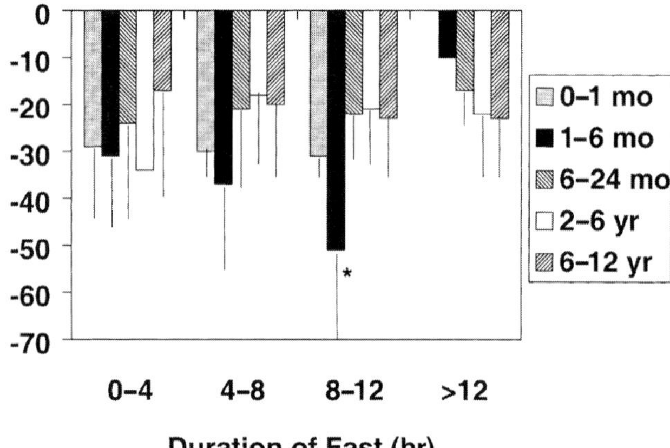

FIGURE 46-3. Blood pressure is lower in children 1 to 6 months of age who fast more than 8 hours, compared with those who fast for less than 4 hours.[16] Illustrated are changes in systolic blood pressure from baseline to the time when 2 minimum alveolar concentration halothane was reached in 250 infants and children. *$P < .05$ vs. 0- to 4-hour fasting group. (Reprinted with permission from Friesen RH, Wurl JL, Friesen RM: Duration of preoperative fast correlates with arterial blood pressure response to halothane in infants. Anesth Analg 95:1572, 2002.)

To ensure patients are optimally medically managed before their outpatient surgery, given the fact that clear liquids can be taken up to 2 hours before surgery, patients should be encouraged to take their chronic medications.

MANAGING THE ANESTHETIC: PREMEDICATION

The outpatient is not that different from the inpatient undergoing surgery. In both, premedication is useful to control anxiety, postoperative pain, nausea, and vomiting, and to reduce the risk of aspiration during induction of anesthesia. Because the outpatient is going home on the day of surgery, the drugs given before anesthesia should not hinder recovery afterward. Most premedicants do not prolong recovery when given in appropriate doses for appropriate indications, although drug effects may be apparent even after discharge.

Controlling Anxiety

Clearly, some patients scheduled to undergo surgery are anxious, and they are probably anxious long before they come to the outpatient area. However, not all outpatients are anxious. For example, insomnia and anxiety are related, and in a study of sleep characteristics of outpatients before elective surgery, no differences in sleep quality between patients before surgery and a community control group was seen.[21] Indeed, physicians often tend to overestimate the level of anxiety that patients are actually experiencing.[22] Some operations can certainly generate more anxiety than others. The need to remove dentures is also associated with increased preoperative stress. If in doubt about patient anxiety, ask the patient: visual analog scales are also easy to use and are an accurate tool to assess anxiety.[23]

Like adults, children should have some idea of what to expect during a procedure. But much of a child's anxiety before surgery concerns separation from a parent or parents. A child is more likely to demonstrate problematic behavior from the time of separation from parents to induction of anesthesia if a procedure has not been explained preoperatively. Parents and children need to be involved in some preoperative discussions together so the anxiety of the parents is not transmitted to the child. The transmission of anxiety is at least as problematic as is the separation itself (e.g., experiences of children being left with baby-sitters). If the parents are calm and can effectively manage the physical transfer to a warm and playful anesthesiologist or nurse, premedication is not necessary. Semisedation may be awkward, and recovery after premedication may be prolonged. If a child is accompanied by a parent during the induction of anesthesia, the child's anxiety can be reduced.

Although historically many classes of drugs (e.g. barbiturates, antihistamines) have been used to reduce anxiety and induce sedation, benzodiazepines are currently the drugs most commonly used. Propofol also has some anxiety reduction properties.

Benzodiazepines

Midazolam is the benzodiazepine most commonly used preoperatively. It can be used intravenously and orally. In adults, it can be used to control preoperative anxiety and, during a procedure alone or in combination with other drugs, for intravenous sedation. For children, oral midazolam in doses as small as 0.25 mg/kg produces effective sedation and reduces anxiety.[24] With this dose, most children can be effectively separated from their parents after 10 minutes and satisfactory sedation can be maintained for 45 minutes.

Fatigue associated with the effects of anxiolytics may delay or prevent the discharge of patients on the day of surgery, although more frequently patients are not discharged because of the effects of the operation. With regard to anesthesia effects, patients normally stay in the hospital not because they are too sleepy but because they are nauseous. In adults, particularly
3 when midazolam is combined with fentanyl, adult patients can remain sleepy for up to 8 hours (Fig. 46-4).[25] Although children may be sleepier after oral midazolam, discharge times are not affected.[26]

Oral diazepam is useful to control anxiety in adult patients, either the day before surgery or the day of surgery and before an intravenous line has been inserted. Indeed, in one study, investigators believed that after 5 mg oral diazepam, it was easier to insert an intravenous catheter.[27]

At proper doses, neither midazolam nor diazepam place patients at any additional risk for cardiovascular and respiratory depression. Decreased oxygen saturation has also been reported after injection of midazolam. Routine administration of supplemental oxygen with or without continuous monitoring of arterial oxygenation is recommended whenever benzodiazepines are given intravenously. This precaution is important not only when midazolam is given as a premedicant, but also when it is used alone or with other drugs for conscious sedation.The potential for amnesia after premedication is another concern, especially for patients undergoing ambulatory surgery. Anterograde amnesia certainly occurs, but benzodiazepines actually facilitate retrograde memory.[28] For midazolam, amnesia is a function of serum concentration and the effects on memory are separate from the effects on sedation.[29] In addition, amnesia is not simply an effect of drug administration, but, among other factors, it is also a function of stimulus intensity.

Opioids and Nonsteroidal Analgesics

Opioids can be administered preoperatively to sedate patients, control hypertension during tracheal intubation, and decrease pain before surgery. Meperidine (but not morphine or fentanyl) is sometimes helpful in controlling shivering in the operating room (OR) or PACU, although treatment is usually instituted at the time of shivering and not in anticipation of the event. The effectiveness of opioids in relieving anxiety is controversial and probably nonexistent, particularly in adults.

Opioids are useful in controlling hypertension during tracheal intubation. Opioid premedication prevents increases in systolic pressure in a dose-dependent fashion. After tracheal intubation, systolic, diastolic, and mean arterial blood pressures sometimes decrease below baseline values.

Preoperative administration of opioids or nonsteroidal anti-inflammatory drugs (NSAIDs) is also useful for controlling pain in the early postoperative period. Controlled-release oxycodone 10 mg, for example, when given before surgery, was

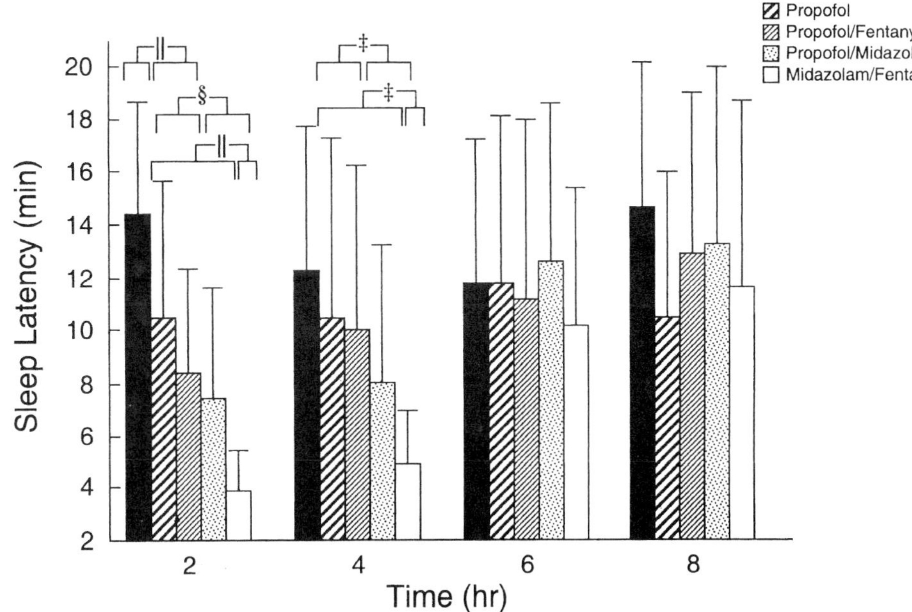

FIGURE 46-4. Patients can remain sleepy after receiving midazolam and fentanyl, even 8 hours after drug administration.[25] The abscissa represents time (hours) after sedation. The ordinate represents sleep latency (i.e., time to fall asleep). Data are the mean time to fall asleep. An individual is sleepier if less time is required to fall asleep. Subjects receiving the midazolam and fentanyl combination were much sleepier than the same subjects receiving other types of sedation. Although not seen in the figure, up to 8 hours after sedation, some subjects were still sleepier than before they received drug. (Reprinted with permission from Lichtor JL, Alessi R, Lane BS: Sleep tendency as a measure of recovery after drugs used for ambulatory surgery. Anesthesiology 96:878, 2002.)

effective in managing pain after laparoscopic tubal ligation surgery and was even associated with less PONV.[30] Celecoxib, up to 400 mg, is effective in reducing postoperative pain.[31] When celecoxib 200 mg was compared with rofecoxib 50 mg, rofecoxib was more effective.[32] Ibuprofen or acetaminophen can be given rectally to children around the time of induction. Nonsteroidal analgesics are associated with less nausea compared with narcotics.[33] If rectal acetaminophen is used, an initial loading dose of 40 mg/kg is appropriate; subsequent doses of 20 mg/kg every 6 hours can be used.[34]

Preoperative sedation is not needed for every patient. The following is our practice when patients require drugs to relieve anxiety. For the patient who has been seen at least 24 hours before a scheduled procedure and expresses a desire for medication to relieve anxiety or has anxiety that cannot be relieved with comforting, oral diazepam, 2 to 5 mg 70 kg^{-1} body weight, is prescribed for the night before and at 6:00 AM on the day of surgery (even if surgery is scheduled for 1:00 PM or later). Patients seen for the first time in the preoperative holding area who seem to need medication, midazolam, 0.01 mg/kg, is administered intravenously, or the patient is brought into the OR and propofol, 0.7 mg/kg, is injected intravenously. For children, when necessary, oral midazolam, 0.5 mg/kg, is administered in the preoperative holding area.

Controlling the Risk of Aspiration

Patients who undergo ambulatory surgery may be at some small risk for aspiration of gastric contents, although this risk is no greater than for inpatients. At greater risk for aspiration are pregnant or morbidly obese patients or patients with hiatal hernia. Preoperative anxiety probably has no effect on gastric acidity for individuals without a history of duodenal ulcer. H_2 receptor antagonists, such as cimetidine and ranitidine, omeprazole, sodium citrate, or metoclopramide, can be used to control the risk of aspiration.

INTRAOPERATIVE MANAGEMENT: CHOICE OF ANESTHETIC METHOD

There are several choices among anesthetic methods: general anesthesia, regional anesthesia, and local anesthesia. Regional and local anesthesia can be used with or without sedation. Except for obstetric cases for which regional anesthesia may be safer than general anesthesia, all three types are otherwise equally safe. However, even for experienced anesthesiologists, there is a failure rate associated with regional anesthesia.

Certainly, some procedures are possible only with a general anesthetic. For others, the preference of patients, surgeons, or anesthesiologists may determine selection. Cost may be a factor: the cost of sedation is usually less than the cost of a general anesthetic. Time to recovery may also influence the choice of anesthetic method. For example, in a study of adult patients undergoing strabismus surgery with either propofol sedation and local anesthesia or general anesthesia with inhalation agents, time to leave the hospital was much less after sedation.[35] For some procedures such as arthroscopy, patients might prefer a regional anesthetic simply because they are curious.[36] Postoperative pain is less after regional anesthesia, and this is discussed in more detail later in this section. Also, with regional anesthesia or sedation, some of the side effects of general anesthesia can be avoided, although no form of medical care is without side effects. Whenever drugs are given that affect memory, patients might have complaints that they do not remember after the procedure. In addition, with regional anesthesia, more time is required to place a block than it takes to induce a general anesthetic, and the success rate with regional anesthesia is not 100%. In one survey of orthopaedic surgeons, the majority of surgeons that direct their patient's choice of anesthetic choose regional anesthesia, yet delay in establishing a block and unpredictable success detracted from their enthusiasm (Fig. 46-5).[37] In most instances after regional anesthesia, PACU time is shorter, and patients can frequently bypass the first phase of the PACU.

One adverse effect associated with spinal anesthesia is headache, but headaches are also experienced by patients after general anesthesia. Especially when smaller spinal needles are used, the incidence of headache after either technique may be similar. In one study, after either method of anesthesia, incidence of headache ranged between 11 and 15%.[38] In that study, backache was higher (26%) after spinal anesthesia than general anesthesia (4%). However, incidence of sore throat (24%) and nausea (22%) was higher after general anesthesia than spinal anesthesia (6% for both). Larger studies of patients undergoing ambulatory surgery are needed that compare sedation with regional and general anesthesia.

Regional Techniques

Local anesthesia and regional anesthesia have long been used for ambulatory surgery. As early as 1963, for example, 56% of ambulatory procedures were performed with the use of these techniques.[39] Regional techniques commonly used for ambulatory surgery, in addition to spinal and epidural anesthesia, include local infiltration, brachial plexus, and other peripheral nerve blocks, and intravenous regional anesthesia. General anesthesia can also be supplemented with regional nerve blocks.

Performing a block takes longer than inducing general anesthesia, and the incidence of failure is higher. Unnecessary delays can be obviated by performing the block beforehand in
4 a preoperative holding area. Because a postoperative nursing intervention, usually associated with general anesthesia, is associated with a 27- to 45-minute delay, the increased setup time may be associated with a shorter time to discharge.[40] Postoperative pain control is best with regional techniques.

An occasional patient may experience syncope when the needle for the regional block is inserted. In the experience of oral and maxillofacial surgeons in Massachusetts in the late 1990s, 1 of 160 patients fainted when local anesthesia was injected.[41] When sedation accompanies local anesthesia injection, the incidence of syncope is reduced. Patients usually experience less postoperative pain when local or regional anesthesia has been used. Patients may still have a numb extremity (e.g., after a brachial plexus block) but otherwise meet all criteria for discharge. In such instances, the extremity must be well protected with a sling, and patients must be cautioned to protect against injury because they are without normal sensations that would warn them of vulnerability. Reassurance that sensation will return should be provided.

Spinal Anesthesia

Spinal anesthesia is useful for ambulatory procedures in children born prematurely. The procedure is best performed with the child in the sitting position, head supported and somewhat extended, to prevent occlusion of the airway. Bupivacaine 0.5% isobaric, 1 mg/kg of tetracaine, 1 mg/kg, mixed with an equal volume of 10% dextrose, is injected into the L4–L5 interspace with a 22-gauge Quincke needle, 3.75 cm long. It is useful to apply a eutectic mixture of lidocaine and prilocaine (EMLA)

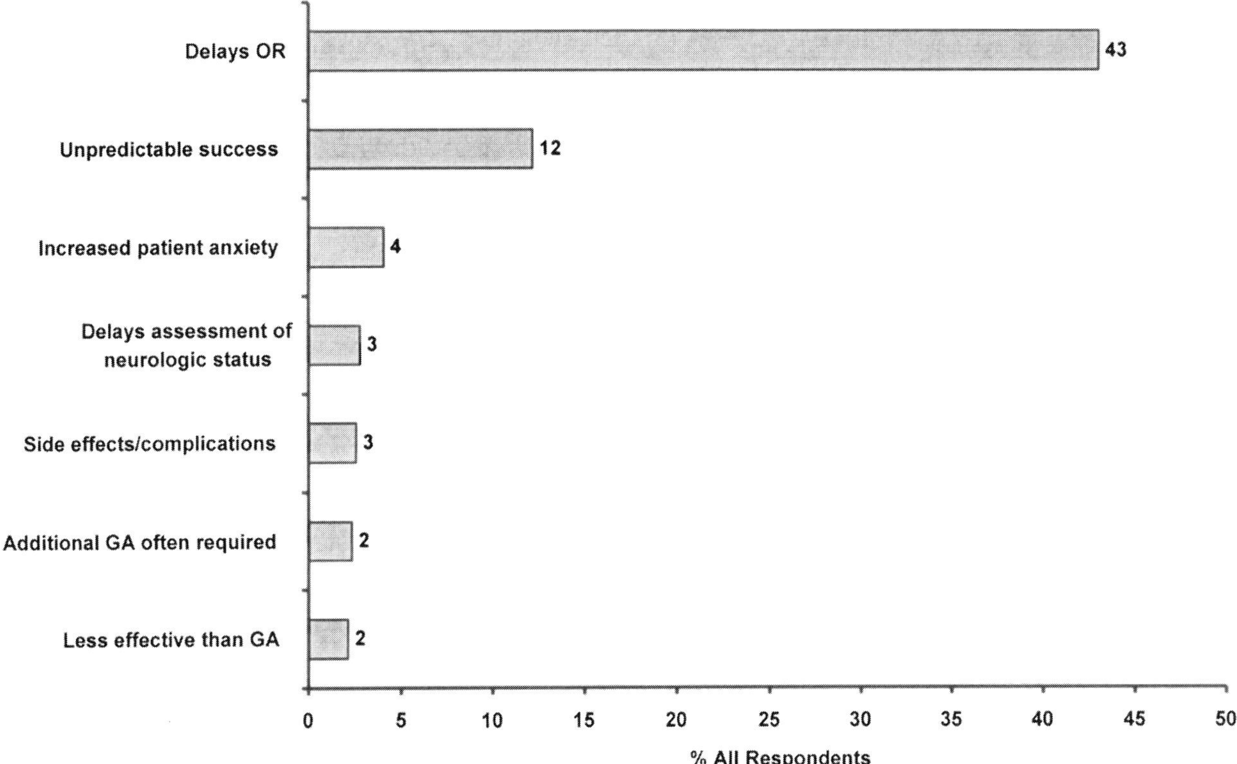

FIGURE 46-5. Operating room (OR) delays are the major reasons orthopaedic surgeons do not favor regional anesthesia.[37] GA, general anesthesia. (Reprinted with permission from Oldman M, McCartney CJ, Leung A *et al*: A survey of orthopedic surgeons' attitudes and knowledge regarding regional anesthesia. Anesth Analg 98:1486, 2004.)

patch to the lumbar puncture site 1 hour before the procedure. Because a leg raised may drive the spinal higher, the child must be kept flat when, for example, the Bovie pad is placed on the back. Hypotension is less common after spinal anesthesia in infants than adults, and when it occurs, typically the spinal is high. An intravenous line can be started in a lower extremity after the spinal is in place, the extremity is anesthetized, and vasodilatation is present. Spinal anesthesia with a local anesthetic alone may not last long enough. In one study, when clonidine was added to bupivacaine, the length of spinal block increased from an average of 67 minutes to 111 minutes after 1 mcg/kg clonidine (Fig. 46-6).[42] See the previous discussion as to whether a neonate should be discharged home on the same day of a spinal anesthetic.

The use of spinal needles with pencil point, noncutting tips has prompted a resurgence of spinal anesthesia for ambulatory

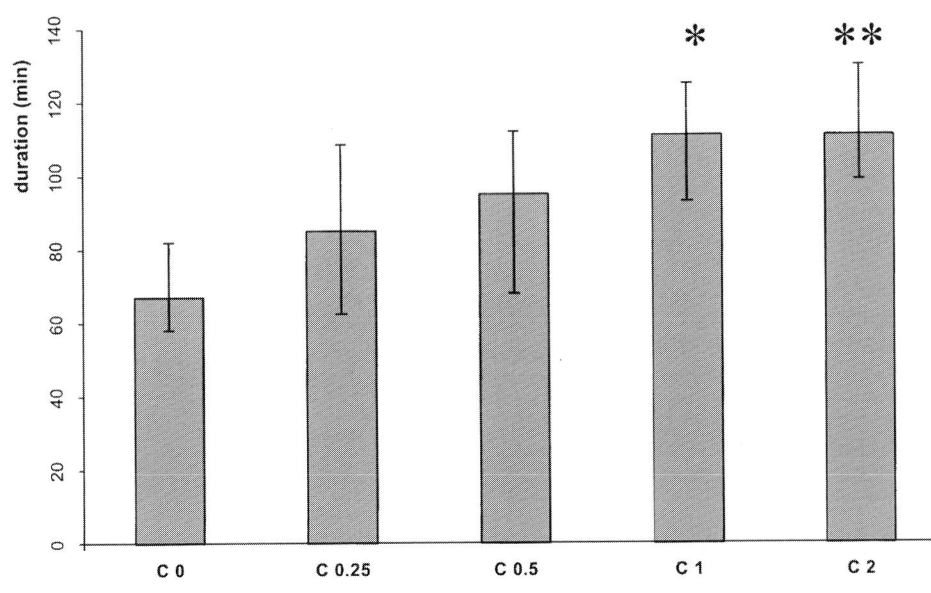

FIGURE 46-6. Clonidine prolongs spinal anesthesia in newborns.[42] Illustrated is the median duration of spinal block with 25 to 75% confidence intervals. C 0, spinal with 0.5% isobaric bupivacaine, 1 mg/kg; C 0.25, bupivacaine with 0.25 mcg/kg clonidine; C 0.5, C 1, and C 2, bupivacaine with 0.5, 1, and 2 mcg/kg clonidine, respectively. $^{*}P < .003$; $^{**}P < .006$ vs. C 0. (Reprinted with permission from Rochette A, Raux O, Troncin R *et al*: Clonidine prolongs spinal anesthesia in newborns: A prospective dose-ranging study. Anesth Analg 98:56, 2004.)

surgery in adults. Epidural or spinal anesthesia is suitable for pelvic, lower abdominal, and lower-extremity surgery, but not for laparoscopic procedures, because most people have difficulty breathing in the head-down position with the abdomen distended with air. Motor block of the legs with either technique may delay a patient's ability to walk. However, the use of a short-acting local anesthetic through an epidural catheter, will minimize this problem while allowing the duration of anesthesia to match the sometimes unpredictable duration of surgery. Nausea is much less frequent after epidural or spinal anesthesia than after general anesthesia.

Different drugs and drug concentrations have been used for spinal anesthesia. Lidocaine and mepivacaine are ideal for ambulatory surgery because of their short duration of action, although lidocaine use has been problematic because of transient neurologic symptoms. In one study comparing patients who underwent knee arthroscopy with either 45 mg 1.5% mepivacaine or 60 mg 2% lidocaine, 22% of patients who received lidocaine had transient neurologic symptoms (back pain or dysesthesia).[43] The symptoms were treated by NSAIDs and resolved within 5 days; no patients who received mepivacaine developed transient neurologic symptoms. Chloroprocaine spinal anesthesia has rapid onset; in a study of nonpatient volunteers, after 40 mg 2-chloroporcaine (2-CP), the study participants could void after 110 minutes.[44] In that study, when 20 μg of fentanyl was included, regression time to L1 was lengthened and tourniquet tolerance was improved, although overall block length was minimally affected. Forty milligrams of preservative-free 2-CP produces a similar onset time and block height when compared with 40 mg lidocaine.[45] In that study, transient neurologic symptoms occurred in seven of eight volunteers who received lidocaine and in none of the volunteers who received 2-CP. Low-dose bupivacaine is useful for some outpatient procedures such as inguinal herniorrhaphy; yet, in one study, patients could not be discharged until almost 7 hours after block initiation.[46]

Although headache is a common complication of lumbar puncture, smaller-gauge needles result in a lower incidence of postdural puncture headache. For those patients who do receive spinal anesthesia, it is incumbent on the anesthesiologist
5 and the facility to have follow-up with telephone calls to ensure no disabling symptoms of headache have developed. If the headache does not respond to bed rest, analgesics, and oral hydration, the patient must return to the hospital for a course of caffeine intravenous therapy or an immediate epidural blood patch.

Spinal anesthesia should not be avoided in ambulatory surgery patients simply because they may be more active postoperatively than inpatients. Bed rest does not reduce the frequency of headache. Indeed, early ambulation may decrease the incidence. Further study is needed to assess the relative risk–benefit ratio of spinal anesthesia as a technique for the ambulatory surgery patient.

Epidural and Caudal Anesthesia

Epidural anesthesia takes longer to perform than spinal anesthesia. Onset with spinal anesthesia is more rapid, although recovery may be the same with either technique. In one study of patients undergoing knee arthroscopy, spinal anesthesia with small-dose lidocaine and fentanyl was compared with 3% 2-CP administered in the epidural space: intraoperative conditions, discharge characteristics and times, and recovery profiles were similar.[47] Also, failure rates for the two techniques, although low, were the same. Some studies suggest that bicarbonate can be added to solutions for faster onset of epidural anesthesia. An advantage of the epidural block is that it can be performed outside the OR, and, after the surgical procedure is completed, the problem of postdural puncture headache is usually avoided.

Caudal anesthesia is a form of epidural anesthesia commonly used in children before surgery below the umbilicus as a supplement to general anesthesia and to control postoperative pain. Bupivacaine, 0.175 to 0.25%, or ropivacaine 0.2%, in a volume of 0.5 to 1.0 mL/kg, may be used; a safe maximal dose is 2.5 mg/kg. Epinephrine, 1:200,000, when added to the anesthetic solution, may allow earlier detection of intravenous, rather than epidural, injection. Other additives useful, albeit controversial, for increasing duration of blockade include narcotics, ketamine, clonidine, and neostigmine.[48] The block may be more difficult in children, particularly those who weigh more than 10 kg and are obese, if landmarks for the block are difficult to locate. The block is usually administered while the child is anesthetized. After injection, the depth of general anesthesia can be reduced. Because of better pain control after a caudal block, children can usually ambulate earlier and be discharged sooner than without a caudal block. Pain control and discharge times are no different whether the caudal block is placed before surgery or after it was completed.

Nerve Blocks

Nerve blocks control pain during a surgical procedure; however, certain procedures are quite painful, and hospitalization can be required to control the pain. An exciting new area in outpatient surgery is where, instead of a needle, a catheter is placed that is then left in after the operation. Paravertebral somatic nerve block can be used for breast surgery followed by a continuous perineural infusion of local anesthetic at home for 24 to 48 hours.[49] Perineural catheters in the sciatic nerve through the popliteal fossa can be used to control pain after foot surgery.[50] Interscalene perineural catheters have been used for patients undergoing moderately painful shoulder surgery.[51] Continuous cervical paravertebral block may also be useful for analgesia after shoulder surgery: early return of motor function in the hand, wrist and elbow, which is seen with this block, may be useful for recovery after shoulder surgery (Fig. 46-7).[52] Patients must be taught about pump function, understand signs of

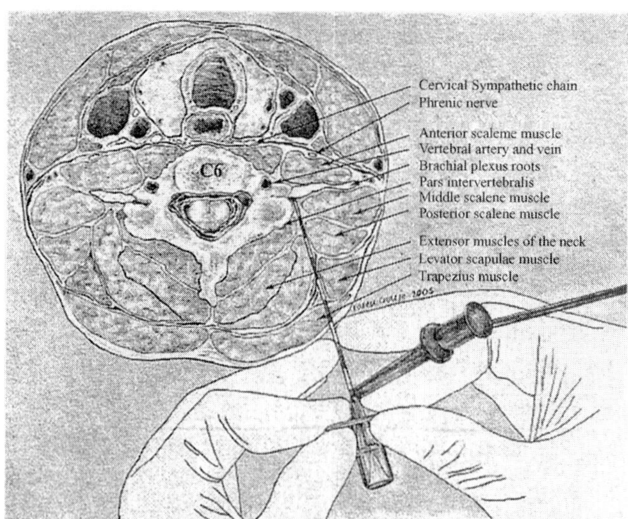

FIGURE 46-7. A continuous cervical paravertebral block can be placed prior to induction of anesthesia for shoulder surgery and can be left in place for up to 7 days after surgery.[52] The figure shows the path that the sheathed Tuohy needle follows, using the posterior approach, from the skin, and then between the trapezius and levator scapulae muscles to the paravertebral space. (Reprinted with permission from Boezaart AP, De Beer JF, Nell ML: Early experience with continuous cervical paravertebral block using a stimulating catheter. Reg Anesth Pain Med 28:406, 2003.)

local anesthesia toxicity, and have someone else at home who can provide assistance. In addition, the patients must be able to communicate with someone by phone. The number of patients who have been sent home with catheters is not large. More study is needed, in order to demonstrate patient safely.

In a survey mailed to members of the Society for Ambulatory Anesthesia in 2001, there was shown to be widespread use of axillary and interscalene blocks for surgery in the upper extremity, and ankle and femoral blocks for lower-extremity surgery.[53] Using different nerve blocks improves postoperative patient satisfaction: PONV and postoperative pain are less. Costs are also less. When nerve block was used for anterior cruciate legament repair reconstruction, one nonrandomized study of outpatients in a university setting showed that PACU admissions, hospital cost, and unexpected hospital admission were all reduced.[54] For knee arthroscopy, psoas compartment block or spinal anesthesia is superior to general anesthesia in terms of postoperative pain management and patient satisfaction.[55] After more complex knee surgery, patients who received femoral-sciatic nerve block required fewer nursing interventions for pain; and, if patients received either that block or only a femoral nerve block, unplanned hospital admissions were less compared with patients who underwent the procedure without a block.[56] In a comparison of patients who underwent either infraclavicular brachial plexus block or general anesthesia for upper-extremity surgery, after brachial plexus block more patients were able to bypass phase I PACU care, had less pain on PACU arrival, and were discharged home much sooner (Fig. 46-8).[57]

Sedation and Analgesia

Many patients who undergo surgery with local or regional anesthesia prefer to be sedated and to have no recollection of the procedure. Sedation is important, in part, because injection with local anesthetics can be painful and lying on a hard OR table can be uncomfortable. Levels of sedation vary from light, during which a patient's consciousness is minimally depressed, to very deep, in which protective reflexes are partially blocked and response to physical stimulation or verbal command may not be appropriate. When patients are unsuitable for outpatient general anesthesia, surgery can often be performed if local or regional anesthesia is supplemented with conscious sedation. However, serious risk, such as death, is probably no different after sedation than after general anesthesia. Children who have surgery usually will not remain immobile unless they are deeply sedated or receive general anesthesia.

For adults, the proper dose might be selected by having the patient control dosage. Yet, at least for ambulatory surgical procedures, patient-controlled sedation is not as popular as patient-controlled analgesia. This may be due to the fact that a member of the anesthesia care team must be continuously present anyway.

General Anesthesia

The drugs selected for general anesthesia determine how long patients stay in the PACU after surgery, and for some patients, whether they can be discharged to go home.

Induction

The popularity of propofol as an induction agent for outpatient surgery in part relates to its half-life: the elimination half-life of propofol is 1 to 3 hours, shorter than that of methohexital (6 to 8 hours) or thiopental (10 to 12 hours). Although the effect of drugs given for induction seems to be transient, these drugs can depress psychomotor performance for several hours. When induction doses of propofol and thiopental were

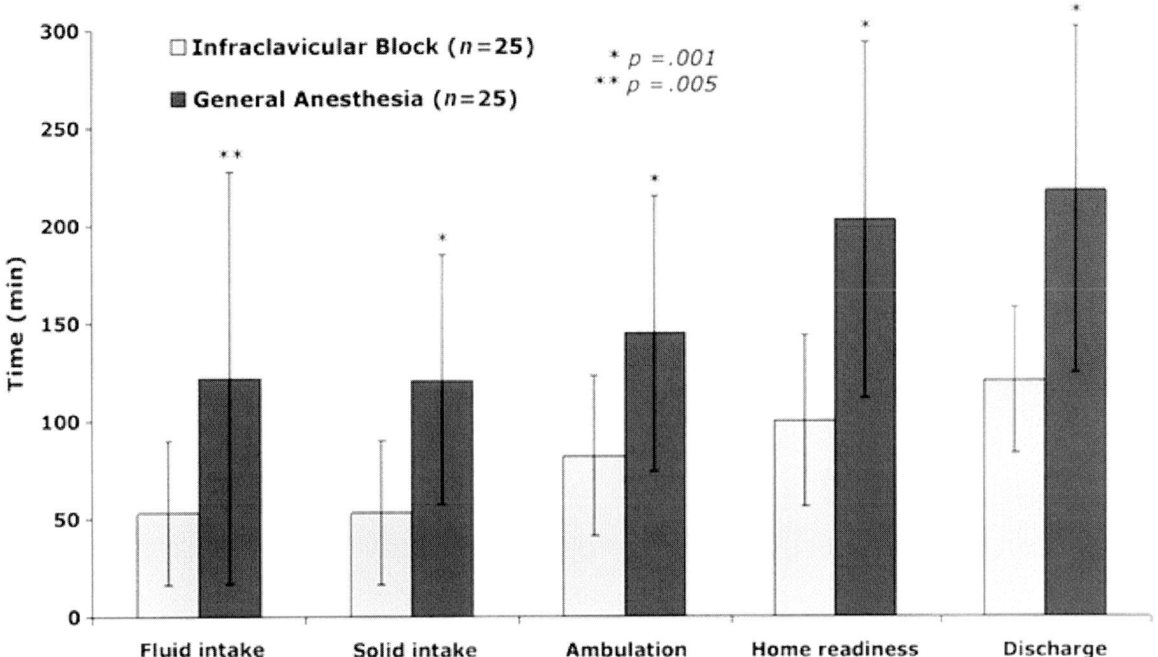

FIGURE 46-8. Recovery was faster when an infraclavicular brachial plexus block with a short-acting local anesthetic was used, compared with general anesthesia and wound infiltration for outpatients undergoing hand and wrist surgery.[57] Times are calculated from the end of anesthesia. (Reprinted with permission from Hadzic A, Arliss J, Kerimoglu B *et al*: A comparison of infraclavicular nerve block versus general anesthesia for hand and wrist day-case surgeries. Anesthesiology 101:127, 2004.)

compared, psychomotor impairment in patients was evident for up to 5 hours after thiopental, but only for 1 hour after propofol.[58]

Pain on injection can be a problem with propofol. Pain is more likely on injection into dorsal hand veins and is minimized if forearm or larger antecubital veins are used. Some individuals, though, experience pain if the drug is injected into proximal larger veins. Nonetheless, thrombophlebitis does not appear to be a problem after intravenous administration of this agent, whereas it can be evident after thiopental. Intravenous lidocaine 0.2 mg/kg or 1% lidocaine mixed with propofol in a 10:1 volume ratio can be used to decrease the incidence and severity of pain.

Most children and some adults prefer not to have an intravenous catheter inserted before the start of anesthesia. Sevoflurane has a relatively low blood-gas partition coefficient and the speed of induction is similar to, albeit somewhat slower than, that of propofol. Induction with sevoflurane can be hastened when the patient is told to breathe out to residual volume, then take a vital capacity breath through a primed anesthesia circuit, and then hold the breath.

Parental presence is becoming more accepted during induction of anesthesia in children, even though scientific evidence of its advantages is not conclusive. Some studies show that children are less upset and have fewer behavioral changes after surgery if a parent is present during induction. Others have suggested that parents can become upset when they see their anesthetized child, who appears to be dead, albeit breathing and with a beating heart. Separation anxiety on the part of the parents is probably no different if the child is awake or asleep.

For short procedures, some patients may not require neuromuscular-blocking drugs; others may need brief paralysis (e.g., with succinylcholine) to facilitate tracheal intubation. Nondepolarizing drugs can be used to facilitate intubation and also during the procedure. Nondepolarizing drugs such as rapacuronium or rocuronium have rapid onset times that are similar to those with succinylcholine. Of course, paralysis is not needed to insert an endotracheal tube: drug combinations such as propofol, alfentanil, and lidocaine obviate the need for paralysis.[59] Succinylcholine should be used with caution in children because of the possibility of cardiac arrest related to malignant hyperthermia or unsuspected muscular dystrophy, particularly Duchenne's disease.

Maintenance

Although many factors affect the choice of agents for maintenance of anesthesia, two primary concerns for ambulatory anesthesia are speed of wake-up and incidence of postoperative nausea and vomiting.

Anesthesia Maintenance and Wake-Up Times. Time to recovery may be measured by various criteria; however, for an ambulatory center, a patient may be considered awake when able to leave the center. Actual discharge from an ambulatory center, though, may depend on administrative issues, such as a written order from a surgeon or anesthesiologist. The time necessary before a patient can be taken from the OR after completion of surgery, or a patient's ability to skip the PACU and go directly to a step-down unit, may be directly related to the anesthetic and result in cost savings for an institution. Does choice of maintenance agent affect recovery after anesthesia? Propofol, desflurane, and sevoflurane have characteristics that make them ideal for maintenance of anesthesia for ambulatory surgery. Propofol has a short half-life and, when used as a maintenance agent, results in rapid recovery and few side effects. Desflurane and sevoflurane, halogenated ether anesthetics with low blood-gas partition coefficients, seem to be ideal for general anesthesia for ambulatory surgery. Sevoflurane, unlike desflurane, facilitates a smooth inhalation induction of anesthesia, the preferred technique to ensure rapid recovery of children in ambulatory surgery centers. For children who receive either sevoflurane or halothane, or halothane and then desflurane, for induction and maintenance of anesthesia, recovery times are significantly shorter after sevoflurane or desflurane.

It is important to distinguish between wake-up time and discharge time. For example, in one study of laparoscopic surgery, patients emerged from anesthesia with desflurane and nitrous oxide significantly faster than after propofol or sevoflurane and nitrous oxide, although the ability to sit up, stand, and tolerate fluids and the time to fitness for discharge were no
6 different.[60] When the bispectral index (BIS) or other guide of anesthetic depth is used, the difference between drugs and wake-up times may not be as great. Conversely, if fast wake-up times can translate to bypass of phase I, there may be cost savings.

Intraoperative Management of Postoperative Nausea and Vomiting. Nausea, with or without vomiting, is probably the most important factor contributing to a delay in discharge
7 of patients and an increase in unanticipated admissions of both children and adults after ambulatory surgery. Patients hate vomiting. In one survey taken before surgery, for example, patients rated vomiting as most undesirable and, if given $100, would spend the most money on that problem to prevent it (Fig. 46-9).[61] Women, especially those who are pregnant, have a higher incidence of PONV. Other risk factors include a previous history of motion sickness or postanesthetic emesis; surgery within 1 to 7 days of the menstrual cycle; not smoking; and procedures such as laparoscopy, lithotripsy, major breast surgery, and ear, nose, or throat surgery. The greater the number of risk factors, the greater risk for nausea or vomiting after surgery.[62] Inhalation agents are associated with an increased
8 risk of PONV, particularly in the early stages of recovery; postoperative narcotic use is associated with PONV more than 2 hours after surgery.[63]

The vomiting pathway starts peripherally, where emetogens through enterochromaffin cells in the GI tract and/or other sensory neurons activate vagal afferents to the group of brainstem nuclei in the area postrema, the nucleus tractus solitarius, and the dorsal motor nucleus of the vagus. This area in the brain is otherwise known as the vomiting center. Although the pathways for vomiting are not completely understood, the area postrema is highly vascular, lacks a complete blood-brain barrier, and has receptors for neurotransmitters and hormones.[64] Receptor antagonists, specifically selective serotonin antagonists (ondansetron, dolasetron, and granisetron), have been shown to have similar efficacy to help alleviate this condition. Dopamine antagonists, antihistamines, and anticholinergic drugs are useful and are generally less expensive, but are associated with extensive side effects. NK_1 receptor antagonists may also be useful to control PONV. At the time of writing, although aprepitant, an NK_1 receptor antagonist, has been shown to be more effective than standard therapy (ondansetron and dexamethasone) after highly emetogenic chemotherapy (Fig. 46-10),[65] no publication has demonstrated the drug's effectiveness to control PONV. Other therapies useful in controlling PONV include acupuncture (Fig. 46-11),[66] supplemental fluid therapy,[67] clonidine (perhaps in part because it decreases anesthesia requirement),[68] and dexamethasone.[69,70] In one study, acupuncture therapy was effective in controlling both PONV and postoperative pain.[71]

Combination therapy is probably the most effective way to
9 control PONV. In one study in children, for example, low-dose ondansetron and dexamethasone was more effective than high-dose ondansetron in reducing PONV.[72] In another study, the need for treatment of symptomatic PONV in the PACU was less when a total intravenous anesthetic without N_2O or paralysis, aggressive intravenous hydration, and three antiemetics

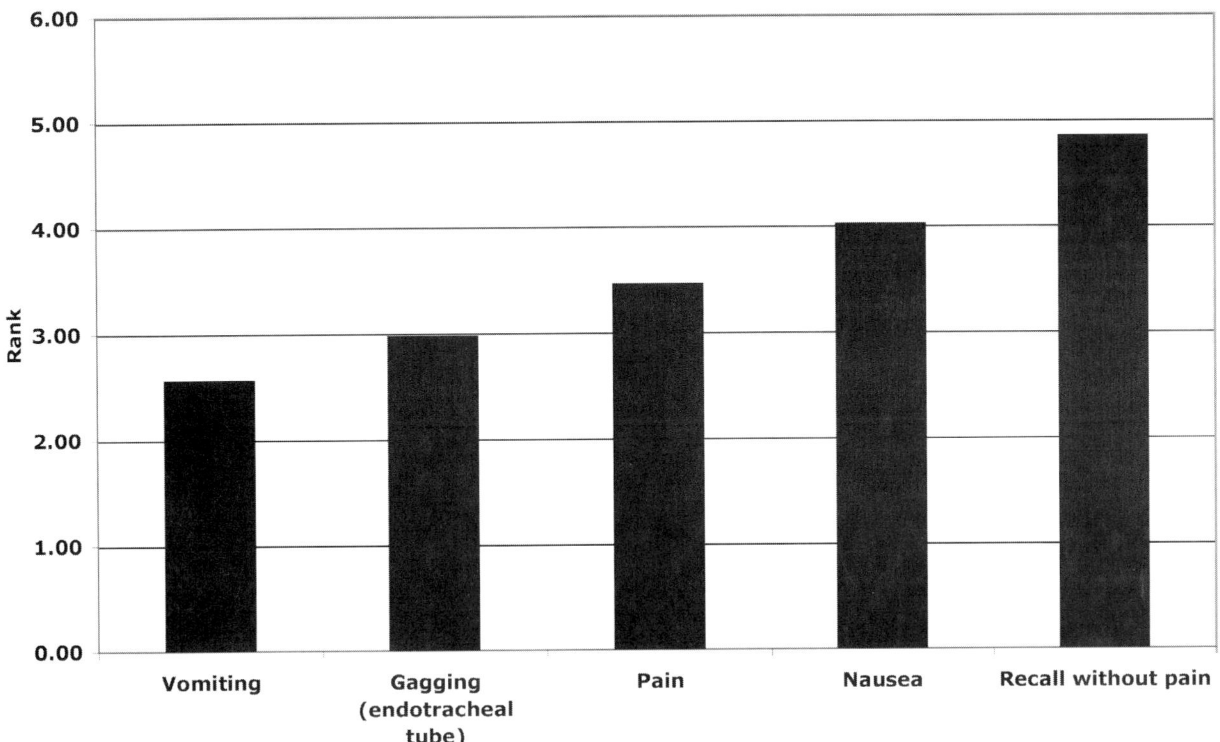

FIGURE 46-9. Patients were asked to rank 10 possible outcomes from most desirable to most undesirable.[61] Illustrated, in relative rank order, are the top 5 undesirable outcomes; the lower the rank, the more undesirable is the outcome. (Adapted with permission from Macario A, Weinger M, Carney S, Kim A: Which clinical anesthesia outcomes are important to avoid? The perspective of patients. Anesth Analg 89:652, 1999.)

were used, compared with an inhalation-based anesthetic with paralysis and ondansetron, and with a third placebo group, which was treated similarly to the previous group but did not receive ondansetron.[73] In a third study of women after laparoscopic surgery, ondansetron with cyclizine was more effective in reducing postoperative vomiting and the need for a rescue antiemetic than ondansetron alone.[74] However, not all have found that combination therapy is more effective. For example, in a study of patients undergoing abdominal surgery, ondansetron with droperidol was not better than ondansetron alone.[75]

Because of its ability to decrease PONV, propofol is the best general anesthetic for ambulatory anesthesia. For example, in a study of 5,161 patients, propofol, compared with a volatile anesthetic, reduced nausea and vomiting by 19%; and nitrogen compared with nitrous oxide reduced the incidence by 12% (Fig. 46-12).[70] Despite the greater initial cost of propofol, overall costs may be less because treatment for nausea and vomiting is eliminated. In one study of patients undergoing office-based surgical procedures, patients received either propofol or sevoflurane for induction and maintenance.[76] Costs of drugs used for anesthesia were the same; yet, when wasted propofol

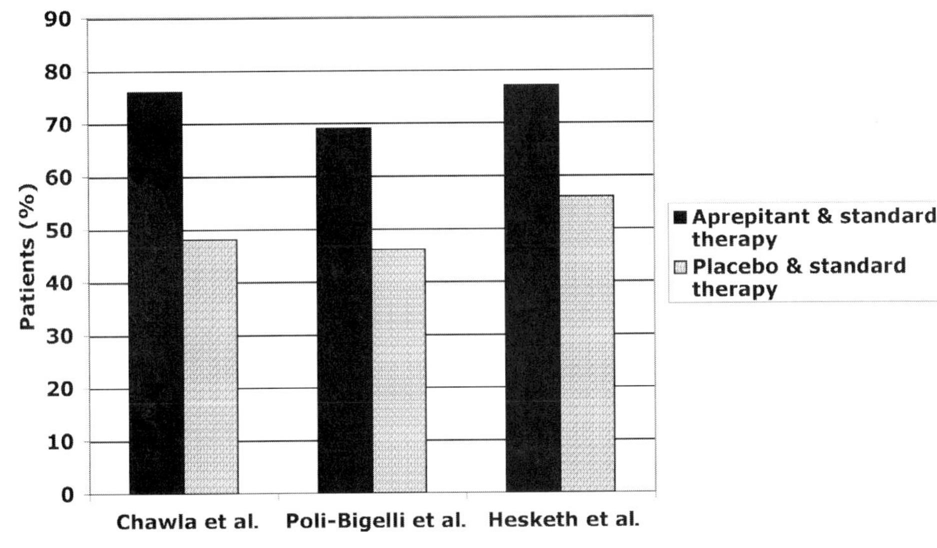

FIGURE 46-10. When oral aprepitant, compared with control, was combined with intravenous ondansetron and oral dexamethasone in adult patients who received one cycle cisplatin-based chemotherapy, based on three different multicenter randomized double-blind studies (Chawla et al,[90] Poli-Bigelli et al,[91] and Hesketh et al[92]); overall emetic events were significantly reduced (all $P < .01$) compared with standard therapy.[65] (Adapted with permission from Dando TM, Perry CM: Aprepitant: A review of its use in the prevention of chemotherapy-induced nausea and vomiting. Drugs 64:777, 2004.)

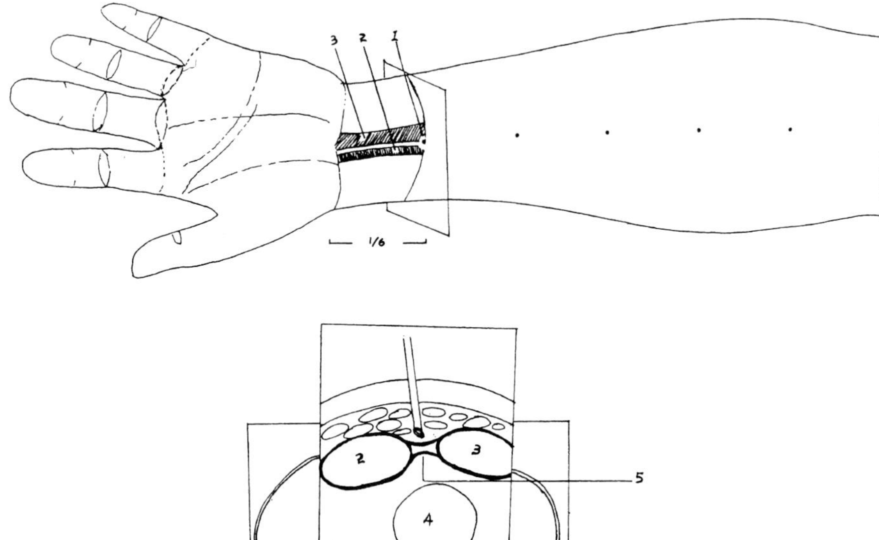

FIGURE 46-11. The P6 acupuncture point in relation to other hand structures is illustrated:[66] (1) P6 acupuncture point, (2) palmrois long tendon, (3) flexor carpi radialis tendon, (4) median nerve, (5) palmar aponeurosis. (Reprinted with permission from Wang SM, Kain ZN: P6 acupoint injections are as effective as droperidol in controlling early postoperative nausea and vomiting in children. Anesthesiology 97:359, 2002.)

was also considered, propofol costs were greater by approximately \$5 per patient. Overall, though, average cost per patient was lowest when propofol was used for both induction and maintenance, primarily because of the costs of treating nausea and vomiting (\$46 for propofol induction and maintenance, \$63 for propofol induction and sevoflurane maintenance, \$72 for sevoflurane induction and maintenance).

The use of nitrous oxide for ambulatory anesthesia is an issue because the incidence of emesis may be greater after nitrous oxide than after other inhalation agents. Yet, many studies have shown that nitrous oxide can be used successfully for ambulatory anesthesia. A meta-analysis, designed to determine if nitrous oxide significantly reduced the odds of PONV, included 26 trials from 24 studies.[77] Overall, the use of nitrous oxide increased the risk of PONV by 28%. The maximal benefit of nitrous oxide avoidance was seen in female patients (46%).

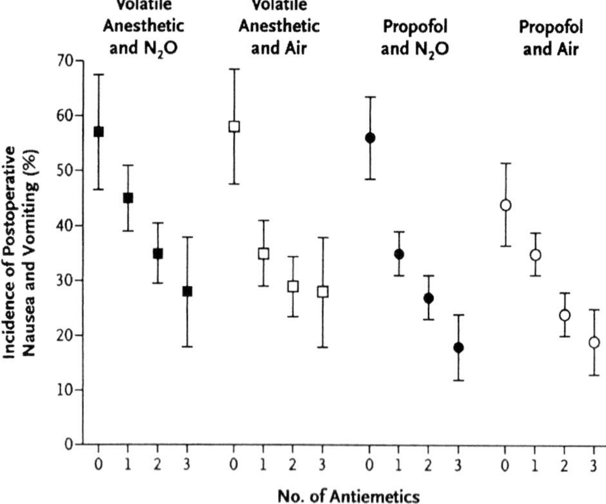

FIGURE 46-12. Postoperative nausea and vomiting (PONV) is least after a propofol anesthetic with air.[70] Illustrated is the incidence of PONV when different anesthetics and different numbers of prophylactic antiemetic treatments are administered. (Reprinted with permission from Apfel CC, Korttila K, Abdalla M *et al*: A factorial trial of six interventions for the prevention of postoperative nausea and vomiting. N Engl J Med 350:2441, 2004.)

Paralysis. Muscle paralysis for ambulatory anesthesia extends beyond the time of paralysis for intubation, particularly when nondepolarizing drugs have been used. The clinical effect of the nondepolarizing agent mivacurium, given as a bolus injection to 25% recovery, lasts 12 to 18 minutes, the shortest duration of effect for the neuromuscular blockers. The duration of action of rocuronium, vecuronium, rapacuronium, and atracurium ranges from 25 to 40 minutes. Because mivacurium depends on plasma cholinesterase for metabolism, recovery can be prolonged in the presence of atypical plasma cholinesterase. In patients with normal plasma cholinesterase levels, postoperative vomiting might be reduced if mivacurium does not have to be reversed. Reversal agents must be used unless there is no doubt that muscle relaxation has been fully reversed. When an ambulatory surgery case is expected to last more than 30 minutes, mivacurium may not be indicated. Particularly for children, in whom muscle relaxants generally have decreased potency, thereby enabling more rapid recovery, longer-acting drugs, such as pancuronium, may be used without sequelae.

Intraoperative Management of Postoperative Pain. Opioids, when given intraoperatively, are useful to supplement both intraoperative and postoperative analgesia. Fentanyl is probably the most popular drug, although all other available narcotics have been tried. All narcotics can cause nausea, sedation, and dizziness, which can delay a patient's discharge. Nonsteroidal analgesics are not effective as supplements during general anesthesia, although they are useful in controlling postoperative pain, particularly when given before skin incision. To control postoperative pain, combination therapy is most useful. For example, in a study of outpatients undergoing inguinal hernia repair under general anesthesia, triple preincisional therapy that included rofecoxib, 50 mg PO, ketamine, 0.2 mg/kg intravenously, and local anesthetic field block reduced pain scores and analgesic use in the first 24 hours after discharge compared with a placebo group.[78] See also the previous discussion on opioids and nonsteroidal analgesics in the Opioids and Nonsteroidal Analgesics section.

Depth of Anesthesia. BIS monitors and entropy or auditory-evoked potential monitors are believed to decrease anesthesia

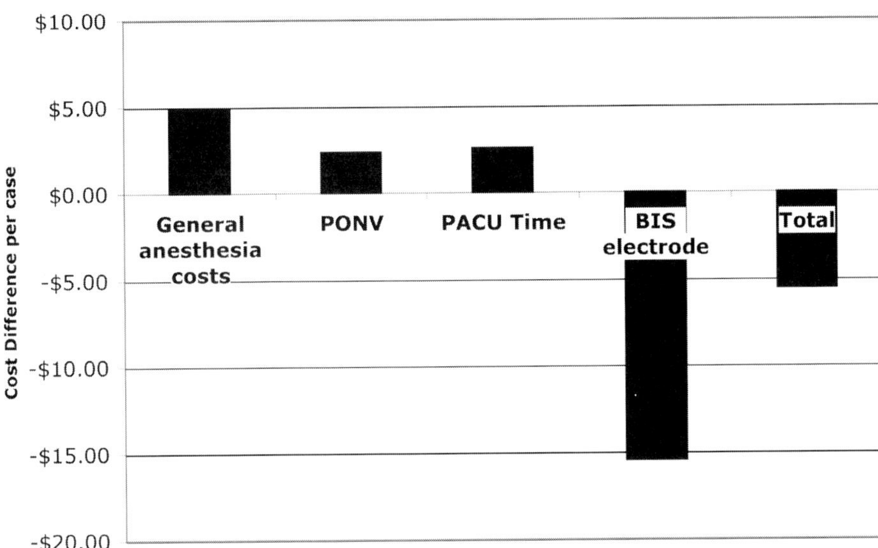

FIGURE 46-13. Bispectral index (BIS) monitoring reduces anesthetic consumption, cost to treat nausea and vomiting, and postanesthesia care unit (PACU) time; the cost of the electrode reverses cost savings.[79] The ordinate represents cost difference per case pooled from three studies (i.e., costs for the control group minus cost for the group that used BIS). The capital cost for the BIS monitor was not included. (Adapted with permission from Liu SS: Effects of bispectral index monitoring on ambulatory anesthesia: A meta-analysis of randomized controlled trials and a cost analysis. Anesthesiology 101:311, 2004.)

requirement without sacrificing amnesia during general anesthesia. Because less anesthesia is used, titration of anesthesia with these monitors results in earlier emergence from anesthesia. In a meta-analysis of BIS monitoring for ambulatory anesthesia, BIS monitoring was shown to reduce anesthetic use by 19%, with more modest decreases in PACU duration (4 min) and PONV (6%) (Fig. 46-13).[79] Results are even more modest, albeit mixed, in terms of later recovery end points. Because these monitors result in less use of anesthesia, there is the possibility that intraoperative awareness and myocardial ischemia might be increased. Sympatholytic drugs, instead of anesthesia, can be used to control autonomic responses to anesthesia. In fact, recovery is faster and side effects are fewer in ambulatory patients whose blood pressure is controlled by sympatholytics instead of inhalation agents.[80] In a study of almost 5,000 patients who underwent general anesthesia and who were paralyzed and/or were intubated, awareness was significantly reduced in the group of patients who were monitored with a BIS
10 compared with the group who were not monitored with the BIS (Fig. 46-14).[81]

Airways. Using a laryngeal mask airway (LMA), or similar type of airway, provides several advantages for allowing a patient to return to baseline status quickly. Muscle relaxants required for intubation can be avoided. Coughing is less than with tracheal intubation. Anesthetic requirements are reduced. Hoarseness and sore throat are also reduced. Overall, cost savings result with the use of LMAs. Because of gastric insufflation, though, nausea and vomiting may be greater. The use of the LMA has been described for laparoscopic procedures, although the potential for aspiration exists because of an inflated abdomen during laparoscopy.

MANAGEMENT OF POSTANESTHESIA CARE

Many recovery issues are part of patient selection and perioperative management and must be considered before the patient enters the PACU. Managing common problems in the PACU quickly and effectively is as important as appropriate patient selection and choice of anesthetic technique if the patient is to return home on the day of surgery. The three most common reasons for delay in patient discharge from the PACU are

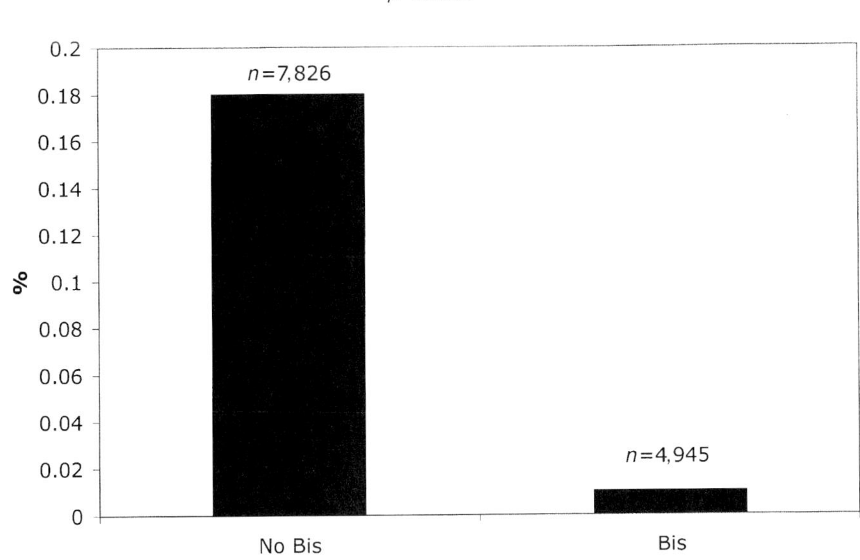

FIGURE 46-14. When a bispectral index (BIS) monitor is used, the incidence of awareness is reduced.[81] (Reprinted with permission from Ekman A, Lindholm ML, Lennmarken C, Sandin R: Reduction in the incidence of awareness using BIS monitoring. Acta Anaesthesiol Scand 48:20, 2004.)

drowsiness, nausea and vomiting, and pain. All three are a function of intraoperative management, but nausea, vomiting, and pain also can be treated in the PACU.

Reversal of Drug Effects

Reversal of muscle relaxants is not unique to the ambulatory surgery patient and is not discussed here. Reversal of opioids may sometimes be necessary. Flumazenil, a benzodiazepine receptor antagonist, has primarily been used to reverse the effects of sedation after endoscopy and spinal anesthesia. Reversal of psychomotor impairment with flumazenil is not complete, and the subjective experience of sedation is not necessarily attenuated. Reversal of amnesia with flumazenil is only partial, and the duration of the reversal effect may not be long enough to be clinically significant. Flumazenil should not be used routinely as a benzodiazepine antagonist, but may be used when sedation appears to be excessive. In addition, reversal of benzodiazepine-induced sedation by flumazenil should not replace appropriate ventilatory assistance and, if necessary, placement of an endotracheal tube.

Nausea and Vomiting

Nausea and vomiting are the most common reasons both children and adults have protracted stays in the PACU or unexpected hospital admission due to anesthesia. Nausea and vomiting are also the most common adverse effect in patients in the PACU. Much research has been undertaken to study prophylactic treatment of this problem before surgery, as well as practice techniques in the OR that can minimize nausea and vomiting in the PACU. The treatment of this problem, once it occurs in the PACU, has not received as much study. Yet, there are a variety of drugs that are effective in treating the problem. The 5-HT3 antagonists seem particularly effective. For example, in one study of children who underwent strabismus surgery and were then nauseous during the first 3 hours after recovery from anesthesia, emesis-free episodes were greater after granisetron 40 mcg/kg (88%), compared with droperidol 50 mcg/kg (63%) or metoclopramide 0.25 mg/kg (58%).[82] Similar findings were seen in a study of patients who underwent laparoscopic cholecystectomy and then experienced PONV during the first 3 hours after their procedure: complete control was more commonly seen after granisetron 40 mcg/kg (88%), compared with droperidol 20 mcg/kg (60%) or metoclopramide 0.2 mg/kg (55%).[83] Hydroxyzine 25 mg is also effective. Midazolam and propofol, although more commonly used for sedation, have antiemetic effects that are longer in duration than their effects on sedation. For example, when patients in the PACU were nauseous and then received either propofol 15 mg, or midazolam 1 mg or 2 mg, subsequent nausea was no different than ondansetron 4 mg.[84] Other authors have also found that propofol 10 mg is effective. When a ReliefBand accustimulation device was compared with ondansetron for patients who were nauseous in the PACU after receiving metoclopramide or droperidol and undergoing laparoscopic surgery, nausea was most effectively treated with both the ReliefBand and ondansetron, although both therapies were equally effective individually in treating PONV.[85] If patients have already received ondansetron prophylaxis in the OR, and then are nauseous in the PACU, another repeat dose might not be effective: in a multicenter study of patients who received ondansetron 4 mg during an outpatient procedure that included nitrous oxide, and who were then nauseous in the PACU, complete response to treatment was no different if patients received either another dose of ondansetron 4 mg or placebo.[86] More work is obviously needed to study effective therapies for treatment PONV in the PACU. Finally, because pain may be associated with nausea, treatment of pain frequently decreases nausea.

Pain

Postsurgical pain must be treated quickly and effectively. It is important for the practitioner to differentiate postsurgical pain from the discomfort of hypoxemia, hypercapnia, or a full bladder. Factors that correlate with greater postoperative pain are younger age of patient, less serious illness, greater body mass index, operative site, and duration of surgery.[87] Medications for pain control should be given in small intravenous doses (e.g., 1 to 3 mg/70 kg morphine or 10 to 25 mcg/70 kg fentanyl). Intramuscular injection of opioid for pain control in the PACU is probably not necessary. Onset of action of drugs is faster after intravenous catheter administration than after oral administration. Control of postoperative pain may include administration of opioid analgesics or NSAIDs, which are not associated with respiratory depression, nausea, or vomiting. Fentanyl is the narcotic frequently used to control postoperative pain, although the effects of morphine last longer. Patients who receive fentanyl for pain control may require additional injections and go home no sooner compared with patients who receive morphine. Nonsteroidal medications, such as ketorolac or ibuprofen, can also effectively control postoperative pain and, compared with narcotics, can give pain relief for a longer period and are associated with less nausea and vomiting. NSAIDs can increase bleeding, although there is no evidence at this time of such a danger for most ambulatory surgery procedures. When swelling and pain are problematic postoperatively, NSAIDs can be more effective than opioids in relieving both.

We manage pain in both adults and children initially either with a short-acting opioid analgesic such as fentanyl (25 mcg/70 kg), or with an injection of ketorolac 30–60 mg/70 kg intramuscularly or intravenously. Fentanyl is repeated at 5-minute intervals until pain is controlled. For children, we also use an elixir of acetaminophen containing codeine (120 mg acetaminophen, 12 mg codeine, in each 5 mL of solution). Five milliliters is administered to children between the ages of 3 and 6, and 10 mL to children between the ages of 7 and 12. Children are returned to parental care as soon as they are awake. We find frequently that infants younger than 6 months of age usually need to be reunited with their mothers for nursing (or bottle feeding) after a procedure not associated with severe pain. For older infants and young children in the PACU, acetaminophen, 60 mg per year of age (given orally or rectally), is commonly used to relieve mild pain. Intravenous fentanyl (up to a dose of 2 mcg/kg) is preferred for more severe pain. Meperidine (0.5 mg/kg) and codeine (1 to 1.5 mg/kg) can be given intramuscularly if an intravenous route has not been established.

Preparation for Discharging the Patient

In addition to the PACU, many ambulatory surgery centers in the United States have another area, often known as a phase II recovery room, where patients may stay until they are able to tolerate liquids, walk, and/or void. With the anesthetics that are typically used in ambulatory surgery ORs, patients who are awakened in the OR and are evaluated as 9 or 10 according to the modified Aldrete scoring system may be transferred directly to phase II recovery from the OR. Patients who undergo procedures under monitored anesthesia care can usually go straight to the phase II area from the OR. After general anesthesia, LMA use and pain control using nonopioid analgesics facilitates fast-tracking. In one study, 35 to 53% of patients who underwent laparoscopic gynecologic surgery were able to bypass the PACU.[88] In that study, residual sedation was the most common reason the PACU was not bypassed. In another study of patients who underwent outpatient knee surgery, in the phase II recovery area, of those who bypassed the PACU, 31% required nursing interventions and were three times more likely to need a nursing intervention, compared with 16% who required a nursing intervention who first went to the PACU. Yet, discharge times were faster and unplanned hospital admissions were fewer if patients were able to bypass the PACU.[89]

Concerning discharge to home, some criteria for discharge have been created without scientific basis. One criterion is the ability to tolerate liquids before being discharged. Postoperative nausea may be greater if patients are required to drink liquids prior to discharge. Even though it is warranted after spinal or epidural anesthesia, the requirement that low-risk patients void before discharge may only lengthen stay in the hospital, particularly if patients are willing to return to a medical facility if they are unable to void. Practical criteria for patient discharge from the OR, from the PACU, and from the phase II recovery area are needed that in no way compromise patient safety. The value of psychomotor tests to measure different phases of recovery (except for research purposes) is questionable.

Although scoring systems may be used to guide transfer from the PACU to the phase II recovery room and from phase II recovery to home, they do little to test higher levels of function, such as the ability to use one's hands, to drive a car, or to remain alert long enough to drive. Patients may feel fine after they leave the hospital, but they should be advised against driving for at least 24 hours after a procedure. Patients and responsible parties should be reminded that the patient should not operate power tools or be involved in major business decisions for up to 24 hours. Once the patient leaves the medical facility, supervision may not be as good as it was in the hospital. Therefore, before a patient is discharged, dressings should be checked. It is wise to include the responsible person in all discharge instructions, which are best made available on printed forms.

Patients should also be informed that they may experience pain, headache, nausea, vomiting, or dizziness and, if succinylcholine was used, muscle aches and pains apart from the incision for at least 24 hours. A patient will be less stressed if the described symptoms are expected in the course of a normal recovery. Written instructions are important. The addition of written and oral education techniques at discharge has a significant impact on improving compliance.

For patients with a language barrier (e.g., in a population with a high percentage of immigrants), consent forms, procedural explanation, and discharge information may have to be written in languages other than English and the services of an interpreter may be necessary. Nursing staff should assess the adult who will take the patient home to determine whether he or she is in fact a responsible person. A responsible person is someone who is physically and intellectually able to take care of the patient at home. Facilities should develop a method of follow-up after the patient has been discharged. At some facilities, staff members telephone the patient the next day to determine the progress of recovery; others use follow-up postcards. Whenever we become innovative in the management of our outpatients, we must assess how a cost-effective, "no frills" approach to care affects patient safety. We must determine what we can do for the patient who lives alone, for the patient whose responsible person is unable to manage his or her needs, for the patient without means of transportation, and for the patient with limited insurance coverage. Hospital beds can be set aside for patients who require observation. Patients in these beds after an ambulatory surgical procedure are still considered outpatients. They are charged for the hours spent in the observation area. Some hospitals have joined with management firms to build a hospital hotel or medical motel close to the hospital itself. The hotel, usually a nonmedical facility, offers the outpatient a comfortable, inexpensive, and convenient place to recuperate while being cared for by family or nurses. Home health care nursing may be appropriate after surgical procedures such as reduction mammoplasty, abdominoplasty, vaginal hysterectomy, and major open ligament repairs of the knee. The various services for management and/or observation of outpatients after surgery stand today where techniques for management of outpatients during surgery stood in the health care delivery system 20 years ago. Prospective studies are needed to assess the quality of care and the effect that these innovative approaches have on patient safety.

Patient, procedure, availability and quality of aftercare, and anesthetic technique must be individually and collectively assessed to determine acceptability for ambulatory surgery. A delicate balance must be maintained between the physical status of the patient, the proposed surgical procedure, and the appropriate anesthetic technique, to which must be added the expertise level of the anesthesiologist caring for a patient.

Anesthesia for ambulatory surgery is a rapidly evolving specialty. Patients once believed unsuitable for ambulatory surgery are now considered to be appropriate candidates. Operations once believed unsuitable for outpatients are now routinely performed in the morning so patients can be discharged in the afternoon or evening. The appropriate anesthetic management before these patients come to the OR, during their operation, and then afterward is the key to success. The availability of both shorter-acting anesthetics and longer-acting analgesics and antiemetics enables us to care for patients in ambulatory centers effectively.

References

1. Packard FR: History of medicine in the United States. New York, Paul B Hoeber, 1931
2. Ford JL, Reed WA: The surgicenter. An innovation in the delivery and cost of medical care. Ariz Med 26:801, 1969
3. Meeks GR, Waller GA, Meydrech EF, Flautt FHJ: Unscheduled hospital admission following ambulatory gynecologic surgery. Obstet Gynecol 80:446, 1992
4. Shenkman Z, Hoppenstein D, Litmanowitz I *et al*: Spinal anesthesia in 62 premature, former-premature or young infants—Technical aspects and pitfalls. Can J Anaesth 49:262, 2002
5. Cote CJ, Zaslavsky A, Downes JJ *et al*: Postoperative apnea in former preterm infants after inguinal herniorrhaphy. A combined analysis. Anesthesiology 82:809, 1995
6. Welborn LG, Hannallah RS, Fink R *et al*: High-dose caffeine suppresses postoperative apnea in former preterm infants. Anesthesiology 71:347, 1989
7. Junger A, Benson M, Klasen J *et al*: Influences and predictors of unanticipated admission after ambulatory surgery. Anaesthesist 49:875, 2000
8. Osborne GA, Rudkin GE: Outcome after day-care surgery in a major teaching hospital. Anaesth Intensive Care 21:822, 1993
9. Twersky R, Fishman D, Homel P: What happens after discharge? Return hospital visits after ambulatory surgery. Anesth Analg 84:319, 1997
10. Chung F, Mezei G, Tong D: Pre-existing medical conditions as predictors of adverse events in day-case surgery. Br J Anaesth 83:262, 1999
11. Ansell GL, Montgomery JE: Outcome of ASA III patients undergoing day case surgery. Br J Anaesth 92:71, 2004
12. Davies KE, Houghton K, Montgomery JE: Obesity and day-case surgery. Anaesthesia 56:1112, 2001
13. Sabers C, Plevak DJ, Schroeder DR, Warner DO: The diagnosis of obstructive sleep apnea as a risk factor for unanticipated admissions in outpatient surgery. Anesth Analg 96:1328, 2003
14. Basu S, Babajee P, Selvachandran SN, Cade D: Impact of questionnaires and telephone screening on attendance for ambulatory surgery. Ann R Coll Surg Engl 83:329, 2001
15. Tait AR, Malviya S, Voepel-Lewis T *et al*: Risk factors for perioperative adverse respiratory events in children with upper respiratory tract infections. Anesthesiology 95:299, 2001
16. Friesen RH, Wurl JL, Friesen RM: Duration of preoperative fast correlates with arterial blood pressure response to halothane in infants. Anesth Analg 95:1572, 2002

17. Brady M, Kinn S, Stuart P: Preoperative fasting for adults to prevent perioperative complications. Cochrane Database Syst Rev 4:CD004423, 2003
18. Practice guidelines for preoperative fasting and the use of pharmacologic agents to reduce the risk of pulmonary aspiration: Application to healthy patients undergoing elective procedures: A report by the American Society of Anesthesiologist Task Force on Preoperative Fasting. Anesthesiology 90:896, 1999
19. Pandit SK, Loberg KW, Pandit UA: Toast and tea before elective surgery? A national survey on current practice. Anesth Analg 90:1348, 2000
20. Evans SM, Griffiths RR: Caffeine withdrawal: A parametric analysis of caffeine dosing conditions. J Pharmacol Exp Ther 289:285, 1999
21. Kain ZN, Caldwell-Andrews AA: Sleeping characteristics of adults undergoing outpatient elective surgery: A cohort study. J Clin Anesth 15:505, 2003
22. Shafer A, Fish MP, Gregg KM *et al*: Preoperative anxiety and fear: A comparison of assessments by patients and anesthesia and surgery residents. Anesth Analg 83:1285, 1996
23. Kindler CH, Harms C, Amsler F *et al*: The visual analog scale allows effective measurement of preoperative anxiety and detection of patients' anesthetic concerns. Anesth Analg 90:706, 2000
24. Cote CJ, Cohen IT, Suresh S *et al*: A comparison of three doses of a commercially prepared oral midazolam syrup in children. Anesth Analg 94:37, 2002
25. Lichtor JL, Alessi R, Lane BS: Sleep tendency as a measure of recovery after drugs used for ambulatory surgery. Anesthesiology 96:878, 2002
26. Richardson MG, Wu CL, Hussain A: Midazolam premedication increases sedation but does not prolong discharge times after brief outpatient general anesthesia for laparoscopic tubal sterilization. Anesth Analg 85:301, 1997
27. Wittenberg MI, Lark TL, Butler CL *et al*: Effects of oral diazepam on intravenous access in same day surgery patients. J Clin Anesth 10:13, 1998
28. Fillmore MT, Kelly TH, Rush CR, Hays L: Retrograde facilitation of memory by triazolam: Effects on automatic processes. Psychopharmacology (Berl) 158:314, 2001
29. Veselis RA, Reinsel RA, Feshchenko VA, Wronski M: The comparative amnestic effects of midazolam, propofol, thiopental, and fentanyl at equisedative concentrations. Anesthesiology 87:749, 1997
30. Reuben SS, Steinberg RB, Maciolek H, Joshi W: Preoperative administration of controlled-release oxycodone for the management of pain after ambulatory laparoscopic tubal ligation surgery. J Clin Anesth 14:223, 2002
31. Recart A, Issioui T, White PF *et al*: The efficacy of celecoxib premedication on postoperative pain and recovery times after ambulatory surgery: A dose-ranging study. Anesth Analg 96:1631, 2003
32. Watcha MF, Issioui T, Klein KW, White PF: Costs and effectiveness of rofecoxib, celecoxib, and acetaminophen for preventing pain after ambulatory otolaryngologic surgery. Anesth Analg 96:987, 2003
33. Wennstrom B, Reinsfelt B: Rectally administered diclofenac (Voltaren) reduces vomiting compared with opioid (morphine) after strabismus surgery in children. Acta Anaesthesiol Scand 46:430, 2002
34. Birmingham PK, Tobin MJ, Fisher DM *et al*: Initial and subsequent dosing of rectal acetaminophen in children: A 24-hour pharmacokinetic study of new dose recommendations. Anesthesiology 94:385, 2001
35. Greenberg MF, Pollard ZF: Adult strabismus surgery under propofol sedation with local versus general anesthesia. J AAPOS 7:116, 2003
36. Pelinka LE, Pelinka H, Leixnering M, Mauritz W: Why patients choose regional anesthesia for orthopedic and trauma surgery. Arch Orthop Trauma Surg 123:164, 2003
37. Oldman M, McCartney CJ, Leung A *et al*: A survey of orthopedic surgeons' attitudes and knowledge regarding regional anesthesia. Anesth Analg 98:1486, 2004
38. Dahl JB, Schultz P, Anker-Moller E *et al*: Spinal anaesthesia in young patients using a 29-gauge needle: Technical considerations and an evaluation of postoperative complaints compared with general anaesthesia. Br J Anaesth 64:178, 1990
39. Cohen DD, Dillon JB: Anesthesia for outpatient surgery. JAMA 196:1114, 1966
40. Williams BA, Kentor ML: Making an ambulatory surgery centre suitable for regional anaesthesia. Best Pract Res Clin Anaesthesiol 16:175, 2002
41. D'eramo EM, Bookless SJ, Howard JB: Adverse events with outpatient anesthesia in Massachusetts. J Oral Maxillofac Surg 61:793, 2003
42. Rochette A, Raux O, Troncin R *et al*: Clonidine prolongs spinal anesthesia in newborns: A prospective dose-ranging study. Anesth Analg 98:56, 2004
43. Liguori GA, Zayas VM, Chisholm MF: Transient neurologic symptoms after spinal anesthesia with mepivacaine and lidocaine. Anesthesiology 88:619, 1998
44. Vath JS, Kopacz DJ: Spinal 2-chloroprocaine: The effect of added fentanyl. Anesth Analg 98:89, 2004
45. Kouri ME, Kopacz DJ: Spinal 2-chloroprocaine: A comparison with lidocaine in volunteers. Anesth Analg 98:75, 2004
46. Gupta A, Axelsson K, Thorn SE *et al*: Low-dose bupivacaine plus fentanyl for spinal anesthesia during ambulatory inguinal herniorrhaphy: A comparison between 6 mg and 7.5 mg of bupivacaine. Acta Anaesthesiol Scand 47:13, 2003
47. Pollock JE, Mulroy MF, Bent E, Polissar NL: A comparison of two regional anesthetic techniques for outpatient knee arthroscopy. Anesth Analg 97:397, 2003
48. de Beer DA, Thomas ML: Caudal additives in children—Solutions or problems. Br J Anaesth 90:487, 2003
49. Buckenmaier CCR, Klein SM, Nielsen KC, Steele SM: Continuous paravertebral catheter and outpatient infusion for breast surgery. Anesth Analg 97:715, 2003
50. Zaric D, Boysen K, Christiansen J *et al*: Continuous popliteal sciatic nerve block for outpatient foot surgery—A randomized, controlled trial. Acta Anaesthesiol Scand 48:337, 2004
51. Ilfeld BM, Morey TE, Wright TW *et al*: Continuous interscalene brachial plexus block for postoperative pain control at home: A randomized, double-blinded, placebo-controlled study. Anesth Analg 96:1089, 2003
52. Boezaart AP, De Beer JF, Nell ML: Early experience with continuous cervical paravertebral block using a stimulating catheter. Reg Anesth Pain Med 28:406, 2003
53. Klein SM, Pietrobon R, Nielsen KC *et al*: Peripheral nerve blockade with long-acting local anesthetics: A survey of the Society for Ambulatory Anesthesia. Anesth Analg 94:71, 2002
54. Williams BA, Kentor ML, Vogt MT *et al*: Economics of nerve block pain management after anterior cruciate ligament reconstruction: Potential hospital cost savings via associated postanesthesia care unit bypass and same-day discharge. Anesthesiology 100:697, 2004
55. Jankowski CJ, Hebl JR, Stuart MJ *et al*: A comparison of psoas compartment block and spinal and general anesthesia for outpatient knee arthroscopy. Anesth Analg 97:1003, 2003
56. Williams BA, Kentor ML, Vogt MT *et al*: Femoral-sciatic nerve blocks for complex outpatient knee surgery are associated with less postoperative pain before same-day discharge: A review of 1,200 consecutive cases from the period 1996–1999. Anesthesiology 98:1206, 2003
57. Hadzic A, Arliss J, Kerimoglu B *et al*: A comparison of infraclavicular nerve block versus general anesthesia for hand and wrist day-case surgeries. Anesthesiology 101:127, 2004
58. Korttila K, Nuotto EJ, Lichtor JL *et al*: Clinical recovery and psychomotor function after brief anesthesia with propofol or thiopental. Anesthesiology 76:676, 1992
59. Jabbour-Khoury SI, Dabbous AS, Rizk LB *et al*: A combination of alfentanil-lidocaine-propofol provides better intubating conditions than fentanyl-lidocaine-propofol in the absence of muscle relaxants. Can J Anaesth 50:116, 2003
60. Song D, Joshi GP, White PF: Fast-track eligibility after ambulatory anesthesia: A comparison of desflurane, sevoflurane, and propofol. Anesth Analg 86:267, 1998
61. Macario A, Weinger M, Carney S, Kim A: Which clinical anesthesia outcomes are important to avoid? The perspective of patients. Anesth Analg 89:652, 1999
62. Apfel CC, Laara E, Koivuranta M *et al*: A simplified risk score for predicting postoperative nausea and vomiting: Conclusions from cross-validations between two centers. Anesthesiology 91:693, 1999
63. Apfel CC, Kranke P, Katz MH *et al*: Volatile anaesthetics may be the main cause of early but not delayed postoperative vomiting: A randomized controlled trial of factorial design. Br J Anaesth 88:659, 2002
64. Saito R, Takano Y, Kamiya HO: Roles of substance P and NK(1) receptor in the brainstem in the development of emesis. J Pharmacol Sci 91:87, 2003
65. Dando TM, Perry CM: Aprepitant: A review of its use in the prevention of chemotherapy-induced nausea and vomiting. Drugs 64:777, 2004
66. Wang SM, Kain ZN: P6 acupoint injections are as effective as droperidol in controlling early postoperative nausea and vomiting in children. Anesthesiology 97:359, 2002
67. Magner JJ, McCaul C, Carton E *et al*: Effect of intraoperative intravenous crystalloid infusion on postoperative nausea and vomiting after gynaecological laparoscopy: Comparison of 30 and 10 ml kg^{-1}. Br J Anaesth 93:381, 2004
68. Oddby-Muhrbeck E, Eksborg S, Bergendahl HT *et al*: Effects of clonidine on postoperative nausea and vomiting in breast cancer surgery. Anesthesiology 96:1109, 2002
69. Henzi I, Walder B, Tramer MR: Dexamethasone for the prevention of postoperative nausea and vomiting: A quantitative systematic review. Anesth Analg 90:186, 2000
70. Apfel CC, Korttila K, Abdalla M *et al*: A factorial trial of six interventions for the prevention of postoperative nausea and vomiting. N Engl J Med 350:2441, 2004
71. Gan TJ, Jiao KR, Zenn M, Georgiade G: A randomized controlled comparison of electro-acupoint stimulation or ondansetron versus placebo for the prevention of postoperative nausea and vomiting. Anesth Analg 99:1070, 2004
72. Splinter WM, Rhine EJ: Low-dose ondansetron with dexamethasone more effectively decreases vomiting after strabismus surgery in children than does high-dose ondansetron. Anesthesiology 88:72, 1998
73. Scuderi PE, James RL, Harris L, Mims GR: Multimodal antiemetic management prevents early postoperative vomiting after outpatient laparoscopy. Anesth Analg 91:1408, 2000
74. Ahmed AB, Hobbs GJ, Curran JP: Randomized, placebo-controlled trial of combination antiemetic prophylaxis for day-case gynaecological laparoscopic surgery. Br J Anaesth 85:678, 2000
75. Bugedo G, Gonzalez J, Asenjo C *et al*: Ondansetron and droperidol in the prevention of postoperative nausea and vomiting. Br J Anaesth 83:813, 1999
76. Tang J, Chen L, White PF *et al*: Recovery profile, costs, and patient satisfaction with propofol and sevoflurane for fast-track office-based anesthesia. Anesthesiology 91:253, 1999

77. Divatia JV, Vaidya JS, Badwe RA, Hawaldar RW: Omission of nitrous oxide during anesthesia reduces the incidence of postoperative nausea and vomiting. A meta-analysis. Anesthesiology 85:1055, 1996
78. Pavlin DJ, Horvath KD, Pavlin EG, Sima K: Preincisional treatment to prevent pain after ambulatory hernia surgery. Anesth Analg 97:1627, 2003
79. Liu SS: Effects of bispectral index monitoring on ambulatory anesthesia: A meta-analysis of randomized controlled trials and a cost analysis. Anesthesiology 101:311, 2004
80. White PF, Wang B, Tang J *et al*: The effect of intraoperative use of esmolol and nicardipine on recovery after ambulatory surgery. Anesth Analg 97:1633, 2003
81. Ekman A, Lindholm ML, Lennmarken C, Sandin R: Reduction in the incidence of awareness using BIS monitoring. Acta Anaesthesiol Scand 48:20, 2004
82. Fujii Y, Tanaka H, Ito M: Treatment of vomiting after paediatric strabismus surgery with granisetron, droperidol, and metoclopramide. Ophthalmologica 216:359, 2002
83. Fujii Y, Tanaka H, Kawasaki T: Randomized clinical trial of granisetron, droperidol and metoclopramide for the treatment of nausea and vomiting after laparoscopic cholecystectomy. Br J Surg 87:285, 2000
84. Unlugenc H, Guler T, Gunes Y, Isik G: Comparative study of the antiemetic efficacy of ondansetron, propofol and midazolam in the early postoperative period. Eur J Anaesthesiol 21:60, 2004
85. Coloma M, White PF, Ogunnaike BO *et al*: Comparison of acustimulation and ondansetron for the treatment of established postoperative nausea and vomiting. Anesthesiology 97:1387, 2002
86. Kovac AL, O'Connor TA, Pearman MH *et al*: Efficacy of repeat intravenous dosing of ondansetron in controlling postoperative nausea and vomiting: A randomized, double-blind, placebo-controlled multicenter trial. J Clin Anesth 11:453, 1999
87. Chung F, Ritchie E, Su J: Postoperative pain in ambulatory surgery. Anesth Analg 85:808, 1997
88. Coloma M, Zhou T, White PF *et al*: Fast-tracking after outpatient laparoscopy: Reasons for failure after propofol, sevoflurane, and desflurane anesthesia. Anesth Analg 93:112, 2001
89. Williams BA, Kentor ML, Williams JP *et al*: PACU bypass after outpatient knee surgery is associated with fewer unplanned hospital admissions but more phase II nursing interventions. Anesthesiology 97:981, 2002
90. Chawla SP, Grunberg SM, Gralla RJ *et al*: Establishing the dose of the oral NK1 antagonist aprepitant for the prevention of chemotherapy-induced nausea and vomiting. Cancer 97:2290, 2003
91. Poli-Bigelli S, Rodrigues-Pereira J, Carides AD *et al*: Addition of the neurokinin 1 receptor antagonist aprepitant to standard antiemetic therapy improves control of chemotherapy-induced nausea and vomiting. Results from a randomized, double-blind, placebo-controlled trial in Latin America. Cancer 97:3090, 2003
92. Hesketh PJ, Grunberg SM, Gralla RJ *et al*: The oral neurokinin-1 antagonist aprepitant for the prevention of chemotherapy-induced nausea and vomiting: A multinational, randomized, double-blind, placebo-controlled trial in patients receiving high-dose cisplatin—The Aprepitant Protocol 052 Study Group. J Clin Oncol 21:4112, 2003

CHAPTER 47 ■ MONITORED ANESTHESIA CARE

SIMON C. HILLIER AND MICHAEL S. MAZUREK

KEY POINTS

1. A comprehensive preanesthetic evaluation is a critical component of any monitored anesthesia care procedure. This is especially important because the patient population that presents for monitored anesthesia care has increasingly complex coexisting disease.
2. There is significant interpatient variability in response to sedative drug administration. Therefore, the safe provision of monitored anesthesia care requires the ability to immediately secure and maintain a patent airway and perform advanced life support techniques.
3. Sedation techniques should be modified to account for interpatient differences in age, general medical condition, and the particular requirements of the procedure. The sedation technique can be conceptually thought of as having hypnotic, anxiolytic, and analgesic components. Each component of the sedation technique should be adjusted as required accordingly.
4. In general, it is preferable to use drugs having a shorter duration of action to facilitate titration, earlier awakening, and a rapid return to street fitness.
5. It is important to titrate drugs carefully, remembering to allow time for the drug to achieve its effect prior to administering supplemental doses. Careful titration of drugs will reduce the likelihood of unintended general anesthesia with an unprotected airway and cardiorespiratory compromise.
6. It is prudent to gain experience and become comfortable with a small armamentarium of drugs. It is particularly important to appreciate the potential adverse synergistic effects of sedative drugs on the respiratory and cardiovascular systems.
7. The institutional standards for monitoring, record keeping and documentation, recovery room practice, quality assurance, and policy and procedure development for sedation and monitored anesthesia care should be no different than those for general anesthesia.
8. Sedation is frequently used as an adjunct to local or regional analgesic techniques. Therefore, it is important to be prepared to recognize and treat local anesthetic toxicity. It should be remembered that the usual premonitory signs of impending local anesthetic toxicity are obscured by concomitant administration of sedative drugs.

Anesthesiologists typically provide monitored anesthesia care to patients undergoing therapeutic or diagnostic procedures that would otherwise be uncomfortable or unsafe. The continuous attention of the anesthesiologist is directed at optimizing patient comfort and safety. Monitored anesthesia care usually involves the administration of drugs with anxiolytic, hypnotic, analgesic, and amnestic properties, either alone or as a supplement to a local or regional technique.

TERMINOLOGY

It is important to distinguish between "monitored anesthesia care" and "sedation/analgesia." *Sedation/analgesia* is the term currently used by the American Society of Anesthesiologists (ASA) in their Practice Guidelines for Sedation and Analgesia by Non-Anesthesiologists.[1] Monitored *anesthesia care* implies the potential for a deeper level of sedation than that provided by sedation/analgesia and is always administered by an anesthesiologist provider. The standards for preoperative evaluation, intraoperative monitoring, and continuous presence of a member of the anesthesia care team are no different from those for general or regional anesthesia.[2]

Conceptually, monitored anesthesia care is attractive because it should invoke less physiologic disturbance and allow a more rapid recovery than general anesthesia. It is instructive to review the ASA position statement approved by the House of Delegates in 1986 and last amended in 1998.[2] The ASA definition of monitored anesthesia care is as follows:

> *Monitored anesthesia care is a specific anesthesia service in which an anesthesiologist has been requested to participate in the care of a patient undergoing a diagnostic or therapeutic procedure.*
>
> *Monitored anesthesia care includes all aspects of anesthesia care—a preprocedure visit, intraoperative care and post procedure anesthesia management.*
>
> *During monitored anesthesia care, the anesthesiologist or a member of the anesthesia care team provides a number of specific services, including but not limited to:*
>
> > *Monitoring of vital signs, maintenance of the patient's airway and continual evaluation of vital functions*
> > *Diagnosis and treatment of clinical problems which occur during the procedure*
> > *Administration of sedatives, analgesics, hypnotics, anesthetic agents or other medications as necessary to ensure patient safety and comfort*
> > *Provision of other medical services as needed to accomplish the safe completion of the procedure*
>
> *Monitored anesthesia care often includes the administration of doses of medications for which the loss of normal protective reflexes or loss of consciousness is likely. Monitored anesthesia care refers to those clinical situations in which the patient remains able to protect the airway for the majority of the procedure. If, for an extended period of time, the patient is rendered unconscious and/or loses normal protective reflexes, then anesthesia care shall be considered a general anesthetic.*
>
> *Because monitored anesthesia care is a physician service provided to an individual patient and is based on medical necessity, it should be subject to the same level of reimbursement as general or regional anesthesia. Accordingly, the ASA Relative Value Guide provides for the use of proper basic procedural units, time units and age and risk modifier units as the basis for determining reimbursement.*

The ASA also states that monitored anesthesia care should be requested by the attending physician and be made known to the patient, in accordance with accepted procedures of the institution. In addition, the ASA states that the service must include the following:

1. Performance of a preanesthetic examination and evaluation
2. Prescription of anesthetic care
3. Personal participation in, or medical direction of, the entire plan of care
4. Continuous physical presence of the anesthesiologist or, in the case of medical direction, of the resident or nurse anesthetist being medically directed
5. Proximate presence, or in the case of medical direction, availability of the anesthesiologist for diagnosis and treatment of emergencies

Furthermore, the ASA states that all institutional regulations pertaining to anesthesia services will be observed, and all the usual services performed by the anesthesiologist will be furnished, including but not limited to:

1. Usual noninvasive cardiocirculatory and respiratory monitoring
2. Oxygen administration, when indicated
3. Administration of sedatives, tranquilizers, antiemetics, narcotics, other analgesics, beta-blockers, vasopressors, bronchodilators, antihypertensives, or other pharmacologic therapy as may be required in the judgment of the anesthesiologist

PREOPERATIVE ASSESSMENT

1 The preoperative evaluation is an essential prerequisite to monitored anesthesia care and should be as comprehensive as that performed prior to any general or regional anesthetic (see Chapter 18). However, in addition to the usual evaluation for the patient who is planned to undergo general anesthesia, there are additional considerations unique to monitored anesthesia care that may ultimately determine the success or failure of the procedure. It is important to evaluate the patient's ability to remain motionless and, if necessary, actively cooperate throughout the procedure. Thus, it is important to evaluate the patient's psychological preparation for the planned procedure. It is also important to elicit the presence of coexisting sensorineural or cognitive deficits. These factors, or the inability to communicate with the patient, may on occasion make general anesthesia a more appropriate alternative. Verbal communication between physician and patient is very important for three reasons: (1) as a monitor of the level of sedation and cardiorespiratory function, (2) as a means of explanation and reassurance for the patient, and (3) as a mechanism of communication when the patient is required to actively cooperate. Although cardiorespiratory disease is often an indication to perform a procedure using monitored anesthesia care rather than general anesthesia, there are occasions when cardiorespiratory disease may reduce the utility of monitored anesthesia care. For example, the presence of a persistent cough may make it difficult for the patient to remain immobile, which can be particularly dangerous during ophthalmologic or awake neurosurgical procedures. Attempts to attenuate coughing with sedation techniques are likely to be unsuccessful and potentially harmful because a significant level of anesthesia is required to abolish the cough reflex. Similarly, some patients with significant cardiovascular disease may experience orthopnea and be unable to lie flat for an extended period.

TECHNIQUES OF MONITORED ANESTHESIA CARE

2 A variety of medications are commonly administered during monitored anesthesia care with the desired end points being providing patient comfort, maintaining cardiorespiratory stability, improving operating conditions, and preventing recall of unpleasant perioperative events. It is helpful to delineate and individualize the goals for each patient to formulate an appropriate regimen that frequently involves the administration of either individual or combinations of analgesic, amnestic, and hypnotic drugs. There should be a minimal incidence of side effects, such as cardiorespiratory depression, nausea and vomiting, delayed emergence, and dysphoria, and there should be a rapid and complete recovery. Ideally, the patient should be able to communicate during the procedure. Clinical experience

suggests that a level of sedation that allows verbal communication is optimal for the patient's comfort and safety. If the level of sedation is deepened to the extent that verbal communication is lost, most of the advantages of monitored anesthesia care are lost, and the risks of the technique approach those of general anesthesia with an unprotected and uncontrolled airway. However, because monitored anesthesia care is provided by anesthesiologists, the range of sedation may be expanded to include significantly deeper sedation techniques than those provided by nonanesthesiologists during sedation/analgesia.

3 The preanesthetic evaluation and plan should strive to identify specific causes of, and provide specific therapy for, pain, anxiety, and agitation. Pain may be treated by local or regional analgesia, systemic analgesics, or removal of the painful stimulus. Anxiety may be reduced by the use of an anxiolytic such as a benzodiazepine and reassurance by the anesthesiologist. Patient agitation may be a result of pain or anxiety, but it is also vitally important to eliminate life-threatening factors such as hypoxia, hypercarbia, impending local anesthetic toxicity, and cerebral hypoperfusion. Other less ominous, but often overlooked, causes of discomfort and agitation include a distended bladder, hypothermia, hyperthermia, pruritus, nausea, positional discomfort, uncomfortable oxygen masks and nasal cannulae, intravenous cannulation site infiltration, a member of the surgical team leaning on the patient, and prolonged pneumatic tourniquet inflation.

Pharmacologic Basis of Monitored Anesthesia Care Techniques—Optimizing Drug Administration

4 The ability to predict the effects of the drugs in our armamentarium demands an understanding of their pharmacokinetic and pharmacodynamic properties. This understanding is a fundamental prerequisite for the design of an effective sedation regimen and greatly increases the probability of producing the desired therapeutic effect. Context-sensitive half-time, effect–site equilibration time, and anesthetic–sedative drug interactions are fundamental concepts that are particularly useful in the context of minimum alveolar concentration (MAC) and are discussed in some detail.

The ultimate objective of any dosing regimen is to deliver a therapeutic concentration of drug to its site of action, which is determined by the unique pharmacokinetic properties of that drug in that particular patient. The therapeutic response to a particular drug concentration is described by the pharmacodynamics of that particular patient–drug combination. There is a large degree of pharmacokinetic and pharmacodynamic variability, producing a significant variability in the dose-response relationship in clinical practice. Excessive sedation may result in cardiac or respiratory depression. Inadequate sedation may result in patient discomfort and potential morbidity due to lack of cooperation. As a general principle, to avoid excessive levels of sedation, drugs should be titrated in small increments or by adjustable infusions rather than administered in larger doses according to predetermined notions of efficacy. In an ideal dosing regimen, an effective concentration of drug is achieved and then adjusted according to the magnitude of the noxious stimulus. If the noxious stimulus is increased or decreased, the concentration is increased or decreased accordingly. By the end of the procedure, the drug concentration should have decreased to a level compatible with rapid recovery. This approach requires the use of drugs that are easily titratable, such as propofol. When using drugs such as propofol, adjustable rate continuous infusions are the most logical method of maintaining a desired therapeutic concentration. When the traditional method of intermittent bolus administration is used, significant fluctuations in drug concentration occur. Under these circumstances, the plasma concentrations are either above or below the desired therapeutic range for a significant proportion of the procedure (Fig. 47-1). Continuous infusions are superior to intermittent bolus dosing because they produce less fluctuation in drug concentration, thus reducing the number of episodes of inadequate or excessive sedation. Administration of drugs by continuous infusion rather than by intermittent dosing also reduces the total amount of drug administered and facilitates a more prompt recovery.[3]

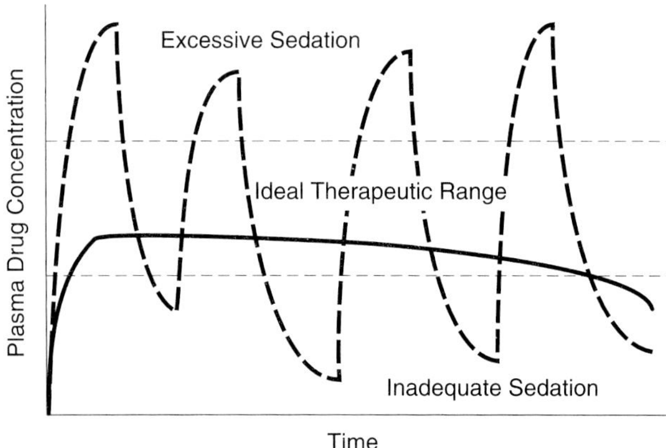

FIGURE 47-1. The changes in drug concentration during differing administration techniques. The *solid line* represents a continuous infusion of a drug. In this situation, the drug is maintained within the therapeutic range for most of the procedure. The *dashed line* represents the drug concentration resulting from intermittent bolus administration. The drug concentration is significantly above or below the desired therapeutic level for most of the procedure.

Distribution, Elimination, Accumulation, and Duration of Action

Following the administration of intravenous anesthetic drugs, the immediate distribution phase causes a brisk decrease in plasma levels as the drug is transported to the rapidly equilibrating vessel-rich group of tissues. There is a simultaneously occurring distribution of drug to the less well perfused tissues such as muscle and skin. Over time, the drug is also distributed to the poorly perfused tissues such as bone and fat. Although the latter compartments are poorly perfused, they may accumulate significant amounts of lipophilic drugs during prolonged administration. This peripheral depot may contribute to a delayed recovery when the drug is eventually released back into the central compartment after its administration is discontinued. Redistributive factors are important determinants of drug effect and influence the plasma concentration of a drug in a time-dependent fashion.

The Elimination Half-Time

Until more recently, the elimination half-time was the predominant pharmacokinetic parameter used as the predictor of an anesthetic drug's duration of action. In everyday clinical practice, however, this parameter has not greatly enhanced our ability to predict anesthetic drug disposition. Only in single-compartment models does the elimination half-time actually represent the time required for a drug to reach half of its initial concentration after administration. This is because in a single-compartment model elimination is the only process that can alter drug concentration. Intercompartmental distribution cannot occur because there are no other compartments for the drug to be distributed to and from. Most drugs in the anesthesiologist's armamentarium are lipophilic and are therefore more suited to multicompartmental modeling than single-compartment modeling. Similarly, other pharmacokinetic parameters such as distribution half-time, distribution volume, intercompartmental rate constants, etc., do not provide us with a practical means of predicting drug disposition. In multicompartmental models, the metabolism and excretion of some intravenous anesthetic drugs may have only a minor contribution to changes in plasma concentration when compared with the effects of intercompartmental distribution.

Context-Sensitive Half-Time

To improve the description and understanding of anesthetic drug disposition, the concept of context-sensitive half-time has been developed.[4] This concept has greatly improved our understanding of anesthetic drug disposition and is clinically applicable. The effect of distribution on plasma drug concentration varies in magnitude and direction over time and depends on the drug concentration gradients that exist between the various compartments. For example, during the early part of an infusion of a lipophilic drug, distributive factors will tend to decrease plasma concentrations as the drug is transported to the unsaturated peripheral tissues. Later, after the infusion is discontinued, drug will return from the peripheral tissues and reenter the central circulation. The relative effect on plasma concentrations of distributive processes versus elimination varies over time and from drug to drug. The context-sensitive half-time describes the time required for the plasma drug concentration to decline by 50% after terminating an infusion of a particular duration. This parameter is calculated by using computer simulation of multicompartmental models of drug disposition (Fig. 47-2). The context-sensitive half-time reflects the combined effects of distribution and metabolism on drug disposition. There are several interesting aspects of these data. First, the data confirm the clinical impression that as the infusion duration increases, the context-sensitive half-time of all the drugs increases; this phenomenon is not described in any way by the elimination half-life. The increase in context-sensitive half-time is particularly marked with fentanyl and thiopental. In the case of fentanyl, drug that is irreversibly eliminated from the plasma by hepatic clearance is immediately replaced by drug returning from the peripheral compartments. Thus, although fentanyl has a shorter elimination half-life than that of sufentanil (462 versus 577 minutes), its context-sensitive half-time is much greater than that of sufentanil after an infusion of duration longer than 2 hours. The storage and later release of fentanyl from peripheral binding sites delay the decline in plasma concentration that would otherwise occur. The context-sensitive half-times of all the drugs bear no constant relationship to their elimination half-times. Also compare the context-sensitive half-times of propofol and thiopental (Fig. 47-2). Although the context-sensitive half-times of propofol and thiopental are comparable following a brief infusion, the context-sensitive half-time of thiopental increases rapidly following all but the shortest infusions. This finding confirms the clinical impression that thiopental is not an ideal drug for continuous infusion during ambulatory procedures. The context-sensitive half-time of propofol is prolonged to a minimal extent as the infusion duration increases. After an infusion of propofol, the drug that returns to the plasma from the peripheral compartments is rapidly cleared by metabolic processes and is therefore not available to retard the decay in plasma levels. This difference between thiopental and propofol is attributable to (1) the high metabolic clearance of propofol compared with thiopental and (2) the relatively slow rate at which propofol returns to the plasma from peripheral compartments.

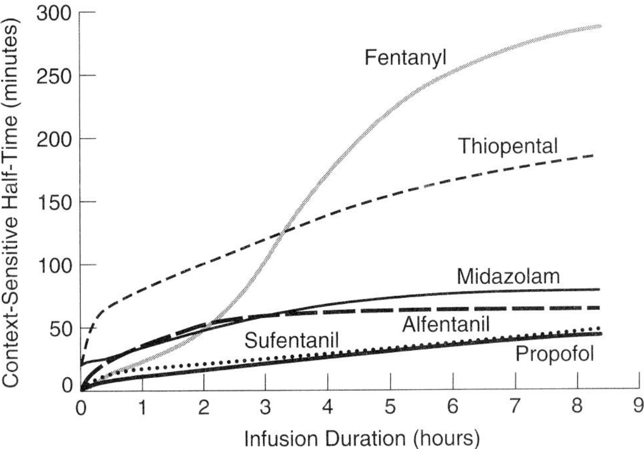

FIGURE 47-2. Context-sensitive half-times as a function of infusion duration. These data were generated from the computer model of Hughes et al.[4] It can be seen that the context-sensitive half-time of propofol demonstrates a minimal increase as the duration of the infusion increases. Also note that for infusions of short duration, sufentanil has a shorter half-time than alfentanil. (Reprinted with permission from Hughes MA, Glass PSA, Jacobs JR: Context-sensitive half-time in multicompartment pharmacokinetic models for intravenous anesthetic drugs. Anesthesiology 76:334, 1992.)

Alfentanil is the opioid that has, until more recently, been most frequently studied, described, and promoted in the context of ambulatory techniques. This is because alfentanil has a short elimination half-time, one-fifth that of sufentanil (111 versus 577 minutes). However, despite the longer elimination half-time of sufentanil, its context-sensitive half-time is actually less than that of alfentanil for infusions up to 8 hours in duration. This phenomenon is explained in part by the huge distribution volume of sufentanil. After termination of a sufentanil infusion, the decay in plasma drug concentrations is accelerated not only by elimination, but also by the continued redistribution of sufentanil into peripheral compartments. In contrast, the small distribution volume of alfentanil equilibrates rapidly; therefore, peripheral distribution of drug away from the plasma is not a significant contributor to the decay in plasma concentration after an infusion. The data derived from computer simulation by Hughes et al[4] show that the plasma decay of alfentanil is slower than that of sufentanil following infusions of similar duration to those used during conscious sedation. Thus, despite its short elimination half-time, alfentanil may not necessarily be superior to sufentanil for ambulatory sedation techniques.

How Does the Context-Sensitive Half-Time Relate to the Time to Recovery? Although the context-sensitive half-time represents a significant advance in our ability to describe drug disposition, this parameter does not directly describe how long it will take the patient to recover from MAC. The context-sensitive half-time merely describes how long it will take for the plasma concentration of the drug to decrease by 50%. The time to recovery depends on other additional factors. The difference between the plasma concentration at the end of the infusion and the plasma concentration below which awakening can be expected is an obvious factor in determining time to recovery. For example, if the drug concentration is maintained at a level just above that required for awakening, the time to recovery will be more rapid than after an infusion during which the drug concentration is much greater than that required for awakening

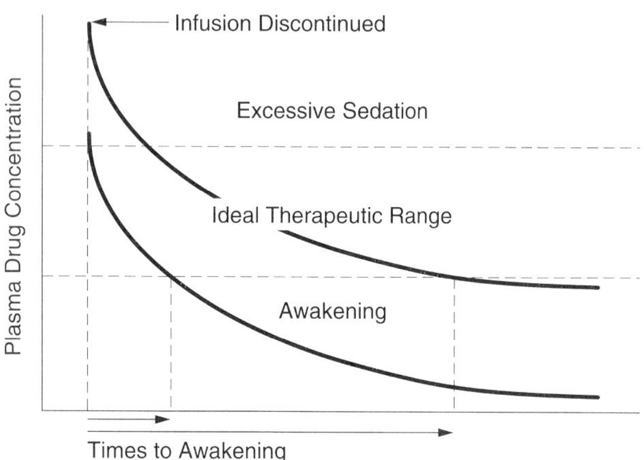

FIGURE 47-3. The context-sensitive half-time is not the sole determinant of the time it takes for the patient to awaken. This parameter merely reflects the time taken for the plasma concentration of a drug to decrease by 50%. The time to awakening is determined in addition by the difference in concentration at the end of the procedure and the concentration below which awakening will occur.

(Fig. 47-3). Furthermore, although context-sensitive half-time is a reflection of plasma drug decay, awakening from anesthesia is actually a function of effect–site (i.e., brain) concentra-
5 tion decay. Changes in effect–site concentration demonstrate a variable time lag behind changes in plasma drug concentration. Effect–site equilibration is a concept that is particularly relevant to intravenous sedation. When a drug is administered intravenously by bolus or infused rapidly, there is a delay before the onset of clinical effect. This delay occurs because the plasma is not usually the site of action but is merely the route by which the drug reaches its effect site. If some parameter of drug effect can be measured (e.g., power spectrum electroencephalographic [EEG] analysis in the case of opioids), the half-time of equilibration between drug concentration in the blood and the drug effect can then be determined.[5] This parameter is abbreviated $t_{1/2}k_{e0}$. Drugs with a short $t_{1/2}k_{e0}$ will equilibrate rapidly with the brain and have a shorter delay in onset than drugs that have a longer $t_{1/2}k_{e0}$. Thiopental, propofol, and alfentanil have short $t_{1/2}k_{e0}$ values compared with midazolam, sufentanil, and fentanyl. The $t_{1/2}k_{e0}$ allows predictions to be made of the time course of equilibration of the drug between the blood and the brain. A distinct time lag between the peak serum fentanyl concentration and the peak EEG slowing can be seen. In contrast, following alfentanil administration, the EEG changes closely parallel serum concentrations. The $t_{1/2}k_{e0}$ for fentanyl is 6.4 minutes compared with a $t_{1/2}k_{e0}$ of 1.1 minutes for alfentanil. If an opioid is required to blunt the response to a single brief stimulus, alfentanil might represent a logical choice over fentanyl. The $t_{1/2}k_{e0}$ is an important determinant of bolus spacing when titrating drugs to clinical effect. In the case of drugs such as midazolam, which have a relatively long equilibration time (midazolam $t_{1/2}k_{e0} = 0.97$ to 5.6 minutes), boluses of drug should be spaced far enough apart to allow the full peak effect to be clinically appreciated before further drug administration to avoid inadvertent overdosing.[6,7] For example, even if the shortest quoted equilibration half-time for midazolam (0.9 minutes) is used, it will take 2.7 minutes for effect–site concentrations to be 87.5% equilibrated. Other factors are also important determinants of bolus size and spacing. For example, a low cardiac output will markedly delay drug arrival at the site of action. If sufficient time is not given for the drug to take effect before giving additional drug increments, significant cardiorespiratory compromise may occur. Furthermore, the effects of initial doses of most drugs in anesthetic practice are terminated by redistribution, which depends on blood flow to redistribution sites. If there is reduced blood flow to redistribution sites because of preexisting and iatrogenic decreases in cardiac output, the dangerous adverse effects of these drugs are likely to be not only delayed, but also markedly prolonged. An example of the previous scenario is the patient with a hemodynamic compromise caused by a tachydysrhythmia that requires sedation for cardioversion. Careful, well-spaced, small boluses of drug should be given to induce the appropriate level of sedation, bearing in mind that it may take several minutes for the full effect of a small bolus dose to become apparent.

DRUG INTERACTIONS IN MONITORED ANESTHESIA CARE

At the present time, no single inhaled or intravenous drug can provide all the components of MAC (i.e., analgesia, anxiolysis, hypnosis) with an acceptable margin of safety or ease of titratability. Therefore, patient comfort is usually maintained with a combination of drugs. By acting synergistically, combinations of drugs enable reductions in the dose requirements of individual drugs. For example, during general anesthesia, the combination of propofol and fentanyl by infusion has been shown to produce a more rapid recovery and better stress response abolition than the use of propofol alone.[8] However, synergistic interaction may also extend to the undesirable interactions of the drugs such as cardiorespiratory depression.

Drug interactions may have both a pharmacodynamic and a pharmacokinetic basis and may vary, depending on the combination of drugs being coadministered, the dose range over which these drugs are administered, and the specific clinical effect that is measured. For example, because fentanyl is primarily an analgesic rather than a hypnotic, it reduces propofol requirements for suppression of response to skin incision to a much greater degree than it reduces propofol requirements for induction of anesthesia.[9] In contrast, because midazolam has significant hypnotic properties, it displays significant synergism with propofol or thiopental when used to induce hypnosis.[10,11]

The plasma concentration of a drug at steady state that is required to abolish purposeful movement at skin incision in 50% of patients ($Cp_{ss}50$) is a measure of potency that is analogous to the familiar parameter of MAC of the volatile inhaled anesthetics. Intravenous anesthetic interactions may be evaluated by their effect on the $Cp_{ss}50$ in a manner analogous to the expression of the effects of opioids on volatile anesthetic requirements in terms of MAC reduction. For example, during general anesthesia, opioid requirements to suppress the responses to noxious stimuli are 10-fold higher when used as the sole agent compared to when they are used in conjunction with a nitrous oxide–potent inhaled vapor technique. This interaction persists at the lighter levels of anesthesia encountered during MAC. Therefore, in an ambulatory conscious sedation setting, it is likely that a rapid recovery would be facilitated by using opioids in combination with other agents (e.g., propofol/midazolam) rather than as the sole drug.

Drug interactions are dose dependent. For example, when fentanyl is combined with isoflurane, the greatest reduction in isoflurane MAC occurs within the analgesic concentration range of fentanyl (i.e., 1 to 2 ng/mL). At a fentanyl concentration of 1.7 ng/mL, the MAC of isoflurane is reduced by 50%.[12] Once the fentanyl concentration is increased beyond 3 ng/mL, there appears to be minimal further reduction with a maximum MAC reduction of 80%. Likewise, the MAC of desflurane is reduced by approximately 50% 25 minutes after a 3-μg/kg intravenous bolus of fentanyl.[13] However, when the fentanyl bolus is increased to 6 μg/kg, there is no significant further decrease in the MAC of desflurane. The interactions between propofol and opioids are important because these agents are frequently used during MAC. When analgesic concentrations of fentanyl (0.6 ng/mL) are used in combination with propofol for anesthesia, the $Cp_{ss}50$ of propofol is reduced by 50% compared with when propofol is used as the sole agent.[11] However, when the dose of fentanyl is increased, there is no significant further reduction of the $Cp_{ss}50$ for propofol beyond a fentanyl concentration of 3 ng/mL.

Although the data presented previously pertain to patients under general anesthesia, these findings have important implications for monitored anesthesia care. These studies demonstrate that the potentiating effects of opioids upon coadministered sedatives are pronounced within the dose range commonly used during MAC. Furthermore, the data suggest that the dose-response curve is likely to be steep within this dose range, thus supporting the clinical impression that significant increases in depth of sedation can occur with only modest increments in opioid or hypnotic/sedative dosage. The following clinical recommendations can be made: during MAC, the maximum benefit of opioid supplementation, in terms of potentiation of other administered sedatives, will accrue when the opioid is used in the analgesic dose range. Within this dose range, there is great potential for adverse cardiorespiratory interaction.

Opioid and benzodiazepine combinations are frequently used to achieve the components of hypnosis, amnesia, and analgesia. This drug combination displays marked synergism in producing hypnosis. Approximately 25% of the ED_{50} for each individual drug is required in combination to induce hypnosis in 50% of patients.[14] If the combination were simply additive, hypnosis would be induced in only approximately 25% of patients. Even subanalgesic doses of alfentanil (3 μg/kg) produce a profound reduction in midazolam requirements for hypnosis.[15] This synergism also extends to the unwanted effects of these drugs, producing the life-threatening complications of respiratory and cardiac depression.[16] Several fatalities have been reported after the use of midazolam, the majority of these being related to adverse respiratory events. In many of these cases, midazolam was used in combination with an opioid. The effects of midazolam and fentanyl upon respiratory function in healthy volunteers have been examined by Bailey et al.[17] Whereas midazolam produced no significant respiratory effects alone and fentanyl alone produced hypoxemia (oxyhemoglobin saturation 95%) in half of the subjects, the combination of midazolam 0.05 mg/kg and fentanyl 2.0 μg/kg resulted in hypoxemia in 11 of 12 subjects and apnea (no spontaneous respiratory effort for 15 seconds) in 6 of 12 subjects. The combination of midazolam and fentanyl places patients at high risk for developing hypoxemia and apnea. The respiratory depressant effects of this drug combination are likely to be even more significant in the patient with coexisting respiratory or central nervous system (CNS) disease or at the extremes of age. In clinical practice, the clinical advantages of the synergy between opioids and benzodiazepines for the maintenance of patient comfort should be carefully weighed against the disadvantages of the potentially adverse effect of this drug combination on the cardiovascular and respiratory systems.

SPECIFIC DRUGS USED FOR MONITORED ANESTHESIA CARE

6

Propofol

Propofol has many of the ideal properties of a sedative-hypnotic for use in MAC. Its pharmacokinetic profile (i.e., a context-sensitive half-time that remains short even after infusions of prolonged duration and a short effect–site equilibration time) makes it an easily titratable drug with an excellent recovery profile. The quality of recovery and the low incidence of nausea and vomiting make propofol particularly well suited to ambulatory MAC procedures. A significant body of experience with the use of propofol for MAC has emerged. Propofol has significant advantages compared with benzodiazepines when used as the hypnotic component of a MAC technique. Although midazolam has a relatively short elimination half-time, its context-sensitive half-time is approximately twice that of propofol. Whereas propofol is noted for the rapid return to clear-headedness, midazolam is often associated with prolonged postoperative sedation and psychomotor impairment, particularly in the elderly. Propofol in typical MAC doses (25 to 75 μg/kg/min) has minimal analgesic properties. However, the unique advantages of propofol can be exploited to the maximum when propofol is used to provide sedation when the analgesic component is provided by a local or regional analgesic technique. The use of propofol (50 to 70 μg/kg/min) to provide sedation (defined as sleep with preservation of the eyelash reflex and purposeful reaction to verbal or mild physical stimulation) as an adjunct to spinal anesthesia for lower limb surgery has been examined.[18] After termination of infusions of approximately 100 minutes in duration, patients regained consciousness in approximately 4 minutes. The authors also noted the ease with which general anesthesia could be induced if necessary by increasing the propofol infusion. The same group also compared propofol (60.5 μg/kg/min) to midazolam (4.3 μg/kg/min) as an adjunct to spinal anesthesia. The propofol group had faster immediate recovery than the midazolam group (2.3 versus 9.2 minutes to spontaneous eye opening). Furthermore, psychomotor function was comparable to baseline values following propofol sedation but did not return to baseline until 2 hours after midazolam administration. White and Negus also compared propofol and midazolam sedation for local and regional anesthesia.[19] These investigators examined several recovery parameters and demonstrated that propofol produced less postoperative sedation, drowsiness, confusion, and clumsiness than midazolam, but that discharge times were similar. It should be noted that most investigators have shown that propofol does not reliably produce amnesia in subhypnotic doses.[20] Although recall of intraoperative events is generally believed to be undesirable, the lack of amnestic properties in propofol may be preferable when patients are required to remember important instructions they are given in the postoperative period.

The use of propofol for sedation has been examined in several diverse clinical settings, including propofol alone for upper gastrointestinal endoscopy[21] and magnetic resonance imaging in children,[22] with fentanyl for extracorporeal shock wave lithotripsy,[23] with alfentanil for transvaginal oocyte retrieval, and for sedation during the dental care to persons with mental and physical disabilities.[24,25]

There is a general clinical impression that patients recovering from propofol not only recover rapidly, but also often experience an increased sense of well-being. However, a study specifically addressing the issue of the subjective effects of low-dose propofol in volunteers could find no evidence for a euphoric effect of propofol.[26] The authors postulate that the sense of well-being arises from the feeling of relief that the procedure is over. This feeling of relief may be inhibited by the prolonged psychomotor impairment that often follows other anesthetic techniques.

General anesthesia with propofol is generally associated with less nausea and vomiting than most other anesthetic techniques. There is now evidence that even subhypnotic doses of propofol (a single 10-mg dose in an adult) also possess direct antiemetic properties.[27] Thus, it is likely that the beneficial effects of propofol on nausea and vomiting will be a feature of MAC techniques using this drug. In contrast, even during

TABLE 47-1

PUBLISHED STRATEGIES FOR REDUCING PAIN ON IV INJECTION OF PROPOFOL

Using larger veins in antecubital fossa
Decreasing the speed of injection
Injection into a fast-running IV
Diluting with 5% glucose or 10% intralipid
Adding lidocaine to propofol
Pretreating with lidocaine and venous occlusion
Pretreatment with opioid
Pretreatment with pentothal
Cooling to 4°C prior to injection
Injecting cooled saline (4°C) prior to injection
Discontinuing IV fluid administration during injection

IV, intravenous(ly).

low-dose infusions used for sedation, pain during injection of propofol may be troublesome in 33 to 50% of patients.[28,29] Several strategies for reducing the pain of propofol administration are described in Table 47-1.[30]

Benzodiazepines

Benzodiazepines are commonly used during MAC for their anxiolytic, amnestic, and hypnotic properties. Midazolam has now displaced diazepam as the most commonly used benzodiazepine for conscious sedation. The important differences between midazolam and diazepam are listed in Table 47-2.[31] Although midazolam has a short elimination half-time, there is often significant and prolonged psychomotor impairment following sedation techniques using midazolam as a significant component. With the more recent availability of propofol, midazolam may be better used in a modified role by using lower doses prior to the start of a propofol infusion to provide the specific amnestic and perhaps anxiolytic component of a "balanced" sedation technique, rather than as the major hypnotic component.[32] This allows the more evanescent and titratable propofol to provide the desired level of conscious sedation in an adjustable manner, according to the specific stimulus. The analgesic component, if required, of a balanced MAC technique could be provided by regional and local techniques or opioids. Again, when using opioids with benzodiazepines, the potential for significant respiratory impairment should be considered.

TABLE 47-2

COMPARISON OF IMPORTANT PROPERTIES OF MIDAZOLAM AND DIAZEPAM

■ MIDAZOLAM	■ DIAZEPAM
Water soluble, does not require propylene glycol for solubilizing	Lipid soluble, requires propylene glycol for solubilizing
Nonvenoirritant, usually painless	Venoirritant, pain on injection
Thrombophlebitis rare	Thrombophlebitis common
Short elimination half-time (1–4 hr)	Long elimination half-time (>20 hr)
Clearance unaffected by H_2 antagonists	Clearance reduced by H_2 antagonists
Inactive metabolites (1-hydroxy-midazolam)	Active metabolites (desmethyl-diazepam, oxazepam)
Resedation unlikely	Resedation more likely

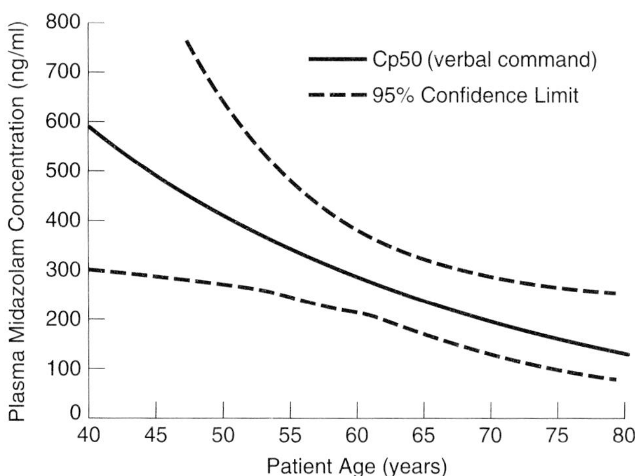

FIGURE 47-4. Midazolam Cp50 (the concentration at which 50% of subjects will fail to respond to a verbal command) as a function of age. There is a marked decrease in midazolam requirements as patient age increases. (Reprinted with permission from Jacobs JR, Reves JG, Marty J *et al*: Aging increases pharmacodynamic sensitivity to the hypnotic effects of midazolam. Anesth Analg 80:143,1995.)

Clinical experience suggests that the dose of a particular benzodiazepine required to reach a desired clinical end point is reduced in the elderly compared with younger patients. This difference in dosing requirements in the elderly is due mainly to pharmacodynamic factors. This is demonstrated by the threefold decrease in plasma concentration of midazolam, at which 50% of patients would be expected not to respond to verbal command (Cp50) at 80 years of age compared with 40 years of age (Fig. 47-4).[33]

Benzodiazepines are valuable components of MAC techniques because they enhance patient comfort, improve operating conditions, and provide amnesia. However, recovery of psychomotor and cognitive function may be significantly prolonged following benzodiazepine sedation, especially when compared with sedative–hypnotic techniques using propofol as the major component.[34] The specific benzodiazepine antagonist flumazenil provides the potential to improve the recovery profile of benzodiazepines by permitting the active termination of their sedative and amnestic effects without invoking adverse side effects. However, the potential for resedation remains an obstacle to the routine use of benzodiazepine reversal, particularly in patients undergoing ambulatory procedures. The effects of midazolam may recur up to 90 minutes following the administration of flumazenil.[35] Thus, it is possible that patients could be discharged prematurely to a less well-monitored area, or even out of the hospital in the case of ambulatory surgery, and later experience recurrence of benzodiazepine effects. An important additional issue is that of cost. The routine use of flumazenil-antagonized benzodiazepine sedation has a significant cost disadvantage. Ghouri et al.[35] demonstrated that flumazenil-antagonized midazolam sedation was more expensive than propofol sedation ($68.67 versus $27.80). Typical dose requirements are listed in Table 47-3.

Opioids

Opioids are most logically used in the context of MAC to provide the specific analgesic component of a "balanced" technique rather than to provide the sedative component. Opioid

TABLE 47-3

RECOMMENDED REGIMEN FOR USE OF FLUMAZENIL TO ANTAGONIZE BENZODIAZEPINE EFFECTS

Initial recommended dose of 0.2 mg
If desired level of consciousness is not achieved in 45 sec, repeat 0.2-mg dose
Doses of 0.2 mg may need to be repeated every 60 sec until a maximum of 1 mg is administered
Be aware of the potential for resedation

analgesics are indicated when regional or local anesthetic techniques are inappropriate or ineffective. Opioids may also play an important role during the initial injection of local anesthetic solution or during other periods of intense patient discomfort. Pain relief may be required for factors other than the procedure itself, such as uncomfortable positioning, propofol injection, pneumatic tourniquet pain, or other pain not relieved by the local anesthetic technique.

A typical circumstance in which the patient must briefly cooperate and remain motionless is during the placement of a retrobulbar block prior to ophthalmic procedures. Patient movement during block placement may increase the incidence of complications such as brainstem anesthesia and cardiac arrest. Retrobulbar block placement affords an excellent opportunity to study the effects of drugs on the response to a standardized, ethically acceptable, brief painful stimulus. The ideal drug for block placement would provide a brief period of intense analgesia, yet allow the patient to be awake and cooperative without causing cardiorespiratory depression, cause minimal nausea and vomiting, and not significantly prolong recovery.[36] Alfentanil (20 μg/kg) has a rapid onset and offset of intense analgesia, and was compared with methohexital (0.5 mg/kg) for retrobulbar block placement.[36] Patients receiving methohexital were unresponsive to verbal command at the time of block placement and demonstrated more movement on injection than those receiving alfentanil, who were mostly (87%) awake and cooperative at the time of injection. The authors noted that 1 of the 15 elderly patients who received alfentanil became apneic for 30 seconds, and suggested that the dose of opioids be reduced in the elderly. They also noted that the personnel performing the block were accustomed to the patient being "asleep" during methohexital sedation, but took some time to become at ease with the awake yet comfortable and cooperative patient who had received alfentanil.

The well-described phenomenon of patient awareness and subsequent recall of intraoperative events following high-dose opioid anesthesia is taken as evidence that opioids lack significant amnestic properties. However, when the effects of low-dose fentanyl on memory were specifically examined in volunteers, it was found that although the subjects appeared to be awake during the fentanyl infusion, there was significant memory impairment.[37] The degree of stimulation was probably less than that experienced by a patient undergoing a painful surgical procedure. Recall for a painful stimulus may not be impaired to the same degree as recall for the less noxious stimuli that the subjects of this study experienced.

Alfentanil appears to have a pharmacokinetic advantage for the treatment of discrete stimuli because of its short effect–site equilibration time, which allows rapid access of the drug to the brain and facilitates titration. However, sufentanil may have a more favorable recovery profile when used over a longer period of time because of its shorter context-sensitive half-time. In clinical practice, however, there is a marked interpatient variability in opioid pharmacokinetics and dynamics. This interpatient variability may be more significant than the interdrug differences, making it difficult to predict with any precision the effects of a given drug dose in an individual patient.

Remifentanil

In the context of monitored anesthesia care, the analgesic properties of opioids are extremely valuable. However, their adverse effects, including respiratory depression, muscle rigidity, and emesis, are undesirable in the spontaneously breathing patient with an unprotected airway and significantly limit the ability to consistently provide effective analgesic doses. A further complicating issue is that the ability to predict the effect of a given dose of opioid in a particular patient is limited by significant interpatient pharmacokinetic and pharmacodynamic variability. This problem is usually overcome in practice by the cautious incremental administration of small, carefully spaced boluses or by titrating infusions to the desired effect.

Remifentanil has pharmacodynamic properties similar to those of other potent μ-opioid receptor agonists such as fentanyl and alfentanil. However, remifentanil is predominantly metabolized by nonspecific esterases generating an extremely rapid clearance and offset of effect.[38] The context-sensitive half-time of remifentanil is consistently short, 3 to 5 minutes, increasing to a minimal degree with the duration of the infusion. Furthermore, remifentanil has a short effect–site equilibration time ($t_{1/2}k_{e0}$) of 1.0 to 1.5 minutes. This $t_{1/2}k_{e0}$ is slightly longer than that of alfentanil (0.6 to 1.2 minutes), but much shorter than that of fentanyl (4 to 5 minutes) and morphine ($\sim$20 minutes), and makes the onset of effect after drug administration rapid, thus facilitating titration of effect during MAC.

In clinical practice, remifentanil has been used successfully as the analgesic component of sedation techniques for regional and local anesthesia. Its unique pharmacokinetic profile makes it well suited for ambulatory MAC techniques. Published experience with the use of remifentanil suggests that it is possible to titrate remifentanil administration to provide effective analgesia with minimal respiratory depression. The published data can be used to generate some practical clinical guidelines,[39] which are discussed as follows:

1. As with other potent opioids used during sedation techniques, the most logical therapeutic end point for remifentanil administration is effective analgesia and patient comfort rather than sedation. When opioids are titrated to preconceived levels of sedation rather than patient comfort, an unacceptable degree of respiratory depression may occur. Drugs such as propofol or midazolam can be used in combination with remifentanil to provide the hypnotic-amnestic component of the sedation technique, remembering that the concomitant administration of midazolam decreases remifentanil dose requirements by up to 50%.[40]
2. Published data suggest that bolus administration of remifentanil is associated with an increased incidence of respiratory depression and chest wall rigidity. Because these side effects are likely to be related to high peak concentrations of drugs, it is recommended that remifentanil boluses be administered slowly (over 30 to 90 seconds) or avoided completely by using a pure infusion technique. Furthermore, the administration of remifentanil boluses during the concomitant administration of remifentanil infusions is also associated with an increased incidence of respiratory depression, the most likely mechanism again being excessive peak drug concentrations. These episodes of respiratory depression are of significant concern, particularly in the spontaneously breathing patient with an

unprotected airway. However, if promptly recognized, and the remifentanil administration is reduced or discontinued, they should resolve within approximately 3 minutes. Thus, despite the pharmacokinetic advantages of remifentanil, the level of vigilance required for its administration should be no different from that for any other potent opioid. Although the offset time of remifentanil is rapid, it still requires the recognition of respiratory depression to trigger a downward adjustment in dosage. Similarly, the short $t_{1/2}k_{e0}$ of remifentanil suggests that sudden respiratory depression may occur in response to upward adjustments in dosage. Despite the potential for respiratory depression, the efficacy of remifentanil boluses during MAC has been investigated by several groups. The most logical scenario in which a bolus dose could be used is immediately prior to a brief but painful stimulus, such as placement of a retrobulbar block.[41] A bolus of 1 μg/kg over 30 seconds was administered 90 seconds prior to block placement. More than three-fourths of patients receiving remifentanil did not report any pain during subsequent block placement. However, 15% of the patients given a single bolus alone had significant respiratory depression (respiratory rates <8 breaths per minute), and 19% of those given a bolus followed by an infusion had significant respiratory depression.

3. The effects of coadministration of benzodiazepines and opioids are well documented. The addition of midazolam to provide the anxiolytic-sedative and amnestic components of a sedation technique has been shown to increase patient satisfaction and significantly reduce remifentanil dose requirements. The combination of remifentanil with midazolam significantly reduces patient anxiety when compared with the use of the opioid alone.[42] Even relatively low-dose midazolam (2 mg intravenously) produces significant reductions in remifentanil requirements and patient anxiety. During breast or lymph node biopsy, remifentanil infusion requirements were 0.065 μg/kg/min when preceded by midazolam compared with 0.123 μg/kg/min when used alone. The advantages of coadministration of small doses of midazolam include increased patient satisfaction, increased amnesia, decreased nausea and vomiting, and decreased anxiety. The disadvantages include a tendency toward increased respiratory depression, apnea, and excessive sedation.
4. Because most painful stimuli are of unpredictable duration and because the risk of adverse respiratory events is increased following bolus administration, the most logical method for the administration of remifentanil during MAC is by an adjustable infusion. This should ideally be preceded by a small bolus of midazolam. Most investigators have used infusion rates that start at 0.1 μg/kg/min approximately 5 minutes prior to the first painful stimulus. This initial "loading" infusion is then weaned to approximately 0.05 μg/kg/min to maintain patient comfort. The maintenance infusion is adjusted upward in response to pain or hemodynamic response or downward in response to excessive sedation, respiratory depression, or apnea. A typical incremental change in infusion rate is 0.025 μg/kg/min. The use of remifentanil infusions of 0.2 μg/kg/min is associated with an increased incidence of respiratory depression that is not necessarily associated with superior analgesia. As in the case of propofol administration, inadvertent interruption of remifentanil administration will result in abrupt offset of effect, which may result in patient discomfort, hemodynamic instability, and even morbidity due to patient movement. It is therefore important to ensure the drug delivery system is monitored carefully during the procedure. Remifentanil is supplied as a powder that must be reconstituted prior to use. It is particularly important when administering this drug to patients with an unsecured airway to ensure there are no errors in drug dilution that would result in inadvertent dosing errors.

TABLE 47-4

TYPICAL DOSE RANGES OF SEDATIVE, HYPNOTIC, AND ANALGESIC DRUGS

■ DRUG	■ TYPICAL ADULT IV DOSE RANGE (TITRATED TO EFFECT IN SMALL INCREMENTS)
■ **BENZODIAZEPINES**	
Midazolam	1–2 mg prior to propofol or remifentanil infusion
Diazepam	2.5–10 mg (in 0.5–2 mg increments)
■ **OPIOID ANALGESICS**	
Alfentanil	5–20-μg/kg bolus 2 min prior to stimulus
Fentanyl	0.5–2.0-μg/kg bolus 2–4 min prior to stimulus
Remifentanil	Infusion 0.1 μg/kg/min 5 min prior to stimulus Wean to 0.05 μg/kg/min as tolerated Adjust up or down in increments of 0.025 μg/kg/min Reduce dose accordingly when coadministered with midazolam or propofol Avoid boluses
■ **HYPNOTICS**	
Propofol	250–500-μg/kg boluses 25–75 μg/kg/min infusion

IV, intravenous(ly).

Typical adult dose recommendations for opioids and other drugs discussed in the text are listed in Table 47-4.

Ketamine

Ketamine is a phencyclidine derivative, is an intense analgesic, and is frequently used as a component of pediatric sedation techniques.[43,44] When used in small doses (0.25 to 0.5 mg/kg), its use is associated with minimal respiratory and cardiovascular depression. Ketamine produces a dissociative state in which the eyes remain open with a nystagmic gaze. However, as the dose of ketamine increases, or when used in combination with other sedatives, a state of deep sedation and/or general anesthesia may be inadvertently achieved. Increased oral secretions make laryngospasm more likely. The fear of laryngospasm is the underlying rationale for the frequent administration of atropine or glycopyrrolate. Ketamine is frequently combined with a benzodiazepine to reduce the incidence of hallucinations associated with its use. However, this practice is controversial.[45] Patient movement may make ketamine less than ideal for procedures requiring a completely motionless patient. Ketamine can elevate intracranial and intraocular pressure and is thus relatively contraindicated in patients with increased intracranial pressure and with glaucoma or open globe injuries. Although it has been suggested that airway reflexes are relatively preserved with ketamine, there is no convincing evidence to support this notion.

Ketamine can be administered orally, intramuscularly, or intravenously. The oral dose of ketamine is 4 to 6 mg/kg. The onset of action typically occurs within 20 to 30 minutes, and the duration of effect is between 60 to 90 minutes. The intramuscular dose is 2 to 4 mg/kg, with an onset of action of 5 to 10 minutes and a duration of action of 30 to 120 minutes. When administered via the intravenous route, ketamine should be given in small (0.25 to 1.0 mg/kg) increments, titrating to effect with an onset of action of 1 to 2 minutes and an approximate duration of 20 to 60 minutes.

Dexmedetomidine

Dexmedetomidine, like clonidine, is a selective alpha-2 receptor agonist. Stimulation of alpha-2 receptors produces sedation and analgesia, a reduction of sympathetic outflow, and an increase in cardiac vagal activity. The use of clonidine in the perioperative period is limited by its long half-life of 6 to 10 hours. However, dexmedetomidine has a much shorter half-life and greater alpha-2 receptor selectivity, thus limiting its peripheral vascular effects. Despite its alpha-2 selectivity, dexmedetomidine may still cause significant bradycardia and hypotension.[46] Dexmedetomidine does not depress respiratory function to the same extent as other classes of sedatives. Furthermore, patients sedated with dexmedetomidine are more easily aroused from a given level of sedation.

Dexmedetomidine has been used as sedative supplementation to regional anesthesia during carotid endarterectomy. Under these circumstances, there were fewer fluctuations from the desired sedation level when compared with the combination of midazolam, fentanyl, and propofol.[47] Dexmedetomidine has also been used successfully in both adult and pediatric patients for MAC during the awake portions of craniotomies requiring patient cooperation during mapping of cortical speech areas.[48,49] When compared with propofol, as a supplement to regional anesthesia, the target sedation level took longer to achieve with dexmedetomidine (25 versus 10 minutes).[50] However, the use of dexmedetomidine resulted in greater sedation, lower blood pressure, and improved analgesia in the recovery room when compared with propofol. Time to PACU discharge was not different between the groups.

Dexmedetomidine is most often delivered as an initial bolus followed by a continuous infusion. Initial bolus doses range from 0.5 to 1.0 μg/kg over 10 to 20 minutes, followed by a continuous infusion of 0.2 to 0.7 μg/kg per hour.

Patient-Controlled Sedation and Analgesia

Techniques that allow the direct patient control of the level of sedation may positively affect patient satisfaction.[51] The degree of sedation desired by the patient varies significantly, and the individual response to drugs is variable. Patient-controlled sedation (PCS) appears to be an attractive solution to this problem. One approach to PCS has been to use a conventional patient-controlled analgesia (PCA) delivery system set to deliver 0.7-mg/kg boluses of propofol with a 3-minute lockout period.[52] Other approaches include fixed-dose combinations of 0.5 mg midazolam and 25 μg fentanyl with a 5-minute lockout interval between doses.[53] This technique was as safe and effective as anesthesiologist-controlled drug delivery, but may be associated with greater postprocedure sedation.[54] The pharmacokinetic profile of alfentanil is ideal for the treatment of short, discrete episodes of pain. These properties have been exploited during vaginal ovum retrieval procedures, when ultrasonically guided needles are passed through the vaginal wall under monitored anesthesia care. Zelcer et al used a PCA delivery system to allow self-administration of alfentanil during this procedure.[55] After midazolam premedication and a loading dose of alfentanil, patients received 5-μg/kg boluses of alfentanil via the PCA pump with a mandatory 3-minute lockout period. Patient acceptability, alfentanil dosage, respiratory variables, and pain scores were similar to those obtained with physician-controlled analgesia. From the limited data that are available, intraoperative PCA during monitored anesthesia care appears to be an effective alternative to physician-administered analgesia.

RESPIRATORY FUNCTION AND SEDATIVE-HYPNOTICS

During monitored anesthesia care, there is significant potential for respiratory compromise mediated via several important mechanisms. These include adverse effects on respiratory drive, either directly as a result of sedative-hypnotic or opioid administration or indirectly as a consequence of brainstem hypoperfusion resulting from hypotension, such as that occurring during spinal or epidural anesthesia. There may also be a marked increase in the work of breathing due to increased resistance to gas flow in the upper airway.[56] During sedation, it is likely that protective airway reflexes will be attenuated. In contrast, sedative doses of benzodiazepines appear to have variable effects on respiratory system mechanics, either decreasing, increasing, or having no effect on functional residual capacity.[57–59]

Sedation and Upper Airway Patency

The upper airway is located outside the thorax. During normal inspiration, the pressure within the upper airway is subatmospheric; thus, there is a tendency for the upper airway to collapse under the influence of the surrounding atmospheric pressure. However, in the normal subject this tendency for airway collapse is opposed by upper airway dilator muscle tone. These muscles probably both increase the diameter and reduce the compliance of the upper airway. An increase in upper airway dilator muscle tone occurs during inspiration, commencing just prior to diaphragmatic contraction.[60] Several studies have confirmed the importance of coordinated activation of the diaphragmatic and upper airway respiratory muscles in maintaining airway patency. Upper airway dilator muscle control appears to be extremely sensitive to sedative-hypnotic drug administration.[61] For example, sedative doses of midazolam have been reported to increase inspiratory subglottic airway resistance three- to fourfold.[62] Sedative doses of diazepam selectively suppress genioglossal muscle activity to a greater degree than diaphragmatic activity; furthermore, this effect is exaggerated in the elderly.[63] In all these examples, the increased upper airway resistance markedly increased the work of breathing. The response to this obstruction is a significant increase in intercostal and accessory muscle activity. However, this response is only partially effective because the increase in inspiratory force will further decrease intraluminal upper airway pressure, predisposing to further airway collapse. It is likely that these effects will be of greatest significance in patients with preexisting respiratory compromise, such as the elderly or those with chronic obstructive pulmonary disease. These patients often have limited respiratory reserve and are unable to increase their respiratory muscle activity in response to the increased work of breathing induced by sedation and may become hypercarbic, acidotic, and hypoxic.

Sedation and Protective Airway Reflexes

Competent laryngeal and upper airway reflexes are required to protect the lower airway from aspiration. It is well documented that protective laryngeal and pharyngeal reflexes are depressed by anesthesia and sedation. Furthermore, it is also well documented that protective airway reflexes are compromised by advanced age and debilitation. Therefore, it is likely that significant depression of airway reflexes could occur during sedation in the patient who is elderly or debilitated. Aspiration of gastric contents could occur either in the operating room or during recovery, particularly if oral intake is allowed before the return of adequate upper airway protective reflexes. The time required for the return of protective reflexes varies considerably. Complete recovery of the swallowing reflex occurs approximately 15 minutes after the return of consciousness following propofol anesthesia.[64] However, the intravenous administration of 15 mg of diazepam has been shown to depress the swallowing reflex for up to 4 hours.[65] The swallowing reflex is significantly depressed for up to 2 hours following the administration of midazolam, despite the return to a normal state of consciousness.[66] In otherwise healthy adult male volunteers, the inhalation of 50% nitrous oxide was associated with marked depression of the swallowing reflex.[67]

It is apparent from the sources quoted previously that the protective airway reflexes alone cannot be relied on to protect the lower airway from aspiration during sedation. Thus, patients who are deemed to be at risk from aspiration of gastric contents should be maintained at the lightest level of sedation possible. Ideally, the patient should be awake enough to recognize the regurgitation of gastric contents and be able to protect his or her own airway. If the ability of the patient to protect his or her own airway cannot be reliably guaranteed and regurgitation/aspiration is believed to be a significant risk, placement of a cuffed endotracheal tube under general or local anesthesia should be seriously considered.

Sedation and Respiratory Control

Clinical experience would lead most anesthesiologists to predict that the administration of sedative-hypnotic drugs is associated with the depression of respiratory drive. However, the findings of scientific studies in this area are often conflicting and confusing, on occasion finding minimal, if any, effects of sedative drugs on ventilatory responsiveness. However, it is important to note that in many cases the methods used to 7
measure respiratory drive may affect the outcome of the study by stimulating the subject, thus attenuating the negative effect of the drug on respiratory drive. In clinical practice, it is likely that during regional anesthesia there is a degree of deafferentation that will potentiate the respiratory depressant effects of sedative-hypnotic drugs.[68] Most studies have demonstrated that opioids depress the ventilatory response to hypercapnia and hypoxia.[69] Reports of the effects of sedative doses of benzodiazepines on carbon dioxide responsiveness have shown variable results, including no significant effect[70] and clinically significant depression.[71] However, when opioids and benzodiazepines are used in combination, there appears to a consistent and marked negative effect on respiratory responsiveness.[17] Initial clinical investigation examining the combination of propofol and opioids has shown little potentiation of the adverse effects of opioids by sedative doses of propofol.[24]

SUPPLEMENTAL OXYGEN ADMINISTRATION

Hypoxia as a result of alveolar hypoventilation is a relatively common occurrence following the administration of sedatives, analgesics, and hypnotics. In the absence of significant lung disease, the administration of only modest concentrations of supplemental oxygen is frequently effective in restoring the patient's oxygen saturation to an acceptable level. This concept is well illustrated by reference to the familiar alveolar gas equation. An extreme example illustrates the point: an otherwise healthy adult male breathing room air receives a dose of an opioid that causes marked alveolar hypoventilation such that his alveolar P_{CO_2} is increased to 80 mm Hg. The alveolar gas equation predicts that his arterial P_{O_2} will fall to approximately 40 mm Hg as shown:

$$P_{AO_2} = P_{IO_2} - P_{ACO_2}/R$$
$$P_{IO_2} = F_{IO_2} \times (P_B - P_{H_2O})$$
$$P_{IO_2} = 0.21 \times (760 - 47) = 150\ \text{mm Hg}$$
$$P_{AO_2} = 150 - 80/0.8$$
$$P_{AO_2} = 50\ \text{mm Hg}$$

Assuming a normal A–a gradient, his Pa_{O_2} will be 40 mm Hg, corresponding to an arterial oxygen saturation of 75%. If while initiating definitive therapy for hypoventilation this patient were to receive only a modest increase in inspired oxygen, a marked improvement in arterial saturation would be achieved:

F_{IO_2} increased to 28%
$$P_{IO_2} = 0.28 \times (760 - 47) - 200\ \text{mm Hg}$$
$$P_{AO_2} = 200 - 80/0.8$$
$$P_{AO_2} = 100\ \text{mm Hg}$$

This theoretical example serves to highlight several points. First, in isolated hypoventilation, modest increases in inspired oxygen are remarkably effective at restoring oxygen saturation to acceptable levels. However, a patient who is receiving minimal supplemental oxygen and has acceptable oxygen saturation may have significant undetected alveolar hypoventilation. Therefore, before making the decision to discharge patients to a less well-monitored environment without supplemental oxygen, it is useful to measure their oxygen saturation while breathing room air.

MONITORING DURING MONITORED ANESTHESIA CARE

American Society of Anesthesiologists Standards

The ASA standards for basic anesthetic monitoring are applicable to all levels of anesthesia care, including monitored anesthesia care. It is useful to review the components of the ASA standards that are pertinent to MAC as approved by the house of delegates on October 21, 1986, and subsequently amended on October 21, 1998.[72] (See Chapter 2, Table 2-1, for the current ASA standards.)

Communication and Observation

A conscientious and well-trained anesthesia caregiver is the single most vital monitor in the operating room. However, his or her effectiveness will be markedly enhanced by the use of the basic quantitative and qualitative monitoring devices, which should be readily available in all operating rooms. It is important that the anesthesiologist continually evaluate the patient's response to verbal stimulation to effectively titrate the level of sedation and to allow the earlier detection of neurologic or cardiorespiratory dysfunction. Continuous visual, tactile, and auditory assessment of physiologic function should include observation of the rate, depth, and pattern of respiration; palpation of the arterial pulse; and assessment of peripheral perfusion by extremity temperature and capillary refill. In addition, the patient should be continually observed for diaphoresis, pallor, shivering, cyanosis, and acute changes in neurologic status.

Auscultation

Auscultation of heart and breath sounds has long been a vital component of monitoring during anesthesia. Placement of a precordial stethoscope near the sternal notch of a nonintubated patient provides important information concerning upper airway patency, as well as a continuous monitor of heart sounds and ventilation. Continuous precordial auscultation is an inexpensive, effective, and essentially risk-free process that serves an additional important purpose by bringing the anesthesia care provider closer to the patient. If access to the patient is limited during the procedure, FM wireless or infrared remote transmission systems are now commercially available.

Pulse Oximetry

No monitor of oxygen transport has had a greater impact on the practice of anesthesiology than the pulse oximeter.[73] Pulse oximetry is noninvasive, safe, and comfortable to the awake patient; it is also technically simple to apply and interpret, and allows continuous real-time monitoring of arterial oxygenation. The use of a quantitative measure of oxygenation is specifically mandated by the ASA standards for intraoperative monitoring. The important mechanisms whereby respiratory function may be compromised during monitored anesthesia care include the effects of sedatives and opioids on respiratory drive, upper airway patency, and protective airway reflexes. Additional important risk factors for arterial desaturation include obesity, preexisting upper airway obstruction and respiratory disease, the extremes of age, and the lithotomy position.[74] The fundamental importance of monitoring oxygenation during monitored anesthesia care can be appreciated from the closed-claim study of Caplan et al,[68] who examined 14 cases of sudden cardiac arrest in otherwise healthy patients who received spinal anesthesia. These major anesthetic mishaps occurred before the routine adoption of pulse oximetry. One of the major findings of this study was that cyanosis frequently heralded the onset of cardiac arrest, suggesting that unappreciated respiratory insufficiency may have played an important role. Further support for the use of pulse oximetry comes from the ASA Committee on Professional Liability analysis of closed anesthesia claims, which reveals that respiratory events constitute the single largest source of adverse outcome. Furthermore, review of these cases suggests that pulse oximetry in combination with capnometry would have prevented the adverse outcome in the vast majority of cases.

Capnography

Although capnography is most effective in the intubated patient, some useful information may be obtained from a spontaneously breathing, nonintubated patient. Sidestream capnographs have been adapted for use with facemasks, nasal airways, and nasal cannulae, and have been used successfully during monitored anesthesia care.[75–78] Nasal cannulae for oxygen delivery have been modified to provide an integral port for respiratory gas sampling and are available commercially. Alternatively, capnograph sampling lines can be attached to shortened intravenous catheters and inserted inside nasal oxygen probes.

Cardiovascular System

At a minimum, the electrocardiogram (ECG) must be continually displayed, and the blood pressure measured and recorded at least every 5 minutes during monitored anesthesia care. The pulse should be monitored by palpation, oximetry, or auscultation. The selection of additional hemodynamic monitoring is usually determined more by the cardiovascular status of the patient than the magnitude of the procedure. Most procedures performed under monitored anesthesia care do not involve major hemorrhage, fluid shifts, or major physiologic trespass. Decisions concerning choice of monitoring for myocardial ischemia and other adverse hemodynamic events will need to be individualized on a case-by-case basis.

Temperature Monitoring and Management During Monitored Anesthesia Care

The value of temperature monitoring is well established during general anesthesia, the perioperative period being frequently complicated by hypothermia and hyperthermia. Although sedation techniques used during monitored anesthesia care do not generally trigger malignant hyperthermia, there is potential for significant inadvertent hypothermia, particularly during neuraxial anesthesia. Even MAC techniques unaccompanied by regional anesthesia are associated with hypothermia at the extremes of age, both the old and very young having impaired thermoregulatory mechanisms. The elderly also have markedly reduced muscle mass and therefore reduced basal heat production. Although the anesthesiologist may be able to exert some control over the ambient temperature in the operating room, he or she may be unable to influence the temperature at remote anesthetizing locations. Radiology suites are often maintained at lower temperatures to accommodate the computer systems that are used to reconstruct images. Radiant heating lamps, forced-air heaters, fluid warmers, or warming blankets, all common items in operating rooms, may be unavailable and unsuitable for use at remote locations. Forced-air heating has been shown to be an effective means of maintaining normothermia and can be combined with intravenous fluid warming.[79] Even mild perioperative hypothermia (i.e., 1 to 2°C) accompanying general anesthesia is associated with adverse myocardial outcomes, increased bleeding tendency and transfusion requirements, wound infections, and delayed wound healing and hospital discharge.[80] There is no evidence suggesting that the morbidity associated with perioperative hypothermia is any less during MAC than during general anesthesia. The morbidity associated with perioperative hypothermia is well described in high-risk patients; this is a group of patients that are likely to undergo procedures under monitored anesthesia care. When hypothermia is significant, shivering may interfere with the planned procedure, markedly increase oxygen requirements, and predispose susceptible patients to myocardial ischemia or respiratory insufficiency. The major thermoregulatory defenses against hypothermia include vasoconstriction, shivering, and behavior. Vasoconstriction and shivering are impaired during major conduction anesthesia. Behavioral thermoregulation is impaired even in the conscious patient. Regional anesthesia

TABLE 47-5

OBSERVER'S ASSESSMENT OF ALERTNESS/SEDATION SCALE

RESPONSIVENESS	SPEECH	FACIAL EXPRESSION	EYES	COMPOSITE SCORE
Responds readily to name spoken in normal tone	Normal	Normal	Clear, no ptosis	5 (Alert)
Lethargic response to name spoken in normal tone	Mild slowing or thickening	Mild relaxation	Glazed or mild ptosis (less than half the eye)	4
Responds only after name is called loudly or repeatedly	Slurring or prominent slowing	Marked relaxation (slack jaw)	Glazed and marked ptosis (half the eye or more)	3
Responds only after mild prodding or shaking	Few recognizable words			2
Does not respond to mild prodding or shaking				1 (Asleep)

Adapted from Chernik DA, Gillings D, Laine H *et al*: Validity and reliability of the observer's assessment of alertness/sedation scale: Study with intravenous midazolam. J Clin Psychopharmacol 10:244, 1990; Liu J, Singh HS, White PF: Electroencephalographic bispectral index correlates with intraoperative recall and depth of propofol induced sedation. Anesth Analg 84:185, 1997.

has major effects on thermoregulation.[81] Lower-extremity vasodilatation causes central cooling via a redistribution of heat from the core to the periphery. Afferent input to the hypothalamus from the warm peripheral compartment counteracts conflicting input from the cooling central compartment, thus delaying the initiation of compensatory thermoregulation. In the absence of reliable temperature monitoring, it is possible that the first indication of hypothermia would be the onset of shivering, by which time considerable central cooling may have occurred.

Frank and coworkers examined the issue of temperature monitoring and management during neuraxial anesthesia and found that temperature monitoring is significantly underused, with only one-third of patients being monitored.[82] Furthermore, the method that was most frequently used to monitor temperature may not accurately reflect core temperature, the most important determinant of thermoregulatory response and perioperative morbidity. Forehead skin surface was the most commonly monitored site. The accuracy of these devices for perioperative temperature monitoring remains controversial; they do not reliably detect malignant hyperthermia and are not sufficiently accurate for fever screening purposes in children.[83] Sessler recommended the use of a properly positioned axillary probe or intermittent oral temperature monitoring during neuraxial anesthetics.[81]

Patients will frequently complain of feeling too warm when covered by heavy drapes. Although malignant hyperthermia is rare during MAC, hyperthermia is still possible as a result of thyroid storm or malignant neuroleptic syndrome. The subjective sensation of hyperthermia may also be the first indicator of important adverse events in evolution such as hypoxia, hypercarbia, cerebral ischemia, local anesthetic toxicity, and myocardial ischemia.

Bispectral Index Monitoring During Monitored Anesthesia Care

The bispectral index (BIS) is a processed EEG parameter that was specifically developed to evaluate patient response during drug-induced anesthesia and sedation. Sedation monitoring is attractive because of the potential to titrate drugs more accurately, avoiding the adverse effects of both overdosing and underdosing. BIS monitoring has some potential advantages over conventional intermittent techniques of patient assessment. Conventional assessment involves patient stimulation at frequent intervals to determine the level of consciousness, requires patient cooperation, and is subject to testing fatigue. An example of a conventional assessment tool is the Observer's Assessment of Alertness/Sedation Scale (OAA/S; Table 47-5).[84] The BIS has been shown to be a useful monitor of drug-induced sedation and of recall in volunteers, and has been shown to correlate with OAA/S scores during propofol-induced sedation in patients undergoing surgery with regional anesthesia.[85] An increasing depth of sedation was associated with a predictable decrease in the BIS. Absence of recall was associated with BIS values less than 80. These findings correspond with those of Kearse et al, who found no intraoperative recall at BIS values less than 79 during midazolam-induced, isoflurane-induced, and propofol-induced sedation.[86] However, the inability to recall a nonnoxious stimulus such as a picture, as used in the previous studies, may not necessarily correspond to amnesia to noxious events such as surgical stimulation. Despite this caveat, Liu and coworkers suggested that using a combination of propofol and midazolam to achieve a BIS value less than 80 will minimize the possibility of intraoperative recall.[85] Although the use of BIS to monitor sedation is appealing, conventional assessment of sedation is an important mechanism whereby continuous patient contact is maintained. Ideally, BIS monitoring will be employed in the future as an adjunct to clinical evaluation rather than as the primary monitor of consciousness.

Preparedness to Recognize and Treat Local Anesthetic Toxicity

8 Monitored anesthesia care is often provided in the context of regional or local anesthetic techniques. It is vitally important that the anesthesiologist responsible for the patient has a high index of suspicion, and is fully prepared to recognize and treat local anesthetic toxicity immediately (see Chapter 17). This point deserves special emphasis, particularly in light of the fact that monitored anesthesia care is often provided to patients who are elderly or debilitated and deemed "unfit" for general anesthesia; these are the patients most likely to suffer adverse reactions to local anesthetic drugs. Even if the anesthesiologist does not perform the block personally, he or she is in a unique position to fulfill an important "preventive" role by advising the surgeon about the most appropriate volume, concentration, and type of local anesthetic drug or technique to be used.

Systemic local anesthetic toxicity occurs when plasma concentrations of drug are excessively high. Plasma concentrations will increase when the rate of entry of drug into the circulation exceeds the rate of drug clearance from the circulation. The clinically recognizable effects of local anesthetics on the CNS are concentration dependent. At low concentrations, sedation and numbness of the tongue and circumoral tissues, as well as a metallic taste, are prominent features. As concentrations increase, restlessness, vertigo, tinnitus, and difficulty of focusing may occur. Higher concentrations result in slurred speech and skeletal muscle twitching, which often herald the onset of tonic-clonic seizures.

The conduct of monitored anesthesia care may modify the individual's response to the potentially toxic effects of local anesthetic administration and adversely affect the margin of safety of a regional or local technique. For example, a patient with compromised cardiovascular function may experience a further decline in cardiac output during sedation. The resultant reduction in hepatic blood flow will reduce the clearance of local anesthetics that are metabolized by the liver and have a high hepatic extraction ratio, thereby increasing the likelihood of achieving toxic plasma concentrations. A patient receiving sedation may experience respiratory depression and a subsequent increase in arterial carbon dioxide concentration. Hypercarbia adversely affects the margin of safety in several ways. By increasing cerebral blood flow, hypercarbia will increase the amount of local anesthetic that is delivered to the brain, thereby increasing the potential for neurotoxicity. By reducing neuronal axoplasmic pH, hypercarbia increases the intracellular concentration of the charged, active form of local anesthetic, thus also increasing its toxicity. In addition, hypercarbia, acidosis, and hypoxia all markedly potentiate the cardiovascular toxicity of local anesthetics. Furthermore, the administration of sedative-hypnotic drugs may interfere with the patient's ability to communicate the symptoms of impending neurotoxicity. However, the anticonvulsant properties of benzodiazepines and barbiturates may attenuate the seizures associated with neurotoxicity. In both of the previous circumstances, it is possible that the symptoms of cardiotoxicity will be the first evidence that an adverse reaction has occurred. Thus, appropriate treatment is delayed or inadvertent intravascular injection is continued because of the absence of any clinical evidence of neurotoxicity. Cardiovascular toxicity usually occurs at a higher plasma concentration than neurotoxicity, but when it does occur, it is usually much more difficult to manage than neurotoxicity. Although cardiotoxicity is usually preceded by neurotoxicity, it may occur de novo when bupivacaine is being used.

Sedation and Analgesia by Nonanesthesiologists

Although anesthesiologists have specific training and expertise to provide sedation and analgesia, in clinical practice these services are frequently provided by nonanesthesiologists. The specific reasons for nonanesthesiologist involvement differ from institution to institution and from case to case, and include convenience, availability, and scheduling issues; perceived lack of anesthesiologist enthusiasm; perceived cost issues; and perceived lack of benefit concerning patient satisfaction and safety when sedation and analgesia are provided by anesthesiologists. Despite our frequent noninvolvement in these cases, anesthesiologists are indirectly involved in the care of these patients by being required to participate in the development of institutional policies and procedures for sedation and analgesia. To assist anesthesiologists in this process, an ASA task force has developed practice guidelines for sedation and analgesia by nonanesthesiologists.[1]

Four levels of sedation are defined in the ASA practice guidelines, and include minimal sedation, moderate sedation, deep sedation, and general anesthesia. The practice guidelines emphasize that sedation and analgesia represent a continuum of sedation where patients can easily pass into a level of sedation deeper than intended. When monitoring a sedated patient during a procedure, it is important to recognize when a patient becomes more deeply sedated than intended so the care team can act appropriately to prevent cardiorespiratory compromise.

The guidelines emphasize the importance of preprocedure patient evaluation, patient preparation, and appropriate fasting periods. The importance of continuous patient monitoring is discussed: in particular, the response of the patient to commands as a guide to the level of sedation. The appropriate monitoring of pulmonary ventilation, oxygenation, and hemodynamics is also discussed, and recommendations are made for the contemporaneous recording of these parameters. The task force strongly suggests that an individual other than the person performing the procedure be available to monitor the patient's comfort and physiologic status. Education and training of providers is recommended. Specific educational objectives include the potentiation of sedative-induced respiratory depression by concomitantly administered opioids, adequate time intervals between doses of sedative/analgesics to avoid cumulative overdosage, and familiarity with sedative/analgesic antagonists. The routine administration of supplemental oxygen is recommended. At least one person with advanced life support skills should be present during the procedure. This individual should have the ability to recognize airway obstruction, establish an airway, and maintain oxygenation and ventilation. The practice guidelines recommend that appropriate patient size emergency equipment be readily available, specifically including equipment for establishing an airway and delivering positive-pressure ventilation with supplemental oxygen, emergency resuscitation drugs, and a working defibrillator. The presence of reliable intravenous access until the patient is no longer at risk for cardiorespiratory depression will improve safety. Adequate postprocedure recovery care with appropriate monitoring must be provided until discharge. Certain high-risk patient groups (e.g., uncooperative patients; extremes of age; severe cardiac, pulmonary, hepatic, renal, or CNS disease; morbid obesity; sleep apnea; pregnancy; drug or alcohol abuse) will be encountered and the guidelines recommend that preprocedure consultation with anesthesiologists, cardiologists, pulmonologists, and so forth be performed *before* administration of sedation and analgesia by nonanesthesiologists.

CONCLUSION

Through the use of monitored anesthesia care, an often terrifying and painful procedure can be made safe and comfortable for the patient. Monitored anesthesia care presents an opportunity for our patients to observe us at work. For the anesthesiologist, monitored anesthesia care can provide a more prolonged and intimate level of care and reassurance to our patients that is in contrast to the more limited exposure that occurs during and after general anesthesia. Our airway management skills and our daily practice of applied pharmacology make us uniquely qualified to provide this service. Monitored anesthesia care presents us with an opportunity to display these skills and increase our recognition in areas outside the operating room. The availability of drugs with a more favorable pharmacologic profile allows us to tailor our techniques to provide the specific components of analgesia, sedation, anxiolysis, and amnesia with minimal morbidity and to facilitate a prompt recovery. As the population ages, increasing numbers of patients will become candidates for monitored anesthesia care. Significant advances in nonsurgical fields (e.g., interventional radiology) will increase the number of procedures that are ideally performed under monitored anesthesia care. It is our responsibility to clearly demonstrate to our nonanesthesia colleagues that anesthesiologist-provided monitored anesthesia care contributes to the best outcome for our patients. If anesthesiologists are not willing or able to provide these services, others who are less qualified are prepared to assume that role.

References

1. American Society of Anesthesiologists Task Force: Practice guidelines for sedation and analgesia by non-anesthesiologists. Anesthesiology 96:1004, 2002
2. American Society of Anesthesiologists (ASA): Position on monitored anesthesia care. In ASA Directory of Members, p 481. Park Ridge, IL, American Society of Anesthesiologists, 1999
3. Ausems ME, Vuyk J, Hug CC Jr, Stanski DR: Comparison of a computer-assisted infusion versus intermittent bolus administration of alfentanil as a supplement to nitrous oxide for lower abdominal surgery. Anesthesiology 68:851, 1988
4. Hughes MA, Glass PSA, Jacobs JR: Context-sensitive half-time in multicompartment pharmacokinetic models for intravenous anesthetic drugs. Anesthesiology 76:334, 1992
5. Scott JC, Ponganis KV, Stanski DR: EEG quantitation of narcotic effect: The comparative pharmacodynamics of fentanyl and alfentanil. Anesthesiology 62:234, 1985
6. Mandema JW, Tuk B, van Stveninck AL *et al*: Pharmacokinetic-pharmacodynamic modeling of the central nervous system effects of midazolam and its main metabolite α-hydroxy-midazolam in healthy volunteers. Clin Pharmacol Ther 51:715, 1992
7. Buhrer M, Maitre PO, Crevoisier C, Stanski DR: Electroencephalographic effects of benzodiazepines. II. Pharmacodynamic modeling of the effects of midazolam and diazepam. Clin Pharmacol Ther 48:555, 1990
8. Glass P, Dyar O, Jhaveri R *et al*: TIVA-propofol and combinations of propofol with fentanyl [Abstract]. Anesthesiology 75:A44, 1991
9. Smith C, McEwan AI, Jhaveri R *et al*: Reduction of propofol Cp50 by fentanyl [Abstract]. Anesthesiology 77:A340, 1992
10. Short TG, Chui PT: Propofol and midazolam act synergistically in combination. Br J Anaesth 67:539, 1991
11. Short TG, Plummer JL, Chui PT: Hypnotic and anesthetic interactions between midazolam, propofol and alfentanil. Br J Anaesth 69:162, 1992
12. McEwan A, Smith C, Dyar O *et al*: MAC reduction of isoflurane by fentanyl [Abstract]. Anesthesiology 75:A43, 1991
13. Sebel PS, Glass PSA, Fletcher JE *et al*: Reduction of the MAC of desflurane with fentanyl. Anesthesiology 76:52, 1992
14. Vinik HR, Bradley EL, Kissin I: Midazolam–alfentanil synergism for anesthetic induction in patients. Anesth Analg 69:213, 1989
15. Kissin I, Vinik HR, Castillo R, Bradley EL: Alfentanil potentiates midazolam-induced unconsciousness in subanalgesic doses. Anesth Analg 71:65, 1990
16. Federal Food and Drug Administration: Warning reemphasized in midazolam labeling. FDA Drug Bull 5,1987
17. Bailey PL, Pace NL, Ashburn MA *et al*: Frequent hypoxemia and apnea after sedation with midazolam and fentanyl. Anesthesiology 73:826, 1990
18. Mackenzie N, Grant IS: Propofol for intravenous sedation. Anaesthesia 42:3, 1987
19. White PF, Negus JB: Sedative infusions during local and regional anesthesia: A comparison of midazolam and propofol. J Clin Anesth 3:32, 1991
20. Smith I, Monk T, White PF, Ding Y: Propofol infusion during regional anesthesia: Sedative, hypnotic and amnestic properties. Anesth Analg 79:313, 1994
21. Dubois A, Balatoni E, Peeters JP, Baudoux M: Use of propofol for sedation during gastrointestinal endoscopies. Anaesthesia 43(Suppl):75, 1988
22. Kain ZN, Gaal D, Jaeger DD, Rimar S: Sedation for MRI in children: Propofol vs. barbiturates [Abstract]. Anesthesiology 79:A1158, 1993
23. Monk TG, Boure B, White PF *et al:* Comparison of intravenous sedative-hypnotic techniques for outpatient immersion lithotripsy. Anesth Analg 72:616, 1991
24. Sherry E: Admixture of propofol and alfentanil: Use for intravenous sedation and analgesia during transvaginal oocyte retrieval. Anaesthesia 47:477, 1992
25. Oei-Lim LB, Vermeulen-Cranch DME, Bouvry-Berends ECM: Conscious sedation with propofol in dentistry. Br Dent J 170:340, 1991
26. Whitehead C, Sanders LD, Oldroyd G *et al*: The subjective effects of low dose propofol. Anaesthesia 49:490, 1994
27. Borgeat A, Wilder-Smith OHG, Saiah M, Rifat K: Subhypnotic doses of propofol possess direct antiemetic properties. Anesth Analg 74:539, 1992
28. White PF, Negus JB: Sedative infusions during local and regional anesthesia: A comparison of midazolam and propofol. J Clin Anesth 3:32, 1991
29. Ghouri AF, Ramirez Ruiz MA, White PF: Effect of flumazenil on recovery after midazolam and propofol sedation. Anesthesiology 81:333, 1994
30. Smith I, White PF, Nathanson M, Gouldson R: Propofol: An update on its clinical use. Anesthesiology 81:1005, 1994
31. Stoelting RK: Benzodiazepines. In Pharmacology and Physiology in Anesthetic Practice, 2nd ed, p 118. Philadelphia, JB Lippincott, 1991
32. Taylor E, Ghouri AF, White PF: Midazolam in combination with propofol for sedation during local anesthesia. J Clin Anesth 4:213, 1992
33. Jacobs JR, Reves JG, Marty J *et al*: Aging increases pharmacodynamic sensitivity to the hypnotic effects of midazolam. Anesth Analg 80:143, 1995
34. Pratila MG, Fischer ME, Alagesan R *et al*: Propofol vs. midazolam for monitored sedation: A comparison of intraoperative and recovery parameters. J Clin Anesth 5:268, 1993
35. Ghouri AF, Ramirez Ruiz MA, White PF: Effect of flumazenil on recovery after midazolam and propofol sedation. Anesthesiology 81:333, 1994
36. Yee JB, Schafer PG, Crandall AS, Pace NL: Comparison of methohexital and alfentanil on movement during placement of retrobulbar nerve block. Anesth Analg 79:320, 1994
37. Veselis RA, Reinsel RA, Feshchenko VA *et al*: Impaired memory and behavioural performance with fentanyl at low plasma concentrations. Anesth Analg 79:952, 1994
38. Glass PSA, Gan TJ, Howell S: A review of the pharmacokinetics and pharmacodynamics of remifentanil. Anesth Analg 89(Suppl):S7, 1999
39. Servin F, Desmonts JM, Watkins WD: Remifentanil as an analgesic adjunct in local/regional anesthesia and monitored anesthesia care. Anesth Analg 89(Suppl):S28, 1999
40. Avramov MN, Smith I, White PF: Interactions between midazolam and remifentanil during monitored anesthesia care. Anesthesiology 85:1283, 1996
41. Ahmad S, Leavell M, Fragen RJ *et al*: Remifentanil versus alfentanil as analgesic adjuncts during placement of ophthalmologic nerve blocks. Reg Analg Pain Med 24:331, 1999
42. Gold MI, Watkins WD, Sung YF *et al*: Remifentanil versus remifentanil/midazolam for ambulatory surgery during monitored anesthesia care. Anesthesiology 87:51, 1997
43. Green SM, Klooster M, Harris T *et al*: Ketamine sedation for pediatric gastroenterology procedures. Pediatr Gastroenterol Nutr 32:26, 2001
44. McCarty EC, Mencio GA, Walker LA *et al*: Ketamine sedation for the reduction of children's fractures in the emergency department. J Bone Surg 82:912, 2000
45. Sherwin TS, Green SM, Khan A *et al*: Does adjunctive midazolam reduce recovery agitation after ketamine sedation for pediatric procedures? A randomized, double blind, placebo-controlled trial. Ann Emerg Med 35:229, 2000
46. Talke P, Richardson CA, Scheinin M *et al*: Postoperative pharmacokinetics and sympatholytic effects of dexmedetomidine. Anesth Analg 85:1136, 1997
47. Bekker AY, Basile J, Gold M *et al*: Dexmedetomidine for awake carotid endarterectomy: Efficacy, hemodynamic profile, and side effects. J Neurosurg Anesthesiol 16:126, 2004
48. Bekker AY, Kaufman B, Samir H *et al*: The use of dexmedetomidine infusion for awake craniotomy. Anesth Analg 92:1251, 2001
49. Ard J, Doyle W, Bekker A: Awake craniotomy with dexmedetomidine in pediatric patients. J Neurosurg Anesthesiol 15:263, 2003
50. Arain SR, Ebert TJ: The efficacy, side effects, and recovery characteristics of dexmedetomidine versus propofol when used for intraoperative sedation. Anesth Analg 95:461, 2002
51. Perry F, Parker RK, White PF *et al*: Role of psychological factors in postoperative pain control and recovery with patient-controlled analgesia. Clin J Pain 10:57, 1994
52. Rudkin GE, Osborne GA, Curtis NJ: Intraoperative patient controlled sedation. Anaesthesia 46:90, 1991
53. Park WY, Watkins PA: Patient-controlled sedation during epidural anesthesia. Anesth Analg 72:304, 1991
54. Cork R, Guillory E, Viswanathan S: Effect of patient-controlled sedation on recovery from ambulatory monitored anesthesia care [Abstract]. Anesthesiology 81:A31, 1994
55. Zelcer J, White PF, Chester S *et al*: Intraoperative patient-controlled analgesia: An alternative to physician administration during outpatient monitored anesthesia care. Anesth Analg 75:41, 1992
56. Montravers P, Duriel B, Molliex S, Desmonts JM: Effects of intravenous midazolam on the work of breathing. Anesth Analg 79:558, 1994
57. Gelb A, Southorn P, Redher K, Didier E: Sedation and respiratory mechanics in man. Br J Anaesth 57:1104, 1983
58. Morel DR, Forster A, Bachmann M, Suter PM: Effect of intravenous midazolam on breathing pattern and chest wall mechanics in humans. J Appl Physiol 55:419, 1983
59. Prato FS, Knill RL: Diazepam sedation reduces functional residual capacity and alters the distribution of ventilation in man. Anesth Analg 61:209, 1982
60. Cohen MI: Phrenic and recurrent laryngeal discharge patterns and the Hering-Breuer reflex. Am J Physiol 228:1489, 1975
61. Gottfried SR, Strohl KP, Van de Graaff W *et al*: Effects of phrenic stimulation on upper airway resistance in anesthetized dogs. J Appl Physiol 55:419, 1983
62. Montravers P, Dureuil B, Desmonts JM: Effects of i.v. midazolam on upper airway resistance. Br J Anaesth 68:27, 1992
63. Leiter JC, Knuth SL, Krol ZRC, Bartlett D: The effects of diazepam on genioglossal muscle activity in normal subjects. Am Rev Respir Dis 132:216, 1985
64. Rimaniol JM, D'Honneur G, Duvaldestin P: Recovery of the swallowing reflex after propofol anesthesia. Anesth Analg 79:856, 1994
65. Groves ND, Rees JL: Effects of benzodiazepines on laryngeal reflexes. Anaesthesia 42:808, 1987
66. Lambert Y, D'Honneur G, Abhay K, Gall O: Depression of swallowing reflex two hours after midazolam [Abstract]. Anesthesiology 75:A891, 1991

67. Nishino T, Takizawa K, Yokokawa N, Hiraga K: Depression of the swallowing reflex during sedation and/or relative analgesia produced by inhalation of 50% nitrous oxide in oxygen. Anesthesiology 67:995, 1987
68. Caplan RA, Ward RJ, Posner K, Cheney FW: Unexpected cardiac arrest during spinal anesthesia: A closed claims analysis of predisposing factors. Anesthesiology 68:5, 1988
69. Weil JV, McCullocugh RE, Kline JS, Sodal IE: Diminished ventilatory response to hypoxia and hypercapnia after morphine in normal man. N Engl J Med 292:1103, 1975
70. Power SJ, Morgan M, Chakrabarti MK: Carbon dioxide response curves following midazolam and diazepam. Br J Anaesth 55:837, 1983
71. Jordan C, Lehane JR, Jones JG: Respiratory depression following diazepam: Reversal with high dose naloxone. Anesthesiology 53:293, 1980
72. American Society of Anesthesiologists: Standards for Basic Intraoperative Monitoring. 1999 Directory of Members, p 462. Park Ridge, IL, American Society of Anesthesiologists, 1999
73. Barker SJ, Tremper KK: Pulse oximetry. In Ehrenworth J, Eisenkraft J (eds): Anesthetic Equipment: Principles and Applications, p 249. St Louis, Mosby, 1993
74. Raemer DB, Warren DL, Morris R *et al*: Hypoxemia during ambulatory gynecologic surgery as evaluated by the pulse oximeter. J Clin Monit 3:244, 1987
75. Pressman MA: A simple method for measuring end-tidal CO_2 during MAC and major regional anesthesia. Anesth Analg 67:900, 1988
76. Norman EA, Zeig NJ, Ahmad I: Better designs for mass spectrometer monitoring of the awake patient [Letter]. Anesthesiology 64:664, 1986
77. Bowe EA, Boysen PG, Brome JA *et al*: Accurate determination of end-tidal CO_2 through nasal cannulae. J Clin Monit 5:105, 1989
78. Goldmann JM: A simple and inexpensive method for monitoring end-tidal CO_2 through nasal cannulae [Letter]. Anesthesiology 67:606, 1987
79. Kurz A, Kurz M, Poeschl G *et al*: Forced-air warming maintains intraoperative normothermia better than circulating-water mattresses. Anesth Analg 77:89, 1993
80. Frank SM, Fleisher LA, Breslow MJ *et al*: Perioperative maintenance of normothermia reduces the incidence of morbid cardiac events: A randomized trial. JAMA 277:1127, 1997
81. Sessler DI: Temperature monitoring and management during neuraxial anesthesia. Anesth Analg 88:243, 1999
82. Frank SM, Nguyen JM, Garcia CM *et al*: Temperature monitoring practices during regional anesthesia. Anesth Analg 88:373, 1999
83. Scholefield JH, Gerber MA, Dwyer P. Liquid crystal forehead temperature strips. Am J Dis Child 136:198, 1982
84. Chernik DA, Gillings D, Laine H *et al*: Validity and reliability of the observer's assessment of alertness/sedation scale: Study with intravenous midazolam. J Clin Psychopharmacol 10:244, 1990
85. Liu J, Singh HS, White PF: Electroencephalographic bispectral index correlates with intraoperative recall and depth of propofol induced sedation. Anesth Analg 84:185, 1997
86. Kearse LA, Manberg P, Chamoun N *et al*: Bispectral analysis of the electroencephalogram correlates with patient movement to skin incision during propofol/nitrous oxide anesthesia. Anesthesiology 81:1365, 1994

CHAPTER 48 ■ TRAUMA AND BURNS

LEVON M. CAPAN AND SANFORD M. MILLER

KEY POINTS

1. Initial evaluation of the trauma patient involves rapid overview, primary survey, and secondary survey.
2. Airway management is tailored to the type of injury, the nature and degree of airway compromise, and the patient's hemodynamic and oxygenation status.
3. Of the several causes that may alter respiration after trauma, tension pneumothorax, flail chest, and open pneumothorax are immediate threats to the patient's life, and therefore, require rapid diagnosis and treatment.
4. Hemorrhage is the most common cause of traumatic hypotension and shock.
5. Approximately 40% of deaths from trauma are caused by head injury.
6. The most important therapeutic maneuvers in head injury patients are aimed at maintaining cerebral perfusion pressure and oxygen delivery.
7. The objective in the evaluation of spinal trauma is to diagnose instability of the spine and the extent of neurologic involvement.
8. Penetrating neck injuries usually present with obvious clinical manifestations, whereas blunt cervical trauma may be more subtle.
9. Patients with three or more fractured ribs have a greater likelihood of pulmonary injury, higher injury severity score, and mortality rate than those with fewer rib fractures.
10. Blunt cardiac injury has replaced "myocardial contusion" and encompasses varying degrees of myocardial damage; coronary artery injury; and rupture of the cardiac free wall, septum, or a valve following blunt trauma.
11. Pelvic fractures result in major hemorrhage in 25% and exsanguination in 1% of patients.
12. Thermal trauma caused by flames in a closed space is likely to be associated with airway damage.
13. In burn victims, carbon monoxide (CO) inhalation is almost always associated with smoke inhalation, which increases the morbidity and mortality compared with CO toxicity alone.
14. Crystalloid solutions are preferred for resuscitation during the first day following a burn injury; leakage of colloids during this phase may increase edema.
15. Evaluation of the multiple trauma patient emergently transported to the operating room involves review of vital signs, oxygenation, preoperative fluid replacement, and confirmation of correct position and patency of a previously inserted endotracheal tube.
16. Anesthetic agents not only have direct cardiovascular depressant effects, but also inhibit compensatory hemodynamic mechanisms such as central catecholamine output and baroreflex (neuroregulatory) mechanisms, which maintain systemic pressure in hypovolemia.
17. Persistent hypotension following trauma is usually the result of one of four mechanisms: bleeding, tension pneumothorax, neurogenic shock, and cardiac injury.
18. The mortality rate after trauma increases with decreasing temperature.
19. Perioperative diagnosis of coagulopathy is often made by observing bleeding from wounds or puncture sites, rather than by interpretation of laboratory tests.
20. Intraoperative hyperkalemia may develop as a result of three mechanisms: alteration of cell membrane permeability, reperfusion injury, and rapid blood transfusion.
21. Reevaluation and optimization of the circulation, oxygenation, temperature, central nervous system function, coagulation, electrolyte and acid-base status, and renal function are the hallmarks of postoperative management.

Injuries are the most common cause of death in Americans between the ages of 1 and 45 years; more than 50% of all deaths in people between 5 and 34 years of age result from trauma.[1] There were nearly 145,000 deaths from trauma in 2001: the fourth most common cause of mortality following heart disease (700,000), malignant neoplasms (554,000), and cerebrovascular disease (164,000).[1] The victim's quality of life may also be affected; approximately 80% of survivors of major trauma have significant functional limitation 12 and 18 months after injury.[2] The economic impact of trauma on society is also enormous. In 2002, the estimated cost of unintentional injuries alone was $586 billion, including the costs of fatal and nonfatal injuries, employer costs, vehicle damage, and fire losses. The additional cost of lost quality of life is estimated as $1,272 billion, bringing the total annual cost of trauma to $1,858 billion.[3]

Approximately 75% of the hospital mortality from trauma occurs within 48 hours after admission,[4–6] most commonly from thoracic, abdominal or retroperitoneal, vascular, or central nervous system (CNS) injuries.[4,5] Hypoxia, systemic air embolism, and cardiac failure may also be direct or contributing factors.[5] Approximately one-third of these patients die within the first 4 hours after admission, representing the majority of operating room (OR) trauma deaths.[6,7] Of the remaining 25% of hospital deaths, 5 to 10% occur between the third and seventh day of admission, usually from CNS injuries,[4,6,7] and the rest in subsequent weeks, most commonly as a result of multiorgan failure.[5] Pulmonary thromboembolism and infectious complications may also contribute to mortality during this phase.[4,5]

INITIAL EVALUATION AND RESUSCITATION

The strategy of initial management can be defined as a continuous, priority-driven process of patient assessment, resuscitation, and reassessment. The general approach to evaluation of the acute trauma victim has three sequential components: rapid
1 overview, primary survey, and secondary survey (Fig. 48-1). Resuscitation is initiated, if needed, at any time during this continuum. *Rapid overview* takes only a few seconds and is used to determine whether the patient is stable, unstable, dead, or dying. The *primary survey* involves rapid evaluation of functions that are crucial to survival. The "ABCs" of airway patency, breathing, and circulation are assessed. Then a brief neurologic examination is performed, and the patient is examined for any external injuries that might have been overlooked.

The *secondary survey* involves a more elaborate systematic examination of the entire body to identify additional injuries. Radiographic and other diagnostic procedures may also be performed if the stability of the patient permits. Within this general framework the anesthesiologist, aside from managing the airway, contributes as part of the team to evaluation and resuscitation, while gathering information needed for possible future anesthetic management.

Injuries may be missed during initial evaluation and even during emergency surgery, resulting in significant pain, complications, residual disability, delay of treatment, or death.[8] Reported missed diagnoses include cervical spine, thoracoabdominal, pelvic, nerve, and external soft-tissue injuries, and extremity fractures. Some of these injuries may present during anesthesia, such as spinal cord damage during airway management in a patient with unrecognized cervical spine injury, massive intraoperative bleeding from an unrecognized thoracoabdominal injury during extremity surgery, or sudden intraoperative hypoxemia in a patient with unrecognized pneumothorax. A *tertiary survey* within the first 24 hours after admission (which may include a period of anesthesia) can potentially diagnose the majority of clinically significant injuries missed during initial evaluation,[8] by repeating the primary and secondary examinations and reviewing the results of radiologic and laboratory testing.

Airway Evaluation and Intervention

2 Airway evaluation involves the diagnosis of any trauma to the airway or surrounding tissues, recognition and anticipation of the respiratory consequences of these injuries, and prediction of the potential for exacerbation of these or other injuries by any contemplated airway management maneuvers. Although nontraumatic causes of airway difficulty, such as preexisting factors, may be present, only the management of trauma-related problems is discussed in this section.

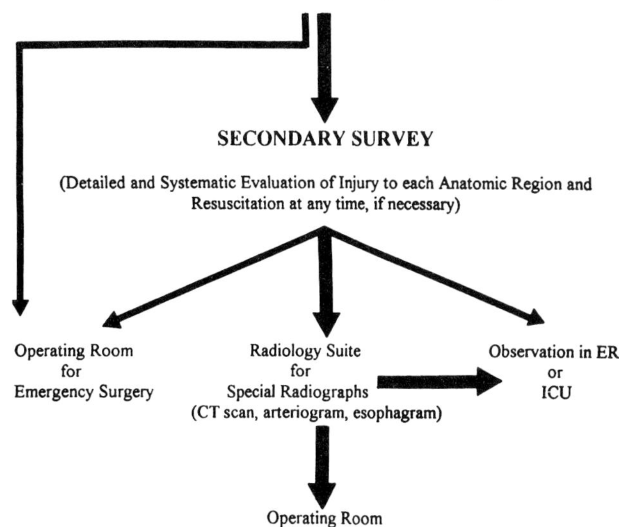

FIGURE 48-1. Clinical sequence for initial management of the major trauma patient. CT, computed tomography; ER, emergency room; ICU, intensive care unit.

Airway Obstruction

Airway obstruction is probably the most frequent cause of asphyxia and may result from posteriorly displaced or lacerated pharyngeal soft tissues, hematoma, bleeding, secretions, foreign bodies, or displaced bone or cartilage fragments. Bleeding into the cervical region may produce airway obstruction not only because of compression by the hematoma, but also from venous congestion and upper airway edema as a result of compression of neck veins. Signs of upper and lower airway obstruction include dyspnea, hoarseness, stridor, dysphonia, subcutaneous emphysema, and hemoptysis. Cervical deformity, edema, crepitation, tracheal deviation, or jugular venous distention may be present before these symptoms appear and may help indicate that specialized airway management techniques are required.

The initial steps in airway management are chin lift, jaw thrust, clearing of the oropharyngeal cavity, placement of an oropharyngeal or nasopharyngeal airway, and in inadequately breathing patients, ventilation with a self-inflating bag.

Immobilization of the cervical spine and administration of oxygen should be applied simultaneously. Blind passage of a nasopharyngeal airway or a nasogastric or nasotracheal tube should be avoided if a basilar skull fracture is suspected; it may enter the anterior cranial fossa.[9] A cuffed oropharyngeal airway or a laryngeal mask airway (LMA) may permit ventilation with a self-inflating bag, although neither provides protection against aspiration of gastric contents. If these measures do not provide adequate ventilation, the trachea must be intubated immediately using either direct laryngoscopy or a cricothyroidotomy, depending on the results of airway assessment.

Maxillofacial, neck, and chest injuries, as well as cervicofacial burns, are the most common trauma-related causes of difficult tracheal intubation. Airway assessment should include a rapid examination of the anterior neck for feasibility of access to the cricothyroid membrane. Tracheostomy is not desirable during initial management because it takes longer to perform than a cricothyroidotomy and requires neck extension, which may cause or exacerbate cord trauma in patients with cervical spine injuries. Conversion to a tracheostomy should be considered later to prevent laryngeal damage if a cricothyroidotomy will be in place for more than 2 to 3 days. Possible contraindications to cricothyroidotomy include age younger than 12 years and suspected laryngeal trauma; permanent laryngeal damage may result in the former, and noncorrectable airway obstruction may occur in the latter situation.

Proper placement by paramedics of devices such as an LMA, esophageal-tracheal combitube, or endotracheal tube should be confirmed by auscultation and capnography as soon as possible after the patient is admitted to the emergency department. Esophageal lacerations presenting as subcutaneous emphysema, pneumomediastinum, or pneumoperitoneum have been described as a result of the use of the combitube.[10]

Full Stomach

A full stomach is a background condition in acute trauma; the urgency of securing the airway often does not permit adequate time for pharmacologic measures to reduce gastric volume and acidity. Thus, rather than relying on these agents, the emphasis should be placed on selection of a safe technique for securing the airway when necessary: rapid-sequence induction with cricoid pressure for those patients without serious airway problems, and awake intubation with sedation and topical anesthesia, if possible, for those patients who may present with serious airway difficulties. Posterior displacement of a vertebral bone fragment, with potential damage to the spinal cord, may result when cricoid pressure and manual inline stabilization (MIS) are applied to patients with cervical spine injuries.[11] Supporting the back of the neck with another hand may alleviate this problem.[12]

The probability of a full stomach precludes the use of an LMA, or any other device that does not protect the trachea, as a definitive airway in trauma patients. However, these devices can serve as a bridge for a brief period to reestablish airway patency or to facilitate intubation aided by a flexible fiberoptic bronchoscope. In patients with maxillofacial injuries, aspiration of pharyngeal blood or secretions is more likely than aspiration of gastric contents. If it can be inserted in these circumstances, an LMA may protect the lungs. Although positive-pressure ventilation may be used with the LMA, patients with pulmonary contusion, edema, or aspiration may be difficult to ventilate with this device. Difficulty may also be encountered when inserting an LMA in the presence of cricoid pressure and MIS of the cervical spine.[12,13] These problems may be somewhat circumvented with the intubating laryngeal mask (ILM); adequate ventilation is more likely, blind tracheal intubation is more successful, and an endotracheal tube as large as 8 mm can be placed through this device, as opposed to the maximum of 6 mm that can be passed through an LMA.[14] An important disadvantage of the ILM is that its metal part may exert considerable pressure against the cervical vertebrae, potentially exacerbating an unstable injury in this region.[15]

The selection of an airway management technique in the trauma patient may be affected by his or her hemodynamic condition. The presence of uncorrectable hypotension from hemorrhage, hypovolemia, or pericardial tamponade may necessitate omitting intravenous anesthetics from the rapid-sequence technique. Muscle relaxants alone may be sufficient. If only a mild to moderate degree of hypovolemia is present, reduced doses (30 to 50%) of intravenous anesthetics should be administered.[16] Although there is no evidence that the choice of intravenous agent affects outcome, ketamine and etomidate may confer advantages over thiopental and propofol. In equipotent doses in normovolemic patients, they produce less cardiovascular depression.[16] Although succinylcholine, with its short onset time and duration, is still the muscle relaxant of choice for rapid-sequence induction, rocuronium (0.9 to 1.2 mg/kg) has almost the same onset time and does not have the undesirable side effects associated with succinylcholine (e.g., increased intragastric, intraocular, and intracranial pressure [ICP]; potassium release in patients with burns and neurologic diseases). Bradycardia, dysrhythmias, and cardiac arrest have been described after succinylcholine in the presence of hypoxia and hypercarbia; some of these complications may also follow apparently uneventful intubation performed without succinylcholine.[17]

In agitated and uncooperative patients, topical anesthesia of the airway may be impossible, whereas administration of sedative agents may result in apnea or airway obstruction, with an increased risk of aspiration of gastric contents and inadequate conditions for tracheal intubation. After locating the cricothyroid membrane and denitrogenating the lungs, a rapid-sequence induction may be used to permit securing the airway with direct laryngoscopy or, if necessary, with immediate cricothyroidotomy. Personnel and material necessary to perform translaryngeal ventilation or cricothyroidotomy must be in place before induction of general anesthesia.[18]

Head, Open Eye, and Contained Major Vessel Injuries

The principles of tracheal intubation are similar for these injuries. Apart from the need to ensure adequate oxygenation and ventilation, these patients require deep anesthesia and profound muscle relaxation before airway manipulation. This helps prevent hypertension, coughing, and bucking, and thereby minimizes intracranial, intraocular, or intravascular pressure elevation, which can result in herniation of the brain, extrusion of eye contents, or dislodgment of a hemostatic clot from an injured vessel, respectively. The preferred anesthetic sequence to achieve this goal includes preoxygenation and opioid loading, followed by relatively large doses of an intravenous anesthetic and muscle relaxant. Hemodynamic responses to the opioid should be carefully monitored and promptly corrected. Systemic hypotension, ICP elevation, and decreased cerebral perfusion pressure (CPP; CPP = mean arterial pressure − ICP) may occur whether cerebral autoregulation is present or absent in patients with head injuries, and if untreated can produce secondary ischemic insults.[19] Ketamine is probably contraindicated in patients with head and vascular injuries because it may increase both intracranial[20] and systemic vascular pressures; however, no significant increase in intraocular pressure (IOP) has been documented.[21] Any muscle relaxant, including succinylcholine, may be used as long as the fasciculation produced by this agent is inhibited by prior administration of an adequate dose of a nondepolarizing muscle relaxant.[22] Alternatively, rocuronium can provide intubating conditions within 60 seconds with a dose of 1.6 to 2.0 mg/kg, although the neuromuscular blockade produced by this dose lasts approximately 2 hours.[23] Intravenous lidocaine has an attenuating effect on the pressor response to airway instrumentation, but it is mild and unpredictable. Of course, neither muscle relaxants nor intravenous anesthetics are indicated when initial assessment suggests a difficult airway. As in any other trauma patient, hypotension dictates either reduced or no intravenous anesthetic administration.

Cervical Spine Injury

Evidence of a serious new spinal cord injury or accentuation of existing neurologic abnormalities has been documented after intubation of patients with unsuspected cervical spine injuries.[24,25] Immobilization of the neck in a neutral position is indicated before airway management in all acute trauma patients with depressed consciousness, cervical pain, posterior midline cervical spine tenderness, extremity paresthesias, or focal neurologic deficits, and whenever the pain of other injuries is likely to mask the neck pain.[26] Additional risk factors that should increase suspicion are high-risk mechanisms of injury (falls, diving, high-speed motor vehicle accidents) and restricted active neck movement, particularly in rotation.[27] The combined use of a semirigid collar, sandbags placed on both sides of the head and neck, bindings, and a backboard provides the most reliable immobilization. For airway management purposes, however, MIS, with assistants holding the head and torso of the patient, is a practical and safe method if the neck is not otherwise reliably stabilized. A semirigid neck collar alone does not provide absolute protection. Protection of the neck should be maintained after tracheal intubation until a cervical spine injury has been ruled out.

Nasotracheal intubation carries the risks of epistaxis, failure of intubation, and the possibility of entry of the endotracheal tube into the cranial vault or the orbit if there is damage to the cranial base or the maxillofacial complex. Absence of the usual signs of cranial base fracture (Battle sign, raccoon eyes, or bleeding from the ear or the nose) cannot be relied on to exclude the possibility of its occurrence because with rapid prehospital transport these signs may not be immediately apparent. Orotracheal intubation with direct laryngoscopy is more desirable, although stabilization of the neck, which limits head extension, may make glottic visualization difficult. The incidence of inadequate exposure of the larynx increases from less than 3% in the general population to approximately 10% with immobilization of the neck.[28,29]

Other devices and techniques, including the McCoy laryngoscope, rigid fiberoptic laryngoscopes (Bullard or WuScope), flexible fiberoptic endoscope, light wand, translaryngeal (retrograde) intubation, and cricothyroidotomy, can be used to secure the airway in patients requiring cervical spine immobilization.[12] In most instances, successful, safe, and rapid tracheal intubation can be achieved with a conventional laryngoscope despite limited visualization of the larynx.[30] The McCoy laryngoscope is able to lift the epiglottis and may improve the laryngeal view: the cuff of a Fogarty catheter attached to the tip of this device may further improve exposure.[12,31] A gum elastic bougie passed through the endotracheal tube, or a satin-sheathed stylet placed through its Murphy aperture, may also be helpful; they can be inserted through the larynx more easily than the tube itself because their small diameter does not block the view of the glottis during direct laryngoscopy.[32] The WuScope provides a consistently good laryngeal view with a high rate of successful intubation and minimal neck movement.[30,33]

Flexible fiberoptic laryngoscopy and translaryngeal guided intubation (see Maxillofacial Injuries section) cause almost no neck movement, but blood or secretions in the airway, a long preparation time, and difficulty in their use in comatose, uncooperative, or anesthetized patients reduce their utility during initial management.

Direct Airway Injuries

Direct airway damage can occur anywhere between the nasopharynx and the bronchi; sometimes more than one site may be involved, resulting in persistent airway dysfunction after one of the problems is corrected.[34]

Maxillofacial Injuries. In addition to soft-tissue edema of the pharynx and peripharyngeal hematoma, blood or debris in the oropharyngeal cavity may be responsible for partial or complete airway obstruction in the acute stage of these injuries. Occasionally, teeth or foreign bodies in the pharynx may be aspirated into the airway, causing some degree of obstruction, which may occur or be recognized only during attempts at tracheal intubation. Another problem is the dynamic nature of soft-tissue injuries in this region. A hematoma or edema in the face, tongue, or neck may expand during the first several hours after injury and ultimately occlude the airway. Serious airway compromise may develop within a few hours in up to 50% of patients with major penetrating facial injuries or multiple trauma, as a result of progressive inflammation or edema resulting from liberal administration of fluids.[35,36] Prophylactic intubation of the trachea or close and repeated examination of the upper airway may avert airway compromise before it occurs.

Fracture-induced encroachment on the airway or limitation of mandibular movement, pain, and trismus may limit mouth opening. Fentanyl in titrated doses of up to 2 to 4 μg/kg over a period of 10 to 20 minutes may produce an improvement in the patient's ability to open the mouth if mechanical limitation is not present.

The selection of an airway management technique in the presence of a maxillofacial fracture is based on the patient's presenting condition. Most patients with isolated facial injuries do not require emergency tracheal intubation. Surgery may be delayed for as long as a week with no adverse effect on the repair. Patients who present with airway compromise may be intubated using direct laryngoscopy; the decision about the use of anesthetics and muscle relaxants is based on the results of airway evaluation. When there is bleeding into the oropharynx, a flexible fiberoptic laryngoscope may be useless because of obstruction of the view. A retrograde technique, using a wire or epidural catheter passed through a 14-gauge catheter introduced into the trachea through the cricothyroid membrane, may be used if the patient can open his or her mouth. A surgical airway is indicated when there is airway compromise, when direct laryngoscopy has failed or is considered impossible, when the jaws will be wired, or when a tracheostomy will be performed anyway after definitive repair of the fracture. Nasogastric or nasotracheal intubation should be avoided when a basilar skull or maxillary fracture is suspected because of the possibility that the tube may enter the cranium or the orbital fossa. Hemorrhagic shock and life-threatening cranial, thoracic, and cervical spine injuries may accompany major facial fractures;[37] airway management must be tailored accordingly.[38] The likelihood of cranial injury increases in midface fractures involving the frontal sinus, as well as the orbitozygomatic and orbitoethmoid complexes.[39]

Cervical Airway Injuries. Injury to the cervical air passages can result from blunt or penetrating trauma. Clinical signs such as escape of air, hemoptysis, and coughing are present in almost all patients with penetrating injuries, facilitating the diagnosis. In contrast, major blunt laryngotracheal damage may be missed, either because the patient is asymptomatic or unresponsive, or because suggestive signs and symptoms are missed in the initial evaluation.[34] The typical presentation includes hoarseness, muffled voice, dyspnea, stridor, dysphagia, odynophagia, cervical pain and tenderness, ecchymosis, subcutaneous emphysema, and flattening of the thyroid cartilage protuberance (Adam's apple).[40] Whether the trauma is blunt or penetrating, attempts at blind tracheal intubation may produce further trauma to the larynx and complete airway obstruction if the endotracheal tube enters a false passage or disrupts the continuity of an already tenuous airway.[41,42] Thus, whenever possible, intubation of the trachea should be performed using a flexible fiberoptic bronchoscope or an airway should be established surgically. A computed tomography (CT) scan of the neck provides valuable information and should be performed before any airway intervention in all stable patients without respiratory and hemodynamic compromise.

The strategy for tracheal intubation depends on the clinical presentation.[42] The tracheas of some patients with penetrating airway injuries, especially stab wounds, may be intubated through the airway defect without the need for anesthetics or optical equipment.[28] Patients with a normal airway on endoscopy can be intubated orotracheally under general anesthesia. The presence of cartilaginous fractures or mucosal abnormalities necessitates awake intubation with a fiberoptic bronchoscope or awake tracheostomy. Laryngeal damage precludes cricothyroidotomy. Tracheostomy should be performed with extreme caution because up to 70% of patients with blunt laryngeal injuries may have an associated cervical spine injury.[42] Uncooperative or confused patients may not tolerate awake airway manipulation. It may be best to transport these patients to the OR, induce anesthesia with inhalational agents, and intubate the trachea without muscle relaxants.[42] Episodes of airway obstruction during spontaneous breathing under an inhalational anesthetic can be managed by positioning the patient upright in addition to the usual maneuvers. In extreme situations such as near-complete transection of the larynx and trachea, femorofemoral bypass or percutaneous cardiopulmonary support may be considered.[43]

Thoracic Airway Injuries. Whereas penetrating trauma can cause damage to any segment of the intrathoracic airway, blunt injury usually involves the posterior membranous portion of the trachea and the mainstem bronchi, usually within approximately 3 cm from the carina. Pneumothorax, pneumomediastinum, pneumopericardium, subcutaneous emphysema, and a continuous air leak from the chest tube are the usual signs of this injury; they occur frequently but are not specific for thoracic airway damage. In patients intubated without the suspicion of a tracheal injury, difficulty in obtaining a seal around the endotracheal tube or the presence on a chest radiograph of a large radiolucent area in the trachea corresponding to the cuff suggests a perforated airway.[44] Other radiographic findings include a radiolucent line along the prevertebral fascia due to air tracking up from the mediastinum, peribronchial air or sudden obstruction along an air-filled bronchus, and the "dropped lung" sign when complete intrapleural bronchial transection causes the apex of the collapsed lung to descend to the level of the hilum.[45] Airway management is similar to that of cervical airway injury. Anesthetics, and especially muscle relaxants, may produce irreversible obstruction, presumably because of relaxation of structures that maintain the airway patent in the awake state; however, airway loss may also occur during attempts at awake intubation, often as a result of further distortion of the airway by the endotracheal tube, patient agitation, or rebleeding into the airway.[46]

After intubation of the trachea, the adequacy of the airway intervention is evaluated by clinical examination, capnography, and pulse oximetry. Pulmonary contusion, atelectasis, diaphragmatic rupture with thoracic migration of the abdominal contents, and pneumothorax may complicate the interpretation of chest auscultation. Likewise, CO_2 elimination may be decreased or absent in shock and cardiac arrest.

Management of Breathing Abnormalities

3 Of the several causes that may alter respiration after trauma, tension pneumothorax, flail chest, and open pneumothorax are immediate threats to the patient's life and therefore require rapid diagnosis and treatment. Hemothorax, closed pneumothorax, pulmonary contusion, diaphragmatic rupture with herniation of abdominal contents into the thorax, and atelectasis from a mucous plug, aspiration, or chest wall splinting can also interfere with breathing and pulmonary gas exchange and deteriorate into life-threatening complications.

Although cyanosis, tachypnea, hypotension, neck vein distention, tracheal deviation, and diminished breath sounds on the affected side are the classic signs of tension pneumothorax, neck vein distention may be absent in hypovolemic patients and tracheal deviation may be difficult to appreciate. The definitive diagnosis is established by chest radiograph; however, in hypoxemic and hypotensive patients, immediate insertion of a 14-gauge angiocatheter through the fourth intercostal space in the midaxillary line or, at times, through the second intercostal space at the midclavicular line is essential. There is no time for radiologic confirmation in this setting.

A flail chest results from comminuted fractures of at least three adjacent ribs or rib fractures with associated costochondral separation or sternal fracture. An underlying pulmonary contusion with increased elastic recoil of the lung and work of breathing is the main cause of respiratory insufficiency or failure, and resulting hypoxemia.[47] It often develops over a 3- to 6-hour period, causing gradual deterioration of the chest radiograph and arterial blood gases (ABGs).[47] Coexisting hemopneumothorax, paradoxical chest wall movement, and/or pain-induced splinting may contribute to the gas exchange abnormalities. Repeated evaluation by physical examination, chest radiograph, and ABG determinations is essential for early recognition of these complications.

Without significant gas exchange abnormalities, chest wall instability alone is not an indication for respiratory support. There is evidence that liberal use of mechanical ventilation in the presence of a flail chest or pulmonary contusion increases the rate of pulmonary complications and mortality, and prolongs the hospital stay.[47] Effective pain relief by itself can improve respiratory function and often avoid the need for mechanical ventilation. For this purpose, continuous epidural analgesia with local anesthetics and opioids, preferably directed to thoracic segments, provides better pain relief and ventilatory function than parenteral opioids, reducing morbidity and mortality in elderly patients with chest wall trauma.[48] Other therapeutic measures include supplemental oxygen, continuous positive airway pressure (CPAP) of 10 to 15 cm H_2O by facemask, airway humidification, chest physiotherapy, incentive spirometry, bronchodilators, airway suctioning (using fiberoptic bronchoscopy, if necessary), and nutritional support.[47] Overzealous infusion of fluids may result in deterioration of oxygenation by worsening underlying pulmonary injury.[47]

In patients with pulmonary contusion, respiratory insufficiency or failure despite adequate analgesia, clinical evidence of severe shock, associated severe head injury or injury requiring surgery, airway obstruction, and significant preexisting chronic pulmonary disease are indications for tracheal intubation and mechanical ventilation. Positive end-expiratory pressure (PEEP) should be used if ventilation is controlled. In intubated, spontaneously breathing patients, airway pressure release ventilation, in which spontaneous breathing is superimposed on mechanical ventilation by intermittent sudden, brief decrease of CPAP, provides improved $\dot{V}/\dot{Q}$ matching and systemic blood pressure, lower sedation requirements, greater O_2 delivery, and shorter periods of intubation.[47,49] Severe unilateral pulmonary contusion unresponsive to these measures may be treated by differential lung ventilation via a double lumen endobronchial tube. In bilateral severe contusions with life-threatening hypoxemia, high-frequency jet ventilation (HFJV) may enhance oxygenation and cardiac function, which may be compromised by concomitant myocardial contusion or ischemia.[50]

Systemic air embolism occurs mainly after penetrating lung trauma and blast injuries, and less frequently after blunt thoracic trauma that produces lacerations of both distal air passages and pulmonary veins[51]; positive-pressure ventilation after tracheal intubation may then result in entrainment of air into the systemic circulation. Hemoptysis, circulatory, and CNS dysfunction immediately after starting artificial ventilation, as well as detection of air in blood from the radial artery, establishes the diagnosis. Air bubbles may also be seen in the coronary arteries during thoracotomy. Surgical management involves immediate thoracotomy and clamping of the hilum of the lacerated lung. Respiratory maneuvers that minimize or prevent air entry into the systemic circulation include isolating and collapsing the lacerated lung by means of a double-lumen tube, or ventilation with the lowest possible tidal volumes via a single-lumen tube.[51] Transesophageal echocardiography (TEE) of the left side of the heart may permit visualization of air bubbles and their disappearance with therapeutic maneuvers.

Management of Shock

4 Hemorrhage is the most common cause of traumatic hypotension and shock. Other causes are abnormal pump function (myocardial contusion, pericardial tamponade, preexisting cardiac disease, or coronary artery or cardiac valve injury), pneumothorax or hemothorax, spinal cord injury, and, rarely, anaphylaxis or sepsis (Table 48-1).

Evaluation of the severity of hemorrhagic shock in the initial phase is based on a few relatively insensitive and nonspecific clinical signs. For example, tachycardia, which is traditionally used as an index of hypovolemia, may be absent in up to 30% of hypotensive trauma patients because of increased vagal tone, chronic cocaine use, or other unknown reasons.[52] In contrast, by increasing catecholamine output, tissue injury, and associated pain may maintain tachycardia and normal or elevated systemic blood pressure in the presence of hypovolemia without necessarily increasing the cardiac index or tissue oxygen delivery.[53] In fact, in this situation an increase in intestinal vascular resistance and a decrease in splanchnic blood flow may occur, and if prolonged, may allow entry of intestinal microorganisms into the circulation and increase the likelihood of subsequent sepsis and organ failure.[54–57] Thus, equating a normal heart rate and systemic blood pressure with normovolemia during initial resuscitation may lead to loss of valuable time for treating an underlying occult hypovolemia or hypoperfusion. Nevertheless, heart rate, systemic blood pressure, pulse pressure, respiratory rate, urine output, and mental status remain the best available early clinical indicators of the severity of hemorrhagic shock[54] (Table 48-2).

Some of the proven markers of organ perfusion can be used during early management to set the goals of resuscitation. Of these, the base deficit, blood lactate level, and probably sublingual P_{CO_2} (SLP_{CO_2}) are the most useful and practical tools during all phases of shock, including the earliest. The base deficit reflects the severity of shock, the oxygen debt, changes in O_2 delivery, the adequacy of fluid resuscitation, and the likelihood of multiple organ failure and survival with reasonable accuracy in *previously healthy* adult and pediatric trauma patients.[58–60] A base deficit between 2 and 5 mmol/L suggests mild shock, between 6 and 14 mmol/L indicates moderate shock, whereas >14 mmol/L is a sign of severe shock. An admission base deficit in excess of 5 to 8 mmol/L correlates with increased mortality.[59,60] Thus, normalization of the base deficit is one of the end points of resuscitation.[61,62]

Elevation of the blood lactate level is less specific than base deficit as a marker of tissue hypoxia because it can be generated in well-oxygenated tissues by increased epinephrine-induced skeletal muscle glycolysis, accelerated pyruvate oxidation, decreased hepatic clearance of lactate, and early mitochondrial dysfunction.[63] All these conditions may be present in the trauma patient. Nevertheless, in most trauma victims an elevated lactate level correlates with other signs of hypoperfusion, rendering it an important marker of dysoxia and an end point of resuscitation.[64,65] The normal plasma lactate concentration is 0.5 to 1.5 mmol/L; levels above 5 mmol/L indicate significant lactic acidosis. The half-life of lactate is approximately 3 hours;[64] thus, the level decreases rather gradually after correction of the cause.[64] Failure to clear lactate within 24 hours after circulatory shock is a predictor of increased mortality.[65,66]

Sublingual capnometry is a new noninvasive addition to organ perfusion monitoring; it appears to indicate gut perfusion as reliably as gastric tonometry in hemorrhage, but with greater ease of use.[67,68] In trauma patients in the early phase of shock, it detected hemorrhage as accurately as base deficit and plasma lactate.[69] The device consists of a sublingual CO_2 sensor that directly measures mucosal P_{CO_2}. The normal value for SLP_{CO_2} is 45 to 50 mm Hg; elevated levels suggest organ hypoperfusion.[69] The gradient between SLP_{CO_2} and Pa_{CO_2} may reflect organ perfusion more accurately, although in young trauma patients hyperventilation or hypoventilation does not seem to affect SLP_{CO_2}.[69]

The response of the pulse and blood pressure to initial fluid therapy also aids in the assessment of hypovolemia.[54] In hypotensive and tachycardic patients, administration of lactated Ringer's (LR) solution, 2,000 mL over 15 minutes in adults or 20 mL/kg in children, should normalize the vital signs if hemorrhage is mild (10 to 20%). A transient improvement after fluid infusion suggests a 20 to 40% decrease in circulating volume or continuing blood loss. More crystalloids and possibly blood transfusion are required in these patients. If the vital signs do not respond to initial fluid resuscitation, there has probably been severe (>40%) severe blood loss or severe volume loss, which must be replaced by rapid infusion of crystalloids, colloids, and blood.

Bickell et al[70] challenged the conventional management of initial shock resuscitation; they showed that delaying fluid resuscitation until surgical control of bleeding in victims of penetrating trauma improved survival to hospital discharge and decreased the length of hospital stay. Vigorous fluid therapy increases arterial and venous pressures, dilutes clotting factors and platelets, and decreases blood viscosity, and thus may reinitiate bleeding already stopped by a soft thrombus. Although many experimental studies have confirmed the findings of Bickell et al, it has also become clear that withholding fluids completely can result in as much harm as vigorous resuscitation.[71] In contrast, slow fluid infusion with isotonic or hypertonic crystalloids, and preferably with packed red blood cells (PRBCs), titrated to lower than normal systemic pressure, had

TABLE 48-1

GUIDELINES FOR MANAGEMENT OF TRAUMATIC SHOCK

	ETIOLOGY					
	HEMORRHAGE OR EXTENSIVE TISSUE INJURY	CARDIAC TAMPONADE	MYOCARDIAL CONTUSION	PNEUMOTHORAX OR HEMOTHORAX	SPINAL CORD INJURY	SEPSIS
Primary Mechanisms	Hypovolemia	Ventricular inflow restriction	Diminished ventricular performance and elevated pulmonary vascular resistance	Lung collapse Mediastinal shift, causing inflow and outflow obstruction of the heart	Vasodilatation and relative hypovolemia caused by loss of sympathetic tone	Intestinal perforation causing peritoneal contamination
Typical Signs and Symptoms	Tachycardia Narrow pulse pressure Cold, clammy skin from vasoconstriction	Tachycardia Hypotension Dilated and engorged neck veins Muffled heart sounds Diminished BP response to fluid challenge	Dysrhythmia Tachycardia Hypotension	Tachycardia Hypotension Dilated and engorged neck veins Absent breath sounds Hyperresonance to percussion Tracheal shift Dyspnea Subcutaneous emphysema	Hypotension without tachycardia, cutaneous vasoconstriction, or narrow pulse pressure	Develops mainly a few hours after colon injury In hypovolemic patients, signs and symptoms indistinguishable from hypovolemic shock In normovolemic patients, fever, modest tachycardia, warm, pink skin, near normal BP, wide pulse pressure Hypotension may develop
Treatment Continuum, from Least to Most Intense	Crystalloids initially Transfusion if 2,000 mL of crystalloid in 15 min does not restore BP	Pericardiocentesis Pericardial window Emergency room thoracotomy	Fluids Fluids and vasodilators Fluids and inotropes	Release of air with 14-gauge catheter Chest tube	Fluids Fluids and vasopressors Fluids, vasopressors, and inotropes, if myocardial damage is present	Fluids and antibiotics Fluids, antibiotics, and inotropes for hypotension

BP, blood pressure.

TABLE 48-2

ADVANCED TRAUMA LIFE SUPPORT CLASSIFICATION OF HEMORRHAGIC SHOCK[a]

	CLASS I	CLASS II	CLASS III	CLASS IV
Blood loss (mL)	≤750	750–1,500	1,500–2,000	≥2,000
Blood loss (% blood volume)	≤15	15–30	30–40	≥40
Pulse rate (per min)	<100	>100	>120	≥140
Blood pressure	Normal	Normal	Decreased	Decreased
Pulse pressure	Normal or increased	Decreased	Decreased	Decreased
Respiratory rate (breaths/min)	14–20	20–30	30–40	>35
Urine output (mL/hr)	≥30	20–30	5–15	Negligible
Mental status	Slightly anxious	Mildly anxious	Anxious and confused	Confused, lethargic
Fluid replacement (3:1 rule)[b]	Crystalloid	Crystalloid	Crystalloid + blood	Crystalloid + blood

[a]For a 70-kg male patient, based on initial presentation.
[b]The 3:1 rule is based on empiric observation that most patients require 300 mL balanced electrolyte solution for each 100 mL blood loss. Without other clinical and monitoring parameters, this guideline may result in excessive or inadequate fluid resuscitation.
Adapted with permission from American College of Surgeons, Committee on Trauma: Shock. In American College of Surgeons (ed): Advanced Trauma Life Support Course for Physicians, p 108. Chicago, American College of Surgeons, 1997.

beneficial effects on animal survival without tissue injury or organ failure.[71] Although there are substantial data to suggest that this "limited resuscitation" may be preferable to the current standard of care, proof of this is lacking. The only clinical study conducted subsequent to Bickell et al failed to demonstrate any decrease in mortality.[72] Thus, although this technique is far from being a standard of care, it emphasizes the useful fact that fluid administration in excess of that needed for achieving normovolemia prior to control of hemorrhage may be deleterious.

A reasonable transfusion threshold is a hematocrit below 25% for young, healthy patients and below 30% for older patients or those with coronary or cerebrovascular disease.[73] Preliminary data suggest that transfusion of PRBC units older than 14 days may prolong the length of hospital stay in moderately injured,[74] and may be an independent risk factor for multiple organ failure in severely injured patients.[75] Normally, type-specific blood can be available in less than 15 minutes for patients with severe hemorrhage. If the situation dictates immediate transfusion, type O, Rh(+) blood is satisfactory in most situations. O, Rh(−) blood should be given to women of childbearing age. However, because of the scarcity of Rh(−) blood, some women require an Rh(+) transfusion. The immunogenicity of the D antigen can be neutralized by administration of Rh immune globulin (anti-Rh antibody).

Rapid establishment of venous access with large-bore cannulae placed in peripheral veins that drain both above and below the diaphragm is essential for adequate fluid resuscitation in the patient who is severely injured. When vascular collapse and extremity injury impair access to arm or leg vessels, percutaneous cannulation of the internal jugular, subclavian, or femoral veins can be performed. Ultrasound guidance may be useful for cannulation of the internal jugular vein and may also be used for an infraclavicular approach to the axillary vein,[76] or to the cephalic or basilic veins at the midarm level.[77] If necessary, a cutdown to a saphenous or arm vein can be rapidly performed in older children and adults. In children younger than 5 years of age, intraosseous cannulation has a high success rate and a low incidence of complications. Infusion rates comparable with those obtained with intravenous lines are possible in small children, although a pressure infusion device may be necessary to achieve adequate flow.[78] A special screw-type needle or the needle of a 16- or 18-gauge angiocatheter is introduced into the bone marrow of the distal femur or proximal tibia at the level of its tuberosity. Care should be taken not to injure the epiphyseal plate during puncture. Proper placement is indicated by loss of resistance to fluid injection or aspiration of marrow.

Patients who arrive in the emergency department in cardiac arrest require advanced cardiac life support. However, the success rate of external cardiac massage in hypovolemic trauma victims is likely to be low.[79] Emergency department thoracotomy not only permits performance of open cardiac massage, but also aids resuscitation efforts by allowing drainage of pericardial blood, control of cardiac and great vessel bleeding, application of a cross-clamp to the aorta, and rapid administration of fluids through a small Foley catheter introduced into the right atrium, or in desperate situations, through a large-bore catheter or introducer in the descending aorta. This procedure is not indicated in blunt torso trauma; the mortality rate is similar regardless of whether it is attempted.[80] In penetrating injuries, depending on the presenting condition of the patient, the initial success rate may be as high as 70%, but the neurologically intact hospital discharge rate is only 10 to 15%.[80,81]

EARLY MANAGEMENT OF SPECIFIC INJURIES

Head Injury

5 Approximately 40% of deaths from trauma are caused by head injury, and indeed, even a moderate brain injury may increase the mortality rate of patients with other injuries.[82] In nonsurvivors, progression of the damaged area beyond the directly injured region (secondary brain injury) can be demonstrated at autopsy.[83] The major factor in secondary injury is tissue hypoxia, which results in lactic acidosis; free radical generation; prostaglandin synthesis and release of excitatory amino acids (primarily glutamate); lipid peroxidation and breakdown of cell membranes; entry of large quantities of sodium, calcium, and water into the cells; and leakage of fluid from the blood vessels into the extracellular space.[84] This process results in brain edema, as well as both regional and global disturbances of the cerebral circulation. Thus, of all the possible insults to the injured brain, decreased oxygen delivery as a result of hypotension and hypoxia has the greatest detrimental impact[85–87] (Table 48-3).

Brain injury by itself does not cause hypotension in adults, except as a preterminal event. However, more than half of patients with severe head trauma have other injuries that render

TABLE 48-3

EFFECTS ON OUTCOME OF SECONDARY INSULTS OCCURRING FROM TIME OF INJURY THROUGH RESUSCITATION[a]

SECONDARY INSULTS	NO. OF PATIENTS	% OF TOTAL PATIENTS	6-MONTH OUTCOME (%)		
			GOOD/ MODERATE	SEVERE/ VEGETATIVE	DEAD
Total cases	717	100	43.0	20.2	36.8
Neither	308	43.0	63.9	10.2	26.9
Hypoxia	161	22.4	50.3	21.7	28.0
Hypotension	62	11.4	32.9	17.1	50.0
Both	166	23.2	20.5	22.3	57.2

[a]Data from hospital emergency departments enrolled in Traumatic Coma Data Bank.
Reprinted with permission from Prough DS, Lang J: Therapy of patients with head injuries: Key parameters for management. J Trauma 42(Suppl):10S, 1997.

approximately 15% of them hypotensive; approximately 30% are hypoxic on admission as a result of central respiratory depression or associated chest injuries.[84] Furthermore, exposure to these insults is likely to occur during any phase of the continuum of hospital care: in the radiology unit, the OR, the recovery room, the intensive care unit, or elsewhere. The most common early complications of head trauma are intracranial hypertension, brain herniation, seizures, neurogenic pulmonary edema, cardiac dysrhythmias, bradycardia, systemic hypertension, and coagulopathy.

Diagnosis

Mental impairment after trauma may have any of several etiologies. However, the possibility of hypoxia and shock must always be considered first. If consciousness remains depressed despite ventilation and fluid replacement, a head injury is assumed to be present, and the patient is managed accordingly. As noted, hypotension is the most important cause of death in the patient with head injury; Chesnut et al[85,88] demonstrated that a single episode of systolic blood pressure <90 mm Hg is associated with a 50% increase in mortality. Therefore, every effort should be made to support the blood pressure with fluids and vasopressors (preferably phenylephrine, which does not constrict cerebral vessels), and ensure adequate oxygenation *before* the unconscious patient is evaluated.[89] A baseline neurologic examination should be performed after initial resuscitation, but before any sedative or muscle relaxant agents are administered, and should be repeated at frequent intervals because the patient's condition may change rapidly. Anesthetic and adjunct drugs render an adequate neurologic examination impossible; thus, long-acting muscle relaxants, opioids, sedatives, or hypnotics should be given selectively.[90,91]

Consciousness can be initially assessed within a few seconds using the AVPU system (*a*lert; responds to *v*erbal stimuli; responds to *p*ain; *u*nresponsive; Table 48-4). More precise information is provided by the Glasgow Coma Scale[92] (GCS; see Table 48-4), which provides a standard means of evaluating the patient's neurologic status. In this test, the sum of the scores obtained for eye opening, verbal response, and motor activity correlates with the state of consciousness, the severity of the head injury, and the prognosis.[90,93] Assessment of motor function should be performed on the extremity that responds best. The limb affected by neurologic injury is examined, but the result is not considered in the GCS.

Dilatation and sluggish response of the pupil is a sign of compression of the oculomotor nerve by the medial portion of the temporal lobe (uncus). A maximally dilated and unresponsive "blown" pupil suggests uncal herniation under the falx cerebri. The presence of similar findings in ocular injuries makes interpretation of pupillary findings difficult when eye and head injuries coexist. However, the pupillary reaction to light is usually more sluggish in the patient with head injury.

CT scanning is used for the diagnosis of most acute head injuries. Positive CT findings after acute head injury include midline shift, distortion of the ventricles and cisterns, effacement of the sulci in the uninjured hemisphere, and the presence of a hematoma at any location in the cranial vault. Subdural hematomas usually have a concave border, whereas epidural hematomas present with a convex outline classically termed a *lenticular* configuration. Patients in coma (GCS < 8) have a 40% likelihood of an intracranial hematoma.[94] Those with a higher GCS score are less likely to have had intracranial bleeding, although it is now evident that the significant incidence

TABLE 48-4

TWO-LEVEL INITIAL EVALUATION OF CONSCIOUSNESS

LEVEL 1. AVPU SYSTEM	
A = Alert	
V = Responds to verbal stimuli	
P = Responds to painful stimuli	
U = Unresponsive	
LEVEL 2. GLASGOW COMA SCALE (GCS)	
Eye opening (E)	
Spontaneous, already open and blinking	4
To speech	3
To pain	2
None	1
Verbal response (V)	
Oriented	5
Answers but confused	4
Inappropriate but recognizable words	3
Incomprehensible sounds	2
None	1
Best motor response (M)	
Obeys verbal commands	6
Localizes painful stimulus	5
Withdraws from painful stimulus	4
Decorticate posturing (upper extremity flexion)	3
Decerebrate posturing (upper extremity extension)	2
No movement	1

GCS ≤ 8 = deep coma, severe head trauma, poor outcome
GCS 9–12 = concious patient with moderate injury
GCS > 12 = mild injury

of this complication even in these patients necessitates a CT study, preferably with contrast enhancement.[87,95] Other benefits of CT scanning include detection of intracranial air and depressed skull fractures.

Management

The primary objective of the early management of brain trauma is to prevent or alleviate the secondary injury process that may follow any complication that decreases the oxygen supply to the brain, including systemic hypotension, hypoxemia, anemia, raised ICP, acidosis, and possibly hyperglycemia (serum glucose >200 mg/dL).[96] These insults cause exacerbation of trauma-induced cerebral ischemia and metabolic derangements, worsening the outcome.[88,97] 6 *The most important therapeutic maneuvers in these patients are aimed at maintaining CPP and oxygen delivery.* The Brain Trauma Foundation and the American Association of Neurological Surgeons have published evidence-based guidelines for the treatment of patients with head injury.[87] Primary therapy includes normalization of the systemic blood pressure (mean blood pressure >80) and arterial oxygenation ($Sa{O_2}$ >95); sedation and paralysis, if necessary; mannitol and possibly a loop diuretic to shrink the brain and decrease the ICP; and drainage of cerebrospinal fluid through a ventriculostomy catheter, if available.

Rapid and adequate restoration of the intravascular volume with isotonic crystalloid and, if necessary, with colloid solutions should be aimed at maintaining the CPP > 60 mm Hg, while attempting to minimize further brain swelling. LR solution, which is slightly hypotonic (Na^+ = 130 mEq/L, osmolality ~255 mOsm/L), may promote swelling in uninjured areas of the brain if it is given in large quantities. Edema tends to occur in injured brain regions regardless of the type of solution administered because of increased permeability of the blood-brain barrier. To minimize edema formation, it is wise to monitor serum osmolality and to replace LR solution with isotonic normal saline. If serum osmolality cannot be measured, this change can be made empirically after 3 L of LR solution.

Effective reduction in ICP can be provided, or at least aided, by administration of mannitol, an important part of the management of severe head injury. It is administered in boluses of 0.25 to 0.5 g/kg, repeated every 4 to 6 hours as needed to control the ICP.[87] In addition to its osmotic diuretic effect, this agent may improve cerebral blood flow (CBF) and O_2 delivery by reducing the hematocrit and thus the blood viscosity.[98] There is a risk of hypovolemia and resultant hypotension when therapeutic doses of mannitol are used. The aim in administration of this agent is a normal volume of mildly hypertonic (~295 mOsm/L) plasma. If the ICP elevation persists, additional doses of mannitol should be given with great care. Acute mannitol toxicity, manifested by hyponatremia, high serum osmolality, and a gap between calculated and measured serum osmolality >10 mOsm/L, may result when the drug is given in large doses (2–3 g/kg) or to patients with renal failure.[99] Hyponatremia in these patients results from intravascular volume expansion rather than sodium loss; thus, treatment with saline solutions is not appropriate. Because of a synergistic action between mannitol and loop diuretics in improving the ICP, addition of furosemide may be a safer and more effective treatment than increasing the dose of mannitol when intracranial hypertension persists.[100]

Until about 1995, hyperventilation to a $Pa{CO_2}$ of 25 to 30 mm Hg was a mainstay of the therapy of head injury. However, brain ischemia, which is probably the most threatening consequence of head injury, is likely to occur during the first 6 hours after trauma,[101–103] even when the CPP is maintained above the generally recommended 60 to 70 mm Hg.[102,104] This hypoperfusion seems to be largely caused by increased cerebral vascular resistance, which may be enhanced by hyperventilation. Ward et al[105] showed that patients ventilated to a $Pa{CO_2}$ of 24 mm Hg had a significantly worse outcome than did those maintained at a $Pa{CO_2}$ of 35 mm Hg. However, some degree of hyperventilation may be necessary for short periods of time in patients who have severe injuries and elevated ICP that does not respond to normal ventilation and diuretics, although this should not be used during the first 24 hours following injury.[87,106] Its use after the initial phase should be based on monitoring of the ICP and, if available, the jugular bulb O_2 saturation ($Sjv{O_2}$) and arteriovenous O_2 difference ($AVD{O_2}$).

Measurement of $Sjv{O_2}$ is used in many centers as a guide to therapy of the patient with head injury.[107] A catheter is passed retrograde into the jugular bulb. The O_2 saturation may be measured with a cooximeter or continuously by means of a fiberoptic sensor. $Sjv{O_2}$ of <50% is considered critical desaturation. $AVD{O_2}$ is a standard measure of the brain's oxygen supply–demand ratio. It is equal to $1.34 \cdot Hgb \cdot (Sa{O_2} - Sjv{O_2})$, and normally, is approximately 6. An increase in this value is a sign of insufficient blood flow, whereas a subnormal level indicates hyperemia. A reduction in ICP with elevation of CPP during treatment is reflected by a rise in $Sjv{O_2}$ and a narrowing of the $AVD{O_2}$, presumably reflecting an improvement in the circulation to the brain.[107,108] Unfortunately, several shortcomings of the technique have hindered its universal acceptance. Because all the cerebral veins drain into the cavernous sinus and from there into the jugular bulbs, $AVD{O_2}$ measures only global O_2 consumption, which may well be different from the situation in the injured region. Indeed, Coles et al[102] demonstrated that a significant increase in the region of critical hypoperfusion resulting from hyperventilation was not necessarily associated with a correspondingly abnormal $Sjv{O_2}$ or $AVD{O_2}$ (Fig. 48-2). Patient or catheter movement may also alter the measured $Pjv{O_2}$. Thus, there may be a high proportion of inaccurate values—as high as nearly two-thirds in one study[109]—although more recent advances in the technique have probably reduced these errors. Cruz[110] suggested that jugular venous monitoring should be used only in sedated, paralyzed patients.

If the ICP remains elevated, pentobarbital (3 to 10 mg/kg given over 0.5 to 2.5 hours, followed by a maintenance infusion of 0.5 to 3.0 mg/kg/hr, aimed at a serum concentration between 2.5 and 4.0 mg/dL) may be required.[87,100] High-dose barbiturates, however, are of no value in the routine therapy of head injury and should be used only for refractory ICP elevation. Whether active normalization of elevated serum glucose (a common occurrence in the patient with head injury) has any salutary effect on outcome is not known. Of course, immediate surgical decompression, especially of epidural hematomas, is an important factor in reducing morbidity and mortality.

If the patient is hemodynamically stable, a CT scan is performed; the strictest attention should be paid to ensuring adequate oxygenation, ventilation, blood pressure, and ICP control during the procedure. If the patient is hemodynamically unstable or requires emergency surgery for associated injuries, and has a history suggesting a head injury even though a significant intracranial hematoma is unlikely on clinical grounds, intraoperative ICP monitoring is indicated to permit rapid detection of ICP elevation. Both intracranial hematomas and hemorrhage in other regions have a high surgical priority. In the multiple trauma victim, prioritization between the two is based on the severity of each injury. Because there is no time to obtain a CT scan of the head in patients with both profuse hemorrhage and brain herniation, the patient is brought directly to the OR for simultaneous control of the bleeding site and evacuation of the intracranial hematoma. The site of the craniotomy can be determined by a ventriculogram or an ultrasound examination with a pencil-tip probe; both tests may be performed under local anesthesia through a frontal burr hole.

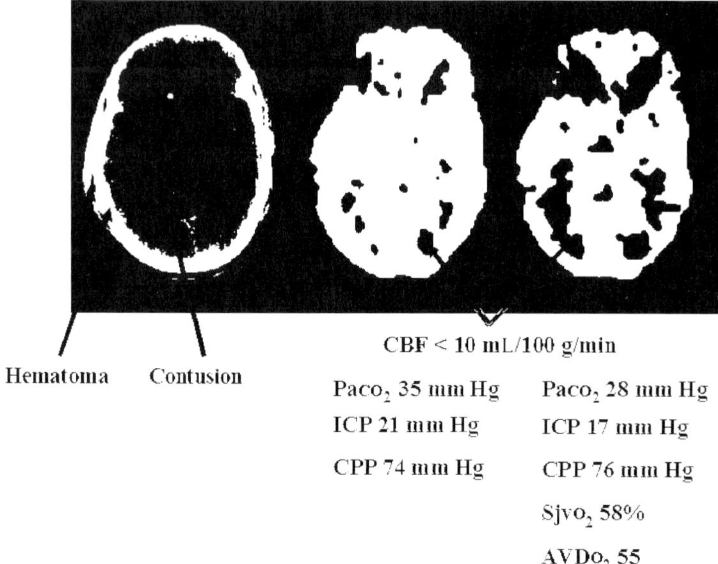

FIGURE 48-2. Effects of hyperventilation on cerebral blood flow (CBF). The left image is a computed tomography scan of the patient whose positron emission tomography scans are shown in the other two images. Note that there is a significant decrease in the CBF and an increase in the areas of hypoperfusion despite improvement in the intracranial pressure (ICP), and normal $Sjvo_2$ and $AVDo_2$. CPP, cerebral perfusion pressure. (Adapted with permission from Coles JP: Regional ischemia after head injury. Curr Opin Crit Care 10:120, 2004.)

The addition of relatively small volumes of hypertonic saline in concentrations between 3% (6 to 8 mL/kg) and 7.5% (4 mL/kg) followed by infusion of LR may be beneficial in multiple trauma patients with head injury.[111,112] Hypertonic saline draws fluid from the intracellular space and, thus, in addition to restoring the blood volume, it reduces brain edema and prevents elevation of the ICP as effectively as 20% mannitol.[113,114] The intravascular volume expansion produced by hypertonic saline is transient; it can be prolonged by addition of 6% dextran-70 or hetastarch to the solution.[115] However, administration of hypertonic saline cannot be maintained for long periods. It may cause hypernatremia, hyperosmolality, or hyperchloremic acidosis, probably from renal bicarbonate loss secondary to increased levels of Cl^-. Serum concentrations of Na^+ and Cl^- and the patient's acid-base status should be followed, and the administration of hypertonic saline should be discontinued if plasma Na^+ reaches 160 mEq/L. Because of these considerations, the use of hypertonic saline is still considered experimental therapy.[116] Resuscitation with colloid solutions (hetastarch, pentastarch, pentafraction, human albumin 5% and 25%, or dextran) provides a sustained improvement in vital signs, but the increase in colloid osmotic pressure produced by these solutions may not have an important role in reducing brain edema.[117]

Several more recent studies seem to indicate that the outlook for patients with brain injury can be improved:

1. Cruz et al[118] and the Lund group[119] used widely different approaches, but the common factor in their treatments was not only maintenance of the CPP, but also avoidance, or at least limitation, of brain swelling. Cruz et al accomplished this by standard therapy augmented by monitoring the cerebral O_2 extraction ($Ceo_2 = Sao_2 - Sjvo_2$). Hyperventilation was used when this value decreased below the normal range of 24 to 42% to constrict the circulation and thus decrease the ICP. The Lund treatment involved a rather complex pharmacological approach, both to control blood pressure and ICP, and to limit edema formation.
2. The earlier definitive treatment is initiated, the better the outcome is likely to be.[120,121] Rudehill et al[120] demonstrated improvement in outcomes in a large series of patients when care was initiated by physicians at the accident scene.
3. Meanwhile, the wide variety of types and severities of injury, and of responses to treatment—both among different patients and in the same patient at different times—imply that therapeutic interventions must be individualized.[122–124] These latter aims may be met, at least partly, by carefully structured intensive care.[125,126] Therapeutic goals should be explicitly set, reviewed, and altered, if necessary, at every change of shift.

Indeed, early intervention and controlled management may explain much of the improvement in outcomes that has been obtained over the past 5 years, including the results obtained by Cruz et al and by the Lund group (Table 48-5). Individualized treatment is likely to result in further advances.

Spine and Spinal Cord Injury

Initial Evaluation

7 The objective in the evaluation of spinal trauma is to diagnose instability of the spine and the extent of neurologic involvement. Not stabilizing the spine in the first hours after a major accident until a definitive diagnosis is established risks converting a neurologically intact patient into a paraplegic or quadriplegic.[127] During transport to the hospital, the patient should be immobilized with a hard collar, a spine board, and tape. After admission, patients should not be left on a rigid spine board for longer than 1 hour, especially when they are paralyzed, because of the risk of decubitus ulcers.

In the conscious patient, the diagnosis is relatively easy: a history of a motor vehicle, industrial, or athletic accident or a fall; penetrating trauma resulting in a neurologic deficit below a specific spinal level; or pain and tenderness over the involved vertebrae strongly suggests a spine injury. Obviously, these symptoms are difficult to elicit in the comatose patient. In these circumstances, flaccid areflexia, loss of rectal sphincter tone, paradoxical respiration, and bradycardia in a hypovolemic patient suggest the diagnosis. In cervical spine trauma, an ability to flex but not to extend the elbow and response to painful stimuli above but not below the clavicle also indicate neurologic injury. Current guidelines consider absence of neck pain or paresthesia and a negative physical examination—lack of tenderness with palpation and during voluntary flexion and extension of the neck—in a neurologically intact, conscious patient as adequate indications for ruling out a cervical spine injury without further radiologic studies.[128–130] Alcohol intoxication and distracting associated injuries do not seem to alter

TABLE 48-5

SIX-MONTH OUTCOMES FOR PATIENTS WITH BRAIN INJURY IN VARIOUS STUDIES

NAME OF STUDY	N	YEAR PUBLISHED	6-MONTH OUTCOME (%) GOOD/ MODERATE	SEVERE/ VEGETATIVE	DEAD	COMMENTS
Three-country (Jennett et al[a])	700	1977	38	11	51	Various treatments, some untreated
Miller et al[b]	158	1981	47	12	40	Vent, surgery, ICP monitoring, and Rx
Traumatic Coma Data Bank (TCDB)[86]	717	1997	43	20	37	Total patients, standard therapy
TCDB[86]	308	1997	54	19	27	Pts without hypotension or hypoxia
Rudehill et al.[120]	1,508	2002	69	11	20	Standard protocol
Cruz[118]	178	1998	74	17	9	CeO_2 group
Eker et al[119]	53	1998	79	13	8	Lund treatment

Results of various treatment protocols for brain injuries. The three-country study surveyed patients who had received a wide variety of treatment; some were untreated. Miller et al. relied on hyperventilation and, when necessary, barbiturates. The TCBD patients were treated similarly; note the difference in outcome of the patients who did not experience hypotension or hypoxia (see Table 48-3). The final three studies are described in the text.
[a]Jennett B, Teasdale G, Galbraith S: Severe head injuries in three countries. J Neurol Neurosurg Psychiatry 40:291, 1977
[b]Miller JD, Butterworth JF, Gudeman SK *et al*: Further experience in the management of severe head injury. J Neurosurg 54:289, 1981

these criteria as long as the patient is alert, conscious, and able to concentrate.[131]

Depending on the degree of deficit, spinal cord injuries are categorized as *complete* or *incomplete.* Intact sensory perception over the sacral distribution and voluntary contraction of the anus (sacral sparing) are present in incomplete, but not in complete, injuries. There is practically no possibility of significant neurologic recovery in complete injury, whereas functional restoration may occur in up to 50% of patients after incomplete injuries.[132] In some patients the development of *spinal shock,* which is manifested by absolute flaccidity and loss of reflexes, precludes distinguishing between complete and incomplete injuries during the initial phase of treatment. Therefore, even in the absence of sacral sparing, the possibility of neurologic recovery dictates that all possible efforts be made at this time to prevent further damage and to preserve cord function. A similar principle applies to the evaluation of the level of injury. After the first few days, spinal cord edema subsides, and the final level is commonly a few segments lower than on initial presentation. Thus, early therapeutic efforts should not be abandoned even in the patient with a high-level injury, which carries a grim functional prognosis.

Spinal shock is probably caused by direct trauma to the spinal cord and usually subsides within days to weeks.[133] The term is frequently used as a misnomer for *neurogenic shock,* which is defined as hypotension and bradycardia caused by the loss of vasomotor tone and sympathetic innervation of the heart as a result of functional depression of the descending sympathetic pathways of the spinal cord. It is usually present after high thoracic and cervical spine injuries and improves within 3 to 5 days.

Radiologic Evaluation

For radiologic diagnosis of the cervical spine, the current strategy is based on the Eastern Association for the Surgery of Trauma guidelines, which recommend a standard three-view (anteroposterior, lateral, and open mouth) series of radiographs and examination of suspect or suboptimally visualized areas with limited, focused CT scans.[134] A more recent trend, however, is to use a helical CT scan with sagittal and coronal reconstruction as the primary diagnostic measure, in conjunction with plain radiographs.[135,136] The advantages of this approach include less reliance on plain films, which are frequently inadequate; almost 100% sensitivity in detecting the injury; the ability to scan other anatomic locations in the same session; and possibly reduced cost. However, the ability of a CT scan to diagnose ligamentous injuries is less than that of detecting fractures. Woodring and Lee[137] found that CT scans detected 90% of the fractures but only 54% of subluxation dislocations, whereas plain films identified only 58% of the fractures but 93% of subluxation dislocations. Newer CT techniques can partially overcome this problem. In fact, it has been suggested that cross-sectional imaging with either CT scanning or magnetic resonance imaging (MRI) should replace the flexion-extension series used to detect ligamentous injury in patients with cervical pain and tenderness but negative spine radiographs.[138] Apart from not being cost effective, flexion-extension films are inadequate when, as in many acute trauma patients, the range of motion of the neck is limited.[138,139]

It is important to recognize that enlargement of the prevertebral space in the neck on lateral films may be due to a retropharyngeal hematoma, which may cause tracheal deviation and tenderness, and complicate airway management.[132] Any radiologic examination should be performed with the patient in the supine position until a spine injury is ruled out, so the risk of displacement of the fracture is minimized. When associated injuries dictate immediate management, radiographic diagnosis may have to be postponed for several hours or days as long as proper immobilization of the spine is maintained.

Initial Management

The spinal cord, a microcosm of the brain, is also vulnerable to a secondary injury process that may be a product of hypotension, hypoxia, and probably other physiologic complications.[140] Prompt recognition and aggressive treatment of these insults, which may also result from associated injuries, may minimize exacerbation of spinal cord lesions and improve the long-term outlook of patients with spinal cord injuries.[93,97,141]

Immobilization and Intubation. Maintenance of immobilization of the injured spine is of paramount importance. If a cervical spine fracture is suspected, immobilization or manual inline stabilization of the neck is necessary before the patient is moved. If the patient has a thoracic or lumbar injury, a careful log-rolling maneuver should be used.[142]

Any intubation technique is safe as long as the neck is held in a neutral position. Thus, a Macintosh laryngoscope may be used if manual inline stabilization of the neck is applied. Inline stabilization, however, decreases the visibility of the larynx in a large proportion of patients. If difficulties occur, it is better to choose an alternate technique rather than manipulate the neck more than a small amount. Cricoid pressure should be applied with great care in the patient with a possible cervical spine injury because it may produce undue motion of the spine if excessive force is used.[93]

Steroids. For several years, high-dose methylprednisolone has been used in many centers in an attempt to improve the outcome from spinal cord injuries. The drug is usually given as a bolus of 30 mg/kg within 8 hours of injury, followed in 1 hour by an infusion of 5.4 mg/kg/hr for the next 23 to 47 hours. The National Acute Spinal Cord Injury Studies (NASCIS-2 and NASCIS-3)[143–145] demonstrated some improvement in motor function in treated patients who had partial sensory and motor loss. The results were best in patients who received 24 hours of therapy starting within 3 hours of injury and those receiving 48 hours of treatment starting within 3 to 8 hours of injury. There was virtually no improvement in sensory scores in any of the groups. There was little or no difference from untreated patients in groups with more severe injuries or in those who were treated after 8 hours, and the long-term improvement in the functional status of most of the patients was at best moderate. Unfortunately, the results of these studies have not been duplicated in any other prospective or retrospective trials.[146–148]

Furthermore, steroid therapy is associated with an increased rate of sepsis, pneumonia, and days of intensive care and positive-pressure ventilation.[143–145,149] Given these results, the *Guidelines for the Management of Acute Cervical Spine and Spinal Cord Injuries*[130] state, "Treatment with methylprednisolone for either 24 or 48 hours is recommended as an option in the treatment of patients with acute spinal cord injuries that should be undertaken only with the knowledge that the evidence suggesting harmful side effects is more consistent than any suggestion of clinical benefit."

Respiratory Complications

Respiratory complications are common in all phases of the care of patients with spinal cord injury, and in the initial period, may be augmented by associated brain, neck, chest, or abdominal injury, alcohol intoxication, or the effects of self-administered or iatrogenic drugs. Injuries at C5 or lower are usually associated with normal tidal volumes because the function of the diaphragm is intact, whereas patients with levels at C4 or above may require permanent ventilatory assistance. Nevertheless, accessory respiratory muscle paresis may cause a significant loss of expiratory reserve even when the injury involves the lower spinal segments.[150,151]

Pulmonary edema is another significant cause of respiratory dysfunction. A severe catecholamine surge follows acute trauma to the spinal cord.[152] Although the resultant hypertension lasts for only a few minutes, its effects persist; it may produce both pulmonary capillary damage, as a result of shifting of a large portion of the blood volume into the pulmonary circulation, and left ventricular dysfunction. Overzealous fluid therapy to treat the patient's initial hypotension may lead to acute pulmonary edema when the sympathetic activity returns approximately 3 to 5 days after the injury.

Paradoxical respiration in the quadriplegic patient results from partial chest wall collapse during inspiration; it may produce limitation of the tidal volume and an increased risk of hypoventilation. The situation is aggravated when the patient is in an upright position. The diaphragm cannot maintain its normal domed shape, which is the only way it can contract efficiently, because the weight of the thoracic contents is not opposed by the normal tone of the abdominal muscles. Thus, in contrast to other diseases that produce respiratory insufficiency, the supine position improves respiration in persons with quadriplegia.[151]

Other causes of inadequate respiration in the early phase of spinal cord injury are aspiration of gastric contents, atelectasis, pneumonia, and bronchoconstriction. Management includes careful observation of the patient's breathing and preparation to ventilate the lungs and intubate the trachea at the first sign of respiratory depression.[151]

Severe bradycardia or dysrhythmias may result from unopposed vagal activity during tracheal intubation or suctioning: the patient must be preoxygenated, and atropine (0.4 to 0.6 mg) should be given before any instrumentation. If bradycardia develops during airway management, treatment includes additional atropine, glycopyrrolate, isoproterenol, or, if necessary, cardiac pacing.

Hemodynamic Management

Hemodynamic management of quadriplegic patients includes a complete assessment, with a pulmonary artery catheter, if necessary, as early as possible after injury. In as many as 25% of patients with cervical spinal cord injuries, left ventricular dysfunction may contribute to the hypotension.[153] Decreased preload can be treated with fluid infusion using cardiac function curves as a guide. In general, volume may be safely replaced to a central venous or pulmonary capillary wedge pressure (PCWP) of 18 mm Hg.[153] This avoids, or at least limits, the severity of the pulmonary edema described previously. Hypotension despite adequate fluid infusion, acidosis, or low mixed venous PO_2 requires treatment with inotropes such as dopamine.

Anesthetic Considerations

Any anesthetic technique compatible with the patient's general condition is satisfactory for the patient with spinal cord injury. Hypotension is common during anesthesia in quadriplegics. Placement of a central venous or pulmonary artery catheter may facilitate management of the patient's volume and blood pressure status.

Succinylcholine may produce a sudden, severe increase in serum K^+ in patients with spine injury. Levels as high as 14 mEq/L may be reached; the result may be irreversible ventricular dysrhythmias and cardiac arrest. Although succinylcholine is probably safe during the first week after injury, it is probably best to avoid it altogether in the paraplegic patient and to use rapid-onset nondepolarizing agents such as rocuronium when a rapid-sequence induction is required.

Neck Injury

Both penetrating and blunt trauma may injure the major structures in the neck: vessels, respiratory and digestive tracts, and nervous system. Hemorrhage, asphyxia, mediastinitis, paralysis, stroke, or death may result if these injuries are not promptly recognized and treated.

8 Penetrating neck injuries usually present with obvious clinical manifestations; blunt cervical trauma may be more subtle. Airway compromise or obstruction, brisk bleeding from the wound site, an expanding pulsatile hematoma, and shock with or without external bleeding are obvious signs of cervical

vascular injury, and dictate immediate airway management and vascular control. Decreased or absent upper-extremity or distal carotid pulses, as well as carotid bruit or thrill, are pathognomonic for cervical arterial injury; however, these often do not require immediate surgery. Hemothorax, pneumothorax, and signs of air embolism are also suggestive. Respiratory distress, cyanosis, or stridor are obvious signs of airway injury and require immediate tracheal intubation. Other signs that strongly suggest airway injury are dysphonia, hoarseness, cough, hemoptysis, air bubbling from the wound, subcutaneous crepitus, laryngeal tenderness, pneumothorax, and hemothorax. Because of their dynamic nature, cervical airway injuries may rapidly progress to obstruction; the patient therefore should be observed carefully and the trachea intubated at the first sign of problems.

Esophageal injuries, whether in the neck or the chest, are insidious and difficult to diagnose. Dysphagia, odynophagia, hematemesis, subcutaneous crepitus, prevertebral air on a lateral cervical radiograph, and major concomitant injuries to other cervical structures suggest an esophageal injury and call for confirmation with an esophagram.

The neurologic manifestations of a penetrating neck injury vary depending on the injured structure. Partial spinal cord transection produces the Brown-Sequard syndrome with ipsilateral motor and contralateral sensory deficit below the injury. Complete spinal cord transection, depending on the level of injury, produces paraplegia or quadriplegia, usually with neurogenic shock. Occasionally, luminal occlusion of the carotid and vertebral arteries may lead to a hemispheric cerebrovascular accident; associated hypotension increases the likelihood of this event.

Patients with severe active bleeding, persistent hypotension, and air bubbling through the wound require immediate surgery without further diagnostic studies.[154] Controversy exists over the indications for surgical management of stable penetrating neck injuries. Mandatory exploration is associated with negative findings in approximately 70% of patients.[154] Thus, in many centers, patients are evaluated with noninvasive diagnostic tests and undergo surgery only when there are positive findings.[154]

Blunt cervical vascular injuries usually present with a hematoma that may compress the cervical veins, displace the airway, and produce pharyngeal and laryngeal congestion. Injury to an artery may produce an intimal tear, pseudoaneurysm, fistula, or thrombosis.[155] If a carotid or vertebral artery is involved, cerebral ischemia may occur. Often thrombosis develops gradually over minutes to a few hours, therefore, the appearance of neurologic symptoms is delayed in approximately 40% of patients.[155] Symptomatic patients may present with a cervical bruit, altered mental status, or lateralizing neurologic deficits including hemiparesis, transient ischemic attacks, amaurosis fugax, or Horner's syndrome. The mortality rate associated with blunt carotid injury varies between 15 and 28%, and 15 to 50% of survivors have neurologic deficits.[155,156] Identification of a blunt carotid injury in an asymptomatic patient using CT, magnetic resonance angiography, or four-vessel arteriography not only allows early institution of antiplatelet therapy, systemic anticoagulation, endovascular intervention, or surgical repair,[156,157] but also occasionally prevents the neurologic deficits that may follow surgery for associated injuries in an unprotected patient.

Airway injuries after blunt trauma are rare, but carry an overall mortality rate of 2%.[158] Their severity varies from a simple mucosal tear or hematoma to a comminuted laryngeal cartilage fracture or complete cricotracheal separation. They frequently require primary laryngeal repair or tracheostomy. Anesthetic management is not only complicated by relatively complex airway management problems[41–43] (discussed in the Airway Evaluation and Intervention section), but also with associated skull base, intracranial, open neck, cervical spine, esophageal, or pharyngeal injuries.[158]

Chest Injury

Although a high percentage of thoracic injuries can be treated conservatively, patients who need surgery may have major intraoperative physiologic disturbances.

Chest Wall Injury

Rib fractures may produce pneumothorax or hemothorax, and both the frequency and severity of visceral injuries increase as
9 the number of fractured ribs increases. Patients with three or more fractured ribs have a greater likelihood of hepatic and splenic injury, a higher mortality rate, a higher injury severity score, and longer intensive care unit (ICU) and hospital stays than those with fewer rib fractures.[159] Patients with lower rib fractures may have an underlying spleen or liver injury. Because of the large amount of energy required to fracture the first rib in its protected location, injury to this bone indicates severe underlying trauma, commonly to the aorta, the subclavian vessels, the heart, or the abdominal viscera, but also to the maxillofacial complex, the brain, or the spinal cord.[160] Scapular fractures also suggest severe injuries in other locations, especially the heart and lungs.[161] Sternal fractures are mainly encountered in elderly motor vehicle occupants wearing seat belts; they are usually not associated with serious trauma to the thoracic or abdominal viscera.[162]

The management principles for these injuries are similar to those previously described for flail chest, although the need for mechanical ventilation is less likely in single rib fractures than in a flail chest. Effective pain relief, preferably with continuous thoracic epidural anesthetics or opioids, is central to management.[48]

Pleural Injury

Closed pneumothorax most commonly develops as a result of lung puncture by a displaced rib fracture after blunt trauma, or by missile injuries or stab wounds. The presence of subcutaneous emphysema suggests coexisting pneumothorax, although this finding alone is not an indication for chest tube placement because it may be the result of other injuries. Tension pneumothorax involving $>50\%$ of a hemithorax presents with dyspnea, tachycardia, cyanosis, agitation, diaphoresis, neck vein distention, tracheal deviation, and displacement of the maximal cardiac impulse to the contralateral side.

The plain chest radiograph, routinely obtained during initial evaluation of all trauma victims, is essential for diagnosis. Although an upright film provides the best opportunity for detection of pneumothorax, this position may be impossible or contraindicated in patients who are experiencing major hemorrhage or those with suspected spine injury. Air in the pleural space tends to accumulate anteriorly in supine or semirecumbent patients, often in the anteromedial sulcus.[163] More recently, transthoracic ultrasound has been used for the diagnosis of pneumothorax. Normally, movement of the lung beneath the chest wall produces "comet tail" artifacts from echodense areas on the lung surface.[164] In the presence of pneumothorax, neither lung motion nor comet tails can be seen.[164] In a more recent study of blunt and penetrating trauma victims, ultrasound was more sensitive than a supine chest film, but did not detect all pneumothoraces. Further, ultrasound detection of rib and sternal fractures also appeared to be more accurate than the chest radiograph.[165] It was recommended that a chest film and the ultrasound can complement each other, but that chest CT be used as the definitive test.[166]

Brasel et al[167] suggested that a small closed pneumothorax can be safely managed by observation alone, without a chest tube, even in those patients who require positive-pressure ventilation, as long as continuing vigilance is maintained. However, based on an earlier study[168] and our own experience, we strongly believe that once diagnosed, a traumatic pneumothorax, no matter how small, should be treated with thoracostomy drainage before tracheal intubation and positive-pressure ventilation.

Bleeding intercostal vessels are responsible for most hemothoraces. Severe airway deviation may be produced by a hemothorax, although it is not as common as it is after a pneumothorax. Treatment consists of drainage with a 30 to 40F chest tube (26 to 32F is used for pneumothorax). Initial drainage of 1,000 mL of blood, or collection of >200 mL/hr for several hours, is an indication for thoracotomy. Additional indications for thoracotomy are a "white lung" appearance on the anteroposterior chest radiograph; a continuous major air leak from the chest tube, which may result from a direct airway injury or major lung laceration; and evidence of pericardial tamponade. Hemodynamically stable patients with persistent bleeding of $<150 \text{ mL} \cdot \text{hr}^{-1}$ are managed with video-assisted thoracoscopic surgery (VATS) to control bleeding.[169] This procedure requires placement of a double-lumen tube to collapse the lung on the involved side; it can also be useful in diagnosis of suspected diaphragmatic, cardiac, or mediastinal injuries; evaluation of some bronchopleural fistulas; and evacuation of clotted blood or an empyema that does not drain with a chest tube.[169] Use of VATS decreases the need for open thoracotomy and the number of negative explorations in trauma patients.[170]

Pulmonary Contusion

This entity often accompanies chest wall injury, but may also develop in isolation. Its management is discussed in the section on flail chest.

Penetrating Cardiac Injury

Pericardial tamponade, cardiac chamber perforation, and fistula formation between the cardiac chambers and the great vessels are the consequences of this type of trauma. Any penetrating wound of the chest, especially one within the "cardiac window" (midclavicular lines laterally, clavicles superiorly, and costal margins inferiorly), can cause this injury. Pneumopericardium visible on a plain chest radiograph after penetrating chest trauma should increase the suspicion, although it is not seen in all patients. Unstable patients require immediate sternotomy or left thoracotomy. Transthoracic echocardiography (TTE) can be used for screening stable patients,[171] but it may be inconclusive in obese patients and in those with pneumothorax; TEE provides an accurate diagnosis in these patients.[172] Of the alternative diagnostic measures, the central venous pressure (CVP) is not always accurate, and a subxiphoid pericardial window is invasive, must be performed in the OR under general anesthesia, takes longer, and cannot detect an intracardiac shunt.

Pericardial Tamponade

The classic findings of pericardial tamponade—tachycardia, hypotension, distant heart sounds, distended neck veins, pulsus paradoxus, or pulsus alternans—are difficult to appreciate or may be absent in a hypovolemic trauma patient. TTE or TEE can demonstrate blood in the pericardial sac and the presence of ventricular "diastolic collapse," which indicates at least a 20% reduction in cardiac output. Initial management consists of intravenous fluids and, if necessary, careful selection and titration of anesthetic agents, such as ketamine and etomidate, which produce relatively little myocardial depression. Evacuation of the pericardial blood by pericardiocentesis or surgery should be performed as soon as possible.

Blunt Cardiac Injury

10 This term has replaced "myocardial contusion" and encompasses varying degrees of myocardial damage; coronary artery injury; and rupture of the cardiac free wall, septum, or a valve following blunt trauma.[173] Myocardial injury consists of myofibrillar disintegration, edema, bleeding, or necrosis that, depending on its severity, presents as minor electrocardiogram (ECG) or enzyme abnormalities, complex arrhythmias, or cardiac failure caused by direct mechanical impact or indirectly by coronary occlusion. Arrhythmias last no more than a few days; ventricular wall motion abnormalities may persist for up to 1 year, but any increased risk of perioperative cardiac complications appears to last for no more than a month.

The prominent clinical findings are angina, sometimes responding to nitroglycerine, dyspnea, chest wall ecchymosis and/or fractures; dysrhythmias of any type; and right-sided or left-sided congestive heart failure. Orliaguet et al[173] proposed an algorithm for the diagnosis and treatment of several clinical scenarios caused by this injury (Fig. 48-3). The diagnosis is based on the 12-lead ECG, troponin I level, and echocardiography. The ECG is very sensitive, although not specific. A normal trace cannot rule out the diagnosis, but it is the best screening test. Common ECG abnormalities include almost any type of arrhythmia, ST or T-wave changes, and conduction delays. Patients with a normal ECG undergoing minor surgery do not require any further testing. Patients with severe injuries need measurement of troponin I and TEE to diagnose any abnormalities caused by the cardiac injury (see Fig. 48-3). Troponin I has replaced serum creatine kinase and its MB fraction (CK-MB) because of its greater specificity for cardiac muscle damage. Echocardiography can demonstrate wall motion abnormalities, valve malfunction, hemopericardium, intracardiac thrombi, venous or systemic embolism, and end-diastolic and fractional ventricular wall area changes. It thus aids not only in the diagnosis of blunt cardiac injury, but also in

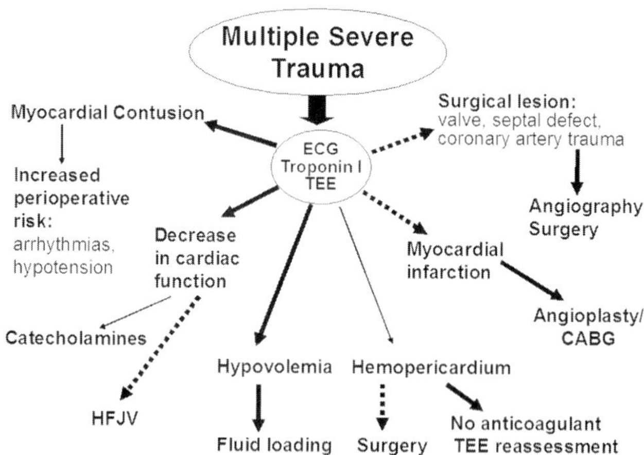

FIGURE 48-3. Algorithm for management of various clinical scenarios produced by severe blunt cardiac injury (BCI). Evaluation of severe multiple trauma induced BCI uses electrocardiogram (ECG), troponin I, and transesophageal echocardiography (TEE). *Arrows* represent the frequency of occurrence of each scenario and the frequency of management measures. *Thick arrows* represent high frequency, *thin arrows* low frequency, and *dotted arrows* very rare occurrences. CABG, coronary artery bypass graft; HFJV, high-frequency jet ventilation. (Adapted with permission from Orliaguet G, Ferjani M, Riou B: The heart in blunt trauma. Anesthesiology 95:544, 2001.)

TABLE 48-6

COMMON CLINICAL, RADIOGRAPHIC, AND ULTRASOUND FEATURES OF THORACIC AORTIC INJURIES

■ CLINICAL	■ RADIOGRAPHIC	■ SPIRAL COMPUTED TOMOGRAPHY	■ ULTRASOUND
Increased arterial pressure and pulse amplitude in upper extremities Decreased arterial pressure and pulse amplitude in lower extremities Absent or weak left radial artery pulse Osler's sign: discrepancy between left and right arm blood pressure Retrosternal or interscapular pain Hoarseness Systolic flow murmur over the precordium or medial to the left scapula Neurologic deficits in the lower extremities	Widened mediastinum Blurring of the aortic contours Widened paraspinal interfaces Opacified pulmonary window Broadened paratracheal stripe Displacement of the left main-stem bronchus Rightward deviation of the esophagus and trachea Left hemothorax Sternal and/or upper rib fractures	Mediastinal hematoma Aortic wall irregularity Intimal flap False aneurysm Pseudocoarctation Intramural hematoma Intraluminal clot or medial flap	Intimal flap Turbulent flow Dilated aortic isthmus Acute false aneurysm Intraluminal medial flap Hemothorax Hemomediastinum

hemodynamic management. Treatment options depend on the diagnosis (see Fig. 48-3). They include antiarrhythmic agents, inotropes, fluid loading, HFJV to optimize cardiac function, and surgery for hemopericardium, valvular, or septal lesions, or coronary artery injury or disease.

Thoracic Aortic Injury

This injury occurs at the isthmus—the junction between the free and fixed portions of the descending aorta—in 90% of cases, and carries an 80% incidence of mortality in the first hour following injury. There may be no clinical findings in the emergency department (Table 48-6). Only 20 to 30% of patients with mediastinal widening actually have this injury, although the negative predictive value of the test is 98%.[174] Measuring the left mediastinal width ($\geq$6 cm) and its fraction of the total mediastinal width ($\geq$0.6) may increase the specificity and positive predictive value of the plain film.[175]

More recent advances in contrast-enhanced spiral CT and ultrasound technologies permit reliable noninvasive diagnosis and have substantially decreased the need for biplanar aortography. Both CT and TEE are equally capable of diagnosing subadventitial aortic injuries that require surgical intervention.[176] CT is more likely to be used for diagnosis because introducing a TEE probe in an awake patient may be undesirable. Lesions of the intima and media that can be treated conservatively, and concomitant blunt cardiac injuries are much more likely to be detectable by TEE than CT.[176] Intraoperative TEE is especially useful for the anesthesiologist when other injuries require immediate surgery without time for CT examination of the chest. Aortography remains the examination of choice when the noninvasive studies are contraindicated or provide equivocal results. It also can demonstrate injuries to the branches of the aorta, which TEE cannot detect.[176]

Surgical prioritization when multiple injuries are present depends on the hemodynamic and neurologic status of the patient. Although the aorta should be repaired as early as possible, control of active hemorrhage from other sites and surgery for intracranial hematomas have a higher surgical priority, unless the aorta is leaking.[177] In most instances, a blood clot between the aorta and the mediastinal pleura occludes the vessel. Any disturbance of the tamponaded region may reinitiate bleeding. A rapid flow of blood in a large artery tends to pull its endothelium with it and thus may rupture an injured vessel that is sealed with a clot or a hematoma. Such an increase in the aortic blood flow is usually caused by increased myocardial contractility; every effort should be made to prevent increased cardiac contractility and hypertension. Endovascular stent grafts have more recently been used in some centers for repair of thoracic aortic injuries, with an apparently reduced risk of paraplegia and the complications associated with thoracotomy.[178]

Diaphragmatic Injury

Injury to the diaphragm may permit migration of abdominal contents into the chest where they may compress the lung, producing abnormalities of gas exchange, or the heart, resulting in dysrhythmias and/or hypotension. Because the defect produced by blunt injury is larger than that resulting from a penetrating injury, migration of abdominal contents, which requires a defect of at least 6 cm in diameter, is also more common after blunt trauma.[179] The liver protects the right side of the diaphragm, thus traumatic herniation is more common on the left side.[179]

The best method of diagnosing a diaphragmatic hernia is laparoscopy, or in selected cases, VATS. Nevertheless, noting that the end of a nasogastric tube is above the diaphragm on the chest radiograph is a certain sign that the stomach is displaced into the chest. A chest radiograph that shows intestinal markings and lung compression, or a contrast-enhanced abdominal CT scan that includes the lower third of the thorax, also provide important information.[180] Failure to retrieve the instilled fluid during diagnostic peritoneal lavage (DPL) or drainage of DPL fluid from a thoracostomy tube also indicates this injury.[180]

Abdominal and Pelvic Injuries

Table 48-7 summarizes the strengths and weaknesses of the currently available diagnostic tools used for abdominal injuries.[181] Because of the unpredictable course of bullets in the body, exploratory laparotomy or, in selected cases, laparoscopy is required after any gunshot wound of the abdomen. Stab wounds may be managed with tractotomy to determine whether the peritoneum is involved. Laparoscopy, laparotomy, or DPL may be indicated after a positive tractotomy. In some hemodynamically stable patients, abdominal and flank gunshot

TABLE 48-7

DIAGNOSTIC TOOLS IN ABDOMINAL TRAUMA: STRENGTHS AND WEAKNESSES

DIAGNOSTIC TOOL	STRENGTH	WEAKNESS
Physical examination	Expeditious, safe, and inexpensive; potential for serial examination	Diagnosis of specific injury (e.g., diaphragm)
Diagnostic peritoneal lavage	Expeditious, safe, and inexpensive	Diagnosis of diaphragmatic injury, hollow viscus injury, retroperitoneal injury; can be oversensitive and nonspecific
Computed tomography	Evaluation of peritoneum and retroperitoneum Staging of solid organ injury	Diagnosis of diaphragmatic injury, hollow viscus injury Expensive; controversial need for contrast
Ultrasonography	Expeditious, safe, and inexpensive; accurate for free peritoneal fluid Potential for serial examinations	Diagnosis of diphragmatic injury, hollow viscus injury Less accurate in the presence of large retroperitoneal hematomas
Laparoscopy	Diagnosis of peritoneal penetration, diaphragmatic injury Evaluation of bleeding or solid organ injury Potential for therapy	Diagnosis of hollow viscus injury, retroperitoneal injury Expensive
Video-assisted thoracic surgery	Evaluation of lung, diaphragm, mediastinum, chest wall, and pericardium; potential for treatment	Requires operating room; expensive

Reprinted with permission from Villavicencio RT, Aucar JA: Analysis of laparoscopy in trauma. J Am Coll Surg 189:11, 1999.

wounds may be managed safely with an initial CT scan.[182] Patients with a negative study are observed, whereas those with positive findings undergo exploratory surgery. Equivocal CT results are followed by a laparoscopy and, if this is positive, by laparotomy.

Patients with blunt abdominal trauma are also evaluated by CT scan unless they are hemodynamically unstable and there are overt abdominal signs such as tenderness, guarding, and gross distention. Absence of abdominal distention, however, does not rule out intra-abdominal bleeding. At least 1 L of blood can accumulate before the smallest change in girth is apparent, and the diaphragm can also move cephalad, allowing further significant blood loss without any change in abdominal circumference.

In hemodynamically stable patients, there are two major diagnostic algorithms: focused approach with sonography for trauma (FAST; Fig. 48-4) and the conventional approach, without ultrasonography (Fig. 48-5). The diagnostic accuracy of these algorithms is similar, but FAST requires one-third of the time and is 3.5 times less expensive than the conventional approach.[183] Screening with abdominal ultrasonography is performed by placing a 3.0 to 5.0 MHz probe on four distinct areas of the abdomen: subxiphoid, to detect pericardial blood; right upper quadrant, for blood in the hepatorenal pouch; left upper quadrant, to detect perisplenic blood; and just above the pubic symphysis, for blood in the rectovesical pouch. FAST is accurate for detection of hemoperitoneum[183,184] and can also identify solid organ injuries, although experience with these is limited. It cannot reliably detect trauma to the intestines unless it is associated with bleeding.[184] Fortunately, isolated intestinal injuries are uncommon after blunt trauma. Depending on the results of FAST, patients are managed with observation, repeat FAST, DPL, abdominal CT, laparoscopy, or laparotomy.[183] Patients managed with the conventional algorithm are evaluated by CT if they are stable, and DPL if they are hemodynamically or neurologically unstable. Depending on the results of these studies, they are observed or undergo surgery.[183]

Laparoscopy is an excellent screening tool in abdominal trauma patients. An analysis showed that it avoided laparotomy in 63% of patients and missed only 1% of the injuries.[181] It is also possible to repair diaphragmatic, bladder, and solid organ injuries with this technique. The complication rate of laparoscopy in trauma is approximately 1%, including pneumothorax, small bowel injury, intra-abdominal vascular injury, and extraperitoneal CO_2 insufflation.[181]

Fractures of the Pelvis

11 Pelvic fractures result in major hemorrhage in 25% and exsanguination in 1% of patients.[185] In most of these fractures,

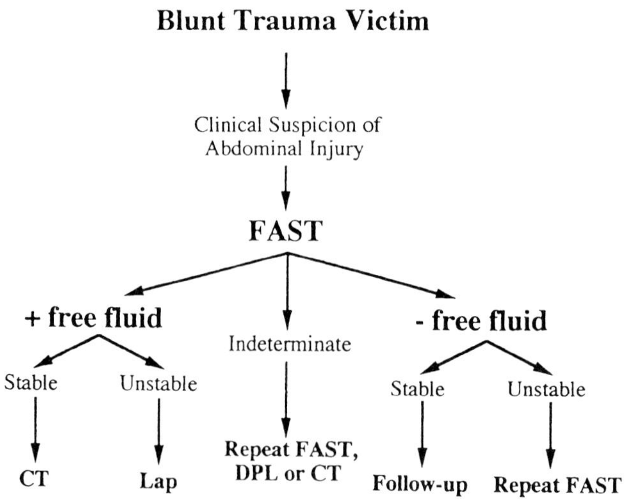

Blunt Trauma Victim

Clinical Suspicion of Abdominal Injury

FAST

+ free fluid | Indeterminate | - free fluid

Stable → CT; Unstable → Lap; Indeterminate → Repeat FAST, DPL or CT; Stable → Follow-up; Unstable → Repeat FAST

FIGURE 48-4. Algorithm for focused assessment with sonography for evaluation of blunt abdominal injury. CT, computed tomography; DPL, diagnostic peritoneal lavage; FAST, focused approach with sonography for trauma; Lap, laparotomy. (Reprinted with permission from Boulanger BR, McLennan BA, Brennemann FD *et al:* Prospective evidence of the superiority of a sonography-based algorithm in the assessment of blunt abdominal injury. J Trauma 47:632, 1999.)

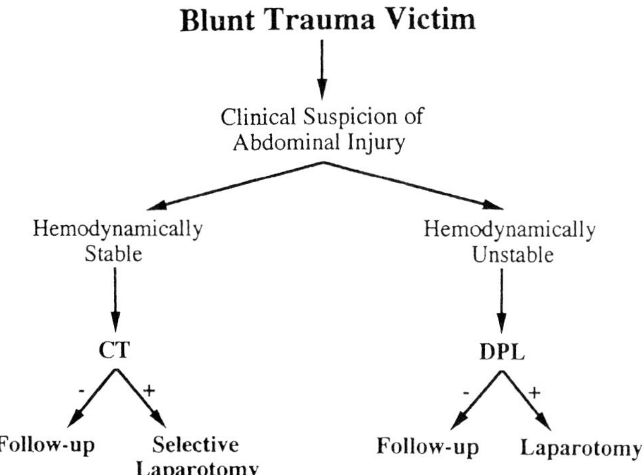

FIGURE 48-5. Conventional algorithm for evaluation of blunt abdominal injury. CT, computed tomography; DPL, diagnostic peritoneal lavage. (Reprinted with permission from Boulanger BR, McLennan BA, Brennemann FD *et al:* Prospective evidence of the superiority of a sonography-based algorithm in the assessment of blunt abdominal injury. J Trauma 47:632, 1999.)

bleeding results from disruption of veins by fragments of bone. Pelvic retroperitoneal bleeding is self-limited in most patients with venous injuries, except those with open fractures, in whom the tamponading effect does not occur. Approximately 18 to 20% of patients have arterial bleeding, which does not stop. The retroperitoneal space in these patients may serve as a distensible container, expanding superiorly and anteriorly toward the abdominal wall and totally obliterating the lower part of the abdominal cavity. Thus, DPL, as in pregnant trauma patients, should be performed above the umbilicus. Large retroperitoneal hematomas may also cause respiratory difficulty because of pressure on the diaphragm.

Following external pelvic fixation, which decreases the mobility of the bone fragments and thus helps control blood loss, angiography can indicate the type and location of bleeding. Arterial bleeding is treated with embolization; the angiography suite should be prepared in advance not only for anesthesia, but also for invasive monitoring and resuscitation. Pelvic fractures may also injure the bladder and the urethra. Thus, an urethrogram should be performed before insertion of a urinary catheter.

Extremity Injuries

Surgical repair of extremity fractures, whether they are open or closed, should be performed as soon as possible. Delayed fracture repair is associated with an increased risk of deep vein thrombosis (DVT), pneumonia, sepsis, and the pulmonary and cerebral complications of fat embolism. In open fractures, an additional important concern is infection. Wounds left unrepaired for more than 6 hours are likely to become septic.

Associated vascular trauma must be recognized early. Most vascular injuries exhibit at least some part of the classic syndrome of *pain, pulselessness, pallor, paresthesias,* and *paresis.* The definitive diagnosis is made with arteriography; in selected patients, a duplex ultrasound study may be used as a screening test.

Compartment syndrome, which is characterized by severe pain in the affected extremity, should be recognized early so emergency fasciotomy can be effective in preventing irreversible muscle and nerve damage. In unconscious patients, swelling and tenseness of the extremity indicate the presence of this complication. The definitive diagnosis is made by measuring compartment pressures, using a transducer attached to a fluid-filled extension tube and a needle inserted into the various compartments of the extremity. A pressure exceeding 40 cm H_2O is an indication for immediate surgery. Caution must be exercised when using epidural or nerve block analgesia for perioperative pain relief in the presence of extremity fractures. Absence of pain could delay the diagnosis of compartment syndrome.

Burns

Determination of the size and depth of a burn sets the guidelines for resuscitation, as well as the indications for surgical intervention.[186] A partial-thickness burn is red, blanches to touch, and is sensitive to painful stimuli and heat. Superficial partial-thickness (first-degree) burns involve the epidermis and upper dermis, and heal spontaneously. Deep partial-thickness (second-degree) burns involve the deep dermis, and require excision and grafting to ensure rapid return of function. A full-thickness (third-degree) burn does not blanch even with deep pressure and is insensate. Complete destruction of the dermis requires wound excision and grafting to prevent wound infection that may lead to local sepsis and systemic inflammation. Fourth-degree burns involve muscle, fascia, and bone, necessitating complete excision and leaving the patient with limited function. The size of the burned area as a fraction of the total body surface area (TBSA) is estimated by the "rule of nines." In an adult, the head contributes to 9%; the upper extremities, 18%; the trunk, 36%; and the lower extremities, 36% of the TBSA. These proportions are somewhat different in children, depending on the age and size. To estimate the size of a burn, the palmar surface of a child (excluding the digits) represents about 0.5% of the TBSA over a wide range of ages.

Information about the mechanism of injury facilitates the di-
12 agnosis of associated clinical abnormalities. For example, thermal trauma caused by flames in a closed space is likely to be associated with airway damage. Burns resulting from motor vehicle, airplane, or industrial accidents may be complicated by other traumatic injuries. Finally, burns caused by electrocution may show little external evidence but may be associated with severe fractures, hematomas, visceral injury, and skeletal and cardiac muscle injury resulting in pain, myoglobinuria, and dysrhythmias or other ECG abnormalities.

Full-thickness burns involving >10% of the TBSA; partial-thickness burns covering >25% of TBSA in adults and over 20% at the extremes of age; burns involving the face, hands, feet, or perineum; inhalation, chemical, and electrical burns; and burns in patients with severe preexisting medical disorders are considered to be major burns.[186] A severe burn is a systemic disease that stimulates the release of mediators such as interleukins, tumor necrosis factor, and neopterins, locally—producing wound edema—and into the circulation, resulting in immune suppression, hypermetabolism, protein catabolism, sepsis, and multisystem organ failure.[186]

Airway Complications

Respiratory distress in the initial phase of a burn is usually caused by airway injury involving the pharynx or the trachea. Singed facial hair, facial burns, dysphonia or hoarseness, cough, soot in the mouth or nose, and swallowing difficulties in patients without respiratory distress should increase the suspicion of upper (frequent) and lower (occasional) airway injury. In the upper airway, glottic and periglottic edema and copious, thick secretions may produce respiratory obstruction. This may be aggravated by fluid resuscitation even in the absence of significant inhalation injury.[187] In lower airway burns, decreased surfactant and mucociliary function, mucosal necrosis and ulceration, edema, tissue sloughing, and secretions produce bronchial obstruction, air trapping, and bronchopneumonia. The development of parenchymal lung injury takes approximately 1 to 5 days and presents with the clinical picture of adult respiratory distress syndrome. Pneumonia and pulmonary embolism (PE) are late complications that occur 5 or more days after burns. The presence of a lung injury markedly increases the mortality rate from thermal injuries.[188]

Administration of the highest possible concentration of O_2 by facemask is the first priority in moderately to severely burned patients with a patent airway. In patients with massive burns, stridor, respiratory distress, hypoxemia, hypercarbia, loss of consciousness, or altered mentation, immediate tracheal intubation is indicated.[189] The intubation technique selected depends on the operator's experience, the age of the patient, and the extent of airway compromise. In adults, awake fiberoptic intubation under adequate topical anesthesia is probably the safest approach, but other techniques (WuScope, intubating LMA, retrograde intubation, or transtracheal jet ventilation) may be used. In most pediatric patients, awake intubation is not possible. An inhalation induction with O_2 and sevoflurane, followed by intubation using a fiberoptic bronchoscope or conventional laryngoscope is appropriate.[186] A surgical airway entails a significant risk of pulmonary sepsis, late upper airway sequelae, and death in burned patients; it should be reserved for those whose airway management cannot be handled in any other way.[186,190] Immediately after securing the airway, ventilation with low levels of PEEP will prevent the pulmonary edema that may develop secondary to loss of laryngeal auto-PEEP in patients with significant airway obstruction before intubation.[191] Airway humidification, bronchial toilet, and bronchodilators if needed for bronchospasm are also indicated.

The pediatric airway is particularly challenging because it may be occluded by minimal amounts of swelling due to its small diameter. Prophylactic intubation may therefore be required in children who are suspected of having an inhalation injury, even though they are not yet in respiratory distress. Prophylactic tracheal intubation may also be indicated in adults when the resources for careful follow-up are insufficient.[191] Information obtained from radiologic, ABG, and endoscopic examinations and pulmonary function testing may be useful to predict which patient will need tracheal intubation and possibly decrease the risks of airway manipulation.[189]

Fiberoptic laryngoscopy is easy to perform and can provide direct information about the glottic and periglottic structures. It may avoid tracheal intubation in patients who would otherwise be considered candidates for this procedure.[189] Fiberoptic bronchoscopy has the additional advantage of providing information about the lower airway, although it is more uncomfortable for the patient and requires topical anesthesia of the tracheobronchial tree.[192] These studies should be performed every 3 to 4 hours for the first 12 hours after injury. In cooperative patients, pulmonary function testing may aid in the evaluation of airway obstruction. A saw-toothed or flattened inspiratory flow and an extrathoracic obstruction pattern on the flow/volume loop suggest upper airway obstruction. Decreased peak expiratory flow, forced vital capacity and pulmonary compliance, and increased airway resistance suggest lower airway injury.

The chest radiograph, ABGs, and pulmonary function tests are usually normal in the immediate postburn period, even in patients with pulmonary complications. However, these tests should be performed at this time for later comparison. As expected, the more extensive the pulmonary edema, the more severe are the functional abnormalities of the lungs. The treatment of smoke inhalation in burns involves ventilatory management, intensive care, and treatment of carbon monoxide (CO) and cyanide (CN^-) toxicity.

Ventilation and Intensive Care

Hypoxemia may persist despite tracheal intubation, ventilation with PEEP, bronchodilators, and suction of airway secretions. In the first 36 hours, this is caused by acute pulmonary edema. From the second to the fifth day, hypoxia may result from atelectasis, bronchopneumonia, and airway edema following mucosal necrosis and sloughing, viscous secretions, and distal airway obstruction. Later there may be nosocomial pneumonia, hypermetabolism-induced respiratory failure, and acute respiratory distress syndrome. Treatment of these complications is individualized, using ventilatory maneuvers such as titrated PEEP, bronchoscopic lavage, antibiotics, chest physiotherapy, and other supportive measures. Lack of response to therapy because of severe ventilation–perfusion mismatching or shunt may be an indication for the use of nitric oxide, a potent, short-acting vasodilator, via the airway.[193] Prophylactic measures against DVT, gastric ulcers, and hypothermia should be used routinely.

Carbon Monoxide Toxicity

13 In burn victims, CO inhalation is almost always associated with smoke inhalation, which increases the morbidity and mortality compared with CO toxicity alone.[194] CO produces tissue hypoxia primarily by its 200-fold greater affinity for hemoglobin than oxygen and by its ability to shift the hemoglobin dissociation curve to the left, impairing O_2 unloading to the tissues. It also interferes with mitochondrial function, uncoupling oxidative phosphorylation and reducing ATP production, thus causing metabolic acidosis. Probably because of this effect on the mitochondria, CO can be a direct myocardial toxin, preventing survival in patients who suffer cardiac arrest, even though they have been resuscitated and treated with hyperbaric oxygen.[195]

A normal oxygen saturation on a pulse oximeter does not exclude the possibility of CO toxicity, although low arterial O_2 saturation measured by a cooximeter should raise the suspicion.[196] Similarly, the mixed venous oximeter catheters that are used for continuous in vivo measurement of $S\bar{v}O_2$ overestimate oxyhemoglobin concentration in the presence of CO.[197] If CO toxicity is not accompanied by a lung injury and thus by decreased PaO_2, tachypnea is absent; the carotid bodies are sensitive to the arterial O_2 tension and not to the O_2 content. The classic cherry-red color of the blood is also absent in most patients because it occurs only at carboxyhemoglobin (COHb) concentrations above 40%, and it may also be obscured by coexistent hypoxia and cyanosis.

The patient's inspired oxygen should be maintained at the highest possible concentration, even when there is no evidence of significant smoke-induced lung injury, until CO toxicity is ruled out by measurement of blood COHb. A high FIO_2 not only improves oxygenation, but also promotes elimination of CO; an FIO_2 of 1.0 decreases the blood half-life of COHb from the 4 hours seen in room air to 60 to 90 minutes, and to 20 to 30 minutes at 3 Atm in a hyperbaric chamber.[186]

The greater the blood concentrations of COHb, the more severe are the presenting symptoms (Table 48-8). Delayed neuropsychiatric disorders have been described in patients exposed to toxic levels of CO, and there is evidence to suggest that early hyperbaric O_2 treatment may prevent these symptoms.[186] The decision to institute this treatment should be based on comparing the risks of transport, decreased patient access, and delay in emergency treatment against the possible neurologic sequelae. Currently, hyperbaric O_2 is recommended for patients with COHb >30% at admission if the treatment of life-threatening problems—shock, neurologic injury, metabolic

TABLE 48-8

SYMPTOMS OF CARBON MONOXIDE TOXICITY AS A FUNCTION OF THE BLOOD COHb LEVEL

■ BLOOD COHb LEVEL (%)	■ SYMPTOMS
<15–20	Headache, dizziness, and occasional confusion
20–40	Nausea, vomiting, disorientation, and visual impairment
40–60	Agitation, combativeness, hallucinations, coma, and shock
>60	Death

COHb, carboxyhemoglobin.

acidosis, myocardial ischemia, infarction, or arrhythmias—will not be compromised.[198]

Cyanide Toxicity

Another cause of tissue hypoxia in burned patients is CN^- toxicity. Cyanide or hydrocyanic acid is produced by incomplete combustion of synthetic materials, and may be inhaled or absorbed through mucous membranes. As in CO toxicity, the usual clinical presentation is unexplained metabolic acidosis. Nonspecific neurologic symptoms such as agitation, confusion, or coma are also common findings. Elevated plasma lactate levels in severe burns may result from hypovolemia, CO toxicity, or CN^- toxicity. However, lactic acidosis after smoke inhalation in a patient without a major burn suggests CN^- toxicity.[199] The definitive diagnosis can be made only by determination of the blood cyanide level, which is toxic above 0.2 mg/L and lethal at levels beyond 1 mg/L.[200] A spectrophotometric assay using methemoglobin as a colorimetric indicator provides a timely and reliable determination of blood CN^-.[201] The pulse oximetry reading will be accurate in the absence of CO toxicity and nitrate therapy-induced methemoglobinemia.[194]

Increased CN^- in the blood can cause generalized cardiovascular depression and cardiac rhythm disturbances, especially in patients with lactic acidosis. Fortunately, the half-life of CN^- is short (approximately 1 hour),[199] and rapid improvement of hemodynamics should be expected after rescue of the victim from the toxic environment. Immediate administration of O_2, which is required for all burn victims, may be lifesaving for this complication. Although there are specific therapies for CN^- toxicity (e.g., amyl nitrate, sodium nitrite, thiosulfate), given the short half-life of the ion, it is not clear whether these measures offer significant help to the patient whose blood CN^- usually decreases to low levels during transport from the field to the hospital.[202] Of course, if circumstances permit, hyperbaric O_2 treatment can be used for all the complications of thermal injury: CO and CN^- poisoning, smoke-induced lung damage, and cutaneous burns.[203]

Fluid Replacement

Immediately after a serious burn, microvascular permeability increases, causing the loss of a substantial amount of protein-rich fluid into the interstitial space. A major burn, a delay in initiation of resuscitation, or an inhalation injury increase the size of the leak.[186] Further, there seems to be a correlation between inhalation injury and cutaneous burns in the production of edema. Pulmonary edema increases cutaneous edema and vice versa.[194] If resuscitation is successful, edema formation stops within 18 to 24 hours.[194] This fluid flux is enhanced by increased intravascular hydrostatic and interstitial osmotic pressures and decreased interstitial hydrostatic pressure. In addition, cardiac contractility may decrease because of circulating mediators, a diminished response to catecholamines, decreased coronary blood flow, and increased systemic vascular resistance.[186] This may result in shock, whose origin is primarily hypovolemic and, to a much smaller extent, cardiogenic.[204] If the hypotension is treated appropriately with fluids, the hemodynamic picture is replaced within 24 to 48 hours by one resembling sepsis or septic shock, with increased cardiac output and diminished systemic vascular resistance caused by the release of inflammatory mediators.[186]

Fluid resuscitation is essential in the early care of the burned patient with an injury >15% of the TBSA. Smaller burns can be managed with replacement at 150% of the calculated maintenance rate and careful monitoring of fluid status. Intravascular volume should be restored with utmost care to prevent excessive edema formation in both damaged and intact tissues resulting from the generalized increase in capillary permeability caused by the injury. Edema from overaggressive resuscitation has many deleterious and potentially life-threatening effects. Mention has already been made of the facilitation of upper airway edema after rapid fluid infusion in large cutaneous burns with or without smoke inhalation.[187] Likewise, chest wall edema may develop after administration of large quantities of fluid, causing respiratory difficulties and necessitating excision of burned tissue from the anterior axillary line to improve breathing. Abdominal edema may also occur, and occasionally increase intra-abdominal pressure and impede venous return. This may be severe enough to produce abdominal compartment syndrome.[205] Edema formation may also increase the tissue pressure in the burned area, resulting in reduction of blood flow to distal sites. This, together with decreased tissue oxygen tension, may produce necrosis of damaged but viable cells, increasing the extent of injury and the risk of infection.

14 Crystalloid solutions are preferred for resuscitation during the first day following a burn injury; leakage of colloids during this phase may increase edema.[186] Nevertheless, crystalloid resuscitation, especially in children, may cause a rapid decline in plasma protein concentration and necessitate administration of 5% albumin in LR[206] after the first day following a >30% burn and/or significant inhalation injury, when the capillary leak stops.[207] It is believed that this will moderate the tendency to edema formation associated with the administration of large amounts of isotonic (0.9% saline or LR) solutions, even though a 6% increase in the risk of mortality has been reported with the use of colloids in patients who are critically injured and burned.[208,209] Alternatively, hypertonic saline solutions draw intracellular water into the bloodstream and thus decrease the fluid volume needed to maintain perfusion, maintain extracellular volume, and limit the severity of edema in patients with burns occupying >50% of the TBSA, circumferential extremity burns, or inhalational injury.[186] Unfortunately, hypertonic solutions cause hypernatremia and intracellular water depletion; patients and experimental animals receiving these fluids for burn therapy often did not show an overall fluid sparing effect, and had an unacceptably high incidence of renal failure and death compared with those receiving LR.[210,211]

Of the many resuscitation formulas available, the Parkland (Baxter) and modified Brooke formulas are tailored to the clinical condition of the patient and are accepted in most centers[207] (Table 48-9). The addition of glucose is not necessary except in children, especially those weighing <20 kg. Albumin 5% may be administered after the first day following injury at a rate of 0.3, 0.4, or 0.5 mL/kg per %burn per 24 hours for burns of 30 to 50%, 50 to 70%, or 70 to 100% of TBSA, respectively. These formulas are guidelines only, and none can be expected to provide adequate restoration of intravascular volume in all burn victims, especially small children and patients with inhalation injuries. Therefore, administration of fluids during the

TABLE 48-9

GUIDELINES FOR INITIAL FLUID RESUSCITATION AFTER THERMAL INJURY

- Adults and children >20 kg
  - Parkland formula[a]
    - 4.0 mL crystalloid/kg/% burn/first 24 hr
  - Modified Brooke formula[a]
    - 2.0 mL lactated Ringer's/kg per % burn per first 24 hr
- Children <20 kg
  - Crystalloid 2–3 mL/kg per % burn per 24 hr[a]
  - Crystalloid with 5% dextrose at maintenance rate
    - 100 mL/kg for the first 10 kg and 50 mL/kg for the next 10 kg for 24 hr
  - Clinical end points of burn resuscitation
    - Urine output: 0.5–1 mL
    - Pulse: 80–140 per min (age dependent)
    - Systolic BP: 60 mm Hg (infants); children 70–90 plus 2x age in years mm Hg; adults MAP > 60 mm Hg
    - Base deficit: <2

BP, blood pressure; MAP, mean arterial pressure.
[a] 50% of calculated volume is given during the first 8 hr, 25% is given during the second 8 hr, and the remaining 25% is given during the third 8 hr.

initial phase should be titrated to specific goals described in Table 48-9; and, if a pulmonary artery catheter is placed, acceptable cardiac output, filling pressures, and a mixed venous oxygen tension ($P\bar{v}O_2$) of 35 to 40 mm Hg. Careful monitoring of the hematocrit may also guide fluid management. An increase in hematocrit during the first day suggests inadequate fluid resuscitation because hemolysis and sequestration are actually expected to cause a decrease in this parameter. Acute anemia, as may occur during excision and grafting of burns, is usually well tolerated. Blood replacement is usually not initiated until the hematocrit is below 15 to 20% in healthy patients requiring limited operations, approximately 25% in those who are healthy but need extensive procedures, and 30% or more when there is a history of preexisting cardiovascular disease.[212]

Although there is evidence that the standard clinical end points of resuscitation often provide inadequate information in major burns and that better information may be obtained from pulmonary artery catheter data,[213,214] there are also practical and methodological problems associated with the latter, especially the risks of infectious complications and the requirement for additional vascular access.

In Europe, the transpulmonary thermodilution technique, which relies on detecting cold fluid dilution in the descending aorta rather than in the pulmonary artery, has been used successfully to determine cardiac output.[215] This technique is less invasive because it uses the arterial and central venous (not pulmonary artery) catheters that are routinely inserted in major burn management. In addition, the double-indicator dilution technique can monitor intrathoracic blood volume—a better indicator of circulatory filling and volume status than central venous or PCWPs—and extravascular lung water.[216] It involves placement of a 5F femoral artery catheter equipped with fiberoptics and a thermostat tip advanced into the descending thoracic aorta, and injection via central venous catheter of 0.3 mg/kg indocyanine green mixed in 10 mL iced glucose, 5%. The resulting dilution curve is subjected to computerized analysis. Comparative studies suggest that this technique is a reliable preload indicator for volume resuscitation of major burn patients. The fluid volume administered with its guidance consistently exceeds that calculated by traditional burn formulas.[215,216]

When in rare instances fluid resuscitation fails despite administration of crystalloids in excess of 6 mL/kg per %TBSA, and invasive or semi-invasive monitoring suggests adequate intravascular volume, vasopressor and/or inotropic agents may be indicated. Dopamine in small doses (5μg/kg/min) and/or beta-adrenergic agents may improve urine output without further need for fluids.[207] Electrolyte abnormalities may occur after the first day for several reasons but are primarily a result of topical agents applied to control pain, decrease vapor loss, prevent desiccation, and slow bacterial growth.[207] Nonaqueous topicals (silver sulfadiazine), if administered without providing free water such as 5% dextrose, may result in hypernatremia and its central nervous system consequences, including intracranial bleeding. In contrast, aqueous topical agents such as 5% silver nitrate solution may cause hyponatremia and its consequences of cerebral edema and seizure secondary to electrolyte leaching. Central pontine demyelination may occur if the hyponatremia is corrected rapidly with salt solutions. Serum ionized calcium and magnesium should also be monitored.

OPERATIVE MANAGEMENT

Overall, nearly 25% of trauma patients present with preexisting conditions such as cirrhosis; cardiovascular, pulmonary, and renal diseases; coagulation disorders; diabetes; and alcohol or drug abuse that may increase trauma-related morbidity and mortality, and require additional care.[217] Premedication is rarely indicated, especially in those who are hypovolemic, head injured, or intoxicated. If needed, small doses of opioid (morphine, 1 to 2 mg; fentanyl, 25 to 50 μg) or sedative (midazolam, 0.5 to 1.0 mg) may be administered with close monitoring of vital signs. Regional analgesia may be provided for stable patients with skeletal injuries awaiting surgery. Femoral nerve block, for example, provides excellent analgesia for femoral
15 shaft fractures. Evaluation of the multiple trauma patient emergently transported to the OR involves reviewing the vital signs, oxygenation, and preoperative fluid replacement, and confirmation of correct position and patency of a previously inserted endotracheal tube.

Monitoring

Table 48-10 lists monitoring techniques currently used in the OR and indicates their relative importance in the intraoperative care of the trauma patient. Clearly, valuable time can be lost if the placement of invasive monitors takes precedence over resuscitation.

Hemodynamic Monitoring

Direct intra-arterial pressure monitoring, which permits beat-to-beat data acquisition and sampling for measurement of blood gases, should be in place before surgery. An ultrasound guided technique or a surgical cut-down may be necessary to facilitate access. The radial artery is the vessel of choice in abdominal or chest trauma in which the aorta may be cross-clamped, making a femoral or dorsalis pedis cannula nonfunctional. The right radial artery is preferred in cases of chest trauma in which cross-clamping of the descending aorta might result in occlusion of the left subclavian artery. In mechanically ventilated patients, the magnitude of systolic pressure variation (the difference between the maximum and minimum systolic pressure over the respiratory cycle) and its Δdown component (the difference between systolic pressure at end expiration and the lowest value during the respiratory cycle) can provide reliable information about the intravascular volume status

TABLE 48-10

TECHNIQUES TO MONITOR PHYSIOLOGIC PARAMETERS AND THEIR IMPORTANCE IN INTRAOPERATIVE MANAGEMENT OF THE TRAUMA PATIENT

PHYSIOLOGIC PARAMETER	DEGREE OF IMPORTANCE	MONITORING EQUIPMENT	SPECIFIC INTRAOPERATIVE USES IN THE TRAUMA PATIENT
Cardiac rate, rhythm, and myocardial ischemia	Essential	Five-lead electrocardiogram system with oscilloscope, digital display, recorder, and printer (three-lead system can be used)	Routine
Arterial blood pressure	Essential	Indirect Blood pressure cuff Doppler system Programmable oscillometric system Direct Pressure transducer with calibrated oscilloscope and recorder	Routine
Central venous pressure	Useful	Pressure transducer with calibrated oscilloscope and recorder	Hypovolemia Pericardial tamponade, myocardial contusion Air embolism Pulmonary contusion
Pulmonary artery pressures	Essential in multiple trauma	Pressure transducer with calibrated oscilloscope and recorder	Blunt chest injury (pericardial tamponade, myocardial contusion) Adult respiratory distress syndrome Differentiation of low-pressure and high-pressure pulmonary edema; traumatic (cardiac contusion) or preexisting heart failure
Cardiac output	Useful in some patients	Thermodilution cardiac output computer with recorder and printer	Same as pulmonary artery pressure measurement
Cardiac wall motion abnormalities, myocardial ischemia, flow through valves or septal defects	Useful in some patients	Transesophageal echocardiograph	Cardic contusion Coronary artery injuries? Septal injuries Air embolism Thoracic aortic rupture Shock
Ventilation	Essential	End-tidal CO_2 monitor with waveform display and recording	Routine Head injury Air embolism
Arterial oxygenation	Essential	Airway pressure Pulse oximeter Arterial blood gases (intermittent or continuous)	Routine
Tissue oxygenation	Useful	Pulmonary artery catheter ($P\bar{v}O_2$) Arterial/venous lactate analyzer Base deficit $SLPCO_2$	Low perfusion states
Renal function	Essential	Foley catheter and graduated container	In all major trauma patients
Temperature	Essential	Esophageal or rectal probe	Routine
Neuromuscular function	Essential	Peripheral nerve stimulator Electromyograph	Head injury Open globe Sealed major vessel injury
Neurologic function	Useful	Intracranial pressure measurement with bolt, catheter, or fiberoptic sensor Jugular bulb O_2 saturation	Head injury
Depth of anesthesia		Bispectral index monitor	Intraoperative awareness
Blood coagulation	Useful	Prothrombin time/partial thromboplastin time/platelet count/fibrinogen, tube test, thrombelastograph	Shock Massive transfusion Preexisting coagulation abnormalities

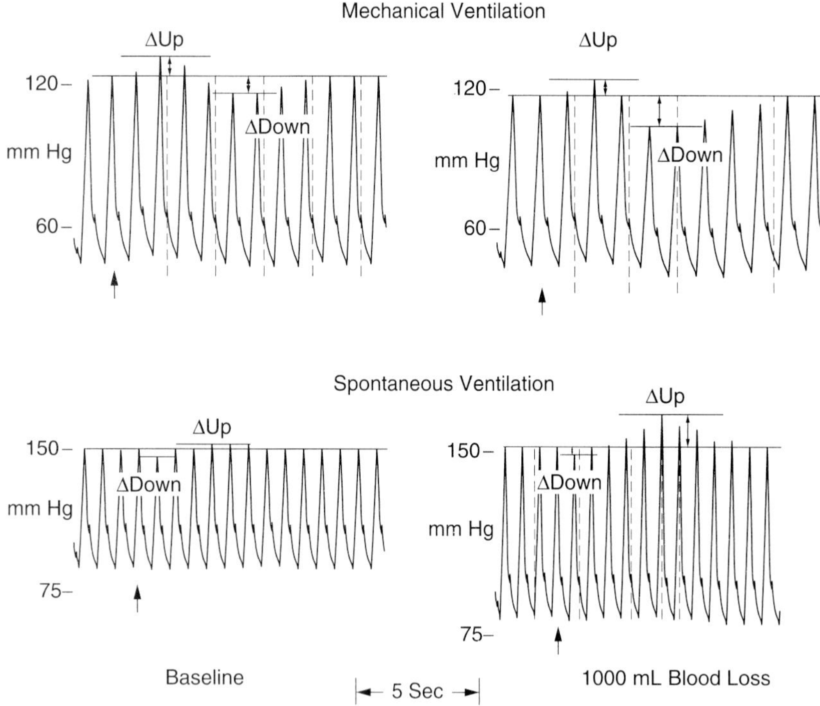

FIGURE 48-6. Arterial pressure records of a mechanically ventilated patient before (*left*) and after (*right*) 1,000 mL blood loss. Note the increase in systolic pressure variation and Δdown component following hemorrhage. Decrease in blood pressure occurs during exhalation with mechanical ventilation and inspiration in spontaneously breathing subjects (*upgoing arrow* defines inhalation). ΔUp is the difference between the end-expiratory systolic pressure and the maximum systolic pressure over a respiratory cycle. See text for definition of systolic pressure variation and Δdown component. (Reprinted with permission from Rooke GA, Schwid HA, Shapira Y: The effect of graded hemorrhage and intravascular volume replacement on systolic pressure variation in humans during mechanical and spontaneous ventilation. Anesth Analg 80:925, 1995.)

(Fig. 48-6). A systolic pressure variation >5 mm Hg and a Δdown >2 mm Hg suggest hypovolemia.[218] Delaying emergent surgery to place a central venous line is rarely indicated unless a large-bore catheter is needed for volume resuscitation. However, if the patient is elderly, there is a likelihood of myocardial damage, or if there is multiple organ damage with requirement for prolonged surgery and massive fluid replacement, early placement of a CVP or pulmonary artery catheter is indicated before the development of coagulopathy renders it hazardous.

Volumetric assessment of preload appears to correlate better with cardiac index than the CVP or PCWP.[219,220] A pulmonary artery catheter equipped with a rapid-response thermistor and intracardiac electrodes is capable of measuring right ventricular (RV) cardiac output and ejection fraction, and calculating RV end-diastolic volume index. The latter appears to correlate with cardiac output better than CVP and PCWP in trauma patients. An RV end-diastolic volume index >130 mL/m^2 is considered optimal for organ perfusion.[219,220]

TEE provides valuable diagnostic information in blunt cardiac injury, cardiac septal or valvular damage, coronary artery injury, pericardial tamponade, and aortic rupture. It also permits assessment of cardiac function, including right and left ventricular volume, ejection fraction, wall motion abnormalities, pulmonary hypertension, and cardiac output, and detects acute ischemia more accurately than either ECG or pulmonary artery pressure monitoring. Monitoring left ventricular volume alone can provide information about the adequacy of the intravascular volume. This technique also allows visualization of fat and air entry into the right heart, or the left heart through a patent foramen ovale, during internal fixation of lower-extremity fractures.[221] In the trauma setting, it is possible that the TEE probe may be introduced into an unrecognized esophageal tear because the insidious nature of esophageal injury makes diagnosis difficult during the first 24 hours after trauma.

Urine Output

Urine output is routinely monitored as an indicator of organ perfusion, hemolysis, skeletal muscle destruction, and urinary tract integrity after trauma. Its reliability for perfusion is decreased by prolonged shock prior to surgery and osmotic diuresis caused by administration of mannitol or radiopaque dye. Dark, cola-colored urine in the trauma patient suggests either hemoglobinuria resulting from incompatible blood transfusion, or myoglobinuria caused by massive skeletal muscle destruction after blunt or electrical trauma. Although the definitive diagnosis is made by serum electrophoresis, rapid differential diagnosis can be made by centrifugation of a blood specimen. Pink-stained serum suggests hemoglobinuria, whereas unstained serum indicates myoglobinuria. Both of these conditions may result in acute renal failure. Prevention involves mannitol diuresis and, in myoglobinuria, alkalinization of the urine with sodium bicarbonate to pH levels above 5.6. Red-colored urine usually is caused by hematuria, which, in the traumatized patient, suggests urinary tract injury. It should be investigated with intravenous pyelography.

Organ Perfusion and Oxygen Utilization

As discussed previously, unrecognized hypoperfusion may lead to splanchnic ischemia with resulting acidosis in the intestinal wall, permitting the passage of luminal microorganisms into the circulation and release of inflammatory mediators, causing sepsis and multiorgan failure.[54–57] Oxygen transport variables, base deficit, blood lactate level, gastric intramucosal pH (pHi), and SLPCO_2 are considered acceptable markers of organ hypoperfusion in the *apparently* resuscitated patient and may be used to set the optimal end points of resuscitation.[57] Gastric intramucosal pH monitoring is too cumbersome to use during surgery and in the immediate postoperative period. Monitoring of base deficit, blood lactate level, and SLPCO_2 has already been discussed in the Management of Shock section.

Oxygen transport variables consist of oxygen delivery (DO_2), O_2 consumption (VO_2), and O_2 extraction ratio. A DO_2 index (DO_2I) of 500 mL/min/m^2 has been shown to be an acceptable goal for optimal shock resuscitation,[222] performing as effectively as the DO_2I of $\geq$600 mL/min/m^2 previously recommended by Bishop et al.[223] Selection of these specific numbers is based on the results of studies in which critically ill patients who could increase DO_2I above this level survived. At $DO_2I \geq 500$ mL/min/m^2, patients received approximately 30% less crystalloids and blood transfusions than were required to attain the higher level.[222] A computerized ICU bedside decision protocol developed to standardize shock resuscitation in some centers uses $DO_2I > 500$ mL/min/m^2 as a goal.[222] This is a particularly useful end point because it integrates three important variables: hemoglobin concentration, arterial oxygen saturation, and cardiac output. The oxygen consumption index (VO_2I) is also an important variable. Subsequent organ failure may occur if it decreases below a value of 170 mL/min/m^2, indicating a flow-dependent phase of O_2 utilization.[57] Increasing DO_2I until VO_2I attains flow independence may prevent organ failure; however, this approach is not practical clinically, mainly because there are also DO_2I-independent regulators of VO_2.[222] Finally a global O_2 extraction ratio >0.25 to 0.3 suggests absence of dysoxia. However, it is possible that dysoxia may be present in an individual organ in the presence of a normal overall O_2 extraction ratio. Monitoring of O_2 transport variables, the most useful of which is DO_2I, is usually done in the ICU when invasive monitoring permits measurement of cardiac output and mixed venous O_2. These values can also be monitored in the OR whenever arterial and pulmonary artery lines are present.

A parameter that has been more recently used intraoperatively as a guide to resuscitation during emergency surgery for trauma patients is the end tidal–arterial CO_2 difference (Pa-ET) CO_2.[224] Values >10 mm Hg after resuscitation predict mortality.[224] It may also be useful in the decision about when to perform damage control surgery, and intraoperatively, in guiding resuscitation with fluids, inotropes, and vasopressors.

Coagulation

Conventional blood coagulation monitoring includes a baseline and subsequent serial measurements of prothrombin time (PT), activated partial thromboplastin time (aPTT), platelet count, blood fibrinogen level, and fibrin degradation products (FDP). Although trauma center laboratories cannot provide results of the standard coagulation tests within an hour, a blood sample should be sent to the laboratory to determine, at least retrospectively, the etiology of any coagulation abnormality. The "tube test," which involves obtaining a tube of blood with no anticoagulant and observing coagulation, clot retraction, and clot lysis, is a practical intraoperative method of coagulation monitoring. If a good-quality clot does not form, or does so only after 10 to 20 minutes, clotting factor deficiency is the most likely cause. Failure of clot retraction within 1 hour after blood sampling suggests platelet depletion or dysfunction. Clot lysis earlier than 6 hours indicates fibrinolysis, which is infrequent in trauma patients.[225] Disseminated intravascular coagulation (DIC) occurs frequently after trauma and is associated with absence of spontaneous clotting in the tube test. In addition to causing bleeding, it may prevent typing and crossmatching of blood.[226]

Thrombelastography (TEG) is similar in principle to the tube test but provides a quantitative, graphic evaluation of clotting function.[227] TEG determines the time necessary for initial fibrin formation, the rapidity of fibrin deposition, clot consistency, the rate of clot formation, and the times required for clot retraction and lysis[227] (Fig. 48-7). Basically, the R and K values are indices of formation, buildup, and cross-linking of fibrin, and depend on the function of coagulation factors. The maximum amplitude (MA) corresponds to the widest portion of the curve and indicates the absolute strength of the fibrin clot. It represents platelet function. The *a* angle is the slope of the external divergence of the tracing from the R value point, indicating the speed of clot formation and fibrin cross-linking. The

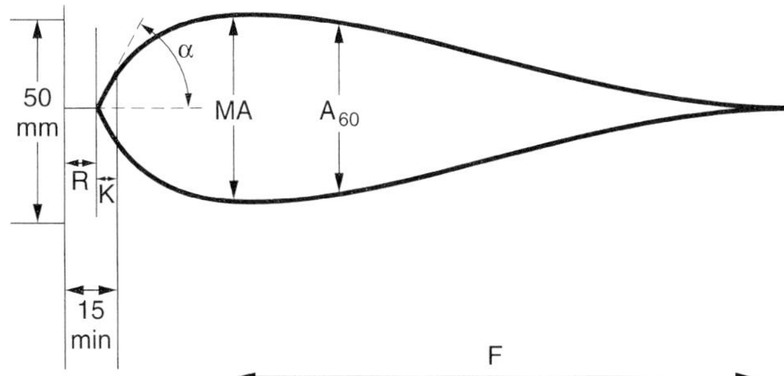

FIGURE 48-7. Thrombelastogram. R, interval from blood deposition in the cuvette to an amplitude of 1 mm on the thrombelastogram; K, time between the end of R and a point with an amplitude of 20 mm on the thrombelastogram; MA, maximum amplitude of thrombelastogram; α angle, slope of the external divergence of the tracing from the R value point; A_{60}, amplitude of thrombelastogram 60 min after maximum amplitude; F, time from MA to return to 0 amplitude (normal >300 min). (Reprinted with permission from Capan LM, Gottlieb G, Rosenberg A: General principles of anesthesia for major acute trauma. In Capan LM, Miller SM, Turndorf H [eds]: Trauma: Anesthesia and Intensive Care, p 259. Philadelphia, JB Lippincott, 1991.)

value of this index is determined by both coagulation factors and platelets. Hypothermia causes coagulopathy by interfering with both platelet and coagulation factor functions.[228–230] When the blood of a cold and coagulopathic patient is placed in the TEG cuvette, which is normally heated to 37°C, a near-normal trace may be obtained.[228] Newer TEG devices are temperature adjustable. Thus, the temperature in the cuvette can be adjusted to that of the patient.

Coagulation test results (PT, aPTT) are often abnormal in major trauma patients. However, these findings do not necessarily indicate that factor and platelet therapy should be initiated, unless there is a clinical indication to do so.[231] The administration of fresh frozen plasma (FFP) is generally recommended when PT and aPTT exceed 1.5 times control,[232] but treatment is based primarily on clinical bleeding (oozing from puncture sites and wound), the amount of blood lost, and the quantity transfused. The likelihood of bleeding, for example, after one blood volume is replaced, increases to 60%, so platelet and factor replacement becomes almost unavoidable once replacement exceeds this volume.[233,234] The results of coagulation tests have little primary impact on treatment. Nevertheless, they should be performed to determine the direction and extent of coagulation dysfunction over time.

Anesthetic and Adjunct Drugs

Apart from regional anesthesia techniques, which are used in patients with minor extremity injuries and stable hemodynamics, anesthetic and adjunct drugs for general anesthesia need to be tailored to five major clinical conditions. The varying contribution of these conditions to the clinical picture of a given patient necessitates priority-oriented planning.

Airway Compromise

Anesthetics and muscle relaxants should be avoided before the airway is secured if there is significant airway obstruction or if there is doubt as to whether the patient's trachea can be intubated because of anatomic limitations. If time permits, lateral neck radiographs, CT scanning, and endoscopy can be used to define the problem better. Topical anesthesia with mild sedation can be used with a flexible fiberoptic scope, Bullard blade,

WuScope, or other aids, and with surgical standby for cricothyroidotomy if intubation attempts are unsuccessful.[235]

Hypovolemia

16 Anesthetic agents not only have direct cardiovascular depressant effects, but also inhibit compensatory hemodynamic mechanisms such as central catecholamine output and baroreflex (neuroregulatory) mechanisms, which maintain systemic pressure in hypovolemia. Hemorrhage and hypovolemia lead to a higher blood concentration following a given dose of intravenous agents, increased sensitivity of the brain to anesthetics, preferential distribution of the cardiac output to the brain and the heart, cerebral hypoxia, dilutional hypoproteinemia, and acidosis, all of which increase the effects of drugs on the brain and the heart.[16] The pharmacokinetic and pharmacodynamic response of intravenous agents to experimental hemorrhagic shock varies. Because of the decrease in size of the central compartment and in systemic clearance, plasma concentrations of fentanyl and remifentanil are increased.[236] A decreased volume of distribution also increases the blood level of etomidate by 20% in shock,[237] and for propofol this effect is substantial.[238]

There is also variation in the extent of brain sensitivity to these agents. Although etomidate pharmacodynamics are unchanged,[237] a significant increase in the sensitivity of the brain and heart to propofol is noted in animals,[238] even after fluid resuscitation.[237] Based on these experimental findings, Shafer[239] calculated that in patients with shock, the dose of propofol should be only 10 to 20% of that given to a healthy patient. The etomidate dose, in contrast, does not require adjustment for shock. Of the opioids, the calculated dose for fentanyl and remifentanil is approximately one-half of that given to healthy patients[239] (Fig. 48-8). Thus, etomidate and fentanyl are the preferred drugs; propofol is not a desirable induction agent in patients with hemorrhagic shock. Of the remaining intravenous agents, thiopental and midazolam are also known to have significant cardiovascular depressant activity,[240,241] whereas ketamine has stimulatory effects when the autonomic nervous system is intact.[242]

There are also differences among anesthetics in the direction and extent of their effects on compensatory mechanisms. For example, the baroreceptor depression produced by intravenous agents is usually milder than that of inhalational agents. Data from animal and human studies have demonstrated that thiopental, propofol, and ketamine depress the baroreflex mechanism most and for approximately 10 minutes, whereas etomidate has little effect; the effects of midazolam, diazepam, and droperidol are intermediate.[243–245] Among inhalational agents, isoflurane has less of an inhibitory effect on the baroreflex mechanism than halothane or enflurane.[246] Opioid agents have little direct cardiovascular or baroreflex depressant effect; however, these agents can cause hypotension by inhibiting central sympathetic activity, especially in the hypovolemic trauma patient whose apparent hemodynamic stability is maintained by hyperactive sympathetic tone.[247]

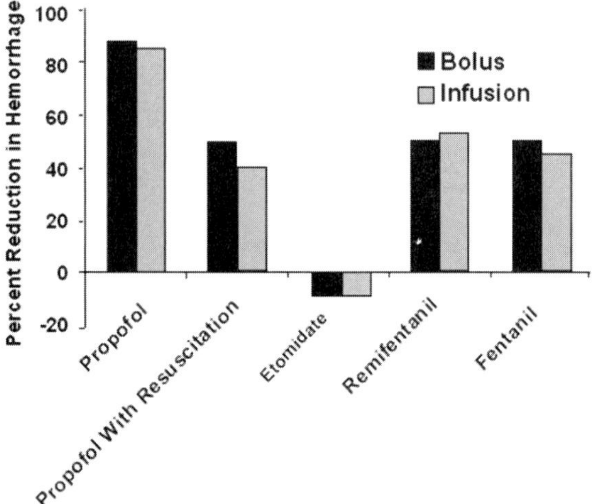

FIGURE 48-8. Calculated dose reduction of various anesthetics administered as a bolus or infusion in moderate hemorrhagic shock. Calculation is based on pharmacokinetic and pharmacodynamic studies performed in experimental hemorrhagic shock. (Reprinted with permission from Shafer SL: Shock values. Anesthesiology 101:567, 2004.)

Two important principles in the use of anesthetic agents are accurate estimation of the degree of hypovolemia and reduction of doses accordingly. The presence of hypotension suggests uncompensated hypovolemia, in which case anesthetics almost invariably produce further deterioration of systemic blood pressure and sometimes cardiac standstill. Intravascular volume, to the extent possible, must be restored before their use. When time constraints or continuing hemorrhage prevent restoration of blood volume, the airway must be secured without the benefit of anesthesia (perhaps using only rapidly acting muscle relaxants and small doses of opioids, etomidate, or ketamine), even though this approach may result in recall of induction and intraoperative events in up to 40% of patients.[248] Hypothermia, alcohol intoxication, drug use before anesthesia, and metabolic disturbances in the acute trauma patient cannot reliably prevent recall. However, scopolamine, 0.6 mg, given before airway management may decrease the likelihood of this complication. Intraoperative use of the bispectral index monitor and, whenever possible, titrating anesthetics to levels <60 may prevent recall in trauma patients.[249]

In normotensive but hypovolemic patients, restoration of volume and selection of an agent with the least cardiovascular depressant effect appears logical. Ketamine and etomidate are the preferred induction agents,[242,250] although at low doses other intravenous anesthetics are also unlikely to produce hypotension. Therefore, the use of any of these drugs in reduced doses is probably more important than the particular agent chosen.[251,252] These principles may become especially important for the anesthesiologist if the concept of delayed fluid resuscitation, with hypovolemia prolonged until hemorrhage is controlled surgically, becomes widely accepted.[70]

Maintenance of anesthesia in the hypovolemic trauma patient raises concerns similar to those pertaining to induction. Although normally nitrous oxide's myocardial depressant effect is somewhat counterbalanced by its ability to increase sympathetic outflow, in acute hemorrhage there is already a dramatic increase in sympathetic activity and stimulation of baroreceptors. Under these circumstances, patients are unlikely to respond to the sympathetic effect of N_2O, and the cardiovascular depressant properties of the gas are unmasked; these may be similar to those of other inhalation agents.[253] In addition, by reducing FIO_2, N_2O incurs a risk of hypoxemia in patients with reduced cardiac output or pulmonary compromise. Despite causing little impairment of reflex tachycardia and having a vasodilatory action that preserves organ blood flow in normovolemic patients, isoflurane can impair cardiac output and organ blood flow in hypovolemia—that is, it can cause cardiovascular depression. Desflurane and sevoflurane are not significantly better than isoflurane in this regard. However, because of their low solubility in blood, severe hemodynamic depression produced by these agents can be rapidly reversed, preventing suboptimal perfusion for a significant period of time.[254]

In summary, in the hypovolemic patient all inhalational agents may reduce both global and regional blood flows, and therefore, should be used only in small concentrations

(<1 minimum alveolar concentration [MAC]). Opioid supplementation is usually well tolerated and often indicated.

Head and Open Eye Injuries

The importance of deep anesthesia and adequate muscle relaxation during airway management of patients with head or open eye injuries has already been discussed. Anesthetic agents selected for management of brain injury should produce the least increase in ICP, the least decrease in mean arterial pressure, and the greatest reduction in cerebral metabolic rate ($CMRO_2$). As demonstrated by intraoperative $Sjvo_2$ measurements in patients with acute head injury, the most important factor in causing cerebral ischemia is increased ICP from intracranial hematoma.[255] Prompt decompression is the most crucial means of ensuring cerebral well-being. Hypotension caused by anesthetics or other factors contributes to the development or progression of cerebral ischemia. Utmost attention should be paid during anesthesia to avoidance of hypotension (mean arterial pressure <60 mm Hg) and, more important, if reliable $Sjvo_2$ monitoring is in place, to avoid values <55 to 60%. With the possible exception of ketamine,[20] all intravenous anesthetics cause comparable degrees of cerebrovascular constriction.[20,256–258] Thiopental, midazolam, propofol, and etomidate therefore also produce a dose-dependent reduction in cerebrospinal fluid formation.[259] Again, with the exception of ketamine, $CMRO_2$ is also reduced by all the available intravenous anesthetics.[20,256–258] An important drawback to these agents is that their cardiovascular depressant effects may reduce CPP.[257,258,260] This problem can be ameliorated by administering pretreatment doses of opioids (fentanyl, 2 to 3 μg/kg), which permit reduction of the anesthetic dose. This may also prevent the myoclonic movements associated with etomidate and occasionally with propofol, and thus reduce the risks of ICP and IOP increase. Nevertheless, myoclonus is best prevented by careful timing of the dose of muscle relaxants.[261] Another measure to preserve CPP during anesthesia is to administer vasopressors, being aware that hypovolemia may be masked by their use.

Ordinarily, administration of succinylcholine should follow pretreatment doses of nondepolarizing agents to prevent fasciculation-induced elevation of ICP and IOP.[22,262] Avoiding succinylcholine usually does not alleviate the problem because laryngoscopy and tracheal intubation produce a greater and longer-lasting increase in IOP and ICP.[263] Rocuronium, at a dose of 0.9 to 1.2 mg/kg has an onset time comparable with that of succinylcholine.[264] Mivacurium has a longer onset time than rocuronium and, unlike rocuronium, can cause vasodilatation and hypotension.[265] None of the nondepolarizing muscle relaxants causes elevation of ICP or IOP in the absence of associated tracheal intubation.

All inhalation anesthetics may increase CBF, cerebral blood volume (CBV), and thus the ICP.[260] Cerebral autoregulation, CO_2 responsiveness, and $CMRO_2$ are reduced. Unlike thiopental, which decreases both CBF and $CMRO_2$ in parallel, inhalational anesthetics decrease $CMRO_2$ while increasing the CBF. The extent of this uncoupling varies with the agent and the dose. Isoflurane has the least vasodilatory effect and thus is the most widely used inhalation anesthetic, although desflurane and sevoflurane have comparable effects on the cerebral circulation.[292] In hyperventilated patients with cerebral tumors or mild edema, isoflurane does not raise the ICP if it is administered at an inspired concentration of <1 MAC.[266] In the presence of severe head injury, when cerebral autoregulation and CO_2 responsiveness are impaired, isoflurane has the potential to increase CBF and ICP even if it is given at levels below 1 MAC and with hyperventilation.[266] Therefore, it may be prudent not to use this agent at high concentrations in the presence of elevated ICP, at least until the skull is opened and the ICP is controlled. In these patients, anesthesia can be maintained initially with opioids plus thiopental, propofol, midazolam, or etomidate.

Nitrous oxide may increase CBF, CBV, and ICP when administered with inhalation anesthetics if the $Paco_2$ is normal or increased.[267] This effect may be eliminated when this agent is administered with adequate doses of barbiturates or hyperventilation. The effect on $CMRO_2$ is variable: both an increase and a decrease have been observed. Thus, N_2O probably is not deleterious in patients with head injury with minimal ICP elevation, if it is used after a bolus dose or during infusion of intravenous anesthetics.

In a spontaneously breathing patient, opioids may produce hypoventilation with an associated increase in CBF and ICP; they should, therefore, be used only in mechanically ventilated patients with head trauma. Some reports suggest that opioids and, to a smaller extent, opiates may interfere with CPP by increasing ICP, decreasing mean arterial pressure, or both.[19,268] Fentanyl and sufentanil are most implicated, and it appears that this phenomenon occurs when the head injury is severe.[269,270] Although the clinical significance of these findings is not yet clear, it is prudent to administer fentanyl or its analogs slowly, when the arterial pressure is normal or slightly elevated, ensuring preservation of systemic blood pressure with vasoactive agents, if necessary.

Cardiac Injury

If there is pericardial tamponade, preload and myocardial contractility should be maintained. Any decrease in these parameters may exacerbate an already existing RV inflow occlusion. A decrease in heart rate should also be treated promptly to maintain adequate cardiac output. Because all the available anesthetics can depress myocardial contractility and cause vasodilation, it is preferable to administer these agents after evacuation of pericardial blood under local anesthesia. If general anesthesia is required to relieve the tamponade, induction should be delayed until the patient is prepared and draped. Both anesthetics and controlled ventilation, particularly with PEEP, impair cardiac output. Deep anesthesia and high airway pressures should be avoided before evacuation of the hemopericardium. In chronic pericardial effusion, ketamine supports the cardiac index better than diazepam.[271] In acute pericardial tamponade, even minor insults can bring cardiac activity to a halt. Ketamine thus remains the agent of choice. It should be given in small doses after adequate fluid infusion. Similar principles apply to the use of maintenance agents, which should be given in the smallest possible doses until the heart is decompressed. TEE monitoring may aid management between induction and pericardiotomy.

In blunt myocardial injury, the objective is not only to maintain cardiac contractility, but also to lower the elevated pulmonary vascular resistance that may result from concomitant pulmonary contusion or aspiration. All anesthetics should preferably be administered after restoration of intravascular volume and titrated to maintain adequate systemic blood pressure and cardiac output. If necessary, inotropes, preferably amrinone or milrinone, which produce some pulmonary vasodilation, may be used. Anesthetic maintenance by infusion of intravenous anesthetics and opioids to avoid the myocardial depression produced by inhalational agents should also be considered.

Burns

Extensive and repeated escharotomies may be required during the initial phase of convalescence after a burn injury, usually between the second day and the second week, often necessitating massive transfusion, temperature control, and management of fluid, electrolyte, and coagulation abnormalities. A hypermetabolic state characterized by tachycardia, tachypnea, catecholamine surge, increased O_2 consumption, and augmented catabolism follows the initial few hours of a burn and continues into the convalescent phase, necessitating increased oxygen, ventilation, and nutrition.[186]

Anesthetic management of escharotomies presents several difficulties. Burned tissue may prevent access for ECG, pulse oximeter, neuromuscular function, and noninvasive blood pressure monitoring; needle electrodes or surgical staples, a reflectance pulse oximeter, and an arterial catheter may be necessary. Large-bore intravenous catheters are essential. Hyperthermia occurs, but hypothermia is more likely in the OR and is to be avoided. Exposure and evaporative fluid loss necessitate maintenance of the OR temperature between 28°C and 32°C, use of countercurrent fluid and blood warming devices, surface heating with forced dry, warm air, and humidified inspired gases. Blood loss can be controlled by restricting the escharotomy to 15 to 20% of TBSA, use of extremity tourniquets, applying dilute epinephrine solution topically (1:10,000) or by injection (0.5 mg per 1,000 mL), and using compression bandages. Epinephrine doses of up to 6.7 mg topically or 0.8 mg by injection into the surgical area are well tolerated;[272] the affinity of beta-adrenergic receptors to ligands is decreased after burns. The administration of a large amount of blood and blood products subjects the patient to complications of transfusion such as coagulopathy. Although citrate-induced hypocalcemia is a relatively rare complication of transfusion,[273] monitoring of Ca^{2+} and administration of calcium chloride (2.5 to 5.0 mg/kg) or gluconate (7.5 to 10.0 mg/kg) should be considered when blood products are administered rapidly.

Shock, hyperdynamic circulation, decreased serum albumin concentration, increased α_1-acid glycoprotein concentration, and altered receptor sensitivity alter the response to various drugs during the resuscitative and convalescent phases.[186] The doses of intravenous anesthetics should be reduced during the resuscitation phase to prevent excessive hemodynamic depression. Burn patients have excruciating pain and exceedingly high opioid requirements. A proven anesthetic regimen for excision and grafting of burns is isoflurane plus large doses of opioid. The response to depolarizing and nondepolarizing muscle relaxants remains unaltered during the first 24 hours after burn injury. However, after the first day, succinylcholine should be avoided for at least 1 year because it can result in a potentially lethal increase of serum K^+ when the burn size exceeds 10% of TBSA. Resistance develops to all nondepolarizing muscle relaxants, except mivacurium in patients with burns of >30% TBSA starting approximately 1 week and peaking 5 to 6 weeks after injury, probably from pharmacodynamic causes, such as an increased number of acetylcholine receptors in the muscle membrane under the burn site and in regions distant from the injury.[186] Increasing the dose can partly overcome this resistance. For instance, rocuronium, which is important for rapid-sequence induction and treatment of laryngospasm when succinylcholine is contraindicated, has an onset time delayed by 30% when a 0.9 mg/kg dose is used. The difference from normal is unchanged at a dose of 1.2 mg/kg, but the onset time is decreased by 30% in burned patients.[274]

For serial wound debridement, ketamine in intermittent doses, neuraxial or peripheral nerve blocks via an indwelling catheter, or sedation with opioids and intravenous agents may be employed.

Management of Intraoperative Complications

Persistent Hypotension

17 Persistent hypotension following trauma is usually the result of one of four mechanisms: bleeding, tension pneumothorax, neurogenic shock, and cardiac injury. Although many other causes, such as citrate intoxication (hypocalcemia), hypothermia, coronary artery disease, allergic reactions, or incompatible transfusion, may be responsible for this complication, they occur infrequently.

Hypotension is most likely due to bleeding. The source may be obvious, such as external bleeding from the skull or an open vessel in the extremities, or hidden. The thoracic and abdominal cavities and the pelvic retroperitoneal space are the most common sites of occult hemorrhage that results in hypotension. Management includes early diagnosis and control of the bleeding site plus effective fluid resuscitation. The latter can best be accomplished using an infusion system with large-diameter tubing (5 mm) and a countercurrent heat exchanger. Up to 1,000 mL/min of crystalloid solution or 600 mL/min of packed cells can be given if a box-type pressure pump and a large-bore intravenous cannula are used.[275] The system should be connected to 14-gauge or larger cannulae, preferably inserted into veins both above and below the diaphragm. The rapid infusor system (Haemonetics, Braintree, MA), which consists of a reservoir, countercurrent heating system, and roller pump, is capable of delivering up to 1,600 mL/min of warm fluids once the rate of infusion is programmed. Although a powerful system, it is costly, difficult to assemble, and infrequently necessary in the trauma patient.

LR solution is the crystalloid of choice in most centers. However, it is slightly hypotonic (273 mOsm/L), acidic (pH 5.1), and contains a small amount of Ca^{2+}, which may counteract the citrate anticoagulant in PRBCs. Normal saline does not cause this problem, but its infusion in large quantities may result in hyperchloremic acidosis. Both Plasma-lyte A and Normosol-R have the advantages of a pH of 7.4, no Ca^{2+}, and a normal osmolarity (295 mOsm). Because of their prolonged intravascular retention and decreased tendency to produce edema, colloid solutions may be used in selected trauma patients such as those with head injury and those in whom edema develops due to inflammatory reactions or prior administration of large amounts of crystalloids. However, consistent evidence for the benefit of colloids over crystalloids is lacking.[208,276] Human serum albumin (5 and 25%) and hydroxyethyl starch are the most commonly used solutions. Hydroxyethyl starch may produce coagulation abnormalities primarily by reducing the levels of fibrinogen, factor VIII, and von Willebrand's factor, and by reducing platelet function. This is especially important in patients with head injury in whom fatal intracranial hemorrhage may develop.[277] The recommended safe dose of this agent as a component of therapy for surgical blood loss is 20 mL/kg, although a review suggests that there is little support for this recommendation.[277]

Neurogenic shock from spinal cord injury may be missed during initial evaluation, especially in unconscious patients. However, differentiation of neurogenic shock from hemorrhagic shock is important;[278] patients with spinal cord injury are often bradycardic and readily respond to catecholamine infusion. Misdiagnosing neurogenic shock for hemorrhagic shock may lead to excessive fluid infusion and pulmonary edema. The reverse error may also occur: depriving patients with hemorrhagic shock of fluids because of misdiagnosis of neurogenic shock.[278] Invasive central hemodynamic monitoring may be indicated in such patients.[153] In some patients, of course, hemorrhagic shock and neurogenic shock may coexist.

Cardiac causes of persistent hypotension include blunt cardiac injury and pericardial tamponade. Intraoperative TEE can be useful in the differential diagnosis. The RV is most commonly involved in blunt cardiac injury. If there is a concomitant increase in pulmonary vascular resistance (e.g., from an associated pulmonary contusion), the RV pressure increases while its output decreases, resulting in an increased CVP. The raised RV pressure causes the interventricular septum to shift toward the left, decreasing left ventricular compliance, increasing its diastolic pressure, and decreasing cardiac output. These alterations in cardiac anatomy and ventricular dynamics can be displayed by TEE, information that can be useful during interpretation of elevated cardiac filling pressures.[279]

In the absence of TEE, a pulmonary artery catheter may be helpful. Equalization of pressures across the cardiac chambers during diastole suggests pericardial tamponade. A similar picture may also be seen in severe blunt cardiac injury, causing difficulty in differential diagnosis. This effect, however, is rare and is usually associated with critical hemodynamic instability. Differential diagnosis in these instances can be established by pericardiocentesis. Septal encroachment into the left ventricle from RV contusion results in an increase in pulmonary artery wedge pressure. Decreasing the rate of fluid infusion in these patients results in a further decrease in cardiac output. Treatment includes fluid infusion, pulmonary vasodilators if the systemic blood pressure is normal, and inotropic support if the systemic blood pressure is low. Absence of response to this treatment is an indication for placement of an intra-aortic balloon pump. Pulmonary artery catheterization may also help detect an oxygen step-up from septal injury. During thoracotomy, a distended RV should also raise the suspicion of a septal defect.

Hypothermia

Shock, alcohol intoxication, exposure to cold, fluid resuscitation, and abnormalities in thermoregulatory mechanisms render the major trauma patient hypothermic during the ini-
18 tial phase of injury. The mortality rate after trauma increases with decreasing temperature. Severe hypothermia, which in the trauma patient is defined as core temperature below 32°C, was associated with a 100% mortality rate in one study.[280] The intraoperative risk of hypothermia is also higher for the trauma victim than for electively operated patients. Heat loss increases in patients with spinal cord, extensive soft-tissue, and burn injuries, and in those who consumed ethanol before surgery.

Hypothermia causes a reduction in cardiac output, cardiac conduction abnormalities, diminished cerebral and renal blood flows, decreased oxygen release from red cells caused by the leftward shift of the O_2 dissociation curve, altered platelet and clotting enzyme function, and abnormalities of K^+ and Ca^{2+} homeostasis.[229] These effects may further compromise poor organ perfusion, oxygenation, blood coagulation, and metabolism.

Aggressive therapy and correction of body temperature to normal within a short time appear to decrease mortality rate, blood loss, fluid requirement, organ failure, and length of ICU stay.[281] Convective warming with forced dry air at 43°C can prevent a temperature drop in most trauma victims but cannot effectively treat severe hypothermia; because of its low specific heat, air has little heat content to give to the cold trauma patient.[281] Airway rewarming can reduce heat loss caused by latent heat of vaporization, but this technique also transfers very little heat.[281] Administration of warm intravenous fluids is the most effective way to prevent and treat hypothermia in the trauma patient, provided that fluids are being administered at a relatively rapid rate. For each liter of fluid given at 40°C to a patient with a body temperature of 33°C, 7 kcal of heat energy is gained. Countercurrent heat exchanging systems are more effective than dry heat or still-water bath warmers. They warm the fluid to 40°C, and the delivered fluid temperature is not affected by rapid rates of administration.[275] The most effective method, however, is continuous arteriovenous rewarming, which can be achieved using a modified level 1 countercurrent system (Fig. 48-9). The blood exits the body from a percutaneously placed femoral arterial catheter at the

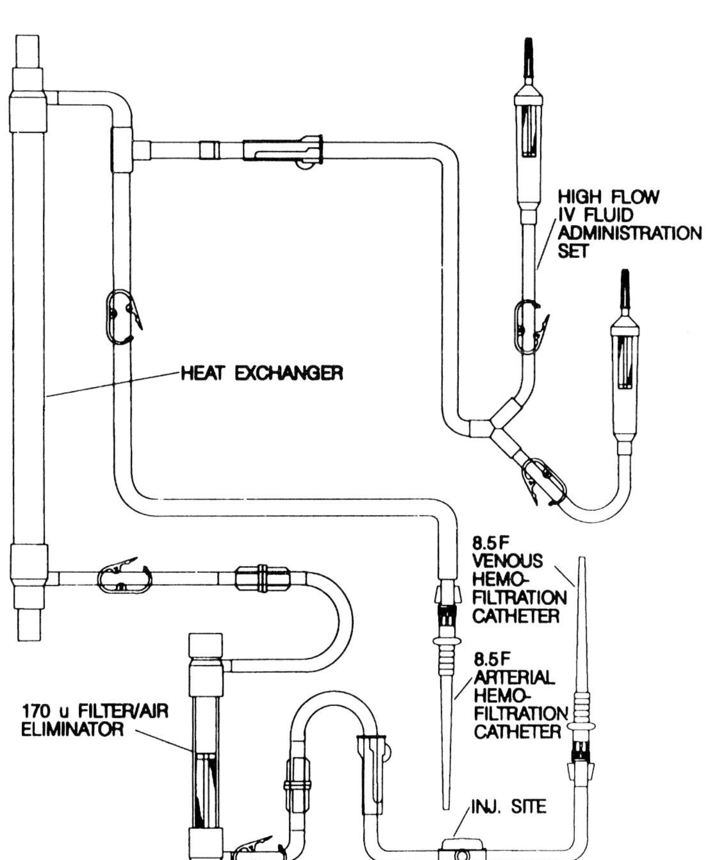

FIGURE 48-9. Schematic drawing of the system used for continuous arteriovenous rewarming. (Reprinted with permission from Gentilello LM, Cobean R, Offner PJ *et al*: Continuous arteriovenous rewarming: Rapid reversal of hypothermia in critically ill patients. J Trauma 32:316, 1992.)

patient's own pressure, and then is warmed in the infusion system and returned to the body through a venous cannula. Because the circuit tubing is heparin bonded, there is no need for heparinization. Experience with this technique in the ICU has been encouraging.[281,282]

Coagulation Abnormalities

In trauma, multiple factors may be responsible for coagulopathy: dilution of platelets and coagulation factors, hypothermia, acidosis, tissue hypoxia, and tissue thromboplastin release. Hypothermia and diminished tissue perfusion aggravate existing coagulation abnormalities,[283] and hypothermia by itself can cause clotting deficiencies in the absence of platelet or factor deficiency.[229] Hypothermia affects platelet morphology, function, and sequestration, and retards enzyme activity, slowing the initiation and propagation of both platelet plug and fibrin clot.[284] Decreased body temperature may also enhance fibrinolytic activity.[284]

The mechanism of hypothermia-induced coagulopathy is complex and depends on the extent of temperature decrease. Down to 33°C there is little alteration in coagulation enzyme activity, explaining the practically unchanged values reported for aPTT.[285] Within this temperature range, coagulopathy results from altered platelet aggregation/adhesion.[285] Both enzymatic activity and platelet aggregation are abnormal below 33°C.[285] Thus, the aPTT at temperatures from 33 to 37°C does not provide any meaningful information about coagulation status, even when the test is performed at the hypothermic patient's temperature, because it does not measure platelet adhesion. In contrast, thrombelastography at the patient's temperature may be reflective of the degree of coagulopathy.

19 Perioperative diagnosis of coagulopathy is often made by observing bleeding from wounds or puncture sites, rather than by interpretation of laboratory tests. However, the differential diagnosis between consumptive and dilutional coagulopathy requires laboratory testing, although the results of these tests are usually delayed. In general, the inability to determine the type of coagulopathy does not present a problem because the initial treatment is similar for both conditions. Nevertheless, the diagnosis of DIC has prognostic significance because its treatment involves elimination of its causes. A blood sample without heparin should be sent for measurement of circulating fibrin degradation products (FDP/fdp). An FDP/fdp level $>$10 mg/mL is suggestive of DIC, whereas a value $>$40 mg/mL is diagnostic. In patients who have not received a large volume of blood products and other fluids, simultaneous determination of fibrinogen level, platelet count, and PT may be helpful in diagnosis of DIC. A fibrinogen level $<$ 150 mg/dL, platelet count $<$ 150,000, and PT $>$ 15 seconds is highly suggestive. If only two of the three are abnormal, FDP/fdp should be measured.

Prompt platelet administration should always be considered once abnormal bleeding is noted. Each unit of platelet concentrate contains 55 billion platelets, which normally increase the platelet count by 5,000 to 10,000 per μL. If there is ongoing surgical bleeding, administration of platelets should perhaps be delayed until it is controlled; otherwise, they will be wasted. In contrast, severe thrombocytopenia may contribute to the bleeding. It has been shown that transfusion of PRBC in elective surgery results in earlier depletion of coagulation factors than of platelets.[232,286] Thus, it is not unreasonable to administer FFP or cryoprecipitate simultaneously with platelets in emergency trauma surgery. The minimum dose of FFP for adults is 2 U ($\sim$600 mL) given within less than 1 hour. Fibrinogen concentration $<$80 mg/dL is an indication for cryoprecipitate administration. Ten units increase plasma fibrinogen concentration by approximately 100 mg/dL.[233]

In the absence of abnormal bleeding, prophylactic administration of platelets, FFP, or cryoprecipitate is unwarranted, even if coagulation tests indicate platelet and factor depletion.[287] However, once transfusion of factor-deficient PRBC and fluids exceeds one blood volume, clinical coagulopathy is likely even in the absence of shock, hypothermia, or other aggravating factors.[233,234] Thus, in trauma patients who receive between one and two blood volume replacements, platelet or factor administration is almost always indicated. In hypothermic patients with clinical coagulopathy, the critical treatment is rewarming rather than platelet and coagulation factor administration, although circumstances may require both.[228,288] Some anecdotal reports suggest that factor VIIa may be useful as an adjunct for control of hemorrhage, especially in coagulopathic patients with liver injuries.[289]

Electrolyte and Acid-Base Disturbances

20 Intraoperative hyperkalemia may develop as a result of three mechanisms. First, in patients with irreversible shock, cell membrane permeability is altered so massive K^+ efflux results in severe hyperkalemia; in this situation, survival is unlikely. Second, after repair of a major vessel, subsequent reperfusion of the ischemic tissues results in a sudden release of K^+. Third, transfusion at a rate faster than 1 U every 4 minutes to an acidotic and hypovolemic patient may cause an increase in plasma K^+ levels.[290] Frequent monitoring of serum K^+, gradual and intermittent unclamping of vascular shunts, and avoiding transfusion at higher rates than needed helps reduce the rate of K^+ increase. If a rise in K^+ is detected, treatment with regular insulin, 10 U intravenously, with 50% dextrose, 50 mL, and sodium bicarbonate, 8.4%, 50 mL is indicated. If there is a dysrhythmia, $CaCl_2$, 500 mg should also be administered.[291] Insulin and dextrose can be repeated two or three times at 30- to 45-minute intervals, if necessary. Hemodialysis may be indicated in desperate situations.

Metabolic acidosis is caused by shock in most trauma patients. Other rare causes of metabolic acidosis in this population are alcoholic lactic acidosis, alcoholic ketoacidosis, diabetic ketoacidosis, and CO or CN^- poisoning after inhalation injuries. The differential diagnosis between hypovolemic, diabetic, and alcoholic acidosis, all of which have anion gaps, requires measurement of blood lactate, urinary ketone bodies, blood sugar, and invasive monitoring to assess intravascular volume. Alcoholic ketoacidosis is treated with intravenous dextrose, whereas diabetic ketoacidosis is managed with insulin. No specific treatment except intravenous normal saline exists for alcoholic lactic acidosis.

Treatment of metabolic acidosis involves correction of the underlying cause: management of hypoxemia, restoration of intravascular volume, optimization of cardiac function, or treatment of CO or CN^- toxicity. Symptomatic treatment with sodium bicarbonate has serious disadvantages, including leftward shift of the oxyhemoglobin dissociation curve causing decreased O_2 unloading, a hyperosmolar state secondary to the excessive sodium load, hypokalemia, further hemodynamic depression, overshoot alkalosis a few hours after giving the drug, and intracellular acidosis if adequate ventilation or pulmonary blood flow cannot be provided. Nevertheless, because of the possibility that severe acidosis can cause dysrhythmias, myocardial depression, hypotension, and resistance to exogenous catecholamines, some clinicians administer bicarbonate to "buy time" if the pH is $<$7.2.

Intraoperative Death

Death is a much greater threat during emergency trauma surgery than it is in any other operative procedure. Approximately 0.7% of patients admitted for acute trauma die in the OR, accounting for approximately 8% of postinjury deaths.[292]

TABLE 48-11

CLINICAL FEATURES ASSOCIATED WITH INTRAOPERATIVE MORTALITY

■ CATEGORY	■ CLINICAL FEATURES
Mechanism of injury	Gunshot wound
	Pedestrian injuries
Injury severity	Mean injury severity score >41
	Mean revised trauma score >3.0
Preoperative physiologic profile	Mean BP in the field <50 mm Hg
	Mean BP on arrival to ED <60 mm Hg
	Best systolic BP in the ED <90 mm Hg
	Circulatory shock time >10 min
	Best mean pH <7.18
	Mean preoperative crystalloid resuscitation >3,850 mL; mean red cell transfusion >834 mL
Type of injury	Significant head, chest, abdominal, and pelvic injuries individually or in combination after blunt trauma
	Significant chest and abdominal injuries individually or in combination after penetrating trauma
Organ injury	Brain
	Liver
	Aorta or other major vascular injury
	Cardiac injury
Operating room resuscitation and physiologic status	Systolic BP <90 mm Hg during first hour
	Systolic BP <90 mm Hg for >30 min
	Deterioration of mean pH from 7.19 to 7.01
	Mean intraoperative blood loss 5,172 mL; mean blood replacement 4,541 mL
	Mean platelet transfusion 784 mL
	Mean fresh frozen plasma 1,418 mL
	Mean intraoperative temperature 32.2°C
	Intraoperative cardiac arrest

BP, blood pressure; ED, emergency department.
Data from Hoyt DB, Bulger EM, Knudson MM *et al:* Death in the operating room: An analysis of a multi-center experience. J Trauma 37:426, 1994.

Uncontrollable bleeding is the cause of approximately 80% of intraoperative mortality; brain herniation and air embolism are the most common causes of death in the remaining patients.[292] A multicenter, retrospective study has defined certain features that increase the likelihood of OR death[292] (Table 48-11). Rapid transport to the OR, rapidly stabilizing life-threatening injuries while deferring definitive surgery ("damage control"), simultaneous thoracotomy and laparotomy for thoracoabdominal injuries, appropriate management of retroperitoneal hematoma, and early correction of hypothermia and shock may reduce intraoperative mortality rates.[292]

Of these measures, the damage control principle has reduced not only the intraoperative, but also the overall mortality from trauma surgery.[293] Originally described in three stages, the current suggestion is that it should be managed in four phases.[293] In the first phase, in the emergency department attention is directed to recognition of the pattern of injury, as well as to the decision to initiate damage control by activating rewarming and blood component replacement. The second phase occurs in the OR where, in addition to efforts to maintain the patient's intravascular volume, near normal temperature, acid-base status, and coagulation, surgeons rapidly control bleeding and leave the abdominal cavity temporarily covered by a Vac-Pac dressing, which allows an enlarged space for edematous organs and controlled egress of fluid from the abdomen. The third phase occurs in the ICU where intravascular volume, hypothermia, acidosis, and coagulation abnormalities are corrected. In the fourth phase, the stabilized patient is returned to the OR for definitive surgery and abdominal closure.

EARLY POSTOPERATIVE CONSIDERATIONS

The concerns in the early postoperative period are similar
21 to those of the intraoperative phase. Reevaluation and optimization of the circulation, oxygenation, temperature, CNS function, coagulation, electrolyte and acid-base status, and renal function are the hallmarks of postoperative management. Pain control in this group of patients may have more than a humanitarian purpose; it can improve pulmonary function, ventilation, and oxygenation in patients with chest injury or a long abdominal incision. For sedation in mechanically ventilated patients, both propofol (25 to 75 μg/kg/min) and midazolam (0.1 to 20 μg/kg/min) infusions alone or in combination are equally effective and safe, although wake-up time in patients receiving midazolam is longer (660 $\pm$ 400 minutes) than in those receiving propofol alone (110 $\pm$ 50 minutes) or in both agents combined (190 $\pm$ 200 minutes).[294] Morphine 0.02 to 0.04 mg/kg/hr or fentanyl 1 to 3 μg/kg/hr may be added for analgesia. Small boluses of midazolam (3 to 5 mg), propofol (50 mg), morphine (2 to 3 mg), or fentanyl (25 to 50 μg) may also be given as required.[294]

Acute Renal Failure

Acute renal failure is a possibility if prolonged shock or crush syndrome occur during early management. Following an episode of shock in patients who have not received an osmotic load (radiopaque material, mannitol) or diuretic, determination of 2- or 6-hour creatinine and free water clearances may help predict the development of posttraumatic renal dysfunction.[295] Creatinine clearance <25 mL/min and free water clearance ≥ -15 mL/hr suggest the likelihood of acute renal failure. Decreased urine flow rate is not a good predictor, and the blood urea nitrogen does not rise until at least 24 hours after surgery or trauma.[295]

The cause of renal failure in crush syndrome is probably rhabdomyolysis-induced myoglobin release into the circulation. Serum CK levels increase in these patients; levels above 5,000 U/L are associated with renal failure.[296] The differentiation of myoglobinuria from hemoglobinuria is described in the Urine Output section. A clear supernatant suggests myoglobin, whereas a rose color indicates hemoglobin. The traditional prophylaxis for renal failure after rhabdomyolysis includes fluids, mannitol, and bicarbonate. However, more recent data suggest that bicarbonate and mannitol are ineffective.[296]

Abdominal Compartment Syndrome

Abdominal compartment syndrome results from intra-abdominal hypertension with organ dysfunction after major abdominal trauma and surgery (primary syndrome), although other patients may develop the syndrome without surgery, for example, during massive fluid resuscitation following major trauma or burns (secondary syndrome).[297–300] It frequently follows hemorrhage.[299] The syndrome results from massive edema of intra-abdominal organs produced by shock-induced inflammatory mediators, fluid resuscitation, and surgical manipulation. The significant cardiac, pulmonary, renal, gastrointestinal, hepatic, and CNS dysfunction caused by this syndrome results in a high mortality rate[298] (Fig. 48-10). A damage control procedure with towel-clip closure of the fascia after laparotomy may increase its incidence from the 17% seen with Bogata bag closure to 80%.[300]

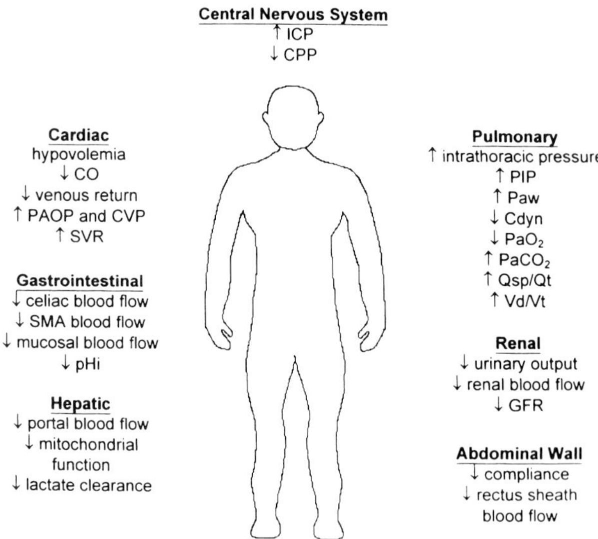

FIGURE 48-10. Physiologic effects of abdominal compartment syndrome. Cdyn, dynamic pulmonary compliance; CO, cardiac output; CPP, cerebral perfusion pressure; CVP, central venous pressure; GFR, glomerular filtration rate; ICP, intracranial pressure; PAOP, pulmonary artery occlusion pressure; Paw, mean airway pressure; pHi, intramucosal pH; PIP, peak inspiratory pressure; Qsp/Qt, intrapulmonary shunt; SMA, superior mesenteric artery; SVR, systemic vascular resistance; Vd/Vt, dead space ventilation. (Reprinted with permission from Cheatham ML: Intra-abdominal hypertension and abdominal compartment syndrome. New Horiz 7:96, 1999.)

Clinically, a tense, distended abdomen should direct the clinician to measure the intravesical pressure (via Foley catheter), which reflects the intra-abdominal pressure (Fig. 48-11).[298] Values >20 to 25 mm Hg indicate inadequate organ perfusion and necessitate abdominal decompression, which, if delayed, results in progression to multiorgan failure and death.[297,300] Use of a volumetric pulmonary artery catheter for assessment of preload by left ventricular end-diastolic volume index determination may be more accurate than measuring CVP or PCWP in these patients.[298] Almost all these patients require mechanical ventilation. Attributing a relatively high PCWP to the ventilator and continuing high-volume fluid infusion may further increase intra-abdominal edema and increase mortality.[301] Interestingly, patients who will develop abdominal compartment syndrome often do not respond to fluid administration with elevated cardiac output despite an increasing PCWP.[301]

Thromboembolism

The overall incidence of DVT in the proximal femoral veins, the major source of PE, is approximately 18% in trauma patients.[302] However, DVT occurs in 24% of lower-extremity injuries, 27% of spine injuries, 20% of major head injuries, and 15% of serious injuries of the face, chest, or abdomen.[302] When injuries involve more than one of these high-risk regions, the likelihood of DVT is even higher.[302] Fortunately, only a relatively small fraction (approximately 0.3 to 2%) of severely injured patients have PE.[302,303] Almost half of all cases of PE occur within the first week, suggesting that DVT develops shortly after trauma.[303] In most instances, DVT is asymptomatic, and in many of those in whom leg swelling develops, concurrent lower-extremity injuries may be implicated. The diagnosis of proximal DVT in symptomatic patients can be made by duplex ultrasonography, but this method has low sensitivity in the absence of symptoms.[304] Venography, which is the gold standard,

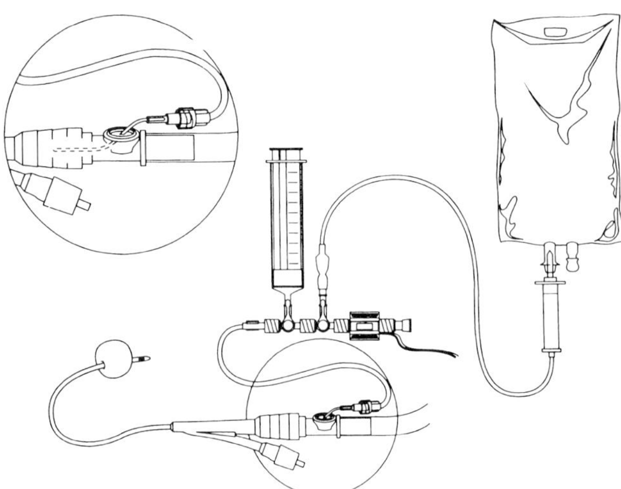

FIGURE 48-11. System used to measure intravesical pressure in abdominal compartment syndrome. (Reprinted with permission from Cheatham ML: Intra-abdominal hypertension and abdominal compartment syndrome. New Horiz 7:96, 1999.)

can be performed in equivocal cases, although it is associated with complications and inherent logistical problems. Hypoxemia, especially when sudden and associated with dyspnea and hemodynamic abnormalities, is highly suggestive of PE. The definitive diagnosis is established by spiral CT and pulmonary angiography. In hemodynamically unstable patients, resuscitation takes precedence over radiologic diagnosis. Management is symptomatic, and includes tracheal intubation, positive pressure ventilation with FIO_2 of 1.0, administration of fluids and inotropes (amrinone or milrinone), and continuous arterial and CVP or pulmonary artery monitoring. TEE is helpful because it may demonstrate RV performance, tricuspid regurgitation, or, in some cases, the thrombus within the pulmonary artery, the right heart chambers, or in transit through a patent foramen ovale to the left atrium.

In patients with relatively minor injuries, PE is treated with anticoagulants. Low-molecular-weight heparin may be used if bleeding is unlikely to exacerbate the injury. Consideration should be given to placement of a vena cava filter if the risk of bleeding is unacceptably high. Removable vena cava filters are now available[305] and are likely to be used prophylactically in high-risk patients more often than permanent filters, which are associated with long-term complications. In patients with severe hemodynamic depression or cardiac arrest unresponsive to resuscitative measures, thrombolytic agents may be considered despite the risk of hemorrhage. The current recommendation for prophylaxis in most trauma patients is low-molecular-weight heparin.[304] Low-dose unfractionated heparin appears to be ineffective in trauma patients.[306] Mechanical devices such as sequential compression boots should be applied as early as possible after injury.

References

1. CDC/NCHS, National Vital Statistics System: LCWK9. Deaths, Percent of Total Deaths, and Death Rates for the 15 Leading Causes of Death: United States and Each State, 2001. Available at: http://www.cdc.gov/nchs/data/dvs/LCWK9_2001.pdf. Accessed March 14, 2005
2. Holbrook TL, Anderson JP, Sieber WJ *et al*: Outcome after major trauma: 12-Month and 18-month follow-up results from the trauma recovery project. J Trauma 46:765, 1999
3. National Safety Council. Injury Facts, 2003 Edition. Chicago, National Safety Council, 2003
4. Acosta JA, Yang JC, Winchell RJ *et al*: Lethal injuries and time of death in a level 1 trauma center. J Am Coll Surg 186:528, 1998
5. Sauaia A, Moore FA, Moore EE *et al*: Epidemiology of trauma deaths: A reassessment. J Trauma 38:185, 1995
6. Trunkey DD, Blaisdell FW: Epidemiology of trauma. Sci Am 4:1, 1988
7. Wyatt J, Beard D, Gray A *et al*: The time of death after trauma. Br Med J 310:1502, 1995
8. Janjua KJ, Sugrue M, Deane SA: Prospective evaluation of early missed injuries and the role of tertiary trauma survey. J Trauma 44:1000, 1998
9. Muzzi DA, Losasso TJ, Cucchiara RF: Complication from a nasopharyngeal airway in a patient with a basilar skull fracture. Anesthesiology 74:366, 1991
10. Vezina D, Lessard MR, Bussieres J *et al*: Complications associated with the use of the esophageal-tracheal combitube. Can J Anaesth 45:76, 1998
11. Gabbott DA: The effect of single handed cricoid pressure on neck movement after application of manual in line neck stabilization. Anaesthesia 52:586, 1997
12. Gabbott DA, Baskett PJF: Management of the airway and ventilation during resuscitation. Br J Anaesth 79:159, 1997
13. Asai T, Neil J, Stacey M: Ease of placement of the laryngeal mask during manual in-line neck stabilization. Br J Anaesth 80:617, 1998
14. Choyce A, Avidan MS, Patel C *et al*: Comparison of laryngeal mask and intubating laryngeal mask insertion by the naive intubator. Br J Anaesth 84:103, 2000
15. Brimacombe J, Keller C: Cervical spine instability and the intubating laryngeal mask—A caution [Letter]. Anaesth Intensive Care 26:708, 1998
16. Weiskopf RB, Bogetz MS: Haemorrhage decreases the anesthetic requirement for ketamine and thiopentone in the pig. Br J Anaesth 57:1022, 1985
17. Schwab TM, Greaves TH: Cardiac arrest as a possible sequela of critical airway management and intubation. Am J Emerg Med 16:609, 1998
18. Ibarra P, Capan LM, Wahlander S, Sutin KM: Difficult airway management in a patient with traumatic asphyxia. Anesth Analg 85:216, 1997
19. de Nadal M, Munar F, Poca MA *et al*: Cerebral hemodynamic effects of morphine and fentanyl in patients with severe head injury. Absence of correlation to cerebral autoregulation. Anesthesiology 92:11, 2000
20. Shapiro HM, Wyte SR, Harris AB: Ketamine anesthesia in patients with intracranial pathology. Br J Anaesth 44:1200, 1972
21. Badrinath SK, Vazeery A, McCarthy RJ, Ivankovich AD: The effect of different methods of inducing anesthesia on intraocular pressure. Anesthesiology 65:431, 1986
22. Stirt JA, Grosslight KR, Bedford RF, Vollmer D: "Defasciculation" with metocurine prevents succinylcholine-induced increases in intracranial pressure. Anesthesiology 67:50, 1987
23. Heier T, Caldwell JE: Rapid tracheal intubation with large-dose rocuronium: A probability based approach. Anesth Analg 90:175, 2000
24. Hastings RH, Kelley SD: Neurologic deterioration associated with airway management in a cervical spine-injured patient. Anesthesiology 78:580, 1993
25. Muckart DJJ, Bhagwanjee S, van der Merwe R: Spinal cord injury as a result of endotracheal intubation in patients with undiagnosed cervical spine fractures. Anesthesiology 87:418, 1997
26. Hoffman JR, Mower WR, Wolfson AB *et al*: Validity of a set of clinical criteria to rule out injury to the cervical spine in patients with blunt trauma. National Emergency X-Radiography Utilization Study Group. N Engl J Med 343:94, 2000
27. Stiell IG, Clement CM, McKnight RD *et al*: The Canadian C-spine rule versus the NEXUS low-risk criteria in patients with trauma. N Engl J Med 349:2510, 2003
28. Hastings RH, Vigil AC, Hanna R *et al*: Cervical spine movement during laryngoscopy with the Bullard, Macintosh and Miller laryngoscopes. Anesthesiology 82:859, 1995
29. Hastings RH, Wood PR: Head extension and laryngeal view during laryngoscopy with cervical spine stabilization maneuvers. Anesthesiology 80:825, 1994
30. Smith CE, Pinchak AB, Sidhu TS *et al*: Evaluation of tracheal intubation difficulty in patients with cervical spine immobilization. Fiberoptic (Wu Scope) versus conventional laryngoscopy. Anesthesiology 91:1253, 1999
31. Mentzelopoulos SD, Tsitsika MV, Balanika MP, Joufi MJ, Karamichali EA: Balloon laryngoscopy reduces head extension and blade leverage in patients with potential cervical spine injury. Crit Care 4:40, 2000
32. Nolan JP, Wilson ME: Orotracheal intubation in patients with potential cervical spine injuries. Anaesthesia 48:630, 1993
33. Sandhu NS, Schaffer S, Capan LM, Turndorf H: Comparison of the Wu-Scope and Macintosh #3 blade in normal and cervical spine stabilized patients. Anesthesiology 91:A480, 1999
34. Cicala RS, Kudsk KA, Butts A *et al*: Initial evaluation and management of upper airway injuries in trauma patients. J Clin Anesth 3:91, 1991
35. Dolin J, Scalea T, Mannor L *et al*: The management of gunshot wounds to the face. J Trauma 33:508, 1992
36. Kihtir T, Ivatury RR, Simon RJ *et al*: Early management of civilian gunshot wounds to the face. J Trauma 35:569, 1993
37. Tung TC, Tseng WS, Chen CT *et al*: Acute life-threatening injuries in facial fracture patients: A review of 1,025 patients. J Trauma 49:420, 2000
38. Davidson JSD, Bindsell DC: Cervical spine injury in patients with facial skeletal trauma. J Trauma 29:1276, 1989
39. Brandt KE, Burruss GL, Hickerson WL *et al*: The management of mid-face fractures with intracranial injury. J Trauma 31:15, 1991
40. Capan LM, Miller SM, Turndorf H: Management of neck injuries. In Capan LM, Miller SM, Turndorf H (eds): Trauma: Anesthesia and Intensive Care, p 409. Philadelphia, JB Lippincott, 1991
41. Deshpande S: Laryngotracheal separation after attempted hanging. Br J Anaesth 81:612, 1998
42. O'Connor PJ, Russell JD, Moriarty DC: Anesthetic implications of laryngeal trauma. Anesth Analg 87:1283, 1998
43. Yamazaki M, Sasaki R, Masuda A, Ito Y: Anesthetic management of complete tracheal disruption using percutaneous cardiopulmonary support system. Anesth Analg 86:998, 1998
44. Rollins RJ, Tocino I: Early radiographic signs of tracheal rupture. Am J Roentgenol 148:695, 1987
45. Klumpe DH, Sang OHK, Wayman SA: A characteristic finding in unilateral complete bronchial transection. Am J Roentgenol 110:704, 1970
46. Shearer VE, Giesecke AH: Airway management for patients with penetrating neck trauma: A retrospective study. Anesth Analg 77:1135, 1993
47. Schweiger JW: The pathophysiology, diagnosis, and management strategies for flail chest injury and pulmonary contusion. Anesth Analg 92(Suppl):86, 2001
48. Karmakar MK, Ho AM: Acute pain management of patients with multiple fractured ribs. J Trauma 54:615, 2003
49. McCunn M, Habashi NM: Airway pressure release ventilation in the acute respiratory distress syndrome following traumatic injury. Int Anesthesiol Clin 40:89, 2002
50. Riou B, Zaier K, Kalfon P *et al*: High-frequency jet ventilation in life-threatening bilateral pulmonary contusion. Anesthesiology 94:927, 2001
51. Ho AMH, Ling E: Systemic air embolism after lung trauma. Anesthesiology 90:564, 1999
52. Demetriades D, Chan LS, Bhasin P *et al*: Relative bradycardia in patients with traumatic hypotension. J Trauma 45:534, 1998

53. Rady MY: Possible mechanisms for the interaction of peripheral somatic nerve stimulation, tissue injury, and hemorrhage in the pathophysiology of traumatic shock. Anesth Analg 78:761, 1994
54. American College of Surgeons Committee on Trauma: InAmerican College of Surgeons (ed): Shock, Advanced Trauma Life Support Instructor Manual, p 97. Chicago, American College of Surgeons, 1997
55. Mackway-Jones K, Foex BA, Kirkman E, Little RA: Modification of the cardiovascular reponse to hemorrhage by somatic afferent nerve stimulation with special reference to gut and skeletal muscle blood flow. J Trauma 47:481, 1999
56. Blow O, Magliore L, Claridge JA *et al*: The golden hour and the silver day: Detection and correction of occult hypoperfusion within 24 hours improves outcome from major trauma. J Trauma 47:964, 1999
57. Porter JM, Ivatury RR: In search of the optimal end points of resuscitation in trauma patients. A review. J Trauma 44:908, 1998
58. Eberhard LW, Morabito DJ, Matthay MA *et al*: Initial severity of metabolic acidosis predicts the development of acute lung injury in severely traumatized patients. Crit Care Med 28:125, 2000
59. Peterson DL, Schinco MA, Kerwin AJ *et al*: Evaluation of initial base deficit as a prognosticator of outcome in the pediatric trauma population. Am Surg 70:326, 2004
60. Randolph LC, Takacs M, Davis KA: Resuscitation in the pediatric trauma population: Admission base deficit remains an important prognostic indicator. J Trauma 53:838, 2002
61. Kincaid EH, Miller PR, Meredith JW *et al*: Elevated arterial base deficit in trauma patients: A marker of impaired oxygen utilization. J Am Coll Surg 187:384, 1998
62. Rutherford EJ, Morris JA, Reed GW, Hall KS: Base deficit stratifies mortality and determines therapy. J Trauma 33:417, 1992
63. James JH, Luchette FA, McCarter FD, Fischer JE: Lactate is an unreliable indicator of tissue hypoxia in injury or sepsis. Lancet 354:505, 1999
64. Mizock BA, Falk JL: Lactic acidosis in critical illness. Crit Care Med 20:80, 1992
65. Abramson D, Scalea TM, Hitchcock R *et al*: Lactate clearance and survival following injury. J Trauma 35:584, 1993
66. McNelis J, Marini CP, Jurkiewicz A *et al*: Prolonged lactate clearance is associated with increased mortality in the surgical intensive care unit. Am J Surg 182:481, 2001
67. Marik PE: Sublingual capnography: A clinical validation study. Chest 120:923, 2001
68. Weil MH, Nakagawa Y, Tang W *et al*: Sublingual capnometry: A new noninvasive measurement for diagnosis and quantitation of severity of circulatory shock. Crit Care Med 27:1225, 1999
69. Baron BJ, Sinert R, Zehtabchi S *et al*: Diagnostic utility of sublingual Pco_2 for detecting hemorrhage in penetrating trauma patients. J Trauma 57:69, 2004
70. Bickell WH, Wall MJ, Pepe PE *et al*: Immediate versus delayed fluid resuscitation for hypotensive patients with penetrating torso injuries. N Engl J Med 331:1105, 1994
71. Stern SA: Low-volume fluid resuscitation for presumed hemorrhagic shock: Helpful or harmful? Curr Opin Crit Care 7:422, 2001
72. Dutton RP, Mackenzie CF, Scalea TM: Hypotensive resuscitation during active hemorrhage: Impact on in-hospital mortality. J Trauma 52:1141, 2002
73. Nacht A: The use of blood products in shock. Crit Care Clin 8:255, 1992
74. Keller ME, Jean R, LaMorte WW, Millham F, Hirsch E: Effects of age of transfused blood on length of stay in trauma patients: A preliminary report. J Trauma 53:1023, 2002
75. Zallen G, Offner PJ, Moore EE *et al*: Age of transfused blood is an independent risk factor for postinjury multiple organ failure. Am J Surg 178:570, 1999
76. Sharma A, Bodenham AR, Mallick A: Ultrasound-guided infraclavicular axillary vein cannulation for central venous access. Br J Anaesth 93:188, 2004
77. Sandhu NP, Sidhu DS: Mid-arm approach to basilic and cephalic vein cannulation using ultrasound guidance. Br J Anaesth 93:292, 2004
78. Neufeld JDG, Marx JA, Moore EE, Light AI: Comparison of intraosseous, central, and peripheral routes of crystalloid infusion for resuscitation of hemorrhagic shock in a swine model. J Trauma 34:422, 1993
79. Luna GK, Pavlin EG, Kirkman T *et al*: Hemodynamic effects of external cardiac massage in trauma shock. J Trauma 29:1430, 1989
80. Durham LA, Richardson RJ, Wall MJ *et al*: Emergency center thoracotomy: Impact of prehospital resuscitation. J Trauma 32:775, 1992
81. Millham FH, Gridlinger GA: Survival determinants in patients undergoing emergency room thoracotomy for penetrating chest injury. J Trauma 34:332, 1993
82. McMahon CG, Yates DW, Campbell FM *et al*: Unexpected contribution of moderate traumatic brain injury to death after major trauma. J Trauma 47:891, 1999
83. Shackford SR, Mackersie RC, Davis JW *et al*: Epidemiology and pathology of traumatic deaths occuring at a level I trauma center in a regionalized system: The importance of secondary brain injury. J Trauma 29:1392, 1989
84. Miller JD, Becker DP: Secondary insults to the injured brain. J R Coll Surg Edinb 27:292, 1982
85. Chesnut RM: Avoidance of hypotension: Conditio sine qua non of successful head injury management. J Trauma 42(Suppl):4S, 1997
86. Chesnut RM, Marshall LF, Klauber MR *et al*: The role of secondary brain injury in determining outcome from severe head injury. J Trauma 34:216, 1993
87. Brain Trauma Foundation/American Association of Neurological Surgeons: Resuscitation of blood pressure and oxygenation. In Florin R, Jagoda A, Kelly JP, Marmarou A, Quinn PC, Rosenberg J, Valadka AB, and European Advisory Committee. Management and Prognosis of Severe Traumatic Brain Injury, p 33. New York, Brain Trauma Foundation, 2000
88. Chesnut RM: The management of severe traumatic brain injury. Emerg Med Clin North Am 15:581, 1997
89. Trauma center descriptions and their role in trauma system. In American College of Surgeons (ed): Resources for Optimal Care of the Injured Patient: 1999. p. 9 Chicago, American College of Surgeons, 1998
90. Head trauma. In American College of Surgeons (ed): Advanced Trauma Life Support Instructor Manual, p 228. Chicago, American College of Surgeons, 1999
91. Brain Trauma Foundation/American Association of Neurological Surgeons: Initial management. In Florin R, Jagoda A, Kelly JP, Marmarou A, Quinn PC, Rosenberg J, Valadka AB, and European Advisory Committee. Management and Prognosis of Severe Traumatic Brain Injury, p 21. New York, Brain Trauma Foundation, 2000
92. Teasdale G, Jennett B: Assessment of coma and impaired consciousness: A practical scale. Lancet 2:81, 1974
93. Miller SM: Management of central nervous system injuries. In Capan LM, Miller SM, Turndorf H (eds): Trauma: Anesthesia and Intensive Care, p 321. Philadelphia, JB Lippincott, 1991
94. Miller JD: Assessing patients with head injury. Br J Surg 77:241, 1990
95. Shackford SR, Wold SL, Ross SE *et al*: The clinical utility of computed tomographic scanning and neurologic examination in the management of patients with minor injuries. J Trauma 33:385, 1992
96. Lam AM, Winn HR, Cullen BF, Sundling N: Hyperglycemia and neurological outcome in patients with head injury. J Neurosurg 75:545, 1991
97. Chesnut RM: Management of brain and spine injuries. Crit Care Clin 20:25, 2004
98. Paczynski RP: Osmotherapy: Basic concepts and controversies. Crit Care Clin 13:105, 1997
99. Huff JS: Acute mannitol intoxication in a patient with normal renal function. Am J Emerg Med 8:338, 1990
100. Wald SL: Advances in the early management of patients with head injury. Surg Clin North Am 75:225, 1995
101. Bouma GJ, Muizelaar P, Choi SC *et al*: Cerebral circulation and metabolism after severe traumatic brain injury: The elusive role of ischemia. J Neurosurg 75:685, 1991
102. Coles JP: Regional ischemia after head injury. Curr Opin Crit Care 10:120, 2004
103. Marion DW, Darby J, Yonas H: Acute regional cerebral blood flow changes caused by severe injuries. J Neurosurg 74:407, 1991
104. Zhuang J, Schmoker JD, Shackford SR, Pictropaol JA: Focal brain injury results in severe cerebral ischemia despite maintenance of cerebral perfusion pressure. J Trauma 33:83, 1992
105. Ward JD, Choi S, Marmarou A *et al*: Effect of prophylactic hyperventilation on outcome in patients with severe head injury. In Hoff JT, Betz AL (eds): Intracranial Pressure II, p 630. Berlin, Springer-Verlag, 1989
106. Yundt KD, Diringer MN: The use of hyperventilation and its impact on cerebral ischemia in the treatment of traumatic brain injury. Crit Care Clin 13:163, 1997
107. Feldman Z, Robertson CS: Monitoring of cerebral hemodynamics with jugular bulb catheters. Crit Care Clin 13:51, 1997
108. Chan KH, Dearden NM, Miller JD *et al*: Multimodality monitoring as a guide to treatment of intracranial hypertension after severe brain injury. Neurosurgery 32:547, 1993
109. Scheinberg M, Kanter MJ, Robertson CS *et al*: Continuous monitoring of jugular venous oxygen saturation in head-injured patients. J Neurosurg 76:212, 1992
110. Cruz J: Jugular venous oxygen saturation monitoring. J Neurosurg 77:162, 1992
111. Ducey JP, Mozingo DW, Lamiell JM *et al*: A comparison of the cerebral and cardiovascular effects of complete resuscitation with isotonic and hypertonic saline, hetastarch, and whole blood following hemorrhage. J Trauma 29:1510, 1989
112. Gunnar W, Jonasson O, Merlotti G *et al*: Head injury and hemorrhagic shock: Studies of the blood brain barrier and intracranial pressure after resuscitation with normal saline solution, 3% saline solution, and dextran-40. Surgery 103:398, 1988
113. Freshman SP, Battistella FD, Mateucci M, Wisner DH: Hypertonic saline (7.5%) versus mannitol: A comparison for treatment of acute head injuries. J Trauma 35:344, 1993
114. Gemma M, Cozzi S, Tommassino C *et al*: 7.5% Hypertonic saline versus 20% mannitol during elective neurosurgical supratentorial procedures. J Neurosurg Anesthesiol 9:329, 1997
115. Hartl R, Ghajar J, Hochleuthner H, Mauritz W: Hypertonic/hyperoncotic saline reliably reduces ICP in severely head-injured patients with intracranial hypertension. Acta Neurochir 70(Suppl):126, 1997
116. Doyle JA, Davis DP, Hoyt DB: The use of hypertonic saline in the treatment of traumatic brain injury. J Trauma 50:367, 2001

117. Kaieda R, Todd MM, Cook LN, Warner DS: Acute effects of changing plasma osmolality and colloid oncotic pressure on the formation of brain edema after cryogenic injury. Neurosurgery 24:671, 1989
118. Cruz J: The first decade of continuous monitoring of jugular bulb oxyhemoglobin saturation: Management strategies and clinical outcome. Crit Care Med 26:344, 1998
119. Eker C, Asgeirsson B, Grande PO *et al*: Improved outcome after severe head injury with a new therapy based on principles for brain volume regulation and preserved microcirculation. Crit Care Med 26:1881, 1998
120. Rudehill A, Bellander B, Weitzberg E *et al*: Outcome of traumatic brain injuries in 1,508 patients: Impact of prehospital care. J Neurotrauma 19:855, 2002
121. Zink BJ: Traumatic brain injury outcome: Concepts for emergency care. Ann Emerg Med 37:318, 2001
122. Cremer OL, van Dijk GW, Amelink GJ *et al*: Cerebral hemodynamic responses to blood pressure manipulation in severely head-injured patients in the presence or absence of intracranial hypertension. Anesth Analg 99:1211, 2004
123. Steiner LA, Czosnyka M, Piechnik SK *et al*: Continuous monitoring of cerebrovascular pressure reactivity allows determination of optimal cerebral perfusion pressure in patients with traumatic brain injury. Crit Care Med 30:733, 2002
124. Warner DS, Borel CO: Treatment of traumatic brain injury: One size does not fit all. Anesth Analg 99:1208, 2004
125. Elf K, Nilsson P, Enblad P: Outcome after traumatic brain injury improved by an organized secondary insult program and standardized neurointensive care. Crit Care Med 30:2129, 2002
126. Ghajar J: Traumatic brain injury. Lancet 356:923, 2000
127. Eismont FJ, Currier BL, McGuire RA Jr: Cervical spine and spinal cord injuries: Recognition and treatment. Instr Course Lect 53:341, 2004
128. American College of Surgeons Committee on Trauma: Spine and spinal cord trauma. In American College of Surgeons (ed): Advanced Trauma Life Support Course Instructor Manual, p 263. Chicago, American College of Surgeons, 1997
129. Pasquale M, Fabian T: Practice management guidelines for trauma from the Eastern Association for the Surgery of Trauma. J Trauma 44:941, 1998
130. Hadley MN, Walters BC, Grabb PA *et al*: Guidelines for the management of acute cervical spine and spinal cord injuries. Clin Neurosurg 49:407, 2002
131. Gonzalez RP, Fried PO, Bukhalo M *et al*: Role of clinical examination in screening for blunt cervical spine injury. J Am Coll Surg 189:152, 1999
132. Sommer RM, Bauer RD, Errico TJ: Cervical spine injuries. In Capan LM, Miller SM, Turndorf H (eds): Trauma, Anesthesia and Intensive Care, p 447. Philadelphia, JB Lippincott, 1991
133. Atkinson PP, Atkinson JL: Spinal shock. Mayo Clin Proc 71:384, 1996
134. Marion DW, Domeier R, Dunham CM *et al*: Practice Management Guidelines for Identifying Cervical Spine Injuries Following Trauma. Eastern Association for the Surgery of Trauma, 1998. Available at: http://www.east.org/tpg/chap3.pdf. Greeneboro, NC Accessed November 14, 2004.
135. Griffen MM, Frykberg ER, Kerwin AJ *et al*: Radiographic clearance of blunt cervical spine injury: Plain radiograph or computed tomography scan? J Trauma 55:222, 2003
136. Widder S, Doig C, Burrowes P *et al*: Prospective evaluation of computed tomographic scanning for the spinal clearance of obtunded trauma patients: Preliminary results. J Trauma 56:1179, 2004
137. Woodring JH, Lee C: Limitations of cervical radiography in the evaluation of acute cervical trauma. J Trauma 34:32, 1993
138. Insko EK, Gracias VH, Gupta R *et al*: Utility of flexion and extension radiographs of the cervical spine in the acute evaluation of blunt trauma. J Trauma 53:426, 2002
139. Anglen J, Metzler M, Bunn P, Griffiths H: Flexion and extension views are not cost-effective in a cervical spine clearance protocol for obtunded trauma patients. J Trauma 52:54, 2002
140. Amar AP, Levy ML: Pathogenesis and pharmacological strategies for mitigating secondary damage in acute spinal cord injury. Neurosurgery 44:1027, 1999
141. Vale FL, Burns J, Jackson AB, Hadley MN: Combined medical and surgical treatment after acute spinal cord injury: Results of a pilot study to assess the merits of aggressive medical resuscitation and blood pressure management. J Neurosurg 87:239, 1997
142. Wardrope J, Ravichandran G, Locker T: Risk assessment for spinal injury after trauma. Br Med J 328:721, 2004
143. Bracken MB, Shepard MJ, Collins WF *et al*: A randomized, controlled trial of methylprednisolone or naloxone in the treatment of acute spinal cord injury. Results of Second National Spinal Cord Injury Study. N Engl J Med 322:1405, 1990
144. Bracken MB, Shepard MJ, Collins WF *et al*: Methylprednisolone or naloxone treatment after acute spinal cord injury. Results of the Second National Acute Spinal Cord Injury Study. J Neurosurg 76:23, 1992
145. Bracken MB, Shepard MJ, Holford TR *et al*: Methylprednisolone or tirilazad mesylate after acute spinal cord injury: Results of the third National Acute Spinal Cord Injury randomized controlled trial. J Neurosurg 89:699, 1998
146. Levy ML, Gans W, Wijesenghe HS *et al*: Use of methylprednisolone as an adjunct in the management of patients with penetrating spinal cord injury: Outcome analysis. Neurosurgery 39:1141, 1996
147. Petitjean ME, Pointillart V, Dixmerias F *et al*: Traitement medicamenteux de la lesion medullaire traumatique au stade aigu. Ann Fr Anesth Reanim 17:114, 1998
148. Poynton AR, O'Farrell DA, Shannon F *et al*: An evaluation of the factors affecting neurological recovery following spinal cord injury. Injury 28:545, 1997
149. Gerndt SJ, Rodriguez JL, Pawlik JW *et al*: Consequences of high-dose steroid therapy for acute spinal cord injury. J Trauma 42:279, 1997
150. Roth EJ, Lu A, Primack S *et al*: Ventilatory function in cervical and high thoracic spinal cord injury. Relationship to level of injury and tone. Am J Phys Med Rehabil 76:262, 1997
151. Winslow C, Rozovsky J: Effect of spinal cord injury on the respiratory system. Am J Phys Med Rehabil 82:803, 2003
152. Theodore J, Robin ED: Pathogenesis of neurogenic pulmonary edema. Lancet 2:749, 1975
153. Mackenzie CF, Shin B, Krishnaprasad D *et al*: Assessment of cardiac and respiratory function during surgery on patients with acute quadriplegia. J Neurosurg 62:843, 1985
154. Demetriades D, Asensio JA, Velmahos G, Thal E: Complex problems in penetrating neck trauma. Surg Clin North Am 76:661, 1996
155. Fabian TC, Patton JH, Croce MA *et al*: Blunt carotid injury. Importance of early diagnosis and anticoagulant therapy. Ann Surg 223:513, 1996
156. Biffl WL, Moore EE, Ryu RK *et al*: The unrecognized epidemic of blunt carotid arterial injuries. Early diagnosis improves neurologic outcome. Ann Surg 228:462, 1998
157. Fabian TC, Cicala RS, Croce MA *et al*: A prospective evaluation of myocardial contusion: Correlation of significant arrhythmias and cardiac output with CPK-MB measurements. J Trauma 31:653, 1991
158. Jewett BS, Shockley WW, Rutledge R: External laryngeal trauma: Analysis of 392 patients. Arch Otolaryngol Head Neck Surg 125:877, 1999
159. Lee RB, Bass SM, Morris JA, Mackenzie EJ: Three or more rib fractures as an indicator for transfer to a level I trauma center. J Trauma 30:689, 1990
160. Philips EH, Rogers WF, Gaspar MR: First rib fracture: Incidence of vascular injury and indications for angiography. Surgery 89:42, 1981
161. McGinnis M, Denton JR: Fractures of the scapula: A retrospective study of 40 fractured scapulae. J Trauma 29:1488, 1989
162. Brookes JG, Dunn RJ, Rogers IR: Sternal fractures: A retrospective analysis of 272 cases. J Trauma 35:46, 1993
163. Tocino IM, Miller MH, Fairfax WR: Distribution of pneumothorax in the supine and semirecumbent critically ill adult. Am J Roentgenol 144:901, 1985
164. Rowan KR, Kirkpatrick AW, Liu D *et al*: Traumatic pneumothorax detection with thoracic US: Correlation with chest radiography and CT—Initial experience. Radiology 225:210, 2002
165. Rainer TH, Griffith JF, Lam E *et al*: Comparison of thoracic ultrasound, clinical acumen, and radiography in patients with minor chest injury. J Trauma 56:1211, 2004
166. Kirkpatrick AW, Sirois M, Laupland KB *et al*: Hand-held thoracic sonography for detecting post-traumatic pneumothoraces: The extended focused assessment with sonography for trauma (EFAST). J Trauma 57:288, 2004
167. Brasel KJ, Stafford RE, Weigelt JA *et al*: Treatment of occult pneumothoraces from blunt trauma. J Trauma 46:987, 1999
168. Enderson BL, Abdalla R, Frame SB *et al*: Tube thoracostomy for occult preumothorax: A prospective randomized study of its use. J Trauma 35:726, 1993
169. Carrillo EH, Heniford BT, Etoch SW *et al*: Video assisted thoracic surgery in trauma patients. J Am Coll Surg 184:316, 1997
170. Mineo TC, Ambrogi V, Cristino B *et al*: Changing indications for thoracotomy in blunt chest trauma after the advent of videothoracoscopy. J Trauma 47:1088, 1999
171. Rozycki GS, Feliciano DV, Ochsner G *et al*: The role of ultrasound in patients with possible penetrating cardiac wounds: A prospective multicenter study. J Trauma 46:543, 1999
172. Porembka DT, Johnson DJ, Hoyt BD *et al*: Penetrating cardiac trauma: A perioperative role for transesophageal echocardiography. Anesth Analg 77:1275, 1993
173. Orliaguet G, Ferjani M, Riou B: The heart in blunt trauma. Anesthesiology 95:544, 2001
174. Richardson JD, Wilson ME, Miller FB: The widened mediastinum. Diagnostic and therapeutic priorities. Ann Surg 211:731, 1990
175. Wong YC, Ng CJ, Wang LJ *et al*: Left mediastinal width and mediastinal width ratio are better radiographic criteria than general mediastinal width for predicting blunt aortic injury. J Trauma 57:88, 2004
176. Vignon P, Boncoeur MP, Francois B *et al*: Comparison of multiplane transesophageal echocardiography and contrast-enhanced helical CT in the diagnosis of blunt traumatic cardiovascular injuries. Anesthesiology 94:615, 2001
177. Wahl WL, Michaels AJ, Wang SC *et al*: Blunt thoracic aortic injury. J Trauma 47:254, 1999
178. Dunham MB, Zygun D, Petrasek P *et al*: Endovascular stent grafts for acute blunt aortic injury. J Trauma 56:1173, 2004
179. Symbas PN, Vlasis SE, Hatcher CR Jr: Blunt and penetrating diaphragmatic injuries with or without herniation of organs into the chest. Ann Thorac Surg 42:158, 1986

180. Kearney PA, Vahey T, Burney RE *et al*: Computed tomography and diagnostic peritoneal lavage in blunt abdominal trauma. Arch Surg 124:344, 1989
181. Villavicencio RT, Aucar JA: Analysis of laparoscopy in trauma. J Am Coll Surg 189:11, 1999
182. Ginzburg E, Carillo EH, Kopelman T *et al*: The role of computed tomography in selective management of gunshot wounds to the abdomen and flank. J Trauma 45:1005, 1998
183. Boulanger BR, McLellan BA, Brenneman FD *et al*: Prospective evidence of the superiority of a sonography based algorithm in the assessment of blunt abdominal injury. J Trauma 47:632, 1999
184. FAST Consensus Conference Committee: Focused assessment with sonography for trauma (FAST): Results from an international consensus conference. J Trauma 46:466, 1999
185. Patel KP, Capan LM, Grant GJ, Miller SM: Musculoskeletal injuries. In Capan LM, Miller SM, Turndorf H (eds): Trauma: Anesthesia and Intensive Care, p 511. Philadelphia, JB Lippincott, 1991
186. MacLennan N, Heimbach DM, Cullen BF: Anesthesia for major thermal injury. Anesthesiology 89:749, 1998
187. Haponik EF, Meyers DA, Munster AM *et al*: Acute upper airway injury in burn patients: Serial changes of flow volume curves and nasopharyngoscopy. Am Rev Respir Dis 135:360, 1987
188. Smith DL, Cairns BA, Ramadan F *et al*: Effect of inhalation injury, burn size and age on mortality: A study of 1447 consecutive burn patients. J Trauma 37:655, 1994
189. Muehlberger T, Kunar D, Munster A, Couch M: Efficacy of fiberoptic laryngoscopy in the diagnosis of inhalation injuries. Arch Otolaryngol Head Neck Surg 124:1003, 1998
190. Jones WG, Madden M, Finkelstein J *et al*: Tracheostomies in burn patients. Ann Surg 209:471, 1989
191. Venus B, Matsuda C, Copozio JB *et al*: Prophylactic intubation and continuous positive airway pressure in the management of inhalation injury in burn patients. Crit Care Med 9:519, 1981
192. Masanes MJ, Legendre C, Lioret N *et al*: Fiberoptic bronchoscopy for the early diagnosis of subglottal inhalation injury: Comparative value in the assessment of prognosis. J Trauma 36:59, 1994
193. Sheridan RL, Hurford WE, Kacmarek RM *et al*: Inhaled nitric oxide in burn patients with respiratory failure. J Trauma 42:629, 1997
194. Miller K, Chang A: Acute inhalation injury. Emerg Med Clin North Am 21:533, 2003
195. Hampson NB, Zmaeff JL: Outcome of patients experiencing cardiac arrest with carbon monoxide poisoning treated with hyperbaric oxygen. Ann Emerg Med 38:36, 2001
196. Vegfors M, Lennmarken C: Carboxyhemoglobinaemia and pulse oximetry. Br J Anaesth 66:625, 1991
197. Haney M, Tait AR, Tremper KK: Effect of carboxyhemoglobin on the accuracy of mixed venous oximetry monitors in dogs. Crit Care Med 22:1181, 1994
198. Hampson NB: Hyperbaric oxygen: A plea for uniform nomenclature. Undersea Hyperb Med 26:267, 1999
199. Baud FJ, Barriot P, Toffis V *et al*: Elevated blood cyanide concentrations in victims of smoke inhalation. N Engl J Med 325:1761, 1991
200. Silverman SH, Purdue GF, Hunt JL, Bost RO: Cyanide toxicity in burned patients. J Trauma 28:171, 1988
201. Tung A, Lynch J, McDade WA: A new biological assay for measuring cyanide in blood. Anesth Analg 85:1045, 1997
202. Breen PH, Isserles SA, Westley J *et al*: Combined carbon monoxide and cyanide poisoning: A place for treatment? Anesth Analg 80:671, 1995
203. Kulig K: Cyanide antidotes and fire toxicology. N Engl J Med 325:1801, 1991
204. Papp A, Uusaro A, Parviainen I *et al*: Myocardial function and haemodynamics in extensive burn trauma: Evaluation by clinical signs, invasive monitoring, echocardiography and cytokine concentrations. A prospective clinical study. Acta Anaesthesiol Scand 47:1257, 2003
205. Ivy ME, Atweh NA, Palmer J *et al*: Intra-abdominal hypertension and abdominal compartment syndrome in burn patients. J Trauma 49:387, 2000
206. Warden GD: Burn shock resuscitation. World J Surg 16:16, 1992
207. Sheridan RL: Burns. Crit Care Med 30:S500, 2002
208. Cochrane Injuries Group Albumin Reviewers. Human albumin administration in critically ill patients: Systematic review of randomised controlled trials. Br Med J 317:235, 1998
209. Wharton SM, Khanna A: Current attitudes to burns resuscitation in the UK. Burns 27:183, 2001
210. Huang PP, Stucky FS, Dimick AR *et al*: Hypertonic sodium resuscitation is associated with renal failure and death. Ann Surg 221:543, 1995
211. Elgjo GI, Poli de Figueiredo LF, Schenarts PJ *et al*: Hypertonic saline dextran produces early (8–12 hrs) fluid sparing in burn resuscitation: A 24-hr prospective, double-blind study in sheep. Crit Care Med 28:163, 2000
212. Mann R, Heimbach DM, Engrav LH, Foy H: Changes in transfusion practices in burn patients. J Trauma 37:220, 1994
213. Bernard F, Guegniaud PY, Bouchard C *et al*: Hemodynamic parameters in the severely burnt patient during the first 72 hours. Ann Fr Anesth Reanim 11:623, 1992
214. Dries DJ, Waxman K: Adequate resuscitation of burn patients may not be measured by urine output and vital signs. Crit Care Med 19: 327, 1991
215. Holm C, Melcer B, Horbrand F *et al*: Arterial thermodilution: An alternative to pulmonary artery catheter for cardiac output assessment in burn patients. Burns 27:161, 2001
216. Holm C, Melcer B, Horbrand F *et al*: Intrathoracic blood volume as an end point in resuscitation of the severely burned: An observational study of 24 patients. J Trauma 48:728, 2000
217. Morris JA, Mackenzie EJ, Edelstein SL: The effect of preexisting conditions on mortality in trauma patients. JAMA 263:1942, 1990
218. Rooke GA, Schwid HA, Shapira Y: The effect of graded hemorrhage and intravascular volume replacement on systolic pressure variation in humans during mechanical and spontaneous ventilation. Anesth Analg 80:925, 1995
219. Chang MC, Blinman TA, Rutherford EJ *et al*: Preload assessment in trauma patients during large-volume shock resuscitation. Arch Surg 131:728, 1996
220. Cheatham ML, Safcsak K, Block EF *et al*: Preload assessment in patients with an open abdomen. J Trauma 46:16, 1999
221. Capan LM, Miller SM, Patel KP: Fat embolism. Anesthesiol Clin North Am 11:25, 1993
222. McKinley BA, Kozar RA, Cocanour CS *et al*: Normal versus supranormal oxygen delivery goals in shock resuscitation: The response is the same. J Trauma 53:825, 2002
223. Bishop MH, Shoemaker WC, Appel PL *et al*: Prospective, randomized trial of survivor values of cardiac index, oxygen delivery, and oxygen consumption as resuscitation endpoints in severe trauma. J Trauma 38: 780, 1995
224. Tyburski JG, Carlin AM, Harvey EH, Steffes C, Wilson RF: End-tidal CO_2-arterial CO_2 differences: A useful intraoperative mortality marker in trauma surgery. J Trauma 55:892, 2003
225. Harrigan C, Lucas CE, Ledgerwood AM: The effect of hemorrhagic shock on the clotting cascade in injured patients. J Trauma 29:1416, 1989
226. Ordog GJ, Wasserberger J, Balasubramanian S: Coagulation abnormalities in traumatic shock. Ann Emerg Med 14:650, 1985
227. Mallett SV, Cox JA: Thromboelastography. Br J Anaesth 69:307, 1992
228. Douning L, Bierig P, Fang X *et al*: Temperature effect on thromboelastograph: A comparative study. Anesth Analg 80:S107, 1995
229. Gubler KD, Gentilello LM, Hassantash SA, Maier RV: The impact of hypothermia on dilutional coagulopathy. J Trauma 36:847, 1994
230. Johnston TD, Chen Y, Reed RL: Functional equivalence of hypothermia to specific clotting factor deficiencies. J Trauma 37:413, 1994
231. Ciavarella D, Reed RL, Counts RB *et al*: Clotting factor levels and the risk of diffuse microvascular bleeding in the massively transfused patient. Br J Haematol 67:365, 1987
232. Miller RD: Coagulation and packed red blood cell transfusions. Anesth Analg 80:215, 1995
233. Murphy WG, Davies MJ, Eduardo A: The haemostatic response to surgery and trauma. Br J Anaesth 70:205, 1993
234. Murray DJ, Olsen J, Strauss R, Tinker JH: Coagulation changes during packed red cell replacement of major blood loss. Anesthesiology 69:839, 1988
235. Capan LM: Airway management. In Capan LM, Miller SM, Turndorf H (eds): Trauma Anesthesia and Intensive Care, p 43. Philadelphia, JB Lippincott, 1991
236. Egar TD, Kuramkote S, Gong G *et al*: Fentanyl pharmacokinetics in hemorrhagic shock. A porcine model. Anesthesiology 91:156, 1999
237. Johnson KB, Egan TD, Kern SE *et al*: Influence of hemorrhagic shock followed by crystalloid resuscitation on propofol: A pharmacokinetic and pharmacodynamic analysis. Anesthesiology 101:647, 2004
238. Johnson KB, Egan TD, Kern SE *et al*: The influence of hemorrhagic shock on propofol: A pharmacokinetic and pharmacodynamic analysis. Anesthesiology 99:409, 2003
239. Shafer SL: Shock values. Anesthesiology 101:567, 2004
240. Adams P, Gelman S, Reves JG *et al*: Midazolam pharmacodynamics and pharmacokinetics during acute hypovolemia. Anesthesiology 63:140, 1985
241. Gauss A, Heinrich H, Wilder-Smith OHG: Echocardiographic assessment of the haemodynamic effects of propofol: A comparison with etomidate and thiopentone. Anaesthesia 46:99, 1991
242. Lippmann M, Appel PL, Mok MS *et al*: Sequential cardiorespiratory patterns of anesthetic induction with ketamine in critically ill patients. Crit Care Med 11:730, 1983
243. Ebert TJ, Kanitz DD, Kampine JP: Inhibition of sympathetic neural outflow during thiopental anesthesia in humans. Anesth Analg 71:319, 1990
244. Ebert TJ, Muzi M, Berens R *et al*: Sympathetic responses to induction of anesthesia in humans with propofol or etomidate. Anesthesiology 76:725, 1992
245. Priano LL, Bernards C, Marrone B: Effect of anesthetic induction agents on cardiovascular neuroregulation in dogs. Anesth Analg 68:344, 1989
246. Takeshima R, Dohi S: Comparison of arterial baroreflex function in humans anesthetized with enflurane or isoflurane. Anesth Analg 69:284, 1989
247. Flacke JW, Davis LJ, Flacke WE *et al*: Effects of fentanyl and diazepam in dogs deprived of autonomic tone. Anesth Analg 64:1053, 1985
248. Bogetz MS, Katz JA: Recall of surgery for major trauma. Anesthesiology 61:6, 1984
249. Lubke GH, Kerssens C, Phaf H *et al*: Dependence of explicit and implicit memory on hypnotic state in trauma patients. Anesthesiology 90:670, 1999

250. Johnson KB, Egan TD, Layman J *et al*: The influence of hemorrhagic shock on etomidate: A pharmacokinetic and pharmacodynamic analysis. Anesth Analg 96:1360, 2003
251. Brown DL: Anesthetic agents in trauma surgery: Are there differences? Int Anesthesiol Clin 25:75, 1987
252. Weiskopf RB, Bogetz MS, Roizen MF, Reid IA: Cardiovascular and metabolic sequelae of inducing anesthesia with ketamine or thiopental in hypovolemic swine. Anesthesiology 60:214, 1984
253. Weiskopf RB, Bogetz MS: Cardiovascular actions of nitrous oxide or halothane in hypovolemic swine. Anesthesiology 63:509, 1985
254. Warltier DC, Pagel PS: Cardiovascular and respiratory actions of desflurane: Is desflurane different from isoflurane? Anesth Analg 75:S17, 1992
255. Gopinath SP, Cormio M, Ziegler J *et al*: Intraoperative jugular desaturation during surgery for traumatic intracranial hematomas. Anesth Analg 83:1014, 1996
256. Modica PA, Tempelhoff R: Intracranial pressure during induction of anesthesia and tracheal intubation with etomidate-induced EEG burst suppression. Can J Anaesth 39:236, 1992
257. Reves JG, Fragen RJ, Vinik R, Greenblatt DJ: Midazolam: Pharmacology and uses. Anesthesiology 62:310, 1985
258. Smith I, White PF, Nathanson M, Gouldson R: Propofol. An update on its clinical use. Anesthesiology 81:1005, 1994
259. Artru AA: Dose-related changes in the rate of cerebrospinal fluid formation and resistance to reabsorption of cerebrospinal fluid following administration of thiopental, midazolam and etomidate in dogs. Anesthesiology 69:541, 1988
260. Shapiro HM: Intracranial hypertension: Therapeutic and anesthetic considerations. Anesthesiology 43:445, 1975
261. Berry JM, Merin RG: Etomidate myoclonus and the open globe. Anesth Analg 69:256, 1989
262. Libonati MM, Leahy MJ, Ellison N: The use of succinylcholine in open eye surgery. Anesthesiology 62:637, 1985
263. Zimmerman AA, Funk K, Tidwell JL: Propofol and alfentanil prevent the increase in intraocular pressure caused by succinylcholine and endotracheal intubation during a rapid sequence induction of anesthesia. Anesth Analg 83:814, 1996
264. Magorian T, Flannery KB, Miller RD: Comparison of rocuronium, succinylcholine, and vecuronium for rapid-sequence induction of anesthesia in adult patients. Anesthesiology 79:913, 1993
265. Savarese JJ, Ali HH, Basta SJ *et al*: The clinical neuromuscular pharmacology of mivacurium chloride (BWB 1090 U). Anesthesiology 68:723, 1988
266. Grosslight K, Coleman A, Bedford RF: Isoflurane anesthesia: Risk factors for increase in intracranial pressure. Anesthesiology 63:533, 1985
267. Field LM, Dorrance DE, Krzeminska EK, Barsoum LZ: Effect of nitrous oxide on cerebral blood flow in normal humans. Br J Anaesth 70:154, 1993
268. Moss E: Alfentanil increases intracranial pressure when intracranial compliance is low. Anaesthesia 47:134, 1992
269. Albanese J, Durbec O, Viviand X *et al*: Sufentanil increases intracranial pressure in patients with head trauma. Anesthesiology 79:493, 1993
270. Sperry RJ, Bailey PL, Reichman MV *et al*: Fentanyl and sufentanil increase intracranial presssure in head trauma patients. Anesthesiology 77:416, 1992
271. Kingston HGG, Bretherton KW, Halloway AM, Downing JW: A comparison between ketamine and diazepam as induction agents for pericardiectomy. Anaesth Intensive Care 6:66, 1978
272. Missavage AE, Bush RL, Kien ND, Reilly DA: The effect of clysed and topical epinephrine on intraoperative catecholamine levels. J Trauma 45:1074, 1998
273. Coté CJ, Drop LJ, Hoaglin DC *et al*: Ionized hypocalcemia after fresh frozen plasma administration to thermally injured children: Effects of infusion rate, duration, and treatment with calcium chloride. Anesth Analg 67:152, 1988
274. Han T, Kim H, Bae J *et al*: Neuromuscular pharmacodynamics of rocuronium in patients with major burns. Anesth Analg 99:386, 2004
275. Uhl L, Pacini D, Kruskail MS: A comparative study of blood warmer performance. Anesthesiology 77:1022, 1992
276. Schierhout G, Roberts I: Fluid resuscitation with colloid or crystalloid solutions in critically ill patients: A systematic review of randomised trials. Br Med J 316:961, 1998
277. Warren BB, Durieux ME: Hydroxyethyl starch: Safe or not? Anesth Analg 84:206, 1997
278. Zipnick RI, Scalea TM, Trooskin SZ *et al*: Hemodynamic responses to penetrating spinal cord injuries. J Trauma 35:578, 1993
279. Johnson SB, Kearney PA, Smith MD: Echocardiography in the evaluation of thoracic trauma. Surg Clin North Am 75:193, 1995
280. Jurkovich GJ, Greiser WB, Luterman A *et al*: Hypothermia in trauma victims: An ominous predictor of survival. J Trauma 27:1019, 1987
281. Gentilello LM: Advances in the management of hypothermia. Surg Clin North Am 75:243, 1995
282. Gentilello LM, Cobean R, Offner PJ *et al*: Continuous arteriovenous rewarming: Rapid reversal of hypothermia in critically ill patients. J Trauma 32:316, 1992
283. Ferrara A, Mac Arthur JD, Wright HK *et al*: Hypothermia and acidosis worsen coagulopathy in the patient requiring massive transfusion. Am J Surg 160:515, 1990
284. Patt A, McCroskey BL, Moore EE: Hypothermia induced coagulopathies in trauma. Surg Clin North Am 68:775, 1988
285. Wolberg AS, Meng ZH, Monroe DM III, Hoffman M: A systematic evaluation of the effect of temperature on coagulation enzyme activity and platelet function. J Trauma 56:1221, 2004
286. Murray DJ, Pennell BJ, Weinstein SL, Olson JD: Packed red cells in acute blood loss: Dilutional coagulopathy as a cause of surgical bleeding. Anesth Analg 80:336, 1995
287. Reed RL, Johnston TD, Hudson JD, Fisher RP: The disparity between hypothermic coagulopathy and clotting studies. J Trauma 33:465, 1992
288. Reed RL, Ciavarella D, Heimbach DM *et al*: Prophylactic platelet administration during massive transfusion: A prospective, randomized, double-blind clinical study. Ann Surg 203:40, 1986
289. Kulkarni R, Daneshmand A, Guertin S *et al*: Successful use of activated recombinant factor VII in traumatic liver injuries in children. J Trauma 56:1348, 2004
290. Linko K, Tigerstedt I: Hyperpotassemia during massive blood transfusions. Acta Anaesthesiol Scand 28:220, 1984
291. Erdmann E, Reuschel-Janetschek E: Calcium for resuscitation? Br J Anaesth 67:178, 1991
292. Hoyt DB, Bulger EM, Knudson MM *et al*: Death in the operating room: An analysis of a multi-center experience. J Trauma 37:426, 1994
293. Johnson JW, Gracias VH, Schwab CW *et al*: Evolution in damage control for exsanguinating penetrating abdominal injury. J Trauma 51:261, 2001
294. Sanchez-Izquierdo-Riera JA, Caballero-Cubedo RE, Perez-Vela JL *et al*: Propofol versus midazolam: Safety and efficacy for sedating the severe trauma patient. Anesth Analg 86:1219, 1998
295. Shin B, Mackenzie CF, Helrich M: Creatinine clearance for early detection of posttraumatic renal dysfunction. Anesthesiology 64:605, 1986
296. Brown CV, Rhee P, Chan L *et al*: Preventing renal failure in patients with rhabdomyolysis: Do bicarbonate and mannitol make a difference? J Trauma 56:1191, 2004
297. Balogh Z, McKinley BA, Cocanour CS *et al*: Secondary abdominal compartment syndrome is an elusive early complication of traumatic shock resuscitation. Am J Surg 184:538, 2002
298. Cheatham ML: Intra-abdominal hypertension and abdominal compartment syndrome. New Horiz 7:96, 1999
299. Maxwell RA, Fabian TC, Croce MA, Davis KA: Secondary abdominal compartment syndrome: An underappreciated manifestation of severe hemorrhagic shock. J Trauma 47:995, 1999
300. Balogh Z, McKinley BA, Holcomb JB *et al*: Both primary and secondary abdominal compartment syndrome can be predicted early and are harbingers of multiple organ failure. J Trauma 54:848, 2003
301. Balogh Z, McKinley BA, Cocanour CS *et al*: Patients with impending abdominal compartment syndrome do not respond to early volume loading. Am J Surg 186:602, 2003
302. Geerts WH, Code KI, Jay RM *et al*: A prospective study of venous thromboembolism after major trauma. N Engl J Med 331:1601, 1994
303. Owings JT, Kraut E, Battistella F *et al*: Timing of the occurrence of pulmonary embolism in trauma patients. Arch Surg 132:862, 1997
304. Jongbloets LM, Lensing AW, Koopman MM *et al*: Limitations of compression ultrasound for the detection of symptomless postoperative deep vein thrombosis. Lancet 343:1142, 1994
305. Morris CS, Rogers FB, Najarian KE *et al*: Current trends in vena caval filtration with the introduction of a retrievable filter at a level I trauma center. J Trauma 57:32, 2004
306. Geerts WH, Jay RM, Code KI *et al*: A comparison of low-dose heparin with low-molecular-weight heparin as prophylaxis against venous thromboembolism after major trauma. N Engl J Med 335:701, 1996

CHAPTER 49 ■ THE ALLERGIC RESPONSE

JERROLD H. LEVY

KEY POINTS

1. Anesthesiologists routinely manage patients during their perioperative medical care where they are exposed to foreign substances, including drugs (antibiotics, anesthetic agents, neuromuscular-blocking agents [NMBAs], sedative/hypnotics), polypeptides (i.e., protamine, aprotinin), blood products, and environmental antigens (i.e., latex).
2. Antibodies are specific proteins called immunoglobulins that can recognize and bind to a specific antigen.
3. Cytokines are inflammatory cell activators that are synthesized to act as secondary messengers and activate endothelial cells and white cells.
4. Immune competence during surgery can be affected by direct and hormonal effects of anesthetic drugs, by immunologic effects of other drugs used, by the surgery, by coincident infection, and by transfused blood products.
5. More than 90% of the allergic reactions evoked by intravenous drugs occur within 5 minutes of administration. In the anesthetized patient, the most common life-threatening manifestation of an allergic reaction is circulatory collapse, reflecting vasodilation with resulting decreased venous return.
6. Many diverse molecules administered during the perioperative period release histamine in a dose-dependent, nonimmunologic fashion.
7. A plan for treating anaphylactic reactions must be established before the event. Airway maintenance, 100% oxygen administration, intravascular volume expansion, and epinephrine are essential to treat the hypotension and hypoxia that result from vasodilation, increased capillary permeability, and bronchospasm.
8. After an anaphylactic reaction, it is important to identify the causative agent to prevent readministration.
9. Health care workers and children with spina bifida, urogenital abnormalities, or certain food allergies have been recognized as people at increased risk for anaphylaxis to latex.
10. NMBAs have several unique molecular features that make them potential antigens.

Allergic reactions represent an important cause of perioperative complications. Anesthesiologists routinely manage patients during their perioperative medical care where they
1 are exposed to foreign substances, including drugs (i.e., antibiotics, anesthetic agents, neuromuscular-blocking agents [NMBAs], sedative hypnotics), polypeptides (protamine, aprotinin), blood products, and environmental antigens (i.e., latex). Anesthesiologists must be able to rapidly recognize and treat anaphylaxis, the most life-threatening form of an allergic reaction.[1]

The allergic response represents just one limb of the pathologic response the immune system that can mount against foreign substances. As part of normal host surveillance mechanisms, a series of cellular and humoral elements monitors foreign structures called *antigens* to provide host defense. These foreign substances (antigens) consist of molecular arrangements found on cells, bacteria, viruses, proteins, or complex macromolecules.[1–4] Immunologic mechanisms (1) involve antigen interaction with antibodies or specific effector cells; (2) are reproducible; and (3) are specific and adaptive, distinguishing foreign substances and amplifying reactivity through a series of inflammatory cells and proteins. The immune system serves to protect the body against external microorganisms and toxins, as well as internal threats from neoplastic cells; however, it can respond inappropriately to cause hypersensitive (allergic) reactions. Life-threatening allergic reactions to drugs and other foreign substances observed perioperatively may represent different expressions of the immune response.[1,2]

BASIC IMMUNOLOGIC PRINCIPLES

Host defense can be divided into cellular and humoral elements.[1–4] The humoral system includes antibodies, complement, cytokines, and other circulating proteins, whereas cellular immunity is mediated by specific lymphocytes of the T-cell series. Lymphocytes have receptors that distinguish between antigens of host and foreign origin. When lymphocytes react with foreign antigens, they respond to orchestrate immunosurveillance, regulate immunospecific antibody synthesis, and destroy foreign invaders. Individual aspects of the immune response and their importance are considered separately.

Antigens

Molecules capable of stimulating an immune response (antibody production or lymphocyte stimulation) are called *antigens*.[4] Only a few drugs used by anesthesiologists, such as polypeptides (protamine) and other large macromolecules (dextrans), are complete antigens (Table 49-1). Most commonly used drugs are simple organic compounds of low molecular weight (approximately 1,000 daltons). For such a small molecule to become immunogenic, it must form a stable bond with circulating proteins or tissue micromolecules to result in a complete antigen (hapten-macromolecular complex). Small molecular weight substances such as drugs or drug metabolites that bind to host proteins or cell membranes to sensitize patients are called *haptens*. Haptens are not antigenic by themselves. Often, a reactive drug metabolite (i.e., penicilloyl derivative of penicillin) is believed to bind with macromolecules to become antigens, but for most drugs this has not been proved.

Thymus-Derived (T-Cell) and Bursa-Derived (B-Cell) Lymphocytes

The thymus of the fetus differentiates immature lymphocytes into thymus-derived cells (T cells). T cells have receptors that are activated by binding with foreign antigens and secrete mediators that regulate the immune response. The subpopulations of T cells that exist in humans include helper, suppressor, cytotoxic, and killer cells.[5] The two types of regulatory T cells are helper cells (OKT4) and suppressor cells (OKT8). Helper cells are important for key effector cell responses, whereas suppressor cells inhibit immune function. Infection of helper T cells with a retrovirus, the human immunodeficiency virus, produces a specific increase in the number of suppressor cells. Cytotoxic T cells destroy mycobacteria, fungi, and viruses. Other lymphocytes, called natural killer cells, do not need specific antigen stimulation to initiate their function. Both the cytotoxic T cells and natural killer cells participate in defense against tumor cells and in transplant rejection. T cells produce a spectrum of mediators that influence the response of other cell types involved in the recognition and destruction of foreign substances.

B cells represent a specific lymphocyte cell line that can differentiate into specific plasma cells that synthesize antibodies, a step controlled by both helper and suppressor T-cell lymphocytes.[5] B cells are also called bursa-derived cells because in birds, the bursa of Fabricius is important in producing cells responsible for antibody synthesis.

TABLE 49-1

AGENTS ADMINISTERED DURING ANESTHESIA THAT ACT AS ANTIGENS

■ HAPTENS	■ MACROMOLECULES
Penicillin and its derivatives	Blood products
Anesthetic drugs(?)	Chymopapain
	Colloid volume expanders
	Muscle relaxants
	Protamine
	Latex

Antibodies

2 Antibodies are specific proteins called *immunoglobulins* (Ig) that can recognize and bind to a specific antigen.[6] The basic structure of the antibody molecule is illustrated in Fig. 49-1. Each antibody has at least two heavy chains and two light chains that are bound together by disulfide bonds. The Fab fragment has the ability to bind antigen, and the Fc, or crystallizable, fragment is responsible for the unique biological properties of the different classes of immunoglobulins (cell binding and complement activation). Antibodies function as specific receptor molecules for immune cells and proteins. When antigen binds covalently to the Fab fragments, the antibody undergoes conformational changes to activate the Fc receptor. The results of antigen-antibody binding depend on the cell type, which causes a specific type of activation (i.e., lymphocyte proliferation and differentiation into antibody-secreting cells, mast cell degranulation, and complement activation).

Five major classes of antibodies occur in humans: IgG, IgA, IgM, IgD, and IgE. The heavy chain determines the structure and the function of each molecule. The basic properties of each antibody are listed in Table 49-2.

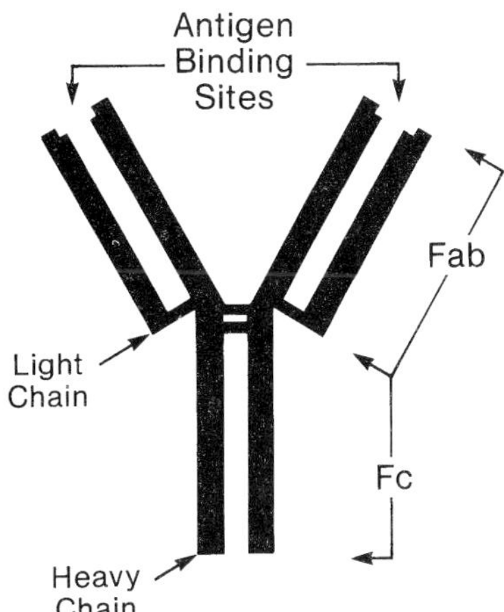

FIGURE 49-1. Basic structural configuration of the antibody molecule representing human immunoglobulin G (IgG). Immunoglobulins are composed of two heavy chains and two light chains bound by disulfide linkages (represented by *crossbars*). Papain cleaves the molecule into two Fab fragments and one Fc fragment. Antigen binding occurs on the Fab fragments, whereas the Fc segment is responsible for membrane binding or complement activation. (Reprinted with permission from Levy JH: Anaphylactic Reactions in Anesthesia and Intensive Care, 2nd ed. Boston, Butterworth-Heinemann, 1992.)

TABLE 49-2

BIOLOGICAL CHARACTERISTICS OF IMMUNOGLOBULINS

	IgG	IgM	IgA	IgE	IgD
Heavy chain	γ	μ	α	ϵ	δ
Molecular weight	160,000	900,000	170,000	188,000	184,000
Subclasses	1,2,3,4	1,2	1,2		
Serum concentration, mg/dL	6–14	0.5–1.5	1–3	$<-0.5 \times 10^3$	<0.1
Complement activation	All but IgG_4	+	–	–	–
Placental transfer	+	–	–	–	–
Serum half-life (days)	23	5	6	1–5	2–8
Cell binding	Mast cells (IgG_4) Neutrophils Lymphocytes Mononuclear cells Platelets	Lymphocytes		Mast cells Basophils Lymphocytes	Neutrophils Lymphocytes

Modified with permission from Levy JH: Anaphylactic Reactions in Anesthesia and Intensive Care, 2nd ed. Boston, Butterworth-Heinemann, 1992.

Effector Cells and Proteins of the Immune Response

Cells

Monocytes, neutrophils (polymorphonuclear leukocytes [PMNs]), and eosinophils represent important effector cells that migrate into areas of inflammation in response to specific chemotactic factors, including lymphokines, cytokines, and complement-derived mediators. The deposition of antibody or complement fragments on the surface of foreign cells is called *opsonization*, a process that facilitates the killing of foreign cells by effector cells. In addition, lymphokines and cytokines produce chemotaxis of other inflammatory cells in a manner described in the following sections.

Monocytes and Macrophages. Macrophages regulate immune responses by processing and presenting antigens to effect inflammatory, tumoricidal, and microbicidal functions. Macrophages arise from circulating monocytes or may be confined to specific organs such as the lung. They are recruited and activated in response to microorganisms or tissue injury. Macrophages ingest antigens before they interact with receptors on the lymphocyte surface to regulate their action. Macrophages synthesize mediators to facilitate both B-lymphocyte and T-lymphocyte responses.

Polymorphonuclear Leukocytes (Neutrophils). The first cells to appear in acute inflammatory reaction are neutrophils that contain acid hydrolases, neutral proteases, and lysosomes. Once activated, they produce hydroxyl radicals, superoxide, and hydrogen peroxide, which aid in microbial killing.

Eosinophils. The exact function of the eosinophil in host defense is unclear; however, inflammatory cells recruit eosinophils to accumulate at sites of parasitic infections, tumors, and allergic reactions.[1]

Basophils. Basophils comprise 0.5 to 1% of circulating granulocytes in the blood.[1] On the surface of basophils are IgE receptors, which function similarly to those on mast cells.

Mast Cells. Mast cells are important cells for immediate hypersensitivity responses. They are tissue fixed and located in the perivascular spaces of the skin, lung, and intestine.[1] On the surface of mast cells are IgE receptors, which bind to specific antigens. Once activated, these cells release physiologically active mediators important to immediate hypersensitivity responses (see IgE-Mediated Pathophysiology section under Anaphylactic Reactions). Mast cells can be activated by a series of both immune and nonimmune stimuli.

Proteins

3 **Cytokines/Interleukins.** Cytokines are inflammatory cell activators that are synthesized by macrophages to act as secondary messengers and activate endothelial cells and white cells.[7] Interleukin-1 and tumor necrosis factor are examples of cytokines considered to be important mediators of the biological responses to infection and other inflammatory reactions. Liberation of interleukin-1 and tumor necrosis factor produces fever, neuropeptide release, endothelial cell activation, increased adhesion molecule expression, neutrophil priming, hypotension, myocardial suppression, and a catabolic state.[7] The term *interleukin* was coined for a group of cytokines that promotes communication between and among ("inter") leukocytes ("leukin"). Interleukins are a group of different regulatory proteins that act to control many aspects of the immune and inflammatory responses. The interleukins are polypeptides synthesized in response to cellular activation; they produce their inflammatory effects by activating specific receptors on inflammatory cells and vasculature. T-cell lymphocytes influence the activity of other immunologic and nonimmunologic cells by producing an array of interleukins that they secrete. Different interleukins of this class have been isolated and characterized; they function as short-range or intracellular soluble mediators of the immune and inflammatory responses. The interleukin family of cytokines has been rapidly growing in number because of advances in gene cloning.

Complement. The primary humoral response to antigen and antibody binding is activation of the complement system.[8] The complement system consists of approximately 20 different proteins that bind to activated antibodies, other complement proteins, and cell membranes. The complement system is an important effector system of inflammation. Complement activation can be initiated by IgG or IgM binding to antigen, by plasmin through the classic pathway, by endotoxin, or by drugs through the alternate (properdin) pathway[8] (Fig. 49-2). Specific fragments released during complement activation include C3a, C4a, and C5a, which have important humoral and chemotactic properties (see NonIgE-Mediated Reactions section). The major function of the complement system is to recognize bacteria both directly and indirectly by attracting phagocytes (chemotaxis), as well as the increased adhesion of phagocytes to antigens (opsonization), and cell lysis by activation of the complete cascade.

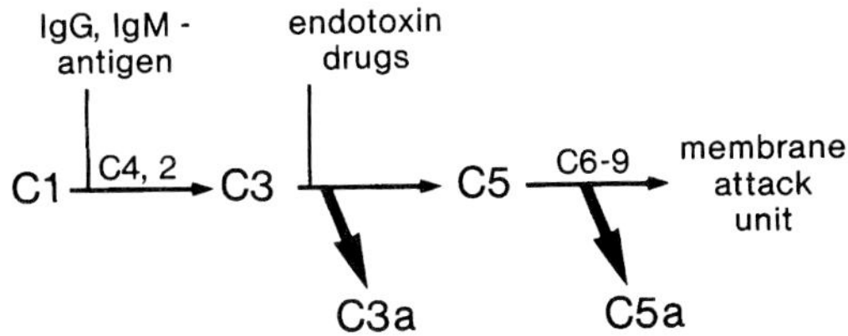

FIGURE 49-2. Diagram of complement activation. Complement system can be activated by either the classic pathway (IgG, IgM–antigen interaction) or the alternate pathway (endotoxin, drug interaction). Small peptide fragments of C3 and C5 called anaphylatoxins (C3a, C5a) that are released during activation are potent vasoactive mediators. Formation of the complete complement cascade produces a membrane attack unit that lyses cell walls and membranes. An inhibitor of the complement cascade, the C1 esterase inhibitor, ensures the complement system is turned off most of the time.

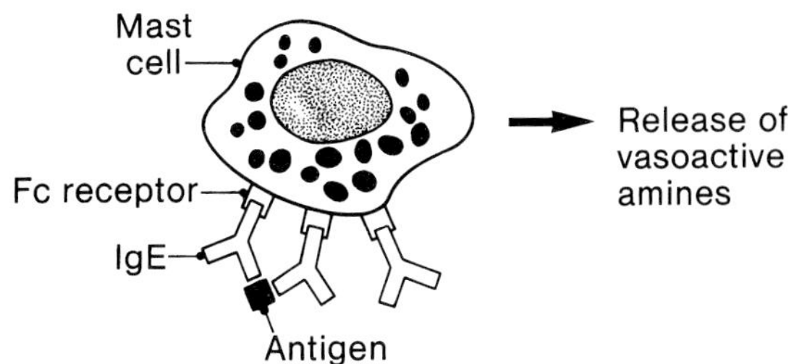

FIGURE 49-3. Type I immediate hypersensitivity reactions (anaphylaxis) involve IgE antibodies binding to mast cells or basophils by way of their Fc receptors. On encountering immunospecific antigens, the IgE becomes cross-linked, inducing degranulation, intracellular activation, and release of mediators. This reaction is independent of complement.

A series of inhibitors regulates activation to ensure regulation of the complement system. Hereditary (autosomal dominant) or acquired (associated with lymphoma, lymphosarcoma, chronic lymphatic leukemia, and macroglobulinemia) angioneurotic edema is an example of a deficiency in an inhibitor of the C1 complement system (C1 esterase deficiency). This syndrome is characterized by recurrent increased vascular permeability of specific subcutaneous and serosal tissues (angioedema), which produces laryngeal obstruction and respiratory and cardiovascular abnormalities after tissue trauma and surgery, or even without any obvious precipitating factor.[9] One of the important pathologic manifestations of complement activation is acute pulmonary vasoconstriction associated with protamine administration.[1]

Effects of Anesthesia on Immune Function

Anesthesia and surgery depress a spectrum of nonspecific host resistance mechanisms, including lymphocyte activation and phagocytosis.[6] Immune competence during surgery can be affected by direct and hormonal effects of anesthetic drugs, by
4 immunologic effects of other drugs used, by the surgery, by coincident infections, and by transfused blood products. Blood represents a complex spectrum of humoral and cellular elements that may alter immunomodulation to various antigens. Although multiple studies demonstrate in vitro changes of immune function, no studies have ever proved their importance.[6] Besides, such changes are likely of minor importance compared with the hormonal aspects of stress responses.

HYPERSENSITIVITY RESPONSES (ALLERGY)

Gell and Coombs[3] first described a scheme for classifying immune responses to understand specific diseases mediated by immunologic processes. The immune pathway functions as a protective mechanism, but can also react inappropriately to produce a hypersensitivity or allergic response. They defined four basic types of hypersensitivity, types I to IV. It is useful first to review all four mechanisms to understand the different immune reactions that occur in humans.

Type I Reactions

Type I reactions are anaphylactic or immediate-type hypersensitivity reactions (Fig. 49-3). Physiologically active mediators are released from mast cells and basophils after antigen binding to IgE antibodies on the membranes of these cells. Type I hypersensitivity reactions include anaphylaxis, extrinsic asthma, and allergic rhinitis.

Type II Reactions

Type II reactions are also known as antibody-dependent cell-mediated cytotoxic hypersensitivity or cytotoxic reactions (antibody-dependent cell-mediated cytotoxic) (Fig. 49-4). These reactions are mediated by either IgG or IgM antibodies directed against antigens on the surface of foreign cells. These antigens may be either integral cell membrane components (A or B blood group antigens in ABO incompatibility reactions) or haptens that absorb to the surface of a cell, stimulating the production of antihapten antibodies (autoimmune hemolytic anemia). The cell damage in type II reactions is produced by (1) direct cell lysis after complete complement cascade activation, (2) increased phagocytosis by macrophages, or (3) killer T-cell lymphocytes producing antibody-dependent cell-mediated cytotoxic effects. Examples of type II reactions in humans are ABO-incompatible transfusion reactions,

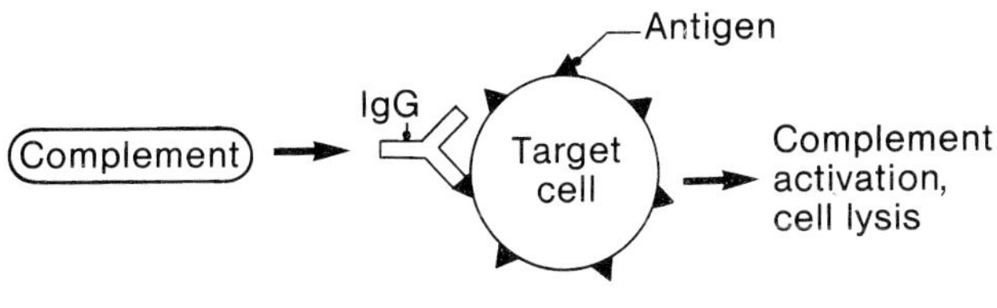

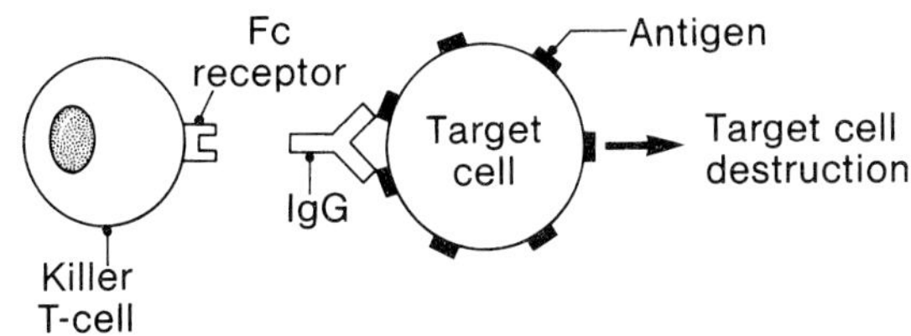

FIGURE 49-4. Type II or cytotoxic reactions. Antibody of an IgG or IgM class is directed against antigens on an individual's own cells (target cell). The antigens may be integral membrane components or foreign molecules that have been absorbed. This may lead to complement activation, including cell lysis (*upper figure*) or to cytotoxic action by killer T-cell lymphocytes (*lower figure*).

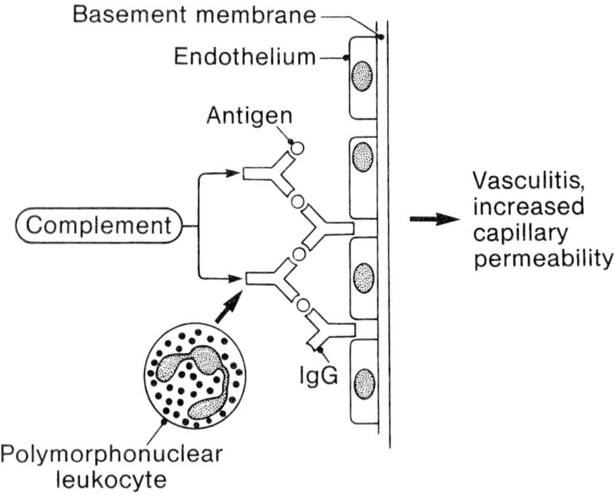

FIGURE 49-5. Type III immune complex reactions. Antibodies of an IgG or IgM type bind to the antigen in the soluble base and are subsequently deposited in the microvasculature. Complement is activated, resulting in chemotaxis and activation of polymorphonuclear leukocytes at the site of antigen-antibody complexes and subsequent tissue injury.

drug-induced immune hemolytic anemia, and heparin-induced thrombocytopenia.

Type III Reactions (Immune Complex Reactions)

Type III reactions result from circulating soluble antigens and antibodies that bind to form insoluble complexes that deposit in the microvasculature (Fig. 49-5). Complement is activated, and neutrophils are localized to the site of complement deposition to produce tissue damage. Type III reactions include classic serum sickness observed after snake antisera or antithymocyte globulin, and immune complex vascular injury, and may occur through mechanisms of protamine-mediated pulmonary vasoconstriction.[1]

Type IV Reactions (Delayed Hypersensitivity Reactions)

Type IV reactions result from the interactions of sensitized lymphocytes with specific antigens (Fig. 49-6). Delayed hypersensitivity reactions are mainly mononuclear, manifest in 18 to 24 hours, peak at 40 to 80 hours, and disappear in 72 to 96 hours. Antigen-lymphocyte binding produces lymphokine synthesis, lymphocyte proliferation, generation of cytotoxic T cells, and attracting macrophages and other inflammatory cells. Cytotoxic T cells are produced specifically to kill target cells that bear antigens identical with those that triggered the reaction. This form of immunity is important in tissue rejection, graft-versus-host reactions, contact dermatitis (e.g., poison ivy), and tuberculin immunity.

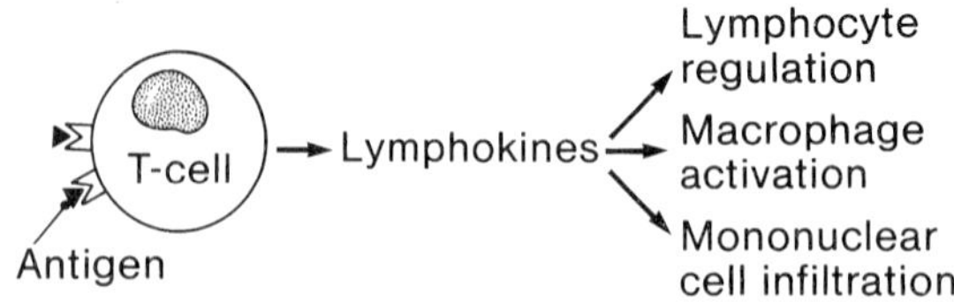

FIGURE 49-6. Type IV immune complex reactions (delayed hypersensitivity or cell-mediated immunity). Antigen binds to sensitized T-cell lymphocytes to release lymphokines after a second contact with the same antigen. This reaction is independent of circulating antibody or complement activation. Lymphokines induce inflammatory reactions and activate, as well as attract, macrophages and other mononuclear cells to produce delayed tissue injury.

Intraoperative Allergic Reactions

Intraoperative allergic reactions occur once in every 5,000 to 25,000 anesthetics, with a 3.4% mortality rate.[10,11] More than
5 90% of the allergic reactions evoked by intravenous drugs occur within 5 minutes of administration. In the anesthetized patient, the most common life-threatening manifestation of an allergic reaction is circulatory collapse, reflecting vasodilation with resulting decreased venous return (Table 49-3). The only manifestation of an allergic reaction may be refractory hypotension.[12] Portier and Richet first used the word *anaphylaxis* (from *ana*, "against," and *prophylaxis*, "protection") to describe the profound shock and resulting death that sometimes occurred in dogs immediately after a second challenge with a foreign antigen.[13] When life-threatening allergic reactions mediated by antibodies occur, they are defined as anaphylactic. Although the term *anaphylactoid* has been used in the past to describe nonimmunologic reactions, this term is now rarely used.[14]

ANAPHYLACTIC REACTIONS

IgE-Mediated Pathophysiology

Antigen binding to IgE antibodies initiates anaphylaxis (Fig. 49-7). Prior exposure to the antigen or to a substance of similar structure is needed to produce sensitization, although an allergic history may be unknown to the patient. On reexposure, binding of the antigen to bridge two immunospecific IgE antibodies found on the surfaces of mast cells and basophils releases stored mediators, including histamine, tryptase, and chemotactic factors.[15–17] Arachidonic acid metabolites (leukotrienes and prostaglandins), kinins, and cytokines are subsequently synthesized and released in response to cellular activation.[18] The released mediators produce a symptom complex of bronchospasm and upper airway edema in the respiratory system, vasodilation and increased capillary permeability in the cardiovascular system, and urticaria in the cutaneous system. Different mediators are released from mast cells and basophils after activation.

Chemical Mediators of Anaphylaxis

Histamine stimulates H_1, H_2, and H_3 receptors. H_1 receptor activation releases endothelium-derived relaxing factor (nitric oxide) from vascular endothelium, increases capillary permeability, and contracts airway and vascular smooth muscle.[1,19,20] H_2 receptor activation causes gastric secretion, inhibits mast cell activation, and contributes to vasodilation.[19] When injected into skin, histamine produces the classic wheal (increased capillary permeability producing tissue edema) and flare (cutaneous vasodilation) response in humans.[21] Histamine undergoes rapid metabolism in humans by the enzymes histamine

TABLE 49-3

RECOGNITION OF ANAPHYLAXIS DURING REGIONAL AND GENERAL ANESTHESIA

SYSTEMS	SYMPTOMS	SIGNS
Respiratory	Dyspnea Chest discomfort	Coughing Wheezing Sneezing Laryngeal edema Decreased pulmonary compliance Fulminant pulmonary edema Acute respiratory failure
Cardiovascular	Dizziness Malaise Retrosternal oppression	Disorientation Diaphoresis Loss of consciousness Hypotension Tachycardia Dysrhythmias Decreased systemic vascular resistance Cardiac arrest Pulmonary hypertension
Cutaneous	Itching Burning Tingling	Urticaria (hives) Flushing Periorbital edema Perioral edema

Reprinted with permission from Levy JH: Anaphylactic Reactions in Anesthesia and Intensive Care, 2nd ed. Boston, Butterworth-Heinemann, 1992.

N-methyltransferase and diamine oxidase found in endothelial cells.[1]

Peptide Mediators of Anaphylaxis

Factors are released from mast cells and basophils that cause granulocyte migration (chemotaxis) and collection at the site of the inflammatory stimulus.[18] Eosinophilic chemotactic factor of anaphylaxis (ECF-A) is a small molecular weight peptide chemotactic for eosinophils.[22] Although the exact role of ECF-A or the eosinophil in acute allergic response is unclear, eosinophils release enzymes that can inactivate histamine and leukotrienes.[18] In addition, a neutrophilic chemotactic factor is released that causes chemotaxis and activation.[18,23] Neutrophil

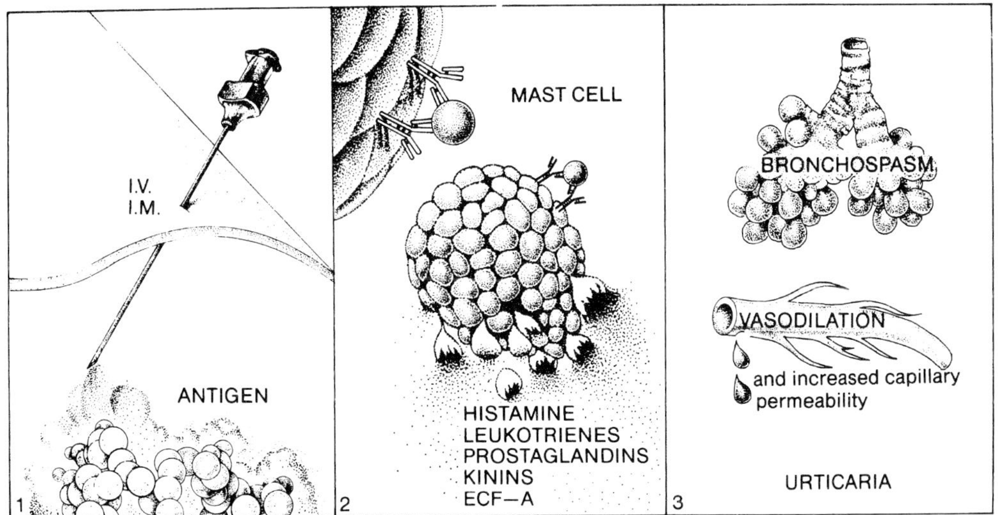

FIGURE 49-7. During anaphylaxis (type I immediate hypersensitivity reaction), (*1*) antigen enters a patient during anesthesia through a parenteral route. (*2*) It bridges two IgE antibodies on the surface of mast cells or basophils. In a calcium-dependent and energy-dependent process, cells release various substances—histamine, eosinophilic chemotactic factor of anaphylaxis, leukotrienes, prostaglandins, and kinins. (*3*) These released mediators produce the characteristic effects in the pulmonary, cardiovascular, and cutaneous systems. The most severe and life-threatening effects of the vasoactive mediators occur in the respiratory and cardiovascular systems. (Reprinted with permission from Levy JH: Identification and Treatment of Anaphylaxis: Mechanisms of Action and Strategies for Treatment Under General Anesthesia. Chicago, Smith Laboratories, 1983.)

activation may be responsible for recurrent manifestations of anaphylaxis.

Arachidonic Acid Metabolites

Leukotrienes and prostaglandins are both synthesized after mast cell activation from arachidonic acid metabolism of phospholipid cell membranes through either lipoxygenase or cyclooxygenase pathways.[24,25] The classic slow-reacting substance of anaphylaxis is a combination of leukotrienes C_4, D_4, and E_4.[25] Leukotrienes produce bronchoconstriction (more intense than that produced by histamine), increased capillary permeability, vasodilation, coronary vasoconstriction, and myocardial depression.[25] Prostaglandins are potent mast cell mediators that produce vasodilation, bronchospasm, pulmonary hypertension, and increased capillary permeability.[18,25] Prostaglandin D_2, the major metabolite of mast cells, produces bronchospasm and vasodilation.[25] Elevated plasma levels of thromboxane B_2 (the metabolite of thromboxane A_2), also a prostaglandin synthesized by mast cells as well as by PMNs, have been demonstrated after protamine reactions associated with pulmonary hypertension.[26,27]

Kinins

Small peptides called *kinins* are synthesized in mast cells and basophils to produce vasodilation, increased capillary permeability, and bronchoconstriction.[18,28] Kinins can stimulate vascular endothelium to release vasoactive factors, including prostacyclin, and endothelial-derived relaxing factors such as nitric oxide.[1]

Platelet-Activating Factor

Platelet-activating factor (PAF), an unstored lipid synthesized in activated human mast cells, is an extremely potent biological material, producing physiologic effects at concentrations as low as 10^{-10} M.[18] PAF aggregates and activates human platelets, and perhaps leukocytes, to release inflammatory products. PAF causes an intense wheal-and-flare response, smooth muscle contraction, and increased capillary permeability.[18]

Recognition of Anaphylaxis

The onset and severity of the reaction relate to the mediator's specific end-organ effects. Antigenic challenge in a sensitized individual usually produces immediate clinical manifestations of anaphylaxis, but the onset may be delayed 2 to 20 minutes.[29,30] The reaction may include some or all the symptoms and signs listed in Table 49-3. Individuals vary in their manifestations and course of anaphylaxis.[31,32] A spectrum of reactions exists, ranging from minor clinical changes to the full-blown syndrome leading to death.[31,33] The enigma of anaphylaxis lies in the unpredictability of happening, the severity of the attack, and the lack of a prior allergic history.

NonIgE-Mediated Reactions

Other immunologic and nonimmunologic mechanisms release many of the mediators previously discussed independent of IgE, creating a clinical syndrome identical with anaphylaxis. Specific pathways important in producing the same clinical manifestations are considered later.

Complement Activation

Complement activation follows both immunologic (antibody-mediated; i.e., classic pathway) or nonimmunologic (alternative) pathways to include a series of multimolecular, self-assembling proteins that release biologically active complement fragments of C3 and C5.[10,34] C3a and C5a are called *anaphylatoxins* because they release histamine from mast cells and basophils, contract smooth muscle, increase capillary permeability, and cause interleukin synthesis (Table 49-4). C5a interacts with specific high-affinity receptors on PMNs and platelets, causing leukocyte chemotaxis, aggregation, and activation.[35] Aggregated leukocytes embolize to various organs, producing microvascular occlusion and liberation of inflammatory products such as arachidonic acid metabolites, oxygen free radicals, and lysosomal enzymes (Fig. 49-8). Antibodies of the IgG class directed against antigenic determinants or granulocyte surfaces can also produce leukocyte aggregation.[36] These antibodies are called *leukoagglutinins*. Investigators have associated complement activation and PMN aggregation in producing the clinical expression of transfusion reactions,[36,37] pulmonary vasoconstriction after protamine reactions,[27] adult respiratory distress syndrome,[36] and septic shock.[38]

TABLE 49-4

BIOLOGICAL EFFECTS OF ANAPHYLATOXINS

BIOLOGICAL EFFECTS	C32	C52
Histamine release	+	+
Smooth muscle contraction	+	+
Increased vascular permeability	+	+
Chemotaxis		+
Leukocyte and platelet aggregation		+
Interleukin release	+	+

Nonimmunologic Release of Histamine

6 Many diverse molecules administered during the perioperative period release histamine in a dose-dependent, nonimmunologic fashion[39–43] (Table 49-5 and Fig. 49-9). The mechanisms involved in nonimmunologic histamine release are not well understood, but represent selective mast cell and not basophil activation[43,44] (Fig. 49-10). Human cutaneous mast cells are the only cell population that releases histamine in response to both drugs and endogenous stimuli (neuropeptides).[1] Nonimmunologic histamine release may involve mast cell activation through specific cell-signaling activation[40] (Fig. 49-11). Different molecular structures release histamine in humans, which suggests that different mechanisms are involved. Histamine release is not dependent on the μ receptor because

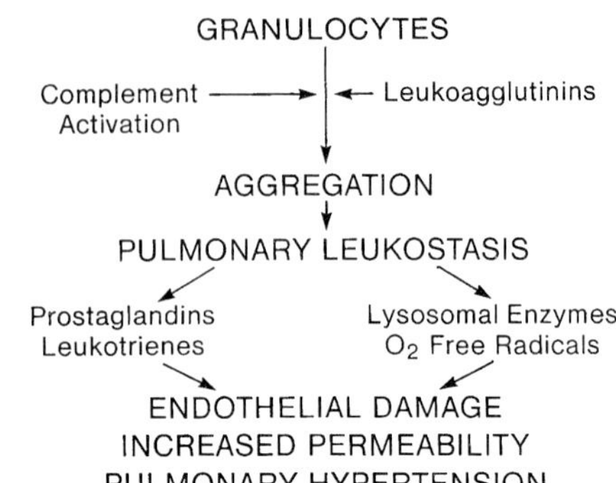

FIGURE 49-8. Sequence of events producing granulocyte aggregation, pulmonary leukostasis, and cardiopulmonary dysfunction. (Reprinted from Levy JH: Anaphylactic Reactions in Anesthesia and Intensive Care, 2nd ed. Boston, Butterworth-Heinemann, 1992.)

TABLE 49-5

DRUGS CAPABLE OF NONIMMUNOLOGIC HISTAMINE RELEASE

Antibiotics (vancomycin, pentamidine)
Basic compounds
Hyperosmotic agents
Muscle relaxants (*d*-tubocurarine, metocurine, atracurium, mivacurium, doxacurium)
Opioids (morphine, meperidine, codeine)
Thiobarbiturates

fentanyl and sufentanil, the most potent μ receptor agonists clinically available, do not release histamine in human skin.[39] Although the newer muscle relaxants may be more potent at the neuromuscular junction, drugs that are mast cell degranulators are equally capable of releasing histamine.[39,40] On an equimolar basis, atracurium is as potent as *d*-tubocurarine or metocurine in its ability to degranulate mast cells.[40] Newer aminosteroidal agents such as rocuronium and rapacuronium at clinically recommended doses have minimal effects on histamine release.[44,45]

Antihistamine pretreatment before administration of drugs that are known to release histamine in humans does not inhibit histamine release; rather, the antihistamines compete with histamine at the receptor and may attenuate decreases in systemic vascular resistance.[1] However, the effect of any drug on systemic vascular resistance may depend on other factors in addition to histamine release.[46,47]

Treatment Plan

7 A plan for treating anaphylactic reactions must be established before the event. Airway maintenance, 100% oxygen administration, intravascular volume expansion, and epinephrine are essential to treat the hypotension and hypoxia that result from vasodilation, increased capillary permeability, and bronchospasm.[1] Table 49-6 lists a protocol for managing anaphylaxis during general anesthesia, with representative doses for a 70-kg adult. The treatment plan is the same for life-threatening anaphylactic or anaphylactoid reactions. Therapy must be titrated to needed effects with careful monitoring.[1] Severe reactions need aggressive therapy and may be protracted, with persistent hypotension, pulmonary hypertension, lower respiratory obstruction, or laryngeal obstruction that may persist 5 to 32 hours despite vigorous therapy.[48] All patients who have experienced an anaphylactic reaction should be admitted to an intensive care unit for 24 hours of monitoring because manifestations may recur after successful treatment.

Initial Therapy

Although it may not be possible to stop the administration of antigen, limiting antigen administration may prevent further mast cell and basophil activation.

Maintain Airway and Administer 100% Oxygen. Profound ventilation–perfusion abnormalities producing hypoxemia can occur with anaphylactic reactions.[49] Always administer 100% oxygen with ventilatory support as needed. Arterial blood gas values may be useful to follow during resuscitation.

Discontinue All Anesthetic Drugs. Inhalational anesthetic drugs are not the bronchodilators of choice in treating bronchospasm after anaphylaxis, especially during hypotension. These drugs interfere with the body's compensatory response to cardiovascular collapse, and halothane sensitizes the myocardium to epinephrine.

Provide Volume Expansion. Hypovolemia rapidly follows during anaphylactic shock.[50] Fisher[50] reported up to 40% loss of intravascular fluid into the interstitial space during reactions. Therefore, volume expansion is important with epinephrine in correcting the acute hypotension. Initially, 2 to 4 L of lactated Ringer's solution, or colloid or normal saline, should be administered, keeping in mind that an additional 25 to 50 mL/kg may be necessary if hypotension persists. Refractory hypotension after volume and epinephrine administration requires additional hemodynamic monitoring. The use of transesophageal echocardiography for rapid assessment of intraventricular volume and ventricular function, and to determine other occult causes of acute cardiovascular dysfunction, can be important for accurate assessment of intravascular volume and guidance of rational therapeutic interventions. Fulminant noncardiogenic pulmonary edema with loss of intravascular volume can occur after anaphylaxis. This condition requires intravascular volume repletion with careful hemodynamic monitoring until the capillary defect improves. Colloid volume expansion has not proved to be more effective

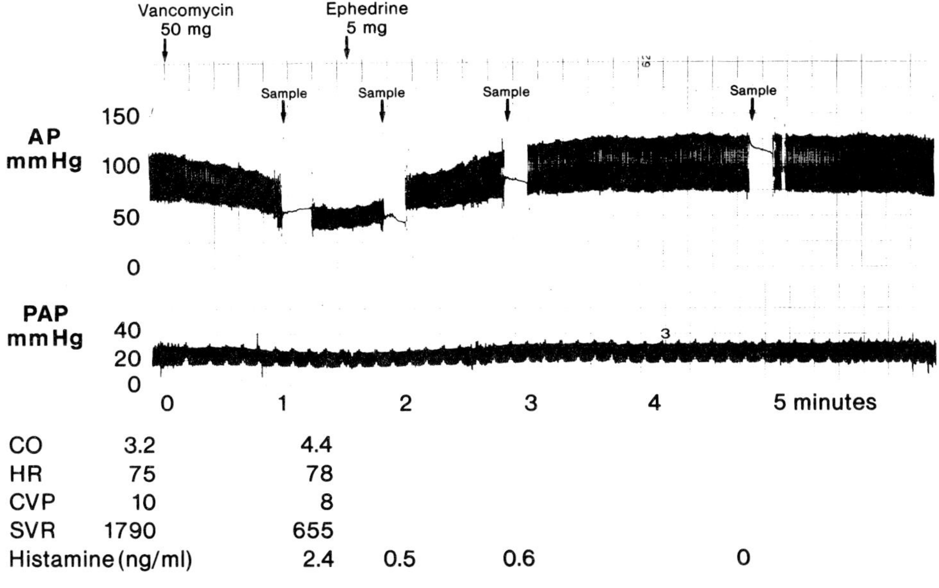

FIGURE 49-9. Example of an anaphylactic reaction after rapid vancomycin administration in a patient. Hypotension is associated with an increased cardiac output and decreased calculated systemic vascular resistance. Plasma histamine levels 1 min after the vancomycin administration were 2.4 ng/mL and subsequently decreased to zero. The patient was given ephedrine, 5 mg, and blood pressure returned to baseline values. (Reprinted from Levy JH, Kettlekamp N, Goertz P *et al*: Histamine release by vancomycin: A mechanism for hypotension in man. Anesthesiology 67:122, 1987.)

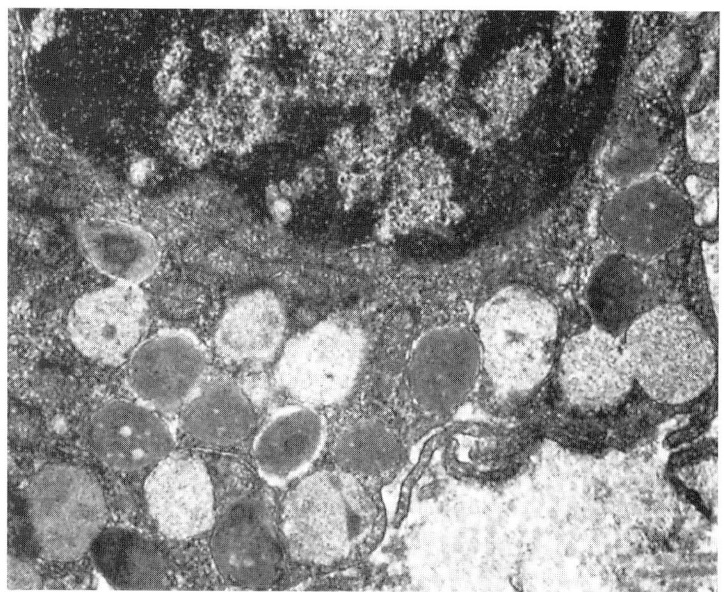

FIGURE 49-10. Electron micrograph of human cutaneous mast cell after injection of dynorphin, a κ opioid agonist. The cell outline is rounded and most of the cytoplasmic granules are swollen, exhibiting varying degrees of decreased electron density and flocculence consistent with ongoing degranulation. The perigranular membranes of the adjacent granules at the periphery of the cell are fused to each other and to plasma membrane. Original magnification ×72,000. (Reprinted from Casale TB, Bowman S, Kaliner M: Induction of human cutaneous mast cell degranulation by opiates and endogenous opioid peptides: Evidence for opiate and nonopiate receptor participation. J Allergy Clin Immunol 73:778, 1984.)

than crystalloid volume expansion for treating anaphylactic shock.

Administer Epinephrine. Epinephrine is the drug of choice when resuscitating patients during anaphylactic shock. α-Adrenergic effects vasoconstrict to reverse hypotension; β_2 receptor stimulation bronchodilates and inhibits mediator release by increasing cyclic adenosine monophosphate (cAMP) in mast cells and basophils.[32] The route of epinephrine administration and the dose depend on the patient's condition. Rapid and timely intervention is important when treating anaphylaxis. Furthermore, patients under general anesthesia may have altered sympathoadrenergic responses to acute anaphylactic shock, whereas the patient under spinal or epidural anesthesia may be partially sympathectomized and may need even larger doses of catecholamines.[51]

In hypotensive patients, 5- to 10-μg boluses of epinephrine should be administered intravenously and incrementally titrated to restore blood pressure. (This dose of epinephrine can be obtained with 0.05 to 0.1 mL of a 1:10,000 dilution [100 μg/mL] or by mixing 2 mg epinephrine with

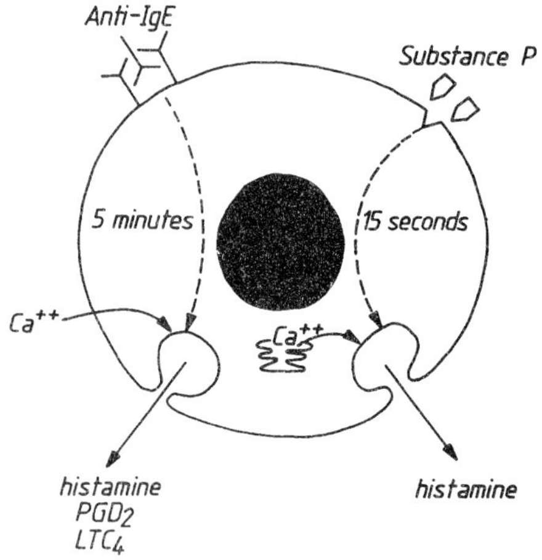

FIGURE 49-11. Different mechanisms of mediator release from human cutaneous mast cells stimulated immunologically by anti-IgE and by nonimmunologic stimuli with substance P. Anti-IgE stimulation, like antigen stimulation, initiates the release of histamine, prostaglandin D_2 (PGD_2), or leukotriene C_4 (LTC_4) by a mechanism that takes 5 minutes to reach completion and requires the influx of intracellular calcium. Nonimmunologic activation with drugs or substance P releases histamine but not PGD_2 or LTC_4 by a mechanism that is complete within 15 seconds and uses calcium mobilized from intracellular sources. (Reprinted from Caulfield JP, El-Lati S, Thomas G, Church MK: Dissociated human foreskin mast cells degranulate in response to anti-IgE and substance P. Lab Invest 63:502, 1990.)

TABLE 49-6

MANAGEMENT OF ANAPHYLAXIS DURING GENERAL ANESTHESIA

■ INITIAL THERAPY

1. Stop administration of antigen
2. Maintain airway and administer 100% O_2
3. Discontinue all anesthetic agents
4. Start intravascular volume expansion (2–4 L of crystalloid/colloid with hypotension)
5. Give epinephrine (5–10 μg IV bolus with hypotension, titrate as needed; 0.1–1.0 mg IV with cardiovascular collapse)

■ SECONDARY TREATMENT

1. Antihistamines (0.5–1 mg/kg diphenhydramine)
2. Catecholamine infusions (starting doses: epinephrine, 4–8 μg/min; norepinephrine, 4–8 μg/min; or isoproterenol, 0.5–1 μg/min as a drip; titrated to desired effects)
3. Aminophylline (5–6 mg/kg over 20 min with persistent bronchospasm)
4. Corticosteroids (0.25–1 g hydrocortisone; alternatively, 1–2 g methylprednisolone)[a]
5. Sodium bicarbonate (0.5–1 mEq/kg with persistent hypotension or acidosis)
6. Airway evaluation (before extubation)

IV, intravenous(ly).

[a] Methylprednisolone may be the drug of choice if the reaction is suspected to be mediated by complement.

Reprinted with permission from Levy JH: Anaphylactic Reactions in Anesthesia and Intensive Care, 2nd ed, p 162. Boston, Butterworth-Heinemann, 1992.

250 mL of fluid to yield an 8 μg/mL solution.) Additional volume and incrementally increased doses of epinephrine should be administered until hypotension is corrected. Although infusion is an ideal method of administering epinephrine, it is usually impossible to infuse the drug through peripheral intravenous access lines during acute volume resuscitation. With cardiovascular collapse, full intravenous cardiopulmonary resuscitative doses of epinephrine, 0.1 to 1.0 mg, should be administered and repeated until hemodynamic stability resumes. Patients with laryngeal edema without hypotension should receive subcutaneous epinephrine. Epinephrine should not be administered IV to patients with normal blood pressures.[52]

Secondary Treatment

Antihistamines. Because H_1 receptors mediate many of the adverse effects of histamine, the intravenous administration of 0.5 to 1 mg/kg of an H_1 antagonist such as diphenhydramine may be useful in treating acute anaphylaxis. Antihistamines do not inhibit anaphylactic reactions or histamine release, but compete with histamine at receptor sites. H_1 antagonists are indicated in all forms of anaphylaxis. The H_1 antagonists available for parenteral administration may have antidopaminergic effects and should be given slowly to prevent precipitous hypotension in potentially hypovolemic patients.[1] The indications for administering an H_2 antagonist once anaphylaxis has occurred remain unclear.

Catecholamines. Epinephrine infusions may be useful in patients with persistent hypotension or bronchospasm after initial resuscitation.[1] Epinephrine infusions should be started at 0.05 to 0.1 μg/kg/min (5 to 10 μg/min) and titrated to correct hypotension. Norepinephrine infusions may be needed in patients with refractory hypotension due to decreased systemic vascular resistance. It may be started at 0.05 to 0.1 μg/kg/min (5 to 10 μg/min) and adjusted to correct hypotension.

Aminophylline. Aminophylline, a nonspecific phosphodiesterase inhibitor, bronchodilates and decreases histamine release from mast cells or basophils in part by increasing intracellular cAMP. In addition, it increases right and left ventricular contractility, and decreases pulmonary vascular resistance. Aminophylline should be considered in patients with persistent bronchospasm and hemodynamic stability, although β_2-adrenergic drugs are the first-line drugs of choice. An intravenous loading dose of 5 to 6 mg/kg of aminophylline given over 20 minutes should be followed by an infusion of 0.5 to 0.9 mg/kg/hr.[1]

Corticosteroids. Corticosteroids have a series of anti-inflammatory effects mediated by multiple mechanisms, including altering the activation and migration of other inflammatory cells (i.e., PMNs) after an acute reaction.[53,54] Corticosteroids may require 12 to 24 hours to work and, despite their unproven usefulness in treating acute reactions, they are often administered as adjuncts to therapy when refractory bronchospasm or refractory shock occurs after resuscitative therapy.[55] Although the exact corticosteroid dose and preparation are unclear, investigators have recommended 0.25 to 1 g intravenously of hydrocortisone in IgE-mediated reactions. Alternately, 1 to 2 g of methylprednisolone (30 to 35 mg/kg) intravenously may be useful in reactions believed to be complement mediated, such as catastrophic pulmonary vasoconstriction after protamine transfusion reactions.[56] Administering corticosteroids after an anaphylactic reaction may also be important in attenuating the late-phase reactions reported to occur 12 to 24 hours after anaphylaxis.[48]

Bicarbonate. Acidosis develops rapidly in patients with persistent hypotension. This diminishes the effect of epinephrine on the heart and systemic vasculature. Therefore, with refractory hypotension or acidemia, sodium bicarbonate, 0.5 to 1 mEq/kg, may be given and repeated every 5 minutes or as dictated by arterial blood gas values.

Airway Evaluation. Because profound laryngeal edema can occur, the airway should be evaluated before extubation of the trachea.[29] Persistent facial edema suggests airway edema. The trachea of these patients should remain intubated until the edema subsides. Developing a significant air leak after endotracheal tube cuff deflation and before extubation of the trachea is useful in assessing airway patency. If there is any question of airway edema, direct laryngoscopy should be performed before the trachea is extubated.

Refractory Hypotension. Based on the efficacy of arginine vasopressin in vasodilatory shock, it should also be considered in therapy of anaphylactic shock not responding to therapy. Vasopressin may attenuate pathologic-induced vasodilation. Further, additional monitoring, including echocardiography and preferably transesophageal, should be considered in patients with refractory hypotension to better evaluate cardiac function or hypovolemia.

PERIOPERATIVE MANAGEMENT OF THE PATIENT WITH ALLERGIES

Allergic drug reactions account for 6 to 10% of all adverse reactions.[57] DeSwarte[58] suggested that the risk of an allergic drug reaction occurring is approximately 1 to 3% for most drugs, and that around 5% of adults in the United States may be allergic to one or more drugs. Unfortunately, patients often refer to adverse drug effects as being allergic in nature. For example, opioid administration can produce nausea, vomiting, or even local release of histamine along the vein of administration. Patients will say they are "allergic" to a specific drug when in fact their adverse reaction is independent of allergy. Approximately 15% of adults in the United States believe they are allergic to specific medication(s) and therefore may be denied treatment with an indicated drug. To understand allergic reactions, the spectrum of adverse reactions to drugs needs to be considered.

Predictable adverse drug reactions account for approximately 80% of adverse drug effects. They are often dose dependent, related to known pharmacologic actions of the drug, and typically occur in normal patients. Most serious, predictable adverse drug reactions are toxic and are directly related to the amount of drug in the body (overdosage) or to an inadvertent route of administration (e.g., lidocaine-induced seizures or cardiovascular collapse). Side effects are the most common adverse drug reactions and are undesirable pharmacologic actions of the drugs occurring at usual prescribed dosages. Most anesthetic drugs present multiple side effects that can produce precipitous hypotension. For example, morphine dilates the venous capacitance bed, thereby decreasing preload; releases histamine from cutaneous mast cells, thereby producing arterial and venous dilation; slows the heart rate; and decreases sympathetic tone. However, the net effects of morphine on blood pressure and myocardial function depend on the patient's blood volume, sympathetic tone, and ventricular function. Hypotension rapidly develops in a volume-depleted trauma patient in pain who is given morphine. Drug interactions also represent important predictable adverse drug reactions. Intravenous fentanyl administration to a patient who has just received intravenous benzodiazepines, or other sedative-hypnotic drugs may produce precipitous hypotension that results from decreased sympathetic tone.[59] This represents a dose-dependent, predictable adverse drug reaction that is independent of allergy.

Unpredictable adverse drug reactions are usually dose independent and usually not related to the drug's pharmacologic actions, but are often related to the immunologic response (allergy) of the individual. On occasion, adverse reactions can be related to genetic differences (i.e., idiosyncratic) in a susceptible individual who has an isolated genetic enzyme deficiency. In most allergic drug reactions, an immunologic mechanism is present or, more often, presumed. Providing that the initiating event involves a reaction between the drug or drug metabolites with drug-specific antibodies or sensitized T lymphocytes is often impractical. In the absence of direct immunologic evidence, criteria that may be helpful in distinguishing an allergic reaction from other adverse reactions include the following: allergic reactions occur in only a small percentage of patients receiving the drug, and the clinical manifestations do not resemble known pharmacologic actions. In the absence of prior drug exposure, allergic symptoms rarely appear after less than 1 week of continuous treatment. After sensitization, the reaction develops rapidly on reexposure to the drug. In general, drugs that have been administered without complications for several months or longer are rarely responsible for producing drug allergy. The time span between exposure to the drug and noticed manifestations is often the most vital information in determining which drugs administered were the cause of a suspected allergic reaction.

Although the reaction may produce a life-threatening response in the cardiopulmonary system (anaphylaxis), a variety of cutaneous manifestations, fever, and pulmonary reactions have been attributed to drug hypersensitivity. Usually, the reaction may be reproduced by very small doses of the suspected drug or other agents possessing similar or cross-reacting chemical structures. On occasion, drug-specific antibodies or lymphocytes have been identified that react with the suspected drug, although the relationship is seldom diagnostically useful in practice. Even when an immune response to a drug is demonstrated, it may not be associated with a clinical allergic reaction. As with adverse drug reactions in general, the reaction usually subsides within several days of discontinuation of the drug.

TABLE 49-7

AGENTS IMPLICATED IN ALLERGIC REACTIONS DURING ANESTHESIA

■ ANESTHETIC AGENTS
Induction agents (cremophor-solubilized drugs, barbiturates, etomidate, propofol)
Local anesthetics (para-aminobenzoic ester agents)
Muscle relaxants (succinylcholine, gallamine, pancuronium, *d*-tubocurarine, metocurine, atracurium, vecuronium, mivacurium, doxacurium)
Opioids (meperidine, morphine, fentanyl)
■ OTHER AGENTS
Antibiotics (cephalosporins, penicillin, sulfonamides, vancomycin)
Aprotinin
Blood products (whole blood, packed cells, fresh frozen plasma, platelets, cryoprecipitate, fibrinin glue, gamma globulin)
Bone cement
Chymopapain
Corticosteriods
Cyclosporin
Drug additives (preservatives)
Furosemide
Insulin
Mannitol
Methylmethacrylate
Nonsteroidal anti-inflammatory drugs
Protamine
Radiocontrast dye
Latex (natural rubber)
Streptokinase
Vascular graft material
Vitamin K
Colloid volume expanders (dextrans, protein fractions, albumin, hydroxyethyl starch)

Reprinted with permission from Levy JH: Anaphylactic Reactions in Anesthesia and Intensive Care, 2nd ed. Boston, Butterworth-Heinemann, 1992.

Immunologic Mechanisms of Drug Allergy

Different immunologic responses to any antigen can occur. Drugs have been associated with all the immunologic mechanisms proposed by Gell and Coombs.[3] Although more than one mechanism may contribute to a particular reaction, any one can occur. Penicillin may produce different reactions in different patients or a spectrum of reactions in the same patient. In one patient, penicillin can produce anaphylaxis (type I reaction), hemolytic anemia (type II reaction), serum sickness (type III reaction), and contact dermatitis (type IV reaction).[58] Therefore, any one antigen has the ability to produce a diffuse spectrum of allergic responses in humans. Why some patients have localized rashes or angioneurotic edema in response to penicillin whereas others sustain complete cardiopulmonary collapse is unknown. Most anesthetic drugs and agents administered perioperatively have been reported to produce anaphylactic reactions[31,39–45,60–81] (Table 49-7). Muscle relaxants are the most common drugs responsible for evoking intraoperative allergic reactions.[67] In this regard, there is cross-sensitivity between succinylcholine and the nondepolarizing muscle relaxants. Unexplained intraoperative cardiovascular collapse has been attributed to anaphylaxis triggered by latex (natural rubber), and certain patients, including those with a history of spina bifida, are at a greater risk for reactions.[1,68] Even vascular graft material has been reported as a cause of intraoperative allergic reactions.[69]

Life-threatening allergic reactions are more likely to occur in patients with a history of allergy, atopy, or asthma. Nevertheless, because the incidence is low, the history is not a reliable predictor that an allergic reaction will occur and does not mandate that such patients should be investigated or pretreated, or that specific drugs be selected or avoided.[60] Although different mechanisms have been proposed, no one theory has been proved.[1] The drugs and foreign substances listed in Table 49-7 may have both immunologic and nonimmunologic mechanisms for adverse drug reactions in humans.

Evaluation of Patients With Allergic Reactions

Identifying the drug responsible for a suspected allergic reaction still depends on circumstantial evidence indicating the temporal sequence of drug administration. Conventional in vivo and in vitro methods of diagnosing allergic reactions to most anesthetic drugs are unavailable or not applicable. The most important factor in diagnosis is the awareness of the physician that an untoward event may be related to a drug the patient received. The physician must always be aware of the capacity of any drug to produce an allergic reaction. The history is important when evaluating whether an adverse drug reaction is allergic and whether the drug can be readministered. Although a prior allergic reaction to the drug in question is important, this is rarely the case. Direct challenge of a patient with a test dose of drug is the only way to establish reaction, but this is potentially hazardous and not recommended. Although the anesthesiologist commonly gives small test doses of anesthetic drugs, these are pharmacologic test doses and have nothing to do with immunologic dosages. The demonstration of drug-specific IgE antibodies is accepted as evidence the patient may be at risk for anaphylaxis if the drug is administered.[58] Different clinical tests are available to confirm or diagnose drug allergy; several are considered in the following section.

Testing for Allergy

8 After an anaphylactoid reaction, it is important to identify the causative agent to prevent readministration. When one particular drug has been administered and there is a clear correlation between the time of administration and the occurrence of a reaction, testing may be unnecessary, and general avoidance of the drug should be instituted. However, when patients have simultaneously received multiple drugs (e.g., an opioid, muscle relaxant, hypnotic, and antibiotic), it is often difficult to prove which particular drug caused the reaction. Further, the reaction might have been caused by the vehicle or by one of the preservatives. For patients who want to know which drug was responsible and for patients scheduled for subsequent procedures, some degree of allergy evaluation should be undertaken to evaluate the drug at risk. Unfortunately, few *laboratory* tests exist for anesthetic drugs; therefore, the available allergy tests are discussed.

Leukocyte Histamine Release. Leukocyte histamine is performed by incubating the patient's leukocytes with the offending drug and measuring histamine release as a marker for basophil activation, although false-positive results can occur.[31] This test is not easy to perform, although variations allow the use of whole blood instead of isolated PMNs, and is generally not available.[76,82]

Radioallergosorbent Test. The radioallergosorbent test (RAST) allows *laboratory* detection of specific IgE directed toward particular antigens.[83] In this test, antigens are linked to insoluble material to make an immunoabsorbent.[83,84] When incubated with the serum in question, antibodies of different classes directed toward the antigen bind to it. After washing, the antigen-antibody complex on the immunoabsorbent is incubated with radiolabeled antibodies directed against human IgE, and counted in a scintillation counter. The concentration of specific IgE in the patient's serum directed toward the allergen is measured. The RAST is more quantitative than skin tests and avoids the potential of reexposure.[84] RAST testing has been used to detect the presence of antibodies to meperidine,[49] succinylcholine,[85] and thiopental.[86] Two major limitations to this test include the commercial availability of the drug prepared as an antigen and false-positive test results in patients with high IgE levels.[87]

Enzyme-Linked Immunosorbent Assay. The enzyme-linked immunosorbent assay (ELISA) measures antigen-specific antibodies. The basis of the ELISA is similar to that of the RAST; however, immunospecific IgE directed against the antigen in question is determined by the addition of an anti-IgE coupled to an enzyme such as peroxidase that acts as a chromogen.[5] A colorless substrate is acted on by peroxidase to produce a colored byproduct. The ELISA has been used to prove IgE antibodies to chymopapain and protamine, and has been developed to screen for other antibodies to diverse agents.

Intradermal Testing (Skin Testing). Skin testing is the method most often used in patients after anaphylactic reaction to anesthetic drugs after the history has suggested the relevant antigens for testing.[88,89] Within minutes after antigen introduction, histamine released from cutaneous mast cells causes vasodilation (flare) and localized edema from increased vascular permeability (wheal). Fisher[67,88] suggested that this is a simple, safe, and useful method of establishing a diagnosis in most cases of anaphylactic reactions occurring in the perioperative period. If the strict protocols established by Fisher[88] are used, intradermal reactions are helpful. Intradermal testing is of no value in reactions to contrast media or colloid volume expanders. Cross-sensitivity between drugs of similar structures can often be evaluated based on skin testing. Skin testing to local anesthetics is considered a direct challenge or provocative dose testing.[90] Local anesthetic drugs are injected in increasing quantities under controlled circumstances. This testing decides if the person can safely receive amide derivatives (e.g., lidocaine) and can also be used to decide if the person is sensitive to the paraaminobenzoic ester agents (e.g., procaine, tetracaine).

Agents Implicated in Allergic Reactions

Multiple agents, including antibiotics, induction agents, muscle relaxants, nonsteroidal anti-inflammatory drugs, protamine, colloid volume expanders, and blood products, are the etiologic agents often responsible for anaphylaxis in surgical patients.[1] However, any agent the patient receives as an injection, infusion, or environmental antigen has the potential to produce an allergic reaction.[1] Almost everything has been reported to produce an allergic reaction at some time, but usually from a case report or small series. The agents most often implicated include antibiotics, blood products, colloid volume expanders, latex, polypeptides, and NMBAs. If patients are allergic to a muscle relaxant, there is a potential for cross-reactivity because of the similarity of the active site, a quaternary ammonium molecule, among the different types of relaxants, and alternatives cannot be chosen without some degree of immunologic testing. Because of the ubiquity of latex as a perioperative environmental antigen, latex allergy is considered separately.

Latex Allergy

For the anesthesiologist, latex represents an environmental agent often implicated as an important cause of perioperative anaphylaxis.[91–99] Latex is the milky sap derived from the tree *Hevea brasiliensis* to which multiple agents, including preservatives, accelerators, and antioxidants are added to make the final rubber product. Latex is present in a variety of different products. In March 1991, the U.S. Food and Drug Administration alerted health care professionals about the potential of severe allergic reactions to medical devices made of latex. The first case of an allergic reaction because of latex was reported in 1979 and was manifested by contact urticaria. In 1989, the first reports of intraoperative anaphylaxis due to latex were reported.

9 Health care workers and children with spina bifida, urogenital abnormalities, or certain food allergies have also been recognized as people at increased risk for anaphylaxis to latex.[91–99] Brown et al[95] reported a 24% incidence of irritant or contact dermatitis and a 12.5% incidence of latex-specific IgE positivity in anesthesiologists. Of this group, 10% were clinically asymptomatic, although IgE positive. A history of atopy was also a significant risk factor for latex sensitization. Brown et al[95] suggested that these people are in their early stages of sensitization and perhaps, by avoiding latex exposure, their progression to symptomatic disease can be prevented. Patients allergic to bananas, avocados, and kiwis have also been reported to have antibodies that cross-react with latex.[96,97] Multiple attempts are being made to reduce latex exposure to both health care workers and patients. If latex allergy occurs, then strict avoidance of latex from gloves and other sources needs to be considered, following recommendations as reported by Holzman.[91]

Because latex is such a common environmental antigen, this represents a daunting task.

More important, anesthesiologists must be prepared to treat the life-threatening cardiopulmonary collapse that occurs after anaphylaxis, as previously discussed. The most important preventive therapy is to avoid antigen exposure; although clinicians have used pretreatment with antihistamine (diphenhydramine and cimetidine) and corticosteroids, there are no data in the literature to suggest that pretreatment prevents anaphylaxis or decreases its severity.[1] Two patients in a series reported by Gold et al[93] were pretreated, yet still had life-threatening reactions to latex. Patients in whom latex allergy is suspected should be referred to an allergist for appropriate evaluation and potential in vitro testing (RAST) for definitive diagnosis. When this is not possible, patients should be treated as if they were latex allergic, and the antigen avoided. Patients with a documented history of latex allergy should wear Medic Alert bracelets.

Muscle Relaxants

NMBAs have several unique molecular features that make them potential allergens. All NMBAs are functionally divalent, and are thus capable of cross-linking cell-surface IgE and causing mediator release from mast cells and basophils without binding or haptenating to larger carrier molecules. NMBAs have also been implicated in epidemiologic studies of anesthetic drug-induced anaphylaxis. Epidemiologic data from France suggest that NMBAs are responsible for 62 to 81% of reactions, depending on the time period evaluated.[100–105]

In more recent years, NMBAs, especially steroid-derived agents, have been reported as potential causative agents of anaphylactic reactions during anesthesia. The data associating NMBAs in the most recent reports from France are mainly based on skin testing; however, studies have previously reported the steroidal-derived NMBAs and other molecules produce false-positive skin tests (i.e., weal and flare). One of the major problems is that anaphylaxis to NMBAs is rare in the United States, but has been reported more often in Europe.[105–107] Although suggestions have been made that this is because of underreporting, the severity of anaphylaxis and its sequelae to produce adverse outcomes clearly make this unlikely based on the current medicolegal climate that exists in the United States. One of the only ways to explain this widely divergent perspective is to understand how the diagnosis is made because the recommended threshold test concentrations have not been defined, resulting in unreliable results.

We previously reported in several studies that steroid-derived agents could induce positive weal and flare responses independent of mast cell degranulation, even at low concentrations, following intradermal injection. This effect is likely because of a direct effect on the cutaneous vasculature that occurs for most NMBAs at concentrations as low as 10^{-5} M using intradermal skin tests in 30 volunteers. A positive cutaneous reaction without evidence of mast cell degranulation was noted at low concentrations (100 mcg/mL) of rocuronium in almost all the volunteers. We have used intradermal injections to compare cutaneous effects of anesthetic and other agents.[106]

Other investigators have also reported similar results. Because prick tests are often used for authenticating NMBAs as causative drugs, Dhonneur et al evaluated 30 volunteers, using prick testing. Each subject received a total of 10 prick tests (50 μL) on both forearms. The investigators studied the weal and flare responses to prick tests with rocuronium and vecuronium, using four dilutions (1/1,000, 1/100, 1/10, and 1) and two controls, and measured weal and flare immediately after and at 15 min. They noted 50 and 40% of the subjects had a positive skin reaction to undiluted rocuronium and vecuronium, respectively.[105] To avoid false-positive results, they suggested that prick testing with rocuronium and vecuronium should be performed in subjects who have experienced a hypersensitivity reaction during anesthesia, with concentrations below that commonly inducing positive reactions in anesthesia-naive, healthy subjects (i.e., for men in a dilution of 1/10 and for women in a dilution of 1/100). Guidelines for prick testing that are internationally agreed on need to be established. Many of these differences may explain the various incidences of allergy to NMBAs among countries. Concentration-skin response curves to rocuronium and vecuronium have showed that prick tests should be performed with dilution of the commercially available preparation. Female volunteers significantly ($P < .01$) reacted to lower vecuronium and rocuronium concentrations than males. In female subjects, positive skin reactions were reported with dilutions of 1/100 of both relaxants. In male subjects, positive skin reactions were noted with the undiluted concentration, except for one volunteer who reacted to rocuronium (1/10 dilution).

SUMMARY

Although the immune system functions to provide host defense, it can respond inappropriately to produce hypersensitivity or allergic reactions. A spectrum of life-threatening allergic reactions to any drug or agent can occur in the perioperative period.[100] The enigma of these reactions lies in their unpredictable nature. However, a high index of suspicion, prompt recognition, and appropriate and aggressive therapy can help avoid a disastrous outcome.

References

1. Levy JH: Anaphylactic Reactions in Anesthesia and Intensive Care, 2nd ed. Boston, Butterworth-Heinemann, 1992
2. deShazo RD, Kemp SF: Allergic reactions to drugs and biologic agents. JAMA 278:1895, 1997
3. Gell PGH, Coombs RRA, Lachmann PJ (eds): Clinical Aspects of Immunology, 3rd ed. Oxford, Blackwell Scientific Publications, 1975
4. Delves PJ, Roitt IM. The immune system (two parts). N Engl J Med 343:37, 108, 2000
5. Kay AB: Allergy and allergic diseases (two parts). N Engl J Med 344:30, 109, 2001
6. Stevenson GW, Hall SC, Rudnick S *et al:* The effects of anesthetic agents on the human immune response. Anesthesiology 72:144, 1990
7. Pober JS, Cotran RS: Cytokines and endothelial cell biology. Physiol Rev 70:427, 1990
8. Walport MJ. Complement (first and second parts). N Engl J Med 344:1058, 1140, 2001
9. Wall RT, Frank M, Hahn M: A review of 25 patients with hereditary angioedema requiring surgery. Anesthesiology 71:309, 1989
10. Fisher MMD, More DG: The epidemiology and clinical features of anaphylactic reactions in anaesthesia. Anaesth Intensive Care 9:226, 1981
11. Weiss ME, Adkinson NF, Hirshman CA: Evaluation of allergic reactions in the perioperative period. Anesthesiology 71:438, 1989
12. Mertes PM, Laxenaire MC, Alla F; Groupe d'Etudes des Reactions Anaphylactoides Peranesthesiques: Anaphylactic and anaphylactoid reactions occurring during anesthesia in France in 1999–2000. Anesthesiology 99:536, 2003
13. Portier MM, Richet C: De l'action anaphylactique de certains venins. C R Seances Soc Biol Fil 54:170, 1902
14. Watkins J: Anaphylactoid reactions to IV substances. Br J Anaesth 51:51, 1979
15. Costa JJ, Weller PF, Galli SJ: The cells of the allergic response: Mast cells, basophils, and eosinophils. JAMA 278:1815, 1997
16. Galli SJ, Wedemeyer J, Tsai M: Analyzing the roles of mast cells and basophils in host defense and other biological responses. Int J Hematol 75(4):363, 2002
17. Winslow CM, Austen KF: Enzymatic regulation of mast cell activation and secretion by adenylate cyclase and cyclic AMP-dependent protein kinases. Fed Proc 41:22, 1982
18. Galli SJ: Mast cells and basophils. Curr Opin Hematol 7:32, 2000
19. MacGlashan D Jr. Histamine: A mediator of inflammation. J Allergy Clin Immunol 112(4 Suppl):S53, 2003

20. Marone G, Bova M, Detoraki A *et al*: The human heart as a shock organ in anaphylaxis. Novartis Found Symp 257:133, 2004
21. Majno G, Palade GE: Studies on inflammation: I. The effect of histamine and serotonin on vascular permeability. An electron microscopic study. J Biophys Biochem Cytol 11:571, 1961
22. Gould HJ, Sutton BJ, Beavil AJ *et al*: The biology of IGE and the basis of allergic disease. *Ann Rev Immunol* 21:579, 2003
23. Mathe AA, Hedqvist P, Strandberg K *et al*: Aspects of prostaglandin function in the lung. N Engl J Med 296:850, 910, 1977
24. Holgate ST, Peters-Golden M, Panettieri RA, Henderson WR: Roles of cysteinyl leukotrienes in airway inflammation, smooth muscle function, and remodeling. J Allergy Clin Immunol 111(1 Suppl):S18, 2003
25. Lazarus SC: Inflammation, inflammatory mediators, and mediator antagonists in asthma. J Clin Pharmacol 38:577, 1998
26. Schulman ES, Newball HH, Demers LM *et al*: Anaphylactic release of thromboxane A2, prostaglandin D2, and prostacyclin from human lung parenchyma. Am Rev Respir Dis 124:402, 1981
27. Morel DR, Zapol WM, Thomas SJ *et al*: C5a and thromboxane generation associated with pulmonary vaso- and bronchoconstriction during protamine reversal of heparin. Anesthesiology 66:597, 1987
28. Tanaka KA, Katori N, Szlam F, Vega JD, Levy JH: Evaluation of a novel kallikrein inhibitor on hemostatic activation in vitro. Thromb Res 113:333, 2004
29. Delage C, Irey NS: Anaphylactic deaths: A clinicopathologic study of 43 cases. J Forensic Sci 17:525, 1972
30. Smith Laboratories: Chymodiactin Post Marketing Surveillance Report. Chicago, Smith Laboratories, 1984
31. Laxenaire MC, Moneret-Vautrin DA, Vervloet D *et al:* Accidents anaphylactoides graves peranesthesiques. Ann Fr Anesth Reanim 4:30, 1985
32. Pumphrey R. Anaphylaxis: Can we tell who is at risk of a fatal reaction? Curr Opin Allergy Clin Immunol 4:285, 2004
33. Pavek K, Wegmann A, Nordström L *et al:* Cardiovascular and respiratory mechanisms in anaphylactic and anaphylactoid shock reactions. Klin Wochenschr 60:941, 1982
34. Atkinson JP, Frank MM: Role of complement in the pathophysiology of hematologic disease. Prog Hematol 10:211, 1977
35. Jacobs HS, Craddock PR, Hammerschmidt DE *et al:* Complement-induced granulocyte aggregation: An unsuspected mechanism of disease. N Engl J Med 302:789, 1980
36. Dubois M, Lotze MT, Diamond WI *et al:* Pulmonary shunting during leukoagglutinin-induced noncardiogenic pulmonary edema. JAMA 244:2186, 1980
37. Teissner B, Brandslund I, Grunnet N *et al:* Acute complement activation during an anaphylactoid reaction to blood transfusion and the disappearance rate of C3c and C3d from the circulation. J Clin Lab Immunol 12:63, 1983
38. Hammerschmidt DE, Weaver LJ, Hudson LD *et al:* Association of complement activation and elevated plasma-C5a with adult respiratory distress syndrome. Lancet 1:947, 1980
39. Levy JH, Brister NW, Shearin A *et al:* Wheal and flare responses to opioids in humans. Anesthesiology 70:756, 1989
40. Levy JH, Adelson DM, Walker BF: Wheal and flare responses to muscle relaxants in humans. Agents Actions 34:302, 1991
41. Veien M, Holdin J, Szlam F *et al:* Mechanisms of non-immunological histamine and tryptase release from human cutaneous mast cells. Anesthesiology 92:1074, 2000
42. Levy JH, Kettlekamp N, Goertz P *et al:* Histamine release by vancomycin: A mechanism for hypotension in man. Anesthesiology 67:122, 1987
43. Caulfield JP, El-Lati S, Thomas G, Church MK: Dissociated human foreskin mast cells degranulate in response to anti-IgE and substance P. Lab Invest 63:502, 1990
44. Casale TB, Bowman S, Kaliner M: Induction of human cutaneous mast cell degranulation by opiates and endogenous opioid peptides: Evidence for opiate and nonopiate receptor participation. J Allergy Clin Immunol 73:775, 1984
45. Levy JH, Davis GK, Duggan J, Szlam F: Determination of the hemodynamics and histamine release of rocuronium (Org 9426) when administered in increased doses under N_2O/O_2-sufentanil anesthesia. Anesth Analg 78:318, 1994
46. Levy JH, Pitts M, Thanopoulos A *et al:* The effects of rapacuronium on histamine release and hemodynamics in adult patients undergoing general anesthesia. Anesth Analg 89:290, 1999
47. Hirshman CA, Downes H, Butler J: Relevance of plasma histamine levels to hypotension. Anesthesiology 57:424, 1982
48. Stark BJ, Sullivan TJ: Biphasic and protracted anaphylaxis. J Allergy Clin Immunol 78:76, 1986
49. Levy JH, Rockoff MR: Anaphylaxis to meperidine. Anesth Analg 61:301, 1982
50. Fisher MM: Blood volume replacement in acute anaphylactic cardiovascular collapse related to anaesthesia. Br J Anaesth 49:1023, 1977
51. Barnett A, Hirshman CA: Anaphylactic reaction to cephapirin during spinal anesthesia. Anesth Analg 58:337, 1979
52. Levy JH: Anaphylactic-anaphylactoid reactions during cardiac surgery. J Clin Anesthesiol 1:426, 1989
53. Schwartz LB. Effector cells of anaphylaxis: Mast cells and basophils. Novartis Found Symp 257:65, 2004
54. Hammerschmidt DE, White JG, Craddock PR *et al:* Corticosteroids inhibit complement-induced granulocyte aggregation: A possible mechanism for their efficacy in shock states. J Clin Invest 63:798, 1979
55. Sin DD, Man J, Sharpe H, Gan WQ, Man SF: Pharmacological management to reduce exacerbations in adults with asthma: A systematic review and meta-analysis. JAMA 292:367, 2004
56. Sheagren JN: Septic shock and corticosteroids (editorial). N Engl J Med 305:456, 1981
57. Borda IT, Slone D, Jick H: Assessment of adverse reactions within a drug surveillance program. JAMA 205:645, 1968
58. DeSwarte RD: Drug allergy: Problems and strategies. J Allergy Clin Immunol 74:209, 1984
59. Tomicheck RC, Rosow CG, Philbin DM *et al:* Diazepam-fentanyl interaction: Hemodynamic and hormonal effect in coronary artery surgery. Anesth Analg 62:881, 1983
60. Fisher MM, Outhred A, Bowey CJ: Can clinical anaphylaxis to anaesthetic drugs be predicted from allergic history? Br J Anaesth 59:690, 1987
61. Christman D: Immune reaction to propanidid. Anaesthesia 39:470, 1984
62. Watkins J, Clarke SJ: Report of a symposium: Adverse responses to intravenous agents. Br J Anaesth 50:1159, 1978
63. Driggs RL, O'Day RA: Acute allergic reaction associated with methohexital anaesthesia: Report of six cases. J Oral Surg 30:906, 1972
64. Watkins J, Salo M, eds. Incidence of immediate adverse response to intravenous anaesthetic drugs. In Trauma, Stress and Immunity in Anaesthesia and Surgery, p 272. London, Butterworth, 1982
65. Schwartz HJ, Sher TH: Bisulfite sensitivity manifesting as allergy to local dental anaesthesia. J Allergy Clin Immunol 75:525, 1985
66. Brown DT, Beamins D, Wildsmith JAW: Allergic reaction to an amide local anesthetic. Br J Anaesth 53:435, 1981
67. Fisher MM, Munro I: Life-threatening anaphylactoid reactions to muscle relaxants. Anesth Analg 62:559, 1983
68. Swartz J, Braude BM, Gilmour RF *et al:* Intraoperative anaphylaxis to latex. Can J Anaesth 37:589, 1990
69. Roizen MF, Rodgers GM, Valone FH *et al*: Anaphylactoid reactions to vascular graft material presenting with vasodilation and subsequent disseminated intravascular coagulation. Anesthesiology 71:331, 1989
70. Laxenaire MC, Moneret-Vautrin DA, Watkins J: Diagnosis of the causes of anaphylactoid anaesthetic reactions. Anaesthesia 38:147, 1983
71. Vervloet D, Nizankowska E, Arnaud A *et al*: Adverse reactions to suxamethonium and other muscle relaxants under general anesthesia. J Allergy Clin Immunol 71:552, 1983
72. Harle DG, Baldo BA, Fisher MM: Detection of IgE antibodies to suxamethonium after anaphylactoid reactions during anaesthesia. Lancet 1:930, 1984
73. Zucker-Pinchoff B, Ramanathan S: Anaphylactic reaction to epidural fentanyl. Anesthesiology 71:599, 1989
74. Gilstad CW. Anaphylactic transfusion reactions. Curr Opin Hematol 10(6):419, 2003
75. Sheffer AL, Pennoyer DS: Management of adverse drug reactions. J Allergy Clin Immunol 74:580, 1984
76. Levy JH, Zaidan JR, Faraj B: Prospective evaluation of risk of protamine reactions in NPH insulin-dependent diabetics. Anesth Analg 65:739, 1986
77. Levy JH, Schwieger IM, Zaidan JR *et al:* Evaluation of patients at risk for protamine reactions. J Thorac Cardiovasc Surg 98:200, 1989
78. Lasser EC: The radiocontrast molecule in anaphylaxis: A surprising antigen. Novartis Found Symp 257:211, 2004
79. Isbister JP, Fisher MM: Adverse effects of plasma volume expanders. Anaesth Intensive Care 8:145, 1980
80. Colman WR: Paradoxical hypotension after volume expansion with plasma protein fraction. N Engl J Med 299:97, 1978
81. Ring K, Messmer K: Incidence and severity of anaphylactoid reactions to colloid volume substitutes. Lancet 1:466, 1977
82. Levy JH: Hemostatic agents and their safety. J Cardiothorac Vasc Anesth 13(4 Suppl 1):6, 1999
83. Thong BY, Yeow-Chan C: Anaphylaxis during surgical and interventional procedures. Ann Allergy Asthma Immunol 92:619, 2004
84. Fisher MM, Baldo BA: Immunoassays in the diagnosis of anaphylaxis to neuromuscular blocking drugs: The value of morphine for the detection of IgE antibodies in allergic subjects. Anaesth Intensive Care 28:167, 2000
85. Baldo BA, Fisher MM: Detection of serum IgE antibodies that react with alcuronium and tubocurarine after life-threatening reactions to muscle relaxants. Anaesth Intensive Care 11:194, 1983
86. Harle DG, Baldo BA, Smal MA *et al:* Detection of thiopentone-reactive IgE antibodies following anaphylactoid reactions during anesthesia. Clin Allergy 16:493, 1986
87. Dueck R, O'Connor RD: Thiopental: False positive RAST in patient with elevated serum IgE. Anesthesiology 61:337, 1984
88. Fisher MM: Intradermal testing after anaphylactoid reaction to anaesthetic drugs: Practical aspects of performance and interpretation. Anaesth Intensive Care 12:115, 1984
89. Fisher MM, Bowey CJ: Intradermal compared with prick testing in the diagnosis of anaesthetic allergy. Br J Anaesth 79:59, 1997

90. Shatz M: Skin testing and incremental challenge in the evaluation of adverse reactions to local anesthetics. J Allergy Clin Immunol 74:606, 1984
91. Holzman RB: Clinical management of latex-allergic children. Anesth Analg 85:529, 1997
92. Kibby T, Akl M: Prevalence of latex sensitization in a hospital employee population. Ann Allergy Asthma Immunol 78:41, 1997
93. Gold M, Swartz JS, Braude BM *et al:* Intraoperative anaphylaxis: An association with latex sensitivity. J Allergy Clin Immunol 87:662, 1991
94. Holzman RS: Latex allergy: An emerging operating room problem. Anesth Analg 76:635, 1993
95. Brown RH, Schauble JF, Hamilton RG: Prevalence of latex allergy among anesthesiologists: Identification of sensitized but asymptomatic individuals. Anesthesiology 89:292, 1998
96. Lavaud F, Prevost A, Cossart C *et al*: Allergy to latex, avocado, pear, and banana: Evidence for a 30 kd antigen in immunoblotting. J Allergy Clin Immunol 95:557, 1995
97. Blanco C, Carrillo T, Castillo R *et al*: Latex allergy: Clinical features and cross-reactivity with fruits. Ann Allergy 73:309, 1994
98. Lebenbom-Mansour MH, Oesterle JR, Ownsby DR *et al:* The incidence of latex sensitivity in ambulatory surgical patients: A correlation of historical factors with positive serum immunoglobin E levels. Anesth Analg 85:44, 1997
99. Suli C, Parziale M, Lorini M *et al:* Prevalence and risk factors for latex allergy: A cross sectional study on health-care workers of an Italian hospital. J Investig Allergol Clin Immunol 14:64, 2004
100. Sampson HA, Munoz-Furlong A, Block SA, et al. Symposium on the definition and management of anaphylaxis: Summary report. J Allergy Clin Immunol 115:584, 2005.
101. Laxenaire MC: Drugs and other agents involved in anaphylactic shock occurring during anaesthesia. A French multicenter epidemiologic inquiry. Ann Fr Anesth Réanim 12:91, 1993
102. Mertes PM, Laxenaire MC, Alla F: Groupe d'Etudes des Reactions Anaphylactoides Peranesthesiques. Anaphylactic and anaphylactoid reactions occurring during anesthesia in France in 1999–2000. Anesthesiology 99:536, 2003
103. Moneret-Vautrin DA, Mouton C: Anaphylaxie aux myorelaxants: Valeur prédictive des intrader-journal moréactions et recherche de l'anaphylaxie croisée. Ann Fr Anesth Réanim 4:186, 1985
104. Monnet-Vautrin DA: Cutaneous tests in anaphylactic reactions to muscular blocking agents. In Reducing the risk of anaphylaxis during anaesthesia: Guidelines for clinical practice. Ann Fr Anesth Réanim 21(1):97, 2002
105. Dhonneur G, Zoffer R, McCall C, *et al*: Skin sensitivity to rocuronium and vecuronium: A randomized controlled prick-testing study in healthy volunteers. Anesth Analg 98:986, 2004
106. Levy JH, Gottge M, Szlam F *et al*: Wheal and flare responses to intradermal rocuronium and cisatracurium in humans. Br J Anaesth 85:844, 2000
107. Levy JH: Anaphylactic reactions to neuromuscular blocking drugs: Are we making the correct diagnosis? Anesth Analg 98:881, 2004

CHAPTER 50 ■ DRUG INTERACTIONS

CARL ROSOW AND WILTON C. LEVINE

KEY POINTS

1. Drug combinations are a useful and necessary part of anesthesia practice, but they are occasionally a source of morbidity. The qualitative nature of most anesthetic interactions is predictable even though the magnitude of the response might not be known with certainty. Drugs that interact to produce a totally unexpected or dangerous effect stand out because of their rarity.
2. A *pharmaceutical* interaction is a chemical or physical interaction that occurs before a drug is administered or absorbed systemically.
3. A *pharmacokinetic* interaction occurs when one drug alters the absorption, distribution, metabolism, or elimination of another.
4. A *pharmacodynamic* interaction occurs when one drug alters the sensitivity of a target receptor or tissue to the effects of a second drug. We commonly classify these interactions by their direction and intensity, that is, additive, antagonistic, or supra-additive (synergistic).
5. *Additive interactions* are most likely to occur when drugs with identical mechanisms are combined.
6. The most common *antagonistic interactions* are those involving deliberate reversal with competitive antagonists. Antagonism that is unintended is a much less common event.
7. *Synergistic interaction* is most likely to occur when drugs with different mechanisms are combined.
8. Most cardiovascular drug–drug interactions are simply extensions of the known pharmacology of the agents. With few exceptions, there is little reason to withhold most vasoactive medications before surgery.
9. Combinations of central nervous system (CNS) depressants almost always produce additive or synergistic increases in CNS effect. These interactions are usually useful and predictable.
10. Among the thousands of herbal preparations available, only a few have been documented to cause problems either through intrinsic toxicity or pharmacokinetic and pharmacodynamic interactions. There are no studies demonstrating specific adverse interactions between herbals and anesthetic drugs.

Modern drug regimens for medical ailments such as hypertension, angina, bronchospasm, or malignancy nearly always involve the use of multiple agents. This strategy is frequently successful because many medical conditions are responsive to groups of drugs that act by different mechanisms and have different dose-limiting toxicities. The goal in each case is to produce an increased therapeutic effect with decreased toxicity compared to treatment with individual agents. Unfortunately, the mixing of drugs is not without risk, and hundreds of research papers on the benefits and drawbacks of drug interactions appear every year. A sizable industry has now evolved to provide clinicians with reference books and computer databases on the subject.

Anesthesiologists face the same dilemma as all other physicians: drug combinations are a useful and necessary part of practice, but they are occasionally a source of morbidity. This chapter reviews the reasons that drugs are combined and the ways in which the combinations can alter either pharmacokinetics or pharmacodynamics. This is *not* a comprehensive list of anesthetic drug interactions—entire books have been devoted to the subject.[1] The examples included have been chosen largely on the basis of proven or likely clinical relevance and the strength of their documentation. When possible, prototypical interactions are illustrated with examples that have direct relevance to anesthesia, although in some cases no such examples are available. The emphasis throughout is on mechanism, but it will quickly be apparent that our understanding of mechanism is incomplete for many pharmacodynamic interactions. Finally, it is important to know how to read the relevant literature, and a short section is devoted to some of the common ways interactions can be studied.

HISTORICAL PERSPECTIVE

Historically, anesthesiologists were trained to regard drug interactions as a danger and something to be avoided. The generations of clinicians who administered open-drop diethyl ether probably had good reason to limit the number of anesthetic drugs administered: ether by itself could produce hypnosis, reasonable levels of analgesia, and muscle relaxation. Ventilation and blood pressure were usually well maintained because ether has respiratory stimulant and sympathomimetic properties. Clinicians could adjust the dose of this single agent fairly accurately using Guedel's criteria for pupil size, respiratory pattern, muscle tone, and so forth. This meant that a patient requiring even major abdominal surgery could be anesthetized using nothing more than a can of ether and a simple mask.

Before World War II, endotracheal intubation and controlled ventilation were usually not options, and muscle relaxants had not been introduced. Clinicians in this era were well served to keep things simple: if an anesthesiologist chose to add morphine to an ether anesthetic, the pupil and respiratory signs would no longer be reliable, muscle relaxation would probably decrease, and ventilatory depression (if it occurred) could not be treated easily.

The introduction of muscle relaxants, opioid-based anesthesia, and modern intravenous and inhaled anesthetics completely changed these considerations. The signs and stages of ether anesthesia are no longer applicable, and controlled or assisted ventilation is often necessary because most of these drugs have profound effects on respiration. Most importantly, clinicians now realize that anesthetics are highly specific drugs, and no single agent can produce all the "desirable" components of anesthesia. There is good evidence that even the potent volatile anesthetics are not sufficient to produce optimal anesthetic conditions when given alone. Zbinden et al[2] showed that even moderately high concentrations of isoflurane in oxygen cannot suppress many cardiovascular responses to surgical stimuli. This finding is reflected in common clinical practice because isoflurane is routinely supplemented with opioids and other drugs to control blood pressure and heart rate.

Our views of what is desirable in anesthesia have also changed markedly. For example, most patients now expect and prefer an intravenous hypnotic, rather than a mask, for anesthetic induction. Similarly, the long emergence after ether is no longer expected or acceptable. A smooth recovery, free of pain or delirium, is now common within minutes after major surgical interventions. These goals are difficult to accomplish without using multiple drugs.

PROBLEMS CREATED BY DRUG–DRUG INTERACTION

There is almost no data on the true incidence of perioperative drug interaction, although there are data on general inpatient populations. It is logical that the probability of drug–drug interaction increases with the number of drugs administered.[3] Many patients are routinely taking three or four antihypertensives, antidepressants, or gastrointestinal drugs in the preoperative period. Most also receive 5 to 10 drugs during general anesthesia, but we do not normally hear about significant complications attributable to drug interaction. There are a number of possible explanations for this:

1. Interactions may occur, but they usually do not present a problem. Toxicity from a drug interaction is likely to become a source of morbidity primarily when it occurs in a setting where it is not rapidly recognized and treated. This happened when opioid and midazolam combinations were first used by nonanesthesia personnel for endoscopic and radiologic procedures. The unexpectedly large sedative and ventilatory effects led to numerous deaths.[4]
2. Many of the effects introduced by mixing drugs are hard to distinguish from clinical "noise." Variability in response to anesthetic drugs is the rule: the data on intravenous opioids[5] and hypnotics,[6] for example, show that different patients may have a three- to fivefold difference in the therapeutic and toxic effects of a given dose—even when the drug is given alone.
3. The qualitative nature of most anesthetic interactions is predictable even though the magnitude of the responses might not be known with certainty. (1) Combining two cardiovascular depressants will produce more hypotension; two central nervous system (CNS) depressants will produce more sedation, and so forth. Drugs that interact to produce a totally unexpected or dangerous effect stand out because of their rarity. A notorious example of such an idiosyncratic interaction is the CNS excitation that may occur when meperidine is administered to patients taking monoamine oxidase inhibitors (MAOIs).
4. Many intravenous anesthetic drugs (diazepam, fentanyl) have large safety margins—especially when respiration is supported—so changes in drug effect have few consequences. The mere fact that a measurable interaction exists does not mean it will cause a difference in outcome or the need for intervention. Dangerous interactions most often involve drugs such as warfarin, digoxin, and theophylline, agents with only small differences between therapeutic and toxic concentrations.
5. Finally, it is likely that many instances of anesthetic drug interaction go unrecognized. Excessive drug effects are often attributed to some ill-defined patient "sensitivity." When a drug *fails* to produce an effect, it is because the patient is "tolerant" or "resistant." It is almost never considered a drug reaction or interaction.

WHY COMBINE DRUGS?

The goal of combining drugs is to decrease toxicity while maintaining or increasing efficacy. It is instructive to see how this principle has been applied in other areas of medicine:

1. Combination therapy can reduce toxicity. For example, a beta-adrenergic antagonist and a vasodilator have at least additive effects on blood pressure, but their side effects are different and (presumably) nonadditive. Lower doses of each drug may be used in combination so dose-related side effects are decreased.
2. Combination chemotherapy for malignancy can increase efficacy. To produce the maximum decrease in tumor burden, each chemotherapeutic drug is given at its maximally tolerated dose, an end-point determined by its toxic effects on some normal cell population. Drugs such as alkylating agents and vinca alkaloids are combined because they have different dose-limiting organ toxicities (bone marrow and nerve, respectively), so each drug can be given at a full tumor-suppressing dose.
3. Single-drug therapy is sometimes preferable. The mainstay drugs for prophylaxis of seizures (phenytoin, carbamazepine) have similar dose-limiting side effects such as

ataxia and drowsiness, so there is little to be gained by combining them.

PHARMACEUTICAL INTERACTIONS

2 A *pharmaceutical* interaction is a chemical or physical interaction that occurs before a drug is administered or absorbed systemically. The most obvious pharmaceutical interactions are the incompatibilities that can occur between drugs in solution:

- Precipitation of thiopental may occur when it is injected together with succinylcholine into the intravenous catheter line.
- Bicarbonate can decrease the solubility of bupivacaine and cause it to precipitate.
- Catecholamine solutions (norepinephrine, epinephrine) can be inactivated if they are alkalinized by the addition of sodium bicarbonate, a circumstance that could occur during cardiopulmonary resuscitation.

The number of these incompatibilities is large, and the anesthesiologist should avoid mixing drugs unless they are known to be compatible. Information on specific intravenous drug incompatibilities is readily available from most hospital pharmacists.

Occasionally, two drugs may interact chemically to form a toxic compound:

- The halogenated anesthetics—desflurane, enflurane, and isoflurane—have been shown to interact with dry soda lime or Baralyme to produce carbon monoxide.[7] Desiccation of soda lime is most likely to occur when oxygen has been left flowing through the canister overnight. Older anesthesiologists recall that trichloroethylene interacted with soda lime to produce the neurotoxin, dichloroacetylene.
- Nitric oxide (NO) is a selective pulmonary vasodilator that has been approved in the United States for treatment of primary pulmonary hypertension in the newborn.[8] If NO is allowed more than fleeting contact with oxygen, it forms nitrogen dioxide (NO_2). The latter compound can be quite toxic, and concentrations >10 ppm can produce pulmonary edema and alveolar hemorrhage. The problem is circumvented by allowing oxygen and NO to mix in the breathing circuit just before administration.

PHARMACOKINETIC INTERACTIONS

3 A *pharmacokinetic* interaction occurs when one drug alters the absorption, distribution, metabolism, or elimination of another. Many of the basic pharmacokinetic principles underlying these interactions are reviewed in Chapter 11.

Absorption

Alteration of absorption may occur because of direct chemical or physical interaction between drugs in the body or because one drug alters the physiologic mechanisms governing absorption of the second:

- Orally administered tetracycline can be inactivated by chelation if it is given together with antacids containing polyvalent cations such as Mg^{2+}, Ca^{2+}, or Al^{3+}.
- Oral antidiarrheal drugs such as kaolin and pectin can physically adsorb digoxin and prevent it from being absorbed.
- The bile acid-binding resin, cholestyramine, can bind to warfarin and prevent its absorption. It can also reduce the absorption of vitamin K and other fat-soluble compounds.

Another interaction of significance to anesthesiologists is the delay of gastric emptying produced by medications such as opioids and anticholinergics. Opioids produce hypertonus of smooth muscle, reduction of peristalsis, and contraction of sphincters throughout the gastrointestinal tract, and it appears that both central and peripheral mechanisms play a role in this effect. Murphy et al[9] gave volunteers 500 mL of distilled water to drink and showed that 0.09 mg/kg of morphine increased the half-time for gastric emptying from 5.5 to 21 minutes. Morphine can also reduce the absorption of orally administered drugs because the primary site for absorption is the small intestine, and gastric emptying is rate limiting. Asai et al[10] demonstrated that morphine significantly reduces the absorption of oral acetaminophen in patients.

Changes in regional blood flow (vasodilators, vasoconstrictors) can affect the absorption of parenterally administered drugs. Shock or congestive heart failure decreases perfusion of peripheral tissues such as skin and muscle, so the onset and intensity of effect may become unpredictable for drugs given by intramuscular or subcutaneous injection:

- Local administration of epinephrine and other vasoconstrictors retard absorption of infiltrated local anesthetics and therefore prolong their effects.
- Drugs that decrease effective pulmonary ventilation have the potential to reduce the uptake of volatile anesthetics. Drugs that increase minute ventilation, reduce intrapulmonary shunting, or relieve bronchospasm can increase the uptake of volatile anesthetics even though the inspired concentration remains constant.
- The rapid uptake of nitrous oxide can increase the alveolar concentration of concomitantly administered volatile anesthetics (the "second gas effect").

Distribution

Many drug–drug interactions occur when one drug alters the distribution of a second. This may occur due to alterations in hemodynamics, drug ionization, or binding to plasma and tissue proteins. Much has been written about the involvement of these mechanisms in drug interactions (particularly the last two), but there are few examples of proven relevance to anesthesia.

Drugs such as volatile anesthetics, beta-blockers, calcium channel blockers, and vasodilators can decrease cardiac output and produce significant changes in drug distribution. A decrease in cardiac output increases the arterial concentrations of other drugs in highly perfused tissues such as the brain and myocardium:[11]

- In a patient with depressed cardiac function, normal doses of intravenous agents such as propofol, thiopental, and remifentanil can produce substantially greater cardiovascular and CNS effects. This can be due to an increase in tissue drug concentrations or an increase in tissue sensitivity to the effects of the drug.[12–14]
- The same effect is seen with volatile anesthetics. Low cardiac output increases end-tidal concentrations and intensifies cardiovascular and CNS effects.

Drug-induced changes in pH in a particular body region or fluid compartment can alter the distribution of other drugs by so-called "ion trapping." Most of our therapeutic agents are weak acids or bases that are partially ionized at normal body pH. It is only the nonionized fraction that can cross lipid membranes and come to equilibrium. The amount ionized can be determined for acids or bases from the general form of the Henderson-Hasselbach equation:

$$\frac{[\text{Protonated}]}{[\text{Unprotonated}]} = 10^{(pK_a - pH)}$$

Recall that an unprotonated acid is ionized, whereas an unprotonated base is nonionized. It is apparent from this relationship that a weak base (fentanyl, lidocaine) will be progressively ionized as the pH decreases, whereas a weak acid (aspirin, phenobarbital) will be more nonionized.

For certain membrane barriers, such as those in the stomach, placenta, or renal tubules, the pH on either side is very different, and this creates the necessary conditions for ion trapping. Consider the case of a weak acid (ionization constant [pK_a] = 3.4) that is distributing between stomach and blood. In stomach acid (pH 2.4),

$$\frac{[\text{Nonionized}]}{[\text{Ionized}]} = 10^{(3.4-2.4)} = 10$$

In blood (pH 7.4),

$$\frac{[\text{Nonionized}]}{[\text{Ionized}]} = 10^{(3.4-7.4)} = 0.0001$$

At equilibrium, the concentrations of nonionized drug must be the same on either side of the gastric membrane barrier. This means that a 10,000-fold concentration gradient is established for total drug (nonionized + ionized):

	■ STOMACH (pH 2.4)	■ BLOOD (pH 7.4)
Nonionized drug	1	1
Ionized drug	0.1	10,000
Total drug	1.1	10,001

It is easy to see why weak acids such as aspirin are well absorbed from the stomach. The potential for drug interaction is great. Even moderate changes in pH can have large effects on this equilibrium: raising intragastric pH to 5.4 decreases the concentration gradient by 100-fold:

- Administration of antacids, histamine type 2 receptor antagonists, or proton pump inhibitors such as omeprazole can reduce the gastric absorption of some acidic drugs. Alteration of pH has been shown to change the oral bioavailability of ketoconazole[15] and midazolam.[16]
- Lipid-soluble basic drugs such as fentanyl and meperidine can diffuse *into* the stomach from the bloodstream. They become ionized and trapped in gastric acid only to be reabsorbed when they enter the more alkaline environment of the proximal jejunum. This gastric "recycling" is believed to be the basis for secondary increases in plasma concentrations of these opioids.[17]
- Alteration of urine pH can markedly affect the renal clearance of certain drugs (described in the Drug Elimination section).

Much has been written about the role of plasma protein binding in drug–drug interaction. The fraction of a dose that remains intravascular is either free or bound to circulating proteins. Acidic drugs usually bind to albumin and various globulin fractions. Many basic drugs such as meperidine, lidocaine, bupivacaine, and propranolol bind to α_1-acid glycoprotein, an acute-phase reactant. Drug binding by α_1-acid glycoprotein can increase after surgery and in certain other conditions such as burns, myocardial infarction, trauma, and malignancies. Conversely, hepatic cirrhosis and the nephrotic syndrome are often accompanied by hypoproteinemia and decreases in both albumin and globulin binding.

The extent to which drug is bound versus free is important because it is only the unbound fraction that is available for crossing membranes, entering tissues, and binding to receptors to produce the pharmacologic effect. Protein-bound drug is not filtered by a normal glomerulus and (for some drugs) is not acted on by drug-metabolizing enzymes. A drug that is highly bound to plasma protein effectively exists in a "depot," not unlike a drug given by deep intramuscular injection. The potential therefore exists that one drug could alter the disposition, clearance, or biological effect of another by affecting its binding:

- The classic example of such an interaction is drug displacement of bilirubin in infants. Premature infants have immature glucuronyl transferase and are unable to conjugate bilirubin formed by destruction of erythrocytes. Much of the load of unconjugated bilirubin is bound to albumin and thus prevented from entering tissues. Sulfonamides and other drugs can compete for albumin-binding sites, and the bilirubin they displace can enter tissues. Excessive levels of bilirubin in the brain can lead to kernicterus, a potentially fatal problem. This effect was discovered accidentally in 1956 during a clinical drug trial. When premature infants were given a penicillin-sulfonamide mixture, the mortality rate increased, and many were found to have kernicterus at autopsy.[18]
- The same mechanism has been postulated for numerous drug–drug interactions. Highly bound, potentially toxic drugs such as warfarin and phenytoin may be displaced by other highly bound drugs. Warfarin is >98% bound to albumin, meaning that only 1 to 2% of the circulating drug accounts for the entire biological effect. Phenylbutazone is a nonsteroidal anti-inflammatory drug (NSAID) that competes effectively for the same binding sites. If phenylbutazone displaces only 2% of warfarin, this theoretically doubles the free (active) fraction and greatly increases the warfarin effect.

This type of drug–drug interaction has been dogma for years, but it is nearly impossible to find documented evidence that it causes harm:[19]

1. Most drugs are widely distributed in the body, so most of the administered dose is *extravascular*—two-thirds of the total dose in the case of warfarin. Even a large change in plasma unbound fraction (e.g., 10%) will therefore release only 3 to 4% of total warfarin in the body.
2. The body acts as a sink or buffer against large changes in unbound fraction (any unbound drug in plasma is rapidly distributed into peripheral tissues).

Some caution is still warranted for anesthesiologists and other clinicians who use intravenous drug regimens with doses often in the toxic range (e.g., high doses of opioids, hypnotics, and muscle relaxants). In these circumstances, it is possible that even a temporary change in free drug concentration can have clinical consequences.

Metabolism

There are numerous examples in anesthesia of drugs that increase or decrease the metabolism of others. Interactions may occur in extrahepatic or hepatic sites of metabolism.

Many drugs—especially those with ester linkages—undergo hydrolysis by specific or nonspecific esterases found in blood and peripheral tissues:

- Drugs given to inhibit acetylcholinesterase at the motor end plate usually inhibit butyrylcholinesterase (pseudocholinesterase) in plasma. Thus, administration of neostigmine or pyridostigmine intensifies and prolongs the effects of succinylcholine and can also theoretically affect ester local anesthetics (procaine, chloroprocaine, tetracaine, cocaine). Enzyme inhibition needs to be substantial (<20% of normal activity remaining) before the clinical effects of these local anesthetics become prolonged.[20,21] The prolongation of effect depends on the specific inhibitor. Neostigmine, for example, can prolong the effect of succinylcholine by several hours. The organophosphate, echothiophate, is a powerful miotic used topically for refractory glaucoma. This compound irreversibly inhibits pseudocholinesterase,[20,22] and the effect persists for weeks, so the risk for interaction is prolonged.
- Drugs such as esmolol and remifentanil are hydrolyzed by so-called "nonspecific" esterases in blood and peripheral tissues. These drugs are not good substrates for cholinesterases, so they are not subject to this interaction.[22] The nonspecific esterases constitute a large group of isozymes with extremely high capacity and low substrate specificity. This enzyme system is not likely to be involved in drug–drug interactions because inhibition of any one isozyme usually does not affect overall drug clearance.

Monamide Oxidase Interactions

The enzyme, monamide oxidase (MAO), is distributed throughout the body, with the largest amounts found in the liver, kidney, and brain. MAO is located on the outer surface of mitochondria in the presynaptic terminals of noradrenergic, dopaminergic, and serotonergic neurons in the CNS and periphery. It acts to regulate the presynaptic pool of norepinephrine, dopamine, epinephrine, and serotonin available for synaptic transmission (see Chapter 12). MAO exists in two isoforms: MAO-A predominates in the gut wall, whereas MAO-B is the major isoform in the CNS.

The MAOIs are used mainly for the treatment of refractory endogenous depression and certain other mood disorders. They have gained some notoriety in medicine because they are the cause of more clinically important drug–drug interactions than almost any other class of drugs. Many of the purported interactions are poorly documented, although they cannot be discounted completely.

There are currently only three MAOIs marketed in the United States. Phenelzine (Nardil) is an older, nonselective MAOI derived from hydrazine. It irreversibly inhibits the enzyme, and synthesis of new enzyme can take 10 to 14 days. Tranylcypromine (Parnate) is a slightly shorter-acting MAOI derived from amphetamine. The newest member of this class is selegiline (deprenyl, Eldepryl), which is used as an adjunct in the treatment of Parkinson's disease. In lower doses, selegiline is relatively selective for MAO-B. The antibiotic furazolidone and the chemotherapeutic drug procarbazine also cause substantial inhibition of MAO and can potentially cause many of the same interactions.

Reported MAOI interactions are broadly of two types: the first group involves drugs that affect sympathetic neurotransmission:

- The well-known interaction with indirect-acting sympathomimetic drugs (ephedrine, amphetamine) occurs because MAOI treatment increases the amount of presynaptic transmitter that can be released by these drugs. Normal doses of ephedrine have produced severe hypertensive crises, occasionally leading to cerebral hemorrhage and death.
- The "wine and cheese" reaction is essentially the same interaction. Many foods such as aged cheese contain tyramine, a phenylethylamine that has ephedrine-like actions at sympathetic nerve endings. Normally, exogenous tyramine is degraded by MAO-A in the gut wall and liver, but patients on an MAOI may achieve high systemic concentrations and consequently have hypertensive crises.
- Paradoxically, a patient who has been taking an MAOI for some time may actually have *decreased* adrenergic responsiveness (some of the older MAOIs were marketed as treatments for hypertension). Even with good dietary compliance, these patients absorb some tyramine. Chronic exposure to low levels of tyramine allows this compound to be taken up by adrenergic terminals (in place of tyrosine), where it is metabolized to octopamine (rather than norepinephrine). Octopamine is a "false transmitter" with little activity, so sympathetic nerve function may eventually be impaired.
- Because MAO plays only a small role in the metabolism of compounds in the synaptic cleft, the response to sympathomimetics that act directly on postsynaptic receptor sites (phenylephrine, norepinephrine, epinephrine) should be affected less by such interactions. In a small study of four healthy volunteers (two receiving tranylcypromine and two receiving phenelzine), there was a moderate (twofold) increase in the response to phenylephrine, but the responses to norepinephrine and epinephrine were not exaggerated.[24] This is reassuring, but any sympathomimetic drug should still be administered with caution to patients on an MAOI.
- Adverse interactions have been described with older MAOIs and levodopa, possibly because both drugs increase dopamine concentrations. Nevertheless, there is some experience that levodopa and selegiline may be combined safely in patients with Parkinson's disease. The MAOI is given in this case to prevent free radical formation believed to be involved in neuronal degeneration.[25]
- Inhibition of norepinephrine reuptake by tricyclic antidepressants (TCAs) increases the amount of neurotransmitter in the synaptic cleft. This would seem to be a recipe for adverse interaction with MAOIs, but with careful monitoring, this combination has been used successfully for therapy.

The second group of MAOI interactions involves CNS depressants. As stated previously, some of these are poorly documented, and the mechanisms are unknown:

- The most important interaction is unquestionably with meperidine. When meperidine is given to a patient on an MAOI, a life-threatening reaction may occur, accompanied by excitation, hyperpyrexia, hypertension, profuse sweating, and rigidity.[26] This may progress to seizures, coma, and death. The reaction does not occur in every instance. It has also been described with selegiline,[27] and one or two case reports suggesting that a toxic interaction may occur with the antitussive, dextromethorphan,[28] and the analgesic, propoxyphene.[29] Other than some poorly documented case reports, the evidence suggests that morphine and fentanyl do not produce this interaction.[30] The mechanism of meperidine–MAOI interaction is unknown, but animal models suggest that it involves elevations in brain concentrations of serotonin.[31]
- Anecdotal reports have appeared regarding adverse MAOI interactions with other psychotropic drugs, including alcohol, phenothiazine, benzodiazepines, and

barbiturates,[32] but the evidence is weak. Some wines, such as Chianti, could be dangerous because they contain tyramine. It is possible (but probably not advisable) to use ketamine for induction of anesthesia in patients taking an MAOI.[33]

Should MAOIs be discontinued before elective surgery? The issue is still a matter of debate,[34] although drug package inserts usually advise an extremely conservative position (i.e., waiting 2 weeks for the enzyme to regenerate). Current clinical opinion probably favors continuing MAOI therapy up to the time of surgery, and our own experience supports this view. Most patients are receiving these drugs for moderate to severe psychiatric disorders that have not responded to other treatments. It is unpleasant and possibly risky for a patient with refractory depression to endure 2 to 3 weeks without effective therapy. If a general anesthetic is planned, it seems prudent to use the fewest possible drugs. Avoiding drugs with substantial sympathetic effects (e.g., pancuronium, cocaine, ketamine) probably makes sense.

There is little doubt that patients taking MAOIs have the potential for perioperative hemodynamic instability, yet beta-blockers, direct vasodilators, and direct-acting pressors appear to be safe and effective treatments in most circumstances. Roizen[35] concluded, "The major problem with continuing MAO inhibitors preoperatively is not the hemodynamic fluctuations that might occur ... but rather the rare instance of hyperpyrexic coma following narcotic administration...." Because opioids such as fentanyl appear safe and there are no major interactions with local anesthetics or NSAIDs, providing analgesia without meperidine should not be a hardship.

Hepatic Biotransformation

Many anesthetic drugs undergo oxidative metabolism by one of the isoforms of cytochrome P450 found in liver microsomes. The P450 isoforms have low substrate specificity, which means that drugs of diverse structures, such as general inhalation anesthetics, meperidine, barbiturates, and benzodiazepines, can be biotransformed by a single group of enzymes. It is not surprising that inhibitors or inducers of these enzymes can also affect the clearance of broad groups of drugs.

The removal of drug from the blood by hepatic biotransformation (hepatic clearance) is a function of two independent variables, the hepatic blood flow and the intrinsic clearance (the maximal ability of the liver to metabolize that drug). The intrinsic clearance is often expressed as the *extraction ratio* (ER)—the fraction of drug that can be metabolized in a single pass through the liver (see Chapter 11).

$$ER = \frac{C_a - C_v}{C_a}$$

where C_a is the drug concentration coming to the liver (mixed portal vein + hepatic artery) and C_v is the drug concentration leaving (hepatic vein). So,

$$\text{Hepatic clearance} = \text{ER} \times \text{hepatic blood flow}$$

Drugs may be classed broadly as "high extraction" and "low extraction," a distinction with important implications for drug interaction:

A high-extraction drug (e.g., lidocaine, propranolol) may have an ER of 0.7 to 0.8 or more (70 to 80% is cleared in one pass through the liver). For these drugs, hepatic blood flow is the rate-limiting factor in overall hepatic clearance, that is, the delivery of drug to the liver determines the amount cleared. Clearance is decreased by drugs or maneuvers that lower hepatic blood flow, such as beta-blockade, cimetidine, halothane, hypotension, and upper abdominal surgery. The clearance of these rapidly metabolized drugs is much less sensitive to changes in enzyme activity. Nor does plasma protein binding have a large effect: the enzymes are so active that a drug such as lidocaine is simply stripped off its binding proteins as it traverses the liver:

- Decreases in hepatic blood flow secondary to decreased cardiac output elevate lidocaine concentrations in humans.[36]
- Pressor administration can also accomplish the same thing. This effect was elegantly demonstrated by Benowitz et al[37] in rhesus monkeys (Fig. 50-1). Steady-state infusions of lidocaine were established, then hepatic blood flow was increased or decreased by infusions of isoproterenol or norepinephrine, respectively. During isoproterenol infusion, the concentration of lidocaine decreased, indicating increased clearance. During norepinephrine infusion, lidocaine concentrations increased.
- Lidocaine clearance is decreased and toxicity is increased when patients are treated chronically with cimetidine.[38] It is not clear whether single-dose premedication with cimetidine produces the same effect.
- Other high-extraction drugs, such as morphine and sufentanil, are affected the same way. The clearance of morphine may be very slow in a patient with decreased hepatic blood flow.

Low-extraction drugs such as diazepam, alfentanil, or mepivacaine have ERs of 0.3 or less. These drugs behave quite differently because hepatic enzyme activity is rate limiting (hepatic clearance is limited by intrinsic clearance). Stimulation or inhibition of enzyme activity can have a large effect on overall pharmacokinetics. Protein binding is also more likely to affect clearance because the bound forms of these drugs are protected from hepatic metabolism. The most common reason for increased intrinsic clearance is enzyme induction. Many drugs of importance in anesthesiology are metabolized by the cytochrome P450 enzymes (so-called microsomal or CYP enzymes). Several families and numerous subfamilies of these enzymes have been identified based on the homology of their amino acid sequences. The most important subfamily appears to be CYP3A, which is found in greatest abundance in human liver and is responsible for the metabolism of a huge number of drugs. Other subfamilies play important roles in drug metabolism, such as CYP2C19 (diazepam) or CYP2E1 (defluorination of volatile anesthetics). There are hundreds of drugs and environmental toxins that can stimulate or "induce" microsomal enzymes. Typically, a single inducer can affect the products of several gene families. For example, phenobarbital can increase the amount of the P450 enzymes CYP2B, 2C, 2E, 3A, and 4B.[39] An increase in the quantity of enzyme protein can therefore increase the clearance of many drugs simultaneously. However, not all inducers affect the same enzymes.

Treatment with an enzyme inducer (Table 50-1) can make an otherwise stable drug regimen ineffective or inconsistently effective:

- A classic example is the interaction between phenobarbital and coumarin-type anticoagulants (Fig. 50-2). Increased metabolism may also result in the production of an active or toxic metabolite.
- In rat microsomal preparations, the liberation of inorganic fluoride by isoflurane, methoxyflurane, and enflurane can be increased by pretreatment with barbiturates,[40] but this interaction appears to be clinically

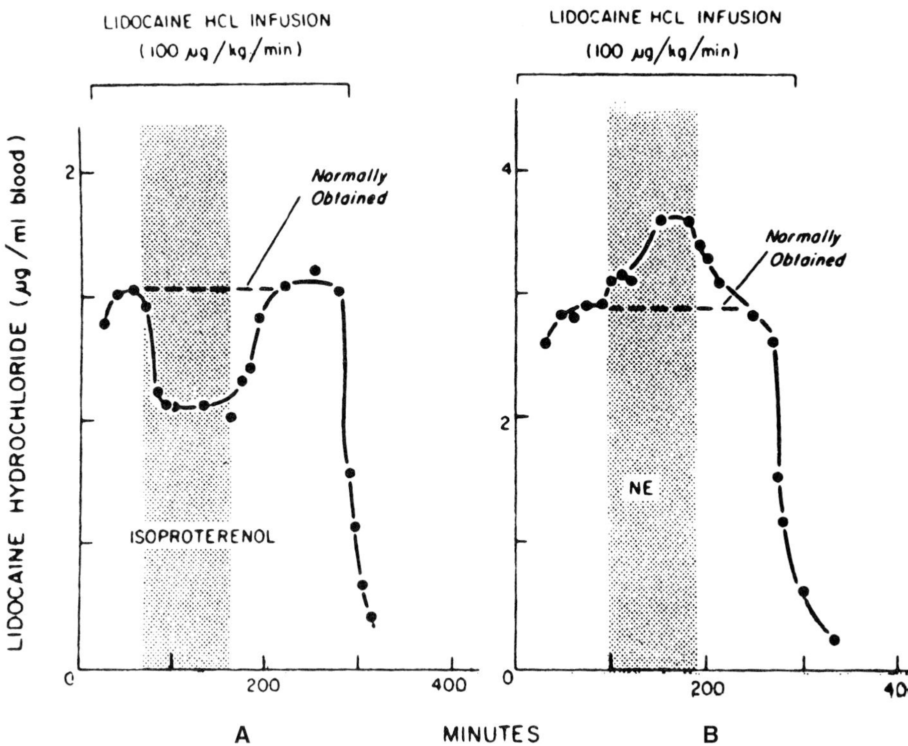

FIGURE 50-1. The effects of increasing or decreasing hepatic blood flow with isoproterenol (A) and norepinephrine (NE) (B) on steady-state arterial lidocaine concentrations in the rhesus monkey. The pressors were administered during the period indicated by the *shaded bar*. The *dashed lines* show the steady-state concentration expected in the absence of pressors. (Reprinted with permission from Benowitz NL, Forsyth RP, Melmon KL *et al*: Lidocaine disposition kinetics in monkey and man: II. Effects of hemorrhage and sympathomimetic drug administration. Clin Pharmacol Ther 16:99, 1974.)

important only for methoxyflurane.[41] In humans, phenobarbital does not induce defluorination of enflurane.

- Reductive pathways also involve P450 enzymes, and the production of toxic reduced intermediates has been postulated as a mechanism for "halothane hepatitis." In animal models, administration of halothane after enzyme inducers can lead to centrilobular necrosis.[42] The clinical relevance of this finding is unknown.

There are many examples of drugs that inhibit the hepatic biotransformation of other drugs (see Table 50-1):

- When two drugs are substrates for the same P450 enzymes, they can interact competitively and reduce the clearance of both. For example, it has been demonstrated that midazolam and fentanyl are competitive inhibitors in vitro of metabolism by CYP3A4.[43] This pharmacokinetic interaction is probably far less important than the pharmacodynamic interaction between these drugs (described later).
- Another study concluded that propofol competitively inhibits CYP3A4, and it can reduce the clearance of midazolam by 37%.[44] Propofol itself appears to be metabolized by a different isoform, CYP2B6.[45]

TABLE 50-1

DRUGS THAT INDUCE OR INHIBIT HEPATIC DRUG METABOLISM IN HUMANS

■ INDUCERS	■ INHIBITORS
Phenobarbital	Cimetidine
Phenytoin	Ketoconazole
Rifampicin	Erythromycin
Carbamazepine	Disulfiram
Ethanol	Ritonavir

- Alfentanil and erythromycin are both metabolized by CYP3A4, and the antibiotic greatly prolongs the effect of the opioid.[46] Sufentanil and fentanyl are also metabolized by CYP3A4,[47] but the clearance of sufentanil is not changed by erythromycin.[48] Perhaps this is because it is a high-clearance opioid.
- Cimetidine has an imidazole group that binds to the heme iron of cytochrome P450 and forms an inactive complex. Cimetidine inhibits the metabolism of many drugs, including warfarin, diazepam, phenytoin, and morphine. Several studies have demonstrated that coadministration

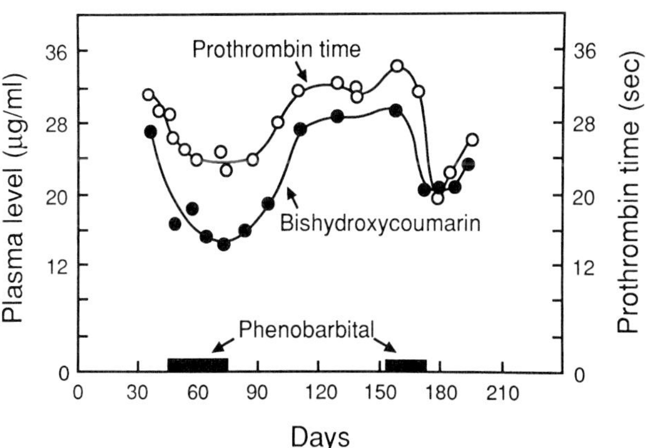

FIGURE 50-2. Effect of phenobarbital on plasma levels of bishydroxycoumarin. The anticoagulant was given at a dose of 75 mg/day. Phenobarbital, 65 mg/day, was given during the periods indicated on the *x*-axis. Induction of hepatic enzymes decreased anticoagulant concentrations and reduced the effect. (Reprinted with permission from Cucinell SA, Conney AH, Sansur M *et al:* Drug interactions in man: I. Lowering effect of phenobarbital on plasma levels of bishydroxy coumarin [dicumarol] and diphenylhydantoin [Dilantin]. Clin Pharmacol Ther 6:420, 1965.)

of cimetidine and diazepam causes clinically significant elevations in the concentration of both diazepam and its active metabolite.[49] As stated previously, cimetidine can decrease hepatic blood flow, so it can also decrease the clearance of high-extraction drugs.[38]

- Protease inhibitors such as saquinavir[50] and ritonavir[51] can inhibit the metabolism of midazolam and fentanyl, respectively, by inhibiting CYP3A4.
- Other imidazole drugs such as the antifungals, ketoconazole and itraconazole, can inhibit a wide variety of microsomal enzymes. They have been shown to decrease the clearance (and increase the toxicity) of glyburide, terfenadine, digoxin, midazolam, theophylline, and warfarin.
- The related benzimidazole, etomidate, blocks the synthesis of cortisol and aldosterone by inhibiting the P450-dependent mitochondrial enzymes, 17α-hydroxylase and 11β-hydroxylase.[52] Etomidate can inhibit the metabolism of other drugs, but the effects do not appear to be clinically important.

Drug Elimination

The final category of pharmacokinetic interaction is through alteration in drug elimination. These interactions usually involve altered renal clearance, but they may also involve changes in pulmonary excretion.

The mechanism for ion trapping was discussed earlier. Ion trapping can be the basis for large changes in renal drug excretion when the pK_a of the drug is close to the normal range of urine pH:

- A weak acid such as phenobarbital ($pK_a = 7.4$) is largely nonionized when the urine pH is 6.0. This means that much of the filtered drug is in a relatively lipid-soluble form and available for tubular reabsorption. If the urine pH is raised to 8 or 9 (e.g., with sodium bicarbonate), most of the phenobarbital becomes ionized, reabsorption decreases, and clearance increases. For a weak base, the reverse situation is true—excretion can be promoted when the urine is acidified. This type of interaction is used therapeutically in certain cases of drug overdose.

Organic anions and cations are actively secreted by separate transporters in the renal tubule. The cation system handles the elimination of atropine, isoproterenol, neostigmine, and meperidine. The anion system is involved in the excretion of salicylate, penicillins, cephalosporins, and most of the potent diuretics. The various anions and cations can compete for their respective transport sites:

- Probenecid inhibits the secretion of penicillin, increasing plasma concentrations and prolonging the duration of action.
- Quinidine has been shown to decrease both the volume of distribution and the renal clearance of digoxin, and plasma digoxin concentrations may increase by two- to fivefold.[53] The renal effect is believed to be due to a reduction in tubular secretion of digoxin.

PHARMACODYNAMIC INTERACTIONS

Up to this point, we have been discussing pharmacokinetic interactions that change the amount of active drug reaching re-
4 ceptor sites. A *pharmacodynamic* interaction occurs when one drug alters the sensitivity of a target receptor or tissue to the effects of a second drug. This means that the dose-response or concentration-response curve for one drug is shifted by another

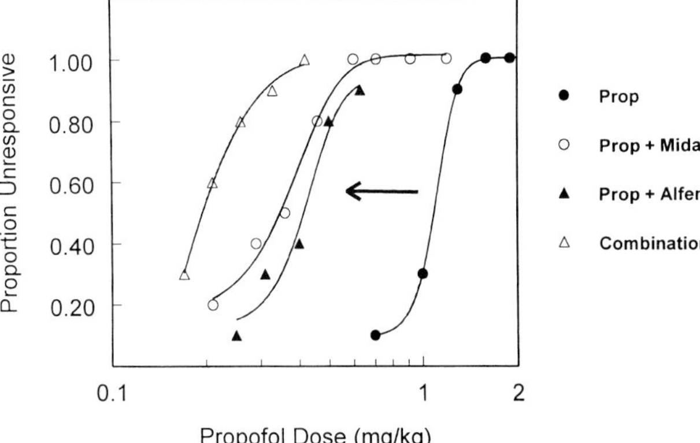

FIGURE 50-3. Dose-response curves for loss of consciousness after an intravenous bolus dose of propofol (Prop) alone, propofol plus midazolam (Midaz), propofol plus alfentanil (Alfent), or all three drugs. Drug combinations were given as constant ratios, based on the measured ED_{50}s of the individual drugs. Both the benzodiazepine and the opioid shifted the dose-response curve for propofol significantly to the left. (Redrawn, with permission, from data in Short TG, Plummer JL, Chui PT: Hypnotic and anaesthetic interactions between midazolam, propofol and alfentanil. Br J Anaesth 69:162, 1992.)

(Fig. 50-3). It is often difficult to assign a specific mechanism to these interactions. We commonly classify them by their direction and intensity, that is, additive, antagonistic, or supra-additive (synergistic).

5 *Additive interactions* are most likely to occur when drugs with identical mechanisms are combined. The clinician normally expects additivity when combining two benzodiazepines, two fentanyl analogs, or two volatile anesthetics. Most additive interactions tend not to be particularly surprising, although some are clinically useful:

- The administration of two aminosteroid nondepolarizing muscle relaxants, such as rocuronium and vecuronium, gives an additive effect[54] (Fig. 50-4). Notably, the

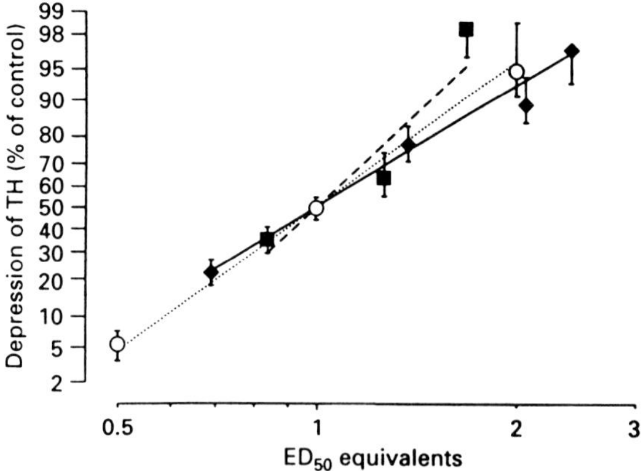

FIGURE 50-4. The interaction of rocuronium and vecuronium is additive in man. Log dose-probit graph plots twitch height (TH) as percentage of control value. Dose is given in terms of ED_{50} multiples. *Dark diamonds, dark squares*, and *open circles* represent rocuronium, vecuronium, and the combination, respectively. The dose–response curve for the combination cannot be distinguished from those of the individual drugs. (Reprinted with permission from Naguib M, Samarkandi AH, Bakhamees HS *et al:* Comparative potency of steroidal neuromuscular blocking drugs and isobolographic analysis of the interaction. Br J Anaesth 75:37, 1995.)

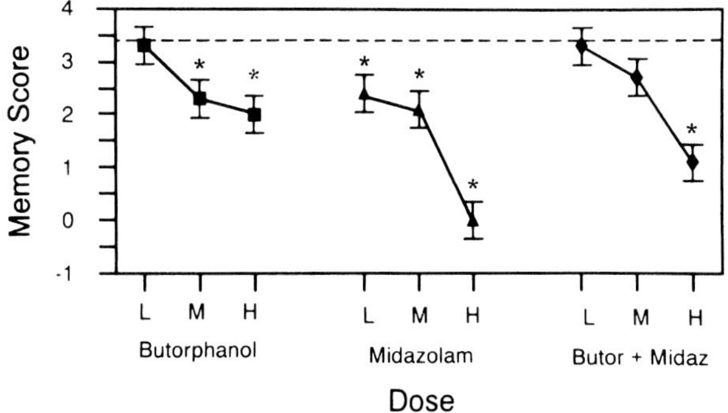

FIGURE 50-5. Memory scores of patients 5 minutes after receiving butorphanol, midazolam, or the combination. L, M, and H signify low, medium, and high doses (7.1, 22.5, and 71.4 μg/kg butorphanol; 4.3, 13.6, and 42.9 μg/kg midazolam; or 3.6 + 2.2, 11.3 + 6.8, and 35.7 + 21.5 μg/kg butorphanol and midazolam in combination). The *dashed line* indicates mean pretreatment value. Midazolam, but not butorphanol, produced a profound anterograde amnestic effect. Giving one-half the dose of each drug in combination produced an effect that was less than that after midazolam alone. (Reprinted with permission from Dershwitz M, Rosow CE, DiBiase PM *et al:* A comparison of the sedative effects of butorphanol and midazolam. Anesthesiology 74:717, 1991.)

interactions between nondepolarizing relaxants of different chemical classes are often synergistic (see later).

- The interaction of two volatile anesthetics or nitrous oxide with volatile anesthetics is additive.[55–57]
- In animals, mixtures of lidocaine-tetracaine or lidocaine-etidocaine produce approximately additive CNS toxicity when given intravenously.[58]

The most common *antagonistic drug interactions* in anes-
6 thesia are those involving deliberate reversal of effect with competitive antagonists such as neostigmine, naloxone, or flumazenil. Pharmacodynamic antagonism that is *unintended* is a much less common event:

- An antagonistic interaction occurs between succinylcholine and the nondepolarizing relaxants.[59]
- When epidural morphine or fentanyl is administered after establishing a block with 2-chloroprocaine, both the duration and the intensity of opioid analgesia are decreased.[60] The mechanism for this interaction is unclear.
- When butorphanol is combined with midazolam, the mixture increases sedation but has less anterograde amnestic effect than midazolam alone (Fig. 50-5). This illustrates the important concept that a drug combination may simultaneously be synergistic and antagonistic for different effects. In the case of the amnestic effect, butorphanol may simply be diluting the effects of midazolam.[61]

The most interesting and clinically important interactions
7 tend to be the *synergistic interactions,* in which small doses of two or more drugs can sometimes produce large effects. Synergy is most likely to occur when drugs of different classes, or even those with slightly different mechanisms, are used to produce the same effects:

- The potentiation of opioids by NSAIDs is a classic and useful interaction between analgesic drugs with completely different mechanisms.[62]
- The potentiation of nondepolarizing relaxants by the various volatile anesthetics is a useful interaction on a daily basis. The exact mechanism is unknown, but several theories have been proposed, including increased blood flow to muscle, depression of centrally mediated muscle tone, decreased neurotransmitter release, and decreased sensitivity of postjunctional or muscle membranes.
- A much more subtle supra-additive interaction occurs between aminosteroid and benzylisoquinolines. Pancuronium and *d*-tubocurarine were shown to produce a synergistic relaxant effect in combination,[63] and this is also seen with similar combinations across these two chemical classes (atracurium and vecuronium, *d*-tubocurarine and vecuronium, mivacurium and rocuronium). Various mechanisms have been proposed, including multiple binding sites[64] (presynaptic for aminosteroid versus postsynaptic for benzylisoquinolines) and allosteric interactions between separate agonist and antagonist binding sites.[65]
- Sedatives and hypnotics with related (but not identical) mechanisms of action usually interact synergistically to produce greater CNS depression. This is discussed in more detail later in this chapter.

STUDYING DRUG INTERACTIONS

As already discussed, a study that demonstrates that a drug–drug interaction exists does not necessarily establish its mechanism, its magnitude, or its clinical relevance. What information is needed to conclude that an interaction is pharmacodynamic rather than pharmacokinetic? How do we know it is really synergistic? Let us consider four clinical experiments to study the interaction of midazolam and thiopental. Given the different mechanisms for these two drugs, we might predict a synergistic interaction: benzodiazepines increase neuronal chloride conductance by facilitating GABA action, whereas barbiturates bind to a separate site and affect the chloride channel more directly:

1. In the simplest study design, two groups of patients are randomly assigned to receive midazolam-thiopental or placebo-thiopental. The percentage that becomes unresponsive in each group is assessed at a standard time after thiopental administration. The data show that midazolam increases the percentage unresponsive.

   Such a study is severely limited: it tells us that an interaction has occurred, but the results cannot be generalized beyond the conditions examined (a single dose of midazolam, a single dose of thiopental). Nothing may be inferred about mechanism.
2. A more complex (but more useful) experiment would be to study a thiopental dose-response curve in the presence and absence of midazolam. This would show that the dose of thiopental required to produce hypnosis in half the patients (ED_{50}) is decreased by midazolam.

   These results allow us to conclude that the interaction occurs over a range of thiopental doses relevant to clinical practice. The data still apply only to a single dose of midazolam, and they tell us nothing about the mechanism of the interaction.
3. A useful modification of this experiment is to administer the thiopental by a constant-rate infusion (with or without midazolam) and measure its concentration over time. The data show that concentrations of thiopental rise at the same rate in both groups, but midazolam decreases the concentration needed to produce hypnosis in 50% of the patients (the EC_{50}).

   This tells us that midazolam has not changed the pharmacokinetics of thiopental, so the interaction must have a pharmacodynamic mechanism.
4. Finally, there are a number of experimental designs for demonstrating synergy, and these have been reviewed

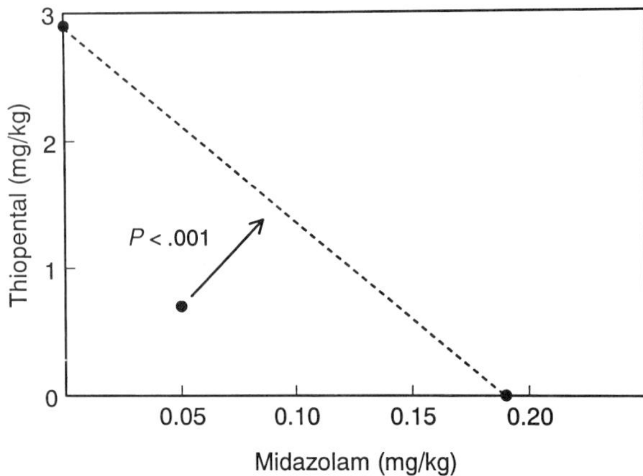

FIGURE 50-6. Isobolographic analysis of the interaction between midazolam and thiopental in humans (see text for details). The ED_{50} of the combination was significantly less than predicted by the dotted "line of additivity." (Redrawn from data of Tverskoy M, Fleyshman G, Bradley EL Jr, Kissin I: Midazolam-thiopental anesthetic interaction in patients. Anesth Analg 67:342, 1988, with permission.)

in the clinical literature.[66] Two of the most common techniques used by experimental pharmacologists are algebraic (fractional)[67] and isobolographic[68,69] analysis, and clinical anesthesia studies using these methods have been appearing frequently. The interaction of thiopental and midazolam was studied with an isobolographic technique, and the results are shown in Fig. 50-6.[70] In general, this analysis requires a minimum of *three* dose-response experiments, one with each drug alone and one with the drugs in combination. The drug combination can be studied as a fixed ratio, or one of the drugs can be given at a fixed dose and the dose of the second drug varied. From these experiments, three estimates of ED_{50} are made, and an isobologram is constructed as shown in Fig. 50-6. The ED_{50}s for thiopental and midazolam alone are graphed on the two axes, and these points are connected by the theoretic "line of additivity." If the two drugs are simply additive when combined, we would expect the ED_{50} of the mixture to fall somewhere along this line. Because the actual ED_{50} of the mixture is significantly less than predicted by this line, the interaction is synergistic (an ED_{50} greater than predicted would signify antagonism).

PHARMACODYNAMIC INTERACTIONS AFFECTING HEMODYNAMICS

The treatment of hypertension, angina, dysrhythmias, and congestive heart failure involves the use of drugs with powerful effects on autonomic function and cardiovascular homeostasis. Until the 1970s, the teaching was generally that cardiovascular depressant or stimulant medications should be discontinued before surgery because they interfered with protective responses to the trauma of anesthesia and surgery. Some older antihypertensives like reserpine and α-methyl dopa altered the depth of anesthesia, and this was believed to be undesirable. There is now a substantial body of evidence showing that most cardiovascular medications need not and should not be stopped before surgery. Hypertensive patients who remain well controlled are less likely to have wide swings in pressure during surgery. Even small doses of beta-blockers given before surgery can reduce the incidence of myocardial ischemia and improve outcome.[71,72] One week of perioperative treatment with atenolol can produce long-term benefits.[73,74] Conversely, the abrupt discontinuation of vasoactive medications can actually increase cardiovascular instability, and in the case of beta-blockers and clonidine, the rebound hypertension and dysrhythmias may be dangerous.

Given the foregoing observations, it is fortunate that most
8 cardiovascular drug–drug interactions are simply extensions of the known pharmacology of the agents (Table 50-2). In short, the hypotensive effects of general or regional anesthesia may be increased by all antihypertensive medications. Using similar logic, antidysrhythmic drugs such as amiodarone or procainamide increase the possibility of bradycardia, hypotension, and decreased cardiac output.

With few exceptions, there is little reason to withhold most vasoactive medications before surgery. It may be prudent to stop diuretic treatment before procedures with large anticipated fluid requirements or significant use of nephrotoxic antibiotics. Some studies suggest that continuation of the angiotensin-converting enzyme inhibitors (ACEIs) and angiotensin receptor blockers (ARBs) leads to a high incidence of severe, sometimes refractory hypotension during induction of general anesthesia.[75,76] These drugs decrease afterload, and they also potentiate anesthetic-induced reduction in preload. The effect on preload may be quite important in hypertensive patients who have preexisting diastolic dysfunction.

Like the baroreceptor reflexes, the renin-angiotensin system is an important way the body can respond to hypovolemia or hypotension. Within minutes after a pressure decrease is sensed by the juxtaglomerular apparatus, angiotensin II causes vasoconstriction by both central and peripheral actions. Chronic blockade of this system not only inhibits the angiotensin response, but it also reduces the vasoconstrictor response to norepinephrine.[77] This may explain why ACEI-induced and ARB-induced hypotension can be so resistant to sympathetic drugs such as phenylephrine, ephedrine, and norepinephrine.[78] Vasopressin and various vasopressin analogs can restore sympathetic response[79] and may be useful pressors in cases of refractory hypotension.

There is currently no consensus on the preoperative management of patients taking ACEI or ARB. Withholding them for 24 hours may decrease hypotension but also make blood pressure extremely labile during surgery. Some have found them to be beneficial during surgery.[80] The considerations are probably different for patients receiving ACEIs for chronic congestive heart failure. ACEIs are given to these patients for afterload reduction; they improve baroreceptor sensitivity, reduce ventricular remodeling, and decrease the mortality rate. Perioperative use of ACEIs in this population may not increase the already high incidence of hypotension during induction.[81]

Most perioperative hemodynamic interactions involve the use of cardiovascular depressants. It is also useful to consider several groups of patients who are treated (or who "self-treat") before surgery with cardiovascular *stimulants*:

1. Patients with bronchospasm may require treatment with rapid-acting β_2 agonists (albuterol, terbutaline), anticholinergics (ipratropium), or phosphodiesterase inhibitors (theophylline). These patients are at increased risk for tachydysrhythmias and ectopic rhythms. Similar considerations apply to the patient receiving the intravenous β_2 agonist, ritodrine, for premature labor.
2. Patients who receive TCAs such as imipramine, desipramine, amitriptyline, and nortriptyline present several possible scenarios for adverse drug interaction. These drugs work by blocking presynaptic reuptake of

TABLE 50-2

EFFECTS OF ANTIHYPERTENSIVE DRUGS DURING ANESTHESIA

■ CLASS	■ DRUGS	■ CLASS EFFECTS
Alpha-blockers	Phenoxybenzamine Phentolamine Prazosin	Hypotension/vasodilation Reflex tachycardia
Beta-blockers	Propranolol Metoprolol Atenolol	Hypotension Decreased contractility Bradycardia AV block
Mixed alpha-/beta-blocker	Labetalol	Hypotension/vasodilation Bradycardia AV block
Calcium channel blockers	Verapamil Diltiazem Nifedipine Nicardipine	Hypotension/vasodilation Decreased contractility Bradycardia AV block
Direct vasodilators	Nitroglycerin Isosorbide Hydralazine	Hypotension/vasodilation Reflex tachycardia
Angiotensin-converting enzyme inhibitors	Captopril Enalapril Lisinopril	Hypotension/vasodilation Hyperkalemia
Angiotensin II blocker	Losartan Valsartan	Hypotension/vasodilation Hyperkalemia
Diuretics	Thiazides Furosemide Bumetanide	Hypovolemia Hypokalemia Possible vasodilation

AV, atrioventricular.

norepinephrine or serotonin, so they can theoretically increase the effects of direct-acting or indirect-acting agonists at these synapses. Most TCAs also have prominent anticholinergic effects. In overdose situations, TCAs can create the entire range of cardiovascular toxicity, including myocardial infarction and sudden death. In spite of this, hypotension and tachydysrhythmias are not common intraoperative problems for patients taking these older antidepressants. It is still reasonable to minimize the use of pancuronium, halothane, ketamine, and other agents with the potential to increase the incidence of dysrhythmias. If TCA-induced hypotension occurs, there is disagreement about the best way to treat it.[82] One case report[83] describes a patient on chronic nifedipine and nortriptyline therapy who had hypotension that was resistant to ephedrine, phenylephrine, and dopamine (norepinephrine was eventually successful).

3. Finally, we must all be prepared to treat patients who are acutely or chronically intoxicated with cocaine. In addition to its local anesthetic properties, cocaine decreases norepinephrine reuptake, like TCAs. Acute intoxication presents a particular challenge. Young, otherwise healthy people may present with fulminant hypertension, tachycardia, and myocardial ischemia (the latter may be severe because cocaine can also induce a thrombotic diathesis). Management of the acute cardiovascular effects is similar to that for pheochromocytoma: these patients need both vasodilators and beta-blockers. A beta-blocker should not be given alone because unopposed α-adrenergic stimulation can cause a further increase in systemic vascular resistance. Patients with chronic cocaine intoxication are less of a problem, but they are still at risk for dysrhythmias (avoiding halothane, pancuronium, atropine, and sympathomimetics still seems like a good idea). Chronic cocaine exposure increases halothane minimum alveolar concentration (MAC) in dogs[84] and isoflurane MAC in sheep,[85] but it may increase the sedative effects of benzodiazepines in humans.[86] This is an interesting contrast to chronic treatment with amphetamine, which appears to decrease MAC in dogs.[87] It might be believed that the adrenergic overactivity induced by cocaine would produce receptor downregulation over time, but several animal studies suggest that chronic cocaine treatment does not decrease brain catecholamine content or sympathetic responsiveness.[88,89] The relevance of these data to human cardiovascular responses remains to be proven.

PHARMACODYNAMIC INTERACTIONS AFFECTING ANALGESIA OR HYPNOSIS

9 Combinations of CNS depressants almost always produce additive or synergistic increases in CNS effect. These interactions are usually useful and predictable. All the common intravenous and inhaled anesthetic agents have been tested in combination in humans. The following sections highlight some of the most important interactions.

Opioid–Hypnotic Interactions

This is arguably the most commonly used synergistic combination in intravenous anesthesia:

- Fentanyl and alfentanil have been shown to reduce the requirement for barbiturates, and there is some evidence that the interaction is beneficial. Reducing the total dose of thiopental[90] or thiamylal[91] during short procedures decreases the time to awakening and orientation.

- Opioids also potentiate propofol, but it has been much more difficult to show that the combination improves recovery compared with propofol alone. Short et al[92] found that a small dose of alfentanil can reduce the induction dose of propofol by 50% (see Fig. 50-3). During total intravenous anesthesia, infusions of remifentanil or alfentanil tremendously reduce the infusion rate of propofol needed to suppress response to voice and movement responses to surgical stimuli.[93,94] Target effect-site concentrations of only 1 to 2 μg/mL of propofol produce adequate anesthesia in many cases. These are routinely achieved with propofol doses used for conscious sedation (25 to 50 μg/kg per minute).

Opioid–Benzodiazepine Interactions

This important interaction was alluded to earlier, and it illustrates why opioids are so commonly used in combination with diazepam or midazolam. Opioids are highly selective CNS depressants; they can produce sedation, but they are relatively weak hypnotics. Even huge doses of fentanyl and its congeners do not dependably produce sleep by themselves.[95] For example, alfentanil doses as high as 100 to 200 μg/kg cannot always induce unconsciousness in unpremedicated patients.[96] Such opioid doses uniformly produce apnea, rigidity, and profound analgesia.

Kissin and coworkers[97] found, however, that a tiny dose of alfentanil (3 μg/kg) is sufficient to reduce the hypnotic ED_{50} of midazolam by 50%. This dose is subanalgesic and subhypnotic when given alone. This means that a small dose of opioid (50 μg fentanyl, 500 μg alfentanil) may have almost no hypnotic effect by itself, but can still be an extremely effective potentiator of other hypnotics. It also means that when fentanyl and midazolam are combined for conscious sedation, the opioid is producing sleep as well as analgesia.

Benzodiazepine–Hypnotic Interactions

The theoretical basis for the interaction between barbiturates and benzodiazepines was discussed earlier, and the thiopental–midazolam interaction is shown in Fig. 50-6.

- Thiopental–midazolam interaction has been studied in humans, and the combination was found to have 1.8 times the expected potency of the individual agents.[70,98] Similar results have been described with the combination of midazolam and methohexital.[99]
- Propofol also acts by modulation of GABA neurotransmission, and its hypnotic effects are potentiated when it is combined with midazolam.[92]

The clinical benefits of benzodiazepine premedication are most obvious during the preoperative period. Intraoperative benefits (i.e., increased efficacy or reduced toxicity) of benzodiazepine–hypnotic combinations have not been demonstrated. The patient premedicated with midazolam needs less thiopental or propofol for induction (or maintenance), but it has not been established that this results in a smoother anesthetic or more rapid awakening.

Volatile Anesthetic–Opioid Interactions

Opioids produce dose-dependent and concentration-dependent decreases in MAC for all the inhalation anesthetics:

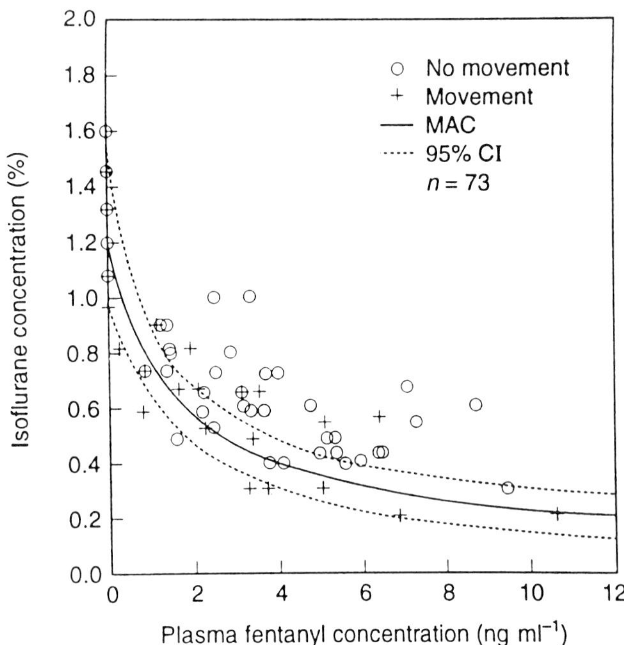

FIGURE 50-7. The interaction between fentanyl and isoflurane. The *solid line* represents the concentration of the two drugs that prevents movement in 50% of patients. MAC, minimum alveolar concentration; CI, confidence interval. (Reprinted with permission from McEwan AI, Smith C, Dyar O *et al*: Isoflurane minimum alveolar concentration reduction by fentanyl. Anesthesiology 78:864, 1993.)

- A steady-state plasma fentanyl concentration of 1.67 ng/mL decreases human isoflurane MAC by 50%[100] (Fig. 50-7).
- Opioid partial agonists such as nalbuphine and butorphanol produce smaller reductions in MAC.[101]
- Animal data consistently show that an approximately 70% reduction in MAC is the maximum effect obtainable with a full agonist like fentanyl.[102] The mechanism for this interaction is unknown, but Licina et al[103] showed that administration of lumbar intrathecal morphine (15 μg/kg) does not alter halothane MAC in humans. This suggests that the effect may be due to supraspinal opioid actions. These findings are particularly interesting in view of the work by Rampil et al[104] who showed that MAC in the rat is not altered when the cerebral cortex and all other precollicular brain structures are removed. MAC therefore appears to reflect an action of the volatile anesthetics on the spinal cord, whereas MAC reduction by opioids is most likely to be mediated by structures in the brainstem or higher. One possible site for interaction is the locus coeruleus.

Opioids and volatile agents are often combined to smooth the intraoperative and postoperative course. In some patients, the combination of opioid and volatile agent is hemodynamically better tolerated than the volatile agent alone. Addition of an opioid may also reduce the incidence of emergence delirium.

Is there any evidence that the combination speeds awakening? Reduction of MAC clearly leads to lower end-tidal concentrations at the end of surgery. Faster emergence occurs only if the concentration of inhaled agent that produces hypnosis (i.e., "MAC awake," the concentration at which 50% of subjects respond to voice) is not reduced by a comparable amount. A few data indicate that MAC awake is not decreased by opioids, suggesting that the combination improves recovery.[105,106]

There have been no studies specifically designed to test this hypothesis.

Other intravenous agents such as lidocaine,[107] midazolam,[108] and α_2 agonists have been shown to decrease MAC in experimental animals. For lidocaine and midazolam, the plasma concentrations required to produce a meaningful decrease in MAC are so high that the interaction is unlikely to have clinical utility. There is some evidence that the simultaneous use of volatile anesthetics and benzodiazepines causes increased cortical binding of the latter.[109]

α_2-Agonist Interactions

It has long been known that drugs that depress CNS sympathetic function can produce sedation and potentiate anesthesia. Older antihypertensives such as reserpine and α-methyldopa can produce drowsiness and reduce halothane MAC.[110] The newer autonomic modulators—α_2 agonists such as clonidine or dexmedetomidine—are powerful sedatives and analgesics in humans.

- In animals, dexmedetomidine produces marked potentiation of opioid analgesia and benzodiazepine-induced hypnosis.[111]
- Dexmedetomidine also lowers halothane MAC by nearly 100% through a specific postsynaptic α_2 mechanism.[112]

Dexmedetomidine interacts with both presynaptic and postsynaptic α_2-adrenergic receptors to decrease central sympathetic tone. Its hypnotic effect is due largely to depression of function in the locus coeruleus (LC), the main adrenergic nucleus in the brain.[113] There is evidence to suggest that the LC is an important site for control of sleep, attention, memory, analgesia, and autonomic function.[114] The LC contains receptors for glutamate, GABA, acetylcholine, opioids, and benzodiazepines, and experimental evidence suggests that it may be the site for some important anesthetic drug effects and interactions:

1. The LC is the rostral portion of an important descending inhibitory pathway, which plays a part in the production of opioid analgesia.[115]
2. In the rat, destroying the LC produces a state of narcolepsy and decreases halothane MAC by 30 to 40%.[116]
3. Agonists at GABA, opioid, and α_2 receptors are all inhibitory when injected into the LC. These drugs all have sedative-hypnotic properties, and all of them lower the requirement for volatile anesthetics.
4. Acetylcholine and glutamate receptor agonists are excitatory in the LC, and antagonists at these receptors (e.g., scopolamine, ketamine) are hypnotics. Some glutamate effects are mediated by NO, and inhibitors of neuronal NO synthase can decrease the requirement for halothane[117] and isoflurane.[118]

Three-Way Interactions

In clinical practice, it is common to combine more than two drugs with sedative-hypnotic effects. We have relatively little information on what happens when a third drug is added to two that already have synergistic effects:

- Short et al[92] performed a clinical study of hypnotic interactions among propofol, midazolam, and alfentanil (see Fig. 50-3). Propofol requirement was reduced by 82% with the three-way combination, but it produced less potentiation than would have been predicted by adding the effects of the two-way combinations.

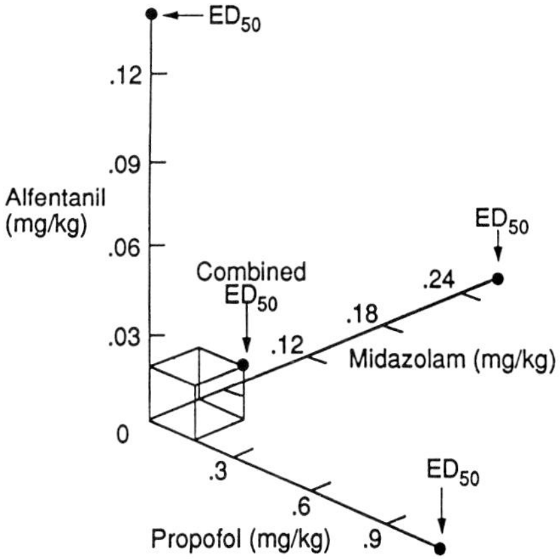

FIGURE 50-8. ED_{50} isobolograms for the three-way hypnotic interactions among midazolam, alfentanil, and propofol. The reader can imagine a triangular "plane of additivity" with its corners at the individual ED_{50} values. The ED_{50} for the triple combination was significantly lower than predicted by additivity. (Reprinted with permission from Vinik HR, Bradley EL Jr, Kissin I: Triple anesthetic combination: Propofol-midazolam-alfentanil. Anesth Analg 78:354, 1994.)

- Vinik et al[119] studied the same combination and also found profound hypnotic synergism: the dose of propofol could be decreased by 86% in the presence of alfentanil and midazolam. The data also suggested that the interaction between midazolam and alfentanil was a marked potentiation, but the addition of propofol did not produce significant additional change. Figure 50-8 shows the data from this experiment analyzed with a three-way isobologram.
- A three-way interaction involving enflurane, dexmedetomidine, and fentanyl was investigated in dogs. Salmenpera et al[120] found that each of the two intravenous agents lowered enflurane MAC, and combining the three drugs produced a MAC reduction that was probably greater than predicted by simple additivity. In this case, the three-way combination produced more bradycardia than enflurane alone.

Herbal Preparations and Drug Interactions

Americans are increasingly using herbal, vitamin, and over-the-counter preparations in an attempt to treat various ailments. In 2003, over-the-counter sales of herbals and vitamins were approximately $62.9 billion, an 8% growth from 2002.[121] A survey of 3,842 patients during preoperative evaluations found that 22% used herbal medications and 51% used vitamins. The most likely patients to use these products were women ages 40 to 60 years.[122] Another survey of 1,017 patients found 32% used one or more herb-related compounds, and 70% did not report this information when asked during routine preanesthetic assessment.[123]

Herbal preparations are classified as dietary supplements in the Dietary Supplement Heath and Education Act of 1994.[124] By this act, herbal preparations are exempt from the safety and efficacy requirements and regulations that prescription and over-the-counter drugs must fulfill. Instead, the U.S. Food and Drug Administration (FDA) must prove lack of safety.[125] There is no regulatory oversight of the specific contents of the herbal preparations, and different batches or brands of the same herbal often do not contain equal amounts of the active compound.

TABLE 50-3

PUBLISHED EVIDENCE FOR HERBAL TOXICITY

NAME(S)	COMMON USE	CLAIMED TOXICITY[127,129,130,132]	PUBLISHED EVIDENCE[a]
Ephedra Ma huang Ephedrine Chinese joint fir	Weight loss Antitussive Bacteriostatic	Halothane: arrhythmias MAOI: enhanced sympathetic effects Oxytocin: hypertension Stroke, hypertension, cardiac arrest	Intravenous ephedrine well characterized Inadequate data on specific interactions with oral ephedra. Oral ephedra known to cause adverse CNS and cardiac events[133]
Echinacea Purple cone flower	Common cold prevention Wounds and burns Urinary tract infections Coughs and bronchitis	Hepatotoxicity Decrease corticosteroid effect	No evidence of hepatotoxicity[130] Lab evidence of macrophage activation and enhanced natural killer cell activation[134,135]
Garlic Ajo	Lipid lowering Hypertension Antiplatelet, antioxidant	Potentiate warfarin	No evidence of interaction with warfarin[136] Decreased platelet aggregation in vitro[137–142]
Ginger	Nausea Antispasmodic	Inhibit thromboxane synthetase	In vitro evidence of thromboxane synthetase inhibition[144–146] No effect on platelet function with 2 g, but inhibition with 5 g[147,148]
Ginkgo Maidenhair tree Fossil tree	Circulatory stimulant	Inhibit PAF	Case reports of increased bleeding in humans[149] In vitro evidence of PAF inhibition[150,151]
Goldenseal Orange root Yellow root Ground raspberry Tumeric root Eye root	Diuretic Anti-inflammatory Laxative Hemostatic	Oxytocic Paralysis in overdose Edema Hypertension	No evidence
Kava Ava/ava pepper Kawa	Anxiolytic	Hepatotoxicity Potentiate barbiturates, benzodiazepines	Case reports of hepatotoxicity[152,153] Clinical and animal studies demonstrating sedation and anxiolysis[154,155]
Licorice Sweet root	Gastric/duodenal ulcer Gastritis Cough and bronchitis	Hypertension Hypokalemia Edema	Licorice abuse can cause hypokalemia Uncontrolled, studies show reductions in ADH, aldosterone, and plasma renin activity[156,157]
St. John's wort Hardhay Amber Goat weed	Depression	Decreased digoxin level Enzyme induction Prolonged anesthesia	Clinical data show decreased digoxin level[158] Clinical evidence for P-glycoprotein and CYP induction[158] Case reports of prolonged emergence, cardiovascular toxicity[159,160]
Valerian All-heal Setwall Vandal root	Sedative Anxiolytic	Potentiate barbiturates	Small controlled clinical trial showed decreased sleep latency[161,162]
Vitamin E	Antiaging Prevent stroke, pulmonary emboli Prevent atherosclerosis Promote wound healing	Increased bleeding Increased hypertension	Decreased platelet aggregation in vitro[163–165] Small clinical trial shows reduction in platelet aggregation[166] No evidence for hypertension

ADH, antidiuretic hormone; CNS, central nervous system; MAOI, monamide oxidase inhibitors; PAF, platelet activating factor;
[a]Based on search of Medline and Cochrane databases, January 1, 1966 to August 15, 2004.

The *Physicians' Desk Reference (PDR) for Herbal Medicines* is now in its third edition,[126] but there is still relatively little peer-reviewed literature addressing herbals and dietary supplements with specific reference to perioperative care.
10 Among the thousands of herbal preparations available, only a few have been documented to cause problems either through intrinsic toxicity or through pharmacokinetic and pharmacodynamic interactions.[127–129] The herbals most commonly cited are echinacea, ephedra (ma huang), garlic, gingko, ginseng, kava, and St. John's wort. As Fugh-Berman noted, many of the papers on herbals contain significant errors and unsubstantiated conclusions.[130] Some commonly mentioned herbal-based interactions are listed in Table 50-3, along with an assessment of the strength of the evidence. We were unable to find clinical trials proving that there are specific adverse interactions between herbals and anesthetic drugs.

MODELS FOR THE FUTURE: DRUG INTERACTION DURING TOTAL INTRAVENOUS ANESTHESIA

Anesthesia must always be titrated to effect, but the clinician usually begins dosing each drug with some notion of a "normal" dose range and a reasonable incremental dose. As additional drugs are added to the anesthetic, these doses need to be modified. Are there any reliable data to guide the administration of anesthetic drugs in combination? The answer for most routine balanced anesthetics is probably "no." As we have seen, almost all anesthetic drugs interact in a nonlinear, synergistic fashion, and the magnitude of the interaction depends on the specific doses of each agent. If the drugs are given by bolus injection or variable-rate infusion, the interaction changes constantly with time. Predicting anesthetic interaction, then, is like aiming at a moving target. Even a relatively simple anesthetic seems to require the analysis of an impossibly large number of potential variables.

In spite of the obstacles, there have been some attempts to apply quantitative models to total intravenous anesthesia (TIVA). The TIVA technique offers several advantages in this regard:

1. Anesthesia is often induced and maintained with only two drugs, a rapid-acting hypnotic (e.g., propofol) and a rapid-acting opioid (e.g., alfentanil, remifentanil). The pharmacokinetics and pharmacodynamics of these drugs are exceptionally well studied.
2. The drugs have pharmacokinetics well suited to administration by continuous infusion with microprocessor-driven pumps. During anesthesia, plasma concentrations of the drugs may be held relatively constant, so blood and brain attain pseudoequilibrium. The researcher may vary the infusion of each drug independently and relate stable plasma concentrations to clinical effects.

In a frequently cited study, Vuyk and colleagues[93] gave computer-controlled infusions of propofol and alfentanil to women undergoing lower abdominal surgery. First, the target concentration of alfentanil was held constant and propofol was varied; then, the reverse experiment was done. The onset of sleep and the time to awakening were measured, as was presence or absence of somatic and hemodynamic responses to laryngoscopy, intubation, incision, and opening of peritoneum. Arterial blood samples were collected, and the EC_{50} of alfentanil for each clinical end point was related to blood propofol concentration. As expected, the data showed that propofol potentiated the analgesic effects of alfentanil, and alfentanil potentiated the hypnotic effects of propofol. More importantly, the authors were able to relate various concentrations of each agent to a given end point.

The interest in these data lie in the way they can be used to model drug interactions.[131] In Fig. 50-9, Vuyk et al simulated the time to regain consciousness at different ratios of propofol and alfentanil. The graph is somewhat complex, but it is worth considering for a few moments. Vuyk and colleagues assume that a 180-minute anesthetic has been given with propofol and alfentanil targeted at various concentrations. Regardless of the ratio of the two drugs, the resulting anesthetic is sufficient to prevent the response to intraabdominal surgery in 50% of patients. The three-axis graph relates the concentrations of each drug to the time after discontinuation of the infusions. At time 0 (the floor of the graph), we see the steady-state concentrations just when the infusions are stopped. The disappearance of both drugs is shown, and the family of plasma decay curves (all possible combinations of propofol and alfentanil) is depicted on the graph surface. The curved line that crosses the time versus concentration surface identifies the time at which a patient has a 50% probability of awakening. The fastest emergence (10 minutes) occurs when propofol and alfentanil are targeted at concentrations of 3.5 μg/mL and 85 ng/mL, respectively. Emergence is significantly longer if the anesthetic is mostly propofol or mostly alfentanil.

How will these data help anyone give an anesthetic? What if the infusion is much shorter or longer than 180 minutes? What if the patients are old and sick? What if the anesthesiologist does not have a computer or an infusion pump? The answer could be another set of questions: "What is the value of knowing that the MAC of halothane is 0.74 vol%, the induction dose of propofol is 2.5 mg/kg, or the analgesic dose of morphine is 0.1 mg/kg?" We all understand that the value of such numbers is to give us a frame of reference for titrating the agents. The value of Vuyk and colleagues' model is not as a "recipe" for a good intravenous anesthetic—it is a way to think about dosing guidelines for two or more drugs simultaneously. It is not farfetched to imagine that the FDA will someday require information on "optimal combinations" for each new pharmacologic agent.

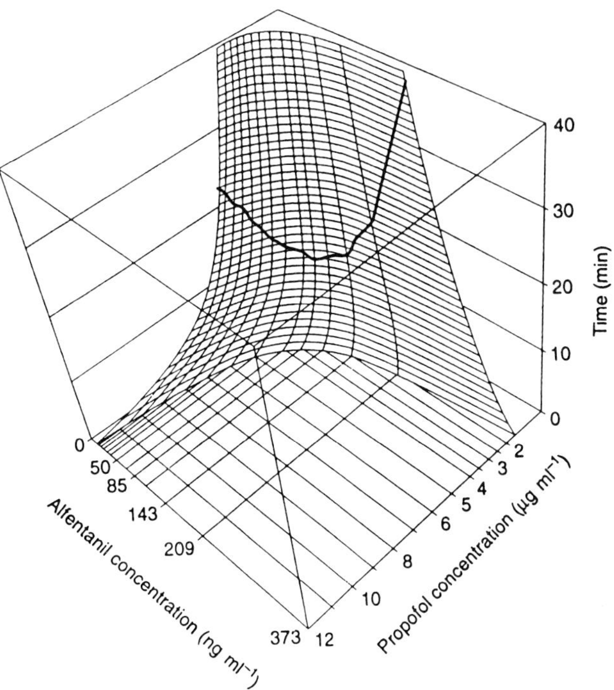

FIGURE 50-9. Computer simulation of the decay in blood propofol and plasma alfentanil concentrations during the first 40 minutes after the termination of a computer-controlled infusion (see text for details). (Reprinted with permission from Vuyk J, Lim T, Engbers FHM *et al*: The pharmacodynamic interaction of propofol and alfentanil during lower abdominal surgery in women. Anesthesiology 83:8, 1995.)

References

1. Smith NT, Corbascio AN (eds): Drug Interactions in Anesthesia, 2nd ed. Philadelphia, Lea and Febiger, 1986
2. Zbinden AM, Petersen-Felix S, Thomson DA: Anesthetic depth defined using multiple noxious stimuli during isoflurane/oxygen anesthesia: II. Hemodynamic responses. Anesthesiology 80:261, 1994
3. Smith JW, Seidl LG, Cluff LG: Studies on the epidemiology of adverse drug reactions: V. Clinical factors influencing susceptibility. Ann Intern Med 65:629, 1966
4. Bailey PL, Pace NL, Ashburn MA *et al*: Frequent hypoxemia and apnea after sedation with midazolam and fentanyl. Anesthesiology 73:826, 1990
5. Ausems ME, Hug CC Jr, Stanski DR *et al*: Plasma concentrations of alfentanil required to supplement nitrous oxide anesthesia for general surgery. Anesthesiology 65:362, 1986
6. Dundee JW, Robinson FP, McCullum JS *et al*: Sensitivity to propofol in the elderly. Anaesthesia 41:482, 1986
7. Baxter PJ, Garton K, Kharasch ED: Mechanistic aspects of carbon monoxide formation from volatile anesthetics. Anesthesiology 89:929, 1998
8. Steudel W, Hurford WE, Zapol WM: Inhaled nitric oxide: Basic biology and clinical applications. Anesthesiology 91:1090, 1999
9. Murphy DB, Sutton JA, Prescott LF *et al*: Opioid-induced delay in gastric emptying: A peripheral mechanism in humans. Anesthesiology 87:765, 1997

10. Asai T, McBeth C, Stewart JIM *et al*: Effect of clonidine on gastric emptying of liquids. Br J Anaesth 78:28, 1997
11. Avram MJ, Krejcie TC, Henthorn TK *et al*: α-adrenergic blockade affects initial drug distribution due to decreased cardiac output and altered blood flow distribution. J Pharmacol Exp Ther 311:617, 2004
12. Johnson KB, Kern SE, Hamber EA *et al*: The influence of hemorrhagic shock on remifentanil: A pharmacokinetic and pharmacodynamic analysis. Anesthesiology 94:322, 2001
13. Adams P, Gelman S, Reves JG *et al*: Midazolam pharmacodynamics and pharmacokinetics during acute hypovolemia. Anesthesiology 63:140, 1985
14. Klockowski PM, Levy G: Kinetics of drug action in disease states: XXV. Effect of experimental hypovolemia on the pharmacodynamics and pharmacokinetics of desmethyldiazepam. J Pharmacol Exp Ther 245:508, 1988
15. van der Meer JWM, Keuning JJ *et al*: The influence of gastric acidity on the bioavailability of ketoconazole. J Antimicrob Chemother 6:552, 1980
16. Elwood RJ, Hildebrand PJ *et al*: Influence of ranitidine on uptake of oral midazolam. Br J Anaesth 55:241, 1983
17. Trudnowski RJ, Gessner T: Gastric excretion of intravenously administered meperidine in surgical patients. Anesth Analg 58:88, 1979
18. Silverman WA, Andersen DH, Blanc WA *et al*: A difference in mortality rate and incidence of kernicterus among premature infants allotted to two prophylactic antibacterial regimens. Pediatrics 18:614, 1956
19. Holford NHG: Pharmacokinetics and pharmacodynamics: Rational dosing and the time course of drug action. In Katzung BG (ed): Basic and Clinical Pharmacology, 9th ed, p 48. New York, McGraw-Hill, 2004
20. Brodsky JB, Campos FA: Chloroprocaine analgesia in a patient receiving echothiophate eye drops. Anesthesiology 48:288, 1978
21. Kuhnert BR, Philipson EH, Pimental R *et al*: A prolonged chloroprocaine epidural block in a postpartum patient with abnormal pseudocholinesterase. Anesthesiology 56:477, 1982
22. Lanks WK, Sklar GS: Pseudocholinesterase levels and rates of chloroprocaine hydrolysis in patients receiving adequate doses of phospholine iodide. Anesthesiology 52:434, 1980
23. Davis PJ, Stiller RL, Wilson AS *et al*: In vitro remifentanil metabolism: The effects of whole blood constituents and plasma butyrylcholinesterase. Anesth Analg 95:1305, 2002
24. Boakes AJ, Laurence DR, Teoh PC *et al*: Interactions between sympathomimetic amines and antidepressant agents in man. Br Med J 1(5849):311, 1973
25. Parkinson's Study Group: Effects of tocopherol and deprenyl on the progression of disability in early Parkinson's disease. N Engl J Med 328:176, 1993
26. Evans-Prosser CDG: The use of pethidine and morphine in the presence of monoamine oxidase inhibitors. Br J Anaesth 40:279, 1968
27. Zornberg GL, Bodkin JA, Cohen BM: Severe adverse interaction between pethidine and selegiline. Lancet 337(8735):246, 1991
28. Rivers N, Horner B: Possible lethal reaction between nardil and dextromethorphan [Letter]. CMAJ 103:85, 1970
29. Zornberg GL, Hegarty JD: Adverse interaction between propoxyphene and phenelzine. Am J Psychiatry 150:1270, 1993
30. Michaels I, Serrins M, Shier NQ *et al*: Anesthesia for cardiac surgery in patients receiving monoamine oxidase inhibitors. Anesth Analg 63:1041, 1984
31. Fahim I, Ismail M, Osman OH: The role of serotonin and norepinephrine in the hyperthermic reaction induced by pethidine in rabbits pretreated with pargyline. J Pharmacol 46:416, 1972
32. Sjoqvist F: Psychotropic drugs (2): Interaction between monoamine oxidase (MAO) inhibitors and other substances. Proc R Soc Med 58:967, 1965
33. Doyle DJ: Ketamine induction and monoamine oxidase inhibitors. J Clin Anesth 2:324, 1990
34. El-Ganzouri AR, Ivankovich AD, Braverman B *et al*: Monoamine oxidase inhibitors: Should they be discontinued preoperatively? Anesth Analg 64:592, 1985
35. Roizen MF: Monoamine oxidase inhibitors: Are we condemned to relive history or is history no longer relevant? J Clin Anesth 2:293, 1990
36. Stenson RE, Constantino RT, Harrison DC: Interrelationship of hepatic blood flow, cardiac output and blood levels of lidocaine in man. Circulation 18:205, 1971
37. Benowitz NL, Forsyth RP, Melmon KL *et al*: Lidocaine disposition kinetics in monkey and man: II. Effects of hemorrhage and sympathomimetic drug administration. Clin Pharmacol Ther 16:99, 1974
38. Feely J, Wilkinson GR, McAllister CB *et al*: Increased toxicity and reduced clearance of lidocaine by cimetidine. Ann Intern Med 96:592, 1982
39. Tukey RH, Johnson EF: Molecular aspects of regulation and structure of the drug-metabolizing enzymes. In Pratt WB, Taylor P (eds): Principles of Drug Action: The Basis of Pharmacology, 3rd ed, p 435. New York, Churchill Livingstone, 1990
40. Greenstein LR, Hitt BA, Mazze RI: Metabolism in vitro of enflurane, isoflurane, and methoxyflurane. Anesthesiology 42:420, 1975
41. Mazze RI, Trudell JR, Cousins MJ: Methoxyflurane metabolism and renal dysfunction: Clinical correlation in man. Anesthesiology 35:247, 1971
42. Sipes JG, Brown BR Jr: An animal model of hepatotoxicity associated with halothane anesthesia. Anesthesiology 45:622, 1976
43. Oda Y, Mizutani K, Hase I *et al*: Fentanyl inhibits metabolism of midazolam: Competitive inhibition of CYP3A4 in vitro. Br J Anaesth 82:900, 1999
44. Hamaoka N, Oda Y, Hase I *et al*: Propofol decreases the clearance of midazolam by inhibiting CYP3A4: In vivo and in-vitro study. Clin Pharmacol Ther 66:110, 1999
45. Oda Y, Hamaoka N, Hiroi T *et al*: Involvement of human liver cytochrome P4502B6 in the metabolism of propofol. Br J Clin Pharmacol 51:281, 2001
46. Bartkowski RR, Goldberg ME, Larijani GE *et al*: Inhibition of alfentanil metabolism by erythromycin. Clin Pharmacol Ther 46:99, 1989
47. Tateishi T, Krivoruk Y, Ueng Y *et al*: Identification of human liver cytochrome P-450 3A4 as the enzyme responsible for fentanyl and sufentanil N-dealkylation. Anesth Analg 82:167, 1996
48. Bartkowski RR, Goldberg ME, Huffnagle S *et al*: Sufentanil disposition. Anesthesiology 78:260, 1993
49. Klotz U, Reimann I: Delayed clearance of diazepam due to cimetidine. N Engl J Med 302:1012, 1980
50. Palkama VJ, Ahonen J, Neuvonen J *et al*: Effect of saquinavir on the pharmacokinetics and dynamics of oral and intravenous midazolam. Clin Pharmacol Ther 66:33, 1999
51. Olkkola KT, Palkama VJ, Neuvonen PJ: Ritonavir's role in reducing fentanyl clearance and prolonging its half life. Anesthesiology 91:681, 1999
52. Wagner RL, White PF, Kan PB *et al*: Inhibition of adrenal steroidogenesis by the anesthetic etomidate. N Engl J Med 310:1415, 1984
53. Leahey EB Jr, Reiffel JA, Drusin RE *et al*: Interaction between quinidine and digoxin. JAMA 240:533, 1978
54. Naguib M, Samarkandi AH, Bakhamees HS *et al*: Comparative potency of steroidal neuromuscular blocking drugs and isobolographic analysis of the interaction. Br J Anaesth 75:37, 1995
55. Quasha AL, Eger EI II, Tinker JH: Determination and applications of MAC. Anesthesiology 53:315, 1980
56. Murray DJ, Mehta MP, Forbes RB *et al*: Additive contribution of nitrous oxide to halothane MAC in infants and children. Anesth Analg 71:120, 1990
57. Eger EI II. Does 1 + 1 = 2? Anesth Analg 41:482, 1989
58. Munson ES, Paul WL, Embro WJ: Central nervous system toxicity of local anesthetic mixtures in monkeys. Anesthesiology 46:179, 1977
59. Kim KS, Na DJ, Chon SU: Interactions between suxamethonium and mivacurium or atracurium. Br J Anaesth 77:612, 1996
60. Eisenach JC, Schlairet TJ, Dobson CE II *et al*: Effect of prior anesthetic solution on epidural morphine analgesia. Anesth Analg 73:119, 1991
61. Dershwitz M, Rosow CE, DiBiase PM *et al*: A comparison of the sedative effects of butorphanol and midazolam. Anesthesiology 74:717, 1991
62. Maves TJ, Pechman PS, Meller ST *et al*: Ketorolac potentiates morphine antinociception during visceral nociception in the rat. Anesthesiology 80:1094, 1994
63. Lebowitz PW, Ramsey FM, Savarese JJ *et al*: Potentiation of neuromuscular blockade in man produced by combinations of pancuronium and metocurine or pancuronium and *d*-tubocurarine. Anesth Analg 59:604, 1980
64. Bowman WC, Prior C, Marshall IG: Presynaptic receptors in the neuromuscular junction. Ann N Y Acad Sci 604:69, 1990
65. Standaert FG: Basic chemistry of acetylcholine receptors. Anesth Clin North Am 11:205, 1993
66. Tallarida RJ: Statistical analysis of drug combinations for synergism. Pain 49:93, 1992
67. Berenbaum MC: Synergy, additivism and antagonism in immunosuppression. J Clin Exp Immunol 28:1, 1989
68. Berenbaum MC: What is synergy? Pharm Rev 41:93, 1989
69. Tallarida RJ, Porreca F, Cowan A: Statistical analysis of drug-drug and site-site interactions with isobolograms. Life Sci 45:947, 1989
70. Tverskoy M, Fleyshman G, Bradley EL Jr, Kissin I: Midazolam-thiopental anesthetic interaction in patients. Anesth Analg 67:342, 1988
71. Stone JG, Foex P, Sear JW: Myocardial ischemia in untreated hypertensive patients: Effect of a single small oral dose of a beta-adrenergic blocking agent. Anesthesiology 68:495, 1988
72. Pasternack PF, Grossi EA, Baumann FG *et al*: Beta blockade to decrease silent myocardial ischemia during peripheral vascular surgery. Am J Surg 158:113, 1989
73. Wallace A, Layug B, Tateo I *et al*: Prophylactic atenolol reduces postoperative myocardial ischemia. Anesthesiology 88:7, 1998
74. Warltier DC: β-Adrenergic-blocking drugs: Incredibly useful, incredibly underutilized. Anesthesiology 88:2, 1998
75. Colson P, Saussine M, Séguin JR *et al*: Hemodynamic effects of anesthesia in patients chronically treated with angiotensin converting enzyme inhibitors. Anesth Analg 74:805, 1992
76. Coriat P, Richer C, Douraki T *et al*: Influence of chronic angiotensin-converting enzyme inhibition on anesthetic induction. Anesthesiology 81:299, 1994
77. Fruncillo RJ, Rotmensch HH, Vlasses PH *et al*: Effect of captopril and hydrochlorothiazide on the response to pressor agents in hypertensives. Eur J Clin Pharmacol 28:5, 1985
78. Boccara G, Ouattara A, Godet G *et al*: Terlipressin versus norepinephrine to correct refractory arterial hypotension after general anesthesia in patients chronically treated with renin-angiotensin system inhibitors. Anesthesiology 98:1338, 2003
79. Noguera I, Medina P, Segarra G *et al*: Potentiation by vasopressin of adrenergic vasoconstriction in the rat isolated mesenteric artery. Br J Pharmacol 122:431, 1997

80. Licker M, Bednarkiewicz M, Neidhart P *et al*: Preoperative inhibition of angiotensin-converting enzyme improves systemic and renal haemodynamic changes during aortic abdominal surgery. Br J Anaesth 76:632, 1996
81. Ryckwaert F, Colson P: Hemodynamic effects of anesthesia in patients with ischemic heart failure chronically treated with angiotensin-converting enzyme inhibitors. Anesth Analg 84:945, 1997
82. Rosenthal JA: American Heart Association recommendations for treating tricyclic antidepressant-induced hypotension [Letter]. Anesthesiology 87:1259, 1997
83. Sprung J, Schoenwald P, Levy P *et al*: Treating intraoperative hypotension in a patient on long-term tricyclic antidepressants: A case of aborted aortic surgery. Anesthesiology 86:990, 1997
84. Stoelting RK, Creasser CW, Martz RC: Effect of cocaine administration on halothane MAC in dogs. Anesth Analg 54:422, 1975
85. Bernards C, Kern C, Cullen BF: Chronic cocaine administration reversibly increases isoflurane minimum alveolar concentration in sheep. Anesthesiology 85:91, 1996
86. Bernards C, Teijeiro A: Illicit cocaine ingestion during anesthesia. Anesthesiology 84:218, 1995
87. Johnston R, Way W, Miller R: Alteration of anesthetic requirement by amphetamine. Anesthesiology 36:357, 1972
88. Seidler F, Slotkin T: Fetal cocaine exposure causes persistent noradrenergic hyperactivity in rat brain regions: Effects on neurotransmitter turnover and receptors. J Pharmacol Exp Ther 263:413, 1992
89. Kelley K, Han D, Fellingham G *et al*: Cocaine and exercise: Physiological responses of cocaine-conditioned rats. Med Sci Sports Exerc 27:65, 1995
90. Epstein B, Levy M-L, Thein M et al: Evaluation of fentanyl as an adjunct to thiopental-nitrous oxide-oxygen anesthesia for short procedures. Anesth Rev 2:24, 1985
91. Rosow CE, Latta WB, Keegan CR *et al*: Alfentanil for use in short surgical procedures. In Estafanous FG (ed): Opioids in Anesthesia, p 93. Boston, Butterworth, 1984
92. Short TG, Plummer JL, Chui PT: Hypnotic and anaesthetic interactions between midazolam, propofol and alfentanil. Br J Anaesth 69:162, 1992
93. Vuyk J, Lim T, Engbers FHM *et al*: The pharmacodynamic interaction of propofol and alfentanil during lower abdominal surgery in women. Anesthesiology 83:8, 1995
94. Smith C, McEwan AI, Jhaveri R *et al*: The interaction of fentanyl on the Cp50 of propofol for loss of consciousness and skin incision. Anesthesiology 81:820, 1994
95. Bailey PL, Wilbrink J, Zwanikken P *et al*: Anesthetic induction with fentanyl. Anesth Analg 64:48, 1985
96. Silbert BS, Rosow CE, Keegan CR *et al*: The effect of diazepam on induction of anesthesia with alfentanil. Anesth Analg 65:71, 1986
97. Kissin I, Vinik HR, Castillo R *et al*: Alfentanil potentiates midazolam-induced unconsciousness in subanalgesic doses. Anesth Analg 71:65, 1990
98. Short TG, Galletly DC, Plummer JL: Hypnotic and anesthetic action of thiopentone and midazolam alone and in combination. Br J Anaesth 66:13, 1991
99. Tverskoy M, Ben-Shlomo I, Finger EJ *et al*: Midazolam acts synergistically with methohexitone for induction of anaesthesia. Br J Anaesth 63:109, 1989
100. McEwan AI, Smith C, Dyar O *et al*: Isoflurane minimum alveolar concentration reduction by fentanyl. Anesthesiology 78:864, 1993
101. Murphy MR, Hug CC Jr: The enflurane sparing effect of morphine, butorphanol and nalbuphine. Anesthesiology 57:489, 1982
102. Murphy RM, Hug CC Jr: The anesthetic potency of fentanyl in terms of its reduction of enflurane MAC. Anesthesiology 57:485, 1982
103. Licina MG, Schubert A, Tobin JE *et al*: Intrathecal morphine does not reduce minimum alveolar concentration of halothane in humans: Results of a double-blind study. Anesthesiology 74:660, 1991
104. Rampil IJ, Mason P, Singh H: Anesthetic potency (MAC) is independent of forebrain structures in the rat. Anesthesiology 78:707, 1993
105. Gross JB, Alexander CM: Awakening concentrations of isoflurane are not affected by analgesic doses of morphine. Anesth Analg 67:27, 1988
106. Katoh T, Ikeda K: The effects of fentanyl on sevoflurane requirements for loss of consciousness and skin incision. Anesthesiology 88:18, 1998
107. Himes RS, DiFazio CA, Burney RG: Effects of lidocaine on the anesthetic requirements for nitrous oxide and halothane. Anesthesiology 47:437, 1977
108. Hall RI, Schwieger IM, Hug CC: The anesthetic efficacy of midazolam in the enflurane-anesthetized dog. Anesthesiology 68:862, 1988
109. Hansen TD, Warner DS, Todd MM *et al*: The influence of inhalational anesthetics on in vivo and in vitro benzodiazepine receptor binding in the rat cerebral cortex. Anesthesiology 74:97, 1991
110. Miller RD, Way WL, Eger EI II: The effects of alpha-methyldopa, reserpine, guanethidine and iproniazide on minimum alveolar anesthetic concentration (MAC). Anesthesiology 29:1156, 1968
111. Salonen M, Reid K, Maze M: Synergistic interaction between α-2-adrenergic agonists and benzodiazepines in rats. Anesthesiology 76:1004, 1992
112. Segal IS, Vickery RG, Walton JK *et al*: Dexmedetomidine diminishes halothane anesthetic requirements in rats through a postsynaptic α-2-adrenergic receptor. Anesthesiology 69:818, 1988
113. Correa-Sales C, Rabin BC, Maze M: A hypnotic response to dexmedetomidine, an α-2-agonist, is mediated in the locus coeruleus in rats. Anesthesiology 76:948, 1992
114. Scheinin M, Schwinn DA: The locus coeruleus: Site of hypnotic actions of α-2-adrenoceptor agonists? [Editorial]. Anesthesiology 76:873, 1992
115. Advokat C: The role of descending inhibition in morphine-induced analgesia. Trends Pharmacol Sci 9:330, 1988
116. Roizen MF, White PF, Eger EI II *et al*: Effects of ablation of serotonin or norepinephrine brain-stem areas on halothane and cyclopropane MACs in rats. Anesthesiology 49:252, 1978
117. Johns RA, Moscicki JC, DiFazio CA: Nitric oxide synthase inhibitor dose-dependently and reversibly reduces the threshold for halothane anesthesia: A role for nitric oxide in mediating consciousness? Anesthesiology 77:779, 1992
118. Pajewski TN, DiFazio CA, Moscicki JC *et al*: Nitric oxide synthase inhibitors, 7-nitro-indazole and nitroG-L-arginine-methyl ester, dose-dependently reduce the threshold for isoflurane anesthesia. Anesthesiology 85:1111, 1996
119. Vinik HR, Bradley EL Jr, Kissin I: Triple anesthetic combination: Propofol-midazolam-alfentanil. Anesth Analg 78:354, 1994
120. Salmenpera M, Szlam F, Hug CC Jr: Anesthetic and hemodynamic interactions of dexmedetomidine and fentanyl in dogs. Anesthesiology 80:837, 1994
121. Nutrition Business Journal. Available at: www.nutritionbusiness.com. Accessed March 15, 2005.
122. Tsen LC, Segal S, Pothier M *et al*: Alternative medicine use in presurgical patients. Anesthesiology 93:148, 2000
123. Kaye AD, Clarke RC, Sabar R *et al*: Herbal medicines: Current trends in anesthesiology practice—a hospital survey. J Clin Anesth 12:468, 2000
124. Dietary Supplement Health and Education Act, 1994, PL 103-417(180 Stat 2126).
125. Marwick C: Growing use of medicinal botanicals forces assessment by drug regulators. JAMA 273:607, 1995
126. Physicians' Desk Reference (PDR) for Herbal Medicines, 3rd ed. Montvale, NJ, Thomson Healthcare, 2004
127. Ang-Lee MK, Moss J, Yuan CS: Herbal medicines and perioperative care. JAMA 286:208, 2001
128. Fugh-Berman A: Herb-drug interactions. Lancet 355:134, 2000
129. Miller LG: Herbal medicinals: Selected clinical considerations focusing on known or potential drug-herb interactions. Arch Intern Med 158:2200, 1998
130. Fugh-Berman A: Herbal medicinals: Selected clinical considerations, focusing on known or potential drug-herb interactions. Arch Intern Med 159:1957, 1999
131. Stanski DR, Shafer SL: Quantifying anesthetic drug interaction. Implications for drug dosing [Editorial]. Anesthesiology 83:1, 1995
132. American Society of Anesthesiologists: Considerations for anesthesiologists: What you should know about your patients' use of herbal medicines and other dietary supplements. ASA pamphlet. American Society of Anesthesiologists, 2003
133. Haller CA, Benowitz NL: Adverse cardiovascular and central nervous system events associated with dietary supplements containing ephedra alkaloids. N Engl J Med 343:1833, 2000
134. See DM, Broumand N, Sahl L *et al*: In vitro effects of echinacea and ginseng on natural killer and antibody-dependent cell cytotoxicity in healthy subjects and chronic fatigue syndrome or acquired immunodeficiency syndrome patients. Immunopharmacology 35:229, 1997
135. Luettig B, Steinmuller C, Gifford GE *et al*: Macrophage activation by the polysaccharide arabinogalactan isolated from plant cell cultures of *Echinacea purpurea*. J Natl Cancer Inst 81:669, 1989
136. Vaes LP, Chyka PA: Interactions of warfarin with garlic, ginger, ginkgo, or ginseng: Nature of the evidence. Ann Pharmacother 34:1478, 2000
137. Bordia A: Effect of garlic on human platelet aggregation in vitro. Atherosclerosis 30:355, 1978
138. Bordia A, Verma SK, Srivastava KC: Effect of garlic (*Allium sativum*) on blood lipids, blood sugar, fibrinogen and fibrinolytic activity in patients with coronary artery disease. Prostaglandins Leukot Essent Fatty Acids 58:257, 1998
139. Ali M, Bordia T, Mustafa T: Effect of raw versus boiled aqueous extract of garlic and onion on platelet aggregation. Prostaglandins Leukot Essent Fatty Acids 60:43, 1999
140. Kiesewetter H, Jung F, Jung EM *et al*: Effect of garlic on platelet aggregation in patients with increased risk of juvenile ischaemic attack. Eur J Clin Pharmacol 45:333, 1993
141. Kiesewetter H, Jung C, Mrowietz G *et al*: Effects of garlic on blood fluidity and fibrinolytic activity: A randomised, placebo-controlled, double-blind study. Br J Clin Pract 69(Suppl):24, 1990
142. Das IKN, Sooranna SR: Potent activation of nitric oxide synthase by garlic: A basis for its therapeutic applications. Curr Med Res Opin 13:257, 1995
143. Bordia A, Verma SK, Srivastava KC: Effect of ginger (*Zingiber officinale Rosc.*) and fenugreek (*Trigonella foenumgraecum L.*) on blood lipids, blood sugar and platelet aggregation in patients with coronary artery disease. Prostaglandins Leukot Essent Fatty Acids 56:379, 1997
144. Srivastava KC: Effect of onion and ginger consumption on platelet thromboxane production in humans. Prostaglandins Leukot Essent Fatty Acids 35:183, 1989
145. Thomson M, Al-Qattan KK, Al-Sawan SM *et al*: The use of ginger (*Zingiber officinale Rosc.*) as a potential anti-inflammatory and antithrombotic agent. Prostaglandins Leukot Essent Fatty Acids 67:475, 2002

146. Lumb AB: Effect of dried ginger on human platelet function. Thromb Haemost 71:110, 1994
147. Janssen PL, Meyboom S, van Staveren WA *et al*: Consumption of ginger (*Zingiber officinale roscoe*) does not affect ex vivo platelet thromboxane production in humans. Eur J Clin Nutr 50:772, 1996
148. Meisel C, Johne A, Roots I: Fatal intracerebral mass bleeding associated with ginkgo biloba and ibuprofen. Atherosclerosis 167:367, 2003
149. Chung KF, Dent G, McCusker M *et al*: Effect of a ginkgolide mixture (BN 52063) in antagonising skin and platelet responses to platelet activating factor in man. Lancet 1:248, 1987
150. Bal Dit Sollier C, Caplain H, Drouet L: No alteration in platelet function or coagulation induced by EGb761 in a controlled study. Clin Lab Haematol 25:251, 2003
151. Russmann S, Lauterburg BH, Helbling A: Kava hepatotoxicity. Ann Intern Med 135:68, 2001
152. Stickel F, Baumuller HM, Seitz K *et al*: Hepatitis induced by Kava (*Piper methysticum rhizoma*). J Hepatol 39:62, 2003
153. Lehrl S: Clinical efficacy of kava extract WS 1490 in sleep disturbances associated with anxiety disorders. Results of a multicenter, randomized, placebo-controlled, double-blind clinical trial. J Affect Disord 78:101, 2004
154. Garrett KM, Basmadjian G, Khan IA *et al*: Extracts of kava (*Piper methysticum*) induce acute anxiolytic-like behavioral changes in mice. Psychopharmacology (Berl) 170:33, 2003
155. Forslund T, Fyhrquist F, Froseth B *et al*: Effects of licorice on plasma atrial natriuretic peptide in healthy volunteers. J Intern Med 225:95, 1989
156. Bernardi M, D'Intino PE, Trevisani F *et al*: Effects of prolonged ingestion of graded doses of licorice by healthy volunteers. Life Sci 55:863, 1994
157. Durr D, Stieger B, Kullak-Ublick GA *et al*: St John's wort induces intestinal P-glycoprotein/MDR1 and intestinal and hepatic CYP3A4. Clin Pharmacol Ther 68:598, 2000
158. Crowe S, McKeating K: Delayed emergence and St. John's wort. Anesthesiology 96:1025, 2002
159. Irefin S, Sprung J: A possible cause of cardiovascular collapse during anesthesia: Long-term use of St. John's wort. J Clin Anesth 12:498, 2000
160. Balderer G, Borbely AA: Effect of valerian on human sleep. Psychopharmacology (Berl) 87:406, 1985
161. Donath F, Quispe K, Diefenbach A *et al*: Critical evaluation of the effect of valerian extract on sleep structure and sleep quality. Pharmacopsychiatry 33:47, 2000
162. Celestini A, Pulcinelli FM, Pignatelli P *et al*: Vitamin E potentiates the antiplatelet activity of aspirin in collagen-stimulated platelets. Haematologica 87:420, 2002
163. Szuwart T, Brzoska T, Luger TA *et al*: Vitamin E reduces platelet adhesion to human endothelial cells in vitro. Am J Hematol 65:1, 2000
164. Pignatelli P, Pulcinelli FM, Lenti L *et al*: Vitamin E inhibits collagen-induced platelet activation by blunting hydrogen peroxide. Arterioscler Thromb Vasc Biol 19:2542, 1999
165. Steiner M: Vitamin E, a modifier of platelet function: Rationale and use in cardiovascular and cerebrovascular disease. Nutr Rev 57:306, 1999

CHAPTER 51 ■ ANESTHESIA PROVIDED AT ALTERNATE SITES

KAREN J. SOUTER

KEY POINTS

1. Alternate sites are locations remote from the operating room.
2. The number of requests for anesthetic services in alternate sites is increasing.
3. A three-step approach is useful in considering an anesthetic at an alternate site: the patient, the procedure, and the environment.
4. The American Society of Anesthesiologists (ASA) has defined guidelines to be applied to the administration of anesthesia at nonoperating room locations.
5. Environmental considerations include hazards such as radiation and the side effects of contrast media.
6. Procedural considerations are both general (e.g., duration, position, and level of discomfort) and specific to individual specialties.
7. Patient considerations include whether the patient will tolerate sedation or require general anesthesia, the ASA grade, significant comorbidities, and the level of monitoring.
8. Patients should receive the same standard of care at an alternate site as they do in the operating room.
9. The anesthetic and monitoring equipment must meet the same standards as equipment provided in the operating room.
10. Following anesthesia at an alternate site, the patient should be transported to an appropriate postanesthesia care unit, accompanied and monitored by anesthesia personnel.

To better understand and develop a systematic approach to providing anesthesia at alternate sites, this chapter discusses the challenges facing the anesthesiologist regarding the procedures, the patients, and the environment. This chapter also describes the special considerations that apply to administering anesthesia at sites other than in the operating room. These sites may be located within a large hospital, such as in a radiology department or endoscopy suite, where the resources of the operating rooms are within the same facility, but are not close at
1 hand. Or, they may include a stand-alone facility such as an office or dental clinic that is remote from the backup of a full surgical hospital. Only the former locations are considered in this section. Office-based anesthesia is described in Chapter 52.

GENERAL PRINCIPLES

2 In more recent years, the number of anesthetics being delivered to patients in areas other than the operating room has steadily increased. This is mainly due to the development of large, complex equipment for both diagnostic and therapeutic procedures that cannot be transported to the operating room. Standards introduced by the Joint Commission on Accreditation of Healthcare Organizations (JCAHO) require that the anesthesia service of a hospital participates with other departments in setting up a uniform quality of care for patients undergoing sedation in all parts of the hospital.[1,2]

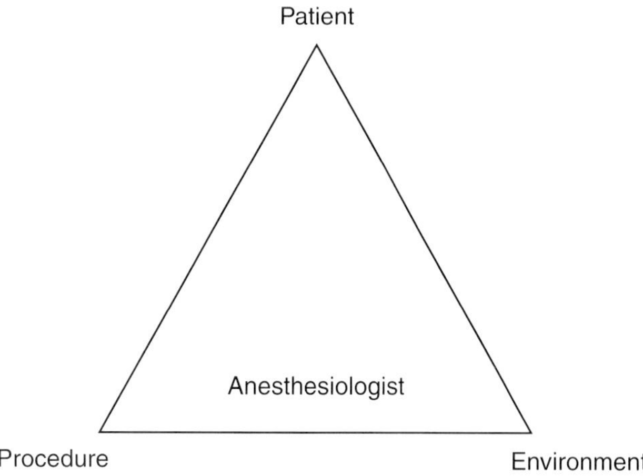

FIGURE 51-1. A three-step paradigm for anesthesia at alternate sites.

3 Anesthesiologists undertake most of their training in the operating room, surrounded by familiar equipment and staff experienced in the care of the anesthetized patient. Away from the operating room, the anesthesiologist may not have this support. A simple three-step paradigm can be used to approach an anesthetic assignment in an alternate site (Fig. 51-1 and Table 51-1).

The Environment

4 The American Society of Anesthesiologists (ASA) has developed standards to apply to anesthesia in remote locations[3] (Table 51-2). Before commencing an anesthetic in an alternate site, it is vital to confirm the presence and proper functioning of all equipment an anesthesiologist would expect to have in the operating room. This equipment includes a central oxygen supply, spare oxygen cylinders, wall suction, overhead lighting, gas scavenging systems, and electrical outlets. Replacement batteries should be available for any equipment that is battery powered. The location of immediately available resuscitation equipment should be noted and plans formulated with the local staff for emergency resuscitation procedures, including cardiopulmonary resuscitation and the management of anaphylaxis.

TABLE 51-1

5 A THREE-STEP APPROACH TO ANESTHESIA AT ALTERNATE SITES

1. Environment	Anesthetic equipment
	Anesthesia monitors
	Suction
	Resuscitation equipment
	Personnel
	Technical equipment
	Radiation hazard
	Magnetic fields
	Ambient temperature
	Warming blankets
2. Procedure	Diagnostic or therapeutic
	Duration
	Level of discomfort/pain
	Position of patient
	Special requirements (e.g., functional monitoring)
	Potential complications
	Surgical support
3. Patient	Ability to tolerate sedation versus general anesthesia
	ASA grade and comorbidity
	Airway assessment
	Allergies—IV contrast
	Monitoring requirements—simple versus advanced

ASA, American Society of Anesthesiologists; IV, intravenous(ly).

TABLE 51-2

AMERICAN SOCIETY OF ANESTHESIOLOGISTS GUIDELINES FOR NONOPERATING ROOM ANESTHETIZING LOCATIONS

1. Oxygen
   - Reliable source
   - Backup E cylinder—full
2. Suction
   - Adequate and reliable
3. Scavenging system if inhalational agents are administered
4. Anesthetic equipment
   - Backup self-inflating bag to deliver positive-pressure ventilation
   - Adequate anesthetic drugs and supplies
   - Anesthesia machine with equivalent function to those in the operating rooms and maintained to the same standards
   - Adequate monitoring equipment to allow adherence to the ASA Standards for Basic Monitoring[9]
5. Electrical outlets
   - Sufficient for anesthesia machine and monitors
   - Isolated electrical power or ground fault circuit interrupters if "wet location"
6. Adequate illumination
   - Battery-operated backups
7. Sufficient space for
   - Personnel and equipment
   - Easy and expeditious access to patient, anesthesia machine, and monitoring
8. Resuscitation equipment immediately available
   - Defibrillator
   - Emergency drugs
   - Cardiopulmonary resuscitation equipment
9. Adequately trained staff to support anesthesia team
10. All building and safety codes and facility standards should be observed
11. Postanesthesia care facilities
    - Adequately trained staff to provide postanesthesia care
    - Appropriately equipment to allow safe transport to main postanesthesia care unit

From American Society of Anesthesiologist (ASA): Standards for postanesthesia care. In ASA Directory of members. Park Ridge, IL, ASA, 2003

Anesthesia Equipment and Monitors. In some alternate sites, anesthesia machines and monitors are provided; in others, it may be necessary to bring anesthesia equipment to the location. Both situations can present problems. Anesthesia machines and monitors that remain in an outside location need to be routinely serviced, as does anesthesia equipment used in the main operating rooms. This equipment is not often used on a daily basis; therefore, before using the equipment, it is vital to conduct a thorough check. For example, attention should be paid to the freshness of the soda lime and whether any pieces of equipment or monitors have been removed or misplaced. Monitoring equipment found in alternate sites is often used by the staff to monitor patients who are not being anesthetized. These monitors may be malfunctioning or different from monitors used in the operating room. Anesthesiologists should be aware of these differences. If more advanced monitors (e.g., an arterial line, central venous pressure or intracranial pressure [ICP] monitoring) are required, these devices should be available to be brought to the alternate site. Small portable anesthesia machines and monitors are available that may be useful to bring into an outside location. A pre-prepared cart containing essential equipment that is checked and restocked after each case is recommended to eliminate the need for anesthesia personnel to move between locations to collect equipment that has been forgotten or that is urgently needed.

Technical Equipment. The complex technical equipment used in alternate sites, particularly in the radiology suites, is often bulky and fixed to the floor so the anesthesia team has to work around it. Ionizing radiation related to both imaging and therapeutic procedures is a hazard to both staff and patients. Magnetic resonance imaging (MRI) creates its own environmental concerns related to magnetic fields. In all these areas, the equipment is kept at low temperatures, and patients may easily develop hypothermia. Warming blankets should be available. Radiotherapy rooms are heavily shielded, and staff are excluded from the room during treatment, requiring the anesthesiology team to monitor patients remotely, often with surveillance cameras.[4]

Procedures

6 Common procedures carried out in alternate sites for which the patient may require anesthesia or sedation are listed in Table 51-3. It is vital for the anesthesiologist to understand the nature of the procedure, the position of the patient, how painful the procedure will be, and how long the procedure will last. This will allow the development of an anesthesia plan to provide safe patient care and facilitate the procedure. Discussions with physicians, dentists, and others performing interventional procedures must include contingencies for adverse outcomes.

TABLE 51-3

COMMON PROCEDURES REQUIRING ANESTHESIA AT ALTERNATE SITES

Radiology
- Computed tomography
- Magnetic resonance imaging
- Interventional radiology (vascular and nonvascular)
- Interventional neuroradiology
- Functional brain imaging

Radiotherapy
- Radiation therapy
- Intraoperative radiotherapy
- Radiosurgery

Gastroenterology
- Upper gastroenterology endoscopy
- Endoscopic retrograde cholangiopancreatography
- Colonoscopy
- Liver biopsy
- Transjugular intrahepatic portosystemic shunt

Cardiology
- Cardiac catheterization
- Radiofrequency ablation
- Cardioversion
- Transesophageal echocardiography

Psychiatry
- Electroconvulsive therapy

TABLE 51-4

PATIENT FACTORS REQUIRING SEDATION OR GENERAL ANESTHESIA AT ALTERNATE SITES

Anxiety and panic disorders
Claustrophobia
Developmental delay and learning difficulties
Cerebral palsy
Seizure disorders
Movement disorders
Severe pain
Acute trauma with unstable cardiovascular, respiratory, or neurologic function
Significant comorbidity
Child

Patients

7 Patients may require anesthesia at alternate sites for a number of reasons (Table 51-4). The patient may have been unable to tolerate the procedure without sedation or has failed with simple sedation administered by a nonanesthesiologist. Children represent a special group of patients who are more likely to require sedation or anesthesia for various diagnostic and therapeutic procedures. Another group is patients who are too ill to tolerate a major surgical procedure, but who may be able to undergo palliative, less invasive procedures at alternate sites. These patients require a thorough preanesthetic assessment and often need invasive monitoring.

ANESTHESIA CARE

The terms *anesthesia, sedation, conscious sedation*, and *deep sedation* are commonly used. They span a continuum that starts
8 with a fully awake patient with a protected, patent airway and ends with general anesthesia and the need for interventions to protect and secure the airway. JCAHO defines *anesthesia care* as the administration of intravenous, intramuscular, or inhalational agents that may result in the loss of the patient's protective reflexes. Patients who receive anesthesia or sedation at alternate sites should expect the same standard of care that they would receive in the operating room. The ASA has published guidelines and standards of care, including those for preanesthesia and postanesthesia care, as well as monitored anesthesia care,[5–7] and definitions of general anesthesia and levels of sedation[8] (Table 51-5). A patient's level of sedation frequently varies during the course of a procedure, and it is important that individuals administering a given level of sedation are able to rescue the patient whose level becomes deeper than initially intended. The ASA basic standards of monitoring should be adhered to in any location where anesthesia or sedation is being performed.[9] Standard I requires a qualified anesthesia provider to be present in the room throughout the
9 conduct of anesthesia. Standard II calls for continual evaluation of the patient's oxygenation, ventilation, circulation, and temperature. The degree of invasive monitoring that should be used will depend on the patient's status and the procedure being undertaken.

At the conclusion of the procedure, patients should recover from anesthesia or sedation in a postanesthesia care unit
10 (PACU) or similar setting. Care should be supervised by personnel who are trained to take care of unconscious patients, and with appropriate monitoring and resuscitation equipment immediately at hand.

TABLE 51-5

DEFINITION OF GENERAL ANESTHESIA AND LEVELS OF SEDATION/ANALGESIA

	■ MINIMAL SEDATION "ANXIOLYSIS"	■ MODERATE SEDATION/ANALGESIA "CONSCIOUS SEDATION"	■ DEEP SEDATION/ ANALGESIA	■ GENERAL ANESTHESIA
Responsiveness	Normal response to verbal stimulation	Purposeful response to verbal or tactile stimulation	Purposeful response following repeated or painful stimulation	Unarousable even with painful stimulus
Airway	Unaffected	No intervention required	Intervention may be required	Intervention required
Spontaneous ventilation	Unaffected	Adequate	May be inadequate	Frequently inadequate
Cardiovascular function	Unaffected	Usually maintained	Usually maintained	May be impaired

RADIOLOGY AND RADIATION THERAPY

Developments in technology have meant that interventional radiologists now perform an increasing number of procedures that were once in the domain of surgeons. Anesthesiologists are increasingly required to take care of patients undergoing both diagnostic and therapeutic interventional procedures. Two important aspects of the radiological environment are the side effects of contrast media, which are commonly used to enhance radiological images, and the hazards of ionizing radiation.

Intravenous Contrast Agents

Intravenous contrast agents are iodinated compounds used for many radiological procedures.[10] MRI contrast media are also now widely used; these agents are chelated metal complexes containing gadolinium, iron, and manganese.

Contrast media are eliminated via the kidneys, and contrast-induced nephropathy is a concern. This condition accounts for 10% of hospital-acquired renal failure[11] and is more likely to occur in patients with preexisting renal insufficiency, diabetes, and those taking nonsteroidal anti-inflammatory drugs.[12] Adequate hydration, careful monitoring of urine output, and the use of low-osmolarity contrast media[13] help reduce the risk of contrast-induced nephropathy. A randomized controlled trial has demonstrated the efficacy of sodium bicarbonate in preventing contrast-induced nephropathy when given by intravenous infusion 1 hour before contrast.[12] In procedures lasting several hours, a urinary catheter is recommended to monitor urine output and prevent restlessness due to a full bladder. Low-osmolarity, nonionic compounds with osmolarities ranging from 290 to 650 mOsm/kg have a lower incidence of adverse reactions compared with the older, high-osmolarity agents.[14,15] The overall incidence of adverse drug reactions with nonionic contrast media is reported as 3.13%, and the incidence of severe reactions is 0.04%.[15] These are shown in more detail in Table 51-6. Reactions are described as mild (e.g., urticaria, chills, fever, facial flushing, nausea, vomiting), moderate (e.g., edema, bronchospasm, hypotension seizures), and severe (e.g., dyspnea, prolonged hypotension, cardiac arrest, loss of consciousness, anaphylactic reactions). Patients with atopy or allergy to shellfish are more prone to contrast-related adverse reactions.[16] Pretreatment with oral methylprednisolone prior to intravenous administration of contrast medium[17] can reduce the incidence of adverse reactions. Treatment of severe reactions should include discontinuing the causative agent and supportive therapy, such as oxygen administration, securing the airway, and cardiovascular support with fluids, vasopressors, and inotropes. Bronchospasm should be treated with appropriate bronchodilators. Adverse reactions to MRI contrast media are similar to those with other contrast media and have a similar incidence.[18] In some cases, there is cross-sensitivity between gadolinium-containing agents and iodinated ones.

Protection From Ionizing Radiation

Patients, physicians, and other health care workers are frequently exposed to ionizing radiation, usually in the form of x-rays. Exposure to gamma radiation, or, rarely, alpha or beta radiation from radioactive isotopes, may also occur during implantation or removal procedures. Ionizing radiation exposure may occur directly from the source, as leakage from the ionizing device, or as scatter from the equipment. Direct exposure must be avoided. A *rad* (radiation-absorbed dose) is a measure of an absorbed dose of radiation. The total dose of x-rays is measured in roentgens, and a *rem* (roentgen-equivalent-man) is the dose of ionizing radiation with the same biological tissue effect as 1 rad of x-rays.[19] The dose of radiation received during a chest radiograph is in the order of 8 mrem, a head computed tomography (CT) scan is 170 mrem, and an abdominal CT is 680 mrem.[20] Radiation exposure with fluoroscopy may be greater than 75,000 mrem.[19] The effective dose received by the patient during intraoperative digital subtraction angiography was calculated as 76.7 mrem.[20] The exposure of health care workers to the radiation emitted from x-ray equipment is several orders of magnitude lower.[20] The National Council on Radiation Protection and Measurements has established guidelines governing medical radiation.[21] The recommended annual occupational exposure is 5,000 mrem. With the routine use of a lead apron, protective goggles, and thyroid shield, exposure to radiation can be kept to a low level. However, this protective clothing is cumbersome, and can result in fatigue and discomfort, which can distract from patient care.

SPECIFIC RADIOLOGICAL PROCEDURES

Cerebral and spinal angiography cause minimal discomfort and may be performed under local anesthesia with or without light sedation administered by nonanesthesiologists. Patients are required to remain completely motionless during these

TABLE 51-6

INCIDENCE OF CONTRAST-RELATED ADVERSE REACTIONS

IODINATED CONTRAST MEDIA		
HIGH-OSMOLARITY CONTRAST MEDIA (%)	ADVERSE REACTIONS	LOW-OSMOLARITY CONTRAST MEDIA (%)
6.0	Nausea and vomiting	1.0
3.0	Urticaria	0.5
2.6	Hoarseness, sneezing, cough, dyspnea, facial edema	0.5
0.1	Hypotension	0.01

MAGNETIC RESONANCE IMAGING CONTRAST MEDIA		
CONTRAST MEDIA	ADVERSE REACTIONS	INCIDENCE (%)
Gadolinium chelates	Mild (nausea and/or vomiting)	2.0
	Moderate	0.1
	Severe	0.01
Ferrous oxide	Aching muscles	8.0
	Others (including allergic-like reactions)	3.0
Manganese fodipir	Injection site discomfort	67.0
	Nausea and/or vomiting	14.0
	Headache	5.0
	Others	<1.0

Reprinted with permission from King BF: Intravascular contrast media and premedication. In Bush WH, Krecke KN, King BF, Bettman MA (eds): Radiology Life Support, p 13. London, Arnold, 1999.

procedures, which may be lengthy, particularly spinal angiography. Neurologic disorders such as recent subarachnoid hemorrhage, stroke, and depressed level of consciousness or raised ICP may make it impossible for patients to tolerate these procedures. Deep sedation or general anesthesia with airway protection is often required. Angiography is usually performed via the femoral artery; the femoral vein may also be accessed when imaging arteriovenous malformations or dural venous abnormalities. Liberal use of local anesthetic at the puncture site precludes the need for intravenous analgesia. The injection of contrast media into the cerebral arteries may cause discomfort, burning, or pruritus around the face and eyes. Hypotension and bradycardia may also occur. Complications following angiography are described as neurologic and nonneurologic, and vary between 1 and 2.5%.[22] During cerebral angiography, the patient is placed on a moving gantry, and the radiologist positions the patient to track catheters as they pass from the groin into the cerebral vessels. It is vital to have extensions on all anesthesia breathing circuits, infusion lines, and monitors to prevent these from being accidentally dislodged as the radiologist swings the x-ray table rapidly back and forth. Care should be taken with positioning of radiopaque pieces of equipment. The electrocardiogram (ECG) electrodes may interfere with imaging during spinal angiography, and little metallic springs in the cuffs of endotracheal tubes can cause interesting and annoying artifacts if they lie over the area being imaged.

Interventional Neuroradiology

A number of neurosurgical conditions may be treated by interventional neuroradiological (INR) techniques.[23] The diseases amenable to endovascular treatment may be classified as emergent or elective; hemorrhagic or occlusive; and definitive, adjunctive, or palliative. Endovascular treatment of intracranial aneurysms with detachable platinum coils (Guglielmi detachable coils)[24] has become an acceptable alternative to surgery for reducing the risk of spontaneous recurrent hemorrhage following subarachnoid hemorrhage.[25] Endovascular treatment avoids the need for craniotomy and is often offered to patients with significant comorbidity or poor prognoses;[26,27] it may also reduce cognitive impairment and frontotemporal brain damage associated with craniotomy.[28] Arteriovenous malformations (AVMs) are increasingly being treated endovascularly, either as the sole therapy or in conjunction with surgical resection or stereotactic radiosurgery.[29] Materials used for INR include occlusive agents; detachable balloons, polyvinyl alcohol particles, coils (pushable, flow directed, and detachable), and liquid agents; and acrylic glues (N-butyl cyanoacrylates), nonadhesive polymerizing agents, and sclerosing agents.[29] For most INR procedures, arterial access is gained using a 6 or 7F sheath via the femoral or, rarely, the carotid or axillary artery[29,30] (Fig. 51-2). The umbilical vessels are an alternative route in neonates. A continuous infusion of heparinized saline is infused into the sheath via a side arm during the procedure. Continuous monitoring of blood pressure and sampling of arterial blood may be performed via the sheath, although most anesthesiologists prefer to insert a dedicated arterial catheter for monitoring the patient. The radiological imaging techniques include high-speed fluoroscopy and digital subtraction angiography. Once the sheath is in place, a guide catheter is advanced through the sheath and a "road mapping" technique is employed, whereby a bolus of contrast medium is injected to outline the vascular anatomy. This image may be superimposed onto the live fluoroscopic imaging to guide the advancement of the microcatheters for placement of embolic materials into an aneurysm or the feeding vessels of an AVM.

Anticoagulation

Anticoagulation with heparin is required during and up to 24 hours after interventional radiological procedures to prevent thromboembolism. The usual dose is between 3,000 and

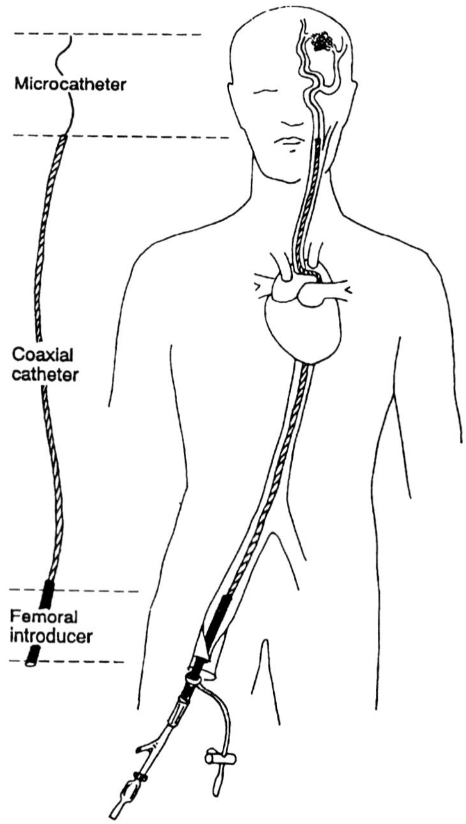

FIGURE 51-2. Representation of a superselective catheter. (Reprinted with permission from Young WL, Pile-Spellman J: Anesthetic considerations for interventional neuroradiology. Anesthesiology 80:427, 1994.)

5,000 U as an initial bolus, and 1,000 U/hour to maintain the activated clotting time at about 2.5 times the patient's baseline.

Complications

Interventional neuroradiological procedures are nonstimulating and generally well tolerated. Particular care should be exerted to prevent air embolism via the femoral sheath. Hematoma or hemorrhage may result from femoral artery puncture. There have also been reports of pulmonary embolic phenomena due to acrylic glues.[31] During angioplasty or stenting of carotid artery stenosis, the anesthesia team should be prepared to treat severe bradycardias or transient asystole. The two most catastrophic complications that can occur are intracranial hemorrhage or thromboembolic stroke. The incidence of these during coiling of cerebral aneurysms is 2.4 and 3.5%, respectively.[32] During embolization of AVMs, the incidence of catastrophic complications is between 1 and 8%.[33] The anesthesia team is vital in the expedient treatment of these life-threatening events (Table 51-7).

Anesthetic Technique

Neuroradiologists are increasingly requesting general anesthesia for interventional procedures.[27,32,34] Anesthetic complications are quite low, although the incidence of complications related to the procedure has been reported as 20%.[34]

General anesthesia is usually conducted with endotracheal intubation and intermittent positive-pressure ventilation, although the laryngeal mask airway is a suitable alternative.[32] Propofol and thiopental are the most commonly used induction agents. Conscious sedation techniques vary. Combinations of a benzodiazepine (usually midazolam) and opioid (usually fentanyl) are popular, as are propofol infusions.[34] Droperidol and dimenhydrinate are less frequently used alternatives. Invasive monitoring is used less often in patients undergoing INR compared with those having neurosurgical procedures.[27] The anesthesia team may facilitate the neuroradiologist in a number of ways by manipulating systemic blood pressure and controlling end-tidal $Paco_2$.[30,32] Controlled hypotension is often requested to facilitate embolization of AVMs. Esmolol, labetalol, metoprolol, and hydralazine are commonly used. Moderate hypertension may help reduce cerebral ischemia by maintaining cerebral perfusion; in this case, phenylephedrine is the agent of choice.

Certain procedures require patients to be awake at least for part of the procedure. A superselective anesthesia functional examination, or SAFE,[30] may be performed prior to therapeutic embolization to determine whether the catheter has been placed in a vessel that supplies an eloquent area of the brain or spinal cord, such as speech or language areas. Following baseline neurologic examination, amobarbital 30 mg (for investigating the gray matter areas) or lidocaine 30 mg (to evaluate the integrity of the white matter tracts) mixed with contrast agent is injected via the catheter. The patient is then reassessed for neurologic deficits in the areas at risk; if the assessment is negative, embolization may proceed. A "sleep-awake-sleep" anesthetic technique using a propofol infusion allows the patient to be rapidly awakened for appropriate neurologic testing; once this is complete, the patient is once again sedated or anesthetized while the definitive procedure is carried out.

TABLE 51-7

ACUTE MANAGEMENT OF NEUROLOGIC CATASTROPHES

Initial resuscitation
- Communicate with radiologists
- Call for assistance
- Secure the airway and hyperventilate with 100% O_2
- Determine if problem is hemorrhagic or occlusive
  - Hemorrhagic: immediate heparin reversal (1 mg protamine for each 100 units heparin given) and low normal pressure
  - Occlusive: deliberate hypertension, titrated to neurologic examination, angiography, or physiologic imaging studies (e.g., TCD, CBF)*

Further resuscitation
- Head up 15° in neutral position
- Titrate ventillation to a $Paco_2$ of 26–28 mm Hg
- 0.5 g/kg mannitol, rapid intravenous infusion
- Anticonvulsants: dilantin (give slowly, 50 mg/min) and phenobarbitol
- Titrate thiopental infusion to electroencephalogram burst suppression
- Allow body temperature to fall as quickly as possible to 33–34°C
- Consider dexamethasone 10 mg

*TCD, Transcranial Dopples; CBF, Cerebral blood flow.
Reprinted from Young WL, Pile-Spellman J: Anesthetic considerations for interventional neuroradiology. Anesthesiology 80:427, 1994.

Computed Tomography and Magnetic Resonance Imaging

CT scanning and MRI are used for a wide array of diagnostic imaging and an increasingly large number of therapeutic procedures. The procedures are similar in that they are relatively painless and most adults can tolerate them without the need for sedation or anesthesia. There is, however, an absolute requirement for the patient to remain motionless while the study is being performed. Children and adults with a variety of psychological or neurologic disorders may require sedation or anesthesia to enable them to tolerate the procedures (see Table 51-4).

Patients with acute thoracic, abdominal, and head trauma often require urgent imaging to facilitate diagnosis. It is not unheard of for these patients to develop hemorrhagic shock, raised intracranial pressure (ICP), depression of consciousness, and cardiac arrest in the CT scanner. Patients must be adequately resuscitated and stabilized before transportation to the radiology department.

Computed Tomography

Modern CT scanners obtain a cross-sectional image in just a few seconds, and spiral scanners can image a slice of the body in less than 1 second, minimizing the problems with motion artifacts. Stereotactic-guided surgery is performed using CT scanning to minimize injury to adjacent structures. Most of these procedures involve biopsy or aspiration of intracranial masses. A radiolucent frame is placed around the head and held in place by pins inserted directly into the skull. This aspect of the procedure is painful. Transient deep sedation or general anesthesia may be necessary in combination with the injection of local anesthetic at the pin insertion sites. Sedation must be used with caution in patients with suspected intracranial hypertension. The frame may completely occlude the patient's airway, so the anesthesia team should have a plan for rapid airway control should the need arise. Such a plan may involve removal of the frame or fiberoptic-assisted tracheal intubation.

Magnetic Resonance Imaging

The physical principles of MRI are described in depth elsewhere.[35] Briefly, when atoms with an odd number of protons in their nuclei, notably hydrogen, are subjected to a powerful static magnetic field, they align themselves with the magnetic field. If they are then intermittently exposed to a radiofrequency wave, the nuclei change their alignment. As the radiofrequency pulses are discontinued, the protons return to their original alignment (i.e., they "relax") within the original magnetic field and, as they do, they release energy. The release of energy over time (the relaxation time) is specific for given tissues and is used to generate the MRI signal. The magnetic field strengths are measured in tesla (T; 1 T = 10,000 gauss). The earth's magnetic field is approximately 0.5 gauss. MRI scanners used for clinical purposes generate a field of 0.15 to 2.0 T,[36] and machines generating magnetic fields from 4 to 8 T are used in research. Despite extensive review,[37] no adverse effects have been described due to human exposure to magnetic fields. Deaths and adverse outcomes in MRI scanners are entirely due to the presence of ferrometallic foreign bodies such as cerebral aneurysm clips or implanted devices such as pacemakers. Before entering the vicinity of the magnet, patients and staff need to complete a rigorous checklist to ensure they have no ferrometallic objects in their bodies. The magnetic field takes several days to establish and is constantly present. It decreases in strength with distance from the center of the magnet, quantified as a number of concentric rings termed "gauss lines." This peripheral or fringe field around the magnet is responsible for malfunction of electrical equipment. The 5 gauss line, for example, is the point beyond which pacemakers will malfunction. Ferromagnetic anesthetic gas cylinders, if brought within the 50 gauss line, become potentially lethal projectiles, and a number of near-miss incidents have been documented.[38] MRI-compatible anesthesia machines and monitors are available, but it is still important to check exactly how close this equipment can be brought to the magnetic field.[39] Standard pulse oximeters will work in the MRI scanner but have been reported to produce burns,[40] and nonferrous or fiberoptically cabled pulse oximeters should be used. The ECG is sensitive to the changing magnetic signals, and it is nearly impossible to eliminate all artifacts. The electrodes should be placed close together and toward the center of the magnetic field. The leads should be insulated from the patient's skin because they may heat up and cause thermal injury. All cables and wires should run a straight path and not be wound in loops to avoid induction heating effects. Noninvasive blood pressure monitors and transducers for invasive pressure monitoring are available. In the absence of MRI-compatible monitors, long sampling tubes can be connected to standard capnographs and anesthetic agent monitors. Most infusion pumps can be used outside the 30 gauss line,[41] and extra lengths of extension tubing should be available. MRI takes upward of 30 minutes, and many patients find it difficult to stay still for long periods. It may become very warm within the coil of the magnate, often reaching 80°F, adding to patient discomfort. The MRI scanner emits a considerable amount of noise, up to 90 dB, and both the patient and the anesthesia team should wear hearing protection. It is important to remember that once a scan sequence is initiated, no one may enter or leave the scan room. In the case of an emergency, the MRI technicians should be notified, the scan sequence stopped, and the patient rapidly removed. Resuscitation attempts should take place outside the scanner because laryngoscopes, oxygen cylinders, cardiac defibrillators, and so on cannot be taken close to the magnet.

Anesthetic Techniques

Thirty percent of adult patients experience some degree of anxiety during MRI scanning,[42] and up to 10% experience severe panic and claustrophobia. Four percent of adult patients will terminate the procedure prematurely,[43] whereas 14% require some form of sedation to tolerate MRI scanning.[44] In most cases, this may be provided as either oral sedation with benzodiazepines or intravenous sedation administered under the supervision of the radiologist. Anesthesiologists are usually only involved with more complex patients, such as those with obesity, obstructive sleep apnea, raised ICP, movement disorders, developmental delay, and the potential for a difficult airway.

Most children younger than the age of 5, and many as old as age 11,[45] require sedation or general anesthesia to tolerate MRI and CT scanning. Twenty-two percent of children undergoing sedation for MRI or CT scans have been found to experience some sort of adverse event; oxygen desaturation occurred in 2.9%, and in 15%, sedation was inadequate.[46] Adverse events are more common in children with higher ASA grades who are undergoing sedation, and preselecting children who are unsuitable for oral sedation improves the efficiency of oral sedation programs. Oral sedation techniques, if appropriately administered, have a success rate of 93%.[45,46] Children who undergo general anesthesia for scans have a very low incidence of adverse reactions (<0.7%).[45,46] Oral chloral hydrate is a popular agent for sedation by nonanesthesiologists, and doses between 80 and 100 mg/kg have shown to be effective for children younger than 3 years of age who are undergoing CT scan.[47] Chloral hydrate can cause excessive sedation, agitation,[48] and respiratory depression; it may also have a prolonged effect in neonates.[49] Benzodiazepines such as midazolam administered either orally (0.25 to 0.75 mg/kg) or intravenously (0.05 to 0.15 mg/kg) are also commonly used for sedation. Deep sedation with propofol infusion, oxygen administration via nasal cannula, and end-tidal CO_2 monitoring are successful techniques.[45] Children are initially sedated with incremental propofol boluses up to 3 mg/kg with or without midazolam, 0.2 to 0.5 mg/kg, and then maintained with an infusion rate of propofol, ~1 to 3 mg/kg/hr with supplemental boluses of 1 mg/kg for movement.

TABLE 51-8

COMMON RADIOSENSITIVE TUMORS

Primary CNS tumor—neuroblastoma, medulloblastoma
Acute leukemia—CNS leukemia
Radiosensitive ocular tumors—retinoblastoma
Intraabdominal tumors—Wilms' tumor
Rhabdomyosarcoma
Other tumors—Langerhans' cell histiocytosis

CNS, central nervous system.

Radiation Therapy

Two different types of radiation therapy commonly require anesthesia care—external beam radiation treatments, usually for children with malignancies, and intraoperative radiation to tumor masses that cannot be completely resected. Radiosensitive malignancies occurring in children are shown in Table 51-8.

Tumors may involve a variety of vital areas, including the airway, thorax, mediastinum, and heart. Patients with central nervous system (CNS) tumors should be assessed for signs of raised ICP. Many children receive cytotoxic or immunosuppressive chemotherapy, as well as radiotherapy. This may result in increased risk of sepsis, thrombocytopenia, and anemia. Patients are typically scheduled for a series of treatments over several weeks. Radiation doses are high, in the range of 180 to 250 cGy, and all medical personnel must leave the room during the actual treatment. Direct observation of the patient is not possible, and an interfaced system of closed-circuit television and telemetric microphones is used with standard monitoring.[4] In the event of a problem, shutdown of the radiation beam and immediate access to the patient are crucial (within 20 to 30 seconds).

The goals of anesthesia for pediatric radiotherapy have been defined as[50]

1. Assurance of immobility
2. Rapid onset
3. Brief duration of action
4. Not painful to administer
5. Prompt recovery
6. Minimal interference with eating or drinking and playing
7. Avoidance of tolerance to the anesthetic agents
8. Maintenance of a patent airway in a variety of body positions

General anesthesia[50] or deep sedation techniques with propofol are preferable to prevent patient movement. The first treatment planning simulation usually lasts 2 hours; following that, treatments usually take 30 minutes several times per week. Most children will have indwelling intravenous access, avoiding the need for repeated intravenous puncture and inhalational induction. Extremely high radiation levels are used as palliation for a variety of tumors.

Intraoperative radiation therapy treatments are provided after the masses are exposed to view. Patients with pancreatic, colon, and rectal cancers; radiation-sensitive sarcomas; and specific types of ovarian cancers receive this form of treatment. Doses of 5,000 to 6,000 cGy may be used during a single, intraoperative treatment. These patients typically suffer from advanced cancers, and may have the attendant nutritional deficiency, dehydration, electrolyte imbalances, and coagulopathies that can complicate anesthetic management. Some hospitals are equipped with combination radiation therapy/operating room suites; however, most centers require that surgical exploration be performed in the traditional operating room. The anesthetized patient is subsequently transported to the radiology suite, which may be at a considerable distance. Portable monitors and methods for delivery of oxygen and agents to maintain general anesthesia during transport are required.[51] Requirements for patient monitoring for intraoperative radiation are comparable to those described for external beam radiation. Personnel must leave the room during the actual treatment. After treatment, patients must be transported back to the operating room for surgical closure. Occasionally, closure can be performed in the radiology suite and the patient taken directly to the PACU.

CARDIAC CATHETERIZATION

Procedures that may require anesthesia in the cardiac catheterization laboratory[52] include diagnostic cardiac catheterization and therapeutic procedures such as percutaneous transluminal coronary angioplasty with coronary stenting, carotid stenting, atherectomy, and valvuloplasty. Electrophysiologic (EP) mapping and ablation studies are also performed. Most adults can tolerate these procedures under light sedation. More complex procedures include laser extraction of automatic implantable cardioverter-defibrillators (AICDs), as well as endovascular stenting of thoracic and abdominal aortic aneurysms. These procedures usually require more invasive monitoring and general anesthesia.

Cardiac catheterization is performed in children with congenital heart disease for both hemodynamic assessment and interventional procedures.[53] Careful cardiac assessment is essential, and the presence of a trained pediatric anesthesiologist is desirable. Patients often present with cyanosis, dyspnea, congestive heart failure, and intracardiac shunts. Hypoxia, hypercarbia, and sympathetic stimulation as a result of anxiety may exacerbate cardiopulmonary abnormalities. In patients with a patent ductus arteriosis, high oxygen tension can lead to premature closure and should be avoided. Prostaglandin infusions are often used to maintain duct patency. Meticulous attention must be paid to preventing air bubbles entering intravenous lines because they may cross to the arterial circulation via a right-to-left shunt. Diagnostic, noninterventional studies are often performed with sedation, and local anesthetic is injected at the site of femoral puncture. Oral sedation techniques include chloral hydrate 75 to 100 mg/kg, or a mixture of meperidine, promethazine, and chlorpromazine.[53] Intravenous agents include midazolam, morphine, and ketamine. General anesthesia is necessary when children cannot tolerate sedation techniques and/or have significant cardiac or other morbidity, and when the procedure involves severe hemodynamic disturbances such as ventricular septal defect occlusion. Ketamine is useful in children with myocardial depression and can be used as an infusion together with propofol.[54] Fentanyl, midazolam, and etomidate are alternatives.

Electrophysiologic Procedures

EP studies and ablation of abnormal conduction pathways are performed for treatment of dysrhythmias caused by aberrant conduction pathways. Cardiac catheters are inserted via the femoral and sometimes internal jugular routes, and multiple stimulations of the cardiac conducting system are carried out. Once identified, the abnormal conduction pathways are ablated using radiofrequency techniques. The volatile anesthetic agents and propofol have been shown not to interfere with cardiac conduction during these procedures.[55] EP studies are lengthy and can be painful; children usually require general anesthesia. Children undergoing radiofrequency ablation experience a high incidence of nausea and vomiting,[56] and this may be reduced using a propofol infusion technique rather than volatile anesthesia. The patient's antidysrhythmic therapy is stopped prior to the procedure, and cardiac dysrhythmias generated by the procedure are usually terminated using overdrive pacing via the catheters or, if unsuccessful, by external cardioversion. External pads should be applied before the procedure.

Automatic Implantable Cardioverter-Defibrillators

In the late 1990s, a number of trials proved the benefit of AICDs in reducing mortality of patients with ventricular tachyarrhythmias and left ventricular dysfunction following myocardial infarction or cardiac arrest.[58,59] AICDs are usually implanted in the EP lab rather than in the operating room, under general anesthesia or sedation. The procedure itself is not particularly painful; however, ventricular fibrillation is induced to test the device during implantation, which is distressing for the patient.

CARDIOVERSION

Atrial fibrillation (AF) affects approximately 0.4% of the general population, its prevalence increasing with age.[60] AF is associated with a number of conditions, particularly hypertension, chronic heart failure, and valvular and ischemic heart disease, and is a frequent sequelal of cardiothoracic surgery.[61] Transthoracic cardioversion is an accepted, often used treatment for atrial fibrillation and atrial flutter.[62] AF is associated with significant morbidity and mortality from thromboembolic stroke. Two strategies are employed to prevent thromboembolism following cardioversion in patients who have been in AF for longer than 48 hours. The conventional approach is to initiate anticoagulation 3 weeks before cardioversion, usually with Coumadin and to continue for 4 weeks after cardioversion.[62,63] More recently, transesophageal echocardiography (TEE) has been recommended to determine whether patients are at low or high risk of thromboembolism.[64,65] In low-risk patients, the dose of anticoagulants can be reduced, whereas in patients considered to be high risk, cardioversion may be postponed to allow adequate anticoagulation.[66] Cardioversion is a brief but distressing procedure that should be carried out using sedation.[67] When TEE is being performed prior to cardioversion, the procedure may take 15 to 30 minutes. Elective cardioversion is often performed in areas near the operating room, usually in the PACU. Alternatively, there may be a requirement for the anesthesia team to provide sedation in the intensive care unit (ICU) for urgent cardioversion in an unstable patient.

The usual anesthetic technique for cardioversion is a small bolus of intravenous induction agent. All currently available induction agents are effective. Propofol produces hypotension more often than etomidate,[68] although this can be attenuated by using an infusion[69] or smaller doses of propofol (1 mg/kg).[70] Etomidate causes a high incidence of myoclonus, which can render interpretation of the ECG difficult.[68,69] Recovery after midazolam tends to be longer than after the other agents, although this may be reversed with flumazenil.[71] Propofol administered by a target-controlled infusion has been compared with inhalational anesthesia with sevoflurane.[72] Sevoflurane was found to provide greater hemodynamic stability than propofol. However, this technique is only practical if there is easy access to a sevoflurane vaporizer and an anesthesia machine. Fentanyl 1.5 mg/kg may also be administered 3 minutes before induction.[68] When TEE is being performed before cardioversion, the patient needs to remain sedated for longer, and a propofol infusion may be useful. In general, patients do not require intubation for cardioversion unless there is a risk of regurgitation. During TEE, local anesthetic is sprayed into the oropharynx to allow easy passage of the TEE probe. A bite block is inserted to prevent the patient from biting down on the probe, damaging both their teeth and the probe. The anesthesiologist can often assist the cardiologists by deepening the level of sedation in the initial stages to allow the TEE probe to be inserted more easily.

GASTROENTEROLOGY

The gastroenterology suite is another location where technology is expanding, and where an increasing number of diagnostic and therapeutic procedures are being performed. Procedures commonly performed in the gastrointestinal (GI) endoscopy suite are shown in Table 51-9.

In the majority of cases, gastroenterologists provide their own sedation for GI endoscopy. Sedation techniques include combinations of benzodiazepine, midazolam, or diazepam with or without an opioid, fentanyl, alfentanil, or meperidine.[73] A greater incidence of side effects is seen when a combination of a benzodiazepine and opioid is used or when patients have significant comorbidity.[74] The incidence of serious cardiorespiratory side effects and death have been reported as 5.4 and 0.3 per 1,000 procedures, respectively.[75] Propofol has been used by gastroenterologists and found to provide excellent conditions for GI endoscopy[76] and endoscopic retrograde cholangiopancreatography (ERCP);[77] however, many gastroenterologists believe it should only be administered by trained anesthesia providers.[78,79]

Upper Gastrointestinal Endoscopy

Upper GI endoscopy is performed for diagnostic procedures, such as biopsy, and for therapeutic procedures, such as retrieval of foreign bodies, treatment of esophageal varices with sclerotherapy or band ligation, dilation of esophageal strictures, and placement of a percutaneous endoscopic gastrostomy. Patients may have a number of comorbidities, including disease of the esophagus and stomach, with a risk of reflux, biliary and hepatic disease with esophageal varices, hepatic dysfunction, coagulopathy, and ascites. The procedure is tolerated without sedation in 66 to 81% of patients,[80] and in the rest, conscious sedation is usually sufficient. With general anesthesia, patients usually require endotracheal intubation to protect the airway and facilitate passage of the endoscope. The laryngeal mask airway has also been used successfully in adults[81] and children[82] as an alternative device for airway management. Local anesthetic is sprayed into the oropharynx to facilitate passage of the

TABLE 51-9

COMMON GASTROENTEROLOGICAL PROCEDURES

Upper endoscopy
Sigmoidoscopy
Colonoscopy
Endoscopic retrograde cholangiopancreatography
Esophageal dilatation
Esophageal stenting
Percutaneous endoscopic gastrostomy tube placement
Transjugular intrahepatic portosystemic shunt

endoscope; this can abolish the gag reflex, increasing the risk of aspiration. A bite block is inserted to prevent the patient from biting down on the endoscope and damaging both their teeth and the endoscope. If the patient has received general anesthesia, care must be taken that the bite block and endoscope do not dislodge or obstruct the endotracheal tube. Procedures are performed in the prone or semiprone position with the patient's head rotated to the side. This position makes the airway less accessible. Care and attention should also be paid to pressure areas, particularly the eyes, lips, and teeth. Extreme rotation of the neck should be avoided. Most procedures are brief, lasting 10 to 30 minutes, and are generally painless.

Endoscopic Retrograde Cholangiopancreatography

ERCP is important in the diagnosis and treatment of both biliary and pancreatic disease. During the procedure, the endoscope is advanced via the mouth into the stomach, and then into the duodenum where the ampulla of Vater is visualized. The biliary and pancreatic duct systems may then be instrumented, and therapeutic maneuvers such as the passage of stents or removal of stones carried out. Sphincter of Oddi manometry (SOM) may also be performed. Patients usually experience discomfort during ERCP, particularly with instrumentation and stenting of the biliary and pancreatic ducts. Conscious or deep sedation techniques are recommended.[83] Only 5 to 8%[81,84] of patients require general anesthesia. The procedure usually lasts between 20 to 80 minutes.[83] The airway and patient positioning considerations are similar to those for GI endoscopy. If SOM is being performed, glycopyrrolate, atropine, and glucagon should be avoided[84] because they effect sphincter pressure. Opioids, particularly morphine[85] and fentanyl, cause spasm of the sphincter of Oddi, which may be relieved with naloxone.[86] Meperidine, in contrast, reduces the frequency of sphincter of Oddi contractions.[85]

Patients presenting for emergency ERCP may have significant comorbidity,[84] including acute cholangitis with septicemia, jaundice with liver dysfunction and coagulopathy, bleeding from esophageal varices resulting in hypovolemia, or biliary stricture following major hepatobiliary surgery, including liver transplantation. Transient bacteremia may occur during endoscopy, and antibiotic prophylaxis is recommended for patients with cardiac valvular abnormalities.

Antispasmodics

Gastroenterologists frequently use antispasmodics to improve operating conditions during endoscopy.[78,87] Intravenous hyoscyamine given as a 0.5-mg bolus before the procedure has been shown to reduce the incidence of spasm, shorten the procedure, and improve patient comfort;[87] however, it can also cause sinus tachycardia.

Transjugular Intrahepatic Portosystemic Shunt

The transjugular intrahepatic portosystemic shunt (TIPS) is created via a catheter inserted in the internal jugular vein and directed into the liver. It connects the right or left portal vein through the liver parenchyma to one of the three hepatic veins.[88] The TIPS functions to decompress the portal circulation in patients with portal hypertension and is often performed in patients who have failed to respond to medical therapy. The TIPS has been found to be equally effective as other therapies in the secondary prophylaxis of bleeding varices and control of refractory cirrhotic ascites,[89] but with no improvement in mortality and an increased risk of development of encephalopathy. The TIPS has been used in children and found to be feasible and safe in providing temporary relief of portal hypertension while awaiting liver transplantation.[90] The TIPS procedure causes minimal stimulation, lasts between 2 to 3 hours, and may be performed under sedation or general anesthesia.[91] Patients presenting for a TIPS procedure, in general, have significant hepatic dysfunction and require careful preoperative assessment. Considerations are outlined in Table 51-10. Chronic liver disease has a number of effects on the pharmacokinetics of anesthetic agents,[91] and the response to anesthetic agents may be unpredictable. Volume of distribution is increased, and protein binding, drug metabolism, and elimination are all decreased. CNS sensitivity is variably affected. Patients need careful monitoring; the use of an arterial catheter to monitor blood pressure, and to allow frequent blood gas and chemistry analysis, is recommended. Blood glucose should be monitored frequently because patients with hepatic disease are at risk for hypoglycemia due to depleted liver glycogen stores. Preoperative use of diuretics and intraoperative fluid shifts make these patients vulnerable to electrolyte abnormalities. Urine output should be closely monitored to prevent worsening of renal function and development of the hepatorenal syndrome.

TABLE 51-10

PREOPERATIVE CONSIDERATIONS IN PATIENTS PRESENTING FOR THE TRANSJUGULAR INTRAHEPATIC PORTOSYSTEMIC SHUNT PROCEDURE

Airway—risk of aspiration	Recent gastrointestinal bleeding Raised intragastric pressure due to ascites Decreased level of consciousness due to hepatic encephalopathy
Respiratory system	Decreased functional residual capacity due to ascites Pleural effusion Intrapulmonary shunts Pneumonia
Cardiovascular system	Associated alcoholic cardiomyopathy Altered volume status Acute hemorrhage from esophageal varices Intraperitoneal hemorrhage
Hematologic system	Coagulopathy Thrombocytopenia
Neurologic system	Hepatic encephalopathy

ELECTROCONVULSIVE THERAPY

Electroconvulsive therapy (ECT) has had an important role in the management of psychiatric disorders since the 1930s. ECT is used to treat depression, mania, and affective disorders in schizophrenic patients, as well as a number of other psychiatric disorders. Its use in the United States is increasing.[92] Typically, ECT is performed three times per week for 6 to 12 treatments, followed by weekly or monthly maintenance therapy to prevent relapses.[93]

Physiologic Response to Electroconvulsive Therapy

The physiologic response to an electrical current applied to the brain includes generalized motor seizures and an acute cardiovascular response. The grand mal seizure lasts several minutes and includes a short, 10- to 15-second tonic phase, followed by a more prolonged clonic phase, lasting 30 to 60 seconds. A minimum seizure duration of 25 seconds is recommended to ensure adequate antidepressant efficacy.[92,94] The cardiovascular response includes increased cerebral blood flow and ICP. Generalized autonomic nervous system stimulation results in an initial 10 to 15 seconds of bradycardia and occasional asystole, followed by a more prominent sympathetic response of hypertension and tachycardia. Occasionally, cardiac dysrhythmias, myocardial ischemia, infarction, or neurologic vascular events may be precipitated. Short-term memory loss is also common following ECT. Other sequelae include muscular aches, fracture-dislocations, headache, emergence agitation, status epilepticus, and sudden death.

Anesthetic Considerations

ECT is usually carried out in the PACU near the operating room; alternatively, psychiatric institutions may have an area set aside for treatments. Psychiatrists place scalp electrodes to monitor the electroencephalogram during the seizure, and a blood pressure cuff is applied to an extremity and inflated before the muscle relaxant is administered to monitor the seizure. Patients with depression presenting for ECT are often elderly with a number of coexisting conditions; therefore, a thorough preoperative assessment and workup should be performed before the patient begins treatment.[95] First-line pharmacotherapeutic agents for the treatment of depression include tricyclic antidepressants, monoamine oxidase inhibitors (MAOIs), and selective serotonin-reuptake inhibitors (SSRIs). Patients may be taking a variety of drugs, which can have important interactions with the anesthetic agent. The MAOIs have the most significant interactions, although more modern drugs are superseding these. The anesthetic requirements for ECT include amnesia, airway management, prevention of bodily injury from the seizure, control of hemodynamic changes, and a smooth, rapid emergence.[93,95] Most of the intravenous induction agents have been used to induce anesthesia for ECT. Methohexital (1 to 1.5 mg/kg) is considered the "gold standard,"[93] although it decreases seizure duration in a dose-dependant way.[96] Etomidate (0.15 to 0.3 mg/kg) is generally associated with longer seizure duration, myoclonus, and delayed recovery,[96] and is useful in patients who experience short seizures.[97] However, etomidate does not depress the cardiovascular system, so hypertensive and tachycardic responses may be accentuated.[93] Propofol is more effective at attenuating the acute hemodynamic responses to ECT,[98] and recovery is rapid. Propofol, however, has anticonvulsant effects, although with a small dose (0.75 mg/kg) seizure duration is usually acceptable,[96] and studies have found that reduction in seizure duration by propofol does not adversely affect the outcome of ECT therapy.[99] Most other induction agents decrease seizure activity. The short-acting opioids alfentanil[100] and remifentanil can be used to decrease the dose of induction agent and prolong seizure duration without reducing the depth of anesthesia.[101] Muscle relaxants are used to prevent musculoskeletal complications such as fractures or dislocations during the seizure. Succinylcholine 0.75 to 1.5 mg/kg is the most commonly used agent and is preferable to the longer-acting nondepolarizing agents.[93] Anesthesia is induced, and the patient is ventilated with 100% oxygen using an oral airway and a self-inflating bag and mask. Moderate hyperventilation is beneficial prior to the ECT to improve the quality and duration of seizures,[97] and it has been suggested that the laryngeal mask airway may be useful to improve ventilation during ECT.[102] Before administrating the seizure, a bite guard is placed to protect the teeth. In younger patients, 15 to 30 mg of intravenous ketorolac helps to reduce ECT-induced myalgia. Older patients, or those in whom ketorolac is contraindicated, may receive aspirin or acetaminophen orally before their treatment.[93] The parasympathetic effects of ECT, salivation, transient bradycardia, and asystole can be prevented by premedication with glycopyrrolate or atropine. Of the two, glycopyrrolate is associated with less tachycardia.[93] A number of drugs have been used to attenuate the hypertensive and tachycardic responses that accompany ECT. Labetalol (0.3 mg/kg) and esmolol (1 mg/kg) both ameliorated the hemodynamic responses, although esmolol has a lesser effect on seizure duration than labetalol.[103] The calcium channel antagonists nifedipine, diltiazem, and nicardipine all attenuate the hemodynamic responses to ECT, particularly in combination with labetalol. Clonidine is also effective in controlling blood pressure without affecting seizure duration.[93]

DENTAL SURGERY

Most dental procedures are performed in the office with no sedation and only local anesthesia. General anesthesia may be required during more complicated or prolonged cases and when patients are uncooperative, phobic, or mentally challenged. Patients may also present for dental clearance prior to undergoing cardiac surgery or heart transplantation with severe cardiomyopathy or valvular abnormalities. A number of genetic diseases result in mental deficiency, psychiatric diagnoses, and aberrant behavior. These patients commonly require sedation or general anesthesia to tolerate dental procedures. Genetic diseases are commonly associated with other medical problems, particularly those related to the cardiovascular system and the airway.[104] Down syndrome is commonly encountered, and the anesthesiologist should be aware of cardiac abnormalities, including conduction abnormalities and structural defects; the risk of atlantooccipital dislocation; and a variety of potential airway problems, including macroglossia, hypoplastic maxilla, palatal abnormalities, or mandibular protrusion. If the patient is positioned head-up in the dental chair, vasodilation and myocardial depressant effects of anesthetics can be pronounced, especially in patients with cardiovascular diseases. Patients with neuromuscular diseases may have a history of aspiration and episodes of chronic recurrent pneumonitis that must be addressed before dental surgery. The most challenging part of anesthesia for dental surgery is induction. Many patients, particularly children, are unable to cooperate due to learning disabilities or mental retardation. Ketamine is a useful induction agent. It may be given by a variety of routes alone or in combination with atropine and midazolam.[105] Doses are as follows: intravenously, 1 to 2 mg/kg; orally, 5 to 10 mg/kg; and intramuscularly, 2 to 4 mg/kg, with an onset time of 5 to 10 minutes. The rectal and intranasal routes have also been used. Ketamine is also advantageous in that it does not abolish upper airway reflexes. Oral midazolam is also popular. A dose of 0.5 mg/kg is dissolved in a small amount of liquid. In children and needle-phobic adults, the use of local anesthetic cream facilitates the placement of intravenous lines. Alternatively, a gaseous induction may be attempted. During and after dental surgery blood, saliva and dental debris are present in the upper airway. A throat pack is used to help protect the airway, and this must be removed at the end of surgery. Tracheal intubation, often via the nasal route is required to protect the airway, although more recently the laryngeal mask airway has been used successfully for both adults[106] and children[107] undergoing dental surgery. Anesthesia can be maintained with intravenous infusions or inhalation anesthesia. Patients need close observation during emergence and recovery. The immediate postoperative complications include bleeding, airway obstruction, and laryngeal spasm. Later complications in ambulatory patients include drowsiness, nausea and vomiting, and pain.[108]

TRANSPORT OF PATIENTS

Patients who receive anesthesia or sedation at alternate sites may need to be transported to the PACU at the end of the procedure; this may be some distance away. During transport, patients should be accompanied by a member of the anesthesia team who should continue to evaluate, monitor, and support the patient's medical condition.[9] Other patients transported within a hospital may require the care of an anesthesiologist for a variety of reasons. For example, surgery patients may be transferred to the ICU or the radiology department for imaging at the end of surgery, or critically ill patients may be transferred to the operating room from the ICU or the emergency room for urgent surgery. In these situations, the anesthesiologist should monitor the patients closely. These patients are often ventilated and receiving a number of drug infusions for both sedation and hemodynamic support. Portable ventilators are useful for transport; however, these are often oxygen powered and adequate supplies of oxygen must be available for the transfer, as well as a manual self-inflating bag to allow hand ventilation in the event of ventilator failure. Similarly, the infusion pumps and portable monitors should have adequate battery power to allow them to continue working in transit. The anesthesiologist should carry spare anesthetic and emergency drugs, equipment for intubation or reintubation, portable suction, and, if the patient's condition requires, a portable defibrillator. It is useful to notify the destination that the patient is in transit so appropriate preparations to receive the patient can be made in advance. It is also useful to send personnel ahead to secure the elevators to prevent delays during transfer.

SUMMARY

The number and complexity of procedures that are performed at alternate sites is steadily increasing. This had led to an expansion of anesthesia services in areas remote from the operating room that may not be familiar to anesthesia providers. In preparing to administer anesthesia or sedation in an alternate site, a simple three-step approach can be followed. This involves giving careful consideration to the needs of the patient, the particular problems posed by the procedure, and the hazards and limitations of the environment. In all cases, the standards of anesthesia care and monitoring should be no different than those provided in the conventional operating room.

References

1. Joint Commission on Accreditation of Healthcare Organizations (JCAHO): Accreditation Manual for Hospitals, p 269. Oakbrook Terrace, IL, JCAHO, 1991
2. Gross JB, Epstein BS: ASA task force on analgesia and sedation by non-anesthesiologists. ASA Newsl 58:22, 1994
3. American Society of Anesthesiologists (ASA): Guidelines for nonoperating room anesthetizing locations. In ASA Directory of Members, p 476. Park Ridge, IL, ASA, 2003
4. Bashein G, Russell AH, Momii ST: Anesthesia and remote monitoring for intraoperative radiation therapy. Anesthesiology 64:804, 1986
5. American Society of Anesthesiologists (ASA): Basic standards for pre-anesthesia care. In ASA Directory of Members. Park Ridge, IL, ASA, 1998
6. American Society of Anesthesiologists (ASA): Standards for postanesthesia care. In ASA Directory of Members. Park Ridge, IL, ASA, 1994
7. American Society of Anesthesiologists (ASA): Position on monitored anesthesia care. In ASA Directory of Members. Park Ridge, IL, ASA, 2003
8. American Society of Anesthesiologists (ASA): Definition of general anesthesia and levels of sedation/analgesia. In ASA Directory of Members. Park Ridge, IL, ASA, 1999
9. American Society of Anesthesiologists (ASA): Standards for basic anesthetic monitoring. ASA Directory of Members, p 462. Park Ridge, IL, ASA, 2003
10. King BF Jr: Intravascular contrast media and premedication. In Bush WH Jr, Krecke KN, King BH Jr, Bettmann MA (eds): Radiology Life Support, p 1. London, Arnold, 1999
11. Briguori C, Tavano D, Colombo A: Contrast agent—Associated nephrotoxicity. Prog Cardiovasc Dis 45:493, 2003
12. Merten GJ, Burgess WP, Gray LV *et al*: Prevention of contrast-induced nephropathy with sodium bicarbonate: A randomized controlled trial. JAMA 291:2328, 2004
13. Lautin EM, Freeman NJ, Schoenfeld AH *et al*: Radiocontrast-associated renal dysfunction: A comparison of lower-osmolality and conventional high-osmolality contrast media. AJR Am J Roentgenol 157:59, 1991
14. Lasser EC, Lyon SG, Berry CC: Reports on contrast media reactions: Analysis of data from reports to the U.S. Food and Drug Administration. Radiology 203:605, 1997
15. Katayama H, Yamaguchi K, Kozuka T *et al*: Adverse reactions to ionic and nonionic contrast media. A report from the Japanese Committee on the Safety of Contrast Media. Radiology 175:621, 1990
16. Goldberg M: Systemic reactions to intravascular contrast media. A guide for the anesthesiologist. Anesthesiology 60:46, 1984
17. Lasser EC, Berry CC, Mishkin MM *et al*: Pretreatment with corticosteroids to prevent adverse reactions to nonionic contrast media. AJR Am J Roentgenol 162:523, 1994
18. Murphy KJ, Brunberg JA, Cohan RH: Adverse reactions to gadolinium contrast media: A review of 36 cases. AJR Am J Roentgenol 167:847, 1996
19. Davies D: Subspeciality monitoring techniques—Miscellaneous. In Gravenstein N (ed): Problems in Anesthesia Monitoring, p 138. Philadelphia, JB Lippincott, 1987
20. Derdeyn CP, Moran CJ, Eichling JO, Cross DT III: Radiation dose to patients and personnel during intraoperative digital subtraction angiography. AJNR Am J Neuroradiol 20:300, 1999
21. National Council on Radiation Protection and Measurements: Recommendations on limits for exposure to ionizing radiation. NCRP Report No. 91. Bethesda, National Council on Radiation, 1987.
22. Dion JE, Gates PC, Fox AJ *et al*: Clinical events following neuroangiography: A prospective study. Stroke 18:997, 1987
23. Armonda RA, Thomas JE, Rosenwasser RH: The interventional neuroradiology suite as an operating room. Neurosurg Clin N Am 11:1, 2000
24. Guglielmi G, Vinuela F, Dion J, Duckwiler G: Electrothrombosis of saccular aneurysms via endovascular approach. Part 2: Preliminary clinical experience. J Neurosurg 75:8, 1991
25. McDougall CG, Halbach VV, Dowd CF *et al*: Endovascular treatment of basilar tip aneurysms using electrolytically detachable coils. J Neurosurg 84:393, 1996
26. Kremer C, Groden C, Hansen HC *et al*: Outcome after endovascular treatment of Hunt and Hess grade IV or V aneurysms: Comparison of anterior versus posterior circulation. Stroke 30:2617, 1999
27. Lai YC, Manninen PH: Anesthesia for cerebral aneurysms: A comparison between interventional neuroradiology and surgery. Can J Anaesth 48:391, 2001
28. Hadjivassiliou M, Tooth CL, Romanowski CA *et al*: Aneurysmal SAH: Cognitive outcome and structural damage after clipping or coiling. Neurology 56:1672, 2001
29. Deveikis JP: Endovascular therapy of intracranial arteriovenous malformations. Materials and techniques. Neuroimaging Clin N Am 8:401, 1998
30. Young WL, Pile-Spellman J: Anesthetic considerations for interventional neuroradiology. Anesthesiology 80:427, 1994
31. Pelz DM, Lownie SP, Fox AJ, Hutton LC: Symptomatic pulmonary complications from liquid acrylate embolization of brain arteriovenous malformations. AJNR Am J Neuroradiol 16:19, 1995
32. Osborn IP: Anesthetic considerations for interventional neuroradiology. Int Anesthesiol Clin 41:69, 2003
33. Martin NA, Khanna R, Doberstein C, Bentson J: Therapeutic embolization of arteriovenous malformations: The case for and against. Clin Neurosurg 46:295, 2000
34. Manninen PH, Gignac EM, Gelb AW, Lownie SP: Anesthesia for interventional neuroradiology. J Clin Anesth 7:448, 1995
35. Menon DK, Peden CJ, Hall AS *et al*: Magnetic resonance for the anaesthetist. Part I: Physical principles, applications, safety aspects. Anaesthesia 47:240, 1992
36. Patteson SK, Chesney JT: Anesthetic management for magnetic resonance imaging: Problems and solutions. Anesth Analg 74:121, 1992
37. Schenck JF: Safety of strong, static magnetic fields. J Magn Reson Imaging 12:2, 2000
38. Chaljub G, Kramer LA, Johnson RF III *et al*: Projectile cylinder accidents resulting from the presence of ferromagnetic nitrous oxide or oxygen tanks in the MR suite. AJR Am J Roentgenol 177:27, 2001
39. Farling P, McBrien ME, Winder RJ: Magnetic resonance compatible equipment: Read the small print! Anaesthesia 58:86, 2003
40. Bashein G, Nessly ML, Bledsoe SW *et al*: Electroencephalography during surgery with cardiopulmonary bypass and hypothermia. Anesthesiology 76:878, 1992

41. Peden CJ, Menon DK, Hall AS *et al*: Magnetic resonance for the anaesthetist. Part II: Anaesthesia and monitoring in MR units. Anaesthesia 47: 508, 1992
42. Melendez JC, McCrank E: Anxiety-related reactions associated with magnetic resonance imaging examinations. JAMA 270:745, 1993
43. Flaherty JA, Hoskinson K: Emotional distress during magnetic resonance imaging. N Engl J Med 320:467, 1989
44. Murphy KJ, Brunberg JA: Adult claustrophobia, anxiety and sedation in MRI. Magn Reson Imaging 15:51, 1997
45. Keengwe IN, Hegde S, Dearlove O *et al*: Structured sedation programme for magnetic resonance imaging examination in children. Anaesthesia 54:1069, 1999
46. Malviya S, Voepel-Lewis T, Eldevik OP *et al*: Sedation and general anaesthesia in children undergoing MRI and CT: Adverse events and outcomes. Br J Anaesth 84:743, 2000
47. Greenberg SB, Faerber EN, Aspinall CL: High dose chloral hydrate sedation for children undergoing CT. J Comput Assist Tomogr 15:467, 1991
48. Merola C, Albarracin C, Lebowitz P *et al*: An audit of adverse events in children sedated with chloral hydrate or propofol during imaging studies. Paediatr Anaesth 5:375, 1995
49. Gooden CK, Dilos B: Anesthesia for magnetic resonance imaging. Int Anesthesiol Clin 41:29, 2003
50. Fortney JT, Halperin EC, Hertz CM, Schulman SR: Anesthesia for pediatric external beam radiation therapy. Int J Radiat Oncol Biol Phys 44:587, 1999
51. Mannaerts GH, Van Zundert AA, Meeusen VC *et al*: Anaesthesia for advanced rectal cancer patients treated with combined major resections and intraoperative radiotherapy. Eur J Anaesthesiol 19:742, 2002
52. Joe RR, Chen LQ: Anesthesia in the cardiac catheterization lab. Anesthesiol Clin North America 21:639, 2003
53. Javorski JJ, Hansen DD, Laussen PC *et al*: Paediatric cardiac catheterization: Innovations. Can J Anaesth 42:310, 1995
54. Kogan A, Efrat R, Katz J, Vidne BA: Propofol-ketamine mixture for anesthesia in pediatric patients undergoing cardiac catheterization. J Cardiothorac Vasc Anesth 17:691, 2003
55. Lavoie J, Walsh EP, Burrows FA *et al*: Effects of propofol or isoflurane anesthesia on cardiac conduction in children undergoing radiofrequency catheter ablation for tachydysrhythmias. Anesthesiology 82:884, 1995
56. Erb TO, Hall JM, Ing RJ *et al*: Postoperative nausea and vomiting in children and adolescents undergoing radiofrequency catheter ablation: A randomized comparison of propofol- and isoflurane-based anesthetics. Anesth Analg 95:1577, 2002
57. Moss AJ, Hall WJ, Cannom DS *et al*: Improved survival with an implanted defibrillator in patients with coronary disease at high risk for ventricular arrhythmia. Multicenter Automatic Defibrillator Implantation Trial Investigators. N Engl J Med 335:1933, 1996
58. Bigger JT Jr, Whang W, Rottman JN *et al*: Mechanisms of death in the CABG patch trial: A randomized trial of implantable cardiac defibrillator prophylaxis in patients at high risk of death after coronary artery bypass graft surgery. Circulation 99:1416, 1999
59. Higgins SL: Impact of the Multicenter Automatic Defibrillator Implantation Trial on implantable cardioverter defibrillator indication trends. Am J Cardiol 83:79D, 1999
60. Kannel WB, Wolf PA, Benjamin EJ, Levy D: Prevalence, incidence, prognosis, and predisposing conditions for atrial fibrillation: Population-based estimates. Am J Cardiol 82:2N, 1998
61. Ommen SR, Odell JA, Stanton MS: Atrial arrhythmias after cardiothoracic surgery. N Engl J Med 336:1429, 1997
62. Kerber RE: Transthoracic cardioversion of atrial fibrillation and flutter: Standard techniques and new advances. Am J Cardiol 78:22, 1996
63. Albers GW, Dalen JE, Laupacis A *et al*: Antithrombotic therapy in atrial fibrillation. Chest 119:194S, 2001
64. Klein AL, Grimm RA, Murray RD *et al*: Use of transesophageal echocardiography to guide cardioversion in patients with atrial fibrillation. N Engl J Med 344:1411, 2001
65. Asher CR, Klein AL: Transesophageal echocardiography to guide cardioversion in patients with atrial fibrillation: ACUTE trial update. Card Electrophysiol Rev 7:387, 2003
66. Troughton RW, Asher CR, Klein AL: The role of echocardiography in atrial fibrillation and cardioversion. Heart 89:1447, 2003
67. Kowey PR: The calamity of cardioversion of conscious patients. Am J Cardiol 61:1106, 1988
68. Canessa R, Lema G, Urzua J *et al*: Anesthesia for elective cardioversion: A comparison of four anesthetic agents. J Cardiothorac Vasc Anesth 5:566, 1991
69. Hullander RM, Leivers D, Wingler K: A comparison of propofol and etomidate for cardioversion. Anesth Analg 77:690, 1993
70. Herregods LL, Bossuyt GP, De Baerdemaeker LE *et al*: Ambulatory electrical external cardioversion with propofol or etomidate. J Clin Anesth 15:91, 2003
71. Coll-Vinent B, Sala X, Fernandez C *et al*: Sedation for cardioversion in the emergency department: Analysis of effectiveness in four protocols. Ann Emerg Med 42:767, 2003
72. Karthikeyan S, Balachandran S, Cort J *et al*: Anaesthesia for cardioversion: A comparison of sevoflurane and propofol. Anaesthesia 57:1114, 2002
73. Donnelly MB, Scott WA, Daly DS: Sedation for upper gastrointestinal endoscopy: A comparison of alfentanil-midazolam and meperidine-diazepam. Can J Anaesth 41:1161, 1994
74. The Standards of Practice Committee of the American Society for Gastrointestinal Endoscopy. ASGE guidelines: Complications of upper GI endoscopy. Gastrointest Endosc 55:784, 2002
75. Arrowsmith JB, Gerstman BB, Fleischer DE, Benjamin SB: Results from the American Society for Gastrointestinal Endoscopy/U.S. Food and Drug Administration collaborative study on complication rates and drug use during gastrointestinal endoscopy. Gastrointest Endosc 37:421, 1991
76. Carlsson U, Grattidge P: Sedation for upper gastrointestinal endoscopy: A comparative study of propofol and midazolam. Endoscopy 27:240, 1995
77. Vargo JJ, Zuccaro G Jr, Dumot JA *et al*: Gastroenterologist-administered propofol for therapeutic upper endoscopy with graphic assessment of respiratory activity: A case series. Gastrointest Endosc 52:250, 2000
78. Bell GD: Premedication, preparation, and surveillance. Endoscopy 32:92, 2000
79. Graber RG: Propofol in the endoscopy suite: An anesthesiologist's perspective. Gastrointest Endosc 49:803, 1999
80. Zaman A, Hapke R, Sahagun G, Katon RM: Unsedated peroral endoscopy with a video ultrathin endoscope: Patient acceptance, tolerance, and diagnostic accuracy. Am J Gastroenterol 93:1260, 1998
81. Osborn IP, Cohen J, Soper RJ, Roth LA: Laryngeal mask airway—A novel method of airway protection during ERCP: Comparison with endotracheal intubation. Gastrointest Endosc 56:122, 2002
82. Gajraj NM: Use of the laryngeal mask airway during oesophago-gastroduodenoscopy. Anaesthesia 51:991, 1996
83. Wehrmann T, Kokabpick S, Lembcke B *et al*: Efficacy and safety of intravenous propofol sedation during routine ERCP: A prospective, controlled study. Gastrointest Endosc 49:677, 1999
84. Etzkorn KP, Diab F, Brown RD *et al*: Endoscopic retrograde cholangiopancreatography under general anesthesia: Indications and results. Gastrointest Endosc 47:363, 1998
85. Thune A, Baker RA, Saccone GT *et al*: Differing effects of pethidine and morphine on human sphincter of Oddi motility. Br J Surg 77:992, 1990
86. Butler KC, Selden B, Pollack CV Jr: Relief by naloxone of morphine-induced spasm of the sphincter of Oddi in a post-cholecystectomy patient. J Emerg Med 21:129, 2001
87. Marshall JB, Patel M, Mahajan RJ *et al*: Benefit of intravenous antispasmodic (hyoscyamine sulfate) as premedication for colonoscopy. Gastrointest Endosc 49:720, 1999
88. Ong JP, Sands M, Younossi ZM: Transjugular intrahepatic portosystemic shunts (TIPS): A decade later. J Clin Gastroenterol 30:14, 2000
89. Boyer TD: Transjugular intrahepatic portosystemic shunt: Current status. Gastroenterology 124:1700, 2003
90. Hackworth CA, Leef JA, Rosenblum JD *et al*: Transjugular intrahepatic portosystemic shunt creation in children: Initial clinical experience. Radiology 206:109, 1998
91. Kelhoffer ER, Osborn IP: The gastroenterology suite and TIPS. Int Anesthesiol Clin 41:51, 2003
92. Thompson JW, Weiner RD, Myers CP: Use of ECT in the United States in 1975, 1980, and 1986. Am J Psychiatry 151:1657, 1994
93. Ding Z, White PF: Anesthesia for electroconvulsive therapy. Anesth Analg 94:1351, 2002
94. American Psychiatric Association: The Practice of Electroconvulsive Therapy: Recommendations for Treatment, Training and Privileging. Washington, DC, American Psychiatric Press, 2000
95. Folk JW, Kellner CH, Beale MD *et al*: Anesthesia for electroconvulsive therapy: A review. J ECT 16:157, 2000
96. Avramov MN, Husain MM, White PF: The comparative effects of methohexital, propofol, and etomidate for electroconvulsive therapy. Anesth Analg 81:596, 1995
97. Datto C, Rai AK, Ilivicky HJ, Caroff SN: Augmentation of seizure induction in electroconvulsive therapy: A clinical reappraisal. J ECT 18:118, 2002
98. Fredman B, d'Etienne J, Smith I *et al*: Anesthesia for electroconvulsive therapy: Effects of propofol and methohexital on seizure activity and recovery. Anesth Analg 79:75, 1994
99. Fear CF, Littlejohns CS, Rouse E, McQuail P: Propofol anaesthesia in electroconvulsive therapy. Reduced seizure duration may not be relevant. Br J Psychiatry 165:506, 1994
100. Nguyen TT, Chhibber AK, Lustik SJ *et al*: Effect of methohexitone and propofol with or without alfentanil on seizure duration and recovery in electroconvulsive therapy. Br J Anaesth 79:801, 1997
101. Smith DL, Angst MS, Brock-Utne JG, DeBattista C: Seizure duration with remifentanil/methohexital vs. methohexital alone in middle-aged patients undergoing electroconvulsive therapy. Acta Anaesthesiol Scand 47:1064, 2003
102. Nishihara F, Ohkawa M, Hiraoka H *et al*: Benefits of the laryngeal mask for airway management during electroconvulsive therapy. J ECT 19:211, 2003
103. Weinger MB, Partridge BL, Hauger R, Mirow A: Prevention of the cardiovascular and neuroendocrine response to electroconvulsive therapy: I. Effectiveness of pretreatment regimens on hemodynamics. Anesth Analg 73:556, 1991

104. Butler MG, Hayes BG, Hathaway MM, Begleiter ML: Specific genetic diseases at risk for sedation/anesthesia complications. Anesth Analg 91:837, 2000
105. Bergman SA: Ketamine: Review of its pharmacology and its use in pediatric anesthesia. Anesth Prog 46:10, 1999
106. Todd DW: A comparison of endotracheal intubation and use of the laryngeal mask airway for ambulatory oral surgery patients. J Oral Maxillofac Surg 60:2, 2002
107. Dolling S, Anders NR, Rolfe SE: A comparison of deep vs. awake removal of the laryngeal mask airway in paediatric dental day-case surgery. A randomised controlled trial. Anaesthesia 58:1224, 2003
108. Enever GR, Nunn JH, Sheehan JK: A comparison of post-operative morbidity following outpatient dental care under general anaesthesia in paediatric patients with and without disabilities. Int J Paediatr Dent 10:120, 2000

CHAPTER 52 ■ OFFICE-BASED ANESTHESIA

LAURENCE M. HAUSMAN AND MEG A. ROSENBLATT

KEY POINTS

1. Prior to administering an anesthetic, the anesthesiologist must determine whether a patient and procedure are appropriate for an office-based setting.
2. Both the surgeon and the anesthesiologist must be appropriately trained and have the proper credentials.
3. Continued medical education, peer review, and performance improvement are critical to the office-based practitioner.
4. An office must be properly designed, constructed, equipped, and staffed to house an office-based anesthetic.
5. All American Society of Anesthesiologists (ASA) standards for preoperative evaluation, and intraoperative and postoperative care and monitoring, must be applied to the office-based practice.
6. Several major organizations currently accredit office-based practices.
7. Many states have laws and regulations in place regarding an office-based anesthetic. The practitioner must be knowledgeable regarding the laws in his or her state of practice.
8. An office-based anesthetic can range from monitored anesthesia care to regional and/or general anesthesia.
9. Anesthetics used should be short acting and have a high safety profile.

Office-based anesthesia (OBA) has become an intrinsic and vital part of our specialty. An office-based anesthetic is one that is performed in a location, such as an office or procedure room, that is not accredited by a state agency as an ambulatory surgery center (ASC) and may, in some states, have no accreditation. In addition, the office must also house nonsurgical activities such as patient consultation and practice administration.

During the 1970s, less than 10% of all surgical and/or diagnostic procedures were performed on an ambulatory basis, and virtually all these were performed in hospitals. In 1987, approximately 25 million procedures, or 40% of all procedures, were performed on an ambulatory basis. In the United States between 1984 and 1990, the number of office-based procedures increased from 400,000 to 1.2 million, and by 1994, 8.5% of all procedures were performed in offices.[1] In the same year, a survey of the membership of the American Society of Plastic Surgeons (ASPS) revealed that 55% of the respondents performed the majority or all their procedures in an office.[2] By the year 2000, approximately 75% of all procedures were performed on an outpatient basis; 17% in freestanding ASCs, and 14 to 25% (approximately 8 to 10 million) in physicians' offices.[3–5] It is estimated that by 2005 approximately 82% of all procedures will be outpatient and, of these, 24% will be office based.[3,6]

Although an OBA practice may be an exciting alternative to the traditional hospital-based one, it requires the anesthesiologist to expand his or her role. Along with providing safe anesthetics across the spectrum of healthy to medically challenged patients undergoing increasingly complex procedures, the anesthesiologist must understand office safety and policy, as well as legal and financial issues such as billing and collection.[5,7]

ADVANTAGES AND DISADVANTAGES

There are several advantages to an office-based procedure when compared with a traditional hospital-based one, the most obvious being cost containment. Several components comprise the cost of a given procedure. In addition to surgical and anesthesia fees, which are usually negotiated prior to an elective procedure, there is a facility fee. This fee covers the associated costs to the office, including equipment and staff, and often constitutes a large component of the patient's overall charge. In an office, this amount is easily predicted and frequently minimized, whereas in a hospital, because of greater overhead costs, it can be both enormous and unpredictable.[3,4,8,9] In 1994, Schultz determined the cost of a laparoscopic inguinal hernia repair, when done in a hospital, to be $5,494.00. When the same procedure was performed in an office, the price decreased to $1,533.84. Similarly, the average cost of an in-hospital open inguinal hernia repair was $2,237.00, whereas the same procedure performed in a private office cost only $894.79.[9] It has been reported that office-based ocular surgery performed under monitored anesthesia care (MAC) can cost 70% less than similar procedures performed in a hospital.[10] Some insurance companies now offer incentives to surgeons who use an office as their surgical venue.[11] Other advantages of office-based procedures over ASCs or traditional hospital-based settings include ease of scheduling, patient and surgeon convenience, a decrease in patient exposure to nosocomial infections, and improved patient privacy and continuity of care because an office is usually staffed by a small and consistent group of personnel.[4,5,7,12,13]

There are potential disadvantages to office-based surgery. These usually relate to issues regarding patient safety and peer review. In most states, no regulations exist regarding certification for the surgeon or anesthesiologist's capabilities, the surgical office's peer review policy, documentation, policies and procedures, and reporting of adverse outcomes. These issues must be considered before selecting an office facility in which to deliver anesthetic care.

OFFICE SAFETY

The earliest questions regarding the safety of office-based procedures were raised by media reports and newspaper articles.[7,14,15] An examination of the data reveals that injuries and deaths occurring in offices are often multifactorial in their causation. Reasons include overdosages of local anesthetics, prolonged surgery with occult blood loss, accumulation of multiple anesthetics, hypovolemia, hypoxemia, and the use of reversal drugs with short half-lives.[14] Both the Anesthesia Patient Safety Foundation and the American Society of Anesthesiologists (ASA) have emerged as leaders in the field of OBA safety and have advocated that the quality of care in an office-based practice be no less than that of a hospital or ASC.[16,17] Thus, it is imperative to ensure all safety precautions one may take for granted in a hospital are present in the surgical office.[14]

In 1990, the mortality rate from anesthesia was approximately 1/10,000. By the year 2000, the rate had decreased to 1/250,000 in hospitals and 1/400,000 in freestanding ASCs.[5,14,18] This can be attributed, in part, to improvements in the training of the anesthesia providers, the safety profiles of the newer anesthetics, and intrinsic safety mechanisms in place within the anesthetizing location. Because the majority of office-based patients are young and healthy, one would expect that an anesthetic performed in an office would be at least equally as safe as an anesthetic performed in a hospital. However, reports of morbidity and mortality within office-based practices vary dramatically. In 1997, Morello et al conducted a survey querying 418 accredited plastic surgeons' offices.[19] They had a 57% response rate and found that, during a 5-year period, 400,675 office procedures were conducted—63.2% cosmetic and 36.8% reconstructive. Several outcomes were reviewed including hemorrhage, hypertension, hypotension, wound infection, need for hospital admission, and reoperation. There was an overall complication rate of 0.24%, and seven deaths occurred. The causes of mortality were both surgery and anesthesia related. They included two cases of myocardial infarction (one following an augmentation mammoplasty, the other one 4 hours after a rhinoplasty), one case of cerebral hypoxia during an abdominoplasty, a tension pneumothorax during a breast augmentation, a cardiac arrest during carpal tunnel surgery, a stroke 3 days following a rhytidectomy and brow lift, and one unexplained death.[19] This represents an overall mortality rate of 1 in 57,000. A report by Hoefflin et al found no complications after 23,000 procedures that occurred in an office under general anesthesia.[20] Similarly, Sullivan et al[21] retrospectively reviewed the results in an office performing more than 5,000 surgical procedures by five independent surgeons. The anesthesia during this time period consisted of deep sedation in conjunction with local anesthesia or regional block, and was performed by an anesthesiologist supervising a certified registered nurse anesthetist (CRNA). No mortalities occurred during the 5-year period. Bitar et al[22] retrospectively studied adverse outcomes in 3,615 consecutive patients undergoing 4,778 procedures in offices between 1995 and 2000, employing MAC with midazolam, propofol, and an opioid. During this time period, no deaths were reported. Dyspnea occurred in 0.05% of patients, and nausea and vomiting occurred in 0.2%. There was a 0.05% rate of hospital admissions.

Other data reveal a significant risk associated with an office-based procedure. Rao et al reported that, according to closed malpractice claims in Florida, 830 deaths and 4,000 injuries were associated with OBA between 1990 and 1999. These claims accounted for 30% of all malpractice claims in that state.[23] In a hospital operating room, the risks of an anesthetic are usually limited to the underlying medical condition of the patient, whereas in an office they may be increased because of factors such as inadequate standards and safeguards.[14] The challenge of acquiring accurate morbidity and mortality data for OBA is complicated by the fact that many offices are not required to report adverse events. In addition, although an anesthesiologist may not even be administering the anesthetic in an office, many complications may still be reported as anesthetic related.[24]

Traditional credentialing procedures, such as board certification and the granting or renewing of hospital privileges based on proficiency and proof of continuing medical education, may not be required in an office.[18] Within and among offices, health care providers of anesthesia may have varying degrees of education and expertise. The provider may be an anesthesiologist, a nurse anesthetist, a dental anesthetist, or a surgeon with little or no training in anesthesia.[25] Furthermore, safety within an anesthetizing location depends on the patient monitoring capabilities that have become the standard of care within hospital operating rooms.[22] There are reported cases of injuries to patients in offices resulting from obsolete and malfunctioning anesthesia machines, as well as resulting from alarms that have not been serviced and/or are not functioning properly.[4] The ASA has created guidelines for defining obsolete anesthesia machines. These guidelines prohibit the use of any anesthesia machine that lacks essential safety features (e.g., oxygen ratio device, oxygen pressure failure alarm), has the presence of unacceptable features (e.g., copper kettles, vaporizers with rotary concentration dials that increase vapor concentration when the dial is turned clockwise), or for which routine maintenance is no longer possible.[26]

A review of ASA Closed Claims Project data reveals safety concerns in office-based practices are more than theoretical.[18] The Closed Claims database incorporates information from 35 liability insurers, which in turn indemnify approximately 50% of the practicing anesthesiologists in the United States. As of 2001, in the Closed Claims Project database there were 753 (13.7%) claims for ambulatory procedures and 14 (0.26%) for office-based ones. This small number of claims is most likely due to the 3- to 5-year time lag in reporting to the Closed Claims Project database.[18] ASA physical status 1 or 2 females who had undergone elective surgery under general anesthesia comprise the majority of claims filed. This statistic parallels the profiles of trends seen in operating rooms and freestanding ASCs. The injuries that occur in offices tend to be of greater severity than those that occur in ASCs. Twenty-one percent of the reported injuries sustained in offices were temporary and nondisabling in nature, and 64% were permanent or led to death, whereas 62% of the injuries sustained in ASCs were temporary and nondisabling, and only 21% were permanent or led to death.[18] A study by Coté et al revealed that the causes for injuries in an office ranged from human error to machine and equipment malfunction (Table 52-1).[27,28]

According to the Closed Claims Project database, injuries during office-based procedures occur throughout the

TABLE 52-1

CAUSES OF INJURY IN THE OFFICE-BASED PRACTICE

Inadequate resuscitation equipment
Inadequate monitoring
- Most commonly no pulse oximetry

Inadequate preoperative or postoperative evaluation
Human error
- Slow recognition of an event
- Slow response to an event
- Lack of experience
- Drug overdosage

Data from Coté CJ, Karl HW, Notterman DA, *et al*: Adverse sedation events in pediatrics: Analysis of medications used for sedation. Pediatrics 106:633, 2000; Coté CJ, Notterman DA, Karl HW, *et al*: Adverse sedation events in pediatrics: A critical incident analysis of contributing factors. Pediatrics 105:805, 2000.

perioperative period and are multifactorial in etiology. The majority, 64%, occurred intraoperatively, whereas 14% occurred in the postanesthesia care unit (PACU) and 21% after discharge.[18] Many of these adverse events (50%) were respiratory in nature and included airway obstruction, bronchospasm, inadequate oxygenation and ventilation, and unrecognized esophageal intubation. The second most common events were drug related, occurring 25% of the time. These events included incorrect agent or dosage, allergy, and malignant hyperthermia. Cardiovascular injuries and equipment-related injuries each occurred in 8% of incidents.[18]

An important point to consider when looking at adverse events is whether they were preventable. Thirteen percent of the events that occurred in ASCs were considered to have been preventable, whereas 46% of the office-based events were deemed so. Furthermore, all the adverse respiratory events that occurred in the PACU of offices could have been prevented if pulse oximetry had been used. Care was considered to be substandard in 50% of OBA claims and in 34% of ASC ones. Claims originating from an office-based procedure resulted in a monetary award 92% of the time, with a median payment of $200,000 (ranging between $10,000 and $2,000,000), whereas claims originating from ASC-based procedures were compensated only 59% of the time with a median payout of $85,000 (ranging between $34 and $14,700,000).[18]

The question of how to make an office-based practice safe has become critical. After several highly publicized office liposuction injuries and deaths in August 2000, the State of Florida attempted to address this problem by placing a 90-day moratorium on all office-based procedures that used anesthetic depths greater than conscious sedation. During that time period, a safety panel that comprised surgeons, anesthesiologists, and other health care professionals was formed and charged with the task of developing recommendations to improve the safety record of office-based procedures. The panel's recommendations concern factors such as patient selection, preoperative evaluation and testing, procedures to be excluded, surgeon qualification, and facility standards.[13,29] Other major organizations that have played a leading role in developing standards for the office-based practitioner include the ASA, the ASPS, the American Association of Nurse Anesthetists, and the American Medical Association.[13,16,25,29–31]

PATIENT SELECTION

1 Prior to presenting for an office-based procedure, the patient must be medically optimized. The patient should have a preoperative history and physical examination recorded within 30 days, all pertinent laboratory tests, and any medically indicated specialist consultation(s). Consent for the procedure and the anesthetic must be in the chart. The anesthesiologist should have access to all this information preoperatively, and when possible, he or she should contact the patient prior to the scheduled procedure. If a patient is an ASA physical status 1 or 2, the surgeon's office should arrange the surgery as per office protocol. However, if a patient has significant comorbid conditions, a preoperative anesthesiology consultation should be obtained before scheduling the patient for surgery.

Patient selection remains a controversial topic among practicing office-based anesthesiologists because little morbidity and mortality data exist to support the inclusion or exclusion of specific patient populations. A study by Meridy in 1982 concluded that patients should not be excluded from undergoing ambulatory procedures based solely on their age, the type of procedure, or the duration of the planned procedure.[32] Similar data are yet to exist regarding office-based practices; however, some recommendations have been made. The ASPS has acknowledged that the ideal patient for an office-based procedure has an ASA physical status of 1 or 2. They recommended that ASA physical status 3 patients undergo an office procedure only after an anesthesia consultation, and patients assigned an ASA physical status greater than 3 should only have an office-based procedure performed under local anesthesia without sedation.[13] The ASA also has developed recommendations regarding patient selection.[33] When determining whether a patient is suitable for OBA it is important to realize that the location is often remote, and the anesthesiologist may be unable to get assistance if required. Anticipated anesthetic problems must be avoided (Table 52-2). Individual anesthesiologists should therefore consider excluding certain patients with significant comorbid conditions to avoid unanticipated problems.[14,34]

The morbidly obese patient and patients with obstructive sleep apnea syndrome (OSAS) present unique and increasingly frequent challenges to the office-based practitioner. Indeed, they are usually the same population, with estimates of 60 to 90% of all OSAS patients being obese (body mass index greater than or equal to 0.30).[35–37] Confounding this problem is that the majority of the patients with OSAS have not been formally diagnosed.[38,39] These patients are likely to present major anesthetic problems throughout the perioperative period.[40] There may be failure to intubate the trachea or ventilate the lungs, or they may have respiratory distress soon after tracheal extubation or suffer from respiratory

TABLE 52-2

COMORBIDITIES THAT CAN PRECLUDE PATIENTS BEING GOOD CANDIDATES FOR AN OFFICE-BASED PROCEDURE

Expected significant blood loss or postoperative pain
History of substance abuse
Seizure disorder
Malignant hyperthermia susceptibility
Potential difficult airway
- Morbid obesity
- Obstructive sleep apnea syndrome

NPO less than 8 hours
No escort
Previous adverse outcome from anesthesia
Significant drug allergies
Pulmonary aspiration risk

NPO, nothing by mouth.

arrest with preoperative sedation or postoperative analgesia.[35] These patients tend to be exquisitely sensitive to the respiratory depressant effects of even small dosages of sedation or analgesics.[37,40,41] Furthermore, respiratory depression may not be reversible with pharmacologic antagonism.[42] One of the first steps in the ASA algorithm for management of the difficult airway is to call for help. In an office, there is usually little or no help available. It has been recommended that an observational unit with close monitoring of oxygen saturation or an intensive care unit setting be used for monitoring the OSAS patient postoperatively.[43] It has also been suggested that outpatient facilities develop specific policies regarding acceptable patients for the outpatient setting, possibly excluding patients with OSAS.[38]

As office-based surgery continues to gain popularity, more subspecialty physicians will begin to perform office-based procedures and older, sicker patients will present for anesthesia. The anesthesiologist must be the patient's advocate in the matter of safety.

SURGEON SELECTION

The relationship between the surgeon and anesthesiologist must be one of mutual trust and understanding. Because the surgeon performing the procedure may also own the office, he or she must not pressure the anesthesiologist to perform an anesthetic if the anesthesiologist believes the patient or procedure is not appropriate for the office-based setting.

The surgeon must have a valid medical license and Drug
2 Enforcement Administration (DEA) number. He or she should be either board eligible or board certified by a recognized member of the American Board of Medical Specialties,[29] and either have privileges to perform the proposed procedure in a local hospital or have training and documented proficiency comparable to a practitioner who does have such privileges. Although this may sound intuitive, there have been cases reported of surgeons performing procedures for which they have little or no training.[4] In addition, the surgeon must have adequate liability insurance, at least equal to that carried by the anesthesiologist. If a lawsuit should arise and the surgeon is inadequately insured, the anesthesiologist may be held financially responsible and become the "deep pocket." Similarly, the facility itself should have adequate liability insurance.

In addition, there should be a system in place for monitoring continuing medical education, as well as peer review and performance improvement, for both the surgeon and anesthesiologist: this is often missing in the office-based practice.[4] If an anesthesia group provides care at more than one office, an overall peer review may be used; however, it does not need to be specific to each office. Solo anesthesia practitioners should not be exempt from this process. They need to align themselves with the offices in which they provide services and either participate in the office's process or help organize an ongoing one. The peer review committee should include surgeons, anesthesiologists, and nursing staff. It should meet regularly and maintain a written record of minutes and recommendations. Similarly, continuing medical education should also be documented and, at a minimum, should be sufficient to meet relicensing requirements.

3 When formulating a quality assurance program, there should be certain sentinel events that trigger a case review (Table 52-3). It is imperative that this review be an open forum to ensure continued quality improvement of care, and not be biased or hindered by fear of litigation. Legal counsel should be sought to determine whether information disclosed at these meetings is discoverable in a court of law if a malpractice claim should arise.

TABLE 52-3

SENTINEL EVENTS THAT SHOULD TRIGGER A CHART REVIEW AND BE PRESENTED AT A PERFORMANCE IMPROVEMENT/QUALITY ASSURANCE MEETING

- Dental injury
- Corneal abrasion
- Perioperative myocardial infarction or stroke
- Pulmonary aspiration
- Reintubation of the trachea
- Return to the operating room
- Peripheral nerve injury
- Adverse drug reaction
- Uncontrolled pain or nausea and vomiting
- Unexpected hospital admission
- Cardiac arrest
- Death
- Incomplete charts
- Controlled substance discrepancy
- Patient complaints

OFFICE SELECTION

4 The anesthesiologist should ensure patients are anesthetized only in a safe location.[25] The office needs to be appropriately equipped and stocked to perform a general anesthetic (Table 52-4). All supplies must be age and size appropriate for the patient population. If an anesthesia machine or ventilator is present, it must be up to date, and regularly maintained and calibrated. If potent inhaled volatile agents or N_2O are used, there must be a functioning waste gas scavenging system. This waste gas system may be exhausted via a window or roof vent. The exhaust must not be vented back into the office or into any other inhabited space and be in accordance with Occupational Safety and Health Administration standards. Air testing

TABLE 52-4

EQUIPMENT REQUIRED FOR SAFE DELIVERY OF OFFICE-BASED ANESTHESIA

- Monitors
  - Noninvasive blood pressure with an assortment of cuff sizes
  - Heart rate/electrocardiogram
  - Pulse oximeter
  - Temperature
- Airway supplies
  - Nasal cannulas
  - Oral airways
  - Facemasks
  - Self-inflating bag-mask ventilation device
  - Laryngoscopes multiple sizes and styles
  - Various sizes of tracheal tubes
  - Intubating stylettes
  - Emergency airway equipment (laryngeal mask airways, cricothyrotomy kit, transtracheal jet ventilation)
- Suction catheters and suction equipment
- Cardiac defibrillator
- Emergency drugs
  - Advanced cardiac life support drugs
  - Dantrolene and malignant hyperthermia supplies
- Anesthetic drugs
- Vascular cannulation equipment

should also be done on a regular basis. In an office without an exhaust system for waste gases, total intravenous anesthesia techniques should be considered. Similarly, all medical and hazardous waste must be disposed of in accordance with state and local laws.

All offices, especially those without ventilators or anesthesia machines, require a method to deliver positive-pressure ventilation to the patient's lungs. This can be achieved using a self-inflating resuscitation device. An adequate supply of compressed oxygen must be present, as well as a backup supply for use in an emergency. In offices that do not have a pipeline supply of oxygen, H cylinders are usually used, with several E cylinders kept in reserve. A policy must be in place describing the transport and storage of gases, consistent with state and local laws. All equipment described in the ASA algorithm for management of the difficult airway should be present.[44] An available means to create an emergency surgical airway and jet ventilation capability may be lifesaving.

Perioperative monitoring must adhere to the ASA standards
5 for basic anesthetic monitoring.[45,46] These include continuous monitoring of heart rate and oxygen saturation, intermittent noninvasive blood pressure monitoring, and the capacity for both temperature and continuous electrocardiogram monitoring. In addition, there must exist a way to monitor respiration either by rate, auscultation, or end-tidal CO_2 ($ETCO_2$). $ETCO_2$ must be monitored in all cases of general anesthesia. Monitors must be routinely serviced, calibrated, and repaired as necessary.

All emergency drugs appearing on the American Heart Association advanced cardiac life support (ACLS) protocol should be available. The expiration dates for these agents should be checked on a regular basis, and outdated drugs replaced. A cardiac defibrillator should also be immediately available and routinely checked, as should a source of suction, including a pharyngeal suction catheter. The office-based anesthesiologist should be prepared to begin the initial treatment of malignant hyperthermia (MH), which requires having at least 12 bottles of dantrolene. A complete listing of MH supplies is available via the Internet at www.mhaus.org.

A protocol for the delivery and secure storage of controlled substances must be in place. A licensed anesthesiologist may supply these drugs in accordance with DEA regulations, as may any licensed physician with a current DEA registration certificate. Instead of transporting drugs, it is often more convenient to store them in the surgeon's office. In this situation, they must be stored in a double-locked storage cabinet, installed in a secure location. Drug accounting must be performed in accordance with state and federal regulations. Individual states have different provisions and regulations regarding the dispensing of controlled substances, and it is the responsibility of the dispensing physician to ensure the office-based practice is in compliance.

A medical director responsible for overall operations should be identified for every office. There must also be a policy and procedures manual that outlines the responsibilities of each staff member, including nurses (circulating/scrub and postop), physician assistants, surgical technicians, and office administrators. The manual should include a description of the infection control policy. All nurses should be licensed by the state and have training and education consistent with their responsibilities. Basic life support certification should be mandatory, and ACLS certification is preferable. In addition, either the anesthesiologist or the physician who supervises the anesthesia care provider must be ACLS or pediatric advanced life support certified, depending on the patient population.

Emergencies can, and do, occur in an office-based setting (Table 52-5). Each office must have a plan in place delineating the responsibilities of each staff member, in the event of such an occurrence. The physical structure of the office is an important consideration. There should be a clear egress that would easily accommodate a stretcher carrying a mechanically ventilated patient. Adequate clearance and room for transport in an elevator must also be considered.

TABLE 52-5

EMERGENCIES THAT MAY OCCUR WITHIN AN OFFICE THAT REQUIRE CONTINGENCY PLANS

Fire
Bomb/bomb threat
Power loss
Equipment malfunction
Loss of oxygen supply pressure
Cardiac or respiratory arrest in the waiting room, operating room, or postanesthesia care unit
Earthquake
Hurricane
External disturbance such as a riot
Malignant hyperthermia
Massive blood loss
Emergency transfer of patient to a hospital

Destinations for a patient in need of hospital admission must be identified. Developing this type of relationship is challenging because hospitals may be reluctant to be involved in office mishaps. However, it is of utmost importance to have a formal written arrangement with a nearby hospital. Telephoning the emergency services number (911) is an acceptable plan for transportation, provided the response time is rapid. If emergency resuscitation personnel are unavailable in a specific city or the response time is slow, the office should have a contractual agreement with an ambulance company.

Ideally, a 1-hour firewall should be in place to provide enough time to awaken and escort a patient to safety in the event of a fire. If a 1-hour firewall is not present, the office should, at a minimum, be in compliance with local fire codes. In addition, the office must be in compliance with commercial construction codes and with maximum occupancy regulations.

There must be contingency plans in the event of a power supply interruption or electrical failure. Each office should have an emergency generator capable of running necessary equipment and monitors; monitors should have battery backup power that is routinely checked. Battery reserve power will usually last for 1.5 hours, but this needs to be verified for each piece of electrically powered equipment.

The office should keep patient records (including anesthesia record) in accordance with local laws, which is usually for a minimum of 5 years. Similarly, the anesthesiologist should maintain his or her own records, which include the preanesthesia history and physical, informed consent, intraoperative documentation, and postoperative care record, as well as discharge orders.

Accreditation

6 One way to objectively evaluate an office is to have it accredited by a nationally recognized agency. The ASA has developed a classification of offices that stratifies them by the level of anesthetic depth that may be offered (Table 52-6).[33] Presently, several states require offices to be accredited, and more are following suit. In states that do not require accreditation of an office, there are benefits to voluntarily obtaining it. Often, this accreditation will allow the facility fee to be reimbursed by a third-party payer in medically necessary procedures.[47] In addition, the patient may be more comfortable undergoing a

TABLE 52-6

AMERICAN SOCIETY OF ANESTHESIOLOGISTS CLASSIFICATION OF SURGICAL OFFICES ACCORDING TO THE ANESTHESIA AND SURGICAL PROCEDURES PERFORMED

- Class A
  - Minor surgical procedures
  - Local, topical, or infiltration of local anesthetic
  - No sedation preoperatively or intraoperatively
- Class B
  - Minor or major surgical procedures
  - Sedation via oral, rectal, or intravenous sedation
  - Analgesic or dissociative drugs
- Class C
  - Minor or major surgical procedures
  - General anesthesia
  - Major conduction block anesthesia

Adapted from ASA Committee on Ambulatory Surgical Care and ASA Task Force on Office-Based Anesthesia: Office-based anesthesia: Considerations for anesthesiologists in setting up and maintaining a safe office anesthesia environment. Available at: http://www.asahq.org/publicationsAndServices/office.pdf. Accessed March 28, 2005.

TABLE 52-7

FACTORS CONSIDERED BY ACCREDITING AGENCIES BEFORE ACCREDITING AN OFFICE

- Physical layout of the office
- Environmental safety and infection control
- Patient and personnel records
- Surgeon qualification
  - Training
  - Local hospital privileges (surgical and admission)
- Office administration
- Anesthesiologist requirements
- Staffing intraoperatively and postoperatively
- Monitoring capabilities, both intraoperatively and postoperatively
- Ancillary care
- Equipment
- Drugs (emergency, controlled substances, routine medications)
- Basic life support and/or advanced cardiac life support/pediatric advanced life support certification
- Temperature
- Neuromuscular functioning
- Patient positioning
- Preanesthesia and postanesthesia care and documentation
- Quality assurance/peer review
- Liability insurance
- Postanesthesia care unit evaluation
- Discharge evaluation
- Emergency procedure (e.g., fire/admission/transfer)

A complete listing of criteria can be obtained from the individual agencies.

procedure in an office that has been accredited. Finally, as more states require accreditation, if a surgeon's office proactively becomes accredited in a state that subsequently requires it, there would be no interruption of services.[7]

Currently, there are three major accrediting bodies for office-based surgery offices, although several other agencies are also recognized. The Accreditation Association for Ambulatory Health Care (AAAHC) was the first major accrediting body, offering certification since 1998. The American Association for Accreditation of Ambulatory Surgical Facilities (AAAASF), originally the Accreditation Association for Ambulatory Plastic Surgical Facilities (AAAPSF), was the second, followed by the Joint Commission for Accreditation of Healthcare Organizations (JCAHO). To date, the most active organization is the AAAASF. Its requirements are simpler than those of AAAHC and JCAHO, and accreditation is less expensive; however, changes are underway to allow AAAHC and JCAHO to be more competitive.[7] Each agency has different criteria for eligibility and different accreditation cycles pertaining to the time limit of a certificate.[48] The agencies deal with issues ranging from office design to patient positioning (Table 52-7). In addition, the AAAHC can accredit not only the surgical office, but also an anesthesia group that provides OBA.

The accrediting agencies were developed, in part, to re-
7 duce some of the variability that exists among offices in regard to safety issues. Several professional societies are encouraging their members to perform procedures only in accredited facilities. The Society for Aesthetic Plastic Surgeons mandates that all its members perform procedures only in offices that have either been accredited by one of the nationally recognized accrediting agencies, have been certified to participate in the Medicare program under Title XVIII, or are licensed by the state. The actual improvement in safety conferred by performing surgery in an accredited office has yet to be determined, and there are those who suggest that it provides no advantage.[19,49] As long as there is no mandatory reporting system in place, it will be impossible to determine true morbidity rates associated with an office-based practice. Clearly, safety in an office depends on more than just accreditation; there must be constant vigilance by all members of the health care team.

PROCEDURE SELECTION

Early in the development of office-based surgery, procedures were generally noninvasive and of short duration. However, as newer surgical and anesthetic techniques have evolved, longer and more invasive procedures have been successfully performed.[25,50–56] Suitable office-based procedures range from incision and drainage of abscesses to microlaparoscopies. There are few data regarding procedure length and suitability for an office; however, the ASPS has recommended that procedures not exceed 6 hours in duration and be completed by 3 PM to allow for recovery time.[29] In addition, when determining the suitability of a procedure one must consider the possibility of hypothermia, blood loss, or significant fluid shifts.[29]

Specific Procedures

Liposuction

Liposuction is the most commonly performed plastic surgery procedure and is performed primarily by plastic surgeons and dermatologists.[57] Liposuction is accomplished by inserting hollow rods into small incisions in the skin and suctioning subcutaneous fat into an aspiration canister. Superwet and tumescent techniques, introduced in the mid-1980s, use large volumes (1 to 4 cc) of infiltrate solution for each 1 cc of fat to be removed. This infiltrate solution consists of 0.9% saline or Ringer's lactate with epinephrine 1:1,000,000 and lidocaine 0.025 to 0.1%. Blood loss is generally 1% of the aspirate with these techniques.[58] The peak serum levels of lidocaine occur 12 to 14 hours after injection and decline over the subsequent 6 to 14 hours.[59,60] Although the maximum dose of lidocaine has been traditionally limited to 7mg/kg, 35 to 55 mg/kg doses have been used safely because the tumescent technique results in a single compartment clearance similar to that of a sustained-release medication.[60,61]

Liposuction is not a benign procedure. In 2000, a census survey of the 1,200 members of the American Society of Aesthetic Plastic Surgeons (ASAPS) revealed an overall mortality rate of 19.1 per 100,000 liposuction procedures, with pulmonary embolism the diagnosis in 23.1% of deaths. Other causes of mortality included abdominal viscus perforation, anesthesia "causes," fat embolism, infection, and hemorrhage; 28.5% of all deaths in this study were reported as unknown or confidential.[62] Risk factors identified included the use of multiliter wetting solution infiltration, large volume aspiration causing massive third spacing, multiple concurrent procedures, anesthetic sedative effects yielding hypoventilation, and permissive discharge policies. The management of the postoperative period, with attention to fluid and electrolyte balance and pain control, is critical to an optimal outcome after liposuction. Generally, it is recommended that an office liposuction be limited to 5,000 mL of total aspirant, which includes supernatant fat and fluid.[29]

Iverson et al developed the following considerations and recommendations regarding office-based liposuction:[13,29]

1. Plastic surgeons should follow the current ASA Guidelines for Sedation and Analgesia.
2. General anesthesia can be used safely in the office setting.
3. General anesthesia has advantages for more complex liposuction procedures that include precise dosing, controlled patient movement, and airway management.
4. Epidural and spinal anesthesia in the office setting is discouraged because of the possibility of vasodilatation, hypotension, and fluid overload.
5. Moderate sedation/analgesia augments the patient's comfort and is an effective adjunct to the anesthetic infiltrate solutions.

Two hundred sixty-one respondents to a survey sent to the membership of The American Society for Dermatologic Surgery reported no mortalities among 66,570 liposuction procedures performed in hospitals, ASCs, and offices. The authors reported adverse events, which mirrored those in the ASAPS survey. They found that serious adverse events occurred more frequently with procedures performed in hospitals and ASCs than those in offices. This may be due to the fact that in hospitals liposuction is performed on sicker patients or that the procedures are associated with removal of a larger amount of fat. Interestingly, 71% of the offices surveyed were nonaccredited. Further, the authors reported that morbidity correlated better with the area of the body suctioned (abdomen and buttocks), than the facility in which the procedure took place.[63]

Aesthetics

Many facial aesthetic procedures such as blepharoplasty, rhinoplasty, and meloplasty are routinely performed in the office, usually under varying depths of MAC, but occasionally under general anesthesia. Facial plastic procedures that require use of a laser, such as facial resurfacing, pose a problem for the anesthesiologist. The use of supplemental nasal oxygen to maintain adequate Spo_2 in patients receiving sedation is a potential fire hazard. Any supplemental oxygen must be turned off during periods of laser or electrocautery use about the face, and this requires vigilance by the anesthesiologist who must be in constant communication with the surgeon. Methods for delivering supplemental oxygen to a patient having a facial procedure include nasal cannula, an oxygen hood, or placement of an oxygen cannula in an oral airway. The latter usually requires a deeper level of sedation.

Breast

Procedures such as breast biopsy or augmentation, implant exchanges, and completion of transverse rectus abdominal muscle flaps are performed in office settings. Breast augmentation entails separating the pectoralis muscles from the chest wall, which is painful and usually requires general anesthesia. This can be accomplished by using either a laryngeal mask airway or tracheal tube. It is likely that patients undergoing breast surgery will require antiemetic medication and postoperative analgesics.[64]

Gastrointestinal Endoscopy

Procedures performed by gastroenterologists include esophageal, gastric, and duodenal endoscopies and colonoscopies. This patient population tends to be older, with significant comorbid conditions. Upper gastrointestinal (GI) procedures rarely require endotracheal intubation because, although many of these patients have gastroesophageal reflux, the stomach is emptied under direct visualization. The endoscopist does require patient participation to aid in insertion of the endoscope, which can usually be accomplished with sedation using midazolam and small doses of propofol.

Colonoscopy is painful secondary to the insertion and manipulation of the endoscope, and may be associated with cardiovascular effects, including dysrhythmias, bradycardia, hypotension, hypertension, myocardial infarction, and death. The mechanism of these cardiovascular effects is not known, but there is evidence that they may be mediated by the autonomic nervous system when stimulated by anxiety or discomfort.[65] Adding an opioid to midazolam during colonoscopy has been shown to improve patient tolerance of the procedure and decrease pain without increasing the frequency of respiratory events.[66] Interestingly, anesthetic techniques consisting of midazolam,[67] remifentanil/propofol, and fentanyl/propofol/midazolam[68] potentiate the low-frequency components of heart rate variability, which reflects sympathetic activation as seen on continuous electrocardiography, and may contribute to the number of cardiovascular events that occur during colonoscopy.

Dentistry and Oral and Maxillofacial Surgery

Nitrous oxide has been used for most of the world's office-based dental anesthetics since 1884, when Horace Wells, himself a dentist, had nitrous oxide administered for a wisdom tooth extraction by a colleague. It was Harry Langa, another dentist, who pioneered the concept of using lower concentrations of nitrous oxide in combination with local anesthetics. This idea of "relative analgesia" was the forbearer of "conscious sedation."[69]

The American Association of Oral and Maxillofacial Surgeons designed a prospective cohort study of patients who underwent oral and maxillofacial surgery (OMS) surgery between January and December 2001. Of the 34,191 patients included, 71.9% received deep sedation/general anesthetics, 15.5% conscious sedations, and 12.6% local anesthesia. The operating surgeon provided anesthesia services in 96% of cases, and anesthesia-specific hospitalization rate was 4 per 100,000, with no reported mortalities. This high level of safety is attributed to the use of pulse oximetry, blood pressure and ventilation monitoring, and administration of supplemental oxygen.[70] As anesthesiologists increase their presence in the dental/OMS arena, one can expect an increased utilization of nontraditional agents for procedures.

Orthopaedics and Podiatry

The orthopaedic office provides an excellent location for the anesthesiologist who practices regional anesthesia. Although knee arthroscopies can be performed with intra-articular local anesthesia and MAC, a three-in-one block of the lumbar plexus with bupivacaine or ropivacaine, supplementing the intra-articular local anesthetic in an arthroscopically assisted anterior cruciate ligament repair will provide long-acting postoperative analgesia. Brachial plexus (interscalene and axillary) regional anesthetics avoid airway manipulations in patients undergoing upper-extremity procedures, whereas ankle blocks or blocks of the sciatic nerve in the popliteal fossa provide anesthesia for operations on the lower extremity. All these blocks can be supplemented with short-acting anxiolytic agents.

Spinal anesthetics in the office-based setting must be of short duration, secondary to limited PACU space. Lidocaine, which provides reliable short-acting analgesia, may be associated with an increased risk of transient neurologic symptoms in the ambulatory patient population,[71] whereas using procaine-fentanyl spinals is associated with nausea and vomiting and pruritus.[72] When the neuraxial anesthetic wears off, issues of postoperative pain management arise; therefore, peripheral regional techniques or general anesthetics may be preferable in this arena.

Gynecology and Genitourinary

Many procedures, such as dilation and curettage, vasectomy, and cystoscopy, have been performed in offices for many years. More recently, there has been an increase in more invasive procedures such as minilaparoscopies, ovum retrieval, prostate biopsies, and lithotripsy, necessitating an anesthesiologist's expertise. A variety of anesthetic options are available for these procedures and the anesthetic choice depends on the surgeon, patient, and anesthesiologist's preferences.

Ophthalmology and Otolaryngology

Ophthalmologic procedures suitable for the office include cataract extraction, lacrimal duct probing, and ocular plastics. Topical anesthesia or periorbital and retrobulbar blocks are frequently used to provide analgesia. Supplemental sedation may be required. Otolaryngology procedures include endoscopic sinus surgery, turbinate resection, septoplasty, and myringotomy. Again, combinations of topical and regional nerve blocks with supplemental sedation are commonly employed, but occasionally general anesthesia is used.

Pediatrics

Although no minimum age requirement for a child to undergo an office-based anesthetic has been established, patients older than 6 months of age and ASA physical status 1 or 2 may be reasonable candidates.[73] Usual OBA pediatric cases are dental. Chloral hydrate with nitrous oxide is the anesthetic choice of many dentists. The use of these agents is associated with significant morbidity. Ross et al found that in children between the ages of 1 and 9 years, 70 mg/kg of chloral hydrate with 30% nitrous oxide resulted in hypoventilation in 94% of patients, which increased to 97% of patients when the chloral hydrate was combined with 50% nitrous oxide.[8] This is significant in view of the findings of Coté et al, who reviewed 95 adverse sedation-related events in pediatric patients. In the 93% of these cases that resulted in permanent neurologic injury or death, the anesthetic was delivered by either an oral surgeon, periodontist, or certified registered nurse anesthetist supervised by a dentist.[27,28]

There are increasing numbers of ophthalmologic (exam under anesthesia, lacrimal duct probing), otolaryngology (myringotomy), cast/dressing changes, and minor plastics procedures being performed on children in offices. The American Academy of Pediatrics, Section on Anesthesiology, has developed guidelines for the pediatric perioperative environment, which should be adhered to in the OBA setting[74] (Table 52-8).

TABLE 52-8

GUIDELINES FOR THE PEDIATRIC PERIOPERATIVE ANESTHESIA ENVIRONMENT

■ **PATIENT CARE FACILITY AND MEDICAL STAFF POLICIES**
Designation of operative procedures
Categorization of pediatric patients undergoing anesthesia
Annual minimal case volume to maintain clinical competence
■ **CLINICAL PRIVILEGES OF ANESTHESIOLOGISTS**
Regular privileges
Special clinical privileges
Pain management
■ **PATIENT CARE UNITS**
Preoperative evaluation and preparation units
Operating room
Anesthesiologists
Other health care providers involved in perioperative care
Clinical laboratory and radiologic services availability and capabilities
Pediatric anesthesia equipment and drugs, including resuscitation cart
Postanesthesia care unit
Nursing staff
Anesthesiologist and physician staff
Pediatric anesthesia equipment and drugs
■ **POSTOPERATIVE INTENSIVE CARE**

ANESTHETIC TECHNIQUES

The ASA recommends that anesthetics be provided or supervised by a fully licensed anesthesiologist.[33] If an anesthesiologist is directing anesthesia care, he or she must be immediately available throughout the entire perioperative period. Regulations in several states have questioned the need for this level of anesthesia training in the delivery of OBA. Some states allow for an anesthetic to be performed by a nonphysician anesthesia provider supervised by a licensed physician. In this situation, the supervising physician must be qualified to perform a preanesthetic focused history and physical examination, as well as be immediately available throughout the perioperative period. He or she must know how to handle anesthetic-related emergencies and complications. The supervising physician must be ACLS certified.

8 OBA may entail any type of anesthesia from MAC through regional and general anesthesia.[75] Anesthesia is, however, a continuum, and it is often impossible to predict how a patient will react. The ASA has developed definitions regarding depths of anesthesia (Table 52-9). The anesthesia provider or supervisor must be able to rescue a patient from a deeper level of anesthetic than is anticipated.

9 When formulating an anesthetic plan, one must consider that all agents and techniques used should be short acting, and the patient should be ready for discharge home soon after the completion of the procedure.[5,75] Furthermore, any agents used should have a high safety profile and be cost effective.[76] In choosing MAC over general anesthesia, one must not be under the false impression that MAC anesthesia is inherently safer than general anesthesia. In 1988, Cohen et al reviewed

TABLE 52-9

DEFINITIONS OF LEVELS OF SEDATION AND ANALGESIA BY THE AMERICAN SOCIETY OF ANESTHESIOLOGISTS

■ MINIMAL SEDATION (ANXIOLYSIS)
Drug-induced sedation Patient responds normally to verbal commands Cognitive and motor function may be impaired Ventilatory and cardiovascular function maintained normally
■ MODERATE SEDATION/ANALGESIA (CONSCIOUS SEDATION)
Drug-induced sedation Patient responds purposefully to verbal commands either alone or with light tactile stimulation Patient maintains a patent airway and spontaneous ventilation Cardiovascular function maintained
■ DEEP SEDATION/ANALGESIA
Drug-induced sedation Patient not easily aroused but can respond purposefully to repeated or painful stimulation Ventilatory function may be impaired, requiring assistance in maintaining a patent airway, and spontaneous ventilation may be inadequate Cardiovascular function usually maintained
■ GENERAL ANESTHESIA
Drug-induced loss of consciousness Patients not aroused by painful stimulation Ventilatory function often impaired; patient may require assistance in maintaining a patent airway Spontaneous ventilation and neuromuscular functioning may be impaired Positive-pressure ventilation often required Cardiovascular function may be impaired

Adapted from ASA 2001 Directory of Members, p 513. Park Ridge, IL: ASA, 2001.

TABLE 52-10

PATIENT INJURIES OCCUR DURING MONITORED ANESTHESIA CARE ACCORDING TO THE CLOSED CLAIMS PROJECT DATABASE

■ PATIENT INJURY	■ PERCENTAGE
Death	34%
Brain damage	19%
Nerve damage	7%
Eye damage	12%
Myocardial infarction	4%
Stroke	4%
Burn	4%
Emotional distress	4%
Aspiration	4%

Adapted from Domino KB: Trends in anesthesia litigation in the 1990's: Monitored anesthesia care claims. ASA Newsl 61:17, 1997.

the data from 100,000 anesthetics. They found that the group with the greatest number of mortalities had undergone procedures with MAC, whereas MAC constituted only 2% of all cases.[77] The complication rate related to MAC anesthetics is increasing as its use expands. The ASA Closed Claims Project database reveals that in the 1970s, MAC cases accounted for 1.6% of the claims; in the 1980s, 1.9%; and by the 1990s, 6%. The injuries sustained in patients receiving MAC ranged from emotional distress to death (Table 52-10). The percentage of claims resulting from mortality was identical for both MAC and general anesthesia cases. When injuries other than death occurred during MAC anesthetics, they were more likely to be permanent, whereas injuries occurring during general anesthetics were more frequently temporary.[78] MAC anesthetics also tend to lead to litigation. Suits were filed in 90% of the MAC claims, 65% were settled, 20% went to judgment, and 15% were discontinued. The range of payout was $2,000 to $6,300,000 with a median of $75,000.[78]

Anesthetic Agents

Intravenous sedation (propofol, barbiturates, midazolam, fentanyl, meperidine) is the most often used anesthetic technique in the OBA setting.[25] When selecting anesthetics for an office-based procedure, one must consider factors such as duration of action, cost effectiveness, and safety profile. The drugs should have a short half-life, be inexpensive, and not be associated with undesirable side effects such as nausea and vomiting. Remifentanil, when combined with propofol for conscious sedation, has been shown to provide discharge readiness within 15 minutes after colonoscopy, which is a marked reduction from the 48 to 80 minutes reported after the traditional meperidine/midazolam technique.[79] Remifentanil, an ultra–short-acting opioid, is an ideal drug for use during many office-based procedures such as facial cosmetic procedures. Facial surgery can be quite painful while the local anesthetic is being injected, after which it is relatively painless. An important caveat to the use of remifentanil is that it may cause nausea and vomiting, in addition to the respiratory depression characteristic of all opioids.

Ketamine has increased in popularity over the past several years in office-based practice.[8] The use of ketamine-propofol sedation has been described as an excellent way to provide a relaxed surgical field in a quiet, immobile patient.[80] Ketamine, a phencyclidine derivative, functions as both an anesthetic and an analgesic. It is particularly useful in that it does not depress respirations and will increase laryngeal reflexes, thus decreasing the risk of aspiration. Furthermore, it is not associated with nausea and vomiting.[81] Ketamine can, however, cause an increase in secretions and cause hallucinations. The latter can be decreased or eliminated by adding propofol and midazolam.[81–84] Glycopyrrolate can be used as an antisialagogue. Another advantage of ketamine is that it is relatively inexpensive.

Clonidine has also been found to be useful in an office. It has long been appreciated that it will help with blood pressure control throughout the perioperative period, thus potentially minimizing blood loss.[85,86] In addition, it may decrease the total propofol usage.[84]

General anesthesia can be administered in an office setting safely. Hoefflin et al reported their 18-year experience using general anesthesia for 23,000 surgical procedures in an accredited office-based plastic surgery facility. There were no intraoperative or postoperative deaths or significant complications.[20] They asserted that general anesthesia decreases the risk of intraoperative airway obstruction, allows the surgeon to focus wholly on the procedure without the distraction of patient movement, and eliminates the "seesaw effect" of intravenous sedation. The inhalational anesthetic agent of choice in their office was desflurane, with or without nitrous oxide. The pharmacokinetics and pharmacodynamics of desflurane and sevoflurane render them good potent inhaled agents for an office-based procedure, although the ability of anesthesia machines to deliver desflurane must be considered. Inhaled anesthetics with poor solubility in blood can be used safely and provide a rapid recovery.

Depth of anesthesia monitoring via a processed electroencephalogram has been shown to decrease the time to tracheal extubation and discharge readiness.[87–89] A depth of anesthesia monitor has been described as useful in the office during MAC procedures, with a possible decrease in total propofol usage.[90] Whether this type of monitoring will prove to be cost effective in the office-based situation remains to be seen.

POSTANESTHESIA CARE UNIT

Following an office-based procedure, it is expected that the patient will be able to sit in a chair or ambulate to an examination room to dress almost immediately. A formal PACU may not be present, and the patient may recover in the surgical suite. Regardless of where the patient recovers, it is important to adhere to all ASA standards for monitoring and documentation throughout the postoperative period.[46] Staffing in the recovery area must be adequate, and the use of a pulse oximeter is imperative.[18,91]

Because PACU space in an office is often limited and the anesthesiologist may have multiple locations to attend in a single day, problems of postoperative nausea and vomiting (PONV) and pain may become particularly troublesome. PONV or pain are not only problems for the patient and anesthesiologist, but they can also have a profound economic impact on an office surgical unit.[92] It is imperative that every anesthetic administered be designed to maximize patient alertness and mobility, and minimize the risks of the need for a prolonged PACU stay.[25] It has been recommended that the postanesthesia discharge scoring system and clinical discharge criteria used in ambulatory surgery are also used in the office-based setting.[93] Interestingly, there is a trend to discharge patients, particularly after colonoscopy, without escorts. This has been sanctioned in some states. In New York, regulations require that all patients undergoing a procedure with anesthesia be "discharged in the company of a responsible adult, unless exempted by a physician".[94] Specific data confirming the safety of this practice do not exist.

Local anesthesia, conscious sedation supplemented by wound infiltration with local anesthetics, or nerve blocks often form the basis for a multimodal strategy for postoperative pain management. These effective pain relief techniques not only decrease the anesthetic and analgesic requirements during surgery, but also reduce the need for more opioid analgesics in the postoperative period, thus facilitating the recovery process.[95] Opioid analgesics are commonly associated with nausea, vomiting, sedation, dysphoria, pruritus, constipation, urinary retention, and respiratory depression. Nonopioid analgesics (e.g., acetaminophen) and nonsteroidal anti-inflammatory drugs (e.g., ketorolac) are routinely used. Ketorolac for postoperative pain decreases the incidence of PONV; patients tolerate oral fluids and meet discharge criteria earlier than those receiving opioids.[96] In an effort to minimize the potential for postoperative bleeding and risk of GI complications, more specific cyclooxygenase-2 inhibitors may be used as nonopioid adjuvants for minimizing postoperative pain.[97] (Recently, some cyclooxygenase-2 inhibitors have been withdrawn from the market in the United States).

An optimal antiemetic regimen for OBA has yet to be established; however, because the causes of PONV are multifactorial, combination therapies may be more beneficial in high-risk patients. Many of the traditional first-line therapies are associated with sedation, drowsiness, and extrapyramidal side effects, and have been supplanted by 5-HT_3 antagonists such as ondansetron, dolasetron, and granisetron.[98] Dexamethasone has been shown to improve the efficacy of both 5-HT_3 antagonists[99] and dopamine antagonists.[100] Routine prophylaxis, though, has not been shown to offer any advantage over symptomatic treatment[101] and has direct costs associated with it. Ensuring adequate hydration (up to 20 mL/kg) to avoid orthostatic hypotension and thus prevent the release of emetogenic chemicals by decreased blood flow to the midbrain emetic centers is an intervention that may be useful in the prevention of PONV.[98]

REGULATIONS

Governmental oversight of office-based surgery varies among states; currently, regulations exist in many states, and others are following (Table 52-11). Whereas accreditation is usually a voluntary certification of an office, regulations are governmental mandates imposed by the local or state government. It is imperative that anesthesiologists embarking on an office-based practice familiarize themselves with any rules and regulations that govern practice in their particular state.

In 1994, California was the first state to adopt legislation regarding office-based anesthesia, followed by New Jersey.[4] A closer look at these two states gives an example of the varied requirements being enforced by states throughout the country. California's regulations pertain to patients undergoing a general anesthetic, and do not address procedures performed under local, peripheral nerve block, or sedation/anxiolysis administered in doses that do not affect a patient's life-preserving reflexes.[102] The regulations deal with issues ranging from office policy and mandatory reporting of adverse outcomes to surgeon and anesthesia provider qualifications.[103] California Health and Safety Code 1248-1248.85 mandates that surgical procedures occur only in offices that have been accredited or have been certified to participate in the Medicare Program under Title XVIII (42 U.S.C. Sec. 1395 et seq.) with few exceptions.[104] In addition, the office must have a written plan in place that deals with issues regarding emergency admissions. The surgeon must have admitting privileges at a local licensed or accredited acute care hospital or have a written transfer agreement with a physician who does have such privileges. The office must have an agreement with the hospital for the admission, in accordance with the hospital's system of quality assurance and peer review. California law also requires that offices have adequate patient monitoring throughout the perioperative period, and have a system in place for the storage and maintenance of patient records. An office that fails to comply with the regulations in place risks sanctions ranging from reprimand with or without monetary penalties through criminal prosecution.

TABLE 52-11

STATES IN WHICH OFFICE-BASED SURGERY AND ANESTHESIA ARE CURRENTLY REGULATED

California	North Carolina
Colorado	Ohio
Connecticut	Oklahoma
Florida	Pennsylvania
Illinois	Rhode Island
Massachusetts	South Carolina
Mississippi	Texas
New Jersey	Virginia

This list is growing, and it is imperative that the anesthesiologist who is considering beginning an office-based practice be familiar with the regulations in place in his or her state.

New Jersey's administrative Code 13:35-4A.1-13:35-4A.18 develops criteria for patient selection. Only ASA physical status 1 and 2 patients may undergo general or regional anesthesia. ASA physical status 3 patients can undergo only conscious sedation. The provider of general anesthesia must have the credentials to do so by a hospital, and only a physician with the appropriate credentials may supervise a certified registered nurse anesthetist. New Jersey law establishes guidelines regarding mandatory monitoring, emergency supplies that must be present, physician credentialing, and peer review. In contrast to California, New Jersey's regulations pertain to all patients undergoing a surgical procedure, regardless of the anesthetic depth. However, similar to California, violations may result in fines ranging from reprimand to license revocation and criminal prosecution.[105]

Although many states have regulations in place regarding office-based surgical procedures, the majority have none. Consequently, any physician who holds a valid medical license may perform any procedure, he or she so chooses, within an office. A surgeon may perform a procedure for which he or she may have had little to no training, and may sedate a patient without any training in anesthesia or airway management. In fact, there have been reported cases of patients undergoing a procedure without a preoperative evaluation, pertinent labs, informed consent, intraoperative or postoperative monitoring, or operative report, and without regard for sterile technique.[4]

Business and Legal Aspects

It is in the anesthesia provider's best interest to seek legal counsel before embarking on a career in OBA. Many OBA groups have formed either professional corporations or limited liability companies. Although not eliminating the need for liability insurance, both of these arrangements serve to protect the private assets of the anesthesiologist in the case of a malpractice claim.[7] Legal counsel will also prove to be beneficial in formulating business plans that follow all state and federal laws regarding billing/collection and antitrust. It is important to have an aboveboard and legal relationship with every office in which one administers anesthesia.

Billing strategies must be legal. In this complex environment of third-party payers, it is quite easy to make errors. Ignorance of the law offers no protection or excuse, and one should seek the advice of expert billing agencies even if one chooses not to outsource this responsibility. In planning prices, one must include all overhead charges such as drugs, equipment, time, and business expenses, including malpractice insurance. A pricing structure with the surgeon must exist before embarking on a business relationship. One must outline specifically what will be provided by the office (e.g., intravenous equipment, antibiotics, monitors) and what will be supplied by the anesthesiologist.

CONCLUSION

OBA continues to rapidly expand and pose unique challenges to anesthesiologists, who must not only provide medical care in new environments, but must also have good business sense and an understanding of operating room management. Although regulations have not kept pace with the growth of OBA, providers must make it their responsibility to ensure every possible safety measure is afforded to their patients. Decisions about appropriate patient selection and equipping anesthetizing locations must be made in conjunction with surgeons, and anesthetics chosen with consideration for the need for rapid turnover and limited PACU availability. The multiple advantages afforded by office-based surgery are fueling its evolution, and as more complex procedures are conducted on patients with increasing numbers of comorbidities, the anesthesiologist's role as patient advocate is vital.

References

1. Lazarov SJ: Office-based surgery and anesthesia: Where are we now? World J Urol 16:384, 1998
2. Courtiss EH, Goldwyn RM, Joffe JM, Hannenberg AA: Anesthetic practices in ambulatory surgery. Plast Reconstr Surg 93:792, 1994
3. Wetchler BV: Online shopping for ambulatory surgery: Let the buyer beware! Ambul Surg 8:111, 2000
4. Quattrone MS: Is the physician office the wild, wild west of health care? J Ambul Care Manage 23:64, 2000
5. Laurito CE: Report of educational meeting: The Society for Office-Based Anesthesia, Orlando, Florida, March 17, 1998. J Clin Anesth 10:445, 1998
6. Johnston DL: Moratorium goes too far. USA Today, August 23, 2000
7. Koch ME, Dayan S, Barinholtz D: Office-based anesthesia: An overview. Anesthesiol Clin North America 21:417, 2003
8. Ross AK, Eck JB: Office-based anesthesia for children. Anesthesiol Clin North America 20:195, 2002
9. Schultz LS: Cost analysis of office surgery clinic with comparison to hospital outpatient facilities for laparoscopic procedures. Int Surg 79:273, 1994
10. Bartamian M, Meyer DR: Site of service, anesthesia, and postoperative practice patterns for oculoplastic and orbital surgeries. Ophthalmology 103:1628, 1996
11. Way JC, Culham BA: Establishment and cost analysis of an office surgical suite. Can J Surg 39:379, 1996
12. Anello S: Office-based anesthesia: Advantages, disadvantages and the nurse's role. Plastic Surg Nurs 22:107, 2002
13. Iverson RE, Lynch DJ. ASPS Task Force on Patient Safety in Office-Based Surgery Facilities: Patient safety in office-based surgery facilities: II. Patient selection. Plast Reconstr Surg 110:1785, 2002
14. Arens J: Anesthesia for office-based surgery: Are we paying too high a price for access and convenience? Mayo Clinic Proc 75:225, 2000
15. Surgeons Leave O.R. and Go to the Office. New York Times, May 16, 1999, 41.
16. American Society of Anesthesiologists: Directory of Members, p 480. Park Ridge, IL: ASA, 2000
17. Anesthesia Patient Safety Foundation: Office based anesthesia growth provokes safety fears. ASA Neswl 65:6, 2001
18. Domino KB. Office-based anesthesia: Lessons learned from the closed-claims project. ASA Newsl 65:9, 2001
19. Morello DC, Colon GA, Fredricks S *et al*: Patient safety in accredited office surgical facilities. Plast Reconstr Surg 99:1496, 1997
20. Hoefflin SM, Bornstein JB, Gordon M: General anesthesia in an office-based plastic surgical facility: A report on more than 23,000 consecutive office-based procedures under general anesthesia with no significant anesthetic complications. Plast Reconstr Surg 107:243, 2001
21. Sullivan PK, Tattini CD: Office-based operatory experience: An overview of anesthetic technique, procedures and complications. Med Health R I 84:392, 2001
22. Bitar G, Mullis W, Jacobs W *et al*: Safety and efficacy of office-based surgery with monitored anesthesia care/sedation in 4778 consecutive plastic surgery procedures. Plast Reconstr Surg 111:150, 2003
23. Rao RB, Ely SF, Hoffman RS: Deaths related to liposuction. N Engl J Med 340:1471, 1999
24. Twersky RS: Updates on office-based anesthesia: Caveats on the professional finger-pointing. ASA Newsl 65:8, 2001
25. Twersky RS: Anaesthetic and management dilemmas in office-based surgery. Ambul Surg 6:79, 1998
26. ASA Committee on Equipment and Facilities: American Society of Anesthesiologists guidelines for determining anesthesia machine obsolescence. Available at: http://www.asahq.org/publicationsAndServices/machineobsolescense.pdf. Accessed March 28, 2005.
27. Coté CJ, Karl HW, Notteman DA *et al*: Adverse sedation events in pediatrics: Analysis of medications used for sedation. Pediatrics 106:663, 2000
28. Coté CJ, Notteman DA, Karl HW *et al*: Adverse sedation events in pediatrics: A critical incident analysis of contributing factors. Pediatrics 105:8, 2000
29. Iverson R, ASPS Task Force on Patient Safety in Office-Based Surgery Facilities: Patient safety in office-based surgery facilities: I. Procedures in the office-based surgery setting. Plast Reconstr Surg 110:1337, 2002
30. Tunajek SK: Office based procedure standards. AANA J 67:115, 1999
31. American Medical Association House of Delegates at the I-01 Meeting: Office-based surgery core principles. ASA Newsl 68:14, 2004
32. Meridy HW: Criteria for selection of ambulatory surgical patients and guidelines for anesthetic management: A retrospective of 1553 cases. Anesth Analg 61:921, 1982

33. ASA Committee on Ambulatory Surgical Care and ASA Task Force on Office-Based Anesthesia: Office-based anesthesia: Considerations for anesthesiologists in setting up and maintaining a safe office anesthesia environment. Available at: http://www.asahq.org/publicationsAndServices/office.pdf. Accessed March 28, 2005.
34. Twersky RS: Increase in office-based procedures begs caution among anesthesiologists. Anesthesiol News 24:9, 1998
35. Benumof JL: Obstructive sleep apnea in the adult obese patient: Implications for airway management. J Clin Anesth 13:144, 2001
36. Bresnitz EA, Goldberg R, Kosinski RM: Epidemiology of obstructive sleep apnea. Epidemiol Rev 16:210, 1994
37. Boushra NN: Anaesthetic management of patients with sleep apnea syndrome. Can J Anaesth 43:599, 1996
38. Benumof JL: Policies & procedures needed for sleep apnea patients. APSF Newsl Winter: 57, 2002/2003
39. Young T, Evans L, Finn L, Palta M: Estimation of the clinically diagnosed proportion of sleep apnea syndrome in middle-aged men and women. Sleep 20:705, 1997
40. Ofsky A: Sleep apnea and narcotic postoperative pain medication: A morbidity and mortality risk. APSF Newsl 17:24, 2002
41. Esclamado RM, Glenn MG, McCulloch TM: Perioperative complications and risk factors in the surgical treatment of obstructive sleep apnea syndrome. Laryngoscope 99:1125, 1989
42. Samuels SI, Rabinov W: Difficulty reversing drug-induced coma in a patient with sleep apnea. Anesth Analg 65:1222, 1986
43. Benumof JL: Creation of observational unit may decrease sleep apnea risk. APSF Newsl 17:39, 2002
44. American Society of Anesthesiologists: Practice guidelines for management of the difficult airway. Available at: http://www.asahq.org/publicationsAndServices/Difficult%20Airway.pdf. Accessed March 28, 2005.
45. American Society of Anesthesiologists (ASA): Standards for basic anesthetic monitoring. In ASA Directory of Members, p 493. Park Ridge, IL: ASA, 2001
46. American Society of Anesthesiologists (ASA): Standards for postanesthesia care. American Society of Anesthesiologists: Standards for basic anesthetic monitoring. In ASA Directory of Members, p 494. Park Ridge, IL: ASA, 2001
47. Moss E: MD office regs stalled in New Jersey. APSF Newsl Winter: 37, 1997
48. Yates JA. American Society of Plastic Surgeons: Office-based surgery accreditation crosswalk. Plastic Surg Nurs 22:125, 2002
49. Coldiron B: Office surgical incidents: 19 months of Florida data. Dermatol Surg 28:710, 2002
50. Bing J, McAuliffe MS, Lupton JR: Regional anesthesia with monitored anesthesia care for dermatologic laser surgery. Dermatol Clin 20:123, 2002
51. Morris KT, Pommier RF, Vetto JT: Office-based wire-guided open breast biopsy under local anesthesia is accurate and cost effective. Am J Surg 179:422, 2000
52. Jones JS, Streem SB: Office-based cystoureteroscopy for assessment of the upper urinary tract. J Endourol 16:307, 2002
53. Friedman O, Deutsch ES, Reilly JS, Cook SP: The feasibility of office-based laser-assisted tympanic membrane fenestration with tympanostomy tube insertion: The duPont Hospital experience. Int J Pediatr Otorhinolaryngol 62:31, 2002
54. Goldblum TA, Summers CG, Egbert JE, Letson RC: Office probing for congenital nasolacrimal duct obstruction: A study of parental satisfaction. J Pediatr Ophthalmol Strabismus 33:244, 1996
55. Jones JS, Oder M, Zippe CD: Saturation prostate biopsy with periprostatic block can be performed in the office. J Urol 168:2108, 2002
56. Goldrath MH, Sherman AI: Office hysteroscopy and suction curettage: Can we eliminate the hospital diagnostic dilatation and curettage? Am J Obstet Gynecol 152:220, 1985
57. American Society of Plastic Surgeons: Information on procedural statistics. Available at: www.plasticsurgery.org/public_education/loader.cfm?url-/commonspots/security/getfile.cfm&pageID-16158. Accessed May 29, 2004
58. Iverson RE, Lynch DJ, American Society of Plastic Surgeons Committee on Safety: Practice advisory on liposuction. Plast Reconstr Surg 113:1478, 2004
59. Fodor PB, Watson JP: Wetting solutions in ultra-sound assisted lipoplasty: A review. Clin Plast Surg 26:289, 1999
60. Klein JA: Tumescent technique for regional anesthesia permits lidocaine doses of 35 mg/kg. J Dermatol Surg Oncol 16:248, 1990
61. Ostad A, Kageyama N, Moy RL: Tumescent anesthesia with lidocaine dose of 55 mg/kg is safe for liposuction. Dermatol Surg 22:921, 1996
62. Grazer FM, deJong RH: Fatal outcome from liposuction: Census survey of cosmetic surgeons. Plast Reconstr Surg 105:436, 2000
63. Housman TS, Lawrence N, Mellen BG *et al*: The safety of liposuction: Results of a national survey. Dermatol Surg 28:971, 2002
64. Jaffe SM, Campbell P, Bellman M, Baildam A: Postoperative nausea and vomiting in women following breast surgery: An audit. Eur J Anaesth 17:261, 2000
65. Vawter M, Vicaroi MD, Moorthy K *et al*: Electrocardiographic monitoring during colonoscopy. Am J Gastroenterol 63:115, 1975
66. Radaelli F, Meucci G, Terruzzi V *et al*: Single bolus of midazolam versus bolus midazolam plus meperidine for colonoscopy: A prospective, randomized trial. Gastrointest Endosc 57:329, 2003
67. Ristikankare M, Julkunen R, Laitinen T: Effect of conscious sedation on cardiac autonomic regulation during colonoscopy. Scand J Gastroenterol 9:990, 2000
68. Petelenz M, Gonciarz M, Macfarlane P *et al*: Sympathovagal balance fluctuates during colonoscopy. Endoscopy 36:508, 2004
69. Finder RL: The art and science of office-based anesthesia in dentistry: A 150-year history. Int Anesthesiol Clin 41:1, 2003
70. Perrott DH, Yuen JP, Andresen RV, Dodson TB: Office-based ambulatory anesthesia: Outcomes of clinical practices of oral and maxillofacial surgeons. J Oral Maxillofac Surg 61:938, 2003
71. Freedman JM, Li DK, Drasner K *et al*: Transient neurologic symptoms after spinal anesthesia: An epidemiologic study of 1,873 patients. Anesthesiology 89:633, 1998
72. Mulroy MF, Larkin KL, Siddiqui A: Intrathecal fentanyl-induced pruritus is more severe in combination with procaine than with lidocaine or bupivacaine. Reg Anesth Pain Med 26:252, 2001
73. Ross AK, Eck JB: Office-based anesthesia for children. Anesthesiol Clin North America 20:195, 2002
74. Hackel A, Badgwell JM, Binding RR *et al*: Guidelines for the pediatric perioperative environment. American Academy of Pediatrics Section on Anesthesiology. Pediatrics 103:572, 1999
75. Tang J, Chen L, White PF *et al*: Use of propofol for office-based anesthesia: Effect of nitrous oxide on recovery. J Clin Anesth 11:226, 1999
76. White PF: Ambulatory anesthesia advances into the new millennium. Anesth Analg 90:1234, 2000
77. Cohen MM, Duncan PG, Tate RB: Does anesthesia contribute to operative mortality? JAMA 260:2859, 1988
78. Domino KB: Trends in anesthesia litigation in the 1990's: Monitored anesthesia care claims. ASA Newsl 61:17, 1997
79. Rudner R, Jalowiecki P, Kawecki P *et al*: Conscious analgesia/sedation with remifentanil and propofol versus total intravenous anesthesia with fentanyl, midazolam, and propofol for outpatient colonoscopy. Gastrointest Endosc 57:657, 2003
80. Friedberg BL: Facial laser resurfacing with the propofol-ketamine technique: Room air, spontaneous ventilation (RASV) anesthesia. Dermatol Surg 25:569, 1999
81. Friedberg BK: Propofol-ketamine technique: Dissociative anesthesia for office surgery (a five year review of 1,264 cases). Aesthetic Plast Surg 23:70, 1999
82. Friedberg BL: Propofol-ketamine technique. Aesthetic Plast Surg 17:297, 1993
83. Friedberg BL: Hypnotic doses of propofol block ketamine-induced hallucinations. Plast Reconstr Surg 91:196, 1993
84. Friedberg BL, Sigl JC: Clonidine premedication decreases propofol consumption during bispectral index (BIS) monitored propofol-ketamine technique for office-based surgery. Dermatol Surg 26:848, 2000
85. Man D: Premedication with oral clonidine for facial rhytidectomy. Plast Reconstr Surg 94:214, 1994
86. Baker TM, Stuzin JM, Baker TJ, Gordon HL: What's new in aesthetic surgery? Clin Plast Surg 23:16, 1996
87. Drover DR, Lemmens JH, Pierce ET *et al*: Patient state index: Titration of delivery and recovery from propofol, alfentanil, and nitrous oxide anesthesia. Anesthesiology 97:82, 2002
88. Gan TJ, Glass PS, Windsor A *et al*: Bispectral index monitoring allows faster emergence and improved recovery from propofol, alfentanil, and nitrous oxide anesthesia. Anesthesiology 87:805, 1997
89. Song D, Joshi GP, White PF: Titration of volatile anesthetics using bispectral analysis index facilitates recovery after ambulatory anesthesia. Anesthesiology 87:842, 1997
90. Friedberg B, Sigl JC: Bispectral index (BIS) monitoring decreases propofol usage during propofol-ketamine office based anesthesia. Anesth Analg 88(S54):54, 1999
91. Singer R, Thomas PE: Pulse oximeter in the ambulatory aesthetic surgical facility. Plast Reconstr Surg 82:111, 1988
92. Tang J, Chen X, White PF *et al*: Antiemetic prophylaxis for office-based surgery—are the 5-HT3 receptor antagonists beneficial? Anesthesiology 98:293, 2003
93. Chung FF, Chan VW, Ong D: A postanesthetic discharge scoring system for home readiness after ambulatory surgery. J Clin Anesth 7:500, 1995
94. Title 10 NYCRR, Section 755.6.f, Volume D. Available at http://www.health.state.ny.us/nysdoh/phforum/nycrr10.htm. Accessed June 4, 2005
95. White PF: The role of non-opioid analgesic techniques in the management of pain after ambulatory surgery. Anesth Analg 94:577, 2002
96. Ding Y, White PF: Comparative effects of ketorolac, dezocine and fentanyl as adjuvants during outpatient anesthesia. Anesth Analg 75:566, 1992
97. Desjardins PJ, Shu VS, Recker DP *et al*: A single preoperative oral dose of valdecoxib, a new cyclooxygenase-2 specific inhibitor, relieves post-oral surgery or bunionectomy pain. Anesthesiology 97:565, 2002
98. Kovac AL: Prevention and treatment of postoperative nausea and vomiting. Drugs 59:213, 2000
99. Henzi I, Walder B, Tramer MR: Dexamethasone for prophylaxis of postoperative nausea and vomiting: A quantitative systematic review. Anesth Analg 90:186, 2000
100. Eberhart LH, Morin AM, Georgieff M: Dexamethasone for prophylaxis of

postoperative nausea and vomiting. A meta-analysis of randomized controlled studies. Anaesthesist 49:713, 2000

101. Scuderi PE, James RL, Harris L, Mims GR: Antiemetic prophylaxis does not improve outcomes after outpatient surgery when compared to symptomatic treatment. Anesthesiology 90:360, 1999
102. California Codes, Business & Professions Code, Division 2. Healing Arts, Chapter 5. Medicine: Article 11.5. Surgery in certain outpatient settings, §2216, Restrictions on use of anesthesia, 2003
103. California Codes, Business & Professions Code, Division 2. Healing Arts, Chapter 5. Medicine: Article 11.5. Surgery in certain outpatient settings. §2215–40, 2003
104. California Health and Safety Code, Division 2. Licensing Provisions, Chapter 1.3. Outpatient settings. §1248.1, Required settings, 2003
105. New Jersey Administrative Code: Title 13. Law and public safety: Chapter 35. Board of medical examiners: Subchapter 4A. Surgery, special procedures, and anesthesia services performed in an office setting. 2003

CHAPTER 53 ■ ANESTHESIA FOR ORGAN TRANSPLANTATION

MARIE CSETE AND KATHRYN GLAS

KEY POINTS

1. Brain death is declared when the clinical picture is consistent with irreversible cessation of all brain function.
2. The preoperative assessment of the donor should include the declaration of brain death, consent for donation, and the donor blood type.
3. The mainstay of donor management is maintenance of euvolemia, oxygenation, perfusion, and normothermia.
4. Immune suppression is associated with severe, life-threatening infections (including recurrence of hepatitis after liver transplantation), increased risk of tumors, and progressive vascular disease.
5. Patients on chronic steroid therapy do not necessarily require large doses of perioperative steroids to cover their stress response, especially for small or local surgical procedures.
6. During transplant evaluation, in addition to history and physical exams, patients are generally screened with electrocardiogram, echocardiography, and pulmonary function tests.
7. For renal transplantation, the major anesthetic consideration is maintenance of renal blood flow. Typical hemodynamic goals during transplant are systolic pressure > 90 mm Hg, mean systemic pressure > 60 mm Hg, and central venous pressure > 10 mm Hg.
8. A kidney graft is defective in concentrating urine and reabsorbing sodium, so attention to electrolytes is important.
9. Patients with end-stage liver disease have multisystem dysfunction with common cardiac, pulmonary, and renal compromise because of their liver disease.
10. Liver transplantation is a complex surgical procedure, traditionally described in three phases: dissection, anhepatic, and neohepatic phases, with reperfusion of the graft marking the start of the neohepatic phase.
11. A major hurdle for small bowel and multivisceral transplantation is line placement adequate for transfusion of blood products and fluids, which may be substantial during these long cases.
12. Use of nitric oxide (NO) for lung transplantation is associated with risks of methemoglobinemia, NO metabolite-related lung injury, and decreased sensitivity of exhaled NO monitoring as a diagnostic tool for acute lung rejection.
13. For nontransplant surgery in solid organ recipients, evaluation of patients is centered on function of the grafted organ.
14. For all transplant recipients, antibiotic, antiviral, antifungal, and immune suppression regimens should be disrupted as little as possible in the perioperative period.

Transplantation is a growth industry in developed countries, and increasingly performed throughout the world. About 87,000 patients are on transplant waiting lists in the United States. As transplant waiting lists grow, organ donation has not increased to meet demand. Consequently, living-related organ donation is increasingly common, and 2001 was the first year in which the number of living-related kidney donors exceeded the number of cadaveric donors in the United States. In addition, use of organs once considered marginal is on the rise, increasing the difficulty of anesthetic management of organ recipients.

The United Network of Organ Sharing (UNOS; www.unos.org) is an important source of information related to organ transplantation for patients and physicians. UNOS was created by the 1984 National Organ Transplant Act to operate the organ procurement and transplant network for efficient and equitable distribution of donated organs. To address local concerns and optimize organ allocation, the United States is divided into 11 regions for purposes of organ distribution, each with its own regional review board. Some 259 transplant centers in the United States perform about 13,000 transplants per year.

Anesthesiologists are involved in the care of organ donors, perioperative management of transplant recipients, and, in major transplant centers, anesthesiologists with special expertise actively participate in the preoperative assessment and optimization of patients for major organ transplant procedures.

ANESTHETIC MANAGEMENT OF ORGAN DONORS

Brain Dead Donors

1 Brain dead heart-beating donors present challenging, unfamiliar management issues to anesthesiologists. Brain death is declared when the clinical picture is consistent with irreversible cessation of all brain function.[1] Legal and medical brain death criteria can differ from state to state and over time, but all require evaluation of both cerebral and brainstem function. Physicians involved in the transplant recipient process should not be involved in declaration of brain death of the donor. Potentially reversible causes of coma or unresponsiveness must be ruled out (hypothermia, hypotension, drugs, or toxins) before declaration of brain death. Brain dead donors are unresponsive to verbal or painful stimuli, and the clinical exam is confirmed by transcranial Doppler or angiography showing no blood flow to the brain. Flat electroencephalogram is consistent with brain death. All brainstem reflexes must be absent, including ventilatory drive with apnea testing.

2 The preoperative assessment of the donor should include the declaration of brain death, consent for donation, and the donor blood type. Brain dead patients may have intact spinal reflexes and some movement, and so may require neuromuscular blockade.

Brain death is associated with hemodynamic instability, hormonal chaos, and diffuse inflammatory changes, all of which may negatively impact donor organ function.[2] Adrenergic surges can cause ischemia. Vasodilation, loss of temperature control, and diabetes insipidus are also surprisingly difficult management issues. Because of the scarcity of randomized controlled trials in brain dead donors, uniform guidelines for managing donors simply are not available. Anesthetic management during organ harvest is guided by the needs of the teams harvesting organs and personnel from organ procurement networks, who may come from several centers, and have discrepant requests, depending on the organs procured. UNOS has created a resource for managing organ donors, in an effort to improve their care, and therefore the function of donated organs (see the Critical Pathway for the Organ Donor form on the Internet at *www.unos.org/resources/pdfs/CriticalPathway Poster.pdf*).

In addition, it is advisable to contact the local representative of the regional organ procurement agency before managing any organ donor in the operating room. The professionals in organ management are aware of the latest management strategies, as well as local preferences and research protocols.

Extrapolation of data from animal models and small clinical studies suggests that donated organs are protected by hormone therapy,[3,4] especially when thoracic organs are procured. A typical regimen is tri-iodothyronine (4 μg intravenously then 3 μg/hour), methylprednisolone 15 mg/kg intravenously q 24 hr, DDAVP 1 U then 0.5 to 4 U/hour to maintain systemic vascular resistance (SVR) at 800 to 1,200 dyne $*$ seconds/cm^5, and insulin infusion to maintain blood glucose 120 to 180 mg/dL.[4] Other medications that should be available are broad spectrum antibiotics, albumin, mannitol and loop diuretics, heparin, dopamine, and norepinephrine.

3 The mainstay of donor management is maintenance of euvolemia. Packed cells are used to maintain hematocrit of 30%, while fresh frozen plasma (FFP) is used to maintain the international normalized ratio (INR) $<$1.5. Arterial catheters and central venous catheters are used to guide fluid and vasopressor therapies. In general, central venous pressure (CVP) is maintained at 6 to 12 mm Hg, and when pulmonary artery catheters are used to assess cardiac function, pulmonary capillary wedge pressure (PCWP) is maintained at $<$12 mm Hg. The goals of volume and hormonal therapies are to minimize the use of vasopressors. Surgeons procuring the lungs will want to keep central filling pressure low and diuretics may be requested just prior to collection of the lungs, whereas those procuring kidneys will request high filling pressures. Obviously, the job of the anesthesiologist is to maintain the donor oxygenation, perfusion, and normothermia, but the targets of therapies require coordination with the various procurement teams, and good communication is essential. Efforts should be made to keep serum Na $<$ 150 mEq/L, and generally arterial pCO_2 is maintained at 30 to 35 mm Hg. Transport of ventilated patients often requires positive end-expiratory pressure (PEEP) valves attached to the ambu bag to maintain oxygenation of the donor. Peak airway pressures should be kept below 30 mm Hg.

Prior to lung removal, surgeons will perform bronchoscopy. An adapter, such as the Portex fiberoptic bronchoscopic swivel adapter (SIMS Portex, Inc., Keene, NH, USA), facilitates ventilation during the procedure. Glucocorticoids are usually administered, and on occasion, prostaglandin E_1 is requested to improve circulation of the preservation solution. Surgical techniques have been developed to allow three recipients from one thoracic donor: two single lung transplants and a heart transplant.[5] The heart is removed first, leaving a small cuff of left atrium attached to the lungs. The harvesting team will ask for systemic heparinization just prior to exsanguination and excision. Cardioplegia is administered, the heart stops ejecting, and the heart is removed. The trachea is transected and the lungs removed en bloc for later separation.

Donor lungs are more susceptible to injury in brain dead patients before procurement than are other organs, likely from contusion, aspiration, or edema with fluid resuscitation. Consequently, only 20% of multiorgan donors meet the current strict criteria for lung donors. These criteria are listed in Table 53-1. A more recent review published by the Pulmonary Council of the International Society for Heart and Lung Transplantation discusses the scientific basis for these criteria.[6] Lungs once considered marginal are being used increasingly because of a severe shortage of donor lungs. Exclusion of donors based on blood gas[7] or CXR findings[6] (see Table 53-1) are based on small single-center trials. With experience, lung transplantation

TABLE 53-1

IDEAL CADAVERIC LUNG DONOR

Age younger than 55 years
ABO compatibility
Clear chest radiograph
PaO_2 >300 on FIO_2 = 1.0, PEEP 5 cm H_2O
Tobacco history <20 pack-years
Absence of chest trauma
No evidence of aspiration or sepsis
Negative sputum Gram's stain
Absence of purulent secretions at bronchoscopy

Adapted from *www.unos.org*, August 2004.

using donors outside these boundaries does not negatively impact the recipient, and most centers rely on bronchoscopy to determine lung suitability for transplantation.[8] A more recent study suggested that aspiration on bronchoscopy, bilateral pulmonary infiltrates, or persistent purulent secretions are criteria for donor exclusion.[9] There is also uniform agreement that advanced donor age (>55 years), together with long ischemic time (>6 hours), is associated with poor transplant outcome. Donors and recipients are matched based on height and/or total lung capacity (TLC) compatibility.

A consensus conference was convened in 2002 in an effort to improve evaluation and utilization of cardiac donors.[10] Mortality on the heart transplant waiting list is 17%, compounded by a donor "yield" of only 42%. The ideal heart donor is younger than 50 years old, and hemodynamically stable. Presence of major chest trauma, known cardiac disease, active infection, prolonged cardiac arrest, malignancy, HIV or HBV positive, or intracardiac injections moves the donor from ideal to marginal status. Overall, health status of the donor prior to determination of brain death can facilitate a directed laboratory evaluation. Electrocardiogram (ECG) is often abnormal in the setting of brain injury/death, and further evaluation with transthoracic echocardiography (TTE) is often necessary. Cardiac catheterization is sometimes requested in older donors, and those with significant personal or family history of coronary artery disease (CAD). Marginal donors are typically used only for high-risk recipients who are at increased risk of waiting list mortality. In recipients with pulmonary hypertension, younger donors, short ischemic time, low donor inotrope requirement, and oversized organs are preferred.

Non–heart-beating donors have been used mostly for kidney transplantation, more recently for livers and islet transplants, and even for lungs.[11–13] These donors usually have severe brain damage but are not brain dead, and death is defined by cessation of cardiac and respiratory function. Life support measures are used to control the timing of death and organ procurement. Guidelines for non–heart-beating donor management, and ethical considerations are available in a study conducted by the Institute of Medicine.[14] Depending on the local hospital protocol, anesthesiologists may not be involved in the care of non–heart-beating donors. The donor may be declared dead just outside the operating room (OR), then quickly taken into the OR for organ procurement without an anesthesiologist in attendance. Other hospitals have developed protocols that involve preparation of the patient in the OR with an anesthesiologist present, and the anesthesiologist may be responsible for removing the patient from ventilatory support and for declaration of death. Despite concerns that non–heart-beating organ donors should be managed throughout by the primary care team without anesthesiologists involved,[15] current federally based recommendations and the success of transplantation using organs from these donors, along with applied research in this area, make it likely that non–heart-beating organ donation will increase. Anesthesiologists should be involved in the design of protocols in their local institution, if they are to be involved in the process.

Living Kidney Donors

Living donors have no significant cardiopulmonary, neurologic, or psychiatric disease, diabetes, obesity, hypertension, history of renal stones, or proteinuria. Renal function must be normal. Living donors are, by definition, quite healthy, and these volunteers deserve exquisite attention to safety and pain management. Historically, open nephrectomy involved a long flank incision and rib resection, a painful procedure. The traditional open procedure was modified to reduce the size of incision, making rib resection unnecessary.[16] The open procedure is still painful, usually requiring postoperative patient-controlled opioid analgesia for at least a day. General anesthesia is used in many centers, but epidural and combined epidural-spinal techniques (supplemented with intravenous propofol) have also been used successfully.[17] For the open procedure, the patient is positioned in the lateral decubitus position with the bed flexed to expose and arch the flank.

Laparoscopic (versus open) donor nephrectomy is increasingly the norm and is generally better tolerated by donors in terms of comfort and shorter hospital stay.[18] However, anesthesiologists must be aware that mastering the technique takes a while, and the first procedures performed by surgeons tend to be long. Anesthetics and insufflation of the peritoneum with CO_2 decrease renal blood flow so fluid repletion is important to maintaining renal perfusion. A reasonable protocol is to administer crystalloid at 10 cc/kg per hour above calculated losses and to maintain urine output at about 100 cc/hour;[19] however, local protocols may rely on CVP for fluid administration or mandate set amounts of fluid. Central venous lines are generally placed after induction of anesthesia for patient comfort.

Virtually all donor tracheas can be extubated in the operating room. Patient-controlled analgesia is common after donor surgery. Some centers admit donors to a step-down or medical intensive care unit (ICU) for a day after surgery, but the total hospital stay is usually only 2 to 4 days. A bladder catheter is removed on postop day 1. Patients should be advised that full recovery (i.e., feeling normal) takes 4 to 6 weeks.

Complications after living donor nephrectomy include atelectasis of the lungs, pneumothorax, arrhythmias, wound pain or infection, urinary tract infection, and mental status changes.[20] Perioperative mortality is rare but cannot be denied as a possible outcome during preoperative patient discussions.[21]

Living Liver Donors

Left lobe liver donation is usually done in the context of parent-to-child donation. Although left lateral segmentectomy is a big operation, it is generally well tolerated. Right lobectomy by comparison is a larger procedure and carries significant risk. Mortality of right liver resection for donation is estimated at 0.4 to 1%.[22,23] A more recent living related donor death that received considerable public scrutiny[24] and the report of the first Japanese donor death[25] highlight the enormity of this operation, the need for experienced teams to manage the patients, and the often neglected need for long-term follow-up of donors. Nonetheless, as donor shortages become more desperate, it is likely that adult-to-adult living related transplantation will be in more demand. Other reported complications of this surgery include air embolism, atelectasis, and pneumonia.[26]

Large liver resections may require virtually complete hepatic venous exclusion (cross-clamping of the hepatic pedicle usually without cava clamping). Not unexpectedly, venous return falls by about 50%. Without the collaterals developed by patients with liver disease, normal donors may experience significant hypotension when the cava or even just the portal vein is cross-clamped. Blood pressure is maintained largely through reflex increases in endogenous vasopressin and norepinephrine levels.[27] For these reasons, volume loading seems a reasonable preparation (often albumin) just prior to clamping and is the practice at our institution. However, some authors have argued that blood loss is reduced if the CVP is kept low during resections.[28] These reports have prompted some centers to not only keep CVP <5 mm Hg by limiting fluids, but also by adding vasodilators and diuretics.[29] Sufficiently powered studies to prove that low CVP benefits (less blood transfusion) outweigh risks (renal compromise and air embolism) are unlikely to be performed, and institutional practices vary widely. If vasopressors are needed, vasopressin and norepinephrine are reasonable choices to enhance normal endogenous reflexes. Most donors do not require vasopressors.

Isovolemic hemodilution has been reported to reduce allogeneic red cell requirements in major hepatic resections.[30] At experienced centers, blood loss is usually less than 1 L, with 20 to 40% of donors requiring transfusion.[31–33] Transesophageal echocardiography, if expertise is available, is ideal and obviates central line placement. Blood salvage is useful, and some centers offer autologous donation programs for donors; both can reduce the need for allogeneic blood transfusions.[34]

The trachea of most donors can be extubated safely in the operating room. Hypothermia is a common reason for not extubating in the OR. Postoperative pain management in these patients is a matter of controversy. Some institutions successfully place epidural catheters, providing excellent analgesia without reported complications.[35] However, with right liver resection, INR rises significantly after surgery, peaking a few days after surgery along with a fall in platelet counts, just when the catheter is usually removed.[32,36] For this reason, many centers will not place epidural catheters in these patients, and rely on intravenous patient-controlled analgesia.

Living Lung Donors

As of March 2004, only 234 living donor lobar lung transplantation (LDLLT) procedures have been reported by UNOS. LDLLT is typically reserved for critically ill recipients unlikely to survive until a cadaveric donor becomes available. Given this, as in all living donors, the inherently coercive conditions must be balanced by numerous visits to review the procedure, allowing the donors multiple opportunities to withdraw from participation. Selection criteria for donors are listed in Table 53-2.[37] No donor mortality has been reported to date, and morbidity remains low. If two donors are used for one recipient, scheduling difficulties are considerable. The surgical procedure is performed in three operating rooms simultaneously, one for each donor and the recipient. Donors receive a general anesthetic with epidural analgesia.

TABLE 53-2

LIVING LUNG DONOR CRITERIA

Member of extended family
Age 18–55 years
No prior thoracic surgery on donor side
Good general health
Taller than recipient preferred
ABO compatible
FVC and FEV_1 $>85\%$ predicted
pO_2 >80 mm Hg on room air
No chronic viral diseases
Normal electrocardiogram and echocardiogram
Normal stress test in donors older than 40 years old

Adapted from *www.unos.org*, August 2004.

IMMUNOSUPPRESSIVE DRUGS

The long-term goal of transplant immunologists is to create recipient tolerance to grafts, but the complexity of immune responses means this goal will be difficult to achieve. Nonetheless, efforts to create hematopoietic chimerism are a major research focus in transplantation. For now, suppression of immune responses is used to blunt reaction to allografts, and drugs powerful enough to suppress the immune system are associated with significant side effects. Immunosuppressed patients who are undertreated can reject an organ. Immune suppression is associated with severe, life-threatening infections (including recurrence of hepatitis after liver transplantation), increased risk of tumors, and progressive vascular disease. Immunosuppression regimens differ considerably from center to center, and anesthesiologists must communicate with the transplant team to obtain the schedule and dose of immunosuppressive agents used for each patient. Considerable variability between patients in intestinal absorption, and genetic and induced differences in metabolism of these drugs require precise individualization of immunosuppressive regimens. It is particularly important to review drug regimens with transplant coordinators when posttransplant patients are scheduled for surgery because the transplant team is likely to have information about peak and trough drug levels that may not be accessible on the hospital chart.

4

All immunosuppression regimens carry major risks: infection and malignancy. Thus, immune-suppressed patients coming to the OR deserve special attention to sterile technique and maintenance of antibiotic/antifungal/antiviral regimens during the perioperative period. Complications of immunosuppression are summarized in Table 53-3. Both a review of immunologic mechanisms of rejection and the various immunosuppressive regimens used for each organ transplant are beyond the scope of this chapter. Rather, the mechanism of each drug's action and information about its use pertinent to anesthesiologists are outlined here.

TABLE 53-3

MULTISYSTEM COMPLICATIONS OF CHRONIC IMMUNE SUPPRESSION

SYSTEM	COMPLICATION
Central nervous system	Lowered seizure threshold
Cardiovascular	Diabetes
	Hypertension
	Hyperlipidemia
Renal/electrolyte	Decreased glomerular filtration rate
	Hyperkalemia
	Hypomagnesemia
Hematologic/immune	Increased risk of infections
	Increased risk of tumors
	Pancytopenia
Endocrine/other	Osteoporosis
	Poor wound healing

Adapted from *www.unos.org*, August 2004.

Calcineurin Inhibitors

The modern transplant era began with the introduction of *cyclosporine*, a calcineurin inhibitor, into the marketplace. These drugs remain a major part of immunosuppression for solid organ transplant recipients.[38] Cyclosporine is still used, but other calcineurin inhibitors are used increasingly in its place. *Tacrolimus* has been particularly important for kidney transplant recipients because of its potency in preventing acute rejection (within 6 months of transplantation), long-term graft survival, and relative lack of side effects compared with historical regimens.[39] Cyclosporine binds cellular cyclophilins and tacrolimus binds the FK binding protein, and these bound complexes interact with the phosphatase, calcineurin. Calcineurin, among other effects, in turn modifies NFAT (nuclear factor of activated T-cells) and frees NF-kB to translocate to the nucleus, where they enhance transcription of T-cell interleukin-2 (IL-2).[40] The (simplified) mechanism of action of calcineurin inhibitors is that they inhibit T-lymphocyte differentiation and cytokine elaboration.

Calcineurin is involved in diverse cellular processes in addition to immune function, and therefore, inhibition of calcineurin is associated with significant side effects. These include hypertension (often requiring therapy), hyperlipidemia, ischemic vascular disease (including in heart recipients), diabetes, and nephrotoxicity.[41] Ischemic cardiac disease is the leading cause of death of kidney transplant recipients, in part due to underlying disease that preceded transplantation, but use of calcineurin inhibitors can exacerbate risk factors for coronary artery disease.[42] It is important to note that end-stage liver disease (ESLD) does not confer protection from coronary artery disease, and liver transplant patients are also at risk for progression of ischemic cardiac disease after transplantation. Neurologic side effects are also common. Most of the side effects of these drugs are dose related, and patients typically require quite a bit of dosage adjustment after transplantation.

An old retrospective review and occasional case report suggested that cyclosporine may prolong the action of pancuronium,[43,44] but these reports have not been followed by clinical experience, suggesting that inability to reverse neuromuscular blockade is common in cyclosporine-treated patients. Cyclosporine increases MAC in rats, but similar studies have not been reported in humans.[45] To switch from oral to intravenous dosing of cyclosporine, usually about one-third the oral dose is used. Usual doses of tacrolimus are 0.15 to 0.3 mg/kg per day given in two doses. To switch from oral to intravenous tacrolimus, a starting dose of about one-tenth the oral dose can be used. For optimal perioperative management, the precise doses of drugs given in the OR should be clearly communicated to the primary care team so immunosuppression is minimally disrupted.

Corticosteroids disrupt expression of many cytokines in T-cells, antigen-presenting cells, and macrophages. These drugs are used both for maintenance immunosuppression and in pulse dosing for acute rejection. Especially for children, corticosteroid-sparing regimens are increasingly popular because growth is negatively affected by steroids and because the drugs are generally not tolerated well. Well-known side effects are hypertension, diabetes, hyperlipidemia, weight gain (including Cushingoid features), and gastrointestinal (GI) ulceration. Patients on chronic steroid therapy do not necessarily
5 require large doses of perioperative steroids to cover their stress response, especially for small or local surgical procedures.[46] Again, communication with the primary transplant service is important in determining steroid coverage that least impacts the delicate balance of immunosuppression.

Antiproliferative drugs rely on the fact that immune activation implies explosive proliferation of lymphocytes. Side effects occur because other proliferating cells (GI tract, bone marrow) are also affected.

mTOR (mammalian target of rapamycin) inhibitors are often used in combination with calcineurin inhibitors to decrease the complications of dose-related side effects ("calcineurin sparing regimens") such as nephrotoxicity.[47] TOR is involved in complex signaling processes that promote synthesis of proteins, including several that regulate cellular proliferation. Thus, mTOR inhibitors such as rapamycin (sirolimus) are antiproliferative, used both in immunosuppression and increasingly in cancer therapies. Similar to cyclosporine and tacrolimus, sirolimus is metabolized in liver via P450CYP3A isoenzymes, but coadministration of sirolimus and a calcineurin inhibitor does not increase calcineurin inhibitor drug requirements. In fact, the combination may be synergistic.[48] Everolimus is a new drug in this category.[49]

Azathioprine is hydrolyzed in blood to 6-mercaptopurine, a purine analog and metabolite with the ability to incorporate into DNA during the S phase of the cell cycle. Because DNA synthesis is a necessary prerequisite to mitosis, azathioprine exerts an antiproliferative effect. The major side effect of azathioprine is repression of bone marrow cell cycling, which can cause pancytopenia. Cardiac arrest and severe upper airway edema are rare complications.[50] The intravenous dose is about half the oral dose.

Mycophenolate mofetil is metabolized into a molecule that inhibits purine synthesis. It too can cause leukopenia and thrombocytopenia as side effects, as well as red cell aplasia.[51] Usual oral dose is 1 to 1.5 g two times a day.

Monoclonal and Polyclonal Antibodies

OKT3 antibody is directed against a component of the T-cell receptor complex and affects immunosuppression by blocking T-cell function. Acute administration of OKT3 in awake patients (especially first administration) may result in generalized weakness, fever, chills, and some hypotension. More severe hypotension, bronchospasm, and pulmonary edema have been reported.[52] Anesthesiologists administering the drug should note that formulations of OKT3 may require filtering before administration (and a syringe filter is supplied with the drug).

"Humanized" antibodies are used with increasing frequency. These are antibodies engineered to contain human constant regions in the immunoglobulin so patients do not develop an antimouse immunologic response against a mouse monoclonal antibody. Muromonab-CD3 is a humanized form of OKT3,[53] usually used for acute rejection. Basiliximab and daclizumab are newer humanized antibodies. These antibodies are both directed against a portion of the IL-2 receptor and work by blocking IL-2-mediated T-cell activation. GI upset is the most commonly cited side effect of these drugs. However, basiliximab was more recently implicated in three cases of pulmonary edema in young renal transplant patients.[54]

Polyclonal antibodies (directed against more than one protein epitope) include *antithymocyte globulin*, used to deplete T-cells from the circulation. Side effects include a serum sickness syndrome, leukopenia and thrombocytopenia, and fever.

RENAL TRANSPLANTATION

Preoperative Considerations

An enormous variety of diseases are treated with renal transplants (Table 53-4). Many of these underlying diagnoses are also risk factors for coronary artery disease, so preoperative evaluation is focused on cardiovascular function. About half the mortality of patients on dialysis is due to heart failure,[55] and

TABLE 53-4

DIAGNOSES OF ADULTS AWAITING RENAL TRANSPLANTS

DISEASE CATEGORY AND EXAMPLES	% OF PATIENTS ON LIST
Glomerular disease	
Chronic glomerulonephritis	4.1
IgA nephropathy	2.3
Systemic lupus erythematosus	2.9
Alport's syndrome	0.5
Membranous nephropathy	1.4
Hemolytic uremic syndrome	0.1
Membranous glomerulonephritis	1.4
Diabetes	
Type 1	6.1
Type 2	20.4
Polycystic kidney disease	5.3
Hypertensive nephrosclerosis	16.4
Renovascular disease	
Malignant hypertension	4.6
Focal glomerular sclerosis	2.8
Polyarteritis	0.03
Scleroderma	0.08
Congenital/metabolic	
Obstructive uropathy	0.5
Cystinosis	0.02
Tubular/interstitial nephritis	0.7
Acquired obstructive nephropathy	0.3
Drug-induced nephropathy	
Analgesics	0.2
Antibiotics	0.03
Cyclosporine	0.05
Chronic pyelonephritis	0.8
Acute tubular necrosis	0.04
Renal graft failure	12.7

Adapted from *www.unos.org*, August 2004.

cardiovascular complications are a leading cause of death after renal transplantation. Therefore, cardiovascular risk factor modification is imperative before and after transplantation.[56]

6 During transplant evaluation, in addition to history and physical exams, patients are generally screened with ECG, echocardiography, and pulmonary function tests (PFTs), which should be reviewed by the anesthesiologist. In addition, patients will be screened for tumors (mammography, Pap test, colonoscopy) and infection (dental evaluation, viral serologies). Patients should have good control of their diabetes before transplantation and have an evaluation for psychiatric stability. Severe heart, lung, or liver disease; most malignancies; and active or untreatable infections such as tuberculosis (TB) are exclusion criteria for renal transplantation. With obesity at epidemic proportions, renal transplantation is commonly performed in obese patients. These patients are at increased risk of surgical complications, including delayed graft function and wound infection.[57]

Dialysis-dependent patients should be dialyzed before surgery. Cadaveric grafts can be safely transplanted after 24 hours of cold ischemia time, and up to 36 hours, allowing scheduling of preoperative dialysis. With preoperative dialysis, severe hyperkalemia during surgery is unusual.

Intraoperative Protocols

Renal transplantation is generally done under general anesthesia, although small studies have suggested good outcomes with epidural anesthesia.[58] Rapid sequence induction is indicated in diabetic patients with gastroparesis[59] (preceded by oral sodium bicitrate). In general, concerns over uremic platelet dysfunction and residual heparin from preoperative dialysis have limited use of regional anesthesia for kidney transplantation. Before incision, antibiotics are given. A central venous catheter (usually triple lumen) is placed for CVP monitoring and drug administration, and a bladder catheter is placed.

Incision is usually in the lower right abdomen to facilitate placement of the graft in the iliac fossa. The recipient iliac artery and vein are used for graft vascularization, followed by connection of the ureter to recipient bladder. If the kidney is too large for the iliac fossa, it can be positioned in the retroperitoneal space; iliac vessels may be used for anastomoses, or the aorta and inferior vena cava may be required.

7 The major anesthetic consideration is maintenance of renal blood flow. No data are available to determine whether inhaled versus intravenous techniques are better at preserving (graft) renal flow. So typical hemodynamic goals during transplant are systolic pressure >90 mm Hg, mean systemic pressure >60 mm Hg, and CVP >10 mm Hg. These goals are usually achieved without use of vasopressors, using isotonic fluids and adjustment of anesthetic doses. (In reality, CVP goals vary considerably from center to center. Some surgeons aim for CVP of about 10 mm Hg, others prefer CVP of about 20 mm Hg, and still others request specified amounts of intravenous fluids and ignore the CVP. Similarly, some programs prefer high mean systemic pressures of 80 to 100 mm Hg.) Because hemodynamic goals vary widely from center to center, close communication between surgeon and anesthesiologist is imperative. If rapid resuscitation of intravascular volume depletion is needed, low molecular weight hydroxyethyl starch is generally recommended by nephrologists and does not compromise coagulation if less than 33 mL/kg are given.[60] Neuromuscular blockade is usually accomplished with cisatracurium.

Once the first anastomosis is started, a diuresis is initiated (mannitol and furosemide are often both given). Heparin and verapamil should also be available in the operating room, and in some centers, anesthesiologists are asked to administer the
8 first doses of immunosuppression. A kidney graft is defective in concentrating urine and reabsorbing sodium, so attention to electrolytes is important. For patients with diabetes, intraoperative administration of insulin to normalize blood glucose has not been formally studied for improving outcome. However, more recent studies in ICU patients suggest that outcome is significantly improved when glucose is tightly controlled.[61] Therefore, optimal management of glucose (80 to 110 mg/dL) seems a reasonable anesthetic goal during renal transplantation. The entire surgery should take about 3 hours. Patient-controlled analgesia is a good choice for postoperative pain management. Nonsteroidal anti-inflammatory agents are contraindicated. Transplant recipients are generally discharged from the hospital within a week of surgery.

Transfusion is rarely required in the OR, although renal transplant patients are often anemic coming to surgery (and may be receiving erythropoietin). Because of immunosuppression, if cytomegalovirus (CMV)-negative patients receiving a CMV-negative organ are to receive transfusion, CMV-negative blood is preferred. Leukocyte filters are also effective in preventing CMV transmission but are probably inferior to CMV-negative blood.[62]

Most surgical complications of renal transplantation are not recognized in the operating room. The common (postoperative) complications are ureteral obstruction and fistulae, vascular thromboses, lymphoceles, and wound complications.[63] Rare complications from self-retaining retractors are bowel perforation and femoral neuropathy.[64]

Pediatric renal transplantation is associated with somewhat lower rates of success than adult transplantation, with vascular thromboses of the grafts more common in young children. Size mismatch may also be a consideration in some small children during the operation. Adult donors to small children require the graft placement in the retroperitoneum. Although chronic peritoneal dialysis may help expand the abdominal volume,[65] attention to peak inspiratory pressures at closure is important and increased pressures should be reported to the surgical team.

LIVER TRANSPLANTATION

Preoperative Considerations

9 Patients with ESLD have multisystem dysfunction with common cardiac, pulmonary, and renal compromise because of their liver disease (Table 53-5). Anesthesiologists should be consulted about liver transplant recipients before they are listed to help surgeons assess candidacy for transplant and to help optimize organ function prior to transplant. Common indications for adult liver transplantation are hepatitis C, Laennec's cirrhosis, and autoimmune diseases.

In an effort to minimize deaths on the liver transplant waiting list with objective factors (rather than "degree of ascites") and to develop a better method for predicting survival after transplantation, the scoring system for allocation of livers was changed in February 2002. Instead of Child's class, adult patients are tracked by the MELD (model for ESLD):[66]

$$\begin{aligned}\text{MELD Score} = {} & 0.957 \times \text{Log}_e\,(\text{creatinine in mg/dL}) \\ & + 0.378 \times \text{Log}_e\,(\text{total bilirubin in mg/dL}) \\ & + 1.12 \times \text{Log}_e\,(\text{INR}) \\ & + 0.643\end{aligned}$$

and pediatric patients using the pediatric end-stage liver disease score (PELD):

$$\begin{aligned}\text{PELD Score} = {} & (0.463[\text{age}^a] - 0.687 \times \text{Log}_e\,[\text{albumin g/dL}] \\ & + 0.480 \times \text{Log}_e\,[\text{total bilirubin mg/dL}] + 1.857 \\ & \times \text{Log}_e\,[\text{INR}] + 0.667\,[\text{growth failure}^b]) \times 10\end{aligned}$$

These scoring systems were adapted from analysis of survival in patients with ESLD independent of transplantation. Ongoing analysis of the MELD/PELD as predictors of transplant survival suggests that this new scoring system helps minimize death on the waiting list.

For adult patients, a major change with MELD is the priority given to patients with renal failure. The hope is that patients will be transplanted at a time when liver transplant can reverse hepatorenal syndrome, and before combined liver-kidney transplantation (associated with poor outcome) is necessary. Nonetheless, because poor renal function is a major risk factor for poor liver transplant outcome,[67] ongoing studies are needed to determine the utility of MELD in prioritizing patients for transplantation. The new system is also designed so ongoing evaluation of MELD/PELD scores is mandated. For example, the sickest patients are required to get laboratory studies for scoring every 48 hours.

Difficult decisions about patient candidacy are common in evaluating liver transplant candidates. Several are discussed here to highlight the need for regular involvement of a transplant anesthesiologist in the candidacy evaluation process. Liver disease does not protect patients from coronary artery disease. Most patients are screened for cardiac problems using dobutamine stress echocardiography.[68] Patients with inducible ischemia are generally evaluated with cardiac catheterization in an effort to identify lesions that can be fixed with percutaneous angioplasty. Patients with severe coronary artery disease are generally not candidates for liver transplantation. (Increasingly, cardiologists are using cardiac positron emission tomography scanning for the evaluation of ischemic disease in transplant candidates.) Significant aortic stenosis also presents a difficult dilemma pretransplant.[69] Because cardiac surgery is considered risky in a patient with ESLD, a new approach is to optimize valve area using valvuloplasty before liver transplantation. Then, after the liver graft is stable, aortic valve replacement can be considered.

Another difficult lesion for which echocardiography is a useful screening tool is portopulmonary hypertension. If screening echo suggests moderate to severe pulmonary hypertension (estimated systolic pulmonary artery [PA] pressure >50 mm Hg), right heart catheterization is suggested to document the severity of disease.[70] Multiple case reports and small retrospective reviews demonstrate that patients with portopulmonary hypertension are at substantial risk of perioperative death. There is general agreement that mean PA pressure >50 mm Hg is an absolute contraindication to liver transplantation. Patients with PA pressures between 35 and 50 mm Hg and pulmonary vascular resistance (PVR) >250 dynes·seconds·cm^{-5} are also likely at increased risk, and should be treated to lower PA pressure before proceeding with transplantation.[71] Epoprostenol is the usual first-line therapy for portopulmonary hypertension

^{a}<1 year old = 1; >1 year old = 0
^{b}>2 SD below mean for age = 1; ≤2SD below median for age = 0

TABLE 53-5

MULTISYSTEM COMPLICATIONS OF END-STAGE LIVER DISEASE

SYSTEM	CONSEQUENCE
Central nervous system	Fatigue
Encephalopathy (confusion to coma)	Blood-brain barrier disruption and intracranial hypertension (acute liver failure)
Pulmonary	Hypoxemia/hepatopulmonary syndrome
Respiratory alkalosis	
Pulmonary hypertension	
Cardiovascular	Reduced systemic vascular resistance
Hyperdynamic circulation	
Diastolic dysfunction	
Prolonged QT interval	
Blunted responses to inotropes	
Blunted responses to vasopressors	
Gastrointestinal	Gastrointestinal bleeding from varices
Ascites	
Delayed gastric emptying	
Hematologic	Hypersplenism (pancytopenia)
Decreased synthesis of clotting factors	
Impaired fibrinolytic mechanisms	
Renal	Hepatorenal syndrome
Hyponatremia	
Endocrine	Glucose intolerance
Osteoporosis	
Nutritional/metabolic	Muscle wasting and weakness
Poor skin integrity	
Increased volume of distribution for drugs	
Decreased citrate metabolism	

and is effective in lowering PA pressures significantly in many patients,[72] but requires home intravenous delivery in the United States. Sildenafil is an alternative for preoperative treatment of portopulmonary hypertension.[73]

PFTs are also used for screening liver transplant candidates. Severe hypoxemia in the setting of liver disease (hepatopulmonary syndrome or HPS) was once a contraindication to liver transplantation. However, if transplants are performed before anatomic changes of the lung are fixed, liver transplantation may cure HPS.[74] Inhaled NO[75] and transjugular intrahepatic portosystemic shunt (TIPS)[76] may help bridge patients with severe HPS to transplantation. (TIPS is also used to stabilize renal dysfunction, severe ascites, and variceal hemorrhages, but similar to surgical shunting, is associated with worsening of encephalopathy.) If HPS is severe and completely unresponsive to oxygen, transplantation is risky because the immediate perioperative period may be complicated by frank graft hypoxia and failure. Fortunately, most patients with HPS have some element of physiologic V/Q mismatch, are oxygen responsive, and with this "room to move" can be safely transplanted.

Intraoperative Procedures

Management of these patients has progressed substantially in the last 5 years with collected experience of transplant teams, such that intraoperative extubation of some patients is routine in busier centers. Nonetheless, intensive preparation for surgery is important because it is difficult to predict which patients are at risk for massive blood loss. We place invasive lines and monitors after induction of general anesthesia. Rapid sequence induction of general anesthesia is indicated because patients with ESLD often have gastroparesis[77] in addition to increased intra-abdominal pressure from ascites. We place two arterial catheters, one in the left radial and one in the right femoral artery. Although venovenous bypass is now rarely used in our center, the left radial catheter serves as a monitor of disruption of arterial flow if the axillary vein is used for bypass, and the right femoral arterial line leaves the left groin free for surgical bypass access. Pulmonary artery catheters or continuous echocardiography are used for monitoring volume status, and at least two large-bore catheters are placed for rapid intravenous infusions (9F each). In many centers, anesthesiologists also place percutaneous lines that can be modified and used for bypass, if necessary.[78,79] Bladder catheters and nasogastric tubes are placed in all patients. A rapid infusion system with the ability to deliver at least 500 mL/minute warmed blood is primed and in the room. Before surgical incision, blood product availability is confirmed and some blood products are in the room and checked (routinely 10 U red cells and 10 U FFP). Normothermia, essential for optimal hemostasis, is maintained with convective warming blankets over the legs and over the upper chest, arms, and head.

10 Liver transplantation is a complex surgical procedure, traditionally described in three phases: dissection, anhepatic, and neohepatic phases, with reperfusion of the graft marking the start of the neohepatic phase. During the dissection phase of surgery, blood loss may be high. The major anesthetic goals of this phase are correction of coagulopathies and maintenance of intravascular volume for renal protection.

Coagulation Management

Similar to any other surgical procedure, FFP is used to maintain INR $\leq$1.5 in any patient with anticipated or ongoing bleeding.[80] With rapid infusion of FFP, citrate binding of ionized calcium often requires treatment. A low dose infusion of $CaCl_2$ is better at maintaining constant Ca^{++} levels than are intermittent boluses (usually 0.5 g $CaCl_2$/hour). Platelet transfusion is used to maintain platelet count higher than 50,000/mm^3. In addition, we use cryoprecipitate concentrates to maintain fibrinogen >150 mg/dL. Cell saver blood may also be used to limit allogeneic transfusions.

Despite the complex coagulopathy in ESLD that makes intraoperative hemostasis difficult, many patients with liver disease simultaneously have a hypercoagulable state. For example, patients with autoimmune liver diseases may have antiphospholipid antibodies (and many other causes of hypercoagulable states are possible in ESLD). So, in addition to monitoring discrete parts of the coagulation profile to guide transfusion therapies, it is important to look at a measure of entire clotting mechanism. Many centers use thrombelastography,[81] others use bedside Lee-White clotting times. Using these tests, normal or hypernormal whole clotting in the presence of high INR, low platelets (and usually elevated D-dimers) should be taken as a caution that the patient may have a clinically significant hypercoagulable state. Under these circumstances, our approach is to maintain transfusion therapies as noted previously and to avoid pharmacologic procoagulant drugs. For the majority of patients with synthetic dysfunction, thrombocytopenia, and hypofibrinogenemia, clotting is delayed. In these patients, many centers supplement transfusion therapy with antifibrinolytic agents.

Worldwide, considerable center-dependent variation in the antifibrinolytic and dose of drug used makes generalizations difficult. The majority of adult patients in our center receive epsilon-aminocaproic acid (EACA; 5 g load and 1 g/hour infusion) to support hemostasis during surgery.[82] Other centers use considerably less drug, less often. Many centers, particularly in Europe, use aprotinin routinely during liver transplantation,[83] but several case reports of fatal pulmonary embolism associated with aprotinin use[84] have made many U.S. centers shy away from the drug during liver transplantation. Fibrinolysis acutely worsens immediately after reperfusion to varying degrees, depending largely on the amount of tissue plasminogen activator (tPA) released from the graft.[85] A (re)bolus of EACA (again doses are highly variable) is helpful to maintain hemostasis once this postreperfusion exacerbation of fibrinolysis is documented.

Activated factor VII (NovoSeven, Novo Nordisk, Copenhagen, Denmark) is approved in Europe and appears to be a safe hemostatic agent during liver transplantation.[86] When this drug is given, INR rapidly normalizes,[87] even though the amount of circulating clotting factors does not change. Although no literature has commented on this resultant inability to use the prothrombin time (PT) to guide FFP transfusion, it must be kept in mind that significant synthesis of coagulation factors may take days after liver transplantation, and a normal PT in this setting does not imply normal coagulation factor reserve. In our center, acute NovoSeven administration has been useful for surgical hemostasis for placement of intracranial pressure monitors in patients with acute liver failure and for selected patients undergoing liver transplantation with difficult red cell cross matches.

Perioperative renal dysfunction is a major problem in liver transplantation, so protection of the kidneys is a critical feature of managing liver transplant patients. Virtually all anesthetics reduce renal blood flow, and it is not uncommon for urine output to decrease dramatically in these patients with induction of anesthesia. Creatinine levels may grossly underestimate the degree of renal dysfunction, especially in ESLD patients with significant muscle wasting.[88] Hepatorenal syndrome (HRS) is a functional renal disorder associated with liver disease and categorized as type 1 (acute severe decompensation, creatinine >2.5 mg/dL), which is usually fatal, and type 2 (chronic, moderate renal failure with Cr >1.5 and GFR <40 mL/min). More recent evidence suggests that albumin may play a role in preventing and treating HRS in the setting of spontaneous bacterial peritonitis.[89] In addition, large volume (>5 L) drainage of ascites with incision is really a paracentesis that should be accompanied by albumin therapy to prevent renal decompensation, with recommended albumin doses of 6 to 8 g/L of ascites drained.[90] Terlipressin (not available in the United States) is a new option for treating HRS.[91] This drug is metabolized into lysine-vasopressin, and for this reason, if hemodynamic support is needed in the setting of HRS, low-dose vasopressin may be a good choice. Other studies suggest that norepinephrine is also well-tolerated and may even improve renal function in patients with type 1 HRS,[92] and for this reason, we use norepinephrine as vasopressor of choice during liver transplantation. There are no prospective trials to support use of one vasopressor over another during transplantation, and anesthesiologists are obligated for now to keep pace with the ICU literature concerning the best treatment for patients with HRS. The most important consideration is to ensure adequate volume replacement before instituting diuresis in the OR.

The *anhepatic phase* begins when the liver is functionally excluded (clamped) from the circulation. Traditionally, the vena cava is clamped above (suprahepatic anastomosis) and below (infrahepatic anastomosis) the liver, the portal vein, and hepatic artery are clamped. With complete cava cross-clamp, venous return falls by 50 to 60%, often resulting in hypotension. Venovenous bypass may be used to increase venous return, improve systemic hemodynamics, increase renal perfusion pressure, and decompress portal pressures for a better surgical field.[93] Venovenous bypass certainly facilitated teaching of a generation of liver transplant surgeons, but experienced centers tend to use it increasingly less. Most patients can be managed without venovenous bypass using some volume loading (vasopressors are rarely required), but other anesthesiologists use vasopressors to support pressures during bypass. Bypass carries potential complications, including arm lymphedema, air embolism, and vascular injury, and its benefit is limited when anhepatic times are short,[94] but it is still used for selected patients in many centers. Furthermore, modification of the surgical technique to preserve caval flow (piggyback technique)[95] clearly results in more stable hemodynamics during the anhepatic period, and venovenous bypass is not needed when this surgical technique is used.

Reperfusion of the graft is the most treacherous time of the liver transplant. Communication between the surgical and anesthesia teams is essential in preparing for reperfusion. Caval clamps are removed first, and the integrity of the caval anastomoses are assured. Caval reperfusion is usually hemodynamically well tolerated. However, portal vein reperfusion (despite flushing of the graft) can often result in hemodynamic instability. The original descriptions of reperfusion syndrome emphasized (often severe) hypotension and bradycardia with portal reperfusion.[96] Now, with flushing techniques that precede reperfusion[97] and changes in preservation solution, bradycardia is uncommon. Typically, reperfusion is associated with hypotension (further drop of already low SVR and increase in CO), which may or may not require treatment.

Our preparation for reperfusion is to give sodium bicarbonate just before unclamping (50 mEq) to meet the acid load from the graft, and 500 mg $CaCl_2$ exactly simultaneous with portal unclamping to counteract the effects of potassium on the heart. If, despite this preparation, T waves (ECG) become elevated, the same treatment is repeated. Other anesthesiologists wait to see T-wave changes before treating. Lidocaine, atropine, and norepinephrine are also available at the time of reperfusion in case of ventricular arrhythmias, bradyarrhythmias, and severe hypotension. Hepatic artery unclamping is usually not hemodynamically significant.

Neohepatic Period

After hemodynamic stability is achieved, the calcium infusion is stopped. One early indication of graft function is the lack of a calcium requirement even when FFP is being infused rapidly. Usually within 30 minutes, the base deficit improves with graft metabolism of citrate. Within the first hour, the CO decreases and SVR increases as the graft metabolizes vasoactive substances. These are early signs of good graft function. In addition, the graft appearance should be noted. It should have a smooth edge, no evidence of engorgement, and bile is made in the first half-hour after reperfusion. Often, renal function improves after reperfusion, probably due to graft metabolism of renal vasoconstrictors.

During the neohepatic period, biliary anastomoses are completed, and sources of surgical bleeding are corrected. Drains are placed, and the abdomen closed. Fast-tracking protocols for liver transplant patients are common in experienced centers.[98]

Pediatric Liver Transplantation

Indications for pediatric liver transplantation differ considerably from adults, with inherited disorders dominating the preop diagnoses (Table 53-6). Children younger than 1 year of age with inherited liver disease are often very small for age. In addition, such a wide variety of metabolic diseases mandates that anesthesiologists consult specialty textbooks for medical management of children with unusual disorders. In small children, a radial artery catheter and at least one large (18 g) peripheral intravenous line are placed after induction of anesthesia. Surgeons may place tunneled central lines before incision, useful for postoperative administration of drugs as well as CVP monitoring during surgery. Children with previous Kasai operations for biliary atresia may have massive bleeding due to adhesions in the dissection phase. Small children receiving large grafts may have respiratory compromise with abdominal closure. Because hepatic artery thrombosis (HAT) is a more common complication in children than adults, some centers choose to have INR at the end of surgery in the 1.8 to 2 range. HAT is

TABLE 53-6

DIAGNOSES LEADING TO LIVER TRANSPLANTATION IN CHILDREN

■ DIAGNOSIS	■ % OF WAITING LIST
Biliary atresia	23.8
Other cholestatic diseases	
Alagille's syndrome	3.8
Inherited metabolic diseases	
α-1-antitrypsin deficiency	2.9
Wilson's disease	1.2
Tyrosinemia	1.1
Glycogen storage diseases	0.6
Acute (fulminant) liver failure	3.1
Chronic active hepatitis	
Neonatal hepatitis	0.6
Autoimmune cirrhosis	3.7
Tumors	
Cystic fibrosis	
Total parenteral nutrition/ hyperalimentation	8.0

Adapted from data from UNOS (*www.unos.org*).

generally recognized to be a technical issue related to the small diameter of arteries in children,[99] and intraoperative reanastomosis may be required if flow is inadequate through the artery. Aortic cross-clamping may be required for these anastomoses.

Acute Liver Failure

Anesthetic considerations for both adults and children with acute liver failure are focused on protection of the brain. Patients with acute or fulminant hepatic failure may have a rapidly progressive course of elevated intracranial pressure (ICP), leading to herniation and death. Intracranial pressure monitoring is useful in managing these patients but risks intracranial bleeding. Vasodilating anesthetics (all inhalation agents) are to be avoided, especially without ICP monitoring. In our experience, pentothal infusion is a good maintenance anesthetic, and acute rises in ICP can be managed with etomidate. When antihypertensive therapy is required, labetalol does not cause significant cerebral vasodilation in these patients.[100] Management of intracranial hypertension is discussed in greater detail in Chapter 27.

PANCREAS AND ISLET TRANSPLANTATION

The majority of pancreas transplants (about three-fourths) are done as simultaneous pancreas/kidney transplants from a single cadaveric donor. Pancreata grafted in these procedures have the best long-term survival, compared with grafts done after kidney transplantation, or (independent) pancreas grafts. Independent pancreas grafts are usually performed for patients with type I diabetes who have frequent metabolic complications (hypoglycemia) but preserved renal function. Living donor partial pancreas grafts are not commonly performed, with the largest ongoing experience at the University of Minnesota.[101]

The preoperative assessment of pancreas transplant recipients focuses on the end-organ complications of diabetes reviewed in Chapter 41. Monitoring will depend on cardiac status, but generally patients do not require PA catheters, and have been evaluated for risk of intraoperative cardiac complications as part of the transplant workup. Nonetheless, cardiovascular disease is present in many patients undergoing pancreas transplantation.

The major difference between pancreas transplantation and other procedures is that strict attention to control of blood glucose is indicated to protect newly transplanted beta cells from hyperglycemic damage. No formula for controlling blood glucose has emerged as a standard of intraoperative management. In general, if adult patients arrive with glucose >250 mg/dL, 10 U of insulin can be given intravenously, followed by an infusion of insulin. The infusion starting rate varies, depending on the initial blood glucose level. Once blood glucose levels are controlled (<150 mg/dL), intravenous 5% dextrose (about 100 mL/ hour) should also be infused as the insulin infusion is continued. The most important issue is to check the response to insulin frequently and adjust infusions as necessary. No literature exists for a patient with an implanted insulin pump, but it seems reasonable to continue to use the pump at basal rates in these patients as long as its operation is reviewed[102] and blood glucoses are monitored regularly during surgery.

Islet transplants were revived by the Edmonton protocol, published in 2000.[103] The major changes introduced included a glucocorticoid-free immunosuppression regimen and immediate transplantation of islets after isolation. Because processing of islets takes only a few hours, the new protocols mean little flexibility in timing islet transplants—the sooner the islets are transplanted, the better they will function. Islets are generally infused into the portal circulation. Acute portal hypertension is a feared complication.[104]

SMALL BOWEL AND MULTIVISCERAL TRANSPLANTATION

In 2003, the American Gastroenterological Association published a medical position statement concerning indications for intestinal transplantation (*http://www.guideline.gov/summary/summary.aspx?ss=15&doc_id=3795&nbr=3021#s23*). Indications for intestinal transplantation include impending liver failure in patients with intestinal failure (or short gut syndromes requiring total parenteral nutrition [TPN]), frequent severe dehydration in patients with intestinal failure, and severe complications of central lines for TPN (sepsis, thrombosis of central veins). Patients who develop liver failure from TPN for intestinal failure are candidates for combined liver-intestine transplantation. In these cases, liver failure should be irreversible, and biopsy findings are often required for this conclusion in patients without overt ESLD,[105] especially because isolated intestinal transplantation may have better results than the combined procedure.[106] In general, intestinal transplantation should only be considered in patients with life-threatening complications of their intestinal failure.

11 For anesthesiologists, a major hurdle for these transplants is line placement adequate for transfusion of blood products and fluids, which may be substantial during these long cases. Anesthesiologists should review angiographic studies to determine patency before attempting central line placement. Ultrasound devices are helpful in identifying the known patent vessels for cannulation, but surgical cutdowns for venous access may be necessary, including transhepatic or intraoperative renal vein catheterization.[107] Superior vena cava or inferior vena cava obstruction may require preoperative intervention (surgical and/or lytic) so adequate vascular access for surgery is possible.[108] Antibiotic regimens should be continued during the surgery. Nitrous oxide, as in liver transplantation, is avoided.

Common complications of intestinal failure include dehydration and electrolyte abnormalities, gastric acid hypersecretion, pancreatic insufficiency, bone disease, and TPN-induced liver failure.[109] Because electrolyte abnormalities are common, they should be monitored continuously during surgery and appropriate replacement instituted. Because enteral feeding will not be possible until weeks after surgery, TPN should be continued in the perioperative period.

Like reperfusion of liver grafts, intestinal reperfusion is associated with an acute release of acid and potassium from the graft. Anticipatory bicarbonate and $CaCl_2$ administration is used to counteract the effects of acid and potassium on the heart. After reperfusion, coagulopathy may worsen, usually managed by reassessment of INR, fibrinogen and platelet counts, and correction with blood products.

LUNG TRANSPLANTATION

Lung transplantation is now accepted therapy for end-stage pulmonary and pulmonary vascular disease, building on successful case series from the early 1980s.[110,111] UNOS reports more than 11,000 lung transplant procedures since 1995, but more than 3,000 patients have died awaiting transplant in this same time frame, due to the shortage of suitable organs. The Registry of the International Society for Heart and Lung Transplantation (ISHLT) lists chronic obstructive pulmonary disease, idiopathic pulmonary fibrosis, cystic fibrosis (CF), and

α_1-antitrypsin deficiency as the most common preoperative diagnoses.[112]

Surgical options for lung transplantation are single lung transplant, en bloc double and sequential double transplants, and heart-lung transplantation. Single and sequential double lung transplants can be performed without cardiopulmonary bypass (CPB), although CPB is often used, especially for recipients with pulmonary hypertension. Bilateral lung transplantation is most commonly used in patients with associated pulmonary vascular disease and CF-related bronchiectasis. Single lung transplantation for emphysema gained favor based on good short-term outcomes, with the added advantage of leaving a donor lung for another recipient. Lung transplant centers vary in their use of single or double lung transplant for varying diagnoses, and the better procedure based on recipient preoperative status and diagnosis is still debated.[113] It is generally agreed that double lung transplantation is indicated in the presence of pulmonary infection (CF), severe bullous emphysema, and primary pulmonary hypertension (PPH). Eisenmenger syndrome is managed with single or bilateral lung transplantation.

Recipient Selection

International Guidelines for the Selection of Lung Transplant Candidates were published in 1988 by consensus agreement
tab 53-7 of several thoracic societies (summarized in Table 53-7).[114] In general, patients should be considered for lung transplantation if they exhibit decline in pulmonary function, despite maximal medical therapy, and expected life span is only 2 to 3 years. Contraindications to lung transplantation are based on their impact on long-term survival. Symptomatic osteoporosis, thoracic musculoskeletal abnormalities, corticosteroid use, nutritional status (<70% or >130% of ideal body weight), active addiction or psychiatric conditions, mechanical ventilation, and colonization with resistant organisms are relative contraindications. Absolute contraindications are significant dysfunction of other organs particularly kidney and heart, HIV or chronic hepatitis B or C, and malignancy (other than basal cell or squamous cell skin carcinoma). Patients with significant cardiac disease can be considered for heart-lung transplantation, but are not candidates for isolated lung transplant.

As for other transplants, patients are screened for malignancy (mammography, Pap test, colonoscopy). Systemic disease processes such as diabetes and hypertension are not considered contraindications, as long as they are clinically stable and medically optimized. Lung transplantation has not been advocated for acute disease processes, such as acute respiratory distress syndrome. PFTs, left and right heart catheterization, and transthoracic echocardiography are routinely used for evaluating recipients. Survival is inversely correlated with patient age, and for these reasons, recommended age limits are

Heart-lung transplant: 55 years
Double lung transplant: 60 years
Single lung transplant: 65 years

A voluntary survey of current clinical practices in North America found remarkable concordance among transplant centers in their patient selection criteria,[115] similar to criteria listed in Table 53-7.

CF is associated with complex pulmonary infections that clearly impact transplant outcomes.[116,117] Patients infected with *Burkholderia cepacia* have poor outcome, and many U.S. centers consider this infection (or some subtypes of the organism) a contraindication to transplantation.[117,118] Twenty-year data by the Toronto group found better long-term survival in CF patients free of *B. cepacia* than in similar patients who were infected.[119]

TABLE 53-7

LUNG RECIPIENT SELECTION GUIDELINES

GENERAL INDICATIONS

End-stage lung disease
Failed maximal medical treatment of lung disease
Age within limits for planned transplant
Life expectancy <2–3 yr
Ability to walk and undergo rehabilitation
Sound nutritional status (70–130% of ideal body weight)
Stable psychosocial profile
No significant comorbid disease

DISEASE-SPECIFIC INDICATIONS

COPD	FEV_1 <25% of predicted value after bronchodilators and/or $PaCO_2$ = 55 mm Hg and/or pulmonary hypertension (especially with cor pulmonale) Chronic O_2 therapy
Cystic fibrosis	FEV_1 <30% predicted Hypoxemia, hypercapnia, or rapidly declining lung function Weight loss and hemoptysis Frequent exacerbations, especially young females Absence of antibiotic-resistant organisms
Idiopathic pulmonary fibrosis	Vital capacity <60–65% of predicted Resting hypoxemia Progression of disease despite therapy (steroids)
Pulmonary hypertension	NYHA functional status class III or IV, despite prostacyclin therapy Mean right atrial pressure >15 mm Hg Mean pulmonary artery pressure >55 mm Hg Cardiac index <2 L/min per m^2
Eisenmenger's syndrome	NYHA class III or IV, despite optimal therapy
Pediatric	NYHA class III or IV Disease unresponsive to maximal therapy Cor pulmonale, cyanosis, low cardiac output

COPD, chronic obstructive pulmonary disease; FEV_1, forced expiratory volume in 1 sec; NYHA, New York Heart Association.

Preanesthetic Considerations

Medical evaluation prior to listing a patient for transplantation encompasses many specialties. Unfortunately, anesthesiologists are not always included in this process. If the patient has been on the waiting list for an extended period, it is important to review lab and functional data because diagnostic testing was performed for transplant listing. It is critical to confirm ABO compatibility of donor and recipient prior to surgery. By definition, lung transplant candidates have poor pulmonary status and are frequently receiving multiple therapies, including oxygen, inhaled bronchodilators, steroids, and vasodilators. These medications should be continued in the perioperative period. Because of the short ischemic times needed for optimal organ function, the procedure must be performed as soon as an organ becomes available, precluding delay of cases for full stomachs.

Although patients are understandably anxious, they also have minimal pulmonary reserve, and sedation must be done carefully under monitored conditions. After determining oxygen saturation, slow, incremental dosing of a short-acting benzodiazepine (0.25 to 1.0 mg midazolam) is used for anxiolysis. Narcotic premedication must be given with extreme care in hypercarbic patients. Premedication with a combination of metoclopramide, histamine-2 antagonists, and a nonparticulate antacid is usually warranted. Many patients are not able to rest supine or in the Trendelenburg position for placement of central access. Placement of large-bore peripheral intravenous catheter and arterial access is usually adequate for initiation of the anesthetic, with central access placed after induction. Placement of a PA catheter with continuous cardiac output and mixed venous oxygenation monitoring provides both rapid assessment of cardiopulmonary status changes and minimizes the fluid administration necessary for frequent cardiac output determinations. Epidural catheters are placed preoperatively at some centers, especially in patients who are believed unlikely to require CPB. (It is not always possible, however, to determine need for CPB preoperatively.) The American Society for Regional Anesthesia Consensus statement on regional anesthesia in the anticoagulated patient[120] states that there is currently insufficient evidence to determine the risk of neuraxial hematoma in patients receiving neuraxial anesthesia and full systemic anticoagulation. Another option is to place the epidural in the early postoperative period after coagulopathies are corrected. This can be done in the lightly sedated patient during weaning of the ventilator, allowing better neurologic monitoring and optimizing pain control prior to extubation. It is currently recommended that recipients receive antibiotics based on donor Gram's stain results, with alteration of therapy as necessary after receipt of culture data.[121]

Intraoperative Management: Single Lung Transplantation

Lung transplant recipients tend to be chronically intravascularly volume depleted, and anesthetic induction can be associated with hypotension. Because fluid restriction is beneficial for postoperative management, small fluid boluses and slow induction with etomidate and narcotics are prudent. These patients remain intubated for hours to days postoperatively, so a fast-track anesthetic technique is unnecessary. A balanced technique combining narcotic and inhalational anesthetics is preferred. Muscle relaxation can be maintained with any nonhistamine-releasing agent. Nitrous oxide is rarely an anesthetic option due to bullous emphysematous disease, pulmonary hypertension, or intraoperative hypoxemia. Lung isolation, preferably with a double-lumen endotracheal tube, is necessary for single and bilateral sequential lung transplantation. The double-lumen endotracheal tube facilitates suctioning of secretions and improved deflation of the operative lung during the initial dissection. A bronchial blocker is more easily dislodged with surgical manipulation, may not provide isolation of the right upper lobe, and requires repositioning midsurgery in the case of a bilateral sequential procedure. Left-sided endotracheal tubes are preferred, due to ease of positioning within the left main-stem bronchus.

A single lung transplant can be performed via posterolateral thoracotomy position. If the surgeon is concerned about possible need for CPB, then the patient must be positioned to allow rapid access to either the aorta and right atrium or the femoral artery and vein. This can be accomplished via either anterior thoracotomy with partial sternotomy or posterolateral thoracotomy with decreased angulation of the hips to allow access to the femoral vessels. Determination of operative side is based on preoperative ventilation-perfusion studies and prior thoracic surgeries. The lung with poorer function is typically the one replaced.

During one-lung ventilation, hypoxemia is common. Strategies to improve oxygenation and ventilation are the same as those discussed in Chapter 29. Introduction of anesthesia machines with pressure-controlled ventilation has diminished the need for ICU ventilators during the operative procedure. Although an ICU ventilator can provide improvement in oxygenation and ventilation, it does not allow concomitant use of inhalational anesthetic, an option available on the newer anesthesia machines.

Lung recipients are susceptible to development of pulmonary hypertension and right ventricular (RV) dysfunction or failure during one-lung ventilation. Optimizing oxygenation and ventilation does not always improve RV function, and vasodilator and/or inotropic support may be required. Some anesthesiologists use inhaled nitric oxide (INO) routinely for lung transplantation,[122] whereas others[123] believe the potential adverse side effects mean its use should be more restricted. Proponents argue that use of INO in the recipient, and possibly even the donor, takes advantage of immunomodulatory and antimicrobial activities of NO that reduce recipient lung injury.[122,124] Opponents argue INO use should be limited to the population at risk for needing CPB during lung transplantation 12 and to patients with reperfusion injury. They cite risks of methemoglobinemia, NO metabolite-related lung injury, and decreased sensitivity of exhaled NO monitoring as a diagnostic tool for acute lung rejection. Further study is needed to confirm the findings in a small cohort suggesting that INO is safe and effective in lung transplantation patients.[125]

NO has an extremely short duration of action in vivo, rapidly inactivated by reacting with heme, producing methemoglobin. INO therapy is used to decrease pulmonary vascular resistance and improve oxygenation. Because INO is preferentially delivered to ventilated areas, vascular relaxation in these areas leads to improved blood flow, and hence improvements in ventilation-perfusion mismatch and improved oxygenation. Rapid inactivation of INO in the pulmonary vasculature prevents systemic vasorelaxation and resulting systolic hypotension.

NO activates NOS in other tissues to produce other clinically beneficial actions. NO activates guanylate cyclase in platelets to attenuate platelet aggregation and adhesion.[126] NO can potentiate microbial killing.[127] INO can thus decrease pulmonary vascular resistance, improve oxygenation, decrease inflammatory response to surgery or trauma, impede microbial growth, and have an effect limited only to the pulmonary system. Its use in successful management of lung transplant patients is well documented.[122,124,125]

CPB is indicated during lung transplantation if adequate oxygenation cannot be maintained, despite ventilatory and pharmacologic maneuvers and PA clamping by the surgeons. Inability to ventilate or development of RV dysfunction is also an indication for CPB. After pneumonectomy, the surgeon will size the donor vascular tissue to the recipient vessels, and sequentially anastomose the atrial/pulmonary vein patch, bronchus, and pulmonary artery. The lung is kept cool with packed ice in the field until reperfusion. Circulation is restored to the donor lung, suture lines are checked for hemostasis, and then ventilation is begun. Systemic hypotension can occur during reperfusion, but it is not as significant as that seen with liver graft reperfusion. Hyperkalemia is also not a common reperfusion event. There can, however, be reperfusion injury to the lung presenting as pulmonary edema. PEEP is useful in this scenario. Bronchoscopy to suction secretions and blood is recommended to improve ventilation and oxygenation, and to examine bronchial suture lines.

Intraoperative transesophageal echocardiography (TEE) has become a valuable tool in the assessment of lung transplant patients. A comprehensive TEE exam should be performed after induction of anesthesia with attention focused on biventricular function, presence of valvular regurgitation, patent foramen ovale (PFO) or atrial septal defect (ASD), and pulse wave Doppler flow patterns in the pulmonary veins. Significant RV dysfunction, valvular regurgitation, or intraatrial shunt may lead the surgeon to plan the operation with CPB. TEE can be helpful in monitoring RV function during initial clamping of the PA for a procedure done without CPB. After reperfusion, another comprehensive TEE exam should be performed. Pulmonary vein anastomotic obstruction can be diagnosed with careful Doppler exam of the pulmonary venous inflow. Because this condition leads to a high incidence of acute graft failure, rapid diagnosis and treatment in the OR are beneficial.

At the completion of the procedure, the patient should be evaluated for exchange of the double-lumen endotracheal tube to a large (8 mm ID or larger) single-lumen endotracheal tube. Significant oropharyngeal edema or high PEEP requirement justify leaving the double-lumen tube in place for 24 hours to allow improvement in clinical status.

Double Lung Transplantation

Bilateral lung transplant is performed in the supine position via the clamshell incision. The arms can be suspended on a padded bar above the patient or tucked at the sides. These cases can also be performed with sternotomy. En bloc double lung transplant requires CPB, and a single-lumen endotracheal tube is sufficient. Bilateral sequential transplantation requires lung isolation, preferably via a double-lumen endotracheal tube. Bilateral sequential transplant is now the preferred procedure because a tracheal anastomosis is unnecessary, and surgical bleeding is less. Most centers electively institute CPB for this procedure in the presence of preoperative pulmonary hypertension, and urgent CPB for indications discussed previously. Serial implantation implies longer ischemic time for the second lung, but this has not adversely affected outcome. The clamshell incision is extensive and can cause significant postoperative pain. Thoracic epidurals are often used to provide pain relief.

Pediatric Lung Transplantation

The Registry of the International Society for Heart and Lung Transplantation Pediatric Report indicates that transplantation of very young children is becoming increasingly uncommon.[128] Instead, adolescents are being transplanted, and the most common diagnoses are cystic fibrosis (CF), congenital heart disease, and primary pulmonary hypertension. Congenital heart disease is the most common indication in infants. Survival is worse for pediatric than for adult lung transplant recipients, and has not improved significantly since 1992, with 5-year survival about 40%. Patients receiving bilateral lung transplants have a better outcome than those receiving single lung transplantation. Only 634 pediatric lung transplants are reported in the UNOS database, and 93 of these are living-related donor lung transplant (LRDLT). The literature regarding pediatric lung transplantation suggests a small increase in life span and an increase in quality of life in the majority of the survivors at 3 years. Cautious optimism appears to be the current status of this procedure.

Most pediatric patients receive double lung transplantation with CPB. Single lung procedures are reserved for larger adolescents with CF. A single-lumen endotracheal tube is adequate. The clamshell incision is used. Central and arterial access is necessary for perioperative monitoring purposes.

Heart-Lung Transplant (Adult and Pediatric)

Heart-lung transplantation is the least common intrathoracic transplant procedure. UNOS lists 834 total procedures to date, with 146 in the pediatric age group. Only 10 cases were reported worldwide in 2001.[128] Bilateral sequential lung transplant has largely replaced heart-lung transplantation, combined with advances in the pharmacologic management of pulmonary hypertension and RV failure. PPH and pulmonary hypertension associated Eisenmenger syndrome are the most common indications for heart-lung transplant. CF is the third most common diagnosis, with the CF native heart usually given to another recipient (domino procedure). Patients with Eisenmenger syndrome have the best survival rates in the adult population (ISHLT adult 2003).[129] Anesthetic management of these patients is similar to that of isolated heart or lung transplantation. Because a tracheal anastomosis is performed, a single-lumen endotracheal tube is adequate. The endotracheal tube is either removed or withdrawn above the suture line during CPB. Inotropes may be needed for RV dysfunction immediately postbypass. Pulmonary reperfusion injury can also occur, requiring PEEP and suctioning, as during isolated lung transplantation.

HEART TRANSPLANTATION

Since Christian Barnard performed the first successful heart transplant in South Africa in 1967, the procedure has moved into the realm of acceptable practice for treatment of heart failure recalcitrant to medical therapy. More than 36,000 individuals have received heart transplants in the United States since 1988. Unfortunately, more than 6,000 patients died while waiting for a donor during that time. Currently, more than 3,000 patients await heart transplants (*www.unos.org*). Overall, 1-year survival has improved from 74% in the early 1980s to 86% in the late 1990s.[130] Ten-year survival was 40% in one study.[131]

The most common diagnoses leading to transplantation are ischemic and idiopathic dilated cardiomyopathies. Less common diagnoses include viral, infiltrative, postpartum, and congenital heart disease-related heart failure.[129] Due to the limited availability of donor organs, technologies that can extend the life of patients waiting for donors have developed. Temporary implantation of a ventricular assist device can provide circulatory support to critically ill patients. Newer versions of the left ventricular assist devices (LVADs) are small enough that some centers are using these devices as permanent treatment for heart failure.[132] Totally implantable artificial hearts are not currently used because of technical issues. Heterotopic heart transplantation has been virtually abandoned.

Recipient Selection

In 1996, the 5-year survival for CHF was reported to be less than 30%.[133] Medical therapy of CHF has improved dramatically in the past 10 years. Current pharmacologic therapy includes angiotensin-converting enzyme (ACE) inhibitors, beta-blockers (specifically carvedilol), diuretics, and digoxin. Cardiac resynchronization therapy can also improve symptoms, exercise tolerance, and quality of life in properly selected patients;[134] however, long-term survival data are not yet available. More than 2 million Americans have CHF, with the incidence increasing with age. Of these, only about 6,000 per year are listed for heart transplantation.

Consensus guidelines for selection criteria were last published in 1993[135] with some recent modifications.[130,136] Patients referred for transplant evaluation should have New York Heart Association class III or IV heart failure, despite optimal medical therapy. Surgical correction of coronary artery disease or valvular heart disease should be undertaken prior to listing. Patients with severe mitral regurgitation and low ejection fraction should be considered for mitral valve repair instead of transplantation because survival is better than with transplantation.[136] Most candidates have severe left ventricular systolic dysfunction; however, transplantation is occasionally indicated for treatment of refractory angina, unmanageable arrhythmias, or diastolic heart failure.

Prognosis in patients with CHF has been linked to functional capacity. Maximal exercise testing with oxygen uptake (VO_2) is an excellent method to determine functional capacity.[136] In patients on a stable medical regimen, maximal VO_2 less than 10 mL/kg/min is associated with a poor prognosis. Patients with VO_2 greater than 10 mL/kg/min have a better 1-year prognosis with medical therapy than transplantation. Patients with Holter monitor evidence of asymptomatic, significant ventricular ectopy should be considered for transplantation to reduce the risk of sudden death.

Pulmonary hypertension is associated with increased perioperative mortality, so severe, irreversible pulmonary hypertension is a contraindication to transplant. Right heart catheterization is performed to determine transpulmonary gradient (the difference between mean PA and PCWP) and pulmonary arteriolar resistance. Transpulmonary gradient >12 indicates significant pathology. Pulmonary arteriolar resistance (the ratio of transpulmonary gradient to cardiac output, expressed as Wood units) >2.5 also indicates a high risk of perioperative RV failure. Patients with elevated transpulmonary gradient or pulmonary arteriolar resistance require management with sodium nitroprusside, prostacyclin, dobutamine, or milrinone in an attempt to decrease pulmonary resistance. Patients unresponsive to these therapies are often considered too high risk for transplantation and may be candidates for LVAD insertion as definitive therapy or bridge to transplant.

Contraindications to cardiac transplantation include significant noncardiac diseases. Because immunosuppressive agents have renal and hepatic side effects, the presence of intrinsic renal or hepatic disease increases perioperative risk of organ dysfunction or failure. Some patients with multiorgan disease can be considered for combined heart-kidney or heart-liver transplant in these cases. Patients with FEV_1 $<50\%$ predicted, despite optimal management of CHF, are at increased risk for ventilatory failure and respiratory infections posttransplant. The presence of significant atherosclerosis is a contraindication due to the increased perioperative morbidity and mortality of atheroembolic phenomenon.

Preanesthetic Considerations

Donor heart function worsens with ischemic times above 6 hours. For this reason, transplantation must occur when the donor surgery can be performed, frequently during night hours. Preoperative evaluation and preparation of the patient must be done quickly. Close communication between the donor and recipient teams facilitates optimal use of donor organs. The goal is to minimize organ ischemic time. Optimally, the recipient heart will be excised when the donor heart arrives. Induction of anesthesia and surgical incision of the recipient begin when the donor team has evaluated the donor and made the final determination that the organ is acceptable. Timing decisions are based on distance and time necessary to transport the donor organ, as well as time it will take to prepare the recipient. History of prior sternotomy or difficult airway can increase recipient preparation time.

When evaluating the recipient, a few issues need special attention: NPO (nothing by mouth) status, level of cardiovascular support (inotropic infusions, chronic medications for heart failure, presence of LVADs), and presence of hemodynamic monitoring lines or antiarrhythmic devices, such as pacemaker or defibrillator. A pacemaker or defibrillator needs to be interrogated and reprogrammed to a mode that will not be affected by electrocautery interference. Due to the emergency nature of these cases, it is common that the patient has recently eaten, and rapid sequence induction may be necessary. Patients are frequently taking ACE inhibitors, which could increase the risk of intraoperative hypotension, or coumadin, which can increase the risk of bleeding. Vasopressin infusions can be beneficial for treatment of ACE inhibitor-induced hypotension, and FFP should be ordered if the INR is elevated. If cardiac status has deteriorated recently, the patient may be receiving infusions of inotropes, such as dobutamine or milrinone. On occasion, patients are receiving chronic dobutamine therapy as outpatients. If patients have had multiple central lines, ultrasound evaluation of the central vessels may be helpful to determine vessel patency. Recent chest films and laboratory studies must be reviewed to assess pulmonary, hepatic, and renal compromise associated with CHF.

Many anesthetic management issues related to the heart transplant patient are similar to those for open heart surgeries (see Chapter 31). The notable differences are strictest attention to sterility and immunosuppression, poorer hemodynamic status of transplant candidates, and issues related to early donor heart function and denervation. The surgical team will request antibiotics specific to donor and recipient infectious patterns, and immunosuppressive medications are given prior to incision.

Placement of the PA catheter prior to anesthetic induction is favored by many centers. Mixed venous saturation (Svo_2) PA catheters are optimal because they provide continuous assessment of CO and Svo_2. If the patient cannot lie flat for central line placement, cautious induction can proceed, but arterial catheters should always be used for blood pressure monitoring during induction. Large-bore intravenous access is necessary for administration of resuscitation medications if no central line is present during induction. Inotropes should be readily available prior to induction. Dobutamine, epinephrine, milrinone, norepinephrine, dopamine, vasopressin, and phenylephrine have all been used effectively in the perioperative management of heart transplant patients.

Presence of an LVAD or prior sternotomy increases the length and the risks associated with the procedure. Aprotinin reduces allogeneic transfusion requirements in patients undergoing repeat sternotomy.[137] Aprotinin has also been used extensively for high-risk procedures, such as LVAD insertion. Where possible, old medical records should be reviewed to determine use of aprotinin during prior operations. Aprotinin is a foreign protein, and its use is associated with anaphylaxis if reexposure occurs within 6 months.[138–140] If aprotinin has been used recently or exposure is uncertain, the test dose should not be administered until such time that the surgeons could rapidly institute CPB for management of hemodynamic collapse. Four units of blood should be immediately available prior to sternotomy for all repeat procedures. Availability of FFP, platelets, and cryoprecipitate should be confirmed at the start of the procedure.

Intraoperative Management

Anesthetic induction in patients with poor ventricular function can be complicated by hemodynamic instability. Instituting inotropes, or increasing those already infusing, can be beneficial in these cases. Choice of anesthetic technique should be focused on minimizing cardiovascular complications. High-dose narcotic techniques have been used for induction and management of cardiac transplantation patients for many years with good results.[139] Balanced anesthetic techniques, using lower doses of narcotics and inhalation anesthetics, can also be used.[136] Neuromuscular blockade with a nondepolarizing agent is recommended. Hypotension may not respond to ephedrine or phenylephrine, and inotrope use should be rapidly instituted or increased if response to phenylephrine is inadequate.

TEE should be performed intraoperatively if there are no contraindications to the procedure. The recipient heart can be monitored prior to CPB for changes in ventricular function or increase in valvular regurgitation. Early diagnosis of deterioration can facilitate rapid therapy and hemodynamic stability. The risk of intracardiac thrombus is increased in the recipient heart. The left atrium and ventricle should be carefully examined. Manipulation of the heart is minimized prior to aortic cross-clamping if thrombus is noted. TEE is also beneficial for evaluation of the donor heart during and after CPB.

Incision is via median sternotomy for orthotopic heart transplantation. The recipient heart is excised, except for the left atrial tissue encompassing the pulmonary veins. In the classic approach, the atria are transected at the grooves. The biatrial approach totally excises both atria, mandating bicaval anastomosis. The biatrial approach is preferred in pediatric recipients.

Heparin dosing is similar to that of other CPB procedures. Cannulation of the aorta is performed high along the ascending aorta, near the aortic arch. The superior and inferior vena cavae are cannulated individually. By encircling the cavae with tourniquets, all blood flow is directed through the cannula into the bypass circuit, and the surgical field is bloodless. Prior to resection of the native heart, the PA catheter should be withdrawn from the surgical field. The catheter can be readvanced after removal of the superior caval cannula. Maintenance of CPB, and weaning from CPB, are associated with the same issues as for other cardiac surgical procedures. Ischemic time for the donor heart starts with aortic cross-clamp during the harvest and ends with removal of the cross-clamp from the recipient aorta. Air should be evacuated prior to weaning from CPB.

Prior to weaning from CPB, the heart is reevaluated with TEE, looking at ventricular and valvular function. Intracardiac shunts should be ruled out. Because the donor heart is denervated, normal physiologic feedback loops controlling inotropy and chronotropy are lost. Isoproterenol is used frequently for its direct effects on cardiac beta-receptors to increase graft heart rate. Use of temporary epicardial pacing is sometimes needed until isoproterenol has had adequate time to reach maximal effect. (Vasoactive drug effects in heart transplantation are reviewed in Table 53-8.) Residual atrial tissue may continue to have electrical activity, seen clinically as two P waves on ECG. The native P wave has no physiologic activity on the donor heart.

Inotrope selection for weaning from CPB is similar to other cardiac surgical procedures. Special consideration should be given to recipients with preoperative pulmonary hypertension, donor hearts with a long ischemic time, or those that were believed to be marginal organs at time of harvest. The risk of donor right heart failure is increased in these cases. The donor right heart is not accustomed to high pulmonary resistance and may fail acutely. Therapy for graft right heart failure is similar to therapy for right heart failure in other cardiac cases. The goal is to improve contractility and decrease pulmonary vascular resistance. If intravenous agents are not adequate support to wean from CPB, inhaled NO and inhaled prostacyclin (Iloprost) have been shown to be beneficial in this population.[141–144]

TABLE 53-8

EFFECT OF DENERVATION ON CARDIAC PHARMACOLOGY

SUBSTANCE	EFFECT ON RECIPIENT	MECHANISM
Digitalis	Normal increase of contractility, minimal effect on atrioventricular node	Direct myocardial effect, denervation
Atropine	None	Denervation
Adrenaline	Increased contractility Increased chronotropy	Denervation hypersensitivity
Noradrenaline	Increased contractility Increased chronotropy	Denervation No neuronal uptake
Isoproterenol	Normal increase in contractility, normal increase in chronotropy	
Quinidine	No vagolytic effect	Denervation
Verapamil	Atrioventricular block	Direct effect
Nifedipine	No reflex tachycardia	Denervation
Hydralazine	No reflex tachycardia	Denervation
Beta-blocker	Increased antagonist effect	Denervation

Reprinted with permission from Deng MC: Cardiac transplantation. Heart 287:177, 2002.

Pediatric Heart Transplantation

UNOS reports 4,054 pediatric heart transplants performed since 1988. Sixty percent are performed on children younger than 1 year of age or children older than 11 years of age. The pretransplant diagnosis was congenital heart disease or idiopathic/viral cardiomyopathy in 75% of these patients. Eight hundred fifty children have died while waiting for a suitable organ. Extracorporeal membrane oxygenation is used as a bridge to transplant at some centers, although it is acknowledged to be only a short-term option.[145] Marginal donors are, not surprisingly, also being used for pediatric heart grafts, including size mismatches of more than three times recipient body weight, high donor inotrope requirement, prolonged ischemic time, and ABO mismatch. (LVADs are currently not available for pediatric patients.) Although ABO incompatible transplantation is contraindicated in the adult population, it is more successful in infant recipients.[146,147] Hyperacute rejection does not occur due to the immaturity of the immune system, and absence of antibodies to various antigens, including blood group antigens. For ABO mismatched grafts, recipient isohemagglutinin titers are obtained pretransplantation, and then plasma exchange is performed during CPB. Four-year follow-up data show similar morbidity and mortality compared with ABO-compatible recipients. Furthermore, waiting list survival is improved due to expansion of the donor pool.

Preoperative evaluation focuses on cardiopulmonary status, and the particulars of the cardiac physiology in congenital heart disease patients. Palliative procedures may have been performed prior to transplant, and reoperation increases surgical risk. Central venous catheters and intraarterial catheters are placed routinely, although frequently after induction. After an inhalation induction, anesthetic management frequently involves high-dose narcotics and intermittent benzodiazepines.

Anesthetic Management of the Transplant Patient for Nontransplant Surgery

As the population of transplant recipients increases, the incidence of elective or emergent nontransplant surgery in this group will also increase.[148] These patients cannot always return to the transplant facility for surgery, so it is incumbent on

TABLE 53-9

DRUGS THAT MAY CAUSE RENAL DYSFUNCTION WHEN COADMINISTERED WITH CALCINEURIN INHIBITORS

Amphotericin	Cotrimoxazole
Cimetidine	Vancomycin
Ranitidine	Tobramycin
Melphalan	Gentamicin
Nonsteroidal anti-inflammatory drugs	

Adapted with permission from Kostopanagiotou G, Smyrniotis V, Arkadopoulos N *et al:* Anesthetic and perioperative management of adult transplant recipients in non-transplant surgery. Anesth Analg 89:613,1999.

all anesthesiologists to review perioperative issues associated with transplantation.[149]

13 For solid organ recipients, evaluation of patients is centered on function of the grafted organ. In renal transplant patients, the level of renal dysfunction will determine choice of drugs, particularly neuromuscular blockers, and dose modification of drugs dependent on renal excretion such as antibiotics. Table 53-9 lists medications that can cause renal dysfunction when administered to a patient receiving immunosuppressive agents. A major consideration for renal transplant recipients is maintenance of renal perfusion with adequate volume replacement. Thus, CVP monitoring is useful for preventing prerenal damage to transplanted kidneys, but CVP lines must be placed using strict aseptic technique.

Similarly failing, rejecting, or reinfected liver grafts are often accompanied by deterioration of renal function. Protection of the kidneys is a central part of anesthesia plans, and CVP or TEE is useful to guide fluid replacement, especially in cases where large fluid shifts are anticipated.

14 For all transplant recipients, antibiotic, antiviral, antifungal, and immune suppression regimens should be disrupted as little as possible in the perioperative period. This may require coordination with the transplant center. Complications of immune suppression are reviewed in Table 53-3, and important drug interactions with calcineurin inhibitors are reviewed in Table 53-10.[149] Significant intraoperative fluid shifts can cause acute decrease in cyclosporine or tacrolimus blood levels, and in these cases, consideration should be given to repeat testing of drug levels during the day of surgery.[149] Nonsteroidal anti-inflammatory medications should be avoided for a number of reasons. First, many patients have underlying renal dysfunction related to immunosuppressives. Second, the risk of GI hemorrhage is increased in patients already at risk for gastritis due to chronic steroids.

Patients who present for surgery with signs of acute rejection or infection may benefit from delay of surgery to optimize status. Both rejection and infection in the face of surgery are associated with increased risk of morbidity and mortality.[149] Regional and general anesthetic techniques have been used successfully in posttransplant patients. In addition to the standard ASA monitors, invasive monitors should be used if warranted based on surgical procedure and general health status of the patient. Invasive monitoring is not indicated solely on the basis of prior transplantation. Nasal intubation should be avoided, due to the potential risk for infection presented by nasal flora.

Lung Transplant Recipients

If the patient had a lung transplant that included a tracheal anastomosis, denervation has occurred below the level of the suture line, and the cough reflex is diminished or absent. These

TABLE 53-10

DRUGS AFFECTING CYCLOSPORINE OR TACROLIMUS BLOOD LEVELS

INCREASE BLOOD LEVELS	DECREASE BLOOD LEVELS
Bromocriptine	Carbamazepine
Chloroquine[a]	Octreotide[a]
Cimetidine[b]	Phenobarbital
Clarithromycin	Phenytoin
Cotrimoxazole	Rifampin
Danazole	Ticlopidine
Erythromycin	
Fluconazole	
Itraconazole	
Ketoconazole	
Metoclopramide	
Nicardipine	
Verapamil	

[a]Reported with cyclosporine; may not interact with tacrolimus.
[b]May not interact with cyclosporine.

patients are at increased risk of retained secretions and pneumonia, and have an increased airway hyperreactivity and bronchospasm. Because most lung transplants are now being done with bronchial instead of tracheal anastomoses, the risk of tracheal suture line stenosis or disruption with manipulation are markedly diminished. Advantages of regional anesthetic techniques in lung transplant patients include minimization of airway manipulation and decreased infectious risk.

Comparison of preoperative PFT, arterial blood gas (ABG), and chest radiograph (CXR) results with prior studies can help diagnose acute infection or rejection. Significant decreases in FEV_1, vital capacity (VC), and total lung capacity (TLC) and an obstructive pattern may indicate acute rejection. ABG in the presence of rejection will show an increased A-a gradient from stable baseline gases, along with perihilar infiltration on CXR. However, rejection and infection can be difficult to distinguish clinically. If the patient is suspected of having an active pulmonary process, consultation with pulmonary medicine for a possible diagnostic bronchoscopy should be considered prior to surgery.

Heart Transplant Recipients

Denervation of the heart has a significant clinical impact on perioperative management. The transplanted heart cannot respond to indirect acting agents, such as ephedrine and even dopamine, or to peripheral attempts to induce hemodynamic changes, such as carotid massage, Valsalva maneuver, or laryngoscopy. Beta effects of epinephrine and norepinephrine are exaggerated in heart transplant recipients (versus alpha effects). Isoproterenol is the mainstay of chronotropic therapy in these patients. ECG analysis may show two P waves, one from the native atrium and one from the implanted atrium. The native P wave will not conduct to the implanted heart, and these nonconducted P waves should not be confused with complete heart block. Isoproterenol should be available as an inotrope and chronotrope. Dobutamine can also be helpful; norepinephrine and epinephrine should be reserved for refractory cardiogenic shock. Because the denervated heart does not reflexively compensate for hemodynamic changes induced by regional anesthetics, general anesthesia is usually preferred.

Preoperative evaluation should focus on cardiac functional status. Significant rejection will present with symptoms of heart failure. All heart transplant patients should be evaluated with ECG and TTE prior to surgery. New findings should be discussed with the cardiology consultant to determine need for stress testing or myocardial biopsy. Invasive monitors should be placed only when warranted by the clinical status and surgical procedure. Use of either TEE or CVP monitoring can be helpful in managing fluid resuscitation and inotropic support.

References

1. A definition of irreversible coma. Report of the Ad Hoc Committee of the Harvard Medical School to Examine the Definition of Brain Death. JAMA 205:337, 1985
2. Nijboer WN, Schuurs TA, van der Hoeven JAB, Ploeg RJ: Effect of brain death and donor treatment on organ inflammatory response and donor organ viability. Curr Opin Organ Transpl 9:110, 2004
3. Salim A, Vassiliu P, Velmahos GC *et al*: The role of thyroid hormone administration in potential organ donors. Arch Surg 136:1377, 2001
4. Rosendale JD, Kauffman HM, McBride MA *et al*: Aggressive pharmacologic donor management results in more transplanted organs. Transplantation 75:482, 2003
5. Todd TR, Goldberg M, Koshal A *et al*: Separate extraction of cardiac and pulmonary grafts from a single donor. Ann Thorac Surg 46:356, 1988
6. Harjula A, Baldwin JC, Starnes VA *et al*: Proper donor selection for heart-lung transplantation. The Stanford experience. J Thorac Cardiovasc Surg 94:874, 1987
7. Orens JB, Boehler A, Perrot M *et al*: A review of lung transplant donor criteria. J Heart Lung Transplant 22:1183, 2003
8. Bhorade SM, Vigneswaran W, McCabe MA, Garrity ER: Liberalization of donor criteria may expand the donor pool without adverse consequence in lung transplantation. J Heart Lung Transplant 19:1200, 2000
9. Sekine Y, Waddell TK, Matte-Martyn A *et al*: Risk quantification of early outcome after lung transplantation: Donor, recipient, operative, and post-transplant parameters. J Heart Lung Transplant 23:96, 2004
10. Maximizing use of organs recovered from the cadaveric donor: Cardiac recommendations. Consensus Conference Report, Crystal City, VA, March 28–29, 2001. Circ 106:836, 2002
11. Moon JI, Nishida S, Butt F *et al*: Multi-organ procurement and successful multi-center allocation using rapid en bloc technique from a controlled non-heart-beating donor. Transplantation 77:1476, 2004
12. Steen S, Sjoberg T, Pierre L *et al*: Transplantation of lungs from a non-heart-beating donor. Lancet 357:825, 2001
13. Nunez JR, Varela A, del Rio F *et al*: Bipulmonary transplants with lungs obtained from two non-heart-beating donors who died out of hospital. J Thorac Cardiovasc Surg 127:297, 2004
14. Committee on Non-Heart-Beating Transplantation II: The Scientific and Ethical Basis for Practice and Protocols, Division of Health Care Services, Institute of Medicine: Non-heart-beating organ transplantation: Practice and protocols.Washington, DC: National Academy Press, 2000
15. Van Norman GA: Another matter of life and death: What every anesthesiologist should know about the ethical, legal, and policy implications of the non-heart-beating cadaver organ donor. Anesthesiology 98:763, 2003
16. Yang S-L, Harkaway R, Badose F, Ginsberg P, Greenstein MA: Minimal incision living donor nephrectomy: Improvement in patient outcome. Urology 59:673, 2002
17. Haberal M, Emirolu R, Arslan G *et al*: Living-donor nephrectomy under combined spinal–epidural anesthesia. Transplantation 34:2448, 2002
18. Perry KT, Freedland SJ, Hu JC *et al*: Quality of life, pain and return to normal activities following laparoscopic donor nephrectomy versus open mini-incision donor nephrectomy. J Urol 169:2018, 2003
19. Biancofiore G, Amorese G, Lugli D *et al*: Laparoscopic live donor nephrectomy: The anaesthesiologist's perspective. Eur J Anaesthesiol 21:74, 2004
20. Blohme I, Fehrman I, Norden G: Living donor nephrectomy. Complication rates in 490 consecutive cases. Scand J Urol Nephrol 26:149, 1992
21. Starzl TE: Living donors: Con Transpl Proc 19:174, 1987
22. Brown RS, Russo MW, Lai M *et al*: A survey of liver transplantation from living adult donors in the United States. N Engl J Med 348:818, 2003
23. Renz JF, Yersiz H, Farmer DG *et al*: Changing face of liver transplantation: Partial-liver grafts for adults. J Hepatobil Pancreat Surg 10:31, 2003
24. Grady D: New Yorker dies after surgery to give liver part to brother. New York Times January 15, 2002
25. Akabayashi A, Slinglby BT, Fujita M: The first donor death after living-related liver transplantation in Japan. Transplantation 77:634, 2004
26. Ayanoglu HO, Ulukaya S, Yuzer Y, Tokat Y: Anesthetic management and complications in living donor hepatectomy. Transplant Proc 35:2970, 2003
27. Eyraud D, Richard O, Borie DC *et al*: Hemodynamic and hormonal responses to the sudden interruption of caval flow: Insights from a prospective study of hepatic vascular exclusion during major liver resections. Anesth Analg 95:1173, 2002
28. Smyrniotis V, Kostopanagiotou G, Theodoraki K, Tsantoulas D, Contis JC: The role of central venous pressure and type of vascular control in blood loss during major liver resections. Am J Surg 187:398, 2004
29. Chen C-L, Chen Y-S, deVilla VH *et al*: Minimal blood loss living donor hepatectomy. Transplantation 69:2580, 2000
30. Johnson LB, Plotkin JS, Kuo PC: Reduced transfusion requirements during major hepatic resection with use of intraoperative isovolemic hemodilution. Am J Surg 176:608, 1998
31. Niemann CU, Roberts JP, Ascher NL, Yost CS: Intraoperative hemodynamics and liver function in adult-to-adult living donor livers. Liver Transpl 8:1126, 2002
32. Cammu G, Troisi R, Cuomo O *et al*: Anaesthetic management and outcome in right-lobe living liver-donor surgery. Eur J Anaesthesiol 19:93, 2002
33. Lentschener C, Ozier Y: Anaesthesia for elective liver resection: Some points should be revisited. Eur J Anaesthesiol 19:788, 2002
34. Lutz JT, Valentin-Gamazo C, Gorlinger K, Malago M, Peters J: Blood transfusion requirements and blood salvage in donors undergoing right hepatectomy for living related liver transplantation. Anesth Analg 96:351, 2003
35. Schumann R, Zabala L, Angelis M *et al*: Altered hematologic profiles following donor right hepatectomy and implications for perioperative analgesic management. Liver Transpl 10:363, 2004
36. Matot I, Scheinin O, Eid A, Jurim O: Epidural anesthesia and analgesia in liver resection. Anesth Analg 95:1179, 2002
37. Barr ML, Baker CJ, Schenkel FA *et al*: Living donor lung transplantation: Selection, technique, and outcome. Transplant Proc 33:3527, 2001
38. Calne RY, Thiru S, McMaster P *et al*: Cyclosporin A in patients receiving renal allografts from cadaver donors. 1978. J Am Soc Nephrol 9:1751, 1998
39. Vicenti F: A decade of progress in kidney transplantation. Transplantation 77:S52, 2004
40. Dumont FJ: FK506, an immunosuppressant targeting calcineurin function. Curr Med Chem 7:731, 2000
41. Heisel O, Heisel R, Balshaw R, Keown P: New onset diabetes mellitus in patients receiving calcineurin inhibitors: A systematic review and meta-analysis. Am J Transplant 4:583, 2004
42. Risaliti A, Baccarani U, Vianello V *et al*: Cardiovascular and metabolic complications after liver transplantation: Neoral-versus tacrolimus-based immunosuppression. Transplant Proc 33:3684, 2001
43. Sidi A, Kaplan RF, Davis RF: Prolonged neuromuscular blockade and ventilatory failure after renal transplantation and cyclosporine. Can J Anaesth 37:543, 1990
44. Crosby E, Robblee JA: Cyclosporine-pancuronium interaction in a patient with a renal allograft. Can J Anaesth 35:300, 1998
45. Niemann CU, Stabernack C, Serkova N *et al*: Cyclosporine can increase isoflurane MAC. Anesth Analg 95:930, 2002
46. Thomason JM, Girdler NM, Kendall-Taylor P *et al*: An investigation into the need for supplementary steroids in organ transplant patients undergoing gingival surgery. A double-blind, split-mouth, cross-over study. J Clin Periodontol 26:577, 1999
47. Neuhaus P, Klupp J, Langrehr JM: mTOR inhibitors: An overview. Liver Transpl 7:473, 2001
48. Barten MJ, Streit F, Boeger M *et al*: Synergistic effects of sirolimus with cyclosporine and tacrolimus: Analysis of immunosuppression on lymphocyte proliferation and activation in rat whole blood. Transplantation 77:1154, 2004
49. Kirchner GI, Meier-Wiedenbach I, Manns MP: Clinical pharmacokinetics of everolimus. Clin Pharmacokinet 43:83, 2004
50. Jungling AS, Shangraw RE: Massive airway edema after azathioprine. Anesthesiology 92:888, 2000
51. Engelen W, Verpooten GA, Van der Planken M *et al*: Four cases of red blood cell aplasia in association with the use of mycophenolate mofetil in renal transplant patients. Clin Nephrol 60:119, 2003
52. Min DI, Monaco AP: Complications associated with immunosuppressive therapy and their management. Pharmacotherapy 11:119S, 1991
53. Wilde MI, Goa KL: Muromonab CD3: A reappraisal of its pharmacology and use as prophylaxis of solid organ transplant rejection. Drugs 51:865, 1996
54. Bamgbola FO, Del Rio M, Kaskel FJ, Flynn JT: Non-cardiogenic pulmonary edema during basiliximab induction in three adolescent renal transplant patients. Pediatr Transplant 7:315, 2003
55. Hunter K: Anesthesiology in renal and pancreas transplantation. Curr Opin Organ Transpl 8:243, 2003
56. Aker S, Ivens K, Guo Z, Grabensee B, Heering P: Cardiovascular complications after renal transplantation. Transplant Proc 30:2039, 1998
57. Espejo B, Torres A, Valentin M *et al*: Obesity favors surgical and infectious complications after renal transplantation. Transplant Proc 35:1762, 2003
58. Akpek EA, Kayhan Z, Donmez A, Moray G, Arslan G: Early postoperative renal function following renal transplantation surgery: Effect of anesthetic technique. J Anesth 16:114, 2002
59. Reissell E, Taskinen MR, Orko R, Lindgren L: Increased volume of gastric contents in diabetic patients undergoing renal transplantation: Lack of effect with cisapride. Acta Anaesthesiol Scand 36:736, 1992
60. Ragaller MJ, Theilen H, Koch T: Volume replacement in critically ill patients with acute renal failure. J Am Soc Nephrol 17:S33, 2001
61. Van den Berghe G, Wouters P, Weekers F *et al*: Intensive insulin therapy in critically ill patients. N Engl J Med 345:1359, 2001

62. Nichols WG, Price TH, Gooley T, Corey L, Boeckh M: Transfusion-transmitted cytomegalovirus infection after receipt of leukoreduced blood products. Blood 101:4195, 2003
63. Parada B, Figueiredo A, Mota Am Furtado A: Surgical complications in 1000 renal transplants. Transplant Proc 35:1085, 2003
64. Noldus J, Graefen M, Huland H: Major postoperative complications secondary to use of the Bookwalter self-retaining retractor. Urology 60:964, 2002
65. Healey PJ, McDonald R, Waldhausen JH, Sawin R, Tapper D: Transplantation of adult living donor kidneys into infants and small children. Arch Surg 135:1035, 2000
66. Freeman RB Jr, Wiesner RH, Harper A *et al*: UNOS/OPTN Liver Disease Severity Score, UNOS/OPTN Liver and Intestine, and UNOS/OPTN Pediatric Transplantation Committees: The new liver allocation system: Moving toward evidence-based transplantation policy. Liver Transpl 8:851, 2002
67. Nair S, Verma S, Thuluvath PJ: Pretransplant renal function predicts survival in patients undergoing orthotopic liver transplantation. Hepatology 35:1179, 2002
68. Plotkin JS, Benitez RM, Kuo PC *et al*: Dobutamine stress echocardiography for preoperative cardiac risk stratification in patients undergoing orthotopic liver transplantation. Liver Transpl Surg 4:253, 1998
69. Pollard RJ, Sidi A, Gibby GL, Lobato EB, Gabrielli A: Aortic stenosis with end-stage liver disease: Prioritizing surgical and anesthetic therapies. J Clin Anesth 10:253, 1998
70. Kim WR, Krowka MJ, Plevak DJ *et al*: Accuracy of Doppler echocardiography in the assessment of pulmonary hypertension in liver transplant candidates. Liver Transpl 6:453, 2000
71. Krowka MJ, Plevak DJ, Findlay JY *et al*: Pulmonary hemodynamics and perioperative cardiopulmonary-related mortality in patients with portopulmonary hypertension undergoing liver transplantation. Liver Transpl 6:443, 2000
72. Kuo PC, Johnson LB, Plotkin JS *et al*: Continuous intravenous infusion of epoprostenol for the treatment of portopulmonary hypertension. Transplantation 63:604, 1997
73. Makisalo H, Koivusalo A, Vakkuri A, Hockerstedt K: Sildenafil for portopulmonary hypertension in a patient undergoing liver transplantation. Liver Transpl 10:945, 2004
74. Lange PA, Stoller JK: The hepatopulmonary syndrome. Ann Intern Med 122:521, 1995
75. Taniai N, Onda M, Tajiri T *et al*: Reversal of hypoxemia by inhaled nitric oxide in a child with hepatopulmonary syndrome after living-related liver transplantation. Transplant Proc 34:2791, 2002
76. Selim KM, Akriviadis EA, Zuckerman E, Chen D, Reynolds TB: Transjugular intrahepatic portosystemic shunt: A successful treatment for hepatopulmonary syndrome. Am J Gastroenterol 93:455, 1998
77. Verne GN, Soldevia-Pico C, Robinson ME, Spicer KM, Reuben A: Autonomic dysfunction and gastroparesis in cirrhosis. J Clin Gastroenterol 38:72, 2004
78. Budd JM, Isaac JL, Bennett J, Freeman JW: Morbidity and mortality associated with large-bore percutaneous venovenous bypass cannulation for 312 orthotopic liver transplantations. Liver Transpl 7:359, 2001
79. Planinsic RM, Nicolau-Raducu R, Caldwell JC, Aggarwal S, Hilmi I: Transesophageal echocardiography-guided placement of internal jugular percutaneous venovenous bypass cannula in orthotopic liver transplantation. Anesth Analg 97:648, 2003
80. Consensus conference. Fresh-frozen plasma. Indications and risks. JAMA 253:555, 1985
81. Kang Y: Thromboelastography in liver transplantation. Semin Thromb Hemost 21(Suppl 4):34, 1995
82. Quach T, Tippens M, Szlam F *et al*: Quantitative assessment of fibrinogen cross-linking by epsilon aminocaproic acid in patients with end-stage liver disease. Liver Transpl 10:123, 2004
83. Molenaar IQ, Legnani C, Groenland TH *et al*: Aprotinin in orthotopic liver transplantation: Evidence for a prohemostatic, but not a prothrombotic, effect. Liver Transpl 7:896, 2001
84. Sopher M, Braunfeld M, Shackleton C *et al*: Fatal pulmonary embolism during liver transplantation. Anesthesiology 87:429, 1997
85. Porte RJ, Bontempo FA, Knot EA *et al*: Systemic effects of tissue plasminogen activator-associated fibrinolysis and its relation to thrombin generation in orthotopic liver transplantation. Transplantation 47:978, 1989
86. Meijer K, Hendriks HG, De Wolf JT *et al*: Recombinant factor VIIa in orthotopic liver transplantation: Influence on parameters of coagulation and fibrinolysis. Blood Coagul Fibrinolysis 14:169, 2003
87. Surudo T, Wojcicki M, Milkiewicz P *et al*: Rapid correction of prothrombin time after low-dose recombinant factor VIIA in patients undergoing orthotopic liver transplantation. Transplant Proc 35:2323, 2003
88. Sherman DS, Fish DN, Teitelbaum I: Assessing renal function in cirrhotic patients: Problems and pitfalls. Am J Kidney Dis 41:269, 2003
89. Sort P, Navasa M, Arroyo V *et al*: Effect of intravenous albumin on renal impairment and mortality in patients with cirrhosis and spontaneous bacterial peritonitis. N Engl J Med 341:403, 1999
90. Runyon BA: Management of adult patients with ascites caused by cirrhosis. Hepatology 27:264, 1998
91. Solanki P, Chawla A, Garg R *et al*: Beneficial effects of terlipressin in hepatorenal syndrome: A prospective, randomized placebo-controlled clinical trial. J Gastroenterol Hepatol 18:152, 2003
92. Duvoux C, Zandirenas D, Hezode C *et al*: Effects of noradrenalin and albumin in patients with type 1 hepatorenal syndrome: A pilot study. Hepatology 36:374, 2002
93. Rettke SR, Chantigian RC, Janossy TA *et al*: Anesthesia approach to hepatic transplantation. Mayo Clin Proc 64:224, 1989
94. Grande L, Rimola A, Cugat E *et al*: Effect of venovenous bypass on perioperative renal function in liver transplantation: Results of a randomized, controlled trial. Hepatology 23:1418, 1996
95. Steib A, Saada A, Clever B *et al*: Orthotopic liver transplantation with preservation of portocaval flow compared with venovenous bypass. Liver Transpl Surg 3:518, 1997
96. Aggarwal S, Kang Y, Freeman JA *et al*: Postreperfusion syndrome: Hypotension after reperfusion of the transplanted liver. J Crit Care 8:154, 1993
97. Millis JM, Melinek J, Csete M *et al*: Randomized controlled trial to evaluate flush and reperfusion techniques in liver transplantation. Transplantation 63:397, 1997
98. Findlay JY, Jankowski CJ, Vasdev GM *et al*: Fast track anesthesia for liver transplantation reduces postoperative ventilation time but not intensive care unit stay. Liver Transpl 8:670, 2002
99. McDiarmid SV: Current status of liver transplantation in children. Pediatr Clin North Am 50:1335, 2003
100. Lidofsky SD, Bass NM, Prager MC *et al*: Intracranial pressure monitoring and liver transplantation for fulminant hepatic failure. Hepatology 16:1, 1992
101. Humar A, Gruessner RW, Sutherland DE: Living related donor pancreas and pancreas-kidney transplantation. Br Med Bull 53:879, 1997
102. Mokshagundam SPL: Perioperative management of diabetes mellitus. Crit Care Nurs Q 27:135, 2004
103. Shapiro AM, Lakey JR, Ryan EA *et al*: Islet transplantation in seven patients with type 1 diabetes mellitus using a glucocorticoid-free immunosuppressive regimen. N Engl J Med 343:230, 2000
104. Mittal VK, Toledo-Pereyra LH, Sharma M *et al*: Acute portal hypertension and disseminated intravascular coagulation following pancreatic islet autotransplantation after subtotal pancreatectomy. Transplantation 31:302, 1981
105. Langnas AN: Advances in small-intestine transplantation. Transplantation 77:S75, 2004
106. Fishbein TM: The current state of intestinal transplantation. Transplantation 79:175, 2004
107. Goldman LJ, Santamaria ML, Gamez M: Anaesthetic management of a patient with microvillus inclusion disease for intestinal transplantation. Paediatr Anaesth 12:278, 2002
108. Mims TT, Fishbein TM, Feierman DE: Management of a small bowel transplant with complicated central venous access in a patient with asymptomatic superior and inferior vena cava obstruction. Transplant Proc 36:388, 2004
109. Goulet O, Ruemmele F, Lacaille F, Colomb V: Irreversible intestinal failure. J Pediatric Gastroenterol Nutr 38:250, 2004
110. Reitz BA, Wallwork JL, Hunt SA *et al*: Heart-lung transplantation. Successful therapy for patients with pulmonary vascular disease. N Engl J Med 306:557, 1982
111. Toronto Lung Transplant Group: Unilateral lung transplantation for pulmonary fibrosis. N Engl J Med 314:1140, 1986
112. Trulock ET, Edwards LB, Taylor DO *et al*: The registry of the International Society for Heart and Lung Transplantation: Twentieth official adult lung and heart-lung transplant report—2003. J Heart Lung Transplant 22:625, 2003
113. Weill D, Keshavjee S: Lung transplantation for emphysema: Two lungs or one. J Heart Lung Transplant 20:739, 2001
114. Joint Statement of the American Society for Transplant Physicians (ASTP)/American Thoracic Society (ATS)/European Respiratory Society (ERS)/International Society for Heart and Lung Transplantation (ISHLT). International guidelines for the selection of lung transplant candidates. Am J Respir Crit Care Med 158:335, 1998
115. Levine SM. Transplant/Immunology Network of the American College of Chest Physicians: A survey of clinical practice of lung transplantation in North America. Chest 125:1224, 2004
116. Sweet S: Pediatric lung transplantation: Update 2003. Pediatr Clin North Am 50:1393, 2003
117. Yankaskas JR, Mallory GB, the Consensus Committee: Lung transplantation in cystic fibrosis—consensus conference statement. Chest 113:217, 1998
118. De Soyza A, McDowell A, Archer L *et al*: *Burkholderia cepacia* complex genomovars and pulmonary transplantation outcomes in patients with cystic fibrosis. Lancet 358:1780, 2001
119. De Perrot M, Chaparro C, McRae K *et al*: Twenty-year experience of lung transplantation at a single center: Influence of recipient diagnosis on long-term survival. J Thorac Cardiovasc Surg 127:1493, 2004
120. Horlocker TT, Wedel DJ, Benzon H *et al*: Regional anesthesia in the anticoagulated patient: Defining the risks (the second ASRA consensus conference on neuraxial anesthesia and anticoagulation). Reg Anesth Pain Med 28:172, 2003
121. Low DE, Kaiser LE, Haydock DA *et al*: The donor lung: Infectious and pathologic factors affecting outcome in lung transplantation. J Thorac Cardiovasc Surg 106:614, 1993

122. Lang JD, Lell W: Pro: Inhaled nitric oxide should be used routinely in patients undergoing lung transplantation. J Cardiothorac Vasc Anesth 15:785, 2001
123. McQuitty CK: Con: Inhaled nitric oxide should not be used routinely in patients undergoing lung transplantation. J Cardiothorac Vasc Anesth 15:790, 2001
124. Meyer KC, Love RB, Zimmerman JJ: The therapeutic potential of nitric oxide in lung transplantation. Chest 113:1360, 1998
125. Cornfield DN, Milla CE, Haddad IY *et al*: Safety of inhaled nitric oxide after lung transplantation. J Heart Lung Transplant 22:903, 2003
126. Beghetti M, Sparling C, Cox PN *et al*: Inhaled NO inhibits platelet aggregation and elevates plasma but not intraplatelet cGMP in healthy human volunteers. Am J Physiol Heart Circ Physiol 285:H637, 2003
127. Hoehn T, Huebner J, Paboura E *et al*: Effect of therapeutic concentrations of nitric oxide on bacterial growth in vitro. Crit Care Med 26:1857, 1998
128. Boucek MM, Edwards LB, Keck BM *et al*: The registry of the International Society for Heart and Lung Transplantation: Sixth official pediatric report—2003. J Heart Lung Transplant 22:636, 2003
129. Taylor DO, Edwards LB, Mohacsi PJ *et al*: The registry of the International Society for Heart and Lung Transplantation: Twentieth official adult heart transplant report—2003. J Heart Lung Transplant 22:616, 2003
130. Deng MC: Cardiac transplantation. Heart 287:177, 2002
131. Shiba N, Chan MC, Valantine HA *et al*: Longer-term risks associated with 10-year survival after heart transplantation in the cyclosporine era. J Heart Lung Transplant 22:1098, 2003
132. Rose EA, Gelijns AC, Moskowitz AJ *et al*: Long-term mechanical left ventricular assistance for end-stage heart failure. N Engl J Med 345:1435, 2001
133. Levy D, Larson MG, Vasan RS *et al*: The progression from hypertension to congestive heart failure. JAMA 275:1557, 1996
134. Seidl K, Rameken M, Vater M, Senges J: Cardiac resynchronization therapy in patients with chronic heart failure. Am J Cardiovasc Drugs 2:219, 2002
135. Hunt SA: Twenty-fourth Bethesda conference: Cardiac transplantation. J Am Coll Cardiol 22(Suppl 1):1, 1993
136. Frantz RP, Olson LJ: Recipient selection and management before cardiac transplantation. Am J Med Sci 314:139, 1997
137. Levy JH, Pifarre R, Schaff HV *et al*: A multicenter, double-blind, placebo-controlled trial of aprotinin for reducing blood loss and the requirement for donor-blood transfusion in patients undergoing repeat coronary artery bypass grafting. Circulation 92:2236, 1995
138. Dietrich W, Spath P, Ebell A, Richter JA: Prevalence of anaphylactic reactions to aprotinin: Analysis of two hundred forty-eight reexposures in heart operations. J Thor Cardiovasc Surg 113:194, 1997
139. Hensley FA, Martin DE, Larach DR, Romanoff ME: Anesthetic management for cardiac transplantation in North America—1986 survey. J Cardiothorac Anesth 1:429, 1987
140. Demas K, Wyner J, Mihm FG, Samuels S: Anaesthesia for heart transplantation. A retrospective study and review. Br J Anaesth 58:1357, 1986
141. Sablotzki A, Czeslick E, Schubert S *et al*: Iloprost improves hemodynamics in patients with severe chronic cardiac failure and secondary pulmonary hypertension. Can J Anesth 49:1076, 2002
142. Ardehali A, Hughes K, Sadeghi A *et al*: Inhaled nitric oxide for pulmonary hypertension after heart transplantation. Transplantation 72:638, 2001
143. Mosquera I, Crespo-Leiro MG, Tabuyo T *et al*: Pulmonary hypertension and right ventricular failure after heart transplantation: Usefulness of nitric oxide. Transplant Proc 34:166, 2002
144. Rajek A, Pernerstorfer T *et al*: Inhaled nitric oxide reduces pulmonary vascular resistance more than prostaglandin E(1) during heart transplantation. Anesth Analg 90:523, 2000
145. Burch M, Aurora P: Current status of paediatric heart, lung, and heart-lung transplantation. Arch Dis Child 289:386, 2004
146. West LJ, Pollock-Barziv SM, Dipchand AI *et al*: ABO-incompatible heart transplantation in infants. N Engl J Med 344:793, 2001
147. Rao JN, Hasan A, Hamilton JRL *et al*: ABO-incompatible heart transplantation in infants: The Freeman Hospital experience. Transplantation 77:1389, 2004
148. Ashary N, Kaye AD, Hegazi AR *et al*: Anesthetic considerations in the patient with a heart transplant. Heart Disease 4:191, 2002
149. Kostopanagiotou G, Smyrniotis V, Arkadopoulos N *et al*: Anesthetic and perioperative management of adult transplant recipients in non-transplant surgery. Anesth Analg 89:613, 1999

SECTION VI ▪ POSTANESTHESIA AND CONSULTANT PRACTICE

CHAPTER 54 ■ POSTOPERATIVE RECOVERY

ROGER S. MECCA

KEY POINTS

1. Choosing a postanesthesia setting based on each patient's individual need can reduce cost, enhance patient satisfaction, and optimize use of scarce postanesthesia care unit (PACU) resources. If doubt exists about the safety of a lower-intensity setting, admit to a "full-service" PACU.
2. Anesthesiology personnel should manage a patient until a PACU nurse secures admission vital signs and attaches appropriate monitors. Ensure a succinct but thorough report is documented that includes sufficient information to allow rapid evaluation and intervention for postoperative complications.
3. Postoperative analgesia remains a top priority for patients and providers. Careful assessment of individual analgesic requirements and implementation of a planned, multimodal approach provides seamless pain control through and beyond the PACU interval.
4. Ideally, an anesthesiologist should evaluate each patient for discharge using a consistent set of criteria. Consider the severity of underlying disease, the anesthetic and recovery course, the likelihood of complications, and the level of care available at the destination
5. Hypovolemia is a common postoperative problem. Evaluate and actively manage intravascular volume status throughout the PACU interval, considering preoperative status, type and duration of surgery, estimated blood loss, fluid replacement, and hemostasis.
6. Risk of postoperative myocardial ischemia and infarction remains high. Control of precipitating factors, as well as timely therapy with analgesia and aggressive use of beta-adrenergic blocking agents and nitrates when appropriate, helps decrease morbidity.
7. In PACU patients, elevated $PaCO_2$ and respiratory acidemia do not necessarily indicate inadequate postoperative ventilation. During early recovery from anesthesia, residual anesthetics, opioids, and sedatives blunt the ventilatory responses to both hypercarbia and hypoxemia.
8. One cannot predict which postoperative patients will become hypoxemic or when hypoxemia will occur. Supplemental oxygen helps prevent or treat hypoxemia; however, oxygen does not address underlying causes of hypoxemia in postoperative patients, and its use does not guarantee that hypoxemia will not occur.
9. The incidence of serious aspiration is relatively low in PACU patients, but the risk is still significant. Preventing aspiration is critical because effective therapy is limited.
10. The ability to void should be assessed because opioids and autonomic side effects of regional anesthesia interfere with sphincter relaxation and promote urine retention.

11 Moderate postoperative hyperglycemia (200 to 300 mg/dL) resolves spontaneously and has little adverse effect. Higher glucose levels cause glycosuria with osmotic diuresis and interfere with serum electrolyte determinations.

12 Avoiding postoperative nausea and vomiting is a high priority. The most effective medications for prophylaxis and treatment are serotonin blocking agents, dexamethasone, and droperidol.

13 Hypothermia complicates care in the PACU. Average PACU stay is increased by 40 to 90 minutes for hypothermic patients

14 A high percentage of elderly patients experience some degree of postoperative confusion, delirium, or cognitive decline.

An individualized, problem-oriented approach to the assessment of surgical patients is essential to optimize outcome and to minimize risk and expense during postoperative recovery.

ASSESSING THE VALUE OF POSTANESTHESIA CARE

Indicators of quality in postanesthesia care now include not only clinical results and patient satisfaction, but also the "value" of the care provided, loosely defined as the improvement in postoperative outcome per dollar spent. The actual impact that postanesthesia care has on clinical outcomes in a surgical population varies with incidence and severity of underlying illness; the frequency, urgency, and type of surgical procedures; and the blend of surgical and anesthetic techniques used. Training, skill, and preferences of surgeons, anesthesia providers, and nurses also affect how important a postanesthesia care unit (PACU) admission is to a patient. The effectiveness with which PACU staff recognize complications, the quality of diagnostic and consultative services, and the efficiency with which physicians institute therapy are also important.

Actual cost of PACU care incorporates costs of staffing, space, and hardware. Triage, admission, and discharge policies affect how many admissions occur and what resources each admission consumes. Nurse staffing is the largest direct cost in the PACU. Mix of nursing staff (e.g., amount of training and experience, salaries and benefit levels), the staffing ratios (e.g., number of patients per caregiver, number of support staff), and the duration of PACU stay affect the overall personnel cost per admission. The level of monitoring provided affects capital expenditure for equipment and operating expenditure for disposable items. Expenditures for staffing, and for equipment such as intravenous pumps and ventilators, are also affected by patient mix. The type of physician coverage (e.g., dedicated versus on-demand coverage, response times) impacts the efficiency of care. Routine postoperative diagnostic testing increases costs for securing, processing, and professionally interpreting tests. Finally, routine use of therapies (e.g., antiemetics, respiratory treatments) increases the expenditure per patient for drugs and disposable items, and can add to the staffing resources required per patient.

Value comparisons among institutions are difficult because factors affecting impact and cost are facility specific and vary over time. Regulatory requirements, standards of care, and medicolegal climates also differ among regions or between facilities in the same locale. Attempts to establish national benchmarks of the "cost effectiveness" of postanesthesia care are fraught with inaccuracy. Despite this complexity, emphasis on reducing health care costs forces each surgical facility to evaluate the value of its PACU care to individual patients.

Innovative PACU practices help postanesthesia care unit directors maintain safe care, optimize clinical outcomes, minimize cost, and fulfill regulatory requirements. Inappropriate PACU admissions should be eliminated. Medical leaders must also identify those interventions that have yield versus those that are "wasteful." The actual impact of many PACU interventions on clinical outcome is not substantiated by controlled scientific analysis, so avoid inappropriate use of expensive therapies or testing. However, using a more expensive therapy can sometimes generate real savings by decreasing length of stay, or avoiding complications or hospital admission. Integration of the PACU service with other elements in the surgical continuum is essential. The most important interface is between the PACU and the intraoperative anesthesiology service. Consumption of PACU resources is definitely linked to anesthetic duration and technique. In one study, 22.1% of 37,000 patients had a minor anesthesia-related event or complication that prolonged PACU stay and consumed PACU resources.[1]

It is important to distinguish between potential and actual cost savings. Improvements in care might create an opportunity to shorten length of stay in the PACU or discharge unit, but the realized change is frequently reduced by transportation delays, persistence of pain or nausea, waiting for space, or surgeon discharge delays.[2] Also, beware of cost-saving measures in other areas that increase the cost of PACU care. For example, use of a cheaper, longer-acting muscle relaxant might trim cost in anesthesiology but increase length of stay, complication rates, and cost in the PACU. Finally, savings are illusory unless an operational change yields a decrease in expenditures for staff, supplies, or equipment. For example, bypassing the PACU creates a savings opportunity that is realized only if paid nursing hours are reduced or if more surgical cases are covered with the same hours. If ineffective scheduling or low-yield clerical or maintenance tasks consume excess staffing hours, then no savings are realized. Finally, trimming costs sometimes entails an increase in risk. Differentiating between cost-effective postanesthesia care and unsafe clinical practice must remain a matter of professional judgment.

SELECTING THE APPROPRIATE LEVEL OF POSTOPERATIVE CARE

For both ambulatory and inpatient surgery, the level of postoperative care that a patient requires is determined by the degree of underlying illness, the duration and complexity of anesthesia and surgery, and the risk of postoperative complications. Less invasive surgical techniques and shorter-duration anesthetic regimens facilitate high levels of arousal and minimal
1 cardiovascular or respiratory depression at the end of surgery. Choosing a less intensive postanesthesia setting based on each patient's individual need can reduce cost of a surgical procedure and allow utilization of scarce PACU resources for patients with greater needs. Also, each patient's impressions during recovery have a major impact on his or her perception of the entire surgical episode. Patients are more satisfied when spared unnecessary assessments and the potentially upsetting environment of intensive PACU care. Earlier reunion with family in a lower-intensity recovery setting that offers amenities such as recliners, reading material, television, music, and food improves perceptions without affecting quality or safety.

Patients must be carefully triaged to receive an appropriate level of postoperative care by evaluating clinical condition and the potential for complications inherent in the specific procedure. Do not use artificial triage categories based on age, American Society of Anesthesiologists (ASA) classification, ambulatory versus inpatient status, or type of insurance. Similarly, the level of postanesthesia care required should not vary depending on where surgery is performed. An individual patient undergoing a specific procedure should receive the same appropriate level of postoperative care whether the procedure is performed in a hospital operating room, an ambulatory surgical center, an endoscopy room, an invasive radiology suite, or an outpatient office. Preserve a wide margin of safety, and observe applicable PACU guidelines when appropriate[3,4]. If doubt exists about the safety of a lower-intensity setting, admit the patient to a "full-service" PACU or provide equivalent services. Always err for patient safety, regardless of cost.

Healthy patients can almost always recover safely with less intensive monitoring and coverage after procedures using local anesthetic infiltration, minor blocks with sedation, or even major plexus anesthesia. Selected ambulatory patients who meet the PACU discharge criteria at the end of general anesthesia can also bypass the PACU and be admitted directly to a discharge area. Use of short-acting anesthetics and bispectral index monitoring help facilitate this fast-track postoperative care.[5] However, inadequate control of pain or postoperative nausea and vomiting (PONV) often derails PACU bypass and reduces potential resource savings. PACU bypass increases capacity and monitoring requirements, as well as workload and complexity of nursing interventions in the phase II discharge area.[6]

Requirements of state and national agencies sometimes impede the implementation of innovative postanesthesia care policies. Regulations are sometimes outdated or poorly substantiated. Flexibility and evidence-based logic need to be incorporated into regulations for complete evolution of postanesthesia care to occur. Also, full-intensity PACU care must always be available, given the unavoidable incidence of complications after anesthesia and surgery.[7]

SAFETY IN THE POSTANESTHESIA CARE UNIT

The PACU medical director must ensure the PACU environment is as safe as possible for both patients and staff. Beyond usual safety policies, maintain staffing and training to ensure appropriate coverage and skill mix are available to deal with unforeseen crises. Incidence of adverse events in the PACU correlates with nursing workload and staff availability.[8] Ideally, all staff should have PACU certification, and staffing ratios should never fall below acceptable standards.[3] Less skilled staff must be appropriately supervised, and a sufficient number of certified personnel must always be available to handle worst-case scenarios.

The PACU staff protects patients who are temporarily incompetent and preserves patients' rights to observance of advanced directives and to informed consent for additional procedures. The staff is obligated to optimize each patient's privacy and dignity, and to minimize the psychological impact of unpleasant or frightening events. Observance of procedures for hand washing, sterility, and infection control should be assiduous.[9] Medical directors must safeguard against potential for personal assault of patients during recovery. Access to the PACU should be strictly controlled, and unobserved coverage of a PACU patient by one staff member for prolonged periods should be avoided, especially if there is a gender difference.

The PACU environment must also be safe for professionals. Air handling should guarantee that personnel are not exposed to unacceptable levels of trace anesthetic gases, although trace gas monitoring is not necessary. Ensure staff members receive appropriate vaccinations, including that for hepatitis B. Practitioners must adhere to policies for radiation safety, infection control, disposal of sharps, universal precautions for bloodborne diseases, and safeguarding against exposure to pathogens such as methicillin-resistant *Staphylococcus* or tuberculosis. Always keep masks, gloves, eye protection, and appropriate personal respiratory equipment available. Ensure sufficient help is available to avoid injury while lifting and positioning patients or while dealing with emergence reactions. Compulsive documentation and clear delineation of responsibility protect staff against unnecessary medicolegal exposure.

ADMISSION TO THE POSTANESTHESIA CARE UNIT

Every patient admitted to a PACU should have heart rate and rhythm, systemic blood pressure, airway patency, oxygen saturation, ventilatory rate and character, and level of pain recorded and periodically monitored.[4] Assessment with contemporaneous recording every 5 minutes for the first 15 minutes and every 15 minutes thereafter is a prudent minimum. Document temperature, level of consciousness, mental status, neuromuscular function, hydration status, and degree of nausea on admission and discharge, and more frequent if appropriate. Every patient should be continuously monitored with a pulse oximeter and a single-lead electrocardiogram (ECG). Capnography is necessary only for patients receiving mechanical ventilation or those at risk for compromised ventilatory function. Transduce and record the output from invasive monitors such as central venous, systemic, or pulmonary arterial catheters. Order diagnostic tests only for specific indications.

2 Anesthesiology personnel should manage the patient until a PACU nurse secures admission vital signs and attaches appropriate monitors. A succinct but thorough report that includes sufficient information to allow rapid evaluation and intervention for postoperative complications (Table 54-1) must be legibly recorded using a standardized format printed on the PACU record. Document the time and amount of all neuromuscular relaxants, respiratory depressant medications, and reversal agents. Outline orders, specific therapeutic end points, and how to contact the responsible anesthesiologist. Never transfer responsibility to PACU personnel until the patient's airway status, ventilation, and hemodynamics are appropriate. Check the function of indwelling cannulae, intravenous catheters, and monitors before leaving.

POSTOPERATIVE PAIN MANAGEMENT

3 Relief of surgical pain with minimal side effects is a high priority during PACU care,[4,10–12] so periodically assess and document level of pain throughout recovery (see Chapter 55). Inadequate postoperative analgesia is a major source of preoperative fear and postoperative dissatisfaction for surgical patients. In addition to improving comfort, analgesia reduces sympathetic nervous system (SNS) response and helps avoid hypertension, tachycardia, and dysrhythmias. In hypovolemic patients relying on SNS activity for cardiovascular homeostasis, analgesics can precipitate hypotension, especially if direct or histamine-induced vasodilation occurs. Assess a tachycardic patient with low or normal blood pressure who complains of pain carefully before giving analgesics that might precipitate or accentuate hypotension.

TABLE 54-1

COMPONENTS OF A POSTANESTHESIA CARE UNIT ADMISSION REPORT

PREOPERATIVE HISTORY

- Medication allergies or reactions
- Pertinent earlier surgical procedures
- Underlying medical illness
- Chronic medications
- Acute problems (e.g., ischemia, acid-base status, dehydration)
- Premedications
- NPO status

INTRAOPERATIVE FACTORS

- Surgical procedure
- Type of anesthetic
- Relaxant/reversal status
- Time and amount of opioids administered
- Type and amount of intravenous fluids administered
- Estimated blood loss
- Urine output
- Unexpected surgical or anesthetic events
- Intraoperative vital sign ranges
- Intraoperative laboratory findings
- Drugs given (e.g., steroids, diuretics, antibiotics, vasoactive medications)

ASSESSMENT AND REPORT OF CURRENT STATUS

- Airway patency
- Ventilatory adequacy
- Level of consciousness
- Level of pain
- Heart rate and heart rhythm
- Endotracheal tube position
- Systemic pressure
- Intravascular volume status
- Function of invasive monitors
- Size and location of intravenous catheters
- Anesthetic equipment (e.g., epidural catheters)
- Overall impression

POSTOPERATIVE INSTRUCTIONS

- Expected airway and ventilatory status
- Acceptable vital sign ranges
- Acceptable urine output and blood loss
- Surgical instructions (e.g., positioning, wound care)
- Anticipated cardiovascular problems
- Orders for therapeutic interventions
- Diagnostic tests to be secured
- Therapeutic goals and end points before discharge
- Location of responsible physician

NPO, nothing by mouth.

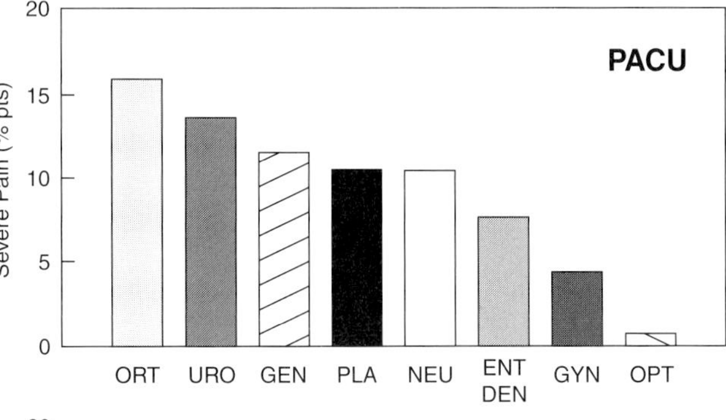

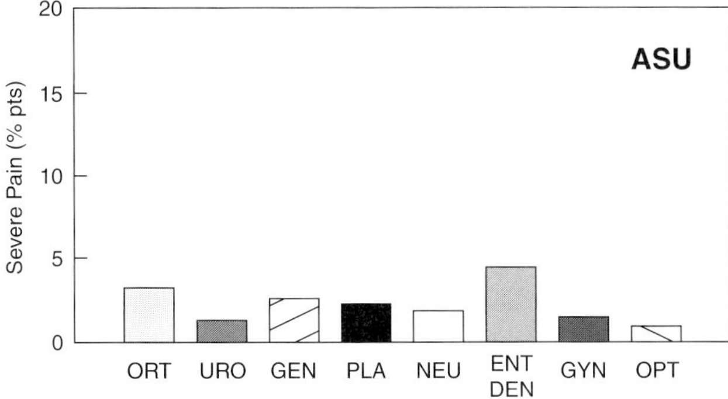

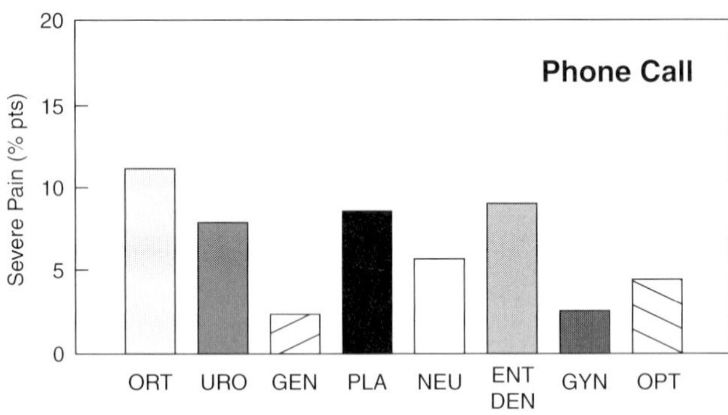

FIGURE 54-1. Percentage of patients experiencing severe pain in the postanesthesia care unit (PACU), the ambulatory surgery unit (ASU), and during a postanesthesia phone call at 24 hours. (Reprinted with permission from Chung F, Ritchie E, Su J: Postoperative pain in ambulatory surgery. Anesth Analg 85:808, 1997.)

The actual degree of postoperative pain can be difficult to establish. Severity of pain varies among surgical procedures and anesthetic techniques. Staff members are relatively ineffective at quantifying level of discomfort. Inexperienced nurses overestimate a patient's pain, whereas more experienced nurses tend to underestimate.[13] Either error leads to inappropriate treatment. Use of a quantitative pain scale yields more reliable results. A wide divergence can exist between a patient's cognitive perception of pain and SNS response, related to psychological, cultural, and cardiovascular differences among individuals. Some patients perceive severe pain with minimal SNS activity, whereas others exhibit hypertension and tachycardia with minimal complaint of discomfort. The best barometer of analgesia is the patient's perception.

Careful identification of patient subgroups, assessment of individual analgesic requirements, and implementation of a planned, multimodal approach will provide seamless pain control through and beyond the PACU interval.[14] In a study of postoperative pain in 10,008 ambulatory patients, only 5.3% related severe pain in the PACU and 1.7% in the discharge area (Fig. 54-1). However, a much higher percentage of patients relate that moderate to severe pain recurs after discharge.[15,16] To avoid masking signs of an unrelated condition or a surgical complication, ascertain that the nature and intensity of pain are appropriate for the surgical procedure. The central nervous system (CNS) signs of hypoxemia, acidemia, or cerebral hypoperfusion often mimic those of pain, especially during emergence. Administration of parenteral analgesics or sedatives can acutely worsen hypoventilation, airway obstruction, or hypotension, causing sudden deterioration. Evaluating orientation, the level of arousal, and cardiovascular or pulmonary status usually identifies such patients.

Incisional pain can be effectively treated with intravenous opioids as part of a planned analgesic continuum that begins prior to the induction of surgical anesthesia and continues throughout the postoperative course. Sufficient analgesia is the end point, even if large doses of opioids are necessary in tolerant patients. Short-acting opioids are useful to expedite discharge and minimize nausea in ambulatory settings,[17] although duration of analgesia can be a problem. During intravenous titration of opioids, assess for incremental respiratory or cardiovascular depression. Disadvantages of intramuscular administration include larger dose requirements, delayed onset, and unpredictable uptake in hypothermic patients. Oral and transdermal analgesics have a limited role in the PACU but are helpful for ambulatory patients after PACU discharge. Rectal analgesics are sometimes useful in small children.

Perioperative oral or intravenous administration of cyclooxygenase-2 (COX-2) inhibitors seems to offer a promising adjunctive therapy that augments postoperative analgesia, probably by reducing the inflammatory components of postoperative pain.[18] Unfortunately, more recent concern about negative cardiac side effects of COX-2 inhibitors, culminating in the withdrawal of rofecoxib, has clouded the overall appropriateness of this approach. Ibuprofen or acetaminophen are also effective, especially when administered orally before surgery. Preoperative administration likely augments the overall level of analgesia rather than offering a substantial preemptive advantage.[19] Ketorolac is an effective analgesic and anti-inflammatory that lowers opioid requirements, although possibility of hemorrhage due to its antiplatelet properties limits its use. Ketorolac might also decrease ischemic events in patients with coronary artery disease through analgesic and antiplatelet actions. Use of clonidine to supplement analgesia is effective but can cause hypotension. Agonist–antagonist analgesics offer little advantage. Interventions such as repositioning, reassurance, or extubation also help minimize discomfort.

Other analgesic modalities provide pain relief in and beyond the PACU.[20] Intravenous opioid loading in the PACU is important for smooth transition to intravenous patient-controlled analgesia. Injection of opioids into the epidural or subarachnoid space during anesthesia or in the PACU yields prolonged postoperative analgesia in selected patients.[21,22] Nausea and pruritus are troubling side effects, and immediate or delayed ventilatory depression can occur, related to vascular uptake and cephalad spread in cerebrospinal fluid. Nausea resolves with antiemetics, whereas pruritus and ventilatory depression often respond to naloxone infusion. Addition of local anesthetic or clonidine enhances analgesia and decreases the risk of side effects from epidural opioids, although local anesthetics add risk of hypotension or motor blockade. Epidural analgesia is effective after thoracic and upper abdominal procedures and helps wean patients with obesity or chronic obstructive pulmonary disease (COPD) from mechanical ventilation. Whether epidural analgesia improves surgical outcomes is debatable.

Placement of long-acting regional analgesic blocks reduces pain, controls SNS activity, and often improves ventilation.[20] After shoulder procedures, interscalene block yields almost complete pain relief with only moderate inconvenience from motor impairment. Paralysis of the ipsilateral diaphragm can impair postoperative ventilation in patients with marginal reserve, although the impact is small in most patients.[23] Suprascapular nerve block might be an alternative to avoid this potentially serious side effect. Percutaneous intercostal blocks reduce analgesic requirements after thoracic or high abdominal incision, although beneficial effects on postoperative pulmonary function are questionable. Caudal analgesia is effective in children after inguinal or genital procedures, whereas infiltration of local anesthetic into joints, soft tissues, or incisions decreases the intensity of pain. Instillation of opioids or neostigmine into joints is also analgesic. Other modalities, such as positive suggestion, hypnosis, transcutaneous nerve stimulation, "white noise," or acupuncture have limited utility for surgical pain.

Use of patient-controlled analgesia, spinal opioids, or neural blockade mandates anticipation of risk beyond the PACU. Plan for extended postoperative analgesia before induction of surgical anesthesia, and orient the anesthetic and PACU care toward that plan. If one analgesic modality proves inadequate, take particular care when implementing a second technique.

Fear, anxiety, and confusion often accentuate postoperative pain during recovery, especially after general anesthesia. Titration of an intravenous sedative such as midazolam attenuates this psychogenic component, although analgesic requirements may increase slightly because benzodiazepines interact with γ-aminobutyric acid receptors. It is important to distinguish between requirements for analgesia and for sedation. Opioids are poor sedatives, whereas benzodiazepines are poor analgesics.

DISCHARGE CRITERIA

When possible before discharge from postoperative care, each patient should be sufficiently oriented to assess his or her physical condition and summon assistance. Airway reflexes and motor function must be adequate to maintain patency and prevent aspiration. Ensure ventilation and oxygenation are acceptable, with sufficient reserve to cover minor deterioration in unmonitored settings. Blood pressure, heart rate, and indices of peripheral perfusion should be relatively constant for at least 15 minutes and appropriately near baseline. Achieving normal body temperature is not an absolute requirement, but resolution of shivering is. Acceptable analgesia must be achieved and vomiting appropriately controlled. Patients should be observed for at least 15 minutes after the last intravenous opioid or sedative is administered to assess peak effects and side effects. After reinforcement of regional anesthetics, longer observation could be appropriate. Monitor oxygen saturation for 15 minutes after discontinuation of supplemental oxygen to detect hypoxemia. Assess likely complications of surgery (e.g., bleeding, vascular compromise, pneumothorax) or of underlying conditions (e.g., hypertension, myocardial ischemia, hyperglycemia, bronchospasm). Document a brief neurologic assessment of orientation, eye signs, facial symmetry, and extremity movement. Review results of diagnostic tests. If these generic criteria cannot be met, postponement of discharge or transfer to a specialized unit is advisable.

There is no demonstrable benefit from a mandatory minimum duration of PACU care. Rather, observe patients until they meet discharge criterion and are no longer at increased risk for cardiorespiratory depression.[4] Fixed PACU discharge criteria must be used with caution because variability among patients is tremendous. Scoring systems that quantify physical status or establish thresholds for vital signs are useful for as-
4 sessment but cannot replace individual evaluation.[24,25] Ideally, each patient should be evaluated for discharge by an anesthesiologist using a consistent set of criteria (Table 54-2), considering the severity of underlying disease, the anesthetic and recovery course, and the level of care at the destination (see Chapter 46). Plan for the continued management of likely post-discharge symptoms such as pain, nausea, headache, dizziness, drowsiness, and fatigue.[16]

CARDIOVASCULAR COMPLICATIONS

Postoperative Hypotension

5 Systemic hypotension, a common postoperative complication, can cause hypoperfusion of vital organ systems. Consequent tissue hypoxia promotes inefficient anaerobic metabolism and lactic acidemia. During hypotension, the SNS diverts blood

TABLE 54-2

GUIDELINES FOR DISCHARGE EVALUATION FROM POSTANESTHESIA CARE UNIT

■ GENERAL CONDITION

- Oriented to time, place, and surgical procedure
- Responds to verbal input and follows simple instructions
- Acceptable color without cyanosis, splotchiness, or paleness
- Adequate muscular strength and mobility for minimal self-care
- Absence or control of specific acute surgical complications (e.g., bleeding, edema, neurologic weakness, diminished pulse)
- Suitable control of nausea and emesis
- Destination unit appropriate for patient's status

■ SYSTEM BLOOD PRESSURE

- Within ±20% of resting preoperative value
- Heart rate and rhythm relatively constant for at least 30 min
- Resolution of any new dysrhythmia
- Acceptable intravascular volume status
- Any suspicion of myocardial ischemia rectified

■ VENTILATION AND OXYGENATION

- Ventilatory rate >10, <30 breaths/min
- Forced vital capacity approximately twice tidal volume
- Adequate ability to cough and clear secretions
- Qualitatively acceptable work of breathing

■ AIRWAY MAINTENANCE

- Protective reflexes (swallow, gag) intact
- Absence of stridor, retraction, or partial obstruction
- No further need for artificial airway support

■ CONTROL OF PAIN

- Ability to localize and identify intensity of surgical pain
- Adequate analgesia, at least 15 min since last opioid
- Safe, appropriate orders for postdischarge analgesics

■ RENAL FUNCTION

- Urine output >30 mL/h (catheterized patients)
- Appropriate color and appearance of urine, evaluation of hematuria
- Follow-up orders in regard to output if spontaneous voiding has not occurred

■ METABOLIC/LABORATORY

- Acceptable hematocrit level in view of hydration, blood loss, and potential for future losses
- Suitable control of blood glucose
- Appropriate electrolyte homeostasis
- Evaluation of chest radiograph, electrocardiogram, and other tests as appropriate

■ AMBULATORY PATIENTS

- Ability to ambulate without dizziness, hypotension, or support
- Suitable control of nausea and vomiting after ambulation

Not all criteria will be satisfied by every patient, especially if discharge is to a critical care unit. Clinical judgment must always supersede established guidelines if the patient's condition is less than optimal in a given area. Whenever doubt exists about diagnosis or patient safety, discharge should be delayed.

flow to preserve the brain, heart, and kidneys, so symptoms of hypoperfusion referable to these organs (e.g., disorientation, nausea, loss of consciousness, angina, reduced urine output) indicate that compensatory mechanisms have been exhausted. Complications of hypotension include ischemia or infarction of the myocardium, cerebrum, renal tubules, spinal cord, or bowel. Reduced venous flow rate increases risk of deep vein thrombosis and pulmonary embolism. Decreased hepatic oxygen delivery might change metabolic pathways for drugs or cause hepatic damage by toxic metabolites. The degree of postoperative hypotension at which risk of complications increases varies with the baseline blood pressure, and is higher in patients with arteriosclerotic disease, stenotic vascular lesions, chronic hypertension, increased intracranial pressure, or renal failure.

Spurious Hypotension

Identifying spurious hypotension avoids unnecessary treatment and iatrogenic hypertension. A blood pressure cuff that is too large yields falsely low values. A transducer system that is improperly zeroed or excessively damped by air bubbles or catheter obstruction yields artificially low readings from an arterial catheter. Arterial constriction caused by hypothermia or alpha-adrenergic agonist drugs can reduce radial or brachial blood pressure below aortic pressure.

Hypovolemia

A reduction in circulating intravascular volume ("absolute" hypovolemia) decreases ventricular filling and cardiac output. SNS-mediated tachycardia, increased systemic vascular resistance (SVR), and venoconstriction might compensate for a 15 to 20% loss of intravascular volume. Greater deficits cause hypotension.

Failure to replace preoperative fluid deficit and fluid or blood lost during surgery frequently causes absolute hypovolemia. In the PACU, ongoing hemorrhage, sweating, and exudation of fluid into tissues (third-space losses) exacerbate hypovolemia. Blood loss is often occult, as with retroperitoneal bleeding, oozing related to coagulopathy, or hemorrhage into muscle after trauma or orthopaedic procedures. Third-space losses can continue for up to 48 hours after surgery and can be massive during high-permeability pulmonary edema or accumulation of ascites. In a hypothermic, venoconstricted patient, a low intravascular volume might maintain cardiac output on PACU admission but cause hypotension when venous capacity increases during rewarming.

Sometimes, a "normal" intravascular volume is inadequate to maintain blood pressure (relative hypovolemia). Sudden decreases in endogenous SNS activity caused by relief of pain or vasovagal responses can acutely increase venous capacity, as can medications that mimic alpha-adrenergic receptor blockade (droperidol, chlorpromazine), release histamine (morphine), or directly dilate veins (nitrates, furosemide). Spinal or epidural anesthesia interferes with SNS regulation of venous tone, increasing venous capacitance and preventing constriction of veins in response to hemorrhage or positional changes. Compression of thoracic veins from positive intrathoracic pressure during mechanical ventilation impedes venous return, as does inferior vena caval compression from a gravid uterus or increased intra-abdominal pressure. Pericardial tamponade or air embolism also impedes ventricular filling.

Evaluate each patient's hydration status on admission and throughout the PACU stay,[4] considering preoperative status, type and duration of surgery, estimated blood loss, fluid replacement, and hemostasis. Monitoring urine output as an index of intravascular volume can be misleading. Surgery and anesthesia impair renal tubular concentrating ability, and glycosuria causes osmotic diuresis, each falsely indicating that intravascular volume is adequate. The variation of systolic blood pressure seen on an arterial catheter or pulse oximeter trace during positive-pressure ventilation provides a qualitative warning of hypovolemia in some patients. Central venous pressure (CVP), pulmonary artery (PA) pressure, or transesophageal echocardiography (TEE) monitoring helps clarify volume status. Manage intravascular volume actively during recovery.

Ventricular Dysfunction

Postoperative hypotension caused by ventricular dysfunction usually indicates that baseline ventricular contractility is reduced. Such patients often need high left ventricular end-diastolic pressure and elevated SNS activity to maintain cardiac output. Excessive fluid administration causes ventricular dilation, decreased cardiac output, and hypotension, often complicated by hydrostatic pulmonary edema. Overhydration may not be evident. If sympathetic blockade during spinal or epidural anesthesia is treated with excessive fluids, ventricular filling pressures can be normal during early recovery, despite hypervolemia. When SNS blockade resolves, a characteristically high level of SNS outflow mobilizes large fluid volumes to the central circulation, precipitating ventricular failure. Depression from residual inhalational anesthetics and opiates contributes to decreased SNS outflow, reducing ventricular contractility during early recovery. Profound metabolic or respiratory acidemia reduces ventricular performance by interfering with catecholamine–receptor interaction and by depressing central SNS outflow. Low ionized calcium levels caused by dilution, chelation, or acute alkalemia also reduce ventricular contractility. Right ventricular dysfunction caused by pulmonary thromboembolism often presents with systemic hypotension.

Myocardial Ischemia

Among patients with coronary disease, risk of postoperative myocardial ischemia and infarction is higher for those with a history of congestive heart failure, valvular disease, low ejection fraction, smoking, anemia, and probably hypertension, and those having emergency surgery.[26,27] Patients are at significant risk after both general and regional anesthetics. Ischemia is often initiated in high-risk patients by tachycardia that reduces diastolic filling time. Postoperative tachycardia is caused by pain, hypotension, acidemia, anxiety, or medications. Diastolic hypotension from hypovolemia, bradycardia, or vasodilation can also precipitate ischemia by decreasing the pressure gradient for coronary perfusion. Increased ventricular wall tension secondary to overhydration, hypertension, or increased SNS activity increases myocardial oxygen consumption. Severe hypoxemia, anemia, or carbon monoxide (CO) poisoning generates ischemia independent of coronary perfusion. The lowest tolerable oxygen saturation value varies among individuals but is usually higher in patients with vascular disease. Postoperative ischemia is often silent and more frequently leads to non–Q-wave infarction. Risk of early morbidity is still high.[28] Postoperative anginal chest pain might be overshadowed by pain from surgical incisions and gastric distention, or masked by analgesia from residual anesthetics or opioids. The incidence of ischemic dysrhythmias is difficult to determine, given the high incidence of benign postoperative dysrhythmias. Hypotension caused by ischemic ventricular dysfunction can quickly cause irreversible infarction. Close evaluation of the hemodynamic responses to fluid challenge, the ST segment and T-wave morphology on the ECG, and the PA pressures can sometimes uncover ischemia before hypotension occurs (Fig. 54-2). However, the predictive
6 value of these indices is controversial. Control of precipitating factors and timely therapy with analgesia, aggressive use of beta-adrenergic blocking agents, and nitrates when appropriate helps decrease morbidity.[29–31] Postoperative use of short-acting beta-adrenergic blockers is generally safe in patients with bronchospastic disease or decreased ventricular contractility. Efficacy is significant even with nearly baseline heart rates and may reflect other benefits of beta-blockade beyond rate control.

Cardiac Dysrhythmias

Preexisting myocardial disease or rhythm disturbances increase the risk of postoperative hypotension caused by cardiac

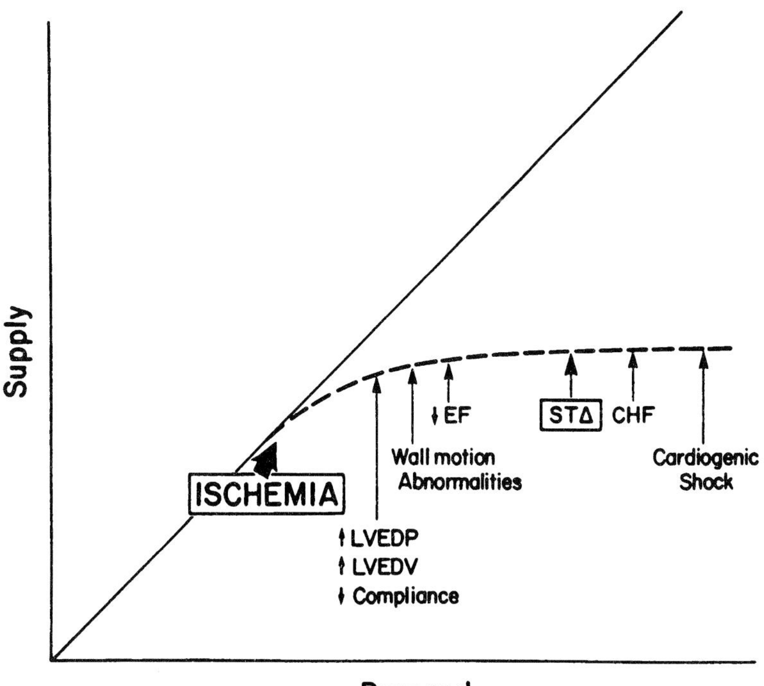

FIGURE 54-2. Physiologic consequences of myocardial ischemia. Note that changes in ventricular pressure and compliance may precede electrocardiographic changes (ST segment). LVEDP, left ventricular end-diastolic pressure; LVEDV, left ventricular end-diastolic volume; EF, ejection fraction; ST, ST segment change; CHF, congestive heart failure. (Reprinted with permission from Barash PG: Monitoring myocardial oxygen balance: Physiologic basis and clinical application. In Barash PG, Deutsch S, Tinker J [eds]: Refresher Courses in Anesthesiology, vol 13, p 21. Philadelphia, JB Lippincott, 1985.)

dysrhythmias. Sinus or nodal bradycardia with ventricular rates below 40 beats/min decreases cardiac output and blood pressure, as do slow ventricular rhythms associated with complete heart block. A tachydysrhythmia that generates ventricular rates of 140 to 150 beats/min can decrease cardiac output because ventricular filling time is compromised. Ventricular fibrillation, asystole, or electromechanical dissociation causes life-threatening reductions of output. Swings in autonomic nervous system activity place patients with critical valvular abnormalities at particular risk of hypotension from rate or rhythm changes. An increased heart rate in patients with aortic stenosis reduces systolic ejection time, whereas tachycardia in patients with mitral stenosis impedes ventricular filling. Both decrease cardiac output and cause hypotension.

Decreased Systemic Vascular Resistance

Hypotension associated with regional anesthesia, alpha-adrenergic receptor blocking drugs, blood components, warming, or systemic sepsis is caused by decreased SVR and by reduced venous return. Severe systemic acidemia decreases SVR by directly dilating vessels and by interfering with the catecholamine–alpha-receptor interaction. Decreased SVR often generates a high-output, low-resistance hypotension.

Postoperative hypotension is occasionally caused by the effects of anesthesia or surgery on baroreceptor function or by intracranial disease. Rarely, hypotension reflects steroid deficiency in patients whose adrenal axis is suppressed by exogenous steroid use. Hypotension secondary to steroid deficiency is often preceded by lethargy, fever, or nausea and by hyponatremia, hyperkalemia, and hypoglycemia.

Treatment of Postoperative Hypotension

In general, symptoms of vital organ hypoperfusion or a 20 to 30% reduction in systolic pressure from preoperative levels is an indication to treat. If risk for complication from hypotension is high, tighter limits for pressure and heart rate should be defined during PACU admission. A low blood pressure determination should be quickly validated. Auscultation of heart sounds and palpation of carotid or femoral pulses are useful qualitative indicators of central blood pressure. Check breath sounds and the cardiac rate and rhythm, and administer supplemental oxygen. Evaluate recent drug administration, and stop infusions that might cause vasodilation. A 12-lead ECG, arterial blood gas, or chest radiography might be indicated.

Direct therapy toward the etiology of reduced blood pressure. Simple maneuvers such as reducing airway pressure, placing pregnant patients in a lateral tilt position, or placing patients with orthostatic changes in a supine position should be used when appropriate. Tension pneumothorax must be evacuated. Increase the intravenous infusion rate to maximum because hypovolemia is the most common etiology. If hypotension is spurious or caused by a reduced SVR or ischemia, the amount of excess fluid infused while these diagnoses are established is usually inconsequential. Infusion of crystalloid solutions is usually sufficient to treat hypovolemia, although plasma expanders or blood facilitate more rapid volume expansion. Sympathomimetic alpha-adrenergic pressors such as phenylephrine that increase SVR and venous return will temporarily maintain systemic pressure until sufficient volume can be infused. Ephedrine is less desirable because increased heart rate and contractility are usually unnecessary.

If fluid administration (300 to 500 mL) does not improve hypotension, myocardial dysfunction should be considered. If hypotension is caused by ischemia, resolution of the ischemia usually restores baseline cardiac function. Heart rate control with analgesics, sedatives, and especially beta-receptor blockers is important. Support of aortic diastolic pressure with an alpha-receptor agonist and reduction of left ventricular end-diastolic pressure with nitroglycerin help maximize the coronary artery pressure gradient. Accurate diagnosis of ischemia is critical because therapy for ischemia can worsen hypotension caused by hypovolemia or other causes. PA catheterization or TEE might be useful to estimate left ventricular filling and cardiac output, although the value of PA readings is questionable. For dysfunction not related to ischemia, drugs that augment contractility, perhaps in conjunction with systemic vasodilators, restore cardiac output and systemic pressure.

If hypotension is caused by metabolic acidemia, intravenous bicarbonate or another alkalinizing agent helps restore pH until the underlying cause is remedied. Hypotension from severe hypoxemia or respiratory acidemia mandates tracheal intubation and mechanical ventilation with supplemental oxygen. Sinus bradycardia unrelated to hypoxemia usually responds to intravenous atropine, glycopyrrolate, or ephedrine. Refractory bradycardia caused by sinus node disease or complete heart block is managed with intravenous epinephrine or isoproterenol, or with cardiac pacing. Beta-adrenergic or calcium channel blockade reduces the ventricular rate from acute-onset atrial fibrillation, whereas reentrant paroxysmal atrial tachycardia often disappears with beta-adrenergic blockade or with maneuvers or drugs that change cardiac conduction rates. If hypotension is severe, immediate low-energy, direct-current cardioversion is indicated.

Hypotension caused by a low SVR is treated with an alpha-adrenergic agent. Sympathectomy from regional anesthesia responds to low levels of alpha stimulation. During advanced sepsis or catecholamine depletion, norepinephrine infusions may be required. If decreased SVR is caused by acidemia, correction of pH is necessary before pressor therapy will be effective.

Postoperative Hypertension

A moderate elevation in systemic blood pressure is common and acceptable in well-hydrated postoperative patients.[7] However, excessively high blood pressure can cause hemorrhage and third-space losses, and might disrupt vascular suture lines. High ventricular intracavitary pressure might lead to myocardial fiber stretch and increased wall tension, precipitating ischemia or dysrhythmias. Elevated intraocular or intracranial pressure, cerebral edema, and intracranial hemorrhage also potentially increase morbidity.

A blood pressure cuff that is too small yields erroneously high readings, especially in obese or very muscular patients. A transducing system that is improperly zeroed or exhibits excessive resonance overestimates systolic pressure. Overshoot does not significantly change the accuracy of diastolic readings. Patients with preexisting hypertension exhibit exaggerated blood pressure responses because they have noncompliant vasculature, elevated peripheral vascular tone, and high levels of baseline endogenous SNS activity. Baroreceptor control of heart rate may be impaired, especially after carotid endarterectomy or anticholinergic administration during reversal of neuromuscular relaxation.

Enhanced SNS activity frequently causes hypertension in PACU patients. Peripheral arteriolar and venous constriction mediated by alpha-adrenergic stimulation increases SVR and venous return, whereas increased β_1 receptor stimulation increases ventricular contractility and heart rate. SNS outflow most often reflects an appropriate response to noxious stimuli or adverse physiologic conditions (Table 54-3). SNS activity might also result from exogenous sympathomimetics, monoamine oxidase inhibition, or pheochromocytoma. Intravascular volume expansion and hypothermia accentuate the

TABLE 54-3

FACTORS THAT INCREASE POSTOPERATIVE SYMPATHETIC NERVOUS SYSTEM ACTIVITY

■ FACTORS INCREASING SYMPATHETIC ACTIVITY
Noxious stimuli
Pain, anxiety, cranial stimulation, full bladder, tracheal intubation
Adverse physiologic conditions
Hypercarbia/acidosis, hypoxemia, hypotension, hypoglycemia, congestive heart failure, increased intracranial pressure, myocardial ischemia
Medications
Beta-mimetic pressors, ephedrine, isoproterenol, epinephrine
Dopamine, dobutamine
Bronchodilators
Terbutaline, aminophylline
Antihypertensives
Hydralazine, nitroprusside
Anesthetics
Ketamine, isoflurane
■ FACTORS DECREASING PARASYMPATHETIC ACTIVITY
Medications
Parasympatholytics
Atropine, glycopyrrolate
Relaxants
Pancuronium

TABLE 54-4

FACTORS THAT INCREASE POSTOPERATIVE PARASYMPATHETIC NERVOUS SYSTEM ACTIVITY

■ FACTORS INCREASING PARASYMPATHETIC ACTIVITY
Vagal reflexes
Carotid sinus massage, Valsalva maneuver, gagging, rectal examination, increased ocular pressure, bladder distention, pharyngeal stimulation
Parasympathomimetic medications
Acetylcholinesterase inhibitors
Neostigmine, edrophonium
Alpha-adrenergic drugs
Neo-Synephrine, norepinephrine
Opioids
Morphine, fentanyl
Succinylcholine
■ FACTORS DECREASING SYMPATHETIC ACTIVITY
High spinal or epidural anesthesia
Withdrawal of stimulus, extubation, emptying bladder
Severe acidemia/hypoxemia
Sympatholytic medications
Beta-receptor blockers (propranolol)
Opioids/sedatives/general anesthetics
Ganglionic blockers
Local anesthetics

effect of SNS activity on blood pressure. Cerebral vascular accidents, hypoxic encephalopathy, increased intracranial pressure, or osmotic changes can interfere with central SNS regulation and cause autonomic dysfunction and severe hypertension.

Indications for treatment of postoperative hypertension include a systolic or diastolic pressure 20 to 30% above baseline, signs or symptoms of complications (e.g., headache, bleeding, ocular changes, angina, ST segment depression), or an unusual risk of morbidity (e.g., increased intracranial pressure, mitral regurgitation, open eye injury). In patients with chronic hypertension, achieving a "normal" systemic pressure could promote vital organ hypoperfusion so blood pressure should be reduced toward preoperative levels. Orient therapy toward causes of increased SNS activity. Administering analgesics or sedatives, correcting acidemia or hypoxemia, and ensuring ability to void are helpful. If hypertension persists, intravenous antihypertensive medications such as labetalol, esmolol, hydralazine with propranolol, or nicardipine yield temporary control. Incorporation of clonidine into the overall regimen may augment analgesia, control blood pressure, and blunt the postoperative SNS response to stimuli. Potent vasodilators (nitroprusside, nitroglycerin) are reserved for refractory or profound hypertension.

Cardiac Dysrhythmias in the Postoperative Period

Asymptomatic Electrocardiographic Abnormalities

General anesthesia causes ECG changes in axis, intraventricular conduction, P-wave and T-wave morphology, and ST segments that are not related to cardiac abnormality (see Appendix – Electrocardiography). These changes reflect electrophysiologic effects of hypothermia, inhalation anesthetics, autonomic nervous system imbalance, and mild electrolyte abnormalities. Changes usually resolve within 3 to 6 hours. If persistent ECG changes indicate ischemia, optimize myocardial oxygen supply and demand, follow serial ECG and enzyme determinations, and monitor as appropriate.

Bradycardia

In the PACU, increased parasympathetic nervous system (PNS) or decreased SNS activity influence promotes sinus bradycardia (Table 54-4). Sick sinus syndrome, sinoatrial nodal ischemia, or severe hypoxemia also reduce sinus rate. Sinus bradycardia is benign unless it causes hypotension, usually when the rate falls below 40 to 45 beats/min. Therapy involves restoring SNS/PNS balance to normal. Bradycardia caused by excess PNS activity usually responds to muscarinic blocking drugs such as atropine or glycopyrrolate. Decreased SNS activity usually responds to a beta-mimetic drug such as ephedrine.

Emergence of a nodal pacemaker in the lower atrioventricular (AV) node or the bundle of His is also usually caused by autonomic imbalance. Factors that stop sinus impulses from reaching the ventricle also promote nodal rhythms. Nodal rhythms are benign unless a low ventricular rate or lack of coordinated atrial contraction reduces cardiac output and blood pressure. If hypotension occurs, atropine or beta-mimetic medications can restore a sinus rhythm. These measures sometimes only increase nodal rate, necessitating support of blood pressure until spontaneous resolution occurs.

Risk of developing complete heart block in patients with bifascicular block or left bundle-branch block is small but real. Idioventricular bradycardia seldom generates adequate cardiac output, and usually indicates life-threatening heart block, hypoxemia, acidemia, or myocardial ischemia. Atropine might improve AV nodal conduction enough to allow supraventricular impulses to reach the ventricles with acute third-degree AV nodal block. Atropine does not increase rate of ventricular pacemaker cells because they lack PNS innervation, but epinephrine, isoproterenol, or cardiac pacing will accelerate the ventricular rate.

Tachycardia

Postoperative sinus tachycardia is nearly always associated with a physiologic increase in SNS influence (see Table 54-3). Tachycardia is usually harmless, but it can precipitate acute myocardial ischemia in patients with coronary artery disease. Sinus tachycardia seldom interferes with ventricular filling but compromises cardiac output in patients with stenotic valvular lesions. Tachycardia exacerbates hypertension and might indicate acidemia, hypoxemia, or malignant hyperthermia. Sinus tachycardia is treated by addressing the underlying cause. Giving analgesics for pain, intravenous fluids for hypovolemia, or sedatives to calm anxiety is usually sufficient. Decompressing a full bladder is helpful. Tachycardia caused by sympathomimetic drugs resolves as drug levels fall. If SNS activity is beyond control or tachycardia presents a threat, beta-blockade helps control rate. Digoxin is ineffective unless ventricular failure is the underlying cause.

Overall incidence of postoperative supraventricular arrhythmia after noncardiac surgery can approach 6%, with atrial fibrillation twice as common as supraventricular tachycardia.[32] Sudden-onset atrial fibrillation sometimes generates ventricular rates greater than 150 beats/min and might appear as a fast, nearly regular tachycardia on the ECG. Patients recovering from thoracic surgical procedures or those with mitral valvular disease or pulmonary emboli have a higher incidence. Rapid ventricular rate might cause hypotension or myocardial ischemia. Once aggravating factors are resolved, control of rate with beta-adrenergic or calcium channel blockers is appropriate to decrease the number of impulses that traverse the AV node per minute. For acute postoperative atrial fibrillation, rate control is more effective than rhythm conversion. Be cautious using adenosine, beta-blockers, digoxin, or calcium channel blockers if there is a possibility that the dysrhythmia is caused by Wolfe-Parkinson-White syndrome. Digoxin should be used for patients who will benefit from increased contractility. If hypotension is serious, direct-current cardioversion can convert fibrillation to sinus rhythm.

Atrial flutter is uncommon in postoperative patients. Treatment decreases the ventricular rate and regularizes atrial electrical activity. Paroxysmal atrial tachycardia usually reflects either circus reentry in a loop of conduction tissue, or discrete, rapidly firing atrial cells causing junctional, ectopic, or multifocal atrial tachycardia. Rapid rates can interfere with ventricular filling and compromise cardiac output. Treatment involves slowing conduction velocities to interrupt reentrant synchrony by increasing PNS influence (see Table 54-4). Beta-adrenergic or calcium channel blockers are useful for rate control, whereas slowing conduction velocities by increasing PNS influence (see Table 54-4) can interrupt reentrant synchrony. Junctional, ectopic or multifocal atrial tachycardices initially slow with adenosine and are subsequently treated with beta-blockers, Ca^{++} channel blockers, or amiodarome. They are not amenable to cardioversion.

Postoperative ventricular tachycardia or fibrillation almost always reflects severe myocardial ischemia, systemic acidemia, or hypoxemia, although reentrant ventricular tachycardia does occur. Cardiopulmonary resuscitation, beta-mimetic pressors, cardioversion, and control of ventilation, oxygenation, and serum pH help restore a synchronized rhythm.

Premature Contractions

An aberrant impulse arising in the atrium, AV node, or upper bundle of His generates an atrial premature contraction (APC), causing an early but otherwise normal QRS complex that is often not preceded by a P wave. In postoperative patients, APCs usually reflect increased SNS activity and seldom cause hemodynamic compromise. Control of stimuli causing increased SNS activity often eliminates APCs (see Table 54-3).

Ventricular ectopy present before surgery usually reappears in the PACU and does not predict postoperative outcome.[33] In postoperative patients, many high-amplitude, wide, and bizarre QRS complexes represent benign, aberrantly conducted APCs or reentrant beats rather than abnormal impulses that originate in the ventricle. If an early supraventricular impulse enters the ventricular conduction system before all pathways have fully recovered excitability, it will generate asynchronous ventricular depolarization and a wide, high-amplitude ECG complex. This aberrantly conducted APC is sometimes preceded by an abnormal P wave, often exhibits a noncompensatory pause, and frequently resembles normal complexes in general shape. If a sinus impulse is delayed in a ventricular conduction pathway long enough to encounter tissue that has recovered excitability, the impulse redepolarizes this tissue and spreads through the entire heart a second time. This "reentrant" depolarization generates uniform, wide, high-amplitude QRS complexes that manifest full compensatory pauses, follow the preceding normal complex by a constant interval (fixed coupling), and often appear in a bigeminal pattern. Delayed recovery of excitability after general anesthesia and increased SNS tone favor both aberrant conduction and reentry.

In postoperative patients, most actual premature ventricular contractions (PVCs) are caused by nonthreatening conditions. PVCs usually occur at varying intervals from a previous normal QRS and often exhibit a full compensatory pause. Benign PVCs often accompany excessive PNS or SNS activity. Increased PNS influence allows emergence of ventricular escape beats. Increased SNS activity accelerates ventricular automatic cells, promoting depolarization between supraventricular impulses, and fosters emergence of parasystolic foci. PVCs resolve when autonomic nervous system balance is restored. Benign postoperative PVCs can also be generated by stretch of myocardial fibers from hypertension and by mechanical stimulation from central vascular catheters. PVCs that reflect myocardial ischemia, electrolyte disturbances, or digitalis toxicity are rare but serious.

If frequent ectopic beats compromise cardiac output, control of autonomic nervous system imbalance usually suffices. Antidysrhythmics are seldom necessary, although beta-receptor blockade might be useful. Elimination of factors that cause conduction delay or nonuniform recovery of excitability will often abolish reentrant impulses.

POSTOPERATIVE PULMONARY DYSFUNCTION

Mechanical, hemodynamic, and pharmacologic factors related to surgery and anesthesia impair ventilation, oxygenation, and airway maintenance.[34] Heavy smoking, obesity, sleep apnea, severe asthma, and COPD increase the risk of postoperative ventilatory events.[35] Preoperative pulmonary function testing has limited predictive value for postoperative complications,[36] perhaps with the exception of postoperative bronchospasm in smokers.[37]

Inadequate Postoperative Ventilation

7 In PACU patients, mild respiratory acidemia is expected, so elevated $Pa{CO_2}$ does not necessarily indicate inadequate postoperative ventilation. Inadequate ventilation should be suspected when (1) respiratory acidemia occurs coincident with tachypnea, anxiety, dyspnea, labored ventilation, or increased SNS activity; (2) hypocarbia reduces the arterial pH below 7.30; or (3) $Pa{CO_2}$ progressively increases with a progressive decrease in arterial pH.

Inadequate Respiratory Drive

During early recovery from anesthesia, residual effects of intravenous or inhalational anesthetics blunt the ventilatory responses to both hypercarbia and hypoxemia. Sedatives augment depression from opioids or anesthetics and reduce the conscious desire to ventilate (a significant component of ventilatory drive). Residual neuromuscular relaxants might also depress cholinergic portions of the hypoxic drive neural arc.

Hypoventilation and hypercarbia can evolve insidiously during transfer and admission to the PACU. Although effects of intraoperative medications are usually waning, but the peak depressant effect of intravenous opioid given just before transfer occurs in the PACU. Coincident depression of medullary centers that regulate the SNS can blunt signs of acidemia or hypoxemia such as hypertension, tachycardia, and agitation, concealing hypoventilation. Patients might communicate lucidly and even complain of pain still while experiencing significant opioid-induced hypoventilation. A balance must be struck between an acceptable level of postoperative ventilatory depression and a tolerable level of pain or agitation. Patients with abnormal CO_2/pH responses from morbid obesity, chronic airway obstruction, or sleep apnea are more sensitive to respiratory depressants.[38] Risk for apnea after anesthesia in preterm infants depends on type of anesthetic, postconceptual age, and preoperative hematocrit. Preterm infants should be monitored for at least 12 hours (see Chapter 43). Children with active or recent upper respiratory infection are more prone to breath holding, severe cough, and arterial desaturations below 90% during recovery, especially if they have a history of reactive airway disease or secondhand smoke exposure or have undergone intubation and/or airway surgery.[39] If hypoventilation from opioids is excessive, forced arousal and titration of intravenous naloxone reverses respiratory depression without affecting analgesia. Flumazenil directly reverses depressant effects of benzodiazepines on ventilatory drive but is usually unnecessary.

The abrupt diminution of a noxious stimulus (e.g., tracheal extubation, placement of a postoperative block) may promote hypoventilation or airway obstruction by altering the balance between arousal from discomfort and depression from medication. Intracranial hemorrhage or edema sometimes presents with hypoventilation, especially after posterior fossa craniotomy. Bilateral carotid body injury after endarterectomy can ablate peripheral hypoxic drive. Chronic respiratory acidemia from COPD alters CNS sensitivity to pH and makes hypoxic drive dominant, but hypoventilation from supplemental oxygen rarely occurs.

Increased Airway Resistance

High resistance to gas flow through airways increases work of breathing and CO_2 production. If inspiratory muscles cannot generate sufficient pressure gradients to overcome resistance, alveolar ventilation fails to match CO_2 production and progressive respiratory acidemia occurs.

In postoperative patients, increased upper airway resistance is caused by obstruction in the pharynx (posterior tongue displacement, change in anteroposterior and lateral dimensions from soft tissue collapse), in the larynx (laryngospasm, laryngeal edema), or in the large airways (extrinsic compression from hematoma, tumor, or tracheal stenosis). Weakness from residual neuromuscular relaxation[40] or myasthenia gravis can contribute, but it is seldom the primary etiology of airway compromise. If the airway is clear of vomitus or foreign bodies, simple maneuvers such as improving the level of consciousness, lateral positioning, chin lift, mandible elevation, or placement of an oropharyngeal or nasopharyngeal airway usually relieve obstruction. A nasopharyngeal airway is better tolerated with functional gag reflexes. Acute extrinsic upper airway compression (e.g., an expanding neck hematoma) must be relieved.

During emergence, stimulation of the pharynx or vocal cords by secretions, foreign matter, or extubation generates laryngospasm.[41] Laryngeal constrictor muscles occlude the tracheal inlet and reduce gas flow. Patients who smoke or are chronically exposed to smoke, have irritable airway conditions, have copious secretions, or have undergone upper airway surgery are at higher risk.[34,39] Laryngospasm can usually be overcome by providing gentle positive pressure in the oropharynx with 100% O_2. Prolonged laryngospasm is relieved with a small dose of succinylcholine (e.g., 0.1 mg/kg). An intubating dosage of succinylcholine should not be used to break postoperative laryngospasm, especially if the alveolar partial pressure of oxygen (PAO_2) is decreased by hypoventilation. Unless assisted ventilation is provided, declining PAO_2 causes serious hypoxemia before spontaneous ventilation resumes[42] (Fig. 54-3). If the functional residual capacity (FRC) is abnormally reduced, the decreased volume of O_2 available in the lungs accelerates the development of hypoxemia. Severe

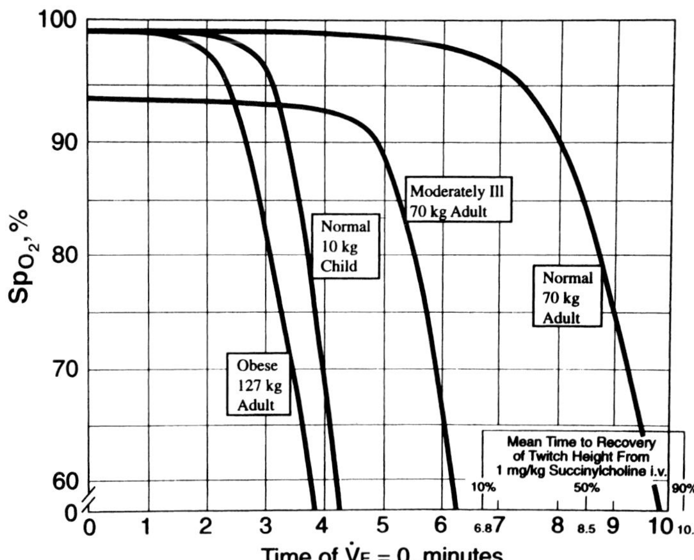

FIGURE 54-3. Rate of SpO_2 decline after onset of apnea. (Reprinted with permission from Benumof JL, Dagg R, Benumof R: Critical hemoglobin desaturation will occur before return to an unparalyzed state following 1 mg/kg intravenous succinylcholine. Anesthesiology 87:979, 1997.)

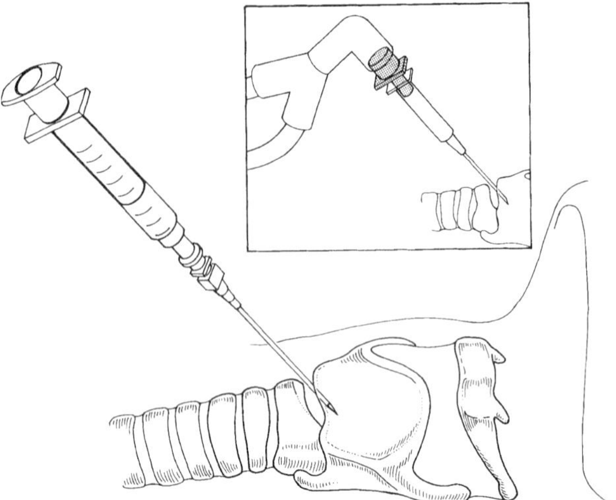

FIGURE 54-4. Cricothyroidotomy using a large-bore (14-gauge) intravenous catheter attached to syringe. After entry into the trachea, the needle is directed toward the carina.

laryngeal obstruction can occur secondary to hypocalcemia after parathyroid excision.

Soft-tissue edema worsens airway obstruction, especially in children and adults recovering from procedures on the neck. Nebulized vasoconstrictors help somewhat, but steroids have little effect. Patients with C1 esterase inhibitor deficiency can develop severe angioneurotic edema after even slight trauma to the airway. Pathologic airway obstruction (e.g., severe edema, epiglottitis, retropharyngeal abscess, encroaching tumors) might require emergency tracheal intubation, but airway manipulation is dangerous because minor trauma from intubation attempts can convert a marginal airway into a total obstruction. Sedatives or muscle relaxants used to facilitate intubation can worsen obstruction by compromising the patient's volitional efforts to maintain the airway and by eliminating spontaneous ventilation. Equipment and personnel necessary for emergency cricothyroidotomy or tracheostomy should be available. Cricothyroidotomy using a 14-gauge intravenous catheter or a commercially available kit permits oxygenation and marginal ventilation until the airway is secured (Fig. 54-4), especially if jet ventilation with 100% oxygen is used.

Reduction of cross-sectional area in small airways increases overall airway resistance because resistance varies inversely with the fourth power of radius during laminar flow and with the fifth power during turbulent flow. Pharyngeal or tracheal stimulation from secretions, suctioning, aspiration, or a tracheal tube can trigger a reflex constriction of bronchial smooth muscle in emerging patients with reactive airways. Histamine release precipitated by medication or allergic reactions also increases airway smooth muscle tone. Decreased radial traction on small airways reduces cross-sectional area in patients with COPD or with decreased lung volume secondary to obesity, surgical manipulation, excessive lung water, or splinting. Preoperative spirometric evidence of increased airway resistance predicts an increased risk of postoperative bronchospasm.[37] Smokers and patients with bronchospastic conditions are at highest risk.[43] If ventilatory requirements are increased by warming, hyperthermia, or work of breathing, high flow rates convert laminar flow to higher-resistance turbulent flow. Prolonged expiratory time or audible turbulent air flow (wheezing) during a forced vital capacity expiration often unmasks subclinical airway resistance. (Resistance is higher during expiration because intermediate-diameter airways are compressed by positive intrathoracic pressure.) High airway resistance does not always cause wheezing because flow might be so impeded that no sound is produced. Signs of increased resistance mimic those of decreased pulmonary compliance. Spontaneously breathing patients exhibit accessory muscle recruitment, labored ventilation, and increased work of breathing with either condition. Mechanically ventilated patients exhibit high peak inspiratory pressures.

The treatment of small airway resistance is directed at an underlying etiology. Eliminate laryngeal or airway stimulation. Patients often respond to their preexisting regimen of albuterol, pirbuterol, or salmeterol inhalers. Isoetharine or metaproterenol nebulized in oxygen resolves postoperative bronchospasm with minimal tachycardia. Intramuscular or sublingual terbutaline can be added. Administration of steroid therapy offers little acute improvement. Adverse side effects of intravenous aminophylline have led to its replacement by other agents. Bronchospasm that is resistant to β_2-sympathomimetic medication may improve with an anticholinergic medication such as atropine or ipratropium. If bronchospasm is life threatening, an intravenous epinephrine infusion yields profound bronchodilation. Increased small airway resistance caused by mechanical factors (e.g., loss of lung volume, retained secretions, pulmonary edema) usually does not resolve with bronchodilators. Restoration of lung volume with incentive spirometry or deep tidal ventilation increases radial traction on small airways. Reducing left ventricular filling pressures might relieve airway resistance caused by increased lung water, although interstitial fluid accumulation can persist. Also, extended contraction of airway smooth muscle obstructs venous and lymphatic flow, leading to airway wall edema that resolves slowly.

Decreased Compliance

Reduced pulmonary compliance accentuates the work of breathing. In the extreme, low compliance causes progressive respiratory muscle fatigue, hypoventilation, and respiratory acidemia. Parenchymal changes also affect compliance. Reduction of FRC leads to small airway closure and distal lung collapse, requiring greater energy expenditure to reexpand the lung. Pulmonary edema increases the lung's weight and inertia, and elevates surface tension by interfering with surfactant activity, making expansion more difficult. Pulmonary contusion or hemorrhage interferes with lung expansion, as do restrictive lung diseases, skeletal abnormalities, intrathoracic lesions, hemothorax, pneumothorax, or cardiomegaly. Obesity affects pulmonary compliance, especially when adipose tissue compresses the thoracic cage or increases intra-abdominal pressure in supine or lateral positions. Extrathoracic factors such as tight chest or abdominal dressings and gas in the stomach or bowel reduce compliance. An intra-abdominal tumor, hemorrhage, ascites, bowel obstruction, or pregnancy impairs diaphragmatic excursion and reduces compliance.

Work of breathing is improved by resolving problems that reduce compliance. Allowing patients to recover in a semisitting position (rather than supine or full sitting) reduces work of breathing. Incentive spirometry and chest physiotherapy help restore lung volume, as does positive end-expiratory pressure (PEEP) or continuous positive airway pressure (CPAP). In patients with COPD and highly compliant lungs, positive airway pressure might force the rib cage and diaphragms toward their excursion limits, accentuating inspiratory muscular effort.

Neuromuscular and Skeletal Problems

Postoperative airway obstruction and hypoventilation are accentuated by incomplete reversal of neuromuscular relaxation. Residual paralysis compromises airway patency, ability to overcome airway resistance, airway protection, and ability to clear secretions.[44] In the extreme, paralysis precludes effective spontaneous ventilation. Intraoperative use of shorter-acting relaxants might decrease the incidence of residual paralysis but does not eliminate the problem. Marginal reversal can be more dangerous than near-total paralysis because a weak, agitated patient exhibiting uncoordinated movements and airway obstruction is more easily identified. A somnolent patient exhibiting mild stridor and shallow ventilation from marginal neuromuscular function might be overlooked, allowing insidious hypoventilation and respiratory acidemia or regurgitation with aspiration to occur. Beware of patients who have received nondepolarizing muscle relaxants but no reversal agents because they often exhibit low levels of residual paralysis.[45] Safety of techniques designed to avoid reversal of short and intermediate duration relaxants has not been substantiated, and reversal of nondepolarizing relaxants is recommended.[4] Patients with neuromuscular abnormalities such as myasthenia gravis, Eaton-Lambert syndrome, periodic paralysis, or muscular dystrophies exhibit exaggerated or prolonged responses to muscle relaxants. Even without relaxant administration, these patients can exhibit postoperative ventilatory insufficiency. Medications potentiate neuromuscular relaxation (e.g., antibiotics, furosemide, propranolol, phenytoin), as does hypocalcemia or hypermagnesemia.

Diaphragmatic contraction is compromised in some postoperative patients, forcing more reliance on intercostal muscles and reducing the ability to overcome decreased compliance or increased ventilatory demands. Impairment of phrenic nerve function from interscalene block, trauma, or thoracic and neck operations can "paralyze" one or rarely both diaphragms.[23] Adequate ventilation will normally be maintained with only one diaphragm and marginal ventilation by external intercostal muscles alone. However, with high work of breathing, muscle weakness, or increased ventilatory demands, a nonfunctional diaphragm impairs minute ventilation. Thoracic spinal or epidural blockade interferes with intercostal muscle function and reduces ventilatory reserve, especially in patients with COPD. Abnormal motor neuron function (e.g., Guillain-Barré syndrome, cervical spinal cord trauma), flail chest, or severe kyphosis or scoliosis can cause postoperative ventilatory insufficiency.

Simple tests help assess mechanical ability to ventilate. The ability to sustain head elevation in a supine position, a forced vital capacity of 10 to 12 mL/kg, an inspiratory pressure more negative than −25 cm H_2O, and tactile train-of-four assessment imply that strength of ventilatory muscles is adequate to sustain ventilation. However, none of these clinical end points reliably predicts recovery of airway protective reflexes,[45] and failure on these tests does not necessarily indicate the need for assisted ventilation.

Occasionally, a clinical picture suggests ventilatory insufficiency when ventilation is adequate. Voluntary limitation of chest expansion to avoid pain (splinting) causes labored, rapid, shallow breathing characteristic of inadequate ventilation. Splinting seldom causes actual hypoventilation and usually improves with analgesia and repositioning. Ventilation with small tidal volumes due to thoracic restriction or reduced compliance seems to generate afferent input from pulmonary stretch receptors, leading to dyspnea, labored breathing, and accessory muscle recruitment in spite of appropriate minute ventilation. (This also occurs during mechanical ventilation with low volumes.) Occasional large, "satisfying" lung expansions often relieve these symptoms. Finally, spontaneous hyperventilation to compensate for a metabolic acidemia might generate tachypnea or labored breathing, which is mistaken for ventilatory insufficiency.

Increased Dead Space

Ventilation of unperfused dead space or of poorly perfused alveoli with high ventilation/perfusion ($\dot{V}/\dot{Q}$) ratios is less effective in removing CO_2. Expansion of dead space volume or reduction of tidal volume increases the fraction of each breath wasted in dead space ($\dot{V}_D/\dot{V}_T$) and the amount of CO_2 from the previous exhalation that is rebreathed. A proportionally larger increase in total minute ventilation is required to meet any increase in CO_2 production. Patients with high $\dot{V}_D/\dot{V}_T$ are at greater risk for postoperative ventilatory failure.

Occasionally, an acute increase in dead space contributes to respiratory acidemia in postoperative patients. Although upper airway dead space is reduced after tracheal intubation and tracheostomy, excessive tubing volume or valve reversal in breathing circuits promotes rebreathing of CO_2. PEEP or CPAP elevates anatomic dead space, especially in patients with high pulmonary compliance. Pulmonary embolization with air, thrombus, or cellular debris increases physiologic dead space, although impact on CO_2 excretion is often compensated by accelerated minute ventilation from hypercorbic and hypoxic drives or reflex responses. Pulmonary hypotension can transiently increase $\dot{V}_D/\dot{V}_T$ by decreasing perfusion to well-ventilated, nondependent lung. Irreversible increases in dead space occur if adult respiratory distress syndrome (ARDS) related to sepsis, massive transfusion, or hypoxia destroys pulmonary microvasculature. Dead space may appear high if an inhalation interrupts the previous exhalation and spent alveolar gas is retained. This "gas trapping" occurs when high airway resistance lengthens the time required to exhale completely, or if improper inspiration/expiration ratios or high ventilatory rates are used during mechanical ventilation.

Increased Carbon Dioxide Production

Carbon dioxide production varies directly with metabolic rate, body temperature, and substrate availability. During anesthesia, CO_2 production falls to approximately 60% of the normal 2 to 3 mL/kg/min as hypothermia lowers metabolic activity and neuromuscular relaxation reduces tonic muscle contraction. Therefore, during recovery, metabolic rate and CO_2 production can increase by 40%. Shivering, high work of breathing, infection, SNS activity, or rapid carbohydrate metabolism during intravenous hyperalimentation accelerate CO_2 production even more. Malignant hyperthermia generates CO_2 production many times greater than normal that rapidly exceeds ventilatory reserve and causes severe respiratory acidemia. Even mild increases of CO_2 production can precipitate respiratory acidemia if low compliance, airway resistance, or neuromuscular paralysis interferes with ventilation. With the exception of adjusting hyperalimentation, improving work of breathing, reducing shivering, or treating hyperthermia, there is little yield from addressing CO_2 production in PACU patients.

Inadequate Postoperative Oxygenation

Systemic arterial partial pressure of oxygen ($Pa{O_2}$) is the best indicator of pulmonary oxygen transfer from alveolar gas to pulmonary capillary blood. Arterial hemoglobin saturation monitored by pulse oximetry yields less information on alveolar-arterial gradients and is not helpful in assessing impact of hemoglobin dissociation curve shifts or carboxyhemoglobin.[46] Evaluation of metabolic acidemia or mixed venous oxygen content yields insight into peripheral oxygen delivery and utilization. Adequate arterial oxygenation does not mean that cardiac output, arterial perfusion pressure, or distribution of blood flow will maintain tissue oxygenation. Sepsis, hypotension, anemia, or hemoglobin dissociation abnormalities can generate tissue ischemia despite adequate oxygenation.

In postoperative patients, the acceptable lower limit for $Pa{O_2}$ varies with individual patient characteristics. A $Pa{O_2}$ below 65 to 70 mm Hg causes significant hemoglobin desaturation, although tissue oxygen delivery might be maintained at lower levels. Maintaining $Pa{O_2}$ between 80 and 100 mm Hg (saturation 93 to 97%) ensures adequate oxygen availability. Little benefit is derived from elevating $Pa{O_2}$ above 110 mm Hg because hemoglobin is saturated and the amount of additional oxygen dissolved in plasma is negligible. During mechanical ventilation, a $Pa{O_2}$ above 80 mm Hg with 0.4 $F{I}{O_2}$ and 5 cm H_2O PEEP or CPAP usually predicts sustained adequate oxygenation after tracheal extubation.

Distribution of Ventilation

Loss of dependent lung volume commonly causes $\dot{V}/\dot{Q}$ mismatching and hypoxemia. A reduction in FRC decreases radial traction on small airways, leading to collapse and distal atelectasis that can worsen for 36 hours after surgery.[47] Reduced ventilation in dependent lung is particularly damaging because gravity directs pulmonary blood flow to dependent areas. Obese patients sustain large decreases in FRC during surgery. Older patients normally exhibit some airway closure at end expiration, and those with COPD have more severe closure that is exacerbated by small reductions in FRC. Retraction, packing, manipulation, or peritoneal insufflation during upper abdominal surgery reduces FRC, as does compression from leaning surgical assistants.[48] Prone, lithotomy, or Trendelenburg positions are disadvantageous, especially in obese patients. Right upper lobe collapse secondary to partial right main-stem intubation is a frequently overlooked cause. During one-lung anesthesia, the weight of unsupported mediastinal contents, pressure from abdominal contents on the dependent diaphragm, and lung compression all reduce dependent lung volume. Gravity and lymphatic obstruction promote interstitial fluid accumulation and further $\dot{V}/\dot{Q}$ mismatching. This "down lung syndrome" may appear as unilateral pulmonary edema on the chest film.

Postoperatively, acute pulmonary edema from overhydration, ventricular dysfunction, or increased capillary permeability leads to hypoxemia by interfering with both $\dot{V}/\dot{Q}$ matching and diffusion of oxygen. Strong inspiratory efforts against an obstructed airway decrease FRC and promote negative-pressure pulmonary edema. Small airway occlusion from compression, retained secretions, or aspiration leads to distal hypoventilation and hypoxemia, as does main-stem intubation. Pneumothorax or hemothorax also reduce lung volume.

Conservative measures that restore lung volume often improve oxygenation. If possible, patients should recover in a semisitting position to reduce abdominal pressure on the diaphragms. Pain with ventilation encourages shallow breathing, so analgesia helps maintain FRC, especially with upper abdominal or chest wall incisions. Deep ventilation, cough, chest physiotherapy, and incentive spirometry seem to help expand FRC, mobilize secretions, and accustom a patient to incisional discomfort, but actual efficacy is debated.[49,50] For serious postoperative reduction of FRC, positive pressure is effective. CPAP (5 to 7 cm H_2O) can be delivered by facemask for several hours until factors promoting loss of lung volume resolve. If hypoxemia is severe or patient acceptance of mask CPAP is poor, tracheal intubation is usually required. Intubation for delivery of CPAP does not mandate positive-pressure ventilation. Ventilatory requirements should be assessed independently, considering $Pa{CO_2}$, arterial pH, and work of breathing. Usually, 5 to 10 cm H_2O of CPAP or PEEP improves $Pa{O_2}$ without risking hypotension, increased intracranial pressure, or barotrauma. If $Pa{O_2}$ does not improve, reevaluate the etiology. During routine postoperative care, airway pressure >10 cm H_2O is transmitted more to thoracic veins and increases incidence of barotrauma. An occasional patient with ARDS or pulmonary contusion might require higher pressures for improved oxygenation.

Tracheal intubation eliminates normal expiratory resistance and the "physiologic PEEP" (2 to 5 cm H_2O) that helps maintain lung volume during spontaneous ventilation. Exposing an intubated trachea to ambient pressure may cause a gradual reduction in FRC. Healthy, slender patients will often tolerate short periods of intubation without positive pressure, but generally it is prudent to allow intubated postoperative patients to exhale against a slight degree of CPAP.

Distribution of Perfusion

Poor distribution of pulmonary blood flow also interferes with $\dot{V}/\dot{Q}$ matching and oxygenation. Flow distribution is primarily determined by hydrodynamic factors (PA and venous pressures, vascular resistance), which are affected by gravity, airway pressure, lung volume, and cardiac dynamics. Flow distribution is modulated by hypoxic pulmonary vasoconstriction (HPV), which diverts flow from air spaces that exhibit low $Pa{O_2}$. In postoperative patients, position affects oxygenation if gravity forces blood flow to areas with reduced ventilation. Placing a poorly ventilated lung in a dependent position can reduce $Pa{O_2}$. Postoperative changes in PA pressure, airway pressure, and lung volume also have complex effects on blood flow distribution that can adversely affect $\dot{V}/\dot{Q}$ matching. Residual inhalational anesthetics, vasodilators, and sympathomimetics directly affect vascular tone and HPV, partially explaining larger alveolar-arterial oxygen gradients after general anesthesia. (Changes in distribution of ventilation also contribute.) Patients with liver cirrhosis exhibit poor $\dot{V}/\dot{Q}$ matching caused by circulating humoral substances related to abnormal hepatic metabolism. Circulating endotoxin impairs HPV, contributing to hypoxemia in septic patients.

In the PACU, few interventions are useful to improve $\dot{V}/\dot{Q}$ matching by changing pulmonary blood flow. Maintain PA and airway pressures within an acceptable range. When possible, avoid placing an atelectatic or diseased lung tissue in a dependent position. Placing poorly ventilated parenchyma in a nondependent position could improve $\dot{V}/\dot{Q}$ matching, but positioning a diseased lung in an "up" position may promote drainage of purulent material into the unaffected lung. Avoiding betamimetic or vasodilatory medications may improve $Pa{O_2}$ but benefits from the medication usually outweigh drawbacks of impaired HPV.

Inadequate Alveolar $P{A}{O_2}$

Postoperative hypoxemia is occasionally caused by a global reduction of $P{A}{O_2}$, usually from inadequate ventilation. If oxygen uptake from alveoli exceeds delivery by ventilation, $P{A}{O_2}$ decreases. Hypoventilation must be severe to cause hypoxemia based on a reduction in oxygen delivery to alveoli. Complete apnea or airway obstruction by a foreign body, soft-tissue edema, or laryngospasm leads to rapid depletion of alveolar oxygen, as does very high small airway resistance, which precludes effective ventilation. If cessation of ventilation does occur, the rate of $P{A}{O_2}$ decline varies with age, body habitus, degree of underlying illness, and initial $P{A}{O_2}$[42] (see Fig. 54-3). Hypoxemia might also occur if opioids or residual anesthetic levels severely depress ventilatory drives. Partial airway obstruction does not usually reduce $P{A}{O_2}$, especially when patients are receiving supplemental oxygen. Increasing the oxygen content of the FRC with supplemental oxygen safeguards against hypoxemia from hypoventilation or airway obstruction. Rarely, excessive concentrations of other gases reduce $P_{A}O_2$. After general anesthesia, rapid outpouring of nitrous oxide displaces alveolar gas and can lower $P_{A}O_2$ if a patient is hypoventilating or breathing ambient air, but this "diffusion hypoxia" would usually occur before PACU admission. Volume displacement of oxygen could also occur during severe hypercarbia in a patient breathing ambient air, although acidemia is often a greater problem.

Reduced Mixed Venous P_{O_2}

Systemic venous partial pressure of oxygen ($P\bar{v}O_2$) is affected by arterial oxygen content, cardiac output, distribution of peripheral blood flow, and tissue oxygen extraction. If arterial oxygen content decreases or tissue extraction increases, $P\bar{v}O_2$ falls. The lower the $P\bar{v}O_2$ in blood that is shunted or flows through low $\dot{V}/\dot{Q}$ units, the greater the reduction of $P_{a}O_2$. Blood with a low $P\bar{v}O_2$ also extracts larger volumes of oxygen from alveolar gas, amplifying the effect of hypoventilation or airway obstruction on $P_{A}O_2$. Very low $P\bar{v}O_2$ increases the risk of resorption atelectasis in poorly ventilated alveoli. In postoperative patients, shivering, infection, and hypermetabolism lower $P\bar{v}O_2$ by increasing peripheral oxygen extraction. Low cardiac output or hypotension also lower $P\bar{v}O_2$ by decreasing tissue oxygen delivery. Supplemental oxygen reduces the impact of low $P\bar{v}O_2$ on alveolar oxygen extraction and on arterial oxygenation.

Carbon Monoxide Poisoning

Carbon monoxide (CO) reversibly binds to hemoglobin with 200 times the affinity of oxygen, reducing oxygen-carrying capacity by impeding both the binding and the dissociation of oxygen. Trauma or burn patients might be poisoned prior to emergency surgery. Patients can also be exposed to CO generated by a reaction between inhalation anesthetics and dry CO_2-absorbing agents during general anesthesia. Risk of intraoperative exposure is low but increases during first cases of the day, especially those performed in peripheral locations. Moderate CO poisoning is difficult to recognize in postoperative patients because symptoms such as headache, nausea, vomiting, irritability, and altered visual or motor skills are nonspecific and common during recovery. CO seldom causes cyanosis and the $P_{a}O_2$ is often high, although $S_{p}O_2$ is low and metabolic acidemia is significant. A pulse oximeter interprets carboxyhemoglobin as oxyhemoglobin, so $S_{p}O_2$ reads falsely high. (A cooximeter is required to differentiate.) Thus, a postoperative patient with CO poisoning can be hypoxemic yet appear well oxygenated. One hundred percent oxygen displaces CO from hemoglobin and accelerates CO elimination. Hyperbaric oxygen therapy may be indicated for severe cases.

Anemia

Preoperative hematocrit and intraoperative hemorrhage determine a patient's red cell mass and oxygen-carrying capacity after surgery. Reduction of hematocrit caused by dilution has less impact. The hematocrit at which oxygen delivery becomes insufficient to match tissue needs varies with cardiac reserve, oxygen consumption, hemoglobin dissociation, $P_{a}O_2$, and blood flow distribution. Each patient has a minimum hematocrit below which tissues use inefficient anaerobic metabolism, generating a lactic acidemia. Patients with vascular disease are at increased risk of vital organ ischemia as hematocrit falls.

Supplemental Oxygen

8 The incidence of hypoxemia in postoperative patients is high. In PACU patients placed on room air, 30% of patients younger than 1 year of age, 20% ages 1 to 3 years, 14% ages 3 to 14 years, and 7.8% of adults had hemoglobin saturations fall below 90%, with many falling below 85%[51] (Fig. 54-5). Clinical observation and assessment of cognitive function do not accurately screen for hypoxemia, so monitoring with oximetry is essential throughout the PACU admission.[46] One cannot predict which patients will become hypoxemic or when hypoxemia will occur. Patients with lung disease or obesity, those recovering from thoracic or upper abdominal procedures, and those with preoperative hypoxemia are at increased risk.[52] Postoperative hypoxemia occurs in children, especially those with respiratory infections or chronic adenotonsillar hypertrophy. Hypoxemia occurs frequently after regional anesthesia.[22]

Supplemental oxygen could be administered only to patients at high risk of hypoxemia or with low $S_{p}O_2$ readings. However, if a patient qualifies for PACU admission, he or she should probably receive oxygen during initial recovery and perhaps during transport to the PACU.[4] Supplemental oxygen improves $P_{a}O_2$ and helps prevent or treat hypoxemia, although its efficacy is variable. However, oxygen does not address underlying causes of hypoxemia in postoperative patients, and its use does not guarantee that hypoxemia will not occur.[53] If hypoxemia is caused by low $\dot{V}/\dot{Q}$, increasing oxygen content in marginally ventilated air spaces improves arterial saturation. Oxygen has a negligible effect on hypoxemia caused by shunting because shunted blood is not exposed to increased $F_{I}O_2$, whereas blood passing ventilated alveoli is already saturated. Increased oxygen content in the FRC delays the onset of serious hypoxemia during airway obstruction or hypoventilation. Cost of supplemental oxygen is minimal, inconvenience to patients is minor, and risk is small. Although oxygen might cause minor mucosal drying, routine humidification is of little benefit unless intubation bypasses natural humidification. Oxygen apparatus might cause corneal abrasion during emergence. An $F_{I}O_2 > 0.8$ promotes resorption atelectasis as inert nitrogen is replaced with oxygen in poorly ventilated alveoli. Inspiration of 100% oxygen for 24 to 36 hours generates early signs of pulmonary oxygen toxicity. Toxicity is accelerated by hyperbaric oxygen therapy. Previous carmustine therapy might increase risk at oxygen toxicity but bleomycin therapy does not.

Perioperative Aspiration

During anesthesia, depression of airway reflexes places patients at risk for intraoperative pulmonary aspiration that causes symptoms in the PACU or for aspiration during recovery. Pulmonary morbidity from perioperative aspiration varies with the type and volume of the aspirate. Although aspiration of gastric contents is most widely feared, surgical patients also experience other aspiration syndromes.

Aspiration of clear oral secretions during induction, facemask ventilation, or emergence is common and usually insignificant. Cough, mild tracheal irritation, or transient laryngospasm are immediate sequelae, although large-volume aspiration predisposes to infection, small airway obstruction, or pulmonary edema. Aspiration of blood secondary to trauma, epistaxis, or airway surgery generates marked changes on the chest radiograph that are out of proportion with clinical signs. Aspirated "sterile" blood causes minor airway obstruction but is rapidly cleared by mucociliary transport, resorption, and phagocytosis. Massive blood aspiration or aspiration of clots obstructs airways, interferes with oxygenation, and leads to fibrinous changes in air spaces and to pulmonary

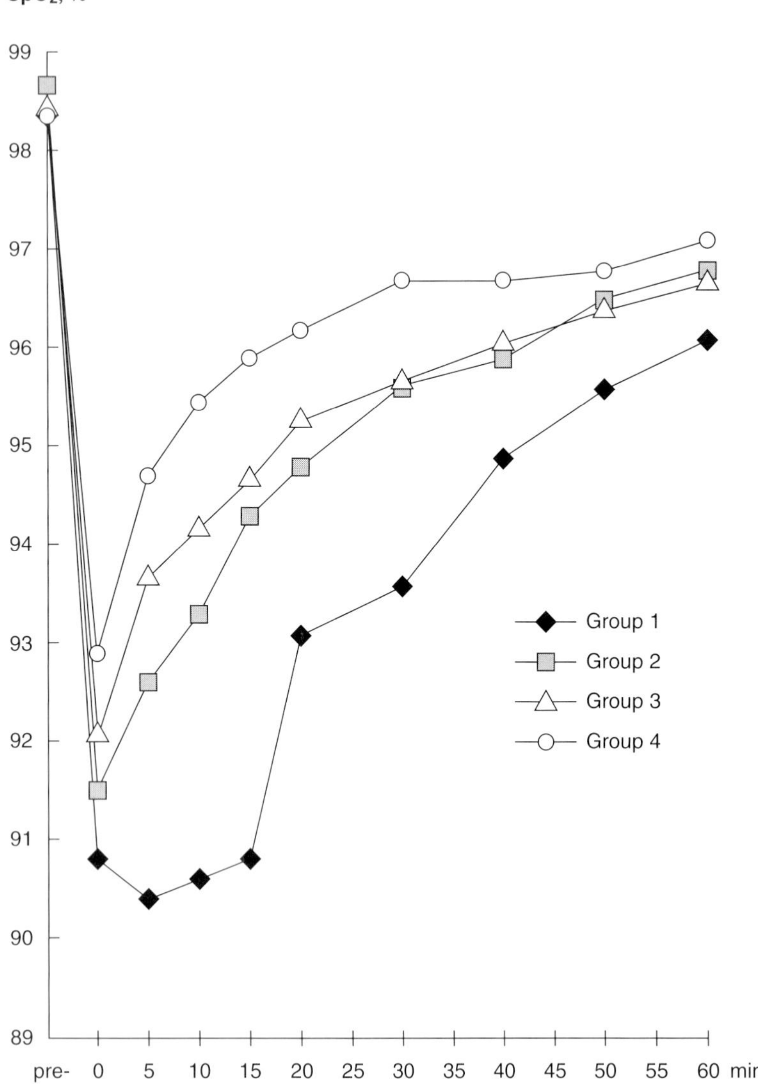

FIGURE 54-5. SpO_2 versus postanesthesia care unit time in patients spontaneously ventilating on room air after general anesthesia (group 1, 0–1 year of age; group 2, 1–3 years; group 3, 3–14 years; group 4, 14–58 years). (Reprinted with permission from Xue FS, Huang YG, Tong SY *et al:* A comparative study of early postoperative hypoxemia in infants, children, and adults undergoing elective plastic surgery. Anesth Analg 83:709, 1996.)

hemochromatosis from iron accumulation in phagocytic cells. Secondary infection is a threat, especially if tissue or purulent matter is also aspirated.

Aspiration of food, small objects, pieces of teeth, or dental appliances causes persistent cough, diffuse reflex bronchospasm, airway obstruction with distal atelectasis, or pneumonia. Complications are often localized and treated with antibiotics and supportive care once the foreign matter is expelled or removed. Secondary thermal, chemical, or traumatic airway injury from aspirated objects can occur. Of course, complete upper airway or tracheal obstruction by an aspirated object is a life-threatening emergency.

Aspiration of acidic gastric contents during vomiting or regurgitation causes chemical pneumonitis characterized initially by diffuse bronchospasm, hypoxemia, and atelectasis.[54] The morbidity increases directly with volume and inversely with the pH of the acidic aspirate. Aspiration of partially digested food worsens and prolongs pneumonitis, especially if vegetable matter is present. Food particles mechanically obstruct airways and are a nidus for secondary bacterial infection. In serious cases, epithelial degeneration, interstitial and alveolar edema, and hemorrhage into air spaces rapidly progresses to ARDS with high-permeability pulmonary edema. Destruction of pneumocytes, decreased surfactant activity, hyaline membrane formation, and emphysematous changes can follow, leading to $\dot{V}/\dot{Q}$ mismatching and reduced compliance. Destruction of microvasculature increases pulmonary vascular resistance and $\dot{V}_D/\dot{V}_T$.

9 The incidence of serious aspiration is relatively low in PACU patients, but the risk is still significant. Frequency of postoperative vomiting remains high, especially if gas has accumulated in the stomach. Protective airway reflexes such as cough, swallowing, and laryngospasm are suppressed by depressant medications such as inhalation anesthetics, barbiturates, and opiates, so observe patients with decreased levels of consciousness carefully. Persisting effects of laryngeal nerve blocks or topical local anesthetics used to reduce airway irritability decrease postoperative airway protection, as does residual sedation. Reflexes are also impaired by residual neuromuscular paralysis.[44,45] Patients can sustain airway patency and spontaneous ventilation, pass a head lift test, have a tactile train-of-four T4/T1 ratio greater than 0.7, and still have impaired airway reflexes from residual paralysis. The T4/T1 ratio might need to exceed 0.9 before reflexes are completely competent.[55] Risk of aspiration also increases if reversal is omitted. Hypotension, hypoxemia, or acidemia cause both emesis and obtundation, increasing aspiration risk.

Preventing aspiration is critical because effective therapy is limited.[56] For patients at high risk, preoperative administration of nonparticulate antacids such as sodium citrate increases the pH of gastric fluid without excessively increasing volume. Avoid particulate antacids. Histamine type 2 receptor blockers such as cimetidine or ranitidine reduce the volume and increase the pH of gastric secretions. Metoclopramide increases gastroesophageal sphincter tone and accelerates gastric emptying. Inserting a nasogastric tube is often ineffective to remove particulate matter and interferes with gastroesophageal sphincter integrity.

In the PACU, vigilance against aspiration is important. Trendelenburg position might promote regurgitation but aids in airway clearance if regurgitation or vomiting occurs. Head elevation in unconscious patients should be avoided because it creates a gravitational gradient from pharynx to lung. High-risk patients should not have the trachea extubated until airway reflexes are fully restored. Aspiration of acidic fluid can still occur around an inflated tracheal tube cuff, so frequently monitor the upper airway for secretions or vomitus. Avoid cuff deflation until extubation because the rigid tube impairs laryngospasm, swallowing, and other protective reflexes. Suction the pharynx completely and extubate at end inspiration with positive airway pressure to promote expulsion of material trapped below the cords but above the inflated cuff. Observation is essential after extubation because airway reflexes might be temporarily impaired. Anatomic distortion in the airway from soft-tissue trauma or surgical intervention interferes with airway protection. Mandibular fixation makes expulsion of vomitus, blood, or secretions difficult, so have equipment for release of mandibular fixation available and ensure patients demonstrate cognitive and physical ability to clear the airway before the trachea is extubated.

Discovery of gastric secretions in the pharynx mandates immediate lateral head positioning (assuming cervical spine integrity) and suction of the airway. If airway reflexes are compromised, tracheal intubation is often appropriate. After intubation, the trachea is suctioned through the tracheal tube before positive-pressure ventilation; this avoids widely disseminating aspirated material into distal airways. Instillation of saline or alkalotic solutions is not recommended. Assessing the pH of tracheal aspirate is useless because buffering is immediate. Checking pharyngeal aspirate pH is more accurate but of little practical value. Suspicion that aspiration has occurred mandates 24 to 48 hours of monitoring for development of aspiration pneumonitis. If the likelihood of aspiration is small in an ambulatory patient, outpatient follow-up can be done, assuming hypoxemia, cough, wheezing, or radiographic abnormalities do not appear within 4 to 6 hours. Give the patient explicit instructions to contact a medical facility at the first appearance of malaise, fever, cough, chest pain, or other symptoms of pneumonitis. If likelihood of aspiration is high, the patient should be admitted to the hospital. Observation includes serial temperature checks, white blood cell counts with differential, chest radiograph, and blood gas determination or pulmonary function testing, if appropriate. Chest physiotherapy, incentive spirometry, and restarting medications for preexisting pulmonary conditions minimize the loss of lung volume, $\dot{V}/\dot{Q}$ mismatching, and infection. Fluffy infiltrates may appear on the chest radiograph any time within 24 hours. Hypoxemia might develop quickly or evolve insidiously as injury progresses, so frequent pulse oximetry monitoring is important.

If hypoxemia, increased airway resistance, consolidation, or pulmonary edema evolves, support the patient with supplemental oxygen, PEEP, or CPAP. Mechanical ventilation is often necessary. Steroids yield little improvement. Bacterial infection does not always follow aspiration, so prophylactic antibiotics merely promote colonization by resistant organisms. If bacterial infection appears, institute antibiotic therapy based on culture results. If cultures are equivocal, use broad-spectrum antibiotics with coverage for gram-negative rods and anaerobes, including *Bacteroides fragilis*. Overall therapy is similar to that for ARDS. Pulmonary edema from increased capillary permeability should not be treated with diuretics unless high filling pressures or hypervolemia exist. Fluid losses into the lung necessitate aggressive hydration.

POSTOPERATIVE RENAL COMPLICATIONS

Ability to Void

10 The ability to void should be assessed because opioids and autonomic side effects of regional anesthesia interfere with sphincter relaxation and promote urine retention. Urinary retention is common after urologic, inguinal, and genital surgery, and frequently delays discharge.[57] Neither the patient nor staff can accurately estimate bladder volume through sensation or palpation, respectively. Avoid the archaic practice of "straight catheterization." An ultrasonic bladder scan helps assess bladder volume before discharge. It is reasonable to discharge selected ambulatory patients from the facility and inpatients to a floor before they void.[4,58,59] However, ensure urination is monitored after discharge to avoid urinary retention. Give ambulatory patients who are discharged without voiding a specific time interval in which to void (i.e., 10 to 12 hours after discharge). If retention persists, the patient must contact a health care facility. High return rates after urologic procedures are related to urinary retention.[60]

Renal Tubular Function

Analysis of urine yields information about postoperative renal tubular function. Urine color is not useful for assessing concentrating ability, but it does assist recognition of hematuria, hemoglobinuria, or pyuria. Urine osmolarity (reflecting the number of particles in solution) is a more reliable index of tubular function than specific gravity, which is affected by molecular weight of solutes. An osmolarity >450 mOsm/L indicates intact tubular concentrating ability. A urine sodium concentration far below or a potassium concentration above serum concentrations also indicates tubular viability, as does acidification or alkalinization of urine. Osmolarity, electrolyte, and pH values close to those in serum may indicate poor tubular function or acute tubular necrosis.

Inorganic fluoride released during metabolism of certain inhalation anesthetics can cause a transient reduction of tubular concentrating ability after long anesthetics. Higher fluoride levels cause renal tubular necrosis. Interaction of sevoflurane with dry carbon dioxide absorbents (often found in first cases or peripheral locations) generates compound A, a vinyl ether that degrades to release inorganic fluoride. Although transient impairment of protein retention and concentrating ability may occur, use of sevoflurane does not seriously affect renal function.

Oliguria

Oliguria ($\leq$0.5 mL/kg/h) occurs frequently during recovery and usually reflects an appropriate renal response to hypovolemia. However, decreased urine output might indicate abnormal renal function. The acceptable degree and duration of oliguria vary with baseline renal status, the surgical procedure, and the anticipated postoperative course. In patients without catheters, assess interval since last voiding and bladder volume to help differentiate oliguria from inability to void. Check indwelling urinary catheters for kinking, for obstruction by blood clots or debris, and for the catheter tip being positioned above the urinary level in the bladder. Aggressively evaluate oliguria if intraoperative events could jeopardize renal function (e.g., aortic cross-clamping, severe hypotension, possible ureteral ligature, massive transfusion). Systemic blood pressure must be adequate for renal perfusion, based on preoperative pressures. Administration of desmopressin for hematologic purposes seldom affects postoperative urinary output. After urine is sent for electrolyte and osmolarity determinations, a 300- to 500-mL intravenous crystalloid bolus helps assess whether oliguria represents a renal response to hypovolemia. If output does not improve, consider a larger bolus or a diagnostic trial of furosemide, 5 mg intravenously. Furosemide increases urine output if oliguria reflects tubular resorption of fluid. Patients on chronic diuretic therapy might require a diuretic effect to maintain postoperative urine output.

Persistence of oliguria despite hydration, adequate perfusion pressure, and a furosemide challenge increases the likelihood of acute tubular necrosis, ureteral obstruction, renal artery or vein occlusion, or inappropriate antidiuretic hormone (ADH) secretion. Cystoscopy, intravenous pyelography, angiography, or radionuclide scanning may help clarify renal status. Osmotic or loop diuretics may be useful to attenuate renal damage. The efficacy of low-dose dopamine or dobutamine is questionable. Consultation with a nephrologist is prudent.

Polyuria

Relying on high postoperative urinary output to gauge intravascular volume status or renal viability can be misleading. Profuse urine output often reflects generous intraoperative fluid administration, but osmotic diuresis caused by hyperglycemia and glycosuria is another common cause, particularly if glucose-containing crystalloid solutions are infusing. Polyuria might also reflect intraoperative diuretic administration. However, sustained polyuria (4 to 5 mL/kg/h) can indicate abnormal regulation of water clearance or high-output renal failure, especially if urinary losses compromise intravascular volume and systemic blood pressure. Diabetes insipidus occurs secondary to intracranial surgery, pituitary ablation, head trauma, or increased intracranial pressure. The diagnosis is made by comparing urine and serum electrolytes with osmolarity. Diagnostic or therapeutic administration of vasopressin is useful.

METABOLIC COMPLICATIONS

Postoperative Acid-Base Disorders

Categorization of postoperative acid-base abnormalities into primary and compensatory disorders is difficult because rapidly changing pathophysiology often generates two or more primary disorders.

Respiratory Acidemia

Respiratory acidemia is frequently encountered in PACU patients because anesthetics, opioids, and sedatives promote hypoventilation by depressing CNS sensitivity to pH and CO_2. In awake, spontaneously breathing patients with adequate analgesia, hypercarbia and acidemia are usually mild ($Paco_2$ 45 to 50 mm Hg, pH 7.36 to 7.32). Deeply sedated patients exhibit more profound acidemia unless supplemental ventilation is administered. Patients with residual neuromuscular paralysis, increased airway resistance, or decreased pulmonary compliance might not sustain adequate ventilation despite an intact CNS drive, especially if CO_2 production is elevated by fever, shivering, or hyperalimentation. The kidneys require hours to generate a compensatory metabolic alkalosis, so compensation for acute postoperative respiratory acidemia is limited.

Symptoms of respiratory acidemia include agitation, confusion, ventilatory dissatisfaction, and tachypnea. SNS response to low pH causes hypertension, tachycardia, and dysrhythmias. Respiratory acidemia caused by CNS depression often produces less intense signs of SNS activity. In patients with head injury, intracranial tumors, or cerebral edema, respiratory acidemia increases cerebral blood flow and intracranial pressure. At very low pH, catecholamines cannot interact with adrenergic receptors, so heart rate and blood pressure decrease precipitously. Treatment consists of correcting the imbalance between CO_2 production and alveolar ventilation. Raising the level of consciousness and judicious reversal of opioids improves ventilatory drive. Improving airway resistance, neuromuscular function, or ventilatory mechanics is useful. If spontaneous ventilation cannot maintain CO_2 excretion, tracheal intubation and mechanical ventilation are necessary. Reducing CO_2 production by controlling fever or shivering may be helpful.

Metabolic Acidemia

Evaluation of acute postoperative metabolic acidemia is relatively straightforward. Occasionally, ketoacidosis occurs in diabetic patients. Serum glucose levels are elevated, and ketones are detectable in blood or urine. Patients with renal failure or renal tubular acidosis usually exhibit a preoperative metabolic acidemia. Excessive saline infusion during surgery can generate a mild hyperchloremic, metabolic acidemia, but use of lactated Ringer's solution avoids this problem. Rarely, a patient manifests acidemia from toxic ingestion of phenformin, aspirin, or methanol. Once these unusual causes are excluded, postoperative metabolic acidemia almost always represents lactic acidemia secondary to insufficient delivery or utilization of oxygen in peripheral tissues. Peripheral hypoperfusion is often caused by low cardiac output (hypovolemia, cardiac failure, dysrhythmia) or decreased SVR (sepsis, catecholamine depletion, sympathectomy). Arteriolar constriction from hypothermia or pressor administration reduces tissue perfusion, as does poor distribution of blood flow. Hypoxemia, severe anemia, impaired hemoglobin dissociation, CO poisoning, and inability to use oxygen in the mitochondria (cyanide or arsenic poisoning) also generate lactic acidemia.

A spontaneously breathing patient will hyperventilate and quickly generate a respiratory alkalosis to compensate for metabolic acidemia, but anesthetics and analgesics interfere with this ventilatory response. The sympathetic response to acute postoperative metabolic acidemia is often milder than the response to respiratory acidemia because hydrogen and bicarbonate ions cross the blood-brain barrier with more difficulty than CO_2. Treatment consists of resolving the condition causing accumulation of metabolic acid. Ketoacidosis is treated with intravenous potassium, insulin, and glucose. Improving cardiac output or systemic blood pressure will reduce lactic acid production, as will rewarming. If conditions causing lactate accumulation are improved and acidemia is mild, renal excretion of hydrogen ions will restore normal pH. For severe or progressive acidemia, intravenous bicarbonate or calcium gluconate helps restore pH.

Respiratory Alkalemia

Pain or anxiety during emergence causes hyperventilation and acute respiratory alkalemia. Excessive mechanical ventilation also generates respiratory alkalemia, especially if hypothermia or paralysis has decreased CO_2 production. Pathologic causes of "central" hyperventilation include sepsis, cerebrovascular accident, or paradoxical CNS acidosis (an imbalance of bicarbonate concentration across the blood-brain barrier caused by prolonged hyperventilation). Acute respiratory alkalemia generates confusion, dizziness, atrial dysrhythmias, or abnormal cardiac conduction. Alkalemia decreases cerebral blood flow, causing hypoperfusion and even stroke in patients with cerebrovascular disease. If the alkalemia is severe, reduced serum ionized calcium concentration precipitates muscle fasciculation or hypocalcemic tetany. Very high pH depresses cardiovascular, CNS, and catecholamine receptor functions. Metabolic compensation for acute respiratory alkalemia is limited because time constants for bicarbonate excretion are large. Treatment necessitates reducing alveolar ventilation, usually by administering analgesics and sedatives for pain and anxiety. Rebreathing of CO_2 has little application in the PACU.

Metabolic Alkalemia

Metabolic alkalemia is rare in PACU patients unless vomiting, gastric suctioning, dehydration, alkaline ingestion, or potassium-wasting diuretics caused an alkalemia that existed before surgery. Excessive intraoperative bicarbonate administration causes postoperative metabolic alkalemia, but alkalemia from metabolism of lactate or citrate usually does not appear within the first 24 hours. Respiratory compensation through retention of CO_2 is rapid but limited because hypoventilation eventually causes hypoxemia. Hydration and correction of hypochloremia and hypokalemia allow the kidney to excrete excess bicarbonate.

Glucose and Electrolyte Disorders

Serum glucose determination is superior to urine glucose measurement for managing blood sugar abnormalities. However, urine glucose concentration helps assess osmotic diuresis and estimate renal transport thresholds by comparison with serum levels.

Hyperglycemia

Glucose infusions and stress responses commonly elevate serum glucose levels after surgery. During anesthesia, the value of including glucose in maintenance intravenous solutions is
11 questionable. Moderate postoperative hyperglycemia (150–250 mg/dL) resolves spontaneously and has little adverse effect. Higher glucose levels cause glycosuria with osmotic diuresis and interfere with serum electrolyte determinations. Severe hyperglycemia increases serum osmolality to a point that cerebral disequilibrium and hyperosmolar coma occur. In diabetic patients, hyperglycemia may indicate insulin deficiency and potential for ketoacidosis. Incremental titration or infusion of intravenous regular insulin adjusts serum glucose rapidly. Potassium replacement and serial blood glucose determinations are essential.

Hypoglycemia

Hypoglycemia in the PACU can be caused by endogenous insulin secretion or by excessive or inadvertent insulin administration. Serious postoperative hypoglycemia is rare and easily treated with intravenous 50% dextrose followed by glucose infusion. Either sedation or excessive SNS activity masks signs and symptoms of hypoglycemia during recovery.

Hyponatremia

Postoperative hyponatremia occurs if free water is infused intravenously during surgery or if sodium-free irrigating solution is absorbed during transurethral prostatic resection or hysteroscopy. Accumulation of serum glycine or its metabolite, ammonia, might exacerbate symptoms. Free water retention is also caused by inappropriate ADH secretion, prolonged labor induction with oxytocin, or respiratory uptake of nebulized droplets. Theoretically, excessive infusion of isotonic saline leads to excretion of hypertonic urine, desalination, and iatrogenic hyponatremia. Symptoms of moderate hyponatremia include agitation, disorientation, visual disturbances, and nausea, whereas severe hyponatremia causes unconsciousness, impaired airway reflexes, and CNS irritability that progresses to grand mal seizures. Therapy includes intravenous normal saline and intravenous furosemide to promote free water excretion. Infusion of hypertonic saline may be useful for severe hyponatremia. Monitor serum sodium concentration and osmolarity.

Hypokalemia

Postoperative hypokalemia is often inconsequential but might generate serious dysrhythmias, especially in patients taking digoxin. A potassium deficit caused by chronic diuretic therapy, nasogastric suctioning, or vomiting often underlies hypokalemia. Urinary and hemorrhagic losses, dilution, and insulin therapy generate acute hypokalemia that worsens during respiratory alkalemia. Excess SNS activity, infusion of calcium, or beta-mimetic medications exacerbates effects of hypokalemia. Adding potassium to peripheral intravenous fluids often restores serum concentration, but concentrated solutions infused through a central catheter may be necessary.

Hyperkalemia

A high serum potassium raises the suspicion of spurious hyperkalemia from a hemolyzed specimen or from sampling near an intravenous catheter containing potassium or banked blood. Postoperative hyperkalemia occurs after excessive potassium infusion or in patients with renal failure or malignant hyperthermia. Acute acidemia exacerbates hyperkalemia. Succinylcholine given in the PACU to patients with burns, severe trauma, or chronic neurologic injuries could increase serum potassium. Treatment with intravenous insulin and glucose acutely lowers potassium, whereas intravenous calcium counters myocardial effects. Beta-mimetic medications might also have a role.

Calcium and Magnesium

Although underlying parathyroid disease or massive fluid replacement reduces total body and ionized calcium, symptomatic hypocalcemia seldom occurs in the PACU. A rare patient might exhibit upper airway obstruction from hypocalcemia after parathyroid excision. Reduction of the ionized fraction by acute alkalemia may cause myocardial conduction and contractility abnormalities, decreased vascular tone, or tetany. Transfusion of blood containing chelating agents (e.g., citrate) rarely causes symptomatic hypocalcemia. Administration of calcium chloride or calcium gluconate to hypocalcemic patients improves cardiovascular dynamics.

Magnesium plays a key role in restoration of neuromuscular function after surgery and in maintenance of cardiac rhythm and conduction.

MISCELLANEOUS COMPLICATIONS

Nausea and Vomiting

12 Avoiding PONV is a high priority for physicians and patients,[10] yet PONV remains a significant problem. Aside from unpleasantness for the patient and staff, PONV poses medical risks. Increased intra-abdominal pressure and forceful vomiting

jeopardize abdominal or inguinal suture lines and risks esophageal rupture, whereas elevated CVP increases morbidity after ocular, tympanic, or intracranial procedures. Risk of aspirating gastric contents increases, especially if airway reflexes or ability to expel secretions are impaired. SNS response elevates heart rate and systemic blood pressure, increasing the risk of myocardial ischemia or dysrhythmias. Movement during PONV worsens postoperative pain and accentuates autonomic responses. Gagging and retching might also elicit PNS responses with bradycardia and hypotension. Finally, PONV delays discharge or necessitates admission of ambulatory patients. Assess the degree of PONV periodically throughout recovery.[4]

The incidence of PONV varies with many factors.[7,61,62] Reported incidence is lower in the PACU than over 24 to 48 hours. A high percentage of patients experience postdischarge PONV,[63] and 36% of those do not experience PONV prior to discharge.[16] Delayed emesis may reflect timing of oral intake, waning effects of antiemetics, or greater postdischarge pain. Risk is low in children younger than age 2, increases thereafter until puberty, and then decreases 13% per decade of age. Women have a higher incidence than men. Ear-nose-throat and dental procedures entail a high risk, followed by orthopaedic and cosmetic surgery. The risk of PONV is also high after procedures involving extraocular muscle traction, middle ear manipulation, peritoneal or intestinal irritation, or testicular traction. However, the predictive value of procedure type is questionable.[64] A history of postoperative emesis or motion sickness predicts PONV. Nonsmokers have a significantly higher risk of PONV than smokers.[65]

Perioperative factors such as starvation, autonomic imbalance, pain, and effects of anesthetics on the chemotactic center probably contribute to emergence of PONV. Conditions that affect the gastroesophageal junction (obesity, hiatal hernia) may increase the likelihood of emesis in the PACU. Swallowed blood or secretions promotes PONV, as does gas in the stomach from facemask ventilation, esophageal intubation, or nitrous oxide diffusion. Incidence of PONV is lower after regional than general anesthesia, although this difference narrows when epinephrine or long-acting axial opioids are included, or once parenteral opioids are needed to control postoperative pain.[66] Exclusion of nitrous oxide from an anesthetic appears to reduce the incidence of PONV.[67,68] The incidence of nausea does not differ greatly among inhalation anesthetics, although desflurane and sevoflurane might generate slightly higher rates. Barbiturate induction seems less offensive than etomidate or ketamine, whereas propofol offers a still lower risk. Use of "pure" inhalational techniques and administration of opioid analgesics increases the incidence PONV, especially after ambulatory surgery. Small doses of shorter-acting opioids might decrease incidence, but short duration of analgesia offsets this advantage. Supplementation with nonopioid analgesics such as ketorolac, acetaminophen, or ibuprofen might reduce the frequency of emesis. It is unclear whether administration of neostigmine or the choice of anticholinergic used to reverse neuromuscular relaxation also increases the incidence.

Several algorithms have been recommended to prevent or treat PONV.[61,64] Evacuation of stomach contents with an orogastric tube is of questionable value. Use of high concentrations of supplemental oxygen and hydration appear to reduce the incidence of PONV, but postoperative drinking is often a triggering event. Need to drink prior to discharge should be determined on a case-by-case basis, so children or high-risk patients can be appropriately discharged before they take oral fluids.[4,68] Whether this decreases incidence of PONV or merely delays onset is unclear. Limiting vestibular stimulation by minimizing brisk head motion seems helpful.

Studies of medications for prophylaxis and treatment of PONV reveal that serotonin blocking agents, dexamethasone, and droperidol are probably equal in efficacy, cost effectiveness, and patient satisfaction.[61,64] Guidelines on postoperative care from the ASA endorse the use of serotonin blocking agents and dexamethasone, and of multiple agents.[4] These antiemetics have different sites of action, so combination therapy might generate better results by simultaneously treating two or more precipitating factors, although their effects appear merely additive rather than synergistic.[64] Prophylaxis should only be used in patients at medium or high risk of emesis, but the unreliability of risk scoring systems mandates use of clinical judgment.

Serotonin receptor blockers are useful in this class for treating PONV, but it is not clear that any particular drug is superior. Optimum intravenous adult dosage of ondansetron, the most widely studied of these drugs, seems to be 4 mg administered near the end of surgery.[69] Serotonin blockers have few side effects and appear to be particularly useful for PONV related to stimulation of gastric enterochromaffin cells. Bothersome headache occurs after intravenous administration, and transient liver enzyme elevation is seen in a small percentage of patients. Serotonin blockers are cost effective if use shortens PACU length of stay, avoids admission, and improves patient satisfaction. However, their cost effectiveness as first-line agents is debatable.

Dexamethasone is a potent agent for PONV prophylaxis, especially during procedures where an inflammation may contribute to postoperative nausea. A dose of 0.05 to 0.1 mg/kg (4 to 8 mg in adults) given intravenously before induction of anesthesia is effective, and offers a low cost and a mild side effect profile. Dexamethasone may be a valuable first-line drug for prophylaxis.

Droperidol decreases the incidence and severity of PONV, although efficacy varies among procedures and patients. A total intravenous dose of 1 to 2 μg/kg (0.625 to 1.25 mg in adults) seems optimal. Droperidol also effectively treats breakthrough nausea after prophylaxis. Although mild sedation might delay discharge slightly, delay from untreated PONV is usually greater. Transient restlessness and rare extrapyramidal side effects are usually inconsequential. The alpha-adrenergic blocking properties of droperidol can precipitate hypotension in hypovolemic patients. Concerns about isolated cases of Q-T interval prolongation and cardiac dysrhythmia have decreased the use of this valuable agent, but the actual risk at doses used for PONV is likely overemphasized. However, the U.S. Food and Drug Administration has issued a "black box warning" relating to Q-T interval prolongation.

Other agents exhibit antiemetic properties. Propofol likely has short-term antiemetic properties and is useful for anesthesia in patients at high risk for PONV, but it does not compare with the three first-line antiemetics. Cimetidine, ranitidine, metoclopramide, dimenhydrinate, and thiethylperazine are relatively ineffective. Intravenous scopolamine causes unacceptable psychogenic reactions, whereas transdermal scopolamine causes postoperative visual disturbances. Efficacy of ephedrine for PONV related to ambulation or motion is unclear. The antiemetic effect of midazolam in children is likely related to the relationship between crying, fear, or agitation and vomiting. P6 acupuncture or acupressure seems a useful adjunct to pharmacologic therapy, especially for cases of refractory nausea.[70,71]

Before treating PONV, serious causes of nausea and emesis such as hypotension, hypoxemia, hypoglycemia, intracranial pressure, or gastric bleeding should be excluded.

Incidental Trauma

Each patient admitted to the PACU should be carefully evaluated for traumatic complications. Discovery of a complication necessitates careful documentation, notification of physicians responsible for extended care, consultation with specialists, and follow-up.

Ocular Injuries and Visual Changes

Corneal abrasion caused by drying or inadvertent eye contact during facemask ventilation or intubation is a common postoperative eye injury. Corneal abrasion occurs more frequently in elderly patients, after long cases, with lateral or prone positioning, and after head or neck surgery.[72] Corneal injury occurs in the PACU if a rigid oxygen facemask rides up on the eye or if the eye is rubbed with a digital pulse oximeter probe. Abrasion causes tearing, decreased visual acuity, pain, and photophobia. Fluorescein staining aids diagnosis. Abrasion usually heals spontaneously within 72 hours without scarring, but severe injury can cause cataract formation and impair vision. Symptomatic treatment includes artificial tears and eye closure.

Visual acuity is often impaired after anesthesia. Autonomic side effects of medications impair accommodation, and residual ocular lubricant clouds vision. Impairment of retinal perfusion by ocular compression generates postoperative visual disturbances ranging from loss of acuity to permanent blindness.[73,74] Ischemic optic atrophy also occurs in the absence of external compression.[75] Risk is higher after long procedures in the prone position, as well as in patients with vascular disease and anemia. A significant percentage of postoperative patients suffer deficits in acuity unrelated to ocular trauma, some of which require permanent refractive adjustment.[76] Be alert for visual impairment and check acuity when assessing patients at higher risk for ischemic optic atrophy.

Hearing Impairment

Hearing impairment after anesthesia and surgery is relatively common.[77] Although impairment is often subclinical, patients sometimes experience decreased auditory acuity, tinnitus, or roaring. Incidence of detectable hearing impairment is particularly high after dural puncture for spinal anesthesia (8 to 16%), and varies with needle size, needle type, and patient age. Impairment can be unilateral or bilateral and usually resolves spontaneously. Hearing loss also occurs after general anesthesia for both noncardiac and cardiac surgery, and is often related to disruption of the round window or tympanic membrane rupture. Eustachian tube inflammation and otitis secondary to endotracheal intubation can also impact hearing.

Oral, Pharyngeal, and Laryngeal Injuries

Laryngoscope blades, surgical instruments, rigid airways, and dentition can all cause trauma of oral soft tissues. Lip, tongue, or gum abrasions are treated with an ice pack and analgesia. Penetrating injuries caused by tissue entrapment between teeth and rigid devices may require topical antibiotics. After a traumatic tracheal intubation, hematoma or edema might cause partial upper airway obstruction. Nebulized racemic epinephrine often improves stridor. Dental damage can occur during airway manipulations or during emergence if a patient bites on a rigid oral airway or forcefully clenches his or her teeth. Document tooth or dental appliance damage, obtain a dental consultation, and observe for signs of foreign body aspiration.[78]

Sore throat and hoarseness after tracheal intubation occur in 20 to 50% of patients, depending on the degree of trauma during laryngoscopy and oropharyngeal suctioning, the duration of intubation, and the type of tube (see Chapter 22). Mucosal irritation also presents as an unquenchable dryness in mouth and throat. The use of local anesthetic ointments to lubricate endotracheal tubes may cause additional mucosal irritation. Topical viscous lidocaine attenuates irritation from nasogastric tubes but may increase risk of aspiration during recovery. In children, the severity of postextubation laryngeal edema or tracheitis varies with age, intubation duration, and degree of trauma or tube movement. Most recover with cool mist therapy, but nebulized racemic epinephrine and dexamethasone are also effective. Laryngoscopy and intubation can also cause hypoglossal, lingual, or recurrent laryngeal nerve damage, vocal cord evulsion, desquamation of laryngeal or tracheal mucosa, edema or ulceration, and tracheal perforation. Postoperative sore throat and dysphagia also occurs without intubation, related to use of laryngeal mask airways,[79] oral airways, trauma from suctioning, or drying from unhumidified gases. Neck and jaw soreness are common after facemask anesthetics.

Nerve Injuries

Nerve injuries caused by improper positioning during anesthesia generate serious long-term complications (see Chapter 23).[80] Spinal cord injury can be caused by positioning for intubation or by hematoma accumulation after placement of regional anesthetics. Peripheral nerve compression during general or regional anesthesia sometimes causes permanent sensory and motor deficits, as do stretch injuries from hyperextension of an extremity.[81] Any bruising or skin breakdown noted postoperatively should prompt evaluation for underlying nerve damage. Many postoperative neuropathies have no identifiable cause. This is particularly true for ulnar neuropathy, which may be related to subtle positioning problems, preexisting impairment, or sensitivity of the nerve to ischemia.[82] Every complaint of nonsurgical pain, numbness, or weakness from a postoperative patient should be carefully evaluated.

Postdural puncture headache sometimes first emerges in the PACU. Headache is more frequent after difficult subarachnoid anesthetics with multiple attempts and after dural puncture during attempted epidural placement. Subarachnoid air bubbles from loss-of-resistance testing may contribute. In the PACU, treatment is supportive with hydration, analgesics, and positioning. In severe cases, an early epidural blood patch might be considered. Nerve injury secondary to needle contact or intraneuronal injection during placement of regional anesthesia is rare but does occur.[81,83] In one study, 6.3% of 4,767 patients experienced paresthesia during placement of spinal anesthesia, but only 0.126% had persisting symptoms.[84] In the PACU, patients complain of pain, focal numbness, residual paresthesia, or dysesthesia. Symptoms are usually transient. Administer analgesia, reassure the patient, document findings, and follow for the possibility of an evolving neurologic deficit.

During recovery from spinal anesthesia, some patients exhibit lower-extremity discomfort, buttock pain, and other signs of sacral or lumbar neurologic irritation. This problem is more common in obese patients, after procedures in lithotomy position, and after spinal anesthesia with 5% lidocaine.[83] Symptoms are transient and treated supportively. Rarely, a patient exhibits headache and meningeal signs caused by chemical meningitis after injection of a spinal drug that is contaminated or outside the acceptable pH range.

Soft-Tissue and Joint Injuries

If pressure points are improperly padded during long procedures, soft-tissue ischemia and necrosis occur, especially with lateral or prone positioning. Prolonged scalp pressure causes localized alopecia, whereas entrapment of ears, breasts, genitalia, or skin folds causes inflammation or necrosis. Regional ischemia from major arterial compression is rare. Thermal, electrical, or chemical burns from cautery equipment, preparatory solutions, or adhesives also occur. Extravasation of intravenous medications or fluids can cause sloughing, localized chemical neuropathy, or compartment syndromes. Excessive joint or muscle extension leads to postoperative backache, joint pain, stiffness, and even joint instability.

Skeletal Muscle Pain

Postoperative muscle pain is caused by many intraoperative factors. Prolonged lack of motion or unusual muscle stretch during positioning often contributes to muscle stiffness and aching. Fasciculation during depolarizing blockade has implicated succinylcholine as a cause of postoperative myalgias. Acute myalgia also occurs after administration of other relaxants and in patients receiving no relaxant. Delayed-onset muscle fatigue can appear days after surgery and resolve spontaneously.

Hypothermia and Shivering

Although intraoperative temperature maintenance is a standard, patients still exhibit postoperative hypothermia. During anesthesia, heat is redistributed and also lost by evaporation during skin preparation, by humidification of dry gases in the airway, and by radiation and convection from the skin and wound. Temperature reduction is accelerated by cold intravenous fluids and low ambient temperatures. The thermoregulatory threshold, below which humans actively regulate body temperature, is decreased during general anesthesia and is less effective under anesthesia. Ability to maintain body temperature is also compromised because paralysis and anesthesia impair shivering and thermoregulatory vasoconstriction, and because nonshivering thermogenesis is ineffective in adults. Rate of heat loss is similar during general or regional anesthesia, but rewarming is slower after regional anesthesia because residual vasodilation and paralysis impede heat generation and retention. Cachectic, traumatized, or burned patients experience greater temperature reduction, as do infants because of a low ratio of body mass-to-surface area.

13 Hypothermia complicates care in the PACU.[85] Average PACU stay is increased by 40 to 90 minutes for hypothermic patients.[86] Postoperative hypothermia increase SNS activity, elevates peripheral vascular resistance, and decreases venous capacitance. Risk of myocardial ischemia[87] and dysrhythmia from mechanical myocardial stimulation is increased. Vasoconstriction interferes with the reliability of pulse oximetry and intra-arterial pressure monitoring. Hypoperfusion jeopardizes marginal tissue grafts, and promotes tissue hypoxia and metabolic acidemia. The alveolar-arterial oxygen gradient increases, and high avidity of hemoglobin compromises oxygen unloading to hypothermic tissues. Platelet sequestration, decreased platelet function, and reduced clotting factor contribute to coagulopathy. Moderate hyperglycemia occurs, cellular immune responses are compromised, and postoperative infection rates increase. A decrease in the minimal alveolar concentration of inhalation anesthetics (5 to 7% per 1°C cooling) accentuates residual sedation. Low perfusion and impaired biotransformation might increase the duration of neuromuscular relaxants and sedatives. Severe hypothermia interferes with cardiac rhythm generation and impulse conduction. On ECG, the PR, QRS, or QT intervals lengthen, and J waves appear. Spontaneous ventricular fibrillation occurs at temperatures <28°C.

During emergence, hypothalamic regulation generates shivering to increase endogenous heat production.[88] Shivering increases the risk of incidental trauma, disrupts medical devices, and interferes with ECG and pulse oximetry monitoring. Oxygen consumption and CO_2 production increase by up to 200%. Associated increases in minute ventilation and cardiac output might precipitate ventilatory failure in patients with limited reserve or myocardial ischemia in those with coronary artery disease.[87] Shivering is accentuated by tremors related to emergence from inhalation anesthesia. Tremors exhibit clonic and tonic components, and likely reflect decreased cortical influence on spinal cord reflexes.

Restoration of normothermia is an important goal during recovery. Forced-air warming devices are most useful for treating hypothermia. For most patients, shivering from mild to moderate hypothermia is uncomfortable but self-limited, and needs no treatment other than rewarming and reassurance. Many medications have been recommended to suppress shivering, but meperidine is most efficacious in conjunction with treatment of hypothermia with rewarming.[4] Other opioid agonists or agonist–antagonists may be useful if meperidine is contraindicated. Withholding reversal of relaxants in ventilated, sedated patients attenuates shivering but increases rewarming time. If temperature is near normal (>96 to 97°F) and shivering is resolved, transfer from PACU to an inpatient floor or a discharge area is acceptable.

Hyperthermia

Hyperthermia is relatively uncommon in the PACU. Occasionally, a patient exhibits short-lived hyperthermia from close draping or aggressive intraoperative heat preservation. Postoperative fever sometimes reflects a preexisting infection (e.g., sinusitis, upper respiratory or urinary tract infection) or an infection exacerbated by the surgical procedure (e.g., resection of infected tonsils or appendix, abscess drainage, urinary tract manipulation). Atelectasis secondary to loss of lung volume, retained secretions, or aspiration is another cause, although fever often appears after PACU discharge. Elevated temperature might indicate a drug or transfusion reaction. Muscarinic blocking agents such as atropine interfere with cooling and might contribute to fever, but they are seldom the cause. Other hypermetabolic states such as thyroid storm must be considered. High fever occurs with malignant hyperthermia, but signs such as tachycardia, muscle rigidity, dysrhythmia, hyperventilation, and acidemia establish the diagnosis first.

Ambient cooling, chest physiotherapy, incentive spirometry, and antipyretics are usually sufficient to treat postoperative fever. Withhold offending medications or blood products if a drug or transfusion reaction is suspected. Notify the physician responsible for extended care to ensure postdischarge evaluation. Therapy for thyroid storm or malignant hyperthermia is well described elsewhere.

Persistent Sedation

Because 90% of patients regain consciousness within 15 minutes of admission to the PACU, unconsciousness persisting for a greater period is considered *prolonged*.[89] Even a highly susceptible patient should respond to a stimulus within 30 to 45 minutes after a reasonably conducted anesthetic. In a patient with prolonged sedation, research the level of preoperative responsiveness to uncover intoxication with drugs and alcohol or preexisting mental dysfunction. Note the time and amount of preoperative and intraoperative sedative medications, and review any unusual intraoperative events. The rate and character of spontaneous ventilation helps judge residual anesthesia depth, whereas the heart rate, rhythm, and blood pressure qualitatively indicate adequacy of cerebral perfusion. Physical assessment should include a tactile stimulus such as a light skin pinch. This elicits greater arousal than verbal stimulation, perhaps because sensory input is amplified through the reticular activating system. Diagnostic value of pupillary size and response is low.

Residual sedation from inhalation anesthetics might cause prolonged unconsciousness, especially after long procedures, in obese patients, or when high concentrations are continued through the end of surgery. This is less likely after anesthesia with low solubility agents such as sevoflurane or desflurane. Long-acting sedatives used for premedication (e.g., pentobarbital, hydroxyzine, promethazine, droperidol, lorazepam, scopolamine) contribute to postoperative somnolence. Sedation from intraoperative opioid or sedative administration is dose related. To assess sedation from opioids, administer low-dose intravenous naloxone (0.04-mg increments every 2 minutes, up to 0.2 mg). With careful titration, respiratory depression and sedation are reversed without dangerous reversal of analgesia. If unconsciousness is related to residual opioid effects, ventilatory rate and arousal will increase with 0.2 mg or less of intravenous naloxone, unless a patient has received a massive opioid overdose. Flumazenil (0.2 mg intravenously per minute to a total of 1.0 mg), a competitive benzodiazepine antagonist, differentiates sedation from midazolam and diazepam, although duration of action is short. Neither naloxone nor flumazenil should be used as a routine element of postoperative care.[4] Administer reversal only for specific indications in individual patients. Administration of intravenous physostigmine (1.25 mg) counteracts but does not reverse sedation caused by inhalation anesthetics and other sedatives. If administration of naloxone, flumazenil, or physostigmine does not elicit a response, unconsciousness is most likely not related to residual anesthetic medications. However, it is still possible that an unrecognized, preoperative overdose with depressant oral drugs is responsible.

Profound residual neuromuscular paralysis might rarely mimic unconsciousness by precluding any motor response to stimuli. This could occur after gross overdosage, if reversal agents are omitted, in patients with unrecognized neuromuscular disease, or with phase II blockade from succinylcholine use in a patient with pseudocholinesterase deficiency. Observation of purposeful motion, spontaneous ventilation, or reflex activity eliminates residual paralysis as an explanation. CNS depression secondary to intravenous local anesthetic toxicity or inadvertent subarachnoid injection can mimic postoperative coma. Children who were exhausted before surgery are often difficult to arouse after anesthesia, especially if sleep patterns are disrupted by emergency surgery at night. Hypothermia below 33°C impairs consciousness and increases the depressant effect of medications. Core temperatures below 30°C can cause fixed pupillary dilation, areflexia, and coma. Check a serum glucose level to eliminate severe hypoglycemia or hyperglycemic, hyperosmolar coma as causes. Suspicion that unresponsiveness is caused by hypoglycemia indicates an immediate empiric trial of intravenous 50% dextrose. Hyposmolar states (<260 mOsm/L) such as acute hyponatremia (Na < 125 mEq/L) are ruled out by checking serum electrolyte and osmolarity. Arterial blood gas analysis reveals CO_2 narcosis ($Paco_2$ > 200 to 250 mm Hg). A patient may also be feigning unresponsiveness or having a hysterical reaction that presents as unconsciousness.

If a diagnosis remains elusive, consult a neurologist for a thorough neurologic evaluation. Occasionally unresponsiveness reflects subclinical grand mal seizures secondary to delirium tremens or an underlying seizure disorder. Cerebral anoxia from intraoperative hypotension, hypoxemia, or CO poisoning must be considered. In injured patients or those recovering from intracranial surgery, evaluate for unrecognized head trauma, intracerebral hemorrhage, or increased intracranial pressure. Patients sometimes awaken very slowly after long intracranial procedures.[90] Cerebral thromboembolism is another possibility in patients who have undergone internal jugular or subclavian cannulation. Patients with atrial fibrillation, carotid bruits, or hypercoagulable states are also at increased risk of thromboembolism. Paradoxical air or fat embolism through a right-to-left intracardiac shunt should be considered. After cardiac, proximal major vascular, or invasive neck surgery, risk of postoperative stroke ranges from 2.2 to 5.2%.[91] Postoperative cerebrovascular accidents in other patients are rare (0.08 to 0.4%) and usually become evident after the PACU interval.

Altered Mental Status

Recovering patients sometimes exhibit inappropriate mental reactions, ranging from lethargy and confusion to physical combativeness and extreme disorientation.

Emergence Reactions

Aside from the disturbance to staff and other patients, a stormy emergence reaction has significant medical consequences. The risk of incidental trauma increases, including contusion or fracture, corneal abrasion, and sprains from struggling. Thrashing jeopardizes suture lines, orthopaedic fixations, vascular grafts, drains, tracheal tubes, and vascular catheters. Agitated patients manifest high levels of SNS tone, tachycardia, and hypertension. Least appreciated is the risk of injury to PACU staff struggling to protect a combative patient.

For a short period after regaining consciousness, some patients appear unable to appropriately process sensory input. Most exhibit somnolence, slight disorientation, and sluggish mental reactions that rapidly clear. Others experience wide emotional swings such as weeping or escalating resistance to positioning and restraint. Predicting which patients will have adverse psychological reactions is difficult. Emergence reactions are prevalent in children and young adults, especially after anesthesia with sevoflurane and desflurane and after ear-nose-throat procedures. In young children, anxiety is heightened by parental separation. Very young children may react inappropriately to sound when hearing acutely improves after myringotomies. Patients with mental retardation, psychiatric disorders, organic brain dysfunction, or hostile preoperative interactions manifest those problems after surgery. Inability to speak secondary to oral fixation or tracheal intubation generates frustration or fear that exaggerates emergence reactions. Ethnic, cultural, and psychological characteristics play some role. A language barrier or a new postoperative hearing impairment accentuates an emergence reaction because input from PACU staff might not be understood. The incidence of stormy emergence is probably higher after procedures with high emotional significance. Recall of intraoperative events can generate severe panic and anxiety during emergence.[92] In patients who abuse alcohol, opioids, cocaine, or other illicit drugs, intoxication or withdrawal elicits bizarre emergence behavior. Disorientation, paranoia, and combativeness occur after use of scopolamine as a premedication or antiemetic. This can be treated with intravenous physostigmine. Ketamine or droperidol can cause dysphoria and hallucination, although acute reactions are rare. Etomidate contributes to restlessness.

Pain amplifies agitation, confusion, and aggressive behavior during emergence;[93] therefore, it is helpful to ensure adequate postoperative analgesia early in the PACU course. Urinary urgency or gastric distention from trapped gas generates discomfort and agitation, as do tight dressings, painful phlebotomy, and poor positioning. Endotracheal or nasogastric tubes and urinary catheters are equally discomforting. Check for unusual pain sources such as corneal abrasion, entrapment of body parts, infiltrated vascular catheters, or small devices left beneath a patient. Nausea, dizziness, and pruritus are distressing during emergence. Some patients struggle to move from a supine into a more comfortable semisitting or lateral position, especially those with gastroesophageal reflux, pulmonary congestion, or obesity. Emerging patients often resist physical restraint. Residual paralysis elicits agitation or uncoordinated motions that make a patient appear disoriented and combative. Observation of weakness or a peculiar flapping nature of voluntary motion help in the diagnosis. However, patients can appear fully recovered by head lift and train-of-four monitoring but still perceive impaired swallowing, visual acuity, and sense of strength.[94]

Combativeness, confusion, or disorientation might reflect respiratory dysfunction. Moderate hypoxemia often presents with clouded mentation, disorientation, and agitation resembling that caused by pain. Respiratory acidemia elicits profound agitation, although acidemia caused by ventilatory center depression generates less agitation because higher CNS functions are also depressed. Hypercarbia without acidemia is usually asymptomatic. Limitation of inspiratory volume by chest dressings, gastric distention, or splinting causes a vague dissatisfaction with lung inflation similar to air hunger. This also occurs during mechanical ventilation with low delivered volumes and is probably mediated by stretch receptors in the lung. Inability to generate a forceful cough or clear secretions causes distress, as does high work of breathing. Interstitial pulmonary edema elicits symptoms of air hunger before airway flooding occurs. Agitation can be profound, even with adequate ventilation and oxygenation.

Metabolic abnormalities interfere with lucidity. Lactic acidemia causes anxiety and mild disorientation, acute hyponatremia clouds the sensorium, and hypoglycemia causes first agitation and then diminished responsiveness. Seizure activity might mimic agitation and combativeness. Suspect seizures in patients with epilepsy, head trauma, and chronic alcohol or cocaine abuse. Cerebral hypoperfusion can produce disorientation, agitation, and combativeness. This is a medical emergency that requires aggressive resolution.

There are few interventions that prevent "stormy" emergence reactions.[95] Use of preoperative sedatives in children does not decrease the incidence of emergence delirium, and preoperative suggestion or reassurance seems ineffective. Altered mental status is treated supportively because most emergence reactions disappear within 10 to 15 minutes. Verbal reassurances that surgery is completed and that the patient is doing well are invaluable. Use the patient's and the surgeon's name frequently, and stress the time and location. When practical, allow patients to choose their own position. Provide adequate analgesia. In selected cases, parenteral sedation relieves fear or anxiety and smooths emergence. Identifying whether a patient is reacting to pain or to anxiety is important. Benzodiazepines and barbiturates are ineffective analgesics, whereas opioids are poor sedatives. Do not administer sedative or analgesic medications if altered mental status might reflect a physiologic abnormality such as hypoxemia, hypoglycemia, hypotension, or acidemia. Use restraint only if a patient's safety is jeopardized.

Delirium and Cognitive Decline

14 A high percentage of elderly patients (5 to 50%) experience some degree of postoperative confusion, delirium, or cognitive decline.[96,97] Patients exhibit fluctuations in level of consciousness and orientation, or deterioration of memory, mental functions, and acquisition of new information. The problem may be related to exacerbation of central cholinergic insufficiency by narcotics, sedatives, or anticholinergics. However, stress of surgery, fever, pain, emesis, sleep deprivation, and loss of routine undoubtedly contribute. Presence of preexisting dementia, cognitive abnormalities, organic brain syndrome, or hearing and visual impairment predicts postoperative delirium, as does evidence of physical infirmity such as high ASA physical status or lack of stress response to surgery. Cognitive dysfunction also occurs at lower incidence (15% greater than control) in younger patients, more frequently resolves within 3 months, and may be related to inactivity during recuperation.[98] Although signs often appear on the first to third postoperative day, onset is sometimes evident in the PACU.

Overall, recovery of cognitive function is slower in the elderly.[99] Because older patients are often skilled at concealing declining capabilities, careful assessment of preoperative capabilities helps identify deficits that affect postoperative status. Postoperative lethargy, clouded sensorium, or delirium sometimes reflect an acute physiologic change. Hyperosmolarity from hyperglycemia or hypernatremia clouds consciousness, as does hyponatremia. Cerebral fluid shifts with decreased mentation occur in patients on dialysis and after rapid correction of severe dehydration. Patients receiving atropine premedication or chronic meperidine therapy might exhibit anticholinergic-induced delirium. Disorientation or clouded sensorium can reflect chronic use of psychogenic drugs, premedication with long-acting sedatives, or unrecognized intoxication. Life-threatening conditions such as seizures, hypoxemia, hypoglycemia, hypotension, acidemia, or cerebrovascular accident sometimes present with confusion, disorientation, inability to vocalize, or reduced level of consciousness, especially if earlier premonitory signs and symptoms are misinterpreted.

References

1. Bothner U, Georgieff M, Schwilk B: The impact of minor perioperative anesthesia related incidents, events and complications on postanesthetic care unit utilization. Anesth Analg 89:506, 1999
2. Pavlin DJ, Rapp SE, Polissar NL *et al:* Factors affecting discharge time in adult outpatients. Anesth Analg 87:816, 1998
3. American Society of PeriAnesthesia Nurses: Standard of peri-anesthesia nursing practice. Cherry Hill, NJ: American Society of Post Anesthesia Nursing, 2002
4. A report by the American Society of Anesthesiologists Task Force on Postanesthetic Care: Practice guidelines for postanesthetic care. Anesthesiology 96:742, 2002
5. Apfelbaum JL, Walawander CA, Grasela TH *et al:* Eliminating intensive postoperative care in same-day surgery patients using short-acting anesthetics. Anesthesiology 97:66, 2002
6. Williams BA, Kentor ML, Williams JP *et al:* PACU bypass after outpatient knee surgery is associated with fewer unplanned hospital admissions but more phase II nursing interventions. Anesthesiology 97:981, 2002
7. Hines R, Barash PG, Watrous G *et al:* Complications occurring in the postanesthesia care unit: A survey. Anesth Analg 74:503, 1992
8. Cohen MM, Obrien-Pallas LL, Copplestone C *et al:* Nursing workload associated with adverse events in the post anesthesia care unit. Anesthesiology 91:1882, 1999
9. Pittet D, Stephen F, Hugonnet S *et al:* Hand-cleansing during postanesthesia care. Anesthesiology 99:530, 2003
10. Macario A, Weinger M, Truong P *et al:* Which clinical anesthesia outcomes are both common and important to avoid? The perspective of a panel of expert anesthesiologists. Anesth Analg 88:1085, 1999
11. Strassels SA, Chen C, Carr DB: Postoperative analgesia: Economics, resource use, and patient satisfaction in an urban teaching hospital. Anesth Analg 94:130, 2002
12. Apfelbaum J, Chen C, Mehta SS *et al:* Postoperative pain experience: Results from a national survey suggest postoperative pain continues to be undermanaged. Anesth Analg 97:534, 2003
13. Rundshagen I, Schnabel K, Standl T *et al:* Patients' vs. nurses' assessments of postoperative pain and anxiety during patient or nurse controlled analgesia. Br J Anaesth 82:374, 1999
14. An updated report by the American Society of Anesthesiologists Task Force on Acute Pain Management. Anesthesiology 100:1573, 2004
15. Chung F, Ritchie E, Su J: Postoperative pain in ambulatory surgery. Anesth Analg 85:808, 1997
16. Wu CL, Berenholtz SM, Pronovost PJ *et al:* Systematic review and analysis of postdischarge symptoms after outpatient surgery. Anesthesiology 96:994, 2002
17. Peng PWH, Sandler AN: A review of the use of fentanyl analgesia in the management of acute pain in adults. Anesthesiology 90:576, 1999
18. Gilron I, Milne B, Hong M: Cyclooxygenase-2 inhibitors in postoperative pain management. Anesthesiology 99:1198, 2003
19. Moiniche S, Kehlet H, Berg J *et al:* A qualitative and quantitative systematic review of preemptive analgesia for postoperative pain relief. Anesthesiology 96:752, 2002
20. White PF: The role of non-opioid analgesic techniques in the management of pain after ambulatory surgery. Anesth Analg 94:577,2002
21. Gwirtz KH, Young JV, Byers RS *et al:* The safety and efficacy of intrathecal opioid analgesia for acute postoperative pain: Seven years experience with

5969 surgical patients at Indiana university hospital. Anesth Analg 88:599, 1999

22. DeLeon-Casasola OA: Postoperative epidural opioid analgesia. Anesth Analg 83:867, 1996
23. Casati A, Fanelli G, Cedrati V *et al:* Pulmonary function changes after interscalene brachial plexus anesthesia with 0.5% and 0.75% ropivacaine: A double blind comparison with 2% mepivacaine. Anesth Analg 88:587, 1999
24. Aldrete JA: The post-anesthesia recovery score revisited. J Clin Anesth 7:89, 1995
25. White PF, Song D: New criteria for fast tracking after outpatient anesthesia: A comparison with the modified Aldrete's scoring system. Anesth Analg 88:1069, 1999
26. Howell SJ, Sear JW, Sear YM *et al:* Risk factors for cardiovascular death within 30 days after anaesthesia and urgent or emergency surgery: A nested, case controlled study. Br J Anaesth 82:679, 1999
27. Sprung J, Abdelmalak B, Gottlieb A *et al:* Analysis of risk factors for myocardial infarction and cardiac mortality after major vascular surgery. Anesthesiology 93:129, 2000
28. Badner NH, Knill RL, Brown JE *et al:* Myocardial infarction after noncardiac surgery. Anesthesiology 88:572, 1998
29. Mangano DT, Layug EL, Wallace A *et al:* Effect of atenolol on mortality and cardiovascular morbidity after noncardiac surgery. N Engl J Med 335:1713, 1996
30. Urban MK, Marlowitz SM, Gordon MA *et al:* Postoperative prophylactic administration of β-adrenergic blockers in patients at risk for myocardial ischemia. Anesth Analg 90:1257, 2000
31. London MJ, Zaugg M, Schaub MC *et al:* Perioperative β-adrenergic receptor blockade. Anesthesiology 100:170, 2004
32. Amar D: Perioperative atrial tachyarrhythmias. Anesthesiology 97:1618, 2002
33. Mahla E, Rotman B, Rehak P *et al:* Perioperative ventricular dysrhythmias in patients with structural heart disease undergoing noncardiac surgery. Anesth Analg 86:16, 1998
34. Rose DK, Cohen MM, Wigglesworth DF *et al:* Critical respiratory events in the postanesthesia care unit: Patient, surgical and anesthetic factors. Anesthesiology 81:410, 1994
35. Schwilk B, Bothner U, Schraag S *et al:* Perioperative respiratory events in smokers and nonsmokers undergoing general anesthesia. Acta Anaesthesiol Scand 41:348, 1997
36. Ballantyne JC, Carr DB, DeFerranti S *et al:* The comparative effects of postoperative analgesic therapies on pulmonary outcome: Cumulative meta-analyses of randomized, controlled trials. Anesth Analg 86:598, 1998
37. Warner DO, Warner MA, Offord KP *et al:* Airway obstruction and perioperative complications in smokers undergoing abdominal surgery. Anesthesiology 90:372, 1999
38. Strauss SG, Lynn AM, Bratton SL *et al:* Ventilatory response to CO_2 in children with obstructive sleep apnea from adenotonsillar hypertrophy. Anesth Analg 89:328, 1999
39. Tait AR, Malviya S, Voepel-Lewis T *et al:* Risk factors for perioperative adverse respiratory events in children with upper respiratory tract infections. Anesthesiology 95:299, 2001
40. D'Honneur G, Lofaso F, Drummond GB *et al:* Susceptibility to upper airway obstruction during partial neuromuscular block. Anesthesiology 88:371, 1998
41. Asai T, Koga K, Vaughan RS: Respiratory complications associated with tracheal intubation and extubation. Br J Anaesth 80:767, 1998
42. Benumof JL, Dagg R, Benumof R: Critical hemoglobin desaturation will occur before return to an unparalyzed state following 1 mg/kg intravenous succinylcholine. Anesthesiology 87:979, 1997
43. Warner DO, Warner MA, Barnes RD *et al:* Perioperative respiratory complications in patients with asthma. Anesthesiology 85:460, 1996
44. Berg H, Viby-Mogensen J, Roed J *et al:* Residual neuromuscular block is a risk factor for postoperative pulmonary complications: A prospective, randomized, and blinded study of postoperative pulmonary complications after atracurium, vecuronium, and pancuronium. Acta Anaesthesiol Scand 41:1095, 1997
45. Debaene B, Plaud B, Dilly MP: Residual paralysis in the PACU after a single intubating dose of nondepolarizing muscle relaxant with an intermediate duration of action. Anesthesiology 98:1042, 2003
46. Moller JT, Johannessen NW, Espersen K *et al:* Randomized evaluation of pulse oximetry in 20,802 patients: Perioperative events and postoperative complications. Anesthesiology 78:445, 1993
47. Rothen HU, Sporre B, Engberg G *et al:* Airway closure, atelectasis and gas exchange during anaesthesia. Br J Anaesth 81:68, 1998
48. Karayiannakis AJ, Makki GG, Mantzioka A *et al:* Postoperative pulmonary function after laparoscopic and open cholecystectomy. Br J Anaesth 77:448, 1996
49. Thomas JA, McIntosh JM: Are incentive spirometry, intermittent positive pressure breathing, and deep breathing exercises effective in the prevention of postoperative pulmonary complications after upper abdominal surgery? A systematic review and meta-analysis. Phys Ther 74:3, 1994
50. Overend TJ, Andersom CM, Levy SD: The effect of incentive spirometry on postoperative pulmonary complications, a systematic review. Chest 120:971, 2001
51. Xue FS, Huang YG, Tong SY *et al:* A comparative study of early postoperative hypoxemia in infants, children, and adults undergoing elective plastic surgery. Anesth Analg 83:709, 1996
52. Xue FS, Li BW, Zhang GS *et al:* The influence of surgical sites on early postoperative hypoxemia in adults undergoing elective surgery. Anesth Analg 88:213, 1999
53. Moller JT, Wittrup M, Johansen SH: Hypoxemia in the postanesthesia care unit: An observer study. Anesthesiology 73:890, 1990
54. Ng A, Smith G: Gastroesophageal reflux and aspiration of gastric contents in anesthetic practice. Anesth Analg 93:494, 2001
55. Eriksson LI, Sundman E, Olsson R *et al:* Functional assessment of the pharynx at rest and during swallowing in partially paralyzed humans: Simultaneous videomanometry and mechanomyography of awake human volunteers. Anesthesiology 78:1035, 1997
56. American Society of Anesthesiologists Task Force on Preoperative Fasting: Practice guidelines for preoperative fasting and the use of pharmacologic agents to reduce the risk of pulmonary aspiration: Application to healthy patients undergoing elective procedures. Anesthesiology 90:896, 1999
57. Pavlin DJ, Rapp SE, Polissar NL *et al:* Factors affecting discharge time in adult outpatients. Anesth Analg 87:816, 1998
58. Mulroy MF, Salinas FV, Larkin KL *et al:* Ambulatory surgery may be discharged before voiding after short-acting spinal and epidural anesthesia. Anesthesiology 97:315, 2002
59. Marshall SI, Chung F: Discharge criteria and complications after ambulatory surgery. Anesth Analg 88:508, 1999
60. Twersky R, Fishman D, Homel P: What happens after discharge? Return hospital visits after ambulatory surgery. Anesth Analg 84:319, 1997
61. Gan TJ, Meyers T, Apfel CC *et al:* Consensus guidelines for managing postoperative nausea and vomiting. Anesth Analg 97:67, 2003
62. Stadler M, Bardiau F, Seidel L *et al:* Difference in risk factors for postoperative nausea and vomiting. Anesthesiology 98:46, 2003
63. Gupta A, Wu CL, Elkassabany N *et al:* Does the routine prophylactic use of antiemetics affect the incidence of postdischarge nausea and vomiting following ambulatory surgery? Anesthesiology 99:488, 2003
64. Apfel CC, Korttila K, Abdalla M *et al:* A factorial trial of six interventions for the prevention of postoperative nausea and vomiting. N Engl J Med 350:2441, 2004
65. Sinclair DR, Chung F, Mezei G: Can postoperative nausea and vomiting be predicted? Anesthesiology 91:109, 1999
66. Borgeat A, Ekatodramis G, Schenker CA: Postoperative nausea and vomiting in regional anesthesia. Anesthesiology 98:530, 2003
67. Hartung J: Twenty four of twenty seven studies show a greater incidence of emesis associated with nitrous oxide than with alternative anesthetics. Anesth Analg 83:114, 1996
68. Fengling J, Norris A, Chung F *et al:* Should adult patients drink fluids before discharge from ambulatory surgery? Anesth Analg 87:306, 1998
69. Tramer MR, Reynolds JM, Moore A *et al:* Efficacy dose response, and safety of ondansetron in prevention of postoperative nausea and vomiting: A quantitative, systematic review of randomized, placebo controlled trials. Anesthesiology 87:1277, 1997
70. Lee A, Done ML: The use of non-pharmacologic techniques to prevent postoperative nausea and vomiting: A meta analysis. Anesth Analg 88:1362, 1999
71. Wang SM, Kain ZN: P6 acupoint injections are as effective as droperidol in controlling early postoperative nausea and vomiting in children. Anesthesiology 97:359, 2002
72. Roth SR, Thisted RA, Erickson JP *et al:* Eye injuries after nonocular surgery: A study of 60,965 anesthetics from 1988–1992. Anesthesiology 85:1020, 1996
73. Myers MA, Hamilton SR, Bogosian AJ: Visual loss as a complication of spine surgery: A review of 37 cases. Spine 22:1325, 1997
74. Warner ME, Warner MA, Garrity JA *et al:* The frequency of perioperative vision loss. Anesth Analg 93:1417, 2001
75. Williams EL, Hart WM, Templehoff R: Postoperative ischemic optic neuropathy. Anesth Analg 80:1018, 1995
76. Warner ME, Fronapfel PJ, Hebl JR *et al:* Perioperative visual changes. Anesthesiology 96:855, 2002
77. Sprung J, Bourke DL, Contreras MG, Warner ME *et al:* Perioperative hearing impairment. Anesthesiology 98:241, 2003
78. Warner ME, Benenfeld SM, Warner MA *et al:* Peri-anesthetic dental injuries: Frequency, outcomes and risk factors. Anesthesiology 90:1302, 1999
79. Brimacombe J, Holyoake L, Keller C *et al:* Pharyngolaryngeal, neck, and jaw discomfort after anesthesia with the face mask and laryngeal mask airway at high and low cuff volumes in males and females. Anesthesiology 96:26, 2000
80. A report by the American Society of Anesthesiologists Task Force on Prevention of Perioperative Peripheral Neuropathies: Practice advisory for the prevention of perioperative peripheral neuropathies. Anesthesiology 92:1168, 2000
81. Cheney FW, Domino KB, Caplan RA *et al:* Nerve injury associated with anesthesia: A closed claims analysis. Anesthesiology 90:1062, 1999
82. Warner MA, Warner DO, Matsumoto JY *et al:* Ulnar neuropathy in surgical patients. Anesthesiology 90:54, 1999
83. Auroy Y, Benhamou D, Bargues L *et al:* Major complications of regional anesthesia in France. Anesthesiology 97:1274, 2002
84. Horlocker TT, McGregor DG, Matsushige DK *et al:* A retrospective review of

4767 consecutive spinal anesthetics: Central nervous system complications. Anesth Analg 84:578, 1997

85. Sessler DI: Complications and treatment of mild hypothermia. Anesthesiology 95:531, 2001
86. Lenhardt R, Marker E, Goll V *et al:* Mild intraoperative hypothermia prolongs post anesthetic recovery. Anesthesiology 87:1318, 1997
87. Frank SM, Fleisher LA, Breslow MJ *et al:* Perioperative maintenance of normothermia reduces the incidence of morbid cardiac events: A randomized clinical trial. JAMA 277:1127, 1997
88. Witte JD, Sessler DI: Perioperative shivering. Anesthesiology 96:467, 2002
89. Zelcer J, Wells DG: Anaesthetic-related recovery room complications. Anaesth Intensive Care 15:168, 1996
90. Schubert A, Mascha EJ, Bloomfield EL *et al:* Effect of cranial surgery and brain tumor size on emergence from anesthesia. Anesthesiology 85:513, 1996
91. Wong GY, Warner DO, Schroeder DR *et al:* Risk of surgery and anesthesia for ischemic stroke. Anesthesiology 92:425, 2000
92. Schwender D, Kunze-Kronawitter H, Dietrich P *et al:* Conscious awareness during general anaesthesia: Patients' perceptions, emotions, cognition and reactions. Br J Anaesth 80:133, 1998
93. Lynch EP, Lazor MA, Gellis JE *et al:* The impact of postoperative pain on the development of postoperative delirium. Anesth Analg 86:781, 1998
94. Kopman AF, Yee PS, Neuman GG: Relationship of the train-of-four fade ratio to clinical signs and symptoms of residual paralysis in awake volunteers. Anesthesiology 86:765, 1997
95. Voepel-Lewis T, Malviya S, Tait AR: A prospective cohort study of emergence agitation in the pediatric postanesthesia care unit. Anesth Analg 96:1625, 2003
96. Cook DJ, Rooke GA: Priorities in perioperative geriatrics. Anesth Analg 96:1823, 2003
97. Zakriya KJ, Christmas C, Wenz JF *et al:* Preoperative factors associated with postoperative change in confusion assessment method score in hip fracture patients. Anesth Analg 94:1628, 2002
98. Johnson T, Monk T, Rasmussen LS *et al:* Postoperative cognitive dysfunction in middle-aged patients. Anesthesiology 96:1351, 2002
99. Dodds C, Allison J: Postoperative cognitive deficit in the elderly surgical patient. Br J Anaesth 81:449, 1998

CHAPTER 55 ■ MANAGEMENT OF ACUTE POSTOPERATIVE PAIN

TIMOTHY R. LUBENOW, ANTHONY D. IVANKOVICH, AND ROBERT L. BARKIN

KEY POINTS

1. Modulation of pain occurs in the brain, spinal cord, and periphery. There are alterations in the excitability of spinal cord neurons as peripheral firing increases.
2. The neurophysiologic response to pain involves endocrine, respiratory, cardiovascular, gastrointestinal, genitourinary, neurologic components, and other organ system such as the coagulation and immune systems.
3. Thoracic epidural analgesia has been shown to diminish cardiovascular and other thrombotic complications after major surgery.
4. Human peripheral nerves that are chronically inflamed synthesize opioid ligands in the dorsal root ganglia and transport them down the nerve axion to the inflamed tissue. This allows opioids to have a local anesthetic type of effect in the periphery.
5. Continuous epidural infusion of an opioid-local anesthetic mixture minimizes side effects and fosters more efficient titration of analgesia.
6. Polymodal pharmacotherapies are designed in a patient specific manner including decisions focused at renal function, liver function, age, comorbidites social history and CYP450 system.

Acute postoperative pain is a complex physiologic reaction to tissue injury, visceral distention, or disease. It is manifested by of autonomic, psychological, and behavioral responses that result in patient-specific unpleasant, unwanted sensory and subjective emotional experience. Patients often perceive postoperative pain as one of the more ominous aspects of undergoing surgical procedures. In the past, the treatment of postoperative pain was given a low priority by both surgeons and anesthesiologists, and pain was considered a requisite part of the comprehensive postoperative experience.

With the development of an expanding awareness of the epidemiology and pathophysiology of pain, more attention has been focused on the polymodal management of pain in an effort to improve quality of life, augment functionality, enhance activities of daily living, and reduce physiological and emotional morbidity. The natural progression of this focus was the formation of the postoperative analgesia service or acute pain service, involving a multidisciplinary group of clinicians who specialize through training and education in pain management and who apply an ever-increasing array of modalities to attenuate postoperative pain. This chapter reviews the pathophysiology of pain; examines some pharmacologic considerations; and compares the use of oral, parenteral, central neuraxial analgesics, and adjuvant pharmacotherapies. Peripheral nerve blocks that have application for postoperative pain relief and some nonpharmacologic interventions are described. Incorporation of this knowledge into clinical practice is the basis and the rationale for the effective management of acute postoperative pain.

FUNDAMENTAL CONCEPTS

Nociception

Nociception refers to the detection, transduction, and transmission of noxious stimuli. Stimuli generated from thermal, mechanical, or chemical tissue damage may activate nociceptors, which are free nerve endings. Nociceptors can be further classified into exteroceptors, which receive stimuli from skin

TABLE 55-1

SOMATOSENSORY RECEPTORS

■ RECEPTOR	■ SENSATION PERCEIVED
Nerve fibers on hair follicles	Touch
Merkel's disks	Touch
Meissner's corpuscles	Touch
Free nerve endings (nociceptors)	Pain
Krause's end bulbs	Cold
Ruffini's endings	Heat
Pacinian corpuscles	Pressure
Golgi-Mazzoni endings	Pressure

surfaces, and interoceptors, which are located in the walls of viscera or deeper body structures. Although nociceptors are free nerve terminals, they are adjacent to small blood vessels and mast cells, with which they operate as a functional unit.[1] In addition to nociceptors, the skin is richly innervated by specialized somatosensory receptors that are sensitive to other forms of stimulation (Table 55-1). Each sensory unit includes an end-organ receptor, accompanying axon, dorsal root ganglion, and axon terminals in the spinal cord. In contrast to other special somatosensory receptors, nociceptors exhibit high response thresholds and persistent discharge to suprathreshold stimuli without rapid adaptation and are associated with small receptive fields and small afferent nerve fiber endings.

Peripheral Nerve Afferent Fibers

Nerve fibers were first described according to their type of covering and the presence or absence of myelination. Neural fibers may be covered with neurolemma or myelin, or both. Speed of conduction is determined by fiber size and the presence or absence of myelination. Small, unmyelinated fibers transmit at slower speed than larger myelinated afferent fibers.

With the invention of the oscilloscope, Erlanger and Gasser[2] were able to describe a more functional classification of peripheral nerve fibers. Nerve fibers were categorized into three classes (A, B, and C), depending on size, degree of myelination, rapidity of conduction, and distribution of fibers. A refinement of this classification is the functional subdivision of the class A fibers into the subtypes of alpha, beta, gamma, and delta.[3]

Class A. These neurons, composed of large myelinated fibers, exhibit a low threshold for activation, conduct impulses at a speed of 5 to 100 m/sec, and measure 1 to 20 μm in diameter. Class A delta fibers mediate pain sensation, whereas class A alpha fibers transmit motor and proprioceptive impulses. Class A beta and gamma fibers are responsible for cutaneous touch and pressure, as well as regulation of muscle spindle reflexes.

Class B. These neurons constitute the medium-size myelinated fibers with a conduction velocity ranging from 3 to 14 m/sec and a diameter less than 3 μm. They have a higher threshold (lower excitability) than class A fibers but a lower threshold than class C fibers. The postganglionic sympathetic and visceral afferents belong to this class.

Class C. These fibers are unmyelinated or thinly myelinated and have conduction velocities in the range of 0.5 to 2 m/sec. This class is composed of preganglionic autonomic fibers and pain fibers. Approximately 50 to 80% of class C fibers modulate nociceptive stimuli.

An additional classification of afferent muscle nerve fibers used by neurophysiologists divides the large myelinated fibers into three functional groups (Ia, Ib, II), placing the thinly myelinated (III) and unmyelinated fibers (IV) into separate groups. The muscle afferents of Erlanger and Gasser's class A alpha fibers are subdivided into two groups, Ia and Ib. Fibers from the annulospiral endings of the muscle spindles compose the Ia group, whereas group Ib fibers emanate from the Golgi tendon organs. Group II consists of the tactile and proprioceptive fibers of classes A beta and gamma, respectively, whereas the primary nociceptive nerve fibers of classes A delta and C are equivalent to groups III and IV, respectively, within this classification.[4]

Spinal Cord and Brain Pathways

The peripheral afferent neuron, termed the *first-order neuron*, has its cell body located in the dorsal root ganglion and sends axonal projections into the dorsal horn and other areas of the spinal cord. At this point, a synapse occurs with a second-order afferent neuron, which can be categorized depending on the afferent input it receives, as a nociceptive-specific or wide dynamic-range neuron. Nociceptive-specific neurons process afferent impulses only from nociceptive afferent fibers, whereas A beta, A delta, and C fibers communicate with wide dynamic-range neurons. In the dorsal horn, further synaptic connections occur between first-order and regulatory internuncial neurons. First-order neurons also communicate with the cell bodies of the sympathetic nervous system and ventral motor nuclei, either directly or through the internuncial neurons.[5] The cell body of the second-order neuron lies in the dorsal horn, and axonal projections of this neuron cross to the contralateral hemisphere of the spinal cord (Fig. 55-1). This second-order afferent neuron ascends from that level in the lateral spinothalamic tract to synapse in the thalamus. Along the way, this neuron divides and sends axonal branches that synapse in the regions of the reticular formation, nucleus raphe magnus, periaqueductal gray, and other areas in the brainstem. In the thalamus, the second-order neuron synapses with a third-order afferent neuron, which sends axonal projections into the sensory cortex.

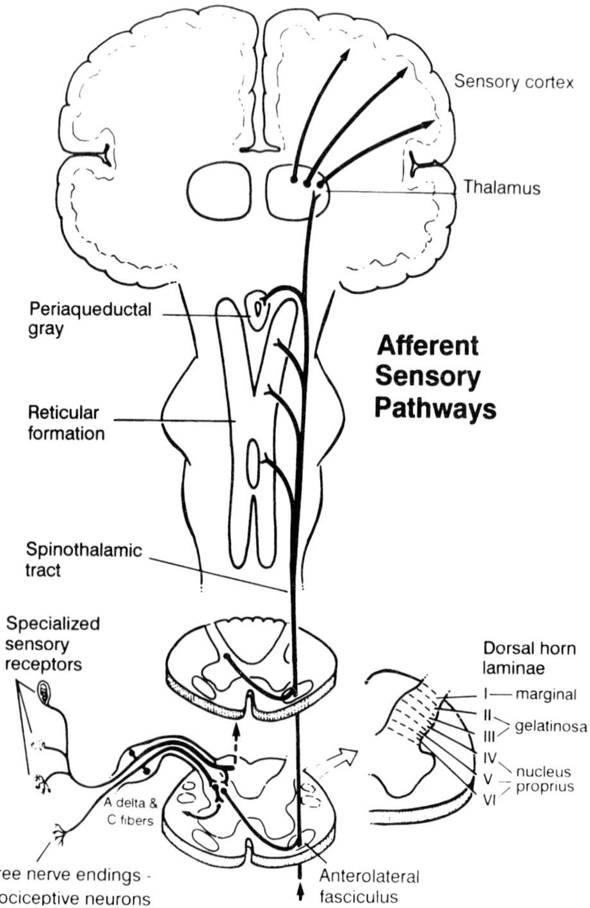

FIGURE 55-1. Afferent sensory pathways for detection and transmission of nociceptive impulses.

Modulation of Nociception

1 Even though nociceptors and the afferent sensory neural pathways detect and transmit noxious stimuli reliably, modulation occurs at several levels in the pathway before perception of the signal at the cortical levels. Modulation can occur either in the periphery or at any point where synaptic transmission occurs.

Peripheral Modulation

Peripheral modulation occurs either by the liberation or elimination of allogeneic substances in the vicinity of the nociceptor. Tissue injury activates nociceptors in the periphery by causing the release of neurotransmitters such as substance P and glutamate, which directly activate nociceptors. Other allogenic mediators—such as potassium and hydrogen ions, lactic acid, serotonin, bradykinin, histamine, and the prostaglandins—further sensitize and excite nociceptors and act as mediators of inflammation. The sources of these substances include ischemic damaged cells and mast cells in the area of the injury, as well as plasma and platelets in the microcirculation surrounding the nociceptors.[1] Aspirin, nonsteroidal anti-inflammatory drugs (NSAIDs), and specific cyclooxygenase-2 (COX-2) inhibitors exert an analgesic effect by inhibiting prostaglandin synthesis and reducing prostaglandin E_1-mediated and prostaglandin E_2-mediated sensitization of peripheral nociceptors. Peripheral terminals of nociceptive sensory neurons contain an excitatory ion channel and are sensitive to heat and the compound capsaicin. This calcium channel receptor, known as the vanilloid or TRPV 1 receptor, is involved in pain sensation and hypersensitivity to noxious stimuli following tissue injury and inflammation.[6] There are also tetrodotoxin-insensitive sodium channels, designated $NA_V1.8$ and $NA_V1.9$, in pain sensing neurons. These channels modulate increased pain hyperexcitability following inflammation, and this may contribute to the effectiveness of use-dependent sodium channel blockers (e.g., local anesthetics) in the treatment of pain.[7–9]

Spinal Modulation

Modulation in the spinal cord results from the action of neurotransmitter substances in the dorsal horn or from spinal reflexes, which convey efferent impulses back to the peripheral nociceptive field. The excitatory amino acid transmitters L-glutamate and aspartate, and several neuropeptides, including vasoactive intestinal peptide, calcitonin gene-related peptide, and neuropeptide Y, are found in central terminals of the first-order neurons and have been shown to modulate transmission of nociceptive afferent signals.[10] Substance P, which is found in the synaptic vesicle of unmyelinated C fibers, is also an important neuromodulator that can enhance or aggravate pain.[11] Prostaglandins produced in response to inflammation play a role in inflammation-evoked central sensitization of spinal cord neurons.[12] The mechanism by which prostaglandin E2 increases inflammatory pain sensitization in the dorsal horn is by decreasing the activity of the $\alpha 3$ subunit of the glycine receptor.[13]

Inhibitory substances involved in the regulation of afferent impulses in the dorsal horn include GABA, glycine, enkephalins, beta-endorphins, norepinephrine, dopamine, and adenosine.[10] Somatostatin, a neuropeptide found in cells that do not contain substance P, may represent another inhibitory neuropeptide involved in afferent modulation. Acetylcholine is also involved in afferent signal processing. Muscarinic receptors of the M_1 and M_2 subtypes have been identified on the nerve terminals of the first-order neurons in laminae II and III of the spinal cord.[14] Cell bodies staining for choline acetyltransferase have been found in laminae III, IV, and V,[15] with dendritic projections into laminae I, II, and III, sites that are primarily involved in processing of nociceptive impulses.[16] Cholinergic agonists have been demonstrated to produce analgesia,[17] as has neostigmine, which inhibits the breakdown of the endogenous neurotransmitter acetylcholine.[18] Acetylcholine acts at muscarinic (M_1 or M_3) receptors that appear to mediate spinal antinociception.[19] The analgesic efficacy of modulating the cholinergic system depends on the tonic release of acetylcholine at muscarinic receptors involved in afferent signal processing because acetylcholine has actions at other spinal sites (inhibition of motor neuron activity, excitation of sympathetic outflow) that produce unwanted side effects.[18]

Afferent modulating mechanisms at the spinal level may also involve spinal reflexes in which afferent signals directly evoke somatic or sympathetic efferent impulses. These impulses discharge in the area of the efferent nociceptive signal. For example, skeletal muscle spasm in an injured area is part of a somatic efferent reflex that is induced as a result of nociceptive afferent signals. Increased skeletal muscle tone initiates more nociceptive signals in a positive feedback loop system from the muscles (Fig. 55-2). In addition, spinal reflexes may involve the discharge of efferent sympathetic signals evoked from the nociceptive impulse (see Fig. 55-2). Efferent sympathetic signals emanate from cell bodies located in the intermediolateral column of the spinal cord. These cell bodies receive internuncial projections from the dorsal horn of the gray matter. This sympathetic reflex produces smooth muscle spasm, vasoconstriction, and liberation of norepinephrine in the vicinity of the wound, thereby generating more pain. Release of norepinephrine has been shown to produce or augment pain after injury.

Neuroplasticity: The Dynamic Modulation of Neural Impulses. The preceding description of the neurophysiology of afferent signal transmission and processing is based on the

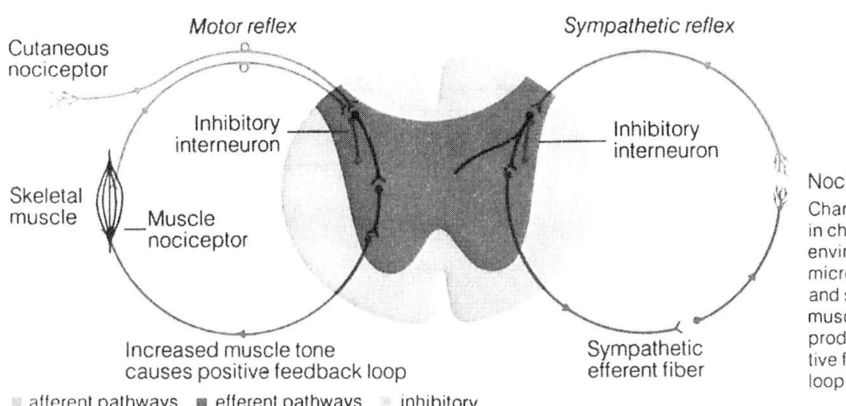

FIGURE 55-2. Schematic representation of spinal reflexes involved in pain modulation. (Reprinted with permission from Bonica JJ, Liebeskind JC, Albe-Fessard DG [eds]: Advances in Pain Research and Therapy, p 3. New York, Raven Press, 1979.)

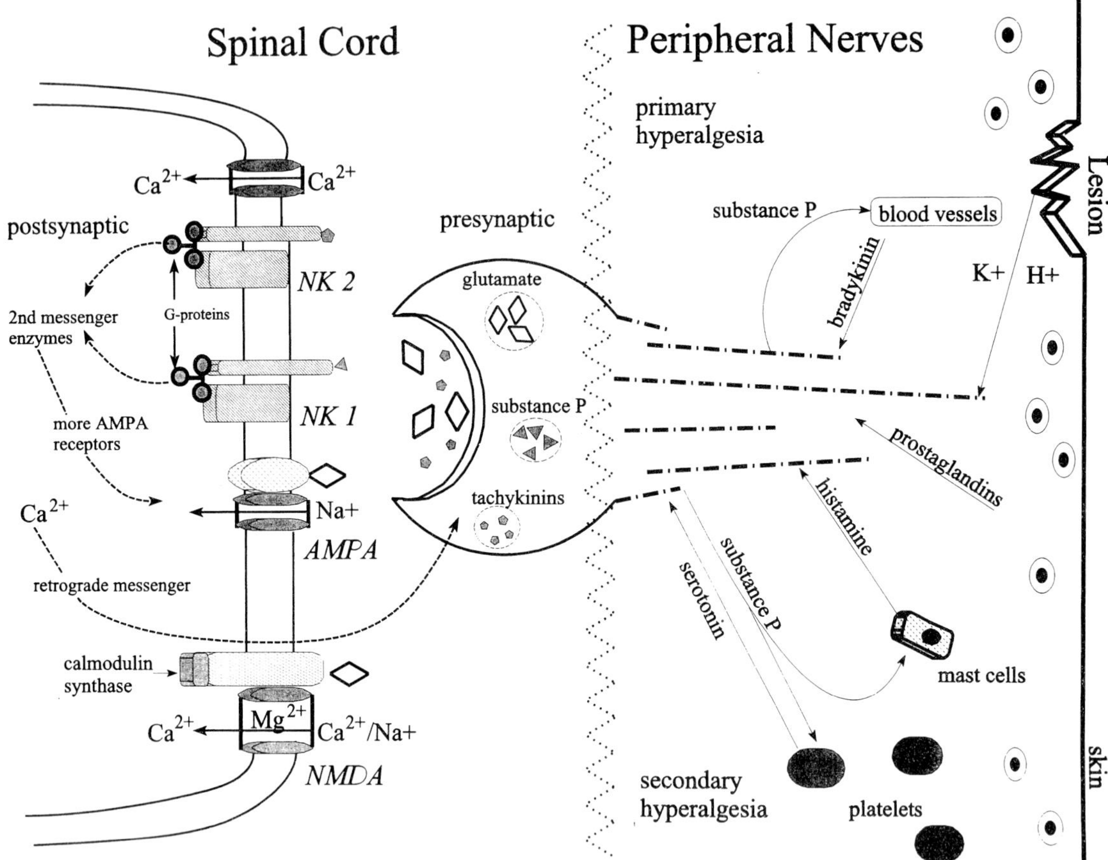

FIGURE 55-3. Schematic representation of peripheral and spinal mechanism involved in neuroplasticity. Primary hyperalgesia results from tissue release of toxic substances. These toxic substances spread to adjacent tissues, prolonging the hyperalgesic state (secondary hyperalgesia). As C fiber terminals increase in frequency of release of neurotransmitters, such as glutamate, substance P, tachykinins, brain-derived neurotrophic factor, and calcitonin gene-related peptide, the effects of these neurotransmitters are summated, resulting in prolonged depolarizations of second-order neurons ("windup"). Function changes at the second-order neuron occur as a result of neurotransmitter binding to postsynaptic receptors, which results in activity-dependent plasticity of the spinal cord. See text for details. AMPA, α-amino-3 hydroxy-5-methyl-4-isoxazole propionic acid; NK, neurokinin; NMDA, N-methyl-D-aspartate.

concept that neural connections involve isolated, unaltered transmission of a single impulse or group of impulses between neurons. Using this model, modulation of noxious afferent signals could be described by gating mechanisms, which formed the initial basis for therapeutic analgesic interventions. Subsequently, however, the description of neural activity-dependent plasticity has enhanced our understanding of the dynamic nature of the nociceptive response to injury. As peripheral nociceptors are sensitized by local tissue mediators of injury (potassium, prostaglandins, and bradykinins), the excitability and frequency of neural discharge increase. This primary hyperalgesia permits previously subnoxious stimuli to generate action potentials and be transduced orthodromically in the spinal cord (Fig. 55-3). The facilitation of impulse transduction in the first-order neuron is partially mediated by noxious substances released from damaged tissues. In addition, axonal reflexes exaggerate this response by releasing substance P. This produces vasodilation and mast cell degranulation, liberating histamine and serotonin, as well as effectively enlarging the peripheral receptive field to include adjacent noninjured tissue, resulting in secondary hyperalgesia.[20]

The increased frequency of impulse transmission to the dorsal horn reduces the gradient between the resting and the critical threshold potential of second-order neurons in the spinal cord. As peripheral nerve firing increases, other changes also occur in the excitability of spinal cord neurons, altering their response to afferent impulses. This central sensitization to afferent impulses results from a functional change in spinal cord processing, termed *neuroplasticity* (see Fig. 55-3). The temporal summation of the number and duration of action potentials elicited per stimulus that occurs in dorsal horn neurons (or in the motor neurons of the ventral horn) has been referred to as the *windup phenomenon.*[21] In general, the windup phenomenon requires a minimum stimulus frequency of 0.5 Hz, arising from C fibers. Once the stimulus frequency reaches a critical threshold, the postsynaptic depolarizing responses of these second-order afferent neurons summate to produce bursts of action potential discharges instead of a single action potential. The windup phenomenon results in a persistence of action potentials for up to 60 seconds after the discontinuance of the stimulus, and results in a change in spinal cord processing that can last for 1 to 3 hours.[22] As this process repeats, more permanent changes in these second-order neurons occur and have been termed *long-term potentiation.*

The cellular mechanisms of spinal cord sensitization involve the relatively slow-onset and long-duration synaptic potentials elicited by A delta and C fibers in dorsal horn neurons.[16] These potentials persist up to 20 seconds (approximately 2,000 times longer than the fast potentials of A beta fibers). These slow potentials are mediated via release by the afferent axon of the excitatory neurotransmitter glutamate, and the neuropeptides substance P and neurokinin A[21,23] (see Fig. 55-3). As peripheral afferent nerve activity increases, progressively more and longer-lasting second-order neuron depolarizations occur because of the accumulation of these excitatory neurotransmitters and summation of these slow potentials. The net result is that a few seconds of C fiber activity can result in several minutes of postsynaptic depolarization.

Spinal cord synaptic plasticity involves the binding of glutamate to the N-methyl-D-aspartate (NMDA) receptor, as well as binding of substance P and neurokinins to tachykinin receptors.[21,24] High-frequency presynaptic activity causes release of glutamate and tachykinins from presynaptic vesicles. Binding of glutamate to NMDA receptors alters a magnesium-dependent block of ion channels, subsequently increasing cellular permeability to all cations, especially calcium and sodium. Glutamate also activates the α-amino-3 hydroxy-5-methyl-4-isoxazole propionic acid (AMPA) and metabotropic receptors on the postsynaptic cell. AMPA receptors control depolarization primarily through modulation of sodium influx into the cell. Neurokinins and substance P, through G protein-linked receptors, increase enzymatic activity, resulting in augmented depolarization and increases in stores of secondary neurotransmitters. Calcitonin gene-related peptide (CGRP) acting through CGRP receptors is involved in central sensitization and mechanical hyperalgesia, although the second-messenger systems have not been clearly identified.[25] Brain-derived neurotrophic factor is released by primary sensory neurons, and its activation of the TrkB receptor mediates postsynaptic excitability.[26,27] In aggregate, stimulation of these receptor groups enhances the excitability of the second-order neuron (see Fig. 55-3).

In addition to modulating augmented excitability, these transmitter and cellular mechanisms mediate changes in the postsynaptic cell, leading to more permanent changes in nerve conduction or long-term potentiation.[22] Extracellular calcium influx enhances release of intracellular calcium stores, initiating a series of intracellular events that include calcium-dependent enzymatic reactions mediated by protein kinase C, calcium-calmodulin, and cyclic adenosine monophosphate-dependent protein kinase A. These enzymes phosphorylate membrane proteins, namely, receptors and ion channels on the postsynaptic cell, which further increases excitability. AMPA receptor density increases on the postsynaptic cell membrane, and a retrograde factor is released that diffuses back to the presynaptic cell, augmenting neurotransmitter release in response to a given presynaptic action potential. Finally, changes in second messengers also activate immediate early gene products, transcription factors that can alter the expression of particular genes, which in turn can result in more persistent changes in neural processing.

Although much of the preceding discussion of altered spinal cord processing in response to nociceptive input has been derived from the study of chronic pain, similar changes in spinal cord processing occur even after a minor surgical incision.[28] These changes result in an increase in primary hyperalgesic response to noxious stimulus that persists for many days in the area of the incision and secondary hyperalgesia of shorter duration in surrounding tissues.[29]

Supraspinal Modulation

Brainstem. Descending inhibitory tracts at the brainstem level originate from cell bodies located in the region of the periaqueductal gray, reticular formation, and nucleus raphe magnus. These inhibitory tracts descend into the dorsolateral fasciculus and synapse in the dorsal horn. Neurotransmitters act presynaptically on the first-order neuron and postsynaptically on the second-order neuron of the spinothalamic tract or on the internuncial neuron pool. Internuncial neurons can be inhibitory and can regulate synaptic transmission between primary and secondary afferent neurons in the dorsal horn. At least two groups of nerve fibers have been identified as participants in this inhibitory modulation. One group of fibers involves the opioid system and contains the neurotransmitters beta-endorphin and the enkephalins, as well as other neuropeptides. Analgesia is produced during electrical stimulation of the periaqueductal gray, and this effect is blocked by naloxone.[30] These opioid projections from the nucleus raphe magnus and reticular formation interface presynaptically with the first-order afferent neurons. Neurotransmitters released from these projections hyperpolarize class A delta and C fibers, which serve to negate or shunt out the depolarizing current that approaches the terminal end plate, thereby diminishing the release of neurotransmitters such as substance P[31] (Fig. 55-4). In addition to this presynaptic modulation, exogenously applied opioids inhibit L-glutamate–evoked discharge of dorsal horn neurons, suggesting that opioids exert a direct postsynaptic effect.[32] In summary, opioids modulate transmission of afferent impulses in the dorsal horn presynaptically at the level of the first-order neuron. The enkephalinergic transmitter that is released from the descending inhibitory pathways hyperpolarizes the afferent terminals to block neurotransmitter release. Opioids also exert a direct inhibitory effect on the postsynaptic membrane potential (see Fig. 55-4).

In addition to the opioid descending inhibitory pathway, a monoamine pathway also originates from locations in the periaqueductal gray and reticular formation. Stimulation of these pathways inhibits synaptic transmission in the dorsal

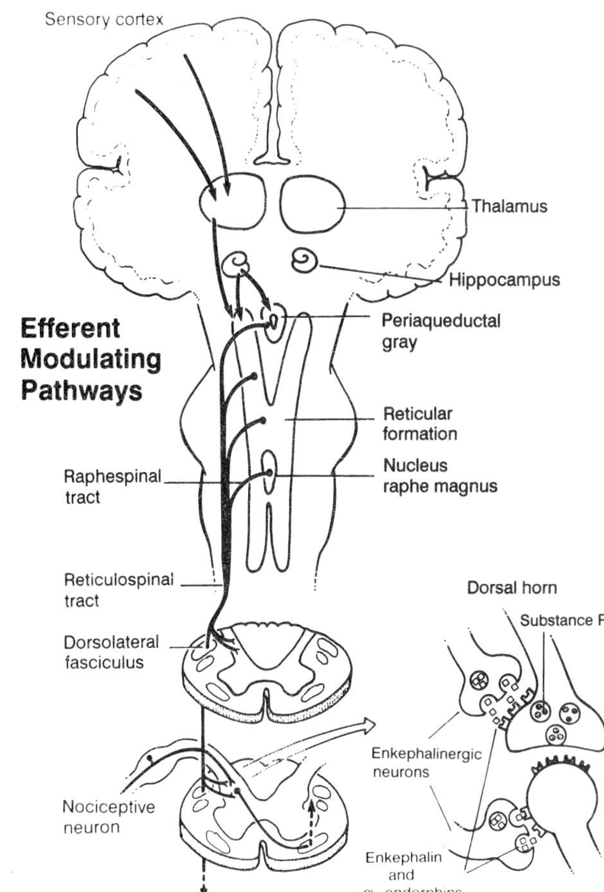

FIGURE 55-4. Efferent pathways involved in nociceptive regulation.

horn, similar to the inhibiton produced by the opioid system. Electrical stimulation of these pathways and intracerebral injections of α_2-adrenergic agonists can inhibit spinal nociceptive reflexes, and this effect can be antagonized by intrathecally administered α_2-adrenergic antagonists.[33] Further evidence of a monoamine pathway stems from the observation that the intrathecal administration of α_2-adrenergic agonists produces analgesia, implying that α_2 adrenoreceptors are responsible for this antinociceptive effect.[34] These fibers descend into the dorsolateral fasciculus, in a manner similar to that of the opioid fibers, and synapse in the substantia gelatinosa region of the dorsal horn. Norepinephrine is released from these nerve terminals and produces hyperpolarization of the first-order neurons, internuncial neurons, and wide dynamic-range neurons in the spinothalamic tract. In addition, there are α_2-adrenoreceptor projections into the ventral gray matter area of the motor nuclei.

The opioid and the α_2 receptors share a common mechanism of action. At the cellular level, these receptors belong to a family of receptors that are coupled to a G protein[35] (Fig. 55-5). The G protein exerts its membrane function through a secondary messenger protein capable of converting guanosine triphosphate to guanosine diphosphate. When the receptor is occupied, the α subunit of the G protein releases from the β and γ subunits and modulates cellular functions, such as ion exchange, adenyl cyclase, and phospholipase C activity. Hyperpolarization of the nerve results in decreased transmission of the action potential and decreased release of stored neurotransmitter. Hyperpolarization of the nerve most likely occurs because of the opening of potassium channels and the inhibition of calcium movement.[35,36]

Nociceptive nerve membrane without alpha-2 activation

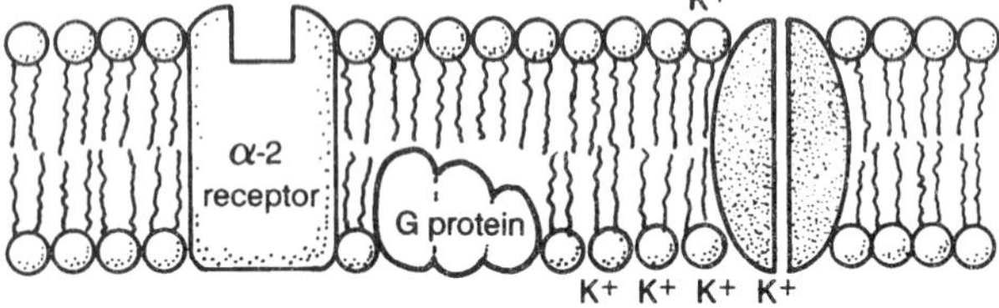

with alpha-2 activation

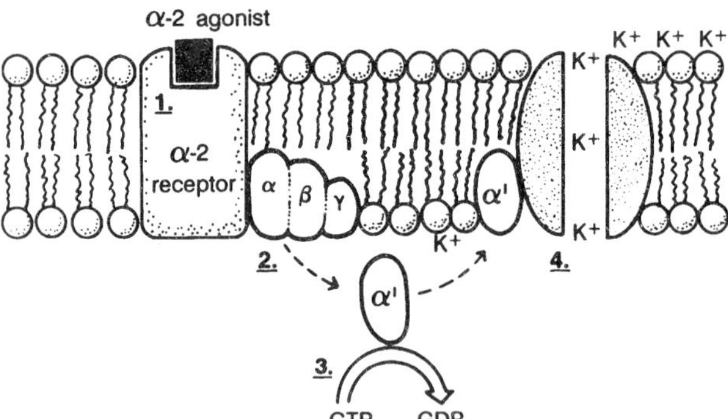

FIGURE 55-5. Schematic representation of cellular mechanisms of G-protein–linked receptor, depicted as an α_2-adrenergic receptor. Binding of agonist at receptor causes conformational change in G protein, allowing for cleavage of α subunit. Activation of α subunit occurs by hydrolysis of guanosine triphosphate (GTP) to active state α', which is capable of increasing K^+ movement and resulting in membrane hyperpolarization. GDP, guanosine diphosphate. (Adapted with permission from Maze M: Alpha-2 adrenoreceptor agonists: Defining the role in clinical anesthesia. Anesthesiology 74:581, 1991.)

Higher Central Nervous System. A basic review of the dimensions of perceptual psychology is required to understand the role of higher cortical function. Perception is the phenomenon by which noxious stimuli reach consciousness. Input from the cerebral cortex is necessary to provide interpretation and to give meaning to the stimuli. Perception can be subdivided into two categories: cognition and attention. Cognitive functions are those abilities that recognize, discriminate, memorize, or judge afferent information that stems from external stimuli. Therefore, cognitive modulation of pain involves the patient's ability to relate a painful experience to another event. For example, pain experienced in a pleasant environment elicits a less intense response than pain experienced in a setting of depression. The other area of perception is attention. Attention operates on the premise that only a fixed number of afferent stimuli can reach cortical centers. If a patient in pain concentrates on a separate and unrelated image, it is possible to reduce the effect of a painful sensation. The positive impact on pain from biofeedback or hypnosis operates on this principle.

PATHOPHYSIOLOGY OF PAIN

Components of the Surgical Stress Response

2 It has been well established that surgical patients receiving routine, intermittent, on-demand opioid analgesics remain in moderate to severe pain. Provision of effective postoperative analgesia is important not only for humanitarian reasons, but also because of the deleterious effects of postoperative pain on specific organ systems and the negative impact on postoperative recovery (Table 55-2).

Neuroendocrine

Surgical stress and pain elicit a consistent and well-defined metabolic response, involving release of neuroendocrine hormones and cytokines, which leads to a myriad of detrimental effects.[33] In addition to the rise in catabolically active hormones such as catecholamines, cortisol, angiotensin II, and antidiuretic hormone, stress causes an increase in adrenocorticotropic hormone, growth hormone, and glucagon.[38] The stress response results in lower levels of anabolic hormones, such as testosterone and insulin. Epinephrine, cortisol, and glucagon produce hyperglycemia by promoting insulin resistance and gluconeogenesis. They induce protein catabolism and lipolysis to provide substrates for gluconeogenesis. The stress response causes a negative postoperative nitrogen balance. Aldosterone, cortisol, and antidiuretic hormone influence water and electrolyte reabsorption by promoting Na^+ and water retention, while expending potassium. This contributes to increases in the extravascular fluid compartment both peripherally and within pulmonary parenchymal tissue. Local release of cytokines such as interleukin-2, interleukin-6, and tumor necrosis factor may contribute to abnormal physiologic responses such as alterations in heart rate, temperature, blood pressure, and ventilation.[39] Finally, catecholamines sensitize peripheral nociceptive endings, which serve to propagate more intense pain and may contribute to a vicious pain–catecholamine release–pain cycle.[40] The magnitude of these neuroendocrine and cytokine responses is related to the severity of tissue injury and correlates with outcome after injury.[41,42]

Cardiovascular

The cardiovascular effects of pain are initiated by the release of catecholamines from sympathetic nerve endings and the adrenal medulla, of aldosterone and cortisol from the adrenal cortex, and of antidiuretic hormone from the hypothalamus,

TABLE 55-2

ADVERSE PHYSIOLOGIC SEQUELAE OF PAIN

■ ORGAN SYSTEM	■ CLINICAL EFFECT
■ RESPIRATORY	
Increased skeletal muscle tension Decreased total lung compliance	Hypoxemia Hypercapnia Ventilation-perfusion abnormality Atelectasis Pneumonitis
■ ENDOCRINE	
Increased adrenocorticotropic hormone	Protein catabolism
Increased cortisol Increased glucagon Increased epinephrine	Lipolysis Hyperglycemia
Decreased insulin Decreased testosterone	Decreased protein anabolism
Increased aldosterone Increased antidiuretic hormone	Salt and water retention
Increased cortisol Increased catecholamines Increased angiotensin II	Congestive heart failure Vasoconstriction Increased myocardial contractility Increased heart rate
■ CARDIOVASCULAR	
Increased myocardial work (mediated by catecholamines, angiotensin II)	Dysrhythmias Angina Myocardial infarction Congestive heart failure
■ IMMUNOLOGIC	
Lymphopenia	Decreased immune function
Depression of reticuloendothelial system Leukocytosis Reduced killer T-cell cytotoxicity	
■ COAGULATION EFFECTS	
Increased platelet adhesiveness Diminished fibrinolysis Activation of coagulation cascade	Increased incidence of thromboembolic phenomena
■ GASTROINTESTINAL	
Increased sphincter tone Decreased smooth muscle tone	Ileus
■ GENITOURINARY	
Increased sphincter tone Decreased smooth muscle tone	Urinary retention

as well as by activation of the renin-angiotensin system. These hormones have direct effects on the myocardium and vasculature, and they augment salt and water retention, which places a greater burden on the cardiovascular system.

Angiotensin II causes generalized vasoconstriction, whereas catecholamines increase heart rate, myocardial contractility, and systemic vascular resistance. The sympathoadrenal release of catecholamines and the effects of angiotensin II may result in hypertension, tachycardia, and dysrhythmias and may lead to myocardial ischemia in susceptible patients as a consequence of increased oxygen demand. In addition, a significant proportion of perioperative myocardial ischemia is related to reductions in myocardial oxygen supply without hemodynamic aberrations. Activation of the sympathetic nervous system may trigger coronary vasoconstriction, which may result in myocardial ischemia in the presence of atherosclerotic coronary artery disease. This may occur through direct activation of cardiac sympathetic nerves,[43] as well as through circulating catecholamines that may contribute to hypercoagulability, a known mediator of adverse outcome in patients with ischemic heart disease. Salt and water retention secondary to aldosterone, cortisol, and antidiuretic hormone, in combination with the previously described effects of catecholamines and angiotensin II, can also precipitate congestive heart failure in patients with limited cardiac reserve.

Respiratory

Increases in extracellular lung water may contribute to ventilation-perfusion abnormalities. For surgical procedures performed on the thorax and abdomen, pain-induced reflex increases in skeletal muscle tension may lead to decreased total lung compliance, splinting, and hypoventilation. These changes promote atelectasis, contribute to further ventilation-perfusion abnormalities, and result in hypoxemia. In major surgical procedures or in high-risk patients, these respiratory effects of pain may lead to a significant reduction in functional residual capacity ranging from 25 to 50% of preoperative values.[44] Hypoxemia stimulates increases in minute ventilation. Although tachypnea and hypocapnia are common initially, prolonged increases in the work of breathing may result in hypercapnic respiratory failure. Pulmonary consolidation and pneumonitis may occur because of hypoventilation and further aggravate the clinical scenario. These sequelae are especially significant in patients with preexisting pulmonary disease, upper abdominal and thoracic incisions,[45] advanced age, or obesity.[44]

Gastrointestinal

Pain-induced sympathetic hyperactivity may cause reflex inhibition of gastrointestinal function.[46] This promotes postoperative ileus, which contributes to postoperative nausea, vomiting, and discomfort, and delays resumption of an enteral diet. Failure to resume early enteral feeding may be associated with postoperative morbidity, including septic complications and abnormal wound healing.[47]

Genitourinary

An increase in sympathetic activity responses to pain causes reflex inhibition of most visceral smooth muscle, including urinary bladder tone. This can result in urinary retention with subsequent urinary tract infections and related complications.

Immunologic

The pain-related stress response suppresses both cellular and humoral immune function[48,49] and results in lymphopenia, leukocytosis, and depression of the reticuloendothelial system. In addition, some anesthetic agents reduce chemotaxis of neutrophils and may be one factor involved in the reduction of monocyte activity. Many known mediators of the stress response are potent immunosuppressants, and both cortisol and epinephrine infusions decrease neutrophil chemotaxis.[50] These effects can lower resistance to pathogens and may be key factors in the development of perioperative infectious complications.[51] When surgical manipulation of neoplasms causes release of tumor cells, the postoperative stress response may reduce the cytotoxicity of killer T cells. Increases in catecholamines, glucocorticoids, and prostaglandins in response to stress may impair immunologic responses important for patients with neoplasms.[52]

Coagulation

Stress-related alterations in blood viscosity, platelet function, fibrinolysis, and coagulation pathways have been described.[53–56] These stress-mediated effects include increased platelet adhesiveness, diminished fibrinolysis, and promotion of a hypercoagulable state. When these effects are coupled with the microcirculatory effects of catecholamines and immobilization of the patient in the postoperative period, thromboembolic events are more likely to occur.

General Well-Being

Pain increases skeletal muscle tone in the area of the surgical field. This postoperative impairment of muscle function may lead to physical immobility and a delayed return to normal function. Poorly controlled pain also contributes to insomnia, anxiety, and a feeling of helplessness. These psychological factors, coupled with the immobilization that occurs because of the increased skeletal muscle tone, create a postoperative scenario feared by many patients.

Attenuation of Central Sensitization and the Stress Response

As discussed earlier, acute tissue injury results in peripheral and central neural sensitization. It is also evident that acute nociceptive stimulation can result in neuroplastic responses that compound the intensity of pain perception in concert with other deleterious systemic effects, including those modulated as part of the stress response. Because most of these events are not manifest until after surgery, most efforts to attenuate the cascade of events precipitated by intraoperative trauma have focused on the postoperative period. These efforts are well founded because of the need to interrupt and limit central sensitization propagated by ongoing tissue injury. However, perioperative anesthetic and analgesic strategies must also consider the temporal relation of nociceptive stimulation to the initiation of central sensitization. The ideal perioperative intervention should focus on preventive, rather than primarily therapeutic measures to control the adverse sequelae of central sensitization and the stress response. Our current understanding of the pathophysiologic consequences of tissue injury has therefore prompted the application of preoperative and intraoperative techniques that prevent or minimize this postinjury hypersensitivity, and has fostered the concept of preemptive analgesia.

The relative importance of preemptive analgesia in preventing adverse sequelae depends on several factors, including preoperative patient status, as well as the magnitude and site of the surgical intervention. It is widely believed that preemptive analgesia has a greater impact in patients with impaired physiologic reserve than in healthier patients who can better tolerate the perturbations induced by surgery. Minor, peripheral surgical procedures performed with the use of local anesthesia usually produce minimal systemic or central neuraxial changes. The more extensive the surgical procedure, the greater the magnitude of the neuroendocrine stress response. Procedures associated with greater degrees of surgical trauma may also contribute to greater central sensitization than less invasive procedures.

From the previous discussion, it is apparent that postoperative physiologic changes are not homeostatic mechanisms but are reproducible adverse responses to tissue injury that result in a myriad of adverse physiologic events that likely modulate perioperative outcome. Research efforts have therefore been focused on the effectiveness of various anesthetic and analgesic strategies targeted to modify the adverse neural and systemic derangements commonly observed after surgery.

Influence of Anesthesia on the Surgical Stress Response and Outcome

General Anesthesia

It has been demonstrated that general anesthesia, either with intravenous or inhalational anesthetics, does not effectively attenuate the neuroendocrine stress response.[57] One exception to this assertion is the administration of high-dose opioid anesthesia. Extremely high doses of certain opioids can inhibit some aspects of the stress response, but lower doses of opioids usually are unable to hinder the neuroendocrine effects of stress.[58,59] The effect of opioids on immune function is controversial because both immune-suppressing and immune-enhancing effects have been described.[60] High doses of inhalational agents (1.5 times minimum alveolar concentration) may suppress the intraoperative catecholamine response but do not diminish the catecholamine response that develops after surgery.

Regional Anesthesia and Analgesia

Mitigation of nociception at the peripheral and central level may be accomplished through a variety of techniques. A regional anesthetic or analgesic modality is ideally suited to produce this desired effect because it diminishes the intensity of afferent impulses reaching the spinal cord. Regional anesthesia and analgesia have been shown to reduce catecholamine and other stress hormone responses during the perioperative period for certain surgical procedures.[38,55,61] The finding that regional anesthesia and analgesia can ablate the neuroendocrine stress responses is not universal. Some studies have demonstrated that central neuraxial techniques have no significant influence on cortisol release. The differing results may be related to the level of the afferent neural blockade. Another confounding variable is the region of the body where the surgical procedure was performed. In studies where regional anesthesia did not have an influence on the cortisol response, surgery was performed in the upper abdomen, whereas in most studies that demonstrate inhibition, surgery was performed on a lower extremity or the lower abdomen. Sensory blocks below L1 usually have no effect on cortisol response. To prevent a cortisol response to surgery, all afferent pathways from the surgical site must be blocked.[62]

Besides reducing the neuroendocrine stress response, regional anesthesia can reduce myocardial work and oxygen consumption by reducing heart rate, arterial pressure, and left ventricular contractility. Left ventricular ejection fraction is not significantly affected by epidural anesthesia in normal patients, whereas patients with chronic stable angina experience a modest but significant improvement in left ventricular ejection fraction and left ventricular wall motion, provided that volume loading is limited.[63] In patients with unstable angina that is refractory to treatment with nitrates, beta-blockers, and Ca^{2+} antagonists, thoracic epidural analgesia alleviates chest pain without changing coronary perfusion pressure, cardiac output, or systemic vascular resistance.[64] Studies evaluating regional myocardial blood flow distribution in intact animals indicate that epidurally administered local anesthetics can improve endocardial-to-epicardial blood flow ratios, shifting blood flow to the area of myocardium at greatest risk of ischemia and infarction.[65] A reduction in infarct size in experimental models of acute coronary occlusion has also been demonstrated.[65]

Administration of epidural local anesthetics or opioids in the postoperative period can reduce the incidence of myocardial ischemia and dysrhythmias compared with systemic opioids.[66,67] Beneficial effects of epidural anesthesia and analgesia on cardiac outcomes have been demonstrated only in high-risk populations undergoing major operations, perhaps because such patients experience a high incidence of complications which may show allowing differences to be detected in relatively small samples. Epidural anesthesia and analgesia was associated with both statistically and clinically significant reductions in serious cardiovascular morbidity when compared with general anesthesia with on-demand opioid analgesia alone in a population of patients undergoing major intrathoracic, intra-abdominal, or vascular surgery,[68] as well as in a series of patients undergoing major peripheral vascular surgery (approximately 45% of operations involving the abdominal aorta).[53] Another study in abdominal aortic reconstructive surgery comparing general anesthesia with combined epidural anesthesia and general anesthesia found no differences in cardiovascular or other outcomes, although postoperative analgesia techniques were not controlled or randomized.[69] In aggregate, these findings are consistent with the hypothesis that outcome improvement requires that intraoperative initiation of central neuraxial blockade be accompanied by postoperative continuation of this modality. Other studies investigating lower-risk patient populations,[70] or less invasive surgical procedures (infrainguinal revascularizations)[71] with a lesser magnitude of surgical insult, had lower incidences of cardiac morbidity and could not demonstrate significant effects on cardiac morbidity, despite other beneficial effects of epidural anesthesia and analgesia. Therefore, the benefits of epidural analgesia on cardiac morbidity remain controversial, and formation of definitive conclusions has been hindered by the absence of studies with sufficient numbers of patients and the multifactorial causation of cardiac morbidity, which mandates a tightly controlled study design. Most studies with negative results have not consistently continued the intraoperative epidural technique for postoperative analgesia.

3 The beneficial effects of epidural anesthesia and analgesia on some aspects of cardiovascular outcome may be intimately related to modulation of the hypercoagulable state that occurs and persists after major surgical trauma, especially in patients with atherosclerotic vascular disease and others with a predisposition to hypercoagulability.[72] General anesthesia with parenteral opioid analgesia has little effect on postoperative hypercoagulability.[53,54,71,73] Epidural anesthesia using local anesthetics with or without opioids enhances fibrinolytic activity,[54,74] hastens the return of antithrombin III from elevated to normal levels, and attenuates postoperative increases in platelet activity. These effects probably occur through multiple mechanisms, including block of sympathetic efferent nerves, reduced levels of circulating catecholamines, and anticoagulant properties of even low levels of systemically absorbed local anesthetics. These reductions in postoperative hypercoagulability appear to reduce the incidence of thromboses of vascular grafts in patients undergoing lower-extremity revascularization,[53,71] and also reduce the incidence of deep venous thromboses and risk of pulmonary thromboembolism in patients undergoing total hip replacements. The reduced incidence of thrombotic phenomena in these settings may be related to an inhibitory effect on platelet aggregation and to improvements in lower limb blood flow.[75] Similar reductions in thromboembolic complications have been reported with the use of epidural anesthesia and analgesia (with local anesthetics) after other procedures, including knee arthroplasty[76] and open prostatectomy.[77] The differences in coagulability associated with epidural anesthesia and analgesia have been observed only in patients inherently at high risk for vaso-occlusive events.

Epidural analgesia is associated with improved pulmonary function after surgery compared with intramuscular and intravenous opioid.[44,78–81] Diaphragmatic function is commonly impaired after abdominal or thoracic surgery, probably as a result of reflex inhibition of phrenic nerve activity.[82,83] Although analgesia provided by parenterally or epidurally administered opioids alone does not significantly improve this dysfunction,[84] thoracic epidural analgesia with local anesthetic may improve postoperative diaphragmatic function by neural blockade of the inhibitory reflex[82,83] and by changing chest wall compliance.

Although epidural and parenteral opioids are associated with similar frequencies of episodic postoperative hypoxemia,[85] epidural analgesia with local anesthetics reduces the frequency and severity of early postoperative hypoxemia. It is likely that reductions in the work of breathing and other beneficial effects of improved analgesia, such as enhanced ability to cough and facilitation of chest physiotherapy, also play an important role in preventing postoperative respiratory complications. The former effects may be related to improved analgesia during activity, particularly when epidural local anesthetics and opioid are combined.[86]

Several studies have demonstrated reductions in the incidence of postoperative pneumonia and respiratory failure in high-risk patients undergoing thoracic or abdominal operations.[44,53] Similar differences in pulmonary morbidity between parenteral postoperative opioids and epidural analgesia have not been observed in healthy patients undergoing low-risk operations or when postoperative analgesia was not managed using well-defined protocols.[63,87–89]

In summary, epidural anesthesia and analgesia can reduce the frequency and severity of postsurgical stress-induced physiologic perturbations. The effect of epidural anesthesia and postoperative analgesia on mediators of the stress response appears to have the greatest impact on perioperative outcome in patients at high risk of complications. The relative importance of preemptive intraoperative initiation compared with postoperative application of epidural local anesthetics (versus opioid alone or in combination), as well as the cost effectiveness of these analgesic techniques compared with other modalities for management of postoperative pain, depends on the patient's preoperative status and the specific operative procedure.

PHARMACOLOGY OF POSTOPERATIVE PAIN MANAGEMENT

Drugs administered orally, parenterally, transdermally, transmucosally, and transnasally for postoperative pain management may be grouped by their mechanism of effect as nonopioid or opioid analgesics and adjuvant pharmacotherapeutic agents.

Nonopioid Analgesics

NSAIDs, COX-1 and COX-2 Inhibitors, and Acetaminophen

Aspirin (ASA), acetaminophen (APAP), the NSAIDs, and the selective COX-2 inhibitors ("coxibs") are the principal nonopioid analgesics used to treat minor or moderate acute postoperative pain (Table 55-3). Although these compounds represent diverse chemical entities, their common mechanism of action is inhibition of prostaglandin-mediated amplification of chemical and mechanical irritants on the sensory pathways peripherally and centrally. Although sensitization or intensification of painful stimuli is mediated by the prostaglandins and lowers the threshold for further activation of the nociceptors, the prostaglandins directly evoke little painful response.

TABLE 55-3

PHARMACOKINETIC PARAMETERS AND MAXIMUM DOSAGE RECOMMENDATIONS OF NONNARCOTIC ANALGESICS

	ROUTE	TIME TO PEAK LEVELS (hr)	HALF-LIFE (hr)	ANALGESIC ACTIONS (hr)		MAXIMUM RECOMMENDED DAILY DOSE (mg)
				ONSET	DURATION	
SALICYLATES						
Aspirin/sodium salicylate	PO	0.5–2	2–3[a]	0.5–1	2–4	3,600
Diflunisal	PO	2–3	8–12	1–2	8–12	2,000
PROPIONIC ACIDS						
Fenoprofen	PO	1–2	2–3	1	4–6	3,200
Flurbiprofen	PO	1.5	5.7	—	4–6	300
Ibuprofen	PO	1–2	1.8–2.5	0.5	4–6	3,200
Ketoprofen	PO	0.5–2	2.4	—	4–7	300
Naproxen	PO	2–4	12–15	1	4–7	1,500
Naproxen sodium	PO	1–2	12–13	1		1,375
ACETIC ACIDS						
Etodolac	PO	1–2	7.3	0.5	4–12	200
Indomethacin	PO	1–2	4.5	0.5	4–6	200
Indomethacin sustained release	PO	2–4	4.5–6	0.5	4–6	150
Ketorolac	IM/PO	1	2.4–6[g]	0.5–1	4–6	120[h]
Nabumetone	PO	2.4–4	5–9[d]	1	4–12	40[i]
Sulindac	PO	2–4	22.5–30[e]	—	—	2,000
Tolmetin	PO	0.5–1	7.8	—	—	400
			(16.4)[e]			2,000
			1–1.5			
FENAMATES (ANTHRANILIC ACIDS)						
Meclofenamate	PO	0.5–1	2 (3.3)[b]	0.5–1	4–6	400
Mefenamic acid	PO	2–4	2–4	1	4–6	1,000
OXICAMS						
Piroxicam	PO	3–5	30–86	1	48–72	20
Meloxicam	PO	5–14	15–20	—	24	15
PHENYLACETIC ACIDS						
Diclofenac sodium	PO	2–3	2	1	1.6	200
p-AMINOPHENOLS						
Acetaminophen	PO	0.5–1	1.4	0.5	2–4	1,200
Phenacetin[f]	PO	1				2,400
		1–2[c]				

[a] Half-life of aspirin dose dependent.
[b] Half-life with multiple dosing.
[c] Time to peak acetaminophen levels.
[d] Half-life in renal failure.
[e] Half-life of active metabolite.
[f] 75–80% of phenacetin converted to acetaminophen.
[g] Half-life in healthy adults.
[h] Daily recommended dose for first day of therapy is 150 mg.
[i] Daily recommended dose for oral dosing.

Two phases of nociceptor sensitization are mediated with the release of potassium, prostaglandin, bradykinins, and substance P from tissues surgically damaged. These substances excite nociceptors and increase their pain sensitivity-hyperalgesia. Substance P, released by axon reflex, induces vasodilation and mast-cell degranulation, leading to histamine and serotonin release. These inflammatory agents sensitize damaged surgical tissue and surrounding nociceptors, further prolonging the hypersensitivity state (secondary hyperalgesia).

Aspirin and Other Nonsteroidal Drugs

Most of these agents modulate prostaglandin synthesis through inhibition of the action of the enzyme prostaglandin endoperoxide synthase (COX-2), which is one of the first steps in the conversion of arachidonic acid into the prostaglandins, thromboxanes, and prostacyclin. By reducing prostaglandin synthesis from tissue damage during surgery, cyclooxygenase inhibitors block the nociceptive response to endogenous mediators of inflammation such as prostaglandins, bradykinin, substance P, potassium, acetylcholine, and serotonin. Such mediators augment nociception and painful sensations up the spinal cord to the brain and pain sensitivity at the surgical site. Although the exact mechanism for the participation of endogenous substances such as prostaglandins in the generation and transduction of nociceptive stimuli is unknown, the effect is greatest in tissues that have been subjected to trauma and inflammation.[90] The prostaglandins represent a diverse group of compounds that mediate many cellular and subcellular functions. The order of the sensitizing or hyperalgesic effect that is usually observed with this group is $PGE_1 > PGE_2 > PGF_{2a}$, whereas PGA_1, PGB_2, and PGI_2 exhibit little sensitizing effect.

Although mediation of the peripheral inflammatory response is an important component of pain, modulation by this group of drugs and inhibition of central mechanisms of hyperalgesia is likely.[91,92] Acetaminophen, ketorolac, and rofecoxib are cyclooxygenase inhibitors that are equipotent to aspirin in inhibiting prostaglandin synthesis in the central nervous system but vastly differ in inhibiting prostaglandin synthesis at peripheral sites. The site of activity of these agents reflects pharmacokinetic factors such as drug distribution, but more important, it reflects differences in the cyclooxygenase enzyme systems throughout the body. Studies in mammalian cells indicate that COX exists as three unique isoenzymes. The most recognized are PGH synthase-1 (COX-1) and PGH synthase-2 (COX-2).[93] Major differences between these isoenzymes involve dissimilar regulation and expression, with COX-1 (PGHS-1) constitutive regulation found in most tissues, especially platelets, stomach, vascular endothelial cells, and renal collecting tubules. Unlike COX-1, under basal conditions COX-2 has inducible regulation and is usually undetectable in most tissues except prostate, central nervous system (CNS), activated macrophages, fibroblasts, synoviocytes, and renal cortex, with expression capability in many tissues by stimulation or induction.[94] The COX-1 isoform primarily produces prostaglandins that regulate renal, gastric, and vascular homeostasis. In the presence of inflammation or tissue injury, inflammatory cytokines induce the expression of the COX-2 enzyme, which generates the prostaglandins involved in pain. Both isoforms of the enzyme are membrane associated and have a long, narrow channel into which arachidonic acid is drawn for conversion to a prostaglandin. NSAIDs block the channel at approximately its midpoint. Although the enzymes are not selective for substrate, a valine amino acid substitution (for isoleucine) in the COX-2 isoform allows for the synthesis of isoform-specific inhibitors. The smaller valine amino acid exposes an area in the channel into which larger side-chain substitutions of the enzyme inhibitor can engage. Because of these bulkier side groups, these same drugs have much less COX-1 activity, resulting in analgesic/anti-inflammatory properties with diminished effects on platelet, gastric mucosal, and renal functions.[95]

Because not all NSAIDs block COX to the same degree, membrane stabilization has also been attributed to these drugs.[96] Membrane stabilization may account for decreased prostaglandin release seen at drug concentrations that are lower than those needed for effective COX inhibition. This theory is supported by the correlation of analgesic potency with the octanol/water partition coefficient in this group.[97] Corticosteroids, which are membrane stabilizers, are known selectively to inhibit the expression of COX-2 during inflammation. NSAIDs, tricyclic antidepressants, and local anesthetics may also function through this mechanism of action, which explains some of their beneficial effects when they are used for acute pain management. Prostaglandin synthesis is known to be catalyzed by not less than 2-cyclooxygenase forms that convert arachidonic acid to multiple prostaglandins. Eiconside synthesis is initiated with arachidonate release from membrane phospholipids by the activity of phospholipase A2 (PLA_2).

Acetaminophen (Paracetamol-APAP)

APAP provides analgesic and antipyretic benefits but in overdose is associated with potentially fatal hepatic necrosis. Analgesic mechanisms of APAP are in part a function of COX-3 inhibition. In certain patients (chronic ethanol users, malnutrition, fasting patients), repeating therapeutic or slightly excessive doses may precipitate hepatotoxicity. A dose of 2,600 to 3,200 mg per day may represent a safer chronic daily dose in the authors' experience. Toxic doses may be a function of baseline glutathione levels and other dose-related factors. APAP is completely and rapidly absorbed following the oral route. Peak serum concentrations are achieved within 2 hours of a therapeutic dose, and therapeutic serum concentrations are 10 to 20 mcg/mL. The $t^1/_2\beta$ (half-life) is 2 to 4 hours when used for acute postoperative pain. About 90% of APAP is hepatically metabolized to sulfate and glucuronide conjugates for renal excretion with a small amount secreted unchanged in the urine. An important minor pathway is phase one metabolism by cytochrome P450 (CYP450, 2E1, 1A2, 3A5). The fraction metabolized by CYP450 produces a reactive intermediate metabolite, N-acetyl-p-benzoquinoneimine (NAPQI), which arylates, binding covalently with hepatocytes, producing oxidative hepatocellular necrotic injury. This CYP450 pathway is engaged during toxicity when NAPQI accumulates, producing hepatic insult. Consumption of three or more alcoholic drinks daily may increase risk of hepatic damage with acetaminophen.

Clinical Uses

Unlike the opioid analgesics, the mechanism of analgesia of the nonopioid analgesics do not specifically involve interrupting the transmission of the nociceptive stimulus. The effectiveness of these agents depends on their ability to modulate the prostaglandin-dependent central and peripheral inflammatory responses to surgical or traumatic tissue injury. They have little or no inhibitory effect on classic catabolic stress hormones, acute-phase proteins, and other immunologic responses.[60] Nonetheless, incorporation of theses drugs into a polymodal, polypharmacotherapeutic pain treatment plan is clinically beneficial. The reduction in prostaglandin-mediated inflammatory response can serve to enhance analgesia when these agents are combined with opioids. Based on their pharmacologic mechanisms, it is predictable that the analgesic effect of nonopioid analgesic drugs are within narrow therapeutic ranges, above which there is little enhancement of analgesia but an increase in end-organ toxicity. Doses of APAP exceeding 3,200 mg chronically may be associated with hepatic toxicity, especially in elderly alcohol users or fasting patients due to glutathione depletion. To reduce the postoperative amplification of the nociceptive response to tissue injury, the most efficacious use of these agents would be presurgical or perisurgical. This is because the effect of COX-2 can last for many hours, and the sensitizing effects of circulating prostaglandins are not completely reversed by COX inhibitors. Unlike the COX-1 agents that affect platelets, the COX-2 agents have no platelet effects, do not increase surgical bleeding and do not have to be discontinued prior to surgery. These agents also appear to be more effective in procedures involving musculoskeletal, post-traumatic, and inflammatory pain, and in conditions such as dysmenorrhea, migraine headache, renal colic, and biliary obstruction, in which prostaglandins are known to be involved in the pathogenesis of the pain. The COX-2 agents additionally have a postoperative opioid-sparing effect. Perioperative administration of a COX-2 inhibitor is an integral component in polymodal analgesic treatment plans. This approach has been shown to improve range of motion after total knee replacement and diminish opioid utilization, pain, and opioid-induced iatrogenic effects such as emesis and insomnia.[98] The COX-2 and COX-1 agents have a dose ceiling effect beyond which there are no

TABLE 55-4

PHARMACOKINETIC PROPERTIES OF COX-2 INHIBITORS

■ PHARMACOLOGIC AGENT	■ CELECOXIB	■ ETORICOXIB	■ VALDECOXIB[a]
Bioavailability (F)	22–40%	100%	83%
Tmax (hr)—time to max concentration	−2.8	~1 hr	3
Cmax (μg/mL)—max serum conc	0.7 (>65 yr, 40% higher)	3.6	—
AUC (μg/hr per mL)—under the plasma conc time curve	6.3 (40% ↑ in African Americans and 50% ↑ in patients ≥65 yr)	37.8	≥65 yr 30% ↑ versus young (plasma concentration 130% ↑ moderate hepatic dysfunction)
(Vd) L/kg	400	120	86
(PPB) %	−97	92	98
(Css) days	≥5	7	4
CYP450 substrate metabolism	2C9	3A4, major; minor 1A2, 2C9/19, 2D6	3A4, 2C9
Inhibition of CYP450	2D6	None	3A4, 2C9, 2C19
Metabolism	Oxidation	Hepatic oxidation	Oxidation (active metabolite 10%)
Elimination of urine (%)	27	70	70
Elimination of feces (%)	57	20	Hepatic (primary)
Kinetics	Linear	Linear	Nonlinear
Sulfonamide allergy	Yes	None	Possible
Chemistry	Sulfonamide	Nonsulfonamide	Sulfonamide
Half-life ($t^1/_2$)	11.2 (fasting) hr	≈22 hr	8–11 hr

[a] Withdrawn from the market.

therapeutic benefits. A pharmacokinetic comparison of the COX-2 agents is provided in Table 55-4.

The FDA asked manufactures of prescription and OTC NAIDs (COX1/COX2) to revise labeling to include a boxed warning and patient medication guide with more specific information about cardiovascular and gastrointestinal bleeding risks.

Opioid Analgesics

Mechanism of Analgesic Effects

4 Morphine and related compounds act as agonists, producing their biologic effects by interacting with stereoselective and saturable membrane-bound receptors that are nonuniformly distributed throughout the CNS. The major sites of opioid activity in the CNS include the periaqueductal and periventricular gray, nucleus reticularis gigantocellularis, medial thalamus, mesencephalic reticular formation, lateral hypothalamus, raphe nuclei, and spinal cord. The endogenous neuromodulating peptides of the enkephalin and beta-endorphin classes also bind to this family of receptors, which are collectively referred to as the *opioid receptors*. The unique properties of the individual drugs of this group are a result of their specific receptor activity and affinity. Three well-characterized classes of opioid receptors have been identified (μ, μ_1, μ_2; κ; δ). Human peripheral nerves contain endogenic opioid ligands and opioid receptors. A peripheral effect of opioids that results in "local analgesia" is more pronounced in chronically inflamed tissues,[99,100] where opioid receptors that are synthesized in the dorsal root ganglia have been transported and activated on primary afferent neurons in response to inflammation.[101] The local analgesic effects of opioids such as morphine have been clinically useful after surgery. Application of morphine at the nerve terminal (e.g., intra-articular injections after orthopaedic procedures) often produces effective, long-lasting analgesia of similar potency to conventional local anesthetics.[102–107] Peripherally acting μ-receptor agonists that do not cross the blood-brain barrier are being investigated.[108]

Affinity and activity at all three of the opioid receptor classes (μ, δ, κ) are responsible for the organ specific pharmacologic effects of the opiates (Table 55-5). The enkephalins and opiates have affinity and activity at the μ_1 receptor, which mediates supraspinal analgesia, prolactin release, and euphoria. Opiate-selective μ_2 receptors appear to mediate respiratory depression and physical dependence. The δ and κ receptors are at least partially responsible for spinal analgesia. Miosis and sedation are a result of κ-receptor activity. Pure opioid agonists (Table 55-6) have affinity, and exhibit at least moderate activity at the μ_1, μ, δ, and κ receptors, which explains their central and spinal analgesic effect, as well as their dose-related side effects and addictive potential. The differences in potency and side effects among drugs in this class are a result of receptor selectivity, affinity, and lipophilicity of the drug.

Tramadol, a synthetic cyclohexanol, 4-phenyl-piperidine chiral racemate analog of codeine, is a centrally acting analgesic that possesses weak affinity for the μ opioid receptor (L-isomer) and modifies transmission of nociceptive impulses through inhibition of monoamine (norepinephrine and serotonin) reuptake (D-isomer), but not production. Receptor-blocking studies have demonstrated that these mechanisms work synergistically to produce the therapeutic analgesic effects of tramadol.[109–111] Tramadol is approximately one-tenth as potent an analgesic as morphine in treating moderately severe pain. At similar analgesic doses, tramadol has less effect on the respiratory center than morphine and has not been associated with a high abuse potential.[112] Analgesic effects are comparable to codeine, hydrocodone, oxycodone, and propoxyphene.

The pharmacologic properties of the mixed agonist–antagonist analgesics are also a result of their affinity for the opioid receptors. Unlike pure agonists, however, not all these agents produce an agonist effect when they interact with the receptor. There are two distinct groupings of the agonist–antagonist drugs based on their receptor affinity and activity. The first of these groups is characterized by high μ receptor affinity with activity less than or similar to that of morphine.

TABLE 55-5

PHARMACOLOGY OF OPIOID RECEPTORS

	μ				
	μ1	μ2	δ	κ	σ
EFFECT					
Analgesia	Supraspinal	Sedation	Spinal	Spinal	Dysphoria, hallucinations
Affect	Euphoria	Depression	Depression		
Pupil	Miosis	Constipation	Nausea/vomiting		
Respiratory	Nausea/vomiting		Urinary retention	Sedation	Mydriasis
Gastrointestinal	Urinary retention		Pruritus	Miosis	Tachypnea
Genitourinary	Increase		Yes	Diuresis	
Temperature	Pruritus		μ	Little	
Other	Yes			No	
Physical	δ				
Dependence/tolerance					
Cross-tolerance					

BINDING PROPERTIES	Affinity	Activity	Affinity	Activity	Affinity	Activity	Affinity	Activity
Agonists	+++	+++	++	++				
Morphine	++	++	++	++			+++	+++
Meperidine	++++	++++	+	+	+	+	++	+
Fentanyl	++	0	++	+	+	+	++	++
Agonist-antagonists	++	0			+++	+++		
Pentazocine	++	0			+++	+++		
Nalbuphine	+++	+			+++	++		
Butorphanol	+++	+			++			
Buprenorphine					+	+		
Dezocine								

Affinity: ++++, very high; +++, high; ++, moderate; +, low activity; 0, no activity; +, low activity; ++, moderate activity; +++, high activity; ++++, very high activity.
Adapted from Benedetti C, Butler SH: Systemic analgesics. In Bonica JJ (ed): The Management of Pain, vol II, 2nd ed, p 1640. LEA and Febiger, 1990.

Agents in this partial agonist category (see Table 55-5) include buprenorphine. The second group of agonist–antagonist analgesics includes pentazocine, butorphanol, and nalbuphine. This group possesses only moderate affinity without activity at the μ receptor, high affinity with at least moderate activity at the κ receptor, and at least moderate affinity and some activity at the σ receptor, which accounts for the highly sedative effects and potential for psychomimetic reactions seen with these drugs. In addition, because of the affinity of both of these classes for the μ receptor, with activity less than that of the pure agonists, the mixed agonist–antagonist drugs have the potential for reversing the effect of an agonist, including precipitation of withdrawal symptoms.

Absorption/Biotransformation/Elimination

Although opioid analgesics are well absorbed from the gastrointestinal tract, differences in analgesic equivalence between oral and parenteral doses result from significant first-pass metabolism by the gut, liver, and lungs (fentanyl). Codeine, oxycodone, and hydrocodone do not undergo extensive first-pass hepatic metabolism owing to the methoxy-substitution of the phenolic component of the phenanthrene ring. These drugs are cytochrome CYP450 2D6 substrates, and they have greater oral-to-parenteral equivalency than morphine. Parenteral administration results in a more rapid onset of effect compared with oral and rectal administration. Fentanyl has a greater lipophilicity than morphine, and consequently, rapidly redistributes to highly perfused tissue (rather than to adipose tissue) and skeletal muscle. Extensive pulmonary first-pass uptake accounts for about 75% of the fentanyl dose absorption. These factors account for the longer duration of action, despite a relatively short elimination half-life ($t^1/_2\beta$). Following redistribution, the slow release into plasma is culminated by CYP450 3A4 hepatic metabolism. Distribution depends on the lipophilicity of the drug; smaller amounts of the more hydrophobic morphine equilibrate in the brain as opposed to more lipophilic agents, such as methadone, meperidine, and codeine. Biotransformation followed by renal elimination of conjugated metabolites is the primary mode of elimination. Active metabolites of morphine (morphine-6-glucuronide, M-3 glucuronide), codeine (morphine), meperidine (normeperidine), hydrocodone (hydromorphone), oxycodone (oxymorphone), and propoxyphene (norpropoxyphene) also contribute to the primary pharmacologic effect. Some of these metabolites (normeperidine, norpropoxyphene) also produce organ-specific toxicity. Morphine is metabolized by phase II glucuronidation yielding both M-3-G (up to 85%) and M-6-G (up to 10%). The active metabolite M-6 glucuronide accumulates with renal compromise (Clcr $\leq$ 30 mL/min) and necessitates cautious utilization of morphine in such patients.

Metabolism of tramadol by CYP450 2D6, including production of its primary metabolite O-dimethyl tramadol and its conjugates, is influenced by debrisoquine polymorphism.[113] This metabolite has a greater affinity for opioid receptors than the parent drug; however, the elimination half-life of this metabolite is not significantly greater than that of tramadol itself.[114] Methadone, a diphenylhetane, is a chiral compound and the S (+) enantiomer is either inactive or less active (weak) at opioid at receptors; however, it is also an NMDA receptor antagonist that blocks morphine tolerance development. The d-isomer and l-isomer of methadone bind to noncompetitive

TABLE 55-6

PHARMACOKINETIC PARAMETERS AND DOSAGE RECOMMENDATIONS OF ORAL AND PARENTERAL OPIOID ANALGESICS

	DOSAGE		HALF-LIFE (hr)	ANALGESIC ACTION (hr)			EQUIVALENCY RATIO
	ROUTE	mg		ONSET	PEAK	DURATION	
AGONISTS							
NATURALLY OCCURRING ALKALOIDS							
Morphine	IV	2.5–15	2–3.5	0.3	0.125	3–4	1
	IM	10–15	3	0.5–1	0.5–1.5	4	6
	PO	30–60		0.25–5	1–2	4–6	12
Codeine	IM	15–60		0.25–1	1–5	3–4	20
	PO	15–60			0.5–2		
PARTIALLY SYNTHETIC DERIVATIVES OF MORPHINE							
Hydromorphone	IM	1–4	2–3	0.3–5	1	2–3	0.2
	PO	1–4	2–3	0.5–1	1	3–4	0.6
Oxymorphone	IM	1–1.5	3.3–4.5	0.5	1	2–4	0.1
Hydrocodone	PO	5–7.5	2–3	—	—	3–8	—
Oxycodone	PO	5		0.5	1–2	3–6	3
SYNTHETIC COMPOUNDS							
Morphons							
Levorphanol	IM	2–3	12–16	1	2	4–6	0.2
	PO	2–4	15–30	1.5	2	4–6	0.4
Phenylheptylamines	IM	2.5–10	3–4	0.25	0.5–1	4–6	1
Methadone	PO	2.5–10	3–4	0.5–1	1.5–2	4–8	1
Propoxyphene HCl	PO	32–65	12–16	0.25–1	1–2	3–6	30
Propoxyphene	PO	50–100		0.12–0.5	1	2–4	100
Napsylate	IM	50–100		0.5–1	1–2	2–3	10
Phenylpiperidines	PO	50–100					
Meperidine							
Normeperidine							
MIXED AGONIST-ANTIAGONISTS							
Buprenorphine	IM	0.3–0.6	2–3	0.12	1	6–8	0.04
	IV	0.03–0.2[a]	2.5–3.5	0.1–0.2	0.5–1	3–4	0.2
Butorphanol	IM	2–4	2.5	0.25–0.5	0.5–1.5	2–4	1
Dezocine	IM	5–20	5	0.25	1	3–6	1
	IV	5–10	2–3	0.25	1–3	3–6	6
Nalbuphine	IM	10–20		0.12–0.5		4–7	18
	IV	1–5[a]					
Pentazocine	IM	30–60					
	PO	50					

[a]Intravenous route usually used for antagonist properties.
Adapted from Intrurrsi DE, Foley KM: Narcotic analgesics in the management of pain. In Kuhar M, Pasternak G (eds): Analgesics Neurochemical, Behavioral and Clinical Perspectives, p 257. New York, Raven Press, 1984.

sites on the NMDA receptor. The d-methadone blocks morphine tolerance and NMDA-induced hyperalgesia.

Renal elimination of the opioids and their metabolites is primarily by glomerular filtration. Only small fractions of the drugs and metabolites are excreted in the feces.

Adverse Effects

With short-term, moderate-dose therapy, CNS and gastrointestinal side effects predominate. Sedation, dizziness, lightheadedness, miosis, nausea, vomiting, and constipation are extensions of the pharmacologic actions of these drugs and occur in dose-dependent fashion. Tolerance to the sedative and other CNS effects develops rapidly over the first few days of therapy or after an increase in dosage. Tolerance to opioids and α_2 agonists may be a paradoxical sensory hypersensitivity that is blocked by NMDA receptor antagonism. Tolerance to the euphorigenic effects of drugs of abuse (prescribed and nonprescribed) develops more insidiously than to the proposed therapeutic effects of these pharmacotherapies. Constipation is a result of decreased bowel peristalsis and decreased secretory actions of the stomach, biliary tract, and pancreas. Spasm of the sphincter of Oddi can increase pressure in the common bile duct and contribute to epigastric distress. This effect may persist for up to 24 hours after a single therapeutic dose of an opioid. Low doses of naloxone and vasodilating agents have been used to relieve this discomfort. Biliary colic tends to occur similarly in patients after morphine administration or after meperidine administration, each producing a similar increase in biliary pressure. The partial agonist–antagonists tend to produce less of a rise in biliary pressure than pure agonists. Stool softeners and colon-specific laxatives may be beneficial if initiated prophylactically to avert severe constipation with opioid therapy. Urinary retention may also result from an increase in sphincter tone. Physical dependence and analgesic tolerance are usually not clinical problems during short-term use, but they may occur following chronic opioid therapy. Unlike the NSAIDs, opioid analgesics do not directly interfere with renal processes or gastric mucosa. Ventilatory depression, apnea, cardiac arrest, circulatory collapse, coma, and death can occur after large parenteral doses. The cardiovascular and hemodynamic opioid effects are not uniform. Opioids may produce dose-dependent bradycardia as a function of vagal nucleus control stimulation that is attenuated by anticholinergic activity. Meperidine has an atropine-like effect that produces tachycardia, and it also has negative inotropic effects. Some opiates (morphine, meperidine, codeine) elicit histamine release that leads to vasodilation-induced hypotension. Clinically significant histamine release is rare with fentanyl, sufentanil, or alfentanil. The propoxyphene metabolite norpropoxyphene produces arrhythmias, QTc prolongation, and pulmonary edema. QTc prolongation is additionally reported with methadone doses (260 mg).

Opioids initially decrease the respiratory rate without affecting tidal volume. Tidal volume diminishes with linear increase of opiate doses, and large doses may precipitate apnea episodes. In general, opioids shift the CO_2 response curve to the right, indicating that a higher serum concentration of CO_2 is required to stimulate ventilatory response.

Clinical Uses

Opioids remain the primary pharmacologic therapy for moderate to severe postoperative pain. Analgesia is achieved by blunting the central response to noxious stimuli without loss of consciousness or affecting tactile, visual, or auditory sensation. Dose-limiting side effects such as nausea, vomiting, constipation, urinary retention, and ventilatory depression can be overcome by proper selection of the agent and route of administration. Sedation and euphoria may be desired in the immediate postoperative period. Analgesic potency is not necessarily of major importance, because at equianalgesic doses there are parallel increases in side effects. Partial agonists and agonist–antagonists can be effective analgesics in the postoperative period and have a ceiling effect for ventilatory depression. Unfortunately, dose escalations with these agents may also produce a ceiling for analgesic effects, while enhancing sedative and dysphoric properties.

Therapeutic approaches using patient request for nursing on-demand administration have been largely replaced with continuous or regularly scheduled dosing methods, and patient-controlled and patient-facilitated analgesia. As postoperative analgesic requirements diminish, the transition from parenteral to oral opioid or transdermal analgesia usually involves replacing the parenteral opioid with oral opioid, NSAID, APAP, and patient-specific adjuvant pharmacotherapy. Tramadol (325 mg)/APAP (325 mg) is indicated for acute pain and may be used in chronic pain (moderate to severe). Codeine, hydrocodone, and oxycodone drug formulations that also contain NSAID or APAP in combination are limited in their analgesic efficacy because of the high incidence of side effects and end-organ toxicities related to the latter coanalgesic components. Meperidine and propoxyphene use is decreasing because of recognition of the potential for neurotoxicity and cardiac/pulmonary toxicity, respectively. Alternative delivery techniques have evolved that may supplant the oral or intravenous delivery of opioids in certain clinical circumstances. Oxymorphone, sufentanil, fentanyl, and morphine dosage forms are being developed to provide greater long-acting analgesic postoperative opportunities. Oral slow release long-acting opioids (e.g., morphine, oxycodone, oxymorphone) that have long been used for chronic pain are finding a role in acute postoperative pain.[115,116]

NEW METHODS OF OPIOID ADMINISTRATION

Fentanyl patient-controlled transdermal analgesia (PCTA) can provide needleless analgesia for moderate to severe pain for $\geq$24 hours, including the postoperative period. A credit card-size PCTA device can deliver up to 80 doses of 40 mcg (μg), each for 10 minutes over a 24-hour period. Fentanyl is embedded in a hydrogel reservoir and delivered transdermally using low-intensity direct current. Due to lack of needle tubing, this delivery system has many potential applications in postoperative pain settings.[117]

Sufentanil (Chronogesic) is currently under investigation for use as a small subcutaneous continuous delivery system with a titanium rod implant that provides up to 90 days of this agent by osmotic pump. This delivery system could prove useful for patients with acute postoperative pain superimposed on chronic pain syndromes.

DepoDur (morphine) is a single 15- to 25-mg epidural injection of sustained release (SR) morphine providing analgesia over 48 hours. The extended release (ER) mechanism is a function of a liposome-capsulated, morphine-based delivery system impregnated within naturally occurring lipid particles (10- to 30-μm diameter) suspended in saline. The lipid particles contain discrete, water-filled chambers dispersed through the synthetic lipid matrix, with activation on metabolism to release morphine.[118]

Oxymorphone is a semisynthetic μ-specific opioid agonist used for moderate to severe pain. This opioid has an oral 12-hour SR dosage form and an immediate release (IR) dosage form available to complement the parenteral and rectal dosage form. The oxymorphone molecule stays in the aqueous phase of the CNS and is highly μ-receptor (especially μ_1) specific. The SR dosage form contains a hydrophilic matrix polysaccharide gel that provides a linear release of oxymorphone without peaks and valleys of blood concentration. Unlike other agonists, the cytochromes CYP450 3A4 and CYP450 2D6 do not significantly metabolize oxymorphone, and there is no oxymorphone induction inhibition of other agents. Uniquely, there appears to be little analgesic tolerance, even after 1 year of administration. The dose-dependent side effects are similar to other opioids. The $t^1/_2\beta$ half-life is 2 hours, and steady-state concentration (Css) is reached in 3 to 4 days for the ER form. The metabolites are 6-OH-oxymorphone and oxymorphone-3-glucuronide. Single dose data reflect dose proportional linear increases for the mean area under the curve (AUC) and Cmax. The median time to maximum concentration (Tmax) for IR is 6.5 hours and 2.5 to 4 hours for the ER version. Clinically, the IR form is administered every 6 hours with low fluctuations in drug levels, whereas the SR form produces consistent drug concentrations over a 12-hour time interval.

Clinical Dosing End Point

Serum concentrations that produce either therapeutic or side effects are a function of multiple dynamic processes that include preoperative opioid tolerance, CYP450 inhibition or induction, plasma albumin binding (acidic drug binding site), α_1 acid glycoprotein binding (basic drug binding site), aging process of essential organs (brain, heart, lung, kidney, liver, hematologic), multiple concurrent disease states, comorbidity, and extent of surgical trauma. Typical therapeutic end points include decreased pain (quality and intensity), increased functionality, and improved activities of daily living. Observing improvements in function is often more useful than analyzing subjective pain scores when titrating opioid and other adjuvant pain medications.

During periods of acute postoperative pain, scheduled administration of opioids, NSAIDs, antiepileptic drugs, antidepressants, lidocaine patch, sedatives, hypnotics, and centrally acting tramadol and acetaminophen are typically more effective than use on an as-needed (PRN) basis. This approach facilitates transition from inpatient to outpatient status in a more time-efficient manner. The addition of a well-structured narrow limit for PRN dosing to treat breakthrough pain may be beneficial.

Adjuvant Analgesia

Lidocaine Topical Patch

Lidocaine topical patch 5% provides relief for some acute postoperative painful conditions, including incisional site pain, and can be useful in combination with polymodal pharmacotherapy for neuropathic and nociception pain states in the immediate postoperative period. No serious systemic adverse effects or drug–drug interactions have been evident with such use. Mechanisms of action include sodium channel blockade, modulation of A delta and C fibers, and inhibition of both nitric oxide expression and T-cell release of proinflammatory cytokines. The patch can be placed 3 inches from intact wound site perimeters (both sides of wound site) and remains in place continuously. The most common side effects are mild local skin reactions (erythema, edema) without sensory changes. Systemic events are unlikely due to minimal absorbed active drug (i.e., one-sixth of concentration for cardiac events, one-twentieth of concentration of toxic events).[119,120] The clinical experience of the authors' indicates that the lidocaine patch can provide an opiate-sparing effect.

METHODS OF ANALGESIA

Pain relief may involve administration of analgesic drugs by various routes or nonpharmacologic application of mechanical, electrical, or psychological techniques. In any patient, the optimal combinations of these techniques depend on the type and degree of pain, the patient's perception of the pain, and the underlying medical, social, emotional, and environmental conditions in which the pain is managed.

Routes of Analgesic Delivery

Oral

Oral analgesics are usually considered less than optimal for moderate to severe acute postoperative pain management because of their lack of immediate titratability and prolonged time to peak effect, and because they require a functional gastrointestinal system. In general, hospitalized inpatients receive systemically administered opioids and then are converted to long-acting and/or short-acting oral or transdermal analgesics when the therapeutic need for rapid adjustments in the level of analgesia has diminished. However, with the focus on more rapid hospital discharge, early use of longer-acting, potent oral opioids facilitates transition of patients from parenteral opioids to oral therapy. Both nonopioid and opioid analgesic agents are available for oral administration, alone or in combination.

Transepithelial (Transdermal, Transmucosal)

With the increased number and complexity of surgical procedures being performed in the outpatient setting, there is a growing need for efficacious analgesic regimens for moderate to severe acute postoperative pain in this subset of patients. Methods of drug delivery such as transdermal[121] or transmucosal[122] administration are available as alternatives to oral analgesics on a patient-specific basis. These techniques permit delivery of potent analgesics that would be less effective when administered orally because of significant first-pass metabolism. Pharmacokinetic characteristics, primarily related to absorption, confer important clinical differences to these routes of administration. For example, to achieve optimal analgesic efficacy, transdermal fentanyl must be applied several hours prior to discontinuation of parenteral analgesics or patient-controlled analgesics. Transmucosal fentanyl is more rapidly absorbed but requires multiple titrations and is not indicated for postoperative pain. As with the oral route, titratability can be problematic and there may be unpredictability of drug absorption. Although transdermal fentanyl combined with patient-controlled analgesia (PCA) using morphine can reduce the number of demand doses, total opioid requirements and side effects are not decreased.[123] The new dosing method of fentanyl (E-Trans) described previously and involving PCTA is gaining increased use for postoperative pain following major surgery.

Parenteral

Parenteral administration of opioid analgesics remains the primary pharmacologic route for the treatment of moderate to severe postoperative pain. The use of computerized, patient-controlled delivery systems has played an important role in refining this method of delivery and reducing side effects of parenterally administered drugs.

Intramuscular. Intramuscular administration of postoperative analgesics produces a more rapid onset and time to peak effect than oral administration. It is also simple to administer analgesics by this route because no special infusion device is needed. However, pain at the injection site, patient apprehensiveness of needle sticks, the potential for delayed ventilatory depression, and wide variability in drug serum concentrations limit the viability of this route. Absorption from intramuscular sites depends on the lipophilicity of the agent and blood flow in the area of the injection. After intramuscular injections of morphine or meperidine, plasma concentrations may vary as much as threefold to fivefold, and time to peak concentration may vary from 4 to 108 minutes.[124] Another limitation is that administration efforts may not actually achieve the intramuscular site but may be deposited in a less perfused adipose tissue site. Conversely, with intramuscular administration, there is less variability in the minimum analgesic plasma concentration for an individual patient.[125] Small changes in plasma concentrations (10 to 20%) for a patient may represent a spectrum of effects from inadequate analgesia to complete pain relief.[126]

The relationship between plasma concentrations, effect, and time is depicted in Fig. 55-6. Plasma concentrations after intramuscular administration of large doses of an opioid analgesic such as morphine at long dosing intervals establish a cyclic pattern of sedation, analgesia, and ultimately inadequate analgesia. When morphine is administered by this route with a 3- or 4-hour dosing interval, plasma concentrations exceed or meet analgesic requirements for only approximately 35% of the dosing interval because of the delayed absorption and narrow therapeutic window. This situation is exacerbated by the patient-specific dynamic nature of analgesic requirements. PCA and continuous epidural infusions, as well as patient-controlled epidural infusions, circumvent many of the challenges of intramuscular administration and may provide more effective analgesia with fewer side effects by maintaining a more uniform control of plasma levels.

Most opioids can be administered by the parenteral route; however, a few NSAIDs, parecoxib, a valdecoxib prodrug, and ketorolac are designed for parenteral injection to manage postoperative pain.

Intravenous. Intermittent intravenous bolus infusions of opioids can be administered in situations when close

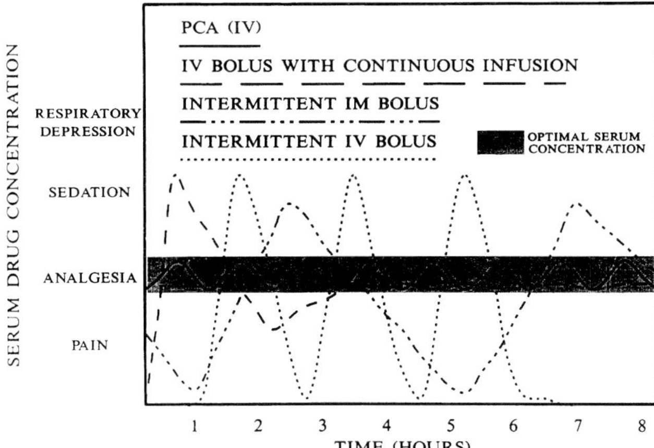

FIGURE 55-6. Relationship between serum drug concentration, pharmacologic effect, and method of administration. IM, intramuscular(ly); IV, intravenous(ly); PCA, patient-controlled analgesia. (Reprinted with permission from Tuman KJ, McCarthy RJ, Ivankovich AD: Pain control in the postoperative cardiac surgery patient. Hosp Formul 23:580, 1988.)

continuous monitoring of the patient is feasible. With a small intravenous bolus, the delay until analgesic effect and the variability in plasma concentrations seen with intramuscular administration can be reduced. Rapid redistribution of the drug shortens the duration of effect after a single intravenous administration compared with intramuscular injections. The numerous personnel needed to supervise frequent administration of boluses and monitoring of responses related to the fluctuations in plasma concentrations in the individual patient has led to the use of continuous intravenous infusions.

Continuous intravenous infusions offer the advantages of maintaining nearly constant plasma drug concentrations and reducing the peak-and-valley effect inherent in intermittent injections. Without the use of an initial bolus loading injection, continuous infusion techniques are inadequate because of the long time required for the drug to reach steady state (four to five elimination half-lives, $t^{1}/_{2}\beta$). Initiating therapy with a loading dose eliminates this problem but still does not allow for rapid dosage adjustments as analgesic requirements change.

Patient-Controlled Analgesia. By combining the advantages of a continuous infusion with the flexibility of interposing small bolus and patient-initiated doses as analgesic requirements vary, PCA appears to effectively address many patients' analgesic needs. This method has evolved as advances in computer technology have met the needs for improved drug delivery. Early PCA devices permitted a patient to titrate analgesic needs by activating a switch to deliver a small bolus dose of an opioid such as morphine sulfate. Limits could be placed on the number of activations per unit time the patient was allowed, as well as the minimum time that would have to elapse between activations (lockout interval). Refinements of this system permit administration of a continuous background infusion superimposed on patient-controlled boluses. Background infusion concomitant with intermittent PCA boluses is advantageous in maintaining serum drug levels within the analgesic range and further attenuates fluctuations in levels, resulting in improved analgesia and patient satisfaction without producing excessive additional unwanted side effects.[127] In addition to combining infusion and bolus dosing, current devices record a profile of the drug administration, including number and time of bolus delivery, number of activations that did not result in drug delivery, and total amounts of the agent that were administered per unit time. Only the patient should be permitted to initiate a bolus dose from a PCA device.

Compared with traditional methods of on-demand analgesic delivery, PCA has been shown to provide superior analgesia, with less total drug use, less sedation, fewer nocturnal sleep disturbances, and a more rapid return to physical activity.[128] Most patients tend to titrate PCA to a level of pain at which they are comfortable and taper their dosage requirements as they convalesce.[129] In addition, patient acceptance of PCA is high because patients believe they have significant control over their therapy.[130]

One limitation to PCA therapy is the selection of agents available for use in the PCA devices (Table 55-7). Ideally, a drug administered by PCA should be highly efficacious, have a rapid onset of action and a moderate duration of effect, should not accumulate or change pharmacokinetic properties with repeated administration, and should have a large therapeutic window. Morphine and fentanyl are the drugs most widely prescribed by this route. The partial agonist and mixed agonist–antagonist drugs are far from ideal, and limitations imposed by the pharmacology of the agonist–antagonist group have made their use in these devices disappointing. Despite theoretic advantages, the use of fentanyl for PCA has not been shown to be a clearly superior analgesic to morphine,[131] although it may improve the initial PCA demand-to-delivery ratio.[132]

Other problems encountered with PCA therapy are primarily a result of operator or mechanical errors.[133] Because patients titrate their own therapy and not third "nonmedical" parties (i.e., family, friends), it is requisite that the patient is capable of understanding the concepts of the device, able to activate the trigger, and willing to participate. This makes the use of PCA devices more difficult in pediatric patients, as well as in patients who are older and debilitated or patients who are cognitively impaired.

Optimum results from PCA therapy are obtained only when the patient's analgesic needs can be met within the prescribed parameters set on the device. The patient's age, end-organ function, surgical procedure, need for a continuous background infusion, number and amount of boluses allowed, and total analgesic requirements are considered. Anesthesiologists must incorporate some flexibility into protocols for ordering PCA therapy to account for the variability introduced by these and other patient-specific factors. Further, the patient's prehospital analgesic burden should be considered in any postoperative analgesic treatment plan. Factors influencing postoperative opiate dosing include use of "recreational" drugs, ethanol use history, pharmacotherapy affecting the cytochrome CYP450 system, and genetic polymorphism.

Genetic Polymorphism. The cytochrome P450 used for metabolism of most pharmacotherapeutic agents has become a clinical challenge. The potential of substrate induction and inhibition by certain drugs used by the patient can importantly influence postoperative analgesic therapy. This is compounded by genetic polymorphism with a CYP450 enzyme deficit and the effect on patient-specific individual pharmacokinetic and pharmacodynamic variances among the extensive metabolites. Genetic polymorphism is displayed primarily by CYP450 2C9, 2C19, 2D6, and 3A4. These account for 80% of the CYP450-mediated reactions. Genetic polymorphism is the presence in the general population of more than one allele at the same locus with the least frequent allele occurring more frequently than can be accounted for by mutation alone. The implication for pharmacotherapeutic dosing and response includes increased risk of therapeutic failure, adverse drug reactions (ADRs), and drug toxicity.

In general, CYP450 induction produces a decrease of therapeutic efficacy, whereas CYP450 inhibition produces an increase in AUC, a decrease in clearance, increase in plasma level

TABLE 55-7

COMMON BOLUS DOSAGES, LOCKOUT INTERVALS, AND CONTINUOUS INFUSIONS FOR VARIOUS PARENTERAL ANALGESICS WHEN USING A PATIENT-CONTROLLED ANALGESIA SYSTEM

DRUG	BOLUS DOSE (mg)	LOCKOUT INTERVAL (min)	CONTINUOUS INFUSION (mg/hr)	4-hr LIMIT (mg)
AGONISTS				
Fentanyl citrate	0.015–0.05	3–10	0.02–0.1	0.2–0.4
Hydromorphone hydrochloride	0.10–0.5	5–15	0.2–0.5	200–300
Meperidine hydrochloride	5–15	5–15	5–40	20–30
Methadone hydrochloride	0.50–3.0	10–20	1–10	
Morphine sulfate	0.50–3.0[a]	5–20	0.1–1	
Oxymorphone hydrochloride	0.20–0.8	5–15		
Sufentanil citrate	0.003–0.015	3–10		
AGONISTS-ANTAGONISTS				
Buprenorphine hydrochloride	0.03–0.2	10–20	1–8	
Nalbuphine hydrochloride	1–5	5–15	6–40	
Pentazocine hydrochloride	5–30	5–15		

[a] For pediatric dosing, see text.

and potential for ADRs, and toxicity of a given substrate drug. This highlights the importance of CYP450 substrate modulation because of concomitant pharmacotherapy. Reduced drug metabolism is associated with genetic polymorphism at the 2C9 allele (6 to 8% Caucasian), 2C19 allele (3 to 5% Caucasian and 12 to 23% Asian), and 2D6 allele (6 to 10% Caucasian, 2 to 5% African American, 1% Asian).

Preoperative Alcohol and Controlled Substance History. Preoperative alcohol, recreational or illicit drug use, and prescription controlled substance use (e.g., opiates, benzodiazepines), as well as history of adverse drug reactions or episodes of abstinence or withdrawal of these agents, are important to assess. Preoperative alcohol, opioid, and benzodiazepine use are factors in postoperative therapeutic selection and in averting withdrawal postoperatively. Alcohol withdrawal may be confused with inappropriate analgesia based on cognitive, behavioral, and other physiologic manifestations. Alcohol and other recreational drug withdrawal may present as autonomic hyperactivity as is seen with inadequate pain relief or side effects of pharmacotherapies (hand tremors, insomnia, psychomotor agitation, nausea, vomiting, anxiety, transient hallucinations, or seizures).

Central Neuraxial Analgesia

5 The technique of spinal analgesia was described by Bier and Tuffler in 1898, and that of sacral epidural analgesia by Sicard and Cathelin in 1901. In 1949, a major advance in the application of central neuraxial analgesia was the description by Cleland[134] of the use of a continuous catheter epidural infusion for postoperative analgesia. Analgesia was maintained for 1 to 5 days after surgery by administering intermittent bolus doses of a local anesthetic. Although effective analgesia was obtained, a significant sympathetic block accompanied the analgesia, and all patients required at least one dose of a vasopressor. Additional shortcomings of this technique, as with any intermittent dosing regimen, were the fluctuating levels of analgesia that occur as the effect of the bolus dissipates and the requirement of the medical staff to reinject the patient every several hours.

Because of the shortcomings of intermittent dosing, the continuous infusion of local anesthetics along the central neuraxis was subsequently recommended as an alternative to the intermittent bolus technique. The continuous infusion of local anesthetics simplifies maintenance of analgesia, but the use of local anesthetics in concentrations sufficient to produce pain relief usually results in sensory and occasional motor blockade. These are unwanted effects in the postoperative period because sensory and, more importantly, motor blockade prohibit ambulation, an important factor in postoperative convalescence.

Although it has long been recognized that application of local anesthetic agents along the spinal canal could provide effective analgesia, the demonstration that opioids could produce analgesia by this route has been responsible for the widespread application of the practice of central neuraxial analgesia. The enthusiasm for this route of administration has also been a direct result of the shortcomings of intramuscular and intravenous therapies. By interrupting pain pathways at the level of communication between the first-order neurons and the second-order neurons, this method can provide effective analgesia without the associated CNS depression and cyclical nature of pain associated with other parenteral routes of administration.

Intrathecal. The intrathecal administration of opioids has the advantage of providing long-lasting analgesia after a single injection. The onset of analgesic effect after the intrathecal administration of an opioid is directly proportional to the lipid solubility of the agent, whereas the duration of the effect is longer with more hydrophilic compounds. Morphine, for example, produces peak analgesic effects in 20 to 60 minutes that last for 2 to 12 hours when doses ranging from 0.25 to 4 mg are administered intrathecally to adults.[135,136] In routine clinical practice, 0.25 to 1 mg morphine can be expected to provide effective analgesia, whereas doses in the range of 0.25 to 0.5 mg generally maintain analgesic efficacy while minimizing the potential for ventilatory depression.[135]

Intrathecal bolus injections share many of the problems of other intermittent techniques, including lack of titratability and extensive time requirements for monitoring and reinjection. In addition, the potential for infection, a greater risk of ventilatory depression owing to rostral spread of the drug, and a higher incidence of side effects make this technique less desirable than epidural administration (Table 55-8). Widespread clinical experience has shown that continuous epidural infusions may be preferable to intrathecal techniques for central neuraxial

TABLE 55-8

COMPLICATIONS OF NEURAXIAL OPIOIDS

■ COMPLICATION	■ REPORTED INCIDENCE (%)[a] ■ SPINAL	■ EPIDURAL	■ TREATMENT
Respiratory depression	5–7	0.1–2	Support ventilation, naloxone
Pruritus	60	1–100	Antihistamine, naloxone
Nausea and vomiting	20–30	20–30	Antiemetic, transdermal scopolamine, naloxone
Urinary retention	50	15–25	Catheterize, naloxone

[a]Reported incidences vary widely, appear to be related to dose, and are higher with spinal than with epidural administration.
Reprinted with permission from Ready LB: Regional analgesics with intraspinal opioids. In Bonica JJ (ed): The Management of Pain, vol II, 2nd ed, p 1976. Philadelphia, Lea & Febiger, 1990.

analgesia. The practical aspects of maintaining a catheter in the intrathecal space for a prolonged period and reports of cauda equina syndrome after continuous spinal anesthesia also may favor the continuous epidural technique.[137] Although intrathecal analgesic techniques are infrequently used outside the setting of labor analgesia, the combination of spinal anesthesia followed by continuous epidural analgesia has gained increasing popularity because it provides the advantages of spinal anesthesia (rapid onset, dense neural blockade), while facilitating the transition to an effective and titratable postoperative analgesia method after major surgery.[138]

Epidural. Epidural administration of opioids and local anesthetics has evolved in parallel with intrathecal techniques. As noted, the advantages of epidural administration of drugs such as opioids and local anesthetics include the reduced incidence of side effects and a diminished propensity for opioid-induced ventilatory depression compared with the intrathecal route. When a drug is placed in the epidural space, it must first cross the dura before it can reach the spinal cord. Besides the physical barrier presented by the dura, the epidural space is highly vascularized, and a significant redistribution of drug to the systemic circulation occurs. The epidural space also contains fat, connective tissues, a lymphatic network, and the dorsal and ventral roots of the spinal nerves, all of which can serve as a repository for lipophilic agents.[139]

The influence of these factors can be demonstrated by an examination of the pharmacokinetics of epidurally administered hydrophilic (morphine) and lipophilic (fentanyl) opioids. Ten milligrams of morphine, given either intravenously or epidurally, produce peak serum levels and decay curves that are nearly identical (Fig. 55-7). Whereas the duration of pain relief from intravenous administration is short lived (1 to 2 hours), epidural morphine can provide 12 or more hours of analgesia. This indicates that, although much of an epidural dose is absorbed into the systemic circulation, a small fraction of the morphine dose (~2 to 10%) diffuses across the dura to bind spinal opiate receptors and produce analgesia. In contrast, when epidural fentanyl 200 μg is given in a similar manner, peak serum levels are only approximately 50% of those after a similar intramuscular injection. However, serum levels of fentanyl 24 hours after a continuous rate epidural infusion are similar to those obtained from a similar intravenous infusion.[140] This implies that with the initial bolus of fentanyl, there is redistribution of the drug to lipophilic tissues, which become saturated after continuous administration. Therefore, only a small fraction of a typically administered epidural dose is necessary to produce spinally mediated analgesia.

Because the diffusion of drugs across the dura is both concentration and time dependent, it is necessary to administer significantly larger amounts of drugs than those that effectively saturate spinal opiate receptors. These higher doses are more likely to produce unwanted side effects from systemic and rostral distribution of the drug, but fewer than those associated with equianalgesic intrathecal doses. When these factors are considered, the margin of therapeutic safety and the decrease in side effects with epidural administration make this route preferred for postoperative analgesia.

Intermittent epidural bolus doses of morphine sulfate ($\leq$15 mg over 24 hours) have been used for postsurgical analgesia.[80] Although this method of administration provides excellent analgesia for up to 12 hours, side effects associated with these bolus doses limit the widespread application of this technique. An intermittent bolus technique also has the disadvantage of limiting the number of usable opioids to the longer-acting drugs (e.g., morphine and hydromorphone).

In an effort to mitigate the frequency and severity of opioid-induced side effects associated with bolus techniques, El-Baz

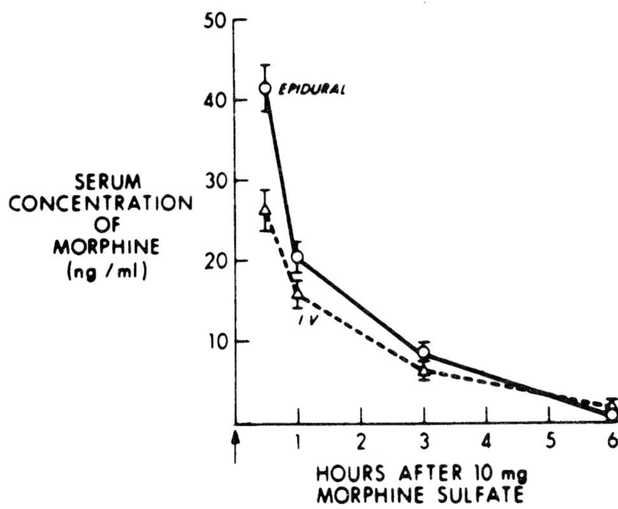

FIGURE 55-7. Serum concentration of morphine (mean ± SEM) after intravenous and lumbar epidural administration of 10 mg of morphine sulfate in 10 subjects. Triangles, intravenous; circles, epidural. (Reprinted with permission from Bromage PR, Camporesi EM, Durant PAC, Nielsen CH: Nonrespiratory side effects of epidural morphine. Anesth Analg 61:490, 1982.)

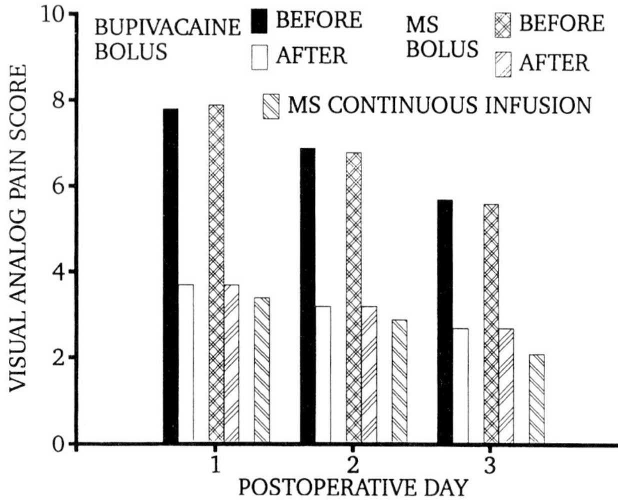

FIGURE 55-8. Analgesic effectiveness of continuous morphine epidural infusion compared with epidural bolus doses of morphine sulfate (MS) or bupivacaine. See text for details. (Adapted from El-Baz NI, Faber LP, Jensik RJ: Continuous epidural infusion of morphine for treatment of pain after thoracic surgery: A new technique. Anesth Analg 63:757, 1984.)

et al[141] described the use of a continuous epidural morphine infusion (100 μg/h) and found equivalent analgesia and fewer side effects than after epidural boluses of either bupivacaine (0.5%) or morphine (5 mg) (Fig. 55-8 and Table 55-9). It is now well accepted that continuous epidural infusions of opioids provide effective analgesia while reducing the side effects associated with bolus administration.[142–144]

Because the laws of mass action apply to diffusion of drugs out of the epidural space to their sites of action, several hours are often required to achieve adequate analgesia when using continuous infusions alone. Effective analgesia with epidural infusions administered at a continuous rate may take as long as 3 to 4 hours to achieve. Delay in onset of effective analgesia can be reduced by adjusting the infusion rate to provide the equivalent of a small (5 to 10 mL) bolus of the epidural solution over 5 to 15 minutes before beginning the maintenance infusion. This allows an adequate concentration of the analgesic drug(s) to be present at their site(s) of action in a shorter time.

In addition to a reduction in adverse effects, another advantage of a continuous epidural infusion over an epidural bolus injection is the ability to titrate the amount of analgesia (Table 55-10). Although morphine usually provides 12 hours of pain relief after a single epidural injection, wide variability has been reported in the duration of effective analgesia (4 to 24 hours), depending on the site and extent of surgical trauma and age of the patient. Because of this variability, it becomes difficult to titrate uniform levels of analgesia. A continuous infusion provides easier analgesic titration, particularly when shorter-acting opioids such as fentanyl are used. Fentanyl has an onset of action within 4 to 5 minutes and a peak effect within 20 minutes.[145,146] Because of the rapid onset, it becomes much easier to adjust dosage, observe the desired effect, and titrate to an optimal intensity of analgesia. Morphine, in contrast, has an onset time of 30 minutes with a time to peak effect ranging from 60 to 90 minutes.

Mirroring the evolution of PCA, a refinement in delivery of analgesics by the epidural route is the use of superimposed patient-controlled bolus doses with a continuous basal infusion. Early application of this technique for delivery of epidural analgesia used relatively large intermittent demand doses alone or combined with a low-rate continuous infusion, and the intermittent demand doses provided the preponderance of analgesia. This dosing paradigm has reduced efficacy because of fluctuations in analgesia occurring as a consequence of large intermittent bolus dosing. Using higher basal infusion rates and smaller patient-activated bolus doses, the continuous infusion maintains a more constant intensity of analgesia, whereas the bolus doses provide supplemental analgesia for transient increases in analgesic requirements[147] (Table 55-11). Patient-controlled epidural analgesia is particularly useful to manage dynamic changes in pain related to patient activity (e.g., coughing, chest physiotherapy).[148] The development of new infusion devices has allowed such combined modes of administration of epidural analgesia to be readily delivered (Appendix 55-1).

Initiation and maintenance of therapy. Based on the preceding considerations, achievement of optimal results with a continuous epidural analgesia technique requires appropriate perioperative planning and assessment. This strategy includes identifying patients who may benefit from epidural analgesia and scheduling the epidural catheter placement as part of the anesthetic plan. At the authors' institution, epidural catheters for postoperative analgesia are commonly placed immediately prior to induction of operative anesthesia. This practice allows the anesthesiologist to administer a test dose of local anesthetic to evaluate while the patient is still awake. The application of bolus administration followed by a continuous infusion mandates that the test dose be administered to an awake patient. This facilitates diagnosis of intrathecal, intravascular, or subdural catheter placement, and allows confirmation of segmental epidural analgesia when the test dose of local anesthetic is administered. This practice also allows the continuous

TABLE 55-9

SIDE EFFECTS WITH POSTOPERATIVE EPIDURAL ANALGESIA

■ SIDE EFFECT	■ GROUP A (BUPIVACAINE 25 mg/5 mL, 0.5%, EPIDURAL BOLUS)	■ GROUP B (MORPHINE 5 mg, EPIDURAL BOLUS)	■ GROUP C (MORPHINE 100 μg/hr EPIDURAL INFUSION)
Urinary retention	30 (100%)	30 (100%)	2 (7%)
Hypotension	7 (23%)	0	0
Weakness of hands	12 (40%)	0	0
Pruritus	0	12 (40%)	1 (3%)
Depressed consciousness	0	8 (27%)	0

Adapted from El-Baz MI, Faber LP, Jensik RJ: Continuous epidural infusion of morphine for treatment of pain after thoracic surgery. A new technique. Anesth Analg 63:757, 1984.

TABLE 55-10

COMPARISON OF EPIDURAL ANALGESIA ADMINISTRATION TECHNIQUES

ADVANTAGES	DISADVANTAGES
CONTINUOUS EPIDURAL INFUSIONS	
1. Less rostral spread so side effects are minimized 2. Provides continuous analgesia avoiding the peaks and nadir seen with intermittent bolus 3. Allows for concomitant use of dilute local anesthetic solutions 4. Allows the use of shorter-acting opiates such as fentanyl or sufentanil 5. Less potential risk of contamination for injection because the catheter system has fewer breaks in sterile technique 6. Simple and easy maintenance; removes the need for anesthesia personnel to inject patients periodically	1. Need for sophisticated infusion device
INTERMITTENT EPIDURAL BOLUS	
1. Simple (providing resident or nursing staff accepts the responsibility of epidural catheter injections) 2. No need for infusion devices	1. Limited number of suitable opioids 2. Higher incidence of side effects 3. Extra effort to inject catheter every 8–12 hr 4. Excludes the use of local anesthesia 5. More difficult to titrate dose

epidural infusion to be started during surgery. Solutions of morphine (0.1 mg/mL) with bupivacaine (1 mg/mL) or fentanyl (10 μg/mL) with bupivacaine (1 mg/mL) are most commonly used. Concentrations of opioid are reduced for patients with increased risk of serious opioid-induced side effects. The infusion is begun during surgery at a rate of 4 to 6 mL/h, augmenting the general anesthetic and providing sufficient time to achieve good analgesia and smooth emergence. If the surgical procedure is relatively short (1 to 2 hours), a 5- to 10-mL bolus of the epidural solution may be given as a rapid infusion as described previously to hasten the onset of analgesia. As an alternative, the patient may be given an epidural bolus of 0.5% bupivacaine combined with either fentanyl (50 to 100 μg) or morphine (2 to 5 mg). If the surgical procedure is expected to exceed 3 to 4 hours, bolus dosing may not be needed because sufficient time is allowed for continuous epidural

TABLE 55-11

EPIDURAL OPIOIDS: LATENCY AND DURATION OF POSTOPERATIVE ANALGESIA

		ANALGESIC EFFECT			CONTINUOUS INFUSION RATE			
AGENT	BOLUS DOSE	ONSET (min)	PEAK (min)	DURATION (hr)	RANGE (mL/hr)	BASE (mL/hr)	PATIENT-ASSISTED BOLUS	INTERVAL (min)
Meperidine	30–100 mg	5–10	12–30	4–6				
Meperidine 0.1–0.25% + bupivacaine 0.1%					2–10	5	1	12
Morphine	5 mg	23.5 ± 6	30–60	12–24				
Morphine 0.01%					1–6			
Morphine 0.01–0.1% + bupivacaine 0.1%					3–6	3	1	20
Methadone	5 mg	12.5 ± 2	17 ± 3	7.2 ± 4.6				
Hydromorphone	1 mg	13 ± 4	23 ± 8	11.4 ± 5.5				
Hydromorphone 0.05%					0.8			
Fentanyl	100 μg	4–10	20	2.6 ± 5.7				
Fentanyl 0.001%					4–12			
Fentanyl 0.001% + bupivacaine 0.1%					4–10	5	1	12
Diamorphine	5 mg	5	9–15	12.4 ± 6.5				
Sufentanil	10–60 μg	7.3 ± 5.6	26.5 ± 8.1	3.9–6.9				
Sufentanil 0.0001%					10			
Alfentanil	15 μg/kg	15		1–2				

Adapted from Cousins MJ, Mather LE: Intrathecal and epidural administration of opioids. Anesthesiology 61:276, 1984.

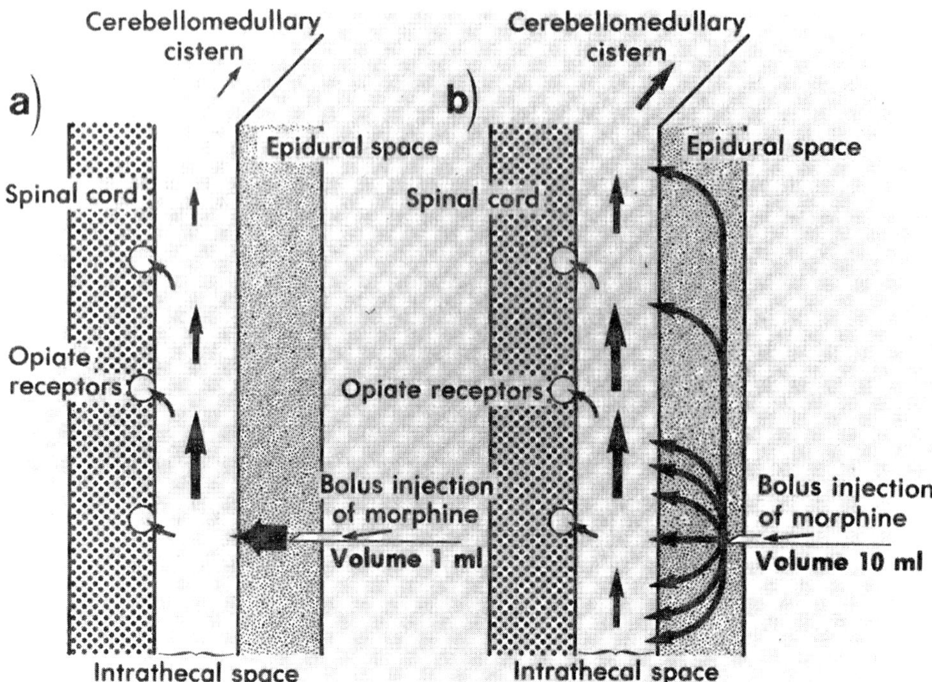

FIGURE 55-9. Rostral spread of central neuraxial morphine. **a.** Spread in small injection volumes of 1 mL after dura penetration into the intrathecal space. **b.** Spread in high injection volumes of 10 mL in the intrathecal and epidural space. (Reprinted with permission from Chrubasik J: Investigations on respiratory repression. In Chrubasik J [ed]: Spinal Infusions of Opiates and Somatostatin, p 19. Obersul, Germany, Verlag Hygeineplan, 1985.)

infusion alone to achieve analgesia at the time of the patient's awakening.

Placement of epidural catheter. Hydrophilic compounds such as morphine, when injected epidurally, result in cerebrospinal fluid concentrations of the drug that allow it to saturate more rostral portions of the spinal cord[149] (Fig. 55-9). Because of this property, epidural morphine may be infused at a lower lumbar level and still provide analgesia for surgical procedures performed on the upper abdomen and thorax. Lipophilic drugs such as fentanyl tend to provide more of a segmental analgesic effect.[150] This may in part be the result of the lipophilic compounds partitioning into lipid compartments in the spinal canal, such as epidural fat and the spinal cord. This segmental nature of analgesia mandates the need to place an epidural catheter in a location to cover the dermatomes included in the surgical field. A general guideline for the catheter locations in various types of surgery is as follows: thoracic surgery—upper to lower thoracic; upper abdominal and renal surgery—low thoracic to high lumbar; orthopaedic procedures of the lower extremities and lower abdominal and gynecologic surgery—lumbar region. Alternatively, catheter placement should be approximately at the dermatomal level that corresponds to a point intersecting the upper one-third and lower two-thirds of the surgical incision. In general, placement of the epidural catheter at a level lower than that described previously necessitates increased epidural drug dosing to achieve effective analgesia, especially when lipophilic opioids are used, and this may lead to an increase in side effects.

Selection of analgesics. The differences among the opioids used for epidural analgesia relate to their duration of action and propensity to produce side effects. Patient factors such as advanced age, small body habitus, morbid obesity, history of sleep apnea, and general debilitation should be considered when initiating epidural analgesia because these conditions are associated with a greater propensity for respiratory complications. Reduced concentrations of opioids should be used when initiating epidural analgesia in such patients (Appendices 55-1 to 54-3).

Pain relief lasts longer with hydrophilic agents such as morphine than with the more lipid-soluble hydromorphone or fentanyl (see Table 55-11). The relatively long duration of action of epidural or intrathecal morphine allows it to be used effectively as an intermittent bolus given every 12 hours, whereas because of a shorter duration of analgesia, fentanyl is better suited for continuous epidural infusions. Morphine can be used as a continuous epidural infusion and has been associated with reduced side effects compared with epidural bolus injections.[141] Hydromorphone, which has a lipid solubility between that of morphine and fentanyl, is 7 to 10 times as potent as morphine. Intermittent epidural bolus administration of hydromorphone provides effective analgesia for 7 to 12 hours, with a reduced incidence of pruritus and nausea compared with morphine.[151]

Lipophilic compounds such as fentanyl, sufentanil, and, to a lesser extent, hydromorphone partition into the spinal cord and lipid structures in the epidural space more than hydrophilic agents, which remain in the cerebrospinal fluid to a greater extent. Therefore, it may be preferable to use lipophilic opioids such as fentanyl, rather than the more hydrophilic morphine, to produce a more segmental level of analgesia. Although the tendency of hydrophilic drugs for rostral ascension facilitates the dermatomal distribution of analgesia, it also can result in a higher incidence of some side effects.[149]

Epidural coadministration of opioids with local anesthetics takes advantage of the desirable properties of each drug. The desired result of these combinations is achievement of potentiated analgesia at lower opioid doses with a concentration of a local anesthetic that does not produce significant motor blockade. This potentiation may be a result of antinociception at different sites in the spinal cord.[152] Opioids produce analgesia by binding to opiate receptors in the substantia gelatinosa, whereas local anesthetics block transmission of afferent impulses at the nerve roots and dorsal root ganglia.[153] Another advantage of the combination using reduced doses is the concomitant decrease in the incidence and severity of side effects. Despite wide acceptance, not all studies have demonstrated analgesic potentiation when bupivacaine and fentanyl have been used in combination.[154]

Adrenergic receptors of the α_2 class modulate nociceptive impulses in the dorsal horn of the spinal cord and throughout the CNS. Agonists of these receptors produce antinociception

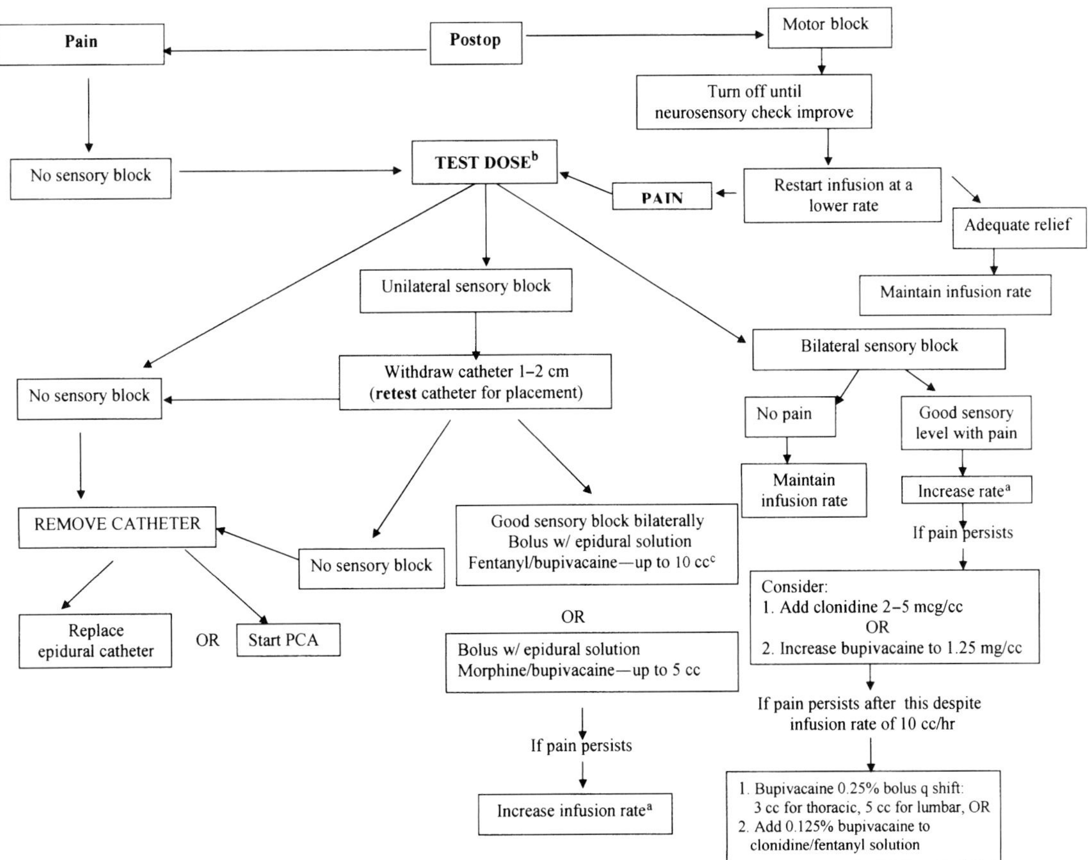

FIGURE 55-10. Postoperative epidural management algorithm. The test dose, given by anesthesia personnel, is 2% lidocaine with epinephrine 1:200,000 (5 mL for lumbar catheters; 3 mL for thoracic catheters). PCA, patient-controlled analgesia. [a]Not to exceed 10 cc/degree with fentanyl or morphine. [b]Test dose: 3 cc 2% lidocaine with epinephrine 1:200,000 for thoracic catheter. Test dose: 5 cc 2% lidocaine epinephrine 1:200,000 for lumbar catheter.

with minimal ventilatory depression compared with opioids.[155] Clonidine has been the most widely used α_2 agonist for epidural analgesia, producing dose-dependent analgesia when given as a bolus.[156,157] Epidural clonidine has been associated with hypotension and with bradycardia because of inhibition of preganglionic sympathetic fibers. This is most prevalent at smaller doses, whereas large doses normalize blood pressure because of systemic vasoconstriction that overrides the central hypotensive effect. Although epidural clonidine has been used as a single agent to provide postoperative analgesia,[158] it has more frequently been used in combination with local anesthetics[159] or opiates[160,161] to potentiate analgesia and minimize side effects. Optimal ratios for combining α_2 agonists with opioid or local anesthetics are yet to be defined[162] because these drugs exhibit nonlinear synergism.[163] Other α_2 agonists that have been used for pain management include dexmedetomidine and tizanidine.[164] Dexmedetomidine is an α_2 agonist with a very high α_2-to-α_1 selectivity (ratio of 1,600) compared with clonidine (ratio of 200).[165] Tizanidine, an analog of clonidine, produces analgesia in a manner similar to clonidine but has fewer cardiovascular effects.[164,166]

Management of inadequate analgesia. Although epidural analgesia is usually effective, patients may occasionally experience inadequate pain relief. A systematic approach is necessary to evaluate and manage inadequate epidural analgesia. The initial step in this process is verification of the integrity of the catheter system, followed by a bolus (5 to 7 mL) of the epidural solution (typically a combination of dilute local anesthetic with opioid), with analgesic assessment after a short interval (15 to 30 minutes). If analgesia remains inadequate, a test dose of a local anesthetic solution, such as 2% lidocaine with 1:200,000 epinephrine, can then be given to evaluate epidural catheter location (Fig. 55-10). The test dose usually yields one of three results. If bilateral sensory block occurs in a few segmental dermatomes, epidural catheter location is confirmed. In this case, volume of the infusion was likely insufficient for adequate dermatomal coverage, resulting in inadequate analgesia, and increasing the rate of infusion may produce effective analgesia. A unilateral sensory block after administration of a test dose of local anesthetic is suggestive of the catheter tip residing laterally in or near a neuroforamen. Withdrawal of the catheter 1 to 2 cm is usually associated with a bilateral sensory block after a subsequent test dose. Once bilateral sensory blockade has been documented, adequate analgesia can be maintained with bolus administration of the epidural solution followed by adjustments of the continuous epidural infusion or patient-controlled epidural infusion parameters.

Finally, a lack of sensory blockade after test dose administration indicates that the epidural catheter does not reside in the epidural space. In this situation, the catheter is removed, and the patient is given the option of having another epidural catheter placed or switching to PCA therapy.

Safety considerations. Serious complications that can occur with a continuous epidural technique include accidental intrathecal administration of drug, infection-related problems, epidural hematoma, and ventilatory depression. To decrease the incidence of these complications, the authors propose the following guidelines:

1. A low concentration of local anesthetic (e.g., 0.1% bupivacaine) in combination with an opioid analgesic allows subarachnoid catheter migration to be identified earlier by the onset of progressive sensory blockade. Low concentrations of local anesthetics do not interfere with neurologic assessments because they do not usually produce significant sensory or motor block when administered epidurally. If sensory or motor deficits are present, discontinuation of the infusion should allow for regression of these anesthetic effects within 2 to 4 hours. Persistent impairment of sensory or motor function should prompt appropriate evaluation to identify potentially serious causes of neurologic dysfunction, especially in anticoagulated patients (see Fig. 55-10).
2. Catheter sites should be examined daily, temperature curves monitored, and the patient periodically evaluated for signs of meningism. Symptoms of epidural abscess include neurologic deficits, elevated body temperature, and back pain, although meningitis is uncommon.[167] If any findings consistent with infection are present, the catheter is removed and cultures performed. In the authors' experience of more than 30,000 cases of postoperative epidural analgesia, only a single case of epidural abscess has been encountered, and this patient was successfully treated without neurologic compromise. In a small number of patients, infections limited to the cutaneous structures have developed and resolved with conservative therapy.
3. Epidural catheters should be placed at least 1 hour before intravenous heparinization in patients without preoperative coagulation defects but requiring intraoperative anticoagulation with unfractionated heparin. At least one published series has shown that if epidural catheters are placed at least 1 hour before heparinization, the incidence of clinically significant epidural hemorrhage does not appear to increase.[168]
4. The risk of epidural hematoma formation related to epidural catheter placement in patients receiving certain forms of perioperative anticoagulation is controversial. Historically, concern for epidural hematoma formation with epidural catheterization has been generated primarily in the setting of intraoperative anticoagulation with unfractionated heparin. With the introduction of low-molecular-weight heparins (LMWHs), increased risk of epidural hematoma formation related to epidural catheterization has been attributed to the perioperative use of such fractionated heparin compounds. Similar to unfractionated heparin, LMWH binds to antithrombin III; however, the resulting complex also diminishes thrombin generation by inhibiting factor Xa. In contrast to unfractionated heparin, the anticoagulating effects of LMWH are of longer duration and not effectively monitored with the activated clotting time or activated partial thromboplastin time.[169] Based on consensus opinion, after assessing the risks and benefits of epidural anesthesia/analgesia on an individual patient basis, it has been recommended that epidural catheterization (as well as removal of epidural catheters) be performed at least 10 to 12 hours after a dose of LMWH.[170] In addition, dosing of LMWH should not occur for at least 2 hours after removal of an epidural catheter to avoid manipulation during the peak anticoagulant effect.[170] Although some clinicians remove epidural catheters before postoperative initiation of LMWH, others continue postoperative epidural analgesia for longer than 24 hours in some patients. In such instances, LMWH administration may be delayed or alternative methods of thromboprophylaxis selected. The risks of spinal hematoma are incrementally increased when LMWH is used concomitantly with other drugs that affect hemostasis, including antiplatelet drugs, standard heparin, and dextran. The entire patient care team must be cognizant of this whenever postoperative epidural analgesia is used, and the postoperative analgesia service should interface with other managing clinicians to determine the optimal management of patients with these considerations. Whenever perioperative anticoagulation is used in patients managed with epidural analgesia, monitoring of anticoagulation and neurologic status is imperative.
5. With appropriate monitoring of coagulation status, epidural catheters may be inserted safely in patients who receive perioperative warfarin.[171] In patients with international normalized ratio values exceeding 1.5, neurologic checks should be continued for at least 24 hours after epidural catheter removal.[172]
6. Respiratory rates and level of sedation should be monitored every hour for the first 24 hours of the epidural infusion and every 4 hours thereafter. Apnea monitors can be used to supplement, but cannot replace, direct patient observation. Patients at increased risk for respiratory compromise include the elderly and those with sleep apnea or any debilitating disease. In the authors' institution, an apnea monitor is commonly used for the first 24 hours when epidural bolus doses of morphine 2 mg or greater are given as loading doses.

   It has become increasingly evident that the patient with obstructive sleep apnea (OSA) is at a greater risk of respiratory depression from opioids, regardless of the route of administration. The expanding knowledge base of OSA also suggests that it is more common than previously appreciated.[173] Patients with a constellation of symptoms (e.g., excessive snoring, hypertension, daytime somnolence) and who have physical findings consistent with OSA should probably be considered to have a provisional diagnosis of OSA and thus managed with appropriate precautions. Patients with sleep apnea should have continuous pulse oximetry monitoring to promote early detection of respiratory depression, and they may benefit from nasal continuous positive airway pressure (NCPAP) after extubation and during periods of sleep.[174]

In summary, a continuous infusion technique alone or in combination with patient-controlled epidural boluses simplifies maintenance of epidural analgesia and allows greater analgesic titratability than intermittent epidural bolus dosing. Proper patient selection, catheter placement, and methods to identify and treat inadequate analgesia are important aspects of postoperative pain management. Patient safety is paramount and guidelines should be established within each facility for prevention, early diagnosis, and treatment of complications.

Caudal. Caudal nerve blocks play a minor role in acute postoperative pain management in adults. Because they are technically more difficult to perform in adults than other efficacious forms of lumbar epidural blocks, they are used less frequently in adults than in the pediatric population. Continuous caudal analgesia for postoperative pain has a limited utility because of the difficulty of securing a catheter, but it may have a role in select patients such as those who have had extensive lumbar or thoracic spine surgery. In those unusual situations where continuous caudal analgesia is used, the standard solutions for lumbar epidural analgesia may be used, although infusion rates may need to be higher than those with a lumbar epidural infusion.

Pediatric ("kiddie") caudals have become popular for intraoperative supplementation and postoperative pain relief. Palpation of the sacral hiatus is much easier in the pediatric population, and a distinct "pop" can be heard as the needle pierces the sacrococcygeal membrane. A short, 22- or 23-gauge needle should be used; the block is usually performed with the child in the lateral position. After needle insertion, needle aspiration should be performed to avoid inadvertent injection into the intrathecal or vascular space. Volumes of local anesthetic ranging from 0.75 to 1 mL/kg body weight of 0.25% bupivacaine should provide analgesia to the T10 level, which is sufficient for procedures in the groin and lower extremities. Although bupivacaine usually provides 4 to 6 hours of effective pain relief, children receiving caudal nerve blocks at the time of surgery exhibit better pain relief and use significantly fewer supplemental opioids during the first 12 postoperative hours.

As with other combined regional and general techniques, a relatively lighter plane of general anesthesia is required to maintain adequate surgical anesthesia when this block is instituted before the surgical incision, and this may represent an advantage over the use of a caudal block placed at the conclusion of the procedure. Blocks placed before surgical incisions also allow the patient to awaken more quickly and to benefit from a smoother emergence from general anesthesia.

Peripheral Nerve Blocks

General Considerations. Peripheral application of local anesthetics to block nociceptive neural transmission can be a useful adjunct in the treatment of acute postoperative pain. Although peripheral neural blocks are simple to perform and have a historical record of safety, the relatively short duration of analgesia and the selective nature of these blocks preclude their general application to all patient populations. With proper selection of the patient and the local anesthetic, the pain relief afforded by regional nerve blocks may be superior to that achievable with systemic opioids.

Mechanism of action of local anesthetics. The electrophysiology of local anesthetics is described in detail elsewhere in this textbook (see Chapter 17). Local anesthetics produce their neuronal blocking effect by diffusing across the nerve membrane and inhibiting sodium channels, thereby preventing the normal influx of sodium ions necessary for depolarization and nerve transmission. Thus, the membrane remains in its normal polarized state, and neither local miniature endplate potentials nor action potentials are generated.

Local Infiltration. Local infiltration, the instillation of local anesthetics in the vicinity of the surgical incision, is a simple technique for providing postoperative analgesia for the first several hours after a minor surgical procedure. Needle aspiration before injection should be performed to avoid intravascular injection or perforation of deep vascular structures. Even when blood has not been aspirated before injection, it is still possible for local anesthetic to be delivered intravascularly during a local infiltration. In addition to intravascular injection, exceeding recommended total volume and dosages of local anesthetic is another factor that can be responsible for untoward reactions.

The primary advantages of the local infiltration technique are simplicity and the ability to block afferent nerve activity in the area of the incision without affecting the general sensorium. A major disadvantage is the limited duration of analgesia, which usually lasts only several hours. The most commonly used local anesthetics for this procedure are bupivacaine and ropivacaine because of their long duration of effect compared with most other local anesthetics.

A special type of local infiltration is the intra-articular injection of local anesthetics after arthroscopic procedures. This technique decreases postoperative discomfort and facilitates postsurgical recuperation.[175] Bupivacaine is the most commonly used local anesthetic, with doses of 100 mg providing effective analgesia while maintaining serum concentrations below toxic levels.[175,176]

Intercostal. Intercostal nerve blocks are useful for providing analgesia after operations of the thorax and upper abdomen. A 22- or 25-gauge needle is advanced at the midaxillary or postaxillary line until a rib is contacted. The needle is then walked off the inferior border and advanced 1 mm. When performing intercostal blocks for large thoracic incisions, it is important to identify the sensory dermatomes supplying the surgical incision so each can be blocked. Dermatomes that supply the area where thoracostomy drainage tubes may be inserted should also be blocked. When abdominal incisions are large and lie in or extend across the midline, a large volume of local anesthetic is needed for optimal pain relief. Providing adequate analgesia for these types of incisions usually requires multiple bilateral intercostal nerve blocks. In general, postoperative pain management for abdominal surgery is better conducted with continuous epidural infusion of opioids or with opioid and local anesthetic solutions. An additional problem with intercostal nerve blocks is the potential for pneumothorax and respiratory compromise. Bupivacaine or bupivacaine with epinephrine is recommended for postsurgical pain relief with an intercostal nerve block. Intercostal blocks should be performed in the midaxillary or posterior axillary line. The site of the injection must be proximal or more posterior to the area of incision. This may occasionally present technical difficulties because the ribs tend to project more anteriorly as they approach the posterior midline. Adequate analgesia for a surgical incision usually requires application of local anesthetic to a minimum of two intercostal segments, and optimal analgesia usually requires that a minimum of three segments be blocked.

An alternative to the injection of local anesthetic on the intercostal nerve is the use of a cryoprobe, which is designed to produce local intercostal nerve freezing (cryoanalgesia).[177] This technique has been reported to produce reversible nerve disruption while preserving intraneural and peridural connective tissues. For optimal results, the cryoprobe should be applied on the intercostal nerve from within the chest by piercing the parietal pleura, and two to three levels above and below the incision should be blocked. Two to 3 weeks after cryoanalgesia, nerve function and structure begin to recover, with complete recovery occurring within 1 to 3 months. Advantages reported with this technique include a low incidence of neuritis or neuroma formation. Because of the extended period of postoperative analgesia, this technique is advantageous when prolonged effective postoperative analgesia is desirable, such as in the patient with chest trauma or significantly limited respiratory function.[178]

Ilioinguinal. An ilioinguinal nerve block is useful for pain relief after inguinal or femoral herniorrhaphy, appendectomy, or procedures involving the scrotum. A simple technique to perform ilioinguinal nerve block involves palpation of the anterior superior iliac spine.[179] Next, a position is located two fingerbreadths medial and two fingerbreadths superior until an imaginary line drawn from the anterosuperior iliac spine to the umbilicus is reached. At this point, a 22-gauge, 8.75-cm spinal needle is advanced perpendicular to the skin. The needle is advanced slowly and bounced every several millimeters until a paresthesia is elicited. This is indicative of needle contact with the fascia immediately outside the external oblique muscle pierced by the ilioinguinal nerve on its path to more superficial structures. Once the needle is in this location, 10 to 15 mL of local anesthetic is injected after aspiration. The needle is then withdrawn by several centimeters and redirected laterally until the tip reaches the medial edge of the anterior superior iliac spine. An additional 10 to 15 mL of local anesthetic solution is then injected. Complications of ilioinguinal nerve blocks include hemorrhage and hematoma at the injection site. Occasionally, numbness in the distribution of the lateral femoral cutaneous nerve can be demonstrated. Ilioinguinal nerve blocks are useful for acute postoperative analgesia after outpatient procedures such as inguinal herniorrhaphy.

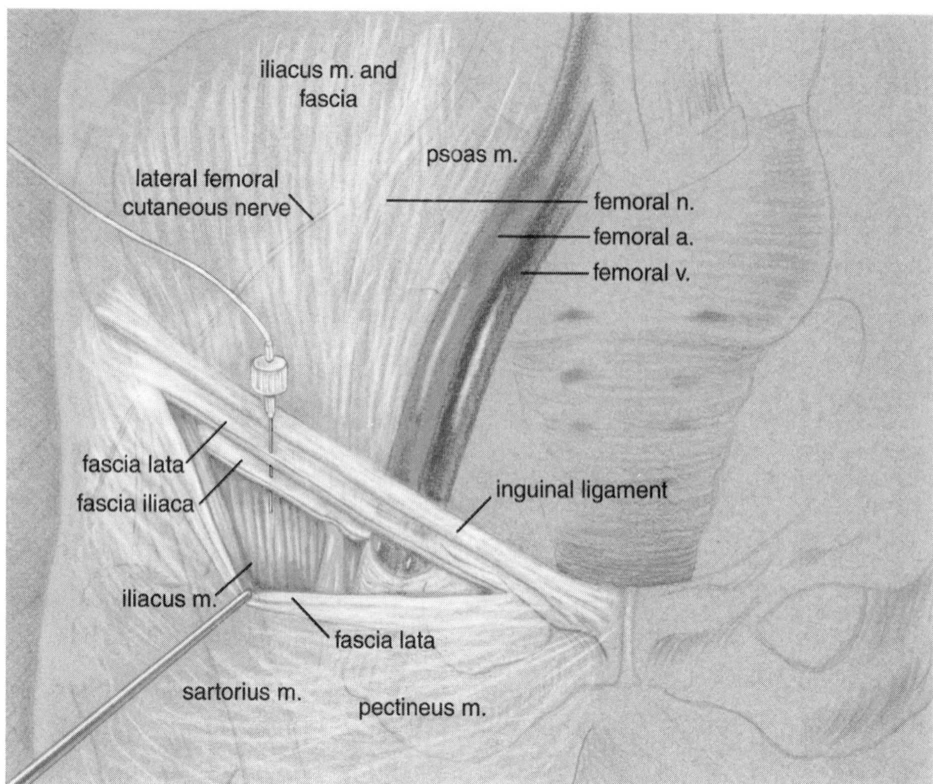

FIGURE 55-11. Anatomic relationships during fascia iliaca block.

Femoral Nerve Block/Fascia Iliaca Blocks

The increased use of new anticoagulant drugs following joint replacement has prompted the use of alternative peripheral regional nerve block techniques. The techniques of femoral nerve block (FNB) and fascia iliaca block (FIB) are particularly useful for managing pain from total knee arthroplasty. Either FNB or FIB technique may be used as a single injection or continuous catheter technique. The FIB is performed with the patient in the supine position. The site of needle entry is typically 1 cm below the junction of the lateral one-third and medial two-thirds of the inguinal ligament (running between the anterior superior iliac spine and the pubic symphysis medially). A 22-gauge, B bevel-type needle is advanced until two "pops" are felt as the needle traverses first the fascia lata and then fascia iliaca (Fig. 55-11). A volume of 20 to 30 mL of local anesthetic is injected after needle aspiration. The technique for a continuous FIB catheter technique is similar to the single injection technique, except that an 18-gauge epidural needle is advanced with a slight cephalad direction after the second "pop" is felt. A catheter is then threaded through the needle and advanced 5 to 6 cm. A stimulating catheter may aid in directional placement. Infusion of 0.2% ropivacaine or 0.25% bupivacaine (with or without clonidine 1.5 to 2 mcg/kg) up to 10 to 15 mL/hour generally provides adequate analgesia.

Penile. A penile nerve block performed with 0.25% bupivacaine can provide effective analgesia after circumcision or orchiopexy. Two techniques are described for performing this block. One involves injecting half of the volume of local anesthetic at the 10 o'clock position at the base of the penis, with the remainder at the 2 o'clock position. An alternative involves placing the local anesthetic in a ring of the subcutaneous tissue 360 degrees around the base of the penis. Epinephrine-containing local anesthetic should not be used for penile blocks because of the risk of vasoconstriction and ischemic necrosis of the skin.

Brachial Plexus. Continuous postoperative brachial plexus analgesia can be achieved using catheters placed by the infraclavicular, supraclavicular, axillary, or interscalene approach. A catheter-over-needle technique using an 18-gauge, 5-cm Teflon-coated intravenous catheter threaded over a 22-gauge, 8.75-cm spinal needle is one method. A nerve stimulator is essential to elicit paresthesias and identify when the neurovascular bundle is contacted. Another method for catheter placement uses the Seldinger technique. With this technique, the needle is positioned with the aid of a nerve stimulator, and after paresthesias are elicited, a guidewire is passed through the needle. Sterile alligator clips connected to the nerve stimulator can then be placed on the guidewire after the needle has been removed to confirm that the guidewire is still contacting the brachial plexus. A 20-gauge catheter is passed over the guidewire, which is then removed. For rapid sequential confirmation of correct catheter placement, the guidewire can be reinserted through the catheter at any time and a nerve stimulator used to determine if paresthesias can be elicited.

Postoperative brachial plexus analgesia has been described using bupivacaine 0.25% at rates ranging from 6 to 10 mL/hr. When infusion rates are maintained in this range, toxic serum levels are unlikely to occur. Application of this regimen does not preclude the use of any commonly used doses and volumes of local anesthetics currently recommended for surgical anesthesia with brachial plexus blockade. Patient-controlled interscalene brachial plexus analgesia has also been used in patients after shoulder surgery.[180] One disadvantage to this technique is postoperative catheter migration, and the infraclavicular and interscalene approaches may be better suited to continuous postoperative analgesia of the upper extremity because there tends to be less catheter migration than with the axillary approach.

Intrapleural. Intrapleural regional analgesia involves the percutaneous placement of a catheter in the thoracic cage between the visceral and parietal pleurae. The procedure is usually performed with the patient in the lateral decubitus position. An intercostal space between the fifth and tenth ribs is usually chosen, and a 17-gauge Touhy needle is inserted in the posterior axillary line over the superior aspect of the rib. A saline-lubricated glass syringe filled with 3 to 4 mL of air is attached to the needle, and the syringe and needle unit is advanced with the needle bevel directed in a cephalad direction. Once the pleural space is entered, the negative interpleural pressure draws the syringe plunger down in a manner analogous to the hanging drop technique of Gutierrez used for locating the epidural space. An epidural catheter may then be advanced 6 cm into the pleural space, rapidly to prevent the development of a clinically significant pneumothorax. If patients are mechanically ventilated, positive-pressure ventilation should be interrupted while the needle and catheter are being inserted to prevent injury to the pulmonary parenchyma. When patients are breathing spontaneously, the needle and catheter procedure should be performed during end exhalation.

Local anesthetics placed in the pleural cavity diffuse across the parietal pleura to the intercostal neurovascular bundle, producing a unilateral intercostal nerve block at multiple levels. A more extensive block may be achieved with placement of two catheters in the interpleural space. Interpleural analgesia using intermittent boluses of local anesthetic may be used to provide postoperative analgesia after upper abdominal surgical procedures, such as open cholecystectomy with subcostal incision and laparoscopic cholecystectomy. Effective postoperative pain relief requires intermittent intrapleural injections every 6 hours with approximately 20 mL of 0.25 to 0.5% bupivacaine. As in other intermittent bolus techniques, peaks and valleys in intrapleural analgesia occur when sequential doses are separated by hours.

Intrapleural analgesia may be less effective for postthoracotomy pain than after other procedures in which the pleura is intact, and there are no pleural drainage tubes to divert the local anesthetic from its site of action. Certain intercostal incisions, particularly those used for anterior thoracotomies, require that pleural drainage tubes be clamped for a short time after each intermittent local anesthetic injection to allow the local anesthetic to cross the parietal pleura and provide effective analgesia. Intermittent clamping of the pleural drainage tube after injection of the local anesthetic may not be tolerated in patients with a moderate or large air leak from the pulmonary parenchyma after thoracotomy. The risk of pneumothorax and the problems of fluctuating levels of analgesia with intermittent dosing of intrapleural catheters suggest that other techniques, such as continuous thoracic epidural analgesia, may be preferable after thoracotomy when there is an anterior intercostal incision.[181,182]

Other Modalities

Psychological Interventions for Postoperative Analgesia

The use of various analgesic techniques involving nerve blocks and opioids applied to the central neuraxis and administered by intravenous infusions has produced dramatic changes in the management of pain. Nevertheless, it is sometimes necessary to augment these techniques with various psychological interventions. Psychological interventions are used widely in the treatment of chronic pain, and the benefit of these behavioral strategies for the management of acute pain is now recognized. This often involves approaching the treatment of pain on a cognitive basis and using interventions such as distraction or imagery that attempt to focus attention away from the painful event. Other, simpler methods consist of educating patients about their surroundings, disease state, treatment plans, and the hospital environment in an effort to reduce fear and anxiety about unknown events or situations in the perioperative period. Despite the banality of this approach, it is a frequently overlooked element when dealing with patients who often are unfamiliar with the hospital environment. Other psychological interventions that may be effective are relaxation techniques such as deep breathing exercises or muscle relaxation training, which can reduce anxiety and muscle tension.

ORGANIZATION OF A POSTOPERATIVE ANALGESIA SERVICE

6 With the increasing number and complexity of modalities for treating postoperative pain, it is logical that an organized, systematic approach involving all members of the health care team has evolved in the form of the postoperative analgesia service. The anesthesiologist is uniquely qualified to lead this team because of his or her knowledge of the neurophysiology, pathophysiology, pharmacology, and anatomic pathways involved in the modulation of acute pain. Furthermore, with the postoperative analgesia service under the direction of the anesthesiologist, continuity of pain care management is enhanced because the anesthesiologist is routinely involved in the preoperative assessment, intraoperative management, and postoperative follow-up of surgical patients. Because anesthesiologists are the logical choice for managing the postoperative analgesia service, it is desirable that each department of anesthesiology assume responsibility for organizing and maintaining efficient operation of the service.

When initiating a postoperative analgesia service (e.g., physician, pharmacologist, nursing, psychologist), it is essential that the department of anesthesiology have one or more members who will assume the position of director or codirector. This ensures at least one person will be responsible for communication with the pharmacy, nursing, and surgical departments, development of policy and procedural protocols, and departmental representation when issues concerning postoperative pain management arise.

The delivery of central neuraxial opioid analgesia requires cooperation among the anesthesiology, nursing, surgery, and pharmacy staffs. Success of such an interdisciplinary program for postoperative analgesia often requires significant flexibility to satisfy the needs of all parties concerned. Each institution must identify the approach that is practical and most beneficial for its patients after considering available resources. With these considerations, protocols that reflect individual practice patterns can be effectively developed. These protocols should include written policy and procedure manuals for nursing staff (see Appendices 55-2 and 55-4), as well as preprinted epidural analgesia orders (see Appendix 55-3). Postoperative pain relief has generated intense interest and fostered the introduction of several new analgesic modalities. Although these techniques have been shown to provide better pain relief than conventional intramuscular administration of opioids, the complexity of these modalities requires the use of an organized approach to maximize efficacy while minimizing potentially adverse effects. The transition phase from the operating room to the recovery area, and then to the patient ward, is a crucial period for intervention by the postoperative analgesia service. Optimization of analgesia (while the effects of anesthesia are dissipating) and potential reduction in the incidence or severity of side effects requires proactive evaluation and management in the recovery area by personnel trained and dedicated to these aspects of patient care.

When formulating the strategy for development and initiation of an epidural analgesia service, consideration must be given to the choice of continuous infusion techniques, intermittent bolus regimens, or combinations of these methods. In addition, with the use of PCA devices, similar protocols outlining the initial parameters for starting therapy should be established to facilitate effective use when these devices are prescribed (see Table 55-7).

The basic goals of the postoperative analgesia service are (1) administering and monitoring postoperative analgesia, and (2) identifying and managing complications or side effects of postoperative analgesic techniques. Implicit in these goals is the inclusion of an active quality assurance program directed at maintaining high-quality patient care while minimizing complications. When the postoperative analgesia service is managed by anesthesiologists, quality assurance monitoring can be applied to the heterogeneous surgical population so the goals of pain management can be refined for the individual patient. This is much more difficult to achieve when individual surgical services are charged with the management of postoperative pain. Nonetheless, successful implementation of these principles requires the cooperation and involvement of health care providers outside the department of anesthesiology, such as surgeons, nurses, and pharmacy personnel.

The foundation of an effective postoperative analgesia service is based on education of all members of the interdisciplinary health care team. This educational process must begin within the department of anesthesiology and, optimally, be directed by physicians with special qualifications in pain medicine and regional anesthesia. A corollary of this educational process is the use of a standardized approach to the initiation of pain management, which may include choices among fixed medication protocols, algorithms to identify and treat inadequate analgesia, and preprinted postoperative orders. The use of such methods increases efficiency, serves as a guideline for health care providers involved with the postoperative analgesia service, and gives the postoperative analgesia service team the flexibility to individualize therapy. This approach also facilitates the education of ancillary personnel, such as nursing staff, necessary to the functioning of the service.

Ideally, all members of each anesthesia department should become well versed in the basic principles necessary for the day-to-day operation of the postoperative analgesia service. Although its management usually is the responsibility of a limited number of anesthesia personnel, education of all members of the department ensures the smooth operation of the service when those key individuals are not available after hours or on weekends. Although patients receiving postoperative analgesia should be seen on a regular basis by the anesthesiologist, it may be necessary for nurse clinicians or anesthesiology residents to assist in performing these functions if the service is very large. It is the responsibility of the anesthesiologist to educate these individuals in the principles of pain management. Nurse clinicians often have excellent rapport with other nursing staff and can act as effective liaisons. In addition, nurse clinicians can facilitate the operation of the postoperative analgesia service by performing tasks such as charting daily progress notes, inspecting epidural catheter sites, removing epidural catheters when therapy is discontinued, notifying the anesthesiologist of any problems pertaining to pain management, and collecting patient data to facilitate quality assurance. The participation of anesthesiology residents in the postoperative analgesia service allows them to gain knowledge and expertise in this area of perioperative care. Depending on the size of the surgical population and the scope of the service, additional support may be required from clinical pharmacologists, nurse anesthetists, psychologists, or other physicians. Developing this solid foundation is an important consideration when establishing a postoperative analgesia service.

In addition to 24-hour per day support from the anesthesia department, a successful postoperative analgesia service requires the cooperation and education of nursing staff so they are responsive to the needs of the patients. In-service training of hospital nurses requires instruction in the principles of analgesic techniques, including appropriate aspects of neuroanatomy, neuropsychopharmacology, side effects and their treatment, monitoring skills, analgesia assessment, and the technical aspects of the operation of PCA and epidural infusion devices. This instruction should also be conducted under the supervision of the anesthesiologist in charge of the postoperative analgesia service, but may also involve a clinical nurse specialist, trained by the anesthesiology department, who may assist in solving nursing problems related to the operation of the service. To minimize dosing and medication errors, and to improve patient comfort by early treatment of inadequate analgesia and complications such as pruritus, nurses must understand the use of the standardized protocols.

One additional benefit of such a model is the ability to transition patients from epidural or PCA techniques to oral or other analgesia delivery systems, facilitating postoperative discharge. This can usually be accomplished for most surgical patients by converting from the parenteral techniques to an orally administered acetaminophen–hydrocodone or acetaminophen–codeine preparation. However, some patients experience difficulty with transition from parenteral therapy and require more potent opioids and other nonopioid adjuvants. Such patients have typically received opioids chronically for pain and have higher analgesic requirements to achieve satisfactory postoperative pain control.[165] Because of their experience with the principles and use of the more potent, longer-acting oral opioid preparations (in the setting of chronic pain management), anesthesiologists can facilitate the management of this complicated set of patients. For example, combining sustained-release forms of long-duration drugs such as oxycodone or morphine sulfate every 6 to 12 hours can be effective in the transition from parenteral analgesic therapy. Using such an approach, this transition may be accomplished more efficiently and potentially hastens postsurgical discharge in patients who have received opioids chronically for pain.

Another key aspect to the initiation of a postoperative analgesia service is the identification of patient populations that are most likely to benefit from improved postoperative pain management. Patients undergoing thoracic and upper abdominal procedures, major orthopaedic operations such as hip surgery, and high-risk vascular surgical procedures are examples of groups in whom effective postoperative pain management produces the most rewarding results. It is often useful to consider a pilot program using PCA or epidural analgesia when surgeons are doubtful or hesitant about the efficacy of these methods. After the utility of the postoperative analgesia service has been demonstrated to surgeons, referring physicians, and others, the service can expand logically to patient populations in which improved analgesia will be obvious, but in which the effects on outcome may be more subtle. Initiation of the service in any subset of patients also requires the education of surgical staff regarding (1) the advantages to their practice of being able to offer patients surgery with less postoperative discomfort, and (2) the potential differences in outcome when using certain methods of postoperative analgesia. Despite the lack of large-scale, randomized studies to demonstrate that improved postoperative analgesia (especially the use of epidural analgesia in high-risk patients) is definitively associated with improved outcomes (such as shorter, less expensive hospital stays, with fewer major complications), there is more than enough evidence currently in the literature to support the important role of epidural anesthesia and analgesia in clinical practice. Surgeons must understand that their patients will receive attentive care and that an essential element of the postoperative analgesia service is the maintenance of a cooperative spirit among disciplines.

Once the appropriate subsets of patients have been identified and educated, the physicians in charge of initiating the postoperative analgesia service must make plans for the provision of the capital resources necessary to operate the service. Plans must be made regarding types of equipment needed for continuous or patient-controlled intravenous catheter or epidural analgesia, whether such devices are to be rented or purchased, types of monitoring equipment deemed necessary, any pharmacy-related factors necessary to prepare solutions of drugs for administration, and the printing of standard orders for the postoperative management of pain and treatment of complications. Decisions regarding funding sources for these capital expenses often must involve discussions with hospital administrators. In the present medical-economic climate, hospital administrators may be opposed to the purchase of new equipment if old methods appear to be functional. It is important to educate administrators who are reluctant to support the concept of a postoperative analgesia service about the potential benefits to some patients in terms of shorter, less complicated, less expensive hospital stays. Not only can the service be cost effective, but sometimes it can be used by hospital administrators as a marketing tool to attract surgical patients. Preprinted order forms usually require approval from the hospital's medical records/forms department. Job descriptions and resources are necessary to define and fund support staff such as nurse clinicians, psychologists, or clinical pharmacologists. Thus, a significant degree of planning, effort, and commitment is necessary to initiate a properly functioning postoperative analgesia service. When such efforts are expended, the establishment of such a service allows the anesthesiologist to play an important role in the postoperative period and to provide a valuable service to patients.

SPECIAL CONSIDERATIONS IN PEDIATRIC ACUTE PAIN MANAGEMENT

Acute pain management in the pediatric patient poses a unique challenge to the anesthesiologist. It is often more difficult to evaluate pain intensity in children because the expression of pain is manifested over a broad emotional spectrum. For instance, some children withdraw and become nonverbal with the onset of pain, whereas others become emotionally labile, with crying, screaming, and violent behavior. Psychological distress is often compounded in children by separation from their parents and by inadequate understanding of their disease and its treatment. Furthermore, depending on age, lack of cognitive development makes it more difficult to communicate relevant concepts to children. In view of these difficulties, a useful monitor of analgesic efficacy in children is behavior observation. Some behavior such as crying can be easily understood, but social withdrawal and the inability to be distracted often indicate that a young patient has distressing pain.

The selection and dosing of analgesic agents also requires special attention in the pediatric patient (Table 55-12). Neonates and infants, because of immature hepatic function and reduced plasma proteins and plasma protein-binding capacity, exhibit a higher fraction of free drug in the central compartment. This effect is offset to some degree by the higher total body water and extracellular fluid, and larger blood volume in this group compared with adults. Increased susceptibility to the respiratory depressant component of opioids may be a result of the increased fraction of cardiac output to the developing brain or of reduced metabolic pathways, leading to accumulation of opioids and their metabolites. Morphine exhibits an increase in half-life and respiratory depressant effect in infants younger than 1 month of age, owing to immature glucuronidation pathways. The half-lives of meperidine and fentanyl are similarly increased during the first 3 months of life. The pharmacokinetics of local anesthetics exhibit a similar pattern of development in neonates and infants. Free fractions of local anesthetics approach those seen in adults by 6 months of age (Table 55-13).

Oral Analgesics

Nonopioid

NSAIDs are useful oral drugs for acute postoperative pain management in the pediatric population. Ibuprofen can be administered at 6- to 8-hour intervals in doses of 8 mg/kg. Contraindications to the use of NSAIDs in the pediatric population are similar to those in adults. The most frequently encountered adverse effects are gastrointestinal. Platelet function alteration can occur with non–COX-2 agents, but this is usually not a significant clinical problem after short-term administration in the postoperative period. Acetaminophen has fewer side effects than ibuprofen and can be administered in doses of 5 to 15 mg/kg orally or 20 mg/kg rectally every 4 to 6 hours. Ketorolac in doses of 0.4 to 1.0 mg/kg is also useful for mild to moderate postoperative pain in children when parenteral administration is desirable, but may be associated with a greater incidence of vomiting than morphine.[183,184]

Opioid

Codeine in combination with acetaminophen is a commonly used oral preparation for moderate postoperative pain in the pediatric population. The recommended oral dosage range is 0.5 to 1 mg/kg every 4 to 6 hours. Internationally, tramadol 1 to 2 mg/kg every 6 hours PRN has been used for pain in pediatric patients.

Patient-Controlled Analgesia

PCA is an opioid delivery system that has been used with increasing frequency to treat acute postoperative pain in children. Morphine sulfate given as a loading dose of 0.1 to 0.2 mg/kg and administered as small incremental boluses of 0.01 to 0.03 mg/kg can be used to initiate PCA therapy. After this, maintenance doses of morphine sulfate (0.01 to 0.015 mg/kg) given every 6 to 10 minutes with a 4-hour limit of 0.25 mg/kg are appropriate. Incorporation of a continuous infusion (0.01 to 0.015 mg/kg/h) into the regimen may be beneficial.[185] Smaller doses of morphine may be used if ketorolac is used in conjunction with PCA.[186] Meperidine maintenance doses of 0.15 to 0.20 mg/kg with a 4-hour limit of 2 to 3 mg/kg has been used but may be associated with neurotoxic side effects.

Epidural Opioids

Similar to other methods of pain control, the use of epidural opioids has not been extensively studied in the pediatric population. Lumbar epidural analgesia has been used for young patients undergoing abdominal, urologic, or orthopaedic procedures. Because lumbar epidural catheters may be more difficult to place in the pediatric patient than in adults, an alternative is to perform a "kiddie caudal" with a mixture of local anesthetic and opioid for postoperative analgesia. Morphine is the preferable drug for single-injection techniques and can be administered as a 0.05 mg/kg bolus in volumes appropriate for the age and weight of the child.[175] Additional information on caudal analgesia is reported in earlier sections of this chapter.

TABLE 55-12

PHARMACOLOGIC CONSIDERATIONS FOR PEDIATRIC PATIENTS

DRUG	DOSE (Age > 6 mo)[a]	INTERVAL (hr)	ROUTE	COMMENTS
NONOPIOID				
Acetaminophen	5–15 mg/kg	4–6	PO	Overdose may cause hepatotoxicity
Ibuprofen	20 mg/kg	4–6	Rectal	
Naproxen	8 mg/kg	6	PO	
	5 mg/kg	8–12	PO	
OPIOID				
Codeine	0.5–1 mg/kg	4–6	PO	Most commonly combined with acetaminophen
Oxycodone	0.005–0.15 mg/kg	4–6	PO	Similar to codeine
		3–4	IM	May cause less constipation, ileus, and urinary retention than morphine
Meperidine	1–1.5 mg/kg	2–3	IV	
	0.8–1 mg/kg	3–4	IM	
Morphine	0.1–0.15 mg/kg	2	IV	
	0.08–0.1 mg/kg	12–24	IV	
	0.05–0.06 mg/kg	12–24	EPI	
	50 μg/kg	12–24	EPI	Continuous infusion
	120–150μg/kg	1–2	Caudal	Abdominal surgery
	50–100 μg/kg		IV	Thoracic surgery
Fentanyl	1–1.5 mg/kg		IV	Diluted in equal volume of normal saline
	2–4 μg/kg/hr			Minimum age, 1 yr
				Continuous infusion

[a]Fractionation of dose is recommended for age < 6 mo.
Caudal, S4–S5; EPI, epidural (L3–L5); IM, intramuscular; IV, intravenous: PO, by mouth.

RELATIONSHIP BETWEEN ACUTE (EUDYNIA) AND CHRONIC PAIN (MALDYNIA)

For an individual patient, the development of a chronic pain syndrome may simply be the extension of inadequately treated acute pain after trauma or surgery. Differentiation between acute (eudynia as a symptom) and chronic pain (maldynia as a syndrome) is important in clinical practice because therapy usually is vastly different. Pain persisting longer than 30 days can be viewed as chronic pain. Acute pain management techniques usually are not effective and may cause other problems when applied to chronic pain. For instance, systemic opioids for long-term use are often associated with the development of tolerance and, occasionally, drug dependency. Chronic pain is not simply the extension of acute pain as an isolated entity but involves multiple additional factors such as altered mechanisms of nociceptive modulation, and centralization and amplification of neural responses that account for the differences in clinical presentation and, more importantly, in choice of therapeutic modality.

TABLE 55-13

MAXIMUM LOCAL ANESTHETIC DOSES IN INFANTS AND CHILDREN

DRUG	INFANT DOSE (mg/kg): AGE	CHILD DOSE (mg/kg)
Lidocaine (plain)	5: from birth on	5
Lidocaine (epinephrine)	7: from birth on	7
Mepivacaine	4: <6 mo	5
Bupivacaine (plain)	2: <3 mo	3
Bupivacaine (epinephrine)	2: <3 mo	4
Chloroprocaine (plain)	4: <6 mo	8
Chloroprocaine (epinephrine)	5: <6 mo	10

Reprinted with permission from Vetter TR: Acute pediatric pain management. Adv Anesth 8:29, 1991.

SUMMARY

This chapter reviews the physiology of nociception and the production of acute postoperative pain, as well as compares and contrastes various methods for analgesia. In addition, the rationale behind the development of a multidisciplinary team of health care personnel aimed at managing postoperative pain has been addressed. Postoperative pain management requires continued study to refine, explore, and open new avenues for further improvement of current techniques.

References

1. Sorkin L, Wallace MS: Acute pain mechanisms. Surg Clin North Am 79:213, 1999
2. Erlanger J, Gasser HS: The compound nature of the action current of nerve as disclosed by cathode ray oscillograph. Am J Physiol 70:624, 1924
3. de Jong RH: Function and diameter of nerve fiber. In de Jong RH (ed): Physiology and Pharmacology of Local Anesthesia, p 97. Springfield, IL, Charles C Thomas, 1970

4. Guyton AC: Sensory receptors: Neuronal circuits for processing information. In Guyton AC (ed): Textbook of Physiology, 8th ed, p 495. Philadelphia, WB Saunders, 1991
5. Kerr FWL: The structured basis of pain: Circulatory and pathway. In Ng LWY, Bonica JJ (eds): Pain, Discomfort and Humanitarian Care, p 49. New York, Elsevier, 1980
6. Caterina MJ, Julius D: The vanilloid receptor: A molecular gateway to the pain pathway. Annu Rev Neurosci 24:487, 2001
7. Waxamn SG, Cummins TR, Dib-Hajj SD, Black JA: Voltage-gated sodium channels and the molecular pathogenesis of pain: A review. J Rehabil Res Dev 37:517, 2000
8. Wood JN, Akopian AN, Baker M *et al*: Sodium channels in primary sensory neurons: Relationship to pain states. Novartis Found Symp 241:159, 2002
9. Lai J, Porreca F, Hunter JC *et al*: Voltage-gated sodium channels and hyperalgesia. Annu Rev Pharmacol Toxicol 44:371, 2004
10. Dougherty PM, Staats PS: Intrathecal drug therapy for chronic pain. Anesthesiology 91:1891, 1999
11. Henry JL: Effects of substance P on functionally identified units in cat spinal cord. Brain Res 114:439, 1976
12. Ebersberger A, Grubb BD, Willingale HL *et al*: The intraspinal release of prostaglandin E2 in a model of acute arthritis is accompanied by an up-regulation of cyclo-oxygenase-2 in the spinal cord. Neuroscience 93:775, 1999
13. Harvey RJ, Depner UB, Wassle H *et al*: GlyR α3: An essestial target for spinal PGE2-mediated inflammatory pain sensitization. Science 304:884, 2004
14. Gilbert PG, Askmark H: Changes in cholinergic and opioid receptors in the rat spinal cord, dorsal root and sciatic nerve after ventral and dorsal root lesion. J Neural Transm 85:31, 1991
15. Barber RP, Phelps PE, Houser CR *et al*: The morphology and distribution of neurons containing choline acetyltransferase in the adult rat spinal cord: An immunocytochemical study. J Comp Neurol 229:329, 1984
16. Ribeiro-Da-Silva A, Cuello AC: Choline acetyltransferase-immunoreactive profiles are presynaptic to primary sensory fibers in the rat superficial dorsal horn. J Comp Neurol 295:370, 1990
17. Iwamoto ET, Marion L: Characterization of the antinociception produced by intrathecally administered muscarinic agonists in rats. J Pharmacol Exp Ther 266:329, 1993
18. Hood DD, Eisenach JC, Tuttle R: Phase I safety assessment of intrathecal neostigmine methylsulfate in humans. Anesthesiology 82:331, 1995
19. Naguib M, Yaksh TL: Characterization of muscarinic receptor subtypes that mediate antinociception in the rat spinal cord. Anesth Analg 85:847, 1997
20. Treede R-D, Meyer RA, Raja SN, Cambell JN: Peripheral and central mechanisms of cutaneous hyperalgesia. Prog Neurobiol 38:397, 1992
21. Thompson SWN, King AE, Woolf CJ: Activity-dependent changes in rat ventral horn neurons in vitro, summation of prolonged afferent evoked depolarizations produce a D-2-amino-5-phosphonovaleric acid sensitive windup. Eur J Neurosci 2:638, 1990
22. Pockett S: Spinal cord plasticity and chronic pain. Anesth Analg 80:173, 1995
23. Urban L, Randic M: Slow excitatory transmission in rat dorsal horn: Possible mediation by peptides. Brain Res 290:336, 1992
24. Nagy J, Maggi CA, Dray A *et al*: The role of neurokinin and N-methyl-s-aspartate receptors in synaptic transmission from capsaicin sensitive primary afferents in the rat spinal cord in vitro. Neuroscience 52:1029, 1993
25. Sun RQ, Tu YJ, Lawand NB *et al*: Calcitonin gene-related peptide receptor activation produces PKA- and PKC-dependent mechanical hyperalgesia and central sensitization. J Neurophysiol 92:2859, 2004
26. Pezet S, Malcangio M, McMahon SB: BDNF: A neuromodulator in nociceptive pathways? Brain Res Brain Res Rev 40:240, 2002
27. Merighi A, Carmignoto G, Gobbo S *et al*: Neurotrophins in spinal cord nociceptive pathways. Prog Brain Res 146:291, 2004
28. Zahn PK, Brennan TJ: Incisional-induced changes in receptive field properties of rat dorsal horn neurons. Anesthesiology 91:772, 1999
29. Zahn PK, Brennan TJ: Primary and secondary hyperalgesia in a rat model for human postoperative pain. Anesthesiology 91:863, 1999
30. Hosobuchi Y, Adams JE, Linchitz R: Pain relief by electrical stimulation of central grey matter in humans and its reversal by naloxone. Science 197:183, 1977
31. Yaksh TL: Multiple opioid receptor systems in brain and spinal cord: Part 2. Eur J Anesthesiol 1:201, 1984
32. Zieglgansberger W, Tulloch IF: The effects of methionine and leucine-enkephalin on spinal neurones of the cat. Brain Res 167:53, 1979
33. Camarata PJ, Yaksh TL: Characterization of the spinal adrenergic receptors mediating the spinal effects produced by microinjection of morphine into the periaqueductal gray. Brain Res 336:133, 1985
34. Reddy SV, Maderdrut JL, Yaksh TL: Spinal cord pharmacology of adrenergic agonist mediated antinociception. J Pharmacol Exp Ther 213:525, 1980
35. Maze M, Tranquilli W: Alpha-2 adrenoreceptor agonists: Defining the role in clinical anesthesia. Anesthesiology 74:581, 1991
36. Sabbe MB, Yaksh TL: Pharmacology of spinal opioids. J Pain Symptom Manage 5:191, 1990
37. Weissman C: The metabolic response to stress: An overview and update. Anesthesiology 73:308, 1990
38. Hagen C, Brandt MR, Kehlet H: Prolactin, LH, FSH, GH and cortisol response to surgery and the effect of epidural analgesia. Acta Endocrinol (Copenh) 94:151, 1980
39. Michie HR, Wilmore DW: Sepsis, signals, and surgical sequelae (a hypothesis). Arch Surg 125:531, 1990
40. Levin JD, Coderne JS, Basbaum AI: The peripheral nervous system and the inflammatory process. In Dubner R, Gebhart GF, Bond MR (eds): Proceedings of the Vth World Congress on Pain, p 33. Amsterdam, Elsevier Science, 1988
41. Marano MA, Fong Y, Moldawer LL *et al*: Serum cachectin/tumor necrosis factor in critically ill patients with burns correlates with infection and mortality. Surg Gynecol Obstet 170:32, 1990
42. Chernow B, Alexander HR, Smallridge RC *et al*: Hormonal responses to graded surgical stress. Arch Intern Med 147:1273, 1987
43. Lee DD, Kimura S, DeQuattro V: Noradenergic activity and silent ischemia in hypertensive patients with stable angina: Effect of metoprolol. Lancet 1:403, 1989
44. Rawal N, Sjostrand U, Christoffersson E *et al*: Comparison of intramuscular and epidural morphine for postoperative analgesia in the grossly obese: Influence on postoperative ambulation and pulmonary function. Anesth Analg 63:583, 1984
45. Rademaker BM, Ringers J, Oddom JA *et al*: Pulmonary function and stress response after laparoscopic cholecystectomy: Comparison with subcostal incision and influence of thoracic epidural analgesia. Anesth Analg 75:381, 1992
46. Livingston E, Passaro E: Postoperative ileus. Dig Dis Sci 35:121, 1990
47. Moore FA, Feliciano DV, Andeassy RJ *et al*: Early enteral feeding, compared with parenteral, reduces postoperative septic complications. Ann Surg 216:172, 1992
48. Saol M: Effects of anesthesia and surgery on the immune response. Acta Anaesthesiol Scand 36:201, 1992
49. Toft P, Svendsen P, Tonnesen E *et al*: Redistribution of lymphocytes after major surgical stress. Acta Anaesthesiol Scand 37:245, 1993
50. Davis JM, Albert JD, Tracy KJ *et al*: Increased neutrophil mobilization and decreased chemotaxis during cortisol and epinephrine infusion. J Trauma 31:725, 1991
51. Akca O, Melischek M, Scheck T: Postoperative pain and subcutaneous oxygen tension [Letter]. Lancet 354:41, 1999
52. Pollock RE, Lotzoua E, Stanford SD: Mechanism of surgical stress impairment of human perioperative natural killer cell cytotoxicity. Arch Surg 126:338, 1991
53. Tuman KJ, McCarthy RJ, March RJ *et al*: Effects of epidural anesthesia and analgesia on coagulation and outcome after major vascular surgery. Anesth Analg 73:696, 1991
54. Rosenfeld BA, Beattie C, Christopherson R *et al*: The effects of different anesthetic regimens on fibrinolysis and the development of postoperative arterial thrombosis. Anesthesiology 79:435, 1993
55. Breslow MJ, Parker SD, Frank SM *et al*: Determinants of catecholamine and cortisol responses to lower-extremity revascularization. Anesthesiology 79:1202, 1993
56. Rosenfeld BA, Faraday N, Campbell D *et al*: Hemostatic effects of stress hormone infusion. Anesthesiology 81:1116, 1994
57. Oyama T: Influence of anesthesia on the endocrine system. In Stoeckel H, Oyama T (eds): Endocrinology in Anaesthesia and Surgery, p 39. New York, Springer-Verlag, 1980
58. Roizen MF, Horrigan RW, Frazer BM: Anesthetic doses blocking adrenergic (stress) and cardiovascular response to incision: MAC BAR. Anesthesiology 54:390, 1981
59. Kehlet H: Modification of response to surgery by neural blockade: Clinical implications. In Cousins MJ, Bridenbaugh PO (eds): Neural Blockade in Clinical Anesthesia and Management of Pain, p 129. Philadelphia, Lippincott-Raven, 1998
60. Kehlet H: Acute pain control and accelerated postoperative recovery. Surg Clin North Am 79:431, 1999
61. Moeller IW, Rem J, Brandt MR, Kehlet H: Effect of posttraumatic epidural analgesia on the cortisol and hyperglycemic response to surgery. Acta Anaesthesiol Scand 26:56, 1980
62. Cosgrove DO, Jenkins JS: The effect of epidural anaesthesia on the pituitary-adrenal response to surgery. Clin Sci Mol Med 46:403, 1974
63. Baron JF, Coriat P, Mundler O *et al*: Left ventricular global and regional function during lumbar epidural anesthesia in patients with and without angina pectoris: Influence of volume loading. Anesthesiology 66:621, 1987
64. Blomberg S, Curelaru I, Emanuelsson H *et al*: Thoracic epidural anaesthesia in patients with unstable angina pectoris. Eur Heart J 10:437, 1989
65. Davis R, DeBoer LWV, Maroko PR: Thoracic epidural analgesia reduces myocardial infarct size after coronary artery occlusion in dogs. Anesth Analg 65:711, 1986
66. Kataja J: Thoracolumbar anesthesia and isoflurane to prevent hypertension and tachycardia in patients undergoing abdominal aortic surgery. Eur J Anaesthesiol 8:427, 1991
67. Breslow MJ, Jordan DA, Christopherson R *et al*: Epidural morphine decreases postoperative hypertension by attenuating sympathetic nervous system hyperactivity. JAMA 261:3577, 1989
68. Yeager MP, Glass DD, Neff RK, Brinck-Johnsen T: Epidural anesthesia and analgesia in high-risk surgical patients. Anesthesiology 66:729, 1987
69. Baron JF, Bertrand M, Barre E *et al*: Combined epidural and general anesthesia versus general anesthesia for abdominal aortic surgery. Anesthesiology 75:611, 1991

70. Hjortso NC, Neumann P, Frosig F *et al*: A controlled study on the effect of epidural analgesia with local anaesthetics and morphine on morbidity after abdominal surgery. Acta Anaesthesiol Scand 29:705, 1985
71. Christopherson R, Beattie C, Frank SM *et al*: Perioperative morbidity in patients randomized to epidural or general anesthesia for lower-extremity vascular surgery. Anesthesiology 79:422, 1993
72. McDaniel MD, Pearce WH, Yao JS *et al*: Sequential changes in coagulation and platelet function following femorotibial bypass. J Vasc Surg 1:261, 1984
73. Lichtenfeld K, Schiffer D, Helrich M: Platelet aggregation during and after general anesthesia and surgery. Anesth Analg 58:293, 1979
74. Modig J, Borg T, Bagge L, Saldeen T: Role of extradural and of general anesthesia in fibrinolysis and coagulation after total hip replacement. Br J Anaesth 55:625, 1983
75. Modig J, Malberg P, Karlstrom G: Effect of epidural versus general anesthesia on calf blood flow. Acta Anaesthesiol Scand 24:305, 1980
76. Jorgensen L, Rasmussen L, Nielsen P *et al*: Antithrombotic efficacy of continuous extradural analgesia after knee replacement. Br J Anaesth 66:8, 1991
77. Hendolin H, Mattila MAK, Poikolainen E: The effect of lumbar epidural analgesia on the development of deep vein thrombosis of the legs after open prostatectomy. Acta Chir Scand 147:425, 1981
78. Cuschieri RJ, Morran CG, Howie JC, McArdle CS: Postoperative pain and pulmonary complications: Comparison of three analgesic regimens. Br J Surg 72:495, 1985
79. Hedolin H, Lahtinen J, Länsimies E *et al*: The effect of thoracic epidural analgesia on respiratory function after cholecystectomy. Acta Anaesthesiol Scand 31:645, 1983
80. Bromage PR, Camporessi E, Chestnut D: Epidural narcotics for postoperative analgesia. Anesth Analg 59:473, 1980
81. Shulman M, Sandler AN, Bradley JW *et al*: Postthoracotomy pain and pulmonary function following epidural and systemic morphine. Anesthesiology 61:569, 1984
82. Pansard J-L, Mankikian B, Bertrand M *et al*: Effects of thoracic extradural block on diaphragmatic electrical activity and contractility after upper abdominal surgery. Anesthesiology 78:63, 1993
83. Mankikian B, Cantineau JP, Bertrand M *et al*: Improvement of diaphragmatic function by a thoracic extradural block after upper abdominal surgery. Anesthesiology 68:379, 1988
84. Simonneau G, Vivien A, Saberne R *et al*: Diaphragm dysfunction induced by upper abdominal surgery: Role of postoperative pain. Am Rev Respir Dis 128:899, 1983
85. Wheatley R, Somerville I, Sapsford D, Jones J: Postoperative hypoxaemia: Comparison of extradural, I.M., and patient-controlled analgesia. Br J Anaesth 64:267, 1990
86. Kehlet H, Dahl JB: The value of multi-modal or balanced analgesia in postoperative pain relief. Anesth Analg 77:1048, 1993
87. Schulze S, Roikjaer O, Hasselstrøm L *et al*: Epidural bupivacaine and morphine plus systemic indomethacin eliminates pain but not systemic response and convalescence after choleystectomy. Surgery 103:321, 1988
88. Jayr C, Thomas H, Rey A *et al*: Postoperative pulmonary complications: Epidural analgesia using bupivacaine and opioids versus parenteral opioids. Anesthesiology 78:666, 1993
89. Jayr C, Mollie A, Bourgain JL *et al*: General anesthesia with postoperative parenteral morphine compared with epidural analgesia. Surgery 104:57, 1987
90. Ferreira SH: Prostaglandins hyperalgesia and the control of inflammatory pain. In Bonta IL, Bray MA, Parnham MJ (eds): Handbook of Inflammation, Vol 5: The Pharmacology of Inflammation, p 108. New York, Elsevier, 1985
91. Malberg AB, Yaksh TL: Hyperalgesia mediated by spinal glutamate substance P receptor blocked by spinal cyclooxygenase inhibition. Science 257:28, 1992
92. Ferreira SH: Prostaglandins: Peripheral and central analgesia. Adv Pain Res Ther 5:627, 1983
93. Hawkey CJ: COX-2 inhibitors. Lancet 353:307, 1999
94. Ehrich EW, Dallob A, DeLepeleire I, *et al*: Characterization of rofecoxib as a cyclooxygenase-2 isoform inhibitor and demonstration of analgesia in the dental pain model. Clin Pharmacol Ther 65:336, 1999
95. Blanco FJ, Guitan R, Moreno J *et al*: Effect of anti-inflammatory drugs on COX-1 and COX-2 activity in human articular chondrocytes. J Rheumatol 26:1366, 1999
96. Lee VC: Non-narcotic modalities for the management of acute pain. Anesthesiol Clin North America 7:101, 1989
97. Jung D, Mroszczak E, Bynum L: Pharmacokinetics of ketorolac tromethamine in humans after intravenous, intramuscular and oral administration. Eur J Clin Pharmacol 35:423, 1988
98. Buvanendran A, Kroin JS, Tuman KJ *et al*: Effects of perioperative administration of a selective cyclooxygenase 2 inhibitor on pain management and recovery of function after knee replacement. JAMA 290:2411, 2003
99. Antonijevic I, Mousa SA, Schäfer M, Stein C: Perineurial defect and peripheral opioid analgesia in inflammation. J Neurosci 15:165, 1995
100. Stein C: Peripheral mechanisms of opioid analgesia. Anesth Analg 76:182, 1993
101. Zhou L, Zhang Q, Stein C, Schafer M: Contribution of opioid receptors on primary afferent versus sympathetic neurons to peripheral opioid analgesia. J Pharmacol Exp Ther 286:1000, 1998
102. Stein C, Comisel K, Haimeri E *et al*: Analgesic effect of intraarticular morphine after arthroscopic knee surgery. N Engl J Med 325:1123, 1991
103. Khoury GF, Chen ACN, Garland DF, Stein C: Intraarticular morphine, bupivacaine, and morphine/bupivacaine for pain control after knee videoarthroscopy. Anesthesiology 77:263, 1992
104. Joshi GP, McCarroll SM, O'Brien TM, Lenane P: Intraarticular analgesia following knee arthroscopy. Anesth Analg 76:333, 1993
105. DeAndres J, Bellver J, Barrera L *et al*: A comparative study of analgesia after knee surgery with intraarticular bupivacaine, intraarticular morphine and lumbar plexus block. Anesth Analg 77:727, 1993
106. Dalsgaard J, Felsby S, Juelsgaard P, Froekjaer J: Low-dose intra-articular morphine analgesia in day case knee arthroscopy: A randomized double-blinded study. Pain 56:151, 1994
107. Heine MF, Tillet ED, Tsueda K *et al*: Intra-articular morphine after arthroscopic knee operation. Br J Anaesth 73:413, 1994
108. Nozaki-Taguchi N, Yaksh TL: Characterization of the antihyperalgesic action of a novel peripheral mu-opioid receptor agonist-loperamide. Anesthesiology 90:225, 1999
109. Raffa RB, Friderichs E, Reimann W *et al*: Opioid and nonopioid components independently contribute to the mechanism of action of tramadol, an "atypical" opioid analgesic. J Pharmacol Exp Ther 260:275, 1992
110. Kayser V, Besson JM, Guilbaud G: Effects of the analgesic agent tramadol in normal and arthritic rats: Comparison with the effects of different opioids, including tolerance and cross-tolerance to morphine. Eur J Pharmacol 195:37, 1991
111. Kayser V, Besson JM, Guilbaud G: Evidence for nonadrenergic component in the antinociceptive effect of the analgesic agent tramadol in an animal model of clinical pain. Eur J Pharmacol 224:83, 1992
112. Lehman KA: Tramadol for management of acute pain. Drugs 47:19, 1994
113. Collart L, Luthy C, Dayer P: Multimodal analgesic effect of tramadol. Annual meeting of the American Society of Clinical Pharmacology and Therapeutics, Honolulu, March 1993. Clin Pharmacol Ther 53:233, 1993
114. Lee CR, McTavish D, Sorkin EM: Tramadol: A preliminary review of its pharmacodynamic and pharmacokinetic properties, and therapeutic potential in acute and chronic pain states. Drugs 46:313, 1993
115. Ginsberg B, Sinatra RS, Adler LJ *et al*: Conversion to oral controlled-release oxycodone from intravenous opioid analgesic in the postoperative setting. Pain Med 4:31, 2003
116. Czarnecki ML, Jandrisevits MD, Theiler SC, Huth MM, Weisman SJ: Controlled-release oxycodone for the management of pediatric postoperative pain. J Pain Symptom Manage 27:379, 2004
117. Viscusi ER, Reynolds L, Chung F, Atkinson LE, Khanna S: Patient-controlled transdermal fentanyl hydrochloride vs intravenous morphine pump for postoperative pain. JAMA 291:1333, 2004
118. Hartrick CT, Manvelian G: Sustained release epidural morphine (DepoDur): A review. Todays Therapeutic Trends 22:167, 2004
119. Saito I, Koshino T, Nakashima K *et al*: Increased cellular infiltrate in inflammatory synovia of osteoarthritic knees. Osteoarthritis Cartilage 10:156, 2002
120. Shiga M, Nishina K, Mikawa K *et al*: The effects of lidocaine on nitric oxide production from an activated murine macrophage cell line. Anesth Analg 92:128, 2001
121. Lehmann LJ, DeSio JM, Radvany T, Bikhazi GB: Transdermal fentanyl in postoperative pain. Regional Anesth 22:24, 1997
122. Lichtor JL, Sevarino FB, Joshi GP *et al*: The relative potency of oral transmucosal fentanyl citrate compared with intravenous morphine in the treatment of moderate to severe postoperative pain. Anesth Analg 89:732, 1999
123. Sevarino FB, Paige D, Sinatra RS, Silverman DG: Postoperative analgesia with parenteral opioids: Does continuous delivery utilizing a transdermal opioid preparation affect analgesic efficacy or patient safety? J Clin Anesth 9:173, 1997
124. Rigg JR, Browne RA, Davis C *et al*: Variation in the disposition of morphine after administration in surgical patients. Br J Anaesth 5:1125, 1978
125. Gourlay GK, Kowalski SR, Plummer JL *et al*: Fentanyl blood concentration–analgesic response relationship in the treatment of postoperative pain. Anesth Analg 67:329, 1988
126. Edwards DJ, Svensson CK, Visco JP, Lalka D: Clinical pharmacokinetics of pethidine: 1982. Clin Pharmacokinet 7:421, 1982
127. Berde CB, Lehn BM, Yee JD *et al*: Patient controlled analgesia in children and adolescents: A randomized, prospective comparison with intramuscular administration of morphine for postoperative pain. J Pediatr 118:460, 1991
128. Egbert AM, Parks LH, Short LM, Burnett ML: Randomized trial of postoperative patient-controlled analgesia vs intramuscular narcotics in frail elderly men. Arch Intern Med 150:1897, 1990
129. Sidebotham D, Dijkhuizen MR, Schug SA: The safety and utilization of patient-controlled analgesia. J Pain Symptom Manage 24:202, 1997
130. Egan KJ, Ready LB: Patient satisfaction with intravenous PCA or epidural morphine. Can J Anaesth 41:6, 1994
131. Woodhouse A, Ward ME, Mather LE: Intra-subject variability in postoperative patient-controlled analgesia: Is the patient satisfied with morphine, pethidine and fentanyl? Pain 80:545, 1999
132. Ginsberg B, Gil KM, Muir M *et al*: The influence of lockout intervals and drug selection on patient-controlled analgesia following gynecological surgery. Pain 62:95, 1995

133. White PF: Mishaps with patient-controlled analgesia. Anesthesiology 66:81, 1987
134. Cleland JG: Continuous peridural caudal analgesia in surgery and early ambulation. N W Med J 48:26, 1949
135. Abboud TK, Dror A, Mosaad P *et al*: Mini-dose intrathecal morphine for the relief of post-cesarean section pain: Safety, efficacy and ventilatory responses to carbon dioxide. Anesth Analg 67:137, 1988
136. Aun C, Thomas D, St. John-Jones L *et al*: Intrathecal morphine in cardiac surgery. Eur J Anaesthesiol 2:419, 1985
137. Rigler ML, Drasner K, Krejcie TC *et al*: Cauda equina syndrome after spinal anesthesia. Anesth Analg 72:275, 1991
138. Eisenach JC: Combined spinal-epidural analgesia in obstetrics. Anesthesiology 1:299, 1999
139. van Lersberghe C, Camu F, de Keersmaecker E, Sacré S: Continuous administration of fentanyl for postoperative pain: A comparison of the epidural, intravenous, and transdermal routes. J Clin Anesth 6:308, 1984
140. Loper KA, Ready LB, Downey M *et al*: Epidural and intravenous fentanyl infusions are clinically equivalent after knee surgery. Anesth Analg 70:72, 1990
141. El-Baz NM, Faber LP, Jensik RJ: Continuous epidural infusion of morphine for treatment of pain after thoracic surgery: A new technique. Anesth Analg 63:757, 1984
142. Chestnut DH, Owen CL, Bates JN *et al*: Continuous infusion epidural analgesia during labor: A randomized double-blind comparison of 0.0625% bupivacaine/0.0002% fentanyl versus 0.125% bupivacaine. Anesthesiology 68:754, 1988
143. Cullen ML, Staren ED, el-Ganzouri A *et al*: Continuous thoracic epidural analgesia after major abdominal operations: A randomized prospective double-blind study. Surgery 98:718, 1985
144. Logas WG, el-Baz N, el-Ganzouri A *et al*: Continuous thoracic epidural analgesia for prospective pain relief following thoracotomy: A randomized prospective study. Anesthesiology 67:787, 1987
145. Cousins MJ, Mather LE: Intrathecal and epidural administration of opioids. Anesthesiology 61:276, 1984
146. Rutter DV, Skewes DG, Morgan M: Extradural opioids for postoperative analgesia: A double blind comparison of pethidine, fentanyl and morphine. Br J Anaesth 53:915, 1981
147. Lubenow TR, Tanck EN, Hopkins EM *et al*: Comparison of patient-assisted epidural analgesia with continuous-infusion epidural analgesia for postoperative patients. Reg Anesth 19:206, 1994
148. Paech MJ, Moore JS, Evans SF: Meperidine for patient-controlled analgesia after cesarean section. Anesthesiology 80:1268, 1994
149. Angst MS, Ramaswamy B, Riley ET, Stanski DR: Lumbar epidural morphine in humans and supraspinal analgesia to experimental heat pain. Anesthesiology 92:312, 2000
150. Hansdottir V, Woestenborghs R, Nordberg G: The cerebrospinal fluid and plasma pharmacokinetics of sufentanil by the lumbar versus thoracic route after thoracotomy. Anesth Analg 78:215, 1994
151. Shulman MS, Wakerlin G, Yamaguchi L, Brodsky JB: Experience with epidural hydromorphone for post-thoracotomy pain relief. Anesth Analg 66:1331, 1987
152. Akerman B, Arwenstrom E, Post C: Local anesthetic potentiates spinal morphine antinociception. Anesth Analg 67:943, 1988
153. Solomon RE, Gebhart GF: Synergistic antinociceptive interaction among drugs administered to the spinal cord. Anesth Analg 78:1164, 1994
154. Badner NH, Reimer EJ, Komar WE, Moote CA: Low-dose bupivacaine does not improve postoperative epidural fentanyl analgesia in orthopedic patients. Anesth Analg 72:237, 1991
155. Eisenach J, Detweiler D, Hood D: Hemodynamic and analgesic actions of epidurally administered clonidine. Anesthesiology 78:277, 1993
156. Eisenach JC, Lysaks Z, Viscomi CM: Epidural clonidine following surgery: Phase I. Anesthesiology 71:640, 1989
157. Eisenach JL, Rauch RL, Buzzanell C, Lysak SZ: Epidural clonidine for intractable cancer pain: Phase I. Anesthesiology 71:647, 1989
158. DeKock M, Gautier P, Pavlopoulou A *et al*: Epidural clonidine or bupivacaine as the sole analgesic agent during and after abdominal surgery. Anesthesiology 90:1354, 1999
159. Klimscha W, Chiari A, Krafft P *et al*: Hemodynamic and analgesic effects of clonidine added repetitively to continuous epidural and spinal blocks. Anesth Analg 80:322, 1995
160. DeKock M, Crochet B, Morimont C, Scholtes JL: Intravenous or epidural clonidine for intra- and postoperative analgesia. Anesthesiology 79:525, 1993
161. Motsch J, Graber E, Ludwig K: Addition of clonidine enhances postoperative analgesia from epidural morphine: A double-blind study. Anesthesiology 73:1067, 1990
162. Curatolo M, Schnider TW, Petersen-Felix S *et al*: A direct search procedure to optimize combinations of epidural bupivacaine, fentanyl, and clonidine for postoperative pain. Anesthesiology 92:325, 2000
163. Tallarida RJ, Stone DJ Jr, McCary JD, Raffa RB: Response surface analysis of synergism between morphine and clonidine. J Pharmacol Exp Ther 289:8, 1999
164. Asano T, Dohi S, Ohta S *et al*: Antinociception by epidural and systemic α2-adrenoceptor agonists and their binding affinity in rat spinal cord and brain. Anesth Analg 90:400, 2000
165. Nagasaka H, Yaksh TL: Pharmacology of intrathecal adrenergic agonists: Cardiovascular and nociceptive reflexes in halothane-anesthetized rats. Anesthesiology 73:1198, 1990
166. McCarthy RJ, Kroin JS, Lubenow TR *et al*: Effect of intrathecal tizanidine on antinociception and blood pressure in the rat. Pain 40:333, 1990
167. Wang LP, Hauerberg J, Schmidt JF: Incidence of spinal epidural abscess after epidural analgesia. Anesthesiology 91:1928, 1999
168. Rao TL, El-Etr AA: Anticoagulation following placement of epidural and subarachnoid catheters: An evaluation of neurologic sequelae. Anesthesiology 56:618, 1981
169. Vandermeulen EP, Van Aken M, Vermylen J: Anticoagulants and spinal epidural anesthesia. Anesth Analg 79:1165, 1994
170. Horlocker TT, Wedel DJ: Neuraxial block and low molecular weight heparin: Balancing perioperative analgesia and thromboprophylaxis. Reg Anesth Pain Med 23(6 Suppl 2):129, 1998
171. Horlocker TT, Wedel DJ, Schlichting JL: Postoperative epidural analgesia and oral anticoagulant therapy. Anesth Analg 79:89, 1994
172. Enneking FK, Benzon HT: Oral anticoagulants and regional anesthesia: A perspective. Reg Anesth Pain Med 23(6 Suppl 2):140, 1998
173. Johnson JT, Braun TW: Preoperative, intraoperative and postoperative management of patients with obstructive sleep apnea syndrome. Otolaryngol Clin North Am 31:1025, 1998
174. Rennotte MT, Bacle P, Aubert G *et al*: Nasal continuous positive airway pressure in the perioperative management of patients with obstructive sleep apnea submitted to surgery. Chest 107:367, 1995
175. Katz JA, Kaeding CS, Hill JR, Henthorn TK: The pharmacokinetics of bupivacaine when injected intraarticularly after knee arthroscopy. Anesth Analg 67:872, 1988
176. Kaeding CC, Hill JA, Katz J, Benson L: Bupivacaine use after knee arthroscopy: Pharmacokinetics and pain control study. Arthroscopy 6:33, 1990
177. Katz J, Nelson W, Forest R *et al*: Cryoanalgesia for postthoracotomy pain. Lancet 1:512, 1980
178. Benumof JL: Management of postoperative pain. In Benumof JL (ed): Anesthesia for Thoracic Surgery, p 467. Philadelphia, WB Saunders, 1987
179. Moore DC: Regional block. In Moore DC (ed): A Handbook for Use in the Clinical Practice of Medicine and Surgery, p 169. Springfield, IL, Charles C Thomas, 1981
180. Singelyn FJ, Seguy S, Gouverneur JM: Interscalene brachial plexus analgesia after open shoulder surgery: Continuous versus patient controlled infusion. Anesth Analg 89:1216, 1999
181. Hamza MA, White PF, Ahmed HE, Ghoname EA: Effect of frequency of transcutaneous electrical nerve stimulation on the postoperative opioid analgesic requirements and recovery profile. Anesthesiology 5:1232, 1999
182. Rapp SE, Ready LB, Nessly ML: Acute pain management in patients with prior opioid consumption: A case-controlled retrospective review. Pain 61:195, 1995
183. Forrest JB, Heitlinger EL, Revell S: Ketorolac for postoperative pain management in children. Drug Saf 16:309, 1997
184. Lieh-Lai MW, Kauffman RE, Uy HG *et al*: A randomized comparison of ketorolac tromethamine and morphine for postoperative analgesia in critically ill children. Crit Care Med 27:2786, 1999
185. Lubenow TR, Ivankovich AD: Patient-controlled analgesia for postoperative pain. Crit Care Nurs Clin North Am 3:35, 1991
186. Sutters KA, Shaw BA, Gerardi JA, Herbert D: Comparison of morphine patient controlled analgesia with and without ketorolac for postoperative analgesia in pediatric orthopedic surgery. Am J Orthop 28:351, 1999
187. Tyler D, Krane E: Postoperative pain management in children. Anesthesiol Clin North America 7:155, 1989

APPENDIX 55-1 SOLUTIONS AND RATES OF PATIENT-CONTROLLED EPIDURAL ANALGESIA

Standard Fentanyl Solutions

Fentanyl 3,000 μg with bupivacaine 300 mg in 300 mL normal saline (NS)—adults <70 yr, >50 kg

Fentanyl 1,500 μg with bupivacaine 300 mg in 300 mL NS—adults $\geq$70 yr, $\leq$50 kg, history of sleep apnea

Maximum continuous rate 10 mL/hr for lumbar epidural catheters (total infusion rate $\leq$40 mL/4 hr)

Examples of Continuous and Demand Dosing Combinations for Fentanyl Solutions

- 4 mL/hr continuous, demand mode 1 mL q10min, 40 mL/4 hr lockout
- 4 mL/hr continuous, demand mode 2 mL q20min, 40 mL/4 hr lockout

- 5 mL/hr continuous, demand mode 1 mL q12min, 40 mL/4 hr lockout
- 6 mL/hr continuous, demand mode 1 mL q15min, 40 mL/4 hr lockout
- 6 mL/hr continuous, demand mode 2 mL q30min, 40 mL/4 hr lockout
- 7 mL/hr continuous, demand mode 1 mL q20min, 40 mL/4 hr lockout
- 8 mL/hr continuous, demand mode 1 mL q30min, 40 mL/4 hr lockout
- 8 mL/hr continuous, demand mode 2 mL q60min, 40 mL/4 hr lockout
- 9 mL/hr continuous, demand mode 1 mL q60min, 40 mL/4 hr lockout
- 10 mL/hr, no demand mode

Morphine Solutions

Morphine 30 mg with bupivacaine 300 mg in 300 mL NS—adults <70 yr, >50 kg

Morphine 15 mg with bupivacaine 300 mg in 150 mL NS—adults ≥70 yr, ≤50 kg, history of sleep apnea

Maximum continuous rate 6 mL/hr for lumbar or thoracic epidural catheters (total infusion rate ≤24 mL/4 hr)

Examples of Continuous and Demand Dosing Combinations for Morphine Solutions

- 3 mL/hr continuous, demand mode 1 mL q20min, 24 mL/4 hr lockout
- 4 mL/hr continuous, demand mode 1 mL q30min, 24 mL/4 hr lockout
- 5 mL/hr continuous, demand mode 1 mL q60min, 24 mL/4 hr lockout
- 6 mL/hr continuous, no demand mode

APPENDIX 55-2 POLICY AND PROCEDURES FOR INITIATION AND NURSING CARE OF PATIENTS WITH POSTOPERATIVE EPIDURAL ANALGESIA

I. Purpose
  A. To list guidelines for initiating and monitoring patients receiving postoperative epidural analgesia and to provide quality assurance and patient safety
II. Candidates
  A. Postsurgical patients who have no previous history of allergy to the ordered analgesics
  B. Patients must not have any contraindications to the placement of an epidural catheter (e.g., sepsis, severe coagulation abnormality, hypovolemia, head injury)
III. Equipment
  A. Epidural infusion pump
  B. Cassette tubing
  C. Epidural catheter tray
  D. Micropore tape
  E. Tegaderm dressing
  F. Apnea monitor (if required)
  G. Naloxone 0.4 mg/mL—two ampules
  H. 3-mL syringes with needles
  I. Alcohol wipes
  J. Epidural solution
    1. Fentanyl 0.001%/bupivacaine 0.1%—300 mL (age <70 yr)
    2. Fentanyl 0.0005%/bupivacaine 0.1%—300 mL (age ≥70 yr, ≤50 kg, history of sleep apnea)
    3. Morphine 0.01%/bupivacaine 0.1%—300 mL (age <70 yr)
    4. Morphine 0.005%/bupivacaine 0.1%—300 mL (age ≥70 yr, ≤50 kg, history of sleep apnea)
IV. Treatment initiation and guidelines
  A. Placement of epidural catheter is performed by the anesthesiologist.
  B. Epidural order sheet must be completed by the anesthesiologist.
    1. Anesthesiologist's written order for epidural solution to include the name and amount of fluid, rate of infusion, name and dosage of any medications added, and supplemental intravenous/intramuscular pain medications as required.
  C. Epidural solution must be administered via designated infusion pump.
  D. Baseline blood pressure and respiratory rate must be documented before initiating epidural infusion.
  E. Blood pressure, heart rate, level of consciousness, and temperature are to be monitored every 4 hours for the first 24 hours of the epidural infusion.
  F. Respiratory monitoring
    1. An apnea monitor is required for patients who received epidural narcotic bolus of MSO_4 ≥2 mg. Patients may receive an epidural bolus of fentanyl 50 to 150 μg without the routine use of an apnea monitor.
    2. Respiratory rate to be monitored every hour for the first 24 hours of the epidural infusion.
      a. Naloxone, syringe, and needle are to be readily available at all times.
  G. The epidural solution bag and volumetric pump cassette are not changed unless otherwise ordered.
V. Nursing responsibilities
  A. Record vital signs (blood pressure, level of consciousness, ambulation, temperature) every 4 hours for first 24 hours of epidural infusion, then as ordered.
  B. Record respiratory rates every 1 hour for the first 24 hours of the epidural infusion and every 4 hours thereafter.
    1. If the respiratory rate falls below 8 per minute, notify the postoperative analgesia service (PAS) and administer naloxone as ordered.
  C. Record all analgesic medications administered on the medication record.
  D. Using the visual analog scale, record patient's subjective level of pain with vital signs on flow sheet.
    1. Scale for pain: 0 to 10, with 0 = no pain and 10 = worst pain ever.
  E. Assess epidural catheter integrity, and check dressing for wetness every shift and as needed.
    1. Reinforce with dry 4 × 4 gauze if dressing is wet.
    2. Cover with clear plastic tape.
    3. Notify PAS if excessive wetness or integrity of catheter is in question.
      a. If epidural catheter becomes dislodged or disconnected:
        i. Notify PAS.
        ii. If catheter is disconnected, cover end of catheter with sterile 4 × 4 gauze (do not reconnect).
        iii. If catheter becomes dislodged, keep for inspection by anesthesiologist.
  F. Assess and document signs and symptoms of side effects.
    1. Pruritus with and without rash
    2. Nausea or vomiting
    3. Paresthesia, numbness, motor weakness

4. Headache
5. Backache
6. Signs of infection around catheter site
7. Urinary retention

G. Assess and document the following if patient is on anticoagulation medication:
1. Notify PAS if patient receiving warfarin has an international normalized ratio (INR) >1.8.
2. Notify PAS if a second anticoagulant is ordered.

H. Record any prescribed treatment administered for side effects or supplemental analgesics on patient care record.

VI. Postoperative analgesia service responsibilities

A. Team members will see patients daily and chart progress notes documenting adequacy of pain relief and the occurrence of side effects or problems associated with epidural use; will adjust therapy or institute test dose algorithm if current protocol is associated with inadequate analgesia, side effects, or complications; and will collect and maintain data for review by anesthesiologist on a weekly basis.

B. Organize and conduct inservice training of hospital nursing staff.

C. Review epidural medication record to ensure adequate documentation of use and disposal of medications.

D. Evaluate and make recommendations regarding new equipment for epidural analgesia.

E. Analyze data, identify problems, propose changes, if any, and evaluate changes for quality assurance purposes.

F. Review anticoagulation medication taken along with coagulation status before epidural catheter removal.
1. The epidural catheter should not be removed for at least 4 hours after the previous dose of subcutaneous standard heparin or discontinuation of intravenous heparin infusion. The next subcutaneous dose or the resumption of the intravenous infusion should be at least 2 hours after catheter removal.
2. The epidural catheter should not be removed for at least 10 hours after the previous dose of a low-molecular-weight heparin. The next dose should not be given for at least 2 hours after catheter removal.
3. Patients receiving warfarin should not have the epidural catheter removed until INR <1.8 and platelet count >80,000 per mm^3. After epidural catheter removal in patients with INR >1.5, order neurosensory assessments to be made every 4 hours for the next 24 hours.

VII. Pharmacy responsibilities

A. Daily log of all patients receiving epidural analgesia with type of solution and amount dispensed.

B. Computer printout of all patients started on epidural analgesia in the last 24 hours. Printout should be available in pharmacy at 8 AM Monday through Saturday. Patients started on epidural analgesia on Saturday or Sunday will be on the Monday morning printout. This list will be picked up by the PAS personnel to aid in identifying those patients started on epidural analgesia.

C. Collaborate with PAS personnel in quality assurance matters.

VIII. Termination

A. Epidural infusions ordinarily will be terminated by the PAS in conjunction with the primary surgical service using guidelines established for the type of surgical procedure and patients' analgesic requirements.

IX. Questions/problems

A. Any questions or problems regarding epidural drip or catheter are referred to the PAS between 8:00 AM and 4:30 PM, or to the anesthesiologist on call after 4:00 PM and weekends.

APPENDIX 55-3 POSTOPERATIVE EPIDURAL ANALGESIA ORDER SHEET

(PLEASE CIRCLE ORDERS TO BE IMPLEMENTED AND COMPLETE BLANKS WHERE APPROPRIATE)
(DATE AND TIME FOR EACH PROCEDURE IS TO BE NOTED)

1. Admit to PACU or SICU, routine PACU or SICU VS.
2. Discharge from PACU per anesthesia care team.
3. On floor (circle):
   a. Monitoring
      1. Apnea monitor
      2. Telemetry
      3. Pulse oximetry
   b. VS q4hr, respiratory rate q1hr for the first 24 hours.
   c. Tape two ampules of naloxone with syringe and needle at bedside.
   d. If respiratory rate <8 per minute, give 0.4 mg naloxone intravenously stat and call anesthesia.
4. Epidural solution (circle one):
   a. Morphine 15 mg with bupivacaine 300 mg in 300 mL NS, rate ____ mL/hr (age ≥70 yr, ≤50 kg, history of sleep apnea)
   b. Morphine 30 mg with bupivacaine 300 mg in 300 mL NS, rate ____ mL/hr
   c. Fentanyl 1,500 μg with bupivacaine 300 mg in 300 mL NS, rate ____ mL/hr (age ≥70 yr, ≤50 kg, history of sleep apnea)
   d. Fentanyl 3,000 μg with bupivacaine 300 mg in 300 mL NS, rate ____ mL/hr
   e. PATIENT-ASSISTED EPIDURAL MODE ____ mL q ____ min, with ____ mL/4 hr lockout
5. Supplemental medications (circle):
   a. Morphine 2 mg intravenously, intramuscularly, or sq q2–4hr PRN VAS > ____
   b. Metoclopramide 10 mg intramuscularly q4–6hr PRN for nausea
   c. Nalbuphine 10 mg intramuscularly or sq q4–6hr PRN for pruritus
   d. Ketorolac 30 mg intramuscularly q6hr × 48 hr PRN for pain; if patient >65 yr or <65 kg, give 15 mg intramuscularly q6hr × 48 hr PRN for pain
6. Nursing staff on floor call postoperative analgesia service × 24 hours per day if any problems arise or if catheter needs to be discontinued.
7. All other preoperative orders, medications, and diet per service with the exception of opioids and sedatives.

Signed ________, MD Date ________

APPENDIX 55-4 PATIENT-CONTROLLED ANALGESIA SERVICE PROTOCOL FOR POSTSURGICAL PAIN RELIEF

I. Purpose

A. To list guidelines to follow when PCA is ordered and to provide quality assurance and patient safety

II. Candidates
   A. Postsurgical patients who have no previous history of allergy to the ordered analgesics
   B. Patients must be mentally alert, understand basic instructions, and be physically capable of operating the PCA infusion device
III. Treatment initiation
   A. Treatment may be initiated by any surgical service and by anesthesia personnel. PCA treatment initiated by surgical services must conform to the guidelines listed as follows.
IV. Postoperative PCA guidelines
   A. The physician's order for PCA must include the following:
      1. Drug (Only morphine and meperidine are available for routine use for postsurgical pain. Fentanyl and other drugs may be used only with the approval of the postoperative analgesia service [PAS] physician or anesthesiologist on call when the PAS service is not available.)
      2. Loading dose (if patient has pain when PCA is ordered)
      3. Maintenance infusion (if desired)
      4. Incremental or maintenance dose
      5. Lockout interval
      6. 4-hr limit
      7. Mode of operation—PCA
   B. Recommended starting parameters
      1. Loading dose, morphine 1–4 mg, meperidine 10–40 mg
      2. Maintenance dose, morphine 1 mg, meperidine 10 mg
      3. Lockout interval, 6–10 min
      4. 4-hr limit, morphine 20 mg, meperidine 200 mg
      5. Mode of operation—PCA
V. Surgical staff
   A. Initiate preprinted order sheet.
   B. Evaluate adequacy of therapy.
   C. Contact PAS personnel if inadequate pain relief or patient has requirements for more complex PCA dosing.
   D. Monitor for complications.
VI. Nursing responsibilities
   A. Obtain and assure prompt delivery of PCA morphine/meperidine vials from pharmacy to nursing units.
   B. Verify proper and patent intravenous line.
   C. Monitor and record vital signs per orders.
   D. Reinforce patient teaching on use of PCA, if needed.
   E. Assess pain level and effectiveness of PCA.
   F. Change PCA tubing every 48 hours.
   G. Document accurate dosage of narcotic used or wasted in separate PCA medication sheets (two signatures needed for drug wasted).
   H. Verify that PCA is programmed to deliver dosage as ordered.
   I. At the change of shift, the incoming and outgoing nurses will check the PCA flow sheet, the pump readout, and the labeled syringe. The amount of drug administered in the previous 8 hours will be recorded on the PCA medication sheet.
   J. Notify PAS personnel and primary surgical service if the patient experiences side effects, complications, or inadequate analgesia.
   K. Assess and document signs and symptoms of side effects.
      1. Pruritus with and without rash
      2. Nausea or vomiting
      3. Sedation/decreased mentation
      4. Decreased respiration
      5. Ileus/constipation
      6. Signs of infection or infiltration around catheter site
      7. Urinary retention
   L. Record any prescribed treatment administered for side effects or supplemental analgesics on patient care record.
VII. Postoperative analgesia service responsibilities
   A. Instruct patients on the use of PCA when ordered by anesthesia and provide additional teaching if PCA is ordered by surgical service.
   B. Team members will see patients daily and chart progress notes documenting adequacy of pain relief and the occurrence of side effects or problems associated with PCA use. Will adjust therapy or substitute with a new protocol if current therapy is associated with inadequate analgesia, side effects, or complications. Will collect and maintain data for review by anesthesiologist on a weekly basis.
   C. Organize and conduct inservice training of hospital nursing staff.
   D. Review PCA medication record to ensure adequate documentation of use and disposal of medications.
   E. Evaluate and make recommendations regarding new equipment for PCA.
   F. Analyze data, identify problems, propose changes, if any, and evaluate changes for quality assurance purposes.
VIII. Pharmacy responsibilities
   A. Daily log of all patients receiving PCA with type of solution and amount dispensed.
   B. Computer printout of all patients started on epidural analgesia in the last 24 hours. Printout should be available in pharmacy at 8 AM Monday through Saturday. Patients started on PCA on Saturday or Sunday will be on the Monday morning printout. This list will be picked up by the PAS personnel to aid in identifying those patients started on epidural analgesia.
   C. Collaborate with PAS personnel in quality assurance matters.
IX. Termination
   A. PCA ordinarily will be terminated by the PAS in conjunction with the primary surgical service using guidelines established for the type of surgical procedure and patients' analgesic requirements.
X. Questions/problems
   A. Any questions or problems regarding PCA are referred to the postoperative analgesia service between 8:00 AM and 4:30 PM or to the anesthesiologist on call after 4:00 PM and weekends.

CHAPTER 56 ■ CHRONIC PAIN MANAGEMENT

STEPHEN E. ABRAM

KEY POINTS

1. Persistent activation of peripheral nociceptors produces sensitization of spinal cord pain transmission systems that is triggered by the prolonged release of glutamate, substance P, and other peptides, and mediated through N-methyl-D-aspartate (NMDA) receptor-dependent mechanisms.
2. Tissue inflammation, nerve injury, and central nervous system (CNS) injury or infection can activate glial cells in the CNS and glia-like elements in peripheral nerves. Activated glia release proinflammatory cytokines and other substances that increase the sensitivity of surrounding neurons to both noxious and nonnoxious stimulation.
3. Central sensitization, whether triggered by neuronal or glial mechanisms, leads to reduced responsiveness to both endogenous and exogenous opioids. Prolonged opioid administration, even in the absence of nerve or tissue injury, can produce central sensitization and hyperalgesia through both NMDA-mediated neuronal mechanisms and glial activation.
4. Interactions between the sympathetic nervous system and pain projections systems can add to the sensitized state of the nervous system seen in a number of chronic pain syndromes. Complex regional pain syndromes are seen in both the presence and absence of significant nerve injury and may or may not have a component of sympathetically mediated pain.
5. Low back pain and cervical pain are associated with multiple physical pain mechanisms, including discogenic, radicular, arthropathic, and myofascial syndromes. Most patients with chronic back or neck pain have more than one active pain mechanism. This is particularly true of patients who have failed multiple surgical procedures.
6. Medication management of chronic pain patients can provide substantial pain reduction for some patients, but rarely produces complete or near-complete relief. Long-term opioid administration should be continued only when there is substantial pain reduction, significant improvement in physical function, minimal dose escalation over time, and minimal side effects.
7. Cancer pain needs to be addressed promptly and aggressively with management, based on careful determination of the site and mechanism of pain. Opioids should be given in adequate doses throughout the course of the disease. Spinal drug administration and neuroablative procedures are considered when tolerance and side effects limit the ability of systemic medications to provide significant pain relief.
8. The great majority of chronic pain patients have significant disability related to loss of physical conditioning and psychopathological changes. Any management program that fails to include rehabilitation, patient education, and psychological therapy will provide suboptimal treatment to most chronic pain patients.
9. New, invasive, and often expensive techniques have expanded the ability of physicians to provide effective nonsurgical treatment of painful conditions. It is essential that these technologies be critically assessed and that they are applied only to those conditions that have a high likelihood of success.

Perhaps the most common factor associated with treatment failure of chronic pain is the assumption that treatment principles that apply to acute pain management are appropriate for chronic pain. It is often assumed that if we can find the source of the pain, the "pain generator," and remove it, denervate it, or modify the pathologic process, the pain will go away. Similarly, we assume the pharmacologic approaches that work for acute pain also apply to chronic pain. For many, perhaps most chronic pain patients, such approaches will invariably fail.

Persistent pain, especially pain associated with nerve injury, produces significant and often permanent changes in the way the nervous system processes sensory information. Activation of peripheral nociceptors, nerve injury, tissue inflammation, and infection can produce dramatic changes in firing thresholds for neurons in the peripheral and central nervous system (CNS). Activation of glial cells leads to the production of substances that greatly enhance the responses to both painful and nonpainful tissue stimulation. Persistent firing of nociceptive afferent fibers leads to high levels of excitatory amino acids in the CNS, which can cause injury to neurons that normally inhibit pain projection neurons.

Persistent pain can also lead to anatomic changes in both the peripheral and CNS. Following nerve injury, a variety of neuronal plasticity changes occur, such as sprouting of dendrites on neurons projecting to the dorsal horn or ingrowth os sympathetic fibers into the dorsal root ganglia. These anatomic deviations undoubtedly produce some of the functional changes characteristic of chronic pain states.

Opioids, the mainstay of acute pain management, behave very differently when given chronically. Daily opioid administration to intact animals consistently produces hyperalgesia within 1 week. This phenomenon occurs more rapidly and more profoundly in animals subjected to peripheral nerve injury. The neurophysiologic mechanisms of these changes are now well characterized. These data lead to concern about the advisability of long-term administration of opioids to those patients who experience minimal relief from high doses.

These recently characterized physiologic changes represent only a portion of the story. Persistent pain leads to inactivity, deconditioning, muscle and tendon shortening and fibrosis, and joint dysfunction. It is also associated with behavioral changes that lead to dramatic and often devastating deterioration in function, and decreased participation in vocational, social, and recreational activities. Depression, which occurs in the majority of patients with chronic pain, can be even more debilitating than the original painful condition.

No two patients share the same constellation of pathologic, physiologic, physical, and psychological changes. Each patient deserves assessment based on a careful medical, social, and psychological evaluation. Evaluation should include both a psychological and a functional assessment, as well as a plan for rehabilitative therapies. This can only be accomplished in a health care environment that includes close cooperation among multiple disciplines. At minimum, medical, rehabilitation, psychological, and social services should be provided in a coordinated fashion. The picture is further complicated by the presence in the chronic pain patient population of individuals whose complaints are related to addiction rather than pain. The practitioner must also confront the reality that drug diversion is a source of income for some individuals whose pain complaints serve only to provide a steady source of medications for resale on the street. Resources should therefore be readily available for identifying and treating addiction.

PAIN PATHWAYS AND MECHANISMS

Pain is most often experienced as a result of injury. Its survival value to an organism is based on the fact that it is initiated by tissue injury or by stimuli that threaten damage, and that it produces sufficient arousal and distress so as to unlikely be ignored. It is tempting to envision pain as a straightforward receptive system, with transducers that respond to intense, tissue-threatening stimuli and neurons that project to areas of the brain capable of processing pain information. Unfortunately, such a view of pain perception fails to explain the tremendous variation in pain sensitivity between individuals or the dramatic shifts in sensitivity that can occur in a single individual. It also fails to explain chronic pain that is experienced without any noxious stimulation. Oversimplified anatomic concepts also predispose to simplistic therapeutic interventions, such as neurectomy or rhizotomy, that may intensify pain or create new and often more distressing pain.

In reality, the nociceptive system is highly complex and highly adaptable. Sensitivity of most of its components can be reset by a variety of physiologic and pathologic conditions. Injury to neural elements may result in loss of ability to perceive pain or may cause spontaneous pain or heightened pain sensitivity.

To understand the pathophysiologic mechanisms involved in chronic pain, it is important to have a sound understanding of acute pain pathways and mechanisms. This requires knowledge of the physiology of receptors that respond to tissue-threatening stimuli, the anatomy of peripheral and CNS pathways that are activated, and the mechanisms by which various components of the pain projection system can be acutely sensitized or suppressed. Mechanisms of chronic pain are even more complex. Chronic injury may lead to irreversible alterations in nociceptor sensitivity, to spontaneous firing of peripheral or central pain projection fibers, and to dramatic changes in the reaction of the CNS to sensory inputs. This section provides an overview of the anatomic pathways, the physiologic modulating mechanisms, and the pathologic alterations that are important to the perception of pain.

ANATOMIC PATHWAYS

Nociceptors

Receptors that respond exclusively to intense, potentially tissue-damaging stimuli are well characterized. Cutaneous nociceptors have been extensively studied. Considerably less is known about receptors responsive to intense stimuli found in deep somatic structures, and still less is known about the physiology of visceral pain.

Cutaneous Nociceptors

Most cutaneous nociceptors respond to both intense mechanical stimulation and to high temperatures and are termed mechanoheat nociceptors.[1] These nociceptors do not respond to low-threshold mechanical stimulation (light touch, pressure) or to warm temperatures below the noxious range. C fiber mechanoheat (CMH) nociceptors respond to temperatures above 43°C. Firing frequency increases in a roughly linear fashion as skin temperature is increased within the noxious range. Repeated or prolonged exposure to suprathreshold stimuli may lead to a reduction in response, or habituation. However, under certain circumstances, previous exposure to a noxious stimulus may lead to an enhanced response (sensitization).

There are two types of A fiber mechanoheat (AMH) nociceptors. Type I AMHs have a very high threshold to thermal stimuli (53°C or greater) and are considered by some investigators to be mechanical nociceptors, or high-threshold mechanoreceptors. These nociceptors are found principally in glabrous skin. Although most have afferent fibers with conduction velocities in the A-delta range (~30 m/sec), some have conduction velocities as high as 55 m/sec, and would be considered A-b fibers. Type II AMHs are activated by temperatures below activation thresholds of type I AMHs and conduct at about 15 m/sec. These nociceptors also have a much shorter delay between stimulus onset and receptor activation. They are generally found in hairy skin and on the face.

The receptive fields for mechanical and thermal nociception are essentially identical for both CMHs and AMHs. However, there may be differences in the transducer mechanisms for mechanical versus thermal nociception. For instance, application of capsaicin to the skin produces analgesia to noxious thermal, but not mechanical stimulation. Cutaneous AMHs and CMHs are poorly responsive to cooling stimuli, and there is some evidence that afferent fibers from vascular structures are capable of signaling cold pain.[2]

A number of chemical mediators that are released following injury are capable of either activating or sensitizing both CMHs and AMHs. These substances include bradykinin, serotonin, prostaglandins, leukotrienes, histamine, and substance P (SP). Bradykinin, which is released locally following tissue injury, is capable of evoking pain on intradermal injection, and has been shown to activate both CMHs and AMHs when administered within a nerve's receptive field. In addition, bradykinin produces hyperalgesia to heat stimuli through receptor sensitization. Serotonin can activate nociceptors and potentiates bradykinin-induced pain. Low pH is also capable of producing pain, both by nociceptor activation and by sensitization to mechanical stimuli.[1]

Nociceptors in Other Somatic Structures

A large number of A-delta and C fibers found in muscle, fascia, and tendons are poorly responsive to normal stretching or contraction and are probably nociceptive in function. Many of the C fibers are responsive to chemical irritants, heat, and strong pressure.[3] A few respond to strong contraction and to ischemia, whereas others fire in response to muscle stretching. Some A-delta fibers in muscle have relatively low sensitivity to mechanical stimuli, responding best to chemicals, such as bradykinin. Others, which tend to be arranged near muscle–tendon junctions, respond to local pressure, stretch, and contractions.[3]

Nociceptors in joints are located in the joint capsule, ligaments, periosteum, and articular fat pads, but probably not in cartilage. Small myelinated and unmyelinated fibers terminate in free nerve endings in joints, and A-delta fibers form a widespread plexus in capsules, fat pads, and ligaments.[4] Some of the A-delta axons respond to noxious stimuli. Intracapsular bradykinin in animals produces generalized nociceptive responses that are enhanced by prostaglandins.

Corneal sensitivity serves a primarily protective function, and most stimuli to corneal epithelium are sensed as pain. Innervation is mainly from A-delta fibers, with fine terminals devoid of Schwann cell covering.[3] These fibers have activation thresholds similar to low-threshold mechanoreceptors in skin,[5] but low-intensity stimulation is capable of evoking pain. Tooth pulp afferents respond to a variety of chemical stimuli, strong heating, cooling, and pressure. Electrical stimulation produces almost exclusively painful sensations.[3]

Visceral Pain Receptors

Because of the infrequency with which visceral structures are exposed to potentially damaging events, it would not seem efficient to provide these structures with receptors designed solely to detect intense stimuli in the environment. Although severe pain of visceral origin is a common clinical phenomenon, there is little evidence that specialized pain receptors exist in visceral structures. Many damaging stimuli, such as cutting, burning, or clamping, produce no pain when applied to visceral structures. In contrast, inflammation, ischemia, mesenteric stretching, or dilation or spasm of hollow viscera may produce severe pain. These stimuli are usually associated with pathologic processes, and the pain they induce may serve a survival function by promoting immobility.

For almost all intrathoracic, intra-abdominal, and pelvic viscera, pain perception is a function of visceral afferent (sometimes termed sympathetic afferent) nerve activity.[3] These neurons accompany sympathetic afferent axons in the sympathetic chain and intra-abdominal and intrathoracic plexuses; but most, like other afferent fibers, have their cell bodies in the dorsal root ganglia and synapse with dorsal horn neurons.

Pain Perception in the Gut

It has been widely accepted that nociceptive-specific fibers do not exist in the gut. Pain is believed to result from intense activation of afferent fibers that serve other functions, such as stretch receptors. High-frequency activation of these visceral afferents in turn activates dorsal horn pain projection neurons, producing pain perceived within cutaneous referral sites. This referred pain is probably the result of viscerosomatic convergence, the phenomenon of a single spinothalamic tract (STT) neuron that can be activated by either visceral or somatic stimuli. Another type of convergence, reported by Bahr et al,[6] is based on the existence of afferent neurons with two sensory branches, one visceral (sympathetic afferent) and one somatic. It is not possible to locate the site of a painful stimulus to the gut with any accuracy because stimulation of widely distant sites can give rise to the same referred sensations.

Cardiac Pain

Cardiac afferent fibers, conducting in the C and A-delta range, have been shown to fire at high rates in response to coronary occlusion or intracoronary bradykinin.[7] However, to designate these nerves as nociceptors, they should respond only to noxious stimuli and should exhibit no background discharge. Malliani[7] showed that these putative nociceptors are tonically active, demonstrate mechanosensitivity, and respond to normal hemodynamic events. It is likely that cardiac afferents that are responsive to tissue-threatening stimuli have physiologic functions under normal circumstances, but give rise to volleys of activity that can cause poorly localized pain referred to somatic structures. Viscerosomatic convergence probably occurs with these fibers.

Other Visceral Structures

Pain associated with gallbladder disease is similar in character and location to angina pectoris.[8] Mechanical stimulation of the gallbladder or the application of chemical stimuli can affect the electrical activity and contractility of the heart.[9] Stretching of the bile ducts and gallbladder activates two populations of afferent fibers, one responding to small changes in pressure and the other responding only to high pressures (>25 mm Hg).[10] The high-threshold stretch receptors may have a nociceptive function. Gallbladder distension activates spinothalamic cells in the T1–T5 portion of the cord, cells that are also activated by cardiac afferents and somatic afferents from the medial aspect of the arm and the chest wall.

Pain from the upper portions of the esophagus is most likely caused by activation of vagal afferents.[3] Heartburn pain may be a vagally mediated phenomenon, but little study of the activation of pain by acids in the esophagus has been carried out.

Distension of the renal pelvis or ureters is known to produce pain, but few studies have characterized afferent responses from the urinary tract. Pain of urethral origin is probably transmitted via sacral nerve roots rather than through sympathetic afferents. Urinary bladder distension is capable of producing cardiovascular responses, but, unlike gallbladder distension, is associated with reduced heart rate and contractility.

Dorsal Horn Mechanisms

The spinal dorsal horn and its analog in the medulla are exceedingly complex sensory processing areas. They contain the central terminals of peripheral afferent fibers, projection neurons of spinothalamic and other ascending tracts, local neurons that activate or inhibit projection neurons, and axon terminals of descending brainstem fibers.

As nerve roots approach the dorsal horn, segregation of fibers according to size takes place, with large myelinated afferents becoming arranged medially and small unmyelinated and thinly myelinated fibers arranged laterally. Most large myelinated fibers enter the cord medial to the dorsal horn. Many of these axons bifurcate, sending one branch rostrally in the dorsal columns. The other branch enters deeper layers of the dorsal horn, sending terminals into laminae IV and V and extensive arborizations into the substantia gelatinosa (laminae II and III).

Most unmyelinated or thinly myelinated afferents pass directly through the outer layer of lamina I, where they synapse with marginal layer cells and send a few branches into the underlying substantia gelatinosa. Some axons pass ventrally through these outer layers to terminate in laminae V and X.[11]

There are two groups of cells in the dorsal horn that respond to noxious stimulation in the periphery. One group, located mainly in lamina I, responds exclusively to noxious stimulation. Most of these cells, termed nociceptive specific, have relatively limited receptive fields, confined to some fraction of a dermatome. The second group of cells, termed wide dynamic range neurons, can be activated by either tactile or noxious stimuli. Most of these cells are located in lamina V. They have large, complex receptive fields that often have a central area of responsiveness to either noxious or tactile stimulation, surrounded by an area of responsiveness only to noxious stimulation. Stimulation just outside the entire receptive field may produce inhibition. It is generally accepted that wide dynamic range neurons contribute to pain perception and that their selective activation is sufficient to cause pain. It is likely that many of the neurons in laminae I and V that respond to noxious stimuli are STT neurons.

Activation of the Dorsal Horn Projection System

There is considerable evidence that excitatory amino acids (EAAs) such as glutamate and aspartate are the principal neurotransmitters responsible for activation of dorsal horn neurons following noxious stimulation. Evidence for this conclusion is based on localization of these substances in nerve terminals in the dorsal horn, detection of release of EAAs following noxious stimulation, and behavioral evidence of hyperalgesia following intrathecal (IT) administration of EAAs in animals.[12]

Several types of EAA receptors are involved in the initiation of neuronal excitation that leads to the transmission of pain information. The AMPA receptor responds briefly (tens of milliseconds) and unconditionally to the release of glutamate.[13] Activation of the N-methyl-D-aspartate (NMDA) receptor results in postsynaptic potentials that may last much longer, on the order of seconds to minutes. The NMDA receptor is normally unresponsive to EAAs because of a voltage-dependent block that occurs at normal resting membrane potentials and physiologic concentrations of Mg^{2+}. Following a period of depolarization of the AMPA receptor or activation of neurokinin (NK-1) receptors by SP (which is released from nociceptive afferent terminals following intense activation), the NMDA receptor becomes responsive to EAAs and produces a relatively prolonged postsynaptic response (Fig. 56-1). In such a way, the brief response to a short-lived stimulus is converted to a prolonged response, one likely to be perceived as pain, following prolonged repetitive stimulation. The phenomenon of "windup,"[14] the progressive increase in response to repetitive, brief C fiber intensity stimulation, appears to be NMDA receptor mediated, and can be blocked by pretreatment with NMDA receptor antagonists. It has been proposed that the NMDA receptor is principally activated by aspartate released from excitatory interneurons in the dorsal horn, whereas the AMPA receptor is usually activated by glutamate released directly from afferent nerve terminals.

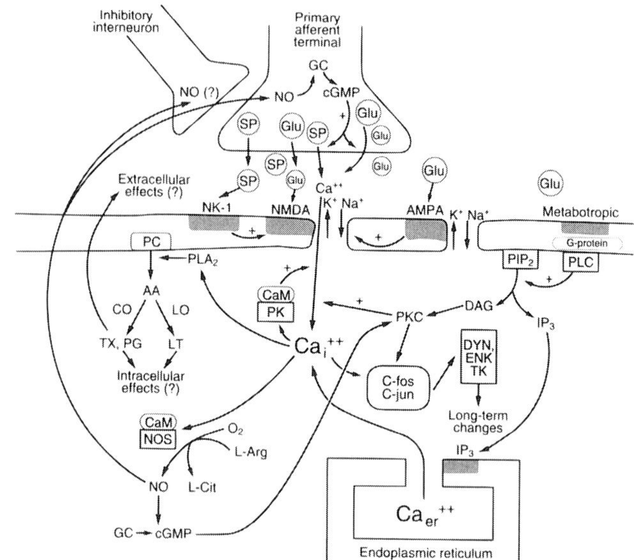

FIGURE 56-1. Sequence of events leading to sensitization of dorsal horn neurons following injury and intense nociceptive stimulation. Intense activation of primary afferent neuron stimulates release of glutamate (Glu) and substance P (SP). The NMDA receptor, at physiologic Mg^{2+} levels, is initially unresponsive to Glu. However, following depolarization of the AMPA receptor by Glu on the metabotropic receptor, it stimulates G protein-mediated activation of phospholipase C (PLC), which catalyzes hydrolysis of phosphatidylinositol 4, 5-biphosphate (PIP_2) to produce inositol triphosphate (IP_3) and diacylglycerol (DAG). DAG stimulates production of protein kinase C (PKC), which is activated in the presence of high levels of intracellular Ca^{2+} (Ca^{2+}). IP_3 stimulates release of intracellular Ca^{2+} from intracellular stores within the endoplasmic reticulum ($Ca^{2+}{}_{er}$). Increased PKC induces a sustained increase in membrane permeability and, in conjunction with increased intracellular Ca^{2+}, leads to increased expression of protooncogenes such as *c-fos* and *c-jun*. The proteins produced by these protooncogenes encode a number of neuropeptides, such as enkephalins (ENK), dynorphin (DYN), and tachykinins (TK). Increased $Ca^{2+}{}_i$ also leads to activation of phospholipase A_2 (PLA_2) and to activation of nitric oxide synthase (NOS) through a calcium/calmodulin mechanism. PLA_2 catalyzes the conversion of phosphatidyl choline (PC) to prostaglandins (PG) and thromboxanes (TX), and by lipoxygenase (LO) to produce leukotrienes (LT). NOS catalyzes the production of protein kinases, such as PKC, and alterations in gene expression. NO diffuses out of the cell to the primary afferent terminal, where, through a GC/cGMP mechanism, it increases the release of glutamate. It is speculated that NO may interfere with release of inhibitory neurotransmitters from inhibitory neurons. (From Hogan QH, Abram SE: Diagnostic and prognostic neural blockade. In Cousins MJ, Bridenbaugh PO [eds]: Neural Blockade in Clinical Anesthesia and Management of Pain, p 837. Philadelphia, Lippincott-Raven, 1998.)

There is evidence for still more prolonged increases in sensitivity of spinal cord neurons to sensory inputs occurring in response to ongoing nociceptor activation. Changes in dorsal horn neural function known as long-term potentiation can occur in the spinal cord and may last hours to days. It has been shown that prolonged excitation and release of EAAs in certain areas of the CNS can lead to damage or loss of neurons, and that such neurotoxicity is mediated at least in part by the NMDA receptor.[15] Following some types of peripheral nerve lesions in animals, the appearance of small darkly staining neurons in the substantia gelatinosa occurs coincidentally with the development of thermal hyperalgesia.[16] It has been proposed that these cells represent degenerating inhibitory interneurons (e.g., GABAergic or glycinergic cells) damaged by the large amounts of EAAs released by barrages of neural discharge from the injured nerve segment.[13]

Several neuropeptides that are released in the dorsal horn in response to noxious stimulation, including SP, neurokinin A, somatostatin, calcitonin gene-related peptide, and galanin, are believed to play a role in modulating the neural responses of dorsal horn cells sensory inputs.[16] The role of SP is perhaps best understood. It activates a postsynaptic NK-1 receptor, resulting in reduction of K^+ efflux (μ-opioids and α_2-adrenergic agonists enhance K^+ efflux), thereby increasing neuronal excitability. Its activity is limited by rapid enzymatic degradation. Neurokinin A also acts as an NK-1 receptor agonist, but it is more slowly broken down and may actively enhance dorsal horn transmission for a period of many minutes to a few hours following injury.[17]

1 Intense or prolonged noxious stimulation produces sustained depolarization of dorsal horn neurons leading to a series of intracellular events that alter cellular responsiveness to subsequent sensory input. Ca^{2+} influx into dorsal horn cells is generated by both membrane depolarization and NMDA receptor activation. Ca^{2+} influx then results in a series of intracellular events. These include the activation of phospholipase A_2 (PLA_2), as well as increased production of intracellular arachidonic acid and the products of the prostaglandin cascade. The resultant spinal cord accumulation of prostaglandins augments the hyperalgesic state through mechanisms not yet identified. Evidence for this proposal is provided by the fact that IT prostaglandins are indeed capable of inducing a hyperalgesic state[18] and that hyperalgesia induced by IT NMDA is inhibited by IT administration of nonsteroidal anti-inflammatory drugs (NSAIDs).[19]

Another mechanism by which Ca^{2+} influx enhances responsiveness to noxious stimulation is through an increase in the production of intracellular nitric oxide (NO). Intracellular Ca^{2+} activates the enzyme nitric oxide synthase through a calcium-calmodulin mechanism. NO is produced by the action of the enzyme on L-arginine. NO, which is rapidly diffusible both within and outside the cell, activates protein kinases through a cyclic guanosine monophosphate (cGMP) mechanism, leading to enhanced release of neurotransmitters from primary afferent terminals and enhanced responsiveness of the NMDA receptor in postsynaptic neurons. IT administration of substances that block the synthesis NO has been shown to inhibit nociceptor-induced spinal sensitization.[20]

Still other intracellular events, triggered by the action of EAAs and neuropeptides on metabotropic receptors, may lead to enhanced sensory processing. The activation of intracellular phospholipase C (PLC) stimulates the formation of inositol triphosphate (IP_3) and diacylglycerol (DAG). IP_3 stimulates release of intracellular Ca^{2+} stores, whereas DAG leads to increased production of protein kinase C (PKC). PKC further enhances NMDA receptor excitation and increases the expression of protooncogenes such as *c-fos* and *c-jun,* which control transcription of genes encoding a variety of neuropeptides that modulate responses to noxious stimuli.[16] Agents that inhibit production of PLC (e.g., neomycin) or PKC (e.g., H-7) reduce the delayed hyperalgesic response to subcutaneous formalin injection in rats (see Fig. 56-1).[21]

PKC is involved in the development of opioid tolerance.[22] Following prolonged occupation of opioid receptors on postjunctional dorsal horn neurons, there is translocation and activation of PKC, which in turn may uncouple the G protein that activates the potassium channel from the opioid receptor, producing tolerance. Thus activated, PKC may also enhance calcium influx through the NMDA receptor, producing sensitization of the cell as described previously. In addition, PKC activated by the activity of EAAs on the NMDA receptor is capable of uncoupling the opiate receptor mechanism, reducing opioid responsiveness (see Fig. 56-1). Thus, prolonged opioid administration can lead to spinal sensitization, and prolonged EAA release, as occurs with neuropathic pain states, and can reduce responsiveness to opioids.[22]

2 More recently, considerable research has been performed to characterize the role of glial, as opposed to neuronal cells, in the processes involved in sensitization of pain projection systems. Glial cells (microglia, astrocytes, oligodendrocytes) represent nearly three-fourths of all the cells in the CNS. It was originally believed that the sole function of these cells was to provide physical support for neurons. It is now known that they have important neuromodulatory and neurotrophic effects, and that they are extremely important in providing immune functions following injury, inflammation, or infection.[23]

Following nerve injury, there is rapid activation of glial cells within the CNS. Microglias, which are normally quiescent, are the first to respond. A triggering mechanism for glial activation is stimulation of toll-like receptors, which respond to membrane proteins of various viral and bacterial pathogens. One of these receptors, TLR4, can respond to substances produced during nerve injury in the absence of pathogens.[23] Following TLR4 upregulation, microglia then exhibit a change in morphology to an amoeboid form, they hypertrophy and proliferate, and they release substances that subsequently activate astrocytes (Fig. 56.2). Microglias initiate the immune response, and astrocytes maintain it. Both types of cells produce proinflammatory cytokines, including the interleukins IL-1β and IL-6 and tumor necrosis factor (TNF), which can diffuse throughout the region and produce functional changes in the surrounding neuronal cells.

Cytokines induce the release of a variety of substances that participate in the sensitization of sensory neurons. These include cyclooxygenase 2 (COX-2), inducible nitric oxide synthase (iNOS), and SP. They also activate chemokines in macrophages and endothelial cells, which initiate extravasation of leukocytes from the blood. Activated glial cells also release glutamate, NO, reactive oxygen species, eicosanoids, and other substances that act via the NMDA receptor to produce spinal sensitization.

A variety of stimuli have been shown experimentally to induce glial activation and the release of proinflammatory cytokines. These include nerve injury, nerve root ligation, tissue inflammation, arthritis, infection, and HIV antigen. Agents that prevent glial activation or that block the effect of cytokines have been shown to reliably prevent the development of hyperalgesia and allodynia in a number of experimental models.[24]

3 A particularly important part of the glial activation story is the observation that neuroimmune activation can occur following the induction of opioid tolerance.[25] Glial activation and upregulation of IL-1β, IL-6, and TNF-α were observed in the lumbar spinal cord of rats after 5 days of twice daily morphine but not saline injections. In addition, hyperalgesia and allodynia occurred following withdrawal of morphine. Chronic administration of morphine to nerve-injured rats produced more rapid development of allodynia and hyperalgesia, as well as greater cytokine production, than was seen in animals exposed to nerve injury but not morphine. The spinal administration of substances that inhibited cytokines restored the antinociceptive

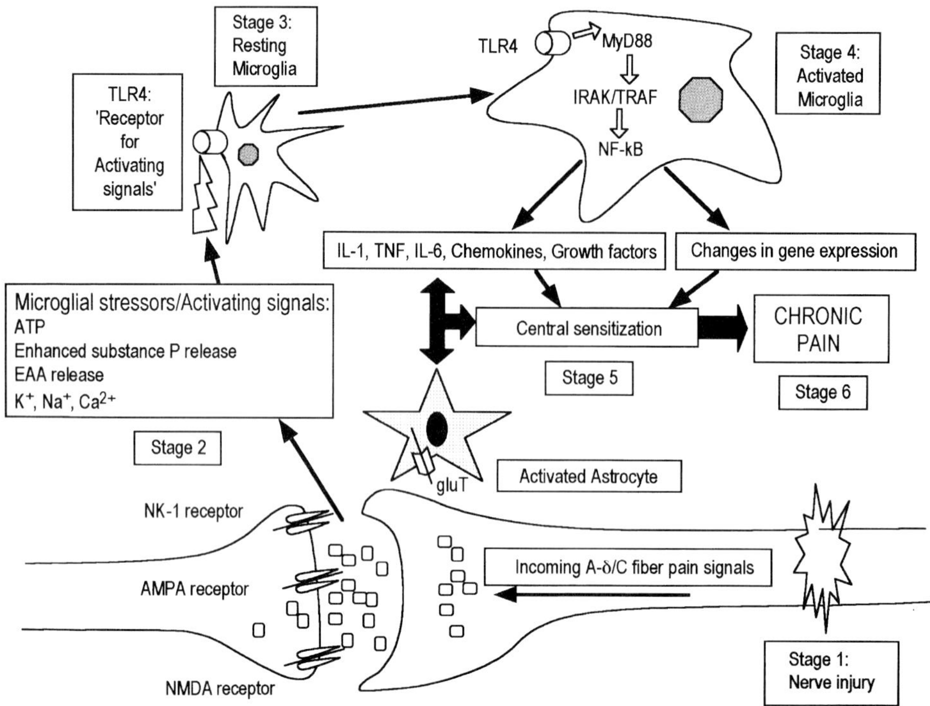

FIGURE 56-2. Proposed schema of TLR4-"receptor for activating signals" cascade in relation to the generation of chronic pain states. Under normal conditions, microglia are quiescent and highly ramified (stage 3). Upon nerve injury (stage 1), "pain" signals arriving from the periphery along a-δ and C fibers cause the release of substance P, excitatory amino acids (EAAs), adenosine triphosphates (ATPs), extracellular ions, and so on (stage 4). The stimulation of TLR4 leads to microglial activation, the recruitment of adaptor proteins (MyD88 and IRAK/TRAF6), the release of growth factors, and proinflammatory cytokines that trigger further cytokine and chemokine transcription and release. Upon release, cytokines contribute to activating astrocytes, which may decrease the efficiency of glutamate transporters (GluT, important for uptake of excess synaptic glutamate), and cause further release of additional cytokines and other algesic mediators. The release of these mediators leads to central sensitization (stage 5) and the clinical manifestation of chronic pain (stage 6). (Reprinted with permission from Deleo JA, Tanga FY, Tawfikk VL: Neuroimmune activation and neuroinflammation in chronic pain and opioid tolerance/hyperalgesia. Neuroscientist 10:40, 2004.)

effects of morphine and reversed the morphine-induced allodynia and hyperalgesia in both nerve-injured and sham-operated animals.[25] One proposed mechanism of opioid-induced hyperalgesia involves direct interference with glutamate transporter mechanisms on primary afferent nerve terminals and glial cells, blocking reuptake of excitatory amino acids and increasing their synaptic levels[23,26] (Fig. 56-3).

There are several systems capable of suppressing activity in STT neurons. There is substantial evidence that both descending and segmental neuronal inputs can inhibit activation of nociceptive-specific and wide dynamic-range neurons. The amino acids glycine and γ-aminobutyric acid (GABA) are known to be inhibitors of synaptic transmission, and there is some speculation that they are important mediators of segmental inhibition of nociception. There are two known GABA recognition sites: $GABA_A$, for which muscimol and isoguvacine are agonists, and $GABA_B$, for which baclofen is an agonist. Benzodiazepines act to enhance the effect of GABA on $GABA_A$ receptors. When administered spinally, they produce a mild analgesic effect and inhibit sympathetic response to noxious stimuli.

Two pentapeptides, leucine enkephalin and methionine enkephalin, appear to be important spinal cord inhibitors of nociception. STT neurons in laminae I and V receive input from enkephalin-containing cells in the dorsal horn. It has been proposed that enkephalins are released in proximity to primary afferent terminals in the dorsal horn, activating presynaptic opiate receptors that prevent release of SP. However, the presence of direct synaptic contact between enkephalin-containing cells and STT neurons suggests that their inhibitory mechanism is, at least in part, postsynaptic. Enkephalins are found in highest concentrations in laminae I and II but are also present in deeper laminae. Most dorsal horn enkephalins originate from intrinsic neurons.

It is not clear whether dorsal horn enkephalins function in a tonic fashion or whether their activity is stimulated for the most part by descending or peripheral segmental activity. If there is significant tonic inhibition by enkephalins, administration of naloxone should markedly increase activity in STT neurons. There is only equivocal evidence for such disinhibition. Release of enkephalins in response to descending neural activity has not been well documented. There is, however, evidence of enkephalin release in response to segmental activity.[27]

Serotonin, or 5-hydroxytryptamine (5-HT), produces analgesia when injected intrathecally, and its antagonist methysergide attenuates the analgesia produced by certain pharmacologic interventions. It is likely that this neurotransmitter is involved in descending control mechanisms that originate in the midbrain and medulla. It has been speculated that the analgesic effect of some of the tricyclic antidepressants may be related to an increase in serotonin availability in the CNS. However, the class of antidepressants known as serotonin-specific reuptake inhibitors (SSRIs) appears to have little or no

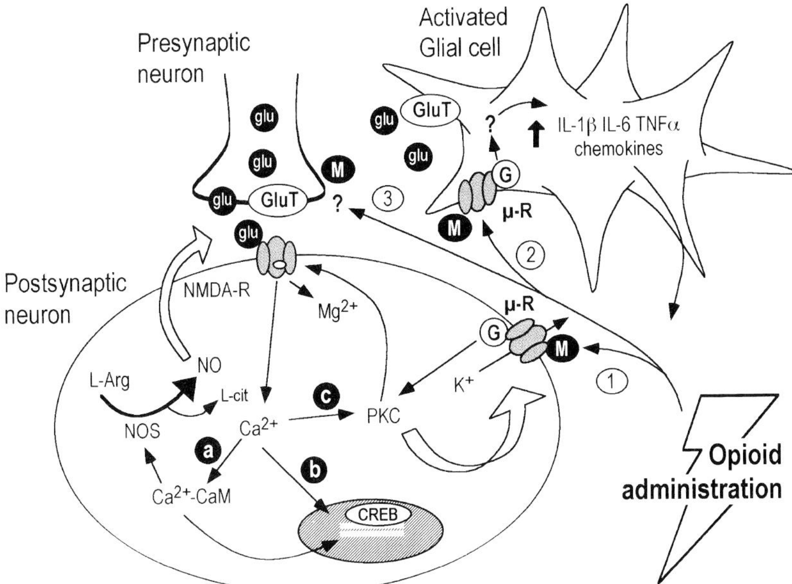

FIGURE 56-3. Cellular mechanisms of morphine tolerance/hyperalgesia. An opioid may act on the postsynaptic neuron (1), on the glial cell network (s), or on the presynaptic neuron (3). On the presynaptic neuron (1), opioid binding (represented by morphine, M) to the neuronal μ-receptor (μ-R) activates G protein-mediated protein kinase C (PKC) translocation and activation promoting removal of the NMDA receptor MG^{2+} plug. The ionotropic NMDA-R then responds to glutamate released from the presynaptic cell by allowing Ca^{2+} influx. This increase in intracellular Ca^{2+} leads to several downstream effects, including activation of Ca^{2+}-CaM (a), changes in gene expression (b), and further activation of PCK (c). Ca^{2+}-CaM in turn initiates the conversion of L-arginine to nitric oxide (NO) by nitric oxide synthase (NOS). NO may then act as a retrograde messenger to enhance glutamate release from the presynaptic neuron. With continual activation of these pathways by opioid receptor occupation, PKC may uncouple the G protein from the μ-R, preventing any downstream signaling upon ligand binding. Chronic opioid administration can act through the μ-R (2) on astrocytes to increase the production and secretion of cytokines and chemokines, or it can act directly on glial and neuronal glutamate transporters (Glu-T) to alter synaptic glutamate levels (3). Once released, cytokines may then act on the presynaptic or postsynaptic neurons to induce tolerance/hyperalgesia, or on the glial cells to promote further neuroimmune activation. G, G protein; glu, glutamate; Ca^{2+}-CaM, calcium-calmodulin. (Reprinted with permission from Deleo JA, Tanga FY, Tawfikk VL: Neuroimmune activation and neuroinflammation in chronic pain and opioid tolerance/hyperalgesia. Neuroscientist 10:40, 2004.)

beneficial effect on those conditions that typically respond to tricyclics.

Norepinephrine is also an important neurotransmitter in descending inhibitory pathways. Spinally administered adrenergic agonists, such as epinephrine, have been shown to have analgesic effects in animals. This analgesic effect is mediated by α_2-adrenergic receptors. Evidence for this is provided by the fact that α_2 agonists such as clonidine and dexmedetomidine produce analgesia when injected spinally and that α_2 antagonists such as yohimbine and idazoxan block their analgesic effects. IT clonidine is now in use for the treatment of intractable cancer pain. It appears to be helpful in some opioid-tolerant patients.

Adenosine receptors appear to play a role in the modulation of nociceptive transmission in the dorsal horn. There are two receptor subtypes: A_1, which inhibits adenyl cyclase activity, and A_2, which stimulates it.[28] Adenosine receptors may play a role in the analgesia provided by transcutaneous electrical stimulation because it has been demonstrated that dorsal horn inhibition induced by high-frequency stimulation is blocked by methylxanthines, which antagonize adenosine receptor activity. The adenosine receptor may also play a role in the mediation of analgesia induced by spinally administered opiates. Adenosine agonists have been shown to reduce the tactile hyperesthesia induced by low-dose spinal strychnine, a glycine receptor antagonist, and may prove to be effective in certain hyperalgesic states.

In summary, the dorsal horn functions as a relay center for nociceptive and other sensory activity. The degree of activation of ascending pain projection systems depends on the degree of activation of segmental and descending inhibitory neurons in the dorsal horn, the preexisting concentration of excitatory neurotransmitters, the level of activation of inhibitory neurotransmitters, the intensity of the noxious stimulus, and the degree of sensitization of nociceptors in the periphery.

Ascending Pathways

The STT has been considered for many years to be the most important pathway transmitting nociceptive stimuli to the brain. Although it is important to normal perception of pain, it is by no means the only pathway with that function. The ability of patients to perceive pain following spinothalamic tractotomy provides evidence that other pathways are involved.

Many of the neurons in laminae I and V that respond to noxious stimulation are probably cells of origin of the STT. The majority of STT fibers cross near their level of origin. There are believed to be two functionally distinct divisions of the STT: the neospinothalamic tract, whose fibers tend to be more lateral, and the paleospinothalamic tract, located in the medial portion of the pathway. The phylogenetically newer neospinothalamic tract projects to posterior nuclei of the thalamus, such as the ventral posterolateral nucleus, and is believed to be involved with discriminative functions (e.g., location, intensity, and duration of noxious stimulation).[29] The paleospinothalamic tract projects to medial thalamic nuclei, and its activation, is probably associated with autonomic and unpleasant emotional aspects of pain. This older portion of the STT is likely to be important in pain associated with denervation dysesthesia. Stimulation of the thalamic projections of the paleospinothalamic tract in patients with denervation dysesthesia reproduces the burning pain these patients experience spontaneously.[30]

The spinoreticular tract is likely to play a role in pain perception. Its cells of origin are unknown. It is believed to produce arousal associated with pain perception, and probably contributes to neural activity underlying motivational, affective, and autonomic responses to pain.[31] The spinomesencephalic tract projects to the midbrain reticular formation. It probably evokes nondiscriminative painful sensations and may be important in the activation of descending antinociceptive pathways.[31]

Following bilateral spinothalamic tractotomy, it is still possible for patients to perceive pain from peripheral stimulation. There must necessarily be pathways in the dorsal portions of the spinal cord that are capable of producing pain perception. The spinocervical tract is a likely candidate for such a function. It is located in the dorsolateral funiculus. Its fibers ascend uncrossed to the lateral cervical nucleus, which serves as a relay, sending fibers to the contralateral thalamus.[31] There is also evidence that some fibers in the dorsal columns are responsive to noxious stimuli.

Descending Control

In the early 1970s, several reports showed that electrical stimulation of the periaqueductal gray (PAG) area of the midbrain could produce widespread analgesia in animals and humans. The PAG was later found to have high concentrations of endogenous opiates and to be rich in opiate receptors. Microinjection of small quantities of morphine into that area produces generalized analgesia. Anatomic connections from the PAG area to the nucleus raphe magnus and to the medullary reticular formation were subsequently described. From the nucleus raphe magnus, serotoninergic fibers descend via the dorsolateral funiculus to spinal cord dorsal horn cells. It is not clear whether serotoninergic fibers produce a direct, postsynaptic inhibition of STT neurons or whether they act by activation of inhibitory neurons that release enkephalins or GABA.

There are also adrenergic fibers that descend in the dorsolateral funiculus that are believed to be inhibitors of pain. The cells of origin of these descending adrenergic pathways are believed to lie in the locus ceruleus and parabrachial regions of the medulla. Stimulation of spinal α_2-adrenergic receptors produces analgesia through G protein-mediated K^+ channel activation.

Multiple environmental factors appear to activate descending pain control mechanisms. Nociceptive inputs and various types of stress can produce generalized increases in pain threshold. Anxiety, depression, and emotional distress can reduce pain threshold. The descending control mechanisms described may respond to such factors. Under normal circumstances, inhibitory and pronociceptive neurons located in the midbrain periaqueductal gray rostral ventromedial medulla (RVM) play an important role in integrating and coordinating behavioral and autonomic responses to noxious stimuli.[32] Following a brief noxious stimulus, certain cells, known as "off-cells," in the RVM abruptly cease firing. It is believed that these cells produce tonic inhibition of nociceptive reflexes, and their cessation is associated with loss of such inhibition. Other cells, known as "on-cells," show a sudden burst of activity just before a behavioral response to a noxious stimulus. Their activation appears to produce a facilitatory influence on nociceptive transmission. At least some on-cells are GABAergic and exert an inhibitory influence on descending inhibitory neurons, including off-cells. On-cell activity is inhibited by local application of opioids, which block their inhibitory effect on pain-inhibitory pathways.

Pain and Nerve Injury

Spontaneous discharge of injured peripheral nerves was demonstrated by Wall and Gutnick,[33] who reported spontaneous neural activity originating from experimentally induced neuromas. It was later demonstrated that sympathetic stimulation or norepinephrine infusion could increase such abnormal firing.[34] There is now considerable evidence that changes in ion channel configuration and distribution are responsible for functional changes in the behavior of injured axons. Following nerve injury, there is an increase in the occurrence of large intramembranous particles, which represent surface proteins such as receptors and channel proteins. In addition, the membrane properties of a regenerating nerve tip differ from those of intact nerves. There is disappearance of the sodium-dependent action potential and an increase in conductance to Na^+, K^+, and Ca^{2+}.[35]

In addition to impulse generation originating from the site of injury, there is considerable evidence that impulse generation occurs at points of membrane instability proximal to the injury. Wall and Devor[36] reported spontaneous discharge originating from dorsal root ganglia in sciatic nerve-sectioned rats. They proposed that the dorsal root ganglia impulses could contribute to pain after peripheral nerve injury.

Another possible mechanism for chronic pain following peripheral nerve lesions involves the short circuiting of action potentials (ephaptic transmission, cross-talk) across demyelinated segments. Several possible types of interaction might exist. Demyelination of large afferent fibers could cause activation of nociceptors at the site of injury in response to stimulation of mechanoreceptors by nonnoxious stimuli. Injury of motor fibers could cause nociceptor activation in response to motoneuron activation. Loss of Schwann cell protection of postganglionic sympathetics could produce nociceptor firing in response to sympathetic discharge.

Intact peripheral nerve pathways are essential for normal function of pain projection neurons and inhibitory interneurons in the dorsal horn. Following loss of peripheral nerve activity, there may be an increase in sensitivity or onset of spontaneous activity in STT neurons. It has been postulated that disruption of large afferents, which send extensive arborizations into the substantia gelatinosa, decreases the activity of inhibitory neurons in those areas.

Spontaneous activity or heightened sensitivity of neurons is also believed to occur at more central locations within the pain projection system. Thalamic cells may undergo such changes following cord injury or some cerebrovascular accidents. Sensitization of central neurons may also occur some time after peripheral nerve injuries.

Sympathetically Maintained Pain

4 There are several mechanisms by which the sympathetic nervous system influences the perception of pain. Interactions between sympathetic outflow and spontaneous depolarization of

injured nerve segments have already been discussed. Following trauma, surgery, and certain illnesses, a syndrome of pain, hyperalgesia, autonomic dysfunction, and dystrophy, known as complex regional pain syndrome (CRPS), can occur. A common explanation is that there is interference with the normal regulatory function of the sympathetics to the affected area induced by pain or injury, hence the former name of the syndrome, reflex sympathetic dystrophy (RSD). Periods of heightened sympathetic activity are believed to result in vasoconstriction, ischemia, changes in interstitial environment, and, perhaps, release of prostaglandins, bradykinin, and other pain-sensitizing substances. This explanation is highly simplistic and is contradicted by several clinical findings: (1) early in the course of the syndrome, the affected limb is usually warm and erythematous; (2) microneurographic recording studies have failed to demonstrate alterations in sympathetic outflow in the affected limb; and (3) venous catecholamine levels in the affected limb are not elevated. However, there may be central dysregulation of autonomic function in these patients. Experimental evidence for interference with sympathetic regulatory function following injury was provided by Blumberg and Janig,[37] who demonstrated loss of the normal reciprocity between skin and muscle vasoconstrictors in animals with peripheral nerve lesions. Skin vasoconstrictors are normally under the influence of hypothalamic centers. They are important in thermoregulation and tend to be inhibited by stimuli that activate muscle vasoconstrictors, which are under medullary control. Following peroneal nerve lesions, skin vasoconstrictors begin to respond like muscle vasoconstrictors and appear to be under medullary control.[37]

Another possible interaction between sympathetic activity and pain perception involves ephaptic transmission, or "cross-talk," between different fiber types at injured nerve segments. Segmental loss of myelin or protective Schwann cell sheaths could lead to depolarization of nociceptor fibers by efferent sympathetic transmission. Although such segmental demyelination has been demonstrated anatomically, physiologic evidence for the phenomenon is scant.

Another proposal is the direct sensitization of nociceptor nerve endings by sympathetic nerve terminals. Again, there is little evidence that such nociceptor sensitization occurs. There is, however, considerable evidence that sympathetic fibers are in direct contact with mechanoreceptors and that sympathetic activity can sensitize mechanosensitive afferents. Roberts[38] proposed that a combination of sensitization of mechanoreceptors plus disinhibition of wide dynamic-range neurons could occur in certain posttraumatic states. Such a situation would lead to high-frequency firing of STT neurons and pain perception in response to nonnoxious mechanical stimulation.

Several studies have demonstrated sprouting of sympathetic neurons following nerve injury. These neurons proliferate to form elaborate arborizations, known as baskets, surrounding neuronal cell bodies.[39] It is not known as yet whether there is synaptic contact between the sympathetic fibers and the cell bodies, nor have the types of afferents whose somata are invaded by sympathetic sprouts been characterized. Nerve growth factor (NGF) and the cytokines leukemia inhibitor factor and IL-6 appear to contribute to the initiation of sympathetic sprouting. There is considerable speculation, although so far no proof, that the interactions between sympathetic sprouts and DRG cell bodies are responsible in part for sympathetically maintained pain in some clinical states.

PSYCHOLOGICAL MECHANISMS

No discussion of chronic pain is complete without some consideration of the psychological factors that are related to pain. In 1986, the International Association for the Study of Pain published a taxonomy of pain-related terms to promote uniformity of usage and to enhance accurate reporting of clinical and experimental phenomena.[40] Pain was defined as "an unpleasant sensory and emotional experience associated with actual or potential tissue damage, or described in terms of such damage." The salient features of that definition are that (1) pain is unpleasant, which is no surprise to most; (2) it may have a sensory component, also not surprising; (3) it has an emotional component, which distinguishes it from other sensory experiences such as touch, pressure, and vibration; and, most important, (4) it is an experience and, as such, is subjective, personal, private, and verifiable only by report of the individual suspected of suffering from pain. This last point cannot be overemphasized. Although much of what a physician does when dealing with pain patients is objectively verifiable by monitors, touch, or direct vision, these clinical tools only allow us to make inferences about another's suffering. The gold standard for determining if a patient is in pain is to ask the patient if he or she hurts. Other observations may aid in formulating a diagnostic impression, but only the patient can tell you if he or she has pain.

Psychological mechanisms can contribute to the pain experience in two general ways. A direct influence is exemplified by a situation in which psychological factors are entirely the cause of a report of pain. An example of this is psychogenic pain, which is considered to be rare. The psychological construct that is invoked to explain this involves the production of a perception of pain as a result of purely psychological factors, such as the need to suffer, a means of assuaging guilt, or a way to resolve some other intrapsychic conflict. This type of condition does exist but is frequently overdiagnosed. In fact, the likelihood of diagnosing psychogenic pain is inversely proportional to the skill and expertise of the physician examining the patient. The histories of these patients present no clear patterns or similarities, making a neat diagnostic algorithm impossible. Dramatic presentations, or conversely, apparent indifference, are not pathognomonic.[41]

Other direct psychological influences are found in the somatization disorders. These are a group of psychiatric disorders that are typified by a preoccupation with bodily function or symptoms. Hypochondriasis is a condition in which the individual is preoccupied with the notion that he or she is sick, despite continual reassurance from physicians. The exact psychological mechanism is not well understood, but this condition should be treated by a psychologist or psychiatrist. In suspecting this diagnosis, it is wise to remember that the term arose from patients describing pain below the right costal margin (hypochondriac) at a time when cholecystitis was not recognized as a bona fide medical entity. Patients with fears or convictions that they are ill do, on occasion, turn out to be right, so a careful history and physical examination coupled with performance of clearly indicated tests is advisable.

Somatization disorder is characterized by an onset of physical symptoms before the age of 30 years and includes at least 12 (for men) or 14 (for women) of 37 symptoms involving various organ systems. These symptoms are of sufficient severity to cause the individual to seek medical attention, to take medicines, or to otherwise alter his or her lifestyle. These patients typically have undergone extensive investigations, usually from multiple physicians, all of which have yielded negative, equivocal, or conflicting results. Frequent surgeries, usually of an exploratory nature, are a common historical feature. These features are superimposed on any genuine somatic diseases suffered by the person, presenting a complex clinical picture. The mechanism for this disorder is not proved, but it is suspected that these persons come from families in which little credence or attention is given to display of emotion, yet care and attention are provided in response to physical symptoms. Thus, the theory goes, the patient learns that the exhibition of a physical symptom results in attention to the patient's needs.

This modus operandi becomes ingrained on a subconscious level and then becomes part of the person's psychic constitution. This condition is not nearly as rare as psychogenic pain and, therefore, is likely to be seen with some frequency by a physician treating patients presenting with pain.

Factitious disorders (Munchausen syndrome) present with reporting of symptoms and the intentional creation of signs that are intended to lead a physician to suspect a medical or surgical disorder. Patients have been known to instrument their urethra to cause hematuria and complain of flank pain or to use tourniquets to induce edema of the limb. The motivation for this behavior appears to be to occupy the role of a patient. The reasons for this goal are poorly understood.

Another similar condition is malingering, which is differentiated only by motivation. In this case, the motivation to assume the role of a patient is driven by the desire to avoid some other alternative that the individual believes is distasteful, such as military service or apprehension by the police, or to achieve financial gain. Fortunately, these charades are usually transparent to the astute physician. The incidence of this disorder in pain clinics is probably low.

Indirect psychological effects that influence the pain experience are common in chronic pain syndromes. At its most basic level, the presence of an ongoing nociceptive process that is not well relieved and produces continual suffering is bound to have some psychological sequelae that will color the whole pain experience. Such secondary effects as sleep deprivation, fatigue, irritability, and anger are commonly observed.[42]

The issue of depression and pain has been discussed by several authors.[41,43] It is not surprising that most patients with chronic pain are likely to show signs of depression. It is difficult at times, however, to clarify the distinction between a set of depressive features that are reactive to having chronic pain and an episode of major depression because there can be so much overlap in symptoms.[43] The *Diagnostic and Statistical Manual of Mental Diseases*[44] includes many somatic and related symptoms in its criteria for diagnosing major depression. Most chronic pain patients will have several of these, but the genesis of the symptom (e.g., insomnia) may be due to the pain itself rather than depression. It is clear, however, that a negative affective state such as depression serves to enhance the suffering of a person with chronic pain.

Another indirect influence is that of pain behavior. Pilowsky et al[45] described the concept of illness behavior as it applies to pain patients. Simply stated, an illness is the individual's reaction or response to a disease. Illness behaviors arise from the patient's underlying physical condition and may consist of active behaviors, such as taking pills and visiting physicians, or passive behaviors, such as not working and lying down or sitting much of the day. In many chronic pain patients, the illness behaviors must become a focus of treatment.

Behaviors of any type are subject to influence by operant factors. Operant conditioning states that the likelihood of a behavior being expressed in a given situation can be altered by the consequences of the behavior. In chronic pain, for example, pain behavior (moaning) may be unwittingly reinforced by a spouse (showing attention), resulting in an increased frequency of the behavioral expression in the presence of the spouse. This is an example of positive reinforcement. By rewarding the behavior, its frequency is increased. The term *secondary gain* is often used to describe the type of paradigm wherein the individual, despite suffering with pain, does receive some benefit from it. Negative reinforcement increases the frequency of the behavior by removing a noxious condition from the environment in response to the behavior. Avoiding taking the garbage out by complaining of back pain is an example. Punishment, or the provision of undesirable consequences in response to a behavior, and extinction, the provision of no consequences, lead to decreased frequency of a behavior.

Cognitive factors also influence a pain experience. The belief that a person has about the meaning of his or her pain can substantially alter the actual perception of the pain. An important issue in this regard is the perceived degree of control over the pain. Using this fact, it is common practice for dentists to tell patients to raise their finger if anything hurts during the procedure. This granting of control allows patients to tolerate procedures with greater comfort. Contrast this with a patient suffering from poorly controlled cancer. Here, every time a pain is experienced, it reminds the patient of the cancer and the likelihood of an imminent and probably painful death.

MANAGEMENT OF COMMON CHRONIC PAIN SYNDROMES

It is beyond the scope of this chapter to consider the entire spectrum of long-term pain problems. Instead, the medical management of several painful conditions that are likely to respond to regional analgesic techniques or other modalities that anesthesiologists are likely to use is discussed. In addition, this section presents, in general terms, the use of some pharmacologic agents that are helpful in certain pain syndromes and provides a brief overview of the psychological principles that are important in managing chronic pain.

Low Back Pain

5 Several low back structures are innervated by nociceptors and act as sources of pain under certain pathologic conditions. The outer third of the annulus of the intervertebral disc has sensory innervation. Pain associated with annular tears is generally thought of as occurring only in the back; however, during discography, distension of the annulus commonly produces pain in the thigh and lower leg.[46] There is also evidence that, in the presence of chronic degenerative or inflammatory conditions, the vertebral bodies and vertebral end plates may become sources of pain.[47] Facet joints receive sensory innervation and, particularly if there are inflammatory changes in the joint, mechanical stimulation or injection of the joint may result in pain that may be localized to the back or may radiate to the buttock, thigh, and lower leg. A study using saline-controlled diagnostic local anesthetic injections of the facet joint indicated that in 40% of patients the facet joint was a source of low back pain.[48] Similarly, the sacroiliac (SI) joint is a source of pain in some patients, and injection of the joint reproduces back and lower-extremity pain in some patients who have evidence of SI joint pathology. Using a rigorous paradigm requiring pain relief after two separate joint injections, Maigne et al[49] concluded that only 20% of patients with clinical symptoms compatible with SI arthropathy had pain of SI joint origin. Mechanical compression or traction on a normal nerve root produces painless paresthesias. However, similar stimulation of a chronically injured or inflamed nerve root produces sciatica or pain in the normal sensory distribution of that nerve root.[50]

Lumbosacral Radiculopathy

Mechanical nerve root compression was originally presumed to be the cause of pain in discogenic radiculopathy. The lack of uniform success with surgical decompression and the fact that many asymptomatic patients demonstrate substantial disc protrusion on myelography or on subsequent postmortem examination suggests that other mechanisms must also be operative. Following a period of mechanical nerve root compression, an acute inflammatory process may ensue, leading to intraneural accumulation of serum proteins and fluid, raised intraneural pressure, ischemia, and axonal degeneration.[51] There is considerable evidence that the contents of the intervertebral disc can produce severe inflammation in the spinal canal. Gertzbein et al[52] found that patients with lumbar disc disease in which sequestration of nucleus pulposus occurred were highly likely to exhibit cellular immune responses to homogenates of lumbar disc material, whereas patients who did not show sequestration were less likely to show such a response. These findings led the authors to propose an inflammatory autoimmune mechanism for the radicular pain associated with disc rupture. Marshall and Trethwie[53] demonstrated the production of antibodies to glycoproteins from nucleus pulposus among patients who suffered from acute lumbar disc disease. They also demonstrated severe inflammatory reaction to nuclear glycoproteins following pulmonary arterial injection in a guinea pig heart-lung preparation.

A different line of evidence for the development of inflammation in response to disc rupture was presented by Saal et al.[54] They collected human disc samples removed at surgery from patients with symptomatic radiculopathy and analyzed the material for PLA_2 activity. They found extremely high levels in this material, 20- to 100-fold higher than activity from human inflammatory synovial effusion. They concluded that the high PLA_2 activity leads to inflammation at the site of disc herniation by action of the enzyme to liberate arachidonic acid from cell membranes.

Cytokines, including interleukins, NGF, interferons, and tumor necrosis factor alpha (TNF-α), are believed to play an important role in the pathophysiology of radiculopathic pain. Intrathecal administration of IL-6 can produce touch-evoked allodynia in rats, and substances that block the effects of TNF-α are capable of blocking the hyperalgesic effect of experimental mononeuropathy or endotoxin.[55]

It has been proposed that epidural or subarachnoid injection of corticosteroids provides beneficial effects by reducing the inflammation initiated by either mechanical or chemical insult to the nerve root.[56] The earliest use of epidural steroids was published by Lievre et al[57] in 1957, who reported good to excellent results in 50% of patients following injection of cortisone acetate plus radiographic dye. Most subsequent series of epidural steroid injections used a combination of local anesthetic and suspensions of insoluble steroids. To determine whether local anesthetic alone provided benefit for patients with sciatica, Coomes[58] compared patients receiving bed rest plus epidural injections of procaine with patients treated with bed rest alone. He found that patients treated with procaine became ambulatory in 11 days, whereas it took the noninjected patients an average of 31 days to regain ambulation. Swerdlow and Sayle-Creer,[59] in a nonrandomized study, found consistently better results among chronic pain patients treated with epidural lidocaine and methylprednisolone than for patients treated with epidural saline or lidocaine injections. There was no difference in success rates among the three treatment groups for patients with acute or recurrent sciatica. Winnie et al[60] compared patients treated with epidural methylprednisolone with patients treated with local anesthetic combined with the steroid. Success was close to 100% in both groups, suggesting that the steroid, rather than the local anesthetic, was providing the benefit.

Reports on more than 7,000 patients appear in the English language literature attesting to the beneficial effects of epidural steroid injections for the treatment of sciatica. However, although there have been anecdotal reports or noncontrolled case series attesting to the beneficial effect of epidural steroids in several thousand patients, only 13 controlled, randomized studies of the use of caudal or lumbar epidural steroid injections have been published. Koes et al[61] found that more than half of these controlled studies had substantial methodologic flaws. Of four studies that had reasonable methodologies, two reported positive (beneficial) results and two reported negative results. Watts and Silagy[62] performed a meta-analysis of nearly the same group of studies (11 randomized studies with 907 patients). In assessing the rate of treatment success, defined as >75% improvement for up to 60 days, they found the odds ratio for success in the steroid treatment group to be 2.61 (95% confidence interval [CI] 1.90 to 3.77). For long-term (>12 months) treatment success, the odds ratio for the steroid treatment group was 1.87 (95% CI 1.31 to 2.68). There was no significant difference in outcomes between the caudal and lumbar route of injection. A more recent controlled study, not included in either of the previous reviews, compared epidural methylprednisolone acetate with epidural saline.[63] The steroid-treated group experienced more improvement in sensory function and flexibility, but only at the 3-week assessment.

Few studies have evaluated the long-term effects of epidural steroids. Abram and Hopwood[64] compared the long-term responses of patients who initially experienced a favorable response to epidural steroid injections to those of patients who were considered treatment failures. After 6 months, patients in the initial success group were significantly more likely to rate their pain level lower, had significantly less sleep disruption, and were significantly less likely to be unemployed as a result of their pain when compared with initial failure patients.

The L5 and S1 nerve roots are most commonly affected by disc disease. Those roots pass through a narrow lateral bony recess as they exit the spinal canal, a circumstance that increases the likelihood of root compression.[65] Symptoms of lumbosacral radiculopathy consist of varying degrees of low back pain, pain radiating a varying distance into the lower extremity, and, in more severe cases, motor and sensory loss consistent with damage to the affected root. Typical signs and symptoms are listed in Table 56-1. As noted previously, the pain typically associated with nerve root pathology is often in the

TABLE 56-1

PAIN DISTRIBUTION AND PHYSICAL SIGNS ASSOCIATED WITH ACUTE DISC HERNIATION

LEVEL OF HERNIATION	PAIN DISTRIBUTION	NUMBNESS	WEAKNESS	REFLEX CHANGES
L3–L4 disc (L4 root)	Low back, buttock, lateral thigh, anterior calf, ankle, and occasionally big toe	Lower anterior thigh and patella	Mid (quadriceps)	Diminished (knee jerk)
L4–L5 disc (L5 root)	Low back, buttock, lateral thigh, calf, ankle, big toe	Lateral calf, web space of first and second toe	Foot (dorsiflexion)	None
L5–S1 disc (S1 root)	Low back, buttock, posterior thigh, and calf	Posterior calf, lateral heel, and foot	Foot (plantar flexion)	Diminished or absent (ankle jerk)

Reprinted with permission from Abram SE: Management of pain. In Cottrell JE, Turndorf H (eds): Anesthesia and Neurosurgery, p 496, St Louis, Mosby, 1986.

same distribution as pain associated with lumbosacral or facet arthropathy or with annular tears without nerve root pathology. The presence of sciatic stretch signs (positive straight leg raising, Lasegue's sign) or single segment sensory, motor, or reflex changes increase the likelihood that the pain is related to radiculopathy.

If bowel and bladder dysfunction are present, indicative of a large midline disc, prompt surgical intervention may be indicated. Otherwise, initial treatment of acute discogenic radiculopathy consists of short periods (a few days) of immobilization and mild analgesics followed by gradual resumption in physical activity. Prolonged immobilization has been shown to be counterproductive. If severe pain persists after reasonable trials of conservative management, epidural steroids may be used.

Methylprednisolone acetate is the most commonly used preparation. The usual dose is 80 mg, but smaller amounts should be considered in diabetic patients. Injections are generally performed as close to the affected nerve root as possible. Injection of a small volume (3 to 4 mL) of local anesthetic (preferably short acting, e.g., 1% lidocaine) will produce considerable analgesia if it reaches the affected nerve root, confirming proper drug placement. The anesthetic may be injected first as a test dose to rule out intrathecal placement. In occasional patients, particularly those with S1 pathology, the drug will not spread adequately to the affected root. In that situation, caudal injection may result in better drug access to the injured nerve.

Fluoroscopic guidance is often used to ensure the drug reaches the target nerve root. For the interlaminar approach, the patient is positioned prone and the appropriate interspace is identified. The needle is introduced slightly off the midline on the affected side, at the lower border of the interlaminar space, and directed slightly cephalad. It is advanced until the ligamentum flavum is engaged, and a loss of resistance technique is used to initially identify the epidural space (Fig. 56-4). A small volume of nonionic radiographic dye is injected "live," and both AP and lateral images are observed (Fig. 56-5). Intravascular injection can be readily identified as the dye is quickly carried away from the injection site. Following observation of appropriate spread of dye, the steroid is injected, either with or without anesthetic. If dye does not spread to the affected nerve root, another approach is attempted, either at a different level or via a transforaminal technique.

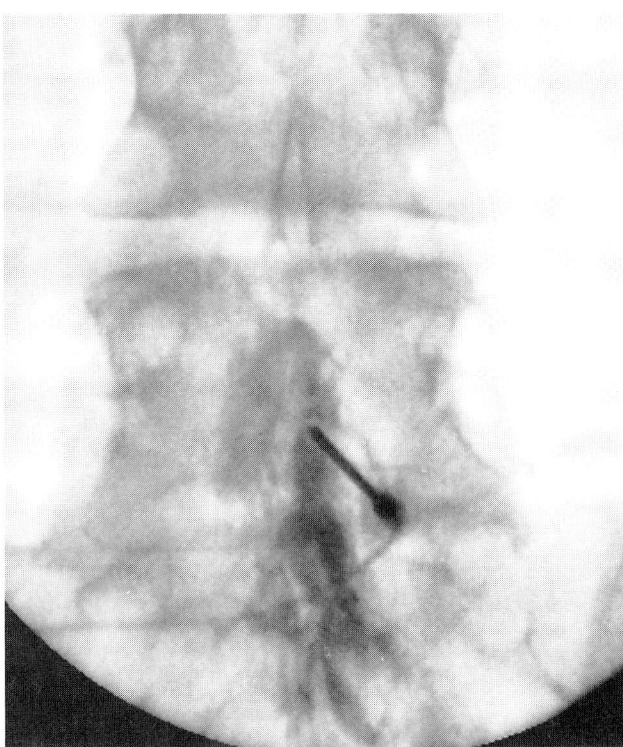
FIGURE 56-5. Epidural injection of 2 mL nonionic radiopaque dye via the L5–S1 interlaminar space.

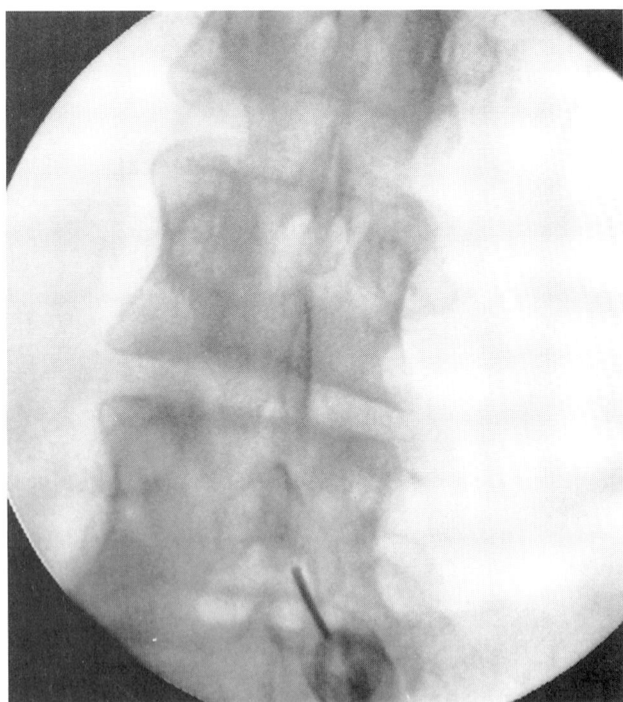
FIGURE 56-4. Fluoroscopic translaminar approach to the epidural space at the L5–S1 level.

The transforaminal approach involves placement of a needle at the exit site of the affected nerve root from the foramen. Using an oblique view (left anterior oblique for a right-sided block), the needle is positioned against the posterolateral aspect of the vertebral body, just below the pedicle. Injection in this so-called "safe triangle" will reduce the risk of intraneural injection, which can result in intrathecal drug spread.[66] Nonionic radiographic dye is injected "live," and should be seen to spread both centrally into the epidural space and peripherally along the nerve root (Fig. 56-6). Careful observation during injection will help rule out intra-arterial injection. Injection of the particulate steroid into a radicular artery could theoretically produce spinal cord or nerve root injury. A small amount of local anesthetic (1 to 2 mL) should be injected to determine if the target nerve root is indeed a pain generator. The usual dose of methylprednisolone acetate is 20 to 40 mg.

Another approach involves passage of a radiopaque caudal catheter under fluoroscopic control. The catheter is advanced epidurally to the foramen of the target nerve root. Injection should be carried out in the same manner as for transforaminal injection.

The fluoroscopically controlled techniques are especially indicated for patients who have had previous surgery or who have anatomic conditions that are likely to make a blind epidural difficult. Although a growing number of physicians use fluoroscopy for all epidural steroid injections, standard techniques may be reasonable for patients who have relatively normal anatomy.

Reassessment should be carried out 1 to 2 weeks after the initial treatment. If the patient has little or no pain at the time

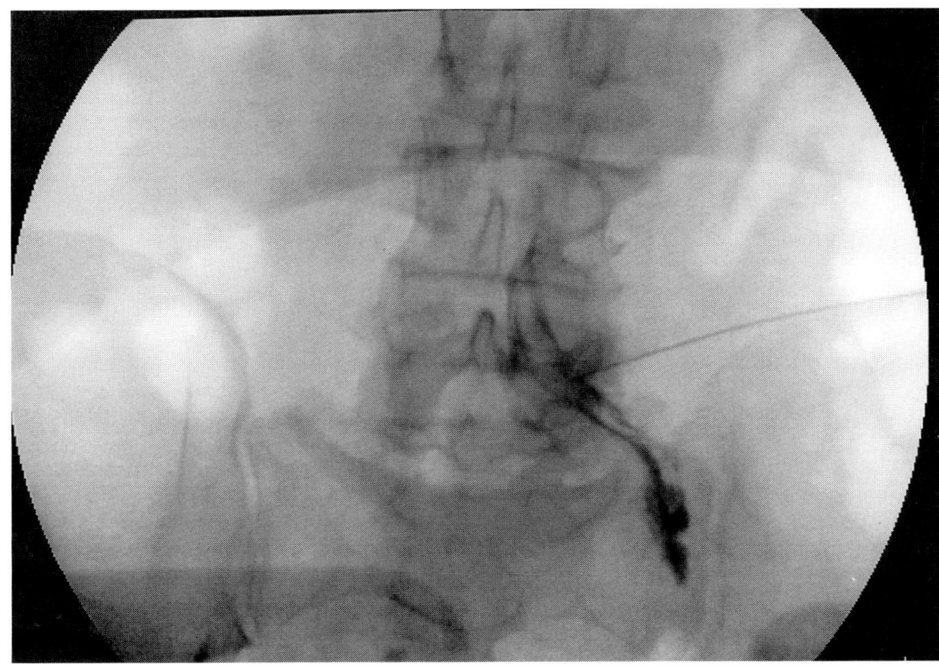

FIGURE 56-6. Right transforaminal epidural injection. Injection of 2 mL nonionic radiopaque dye demonstrates spread of injectate proximally into the epidural space and distally along the nerve root. The nerve root can be visualized as lucency outlined by the dye.

of the return visit, repeating the injection is relatively unlikely to be of benefit. However, if it was believed that the drug may not have reached the affected root at the time of the initial injection, a repeat procedure is a reasonable option. If symptoms are improved at the time of the follow-up visit, but some pain is still present, it is likely that a repeat injection will produce further improvement. A third block can be performed 1 to 2 weeks later if some symptoms persist. An algorithm for epidural steroid treatment is shown in Fig. 56-7.

There appears to be extremely little risk of serious complications associated with the use of epidural steroid injections. Animal studies tend to confirm the safety of neuraxial administration of depo steroids.[67,68] Allegations that the 3% polyethylene glycol vehicle of methylprednisolone acetate (MPA) and triamcinolone diacetate (TD) is capable of producing neurologic damage[69] are based on studies of high concentrations of propylene glycol (80 to 100%), and appear to be unfounded. The doses of corticosteroids commonly used for the treatment

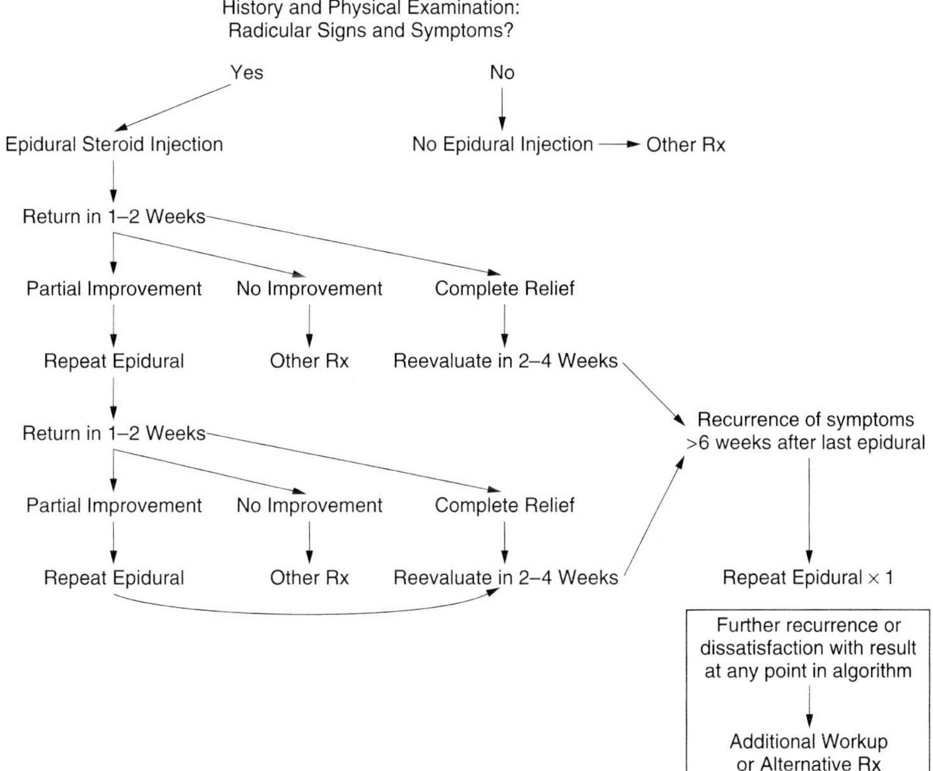

FIGURE 56-7. Algorithm for treatment of sciatica with epidural steroid injections.

of sciatica are capable of producing adrenal suppression for up to several weeks, and there are occasional reports of cushingoid side effects, sometimes lasting for weeks or longer. For example, a single injection of triamcinolone into the epidural space for the treatment of low back pain in adult patients has been shown to acutely suppress the hypothalamic-pituitary-adrenal (HPA) axis as reflected by decreased plasma cortisol and adrenocorticotrophic hormone levels in response to a provocative stimulus.[70] When three epidural triamcinolone injections were administered at 7-day intervals, the median suppression of the HPA axis was less than 1 month following the last injection, and all patients had recovered by 3 months. Sedation with midazolam in conjunction with the epidural steroid injection accentuates the suppression of the HPA axis.[70] These observations suggest the possible need for exogenous steroid coverage in patients undergoing major stress during the period that the HPA axis may be suppressed by epidural steroids. Epidural steroid injections should be used with caution in diabetic patients, who may be at added risk for epidural infections, and whose glucose control may be compromised. Of the several cases of epidural abscess reported following epidural steroids, most occurred in diabetic patients.[71] Because of the immunosuppression associated with the steroid, aseptic technique should be meticulous.

Most of the literature documenting the safety of epidural steroids comes from reports on the use of a small number of injections, usually one to three, and with modest doses, usually 40 to 80 mg MPA or 50 mg TD. There are few data to support the safety of this treatment when higher doses are used.

There is some evidence that complications can occur following intrathecal steroid injections. Accidental injection of substantial doses of local anesthetic can result in high or total spinal. No cases of death or brain damage were reported following epidural steroid injections by the ASA Closed Claims Project,[72] all of which undoubtedly involved intrathecal local anesthetic placement. Aseptic meningitis[73] and bacterial meningitis[74] appear to be uncommon but real risks. Arachnoiditis[75] and cauda equina syndrome[76] have been reported, but these cases are rare and have occurred after multiple injections over a prolonged time interval. Nevertheless, it may be reasonable to use a test dose of local anesthetic prior to injection of steroid, or to use fluoroscopy and radiographic dye to rule out intrathecal placement of the needle.

Patients with chronic radicular low back pain are much less likely to benefit from epidural steroid injections than are patients with more acute symptoms. Abram and Anderson[77] reported in a retrospective study that patients with long-standing symptoms were much less likely to experience even transient relief from epidural steroid injections. Similar findings were seen in a subsequent prospective study.[64] Patients who had undergone previous back surgery also had a much lower success rate. Several mechanisms may lead to chronic radicular pain that is unresponsive to steroid injections. Spontaneous activity or ephaptic transmission may occur from the injured, demyelinated root. Scarring of the root, with replacement of neural elements with fibrous tissue, causes inelasticity of the nerve. The nerve root can no longer stretch with leg motion, and chronic mechanical irritation ensues.[51] Loss of large afferent fibers may lead to disruption of dorsal horn gating mechanisms and disinhibition of spinothalamic projection cells. Loss of disc height following herniation can lead to narrowing of intervertebral foramina, with subsequent root irritation laterally, or may cause redundancy and buckling of the posterior longitudinal ligament, which can effectively narrow the spinal canal. Loss of disc height can lead to facet joint subluxation and degeneration, producing pain from the joint itself and to osteophyte formation, which can narrow foramina or the central canal. Injury to the vertebral plate, the cartilaginous portion of the vertebral body adjacent to the disc, often accompanies disc disease and may lead to osteophytic growth into the central canal.

Some patients with chronic radicular pain do experience relief for several weeks to months after epidural steroids, and a growing number of physicians are willing to repeat the injections at 3- to 4-month intervals. Such treatment appears to be relatively safe, although no prospective studies have been carried out in this treatment population.

Lumbosacral Arthropathies

Degeneration and inflammation of the lumbar facet joints and sacroiliac joints can produce low back pain that is often difficult to distinguish from radicular pain. Both conditions may cause pain that radiates to the lower extremities. Computed tomography scanning is a fairly reliable method of demonstrating pathology in these joints. Bone scans, particularly single-photon emission computed tomography (CT) scanning, may also be useful diagnostically.

When facet arthropathy is the suspected cause of low back pain, the diagnosis can be confirmed by injection of local anesthetic into the facet joint. The procedure can be done easily under fluoroscopic control. The patient is placed prone, and the affected side is tilted upward until the joint space is visualized. Proper needle placement can be confirmed by injection of 0.5 to 1 mL of nonionic contrast (Fig. 56-8). The injection should transiently reproduce the patient's pain, and the dye will outline the extent of the capsule. Injection of 0.5 mL of local anesthetic should produce dramatic relief of arthropathic pain. Injection of a small volume of insoluble corticosteroid into an affected joint has been reported to produce analgesia lasting 6 months or longer in about one-third of patients who experience relief from the local anesthetic. NSAIDs may be of some benefit.

When sacroiliac pathology is demonstrated, injection of the joint with local anesthetic will help confirm the diagnosis. In an uncontrolled study, we found that 25 of 35 patients with suspected sacroiliac disease experienced pain relief from local anesthetic injection of the joint. After injection of triamcinolone diacetate, 7 of 20 patients who were followed long-term experienced at least 6 months of moderate to complete pain relief (Abram SE, unpublished data, 1982). As noted previously, a more rigorous local anesthetic treatment paradigm showed only a 20% response to local anesthetic injection.[49] Injection is performed in the lower one-third of the joint, within the diarthrodial portion. A slightly posterior oblique view permits alignment of the anterior and posterior joint lines, giving a view along the plane of the joint. Correct positioning of the needle can be confirmed with the injection of a small volume of dye, which will be seen spreading along the joint space (Fig. 56-9).

Myofascial Pain

The myofascial syndrome is an extremely common cause of somatic pain. It is associated with marked tenderness of discrete points (trigger points) within affected muscles, pain that is referred to areas some distance from the trigger point, and the appearance of tight, ropy bands of muscle. Autonomic changes, such as vasoconstriction and skin conductivity changes, may occur some distance from the affected muscle.[78] Biopsies of trigger points have been reported to show little or no change or to show degenerative changes, the severity of which corresponds to the intensity of the symptoms.[78] Although the pathophysiology of the condition has not been clearly defined, Travell and Simons[78] proposed the following explanation: acute muscle strain causes disruption of sarcoplasmic reticulum and release of calcium, which in turn produces sustained or

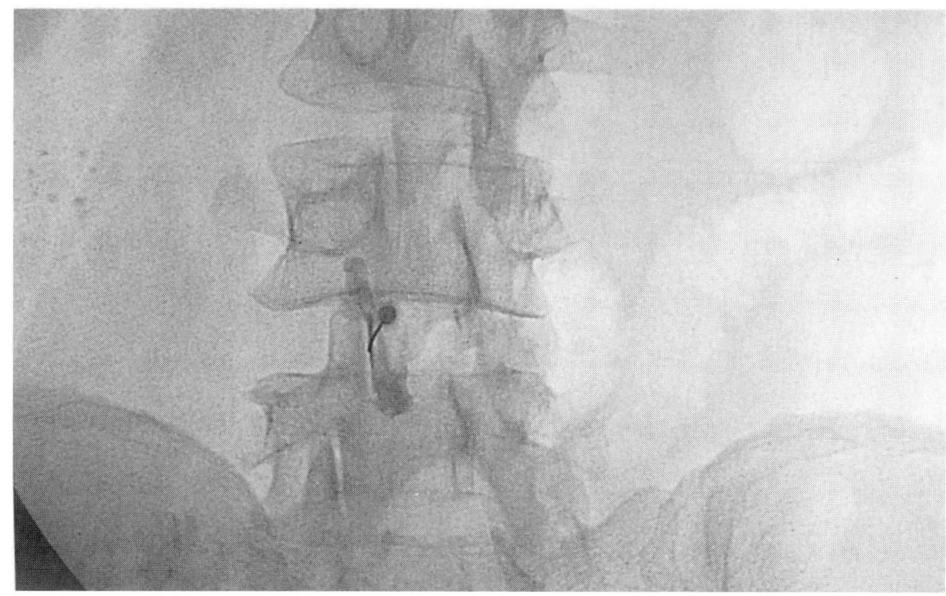

FIGURE 56-8. Left L4–L5 facet injection. Injection of 0.5 mL nonionic radiopaque dye demonstrates the extent of the joint capsule.

repeated contraction and fatigue. Blood flow becomes inadequate for the degree of metabolic activity occurring locally. Adenosine triphosphate becomes depleted, preventing release of myosin from actin, causing sarcomeres to become rigid and affected muscles to become taut. Nociceptor-sensitizing substances, such as prostaglandins, bradykinin, and serotonin, are released from platelets and mast cells, causing increased firing of muscle nociceptors.

Many of the commonly affected muscles, the sites of their trigger points, and their zones of referred pain have been mapped out. The scapulocostal syndrome, one of the most common patterns of myofascial pain, is characterized by a trigger point located just medial and superior to the upper portion of the scapula and pain that can radiate to the occipital region, shoulder, medial aspect of the arm, or anterior chest wall.[79] Myofascial pain involving gluteal muscles produces pain referred into the posterior thigh and calf, mimicking S1 radiculopathy. Myofascial pain involving the piriformis muscle, which overlies the sciatic nerve, can produce sciatic irritation and, occasionally, hypoesthesia, again resembling radiculopathy.

The most important aspect of treatment for myofascial pain is to regain muscle length and elasticity. This is best done by maneuvers that gently stretch affected muscles. Because of the sensitization of muscle afferents, appropriate physical therapeutic maneuvers are often painful and may reinitiate muscle contraction. Therapy aimed at reducing muscle pain and sensitivity should therefore be employed before stretching exercises. Trigger point injection, infiltration of local anesthetic directly into the trigger point, is a valuable initial therapy. Pain relief following injection confirms the diagnosis of myofascial

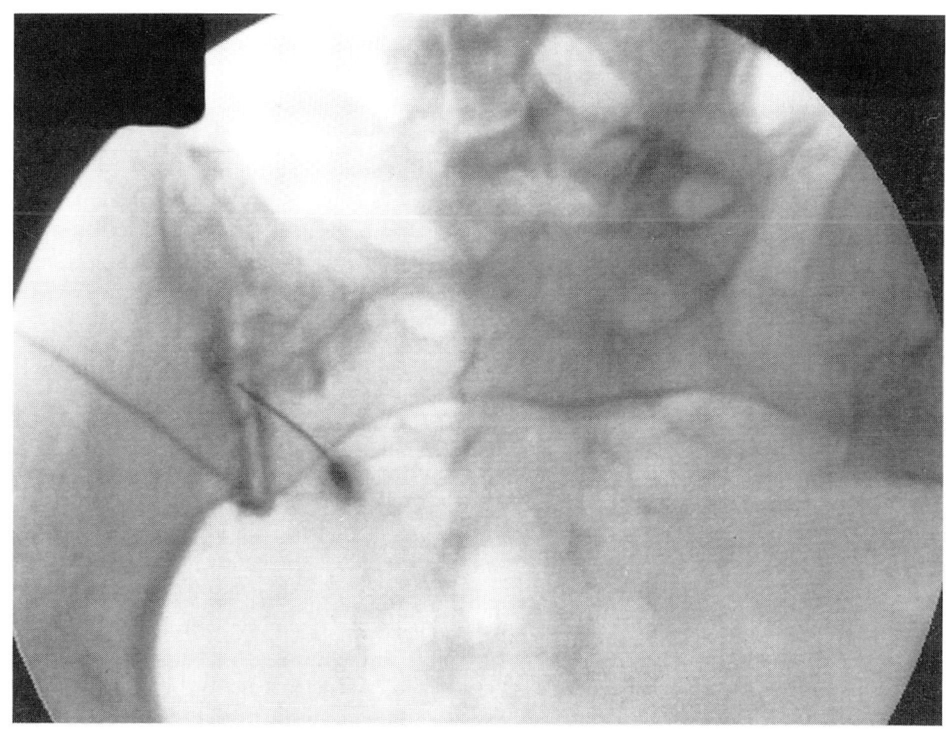

FIGURE 56-9. Sacroiliac joint injection. Radiopaque dye injection outlines the cartilaginous portion of the joint.

syndrome, and a series of several injections performed daily or every several days can markedly reduce muscle sensitivity. Fairly vigorous therapy can be carried out during the analgesic period after each injection. Ultrasound therapy applied over the affected muscle may also produce periods of analgesia.

Trigger point injections and ultrasound require the participation of trained personnel, precluding their use on a frequent regular basis (e.g., several times per day). Several treatment modalities can be used by the patient alone or with the help of family members. Transcutaneous electrical nerve stimulation (TENS), applied directly over the trigger points, may produce analgesia during stimulation and often for some time afterward. Stimulation should be carried out for 20 to 30 minutes prior to stretching exercises. Some patients who do not respond to the usual high-frequency TENS may benefit from a brief period (about 5 to 10 minutes) of low-frequency (2 to 4 Hz), high-intensity TENS. The current should be high enough to cause muscle contraction and mild discomfort. Vapocoolant spray (e.g., fluoromethane) sprayed over the affected muscle may produce transient analgesia sufficient to facilitate physical therapy. Massage of the affected muscle with ice may also be of some benefit.

Injection of myofascial trigger points with botulinum toxin, which produces a long-lasting block of acetylcholine release from peripheral nerves, has been shown to provide lasting pain relief in myofascial syndrome.[80] Pain relief begins within 1 to several days after injection and generally lasts several weeks. The principal side effect is weakness in the injected and adjacent muscles.

Myofascial pain often develops in patients whose response to stress is an increase in muscle tone. This mechanism frequently contributes to the pathophysiology of tension headache. Surface measurement of electromyography in such patients will often demonstrate extremely high activity at rest. Electromyographic biofeedback is a useful added therapy for such patients and appears to be helpful in preventing future painful episodes for patients with recurrent problems.

Complex Regional Pain Syndromes

The term *reflex sympathetic dystrophy* (RSD) has been widely used to describe a group of conditions associated with burning pain in an extremity; dystrophic changes in skin, hair, nails, and joints; allodynia; and signs of autonomic dysfunction, including skin temperature changes and alterations of sweat gland activity. The term *causalgia* has been used to describe a syndrome with similar clinical features following injury to a major nerve trunk. The term *sympathetically maintained pain* (SMP) has been used synonymously with both of these syndromes, implying that the autonomic nervous system is somehow involved in the pathophysiology of these conditions. Although autonomic dysfunction is clearly evident in some cases of causalgia and RSD, it is not a prominent feature in some cases, and many patients with these conditions fail to respond to blockade or ablation of sympathetic fibers. Therefore, the term *complex regional pain syndrome* (CRPS) has become widely accepted.[81] Complex regional pain syndrome type I (CRPS-I) has replaced the term RSD, and CRPS-II is now used in place of the term causalgia. SMP describes that component of pain that is initiated or maintained by activity in the sympathetic nervous system, including both efferent sympathetic nervous system activity and circulating catecholamines. Painful conditions that are not typical of CRPS may have a sympathetically mediated component. Patients with certain types of neuropathic pain do not exhibit the typical clinical features of CRPS and yet experience significant pain relief following sympathetic blockade. Likewise, some patients with typical features of CRPS experience no relief from sympathetic denervation. Pain that does not appear to be sympathetically mediated is termed *sympathetically independent pain.*

CRPS-I

Common antecedents to the development of this syndrome include crush injuries, lacerations, fractures, sprains, and burns. Many postoperative cases occur after surgery involving the median nerve distribution, such as carpal tunnel release or palmar fasciectomy. The syndrome occasionally occurs after cerebrovascular accident or myocardial infarction. The pain is usually burning in quality and is often accompanied by diffuse tenderness and pain on light touch. The hand or foot are commonly the major sites of pain. The pain and hypersensitivity often spread beyond the original sites of pain.

Autonomic dysfunction is manifested as changes in skin temperature, cyanosis, edema, and hyperhydrosis. The skin may be warm and erythematous, with occasional to frequent bouts of intense vasoconstriction. In more severe, rapidly progressive cases the involved extremity is predominantly cool and pale or cyanotic. The vascular phase of bone scanning often demonstrates differences in flow between the normal and the affected extremity. Thermography or local measurement of skin temperature using surface thermistors is useful in documenting differences in skin blood flow.

Dystrophic changes become increasingly evident with time if the condition is untreated. Skin of the affected area becomes smooth and glossy. Bone demineralization takes place to a much greater extent than would be expected on the basis of reduced activity. Joints in the affected extremity become stiff and painful as a result of synovial edema, hyperplasia, fibrosis, and perivascular inflammation.

Local anesthetic blockade of the sympathetic chain is useful diagnostically, particularly when only a portion of the spectrum of possible symptoms is present. Cervicothoracic sympathetic block is usually carried out by injection of local anesthetic on the anterior tubercle of C6 (see Fig. 56-10) or on the medial portion of the transverse process of C7. Unfortunately, a moderate number of patients experience Horner's syndrome but fail to demonstrate evidence of sympathetic denervation of the upper extremity. Using magnetic resonance imaging (MRI) scans, Hogan et al[82] demonstrated that solutions injected paratracheally at the C6 or C7 anterior tubercle often fail to spread to the stellate ganglion. Subsequently, he and his colleagues described a CT-guided technique for direct injection of the stellate ganglion just anterior to the head of the first rib.[83] Using this technique, evidence of sympathetic denervation of the extremity is often seen after injection of as little as 1 mL of local anesthetic. Lumbar sympathetic block is performed by injecting local anesthetic at the anterolateral aspect of the lumbar spine (see Fig. 56-11). Placement of the needle at the lower border of the L2 vertebral body minimizes needle contact with the nerve root and places the needle tip in the plane of the sympathetic chain.

Pain relief following sympathetic blockade does not guarantee that there is a sympathetically mediated component to the patient's pain. Pain relief may be the result of a placebo effect, spread of anesthetic to somatic afferent fibers, blockade of afferent fibers located in the sympathetic chain, or the systemic effect of absorbed local anesthetic.[84] Similarly, failure to achieve pain relief following sympathetic block does not guarantee that the pain is not sympathetically mediated. There may be sympathetic efferent fibers to the limb that do not travel with that portion of the sympathetic chain that has been interrupted.[84]

Once it has been established that there is a sympathetically mediated component to the patient's pain, treatment consists of a series of local anesthetic sympathetic blocks. For patients with lower-extremity pain, if lumbar sympathetic block is

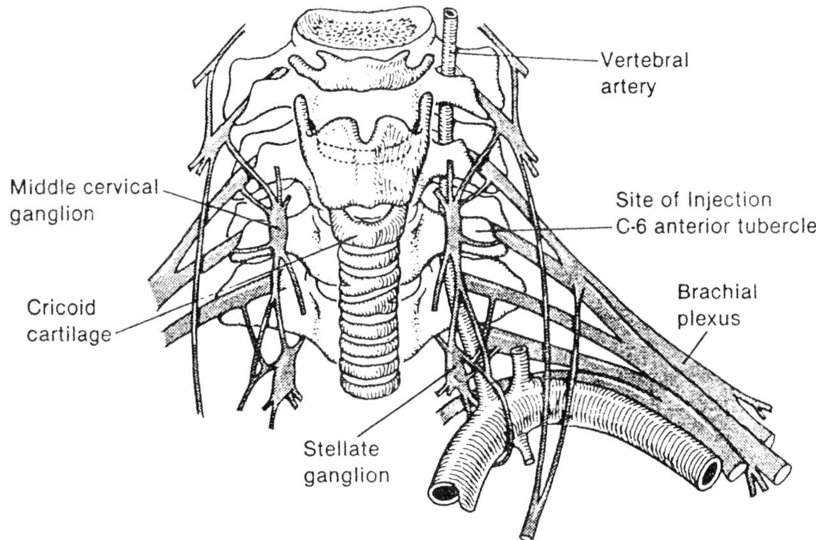

FIGURE 56-10. Site of injection for the C6 paratracheal approach to the cervicothoracic sympathetic chain. (From Abram SE, Boas RA: Sympathetic and visceral nerve blocks. In Benumof JL [ed]: Clinical Procedures in Anesthesia and Intensive Care, p 787. Philadelphia, JB Lippincott, 1992.)

technically difficult or is particularly painful to the patient, repeated or continuous lumbar epidural blockade can be used instead. Injections are generally continued until symptoms are minimal or until there is no further progression of benefit. Physical therapy, consisting of desensitizing techniques and active or active-assisted range of motion, is usually indicated and should be carried out immediately after each sympathetic block. Vigorous passive range of motion and heavy weights should be avoided because they may retrigger symptoms. Patients whose condition is diagnosed and treated early are more likely to respond to sympathetic blocks. Success rates of 90% or more have been reported.[85] Unfortunately, few if any controlled studies documenting the long-term effects of sympathetic blockade exist, and the high success rates associated with early intervention may simply reflect the natural history of the process.

The use of systemic sympathetic blocking drugs is occasionally useful clinically. Prazosin and phenoxybenzamine, both α-adrenergic blocking agents, provide partial symptomatic relief in some patients, particularly those patients exhibiting signs of vasoconstriction.[86] Intravenous phentolamine, given in small incremental doses up to 30 mg maximum, is helpful in predicting response to oral α-adrenergic blockers.[87] Oral and transdermal clonidine are also occasionally useful. Other systemic medications that have been used with variable success include calcium channel blockers, tricyclic antidepressants, and anticonvulsants. Gabapentin has been used with some success and is better tolerated than most of the older anticonvulsants.

Kozin et al[88] reported substantial benefit from treatment of RSD with a brief course of high-dose corticosteroids. Their success rate was 82%, which is particularly impressive in that many of their patients had experienced long-term symptoms. However, it is not clear whether improvement was permanent in these patients. In addition, their criteria for diagnosing RSD were somewhat vague and did not include response to sympathetic block, allodynia, hyperpathia, or burning pain. Side effects from high-dose systemic steroids are often troublesome. An alternative treatment is the intravenous regional injection of soluble steroids in the affected limb.[89] TENS can be a useful adjunctive treatment for CRPS-I. Increased skin temperature during stimulation has been documented in patients who experience pain relief following treatment,[90] and TENS has been reported to provide substantial clinical benefit when used as the sole therapy.[91]

Patients with long-standing symptoms of CRPS-I, who develop dystrophic changes and, frequently, the behavioral and psychological profiles typical of chronic pain patients, are extremely resistant to the types of intervention described previously. Surgical or neurolytic sympathectomy has been suggested as a treatment for patients who respond only transiently to sympathetic blocks. It is the authors' experience, however, that most patients with chronic CRPS-I get no relief or only a few days to weeks of benefit from sympathetic ablation. Therapy instead should be directed toward extinguishing pain behavior, increasing strength and mobility, and developing coping strategies.

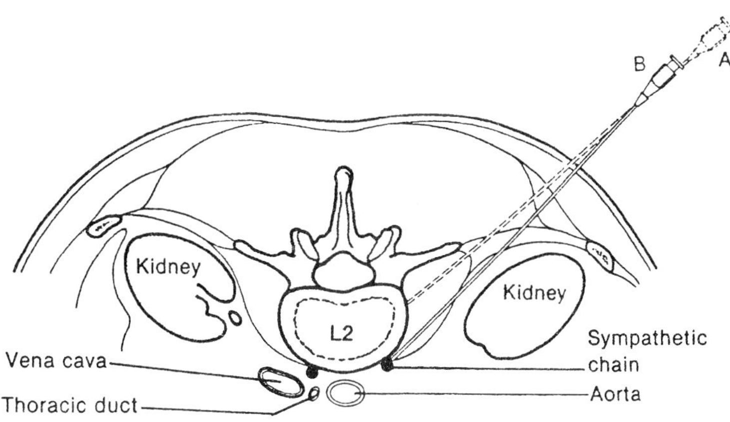

FIGURE 56-11. Initial needle position (A) and final needle position (B) for lumbar sympathetic block. Contact should be made at the lower portion of the L2 vertebral body, just cephalad to the L2–L3 disc. (Reprinted with permission from Stanton-Hicks M, Abram SE, Nolte H: Sympathetic blocks. In Raj PP [ed]: Practical Management of Pain, p 674. Chicago, Year Book, 1986.)

CRPS-II

The term *causalgia*, which has been used to indicate a specific syndrome of burning pain and autonomic dysfunction associated with major nerve trunk injury,[85] has been replaced by the term *complex regional pain syndrome type II* (CRPS-II). Most cases of CRPS-II are caused by gunshot wounds. Rapid, violent deformation of the nerve seems to play a major pathophysiologic role. Most cases involve partial injury to the brachial plexus, median nerve, or tibial division of the sciatic nerve proximal to the elbow or knee. Pain often begins immediately after injury and may spread to involve previously unaffected areas. There is usually severe burning pain, allodynia, and hyperpathia, often accompanied by deep shooting, crushing, or stabbing pains. The pain is aggravated by movement or any physical stimulation, such as light touch or pressure. Stimuli that increase sympathetic activity, such as a loud noise, a flash of light, or anxiety, often increase the severity of the pain. Pain may persist for many years in inadequately treated patients. There is usually evidence of reduced sympathetic activity in the affected extremity, which is generally warm, dry, and venodilated. Vasoconstriction, hyperhydrosis, cyanosis, and edema are occasionally seen. Dystrophic changes of skin, bone, and joints, similar to those encountered in CRPS-I patients, often begin early.

Reports on the therapy of causalgia from the early 1900s described surgical destruction of peripheral nerves, which was uniformly unsuccessful. Opioid analgesics were likewise ineffective. In 1930, Spurling[92] published encouraging results of treatment with sympathetic ganglionectomy. Since then, numerous reports have documented the efficacy of such treatment. Mayfield[93] reported complete relief of symptoms in 91% of 105 causalgia victims treated with surgical sympathectomy. Bonica,[85] in a review of 500 cases, found that 80% of patients responded to sympathectomy.

More recently, less invasive therapy has been undertaken in the management of CRPS-II. Neurolytic lumbar sympathetic block has been proposed as an alternative to surgical lumbar sympathectomy and has been shown to produce long-term sympathetic denervation in the large majority of patients.[94] Aggressive treatment with local anesthetic sympathetic blockade has met with some success. Bonica[85] reported success in 10 of 17 causalgia patients managed with frequent local anesthetic blocks. The authors have treated three patients with early, severe causalgia who responded dramatically to continuous-infusion lumbar epidural blockade or continuous-infusion brachial plexus block that was maintained for 5 to 7 days (unreported findings Abram SE, 1986).

Herpes Zoster

Herpes zoster is caused by the varicella zoster virus, which, following a chickenpox infection, lies dormant in dorsal root ganglia. As immunity to the virus declines with advancing age or immunosuppression, the virus becomes active again. In patients with normal immune systems, the infection is confined to a single dermatomal segment. In immunocompromised patients, multiple segments may be involved.

Herpes zoster most commonly involves the thoracic and trigeminal dermatomes, with the ophthalmic division of the trigeminal nerve being second most common.[95] Autopsy studies have shown evidence of viral DNA in trigeminal ganglia in 87% of patients and in thoracic dorsal root ganglia in 53% of patients.

The incidence of herpes zoster in the general population is 1 to 2/1,000 per year. It is higher among older patients, whose incidence is 5 to 10/1,000 per year. Postherpetic neuralgia has been defined as pain persisting well beyond healing of the skin rash (4 weeks to 6 months). Overall incidence among patients with herpes zoster infection has been reported to range from 9 to 34%.[96] Incidence is considerably higher in older patients (16% in patients younger than 60 years of age, 47% in patients older than 60 years of age).[97] Patients with severe pain during the acute phase of the disease are more likely to develop postherpetic neuralgia.

As the latent virus in the sensory ganglion becomes active, it causes a vesicular skin eruption characterized by inflammation, intranuclear inclusion bodies, and giant cell formation. Severe inflammation, hemorrhage, and necrosis occur in the dorsal root ganglia, dorsal horn, and adjacent meninges. Changes in the peripheral nerve include demyelinization, Wallerian degeneration, fibrosis, and cellular infiltration.[98] Noordenbos proposed that pain of postherpetic neuralgia is associated with loss of large afferent fibers with relative preservation of C fibers.[99] In subsequent studies, however, examination of biopsy and autopsy specimens from patients with or without persistent pain failed to show differences in populations of different fiber types.[98,100] Some specimens showed predominantly large fiber loss, but this was seen in patients with and without postherpetic neuralgia. In contrast, atrophy of the dorsal horn appears to be a regular autopsy feature in patients who had postherpetic neuralgia at the time of death. Persistence of inflammatory cells has been described in patients with long-standing postherpetic pain.[100]

Because of anecdotal evidence that sympathetic blocks provide lasting pain relief in patients with acute herpes zoster,[101] there has been speculation that intense sympathetic stimulation initiated by the virus is, at least in part, responsible for the pathologic changes that lead to postherpetic neuralgia. Winne[102] proposed that the increased sympathetic discharge initiated by the virus produces perineural ischemia that results in loss of large afferent fibers and persistence of small, unmyelinated neurons. There are several problems with the theory, including a lack of evidence that there is a local increase in sympathetic activity or that neural ischemia results from sympathetic discharge. In addition, the Noordenbos theory that pain is associated with small fiber predominance does not appear to be valid, nor is there substantial evidence that early sympathetic blockade reduces the incidence of postherpetic neuralgia.

A variety of treatments have been advocated for managing patients with acute herpes zoster. The goal of management is to control the pain associated with the acute eruption and, if possible, prevent the occurrence of persistent pain or postherpetic neuralgia. Antiviral agents have been advocated for management of the acute stage of the disease. Acyclovir has been widely used and has been shown to modestly accelerate the rate of cutaneous healing and to reduce the severity of the acute pain, but there is little evidence that it reduces the incidence of postherpetic neuralgia.[103] In contrast, one of the newer antiviral agents, famciclovir, does appear to reduce the incidence and severity of postherpetic neuralgia if initiated soon after the eruption begins.[104]

Corticosteroids have enjoyed some popularity for the treatment of the pain of acute herpes zoster. Eaglestein,[105] in a double-blind, controlled study, demonstrated that systemic triamcinolone reduced the duration of acute pain in patients older than 60 years of age. Several other studies have failed to demonstrate a reduction in the incidence of postherpetic neuralgia. Likewise, subcutaneous steroid infiltration[106] and epidural steroid injection[107] have been shown to reduce the acute pain intensity and/or duration, but there have been no controlled trials to determine whether they influence the incidence of postherpetic neuralgia. Although there is some concern over the possibility that steroids may increase the risk of dissemination of the virus, there is little evidence that this is likely to occur.[95]

Rosenak[108] was the first to report a beneficial effect of local anesthetic blocks on the pain of herpes zoster infection. He found that paravertebral sympathetic blocks or gasserian ganglion blocks with procaine resulted in dramatic relief of pain and rapid drying of vesicles. A number of subsequent uncontrolled studies also attest to the beneficial effect of sympathetic blockade. A single controlled study[109] attests to the ability of sympathetic blocks done early in the acute stage to prevent postherpetic neuralgia. The study contained only 10 patients in each treatment arm, and there have been no subsequent controlled studies to confirm these findings.

There is substantial evidence that local anesthetic blocks are ineffective in the management of postherpetic neuralgia. At best, they provide temporary relief, often only for the duration of the anesthetic agent. Winnie[102] more recently confirmed this observation in a study that showed a low incidence of lasting benefit from sympathetic blocks instituted more than a few months after the eruption. It is unclear whether the apparently favorable response to blocks instituted early in the course of the disease represents a real benefit from treatment or simply the natural history of the disease in the majority of patients.

The management of postherpetic neuralgia is often frustrating because some patients respond poorly to nearly every therapy provided. Tricyclic antidepressants provide the best chance of relief with the fewest side effects, although drowsiness, xerostomia, dysphoria, arrhythmias, and ataxia are potential problems. The onset of analgesia is slow (often requiring 2 to 3 weeks) and the relief is rarely complete, so many patients fail to realize they are experiencing much relief until they discontinue the drug and the pain returns to its former intensity. The addition of a second drug, such as an anticonvulsant (carbamazepine, valproic acid, phenytoin), may provide some additional benefit, but one must follow patients closely for the possibility of liver dysfunction or bone marrow depression. Gabapentin has been shown to be significantly more effective than placebo for the management of postherpetic neuralgia.[110] The majority of patients required 3,600 mg per day. Side effects of gabapentin are usually mild, there are few significant drug interactions, and it does not carry the risk of organ dysfunction seen with older anticonvulsants. Opioids rarely provide dramatic relief and cause major problems with constipation in older patients. Most studies fail to show much benefit from spinal cord stimulation. TENS may help in occasional patients, but cause aggravation of pain in patients with severe allodynia, and is not beneficial if there is considerable cutaneous sensory loss. Topical capsaicin is occasionally helpful, but can aggravate the pain in some individuals. Transdermal lidocaine patches can be helpful in some patients.

PHARMACOLOGIC TREATMENT OF CHRONIC PAIN

6 The long-term use of systemic opioids in patients who have noncancer pain continues to cause concern for many physicians. Although most pain management physicians are comfortable with the use of opioids for patients who do not have a terminal illness, there is much disagreement regarding appropriate dosage, patient selection, and choice of drug. Among primary care practitioners, there remains much resistance to prescribing opioids for noncancer pain for a variety of reasons. These include the following concerns:

1. Addiction will occur.
2. Tolerance will develop, leading to loss of efficacy and increasing drug side effects.
3. Drug regulatory agencies will take action against the prescribing physician.
4. Patients may be diverting (selling) drugs.

The reality is that certain patients experience good pain control over long periods of time with minimal tolerance and few side effects. Others have pain that is poorly controlled by opioids or have rapid reduction in efficacy requiring substantial dose escalation and eventual treatment failure. Although it is difficult to predict response to opioids in a given patient, there are some predictors of poor response. Patients with neuropathic pain are less likely to experience good pain control, and phasic pain (e.g., incident pain) is more difficult to control than constant or tonic pain. Patients with cognitive impairment or high levels of psychological distress are more likely to experience suboptimal pain control from opioids. A history of substance abuse is associated with a high risk of treatment failure and is believed by some physicians to represent a contraindication to opioid use.

The decision to prescribe opioids for patients with chronic pain should be based on the answers to three questions:

1. Is there a history of significant substance abuse?
2. Is there a good therapeutic effect? The selected medication should provide complete or substantial analgesia. There should be minimal dose escalation over time, and there should be measurable improvement in functional activity.
3. Are there substantial side effects? These should be minimal or tolerable.

Side effects should be monitored closely. Cognitive impairment is often insidious and may not be recognized by the patient or family members during treatment, but becomes obvious when the medication is withdrawn. Sedation, nausea, constipation, insomnia, and sexual dysfunction are common problems.

As noted in the section on pain mechanisms, there is substantial theoretical evidence that chronic opioid use may lead to a state of hyperalgesia or sensitization of spinal pain projection systems. Persistent opioid administration may lead to loss of responsiveness to both endogenous and exogenous opioids, as well as to hypersensitivity of systems that respond to noxious stimulation. Therefore, it is reasonable to withdraw and discontinue opioid administration for those patients who have evidence of central facilitation (allodynia, hyperalgesia, hyperpathia) and who exhibit poor responsiveness to opioids. Occasionally, such patients experience gradual improvement in pain, generally beginning a few weeks after drug withdrawal. Often, they will experience a reduction in adverse effects, especially cognitive impairment, sedation, constipation, and sexual dysfunction. Opioid withdrawal is commonly incorporated into chronic pain rehabilitation programs. All but 3 of 135 patients who had been on chronic opioid therapy were able to discontinue opioids during a comprehensive pain rehabilitation program at the Mayo Clinic.[111] The group demonstrated significant reduction in pain ratings, affective distress and depression, and increases in activity despite the discontinuation of opioids. Patients who had been on high doses did as well as those on low doses.

Few patients with chronic pain are addicted to opioids. Addiction is defined as compulsive use of a drug or substance resulting in physical, psychological, or social harm to the user, and continued use despite that harm.[112] It may be difficult to recognize addiction in patients with persistent pain. Signs of addiction include:

1. Intense desire for the drug and unfounded concerns over availability
2. Unsanctioned dose escalation
3. Use of drug when pain is absent or treatment of nonpain symptoms (anxiety, depression)
4. Aberrant drug-related behaviors

Drug diversion, or sale of drugs for recreational or street use, is difficult to document or to disprove. Occasionally, an acquaintance or a family member will report such activity. Documentation depends on a negative drug screen. The patient is asked whether he or she has taken the prescribed drug in the past several hours. If the answer is yes, a urine sample is obtained immediately and analyzed for the prescribed drug. If it is absent, diversion is likely.

When opioids are prescribed over long intervals, there should be an agreement, either informal or written, outlining the physician's obligation to continue treatment and the patient's obligation to meet several expectations of behavior. For patients who have previously failed to meet behavioral expectations, a written agreement, or "opioid contract," may be helpful. Under such a contract, the patient agrees to obtain prescriptions from one physician source and to fill prescriptions at one pharmacy, and to discontinue use if there is rapid tolerance development, minimal therapeutic effect, substantial side effects, or failure to achieve improved physical function. The patient agrees to take medications only as prescribed and is not to request early refills. The patient agrees that no prescription will be issued in the event that drugs are lost, stolen, or accidentally destroyed. The physician, however, should be willing to adjust dosage as needed, within reason, particularly in the early stages of treatment. The patient should agree to unannounced random drug screening and to allow the physician access to all other medical records. The patient understands that violation of this agreement could result in discontinuation of opioid therapy and/or referral to an addiction specialist.

Adjuvant Analgesics

Imipramine was shown to be useful in treating chronic pain in 1960.[113] Since then, the tricyclic antidepressants have come into widespread use in the management of certain chronic pain conditions, particularly neuropathic pain. The most popular explanation of the analgesic property of these drugs is that reuptake inhibition of serotonin and norepinephrine increases the levels of these inhibitory neurotransmitters in the brainstem and spinal cord.

The clinically relevant benefits to be expected from judicious use of these drugs in patients with chronic pain syndromes are normalization of sleep patterns, reduction in anxiety and depression (if present), and reduction of the patient's perception of pain. Although the antidepressant and pain-relieving effects are often delayed in onset, the improvement in sleep patterns provided by these drugs usually occurs promptly, often with the initial dose. Tricyclics suppress rapid eye movement sleep, and abrupt cessation can be associated with rebound in the form of restless sleep, with excessively vivid and pervasive dreams.

The common side effects of the tricyclics include the antimuscarinic effects of xerostomia, impaired visual accommodation, urinary retention, and constipation. Antihistaminic effects occur via blockade of both H_1 and H_2 receptors, and include sedation and an increase in gastric pH. Orthostatic hypotension is mediated through the blockade of peripheral α_1-adrenergic receptors. Cardiac conduction effects mimic the actions of quinidine but in general are of little clinical relevance, except in the case of overdosage. The lethal potential of these drugs in overdose is substantial, especially when doses exceed 2,000 mg of amitriptyline or the equivalent.

Most studies of efficacy of these drugs in pain syndromes are open and are not controlled for placebo effects or for the presence of depression. Since the first double-blind placebo-controlled study by Watson et al in 1982,[114] several well-designed studies have been conducted. They studied the effects of gradually increasing doses of amitriptyline in patients suffering from postherpetic neuralgia. After 3 weeks, 16 of 24 patients had obtained good to excellent relief, with doses below the norm for treatment of depression and with no change in a standard psychometric instrument assessing the presence and severity of depression. Getto et al[115] reviewed 24 studies and found 19 to report some degree of benefit. Four double-blind placebo studies with a combined enrollment of 107 subjects yielded a 68% response rate with the active drug, as compared with a 13% response with placebo. Studies of a double-blind placebo crossover design included 140 subjects in five reports and revealed an aggregate response rate of 61%.

Beginning in 1987, Max et al[116,117] published a series of double-blind, placebo-controlled trials that assessed the efficacy of antidepressants in certain painful syndromes. They showed that tricyclic antidepressants had analgesic effects independent of their effects on mood in neuropathic pain states (diabetic neuropathies and postherpetic neuralgia), although not all subjects had a beneficial response.

With the introduction of the SSRI fluoxetine, there was hope that the new class of drugs would provide pain relief at least comparable to the tricyclics. Clinical experience and research into this have yielded mixed results. In 1989, Diamond and Freitag reported their somewhat positive experience with the use of fluoxetine in the treatment of headache.[118] This prompted numerous reports of fluoxetine use in pain, some of which purport to demonstrate some benefit.[119,120] Max compared desipramine, amitriptyline, fluoxetine, and placebo in the treatment of diabetic neuropathy pain and found that, whereas both amitriptyline and desipramine were beneficial, fluoxetine had no more effect than placebo.[121] Paroxetine has, however, been shown to be of benefit in the treatment of diabetic neuropathy pain.[122]

As noted previously, the pain-relieving effect of antidepressants has been attributed to the ability to block reuptake of serotonin and norepinephrine. Because serotonin is believed to be an important inhibitory neurotransmitter in descending pain inhibitory pathways, it was anticipated that the SSRIs would be at least as effective as the tricyclics, but with fewer side effects. This has not generally been the case. It is now postulated that the tricyclic antidepressants may exert their analgesic and antihyperalgesic effects through other mechanisms. These drugs have been shown to bind at NMDA receptors and can block NMDA-mediated synaptic activity.[123] This property, which may not be shared by many of the SSRIs, may be the principal mechanism of analgesic action.

Another class of agents said to have some efficacy in the treatment of chronic pain syndromes are the anticonvulsants. Unlike the antidepressants and neuroleptics, the pharmacology of this group varies substantially from one drug to another. The older members of this class that have some benefit in pain patients are phenytoin, valproic acid, carbamazepine, and clonazepam. The first three affect sodium, potassium, or calcium flux across the neuronal membrane, whereas clonazepam is a benzodiazepine and works via the benzodiazepine-GABA-chloride channel receptor complex.

The side effect profiles of these drugs are also variable, with nausea and ataxia being commonly seen with any of them. Phenytoin can cause vitamin D and K and folate deficiencies, hirsutism, and gingival hyperplasia. Valproic acid use is associated with hepatic enzyme elevations, rare but occasionally fatal hepatic necrosis in children, and significant gastrointestinal effects that can be modified by the use of the enteric-coated form of the drug. Carbamazepine can cause a clinically significant decrease in any of the blood elements selectively or can induce pancytopenia. Clonazepam is occasionally associated with disinhibition, leading to hostility and aggression or emotional lability.

Several newer anticonvulsants appear to have some efficacy in treating painful conditions, particularly neuropathic pain. Gabapentin has been shown to provide significant pain relief for patients with reflex sympathetic dystrophy,[124] diabetic neuropathy,[125] and postherpetic neuralgia.[110] It has antihyperalgesic effects in rat mononeuropathy models when administered spinally.[126] Although it is a structural analog of GABA, its action does not appear to be limited to its effects on GABA receptors. Inhibition of voltage-gated calcium currents may be an important mechanism. It may also have anti-inflammatory properties.[127] It has fewer side effects and drug interactions than most of the older anticonvulsants, but somnolence, dizziness, ataxia, and peripheral edema are occasional problems.

Lamotrigine acts by inhibition of a sodium channel subtype and has been shown to inhibit glutamate release. Although there are a few reports of beneficial effects on neuropathic pain,[128] there are few controlled studies demonstrating efficacy. Rashes are fairly common and can progress to Stevens-Johnson syndrome or toxic epidermal necrolysis.

The mechanism of topiramate has not been fully investigated. Proposed mechanisms of action include sodium channel blockade, GABA potentiation, and blockade of some excitatory amino acid receptors. There are anecdotal reports of beneficial effects in a variety of neuropathic pain states. Weight loss is a common side effect.

Oxcarbazepine has mechanisms of action similar to those of carbamazepine, including sodium channel blockade and suppression of synaptic transmission. It is better tolerated than carbamazepine and appears to lack the potential for producing blood dyscrasias. It has been proposed as a first-line drug for treating trigeminal neuralgia. Its benefits in other neuropathic pain states are not as well documented.

Other drugs that are being used with increasing frequency in the management of neuropathic pain include zonisamide, levetiracetam, pregabalin, and tiagabine. There have been few studies comparing efficacy of the large number of antidepressants currently available, and there are essentially no studies that have examined the combined effects of multiple drugs. Although there appears to be some rationale for switching to another drug following the failure of the first anticonvulsant, the process so far has been totally empirical.

Use-dependent sodium channel blocking drugs have a role in the management of neuropathic pain. Systemically administered lidocaine is capable of suppressing spontaneous activity originating from experimentally induced neuromas at blood levels that produce no adverse effects.[129] Intravenous lidocaine and oral mexiletine have analgesic properties in some patients with neuropathic pain.[130] The analgesic effects of lidocaine are generally transient unless a continuous infusion is used. Lidocaine is commonly used to predict response to oral mexiletine, although its prognostic utility has not been well established. Lidocaine is given as a slow intravenous bolus at 1.5 mg/kg over 5 minutes followed by an infusion of 50 μg/kg/min. The infusion is adjusted downward if symptoms of systemic toxicity become evident.

CANCER PAIN

In assessing patients with malignant disease who seek treatment for pain, it is essential to determine the specific site and mechanism of their pain. It is not enough to make a diagnosis of cancer pain. The entire range of acute and chronic pain mechanisms is encountered among patients with malignancy. It is also essential to know the stage of the patient's malignant disease. The approach to a given pain for a terminal patient may vary greatly from the approach to the same type of pain in a patient whose cancer is curable.

It is useful to determine whether the patient's pain is acute or chronic, and whether it is related to tumor progression, therapeutic intervention, or, as is occasionally the case, factors unrelated to the patient's malignant disease (arthritis, herniated disc, etc.). It is also useful to know whether the patient has a history of chronic pain or drug abuse predating the onset of malignant disease. Pain caused by tumor progression can result from compression or infiltration of peripheral nerves, nerve root, or spinal cord; infiltration of bone and soft tissue; obstruction or distension of visceral structures; and vascular occlusion. Surgical intervention may lead to scar pain, neuroma formation, sympathetic dystrophy, and venous or lymphatic obstruction. Chemotherapy may be associated with peripheral neuropathies. Therapy with steroids can cause aseptic bony necrosis or rheumatoid-like symptoms when therapy is withdrawn. Herpes zoster is associated with agents that suppress immune function. Radiation therapy sometimes results in esophagitis, plexopathy and myelopathy, and bone necrosis.

7 A substantial range of therapeutic options is available to the cancer patient. A major consideration in approaching the patient with severe pain is when to institute a particular modality. It is generally advisable to consider less invasive, lower-risk options initially, progressing to procedures that are more invasive, more painful to perform, and carry a higher risk of complications only when the more benign procedures are ineffective. Occasionally, it is prudent to select a more invasive procedure early in the course of management if it is believed that it will provide the patient maximum comfort or if the patient's pain level has progressed to a crisis state.

Pharmacologic Therapy

The use of oral analgesic agents is the mainstay of treatment for cancer pain. Adequate analgesia can be achieved in the large majority of patients with cancer-related pain if sound pharmacologic principles are employed. Several guidelines are essential to cancer pain management:

1. *Use agents appropriate for the nature and severity of the patient's pain.* Weaker opioids such as codeine may be adequate for mild to moderate pain. For severe pain, more efficacious agents such as morphine, hydromorphone, or methadone should be employed. Agonist–antagonist agents such as pentazocine and buprenorphine have a ceiling effect on their analgesic efficacy and are generally effective only for mild to moderate pain. Meperidine is a poor drug for repetitive dosing because accumulation of its metabolite normeperidine can cause CNS stimulation manifested as anxiety, tremors, or seizures. Be aware of the oral bioavailability of the drug used. The oral dose of morphine, for instance, is about three times the parenteral dose. When peripheral nociceptive processes are involved (e.g., bony or soft-tissue invasion), the addition of NSAIDs may be helpful.
2. *Use adequate doses.* The dose of opioid analgesic should be escalated until satisfactory analgesia occurs (usually the case) or until problematic side effects occur. The dose required varies tremendously. It is not unusual for cancer patients to require 100 to 200 mg of oral morphine or its equivalent every 3 to 4 hours.
3. *Maintain steady blood and tissue levels of analgesic.* All analgesics should be given by the clock. As-needed administration may result in periods of inadequate relief. The time interval for administration should be consistent with the duration of action of the drug. When possible, use long-acting agents. Methadone, whose plasma half-life is 24 to 36 hours, can be given twice per day, avoiding the need for nighttime awakening for analgesic administration. Morphine is available in a time-release form that can be administered once or twice per day. Transdermal fentanyl provides prolonged, steady release that achieves fairly constant blood levels.

4. *Consider the use of adjuvant drugs.* Tricyclic antidepressants are frequently beneficial for postherpetic neuralgia, may be helpful for some patients with other types of neuralgic pain or denervation dysesthesia, and can be effective for treating concomitant depression. Some anticonvulsants may be beneficial for neuralgic pain. Phenothiazines or butyrophenones have been shown to reduce symptoms of nausea, agitation, and pain when used in conjunction with narcotic analgesics. Corticosteroids should be considered for increased intracranial pressure, cord compression, severe bone pain, or pain from liver metastases. Calcitonin is effective in some patients with bone pain.
5. *Anticipate and promptly treat side effects.* Constipation, which may become a major problem, occurs in most patients on opiates. Prophylactic management is essential. Nausea is a common opiate side effect, and concomitant administration of antiemetics may be necessary. Respiratory depression is unusual in tolerant patients. When it occurs in opioid-naive patients, it should be treated with small incremental doses of intravenous naloxone (e.g., 0.05 to 0.1 mg) until the respiratory rate increases to an acceptable range. Large doses precipitate withdrawal, reverse much of the patient's analgesia, and initiate vomiting. Patients who are unable to take analgesics orally can often be satisfactorily managed with parenteral opiate administration. Some patients who do not achieve satisfactory analgesia with oral drugs may have adequate control with parenteral agents, possibly because enteric absorption is poor. When the parenteral route is chosen, a constant-infusion technique or infusion plus patient-controlled analgesia (PCA) is usually superior to intermittent intramuscular injections. Many cancer patients have long-term venous access ports for chemotherapy that can be used for narcotic infusion.

When beginning opiate infusions, it is generally prudent to start with a relatively low-dose bolus injection and a modest infusion rate. If analgesia is inadequate after 1 to 2 hours, a small bolus is repeated, and the infusion rate is increased. The process is repeated until the infusion rate is adequate. An alternative, less labor-intensive method is to use a PCA device. Once the daily opiate requirement is established, the patient can be switched to a portable, battery-powered, constant-infusion device or portable PCA. When venous access is not available, portable external infusion devices can be used to deliver opiates subcutaneously through a "butterfly"-type needle. The infusion site is changed every few days or when soreness occurs. When large doses are required, the use of a concentrated preparation of hydromorphone (10 mg/mL) allows for longer intervals between refilling the portable infusion pump and reduces the mass of fluid injected.

Patients may experience diminishing analgesic effects from oral or parenteral opioids, either from tolerance development or from increasing noxious stimulation related to tumor spread. A study by Collin et al[131] suggests that increasing dose requirement is nearly always associated with spread of disease. In either event, there may be a rationale for changing from morphine to a more potent drug such as fentanyl or sufentanil. This rationale is related to the concept of intrinsic activity (IA) of analgesics (i.e., the fractional receptor occupancy [FRO]) required to produce a given effect. A drug with relatively low IA, such as morphine or meperidine, requires a higher FRO than a drug with a high IA, such as fentanyl or sufentanil. Under conditions of tolerance, some receptors become unresponsive, and a drug with low IA may not be capable of interacting with enough of the remaining receptors to achieve adequate analgesia. Likewise, if the level of noxious stimulation increases, a greater number of receptors must be activated to produce a given analgesic effect, and a drug with a low IA may not interact with sufficient receptors to provide a reasonable analgesic response. Chronic infusion of morphine or meperidine in animals is associated with rapid development of tolerance to subsequent doses of morphine or meperidine, but not fentanyl or sufentanil.[132]

Transdermal fentanyl offers an alternative to parenteral opioids for patients who are unable to take medications orally. It is available in four dosage forms, which deliver 25, 50, 75, or 100 μg/hr of fentanyl. The continuous use of the 100-μg/hr form offers roughly the same analgesia as 360 mg of oral morphine or 60 mg of parenteral morphine per 24 hours. If higher delivery rates are required, multiple patches can be used simultaneously. Several hours are required for analgesia to develop following application of the transdermal patch and for analgesia to dissipate following its removal. An oral transmucosal preparation of fentanyl is available in doses up to 1,600 μg. The onset of analgesia is much more rapid with this form of administration, with peak levels occurring at about 20 minutes.

Intraspinal Opioids

Some cancer patients do not achieve satisfactory analgesia with systemic opiates without pushing the doses to the point of marked sedation or confusion. Less conventional methods of opiate administration may be effective for some of these patients. The discovery of spinal cord opiate receptors led to speculation regarding the feasibility of intraspinal administration of opioids. Most experience with chronic intraspinal opioid administration has been with morphine, probably because it has a long duration, allowing bolus and continuous administration, and because it has been approved by the U.S. Food and Drug Administration (FDA) for intraspinal use. The use of intraspinal opioids in patients who had not previously been on systemic opioids (e.g., postoperative patients and volunteers) was associated with nausea and vomiting, urinary retention, pruritus, and respiratory depression. As more experience with cancer patients accumulated, it became evident that these problems were, indeed, uncommon in this population, probably because the patients had been on systemic opioids chronically and had become tolerant to these side effects.

Intraspinal opioids have been chronically administered by both the epidural and IT routes. IT administration has the advantage of allowing use of much lower doses, potentially minimizing systemic side effects, but carries the risks of cerebrospinal fluid leak, headache, meningitis, and arachnoiditis. With either epidural or IT administration, the drug may be administered as a bolus, by infusion via an external pump, or by infusion via a totally implanted pump.

Percutaneous placement of an epidural catheter followed by bolus administration of opioid constitutes the simplest method of administration. The principal drawback of this technique is the risk of infection, which may spread to the epidural space. Such a technique is useful as a temporary measure to evaluate efficacy of epidural narcotics and is a reasonable method of administration for patients whose life expectancy is relatively short. The simple expedient of tunneling the catheter subcutaneously to the flank decreases the incidence of catheter dislodgment, allows the patient access to the catheter exit site to facilitate dressing changes, and may reduce the risk of epidural infection.

The decision to use an external pump is based on pharmacokinetic, technical, and financial considerations. There is some evidence that lower doses of morphine can be employed when using a continuous infusion. Coombs et al[133] were able to provide good analgesia for a group of cancer pain patients using a mean dose of 2 mg/day initially and

6.6 mg/day at the end of 12 weeks. Reports of studies that use bolus injection describe much higher daily doses. Bolus injection produces much higher peak cerebrospinal fluid levels,[134] which may predispose to more cephalad migration of the drug. Another advantage to continuous-infusion techniques is the lower incidence of catheter occlusion. Inability to inject is a fairly common problem with bolus injection technique. When an obstructed catheter is removed, it is common to find fibrin material in the lumen. However, the use of large-bore silicone rubber catheters should minimize that possibility. Patients with epidural metastases may have severe pain with bolus injection but tolerate continuous infusion well. Perhaps the biggest drawback to continuous-infusion techniques is the expense. Portable pumps cost up to several thousand dollars, and the use of implantable systems adds several thousand dollars in additional physician and operating room expenses.

The totally implantable infusion pump is the most elegant and expensive drug delivery system. The Infusaid pump is a freon-driven device with a 50-mL, percutaneously filled drug chamber and a constant infusion rate. Pumps with a 2 to 3 mL/day flow rate will run for 15 to 20 days between refills. Daily dose is adjusted by changing the drug concentration. A separate drug injection septum allows injection directly into the catheter, bypassing the drug chamber. The technique is most appropriate for patients with a relatively long life expectancy (months rather than weeks). Medtronic produces an electronically driven, externally programmable implanted pump that allows variations in rate plus the administration of intermittent bolus injections.

Perhaps the most frustrating problem associated with intraspinal opioid administration is the development of marked resistance or tolerance to the medication. Although most patients develop tolerance slowly and to a limited degree, some demonstrate rapid escalation of doses. Woods and Cohen[135] reported a patient who had been on 280 mg of morphine intravenously and 90 mg of methadone orally per day who was initially comfortable on 5 mg/day of epidural morphine. However, by the fifth day of epidural morphine administration, the dose had increased to 7 to 10 mg/hr. One of the reported side effects of such high doses, particularly with high-dose IT morphine, is the paradoxical development of segmental allodynia, which has been reported in patients[136] and in animal studies.[137]

Neuraxial administration of nonopioid analgesics, either alone or in combination with opioids, may be effective when opioids alone are ineffective. Limited trials of the α_2-agonist clonidine injected epidurally and intrathecally have proved at least temporarily effective. Animal studies suggest that there is a synergistic interaction between spinally administered α_2-adrenergic agonists and opioids. Eisenach et al[138] found a dose-related analgesic effect from epidural clonidine in a series of nine cancer patients. They reported dose-related decreases in heart rate and blood pressure, as well as somnolence. Seven patients were maintained on clonidine plus morphine infusions at home for periods of up to 5 months. These patients reported satisfactory analgesia, as well as less nausea and sedation than they experienced with systemic morphine. There was minimal escalation of either clonidine or morphine during the combined infusions.

The intrathecal administration of baclofen has been used to treat patients with spasticity associated with multiple sclerosis and spinal cord injury. However, baclofen appears to have some potential as a spinal analgesic in patients without increased muscle tone who are resistant or tolerant to opioids. Intrathecal L-baclofen is antinociceptive in several animal models at doses that produce no discernible motor blockade.[139] It has been shown to produce substantial lasting analgesia in opioid-tolerant patients with neuropathic and radiculopathic pain at doses devoid of motor effects.[140]

Another approach to the patient who has become resistant to neuraxial opioids is to use combinations of opioids and dilute local anesthetics. The combined use of these agents makes sense because the local anesthetic, even at subblocking concentrations, can reduce the maximum firing rates of nociceptor fibers, and the opiate reduces the sensitivity of wide dynamic-range and nociceptive-specific neurons in the dorsal horn to activation by nociceptors. Hogan et al[141] found that 10 of 16 patients, selected from a total of 1,205 cancer admissions, required local anesthetic infusions along with epidural morphine to achieve satisfactory analgesia. Du Pen et al[142] found that 68 of 375 patients (18%) failed to achieve satisfactory analgesia with neuraxial opioids alone. Sixty-one of those 68 patients experienced satisfactory analgesia with the addition of local anesthetics.

Nonneurolytic Nerve Blocks

Myofascial pain is common among cancer patients. It is often associated with bony infiltration, neural compression, or visceral pain. Local anesthetic injections of trigger points may be surprisingly effective. Fluoromethane spray of trigger points combined with gentle stretching of affected muscles can be helpful. TENS is also likely to be of benefit.

Tumor compression of nerve roots, brachial or femoral plexus, or peripheral nerves sometimes responds dramatically to perineural injection of insoluble steroids. Pain relief can be achieved for up to 1 month in many instances. When radicular pain is caused by epidural tumor spread, epidural injections of triamcinolone diacetate are likely to be of benefit. Tumor compression of the brachial plexus may respond to brachial plexus block with a combination of depo steroid and local anesthetic. The interscalene, supraclavicular, infraclavicular, or axillary approaches may all be used, the choice depending on the site of pathology. Femoral plexopathy can be treated with a paravertebral approach (psoas compartment block) to the femoral plexus, again using depo steroids and local anesthetic. Steroid local anesthetic blocks of peripheral nerves that are irritated or compressed by tumor are occasionally beneficial, particularly if they are performed reasonably soon after the onset of pain. Patients with severe neurogenic pain should be warned that if the injections are successful in producing pain relief, they are likely to be left with some numbness, not from the injections, but from the already present neural pathology.

Acute herpes zoster is a relatively common and often debilitating source of pain in patients with malignancy. There is some evidence that local anesthetic blockade of sympathetic fibers, using either paravertebral sympathetic blocks or epidurals, will promptly relieve pain and may shorten the acute phase of the illness.[109] Even if the overall course of the illness is not dramatically affected, patients are usually extremely grateful for any respite from the severe pain associated with this condition.

Occasionally, patients with severe cancer pain are refractory to any opioid intervention. These patients may progress to psychological decompensation without reasonably prompt intervention. The use of continuous-infusion local anesthetic blockade may be the best answer for patients who reach such a crisis. Continuous epidurals with dilute local anesthetics can be performed at any level of the neuraxis. When upper thoracic or cervical approaches are used, close monitoring of blood pressure and respiratory function is necessary.

Neurolytic Blocks

There is a much greater willingness among anesthesiologists to perform neurolytic blocks for terminal cancer patients with pain than for patients with nonmalignant causes of pain.

Reluctance to use neurolytic blocks for noncancer pain is certainly justified. The extent and duration of analgesia from neurodestructive procedures is limited by regrowth of axons and development of central pain mechanisms (denervation dysesthesia). Although neurolytic blocks can produce dramatic relief for some cancer pain patients, there are some serious potential drawbacks to the technique, and overzealous use of neurodestructive procedures should be avoided.

The principal disadvantage of neurolytic blocks is the inability to precisely control the spread of the destructive agents. Loss of motor function and inability to control bowel or bladder function following neurolysis can be devastating to a patient and will greatly impair the quality of remaining life. The expected analgesia may not always result from destruction of the intended neural structures, even when prognostic local anesthetic blocks have been performed. If CNS mechanisms play a major role in a patient's pain, neurolysis is unlikely to be of benefit. In some cases, tumor progression rapidly produces pain beyond the confines of the block. With the advent of improved methods of cancer therapy, more patients survive well beyond the efficacy of the block. Overall, the incidence of fair to good results following neurolytic blockade is estimated at 50 to 60%.

Alcohol and phenol are the agents most commonly used for prolonged interruption of neural function. There is relatively little difference in overall efficacy between these agents, but there are major differences in the initial responses. Phenol produces no pain on injection, has an initial anesthetic effect, and takes about 15 minutes to exert its neurolytic effect. Alcohol causes significant pain on injection and produces neurolysis promptly. When used for IT neurolysis, alcohol is hypobaric, whereas phenol in glycerine, the usual IT preparation, is hyperbaric.

IT neurolysis with small volumes of alcohol or phenol requires careful positioning to place the affected sensory root uppermost (for alcohol) or in the most dependent position (for phenol). In such a way, only the involved sensory roots are affected. Patient movement during or shortly after injection can produce spread of drug to the cord, other dermatomes, or motor roots. Papo and Visca[143] published results in a large series of patients who underwent phenol rhizotomy. They reported good results (pain free until death) in 40% of 290 patients and fair results (reduced analgesic requirements or temporary complete relief) in 35%. Patients whose pain was localized to sacral dermatomes had the best results, whereas patients with pain in the upper thoracic area or upper or lower extremities had poor analgesia and more frequent complications. Swerdlow[144] reviewed 13 reports of the results of phenol and alcohol rhizotomies and found good relief of pain in about 60% of patients. In reviewing results on his own patients, he found that analgesia lasted less than 2 months in 50% the patients and less than 1 month in 25% of patients. Complications lasting longer than a week occurred in 15% of patients.

Patients with severe, localized perineal pain are likely to experience relief with IT blocks with phenol in glycerine. Phenol 7% in glycerine is injected in 0.25-mL increments up to a maximum of 2 mL, with the patient in the sitting position. Injection is stopped at a lower dose if the patient experiences any lower-extremity sensory changes. This treatment is limited to patients who have undergone fecal and urinary diversion procedures.

Celiac plexus block for pain associated with upper abdominal malignancy is the most successful and rewarding of the neurolytic blocks. Thompson et al[145] reported that 94% of 97 patients who underwent celiac plexus block for pain of upper abdominal cancer had good-to-excellent pain relief. Injections were performed with 50 mL of 50% alcohol. Survival from the cancer ranged from 2 days to 14 months. Fourteen patients required repeat injections for recurrent pain. Ten patients experienced transient orthostatic hypotension, and one patient had partial motor loss in one leg.

The classical technique for percutaneous injection of the celiac plexus involves bilateral placement of block needles just anterior to the body of L1, and posterior to the aorta and diaphragmatic crura. More recently, techniques have been described that involve more anterior positioning of the needle tip with CT assistance so it lies anterior to the diaphragmatic crura.[146] The injected solution can be seen to spread more anteriorly, surrounding the aorta. There is much less tendency of the injected solution to spread posteriorly to the paravertebral nerve roots or sympathetic chain, minimizing risk of paresis or orthostatic hypotension. Ischia et al,[147] using such a technique, reported 93% success in relieving pain in 28 patients with cancer pain. Similar placement can be achieved with the use of biplane fluoroscopy. Five-inch 22-gauge needles are advanced from both sides at a point 7 cm from the midline, at the lower border of the twelfth rib toward the midpoint of the L1 vertebral body, and advanced under anteroposterior fluoroscopy until they are just past the lateral border of the body. Under lateral fluoroscopy, the right-sided needle is advanced 1 cm beyond the anterior border of the body. It will probably lie between the aorta and vena cava. The left-sided needle is advanced the same distance, but it will usually enter the aorta at this point. If so, it is advanced through the aorta until negative aspiration occurs. Half the total alcohol dose is then injected through each needle (see Fig. 56-12). Alternatively, deafferentation of the upper abdominal viscera can be accomplished with the use of splanchnic block. With this technique, the neurolytic agent is injected over the anterolateral surface of the T12 and/or T11 vertebral body (see Fig. 56-12). This technique may be more effective than the transcrural approach if there is dense, widespread tumor invasion around the celiac plexus.

Patients with pelvic pain associated with gynecologic, rectal, and genitourinary malignancies may benefit from interruption of pelvic visceral innervation at the level of the superior hypogastric plexus. The technique of needle placement just anterior to the upper portion of the sacrum originally described by Plancarte et al[148] allows for interruption of afferents from the pelvic viscera with minimal risk of somatic blockade. The block is performed by introducing bilateral needles medially and caudally through the space between the L5 spinous process and the upper border of the sacrum under fluoroscopic control. Eight milliliters of phenol introduced through each needle is generally sufficient to provide reduction in pain and opioid requirement[149] (see Fig. 56-13). Bladder pain and spasm have been successfully treated with transsacral phenol injections.[150] If blocks are confined to one or two roots, there is little risk of disrupting bladder function.

Other Modes of Therapy

There are a number of therapeutic options that are relatively specific for the type of malignancy with which one is dealing. When dealing with tumors that are extremely radiosensitive, radiation therapy is often the most effective form of intervention. If chemotherapeutic options are available, they may provide analgesia through reduction of tumor mass. Pain caused by hormonally sensitive tumors may be best treated by appropriate manipulation of the patient's hormonal environment. Surgical debulking of a large tumor will sometimes relieve pain of obstruction or abdominal distension. Stabilization of an isolated pathologic fracture can be an extremely effective pain-relieving procedure. Certain neurosurgical procedures, such as spinal cord stimulation, cordotomy, or hypophysectomy, may afford months of profound relief in certain types of cases. Some patients benefit considerably from psychological interventions

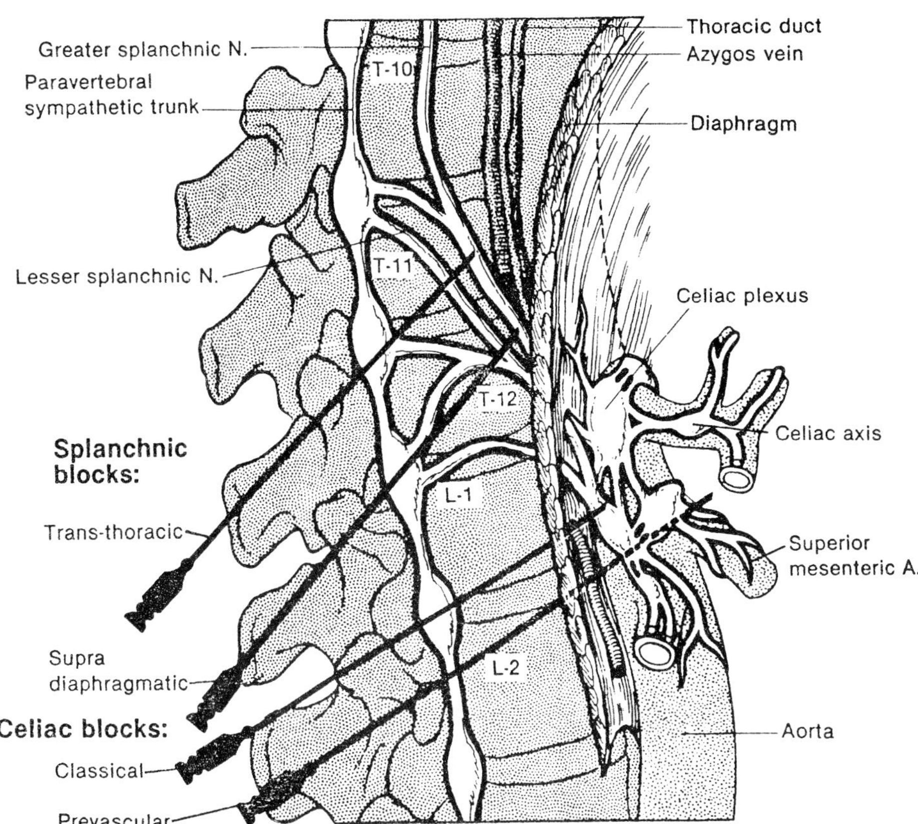

FIGURE 56-12. Lateral projection showing the splanchnic nerves and celiac plexus in relation to the diaphragm, vertebrae, and aortic vessels. Placement of needles for two approaches to the celiac plexus and two approaches to the splanchnic nerves is shown. (From Abram SE, Boas RA: Sympathetic and visceral nerve blocks. In Benumof JL [ed]: Clinical Procedures in Anesthesia and Intensive Care, p. 787. Philadelphia, JB Lippincott, 1992.)

such as hypnosis or other cognitive strategies. With the complexity of the disease processes involved with cancer-related pain and the number of pain mechanisms and therapeutic interventions that are possible, it is essential that the full range of medical and behavioral science disciplines be made available to this group of patients.

PAIN IN HIV/AIDS

Knowledge of the syndromes in HIV disease is the fundamental prerequisite for diagnosis of HIV disease pain. HIV disease pain can be divided into three classifications: nociceptive pain, neuropathic pain, and idiopathic pain. The most common pain sources associated with HIV disease-related pain are abdominal pain 26%, peripheral neuropathy 25%, throat pain 20%, HIV disease-related headaches 17%, AZT-induced headache 16%, arthralgia 5%, back pain 5%, and herpes zoster 5%.[151]

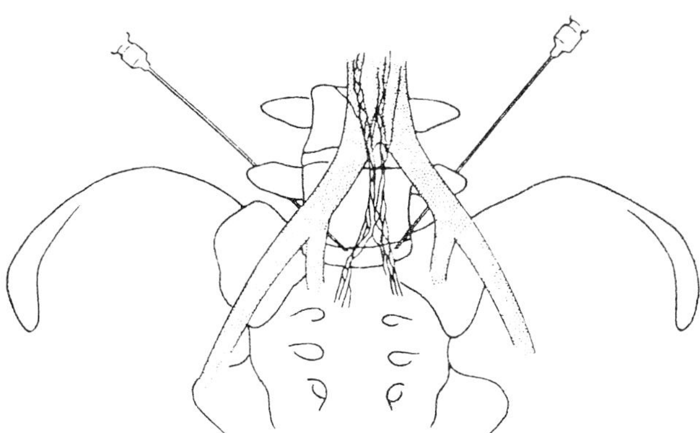

FIGURE 56-13. Anterior view of the pelvis showing location of the hypogastric plexus and suggested bilateral needle placement. (Reprinted with permission from Plancarte R, Amescua C, Patt RB, Aldrete A: Superior hypogastric plexus block for pelvic cancer pain. Anesthesiology 73:236, 1990.)

Pain in HIV disease varies, depending on the stage of HIV disease progression with acute phase evidenced by mononeuritides, brachial plexopathy, and acute demyelinating polyneuropathy, such as Guillain-Barré syndrome. As the disease progresses, pain will be associated with chronic inflammatory demyelinating polyneuropathy, herpes zoster, and mononeuritis multiplex. Late-stage HIV disease pain arises out of sensory polyneuropathy, cytomegalovirus polyradiculopathy, progressive mononeuritis multiplex, aseptic meningitis, lymphomatous meningitis, and nucleoside toxicity. As discussed earlier in this chapter, sensitization of neurons and activation of glial cells in the CNS undoubtedly play a major role in the pathophysiology of AIDS neuropathy. For instance, HIV envelope proteins have been shown to induce glial activation. Much clinical research is now focused on drugs that inhibit glial activation or that block the effects of proinflammatory cytokines.

Pain at any stage is influenced by perception, and by psychological, social, and even spiritual anxieties.[152] The psychological sequelae of HIV disease pain are essentially similar to cancer pain, where there is the constant threat of severity and persistence. Optimal HIV disease treatment should incorporate psychological treatment strategies because patient mood, depression, and beliefs about pain, as well as the significance (meaning) of pain influence pain perception.

Pharmacologic treatment for HIV disease pain should follow the World Health Organization analgesic pain treatment protocol developed for cancer, beginning with acetaminophen and NSAIDs, with appropriate caution related to possible drug interaction with acetaminophen and AZT. Weak opioids are then used, including codeine, oxycodone, and hydrocodone added to acetaminophen. Concerns over use of opioid treatment in substance abusers presents difficulties that require firm limits and contractual, written agreement on the use of narcotic analgesics.

The overall course of treatment and ability of the patient to cooperate in treatment may be compromised by the impact of HIV disease dementia. As the disease progresses, the risks of associated pain and dementia increase. Some studies have found that dementia is the initial AIDS-defining illness, viz. 4% followed by an increased incidence of 7% after a second AIDS-defining illness and a cumulative risk of 25%.[153] Nonpharmacologic treatment such as physical therapy and psychological interventions may be difficult in the presence of apathy, psychomotor retardation, decreased attention span, and short-term memory loss.

Nerve blocks, including injection of local anesthetic or neurolytic agents, are not typically applicable to HIV disease pain. However, temporary relief from pain may facilitate physical therapy, and frequently, sympathetic or somatic blocks may result in relief of pain that exceeds the actual anesthetic action.

PSYCHOLOGICAL INTERVENTIONS FOR CHRONIC PAIN

Psychological input into the diagnosis and treatment of chronic pain has become an accepted part of any comprehensive team approach to the management of this class of patients. Because the psychological influences on pain experiences are myriad, the regular consultation of a specialist in behavioral medicine is invaluable. In addition to helping understand some of the psychological influences mentioned earlier, the psychologist has at his or her disposal a number of specific techniques that prove useful as part of a multidisciplinary treatment plan for chronic pain management.

8 Psychodynamic approaches to the patient in chronic pain are typified by an attempt to understand the patient in terms of personality structure, biological drives, social contexts, desires, and expectations. This leads to a psychodynamic formulation that posits a relationship between any or all these factors and the presenting problem. Therapy is usually done on an individual basis and is aimed at establishing a therapeutic alliance with the patient, providing an interpretation of relevant symptoms, leading the individual to new levels of understanding about the derivation of their symptoms, and enhancing symptom resolution through the patient–therapist relationship, with termination of that relationship as the ultimate goal. To engage in this sort of approach requires a knowledge of fundamental psychoanalytic and therapeutic principles, training in the particulars of psychotherapy with chronic pain patients, and the time to engage in weekly or more frequent sessions with the patient for months to years of therapy. Clearly, this is out of the realm of expertise or desire of most anesthesiologists, and is typically so labor intensive that it is not practical for many psychologists. In general, a small proportion of patients in a given clinic population would be either amenable or appropriate to involvement in this style of therapy.

Much more common is the use of cognitive therapies. This group of strategies focuses on the cognitive or thought processes that are found in chronic pain patients. Often, the thinking style of an individual has a great deal of effect on how he or she copes with pain. As mentioned earlier, the meaning of the pain experience can greatly influence the suffering. A classic example of this is the often quoted observation by Beecher[154] that injured soldiers on the battlefront in World War II often complained of pain far less than would be expected from the severity of their wounds. When they were safely behind the lines, however, they would complain just as loudly as anyone else when multiple venipunctures or other mildly painful procedures were required, disproving the notion that these people were stoic by nature. Beecher[154] reasoned that the meaning of the pain was making the difference in that a significant injury meant that one would be taken back home and, therefore, would survive the war. A common clinical example in a pain clinic would be the individual who is convinced that he or she cannot cope with a flare-up of pain. Such an individual will frequently think catastrophic thoughts such as "If this pain gets real bad, I don't know what I'll do!" These thoughts can become the focus of treatment and can, with motivation and practice on the part of the patient, be changed to more adaptive thoughts. This in time will give the individual some degree of control over the situation and will prevent him or her from engaging in self-defeating destructive thought patterns. Coping ability is thereby improved.[155]

Behavioral therapies involve efforts to reshape behaviors, rather than the sensory or emotional conditions that underlie them. This is a direct outgrowth of the work of Fordyce et al,[156] who adapted B. F. Skinner's operant model of behavior to the human pain patient. As previously discussed, this model states that behaviors can be cued by certain stimuli and can be modified by conditions that follow the emission of the behavior. Taking this antecedent-behavior-consequence paradigm view of pain behaviors, such as limping, groaning, seeking dependence on others, and taking inappropriate analgesics, Fordyce and colleagues imposed strict control on the environment into which the chronic pain patient was placed. No reinforcement of pain behaviors was forthcoming from the staff (extinction), and positive reinforcement for wellness behaviors was instituted. This resulted in a significant decrease in pain behaviors. A critique of this method was that only the behaviors were decreased, but Fordyce et al argued that many patients state that after a largely behavioral treatment program they perceive less pain.[157] The principles of behavior modification extend to the staff of a pain clinic, the patient's workplace, and the home, in that solicitous responses from a spouse in response to pain behaviors by the patient may sabotage an otherwise intact and appropriate treatment plan.

Biofeedback is the providing of information to an individual about bodily functions that are commonly held to be inaccessible to the conscious mind. Commonly used devices measure surface electromyographic activity, temperature, or electrodermal activity. When feedback from these systems is provided, a patient can frequently be taught to control those functions at will. Originally, the logical assumption was made that teaching an individual to reduce muscle tone in a specific muscle would reduce the pain by the mechanism of muscle relaxation. Although the outcome is generally that which is expected, the mechanism is not universally accepted to be reduction in muscle tone, leading to decreased activation of muscle nociceptive afferent neurons. The same statement can be made for the other modes of biofeedback. This does not, however, detract from the usefulness of the techniques, and they remain a valuable psychological intervention for some patients.

Numerous strategies have evolved for the induction of a state of relaxation in chronic pain. The theory is that relaxation induces both positive mental and physical changes in the individual that promote a sense of well-being, decrease muscle tone, and enhance coping. Jacobson[158] developed the first standardized approach to relaxation using the progressive contraction and relaxation of muscle groups in an ascending sequence from feet to head. There have been numerous procedures since then that can be learned to induce relaxation. These techniques rely on conscious manipulation of the body to induce a relaxed state, not merely getting comfortable on the couch and propping up one's feet. Benson[159] studied the physiologic concomitants of a relaxed state and found commonalities to the conditions induced by a variety of methods. These included a decrease in sympathetic tone, regularity in respiratory pattern, decreased skeletal muscle tone, and a feeling of well-being. He termed this physiologic pattern the *relaxation response*, postulated that the means of achieving it was unimportant, and developed a simple and straightforward induction method. This and similar techniques find great applicability to chronic pain patients, especially those with muscular involvement such as myofascial pain syndromes.

Hypnosis has long been used to help alleviate surgical and other acute pains. It also has some utility in the chronic pain population. For an individual to become hypnotized, several conditions must exist: (1) an ability to concentrate, (2) a belief in the process, and (3) some motivation for the process to ensue. The trance state is believed to be a naturally occurring phenomenon in most people, although there is great variability in the population with regard to frequency and ease of occurrence. Trance state can be defined as an altered state of awareness characterized by extremely focused attention, relaxation, and responsiveness to suggestion. It is believed by most modern practitioners that the hypnotist does not hypnotize the subject but rather facilitates entry into trance by directing and guiding the individual's attention. The use of hypnosis can, in the properly selected individual, be a useful adjunct to therapy of chronic pain. It has found particular utility in the treatment of patients with cancer pain, possibly because these patients are so profoundly motivated. The mechanism of analgesia associated with hypnosis is unclear, but it does not appear to be due to endogenous opiates or to be solely due to placebo effect.

Group therapy, supportive therapy, education, and family therapy are other types of psychological interventions that have utility in the management of chronic pain patients. A skilled practitioner of behavioral medicine will aid the anesthesiologist in the diagnosis, conceptualization, and treatment of patients presenting with chronic pain by selecting evaluation and therapeutic strategies that are tailored to each individual's presentation.

INTERVENTIONAL PAIN MANAGEMENT

9 Over the past two decades, there has been rapid technological development in the field of pain management. Reliable and sophisticated intraspinal drug delivery devices can provide complex patterns of infusion over long periods of time. Totally implanted spinal cord stimulation devices can now access multiple electrodes simultaneously. Techniques for radiofrequency denervation have been developed for many neurologic structures. Miniaturized endoscopic devices permit more accurate perineural injection of medications within the spinal canal. Systems have been developed for thermocoagulation of annular tears of intervertebral discs and for stabilization of vertebral compression fractures. Although these interventional techniques are not appropriate for the majority of patients with chronic pain, they have extended our capability for managing some of the most intractable problems. The following discussion describes a few of these systems.

Intrathecal Drug Delivery Devices

The discovery of opioid receptors and endogenous opioids in the late 1970s[160] led to early experiences with intraspinal opioids in animals[161] and eventually patients with chronic pain.[162] The original research with spinal opioids was fueled by the search for alternatives to irreversible neurodestructive techniques. The advantage of spinal opioid analgesia was believed to lie in the potential for obtaining more potent analgesia and fewer side effects due to higher drug concentrations at spinal opioid receptors. What made intraspinal opioids suited for continuous administration and eventually outpatient use was the selective nature of its action compared with local anesthetics, avoiding sensory, motor, and sympathetic blockade.

The original use of spinal narcotics for continuous drug delivery focused on cancer pain, proving its safety and efficacy in multiple studies.[163,164] A subsequent development was the successful utilization of intrathecal baclofen for the treatment of spasticity and rigidity in patients with spinal cord injuries.[165] Utilization of spinal opioids for nonmalignant pain remains controversial but is gaining acceptance. More recent studies in this patient population seem to suggest a lower incidence of tolerance and iatrogenic addiction than first feared.[166]

Opioids administered by the spinal route act preferentially on receptors in the dorsal horn. Pain relief is produced through modulation of incoming A-delta and C fiber sensory input.[167] In part, opioids also travel rostrally and act on supraspinal opiate receptors.

In selecting patients for chronic intrathecal opioid therapy, one must distinguish between neuropathic and nociceptive pain syndromes. Nociceptive pain is generally opioid responsive; neuropathic pain, however, may not respond or may require much larger opioid doses.[168] The latter may respond to the spinal administration of α_2-receptor agonists such as clonidine or local anesthetic/opioid combinations. Although intrathecal baclofen is currently used mainly for the treatment of spasticity, it has been shown to provide persistent pain relief in patients who have failed intrathecal morphine treatment.[169] Success has been reported among patients with persistent postlaminectomy pain[140] and CRPS-I.[170]

Selection of patients with nonmalignant pain for chronic spinal drug administration remains difficult, with no clear selection criteria identified. Prior to considering these patients for candidacy, every effort must be made to establish a diagnosis of the pain syndrome at hand. All available surgical and medical alternatives should be explored, including trials of long-acting opioids. These should be escalated until side effects are encountered or inadequate benefit is established. Psychological evaluation and psychometric testing should be considered to investigate the possibility of primary psychological pain states. Contraindications to the placement of implantable infusion devices include, among other things, the presence of sepsis, anticoagulation, severe immune suppression, and drug addiction.

Morphine continues to be the most widely used agent for long-term spinal administration. It remains the only FDA-approved intraspinal analgesic. Its high water solubility and receptor affinity provide for prolonged duration predictability and a widespread distribution throughout the cerebrospinal fluid compartment. Substances with higher lipid solubility, such as fentanyl, sufentanil, and meperidine, not only reduce supraspinal effects through limited spread, but also require accurate catheter placement adjacent to the spinal cord level associated with the specific pain syndrome. Opioid rotation is commonly done in long-term use because tolerance and drug side effects can develop. Owing to the phenomenon of incomplete cross-tolerance among opioids, a lower dose of a different opioid can often be substituted.

Efficacy trials are essential to pump implantation. Different methods are in clinical use, ranging from single-shot outpatient drug administration to titration of a continuous epidural or intrathecal infusion in the inpatient setting. Prior oral or systemic opioid needs will determine trial doses of intrathecal drugs. The patient is then observed for analgesic efficacy and drug side effects. The minimum analgesic response is controversial, but often a minimum of 50% reduction in pain scores and duration twice the half-life of the agent is sought. Response to placebo injections should be compared with responses to active drug. The development of early side effects such as intractable pruritus or nausea is often discouraging, even though tolerance to them may develop with longer-term administration. Efficacy of intrathecal baclofen for treatment of spasticity is assessed using the Ashworth muscle rigidity/tone scale.

Intrathecal drug delivery systems vary from simple percutaneous catheters to totally implantable and programmable infusion pumps. Implanted systems have gained in popularity for long-term infusions, both in cancer pain states with long survival times and in nonmalignant pain states. These systems provide for a broad range of delivery rates and modes, and hence flexibility. Refill periods range from weeks to months, depending on drug concentrations and tolerance.

Examples of postoperative complications include bleeding, infection, seroma formation, and cerebrospinal fluid leakage. Infection is usually localized; however, epidural or intrathecal sepsis is disastrous, requiring the removal of all hardware and administration of systemic antibiotics.[171] Long-term complications related to the implanted equipment include catheter disconnects, obstruction, or breakage as well as pump failure among other things. Pump malfunction is uncommon, but errors in refilling and reprogramming have resulted in serious morbidity and mortality.[172]

A serious potential complication reported with the use of high doses of spinal morphine or hydromorphone is the formation of intrathecal mass lesions. North et al[173] first reported this complication in a 42-year-old woman who had been receiving 25 mg/day of IT morphine (50 mg/mL) for 2 months and who presented with paraplegia and incontinence. At laminectomy, a soft-tissue mass containing chronic inflammatory cells surrounding the catheter tip was found and removed, but the patient remained paraplegic.

Coffey and Burchiel[174] provided a review of the known cases of this complication in 2002. They found 41 cases, most of whom were receiving >10 mg/day morphine at concentrations of 25 to 50 mg/mL or >10 mg/day hydromorphone at concentrations of 10 to 100 mg/mL. Most had been receiving IT medications for more than 6 months. Seven patients presented with new or increased pain complaints, whereas 34 presented with neurologic dysfunction. Thirty patients underwent surgical resection, nine of whom had persistent neurologic defects. The pathologic diagnosis in most cases was granuloma. No cases have been reported in patients receiving baclofen alone.

Spinal Cord Stimulation

The gate control theory, introduced by Melzack and Wall in 1965, provided the theoretical foundation for the use of implanted electrical stimulation. Several years later, Shealy[175] was the first to describe what was initially known as dorsal column stimulation and eventually spinal cord stimulation (SCS). Electrical stimulation in proximity of the dorsal columns through epidural lead placement was believed convenient because sensory pathways there are segregated from motor pathways. Initially, however, poor patient selection and technological limitations led to disappointing results. Patient selection improved through work done in the late 1980s and early 1990s.[176] At the same time, new technology became available, including the arrival of multichannel leads, dual-lead configurations, totally implantable generators, and expanded programming options. The specific mechanism of action of SCS remains elusive. Neural and neurochemical changes, perhaps resulting from stimulation in the dorsal roots, dorsal root entry zone, or dorsal columns, have been implicated.[177] The efficacy of SCS is greatest for certain types of ischemic and neuropathic pain syndromes with primarily causalgic and dysesthetic features.[178]

Conditions that have favorably responded to SCS include lumbosacral fibrosis and arachnoiditis,[179]complex regional pain sydromes,[180] and more recently, pain associated with peripheral vascular disease[181] and angina pectoris.[182] Failed back surgery patients with predominantly radicular pain elements have shown response rates of 50 to 60% at 5 years in more recent studies.[183,184] Patients with peripheral vascular disease have also responded favorably, with significant limb salvage rates reported.[181,185] Patients with medically refractory angina pectoris who were not candidates for revascularization have experienced pain relief and improvement in cardiac function and stress testing.[182] Significant improvement in anginal symptoms and improvement in functional class was shown to occur in more than 70% of patients with severe coronary artery disease and intractable angina.[186]

The most critical issues in patient selection consist of identifying a well-founded diagnosis and the presence of specific neuropathic or ischemic pain states. A multidisciplinary approach including a psychological evaluation is recommended. High scores on the Minnesota Multiphasic Personality Inventory's depression scale have been associated with SCS failure.[187] Other contraindications such as the presence of localized infection, systemic sepsis, severe immune suppression, and coagulopathy are similar to other implantable devices.

The systems in current use employ a totally implantable generator system that employs an implantable receiver and external transmitter. Either system is adaptable to multiple leads, depending on the need for bilateral extremity stimulation or wider unilateral coverage. Similarly, different electrode configurations exist, varying in number and spacing of electrodes. One can also take advantage of complex programming options to fine-tune or change stimulation patterns.

Prior to permanent placement, a trial stimulation is performed. Generally, temporary percutaneous stimulator leads are used for this purpose. Once an appropriate stimulation pattern is produced, most protocols will require at least a 50% improvement in pain scores. The length of trial screening is controversial, varying from days to weeks.

Lead migration and breakage are common problems with long-term stimulation. Lead migration may produce unwanted paresthesias or diminish benefit in the original area of stimulation. This can sometimes be overcome by reprogramming of the electrode but may require lead replacement. Serious infection, bleeding, and nerve injury are uncommon complications.[183] Generator or transmitter failure is unlikely; however, fully implantable generators will require replacement, depending on use.

Radiofrequency Lesioning

Radiofrequency (RF) technology was first used to produce nervous system lesions in the 1950s. The technique was further refined in the 1970s by the invention of the RF probe, leading to the technique of facet joint denervation. Modern RF thermocoagulation has been used to ablate pain pathways in the spinal cord, dorsal root entry zone, dorsal root ganglion, trigeminal ganglion, sympathetic chain, and peripheral nerves.

An insulated probe with an uninsulated tip is placed in proximity of the target tissue and RF current is allowed to flow from a generator. As the current encounters resistance in the tissue, heat is generated, creating a lesion. Lesion size is directly proportional to tissue temperature at thermal equilibrium between the probe tip and the surrounding tissue. This equilibrium is generally achieved in 1 minute. Prior to lesioning, the target structure must be localized. This is accomplished by electrical stimulation. High frequencies and lower voltages are used to elicit a paresthesia in the desired distribution, whereas low frequencies and higher voltages are used to test for motor stimulation. Temperatures specific for the target nerve can be selected.

Patient selection requires a firm diagnosis verified by prognostic blocks with local anesthetics. RF lesioning is by definition neurodestructive and can be considered only after more conservative options have failed. Patients may require psychological screening and should be aware of all potential adverse sequelae, including neurologic impairment. Thorough knowledge of neuroanatomy and the use of fluoroscopy are mandatory for the pain physician.

The lumbar spine is an area where RF lesioning is often applied. Specific techniques have been developed for pain originating from the facet joints, nerve roots, annulus fibrosis, and sacroiliac joints. Approximately 50 to 60% of carefully selected patients with mechanical low back pain due to facet arthropathy achieve at least moderate reduction in pain following RF lesioning of the medial branches of the posterior primary divisions (i.e., the nerves that supply the facet joints).[188] A randomized, double-blind, controlled trial of RF facet denervation versus a sham procedure using no RF current showed a significantly better response in the RF group 8 weeks after the procedure. Ten of 15 RF subjects and 6 of 16 control subjects met criteria for treatment success.[189]

Lesions for discogenic pain are performed at the ramus communicans and intradiscally.[198] Owing to the complexity of disc innervation and disc pathology, this procedure is not nearly as successful as for medial branch denervation. RF applications for cervical spine pain are primarily oriented toward facet joint denervation, and results are similar to those for lumbar facet arthropathy. Lesions of the sphenopalatine and trigeminal ganglia[190] have been successfully used for select patients for the treatment of migraine headaches and trigeminal neuralgia, respectively. RF neurolysis of the sympathetic chain, although not in widespread use, has been helpful in some patients with type II complex regional pain syndrome and vasoocclusive disorders.

Patients can experience postoperative pain or dysesthesia for days to weeks after the procedure as a result of low-level heat injuries to tissue. Subsequently, judging the efficacy of the procedure is often difficult in the short term. More permanent nerve injuries and disc infections have been described.[191] Duration of benefit from RF lesioning is usually no more than 6 to 8 months because nerve regeneration usually occurs, but the procedure may offer more prolonged analgesia than nerve blocks. For patients who experience several months of relief from facet joint steroid injections, repeating that procedure may be a more appropriate alternative.

Minimally Invasive Treatment for Disc Pathology

Discography

Discography is a purely diagnostic procedure that incorporates provocative injection to determine whether a particular disc is a source of pain with radiographic imaging using radiographic dye. Using a combination of oblique, PA and lateral views, a needle is placed into the central portion of the disc. A two needle technique is often used to reduce the risk of bacterial discitis, advancing a larger needle into close proximity to the disc and passing a finer needle through it into the disc. A small volume (0.5 to 3 mL) is slowly injected until resistance to injection or pain is elicited. Anteroposterior and lateral views are observed for the pattern of dye spread. Commonly seen defects include annular tears and extravasation into the epidural space. Subsequent CT scan provides more detailed imaging of anatomic defects. Often, an adjacent, presumably normal disc is injected. Concordant pain in the affected disc and lack of pain in the adjacent, normal disc helps confirm the abnormal disc as the source of pain.

Percutaneous Annuloplasty

Intradiscal electrothermal therapy (IDET) is a treatment system that permits the controlled delivery of electrothermal heat to the intervertebral disc via a thermal resistive coil. The electrode is navigated circumferentially around the inner surface of the disc annulus. By then heating the electrode, annular collagen is denatured and nerve endings innervating the disc are coagulated. A similar system uses RF heating of the annulus. The target diagnoses for these procedures are discogenic pain with internal disc disruptions secondary to small contained disc herniations, posterior annular fissures, and degenerated disc with relatively preserved disc height. Patients with these diagnoses are likely to fail conservative therapy, whereas discectomy and fusion surgery have shown mixed results. MRI evidence of disc disruption and a positive discogram are usually required for patient selection. A review of the available literature published in 2002 indicated that several prospective studies showed significant improvement lasting a year or longer.[192] One nonrandomized study that compared IDET with a control group treated with a physical rehabilitation program showed better outcomes after 1 year in the IDET group.[193] Randomized controlled trials are needed.

Percutaneous Disc Decompression

Several minimally invasive techniques have been introduced that are designed to reduce intradiscal pressure, thus reducing tension on the outer layers of the annulus fibrosus and decreasing compression of the adjacent nerve root. Chymopapain chemonucleolysis was first used in the 1960s. Although successful in some patients, the process was not controllable, and resulted in overdecompression with disc collapse and spine instability in some individuals. In addition, there were a number of reports of serious complications, including anaphylaxis and transverse myelitis.[194] Percutaneous laser discectomy has had limited success, and may produce complications related to overdecompression and injury to surrounding tissues, especially nerve roots, because of the high temperatures generated.

Nucleoplasty is a newer technology that produces vaporization of small volumes of material in the nucleus followed by RF thermocoagulation. Relatively low temperatures are used, and small amounts of tissue are eliminated, making it a fairly safe procedure.[194] A similar decompressive procedure involves the use a small percutaneous motorized augur, which removes measurable amounts of nuclear tissue percutaneously. For both procedures, treatment appears to be more useful for radiculopathy associated with disc bulge than for discogenic pain. Neither procedure has been subjected to randomized controlled trial.

CONCLUDING REMARKS

During the 1970s and 1980s, there was dramatic evolution of pain management toward a multidisciplinary approach. The biopsychosocial model was introduced, combining medical and behavioral and management, while addressing important issues regarding financial, vocational, recreational, and social aspects of the patient's life. There was a strong emphasis on reducing or eliminating opioid and sedative medications. Although these programs were expensive, results were often dramatic. Few such programs exist any longer. Perhaps the primary reason has been the devolution of much of the health insurance industry to programs that require participation of separate, selected providers for medical, psychological, and rehabilitation services. The opportunities for obtaining reimbursement for all three types of services in a coordinated fashion within a single institution are almost nonexistent. At the same time, new technologies have been introduced that, while apparently beneficial for selected individuals, are rarely of lasting benefit for patients with truly chronic pain. Nevertheless, the same third-party payers that fail to reimburse a multidisciplinary approach that addresses the entire spectrum of a chronic pain patient's needs may provide payment for expensive interventions or surgeries without hesitation.

Above all, the practice of pain medicine requires a comprehensive and meticulous assessment of all aspects of each patient's problem. There are indeed problems that can be managed expeditiously, particularly for patients whose duration of symptoms has been relatively short and for whom specific procedures can be of substantial benefit. However, the patient who has had back and leg pain for 7 years, is unemployed, has had five back surgeries, and is on three opioid medications is unlikely to experience a quick cure from an injection, a device, or another operation. Such a patient requires the services of multiple health care professionals who can address his medical, behavioral, and rehabilitation needs.

References

1. Raja SN, Meyer RA, Campbell JN: Transduction properties of the sensory afferent fibers. In Yaksh TL *et al* (eds): Anesthesia: Biologic Foundations, p 513. Philadelphia, Lippincott-Raven, 1997
2. Klement W, Arndt JO: The role of nociceptors of cutaneous veins in the mediation of cold pain in man. J Physiol (Lond) 449:73, 1992
3. Lynn B: The detection of injury and tissue damage. In Melzack R, Wall PD (eds): Textbook of Pain, p 19. New York, Churchill Livingstone, 1984
4. Freeman MAR, Wyke B: The innervation of the knee joint: An anatomical and histological study of the cat. J Anat 101:505, 1967
5. Tanelian DL, Beuerman RW: Responses of rabbit corneal nociceptors to mechanical and thermal stimulation. Exp Neurol 84:165, 1984
6. Bahr R, Blumberg H, Janig W: Do dichotomizing afferent fibers exist which supply visceral organs as well as somatic structures? Neurosci Lett 24:25, 1981
7. Malliani A: Cardiovascular sympathetic afferent fibers. Rev Physiol Biochem Pharmacol 94:11, 1982
8. Foreman RD: Organization of visceral output. In Yaksh TL *et al* (eds): Anesthesia: Biologic Foundations, p 663. Philadelphia, Lippincott-Raven, 1997
9. Ordway GA, Longhurst JC: Cardiovascular reflexes arising from the gallbladder of the cat. Circ Res 52:26, 1983
10. Cervero F: Afferent nerve activity evoked by natural stimulation of the biliary system in the ferret. Pain 13:137, 1982
11. Light AR, Perl ER: Spinal termination of functionally identified primary afferent neurons with slowly conducting myelinated fibers. J Comp Neurol 168:133, 1979
12. Malmberg AB, Yaksh TL: Hyperalgesia mediated by spinal glutamate or SP receptor blocked by spinal cyclooxygenase inhibition. Science 257:1276, 1992
13. Wilcox GL: Excitatory neurotransmitters and pain. In Bond MR, Charlton JE, Woolf CJ (eds): Proceedings of the Sixth World Congress on Pain, p 97. Amsterdam, Elsevier, 1991
14. Mendell LM: Physiological properties of unmyelinated fibre projections to the spinal cord. Exp Neurol 16:316, 1966
15. Meldrum B, Garthwaite J: Excitatory amino acid neurotoxicity and neurodegenerative disease. Trends Pharmacol Sci 11:379, 1990
16. Coderre TJ, Katz J, Vaccarino AL, Melzack R: Contribution of central neuroplasticity to pathological pain: Review of clinical and experimental evidence. Pain 52:259, 1993
17. Hope PJ, Schaible HG, Jarrott B, Duggan AW: Release and persistence of immunoreactive neurokinin A in the spinal cord is associated with chemical arthritis. Pain 5:S230, 1990
18. Malmberg AB, Yaksh TL: Antinociceptive actions of spinal nonsteroidal anti-inflammatory agents on the formalin test in the rat. J Pharmacol Exp Ther 263:136, 1992
19. Meller ST, Gebhart GF: Nitric oxide (NO) and nociceptive processing in the spinal cord. Pain 52:127, 1993
20. Malmberg AB, Yaksh TL: Spinal nitric oxide synthesis inhibition blocks NMDA-induced thermal hyperalgesia and produces antinociception in the formalin test in rats. Pain 54:291, 1993
21. Coderre TJ: Contribution of protein kinase C to persistent nociception following tissue injury in rats. Neurosci Lett 140:181, 1992
22. Mayer DJ, Mao J, Holt J, Price DD: Cellular mechanisms of neuropathic pain, morphine tolerance and their interactions. Proc Natl Acad Sci U S A 96:7731, 1999
23. Deleo JA, Tanga FY, Tawfik VL: Neuroimmune activation and neuroinflammation in chronic pain and opioid tolerance/hyperalgesia. Neuroscientist 10:40, 2004
24. Raghavendra V, DeLeo J: The role of astrocytes and microglia in persistent pain. Adv Molecular Cell Biol 31:951, 2004
25. Raghavendra V, Rutkowski MD, DeLeo JA: The role of spinal neuroimmune activation in morphine tolerance/hyperalgesia in neuropathic and sham-operated rats. J Neurosci 22:9980, 2002
26. DeLeo JA, Tanga FY, Tawfik VL: Neuroimmune activation and neuroinflammation in chronic pain and opioid tolerance/hyperalgesia. Neuroscientist 10:40, 2004
27. Yaksh TL, Elde RP: Factors governing release of methionine enkephalin-like immunoreactivity from mesencephalon and spinal cord of the cat *in vivo*. J Neurophysiol 46:1056, 1981
28. Van Calker P, Muller M, Hemprecht B: Adenosine regulates via two different types of receptors the accumulation of cAMP in cultured brain cells. J Neurochem 33:999, 1979
29. Yaksh TL, Hammond DL: Peripheral and central substrates involved in the rostrad transmission of nociceptive information. Pain 13:1, 1982
30. Tasker RR: Deafferentation. In Melzack R, Wall PD (eds): Textbook of Pain, p 119. New York, Churchill Livingstone, 1984
31. Willis WD: The origin and destination of pathways involved in pain transmission. In Melzack R, Wall PD (eds): Textbook of Pain, p 88. New York, Churchill Livingstone, 1984
32. Heinricher MM: Organizational characteristics of supraspinally mediated responses to nociceptive inputs. In Yaksh TL *et al* (eds): Anesthesia: Biologic Foundations, p 643. Philadelphia, Lippincott-Raven, 1997
33. Wall PD, Gutnick M: Ongoing activity in peripheral nerves: The physiology and pharmacology of impulses originating from a neuroma. Exp Neurol 43:580, 1974
34. Blumberg H, Janig W: Discharge pattern of afferent fibers from a neuroma. Pain 20:335, 1984
35. Garry MC, Tanelian DL: Afferent activity in injured afferent nerves. In Yaksh TL *et al* (eds): Anesthesia: Biologic Foundations, p 531. Philadelphia, Lippincott-Raven, 1997
36. Wall PD, Devor M: Sensory afferent impulses originate from dorsal root ganglia as well as from the periphery in normal and nerve injured rats. Pain 17:321, 1983
37. Blumberg H, Janig W: Changes in vasoconstrictor neurons supplying cat hindlimb following chronic nerve lesions: A model for studying mechanisms of reflex sympathetic dystrophy? J Auton Nerve Syst 7:399, 1983
38. Roberts WJ: A hypothesis on the physiological basis for causalgia and related pains. Pain 24:297, 1986
39. Ramer MS, Thompson SWN, McMahon SB: Causes and consequences of sympathetic basket formation in dorsal root ganglia. Pain 6(Suppl):S111, 1999
40. Merskey H: Pain terms: A list with definitions and notes on usage. Pain 6:249, 1979
41. Engel GL: "Psychogenic" pain and the pain-prone patient. Am J Med 26:899, 1959
42. Haddox JD: Psychological aspects of pain. In Abram SE, Haddox JD, Kettler RE (eds): The Pain Clinic Manual, p 31. Philadelphia, JB Lippincott, 1990
43. Turk DC, Rudy TE, Steig RL: Chronic pain and depression. Pain Management 1:18, 1987
44. Williams JBW (ed): Diagnostic and Statistical Manual of Mental Disorders, 3rd ed. Washington, DC, American Psychiatric Association, 1987
45. Pilowsky I, Chapman CR, Bonica JJ: Pain, depression and illness behavior in a pain clinic population. Pain 4:183, 1977
46. Ohnmeiss DD, Vanharanta H, Ekholm J: Degree of disc disruption and lower extremity pain. Spine 22:1600, 1997
47. Brown MF, Hukkanen MVJ, McCarthy ID *et al*: Sensory and sympathetic innervation of the vertebral endplate in patients with degenerative disc disease. J Bone Joint Surg Br 79:147, 1997
48. Dreyer SJ, Dreyfuss PH: Low back pain and the zygapophyseal (facet) joints. Arch Phys Med Rehabil 77:290, 1996
49. Maigne J-Y, Avaliklis A, Pfefer F: Results of sacroiliac joint double block and value of sacroiliac pain provocation tests in 54 patients with low back pain. Spine 21:1889, 1996
50. Kuslich SD, Ulstrom CL, Michael CJ: The tissue origin of low back pain and sciatica: A report of pain response to tissue stimulation during operation on the lumbar spine using local anesthesia. Orthop Clin North Am 22:181, 1991
51. Murphy RW: Nerve roots and spinal nerves in degenerative disc disease. Clin Orthop 129:46, 1977
52. Gertzbein SD, Tile M, Gross A, Falk R: Autoimmunity in degenerative disc disease of the lumbar spine. Orthop Clin North Am 6:67, 1975
53. Marshall LL, Trethwie ER: Chemical irritation of nerve roots in disc prolapse. Lancet 2:230, 1973
54. Saal JS, Franson RC, Dobrow R *et al:* High levels of phospholipase A_2 activity in lumbar disc herniations. Spine 15:674, 1990
55. Gordon SL, Weinstein JN: A review of basic science issues in low back pain. Phys Med Rehabil Clin North Am 9:323, 1998

56. Benzon HT: Epidural steroid injections for low back pain and lumbosacral radiculopathy. Pain 24:277, 1986
57. Lievre JA, Block-Michael H, Attali P: L'injection transsacré: Etude Clinique et Radiologique. Bull Soc Med 73:1110, 1957
58. Coomes EN: A comparison between epidural anesthesia and bedrest in sciatica. Br Med J 1:20, 1961
59. Swerdlow M, Sayle-Creer W: A study of extradural medication in the relief of the lumbosciatic syndrome. Anaesthesia 25:341, 1970
60. Winnie AP, Hartman JT, Myers HL Jr., Ramamurthy S, Barangan V; Pain clinic: II. Intradural and extradural corticosteroids for sciatica. Anesth Analg 51:990, 1972
61. Koes BW, Scholten RJPM, Mens JMA, Bouter LM: Efficacy of epidural steroid injections of low-back pain and sciatica: A systematic review of randomized trials. Pain 63:279, 1995
62. Watts RW, Silagy CA: A meta-analysis on the efficacy of epidural corticosteroids in the treatment of sciatica. Anaesth Intensive Care 23:564, 1995
63. Carette S, Leclaire R, Marcoux S *et al:* Epidural corticosteroids injections for sciatica due to herniated nucleus pulposus. N Engl J Med 336:1634, 1997
64. Abram SE, Hopwood MB: What factors contribute to outcome with lumbar epidural steroids? In Bond MR, Charlton JE, Woolf CJ (eds): Proceedings of the Sixth World Congress on Pain, p 491. Amsterdam, Elsevier, 1991
65. Finneson BE: Low Back Pain. Philadelphia, JB Lippincott, 1973
66. Sitzman BT: Epidural injections. In Fenton DS, Czervionke LF (eds): Image-Guided Spine Intervention, p 99. Philadelphia, WB Saunders, 2003
67. Cicala RS, Turner R, Moran E *et al:* Methylprednisolone acetate does not cause inflammatory changes in the epidural space. Anesthesiology 72:556, 1990
68. Abram SE, Marsala M, Yaksh TL: Analgesic and neurotoxic effects of intrathecal corticosteroids in rats. Anesthesiology 81:1198, 1994
69. Nelson DA: Dangers from methylprednisolone acetate therapy by intraspinal injection. Arch Neurol 45:804, 1988
70. Kay J, Findling JW, Raff H: Epidural triamcinolone suppresses the pituitary adrenal axis in human subjects. Anesth Analg 79:501, 1994
71. Abram SE, O'Connor TC: Complications associated with epidural steroid injections: A review. Regi Anesth 21:149, 1996
72. Fitzgibbon DR, Posner KL, Domino K *et al:* Chronic pain management: American Society of Anesthesiologists Closed Claims Project. Anesthesiology 100:98, 2004
73. Plumb VJ, Dismukes WE: Chemical meningitis related to intrathecal corticosteroid therapy. South Med J 70:1241, 1977
74. Dougherty JH, Fraser RAR: Complications following intraspinal injection of steroids. J Neurosurg 48:1023, 1978
75. Ryan MD, Taylor TKF: Management of lumbar nerve root pain by intrathecal and epidural injection of depot methylprednisolone acetate. Med J Aust 2:532, 1981
76. Cohen FL: Conus medullaris syndrome following multiple intrathecal corticosteroid injections. Arch Neurol 36:228, 1979
77. Abram SE, Anderson RA: Using a pain questionnaire to predict response to steroid epidurals. Reg Anaesth 5:11, 1980
78. Travell JG, Simons DG: Myofascial Pain and Dysfunction. Baltimore, Williams & Wilkins, 1983
79. Berges PV: Myofascial pain syndromes. Postgrad Med 53:161, 1953
80. Cheshire WP, Abashian SW, Mann JD: Botulinum toxin in the treatment of myofascial pain syndrome. Pain 59:65, 1994
81. Stanton-Hicks M, Janig W, Hassenbusch S *et al:* Reflex sympathetic dystrophy: Changing concepts and taxonomy. Pain 63:127, 1995
82. Hogan QH, Erickson SJ, Haddox JD, Abram SE: The spread of solutions during stellate ganglion block. Reg Anesth 17:78, 1992
83. Hogan QH, Erickson SJ, Abram SE: Computerized tomography-guided stellate ganglion blockade. Anesthesiology 77:596, 1992
84. Hogan QH, Abram SE: Neural blockade for diagnosis and prognosis. Anesthesiology 86:216, 1997
85. Bonica JJ: Causalgia and other reflex sympathetic dystrophies. In Bonica JJ, Albe-Fessard D (eds): Advances in Pain Research and Therapy, vol 1, p 141. New York, Raven Press, 1979
86. Abram SE, Lightfoot RW: Treatment of long standing Cau Salgia with prazosin. Reg Anesth, 6:79, 1981
87. Raja SN, Treede RD, Darts KD, Campbella JN: Systemic alpha-adrenergic blockade with phentolamine: a diagnostic test for sympathetically maintained pain. Anesthesiology, 74:691, 1991
88. Kozin F, Ryan LM, Carrera GF, Soin JS, Wortmann RL: The reflex sympathetic dystrophy syndrome (RSDS): III. Scintigraphic studies, further evidence for the therapeutic efficacy of systemic corticosteroids, and proposed diagnostic criteria. Am J Med 70:23, 1981
89. Poplawski ZJ, Wiley AM, Murray JF: Post-traumatic dystrophy of the extremities. J Bone Joint Surg Am 65:642, 1983
90. Abram SE, Asiddao CB, Reynolds AC: Increased skin temperature during transcutaneous electrical stimulation. Anesth Analg 59:22, 1980
91. Stilz RJ, Carron H, Sanders DB: Reflex sympathetic dystrophy in a 6 year old: Successful treatment by transcutaneous nerve stimulation. Anesth Analg 56:438, 1977
92. Spurling RG: Causalgia of the upper extremity: Treatment by dorsal sympathetic ganglionectomy. Arch Neurol Psychiatry 23:784, 1930
93. Mayfield FH: Causalgia. Springfield, IL, Charles C Thomas, 1951
94. Boas RS, Hatangdi VS, Richards EG: Lumbar sympathectomy: A percutaneous technique. In Bonica JJ, Albe-Fessard D (eds): Advances in Pain Research and Therapy, vol 1, p 485. New York, Raven Press, 1976
95. Loeser JD: Herpes zoster and postherpetic neuralgia. Pain 25:149, 1986
96. Watson CP, Watt VR, Chipman M, Birkett N, Evans RJ: The prognosis with postherpetic neuralgia. Pain 46:195, 1991
97. Rogers RS, Tindall JP: Geriatric herpes zoster. J Am Geriatr Soc 19:495, 1971
98. Zacks SI, Langfitt TW, Elliott FA: Herpetic neuritis, a light and electron microscopic study. Neurology 14:774, 1964
99. Noordenbos W: Pain, p 182. Amsterdam, Elsevier, 1959
100. Watson CP, Deck JH, Morshead C, Van der Kooy D, Evans RJ: Postherpetic neuralgia: Further post-mortem studies of cases with and without pain. Pain 44:105, 1991
101. Rosenak S: Procaine injection treatment of herpes zoster. Lancet 2:1056, 1938
102. Winnie AP, Hartwell PW: The relationship between the time of treatment of acute herpes with sympathetic blockade and post-herpetic neuralgia: Clinical support for a new theory of the mechanism by which sympathetic blockade provides therapeutic benefit. Reg Anesth 18:277, 1994
103. Whitley RJ, Gnann JW: Acyclovir: A decade later. N Engl J Med 327:782, 1992
104. Tyring S, Barbarash RA, Nahlik JE *et al:* Famcyclovir for the treatment of acute herpes zoster: A randomized, controlled, double blind trial. Ann Int Med 123:89, 1995
105. Eaglestein WH, Katz R, Brown JA: The effects of early corticosteroid therapy on the skin eruption and pain of herpes zoster. JAMA 211:1681, 1970
106. Epstein E: Herpes zoster and post-zoster neuralgia: Intralesional triamcinolone therapy. Cutis 12:898, 1973
107. Schreuder M: Pain relief in herpes zoster. S Afr Med J 63:820, 1983
108. Rosenak S: Procaine injection treatment of herpes zoster. Lancet 2:1056, 1938
109. Tenicela R, Lovasik D, Eaglestein W: Treatment of herpes zoster with sympathetic blocks. Clin J Pain 1:63, 1985
110. Rowbotham M, Harden N, Stacey B *et al:* Gabapentin for the treatment of postherpetic neuralgia. JAMA 280:1837, 1998
111. Rome JD, Townsend CO, Bruce BK *et al:* Chronic noncancer pain rehabilitation with opioid withdrawal: Comparison of treatment outcomes based on opioid use status at admission. Mayo Clin Proc 79:759, 2004
112. Portenoy RK: Opioid therapy for chronic non-malignant pain: Current status. In Fields HL, Liebeskind JS (eds): Progress in Pain Research and Management, vol 1, p 247. Seattle, IASP Press, 1994
113. Paoli F, Darcourt G, Corsa P: Note preliminare sur l'action de l'imipramine dans les etats douloureaux. Rev Neurol 102:503, 1960
114. Watson CP, Evans RS, Reed K *et al:* Amitriptyline versus placebo in postherpetic neuralgia. Neurology 32:671, 1982
115. Getto CJ, Sorkness CA, Howell T: Antidepressants and chronic nonmalignant pain: A review. J Pain Symptom Manage 2:9, 1987
116. Max MB, Culane M, Schafer SC *et al:* Amitriptyline relieves diabetic neuropathy pain in patients with normal or depressed mood. Neurology 37:589, 1987
117. Max MB, Schafer SC, Culane M *et al:* Amitriptyline, but not lorazepam, relieves postherpetic neuralgia. Neurology 38:1427, 1988
118. Diamond S, Freitag FG: The use of fluoxetine in the treatment of headache. Clin J Pain 5:200, 1989
119. Camran A, Staumanis J, Chesson A: Fluoxetine prophylaxis of migraine. Headache 32:101, 1991
120. Power-Smith P, Turkington D: Fluoxetine in phantom limb pain. Br J Psychiatry 163:105, 1993
121. Max MB, Lynch SA, Muir J *et al:* Effects of desipramine, amitriptyline and fluoxetine on pain in diabetic neuropathy. N Engl J Med 326:1250, 1992
122. Sindrup SH, Gram LF, Brsen K *et al:* The selective serotonin reuptake inhibitor paroxetine is effective in the treatment of diabetic neuropathy symptoms. Pain 42:135, 1990
123. Reynolds IJ, Miller RJ: Tricyclic antidepressants block *N*-methyl-D-aspartate receptors: Similarities to the action of zinc. Br J Pharmacol 95:95, 1988
124. Mellick GA, Mellicy LB, Mellick LB: Gabapentin in the management of reflex sympathetic dystrophy. J Pain Symptom Manage 10:265, 1995
125. Backonja M, Beydoun A, Edwards KR *et al:* Gabapentin for the symptomatic treatment of painful neuropathy in patients with diabetes mellitus. JAMA 280:1831, 1998
126. Xiao W-H, Bennett GJ: Gabapentin has an antinociceptive effect mediated via a spinal site of acion in a rat model of painful peripheral neuropathy. Pain 2:267, 1996
127. Stanfa LC, Singh L, Williams RG, Dickenson AH: Gabapentin, ineffective in normal rats, markedly reduces C-fiber evoked responses after inflammation. Neuroreport 8:587, 1997
128. Eisenberg E, Alon N, Ishay A *et al:* Lamotrigine in the treatment of painful diabetic neuropathy. Eur J Neurol 5:167, 1998
129. Chabal C, Russell LC, Burchiel KJ: The effect of intravenous lidocaine, tocainide, and mexiletine on spontaneously active fibers originating in rat sciatic neuromas. Pain 38:333, 1989
130. Tanelian DL, Brose WG: Neuropathic pain can be relieved by drugs that are use-dependent sodium channel blockers: Lidocaine, carbamazepine, and mexiletine. Anesthesiology 74:949, 1991

131. Collin E, Poulain P, Gauvin-Piquard A, Petit G, Pichard-Leandri E: Is disease progression the major factor in morphine 'tolerance' in cancer pain treatment? Pain 55:319, 1993
132. Paronis CA, Holtzman SG: Development of tolerance to the analgesic activity of μ agonists after continuous infusion of morphine, meperidine or fentanyl in rats. J Pharmacol Exp Ther 262:1, 1992
133. Coombs DW, Saunders RL, Gaylor MS *et al:* Relief of continuous chronic pain by intraspinal narcotics infusion via an implanted reservoir. JAMA 250:2336, 1983
134. Jorgensen BC, Andersen HB, Engquist A: CSF and plasma morphine after epidural and intrathecal application. Anesthesiology 55:714, 1981
135. Woods WA, Cohen SE: High-dose epidural morphine in a terminally ill patient. Anesthesiology 56:311, 1982
136. Stillman MJ, Moulin DE, Foley KM: Paradoxical pain following high dose spinal morphine. Pain 4:S389, 1987
137. Yaksh TL, Harty GJ: Pharmacology of the allodynia in rats evoked by high dose intrathecal morphine. J Pharmacol Exp Ther 244:501, 1988
138. Eisenach JC, Rauck RL, Buzzanell C *et al:* Epidural clonidine for intractable cancer pain. Anesthesiology 71:647, 1989
139. Wilson PR, Yaksh TL: Baclofen is antinociceptive in the spinal intrathecal space of animals. Eur J Pharmacol 51:323, 1978
140. Zuniga RE, Schlicht CR, Abram SE: Intrathecal baclofen is analgesic in patients with chronic pain. Anesthesiology 92:876, 2000
141. Hogan Q, Haddox JD, Abram SE *et al:* Epidural opiates for the management of cancer pain. Pain 42:271, 1991
142. Du Pen SL, Kharasch ED, Williams A *et al:* Chronic epidural bupivacaine-opioid infusion in intractable cancer pain. Pain 49:293, 1992
143. Papo I, Visca A: Phenol subarachnoid rhizotomy for the treatment of cancer pain: A personal account of 290 cases. In Bonica JJ, Ventafridda V (eds): Advances in Pain Research and Therapy, vol 2, p 339. New York, Raven Press, 1979
144. Swerdlow M: Subarachnoid and extradural neurolytic blocks. In Bonica JJ, Ventafridda V (eds): Advances in Pain Research and Therapy, vol 2, p 325. New York, Raven Press, 1979
145. Thompson GE, Moore DC, Bridenbaugh LD, Artin RY: Abdominal pain and alcohol celiac plexus nerve block. Anesth Analg 56:1, 1977
146. Singler RC: An improved technique for alcohol neurolysis of the celiac plexus. Anesthesiology 56:137, 1982
147. Ischia S, Luzzani A, Ischia A *et al:* A new approach to the neurolytic block of the celiac plexus: The transaortic technique. Pain 16:333, 1983
148. Plancarte R, Amescua C, Patt RB, Aldrete A: Superior hypogastric plexus block for pelvic cancer pain. Anesthesiology 73:236, 1990
149. de Leon-Casasola OA, Kent E, Lema MJ: Neurolytic superior hypogastric plexus block for chronic pelvic pain associated with cancer. Pain 54:145, 1993
150. Simon DL, Carron H, Rowlingson JC: Treatment of bladder pain with transsacral nerve block. Anesth Analg 61:46, 1982
151. Bouhassira D, Lefkowitz M, Meynadier J, Serrie A: Origins of pain in HIV/AIDS. In Pain in HIV/AIDS, p 1. Chicago, Addison, 1994
152. O'Neill W, Sherrard S: Pain in human immunodeficiency virus disease: A review. Pain 54:3, 1993
153. McArthur JC, Hoover DR, Bacellar H: Dementia in AIDS patients: Incidence and risk factors. Neurology 43:2245, 1993
154. Beecher HK: The Measurement of Subjective Responses: Quantitative Effects of Drugs. New York, Oxford University Press, 1959
155. Taylor ML: Psychological treatment of chronic pain. In Abram SE, Haddox JD, Kettler RE (eds): The Pain Clinic Manual, p 225. Philadelphia, JB Lippincott, 1990
156. Fordyce WE, Fowler RS, Lehman JF *et al:* Operant conditioning in the treatment of chronic clinical pain. Arch Phys Med Rehabil 54:399, 1973
157. Fordyce WE, Roberts AH, Sternbach RA: The behavioral management of chronic pain: A response to critics. Pain 22:113, 1985
158. Jacobson E: Progressive Relaxation. Chicago, University of Chicago Press, 1929
159. Benson H: The Relaxation Response. New York, William Morrow, 1975
160. Hughes J, Smith TW, Kosterlitz HW *et al:* Isolation of two related pentapeptides from brain with potent opiate activity. Nature 258:577, 1975
161. Yaksh TL, Rudy TA: Studies on the direct spinal action of narcotics in the production of analgesia in the rat. J Pharmacol Exp Ther 202:411, 1977
162. Bahar M, Magora F, Olshwang D, Davidson JT: Epidural morphine in the treatment of pain. Lancet i:527, 1979
163. Krames ES, Gershow J, Galssberg A *et al:* Continuous infusion of spinally administered narcotics for the relief of pain due to malignant disorders. Cancer 56:696, 1985
164. Shetter AG, Hadley MN, Wilkinson E: Administration of intraspinal morphine for the treatment of cancer pain. Neurosurgery 18:740, 1986
165. Penn RD, Kroi JS: Long-term intrathecal baclofen infusion for treatment of spasticity. J Neurosurg 66:181, 1987
166. Protenoy RK, Foley KM: Chronic use of opioid analgesics in nonmalignant pain: Report of 38 cases. Pain 25:171, 1986
167. Yaksh TL: Spinal opiates: A review of their effect on spinal function with an emphasis on pain processing. Acta Anaesthesiol Scand 31(Suppl):25, 1987
168. Arner S, Meyerson B: Lack of analgesic effect of opioids on neuropathic and idiopathic forms of pain. Pain 33:11, 1988
169. Slonimski M, Abram SE, Zuniga RE: Intrathecal baclofen for chronic pain management. Reg Anesth Pain Med 29:269, 2004
170. Zuniga RE, Perera S, Abram SE: Intrathecal baclofen: A useful agent in the treatment of well-established complex regional pain syndrome. Reg Anesth Pain Med 27:90, 2004
171. Patt RB: Implantable technology for pain control: Identification and management of problems and complications. In Waldman S, Winnie A (eds): Interventional Pain Mangement, p 438. Philadelphia, WB Saunders, 1996
172. Wu C, Patt RB: Accidental overdose of systemic morphine during intended refill of intrathecal infusion device. Anesth Analg 75:130, 1992
173. North RB, Cutchis PN, Epstein JA, Long DM: Spinal cord compression complicating subarachnoid infusion of morphine: Case report and laboratory experience. Neurosurgery 29:778, 1991
174. Coffey RJ, Burchiel K: Inflammatory mass lesions associated with intrathecal drug infusion catheters: Report and observations on 41 patients. Neurosurgery 50:78, 2002
175. Shealy C, Mortimer J, Reswik J: Electrical inhibitors of pain by stimulation of the dorsal column. Preliminary clinical reports. Anesth Analg 46:489, 1967
176. North R, Kidd D, Fabarch M *et al*: Spinal cord stimulators for chronic, intractable pain: Experience over two decades. Neurosurgery 32:384, 1993
177. Campbell JN: Examination of possible mechanisms by which stimulation of the spinal cord in man relieves pain. Appl Neurophysiol 44:181, 1981
178. Tasker RR, de Carvalho GTC, Dolan EJ: Intractable pain of spinal cord origin: Clinical features and implications for surgery. J Neurosurg 77:373, 1992
179. De la Porte C, Siegfried J: Lumbosacral spinal fibrosis (spinal arachnoiditis): Its diagnosis and treatment by spinal cord stimulation. Spine 8:593, 1983
180. Barolat G, Schwartzman R, Woo R: Epidural spinal cord stimulation in the management of reflex sympathetic dystrophy. Stereotact Funct Neurosurg 53:29, 1989
181. Horsh S, Cleyes L: Epidural spinal cord stimulation in the treatment of severe peripheral artery vascular disease. Ann Vasc Surg 8:468, 1994
182. Houtuast R, Blanksira P, DeJongsle M *et al*: Effect of spinal cord stimulation on myocardial blood flow assessed by positive emission and tomography in patients with refractory angina. Am J Cardiol 77:462, 1996
183. Turney J, Loeser J, Bell K: Spinal cord stimulation for chronic low back pain: A systematic literature synthesis. Neurosurgery 37:1088, 1995
184. North R, Kidd D, Lee M, Piartodosi S: A prospective randomized study of spinal cord stimulation versus reoperation for failed back surgery syndrome: Initial results. Stereotactic Funct Neurosurg 74:267, 1994
185. Gersback P, Hasdemir M, Stevens R *et al:* Discriminative microcirculatory screening of patients with refractory limb ischemia for dorsal column stimulation. J Endovasc Surg 13:464, 1997
186. Di Pede F, Lanza GA, Zuin G *et al*: Immediate and long-term clinical outcome after spinal cord stimulation for refractory stable angina pectoris. Am J Cardiol 91:951, 2003
187. Brandwin MA, Kewman DG: MMPI indicators of treatment response to spinal cord stimulation in patients with chronic pain and patients with movement disorders. Psychol Rep 51:1059, 1982
188. North RB, Zahurak M, Kidd D: Radiofrequency lumbar facet denervation: Analysis of prognostic factors. Pain 57:77, 1994
189. van Kleef M, Barendse GA, Kessels A *et al*: Randomized trial of radiofrequency lumbar facet denervation for chronic low back pain. Spine 24:1937, 1999
190. Broggi G, Franzini A, Lasio G *et al*: Long-term results of percutaneous retrogasserian thermorhizotomy for "essential" trigeminal neuralgia. Instituto Neurologico 26:26, 1990
191. Savitz MH: Percutaneous radiofrequency rhizotomy of the lumbar facets: Ten years' experience. Mt Sinai J Med 58:177, 1991
192. Wetzel FT, McNally TA, Phillips FM: Intradiscal electrothermal therapy used to manage chronic discogenic low back pain: new directions and interventions. Spine 27:2621, 2002
193. Karasek M, Bogduk N: Twelve month followup of a controlled trial of intradiscal thermal annuloplasty for back pain due to internal disc disruption. Spine 25:2601, 2000
194. Baker RM, Cole AJ: Percutaneous intradiscal therapies. In Cole AJ, Herring SA (eds): The Low Back Pain Handbook, p 375. Philadelphia, Hanley and Belfus, 2003

CHAPTER 57 ■ ANESTHESIA AND CRITICAL CARE MEDICINE

MIRIAM M. TREGGIARI AND STEVEN DEEM

KEY POINTS

1. Administration of high-dose corticosteroids to patients presenting with traumatic brain injury is associated with a 20% increase in the relative risk of death.
2. Administration of thrombolytic therapy (rt-PA) to patients presenting within 3 hours of onset of acute ischemic stroke results in improved neurologic outcome.
3. Patients who are resuscitated from cardiac arrest due to ventricular fibrillation have improved neurologic outcome and possibly reduced mortality when treated with mild therapeutic hypothermia (32 to 34°C) for 12 to 24 hours after hospital admission.
4. In patients with severe sepsis or septic shock, activated protein C is associated with a 6% absolute 28-day mortality reduction, and early goal-directed therapy, targeting an $Scvo_2$ >70% in the first 6 hours after admission to the emergency department, has been associated with an even greater reduction in mortality.
5. Separation from mechanical ventilation in patients who are recovering from respiratory failure is accelerated by respiratory therapy-driven protocols and daily trials of spontaneous breathing.
6. Ventilation with low tidal volume (6 mL/kg) in patients with acute lung injury and acute respiratory distress syndrome reduces mortality, compared with traditional tidal volumes (12 mL/kg).
7. Tight glycemic control using intensive insulin therapy (goal glucose <110 mg/dL) reduces intensive care unit (ICU) mortality by approximately 50% compared with more conventional therapy (goal glucose <215).
8. Red blood cell transfusion in the ICU should be restricted (transfusion threshold hemoglobin <7 g/dL) with the possible exception of patients with a diagnosis of active bleeding, early septic shock, acute myocardial infarction or unstable angina, or with primarily neurologic or neurosurgical problems.
9. Nurse-driven sedation protocols and daily interruption of sedative infusions reduce the duration of mechanical ventilation and ICU length of stay.
10. The incidence of ventilator-associated pneumonia (VAP) can be reduced with strict hand washing during patient care and semirecumbent positioning of the patient. Antibiotic therapy of VAP should use a "deescalating" strategy and can be limited to an 8-day course in uncomplicated cases.

ANESTHESIOLOGISTS AND CRITICAL CARE MEDICINE

Historically, critical care medicine evolved as a specialty nearly simultaneously in Europe and North America, but it has followed strikingly different models in regard to the involvement of anesthesiologists. The first intensive care unit (ICU) in Europe may have been located in Denmark in the 1950s, and concurrently, the first critical care physician, or "intensivist," may well have been an anesthesiologist.[1] Anesthesiologists continued to play a defining role in the development of critical care medicine in most of Europe, Australia, New Zealand, Japan, and elsewhere, and comprise the majority of intensivists in many countries around the world today. In North America, anesthesiologists were also integral to the development of critical care medicine as a specialty. However, in contrast to other countries, in the United States anesthesiologists have played an ever-diminishing role in the specialty, and today comprise a small minority of the intensivist workforce.[2]

Although it has been suggested that the first ICU in North America was established at Johns Hopkins in 1923 to care for postoperative neurosurgical patients, it was not until the late 1950s and early 1960s that true multidisciplinary ICUs began to appear. The driving forces behind ICU development included advances in surgical techniques; polio epidemics, which resulted in widespread respiratory failure; and later the recognition of acute respiratory distress syndrome (ARDS). Anesthesiologists played a natural role in the evolution of ICUs, given their familiarity with surgical resuscitation and mechanical ventilation. Early on, however, the concept of "intensivists" did not exist, and patients were often managed by their primary physician (be it surgeon or internist) and nurses, with formal or informal consultation given by specialists, including anesthesiologists.

In the early 1960s, the first critical care medicine training program was established at the University of Pittsburgh under the direction of an anesthesiologist, Peter Safar. At this point, the concept of "intensivist" was born; as defined by Dr. Safar, the qualities and qualifications of such an individual should include inquisitiveness, thoughtfulness, high motivation level, action orientation, diplomacy, and scientific training. In the late 1960s, a group that included Dr. Safar and another anesthesiologist, Ake Grenvik, were instrumental in inaugurating the Society of Critical Care Medicine (SCCM). Anesthesiologists working through SCCM were instrumental in developing the board certification process for critical care medicine, and in 1986, the first critical care medicine certification examination was administered by the American Board of Anesthesiology.[3] From the 1960s until now, numerous anesthesiologists made important contributions to the development of the specialty, to critical care-related research, and to improvements in the care of critically ill patients. However, as of 2004, only about 1,100 anesthesiologists had completed the certification process in critical care medicine in the United States.[4]

Anesthesiology and Critical Care Medicine: The Future

Although it seems certain that anesthesiologists will continue to play an important role in critical care medicine worldwide, in the United States, anesthesiology is currently at a crossroads in regard to its continued involvement in critical care medicine. There are several forces that will shape the evolution of the specialty of critical care medicine as a whole and the contribution that anesthesiologists will make to this evolution. These forces are (1) quality of care issues and the contribution of intensivists to improved ICU outcomes, (2) business/economic factors, and (3) the aging population and increasing demand for critical care services.

Intuitively, the involvement of intensivists in the management of critical illness makes sense. This has become increasingly clear as advances in medical and surgical therapeutics have increased the complexity of care for an aging and increasingly ill population of patients. However, debates over loss of physician autonomy, economic and training considerations, and a lack of hard evidence of the benefit of intensivists has hindered the development of an intensivist-centered ICU paradigm in the United States. More recently, however, several studies have suggested that mortality and other intermediate endpoints such as ICU length of stay can be reduced when "high-intensity" physician staffing models that mandate management or comanagement by intensivists are used.[5] These studies, as summarized in a meta-analysis by Pronovost et al,[5] have provoked a reconsideration of the ideal staffing model for ICUs in the United States, particularly among the business community.

TABLE 57-1

LEAPFROG INTENSIVE CARE UNIT PHYSICIAN STAFFING STANDARD

Hospitals fulfilling the IPS standard will operate adult and/or pediatric ICUs that are managed or comanaged by intensivists who

1. Are present during daytime hours and provide clinical care exclusively in the ICU and,
2. At other times can, at least 95% of the time,
   i. Return ICU pages within 5 minutes
   ii. Arrange for a FCCS-certified nonphysician effector to reach ICU patients within 5 minutes

IPS, intensive care unit physician staffing; ICU, intensive care unit; FCCS, fundamental critical care support (course training sponsored by the Society of Critical Care Medicine to prepare nonintensivists to manage the first 24 hours of critical illness).
Data from http://www.leapfroggroup.org/for_consumers/hospitals asked what

The Business Roundtable, a national association of CEOs of Fortune 500 companies, formed the Leapfrog Group in 1999. The Leapfrog Group is a coalition of more than 150 purchasers and providers of health care benefits, including large companies such as General Motors, Motorola, and Merck, and insurers such as Aetna. The stated goal of the Leapfrog Group is to improve health care, in particular by reducing deaths due to medical error. To accomplish this aim, the group formulated the Leapfrog Initiative, which includes a series of "safety standards" that health care providers (largely meaning hospitals) should strive for if they are to provide care for Leapfrog Group employees. Prompted by the more recent data associating intensivists with improved outcomes, the Leapfrog Initiative included an ICU physician staffing (IPS) standard that promotes the continuous involvement of intensivists in the care of critically ill patients (Table 57-1). Given that only an estimated 10% of hospitals met this standard when it was initially published, the Leapfrog Initiative has moved the discussion of ICU staffing models from academic debate to the administrative boardroom. Although many hospitals may be able to meet the IPS standards by simple reconfiguration of current care models, meeting the standards in full will certainly increase the demand for intensivists.

A final, important force driving the evolution of critical care medicine in the United States is the aging population, which will place increasing demands on the health care system. Increased demand will result in a shortage of intensivists starting in 2007 that will grow to a greater than 20% deficit by the year 2020, given current training levels.[2] This prediction does not take into account any additional demands placed on the health care system, if any, by the Leapfrog Initiative, and thus is likely an underestimate of the true future need for intensivists.

Given the previous observations, it is clear that opportunities for careers in critical care medicine will be amply available in the coming years. Anesthesiology as a specialty would seem ideally suited to help satisfy the increasing demand for intensivists. Anesthesiologists are hospital based; have sound fundamental training in physiology, pharmacology, and invasive procedures and monitoring; and have excellent historical and concurrent (see Europe, etc.) role models for the anesthesiologist as intensivist. However, economic and lifestyle incentives have recently dissuaded residents from pursuing further training and careers in critical care medicine. Critical care services are currently not reimbursed at rates commensurate with surgical anesthesia, and critical care practice is accurately perceived as more time-consuming and unpredictable than an operating room-based practice. However, these factors may change in the coming years, as reimbursement for surgical anesthesia and critical care services equalize and the lifestyle constraints associated with critical care are moderated by creative organizational strategies, including the use of physician extenders and other mechanisms for reducing the "24-7" workload. Last, more recent proposals to expand the anesthesiology residency training requirement to include 6 months of intensive care may imbue trainees with a greater interest in critical care medicine as a career choice. As stated previously, anesthesiology in the United States is at a crossroads—with the proper imagination, emphasis, support, and training, the specialty can reassert itself as a leader in the field of critical care medicine. The alternative is that the percentage of anesthesiologists involved in critical care medicine will continue to decline and anesthesiology will become little more than a historical footnote in this field.

Critical Care Medicine: A Systems and Evidence-Based Approach

Critical care encompasses all disciplines of medicine. It is clearly beyond the scope of a single chapter to provide detailed coverage of all aspects of critical illness, including physiology, pathophysiology, mechanisms, and management of disease. In addition, many critical care issues are commonly faced by anesthesiologists that practice solely in the operating room, and are covered in detail elsewhere in this text. Thus, this chapter focuses on issues that are relatively unique to the ICU, on therapeutic approaches, and on practices for which strong evidence exists. Where appropriate, the level of evidence supporting treatment regimens is graded according to commonly accepted methodology (Table 57-2).[6]

TABLE 57-2

EVALUATING EVIDENCE FOR MEDICAL THERAPIES

■ LEVELS OF EVIDENCE

I. Large, randomized trials with clear-cut results; low risk of false-positive (alpha) error or false-negative (beta) error
II. Small, randomized trials with uncertain results; moderate-to-high risk of false-positive (alpha) and/or false-negative (beta) error
III. Nonrandomized, contemporaneous controls
IV. Nonrandomized, historical controls and expert opinion
V. Case series, uncontrolled studies, and expert opinion

■ GRADES OF RECOMMENDATION BASED ON EXPERT CONSENSUS[a]

A. Supported by two or more level I studies
B. Supported by only one level I study
C. Supported by level II studies
D. Supported by level III studies
E. Supported by level IV or V studies

[a] The grades assigned in this chapter are taken directly from consensus conference statements. However, consensus grading systems are not consistent between conferences. This grading scale is one that is objective and widely used, but it may not directly reflect the criteria used to derive the individual grades reported here.
Adapted from Sackett DL: Rules of evidence and clinical recommendations on the use of antithrombotic agents. Chest 95:2S, 1989.

NEUROLOGIC AND NEUROSURGICAL CRITICAL CARE

Neuromonitoring

Several neuromonitoring devices used in the ICU setting may help in assessing pathophysiologic processes and adjusting therapy. The following section discusses some commonly used neuromonitoring devices, including transcranial Doppler ultrasonography, brain tissue oxygenation, and microdialysis. Intracranial pressure (ICP) monitoring and jugular venous oximetry are discussed in chapters on monitoring the anesthetized patient, anesthesia for neurosurgery, and burns and trauma, and are not discussed in detail here.

Transcranial Doppler Ultrasonography

Transcranial Doppler (TCD) measures mean, peak systolic, and end-diastolic flow velocities, and indirectly estimates cerebral blood flow (CBF). In patients with subarachnoid hemorrhage or traumatic brain injury (TBI), TCD can be used as a tool to identify vasospasm. Despite some technical limitation due to the quality of the bone window and the fact that increased velocity needs to be interpreted either in the context of vasospasm or hyperdynamic flow patterns, TCD remains a valuable monitoring device to follow trends over time. In patients with TBI, flow velocities are depressed, and impaired autoregulation and vascular reactivity are common. In these patients, monitoring of TCD and jugular venous oxygen saturation (Sjo_2) may be used to define the optimum cerebral perfusion pressure (CPP) level.[7] Patients with subarachnoid hemorrhage are at high risk of cerebral vasospasm, and serial TCD can monitor changes in blood velocities, detecting occurrence of ischemic flow patterns.

Brain Tissue Oxygenation

Brain tissue oxygen pressure ($Pbro_2$) measurements are performed by introducing a small, oxygen-sensitive catheter into the brain tissue. The device monitors a very local area of the brain tissue, and this technique is increasingly used for evaluation of cerebral oxygenation (normal $Pbro_2$ values: 25 to 30 mm Hg).[8] Monitoring may be performed in relatively undamaged parts of the brain or, preferably, in the penumbra region of an intracerebral lesion. Various studies have shown that an increase in ICP and a decrease in CPP or arterial oxygenation, as well as hyperventilation, may result in decreased $Pbro_2$. In patients with TBI, ischemic episodes defined as $Pbro_2$ <10 mm Hg for longer than 15 minutes in the first week after the injury were found to be associated with unfavorable neurologic outcome. CPP >60 mm Hg has been identified as the most important factor determining sufficient brain tissue oxygenation.

Microdialysis

Microdialysis uses a probe as an interface to the brain to continuously monitor the chemistry of a small focal volume of the cerebral extracellular space. This method uses internally perfused semipermeable membrane probes, which allow neurochemical water-soluble substances to be collected outside the brain for further analysis. Microdialysis monitoring in neurointensive care allows measurement of chemical substances such as lactate, pyruvate, glucose, glutamate, glycerol, and metabolites of several biochemical pathways and electrolytes, and thus provides insight into the bioenergetic status of the brain. Increased lactate, decreased glucose, and an elevated lactate/glucose ratio indicate accelerated anaerobic glycolysis. This metabolic pattern commonly occurs with cerebral ischemia or hypoxia, and increased glycolysis in this setting is associated with a poor outcome. Extracellular excitatory amino acids such as glutamate may provide a marker for secondary brain insults, as indicated by elevation during periods of hypoxia and intracranial hypertension. However, metabolism can be altered without changes of cerebral oxygenation and may not correlate with high ICP or low CPP.[9] In addition, lack of equilibration with the extracellular space may introduce sampling error.

Diagnosis and Clinical Management of the Most Common Types of Neurologic Failure

Traumatic Brain Injury

1 TBI is the leading cause of death from blunt trauma, with an incidence of approximately 10 per 100,000 per year. With a proportion of 20% of deaths occurring in patients between the age of 5 and 45 years, TBI represents the leading cause of death in this age group. The most powerful predictors of poor outcome from injury through resuscitation are age older than 55 years, poor pupillary reactivity, postresuscitation Glasgow Coma Scale (GCS), hypotension, hypoxia, and unfavorable intracranial diagnosis as established by radiologic features (computed tomography [CT] scan). In addition, early hyperglycemia (>200 mg/dL) is a reliable independent predictor of poor outcome.

The GCS (see Chapter 48) is the most widely used clinical measure of injury severity in patients with TBI. The advantages of this scale are that it provides an objective method of measuring consciousness, it has high intrarater and interrater reliability across observers with a wide variety of experience, and it has an excellent correlation with outcome. However, the GCS is unmeasurable in up to 25 to 45% of the patients at admission and is inaccurate when only the partial score is used, such as in patients with endotracheal intubation whose verbal response cannot be assessed. TBI qualifies as severe when the GCS is 8 or less after cardiopulmonary resuscitation. The predictive value of the GCS at admission is about 69% for good neurologic outcome and 76% for unfavorable outcome. After 7 days, these figures approximate 80% for both favorable and unfavorable outcome.[10]

Pupillary dilatation and light reactivity are also useful predictors of neurologic outcome. When both pupils are dilated and unreactive, the likelihood of poor neurologic outcome or death is as high as 90 to 95%. When both pupils are reactive, the likelihood of poor neurologic outcome is approximately 30 to 40%, whereas the probability of good outcome is 50 to 70%.

Hypotension is a strong predictor of poor outcome in TBI. Chesnut et al reported that there was a 15-fold increased risk of mortality in patients with early hypotension and an 11-fold increase in mortality in patients with late hypotension.[11]

Radiologic imaging is important in the diagnosis and in assessing the prognosis of patients with TBI. Based on the CT scan, TBI can be classified according to the severity of the intracranial lesion: diffuse injury I (no visible intracranial pathology); diffuse injury II (cisterns are present with midline shift 0 to 5 mm, no high-density or mixed-density lesion >25 cc); diffuse injury III (swelling; cisterns are compressed or absent with midline shift 0 to 5 mm, no high-density or mixed-density lesion >25 cc); diffuse injury IV (shift; midline shift >5 mm, no high-density or mixed-density lesion >25 cc); evacuated mass lesion (any lesion surgically evacuated); nonevacuated mass lesion (high-density or mixed-density lesion >25 cc, not surgically evacuated). The CT classification of TBI is correlated with neurologic outcome, with diffuse injury I having a 38% rate of unfavorable (death, vegetative, or severe disability) outcome, increasing to a 94% rate in patients with a grade IV diffuse injury. In addition, it should be noted that about one-third to one-half of the patients present with no lesion at admission and develop new lesions secondarily, which is associated with substantially worse neurologic outcome.

The goal of resuscitation in TBI and other types of brain injury is to prevent continuing cerebral insult after a primary injury has already occurred. The extent of the primary cerebral injury is usually determined by the mechanism of the trauma, the cause, and duration of cerebral ischemia. A primary insult is often associated with intracranial hypertension and systemic hypotension, leading to decreased cerebral perfusion and brain ischemia. Concomitant hypoxemia aggravates brain hypoxia, especially in the presence of hyperthermia, which increases brain metabolic demand. The combined effect of these factors leads to secondary brain injury characterized by excitotoxicity, oxidative stress, and inflammation. The resulting cerebral ischemia may be the single most important secondary event affecting outcome following a cerebral insult. Prevention of secondary injury is the main goal of resuscitative efforts.

Traumatized areas of the brain manifest impaired autoregulation, with increased dependency of flow on perfusion pressure, and disruption of the blood-brain barrier. If space-occupying lesions or edema are present, they will contribute to reduced brain compliance, leading to increased ICP and consequent deleterious effect on CBF. The rationale for attempting to optimize CPP arises from the fact that cerebral regions surrounding the primary lesion may be close to the ischemic threshold. Therefore, the goals of neuroresuscitation are oriented at restoration of CBF by maintenance of adequate CPP, reduction of ICP, evacuation of space-occupying lesions, and initiation of therapies for cerebral protection and avoidance of hypoxia.

Unfortunately, the ICU treatment of TBI is hindered by a lack of rigorous, randomized, controlled trials to prove benefit, or lack thereof, for many of the management strategies used today. Thus, treatment is based largely on pathophysiologic principles and uncontrolled trials (level III evidence or less). A general guideline for management of patients with severe TBI appears in Table 57-3. Basic principles of management of acute TBI, including osmotherapy, are discussed further in Chapter 48, whereas sedation, hyperventilation, hypothermia, corticosteroids, and antiseizure prophylaxis are discussed in further detail in this chapter.

Sedation of neurologically impaired patients should typically be achieved with short-acting sedatives to allow for frequent assessment of neurologic examination.[12] Although no studies have investigated the effect of sedation on outcome in patients with neurologic disorders, a common practice is to provide sedation with propofol or benzodiazepines in patients following TBI. These agents have favorable effects on cerebral oxygen balance, although propofol is more potent in this regard. Undesirable effects of sedatives are those leading to a reduction in CPP due to hemodynamic depression, or to an increase in CBF accompanied by a simultaneous increase in ICP, a condition occurring, for example, with the use of ketamine.

Propofol rapidly penetrates the central nervous system and has rapid elimination kinetics. Despite the induction of systemic hypotension, propofol decreases cerebral metabolism resulting in a coupled decline in CBF, with consequent decrease in ICP. Propofol's favorable pharmacologic and neurophysiologic profile has lead to its widespread use in neurointensive care, and high-dose propofol has been advocated as a substitute for barbiturate therapy in patients with refractory intracranial hypertension. However, prolonged (>24 hours), high-dose (>80 μg/kg per minute) propofol administration has been associated with lactic acidosis, cardiac failure, and death (propofol infusion syndrome) in children and adults with TBI.[13] Thus, the use of high-dose propofol to control refractory intracranial

TABLE 57-3

INTENSIVE CARE UNIT MANAGEMENT OF PATIENTS WITH SEVERE TRAUMATIC BRAIN INJURY

Basic principles applied to all patients, assuming initial surgical management	• Head elevation 30–45°[a] • CPP > 60 mm Hg o Euvolemia, vasopressors as needed • ICP < 20 mm Hg o Mannitol, hypertonic saline o CSF drainage • Sao_2 ≥95%; $Paco_2$ 35–40 mm Hg • Temperature ≤37°C • Glucose < 180 mg/dL[b] • Sedation and analgesia • Early enteral nutrition • Seizure, stress ulcer, and DVT prophylaxis
Refractory intracranial hypertension Consider one or all these interventions, depending on individual circumstances	• Optimized hyperventilation with Sjo_2 and/or $Pbro_2$ monitoring • Barbiturate coma • Mild therapeutic hypothermia (33–35°C) • Decompressive craniectomy

CSF, cerebrospinal fluid; CPP, cerebral perfusion pressure; DVT, deep venous thrombosis; ICP, intracranial pressure.
[a]Unless contraindicated by spine injury, hemodynamic instability, or otherwise.
[b]Consider intensive control (glucose < 110 mg/dL).[96]

hypertension is not recommended, and barbiturates should be considered if ICP is not controlled by moderate doses of propofol.

The mechanisms by which barbiturates exert their cerebral protective effect appear to be mediated by a reduction in ICP via alteration in vascular tone, reduction of cerebral metabolic rate, and inhibition of free radical peroxidation. Although barbiturates are effective at reducing ICP, their routine use in TBI does not appear beneficial, and may in fact result in excess mortality in patients with diffuse brain injury (level II evidence).[14,15] This effect may in part relate to the profound cardiovascular depressant effects of barbiturates. Based on one small randomized trial, barbiturates do appear to reduce mortality in patients with refractory high ICP (level II evidence).[16] Thus, high-dose barbiturate therapy may be considered in hemodynamically stable severe TBI patients with intracranial hypertension refractory to maximal medical and surgical ICP-lowering therapy. In some patients, pentobarbital may induce hypoxia by reducing CBF in excess of metabolism, and therefore, Sjo_2 monitoring should be considered during barbiturate therapy.

Although neuromuscular blockade may result in a fall in ICP, the routine use of neuromuscular blockade is discouraged because its use has been associated with longer ICU course, a higher incidence of pneumonia, and a trend toward more frequent sepsis without any improvement in outcome.

Hyperventilation effectively reduces ICP by reducing CBF. However, the role that hyperventilation should play in routine management of TBI is not clear. Primarily, this is related to concerns that hyperventilation may lead to dangerously low CBF, resulting in worsening cerebral ischemia.[17] In small randomized trials, prophylactic hyperventilation has not proven to be beneficial in TBI.[18] In contrast, it has been proposed that "optimized hyperventilation" in the presence of "luxury perfusion" (excess CBF) may increase global cerebral oxygen metabolism and help normalize global cerebral glucose extraction. Cruz reported that an optimized hyperventilation strategy resulted in a reduction in mortality compared with CPP management in concurrent matched control patients, although this was not a randomized trial (level III evidence).[19] Based on the available evidence, prolonged or prophylactic hyperventilation should be avoided after severe TBI. Hyperventilation may be necessary for brief periods to reduce intracranial hypertension refractory to sedation, osmotic therapy, and CSF drainage, and should be guided by Sjo_2 and/or $Pbro_2$. A marked fall in either of these values suggests a harmful effect of hyperventilation, and it should be discontinued.

Experimentally, hypothermia causes a reduction in cerebral metabolism by decreasing all cell functions, both related to neuronal electric activity and those responsible for cellular integrity. In addition, mild hypothermia has been shown to decrease the release of substrates associated with tissue injury such as glutamate and aspartate. A meta-analysis of eight randomized trials using mild hypothermia (33 to 35°C) in 748 patients with TBI indicated that, despite a marginal improvement in poor neurologic outcome, there was no mortality advantage and an increased risk of pneumonia.[20] Therefore, there is insufficient evidence to provide recommendations for the use of moderate hypothermia in patients with TBI. In patients with TBI, mild iatrogenic hypothermia should be differentiated from spontaneous hypothermia, which indeed carries a poor prognosis, and is characterized by markedly abnormal brain metabolic indices. In contrast, immediate rewarming of TBI patients with spontaneous hypothermia may further worsen outcome.[21]

Corticosteroids to reduce posttraumatic inflammatory injury in TBI have been advocated for 30 years or more, but without convincing evidence of benefit. However, a more recent large, prospective, randomized trial confirms that corticosteroids in this setting are harmful. The CRASH study randomized more than 10,000 patients presenting with acute TBI to receive high-dose methylprednisolone or placebo for 48 hours after hospital admission. Methylprednisolone administration was associated with an approximately 20% increase in the relative risk of death at 2 weeks in the entire cohort, and detriment was evident across subgroups divided by severity and type of injury (level I evidence).[22] Thus, high-dose corticosteroids should not be administered as therapy for acute TBI.

Antiseizure prophylaxis is not recommended for preventing posttraumatic late seizures. Anticonvulsants may be used to prevent early posttraumatic seizures following head trauma. However, the evidence does not indicate that prevention of early seizures improves outcome following TBI.[23]

Subarachnoid Hemorrhage

The incidence of subarachnoid hemorrhage (SAH) in the United States varies from 7.5 to 12.1 cases per 100,000 population. SAH is most commonly caused by the rupture of an intracranial aneurysm. Other causes of SAH include trauma, vertebral and carotid artery dissection, dural and spinal arteriovenous malformations, mycotic aneurysms, sickle cell disease, cocaine abuse, coagulation disorders, and pituitary apoplexy. SAH is associated with considerable morbidity and mortality, with only one-third of the patients suffering from SAH being functional survivors. The leading causes of death and disability are the direct effect of the initial bleed, cerebral vasospasm, and rebleeding. The Report of the Cooperative Study of Intracranial Aneurysms and SAH estimated that 33% of the patients would die before receiving medical attention. Another 27% would either die during hospitalization or become severely disabled, leaving only about 30% to survive without major disability.[24,25] Severity of the initial bleed is the most important determinant of SAH outcome.

At the time of aneurysm rupture, there is a critical reduction in CBF due to increase in ICP toward arterial diastolic values. The persistence of a no-flow pattern is associated with acute vasospasm and swelling of perivascular astrocytes, neuronal cells, and capillary endothelium. After SAH, injury to the posterior hypothalamus may stimulate release of norepinephrine from the adrenal medulla and sympathetic cardiac efferent nerves. The release of norepinephrine has been associated with ischemic changes in the subendocardium (neurogenic stunned myocardium), cardiac dysrhythmias, and pulmonary edema.

In survivors of the initial bleed, emphasis has been placed on early aneurysm securing with either surgery or interventional neuroradiology (coiling). Approximately 10 to 23% of unsecured aneurysms will rebleed in the first 2 weeks, most within the first 6 to 12 hours after the initial hemorrhage, and rebleeding is associated with mortality approximating 80%. Early aneurysm occlusion substantially reduces the risk of this complication. However, with the improvement of the operative management, delayed complications have become increasingly important causes of death and disability.

Cerebral vasospasm after SAH, consisting of intracerebral arterial narrowing, has been identified by angiography in up to 60% of patients, and is correlated with the amount and location of subarachnoid blood. A reduction in CBF is ultimately responsible for the appearance of *delayed ischemic neurologic deficits (DINDS)*. DINDS occur in approximately one-third of patients suffering from SAH. In a systematic review of the literature, Dorsch et al found an overall death rate of 31% (versus 17% in patients without vasospasm), permanent deficits in 35%, and good outcome in 34% of the patients who developed symptomatic vasospasm.[26] DINDS typically presents as alteration in consciousness and/or transient focal neurologic deficits that rarely occur within the first 3 days after aneurysm rupture, typically peak in 7 to 10 days, and resolve over 10 to 14 days. If severe, vasospasm can result in cerebral infarction and persistent neurologic deficits, which contribute to considerable long-term morbidity.

TCD has been used to identify and quantify cerebral vasospasm on the basis that velocity profiles increase as the diameter of the vessel decreases. Changes in measured velocities over time may be more reliable than absolute values in predicting symptomatic vasospasm. Velocities greater than 200 cm/second have been associated with a high risk of infarction, but there is a poor correlation between the TCD velocities and angiographic findings, especially for the anterior cerebral artery and the posterior circulation. Single photon emission CT may provide a more accurate means of identifying patients at risk for delayed ischemia.

Oral nimodipine (60 mg every 4 hours for 21 days) as prophylaxis for cerebral vasospasm is recognized as an effective treatment in improving neurologic outcome (reduction of cerebral infarction and poor outcome) and mortality from cerebral vasospasm in patients suffering from SAH (level I evidence).[27] Although angiographic studies did not demonstrate a difference in the frequency of vasospasm compared with a placebo treated group, the benefits of nimodipine have been attributed to a cytoprotective effect related to the reduced availability of intracellular calcium and improved microvascular collateral flow. No other pharmacologic therapies to prevent or treat cerebral vasospasm have demonstrated effective results in clinical trials.

Hypervolemic/hypertensive and hemodilution (triple H) therapy is one of the mainstays of treatment for cerebral ischemia associated with SAH-induced vasospasm, despite the lack of evidence for its effectiveness, especially for its prophylactic use.[28] The rationale for this therapy is that hypovolemia is present because of blood loss, and also induced by hypothalamic dysfunction and secretion of natriuretic peptides. Volume expansion is therefore considered beneficial to optimize the hemodynamic profile. The rationale for hypertension derives from the concept that a loss of cerebral autoregulation associated with vasospasm results in pressure-dependent blood flow. Finally, hemodilution is a consequence of hypervolemic therapy, and is believed to optimize the rheologic properties of the blood, thereby improving microcirculatory flow. There is no consensus with regard to the goals of therapy, and it is unclear which component of this therapy is necessary or sufficient to treat vasospasm. Common complications of treatment are pulmonary edema and myocardial ischemia. Because the blood-brain barrier may be disrupted, aggravation of vasogenic edema or hemorrhagic infarction have also been described.[29]

Interventional neuroradiology with the use of balloon angioplasty can reverse or improve vasospasm-induced neurologic deficits. Patients treated within 6 to 12 hours after the development of ischemic symptoms have better results than those receiving delayed intervention. The risks of angioplasty include intimal dissection, vessel rupture, ischemia, and infarction.

Hydrocephalus is another cause of neurologic dysfunction after SAH, occurring in 25% of patients surviving the hemorrhage. The presence of blood in the ventricular system obstructs ventricular drainage and CSF absorption sites (subarachnoid villi). Ventricular drainage is usually successful in improving neurologic symptoms due to hydrocephalus. A minority of patients will require a permanent ventriculoperitoneal shunt. Seizures occur in 13% of patients with SAH, and are more common in patients with a neurologic deficit; thus, prophylactic anticonvulsant therapy is recommended.

A relatively common complication after SAH (10 to 34%) is hyponatremia. Hyponatremia usually develops several days after the hemorrhage, and is attributed to two main causes: (1) a syndrome of inappropriate antidiuretic hormone (SIADH), which is associated with euvolemia or mild hypervolemia and an excess of free water; or (2) cerebral salt wasting, which is marked by depletion of sodium and water. The differentiation of these two entities can be difficult but is theoretically important, in that SIADH is treated by free water restriction, and cerebral salt wasting with volume expansion and sodium administration. Thus, assessment of intravascular volume status is a key component when deciding on the treatment regimen for hyponatremia associated with SAH. Other medical complications of SAH include pneumonia, neurogenic pulmonary edema and acute lung injury, sepsis, gastrointestinal (GI) bleeding, deep venous thrombosis (DVT), and pulmonary embolism (PE).

Acute Ischemic Stroke

Although evidence indicates that the incidence of stroke has declined during the past 30 years, stroke remains one of the leading causes of disability and death in the United States. More than one-half of all strokes can be attributed to a thrombotic mechanism. Other major causes of stroke are embolism, lacunar infarct, cerebellar infarction, and hemorrhage. Transient ischemic attacks may precede stroke and thus should be considered a warning sign. The prognosis of stroke patients varies, depending on the size of the lesion. In patients with acute ischemic stroke, the duration of coma appears to be the most important predictor of outcome and successful therapy.

Rapid clot lysis and restoration of circulation have been
2 proposed as measures to limit the extent of brain injury and improve outcome after stroke. In accordance with the American Heart Association guidelines, systemic thrombolysis using alteplase (rt-PA) should be provided within 3 hours of stroke onset (level I evidence, grade A recommendation).[30] Thrombolytic therapy has been shown to recanalize both the carotid and the vertebrobasilar territories in 21 to 93% of cases when provided within 3 hours after the onset of symptoms, and to improve 24-hour and 3-month neurologic outcome, but not

mortality. A more recent placebo-controlled study provided evidence of a sustained benefit at 1 year from systemic thrombolysis in patients with acute ischemic stroke. The overall rate of recurrent stroke was 6.6%, and the transient ischemic attack rate 3.3% at 1 year. Regional or local intra-arterial administration of a thrombolytic agent within 6 hours of symptom onset demonstrated a high recanalization rate, but a potential limitation to the use of intra-arterial treatment is the time required to mobilize a team to perform angiography (level II evidence). There is no evidence that intra-arterial thrombolysis is superior or inferior to intravenous administration. Intravenous streptokinase is not indicated for the management of ischemic stroke (grade A recommendation).

Concerns persist regarding the safety of rt-PA therapy for acute ischemic stroke, primarily related to hemorrhage. The symptomatic intracerebral hemorrhage rate has been reported to be around 5 to 6%, and is greater than in patients receiving thrombolytic therapy for management of myocardial ischemia (level I evidence).[31] Patients receiving systemic rt-PA should not receive aspirin, heparin, warfarin, ticlopidine, or other antithrombotic or antiplatelet aggregating drugs within 24 hours of treatment (grade A recommendation).

Unfractionated and low-molecular-weight heparin (LMWH) have not been shown to prevent progression or reduce the rate of stroke recurrence when administered within 48 hours of the acute event; therefore, their use is not recommended (grade A recommendation). In general, heparin is only recommended for early secondary prophylaxis in patients with suspected cardiac embolism. Aspirin (160 to 325 mg/day) has been shown to reduce the risk of early recurrent ischemic stroke when given within 48 hours of stroke onset, but increases the risk of hemorrhagic stroke. The frequency of deep venous thrombosis (DVT) in acute stroke is reduced by anticoagulants, especially LMWH, but not by antiplatelet agents. However, it is unclear if the frequency of pulmonary embolism (PE) is also reduced.

The majority of patients with acute ischemic stroke present with severe arterial hypertension. If intracerebral hemorrhage is excluded, treatment of hypertension should be delayed because reduction of the perfusion pressure could compromise the viable brain surrounding the ischemia (ischemic penumbra). However, severe hypertension (systolic blood pressure >220 mm Hg, or mean arterial blood pressure of >130 mm Hg, or diastolic >120 mm Hg) should be controlled because of increased risk of hemorrhagic transformation in anticoagulated patients or after thrombolysis. Although there is no evidence for an optimal level of blood pressure, there is general consensus that the systolic pressure should not be lowered below 150 to 160 mm Hg. If the event is accompanied by raised ICP due to cerebral edema, the principles of treatment of raised ICP discussed previously with regard to TBI similarly apply. Cytotoxic brain edema usually occurs 24 to 96 hours after acute ischemic stroke, and osmotherapy constitutes the basis of ICP reduction. Steroids are of no value in the treatment of ischemic stroke. Because hyperglycemia is associated with poor outcome in ischemic stroke, tight glucose control is recommended.

Space-occupying middle cerebral artery (malignant MCA syndrome) and cerebellar infarctions have a high mortality rate and, in selected cases where signs of intractable intracranial hypertension are present, hemicraniectomy or decompressive surgery of the posterior fossa, respectively, could be lifesaving and improve outcome.

Anoxic Brain Injury

Anoxic brain injury most commonly occurs as a result of cardiac arrest, either in-hospital or out-of-hospital. Of patients who survive their initial cardiac arrest, in-hospital mortality ranges from approximately 50 to 90%, and a high percentage of survivors suffer brain injury with significant long-term disability. The pathophysiology of anoxic brain injury is multifactorial and includes excitatory neurotransmitter release, accumulation of intracellular calcium, and oxygen-free radical generation. Unfortunately, pharmacologic therapies aimed at several of these pathways, including barbiturates, benzodiazepines, corticosteroids, calcium channel antagonists, and free radical scavengers have failed to improve the outcome of anoxic brain injury.

A strong experimental literature supports a role for mild therapeutic hypothermia in anoxic brain injury. Two more recently published prospective, randomized trials of mild hypothermia (temperature 32 to 34°C) in survivors of out-of-hospital ventricular fibrillation have provided some encouragement for survivors of cardiac arrest.[32,33] Hypothermia was associated with a relative increase in patients with a favorable neurologic outcome (moderate disability or less) of 40 to 50%, and in one study was also associated with relative 6-month
3 mortality reduction of approximately 25% (level II evidence).[32]
Thus, mild therapeutic hypothermia should be routinely applied to comatose survivors of out-of-hospital cardiac arrest due to ventricular fibrillation; it should also be considered in other scenarios, including in-hospital cardiac arrest and cardiac arrest due to asystole and pulseless electrical activity.

CARDIOVASCULAR AND HEMODYNAMIC ASPECTS OF CRITICAL CARE

Principles of Monitoring and Resuscitation

Shock states are associated with impairment of adequate oxygen delivery resulting in decreased tissue perfusion and tissue hypoxia. It is important to emphasize that global hemodynamic monitoring may not reflect regional perfusion or the peripheral tissue energy status. Occasionally, despite increased cardiac output and oxygen delivery, peripheral tissues suffer from hypoxia due to blood flow maldistribution, as well as uncoupling between oxygen delivery and oxygen utilization from mitochondrial dysfunction and energetic failure.

Invasive monitoring in shock states provides insight into the circulatory status, organ perfusion, tissue microcirculation, and cellular metabolic status of the critically ill patient. Hemodynamic monitoring ranges from the simple monitoring of electrocardiogram and pulse oximetry, to continuous arterial pressure via an arterial catheter and the monitoring of cardiac filling pressures with central venous or pulmonary artery catheters, to cardiac echocardiography. Several experimental monitoring devices detecting microenvironmental conditions at the tissue level are under continuous investigation.

Functional Hemodynamic Monitoring

Pulmonary Artery Catheter

The pulmonary artery catheter (PAC) measures hemodynamic indices, including central venous pressure (CVP), pulmonary artery pressure and occlusion pressure (PaOP), cardiac output (thermodilution method), systemic and pulmonary vascular resistances, and mixed venous oxygen saturation (SvO_2), and provides data for deriving oxygenation variables (oxygen delivery [DO_2], consumption [VO_2], and extraction [O_2ER]). The information provided by the PAC may assist in the differentiation of cardiogenic and noncardiogenic circulatory and respiratory failure, and help guide fluid, inotropic, and vasopressor therapy. The technical and physiologic principles of the PAC are discussed in detail in other chapters in this text.

Despite the theoretical benefits of pulmonary artery catheterization, there are few data to support a positive effect of the PAC on mortality or other substantive outcome variables, leading some experts to call for a moratorium in PAC use until more definitive evidence of benefit is made available. In a retrospective analysis using propensity scores, Connors et al suggested that the use of the PAC within 24 hours following ICU admission was associated with increased mortality, length of stay, and health care costs in postoperative patients.[34] However, this study may have overestimated the mortality in the group with the PAC because of residual confounding despite patient matching. Vieillard-Baron et al. suggested that right heart catheterization may be associated with increased mortality, but after adjustment for the use of vasopressors, there was no increased mortality associated with the use of the PAC.[35] As a consequence of these studies questioning the benefits of the PAC, the frequency of use of the PAC has substantially decreased in the management of patients with cardiogenic shock and in other ICU settings.[36] More recently, a randomized controlled trial assigning patients with shock, ARDS, or both to receive a PAC or not did not find any differences in mortality, organ system failures, renal support, and use of vasoactive agents between the two groups.[37] Similarly, there was no benefit to therapy directed by PAC over standard therapy in elderly, high-risk surgical patients requiring intensive care.[38]

Some or all the following factors may be responsible for the observed lack of benefit associated with PAC use: (1) device or procedure-related complications, (2) inaccurate data, (3) fundamentally incorrect assumptions about the meaning of the measured data, (4) inappropriate decisions resulting from misinterpretation of the data, and (5) harmful effects of well-intended therapies. As an example of the third factor, there is increasing evidence that CVP and pulmonary artery pressure do not predict the hemodynamic response to intravenous fluid administration in normal subjects or patients with shock.[39,40] As an example of the fifth factor, the ability to increase DO_2 with fluid resuscitation and inotropic therapy in patients with septic shock identifies a better prognosis. This observation led to a therapeutic strategy known as "supraphysiologic resuscitation" to defined end points (cardiac index >4.5 L/min, DO_2 >600 mL/m^2 per minute, and VO_2 >170 mL/m^2 per minute) in patients with septic and surgical/trauma-related shock. However, a large, randomized, prospective study found that this approach was associated with increased mortality in patients with septic shock.[41] As a result, supraphysiologic resuscitation has generally fallen out of favor, although it is still used in some centers. However, this example shows how information derived from the PAC can lead to patient harm, despite the best of intentions.

In summary, although the PAC remains a commonly used tool in critical care medicine, the evidence supporting its benefit is scant. A consensus conference on the use of the PAC concluded that the catheter should only be used when noninvasive methods are not available to provide the information required.[42] The decision to insert a PAC must weigh the risks of monitoring versus the potential benefits in terms of adaptation of treatment to the information obtained from the monitoring. In this regard, the PAC may be most useful as a tool to allow interpretation of the relationship between cardiac output and the peripheral demand for oxygen, and to direct therapy accordingly, rather than as a measure of intravascular volume status. Clearly, further research is necessary to establish the utility, if any, of the PAC in critically ill patients.

A somewhat less invasive and less costly alternative to placing a PAC for the measurement of SvO_2 is to measure central venous oxygen saturation ($ScvO_2$) via a fiberoptic central venous catheter. $ScvO_2$ is typically approximately 5 mm Hg higher than SvO_2, but it appears to correlate well with SvO_2 during changes in hemodynamic status.[43] Targeting an $ScvO_2$ >70% as a component of early goal-directed therapy in patients with septic shock has been associated with a reduction in mortality.[44]

Arterial Pressure Waveform Analysis

In addition to static pressure measurements such as CVP and PaOP, dynamic indicators of preload include respiratory variation in systolic pressure and pulse pressure, both of which can be derived from the analysis of the waveform generated by a peripherally placed arterial catheter. In addition, techniques for deriving stroke volume, cardiac output, and intrathoracic blood volume have more recently become available. These techniques present a less invasive and perhaps superior approach to hemodynamic monitoring of critically ill patients.

The variation in systolic blood pressure and pulse pressure during positive-pressure ventilation is highly predictive of the response to intravascular fluid administration in both normal subjects and critically ill patients. During positive-pressure ventilation, there is an inspiratory reduction in right ventricular stroke volume due to decreased venous return and a subsequent reduction in left ventricular end-diastolic volume appearing during the expiratory phase of the respiratory cycle. Therefore, the left ventricular stroke volume varies cyclically with ventilation, and is paralleled by a similar variation in systolic blood pressure and pulse pressure. These effects are exaggerated during absolute and relative hypovolemia. Systolic and pulse pressure variation are superior predictors of fluid responsiveness (compared with static measures such as CVP and PaOP) in patients with a variety of critical illnesses, including septic shock, acute lung injury, and following cardiac surgery.[45]

Analysis of the systemic arterial pulse contour allows derivation of cardiac output after initial calibration using an indicator dilution technique. Two commercially available devices use either lithium (injected through a peripheral intravenous catheter; LiDCO) or thermal dilution (injected through a central venous catheter; PiCCO) for initial calibration. Cardiac output derived using pulse contour analysis correlates well with thermodilution cardiac output in a variety of conditions and has the advantage of providing continuous measurement without necessitating the placement of a PAC. The PiCCO device also allows for measurement of intrathoracic blood volume using transpulmonary thermodilution; the latter may be a more accurate reflection of preload than static central pressure measurements. Although further validation of these techniques in critically ill patients is necessary, the use of pulse contour analysis may potentially obviate the need for pulmonary artery catheterization to measure cardiac output, particularly if combined with the measurement of $ScvO_2$ as an indicator of the balance between oxygen delivery and consumption.

Echocardiography

An even less invasive hemodynamic monitoring tool is echocardiography. Transthoracic and transesophageal echocardiography provide accurate diagnostic information with regard to right and left ventricular function, valve function, pericardium anatomy, traumatic vascular injury, and PE (direct and indirect signs). Transesophageal echocardiography can also be used to assess volume status or preload via measurement of left ventricular end-diastolic volume and/or area. The major limitation of echocardiography is that it does not provide continuous monitoring, is associated with high initial cost, and requires a high standard of training and experience.

Transesophageal Doppler sonography using a small probe in a large nasogastric tube (6 mm) monitors descending aortic flow velocity continuously and allows noninvasive monitoring of cardiac output. The disadvantages of this technique are that it is inaccurate if not positioned correctly, ideally at an angle with the aorta of 45 degrees (minimal error in flow measurement), and that it does not measure the supra-aortic output or the aortic cross-sectional area, which is determined using a nomogram and assumed to remain constant throughout the systole.[46] Two cases of intrabronchial displacement of the probe have been reported.

Although the role of echocardiography in routine critical care management remains undefined, it has been suggested that this technique can replace pulmonary arterial catheterization in the ICU without adversely affecting outcomes.[47]

Definition and Types of Circulatory Failure

The common denominator of shock is circulatory instability characterized by severe hypotension and inadequate tissue perfusion. Shock states are classified according to the primary cause of circulatory failure. Distributive or vasodilatory shock results from a reduction in systemic vascular resistance, often associated with an increased cardiac output, whereas cardiogenic (left or right cardiac failure) and hypovolemic shock are low cardiac output states usually characterized by increased peripheral resistance. The most common forms of shock encountered in the ICU are cardiogenic, septic, and hypovolemic shock. Despite extensive research and aggressive management, the mortality from shock remains staggeringly high; approximately 35 to 40% of patients die within 28 days of the onset of septic shock, and the mortality rate is 70 to 80% for patients with cardiogenic shock. The mortality from hypovolemic shock is highly variable and depends on the etiology and the rapidity of recognition and treatment. Cardiogenic and septic shock are discussed in more detail in the following section; the causes and treatment of traumatic shock, including hypovolemic shock, are discussed in Chapter 48.

Cardiogenic Shock

The initiating event in cardiogenic shock is a primary pump failure. Heart failure may result from extensive myocardial infarction, cardiomyopathy, arrhythmias, mechanical complications (mitral regurgitation, ventricular septal defect), tamponade, and so on. The pathophysiologic characteristics include reduction in contractility, usually accompanied by dilatation of cardiac cavities and venous congestion. Absence of pulmonary congestion at initial clinical evaluation does not exclude a diagnosis of cardiogenic shock due to predominant left ventricular failure and is not associated with a better prognosis. The onset of pump failure is associated with two compensatory mechanisms: (1) a reflex vasoconstriction in systemic vessels, causing an increase in left ventricular workload and myocardial oxygen demand; and (2) a redistribution of blood volume toward the heart and the lungs. However, cardiogenic shock developing within 36 hours of an acute myocardial infarction has been associated with variably decreased systemic vascular resistances, possibly mediated by the presence of a systemic inflammatory response.

Several studies demonstrated that the incidence and severity of left ventricular failure complicating acute myocardial infarction were directly related to the extent of ventricular mass necrosis. Consequently, therapy should minimize myocardial oxygen demand and raise oxygen delivery to the ischemic area; this goal is complicated by the fact that many resuscitative approaches to correct hypotension (preload augmentation, inotropes, and vasopressors) increase myocardial oxygen consumption. In patients without hypotension, pharmacologic vasodilatation using nitrates or sodium nitroprusside may reduce myocardial oxygen consumption and improve ventricular ejection by reducing left ventricular afterload, and possibly produce a shift of blood from the lungs to the periphery by reducing venous tone. B-type natriuretic peptide (human recombinant form of BNP, nesiritide) and fenoldopam have similar effects, and have an additional beneficial diuretic effect.[48] When pharmacologic interventions are not sufficient to restore hemodynamic stability, the use of mechanical support with the insertion of intra-aortic balloon pump counterpulsation and ventricular assist devices can help unload the ventricles.

In patients with myocardial infarction, coronary reperfusion can be achieved with thrombolysis or, preferably, primary percutaneous coronary intervention (PCI). A randomized trial comparing emergency revascularization with primary PCI or coronary artery bypass surgery to a regimen of thrombolysis did not demonstrate a mortality difference at 30 days. However, at 6 months and 1 year, there was a significant mortality reduction with emergency revascularization in patients younger than 75 years of age.[49] The use of primary PCI in patients younger than 75 years with acute ST elevation and myocardial infarction complicated by cardiogenic shock who can be treated within 18 hours of the onset of shock is a grade A recommendation.

Septic Shock

Septic shock is a form of distributive shock associated with the activation of the systemic inflammatory response, and is usually characterized by a high cardiac output, low systemic vascular resistance, hypotension, and regional blood flow redistribution, resulting in tissue hypoperfusion. Other forms of distributive shock include pancreatitis, burns, fulminant hepatic failure, multiple traumatic injuries, toxic shock syndrome, anaphylaxis and anaphylactoid reactions, and drug or toxin reactions, including insect bites, transfusion reactions, and heavy metal poisoning. In patients with systemic infections, the physiologic response can be staged on a continuum from a systemic inflammatory response syndrome (SIRS), to sepsis, severe sepsis, and septic shock (Table 57-4). The hemodynamic profile of septic shock is influenced by several sepsis-induced physiologic changes, including hypovolemia and vasodilation, in addition to cardiac depression. Sepsis is associated with a global decrease in cardiac contractility, and echocardiographic measurements of the left ventricle size demonstrate an inability of the ventricle to dilate in septic patients.[50]

In endotoxemia and sepsis, metabolic needs are increased, and the ability of the tissues to extract and use oxygen may be impaired. Thus, a metabolic acidosis may be present despite normal levels of oxygen transport. A decrease in cellular O_2 extraction capacity may result from factors other than hypoperfusion, such as direct cellular damage by toxins and/or mediators or maldistribution of blood flow. The impact of impaired perfusion on organ function depends on individual susceptibility to hypoxia. The peculiar anatomy and the microcirculatory structure of intestinal villi with their countercurrent flow mechanism render the superficial layers of the mucosa particularly vulnerable to ischemia. The GI tract has been implicated as the "motor" of multiple organ dysfunction syndrome (MODS), and "splanchnic resuscitation" has been advocated as a central objective in patients with septic shock. Intramucosal pH and P_{CO_2} monitoring has been proposed as a technique to assess the splanchnic metabolic state.

Although hypoperfusion is the dominant cause of lactic acidosis in sepsis, various degrees of intermediary metabolic alterations may contribute to the increased lactate production independent of perfusion. Normally, lactate is cleared by the liver metabolic activity via the Cori cycle. Subsequently, with the development of liver perfusion impairment, this organ may turn to a net lactate producer. Furthermore, the increase in the rate of glucose metabolism may also occur due to inhibition of the step-limiting enzyme, pyruvate dehydrogenase, for pyruvate to enter the Krebs cycle. An increase in the relative proportion of

TABLE 57-4

DEFINITIONS OF SEPSIS AND ORGAN FAILURE

Clinical evidence of infection:
Infection: Microbial phenomenon characterized by an inflammatory response to the presence of microorganisms or the invasion of normally sterile tissue by those organisms.
Bacteremia: The presence of viable bacteria in the blood.
Systemic inflammatory response syndrome (SIRS): Systemic inflammatory response to a variety of severe clinical insults. The response is manifested by two or more of the following conditions:
- Core temperature <36°C or >38°C
- Tachycardia >90 beats/min
- Tachypnea >20 breaths/min while breathing spontaneously, or $PaCO_2$ <32 mm Hg
- White blood count >12,000 cells/mm^3, <4,000 cells/mm^3, or >10% immature forms

Sepsis: The systemic response to infection. This systemic response is manifested by three or more of the conditions described previously (SIRS) and presented clinical or microbiological evidence of infection.
Severe sepsis: Sepsis associated with organ dysfunction, hypoperfusion, or hypotension. Hypoperfusion and perfusion abnormalities may include, but are not limited to, lactic acidosis, oliguria, or an acute alteration in mental status.
Septic shock: Sepsis with hypotension, despite adequate fluid resuscitation, along with the presence of perfusion abnormalities that may include, but are not limited to, lactic acidosis, oliguria, or an acute alteration in mental status. Patients who are on inotropic or vasopressor agents may not be hypotensive at the time perfusion abnormalities are measured.
Sepsis-induced hypotension: A systolic blood pressure of <90 mm Hg or a reduction of >40 mm Hg from baseline in the absence of other causes for hypotension.
Multiple organ dysfunction syndrome: Presence of several altered organ function in an acutely ill patient, such that homeostasis cannot be maintained without intervention.

From American College of Chest Physicians/Society of Critical Care Medicine Consensus Conference Committee. American College of Chest Physicians/Society of Critical Care Medicine Consensus Conference: Definitions for sepsis and organ failure and guidelines for the use of innovative therapies in sepsis. Crit Care Med 20:864, 1992.

inactive to active enzyme results in pyruvate accumulation and lactate production.

MODS refers to the presence of altered organ function in an acutely ill patient such that homeostasis cannot be maintained without intervention.[51] The exact pathophysiology of MODS is not yet fully understood, although alterations in systemic hemodynamics, organ perfusion, and tissue microcirculation resulting in tissue hypoxia play a role in initiating and maintaining the syndrome. MODS accounts for most deaths in the ICU.

Although organ failure only qualifies a dichotomous event that is either present or absent, organ dysfunction represents a continuum of physiologic derangements. Different severity scores have been proposed to quantify the range of severity of MODS. A commonly used score that correlates with a higher mortality in the ICU was developed by Marshall et al.[52] This scoring system assigns increasingly high values based on markers of increasing respiratory, renal, cardiovascular, hepatic, hematologic, and central nervous system dysfunction.

Based on the etiology, MODS can be classified as either primary or secondary. Primary MODS is the result of a well-defined insult in which a primary organ dysfunction occurs early and can be directly attributable to the insult itself (e.g., ARDS due to pulmonary contusion). Secondary MODS represents an abnormal host response (e.g., ARDS in patients with sepsis) and is the result of a systemic inflammatory response initiated by a primary insult involving another organ system.

Clinical Management of Shock/Circulatory Failure Based on Hemodynamic Parameters

The mainstay of treatment of hemodynamic instability is correction of hypotension and restoration of regional blood flow with intravascular volume expansion and vasopressors, and/or inotropes. Adequacy of regional perfusion is usually assessed by evaluating indices of organ function, including myocardial ischemia, renal dysfunction (urine output and renal function tests), arterial lactate levels as an indicator of anaerobic metabolism, central nervous system dysfunction as indicated by abnormal sensorium, and hepatic parenchymal injury by liver function tests. However, these functional assessments of satisfactory organ perfusion may not allow rapid adjustments in therapy compared with more direct continuous monitoring of global and/or regional perfusion. Therefore, additional end points of treatment consist of mean arterial pressure and Do_2, or some surrogate of the latter (SvO_2 or $ScvO_2$).

Management of Hypotension With Fluid Replacement Therapy

Intravascular volume expansion is the first line of therapy in all forms of shock. Clinical indicators of the response to a fluid challenge (bolus fluid therapy of 250 to 1,000 mL crystalloids over 5 to 15 minutes) are heart rate, blood pressure, and urine output, as well as invasively acquired measures, including CVP, PaOP, systolic and pulse pressure variation, and cardiac output. An increase in cardiac output following volume expansion unmasks an absolute or relative hypovolemic state (preload dependency). Lack of change or a decrease in cardiac output following volume expansion suggests a euvolemic status, volume overload, or cardiac failure.

The choice of crystalloids versus colloids for volume expansion has been debated for decades, without clear resolution. Two meta-analyses examined how the choice of crystalloid or colloid solutions affects survival in critically ill patients. Results from these analyses were conflicting, demonstrating either noninferior or increased mortality with the use of albumin-containing fluids.[53,54] A more recent multicenter, randomized, double-blind trial compared the effect of fluid resuscitation with albumin or saline on mortality in ICU patients.[55] The study indicated that use of either 4% albumin or normal saline for fluid resuscitation resulted in similar outcomes at 28 days (level II evidence).

Management of Shock With Vasopressors/Inotropes

If patients remain persistently hypotensive despite volume expansion and markers of adequate preload, the use of vasopressors is indicated. Pharmacologic agents include adrenergic agonists with inotropic and vasoconstrictor effects (norepinephrine, dopamine, dobutamine, epinephrine, phenylephrine); other vasoconstrictors are vasopressin and nitric oxide synthase inhibitors. Select agents are discussed in the following sections.

Norepinephrine. Norepinephrine (NE) increases systemic arterial pressure, with variable effects on cardiac output and heart rate. This effect is mainly mediated by α-adrenergic and β-adrenergic receptor agonism. Studies comparing the hemodynamic and splanchnic effects of NE to dopamine in patients with sepsis indicate that NE improves organ perfusion by an increase in systemic vascular resistance and oxygen consumption accompanied by a decrease in lactate levels, whereas dopamine acts largely by increasing cardiac performance, with an unfavorable effect on the oxygen delivery and consumption relationship.[56,57]

A concern that NE may compromise renal perfusion has led to some hesitancy to use this drug; however, the majority of available evidence suggests that NE improves renal function in volume-resuscitated, hypotensive patients with septic shock. It is worth noting that the combination of excessively high doses of NE with inadequate effective plasma volume expansion may reduce organ perfusion and should be avoided.

In summary, provided adequate fluid replacement therapy, NE restores perfusion pressure, improves organ function, and corrects splanchnic ischemia in hypotensive patients. Because of its favorable hemodynamic profile, NE is the drug of first choice in the management of septic shock.[56,57] In addition, in the only large, prospective evaluation of vasopressor therapy for septic shock, norepinephrine administration was associated with a reduction in mortality compared with dopamine or epinephrine, although this was not a randomized or blinded trial (level III evidence).[58]

Dopamine. Dopamine raises mean arterial pressure by increasing cardiac index and, to a lesser degree, systemic vascular resistance. Dopamine does not have selective dopaminergic effects on renal blood flow, but rather improves urine output by either by improving overall hemodynamics, a direct diuretic effect, or by decreasing the release of antidiuretic hormone via baroreceptor responses.[56] Further, a large randomized trial and a meta-analysis comparing low-dose dopamine to placebo in critically ill patients found no differences in either renal function tests or survival, and the use of low-dose dopamine is therefore not recommended (level II evidence, grade B recommendation).[59] In addition, dopamine may have detrimental effects on the splanchnic circulation. Marik et al showed that dopamine increased splanchnic oxygen consumption, which was not compensated by an increase in oxygen delivery and therefore resulted in increased oxygen debt, and suggested that dopamine might redistribute flow within the intestinal wall and ultimately reduce mucosal blood flow.[57] Last, the response to receptor activation by dopamine administration is highly unpredictable at any dopamine dosage. In patients with septic shock, even low doses of dopamine have consistent inotropic effects and, despite an increased oxygen transport, dopamine may adversely affect gastric mucosal perfusion.

Dobutamine. Dobutamine is a β-1 and β-2 receptor agonist that demonstrates potent inotropic and chronotropic effects, as well as mild peripheral vasodilatation, with the ultimate effect of increasing oxygen delivery and consumption. Dobutamine is the drug of choice in patients with circulatory failure primarily due to cardiac pump failure (cardiogenic shock). However, dobutamine should not be used as first-line single therapy when hypotension is present. In patients with septic shock, dobutamine may be useful in the presence of impaired cardiac contractility with resulting inadequate cardiac output and oxygen delivery. Several studies show that dobutamine alone or added to standard vasopressor regimens increases both oxygen delivery and consumption in septic and elderly septic patients.[60] In patients with septic shock, the combination of NE plus dobutamine resulted in increased gastric mucosal perfusion compared with NE alone.[61] Other studies comparing the effects of NE plus dobutamine versus epinephrine or dopamine alone suggested an improved balance between oxygen delivery and consumption with the combination therapy.

Despite these physiologic benefits of dobutamine in septic shock, detrimental effects have been observed when therapy is oriented to supranormal cardiac output, DO_2 and VO_2 in critically ill patients, as discussed previously.[41] Based on this and other studies, the use of aggressive strategies, such as high-dose dobutamine to drive cardiac index above a predefined supraphysiologic level, is not recommended as routine therapy in the critically ill (grade A recommendation). In contrast, a more recent clinical trial of early goal-directed therapy during the first 6 hours of septic shock to maintain central venous oxyhemoglobin saturation ($ScvO_2$) of 70% or greater with volume resuscitation, packed red blood cell transfusion to a hematocrit of 30%, and, if not sufficient, with dobutamine up to 20 μg/kg per minute demonstrated a 16% absolute reduction in 28-day mortality compared with standard therapy (level II evidence).[44] It is not clear whether the observed benefits of early goal-directed therapy were due to the early initiation of treatment, achievement of the goal end points, or specific elements of treatment (e.g., blood transfusion or dobutamine). However, this early approach of increasing oxygen delivery in septic shock patients by targeting an indicator of supply–demand relationship is substantially different from the supraphysiologic resuscitation in general ICU populations previously described.

In summary, dobutamine treatment is the first line of treatment in patients with shock and decreased cardiac contractility and performance. In patients with septic shock, dobutamine may be useful as a second-line agent, after adequate fluid resuscitation and if introduction of vasopressors has not restored sufficient levels of oxygen delivery, reflected by an $ScvO_2$ of $>70\%$ (which approximates a mixed venous oxygen saturation, SvO_2, of $>65\%$) and increased lactate clearance. However, further corroborating data are necessary to determine the true benefits of early optimization of oxygen delivery. Targeting supranormal levels of oxygen delivery and consumption is not recommended.

Epinephrine. Epinephrine increases cardiac index by increasing contractility and heart rate, and also increases systemic vascular resistance. The response to stepwise dose increments of epinephrine on hemodynamic variables confirms that this drug is a strong inotropic agent even in patients with septic shock, and increases mean arterial blood pressure, cardiac output, DO_2, and VO_2. Epinephrine also increases VO_2 via activation of metabolic pathways.

In patients with septic shock, epinephrine may reduce splanchnic perfusion despite an increase in global hemodynamic and oxygen transport.[62,63] In addition, epinephrine therapy consistently increases plasma lactate levels in septic shock. Whether this reflects a reduction in vital organ perfusion with resulting anaerobic metabolism, increased production consequent to a thermogenic effect in skeletal muscle, or reduced clearance remains to be defined. However, epinephrine treatment at best brings no additional benefit to other catecholamine therapy in the management of patients with septic shock.

Vasopressin. Vasopressin is a potent vasoconstrictor when administered in low doses to patients in shock, particularly those with distributive shock due to sepsis or hepatic failure, or with circulatory failure following cardiopulmonary bypass.[64] This may be in part related to a relative deficiency of vasopressin in these settings. Vasopressin may also be useful in resuscitation from cardiac arrest, particularly if due to asystole, and is offered as an option in the current advanced cardiac life support algorithm for treatment of ventricular fibrillation (level II evidence).[65]

Vasopressin administration during shock typically results in dramatically increased systemic blood pressure, with either no effect or a mild decrease in cardiac output, little change in heart rate, and no effect on pulmonary vascular resistance. Although vasopressin has the potential to reduce mesenteric and renal blood flow, it does not appear to do so when administered at low dose during vasodilatory shock.[66,67] In addition, vasopressin and its analogs have been shown to improve urine output in the hepatorenal syndrome, supporting a positive effect of vasopressin on renal blood flow in vasodilatory states. However, because there are no outcome data to suggest the superiority of vasopressin in the management of septic shock at this time, its use should be reserved for cases of catecholamine refractory shock; in addition, it should be used as a fixed, low-dose infusion (0.01 to 0.1 U/minute) to avoid possible deleterious vasoconstrictor effects associated with higher doses.[64]

Additional Treatment Considerations for Critically Ill Patients With Septic Shock

Activated Protein C. Clinical or subclinical manifestations of intravascular disseminated coagulation and consumption coagulopathy (increase in D-dimers, decreased protein C, thrombocytopenia, and increased prothrombin time) are present in essentially all patients with septic shock. The activation of protein C is believed to be an important mechanism for modulating sepsis-induced consumption coagulopathy. Activated protein C works as an antithrombotic agent by inactivating factors Va and VIIIa. Activated protein C also facilitates clot lysis by inhibiting plasminogen activator inhibitor 1. In patients with sepsis, inflammatory cytokines (TNF-α, IL-1β) downregulate two key components of the protein C activation complex, thrombomodulin and the endothelial cell protein C receptor, resulting in decreased protein C activation. In addition, activated protein C inhibits the generation of inflammatory cytokines from monocytes, and reduces the expression of adhesion receptors and inflammatory mediators from the endothelium. The rationale for replacing activated protein C relates to its anticoagulant and profibrinolytic properties, which interrupt the consumption coagulopathy and are particularly effective at preventing microvascular thrombosis. Drotrecogin-alfa, a human recombinant-activated protein C, administrated intravenously for 96 hours at the rate of 24 μg/kg per hour to patients with severe sepsis, has been investigated in a large randomized trial.[68] Infusion of activated protein C decreased the circulating D-dimers and decreased IL-6 levels. The study showed a 6.1% absolute 28-day mortality reduction (30.8%
4 versus 24.7%). Given the risk of drug-induced bleeding, activated protein C is only approved in patients with severe sepsis and high risk of death as indicated by an APACHE II score >25 (grade B recommendation). In addition to the latter indication, small reports suggest that protein C supplementation can be beneficial in treating purpura fulminans-associated meningococcemia.

Corticosteroids. Although high-dose corticosteroids for the treatment of septic shock are of no benefit, more recent evidence suggests that lower doses, on the order of hydrocortisone 200 to 300 mg per day, can reduce dependency on vasopressors and confer a mortality benefit (level II evidence);[69] this issue is discussed in depth in the Endocrinology section.

Treatment of Infection. Identifying the source of the infection, source control, and early initiation of appropriate antibiotic therapy are critical priorities in addition to hemodynamic support. Appropriate cultures should always be obtained before antimicrobial therapy is initiated. At least two blood cultures (one drawn percutaneously and one drawn through a vascular access device), and cultures of respiratory secretions, urine, cerebrospinal fluid, wounds, or fluid collection should be obtained as indicated by the clinical scenario (grade D recommendation). Diagnostic studies should be performed promptly to assist with the identification of the source of infection and the causative organism, especially for foci amenable to source control measures (e.g., abscess drainage) (grade E recommendation). Empiric antibiotic therapy should be started as soon as possible after appropriate culture collection (grade E recommendation). Initial empiric therapy should be broad enough, and should include one or more drugs that have activity against the likely pathogens and that penetrate into the presumed site of infection. After antibiotic susceptibility testing is available, restricting the number of antibiotics and narrowing the spectrum of antimicrobial treatment is appropriate. For a more detailed discussion and specific sites of infection, see the Nosocomial Infections section.

ACUTE RESPIRATORY FAILURE

Acute respiratory failure is a generic term that encompasses the need for mechanical ventilation and/or airway intubation, independent of cause. Indeed, in some cases respiratory failure may be caused by nonrespiratory issues (e.g., coma that results in the inability to protect the airway). Acute respiratory failure is a relatively common phenomenon; depending on the type of ICU, the majority of patients may be mechanically ventilated at any given time, and virtually all critically ill patients are mechanically ventilated for some portion of their ICU stay. Suffice it to say that the treatment of acute respiratory failure is primarily supportive, and the need for mechanical ventilation and airway intubation typically resolves when the initiating condition is adequately treated. The following sections discuss basic principles of mechanical ventilation, some of the more challenging types of respiratory failure, and potential therapeutic approaches to respiratory failure.

Principles of Mechanical Ventilation

Mechanical ventilation in the ICU is provided through the application of positive pressure to the airway; commonly, a preset tidal volume and rate are provided, and any breathing that the patient does above this set minute ventilation is either supported (assist control or AC) or not (intermittent mandatory ventilation or IMV). However, beyond this simplest level, ICU ventilators have become increasingly powerful and complex, and are high-flow capacity, microprocessor-based systems that offer multiple modes of ventilation and computer-compatible monitoring or control. Thus, ventilatory modes used today (in addition to the traditional "volume" modes AC and IMV) include pressure support ventilation, pressure control ventilation, volume support ventilation, pressure-regulated volume control, high-frequency ventilation, proportional assist ventilation, and airway pressure release ventilation. In reality, there is little evidence to suggest that the mode of mechanical ventilation contributes significantly to any major outcome measure, and the choice of mode is at this point one of clinician preference. Thus, this discussion does not dwell on specific modes of ventilation.

As indicated previously, mechanical ventilation is a supportive therapy that is applied until the initiating cause of respiratory failure improves sufficiently such that the patient can breathe unassisted. Moreover, more recent evidence suggests that mechanical ventilation may be injurious in certain settings. Traditionally, tidal volumes of 10 to 15 mL/kg have been routinely used to ventilate patients in the ICU. The use of such supraphysiologic tidal volumes (normal resting tidal volumes are 5 to 7 mL/kg) evolved from the observation that the use of smaller-size volumes was associated with the development of atelectasis and hypoxemia in anesthetized patients in the operating room. However, in certain patients, large tidal volumes can result in cardiovascular compromise, barotrauma, ventilator-induced lung injury (VILI) or ventilator-associated lung injury (VALI), and excess mortality.

Positive-pressure ventilation results in increased intrathoracic pressure, which reduces venous return, and in turn results in reduced cardiac output and blood pressure. In addition, positive-pressure ventilation can result in alveolar overdistention and alveolar rupture, which manifests as pneumothorax and pneumomediastinum (barotrauma). Both these effects are amplified in patients with obstructive lung disease (asthma and chronic obstructive lung disease [COPD]). In these patients, limitation of expiratory flow leads to air trapping and the development of intrinsic positive end-expiratory pressure, or auto-PEEP. Air trapping results in alveolar overdistention and increases the risk of barotrauma, and auto-PEEP can contribute substantially to increased intrathoracic pressure and cardiovascular depression. Auto-PEEP cannot be detected without holding exhalation for a prolonged interval (expiratory pause), with both inspiratory and expiratory ventilator valves closed; thus, auto-PEEP may not be appreciated unless actively looked for.

The development of air trapping and auto-PEEP leads to significant morbidity and mortality in patients with obstructive lung disease. Thus, the ventilatory strategy in these patients should focus on prolongation of expiratory time by limiting minute ventilation by using low tidal volumes ($\leq$6 to 8 mL/kg) and a low rate (8 to 12 breaths per minute), and by reducing the inspiratory time of the respiratory cycle. Low minute ventilation is often associated with hypercapnia and respiratory acidosis (permissive hypercapnia); however, this does not appear to be harmful, and the benefits of reduced air trapping and auto-PEEP far outweigh any possible detriment. The reduction of inspiratory time is accompanied by increasing inspiratory flow; this results in increased peak airway pressure. However, most of the peak pressure is dissipated in the endotracheal tube and large airways, and more important, end-expiratory, static or plateau, and mean airway pressures will fall with increased expiratory time. To accomplish the previous goals, deep sedation is often required, and rarely, neuromuscular blockade must be used. The adoption of this type of ventilatory strategy in the 1980s and 1990s was associated with a dramatic reduction in mortality due to acute, severe asthma and respiratory failure, from as high as 23% to less than 5% (level IV evidence).[70]

In contrast to barotrauma, VILI or VALI refers to microscopic injury to the lung due to overdistention and cyclic reopening of alveoli. VALI has been well-demonstrated in numerous experimental models, and is histologically similar to the features seen in acute lung injury of other causes, with diffuse alveolar damage and increased microvascular permeability.[71] In addition, VALI is associated with the systemic release of inflammatory mediators that may contribute to multiple organ failure. Clinically, patients believed to be at risk for VALI are those with abnormally low recruitable lung volumes, in particular those with acute lung injury (ALI) and ARDS. Thus, a "lung-protective" ventilatory strategy using low tidal volume ventilation has been proven to save lives when applied to patients with ALI/ARDS.

In summary, although tidal volumes of 10 to 12 mL/kg may still be appropriate for some patients, the choice of tidal volume should be carefully individualized, and volumes as low as 4 mL/kg may be appropriate in some cases. In addition, because lung volumes correlate with height rather than weight, tidal volume selection should be based on predicted body weight (PBW) or ideal body weight, rather than on actual weight, to avoid lung overdistention. PBW can be calculated from the following formula:

$$\begin{aligned} \text{PBW} &= 50 + 2.3(\text{height [in.]} - 60) \text{ (males), or} \\ &\quad 45.5 + 2.3(\text{height [in.]} - 60) \text{ (females)} \end{aligned}$$

Although mechanical ventilation generally implies airway intubation, either translaryngeal or via tracheotomy, noninvasive positive-pressure ventilation (NPPV) or continuous positive airway pressure (CPAP) can be delivered via a tight sealing nasal or full facemask. NPPV is applied using either standard ICU ventilators (typically set to pressure support or pressure control modes, with or without positive end-expiratory pressure [PEEP]), or specially designed ventilators that deliver CPAP or bilevel positive airway pressure (Bi-PAP). These dedicated noninvasive ventilators generate high gas flow, can cycle between a high inspiratory pressure and a lower expiratory pressure, and can sense and respond to patient inspiratory effort. Originally developed for home ventilation in patients with obstructive sleep apnea and chronic respiratory failure, newer models are targeted for use in the ICU by incorporating monitoring packages that allow assessment of delivered tidal volumes and respiratory patterns. However, there is no evidence that the type of ventilator used for NPPV affects patient outcome, and the choice of equipment is typically based on availability and familiarity.

NPPV compared with standard therapy has been associated with improved outcomes in a variety of causes of respiratory failure, including cardiogenic pulmonary edema, COPD, and acute lung injury in immunosuppressed patients (level II evidence).[72,73] Improved outcomes include the avoidance of endotracheal intubation; a reduction in complications associated with intubation, including ventilator-associated pneumonia; and reduced mortality. However, NPPV is not without risk and has been associated with increased complications in some studies, including a higher rate of myocardial infarction in patients with cardiogenic pulmonary edema and increased mortality in patients with respiratory failure after extubation.[74,75] Therefore, NPPV is best and most safely used when patient characteristics are ideal, including an awake, cooperative patient (with the exception of rapidly reversible obtundation due to high PCO_2), a low risk for regurgitation and aspiration of gastric contents, and a high likelihood that the process resulting in respiratory failure is rapidly reversible. Further research including larger, randomized trials of NPPV is necessary to better define the particular subgroups of patients who will benefit from this approach.

Weaning from mechanical ventilation is better termed "liberation" or "separation" from ventilation because "weaning" implies that ventilation must be gradually withdrawn to allow respiratory muscle and patient adaptation to the process. In reality, separation from mechanical ventilation is more a function of the resolution of the cause of respiratory failure, rather than the technique used to withdraw ventilatory support. This is supported by a study showing that daily trials of unassisted ventilation (T-piece trials) resulted in more rapid separation from ventilation than other more gradual approaches, in particular, IMV weaning (level I evidence).[76] In addition, so-called "weaning parameters" are inadequate predictors of the success or failure of withdrawal of ventilatory support, adding little to routine management. Thus,
5 the process of separation from mechanical ventilation is expedited when respiratory therapy-driven protocols are used that focus on daily assessment of the ability to breath without assistance, assuming improvement of the inciting process, adequate oxygenation, and hemodynamic stability (grade A recommendation).[77] Once the patient can breath comfortably for 30 to 120 minutes without support, the trachea can be extubated, assuming there are no other precluding factors such as airway abnormalities, coma, etc.

Acute Lung Injury and Acute Respiratory Distress Syndrome

ALI and ARDS are syndromes of acute, hypoxemic respiratory failure marked pathologically by diffuse alveolar damage (DAD), with resulting increased lung permeability and diffuse alveolar edema.[78] ARDS can occur as a result of direct injury to the lung (e.g., aspiration or pneumonia) or in association with extrapulmonary infection (sepsis) or injury (e.g., multiple trauma). ARDS/DAD are associated with an inflammatory cell infiltration of the lung; increased systemic markers of inflammation; and progression through exudative, fibroproliferative, and fibrotic phases of injury over days to weeks.

TABLE 57-5

CONSENSUS CRITERIA FOR THE DIAGNOSIS OF ACUTE LUNG INJURY AND ACUTE RESPIRATORY DISTRESS SYNDROME

1. Identifiable cause
2. Acute onset
3. Hypoxemia[a]
4. Diffuse, bilateral radiographic opacities
5. PaOP $\leq$18, or no clinical evidence of left atrial hypertension

PaOP, pulmonary artery occlusion pressure.
[a]Acute lung injury: $Pa{O_2}/F{IO_2}$ ratio $\leq$300; acute respiratory distress syndrome: $Pa{O_2}/F{IO_2}$ ratio $\leq$200.
Adapted from Bernard GR, Artigas A, Brigham KL *et al*: Report of the American-European consensus conference on ARDS: Definitions, mechanisms, relevant outcomes and clinical trial coordination. The Consensus Committee. Intensive Care Med 20:225, 1994.

To better standardize the definition of ARDS for epidemiologic and research purposes, in 1994, a joint American–European conference proposed criteria for characterizing ARDS according to the severity of gas exchange abnormality.[79] Despite some controversy, these criteria have been generally accepted (Table 57-5).[78] Thus, ALI is identical to ARDS in all aspects, except for the ratio of $Pa{O_2}$ to $F{IO_2}$ (P/F ratio) at the time of diagnosis. The rationale for characterizing ALI/ARDS according to gas exchange abnormality was that this might allow identification of patients at lower and higher risk of death. However, this does not appear to be the case, because more recent evidence suggests that the P/F ratio is not a risk factor for mortality in ARDS, and mortality in ARDS and ALI appear to be similar.[80]

ALI/ARDS is highly prevalent in the ICU population. A more recent prospective, multicenter study of ICUs in France found that patients with ALI/ARDS comprised approximately 9% of all ICU patients and approximately 40% of all patients with hypoxemic respiratory failure.[81] Of predisposing factors, sepsis carries the highest risk (approximately 30%) and is the most common cause of ALI/ARDS. Mortality associated with ARDS has fallen substantially since the mid-1980s, and is currently in the 30 to 40% range overall. However, ARDS mortality varies greatly with the population of patients studied (e.g., ARDS mortality in trauma patients is in the 10 to 15% range, whereas mortality in medical ICU patients is as high as 60%). Moreover, patients with ARDS continue to die primarily as a result of associated conditions (e.g., sepsis, multiple organ failure), and uncommonly die of hypoxemia per se.

Clinically, ARDS and ALI are characterized by reduced static thoracic (lung and chest wall) compliance and severe impairment of gas exchange, including high intrapulmonary shunt and dead space fraction. These mechanics and gas exchange abnormalities create a challenge in terms of optimizing mechanical ventilation because maintenance of adequate oxygenation and CO_2 elimination are both problematic. In addition, although the P/F ratio does not appear to predict mortality, high dead space fraction does, and may reflect the extent of pulmonary vascular injury.[82] Pulmonary hypertension often develops as the syndrome progresses and can complicate hemodynamic management.

Although ALI/ARDS appears to be a diffuse process by chest radiography, lung opacification is surprisingly heterogeneous when the lung is imaged by CT. Areas of dense opacification are frequently confined to the posterior, dependent portion of the lung, leaving a small, relatively normal, recruitable volume available for ventilation. This low recruitable lung volume has been termed the "baby lung" and has important implications for ventilatory management in ARDS.[71]

The treatment of ALI/ARDS is largely supportive, and includes aggressive treatment of inciting events, avoidance of complications, and mechanical ventilation. In regard to the latter, it is critical that tidal volumes and static ventilatory pressures are minimized to avoid further injury to the remaining relatively uninjured lung (VALI). A more recent large, randomized, prospective trial found that a strategy that used tidal volumes of 6 mL/kg or less and maintained static (plateau) airway pressure at $\leq$30 cm H_2O resulted in a relative mortality reduction of 22% when compared with a control group ventilated with tidal volumes of 12 mL/kg (level I evidence).[83] This is the only intervention that has been unequivocally proven to reduce mortality in patients with ARDS.

6

Because ARDS is marked by high intrapulmonary shunt, hypoxemia is relatively unresponsive to oxygen therapy. Thus, strategies to recruit collapsed lung are necessary. This is most commonly achieved by using PEEP. The optimal balance between PEEP and $F{IO_2}$ has been long debated, but at this point there is no strong evidence to favor either a "high PEEP, low $F{IO_2}$" versus a "minimal PEEP, high $F{IO_2}$" strategy (level II evidence).[84] Other maneuvers to promote recruitment of lung include the use of intermittent, high-level, end-expiratory pressure or sigh breaths, pressure-controlled ventilation, inverse ratio ventilation (prolonged inspiratory time), prone positioning, and high-frequency ventilation. However, although each intervention has been temporally associated with improved oxygenation, none have been shown to result in significant outcome differences when compared with standard approaches (level II and III evidence).

Inhaled nitric oxide (iNO) also variably and transiently improves oxygenation in ALI/ARDS by improving blood flow to ventilated alveoli. However, several randomized, prospective trials have failed to show any relevant long-term outcome benefits associated with iNO administration to patients with ALI/ARDS (level I evidence).[85,86] iNO may still be useful as "rescue" therapy in selected patients with severe, refractory hypoxemia, although its benefits in this setting have not been rigorously tested.

Given that ALI/ARDS are marked by high-permeability pulmonary edema, it is intuitive that administration of excessive fluids be avoided. However, the correct balance between adequate resuscitation and aggressive diuresis is controversial. Furthermore, the level of hemodynamic monitoring, specifically the utility of the PAC, in the management of patients with ARDS is the subject of great debate. These issues are addressed in an ongoing prospective, randomized, multicenter trial sponsored by the National Institutes of Health.

Multiple therapies have been tested in an effort to halt the inflammatory and proliferative phases of injury, with little success. Yet, although corticosteroid administration early in the course of ARDS is of no benefit or even harmful, administration during the fibroproliferative phase (day 3 and beyond) has been associated with reduced mortality in small trials (level II evidence).[87] Preliminary results from a large, multicenter randomized trial of corticosteroid therapy for "late-phase" ARDS are less encouraging, however.

ACUTE RENAL FAILURE

Acute renal failure (ARF) is reported to occur in as many as 25% of critically ill patients. Unfortunately, the true incidence is difficult to pinpoint due to variability in patient populations and the use of multiple diagnostic criteria. More recently, a consensus group proposed standard criteria for the diagnosis of renal risk, injury, and failure, which is expected to improve the ability to identify, study, and treat renal failure in the ICU.[88]

Despite these caveats regarding the diagnosis of ARF, since the mid-1980s, the incidence appears to be fairly stable.[89]

TABLE 57-6

URINALYSIS, URINE CHEMISTRIES, AND OSMOLALITY IN ACUTE RENAL FAILURE

	HYPOVOLEMIA	ACUTE TUBULAR NECROSIS	ACUTE INTERSTITIAL NEPHRITIS	GLOMERULONEPHRITIS	OBSTRUCTION
Sediment	Bland	Broad, brownish granular casts	WBCs, eosinophils, cellular casts	RBCs, RBC casts	Bland or bloody
Protein	None or low	None or low	Minimal but may be ↑ with NSAIDs	Increased, >100 mg/dL	Low
Urine Na^+, mEq/L[a]	<20	>30	>30	<20	<20 (acute) <40 (days)
Urine osmolality, mOsm/kg	>400	<350	<350	>400	<350
$FENa^+$, %[b]	<1	>1	Varies	<1	<1 (acute) >1 (days)

NSAIDs, nonsteroidal anti-inflammatory drugs; RBCs, red blood cells; WBCs, white blood cells.
[a]The sensitivity and specificity of urine sodium of less than 20 in differentiating prerenal azotemia from acute tubular necrosis are 90% and 82%, respectively.
[b]$FENa^+$: The fractional excretion of sodium is the urine to plasma (U/P) of sodium divided by U/P of creatinine × 100. The sensitivity and specificity of fractional excretion of sodium of less than 1% in differentiating prerenal azotemia from acute tubular necrosis are 96% and 95%, respectively.
Adapted from Singri N, Ahya SN, Levin ML: Acute renal failure. JAMA 289:747, 2003.

Moreover, the mortality associated with ARF requiring dialysis has remained approximately 60% since the mid-1950s .[89] This is discouraging when one considers reductions in mortality in association with other organ failures over the same time interval. The reasons for the lack of improvement in outcome are unclear, but likely include insensitive means for identifying patients with incipient renal failure, and lack of effective preventive and therapeutic measures.

In the ICU, ARF occurs due to prerenal causes and tubular injury (acute tubular necrosis) in the vast majority of cases.[89] Other potential causes of ARF in the ICU include glomerulonephritis, vasculitis, interstitial nephritis, macrovascular and microvascular disease (e.g., thrombotic thrombocytopenic purpura), toxins (e.g., nonsteroidal anti-inflammatory drugs, cisplatin, aminoglycosides, myoglobin, hemoglobin), and urinary tract obstruction. The initial evaluation of ARF should focus on identifying easily correctable causes; thus, urine sodium concentration and fractional excretion of sodium can help identify prerenal azotemia, urinalysis can identify possible glomerulonephritis or interstitial nephritis, and ultrasonography can rule out postrenal or obstructive sources of ARF (Table 57-6).

In incipient and established ARF, supportive care is the rule, with the focus on maintenance of euvolemia, avoidance of renal toxins, adjustment of medication doses, and monitoring of electrolytes and acid-base status. Pharmacologic approaches to the prevention and treatment of ARF have been uniformly disappointing; these include low-dose dopamine[59] (level II evidence), anaritide (recombinant atrial natriuretic peptide) (level I evidence), and diuretics. More recent evidence suggests that diuretics may in fact be harmful in early ARF, and their use should probably be restricted to the treatment of hypervolemia prior to the institution of dialysis or ultrafiltration (level III evidence).[90] Although N-acetylcysteine has been advocated for the prevention of contrast-induced nephropathy, the evidence supporting significant benefit for this agent is limited, and there is no evidence that this drug prevents ARF in the ICU.

Although hemodialysis (renal replacement therapy or RRT) is typically considered a supportive measure in ARF, more recent interest has focused on the potential for RRT to improve renal recovery and reduce mortality. Research on RRT in the ICU has focused on the type and intensity or dose of dialysis. Although the timing of initiation of RRT is also of interest, it has not been rigorously studied in this setting.

The intensity of RRT is determined by both the frequency of treatment and the degree of solute clearance per time. Increased intensity of dialysis improves outcome in patients with end-stage renal disease, and more recent studies suggest similar benefits in ARF. Daily dialysis has been associated with reduced mortality and faster recovery of renal function compared with alternate day dialysis in ARF (level II evidence).[91] Likewise, increased clearance during continuous RRT (CRRT) is also associated with reduced mortality (level I evidence).[92]

CRRT (including continuous venovenous hemofiltration and hemodialysis) has been long known as a useful technique when hemodynamic instability is present; in contrast to intermittent hemodialysis, effective solute removal is possible with CRRT in the presence of arterial hypotension. However, given the previous considerations regarding dialysis dose, the routine use of CRRT to increase the intensity of dialysis in ARF has been proposed as a means of improving outcome. Studies comparing CRRT to intermittent RRT have been inconclusive, although meta-analyses suggest a mortality benefit and a trend toward improved recovery of renal function with CRRT (level II evidence).[93] CRRT is used much more commonly than intermittent hemodialysis for ARF in Europe and Australia compared with the United States. Additional large, randomized trials are necessary to determine whether CRRT is indeed associated with the outcome benefits suggested in meta-analyses. In the interim, the weight of evidence supports an increased intensity of dialysis, using either daily standard hemodialysis, CRRT, or extended daily hemodialysis (slow dialysis).

ENDOCRINE ASPECTS OF CRITICAL CARE MEDICINE

Glucose Management in Critical Illness

Hyperglycemia is commonly encountered in critically ill patients, and occurs in both diabetics and nondiabetics. Hyperglycemia results primarily because of increased glucose production and insulin resistance caused by inflammatory and hormonal mediators that are released in response to injury. Hyperglycemia may also be aggravated by various therapeutic and supportive interventions, including the use of corticosteroids and total parenteral nutrition. Although the risks of hyperglycemia for patients with diabetes who are ketosis prone have long been appreciated, mounting evidence suggests that hyperglycemia is detrimental to critically ill patients in a broader sense. Hyperglycemia is associated with increased risk of postoperative wound infection, and poor outcome in patients with stroke or TBI.[94] In addition, the blood glucose level is a risk factor for mortality in diabetic patients admitted with acute myocardial infarction.[95]

Strict glycemic control in critically ill patients is likely to confer substantial outcome benefits. A more recent prospective, randomized trial in surgical patients found that inten-
7 sive insulin therapy (goal glucose <110 mg/dL) reduced ICU mortality by approximately 50% compared with more conventional therapy (goal glucose <215) (level I evidence).[96] The benefit was most pronounced in patients who were in the ICU for more than 5 days. Intensive insulin therapy reduced multiple organ failure, bloodstream infection, the need for dialysis, and the incidence of polyneuropathy. A later retrospective analysis of the data generated from this study suggested that the mortality and morbidity benefits occurred because of blood glucose reduction, rather than insulin administration per se.[97] Another study found a significant long-term mortality reduction when diabetic patients with acute myocardial infarction were managed with intensive insulin therapy.[98] Thus, although questions remain as to the optimal goal glucose threshold and whether intensive insulin therapy confers similar benefits to a general population of medically ill patients, the data clearly favor an aggressive approach to blood glucose control in the ICU.

Adrenal Function in Critical Illness

The stress response to injury includes an increase in serum cortisol levels in most critically ill patients.[99] However, adrenal insufficiency may also occur in critically ill patients for several reasons, including inhibition of adrenal stimulation or corticosteroid synthesis by drugs or cytokines, and direct injury to or infection of the pituitary or adrenal glands.[100] Thus, adrenal insufficiency has been reported to occur with increased frequency in critically ill patients with trauma, burns, sepsis, and other conditions in comparison with the general population.

The diagnosis of adrenal insufficiency in critical illness is complicated by limitations of commonly used tests of adrenal function. Cortisol is highly protein bound, and serum proteins, including albumin, are commonly depressed in critically ill patients. A more recent study found that although total serum cortisol levels are low in critically ill patients with hypoproteinemia, free cortisol levels are elevated.[101] This suggests that earlier reports that used total serum cortisol levels in critically ill patients may have overestimated the incidence of adrenal insufficiency. However, until free cortisol assays are more widely available, the diagnosis of adrenal insufficiency in critical illness must be based on clinical suspicion and total cortisol levels.

In addition to absolute adrenal insufficiency (low baseline cortisol and poor response to adrenocorticotropic [ACTH] administration/stimulation), a condition of relative adrenal insufficiency (poor response to ACTH independent of the baseline cortisol level) has been described in patients in septic shock. In these patients, both a high baseline cortisol level and a poor response to ACTH are predictors of increased mortality, with a combination of the two being particularly ominous.[102]

Although high-dose corticosteroids for the treatment of septic shock are of no benefit, more recent evidence suggests that lower doses, on the order of hydrocortisone 200 to 300 mg per day, can reduce dependency on vasopressors and confer a mortality benefit (level II evidence). A more recent prospective, randomized trial suggests that these benefits are limited to those patients with relative adrenal insufficiency, defined as an increase in serum cortisol of ≤ 9 μg/dL after ACTH administration.[69] Although the precise role of corticosteroid administration in septic shock and other acute conditions remains undefined, adrenal insufficiency should be considered in all critically ill patients with pressor-dependent shock. A reasonable approach in these patients is to administer "stress-dose" corticosteroids to such patients while awaiting results of adrenal testing (baseline and ACTH-stimulated serum cortisol levels), and continue steroids in only those patients with confirmed absolute or relative adrenal insufficiency. However, this approach has not been prospectively tested.

Thyroid Function in Critical Illness

Measures of thyroid function, including levels of thyrotropin (TSH), T_3, and T_4, are deranged in the majority of critically ill patients. Depression of T_3 occurs within hours of injury or illness and can persist for weeks. TSH levels may be normal initially, but they fall to inappropriately low levels as illness progresses. T_4 levels are also often low, but they can be normal or high. Low hormone levels may occur for a variety of reasons, including altered binding and metabolism early in the course of illness, and depressed neuroendocrine function with more prolonged courses. In addition, certain drugs, in particular the vasopressor dopamine, can depress thyroid function through central mechanisms.[103] Low thyroid hormone levels, particularly for T_3, correlate with the severity of illness and are associated with an increased risk of death.[99]

It is controversial as to whether the observed abnormalities in thyroid hormones represent an appropriate response to illness or true hypothyroidism; thus, the terms "euthyroid sick syndrome" or "nonthyroidal illness" have been coined to describe thyroid function abnormalities in critical illness.[104] Furthermore, it is not clear whether replacement of thyroid hormones is indicated or beneficial in critical illness. T_3 administration to brain dead organ donors appears to improve hemodynamic stability (level IV evidence), although randomized trials found minimal or no benefit to T_3 or T_4 administration in patients undergoing cardiopulmonary bypass and cardiac surgery (level II evidence).[105] In addition, several small studies have found no benefit to T_3 or T_4 administration to patients with a variety of critical illnesses (level II evidence). Larger, randomized prospective trials are necessary to define the role of routine thyroid hormone supplementation in nonthyroidal illness.

Importantly, true hypothyroidism may be present in the critically ill, particularly in the geriatric population, and should be considered in the face of refractory shock, adrenal insufficiency, unexplained coma, and prolonged, unexplained respiratory failure. True hypothyroidism is marked by an elevation of TSH (usually >25 mU/L) in the face of a low T_4 level.

Somatotropic Function in Critical Illness

Growth hormone (GH) levels are low in prolonged critical illness, and it has been conjectured that deficiencies of GH and insulin-like growth factor-1 (IGF-1) contribute to the muscle wasting seen in acute illness.[99] However, although small trials have found that GH administration can attenuate muscle catabolism in critical illness, a large, randomized prospective trial found that administration of large doses of GH to critically ill patients resulted in increased mortality (level I evidence).[106] Thus, GH administration during critical illness cannot be advocated at this time, although further exploration of the benefits of smaller doses of GH may be warranted.

ANEMIA AND TRANSFUSION THERAPY IN CRITICAL ILLNESS

Anemia is a frequent, if not obligate, accompaniment of critical illness. The vast majority of patients admitted to the ICU are anemic at some point in their hospital stay, and more than one-third of them will receive transfused blood.[107,108] Importantly, both anemia (Hb <9 g/dL) and the amount of transfused blood are independently associated with mortality.[107,108] This association does not denote cause and effect, however, particularly for anemia, which may just be a marker of the severity of illness.

The cause of anemia in critical illness is multifactorial, and related to blood loss from the primary injury or illness, iatrogenic blood loss due to daily blood sampling, and nutritional deficiencies.[109] Given that approximately 13% of ICU patients may have iron, folate, or vitamin B12 deficiencies, these parameters should be checked prior to blood transfusion.

Treatment of anemia in critical illness is the source of considerable debate. In unstressed subjects, severe anemia (Hb of ≤5 g/dL) is amazingly well tolerated due to physiologic compensations that maintain oxygen delivery and extraction. However, it has long been assumed that critically ill patients have less efficient compensatory mechanisms and reduced physiologic reserve, and thereby require a higher Hb concentration than unstressed individuals. Historically, this has translated to a transfusion threshold at an Hb concentration of approximately 10 g/dL. However, a large, randomized, prospective trial of transfusion requirements in critical illness (the TRICC study) found that 30-day mortality was not affected when a restrictive transfusion threshold (Hb <7 g/dL) was used, compared with a more conventional threshold of <10 g/dL (level I evidence).[110] Furthermore, a trend in mortality reduction favored the restrictive group, and various subgroups of patients (younger than 55 years of age and less severely ill by APACHE scoring) had a significantly lower mortality when they were transfused using the restrictive strategy. These data
8 strongly suggest that routine transfusion of critically ill patients is not necessary and may be harmful unless the Hb concentration is less than 7 g/dL. Unfortunately, data collected from ICUs at multiple centers in the United States since the publication of the TRICC study suggests that the transfusion threshold remains substantially higher, at a mean Hb of 8.6 g/dL.[107]

There are multiple possible reasons for the persistence of a high transfusion threshold in the ICU. Although the TRICC study included a broad spectrum of critically ill patients, some groups were excluded (active bleeding) or underrepresented (neurologic or neurosurgical injury). Furthermore, although a retrospective analysis of the TRICC data suggested that patients with coronary artery disease did not benefit from more liberal transfusion unless they had unstable angina or acute myocardial infarction, concern remains about the tolerance for anemia in this group of patients. Last, Hb is an important determinant of oxygen delivery (Do_2), and transfusion is an integral component of goal-directed therapeutic strategies that aim to optimize Do_2 in early shock states.[44] In the absence of these possible exclusions (active bleeding, acute neurologic injury, active myocardial ischemia, or the early resuscitation of septic shock), restriction of blood transfusion to a threshold of <7.0 g/dL should be considered the standard of care and as potentially lifesaving.

Alternatives to the transfusion of red cells for treatment of anemia are not currently available for widespread use. Several hemoglobin-based oxygen carriers (HBOCs) have been studied in clinical trials involving trauma and surgery, but results have been mixed, and none are currently U.S. Food and Drug Administration (FDA) approved for use. Compassionate use of HBOCs in patients that have refused blood transfusion for religious reasons has been reported.

Prevention of anemia in critical illness is an appealing alternative to transfusion. One simple and potentially cost-saving approach is to reduce the volume and frequency of blood draws in the ICU. As noted earlier, iatrogenic blood loss is a major factor in the development of anemia of critical illness. Another potential approach is the administration of recombinant erythropoietin and iron. A more recent large, randomized, prospective trial found that administration of erythropoietin to critically ill patients on day 3 of ICU stay and every week thereafter reduced transfusion requirements significantly, without affecting mortality or other outcome variables (level I evidence).[111] However, the threshold for transfusion in this study was high (Hb of 8.5) and the mean amount of transfused blood saved per patient was quite small (approximately 0.5 U); it is possible that with a lower transfusion threshold there would have been no difference between groups. Given the current high cost of erythropoietin, it is not a cost-effective alternative at this time.

NUTRITION IN THE CRITICALLY ILL PATIENT

Critical illness can lead to hypermetabolic states and if nutritional support is inadequate or delayed, patients are at immediate risk of malnutrition. Poor nutritional status is associated with increased mortality and morbidity among critically ill patients. Therefore, appropriate nutrition is an important aspect of critical care, and adequate nutritional support should be considered a standard of care. The American College of Chest Physicians recommends that the daily caloric intake be based on the patient's ideal body weight (25 kcal/kg or 27.5 kcal/kg in the presence of SIRS), of which 15 to 20% should be represented by proteins (1.5 to 2 g/kg per day).

Patient metabolic requirements should be established early after ICU admission and, enteral feeding tolerance evaluated without delay (within 24 hours of admission). A more recent small randomized trial indicated that early enteral nutrition (EN) initiated within 4.4 hours after ICU admission resulted in less organ dysfunction than delayed feeding (36.5 hours after ICU admission) (level II evidence).[112] Feeding intolerance due to high gastric residual volume can be improved by the administering gastric prokinetic agents, and positioning the tube postpyloric. However, a systematic review comparing gastric versus postpyloric feeding did not suggest a clinical benefit from postpyloric tube feeding with regard to pneumonia, ICU length of stay, and mortality.[113] Because gastric feeding was initiated sooner, no advantages in terms of overall caloric goal achievement were observed.

Most of the trials evaluating parenteral nutrition (PN) do not demonstrate any favorable impact on outcome (level II evidence). More recent reviews suggest that enteral nutrition is associated with lower infection risk, and that PN is associated with increased rates of complications and death. Animal studies show that endotoxin-induced ischemia can be prevented by early EN, and adding EN to parenteral nutrition has favorable effects on bacterial translocation and nitrogen balance, independent of total energy and protein intake. Therefore, EN is preferred over PN whenever possible because of its lower cost, and less frequent complications. Although not rigorously investigated, PN is preferable to no nutrition in patients who cannot tolerate enteral feedings. However, it is unclear how long of a delay in initiating PN is acceptable, assuming EN is contraindicated or not tolerated despite vigorous attempts.

Complications associated with enteral feedings include aspiration of gastric feeding, diarrhea, and fluid and electrolyte imbalance. To prevent aspiration with gastric feeding, the head of the patient's bed should be raised 30 to 45 degrees during feeding; jejunal access can be considered in patients with recurrent tube feeding aspiration. Diarrhea is a common complication during enteral feeding associated with many potential causes, including medications (antibiotics or sorbitol-containing products), altered bacterial flora (*Clostridium difficile*), formula composition (including osmolality), infusion rate, hypoalbuminemia, bacterial contamination of the enteral fluid, and the patient's related conditions. To prevent or reduce diarrhea, all potential etiologies should be considered and corrected. Exchanging a polymeric formula with fiber with a more expensive elemental amino acid diet may improve feeding tolerance. However, animal studies demonstrated that elemental diets promote bacterial overgrowth and may result in greater bacterial translocation (level V evidence).

Among special formulations, immunonutrition has been hypothesized to influence infectious morbidity and mortality in critically ill patients via a beneficial effect on GI immunologic function. Specific enteral formulations, particularly those with high concentrations of branch chain amino acids (isoleucine, leucine, valine), arginine, glutamine, nucleotides, or omega-3 fatty acids, have been suggested to improve mortality and decrease infectious complications in burn and postoperative cancer patients.[114] A more recent meta-analysis indicates that immune-enhancing diets may be beneficial for elective surgical patients but have no demonstrated benefit and may be deleterious in critically ill patients (level II evidence).[115] Use of special formulations may be beneficial in patients with renal or liver disease.

SEDATION OF THE CRITICALLY ILL PATIENT

Critically ill patients are often deeply sedated, in part due to concerns for patient comfort, but also because of potential benefits afforded by a reduction in the sympathoadrenal response to injury. In addition, complications associated with undersedation include ventilator dyssynchrony, patient injury, agitation, anxiety, stress disorders, and, possibly, unplanned extubation.

Several more recent studies have tempered the enthusiasm for deep sedation in the ICU. In a prospective cohort study, Kollef et al observed that patients who received continuous infusions of sedatives had nearly twice the duration of mechanical ventilation compared with patients not receiving continuous intravenous sedation (level III evidence).[116] Furthermore,
9 the implementation of nurse-driven sedation protocols that discourage the use of continuous infusions has been demonstrated to reduce the duration of mechanical ventilation, the ICU length of stay, and the requirement for tracheostomy (level I evidence).[117] In a randomized trial of critically ill patients receiving continuous sedative and analgesic drug infusions, daily interruption of these infusions was effective in reducing the length of mechanical ventilation and length of ICU stay (level I evidence).[118] Length of ICU stay was reduced by 3.5 days, and no incremental complications were observed in the intervention group. Beyond longer duration of mechanical ventilation, other complications are associated with oversedation, such as excessive cardiovascular and respiratory depression, as well as infectious complications.[119]

The depth of sedation may also play a role in long-term outcomes after discharge from the ICU and hospital. Increasing evidence suggests that patients admitted to the ICU are at risk of developing symptoms of posttraumatic stress disorder and of experiencing delusional memories. More recently, Kress et al followed-up long-term psychological effects in those subjects that were enrolled in the daily sedative interruption trial. Although the loss to follow-up was negligible and the design was exploratory in nature, the study suggested that daily interruption of sedation tended to be protective for subsequent development of posttraumatic stress disorder, or at least did not result in adverse psychological outcomes (level III evidence).[120]

Several factors such as interindividual variability, changes over time, severity of disease, intensity of painful stimuli, drug interactions, and organ dysfunction influence the analgesic and sedative needs of ICU patients. Therefore, it is important to titrate medications according to established therapeutic goals and to reevaluate the sedation requirements frequently. Several scales are available to assess sedation levels over time. The most commonly used scales are the Ramsay sedation scale, the sedation-agitation scale, and the Richmond agitation-sedation scale. Common features to all these scales are the grading of sedation over different depths and allowance for indicators of agitation. There is no evidence that one scale is superior to another at this time.

Confusion and agitation are common in ICU patients and could have unfavorable consequences on patient outcome. Patients experiencing agitation have been reported to have a higher incidence of major complications, higher admission to rehabilitation centers, and increase duration of hospital stay. Agitation is also a predictive factor for mortality. Agitation needs to be distinguished from delirium, which is relatively common in ICU patients and equally associated with increased length of stay, morbidity, and mortality.[121] Delirium can be difficult to diagnose in ICU patients because features of delirium, such as altered status of consciousness, are shared with several disorders typical of ICU patients. The distinguishing characteristics of delirium include acute onset and fluctuating course, inattention, disorganized thinking, and altered level of consciousness. An ICU delirium diagnostic scale (CAM-ICU scale) has been more recently proposed and is a valid instrument to diagnose delirium in the ICU.[122]

Nonpharmacologic and pharmacologic means can be used to provide comfort and safety to ICU patients. The former include communication and frequent reorientation, maintenance of a day–night cycle, noise reduction, and ensuring ventilation synchrony. Pharmacologic agents include hypnotics-anxiolytics, opioids, and antipsychotics. Hypnotics most commonly used are propofol, midazolam, and lorazepam; each drug has its own particular advantages, but there are insufficient data at this time to suggest a difference in relevant patient outcomes among them. A prospective, randomized, nonblinded trial compared a continuous infusion of lorazepam, midazolam, and propofol in trauma patients.[123] Midazolam appeared to be the most titratable drug, with the lowest incidence of oversedation and undersedation. Lorazepam was the most cost-effective choice for sedation, despite the observation that oversedation occurred twice as often with lorazepam than with propofol or midazolam. A meta-analysis including 27 randomized trials comparing propofol versus midazolam suggested that extubation occurred earlier with the use of propofol for patients that were ventilated for less than 36 hours.[124] However, no differences were found with regard to the ICU length of stay or mortality. Greater levels of hypotension and elevated triglyceride levels were observed with the use of propofol.

Adverse effects unique to hypnotic-anxiolytic drugs include a hyperosmolar acidosis due to the diluent mixed with lorazepam (propylene glycol), and the potentially lethal "propofol infusion syndrome" (for more details, see Traumatic Brain Injury section).[13] Both complications can be avoided by minimizing the administered dose of the respective agent.

Dexmedetomidine is a unique sedative agent for several reasons: (1) mechanistically, it is an α-2 adrenergic receptor agonist, similar to clonidine; (2) it provides sedation without inducing unresponsiveness or coma; (3) it has some analgesic effect; and (4) it has little effect on respiratory drive. Dexmedetomidine has been effectively used as a single agent or in combination with other drugs in postsurgical and medical ICU patients. Although, the acquisition costs of dexmedetomidine are high, it is currently FDA approved for use for only up to 24 hours, and there is insufficient evidence to recommend its routine use at the current time.[125]

Morphine and fentanyl are the most commonly used opioids to provide analgesia in the ICU. Morphine should be avoided in patients with renal failure due to active metabolites that accumulate in the presence of impaired renal elimination.

Delirium in the ICU is commonly treated with antipsychotic agents such as haloperidol, and more recently, newer antipsychotics such as olanzapine and risperidone. However, none of these agents has been proven effective for the treatment of ICU-associated delirium in a randomized, placebo-controlled trial, and it is not clear that the newer agents, which are also more expensive, are more effective than haloperidol.

Neuromuscular blockade may be occasionally indicated in ICU patients with severe TBI or respiratory failure, but routine use is discouraged because of concerns that this practice may predispose to critical illness polyneuropathy and myopathy (see Acquired Neuromuscular Disorders in Critical Illness section), and because of an increased risk of nosocomial pneumonia in patients receiving these agents.

In summary, sedation and analgesia should be provided in the ICU population to ensure patient comfort and safety. In establishing treatment algorithms, analgesia should be prioritized over sedation. Titration and assessment of analgesia and sedation should be an integral part of the ICU monitoring so oversedation and undersedation can be avoided. The establishment of nurse-guided sedation protocols and daily interruption of sedation have been shown to be effective in reducing the length of mechanical ventilation and ICU stay.

COMPLICATIONS IN THE ICU: DETECTION, PREVENTION, AND THERAPY

Nosocomial Infections

Nosocomial infections are a major source of morbidity and mortality in the critically ill. At some level, nosocomial infections are unavoidable and occur because of the nature of intensive care: patients are critically ill with altered host defenses; they require invasive devices (e.g., endotracheal tubes, intravascular catheters) for support, monitoring, and therapy that provide portals of entry for infectious organisms; and they receive therapies that increase the risk of infection (glucocorticoids, parenteral nutrition). In contrast, many nosocomial infections are preventable with relatively simple interventions.[126]

Several types and sources of infections are relatively unique to ICU care and should be included in the differential diagnosis when signs suggestive of infection arise. These infections include sinusitis, ventilator-associated pneumonia, intravascular catheter-associated bacteremia, catheter-associated urinary tract infection, and invasive fungal infection. The diagnosis, prevention, and treatment of these infections are discussed in this section.

Sinusitis

Radiographic sinusitis is common in critically ill patients with indwelling oral and nasal tubes. Nasal intubation confers a greater risk than oral intubation of radiographic sinusitis, occurring in approximately 95% and 25% of patients with nasal and oral tubes after 1 week of intubation, respectively.[127] Approximately 10% of radiographically diagnosed sinusitis is infected as determined by quantitative cultures, with the cultured organisms representing those that are responsible of other nosocomial infections, particularly ventilator-assisted pneumonia (VAP) (*Staphylococcal* species, enteric Gram-negative bacteria, nonlactose fermenting Gram-negative rods such as *Pseudomonas* and *Acinetobacter*). Bacterial sinusitis may predispose to the development of VAP, possibly because of microaspiration of infected secretions.

Prevention of sinusitis should focus on efforts to improve sinus drainage, including semirecumbent positioning and avoidance of nasal tubes. Bacterial sinusitis should be considered in patients with unexplained fever and leukocytosis in the ICU. If radiographic sinusitis is documented, any nasal tubes should be removed, and nasal irrigation and short-term administration of nasal decongestants should be considered. If the patient is severely ill, broad-spectrum antibiotic coverage should be considered. If these maneuvers do not result in resolution of signs and symptoms of infection in 2 to 3 days, and in the absence of infection elsewhere, otolaryngologic consultation and consideration of sinus drainage procedures should be undertaken.

Ventilator-Associated Pneumonia

Endotracheal intubation and mechanical ventilation increase the risk of nosocomial pneumonia, in this situation termed VAP. The likelihood of developing VAP increases with the duration of mechanical ventilation, although the incremental risk may fall over time from a high of 3% per day in the first week of intubation/ventilation, to 1% per day after 15 days in the ICU.[128] The quoted incidence of VAP depends on the criteria used to diagnose pneumonia (clinical versus invasive technique); traditional clinical criteria are likely to be both insensitive and nonspecific, and may lead to a falsely high or low incidences of VAP. For example, in a more recent study comparing an invasive diagnostic technique with traditional clinical criteria in patients suspected of having VAP, only 50% of the patients in the invasive group met criteria for VAP compared with the clinical diagnostic group.[129] Given this caveat, studies that solely or primarily relied on invasive techniques to diagnose VAP suggest an incidence greater than 15% at 1 week of ICU stay and greater than 20% at 2 weeks.[128]

Although the mortality in patients with VAP ranges between 30 to 70%, the attributable mortality—the number of patients who die because of VAP rather than with VAP—is more difficult to pinpoint. This may be due to differences in the type of ICU, patient factors, diagnostic techniques across studies or differences in the virulence of the causative pathogens. Thus, some investigators have been unable to find any mortality attributable to VAP, whereas others have suggested a rate greater than 40%.[130]

VAP can be categorized as "early onset," occurring within the first 48 to 72 hours of intubation/ventilation, or "late onset," occurring thereafter. Early-onset VAP is generally caused by organisms such as *Haemophilus influenza*, *Streptococcus pneumonia*, methicillin-sensitive *Staphylococcus aureus*, and other relatively antibiotic-sensitive oral flora that enter the trachea around the time of intubation. Late-onset VAP is associated with more virulent and antibiotic-resistant organisms such as methicillin-resistant *S. aureus*, *Pseudomonas aeruginosa*, and *Acinetobacter*. In general, early-onset organisms are associated with zero or low attributable mortality, whereas late-onset organisms, particularly *Pseudomonas* and *Acinetobacter* species, are associated with high mortality.[130]

There are a number of interventions that can reduce the incidence of VAP, some of which are relatively simple and inexpensive, and others of which are more costly and/or associated with some risk. The simplest and least expensive, yet very effective, interventions are strict hand washing between patients, and semirecumbent positioning of the patient (head height at 30 degrees or greater from horizontal) (level II evidence). These practices should be rigorously applied in all ICUs (granted that semirecumbent positioning is not possible in all patients).

A somewhat more controversial subject involves the use of prophylaxis to prevent GI bleeding. As mentioned previously, acid-suppression therapies have been associated with an increased risk of VAP because they allow bacterial overgrowth in the stomach. Further, the risk of significant GI bleeding is low in the ICU, even in high-risk patients (those with coagulopathy or those on mechanical ventilation). Thus, GI prophylactic therapy should be reserved for only these high-risk patients, and sucralfate should be considered as an alternative agent to acid-suppressive regimens despite its potentially reduced effectiveness.

Somewhat more expensive interventions to reduce VAP that may be useful in certain patients include subglottic suctioning and oscillating beds.[131] Intermittent subglottic suctioning using specially designed tracheal tubes has been shown to reduce the incidence of VAP in two small studies (level II evidence). However, these tubes are more expensive than conventional tracheal tubes, and their cost effectiveness has not been established, particularly if their use is instituted in all intubated patients. Oscillating beds have been shown to reduce the incidence of VAP in surgical populations and patients with neurologic injury (level II evidence). However, these beds are quite costly and cannot be recommended for routine use.[131] In patients who do not tolerate semirecumbent positioning because of fractures, hemodynamic instability, etc, the use of oscillating beds should be considered.

Given that gastric and oropharyngeal colonization with resistant organisms appears to be a risk factor for the development of VAP, intervention to "decontaminate" these sites have been investigated. Selective digestive decontamination (SDD) typically involves the application of a mix of nonabsorbable antimicrobial agents, such as polymyxin, amphotericin, and aminoglycoside, in paste form to coat the oropharynx, and as an elixir applied orally and via a nasogastric tube to decontaminate the GI tract, with or without the concomitant administration of systemic antibiotics. SDD does reduce the incidence of VAP and has been associated with variable mortality reduction in some studies (level II evidence). However, SDD is also associated with the development of antibiotic resistance, and concerns regarding the long-term impact of resistance have limited the widespread adoption of SDD.[131]

An additional and important approach to reduce the overall mortality from VAP involves refinement of the diagnostic process and limitation of antibiotic therapy to avoid the development of antibiotic resistance. As mentioned previously, an invasive diagnostic strategy is likely more accurate than traditional clinical criteria to diagnose VAP. Invasive strategies typically involve collection of bronchial-alveolar specimens using lavage or protected brushes, and then quantitating bacterial growth in the laboratory. Thus, VAP is diagnosed only when bacteria are seen within bronchoalveolar cells microscopically, or when bacterial growth exceeds specific thresholds ($\geq 10^4$ colony-forming U/mL for bronchoalveolar lavage and $\geq 10^3$ colony-forming U/mL for protected brush specimens). Specimens have typically been obtained bronchoscopically, although more recent data suggest that specimens obtained by direct aspiration through the tracheal tube are comparable to bronchoscopic specimens, suggesting it is quantitation of bacterial growth rather than the "invasiveness" of the technique that is important (level II evidence).[132] The important adjunct to this diagnostic approach is that although antibiotics may be started at the time clinical criteria for pneumonia are met and quantitative cultures are sent, they are stopped if the threshold values for VAP are not reached.

A more recent, moderately sized, randomized, prospective trial of invasive versus noninvasive strategies to diagnose and treat VAP found that the invasive approach resulted in a mortality reduction at 14 days and a trend toward mortality reduction at 28 days (level II evidence).[129] In addition, the invasive strategy was associated with less multiple organ failure and reduced antibiotic use. Surprisingly, the invasive strategy did not result in a reduced incidence of emergence of resistant bacteria, although the incidence of *Candida* growth was reduced. However, these data suggest that an invasive strategy to diagnose VAP should be used when and if possible.

It is clear that delay in treatment of nosocomial infections, including VAP is associated with increased mortality. Thus, treatment should not be delayed pending diagnostic evaluation; rather treatment should be started after culture specimens are sent if the clinical suspicion of VAP is high. Antibiotics can then be narrowed in spectrum or discontinued, depending on the results from quantitative cultures after 48 to 72 hours. This approach is known as "deescalating therapy", and is designed to ensure adequate antibiotic treatment up front but avoid overuse of antibiotics in the long run.[130] Antibiotic selection should be predicated on hospital bacterial growth and resistance patterns. In general, for patients with early-onset VAP, antibiotics can be relatively narrow in spectrum and limited to a single agent. For late-onset VAP, broader spectrum antibiotics should be initiated. These should include agents from two different classes directed toward resistant Gram-negative organisms, and in many cases, an agent directed against methicillin-resistant *S. aureus* (Table 57-7).

The optimal duration of antibiotic therapy for VAP is not
10 well defined. A more recent, moderately sized, prospective, randomized trial found that 8 days of antibiotic therapy was comparable for treatment of VAP in terms of mortality and recurrent infections, and resulted in more antibiotic-free days (level II evidence).[133] However, patients who had VAP caused

TABLE 57-7

EMPIRIC THERAPY OF VENTILATOR-ASSOCIATED PNEUMONIA

■ COMMON ORGANISMS	■ ANTIBIOTICS
■ EARLY-ONSET VAP	
Enteric Gram-negative rods • *Escherichia coli* • *Enterobacter* species • *Proteus* species • *Klebsiella* species • *Haemophilus influenzae* • Methicillin-sensitive *Staphylococcus aureus* • *Streptococcus pneumoniae*	β-lactam/β-lactamase inhibitor combination, *or* second-generation cephalosporin, *or* fluoroquinolone
■ LATE-ONSET OR SEVERE EARLY-ONSET VAP	
Above, plus • *Pseudomonas aeruginosa* • *Acinetobacter* species • Methicillin-resistant *S. aureus*	β-lactam/β-lactamase inhibitor combination, *or* third-generation or fourth-generation cephalosporin, *or* fluoroquinolone *plus* aminoglycoside, *or* second, structurally unrelated agent with antipseudomonal activity *plus*, vancomycin or linezolid[a]

VAP, ventilator-assisted pneumonia.
[a]If likelihood of methicillin-resistant *S. aureus* is high.

by nonlactose fermenting Gram-negative rods (including *Pseudomonas*) had a higher infection recurrence rate if they received an initial 8-day course of therapy. It is unclear whether intermediate courses of therapy would have avoided infection recurrence. Thus, it is reasonable to choose an 8-day course of therapy for many patients with VAP; however, if there is an inadequate early clinical response or infection with nonlactose fermenting Gram-negative rods a longer course should be considered.

Intravascular Catheter-Associated Bacteremia

Intravascular catheter-associated bacteremia as strictly defined by the Centers for Disease Control and Prevention (CDC) includes the following criteria: (1) clinical suspicion of catheter-related infection (including low likelihood of infection elsewhere); (2) positive culture of blood drawn from the catheter or of a segment of catheter; and (3) matching positive blood culture drawn from another site, preferably by direct venotomy or arterial puncture. Given this strict definition, the incidence of catheter-associated bacteremia is less than 5% in most studies. However, the incidence of bacteremia is affected by several factors, including the conditions and technique of insertion, type and location of catheter, and the duration of catheterization, and can vary widely from study to study. The attributable mortality of catheter-associated bacteremia is approximately 11%, which is much lower than that for primary bacteremia or bacteremia associated with another site of infection.[134]

Catheter infection is more likely when placement occurs under emergency conditions and is reduced by the use of strict aseptic technique with full barrier precautions. This includes preinsertion hand washing, full gown and gloves, and the use of a large barrier drape.[135] In addition, skin cleansing with chlorhexidine is more effective than other agents at reducing catheter-related infection. These simple interventions should be considered as standards of care and are recommended by the CDC.

Catheter-related infection and bacteremia increase with the duration of catheterization, particularly for durations of greater than 2 days. However, routine catheter replacement at 3 or 7 days does not reduce the incidence of infection and results in increased mechanical complications. Thus, routine guidewire change of catheters is not recommended.

Catheters coated with either antiseptics (chlorhexidine and silver sulfadiazine) or antibiotics (rifampin and minocycline) reduce catheter-related infection and bacteremia (level I evidence).[135] Antibiotic-coated catheters appear to be more effective than antiseptic-coated catheters at reducing infection and bacteremia (level I evidence).[136] Coated catheters are relatively expensive compared with conventional catheters, but they should be considered when insertion is predicted to be for longer than 2 days.

Catheter-related infection is insertion site dependent, increasing in frequency from subclavian to internal jugular to femoral vein sites, respectively. In addition, infection appears to be less likely for arterial versus venous catheters. Thus, the subclavian site should be used when possible if the duration of catheterization is predicted to be longer than 2 days.[135]

Catheter-related venous thrombosis occurs commonly and is associated with an increased risk of infection. Routine flushing of catheter ports with heparin reduces both the incidence of thrombosis and infection (level II evidence).[135]

Organisms commonly responsible for catheter-related bacteremia include *Staphylococcus epidermidis* and *S. aureus*, enteric Gram-negative bacteria, *P. aeruginosa*, *Acinetobacter*, and occasionally, *Enterococcal* species. When catheter-related bacteremia is confirmed, the offending catheter should be removed and appropriate antibiotics continued for a minimum of 7 days; longer courses should be considered for *S. aureus* bacteremia, given the predilection for this organism to cause endocarditis. Suspected catheter-related infections can be addressed by sending screening cultures drawn through the catheter and from a peripheral site; guidewire exchange of the catheter with culture of the intracutaneous segment and tip can also be considered in this situation. Depending on the patient's severity of illness, a strong suspicion of catheter-related bacteremia should trigger the institution of broad-spectrum antibiotic coverage, including coverage for methicillin-resistant *Staphylococcal* species and nonlactose fermenting Gram-negative rods until culture results return, with subsequent deescalation of therapy. Similar to VAP, early appropriate antibiotic coverage of catheter-related bacteremia will likely reduce mortality, although this has not been systematically studied.

Urinary Tract Infection

The urinary tract is the second most common source of infection in the ICU, with infections occurring in up to one-third of patients. The incidence of urinary tract infection (UTI) increases with the duration of bladder catheterization.[126,137] The responsible organisms are similar to those causing other nosocomial infections, and include *Staphylococcal* species, *Enterococcus*, enteric Gram-negative bacteria, and nonlactose fermenting Gram-negative bacteria such as *Pseudomonas*. Bacteruria is associated with bacteremia about 5% of the time. Similar to other ICU-acquired infections, UTIs are associated with increased mortality, although the attributable mortality is not clear.

Prevention of ICU-acquired UTIs includes using careful hand washing and aseptic technique during catheter insertion and minimization of catheterization duration. The use of silver-alloy and antibiotic-coated catheters may also reduce the incidence of UTI, although the evidence is insufficient at this point to recommend general use of coated catheters.[126,137]

Invasive Fungal Infections

Invasive fungal infection in non-neutropenic patients is caused by *Candida* species in the vast majority of cases. It is increasingly common in the ICU population, and accounts for 5 to 10% of all bloodstream infections in the ICU.[134,138] Other than neutropenia, risk factors for *Candida* bloodstream infection include the presence of central venous catheters; uremia and dialysis-dependent renal failure; and administration of parenteral nutrition, multiple broad-spectrum antibiotics, and steroids. In addition, colonization of multiple sites by *Candida* is a risk factor for the development of fungemia.[139] The attributable mortality due to *Candida* bloodstream infection is high, approaching 40%, and mortality appears to be much higher in medical versus surgical ICU patients. Invasive *Candida* infection is also associated with increased duration of mechanical ventilation, as well as with ICU and hospital length of stay.

In addition to simple bloodstream infection, *Candida* species are associated with UTI, postoperative peritonitis, and disseminated bloodborne infection. *Candida* is frequently cultured from the urine of catheterized patients, and candiduria is associated with the development of bloodstream infection. True *Candida* peritonitis is also difficult to separate from contamination of culture specimens, but given that the mortality associated with *Candida* peritonitis is approximately 50%, treatment is warranted if clinical signs suggest infection. Disseminated bloodborne infection can result in endophthalmitis, endocarditis, and hepatic and pulmonary abscesses; is likely to occur when initial treatment of candidemia is delayed; and is associated with a high mortality. Last, although *Candida* is frequently grown from sputum cultures, true *Candida* pneumonia is unlikely. However, sputum colonization is a risk factor for bloodstream infection.

Candida albicans is responsible for approximately 50% of invasive *Candida* infections in critically ill patients. *Candida tropicalis*, *Candida parapsilosis*, *Candida glabrata*, and *Candida krusei* account for the remainder, in descending order of frequency. Speciation is important because *C. glabrata* and, particularly, *C. krusei* are resistant to treatment with the most commonly used therapeutic agent, fluconazole.

Prevention of invasive *Candida* infection involves avoidance of risk factors, including limitation of intravascular catheterization, parenteral nutrition, and antibiotic regimens. Prophylactic therapy with fluconazole is effective at reducing the risk of invasive *Candida* infection in high-risk patients, but this strategy has been studied most extensively in the neutropenic population. Prophylactic fluconazole appears to increase the incidence of invasive infection with more resistant species, such as *C. glabrata* and *C. krusei*; thus, prophylactic therapy should be reserved for only the highest risk patients.[140]

Candida grows slowly in blood culture medium, and invasive infection can be indolent, making diagnosis of invasive candidiasis difficult. Serologic and molecular tests for *Candida* infection are not currently clinically available. Thus, a high level of suspicion for invasive *Candida* infection in critically ill patients is necessary, particularly in patients with multiple risk factors, including multiple site colonization. While awaiting blood culture results, "preemptive" therapy should be considered in patients with a high likelihood of invasive *Candida* infection because delay in treatment is associated with increased mortality. Unfortunately, many cases of invasive candidiasis are identified only at autopsy.[138]

Documented *Candida* bloodstream infection should be treated aggressively, with therapy started promptly (or preemptively, as described previously) and continued for at least 2 weeks after the last positive blood culture. An ophthalmologic exam is warranted in patients with documented or suspected bloodstream infection because patients with endophthalmitis may require longer courses of therapy. Intravascular catheters that are potential sources of bloodstream infection should be removed.

It is not clear that routine treatment of candiduria is warranted because it often clears without treatment or with discontinuation of the bladder catheter; in addition, candiduria often recurs after initially successful antifungal therapy.[140] However, if candiduria is associated with signs of systemic infection, antifungal treatment should be considered; a similar approach can be taken when *Candida* is cultured from the peritoneal space.

Organisms sensitive to the azole derivative fluconazole cause the majority of invasive *Candida* infections in the ICU, and fluconazole is the first-line treatment given its reasonable efficacy and limited toxicity. Infections caused by resistant organisms such as *C. glabrata* and *C. krusei* may respond to newer-generation azoles such as voriconazole, although there are limited data on these agents at present. Caspofungin is another new antifungal agent with broad-spectrum activity and seemingly limited toxicity that is a reasonable alternative for infection due to resistant species. Amphotericin B is generally reserved for refractory, life-threatening infections due to its toxicity. The reader is directed elsewhere for a more detailed discussion of antifungal agents.[140]

Stress Ulceration and Gastrointestinal Hemorrhage

Gastric mucosal breakdown with resulting gastritis and ulceration (often called stress ulceration) can lead to GI bleeding in the ICU. Clinically significant GI bleeding is that which results in hemodynamic instability and/or a sudden fall in hematocrit that results in blood transfusion. The incidence of clinically significant stress-related GI bleeding was once believed to be quite high (20% or greater), but large studies from the past 10 years suggest that the incidence is much lower at less than 5% in high-risk patients and less than 1% in low-risk patients.[141] The major risk factors for stress-related GI bleeding are mechanical ventilation and coagulopathy; secondary risk factors among mechanically ventilated patients include renal failure, thermal injury, and possibly head injury, although the latter two factors have not been recently evaluated.[141–143] Enteral nutrition may protect against significant GI bleeding.[143]

Agents used to prevent stress ulceration and GI bleeding include methods to suppress acid production (H_2 blockers and proton pump inhibitors [PPIs]) and cytoprotective agents (sucralfate). However, the agent of choice—and whether any prophylaxis is beneficial or indicated—is somewhat controversial for the following reasons. Although ranitidine was shown to be more effective than sucralfate in preventing clinically significant GI bleeding in high-risk patients in a large, randomized prospective trial (level I evidence), the incidence of bleeding with both agents was quite low (1.7 vs. 3.8%).[144] Furthermore, a more recent meta-analysis suggests that neither ranitidine nor sucralfate are superior to placebo in reducing clinically important bleeding.[145] Acid suppression may favor gastric colonization with enteric flora, which may in turn increase the risk of nosocomial pneumonia. Multiple small, randomized trials suggested a higher incidence of VAP when ranitidine was compared with sucralfate, and in the previously quoted large trial, there was a trend toward increased VAP in the ranitidine group (level II evidence). It appears that stress ulcer prophylaxis is more widely used than necessary, is often administered to low-risk patients, and results in an overall cost that may be higher than the benefit. Thus, although stress ulcer prophylaxis, predominantly with ranitidine, is commonly used in critically ill patients, the utility of this intervention is unclear.

PPIs are quite effective at suppressing gastric acid production and have been shown to be as effective as ranitidine at reducing stress ulcer-related bleeding in the ICU. In addition, PPIs may be more effective than ranitidine in preventing rebleeding due to stress ulceration (level II evidence).[146] However, PPIs cannot be recommended for routine use as prophylactic agents due to insufficient data and cost considerations. In addition, PPIs have the potential to increase the risk of VAP, given their effective suppression of gastric acid secretion.

Venous Thromboembolism

Venous thromboembolism (VTE) occurs frequently in critically ill patients, with incidences of DVT of 10 to 30% and of PE of 1.5 to 5%. However, the reported incidence varies widely, depending on study design, tests used to detect DVT, and the patient population studied. Virtually all critically ill patients have one or more risk factors for VTE. Risk factors can be grouped according to their importance, as described by Anderson and Spencer (Table 57-8).[147] Determination of VTE risk is important in that it will help in choosing prophylactic therapy and in determining the level of suspicion for VTE in individual patients.

In addition to classic lower-extremity DVT, upper-extremity DVT occurs with increased frequency in the ICU population. This is directly associated with the use of central venous catheters in the subclavian and internal jugular sites. Upper-extremity DVT can result in PE in up to two-thirds of cases, with occasional fatalities. Catheter-related thrombosis is also associated with increased risk of catheter-associated infection and bacteremia. Finally, upper-extremity DVT is associated

TABLE 57-8

RISK FACTORS FOR VENOUS THROMBOEMBOLISM

Strong risk factors (odds ratio >10)
Fracture (hip or leg)
Hip or knee replacement
Major trauma
Spinal cord injury
Moderate risk factors (odds ratio 2–9)
Arthroscopic knee surgery
Central venous lines
Chemotherapy
Congestive heart or respiratory failure
Hormone replacement therapy
Malignancy
Oral contraceptive therapy
Paralytic stroke
Pregnancy/postpartum
Previous venous thromboembolism
Thrombophilia
Weak risk factors (odds ratio <2)
Bed rest >3 days
Immobility due to sitting (e.g., prolonged car or air travel)
Increasing age
Laparoscopic surgery (e.g., cholecystectomy)
Obesity
Pregnancy/antepartum
Varicose veins

Reprinted with permission from Anderson FA Jr, Spencer FA: Risk factors for venous thromboembolism. Circulation 107:19, 2003.

with considerable long-term morbidity, particularly related to postthrombotic syndrome.[148]

The literature supporting prophylactic measures to prevent VTE in the ICU population is relatively poor and marked by small, heterogeneous studies. In addition, studies supporting VTE prophylaxis in the ICU generally show differences only in intermediate end points, such as asymptomatic DVT, with no differences in the incidence of PE or death. This is particularly true for VTE prophylaxis in patients with traumatic injury and makes evidence-based recommendations for prophylaxis difficult. Finally, the risks of VTE prophylaxis, including heparin-induced thrombocytopenia and bleeding, must be weighed when considering prophylaxis in the ICU population. Nonetheless, it is generally agreed that high-risk patients without contraindications should receive prophylaxis with LMWH, and that patients with low-to-moderate risk should receive low-dose unfractionated heparin (UFH) (see Table 57-8). Patients with contraindications to LMWH or UFH should probably receive prophylaxis with mechanical devices (serial compression devices), although there is no compelling evidence to suggest that they are effective in the ICU population.[149] Fondaparinux has not been studied in critically ill patients, and there is no evidence to support the preventive placement of vena cava filters in the critically ill. To reduce central venous catheter-associated thrombosis and infection, catheter tips should be positioned in the superior vena cava, and catheters should be flushed with a dilute heparin solution (level II evidence). Heparin bonding of catheters may also reduce local thrombosis. Importantly, it should be recognized that the incidence of VTE in patients receiving pharmacologic prophylaxis remains substantial, ranging between 5 to 30%, depending on the therapy and population studied.

Given the high incidence of asymptomatic DVT in critically ill patients, a high index of suspicion for VTE must be maintained in the ICU. However, despite the high incidence of DVT, routine screening studies for DVT do not appear to improve clinical outcomes in the ICU. Thus, VTE should be considered in critically ill patients in the face of relatively nonspecific findings, such as unexplained tachycardia, tachypnea, fever, asymmetric extremity edema, and gas exchange abnormalities, including high dead space ventilation. Compression Doppler ultrasonography is the most commonly used test for diagnosis of DVT, and has good positive and negative predictive value compared with contrast venography.[150] Helical CT has supplanted radionuclide ventilation-perfusion scanning as the primary test for the diagnosis of PE.[151] CT scanning can also be extended to include the extremities to diagnose DVT. However, ventilation-perfusion scanning and/or pulmonary angiography may have utility in specific circumstances, including in the presence of renal insufficiency (concerns about contrast-induced nephrotoxicity) or equivocal results on CT scan. In addition, pulmonary angiography may be the test of choice when the likelihood of PE is high and anticoagulation is contraindicated, necessitating immediate placement of a vena cava filter. Although low D-dimer levels have a high negative predictive value in ruling out venous thromboembolism in outpatients, this test appears to have less utility in the ICU setting due to the frequent occurrence of high levels in critically ill patients.[152]

The mainstay of treatment for VTE is heparin, which should be started prior to confirmatory studies if clinical suspicion is high. LMWH may be superior to UFH in efficacy, with comparable rates of bleeding for the treatment of VTE (level II evidence). The choice of drug should be based on clinical circumstances and availability. The advantage of UFH in the ICU population is its titratability and rapid reversibility, which may be desirable in patients at high risk for bleeding. In patients with PE and hemodynamic instability, thrombolytic therapy should be considered if not contraindicated. Although the data supporting thrombolytic therapy for treatment of PE are limited, patients with massive PE and/or shock are likely to benefit from thrombolysis; patients with more subtle signs of instability, including right ventricular dilation may also benefit.[153]

For patients who have contraindications to anticoagulation or who have recurrent PE despite anticoagulation, vena cava filters can be placed in the SVC or IVC, depending on DVT location. Ultimately, given the long-term thrombotic complications associated with these devices, patients with vena cava filters should be anticoagulated when no longer contraindicated. Another attractive option is to place a retrievable vena cava filter and remove it once anticoagulation can be started.[153] The timeframe for safe removal varies with filter type; they can remain permanently, if necessary.

Acquired Neuromuscular Disorders in Critical Illness

Neuromuscular abnormalities developing as a consequence of critical illness can be found in the majority of patients hospitalized in the ICU for 1 week or more. The spectrum of illness ranges from isolated nerve entrapment with focal pain or weakness, to disuse muscle atrophy with mild weakness, to severe myopathy or neuropathy with associated severe, prolonged weakness. In particular, so-called critical illness polyneuropathy and myopathy (CIPNM) and a similar and likely related disorder, acute quadriplegic myopathy (AQM), produce significant morbidity and are associated with increased mortality in critically ill patients.[154]

CIPNM is the most common acquired neuromuscular disorder in the ICU. Prospective studies have shown that 25 to 36% of patients receiving intensive care are weak by clinical evaluation. Electrodiagnostic studies (nerve conduction and electromyography) suggest that CIPNM is present in 42 to 47% of patients in the ICU for 7 days or more, and in 68 to 100% of patients with sepsis or the SIRS. In addition to sepsis, factors associated with the development of CIPNM include duration of illness, hyperglycemia, and corticosteroid and neuromuscular blocking drug administration.

AQM was initially described in asthmatics with respiratory failure that were receiving high-dose corticosteroids and neuromuscular blocking drugs, but has since been described in other patients receiving similar therapeutic regimens. It is likely that the combination of these two drugs, in addition to as yet undefined patient factors, results in toxic injury to muscle that can range from a mild myopathy to rhabdomyolysis. It is also likely that CIPNM and AQM overlap, and it is often difficult to differentiate one from the other in published studies.

CIPNM and AQM can result in severe weakness with flaccid quadriplegia that lasts for weeks or months. It is likely that CIPNM and AQM prolong the duration of mechanical ventilation, ICU stay, and hospitalization, and provide a significant impediment to long-term functional recovery from critical illness.[154,155] In addition, acquired weakness in the ICU may be a significant contributor to ICU and hospital mortality.

Prevention of acquired neuromuscular disorders in the ICU centers on avoidance or minimization of contributory risk factors, including high-dose steroids, prolonged administration of neuromuscular blockade, and hyperglycemia. In regard to the latter, the only prospectively proven intervention for prevention of CIPN is tight glycemic control using intensive insulin therapy (goal glucose <110 mg/dL).[96] In addition, efforts to reduce the risk of infection and ICU length of stay, including rigorous hand washing and infection control procedures, semirecumbent positioning, careful aseptic technique and barrier protection for central venous catheter placement, and lung protective ventilation, will likely result in a reduction in the incidence and ramifications of CIPNM.

The diagnosis of CIPNM and/or AQM should be entertained in all critically ill patients with unexplained weakness. Electrodiagnostic studies can help confirm the diagnosis and rule out other, potentially treatable causes of weakness such as Guillain-Barré syndrome. Muscle biopsy is confirmatory in cases of myopathy, but given its invasive nature, biopsy is not warranted outside research settings. Unfortunately, no treatment for either CIPNM or AQM has been identified; avoidance of potentially contributing agents and aggressive physical therapy are warranted. Discharge planning should include the potential need for long-term nursing and rehabilitative care.

References

1. Berthelsen PG, Cronqvist M: The first intensive care unit in the world. Copenhagen 1953. Acta Anaesthesiol Scand 47:1190, 2003
2. Angus DC, Kelley MA, Schmitz RJ *et al*: Caring for the critically ill patient. Current and projected workforce requirements for care of the critically ill and patients with pulmonary disease: Can we meet the requirements of an aging population? JAMA 284:2762, 2000
3. Spielman FJ: Critical care medicine: Anesthesiology steps forward. Bull Anesth Hist 21:12, 2003
4. Kummer HB: Is the U.S. the odd one out? An international perspective on anesthesiologist-intensivists. ASA Newsl 68:8, 2004
5. Pronovost PJ, Angus DC, Dorman T *et al*: Physician staffing patterns and clinical outcomes in critically ill patients: A systematic review. JAMA 288:2151, 2002
6. Sackett DL: Rules of evidence and clinical recommendations on the use of antithrombotic agents. Chest 95:2S, 1989
7. Chan KH, Miller JD, Dearden NM *et al*: The effect of changes in cerebral perfusion pressure upon middle cerebral artery blood flow velocity and jugular bulb venous oxygen saturation after severe brain injury. J Neurosurg 77:55, 1992
8. Haitsma IK, Maas AI: Advanced monitoring in the intensive care unit: Brain tissue oxygen tension. Curr Opin Crit Care 8:115, 2002
9. Peerdeman SM, Girbes AR, Polderman KH, Vandertop WP: Changes in cerebral interstitial glycerol concentration in head-injured patients: Correlation with secondary events. Intensive Care Med 29:1825, 2003
10. Thatcher RW, Cantor DS, McAlaster R *et al*: Comprehensive predictions of outcome in closed head-injured patients. The development of prognostic equations. Ann N Y Acad Sci 620:82, 1991
11. Chesnut RM, Marshall SB, Piek J *et al*: Early and late systemic hypotension as a frequent and fundamental source of cerebral ischemia following severe brain injury in the Traumatic Coma Data Bank. Acta Neurochir Suppl (Wien) 59:121, 1993
12. Mirski MA, Muffelman B, Ulatowski JA, Hanley DF: Sedation for the critically ill neurologic patient. Crit Care Med 23:2038, 1995
13. Cremer OL, Moons KG, Bouman EA *et al*: Long-term propofol infusion and cardiac failure in adult head-injured patients. Lancet 357:117, 2001
14. Schwartz ML, Tator CH, Rowed DW *et al*: The University of Toronto head injury treatment study: A prospective, randomized comparison of pentobarbital and mannitol. Can J Neurol Sci 11:434, 1984
15. Ward JD, Becker DP, Miller JD *et al*: Failure of prophylactic barbiturate coma in the treatment of severe head injury. J Neurosurg 62:383, 1985
16. Eisenberg HM, Frankowski RF, Contant CF *et al*: High-dose barbiturate control of elevated intracranial pressure in patients with severe head injury. J Neurosurg 69:15, 1988
17. Robertson CS, Valadka AB, Hannay HJ *et al*: Prevention of secondary ischemic insults after severe head injury. Crit Care Med 27:2086, 1999
18. Muizelaar JP, Marmarou A, Ward JD *et al*: Adverse effects of prolonged hyperventilation in patients with severe head injury: A randomized clinical trial. J Neurosurg 75:731, 1991
19. Cruz J: The first decade of continuous monitoring of jugular bulb oxyhemoglobin saturation: Management strategies and clinical outcome. Crit Care Med 26:344, 1998
20. Henderson WR, Dhingra VK, Chittock DR *et al*: Hypothermia in the management of traumatic brain injury. A systematic review and meta-analysis. Intensive Care Med 29:1637, 2003
21. Clifton GL, Miller ER, Choi SC *et al*: Hypothermia on admission in patients with severe brain injury. J Neurotrauma 19:293, 2002
22. Roberts I, Yates D, Sandercock P *et al*: Effect of intravenous corticosteroids on death within 14 days in 10,008 adults with clinically significant head injury (MRC CRASH trial): Randomised placebo-controlled trial. Lancet 364:1321, 2004
23. Temkin NR, Dikmen SS, Wilensky AJ *et al*: A randomized, double-blind study of phenytoin for the prevention of post-traumatic seizures. N Engl J Med 323:497, 1990
24. Kassell NF, Torner JC, Jane JA *et al*: The international cooperative study on the timing of aneurysm surgery. Part 2: Surgical results. J Neurosurg 73:37, 1990
25. Kassell NF, Torner JC, Haley EC Jr *et al*: The international cooperative study on the timing of aneurysm surgery. Part 1: Overall management results. J Neurosurg 73:18, 1990
26. Dorsch NW: Cerebral arterial spasm—a clinical review. Br J Neurosurg 9:403, 1995
27. Barker FG II, Ogilvy CS: Efficacy of prophylactic nimodipine for delayed ischemic deficit after subarachnoid hemorrhage: A metaanalysis. J Neurosurg 84:405, 1996
28. Treggiari MM, Walder B, Suter PM, Romand JA: Systematic review of the prevention of delayed ischemic neurological deficits with hypertension, hypervolemia, and hemodilution therapy following subarachnoid hemorrhage. J Neurosurg 98:978, 2003
29. Shimoda M, Oda S, Tsugane R, Sato O: Intracranial complications of hypervolemic therapy in patients with a delayed ischemic deficit attributed to vasospasm. J Neurosurg 78:423, 1993
30. The National Institute of Neurological Disorders and Stroke rt-PA Stroke Study Group. Tissue plasminogen activator for acute ischemic stroke. N Engl J Med 333(24):1581, 1995
31. Adams HP Jr, Brott TG, Furlan AJ *et al*: Guidelines for thrombolytic therapy for acute stroke: A supplement to the guidelines for the management of patients with acute ischemic stroke. A statement for healthcare professionals from a Special Writing Group of the Stroke Council, American Heart Association. Circulation 94:1167, 1996
32. Hypothermia after Cardiac Arrest Study Group. Mild therapeutic hypothermia to improve the neurologic outcome after cardiac arrest. N Engl J Med 346:549, 2002
33. Bernard SA, Gray TW, Buist MD *et al*: Treatment of comatose survivors of out-of-hospital cardiac arrest with induced hypothermia. N Engl J Med 346:557, 2002
34. Connors AF Jr, Speroff T, Dawson NV *et al*: The effectiveness of right heart catheterization in the initial care of critically ill patients. SUPPORT Investigators. JAMA 276:889, 1996
35. Vieillard-Baron A, Girou E, Valente E *et al*: Predictors of mortality in acute respiratory distress syndrome. Focus on the role of right heart catheterization. Am J Respir Crit Care Med 161:1597, 2000
36. Carnendran L, Abboud R, Sleeper LA *et al*: Trends in cardiogenic shock: Report from the SHOCK study. Should we emergently revascularize occluded coronaries for cardiogenic shock? Eur Heart J 22:472, 2001
37. Richard C, Warszawski J, Anguel N *et al*: Early use of the pulmonary artery catheter and outcomes in patients with shock and acute respiratory distress syndrome: A randomized controlled trial. JAMA 290:2713, 2003
38. Sandham JD, Hull RD, Brant RF *et al*: A randomized, controlled trial of the use of pulmonary-artery catheters in high-risk surgical patients. N Engl J Med 348:5, 2003

39. Kumar A, Anel R, Bunnell E *et al*: Pulmonary artery occlusion pressure and central venous pressure fail to predict ventricular filling volume, cardiac performance, or the response to volume infusion in normal subjects. Crit Care Med 32:691, 2004
40. Michard F, Boussat S, Chemla D *et al*: Relation between respiratory changes in arterial pulse pressure and fluid responsiveness in septic patients with acute circulatory failure. Am J Respir Crit Care Med 162:134, 2000
41. Hayes MA, Timmins AC, Yau EH *et al*: Elevation of systemic oxygen delivery in the treatment of critically ill patients. N Engl J Med 330:1717, 1994
42. Pulmonary Artery Catheter Consensus Conference: Consensus statement. Crit Care Med 25:910, 1997
43. Reinhart K, Kuhn HJ, Hartog C, Bredle DL: Continuous central venous and pulmonary artery oxygen saturation monitoring in the critically ill. Intensive Care Med 30:1572, 2004
44. Rivers E, Nguyen B, Havstad S *et al*: Early goal-directed therapy in the treatment of severe sepsis and septic shock. N Engl J Med 345:1368, 2001
45. Michard F, Teboul JL: Predicting fluid responsiveness in ICU patients: A critical analysis of the evidence. Chest 121:2000, 2002
46. Baillard C, Cohen Y, Fosse JP *et al*: Haemodynamic measurements (continuous cardiac output and systemic vascular resistance) in critically ill patients: Transesophageal Doppler versus continuous thermodilution. Anaesth Intensive Care 27:33, 1999
47. Vieillard-Baron A, Prin S, Chergui K *et al*: Hemodynamic instability in sepsis: Bedside assessment by Doppler echocardiography. Am J Respir Crit Care Med 168:1270, 2003
48. Silver MA, Horton DP, Ghali JK, Elkayam U: Effect of nesiritide versus dobutamine on short-term outcomes in the treatment of patients with acutely decompensated heart failure. J Am Coll Cardiol 39:798, 2002
49. Hochman JS, Sleeper LA, Webb JG *et al*: Early revascularization in acute myocardial infarction complicated by cardiogenic shock. SHOCK investigators. Should we emergently revascularize occluded coronaries for cardiogenic shock? N Engl J Med 341:625, 1999
50. Vieillard Baron A, Schmitt JM, Beauchet A *et al*: Early preload adaptation in septic shock? A transesophageal echocardiographic study. Anesthesiology 94:400, 2001
51. American College of Chest Physicians/Society of Critical Care Medicine Consensus conference: Definitions for sepsis and organ failure and guidelines for the use of innovative therapies in sepsis. Crit Care Med 20:864, 1992
52. Marshall JC, Cook DJ, Christou NV *et al*: Multiple organ dysfunction score: A reliable descriptor of a complex clinical outcome. Crit Care Med 23:1638, 1995
53. Wilkes MM, Navickis RJ: Patient survival after human albumin administration. A meta-analysis of randomized, controlled trials. Ann Intern Med 135:149, 2001
54. Cochrane Injuries Group Albumin Reviewers. Human albumin administration in critically ill patients: Systematic review of randomised controlled trials. BMJ 317:235, 1998
55. Finfer S, Bellomo R, Boyce N *et al*: A comparison of albumin and saline for fluid resuscitation in the intensive care unit. N Engl J Med 350:2247, 2004
56. Martin C, Papazian L, Perrin G *et al*: Norepinephrine or dopamine for the treatment of hyperdynamic septic shock? Chest 103:1826, 1993
57. Marik PE, Mohedin M: The contrasting effects of dopamine and norepinephrine on systemic and splanchnic oxygen utilization in hyperdynamic sepsis. JAMA 272:1354, 1994
58. Martin C, Viviand X, Leone M, Thirion X: Effect of norepinephrine on the outcome of septic shock. Crit Care Med 28:2758, 2000
59. Bellomo R, Chapman M, Finfer S *et al*: Low-dose dopamine in patients with early renal dysfunction: A placebo-controlled randomised trial. Australian and New Zealand Intensive Care Society (ANZICS) Clinical Trials Group. Lancet 356:2139, 2000
60. Shoemaker WC, Appel PL, Kram HB: Hemodynamic and oxygen transport effects of dobutamine in critically ill general surgical patients. Crit Care Med 14:1032, 1986
61. Duranteau J, Sitbon P, Teboul JL *et al*: Effects of epinephrine, norepinephrine, or the combination of norepinephrine and dobutamine on gastric mucosa in septic shock. Crit Care Med 27:893, 1999
62. Meier-Hellmann A, Reinhart K, Bredle DL *et al*: Epinephrine impairs splanchnic perfusion in septic shock. Crit Care Med 25:399, 1997
63. Levy B, Bollaert PE, Charpentier C *et al*: Comparison of norepinephrine and dobutamine to epinephrine for hemodynamics, lactate metabolism, and gastric tonometric variables in septic shock: A prospective, randomized study. Intensive Care Med 23:282, 1997
64. Holmes CL, Patel BM, Russell JA, Walley KR: Physiology of vasopressin relevant to management of septic shock. Chest 120:989, 2001
65. Wenzel V, Krismer AC, Arntz HR *et al*: A comparison of vasopressin and epinephrine for out-of-hospital cardiopulmonary resuscitation. N Engl J Med 350:105, 2004
66. Patel BM, Chittock DR, Russell JA, Walley KR: Beneficial effects of short-term vasopressin infusion during severe septic shock. Anesthesiology 96:576, 2002
67. Dunser MW, Mayr AJ, Ulmer H *et al*: Arginine vasopressin in advanced vasodilatory shock: A prospective, randomized, controlled study. Circulation 107:2313, 2003
68. Bernard GR, Vincent JL, Laterre PF *et al*: Efficacy and safety of recombinant human activated protein C for severe sepsis. N Engl J Med 344:699, 2001
69. Annane D, Sebille V, Charpentier C *et al*: Effect of treatment with low doses of hydrocortisone and fludrocortisone on mortality in patients with septic shock. JAMA 288:862, 2002
70. Feihl F, Perret C: Permissive hypercapnia. How permissive should we be? Am J Respir Crit Care Med 150:1722, 1994
71. Moloney ED, Griffiths MJ: Protective ventilation of patients with acute respiratory distress syndrome. Br J Anaesth 92:261, 2004
72. Nava S, Carbone G, DiBattista N *et al*: Noninvasive ventilation in cardiogenic pulmonary edema: A multicenter randomized trial. Am J Respir Crit Care Med 168:1432, 2003
73. International Consensus Conferences in Intensive Care Medicine: Noninvasive positive pressure ventilation in acute respiratory failure. Am J Respir Crit Care Med 163:283, 2001
74. Esteban A, Frutos-Vivar F, Ferguson ND *et al*: Noninvasive positive-pressure ventilation for respiratory failure after extubation. N Engl J Med 350:2452, 2004
75. Mehta S, Jay GD, Woolard RH *et al*: Randomized, prospective trial of bilevel versus continuous positive airway pressure in acute pulmonary edema. Crit Care Med 25:620, 1997
76. Esteban A, Frutos F, Tobin MJ *et al*: A comparison of four methods of weaning patients from mechanical ventilation. Spanish Lung Failure Collaborative Group. N Engl J Med 332:345, 1995
77. MacIntyre NR, Cook DJ, Ely EW Jr *et al*: Evidence-based guidelines for weaning and discontinuing ventilatory support: A collective task force facilitated by the American College of Chest Physicians; the American Association for Respiratory Care; and the American College of Critical Care Medicine. Chest 120:375S, 2001
78. Schuster DP: What is acute lung injury? What is ARDS? Chest 107:1721, 1995
79. Bernard GR, Artigas A, Brigham KL *et al*: Report of the American-European consensus conference on ARDS: Definitions, mechanisms, relevant outcomes and clinical trial coordination. The Consensus Committee. Intensive Care Med 20:225, 1994
80. Bersten AD, Edibam C, Hunt T, Moran J: Incidence and mortality of acute lung injury and the acute respiratory distress syndrome in three Australian states. Am J Respir Crit Care Med 165:443, 2002
81. Roupie E, Lepage E, Wysocki M *et al*: Prevalence, etiologies and outcome of the acute respiratory distress syndrome among hypoxemic ventilated patients. SRLF Collaborative Group on Mechanical Ventilation. Societe de Reanimation de Langue Francaise. Intensive Care Med 25:920, 1999
82. Nuckton TJ, Alonso JA, Kallet RH *et al*: Pulmonary dead-space fraction as a risk factor for death in the acute respiratory distress syndrome. N Engl J Med 346:1281, 2002
83. The Acute Respiratory Distress Syndrome Network. Ventilation with lower tidal volumes as compared with traditional tidal volumes for acute lung injury and the acute respiratory distress syndrome. N Engl J Med 342:1301, 2000
84. Brower RG, Lanken PN, MacIntyre N *et al*: Higher versus lower positive end-expiratory pressures in patients with the acute respiratory distress syndrome. N Engl J Med 351:327, 2004
85. Taylor RW, Zimmerman JL, Dellinger RP *et al*: Low-dose inhaled nitric oxide in patients with acute lung injury: A randomized controlled trial. JAMA 291:1603, 2004
86. Sokol J, Jacobs SE, Bohn D: Inhaled nitric oxide for acute hypoxic respiratory failure in children and adults: A meta-analysis. Anesth Analg 97:989, 2003
87. Meduri GU, Headley AS, Golden E *et al*: Effect of prolonged methylprednisolone therapy in unresolving acute respiratory distress syndrome: A randomized controlled trial. JAMA 280:159, 1998
88. Bellomo R, Ronco C, Kellum J *et al*: Acute renal failure-definition, outcome measures, animal models, fluid therapy, and information technology needs: The second international consensus conference of the Acute Dialysis Quality Initiative (ADQI) group. Crit Care 8:R204, 2004
89. Singri N, Ahya SN, Levin ML: Acute renal failure. JAMA 289:747, 2003
90. Mehta RL, Pascual MT, Soroko S, Chertow GM: Diuretics, mortality, and nonrecovery of renal function in acute renal failure. JAMA 288:2547, 2002
91. Schiffl H, Lang SM, Fischer R: Daily hemodialysis and the outcome of acute renal failure. N Engl J Med 346:305, 2002
92. Ronco C, Bellomo R, Homel P *et al*: Effects of different doses in continuous veno-venous haemofiltration on outcomes of acute renal failure: A prospective randomised trial. Lancet 356:26, 2000
93. Kellum JA, Angus DC, Johnson JP *et al*: Continuous versus intermittent renal replacement therapy: A meta-analysis. Intensive Care Med 28:29, 2002
94. McCowen KC, Malhotra A, Bistrian BR: Stress-induced hyperglycemia. Crit Care Clin 17:107, 2001
95. Malmberg K, Norhammar A, Wedel H, Ryden L: Glycometabolic state at admission: Important risk marker of mortality in conventionally treated patients with diabetes mellitus and acute myocardial infarction: Long-term results from the Diabetes and Insulin-Glucose Infusion in Acute Myocardial Infarction (DIGAMI) study. Circulation 99:2626, 1999

96. van den Berghe G, Wouters P, Weekers F *et al*: Intensive insulin therapy in the critically ill patients. N Engl J Med 345:1359, 2001
97. Van den Berghe G, Wouters PJ, Bouillon R *et al*: Outcome benefit of intensive insulin therapy in the critically ill: Insulin dose versus glycemic control. Crit Care Med 31:359, 2003
98. Malmberg K: Prospective randomised study of intensive insulin treatment on long term survival after acute myocardial infarction in patients with diabetes mellitus. DIGAMI (Diabetes Mellitus, Insulin Glucose Infusion in Acute Myocardial Infarction) study group. BMJ 314:1512, 1997
99. Van den Berghe G, de Zegher F, Bouillon R: Clinical review 95: Acute and prolonged critical illness as different neuroendocrine paradigms. J Clin Endocrinol Metab 83:1827, 1998
100. Cooper MS, Stewart PM: Corticosteroid insufficiency in acutely ill patients. N Engl J Med 348:727, 2003
101. Hamrahian AH, Oseni TS, Arafah BM: Measurements of serum free cortisol in critically ill patients. N Engl J Med 350:1629, 2004
102. Annane D, Sebille V, Troche G *et al*: A 3-level prognostic classification in septic shock based on cortisol levels and cortisol response to corticotropin. JAMA 283:1038, 2000
103. Van den Berghe G, de Zegher F, Lauwers P: Dopamine and the sick euthyroid syndrome in critical illness. Clin Endocrinol (Oxf) 41:731, 1994
104. De Groot LJ: Dangerous dogmas in medicine: The nonthyroidal illness syndrome. J Clin Endocrinol Metab 84:151, 1999
105. Bennett-Guerrero E, Jimenez JL, White WD *et al*: Cardiovascular effects of intravenous triiodothyronine in patients undergoing coronary artery bypass graft surgery. A randomized, double-blind, placebo-controlled trial. Duke T3 study group. JAMA 275:687, 1996
106. Takala J, Ruokonen E, Webster NR *et al*: Increased mortality associated with growth hormone treatment in critically ill adults. N Engl J Med 341:785, 1999
107. Corwin HL, Gettinger A, Pearl RG *et al*: The CRIT study: Anemia and blood transfusion in the critically ill—current clinical practice in the United States. Crit Care Med 32:39, 2004
108. Vincent JL, Baron JF, Reinhart K *et al*: Anemia and blood transfusion in critically ill patients. JAMA 288:1499, 2002
109. Rodriguez RM, Corwin HL, Gettinger A *et al*: Nutritional deficiencies and blunted erythropoietin response as causes of the anemia of critical illness. J Crit Care 16:36, 2001
110. Hébert PC, Wells G, Blajchman MA *et al*: A multicenter, randomized, controlled clinical trial of transfusion requirements in critical care. N Engl J Med 340(6):409, 1999
111. Corwin HL, Gettinger A, Pearl RG *et al*: Efficacy of recombinant human erythropoietin in critically ill patients: A randomized controlled trial. JAMA 288:2827, 2002
112. Kompan L, Kremzar B, Gadzijev E, Prosek M: Effects of early enteral nutrition on intestinal permeability and the development of multiple organ failure after multiple injury. Intensive Care Med 25:157, 1999
113. Marik PE, Zaloga GP: Gastric versus post-pyloric feeding: a systematic review. Crit Care 7:R46, 2003
114. Heyland DK, Cook DJ, Guyatt GH: Does the formulation of enteral feeding products influence infectious morbidity and mortality rates in the critically ill patients? A critical review of the evidence. Crit Care Med 22:1192, 1994
115. Heyland DK, Novak F, Drover JW *et al*: Should immunonutrition become routine in critically ill patients? A systematic review of the evidence. JAMA 286:944, 2001
116. Kollef MH, Levy NT, Ahrens TS *et al*: The use of continuous i.v. sedation is associated with prolongation of mechanical ventilation. Chest 114:541, 1998
117. Brook AD, Ahrens TS, Schaiff R *et al*: Effect of a nursing-implemented sedation protocol on the duration of mechanical ventilation. Crit Care Med 27:2609, 1999
118. Kress JP, Pohlman AS, O'Connor MF, Hall JB: Daily interruption of sedative infusions in critically ill patients undergoing mechanical ventilation. N Engl J Med 342:1471, 2000
119. Schweickert WD, Gehlbach BK, Pohlman AS *et al*: Daily interruption of sedative infusions and complications of critical illness in mechanically ventilated patients. Crit Care Med 32:1272, 2004
120. Kress JP, Gehlbach B, Lacy M *et al*: The long-term psychological effects of daily sedative interruption on critically ill patients. Am J Respir Crit Care Med 168:1457, 2003
121. Ely EW, Shintani A, Truman B *et al*: Delirium as a predictor of mortality in mechanically ventilated patients in the intensive care unit. JAMA 291:1753, 2004
122. Ely EW, Inouye SK, Bernard GR *et al*: Delirium in mechanically ventilated patients: Validity and reliability of the confusion assessment method for the intensive care unit (CAM-ICU). JAMA 286:2703, 2001
123. McCollam JS, O'Neil MG, Norcross ED *et al*: Continuous infusions of lorazepam, midazolam, and propofol for sedation of the critically ill surgery trauma patient: A prospective, randomized comparison. Crit Care Med 27:2454, 1999
124. Walder B, Elia N, Henzi I *et al*: A lack of evidence of superiority of propofol versus midazolam for sedation in mechanically ventilated critically ill patients: A qualitative and quantitative systematic review. Anesth Analg 92:975, 2001
125. Coursin DB, Maccioli GA: Dexmedetomidine. Curr Opin Crit Care 7:221, 2001
126. Vincent JL: Nosocomial infections in adult intensive-care units. Lancet 361:2068, 2003
127. Rouby JJ, Laurent P, Gosnach M *et al*: Risk factors and clinical relevance of nosocomial maxillary sinusitis in the critically ill. Am J Respir Crit Care Med 150:776, 1994
128. Cook DJ, Walter SD, Cook RJ *et al*: Incidence of and risk factors for ventilator-associated pneumonia in critically ill patients. Ann Intern Med 129:433, 1998
129. Fagon JY, Chastre J, Wolff M *et al*: Invasive and noninvasive strategies for management of suspected ventilator-associated pneumonia. A randomized trial. Ann Intern Med 132:621, 2000
130. Hoffken G, Niederman MS: Nosocomial pneumonia: the importance of a de-escalating strategy for antibiotic treatment of pneumonia in the ICU. Chest 122:2183, 2002
131. Collard HR, Saint S, Matthay MA: Prevention of ventilator-associated pneumonia: An evidence-based systematic review. Ann Intern Med 138:494, 2003
132. Wood AY, Davit AJ II, Ciraulo DL *et al*: A prospective assessment of diagnostic efficacy of blind protective bronchial brushings compared to bronchoscope-assisted lavage, bronchoscope-directed brushings, and blind endotracheal aspirates in ventilator-associated pneumonia. J Trauma 55:825, 2003
133. Chastre J, Wolff M, Fagon JY *et al*: Comparison of 8 vs 15 days of antibiotic therapy for ventilator-associated pneumonia in adults: A randomized trial. JAMA 290:2588, 2003
134. Renaud B, Brun-Buisson C: Outcomes of primary and catheter-related bacteremia. A cohort and case-control study in critically ill patients. Am J Respir Crit Care Med 163:1584, 2001
135. Polderman KH, Girbes AR: Central venous catheter use. Part 2: Infectious complications. Intensive Care Med 28:18, 2002
136. Darouiche RO, Raad II, Heard SO *et al*: A comparison of two antimicrobial-impregnated central venous catheters. Catheter Study Group. N Engl J Med 340:1, 1999
137. Di Filippo A, De Gaudio AR: Device-related infections in critically ill patients. Part II: Prevention of ventilator-associated pneumonia and urinary tract infections. J Chemother 15:536, 2003
138. Eggimann P, Garbino J, Pittet D: Epidemiology of *Candida* species infections in critically ill non-immunosuppressed patients. Lancet Infect Dis 3:685, 2003
139. Verduyn Lunel FM, Meis JF, Voss A: Nosocomial fungal infections: Candidemia. Diagn Microbiol Infect Dis 34:213, 1999
140. Eggimann P, Garbino J, Pittet D: Management of *Candida* species infections in critically ill patients. Lancet Infect Dis 3:772, 2003
141. Cook DJ, Fuller HD, Guyatt GH *et al*: Risk factors for gastrointestinal bleeding in critically ill patients. Canadian Critical Care Trials Group. N Engl J Med 330:377, 1994
142. Metz CA, Livingston DH, Smith JS *et al*: Impact of multiple risk factors and ranitidine prophylaxis on the development of stress-related upper gastrointestinal bleeding: A prospective, multicenter, double-blind, randomized trial. The Ranitidine Head Injury Study Group. Crit Care Med 21:1844, 1993
143. Cook D, Heyland D, Griffith L *et al*: Risk factors for clinically important upper gastrointestinal bleeding in patients requiring mechanical ventilation. Canadian Critical Care Trials Group. Crit Care Med 27:2812, 1999
144. Cook D, Guyatt G, Marshall J *et al*: A comparison of sucralfate and ranitidine for the prevention of upper gastrointestinal bleeding in patients requiring mechanical ventilation. Canadian Critical Care Trials Group. N Engl J Med 338:791, 1998
145. Messori A, Trippoli S, Vaiani M *et al*: Bleeding and pneumonia in intensive care patients given ranitidine and sucralfate for prevention of stress ulcer: Meta-analysis of randomised controlled trials. BMJ 321:1103, 2000
146. Morgan D: Intravenous proton pump inhibitors in the critical care setting. Crit Care Med 30:S369, 2002
147. Anderson FA Jr, Spencer FA: Risk factors for venous thromboembolism. Circulation 107:19, 2003
148. Joffe HV, Goldhaber SZ: Upper-extremity deep vein thrombosis. Circulation 106:1874, 2002
149. Geerts W, Selby R: Prevention of venous thromboembolism in the ICU. Chest 124:357S, 2003
150. Kearon C, Ginsberg JS, Hirsh J: The role of venous ultrasonography in the diagnosis of suspected deep venous thrombosis and pulmonary embolism. Ann Intern Med 129:1044, 1998
151. Goldhaber SZ, Elliott CG: Acute pulmonary embolism: Part I: Epidemiology, pathophysiology, and diagnosis. Circulation 108:2726, 2003
152. Kollef MH, Zahid M, Eisenberg PR: Predictive value of a rapid semiquantitative D-dimer assay in critically ill patients with suspected venous thromboembolic disease. Crit Care Med 28:414, 2000
153. Goldhaber SZ, Elliott CG: Acute pulmonary embolism: Part II: Risk stratification, treatment, and prevention. Circulation 108:2834, 2003
154. Deem S, Lee CM, Curtis JR: Acquired neuromuscular disorders in the intensive care unit. Am J Respir Crit Care Med 168:735, 2003
155. Herridge MS, Cheung AM, Tansey CM *et al*: One-year outcomes in survivors of the acute respiratory distress syndrome. N Engl J Med 348:683, 2003

CHAPTER 58 ■ CARDIOPULMONARY RESUSCITATION

CHARLES W. OTTO

KEY POINTS

1. Early uninterrupted basic life support and rapid defibrillation are necessary to obtain the best possible rates of resuscitation.
2. For arrests due to ventricular fibrillation/tachycardia, ventilation is probably not necessary for the first 10 minutes. Bystanders should be encouraged to provide chest compressions with or without mouth-to-mouth ventilation.
3. No alternative method of closed-chest compression has been shown to improve outcome from cardiac arrest when compared with the standard technique.
4. Restoration of spontaneous circulation depends on restoring oxygenated blood flow to the myocardium. Arterial diastolic pressure of 40 mm Hg and/or end-tidal carbon dioxide of >10 mm Hg indicate adequate blood flow for resuscitation, and should be used to guide resuscitation efforts whenever possible.
5. Public access defibrillation improves outcome from cardiac arrest by allowing definitive treatment of ventricular fibrillation within the first few minutes of collapse. If more than 4 to 5 minutes have elapsed since collapse, 2 to 3 minutes of chest compressions should be performed before defibrillation.
6. Epinephrine aids resuscitation through its alpha-adrenergic effects, causing vasoconstriction leading to increased coronary perfusion pressure and myocardial blood flow. Experimentally, all strong vasoconstrictors are equally effective.
7. High-dose epinephrine and vasopressin have not been found superior to epinephrine in aiding resuscitation from cardiac arrest.
8. Amiodarone, when administered during out-of-hospital cardiac arrest resistant to initial defibrillation, has been shown to improve initial resuscitation but not to improve survival to discharge from the hospital.
9. Comatose survivors of cardiac arrest had improved neurologic outcome when mild therapeutic hypothermia (32 to 34°C) was induced for 24 hours. No specific pharmacologic agent has been found to improve neurologic outcome following cardiac arrest.

Treatment of cardiac and respiratory arrest is an integral part of anesthesia practice. The American Board of Anesthesiology indicates in its *Booklet of Information* that the "clinical management and teaching of cardiac and pulmonary resuscitation" are some of the activities that define the specialty of anesthesiology. The cardiopulmonary physiology and pharmacology that form the basis of anesthesia practice are applicable to treating the victim of cardiac arrest. However, there is specialized knowledge relating to blood flow, ventilation, and pharmacology under the conditions of a cardiac arrest that must be understood to maintain leadership of the modern cardiopulmonary resuscitation (CPR) team. This chapter concentrates on those aspects of CPR that are different from the more common circumstances requiring cardiovascular support (e.g., shock, dysrhythmias).

HISTORY

Anesthesiologists have contributed many of the elements of modern CPR and continue to be active investigators and teachers in the field. Discoveries leading to current CPR practice have a long history recorded in many famous works.[1,2] The earliest reference may be the Bible story of Elisha breathing life back into the son of a Shunammite woman (II Kings 4:34). In 1543, Andreas Vesalius described tracheotomy and artificial ventilation.[3] William Harvey's manual manipulation of the heart is well known. Early teaching of resuscitation was organized by the Society for the Recovery of Persons Apparently Drowned, founded in London in 1774. The combined techniques of modern CPR developed primarily from the fortuitous assemblage of innovative clinicians and researchers in Baltimore in the 1950s and early 1960s. Building on the long history of contributions from around the world, these investigators laid the framework for current CPR practice. In the late 1950s, mouth-to-mouth ventilation was established as the only effective means of artificial ventilation.[4–7] The internal defibrillator was developed in 1933,[8] but it was not applied successfully until 1947.[9] It was another decade before general use was made possible by the development of external cross-chest defibrillation.[10,11] Despite these advances, widespread resuscitation from cardiac arrest was not possible until Kouwenhoven et al described success with closed-chest cardiac massage in a series of patients.[12] The final major component of modern CPR was added in 1963, when Redding and Pearson described the improved success obtained by administering epinephrine or other vasopressor drugs.[13]

SCOPE OF THE PROBLEM

Cardiovascular disease remains the most common cause of death in the industrialized world. Although cardiovascular mortality has been declining in the United States since the mid-1960s, nearly 50% of all deaths are due to cardiovascular causes.[14] Of the 1 million annual cardiovascular deaths, approximately half are related to coronary artery disease and the majority of these are sudden deaths. Thus, CPR teaching and research tend to focus on myocardial ischemia as the primary cause of cardiac arrest. However, anesthesiologists are more likely than other practitioners to deal with etiologies other than myocardial infarction. CPR is symptomatic therapy, aimed at sustaining vital organ function until natural cardiac function is restored. The details of effective resuscitation technique are important. However, search for a remediable cause of the arrest must not be lost in excessive attention to mechanics.

Brain adenosine triphosphate (ATP) is depleted after 4 to 6 minutes of no blood flow. It returns nearly to normal within 6 minutes of starting effective CPR. Studies in animals suggest that good neurologic outcome may be possible from 10- to 15-minute periods of normothermic cardiac arrest if good circulation is promptly restored.[15,16] In clinical practice, the severity of the underlying cardiac disease is the major determining factor in the success or failure of resuscitation attempts. Of those factors under control of the rescuers, poor outcomes are associated with long arrest times before CPR is begun, prolonged ventricular fibrillation without definitive therapy, and inadequate coronary and cerebral perfusion during cardiac massage. Survival from out-of-hospital cardiac arrest is improved when
1 CPR is begun by bystanders.[17] Optimum outcome from ventricular fibrillation is obtained only if basic life support is begun within 4 minutes of arrest and defibrillation applied within 8 minutes.[18,19] The importance of early defibrillation has been known for some time and is emphasized in CPR practice.[20,21] What is not as well recognized is the tendency to interrupt chest compressions frequently during a resuscitation attempt. Studies of emergency medical systems suggest that chest compressions are performed for less than 50% of the time during a typical out-of-hospital resuscitation, being interrupted for pulse checks, intubations, starting intravenous catheters, defibrillation attempts, and moving the victim. Because blood flow falls rapidly with cessation of compressions and resumes slowly with reinstitution of compressions, these interruptions undoubtedly contribute to the poor survival rates.

With an effective rapid response emergency medical system, initial resuscitation rates of 40% and survival to hospital discharge of 10 to 15% are reported after out-of-hospital arrests.[19,21] A better outcome might be expected for in-hospital arrests because of rapid response times and expert personnel. However, overall rates for initial resuscitation and survival to discharge from in-hospital arrest are about 40% and 10%, respectively.[22] Intercurrent illnesses of hospitalized patients reduce the likelihood of survival and the arrest victim is more likely to be elderly, a factor that may reduce survival. Within the hospital, the operating room is the location where CPR has the highest rate of success. Cardiac arrest occurs approximately 7 times for every 10,000 anesthetics.[23] The cause for the arrest is anesthesia related, ~4.5 times for every 10,000 anesthetics, but mortality from these arrests is only 0.4 per 10,000 anesthetics. Thus, resuscitation is successful ~90% of the time in anesthesia-related cardiac arrests. Outside the operating suite, the best initial resuscitation rates are found in the intensive care unit (ICU), whereas the best survival rates are for patients arresting in the emergency department.[22]

ORGANIZING A SOLUTION

Since the mid-1970s, CPR has become widely practiced, facilitated by the efforts of the American Heart Association, the International Red Cross, the European Resuscitation Council, and many other organizations around the world. Specific guidelines for the teaching and practice of CPR are published periodically.[24] These guidelines were developed because numerous individuals with varying levels of expertise (laypersons, emergency personnel, nurses, and physicians) need to be trained if CPR is to be effective in saving lives. For training to be effective, a standardized approach is needed (Table 58-1). The organizations also develop and sponsor courses at different levels of complexity for teaching CPR. The two levels of CPR care are referred to as basic life support (BLS) for ventilation and chest compressions without additional equipment, and advanced cardiac life support (ACLS) for using all modalities available for resuscitation. Medical personnel need to be well versed in both levels of care. BLS is also appropriate for laypersons.

The American Heart Association, in conjunction with the International Liaison Committee on Resuscitation (ILCOR), periodically coordinates an International Conference on CPR and emergency cardiac care, during which worldwide experts evaluate the scientific data regarding CPR. The recommendations resulting from the conference comprise the most complete compilation of guidelines for CPR practice.[24] International contributions to the most recent conferences in 1992 and 2000 produce similar CPR practices worldwide. However, no common infrastructure exists that allows adoption of true international guidelines for CPR. The algorithms for approaching the patient with cardiac arrest published in the guidelines are familiar to all physicians and are reproduced throughout this chapter. However, the major purpose of this chapter is not

TABLE 58-1

STANDARD APPROACH TO THE UNCONSCIOUS PATIENT

1. Determine unresponsiveness.
2. Activate emergency medical services or team.
3. Position victim supine on firm surface.
4. Open airway.
5. Determine absence of breathing.
6. Perform ventilation by giving 2 breaths.
7. Determine absence of pulse.
8. Initiate chest compressions.
9. Alternate 15 compressions with 2 breaths.

to reiterate the standard approach but to provide the scientific background, where it exists, that led to adoption of the standard approach; to point out areas of continuing controversy; and to suggest areas of possible future development.

ETHICAL ISSUES: DO NOT RESUSCITATE ORDERS IN THE OPERATING ROOM

Institution of CPR is standard medical care when an individual is found to be apparently dead. In more recent years, terminally ill patients have become increasingly concerned about inappropriate application of life-sustaining procedures, including CPR. Through living wills and other instruments, patients have begun placing limitations on medical treatment to include do not resuscitate (DNR) orders. Such requests are generally accepted, even welcomed, by health care workers. However, the operating room is one area of the hospital where DNR orders continue to cause ethical conflicts between medical personnel and patients.[25,26] There are ethically sound arguments on both sides of the issue as to whether DNR orders should be upheld in the operating room.

The patient's right to limit medical treatment, including refusing CPR, is firmly established in modern medical practice based on the ethical principle of respect for patient autonomy. A terminally ill patient can reject heroic measures such as resuscitation and still choose palliative therapy. If a surgical intervention will ameliorate symptoms or cure a problem that improves quality of life, there is no reason to withhold this treatment. During surgery, the patient reasonably may want to maintain the DNR status to avoid heroic measures that serve only to prolong death. Operative intervention increases the risk of cardiac arrest, and the patient may not want the burden of surviving in a worse condition than previously. Thus, the time that the DNR order provides the greatest protection against unwanted intervention is during surgery. The possibility of death under anesthesia may be viewed as especially peaceful.

Despite these rather strong arguments for treating a DNR status in the operating room the same way it is treated elsewhere in the hospital, most operating room personnel are at least a little uneasy caring for these patients. Many surgeons require that DNR orders be suspended during the perioperative period or assume consent to surgery includes such suspension. There are multiple reasons for the reluctance to accept DNR status during surgery and anesthesia. Approximately 75% of cardiac arrests in the operating room are related to a surgical or anesthetic complication, and resuscitative attempts are highly successful.[23] Ethically, surgeons and anesthesiologists feel responsible for what happens to patients in the operating room: primum non nocere (first, do no harm). Although the physicians are highly diligent in monitoring and managing changes in the patient's status, complications and arrests do occur. Honoring a DNR under these circumstances is frequently viewed as failure to treat a reversible process, and hence, tantamount to killing. This is an ethically sound view if the cause of arrest is readily identifiable and easily reversible, and if treatment is likely to allow the patient to fulfill the objectives of coming to surgery.[25]

Institutionally, these ethical conflicts should be addressed by adoption of clear policies by hospitals.[27] For the individual patient, conflicts can be resolved by communication among the patient, family, and caregivers. A mutual decision can often be reached to suspend or severely limit a DNR order in the perioperative period if the patient understands the special circumstances of perioperative arrest, that interventions are brief and usually successful, and that the physicians support the patient's goals in coming to surgery and values in desiring not to prolong death. Many interventions commonly used in the operating room (mechanical ventilation, vasopressors, antidysrhythmics, blood products) may be considered forms of resuscitation in other situations. The only modalities that are not routine anesthetic care are cardiac massage and defibrillation. Therefore, the specific interventions included in a DNR status must be clarified with specific allowance made for methods necessary to perform anesthesia and surgery.

BASIC LIFE SUPPORT

BLS consists of those elements of resuscitation that can be performed without additional equipment: basic airway management, rescue breathing, and manual chest compressions. Common practice is to approach a victim with the airway, breathing, and circulation (ABC) sequence, although the circulation, airway, and breathing (CAB) sequence has been used in some countries with comparable results. Table 58-1 itemizes the standard approach to an unconscious victim.

Airway Management

The problem of airway obstruction by the tongue in the unconscious patient is familiar to the anesthesiologist. The techniques used for airway maintenance during anesthesia are applicable to the cardiac arrest victim. The primary method recommended to the public is the same "head tilt–chin lift" method commonly employed in the operating room.[28] The head is extended by pressure applied to the brow while the mandible is pulled forward by pressure on the front of the jaw, lifting the tongue away from the posterior pharynx. The "jaw thrust" maneuver (applying pressure behind the rami of the mandible) is an effective alternative. Properly inserted oropharyngeal or nasopharyngeal airways can be useful before intubation, recognizing the danger of inducing vomiting or laryngospasm in the semiconscious victim. Tracheal intubation provides the best airway control, preventing aspiration and allowing the most effective ventilation. Intubation is indicated in any resuscitation lasting more than a few minutes, but it should not be performed until adequate ventilation (preferably with supplemental oxygen) and chest compressions have been established. A number of alternative airways designed for blind placement by individuals who are not skilled laryngoscopists have been described.[24] These include the laryngotracheal mask, pharyngotracheal lumen airway, esophageal obturator airway, esophageal gastric tube airway, and combination esophageal tracheal tube. None ensures airway control as well as an endotracheal tube. When other methods of establishing an airway are unsuccessful, translaryngeal ventilation or tracheotomy by cricothyroid puncture may be necessary.

Foreign Body Airway Obstruction

It is estimated that foreign body airway obstruction accounts for 1% of all sudden deaths (~3,900 deaths in the United States in 1989).[24] Airway occlusion by a foreign object must be considered in any victim who suddenly stops breathing and becomes cyanotic and unconscious. It occurs most commonly during eating and is usually due to food, especially meat, impacting in the laryngeal inlet, at the epiglottis or in the vallecula. Sudden death in restaurants from this cause is frequently mistaken for myocardial infarction, leading to the label "cafe coronary." Poorly chewed pieces of food, poor dentition or dentures, and elevated blood alcohol are the most common factors contributing to choking. The signs of total airway obstruction are the lack of air movement despite respiratory efforts and the inability of the victim to speak or cough. Cyanosis, unconsciousness, and cardiac arrest follow quickly. Partial airway obstruction will result in rasping or wheezing respirations accompanied by coughing. If the victim has good air movement and is able to cough forcefully, no intervention is indicated. However, if the cough weakens or cyanosis develops, the patient must be treated as if there were complete obstruction.

Mothers and friends have been pounding on the backs of choking victims for centuries. In 1974, Heimlich proposed abdominal thrusts as a better method of relieving airway obstruction and, in 1976, Guildner et al reported that sternal thrusts were just as effective.[29,30] Subsequently, there were multiple studies of these maneuvers. In clinical practice, Redding[31] observed that no maneuver was always successful and that each occasionally was successful when another had failed. To minimize confusion from teaching multiple techniques (especially to the lay public), the American Heart Association has elected to emphasize the abdominal thrust maneuver (with chest thrusts as an alternative for the pregnant and massively obese) and the finger sweep.[24] This recommendation is made on the twofold premise that the abdominal thrust is at least as effective as other techniques and that teaching one method simplifies education.

For the awake victim, abdominal thrusts are applied in the erect position (sitting or standing). The rescuer reaches around the victim from behind, placing the fist of one hand in the epigastrium between the xiphoid and umbilicus. The fist is grasped with the other hand and pressed into the epigastrium with a quick upward thrust. In the unconscious, thrusts are applied by kneeling astride the victim, placing the heel of one hand in the epigastrium and the other on top of the first. Care must be taken to ensure the xiphoid is not pushed into the abdominal contents and that the thrust is in the midline. Sternal thrusts are valuable in the massively obese or in women in advanced pregnancy. In the erect victim, the chest is encircled from behind as in the abdominal maneuver but the fist is placed in the midsternum. For the unconscious, thrusts are applied from the side of the supine victim with a hand position the same as for external cardiac compression. Back blows are applied directly over the thoracic spine between the scapulae. They must be delivered with force. Placing the victim in a head-down position (e.g., leaning over a chair) may help move the obstruction into the pharynx.

Whatever technique is used, each individual maneuver must be delivered as if it will relieve the obstruction. If the first attempt is unsuccessful, repeated attempts should be made because hypoxia-related muscular relaxation may eventually allow success. Complications of thrust maneuvers include laceration of the liver and spleen, gastric rupture, fractured ribs, and regurgitation.

In the unconscious victim, if these maneuvers are unsuccessful, manual dislodgment of the obstruction should be tried. The mouth is opened, and the tongue and jaw are grasped between the thumb and fingers and pulled forward. A finger of the other hand is inserted along the buccal mucosa, attempting to dislodge the object laterally. Care must be taken not to push the foreign body deeper into the larynx. Direct visualization of the object may also be successful. In the absence of a laryngoscope and Magill forceps, ordinary instruments (e.g., a tablespoon and ice tongs) may be used. However, blind grasping with instruments is rarely successful and may cause damage to tonsils or other tissue. Finally, if the object cannot be dislodged, a cricothyroidotomy can be lifesaving.

Ventilation

The standard approach to the unresponsive victim is to follow opening the airway with ventilation (see Table 58-1). If the airway remains patent, chest compressions cause substantial air exchange. Early studies in anesthetized humans suggested that the airway would not remain open in the unconscious,[6,7] leading to the teaching that airway control and artificial ventilation must accompany chest compressions. However, data from the Belgian CPCR Registry have demonstrated that 14-day survival and neurologic outcome are the same if bystanders initiate full BLS or do only chest compressions. Both lead to substantially better survival than if the bystanders do only mouth-to-mouth ventilation or do not attempt CPR.[32,33] Studies in the more controlled setting of the animal laboratory also raise questions about the importance of ventilation during assisted ventilation during the first 10 minutes of BLS. A cumulative series of more than 170 swine in ventricular fibrillation have been studied, and no differences in 24- to 48-hour survival or neurologic outcome have been found between those provided with assisted ventilation and those not provided with assisted ventilation during simulated bystander CPR prior to the application of ACLS.[34–37] Another study using an asphyxial cardiac arrest model found a markedly improved 24-hour outcome when
2 ventilation was added to chest compressions during BLS.[38] These observations suggest that when arrest is witnessed, likely to be of cardiac (rather than respiratory) cause, and when intubation is available within a short time, closed-chest compressions alone may be as efficacious as compressions and mouth-to-mouth ventilation. If these preliminary studies are confirmed, BLS teaching could be considerably simplified, potentially resulting in improved rates of bystander CPR because studies show that many people are reluctant to provide mouth-to-mouth ventilation.[39–41] Currently, airway management and ventilation remain the standard first steps of CPR. Mouth-to-mouth or mouth-to-nose ventilation is the most expeditious and effective method immediately available. Although inspired gas with this method will contain ~4% carbon dioxide and only ~17% oxygen (composition of exhaled air), it is sufficient to maintain viability.

Physiology of Ventilation During CPR

In the absence of an endotracheal tube, the distribution of gas between the lungs and stomach during mouth-to-mouth or mask ventilation will be determined by the relative impedance to flow into each (i.e., the opening pressure of the esophagus and the lung-thorax compliance). It is likely that esophageal opening pressure during cardiac arrest is no more than that found in anesthetized individuals (~20 cm H_2O), and lung-thorax compliance is likely reduced. To avoid gastric insufflation, inspiratory airway pressures must be kept low.

Insufflation of air into the stomach during CPR leads to gastric distension, impeding ventilation and increasing the risk of regurgitation and gastric rupture. Avoiding gastric insufflation requires that peak inspiratory airway pressures stay below esophageal opening pressure. Partial airway obstruction by the tongue and pharyngeal tissues is a major cause of increased airway pressure contributing to gastric insufflation during CPR. Meticulous attention to airway management is necessary during rescue breathing. Recommended tidal volumes to cause a noticeable rise in the chest wall in most adults is 0.8 to 1.2 L. To achieve these tidal volumes with low inspiratory pressures, a slow inspiratory flow rate and long inspiratory time are needed, even with an open airway. Therefore, rescue breaths should be given over 1.5 to 2 seconds during a pause in chest compressions.

A useful adjunct for preventing gastric insufflation during positive-pressure ventilation without an endotracheal tube is cricoid pressure (Sellick maneuver).[42] Properly applied pressure to the anterior arch of the cricoid causes the cricoid lamina to seal the esophagus and can prevent air from entering the stomach at airway pressures up to 100 cm H_2O.[43] Pressure on the thyroid cartilage is useless. Cricoid pressure should be used during rescue breathing without an endotracheal tube, but this inevitably involves the need for an additional rescuer.

Techniques of Rescue Breathing

While maintaining an open airway with the head tilt–jaw lift technique, the hand on the forehead pinches the nose, the rescuer takes a deep breath and seals the victim's mouth with the lips and exhales, watching for the chest to rise, indicating effective ventilation. For exhalation, the rescuer's mouth is removed from the victim, listening for escaping air and taking a breath. When both hands are being used in the jaw thrust maneuver of opening the airway, the cheek is used to seal the nose. For mouth-to-nose ventilation, the rescuer's lips surround the nose and the victim's lips are held closed. In some patients, the mouth must be allowed to open for exhalation with this technique. On initiation of resuscitation, two consecutive breaths should be given and breathing continued at a rate of 10 to 12 minutes^{-1}. During a one-rescuer CPR, a pause for two breaths should be made after each 15 chest compressions. When there are two rescuers, a 1.5- to 2-second pause after every fifth chest compression will allow a breath to be given. Exhalation can occur during subsequent compressions.

Several adjuncts to ventilation are available. An oropharyngeal airway with mouthguard and external extension mouthpiece has been used, but obtaining a good mouth seal is often difficult. Perhaps the most useful adjunct is a common mask, such as that used for anesthesia. The mask can be applied to the face and held in place with the thumbs and index fingers while the other fingers are used to apply jaw thrust. Breathing into the connector port of the mask provides ventilation. Mouth-to-mask ventilation may be more aesthetic than mouth-to-mouth ventilation and can be just as effective in trained hands. Masks are also available with one-way valves that direct the victim's exhaled gas away from the rescuer. Masks with integral nipple adapters are useful for providing supplemental oxygen. An oxygen flow of 10 L/min can raise the inspired concentration to 50%.

The self-inflating resuscitation bag and mask are the most common adjuncts used in rescue vehicles and hospitals. Although these devices have the advantages of noncontact and ability to use supplemental oxygen, they have been shown to be difficult for a single rescuer to apply properly, preventing substantial gas leak while maintaining a patent airway.[44] Tidal volumes with mouth-to-mouth and mouth-to-mask ventilation are often greater than with the resuscitation bag. It is now recommended that if this device is to be used, two individuals manage the airway: one to hold the mask and maintain head position, and one to squeeze the bag using both hands.[45] Finally, tracheal intubation provides the best control of ventilation. With a tube in place, breathing can proceed without concern for gastric distension or synchronizing ventilation with chest compressions. Blood flow during CPR slows rapidly when chest compressions are stopped and recovers slowly when they are resumed. Consequently, following intubation, no pause should be made for ventilation, and ventilation should be delivered without regard for the compression cycle.

Circulation

Physiology of Circulation During Closed-Chest Compression

Two theories of the mechanism of blood flow during closed-chest compression have been suggested.[12,46] They are not mutually exclusive, and which theory predominates in humans continues to be the subject of controversy.

Cardiac Pump Mechanism. The cardiac pump mechanism was originally proposed by Kouwenhoven et al.[12,47] According to this theory, pressure on the chest compresses the heart between the sternum and the spine. Compression raises the pressure in the ventricular chambers, closing the atrioventricular valves and ejecting blood into the lungs and aorta. During the relaxation phase of closed-chest compression, expansion of the thoracic cage causes a subatmospheric intrathoracic pressure, facilitating blood return. The mitral and tricuspid valves open, allowing blood to fill the ventricles. Pressure in the aorta causes aortic valve closure and coronary artery perfusion.

Thoracic Pump Mechanism. In 1976, Criley et al[48] reported a patient undergoing cardiac catheterization who simultaneously developed ventricular fibrillation and an episode of cough-hiccups. With every cough-hiccup, a significant arterial pressure was noted. This observation of self-administered "cough CPR" prompted further investigations on the mechanism of blood flow, and these studies produced the theory of a thoracic pump mechanism for blood flow during closed-chest compressions.[46] According to this theory, blood flows into the thorax during the relaxation phase of chest compressions in the same manner as that described for the cardiac pump mechanism. During the compression phase, all intrathoracic structures are compressed equally by the rise in intrathoracic pressure caused by sternal depression, forcing blood out of the chest. Backward flow through the venous system is prevented by valves in the subclavian and internal jugular veins, and by dynamic compression of the veins at the thoracic outlet by the increased intrathoracic pressure. Thicker, less compressible vessel walls prevent collapse on the arterial side, although arterial collapse will occur if intrathoracic pressure is raised enough.[49] The heart is a passive conduit with the atrioventricular valves remaining open during chest compression. Because there is a significant pressure difference between the carotid artery and jugular vein, blood flow to the head is favored. The lack of valves in the inferior vena cava results in less resistance to backward flow, and pressures in the arteries and veins below the diaphragm are nearly equal. This is consistent with the fact that there is little blood flow to organs below the diaphragm.[50,51]

It seems clear that fluctuations in intrathoracic pressure plays a significant role in blood flow during CPR. It is also likely that compression of the heart occurs under some circumstances. Factors that influence the mechanism probably include the compliance and configuration of the chest wall, size of the heart, force of the sternal compressions, duration of cardiac arrest, and other undiscovered factors. Which mechanism predominates varies from victim to victim and even during the resuscitation of the same victim.

Distribution of Blood Flow During CPR. Whatever the predominant mechanism, total body blood flow (cardiac output) is reduced to 10 to 33% of normal during experimental closed-chest cardiac massage. Similar severe reductions in flow are likely during clinical CPR in humans. Nearly all the blood flow is directed to organs above the diaphragm.[50,51] Myocardial perfusion is 20 to 50% of normal, whereas cerebral perfusion is maintained at 50 to 90% of normal. Abdominal visceral and lower-extremity flow is reduced to 5% of normal. Total flow tends to decrease with time during CPR, but the relative distribution is not altered. Changes in CPR technique and the use of epinephrine may help sustain cardiac output over time.[51] Epinephrine improves flow to the brain and heart, whereas flow to organs below the diaphragm is unchanged or further reduced.

Gas Transport During CPR. During the low flow state of CPR, excretion of carbon dioxide (CO_2) (mL of CO_2/minute in exhaled gas) is decreased from prearrest levels to approximately the same extent as cardiac output is reduced. This reduced CO_2 excretion is due primarily to shunting of blood flow away from the lower half of the body. The exhaled CO_2 reflects only the metabolism of the part of the body that is being perfused. In the nonperfused areas, CO_2 accumulates during CPR. When normal circulation is restored, the accumulated CO_2 is washed out, and a temporary increase in CO_2 excretion is seen.

Although CO_2 excretion is reduced during CPR, measurement of blood gases reveals an arterial respiratory alkalosis and a venous respiratory acidosis with a markedly elevated arteriovenous CO_2 difference.[52,53] The primary cause of these changes is the severely reduced cardiac output. Two factors account for the elevation of the venous partial pressure of CO_2 ($Pv{CO_2}$). Buffering acid causes a reduction in serum bicarbonate so the same blood CO_2 content results in a higher $Pv{CO_2}$. In addition, the mixed venous CO_2 content is elevated. When flow to a tissue is reduced, all the CO_2 produced fails to be removed and CO_2 accumulates, raising the tissue partial pressure of CO_2. This allows more CO_2 to be carried in each aliquot of blood and mixed venous CO_2 content increases. If flow remains constant, a new equilibrium is established where all CO_2 produced in the tissue is removed but at a higher venous CO_2 content and partial pressure. In contrast to the venous blood, arterial CO_2 content and partial pressure ($Pa{CO_2}$) are usually reduced during CPR. This reduction accounts for most of the observed increase in arteriovenous CO_2 content difference. Even though venous blood may have an increased CO_2, the marked reduction in cardiac output with maintained ventilation results in efficient CO_2 removal.

Decreased pulmonary blood flow during CPR causes lack of perfusion to many nondependent alveoli. The alveolar gas of these lung units has no CO_2. Consequently, mixed alveolar CO_2 (i.e., end-tidal CO_2) will be low and correlate poorly with arterial CO_2. However, end-tidal CO_2 does correlate well with cardiac output during CPR. As flow increases, more alveoli become perfused, there is less alveolar dead space, and end-tidal CO_2 measurements rise.

Technique of Closed-Chest Compression

In an unconscious apneic patient, cardiac arrest must be assumed in the absence of a pulse in a major artery (carotid, femoral, axillary). Because a systolic pressure of ~50 mm Hg is necessary for a palpable pulse, some circulation may remain in the "pulseless" patient with primary respiratory arrest. Opening the airway and ventilation may be sufficient for resuscitation in such circumstances. Therefore, further search for a pulse should always be made following artificial ventilation and before beginning sternal compressions.

Important considerations in performing closed-chest compressions are the position of the rescuer relative to the victim, the position of the rescuer's hands, and the rate and force of compression. The victim must be supine, the head level with the heart, for adequate brain perfusion. The victim must be on a firm surface. The rescuer should stand or kneel next to the victim's side. Compressions are performed most effectively if the rescuer's hips are on the same level, or slightly above the level of, the victim's chest.

Standard technique consists of the rhythmic application of pressure over the lower half of the sternum. The heel of one hand is placed on the lower sternum, and the other hand is placed on top of the first. Great care must be taken to avoid pressing the xiphoid into the abdomen, which can lacerate the liver. Even with properly performed CPR, costochondral separation and rib fractures are common. Applying pressure on the ribs by improper hand placement increases these complications and risks puncturing the lung. Pressure on the sternum should be applied through the heel of the hand only, keeping the fingers free of the chest wall. The direction of force must be straight down on the sternum, with the arms straight and the elbows locked into position so the entire weight of the upper body is used to apply force. During relaxation, all pressure should be removed from the hands, but they should not lose contact with the chest wall.

The sternum must be depressed 3.5 to 5.0 cm in the average adult. Occasionally, deeper compressions are necessary to generate a palpable pulse. The duration of compression should be equal to that of relaxation, and the compression rate should be 80 to 100 times/min. This rate seems to be optimal for both possible mechanisms of blood flow. The faster rate makes it easier to maintain a 50% compression–relaxation ratio, important in the thoracic pump mechanism. It also requires a rapid, more forceful compression that may be important in the cardiac pump mechanism.[70] A fast rate also allows time to pause for ventilations. With a single rescuer, two ventilations should be given following every 15 compressions. With two rescuers, a 1.5- to 2.0-second pause for ventilation should occur every 5 compressions. With an endotracheal tube in place, ventilations at a rate of 12 breaths/min should be interposed between compressions without a pause.

Alternative Methods of Circulatory Support

As currently practiced, CPR has limited success, with only ~40% of victims being admitted to the hospital and 10% surviving to discharge. Despite the occasional success of prolonged resuscitation, standard CPR will sustain most patients for only 15 to 30 minutes. If return of spontaneous circulation has not been achieved in that time, the outcome is dismal. Recognition of these limits and improved understanding of circulatory physiology during CPR have led to several proposals for alternatives to the standard techniques of closed-chest compression. Most, but not all, are based on the thoracic pump mechanism of blood flow. The goals of the new methods are to provide better hemodynamics during CPR and thus improve survival and/or to extend the duration during which CPR can success-
3 fully support viability. Unfortunately, none of the alternatives has proved reliably superior to the standard technique.

Simultaneous Ventilation–Compression CPR and Abdominal Binding. According to the thoracic pump theory, elevation of intrathoracic pressure during chest compression should improve blood flow and pressure.[49] Initial studies with techniques that raise intrathoracic pressure (abdominal binding, simultaneous ventilation/compression) were encouraging because the increased aortic pressure suggested better myocardial and cerebral perfusion.[54,55] Subsequent investigations have demonstrated that right atrial pressure and intracranial pressure are elevated as much as, or more than, the arterial pressures.[56–59] Thus, no improvement in myocardial or cerebral blood flow is found. Most important, survival from cardiac arrest is not improved when these techniques are compared with standard CPR in experimental animals or limited human trials.[59–63]

Interposed Abdominal Compression CPR. Interposed abdominal compression (IAC) is fundamentally different from abdominal binding. With this technique, an additional rescuer applies abdominal compressions manually during the relaxation phase of chest compression.[64] Abdominal pressure is released when chest compression begins.[65] One large randomized trial of out-of-hospital cardiac arrest with IAC CPR found no improvement in survival compared with standard CPR,[66] but a subsequent in-hospital study demonstrated improved outcome.[67] The safety of IAC CPR has been established and is recommended as an alternative to standard CPR for in-hospital resuscitation. Further studies will be needed to establish out-of-hospital efficacy.

Pneumatic Vest CPR. Following the description of "cough CPR" and the development of the thoracic pump theory, a pneumatic vest device was developed that would simulate the events of vigorous coughing.[68,69] With the original method, thoracic and abdominal vests containing pneumatic bladders inflate simultaneously with positive-pressure ventilation. The technique continues to be investigated with a number of modifications from the original method. In a preliminary clinical study, aortic and coronary perfusion pressure was better with the vest than with standard CPR, but survival was not significantly improved.[70] Randomized human trials are now being conducted.

Active Compression–Decompression CPR. The newest proposed alternative technique developed from the anecdotal report of CPR performed with a plumber's helper applied to the anterior chest wall.[71] This suggested that active decompression of the chest wall might reduce intrathoracic pressure during the relaxation phase of chest compressions, leading to improved venous return, increased stroke volume with compression, and better blood flow. A suction device that can be applied to the chest wall to enable active compression and decompression was developed.[72] Hemodynamic studies in animals and humans with this technique have shown that coronary and cerebral perfusion may be somewhat improved with this method compared with standard CPR, although when epinephrine is used there is no difference between techniques.[72,73] Early clinical trials of this technique were discouraging, but more recent reports have had conflicting results.[74–76] A large randomized trial in France found improved outcome in out-of-hospital arrest.[77] However, a large study in Canada involving in-hospital and out-of-hospital arrests found no difference in immediate resuscitation or survival.[78]

Invasive Techniques. In contrast to the closed-chest techniques, two invasive methods have been able to maintain cardiac and cerebral viability during long periods of cardiac arrest. In animal models, open-chest cardiac massage and cardiopulmonary bypass (through the femoral artery and vein using a membrane oxygenator) can provide better hemodynamics, as well as better myocardial and cerebral perfusion, than closed-chest techniques.[57,79] Preliminary trials of percutaneous cardiopulmonary bypass for refractory human cardiac arrest have been reported.[80–82] Prompt restoration of blood flow and perfusion pressure with cardiopulmonary bypass can provide resuscitation with minimal neurologic deficit after 20 minutes of fibrillatory cardiac arrest in canines.[15] However, these techniques must be instituted relatively early (probably within 20 to 30 minutes of arrest) to be effective.[16,83] If open chest massage is begun after 30 minutes of ineffective closed-chest compressions, survival is no better even though hemodynamics are improved.[84] The need to apply these maneuvers early in an arrest obviously limits the application. Before invasive procedures play a greater role in modern CPR, a method must be developed to predict, early in resuscitation, which patients will and will not respond to closed-chest compressions.

Assessing the Adequacy of Circulation During CPR

The adequacy of closed-chest compression is usually judged by palpation of a pulse in the carotid or femoral vessels. The palpable pulse primarily reflects systolic pressure. Cardiac output correlates better with mean pressure and coronary perfusion with diastolic pressure. In the femoral area, the palpable pulse is as likely to be venous as arterial. Despite these shortcomings, palpating the pulse remains the only monitor available during BLS.

4 Return of spontaneous circulation with an arrested heart greatly depends on restoring oxygenated blood flow to the myocardium. In experimental models, a minimum blood flow of 15 to 20 mL/min/100 g of myocardium has been shown to be necessary for successful resuscitation.[85] Obtaining such flow depends on closed-chest compressions developing adequate cardiac output and coronary perfusion pressure. Similar to the beating heart, coronary perfusion during CPR occurs primarily in the relaxation phase (diastole) of chest compressions. In 1906, Crile and Dolley suggested that a critical coronary perfusion pressure was necessary for successful resuscitation.[86] This concept has been confirmed in numerous other reports.[51,85–95] During standard CPR, critical myocardial blood flow is associated with aortic diastolic pressure exceeding 40 mm Hg. Because right atrial pressure can be elevated with some techniques, the aortic diastolic pressure minus the right atrial diastolic pressure is a more accurate reflection of coronary perfusion pressure. The critical coronary perfusion pressure is 15 to 25 mm Hg. When invasive monitoring is available during CPR, adjustments in chest compression technique and epinephrine should be used to ensure critical perfusion pressures are exceeded. Damage to the myocardium from underlying disease may preclude survival no matter how effective the CPR efforts. However, vascular pressures below critical levels are associated with poor results even in patients who may be salvageable (Table 58-2).

TABLE 58-2

CRITICAL VARIABLES ASSOCIATED WITH SUCCESSFUL RESUSCITATION

VARIABLE	AMOUNT
Mycocardial blood flow (mL/min/100 g)	>15–20
Aortic diastolic pressure (mm Hg)	>40
Coronary perfusion pressure (mm Hg)	>15–25
End-tidal carbon dioxide (mm Hg)	>10

Although invasive pressure monitoring may be ideal, it is rarely available during CPR. End-tidal CO_2 also has been found to be an excellent noninvasive guide to the adequacy of closed-chest compressions.[96] Carbon dioxide excretion during CPR with an endotracheal tube in place is flow dependent rather than ventilation dependent. Because alveolar dead space is large in low-flow states, end-tidal CO_2 is very low (frequently <10 mm Hg). If blood flow improves with better CPR technique, more alveoli are perfused and end-tidal CO_2 rises (usually to >20 mm Hg with successful CPR). The earliest sign of return of spontaneous circulation is frequently a sudden increase in end-tidal CO_2 to >40 mm Hg. Within a wide range of cardiac outputs during CPR, end-tidal CO_2 correlates well with cardiac output,[97] coronary perfusion pressure,[98] and initial resuscitation.[99] End-tidal CO_2 correlates with survival in human CPR and can predict outcome.[100,101] Patients with end-tidal CO_2 <10 mm Hg will not be resuscitated successfully. In the absence of invasive monitoring, end-tidal CO_2 should be used to judge the effectiveness of chest compressions, whenever possible.[102] Attempts should be made to maximize the measured end-tidal CO_2 by alterations in technique or drug therapy. It should be remembered that sodium bicarbonate administration liberates CO_2 into the blood and causes a temporary increase in end-tidal CO_2. The elevation returns to baseline within 3 to 5 minutes of drug administration and end-tidal CO_2 monitoring can again be used for monitoring effectiveness of closed-chest compressions.

ADVANCED CARDIAC LIFE SUPPORT

ACLS encompasses all the cognitive and technical skills that are necessary to restore spontaneous circulatory function when simple support does not result in resuscitation. In addition to BLS skills, it includes use of adjunctive equipment and techniques for assisting ventilation and circulation, electrocardiogram (ECG) monitoring with dysrhythmia recognition and defibrillation, establishment of intravenous access, and pharmacologic therapy. A number of aspects of ACLS have been discussed in previous sections. The following sections concentrate on electrical and drug treatment, as well as the generalized

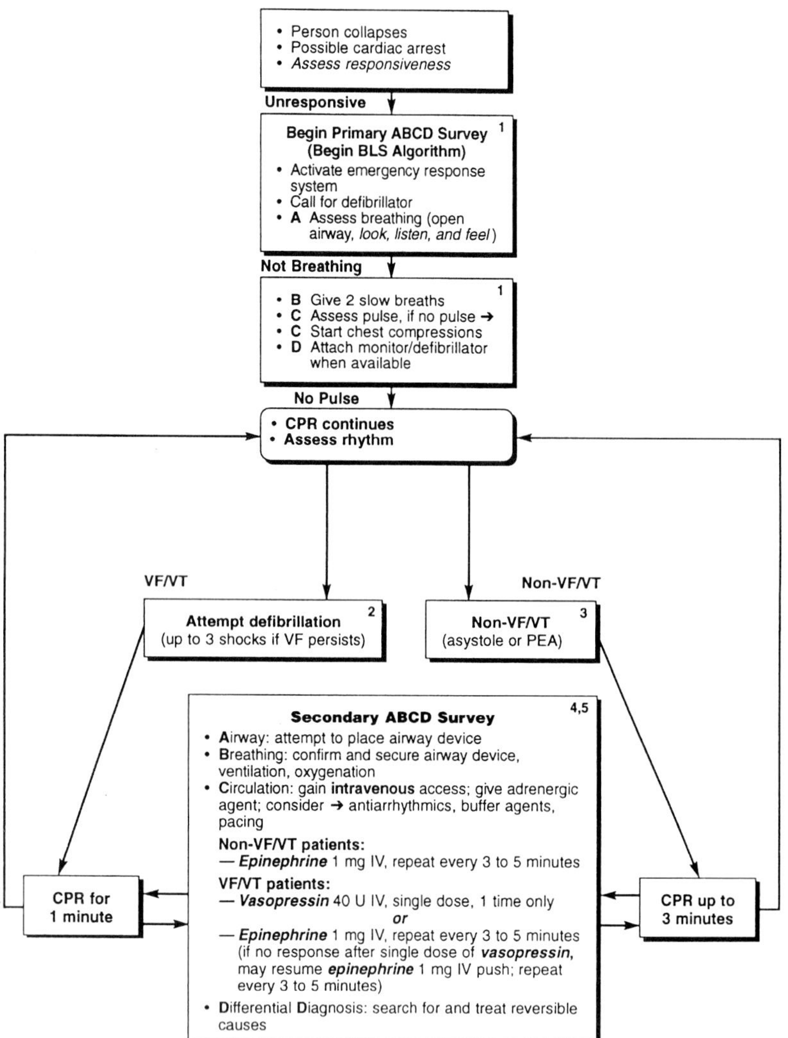

FIGURE 58-1. Comprehensive emergency cardiac care algorithm. BLS, basic life support; CPR, cardiopulmonary resuscitation; IV, intravenous(ly); PEA, pulseless electrical activity; VF, ventricular fibrillation; VT, ventricular tachycardia. (Reprinted with permission from American Heart Association: Guidelines 2000 for cardiopulmonary resuscitation and emergency cardiovascular care: International consensus on science. Circulation 102:I-144, 2000.)

ACLS algorithms. Figure 58-1 demonstrates the universal algorithm for adult emergency cardiac care.

Defibrillation

Electrical Pattern and Duration of Ventricular Fibrillation

Ventricular fibrillation is the most common ECG pattern found during cardiac arrest in adults. The only consistently effective treatment is electrical defibrillation. The most important controllable determinant of failure to resuscitate a patient with ventricular fibrillation is the duration of fibrillation.[103] Other important factors, such as underlying disease and metabolic status, are largely beyond the control of rescuers. The fibrillating heart has high oxygen consumption, increasing myocardial ischemia and decreasing the time to irreversible cell damage. The longer ventricular fibrillation continues, the more difficult it is to defibrillate and the less likely is successful resuscitation.[83,104] If defibrillation occurs within 1 minute of fibrillation, CPR is unnecessary for resuscitation. Initial resuscitation success following out-of-hospital fibrillation and survival to hospital discharge are improved the earlier that defibrillation is accomplished.[18,20,105]

The coarseness of the fibrillatory waves on the ECG may reflect the severity and duration of the myocardial insult, and thus, have prognostic significance.[106] However, the fibrillation amplitude seen on any one ECG lead varies with the orientation of that lead to the vector of the fibrillatory wave.[107] If the lead is oriented at right angles to the fibrillatory wave, a flat line can be seen. For this reason, the trace from a second lead or from a different position of paddle electrodes should always be inspected before a decision is made not to defibrillate. Low-*amplitude* fibrillatory waveforms are less likely to be associated with successful resuscitation and more likely to convert to asystole following defibrillation.[106] Similarly, low-*frequency* fibrillatory waveforms are associated with poor outcome, and the median frequency of the waveform correlates with myocardial perfusion during CPR and with success of defibrillation.[108,109] Catecholamines with β-adrenergic activity increase the vigor of fibrillation and the amplitude of the electrical activity, leading to the practice of administering epinephrine to make it "easier" to defibrillate. However, experimental work has shown that manipulation of the electrical pattern with epinephrine does not influence the success of defibrillation or reduce the energy needed for defibrillation.[104,110] Consequently, defibrillation should not be delayed for drug administration. The algorithm for managing ventricular fibrillation–tachycardia is illustrated in Fig. 58-2.

Current CPR guidelines recommend that defibrillation should not be postponed for any other therapy but should be carried out as soon as fibrillation is diagnosed and the equipment is available. The application of this principle has been made much easier by the development of automatic external defibrillators that recognize ventricular fibrillation, charge

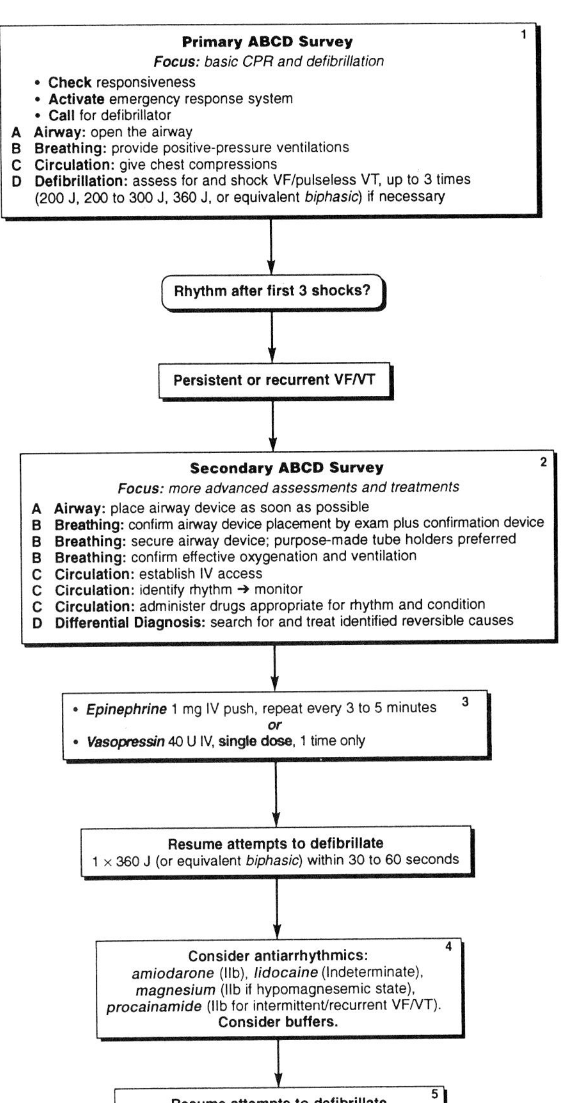

Primary ABCD Survey
1
Focus: basic CPR and defibrillation
• Check responsiveness
• Activate emergency response system
• Call for defibrillator
A Airway: open the airway
B Breathing: provide positive-pressure ventilations
C Circulation: give chest compressions
D Defibrillation: assess for and shock VF/pulseless VT, up to 3 times (200 J, 200 to 300 J, 360 J, or equivalent biphasic) if necessary
Rhythm after first 3 shocks?
Persistent or recurrent VF/VT
Secondary ABCD Survey
2
Focus: more advanced assessments and treatments
A Airway: place airway device as soon as possible
B Breathing: confirm airway device placement by exam plus confirmation device
B Breathing: secure airway device; purpose-made tube holders preferred
B Breathing: confirm effective oxygenation and ventilation
C Circulation: establish IV access
C Circulation: identify rhythm → monitor
C Circulation: administer drugs appropriate for rhythm and condition
D Differential Diagnosis: search for and treat identified reversible causes
• Epinephrine 1 mg IV push, repeat every 3 to 5 minutes
3
or
• Vasopressin 40 U IV, single dose, 1 time only
Resume attempts to defibrillate
1 × 360 J (or equivalent biphasic) within 30 to 60 seconds
Consider antiarrhythmics:
4
amiodarone (IIb), lidocaine (Indeterminate),
magnesium (IIb if hypomagnesemic state),
procainamide (IIb for intermittent/recurrent VF/VT).
Consider buffers.
Resume attempts to defibrillate
5

FIGURE 58-2. Ventricular fibrillation (VF)/pulseless ventricular tachycardia (VT) algorithm. CPR, cardiopulmonary resuscitation; IV, intravenous(ly). (Reprinted with permission from American Heart Association: Guidelines 2000 for cardiopulmonary resuscitation and emergency cardiovascular care: International consensus on science. Circulation 102:I-147, 2000.)

automatically, and give a defibrillatory shock.[111] This device has allowed the introduction of public access defibrillation because minimally trained individuals can incorporate defibrillation into BLS skills, improving survival in out-of-hospital arrest by reducing time to delivery of the first shock.[18–21,112] The algorithms these devices use to detect ventricular fibrillation are accurate with nearly perfect specificity. They will not defibrillate a nonfibrillatory rhythm. Sensitivity rates are somewhat lower. They sometimes have trouble recognizing low-amplitude ventricular fibrillation and can misinterpret pacemaker spikes as QRS complexes. Unfortunately, rhythm analysis can require up to 90 seconds during which chest compressions are not being given. This may adversely influence outcome in some circumstances. The improved success with public access defibrillation was dramatically demonstrated by the results of installing automatic external defibrillators (AEDs) in Chicago airports where, over the first 2 years, there was a 55% 1-year neurologically intact survival.[113] Similarly, when AEDs were installed in Las Vegas casinos and security personnel instructed in their use, there was a 53% survival to discharge (74% in patients who received the shock within 3 minutes of collapse).[114]

However, what if defibrillation is not really applied early after collapse? In the usual out-of-hospital rescue with emergency medical technicians or paramedics doing the defibrillation, a rapid response is to apply the first shock in 6 to 7 minutes and frequently it may be more than 10 minutes. In Seattle, it has been noted that patients who had CPR prior to defibrillation had a better survival, and the improvement was accounted for by better results in the group of patients in whom the response time was greater than 4 minutes.[115] In a randomized trial of 200 out-of-hospital cardiac arrests in Oslo, there was a highly significant improvement in outcome if CPR was provided before defibrillation when the response time was greater than 5
5 minutes.[116] Consequently, it now appears that immediate defibrillation is only effective if applied within 4 to 5 minutes of collapse. Otherwise, a brief period of 2 to 3 minutes of chest compressions before defibrillation is necessary. The precordial thump, although rarely successful, can be tried while awaiting a defibrillator. It should not be used for the conscious patient with ventricular tachycardia unless a defibrillator is immediately available. It is as likely to induce fibrillation as normal rhythm. Blind defibrillation should no longer be necessary because modern defibrillators have built-in monitoring capability using the paddles as electrodes.

Defibrillators: Energy, Current, and Voltage

Defibrillators derive power from a line source of alternating current or an integral battery. The typical defibrillator consists of a variable transformer that allows selection of a variable voltage potential, an AC/DC converter to provide a direct current that is stored in a capacitor, a switch to charge the capacitor, and discharge switches to complete the circuit from capacitor to electrodes. Until more recently, the current waveform of most clinically used defibrillators was a damped half-sinusoid, although some delivered trapezoidal or near-square waves. Implantable defibrillators use multipulse, multipathway defibrillation, but such techniques have had conflicting results in transthoracic defibrillation. Many newer defibrillators deliver a biphasic, truncated, exponential waveform for transthoracic defibrillation. This is the waveform used in AEDs and allows successful defibrillation at lower energies than MDS waveforms.[117]

Defibrillation is accomplished by current passing through a critical mass of myocardium causing simultaneous depolarization of the myofibrils. However, the output of most defibrillators is indicated in energy units (joules or watt-seconds), not current (amperes). The relationships among energy, current, and impedance (resistance) are given by the following equations (standard units are indicated):

$$\text{Energy (joules)} = \text{Power (watts)} \times \text{Duration (seconds)} \tag{58.1}$$

$$\text{Power (watts)} = \text{Potential (volts)} \times \text{Current (amperes)} \tag{58.2}$$

$$\text{Current (amperes)} = \text{Potential (volts)/Resistance (ohms)} \tag{58.3}$$

$$\text{Current (amperes)} = \{\text{Energy (joules)/[Resistance (ohms)} \times \text{Duration (seconds)]}\}^{1/2} \tag{58.4}$$

From these equations, it can be determined that as the impedance between the paddle electrodes increases, the delivered energy will be reduced. Because internal resistance is low, the primary determinant of delivered energy will be transthoracic impedance. For consistency, the energy level indicated on most commercially available defibrillators is the output when discharged into a 50-ohm load. When transthoracic impedance is higher than that standard, actual delivered energy will be lower. Even at a constant delivered energy, Eq. (58-4) indicates that delivered current (the critical determinant of defibrillation) will be reduced as impedance increases. At high impedance and relatively low energy levels, current could be too low for defibrillation. Optimal success of defibrillation is obtained by keeping impedance as low as possible.

Transthoracic Impedance

Transthoracic impedance has been measured between 15 to 143 ohms in human defibrillation.[118] Many of the important factors in minimizing transthoracic impedance are under the control of the rescuers. Resistance decreases with increasing electrode size, and studies suggest that optimal paddle size may be 13 cm in diameter.[119,120] Concern has been expressed that a paddle this large may diffuse the current over too great an area for effective defibrillation. The most common paddle size remains 8 to 10 cm in diameter. The high impedance between metal electrode and skin can be reduced somewhat by use of saline-soaked gauze pads or creams, such as those used for recording ECGs. However, resistance is least when a gel or paste specifically designed to conduct electricity in the defibrillation setting is used.[119,120] Self-adhesive defibrillation/monitor pads also work well when carefully applied. When paste is used, it should be applied liberally to the paddle surface, especially the edges, to prevent burns and to obtain the maximum reduction in impedance. In experimental models, transthoracic impedance decreases with successive shocks.[121] Although the clinical significance has been questioned,[118] this factor may partially explain why an additional shock of the same energy can cause defibrillation when previous shocks have failed. Transthoracic impedance is slightly, but significantly, higher during inspiration than during exhalation.[122] Air is a poor electrical conductor. Firm paddle pressure of at least 11 kg reduces resistance by improving paddle-to-skin contact and by expelling air from the lungs.[118]

The average transthoracic impedance in human defibrillation is 70 to 80 ohms. Resistance is probably of little clinical significance when reasonably proper technique and high energy (300 J) shocks are used. For lower energy shocks, great care should be taken to minimize resistance. Defibrillators have been developed that measure transthoracic impedance prior to the shock by passing a low-voltage current through the chest during the charge cycle.[123,124] This allows the use of low-energy shocks in appropriate patients and identification of victims needing higher energy. Although not widely used, this technology allows current-based defibrillation by adjusting the delivered energy for the measured resistance.[125]

Adverse Effects and Energy Requirements

Repeated defibrillation with high energy in animals can be associated with dysrhythmias, ECG changes suggesting myocardial damage, and morphologic evidence of myocardial necrosis.[126,127] Whether similar injuries occur in humans is less certain. Slight elevations in creatine kinase MB fractions have been measured in patients following cardioversion with high energies.[128] A higher incidence of atrioventricular block has been observed in patients receiving high-energy shocks than in patients receiving low-energy shock.[129] It seems likely that high-energy shocks, especially if repeated at close intervals, may result in myocardial damage. Therefore, it would be prudent to keep energy levels as low as possible during defibrillation attempts. However, if energy is too low, the delivered current may be insufficient for defibrillation, especially when transthoracic impedance is high.

When using monophasic waveforms, there is a general relationship between body size and energy requirements for defibrillation. Geddes et al observed that the current necessary for defibrillation in animals increased with increasing body mass.[130] Children need less energy than adults, perhaps as low as 0.5 J/kg,[131] although the recommended dose is 2.0 J/kg.[24] However, over the size range of adults, weight variability is not clinically significant and other factors are more important.[132] Multiple studies have demonstrated high rates of successful defibrillation using relatively low levels (160 to 200 J) of delivered energy.[133–136] Studies of out-of-hospital and in-hospital arrests have demonstrated equal success when using ≤200 J initial energy compared with administering all shocks at energies ≥300 J.[129,137] Therefore, when using defibrillators with a monophasic waveform, current recommendations are to use 200 J for the initial shock followed by a second shock at 200 to 300 J if the first is unsuccessful. If both fail to defibrillate the patient, additional shocks should be given at 300 to 360 J (see Fig. 58-2).[24] When using defibrillators with a biphasic waveform, 150 J shocks provide similar success to the escalating energies used with monophasic waveforms. It is not yet clear if escalating biphasic energies improve success in difficult defibrillation.

Pharmacologic Therapy

This discussion of drug therapy is confined to the use of drugs during CPR attempts to restore spontaneous circulation. The use of drugs to support the circulation when there is mechanical cardiac function is discussed elsewhere (see Chapters 12 and 32). During cardiac arrest, drug therapy is secondary to other interventions. Chest compressions, airway management, ventilation, and defibrillation, if appropriate, should take precedence over medications. Establishing intravenous access and pharmacologic therapy should come after other interventions are established. The most common drugs and the appropriate adult doses are shown in Table 58-3. Of the drugs given during CPR, only vasopressors are usually acknowledged as being helpful in restoring spontaneous circulation.[138] Asystole and pulseless electrical activity (PEA), also called electromechanical dissociation (EMD), are circumstances in which drugs are

TABLE 58-3

ADULT ADVANCED CARDIAC LIFE SUPPORT DRUGS AND DOSES (INTRAVENOUS)

	DOSE	INTERVAL	MAXIMUM
Epinephrine	1 mg	Every 3–5 min	None
If dose fails, consider	3–7 mg	Every 3–5 min	None
Amiodarone	300 mg	Repeat in 3–5 min	2 g
Lidocaine	1.5 mg/kg	Repeat in 3–5 min	3.0 mg/kg
Bretylium tosylate	5 mg/kg	Repeat in 5 min	10 mg/kg
Atropine	1 mg	Every 3–5 min	0.04 mg/kg
Sodium bicarbonate	1 mEq/kg	As needed	Check pH

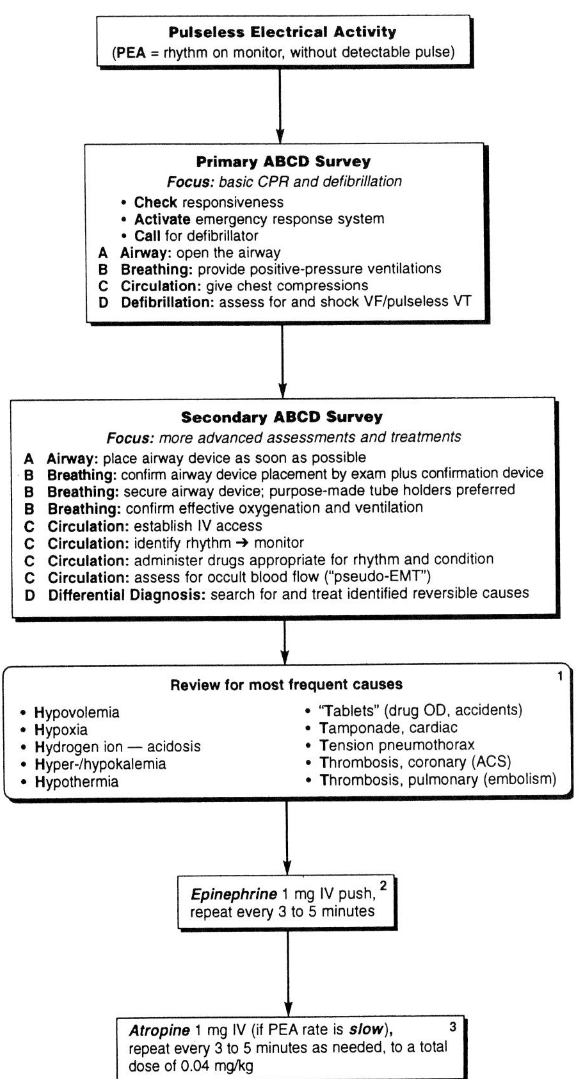

FIGURE 58-3. Pulseless electrical activity (PEA) algorithm. ACS, acute coronary syndrome; CPR, cardiopulmonary resuscitation; EMT, emergency medical technician; IV, intravenous(ly); OD, overdose; VF, ventricular fibrillation; VT, ventricular tachycardia. (Reprinted with permission from American Heart Association: Guidelines 2000 for cardiopulmonary resuscitation and emergency cardiovascular care: International consensus on science. Circulation 102:I-151, 2000.)

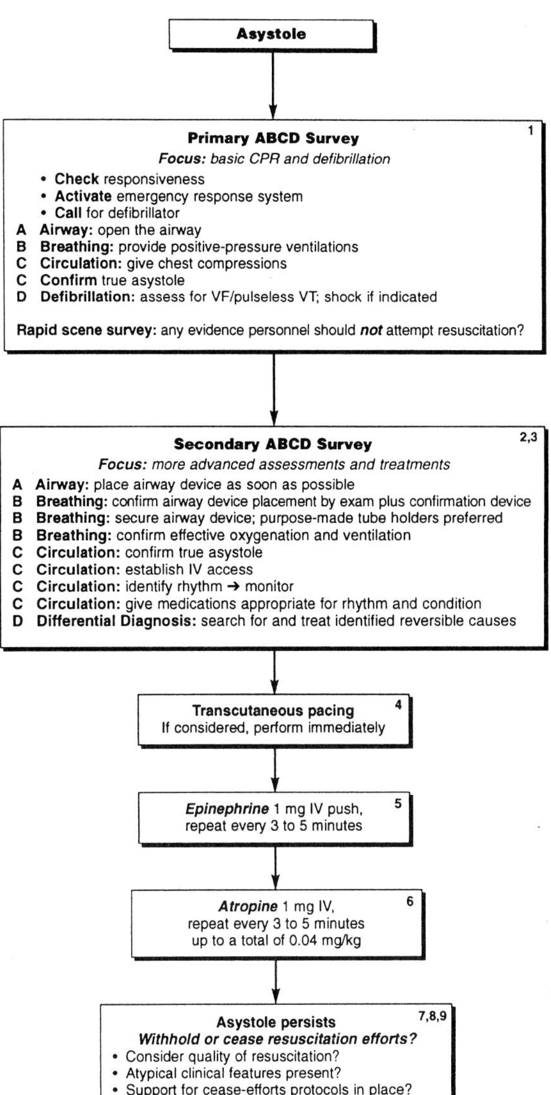

FIGURE 58-4. Asystole: The silent heart algorithm. CPR, cardiopulmonary resuscitation; IV, intravenous(ly); VF, ventricular fibrillation; VT, ventricular tachycardia. (Reprinted with permission from American Heart Association: Guidelines 2000 for cardiopulmonary resuscitation and emergency cardiovascular care: International consensus on science. Circulation 102:I-153, 2000.)

most frequently given. The standard algorithms for management of these types of cardiac arrest are shown in Figs. 58-3 and 58-4. In addition, the algorithms for the American Heart Association protocols for bradycardia, tachycardia, shock, and synchronized cardioversion are included (Figs. 58-5 to 58-8).

Routes of Administration

The preferred route of administration of all drugs during CPR is intravenous. The most rapid and highest drug levels occur with administration into a central vein. However, peripheral intravenous administration is also effective. The antecubital and external jugular veins are the sites of first choice for starting an infusion during resuscitation because inserting a central catheter usually necessitates stopping CPR. Because of poor blood flow below the diaphragm during CPR, drugs administered in the lower extremity may be extremely delayed or not reach the sites of action. Even in the upper extremity, drugs may require 1 to 2 minutes to reach the central circulation. Onset of action may be speeded if the drug bolus is followed by a 20- to 30-mL bolus of intravenous fluid. If intravenous access cannot be established, the endotracheal tube is an alternative route for administration of epinephrine, lidocaine, and atropine. (Sodium bicarbonate should not be given endotracheally.) The time to effect and drug levels achieved are inconsistent using this route during CPR. Better results may be obtained by administering 5- to 10-mL volumes. It is unclear whether deep injection is better than simple instillation into the endotracheal tube. Doses 2 to 2.5 times higher than the recommended intravenous dose should be administered when this route is used.

Catecholamines and Vasopressors

Mechanism of Action. Epinephrine has been used in resuscitation since the 1890s and has been the vasopressor of choice in modern CPR since the studies of Redding and Pearson in the 1960s.[13,139] The efficacy of epinephrine lies entirely in its α-adrenergic properties.[92] Peripheral vasoconstriction leads to an increase in aortic diastolic pressure, causing

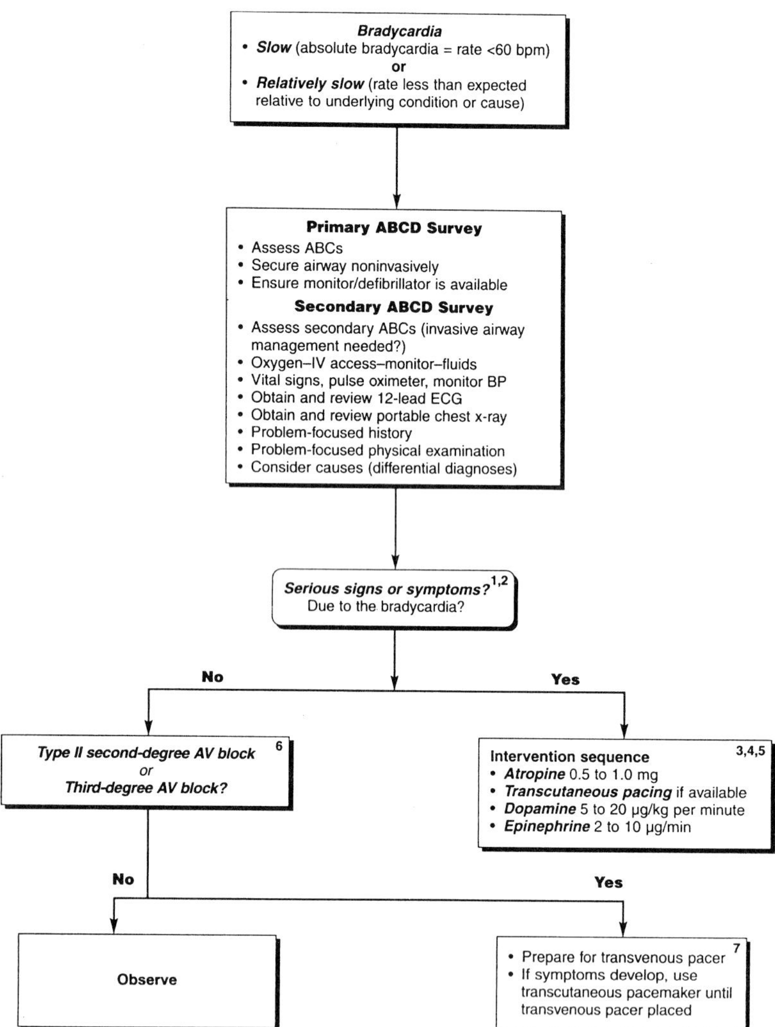

FIGURE 58-5. Bradycardia algorithm. ABCs, airway, breathing, and circulation; AV, atrioventricular; BP, blood pressure; ECG, electrocardiogram; IV, intravenous(ly). (Reprinted with permission from American Heart Association: Guidelines 2000 for cardiopulmonary resuscitation and emergency cardiovascular care: International consensus on science. Circulation 102:I-156, 2000.)

an increase in coronary perfusion pressure and myocardial
6 blood flow.[51,140,141] All strong α-adrenergic drugs (epinephrine, phenylephrine, methoxamine, dopamine, norepinephrine), regardless of β-adrenergic potency, are equally successful in aiding resuscitation, as are strong nonadrenergic vasopressors (vasopressin, endothelin-1).[13,139,142,143] β-Adrenergic agonists without α activity (isoproterenol, dobutamine) are no better than placebo. α-Adrenergic blockade precludes resuscitation, whereas β-adrenergic blockade has no effect on the ability to restore spontaneous circulation.[89,90]

The β-adrenergic effects of epinephrine are potentially deleterious during cardiac arrest. In the fibrillating heart, epinephrine increases oxygen consumption and decreases the endocardial–epicardial blood flow ratio, an effect not seen with methoxamine. Myocardial lactate production in the fibrillating heart is unchanged after epinephrine administration during CPR, suggesting that the increased coronary blood flow does not improve the oxygen supply–demand ratio. Large doses of epinephrine increase deaths in swine early after resuscitation due to tachyarrhythmias and hypertension, an effect partially offset by metoprolol treatment. Despite these theoretical considerations, survival and neurologic outcome studies have shown no difference when epinephrine is compared with a pure α-agonist (methoxamine or phenylephrine) during CPR in animals[139,144] or humans.[145]

Epinephrine. When added to chest compressions, epinephrine helps develop the critical coronary perfusion pressure necessary to provide enough myocardial blood flow for restoration of spontaneous circulation. With invasive monitoring present during CPR, an arterial diastolic pressure of 40 mm Hg or coronary perfusion pressure of 20 mm Hg must be obtained with good chest compression technique and/or epinephrine therapy (see Table 58-2). In the absence of such monitoring, the dose of epinephrine must be chosen empirically. For many years, the empiric standard intravenous dose used has been 0.5 to 1.0 mg. However, animal studies in the 1980s suggested that higher doses of epinephrine in human CPR might improve myocardial and cerebral perfusion, and improve success of resuscitation. Case reports and a series of children with historical controls were published of return of spontaneous circulation when large doses (0.1 to 0.2 mg/kg) of epinephrine were given to patients who had failed resuscitation with standard doses.

Subsequent outcome studies have not demonstrated conclusively that higher doses of epinephrine will improve survival. Eight adult prospective randomized clinical trials involving more than 9,000 cardiac arrest patients have found no improvement in survival to hospital discharge or neurologic outcome, even in subgroups, when initial high-dose epinephrine (5 to 18 mg) is compared with standard doses (1 to 2 mg).[146–153] Some of the studies (and the cumulative data) suggest that there may be an improvement in immediate resuscitation with high-dose epinephrine. None of the studies found improvement in survival to hospital discharge. Retrospective studies of epinephrine dosing have suggested that higher doses may be associated with impaired postresuscitation

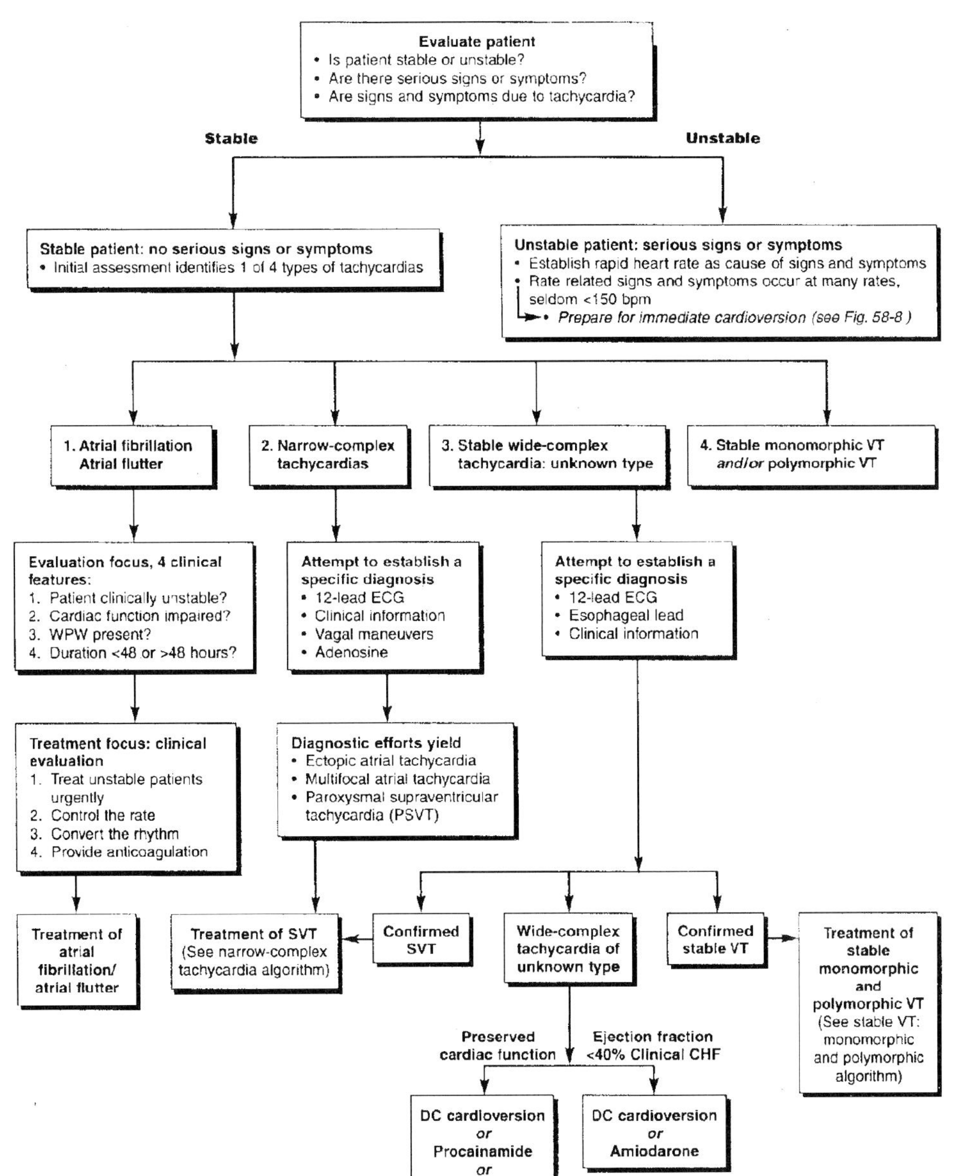

FIGURE 58-6. The tachycardia overview algorithm. CHF, congestive heart failure; DC, direct current; ECG, electrocardiogram; SVT, supraventricular tachycardia; VT, ventricular tachycardia. (Reprinted with permission from American Heart Association: Guidelines 2000 for cardiopulmonary resuscitation and emergency cardiovascular care: International consensus on science. Circulation 102:I-159, 2000.)

cardiovascular function and worse neurologic outcome.[154,155] None of the prospective studies found lower survival or worse neurologic outcome with higher epinephrine dosing.

It should be noted that these outcome studies used high-dose
7 epinephrine as initial therapy. High doses apparently are not needed early in most cardiac arrests and could be deleterious under some circumstances. The successful case reports were in patients who had failed conventional treatment. The high doses were given late in prolonged CPR when the vasculature may not be as responsive to catecholamines. Although the use of high-dose epinephrine as rescue therapy when standard doses have failed has not been rigorously studied, this may be its appropriate place in CPR practice. Current recommendations are to give 1 mg intravenously every 3 to 5 minutes in the adult. If this dose seems ineffective, higher doses (3 to 8 mg) should be considered (see Figs. 58-2 to 58-4).

Vasopressin. The newest addition to the pharmacologic armamentarium in CPR is arginine vasopressin. It is currently recommended as an alternative to epinephrine in a dose of 40 units intravenously one time only. If additional vasopressor doses are needed, epinephrine should be used. Vasopressin is a naturally occurring hormone (antidiuretic hormone) that, when administered in high doses, is a potent nonadrenergic vasoconstrictor, acting by stimulation of smooth muscle V_1 receptors. It is usually not recommended for conscious patients with coronary artery disease because the increased peripheral vascular resistance may provoke angina. The half-life in the intact circulation is 10 to 20 minutes and longer than epinephrine during CPR. Animal studies have demonstrated that vasopressin is as effective as or more effective than epinephrine in maintaining vital organ blood flow during CPR. Repeated doses during prolonged CPR in swine were associated with significantly improved rates of neurologically intact survival compared with epinephrine and placebo. Postresuscitation myocardial depression and splanchnic blood flow reduction are more marked with vasopressin than epinephrine, but they are transient and can be treated with low doses of dopamine.[156] Preliminary clinical studies indicate that vasopressin is as effective as epinephrine, but have not definitively shown it to be superior. A small randomized, blinded study comparing vasopressin and standard dose epinephrine in 40 patients with out-of-hospital ventricular fibrillation found improved 24-hour survival with vasopressin, but no difference in return of spontaneous circulation or survival to hospital discharge.[157] A larger,

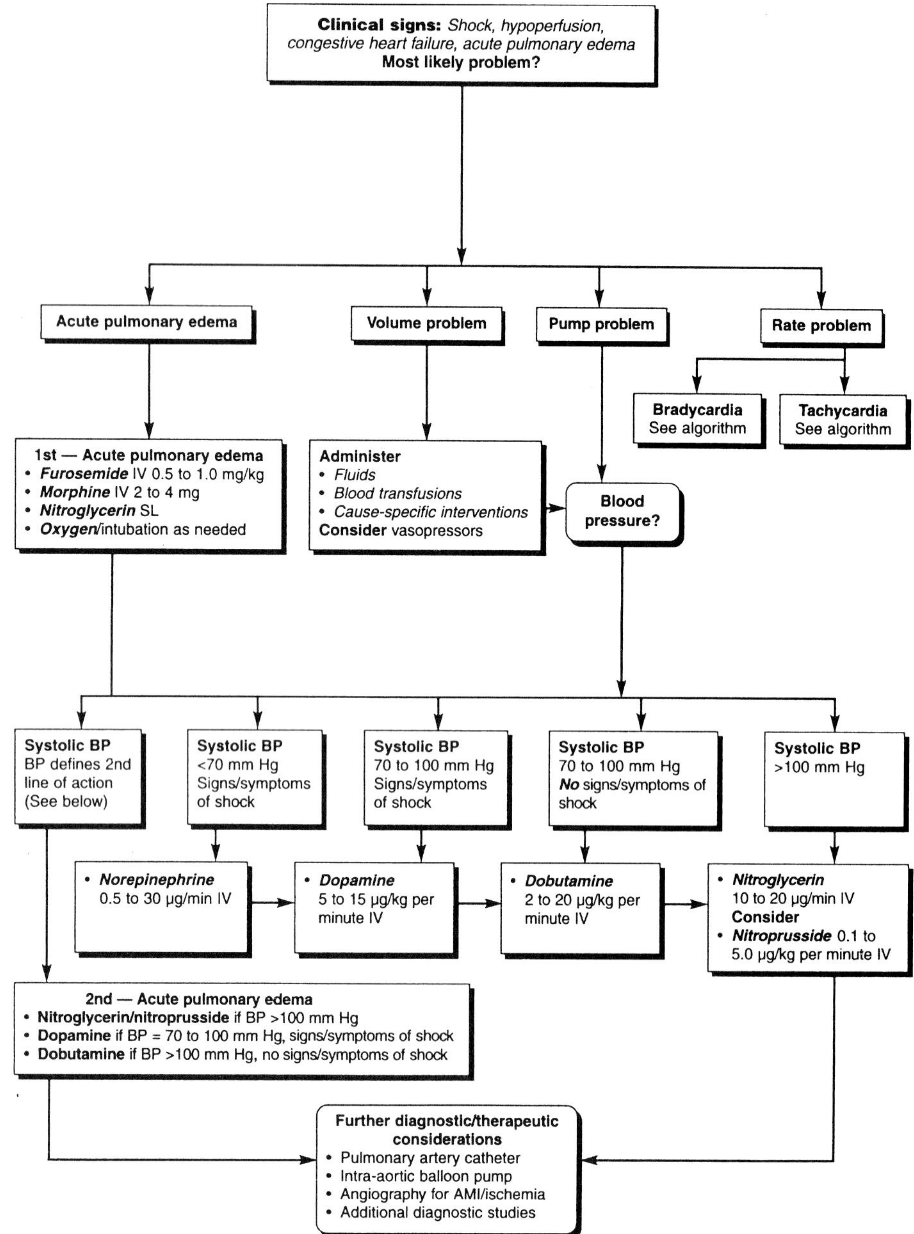

FIGURE 58-7. The acute pulmonary edema, hypotension, and shock algorithm. AMI, acute myocardiol infarction; BP, blood pressure; IV, intravenous(ly); SL, sublingucal. (Reprinted with permission from American Heart Association: Guidelines 2000 for cardiopulmonary resuscitation and emergency cardiovascular care: International consensus on science. Circulation 102:I-189, 2000.)

clinical trial of 200 in-patients found no difference between the drugs in survival for 1 hour or to hospital discharge.[158] In this study, response times were short, indicating that CPR outcome achieved with both vasopressin and epinephrine in short-term cardiac arrest may be comparable. The hemodynamic effects of vasopressin, compared with epinephrine, are especially impressive during long cardiac arrests. Thus, vasopressin may find most use in CPR during prolonged resuscitation. A multicenter, randomized study of 1,186 patients comparing vasopressin 40 U and epinephrine 1 mg for the first two doses of vasopressor during resuscitation from out-of-hospital cardiac arrest found no overall difference in survival to hospital admission (36% versus 31%) or discharge (10% versus 10%).[159] However, in subgroup analysis, in patients presenting in asystole, there was a significant improvement in survival to hospital admission (29% versus 20%) and discharge (4.7% versus 1.5%). In those patients who did not resuscitate following two doses of study drug, approximately 60% received additional epinephrine. In these difficult to resuscitate patients, irrespective of presenting rhythm, those that received vasopressin followed by epinephrine had better outcomes than those that received only epinephrine, suggesting that the combination of the drugs may have advantages. Overall, evidence currently suggests that, like other potent vasopressors, vasopressin is equivalent to but not better than epinephrine for use during CPR.

Amiodarone and Lidocaine

After epinephrine, the most effective drugs during CPR are those that help suppress ectopic ventricular rhythms. Amiodarone and lidocaine are used during cardiac arrest to aid defibrillation when ventricular fibrillation is refractory to electrical countershock therapy or when fibrillation recurs following successful conversion. Bretylium used to be included in this category but is no longer available for clinical use. Lidocaine, primarily an antiectopic agent with few hemodynamic effects, tends to reverse the reduction in ventricular fibrillation

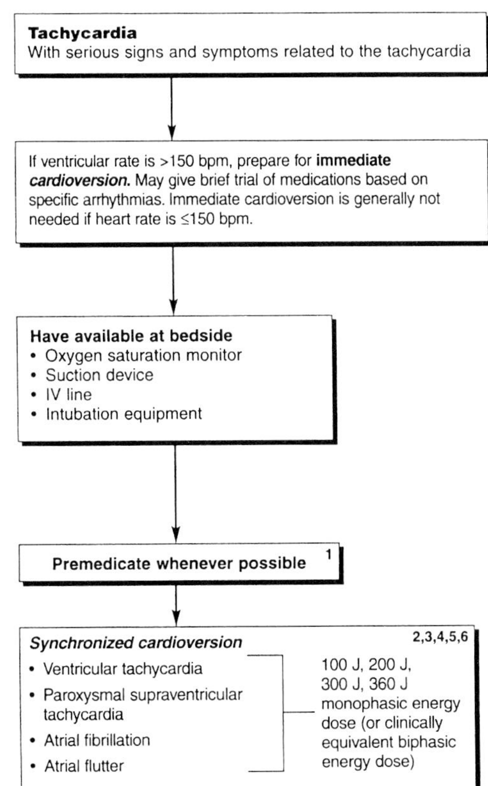

Tachycardia
With serious signs and symptoms related to the tachycardia
If ventricular rate is >150 bpm, prepare for **immediate *cardioversion.*** May give brief trial of medications based on specific arrhythmias. Immediate cardioversion is generally not needed if heart rate is ≤150 bpm.
Have available at bedside
• Oxygen saturation monitor
• Suction device
• IV line
• Intubation equipment
Premedicate whenever possible 1
Synchronized cardioversion 2,3,4,5,6
• Ventricular tachycardia
• Paroxysmal supraventricular tachycardia
• Atrial fibrillation
• Atrial flutter
100 J, 200 J, 300 J, 360 J monophasic energy dose (or clinically equivalent biphasic energy dose)

FIGURE 58-8. Synchronized cardioversion algorithm. IV, intravenous. (Reprinted with permission from American Heart Association: Guidelines 2000 for cardiopulmonary resuscitation and emergency cardiovascular care: International consensus on science. Circulation 102: I-164, 2000.)

threshold caused by ischemia or infarction. It depresses automaticity by reducing the slope of phase 4 depolarization and reducing the heterogeneity of ventricular refractoriness. Amiodarone is a pharmacologically complex drug with sodium, potassium, calcium, and α-adrenergic and β-adrenergic blocking properties that is useful for treatment of atrial and ventricular arrhythmias. Amiodarone can cause hypotension and bradycardia when infused too rapidly in patients with an intact circulation.[160] This can usually be prevented by slowing the rate of drug infusion, or it can be treated with fluids, va-
8 sopressors, chronotropic agents, or temporary pacing. There are two randomized, blinded, placebo-controlled clinical trials in shock-resistant cardiac arrest victims demonstrating improved admission alive to hospital with amiodarone treatment, although there was no difference in survival to discharge.[161,162] Although weak, this is more evidence of efficacy than exists for lidocaine.

When ventricular fibrillation or pulseless ventricular tachycardia is recognized, defibrillation should be attempted as soon as possible (see Fig. 58-2). No antiarrhythmic agent has been shown to be superior to electrical defibrillation or more effective than placebo in the treatment of ventricular fibrillation. Consequently, defibrillation should not be withheld or delayed to establish intravenous access or to administer drugs. When ventricular tachycardia or ventricular fibrillation has not responded to or recurred following BLS, epinephrine, and defibrillation, amiodarone should be administered. In cardiac arrest, amiodarone is initially administered as a 300-mg rapid infusion. Supplemental infusions of 150 mg can be repeated as necessary for recurrent or resistant arrhythmias to a maximum total daily dose of 2 g. (For dysrhythmias with an intact circulation, amiodarone is usually administered as 150 mg intravenously over 10 minutes, followed by 1 mg/min infusion for 6 hours and 0.5 mg/min thereafter.) Lidocaine is an alternative therapy in refractory fibrillation. To rapidly achieve and maintain therapeutic blood levels during CPR, relatively large doses are necessary. An initial bolus of 1.5 mg/kg should be given and additional boluses of 0.5 to 1.5 mg/kg can be given every 5 to 10 minutes during CPR up to a total dose of 3 mg/kg. Only bolus dosing should be used during CPR, but an infusion of 2 to 4 mg/min can be started after successful resuscitation.

Sodium Bicarbonate

Although sodium bicarbonate was used commonly during CPR in the past, little evidence supports its efficacy. Use of sodium bicarbonate during resuscitation has been based on the theoretical considerations that acidosis lowers fibrillation threshold[163] and impairs the physiologic response to catecholamines.[164] But most studies have failed to demonstrate improved success of defibrillation or resuscitation with the use of bicarbonate.[165–167] The lack of effect of buffer therapy may be partially explained by the slow onset of metabolic acidosis during cardiac arrest. As measured by blood lactate or base deficit, acidosis does not become severe for 15 or 20 minutes of cardiac arrest.[52,53,168]

In contrast to the lack of evidence that buffer therapy during CPR improves survival, the adverse effects of excessive sodium bicarbonate administration are well documented. In the past, metabolic alkalosis, hypernatremia, and hyperosmolarity were common after administration of bicarbonate during resuscitation attempts.[168,169] These abnormalities are associated with low resuscitation rates and poor outcome. However, if sodium bicarbonate is given judiciously according to standard recommendations, no significant metabolic abnormalities should occur.[170]

Intravenous sodium bicarbonate combines with hydrogen ion to produce carbonic acid that dissociates into CO_2 and water. The P_{CO_2} in blood is temporarily elevated until the excess CO_2 is eliminated through the lungs. Tissue acidosis during CPR is caused primarily by the low blood flow and accumulation of CO_2 in the tissues.[52,53] Therefore, concern has been expressed that the liberation of CO_2 by bicarbonate administration would only worsen the existing problem. This is of particular concern within myocardial cells and the brain. Carbon dioxide readily diffuses across cell membranes and the blood-brain barrier, whereas bicarbonate diffuses much more slowly. Thus, it is possible that sodium bicarbonate administration could result in a paradoxical worsening of intracellular and cerebral acidosis by further raising intracellular and cerebral CO_2 without a balancing increase in bicarbonate. Direct evidence for this effect has not been found. One study demonstrated an elevation in cerebral spinal fluid P_{CO_2}, and reduction in pH could occur when very large doses of bicarbonate were given.[171] However, with clinically relevant doses, another study found no changes in spinal fluid acid-base status.[172] Measurement of myocardial intracellular pH during bicarbonate administration has also not detected a worsening in acidosis.[173] Therefore, paradoxical acidosis from sodium bicarbonate therapy remains a concern primarily on theoretical grounds.

Current practice restricts the use of sodium bicarbonate primarily to arrests associated with hyperkalemia, severe preexisting metabolic acidosis, and tricyclic or phenobarbital overdose. It may be considered for use in protracted resuscitation attempts after other modalities have been instituted and failed. When bicarbonate is used during CPR, the usual dose is 1 mEq/kg initially with additional doses of 0.5 mEq/kg every 10 minutes. However, dosing of sodium bicarbonate should be guided by blood gas determination whenever possible.

Atropine

Atropine sulfate enhances sinus node automaticity and atrioventricular conduction by its vagolytic effects. Although atropine is frequently given during cardiac arrest associated with an ECG pattern of asystole or slow PEA, neither animal nor human studies provide evidence that it actually improves outcome from asystolic or bradysystolic arrest.[174,175] The predominant cause of asystole and EMD is severe myocardial ischemia. Excessive parasympathetic tone probably contributes little to these rhythms during cardiac arrest in adults. Even in children, it is doubtful that parasympathetic tone plays a significant role during most arrests. Therefore, the most important treatment for asystole and EMD is effective chest compressions, ventilation, and epinephrine to improve coronary perfusion and myocardial oxygenation. However, cardiac arrest with these rhythms has a poor prognosis.[24] Because atropine has few adverse effects, it is recommended in arrest with asystole or PEA and refractory to epinephrine and oxygenation. The dose is 1.0 mg intravenously, repeated every 3 to 5 minutes up to a total of 0.04 mg/kg, which is totally vagolytic.[176] Full vagolytic doses may be associated with fixed mydriasis, following successful resuscitation confounding neurologic examination. Occasionally, a sinus tachycardia following resuscitation may be due to the use of atropine during CPR.

Calcium

With normal cardiovascular physiology, calcium increases myocardial contractility and enhances ventricular automaticity. Consequently, it has been advocated as a treatment for asystole and PEA. Early animal studies showed moderate success with calcium chloride in asphyxial arrest, although vasopressors were better.[13] In 1981, Dembo reported dangerously high serum calcium levels (up to 18.2 mg/dL) during CPR and questioned the efficacy of calcium in cardiac arrest.[177] Subsequently, several retrospective studies and prospective clinical trials during out-of-hospital cardiac arrest showed that calcium was no better than placebo in promoting resuscitation and survival from asystole or EMD.[178–183] Consequently, because of potentially deleterious effects, calcium is not recommended during CPR unless specific indications exist. Calcium may prove useful if hyperkalemia, hypocalcemia, or calcium channel blocker toxicity is present. There are no other indications for its use during CPR. When calcium is administered, the chloride salt is recommended because it produces higher and more consistent levels of ionized calcium than other salts. The usual dose is 2 to 4 mg/kg of the 10% solution administered slowly intravenously. Calcium gluconate contains one-third as much molecular calcium as does calcium chloride and requires metabolism of gluconate in the liver.

PEDIATRIC CARDIOPULMONARY RESUSCITATION

The principles of CPR discussed previously apply to the child in cardiac arrest. Arrest is less likely to be a sudden event and more likely related to progressive deterioration of respiratory and circulatory function in the pediatric age group. Airway

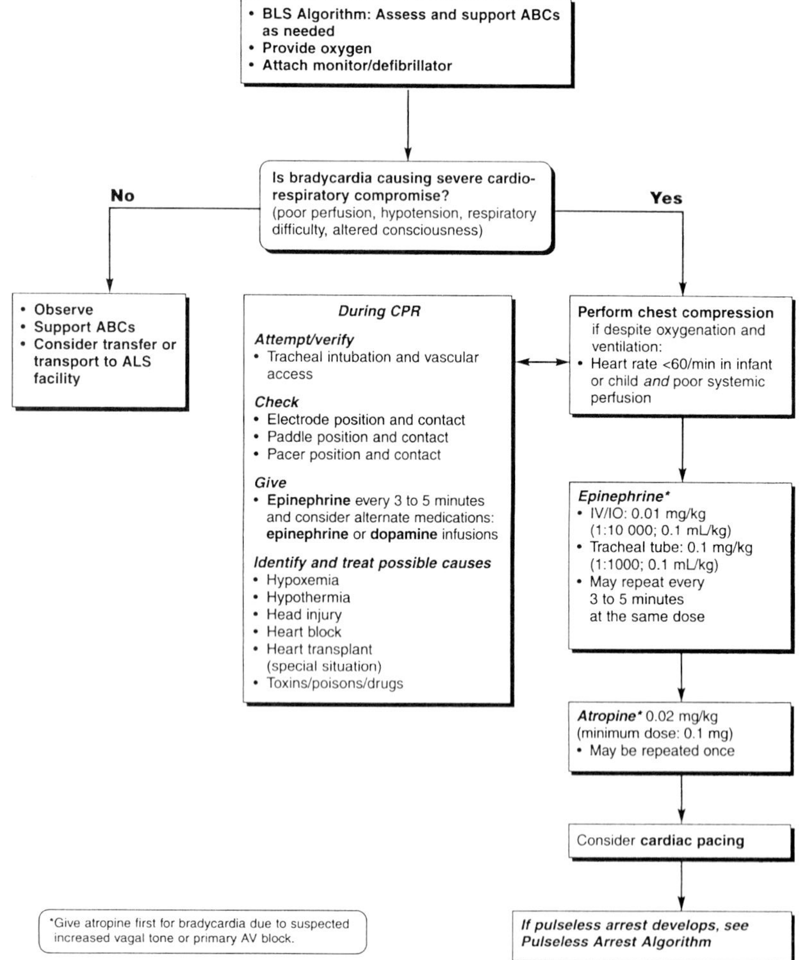

FIGURE 58-9. Pediatric advanced life support (PALS) bradycardia algorithm. ABCs, airway, breathing, and circulation; ALS, advanced life support; BLS, basic life support; CPR, cardiopulmonary resuscitation; IV, intravenous(ly); IO, intraosseous(ly). (Reprinted with permission from American Heart Association: Guidelines 2000 for cardiopulmonary resuscitation and emergency cardiovascular care: International consensus on science. Circulation 102:I-313, 2000.)

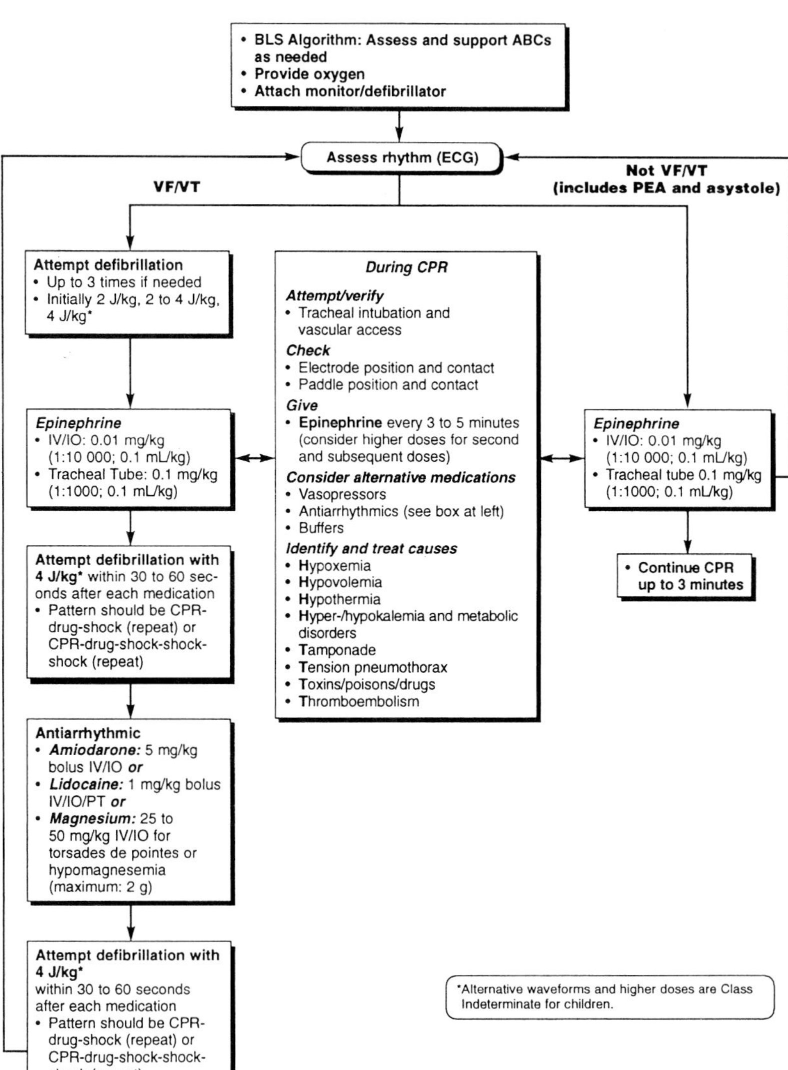

FIGURE 58-10. Pediatric advanced life support (PALS) pulseless arrest algorithm. ABCs, airway, breathing, and circulation; BLS, basic life support; CPR, cardiopulmonary resuscitation; ECG, electrocardiogram; IV, intravenous(ly); IO, intraosseous(ly); PEA, pulseless electrical activity; PT, per trachea; VF, ventricular fibrillation; VT, ventricular tachycardia. (Reprinted with permission from American Heart Association: Guidelines 2000 for cardiopulmonary resuscitation and emergency cardiovascular care: International consensus on science. Circulation 102:I-311, 2000.)

and ventilation problems lead to asystole and PEA as the most common presenting rhythms. However, the consequences of myocardial and cerebral ischemia are the same as for the adult. The basic approach to the arrest victim is the same (see Table 58-1). The specific anatomic and physiologic considerations necessary for the child will be familiar to anesthesiologists. The special circumstance of neonatal resuscitation has been discussed in other chapters.

The problem of airway management in the infant is well known to the anesthesiologist. Effective ventilation is especially critical because respiratory problems are frequently the cause for arrest. Mouth-to-mouth or mouth-to-nose and mouth (for infants) can be used as well as bag-valve-mask devices until intubation is possible. Cardiac compression in the infant is provided with two fingers on the midsternum or by encircling the chest with the hands and using the thumbs to provide compression. For the small child, compression can be provided with one hand on the midsternum.

The algorithm for ACLS in the pediatric patient is shown in Figs. 58-9 and 58-10. Although defibrillation is less frequently necessary in children, the same principles apply as in the adult. However, the recommended starting energy is 2 J/kg, which is doubled if defibrillation is unsuccessful. Considerations for drug administration are the same as for the adult, except that the interosseous route in the anterior tibia provides an additional option in small children. Drug therapy is similar to the adult but plays a larger role because electrical therapy is less often needed (see Figs. 58-9 and 58-10; Table 58-4).

POSTRESUSCITATION CARE

The major factors contributing to mortality following successful resuscitation are progression of the primary disease and cerebral damage suffered as a result of the arrest. There is growing awareness that any cardiac arrest, even of brief duration, causes a generalized decrease in myocardial function similar to the regional hypokinesis seen following periods of regional ischemia. This is usually referred to as global myocardial stunning and can be mitigated with inotropic agents, if necessary. Active management following resuscitation appears to mitigate post-ischemic brain damage and improve neurologic outcome.[184] Although a significant number of patients have severe neurologic deficits following resuscitation, aggressive brain-oriented support does not seem to increase the proportion surviving in vegetative states. Most severely damaged victims die of multisystem failure within 1 to 2 weeks.

When flow is restored following a period of global brain ischemia, three stages of cerebral reperfusion are seen in the ensuing 12 hours. Immediately following resuscitation, there are multifocal areas of the brain with no reflow. Within 1 hour, there is global hyperemia followed quickly

TABLE 58-4

PEDIATRIC ADVANCED LIFE SUPPORT MEDICATION FOR CARDIAC ARREST AND SYMPTOMATIC ARRHYTHMIAS

DRUG	DOSAGE (PEDIATRIC)	REMARKS
Adenosine	0.1 mg/kg Repeat dose: 0.2 mg/kg Maximum single dose: 12 mg	Rapid IV/IO bolus Rapid flush to central circulation Monitor ECG during dose.
Amiodarone for pulseless VF/VT	5 mg/kg IV/IO	Rapid IV bolus
Amiodarone for perfusing tachycardias	Loading dose: 5 mg/kg IV/IO Maximum dose: 15 mg/kg per day	IV over 20 to 60 min Routine use in combination with drugs prolonging QT interval is *not* recommended. Hypotension is most frequent side effect.
Atropine sulfate[a]	0.02 mg/kg Minimum dose: 0.1 mg Maximum single dose: 0.5 mg in child, 1.0 mg in adolescent. May repeat once.	May give IV, IO or ET Tachycardia and pupil dilation may occur but *not* fixed dilated pupils.
Calcium chloride 10% =100 mg/mL (=27.2 mg/mL elemental Ca)	20 mg/kg (0.2 mL/kg) IV/IO	Give slow IV push for hypocalcemia, hypermagnesemia, calcium channel blocker toxicity, preferably via central vein. Monitor heart rate; bradycardia may occur.
Calcium gluconate 10%= 100 mg/mL (=9 mg/mL elemental Ca)	60–100 mg/kg (0.6–1.0 mL/kg) IV/IO	Give slow IV push for hypocalcemia, hypermagnesemia, calcium channel blocker toxicity, preferably via central vein.
Epinephrine for symptomatic bradycardia[a]	IV/IO: 0.01 mg/kg (1:10,000, 0.1 mL/kg) ET: 0.1 mg/kg (1:1,000, 0.1 mL/kg)	Tachyarrhythmias, hypertension may occur.
Epinephrine for pulseless arrest[a]	First dose: IV/IO: 0.01 mg/kg (1:10,000, 0.1 mL/kg) ET: 0.1 mg/kg (1:1,000, 0.1 mL/kg) Subsequent doses: Repeat initial dose or may increase up to 10 times (0.1 mg/kg, 1:1,000, 0.1 mL/kg) Administer epinephrine every 3 to 5 min. IV/IO/ET doses as high as 0.2 mg/kg of 1:1,000 may be effective.	
Glucose (10% or 25% or 50%)	IV/IO: 0.5–1.0 g/kg • 1–2 mL/kg 50% • 2–4 mL/kg 25% • 5–10 mL/kg 10%	For suspected hypoglycemia; avoid hyperglycemia.
Lidocaine[a]	IV/IO/ET: 1 mg/kg	Rapid bolus
Lidocaine infusion (start after a bolus)	IV/IO: 20–50 μg/kg per minute	1 to 2.5 mL/kg per hour of 120 mg/100 mL solution or use "rule of 6"
Magnesium sulfate (500 mg/mL)	IV/IO: 25–50 mg/kg. Maximum dose: 2 g per dose	Rapid IV infusion for torsades or suspected hypomagnesemia; 10- to 20-min infusion for asthma that responds poorly to β-adrenergic agonists.
Naloxone[a]	≤5 years of ≤20 kg: 0.1 mg/kg >5 years or >20 kg: 2.0 mg	For total reversal of narcotic effect. Use small repeated doses (0.01 to 0.03 mg/kg) titrated to desired effect.
Procainamide for perfusing tachycardias (100 mg/mL and 500 mg/ mL)	Loading dose: 15 mg/kg IV/IO	Infusion over 30 to 60 min; routine use in combination with drugs prolonging QT interval is *not* recommended.
Sodium bicarbonate (1 mEq/mL and 0.5 mEq/mL)	IV/IO: 1 mEq/kg per dose	Infuse slowly and only if ventilation is adequate.

ECG, electrocardiogram; ET, endotracheal; IO, intraosseous; IV, intravenous; VF, ventricular fibrillation; VT, ventricular tachycardia.

[a]For endotracheal administration use higher doses (2 to 10 times the IV dose); dilute medication with normal saline to a volume of 3 to 5 mL and follow with several positive-pressure ventilations.

Adapted from American Heart Association: Guidelines 2000 for cardiopulmonary resuscitation and emergency cardiovascular care: International consensus on science. Circulation 102:I-308, 2000.

by prolonged global hypoperfusion. Elevation of intracranial pressure is unusual following resuscitation from cardiac arrest. However, severe ischemic injury can lead to cerebral edema and increased intracranial pressure in the ensuing days.

Postresuscitation support is focused on providing stable oxygenation and hemodynamics to minimize any further cerebral insult. A comatose patient should be maintained on mechanical ventilation for several hours to ensure adequate oxygenation and ventilation. Restlessness, coughing, or seizure activity should be aggressively treated with appropriate medications, including neuromuscular blockers, if necessary. Arterial Pa_{O_2} should be maintained above 100 mm Hg, and hypocapnia (Pa_{CO_2} <30 mm Hg) should be avoided. Blood volume should be maintained normal, and moderate hemodilution to a hematocrit of 30 to 35% may be helpful. A brief, 5-minute period of hypertension to mean arterial pressure of 120 to 140 mm Hg may help overcome the initial cerebral no reflow. This frequently occurs secondary to the effects of epinephrine given during CPR. Because cerebral autoregulation of blood flow is severely attenuated, both prolonged hypertension and hypotension are associated with a worsened outcome. Therefore, mean arterial pressure should be maintained at 90 to 110 mm Hg. Hyperglycemia during cerebral ischemia is known to result in increased neurologic damage. Although it is unknown if high serum glucose in the postresuscitation period influences outcome, it seems prudent to control glucose in the 100 to 250 mg/dL range. Specific pharmacologic therapy directed at brain preservation has not been shown to have further benefit. Some animal trials of barbiturates were promising, but a large multicenter trial of thiopental found no improvement in neurologic status when this drug was given following cardiac arrest.[184] Similar results were found with calcium channel blockers. Animal studies were encouraging, but a clinical trial found no improvement in outcome.[185]

9 In contrast to pharmacologic therapy, two more recent studies have demonstrated improved neurologic outcome when mild therapeutic hypothermia (32 to 34°C) was induced for 12 to 24 hours in cardiac arrest survivors who remained comatose after admission to the hospital.[186,187] Both investigations studied only patients whose initial rhythm was ventricular fibrillation, and the larger of the trials included only witnessed arrests. Nevertheless, these are the first studies to document improved neurologic outcome with a specific postarrest intervention. ILCOR now recommends "unconscious adult patients with spontaneous circulation after out-of-hospital cardiac arrest should be cooled to 32 to 34°C for 12 to 24 hours when the initial rhythm was ventricular fibrillation. Such cooling may also be beneficial for other rhythms or in-hospital cardiac arrest."

Prognosis

For the comatose survivor of CPR, the question of ultimate prognosis is important. One retrospective study demonstrated that the admission neurologic examination of comatose victims is highly correlated with the likelihood of awakening.[188] If there were no pupillary light response and no spontaneous eye movement, and if the motor response to pain were absent or extensor posturing, there was only a 5% chance the patient would ever awaken. A companion study demonstrated that the chance of ever awakening fell rapidly in the days following arrest.[189] If the patient was not awake by 4 days following arrest, the chance of ever awakening was 20%, and all those awakening had marked neurologic deficits. Most patients who completely recover show rapid improvement in the first 48 hours. There is also a high correlation between severity of neurologic injury and the level of creatine kinase-BB found in the cerebrospinal fluid.[190,191] Peak values of ≥25 IU are associated with severe neurologic damage and are reached 48 to 72 hours following arrest.

References

1. Wood Library Museum: Resuscitation: An Historical Perspective. Park Ridge, IL,Wood Library Museum, 1976
2. Brooks DK: Resuscitation: Care of the Critically Ill. London, Edward Arnold, 1986
3. Vesalius A: De Humani Corporis. Basel, Fabrica, 1543
4. Elam JO, Brown ES, Elder JD Jr: Artificial respiration by mouth to mask method: A study of the respiratory gas exchange of paralyzed patients ventilated by operator's expired air. N Engl J Med 250:749, 1954
5. Gordon AS, Frye CS, Gittelson L *et al*: Mouth-to-mouth versus manual artificial respiration for children and adults. JAMA 167:320, 1958
6. Safar P, Escarraga LA, Elam JO: A comparison of the mouth-to-mouth and mouth-to-airway methods of artificial respiration with the chest-pressure arm-lift methods. N Engl J Med 258:671, 1958
7. Safar P: Failure of manual respiration. J Appl Physiol 14:84, 1959
8. Hooker DR, Kouwenhoven WB, Langworthy OR: The effects of alternating current on the heart. Am J Physiol 103:444, 1933
9. Beck CS, Pritchard WH, Feil HS: Ventricular fibrillation of long duration abolished by electric shock. JAMA 135:985, 1947
10. Zoll PM, Linenthal AJ, Gibson W *et al*: Termination of ventricular fibrillation in man by an externally applied electric shock. N Engl J Med 254:727, 1956
11. Kouwenhoven WB, Milnor WR, Knickerbocker GG, Chestnut WR: Closed-chest defibrillation of the heart. Surgery 42:550, 1957
12. Kouwenhoven WB, Jude JR, Knickerbocker GG: Closed-chest cardiac massage. JAMA 173:1064, 1960
13. Redding JS, Pearson JW: Evaluation of drugs for cardiac resuscitation. Anesthesiology 24:203, 1963
14. National Heart Lung and Blood Institute: Morbidity and Mortality Chartbook on Cardiovascular, Lung and Blood Diseases 1990. Bethesda, MD, National Heart Lung and Blood Institute, 1990
15. Angelos M, Safar P, Reich H: A comparison of cardiopulmonary resuscitation with cardiopulmonary bypass after prolonged cardiac arrest in dogs: Reperfusion pressures and neurologic recovery. Resuscitation 21:121, 1991
16. Kern KB, Sanders AB, Janas W *et al*: Limitations of open-chest cardiac massage after prolonged, untreated cardiac arrest in dogs. Ann Emerg Med 20:761, 1991
17. Copley DP, Mantle JA, Rogers WJ *et al*: Improved outcome for prehospital cardiopulmonary collapse with resuscitation by bystanders. Circulation 56:901, 1977
18. Eisenberg MS, Bergner L, Hallstrom A: Cardiac resuscitation in the community: Importance of rapid provision and implications for program planning. JAMA 241:1905, 1979
19. Weaver WD, Cobb LA, Hallstrom AP *et al*: Factors influencing survival after out-of-hospital cardiac arrest. J Am Coll Cardiol 7:752, 1986
20. Eisenberg MS, Copass MK, Halstrom AP *et al*: Treatment of out-of-hospital cardiac arrest with rapid defibrillation by emergency medical technicians. N Engl J Med 302:1379, 1980
21. Weaver WD, Hill D, Fahrenbruch CE *et al*: Use of the automatic external defibrillator in the management of out-of-hospital cardiac arrest. N Engl J Med 319:661, 1988
22. Taffet BE, Teasdale TA, Luchi RJ: In-hospital cardiopulmonary resuscitation. JAMA 260:2069, 1988
23. Olsson GI, Hallen B: Cardiac arrest during anaesthesia: A computer-aided study of 250,543 anaesthetics. Acta Anaesthesiol Scand 32:653, 1988
24. American Heart Association: Guidelines 2000 for Cardiopulmonary Resuscitation and Emergency Cardiovascular Care: International Consensus on Science. Circulation 102(8):I-1, 2000
25. Cohen CB, Cohen PJ: Do-not-resuscitate orders in the operating room. N Engl J Med 325:1879, 1991
26. Walker RM: DNR in the OR: Resuscitation as an operative risk. JAMA 266:2407, 1991
27. Margolis JO, McGrath BJ, Kussin PS, Schwinn DA: Do no resuscitate (DNR) orders during surgery: Ethical foundations for institutional policies in the United States. Anesth Analg 80:806, 1995
28. Guildner CW: Resuscitation. Opening the airway: A comparative study of techniques for opening an airway obstructed by the tongue. JACEP 5:588, 1976
29. Heimlich HJ: Pop goes the cafe coronary. Emerg Med 6:154, 1974
30. Guildner CW, Williams D, Subtich T: Airway obstructed by foreign material: The Heimlich maneuver. JACEP 5:675, 1976
31. Redding JS: The choking controversy: Critique of evidence on the Heimlich maneuver. Crit Care Med 7:475, 1979
32. Bossaert L, Van Hoeyweghen R: The cerebral resuscitation study group: Bystander cardiopulmonary resuscitation (CPR) in out-of-hospital cardiac arrest. Resuscitation 17(Suppl):S55, 1989
33. Van Hoeyweghen RJ, Bossaert LL, Mullie A *et al*: Quality and efficiency of bystander CPR. Resuscitation 26:47, 1993

34. Berg RA, Kern KB, Sanders AB *et al*: Bystander cardiopulmonary resuscitation: Is ventilation necessary? Circulation 88:1907, 1993
35. Berg RA, Wilcoxson D, Hilwig RW *et al*: The need for ventilatory support during bystander cardiopulmonary resuscitation. Ann Emerg Med 26:342, 1995
36. Berg RA, Kern KB, Hilwig RW *et al*: Assisted ventilation does not improve outcome in a porcine model of single-rescuer bystander cardiopulmonary resuscitation. Circulation 95:1635, 1997
37. Berg RA, Kern KB, Hilwig RW *et al*: Assisted ventilation during 'bystander' CPR in a swine acute myocardial infarction model does not improve outcome. Circulation 96:4364, 1997
38. Berg RA, Hilwig RW, Kern KB *et al*: Simulated mouth-to-mouth ventilation and chest compressions ('bystander' CPR) improves outcome in a swine model of prehospital pediatric asphyxial cardiac arrest. Crit Care Med 27:1893, 1999
39. Ornato JP, Hallagan LF, McMahan SB *et al*: Attitudes of BCLS instructors about mouth-to-mouth resuscitation during the AIDS epidemic. Ann Emerg Med 19:151, 1990
40. Brenner BE, Kauffman J: Reluctance of internists and medical nurses to perform mouth-to-mouth resuscitation. Arch Intern Med 153:1763, 1993
41. Locke CJ, Berg RA, Sanders AB *et al*: Bystander cardiopulmonary resuscitation: Concerns about mouth-to-mouth contact. Arch Intern Med 155:938, 1995
42. Sellick BA: Cricoid pressure to control regurgitation of stomach contents during induction of anaesthesia. Lancet 2:404, 1961
43. Salem MR, Wong AY, Fizzotti GF: Efficacy of cricoid pressure in preventing aspiration of gastric contents in paediatric patients. Br J Anaesth 44:401, 1972
44. Harrison RR, Maull KI, Keenan RL, Boyan CP: Mouth-to-mask ventilation: A superior method of rescue breathing. Ann Emerg Med 11:74, 1982
45. Jesudian MCS, Harrison RR, Keenan RL, Maull KI: Bag-valve-mask ventilation: Two rescuers are better than one: Preliminary report. Crit Care Med 13:122, 1985
46. Babbs CF: New versus old theories of blood flow during CPR. Crit Care Med 8:191, 1980
47. Jude JR, Kouwenhoven WB, Knickerbocker GG: Cardiac arrest: Report of application of external cardiac massage on 118 patients. JAMA 178:1063, 1961
48. Criley JM, Blaufuss AH, Kissel GL: Cough-induced cardiac compression: Self-administered form of cardiopulmonary resuscitation. JAMA 236:1246, 1976
49. Rudikoff MJ, Maughan WL, Effrom M *et al*: Mechanisms of blood flow during cardiopulmonary resuscitation. Circulation 61:345, 1980
50. Holmes HR, Babbs CF, Voorhees WD *et al*: Influence of adrenergic drugs upon vital organ perfusion during CPR. Crit Care Med 8:137, 1980
51. Michael JR, Guerci AD, Koehler RC *et al*: Mechanisms by which epinephrine augments cerebral and myocardial perfusion during cardiopulmonary resuscitation in dogs. Circulation 69:822, 1984
52. Weil MH, Rackow EC, Trevino R *et al*: Difference in acid–base state between venous and arterial blood during cardiopulmonary resuscitation. N Engl J Med 315:153, 1986
53. Weil MH, Grundler W, Yamaguchi M *et al*: Arterial blood gases fail to reflect acid-base status during cardiopulmonary resuscitation: A preliminary report. Crit Care Med 13:884, 1985
54. Chandra N, Rudikoff M, Weisfeldt ML: Simultaneous chest compression and ventilation at high airway pressure during cardiopulmonary resuscitation. Lancet 1:175, 1980
55. Chandra N, Snyder LD, Weisfeldt ML: Abdominal binding during cardiopulmonary resuscitation in man. JAMA 246:351, 1981
56. Luce JM, Ross BK, O'Quinn RJ *et al*: Regional blood flow during cardiopulmonary resuscitation in dogs using simultaneous and nonsimultaneous compression and ventilation. Circulation 67:258, 1983
57. Bircher N, Safar P, Stewart R: A comparison of standard, MAST-augmented, and open-chest CPR in dogs: A preliminary investigation. Crit Care Med 8:147, 1980
58. Niemann JT, Rosborough JP, Ung S, Criley JM: Coronary perfusion pressure during experimental cardiopulmonary resuscitation. Ann Emerg Med 11:127, 1982
59. Sanders AB, Ewy GA, Alferness CA *et al*: Failure of one method of simultaneous chest compression, ventilation and abdominal binding during CPR. Crit Care Med 10:509, 1982
60. Kern KB, Carter AB, Showen RL *et al*: Twenty-four-hour survival in a canine model of cardiac arrest comparing three methods of manual cardiopulmonary resuscitation. J Am Coll Cardiol 7:859, 1986
61. Kern KB, Carter AB, Showen RL *et al*: Comparison of mechanical techniques of cardiopulmonary resuscitation: Survival and neurologic outcome in dogs. Am J Emerg Med 5:190, 1987
62. Niemann JT, Rosborough JP, Ung S, Criley JM: Hemodynamic effects of continuous abdominal binding during cardiac arrest and resuscitation. Am J Cardiol 53:269, 1984
63. Kirscher JP, Fine EG, Weisfeld ML *et al*: Comparison of prehospital conventional and simultaneous compression–ventilation cardiopulmonary resuscitation. Crit Care Med 17:1263, 1989
64. Ohomoto T, Miura I, Konno S: A new method of external cardiac massage to improve diastolic augmentation and prolong survival time. Ann Thorac Surg 21:284, 1976
65. Babbs CF, Tacker WA: Cardiopulmonary resuscitation with interposed abdominal compression. Circulation 74(Suppl 4):37, 1986
66. Mateer JF, Stueven HA, Thompson BM *et al*: Pre-hospital IAC-CPR versus standard CPR: Paramedic resuscitation of cardiac arrests. Am J Emerg Med 3:143, 1985
67. Sack JB, Kesselbrenner MB, Bregman D: Survival from in-hospital cardiac arrest with interposed abdominal counterpulsation during cardiopulmonary resuscitation. JAMA 267:379, 1992
68. Criley JM, Niemann JT, Rosborough JP, Hausknecht M: Modifications of cardiopulmonary resuscitation based on the cough. Circulation 74(Suppl 4):42, 1986
69. Niemann JT, Rosborough JP, Criley JM, Niskanen RA: Circulatory support during cardiac arrest using a pneumatic vest and abdominal binder with simultaneous high pressure airway inflation. Ann Emerg Med 13:767, 1984
70. Halperin HR, Tsitlik JE, Belfand M *et al*: A preliminary study of cardiopulmonary resuscitation by circumferential compression of the chest with use of a pneumatic vest. N Engl J Med 329:762, 1993
71. Lurie KG, Lindo C, Chin J: CPR: The P stands for plumber's helper (Letter). JAMA 264:1661, 1990
72. Cohen TJ, Tucker KJ, Lurie KG *et al*: Active compression–decompression. A new method of cardiopulmonary resuscitation. JAMA 267:2916, 1992
73. Linder KH, Pfenniger EG, Lurie KG *et al*: Effects of active compression–decompression resuscitation on myocardial and cerebral blood flow in pigs. Circulation 88:1254, 1993
74. Cohen TJ, Goldner BG, Maccaro PC *et al*: A comparison of active compression-decompression cardiopulmonary resuscitation for cardiac arrests occurring in the hospital. N Engl J Med 329:1918, 1993
75. Lurie KG, Shultz JJ, Callaham ML *et al*: Evaluation of active compression-decompression CPR in victims of out-of-hospital cardiac arrest. JAMA 271:1405, 1994
76. Schwab TM, Callaham ML, Madsen CD *et al*: A randomized clinical trial of active compression–decompression CPR vs standard CPR in out-of-hospital cardiac arrest in two cities. JAMA 273:1261, 1995
77. Plaisance P, Lurie KG, Vicaut E *et al*: A comparison of standard cardiopulmonary resuscitation and active compression-decompression resuscitation for out-of-hospital cardiac arrest. N Engl J Med 341:569, 1999
78. Stiell IG, Herbert PC, Wells GA *et al*: The Ontario trial of active compression-decompression cardiopulmonary resuscitation for in-hospital and prehospital cardiac arrest. JAMA 275:1417, 1996
79. DeBehnke DJ, Angelos MG, Leasure JE: Comparison of standard external CPR, open-chest CPR, and cardiopulmonary bypass in a canine myocardial infarct model. Ann Emerg Med 20:754, 1991
80. Reichman RT, Joyo CI, Dembitsky WP *et al*: Improved patient survival after cardiac arrest using a cardiopulmonary support system. Ann Thorac Surg 49:101, 1990
81. Hartz R, LoCicero J, Sanders JH *et al*: Clinical experience with portable cardiopulmonary bypass in cardiac arrest patients. Ann Thorac Surg 50:437, 1990
82. Mooney MR, Arom KV, Joyce LD *et al*: Emergency cardiopulmonary bypass support in patients with cardiac arrest. J Thorac Cardiovasc Surg 101:450, 1991
83. Sanders AB, Kern KB, Atlas M *et al*: Importance of the duration of inadequate coronary perfusion pressure on resuscitation from cardiac arrest. J Am Coll Cardiol 6:113, 1985
84. Kern KB, Sanders AB, Badylak SF *et al*: Long term survival with open-chest cardiac massage after ineffective closed-chest compression in a canine preparation. Circulation 75:498, 1987
85. Ralston SH, Voorhees WD, Babbs CF: Intrapulmonary epinephrine during prolonged CPR: Improved regional blood flow and resuscitation in dogs. Ann Emerg Med 13:79, 1984
86. Crile G, Dolley DH: Experimental research into resuscitation of dogs killed by anesthetics and asphyxia. J Exp Med 8:713, 1906
87. Redding JS: Abdominal compression in cardiopulmonary resuscitation. Anesth Analg 50:668, 1971
88. Pearson JW, Redding JS: Influence of peripheral vascular tone on cardiac resuscitation. Anesth Analg 44:746, 1965
89. Yakaitis RW, Otto CW, Blitt CD: Relative importance of alpha and beta adrenergic receptors during resuscitation. Crit Care Med 7:293, 1979
90. Otto CW, Yakaitis RW, Blitt CD: Mechanism of action of epinephrine in resuscitation from asphyxial arrest. Crit Care Med 9:321, 1981
91. Ditchey RV, Winkler JV, Rhodes CA: Relative lack of coronary blood flow during closed-chest resuscitation in dogs. Circulation 66:297, 1982
92. Otto CW, Yakaitis RW: The role of epinephrine in CPR: A reappraisal. Ann Emerg Med 13:840, 1984
93. Sanders AB, Ewy GA, Taft TV: Prognostic and therapeutic importance of the aortic diastolic pressure in resuscitation from cardiac arrest. Crit Care Med 12:871, 1984
94. Niemann JT, Criley JM, Rosborough JP *et al*: Predictive indices of successful cardiac resuscitation after prolonged arrest and experimental cardiopulmonary resuscitation. Ann Emerg Med 14:521, 1985
95. Paradis NA, Martin GB, Rivers EP *et al*: Coronary perfusion pressure and the return of spontaneous circulation in human cardiopulmonary resuscitation. JAMA 263:1106, 1990
96. Kalenda Z: The capnogram as a guide to the efficacy of cardiac massage. Resuscitation 6:259, 1978

97. Weil MH, Bisera J, Trevino RP: Cardiac output and end tidal carbon dioxide. Crit Care Med 13:907, 1985
98. Sanders AB, Atlas M, Ewy GA *et al*: Expired P_{CO_2} as an index of coronary perfusion pressure. Am J Emerg Med 3:147, 1985
99. Sanders AB, Ewy GA, Bragg S *et al*: Expired P_{CO_2} as a prognostic indicator of successful resuscitation from cardiac arrest. Ann Emerg Med 14:948, 1985
100. Sanders AB, Kern KB, Otto CW *et al*: End-tidal carbon dioxide monitoring during cardiopulmonary resuscitation: A prognostic indicator for survival. JAMA 262:1347, 1989
101. Levine RL, Wayne MA, Miller CC: End-tidal carbon dioxide and outcome of out-of-hospital cardiac arrest. N Engl J Med 337:301, 1997
102. Kern KB, Sanders AB, Raife J *et al*: A study of chest compression rates during cardiopulmonary resuscitation in humans: The importance of rate-directed compressions. Arch Intern Med 152:145, 1992
103. Kerber RE, Sarnat W: Factors influencing the success of ventricular defibrillation in man. Circulation 60:226, 1979
104. Yakaitis RW, Ewy GA, Otto CW *et al*: Influence of time and therapy on ventricular defibrillation in dogs. Crit Care Med 8:157, 1980
105. Weaver WD, Copass MD, Bufi D *et al*: Improved neurologic recovery and survival after early defibrillation. Circulation 69:943, 1984
106. Weaver WD, Cobb LA, Dennis D *et al*: Amplitude of ventricular fibrillation waveform and outcome after cardiac arrest. Ann Intern Med 102:53, 1985
107. Ewy GA, Dahl CF, Zimmermann M, Otto CW: Ventricular fibrillation masquerading as ventricular standstill. Crit Care Med 9:841, 1981
108. Stewart AJ, Allen JD, Adgey AAJ: Frequency analysis of ventricular fibrillation and resuscitation success. Q J Med 306:761, 1992
109. Brown CG, Griffith RF, Ligten PV *et al*: Median frequency—a new parameter for predicting defibrillation success rate. Ann Emerg Med 20:787, 1991
110. Otto CW, Yakaitis RW, Ewy GA: Effects of epinephrine on defibrillation in ischemic ventricular fibrillation. Am J Emerg Med 3:285, 1985
111. Cummins RO, Eisenberg MS, Bergner L, Murray JA: Sensitivity, accuracy and safety of an automatic external defibrillator: Report of a field evaluation. Lancet 1:318, 1984
112. Cummins RO, Eisenberg MS, Graves JR *et al*: Automatic external defibrillators used by emergency medical technicians: A controlled clinical trial. Circulation 72(Suppl 3):8, 1985
113. Caffrey SL, Willoughby PJ, Pepe PE *et al*: Public use of automated external defibrillators. N Engl J Med 347:1242, 2002
114. Valenzulea TD, Roe DJ, Nichol G *et al*: Outcomes of rapid defibrillation by security officers after cardiac arrest in casinos. N Engl J Med 343:1206, 2000
115. Cobb LA, Fahrenbruch CE, Walsh TR *et al*: Influence of CPR prior to defibrillation in out-of-hospital ventricular fibrillation. JAMA 281:1182, 1999
116. Wik L, Hansen TB, Fylling F *et al*: Delaying defibrillation to give basic cardiopulmonary resuscitation to patients with out-of-hospital ventricular fibrillation. JAMA 289:1389, 2003
117. Bardy GH, Marchlinski FE, Sharma AD *et al*: Multicenter comparison of truncated biphasic shocks and standard damped sine wave monophasic shocks for transthoracic ventricular defibrillation. Circulation 94:2507, 1996
118. Kerber RE, Grayzel J, Hoyt R *et al*: Transthoracic resistance in human defibrillation: Influence of body weight, chest size, serial shocks, paddle size and paddle contact pressure. Circulation 63:676, 1981
119. Connel PN, Ewy GA, Dahl CF, Ewy MD: Transthoracic impedance to defibrillation discharge: Effect of electrode size and electrode-chest wall interface. J Electrocardiol 6:313, 1973
120. Ewy GA, Taren D: Comparison of paddle electrode pastes used for defibrillation. Heart Lung 6:847, 1977
121. Dahl CF, Ewy GA, Ewy MD, Thomas ED: Transthoracic impedance to direct current discharge: Effect of repeated countershocks. Med Instrum 10:151, 1976
122. Ewy GA, Hellman DA, McClung S, Taren D: Influence of ventilation phase on transthoracic impedance and defibrillation effectiveness. Crit Care Med 8:164, 1980
123. Kerber RE, Kouba C, Marines J *et al*: Advance prediction of transthoracic impedance in human defibrillation and cardioversion: Importance of impedance in determining the success of low energy shocks. Circulation 70:303, 1984
124. Kerber RE, McPherson D, Charbonnier R *et al*: Automatic impedance-based energy adjustment for defibrillation: Experimental studies. Circulation 71:136, 1985
125. Lerman BB, DeMarco JP, Haines DE: Current-based versus energy-based ventricular defibrillation: A prospective study. J Am Coll Cardiol 12:1259, 1988
126. Dahl CF, Ewy GA, Warner ED, Thomas ED: Myocardial necrosis from direct current countershock. Circulation 50:956, 1974
127. Warner ED, Dahl CF, Ewy GA: Myocardial injury from transthoracic defibrillator countershock. Arch Pathol 99:55, 1975
128. Ehsani A, Ewy GA, Sobel BE: Effects of electrical countershock on serum creatine phosphokinase (CPK) isoenzyme activity. Am J Cardiol 37:12, 1976
129. Weaver WD, Cobb LA, Copass MK *et al*: Ventricular defibrillation: A comparative trial using 175-J and 320-J shocks. N Engl J Med 307:1101, 1982
130. Geddes LA, Tacker WA, Rosborough JP *et al*: Electrical dose for ventricular defibrillation of large and small animals using precordial electrodes. J Clin Invest 53:310, 1974
131. Gutgesell HP, Tacker WA, Geddes LA *et al*: Energy dose for defibrillation in children. Pediatrics 58:898, 1976
132. Kerber RE, Sarnat W: Factors influencing the success of ventricular defibrillation in man. Circulation 60:226, 1979
133. Pantridge JR, Adgey AAJ, Webb SW, Anderson J: Electrical requirement for ventricular defibrillation. BMJ 2:313, 1975
134. Adgey AA: Electrical energy requirement for ventricular defibrillation. Br Heart J 40:1197, 1978
135. Crampton JA, Crampton RS, Sipes JN, Cherwek ML: Energy levels and patient weight in ventricular defibrillation. JAMA 242:1380, 1979
136. Gascho JA, Crampton RS, Cherwek ML *et al*: Determinants of ventricular defibrillation in adults. Circulation 60:231, 1979
137. Kerber RE, Jensen SR, Gascho JA *et al*: Determinants of defibrillation: Prospective analysis of 183 patients. Am J Cardiol 52:739, 1983
138. Otto CW: Cardiovascular pharmacology II: The use of catecholamines, pressor agents, digitalis, and corticosteroids in CPR and emergency cardiac care. Circulation 74(Suppl 4):80, 1986
139. Redding JS, Pearson JW: Resuscitation from ventricular fibrillation (drug therapy). JAMA 203:255, 1968
140. Schleien CL, Dean JM, Koehler RC *et al*: Effect of epinephrine on cerebral and myocardial perfusion in an infant animal preparation of cardiopulmonary resuscitation. Circulation 73:809, 1986
141. Schleien CL, Koehler RC, Gervais H *et al*: Organ blood flow and somatosensory-evoked potentials during and after cardiopulmonary resuscitation with epinephrine or phenylephrine. Circulation 79:1332, 1989
142. Otto CW, Yakaitis RW, Redding JS, Blitt CD: Comparison of dopamine, dobutamine, and epinephrine in CPR. Crit Care Med 9:640, 1981
143. Lindner KH, Prengel AW, Pfenniger EG *et al*: Vasopressin improves vital organ blood flow during closed-chest cardiopulmonary resuscitation in pigs. Circulation 91:215, 1995
144. Brillman JC, Sanders AB, Otto CW *et al*: A comparison of epinephrine and phenylephrine for resuscitation and neurologic outcome of cardiac arrest in dogs. Ann Emerg Med 16:11, 1987
145. Silvast T, Saarnivaara L, Kinnunen A *et al*: Comparison of adrenaline and phenylephrine in out-of-hospital CPR: A double-blind study. Acta Anaesthesiol Scand 29:610, 1985
146. Linder KH, Ahnefeld FW, Prengel AW: Comparison of standard and high-dose adrenaline in the resuscitation of asystole and electromechanical dissociation. Acta Anaesthesiol Scand 35:253, 1991
147. Stiell IB, Hebert PC, Weitzman BN *et al*: High-dose epinephrine in adult cardiac arrest. N Engl J Med 327:1045, 1992
148. Brown CG, Martin DP, Pepe PE *et al*: A comparison of standard-dose and high-dose epinephrine in cardiac arrest outside the hospital. N Engl J Med 327:1051, 1992
149. Callaham M, Madsen CD, Barton CW *et al*: A randomized clinical trial of high-dose epinephrine and norepinephrine vs standard-dose epinephrine in prehospital cardiac arrest. JAMA 268:2667, 1992
150. Choux C, Gueugniaud P-Y, Barbieux A *et al*: Standard doses versus repeated high doses of epinephrine in cardiac arrest outside the hospital. Resuscitation 29:3, 1995
151. Gueugniaud P-Y, Mols P, Goldstein P *et al*: A comparison of repeated high doses and repeated standard doses of epinephrine for cardiac arrest outside the hospital. N Engl J Med 339:1595, 1998
152. Lipman J, Wilson W, Kobilski S *et al*: High-dose adrenaline in adult in-hospital asystolic cardiopulmonary resuscitation: A double-blind randomized trial. Anaesth Intensive Care 21:192, 1993
153. Sherman BW, Munger MA, Foulke GE *et al*: High-dose versus standard-dose epinephrine treatment of cardiac arrest after failure of standard therapy. Pharmacotherapy 17:242, 1997
154. Rivers EP, Wortsman J, Rady MY *et al*: The effect of the total cumulative epinephrine dose administered during human CPR on hemodynamic, oxygen transport, and utilization variables in the postresuscitation period. Chest 106:1499, 1994
155. Behringer W, Kittler H, Sterz F *et al*: Cumulative epinephrine dose during cardiopulmonary resuscitation and neurologic outcome. Ann Intern Med 129:450, 1998
156. Prengel AW, Lindner KH, Keller A, Lurie KG: Cardiovascular function during the postresuscitation phase after cardiac arrest in pigs: A comparison of epinephrine versus vasopressin. Crit Care Med 24:2014, 1996
157. Lindner KH, Dirks B, Strohmenger HU *et al*: Randomized comparison of epinephrine and vasopressin in patients with out-of hospital ventricular fibrillation. Lancet 349:535, 1997
158. Stiell IG, Hebert PC, Wells GA *et al*: Vasopressin versus epinephrine for inhospital cardiac arrest: A randomized controlled trial. Lancet 358:105, 2001
159. Wenzel V, Krismer AC, Arntz HR *et al*: A comparison of vasopressin and epinephrine for out-of-hospital cardiopulmonary resuscitation. N Engl J Med 350:105, 2004
160. Kowey PR, Levine JH, Herre JM *et al*: Randomized, double-blind comparison of intravenous amiodarone and bretylium in the treatment of patients

with recurrent hemodynamically destabilizing ventricular tachycardia or fibrillation. Circulation 92:3255, 1995

161. Kudenchuk PJ, Cobb LA, Copass MK *et al*: Amiodarone for resuscitation after out of hospital cardiac arrest due to ventricular fibrillation. N Engl J Med 341:871, 1999
162. Dorian P, Cass D, Schwartz B *et al*: Amiodarone as compared with lidocaine for shock-resistant ventricular fibrillation. N Engl J Med 346:884, 2002
163. Gerst PH, Fleming WH, Malm JR: Increased susceptibility of the heart to ventricular fibrillation during metabolic acidosis. Circ Res 19:63, 1966
164. Houle DB, Weil MH, Brown EB, Campbell GS: Influence of respiratory acidosis on ECG and pressor response to epinephrine, norepinephrine, and metaraminol. Proc Soc Exp Biol Med 94:561, 1957
165. Guerci AD, Chandra N, Johnson E *et al*: Failure of sodium bicarbonate to improve resuscitation from ventricular fibrillation in dogs. Circulation 74(Suppl 4):75, 1986
166. Federiuk CS, Sanders AB, Kern KB *et al*: The effect of bicarbonate on resuscitation from cardiac arrest. Ann Emerg Med 20:1173, 1991
167. Vukmir RB, Bircher NG, Radovsky A, Safar P: Sodium bicarbonate may improve outcome in dogs with brief or prolonged cardiac arrest. Crit Care Med 23:515, 1995
168. Bishop RL, Weisfeldt ML: Sodium bicarbonate administration during cardiac arrest: Effect on arterial pH, P_{CO_2}, and osmolality. JAMA 235:506, 1976
169. Mattar JA, Weil MH, Shubin H *et al*: Cardiac arrest in the critically ill: II. Hyperosmolal states following cardiac arrest. Am J Med 56:162, 1974
170. White BC, Tintinalli JE: Effects of sodium bicarbonate administration during cardiopulmonary resuscitation. JACEP 6:187, 1977
171. Berenyi KG, Wolk M, Killip T: Cerebrospinal fluid acidosis complicating therapy of experimental cardiopulmonary resuscitation. Circulation 52:319, 1975
172. Sanders AB, Otto CW, Kern KB *et al*: Acid–base balance in a canine model of cardiac arrest. Ann Emerg Med 17:667, 1988
173. Kette F, Weil MH, von Planta MS *et al*: Buffer agents do not reverse intramyocardial acidosis during cardiac resuscitation. Circulation 81:1660, 1990
174. Stueven HA, Tonsfeldt DJ, Thompson BM *et al*: Atropine in asystole: Human studies. Ann Emerg Med 13:815, 1984
175. Coon GA, Clinton JE, Ruiz E: Use of atropine for brady-asystolic prehospital cardiac arrest. Ann Emerg Med 10:462, 1981
176. O'Rourke GW, Greene NM: Autonomic blockade and the resting heart rate in man. Am Heart J 80:469, 1970
177. Dembo DH: Calcium in advanced life support. Crit Care Med 9:358, 1981
178. Harrison EE, Amey BD: The use of calcium in cardiac resuscitation. Am J Emerg Med 1:267, 1983
179. Harrison EE, Amey BD: Use of calcium in electromechanical dissociation. Ann Emerg Med 13:844, 1984
180. Stueven HA, Thompson BM, Aprahamian C, Darin J: Use of calcium in prehospital cardiac arrest. Ann Emerg Med 12:136, 1983
181. Stueven HA, Thompson BM, Aprahamian C *et al*: Calcium chloride: Reassessment of use in asystole. Ann Emerg Med 13:820, 1984
182. Stueven HA, Thompson BM, Aprahamian C *et al*: The effectiveness of calcium chloride in refractory electromechanical dissociation. Ann Emerg Med 14:626, 1985
183. Stueven HA, Thompson BM, Aprahamian C *et al*: Lack of effectiveness of calcium chloride in refractory asystole. Ann Emerg Med 14:630, 1985
184. Abramson NS, Safar P, Detre KM *et al*: Randomized clinical study of cardiopulmonary-cerebral resuscitation: Thiopental loading in comatose cardiac arrest survivors. N Engl J Med 314:397, 1986
185. Brain Resuscitation Clinical Trial II Study Group: A randomized clinical study of a calcium-entry blocker (lidoflazine) in the treatment of comatose survivors of cardiac arrest. N Engl J Med 324:1225, 1991
186. Holzer M, The Hypothermia After Cardiac Arrest Study Group: Mild therapeutic hypothermia to improve the neurologic outcome after cardiac arrest. N Engl J Med 346:549, 2002
187. Bernard SA, Gray TW, Buist MD *et al*: Treatment of comatose survivors of out-of-hospital cardiac arrest with induced hypothermia. N Engl J Med 346:557, 2002
188. Longstreth WT, Diehr P, Inui TS: Prediction of awakening after out-of-hospital cardiac arrest. N Engl J Med 308:1378, 1983
189. Longstreth WT, Inui TS, Cobb LA, Copass MK: Neurologic recovery after out-of-hospital cardiac arrest. Ann Intern Med 98:588, 1983
190. Mullie A, Lust P, Penninck J *et al*: Monitoring of cerebrospinal fluid enzyme levels in post-ischemic encephalopathy after cardiac arrest. Crit Care Med 9:399, 1981
191. Edgren E, Terent H, Hedstrand U, Ronquist G: Cerebral spinal fluid markers in relation to outcome in patients with global cerebral ischemia. Crit Care Med 11:4, 1983

CHAPTER 59 ■ DISASTER PREPAREDNESS AND WEAPONS OF MASS DESTRUCTION

MICHAEL J. MURRAY

KEY POINTS

1. Emergency preparedness is a way of life in many countries. It needs to become much more a part of life in the United States than it is today. What we need to do as healthcare leaders is to call the first meeting to prepare a community response, or if it already exists, become familiar with the community's response plan.
2. When caring for patients with severe acute respiratory syndrome in both Canada and in several countries in Asia, not only many healthcare providers become patients, but several also became fatalities. To maintain surge capacity, it is imperative that each healthcare provider recognize the importance of protecting himself or herself.
3. The reality is that we are far more likely to have to manage patients and healthcare facilities that are victims of natural and unintentional disasters. These are most often related to extreme weather, earthquakes, and industrial accidents.
4. Physicians avoided neuromuscular blockade to intubate the tracheas of patients with inhalation injuries and were glad they did because several patients had significant airway edema that may have made intubation difficult, if not impossible.
5. The Federal Emergency Management Agency is the lead agency for management assistance to state and local governments, providing emergency relief to affected individuals and businesses, decontaminating affected areas, and helping ensure public health safety.
6. The anesthesiologist, depending on where he or she practices, may be called on to manage situations that are unimaginable by current standards. However, with their basic understanding of physiology and pharmacology, their airway skills, their fluid-resuscitation expertise, and their ability to manage ventilators and to provide anesthesia in the field environment, emergency department, operating room, and intensive care units will be invaluable.
7. The experience from Chernobyl should indicate the kind of injuries and results that anesthesiologists can anticipate from nuclear accidents, including radiation burns, bone marrow suppression, the destruction of the lining of the gastrointestinal tract, gastrointestinal bleeding with translocation of bacteria, infection, sepsis, septic shock, and death.
8. Because of the possibility of exposure to ionizing radiation from nuclear power plants and so on, the American Academy of Pediatrics has recommended that at least two tablets of potassium iodide be available for all inhabitants within 10 miles of any nuclear power plant.
9. With any nuclear explosion, many individuals will be injured or die from building collapse or the thermal pulse. Patients could have burn, crush, radiation injury, or any combination thereof.
10. Influenza has killed more people in the 20th century than any other infectious disease. There have been three large pandemics, including one in 1918 when an avian virus infected humans, creating the deadliest outbreak of disease in U.S. history.
11. In the event of a documented case of smallpox, the Centers for Disease Control and Prevention has plans to quarantine the patient and then immunize immediate contacts of patients within a certain geographic radius.

Since antiquity, physicians have cared not only for individuals, but also for the welfare of the state. In the former role, they functioned not only as doctors, but also as priests. Because so little was known of science, supernatural forces were often invoked to help heal the patient. In the latter role, as the guardian and advisor to state and public health issues, the same was often true. During the Middle Ages, physicians became more focused on science and less on the supernatural. After September 11, 2001, however, physicians have been faced with a prospect that challenges their scientific training. Although, during war, catastrophic events occur on a daily basis, we are now in an era in which the unimaginable can happen at any time. We must confront the possibility that terrorists can attack our cities with conventional, nuclear, biological, and chemical weapons. As anesthesiologists, we must now be prepared at any time to care for the victims of such assaults and to protect our own welfare so that we do not become casualties and an additional burden to the healthcare system. We must use our scientific training to manage events that will likely evoke widespread fear and panic.

JOINT COMMISSION ON ACCREDITATION OF HEALTHCARE ORGANIZATIONS

Following the events of September 11, 2001, and subsequent anthrax attacks, the Joint Commission on Accreditation of Healthcare Organizations (JCAHO) published a "white paper" to help hospitals develop systems to create and sustain community-wide emergency preparedness.[1] The JCAHO recognizes that there has been a change in healthcare delivery in the United States over the last several years and decades, reflective of similar problems faced worldwide, that has left the healthcare system underfunded with limited resources[2] and ever-increasing demand. However, the JCAHO also recognizes that despite the best effort of law enforcement, fire and rescue, and emergency medical agencies, hospitals will continue to play a vital role in helping communities respond to catastrophic events, whether natural, unintentional, or terrorist initiated. The JCAHO's initiative was proactive in recognition of the fact that, "It is no longer sufficient to develop disaster plans and dust them off if a threat appears imminent. Rather, a system of preparedness across communities must be in place everyday."[1] The JCAHO acknowledged the need, despite decreasing healthcare resources, for what it describes as "surge capacity" within healthcare systems to handle the potentially hundreds, if not thousands or more, of patients who might be victims of catastrophic events. By being prepared, the JCAHO wants to reduce the appeal to terrorists of using weapons of mass destruction as an effective means of warfare and to help communities to better respond to natural disasters. The JCAHO white paper focuses on three major areas:

1. *Enlisting the community* to develop the local response
2. *Focusing on the key aspects of the system* that prepares the community to mobilize to care for patients, protect its staff, and serve the public
3. *Establishing* the accountability, oversight, leadership, and sustainability of *a community-preparedness system*

Although JCAHO guidelines are just that—guidelines that are not mandatory or required by law—all hospitals aspire to have JCAHO accreditation. From that perspective, the white paper is an important step in helping prepare the medical community to deal with catastrophic events that could inundate the healthcare system. It is incumbent on physicians to be familiar with what their hospital has done to comply with the JCAHO standards, in anticipation of what their roles may be.

Enlisting the Community

In the past, the JCAHO required that hospitals test their disaster plans twice per year. Often, organizations went through the motions without truly embracing the idea of planning for a catastrophe; however, even these minimal events did have benefit if the hospital was confronted with an actual disaster. However, with the World Trade Center and Pentagon bombings and the anthrax attacks, the JCAHO recognized how deficient most hospitals' plans were. By serendipity, prior to the events of 2001, the JCAHO had been reworking its disaster preparedness standards. Their requirements were introduced in January 2002 and have been updated since then (Table 59-1). Central to these is the recognition that the response needs to be a local response; most hospitals and communities may have to deal with whatever they are confronted with during the first 24 to 72 hours. In addition, there needs to be a better framework for integrating community resources.

The aforementioned terrorist events of 2001 and 2002, the 2001 Houston flood experience, and the 2004 Florida hurricane experiences underscored the fact that healthcare-provider organizations need to communicate more effectively with one another. There has traditionally been poor communication between law enforcement agencies, fire and rescue services, and emergency medical services. The medical community does no better in its interactions with the public health

TABLE 59-1

2004 EMERGENCY MANAGEMENT STANDARDS OF THE JOINT COMMISSION ON ACCREDITATION OF HEALTHCARE ORGANIZATIONS HOSPITAL ACCREDITATION STANDARDS

1. Develop a management plan that addresses emergency management (Standards EC.4.10–4.110). The four phases of emergency management activities are as follows:
   - Mitigation
   - Preparedness
   - Response
   - Recovery
2. Perform a hazard vulnerability analysis.
   - Establish emergency procedures in response to a hazard vulnerability analysis.
   - Define the organization's role with that of other community agencies.
   - Notify external authorities of emergencies.
   - Notify hospital personnel when emergency procedures are initiated.
   - Assign available personnel to cover necessary positions.
   - The following activities must be managed:
     - Patient/resident activities
     - Staff activities
     - Staff/family support
     - Logistics of critical supplies
     - Security
     - Evacuation of the facility, if necessary
   - Establish internal/external communication systems
   - Establish an orientation/education program
   - Monitor ongoing drills and real emergencies
   - Determine how an annual evaluation will occur
   - Provide alternate means of meeting essential building and utility needs
   - Identify radioactive and biological isolation decontamination sites
   - Clarify alternate responsibility of personnel
3. Involve community-wide response.
4. Reestablish and continue operations following a disaster.

community. They have different priorities—the medical community focuses on the individual, and public health personnel focus on the community at large. As is often the case, rarely have these five "agencies" come together to prepare a community-wide response, often expecting the local, state, or federal government to provide coordination. However, there is a fundamental need to formalize an organization of community resources of which hospitals and physicians are but one component.

Community-wide emergency response plans are in place in some large cities. However, the majority of metropolitan areas do not have such an organizational structure, and many hospitals and physicians are waiting for someone to take the first step in organizing such a response plan. The JCAHO, in publicizing its white paper, wanted to stimulate hospitals and hospital leadership to initiate a discussion of the responsibility of "the community" in preparing a response and to stimulate hospitals and healthcare providers to forge new partnerships in addressing this critical need.

In New York City, the Greater New York Hospital Association took a leadership role in forging a cross-disciplinary, cross-jurisdictional partnership to prepare an integrated response plan to any future disaster. Obviously, New York City had a vested interest in doing so, but the entire world watched the World Trade Center buildings collapse, and the anthrax attacks affected people in several states and received widespread media coverage.

Although the average layperson may conclude that the healthcare system seemed to respond adequately to the events of September 11 and the anthrax attacks, but in essence the healthcare system was not significantly challenged. Both New York City and Oklahoma City (with the bombing of the Federal Building on April 19, 1995) had a much higher fatality rate than is normal for mass casualties in which the ratio is between 5 and 10 casualties to 1 fatality. In both New York City and Oklahoma City, the ratio was reversed, with approximately 10 fatalities for every 1 casualty. In the post-hoc analysis, there were multiple problems identified to which the revised New York City disaster plan responded in anticipation of what the future might hold. Communications were one major problem that needed resolution. In New York City on September 11, pilots in helicopters recognized shortly after the South Tower collapsed that the North Tower would also collapse and radioed that warning to rescuers on the ground 21 minutes before the building fell. The message was relayed to police over their radios, and most managed to escape. Unfortunately, firefighter radios used a different frequency and did not pick up the warning, and at least 121 firefighters died because of the telecommunication breakdown.[3]

As the building fell, the entire telecommunications infrastructure in the area became nonfunctional. Communication throughout most of lower Manhattan had to be person-to-person or with hand-delivered notes within hospitals.

However, communication involves not only communicating within the hospital when a healthcare facility is inundated with casualties, but it also involves communication with other hospitals and healthcare and government agencies before and after a disaster. The anthrax letters of October 2001 were the first bioterrorism attack in this country to which the Centers for Disease Control and Prevention (CDC) had to respond. Twenty-two cases were confirmed or suspected—11 inhalation and 11 cutaneous attacks with 5 deaths. The first diagnosis of anthrax was made by a physician who suspected the disease, with confirmation by a laboratory technician who had trained in bioterrorism preparedness. But the general unfamiliarity of many healthcare professionals with biological agents contributed to misdiagnoses and delayed treatment for some patients. Even when the diagnosis was made, there was reluctance of hospitals and healthcare agencies to notify others. After the Brentwood postal worker was diagnosed at a hospital in the District of Columbia and the case was reported to public health care officials, the latter did not immediately act to notify other area hospitals.[4] It seems incredible that just months after the attacks on the World Trade Center that people were still doubtful that the United States could be attacked in yet another format.

1 Whereas emergency preparedness is a way of life in many countries, it very much needs to become much more a part of life in the United States than it is today. What we need to do as healthcare leaders is to call the first meeting to prepare a community response, or if it already exists, become familiar with the community's response plan. Community planning needs to occur, and the results of that planning need to be widely disseminated to as many potential partners in implementing the plan as possible.

Focusing on the Key Aspects of the System

To respond to a mass casualty event, an emergency medical system must be able to assess and expand its surge capacity—the ability to provide care for and transport countless numbers of patients to facilities with appropriate capacity, resources, and staff. To anticipate surge capacity, one must know which beds are available for patients, if there is space available for triaging and decontaminating patients, and if there are personnel available to provide first aid and more-comprehensive care. Because many emergency departments are already overwhelmed and there are fewer hospitals today than there were 10 years ago, the U.S. healthcare system has less surge capacity. However, we need to be proactive, recognize that standards may change, and plan accordingly. Patients may be cared for in hallways, and decontamination may not even take place in the hospital. It may be best done outside the hospital (e.g., near a loading dock or in an emptied parking lot between two fire trucks).

To preserve the functionality of the system, the staff must also protect themselves. In the Tokyo sarin attacks of 1995, several healthcare providers were contaminated with sarin when they cared for patients who had not been decontaminated,[5] thereby becoming patients themselves and further burdening the health care system. Similarly, when caring for patients with severe acute respiratory syndrome (SARS) in Canada and
2 in several countries in Asia, not only did many healthcare providers not only became patients,[6] but also several became fatalities. To maintain surge capacity, it is imperative that every healthcare provider recognize the importance of protecting himself or herself.

Also in these situations, one cannot forget about the patients for whom one is already caring. Patients who are healthy enough need to be discharged immediately, but more critically ill patients may need to be moved to other hospitals. This may occur if a hospital is inundated with patients from a disaster or as a result of the hospital being affected by the catastrophe such as occurred in Houston during the 2001 flood[7] or in Florida in 2004 when some hospitals lost power and patients had to be transported elsewhere.

After having established the basics, the most important aspect of managing a mass casualty event, again whether it is natural, unintentional, or intentional, is having a command and control structure with which everyone is familiar. In the Northridge, California, earthquake in 1994, many healthcare providers coming into the hospital, which lacked electricity and was severely damaged itself, had difficulty finding the command and control center. As a result, efforts were not coordinated and were slow to be implemented.

Healthcare providers also need to be concerned not only about their personal safety, but also about their psychological safety. That is, they should have plans in place for their families if they are required to stay at hospitals for an extended length of time. Because of natural catastrophes that have occurred throughout the United States with hurricanes, floods, tornados, earthquakes, and so on, most healthcare providers have had the opportunity to establish a plan for their families while they provide care during mass casualty situations.

Finally, in addressing these issues, the public must be mobilized to participate in the response. As part of this response, the health care system and its leaders must identify communication and information needs. During the synagogue and business bombings in Istanbul, Turkey, in 2003, the hospital at which most victims were admitted was ill prepared to handle the information needs of multiple governments, their healthcare agencies, and their intelligence and law enforcement agencies.

Hospital and healthcare providers must be able to manage not only the external, but also the internal communication needs of the hospital and have a plan to address them, especially if any aspect of the system fails, as occurred at the World Trade Center site on September 11, 2001. Finally, one must test, learn, improve, and be ready to address deficiencies in the plan. JCAHO requires two drills annually, with one of them expected to be a community-wide drill. These situations provide healthcare providers an opportunity to hone their skills and anticipate problems they might confront in the future in dealing with natural disasters and terrorist attacks.

Establishing a Community-Preparedness System

At this level, most of the responsibility for preparedness is with local, state, and federal governments inconjunction with hospitals and hospital organizations. As physicians, we should be familiar with the clinical competencies for emergency preparedness in bioterrorism developed through the Association of Teachers of Preventive Medicine in collaboration with the Center for Health Policy, Columbia University School of Nursing (Table 59-2).[8]

TABLE 59-2

CLINICAL COMPETENCIES FOR CLINICIANS AND EMERGENCY PREPAREDNESS

Clinicians should be able to

- Describe their role in the emergency response.
- Respond to an emergency event within the emergency management system.
- Recognize an illness or injury as potentially resulting from exposure to weapons of mass destruction.
- Institute appropriate steps to limit the spread of the offending agent.
- Report identified cases or events through the public health care system.
- Initiate patient care within their professional skill.[a]
- Use reliable information sources.
- Provide reliable information to others.
- Communicate risks and actions to patients.
- Identify and manage expected stress and anxiety.
- Participate in postevent feedback (after action report).

[a]Remember that anyone can provide rudimentary first aid if the situation warrants.

Modified from Association of Teachers of Preventive Medicine and Centers for Disease Control and Prevention: Clinician Competencies for Emergency Preparedness and Bioterrorism. July 2003. Available at: http://cumc.columbia.edu/dept/nursing/institutes/chphsr/clincomp.pdf. Accessed June 9, 2005.

DISASTER PREPAREDNESS

3 Although we recognize the critical importance for planning and preparing to deal with the use of weapons of mass destruction, the reality is that we are far more likely to have to manage patients and healthcare facilities that are victims of natural and unintentional disasters. These are most often related to extreme weather, earthquakes, and industrial accidents (Table 59-3).

Among weather-related events, hurricanes, tsunamis, tropical storms, and tornadoes are the most likely to wreak havoc, creating mass casualty situations (Table 59-4). Hurricane Andrew, which came ashore in south Florida on August 24, 1992, killed 40 people, injured scores more, left 250,000 people homeless, and severely compromised the ability of hospitals to provide care because healthcare workers were unable to get to work, electricity and water supplies were jeopardized, and many hospitals suffered direct damage.[9] Similar events occurred in Houston in June 2001 when tropical storm Allison destroyed the ability of many hospitals to provide care. Hospitals had to be evacuated, with critically ill patients going to other facilities, many of which were attempting to deal with the city's "normal", if not increased, number of emergencies.[7]

Although many die in such catastrophic events, the sequelae to survivors are often unimaginable. The Indian Ocean tsunami of December 26, 2004, killed many healthcare workers and destroyed countless numbers of healthcare facilities, and surging flood water with huge debris crushed and fractured extremities, resulting in many amputations. Survivors had to contend with lack of potable water, sanitation issues, rotting corpses, and incipient disease. Cholera, typhoid, and other communicable diseases were rampant in multiple countries.

Hospitals are often destroyed or, if not, need to evacuate because of an earthquake. In the January 17, 1994, earthquake affecting Northridge, California, 8 of 91 acute care hospitals had to be evacuated. Six of the hospitals evacuated within the first day because of water damage and loss of electrical power. Two of the eight hospitals evacuated within 72 hours when major structural damage was found, despite the fact that

TABLE 59-3

DISASTERS THAT RESULT IN MASS CASUALTIES

Natural
- Hurricanes
- Tornados
- Floods
- Earthquakes
- Fires

Unintentional
- Public transportation accident
- Boat accident
- Nuclear accident
- Industrial accident
- Building collapse/sports stadium disaster

Intentional
- Bombing
- Nuclear
- Biological
- Chemical

TABLE 59-4

FATALITIES FROM NATURAL DISASTERS

NATURAL DISASTER	DATE	NO. OF FATALITIES
Galveston hurricane	September 8, 1900	6,000
Bangladesh floods	November 12, 1970	300,000
Mount St. Helen's volcanic eruption	May 18, 1980	57
Bam, Iran earthquake	December 26, 2003	41,000
Indian Ocean tsunami	December 26, 2004	155,000

initial inspections of the hospitals did not reveal significant damage. Both hospitals ultimately had to be demolished and rebuilt.[10]

Much can be learned in preparing for disaster management from a risk assessment of major earthquakes. The Marmara earthquake that struck northwest Turkey on August 17, 1999, killed approximately 16,000 people, injured 44,000 (many healthcare workers were killed or injured), and demolished the majority of healthcare facilities. Patients had to be taken from Marmara to 35 hospitals outside the earthquake zone that were not affected. Of the thousands of injuries, there were many patients who were crushed and lay in the rubble for hours to days. Surprisingly, the time under the rubble did not correlate with morbidity and mortality. Most of these patients had amputations, but the incidence of renal failure did not increase as the time under the rubble increased.[11] Individuals involved in management of the disaster concluded that rescuers should try to find and uncover victims for at least 5 days after an earthquake.[11]

The earthquake that struck Bam, Iran, on December 26, 2003, killed 41,000 people and tens of thousands were injured. Because so many medical facilities were destroyed, Iran relied on 40 international teams to help provide search-and-rescue services, as well as evacuation and treatment of casualties. Mortuary teams had to deal with thousands of corpses, and public health agencies addressed sanitation needs and had to provide potable water, food, and shelter.[12]

Most casualties in earthquakes are from crush injuries, but a number of patients will also experience burn injuries. Obviously, the greatest likelihood of dealing with patients with burns involves fires, as evidenced from the Rhode Island nightclub fire on February 20, 2003, that killed 100 people immediately and left more than 200 injured. There are important lessons from that fire, especially for anesthesiologists, because one of the greatest challenges faced by physicians and healthcare workers at the small community hospital only 2 miles away was how to manage the airway. Physicians avoided neuromuscular blockade to intubate the tracheas of patients with inhalation injuries and were glad they did be-
4 cause several patients had significant airway edema that may have made intubation difficult, if not impossible. Several patients were given local nerve blocks with small amounts of sedatives and intubated awake.[13]

In situations in which area hospitals are completely destroyed or nonfunctional, the government may have to establish healthcare facilities such as field hospitals[14] or, if close to a body of water, bring in one of the U.S. Navy's hospital ships as they did in New York City after the World Trade Center collapsed.

Finally, healthcare facilities near large industrial complexes must anticipate chemical injuries, explosions, and fires. The Bhopal gas tragedy of December 3, 1984, is but one example. Methyl isocyanate gas leaked from a tank, killing approximately 3,800 people and injuring several thousand.[15] Four years later, an independent investigation concluded that the event could have only been the result of sabotage; that is, a person or persons deliberately attached a water hose to the gas storage tank, initiating a massive chemical reaction.[15]

Role of Government

The initial response to any disaster, whether natural, unintended, or terrorist initiated, begins at the local level and involves law enforcement agencies, especially if there is criminal activity suspected; firefighters; and paramedics. Depending on the nature of the disaster, local passersby might also become involved, as is often the case. Fire departments are trained to deal with toxic chemicals, and, depending on the size of the municipality, many have hazardous materials teams, which are trained to deal with chemical and toxic agent spills. Unfortunately, many other first responders may not have had such training and are at risk of becoming casualties themselves, as has happened several times in the past.

If the incident is more than local agencies can handle, not only from a government perspective but also from the hospitals perspective, then state emergency management systems are called into play. The governor of the state could call up the National Guard to provide medical decontamination, transportation, and other services. Within the National Guard, there are a total of 32, with 11 more planned, chemical defense units stationed around the United States. Unfortunately, these units require many hours to mobilize and deploy to a site.[16] The Marine Chemical Biological Incident Response Force at Camp LeJuene, North Carolina, could likewise be activated.[17]

If the event supersedes the state's ability to respond, the federal government would become involved. The federal government's actions are predicated on multiple presidential decision directives, many of which have been established following September 11.[18] The Federal Bureau of Investigation has the responsibility for domestic terrorism and crisis management, investigating and preparing documentation for any criminal proceedings that might be conducted within the judicial system. The Federal Emergency Management Agency (FEMA) is
5 the lead agency for management assistance to state and local governments, providing emergency relief to affected individuals and businesses, decontaminating affected areas, and helping ensure public health safety.[19]

In addition to FEMA, the Department of Health and Human Services is the lead agency under the federal response plan to help provide health and health-related services, as well as medical services.[20] The Public Health Service would, in turn, activate the National Disaster Medical System,[21] which helps prepare direct relief to disaster survivors in the field. The National Disaster Medical System has three components—prehospital treatment, hospital evacuation, and in-hospital care. The prehospital treatment is provided by disaster medical assistance teams,[22] which are teams of about 40 individuals to include physicians, nurses, paramedics, and so on, who are responsible for first aid, casualty-clearing medical station, and field surgical intervention. As with the National Guard, however, these activities take a minimum of 12 to 24 hours to organize and implement. The Department of Health and Human Services has a number of other specialized teams that help respond.

The Department of Defense (DD) is also in a position to assist with incidents of biological or chemical terrorism, providing technical assistance, bomb disposal, decontamination, security, and other services to federal, state, and local authorities. The DOD can assign a military support liaison officer who works with FEMA to coordinate interagency efforts between FEMA and the branches of the Armed Forces.[23,24]

What the anesthesiologist in his or her worksite needs to know is that while he or she is managing a disaster, there are a number of local, state, and federal agencies that are mobilizing to help him or her handle the situation, depending on the gravity and number of casualties. The individual physician-anesthesiologist needs to focus his or her activities on dealing with individual patients, as outlined in this section.

The CDC has established a National Pharmaceutical Stockpile program as a national repository of antibiotics, chemical antidotes, life-support medications, intravenous administration and airway maintenance supplies, and medical/surgical items. There are two phases to this program. The first phase is the provision of eight separate, yet identical, prepackaged caches of medical materials called 12-hour "push packages," which are deployed throughout the United States. The second phase is, if the incident requires a larger response, that vendor management inventories are sent to arrive within 24 to 36 hours after the initial cache of materials arrives. Unfortunately, as with many of these initiatives, there are problems with the adequacy of the response plan.[25]

Military installations have also developed, and have provided when asked by FEMA, critical incident stress management teams, as they did following the attacks on the World Trade Center on September 11, 2001. These teams are designed to help individuals, both patients and healthcare providers, cope with traumatic stress and provide grief management.[26]

Role of Anesthesiologist in Managing Mass Casualties

It is probably difficult to anticipate all the ways in which anesthesiologists could be asked to assist in managing mass casualty situations. For example, on October 26, 2002, terrorists held 750 hostages at the Nord-Ost theater in Moscow. Many believe that the authorities instilled nebulized or volatile carfentanil into the air ducts of the opera house, thereby immobilizing the terrorists.[27] Unfortunately, because of the incapacitating effect of carfentanil, the hostages also became victims. Patients were transported from the theater to hospitals without any treatment prior to arrival. Ideally, anesthesiologists or other healthcare providers with an opioid antagonist such as naloxone should have been readily available and present at the site to manage both hostages and the terrorists themselves. Unfortunately, this was not the case.

6 As unusual as this scenario is, the anesthesiologist, depending on where he or she practices, may be called to manage situations that are unimaginable by current standards. However, with their basic understanding of physiology and pharmacology, their airway skills, their fluid-resuscitation expertise, and their ability to manage ventilators and to provide anesthesia in the field environment, in the emergency department, in the operating room, and in intensive care units (ICUs) will be invaluable. In these mass-casualty situations, many patients suffer burns, fractures, lacerations, soft-tissue trauma, and amputations that will require triage, stabilization in the emergency room or in some other facility near the emergency room, and more-definitive treatment in the operating room or ICU.

In previous industrial accidents and fires, appropriate management of the airway has been critical. Patients with large-area burns will require establishment of intravenous access for provision of intravascular volume resuscitation. Depending on the event (burn versus a crush injury—protocols for fluid resuscitation vary), in patients with extensive soft-tissue and skeletal muscle damage, alkalinization of the urine with volume resuscitation and diuresis may be organ saving and life saving.[28,29]

If chemical weapons are also used, again depending on the severity of the injury, not only may tracheal intubation be required, but ventilator management may also be necessary. The correct antidotes for managing patients who are victims of industrial chemical accidents and/or chemical warfare agents are discussed subsequently.

NUCLEAR ACCIDENTS

The likelihood of dealing with patients who are exposed to ionizing radiation—from most likely to least likely—would be from a nuclear power plant or reactor accident, terrorist action, and detonation of a nuclear bomb (Table 59-5). Unfortunately, this has happened too often in the past, with Chernobyl being the best example. On April 26, 1986, workers at the Chernobyl nuclear power plant did not recognize or respond to evidence of one of the reactors malfunctioning, with loss of cooling capacity and an explosion of the nuclear reactor.[30] Two workers died as a direct effect of the explosion, whereas those who remained in shielded areas survived unless they went to fight the fire, in which case they eventually died of radiation exposure. Short-term gamma and beta emissions from the explosion, as well as subsequent gamma and beta radiation from the reactor-core debris, killed many more and caused long-term health effects to the entire community. Because of a lack of protective clothing and respirators, the radioactive material that exploded into the atmosphere rained down for several hours and days, affecting many more workers and thousands of civilians. Primary sources of radiation were iodine-131, strontium-90, and cesium-137. During the next 24 hours, 140,000 people were evacuated, and potassium iodide tablets were distributed to as many people in the area as possible. Two hundred and thirty patients were subsequently hospitalized, with many patients succumbing to infections because of bone marrow suppression; and, in those patients in whom bone marrow transplantation was attempted, 17 of 19 died because of associated radiation burns. All told, radiation burns caused 21 deaths. Oropharyngeal burns occurred in 28 patients.

Over the next several years, the average exposure around Chernobyl was four times normal due to residual ground contamination. Almost two decades later, the effects of Chernobyl

TABLE 59-5

NUCLEAR THREATS IN DECREASING ORDER OF PROBABILITY

Accidents (nuclear power plants, reactors)
Terrorist action
Single nuclear bomb detonation
Theater nuclear war
Strategic nuclear war

continue to be felt in the immediate vicinity and in the area downwind from the reactor site.[30,31] The experience from 7 Chernobyl should indicate the kind of injuries and results that anesthesiologists can anticipate from nuclear accidents, including radiation burns, bone marrow suppression, the destruction of the lining of the gastrointestinal (GI) tract, GI bleeding with translocation of bacteria, infection, sepsis, septic shock, and death. The sequelae of infection and sepsis are best managed using the evidence-based medicine guidelines promulgated by 11 international groups.[32] As evidenced by the experiences in Chernobyl, potassium iodide is indicated to protect the thyroid gland from taking up iodine-131 and the use of other drugs are being considered, such as 5-androstenediol.

There have also been other situations, from which we can learn, during which people have been exposed to ionizing radiation. On March 28, 1979, at the Three Mile Island nuclear power plant, the number 2 nuclear reactor overheated, and, because the pressure-relief valve failed to close, radioactive coolant was released into the containment facility.[33] As is often the case, there were numerous communication missteps, which resulted in the release of inconsistent information, generating genuine fear among individuals living nearby the nuclear power plant. There were no biological effects of the event, but severe psychological sequelae did result.

On September 13, 1987, in Goiania, Brazil, a lead canister containing between 1,400 and 1,600 curies of cesium-137 was opened, contaminating 250 people. Four people died, but multiple individuals had short-term and long-term health sequelae.[34] Mitigation efforts required the removal of 6,000 tons of clothing, furniture, dirt, trees, and other materials.[35] The cesium had been left in a building in a lead canister when it was abandoned by its occupants; the canister was taken and opened by looters, and children played with the material.

Because of the possibility of exposure to ionizing radiation 8 from nuclear power plants and so on, the American Academy of Pediatrics has recommended that at least two tablets of potassium iodide be available for all inhabitants within 10 miles of any nuclear power plant.[36]

Potential Sources of Ionizing Radiation Exposure

We are exposed to radiation on an annual basis from cosmic radiation, radon, medical devices, and in multiple stores, factories, and so on. Even an air flight is associated with cosmic radiation exposure. A chest radiograph leads to 5 to 10 mrem of exposure, whereas a computed tomography scan can lead to up to 5,000 mrem of exposure.[37]

Obviously, the greatest concern is the exposure to ionizing radiation that is unintentional, such as occurred at the Chernobyl nuclear power plant, or intentional. Intentional threats are the result of military conflict or terrorism, two occurres of intental exposure were in Hiroshima and Nagasaki in 1945. It is important to remember that in Hiroshima, the bomb ("little boy") was only a 12.5-kiloton bomb, which killed an estimated 66,000 people and injured 69,000 more.[38] The bomb that fell at Nagasaki ("fat boy") was a 22-kiloton plutonium implosion-type bomb, which killed between 39,000 and 74,000 people, with 75,000 people sustaining severe injuries.[38] We learned in that experience that the majority of casualties are from the initial blast, from fire, and from the collapse of 9 buildings. Radiation exposure subsequently kills many more. With any nuclear explosion, then, many individuals will be injured or die from building collapse or the thermal pulse. Patients could have burn, crush, or radiation injury, or any combination thereof.

TABLE 59-6

TYPES OF RADIATION

TYPE	DESCRIPTION
Ionizing radiation	A high-frequency, low-amplitude form of radiation that interacts significantly with biological systems.
Alpha particle (α-particle)	A particle emitted from the nucleus of an atom. It contains two protons and two neutrons and is identical to the nucleus of a helium atom, without the electrons. Having a very large mass, α-particles have poor penetration and pose little hazard after external exposure but can produce tissue injury when inhaled or ingested.
Beta particle (β-particle)	A high-speed particle, identical to an electron, emitted from the nucleus of an atom.
Neutrons	A powerful but uncommon type of radiation, emitted only after a nuclear detonation. Neutrons are highly destructive, producing 10 times more tissue damage than gamma rays.
Gamma rays (γ-rays)	A form of ionizing radiation having no mass. Like visible light, γ-rays are made of photons, have significant penetrance, and are the most important external radiation hazard after a radiation disaster. γ–Rays are emitted from nuclei.
X-rays	Like γ-rays, x-rays have no mass; their energy is emitted from electrons.

More recently, we recognize that exposure to ionizing radiation may be as a result of terrorism. The most likely event will be the use of a dispersion device such as a conventional weapon (i.e., a bomb), surrounded with radionuclides such as cesium or strontium. In fact, in 1987, Iraq tested a one-ton "dirty" bomb, and, in 1996, Islamic terrorists in Chechnya placed a bomb packed with cesium-137 that did not explode in a Moscow park.[39] Although a radiologic dispersion device remains the most likely event, terrorists could also target a nuclear power plant using a commercial jet, munitions, or internal sabotage.

Although a blast, crush, or thermal injury is readily apparent, the effects of ionizing radiation are usually not apparent. Individuals should be familiar with types of ionizing radiation that include alpha particles, beta particles, gamma rays, x-rays, and neutrons (Table 59-6).[40] It is also helpful to understand how radiation is measured (Table 59-7). There are several methods that take into account the decay rate of a radioactive isotope (becquerel or a curie) or the dose absorbed, usually quantified as the amount absorbed by any type of tissue or material. The radiation-absorbed dose (rad) = 0.01 Gray (Gy), which is the international system of units (SI) for denoting the amount of energy deposited in joules per kilogram. One Gy equals 100 rad. A Sievert (Sv) is the SI unit for measurement of *human* exposure to radiation in joules per kilogram, with 1 Sv = 100 rem, the latter being a roentgen equivalent for man (rem).

In a nuclear accident or catastrophe, patients could have several types of radiation exposure, such as external radiation from an x-ray–emitting device or from gamma rays or beta particles. They can also be contaminated with debris-emitting ionized radiation, or they can inhale or ingest gaseous

TABLE 59-7

RADIATION EXPOSURE TERMS

TERM	DEFINITION	COMPARISON
Becquerel (Bq)	International system of units (SI) measurement of radioactivity, defined as decay events per second	1 Bq = 1 disintegration/sec
Curie (Ci)	Traditional measure of radioactivity, as measured by radioactive decay	1 Ci = 2.7×10^{10} disintegrations/sec
Radiation-absorbed dose (rad)	Energy deposited by any type of radiation to any type of tissue or material	1 rad = 0.01 Gy
Gray (Gy)	SI unit for the energy deposited by any type of radiation, in joules per kilogram	1 Gy = 100 rad
Roentgen equivalent man (rem)	Unit of *human* exposure to radiation	1 rem = 0.01 Sievert
Sievert (Sv)	SI unit for measurement of *human* exposure to radiation, in joules per kilogram	1 Sv = 100 rem

radioactive material. Some of this material can become incorporated into tissue, such as with radioactive iodine isotopes. To protect individuals, the distance from the source or explosion is the amount of shielding, the time one is exposed, and the amount of radioactive material to which one is exposed are important. Human tissue will block alpha particles (although, if inhaled, alpha particles can penetrate up to 50 μm into the pulmonary epithelium material, leading to the development of lung cancer) but will not stop beta particles or gamma rays. Beta particles can be stopped by aluminum shields, but gamma rays can penetrate even concrete walls, and, from that perspective, therefore, lead is required to shield for both gamma rays and x-rays.

The most likely injury from ionizing radiation is to those tissues that have the greatest turnover rate (i.e., the sensitivity of tissues to radiation is greatest for lymphoid tissues and greater for GI, reproductive, dermal, bone marrow, and nervous system tissue than for other types of tissue). In reality, the response of lymphoid and bone marrow to ionizing radiation causes the most problems. The thrombocytopenia, granulocytopenia, and GI injury lead to bleeding and bacterial translocation across the GI epithelium, the net result of which is sepsis and bleeding, the hallmarks of acute radiation syndrome, which lead to death.

Because ionizing radiation is invisible, individuals may appear normal or may present with nausea, vomiting, diarrhea, fever, hypotension, erythema, and central nervous system (CNS) dysfunction. Patients who present with nausea, vomiting, diarrhea, and fever are likely to have severe acute radiation syndrome. Hypotension, erythema, and CNS dysfunction will manifest later. "Short-term" effects such as these, however, may not appear until days to weeks after the exposure, depending on the amount of exposure (as little as 0.75 to 1.0 Gy), whereas hematopoietic syndrome (severe lymphoid and bone marrow suppression) results from exposure to 3 to 6 Gy and may lead to death within 8 to 50 days.[39] Long-term effects include thyroid cancer and psychologic injury, as has been documented many times in the past.

Management of Ionizing Radiation Exposure

If a radiation disaster occurs, it would be followed by a huge coordinated local, state, and federal response, which, at the federal level, would include the U.S. Department of Homeland Security, the Department of Energy, the Department of Justice, FEMA, the Environmental Protection Agency, and the Nuclear Regulatory Commission.

Of most importance, depending on the type of event, would be the immediate evacuation of the area. If evacuation is impossible, a safe place should be sought within the home or building. The principle of disaster management always involves containment (avoid bringing patients with material emitting ionizing radiation to the hospital). Therefore, as part of the containment process—to the extent possible—patients should be decontaminated at the site of exposure. Removal of clothing is important. Beta and gamma rays and neutrons will be gone unless there is still material emitting this radiation on patients' clothing. Rather than guess, it is best to disrobe. In previous mass casualty situations, maintenance of patients' privacy has been a concern, but not one that is readily solved, depending on the number of casualties. Afterward, patients' skin should be washed with warm soapy water. Depending on the number of casualties, decontamination areas may have to be set up outside hospitals, with care taken to isolate belongings. The same consideration must also be given to biological fluids as for clothing, including saliva, blood, urine, and stool, because they may be contaminated with radioisotopes and require special handling precautions.

As mentioned earlier, potassium iodide can prevent radiation-induced thyroid effects but must be given as quickly as possible; within 24 hours, if not given it has little protective effect.[36] Other drugs under investigation for prophylaxis of radiation-induced injuries include vitamin E, 5-androstenediol, nitroxides,[41–43] and a new compound, HE2100, which is a naturally occurring synthetic adrenal steroid hormone that has been found to have protective effects against radiation injury in nonhuman primates.[44] Currently, though, treatment is largely supportive because these patients will develop, based on their acute exposure, acute radiation syndrome manifested by bleeding and sepsis.

Treatment guidelines for management of postirradiation sepsis have been developed and advocated by the military.[45] The use of granulocyte colony-stimulating factor and so on may be of benefit.[39] Other treatments would include oral and GI decontamination using nasopharyngeal lavage, oral lavage and brushing; early stomach lavage; or administration of emetics and osmotic laxatives. Blocking agents include potassium iodide and strontium lactate. Mobilizing agents include ammonium chloride, calcium gluconate, and diuretics, which may enhance renal excretion. Chelation therapy that has been recommended includes calcium diethylenetriamine pentaacetic acid (DTPA) as an initial dose and then zinc DTPA.[46] The use of granulocyte macrophage colony-stimulating factor and thrombopoietin or interleukin 11, although postulated, has not been proven to be of benefit. For individuals with a contaminated GI tract, selective decontamination may be helpful although, again, has not been demonstrated to be of benefit in this situation.[46]

Unfortunately, because of the possibility of blast, thermal, and crush injury, along with the radiation injury, the care of the injured may require the care of patients who have multiple combined injuries. The initial response should be as per the advanced trauma life support guidelines, which include an assessment of the airway, breathing, and circulation, as well as extent of trauma, and then decontamination of the patient, after which the patient is stabilized and further evaluated. Wounds must be considered contaminated. "Dirty wounds" should not be closed but cleaned and débrided, excised, and observed. Unfortunately, in this situation, there is also the possibility that there may be the combined effects of a radiation-releasing event and the use of chemical or biological weapons.[47]

BIOLOGICAL DISASTERS

Although the threat of biological warfare has existed for some time, following the anthrax attacks of 2001 and 2002, we have had to confront the specter of terrorists using biological weapons to attack the United States, creating widespread panic and, based on what they used and how it was dispersed, large numbers of casualties and deaths.

Even with this heightened awareness of biological terrorism, as in every other area, the reality is that anesthesiologists need to be familiar with contagious diseases that are not initiated by terrorist groups (i.e., influenza, severe acute respiratory syndrome (SARS), West Nile virus). Influenza has killed more people in the twentieth century than any other infectious disease. There have been three large pandemics, including one in 1918 when an avian virus infected humans, creating the dead-
10 liest outbreak of disease in U.S. history. Somewhere between 25 and 50 million people, if not more, died, half of whom were otherwise healthy young adults. There were so many deaths in some communities that mass graves were dug to accommodate all the corpses.[48]

The Spanish flu was caused by a subtype of influenza A (there are three types of human influenza viruses: A, B, and C). Only subtypes of influenza A virus normally infect people: H1N1, H1N2, H3N2, H2N2, and now H1N5. All subtype of influenza A viruses infect birds, although birds. Typically, birds do not get sick when they are infected, but avian viruses can transform and infect humans, with subsequent human to human transmission in which case a pandemic could result. Alternately, current human influenza A viruses could have antigenic drift or shift, in which case a virus for which there is already a vaccine could transform such that populations would be naive and another pandemic would develop. This was the case in 1957 and 1958, when the Asian flu (H2N2) caused some 70,000 deaths in the U.S., and in 1968 to 1969, when the Hong Kong flu (H3N2) caused approximately 34,000 deaths in the United States.[49] Usually, the new pathogenic virus is detected several months in advance of major outbreaks and, hopefully, could allow sufficient time for the preparation of vaccines for entire populations. However, currently in the U.S., there is a shortage of vaccines, a shortage that is unlikely to be resolved because of manufacturing liability issues, in which case the government may have to become more involved. There are four antiviral drugs that currently have benefit in patients with the flu, including amantadine, rimantadine, zanamivir, and oseltamivir. If there were another flu pandemic, the World Health Organization (WHO) acknowledges that it could kill up to 50 million people worldwide.[49a] Because of their airway and ventilator-management skills, anesthesiologists will be involved in providing care for many of these patients.

Of greater worry is a recurrence of SARS. This is a viral illness, a coronavirus, that first presented in February 2003, infecting thousands of people worldwide, and almost 1,000 died (almost a 10% fatality rate).[50] Healthcare workers were significantly at risk, especially because they were called on to manage these patients in emergency departments, operating rooms, and ICUs. Because the virus was airborne and some healthcare workers wore ineffective isolation equipment, such as standard facemasks and so on, some of these individuals inhaled virions, became sick, and died.[51] Entire hospitals had to be quarantined, with no individuals allowed to leave or enter for fear of spreading the virus. Although this seems draconian, the action of several governments in enforcing this strict quarantine was one of the most important ways that the disease was limited. At this time, treatment of SARS is supportive, without any definitive therapy. In 2004, there were several isolated cases reported, but, as of December 2004, no further cases are currently being reported.[52]

The West Nile virus, a mosquito-borne encephalitis, had killed 87 of 2,432 infected people in 2004.[53] The death rate was relatively high, although the number of individuals infected was relatively small. The reason to highlight the West Nile virus is to underscore the importance of public health measures in controlling mosquito-borne diseases.

Biological Terrorism

History

Infectious agents have been used as biological weapons since the dawn of history. Ghengis Khan is reported to have used cats infected with fleas bearing the plague to destroy towns in his conquest of Asia. British forces distributed blankets that had been used by smallpox patients to Native Americans, killing more than 50% of the infected tribes.[54] In World War II, Unit 731, a Japanese military unit, is reported to have dropped plague-infected fleas over populated areas of China, causing outbreaks of plague and killing several hundred thousand people.[54]

The ideal biological agent is one that has the greatest potential for adverse public health impact, generating mass casualties and with potential for easy large-scale dissemination that could cause mass hysteria and civil disruption.[55] Such weapons should be relatively easy to produce, inexpensive, highly infectious, and contagious, resulting in widespread morbidity and mortality. To be effective, there needs to be no natural immunity, which is currently the case with diseases such as smallpox, for which we no longer routinely vaccinate individuals, except in the military and in high-risk public-health areas. There are three categories of biological weapons (Table 59-8). Category A are those weapons that are highly contagious and that fit all the characteristics of a relatively ideal biological agent.

Smallpox

The last case of naturally occurring smallpox in the world was reported in 1977 in Somalia.[56] In 1978, two laboratory workers in the United Kingdom were infected with smallpox.[56] In 1980, the WHO announced that the world was free of this scourge. In 1972, routine vaccination for smallpox was discontinued in the United States.[56] It is precisely because of this that we are at most risk for terrorists using smallpox as a biological weapon. Forty percent to 80% of patients exposed to the smallpox virus will come down with the disease. Smallpox is highly infective, requiring only 10 to 100 organisms to infect an individual. The mortality rate is approximately 30% in unvaccinated patients, and as high as 50% if smallpox occurs in communities that have no native immunity against smallpox. The protective effect of the smallpox vaccine decreases with time, but, even at 20 years, the vaccine would provide some protection.

TABLE 59-8

BIOLOGICAL AGENTS USED FOR WARFARE

■ CATEGORY A	■ CATEGORY B	■ CATEGORY C
Bacillus anthracis (anthrax)	*Coxiella brunetti* (Q fever)	Various equine encephalitic viruses
Variola major (smallpox)	*Vibrio cholerae* (cholera)	
Yersinia pestis (plague)	*Burkholderia mallei* (glanders)	
Clostridium botulinum (botulism)	Enteric pathogens (*Escherichia coli* O157:H7, salmonella, shigella)	
Francisella tularensis (tularemia)	Cholera, cryptosporidium	
Viral hemorrhagic fever (Ebola, Lassa, Marburg, Argentine)	Various encephalitic viruses	
	Various biological toxins	

When an unvaccinated person is initially infected, he or she develops a prodrome of malaise, headache, and backache with the onset of fever to as high as 40°C. The fever decreases over the next 3 or 4 days, at which time a rash develops. This is in contradistinction to chickenpox, in which the rash develops at the same time as the fever. Unlike chickenpox, smallpox has a predilection for the distal extremities and face, although no part of the body is spared (Fig. 59-1). Also, all lesions in a patient with smallpox are at the same stage, whereas, with chickenpox, lesions are at multiple stages, including papules, vesicles, pustules, and scabs (Table 59-9). Most cases of smallpox are transmitted through aerosolized droplets that are inhaled, but clothes and blankets that have come in contact with pustules, until the scab falls off, are infectious; the organism can be transmitted in these linens.

Smallpox has probably been present in humans since 10,000 BC. It is transmitted human to human, and, if used as a bioterrorism agent, would likely be dispersed by aerosols in the environment with the hope that multiple humans would be infected and would transmit it to other humans. There is evidence that the former Soviet Union has developed transgenic smallpox viruses that are very infectious and for which the U.S. vaccine may not be completely protective. The onset of such a virus might be very short. Currently, there are only two WHO-approved depositories of smallpox, at the CDC in Atlanta, Georgia, and at the Institute of Virus Preparations in Russia. With the collapse of the Soviet Union, there was concern that some stores of smallpox made it into rogue countries that may have developed their own biological weapons.

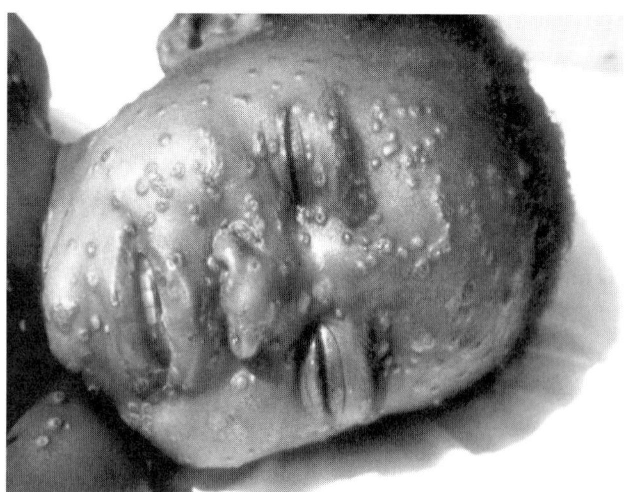

FIGURE 59-1. Smallpox.

A look at how the WHO eradicated smallpox might be helpful in understanding how the United States has prepared to respond to smallpox as a biological weapon. It must be remembered that, in the eighteenth century, 400,000 Europeans per year were dying from smallpox. Although only 1% of patients who survive smallpox become blind, it accounted for one third of all cases of blindness in Europe. The WHO eradicated smallpox by identifying patients with smallpox and placing them in strict quarantine. Such patients are readily identified because of the presence of smallpox lesions on the face. Not only were patients isolated, but all their contacts were vaccinated because there was a 3- to 7-day window with the naturally occurring virus before the patient developed symptoms and signs of smallpox.[57]

Vaccination against smallpox is controversial. The vaccine is made from a live vaccinia virus developed in calf lymph, but it is not an attenuated smallpox virus itself. Smallpox is a member of the *Orthopox* genus of the *pox varidae* family of double-stranded DNA viruses that also contain cowpox, monkeypox, vaccinia, and so on. In the event of a documented case of smallpox, the CDC has plans to quarantine the patient and then vaccinate immediate contacts of patients within a certain geographic radius. There are stockpiles of vaccines placed strategically throughout the U.S. for just such an event. A bifurcated needle is dipped into the reconstituted vaccine and then 10 to 15 jabs are made into the dermis of the upper deltoid. Because of the side effects of smallpox vaccinations, people with immunologic disorders or eczema (active or with a history of severe eczema) and pregnant or nursing women will not be administered the vaccine. As of 2003, with the use of

TABLE 59-9

DIFFERENTIAL OF PUSTULAR LESIONS

	■ SMALLPOX	■ CHICKENPOX
Fever	2–4 days before rash	Simultaneous with rash
Rash	All lesions have same-stage development	Lesions at various stages (papules, pustules, scabs all present)

vaccination in the U.S. Armed Forces and for healthcare workers, 11 the CDC reported several nonserious adverse events such as fever, rash, and malaise, and two cases of cardiomyopathy.[58] Because of this, there is no plan to routinely vaccinate the U.S. population. The CDC and the state departments of health will implement their quarantine and vaccination plans should an index case or several cases (a cluster) occur.

Anthrax

Bacillus anthracis (anthrax) was probably used as a biological weapon in the Middle Ages when troops laying siege to a town would catapult infected animal carcasses over the ramparts and into the inhabited areas. For reasons discussed later, this was not a particularly effective way of infecting the native population. During the 20th century, several countries, including the U.S., Great Britain, Russia, and Iraq, studied ways to weaponize anthrax. Anthrax has appeal as a bioterrorism agent because, if it can be "weaponized" (normally, if anthrax spores are inhaled, they clump in the nasal pharynx), *B. anthracis* must be finely ground so it readily aerosolizes and can get to and deposit in the terminal bronchioles and alveoli.[59] Inhalation anthrax, which was relatively uncommon in the past, has an 80% fatality rate. One of the letters that was mailed in the anthrax attacks of 2001 contained 2 g of weapons-grade anthrax. With an LD50 of 1,000 spores under optimum conditions, this was enough material to infect 50 million individuals. Most countries that have weaponized anthrax would either aerosolize it using airplanes or deliver it through a dispersion device mounted on top of a missile. The attacks on North America in 2001, as well as the dispersion of anthrax spores from the accidental release at a biological facility in the city of Sverdlovsk in the former Soviet Union in 1979, are illustrative of the potential of anthrax as a weapon. In the U.S., 5 of 11 cases died (50% mortality rate); in the former Soviet Union, 66 of 77 died (86% mortality rate).[60] The Aum Shinrikyo also released anthrax spores in Tokyo in 1993. Fortunately, they used a nonpathogenic strain of anthrax and so there were no casualties.[59] As demonstrated in 2001 in the U.S., smarter terrorists will be far more successful in using infectious weapons-grade anthrax. Such attacks, even if detected, create mass hysteria and greatly impact the public healthcare system.[61]

Anthrax is a Gram-positive, spore-forming bacillus that is transmitted to humans from contaminated animals, their byproducts, or their carcasses. Spores may persist in soil for years. The disease is all but gone from North America, but it is still prevalent in many developing countries, and herbivores, especially cattle, usually die within 24 to 48 hours of contracting the disease. The dead carvs has such a huge number of organisms that humans, who are relatively resistant to infection, can be exposed and contract the disease.[62]

There are three primary types of anthrax infection: cutaneous, inhalation, and GI. Ninety-five percent of cases are cutaneous. From a public-health perspective, we are worried most about inhalation anthrax, which worldwide usually affects 2,000 to 20,000 people per annum. People can be exposed through contact with animals in an agricultural setting or in an industrial setting (e.g., a rendering plant or tanning facility) or, as mentioned previously, in the production of biological weapons.[63]

Anthrax has additional appeal to bioterrorists because inhalation anthrax is hard to detect. It manifests as an influenza-like disease with fever, myalgias, malaise, and a nonproductive cough with or without chest pain.[64] After a few days, the patient appears to get better, but then a couple of days later the patient becomes much sicker with dyspnea, cyanosis, hemoptysis, stridor, and chest pain. The most notable finding on physical examination and laboratory testing is a widened mediastinum. Usually, when a patient develops profound dyspnea, death ensues within 1 to 2 days. In the past, penicillin G was the treatment of choice, but, because weaponized anthrax has been engineered to be resistant to penicillin G, ciprofloxacin or doxycycline is more commonly used. In the outbreaks in Florida; and New Jersey, the District of Columbia contacts of infected patients or people exposed to the spores were treated with ciprofloxacin or doxycycline.

Plague

The oldest cases of *Yersinia pestis* (plague) were documented in China in the third century. It created multiple epidemics throughout the world in subsequent years. In the 14th century alone, plague killed one third of the European population. The first documented use of plague as a biological weapon was in 1346 when the Tartars in their siege of the fortress at Kaffa catapulted infected corpses into the city.[54] The plague was used by Unit 731 to infect large areas of China, and as many as 200,000 Chinese may have died. More recently, the U.S. and Russia have studied *Y. pestis* as a bioagent, examining ways to aerosolize it and ways to distribute it. It is viable for approximately 60 minutes after being distributed, and, if spread by an airplane, could remain viable on wind currents for up to 10 km from the dispersion site.

Y. pestis is a nonmotile, Gram-positive bacillus.[55] Rodents and fleas are its natural hosts, and they reinfect each other by fleas biting infected rodents, or, because the soil can be contaminated, rodents can acquire the disease simply by digging in an infected area. Humans are an accidental host, and they acquire the disease usually from a flea bite, although rarely there can be direct inoculation of infected material into a person. Direct person-to-person transmission occurs with pneumonic plague.

There are two types of plague: bubonic and pneumonic. With bubonic plague, after a flea bite, there is a 2- to 6-day incubation period, at which time there is the sudden onset of fever, chills, weakness, and headache. Intense painful swelling occurs in the lymph nodes, usually in the groin, axilla, or neck. This swelling or buboes is typically oval in nature, 1 to 10 cm in diameter and extremely tender. Up to 25% of patients will have pustules, papules, or skin lesions near this buboe. Without treatment, patients become septic and develop septic shock with cyanosis and gangrene in peripheral tissues, leading to the "black death" descriptor that was used during the epidemics in Europe. As mentioned, material from these buboes is infective only if inoculated into human tissue. However, patients who have bubonic plague can seed their lungs, in which case they develop pneumonic plague. During coughing, they aerosolize *Y. pestis*, which is highly contagious. Mortality for either form of the disease is more than 50%. Diagnosis is made with a Gram stain or culture of organisms from blood, sputum, or buboe.

The treatment of choice is streptomycin, but chloramphenicol and tetracycline are acceptable alternatives. These patients with pneumonic plague should be managed as one would manage a patient with drug resistance to tuberculosis because the respiratory secretions are highly infectious.

There was one formal and fixed whole organism vaccine that has been removed from the market, but the U.S. government continues to develop vaccines to *Y. pestis*.[65]

Tularemia

Francisella tularensis (tularemia) has some similarities to anthrax and plague, but it is not nearly as dangerous. It was studied as a biological weapon in the 20th century because it is highly infectious, requiring an inoculum of perhaps as small as only 10 organisms.[66] During World War II, tularemia developed in soldiers along the German-Russian front that was believed secondary to the use of *F. tularensis* as a biological weapon. The fact that both armies were infected underscores one of the dangers of using infectious agents as biological weapons. Often these are dispersed with aerosols, and, despite the best predictions of air currents, they are notoriously unpredictable; with the shifting air currents, one's own troops could become infected. Unit 731 of the Japanese army also studied the use of *F. tularensis* as a biological weapon, and the U.S. and Russia were known to have grown large quantities of *F. tularensis* and stored it.

F. tularensis is a gram-negative, pleomorphic rod.[55] There are several animal hosts, with the cotton-tailed rabbit being one of the most susceptible. Normally, humans acquire *F. tularensis* with direct contact with an infected animal or from the bite of an infected tick or deerfly.[66] Occasionally, the ingestion of infected food or inhalation of a small amount of aerosol will initiate the disease. There are two strains of *F. tularensis,* Jellisoni A and B, with the B strain being relatively innocuous, and, in North America, the A strain is quite virulent. Normally, a patient will develop a cutaneous ulcer at the site of entry after contact with an animal. As few as 10 or 50 organisms can invade the body, either through hair follicles or miniabrasions. The incubation period is 2 to 6 days, at which time there is swelling and ulceration at the site of entry. As the swelling continues, the skin eventually breaks and creates an ulcer, which develops a necrotic base that becomes black as it scars.

It is most likely that *F. tularensis* would be delivered from an aerosol via an airplane, in which case, following inhalation, there is a 3- to 5-day incubation period, and then the onset of disease is marked with fever, pharyngitis, bronchitis, pneumonia, pleuritis, and hilar lymphadenopathy. Mortality rate for pneumonic tularemia is 5 to 15%.[67]

The treatment of choice for tularemia is streptomycin, although gentamicin, tetracycline, and chloramphenicol have been used. There is concern that the former Soviet Union, and perhaps the U.S. and terrorists, have engineered *F. tularensis* to be resistant to a number of agents. Prophylaxis with streptomycin, ciprofloxacin, or doxycycline has been recommended in the past for individuals exposed to the organism. There was a vaccine that was comprised of an attenuated whole organism strain, but it is no longer available. The U.S. Army Medical Research Institute of Infectious Diseases continues to work on vaccines to tularemia.[68]

Botulism

The first known work with *Clostridium botulinum* (botulism) as a biological weapon was in World War II. Both the Germans and Japanese military and scientific communities experimented with *C. botulinum*. Unit 731 fed pure cultures of *C. botulinum* to Chinese captives with devastating effects. Both the United States and the former Soviet Union are known to have produced large quantities of *botulinum* toxin, as has Iraq, Iran, Syria, and North Korea. In fact, after the first Gulf War, Iraq admitted to having more than 19,000 L of concentrated *botulinum* toxin, of which almost half was loaded on military weapons.[69] Nineteen thousand liters of *botulinum* toxin is enough to kill the world's population three times over. More recently, the Aum Shinrikyo cult in Japan dispersed aerosols of *C. botulinum* toxin on three different occasions in their country. Fortunately, their dispersal methods and the agent were associated with multiple problems, and no one was injured. Of concern is if a terrorist organization working with a rogue state acquired and used *C. botulinum* as a bioterrorist weapon.

Botulism is a neuroparalytic disease caused by the toxin from *botulinum*. Unlike all the other bioterrorist agents mentioned previously, it is not caused by a live organism and is, therefore, not contagious. The organism from which *botulinum* toxin is derived is a gram-positive spore, which is an obligatory anaerobe widely distributed in nature in soil and in marine and agriculture products. Humans ingest *C. botulinum* without apparent effects. It is the toxin that produces toxicity. *C. botulinum* has seven distinct toxins, and, once ingested or inhaled, the toxins are distributed in the bloodstream to the cholinergic receptor, where they block the release of acetylcholine by inhibiting the intracellular fusion of the acetylcholine vesicle to the membrane for release. Victims develop progressive weakness, a flaccid paralysis that begins in the extremities and progresses until the respiratory muscles are paralyzed. Of note, *C. botulinum* toxin is the most potent poison known to humans; the LD100 dose is only 1 picogram.[70]

Shortly after ingestion or inhalation of the toxin, the incubation period is between 2 hours and 8 days but most commonly between 12 and 36 hours.[71] It is manifested, as muscles become weak as diplopia, dysphonia, dysarthria, dysphagia, and eventually dyspnea and frank paralysis. Along with the effects in the skeletal muscular system caused by dysfunction of the nicotinic receptor, muscularinic blockade results in decreased salivation, ileus, and urinary retention. The toxin can be removed through gastric lavage, and the use of cathartics with enemas. The treatment of patients includes the use of a trivalent antitoxin. Patients with profound respiratory embarrassment should have their trachea protected and mechanical ventilation initiated. Without the use of antitoxin, it takes the patient 2 to 8 weeks to recover. From past experience, the mortality rate is quoted as 5 to 10%.

Hemorrhagic Fevers

There are a number of viral hemorrhagic fevers that are listed as category A agents, including the arena viruses (e.g., Lassa fever), bunya viruses (e.g., Hanta), flaviruses (e.g., Dengue), and filoviruses (e.g., Ebola, Marburg). There are at least 18 viruses that cause human hemorrhagic fevers, which form a special group of viruses characterized by viral replication in lymphoid cells, after which patients develop fever and myalgia with an incubation of anywhere from 2 to 18 days, depending on the agent itself and the amount of the agent that is inhaled or inoculated across the dermis.[70] They encompass syndromes that vary from febrile hemorrhagic fever with edema to distributive shock, which rapidly leads to death. Both the U.S. and the former Soviet Union have experimented with and weaponized several of these viruses. Studies in nonhuman primates suggest that the agents are highly infectious, requiring only a few virions to produce illness.[71] As mentioned, several governments have weaponized hemorrhagic fever viruses, and the Aum Shinrikyo cult in Japan went to Africa in the 1990s to try to obtain an Ebola virus that they could weaponize. There is no known incident in which these agents have been used as a biological weapon, but there is clear interest and potential for this use.

The viruses are single-stranded, RNA viruses that have a rodent or insect reservoir and are communicated to humans by inhalation of an aerosol or, as mentioned, contact with an infected animal or through a bite. Humans are not a reservoir for the virus but become infected through contact with infected animals or the bite of an infected insect. The diseases are contagious, and person-to-person transmission in Africa has been documented with several of these viruses.[68] As mentioned, the incubation period is within several days of contact or inhalation of the agent, at which time patients present with fever, myalgia, and evidence of capillary leak (peripheral or pulmonary edema), disseminated intravascular coagulation, and thrombocytopenia, which is one of the hallmarks of the illnesses. The fatality rate, depending again on the specific virus used, is anywhere from 2 to 60%.[68] There are no specific antiviral therapies for this class of viruses, but there have been anecdotal reports of ribavirin, interferon-alpha, and hyperimmune globulin as being protective, but there is simply not enough experience to know for sure.

There is a live attenuated virus vaccine for yellow fever, but there are none for any of the other agents, although there is extensive, ongoing testing with the development of vaccines for several of these most dangerous viruses.

Role of the Anesthesiologist in Bioterrorism

It is unlikely that an ICU physician or anesthesiologist would be at the initial site of origin of a biological attack, but it could happen. Most likely, they will become involved if the hospital at which they work ends up providing care for a number of these patients.[55] As in the previous situations, anesthesiologists could find themselves being involved in triage in the emergency room, operating room, or ICU.[72] As suggested for several of these situations, airway management and ventilator management may be critical, as would the establishment of intravascular access and volume resuscitation. There is anecdotal evidence from Asia that, with infectious agents, healthcare workers are better protected if they use a neuromuscular blocker when intubating the trachea for the obvious reason that when the anesthesiologist intubates the trachea, they are less likely to be subjected to any aerosolized particles (S. F. Yim, personal communication June 1, 2003). However, this argument is somewhat specious because, whenever dealing with a patient with a suspected pulmonary contagious disease such as anthrax, plague, hemorrhagic virus, tularemia, or drug-resistant tuberculosis, anesthesiologists must protect themselves by using 100% effective respiratory protection, going so far as to consider an oxygen-rebreathing system. (With a burn injury to the airway, however, neuromuscular blockers are not recommended in managing the casualties of a major disaster.)

Obviously, it is critical to have a high index of suspicion if you are managing the index case or two or more patients with presenting signs and symptoms that are suggestive of the use of a biological weapon. The individual who is the point of contact for the index case should notify the hospital infectious disease specialist and the local and state health departments. Factors that might indicate the intentional release of a biological agent would include unusual temporal or geographic clustering of cases, an uncommon age distribution, or a significant number of cases (more than one) of acute flaccid paralysis that might suggest use of *botulinum* toxin.

If called to the hospital to be involved in managing such a catastrophe, the anesthesiologist must review basic decontamination and isolation techniques and, as commented previously, must follow those guidelines scrupulously.

CHEMICAL

Emergency management teams in the U.S. have traditionally prepared to respond to chemical spills and industrial accidents. Many communities have hazardous materials teams that would respond to a chemical spill and exposure at an industrial or commercial site, and communities that have large industrial/chemical plants have emergency plans and systems in anticipation of an accident in their community. It is more difficult to prepare for accidents that involve derailments of railroad tank cars containing chemical agents, but, in this circumstance, state and federal agencies would respond in assisting local communities.

Prior to the mid-1980s, it was unthinkable that chemical agents would be used by rogue states or terrorists, but much has changed. In the 20th century, during World War I, more than 1 million soldiers and civilians were exposed to chemical (gas) injuries, with more than 100,000 of them dying. In 1935, Italy invaded Abyssinia (Ethiopia) and, during that invasion, sprayed mustard gas from aircraft. When Japan invaded China, mustard gas, phosgene, and hydrogen cyanide were used. In that same year, German chemical laboratories produced the first nerve agent, tabun. From 1963 to 1967, Egypt used phosgene and mustard agents in support of South Yemen during the civil war in that country. When Iraq attacked Iran in the 1980s, mustard gas and nerve agents were used. In all these examples,[73] chemical agents were used by the military during armed conflict. In 1994 and 1995, the use of nerve agents by the Japanese cult Aum Shinrikyo was a major turning point.[74] As outlined previously in this chapter, the cult had tried to use anthrax and *botulinum* spores and, as noted, tried to obtain specimens of hemorrhagic viruses for use as biological weapons. They were not successful with any of these enterprises, but it was their use of sarin in Tokyo that had major healthcare consequences and far-reaching ramifications. As a result of the attack, more than 5,000 persons required emergency medical evaluation, with approximately 1,000 of them likely exposed to the agent, resulting in at least 11 deaths.

Since then, and because of the events of September 11 and the anthrax attacks of 2001, we have had to prepare for the possibility that terrorists would use chemical weapons to attack the United States. Chemical weapons make sense because they are relatively inexpensive compared with conventional and nuclear weapons, they are relatively easy to use, and when used against a population, create major fear and panic and incredible demands on healthcare systems.[73] A well-planned attack would severely cripple a U.S. city, as well as inflict considerable morbidity and mortality. In this section, we discuss some of the different chemical agents that have been developed (Table 59-10).

TABLE 59-10

POTENTIAL CHEMICAL WEAPONS

Nerve
GA (tabun)
GB (sarin)
GD (soman)
GF
VX
Pulmonary
Chlorine
Phosgene
Blood
AC (hydrogen cyanide)
CK (cyanogen chloride)
Vesicants
H, HD (sulfur mustard)
HN_1, HN_2, HN_3 (nitrogen, mustard)
Lewisite (chlorovinyldichloroarsine)

Nerve Agents

The nerve agents are chemicals that affect nerve transmission by inhibiting acetylcholinesterase so that acetylcholine accumulates at the muscarinic and nicotinic acetylcholine receptor and within the CNS. Their effects are due to excess catecholamine. Examples of nerve agents that anesthesiologists use on a regular basis are the carbamates, which include physostigmine, neostigmine, and pyridostigmine. Savin is a carbamate compound that is an insecticide. The rest of the anticholinesterases are the organophosphates, which include the insecticides malathion and diazinon and the nerve agents.

Nerve agents were developed by Germany before World War II but were not used in World War II. They include GA, GB, GD,

TABLE 59-11

TOXICITY OF NERVE AGENTS

	LCT_{50} mg/min per m^3	LD_{50} mg/70 kg
GA	400	1,000
GB	100	1,700
GD	70	50
GF	50	30
VX	10	10

GF, and VX in increasing potency and toxicity. These five agents are clear, colorless liquids, which vaporize at room temperature and can then penetrate skin, clothing, or the epithelium of the lung or GI tract. As the agents bind to acetylcholinesterase, acetylcholine accumulates, and one sees the sequelae of excess acetylcholine.

With muscarinic receptor activation, patients experience airway, pupillary, and GI constriction; bradycardia; and activity of the glands within the eyes, nose, and mouth and sweat glands. Nicotinic stimulation leads to tachycardia and hypertension from stimulation at the preganglionic site and, from stimulation of the nicotinic acetylcholine receptor on the neuromuscular junction, fasciculations, twitching, fatigue, and flaccid paralysis. Excess parasympathetic activity leads to miosis and loss of accommodation, so patients complain of blurred vision. Within the respiratory system, the increased parasympathetic activity leads to bronchospasm, dyspnea, and rhinorrhea. The agent on the skin will produce localized sweating, and fasciculations can be observed. Within the cardiovascular system, activity within the muscarinic system leads to bradycardia, and, at the nicotinic site, preganglionic nodes and increase in heart rate. The net effect is difficult to anticipate; the patient's heart rate may be low, normal, or high. Within the GI tract, the increased parasympathetic activity leads to nausea, vomiting, diarrhea, and incontinence. This overall unopposed parasympathetic activity leads to a pneumonic of DUMBELS (diarrhea, urination, miosis, bronchorrhea and bronchoconstriction, emesis, lacrimation, and salivation).

The toxicity of the nerve agents depends on the compound delivered, the dose that is delivered, and the time that an individual is exposed to that dose. Toxicity of the compounds is demonstrated in Table 59-11, where LCt_{50} is a measure of the concentration versus the time (Ct) of exposure. For example, a patient exposed to 10 mg/m^3 of an agent for 10 minutes would have a Ct of 100 mg/min per m^3. The same could be achieved by being exposed to a concentration of 100 mg/m^3 for only 1 minute.

The treatment for nerve agent poisoning is one with which every anesthesiologist is familiar. Atropine is a competitive muscarinic blocker. Pralidoxime chloride is the better long-term treatment because it reactivates acetylcholinesterase by removing the organophosphate compound. Atropine is administered at a dose of 2 to 6 mg or more and is repeated every 5 to 10 minutes until secretions begin to decrease (the patient is not salivating) and ventilation is improved. In severe casualties, 15 to 20 mg would not be unusual, and some casualties have required over 1000 mg of atropine.[75] The U.S. military travels with automatic injectors containing 2 mg of atropine and 600 mg of 2-PAM CL (pyridostigmine) or pralidoxime chloride.

Depending on the extent of exposure, treatment is different. For minimal exposure, often seen with brief exposure to nerve agent vapor, patients may complain of headache and tightness in the chest and manifest miosis, rhinorrhea, and salivation. Individuals must be removed from further exposure, clothing removed, topical atropine instilled in the eye if pain is significant, and wet decontamination provided if there was any liquid exposure. With moderate exposure, the same signs are present, but now the patient demonstrates more severe rhinorrhea, complains of dyspnea, and on examination, there is evidence of bronchospasm and muscular fasciculations. Patients should now be treated with atropine and 2-PAM CL intramuscularly. Casualties again must have their clothing removed, and, if they were exposed to liquid nerve agent, they need to go through a wet decontamination process. With severe exposure, the same symptoms as mentioned previously are present, but now the patient manifests severe respiratory compromise, flaccid paralysis, incontinence, convulsions, and arrhythmias. The patient should receive aggressive atropine, along with 2-PAM CL to a maximum of 1,500 mg intravenously or intramuscularly, and the patient should go through a wet decontamination, with ventilatory assistance provided if necessary.

For situations in which one is anticipating nerve agent exposure, pyridostigmine is a long-acting agent that binds with acetylcholinesterase, allowing the enzyme to spontaneously regenerate. It does not cross the blood-brain barrier and, if used, must be taken more than 30 minutes prior to exposure.

With nerve injury casualties, decontamination is critical. It needs to be done as quickly as possible, first as mentioned previously by leaving the area of exposure, whether to liquid or vapor. As commented on at the beginning of this chapter, healthcare and emergency workers in Japan became victims themselves by standing unprotected in the subway cars in which there was liquid sarin with some vapor.[5] Patients are decontaminated by removing their clothing and by pouring on them copious amounts of water in 5% hypochlorite (household bleach). The bleach is not as critical as washing with copious amounts of water. Depending on the number of casualties, emergency departments have plans in place to set up fire trucks side by side, with a "chamber" established between the two trucks in which individuals would disrobe as they came into the chamber and be exposed to water sprays as they walked through the chamber to the other side.[76] From there, depending on the severity of the symptoms, they would receive atropine, 2-PAM CL, and further treatment (e.g., assisted ventilation, benzodiazepines, oxygen procedures).

Pulmonary Agents

The pulmonary or choking agents were probably the first chemicals to be used in warfare during World War I. On April 22, 1915, near Ypres, Belgium, the Germans released about 160 tons of chlorine gas from 6,000 pressurized cylinders along their lines with the wind blowing toward the Allies. The chlorine floated on huge clouds toward the Allied lines, causing eye, nose, and throat burning and, as it was inhaled, created pulmonary edema. Casualties began to cough up yellow-tinged pulmonary secretions. Approximately 5,000 soldiers died in that attack, and 2 days later, in a second attack, another 500 soldiers died. In all, more than 15,000 men were wounded. By late 1915, chlorine was replaced by phosgene, which was more deadly than the chlorine gas previously used.[77] During World War II, no chemical weapons were used, but, as mentioned previously, prior to the war, the Germans discovered the chemical weapons known as nerve agents. Following the war, both the Allies and the former Soviet Union used German chemists to develop their own chemical weapons programs.

There are primarily four pulmonary agents: chloropicrin, chlorine, phosgene (CG), and diphosgene. Phosgene is a prototypical agent because, as stated, it is deadlier than any of the other compounds.[78] Its chemical formula is $COCL_2$ with a molecular weight of 98 and a boiling point of 8.2°C. It is a colorless gas and has an odor of recently cut hay at 22 to 28°C and normal pressure conditions. Because of a vapor density of 3.4, it stays in the air for a long period of time, congregating in low-lying places. It is highly soluble in lipids and, therefore, can easily penetrate pulmonary epithelium and the cells lining the alveoli. Although it is very lipid soluble, it reacts rapidly with water to form hydrochloric acid and carbon dioxide. This may explain how it works because, when it reaches the alveoli, it may produce hydrochloric acid, which is itself extremely toxic to tissues, causing a capillary leak and the development of acute lung injury, which would progress to acute respiratory distress syndrome. Depending on the amount of gas inhaled, hypoxia from low FIO_2 would also complicate this picture. Immediately on exposure to phosgene, patients begin coughing because of the noxious nature of the gas and also exhibit nausea, vomiting, choking, and chest tightness. Following the initial exposure, depending on the amount of gas inhaled, there is a 1- to 24-hour period in which the individual seems relatively free of abnormalities, but during this period of time the pulmonary capillary membranes are being injured with leakage of fluid into the alveoli.

For individuals who are exposed, gas masks provide the best protection. If gas masks are not available, individuals need to remove themselves from exposure as quickly as possible. For those individuals who inhale sufficient quantities of gas who then develop acute lung injury or acute respiratory distress syndrome, the management is similar to patients who develop this syndrome for other reasons. In this circumstance, the anesthesiologists should be relatively at ease because this is a situation in which they have the physiologic and pharmacologic experience to manage the airway, ventilators, and hemodynamic monitoring to optimize care for patients with noncardiogenic pulmonary edema.

Blood Agents

The so-called blood agents are cyanogens, which are inhaled and release hydrogen cyanide, which impairs cytochrome oxidase and aerobic metabolism at the level of the mitochondria. The blood agents are hydrogen cyanide (AC), hydrocyanic acid, cyanogen chloride, and arsine.[78] At 22 to 27°C, AC is a colorless liquid and can be taken up through the skin as a liquid or inhaled. Its boiling point is 25.7°C, and it is difficult to use as a biological weapon because it is so highly volatile and, therefore, is not persistent. If released in an open area, high concentrations are hard to obtain. In a closed area, high concentrations, which are lethal, can readily be obtained. It is lethal because it interferes with cytochrome oxidase and cellular respiration. Patients quickly develop metabolic acidosis and all the sequelae associated with cellular hypoxemia.

Patients who present with AC exposure have a variety of symptoms, depending on the amount to which they were exposed, the root of poisoning, and as in previous examples, the exposure time. The patient will appear restless, tachypneic, and occasionally will complain of headaches, palpitations, and dyspnea. As time progresses, depending on the severity of the inhalation, nausea, vomiting, convulsions leading to coma, and respiratory failure manifest themselves. If the AC dosage is high, patients may not have any of these symptoms and simply collapse within seconds to minutes of exposure, which would be followed within 1 to 2 minutes by convulsions and cardiac arrest.

Treatment for AC toxicity is another problem for which anesthesiologists are quite familiar because of their use of nitroprusside, which at high doses and for extended periods of time also releases cyanide ions that can poison the cellular respiration. Cyanide ions are normally metabolized by the body by the rhodanese enzyme in the liver, which is a sulfur-requiring step that leads to the bioformation of methemoglobin. Often, there is an insufficient quantity of sulfur present for rhodanese to operate efficiently; therefore, treatment involves the administration of sodium thiosulfate, with supportive care in terms of tracheal intubation, ventilation, 100% oxygen, and cardiac support with ionotropes and vasopressors. If the number of casualties is too great and there is insufficient means to manage casualties, then mortality could be quite high.

Again, for the reasons mentioned, it would be difficult to use AC as an effective chemical weapon by terrorists that would affect large numbers of persons in civilian areas. It is mentioned primarily because of its historical interest and because there may be situations in which in could be used in the future.

Vesicants

During World War I, not only were chlorine and phosgene used, but sulfur mustard was also widely used on both sides of the conflict. Sodium mustard and related compounds such as nitrogen mustard, phosgene oxime, and lewisite, also known as "blister agents," get their names from the burns and blisters produced by these compounds on contact with the skin. Although these blisters are the most readily apparent manifestations, these compounds are also inhaled and can inflict severe damage to the respiratory system and the eyes and produce multiple organ dysfunction syndrome. Vesicants are often used by warring factions to force enemy troops to wear protective equipment, which makes them less mobile and able to fight less efficiently.[78] Blister agents are colorless and almost odorless. If the temperature is high enough, an odor that smells like rotten onions or mustard is present.

Sulfur mustard is a bifunctional alkylating agent that contains two reactive chloroethyl moieties. These chloroethyl compounds are extremely reactive and allow them to bind to other substances such as nucleic acids, proteins, and nucleotides. For individuals exposed to sulfur mustard, it readily penetrates clothing and infiltrates the skin and the eyes. As it volatilizes, it can be inhaled or ingested through the GI tract. Symptoms of sulfur poisoning do not show up for 1 to 24 hours after the initial exposure occurs, depending on the amount of material to which an individual is exposed. By this point in time, the majority of damage has already been done. Mild poisoning with sulfur mustard results in such symptoms as eye pain with extensive tearing, erythema and inflammation of the skin, irritation of the mucous membranes, cough, sneezing, and hoarseness. Mild poisoning does not warrant anything other than supportive care and will pass with time.

Exposure to larger amounts of sulfur mustard cause considerable dysfunction, incapacitating individuals and requiring emergency medical care. Individuals often lose their sight, as was common in World War I. Lines of soldiers were led around by one individual with good vision at the front and subsequent individuals in the chain following the soldier ahead of them, with one arm extended onto the shoulder of the soldier in front of them. Nausea, vomiting, and diarrhea develop along with severe respiratory difficulty because the same thing that happens to the skin can occur to the pulmonary epithelium.

A nuclear-biological-chemical protective suit and gas mask provide the best protection against sulfur mustard. Individuals who are exposed should be decontaminated as they would be

TABLE 59-12

ANESTHESIA AND MASS CASUALTIES

- Consider injuries that are or will become life threatening if untreated.
- Aim for anesthesia and surgery that are quick and effective.
- Perioperative deaths are to be expected.
- Many patients are at high risk.
- The usual standard of care is likely to be impossible.
- A vaporizer is unnecessary if total intravenous anesthesia is used. A draw over vaporizer is the most versatile inhalation device.

TABLE 59-13

FUNCTIONS OF ANESTHESIOLOGIST AT COMMAND AND CONTROL CENTER DURING IMPENDING MASS CASUALTY

Report to command and control center (may be difficult to get to, hospital may be secure) and perform the following functions:

- Decontamination
- Triage
  - Dead
  - Expectant
  - Minor
  - Operating room
  - Stabilize—floor
  - Intensive care unit (ICU)—to operating room later
- Operating room—intervention
- ICU—burns, flail chests, traumatic amputations

if they were exposed to a nerve agent (i.e., clothing is removed and they are washed with warm soapy water with or without 0.5% hypochlorite). Those patients who develop respiratory compromise are managed as they would be with the inhalation of a pulmonary agent.

CONCLUSION

It is difficult to anticipate the role anesthesiologists might play in managing patients who are victims of natural disasters or casualties of a terrorist attack with weapons of mass destruction. What is clear is that anesthesiologists have the requisite training and experience to be of vital importance in managing such casualties. However, based on their training, they may not be emotionally prepared to manage these patients. They must remember that, unlike in their normal practice, they may have to triage patients, accept the fact that the standard of care may be changed, and focus their efforts on interventions that will carry the greatest benefit for the greatest number of casualties (Table 59-12).

This process begins when the anesthesiologist receives the call at home or in the hospital of an impending mass casualty. He or she must first report to the command and control center and, although will most likely work in the operating room, he or she could also be used in the triage area in the emergency department or in the ICU (Table 59-13). Of utmost importance is familiarity with the hospital's disaster plan. The anesthesiologist, like other healthcare personnel, must also develop their own family care plan in anticipation of absence from the home for extended periods of time. Ensuring the safety of healthcare personnel through the appropriate use of protective devices to serve as barriers against radiologic, biological, and chemical weapons is also of vital importance.

References

1. Joint Commission on Accreditation of Healthcare Organizations: Health Care at the Crossroads: Strategies for Creating and Sustaining Community-Wide Emergency Preparedness Systems [White paper]. Available at: http://www.jcaho.org/about+us/public+policy+initiatives/emergency.htm. Accessed April 4, 2005.
2. Chen L, Evans T, Anand S *et al*: Human resources for health: overcoming the crisis. Lancet 364:1984, 2004
3. Combs CD: Preparing Health Professionals for the Unthinkable. Washington, DC: Association of Academic Health Centers, 2003
4. Chen K, Hitt G, McGinley L, Petersen A: Seven days in October spotlight weakness of U.S. response to threat of bioterrorism. Wall Street Journal, November 2, 2001
5. Okumura T, Suzuki K, Fukuda A *et al*: The Tokyo subway sarin attack: Disaster management, Part 1: Community emergency response. Acad Emerg Med 5:613, 1998
6. Ofner M, Lem M, Vearncombe M *et al*: Cluster of severe acute respiratory syndrome cases among protected health-care workers—Toronto, Canada, April 2003. Morbid Mortal Wkly Rep 52:433,2002. Available at: www.cdc.gov/mmwr/preview/mmwrhtml/mm5219a1.htm. Accessed June 18, 2003.
7. Copeland L: Houston drying out after deluge. USA Today, June 13, 2001. Available at: http://www.usatoday.com/weather/news/2001/2001-06-14-houston-allison.htm. Accessed April 4, 2005.
8. Association of Teachers of Preventive Medicine and Center for Health Policy, Columbia University School of Nursing: Emergency Response. Clinician Competencies in Initial Assessment and Management. July 2003. Available at: http://cumc.columbia.edu/dept/nursing/institutes/chphsr/clincomp.pdf. Accessed June 9, 2005.
9. Hurricane Andrew: After the storm: Ten years later. A special report. St. Petersburg Times, 2002. Available at: http://www.sptimes.com/2002/webspecials02/andrew/. Accessed April 4, 2005.
10. Schultz C, Koenig K, Lewis RJ: Implications of hospital evacuation after the Northridge, California, earthquake. N Engl J Med 348:1349, 2003
11. Sever MS, Erek E, Vanholder R *et al*: Lessons learned from the Marmara disaster: Time period under the rubble. Crit Care Med 30:2443, 2002
12. Schnitzer JJ, Briggs SM: Earthquake relief—the U.S. medical response in Bam, Iran. N Engl J Med 350:1174, 2004
13. Dacey MJ: Tragedy and response—the Rhode Island nightclub fire. N Engl J Med 349:1990, 2003
14. Halpern P, Rosen B, Carasso S *et al*: Intensive care in a field hospital in an urban disaster area: Lessons from the August 1999 earthquake in Turkey. Crit Care Med 31:1410, 2003
15. Union Carbide Corporation: Chronology of Key Events Related to the Bhopal Incident. October 2004. Available at: www.bhopal.com/pdfs/chrono.pdf. Accessed April 4, 2005.
16. Robinson C. Terrorism: The Army National Guard's restructuring for homeland security. Washington, DC: Center for Defense Information, August 1, 2003. Available at: www.cdi.org/friendlyversion/printversion.cfm?documentID=1568. Accessed April 4, 2005.
17. United States Marine Corps College of Continuing Education: Chemical Biological Incident Response Force. Available at: www.cbirf.usmc.mil. Accessed April 4, 2005.
18. Homeland Security Presidential Directives. Available at: www.mipt.org/Presidential-decision-directives.asp. Accessed April 4, 2005.
19. Federal Emergency Management Agency (FEMA). Available at: www.fema.gov. Accessed April 4, 2005.
20. United States Department of Health & Human Services: Disasters and Emergencies. Biological, Chemical and Radiological Weapons. Available at: www.hhs.gov/emergency/index.shtml. Accessed April 4, 2005.
21. U.S. Department of Homeland Security: National Disaster Medical System. Available at: www.ndms.dhhs.gov/dmat.html. Accessed April 4, 2005.
22. Mahoney LE, Whiteside DF, Belue HE *et al*: Disaster medical assistance teams. Ann Emerg Med 16:354, 1987
23. United States Department of Defense: Military Support. Section DL1.1.61, page 18. Available at: www.dtic.mil/whs/directives/corres/text/p30251m.txt. Accessed April 4, 2005.
24. Bacon LM: Chemical and biological incident response force. Surface Warfare 21:18, 1996
25. House Select Committee on Homeland Security: Bioterrorism: America Still Unprepared. October 2004. www.house.gov/hsc/democrats/pdf/hsc-docs/finalreportwithcover.pdf. Accessed December 20, 2004.
26. Carcia E, Horton DA: Supporting the Federal Emergency Management Agency rescuers: A variation of critical incident stress management. Mil Med 168:87, 2003
27. Dreyfus M: The war against terrorism collides with anesthesia. Anesthesiol New March: 46, 2003
28. Hardman JG, Wilson MJA, Yeoman PM, Riley B: Anaesthetic management of severely injured patients: General issues. Br J Hosp Med 58:19, 1997
29. Barker SJ: Anesthesia for trauma. International Anesthesia Research Society (IARS) 2004 Review Course Lectures, 1.
30. Shibata Y, Yamashita S, Masyakin VB *et al*: 15 years after Chernobyl: New evidence of thyroid cancer. Lancet 358:1965, 2001
31. United Nations General Assembly: Optimizing the international effort to study, mitigate and minimize the consequences of the Chernobyl disaster. Report of the Secretary-General. August 29, 2003. Available at: http://ods-dds-ny.un.org/doc/UNDOC/GEN/N03/485/92/PDF/N0348592.dpf?OpenElement.
32. Dellinger RP, Carlet JM, Masur H, Gerlach H: Introduction. Crit Care Med 32:S445, 2004
33. Collins DL: Human responses to the threat of or exposure to ionizing radiation at Three Mile Island, Pennsylvania, and Goiania, Brazil. Mil Med 167:137, 2002
34. Collins DL, de Carvalho AB: Chronic stress from the Goiania 137Cs radiation accident. Behav Med 18:149, 1993
35. Niefert A: Case study: Accidental leakage of cesium-137 in Goiania, Brazil, in 1987. Available at: www.nbc-med.org/sitecontent/medref/onlineref/casestudies/csgoiania.html. Accessed April 4, 2005.

36. American Academy of Pediatrics Committee on Environmental Health: Radiation disasters and children. Pediatrics 111:1455, 2003
37. American Academy of Pediatrics, Committee on Environmental Health: Risk of ionizing radiation exposure to children: A subject review. Pediatrics 101:717, 1998
38. The Avalon Project at Yale Law School: Total casualties. In: The Atomic Bombings of Hiroshima and Nagasaki: Documents in Law, History, and Diplomacy. New Haven, CT: The Avalon Project at Yale Law School, 2002. Available at: http://www.yale.edu/lawweb/avalon/abomb/mp10.htm. Accessed April 4, 2005.
39. Mongan PD, Shields C, Via D: Threat of radiologic terrorism increases. Unfamiliar patient care and safety issues mandate preparedness. APSF Newsletter 17:9, 2002. Available at: www.apsf.org/resourcecenter/newsletter/2002/spring/oqradiation.htm. Accessed June 9, 2005
40. O'Neill K: The Nuclear Terrorist Threat. Washington, DC: Institute for Science and International Security; 1997. Available at: www.isis-online.org/publications/terrorism/threat.pdf. Accessed April 4, 2005.
41. Kumar KS, Srinivasan V, Toles R, Jobe L, Seed TM: Nutritional approaches to radioprotection: Vitamin E. Mil Med 167:57, 2002
42. Whitnall MH, Elliott EB, Landauer MR *et al*: Protection against γ-irradiation and 5-androstenediol. Mil Med 167:64, 2002
43. Mitchell JB, Krishna M: Nitroxides as radiation protectors. Mil Med 167:49, 2002
44. Stickney DR, Dowding C, Reading C, Frincke J: HE2100 and HE3204 protect Rhesus Macaques from chemotherapy or radiation-induced myelosuppression. J Clin Oncol 22:6668, 2004
45. Brook I, Elliott TB, Ledney GD, Knudson GB: Management of postirradiation sepsis. Mil Med 167:105, 2002
46. Reeves GI: Radiation injuries. Crit Care Clin 15:457, 1999
47. Knudson GB, Elliott TB, Brook I *et al*: Nuclear, biological, and chemical combined injuries and countermeasures on the battlefield. Mil Med 167:95, 2002
48. Barry JM: Viruses of mass destruction. FORTUNE November 1:74, 2004
49. Centers for Disease Control and Prevention: Influenza pandemics. Available at: www.cdc.gov/flu/avian/gen-info/pdf/pandemic_factsheet.pdf. Accessed December 16, 2004.
49a. Enserink M: WHO adds more "1918" to pandemic predictions. Science 306:1025, 2004
50. Centers for Disease Control: Fact Sheet: Basic Information About SARS. January 13, 2004. Available at: www.cdc.gov/ncidod/sars/factsheet.htm. Accessed April 4, 2005.
51. Kamming D, Gardam M, Chung F: Anaesthesia and SARS. Br J Anaesth 90:715, 2003
52. Centers for Disease Control and Prevention: Current SARS Situation. October 6, 2004. Available at: www.cdc.gov/ncidod/sars/situation.htm. Accessed April 4, 2005.
53. Centers for Disease Control: Statistics, Surveillance, and Control: 2004 West Nile Virus Activity in the United States (reported as of January 11, 2005). Available at: www.cdc.gov/ncidod/dvbid/westnile/surv&controlCaseCount04_detailed.htm. Accessed April 4, 2005.
54. Beeching NJ, Dance DAB, Miller ARO, Spencer RC: Biological warfare and bioterrorism. BMJ 324:336, 2002
55. Coursin DB, Ketzler JT, Kumar A, Maki DG: Bioterrorism may overwhelm medical resources: New and different patient safety challenges must be anticipated. APSF Newsl 17:4, 2002
56. Breman JG, Henderson DA: Diagnosis and management of smallpox. N Engl J Med 346:1300, 2002
57. The smallpox eradication programme. WHO Chron. 22:354, 1968
58. Centers for Disease Control and Prevention: Smallpox vaccine adverse events among civilians—United States, January 24–February 18, 2003. JAMA 289:1497, 2003
59. Inglesby TV, Henderson DA, Bartlett JG *et al*: Anthrax as a biological weapon. Medical and public health management. JAMA 281:1735, 1999
60. Kalamas AG: Anthrax. Anesthesiol Clin North Am 22:533, 2004
61. Martin G: Anthrax: Lessons learned from the U.S. Capitol experience. Mil Med 168:9, 2003
62. Swartz MN: Recognition and management of anthrax—an update. N Engl J Med 345:1621, 2001
63. Dixon TC, Meselson M, Guillemin J, Hanna PC: Anthrax. N Engl J Med 341:815, 1999
64. Shafazand S, Doyle R, Ruoss S *et al*: Inhalational anthrax. Epidemiology, diagnosis, and management. Chest 116:1369, 1999
65. National Institute of Allergy and Infectious Diseases: Plague. February 2003. Available at: www.niaid.nih.gov/factsheets/plague.htm. Accessed April 4, 2005.
66. Zietz BP, Dunkelberg H: The history of the plague and the research on the causative agent Yersinia pestis. Int J Hygiene Environ Health 207:165, 2004
67. Cronquist SD: Tularemia: The disease and the weapon. Dermatol Clin 22:313, 2004
68. USAMRIID's Medical Management of Biological Casualties Handbook, 5th ed. Ft Detrick, Frederick, MD: U.S. Army Medical Research Institute of Infections Diseases. Available at: http://usamriid.detrick.army.mil/education/bluebookpdf/USAMRIID%20Blue%20Book%205th%20 Edition.pdf. Accessed April 4, 2005.
69. Josko D: Botulin toxin: A weapon in terrorism. Clin Lab Sci 17:30, 2004
70. Franz DR, Jahrling PB, Friedlander AM *et al*: Clinical recognition and management of patients exposed to biological warfare agents. JAMA 278:399, 1997
71. Bhalla DK, Warheit DB: Biological agents with potential for misuse: A historical perspective and defensive measures. Toxicol Appl Pharmacol 199:71, 2004
72. Baker DJ: Management of casualties from terrorist chemical and biological attack: A key role for the anaesthetist. Br J Anaesth 89:211, 2002
73. Evison D, Hinsley D, Rice P: Chemical weapons. BMJ 324:332, 2002
74. De Jong RH: Nerve gas terrorism: A grim challenge to anesthesiologists. Anesth Analg 96:819, 2003
75. Brennan RJ, Waeckerle JF, Sharp TW, Lillibridge SR: Chemical warfare agents: Emergency medical and emergency public health issues. Ann Emerg Med 34:191, 1999
76. Lake WA, Fedele PD, Marshall SM: Guidelines for mass casualty decontamination during a terrorist chemical agent incident. U.S. Army Soldier and Biological Chemical Command (SBCCOM), January 2000
77. Duffy M: Weapons of War: Poison Gas. May 5, 2002. Available at: www.firstworldwar.com/weaponry/gas.htm. Accessed April 4, 2005
78. Lung-damaging agents (choking agents). In: Treatment of chemical Agent Casualties and Conventional Military Chemical Injuries. Washington: Departments of the Army, the Navy, the Air Force, and Commandant Marines. Field manual No. 8-285. Available at: http://www.nbmed.org/sitecontent/medref/onlineref/fieldmanuals/fm8-285/new/toc.pdf. Accessed June 9, 2005.

APPENDIX ■ ELECTROCARDIOGRAPHY

JAMES R. ZAIDAN AND PAUL G. BARASH

ELECTROCARDIOGRAM

LEAD PLACEMENT

	■ ELECTRODE	
	■ POSITIVE	■ NEGATIVE
BIPOLAR LEADS		
I	LA	RA
II	LL	RA
III	LL	LA
AUGMENTED UNIPOLAR		
aVR	RA	LA, LL
aVL	LA	RA, LL
aVF	LL	RA, LA
	■ POSITION	
PRECORDIAL		
V_1	4 ICS–RSB	
V_2	4 ICS–LSB	
V_3	Midway between V_2 and V_4	
V_4	5 ICS–MCL	
V_5	5 ICS–AAL	
V_6	5 ICS–MAL	

THREE-LEAD SYSTEMS

■ BIPOLAR LEAD SYSTEM	■ ELECTRODE PLACEMENT	■ ECG LEAD*	■ ADVANTAGE
II	RA R–clavicle LA L–10th rib (midclavicular line) LL Ground	II (II)	Dysrhythmias
MCL 1	RA Ground LA L–clavicle LL V_1	III (V_1)	Dysrhythmias and conduction defects
CS 5	RA R–clavicle LA V_5 LL Ground	I (V_5)	Precordial ischemia
CB 5	RA R–scapula LA V_5 LL Ground	I (V_5)	Precordial ischemia and dysrhythmias

MCL = modified central lead; CB = central back; CS = central subclavian.
*Selected lead on monitor: ( ) = simulated ECG lead.

We wish to thank Dr. Malcom S. Thaler for graciously permitting reproduction of electrocardiographic tracings from his book, *The Only EKG Book You'll Ever Need* (Philadelphia, JB Lippincott, 1988).

THE NORMAL ELECTROCARDIOGRAM—CARDIAC CYCLE

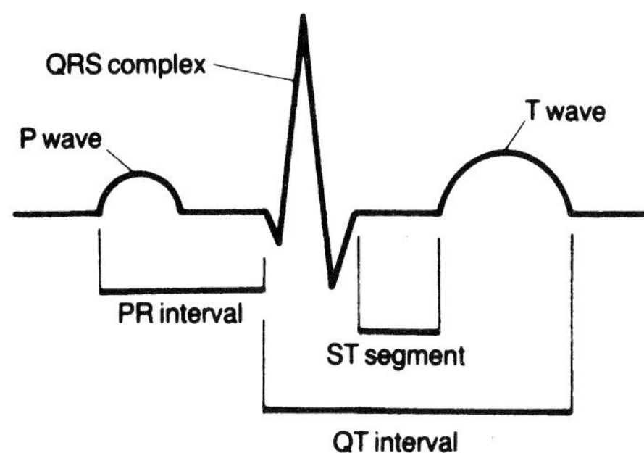

In this section the ECG complex is divided into the atrial (PR interval) and ventricular (QT interval) components.

ASHMAN BEATS

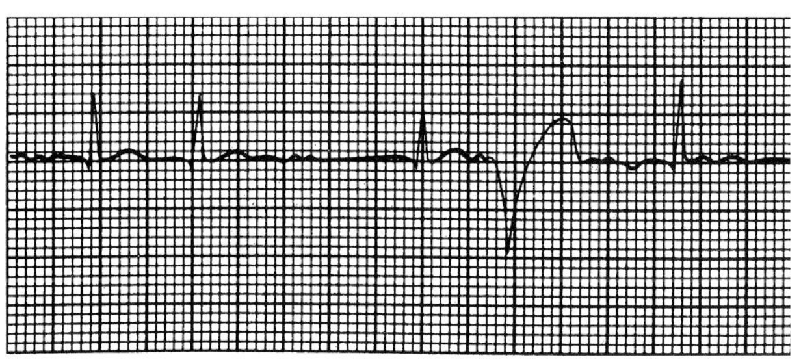

Rate: Variable.

Rhythm: Irregular.

PR interval: P wave may be present if supraventricular premature beat.

QT interval: QRS prolonged (>0.12 s) and altered, revealing bundle-branch pattern, most commonly right bundle. ST segment abnormal.

Note: Ashman beats are often confused with ventricular premature contractions. Ashman beats, usually seen with atrial fibrillation, have no compensatory pause and are a benign ECG finding requiring no treatment.

ATRIAL FIBRILLATION

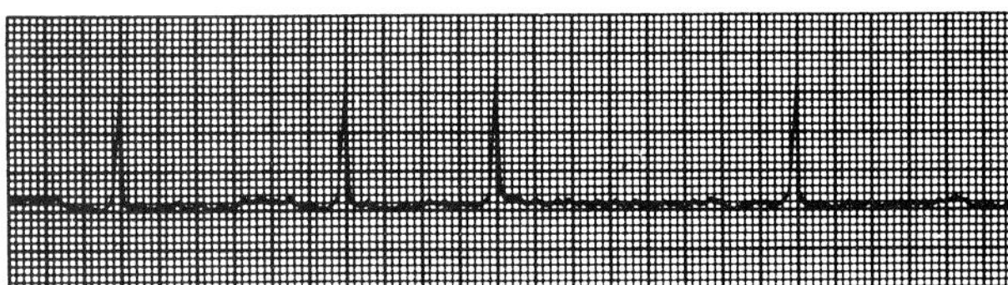

Rate: Variable (~150–200 beats/min).

Rhythm: Irregular.

PR interval: No P wave, and PR interval not discernible.

QT interval: QRS normal.

Note: Must be differentiated from atrial flutter: (1) absence of flutter waves and presence of fibrillatory line; (2) flutter usually associated with higher ventricular rates (>150 beats/min). Loss of atrial contraction reduces cardiac output (10–20%). Mural atrial thrombi may develop. Considered controlled if ventricular rate <100 beats/min.

ATRIAL FLUTTER

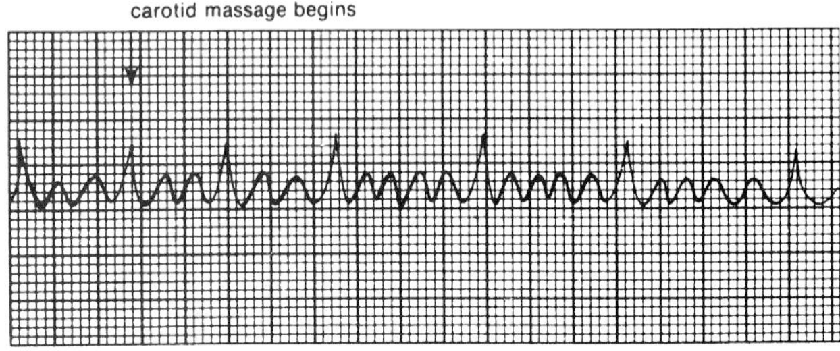

Rate: Rapid, atrial usually regular (250–350 beats/min); ventricular usually regular (<100 beats/min).

Rhythm: Atrial and ventricular regular.

PR interval: Flutter (F) waves are saw-toothed. PR interval cannot be measured.

QT interval: QRS usually normal; ST segment and T waves are not identifiable.

Note: Carotid massage will slow ventricular response, simplifying recognition of the F waves.

ATRIOVENTRICULAR BLOCK (First-Degree)

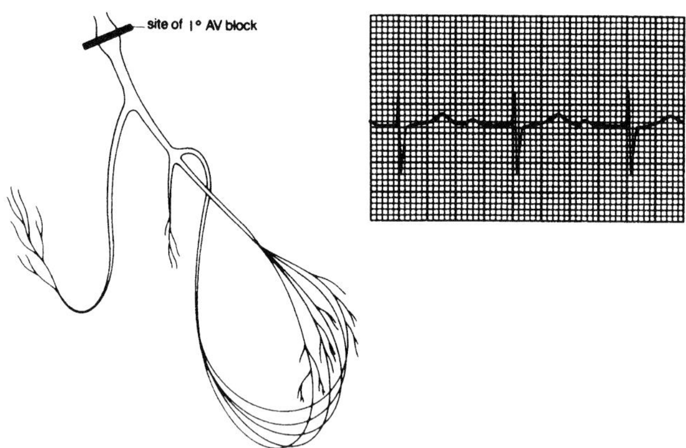

Rate: 60–100 beats/min.

Rhythm: Regular.

PR interval: Prolonged (>0.20 s) and constant.

QT interval: Normal.

Note: Usually clinically insignificant; may be early harbinger of drug toxicity.

ATRIOVENTRICULAR BLOCK (Second-Degree), Mobitz Type I/ Wenckebach Block

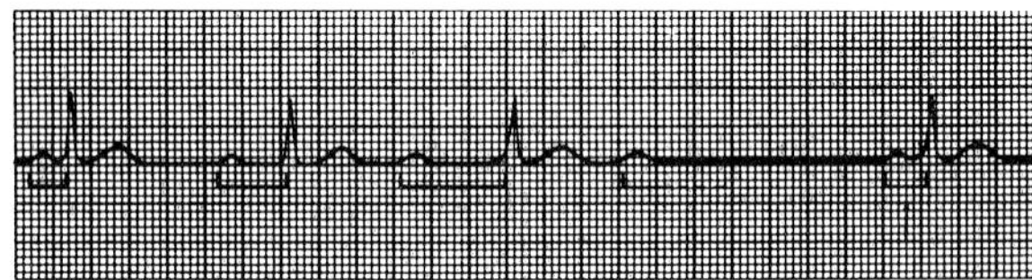

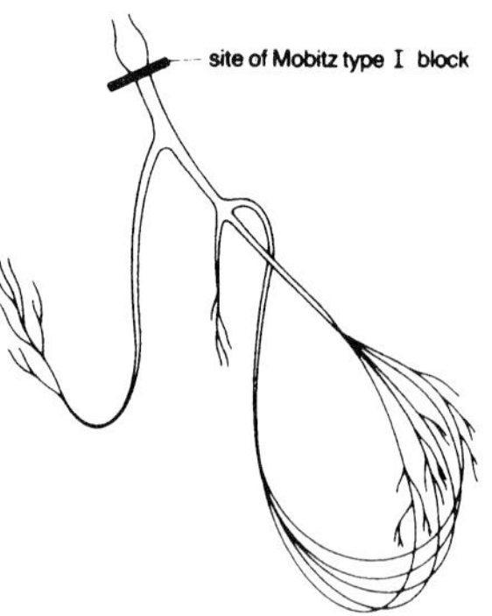

Rate: 60–100 beats/min.

Rhythm: Atrial regular; ventricular irregular.

PR interval: P wave normal; PR interval progressively lengthens with each cycle until QRS complex is dropped (dropped beat). PR interval following dropped beat is shorter than normal.

QT interval: QRS complex normal but dropped periodically.

Note: Commonly seen (1) in trained athletes and (2) with drug toxicity.

ATRIOVENTRICULAR BLOCK (Second-Degree), Mobitz Type II

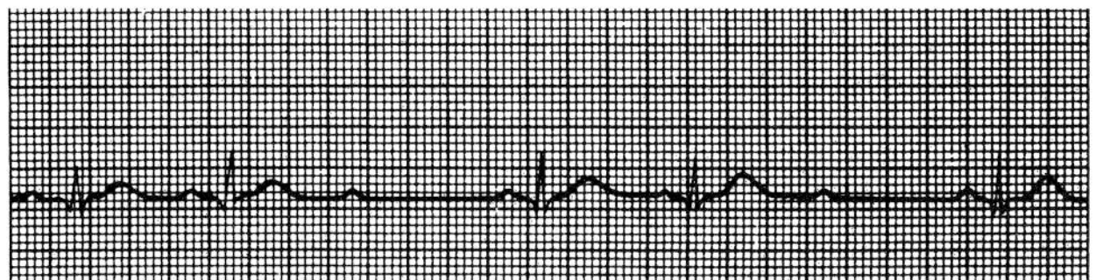

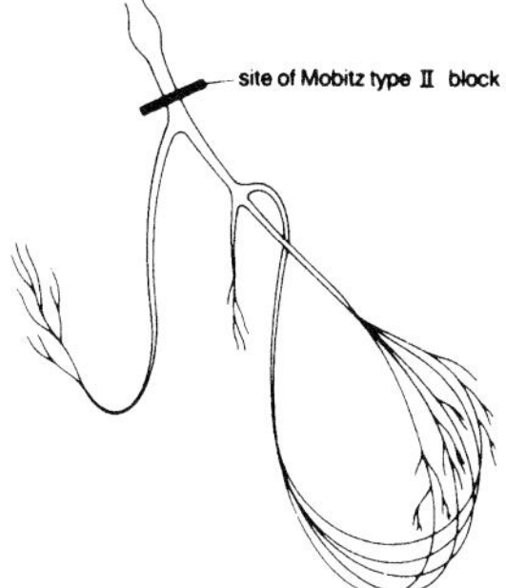

Rate: <100 beats/min.

Rhythm: Atrial regular; ventricular regular or irregular.

PR interval: P waves normal, but some are not followed by QRS complex.

QT interval: Normal but may have widened QRS complex if block is at level of bundle branch. ST segment and T wave may be abnormal, depending on location of block.

Note: In contrast to Mobitz type I block, the PR and RR intervals are constant and the dropped QRS occurs without warning. The wider the QRS complex (block lower in the conduction system), the greater the amount of myocardial damage.

ATRIOVENTRICULAR BLOCK (Third-Degree), Complete Heart Block

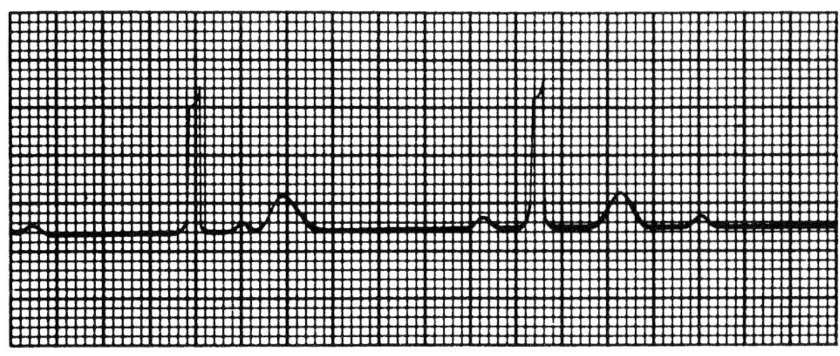

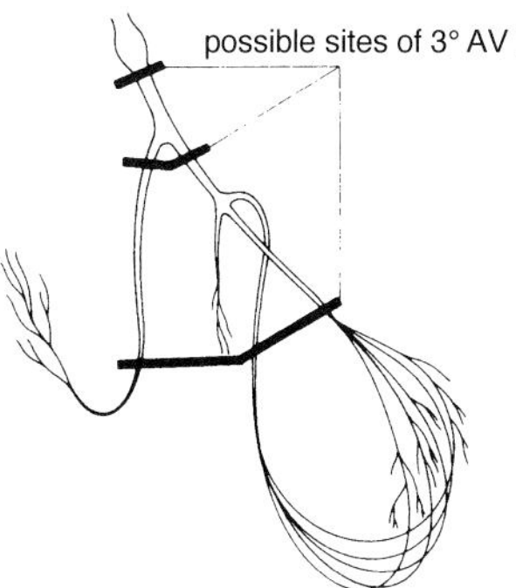

Rate: <45 beats/min.

Rhythm: Atrial regular; ventricular regular; no relationship between P wave and QRS complex.

PR interval: Variable because artia and ventricles beat independently.

QT interval: QRS morphology variable, depending on the origin of the ventricular beat in the intrinsic pacemaker system (atrioventricular junctional versus ventricular pacemaker). ST segment and T wave normal.

Note: Immediate treatment with atropine or isoproterenol is required if cardiac output is reduced. Consideration should be given to insertion of a pacemaker. Seen as a complication of mitral valve replacement.

ATRIOVENTRICULAR DISSOCIATION

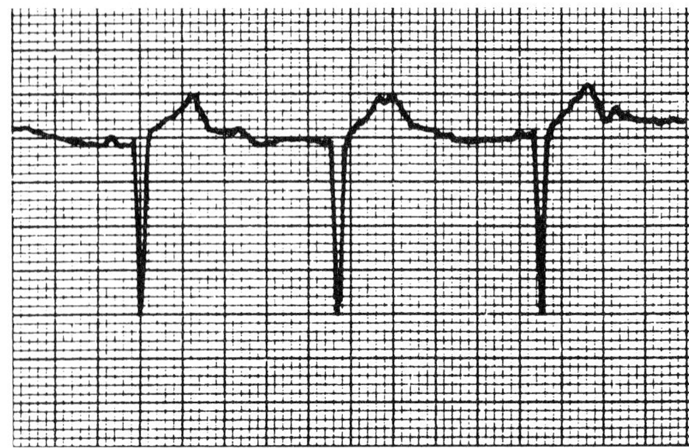

Rate: Variable.

Rhythm: Atrial regular; ventricular regular; ventricular rate faster than atrial rate; no relationship between P wave and QRS complex.

PR interval: Variable because atria and ventricles beat independently.

QT interval: QRS morphology depends on location of ventricular pacemaker. ST segment and T wave abnormal.

Note: Digitalis toxicity can present as atrioventricular dissociation.

BUNDLE-BRANCH BLOCK—RIGHT (RBBB)

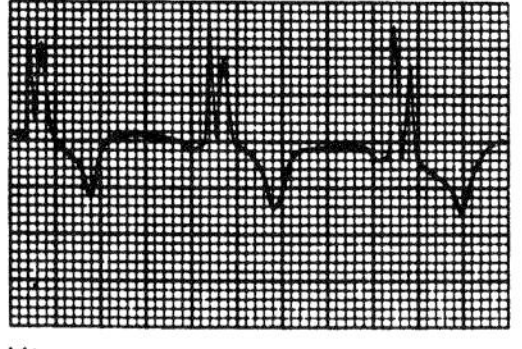

V1

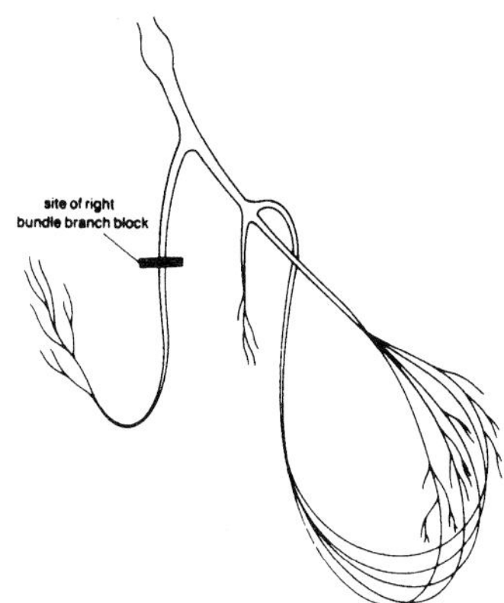

Rate: <100 beats/min.

Rhythm: Regular.

PR interval: Normal.

QT interval: Complete RBBB (QRS >0.12 s); incomplete RBBB (QRS = 0.10–0.12 s). Varying patterns of QRS complex; rSR (V_1); RS, wide R with M pattern. ST segment and T wave opposite direction of the R wave.

Note: In the presence of RBBB, Q waves may be seen with a myocardial infarction.

BUNDLE-BRANCH BLOCK—LEFT (LBBB)

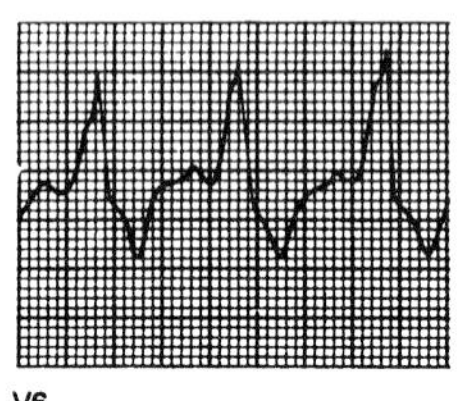

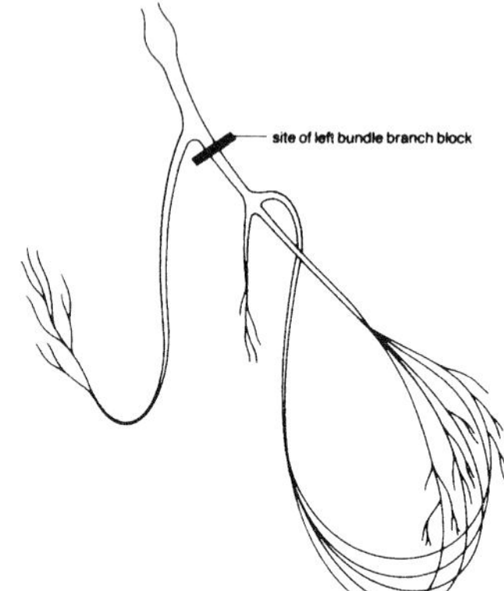

Rate: <100 beats/min.

Rhythm: Regular.

PR interval: Normal.

QT interval: Complete LBBB (QRS >0.12 s); incomplete LBBB (QRS = 0.10–0.12 s); Lead V_1 negative rS complex; I, aVL, V_6 wide R wave without Q or S component. ST segment and T wave defection opposite direction of the R wave.

Note: LBBB does not occur in healthy patients and usually indicates serious heart disease with a poorer prognosis. In patients with LBBB, insertion of a pulmonary artery catheter may lead to complete heart block.

ELECTROLYTE DISTURBANCES

	■ ↓ Ca^{2+}	■ ↑ Ca^{2+}	■ ↓K^+	■ ↑K^+
Rate	<100 beats/min	<100 beats/min	<100 beats/min	<100 beats/min
Rhythm	Regular	Regular	Regular	Regular
PR interval	Normal	Normal/ increased	Normal	Normal
QT interval	Increased	Decreased	T flat U wave	T peaked QT decreased

Note: ECG changes usually do not correlate with serum calcium. Hypocalcemia rarely causes dysrhythmias in the absence of hypokalemia. In contrast, abnormalities in serum potassium concentration can be diagnosed by ECG.

DIGITALIS EFFECT

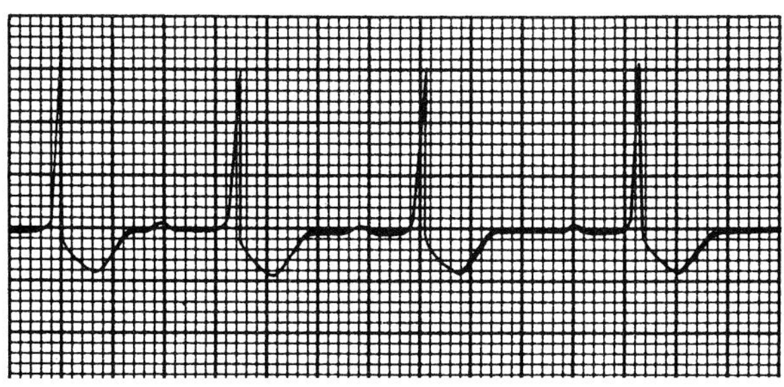

Rate: <100 beats/min.

Rhythm: Regular.

PR interval: Normal or prolonged.

QT interval: ST segment sloping ("digitalis effect").

Note: Digitalis toxicity can be the cause of many common dysrhythmias (*e.g.*, premature ventricular contractions, second-degree heart block). Verapamil, quinidine, and amiodarone cause an increase in serum digitalis concentration.

CORONARY ARTERY DISEASE—
Myocardial Infarction

ANATOMIC SITE	LEADS	ECG CHANGES	CORONARY ARTERY
Inferior	II, III, aVF	Q, ST, T	Right
Lateral	I, aVL, V_5–V_6	Q, ST, T	Left circumflex
Anterior	I, aVL, V_1–V_4	Q, ST, T	Left
Anteroseptal	V_1–V_4	Q, ST, T	Left anterior descending

SUBENDOCARDIAL MYOCARDIAL INFARCTION (SEMI)

Persistent ST segment depression and/or T-wave inversion in the absence of Q wave. Usually requires additional laboratory data (*e.g.*, isoenzymes) to confirm diagnosis.

TRANSMURAL MYOCARDIAL INFARCTION (TMI)

Q waves seen on ECG useful in confirming diagnosis. Associated with poorer prognosis and more significant hemodynamic impairment; dysrhythmias frequently complicate course.

CORONARY ARTERY DISEASE—Ischemia

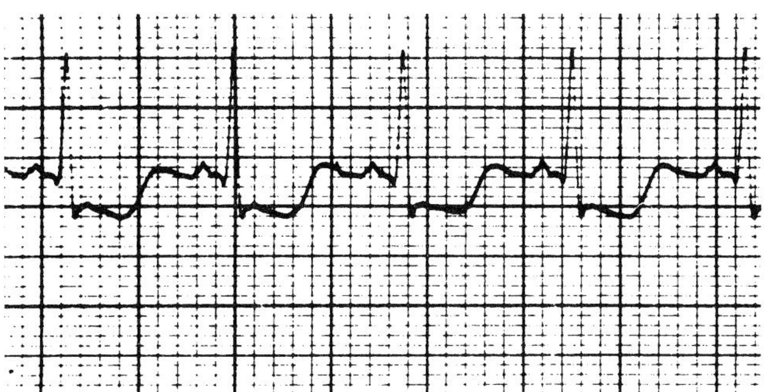

Rate: Variable.

Rhythm: Usually regular, but may show atrial and/or ventricular dysrhythmias.

PR interval: Normal.

QT interval: ST segment depressed; J point depression; T-wave inversion; conduction disturbances. Coronary vasospasm (Prinzmetal) ST segment elevation.

Note: Intraoperative ischemia is usually seen in the presence of "normal" vital signs (*e.g.*, ±20% of preinduction values).

PAROXYSMAL ATRIAL TACHYCARDIA (PAT)

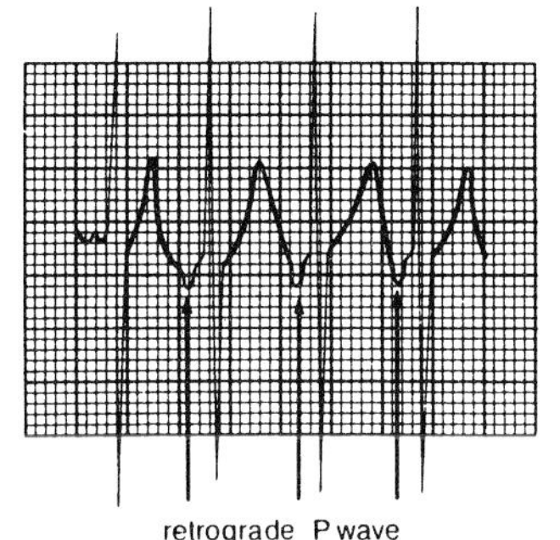

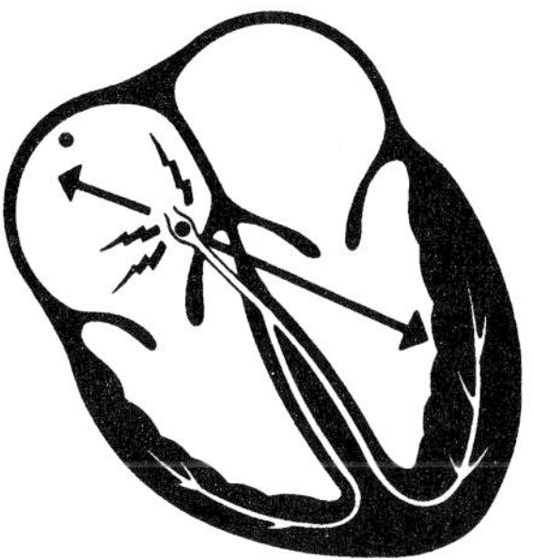

Rate: 150–250 beats/min.

Rhythm: Regular.

PR interval: Difficult to distinguish because of tachycardia obscuring P wave. P wave may precede, be included in, or follow QRS complex.

QT interval: Normal, but ST segment and T wave may be difficult to distinguish.

Note: Therapy depends on degree of hemodynamic compromise. In contrast to management of PAT in awake patients, synchronized cardoversion rather than pharmacologic treatment is preferred in hemodynamically unstable anesthetized patients.

PREMATURE ATRIAL CONTRACTION (PAC)

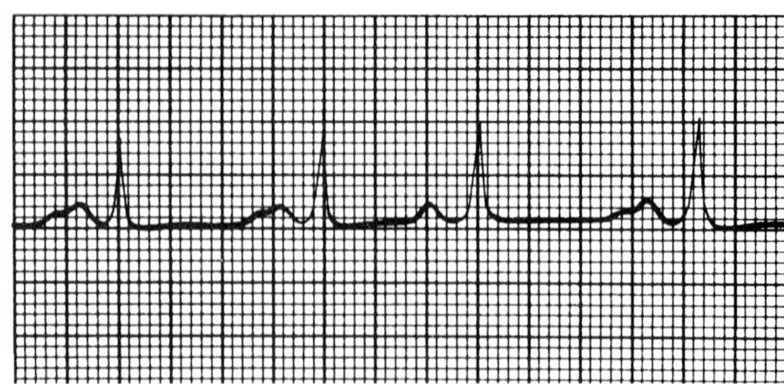

Rate: <100 beats/min.

Rhythm: Irregular.

PR interval: P waves may be lost in preceding T waves. PR interval is variable.

QT interval: QRS normal configuration; ST segment and T wave normal.

Note: Nonconducted PAC appearance similar to that of sinus arrest; T waves with PAC may be distorted by inclusion of P wave in the T wave.

SINUS TACHYCARDIA

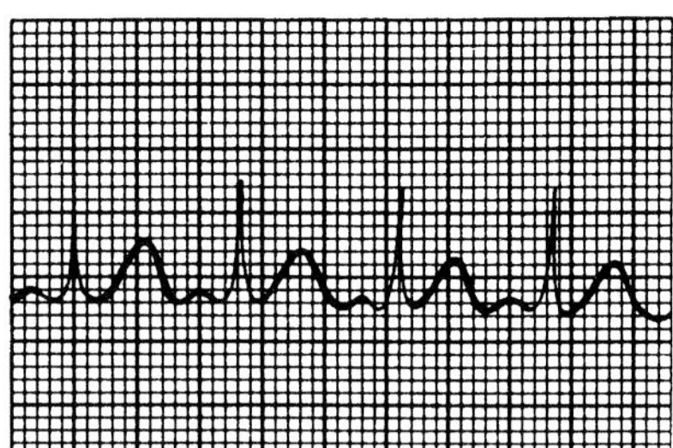

Rate: 100–160 beats/min.

Rhythm: Regular.

PR interval: Normal; P wave may be difficult to see.

QT interval: Normal.

Note: Should be differentiated from paroxysmal atrial tachycardia (PAT). With PAT, carotid massage terminates dysrhythmia. Sinus tachycardia may respond to vagal maneuvers but reappears as soon as vagal stimulus is removed.

PREMATURE VENTRICULAR CONTRACTION (PVC)

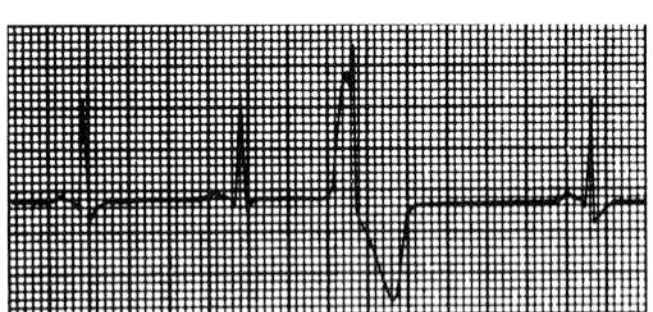

A

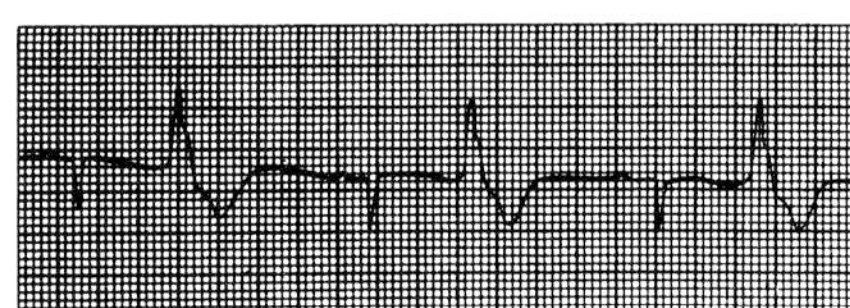

B

Rate: Usually <100 beats/min.

Rhythm: Irregular.

PR interval: P wave and PR interval absent; retrograde conduction of P wave can be seen.

QT interval: Wide QRS (>0.12 s); ST segment cannot be evaluated (*e.g.*, ischemia); T wave opposite direction of QRS with compensatory pause (*A*). Bigeminy: every other beat a PVC (*B*); trigeminy: every third beat a PVC. R-on-T occurs when PVC falls in the T wave and can lead to ventricular tachycardia or fibrillation.

Note: If compensatory pause is not seen following an ectopic beat, the complex is most likely supraventricular in origin.

TORSADES DE POINTES

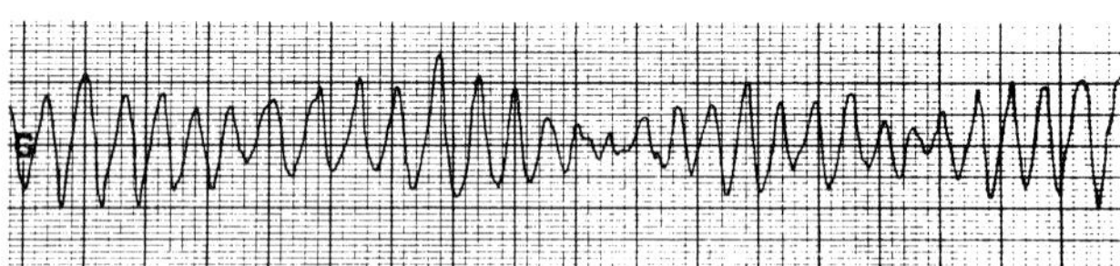

Rate: 150–250 beats/min.

Rhythm: No atrial component seen; ventricular rhythm regular or irregular.

PR interval: P wave buried in QRS complex.

QT interval: QRS complexes usually wide and with phasic variation twisting around a central axis (a few complexes point upward then a few point downward). ST segments and T waves difficult to discern.

Note: Type of ventricular tachycardia associated with prolonged QT interval. Seen with electrolyte disturbances (*e.g.*, hypokalemia, hypocalcemia, and hypomagnesemia) and bradycardia. Administering standard antidysrhythmics (lidocaine, proeain-amide, etc.) may worsen Torsades de Pointes. Treatment includes increasing heart rate pharmacologically or by pacing.

VENTRICULAR FIBRILLATION

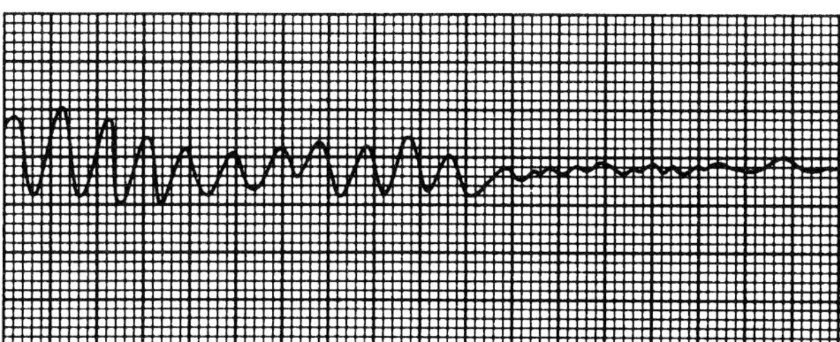

Rate: Absent.

Rhythm: None.

PR interval: Absent.

QT interval: Absent.

Note: "Pseudoventricular fibrillation" may be the result of a monitor malfunction (*e.g.*, ECG lead disconnect). Always check for carotid pulse before instituting therapy.

VENTRICULAR TACHYCARDIA

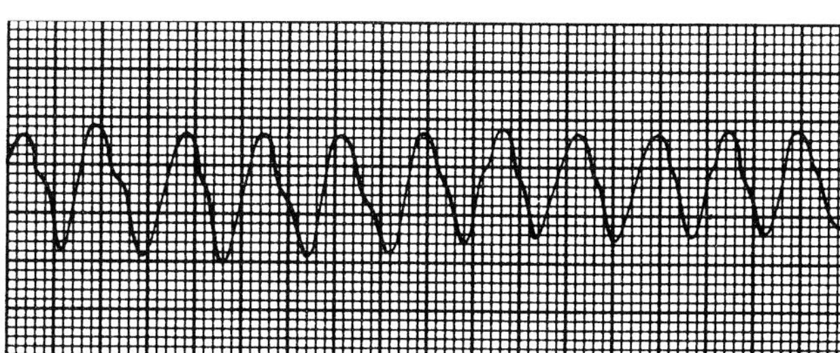

Rate: 100–250 beats/min.

Rhythm: No atrial component seen; ventricular rhythm irregular or regular.

PR interval: Absent; retrograde P wave may be seen in QRS complex.

QT interval: Wide, bizarre QRS complex. ST segment and T wave difficult to determine.

Note: In the presence of hemodynamic compromise, immediate DC synchronized cardioversion is required. If the patient is stable, with short bursts of ventricular tachycardia, pharmacologic management is preferred. Should be differentiated from supraventricular tachycardia with aberrancy (SVT-A). Compensatory pause and atrioventricular dissociation suggest a PVC. P waves and SR' (V_1) and slowing to vagal stimulus suggest SVT-A.

WOLFF-PARKINSON-WHITE SYNDROME (WPW)

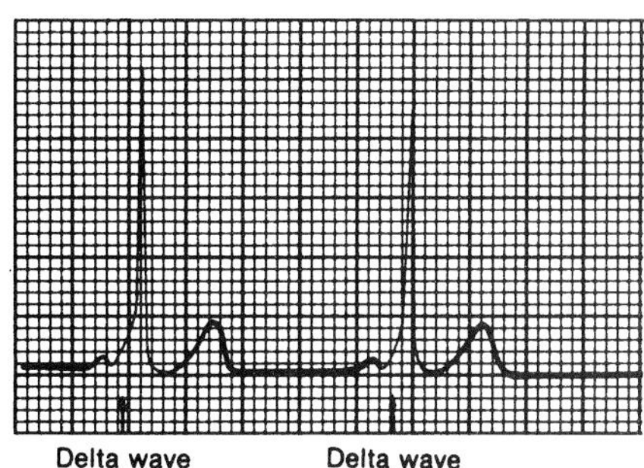

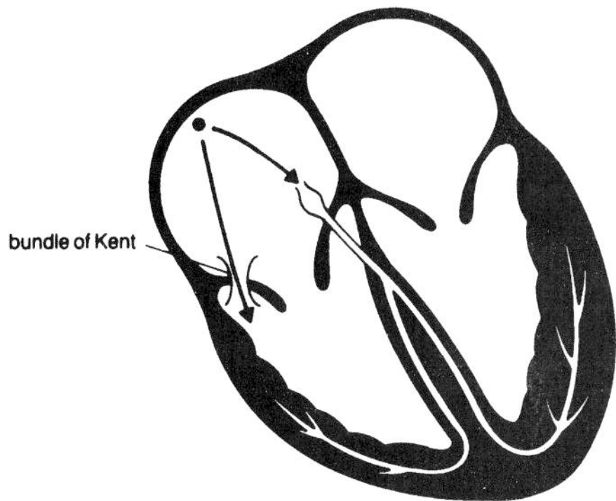

Rate: <100 beats/min.

Rhythm: Regular.

PR interval: P wave normal; PR interval short (<0.12 s).

QT interval: Duration (>0.10 s) with slurred QRS complex. Type A has delta wave, RBBB, with upright QRS complex V_1. Type B has delta wave and downward QRS-V_1. ST segment and T wave usually normal.

Note: Digoxin should be avoided in the presence of WPW because it increases conduction through the accessory bypass tract (bundle of Kent) and decreases atrioventricular node conduction; consequently, ventricular fibrillation can occur.

PACEMAKER

GENERIC PACEMAKER CODE (NBG*): NASPE/BPEG REVISED (2002)

■ POSITION I, PACING CHAMBER(S)	■ POSITION II, SENSING CHAMBER(S)	■ POSITION III, RESPONSE(S) TO SENSING	■ POSITION IV, PROGRAMMABILITY	■ POSITION V, MULTISITE PACING
O = none A = atrium V = ventricle D = dual (A+V)	O = none A = atrium V = ventricle D = dual (A+V)	O = none I = Inhibited T = triggered D = dual (T+I)	O = none R = rate modulation	O = none A = atrium V = ventricle D = dual (A+V)

ICD, implanted cardioverter defibrillator.
*NBG: N refers to North American Society of Pacing and Electrophysiology (NASPE), now called the Heart Rhythm Society (HRS), B refers to British Pacing and Electrophysiology Group (BPEG), and G refers to generic.
From practice advisory for perioperative management of patients with cardiac rhythm management devices: Pacemakers and implantable cardioventer defibrillators. Anesthesiology, 103:186, 2005.

GENERIC DEFIBRILLATOR CODE (NBD): NASPE/BPEG

■ POSITION I, SHOCK CHAMBER(S)	■ POSITION II, ANTITACHYCARDIA PACING CHAMBER(S)	■ POSITION III, TACHYCARDIA DETECTION	■ POSITION IV,* ANTIBRADYCARDIA PACING CHAMBER(S)
O = none A = atrium V = ventricle D = dual (A+V)	O = none A = atrium V = ventricle D = dual (A+V)	E = electrogram H = hemodynamic	O = none A = atrium V = ventricle D = dual (A+V)

*For robust identification, position IV is expanded into its complete NBG code. For example, a biventricular pacing–defibrillator with ventricular shock and antitachycardia pacing functionality would be identified as VVE-DDDRV, assuming that the pacing section was programmed DDDRV. Currently, no hemodynamic sensors have been approved for tachycardia detection (position III).
From practice advisory for perioperative management of patients with cardiac rhythm management devices: Pacemakers and implantable cardioventer defibrillators. Anesthesiology, 103:186, 2005.

EXAMPLE OF A STEPWISE APPROACH TO THE PERIOPERATIVE TREATMENT OF THE PATIENT WITH A CARDIAC RHYTHM MANAGEMENT DEVICE (CRMD)

■ PERIOPERATIVE PERIOD	■ PATIENT/CRMD CONDITION	■ INTERVENTION
Preoperative evaluation	Patient has CRMD	• Focused history • Focused physical examination
	Determine CRMD type (pacemaker, ICD, CRT)	• Manufacture's CRMD identification card • Chest x-ray studies (no data available) • Supplemental resources*
	Determine whether patient is CRMD-dependent for pacing function	• Verbal history • Bradyarrhythmia symptoms • Atrioventricular node ablation • No spontaneous ventricular activity †
	Determine CRMD function	• Comprehensive CRMD evaluation ‡ • Determine whether pacing pulses are present and create paced beats
Preoperative preparation	EMI unlikely during procedure	• If EMI unlikely, special precautions are not needed
	EMI likely: CRMD is pacemaker	• Reprogram to asynchronous mode when indicated • Suspend rate-adaptive functions§
	EMI likely: CRMD is ICD	• Suspend antitachyarrhythmia functions • If patient is dependent on pacing function, after pacing functions as above
	EMI likely: all CRMD	• Use bipolar cautery; ultrasonic scalpel • Temporary pacing and external cardioversion–defibrillation available
	Intraoperative physiologic changes likely (*e.g.*, bradycardia, ischemia)	• Plan for possible adverse CRMD–patient interaction

EXAMPLE OF A STEPWISE APPROACH TO THE PERIOPERATIVE TREATMENT OF THE PATIENT WITH A CRMD (CONTINUED)

■ PERIOPERATIVE PERIOD	■ PATIENT/CRMD CONDITION	■ INTERVENTION
Intraoperative management	Monitoring	• Electrocardiographic monitoring per ASA standard • Peripheral pulse monitoring
	Electrocautery interference	• CT/CRP—no current through PG/leads • Avoid proximity of CT to PG/leads • Short bursts at lowest possible energy • Use bipolar cautery; ultrasonic scalpel
	Radiofrequency catheter ablation	• Avoid contact of radiofrequency catheter with PG/leads • Radiofrequency current path far away from PG/leads • Discuss these concerns with operator
	Lithotripsy	• Do not focus lithotripsy beam near PG • R wave triggers lithotripsy? Disable atrial pacing[‖]
	MRI	• Generally contraindicated • If required, consult ordering physician, cardiologist, radiologists, and manufacturer
	RT	• PG/leads must be outside of RT field • Possible surgical relocation of PG • Verify PG function during/after RT course
	ECT	• Consult with ordering physician, patient's cardiologist, a CRMD service, or CRMD manufacturer
Emergency defibrillation–cardioversion	ICD: magnet disabled	• Terminate all EMI sources • Remove magnet to reenable therapies • Observe for appropriate therapies
	ICD: programming disabled	• Programming to reenable therapies or proceed directly with external cardioversion–defibrillation
	ICD: either of above	• Minimize current flow through PG/leads • PP as far as possible from PG • PP perpendicular to major axis PG/leads • To extent possible, PP in anterior–posterior location
	Regardless of CRMD type	• Use clinically appropriate cardioversion/defibrillation energy
Postoperative management	Immediate postoperative period	• Monitor cardiac R&R continuously • Backup pacing and cardioversion/defibrillation capability
	Postoperative interrogation and restoration of CRMD function	• Interrogation to assess function • Setting appropriate?# • Is CRMD an ICD?** • Use cardiology/pacemaker–ICD service if needed

*Manufacturer's databases, pacemaker clinic records, cardiology consultation. †With cardiac rhythm management device (CRMD) programmed WI at lowest programmable rate. ‡Ideally CRMD function assessed by interrogation, with function altered by reprogramming if required. §Most times this will be necessary; when in doubt, assume so. ‖Atrial pacing spikes may be interpreted by the lithotriptor as R waves, possibly inciting the lithotriptor to deliver a shock during a vulnerable period in the heart. #If necessary, reprogram appropriate setting. **restore all antitachycardia therapies.

CRP, current return pad; CRT, cardiac resynchronization therapy; CT, cautery tool; ECT, electroconvulsive therapy; EMI, electromagnetic interference; ICD, internal cardioverter–defibrillator; MRI, magnetic resonance imaging; PG, pulse generator; PP, external cardioversion–defibrillation pads or paddles; R&R, rhythm and rate; RT, radiation therapy.

From practice advisory for perioperative management of patients with cardiac rhythm management devices: Pacemakers and implantable cardioventer defibrillators. Anesthesiology, 103:186, 2005.

TREATMENT OF PACEMAKER FAILURE

■ RATE	■ POSSIBLE RESPONSE
Adequate to maintain blood pressure	1. Oxygen, airway control 2. Place magnet over pacemaker 3. Atropine if sinus bradycardia
Severe bradycardia and hypotension	1. Oxygen, airway control 2. Place magnet over pacemaker 3. Other types of pacing if magnet does not activate the pacemaker (transcutaneous, esophageal, or transvenous) 4. Atropine if sinus bradycardia 5. Isoproterenol to increase ventricular rate
No escape rhythm	1. Cardiopulmonary resuscitation 2. Place magnet over pacemaker 3. Other types of pacing if magnet does not activate the pacemaker (transcutaneous, esophageal, or transvenous) 4. Isoproterenol to increase ventricular rate

Adapted from Zaidan JR: Pacemakers. In Youngberg JA, Lake CL, Roizen MF, Wilson KS (eds): Cardiac, Vascular and Thoracic Anesthesia. New York, Churchill Livingstone, 2000.

ATRIAL PACING

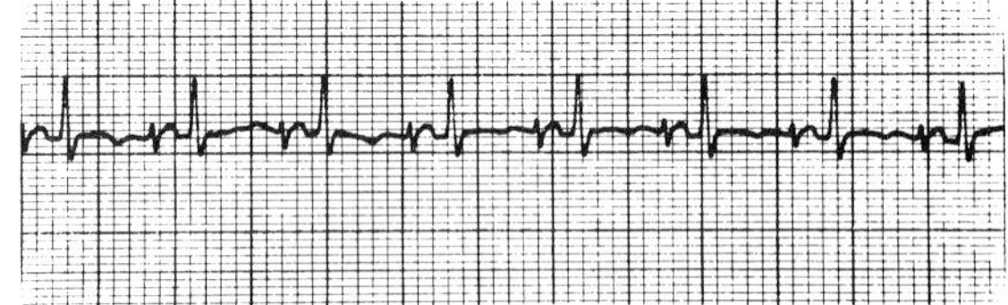

Atrial pacing as demonstrated in this figure is used when the atrial impulse can proceed through the AV node. Examples are sinus bradycardia and junctional rhythms associated with clinically significant decreases in blood pressure.

VENTRICULAR PACING

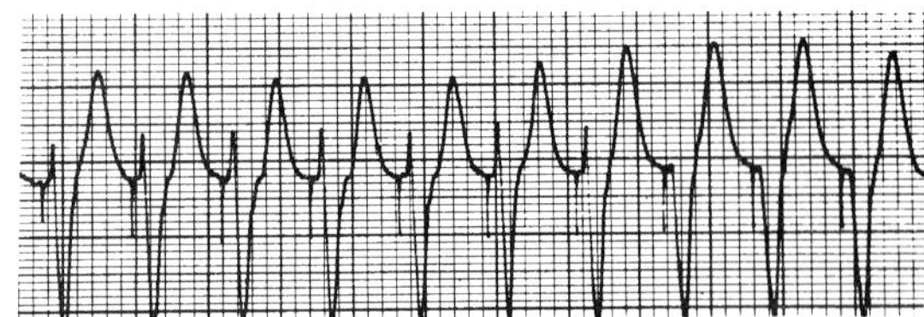

In this tracing ventricular pacing is evident by absence of atrial wave (P wave) and pacemaker spike preceding QRS complex. Ventricular pacing is employed in the presence of bradycardia secondary to AV block or atrial fibrillation.

DDD PACING

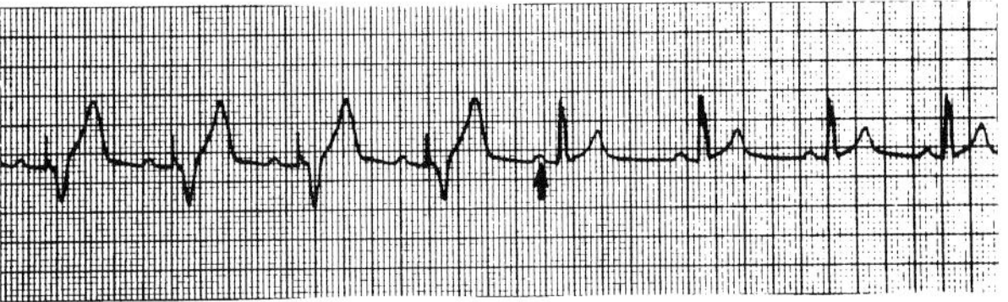

The DDD pacemaker (generator), one of the most commonly used, paces and senses both atrium and ventricle. In the first four beats, the P waves were not followed by a QRS complex within the programmed PR interval. Therefore, a ventricular pacing spike and a ventricular paced beat occurred. In the last four beats (after the arrow), atrial activity proceeded through the AV node in the allotted amount of time; therefore, ventricular pacing was inhibited.

ATRIAL ELECTROGRAM (AEG)

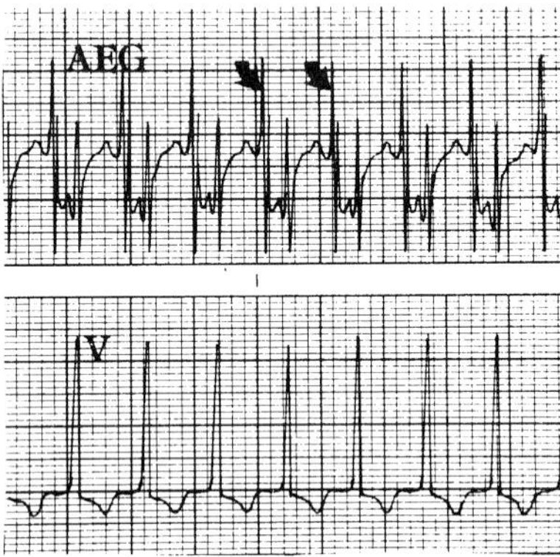

The AEG is useful in differentiating various atrial dysrhythmias. The AEG is obtained from an intracardiac or esophageal lead, if P waves are not clearly seen on the surface ECG. In this trace the V lead does not have obvious P waves; however, the AEG reveals large P waves (arrows) that precede each QRS complex. Locate the QRS on the AEG by matching the R wave on the surface ECG to the AEG. The surface and AEG must be simultaneously recorded.

GUIDELINES FOR USING THE ELECTROCAUTERY

1. Electromagnet interference created by an electrocautery can cause a number of problems with pacemaker or ICD function including, but not limited to, reprogramming, inhibition, noise reversion mode, electrical reset, myocardial burns, increase in threshold, rate increment changes in rate adaptive pacemakers, and inappropriate sensing and charging in ICDs.[2,3]
2. When positioning the return plate of the electrocautery,
   a. Ensure it is located so the pacemaker or ICD is not between this return plate and the active electrode.
   b. Ensure the plane described by the return plate and the active electrode of the electrocautery is perpendicular to a plane described by the pacemaker or ICD and the pacemaker's electrodes.
3. Use the smallest current required to cut or coagulate.
4. Use the electrocautery in short bursts.
5. Avoid using the electrocautery within 6 in. of the device or leads.
6. Consider using the bipolar electrocautery or the ultrasonic scalpel[4,5] to minimize interference with pacemaker or ICD function.
7. Activating the electrocautery in the area of the pacemaker or ICD, even if the active electrode is not touching the patient, will cause interference.
8. Do not use the electrocautery when an ICD is programmed to sense and deliver therapy.
9. Convert the ICD to no response either by programming or by using the magnet, depending on the manufacturer of the ICD so the device will not deliver therapy secondary to misinterpretation of signals from the electrocautery as a dysrhythmia. These maneuvers will not change the program of a pacemaker that is incorporated into an ICD.
10. If desired, convert a pacemaker that does not have an ICD to the asynchronous mode so it is not inhibited by the electrocautery.
11. A magnet will not change bradycardia-related pacing parameters in the ICD.
12. ICDs must be programmed to respond to a magnet.

ICD, implanted cardioverter defibrillator.

ADDITIONAL ISSUES FOR PATIENTS WITH IMPLANTED CARDIOVERTER DEFIBRILLATORS

1. All ICDs have pacemakers incorporated into the circuitry.
2. Preoperative assessments should include those procedures that are standard for patients with heart disease.
3. Obtain a cardiology consult to help assess the patient, interrogate the ICD, program the device to no response, and program the device to respond to the magnet.
4. There is no particular anesthetic technique that is clearly right or wrong for a patient who has an ICD.
5. Apply patches for external defibrillation when the ICD is programmed to no response. Ensure these external patches are as far away as possible from the device and, if possible, not in the same plane as the device and electrodes.
6. Monitor as required for patient care. If monitoring with a pulmonary arterial catheter, discuss the issues of dislodgment of the ICD's electrodes with the patient and cardiologist. Document in the chart your discussions and the logic supporting the necessity for a pulmonary arterial catheter. Maintain sterile technique, and consider administering antibiotics just before inserting central lines.
7. Continue antidysrhythmic agents until the time of surgery. Discuss with the cardiologist the necessity of administering an additional dose of an antidysrhythmic agent if the patient experiences an intraoperative dysrhythmia.
8. Intraoperative dysrhythmias:
   a. If the patient has a dysrhythmia, rule out and treat the usual intraoperative causes to prevent a recurrence.
   b. If the dysrhythmia continues and a magnet has been used to create the no response mode, remove the magnet from the ICD and allow the ICD to charge and deliver a response.
   c. If the ICD has been programmed to the no response mode, then either quickly reprogram the ICD to deliver a response or proceed directly to external defibrillation.
   d. If external defibrillation or cardioversion is required, apply the defibrillator paddles in an anterior-posterior position if possible and deliver the shock at a level sufficient to terminate the dysrhythmia.
   e. External pacing might be required if the pacemaker/ICD is damaged with the shock.
9. Monitor the patient's ECG and be prepared to deliver an external defibrillation when transporting the patient to and from the operating room.
10. Interrogate and reprogram the ICD when the patient has entered the postoperative care unit.

ECG, electrocardiogram; ICD, implanted cardioverter defibrillator.

References

1. Practice advisory for perioperative management of patients with cardiac rhythm management devices: Pacemakers and implantable cardioverter-defibrillators. A Report by the American Society of Anesthesiologists Task Force on Perioperative Management of Patients with Cardiac Rhythm Management Devices. Anesthesiology, 103:186, 2005
2. Hayes DL, Strathmore NF: Electromagnetic interference with implantable devices. In Ellenbogen KA, Kay GN, Wilkoff BL (eds): Clinical Cardiac Pacing and Defibrillation, 2nd ed, p 939. Philadelphia, WB Saunders, 2000
3. Atlee JL, Bernstein AD: Cardiac rhythm management devices (part II): Perioperative management. Anesthesiology 95:1492, 2001
4. Epstein MR, Mayer JE Jr, Duncan BW: Use of an ultrasonic scalpel as an alternative to electrocautery in patients with pacemakers. Ann Thorac Surg 65:1802, 1998
5. Ozeren M, Dogan OV, Duzgun C, Yucel E: Use of an ultrasonic scalpel in the open-heart reoperation of a patient with pacemaker. Eur J Cardiothorac Surg 21:761, 2002

Page numbers followed by f indicate figures; page numbers followed by t indicate tabular material.

C

J

O

P